Oxford Textbook
of Pathology

Oxford Textbook of Pathology

Volume 2b
Pathology of Systems

Edited by

James O'D. McGee
Nuffield Department of Pathology
and Bacteriology
University of Oxford

Peter G. Isaacson
University College and Middlesex
School of Medicine
University College, London

Nicholas A. Wright
Royal Postgraduate Medical School
Hammersmith Hospital

Associate editors
Heather M. Dick
Department of Medical Microbiology
University of Dundee

Mary P. E. Slack
Nuffield Department of Pathology
and Bacteriology
University of Oxford

OXFORD   NEW YORK   TOKYO
Oxford University Press
1992

Oxford University Press, Walton Street, Oxford OX2 6DP

Oxford   New York   Toronto
Delhi   Bombay   Calcutta   Madras   Karachi
Petaling Jaya   Singapore   Hong Kong   Tokyo
Nairobi   Dar es Salaam   Cape Town
Melbourne   Auckland

and associated companies in
Berlin   Ibadan

Oxford is a trade mark of Oxford University Press

Published in the United States
by Oxford University Press, New York

© *Oxford University Press and the editors, James O'D. McGee, Peter G. Isaacson, and Nicholas A. Wright*

A catalogue record for this book is available from the British Library

Library of Congress Cataloging-in-Publication Data
(Cataloging data is available)
ISBN 0–19–261976–4 (hbk. : set)
ISBN 0–19–261973–X (hbk. Vol. 1)
ISBN 0–19–261975–6 (hbk. Vol. 2a) } *Available as part of set only*
ISBN 0–19–262273–0 (hbk. Vol. 2b)
ISBN 0–19–261972–1 (pbk. Vol. 1)
ISBN 0–19–261974–8 (pbk. Vol. 2)
ISBN 0–19–262274–9 (pbk. Vol. 2a) } *Available as part of Vol. 2 'set' only*
ISBN 0–19–262275–7 (pbk. Vol. 2b)

Typeset by
Cotswold Typesetting Ltd, Gloucester
Printed in Great Britain by
William Collins Sons and Company Ltd, Glasgow

List of chapters

Contents

25 The nervous system

29   Pathology of tropical infections

Protozoan infections

23

Blood and bone marrow

23

Blood and bone marrow

23.1 Normal structure and function

T. M. Dexter

23.1.1 Introduction

All mature blood cells are derived from stem cells, which, although few in number, persist throughout life by virtue of their ability to undergo proliferation to produce more stem cells: a process known as self-renewal. These stem cells arise during early embryonic development and migrate from the yolk sac to the fetal liver. From the fetal liver they then migrate to and colonize the developing bones and establish the various haemopoietic lineages. The bone marrow subsequently constitutes the major site of myelopoiesis and B-lymphocyte development throughout adult life and contributes the pre-T cells which migrate to the thymus. Under the influence of the thymic microenvironment, the pre-T cells are subsequently processed and selected and eventually leave the thymus as mature T-lymphocytes which circulate and colonize the various lymphoid organs to establish (along with B-cells and antigen-presenting cells) the various arms of the immune response. Once they are produced, many of the mature myeloid cells and lymphocytes have a short life-span: granulocytes, for example, persist for only a few hours, while mature erythrocytes are functionally active for only a few weeks before being sequestered and destroyed by the phagocytic system. When the destruction of these mature cells is taken into consideration, it has been estimated that, to maintain normal circulating levels of myeloid cells, the average human must produce something in the order of 3.7×10^{11} myeloid cells each day. Since the capacity of the haemopoietic system to produce mature cells does not apparently decline with age (indeed, in mice the haemopoietic reserve seems to increase), it is obvious that mechanisms must exist to ensure that the processes of birth and death are balanced, and that the founder cells (the stem cells) do not become exhausted as a result of the proliferative demands continually placed upon the system.

Furthermore, because production of one or more of the cell lineages needs to adjust to changing circumstances (recruitment of more red cells during periods of oxygen deficiency, or of granulocytes and lymphocytes during episodes of infection), it is clear that a degree of flexibility needs to be built into the system to meet the changing demands. Our understanding of how this is achieved has advanced considerably in the past decade and the knowledge is now beginning to have a considerable practical and clinical impact.

23.1.2 The pluripotent stem cells

That the various mature blood cell elements, granulocytes, platelets, erythrocytes, monocytes, and lymphocytes, are all derived from a common stem cell is suggested by several lines of work. First, unique radiation-induced chromosome markers have been detected in both myeloid and lymphoid cells, showing that they are the progeny of a single cell. Secondly, the ability of retroviruses to insert randomly into the genome of infected cells has been used as a way of following the proliferative and differentiation potential of 'marked' cells. Using this approach, cells with extensive proliferative ability, as well as the potential to produce myeloid and lymphoid cells, have been clearly demonstrated following transplantation of suitable virus-infected cells. Thirdly, in the human myeloproliferate disease, chronic myeloid leukaemia (CML), the distinctive Ph′ chromosome marker can be detected in both the myeloid and lymphoid cells in such patients—again indicating the existence of cells with myelo-lymphoid potential (presumably the 'target' cells for most, if not all, CMLs). Thus, that pluripotent stem cells exist is beyond doubt. However, what is still unclear is whether or not these are the *only* primitive haemopoietic cells that have an ability to self-renew. Both the chromosome-marker studies and the retrovirus-insertion models indicate the existence of cells, with extensive proliferative ability, which are restricted in their capacity to produce mature haemopoietic cells. For example, it has been shown that, following transplantation, primitive cells exist which may give rise only to myeloid cells and B-lymphocytes, but not T-lymphocytes. Also, examples have been recorded where only T-lymphocytes or only myeloid cells are produced from transplanted cells. From these data, it can be argued that the stem-cell population is heterogeneous with respect to the ability of cells to undergo differentiation into the various lineages. However, whether or not these cells can undergo extensive and prolonged self-renewal is unclear.

What is clear, however, is that the proliferative potential of the bone marrow (or stem-cell reserve) far exceeds the requirements of a normal life-span. For example, injection of only 10^5 bone marrow cells into a potentially lethally irradiated mouse will rescue the haemopoietic system and fully reconstitute the bone marrow of the recipient. The transplanted recipient then lives a near normal life-span, producing normal numbers of all the mature cells. Since 10^5 marrow cells represents only about 0.03 per cent of the total marrow revenue, then it follows that an individual mouse must possess at least a number of stem cells sufficient to reconstitute at least 3000 mice. Moreover, each of these recipients will then possess sufficient stem cells to reconstitute 3000 secondary recipients. In other words, for practical purposes the stem cell is 'immortal'. A similar conclusion is reached from data showing the recovery of the haemopoietic system in mice that have been repeatedly treated with cell-cycle-specific cytotoxic agents.

Self-renewal and differentiation of stem cells

When animals are potentially lethally irradiated (to destroy endogenous haemopoiesis) and then transplanted with a min-

imal number of bone marrow cells, the donated stem cells fully reconstitute the haemopoietic system. The remarkable feature here is that in order to reconstitute haemopoiesis and amplify the numbers of stem cells, the transplanted stem cells must initially undergo preferential self-renewal rather than differentiation. Yet this occurs in a situation where the lack of production of mature cells, in the short term, is life threatening and the 'pressure' for differentiation should be an overriding feature. Thus, there must exist some mechanism to ensure that the *probability* of differentiation never exceeds the probability of self-renewal. How this is achieved is unknown.

Differentiation of stem cells and the generation of committed cells

The stem cells represent only a minor population (comprising 0.01–0.001 per cent) of total bone marrow cells. Therefore, in order to achieve production of the mature cells (most of which are post-mitotic 'end' cells) extensive proliferation (or amplification) must occur in intermediate cell compartments. This is achieved via the generation and subsequent proliferation and development of committed progenitor cells (Fig. 23.1).

Although the fundamental mechanisms which lead to differentiation of stem cells are unknown, many of the differentiated progenitor cells can be easily recognized using *in vitro* or *in vivo*

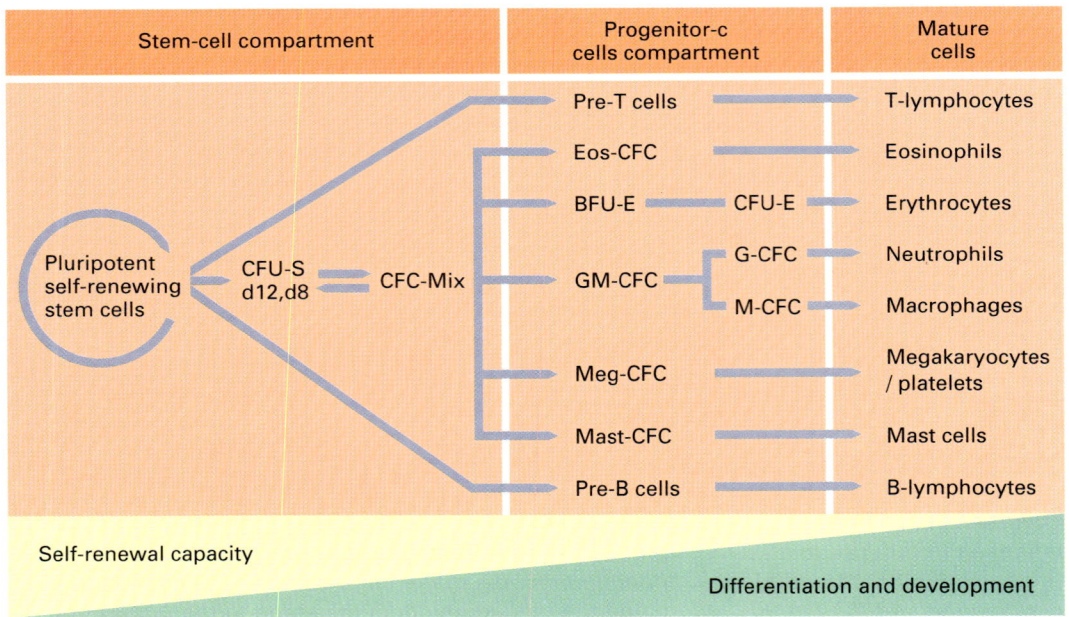

Fig. 23.1 The structure of the haemopoietic system. CFU-S, cells able to form colonies in the spleens of potentially lethally irradiated mice—those cells producing colonies 12 days post-transplantation are more primitive than the cells forming colonies 8 days post-injection; CFC-Mix, multipotent cells with an ability to produce colonies *in vitro* containing cells of various myeloid lineages; GM-CFC, bipotent cells able to produce both macrophages and rentrophils—these give rise to neutrophil restricted (G-CFC) and macrophage restricted (M-CFC) progenitor cells; BFU-E, primitive erythroid progenitor cells which undergo proliferation and development *in vitro* to produce cells (CFU-E) which can respond to erythropoietin; subsequent proliferation and development of the CFU-E result in the production of mature erythrocytes; Eos-CFC, progenitor cells which give rise to colonies *in vitro* containing mature eosinophils; Meg-CFC, diploid progenitor cells which proliferate and develop into polyploid megakaryocytes *in vitro*; Mast-CFC, progenitor cells developing *in vitro* into mast cells. The production and development of all these cells takes place in the bone marrow. Pre-T cells migrate to the thymus, where they proliferate and develop into mature immune-reactive T-lymphocytes. Pre-B cells develop in the bone marrow.

assay systems. For example, when marrow cells are cultured *in vitro* in semi-solid growth medium containing a suitable growth factor, some of the cells undergo proliferation and development to produce colonies of mature cells some days later. Using various techniques it can be shown that such colonies are clonally derived from a single cell and can vary in cellularity from aggregates of a few cells to large foci containing up to 10^5 cells. Furthermore, some of the colonies contain cells of multiple lineages and are obviously derived from a multipotent cell whereas other colonies contain cells of only one or two cell lineages—presumably reflecting their origin from a more developmentally restricted colony-forming cell. The size and developmental nature of the colonies produced are a reflection of both the growth factors present and the heterogeneity of target cells within the marrow sample. For example, colony-forming cells (CFC) have been described which, under appropriate circumstances, can produce colonies *in vitro* containing erythrocytes, granulocytes, eosinophils, macrophages, and megakaryocytes. Since these cells produce a mixed myeloid colony, they are commonly referred to as CFC-Mix. Other CFC produce only granulocytes and macrophages (GM-CFC), eosinophils (Eos-CFC), megakaryocytes (Meg-CFC), large 'bursts' of erythroid cells (BFU-E), small colonies of erythroid cells (CFU-E), or colonies containing B-lymphocytes or T-cells. The bipotent GM-CFC can undergo further development to produce granulocyte (G-CFC) or macrophage (M-CFC) restricted precursor cells. Furthermore, the variation in final cellularity of the colonies produced from all of these progenitor cells seems to be a reflection (at least in part) of a 'continuum' of development where, as development proceeds, proliferate capacity is progressively lost. In other words, the production of mature cells is being met by proliferation (and ultimately clonal extinction) of the committed progenitor cells. It seems reasonable to assume that it is in this 'amplifying' compartment that most flexibility occurs, either by increasing or decreasing the number of divisions before the post-mitotic cells are finally formed. *In vivo* evidence to support this comes from studies in the erythroid-cell compartment following perturbation in the production of erythropoietin (the hormone required for proliferation and haemoglobinization of the mature erythroid progenitor cells).

The point at which cells committed to lymphopoiesis branch off from the pluripotent stem cell is still a matter of some controversy. However, it has been difficult to demonstrate unequivocally the presence of pre-T, pre-B, or mature lymphoid cells in *in vitro* colonies derived from the CFC-Mix. Because of this, it is likely that lymphoid commitment occurs at a very early stage of differentiation. Indeed, it seems that many of the primitive spleen colony forming cells (CFU-S) are also unable to produce lymphoid progeny. However, marker analysis (using either radiation-induced unique chromosome markers or retroviral insertion) indicates a closer lineage relationship between B-cells and myeloid cells, than between T-cells and myeloid cells, suggesting that T-lymphocyte restriction occurs as one of the earliest events in stem-cell commitment.

23.1.3 Growth factors involved in haemopoiesis

Growth factors are *absolutely* required *in vitro* for the survival, proliferation, and development of dispersed CFC: in the absence of growth factors, the cells die. Until recently, most of the growth factors were ill-defined entities present in 'conditioned media'. Since they were present in only minute amounts, it was difficult to address the fundamental questions concerning their nature, origin, and mode of action. In the past few years, however, many of these growth factors have been molecularly cloned and purified to homogeneity and are being produced in large amounts in prokaryotic expression systems. They are summarized in Table 23.1.

Some of these growth factors (e.g. IL-3 and GM-CSF) can influence the growth and differentiation of multiple target cells, including multipotent stem cells, some (e.g. IL-2, G-CSF, and M-CSF) have direct effects only one cell population, while yet others influence mainly *maturation* of cells rather than proliferation of the progenitor cells, e.g. IL-5 for eosinophil development. Simplistically it may be thought that haemopoiesis is regulated

Table 23.1 Growth factors in haemopoiesis

Growth factor	CFU-S/ CFC-Mix	B-cell/ pre-B cell	T-cell/ pre-T cell	GM-/M-/ G-CFC	BFU-E	CFU-E	Meg-CFC	Mast cells	Eos-CFC	Mature cells
IL-1	(+)	+	+	?(+)	?	?	?	?	?	+
IL-2	?	+	+	−	−	−	−	−	−	+
IL-3	+	−/+	−/+	+	+	+	+	+	+	+
IL-4	(+)	+	+	(+)	(+)	(+)	(+)	+	?	?
IL-5	−	+	−	−	−	−	−	−	+	+
IL-6	(+)	+	?	?	?	?	?	?	?	?
GM-CSF	−/+	−	−	+	+/−	−	+	−	+	+
M-CSF	−	−	−	+	−	−	−	−	−	+
G-CSF	−	−	−	+	−	−	−	−	−	+
Meg-CSF	−	−	−	−	−	−	+	−	−	+
Erythro-poietin	−	−	−	−	−	+	+/−	−	−	+

IL-1, Interleukin; G, granulocyte; M, macrophage; Meg, megakaryocyte; CSF, colony stimulating factor; see also Fig. 23.1.

by modulation of the production of these directly acting growth factors, i.e. recruiting multipotent stem cells and other committed cells with the pan-stimuli such as IL-3 or GM-CSF or facilitating the production of mature neutrophils or T-cells by producing G-CSF or IL-2, as required. However, control is exerted at a more complex level than this since (apart from the directly acting growth factors) there are other regulatory molecules which do not, by themselves, stimulate proliferation or development of haemopoietic cells, but which can act in synergy with other growth factors to recruit cell populations that were previously inaccessible. For example, multipotent stem cells do not respond to IL-1 or to M-CSF in terms of colony formation *in vitro*. However, when these two stimuli are combined, then the multipotent cells proliferate and develop into mature macrophages. Indeed, the combination of IL-1 and M-CSF is as potent a stimulus for development of the multipotent stem cells as IL-3. But the outcome of the response obviously differs: with IL-3, mixed myeloid colonies develop, whereas with IL-1 plus M-CSF, only macrophages are found. In recent work in our laboratory, we have also shown a dramatic synergy between G-CSF and M-CSF in terms of the recruitment of multipotent stem cells— giving a proliferative stimulus at least as good as IL-1 plus M-CSF. Similarly, it has been shown that IL-4 (originally described as a B-cell growth factor) can synergize with IL-3 in stimulating the proliferation of mast cells, and that IL-6 (also described as a B-cell factor) can influence the growth of multipotent cells in response to other growth factors. Since IL-1 is also the stimulus for IL-2 production from T-cells as well as for the expression of the IL-2 receptor and the associated T-cell proliferative response, it is obvious that growth-promoting agents are not servants of only one target cell. What is apparent, then, is that neither the receptors for these various growth factors nor the capacity of the haemopoietic cells to respond to the factors, are as restricted as previously thought. Rather, regulation of proliferation and development is mediated by an interactive network and the outcome of a response will depend upon the previous history of the cells, and the various factors that the cells are exposed to during development.

The role of growth factors *in vivo*

While growth factors are obviously necessary for the proliferation and development of haemopoietic cells *in vitro*, their role *in vivo*, in the bone marrow, is equivocal. Within the bone marrow, the haemopoietic cells are found in association with a complex stromal cell meshwork, which provides the infrastructure in which haemopoiesis occurs. That these stromal cells are not simply supplying a physical matrix for the lodgement and development of stem cells is indicated by several lines of research, but particularly from using long-term marrow cultures—where both myelopoiesis and B-lymphocyte development can be supported for months *in vitro*—and from using thymus explants, which facilitate the growth and differentiation of early pre-T cells (and perhaps even multipotent stem cells) *in vitro*.

It has been shown conclusively that *in vitro* cultures of marrow stromal cells can support the proliferation and differentiation of stem cells for many months. Furthermore, the committed progenitor cells produced can undergo full terminal development to produce mature cells. Significantly, haemopoiesis in this case occurs in the absence of added growth factors, which presumably means that the growth factors (and/or other molecules that are essential for haemopoiesis) are being produced by the stromal cells. An important characteristic of these cultures is that myelopoiesis or lymphopoiesis only occurs when the haemopoietic cells are in intimate association with the stromal cells—stressing the importance of direct cell-to-cell contact. In other words, the haemopoietic cells are responding to membrane-bound molecules. But the nature of these molecules remains an enigma. Extensive investigations have failed to demonstrate the production of IL-3 from marrow stromal cells, although the stromal cells will constitutively produce IL-1, IL-4, small amounts of M-CSF, and ill-defined molecules that influence DNA synthesis in multipotent cells. However, little or no GM-CSF or G-CSF is constitutively produced or released from the marrow stromal cells unless stressed by radiation. In this case, GM-CSF is apparently produced at a high level. Since all of these growth factors are primarily developmental stimuli, it is difficult to envisage how homeostasis is maintained. Perhaps many other growth regulatory molecules still await discovery?

However, the role of growth factors is much more obvious when we consider their effects upon the mature circulating cells. Growth factors such as GM-CSF, G-CSF, and M-CSF, for example, do not only stimulate proliferation and development of the earliest blood precursor cells, they also activate the function of mature monocytes, macrophages (in the case of GM-CSF and M-CSF), and mature neutrophils (GM-CSF and G-CSF). In this way, the ability of the cells to generate superoxide (a powerful bactericidal agent) to phagocytose bacteria and protozoa such as *Leishmania* spp. is enhanced. Similarly, IL-5 is important for the functional maturation of eosinophils. IL-1 and IL-2 are important regulatory molecules for T-cell activation, and IL-4 and IL-6 for B-lymphocyte maturation and response to antigen. Since many of these growth factors are produced by a variety of connective tissue cells (at least *in vitro*), either constitutively or in response to agents such as bacterial endotoxins or cytotoxic damage, they are likely to play a local role in recruiting and activating cells at sites of tissue damage.

However, while a role for many of these growth factors in terms of regulating cell development in the marrow and lymphoid organs has not been clearly established, this is not the case for erythropoietin. This growth factor is intimately concerned with stimulating the proliferation and development of fairly mature erythroid progenitor cells (the CFU-E or 'erythropoietin-responsive cells'), allowing them to mature into the haemoglobinized red blood cells. However, unlike most of the other growth factors described, erythropoietin is a classic hormone, being produced by cells in the kidney in response to the prevailing oxygen tension and having an effect upon cells in the marrow. Thus, when animals are rendered polycythaemic, the production of erythropoietin is switched off: and during periods of hypoxia or following severe bleeding or induced haemolysis, erythropoietin production is increased.

23.1.4 The haemopoietic environment

The previous discussion has emphasized the putative role of soluble growth and developmental factors. Probably of equal importance, however, in the regulation of haemopoietic cell development, is the influence of the stromal cell matrix in the various sites of haemopoiesis. For many years the role of stromal cells has been controversial. On the one hand, many workers considered that the stromal cells of the bone marrow and thymus were simply supplying a supportive matrix in which the developing haemopoietic cells could respond to externally derived regulatory molecules. Other workers suggested that the stromal cells were acting as an 'inductive microenvironment', directly regulating the processes of self-renewal and differentiation of the stem cells and their progeny. As discussed previously (and emphasized later) the influence of soluble mediators of growth and development cannot be discounted: neither, however, can the importance of stromal cells.

Classical work by developmental biologists has clearly shown the influence of stromal cells; the thymic epithelial cells in T-cell development, the Bursa of Fabricius in B-cell development, and the bone marrow in myelopoiesis. The absence of T-lymphocytes seen in athymic nude mice and in animals subjected to neonatal thymectomy are well-known examples. Similarly, the maintenance of myelopoiesis and B-lymphopoiesis seen in association with marrow stromal cells *in vitro* in the absence of *added* growth factors suggests an important role for these cells at the mechanistic level. Furthermore, the importance of the stromal cells in myelopoiesis has been well documented in mice carrying mutations at the Steel locus. Such animals have a severe macro-

cytic anaemia which is clearly associated with a defect at the level of the stromal cell environment.

The nature of the interactions between the haemopoietic cells and stromal cells has been shown in both *in vivo* and *in vitro* studies. Examination of the bone marrow demonstrates that this tissue is not as randomly organized as once thought (Fig. 23.2): although appreciation of the organization is complicated by the three-dimensional structure. Within the marrow, three main stromal cell types can be recognized. The endothelial cells, which line the marrow sinuses; the adventitial reticular cells, which branch into the marrow spaces to form a sponge-like matrix enclosing islands of haemopoiesis; and the marrow adipocytes. These cells can be clearly distinguished using cytochemical techniques. Within the marrow, associations are commonly seen between the alkaline-phosphatase-positive reticular cells and developing granulocytes, and between the macrophages and developing erythroid cells producing the characteristic 'erythroblastic islands'. Similar associations can be seen *in vitro* in the long-term bone marrow cultures (Figs 23.2, 23.3). These intimate cell associations are clearly important: if developing haemopoietic cells are prevented from attaching to the stromal cells, they rapidly die.

The origin of the stromal cells and their relationships with each other is still a matter of conjecture. We have shown, using *in vitro* culture systems, that a single cell is able to generate a clone of stromal cells of appreciable phenotypic diversity in terms of alkaline phosphatase production, laminin, collagen, and fibronectin secretion, and lipid accumulation. Thus, it is likely that a single precursor cell can give rise to the connective tissue cells, the reticular cells, and to the marrow adipocytes.

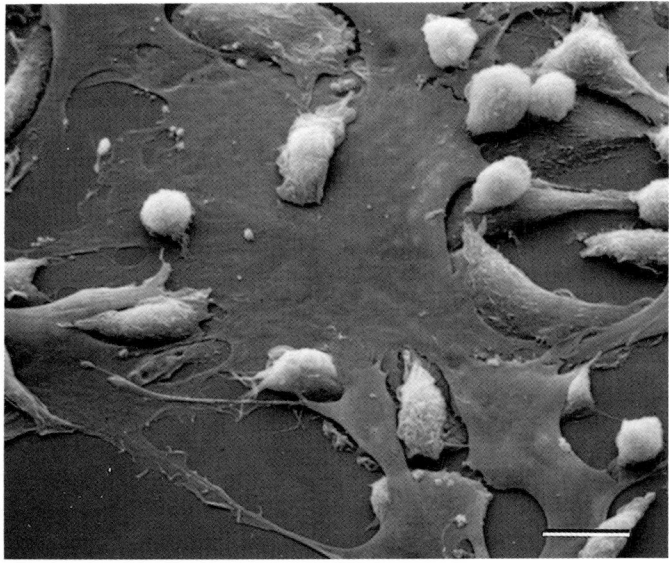

(a)

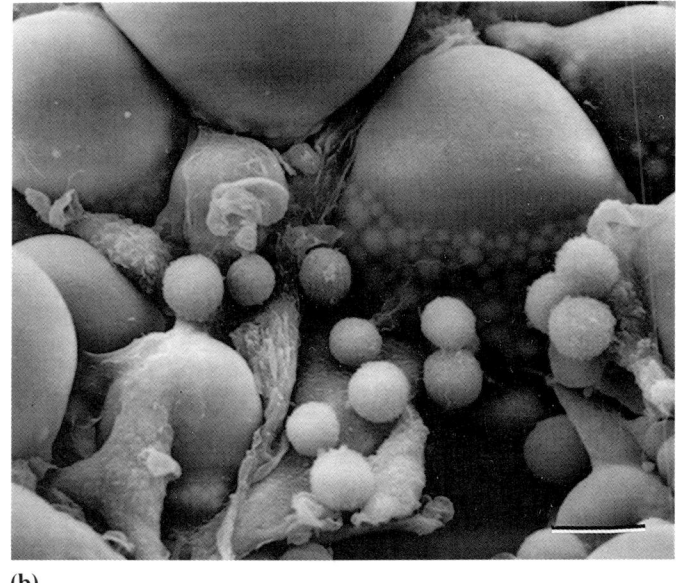

(b)

Fig. 23.2 Ultrastructural characteristics of the marrow stromal cells. (a) A typical 'blanket' or reticular cell in association with macrophages (scale bar = 20 μm); (b) a collection of adipocytes in association with developing granulocytic cells (scale bar = 10 μm). These scanning electron micrographs were derived from actively haemopoietic long-term *in vitro* bone marrow cultures, and were supplied by Dr T. D. Allen, Paterson Institute for Cancer Research, Manchester.

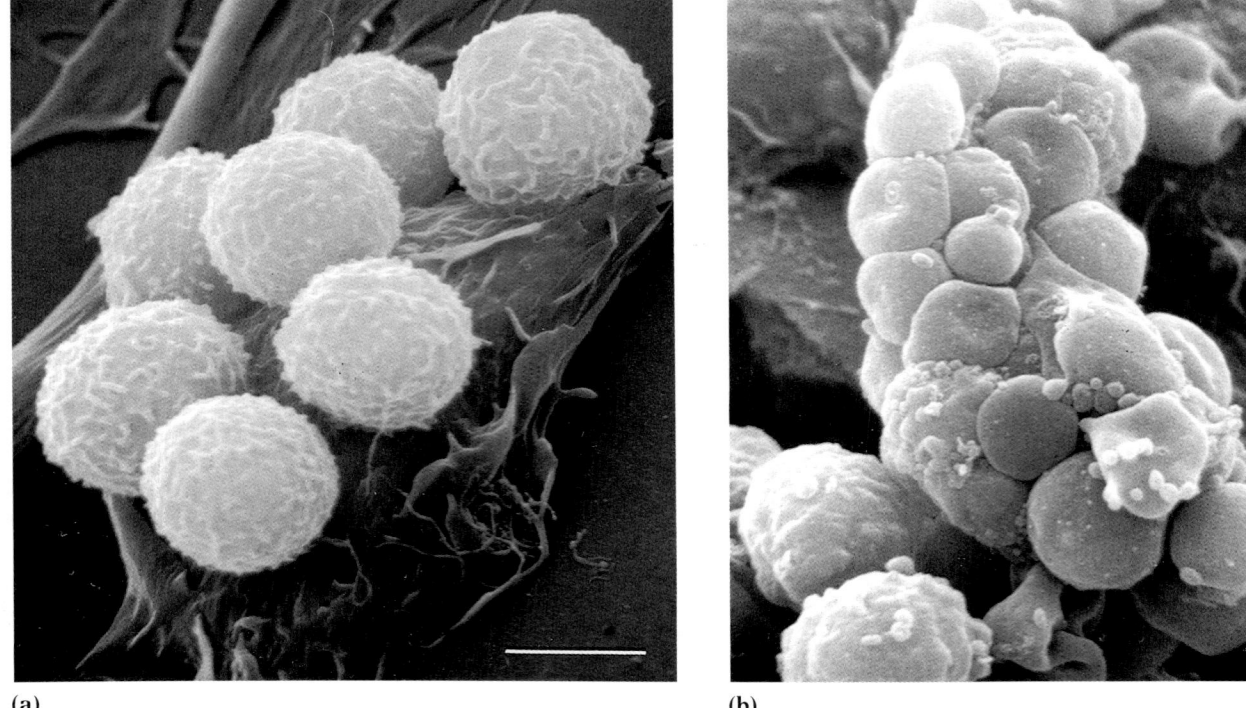

(a)   (b)

Fig. 23.3 Ultrastructural aspects of haemopoietic cells. (a) Developing, immature, granulocytes (scale bar = 5 μm); (b) developing erythroid cells (scale bar = 5 μm). Both granulocytes and erythroid cells develop as 'islands' in the bone marrow. Of particular significance is the synchrony of development seen in individual colonies, such that whole clusters of cells are seen at the same stage of maturation. In both these examples, taken from long-term *in vitro* bone marrow cultures, the developing granulocytes and erythroid cells are intimately associated with macrophages [seen clearly in (a)]. (Kindly supplied by Dr T. D. Allen, Paterson Institute for Cancer Research, Manchester.)

This phenotypic diversity is also associated with functional diversity, since myelopoiesis *in vitro* occurs primarily in association with the large reticular cells, or 'blanket' cells—so named because they overlay areas of granulocyte development.

The ability of marrow stromal cells to support haemopoiesis in the absence of added growth factors infers that the stromal cells themselves are producing whatever is necessary for promoting proliferation and differentiation of the haemopoietic cells. Furthermore, the absolute requirement for intimate cell-to-cell association suggests that the growth stimuli are present only on the *surface* of the stromal cells and are not normally released as diffusible regulatory molecules. The nature of these molecules is, however, unclear, since careful examination of supportive stromal cells has failed to detect the presence of growth factors such as IL-3, GM-CSF, or G-CSF, although molecules such as M-CSF and IL-1 are certainly present. Assuming that the growth factors are indeed *not* being produced by the stromal cells (rather than being below the limits of detection) this presumably means that other growth factors (yet to be characterized) are being produced by the stroma. Alternatively, haemopoiesis mediated by stromal cells may be facilitated by a growth-factor-independent mechanism. Recent work, however, suggesting the involvement of growth factors has come from studies showing that haemopoietic growth-stimulating molecules can be extracted from the surface of

marrow stromal cells. It seems likely that, upon synthesis and export of the growth factor(s) from the stromal cells, the material is then sequestered by heparan sulphate proteoglycan (present on the surface of the stromal cells) and presented in a biologially active form to the developing haemopoietic cells. Such a sequestration of growth factor may well represent a general mechanism for 'localizing' growth factor, thus ensuring that the biological effects are spatially restricted. Furthermore, growth factors bound to extracellular matrix molecules, such as heparan sulphate, have been shown to be protected from attack by proteolytic enzymes, i.e. this may be a way of increasing the biological half-life of growth-promoting agents—an idea that may be relevant to the succeeding section.

23.1.5 Clinical studies

The *in vitro* culture systems outlined previously are useful models for investigating the mechanism underlying various haemopoietic disorders. Clearly, defective production of blood cells may be related to intrinsic defects in stem cells and/or progenitor cell production or to defective control of these cell populations by growth factors and/or the stromal cell milieu. Examples have been reported where either or both of these mechanisms has been shown to be responsible for perturbed haemopoiesis. In such cases, it is reasonable to ask if it is possible to rectify the defect by the use of biological response modifiers, i.e. to exploit the normal physiological regulation of growth and development to either enhance or suppress the production of one or the other cell types as appropriate. Recent work suggests that this may well be the case.

The molecular cloning of growth factor genes and their subsequent expression in prokaryotic systems has made available large amounts of 'recombinant' material. This, in turn, has allowed preclinical and clinical studies to be undertaken with these agents. The results have been dramatic. Treatment of normal animals with recombinant G-CSF or GM-CSF was shown to lead to a marked increase in circulating leucocytes. In the case of G-CSF, the cells recruited were mainly neutrophils; while GM-CSF recruited neutrophils, eosinophils, and monocytes. Furthermore, the marrow of these animals showed evidence for increased proliferative activity and became hypercellular. It should be noted that in order to elicit these responses, only exquisitely low doses of growth factor were required (in the order of μg/kg), thus demonstrating the potency of these agents. Significantly, even when animals were maintained on growth factor for many months, there was no desensitization of the response (the leucocyte count remained elevated throughout the treatment). Furthermore, when growth factor treatment

was stopped, the counts returned to normal levels, and, upon autopsy, no pathological changes were observed in the organs examined. These studies set the scene for the first clinical trials—initially with an emphasis on alleviating anaemia seen in patients with kidney damage (by infusion of erythropoietin) and the neutropaenia seen in patients with acquired immunodeficiency syndrome (AIDS), and in patients with neutropaenia consequent upon treatment with chemotherapy for malignant disease. This type of study is worthy of attention since it makes some important points about the possible usefulness of growth factors.

Following treatment of malignant disease with cytoreductive agents, the patients usually become neutropaenic. The degree and longevity of the neutropaenia obviously depends upon the marrow reserve, the number of courses of chemotherapy, and the aggressiveness of treatment. But the current trend is to treat patients as aggresively as possible and with the shortest time interval between treatments—before rapid recovery of the tumour cell population and the acquisition of resistance to the chemotherapeutic agents has occurred. Because of this, not only is the neutropaenia dose-limiting, but the opportunistic infections that arise as a consequence of the neutropaenia are a major cause for concern. Infective episodes often require

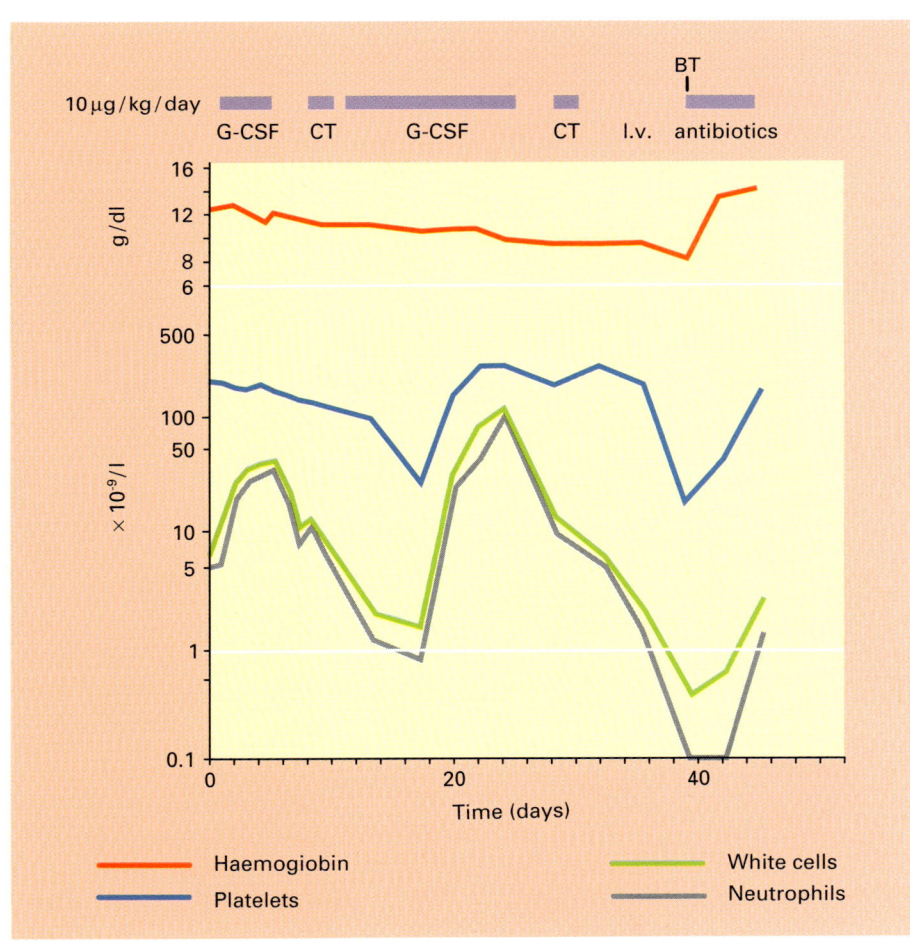

Fig. 23.4 Haematological response to rhG-CSF during phase I and after chemotherapy. This response to recombinant human (rh) G-CSF is representative of the response achieved in a group of patients with small cell lung carcinoma. During the phase I part of the treatment, circulating leucocytes (predominantly neutrophils) increased eightfold, following continuous i.v. infusion of G-CSF (10 μg/kg/day) for 5 days. Following the first course of chemotherapy (adriamycin, etoposide, ifosfamide, mesna) 10 μg/kg/day G-CSF was given continuously for 14 days. Note that the blood count did not fall below the 'critical' level of 1×10^{-9}/l. Following the second course of chemotherapy, when no G-CSF was given, a prolonged neutrophil nadir was observed and the patient required hospitalization and treatment with antibiotics for an acute infection. (Drawn after Bronchud *et al.* 1987, with permission.)

hospitalization and sometimes lead to death. Therefore, any treatment that more rapidly recruits neutrophils into the circulation has many benefits for the clinical management of patients. In a recent study, it has been shown clearly that infusion of G-CSF following treatment of patients with aggressive combination chemotherapy for small cell lung carcinoma led to a reduction in the neutrophil nadir and a much more rapid recovery (Fig. 23.4). Furthermore, patients who received G-CSF following chemotherapy only occasionally had infections requiring antibiotic therapy, whereas in those patients who received no G-CSF, infections requiring hospitalization were commonly observed. These encouraging results have been confirmed in several more clinical trials.

Taken together with the successful use of recombinant erythropoietin for the treatment of the anaemia of patients with kidney damage, such data perhaps indicate that we are at the start of a new era in the management of the haematological diseases that will be discussed in the succeeding sections.

23.1.6   Further reading

Abramson, S., Miller, R. G., and Phillips, R. A. (1979). The identification in adult bone marrow of pluripotent and restricted stem cells of the myeloid and lymphoid systems. *Journal of Experimental Medicine* **145**, 1567.

Allen, T. D. and Dexter, T. M. (1984). The essential cells of the haemopoietic microenvironment. *Experimental Hematology* **9**, 305.

Bronchud, M. H., *et al.* (1987). Phase I/II study of recombinant human granulocyte colony stimulating factor in patients receiving intensive chemotherapy for small cell lung cancer. *British Journal of Cancer* **56**, 809.

Cronkite, E. P. and Feinendegen, L. E. (1976). Notions about human stem cells. *Blood Cells* **2**, 263.

Dexter, T. M. (1984). The message in the medium. *Nature* **309**, 746.

Dexter, T. M. (1987a). Stem cells in normal growth and disease. *British Medical Journal* **295**, 1192.

Dexter, T. M. (1987b). Growth factors involved in haemopoiesis. *Journal of Cell Science* **88**, 1.

Dexter, T. M. and Boettiger, D. (1991). Gene transfer into haematopoietic cells by retroviral vectors. In *ISI atlas of immunology,* in press.

Gabrilove, J. L., *et al.* (1988). Effect of granulocyte colony-stimulating factor on neutropenia and associated morbidity due to chemotherapy for transitional-cell carcinoma of the urothelium. *New England Journal of Medicine* **319**, 1414.

Groopman, J. G., Mitsuy Asu, R. T., Deteo, M. J., Oette, D. H., and Golde, D. W. (1987). Effect of recombinant human granulocyte macrophage colony-stimulating factor on myelopoiesis in the acquired immunodeficiency syndrome. *New England Journal of Medicine* **317**, 593.

Metcalf, D. (1977). *Hemopoietic colonies.* Springer-Verlag, Berlin.

Metcalf, D. (1984). *The hemopoietic colony stimulating factors.* Elsevier, Amsterdam.

Metcalf, D. and Moore, M. A. S. (1971). *Hemopoietic cells.* North Holland, Amsterdam.

Morstyn, G., *et al.* (1988). Effect of granulocyte colony stimulating factor on neutropenia induced by cytotoxic chemotherapy. *Lancet* **i**, 1414.

Testa, N. G. and Gale, R. P. (1988). *Hematopoiesis: long-term effects of chemotherapy and radiation.* Marcel Dekker, New York.

Weiss, L. (1965). The structure of bone marrow. *Journal of Morphology* **117**, 467.

Wolf, N. S. (1979). The haemopoietic microenvironment. *Clinical Haematology* **8**, 469.

Zucker-Franklin, D., Greaves, M. F., Grossi, C. F., and Marmont, A. M. (1981). *Atlas of blood cells*, Vols 1 and 2. E. E. Edi. Ermes, Milan.

23.2   Anaemia and red blood cell hyperplasia

I. Chanarin

23.2.1   Introduction

In the new-born, blood formation takes place in the bone marrow of virtually all bones; in adults haemopoiesis is confined to the central skeleton, that is, vertebral column, pelvis, skull, ribs and sternum, and upper ends of the femora and humeri. In these parts there is normally an admixture of adipose cells and haemopoietic tissue. When there is an increased demand for making blood, active blood formation returns to marrow previously occupied by fat and throughout there is replacement of adipose cells by dividing haemopoietic cells.

Although anaemia refers to a fall in haemoglobin concentration (or red cell count) to below the normal range, it is usual to use the term for qualitative abnormalities of the red cell even when the haemoglobin level is still maintained within the normal range.

Polycythaemia is an increase in the total amount of blood (Fig. 23.5). An adult male has a blood volume of 4.8 litres, of which 2.1 litres are red cells, and an adult woman 4.5 litres of blood, of which 1.7 litres are red cells. Polycythaemia refers to the situation where there is an absolute increase in the red cell volume, usually with some accompanying fall of plasma volume. This can be *physiological* in those living at high altitudes, *secondary* to an impairment of oxygen transport, or *primary* due to increased marrow production of red cells in the absence of an obvious stimulus.

Requirements for red cell production (erythropoiesis)

The requirements for nutrients and hormones are similar to those of any growing tissue. The regulatory growth factors concerned with development from stem cell to normoblast are described earlier in this chapter. The absence of several important nutrients may lead to considerable limitation in blood formation and are important causes of anaemia in man. These are iron, folic acid, and cobalamin (vitamin B_{12}). Iron is part of the haemoglobin molecule. Folic acid and cobalamin are required for normal single-carbon-unit transfer essential for the synthesis of nucleic acids. Rarely, deficiency of protein, ascorbic acid, vitamin E, pyridoxine, riboflavin, and copper may be associated with anaemia.

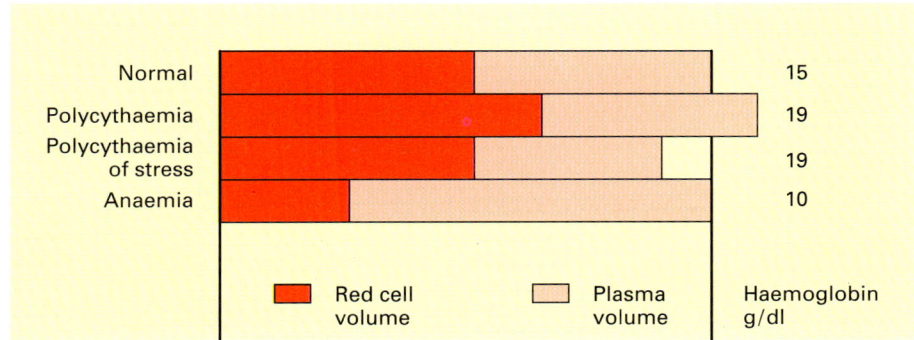

Fig. 23.5 The concentration of haemoglobin and the red cell count increases in polycythaemia and decreases in anaemia. In stress polycythaemia haemoconcentration results from a fall in plasma volume.

Development in the marrow

In normal marrow the majority of cells are white blood cell (granulocyte) precursors and these outnumber red blood cell (erythroblast) precursors by two- to eightfold. When there is a demand for increased red cell production erythroblasts increase in number and become the dominant marrow cell. The earliest recognizable red cell precursor, the pro-erythroblast, is a large cell with a rim of basophilic cytoplasm surrounding a large nucleus which contains nucleoli. Further cell division and maturation is accompanied by the appearance of haemoglobin in the cytoplasm and shrinkage of the nucleus during some three cell divisions over 6 days. The cell is called a normoblast. In the final stage a small pyknotic nucleus is extruded from the cell leaving an erythrocyte which still has considerable amounts of RNA in the cytoplasm (a reticulocyte). After a further sojourn of 1–2 days in marrow the erythrocyte enters the marrow sinusoid and so reaches the circulation. These young red cells can be recognized in a blood film because they tend to stain grey with Romanowsky stains rather than the pink-stained older erythrocytes. This is called polychromasia. The residual RNA disappears after some 20 hours. The normal reticulocyte count is less than 2 per cent of all erythrocytes.

23.2.2 The anaemias

A broad grouping of anaemia is shown in Table 23.2. The anaemias may also be grouped in terms of the size of the red blood cells. The mean corpuscular volume (MCV) normally varies between about 80–94 femtolitres.

Anaemias with small red cells are:

1. iron deficiency;
2. thalassaemia;
3. anaemia of chronic disorders.

Anaemias with large red cells include:

1. megaloblastic anaemia;
2. marrow failure;
3. hypothyroidism;
4. alcoholism;
5. myelodysplastic syndrome;
6. haemolytic anaemias.

Finally, anaemias with normal-sized red cells include:

1. some haemolytic anaemias;
2. haemoglobinopathies;
3. some anaemias of chronic disorders.

Table 23.2 The anaemias

Iron-deficiency anaemias
Megaloblastic anaemias
Haemolytic anaemias
Haemoglobinopathies
Thalassaemias
Anaemia of chronic disorders
Marrow failure

23.2.3 Iron-deficiency anaemia

Adult stores of iron are some 3–4 g. Between 80 and 95 per cent of the iron is present in the haemoglobin of red blood cells. A small amount is in iron-containing enzymes and the remainder is storage iron linked to ferritin. Whereas most men have significant amounts of storage iron, women, because of heavier iron losses as the result of menstruation, often have little or no iron reserves. The red cell has a life-span of about 110 days and at the end of this time the effete red cell is removed by macrophages, generally in the spleen. The iron is carefully conserved within the macrophage and any free haemoglobin reaching plasma is taken up by a protein called haptoglobin, which again is taken up by macrophages. Indeed, some 22 mg of iron is required each day for haemoglobin synthesis and almost all of this comes from recycled iron, as only about 1 mg of dietary iron is absorbed each day.

It is by regulating the amount of iron absorbed in the upper gut that the body regulates its iron requirements. In time of need the amount of iron absorbed can increase to about 4–5 mg daily from a norm of 1–2 mg. Iron losses in excess of 4–5 mg cannot be compensated and a negative iron balance ensues.

Development of iron deficiency

At first the negative iron balance is compensated by using iron reserves attached to ferritin and haemosiderin (iron attached to partially degraded ferritin) and when these stores are exhausted the serum iron levels falls below 12 nmol/l and transferrin (the specific iron-transporting protein in plasma) rises above 75 nmol/l (Fig. 23.6). At this stage there is insufficient iron to maintain haemoglobin formation. Anaemia develops with a fall in the haemoglobin concentration below normal levels (12 g/dl in women and 13 g/dl in men). At the same time the red cells become smaller in size, that is the MCV falls below the lower limit of 80 fl. This process continues until anaemia can become severe with haemoglobin levels below 5 g/dl and the MCV approaching 60 fl. As the anaemia develops there is impairment of iron supply to a variety of enzymes and a failure to maintain epithelial surfaces, resulting in a smooth and sometimes painful tongue, angular stomatitis (cracks at the angle of the mouth), and a pale, smooth, dry skin.

Causes

There are four groups of factors that can lead to iron deficiency:

1. blood loss;
2. poor diet;
3. increased demand;
4. malabsorption.

Blood loss is by far the most important single factor leading to loss of iron from the body. Until proved otherwise iron deficiency must be regarded as due to blood loss. The investigation of iron deficiency is a search for the site of blood loss. The two major sites of blood loss are the uterus in women and the gastrointestinal tract in both sexes.

In women increased menstrual blood loss (menorrhagia) is by far the most important single cause for the development of iron-deficiency anaemia.

Lesions in the gut that may be associated with chronic persistent blood loss include:

1. Gastric causes: ulceration associated with hiatus hernia; oesophageal varices; peptic ulcer; acute ulcer due to aspirin or non-steroidal anti-inflammatory agents; carcinoma.
2. Small intestine: hookworm; neoplasm; angioma; Crohn's; duodenal ulcer.

3. Large intestine: diverticulitis; carcinoma; ulcerative colitis; haemorrhoids; angioma.

Hereditary telangiectasia is transmitted as a simple dominant trait affecting both sexes. There are multiple subcutaneous and submucosal dilated fragile capillaries. Those in the nasal and gut mucosa may bleed profusely.

The important test in detection of gut haemorrhage is that for occult blood in faecal samples. Only rapid passage of large volumes of blood will be recognizable in a stool sample. Smaller volumes of blood are not detectable by eye. Since intestinal blood loss may be intermittent, repeated testing is necessary.

Diet Iron present as dietary haem is absorbed as haem. The availability for absorption of other forms of iron depend on the overall composition of the diet. Iron is poorly absorbed from a vegetarian diet but well absorbed from a meat-containing diet. Animal products contain promoters of iron absorption. Tea and other foods contain inhibitors to iron absorption. Clinical iron deficiency is much more frequent among those on vegetarian diets. Reducing substances, such as ascorbate, which maintain iron as the ferrous salt, promote iron absorption.

Increased demand for iron occurs primarily in pregnancy in order to expand the mother's red cell mass and provide for the fetus.

Absorption Poor iron absorption is a factor in producing iron deficiency after partial gastrectomy and in intestinal disease such as gluten-sensitive enteropathy (coeliac disease).

Blood and marrow

The blood film in iron-deficiency anaemia shows poorly haemoglobinized red blood cells, i.e. there is only a thin rim of haemoglobin at the edge of the cell (Fig. 23.7). The characteristic change in the marrow is the presence of small late normoblasts with an irregular nucleus and a ragged edge to the cytoplasm (micronormoblast). There is no stainable iron in aspirated marrow fragments.

Changes in epithelial surfaces may result in irregular (spoon-shaped) nail formation (koilonychia) and protrusion of pharyn-

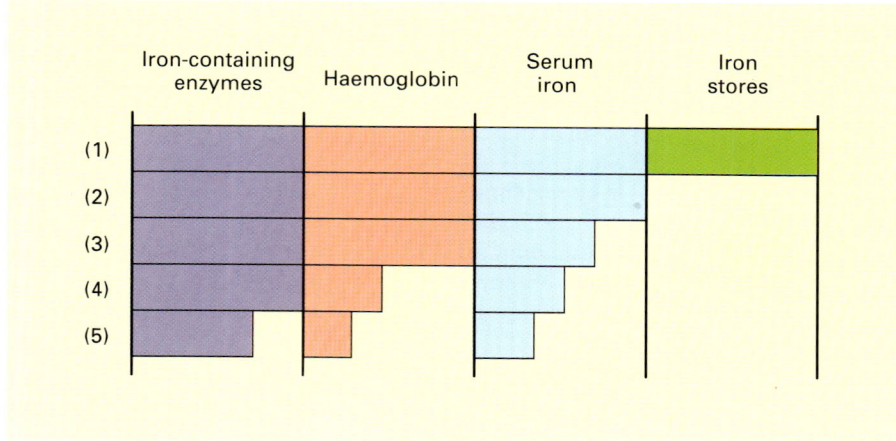

Fig. 23.6 The sequence of change in the development of iron-deficiency anaemia. (1) Normal; (2) loss of iron reserves; (3) fall in serum iron; (4) fall in haemoglobin level; (5) finally, inadequate iron to maintain iron-containing enzymes.

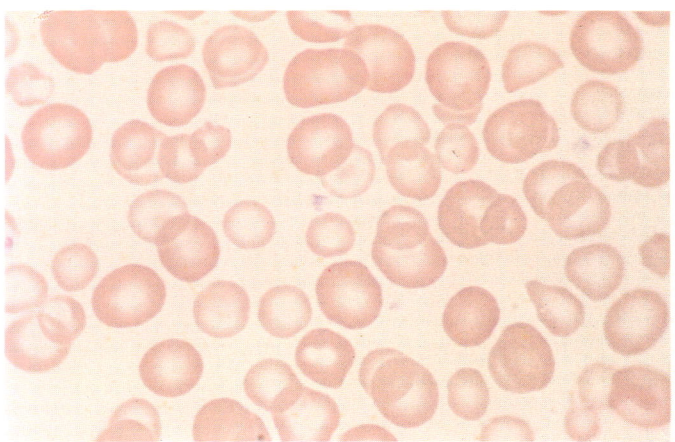

Fig. 23.7 The peripheral blood film in a patient with iron deficiency 6 weeks after treatment with iron. The small pale cells are iron-deficient red cells. The larger fully haemoglobinized cells were produced after iron became available as a result of treatment with iron.

geal mucosa to give the appearance of a pharyngeal web on a barium swallow and radiograph. Such patients may complain of a lump in the throat and have discomfort on swallowing.

23.2.4 Megaloblastic anaemia

The blood

These disorders have abnormally large red blood cells, a low white blood cell count, neutrophil polymorphs which have an increased number of nuclear lobes, and a reduced platelet count. All these changes are present in the severe cases. At an early stage in the disease, only a modest increase in red cell size is detectable in a blood count.

These changes in the peripheral blood (Fig. 23.8) are accompanied by changes in the marrow. There is increased cellularity

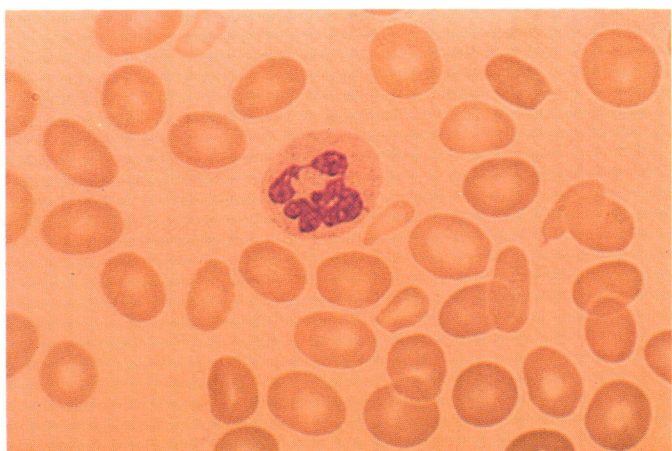

Fig. 23.8 The peripheral blood film in a patient with megaloblastic anaemia. The red cells show variation in size (misocytosis), large red oval cells predominate (macrocytosis), and there are some red cell fragments. The while blood cells have more nuclear lobes than usual (hypersegmented neutrophil).

and replacement of normal erythropoiesis, termed normoblastic, with an abnormal form, termed megaloblastic. This is seen as a very open nuclear chromatin pattern in erythroblasts (Fig. 23.9) and abnormal late white blood cell precursors wherein the nucleus assumes a large horseshoe shape (Fig. 23.10). This latter cell is called a giant metamyelocyte. Many cells fail to complete development and die in the marrow. This is termed ineffective haemopoiesis.

Causes of megaloblastic anaemia

Megaloblastic anaemia is usually due to either deficiency of cobalamin (vitamin B_{12}) or folate, but therapeutic substances that interfere with nucleic acid synthesis or assembly (hydroxyurea, cytosine arabinoside, etc.) can have similar effects.

Folate

Folate is concerned with single-carbon-unit transfer into carbons 2 and 8 of the purine nucleus and into the 5-methyl group

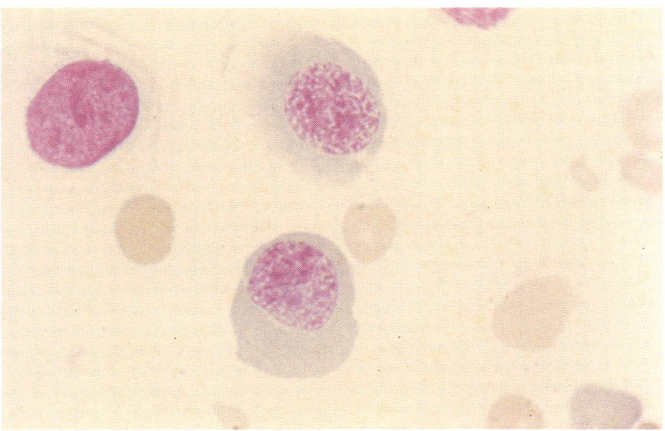

Fig. 23.9 Two narrow megaloblasts. These cells are unusually large, and the nucleus has a characteristically open nuclear pattern.

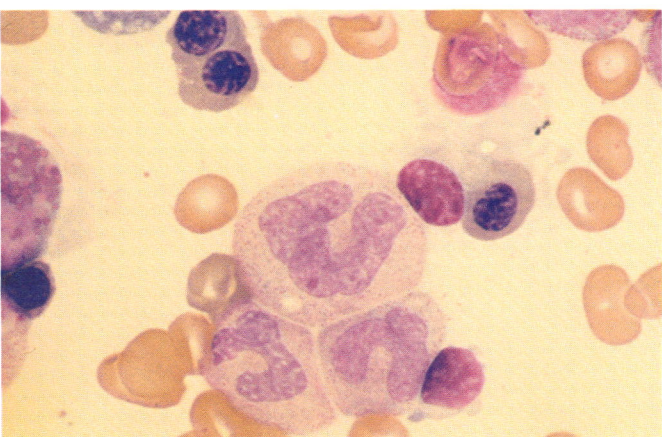

Fig. 23.10 Large granulocytes in the marrow with horseshoe-shaped nuclei. These are called giant metamyelocytes. They are cells that have failed to double their DNA preceding mitosis and undergo phagocytosis in the marrow.

of thymidine. Three of the four nucleic acid bases of DNA and two of four in RNA are dependent on normal folate function.

Cobalamin

This (with folate) is concerned in methionine synthesis. Methionine in turn is a source of active-formate, which is an important carbon-unit transferred by folate. Cobalamin is also concerned in the conversion of methylmalonic acid to succinic acid.

Causes of cobalamin deficiency

Cobalamin is present only in animals and micro-organisms but is entirely absent from the plant kingdom. It follows that a strictly vegetarian diet is devoid of cobalamin. This is the reason for a high incidence of nutritional cobalamin deficiency in life-long vegetarians such as strict Hindu Indians. Apart from strict vegetarians, cobalamin deficiency always arises from impairment of its intestinal absorption.

Dietary cobalamin is freed from protein by proteolytic enzymes in the gut lumen and binds to a specific glycoprotein (intrinsic factor) secreted by the gastric parietal cell in man. Thereafter, the intrinsic factor–cobalamin complex binds to specific receptors on the brush borders of the ileal enterocyte and is internalized by endocytosis. Cobalamin alone then binds to a specific transport protein, transcobalamin II, and a transcobalamin II–cobalamin complex enters the portal blood. Cells have specific receptors on their surface for transcobalamin II and this allows cobalamin to enter cells again by endocytosis of the complex.

There are a variety of lesions that produce impaired cobalamin absorption.

Gastric causes

Atrophic gastritis Severe atrophy of the gastric mucosa with almost total loss of parietal and oxyntic cells (Figs 23.11, 23.12) occurs accompanied by the appearance of auto-antibodies against gastric–parietal cells and against intrinsic factor. Loss of intrinsic factor leads to failure of cobalamin absorption. This condition, described by Thomas Addison in 1855 and possibly earlier by Coombe in 1822, is called Addisonian pernicious anaemia. It is the common form of megaloblastic anaemia in Caucasians, but is equally common in Asiatic Indians and probably other races. The loss of parietal cells also leads to total loss of acid from the gastric secretion—a histamine or pentagastrin-fast achlorhydria.

Gastrectomy If sufficiently extensive, this will also lead to loss of parietal cells and intrinsic factor. Often remaining secreting cells in the gastric remnant undergo atrophy.

Intestinal causes

Disease that leads to the development of an abnormal intestinal bacterial flora in the small gut can result in cobalamin deficiency. The bacteria, particularly anaerobes such as bacteroides, abstract cobalamin from the luminal contents. Such gut lesions are small intestinal diverticulosis (Fig. 23.13), scleroderma, gut strictures (which may be the result of healed tuberculosis), entero–entero fistulae, and non-emptying blind loops.

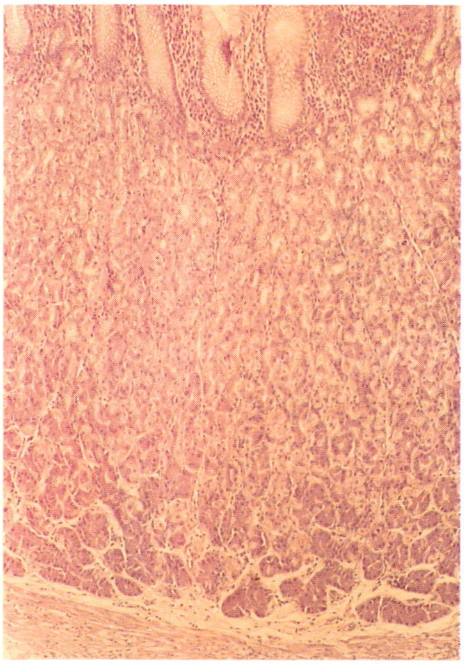

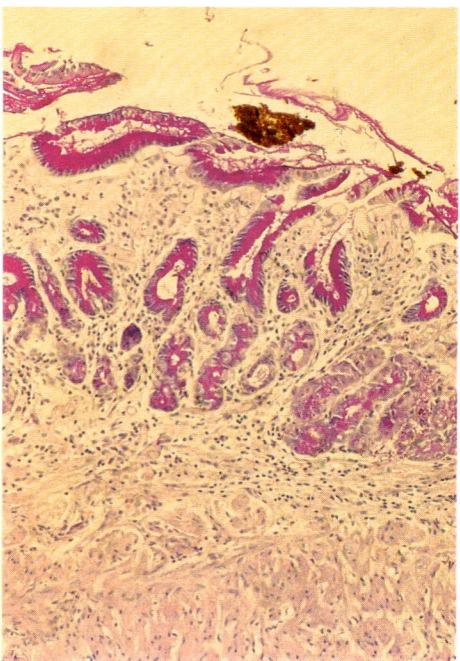

Fig. 23.11   Normal gastric biopsy. The cells with clear pale cytoplasm are parietal cells which secrete both hydrochloric acid and intrinsic factor.

Fig. 23.12   Gastric biopsy from a patient with pernicious anaemia. There is complete loss of parietal cells and replacement by mucus secreting cells (intestinal metaplasia). (PAS stain.)

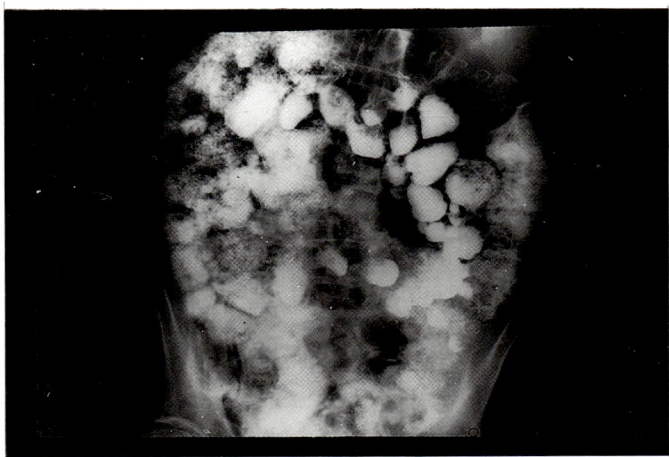

Fig. 23.13 A radiograph after a barium swallow showing multiple small intestinal diverticula. These have a bacterial flora which removes cobalamin from the intestinal contents.

Tropical sprue probably also falls into this group. The fish tapeworm, *Diphyllobothrium latum*, present in Finland, also abstracts cobalamin from the diet at the expense of the host.

A recessively transmitted disorder (Imerslund-Gräsbeck syndrome) results in a defective ileal receptor for cobalamin–intrinsic factor, which prevents cobalamin absorption. Irradiation of the pelvis for treatment of a carcinoma of the cervix uteri may inadvertently affect the distal gut, damage the mucosa, and cause cobalamin malabsorption.

Causes of folate deficiency

Folates (pteroylglutamic acid and related compounds) are present in all foodstuffs. Folates are labile, being readily lost on cooking and storage of food. Deficiency arises from the following.

Nutritional deficiency

An inadequate intake of poor-quality food.

Increased demand

Increased cell proliferation is accompanied by an increased requirement for folate. This occurs in pregnancy and in haemolytic anaemia where there is rapid replacement of short-lived red blood cells.

Malabsorption

Almost all patients with coeliac disease malabsorb folate. Folate is absorbed mainly in the upper gut, which is most severely affected in the gluten sensitivity of coeliac disease. Extensive gut disease of whatever cause will be accompanied by folate malabsorption.

Drugs

Various therapeutic agents such as anticonvulsants (Phenytoin, Mysoline, etc.) and folate antagonists, such as Methotrexate and pyrimethamine, will interfere with folate function and lead to deficiency.

The development of megaloblastic anaemia

Cobalamin deficiency

Stores of cobalamin are relatively large and with a daily requirement of 1–2 μg daily it takes 5 years or more for stores of 3000 μg or more to be depleted should absorption cease. Whereas abrupt cessation of cobalamin absorption occurs after total gastrectomy, in pernicious anaemia there is a relatively gradual decline in cobalamin absorption, and many years elapse before deficiency emerges. Thus pernicious anaemia is a disease of later life. Macrocytosis (large red blood cells) and anaemia appear gradually.

Epithelial surfaces require cobalamin and folate for normal cell renewal, and a smooth, sometimes red, tongue (Fig. 23.14) is usual at diagnosis. Megaloblastic-like changes are recognizable in epithelial squames, cells from the cervix uteri, lung macrophages, etc.

In addition to an effect on dividing cells, cobalamin is required to maintain the integrity of nerve cells. The biochemical pathways are not known. Patients complain of pins and needles sensation in hands and feet and loss of lateral and posterior spinal cord functions, such as loss of vibration sense, appreciation of passive movement, and have extensor plantars. Histologically there is demyelination in both peripheral nerves and in posterior, lateral, and pyramidal tracts.

Folate deficiency

Stores of folate are smaller relative to requirement than cobalamin. With a requirement of about 100–150 μg daily, deficiency can arise within 3–4 months of curtailing intake. The nervous system is not involved in the way that it is with cobalamin deficiency, but similar changes occur in blood, marrow, and epithelial surfaces.

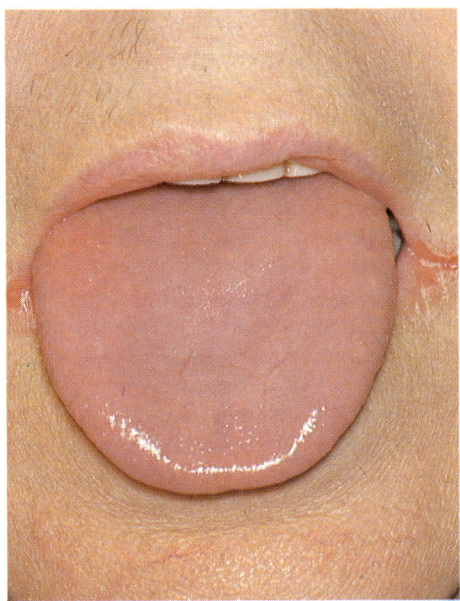

Fig. 23.14 Smooth shiny mucosa of the tongue in untreated pernicious anaemia with angular stomatitis.

Diagnosis

Diagnosis of a megaloblastic anaemia is made by examining the peripheral blood and by demonstrating megaloblastic haemopoiesis in marrow cells obtained by needle aspiration. The cause of the megaloblastosis is determined by measuring the concentration of cobalamin in serum and that of folate in both serum and red cells. The levels are reduced in deficiency states. In the case of cobalamin deficiency, tests for the absorption of isotopically labelled cobalamin, with ^{57}Co replacing the cobalt atom in the molecule, are performed.

In pernicious anaemia there is malabsorption of cobalamin. When the test is repeated with a preparation containing gastric intrinsic factor the absorption of cobalamin is corrected. However, in intestinal disease absorption of cobalamin remains abnormal even when additional intrinsic factor is supplied.

23.2.5   Pernicious anaemia

Pernicious anaemia is a disorder due to cobalamin deficiency, the result of severe gastric atrophy, accompanied by a megaloblastic anaemia and/or a neuropathy. Its frequency is 127 per 100 000 in the UK, but above the age of 60 it affects 1 per cent of the population. As with other auto-immune disorders, women are more often affected than men, in a ratio of 10 : 7.

In one-third of patients there is a history of an affected relative, and in such families there is often a history of other auto-immune disorders, particularly hypothyroidism. In families with a history of pernicious anaemia the age of onset of the disease is earlier than in patients without a family history. At the most extreme end of the spectrum, pernicious anaemia can be part of an auto-immune polyendocrinopathy syndrome in the first and second decades of life, wherein patients may have, in addition, hypoparathyroidism, adrenal atrophy, ovarian failure, and/or candidiasis.

Patients usually complain of loss of well-being, shortness of breath, a sore mouth or tongue, and pins and needles sensation in the feet and/or hands. The blood is macrocytic (Fig. 23.8) and the marrow shows megaloblastic haemopoiesis (Fig. 23.9). The serum cobalamin level is low and the patients are unable to absorb cobalamin unless an additional source of intrinsic factor is provided. In addition to these changes there is loss of secretion of both acid and intrinsic factor in the gastric juice due to severe gastric atrophy (Fig. 23.12). In one-third of patients there may be a few remaining parietal cells in the gastric mucosa, but in the majority these have disappeared completely. There is intestinal metaplasia and considerable lymphocytic infiltration.

Severe gastric atrophy is common in elderly subjects but the majority of such subjects do not develop pernicious anaemia even though in some there is evidence of diminished intrinsic factor production both on direct assay and as seen by somewhat depressed cobalamin absorptions. Nevertheless, even after many years of observation their blood remains normal.

The transition from severe simple atrophic gastritis to the situation in pernicious anaemia wherein a strongly negative cobalamin balance ensues, appears to be related to auto-immune factors. The pernicious anaemia patient generally has evidence of auto-immune factors.

1. Gastric parietal-cell antibodies in both serum and gastric secretion are present in about 90 per cent of patients with pernicious anaemia. Such parietal-cell antibodies are quite common in patients without pernicious anaemia, the highest frequency of about 16 per cent being present in elderly women. All patients with parietal-cell antibodies have biopsy evidence of gastritis.

2. Intrinsic-factor antibodies, usually IgG immunoglobins, are present in serum in 57 per cent of patients with pernicious anaemia. In addition, an intrinsic-factor antibody, an IgA immunoglobulin, is present in the gastric secretion of almost half the patients. In all, about 75 per cent of patients have an antibody against intrinsic factor in either serum, gastric juice, or both.

3. Evidence of cell-mediated immunity against intrinsic factor is demonstrable in about 80 per cent of pernicious anaemia patients. The importance of cell-mediated immunity in the development of pernicious anaemia is highlighted by the observation that 30 per cent of patients with acquired hypogamma-globulinaemia who are unable to form humoral antibodies, nevertheless have pernicious anaemia.

4. There is an increase in lymphocytes in the gastric mucosa, most marked for B-lymphocytes. The ratio of T-helper to T-suppressor cells in the gastric mucosa was no different from that in gastric biopsies from control subjects. In peripheral blood, however, there is a significant decline in the number of T-suppressor lymphocytes in patients who have humoral antibody against intrinsic factor. This would support the hypothesis that failure of T-cell suppression allows clones of B-lymphocytes to develop against gastric as well as thyroid and other antigens.

Experimental development of 'pernicious anaemia'

Treatment of pernicious anaemia by replacement of the missing endogenous intrinsic factor by an oral preparation of intrinsic factor obtained from hog mucosa, offered an interesting parallel to events in the development of the disease. Giving hog intrinsic factor by mouth restored the capacity of the patient to absorb his dietary cobalamin. As a result a normal blood count was restored and the serum cobalamin level became normal. However, after a variable period of time the serum cobalamin fell again, followed by the reappearance of megaloblastic anaemia (Fig. 23.15). Tests for the absorption of cobalamin now showed that hog intrinsic factor was no longer able to promote cobalamin absorption, although human intrinsic factor remained effective. In addition, such patients generally had an antibody in serum that reacted with hog intrinsic factor and prevented hog intrinsic factor from binding cobalamin. Thus it appeared that the failure of intrinsic factor was due to the appearance of a specific antibody against the intrinsic factor molecule.

In the pathogenesis of the disease the transition from simple severe atrophic gastritis to pernicious anaemia is similarly due

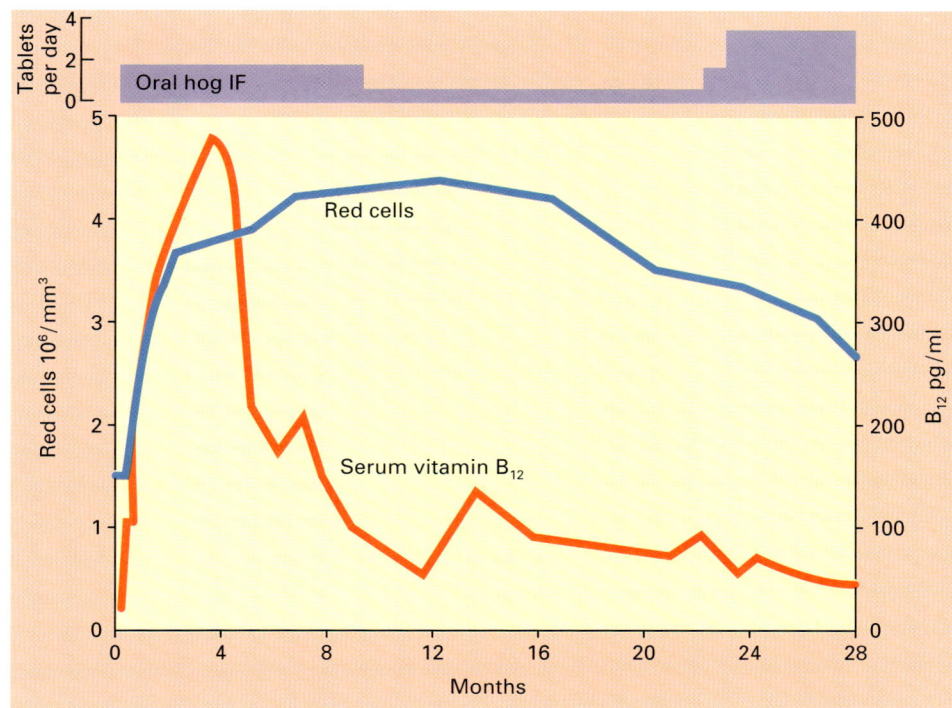

Fig. 23.15 This patient with pernicious anaemia presented with a red cell count of 1.4 million/mm^3 and a serum cobalamin (B$_{12}$) level of 25 pg/ml. He was treated by replacing the intrinsic factor (IF) missing from his own gastric secretion with IF from hog stomach in the form of tablets. As a result he once again was able to absorb cobalamin from his diet. The level of serum cobalamin rose, and the blood responded as shown by the rise of the red cell count to over 4.0 million/mm^3. However, after 5 months, the serum B$_{12}$ level fell and this was followed by a fall in the red cell count. The relapse was due to the formation of antibodies against hog IF so that it was no longer able to potentiate cobalamin absorption.

to the development of immunity against intrinsic factor as well as to the cells secreting intrinsic factor. This converts a just adequate intrinsic factor secretion to an inadequate one.

Finally, there is an increased frequency of carcinoma of the stomach and of carcinoid tumours in the stomach in patients with pernicious anaemia.

23.2.6 Haemolytic anaemia

New red blood cells delivered to the circulation from the marrow survive for about 110 days. In a variety of situations red cell survival may be shortened very significantly and if the marrow cannot compensate by increasing production of red cells, anaemia results. Such an anaemia is termed a haemolytic anaemia.

Healthy marrow can augment erythropoiesis some eight- to tenfold. Thus modest reduction of red cell survival is not uncommon, and occurs in many disorders not necessarily associated with anaemia. Such disorders include hepatic cirrhosis, anaemia of chronic disorders, and megaloblastic anaemia. Similarly, a disorder present in a mild form can be fully

compensated by a responding marrow but when present in a severe form is accompanied by severe anaemia.

Evidence of haemolysis

Increased red cell destruction, either by macrophages or in the circulation, results in an increase in plasma unconjugated bilirubin from haemoglobin catabolism and the patient may be clinically jaundiced. The urine may be dark due to increased urobilinogen, but it does not contain bile. Urobilinogen arises from conjugated bilirubin excreted into bile and altered in the gut, its reabsorption from gut to plasma and its re-excretion in the urine.

One of the methene bridges between the pyrrole rings of haemoglobin is exhaled as carbon monoxide during haemoglobin breakdown and this, too, increases with increased red cell breakdown. It has been used as a means of quantitation of red cell breakdown.

Any haemoglobin reaching the plasma binds to a protein, haptoglobin, and the haptoglobin–haemoglobin complex is taken up by macrophages. Haemolysis with increased release of haemoglobin results in a rapid disappearance of haptoglobin from the plasma, further evidence for a haemolytic process. Another plasma protein, termed haemopexin, takes up free haem.

Evidence of increased erythropoiesis

Increased production of red cells by the marrow is indicated by a rise in reticulocyte count above 2 per cent and by an increase in the mean corpuscular volume since young red cells are larger than mature ones. The marrow shows erythroid hyperplasia.

Consequence of long-standing haemolysis

Long-standing haemolysis may lead to the formation of pigment gallstones and repeated attacks of gallstone colic.

Parvovirus infection can cause abrupt failure of erythropoiesis with disappearance of all erythroblasts from the marrow. There is recovery in 10–12 days. When red cell life-span is normal there may be only a minor fall in the red cell count during the course of a parvovirus infection but in haemolytic anaemia when the red cell survival is of the order of 10 days, the red cell count can fall from 5 million to 1 million per μl with severe symptoms which may require blood transfusion.

The high red cell turnover results in increased nucleic acid synthesis and an increased requirement for folic acid. If this cannot be met from the diet, folic-acid deficiency can develop and the resulting megaloblastic anaemia can produce a failure of haemopoiesis. This is more likely to occur if a further factor which increases folate requirement, such as pregnancy, supervenes.

Increased haemolysis augments intestinal iron absorption and increased iron stores are usual. Clinically, splenomegaly is common and this can give rise to painful splenic infarcts.

The disorders that give rise to haemolytic anaemia include:

1. Congenital haemolytic anaemia:
   erythrocyte membrane defects;
   erythrocyte enzyme defects; and
   haemoglobin defects.

2. Acquired haemolytic anaemia:
   antibody mediated (auto-immune);
   others—drug-induced, mechanical, infections, burns, hypersplenism, vitamin E deficiency, paroxysmal nocturnal haemoglobinuria.

Hereditary spherocytosis

This is the prototype of defects in the structure of the red cell membrane. There are four major proteins forming a lattice inside the red cell membrane. These four are spectrin, actin, protein 4.1, and ankyrin. The most abundant is spectrin, an elongated protein linked to other spectrin dimers at its head and connected to other spectrin dimers distally through actin and protein 4.1. The lattice is attached to the lipid layers of the membrane by the fourth protein, ankyrin. In these disorders (hereditary spherocytosis, elliptocytosis, and pyropoikilo-

cytosis) there is deficiency or dysfunction of one of these membrane proteins.

The commonest form of hereditary spherocytosis is inherited as an autosomal dominant and involves spectrin deficiency, the severity of deficiency correlating well with the severity of the disease; hereditary elliptocytosis is associated with protein 4.1 deficiency.

Those suffering from hereditary spherocytosis may present at birth or in later life with jaundice, with gallstone colic, sometimes with anaemia, leg ulceration, or with splenomegaly. A family history is present in some two-thirds of patients.

The blood film shows rounded globular red cells (Fig. 23.16) replacing the usual biconcave disc; such cells are termed spherocytes. Such cells tend to be held up during their circulation through the spleen where attempts at phagocytosis may result in loss of red cell membrane. Additionally, portions of the membrane that are not adequately supported by protein may form microvesicles which are lost. Whatever the mechanism, there is a reduced surface area relative to volume in a spherocyte. This leads to a loss of deformability which is a prerequisite for easy passage of red cells through narrow capillaries.

The membrane defects are associated with increased monovalent cation (Na^+ and K^+) passage across the red cell membrane and this is accompanied by an increased glucose requirement. Stasis in the spleen, both by virtue of exposure to macrophages and impairment of glucose supply, may further damage these cells leading to their ultimate demise.

Glucose-6-phosphate dehydrogenase deficiency

Deficiency of glucose-6-phosphate dehydrogenase (G6PD) is common; deficiency of other enzymes involved in the Embden–Myerhof pathway of glucose catabolism, rare. Deficiency of most enzymes can lead to a haemolytic anaemia.

The gene for G6PD is carried on the X-chromosome. Females (XX) can pass on a normal X or a deficient X-chromosome to their sons. The latter have clinical G6PD deficiency. In females,

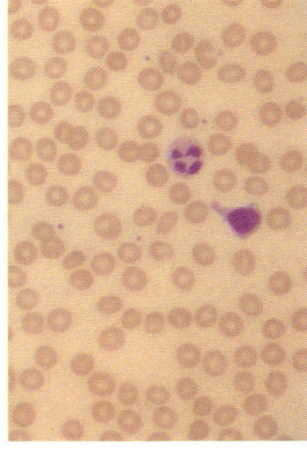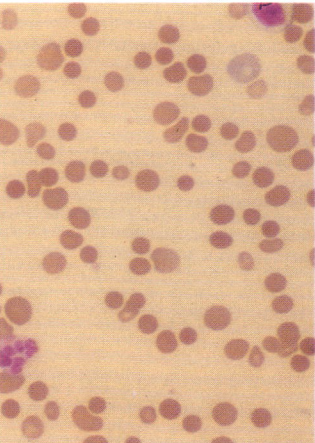

Fig. 23.16 A normal peripheral blood film is shown on the left. On the right is a blood film from a patient with hereditary spherocytosis showing red cells rounding up into densely staining spheres.

one of two X-chromosomes in each cell is inactivated by methylation of DNA cytosine. A cell with a normal functional X-chromosome will have a normal level of G6PD activity. A cell in which the functional X-chromosome carries the defective gene will have a very low level of G6PD. Thus about half the red cells in carrier women have normal levels of G6PD and the other half low levels of G6PD.

Glucose-6-phosphate can be metabolized by either an anaerobic pathway (Embden–Myerhof) or by the aerobic pathway (pentose phosphate shunt). The latter pathway provides reduced NADPH and reduced glutathione and these, with other reducing systems, convert methaemoglobin to oxyhaemoglobin. Oxidant drugs increase the amount of methaemoglobin formed. However, the G6PD-deficient cell cannot produce enough NADPH to cope with the increased amounts of methaemoglobin formed. As a result, globin becomes oxidized and precipitated out of solution. Precipitated globin is visible on methyl-violet staining as large dark blobs in red cells and these are termed Heinz bodies. These cells are destroyed and a haemolytic process ensues.

The classical presentation of G6PD deficiency is that of a child given a meal of beans (*Vicia fava*). A few hours later he develops haemoglobinuria (black urine) and even peripheral vascular collapse. There is a rapid fall in haemoglobin and a rise in free plasma haemoglobin, a rise in unconjugated bilirubin and a fall in haptoglobin. The episode lasts a few days and resolves spontaneously. More usually the onset is less dramatic, coming 1–3 days after starting on oxidant drugs such as an anti-malarial or sulphonamide. Older red cells are most susceptible; younger red cells have higher levels of G6PD and can resist the drug. Thus once the older red cell population has been destroyed the episode ceases.

Rarely, G6PD deficiency can present as neonatal jaundice and, with some molecular variants of the enzyme, as a chronic haemolytic state. G6PD deficiency is commonest in Mediterranean and Negro populations.

The high frequency of G6PD deficiency in Africa has been attributed to a protection of such persons against malaria. Falciparum malaria is less able to enter a G6PD-deficient red cell than a normal cell. This phenomenon is called balanced polymorphism—something bad provides protection against something worse!

Thalassaemia and haemoglobinopathies

These are discussed in Chapter 2.

Auto-immune haemolytic anaemia

In these disorders antibodies are formed against components of the red cell membrane. Usually such antibody-coated red cells are cleared rapidly by macrophages in the spleen and liver so that a brisk haemolytic anaemia ensues.

Haemolytic anaemia due to warm antibodies

The test that is used to demonstrate an antibody on the red cell surface is the antiglobulin test. The antiserum against human gammaglobulin is prepared in either goat or rabbit. When such an antiserum is added to normal red blood cells there is no effect. When added to red cells that have immunoglobulin on the surface, the antiserum reacts with the immunoglobulin and produces a brisk agglutination reaction. The antibody causing warm haemolytic anaemia is usually an IgG immunoglobulin reacting best at 37 °C.

Clinically, the patient is jaundiced, splenomegaly is usual, and there may be evidence of lymphoma. The blood film from a patient is similar to that in hereditary spherocytosis. There is spherocytosis and polychromasia due to the meta-chromatic staining of young red cells (reticulocytes).

Haemolytic anaemia due to cold antibodies

Another type of auto-immune haemolytic anaemia is due to an IgM immunoglobulin directed against the red blood cell. Unlike the IgG immunoglobulin, IgM produces agglutination of red cells in the circulation. The antibody is termed a cold antibody. It reacts best at low temperatures and at higher temperatures the red cell–antibody complex dissociates. Thus the clinical effect of the antibody depends on its thermal amplitude. An antibody that is active at the temperature normally reached in the body extremities (limbs, ears, nose) will result in intravascular agglutination, stasis of blood in small vessels, and vasospasm. The antibody–red cell complex binds complement and this causes disruption of the red cell with release of haemoglobin (haemolysis).

Patients suffer from blue-cyanosed extremities and severe anaemia. The marrow response is often inadequate so that reticulocyte levels do not often exceed 10 per cent as compared to 30–40 per cent in warm-antibody haemolytic anaemia. Often cold antibody is associated with an underlying lymphoma. In the majority of patients there is no underlying disease, although marrow plasma cells show the presence of a monoclonal antibody. Similar antibodies may appear 2–3 weeks after *Mycoplasma* pneumonia when acute haemolysis supervenes.

Other acquired haemolytic anaemias

Drug-induced haemolytic anaemias

Drugs can induce haemolysis in a variety of ways.

1. Some, such as dapsone, damage red cells directly, the severity of the anaemia being dose related.

2. Other drugs may only affect abnormal red cells, such as those with G6PD deficiency or unstable haemoglobins.

3. Quinine and Phenacetin bind to plasma protein and an antibody forms against the complex. The drug–plasma protein complex may adhere to the red cell surface and further binding of antibody and complement causes haemolysis.

4. Penicillin and cephalosporin bind directly to the red cell surface and the antibody is directed against the red cell–drug complex.

5. Aldomet, possibly by reducing numbers of T-suppressor

cells, allows IgG antibodies to appear which lead to a positive antiglobulin test in 20 per cent of patients taking the drug and to haemolytic anaemia in about 1 per cent of patients.

In all cases a history of medication must raise the possibility that the drug is responsible.

23.2.7   Anaemia of chronic disorders

Moderate, occasionally severe, anaemia is common in a variety of disorders not primarily affecting the haemopoietic system. These disorders include rheumatoid arthritis, polymyalgia rheumatica, renal and hepatic failure, tuberculosis and chronic sepsis, neoplasia, and others.

Apart from anaemia the blood picture may be unremarkable, but in others it closely resembles the picture seen in iron deficiency. The red cells are small (low MCV) and there is a low serum iron level. However, unlike iron deficiency, the serum iron-binding capacity is low (elevated in iron deficiency), the serum ferritin level is normal (low in iron deficiency), and there are ample marrow iron stores (absent in iron deficiency).

In renal failure the anaemia is due to lack of the hormone erythropoietin and responds to treatment with the hormone. The kidney is the normal source of erythropoietin. In other conditions it is more complex. Iron tends to be retained in macrophages and is not available to developing normoblasts. There is a modest shortening of red cell survival to which the marrow is unable to respond. Clinically its importance lies in not confusing it with iron deficiency. The anaemia responds only to treatment of the underlying disease.

23.2.8   Aplastic and hypoplastic anaemia

Failure of the marrow to produce enough cells usually affects all three cell lines, erythrocytes, granulocytes, and platelets, but rarely an auto-immune process can suppress only red cell production (pure red cell aplasia). The blood count shows anaemia which is almost invariably macrocytic, low white cell count (leucopenia), and a low platelet count (thrombocytopenia). Usually one or two cell lines are depressed to a greater extent that others.

Causes

Drugs

Therapeutic drugs are an important cause of marrow failure. Drugs such as chloramphenicol, aspirin, penicillin, sulphonamide, gold compounds, and many others are well tolerated by the vast majority of patients but a very small number suffer transient or more prolonged marrow damage. Chemotherapeutic agents in larger dose commonly suppress marrow and some, such as busulphan, are known stem-cell poisons. The mechanism of drug action is not known.

Radiation exposure

This may produce marrow failure and a heavily irradiated area is devoid of haemopoietic activity.

Congenital

Congenital marrow aplasia occurs in Fanconi's anaemia. Presenting usually after the age of 4 years, it accompanies other congenital abnormalities and chromosomal analysis reveals breaks and gaps in the chromosomes.

Viral

Aplasia may follow hepatitis. Transient marrow failure recovering in 10 days can be due to parvovirus infection (Fifth disease).

Idiopathic

In more than half the patients a cause is not identified. An immune factor may have a role in many, since there is often a response to antilymphocyte globulin. Further, a marrow transplant from an identical twin is often rejected unless it is accompanied by immunosuppressive therapy.

Marrow

The marrow simply contains fat spaces, a few plasma cells, lymphocytes, and macrophages (Fig. 23.17). Depending on the severity, an occasional residual normoblast or myelocyte is present. Occasionally one is surprised to aspirate marrow fragments with haemopoietic activity in a patient with pancytopenia. Aspiration at another site invariably shows hypoplasia and a trephine confirms the diagnosis.

Clinically, the patient complains of either shortness of breath, infections, or bruising. The serum iron is abnormally high but there are few other significant findings.

In pure red cell aplasia, immunity against erythroblasts appears. About half the patients have a thymoma, benign or malignant, and there is an association with other auto-immune disorders, such as pernicious anaemia. The marrow shows normal granulopoiesis and normal megakaryocytes but erythroblasts are either completely absent or very scanty.

23.2.9   Hyperplasia of red blood cells

An increase in red cell mass occurs as a result of a primary increase in production of red cells or as a compensation for intpaired delivery of oxygen to the tissues. These disorders known as polycythaemia include:

1. polycythaemia rubra vera;
2. secondary polycythaemia;
3. high oxygen-affinity haemoglobins;
4. familial polycythaemia; and
5. increased carboxyhaemoglobin.

In addition there is a disorder termed stress polycythaemia (Gaisbock's disease) in which there is a reduction in plasma volume so that there is haemoconcentration (Fig. 23.5). The red cell mass, however, is normal. These patients are usually very plethoric with a high haemoglobin concentration. The explanation for the reduction in plasma volume is not known. Residence at high altitude is accompanied by an elevated red cell count as a result of low oxygen tension.

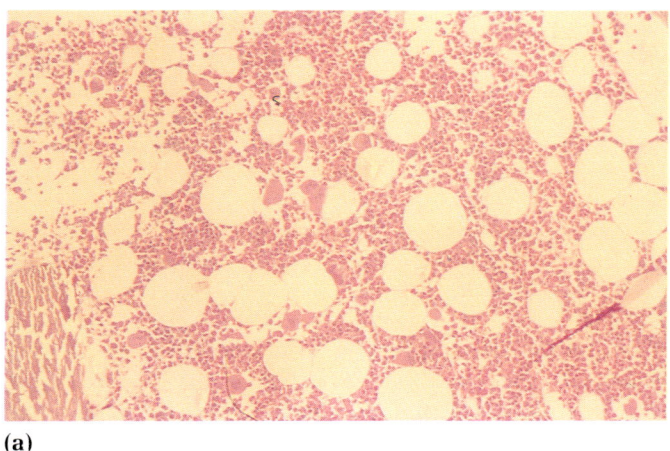

(a)

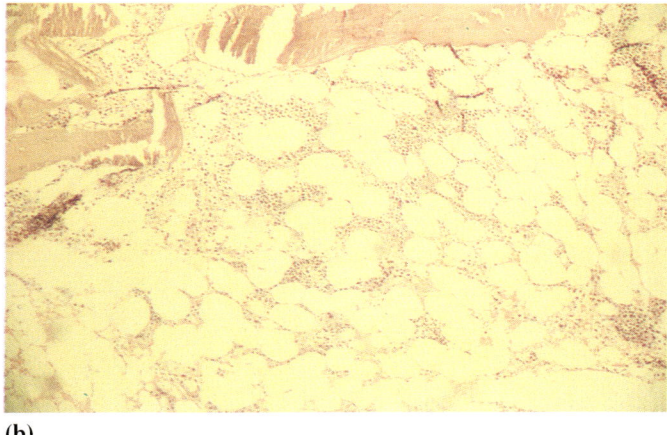

(b)

Fig. 23.17 (a) A normal section of marrow showing adipose cells and haemopoietic cells, and (b) a marrow from a patient with hypoplastic anaemia showing severe loss of haemopoietic cells.

Polycythaemia rubra vera

This disorder is discussed later in this chapter (see Section 23.5.4).

Secondary polycythaemia

Polycythaemia is commonly present in patients with right to left cardiac shunts associated with low oxygen saturation of arterial blood and with cyanosis. Less severe polycythaemia occurs in patients with chronic pulmonary disease similarly associated with impaired oxygenation. This polycythaemia is probably better referred to as erythrocytosis since it does not affect leucocytes or platelets.

It is important to ask a patient with polycythaemia whether any other relative has similar problems. Familial polycythaemia is present in those with high oxygen affinity haemoglobins which do not release their oxygen readily at the normal capillary oxygen tension of tissue. These haemoglobins may have amino-acid substitutions in the region of contact between globin chains and prevent the opening up of the pocket carrying oxygen molecules within the tetramer, that is, there is absence of a haem–haem interaction. Such haemoglobins include Hb Chesapeake, Hb Capetown, Hb San Diego, etc. High oxygen affinity is detected by measuring the PO_{50} (normal about 12 mm Hg) but in these patients values of 20–25 are found.

Familial polycythaemia may also occur in rare families with permanently elevated erythropoietin levels, and these may show a dominant autosomal inheritance. Other familial polycythaemias have normal erythropoietin levels and the mechanism is not understood.

Certain tumours may be associated with polycythaemia by virtue of erythropoietin excretion and these include patients with renal cysts, some hypernephromas, uterine myomas, hepatomas, cerebellar haemangioma, some adenomas, and pheochromocytoma.

Finally, so called smoker's polycythaemia is due to elevated carboxyhaemoglobin levels in heavy smokers, which cause impaired oxygen release at normal oxygen tension in tissue. Such patients may have not only a modest increase in red cell mass but also some shrinkage of plasma volume.

23.2.10 Further reading

Chanarin, I., Brozovic, M., Tidmarsh, E., and Waters, D. A. W. (1984). *Blood and its diseases* (3rd edn). Churchill Livingstone, Edinburgh.

Kaye, M. D., Whorwell, P. J., and Wright R. (1983). Gastric mucosal lymphocyte subpopulations in pernicious anemia and in normal stomach. *Clinical Immunology and Immunopathology* 28, 431–40.

Williams, W. J., Beutler, E., Erslev, A. J., and Lichtman, M. A. (1983). *Hematology* (3rd edn). McGraw-Hill, New York.

Wodzinski, M. A., Forrest, M. J., Barnett, D., and Lawrence A. C. K. (1985). Lymphocyte subpopulations in patients with hydroxo-cobalamin responsive megaloblastic anaemia. *Journal of Clinical Pathology* 38, 582–4.

23.3 Non-neoplastic white cell disorders

K. Patterson

23.3.1 Quantitative abnormalities

Introduction

The total white cell count is measured in units of thousand millions of cells per litre of blood, invariably abbreviated to $10^9/l$. The normal total white cell count is $3.5–10 \times 10^9/l$.

The white cells may be sub-classified into neutrophils, lymphocytes, monocytes, eosinophils, and basophils, usually expressed as a percentage. By multiplying this percentage by the total white cell count an absolute count of neutrophils, lymphocytes, etc. may be obtained. Children have a lymphocytosis compared to adults. The leucocytes are usually identified by their morphological appearances on Romanovsky-stained blood films. A Romanovsky stain will stain acid substances one colour and basic substances a different colour. Examples are May–Grunwald, Giemsa, Wright's, and Leishman stains. The granulocytes are identified by the staining of their specific granules. Eosinophils have orange granules, basophils blue granules, and neutrophils neutral (weakly staining) granules. Examples are shown in Fig. 23.18.

Immature white cells such as metamyelocytes, myelocytes, promyelocytes, and blast cells are not usually found in the blood though they may appear in a variety of disease states.

23.3.2   Leucopenia

A leucopenia may be defined as a total white cell count less than $3.5 \times 10^9/l$. All types of leucocyte may be reduced, or particular types of leucocyte may be reduced in number. Neutropenia refers to a reduction in the count of neutrophils, lymphopenia a reduction in lymphocytes. The term leucopenia, if unqualified, usually implies neutropenia.

When the bone marrow is involved by haematological disease, such as leukaemia, lymphoma, or megaloblastic anaemia, thrombocytopenia and anaemia frequently accompany the leucopenia. Neutrophils are particularly responsible for defences against pyogenic organisms, and a neutrophil count of less than $1.0 \times 10^9/l$ is associated with increased risk of infection; this may be life-threatening when the count is less than $0.5 \times 10^9/l$.

Monocytes, eosinophils, and basophils are present in small numbers in the blood, and the recognition of reduced numbers of these cells (monocytopenia, eosinophilopenia) is technically difficult, requiring very large numbers of cells to be counted. The use of automated blood cell counters allows the easy recognition of variation in these minor components of the differential, but they are of limited clinical significance.

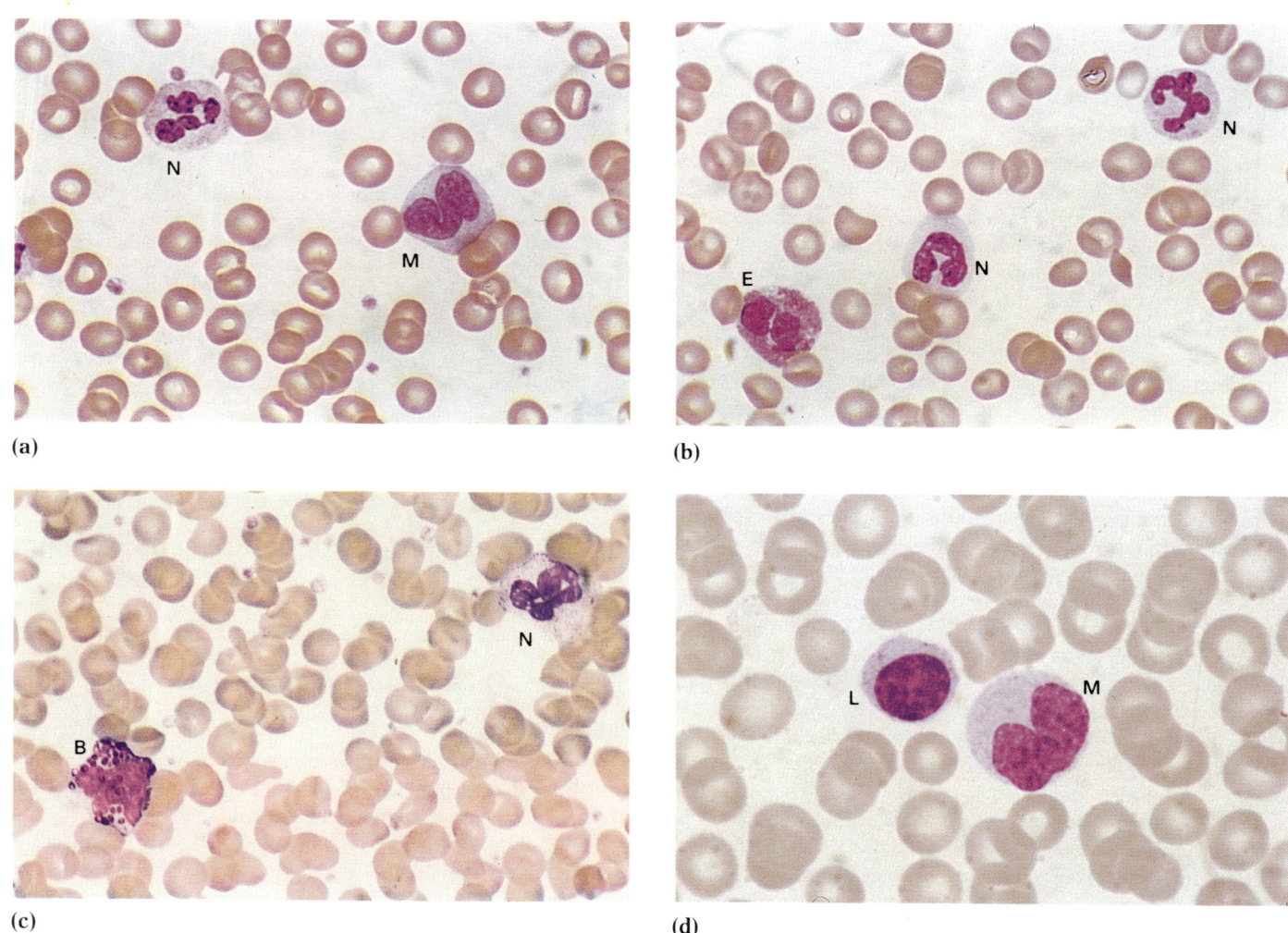

(a)

(b)

(c)

(d)

Fig. 23.18 Normal blood leucocyte morphology. (a) A neutrophil (N) and monocyte (M); (b) an eosinophil (E) and two neutrophils (N); (c) a basophil (B) and neutrophil (N); (d) a monocyte (M) and lymphocyte (L).

Isolated leucopenia

Racial leucopenia

Non-Caucasian persons, particularly Blacks and Arabs tend to have a lower white cell count than Caucasians. Even so, the total white cell count is rarely below $2 \times 10^9/l$, and the neutrophil count is usually over $1.5 \times 10^9/l$. These healthy persons appear to mount a normal neutrophil response to infection, many of their neutrophils being held in the marginating pool rather than in the circulating blood. The administration of steroids causes a transient neutrophilia in normal persons and in racial neutropenia, and this has been used as the basis of a diagnostic test to distinguish racial neutropenia from other more worrying forms of neutropenia.

Leucopenia after viral infection

Modest leucopenia may be seen during common viral infections, such as influenza, and resolves after clinical recovery.

The lymphocytes may show reactive changes, shown in Fig. 23.19.

Infection with human immunodeficiency virus (HIV) commonly causes lymphocytopenia and neutropenia. The lymphocytopenia is because HIV is cytotoxic to its target cell, the T-4 (helper) lymphocytes. The mechanism of the neutropenia is less clear, though antibody-mediated neutrophil destruction frequently occurs and, in some cases, the virus may multiply within and suppress myeloid progenitor cells.

Drug-induced leucopenia

Cytotoxic agents As might be expected, cytotoxic agents cause leucopenia, often with anaemia and thrombocytopenia. Very careful monitoring of the blood count is important during treatment with these agents. For example, the treatment of acute lymphoblastic leukaemia with maintenance chemotherapy (see Section 23.4.1) of mercaptopurine and methotrexate requires

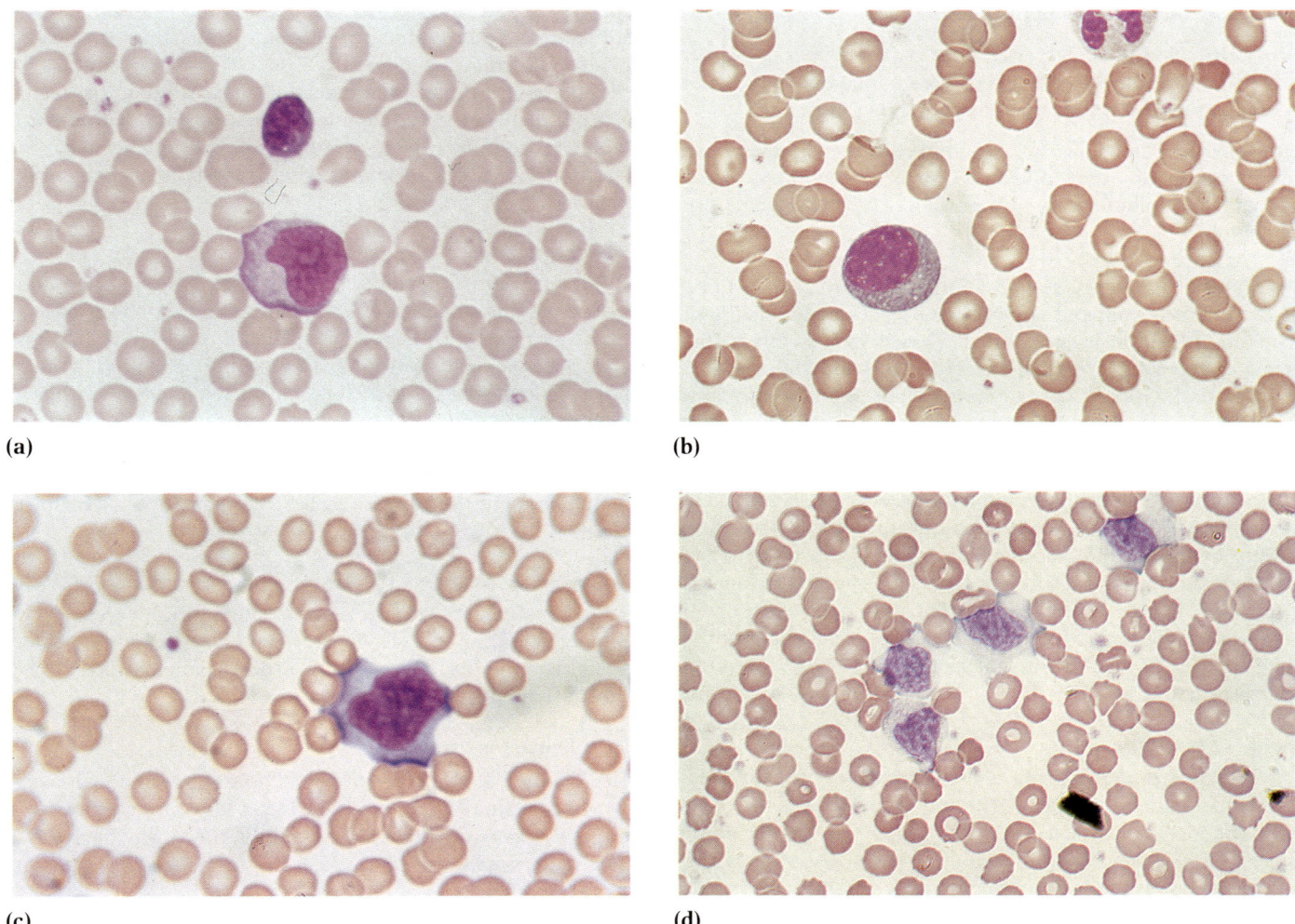

(a)   (b)

(c)   (d)

Fig. 23.19 Examples of reactive lymphocytes. (a) A large reactive lymphocyte with irregular primitive nucleus and a small normal lymphocyte; (b) a typical 'ameoboid' type of reactive lymphocyte with indentation of the cytoplasm by surrounding red cells; (c) a Turk cell, a reactive lymphocyte resembling a small plasma cell, with eccentric nucleus; (d) a collection of reactive lymphocytes from a case of glandular fever.

the dosage of these drugs to be adjusted according to the white cell count.

Antithyroid drugs These drugs, particularly carbimazole, may cause severe and sudden neutropenia associated with life-threatening infections—agranulocytosis.

Sulphonamides and co-trimoxazole may cause leucopenia, particularly when used in the elderly or in high doses, such as those employed in *Pneumocystis carinii* infections. Interference with folate metabolism is a likely cause of the leucopenia.

Chloramphenicol This may cause leucopenia, but is more commonly associated with aplastic anaemia.

The aminopyrone group This group of analgesics have largely been withdrawn from use because of the high incidence of agranulocytosis associated with their use, but it is still possible to purchase them over the counter in some countries. Antibodies are produced against the drug and the neutrophils become coated with the drug–antibody complexes and phagocytosed by the reticuloendothelial system.

Anti-arthritis drugs Such drugs that are sometimes associated with neutropenia are phenylbutazone, indomethacin, gold, penicillamine, ibuprofen, and (very rarely) aspirin.

Other drugs The following drugs have been reported to cause agranulocytosis: the phenothiazines, cimetidine, chlorpropamide, tolbutamide, allopurinol, procainamide, and phenytoin.

A careful drug history should be taken in any case of unexplained neutropenia and any unnecessary medication stopped. The complete list of drugs reported to be associated with neutropenia is too long to be reproduced here, and the reader is referred to the reports of the Committee of Safety in the Use of Drugs.*

Auto-immune leucopenia

Auto-immune cytopenias commonly affect red cells and platelets. The recognition of auto-immune leucopenias has been limited by the difficult laboratory tests that are required to substantiate the diagnosis. Auto-antibodies may be directed against peripheral blood neutrophils, resulting in neutropenia with active granulopoiesis in the bone marrow, or against granulocyte precursors, resulting in leucopenia with a lack of granulocyte precursors.

Felty's syndrome

This consists of neutropenia and splenomegaly in association with rheumatoid arthritis. The neutropenia is caused by immune-mediated destruction of mature neutrophils in the spleen. The bone marrow usually shows a compensatory granulocytic hyperplasia. Splenectomy usually restores the

* Reports on adverse drug reactions are published by the Committee on Safety of Medicines, 1 Nine Elms Lane, London SW8 5NQ. These are available in most hospital pharmacies.

neutrophil count to normal, at least initially, but may also render the patient more liable to infections.

Cyclical neutropenia

This condition is inherited in an autosomal dominant fashion, but not all are clinically affected. Approximately every four weeks a period of profound neutropenia occurs and may be associated with fever, ulceration of mouth and perianal region, and sometimes other infective manifestations. In some cases the periodicity of the neutropenia may be related to the menstrual cycle. If suspected as a cause of neutropenia, blood counts should be repeated fortnightly for 6 weeks. Examination of the marrow will usually show granulocytic hyperplasia or the absence of the more mature myeloid precursors. The neutropenia resolves spontaneously after 3–4 days. In some patients with this disorder the red cells and platelets are also affected and cycle synchronously with the neutrophils. There may be a compensatory monocytosis. This disorder is thought to result from a failure of the usual smooth autoregulatory mechanism that controls granulocyte production. The bone marrow is only stimulated into producing granulocytes when the blood neutrophil count is extremely low. The administration of recombinant human granulocyte colony-stimulating factor (G-CSF) reduces the period of severe neutropenia, but does not totally prevent the cycling. Prompt treatment of infective complications is most important. The disorder not infrequently improves spontaneously over the years.

Hypersplenism

Hypersplenism usually affects all cell lines, resulting in a pancytopenia, but on occasions one cell type may be more affected than the others. To cause cytopenias the spleen will almost always be palpable. Causes of splenic enlargement which may result in hypersplenism include portal hypertension, tropical splenomegaly, chronic haemolytic anaemias, and storage diseases. An element of hypersplenism may be present in myelofibrosis, chronic granulocytic leukaemia, and splenic lymphoma, but the marrow is also commonly affected by these diseases.

Neutropenia associated with excess of T-8 lymphocytes

Some patients with chronic neutropenia have an excess of T-8 (suppressor) lymphocytes, often of granular type, in their blood or marrow. Many, but not all, of these patients have T-cell chronic lymphocytic leukaemia.

Lazy leucocyte disease

This is a disorder of neutrophil mobilization which may be congenital or acquired. Although the blood shows a severe neutropenia, the marrow shows normal numbers of granulocytes and their precursors.

Neutropenia with pancreatic exocrine failure (Schwachman–Diamond syndrome)

This rare autosomal recessive inherited disorder commonly presents with failure to thrive and steatorrhoea in childhood, a clinical picture similar to fibrocystic disease, but without pulmonary disease. Although the blood commonly shows a severe neutropenia, the bone marrow usually shows granulocytic hyperplasia.

Infantile genetic agranulocytosis (Kostmann's disease)

This rare group of congenital severe neutropenias present in early childhood with severe recurrent infections. The blood shows very low neutrophil counts but often a monocytosis or eosinophilia. The marrow usually has normal numbers of myelocytes and promyelocytes, which fail to mature. Family consanguinity and associated congenital malformations are common. There appears to be a major defect in neutrophil maturation in this disorder. The disorder can be corrected in at least some patients by administration of G-CSF but not GM-CSF.

Management of the neutropenic patient

Patients with neutrophil counts less than 0.5×10^9/l, for whatever reason, are at serious risk of infection. Although avoiding exposure to sources of pathogenic organisms, such as infected patients or relatives, is sensible, it is commonly the neutropenic patient's own commensal flora that is the cause of serious infection. Reverse barrier isolation is therefore only of value when accompanied by decontamination of the gastrointestinal tract with broad-spectrum antibiotics and antifungals, the provision of sterile food, and nursing in an environment of filtered air. Such measures are generally only employed in the management of the most severely neutropenic patients, such as those receiving a bone marrow transplant.

For the majority of neutropenic patients, such as those receiving cytotoxic chemotherapy, the mainstay of management is close observation of the temperature and sites of potential infection such as mouth, intravenous access sites, and perineum. Topical antifungals (e.g. nystatin suspension) and antiseptic mouthwashes are employed as a routine precaution against oral infections. At the first sign of infection or pyrexia, blood cultures, mid-stream specimens of urine, and swabs of throat and any infective lesion are taken. Broad-spectrum antibiotics are then started while awaiting the results of microbiological investigations. Suitable antibiotics would be a combination of an aminoglycoside (gentamycin) and a broad-spectrum cephalosporin (e.g. cephtazidine) or a ureido penicillin (e.g. piperacillin). The advice of the microbiology laboratory in the choice of antibiotic policy should be sought at an early stage.

23.3.3 Leucocytosis

Introduction

A leucocytosis is defined as a total white cell count $> 10 \times 10^9$/l. This is most commonly due to an increase in neutrophils (neutrophilia), and more rarely to an increase in lymphocytes (lymphocytosis). Other components of the differential may be increased both in relative and absolute terms, but this increase is not usually reflected by an increase in the total white cell count.

A leucocytosis is a feature of the leukaemias and myeloproliferative disorders. These are distinguished from the reactive leukocytoses considered in this section because the leucocytes are often abnormal and there are associated abnormalities of the red cells and platelets.

Neutrophilia

A neutrophilia is the commonest white cell abnormality found in the blood count. Trauma and bacterial infection are the most frequent causes. Physical trauma may include accident, surgical operations, or thermal burns. Acute inflammation of any type, including chemical irritation, and infarction of tissue, for example myocardial infarction, also result in neutrophilia. The presence of necrotic tissue, such as a tumour, may stimulate a neutrophilia.

In bacterial infections the height of the neutrophil count is roughly proportional to the severity of infection, although occasionally patients with severe sepsis will have a low white cell count due to marrow depression and rapid transit of neutrophils to the infected area.

A neutrophilia is a normal finding in pregnancy, and total white cell counts of $12–13 \times 10^9$/l are not unusual. This may be related to the increased steroid hormone levels during pregnancy. The therapeutic administration of steroids such as hydrocortisone or prednisone will also cause a neutrophilia. Other drugs recognized to cause a neutrophilia are adrenaline and the lithium salts employed in the treatment of mania.

Physical and emotional stress may cause a neutrophilia. This may be seen after exercise, circulatory arrest, or anaphylactic reaction. When blood taking has been a difficult, traumatic, or tearful procedure in children a mild neutrophilia may be noted.

Neutrophilia usually accompanies the four myeloproliferative diseases—polycythaemia rubra vera, essential thrombocythaemia, myelofibrosis, and chronic granulocytic leukaemia. In polycythaemia, the finding of a neutrophilia helps to confirm the diagnosis of polycythaemia rubra vera as opposed to secondary polycythaemia. Chronic granulocytic leukaemia is manifested as a massive leucocytosis with left shift (the presence of immature granulocyte cells). In addition, there is usually an increase in eosinophils and basophils. Some cases of reactive neutrophilia may be difficult to distinguish from early chronic granulocytic leukaemia. The neutrophil alkaline phosphatase score may be used to distinguish between these disorders. The technique involves staining the neutrophils cytochemically for alkaline phosphatase activity and scoring the intensity of staining. Infections are associated with a high alkaline phosphatase score, acute and chronic myeloid leukaemia with a low one (Fig. 23.20).

Lymphocytosis

Children have a relative and absolute lymphocytosis in comparison to adults, from the first week of life to 7 years of age when adult values are attained.

Viral infections are the commonest cause of a reactive lymphocytosis, which may be found in the common cold,

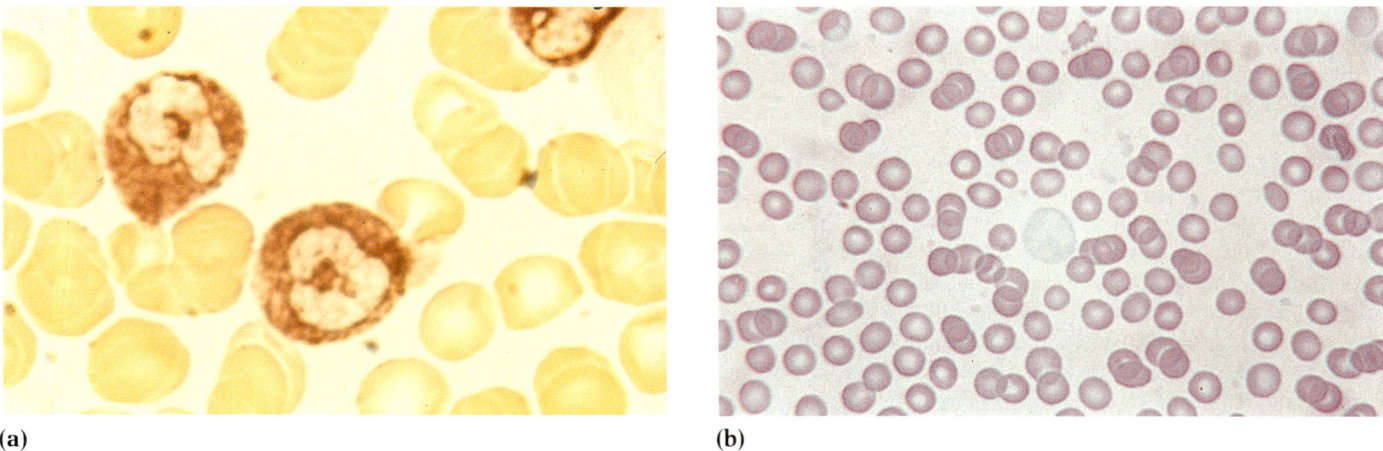

(a)   (b)

Fig. 23.20 Examples of neutrophils stained for the enzyme alkaline phosphatase. The presence of the enzyme is indicated by a brown precipitate in this method. (a) A high neutrophil alkaline phosphatase (NAP) score; (b) a low score, with absent staining.

influenza, cytomegalovirus, viral hepatitis, and glandular fever. The lymphocytes in these infections commonly show morphological abnormalities termed 'reactive changes'. These include enlargement and irregularity of the nucleus, cytoplasmic basophilia, increase in cytoplasmic volume, and indentation of the cytoplasm by surrounding red cells on the blood film. These atypical lymphocytes are most marked in glandular fever, considered in detail below.

Whooping cough (pertussis) infection is one of the few bacterial causes of a lymphocytosis, which may on occasions be sufficiently marked to produce white cell counts of over $50 \times 10^9/l$, mimicking leukaemia (a 'leukaemoid' reaction).

The commonest cause of a lymphocytosis in middle-aged and elderly people is chronic lymphocytic leukaemia. The small lymphocytes seen in the blood in this condition are fragile cells and easily crushed during the spreading of the blood film. They are seen on the blood film as 'smear' or 'smudge' cells (see Section 23.4.2).

Glandular fever (infectious mononucleosis)

This common, self-limiting viral disease is caused by the Epstein–Barr virus (EBV). It is transmitted by saliva or sexually and is commonest in adolescence (the 'kissing disease'). Presentation is commonly with malaise, fever, and cervical or generalized lymphadenopathy. There is usually sore throat, sometimes severe with membrane formation. The disease usually lasts from 1 to 4 weeks, though malaise and easy-tiring may persist for some months. Rarely, meningitis or encephalitis may be the predominant clinical feature. Some patients have a clinical syndrome indistinguishable from infectious hepatitis, and most have elevated transaminases.

The blood shows a lymphocytosis with reactive lymphocytes on the blood film. Occasionally the patient may be thrombocytopenic. Distinction from the other causes of a reactive lymphocytosis is made by detection of heterophile antibodies in the patient's serum, which are characteristic of the disease. These antibodies have the characteristic of agglutinating the cells of other animal species. The Paul–Bunnell test detects the presence of antibodies against sheep red blood cells. A nonspecific heterophile antibody may be found in the serum in infectious diseases other than glandular fever. This is removed from the serum by absorption against ox red blood cells before testing against sheep red blood cells. A rapid slide test (e.g. Monospot) is available in which the non-specific antibody is absorbed by an homogenate of guinea-pig kidney before the sheep red cells are added. Although a positive slide test for glandular fever is not completely specific for this disease, this is not usually of clinical importance as related viral illnesses usually pursue a similar clinical course. Early in the course of the illness a reactive lymphocytosis may be found in the blood without heterophile antibody. In cases with a strong clinical suspicion of glandular fever the Paul–Bunnell test should be repeated in a week. The test will remain positive after clinical recovery for weeks or months.

The blood film may show cold agglutinates due to an autoreacting anti-i. This antigen is present on all red cells but strongest on fetal red cells. It may be detected by making serial dilutions of the serum in saline and incubating them with adult (I antigen) and cord (i antigen) red cells at 4 °C. A high titre of anti-I may be found in idiopathic cold haemagglutinin disease (see Section 23.2.6) and *Mycoplasma pneumoniae* infection. Rarely the anti-i found in glandular fever may cause a cold auto-immune haemolytic anaemia.

Monocytosis

An increased count of monocytes is often found in conditions associated with a neutrophilia. An isolated monocytosis is unusual. It is seen during recovery from cytotoxic chemotherapy when the monocytes may be *en route* to damaged tissues to participate in the repair mechanism and phagocytose debris. Chronic tuberculous infection may also cause a monocytosis. The commonest cause of a chronic monocytosis is chronic myelomonocytic leukaemia and the other myelodysplastic states (see Section 23.5.2).

Eosinophilia

An eosinophilia is defined as an absolute eosinophil count over $0.5 \times 10^9/l$. Eosinophils are easily recognized in blood films because of their orange granulation when stained by conventional Romanovsky stains (Fig. 23.15b). They are the hallmark of allergic disorders, being increased in asthma, hayfever, eczema, allergic dermatitis, and drug reactions. In tropical countries parasitic infection (e.g. hookworms) is a very common cause of eosinophilia. Rarer causes include Hodgkin's disease and polyarteritis nodosa.

When the eosinophilia is very marked ($> 1.5 \times 10^9/l$) and not clearly related to one of the above disorders, the term hypereosinophilic syndrome is often applied. When associated with pulmonary infiltrates it is termed Loeffler's syndrome. Prolonged hypereosinophilia may result in tissue damage due to the release of toxic substances, such as eosinophil cationic protein, lysozomal enzymes, and eosinophil neurotoxin, from disintegrating eosinophils. The heart is particularly likely to be affected, with endomyocardial fibrosis and mural thrombi. Some cases of hypereosinophilia are associated with chromosomal abnormalities in the marrow cells and qualify as cases of eosinophilic leukaemia (see Section 23.5.3)

Basophilia

A basophilia is defined as an absolute basophil count over $0.1 \times 10^9/l$. Basophils are recognized by their deep-blue staining on Romanovsky stains (Fig. 23.18c). The commonest cause of a basophilia is one of the myeloproliferative disorders (pp. 1717–1731). Other causes are rare but include allergic disorders, colitis, rheumatoid arthritis, myxoedema, and after splenectomy.

23.3.4 Qualitative disorders of neutrophil function

Qualitative abnormalities of neutrophil function may affect any stage of microbial elimination. These stages include recognition, adhesion, phagocytosis, killing, and digestion. Laboratory investigation of neutrophil function is laborious and consequently acquired qualitative disorders of neutrophils are rarely recognized. The majority of neutrophil functional disorders are congenital.

Congenital neutrophil dysfunction

Chediak–Higashi syndrome

This autosomal recessive disorder is characterized by defects in the cell membranes and granule-limiting membranes within cells. The neutrophils, monocytes, and lymphocytes have characteristic giant cytoplasmic granules.

Failure of the correct dispersion of melanin pigment granules in melanocytes leads to albinism, the patient having pale skin, silvery hair, and photophobia. A peripheral neuropathy is sometimes present.

Besides the morphological and functional abnormalities of white cells, there is also leucopenia, thrombocytopenia, and a deficiency of natural killer cells. The bleeding tendency is ex-acerbated by lack of ADP and serotonin in platelet granules—one variety of storage-pool deficiency (see Section 23.6.2).

The disease is subject to exacerbations resembling malignant proliferations of lymphocytes and monocytes—'accelerated phase'. Some clinical improvement has been reported with high doses of vitamin C.

Chronic granulomatous disease (CGD)

A variety of abnormalities at the genetic molecular level may result in failure of neutrophils to generate sufficient superoxide and hydrogen peroxide, which are responsible for the killing of phagocytosed bacteria. The neutrophils from affected patients fail to consume oxygen after phagocytosis (the 'respiratory burst'). Some bacteria, such as *Pseudomonas* and *Serratia marcescens* contain catalase, an enzyme that breaks down hydrogen peroxide formed in phagocytic vacuoles. Normal neutrophils generate enough hydrogen peroxide to overwhelm this enzyme and, in the presence of myeloperoxidase, the hydrogen peroxide kills the organism. In CGD the catalase is sufficient to neutralize the small amounts of hydrogen peroxide produced, allowing the organism to multiply in the neutrophil where it is protected from circulating immunoglobulin. Patients with CGD are particularly susceptible to infections by these bacteria. Chronic granulomatous disease may be inherited as an X-linked, autosomal recessive, or autosomal dominant disorder. The enzyme system responsible for the respiratory burst, NADP oxidase, may show a variety of abnormalities, causing different clinical variants of the disease. Cytochrome b, part of this enzyme system, is absent in all cases of classic sex-linked CGD, but present in autosomally inherited variants.

CGD presents with recurrent mucocutaneous infections in childhood (with organisms such as the staphylococcus or streptococcus) which fail to heal, forming chronic granulomatous lesions. Lymphadenopathy with abscess formation, hepatic abscesses, and osteomyelitis are common. The white cell count is usually normal but the neutrophils fail to kill ingested organisms. Diagnosis is commonly based on the nitroblue-tetrazolium (NBT) test. In this test the patient's neutrophils are incubated with the clear yellow NBT solution. If the neutrophils are capable of the chemical reactions required to form a functioning phagocytic vacuole, they will reduce the clear yellow NBT solution to insoluble blue formazan granules, which are viewed microscopically. In chronic granulomatous disease there is failure to reduce NBT to formazan.

The anaemia of chronic disease which accompanies the recurrent infections characteristic of this disorder may be severe enough to merit transfusion. Difficulties in obtaining compatible blood may be experienced because some of these patients have an unusual Kell blood group termed 'Kell null' or the McLeod phenotype. After the first transfusion with blood bearing the usual Kell antigens the patient may make atypical antibodies against these antigens, which may result in the haemolysis of further transfusions.

Prompt and appropriate antibiotic treatment of infections is the mainstay of treatment, and continuous prophylactic cotrimoxazole treatment is useful in many cases.

CD11/CD18 glycoprotein deficiency

This rare congenital (usually autosomal recessive) defect of neutrophil function is associated with the absence of a number of cellular adhesion molecules from the cell surface. These include the CD11 and CD18 antigens and the complement receptor C3R. The adhesion molecules help the neutrophil move and stick to target structures. Treating leucocytes with antibodies raised in animals against the CD11/CD18 antigens mimics the functional defects found in the leucocytes from patients with this disease.

Diagnosis is made in early childhood. Besides suffering repeated skin, mouth, ear, and chest infections, these children have delayed wound healing, which is often first manifest as delayed separation of the umbilical cord. They usually have a neutrophil leucocytosis. Bone marrow transplantation is probably the treatment of choice if an HLA-matched sibling donor is available.

23.3.5 Further reading

Baranski, B. and Young, N. (1987). Hematologic consequences of viral infections. *Hematology/Oncology Clinics of North America* **1** (2), 167–83.

Bowdler, A. J. (1983). Splenomegaly and hypersplenism. *Clinics in Haematology* **12** (2), 467.

Carter, R. L. (1969). *Infectious mononucleosis.* Blackwell Scientific Publications, Oxford.

Cline, M. J. and Golde, D. W. (1977). Granulocytes and monocytes: function and functional disorders. In *Recent advances in haematology* (ed. A. V. Hoffbrand, M. C. Brain, and J. Hirsh). Churchill Livingstone, London.

Dale, D. C. and Hammond, W. P. IV (1988). Cyclical neutropenia, a clinical review. *Blood Reviews* **2** (2), 178–85.

Forrest, C. B., Forehand, J. R., Axtell, R. A., Roberts, R. L., and Johnston Jr., R. B. (1988). Clinical features and current management of chronic granulomatous disease. *Hematology/Oncology Clinics of North America* **2** (2), 253.

Kostmann, R. (1956). Infantile genetic agranulocytosis. A new recessive lethal disease in man. *Acta Paediatrica Scandinavica* **105**, 45–9.

Logue, G. L. and Shimm, D. S. (1980). Auto-immune granulocytopenia. *Annual Review of Medicine* **31**, 191–200.

Mowat, A. G. (1971). Haematological abnormalities in rheumatoid arthritis. *Seminars in Arthritis and Rheumatism* **1**, 195–219.

Newland, A. C. *et al.* (1984). Chronic T cell lymphocytosis, a review of 21 cases. *British Journal of Haematology* **58**, 433–46.

Prentice, H. G. (ed.) (1984). Infections in haematology. *Clinics in Haematology* **13**, (3).

23.4 Neoplastic lymphoproliferative disorders

D. C. Linch

23.4.1 Acute lymphoblastic leukaemia

Epidemiology

The annual incidence of acute lymphoblastic leukaemia (ALL) in the UK is approximately 1.2 per 100 000. The incidence peaks in childhood between the ages of 1 and 6 years, falls during adolescence, and then remains low throughout adulthood.

Pathogenesis

In ALL the malignant change occurs in a lymphoid cell at an early stage of differentiation and there is an accumulation in the blood and marrow of primitive lymphoid cells (lymphoblasts). The lymphoblasts may be of T-cell or B-cell origin. In the West, T-cell ALL accounts for 10–15 per cent of cases, whereas in underdeveloped countries the incidence of T-ALL is apparently higher. B-cell ALL can be subdivided into three types according to the stage of differentiation at which the lymphoblasts are arrested; early, intermediate, and late. These types of ALL are recognized by immunophenotyping (Table 23.3) and are referred to as 'null ALL', common ALL, and the rare B-cell ALL. The antigens detected are normal differentiation stage-associated antigens and are not leukaemia specific. In childhood the large majority of cases are of the 'common type' whereas in adults only half the cases are of the common type, nearly 40 per cent being 'null ALL'. Cytogenetic abnormalities are found in about two-thirds of cases. Hyperdiploidy is common. The Philadelphia chromosome (9;22 translocation) is found in about 5 per cent of childhood ALL and 20 per cent of adult cases. An 8;14 translocation is found in most cases of B-cell ALL as in Burkitt's lymphoma. The accumulation of lymphoblasts within the bone marrow results in failure of normal haemopoiesis. Infiltration and enlargement of the lymph nodes, liver, and spleen also occurs frequently. Involvement of the central nervous system is rare at presentation but is a common site of relapse if no specific CNS prophylaxis is given.

Table 23.3 Subcategories of ALL based on lineage and differentiation stage

Cell lineage	Differentiation stage	Alternative name	Terminal deoxynucleotidyl transferase (Tdt)	HLA-DR	CD10 (common ALL)	CD19 (pan B antigen)	CD7 (pan T antigen)	Surface Ig	Ig gene rearrangement	T-cell receptor gene rearrangement
B-lineage	Very early	Null cell ALL	+	+	−	+	−	−	+	−
	Early	Common ALL	+	+	+	+	−	−	+	−
	Late	B-cell ALL	−	+	−	+	−	+	+	−
T-lineage		T-cell ALL	+	−	+/−	−	+	−	−	+

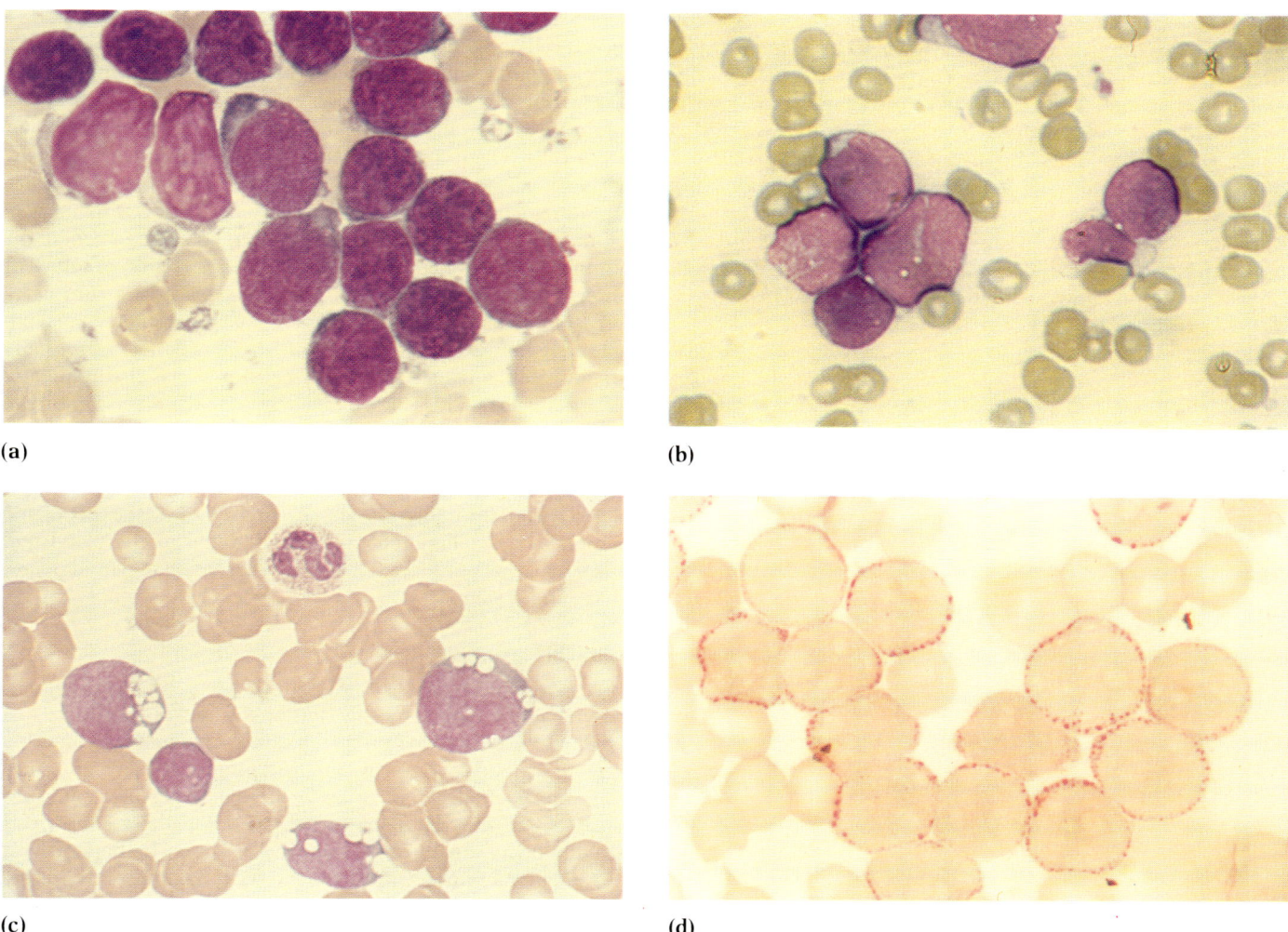

(a)

(b)

(c)

(d)

Fig. 23.21 (a) The bone marrow in a case of acute lymphoblastic leukaemia type L_1. The blast cells tend to be more uniform and smaller than in the L_2 type, shown in (b). Type L_3 is distinguished by blast cells with deep-blue cytoplasm and cytoplasmic vacuoles (c). Immunologic surface typing of these blasts shows them to be of B-cell lineage. Cytochemical stains may assist in the diagnosis of acute lymphoblastic leukaemia and its distinction from acute myeloid leukaemia. Dot and necklace staining for periodic acid–Schiff staining is characteristic (d).

Clinical presentation

Most patients present with the features of marrow failure, namely anaemia, infection, and bleeding. There is no 'preleuk-aemic phase' in ALL [cf. acute myeloid leukaemia (AML)] except that a small proportion of patients present with transient aplastic anaemia with no evidence of a leukaemic proliferation. Bone and joint pain may occur, especially in children, and a mistaken diagnosis of arthritis may be made. On examination an element of lymphadenopathy and hepatosplenomegaly is common. In T-cell ALL a chest X-ray reveals a thymic mass in 50 per cent of cases.

Haematological features

The hallmark of ALL is the presence of lymphoblasts in the bone marrow and usually in the blood. Lymphoblasts can usually be discriminated from myeloblasts by light microscopy. Lympho-blasts tend to have less cytoplasm than myeloblasts and do not contain Auer rods. The nuclei contain only one or two nucleoli, whereas more than this are often seen in myeloblasts. In diffi-cult cases cytochemistry and immunophenotyping are usually diagnostic. Lymphoblasts are peroxidase and Sudan black negative (cf. AML) and usually PAS positive. The phenotypes of the different types of ALL are shown in Table 23.3. Lympho-blasts vary in their appearance (Fig. 23.21) and have been arbi-trarily divided into L_1, L_2, and L_3 types. L_1 lymphoblasts are relatively small blasts with little cytoplasm and regular shaped nuclei, and L_2 blasts are more pleomorphic and irregular. L_3 blasts are very rare and correspond to the B-cell-type ALL. They have relatively abundant dark-blue vacuolated cytoplasm. Normocytic anaemia is frequently seen.

Treatment and prognosis

The first stage of treatment is the 'induction of remission', defined as a normal blood count and < 5 per cent blasts in the marrow. Vincristine and prednisone have been the mainstay of therapy, but most regimes now contain anthracyclines and often other agents. With these types of regimes remission is obtained in over 95 per cent of children and over 90 per cent of adults. Once remission is obtained it is usual to give a further intensive course of therapy referred to as 'consolidation', followed by more gentle 'maintenance therapy'. This is usually given for at least 2 years. In some centres maintenance therapy is interrupted after about 6 months by a further course of intensive therapy known as 'late intensification'. This may be particularly useful in 'poor prognosis' cases.

Craniospinal prophylaxis must also be given during remission to prevent CNS relapse. It is usual to give a combination of cranial irradiation and intrathecal cytoxic therapy. Spinal irradiation is avoided in children as it arrests vertebral growth.

Bone marrow transplantation (BMT) is not usually employed as a first treatment option in ALL because it is associated with a high risk of leukaemia recurrence if the patient is not in remission and the procedure is associated with a significant mortality. Also, 60 per cent of children may be cured by conventional chemotherapy alone, so BMT is usually employed during second remission. In adults bone marrow transplantation in first remission may be appropriate.

The overall long-term survival of children with ALL now exceeds 60 per cent, whereas in adults it is still less than 30 per cent. Factors adversely influencing outcome, in addition to age, are a high peripheral blood blast cell count at presentation and male sex. A normal chromosome pattern or hyperdiploidy is associated with a relatively good prognosis, whereas most other chromosome changes are indicative of a poor prognosis. T-cell-ALLs have a worse prognosis than null ALLs, and common ALLs fare best of all. The phenotype correlates with the presenting white count, however, and provides little independent prognostic information. By use of such factors it is possible to define 'high-risk' cases for relapse, but the use of more intensive therapy in such childhood patients may result in a similar long-term survival to the 'low-risk' group.

23.4.2 Chronic lymphocytic leukaemia

Epidemiology

Chronic lymphocytic leukaemia (CLL) has an incidence in the UK of approximately 6 per 100 000 per annum. The disease does not occur in children and the incidence rises steeply in the later decades of life. It is nearly twice as common in males as in females.

Pathogenesis

At least 95 per cent of cases of CLL are B-cell neoplasms. No specific causes have been identified. CLL has an unusual characteristic in that it is one of the few haematological malignancies in which the incidence does not rise following exposure to irradiation. The normal counterpart of the cell that accumulates in CLL has not been clearly defined but is probably a relatively 'early' resting B-cell. The CLL cell expresses the CD19 and CD20 pan B-cell antigens, and the CD5 antigen which is expressed on T-cells and a limited differentiation stage of B-lymphocytes. B-CLL cells also express receptors that bind mouse erythrocytes to form rosettes, in contrast to T-cells and many natural killer (NK) cells which form rosettes with sheep erythrocytes. Low levels of surface immunoglobulin are present and the surface immunoglobulin is light-chain restricted, which is a hallmark of clonal B-cell proliferations. There is clonal rearrangement of the immunoglobulin heavy and light chains. Secretion of sufficient monoclonal immunoglobulin to be detected as a serum paraprotein band is rare (approximately 5 per cent of cases). Hypogammaglobulin occurs in about one-third of patients, especially in those with advanced disease. T-cell function is also frequently abnormal but there is little agreement as to the precise nature of the defect. The number of CD8$^+$ T-cells is commonly raised. Auto-immune haemolysis is a not infrequent feature of the immunodysregulation. The offending auto-antibodies are not derived from the malignant B-cells. In the early stages of CLL the lymphocyte proliferation may be restricted to the blood and bone marrow, but there is usually enlargement of lymph nodes, liver, and spleen.

Clinical features

CLL typically presents because the patient discovers lymphadenopathy or splenomegaly, although the disease may be discovered on an incidental blood count. Anaemia may develop due to extensive marrow infiltration, hypersplenism, auto-immune haemolysis, or due to cytotoxic drug therapy. Similarly, there may be a low neutrophil or platelet count, this usually being a feature of advanced disease. The patient with CLL is often immunosuppressed and bacterial infections are frequently the terminal event.

Lymph node histology

There is diffuse infiltration and effacement of the nodal architecture by small mature lymphocytes. Also, within the node are foci of larger cells containing nucleoli and referred to as proliferation centres. These are the features of malignant lymphoma: lymphocytic, which may occur without an overt leukaemic element. Similar infiltration is seen in other organs if affected.

Blood film

The lymphocyte count is variably raised from just above the upper limit of normal to over 300×10^9/l. Most of the lymphocytes are small with nuclear condensation and little cytoplasm, although a few cells are larger with a detectable nucleolus (prolymphocytes). Smudge cells are usually numerous on the blood film (Fig. 23.22a).

Treatment and prognosis

Treatment is only indicated if the patient is symptomatic or has critical organ dysfunction, as the disease is incurable. Therapy is usually commenced with an oral alkylating agent such as chlorambucil. Corticosteroids are of value if there is immune haemolysis or thrombocytopenia. There is usually a good initial response but ultimately there is disease progression despite increased therapy. The clinical progression may be associated with increasing numbers of prolymphocytes on the blood film and, rarely, there is a transformation to a high grade, usually retroperitoneal, non-Hodgkin's lymphoma. The median survival from diagnosis is approximately 5 years, although many patients presenting with early disease survive for much longer periods.

23.4.3   Variants of chronic lymphocytic leukaemia

T-cell chronic lymphocytic leukaemia

The chronic T-cell lymphoproliferative disorders include several distinct clinicopathological entities. A monoclonal proliferation of large granular CD8$^+$ lymphocytes is usually a very low-grade malignancy (Fig. 23.22b). It is often associated with rheumatoid arthritis and severe cytopenias that may have an immune basis. By contrast, the proliferation of CD4$^+$ lymphocytes, including Sezary's syndrome (Fig. 23.22c), is usually far more aggressive.

Prolymphocytic leukaemia (PLL)

In this variant of chronic lymphocytic leukaemia, the proportion of prolymphocytes on the blood film is high (Fig. 23.22d). The majority of cases are of B-cell origin, although the B-PLL cells differ from B-CLL cells, not only morphologically but also in immunophenotyping. They express more surface immunoglobulin and not the CD5 antigen or mouse erythrocyte receptor. In prolymphocytic leukaemia the peripheral lymphocyte count is often extremely elevated and sufficient to cause hyperviscosity. The spleen may be enormous. The prognosis is less favourable than in typical CLL.

Hairy-cell leukaemia

Hairy-cell leukaemia is a chronic B-cell lymphoproliferative disorder in which the malignant cells in the blood and marrow typically have fine cytoplasmic projections (Fig. 23.22e). The peripheral lymphocyte count is not usually high but there may be a heavy infiltration of the marrow with marked reactive fibrosis. A marrow aspirate usually reveals a 'dry tap'. Biopsy of the marrow shows a diffuse infiltration of widely spaced mononuclear cells forming a 'lacey' or 'web-like' network with increased reticulin. This, together with hypersplenism, commonly leads to severe neutropenia and monocytopenia with its concomitant infective complications.

Good responses can be achieved with the adenosine deaminase inhibitor deoxycorformycin and α-interferon. Splenectomy may also be of value. The prognosis is similar to CLL.

Waldenstrom's macroglobulinaemia

This is a rare low-grade malignancy that occurs predominantly in the elderly. There may be a moderate lymphocytosis in the blood or the presentation may be of a lymphomatous type with lymphadenopathy and hepatosplenomegaly. Biopsy of involved tissue shows a diffuse infiltration of small lymphocytes with plasmacytoid differentiation (malignant lymphoma: lymphoplasmacytoid). Similar cells are seen in the blood and bone marrow (Fig. 23.22f). The major feature of Waldenstrom's macroglobulinaemia is the production of large quantities of IgM paraprotein which may lead to a hyperviscosity syndrome, cold sensitivity if the paraprotein is a cryoglobulin, and haemorrhagic tendencies.

No specific therapy is needed in asymptomatic patients. When symptoms arise, a good, albeit partial, response may be obtained with an oral alkylating agent. Hyperviscosity may necessitate plasmapheresis until the disease is brought under control with chemotherapy.

23.4.4   Multiple myeloma

Epidemiology

Multiple myeloma has an annual incidence of approximately 6 per 100 000. It occurs predominantly in the elderly and is very rare below the age of 30 years.

Pathophysiology

Multiple myeloma is a malignant B-cell proliferation within the bone marrow in which the predominant cell type to accumulate is the plasma cell. The stage of differentiation at which malignant transformation occurs is not known but is likely to be earlier than the plasma cell.

Although primarily a marrow disorder, multiple myeloma results in multiple systemic disturbances (Fig. 23.23). Osteoclast activating factors are released from the diseased marrow and lead to osteoporosis, the formation of osteolytic lesions and hypercalcaemia in some cases. The nature of the osteoclast activating factor is uncertain but interleukin-I (IL-1) and transforming growth factor-β_1 (TFG-β) have been implicated as candidate molecules. The osteoporosis and lytic lesions frequently lead to spinal collapse and fractures of weight-bearing bones on minimal trauma. Lytic lesions of the skull are common but rarely cause clinical problems. The X-ray appearances of the lytic lesions and fractures are typically characterized by absence of sclerosis due to lack of an osteoblastic reaction. In accordance with this, the serum alkaline phosphatase level is not usually raised.

Hypercalcaemia occurs in 30 per cent of patients at some stage of the disease and produces the same symptomatology as other forms of hypercalcaemia. Hypercalcaemia is often reversible and does not necessarily imply a poor progress, although it can cause or exacerbate any renal impairment.

The proliferation of excessive plasma cells within the marrow (Fig. 23.24) may lead to anaemia and other cytopenias with their concomitant infective complications. This is partly due to marrow replacement and partly due to a poorly understood myelosuppressive effect of the malignant proliferation. The anaemia may be augmented by a dilutional element due to a

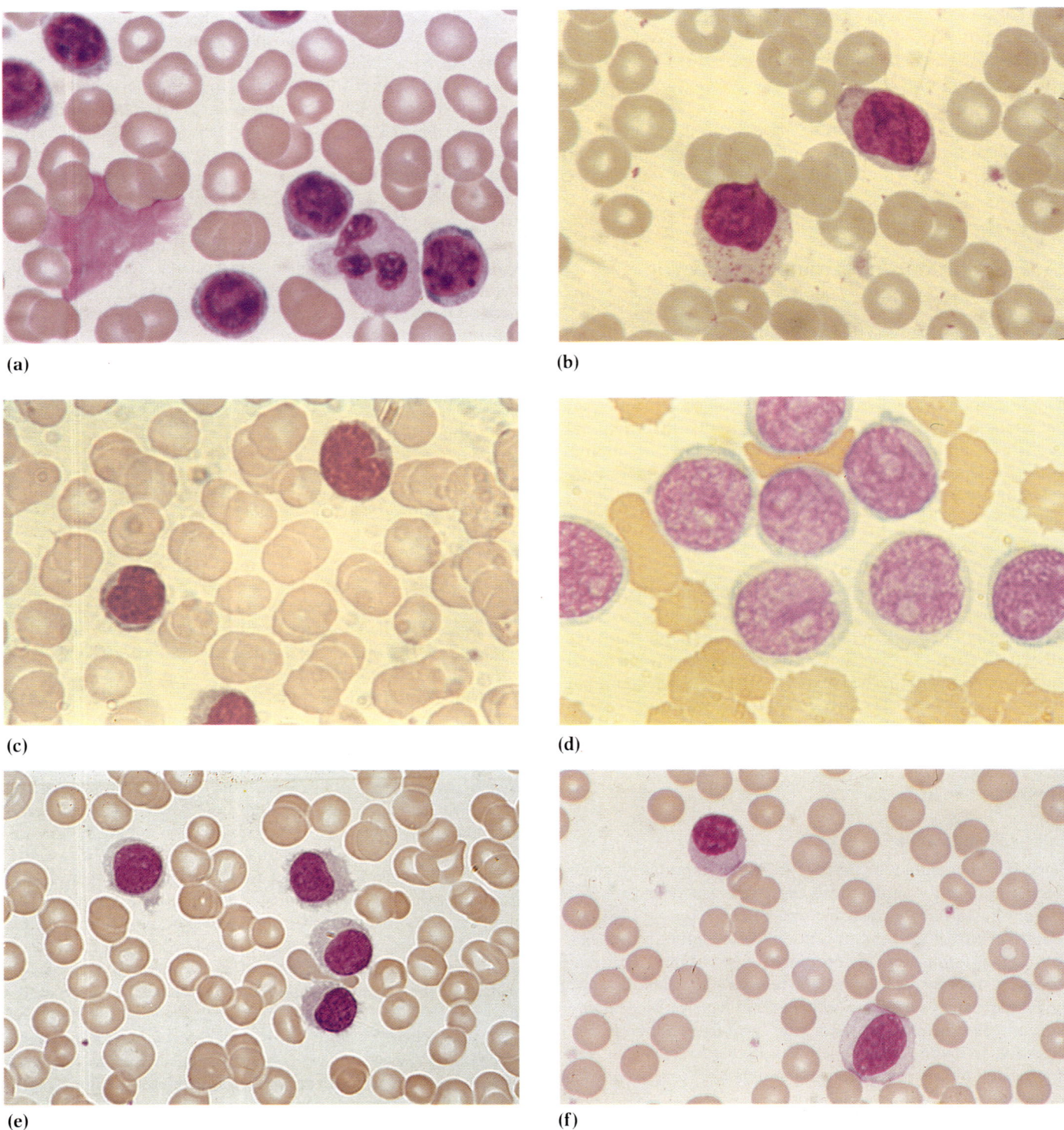

Fig. 23.22 (a) The peripheral blood in chronic lymphocytic leukaemia. The major cell type is the small lymphocyte. One of these has become crushed during the making of the blood film—a smear or smudge cell (bottom left). (b) An example of a large granular T-lymphocyte. A large non-granular lymphocyte is also present. (c) Lymphocytes from a case of Sezary's syndrome. The majority of lymphocytes in this T-cell disorder are clefted. (d) Prolymphocytes from a case of prolymphocytic leukaemia. These cells have prominent nucleoli but are distinguished from blast cells by their relatively voluminous cytoplasm. (e) Hairy cells from a case of hairy-cell leukaemia. These cells have fine hair-like projections from the cytoplasmic surface. (f) Lymphoplasmacytoid lymphocytes from a case of Waldenstrom's macroglobulinaemia. The cells have an eccentric nucleus and resemble small plasma cells.

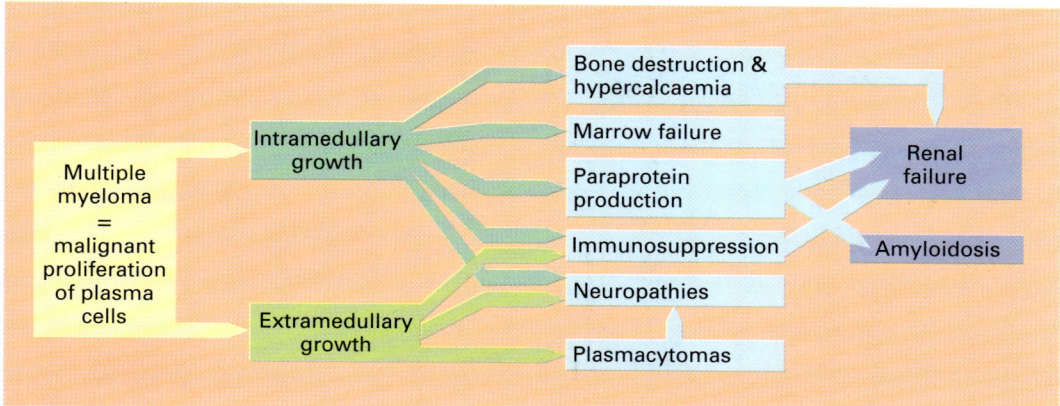

Fig. 23.23 Pathophysiology of multiple myeloma.

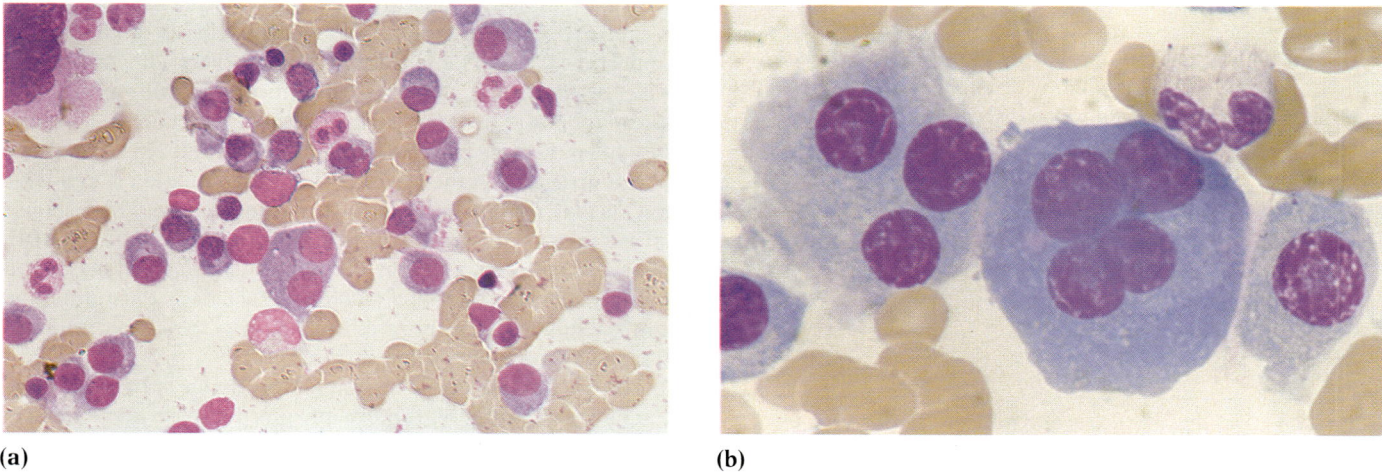

(a)   (b)

Fig. 23.24 (a) The bone marrow in a case of myeloma. There is an excess of plasma cells, which normally constitute less than 5 per cent of nucleated cells. Plasma cells are distinguished by their eccentric nuclei, blue cytoplasm, perinuclear halo, and 'clock-face' nuclear chromatin pattern. In myeloma the plasma cells may show morphological abnormalities such as multinuclearity, shown in (b).

raised plasma volume, which not infrequently occurs if there is a large quantity of circulating paraprotein. Cytopenias are also exacerbated by cytotoxic therapy.

A paraprotein is detectable on serum electrophoresis in over 75 per cent of cases and is most commonly of IgG type (Fig. 23.25). A further 20 per cent of patients have an excess of free light-chains within the urine without evidence of a circulating paraprotein. These light-chains are known as Bence–Jones protein (BJP). A non-secretory myeloma (without paraprotein or BJP) is rare. The paraprotein itself does not usually cause symptoms but may give rise to a hyperviscosity syndrome, especially with IgA paraproteins which have a tendency to polymerize. Other paraproteins may be cryoglobulins and give rise to Raynaud's phenomena, and occasionally paraproteins may contribute to a bleeding diathesis by non-specific coating of platelets which impairs their function. Some paraprotein light-chains are amyloidogenic and readily form amyloid deposits

(see Section 5.5). The properties of the light-chain that contribute to the formation of amyloid are poorly understood.

Renal dysfunction is not infrequent at presentation and with advancing disease. The causes are multiple and include light-chain precipitation in the renal tubules, deposition of amyloid in the glomeruli, hypercalcaemia, infection, and, less commonly, hyperuricaemia and plasma cell infiltration. Most importantly, there is often a prerenal element that can be corrected with prompt and vigorous rehydration.

Myeloma deposits in vertebral bodies may cause cord compression or root lesions. In addition, peripheral neuropathies may arise as a non-metastatic manifestation of malignancy.

Plasmacytomas are localized accumulations of plasma cells which form distinct tumours. They may occur on the background of multiple myeloma or may arise without apparent disseminated disease. They may arise in almost any site but are particularly common in skin, pleura, lung, retroperitoneal, and

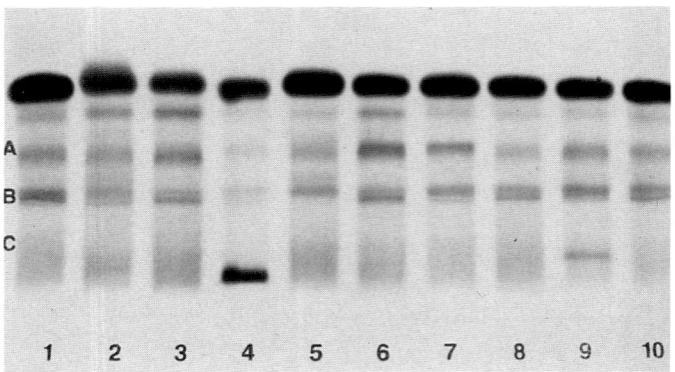

Fig. 23.25 Examples of protein electrophoretic strips. Electrophoresis of the plasma proteins separates them into albumin (top), alpha$_1$, alpha$_2$, beta, and gammaglobulin (bottom). Sample number four shows the presence of a dense band in the gammaglobulin region—a paraprotein.

retro-orbital tissues. Solitary plasmacytomas may be associated with a paraprotein. This should disappear after radical local radiotherapy; if not, disseminated disease can be assumed.

Diagnostic criteria

Most cases of multiple myeloma are readily diagnosed. Occasionally difficulties arise and strict diagnostic criteria must be adhered to (Table 23.4). Two of the three major criteria should be present, and when there is significant doubt it is often advis-

Table 23.4 Diagnostic criteria and differential diagnosis of multiple myeloma

Major criteria	Differential diagnosis
Bone marrow plasmacytosis (>20 per cent, or less if monoclonality proven)	Chronic infections* and inflammatory disorders
	Liver disease*
	Other tumours*
Lytic bone lesions	Multiple metastases
	Spotty osteoporosis†
	Hyperparathyroidism
	Multiple granuloma
	Hydatid disease
	Fibrous dysplasia
Paraprotein in blood or urine	Benign monoclonal gamnopathies
	Malignant lymphoproliferative disorders
	Some other tumours
	Auto-immune disease
	Infections
	Liver disease

* Plasmacytosis rarely at 20 per cent level.
† Differential diagnosis in italics are unusual.

able to adopt an expectant policy. The infiltration of bone marrow plasma cells may be patchy, and occasionally a repeat aspirate is necessary. Some difficulty can arise with benign monoclonal gammopathies (BMGs), which can only be diagnosed with certainty in retrospect. It is initially a diagnosis of exclusion. The haemoglobin should be normal, there should be < 10 per cent plasma cells in the marrow, little or no Bence–Jones protein in the urine and no osteolytic lesions. The paraprotein level should remain constant and below 35 g/l for IgG and 20 g/l for IgA. Other immunoglobulins should not be suppressed. BMG is very common in the elderly being present in 3 per cent of individuals in the eighth decade of life and 15 per cent of individuals in the tenth decade.

Treatment and prognosis

Most patients are symptomatic at presentation and require urgent treatment. Supportive therapy including rehydration, treatment of hypercalcaemia, and pain relief is of paramount importance. Local radiotherapy is often very effective in the relief of bone pain. Hyperviscosity, if present, may necessitate plasmapheresis. Specific therapy is usually with an oral alkylating agent such as melphalan, with or without corticosteroids, although there is some evidence that a combination of cytotoxic agents may slightly improve the tumour response. The response is usually partial and in a proportion of patients a 'plateau phase' is achieved, whereby the reduced plasma cell mass (and paraprotein level) become stable. At this stage chemotherapy can be stopped until progression again occurs. The unmaintained plateau may last for many months.

The median survival in multiple myeloma is only 2 years. Patients presenting with more advanced disease have a worse prognosis. Poor prognostic indicators at presentation are anaemia, renal failure, reduced performance status, and a markedly raised serum β_2 microglobulin level.

23.4.5 Cryoglobulinaemia

Cryoglobulins are immunoglobulins which precipitate when cooled. They may be monoclonal, polyclonal, or mixed. The monoclonal cryoglobulins are usually indicative of a lymphoproliferative disease and the polyclonal varieties are usually reactive. A mixed monoclonal and polyclonal cryoglobulin is not infrequently associated with auto-immune disease. Clinically, their presence may give rise to peripheral cyanosis, Raynaud's phenomenon, vascular purpura, arthralgia, and, in the most severe cases, renal failure, hepatic failure, and isolated neurological lesions.

The blood film typically shows marked agglutination of red cells and the ESR may be spuriously low at room temperature but normal if performed at 37 °C.

The mainstay of treatment is avoidance of cold, and treatment of any underlying conditions such as a lymphoma. Plasmapheresis may have a role if there are severe symptoms.

23.5 Myeloproliferative disorders

J. M. Goldman

23.5.1 Acute myeloid leukaemia

The existence of an apparently primary or autonomous proliferation of immature cells in the haemopoietic system, originally termed 'leukocythaemia' and subsequently abbreviated to 'leukaemia', was recognized more than 100 years ago. For many of these intervening years, however, the disease was regarded as basically untreatable and therefore incurable and was, as a consequence, of only passing interest to clinicians and haematologists. Much has changed in the past 30 years. Something is now known of the epidemiology and factors predisposing to development of the acute leukaemias; considerable progress has been made in distinguishing the two major types of acute leukaemia, myeloid and lymphoblastic, and the methods for sub-classifying the leukaemic cells are now very sophisticated. Progress has been made in treatment also. In specialist centres 70–80 per cent of younger patients (aged less than 60 years) with acute myeloid leukaemia (AML) may expect to achieve complete remission and about 25 per cent of these may be cured. Results of treating older patients and those too sick for referral to specialist centres are still much less encouraging.

Epidemiology

Statistics on the incidence, mortality, and demographic aspects of acute myeloid leukaemia (AML) are still rather incomplete. The problem relates, in part, to the difficulties in obtaining accurate diagnostic information, the difficulties in ensuring that data for a particular geographical area are complete and the variations in the data collection methods used in different countries. In the United States the death rate from AML in the 1970s was about 2.1 per 100 000 people per annum; the diagnosis is comparatively rare in children and young adults and becomes progressively more frequent with advancing age.

Aetiology

In the great majority of cases of AML no predisposing cause can be identified. In selected cases, however, there are congenital or environmental factors that are believed to have contributed to leukaemogenesis. It is likely, however, in every case that leukaemogenesis is multifactorial and multistep, and the precise contribution of these identifiable factors cannot be quantitated.

A number of congenital or constitutional conditions predispose to development of AML. Children with Down's syndrome may develop a haematological picture resembling AML that then remits spontaneously, but may also develop a progressive leukaemia that proves fatal. Patients with Fanconi's anaemia also have an increased risk of developing AML, as do patients with Bloom's syndrome and ataxia telangiectasia.

It has been known for some years that exposure to high levels of irradiation may induce leukaemia. Individuals who survived the atomic bombs at Hiroshima and Nagasaki (1945) had a ten- to fifteenfold increased risk of developing any type of leukaemia compared with a control population. The peak incidence was 4–7 years after exposure but the excess risk persisted longer. Persons exposed to high levels of irradiation in their occupation, such as radiologists, had a significantly increased risk of leukaemia, as did patients exposed to radioactive thorotrast used at one time as a contrast agent in radiology. The most convincing evidence for the leukaemogenic potential of radiation in clinical practice came from a study of patients who had been irradiated for ankylosing spondylitis. They had a tenfold increase in risk of leukaemia, and the commonest type of leukaemia was AML.

Two groups of chemical agents are implicated in the aetiology of AML, benzene, and certain cytotoxic drugs. Exposure to benzene produces chromosomal abnormalities and it has been known for many years that industrial exposure, as occurs in the leather industry in Turkey and other Mediterranean countries, may lead to AML. Benzene has also been a component of synthetic glues, dry-cleaning fluids, and petroleum spirit but its contribution to leukaemogenesis for persons less regularly exposed to these agents is uncertain. Various cytotoxic drugs, including alkylating agents, nitrosoureas and procarbazine, are mitogenic in experimental animals and seem to increase the risk of leukaemia in patients treated for other malignant disease. For example, the incidence of 'secondary' leukaemias in patients apparently cured of Hodgkin's disease by chemotherapy or chemotherapy plus radiotherapy may be as high as 6 per cent in some series. The cytotoxic drug combinations in these cases have usually included nitrogen mustard and procarbazine. AML also occurs as a complication of treatment of myeloma with cyclophosphamide or melphalan and of polycythaemia vera with chlorambucil. The mechanism by which cytotoxic drugs exert their leukaemogenic effect is unknown, but the AMLs secondary to exposure to drugs usually differ haematologically from AML arising *de novo* (see below).

Though various retroviruses cause different kinds of acute leukaemia in experimental animals and two well-characterized viruses (EB virus and HTLV-I) are implicated in the aetiology of haemopoietic neoplasia in man, no virus has been identified that contributes to AML.

Pathogenesis and cell kinetics

Acute myeloid leukaemia, in common with other malignant diseases of the haemopoietic system, is regarded as a clonal disease originating in a single stem cell already committed to myeloid differentiation. This concept is based on the demonstration by morphological, cytogenetic, or enzymological methods that the whole leukaemic cell population seems to be clonally derived. More specifically, the leukaemic cells from a patient with AML may have morphological abnormalities in all three myeloid lineages, and in some cases the same cytogenetic abnormality can be demonstrated throughout the myeloid series. Moreover, studies in black females heterozygous for the two isoenzymes of glucose-6-phosphate dehydrogenase (G6PD) have revealed that the whole leukaemic population is exclusively of one or other (but not both) isoenzyme types. Non-clonal haemopoiesis is usually restored when the patient achieves haematological remission.

In practice, the view that all leukaemic cells in a patient with AML are derived from a single progenitor must be an oversimplification. It is far more likely that the clinical manifestations of leukaemia are the result of a multistep process, with the result of each step being continued expansion of one clone of malignant cells at the expense of another.

Methods for the study of the earlier stages of leukaemogenesis are still inadequate, and will depend in part on recognition of specific molecular changes preceding overt leukaemia.

Although examination of the blood or marrow of a patient with AML might suggest that the rate of production of leukaemic cells is much greater than that of their normal counterparts, this is not in fact the case. Studies involving infusion of [³H]-thymidine into untreated patients have shown that the mean generation time for leukaemic myeloblasts ranges between 36 and 96 h and is thus considerably longer than that of normal cells; moreover, the growth fraction is smaller than that of comparable cells in a regenerating normal marrow. These findings emphasize the fact that the essential defect in AML at diagnosis is a failure of cell maturation leading to accumulation of leukaemic blast cells and the disease only assumes features of excessive proliferation at later stages in its evolution.

Clinical features

The clinical findings in a patient with AML at presentation are not specific. An increasing number of patients are diagnosed as a result of routine blood tests before the onset of symptoms. Symptoms when present are usually non-specific and include those due to anaemia (weakness, lethargy, dyspnoea, ankle swelling), those attributable to thrombocytopenia (purpura, retinal haemorrhages, bleeding from nose, gums, intestine, urinary tract, etc.), or those attributable to infection (fever, pneumonia, urinary tract infections, skin infections, etc.). Physical findings are also non-specific. The patient may show signs of haemorrhage. The gums may be hypertrophied (suggesting a monocytic component). The liver and spleen may be enlarged but the degree of enlargement is seldom great. There may be tenderness on palpation of the sternum and other accessible bones. Patients with disseminated intravascular coagulation may present with extensive purpura and bleeding from multiple sites.

Haematology

The diagnosis of AML is based on examination of the peripheral blood and marrow (Figs. 23.26–23.36). The total leucocyte count may be low, normal, or raised but the finding of diagnostic importance is of blast cells. These may vary in proportion from very occasional (< 1 per cent) to 85 per cent or more of the differential count. The blast cells may have the appearances of myeloblasts, monoblasts, erythroblasts, or

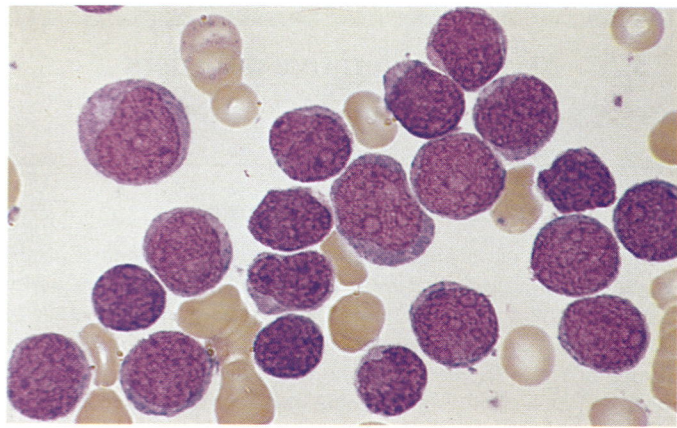

Fig. 23.26 Photomicrograph of blast cells from a patient with acute myeloid leukaemia, FAB type M1 (May–Grünwald Giemsa). (Kindly provided by Professor Daniel Catovsky.)

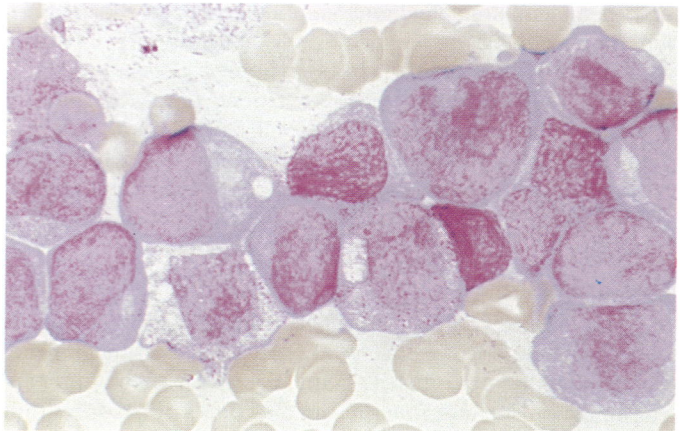

Fig. 23.27 Photomicrograph of blast cells from a patient with acute myeloid leukaemia, FAB type M2 (May–Grünwald Giemsa). (Kindly provided by Professor Daniel Catovsky.)

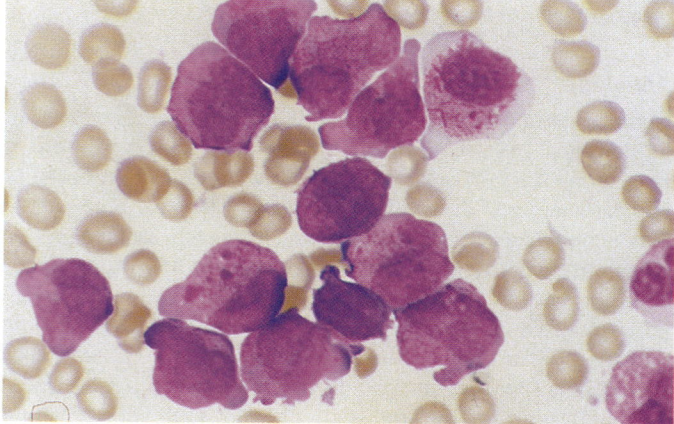

Fig. 23.28 Photomicrograph of blast cells from a patient with acute myeloid leukaemia, FAB type M3 (May–Grünwald Giemsa). (Kindly provided by Dr David Swirsky.)

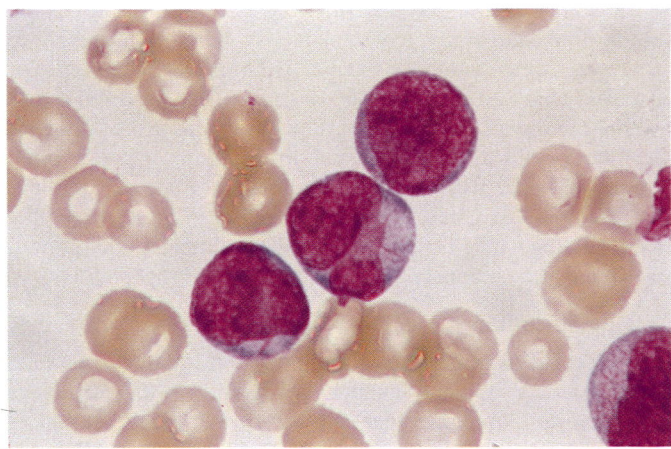

Fig. 23.29 Photomicrograph of blast cells from a patient with acute myeloid leukaemia, FAB type M4 (May–Grünwald Giemsa). Note presence of Auer rods in the cytoplasm of two cells. (Kindly provided by Dr David Swirsky.)

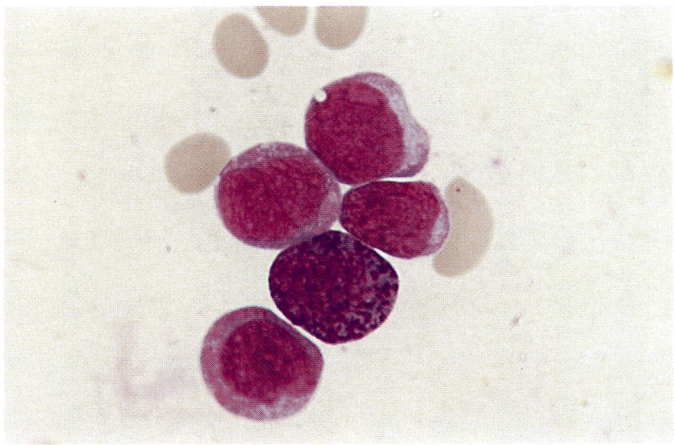

Fig. 23.31 Photomicrograph of blast cells from a patient with acute myeloid leukaemia, FAB type M4 Eo (May–Grünwald Giemsa). Note presence of abnormal eosinophils. This type of leukaemia is usually associated with a specific chromosomal abnormality, inv(16). (Kindly provided by Professor Daniel Catovsky.)

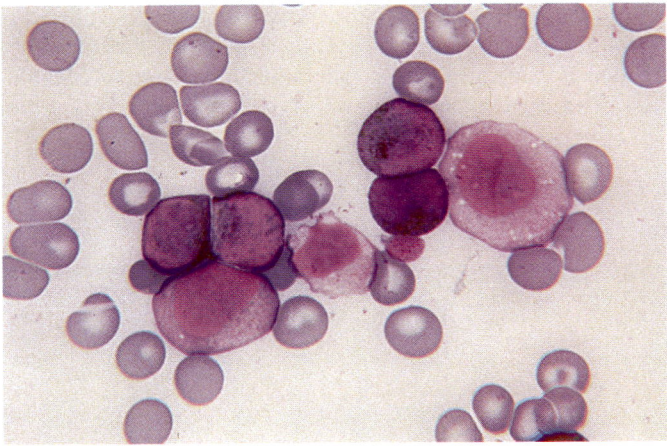

Fig. 23.30 Photomicrograph of blast cells from a patient with acute myeloid leukaemia, FAB type M4, stained with Sudan black. Note the presence of black stain in the cytoplasm of monocytoid cells. (Kindly provided by Dr David Swirsky.)

megakaryoblasts, or various combinations. The identification of rod-like crystalline azurophilic inclusions (Auer rods) in the cytoplasm of occasional cells clinches the diagnosis of AML (Fig. 23.29). With Romanowsky-stained films it is usually possible to make a confident diagnosis of AML and to ascribe a subtype (see below). Cells at stages of maturation between blasts (or promyelocytes) and mature granulocytes are usually absent from the peripheral blood. Mature granulocytes may be normal in appearance or may show various dysplastic changes, including pseudo-Pelger formation (failure of nuclear lobulation) and loss of secondary granules normally visible in the cytoplasm (hypogranularity). The patient may or may not be anaemic at diagnosis. The platelet count may be normal or reduced to variable degrees. Occasionally nucleated red cells may be present in the blood but red cell morphology is usually normal.

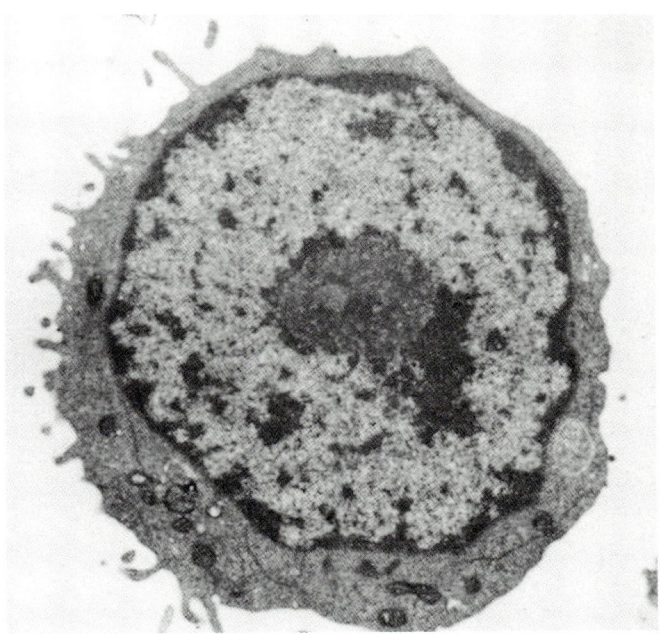

Fig. 23.32 Transmission electron micrograph of an immature leukaemic blast cell without any signs of differentiation. The cell is rounded with a high nuclear–cytoplasmic ratio, a prominent nucleolus and marginated peripheral chromatin. Some organelles are present in the cytoplasm but without primary or secondary granules. This ultrastructural appearance does not permit a diagnosis of AML-M1 according to the FAB classification, and is consistent with acute 'undifferentiated' or unclassified leukaemia. (Kindly provided by Professor Aaron Polliack.)

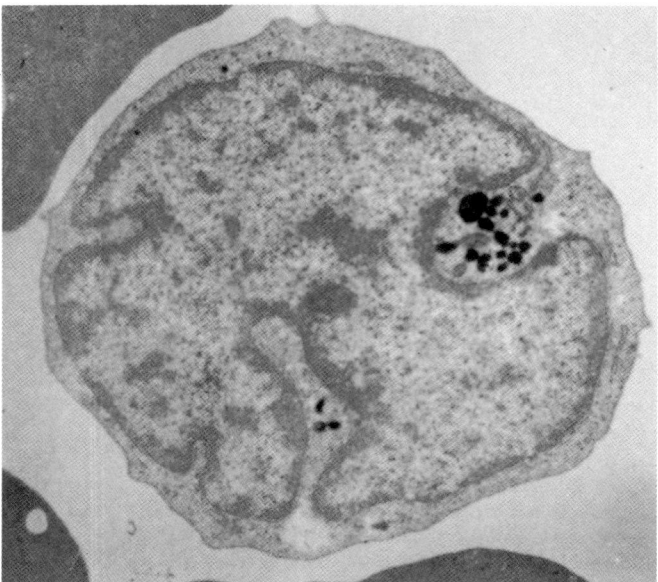

Fig. 23.33 Transmission electron micrograph of a cell from a patient with acute leukaemia without signs of differentiation (as in Fig. 23.29) but showing dense myeloperoxidase (MPO) positive granules in the cytoplasm. This feature shows the cell to be an early acute myeloid leukaemia, i.e. FAB M1. (Kindly provided by Professor Aaron Polliack.)

The bone marrow may be examined by aspiration through a standard needle or by trephine biopsy with a Jasmshidi or other percutaneous biopsy needle. The marrow fragments (or particles) obtained by aspiration are usually hypercellular and trails show a vast excess of blasts or blasts and promyelocytes. Megakaryocytes may be normal in number or more often reduced. There may be abnormalities in nuclear lobation. Erythroid precursors are usually reduced in number; they may be morphologocially normal or may show abnormalities in nuclear shape and cytoplasmic maturation (dyserythropoiesis).

FAB classification

In most cases examination of the blood (and marrow) enables an experienced haematologist to subclassify AML into one of seven major categories defined by the French–American–British (FAB) Collaborative Study Group (Table 23.5). M0 is not formally included in the FAB classification but describes cases with myeloid membrane markers but negative cytochemistry. M1 and M5A require confirmation by cytochemistry. M2 cases may have prominent promyelocytes with coarse granules and frequent Auer rods. M3 cases (also referred to as acute promyelocytic leukaemia or hypergranular promyelocytic leukaemia) represent 5–7 per cent of all cases of AML and are frequently associated with disseminated intravascular coagulation. The predominant promyelocyte may show very dense

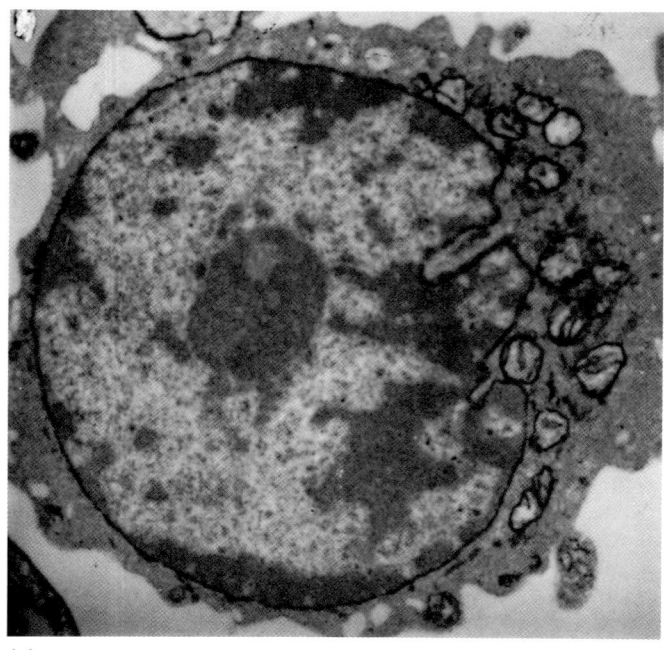

(a)

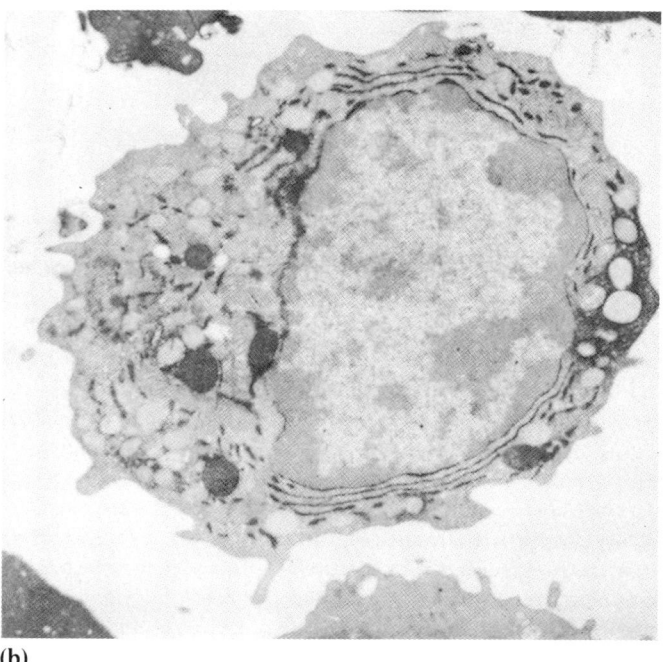

(b)

Fig. 23.34 (a) Transmission electron micrograph showing the typical staining pattern of nuclear and cytoplasmic membranes for platelet peroxidase (PPO). There are no positively stained cytoplasmic granules. These findings confirm the diagnosis of AML-M7 (acute megakaryoblastic leukaemia). (b) Typical staining pattern of a myeloblast (AML-M1) which shows PPO positivity in the membranes but also in the dense granules, a feature that distinguishes this cell from AML-M7. (Kindly provided by Professor Aaron Polliack.)

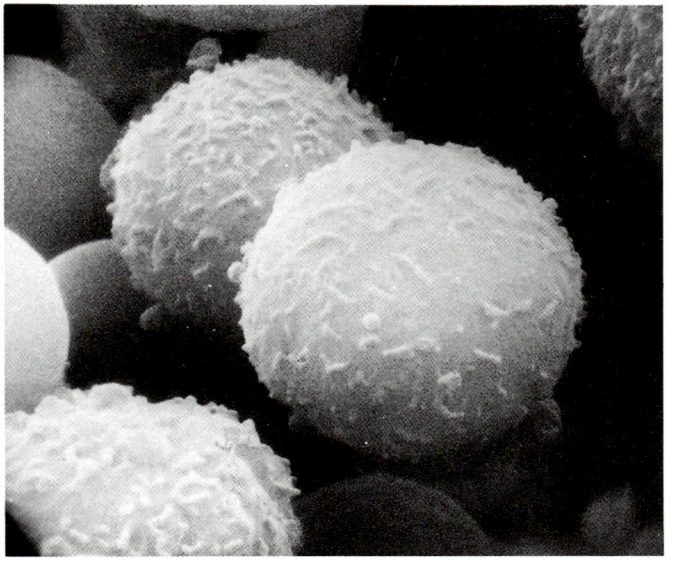

(a)

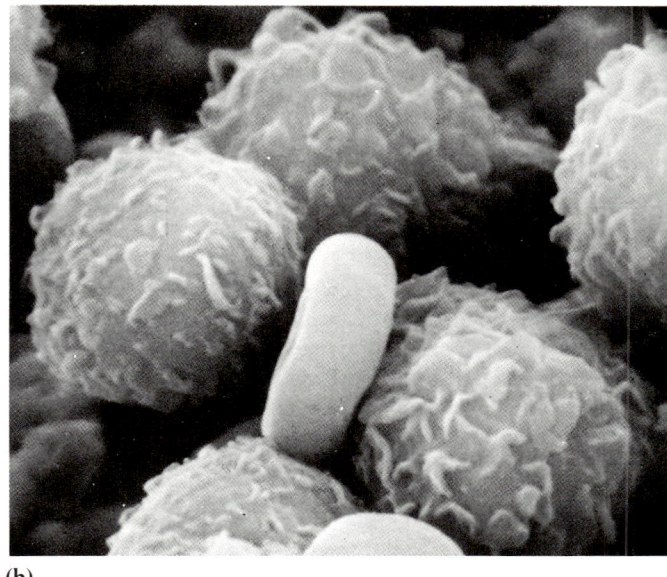

(b)

Fig. 23.35 Typical scanning electron micrograph showing the surface architecture of AML cells. (a) Transverse ridge-like folds are seen on the surface of an AML-M2 cell; and (b) broader, well-developed ruffles characterize the surface of a monoblastic leukaemia cell (AML-M5). (Kindly provided by Professor Aaron Polliack.)

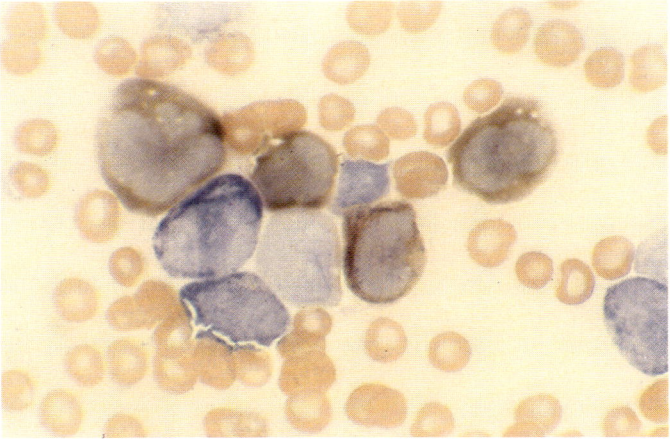

Fig. 23.36 Photomicrograph of blast cells from a patient with acute myeloid leukaemia, FAB type M4, stained with combined esterase stain. Granulocyte precursors show blue staining (naphthol-AS-Dchloroacetate) and monocyte precursors show green–brown stain (α-naphthyl butyrate). (Kindly provided by Dr David Swirsky.)

Table 23.5 Morphological classification of acute myeloid leukaemia based on the proposals of the French–American–British (FAB) group

M0	Undifferentiated*
M1	Myeloblastic without maturation
M2	Myeloblastic with maturation
M3	Hypergranular promyelocytic M3-variant: hypogranular bilobed promyelocytes
M4	Myelomonocytic
M5	A: Monoblastic B: Monocytic
M6	Erythroleukaemia with >50 per cent erythroblasts or >30 per cent less-differentiated blasts
M7	Megakaryoblastic†

* Classification based on the results of membrane markers, e.g. CD34 positivity.
† Classification based on the results of membrane markers, e.g. CD41/42 positivity, or demonstration of membrane platelet peroxidase at ultrastructural levels.

granulation, partially occluding the nucleus, and variable numbers of cells may show multiple Auer-like rods arranged in bundles ('faggot' cells). The nuclei of these cells are often bilobed. About 15 per cent of M3 cases are classified as 'M3-variant' when the predominant cell in the blood lacks abnormal granules and resembles a monocyte more than a promyelocyte. Faggot cells may still be found, as may cells with bilobed nuclei. Both M3 and M3-variant cells have the translocation t(15;17) (see below). M4 (myelomonocytic leukaemias) describes cases midway between M2 and M5, in which cells with features of immature granulocytes and monocytes coexist in the blood and/or marrow. In M5 monocytic differentiation predominates; M5A is monoblastic and M5B includes cases where more mature monocytes predominate. M6 describes erythroleukaemias (also known as Di Guglielmo's disease). M7 describes acute leukaemias in which megakaryoblasts predominate. The latter are usually scanty in the peripheral blood and may be associated with moderate or extensive marrow fibrosis; when blast cells in the marrow are inconspicuous, differentiation from primary myelofibrosis may be difficult.

Cytochemistry

Whereas cytochemical methods were the mainstay for distinguishing AML from acute lymphoblastic leukaemia, and to a lesser extent for subclassifying the AMLs, they have been displaced to a certain degree by the advent of monoclonal antibody technology (Table 23.6). In general, stains for peroxidase and Sudan black B may be positive in M1, M2, M3, and M4 (Fig. 23.30) and always negative in lymphoblasts. Non-specific esterases (α-naphthyl acetate esterase, α-naphthyl butyrate esterase, or naphthol-AS acetate esterase) give strong diffuse reactions in the monocytic leukaemia (M4 and M5); the reactions are inhibited by sodium fluoride. Conversely, naphthol-AS chloroacetate esterase may give positive results with M1, M2, M3, and some cases of M4 (Fig. 23.36); it is usually negative in M5. The cytobacterial test for lysozyme production (using a lysozyme-sensitive micro-organism, *Micrococcus lysodeikticus*) may be positive in M4 and M5 AMLs.

Table 23.6 Cell markers of diagnostic value in AML

Marker	FAB Type					
	M0	M1	M2/M3	M4/M5	M6	M7
CD34	+	+	+	+	−	−
CD13	+	+	+	+	+	+
CD33	+	+	+	+	+	+
CD11b	−	−	+	+	−	−
CD14	−	−	−	+	−	−
Glycophorin	−	−	−	−	+	−
CDw41/42	−	−	−	−	−	+
TdT	(+)	(+)	−	−	−	−

TdT, Terminal deoxynucleotidyl transferase; +, sometimes positive; (+), may rarely be positive.

Cell markers and gene rearrangements

The recognition in the 1970s that ALL blast cells consistently expressed the c-ALL antigen (see Section 23.4.1) gave ephemeral support to the concept that leukaemic cells in general might express specific antigens. Though this appears not be true, the advent first of specific polyclonal antisera and, more recently, of monoclonal antibodies shows that leukaemic blast cells routinely express a pattern of surface (and nuclear) molecules that is relatively consistent in any one patient and usually parallels a pattern present on rare cells in normal bone marrow. This provides support for the notion that leukaemic proliferations are clonal expansions derived (at some point) from a single progenitor cell.

The pattern of surface antigen expression is extremely helpful for differentiating AML from ALL and for classifying undifferentiated leukaemias, which may be positive with the 'early myeloid' CD33 antigen (Table 23.6). Surface antigen characterization also provides diagnostic information in M6 and M7 types of AML. In general, efforts to discriminate between M2, M3, and M5 by analysis of surface membrane characteristics have not provided information over and above what can be obtained by routine morphology and cytochemistry.

The nuclear enzyme, terminal deoxynucleotidyl transferase, at one time thought to be specific for the lymphoid lineage, is occasionally identified in M0 and M1 AMLs. In these cases the myeloid nature of the leukaemia may be documented by the presence of conventional myeloid surface antigens (e.g. CD13, CD33) and the absence of other lymphoid markers or Ig or T-cell receptor (TCR) gene rearrangements.

There are two situations in which the precise classification of a case of acute leukaemia is ambiguous, even when all immunological markers and genotypic data are available. Some patients have blast cells that are typical myeloblasts or typical lymphoblasts by most criteria but, unexpectedly, express one or more antigens of the opposite lineage. These cases have been designated 'hybrid' or 'biphenotypic' and presumably represent the progeny of an abnormal (=neoplastic) differentiation programme or persistence of a very rare but normal immature cell (reflecting 'lineage' promiscuity) that was destined for extinction. In other cases, markers for myeloid and lymphoid are identified on separate cells in a mixed population of blasts; these cases are examples of 'mixed' or 'bilineage' acute leukaemia. The two lineages are probably derived from the same malignant progenitor cell.

The demonstration of clonal rearrangement of Ig or T-cell receptor α/β or γ/δ genes has proved most useful in subclassification of the lymphoid malignancies (see Chapter 22). Occasional patients with AML show clonal rearrangement of TCR genes (though very rarely of Ig genes). Such patients are presumably examples of biphenotypic disease, described above.

Chromosomes

Using conventional methods to examine leukaemic cells from the marrow (or peripheral blood) of patients with AML, clonal cytogenetic abnormalities are found in about 50 per cent of cases. However, recent results suggest that if specialized methods are used to obtain high-resolution banding and extended metaphases preparations, then the proportion of patients with cytogenetic abnormalities may rise to 80 per cent. In general, the cytogenetic changes in AML can be classified into three groups:

1. consistent (or 'non-random') abnormalities that correlate to a greater or lesser extent with morphology as defined, for example, by the FAB group;

2. consistent or non-random abnormalities that have no particular morphological associations; and

3. random abnormalities.

Groups 1 and 2 are summarized in Table 23.7. Group 3 abnormalities may constitute the commonest type of abnormalities but will not be considered further.

The observation that some cytogenetic abnormalities correlate with FAB subtype is strong evidence for a causal association. For example, the t(15;17) is consistently associated with a break in the first intron of the retinoic acid receptor alpha gene on chromosome 17. This leads to the formation of a chimeric gene on chromosome 15 which is expressed as a fusion protein.

Table 23.7 Cytogenetic abnormalities associated with AML

Chromosomal abnormalities	Associated FAB type	Specific morphological features
t(8;21)	M2	Myeloblasts, monocytes
t(15;17)	M3	Promyelocytes
	M3-variant	Promyelocytes with microgranules
inv(16) (p13q22) del(16)q22	M4	Abnormal eosinophils
del or t(11) (q23)	M5	Monoblasts
t(11) (q13)	M5	Monocytes
t(9;11) (p22;q23)	—	Nil
t(9;22) (q34;q11)	—	Distinct from CML
t(6;9) (p23;q24)	—	Basophilia
inv(3) (q21;q26)	—	Thrombocytosis
t(3;3) (q21;q26)	—	Abnormal megakaryocytes
−5 or 5q−	—	Dysplastic features
−7 or 7q−		Dysplastic features
+8		Nil

The rarer t(6;9) translocation also leads to formation of a novel chimeric gene on chromosome 6 with associated transcript and fusion protein. The Ph chromosome [t(9;22)], characteristic of chronic myeloid leukaemia (CML), is also found in 1–2 per cent of patients with AML; by definition such patients cannot be classified as CML presenting in transformation but molecular studies have none the less revealed the formation of a BCR/ABL chimeric gene identical to that found in CML or Ph-positive ALL. It is extremely likely that each of these molecular changes is involved in the pathogenesis of the corresponding form of acute leukaemia. It is likely also that other non-random cytogenetic abnormalities, not yet characterized at the molecular level, such as t(8;21), inv(16q), and loss of parts of chromosomes 5 and 7, will also prove to be associated with specific deletions or juxtapositions of oncogenes that are critical in the pathogenesis of the acute leukaemia.

Further support for the concept that some, at least, of the cytogenetic changes described above have pathogenetic significance derives from the observation that their presence may correlate with prognosis in individual patients. Thus AML patients with inv(16), t(8;21), and t(15;17) may have relatively long remissions while patients with complex defects or those with t(6;9) or involvement of chromosomes 5 or 7 may fare worse than average.

Abnormalities of chemistry and coagulation

Serum electrolytes are usually normal in patients with AML at diagnosis but occasional patients with M4 or M5 disease have hypokalaemia due to renal tubular damage by high serum lysozyme (muramidase) levels. Uric acid levels are usually normal but may rise abruptly when chemotherapy is administered. Such hyperuricaemia may be asymptomatic or may lead to urate nephropathy and acute renal failure. It can be prevented by administration of the xanthine oxidase inhibitory drug, allopurinol, in full dosage. Liver enzymes are usually normal but some patients have increased levels of lactate dehydrogenase, a finding associated in some series with poor prognosis.

Almost all patients with M3 and M3-variant AML, and a small proportion of patients with other subtypes of AML, have biochemical features of disseminated intravascular coagulation (DIC). These include low levels of fibrinogen (< 1.0 g/l), increased levels of fibrin degradation products (> 100 μg/ml, N < 10 μg/ml) and reduced levels of factors II, V, and VIII, and fibronectin. Platelet numbers are also typically low or very low as a result of consumption. The best screening tests to identify DIC and to assess its severity are therefore the thrombin time, the prothrombin time, a measure of clottable fibrinogen, and some measure of fibrin degradation products.

23.5.2 Myelodysplastic syndromes

The term myelodysplastic syndromes (MDS) is applied to a group of acquired conditions characterized by progressive bone marrow failure associated with normocellularity or hypercellularity of the marrow and variable degrees of anaemia, leucopenia, and/or thrombocytopenia. The severity of the cytopenia usually progresses over months or years and death is due either to the consequences of marrow failure or to transformation to acute myeloid leukaemia. In most cases no primary cause can be identified but cytotoxic drugs, especially alkylating agents, are incriminated with increasing frequency. In the UK the term MDS has replaced the less descriptive and less accurate terms 'preleukaemia' or 'smouldering leukaemia', but the latter are sometimes used by some to apply to those forms of MDS in which features suggestive of leukaemia are already present at diagnosis.

Classification of the MDS

The MDS are an extremely heterogeneous group of conditions, ranging at the one extreme from a refractory anaemia (RA) without obvious numerical deficiency of granulocytes or platelets, in which the marrow is hypercellular but without an excess of blast cells, to the other extreme represented by refractory anaemia with an excess of blasts in transformation (RAEB-t), a condition in which the distinction from an AML arising *de novo* is based largely on the facts that the proportion of blasts in the marrow is still relatively low and dysplastic changes in all three myeloid lineages are prominent. The full classification proposed by the FAB group in 1982 is summarized in Table 23.8.

The term refractory anaemia with ringed sideroblasts describes a condition in which the anaemia is prominent and unresponsive to haematinic therapy. The defining feature is the presence of 15 per cent or more of erythroid cells containing siderotic granules partially ringing the nucleus. The major difference between RA and RAEB is the finding that blast cells number between 5 and 15 per cent in the latter condition. Any increase above 15 per cent, or the finding of Auer rods in some of the blast cells, justifies the designation RAEB-t.

Haematology

Patients with MDS may have varying degrees of pancytopenia. The marrow is characteristically hypercellular but may be normocellular. The most important unifying feature of MDS is the consistent presence of distinctive morphological abnormalities in the myeloid series in both blood and marrow (Fig. 23.37). The dyserythropoiesis has perhaps the least diagnostic value. Features include the presence of ringed sideroblasts (Fig. 23.38), often associated with a dimorphic population of red cells in the blood, the presence of bilobed, trefoil, or tetrafoil nuclei in late normoblasts, and occasionally internuclear bridging and nuclear fragmentation. In addition, non-haemoglobinized pale areas may be seen in the cytoplasm of intermediate and late normoblasts. The dysgranulopoiesis is characterized by agranular or hypogranular neutrophils. The granulocyte nucleus may show acquired Pelger formation—the nucleus is round or bilobed and has mature-type chromatin condensation. Multisegmented nuclei, distinct from those that characterize megaloblastosis, may also be seen. The three types of abnormal megakaryocyte are perhaps most characteristic of

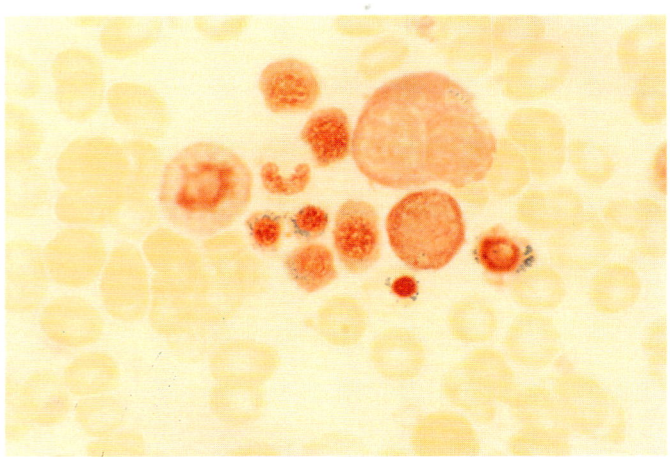

Fig. 23.38 Photomicrograph of ringed sideroblasts from a patient with refractory anaemia (Perl's iron stain). (Kindly provided by Dr David Swirsky.)

MDS (Fig. 23.37). The micromegakaryocyte is small, about the size of a monocyte, and has a single, small, round, centrally placed nucleus. It is recognized by its characteristic cytoplasm. In contrast, the polynuclear megakaryocyte has 2–12 or more small, round, separate nuclei. A third type of abnormal megakaryocyte is the large mononuclear form with a single large round or ovoid nucleus.

Cytogenetic studies of marrow cells from patients with MDS show that abnormal karyotypes are present in 40–60 per cent of cases where no primary cause has been identified and in more than 90 per cent of cases of MDS secondary to use of cytotoxic drugs. These abnormalities may be similar to those found in AML presenting *de novo*. The commonest single abnormalities are 5q − or monosomy 7, which appear less commonly in AML. In general, multiple abnormalities in a myeloid clone are more common than single changes.

23.5.3   Chronic myeloid leukaemia

The term chronic myeloid leukaemia (CML) describes a group of diseases characterized by autonomous, presumably malignant, proliferation of myeloid cells in the bone marrow, peripheral blood, and other sites. In most cases CML after diagnosis evolves

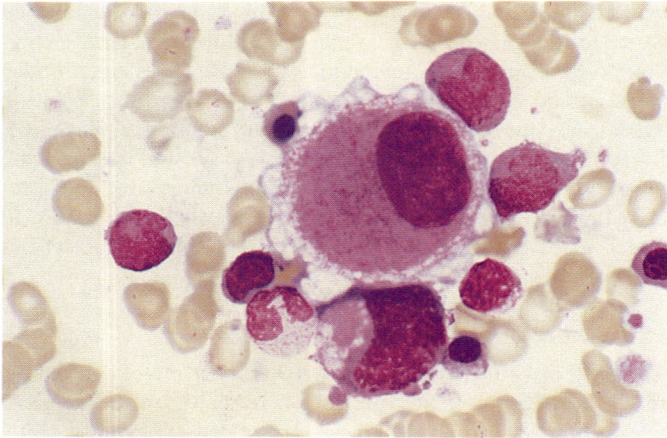

Fig. 23.37 Photomicrograph of abnormal megakaryocytes from a patient with myelodysplastic syndrome (May–Grünwald Giemsa). (Kindly provided by Dr David Swirsky.)

Table 23.8   Classification of the myelodysplastic syndromes

Refractory anaemia (RA)	Usually in patients aged >50 yr; presentation with anaemia; blast cells <1% in blood and <5% in marrow; dysmyelopoiesis
Refractory anaemia with ringed sideroblasts	Acquired idiopathic sideroblastic anaemia; ringed sideroblasts account for >15% of marrow nucleated cells; other features resemble RA
Refractory anaemia with excess of blasts (RAEB)	Anaemia; cytopenia affecting at least 2 myeloid lineages; dysgranulopoiesis prominent; marrow hypercellular with 5–20% blasts
Refractory anaemia with excess of blasts in transformation (RAEB-t)	Cytopenia with blast cells in blood or marrow not classifiable as AML or as RA or RAEB; morphology similar to RAEB; usually 20–30% blasts in marrow
Chronic myelomonocytic leukaemia	Absolute monocytosis (>1.0 × 10⁹/l); granulocytes may show morphological abnormalities; marrow may resemble RAEB; percentage blasts usually <5%, may be up to 20%

slowly over a number of years, which distinguishes it from the acute leukaemias, in which survival is often measured in months. The classification of the chronic myeloid leukaemias is somewhat controversial at present but a reasonable approach is summarized in Table 23.9. Philadelphia (Ph) chromosome positive CML is by far the commonest form of CML.

Table 23.9 Classification of the chronic myeloid leukaemias

Chronic myeloid leukaemia: Ph-positive

Chronic myeloid leukaemia: Ph-negative

Juvenile chronic myeloid leukaemia

Chronic neutrophilic leukaemia

Eosinophilic leukaemia

Chronic myelomonocytic leukaemia (alternatively classified as amyelodysplastic syndrome)

Epidemiology

CML is a rare disease. It constitutes about 15 per cent of all leukaemias. Its annual incidence is about 1 per 100 000 of the population in all countries for which adequate statistics exist, which corresponds to about 500 new cases per year in the UK and 2500 in the US. CML occurs in patients of all ages but is somewhat less common before the age of 40 than after. It is slightly more common in males than in females.

Aetiology and pathogenesis

The cause of CML is unknown in most cases. Exposure to ionizing radiation, as occurs in patients who receive radiotherapy for diseases such as ankylosing spondylitis, or in survivors of the atomic bomb detonations in Japan in 1945, is associated with a small but significantly increased risk of sustaining CML. Whether low levels of 'cosmic' radiation play any role in the aetiology of the sporadic case of CML is unknown.

CML is thought to arise as a result of an acquired somatic mutation in a single pluripotential haemopoietic stem cell which then expresses a proliferative advantage and gradually displaces normal haemopoiesis in the bone marrow. The evidence for this conclusion derives from a number of sources:

1. The Philadelphia chromosome, regarded as a specific marker for the leukaemic clone, can be identified in metaphases not only from cells of granulocyte and monocyte lineages but also in erythroid, megakaryocytic, and some B-lymphoid precursors.

2. Studies of G6PD heterozygotes with CML, whose somatic cells each express one or other (but not both) isoenzymes, have shown that the whole leukaemic cell population is of one or other isoenzyme type, a finding consistent with the notion that the leukaemic clone was derived from a single stem cell.

3. The observation that the cells that characterize acute transformation may be predominantly myeloid or lymphoid, and that the latter are usually B-lymphoid but occasionally T-lymphoblastic, is further circumstantial evidence for pluripotential stem cell involvement.

Cytogenetics and molecular biology

In 1960 Nowell and Hungerford in Philadelphia discovered an abnormal G-group chromosome in the leukaemic cells of patients with CML. There was consistent loss of part of the long arms of one member of the pair. This abnormality became known as the Philadelphia (Ph[1] or just Ph) chromosome (Table 23.10). The chromosome pair involved was distinct from the chromosome involved in Down's syndrome and the abnormality was therefore later designated 22q−. In 1973 Janet Rowley showed that the material apparently lost from chromosome 22q− had, in fact, been translocated to chromosome 9. A small quantity of chromosomal material is also translocated from chromosome 9 to chromosome 22 and the translocation is therefore reciprocal, usually described as t(9;22) (q34;q11) (Fig. 23.39). In Ph-chromosome-positive CML all dividing cells in the myeloid series carry the Ph chromosome; because only a minority of lymphoid cells are Ph positive, cytogenetic examination of the blood of treated patients is usually normal. Other somatic cells, such as skin fibroblasts, are not involved in the leukaemic process and are therefore also cytogenetically normal.

Table 23.10 History of the Ph chromosome and associated molecular findings

Year	Discovery	Investigators
1960	Ph chromosome, G group	Nowell and Hungerford
1970	Ph chromosome is 22q−	Caspersson et al.
1973	Ph due to translocation designated t(9;22)	Rowley
1982	Demonstration of ABL oncogene translocation from chr. 9 to chr. 22	De Klein et al.
1984	Description of the 'breakpoint cluster region' (BCR) on chr. 22	Groffen et al.
1984	Localization of breakpoint at subregions t(9;22) (q34.1;q11.21)	Prakash and Yunis
1984	Discovery of abnormal ABL transcript	Gale and Canaani
1984	Discovery of P210$^{BCR/ABL}$	Konopka et al.
1985	Confirmation of BCR/ABL chimeric gene	Shtivelman et al.

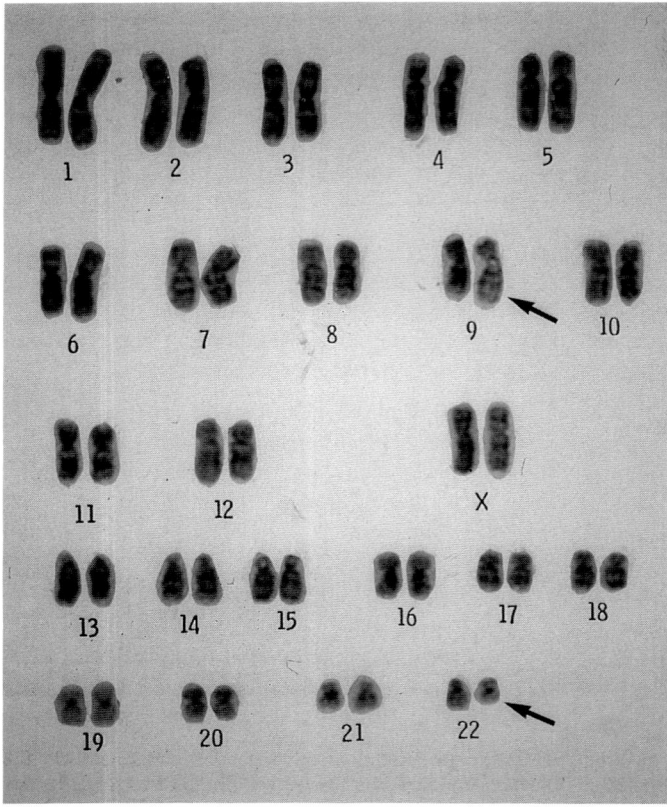

Fig. 23.39 Karyotype of metaphase from leukaemic cell in chronic myeloid leukaemia. Note the shortened chromosome 22 and the lengthened chromosome 9, which is usually described as t(9;22) (q34;q11).

There have been considerable advances recently in knowledge of the molecular changes that characterize CML. The cellular oncogene or proto-oncogene homologous with the transforming sequence of the Abelson strain of Moloney murine leukaemia virus is located on the long arm of chromosome 9 in all normal human nucleated cells. In leukaemic cells from patients with Ph-positive CML this oncogene (ABL) is translocated to chromosome 22, where it comes into juxtaposition with the 5′ portion of a functional gene designated BCR (for breakpoint cluster region). The translocation results in formation of a new chimeric gene (BCR/ABL) with 5′ components derived from chromosome 22 and 3′ components from chromosome 9. The gene expressed a novel 8.5 kb mRNA and a protein of M_r 210 000 (P210). The normal functions of the ABL and BCR genes are unknown but the ABL gene product has weak tyrosine kinase activity. The consistent finding of P210[BCR/ABL] in leukaemic cells (and only in leukaemic cells) from almost every patient with Ph-positive CML, and in a proportion of patients with Ph-negative CML, suggests that it must play a central role in pathogenesis. The observation that the P210 shows very greatly enhanced kinase activity suggests that it may perturb normal stem cell kinetics by an abnormal action within the second messenger system.

Further oncogene events probably determine the evolution of CML after the chronic phase. There are reports of further genomic changes in the BCR gene, of MYC amplification and rearrangement, of point mutations in RAS, and of rearrangement of P53 but no consistent pattern has yet emerged.

Clinical features and natural history

The clinical evolution of CML may be divided into two or three distinct phases. Most patients present in the chronic or stable phase, which usually continues for a median of about 3 yr (range < 1 to > 10 yr). Some patients pass abruptly and unpredictably from chronic phase to a phase of blastic transformation but more often an intermediate phase, termed acceleration, precedes overt blastic transformation.

Chronic phase

The presenting features of CML are often non-specific. About one-third of patients in Western countries have no symptoms when first seen but are diagnosed as a result of routine blood tests performed for other reasons. When present, symptoms may be attributable to anaemia, such as weakness, lethargy, or shortness of breath, or to splenomegaly, including a feeling of fullness in the abdomen, left upper abdominal pain, or early satiety. Undue sweating at diagnosis may occur but fever is unusual and raises the possibility that the disease may already have evolved to acceleration. Patients may have noticed excessive bleeding or the formation of spontaneous haematomas or retinal haemorrhages. Priapism is a rare presenting feature of CML and gout even rarer.

On physical examination pallor may be prominent if the patient is anaemic. About 70–80 per cent of patients have splenomegaly. The liver is palpably enlarged in about 50 per cent of cases but the liver edge is often soft and difficult to define. Patients may have varying amounts of purpura but other abnormalities at diagnosis are unusual.

The median duration of survival after diagnosis is 3–4 yr but the onset of transformation seems to be largely unpredictable in individual patients. A number of attempts have been made to define features assessable at diagnosis that may correlate with survival. Sokal and colleagues devised an equation to calculate a prognostic index based on the patient's age, spleen size, peripheral blood blast cell and platelet counts at diagnosis, but the general applicability of this approach has not yet been confirmed. It is, however, generally accepted that patients whose disease can be controlled with small amounts of cytotoxic drugs, or patients whose disease remains stable for many months or years without treatment, seem to survive longer with those who appear to have more aggressive chronic-phase disease.

Accelerated phase

Sooner or later most patients develop clinical or haematological features that are no longer strictly consistent with chronic phase disease yet fall short of frank blastic transformation. Such features include increasing splenomegaly or leucocytosis resistant to cytotoxic drugs that were previous effective, increasing basophilia or thrombocytosis, or increasing numbers of blast cells. The finding of new cytogenetic changes in addition to the Ph chromosome is usually taken as evidence of acceleration. The phase of acceleration typically lasts a few months but can be prolonged.

Blastic transformation

In about 80 per cent of cases CML terminates in a phase of overt blastic transformation, with or without a preceding phase of acceleration. This phase is also referred to as 'blast crisis' (BT). Patients in BT may initially be entirely free of symptoms or may have fevers, sweating, anorexia and weight loss, bleeding from various sites, or bone pain of variable intensity. There may be a rapid increase in the size of the spleen and generalized lymphadenopathy may appear. Cutaneous and subcutaneous nodules of variable size may be due to infiltration of leukaemic cells. X-ray examination of areas of bone pain may show single or occasionally multiple lytic lesions; a radionuclide bone scan may show one or more 'hotspots' even when conventional radiology is negative. Patients in blastic transformation may respond temporarily to treatment but survival is usually only a question of months.

Haematology

The diagnosis of CML is usually made readily from examination of the peripheral blood alone (Fig. 23.40). In patients with symptoms the leucocyte count often exceeds $200 \times 10^9/l$ and may on occasion be as high as $900 \times 10^9/l$ at diagnosis. In asymptomatic patients counts as low as $15 \times 10^9/l$ or $20 \times 10^9/l$ may lead to further investigations that establish the diagnosis. The leucocyte differential typically shows increased numbers of granulocytes at all stages of differentiation with 'peaks' of mature granulocytes, myelocytes, and blast cells. The percentage of blast cells rises in proportion to the leucocyte count, and as many as 12 per cent of blast cells are still consist-

ent with chronic-phase disease. The absolute numbers of basophils and eosinophils are usually increased. Monocyte numbers are relatively low. Platelet numbers are usually increased (range $350-700 \times 10^9/l$) but occasionally decreased. Some degree platelet anisocytosis may be seen. Occasional nucleated red cells may be present in the peripheral blood.

The bone marrow in a newly diagnosed patient usually shows greatly increased cellularity with complete obliteration of normal fat spaces (Fig. 23.41). Megakaryocytes may be greatly increased in number and relatively small with hypolobulation. Blast cells may number up to 10 or 12 per cent. Occasionally Gaucher-like cells are identified. Reticulin formation may be normal or slightly increased; major increases or overt collagen deposition, as may occur during the course of the disease, are rare at diagnosis. Examination of the marrow is not strictly necessary to confirm the diagnosis of CML, but it may be useful to document the absence of fibrosis, and cytogenetic preparations are often more successful with marrow than with peripheral blood cells.

A number of additional changes are characteristic in the newly diagnosed patient. The alkaline phosphatase content of the neutrophil cytoplasm is almost always strikingly reduced, possibly due to an absence of G-CSF production. This deficiency can be demonstrated readily by biochemical or cytochemical methods and forms the basis for a simple test to differentiate CML from other causes of leucocytosis. The vitamin B_{12} and B_{12}-binding capacity are usually greatly increased as a result of increased synthesis of transcobalamins I and III by the expanded total granulocyte mass. The serum uric acid is sometimes increased above normal. The serum alkaline phosphatase and lactic dehydrogenase levels may be raised, both presumably due to liver infiltration by myeloid cells.

Blast-cell transformation is usually defined by the finding of 25 per cent or more of blast cells or blasts plus promyelocytes in the peripheral blood and/or bone marrow. This figure may be

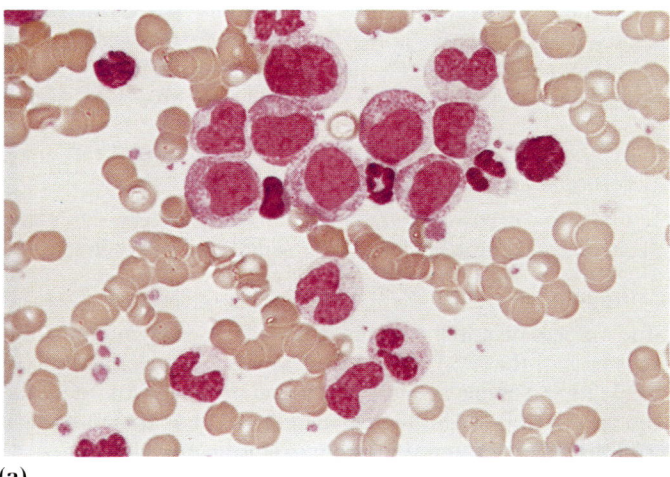

(a)

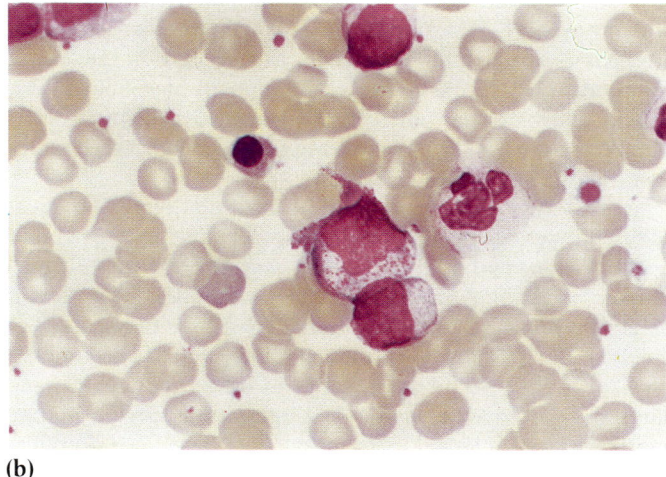

(b)

Fig. 23.40 Photomicrograph of peripheral blood from a patient with CML. (a) There is leucocytosis with promyelocytes, myelocytes, and more mature cells in the granulocyte series. Note also the thrombocytosis. (b) Note immature granulocytes, a nucleated red cell, and platelet anisocytosis.

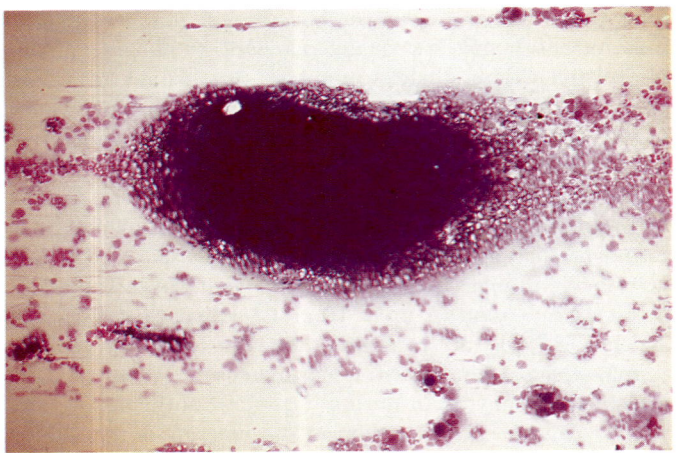

Fig. 23.41 Photomicrograph of marrow fragment aspirated from a patient with chronic myeloid leukaemia. Note the dense cellularity and complete absence of fat spaces (May–Grünwald Giemsa).

achieved abruptly in a patient whose leucocyte count was adequately controlled by chemotherapy only a few days earlier, or more insidiously with a preceding phase of acceleration. Morphologically the blast cells may vary greatly from one patient to another. They may resemble the myeloblasts that characterize AML (M2) or have monoblastic features (M4 or M5). Cells with erythroblastic, megakaryoblastic, basophilic, and eosinophilic features are sometimes seen. In about 20 per cent of cases the predominant blast has lymphoid features. In general, the FAB classification based on morphology of the acute leukaemias presenting *de novo* cannot readily be applied to blastic transformation of CML.

Cytochemical and marker studies confirm that blastic transformation of CML may be predominantly myeloid or lymphoid. Thus myeloid blasts may stain positively for myeloperoxidase, Sudan black, or non-specific esterase, while lymphoid cells may show block positivity for periodic acid–Schiff. The myeloid cells show appropriate membrane markers (positive for My9 (CD33) and granulocytic, monocytic, megakaryocytic, or erythroid antigens), while lymphoid cells express pre-B, DR, and common-ALL antigens. Cells with lymphoid morphology also usually show nuclear positivity for terminal deoxynucleotidyl transferase (TdT). Very rarely, lymphoblasts with T-cell membrane features have been reported.

About 80 per cent of patients in transformation of CML have additional cytogenetic changes in their leukaemia cells; more than one clone of new abnormalities may be present. The 'non-random' additional changes include acquisition of a second Ph chromosome (+Ph), usually regarded as a duplication of the first Ph, trisomy 8, formation of an isochromosome 17 (iso17q), and +19. A large series of other new cytogenetic abnormalities have been described but no one specific change appears to have clinical or morphological relevance. Patients with lymphoid transformations may have rearrangement of Ig heavy-chain or heavy- plus light-chain genes consistent with clonal expansion, but there is no suggestion that the changes

are pathogenetically relevant. Occasional patients with clonal changes in T-cell-receptor genes have been described.

About 10 per cent of patients proceed ultimately to a myelofibrotic termination of their disease. This is usually associated with increasing splenomegaly resistant to conventional treatment associated with a leuco-erythroblastic blood picture or gradually increasing pancytopenia. The marrow appearances at this stage are variable. There may be dense collagen fibrosis or, indeed, evidence of new bone formation (osteosclerosis). Residual myeloid tissue may resemble chronic phase disease or may show an increased number of blasts (often megakaryoblasts) and megakaryocytes. Dysplastic changes in the granulocytic and erythroid series are seen. Myelofibrotic transformation of CML progresses at very different rates in different patients.

Variants of Ph-positive CML

A number of variant forms of CML are now well characterized. All are much rarer than Ph-positive CML and usually respond less well to conventional treatment. These variants are summarized in Table 23.11.

Table 23.11 Variants of the t(9;22) translocation

Complex variants	involve chromosomes 9 and 22 and at least one (some more) additional chromosome(s)
Simple variants	involve movement of the distal part of chromosomal 22 (22q11–qter) without apparent involvement of either chromosome 9
Masked Ph	The Ph chromosome has lost its typical 22q– appearance as a result of translocation of additional material to the q arm

23.5.4 Polycythaemia rubra vera

The term polycythaemia usually refers to a raised haematocrit or packed-cell volume (PCV) and may be classified as relative when the red cell mass is normal or absolute when the red cell mass is raised. Relative polycythaemia is due to a reduction in the plasma volume, which may arise from a variety of causes. Absolute polycythaemia may be divided into three major types:

1. polycythaemia rubra vera (PRV);

2. secondary polycythaemias; and

3. idiopathic erythrocytosis, a term used to describe cases that do not fit the criteria for PRV or secondary polycythaemias.

Pathogenesis

Study of female patients heterozygous for isoenzymes of G6PD have shown that PRV, like AML and CML, is a clonal disorder involving the whole myeloid series, and the alternative designation 'primary proliferative polycythaemia' has therefore been proposed to divert attention from exclusive involvement of the red cell series. The disease presumably results from an acquired change in haemopoietic stem cells, whereby they escape, in a subtle manner, normal homeostatic control mechanisms. Apart from the numerical increase in cellular components, the principal manifestation of this abnormality is the generation *in vitro* of 'spontaneous' erythroid colonies. Thus, normal bone marrow contains a small proportion of cells (burst-forming units, BFU-E) that can proliferate *in vitro* in the presence of erythropoietin and form visible colonies of haemoglobinized cells. No such colonies are formed in the absence of erythropoietin. In PRV, however, a proportion of marrow-derived BFU-E form colonies in the absence of added erythropoietin, presumably stimulated by the minute quantities of erythropoietin already present in the culture medium. Thus BFU-E in PRV are thought to be supersensitive to erythropoietin and possibly also to other haemopoietic growth factors.

Clinical features at diagnosis

Patients are typically diagnosed in the sixth decade of life, but there are rare, well-documented cases in persons under the age of 40 and even in childhood. There are reports of PRV occurring more than once in the same family. There is a slight male preponderance. Some patients are identified as a result of blood tests performed for unrelated reasons. Symptoms, when present at diagnosis, include vascular complications, such as cerebral ischaemic attacks or thrombosis of cerebral retinal or mesenteric arteries. Retinal haemorrhages may be present. They may have non-specific symptoms such as headache, a 'full' feeling in the head, or impaired mental function. Patients may bleed excessively as a consequence of abnormal platelet function. The incidence of peptic ulceration is probably not increased in PRV, but bleeding from an existing ulcer may be exacerbated and lead to iron deficiency, which may then mask the PRV. About 25 per cent of patients have pruritus which may be aggravated by heat or hot baths. Rare patients have pruritus triggered by contact with water of any temperature (aquagenic pruritus). Pruritus may or may not improve when treatment reduces the red cell mass. A few patients present with symptoms of gout.

Physical findings serve to support the diagnosis. The patient may have a plethoric facies and acne rosacea. The conjunctival vessels may be prominent. About 50 per cent of patients have splenomegaly, which is usually moderate in degree.

Haematology

The haemoglobin concentration and PCV are raised at diagnosis. The number of red cells (per litre) is increased but their morphology and life-span are normal in the absence of iron deficiency. There may occasionally be macrocytosis due to folate deficiency. Leucocyte numbers are increased in the majority of patients ($12–25 \times 10^9$/l) with granulocytes predominating. Eosinophil and basophil numbers may be increased. In contradistinction to CML, the neutrophil alkaline phosphatase score is usually raised in PRV. Platelet numbers are often raised, typically $400–800 \times 10^9$/l or higher. There may be platelet anisocytosis with increased numbers of large forms.

The bone marrow is hypercellular with loss of normal fat spaces and increased numbers of erythroid, granulocytic, and megakaryocytic cells. The reticulin pattern is normal initially but may become increased in the course of the disease. Serum B_{12} and B_{12}-binding capacity are high in PRV, reflecting increased production of transcobalamins I and III by the increased total granulocyte mass. The level of erythropoietin in the serum is usually reduced or absent but normal levels are detected in some patients. The serum uric acid level may be raised.

Because the diagnosis of PRV is not always straightforward, the Polycythemia Vera Study Group in the United States has established a series of criteria. In the presence of splenomegaly the diagnosis of PRV also requires:

1. An absolute polycythaemia with a red cell mass > 36 ml/kg body weight in males and > 32 ml/kg in females;
2. No evidence of any cause for secondary polycythaemia and an arterial saturation > 92 per cent.

In the absence of splenomegaly, the diagnosis of PRV requires, in addition to the two criteria above, two of the three secondary features:

1. platelet count $> 400 \times 10^9$/l;
2. leucocyte count $> 12 \times 10^9$/l; and
3. raised neutrophil alkaline phosphatase and raised serum B_{12} and B_{12}-binding capacity.

Clinical course

PRV pursues a relatively indolent course and some patients die of natural causes. In other cases the disease transforms to myelofibrosis with progressive anaemia, splenomegaly, and extramedullary haemopoiesis. A small proportion of patients develop a haematological picture resembling AML, and although this may be more common in those who have received treatment with ^{32}P or alkylating agents, it is seen also, though less commonly, in patients treated by venesection only. The overall duration of survival from diagnosis is unpredictable, but median figures ranging from 8 to 15 years have been reported in different series.

23.5.5   Primary myelofibrosis

Primary myelofibrosis, also known as chronic myelofibrosis or agnogenic myeloid metaplasia, is in most cases a slowly progressive disease of older patients, characterized by splenomegaly, marrow fibrosis, and gradual onset of marrow failure. On occasion it may be preceded by polycythaemia rubra vera.

Pathogenesis

Although not yet conclusively proved, the key defect in primary myelofibrosis is believed to be the malignant proliferation of a myeloid progenitor cell committed to megakaryoblastic differentiation associated with expansion of the megakaryocyte pool and ineffective megakaryocytopoiesis. The latter leads presumably to intramedullary release of a well-characterized protein termed 'platelet-derived growth factor' which stimulates fibroblast proliferation *in vitro* and probably exerts the same function *in vivo.* Simultaneously, the release from megakaryocytes and platelets of platelet factor 4 inhibits 'physiological' collagenase activity. These two pathological processes combine to promote the excessive marrow reticulin and collagen deposition. The fibrosis consists initially of excess reticulin, but later various types of collagen, especially type III, are deposited in excess. At first the collagen deposition is reversible but at later stages the proline residues in the collagen molecule are hydroxylated and this leads to production of a polymeric form that is relatively stable and insoluble. In some cases new bone formation, so-called osteosclerosis, is also prominent.

The basis for the extramedullary haemopoiesis that underlies the splenomegaly is unknown. The amount of myeloid tissue in the spleen increases very gradually and collagen deposition leads to progressive fibrosis. The spleen may achieve an enormous volume and come to occupy the whole of the left side of the abdomen. The liver also may enlarge and shows progressive infiltration with myeloid tissue.

Clinical features at diagnosis

The disease usually presents in late middle age or later but may very occasionally prove to be the cause of asymptomatic splenomegaly recognized in the fifth decade of life or earlier. The patient may have non-specific symptoms attributable to anaemia, or may present with symptoms due to splenomegaly, including abdominal fullness, early satiety, or left upper quadrant pain. Constitutional symptoms may be prominent, including night sweats, fevers, weight loss, or itching. Hyperuricaemia is not uncommon in primary myelofibrosis and occasional patients present with gout or ureteric colic. The most prominent physical findings are splenomegaly and hepatomegaly. Rare patients have ascites at presentation or during the course of the disease. Lymphadenopathy also occurs occasionally.

Haematology

Patients are typically anaemic at presentation and the red cells are usually normocytic. There may be some anisocytosis, and characteristic 'tear-drop' cells may be prominent. Microcytosis with hypochromia may be present if the patient has been bleeding or macrocytosis may occur in the case of folate deficiency. The reticulocyte count is often increased and nucleated red cells may be present in the peripheral blood. The leucocyte count may be normal, increased, or reduced, but the presence in the film of occasional blast cells justifies the term 'leuco-erythroblastic anaemia'. When leucocytosis is present the leucocytes are predominantly neutrophils, metamyelocytes, and blast cells and the absence of myelocytes, basophilia, and eosinophilia distinguishes the blood film from that of CML. Moreover, the neutrophil alkaline phosphatase is usually normal or raised, unlike CML. In the early stages of myelofibrosis the platelet count is often raised, sometimes as high as $1000 \times 10^9/l$, but later it may be normal or reduced. Platelet function, as assessed by measurement of aggregation in response to adrenaline or adenosine diphosphate, is often defective.

Attempts at marrow aspiration usually yield only 'dry taps' but occasionally normal or hypercellular marrow fragments are obtained; the latter may show gross increases in the number of megakaryocytes, which may be grouped in clusters. A trephine biopsy is essential to confirm the diagnosis. This will show increased thickness and density of reticulin fibres in conjunction with deposition of collagen and sometimes osteosclerosis. Though the myeloid tissue is hypercellular in the initial phases of the diseases, in later stages only discrete islands of hypercellular tissue are identified and in most advanced cases the biopsy may show almost exclusively fibrous tissue.

Ferrokinetic studies with ^{59}Fe show very rapid clearance of injected iron from the circulation and very rapid plasma iron turnover. Surface counting shows evidence of erythropoiesis in the spleen and liver as well as in the marrow. The use of ^{52}Fe obtained from a cyclotron enables the clinician to study the distribution of labelled iron within the body. Much of the iron localizes to the liver and spleen; uptake by marrow in the central skeleton may be reduced and the isotope may be localized disproportionately in the limbs.

Natural history

The disease progresses slowly and the median survival is 3–5 years, although some patients may survive with few problems for 10 years or longer. The major causes of death are infection or haemorrhage associated with leucopenia or thrombocytopenia due to marrow failure. In about 10 per cent of cases the proportion of blast cells in the blood rises inexorably and the haematological picture resembles one of acute leukaemia. This leukaemic transformation responds very poorly to cytotoxic drugs and remissions cannot usually be obtained.

23.5.6   Primary thrombocythaemia

The term primary thrombocythaemia describes a now relatively well-defined myeloproliferative disorder characterized by autonomous increase in the number of platelets in the peripheral blood associated with megakaryocytosis in the marrow and a variable degree of splenomegaly. The condition is also known as essential or idiopathic thrombocytosis or thrombocythaemia.

Pathogenesis

Primary thrombocythaemia is a clonal disease of the pluripotential haemopoietic stem cell with preferential involvement of the megakaryocyte lineage. The number of megakaryoblast progenitors (CFU-Mk) may be increased in the marrow and blood of newly diagnosed patients. Erythroid burst-forming cells (BFU-E) from the patient's peripheral blood or marrow may proliferate *in vitro* in the absence of added erythropoietin, a phenomenon also observed in polycythaemia rubra vera.

Clinical features

The mean age at presentation is about 60 years, but occasionally the disease is diagnosed in young or middle-aged adults. Some patients are entirely asymptomatic when the thrombocytosis is identified in the course of investigations for unrelated causes or as a result of routine blood tests. In other cases symptoms attributable to haemorrhage or occlusion of small or medium-sized blood vessels are prominent. There may be spontaneous bleeding or excessive bleeding after minor trauma or surgical operations. When bleeding occurs from the gastro-intestinal tract, the associated iron deficiency may delay the diagnosis of primary thrombocythaemia. The earliest features of small-vessel occlusion include erythromelalgia and ischaemia of the fingers or toes, which may proceed to pregangrenous or frank gangrenous change. Transient neurological symptoms are not uncommon, and transient episodes of visual loss (amaurosis fugax) may occur. The vascular phenomena are usually, but not always, reversible. They are presumably due to spontaneous platelet aggregation or blockage of blood vessels by platelet thrombi. Physical examination at diagnosis may reveal signs of haemorrhage or minor degrees of splenomegaly. Many patients have no abnormal signs.

Haematology

The major haematological finding is the presence of thrombocytosis, with platelet numbers in the range $600 \times 10^9/l$ to more than $2500 \times 10^9/l$. The platelets show considerable variation in size and shape. The leucocyte count is moderately raised in about one-third of patients. Occasional immature granulocytes may be present in the film, and eosinophil and basophil numbers may be increased. The neutrophil alkaline phosphatase may be normal, low, or high. The haemoglobin is normal unless bleeding complicates the picture. The marrow may be difficult to aspirate on account of increased reticulin. When marrow fragments are obtained, these are usually hypercellular with decreased fat spaces and increased numbers of megakaryocytes, the majority of which are larger than is characteristic in reactive thrombocytoses.

Chromosome studies may show a normal karyotype or a variety of non-specific abnormalities. When a Ph chromosome is identified in a patient with otherwise typical primary thrombocythaemia, the patient's disease must be regarded as lying midway between a standard primary thrombocythaemia and Ph-positive CML.

Clinical course

The clinical course for patients with primary thrombocythaemia is typically indolent. The median survival is of the order of 10 years from diagnosis and because of their advanced age at diagnosis many patients die of apparently unrelated causes. In some patients the marrow becomes increasingly fibrotic and marrow failure leads to anaemia and thrombocytopenia. Rarely, there is a transformation to acute leukaemia.

23.5.7 Further reading

Bellucci, S., Janvier, M., Tobelem, G., Flandrin, G., Charpak, Y., Berger, R., et al. (1986). Essential thrombocythemias. *Cancer* 58, 2440–7.
Bennett, J. M., Catovsky, D., Daniel, M. T., Flandrin, G., Galton, D. A. G., Gralnick, H. R., et al. (1976). Proposals for the classification of the acute leukaemias: French–American–British Co-operative Group. *British Journal of Haematology* 33, 451–3.
Bennett, J. M., Catovsky, D., Daniel, M. T., Flandrin, G., Galton, D. A. G., Gralnick, H. R., et al. (1982). Proposals for the classification of the myelodysplastic syndromes. *British Journal of Haematology* 51, 189–99.
Gale, R. P. and Hoffbrand, A. V. (eds) (1986). Acute leukaemia. *Clinics in Haematology* 15, 567–908.
Galton, D. A. G. (1984). The myelodysplastic syndromes. *Clinical and Laboratory Haematology* 6, 99–112.
Goldman, J. M. (ed.) (1987). Chronic myeloid leukaemia. *Baillieres Clinical Haematology* 1, 869–1077.
Lewis, S. M. (ed.) (1985). *Myelofibrosis: pathophysiology and clinical management*. Marcel Dekker, New York.
Manoharan, A. (1988). Myelofibrosis: prognostic factors and treatment. *British Journal of Haematology* 69, 295–8.
Pearson, T. C. (1991). Primary thrombocythaemia: diagnosis and management. *British Journal of Haematology* 78, 145–8.
Shaw, M. T. (ed.) (1982). *Chronic granulocytic leukaemia*. Praeger Scientific, Eastbourne.
Tricot, G., Mecucci, C., and van den Berghe, H. (1986). Evolution of the myelodysplastic syndromes. *British Journal of Haematology* 63, 609–14.

23.6 Defects of blood coagulation and haemostasis

C. R. Rizza

The mechanisms of blood coagulation and haemostasis have been described in Chapter 7. Defective haemostasis may result from a quantitative or qualitative deficiency of one or more components of the normal mechanism and may be inherited or acquired. These defects may occur in the primary phase of haemostasis involving vascular and platelet function or in the secondary phase when the blood coagulation process makes its contribution. Broadly speaking, failure of the primary phase is characterized by prolonged bleeding which continues from the moment of injury, usually involves mucous membranes and skin surfaces, and may be controlled by gentle pressure. In general, this type of bleeding disorder is more mild than that encountered when the secondary phase of haemostasis is defective. Failure of the secondary phase is seen typically in severe haemophilia. In this condition, bleeding following injury usually stops initially in the normal time but restarts several hours or even days later and then persists for days or weeks unless treated. Some of the important differences between coagulation factor deficiencies and platelet deficiencies are shown in Table 23.12.

23.6.1 Haemostatic defects due to vascular abnormalities

Vascular defects leading to bleeding disorders may be inherited or acquired. Some of the commoner conditions are listed in Table 23.13.

Table 23.12 Comparison of clinical features in coagulation factor defects and platelet defects

Clinical features	Coagulation defect	Platelet defect
Spontaneous bruising	Large and spreading; often deep	Small, superficial often multiple
Bleeding from superficial wounds	Not excessive, except perhaps in the very young	Often profuse and prolonged
Haemarthrosis and muscle haemorrhages	Common in severely affected patients.	Very rare
Post-operative bleeding	Usually delayed; not easily controlled by pressure; may persist for many days	Usually immediate; pressure often controls it; seldom continues for more than a few hours
Commonest bleeding	Deep tissue haemorrhages into joints and muscles; life endangering bleeding after injury	Petechiae and ecchymoses; bleeding from mucosa of nose, GI tract, and uterus

Table 23.13 Some vascular abnormalities that may be associated with haemorrhage

Congenital disorders	Hereditary haemorrhagic telangiectasis Ehlers–Danlos syndrome Pseudoxanthoma elasticum Marfan's syndrome
Acquired disorders	Henoch–Schönlein purpura Purpura fulminans Scurvy Amyloidosis Senile purpura

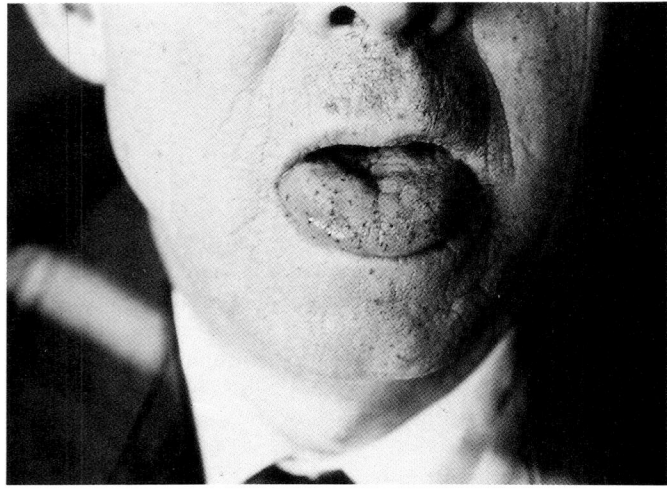

Fig. 23.42 Hereditary haemorrhagic telangiectasia. Note the telangiectatic lesions on the tongue and around the mouth.

Inherited vascular disorders

Hereditary haemorrhagic telangiectasia (Osler–Weber–Rendu disease)

This is the most common inherited vascular bleeding disorder. Transmission is autosomal dominant, both sexes being equally affected. The condition is characterized by localized anatomical abnormalities in the blood vessels of skin and mucous membranes. The lesions consist of dilated and tortuous thin-walled arterioles and capillaries that bleed easily when injured.

Apart from these localized lesions, the blood vessels elsewhere seem to be normal and bleeding takes place only from abnormal vessels. For this reason the skin bleeding time test is usually normal unless by accident an abnormal vessel is punctured. Other laboratory tests of blood coagulation and haemostasis are usually normal.

The defect may not be prominent in early life but becomes apparent in adolescence and early adulthood as the lesions increase in size and in number. The characteristic defects are seen in the mucous membranes of mouth and nose and in the skin of the face and hands (Fig. 23.42). Epistaxis and gastrointestinal bleeding are the commonest symptoms. Patients often develop arteriovenous malformations in the lungs which may cause haemoptysis. In one large family study 15 per cent of those affected were found to have arteriovenous fistulae. Shunting of blood in the lungs may be sufficient to cause anoxia, finger clubbing, and polycythaemia. Vascular malformations in brain, liver, and spleen have also been reported.

Ehlers–Danlos syndrome

This is an uncommon inherited disorder of connective tissue. As a consequence, capillaries are poorly supported and rupture easily. The condition may be autosomal dominant, recessive, or sex-linked in its mode of inheritance. Several types of collagen abnormality have been described and bleeding is particularly severe in what has been called type IV disease in which type III collagen is defective. Platelet abnormalities have also been described in some patients. The clinical features include soft, hyperextensible skin, hyperextensibility of the joints, particularly of fingers and elbows, and 'tissue paper' scars over knees and elbows. Large patchy bruises in the skin, prolonged bleeding from cuts, gastrointestinal bleeding, and prolonged bleeding following dental extraction are common. Laboratory tests of blood coagulation are normal and the diagnosis rests on the clinical and histological features in the skin.

Pseudoxanthoma elasticum

This is a rare condition in which the elastic fibres of skin and blood vessels are abnormal. Transmission is usually autosomal recessive. The skin hangs in loose folds, especially about the neck, axilla, and medial aspect of the thighs, contains tel-angiectases, and bruises easily. Bleeding occurs most commonly into skin, eyes, joints, kidneys, gastrointestinal tract, and uterus. Subarachnoid haemorrhage is a common cause of death.

Marfan's syndrome

This condition is thought to be due to defective cross-linking of collagen. Transmission is autosomal dominant. The clinical features include long extremities with arachnodactyly, aortic wall defects, dislocation of the lens of the eye, spontaneous bruising, and prolonged bleeding after surgery.

Acquired vascular disorders

Henoch–Schönlein (anaphylactoid) purpura

This is an acquired disorder in which haemorrhage may be an important feature. The condition is an acute allergic vasculitis which may involve the gut (described by Henoch), the joints (described by Schönlein), the kidneys, and the skin. The trigger is often unknown but may include bacterial infection, drugs, or food. Purpura is usually preceded by fever and a macular or urticarial rash, and typically affects the arms, legs, and buttock (Fig. 23.43). Haemorrhage or oedema into the gut wall may cause severe abdominal pain and bloody diarrhoea. The condition is self-limiting in the majority of cases, although a small number of patients may go on to develop chronic renal failure as a consequence of damage to renal blood vessels.

Scurvy

This condition, which is due to vitamin C deficiency, is rarely seen now in developed countries, but it is still common in the poorer countries where it is a feature of malnutrition and multiple vitamin deficiency.

Ascorbic acid (vitamin C) activates the enzyme proline hydroxylase, which hydroxylates proline and lysine residues in collagen and thereby stabilizes its helical structure. Deficiency of ascorbic acid results in qualitative and quantitative deficiencies in collagen. As a consequence, small vessels lack support, become fragile, and bleed easily.

Bleeding symptoms include perifollicular haemorrhage in the skin, gingival bleeding, gastrointestinal bleeding, and intracranial bleeding. Subperiosteal haemorrhage in long bones is seen in the young.

Amyloidosis

Both primary and secondary amyloidosis may be complicated by haemorrhage. This mechanism is not fully understood but may be due to amyloid deposits in vessel walls weakening them, or to immune complexes directed against the vessel wall. Occasionally there may be a deficiency of factor X or factor IX. Superficial bruising involving the face and upper trunk may be seen, and there may also be spontaneous internal bleeding.

23.6.2   Haemorrhagic conditions due to platelet defects

Platelets play an important role in haemostasis and a quantitative or qualitative defect affecting them may result in bleeding. As already mentioned above, the clinical features of platelet defects are different from those seen in coagulation defects (Table 23.12).

Inherited disorders of platelet function

Inherited abnormalities of platelets may result in failure of the platelets to participate fully in the haemostatic process because of impaired adhesion, aggregation, thromboxane synthesis, release of stored contents, or the impaired contribution of platelets to the coagulation mechanism.

Inherited disorders can be classified broadly into defects of the platelet membranes, defects of the storage organelles, and defects of the prostaglandin–endoperoxide system (Table 23.14).

Bernard–Soulier syndrome

This is an autosomal recessive disorder which shows a variable degree of thrombocytopenia with giant platelets. The bleeding time is prolonged and superficial bruising and bleeding from mucous membranes is common. The basic defect is thought to

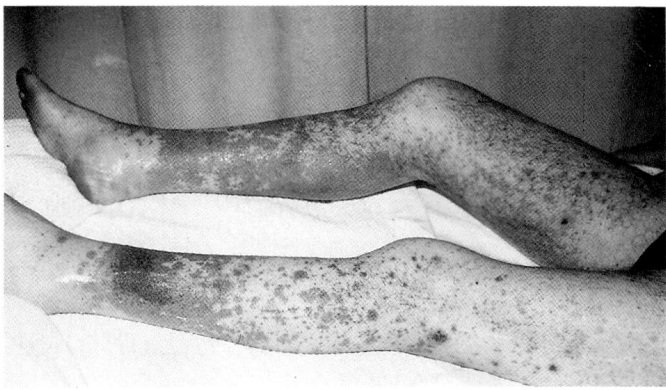

Fig. 23.43   Allergic purpura in a middle-aged man.

Table 23.14   Inherited platelet defects

Defects of platelet membranes
  Bernard–Soulier syndrome
  Thrombasthenia (Glanzmann's disease)

Deficiency of storage organs (storage pool disease)
  Dense-body deficiency
    Hermansky–Pudlak syndrome
    Wiskott–Aldrich syndrome
    Chediak–Higashi syndrome
    idiopathic storage pool disease
  α-Granule deficiency
    Gray platelet syndrome

Defects of the prostaglandin–endoperoxide pathway
  Cyclo-oxygenase deficiency
  Thromboxane synthetase deficiency

---

be a deficiency of platelet membrane glycoprotein I (GPI) and glycoprotein Ib (GPIB), which are important for the interaction of platelets with von Willebrand's factor (vWF) and for adhesion to subendothelium. The diagnosis is made from the clinical history, the appearance of the platelets, and failure of the platelets to aggregate *in vitro* with the antibiotic ristocetin. Aggregation with ADP, collagen, and arachidonic acid is normal.

Thrombasthenia (Glanzmann's disease)

Thrombasthenia is probably the best-known of the inherited platelet disorders. It is an autosomal recessive trait. The bleeding disorder is moderately severe and the bleeding symptoms include multiple superficial bruises (Fig. 23.44), epistaxis, and menorrhagia. Bleeding from superficial cuts is prolonged. The haemorrhagic symptoms tend to be at their most severe in childhood and gradually improve as the patient grows older. The bleeding time is prolonged and clot retraction is abnormal. The platelet count and morphology are normal. The most striking laboratory feature is failure of platelet aggregation on addition of ADP, 5-HT, collagen, or thrombin. The defect is thought to be due to a deficiency of glycoproteins IIb and IIIa in the platelet membrane. These closely associated glycoproteins are thought to provide binding sites for fibrinogen, which is necessary for platelet aggregation by ADP.

Storage pool disease

Failure of secretion of the contents of platelet granules is now known to cause mild bleeding disorders. The deficiency may lie in the granules themselves or in the platelet mechanisms that are necessary for the release of the granules from platelets.

In dense-body deficiency there is a failure of platelets to aggregate in response to collagen. Aggregation with ADP is normal initially but is followed by disaggregation. Dense-body deficiency can be demonstrated by electron microscopy as the dense bodies are electron-opaque.

Acquired disorder of platelets

Acquired platelet disorders are much more common than the inherited defects (Table 23.15).

Secondary thrombocytopenia

Secondary thrombocytopenia is the commonest form of acquired thrombocytopenia and may be brought on by the effect of drugs, ionizing radiation, chemical poison, or bacterial toxins on the bone marrow. These agents may act by damaging the megakaryocytes, the platelet precursors, in the marrow, or by triggering an immune response that results in platelet destruction in the circulation. Invasion of the bone marrow by neoplastic cells and leukaemia are also important causes of thrombocytopenia. Bleeding in thrombocytopenia does not usually occur until the platelet count falls to less than $50 \times 10^9/l$. Counts of less than $25 \times 10^9/l$ may be accompanied by bleeding after trauma. Counts less than $10 \times 10^9/l$ are usually associated with spontaneous severe bleeding from the mucous membranes. Treatment is aimed at trying to cure the underlying condition.

Idiopathic thrombocytopenia

Acute idiopathic thrombocytopenic purpura (ITP) occurs mainly in children between the ages of 2 and 10 years, often 1–6 weeks after a viral illness. It affects the sexes equally. Onset is acute with the sudden appearance of petechial haemorrhages and bleeding from the mucous membranes of nose and gastrointestinal tract. Examination of the blood shows marked thrombocytopenia, usually less than $20 \times 10^9/l$. Platelet-associated IgG is usually increased. The pathophysiology of acute ITP is still not clear. The most commonly accepted hypothesis is that the sufferer makes an antibody against the virus or a virus product which then forms an immune complex. These immune complexes then attach themselves to platelets and

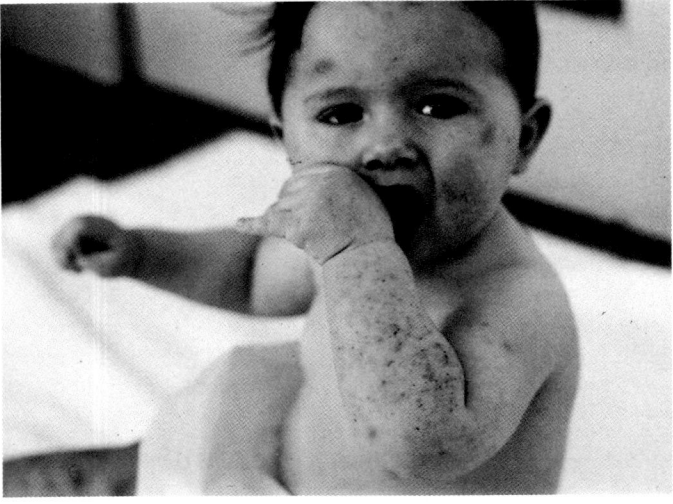

Fig. 23.44 Glanzmann's thrombasthenia.

Table 23.15 Classification of thrombocytopenia

Primary idiopathic thrombocytopenia
  Acute
  Chronic

Secondary thrombocytopenia
  Toxic chemicals and drugs
    fertilizers, insecticides, cytostatic drugs, barbiturates, chloramphenicol, thiazides
  Ionizing radiation
  Aplastic anaemia
  Leukaemia
  Marrow infiltration, e.g. multiple myeloma, lymphoma, carcinomatosis, myelofibrosis
    Gaucher's disease
  Infection
    Hepatitis
    Miliary tuberculosis, etc.
  Artificial surface, e.g. artificial heart valves
  Disseminated intravascular coagulation
  Other
    Paroxysmal nocturnal haemoglobinuria
    haemolytic–uraemic syndrome
    bite of certain snakes

bring about premature destruction or removal of platelets from the circulation. The majority of cases of acute ITP remit spontaneously.

Chronic idiopathic thrombocytopenic purpura

This condition presents with insidious onset of easy bruising, nosebleeds, menorrhagia, and gastrointestinal bleeding. Apart from having a different mode of onset, chronic ITP differs from acute ITP in that it occurs mainly in adults aged 20–50 and is rare in children; women are affected much more often than men (approximately 5 : 1) whereas the sex ratio of acute ITP is 1 : 1. There is rarely a preceding viral illness and, finally, the condition, unlike acute ITP, may last for years. The pathogenesis of the disorder is still not clear. The blood of patients with chronic ITP contains antibodies directed against platelets and transfusion of plasma from these patients into normal individuals causes thrombocytopenia in the recipient. Subsequent studies have shown that antibody-coated platelets are selectively removed by the reticuloendothelial system.

23.6.3 Coagulation disorders

A quantitative or qualitative deficiency of one or more of the coagulation factors is usually accompanied by faulty haemostasis, the severity of the haemostatic disorder usually being related to the severity of the coagulation factor deficiency. Factor XII deficiency is unusual in this respect and is rarely associated with bleeding despite the fact that the whole blood-clotting time may be greatly prolonged *in vitro*.

Deficiencies of blood coagulation factors may be either congenital or acquired. Congenital deficiencies usually present as single factor deficiencies whereas acquired deficiencies are usually multiple factor defects.

Inherited coagulation factor deficiencies

Inherited blood coagulation defects are relatively uncommon, but they have been studied extensively and it is largely from such studies that our knowledge of blood coagulation has developed.

Those clotting factor deficiencies will now be discussed, starting with the more common and more severe disorders.

Haemophilia A (classic haemophilia)

Haemophilia A is the commonest of the severe inherited bleeding disorders. Bleeding is due to a partial or complete deficiency of factor VIII coagulant activity, resulting from a gene defect on the X-chromosome. Being X-linked, haemophilia affects males and is carried by females who sometimes themselves show a lesser tendency to bleed. The absent or lesser bleeding in carrier women is explained by the fact that women have two X-chromosomes in their cells, one bearing the defective gene producing no factor VIII and the other a normal gene producing a normal complement of factor VIII. During early embryogenesis one or other of these chromosomes is randomly inactivated. If inactivation is truly random, the woman will end up with a factor VIII level of 50 per cent of that of the average normal

woman. Inactivation, however, may not be random and more normal chromosomes than abnormal chromosomes may be inactivated, in which case the woman may have a level of factor VIII sufficiently reduced to cause bleeding following injury.

A man with haemophilia does not transmit the condition to his sons but all of his daughters are carriers. Carriers, when they conceive a son, have a 50 : 50 chance of having a haemophiliac and, when they conceive a daughter, have a 50 : 50 chance of having a carrier daughter.

Incidence Classic haemophilia has been described in most human ethnic groups, as well as several species of lower animals. Its incidence in the UK is approximately 90 per million of population.

Clinical features Severe haemophilia is characterized by repeated episodes of bleeding into joints and muscles, often with no apparent preceding injury. Superficial injury, if not treated, may result in persistent bleeding for days or even weeks, although minor cuts and scratches stop bleeding in the normal time and usually do not bleed again unless disturbed. Surgical operations usually result in severe and prolonged bleeding if the patient is not given factor VIII replacement therapy. In general, the severity of bleeding symptoms in a haemophiliac reflects the severity of his factor VIII deficiency. Patients with less than 1 per cent of the average normal amount may bleed spontaneously into joints and muscles.

Bleeding into the joints is a striking feature of severe haemophilia. The knees, ankles, and elbows are particularly affected; wrists, shoulders, and hips less so. It is thought that the knees and ankles are predisposed to bleeding because they are weight-bearing joints, and the knee joint in particular because it is a hinge joint of a relatively unstable nature. It is difficult to understand why the elbow joint should be so predisposed to bleeding, except again that it is a hinge joint with a complex action and has little surrounding tissue to protect it or to prevent twisting and strain.

Bleeding inside a joint is contained within the joint capsule and, as the bleeding progresses, increasing pressure in the joint gives rise to pain which can be very severe. The site of the bleeding is thought to be small synovial vessels that have been injured or have ruptured spontaneously. The effect of blood within the joint space is to cause an inflammatory response in the synovial membrane, with release of several proteolytic enzymes, including cathepsin, plasmin, and collagenase. The synovial membrane shows increased vascularity and, as a consequence, increased tendency to further bleeding. Eventually, after repeated episodes of bleeding, the synovial membrane becomes thickened and fibrotic, with large villous projections and heavily stained with blood pigments (Fig. 23.45). The joint cartilage, which may be stained with haemosiderin, is eroded with consequent loss of joint space. Subchondral cysts form and osteoporosis develops. Movement in the joint becomes progressively limited, fibrous ankylosis develops, followed by bony ankylosis in a position of partial flexion. The above changes are not specific for haemophilia and are very similar to those seen in degenerative osteoarthritis from other causes. The joint

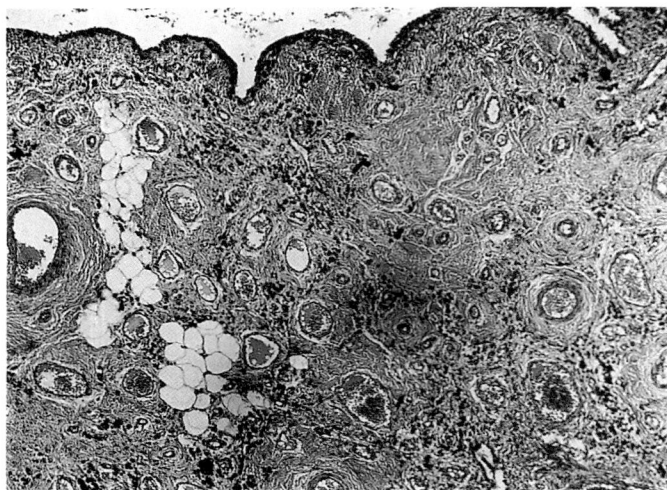

Fig. 23.45 Synovial membrane from the medial aspect of the knee joint of a 26-year-old haemophiliac. The lining layer shows a few folds. Haemosiderin deposits stand out clearly in the lining layer and in the subsynovial tissue. There is also fibrosis and an angiomatoid reaction.

changes can be seen clearly on radiological examination (Fig. 23.46).

The above sequence of events is accompanied by varying degrees of pain.

Bleeding into muscles, with or without obvious trauma, is common in severe haemophilia, less so in mild haemophilia. Practically any muscle mass can be affected but the muscles of the forearm, calf, thigh, or buttock are the main sites of haemorrhage. Bleeding into muscle is important not only because of the damage done to the muscle by the haemorrhage, but also because of the pressure that such haemorrhage may exert on important structures lying nearby, such as nerves and arteries. Bleeding into the muscles of the forearm, calf, and buttock is particularly prone to cause nerve damage by pressure. Volkmann's ischaemic necrosis was one of the dreaded complications of this type of bleeding before the days of effective factor replacement therapy.

Bleeding into muscle is usually associated with pain and swelling, and diminished movement of the associated joint.

Bleeding into the iliacus muscle is of particular importance as it is not uncommon and may be missed if not carefully sought. The iliacus muscle lies on the inner wall of the pelvis enclosed within a tough fibrous sheath with the femoral nerve running on the surface of the muscle under the sheath. Because of the enclosed nature of the muscle, haemorrhage into the muscle may quickly produce pain, pressure on the femoral nerve, and impairment of femoral nerve function.

On examination, the limb on the affected side is held flexed at the hip, a tender mass is palpable at the pelvic brim, and there is diminished sensation down the front of the thigh and diminished or absent knee reflex. If the haematoma is on the right side, the condition may be diagnosed as appendicitis or appendix abscess, as the patient may have a slight temperature

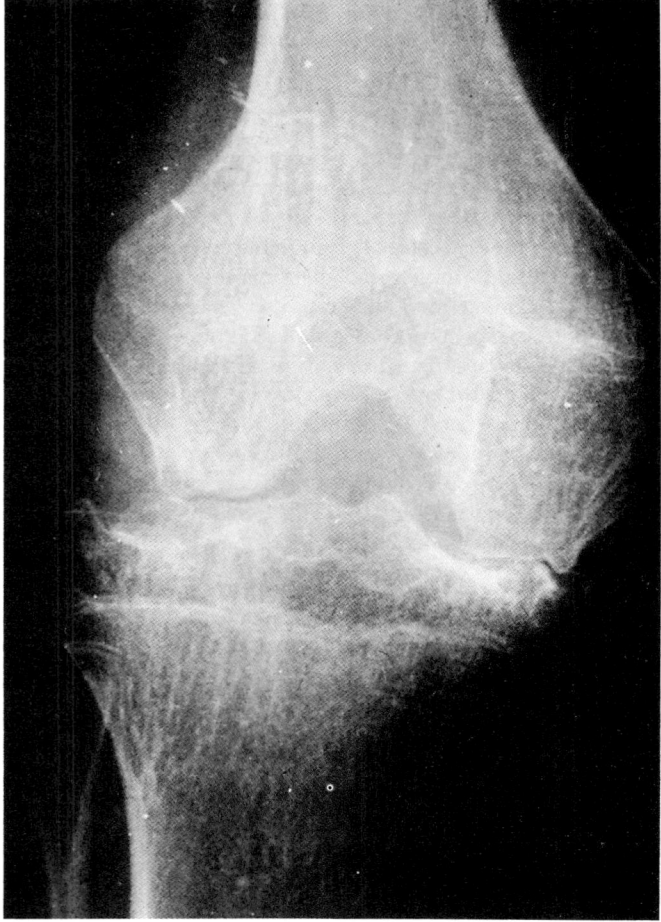

Fig. 23.46 X-ray of knee joint of a severely affected haemophiliac showing loss of joint space, widening of the intercondylar notch, and marked irregularity of the joint surface.

and a raised white cell count. The presence of the femoral nerve palsy should make the diagnosis clear. Ultrasound examination or CAT scan, although useful, are rarely required as the diagnosis can usually be made by clinical examination.

Muscle haemorrhages are prone to recur at the same site if not treated adequately or if the muscle is exercised too early. Occasionally muscle haematomas progress to form muscle cysts, the iliopsoas, buttock, thigh, and calf muscles being most frequently affected. Repeated bleeding into the muscle results in destruction of muscle tissues and formation of a cyst lined by a thick fibrotic capsule and containing old blood and clots and dead muscle. Muscle cysts can attain a large size and may cause damage to adjacent structures by pressure. It is not uncommon for muscle cysts to bring about erosion and fracture of bone.

Occasionally cysts may start in bone. These are thought to be caused by bleeding in the bone or under the periosteum with stripping of periosteum. Clinically the condition presents as a painful expanding lesion. On radiological examination the appearances are sometimes similar to those of osteogenic sarcoma, hence the name 'haemophilic pseudotumour'

(Fig. 23.47). Muscle and bone cysts tend to increase in size unless treated vigorously with factor replacement and complete immobilization of the part. Even then conservative treatment may fail and it may be necessary to excise them surgically.

Intracranial bleeding was, until the appearance of AIDS, perhaps the commonest cause of death in haemophilia, accounting for about 25 per cent of all deaths, and may follow quite minor injury. Bleeding may be subdural or into the brain substance, and may be delayed 24 hours or more following the injury. The diagnosis can usually be made clinically but in difficult cases computer-assisted tomography is of great help.

Haematuria, once the second most common form of bleeding in haemophiliacs, seems now to be much less common. The reason for this reduction in incidence of haematuria is not known but may be related to the fact that aspirin is now no longer used as an analgesic by haemophiliacs, or to the more prompt and frequent use of potent factor VIII preparation for treating this and other forms of bleeding.

The source of bleeding in haematuria is thought to be the kidney itself, probably the glomerular vessels. If bleeding is profuse and the patient is not drinking freely, clots may form in the renal pelvis and ureter, causing ureteric colic, obstruction of urinary outflow, back pressure, and pain, which may be very severe. The amount of blood lost is usually small and rarely causes anaemia. Long-term effects of repeated episodes of haematuria and clot obstruction on renal function have been sought. Some workers have found evidence of obstructive nephropathy as well as evidence of papillary necrosis, but others have observed no long-term effects on renal function.

Haemophilia B (Christmas disease)

Haemophilia B or Christmas disease is due to a deficiency of factor IX. It is clinically indistinguishable from haemophilia A and, as in haemophilia A, bleeding symptoms include deep-tissue haemorrhages and haemarthroses. The condition is transmitted as a sex-linked recessive disorder and affects males.

It is less common than haemophilia A and its prevalence in the UK is approximately 18 per million of population. Using a variety of immunological techniques, including antibody neutralization tests, counter immunoelectrophoresis, electro-immuno assays, and immunoradiometric assays, several variant forms of haemophilia B have been described. These variants can be classified broadly into three groups;

1. those with no detectable factor IX coagulant activity and no detectable factor IX antigen cross-reacting material (CRM−);

2. those with reduced amounts of coagulant activity but normal antigen (CRM+); and

3. those in whom factor IX coagulant activity and factor IX antigen are reduced to the same extent (CRM reduced).

The CRM+ group accounts for approximately 40 per cent of patients with haemophilia B and can be further subdivided depending on the reaction of the patient's plasma to ox brain in the prothrombin time test, binding of factor IX to Ca^{2+} or phospholipid, and electrophoretic mobility of factor IX.

von Willebrand's disease

von Willebrand's disease is an inherited bleeding disorder which affects both sexes and is transmitted as an autosomal dominant condition. It was first described by E. A. von Willebrand (1926) in inhabitants of the Aland Islands in the Gulf of Bothnia. Bleeding from mucous membranes is a notable feature of the condition, and because of this and the prolonged skin bleeding time the defect in von Willebrand's was thought to be in the platelets or in the capillary vessels. von Willebrand in his original paper called the disease 'pseudo haemophilia'.

Pathogenesis von Willebrand's disease has been intensively studied in the past 30 years and it has been shown that the haemostatic defect is due to an abnormality in the factor VIII complex. The factor VIII complex, as has been discussed in Chapter 7, is composed of two distinct molecules, one large and one small, which are linked by non-covalent bonds. The smaller of the two molecules, which contains the procoagulant activity (factor VIII), is coded for by a gene on the X-chromosome and is

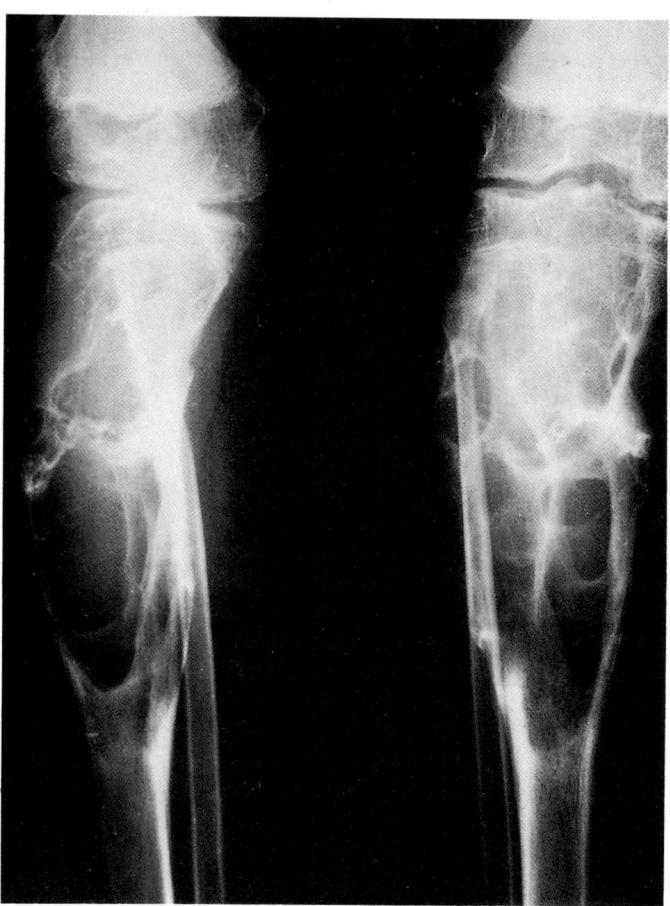

Fig. 23.47 X-ray showing haemophilic pseudotumour of bone affecting the upper end of the tibia. Lateral (left) and anteroposterior (right) views. The normal architecture of the bone has been destroyed and is replaced by numerous cysts.

defective in patients with haemophilia A or classic haemophilia. The large molecule is a multimeric structure (von Willebrand's factor (vWF)) that has an important function in primary haemostasis as it is involved in the interaction between platelets and the vessel wall. von Willebrand's disease is due to either a quantitative or qualitative deficiency of von Willebrand's factor. Since vWF seems to act as a carrier and a protective agent for the small molecular procoagulant component, defective synthesis of vWF is accompanied by a reduction of factor VIII coagulant activity. Patients with von Willebrand's disease therefore suffer from a defect in both the primary and secondary stage of the haemostatic process. von Willebrand's disease is inherited as an autosomal dominant and affects men and women equally. Characteristically, bleeding takes place from superficial injuries to the skin and mucous membranes. Bleeding from the nose, gastrointestinal tract, and uterus is particularly common. Several variants of von Willebrand's disease have been described, and the condition has been classified broadly into three types (Table 23.16). Patients with type III von Willebrand's disease usually have severe bleeding symptoms with undetectable levels of vWF or factor VIII coagulant activity. Haemarthrosis and muscle haemorrhage may occur, as in severe haemophilia. Investigation of variants may show a prolongation of the skin bleeding time, a variable reduction of vWF, vWF-antigen, and factor VIII coagulant activity. Analysis of the multimer by gel electrophoresis gives important additional information about the specific type.

Prothrombin deficiency

Hereditary deficiency of prothrombin is extremely rare and is usually transmitted in an autosomal recessive manner. Approximately 30 families have been described, some with true prothrombin deficiency (hypoprothrombinaemia), with reduced biological activity, and reduced prothrombin-related antigen, and others with abnormal molecular variants of prothrombin (dysprothrombinaemia). Several different prothrombin variants have been described and studied in detail, and have been named after the city where they originated. The variants

are characterized largely on their reactions and their ability to be activated with different snake venoms, brain thromboplastin, and staphylocoagulase. Further information is given by immuno assays and crossed immuno electrophoresis. For example, prothrombin Molise and Brussels show abnormal conversion to thrombin in the presence of the venom of *Echis carinatus*, whereas prothrombin Padua and Barcelona show normal conversion with that venom. Homozygous individuals usually bleed excessively and show easy bruising, bleeding from mucous membranes, and bleeding after surgery. Heterozygotes rarely bleed excessively.

On laboratory testing, the patient's prothrombin time is prolonged and is not corrected on addition of serum or alumina-adsorbed normal plasma (which contains fibrinogen, factor V, and factor VIII only). Specific factor assays reveal deficiency of prothrombin.

Factor V deficiency

Factor V deficiency is rare and was first described by Owren in 1947. The inheritance pattern is usually autosomal recessive, although some cases seem to be partially dominant. Several cases have been the result of consanguineous marriages. A variety of congenital malformations involving the skeletal, cardiovascular, or renal system have been described in association with this coagulation defect. The diagnosis is suggested by a prolongation of the prothrombin time and the activated partial thromboplastin time, which can be corrected by addition of alumina-adsorbed normal plasma but not by normal aged serum. In a proportion of patients the bleeding time is prolonged. Bleeding symptoms include easy bruising, epistaxis, muscle haematomas, menorrhagia, and postoperative bleeding.

Factor VII deficiency

Congenital deficiency of factor VII is very rare. Approximately 100 cases have been described, and the deficiency is thought to be autosomal recessive in inheritance. The condition may be a manifestation of a true deficiency of the factor VII protein or an

---

Table 23.16 Variants of von Willebrand's disease

Disease type	Bleeding time	vWF*	vWF-antigen	VIII-coagulant activity	Pattern of vWF multimers on gel electrophoresis
I	Prolonged	Reduced	Reduced	Reduced	Normal in composition but reduced in amount
II A	Prolonged	Reduced	Reduced but not as much as vWF	Usually reduced	Abnormal with loss of large and intermediate forms
II B	Prolonged	Variable, may be normal	Variable, may be normal	Normal or low	Large multimers absent
II C	Prolonged	Normal or reduced	Normal or reduced	Normal or reduced	Large and intermediate multimers present but small multimers very prominent
III	Prolonged	Undetectable	Undetectable	Undetectable or only a trace	No multimers seen

* Assayed by ability to bring about aggregation of normal platelets in the presence of ristocetin.

abnormal variant of the protein. On the basis of antibody neutralization tests and factor VII assays carried out using thromboplastin from different species of animals, it has been possible to define several variants of factor VII. Bleeding manifestations in factor VII deficiency are usually milder than those seen in severe haemophilia, although some deficient patients have bled quite severely. Easy bruising, epistaxis, and gastrointestinal haemorrhages occur, as well as menorrhagia in the female. Haemarthroses may occur and, as in haemophilia, may cause joint damage and deformity.

Laboratory investigations show a prolonged one-stage prothrombin time, with a normal whole-blood clotting time, activated partial thromboplastin time, and Russell's viper venom time. The diagnosis is confirmed by means of a factor VII assay using known factor VII deficient substrate.

Factor X deficiency

Factor X (Prower–Stuart factor) deficiency is very rare and was originally described in the Prower family and the Stuart family.

The inheritance of the condition is autosomal recessive. By means of immunological methods, such as antibody neutralization tests, and by using tissue thromboplastin and Russell's viper venom in the assay systems, it has been shown that numerous variants of factor X exist. Laboratory tests show a prolonged one-stage prothrombin time when either brain thromboplastin or Russell's viper venom is used, and a prolonged activated partial thromboplastin time. These abnormal tests can be corrected by the addition of normal plasma or aged normal serum, but not by alumina-adsorbed normal plasma.

Patients with factor X deficiency bruise easily and bleed excessively after surgery and accidental injury. Women may suffer from menorrhagia and bleed excessively after childbirth. Haemarthroses have been described.

Factor XI deficiency

This is a condition that affects many people of Ashkenazi Jewish extraction. It is inherited as an autosomal recessive condition and the bleeding manifestations are usually mild, even in homozygotes. Bleeding usually follows surgery or accidental injury and is rarely spontaneous. Easy bruising, epistaxis, and menorrhagia are common. Haemarthroses and muscle haematomas are extremely rare. The severity of bleeding may not be closely correlated with the severity of the factor deficiency, and for this reason it is difficult to define the level of factor XI required for haemostasis. Laboratory tests show a normal one-stage prothrombin time, a prolonged whole-blood clotting time, and prolonged activated partial thromboplastin time. Specific assay of factor XI using factor XI-deficient substrate distinguishes this deficiency from other defects in the early stage of the intrinsic coagulation pathway.

Factor XII (Hageman factor) deficiency

Factor XII deficiency is transmitted as an autosomal recessive trait. Bleeding symptoms are rare in factor XII deficiency; indeed, thromboembolism has been described in several cases, including that of Mr Hageman himself, the original case described by Ratnoff and Colopy. The plasma of factor XII-deficient patients usually lacks protein immunologically recognizable as factor XII, although cross-reacting material has been detected by means of radioimmunoassay in two affected individuals.

Laboratory tests show a prolongation of the whole-blood clotting time and activated partial thromboplastin time. The one-stage prothrombin time is normal.

Deficiency of plasma pre-kallikrein (Fletcher factor) and high molecular weight kininogen (Fitzgerald factor)

Deficiency of Fletcher factor was first described in four siblings of a consanguineous marriage.

Laboratory findings consisted of a prolonged whole-blood clotting time and a prolonged activated partial thromboplastin time. The activated partial thromboplastin time becomes shorter on prolonged incubation with the surface activating agent. Despite significant abnormalities in the early stage of the contact phase of blood coagulation, the patients do not bleed.

Deficiency of high molecular weight kininogen (HMWK Fitzgerald factor, Williams factor, Flaujeac factor) is very rare. The whole-blood clotting time is prolonged, as is the activated partial thromboplastin time. The deficiency is not accompanied by bleeding symptoms.

Plasma pre-kallikrein deficiency and high molecular weight kininogen deficiency are inherited as autosomal recessive conditions.

Fibrinogen deficiency

Inherited deficiency of fibrinogen is rare and may be due to lack of production of the normal protein (afibrinogenaemia or hypofibrinogenaemia). or to production of structurally abnormal protein (dysfibrinogenaemia).

Afibrinogenaemia seems to be inherited in an autosomal manner, with only the homozygotes showing bleeding symptoms. Heterozygotes, if carefully tested, may show reduced levels of fibrinogen but without bleeding problems. There is often a history of consanguinity in the parents. In spite of the fact that the blood may be completely incoagulable *in vitro*, bleeding symptoms are relatively mild when compared with those seen in severe haemophilia. Symptoms may start early in life, with prolonged bleeding from the umbilical cord. Easy bruising and excessive bleeding from cuts and scratches are common, as are muscle haematomas, usually after injury and mucous-membrane bleeding. Bleeding into joints is uncommon, and crippling deformities of the type seen in severe haemophilia are extremely rare. Menorrhagia and postpartum bleeding may be troublesome. The laboratory findings are characteristic with an infinitely prolonged whole-blood clotting time, activated partial thromboplastin time and one-stage prothrombin time, and failure of clotting on the addition of strong thrombin, or the snake venoms ancrod (Arvin) or batroxobin (Reptilase). Immunological tests using specific antibodies show absence of fibrinogen.

Dysfibrinogenaemia

This name represents a qualitative defect in the fibrinogen molecule. Many variants have been described, each named after the city in which the defect was found. Since all of the cases have not been studied in detail, it is not yet known how many of the named variants are identical. The condition is inherited in an autosomal manner; most patients described have been heterozygous for the condition, although some have been homozygous.

Mild bleeding symptoms are seen in a proportion of patients. The symptoms include bleeding from mucous membranes, with epistaxis and menorrhagia. Bleeding may occur after surgery and may be accompanied by abnormal healing and breakdown of wounds. Spontaneous abortion has also been noted. A significant number of patients show a tendency to thrombosis. This is thought to be due to the inability of the abnormal fibrinogen to act as an antithrombin, and possibly also to the fact that some abnormal fibrinogens show resistance to fibrinolysis. The most consistent laboratory finding is a prolonged clotting time on addition of thrombin to the plasma.

Factor XIII deficiency

More than 100 cases of this disorder have so far been described. The condition in most families seems to be autosomal recessive, and there is often a history of consanguinity. Factor XIII is necessary for stabilization of the fibrin clot. Bleeding can be severe and may result in death in early life. Excessive bleeding from the umbilical cord is common, as are easy bruising and muscle haemorrhages. Postoperative bleeding and delayed wound healing and scar formation are characteristic features. Repeated spontaneous abortion has been described, and there is an increased incidence of intracranial haemorrhage. In laboratory testing, all the tests of blood coagulation that reflect fibrin formation are normal. The bleeding time is also normal. The diagnosis is made by demonstrating instability of the fibrin clot in 5 M urea or 1 per cent monochloroacetic acid. These methods are relatively insensitive and are not quantitative. Accurate assays are now available using the covalent incorporation of labelled synthetic amines, such as fluorescent dansylcadaverine or radioactive putrescine.

Acquired deficiencies of blood coagulation factors

Acquired disorders of blood coagulation are more common than inherited deficiencies and arise in people with no previous history of bleeding, usually as a feature of some generalized disease process. In addition to deficiencies of blood coagulation factors, the platelets may be affected, there may be evidence of vessel wall damage, and the fibrinolytic system may be activated. In this respect the acquired bleeding disorders are different from the inherited defects, which usually involve only one coagulation factor.

Vitamin K-dependent clotting factors

Vitamin K is the generic name for a group of eight naphthoquinone derivatives essential for the synthesis of prothrombin, factors VII, IX, and X by the liver. It acts as a cofactor for a hepatic enzyme that inserts a carboxyl group at the γ position in certain glutamic acid residues of the precursors of the above clotting factors. In the absence of vitamin K these clotting factors continue to be synthesized but are unable to bind Ca^{2+} and are biologically inactive. Vitamin K is a fat-soluble substance found in the chloroplasts of many plant leaves and in some vegetable oils. Human requirements are met by the average diet but, in addition, considerable amounts of the vitamin are synthesized by intestinal bacteria. Vitamin K is absorbed from the intestine only if adequate amounts of bile salts are present. Requirements normally sufficient for several days are stored in the liver. A deficiency of vitamin K can result from:

1. poor dietary intake, although this is rare;
2. poor absorption (biliary obstruction, sprue, regional enteritis, fibrocystic disease); and
3. failure of utilization of the vitamin (hepatitis, cirrhosis of liver).

Finally, the action of vitamin K is antagonized by drugs, such as coumarin anticoagulants.

Haemostatic disorders and liver diseases

It has long been known that generalized bleeding may occur in patients suffering from cirrhosis of the liver, acute fulminant hepatitis, or long-standing biliary obstruction. The underlying cause of bleeding in these conditions varies. In chronic obstruction of the biliary tract there is failure of absorption of vitamin K from the gastrointestinal tract with consequent defective synthesis of factors II (prothrombin), VII, IX, and X. In hepatocellular disease impaired synthesis of the above clotting factors may be associated with reduced levels of factor V, increased fibrinolysis, diffuse intravascular clotting (DIC), and impaired clearance of activated clotting factors. Platelets may be reduced as a result of impaired thrombopoiesis or increased destruction in the periphery. All of these contribute to the haemostatic disorder. Laboratory tests reveal a prolongation of the one-stage prothrombin time and activated partial thromboplastin time. Specific factor assays show a varied deficiency of prothrombin and factors VII, IX, and X. Factor V may also be reduced, especially in severe hepatocellular disease. The thrombin clotting time is often prolonged, and this may be due to synthesis of functionally abnormal variants of fibrinogen or to the presence of circulating anticoagulants. In patients with DIC, fibrin degradation products may impede the thrombin–fibrinogen reaction or fibrin polymerization and thereby prolong the thrombin clotting time.

Haemorrhagic disease of the new-born

This is a self-limiting disease of the new-born. Bleeding symptoms typically appear on the second or third day after birth and include extensive bruising, bleeding from the gastrointestinal tract, nose, and umbilical cord. In severe cases, bleeding may take place into the central nervous system or adrenal glands.

Laboratory investigations show that the levels of factors II,

VII, IX, and X are reduced in the new-born. There is a further fall during the first few days of life and adult levels of these factors may not be reached in the normal child for several weeks. Children fed cow's milk instead of human milk are less likely to be deficient in the vitamin K-dependent clotting factors. This is because cow's milk contains 4–5 times more vitamin K than human milk. Also, the feeding of cow's milk probably encourages the colonization of the infant gut by organisms that synthesize vitamin K, thereby providing an endogenous source of the vitamin. The severity of the bleeding disorder may be increased if the mother has been taking anticonvulsants, such as phenobarbitone, phenytoin, and primidone, during pregnancy. The risk of haemorrhagic disease of the new-born may be reduced by a single injection of 0.5–1.0 mg of vitamin K, intramuscularly at birth, especially to high-risk neonates.

Kidney disease

Bleeding is sometimes seen as a complication of renal disease. The severity of bleeding is variable and is usually related to the level of urea in the blood. The precise mechanism of the haemostatic defect is not known but it is thought that failure to excrete certain products of metabolism results in qualitative platelet defects and impaired reaction between platelets and the vessel wall. The platelet defects manifest themselves in a prolongation of the skin bleeding time, poor clot retraction, and abnormal prothrombin consumption during coagulation of blood. Platelet aggregation studies show a variable defect in aggregation when collagen, ADP, or adrenaline is added to the patient's platelet-rich plasma. Attempts to show that retained metabolites may be the cause of the prolonged bleeding time and impaired platelet function have met with little success, although it has been shown that guanidinosuccinic acid, which is increased in uraemic plasma, inhibits the second wave of platelet aggregation with ADP. Other retained products, such as hydroxyphenolic acid, may have a part to play. Deficiency of blood coagulation factors is uncommon in renal disease, although factor IX deficiency has been described in patients with nephrotic syndrome and massive proteinuria.

Bleeding with infection

Many infectious diseases may be accompanied by bleeding symptoms. The mechanism of the bleeding is usually complex and reflects damage to one or more of the three components of normal haemostasis, namely, platelets, vessel wall, and blood coagulation mechanism.

Thrombocytopenia may occur in severe infections with Gram-negative or Gram-positive bacteria, viruses (rubella, dengue, infectious mononucleosis), Rickettsiae (typhus, Rocky Mountain Spotted Fever), and Protozoa (malaria, trypanosomiasis).

In most instances the degree of thrombocytopenia is not severe and is rarely sufficient by itself to cause bleeding. The mechanism of the thrombocytopenia is thought to be a combination of impaired platelet production, damaged vessel walls with consequent platelet adhesion, and direct damage to platelets by viral or bacterial components or by circulating immune complexes. Platelets may also be reduced if diffuse intravascular coagulation is present.

Disseminated intravascular coagulation

Disseminated intravascular coagulation (DIC) is seen in diverse pathological conditions. The process is accompanied by deposition of fibrin in small blood vessels and depletion of several coagulation factors, including fibrinogen, factor II, factor V, and factor VIII. Platelet numbers are often reduced. As a consequence the patients may have signs and symptoms of haemorrhage and thrombosis at the same time, as well as the features of the underlying disease.

The pathophysiology of DIC has been intensively studied since 1834 when de Blainville showed that rapid intravenous injection of brain tissue into animals was followed by widespread intravascular coagulation and death. Slow injection of thromboplastin led to incoagulability of the blood, with the animals surviving. Gross thrombi were usually absent although microthrombi composed of platelets and fibrin could often be found in the small vessels of kidneys, lungs, and liver. Subsequently, it was shown that there was a fall in the concentration of fibrinogen as well as of factor II, factor V, and factor VIII. In addition, the animals became thrombocytopenic. There was also evidence of increased fibrinolytic activity and the appearance of breakdown products of fibrin or fibrinogen. Similar results were obtained following injection of thromboplastin from different tissues, thrombin, and certain snake venoms.

In acute DIC, skin bruising, typically large and spreading, may be very marked and troublesome. Bleeding may take place at sites of venepuncture. Bleeding from the nose and gastrointestinal tract may be severe. If large clots form in the pulmonary vascular tree, the patient develops, in addition, shock, shortness of breath, cough, and cyanosis. In subacute DIC, haemorrhage may still occur but is less prominent. On the other hand, thrombosis may be more pronounced, with arteries and

Table 23.17 Some conditions in which DIC may occur

Acute	Haemorrhagic or post-traumatic shock; septicaemia due to Gram-negative or Gram-positive organisms Anaphylactic shock Intravascular haemolysis, mismatched blood transfusion Amniotic fluid embolism, abruptio placentae Acute viral infection Surgical operation, especially on lungs Burns Snake bite: *Ankistrodon rhodostoma* and Russell's viper Heat stroke
Subacute	Retained dead fetus Disseminated carcinoma Acute promyelocytic leukaemia and other acute leukaemias
Chronic	Liver disease, renal disease Eclampsia Giant haemangioma (Kasabach–Merritt syndrome)

veins being involved with consequent local signs and symptoms.

In the chronic forms of DIC the coagulation defect is often very slight, with few clinical symptoms, and may escape detection for many years. Table 23.17 shows some of the commoner conditions that may be associated with DIC.

Once the diagnosis of DIC is suspected on clinical grounds, it is usually easy to confirm, especially in the acute cases. In severe cases the thrombin time is prolonged, fibrinogen concentration is reduced, as are the levels of factor V, factor VIII, prothrombin, and platelets. Fibrin degradation products in serum are increased. The prothrombin time and activated partial thromboplastin time are prolonged and the clots formed are small, fragile, and break up easily.

In the less severe form of DIC, laboratory diagnosis may be difficult. The thrombin clotting time may be only slightly prolonged and fibrinogen and the other coagulation factors reduced only slightly, if at all. In such cases tests for fibrin degradation products should be carried out, or assay of fibrin peptide A which is released into the plasma when fibrinogen is acted on by thrombin.

23.6.4   Further reading

Biggs, R. and Rizza, C. R. (eds) (1984). *Human blood coagulation haemostasis and thrombosis*. Blackwell Scientific Publications, Oxford.

Bloom, A. L. and Thomas, D. P. (eds) (1987). *Haemostasis and thrombosis* (2nd edn). Churchill Livingstone, Edinburgh.

Bowie, E. J. W. and Sharp, A. A. (eds) (1985). *Haemostasis and thrombosis*. Butterworths, London.

Ratnoff, O. D. and Forbes, C. D. (eds) (1984). *Disorders of hemostasis*. Grune and Stratton, Orlando, Florida.

24

Lymphoreticular tissues

24

Lymphoreticular tissues

24.1 Normal structure and function of lymph nodes

P. G. Isaacson

24.1.1 Introduction

The term 'lymphoreticular system' refers to specific solid organs, such as the lymph nodes, spleen, and thymus, or foci within certain non-lymphoid organs, such as the intestinal tract, in which lymphocytes are aggregated in an organized fashion. The organization of the lymphocytes is dependent on the nature of the reticular framework and the distribution of blood vessels and lymphatics. Specific accessory cells, most of which are part of the mononuclear phagocyte system, are an integral component of the lymphoreticular system. The principal organs of the lymphoreticular system are the lymph nodes, spleen, gut-associated lymphoid tissue (GALT), thymus, and bone marrow. Disorders of the bone marrow have already been covered in Chapter 23, and this chapter will address itself principally to the pathology of the lymph nodes together with that of the spleen, thymus gland, and GALT. An understanding of the lymphoreticular system and its disorders is naturally dependent on knowledge of the properties of its constituent cells, and the reader is referred to Chapter 4 where these are discussed in detail.

24.1.2 The normal lymph node

General concepts and overall structure

The lymph nodes are situated at intervals along the lymphatics throughout the body, with well recognized concentrations at certain sites, such as the cervical region, axillae, groin, etc. Their position is in accordance with their function as a major part of the body's defences. Thus, the nodes serve to filter the lymph draining from a wide area and, in particular, to remove any micro-organisms which may be present. This function is accomplished by the resident mononuclear phagocytes and is an important factor in limiting the spread of infection. In the same way, lymph nodes are strategically placed to perform the function of immune surveillance. As antigens enter the node they encounter accessory cells, which process and 'present' them to a large concentration of lymphocytes (the effector cells). This, together with the fact that the lymphocytes are constantly recirculating, helps greatly to increase the chances of a lymphocyte encountering its specific antigen within a lymph node. Such encounters result in increased traffic of lymphocytes to the lymph node concerned and also in lymphocyte proliferation within the node; both these factors cause lymph node enlargement (lymphadenopathy) and characteristic histopathological changes.

In order to understand the histological and cytological features of the various diseases of the lymphoreticular system it is essential to be familiar with the histology of the normal lymph node. For this purpose it is preferable to study the reactive lymph node, which is not strictly normal, since it is only in this sort of node that all the cell types and structures that characterize lymphoproliferative disorders are represented. The overall structure of lymph nodes is shown diagrammatically in Fig. 24.1. The lymph node is surrounded by a thin fibrous capsule from which fibrous trabeculae penetrate the parenchyma, forming an extracellular matrix of collagen fibres. This matrix is probably an important factor in assisting the directional movement of lymphocytes and other cells within the node. The fibrous capsule is penetrated by afferent lymphatics which communicate with the marginal sinus. From the marginal sinus cortical sinuses branch off into the node as an arborizing network before being gathered into the large medullary sinuses, which in turn enter the single efferent lymphatic vessel. The sinuses are lined by specialized endothelial cells, which are phagocytic, and are traversed by fine collagen bands which are also covered by these cells. Large numbers of phagocytic macrophages are present within the sinuses and these reinforce the filtering function of the lymph node sinuses. The blood supply of the lymph node is usually via a single artery, which enters the node at the hilum, forming an arcade of smaller vessels before dividing into arterioles which then supply the rich capillary network permeating throughout the node. The capillaries drain into the highly characteristic post-capillary venules, also called

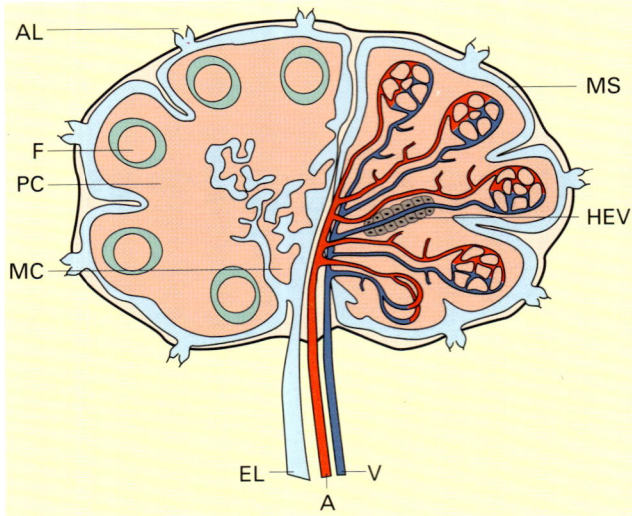

Fig. 24.1 Diagrammatic representation of a lymph node. Lymph enters the node through the afferent lymphatics (AL) which enter the marginal sinus (MS). The sinuses then arborize throughout the node and collect together between the medullary cords (MC) leaving the node at the efferent lymphatic (EL). The B-cell areas of the node comprise the follicle (F) and the medullary cords (MC) which contain a high proportion of plasma cells. The T-cell area consists of the paracortex (PC). Lymphocytes enter the node through the artery (A) which breaks up into capillaries supplying the paracortex and the follicles. The post-capillary venules then coaslesce to form the high endothelial venules (HEV) in the paracortex and it is here that lymphocytes leave the bloodstream, enter the node and home to their respective area. Lymphocytes leave the node via the efferent lymphatic (EL). The venules then collect together to leave the node through the main vein (V).

high endothelial venules after their plump tall endothelium. These specialized blood vessels, which play an important role in lymphocyte traffic, lose their high endothelium as they enter larger veins in the lymph node medulla, which in turn fuse together at the hilum of the node. The different cells that comprise lymphoid tissue are conveniently descibed in three groups which, to a certain extent, are situated in different regions of the lymph node. These are the B-cells, T-cells, and accessory cells.

Most of the lymph node B-cells are present in the cortex, where they are concentrated in follicles (Fig. 24.2). In unstimulated or resting lymph nodes, the follicles, known as primary follicles, are inconspicuous and consist simply of aggregates of small lymphocytes without a centre. In reactive nodes, however, the follicles, known as secondary follicles, are prominent structures consisting of a zone of small lymphocytes, known as the mantle zone, partially surrounding the follicle centre at its capsular aspect, and a follicle centre (Fig. 24.3). The follicle centre is populated principally by two types of cell, the centroblast and centrocyte (Fig. 24.4). Centroblasts are large cells with a small rim of cytoplasm surrounding a round nucleus. The nucleus is characterized by evenly staining chromatin and usually contains two or more nucleoli which are in apposition to the nuclear membrane. Centroblasts are actively dividing

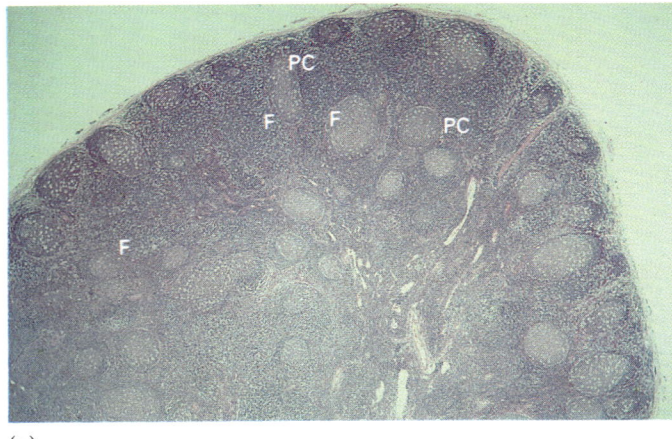

(a)

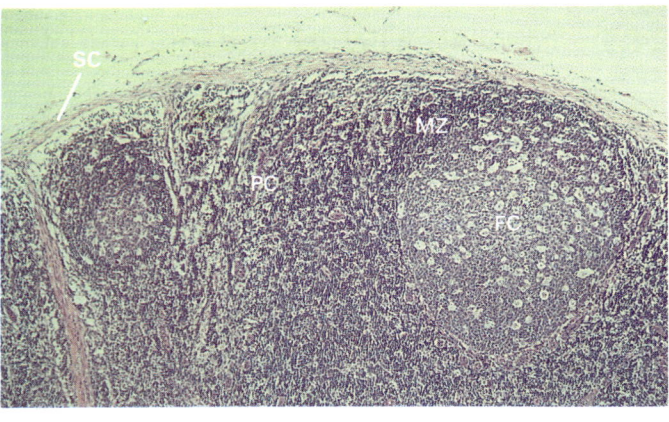

(b)

Fig. 24.2 (a) A lower power photomicrograph of a lymph node showing follicles (F) and intervening paracortex (PC). The medullary chords (MC) are outlined by dilated sinuses. (b) Higher power photomicrograph of lymph node showing follicles, consisting of a follicle centre (FC) and mantle zone (MZ). Large venules can be seen within the paracortex (PC), and the subcapsular sinus (SC) is clearly seen.

cells, as shown by the presence of mitotic figures, and tend to be grouped together at the pole of the follicle furthest from the capsule. Centrocytes are smaller than centroblasts and contain irregularly shaped nuclei with coarse chromatin and inconspicuous nucleoli; their cytoplasm is ill-defined. Macrophages are a conspicuous component of follicle centres and characteristically contain phagocytosed nuclear debris. The follicle centre also contains a population of cells known as dendritic reticulum cells (follicular dendritic cells). These cells can hardly be seen with the light microscope unless special techniques are used, but can be easily identified in electron micrographs. The nucleus and cytoplasm of dendritic reticulum cells are small and inconspicuous, but what distinguishes these cells is the interlacing network formed by their fine processes. The possible origins and the function of these interesting cells, as well as techniques of demonstrating them in histological sections, will be described later. Scattered B-cells are found outside follicles,

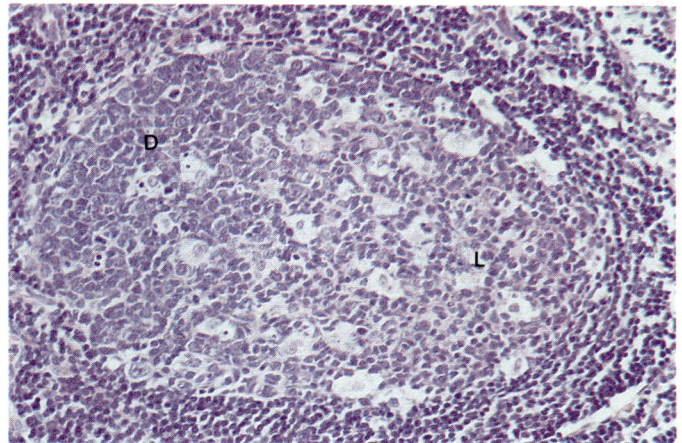

Fig. 24.3 Detail of follicle showing the dark zone (D) consisting principally of centroblasts, and the light zone (L), consisting principally of centrocytes. Macrophages with clear cytoplasm, some of which contain nuclear debris, are scattered through the follicle centre. These are the so-called tingible body macrophages.

presumably as part of the trafficking population, but the other site where cells of B lineage concentrate is in the medulla of the node. Here the medullary chords contain large numbers of plasma cells, which are the immunoglobulin-secreting B-cells (Fig. 24.5).

The lymphoid tissue between the B-cell follicles and impinging on the medulla is known as the paracortex (Fig. 24.6) and it is here that the T-cells are found. These T-cells are not cytologically distinctive, appearing simply as small lymphocytes. The paracortex is distinguished by the presence of high endothelial venules (Fig. 24.6) from which both B- and T-lymphocytes leave the blood after adhering to specific molecules on the specialized endothelium. Larger transformed (or blast) cells, which may be either B- or T-cell derived, can be seen in the paracortex. Also present in the paracortex is a population of specialized macrophages known as interdigitating reticulum cells (Fig. 24.7). These cells have pale vesicular nuclei, which are often rather tortuously shaped, and abundant pale-staining cytoplasm. As their name implies, interdigitating reticulum cells 'interdigitate' with each other and the T-lymphocytes around them via long delicate processes.

The non-lymphoid cells in lymph nodes are known as accessory cells. Many of these are part of the mononuclear phagocyte system, including sinus macrophages (Fig. 24.8) and the 'tingible body' macrophages in follicle centres, named for the phagocytosed nuclear fragments within their cytoplasm. Together with their phagocytic function, these cells participate in the immune response as described in Chapter 4. Interdigitating reticulum cells are also a part of the mononuclear phagocyte system, but their main role appears to be one of antigen presentation to surrounding T-cells. There is no agreement about the origin of dendritic reticulum cells (follicular dendritic cells), although some workers believe that these, too, are bone-marrow derived. Their processes are heavily coated with antigen–antibody complexes and, in forming a dense network

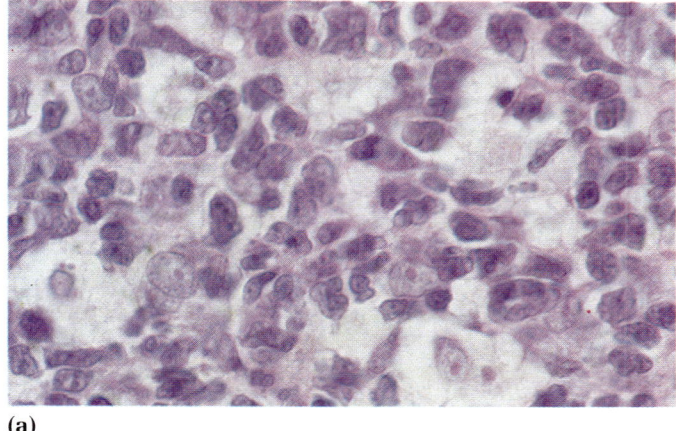

(a)

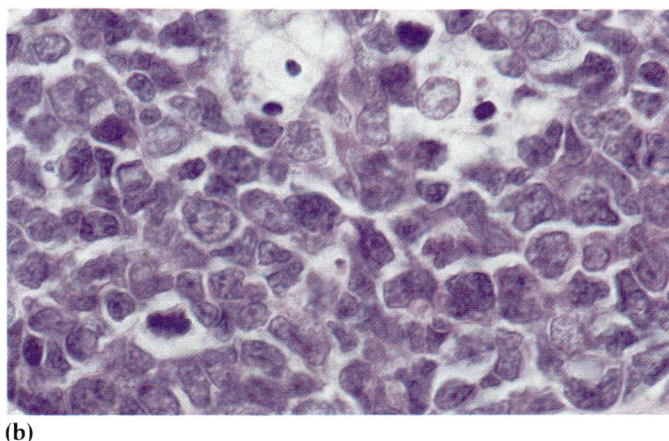

(b)

Fig. 24.4 (a) Detail of the light zone of a follicle centre showing the irregular (cleaved) outline of the nuclei of centrocytes. Larger pale nuclei are those of tingible body macrophages. (b) Detail of the dark zone showing the regular contour of centroblast nuclei in which nucleoli can be seen sometimes apposed to the nuclear membrane.

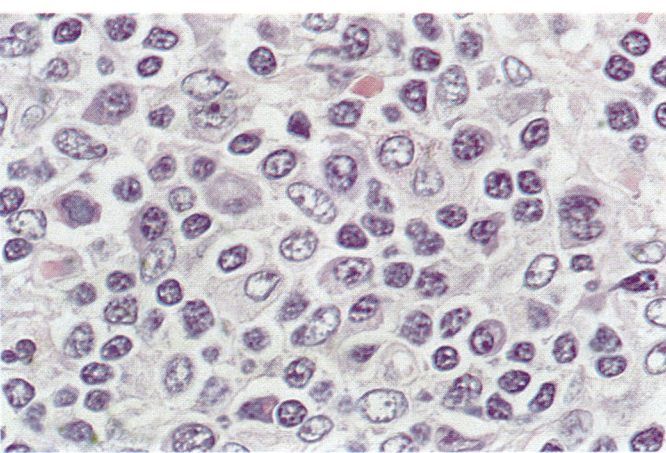

Fig. 24.5 Detail of medullary cords showing numerous plasma cells.

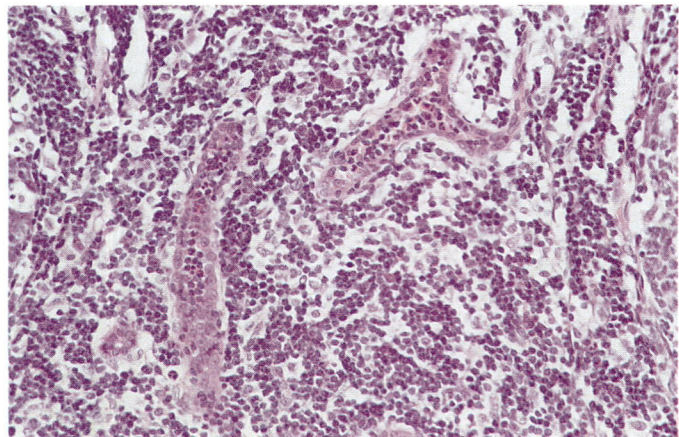

Fig. 24.6 Paracortex showing small lymphocytes, larger cells with pale cytoplasm, and prominent high endothelial venules filled with lymphocytes and other cells.

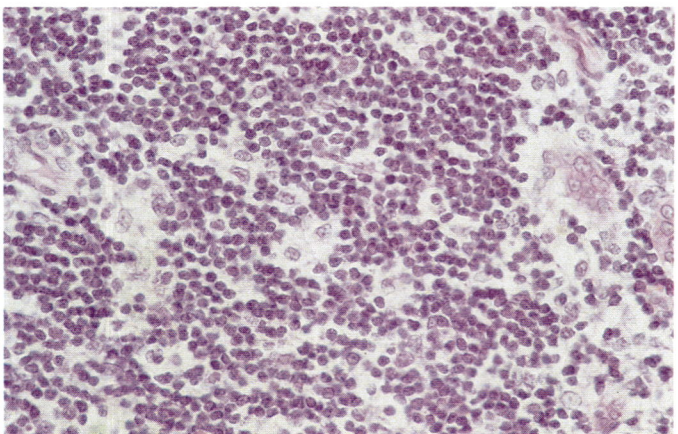

Fig. 24.7 Detail of the paracortex showing interdigitating reticulum cells with clear cytoplasm and irregularly shaped nuclei scattered amongst small lymphocytes. High endothelial venules are seen to the right.

amidst the B-cells of the follicle centre, it would appear that dendritic reticulum cells are concerned with presentation of antigen to B-cells. Other accessory cells in lymph nodes include those of the granulocyte series, mast cells, and natural killer cells.

Immunocytochemistry of lymph nodes

Our knowledge of the different cell types in lymphoid tissue has been greatly enhanced by newly developed techniques whereby the phenotype of morphologically similar cells can be discriminated using monoclonal antibodies that react with distinctive molecules on the cell membrane or in the cytoplasm. This is accomplished by conjugating the antibodies to a label that can be rendered visible under either normal or ultraviolet light (see Appendix 5 for details of the technique).

These techniques are particularly valuable in the analysis of

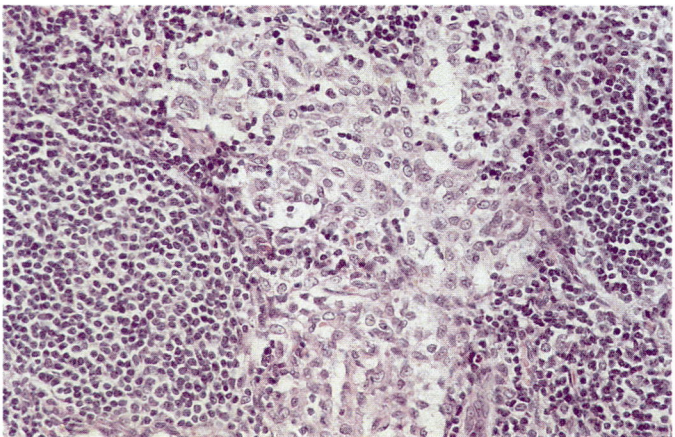

Fig. 24.8 A lymph node sinus containing sinus macrophages.

lymphoproliferative diseases where architectural landmarks such as follicles may be lost. Many antibodies are now available that recognize antigenic determinants specific for the different lymphoid cells described above. Indeed, so many of these antibodies have been reproduced that it has become necessary to convene special international meetings, or 'workshops', for the specific purpose of grouping closely similar antibodies together; as a result of these workshops an international classification of antibodies that recognize lymphoreticular cells has been formulated. Each group (or 'cluster') of antibodies that recognizes the same antigen indicative of a certain type of cell differentiation receives a number. Hence, for example, the designation CD3 (cluster of differentiation 3) has been agreed for all those antibodies that recognize a certain T-cell receptor molecule present on almost all T-cells. There are to date more than 70 recognized clusters. Not all antibodies in common use have necessarily been clustered, and until sufficient numbers of other antibodies with similar specificity are produced, they retain their proprietary names. As well as antibodies that recognize molecules that are an integral part of the cell, antibodies to the different types of immunoglobulin secreted by B-cells are particularly useful in the study of lymphoreticular tissue. A list of some of the most commonly used antibodies and their specificities is given in Table 24.1.

Table 24.1   Antibodies in common use for immunocytochemistry of lymphoreticular tissues

Antibody	Specificity
CD1	Early 'thymic' T-cells
CD2	T-cells
CD3	T-cells
CD4	T-helper cells
CD5	T-cells and some B-cells
CD8	T-suppressor/cytotoxic cells
CD20	B-cells
CD45	Leucocyte common antigen
Anti-immunoglobulins	α, γ, and μ heavy chains
	κ and λ light chains

Using antibodies that recognize all B-cells (pan B antibodies) and all T-cells (pan T antibodies) the detailed distribution of these cells in the normal lymph node can be mapped (Fig. 24.9). The B- and T-cell populations can then be further subdivided with appropriate antibodies. The B-cells of the follicular mantle, for example, express both immunoglobulin (Ig) M and IgD, and in this way they differ from follicle centre B-cells, which express only IgM. The Ig expressed by each B-cell is of either κ or λ light chain isotype and thus mixed, or polytypic, light chain expression by a population of B-cells is indicative of polyclonal proliferation. B-cell neoplasms, on the other hand, are, by definition, monoclonal and therefore express only one type of light chain, a property known as light chain restriction. The different subsets of T-cells can also be recognized with appropriate antibodies, but it is important to bear in mind that the expression of T-cell subset antigens does not have the same meaning with regard to clonality as that of κ and λ light chains by B-cells. The accessory cells in lymphoid tissue can also be

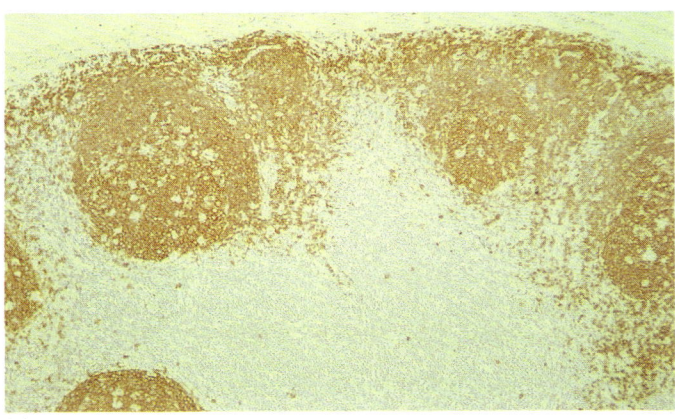

(a)

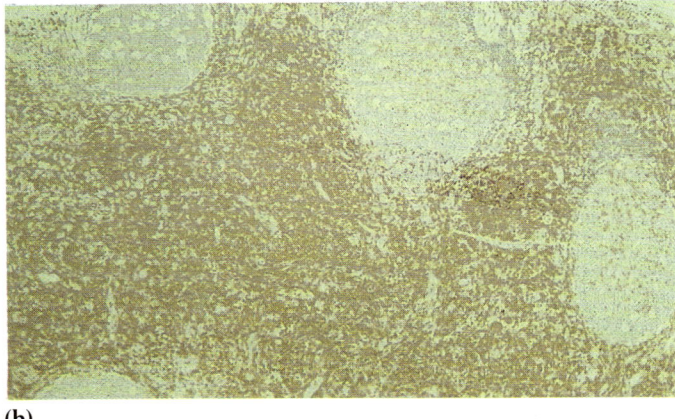

(b)

Fig. 24.9 Lymph node stained with the immunoperoxidase method using (a) antibody to B-cells and (b) antibody to T-cells. Positive staining is brown and the counterstain is blue. The B-cell antibody outlines the follicles and occasional cells beyond them. The T-cell antibody stains the paracortex heavily but scattered cells within the follicles are also marking as T-cells.

distinguished using immunocytochemistry. The striking dendritic reticulum cell network is especially well shown in this way (Fig. 24.10) and the presence of immunoglobulin on the cell processes forming this network can be confirmed. Macrophages and interdigitating reticulum cells are equally demonstrable (Fig. 24.11).

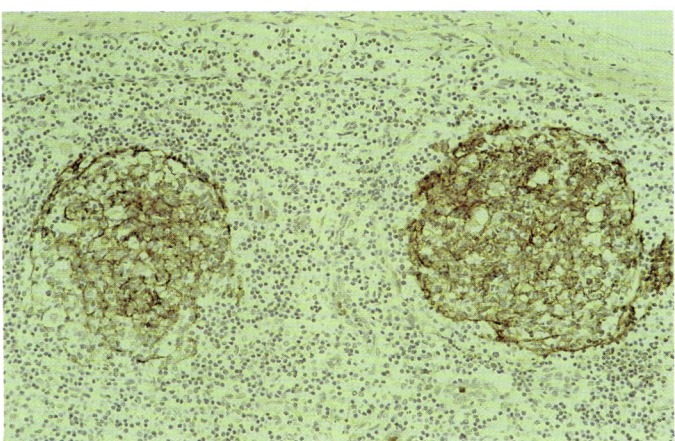

Fig. 24.10 Lymph node stained with an antibody to dendritic reticulum cells. The dense network of these cells and their processes can be seen filling the follicle centres.

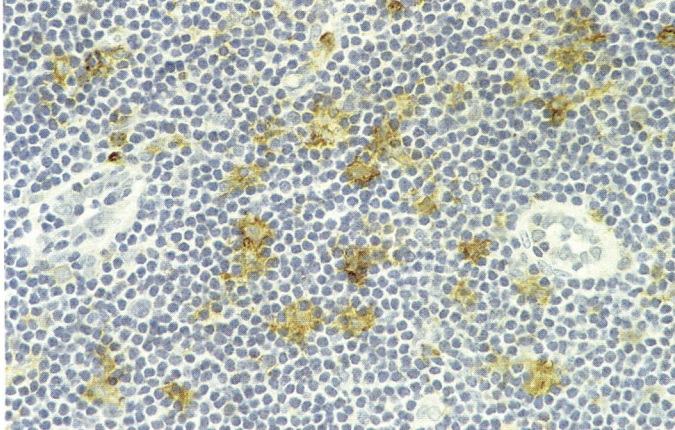

Fig. 24.11 The paracortex of a lymph node stained with an antibody that recognizes interdigitating reticulum cells. Amidst the background of small lymphocytes (T-cells) and high endothelial venules the interdigitating reticulum cells with their complex processes can be seen.

24.1.3 The relation of lymph node structure to function

Given the intimate relationship that exists in lymph nodes between lymphatic sinuses carrying antigens, accessory cells capable of presenting the antigens, and lymphocytes whose function it is to respond to antigens, it is quite clear that the reason for the complexity of the structure of lymph nodes is to ensure effective immune responses to the antigens delivered to them. The interrelated functions of lymphoreticular cells are, however, sufficiently complex that it is impossible to establish with certainty the precise pathways that lead to the formation of antibody-producing B-cells and immunocompetent T-cells. For this reason, too, the mechanism of follicle-centre formation and the exact function of these structures remains poorly understood; nevertheless, there is a wealth of experimental data from which it is worth attempting to construct an outline of the functional and structural changes that occur in lymph nodes exposed to antigen.

Antigen arrives at a lymph node in the afferent lymphatics and, in the process of diffusing through the sinuses and across their walls into the parenchyma, is modified by macrophages and sinusoidal endothelium. The antigen then encounters B- and T-lymphocytes which are constantly recirculating through the node, entering it across the high endothelium of the post-capillary venules and leaving via the efferent lymphatics. There appear to be specific receptors on the high endothelium to which lymphocytes bind, together with mechanisms for guiding them between the endothelial cells into the lymph node parenchyma. Differences in the receptors may be responsible for the selection of different lymphocyte populations depending on the particular anatomical site of the lymph node. Antigen-presenting cells, including interdigitating reticulum cells, then co-operate with lymphocytes that have entered the node and these undergo transformation into large nucleolated cells (blasts) which are capable of further division into immuno-logically effective T-cells, antibody-secreting plasma cells, or memory cells of either T- or B-cell lineage. When secreted antibody encounters more antigen, the resulting antigen–antibody complexes are trapped by dendritic reticulum cells within primary B-cell follicles. These complexes are highly immunogenic and result in transformation of the B-cells with the formation of the follicle centres which characterize secondary follicles. These B-cells are rapidly dividing and leave the follicle either as plasma cell precursors, or memory cells. In this rapidly dividing population many cells die and it is their remnants that are phago-cytosed by the intrafollicular (tingible body) macrophages. Exposure of a lymph node to antigens which react with T-cells (most viruses, for example) result in paracortical hyperplasia, while antigens to which B-cells are sensitive (pyogenic bacteria, for example) cause follicular hyperplasia. A lymph node drain-ing a site of infection is usually exposed to many antigens and will therefore show generalized hyperplasia.

24.1.4   Laboratory methods for studying lymph node diseases

The diagnosis of lymph node disorders is highly dependent on the histopathology laboratory and the availability of an increas-ing number of special techniques. While by no means all of these techniques are a part of routine practice, it is important to be familiar with their application in order to understand the scientific basis of modern lymphoreticular pathology. Lymph nodes should be carefully excised by an experienced surgeon and submitted fresh to the laboratory with as little delay as possible. The following techniques are then applicable.

Routine histology This remains the mainstay of the diagnosis of lymphoreticular disease. One or more 2–3 mm blocks are taken across the equator of the node and placed in fixative for an optimum period. The nature of the fixative varies from labora-tory to laboratory. After routine processing and embedding in wax 3–4 μm sections are cut and stained with haematoxylin and eosin. A variety of special stains can then be applied as required. To an increasing extent, immunohistochemical tech-niques can be performed on routinely processed tissue.

Electron microscopy Small (1 mm cubes) fragments of the node are placed in an appropriate fixative. After special processing and embedding in resin 'thick' (1 μm) sections are cut from which selection is made for cutting 'thin' (60 nm) sections. These are placed on minute metal grids and viewed with the electron microscope. Photographs (electron micrographs) form the permanent record.

Touch preparations The cut surface of the lymph node is lightly touched on a glass slide or several slides. This type of prep-aration is suitable for studying detailed cytology and for per-forming histochemical techniques.

Cell suspension A small fragment of the node is gently teased apart into tissue culture fluid. These cells can be separated in different ways, for example according to their density, and used for phenotypic studies, or to establish short- or long-term cul-tures, either of which is suitable for performing chromosome analysis (karyotyping).

Freezing Blocks of the node are snap frozen, usually in liquid nitrogen. Frozen sections prepared from this tissue are used for immunohistochemistry. Frozen tissue is also used for the extraction of DNA suitable for genotypic studies using Southern blot analysis.

DNA analysis A number of molecular biological techniques are now frequently, if not routinely, employed in the assessment of cases of non-Hodgkin's lymphoma. The most important of these, the technique of Southern blotting, can be used to detect clonal populations of B- or T-cells when the histological and immunohistochemical results are in doubt. DNA is extracted from the frozen tissue and digested with specific restriction enzymes. The resulting fragments are electrophoresed and then 'blotted' on to nylon membranes. The membrane is then 'probed' using radiolabelled probes to known segments of the immunoglobulin or T-cell receptor genes. An autoradiograph is then prepared on X-ray film. Following the arguments set out in Chapter 4, the probe will always recognize the germline genes in accompanying non-lymphoid tissue and this will appear as a dense band on the blot (Fig. 24.12). Since each lymphocyte has differently rearranged genes with different molecular weights, the result of probing will be a continuous, light, hardly detect-able smear. If, however, a significant number of cells have iden-tically rearranged genes (i.e. a clone is present) an additional

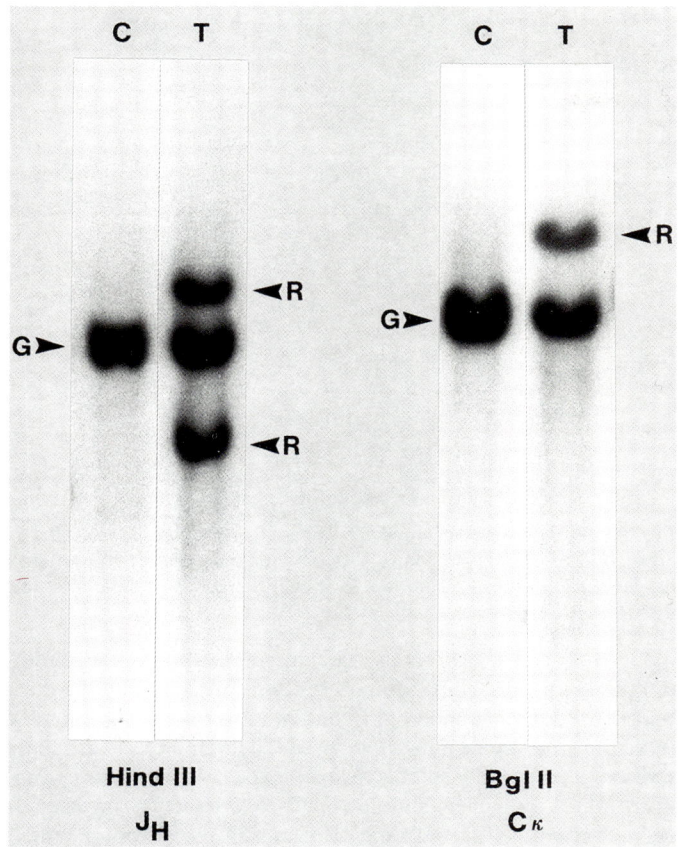

C T   C T

G ▶   ◀R

◀R

G ▶

◀R

Hind III   **Bgl II**

J$_H$ Cκ

Fig. 24.12 Southern blots prepared from placental (C) and lymphoma (T) DNA which has been digested with the restriction enzymes *Hind*III and *Bgl*II. The *Hind*III digest has been probed for J$_H$ rearrangement, while the *Bgl*II digest has been probed for C$_\kappa$ rearrangement. Placental (C) DNA reveals the germline band only (G), while the tumour DNA reveals both germline and clonal rearrangement of J$_H$ and C$_\kappa$ genes. The rearranged genes appear as additional bands (R).

an additional band or bands will appear on the autoradiograph of the Southern blot (Fig. 24.12).

24.1.5 General features of lymph node disorders

With the exception of some of the immunodeficiencies, which are fully discussed in Chapter 4, pathological lymph nodes are enlarged. Hence the term 'lymphadenopathy' which, in referring to an enlarged lymph node or group of nodes, is the commonest physical sign of lymph node disease. Lymphadenopathy always requires an explanation. It may be caused simply by reaction to an immune stimulus, and in those circumstances the pathology must be sought in the area drained by that particular node. Other non-neoplastic conditions may be responsible for lymphadenopathy or the lymph node enlargement may be due to secondary spread of a neoplasm. Finally, neoplastic proliferation lymphoreticular cells themselves may be the cause of lymphadenopathy; this is known as malignant lymphoma.

24.1.6 Further reading

Griesser, H., Tkachuk, D., Reis, M. D., and Mak, T. W. (1989). Gene rearrangements and translocations in lymphoproliferative diseases. *Blood* **73**, 1402–15.

Knapp, W., Dörken, B., Gilks, W. R., Rieber, E. P., Schmidt, R. E., Stein, H., and von dem Borne, A. E. G. (eds) (1989). *Leucocyte typing IV—white cell differentiation antigens*. Oxford University Press.

Nieuwenius, P. and Lennert, K. (1980). Histopathology of normal lymphoid tissue and the immune reactions. In *Malignant proliferative disease* (ed. J. G. van der Tweel), pp. 3–12. Leiden University Press, The Hague.

Norton, A. J. and Isaacson, P. G. (1989). Lymphoma phenotyping in formalin-fixed and paraffin wax-embedded tissues. I. Range of antibodies and staining patterns. *Histopathology* **14**, 437–46.

Norton, A. J. and Isaacson, P. G. (1989). Lymphoma phenotyping in formalin-fixed and paraffin wax-embedded tissues. II. Profiles of reactivity in the various tumour types. *Histopathology* **14**, 557–79.

Southern, E. M. (1975). Detection of specific sequences among DNA fragments separated by gel electrophoresis. *Journal of Molecular Biology* **98**, 503.

Stansfeld, A. G. (ed.). (1985). *Lymph node biopsy interpretation*. Churchill Livingstone, London.

Stein, H., Bonk, A., Tolksdorf, G., Lennert, K., Rodt, H., and Gerdes, J. (1980). Immunohistologic analysis of the organisation of normal lymphoid tissue and non-Hodgkin's lymphomas. *Histochemistry and Cytochemistry* **28**, 746.

24.2 Normal structure and function of the mucosa-associated lymphoid tissue (MALT)

Jo Spencer and P. G. Isaacson

24.2.1 Introduction

The anatomical site and histological structure of lymph nodes are adapted to deal with antigens carried to the node in the afferent lymphatics which drain sites at various distances from the node. However, the vulnerability of mucosal surfaces, such as the gastrointestinal tract and the respiratory tract, which are frequently in contact with external antigens is such that specialized lymphoid tissue has evolved to protect these sites. This is known as mucosa-associated lymphoid tissue (MALT), and is found in the gastrointestinal tract, bronchi, and in smaller quantities in other mucosae.

There is some evidence that the mucosae are united as a common mucosal immune system. They share a system of immunoglobulin transport to the luminal surface, so that immunoglobulins synthesized in one mucosal site may be secreted at another, thus transferring specific immunity to mucosal pathogens. It has also been suggested that the mucosae share a common pool of lymphocytes which preferentially migrate between the mucosae rather than through peripheral somatic lymphoid tissue, but evidence for this is incomplete. Quantitatively, gut-associated lymphoid tissue (GALT) is the most significant component of MALT and it has therefore been characterized most thoroughly. It is assumed that other components of MALT share the same basic features.

The gastrointestinal tract is in direct communication with the external environment and its surface lining has the specific function of absorbing constituents of the environment (food) into the body. Clearly, there must be mechanisms to exclude unwanted factors in the environment, especially harmful micro-organisms. While non-specific mechanisms, such as gastric acidity, are helpful, the principal protection is provided by GALT. GALT is composed of three lymphoid compartments, which have no direct equivalent outside the mucosae. These are:

1. Peyer's patches in the small intestine, and similarly organized lymphoid tissue in the colon;

2. mucosal lamina propria;

3. lymphocytes within the gut epithelium (intra-epithelial lymphocytes).

The interrelationships between the compartments of GALT have been studied extensively in experimental animals; however, it is not clear how the mucosal immune system in man relates to the animal models. The application of immunohistochemistry in recent years has advanced our knowledge of the microanatomy and cell types in human GALT and has allowed comparison with similar studies in laboratory animals.

24.2.2   Histology and immunology of GALT

Peyer's patches

Peyer's patches are organized lymphoid structures concentrated in the ileal mucosa. In man they are macroscopically visible from the luminal side only in individuals up to around 14 years of age, after which they atrophy. Peyer's patch cells are easy to isolate from experimental animals, therefore, most of the information on the function of Peyer's patch has come from animal studies, but, as will be emphasized later, fundamental special differences exist. Results derived from animal experiments should not therefore be uncritically extrapolated to man.

Peyer's patches are unencapsulated clusters of lymphoid cells which bear a certain resemblance to lymph nodes (Fig. 24.13). In the human adult, each Peyer's patch follicle consists of a B-cell follicle centre containing, as in the lymph node, morphologically diverse cells, including large centroblasts with ovoid, euchromatic nuclei and nucleoli on the nuclear membrane, and centrocytes with smaller, cleaved, heterochromatic nuclei. Tingible body macrophages with engulfed particulate material in their cytoplasm are also often present. The follicle centre is surrounded by a mantle of small B-lymphocytes, which is broadest on the mucosal aspect of the follicle. A population of marginal zone B-cells, which morphologically resemble the centrocytes in the follicle centre, surround the mantle zone. The marginal zone extends towards the mucosa and some of the cells characteristically infiltrate the Peyer's patch dome epithelium as intra-epithelial B-lymphocytes. The follicle-

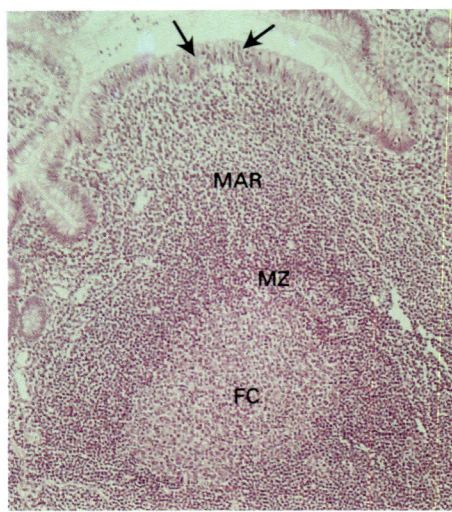

Fig. 24.13   Histology of Peyer's patches showing two B-cell follicles consisting of the follicle centre (FC), mantle zone (MZ), and a broad marginal zone (MAR). Marginal-zone cells can just be seen infiltrating the dome epithelium (arrows).

associated epithelium is a specialized structure containing microfold cells (M-cells) which are thought to sample the contents of the gut. Sampled gut contents are thought to interact with the underlying lymphoid tissue. The ability of antigenic molecules, especially soluble antigens, to cross the villus epithelium intact, however, should not be overlooked. The zone of cells containing the high endothelial venules through which lymphoid cells traffic, which is equivalent to the paracortical T-cell zone of the lymph node, is situated on the serosal aspect of the B-cell follicle lateral to the B-cell area, often abutting the muscularis mucosae (Fig. 24.14).

Human Peyer's patches have recently been studied using immunohistochemistry. It has been shown that the follicle centre, as in lymph nodes, contains follicular dendritic cells with a network of immunoglobulin of all isotypes except IgD on their surface. Cytoplasmic immunoglobulin is present in some

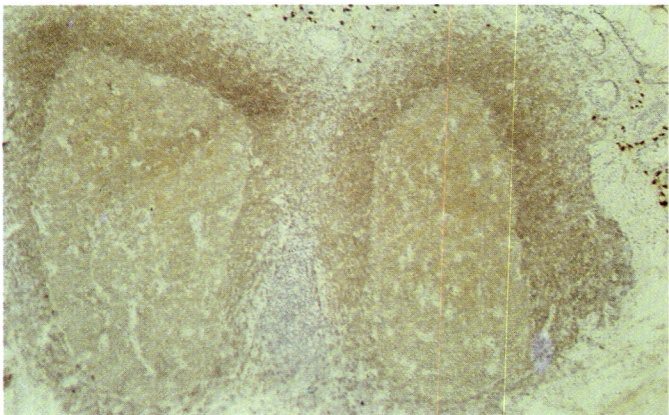

Fig. 24.14   Peyer's patch containing two B-cell follicles stained with a monoclonal antibody to B-cells. The antibody stains the follicle centre, mantle, and marginal zone, leaving the intervening T-cell area.

centrocytes within the follicle centre, but the number of cells and the isotype they express, varies between individual follicles. The follicle centre is surrounded by a mantle zone of small B-cells which express surface IgM and IgD. The marginal zone B-cells that surround the mantle zone are IgD-ve expressing either surface IgM or IgA1, and in other ways are phenotypically distinct from both follicle-centre B-cells and mantle-zone B-cells. Cells which are morphologically and phenotypically identical to the Peyer's patch marginal zone cells are, however, present in the normal splenic marginal zone (see Section 24.7.2).

A few immunoblasts with cytoplasmic immunoglobulin, including IgA, are present in the T-cell zone human Peyer's patches, which contains the high endothelial venules. This observation is significant when considering the migratory route of immunoglobulin-producing B-cells, to be discussed more fully later. B-cells with cytoplasmic immunoglobulin of all isotypes except IgD, some of which have classical plasma-cell morphology, are present in the dome regions of normal human Peyer's patches.

Lamina propria

In the lamina propria there is a diffuse infiltrate of lymphoreticular cells, consisting principally of plasma cells and macrophages. Small B- and T-lymphocytes and polymorphs are also present.

Immunohistochemical studies have shown that human adult lamina propria plasma cells secrete predominantly IgA. In man, IgA exists as two subclasses, IgA1 and IgA2. There is a ratio of 4 : 1 IgA1:IgA2 in the blood. At mucosal surfaces, however, the proportion of IgA2-subclass-secreting plasma cells increases from approximately 20 per cent to 50 per cent of the total IgA-secreting plasma cells. The proportion of IgA1:IgA2 : IgG:IgE: IgM secreting plasma cells in the lamina propria is approximately 10 : 10 : 3 : 3 : 2. IgA is secreted in dimeric form. In dimeric IgA the two IgA molecules are linked by a joining (J) chain. The proportion of IgA-dimer-secreting plasma cells increases from 30 per cent in non-mucosal to 65 per cent in mucosal sites. The J chain of IgA binds to the glycoprotein secretory component (SC) that is expressed on enterocytes. This IgA–J chain–SC complex is actively transported in vesicles, across the enterocytes, into the lumen of the gut (see Fig. 24.15). The increased amount of dimer produced in the lamina propria is, therefore, of obvious functional significance, considering that only dimeric IgA can bind to SC on the enterocytes prior to being transported into the lumen. This IgA probably functions by agglutinating and thus excluding antigenic particles (immune exclusion). SC has an affinity for mucus, which would aid the process of antigen agglutination and expulsion. IgA is adapted to function in an acellular environment; it does not opsonize antigen and it does not fix complement.

Intra-epithelial lymphocytes

Intra-epithelial T-lymphocytes are found between the epithelial cells throughout the small and large intestine. In adult gut,

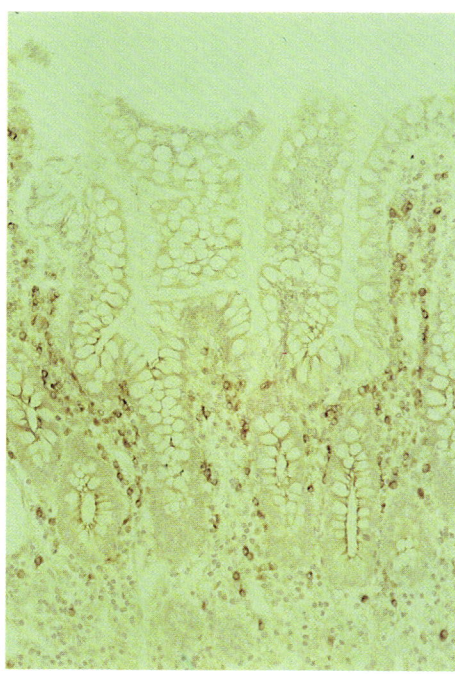

Fig. 24.15 Lamina propria of small intestine stained by the immunoperoxidase method with an antibody to IgA. IgA-containing plasma cells are seen throughout the lamina propria. The IgA secreted by these cells becomes attached to secretory component, produced by epithelial cells, and the secretory component–IgA complex is transported across the epithelial cells and is seen staining positively as an apical lining, most marked in the intestinal crypts.

intra-epithelial lymphocytes are most concentrated in the small intestine, where there are approximately 20 intra-epithelial lymphocytes/100 epithelial cells in the jejunum and 13/100 epithelial cells in the ileum. They are small, round cells with heterochromatic nuclei and are found generally adjacent to the basement membrane in the bottom two-thirds of the total epithelial height. These intra-epithelial T-cells must be distinguished from the population of intra-epithelial B-cells that is restricted to the dome epithelium of Peyer's patches (see p. 1752).

It has been shown, using immunohistochemistry, that intra-epithelial lymphocytes throughout the villi and crypts of the large and small intestine almost all express the CD3 and CD8 antigens. The majority are distinct from peripheral blood T-cells in that they do not express the CD5 antigen. The predominance of the CD8+ phenotype is in contrast with the 4 : 1 ratio of CD4+ :CD8+ T-cells in the lamina propria (Fig. 24.16). Monoclonal antibodies have been raised against human intra-epithelial lymphocytes. These antibodies recognize the majority of intra-epithelial lymphocytes, approximately 50 per cent of lamina propria lymphocytes, but stain very few T-cells outside the gut. This is direct evidence supporting the existence of a mucosal T-cell population different to that in peripheral tissue.

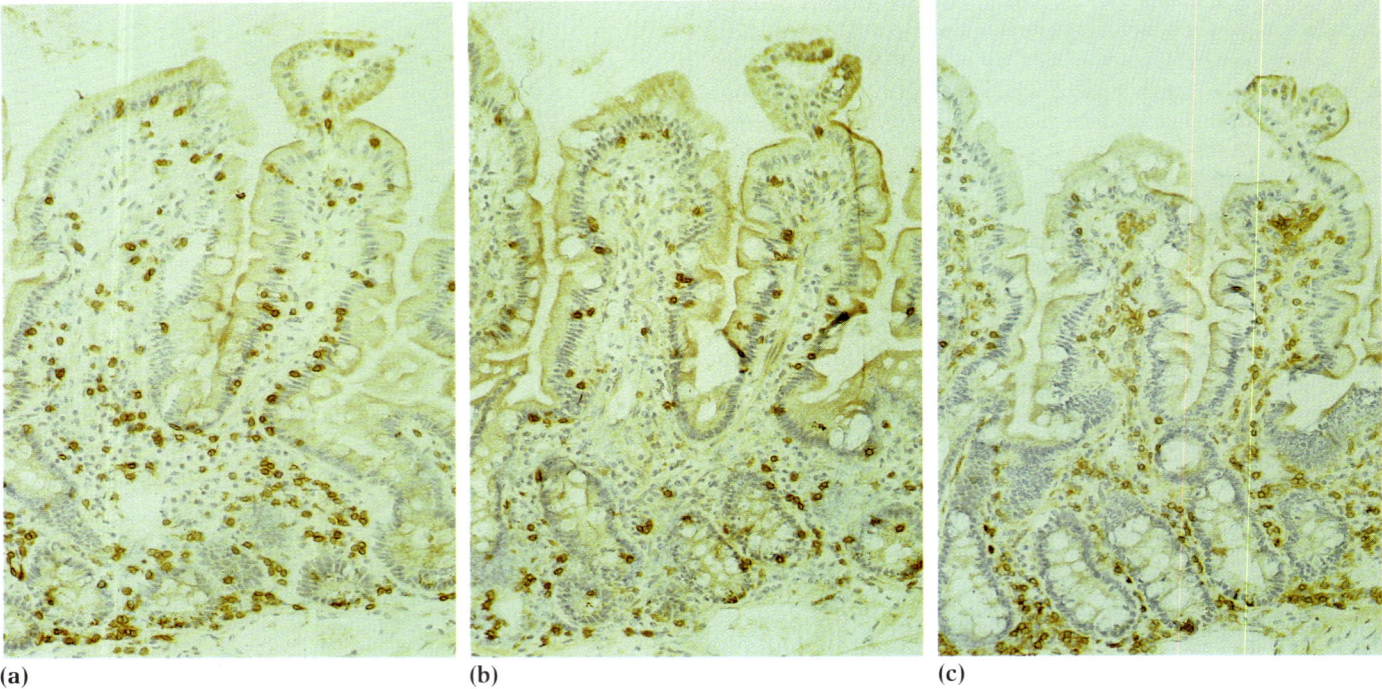

(a)   (b)   (c)

Fig. 24.16 The small intestinal mucosa stained with monoclonal antibodies: (a) CD3, (b) CD8, and (c) CD4. Mucosal T-cells, many of which are in an intra-epithelial position, are CD3-positive. The antibody CD8 selectively stains intra-epithelial lymphocytes, few of which stain with antibody CD4.

24.2.3   Function of normal human GALT

In 1968 Ogra and co-workers were the first to demonstrate antigen-specific IgA in intestinal fluid in the absence of specific serum IgA antibodies in man. The bulk of recent research into functional aspects of mucosal immunity has, however, been in experimental animals, usually rats, rabbits, or sheep. It is important to be aware of differences between species, especially when directly comparable experiments are not possible and when considering the results in the context of human mucosal immunity.

Peyer's patches; a source of IgA plasma cells

In 1964, Gowans and Knight showed that dividing cells from thoracic duct lymph, which is composed largely of lymph from the gut, are able to localize in the lamina propria of the gut after radiolabelling and intravenous injection into syngeneic recipient rats. It was then shown that labelled dividing cells taken either from the thoracic duct or the mesenteric lymph nodes of rats, or the intestinal lymph of sheep, localized in the gut and differentiated into IgA-producing plasma cells in the lamina propria. Activated B-cells derived from GALT migrate to the blood via the local lymphatics, mesenteric lymph nodes, and the thoracic duct. They then extravasate into the gut and differentiate to produce IgA plasma cells. The cellular events that ultimately lead to the synthesis and secretion of antigen-specific IgA into the gut lumen are represented schematically in Fig. 24.17.

Immunohistochemical studies of rats' Peyer's patches have shown that immunoblasts with cytoplasmic IgA are abundant in the zone of cells containing the high endothelial venules, suggesting that this is an important site of traffic, probably extravasation, of IgA-containing immunoblasts. In addition, radiolabelled dividing cells derived from GALT form a 'halo' around the Peyer's patches approximately 20 hours after intravenous infusion, as well as lodging in other sites in the lamina propria.

Experiments involving the removal of Peyer's patches from the ileum and the use of isolated segments of gut lacking Peyer's patches show that Peyer's patches are not essential for extravasation of immunoblasts into the ileum of rats. The presence of Peyer's patches are a significant, but not the only site of extravasation of immunoblasts into the small intestines of rats. It should be noted that a similar population of immunoblasts, predominantly secreting IgA, cannot be detected around the high endothelial venules of human Peyer's patches.

It has been suggested recently that endothelial molecules, termed vascular addressins, communicate the site of endothelium to lymphocytes expressing appropriate receptors. This putative receptor–ligand system permits tissue-specific extravasation of lymphocytes into certain sites, such as the gut, peripheral lymph nodes, and inflamed joints. Not all of the data from experiments *in vivo* support the existence of such a system. However, this is a rapidly developing area and undoubtedly differences will be resolved in the near future.

There is evidence to suggest that the epithelium may play a

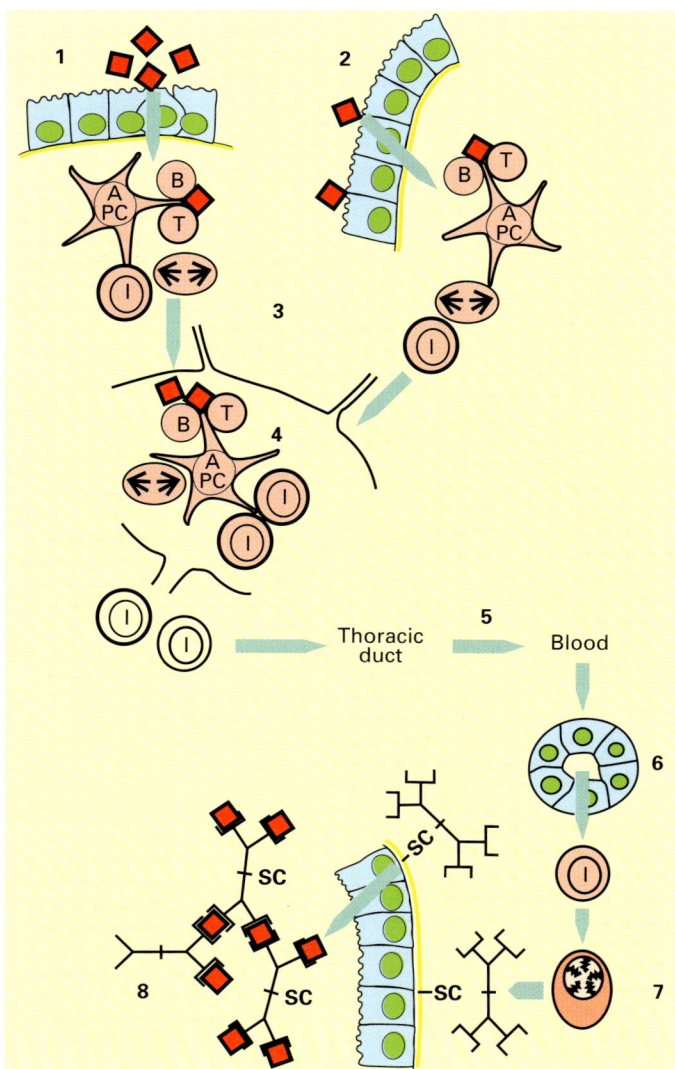

Fig. 24.17 Cellular events leading to the synthesis and secretion of antigen-specific IgA into the gut lumen:

1. Luminal antigen may be sampled by the M-cells in the dome epithelium of the Peyer's patches.
2. Antigen may enter the lamina propria across the villus epithelium.
3. Antigen is presented by the antigen-presenting cells (APC) to the lymphocytes ('B' or 'T' cells) in the Peyer's patches, or the lamina propria, resulting in lymphoid cell division. Dividing cells (immuno-blasts, 'I') and antigen travel via the regional lymphatics to the mesenteric lymph nodes.
4. Further stimulation by antigen and further cell division occur in the mesenteric lymph node. Activated cells acquire the ability to 'home' to the gut.
5. Immunoblasts travel through the intestinal lymphatics, via the thor-acic duct into the blood.
6. Immunoblasts extravasate either through the high endothelial venules, or the capillary network in the villi. Local antigen may stimulate more proliferation.
7. Immunoblasts differentiate into plasma cells, secreting predomin-antly IgA.
8. Dimeric IgA combines with secretory component on the enterocytes and is actively transported into the lumen. Antigen-specific IgA in the lumen then agglutinates the pathogen and it is eliminated from the gut.

role in the retention of GALT-derived cells in the mucosa by the secretion of chemotactic factor. In addition, it has been observed that well-differentiated human carcinomas which express SC are surrounded by a plasma cell infiltrate as in nor-mal gut. However, less-well-differentiated tumours, which do not express SC, do not have an adjacent population of plasma cells. This implies that localization of plasma cells in the lamina propria is dependent upon a function of epithelial cells.

Functional aspects of intra-epithelial lymphocytes

Intra-epithelial T-lymphocytes are the most mysterious lymphoid cell population in the gut. They are unique to mucosal epithelium, have a wide species distribution, and are present in fetal human gut *in utero*, suggesting that they play an important role in the gut immune system, but as yet their func-tion is not known. In the course of a parasitic infection and, most dramatically, in food-induced enteropathies such as coe-

liac disease, intra-epithelial lymphocytes increase in density, i.e. in number per 100 epithelial cells, though not necessarily in total number, because the increase in intra-epithelial cell fre-quency is often accompanied by villus atrophy, resulting in a reduction of the total epithelial surface.

Intra-epithelial lymphocytes divide *in situ*, and dividing T-immunoblasts from thoracic duct lymph have been shown to localize in the intestinal epithelium. In experiments *in vitro*, however, the majority of intra-epithelial lymphocytes do not divide or produce lymphokines in response to mitogens that are stimulatory to most T-cells. In rodents a proportion of intra-epithelial lymphocytes contain metachromatic granules, lead-ing to the suggestion that they are mast-cell like, or have natural killer activity. However, they do not contain histamine, and the natural killer activity of intra-epithelial lymphocytes in rodents is very low, and is absent in the intra-epithelial lympho-cytes of man.

The T-cell receptor for antigen associated with the CD3 complex is present on most intra-epithelial lymphocytes. The T-cell receptor, however, exists in two alternative forms; an α/β heterodimer (TCR α/β) and a γ/δ heterodimer (TCR γ/δ). The expression of TCR γ/δ in mice is more frequent in the intra-epithelial lymphocyte population than in the peripheral T-cell population, suggesting that TCR γ/δ may have a unique function on mucosal surfaces. In contrast, in man 10 per cent of both intra-epithelial lymphocytes and peripheral T-cells which express the T-cell receptor express TCR γ/δ. However, human TCR γ/δ may exist in either a disulphide-linked or a non-disulphide-linked form. Whereas the disulphide-linked form predominates in the peripheral TCR γ/δ population, the non-disulphide-linked form predominates in the intra-epithelial lymphocyte TCR γ/δ population, suggesting that in man, T-cells expressing TCR γ/δ in the non-disulphide-linked form may have a unique mucosal function. The percentage of intra-epithelial lymphocytes expressing TCR γ/δ is increased in coeliac disease and in severe cows' milk sensitive enteropathy in childhood, though not in other enteropathies involving mucosal flattening studied to date. Although this may be of diagnostic use, the functional significance of this observation remains unknown.

24.2.4   Further reading

Bienenstock, J. and Befus, A. D. (1980). Review: mucosal immunology. *Immunology* 41, 249–70.

Brandtzaeg, P., *et al.* (1988). Progress report: lymphoepithelial interactions in the mucosal immune system. *Gut* 29, 1116–30.

Dobbins, A. O. (1986). Progress report: human intestinal intraepithelial lymphocytes. *Gut* 27, 972–85.

Gowans, J. L. and Knight, E. J. (1964). The route of recirculation of lymphocytes in the rat. *Proceedings of the Royal Society of London* B159, 257–82.

Ogra, P. L., Karzon, D. T., Righthand, F., and MacGillivray, M. (1968). Immunoglobulin response in serum and secretions after immunization with live and inactivated polio vaccine and natural infection. *New England Journal of Medicine* 279, 893–900.

Streeter, P. R., Berg, E. L., Rousse, B. T. N., Bargatze, R. F., and Butcher, E. C. (1988). A tissue specific endothelial molecule involved in lymphocyte homing. *Nature (London)* 331, 41–6.

24.3   Non-neoplastic lymphoproliferative disorders

A. G. Stansfield

24.3.1   Introduction

In this section the ways in which the lymphoreticular system responds to injurious stimuli will be considered. It is in the very nature of the immune system, in its role as a defence against microbial attack, that its constituent cells should be exposed to a wide variety of potentially harmful agents, both animate and inanimate. The reactions evoked by these diverse agents show many features in common with one another, so that few of the resultant histological pictures can be said to be 'specific' for any one aetiological agent. Nevertheless, lymph node biopsy is often useful in a case of lymphadenopathy (in a clinical sense = lymph node enlargement), not only in excluding the presence of malignant disease, but in narrowing the field of possibilities and suggesting differential diagnoses. Here I shall discuss first the common, 'non-specific' types of reaction pattern, in which both the lymphoid cells and the associated cells of the mononuclear phagocyte system may play a part. Secondly, I shall approach the subject in reverse, from the standpoint of the aetiological agents concerned, and examine the type of reaction which each provokes. From what has been already said, it will be obvious that the aetiological agent can seldom be identified immediately from the changes seen under the microscope in a lymph node biopsy. The patient's history, the findings on examination, the site of the biopsy, and the results of other investigations all contribute to the final diagnosis. Finally, I shall discuss some types of lymphadenopathy, of unknown aetiology, in which proliferation of lymphoid or reticulum cells occurs without the intervention of any hitherto demonstrable agent, but which do not fulfil the criteria for a neoplasm.

24.3.2   The response of lymphoreticular tissues to injurious stimuli

Lymphoreticular tissue may be envisaged as reacting to noxious stimuli in two ways:

1. the sequence of vascular and cellular events which are common to inflammation in any site; and

2. the specific responses which are peculiar to the immune system and which involve activation and proliferation of lymphoid cells, as well as the participation of macrophages.

In practice, the two types of response are usually inextricably mixed, for it is almost inevitable that any stimulus which excites an inflammatory reaction in lymphoreticular tissue will, at the same time, evoke an immune response of some degree. The *intensity* of the reaction, of course, varies greatly, depending chiefly on the nature and duration of the stimulus, but also on the immune status and perhaps other peculiarities of the individual concerned. The *pattern* of the reaction varies too, being determined largely by the nature of the antigenic stimulus. Thus, many bacterial antigens and some inanimate antigens stimulate chiefly the B lymphocyte system to produce antibodies (immunoglobulins), while many viral antigens and sensitizing drugs evoke a 'cellular' immune response, in which the T-lymphocytes are the main participants. This is, of course, an oversimplification since the B- and T-lymphocyte systems are interdependent and act in concert, so that in the resulting immune reaction one may usually detect elements of both B- and T-reactivity, even when one or other is predominant. The combination of inflammatory and immunological reactive changes in a lymph node is covered by the term 'lymphadenitis'.

It will be apparent already that it is not always possible to distinguish forms of lymphadenitis which are due to an infective agent from similar reactions which are not infective in origin. Furthermore, there are certain types of lymphadenitis in which the histological features, and sometimes the clinical features also, strongly suggest an infective process, although no infective agent has yet been demonstrated. In the following account, conditions of unknown aetiology are discussed in the text where it seems most appropriate to place them, and a sharp separation of infective from non-infective lesions will not be attempted.

24.3.3 Predominantly B-lymphocyte immune response—follicular hyperplasia and plasmacytosis

Although these changes may also affect extranodal lymphoreticular tissue, they are most frequently encountered and most easily recognized in lymph nodes or tonsils and are commonly found in biopsies of enlarged nodes from superficial sites such as the neck, axilla, or groin. There may be some readily identifiable cause of the reaction, such as infected tonsils in the case of enlarged cervical nodes. However, it is often the case that there is no obvious explanation for the lymphadenopathy and in such circumstances biopsy is more likely to be performed. In addition to local factors that can evoke an immune reaction in the draining lymph nodes, some systemic diseases, notably rheumatoid arthritis, may be associated with follicular hyperplasia in a number of superficial lymph nodes. However, an underlying cause is not always discernible even when multiple nodes show striking reactive hyperplasia.

In follicular hyperplasia the follicles may increase both in size and in number, but the chief characteristic of a hyperplastic follicle is the presence of an enlarged germinal centre, the paler cells of which are thrown into relief by the 'mantle zone' of darkly staining small lymphocytes that surround the centre or form a crescent around one pole (Fig. 24.18). Single 'secondary follicles' of this type may attain a very large size and are sometimes quite irregular in shape. Within the germinal centre mitoses are often very numerous and the rate of cell turnover can also be gauged by the number of large, 'tingible-body' macrophages, containing engulfed nuclear fragments. The cellular composition and function of germinal centres have already been discussed (Section 24.1.2).

The presence of hyperplastic follicles and the accumulation of plasma cells in a node are both indications of B-lymphocyte stimulation and the two are commonly found together, but in varying proportions. In some instances follicular hyperplasia is the dominant change and the lymph node may then be largely occupied by follicles with big germinal centres, whereas the plasma cell component is relatively insignificant. At the other extreme, there may be a massive infiltration of the node by plasma cells which are not just confined to the medullary cords, where the process begins, but which fill and expand the interfollicular pulp (Fig. 24.19). These plasma cells are, of course, polytypic and the absence of 'light chain restriction' on

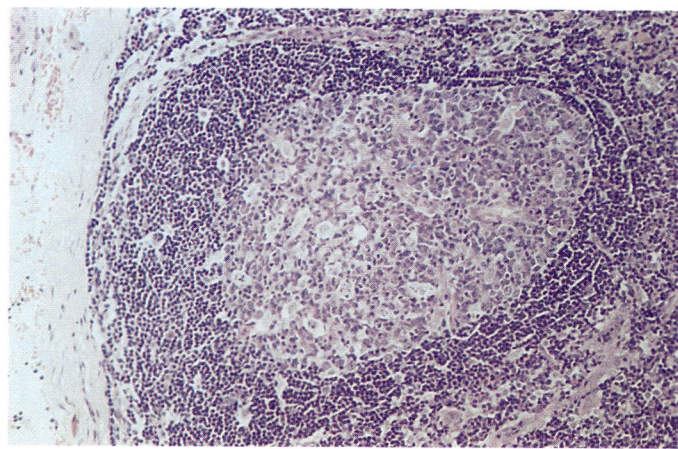

Fig. 24.18 Hyperplastic secondary follicle showing the germinal centre, containing scattered pale-staining macrophages, and the surrounding mantle of small lymphocytes.

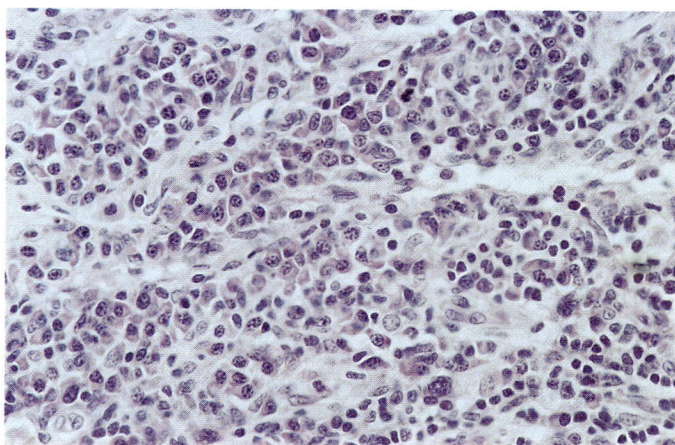

Fig. 24.19 Reactive plasmacytosis. Plasma cells have displaced most of the lymphocytes in the node pulp.

immunostaining distinguishes this reactive plasmacytosis from a neoplasm, i.e. plasmacytoma.

Follicular hyperplasia is particularly striking in childhood, when the individual follicles may at times grow to such a large size that they merge into one another with disappearance of the mantle zone. In some instances of protracted follicular hyperplasia, a proportion of the enlarged germinal centres appear to disintegrate, leaving an expanded nodule occupied predominantly by small lymphocytes with a scattering of large lymphoid cells—a process known as 'progressive transformation of germinal centres'.

Reactive follicular hyperplasia, which is an entirely benign condition, has, of course, to be distinguished from a malignant lymphoma with a follicular pattern, and the distinction is not always easy (see p. 1779).

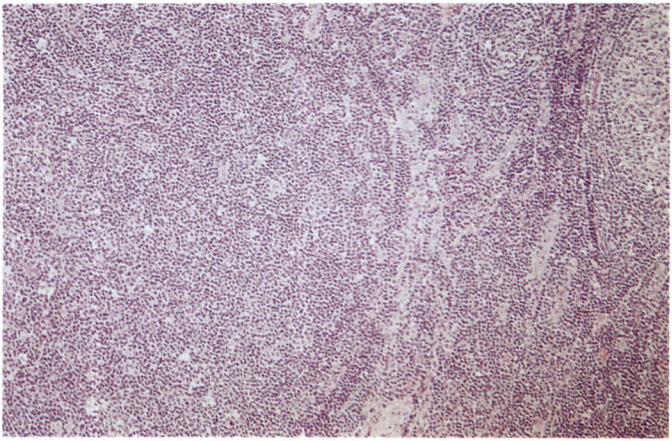

Fig. 24.20 Part of a 'progressively transformed' germinal centre is seen beside a normal germinal follicle.

24.3.4 Predominantly T-cell immune response—paracortical hyperplasia

As indicated above, this type of immunological reaction is particularly characteristic of many viral infections but is also seen in the lymphadenopathy associated with drug hypersensitivity. As with follicular hyperplasia, the intensity and details of the reaction vary greatly, but typically the paracortex of the lymph node expands due to cellular proliferation and accumulation within it, while the follicles diminish and may disappear altogether. The cellular constituents of the enlarged paracortex are often a mixture of small T-lymphocytes with large, transformed 'immunoblasts', frequently seen in mitosis (Fig. 24.21). Along with the lymphocyte population, one often sees other, associated cells, such as the so-called interdigitating reticulum cells, eosinophil leucocytes, and sometimes epithelioid cells. Activation of T-lymphocytes is commonly associated with increased prominence of the high endothelial (post-capillary) venules,

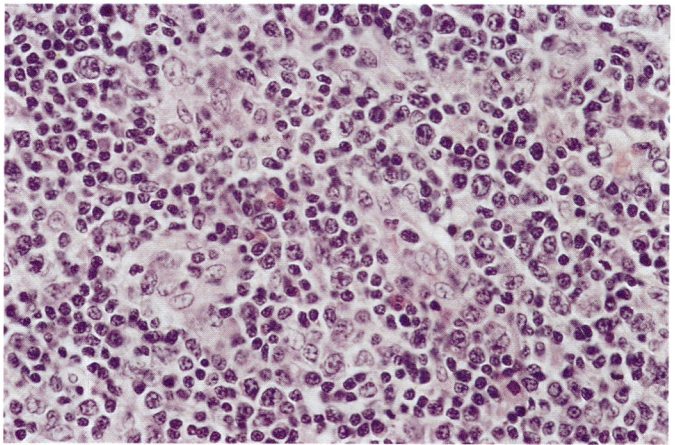

Fig. 24.21 Paracortical hyperplasia with immunoblasts dispersed amongst a mixed cellular infiltrate. Note the high endothelial venules.

which are a characteristic feature of the paracortex. The frequent observation of lymphocytes within the walls of these vessels testifies to the importance of this migration pathway for the lymphocytes of the circulating pool. Whereas the follicles and the resting B-cell population of such nodes are often suppressed, plasma cells are quite frequently found and their presence may perhaps be attributed to the 'helper' function of many T-lymphocytes.

Occasionally the degree of blast-cell transformation in paracortical hyperplasia may be so great as to lead to a mistaken diagnosis of a high-grade malignant lymphoma of diffuse pattern. This is particularly liable to happen in infectious mononucleosis and in some drug reactions.

24.3.5 Macrophage response—reactive histiocytosis

The large number of phagocytic cells of the mononuclear macrophage system which inhabit the lymphoreticular tissues has already been mentioned (p. 1747). Not only do macrophages play a crucial role in initiating immune responses by 'processing' bacterial and other antigens, they are also concerned in the removal and storage of insoluble or only slightly soluble substances that pass through the filters of the various lymphoreticular tissues. Macrophages are a prominent ingredient of lymph nodes in lymphadenitis, both acute and chronic, and their true numbers can best be appreciated by specific immunostaining with a macrophage marker.

Sinus histiocytosis

The highest concentration of histiocytic cells in a lymph node is to be found in the lymph sinuses and, in the resting state, these cells are anchored to the slender reticulin fibres which traverse and form the 'walls' of the sinuses. When stimulated these littoral ('on the shore') cells enlarge and become avidly phagocytic (macrophages). In more prolonged stimulation, the littoral cells increase in number, mainly by recruitment of marrow-derived monocytes and, in time, the lymph sinuses may appear choked by the accumulation of histiocytic cells (Fig. 24.22). Such a reactive sinus histiocytosis is commonly seen in both superficial and deep lymph nodes. The phagocytic propensity of the littoral cells is often evident from the presence in their cytoplasm of engulfed red cells, haemosiderin pigment, or lipid droplets. In infections, intracellular organisms are sometimes seen. It has been claimed, but has never been convincingly proved, that when sinus histiocytosis is found in the axillary nodes of women undergoing mastectomy for breast carcinoma the prognosis is better than when this change is absent.

So-called 'immature sinus histiocytosis' is a misnomer, since the monocyte-like cells that accumulate in the lymph sinuses in these circumstances have been shown to be B-lymphocytes of a distinctive phenotype. The condition is seen in a variety of infections, but is particularly frequent in toxoplasmic lymphadenitis and in acquired immunodeficiency syndrome (AIDS).

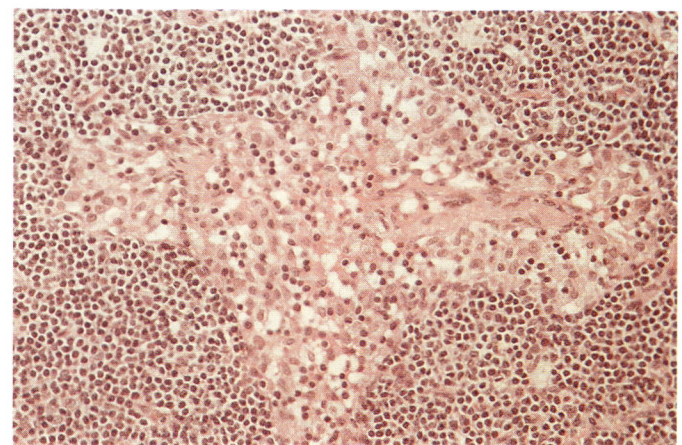

Fig. 24.22 Reactive sinus histiocytosis.

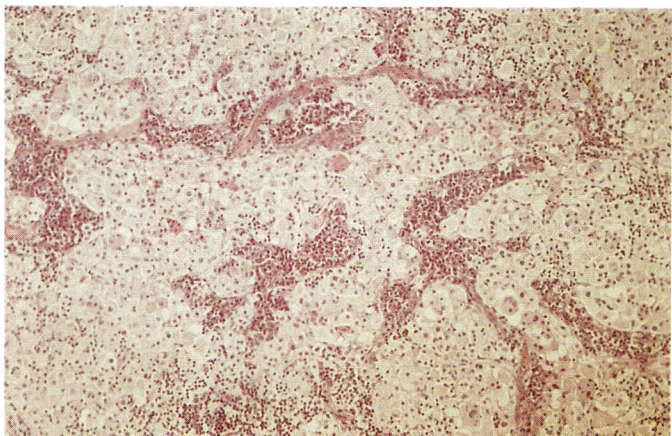

(a)

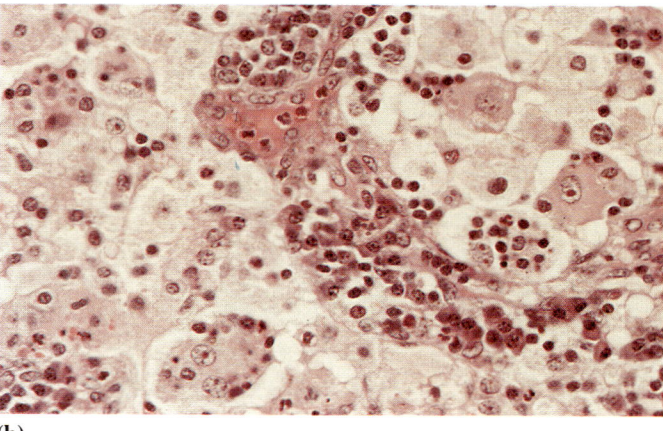

(b)

Fig. 24.23 'Sinus histiocytosis with massive lymphadenopathy.' (a) Low-power and (b) high-power pictures showing the characteristic giant macrophages, some containing engulfed cells.

Sinus histiocytosis with massive lymphadenopathy (Rosai–Dorfman disease)

Is an uncommon entity of unknown aetiology in which the sinuses of the affected nodes (usually cervical) are filled with very large and distinctive macrophages, frequently containing engulfed lymphocytes in their abundant cytoplasm (Fig. 24.23). There is an accompanying reactive plasmacytosis, often of marked degree, which may be reflected in a polyclonal hypergammaglobulinaemia. As implied in the name, the involved nodes may reach a very large size and lymphadenopathy may persist for a long time, but it eventually resolves spontaneously in most cases. The disease has many features of an infective process and it may be associated with fever and a polymorph leucocytosis, but no organism has yet been isolated. The condition is more frequent in Blacks, whether in the tropics or in the UK, than in Whites, and it is now appreciated that the same pathological process may sometimes affect skin, salivary glands, bones, and other tissues, as well as lymph nodes.

Pulp histiocytosis

In circumstances where macrophages are engaged in phagocytosis of lymph-borne insoluble or colloid substances, they tend to accumulate in the dense pulp of lymph nodes rather than, or as well as, in the sinuses. This is seen, for instance, in the mediastinal and bronchopulmonary nodes of workers in dusty occupations. A somewhat similar picture may be seen in leprosy, where the macrophages are stuffed with *Mycobacterium leprae* (globi). In Whipple's disease and in 'storage' diseases, such as Gaucher's disease, characteristic large, pale macrophages accumulate both in the sinuses and the node pulp. Although the abdominal nodes usually show maximal involvement, peripheral nodes may be affected later on. The mesenteric nodes in Whipple's disease may, in addition, show fat globules in the sinuses due to chylous obstruction. A superficially similar picture may be found in abdominal nodes as a result of lymphangiography.

Dermatopathic lymphadenitis

A distinctive form of reactive pulp histiocytosis is found in the superficial lymph nodes of patients with diffuse chronic skin disorders, especially in chronic exfoliative dermatitis, psoriasis, and mycosis fungoides. In this condition the cortical follicles are preserved and may show hyperplastic germinal centres, whereas the paracortex is expanded by masses of pale-staining histiocyte-like cells which progressively replace the lymphocyte population of the pulp (Fig. 24.24). Some of the infiltrating cells are true macrophages and these may contain phagocytosed lipid and melanin pigment; however, the majority are nonphagocytic, interdigitating reticulum cells—the characteristic antigen-presenting reticulum cells of the paracortex. These are intimately mingled with T-lymphocytes and often eosinophils. The distinction between this condition and histiocytosis X is discussed on page 1768.

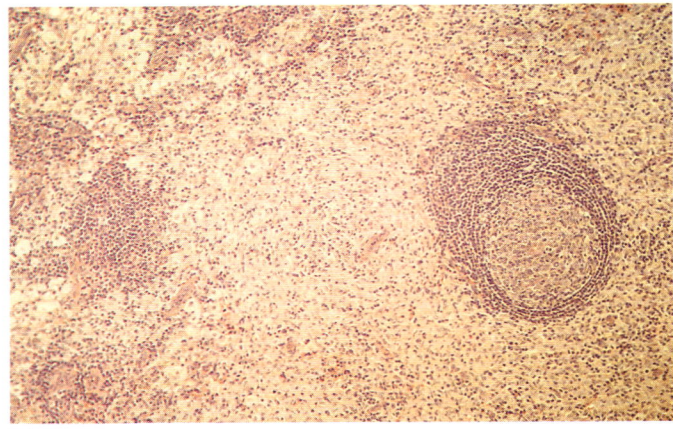

(a)

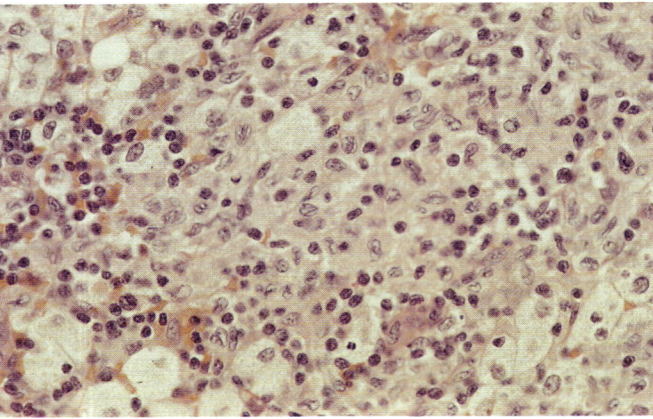

Fig. 24.24 Dermatopathic lymphadenitis. (a) Low power, showing well-preserved follicles and diffuse paracortical infiltration by pale-staining cells; (b) higher magnification of paracortical infiltrate, consisting of interdigitating reticulum cells with grooved nuclei (above) and lipid-containing macrophages (below).

24.3.6   Epithelioid-cell transformation and granuloma formation

In some forms of pulp histiocytosis the macrophages that accumulate in the nodes remain discrete, single cells of rounded contour with well-defined cell boundaries. Quite commonly, however, in circumstances that are not fully understood, macrophages undergo transformation into epithelioid cells. In the process, the cells lose their capacity for phagocytosis to a large extent and instead acquire cytoplasmic organelles characteristic of secretory cells. These functional alterations are matched by changes in the light-microscopic appearance of the cells. The copious cytoplasm becomes more acidophilic, the cell boundaries more irregular and less clearly defined. Furthermore, there is usually a tendency of epithelioid cells to form clusters and not infrequently individual cells fuse together into multinucleate giant cells. Clustered masses of epithelioid cells, with or without giant cells, are often spoken of as 'granulomas'

and conditions in which granulomas commonly form are grouped together as 'granulomatous diseases'.

The classic granulomatous disease is, of course, tuberculosis, but granulomas may be found in lymph nodes in a great variety of conditions, infective and non-infective, including some neoplasms.

Sarcoidosis

One of the most remarkable of the granulomatous diseases is sarcoidosis. Of unknown aetiology, but often suspected of being infective, sarcoidosis has been described as occurring in almost every tissue of the body. Indeed the manifestations of the disease are so diverse that initially several different diseases were independently described (Boeck's sarcoid, uveoparotid syndrome, etc.) before it was recognized that these were different manifestations of one disease. It is convenient to describe sarcoidosis here, since lymph node involvement is common and the diagnosis is frequently made by lymph node biopsy. The pathological lesion underlying the numerous clinical manifestations of sarcoidosis is a small, focal granuloma, which sometimes shows a loss of structure centrally due to necrosis, but in which the characteristic 'caseous' necrosis of tuberculosis is lacking (Fig. 24.25). Giant cells may or may not be present in the granulomas, but these are generally a less conspicuous feature than they are in tuberculosis. When present, the giant cells may contain calcified conchoidal structures (Schaumann bodies) or star-shaped 'asteroid' bodies, but neither of these cytoplasmic inclusions is specific for sarcoidosis. Mediastinal and cervical nodes are common sites of presentation, but almost any group of lymph nodes may be affected. On biopsy, the node is often found to be more or less filled with granulomas of a rather uniform size which are frequently discrete and which retain their focal character even when confluent. The granulomas of sarcoidosis are remarkably persistent, but in time they tend to undergo replacement by hyaline fibrous tissue.

Many theories have been advanced to explain the manifold

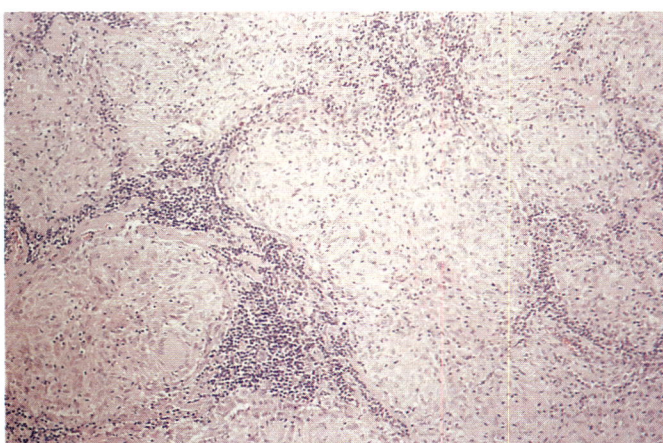

Fig. 24.25 Multiple granulomas in a lymph node in sarcoidosis, showing typical features. Necrosis is seen at the centres of some of the granulomas.

features of sarcoidosis and many attempts made to discover the aetiology. Whether or not there is a single aetiological agent, it is evident that the disease is accompanied by a state of impaired cell-mediated immunity and it has been known for a long time that patients with sarcoidosis have a negative tuberculin reaction, even when the reaction was positive before the onset of the disease. In the Kveim test for sarcoidosis, injection into the skin of a small quantity of Kveim antigen, derived from lesions of a known case of the disease, elicits granulomatous lesions at the site of inoculation, which may be detected on skin biopsy 6 weeks later. A negative result, i.e. absence of granulomas in the skin biopsy, is fairly reliable evidence that the patient is not suffering from sarcoidosis.

Sarcoid-type reactions

Focal granulomas very similar to those of sarcoidosis may be found from time to time in other conditions, in which it is clear that the patient is not suffering from true sarcoidosis. Apart from tuberculosis, which is an important differential diagnosis, granulomas of similar type may occur in other infections, including brucellosis, some fungal infections, leishmaniasis, and chronic tularaemia. Likewise, sarcoid-type granulomas may be seen in berylliosis and in reactions to some other mineral substances including silicones. Hodgkin's disease and less frequently non-Hodgkin's lymphomas and carcinomas may provoke a similar type of reaction in lymph nodes from time to time. The focal granulomas that are seen in the intestinal wall and mesenteric lymph nodes in Crohn's disease are also somewhat similar to those of sarcoidosis. It is generally not difficult to distinguish these various lesions from sarcoidosis when the clinical history, location of the lesions, and associated findings are taken into account.

24.3.7   Acute lymphadenitis

This is most frequently seen in acute bacterial infections, especially those caused by β-haemolytic streptococci and staphylococci. The former organisms are a frequent cause of acute tonsillitis with secondary lymphadenitis in the upper cervical nodes, while staphylococcal infection is common in the skin and in infected wounds, with consequent lymphadenitis in the draining lymph nodes. The nodes enlarge rapidly and are often tender or even painful, sometimes with accompanying lymphangitis, indicated by red lines in the skin along the course of the lymphatics. Rarer infections such as diphtheria and anthrax are occasionally implicated as a cause of acute lymphadenitis.

In all such acute infections the patient is ill and generally pyrexial, so that the diagnosis is obvious and lymph node biopsy is unlikely to be performed. The histological picture is dominated by acute inflammatory changes in the node—hyperaemia, fibrinous exudation, perinodal oedema, and polymorph infiltration. In severe cases the process may progress to suppuration and abscess formation with partial or even total destruction of the node. Today, of course, such infections are more usually cut short by administration of an appropriate antibiotic, with rapid

resolution of the lymphadenitis if suppuration has not occurred. Certain tropical infectious agents, notably *Pasteurella pestis* (bubonic plague) and *Francisella tularensis* (tularaemia) cause a predominantly necrotizing form of acute lymphadenitis, which may or may not progress to actual suppuration in the nodes. The latter infection may sometimes cause a more chronic necrotizing lymphadenitis with granuloma formation, simulating tuberculous lymphadenitis. Focal necrosis is also seen in the acute mesenteric lymphadenitis of typhoid fever, but here there is a mononuclear cell reaction and polymorphs are conspicuously absent.

Much milder forms of acute lymphadenitis are commonly encountered in situations where no pathogenic infectious agent can be incriminated, but where the affected lymph nodes are draining a site of inflammation. A good example is seen in the mesocolic lymph nodes in active ulcerative colitis. Such nodes may show pronounced hyperaemia, but the dominant change is often dilatation of the lymph sinuses—so-called 'sinus catarrh'—which is frequently accompanied by the presence of free-floating macrophages in the contained lymph and sometimes polymorphs as well. The presence of sinus catarrh is evidence of an increased flow of lymph through the node, and this is a commonly occurring feature in 'non-specific' lymphadenitis.

24.3.8   Chronic lymphadenitis

This may be a sequel of an acute lymphadenitis, in which case scarring of the node may be found in addition to sinus histiocytosis and perhaps cellular changes indicative of an immune reaction. Because of the frequent occurrence of such changes in the inguinal nodes, biopsy of nodes in this site is to be avoided if possible, when generalized lymphadenopathy is present and other enlarged superficial nodes are equally accessible. On the other hand, many infections—bacterial, fungal, and protozoal—present initially with a chronic type of inflammation, in which lymph node enlargement is more gradual and persistent and usually painless. There is, of course, no sharp dividing line between acute and chronic stages of inflammation in lymph nodes, as in other tissues. Nevertheless, many forms of chronic lymphadenitis are marked by a greater prominence of immunological reactive changes, as described above. These are often attended by a pronounced macrophage response, with or without granuloma formation. The lymphadenitis of chronic brucellosis may be cited as an example of such changes. Necrosis is common in some types and even localized abscess formation.

Eosinophil granulocytes are a variable component of chronic lymphadenitis, often being found in small numbers along with an increase of mast cells. Occasionally a massive increase of eosinophils is found, which should arouse a suspicion of those types of hypersensitivity which are known to be associated with IgE production—helminthic infestation and some forms of food or drug hypersensitivity. It is important to remember, too, that Hodgkin's disease, some T-cell malignant lymphomas, and occasionally other neoplasms may provoke a considerable eosinophilia. In so-called 'eosinophilic granuloma' of bones or lymph nodes, large numbers of eosinophils are associated with a distinctive type of histiocyte, related to the Langerhans cells of the epidermis.

Having discussed in general terms the features of acute and chronic lymphadenitis, we may now turn to consider the types of reaction associated with specific infectious agents. The reactions evoked by pyogenic cocci, *Corynebacterium diphtheriae*, *Bacillus anthracis*, *P. pestis*, *F. tularensis* and *Salmonella typhi* have been briefly described above and will not be further discussed.

24.3.9 Chronic lymphadenitis of infective origin

Yersinial lymphadenitis (Pseudotuberculosis)

Two species of *Yersinia*, *Y. pseudotuberculosis* and *Y. enterocolitica*, are responsible for infections of the gut, associated with a characteristic type of mesenteric lymphadenitis which generally overshadows the frequently insignificant primary lesions in the intestine itself. Children or adults may be affected and the disease is most frequently seen in country districts in the UK, for the organisms are carried by rats and wood pigeons. The portal of entry is probably through the Peyer's patches of the terminal ileum and the lymphoid follicles of the large intestinal mucosa, so that the ileocolic nodes are frequently involved.

The affected nodes are swollen and the histological lesions, which are similar with the two organisms, show a combination of chronic inflammatory changes and immune reaction. In the fully developed lesion the node contains multiple small foci of necrosis or microabscesses, each surrounded by a zone of granulomatous reaction. Occasionally giant-cells are seen, but the resemblance to tuberculosis is not close. Before total destruction of the node occurs, there are large, hyperplastic germinal follicles in the cortex and the patent lymph sinuses often contain large, basophilic immunoblasts.

The disease is rarely fatal, but its presentation with right iliac fossa pain may lead to a diagnosis of acute appendicitis. Biopsy of the enlarged nodes, if laparotomy is undertaken, will distinguish the condition from viral forms of mesenteric adenitis which also occur in childhood. If the diagnosis is suspected before laparotomy the diagnosis may be confirmed serologically.

Tuberculous lymphadenitis

The dramatic decline in the incidence of tuberculosis in developed countries in the past 50 years has meant that this disease, formerly common, is nowadays rarely seen in Britain except in Asian immigrants. Tuberculous lymphadenitis is a regular feature of the 'primary complex' of tuberculosis—a term which refers to the initial lesion at the portal of entry of *Mycobacterium tuberculosis* into the body, together with the lesions which develop in the regional nodes to which the organisms are carried by macrophages. Lymph node lesions are seldom seen in re-infection tuberculosis, but in rare instances, when there is

exceptional susceptibility to the disease, widespread nodal involvement may be seen.

The primary portal of entry is generally in the lung, due to spread by droplet infection from an individual with 'open' pulmonary tuberculosis. In these circumstances nodal tuberculosis may be found in the pulmonary hilar nodes. Before the stringent control of tuberculosis in cattle and the universal pasteurization of milk the primary lesion was often in the tonsils (with cervical lymphadenitis) or in the gut (with mesenteric lymphadenitis). In many, but not all, such cases the infecting organism is of the bovine strain.

The lesions seen in the lymph nodes are similar to those found in other sites of *M. tuberculosis* infection—a slowly evolving granulomatous inflammation with caseous necrosis appearing at the centres of the focal granulomas or 'tubercles' after a week or two (Fig. 24.26). Coalescence of individual tubercles may lead to eventual replacement of the whole node by a necrotic cheesy mass, but the process is frequently halted before this occurs, the granulomas becoming 'walled-off' by fibrous tissue. In this event the caseous foci frequently become calcified and persist indefinitely in this state. It is doubtful whether such 'arrested' lesions ever become re-awakened, but of course re-infection can occur.

Depending upon the patient's susceptibility, in which immunity, nutritional status, and perhaps other factors play a part, the rate of progression of tuberculosis varies and the type of lesion varies accordingly. The rapid spread of caseation and multiplication of *M. tuberculosis* in the nodes may result in ulceration through the walls of adjacent blood vessels and dissemination of infection by the bloodstream, resulting in miliary tuberculosis. The development of caseation is closely linked with the appearance of hypersensitivity to tuberculoprotein. In some individuals who have altered cellular immunity, such hypersensitivity does not develop, their Mantoux reaction remains negative in the face of a tuberculous infection and the granulomatous foci fail to caseate and thus closely resemble the

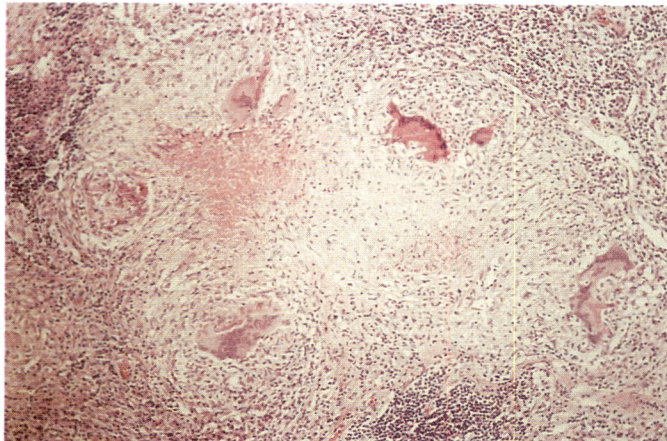

Fig. 24.26 Tuberculous lymphadenitis, showing a typical 'tubercle' with early caseation at its centre, ringed round by 'giant-cell systems'. (Compare with Fig. 24.25.)

focal granulomas of sarcoidosis. Indeed, one theory of the aetiology of sarcoidosis attributes the lesions to this type of tuberculous infection, in which *M. tuberculosis* is notoriously difficult to demonstrate.

Other types of mycobacterial lymphadenitis

From time to time a caseating granulomatous type of lymphadenitis results from infection by other 'atypical' mycobacteria. *M. scrofulaceum* was formerly seen in Britain as a cause of cervical lymphadenopathy in childhood; nowadays it is rare.

A florid proliferation of *Mycobacterium avium intracellulare* resulting in a non-caseating granulomatous reaction (mycobacterial histiocytosis), has been seen in recent years in the lymph nodes of some AIDS sufferers and, very rarely, a similar type of reaction has been observed in the axillary nodes of children who have been inoculated with BCG.

Although a granulomatous reaction may be seen in lymph nodes in tuberculoid leprosy, nodal enlargement is more often seen in lepromatous leprosy where the reaction is quite different.

Fungal diseases (Mycoses)

Most of the fungal infections which are liable to cause lymphadenitis are essentially tropical diseases and are rarely encountered in the UK except in those coming from overseas. The most important of these are histoplasmosis and cryptococcosis. *Histoplasmosis* is common in some parts of southern USA where it leads to forms of illness similar in many respects to tuberculosis. The primary lesions are usually in the lung, but spread occurs to lymph nodes and other organs. Necrotizing granulomatous lesions are found which, on healing, undergo calcification. The organisms (*Histoplasma capsulatum*) are, however, readily demonstrated in sections stained by the PAS or hexamine silver methods and in florid infections they can be seen within macrophages, even in haematoxylin- and eosin-stained sections. Another form of histoplasmosis is seen in tropical Africa.

Cryptococcosis is common in Australia and is again largely a disease of hot climates, although it occasionally occurs in the UK as an opportunistic infection in Hodgkin's disease and other conditions of impaired immunity. *Cryptococcus neoformans* grows readily in the tissues in these circumstances, but evokes very little cellular response. Occasionally poorly developed granulomas are seen. In some primary cutaneous mycoses, such as Madura foot, the regional lymph nodes enlarge as a result of the inflammatory reaction and secondary infection, but do not show evidence of actual fungal infection.

Lymphogranuloma venereum (LGV; lymphogranuloma inguinale)

In this venereally transmitted disease lymphadenitis is a conspicuous feature, although the area of involvement differs in the two sexes. In the male the primary lesion is usually on the penis, although it is often overlooked, but the inguinal nodes enlarge to form bilateral 'buboes' which may break down and discharge through the skin. In the female the transitory primary lesion is generally on the cervix, and secondary inflammation in the pelvic lymph nodes is accompanied by a deep pelvic cellulitis which subsequently heals with much scarring and may lead to rectal stricture.

LGV is caused by a *Chlamydia*, formerly classified as a virus but now recognized as a very small bacterium, which is none the less an obligate intracellular parasite. The affected lymph nodes show chronic inflammation, characterized by the development of multiple, small, stellate abscesses, each surrounded by a zone of histiocytic reaction and fibrosis and filled with degenerate polymorphs. There is a striking accompanying plasmacytosis in the neighbourhood of the lesions which eventually heal with considerable scarring. The diagnosis may be confirmed by intradermal skin testing, using killed *Chlamydia* which have been cultured on chicken yolk sac (Frei test).

Cat-scratch disease (CSD)

The lesions in this disease are very similar to those of LGV and there is now substantial evidence that CSD is also caused by a small Gram-negative bacillus. Patients with AIDS, infected with this organism, may develop focal, angioma-like, proliferative vascular lesions (bacillary angiomatosis). Affecting children or adults, the disease is generally found where cats are kept as domestic pets, although it is not necessary to be scratched or bitten by a cat to acquire CSD. There may or may not be a visible skin lesion, but it is generally assumed that infection enters through the skin. The lymphadenitis which then develops most commonly affects the parotid, cervical, or axillary nodes—drainage sites of skin most liable to be exposed to infection in cat-fondlers. Biopsy of the node shows focal 'microabscesses' or small areas of necrosis with surrounding histiocytic reaction and sometimes granuloma formation—a picture which is characteristic enough to suggest the diagnosis (Fig. 24.27). Confirmation may be obtained by a positive intradermal skin test similar to the Frei test for LGV but using, as the test antigen, material obtained from a known case of CSD. Rarely, there may be fever and other signs of systemic illness in CSD.

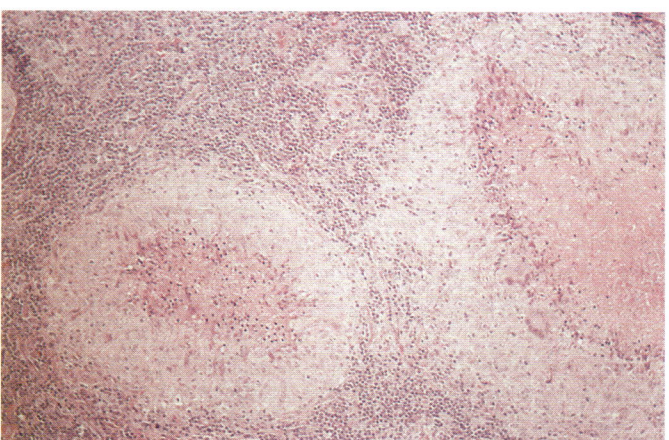

Fig. 24.27 Lymph node in cat-scratch disease, showing focal granulomatous inflammation around necrotic centres. There is a certain similarity to tuberculosis.

Other types of necrotizing lymphadenitis presumed to be infectious

Two diseases fall into this category. In both of them the aetiology is still unknown, although both bear the stamp of an infective process.

Kawasaki's disease (mucocutaneous lymph node syndrome)

Is a disease of infancy and early childhood, characterized by fever, erythematous skin rashes, peripheral oedema, conjunctivitis, oral ulcers, cervical lymphadenopathy, and coronary arteritis, which may prove fatal. The enlarged lymph nodes show irregular areas of necrosis, with relatively mild attendant reactions, but with thrombi in small vessels. It has been suggested that the necrotic foci are infarcts.

Kikuchi's disease (histiocytic necrotizing lymphadenitis without granulocytic infiltration)

Was first described in Japan, but appears to be not uncommon in Europe and the USA. Young women are chiefly affected and the disease presents with enlargement of one or more cervical nodes, sometimes accompanied by malaise and mild pyrexia. Biopsy reveals irregular foci of necrosis in the nodes, apparently arising within areas of lymphoid blast cell transformation and histiocytic infiltration. The necrotic areas are littered with nuclear fragments, giving at first sight an impression of polymorph infiltration, but, as the subtitle implies, polymorphs are conspicuously absent. A rather similar picture is sometimes seen in lymph nodes in florid systemic lupus erythematosus, but here plasma cells are a much more conspicuous feature and haematoxylin bodies may also be found.

Syphilitic lymphadenitis

Lymphadenitis is a feature of both the primary and the secondary stages of syphilis. In the *primary* stage, the regional nodes (usually inguinal with a primary sore on the external genitalia) exhibit an often painless enlargement. If nodes are taken for biopsy, these show a prominent immune reaction with follicular hyperplasia as well as paracortical expansion and blast-cell transformation. Small clusters of epithelioid cells are often present in the paracortex. Polymorphs may also be found in the sinuses, especially when the primary sore has become secondarily infected. *Treponema pallidum* can often be demonstrated by appropriate silver staining or in a wet film prepared from the cut surfaces of fresh unfixed node and examined by dark-field illumination.

In the *secondary* stage, nodal enlargement may be widespread, involving even sites like the epitrochlear nodes. The changes are similar to those found in the primary stage, but sometimes with more striking plasma-cell infiltration. As in the primary stage, lymphocytes and plasma cells often show 'cuffing' of small vessels, especially venules, in the node and in surrounding fat (periadenitis).

24.3.10   Protozoal diseases

Lymphadenitis is an important feature of three protozoal diseases, namely, toxoplasmosis, leishmaniasis, and trypanosomiasis. The first, toxoplasmosis, is of world-wide distribution, whereas the others are confined to tropical or subtropical regions. With the present facilities for air travel, however, even tropical diseases may be encountered in Britain.

Toxoplasmosis

The protozoon *Toxoplasma gondii* is an extremely common parasite, both in man and in many animal species. It has been established that the main reservoir of infection in the UK is the domestic cat, in which the life cycle of the parasite has been worked out. Many human infections are subclinical, as has been shown by the high incidence in the adult population of antibodies to *T. gondii*. Women who acquire the parasite during pregnancy are at risk of passing the infection to the fetus and babies thus infected may be born with ocular or cerebral damage, the latter often proving fatal. Serious or fatal infections are also seen in patients with immune impairment. The commonest clinical presentation of the disease, however, is the development of a localized painless lymphadenopathy, with or without mild constitutional symptoms.

Toxoplasmic lymphadenitis is usually seen in children or young adults. One or several nodes may be involved, often in the cervical region, but any of the superficial groups, e.g. parotid, occipital, axillary, or even inguinal nodes, may be affected. A high or rising titre of antibodies, shown by the dye test, or the presence of complement-fixing antibodies in the patients' serum, provide confirmatory evidence of a recent infection. On biopsy, the nodes show a characteristic picture with prominent follicles containing active germinal centres, asociated with small clusters of epithelioid cells, dotted through the cortex and often infiltrating the germinal follicles (Fig. 24.28). When epithelioid cells are numerous they may also be found in the

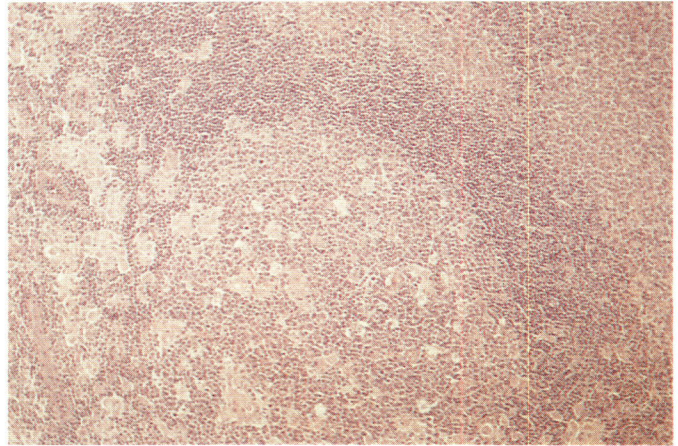

Fig. 24.28 Toxoplasmic lymphadenitis. Small clusters of epithelioid cells have penetrated into a hyperplastic germinal follicle (lower left). Monocytoid B-lymphocytes can be seen in a dilated sinus (top right).

marginal sinus, but the sinuses more often contain closely packed collections of 'monocytoid' B-cells—so-called 'immature sinus histiocytosis' (see p. 1758). This combination of changes provides strong presumptive evidence of toxoplasmic infection, but it may be mimicked by other infections, including infectious mononucleosis, and also occasionally by Hodgkin's disease. On rare occasions a pseudocyst of *T. gondii* may be found in the node.

Leishmaniasis

The form of leishmaniasis with which we are concerned here is visceral leishmaniasis (kala-azar) which is caused by the protozoon *Leishmania donovani*. This parasite is transmitted by the bites of sandflies and the disease is endemic throughout large areas of the Middle East and the Mediterranean region. While hepatosplenomegaly and anaemia are typical of the chronic disease, lymphadenopathy is quite frequently a presenting feature. *L. donovani* may be recognized as small, uniform, haematoxyphil dots within macrophages, which are dispersed throughout the node pulp, along with many plasma cells. Occasionally frank granulomas, with or without necrosis, are seen.

Lymphadenopathy is also a prominent feature of both the African and the South American forms of trypanosomiasis, but these diseases are unlikely to be seen in Britain.

24.3.11   Viral diseases

A number of diseases, caused by both DNA and RNA viruses, are associated with lymphadenopathy, the most important being infectious mononucleosis and the acquired immunodeficiency syndrome (AIDS).

Infectious mononucleosis

Infectious mononucleosis (glandular fever) is caused by a herpes-type DNA virus—the *Epstein–Barr virus* (EBV), which is also known to be associated with Burkitt's lymphoma and nasopharyngeal carcinoma (NPC). The role of this virus in the causation of infectious mononucleosis (IM) was discovered by chance when one member of a research team working on Burkitt's lymphoma developed IM. Infection by EBV is extremely common and the high incidence of EBV antibodies in the adult population indicates that most infections are subclinical. There is evidence that when the virus is acquired early in life, as happens in crowded communities, no disease ensues, unless conditions prevail that favour the development of Burkitt's lymphoma or NPC. However, when the acquisition of the virus is delayed until later childhood or adolescence, infection is likely to lead to an attack of IM. Transmission of the infection at this age is promoted by passionate kissing.

Cervical lymphadenopathy often accompanies the sore throat, with tonsillar swelling and fever that occurs in the acute stage. The lymph node enlargement is not confined, however, to the cervical nodes, other superficial nodes may be involved and the presentation may be abdominal, simulating acute ap-

pendicitis. The spleen is often enlarged and may rarely rupture. Hepatitis can also occur. Concurrently with these changes, abnormal lymphoid cells (earlier misinterpreted as monocytes) appear in the blood and an incorrect diagnosis of acute leukaemia may be made by the inexperienced. Quite soon, the Paul–Bunnell heterophil antibody test, or simpler, monospot test, become positive, pointing to the correct diagnosis. If the diagnosis is not made first, a node may be taken for biopsy, or occasionally tonsillectomy may be performed to relieve obstruction caused by greatly swollen tonsils. The histological changes in lymphoreticular tissues in IM may be extremely dramatic, for there is often widespread blast-cell transformation of lymphocytes with many mitoses and blurring of the normal architectural features. Follicles may or may not be preserved. The mimicry of a high-grade malignant lymphoma is made greater in some cases by the presence of atypical blast cells which sometimes resemble Reed–Sternberg cells. The disturbance of nodal architecture is, however, more apparent than real and the sinuses, filled with basophilic immunoblasts, can still be made out (Fig. 24.29).

It is now known that in the early stages of the reaction T-cells predominate, but as the disease progresses more and more of the blast cells are B-cells and these often show plasmacytoid differentiation.

Boys who have congenital agammaglobulinaemia and who then become infected with EBV may develop a fatal disease with uncontrolled proliferation of lymphoid cells (Duncan's disease). Other herpes-type viruses (*herpes zoster, vaccinia, cytomegalovirus*) from time to time cause lymphadenitis with broadly similar, though generally much milder immunoblastic proliferation in the nodes, accompanied by the presence of atypical lymphoid cells in the bloodstream.

Acquired immunodeficiency syndrome (AIDS)

This grave disease, which has come into prominence in the past decade, is now known to be caused by a type C retrovirus—the *human immunodeficiency virus* (HIV). The virus is generally transmitted by blood or blood products from an infected individual, and most of the reported cases have been in male homosexuals, drug addicts who have shared syringes or needles, or in haemophiliacs who have received infected blood products. More recently, heterosexual transmission has been recognized. Once acquired, HIV proliferates in the T-lymphocytes of the host indefinitely, leading to reversal of the T-helper–T-suppressor cell (TH/TS) ratio and ultimately to complete immune paresis and death from intercurrent infection. There is also an increased risk of malignant lymphoma and possibly other malignant diseases developing. The time sequence in this evolution seems to be variable and it is not known whether or not untreated HIV infection invariably terminates fatally.

Typically, widespread painless lymphadenopathy develops in the early stages of HIV infection, when the patient, often an adult male, may also complain of malaise and listlessness. This stage is commonly referred to as persistent generalized lymphadenopathy (PGL), a term which emphasizes the frequently

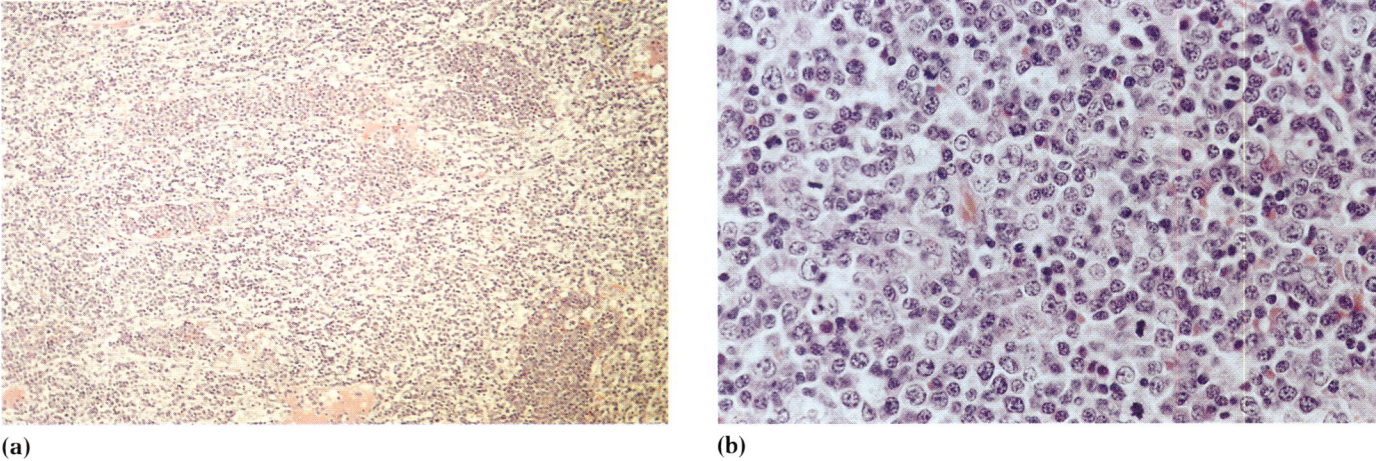

(a)   **(b)**

Fig. 24.29 Mesenteric lymph node in infectious mononucleosis. (a) Low magnification, showing loss of normal pattern but dilated sinuses stuffed with cells; (b) high magnification, showing huge numbers of transformed cells (immunoblasts), some with plasmacytoid features. Note mitoses.

long duration of the lymph node enlargement. Immunological function is still preserved, although a progressive reversal of the TH/TS ratio may be observed and, in some cases, lesions of Kaposi's sarcoma may appear either in the skin or in the nodes. After an interval of months or years, clinical lymphadenopathy disappears and is superseded by the phase of immune deficiency when loss of weight, diarrhoea, and cerebral impairment are common symptoms. At this stage, opportunistic infections such as *Pneumocystis* pneumonia are very frequent. The lymph nodes in the terminal stages of the disease are very small and may be difficult to find on post-mortem examination.

Biopsy of a lymph node in PGL shows striking follicular hyperplasia, out of all proportion to the reaction in the paracortex. Indeed, the latter may appear relatively depleted of lymphocytes, although plasma cells may be plentiful. The very large, and sometimes irregular, germinal centres (Fig. 24.30) show a poorly developed mantle zone and the edges of the centres themselves may show a 'moth-eaten' appearance before the follicles start to shrink or disintegrate and finally disappear. Sometimes small granulomas are seen and so-called 'immature sinus histiocytosis' is often present, so that the picture has to be distinguished from that of toxoplasmosis. The high endothelial venules are unduly conspicuous when the paracortex shows cell depletion, and as the node atrophies proliferation of these vessels may be noted. In the later stages of AIDS, the shrunken lymph nodes show fibrosis and gross cellular depletion in which scanty aggregates of B-lymphocytes show where follicles have been.

Other viral diseases

Of other viral diseases in which lymphadenopathy is encountered, measles deserves mention, since the histological reaction evoked in the lymphoreticular tissues by this RNA virus is pathognomonic of the disease. In particular, the tonsils or appendix may be excised and subjected to examination in children during the incubation period of measles, when the

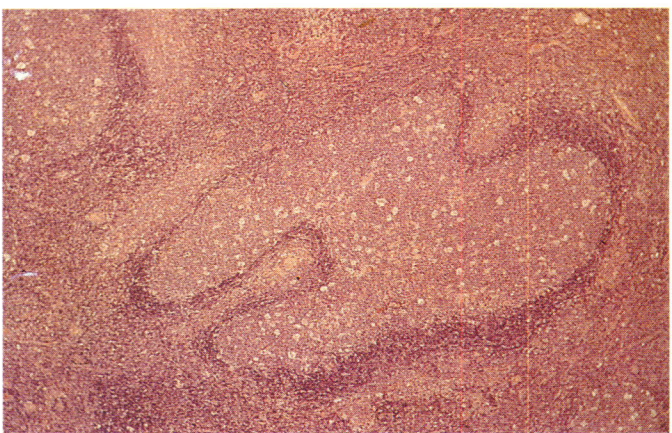

Fig. 24.30 Lymph node in the 'persistent generalized lymphadenopathy' stage of HIV infection, showing disproportionately large germinal follicles of irregular shape. Note the 'starry sky' pattern of the germinal centres.

lymphoid tissues are hyperplastic, but before the appearance of the rash. The hyperplastic lymphoid tissue of these sites is characterized by the presence of distinctive syncitial, Warthin–Finkeldey giant-cells which are seen within the germinal centres. Viral inclusion bodies are not seen and somewhat similar cells have been described in other conditions, but in a different setting.

24.3.12   Drug reactions

Lymphadenopathy is a well-known feature of serum sickness and there are a number of commonly used drugs which may cause a similar type of hypersensitivity reaction in certain individuals. These include some antibiotics (notably penicillin), sulphonamides, some antimalarials, and non-steroidal anti-inflammatory agents. In many instances the relationship of the patient's symptoms (rash, fever, joint pains, and lymphadeno-pathy) to the taking of a drug is obvious and the symptoms rapidly subside when the drug is withdrawn, or an alternative is substituted. Serious illness, or even death, is only liable to occur if for some reason the patient continues to take the offending drug. Difficulty may arise over the use of anticonvulsant drugs in epileptics, for the hydantoin derivatives, which are thera-peutically very effective, are also notoriously liable to cause gum hypertrophy and lymphadenopathy as side effects.

In all these cases the lymphadenopathy is generalized, but the histological findings vary markedly from case to case, depend-ing on the nature of the drug and the duration and severity of the reaction. Typically, the immune reaction involves the T-cells of the paracortex, which may show widespread blastic transformation, while the follicles are inactive or totally sup-pressed. In this respect there are close similarities to the changes of infectious mononucleosis, including the presence of atypical blast cells. The latter have been reported most frequently in hydantoin-associated lymphadenopathy, in which the picture may go on to resemble that of angioimmunoblastic lymph-adenopathy. In rare instances true malignant lymphomas have developed in these patients. On the other hand, in more acute reactions, eosinophilia and vasculitic changes often dominate the histological picture, and focal necrosis is common.

24.3.13　Disorders of unknown nature

Two further conditions remain to be described; in each of which the nature of the process involved is obscure, while the aeti-ology is entirely unknown.

Castleman's disease (giant lymph node hyperplasia, angiofollicular lymph node hyperplasia, lymph nodal hamartoma, pseudothymoma)

The number of proposed synonyms, of which the above are merely a selection, is an indication of the uncertainty surround-ing the nature of this uncommon disorder, and it is not even known whether or not the several forms of Castleman's disease are related to one another. Most frequent is the localized *hyaline vascular type*, which presents as a solitary, asymptomatic, tumour-like mass in the mediastinum, retroperitoneum, or else-where. The occurrence of such tumours in the young supports the hamartomatous theory of their origin, and their peculiar structure has been taken to lend further weight to this sugges-tion. The encapsulated tumour lacks lymph sinuses but has a rich network of blood vessel between the many 'pseudofollicles'. These show at their centres a small vessel surrounded by an 'onion-skin' arrangement of proliferated endothelial cells and hyaline material. This 'hyaline vascular' structure, superficially resembling a Hassall's corpuscle, is surrounded by concentric-ally packed layers of small lymphocytes (Fig. 24.31). Occasion-ally, some follicles with germinal centres are also present. The structure of the fully developed lesion is certainly very different from that of a lymph node, but on occasions 'follicles' of the type described may be seen developing within pre-existing lymph

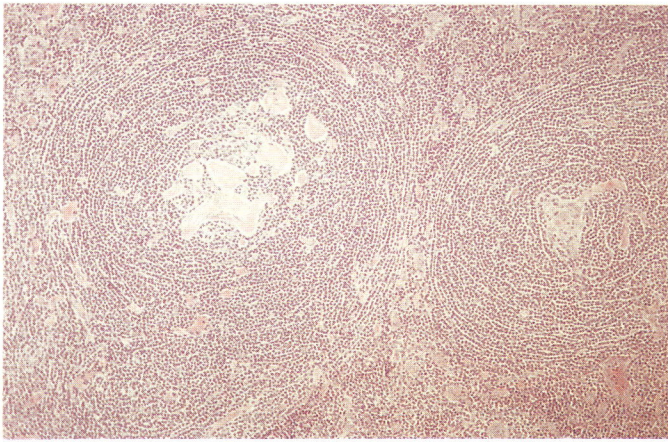

Fig. 24.31　Castleman's disease, showing parts of two hyaline vascu-lar 'follicles' with a rich network of sinusoidal vessels lying between.

nodes of otherwise normal appearance—an observation that runs counter to the hamartomatous theory cited.

The rarer *plasma-cell type* of Castleman's disease has been described in localized and generalized forms. These have many features in common but, as implied in the names, the *localized* form presents with a solitary tumour-like mass, similar to that of the hyaline vascular type, whereas the *generalized* or *multicentric* form presents with a more or less widespread lymphadenopathy. Clinically, both types of disease are often accompanied by fever, anaemia, and a variety of other systemic manifestations. Polyclonal hypergammaglobulinaemia is com-mon. That these systemic effects are related to the 'tumour' is evident from the often reported observation that removal of the 'tumour' in the localized form leads to rapid disappearance of the symptoms and signs of systemic disease.

Histologically the presence of 'hyaline vascular' follicles links these rarer types of Castleman's disease with the localized hyal-ine vascular type. True germinal follicles are, however, more frequently seen, especially in the multicentric type. The chief difference in both types lies in the presence of huge numbers of plasma cells in the interfollicular tissue. In many instances these cells are polytypic, but in some cases of identical mor-phology the plasma cells are monotypic. The significance of these findings has yet to be explained but, whatever the nature of the condition, there is little support for the idea that it is a neoplasm.

Histiocytosis X (Langerhans cell histiocytosis)

The above names embrace a triad of related disorders, charac-terized by focal or more widespread proliferation of distinctive histiocyte-like cells with features similar to those of the Langer-hans cells of the epidermis, whence, it has been suggested, the cells have migrated. The cells have abundant pale-staining cytoplasm and somewhat irregular, folded or grooved nuclei (Fig. 24.32), but their chief distinguishing feature is the presence in the cytoplasm at ultrastructural level of Birbeck granules.

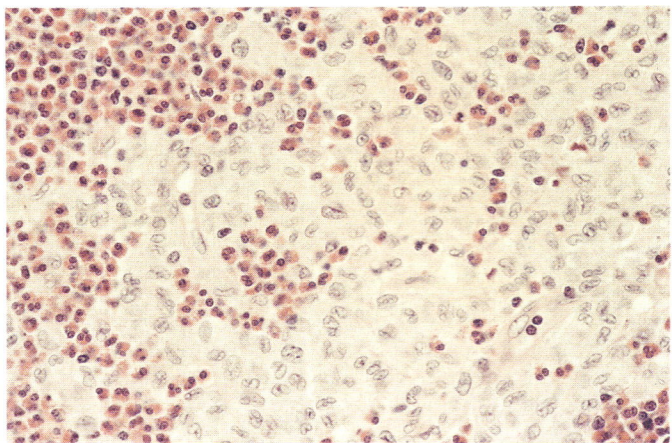

Fig. 24.32 Lymph node in histiocytosis X (eosinophilic granuloma) showing characteristic Langerhans-type cells and eosinophils in a lymph sinus. Note the grooved nuclei of the Langerhans cells.

The rare, acute form of histiocytosis X, *Letterer–Siwe disease*, is seen in infancy and is a systematized, febrile, and generally fatal disorder. The typical skin rash, hepatosplenomegaly, generalized lymphadenopathy, lytic bone lesions, and pulmonary infiltrates are all due to the accumulation in these tissues of histiocyte-like cells having abundant eosinophilic cytoplasm. Although the condition is generally believed not to be a neoplasm, the cells in Letterer–Siwe disease have larger, more hyperchromatic nuclei and appear more 'malignant' than those of the other, more localized forms of histiocytosis X.

The other two disorders, namely *Hand–Schüller–Christian syndrome* (HSCS) and *eosinophilic granuloma*, are closely allied to one another and are generally seen in somewhat older children or even in adults. Focal accumulations of the characteristic cells, often accompanied by numerous eosinophils, are found in bones, where they cause lytic lesions, and in skin, brain (HSCS), lungs, or lymph nodes. In the lymph nodes the cells predominantly occupy the lymph sinuses, in contradistinction to dermatopathic lymphadenitis where similar-looking cells are seen in the paracortex. The extent of involvement of different tissues is variable and in some instances isolated lymph nodes or bones (especially skull and vertebrae) are the only sites of disease.

In the nodes the cells tend to fill and expand the lymph sinuses, but the distinctive character of the 'histiocytes' and the presence of many eosinophils serve to distinguish the picture from that of 'sinus histiocytosis with massive lymphadenopathy' (p. 1759). The cellular infiltrate may be modified by the presence of multinucleate giant-cells with similar nuclei, by lipid in the cell cytoplasm, or by such massive eosinophilia that the Langerhans-type cells are obscured. In many instances, especially in childhood, the disease appears to be self-limiting and the lesions heal spontaneously with resultant fibrosis.

24.3.14 Further reading

Schnitzer, B. (1985). In *Surgical pathology of the lymph nodes and related organs* (ed. E. S. Jaffe), pp. 22–56. Saunders, Philadelphia.
Stansfeld, A. G. (1985). *Lymph node biopsy interpretation*, pp. 85–141, 184–90, 345–66. Churchill Livingstone, Edinburgh.
Wright, D. H. and Isaacson, P. G. (1983). Biopsy pathology of the lymphoreticular system, pp. 26–88. Chapman and Hall, London.

24.4 Hodgkin's disease

D. H. Wright

24.4.1 Introduction

Thomas Hodgkin, a physician at Guy's Hospital London and curator of the Anatomical Museum, published a paper in the *Journal of the Medical and Chirurgical Society* in 1832 'on some morbid appearances of the absorbent glands and spleen'. It is on this description of the gross pathology of six cases of lymphadenopathy, together with a seventh case drawn to his attention by his friend, Robert Carswell, that the eponym Hodgkin's disease (HD) rests. Hodgkin's contribution would probably have been lost in history had it not been publicized in later years by Dr Samual Wilkes, one of his successors at Guy's Hospital, who described further cases and drew attention to Hodgkin's original description. In 1926, Herbert Fox, a pathologist, subjected tissue from Hodgkin's six cases to histopathological analysis. He found microscopical features of HD in three cases and in one case each of tuberculosis, syphilis, and non-Hodgkin's lymphoma.

Various histopathological descriptions of HD were made at the turn of the last century. The characteristic giant cell seen in this disease was described by Carl Sternberg of Vienna, in 1898, and Dorothy Reed of Baltimore, Maryland, in 1902, and is known as the Reed–Sternberg (RS) cell, although W. S. Greenfield, of the University of Edinburgh, probably deserves precedence for his description of this cell in 1878. The diagnosis of HD is now based on the histopathological features of this disease, and the recognition of RS cells and their variants is central to this diagnosis.

Jackson and Parker (1947) introduced a histological classification of HD, dividing the disease into paragranuloma, granuloma, and sarcoma. Although widely adopted, this classification had the disadvantage that, although paragranuloma had a good prognosis and sarcoma a poor prognosis, over 90 per cent of patients fell into the granuloma category, making the prognostic discrimination of little value overall. The modern classification of HD was introduced by Lukes *et al.* (1966). It had six categories, which were shown to be prognostically significant when used in a retrospective analysis of cases. The six categories proposed by Lukes *et al.* were reduced to four in the Rye classification which is now used throughout the world (Rappaport *et al.* 1971). Lukes *et al.* postulated that HD is a single disease and that the various subtypes represent different host reactions against the neoplastic process. It now appears that this is not so, and that the histological subtypes of HD encompass at least two diseases and perhaps more.

24.4.2 Epidemiology

HD accounts for approximately 1 per cent of all cases of cancer in developed countries, and has half the frequency of non-Hodgkin's lymphomas. The annual incidence is in the region of 3 per 100 000 in England and Wales and appears to have increased slightly in the past two decades. An unusual feature of the age incidence of HD is that it is bimodal, with a peak in young adults followed by a plateau in middle age and a steep rise in old age. This double peak has led to the suggestion that HD is, in fact, two diseases. In the underdeveloped world, where HD generally has a lower incidence, the disease occurs more frequently in children, and the young adult peak is absent or attenuated.

There appears to be an increased risk of HD, particularly of the nodular sclerosis subtype, in people of higher social class. This, together with the different age distribution in the developing world, has been interpreted as suggesting that HD is caused by a common environmental agent to which those in poor socio-economic circumstances are exposed in childhood with a low risk of developing HD, whereas those in better circumstances are not exposed until later life and have a higher risk of developing HD; a model analogous to that of paralytic poliomyelitis. The Epstein–Barr virus has been considered as a possible aetiological agent for HD. This hypothesis is based on the observation that patients with previous infectious mononucleosis have a threefold increased risk of developing HD. Patients with HD also have an increased incidence and titre of antibodies to EBV. This latter observation may, of course, merely reflect the impaired T-cell immunity associated with HD, allowing greater viral replication to occur. EBV DNA has been detected in Hodgkin's tissue by filter nucleic acid hybridization (Southern blotting) in up to 35% of cases. The use of the polymerase chain reaction has identified EBV DNA in an even higher proportion of cases. Analysis of the terminal repeat portions of EBV genomes suggests that the EBV infected cells are monoclonal and *in situ* hybridization has localized the EBV DNA to Reed–Sternberg cells. EBV encoded latent gene products, including the latent membrane protein, which is thought to have an important role in EBV induced cell transformation, have been detected in Reed–Sternberg cells using immunohistochemistry. Familial cases of HD, although not common, are well recognized. Siblings of patients with HD have been shown to have a greater risk of developing HD than the general population. This may reflect exposure to an environmental influence, or be associated with genetic factors controlling immunocompetence, such as HLA haplotypes.

24.4.3 Clinical features

Presentation

Although there is overlap between the clinical features of HD and non-Hodgkin's lymphoma (NHL), HD has a distinctive clin-ical presentation and progression. The most frequent presentation is with painless lymphadenopathy (cervical 60 per cent, axillary 20 per cent, inguinal and femoral 15 per cent). Occasional patients experience pain or discomfort in the enlarged lymph nodes following alcohol ingestion. Initial complaints also include systemic symptoms of fever, drenching night sweats, weight loss, or itching. Extranodal and intra-abdominal tumours are very rare as presenting features, and are much more frequently encountered as features of NHL. The diagnosis of HD is almost invariably established by lymph node biopsy.

Staging

A system for the anatomical staging of HD was established in 1971 and is known as the Ann Arbor staging system (Table 24.2). The anatomical stage is further modified by the absence (A) or presence (B) of systemic symptoms (fever, night sweats, weight loss). Treatment protocols are based on this system with most stage 1 and 2 patients being treated by radiotherapy and most stage 3 and 4 patients with chemotherapy. Stage is a strong indicator of prognosis. The high success rate achieved in the treatment of HD has been, in part, due to the accurate staging of the disease. Prior to this, relapse was often due to the failure to identify and treat clinically occult tumours. Staging procedures include a full clinical examination, liver function tests, full blood count, and ESR, followed by bone marrow trephine biopsy and aspiration. Radiological staging includes chest radiographs (Fig. 24.33), bipedal lymphogram, and intravenous pyelogram (Fig. 24.34). Isotopic scans, CT scan, NMR, and ultrasound have a role in selected cases.

Until recently, staging laparotomy with splenectomy, liver biopsy, and biopsy of selected lymph nodes was included as part of the staging investigation of most patients with HD. The rationale of this approach was that fine slicing of the spleen is the only way to determine whether it is involved by HD, since this is

---

Table 24.2 Ann Arbor staging system for Hodgkin's disease

Stage 1
Involvement of a single lymph node region (1) or a single extralymphatic organ or site (1E)

Stage 2
Involvement of two or more lymph node regions on the same side of the diaphragm (2) or localized involvement of an extralymphatic organ or site and one or more lymph node regions on the same side of the diaphragm (2E)

Stage 3
Involvement of lymph node regions on both sides of the diaphragm (3) which may also be accompanied by localized involvement of an extralymphatic organ or site (3E) or by involvement of the spleen (3S) or both (3SE)

Stage 4
Diffuse or disseminated involvement of one of more extralymphatic organs or tissues with or without associated lymph node enlargement; the reason for classifying the patient as Stage 4 should be identified further by defining the site with symbols (e.g. 4 H + M + : liver and bone marrow involved)

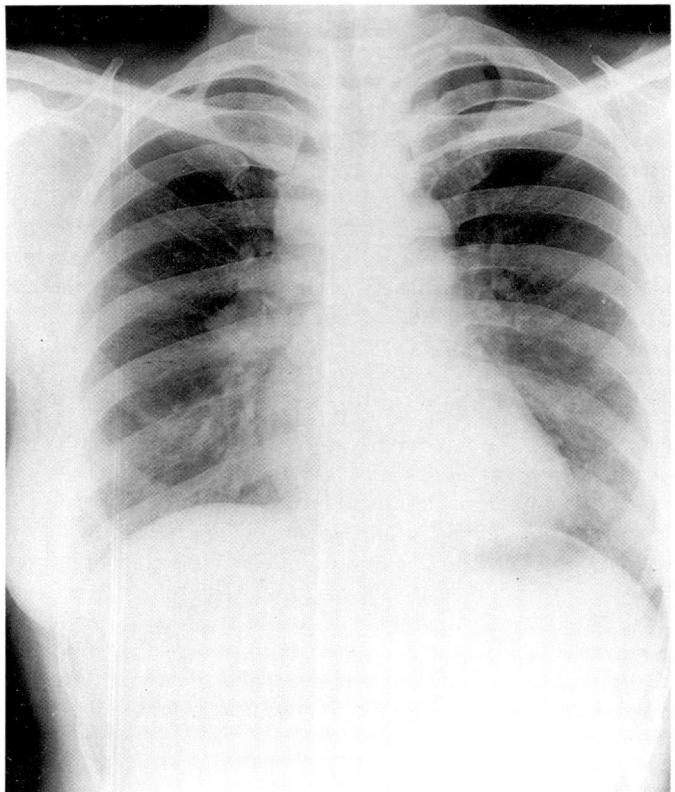

Fig. 24.33 Chest X-ray from a patient with nodular sclerosing Hodgkin's disease, showing marked widening of the superior mediastinum and some right hilar node enlargement. (By kind permission of Dr P. Guyer.)

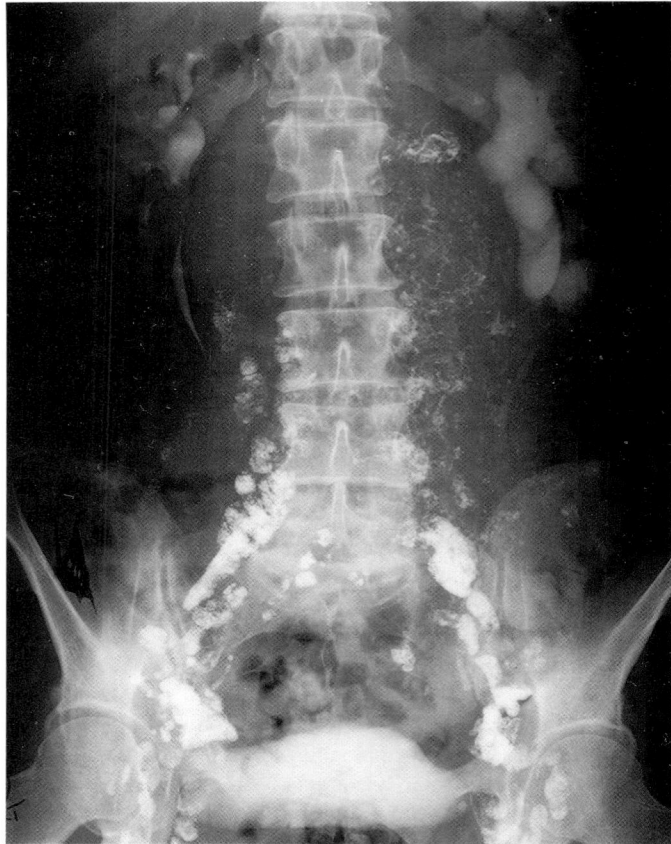

Fig. 24.34 A 24-hour lymphangiogram film with an intravenous pyelogram in a patient with Hodgkin's disease. The inguinal lymph nodes, overlying the femoral heads medially, are normal. The iliac nodes are enlarged, although with a normal pattern. There is massive enlargement of the para-aortic nodes with gross architectural disturbance, indicating involvement by lymphoma. They are displacing the right ureter laterally and causing a left hydronephrosis due to pressure on the pelvi-ureteric junction. (By kind permission of Dr P. Guyer.)

not accurately predicted by the size of the organ. Upper abdominal lymph nodes are not seen on lymphogram, and these could be directly sampled at laparotomy. Clearly, staging laparotomy would not be performed in patients in whom chemotherapy had already been selected as the treatment of choice. Staging laparotomy identified the precise anatomical distribution of HD in a large number of cases (pathological stage, Fig. 24.35). Staging laparotomy is now rarely used. This is partly because so much more is known about the disease that optimal treatment schedules can be predicted from clinical, radiological, and biopsy data, thus avoiding the mortality and morbidity of laparotomy and splenectomy.

Staging investigations, in general, support the concept that HD disseminates in a predictable manner, between contiguous lymph node groups. Haematogenous spread appears to occur mainly from the spleen. Involvement of the liver and bone marrow almost never occurs in the absence of splenic tumour.

24.4.4 Immunology

The association of HD with infectious disease, particularly tuberculosis, was well recognized at the beginning of this century. Even patients with untreated HD appear to have impairment of their T-cell function. This immunodeficiency caused by

the disease itself is exacerbated by splenectomy, radiotherapy, and chemotherapy. Splenectomy, performed as part of the staging procedure, leaves patients susceptible to infection by capsulated bacteria, particularly pneumococcus, meningococcus, and *Haemophilus influenzae*. Heavily treated patients, often those with persistent disease, are susceptible to a number of opportunistic infections, including atypical mycobacteria, fungi (*Candida* sp., *Aspergillus* sp., *Cryptococcus neoformans*, *Pneumocystis carinii*), protozoa (*Toxoplasma gondii*), and viruses (varicella, *Herpes zoster*, *Herpes simplex*, cytomegalovirus). A demyelinating disease, progressive multifocal leukoencephalopathy, caused by the polyoma virus, is a rare complication.

24.4.5 Pathology

Gross pathology

Lymph nodes involved by Hodgkin's disease may attain a considerable size. They usually remain discrete and do not become

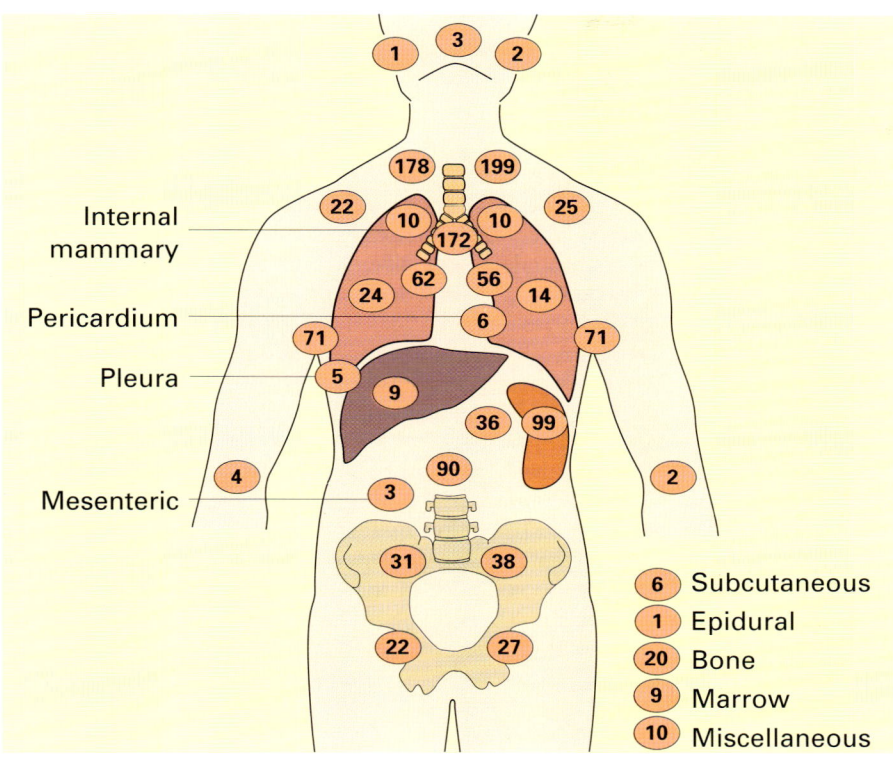

Fig. 24.35 Hodgkin's disease showing the anatomic distribution of sites of involvement in 285 consecutive, unselected, previously untreated cases (285 cases, 272 laparotomies). (Drawn after Kaplan *et al.* (1973), with permission of Dr S. Rosenberg.)

matted together as in tuberculosis and some infective processes. The cut surface will vary in consistency, depending on the subtype of Hodgkin's disease. Nodes involved by nodular sclerosing Hodgkin's disease may be firm and fibrous and the nodularity may be discernible to the naked eye. The cut surface of Hodgkin's tissue sometimes exhibits a pale tan coloration. In the spleen the tumour forms irregular nodules that may become confluent. Small areas of necrosis, within these nodules, are common.

Histopathology

The histopathological diagnosis of Hodgkin's disease is based on the recognition of the Reed–Sternberg cell in an appropriate cellular setting for one of the subtypes of Hodgkin's disease. The classic Reed–Sternberg cell has a bilobed nucleus with large eosinophilic nucleoli separated by a clear space from a thickened nuclear membrane, giving the cell an 'owl's eye' appearance. The cytoplasm is usually well defined and stains either deeply eosinophilic or amphophilic (Fig. 24.36).

Mononuclear cells, with similar nuclear characteristics, are frequently seen in Hodgkin's disease and are referred to as Hodgkin's cells. They may represent Reed–Sternberg cells cut in a plane that shows only one lobe of the nucleus. Similar cells are seen in a number of reactive and neoplastic conditions, so that the finding of Hodgkin's cells is not, in itself, sufficient for the diagnosis of Hodgkin's disease.

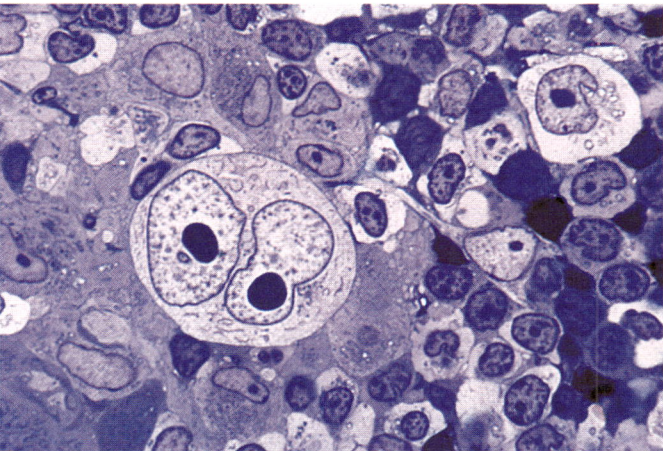

Fig. 24.36 Sections of Hodgkin's disease tissue showing a classic Reed–Sternberg cell. The binucleate cell shows large nucleoli, relatively clear nuclear chromatin, and a thick nuclear membrane. Plastic embedded sections, stained with toluidin blue.

Nodular lymphocyte/histiocyte-predominant Hodgkin's disease (NLPHD)

Histopathologically, this disease is characterized by a nodular proliferation (Fig. 24.37) consisting predominantly of small lymphocytes with a variable number of histiocytes. Histiocytes

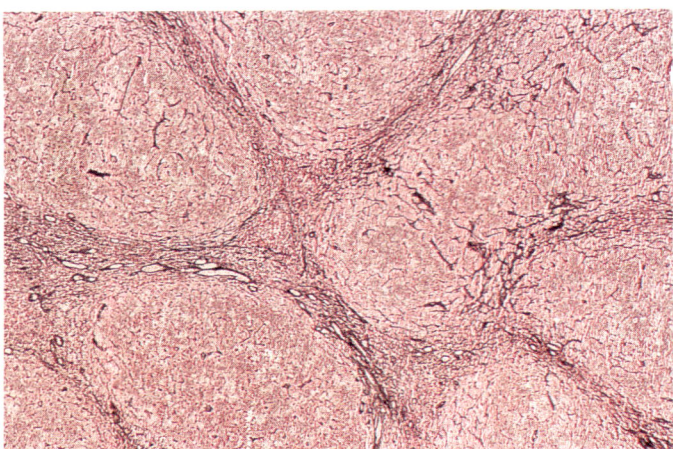

Fig. 24.37 Nodular lymphocyte predominant Hodgkin's disease. This reticulin-stained section shows the nodular structure of this lesion. Gordon and Sweet reticulin stain.

are usually less frequent in NLPHD than in diffuse LPHD. The RS cells that characterize this type of HD (polylobated RS cells, 'popcorn' cells) differ from the classic RS cells in their morphology (Fig. 24.38). They are usually scattered amongst the lymphocytes and histiocytes but, in some cases, are more abundant, particularly at the centre of nodules. Polylobated RS cells express B-cell markers and synthesize cytoplasmic immunoglobulin, in contrast to the uptake of immunoglobulin shown by some classic RS cells. They are, however, polytypic with respect to light chain expression, suggesting that NLPHD is not a neoplastic proliferation.

Patients with NLPHD usually present with enlargement of a single lymph node or group of nodes (stage 1). The disease has a good prognosis, even when untreated, although relapse is frequent (Regula *et al.* 1988); between 3–5 per cent of patients go on to develop large cell, non-Hodgkin's lymphomas or, rarely,

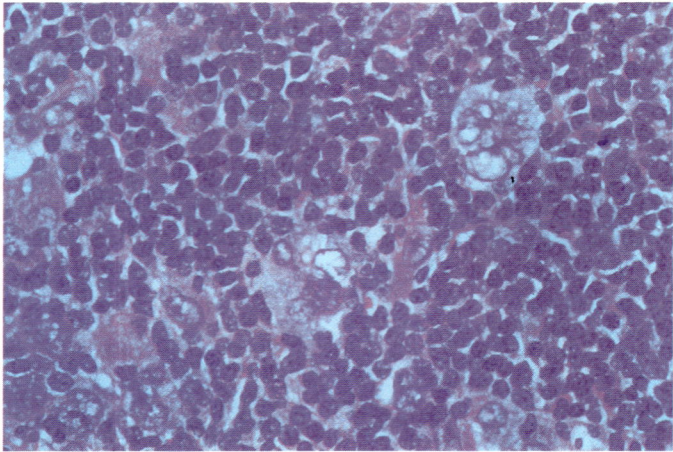

Fig. 24.38 Polylobated Reed–Sternberg cells (popcorn cells) from a case of lymphocyte predominant Hodgkin's disease. The appearance of the multilobated nucleus is different from that of classic Reed–Sternberg cells.

other types of HD. This progression occurs in untreated as well as treated patients, indicating that these are not secondary, therapy-induced neoplasms.

Occasional biopsies of reactive lymph nodes show an expansion of one or more germinal follicles due to an influx of small lymphocytes that disrupt the germinal centre. This condition has been called 'progressive transformation of germinal centres'. The transformed centres may closely mimic NLPHD in their morphology, the difference being that NLPHD contains polylobated RS cells whereas progressively transformed germinal centres contain isolated, morphologically normal germinal centre cells. A number of reports have noted an association between progressive transformation of germinal centres and NLPHD, and it is possible that some cases of progressive transformation of germinal centres may progress to NLPHD.

NLPHD differs from other types of HD in its histopathological features, immunohistochemistry, clinical presentation, and progression. It is unfortunate that it bears the name HD since, if it is not identified as a separate entity, it could confuse studies of that disease. The use of the term 'nodular paragranuloma', rather than NLPHD, might help to emphasize the different nature of this disease.

Diffuse lymphocyte/histiocyte-predominant Hodgkin's disease (DLPHD)

DLPHD differs from NLPHD in its diffuse growth pattern and often by the presence of larger numbers of histiocytes, which may be the predominant cell type in some cases. Although Lukes *et al.* (1966) identified NLPHD and DLPHD as separate entities, in the Rye classification they were combined in the category of lymphocyte-predominant HD. This might appear to be justified, in view of their histological similarities and the fact that some cases of NLPHD show areas with a diffuse growth pattern. Recent studies, however, indicate that there are differences between these two diseases, as reported. In only a minority of cases of DLPHD do the RS cells express B-cell markers, in contrast with NLPHD. Clinically, patients with DLPHD frequently present with stage 3 or 4 disease, whereas NLPHD is almost invariably stage 1. These reports probably reflect the difficulty encountered in the histopathological identification of DLPHD. It is probable that many cases placed in this category are, in fact, examples of histiocyte-rich T-cell lymphomas (Lennert's lymphoma) or of mixed-cellularity Hodgkin's disease.

Nodular sclerosing Hodgkin's disease (NSHD)

As its name implies, NSHD is characterized by bands of fibrous tissue that extend in from the thickened capsule dividing the Hodgkin's tissue into nodules. The disease is also characterized by the presence of lacunar RS cells, classic RS cells often being difficult to find. Lacunar RS cells have complex, often multilobated, nuclei with nucleoli that are usually much smaller than those seen in classic RS cells (Fig. 24.39). In cytological and electron microscopical preparations they are seen to have voluminous and relatively clear cytoplasm. In routinely processed histopathological preparations this cytoplasm retracts, leaving a clear space, or lacuna, around the cell (Fig. 24.39).

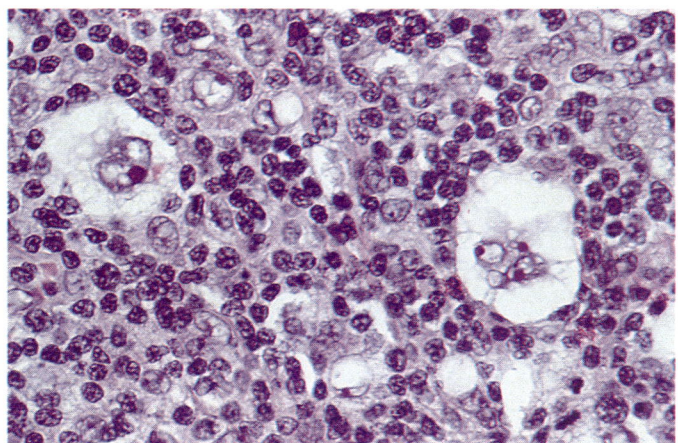

Fig. 24.39 Lacunar Reed–Sternberg cells from a case of nodular sclerosing Hodgkin's disease. These cells have an abundant, pale cytoplasm that often shrinks during processing, leaving a clear space around the cell.

The amount of fibrous tissue found in NSHD varies. In extreme cases, almost the whole node is replaced by collagen. At the other end of the spectrum, collagen may be scanty and pathologists are divided as to whether such cases should be categorized as NSHD or not. Biopsies showing lacunar RS cells, but little or no fibrosis, have been categorized as cellular-phase nodular sclerosis (NS). The justification for this categorization is that patients with cellular-phase NS have been shown to have classic NSHD at other sites or to show typical sclerosis in later biopsies. These studies suggest that cellular phase is part of the spectrum of NSHD. However, difficulties arise when biopsies are encountered that show only occasional lacunar cells in a node that would otherwise be called mixed-cellularity HD. From a clinical point of view this difficulty may not be of importance, since cellular-phase NS has been shown to have a similar prognosis to mixed-cellularity HD (Colby *et al.* 1981).

One of the disadvantages of the Jackson and Parker classification of HD was that most patients fell into the category of Hodgkin's granuloma, so that prognostically significant subtypes could not be identified. Although the Rye classification appeared initially to identify subtypes of prognostic significance, advances in therapy, together with the high proportion of cases in the NSHD category in many studies, has tended to blur these differences. Attempts have, therefore, been made to subdivide the NS subgroup. A large study from the American National Institutes of Health found that the only prognostically significant feature, within the NS subgroup, was the amount of sclerosis that was positively correlated with survival (Colby *et al.* 1981). A large study in England, however, showed that NS could be subdivided into a good prognosis group (grade 1) and a bad prognosis group (grade 2), the latter showing areas of lymphocyte depletion or of large numbers of RS cells and Hodgkin's cells, often forming confluent masses. Since grade 2 NS accounts for 22 per cent of all cases of HD, this subdivision would, if confirmed by further study, be of clinical value.

Other workers have drawn attention to the presence of sheets of RS and HD cells in NSHD, not so much from a prognostic point of view but to highlight the diagnostic difficulty that these cases may pose. Pathologists can easily confuse these sheets of cells with NHL or metastatic tumours. Areas of necrosis are often found within these sheets of RS and HD cells.

Mixed-cellularity Hodgkin's disease (MCHD)

MCHD shows a spectrum of appearances from abundant lymphocytes at one extreme and lymphocyte-depleted Hodgkin's disease (LDHD) at the other. The exact cut-off point between these subtypes is, to some extent, subjective. Lymphocytes, histiocytes, eosinophils, plasma cells, fibrosis, and necrosis are present in variable proportions. In MCHD, classic RS cells (Fig. 24.40) should be easy to find. Biopsies showing prominent follicular hyperplasia with areas of MCHD in the paracortex have been described as interfollicular HD. Such cases are of importance to histopathologists who might overlook the interfollicular HD and report the node as reactive. This presumed early involvement of the T-dependent areas is also of interest in relation to the histogenesis and pathogenesis of HD.

Hodgkin's disease, lymphocyte-depleted reticular

Reticular Hodgkin's disease is equivalent to Hodgkin's sarcoma of the Jackson and Parker classification. The tumour is composed of sheets of RS and HD cells with few lymphocytes and other reactive cells (Fig. 24.41), although immunohistochemistry may show large numbers of histiocytes. Recent studies have shown a high rate of mis-diagnosis of reticular HD, with many cases being subsequently diagnosed as large-cell, non-Hodgkin's lymphoma. The differentiation between reticular HD and large-cell NHL, particularly of the T-cell phenotype, can be extremely difficult. Reticular HD is categorized as a poor prognosis subtype. However, if cases of NHL are excluded, the prognosis more closely approximates to that of other types of HD.

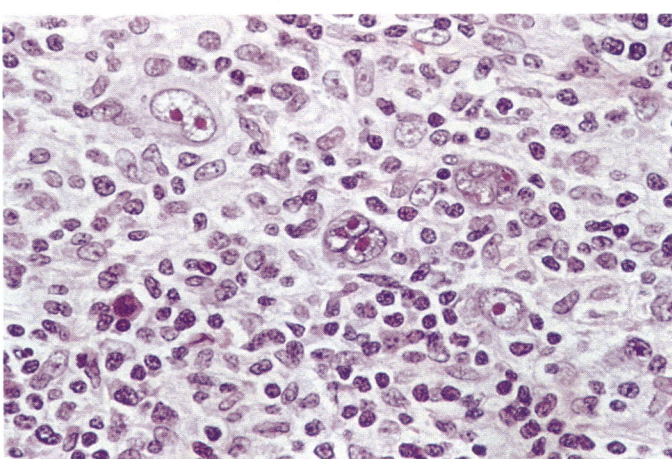

Fig. 24.40 Mixed-cellularity Hodgkin's disease showing Reed–Sternberg cells and mononuclear Hodgkin's cells. The background population is composed predominantly of lymphocytes and histiocytes.

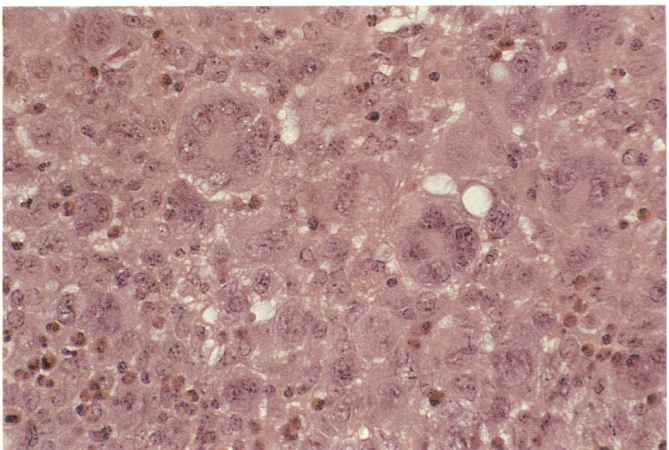

Fig. 24.41 Lymphocyte-depleted Hodgkin's disease, reticular type. The section shows numerous multinucleated cells, resembling Reed–Sternberg cell variants. The sparse background population includes histiocytes and eosinophils.

Hodgkin's disease, lymphocyte-depleted, diffuse fibrosis

This type of HD is characterized by scanty RS cells and HD cells in a cell-poor stroma of amorphous eosinophilic tissue. The term 'diffuse fibrosis' is a misnomer since there is little mature collagen in the stroma. Patients with LDHD diffuse fibrosis often present with fever, anaemia, jaundice, and hepatosplenomegaly without significant lymph node enlargement. The diagnosis is often established on the basis of bone marrow or liver biopsy or at post-mortem examination.

Diagnosis of Hodgkin's disease at other sites

In lymph node biopsy and splenic tissue the diagnosis of Hodgkin's disease is based on the finding of Reed–Sternberg cells in an appropriate cellular environment. When dealing with bone marrow trephine biopsies and liver biopsies less tissue is available for examination and this rule may be relaxed in a patient who has already had a diagnosis of Hodgkin's disease at another site. For example, in a liver biopsy, the finding of mononuclear Hodgkin's cells in an appropriate setting would be acceptable as evidence of involvement in a patient with known Hodgkin's disease. Occasionally, in tissue obtained at staging laparotomies, epithelioid cell granulomas are found in the T-dependent areas of the spleen and in the portal tracts of the liver. The cause of these granulomas is unclear. They do not, however, represent involvement by Hodgkin's disease; indeed, some studies have shown that patients with such granulomas have a better prognosis than those without.

24.4.6   The nature of the Reed–Sternberg cell

The histogenesis of the RS cell, central to our understanding of the nature of HD, has been the subject of intense research in recent years. Paradoxically, many of the techniques that have done so much to unravel the mysteries of NHL appear to have increased the confusion surrounding HD.

Immunohistochemistry

This technique has shown that the polylobated RS cells of NLPHD express B-cell markers and synthesize immunoglobulin. Some reports claim that they do not show light chain restriction, suggesting that they may not be neoplastic. The phenotype of these cells differs from that of classic RS cells and lacunar RS cells. These have been shown to express B- and/or T-cell markers in a variable manner, but to express more consistently the CD15 antigen that is also strongly expressed by cells of the granulocyte lineage. RS cells also possess an antigen (CD30) identified by an antibody raised to an HD cell line. This antigen was, at one stage, thought to be specific for RS cells and their precursors but is now regarded as an activation marker expressed on reactive and neoplastic lymphoid cells. The immunophenotype of RS cells does not appear to correspond to that of any potential benign analogue.

Gene rearrangement studies

These studies are complicated by the fact that RS cells may account for a very small part of the DNA extracted from HD tissue. This may explain the failure of many workers to identify a clonal gene rearrangement in most cases of HD. Clonal rearrangements of immunoglobulin or T-cell receptor genes have been identified in some cases of HD. These results do not yet allow us to form a coherent view of the identity of the RS cell or the nature of the Hodgkin's proliferation.

Cell culture

Several cell lines have been established from effusions and biopsies obtained from patients with HD. Some of these cell lines have been of the B-cell, and some of the T-cell, lineage. They have many interesting properties but their exact relationship to RS cells is debatable.

Cytogenetics

The mixed cellular composition of most HD biopsies, with a relatively small number of RS cells and HD cells in most, has made cytogenetic studies difficult. A variety of chromosomal abnormalities have been described but no chromosomal abnormality specific for HD has been detected.

24.4.7   Second malignancies in Hodgkin's disease

Patients treated for HD by chemotherapy with, or without, radiotherapy have an increased risk of developing acute granulocytic leukaemia. There is a smaller and less definite risk of developing solid tumours. Children are at greater risk of developing second malignancies than adults. The increased risk of second malignancies is presumably due to the carcinogenic action of the drugs used to treat Hodgkin's disease. Immunodeficiency, associated with the disease and its treatment, might possibly also play a causative role. Although a serious complication, second malignancies are relatively uncommon in long-term survivors in comparison with deaths due to persistent Hodgkin's disease and infections.

24.4.8 Bibliography

Colby, T. V., Hoppe, R. T., and Warnke, R. A. (1981). Hodgkin's disease: A clinicopathologic study of 659 cases. *Cancer* **49**, 1848–58.

Jackson, H., Jr and Parker, F., Jr (1947). *Hodgkin's disease and allied disorders*. Oxford University Press, New York.

Kaplan, H. S., Dorfman, R. F., Nelsen, T. S., and Rosenberg, S. A. (1973). Staging laparotomy and splenectomy in Hodgkin's disease: Analysis of indications and patterns of involvement in 285 consecutive, unselected patients. *National Cancer Institute Monograph* **36**, 291–301.

Lukes, R. J. and Butler, J. J. (1966). The pathology and nomenclature of Hodgkin's disease. *Cancer Research* **26**, 1063–81.

Lukes, R. J., Butler, J. J., and Hicks, E. B. (1966). Natural history of Hodgkin's disease as related to its pathologic picture. *Cancer* **19**, 317–44.

Rappaport, H., Berard, C. W., Butler, J. J., Dorfman, R. F., Lukes, R. J., and Thomas, L. B. (1971). Report of the committee on histopathological criteria contributing to staging of Hodgkin's disease. *Cancer Research* **31**, 1864–5.

Regula, D. P., Hoppe, R. T., and Weiss, L. M. (1988). Nodular and diffuse types of lymphocyte predominance Hodgkin's disease. *New England Journal of Medicine* **318**, 214–19.

24.5 The non-Hodgkin's lymphomas

P. G. Isaacson

24.5.1 Introduction

It is a testament to the genius of Thomas Hodgkin that the disease he described in 1832, 16 years before Virchow established the cellular basis of disease, has survived as a clinicopathological entity through the development of the microscope and all the subsequent histopathological techniques. While it has long been evident that neoplasms other than Hodgkin's disease arise in the lymphoreticular system and the heterogeneous nature of these tumours has been recognized, none has come near to acquiring an identity as distinctive as that of Hodgkin's disease. For this reason they have come to be known collectively as the non-Hodgkin's lymphomas. The separation of this group of malignant tumours into distinct entities, as a basis for rational therapy, has been a long-standing objective which has been given great impetus by the therapeutic successes in Hodgkin's disease. There is considerable geographical variation in the incidence and relative incidence of Hodgkin's disease and non-Hodgkin's lymphoma. In less-developed countries there is a higher incidence of lymphoma generally and Hodgkin's disease accounts for well over 50 per cent of all cases. In the United Kingdom, and countries of a similar level of development, lymphomas comprise 3–5 per cent of all malignancies with non-Hodgkin's lymphoma accounting for 60 per cent of cases. Unlike Hodgkin's disease, which rarely arises outside lymph nodes, up to 40 per cent of non-Hodgkin's lymphomas (again depending on geographical location) arise in extranodal sites. These extranodal lymphomas, although broadly similar, behave somewhat differently from their nodal cousins and will be discussed in a separate section in this chapter. Confusion sometimes arises from the use of the terms 'lymphoma' and 'malignant lymphoma'; these terms are synonymous, there being no such recognized entity as a benign neoplasm of the lymphoreticular system.

24.5.2 The classification of non-Hodgkin's lymphoma

To the early pathologists the histological appearances of all non-Hodgkin's lymphomas were alike, consisting of replacement of the normal lymph node architecture by sheets of small dark-staining cells. However, it was quite clear that not all cases behaved alike and pathologists were increasingly asked by their clinical colleagues to attempt to predict the natural course of the individual case since, even without treatment, the survival of patients with non-Hodgkin's lymphoma varied from a few months to many years. As more effective means of therapy were developed and therapeutic successes with Hodgkin's disease (itself diagnosed on histological grounds) began to emerge, the demand for a more meaningful histological diagnosis of non-Hodgkin's lymphoma grew to a clamour. In response to this, the first clinically relevant histological classification of the non-Hodgkin's lymphomas was formulated in 1966 by Henry Rappaport, one of the great lymphoreticular pathologists. Broadly speaking, the Rappaport classification divided lymphomas into those composed of small cells and those composed of large cells, each of which could be further subdivided into those with a follicular (or nodular) pattern and those that were diffuse. The follicular and small-celled tumours were biologically less aggressive; therefore, a better survival could be expected and, importantly, less potent and, therefore, less toxic therapy was suitable for these cases. The converse applied to cases with a diffuse pattern, especially if composed of large cells. As histological techniques improved, allowing finer discrimination between cells, so more detailed classifications emerged. In parallel with these improvements it was becoming possible to identify the phenotype of the lymphoma cells using immunological techniques, first in cell suspensions and later on the tissue sections themselves. It soon became evident that the lymphoma cells were closely related to normal lymph node cells and that most (50 per cent or more) non-Hodgkin's lymphomas were derived from B-cells of the follicle centre. It was also clear, however, that there was an alarmingly wide variety of lymphoreticular neoplasms. A whole host of soundly based classifications sprung up, causing so much confusion that a series of special international meetings were convened to decide on a single clinically relevant classification that could be used throughout the world. The result was the so-called Working Formulation for Clinical Use (Table 24.3) which divides lymphomas up into three grades of malignancy on strictly

Table 24.3 A working formulation of non-Hodgkin's lymphomas for clinical usage

Low grade
  A. Malignant lymphoma, small lymphocytic
      consistent with CLL
      plasmacytoid
  B. Malignant lymphoma, follicular
      Predominantly small cleaved cell
        diffuse areas
        sclerosis
  C. Malignant lymphoma, follicular
      Mixed small cleaved and large cell
        diffuse areas
        sclerosis

Intermediate grade
  D. Malignant lymphoma, follicular
      Predominantly large cell
        diffuse areas
        sclerosis
  E. Malignant lymphoma, diffuse
      Small cleaved cell
        sclerosis
  F. Malignant lymphoma, diffuse
      Mixed, small and large cell
        sclerosis
        epithelioid cell component
  G. Malignant lymphoma, diffuse
      Large cell
        cleaved cell
        non-cleaved cell
        sclerosis

High grade
  H. Malignant lymphoma
      Large cell, immunoblastic
        plasmacytoid
        clear cell
        polymorphous
        epithelioid cell component
  I. Malignant lymphoma
      Lymphoblastic
        convoluted cell
        non-convoluted cell
  J. Malignant lymphoma
      Small non-cleaved cell
        Burkitt's
        follicular areas

Miscellaneous
  Composite
  Mycosis fungoides
  Histiocytic
  Extramedullary plasmacytoma
  Unclassifiable
  Other

ideal is constantly changing as new diagnostic and therapeutic techniques evolve. The classification given in Table 24.4 is the updated Kiel classification. It has the virtue of simplicity, is partly biologically and immunologically based (which lends a degree of objectivity), and, in dividing lymphomas into those of low and high grade, has therapeutic relevance. While the Kiel classification is in common use throughout Europe, the working formulation is still preferred in the United States of America. For this reason, in this section, comparable terms from the working formulation are given as subheadings to those from the Kiel classification under which each category of non-Hodgkin's lymphoma is described.

Strictly the terms 'low grade' and 'high grade' as used in the Kiel classification refer to histological appearances and not clinical behaviour. However, they also have clinical relevance. Thus 'low-grade' lymphomas are slowly progressive, usually over a period of years, and respond to less potent and, therefore, less toxic forms of therapy, be it radiotherapy or chemotherapy. 'High-grade' lymphomas, on the other hand, are rapidly progressive and can result in death of the patient within a few months. Paradoxically, high-grade lymphomas may be more curable with modern forms of therapy than the low-grade tumours, which are slowly but relentlessly progressive. In evaluating the prognosis of an individual case of lymphoma, the clinical stage as well as the histological grade of the tumour has to be taken into account.

24.5.3 Non-Hodgkin's lymphoma of B-cell type

The majority of non-Hodgkin's lymphomas are derived from B-cells. A B-cell phenotype is often obvious from the morphological features of the lymphoma which, for example, may show a B-cell pattern in the form of follicle formation, or the cytological features of B-cells such as those of centrocytes, centroblasts, or plasma cells. While in most instances it is not difficult to discriminate between a neoplastic and a reactive B-cell proliferation, at times this can be extremely difficult and have very serious consequences for the management of the patient concerned. Immunocytochemistry is particularly helpful in this respect, as demonstration of light chain restriction (see p. 1749) indicates a monoclonal B-cell proliferation (Fig. 24.42); indeed, it is the only true tumour marker that there is. B-cell lymphomas, especially those showing differentiation into plasma cells, may secrete this light chain restricted immunoglobulin in amounts sufficient for detection in the circulation, or, as light chains, in the urine. Thus, careful analysis of plasma or urine proteins can be a useful adjunct of the diagnosis and in following the response to treatment. On occasion, for technical reasons, or because of an admixture of polyclonal B-cells in the lymphoma, it is impossible to use immunocytochemistry to demonstrate light chain restriction. Evidence for a monoclonal B-cell proliferation can then be obtained by analysing the tumour DNA for clonal immunoglobulin gene rearrangement, using the Southern blotting technique.

morphological grounds. Needless to say, there is not universal agreement over the working formulation. European pathologists, in particular, led by the prestigious group from Kiel in Germany, criticize the working formulation as not being sufficiently biologically based and, therefore, lacking objectivity. The ideal classification should be as simple as possible, be reproducible, so that comparable clinical trials can be performed in different centres, and give some guidance as to the most suitable treatment for any particular category. The problem is that this

Table 24.4 The updated Keil classification of non-Hodgkin's lymphoma

Low grade	Low grade
Lymphocytic–chronic lymphocytic and prolymphocytic leukaemia; hairy-cell leukaemia	Lymphocytic–chronic lymphocytic and prolymphocytic leukaemia
	Small, cerebriform cell-mycosis fungoides, Sezary's syndrome
Lymphoplasmacytic/cytoid (immunocytoma)	Lymphoepithelioid (Lennert's lymphoma)
Plasmacytic	Angioimmunoblastic (AILD)
Centroblastic/centrocytic follicular ± diffuse diffuse	T zone
Centrocytic	Pleomorphic, small cell (HTLV-1 ±)
High grade	High grade
Centroblastic	Pleomorphic, medium and large cell (HTLV-1 ±)
Immunoblastic	Immunoblastic (HTLV-1 ±)
Large cell anaplastic (Ki-1 ±)	Large cell anaplastic (Ki-1 +)
Burkitt lymphoma	
Lymphoblastic	Lymphoblastic
Rare types	Rare types

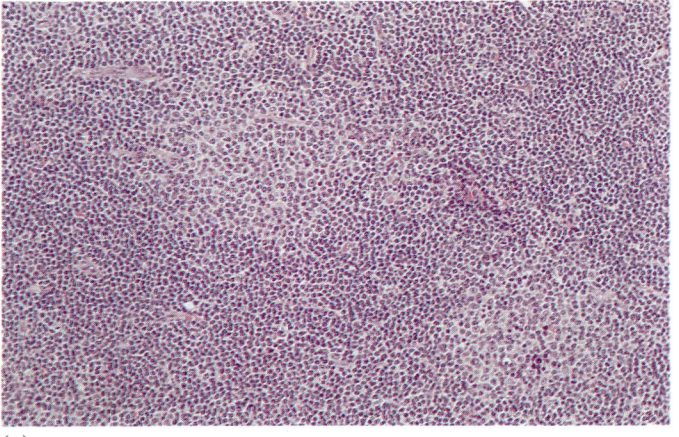 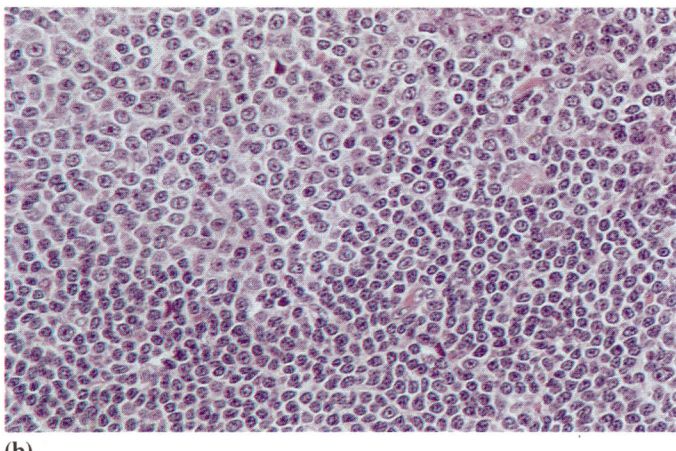

(a)　　　　　　　　　　　　　　　　　　　　　　(b)

Fig. 24.42 Malignant lymphoma lymphocytic. Low power (a) shows a diffuse infiltration of small lymphocytes within which there are ill-defined nodules of larger cells, the so-called proliferation centres. At high power (b) the cells of the proliferation centre, upper right, can be seen to be larger, with larger nuclei containing prominent nucleoli.

Malignant lymphoma lymphocytic

(ML small lymphocytic)

As its name suggests, this type of lymphoma is composed of small lymphocytes morphologically similar to those which form the mantle zone of the B-cell follicle in normal lymph nodes. Most cases are associated with chronic lymphocytic leukaemia, but in a minority the disease is confined to the lymph nodes at presentation. It is one of the commonest types of lymphoma, characteristically occurring in adults past middle age. Lymphadenopathy is usually generalized and the bone marrow is almost always involved. ML lymphocytic is a slowly progressive disease and many patients die of other causes unrelated to the disease itself, or from complications resulting from impaired immunity which is commonly present. Death directly attributable to the lymphoma usually follows transformation into a

tumour of much higher grade; this is sometimes known as Richter's syndrome.

Histology The normal architecture of the lymph node is usually completely effaced by an infiltrate of small lymphocytes, although in some instances occasional follicles are preserved. The monotony of this infiltrate is interrupted by focal collections of larger nucleolated cells; the so-called proliferation centres (Fig. 24.42). A similar infiltrate is seen in the spleen, the bone marrow, and may be found in almost any other organ, especially if the patient has chronic lymphocytic leukaemia. In those cases where the lymphoma transforms into a high-grade tumour, there is striking pleomorphism of large bizarre cells, which are often multinucleated and which are characterized by prominent nucleoli. Immunohistochemistry is helpful in the diagnosis of ML lymphocytic. The B-cell nature of the cells can

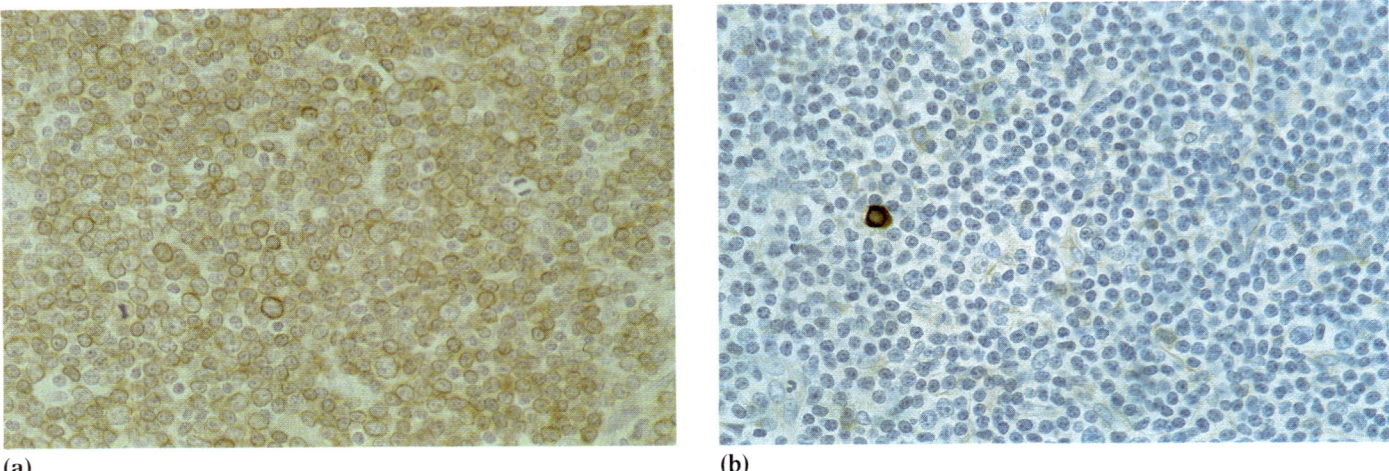

(a)   **(b)**

Fig. 24.43 Malignant lymphoma lymphocytic. The tumour has been stained with antibodies to κ (a) and λ (b) light chains, using the immunoperoxidase technique. Clear perinuclear space staining of the cells for κ light chain is evident. A single cell stains for λ light chain.

be confirmed using pan B-cell antibodies. Paradoxically, however, these neoplastic B-cells also express an antigen (CD5 antigen) which is present on most T-cells. The neoplastic (i.e. clonal) nature of the B-cells can be confirmed further by showing that the immunoglobulin they express is restricted to a single light chain type (Fig. 24.43).

Another entity included in the category of ML lymphocytic is the rare condition known as hairy-cell leukaemia. This condition is discussed in detail (see p. 1804). The lymph nodes are not usually significantly enlarged in this disease and so are seldom biopsied, but when they are, the biopsy shows a diffuse infiltrate of small cells with clear cytoplasm and rather featureless nuclei. Infiltration of the spleen, liver, and bone marrow results in a more distinctive picture caused by dilation of blood-filled sinuses lined by neoplastic hairy cells. These appearances are described in greater detail later in this chapter in the section on splenic disorders.

Malignant lymphoma lymphoplasmacytic

(ML small lymphocytic plasmacytoid)

This type of lymphoma is closely similar to the ML lymphocytic from which it is distinguished by differentiation of a proportion of the small lymphocytes into plasma cells (lymphoplasmacytic) or cells with some plasma cell features (lymphoplasmacytoid). ML lymphoplasmacytic is much less common than ML lymphocytic, but occurs in patients of the same age group, who also often present with chronic lymphocytic leukaemia. Presentation with isolated or generalized lymphadenopathy, without leukaemia, is more frequent than in ML lymphocytic, however. A significant proportion of cases present with a hyperviscosity syndrome, reflecting the secretion of large amounts of immunoglobulin (usually IgM) by the tumour; this syndrome is known as Waldenstrom's macroglobulinaemia. The prognosis of ML lymphocytic plasmacytoid is highly variable, but overall is slightly worse than that of ML lymphocytic.

Histology In the early stages of this disease the lymph node architecture may not be completely effaced and surviving reactive follicles can be seen trapped within the neoplastic infiltrate. Even in later stages the lymph node sinuses are often preserved as widely dilated structures. The infiltrate consists of small lymphocytes with variable numbers of mature plasma cells, showing the typical eccentrically placed 'clock-faced' nucleus and abundant cytoplasm with a prominent perinuclear 'hof' (Fig. 24.44) Plasmacytoid differentiation is also present and may be the predominant feature, with plasma cells hardly in evidence. These cells have the nucleus of a small lymphocyte with increased amounts of cytoplasm resembling that of plasma cells. Usually, occasional large transformed lymphocytes (immunoblasts) can be seen and increased numbers of mast cells are characteristic. The plasma cells often contain immuno-

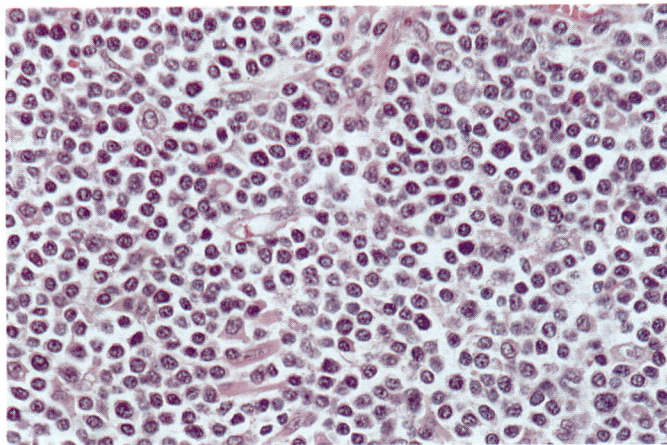

Fig. 24.44 Malignant lymphoma lymphoplasmacytic. The tumour comprises small lymphocytes that possess more cytoplasm and resemble plasma cells. Some frankly plasmacytic cells are present.

globulin inclusions in the form of Russell bodies, or crystals. Small dot-like inclusions of immunoglobulin, which sometimes appear to be intranuclear, are characteristically found in lymphoplasmacytoid cells and are known as Dutcher bodies. The large amount of immunoglobulin synthesized by this tumour is best shown immunocytochemically, using antibodies to immunoglobulin heavy and light chains. In this way, light chain restriction can be demonstrated, thus confirming the neoplastic nature of the process which otherwise may be confused with a reactive B-cell proliferation.

Rarely, a lymph node may show infiltration by a pure population of mature plasma cells (Fig. 24.45). This condition is known as ML plasmacytic, or extramedullary plasmacytoma to distinguish it from the much more common plasma cell neoplasm, multiple myeloma (see Chapter 23). The disease is often confined to a single lymph node, but even in these circumstances, a paraprotein may be present in the peripheral blood. ML plasmacytic is usually an extremely indolent disease and may be cured by simple excision of the involved node. Progression with eventual bone marrow involvement, even after a long disease-free interval, sometimes occurs.

Malignant lymphoma centroblastic/centrocytic

(ML follicular, mixed small cleaved and large cell)

This is the commonest type of non-Hodgkin's lymphoma in Western countries, accounting for approximately 50 per cent of all cases. The follicles in this tumour are neoplastic equivalents of the normal reactive follicles of lymph nodes. It is characteristically a tumour of late adult life and, although it can occur in younger adults, childhood cases are extremely rare. ML centroblastic/centrocytic (cb/cc) usually presents as a group of enlarged lymph nodes or, less commonly, as generalized lymphadenopathy. Peripheral blood involvement, when it occurs, represents 'spillover' of cells from the lymph nodes, rather than a primary phenomenon, and is uncommon. Even when ML cb/cc presents in a single group of nodes, it has usually already disseminated and trephine biopsy of the bone

marrow shows involvement. As a low-grade lymphoma, ML cb/cc may remain static, producing few symptoms, for long periods. It is exquisitely sensitive to therapy, but recurrence of the disease is almost inevitable. Thus, the clinical course is usually a long one, punctuated by numerous therapeutically induced remissions followed by recurrences. The histology of the tumour tends to alter during the course of the disease, gradually moving towards that of a higher-grade lymphoma, both in terms of its cytology and the assumption of a diffuse growth pattern. ML cb/cc is only rarely cured.

Histology This can be quite variable. Typically the lymph node architecture is effaced by closely packed follicles with moderately vascular lymphoid tissue between them and there is complete loss of the sinuses (Fig. 24.46). Unlike the follicles of the reactive lymph node, the follicles in ML cb/cc are surrounded by poorly formed mantle zones, or lack mantle zones altogether. Cytologically they consist principally of centrocytes, and centroblasts can be difficult to find; tingible body macrophages are few in number (Fig. 24.47). Variations which indicate a higher grade of malignancy include increased numbers of centroblasts, larger and pleomorphic centrocytes, and loss of the follicular pattern. In evaluating the grade of the lymphoma, foci of high-grade cytology are more ominous than areas showing a diffuse pattern of infiltration. Finally, most cases of ML cb/cc transform into a high-grade tumour consisting of a diffuse infiltrate of centroblasts and/or immunoblasts. This change usually heralds resistance to all forms of therapy and, thus, the terminal stages of the disease.

Immunocytochemical studies have been important in establishing the relationship of the follicles of ML cb/cc to the normal reactive follicle. They are also of great help in establishing the diagnosis especially when, as is often the case, the differential diagnosis lies between lymphoma and benign reactive follicular hyperplasia. Like the reactive follicle, the follicles of ML cb/cc contain a characteristic network of dendritic reticulum cells. The B-cells of both normal and neoplastic follicles express CD10, but not CD5 antigen. T-cells, almost exclusively T-helper

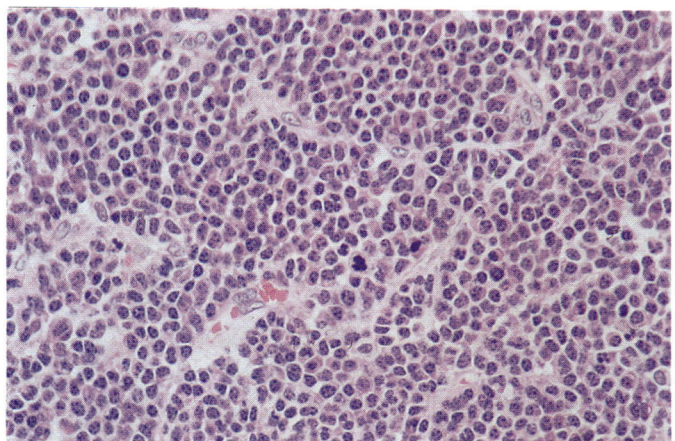

Fig. 24.45 Malignant lymphoma plasmacytic. The lymphoma is composed entirely of plasma cells.

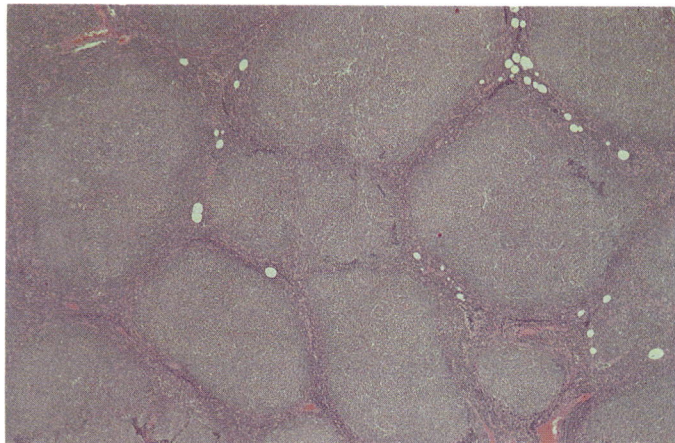

Fig. 24.46 Malignant lymphoma centroblastic/centrocytic, follicular. The lymphoma is composed of tightly packed follicles.

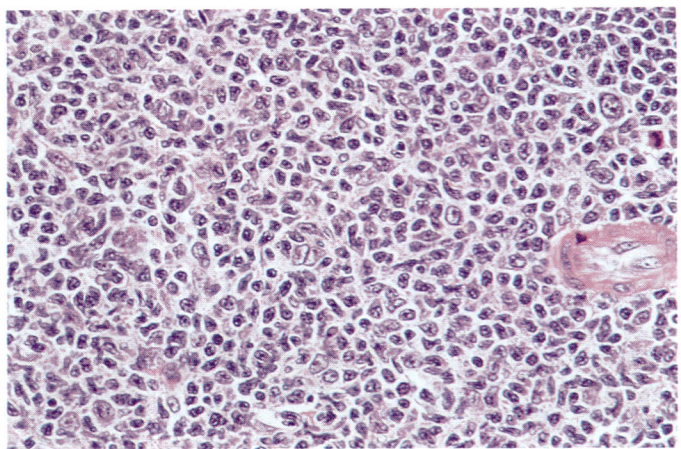

Fig. 24.47 Malignant lymphoma centroblastic/centrocytic. Detail of one of the follicles seen in Fig. 24.46, showing that it consists principally of centrocytes with only scattered centroblasts.

(CD4-positive) cells, are present in both benign and neoplastic follicles. In ML cb/cc T-cells, which in the interfollicular areas are of both CD4 and CD8 phenotypes, are characteristically numerous and may even outnumber the B-cells.

The close similarity between the follicles of ML cb/cc and benign reactive hyperplasia can lead to considerable difficulty in the differential diagnosis between them. This has led to the formulation of detailed histological criteria characteristic, but never diagnostic, of either condition. The advent of immunocytochemistry has greatly simplified matters in that the B-cells of the neoplastic follicle will show light chain restriction as opposed to those of the reactive follicle which will express both κ and λ light chains.

Between 60 and 90 per cent of cases of ML cb/cc show a characteristic translocation between chromosomes 14 and 18. In this t(14;18) translocation the bcl 2 oncogene from the long arm of chromosome 18 is translocated to the long arm of chromosome 14 adjacent to the heavy chain immunoglobulin gene. Approximately 30 per cent of diffuse high-grade B-cell lymphomas, most of which are secondary to ML cb/cc also show this translocation. The translocation can be shown by Southern blotting since the bcl 2 gene rearranges clonally along with the immunoglobulin heavy chain gene, and this rearrangement can be shown with appropriate probes.

Malignant lymphoma centrocytic

(ML diffuse, small cleaved cell)

The cells that comprise this type of lymphoma are cytologically indistinguishable from the centrocytes found in reactive follicle centres and this explains the name chosen for this tumour by Lennert when he first described it in 1975. At that time it was thought that ML centrocytic was indeed a neoplasm of follicle-centre cells, but subsequent immunophenotypic studies have shown important differences between the tumour cell and its supposed benign equivalent. These will be discussed in greater detail below, but suffice it to say that ML centrocytic, while

retaining its name, is no longer thought to be derived from the follicle-centre centrocyte. ML centrocytic occurs with approximately the same frequency as ML lymphoplasmacytic and, similarly, may present with a leukaemic blood picture, or with lymphadenopathy alone, the latter being much more common. It can also present as a primary lymphoma of the spleen, or the gastrointestinal tract, as will be discussed in later sections of this chapter. Although grouped with the low-grade lymphomas, ML centrocytic carries a graver prognosis than the other B-cell tumours described above, including ML centroblastic/centrocytic. The initial response to treatment is often gratifying, but relapse with death due to dissemination of lymphoma is the rule.

Histology The lymph node may be replaced by a uniform diffuse infiltrate of small centrocytes, but not infrequently there is a distinctly nodular pattern which may approach that of true 'follicular' lymphoma. Benign reactive follicles are often trapped within the tumour and the neoplastic cells have a tendency to replace selectively the mantle zones of these follicles; this has given rise to the term 'mantle-zone lymphoma' which is commonly used in the American literature to describe this tumour. The individual cells are slightly larger than small lymphocytes and their irregularly shaped heterochromatic nuclei are quite distinctive (Fig. 24.48). The cells tend to be of remarkably uniform size and larger transformed nucleolated blasts are conspicuously absent. Immunocytochemistry has been pivotal in the characterization of ML centrocytic and in accounting for its perplexing histological appearances. Unlike follicle-centre centrocytes, which express surface (S) IgM but not SIgD, and express the CD10 but not the CD5 antigen, the cells of ML centrocytic express both SIgM and SIgD (of single light chain type) and CD5 but not CD10 antigen. Antibodies with specificity for dendritic reticulum cells show that many of these cells are present and they appear to be derived from pre-existing follicle centres that have been selectively invaded by the neoplastic cells which at first occupy the mantle zone of the follicle. The

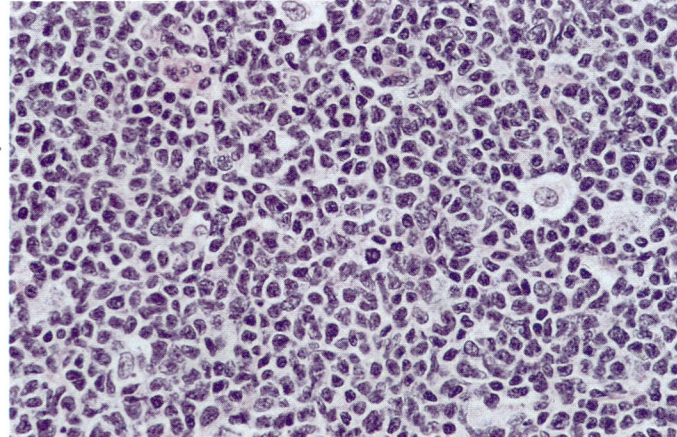

Fig. 24.48 Malignant lymphoma centrocytic. The lymphoma consists of a diffuse infiltrate of cells resembling centrocytes. No centroblasts are seen.

tight meshwork of dendritic reticulum cells then looses its integrity to a variable extent and it is these loose aggregates of dendritic reticulum cells that impose a nodular appearance on the tumour in some cases.

Malignant lymphoma centroblastic

(ML diffuse large non-cleaved cell)

This high-grade B-cell lymphoma is composed of a diffuse infiltrate of cells, the majority of which are morphologically identical, or closely similar, to centroblasts as described in the reactive follicle centre. These features may be present from the time that the tumour is diagnosed, in which case it is termed a primary centroblastic lymphoma, or result from transformation of a centroblastic/centrocytic lymphoma, when it is called secondary centroblastic lymphoma. ML centroblastic is a tumour of adults, and accounts for approximately 5 per cent of non-Hodgkin's lymphomas. The most usual presentation is one of regional lymphadenopathy, although the tumour has often already disseminated to the bone marrow and spleen; peripheral blood involvement is rare. While previously ML centroblastic was associated with rapid progression and death, a significant percentage of cases can now be cured with modern chemotherapy.

Histology The lymph node is completely, or sometimes partially, effaced by a diffuse, uniform infiltrate of large blasts with round nuclei containing 2–5 nucleoli, some of which are apposed to the nuclear membrane (Fig. 24.49). The cells have a clearly identifiable narrow rim of cytoplasm. In secondary centroblastic lymphoma a residual follicular pattern may be present. The cytology is not always so homogeneous and considerable numbers of larger cells with prominent central nucleoli (immunoblasts) are often seen together with a proportion of centrocytes. These cases are sometimes referred to as the polymorphic variety of centroblastic lymphoma. A further subtype is the so-called pleomorphic variant in which the centroblasts

themselves are irregular in size and shape and may have polylobated nuclei. Immunocytochemistry is useful in confirming the B-cell nature of these lymphomas and, once more, in demonstrating light chain restriction in the immunoglobulin that is synthesized by the centroblasts, sometimes in surprisingly high amounts.

Malignant lymphoma immunoblastic (B-cell type)

(ML large cell immunoblastic)

This type of lymphoma, sometimes known as immunoblastic sarcoma, is the commonest high-grade lymphoma. The term 'immunoblast' refers to a large cell with abundant cytoplasm and a large, prominent, and often central nucleolus. A lymphoma may be immunoblastic from the outset, or may evolve as a result of transformation of either ML lymphocytic (Richter's syndrome), lymphoplasmacytic, centroblastic/centrocytic, or centroblastic. Whether it arises *de novo* or following transformation of a lymphoma of lower grade, ML immunoblastic carries a grave prognosis, worse than any of the other high-grade B-cell lymphomas.

Histology The tumour usually consists of a monomorphic infiltrate of immunoblasts, which sometimes resemble plasmablasts and occasionally show frank plasma cell differentiation (Fig. 24.50). In some cases there is striking pleomorphism with large bizarre multinucleated cells predominating and this can lead to confusion with Hodgkin's disease. The B-cell nature of the tumour can, however, be confirmed immunocytochemically.

Malignant lymphoma Burkitt type

(ML small non-cleaved cell, Burkitt's)

This entity was first reported by Burkitt in 1959 as a tumour arising primarily in the jaws of African children. It also involved the retroperitoneum and the viscera, especially the kidneys and, in girls, the ovaries. This disorder, now known as endemic Burkitt's lymphoma, is also seen in other tropical countries where

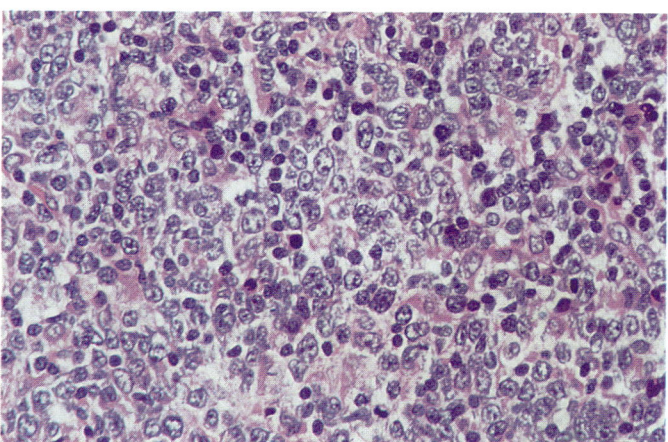

Fig. 24.49 Malignant lymphoma centroblastic. The tumour is composed almost entirely of centroblasts, large cells with nucleoli apposed to the nuclear membrane.

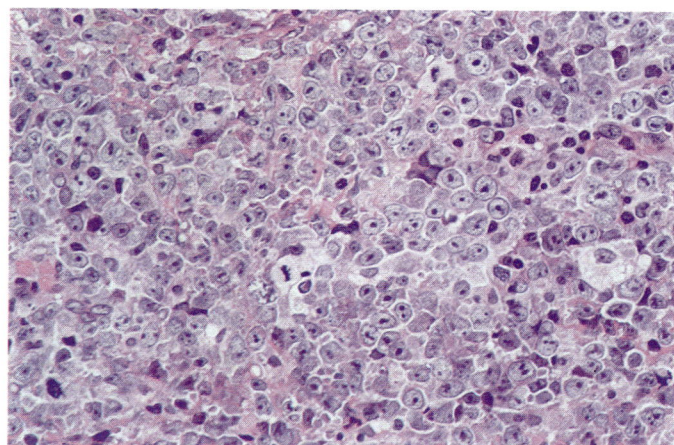

Fig. 24.50 Malignant lymphoma immunoblastic (B). This lymphoma is composed of a uniform infiltrate of centroblasts identified by large nuclei with prominent central nucleoli.

there is a high incidence of malaria, such as Papua New Guinea. The Epstein–Barr (EB) virus is thought to be implicated in the aetiology of endemic Burkitt's lymphoma. The virus can immortalize B-cells in culture and there is evidence of past infection in all cases of endemic Burkitt's lymphoma. Furthermore, the viral genome has been shown to be incorporated into the nuclei of the tumour cells themselves. Since infection with EB virus (the cause of infectious mononucleosis) is so common, some other factor must be operating in Burkitt's lymphoma. It is thought that the combination of malaria, which may depress immunity, and exposure to the virus in infancy rather than in young adulthood is important. Lymph node involvement in endemic Burkitt's lymphoma, while it occurs, is insignificant compared to extranodal disease of the jaws, retroperitoneum, and viscera. In approximately 90 per cent of cases of endemic Burkitt's lymphoma an abnormal karyotype consisting of an 8,14 translocation is present in the malignant cells. It has been shown that this involves translocation of the *c-myc* oncogene from chromosome 8 to the immunoglobulin heavy chain gene locus on chromosome 14. In the remaining 10 per cent of cases similar translocations involving *c-myc* and the light chain loci occur. Before the advent of chemotherapy Burkitt's lymphoma was rapidly fatal. The tumour responds dramatically to chemotherapy, however, and up to 40 per cent of cases can now be cured in this way.

A malignant lymphoma histologically indistinguishable from Burkitt's lymphoma occurs as a non-endemic tumour throughout the world. Again, it is children who are affected principally, but in non-endemic Burkitt's lymphoma the pattern of the disease is quite different, with a higher incidence of lymph node, gastrointestinal, and bone marrow involvement; jaw tumours are comparatively rare. The majority of cases of non-endemic Burkitt's lymphoma do not show incorporation of the EB virus genome into the tumour cell nuclei. The same karyotypic abnormalities are, however, described.

Histology In Burkitt's lymphoma there is a diffuse monomorphic infiltrate of medium-sized round blast cells. The cells have round nuclei with 2–3 nucleoli usually apposed to the nuclear membrane and a narrow rim of cytoplasm. A rapid rate of cell division is evident from the numerous mitotic figures present and the high turnover of cells results in much cell death. In response to this there are large numbers of phagocytic macrophages in the tumour, many of which have engulfed the debris of dead tumour cells. These macrophages, with their pale-staining cytoplasm, scattered among the tumour cells, which have dark blue-staining nuclei, produce the well-described 'starry sky' effect (Fig. 24.51). The extreme monomorphism of Burkitt's lymphoma and lack of any differentiation of the tumour cells suggests that the cells have been 'frozen' at a certain stage of maturation, perhaps, in the case of the endemic form, due to the effects of the EB virus. There is considerable debate as to the nature of the cell from which Burkitt's lymphoma is derived. Most workers favour an origin from the follicle-centre centroblast, but it has to be said that these tumours bear no resemblance to centroblastic or other follicle-centre cell

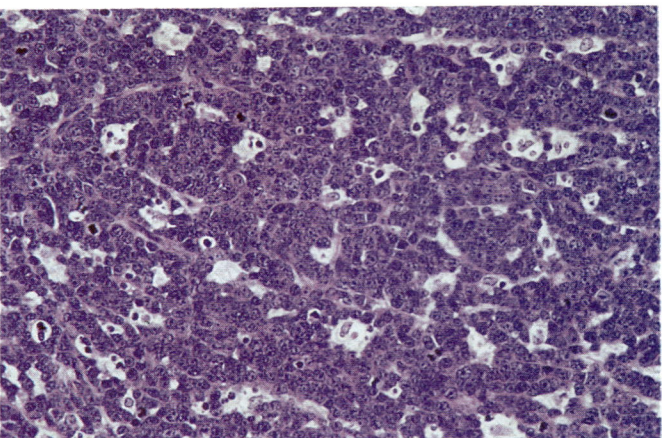

Fig. 24.51 Malignant lymphoma, Burkitt's type. The lymphoma is composed of medium-sized cells with very little cytoplasm and darkly basophilic nuclei within which two or more nucleoli are present. Throughout the tumour macrophages with clear cytoplasm, some of which contain dead tumour cell nuclei, can be seen. This gives an overall 'starry sky' appearance to this tumour.

lymphomas. Peripheral blood involvement may occur as a spill-over phenomenon and should not be confused with B-cell lymphoblastic leukaemia (see below).

The designation 'Burkitt-like' is used for a type of lymphoma which resembles Burkitt's lymphoma, but does not quite meet the stringent histological criteria for that diagnosis. The clinical setting may be similar and these tumours are seen in both endemic and non-endemic areas, but the pattern of disease is more that of non-endemic Burkitt's lymphoma. Histologically there is not the same monomorphism and there is evidence of different degrees of differentiation, with irregularity of nuclear size and shape and accumulation of cytoplasmic immunoglobulin in some cells. This is an ill-defined group of tumours at present.

Malignant lymphoma lymphoblastic (B-cell type)
(ML lymphoblastic)

Patients with B-cell lymphoblastic lymphoma are usually, but not always, children and either have, or soon develop, acute lymphoblastic leukaemia (ALL). This type of leukaemia is known as 'common' ALL (C-ALL), a term coined before the advent of monoclonal antibodies and DNA analysis which established the B-cell phenotype of the cells. The clinical and cytological features of this disease are discussed in greater detail in Chapter 23. In some cases nodal or extranodal (non-leukaemic) disease is the principal or sole manifestation.

Histology The cells of lymphoblastic lymphoma tend to infiltrate in a non-destructive manner along the natural tissue planes, thus, in lymph nodes, preserving the basic architecture of the node (Fig. 24.52). The cells themselves are moderately larger than small lymphocytes, with scant cytoplasm and round to oval nuclei characterized by smooth chromatin and 1–3 small nucleoli.

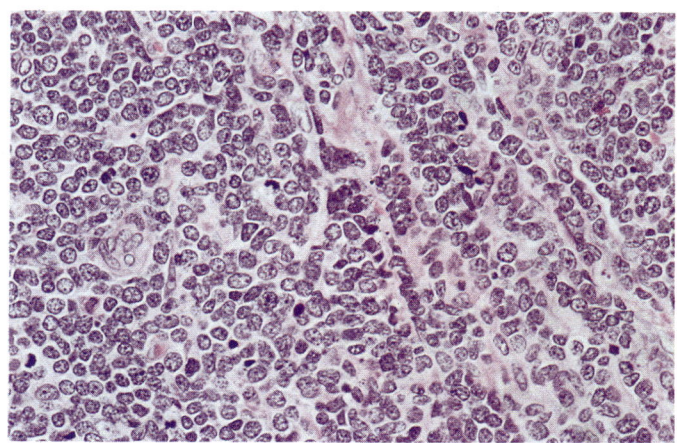

Fig. 24.52 Malignant lymphoma, lymphoblastic (B). The lymphoblasts are characterized by grey, uniform nuclei and 'Indian filing' along tissue planes.

Malignant lymphoma large cell anaplastic

(ML large immunoblastic)

This is a rare variant of high-grade B-cell lymphoma, clinically and histologically identical to the more common T-cell variant which is discussed in detail on p. 1786.

Malignant lymphoma unclassified

(ML unclassifiable)

Inevitably, when dealing with a disease as complex as non-Hodgkin's lymphoma there will be cases which do not fit into any of the categories described above, even though it is possible to demonstrate a B-cell phenotype. As experience accumulates these cases will either be recognized as variants of established conditions, or new categories will be formulated.

24.5.4   Non-Hodgkin's lymphoma of T-cell type

T-cell lymphomas are much less common than those of B-cell origin, comprising 10–15 per cent of all non-Hodgkin's lymphomas in Europe and North America. In Japan, however, close to 40 per cent are T-cell derived, this being a reflection of the prevalence of the human T-cell lymphotrophic virus (HTLV-1) in that country. T-cell lymphomas can be divided into two main groups, those arising from early T-cell precursors, either prethymic or thymic, and those arising from mature T-cells, the so-called peripheral T-cell lymphomas. The former group, known as the T-lymphoblastic lymphomas, are well characterized, but the peripheral T-cell lymphomas remain a challenge to diagnostic histopathologists, immunologists, and clinicians. Some entities, such as the cutaneous lymphomas consisting of small cerebriform cells, are well defined, but any classification of the remainder can only be tentative, particularly with respect to their clinical behaviour which is only beginning to be understood. The morphology of T-cell lymphomas is highly variable and the tumours tend to change their morphology in an unpredictable way, often defying classification. Furthermore, unlike

B-cell lymphomas, there is no convenient method of establishing clonality using immunocytochemistry. Although some T-cell lymphomas show restriction of their phenotype, this is not consistent and is no reflection of clonality. Others may show abnormal distribution of T-cell markers or deletion of certain antigens. Hence, distinguishing between reactive and neoplastic T-cell proliferation depends on the demonstration of T-cell antigens on cells judged to be malignant on morphological grounds or, more specifically, on the demonstration of clonal T-cell receptor gene rearrangements using the Southern blotting technique on DNA extracted from the fresh tissue.

Malignant lymphoma lymphoblastic (prethymic and thymic T-cell lymphoma)

(ML lymphoblastic convoluted or non-convoluted)

This is a highly aggressive tumour carrying a grave prognosis. It occurs predominantly in children and adolescents and is often associated with T-cell acute lymphoblastic leukaemia (T-ALL). Lymphadenopathy with or without a mediastinal (thymic) mass is the common presenting feature.

Histology The pattern of infiltration is similar to that of B-cell lymphoblastic lymphoma (see Fig. 24.52), but in early lymph node involvement the paracortex may be selectively involved. The individual cells are slighly larger than small lymphocytes and in a proportion of the cases show delicate convolutions of their nuclei; it was this feature that gave rise to the term 'convoluted-cell lymphoma' previously thought to be synonymous with T-lymphoblastic lymphoma. T-cell lymphoblastic lymphoma cases vary in their expression of T-cell markers depending on the maturity of the cells, and the pattern of the markers expressed can be correlated with the stages of intrathymic T-cell maturation.

Malignant lymphoma lymphocytic

(ML small lymphocytic)

Almost all cases of this type of lymphoma are accompanied by T-cell lymphocyte leukaemia and are, therefore, essentially haematological disorders (see Chapter 23). The leukaemia can be subclassified into different entities according to both morphology and phenotype and these differ somewhat in their clinical behaviour. The lymph nodes show infiltration by small lymphocytes which usually show more nuclear irregularity than the cells of B-cell lymphocytic lymphoma.

Malignant lymphoma, small cerebriform cell

(Mycosis fungoides; Sezary's syndrome)

The cerebriform T-cell is named for its nucleus which has a strikingly irregular, folded appearance best seen in electron micrographs. These cells, sometimes known as Lutzner's cells, are seen in two clinically distinct lymphomas both of which selectively involve the skin, namely mycosis fungoides and Sezary's syndrome. Although these are strictly extranodal lymphomas, they are more conveniently considered together with the other T-cell lymphomas.

Mycosis fungoides

This is a slowly evolving cutaneous T-cell lymphoma which, over a number of years (up to 20 or more), passes through so-called premycotic, infiltrative, and tumour phases. The first two phases are characterized respectively by flat, slightly reddened and rough patches on the skin and slightly thickened violaceous patches. In the third stage large ulcerating plaques of tumour appear. Eventually the lymph nodes are involved and the tumour transforms into a high-grade T-cell lymphoma.

Histology The upper dermis is infiltrated by cerebriform cells accompanied by variable numbers of reactive macrophages, eosinophils, and other cells. The epidermis is also infiltrated by cerebriform cells either singly, or in clusters, forming so-called Pautrier's microabscesses (Fig. 24.53). Within the infiltrate scattered larger cells with hyperchromatic nuclei are present and these are referred to as mycosis cells. Lymphadenopathy is common in patients with mycosis fungoides and may be due to dermatopathic lymphadenopathy (see p. 1759) or lymphomatous involvement. It may be impossible to differentiate between the two on histological grounds alone and analysis of the lymph node DNA for T-cell receptor β-chain rearrangements frequently indicates the presence of a tumour despite negative histology. The cerebriform cells in mycosis fungoides are, with very few exceptions, positive with CD3 and CD4, and negative with CD8.

Sezary's syndrome

In this disease patients present with diffuse reddening of the skin, alopecia, and a leukaemic blood picture due to circulating cerebriform cells. Sezary's syndrome is, in effect, a leukaemic form of mycosis fungoides, but in contrast to other leukaemias, bone marrow involvement is uncommon. The histological appearances of the skin are similar to those of mycosis fungoides.

Malignant lymphoma lymphoepithelioid type (Lennert's lymphoma)

(ML large cell immunblastic, epithelioid cell component)

Lennert's lymphoma usually presents with regional lymphadenopathy commonly accompanied by tonsillar involvement. Although classified as a low-grade lymphoma, the prognosis of Lennert's lymphoma is less favourable than that of low-grade B-cell lymphomas and in the working formulation it is considered as a high-grade tumour.

Histology The lymph node is replaced by a mixed-cell infiltrate in which small T-cells predominate (Fig. 24.54). A variable number of larger neoplastic T-cells are seen and these may resemble Reed–Sternberg cells. As implied by its name, the characteristic feature of Lennert's lymphoma is the presence of numerous clusters of epithelioid cells. These features can lead to great difficulty in the diagnosis, and differential diagnosis of Lennert's lymphoma and careful immunocytochemistry or DNA analysis are often necessary to make the diagnosis.

Malignant lymphoma angioimmunoblastic

(ML large cell immunoblastic, polymorphous)

The condition angioimmunoblastic lymphadenopathy with dysproteinaemia (AILD) was first described in 1975 and was thought to be a non-neoplastic disease which either resolved spontaneously, caused death due to the associated immunodeficiency, or was complicated by the evolution of lymphoma. Careful study of large numbers of cases in Japan, together with DNA analysis, has shown that most, if not all, cases of AILD are in fact T-cell lymphomas. The clinical presentation is usually acute with generalized lymphadenopathy, a skin rash, hepatosplenomegaly, and severe constitutional symptoms. Hyperglobulinaemia and associated autoimmune phenomena are characteristic. Response to treatment is initially good, but long-term survival is poor.

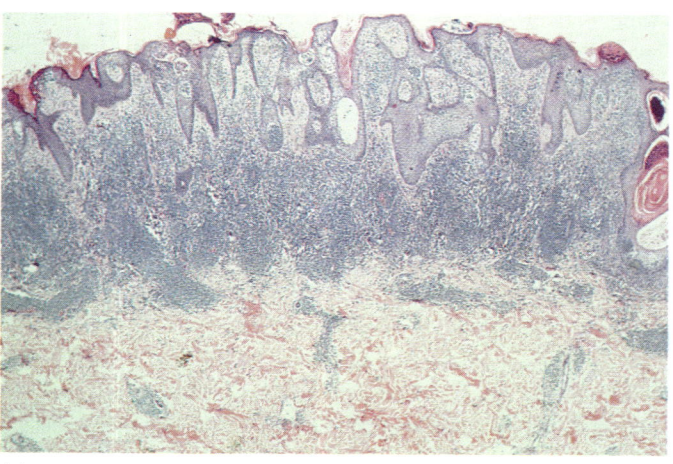
(a)

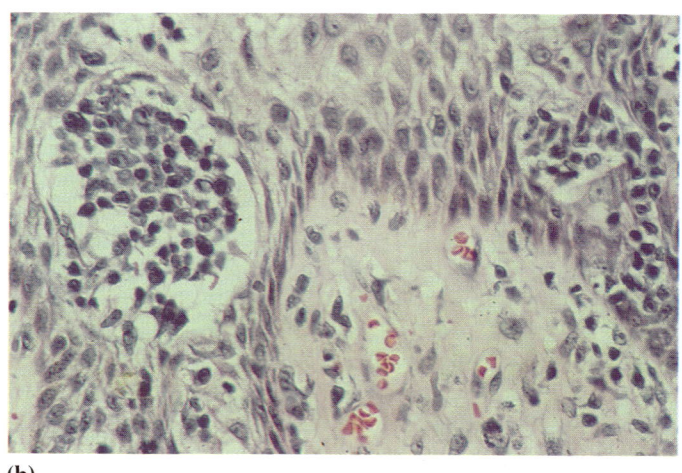
(b)

Fig. 24.53 T-cell lymphoma, small cerebriform cell type (mycosis fungoides). At low power (a) the lymphomatous infiltrate can be seen hugging the epidermis and forming small collections of cells within it. Higher power (b) shows the detail of this epidermal infiltrate, forming so-called 'Pautrier's' microabscesses.

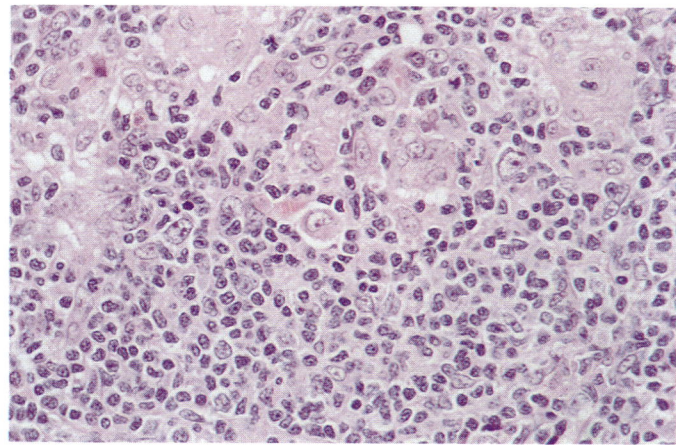

Fig. 24.54 T-cell lymphoma of 'Lennert's' (lymphoepithelioid) type. Large numbers of epithelioid cells are seen at the top of the illustration. The lymphocytes are small to medium sized with irregularly shaped nuclei. Some larger blast forms are present.

Histology The most striking feature is the network of proliferating high endothelial venules, leading to the impression that the whole node consists of paracortical tissue (Fig. 24.55). The T-cells between these venules are small to medium sized with intermingled blast forms and clusters of large cells which often have clear cytoplasm. Characteristically, numerous plasma cells are present, but B-cell follicles are absent or seen only as small atrophic structures. The T-cells are predominantly CD4 positive, but there is usually an admixture of CD8-positive cells as well.

Malignant lymphoma T-zone type

(ML large cell immunoblastic, polymorphous)

The infiltrate in this type of T-cell lymphoma is very similar to the AILD type, except for the presence of numerous, well-

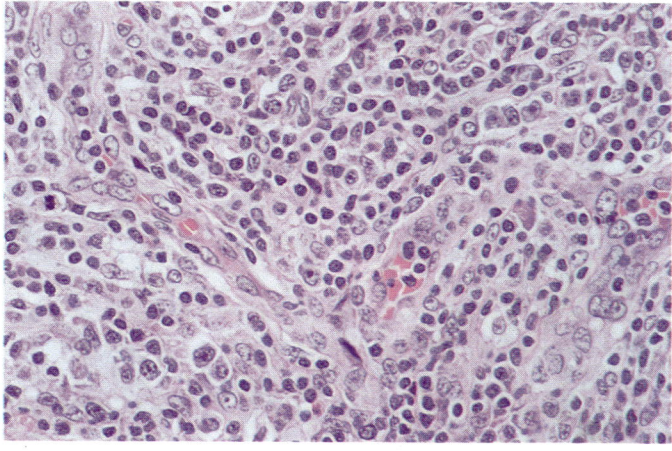

Fig. 24.55 T-cell lymphoma angioimmunoblastic type. Numerous interlacing high endothelial venules are evident between which the lymphoma cells are small to medium sized.

preserved, and often hyperplastic B-cell follicles. Thus in some cases, unless careful attention is given to the 'paracortex', the lymphoma may be confused with lymph node hyperplasia. T-zone lymphoma may progress into a diffuse high-grade lymphoma or become indistinguishable from AILD lymphoma.

Malignant lymphoma pleomorphic (HTLV-1 positive or negative)

(ML large cell immunoblastic, polymorphous)

This group of T-cell lymphomas is divided into large- and small-cell variants (Table 24.4) but, although those composed of smaller cells have a significantly better prognosis, for the purposes of discussion the group is more conveniently subdivided into those cases in which there is evidence of infection with the human T-cell lymphoma virus 1 (HTLV-1) and those in which there is not.

The retrovirus HTLV-1 was first isolated from a cell line derived from an American patient with T-cell lymphoma. A similar virus, called adult T-cell lymphoma virus (ATLV), was identified in south-western Japan as the agent responsible for an endemic form of T-cell lymphoma/leukaemia. It was later established that these two agents were identical. T-cell lymphoma/leukaemia is also endemic in certain areas in the Caribbean and cases have been reported from the United States and Europe. In endemic areas many more people are infected with the virus, as shown by antibody studies, than have lymphoma and in some patients the virus produces a chronic grumbling illness which may later be complicated by lymphoma. The virus preferentially infects CD4-positive T-cells, resulting in transformation and the evolution of 'immortal' cell lines which overexpress interleukin-2 (IL-2) receptors (R) and IL-2 itself. This uncontrolled polyclonal T-cell proliferation then becomes monoclonal. The mechanism appears to be that the transactivating (tat) gene product of HTLV acts on the enhancer sequences of both the IL-2 and IL-2R genes.

T-cell lymphoma caused by HTLV is often, but not always, accompanied by leukaemia. The disease affects adults, usually of late middle-age, and the typical presentation is with generalized lymphadenopathy, splenomegaly, and a skin rash resembling that of mycosis fungoides. Hypercalcaemia is common and there may be profound hypogammaglobulinaemia together with defective cell-mediated immunity. The prognosis is grave with a median survival of only a few months. Less commonly there is a chronic course with slow evolution through a pre-lymphomatous phase to lymphoma involving primarily the skin, producing only mild symptoms and no hypercalcaemia.

Histology The lymph node is replaced by medium-sized to large tumour cells, which have highly pleomorphic nuclei with prominent nucleoli (Fig. 24.56). Polylobated nuclei are common and many cells are multinucleated. These features are reflected in the leukaemic cells in the peripheral blood where the picture is characteristic (see Chapter 23). The infiltrate in the skin is similar to that seen in mycosis fungoides. Immunohistochemistry shows that the cells are consistently CD4 positive, CD8 negative, and CD7 negative. In the chronic cases the cells

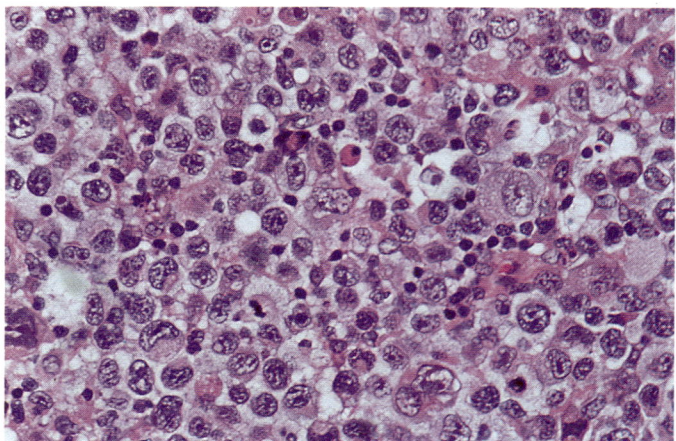

Fig. 24.56 T-cell lymphoma, large-cell pleomorphic type, HTLV-1 positive. Large bizarre lymphoma cells characterize this lymphoma.

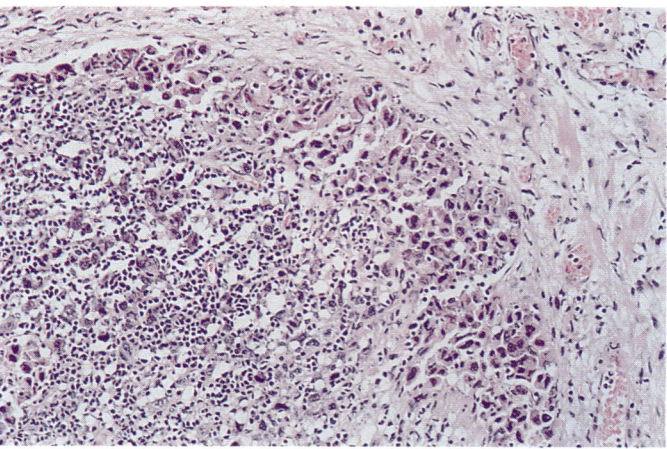

Fig. 24.57 T-cell lymphoma, large cell anaplastic. Note the infiltrate of bizarre lymphoma cells within the sinuses of this lymph node. These cells are positive for the Ki-1 antigen.

are much smaller, but nevertheless show considerable nuclear irregularity and pleomorphism.

HTLV-negative cases of pleomorphic T-cell lymphoma are marginally less aggressive than the virus-positive cases. They are less frequently accompanied by leukaemia and are seldom associated with hypercalcaemia. Most cases share the same phenotype as HTLV-positive lymphoma, but CD8 and CD7 antigen expression is more frequent.

Malignant lymphoma immunoblastic

(ML large cell immunoblastic)

These tumours consist of large cells containing large round nuclei with prominent nucleoli. The cells are uniform in size, unlike the pleomorphic variants described above. A minority of the cases are HTLV-1 positive.

Malignant lymphoma large cell anaplastic

(ML large immunoblastic)

This type of T-cell lymphoma has been recognized since the discovery of the monoclonal antibody Ki-1 (CD30) which recognizes an activation antigen expressed by lymphocytes. While many T-cell (and B-cell) lymphomas contain some large activated cells which are Ki-1 positive, the cells of large-cell anaplastic T-cell lymphomas are uniformly positive with this antibody. In comparison to the other high-grade T-cell lymphomas this tumour occurs in patients of a slightly younger age group, and many cases have been described in children. It also has a slightly better prognosis.

Histology Anaplastic T-cell lymphoma is composed of very large cells with pale-staining cytoplasm and bizarre pleomorphic nuclei (Fig. 24.57). The tumour cells tend to infiltrate lymph node sinuses and not infrequently show phagocytosis of red cells and other particles. Because of these features, in the past cases were often misdiagnosed as examples of malignant histiocytosis. The tumour cells are very variable in their expression of T-cell antigens, often failing to express many, or

even all, T-cell markers. However, all cases express CD30 antigen. A characteristic t(2;5) translocation is present in most cases.

Malignant lymphoma of T-cells, unclassified

The classification of T-cell lymphoma given above is, with few exceptions such as the cerebriform cell type, only tentative at the present time. Many cases defy classification and, typically, T-cell lymphomas can change their histological appearances in sequential biopsies taken within a short time, and even appear different in two biopsies taken at the same time. It is conceivable that systematic karyotyping of this group of tumours may help to rationalize their classification in the future.

24.5.5   Malignant lymphoma of rare and unusual types

Malignant lymphoma histiocytic

(ML miscellaneous, histiocytic)

Malignant tumours of tissue macrophages (histiocytes) were undoubtedly much overdiagnosed in the past; many of these cases were, in fact, examples of peripheral T-cell lymphoma, especially of the anaplastic (Ki-1 positive) variety. Such neoplasms do occur, however, either as a disseminated malignancy throughout the monocyte macrophage system, so-called malignant histiocytosis, or as a localized tumour usually in lymph nodes. Stringent immunocytochemical requirements must be fulfilled before a diagnosis of true histiocytic malignancy is made. The malignant cells should react with one or more of the established macrophage-specific monoclonal antibodies and in most cases can be shown to synthesize lysozyme. Particular care must be taken to ensure that reactive macrophages, which may be present in huge numbers in both B- and T-cell lymphomas, especially the latter, are not mistaken for the tumour cell population.

Malignant histiocytosis This was first described as a clinico-pathological syndrome in 1935, when it was called histiocytic medullary reticulosis (HMR). The presentation is that of an abrupt febrile illness with hepatosplenomegaly and anaemia. The prognosis is poor. Histology shows clearly malignant phagocytic macrophages infiltrating the sinuses throughout the monocyte/macrophage system, including the lymph nodes, spleen, liver, and bone marrow. These cases are readily confused with anaplastic (Ki-1 positive) T-cell lymphoma and can often only be distinguished using immunocytochemistry.

Histiocytic lymphoma This is sometimes called histiocytic sarcoma. It presents with lymphadenopathy, but can transform into a generalized disease undistinguishable from malignant histiocytosis. The clinical behaviour is that of a high-grade lymphoma. The histological appearances of this tumour are very variable and may show features of both phagocytic macrophages and interdigitating reticulum cells, thus suggesting a common origin for these cells. Again, care must be taken not to mistake T-cell lymphoma for this condition.

Granulocytic sarcoma

This rare condition is not strictly speaking a lymphoma at all, but is so readily confused with lymphoma that it is as well to mention it briefly here. As its name suggests, a granulocytic sarcoma results from the infiltration of solid tissue, often lymph nodes, by the cells of acute granulocytic (myeloid) leukaemia. This tumour, in the fresh state, often has a green colour due to the myeloperoxidase in the myeloid cells and, on this account, the term chloroma was often used in the past. Any organ may be involved, but the lymph nodes and gastrointestinal tract are the most common sites. While there is usually evidence of leukaemia at the time of diagnosis, either in the blood or bone marrow, this is not always the case, the granulocytic sarcoma may precede overt leukaemia by as much as several years. It is, therefore, important to make the correct diagnosis at the time of biopsy. Depending on the degree of maturity of the myeloid cells, they can mimic various lymphoid cells, especially lymphoblasts, immunoblasts, and plasma cells. Careful search will often reveal a scattering of eosinophilic myelocytes within the tumour and positive staining of the cells for ASD chloracetate esterase, a granulocyte-specific enzyme that is preserved in formalin-fixed tissue, is helpful. Immunocytochemical stains with antibodies to lysozyme and neutrophil elastase are particularly useful in identifying the myeloid nature of the cells.

24.5.6 Further reading

Blatter, W. A., Gibbs, W. N., Saxinger, C., *et al.* (1983). Human T-cell leukaemia/lymphoma virus-associated lymphoreticular neoplasia in Jamaica. *Lancet* **i**, 61–4.

Croce, C. M., Tsujimoto, Y., Erikson, J., and Nowell, P. (1984). Chromosome translocations and B-cell neoplasia. *Laboratory Investigations* **51**, 258.

Feller, A. C., Griesser, H., Schilling, C. V., *et al.* (1988). Clonal gene rearrangement patterns correlate with immunophenotype and clinical parameters in patients with angioimmunoblastic lymphadenopathy. *American Journal of Pathology* **133**, 549–56.

Kiel lymphoma study group of 1984. Clinical and prognostic relevance of the Kiel classification of non-Hodgkin's lymphomas. Results of a multicentre study. *Haematological Oncology* **2**, 269–306.

Lennert, K., Stein, H., and Kaiserling, E. (1975). Cytological and functional criteria for the classification of malignant lymphoma. *British Journal of Cancer* **31** (Suppl II), 29–43.

Lukes, R. J., and Collins, R. D. (1975). New approaches to the classification of the lymphomata. *British Journal of Cancer* **31** (Suppl II), 1–28.

Mason, D. Y., Bastard, C., Rimokh, *et al.* (1990). CD30 positive large cell lymphomas ('Ki-1 lymphoma') are associated with a chromosomal translocation involving 5q35. *British Journal of Haematology* **74**, 161–8.

Norton, A. J. and Isaacson, P. G. (1989). Lymphoma phenotyping in formalin-fixed and paraffin wax-embedded tissues: I. Range of antibodies and staining patterns. *Histopathology* **14**, 437–46.

Norton, A. J. and Isaacson, P. G. (1989). Lymphoma phenotyping in formalin-fixed and paraffin wax-embedded tissues: II. Profiles of reactivity in the various tumour types.

Rappaport, H. (1966). Tumours of the haematopoietic system. In *Atlas of tumour pathology*, Section 3: Fascicle 8. US Armed Forces Institute of Pathology, Washington DC.

Stansfeld, A. G., Diebold, J., Noel, H., *et al.* (1988). Updated Kiel classification for lymphomas. *Lancet* **i**, 292–3.

Stein, H., Mason, D. Y., Gerdes, J., *et al.* (1985). The expression of the Hodgkin's disease associated antigen Ki-1 in reactive and neoplastic lymphoid tissue. *Blood* **66**, 848–58.

Suchi, T., Lennert, K., Tu, L.-Y., *et al.* (1987). Histopathology and histochemistry of peripheral T-cell lymphomas: a proposal for their classification. *Journal of Clinical Pathology* **40**, 995–1015.

Tajima, K., Tominga, S., and Suchi, T. (1986). Malignant lymphomas in Japan: epidemiological analysis on adult T-cell leukaemia/lymphoma. *Haematology Oncology* **4**, 31–44.

Taub, R., Kirsch, I., Morton, C., *et al.* (1982). Translocation of the c-myc gene into the immunoglobulin heavy chain locus in human Burkitt lymphoma and murine plasmacytoma cells. *Proceedings of the National Academy of Sciences, USA* **79**, 7837.

The non-Hodgkin's lymphoma pathological classification project. (1982). National Cancer Institute sponsored study of lymphomas: Summary and description of a working formulation of clinical usage. *Cancer* **49**, 2112–35.

Tsujimoto, Y., Cossman, J., Jaffe, E., and Croce, C. M. (1985). Involvement of the bcl-2 gene in human follicular lymphoma. *Sciences* **228**, 1440.

Van der Valk, P., Willemze, R., and Meijer, C. J. L. M. (1986). Peripheral T-cell lymphomas: a clinico-pathological and immunological study of 10 cases. *Histopathology* **10**, 235–49.

Yunis, J. J., Oken, M. M., Kaplan, M. E., Ensrud, K. M., Howe, R. R., and Theologides, A. (1982). Distinctive chromosomal abnormalities in histologic subtypes of non-Hodgkin's lymphoma. *New England Journal of Medicine* **307**, 1231–6.

24.6 Extranodal lymphomas

P. G. Isaacson

24.6.1 Introduction

The term 'extranodal lymphoma' is usually reserved for those lymphomas which do not arise from lymph nodes or other recognized lymphoid organs such as the spleen, the thymus gland, or Waldeyer's ring. As many as 40 per cent of lymphomas arise from these extranodal sites. The most common site is the gastrointestinal tract and this is followed by the skin, orbit, lung, thyroid, and salivary glands. Less common sites include the brain, bone, gonads, breast, and soft tissues. Hodgkin's disease only rarely arises in extranodal sites and therefore the term 'extranodal lymphoma', with few exceptions refers to non-Hodgkin's lymphoma. Lymphomas of the gastrointestinal tract exhibit distinctive features which are related to those of gut-associated lymphoid tissue (GALT). Similarly, organized lymphoid tissue is present in other mucosal sites, either naturally, as in the bronchi, or acquired in the course of chronic inflammation, which is most often caused by an auto-immune disorder. Examples of the latter include Sjögren's syndrome affecting the salivary gland and Hashimoto's disease of the thyroid gland. This type of lymphoid tissue is collectively known as mucosa-associated lymphoid tissue (MALT). All lymphomas arising in MALT share certain clinical and pathological features and thus these tumours are usefully considered together as a group.

24.6.2   Malignant lymphomas of mucosa-associated lymphoid tissue (MALT)

Included in this group are lymphomas of the gastrointestinal tract, lung, salivary gland, and thyroid. Orbital lymphomas show many similarities to the MALT tumours, but are not entirely typical. The features of gut-associated lymphoid tissue (GALT) have been described in detail in Section 24.2.2, and can be generalized to include those of MALT at whatever site. Lymphomas arising in this type of lymphoid tissue appear to be derived from the 'centrocyte-like' cells that surround the B-cell follicles. The tumour cells resemble these cells and share their phenotypic and functional properties. The most striking example of this is the tendency of the cells to infiltrate epithelium, forming the so-called lymphoepithelial lesions which are characteristic of MALT lymphomas. There are also certain clinical features which are common to lymphomas of MALT. As mentioned previously, there is a tendency for this type of

lymphoma to be preceded by auto-immune disease of the organ concerned and the distinction between this disease and the complicating lymphoma may be difficult to make. For reasons that are uncertain, MALT lymphomas tend to remain localized for long periods and when they do disseminate it is often to other mucosal organs. These features may be related to the normal behaviour of MALT lymphocytes, which possess the property of 'homing' to mucosal sites (see Section 24.2.2). The result is that, in comparison to lymphomas of peripheral lymph nodes, MALT lymphomas have a much better prognosis and can often be treated conservatively using local measures alone.

24.6.3   Malignant lymphoma of the gastrointestinal tract

Lymphoma of peripheral lymph nodes commonly spreads to involve the gastrointestinal tract secondarily and, therefore, a diagnosis of primary gastrointestinal lymphoma should not be made until this possibility has been excluded. Although they comprise the commonest group of extranodal lymphomas, gastrointestinal lymphomas are comparatively uncommon in Western countries. The reverse is true of the Middle East, where they rate as one of the most frequent malignant tumours. While in the West the stomach is the commonest site, in the Middle Eastern countries most of these tumours arise in the small intestine. The great majority of gastrointestinal lymphomas are typical MALT tumours, being derived from the 'centrocyte-like' B-cells of GALT. A minority of these lymphomas are derived from other GALT lymphocytes, including T-cells. The principal types of gastrointestinal lymphoma are listed in Table 24.5.

Lymphomas of mucosa-associated lymphoid tissue

Low-grade B-cell lymphoma of MALT

Although these lymphomas can occur at any site in the gastrointestinal tract, the stomach is the most common site. The normal stomach is devoid of lymphoid tissue. Mucosal lymphoid nodules are almost always associated with chronic gastritis caused by helicobacter pylori infection. The exact relationship between chronic gastritis and lymphoma, if any, is uncertain

---

Table 24.5   Primary gastrointestinal non-Hodgkin's lymphoma

B-cell
    Lymphomas of mucosa-associated lymphoid tissue (MALT)
        (a) Low-grade B-cell lymphoma of MALT
        (b) High-grade B-cell lymphoma of MALT with or without a low-grade component
        (c) Immunoproliferative small intestinal disease (IPSID) low-grade, mixed or high-grade
    Malignant lymphoma centrocytic (lymphomatous polyposis)
    Burkitt's or Burkitt-like lymphoma
    Other types of low- or high-grade lymphoma corresponding to peripheral lymph node equivalents

T-cell
    Enteropathy associated T-cell lymphoma (EATL)
    Other types unassociated with enteropathy

but, interestingly heliobacter can be found in almost all cases of low grade gastric MALT lymphoma. Patients with gastric lymphoma are usually over 50 years old, but the disease is being recognized increasingly at an earlier age. Presenting symptoms are those of gastritis and peptic ulcer, often with an intermittent response to anti-ulcer therapy. Abdominal pain and weight loss are symptoms of advanced disease. Endoscopy usually reveals antral lesions (although the tumour may occur elsewhere in the stomach) often of indeterminate type, suggesting inflammation rather than a neoplasm. Unless the pathologist is aware of the condition, endoscopic biopsies are frequently interpreted as showing gastritis, perhaps with an unusually heavy lymphocytic infiltrate, and a history of repeated endoscopic biopsies is common. The prognosis of primary gastric lymphoma is closely related to the stage of the tumour. For those tumours confined to the mucosa and submucosa, complete excision is usually curative. When the lymphoma has extended to the serosa, or involves the lymph nodes, chemotherapy is indicated with long-term survival rates being in the order of 50 per cent.

The histological features of gastric lymphoma closely resemble those of normal GALT. Reactive follicles are present and these are surrounded by neoplastic centrocyte-like cells which invade the mucosa and form the characteristic lymphoepithelial lesions (Fig. 24.58a,b). The centrocyte-like cells can vary in their appearance, resembling small lymphocytes, centrocytes, or so-called monocytoid B-cells. Plasma-cell differentiation is common and usually occurs as a band of cells just below the surface epithelium. When the lymph nodes becomes involved, the centrocyte-like cells are seen infiltrating around the follicles, in the same distribution as in the mucosa (Fig. 24.58c). Immunocytochemistry is particularly useful in the diagnosis of these tumours as often only the presence of light-chain restriction can definitely distinguish between the reactive and neoplastic components of the lymphoid infiltrate.

High-grade B-cell lymphoma of MALT, with or without a low-grade component

Most primary gastrointestinal lymphomas are high-grade B-cell tumours. In many, but by no means all, cases a low-grade component of MALT lymphoma can be detected, suggesting that the high-grade lymphoma has arisen from the low-grade lesion (Fig. 24.58d). Where no low-grade component is present it is not possible to be certain that the lymphoma is of MALT type since the cytology of the high-grade cells is not distinctive and lympho-epithelial lesions are not present.

Intestinal lymphoma

Primary intestinal lymphoma, similar to gastric lymphoma, is exceedingly common in the Middle East, where it is sometimes known as 'Western' lymphoma to distinguish it from immuno-proliferative small intestinal disease (IPSID). This latter disease is virtually restricted to the Middle East and is discussed below. The 'Western' type of intestinal lymphoma occurs as a single tumour, usually in the ileum, where it causes obstructive symptoms. The histological features are the same as those described above for gastric lymphoma.

Immunoproliferative small intestinal disease (IPSID)

This disorder is especially common in Iran, Iraq, and Algeria and is well described in other North African countries and Turkey. Occasional cases are reported from other regions and there is a small focus of high incidence in the Cape region of South Africa. The disease occurs in young adults who present with malabsorption, which may be extremely severe. No obvious tumour masses may be present at this time and these may not appear for many years. In a proportion of cases the neoplastic infiltrate in the intestinal mucosa synthesizes and secretes the heavy chain of IgA without accompanying light chain. These cases have sometimes been designated 'alpha chain disease' which is not a good term for this disorder. The histological features of IPSID have been divided into three stages and it is convenient to consider the disease at each stage.

In stage A there is lymphoplasmacytic infiltration confined to the mucosa of the small intestine, which extends distally from the duodenum for varying distances. This infiltrate consists mostly of plasma cells which can be shown to synthesize α heavy chain (Fig. 24.58e). Also present to a variable extent are small aggregates of centrocyte-like cells forming, lymphoepithelial lesions (Fig. 24.58f). The appearances are, thus, similar to those of gastric lymphoma described above, except that plasma cell differentiation is much more marked. At this stage treatment with broad-spectrum antibiotics is often effective, resulting in long remission or even 'cure'. This has led to some doubt whether the mucosal infiltrate is truly neoplastic at this stage, or merely represents polyclonal immunoproliferation, hence the term immunoproliferative small intestinal disease (IPSID). In a few cases of IPSID, light chains are synthesized by the plasma cells and these cases have shown light-chain restriction. This finding, together with demonstration of clonal Ig gene rearrangement, shown by Southern blot hybridization studies, in some cases establishes that the immunoproliferation in stage A IPSID is monoclonal and, therefore, most likely neoplastic. The mechanism whereby IPSID responds to antibiotics appears to be related to removal of lumenal (bacterial) stimulation and implies that the neoplastic cells at this stage are still capable of responding to normal stimuli.

In stage B the mucosal infiltrate extends below the *muscularis mucosae* and cytological atypia is evident. The response to antibiotics at this stage is much less favourable. In stage C, tumour masses are present and the lymph nodes are usually involved. The tumour is composed of centrocyte-like cells which often show blast transformation. Like other MALT lymphomas, spread outside the gastrointestinal tract occurs late if at all.

Although IPSID is essentially similar to other B-cell tumours of GALT, being derived from centrocyte-like cells, its curious epidemiology, extreme plasma-cell differentiation and pattern of Ig synthesis, distinguish it and await explanation.

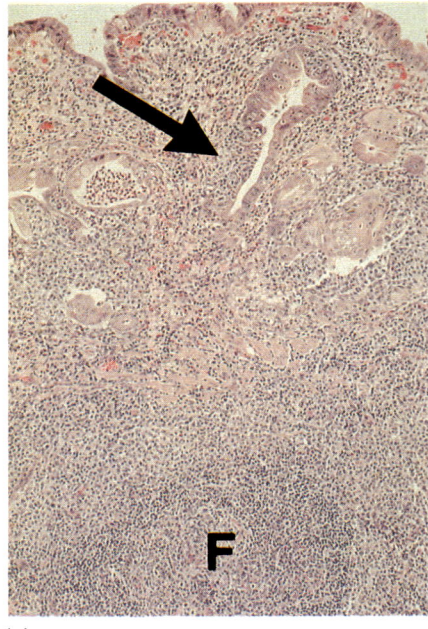

(a)

Fig. 24.58 (a) Low-grade B-cell gastric lymphoma showing reactive follicles (F) surrounded by centrocyte-like cells wich form lymphoepithelial lesions (arrow).

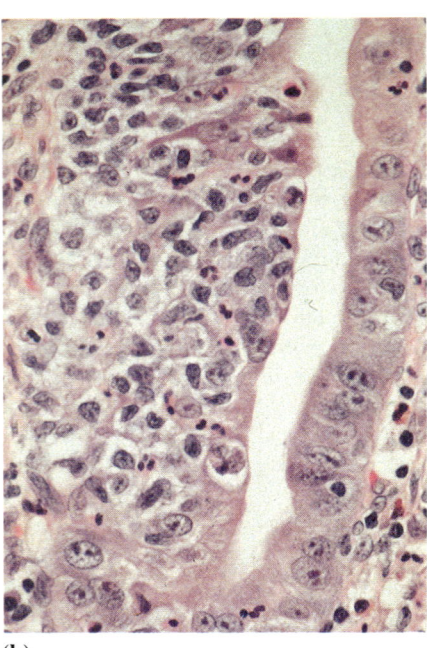

(b)

Fig. 24.58 (b) Detail of lymphoepithelial lesion showing characteristic centrocyte-like cells invading glandular epithelium.

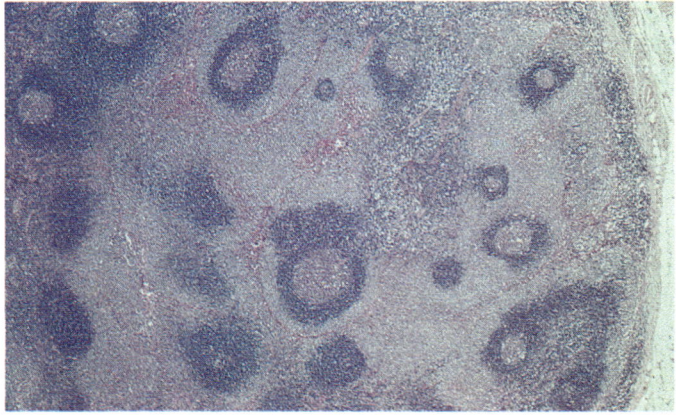

(c)

Fig. 24.58 (c) Involved lymph node from a case of low-grade B-cell gastric lymphoma showing peri and interfollicular infiltration of centrocyte-like cells.

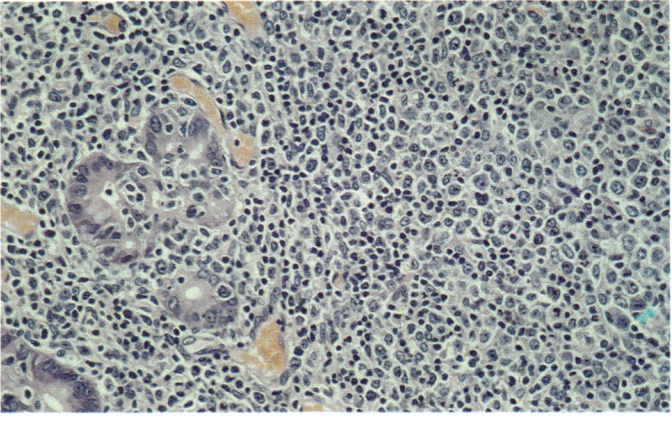

(d)

Fig. 24.58 (d) High grade transformation in a low-grade B-cell MALT lymphoma. The low-grade lymphoma at left forms lymphoepithelial lesion contrasting with the diffuse sheets of high-grade cells at right.

Malignant lymphoma, centrocytic (lymphomatous polyposis)

This is a rare type of lymphoma which, as its name suggests, manifests as multiple polyps throughout the gastrointestinal tract, although often involving one region, particularly the ileocaecal region, more than another. The lymphoma in this disease has been shown to be identical to ML centrocytic (see p. 1780) and it is quite different from B-cell MALT lymphomas in that it is not derived from centrocyte-like cells, does not form lymphoepithelial lesions, and rapidly spreads outside the gastrointestinal tract to involve peripheral lymphoid tissues. Lymphomatous polyposis should not, strictly speaking, be classified with the MALT lymphomas. B-cells with the same phenotype as those in multiple lymphomatous polyposis are found in fetal gut and it is conceivable that the tumour is derived from remnants of this population.

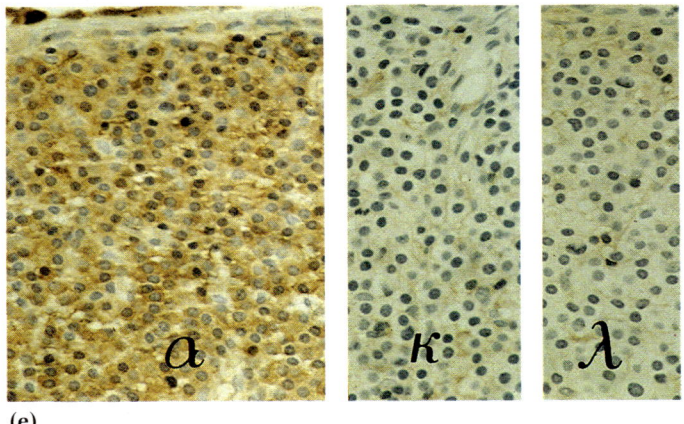

(e)

Fig. 24.58 (e) Plasma cell infiltrate from a case of IPSID. Immuno-stained for α heavy chain and κ and λ immunoglobulin light chain. Only α heavy chain is synthesized by the plasma cells.

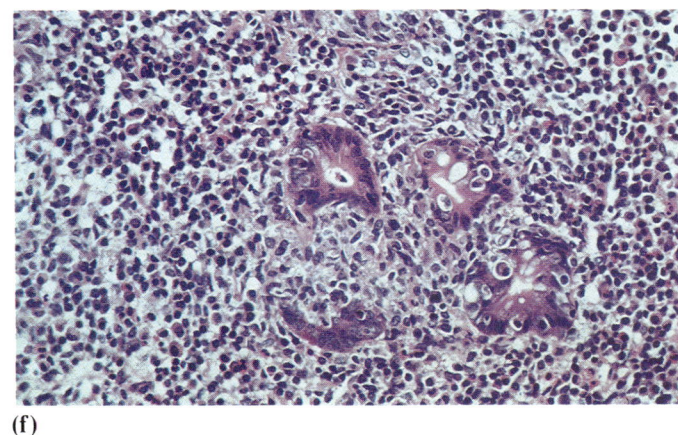

(f)

Fig. 24.58 (f) Mucosal infiltrate from a case of IPSID showing lymphoepithelial lesions formed by centrocyte-like cells within a pre-dominantly plasma cell infiltrate.

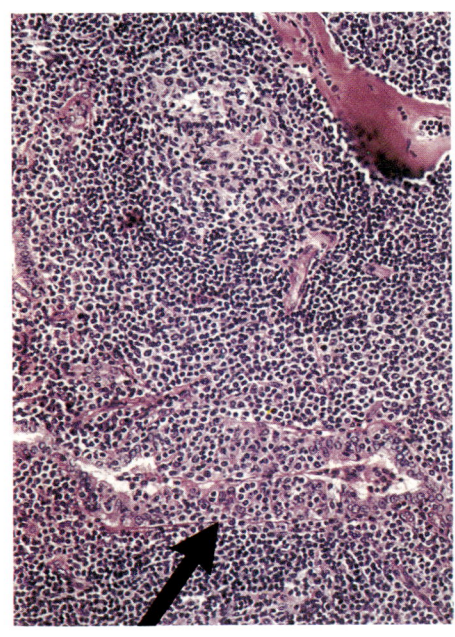

(g)

Fig. 24.58 (g) Low-grade B-cell pulmon-ary lymphoma showing a reactive follicle centre surrounded by centrocyte-like cells which form a lymphoepithelial lesion with bronchiolar epithelium (arrow). Note simil-arity to Fig. 24.58a.

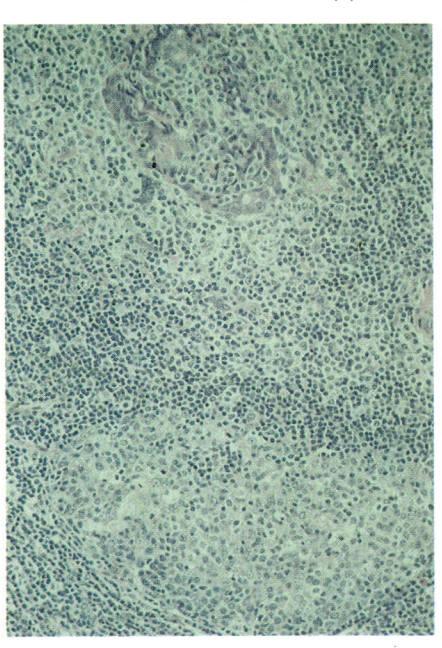

(h)

Fig. 24.58 (h) Low-grade B-cell salivary gland lymphoma showing a reactive follicle below surrounded by centrocyte-like cells which invade salivary gland epithelium. Note similarity to Figs 24.58a and g.

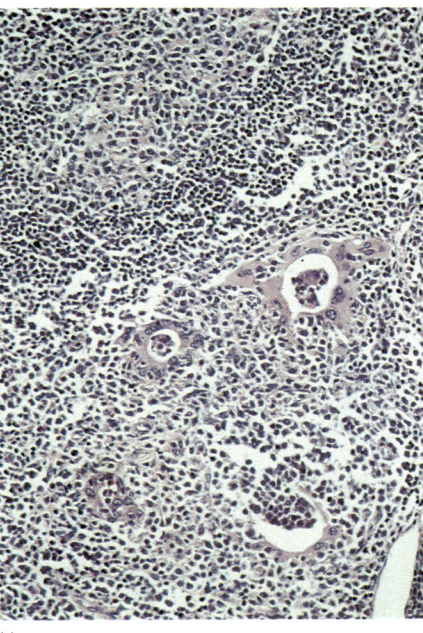

(i)

Fig. 24.58 (i) Low-grade B-cell lymphoma of thyroid showing reactive follicle below with an infiltrate of centrocyte-like cells above forming lymphoepithelial lesions with thyroid acini. Note similarity to Figs 24.58a, g, and h.

Enteropathy-associated T-cell lymphoma

An association of intestinal lymphoma with coeliac disease has been recognized for many years. The lymphoma may complic-ate long-standing childhood-onset coeliac disease, adult coeliac disease, or occur without a preceding history of the disease, but with the typical changes of villous atrophy and crypt hyper-plasia present in the jejunal mucosa. A long latent period, in which there is loss of response to a gluten-free diet, severe malabsorption, and sometimes intestinal ulceration, may pre-cede the onset of overt lymphoma, but other cases may present in a previously well patient. The tumour is often multifocal and commonly presents as an acute abdominal emergency because of perforation or haemorrhage. Frequently, dissemination to mesenteric lymph nodes, liver, spleen, and bone marrow has occurred by the time the tumour is diagnosed, and this type of lymphoma has a poor prognosis.

The histology of this tumour varies from a monomorphic tumour of medium-sized cells to a highly pleomorphic tumour characterized by the presence of multinucleated giant cells. Phenotypic and genotypic studies have confirmed the T-cell phenotype of this tumour. Moreover, the cells share phenotypic properties with intra-epithelial T-cells (see Section 24.2.2) and this, together with the occasional finding of tumour cells within the epithelium, suggests that the tumour is derived from this population which, interestingly, is characteristically increased in coeliac disease. Thus, enteropathy-associated T-cell lymphoma can be considered to be a lymphoma of MALT T-cells.

24.6.4 Pulmonary lymphoma

MALT is well recognized in the lung where it is known as bronchus-associated lymphoid tissue (BALT). There are close similarities between primary B-cell lymphoma of the lung and gastric lymphoma as described above. The lymphomas have a long history and remain localized for prolonged periods. A proportion of cases evolve in a setting of a lymphoproliferative, possibly auto-immune disorder, known as lymphocytic interstitial pneumonia.

The anatomy of the lung dictates that the histological features of pulmonary lymphoma, on superficial examination, are different from those of gastric lymphoma, but a more critical examination reveals the same three components of reactive follicle centres, centrocyte-like cells, and, more rarely, plasma cells (Fig. 24.58g). The centrocyte-like cells form lymphoepithelial lesions with bronchiolar epithelium and may constitute the bulk of the tumour.

24.6.5 Malignant lymphoma of salivary glands

The salivary glands do not normally contain lymphoid tissue, but in the condition known as myoepithelial sialadenitis (MESA) lymphoid tissue accumulates around ducts where it comes to resemble Peyer's patches in all respects, including the presence of small intraepithelial collections of B-cells corresponding to those in the dome region of Peyer's patches. A large proportion of cases of MESA occur as a manifestation of Sjögren's syndrome, which is an auto-immune condition (see Chapter 14). As the lymphoid infiltrate of MESA expands the ducts are reduced to collections of epithelial and myoepithelial cells containing lymphocytes, which are predominantly B-cells; these are known as epimyoepithelial islands. It is in this setting that salivary gland lymphoma arises. These tumours tend to be extremely indolent and remain localized for prolonged periods. In an unpredictable minority of cases, however, transformation into a high-grade lymphoma occurs and the tumour may disseminate widely.

Histologically, salivary gland lymphoma shares the features of other MALT lymphomas, with reactive lymphoid follicles and sheets of neoplastic centrocyte-like cells centred around epimyoepithelial islands, which they infiltrate, forming lymphoepithelial lesions (Fig. 24.58h). Plasma-cell differentiation is a feature of a proportion of cases. High-grade B-cell lymphomas may evolve from these low-grade lymphomas or occur de novo,

in which case they are similar to those occurring in other mucosal sites.

24.6.6 Malignant lymphoma of the thyroid

While the thyroid is not strictly a mucosal organ and, furthermore, contains no native lymphoid tissue, the lymphomas that arise within it closely resemble those of mucosal sites. This may be explained by the fact that the thyroid is derived from the foregut and commonly acquires lymphoid tissue, especially in Hashimoto's disease. Indeed, lymphomas of the thyroid virtually always arise in the setting of Hashimoto's thyroiditis. The lymphoid infiltrate in Hashimoto's thyroiditis, like that in Sjögren's syndrome, is very similar to normal GALT in its cytology and architecture. Lymphoid follicles are prominent, each with a surrounding zone of centrocyte-like cells which infiltrate isolated thyroid acini. Characteristically, plasma cells are present in large numbers reminiscent of the gut lamina propria. Thyroid lymphoma, since it arises in Hashimoto's thyroiditis, occurs predominantly in women. In most cases the tumour is low grade and is very similar in its behaviour to lymphoma of the salivary gland, remaining localized for long periods and responding well to local excision sometimes followed by radiotherapy. The prognosis of the high-grade tumours that may evolve is also favourable provided that the tumour has not spread beyond the thyroid capsule.

The histological features of lymphoma of the thyroid are virtually identical to those of MALT lymphomas. Lymphoepithelial lesions are especially prominent and plasmacytic differentiation is common (Fig. 24.58i). When transformation to a high-grade lymphoma occurs the features are those of other MALT tumours.

24.6.7 Malignant lymphoma of the orbit

Lymphomas presenting in the orbit may arise in the lacrimal gland, the periorbital tissues, or the conjunctiva. Only the latter has native lymphoid tissue, the setting for lymphoma being provided by reactive lymphoid infiltrates which occur in the lacrimal gland and periorbital fat. Despite their different sites of origin, orbital lymphomas are homogeneous both clinically and histologically. These tumours show many similarities to MALT lymphomas, but also exhibit important differences, the most significant of which is their tendency to disseminate even though they are histologically low grade. The pattern of their spread is unusual, however, with a tendency to involve mucosal organs, especially the lung, and the abdominal lymph nodes, with sparing of the bone marrow.

The histology of orbital lymphomas is very similar to that described for lymphomas of MALT, but not absolutely identical. Reactive follicles are a prominent feature of all cases, but the neoplastic cells surrounding them show fewer 'centrocyte-like' features and are often more like small lymphocytes which show variable degrees of plasmacytic differentiation. Lymphoepithelial lesions may occur in those cases where epithelium is adjacent to the tumour. High-grade lymphomas also occur in the orbit.

24.6.8   Malignant lymphoma of the skin

While secondary spread of lymphoma to the skin is common and causes little diagnostic difficulty, primary cutaneous lymphoma is relatively rare and is a source of confusion and controversy for pathologists. There are many chronic inflammatory conditions of the skin that produce dense lymphocytic infiltrates that on histological grounds alone may be impossible to differentiate from lymphoma. Conversely, the natural history of many cutaneous lymphomas is one of extreme indolence, so that they are readily confused with non-neoplastic chronic inflammatory conditions. Following the advent of immunohistochemistry and the Southern blotting technique for detecting Ig and T-cell receptor β-chain gene rearrangements, some order is at last entering the chaos of cutaneous lymphoproliferative lesions.

B-cell cutaneous lymphomas

There are close parallels between B-cell lymphomas of the skin and mucosal sites, such as the stomach. Thus, most cutaneous B-cell tumours present as a slowly growing papule, and a history of multiple local recurrences after excision is characteristic. Spread outside the skin, if it occurs at all, is a late phenomenon and usually follows the transformation of the lymphoma into a high-grade tumour.

Histologically these lesions may resemble lymphomas of MALT. The low-grade tumour cells are often cytologically very similar to the centrocyte-like cells of mucosal lymphomas. Plasmacytic differentiation is a frequent finding, but lymphoepithelial lesions are not seen. There is usually a marked reactive lymphocytic infiltrate accompanying the lymphoma, including reactive B-cell follicles, and without immunohistochemistry it may be impossible to detect the tumour. The high-grade lymphomas consist of larger transformed B-cells, resembling centroblasts or immunoblasts, and these cells tend to overwhelm the reactive lymphoid population, making the diagnosis less difficult.

T-cell cutaneous lymphomas

The commonest lymphoma of the skin is the cerebriform T-cell lymphoma (mycosis fungoides and Sezary's syndrome) already described on p. 1784. Any of the other T-cell lymphomas that usually occur in lymph nodes may occur in the skin either as a primary site, or together with lymph node involvement. There are two distinctive cutaneous T-cell lymphomas which, although rare, are worth discussing briefly. These are lymphomatoid papulosis and the condition inappropriately named regressing atypical histiocytosis.

Lymphomatoid papulosis occurs as an acute eruption of a single papule or, occasionally, multiple papules, usually on the trunk. These papules are clinically benign and heal spontaneously, but appear malignant histologically. They are characterized by scattered, large, bizarre, transformed lymphoid cells within a mixed lymphoproliferative background. Despite their benign behaviour, something over 10 per cent of cases eventually evolve, over a number of years, into frank T-cell lymphoma.

The entity known as regressing atypical histiocytosis is, in some ways, similar to lymphomatoid papulosis. The skin tumours in this condition develop rapidly into large violacious papules which regress spontaneously. This sequence of events recurs often over many years, evolving in some cases into a disseminated high-grade T-cell lymphoma. The histology of these skin tumours is most alarming, showing sheets of large, bizarre T-cells (previously thought to be atypical histiocytes) that express the CD30 (Ki-1) antigen. Therefore, the appearances are those of an anaplastic (CD30+) T-cell lymphoma which, in lymph nodes, carries a poor prognosis (see p. 1786). Both lymphomatoid papulosis and regressing atypical histiocytosis appear to represent the curious phenomenon of a lymphoid neoplasm under some sort of biological control, and are considered by some to represent different morphological expressions of the same biological entity. Clearly the mechanism underlying this control is of great interest.

24.6.9   Extranodal lymphomas of other sites

Primary lymphoma has been reported from almost every site in the body. The more frequent sites include the brain, testis, breast, and bone. Less common are lymphomas of the liver, kidney, female reproductive organs, heart, and soft tissues. Most of these lymphomas are of B-cell phenotype and demonstrate high-grade histology with a diffuse growth pattern.

24.6.10   Malignant lymphoma in immunocompromised patients

There is an increased incidence of lymphoma in immunocompromised individuals, including patients with congenital immunodeficiency, therapeutically induced immunodeficiency, and the acquired immunodeficiency syndrome (AIDS). In the majority of cases these are non-Hodgkin's lymphomas, although Hodgkin's disease also occurs. Extranodal presentation is highly characteristic of this group of patients, in whom gastrointestinal and central nervous system lymphoma are particularly common. Almost all the cases are B-cell tumours with high-grade histology of either immunoblastic, Burkitt-like, or true Burkitt's lymphoma. In many of the cases there seems to be a close association between Epstein–Barr virus infection and the tumour, and it is thought that these lymphomas arise as the result of suppression of immunity against the virus, which then causes unrestricted B-cell proliferation. Initially this proliferation is polyclonal, but a monoclonal population (i.e. lymphoma) then emerges.

24.6.11   Further reading

Addis, B. J., Hyjek, E., and Isaacson, P. G. (1988). Primary pulmonary lymphoma. A re-appraisal of its histiogenesis and its relationship to pseudolymphoma and interstitial pneumonia. *Histopathology* **13**, 1–17.

Beljaards, R. C., Meijer, C. J. L. M., Scheffer, E., *et al.* (1989). Prognostic significance of CD30 (ki-1/Ber-H2) expression in primary cutaneous large-cell lymphomas of T-cell origin. *American Journal of Pathology* **135**, 1169–78.

Freeman, C., Berg, J. W., and Cutler, S. J. (1972). Occurrence and prognosis of extranodal lymphomas. *Cancer* **29**, 252–60.

Hyjek, E. and Isaacson, P. G. (1988). Primary B-cell lymphoma of the thyroid and its relationship to Hashimoto's thyroiditis. *Human Pathology* **19**, 1315–26.

Hyjek, E., Smith, W. J., and Isaacson, P. G. (1988). Primary B-cell lymphoma of the salivary gland and its relationship to myoepithelial sialadenitis (MESA). *Human Pathology* **19**, 766–76.

Isaacson, P. G., Dogan, A., Price, S. K., and Spencer, J. (1989). Immunoproliferative small-intestinal disease: an immunohistochemical study. *American Journal of Surgical Pathology* **13**(12), 1023–33.

Isaacson, P. and Wright, D. H. (1978). Malignant histiocytosis of the intestine. Its relationship to malabsorption and ulcerative jejunitis. *Human Pathology* **9**, 661–77.

Isaacson, P. and Wright, D. H. (1984). Extranodal lymphoma arising from mucosa-associated lymphoid tissue. *Cancer* **53**, 2512–24.

Isaacson, P. G., MacLennan, K. A., and Subbuswamy, S. G. (1983). Multiple lymphomatous polyposis of the gastrointestinal tract. *Histopathology* **8**, 641–56.

Isaacson, P. G., O'Connor, N. T. J., Spencer, J., *et al.* (1985). Malignant histiocytosis of the intestine: a T-cell lymphoma. *Lancet* **ii**, 688–91.

Isaacson, P. G. and Spencer, J. (1987). Malignant lymphoma of mucosa-associated lymphoid tissue. *Histopathology* **11**, 445–62.

Knowles, D. M., Chamulak, G. A., Subar, M., *et al.* (1988). Lymphoid neoplasia associated with AIDS: the New York University Medical Center experience with 105 cases (1981–1986). *Annals of Internal Medicine* **108**, 744.

Locker, J. and Nalesnik, M. (1989). Molecular genetic analysis of lymphoid tumors arising after organ transplantation. *American Journal of Pathology* **135**, 977–87.

Slater, D. (1990). Editorial—clonal dematoses: a conceptual and diagnostic dilemma. *Journal of Pathology* **162**, 1–3.

Weiss, L. M., Wood, G. S., Trela, M., Warnke, R. A., and Sklar, J. (1986). Clonal T-cell populations in lymphomatoid papulosis. Evidence of a lymphoproliferative origin for a clinically benign disease. *New England Journal of Medicine* **315**, 475–9.

Wood, G. S., Ngan, B. Y., Tung, R., *et al.* (1989). Clonal rearrangements of immunoglobulin genes and progression to B-cell lymphoma in cutaneous lymphoid hyperplasia. *American Journal of Pathology* **135**, 13–19.

24.7   The spleen

I. A. Lampert

24.7.1   Introduction

The role of the spleen has always been enigmatic and as far back as the second century AD Galen had named it 'the organ of mystery'. He believed that the humour of melancholy was extracted from the blood and liver, purified by the spleen and ultimately excreted by the stomach. It was only in the seventeenth century that the structure of the organ was described by Harvey, Glisson, Morton, and Malpighi. In the eighteenth century Hewson recognized its association with the lymphatic system. Almost a century later Virchow demonstrated that the Malpighian corpuscle was concerned with the formation of white blood cells. In 1895, Pontfitch recognized the spleen's capacity to remove particles from the blood and realized that it was concerned with blood destruction by removal of erythrocytes.

Enlargement of the spleen has been of concern to physicians as far back as Ancient Greece, when it was almost certainly associated with endemic malaria. The more recent observations of how often an enlarged spleen was associated with various blood diseases confirmed the relationship between the spleen and the haemopoietic system. In some of these diseases the effect of splenectomy made this relationship even more apparent. In 1887 Spencer Wells removed an abdominal tumour from a 27-year-old woman whom he thought had a fibroid. She had a history of dark urine and attacks of jaundice since the age of 9. Instead, he removed an enlarged spleen and the jaundice and dark urine disappeared for the rest of her life. The condition was probably hereditary spherocytosis, first clearly defined in 1931 by Lord Dawson of Penn.

The function of the spleen continues to fascinate as its role in a variety of disease states becomes apparent.

24.7.2   Normal splenic structure

Spleen size

Splenic weight varies in normal people with sex and age and is in proportion to body weight, height, and body surface area. At 29 years mean weight for males is 125 g and for females 103 g (the standard deviation is approximately 25 per cent of the mean, reflecting the considerable variation between individuals). Weight is relatively constant until the seventh decade, after which there is a progressive decrease in size. The mechanisms controlling splenic size are unknown; the direct relationship to body mass suggests that there may be a functional controlling mechanism of size.

Splenic structure

The spleen is essentially a filter inset on the blood circulation. Thus it contains vascular channels, lymphatic tissue, and cells of the lymphatic and haemopoietic system. Structurally it is organized into two major compartments, namely the red pulp and the white pulp (Fig. 24.59). The former is concerned with filtration and linked to the circulatory system. The white pulp is linked to the immune system.

Splenic vasculature

The splenic artery divides into 4–6 terminal branches which continue in the trabeculae as trabecular arteries, sending branches from the trabeculae directly into the white pulp. From the site where the artery leaves the trabecula it is called the central artery. The central artery is invested by lymphoid tissue, which in some places has pronounced, eccentric nodules con-

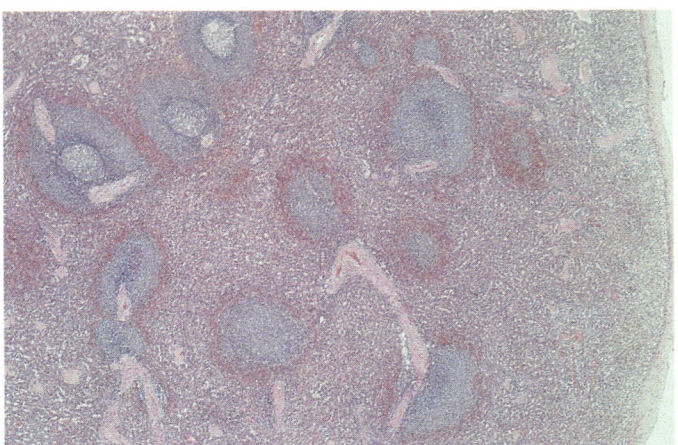

Fig. 24.59 Low-power view of spleen showing the splenic capsule at right, the white pulp, consisting of lymphoid aggregates, and the intervening red pulp. The thick-walled splenic arteries are evident.

taining the germinal centres. Each central artery divides into 4–10 central arterioles, also called the penicillar arteries. Each arteriole also has a lymphoid sheath containing, in places, germinal centres. The central arterioles terminate either directly in the splenic sinusoids, or in the splenic arterial end capillaries; the latter are characterized by the absence of a lymphoid sheath and terminate in the pulp cords. Thus, the blood may remain intravascularly by flowing into the sinusoids (*closed circulation*) or it may pass to the extravascular space via arterial end capillaries terminating in the pulp cords (*open circulation*) (Fig. 24.60).

Organization of the red pulp

Two forms of red pulp organization are recognized:

1. The spleen such as is seen in rodents, where arteriole branches terminate in the pulp space and blood is then collected into pulp veins.

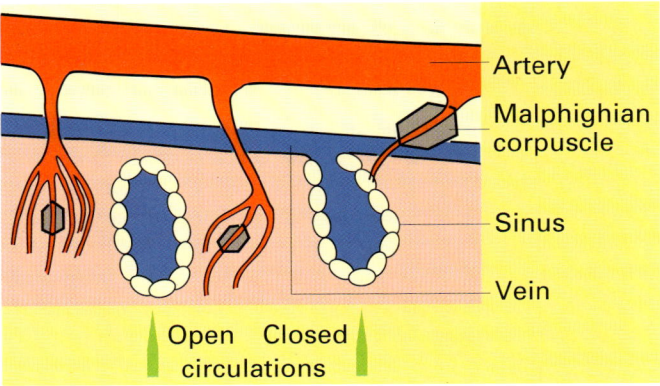

Fig. 24.60 (a) Open circulation, in which the arteriolar branches enter the substance of the splenic chords (crosshatched); (b) closed circulation, in which the arteriolar branches enter directly into the branching sinuses.

2. The *sinusal* spleen, the form seen in man, in which there is a distinctive branching system of sinuses extending from around the white pulp and distally draining into the pulp veins. As a result the red pulp space is reduced to a system of branching anastomosing plates lying between the vascular sinuses called the 'cords of Billroth'. The cords are lined by stromal cells and contain macrophages.

The structure of the sinuses

The walls of the splenic sinus are made up of 3 layers, endothelium, basement membrane and adventitia (Fig. 24.61). The endothelial or sinus littoral cells (Fig. 24.62) lie side by side, joined by junctional complexes. The interendothelial slits of the wall of the sinus constitute an intrinsic part of the vascular pathway. Blood brought into the red pulp by the arterial terminations empties into the splenic cords and, in order to empty into the sinuses, has to pass between these slits. The basement membrane is fenestrated, so that it does not impede the passage of red cells. The adventitial cells are thought to be contractile and regulate blood flow in the spleen: thus by covering a slit they may impede flow; alternatively, by drawing an arterial twig in apposition to a sinus they may enhance flow and, in effect, create an arteriovenous connection.

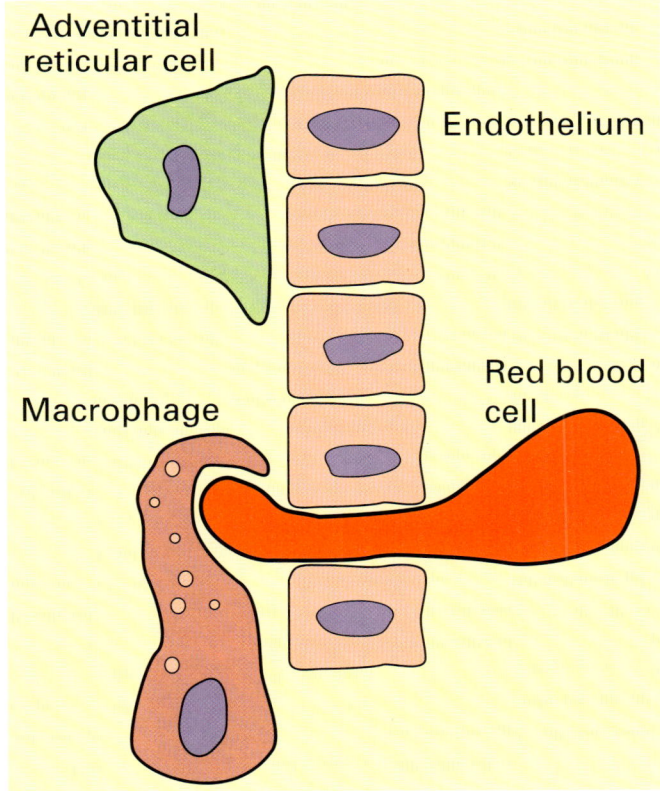

Fig. 24.61 Diagram showing the structure of the lining of a splenic sinus. Blood flow through the pulp chords is regulated by adventitial cells. Red blood cells have to distort to squeeze between the endothelial cell lining of the sinus. Abnormally rigid fragments are phagocytosed by cordal macrophages.

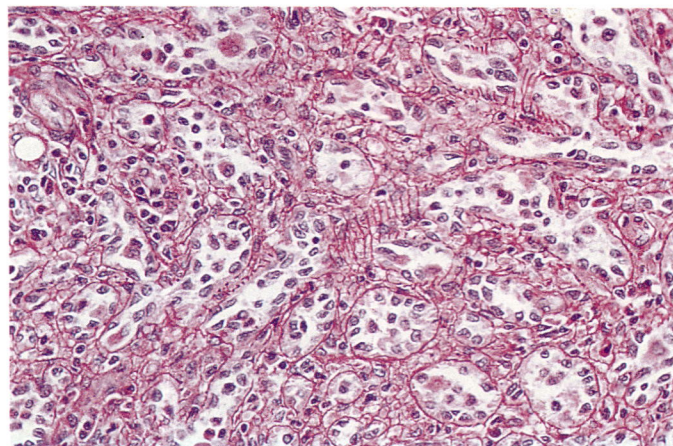

Fig. 24.62 Detail of red pulp of spleen. The sinuses are lined by specialized endothelial cells 'the sinus littoral cells'. They rest on a specialized fenestrated basement membrane system, seen here in a PAS stain, forming a stave-like arrangement around the sinuses.

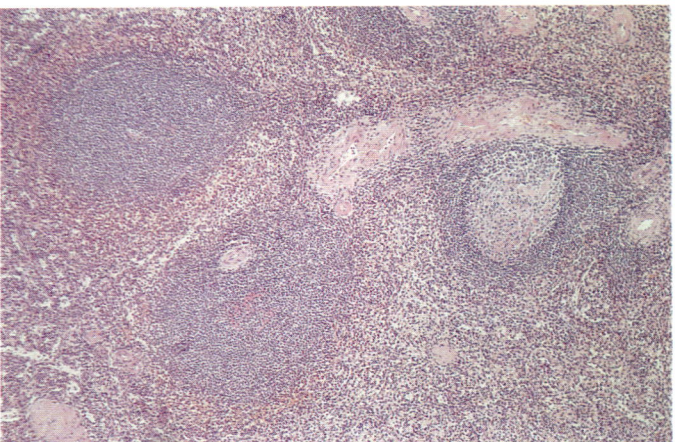

Fig. 24.63 The white pulp of the spleen consists of B-cell follicles and the adjacent peri-arteriolar lymphocyte sheath.

As a consequence of the presence in the spleen of two vascular systems (Fig. 24.60), there is both a rapid and a slow transit of components in the splenic circulation.

Haemoconcentration in the splenic pulp

At right angles to the central arterioles, arterial capillaries depart, communicating with the venous system via sinusoids around the white pulp. As the blood flows through the spleen, the plasma, together with leucocytes, passes preferentially to the white pulp by a process of 'plasma skimming', while the red cells remain in the axial bloodstream of the central arteriole, as reflected by an increased haematocrit measurement. As a consequence, the blood becomes increasingly viscous as it passes into the cords and sinuses of the red pulp. This results in a slowing of flow to a point of stasis, which has important consequences for the filtration and phagocytic function of the organ.

The lymphoid system of the spleen (the white pulp)

The white pulp possesses a definite structural organization (Fig. 24.63). The area adjacent to the central arteriole, called the peri-arteriolar lymphoid sheath (PALS) is essentially a zone of T-lymphocytes (Fig. 24.64). The cells in this zone show the usual markers for T-cells, i.e. CD2, CD3, CD4 (70 per cent of cells), and CD8 (30 per cent of cells), these cells are associated with class II MHC (HLA-DR) positive dendritic cells (the interdigitating reticulum cells) responsible for antigen presentation. T-cells are often seen in smaller numbers in the marginal zone and germinal centres. While CD4$^+$ T-cells predominate in the white pulp, in the red pulp the T-cells are mainly CD8$^+$ cells.

It is to be noted that in staining the spleen for CD8 the sinus littoral cells are positive. It is interesting to note that these cells are negative in fetal life. Adjacent to this is the B-lymphoid area consisting principally of the germinal centre and the corona (Figs. 24.63, 24.65). Surrounding this is a zone composed of a

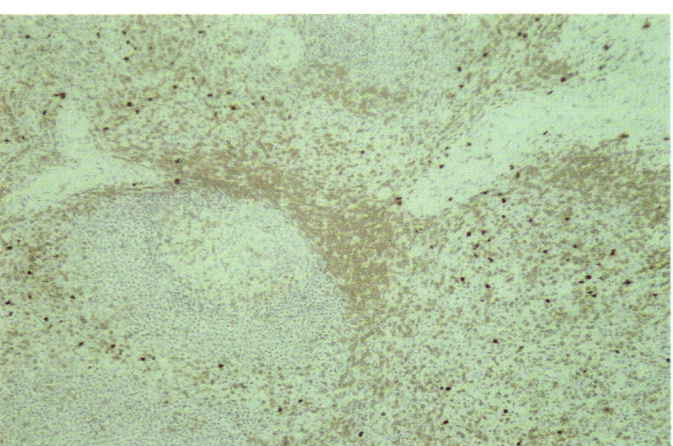

Fig. 24.64 Spleen stained with a monoclonal antibody to T-cells, showing positive brown staining of the cells in the peri-arteriolar lymphocyte sheath. The B-cell areas are unstained.

reticular fibre meshwork, which contains a population of medium-sized and loosely aggregated lymphocytes and appears to communicate both with the red and the white pulp (Fig. 24.66). In man this has variously been called the perifollicular zone or marginal zone, and is thought to be analogous to the marginal zone of rodents. The zone consists predominantly of B-lymphocytes, although T-lymphocytes are present as well. The majority of the marginal-zone B-lymphocytes are distinguishable from coronal lymphocytes by only having IgM on their surface (coronal lymphocytes have IgM and IgD). (Figs. 24.67, 24.68). It is likely that these are activated B-lymphocytes destined to become antibody-producing plasma cells.

Lymphocyte trafficking

While most formed elements pass through the pulp cords and on into the venous system, lymphocytes have the property of

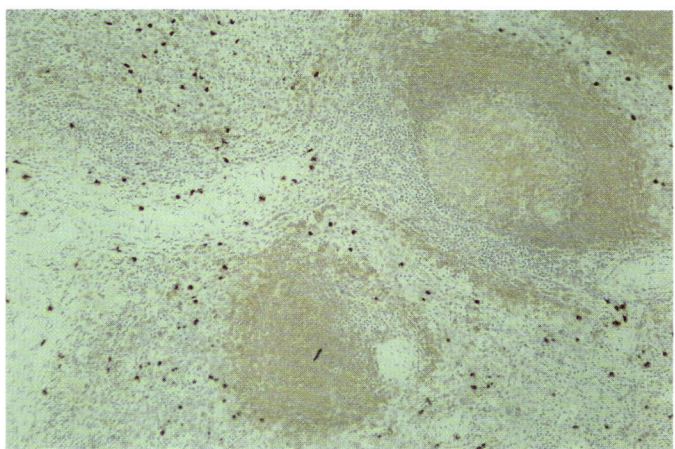

Fig. 24.65 Spleen stained with a monoclonal antibody to B-cells. The B-cell follicles stain strongly while the T-cells in the peri-arteriolar lymphocyte sheath are unstained.

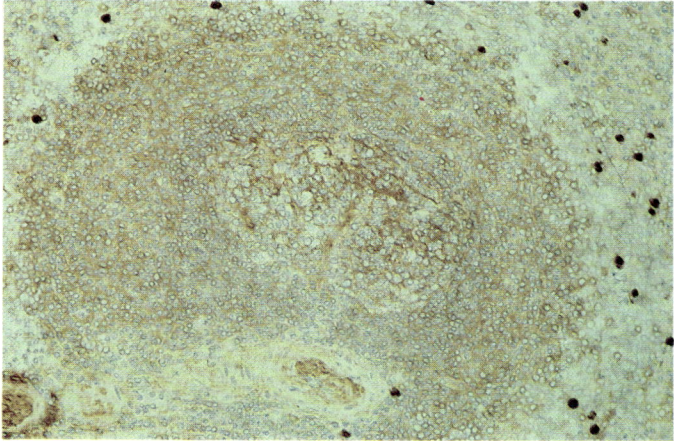

Fig. 24.67 B-cell area of spleen stained with an antibody to IgM, showing expression of surfaces IgM by both mantle-zone (coronal) and marginal-zone cells. The dendritic reticulin cell network of the follicle centre is also outlined.

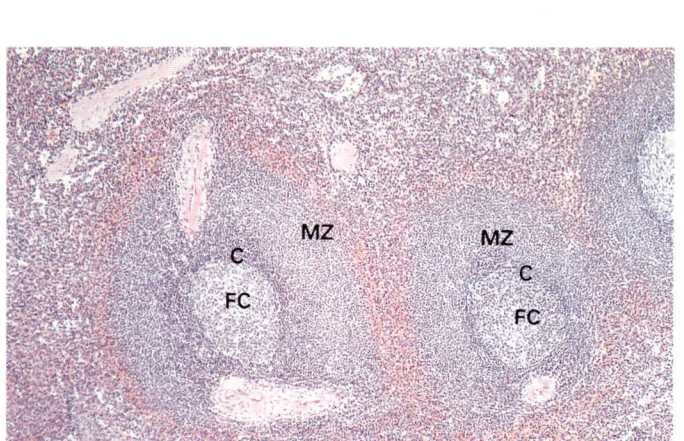

Fig. 24.66 Detail of the white pulp showing the follicle centre (FC) the mantle zone or corona (C) and the marginal zone (MZ) around which there is a zone of congested red pulp.

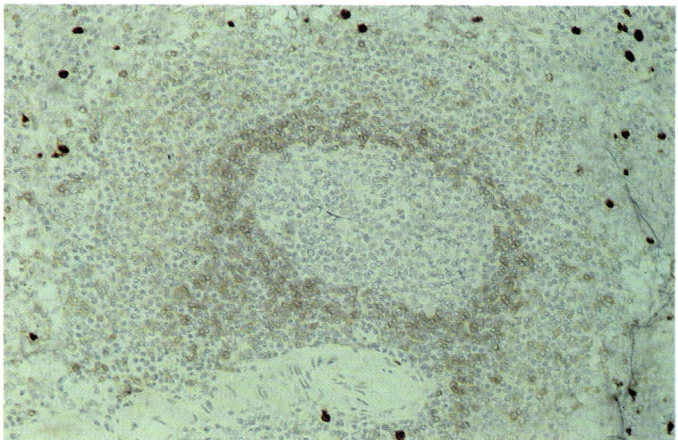

Fig. 24.68 The same area as in Fig. 24.67 stained with an antibody to IgD, showing restriction of staining to the mantle-zone cells. Marginal-zone cells do not express IgD.

migrating into the peri-arterial white pulp areas. This process is an active one since lymphoid migration is against the general flow in the spleen. The point of entry of lymphoid cells into the white pulp is via the marginal sinus (Fig. 24.66) or marginal zone, which is functionally analogous to the high endothelial post-capillary venules of the lymph node.

Kinetic studies using labelled cells in humans have shown that the spleen contains about 25 per cent of the exchangeable T-lymphocyte pool and about 10–15 per cent of the exchangeable B-lymphocyte pool. Studies in experimental animals show that about 50 per cent of the lymphocytes carried to the spleen in the peripheral blood actually enter the white pulp. Once they have left the red pulp the B- and T-cells remain together for between 1 and 6 hours in T-dependent areas. B-lymphocytes move into the follicles, especially to the corona about the germinal centres. The T-lymphocytes leave the peri-arteriolar

sheath to the venous circulation via the red pulp. How the B-lymphocytes leave the corona is unclear. The time spent by the B- and T-cells in the spleen is quite different, T-cells stay from 4 to 6 hours, B-cells four times as long. The duration of lymphoid stay in the spleen suggests that this organ has an important role in lymphoid activity.

Lymphocyte production

Lymphocytopoiesis in the spleen is not restricted to the follicles, but also occurs in the PALS, corona, and red pulp. Large numbers of these splenic lymphocytes migrate out of the spleen to all the lymphoid organs. These emigrating cells include T- and B-cells, of which the latter are probably precursors of antibody-producing cells. The immune functions of the spleen will be referred to later.

24.7.3 Functions of the spleen

The spleen as a filter

The spleen removes unwanted red cells and particles in the blood by three processes.

Phagocytosis

In common with the liver, the spleen contains large numbers of macrophages, which phagocytose unwanted formed elements. As they circulate slowly between the macrophages, bacteria, particularly encapsulated organisms that are not opsonized by antibody or complement, are removed from the circulation, and the spleen is probably the site at which the primary immunological response to those organisms is mounted. If the spleen is removed, there is the danger of death from overwhelming infections by these organisms (see below). The spleen is the site of the removal of red cells coated with IgG antibody, probably because the interaction of IgG and its Fc receptor on phagocytic cells of the immune system is so weak that it is only effective in the slow circulating environments of the spleen.

Mechanical structure of the sinus lining

Red cells may be removed from the circulation simply because they are not sufficiently deformable and thus are not able to pass through the slits between the endothelial cells of the splenic sinus. Thus, spherocytes and red cells containing sickle haemoglobin are not deformable and cannot squeeze through the slits between the sinus littoral cells. They accumulate in the cords and are phagocytosed. Red cells containing malarial organisms also loose deformability and are removed. Reticulocytes are somewhat less deformable than mature red cells and they spend about 1–2 days in the spleen before they circulate. The spleen plays a major role in the maturation of the reticulocyte into the mature biconcave erythrocyte. After delivery from the marrow, red cells become smaller in volume.

Pitting

This removes siderotic granules, Howell–Jolly and Heinz bodies from the red cells. This process occurs as the pliant red cells squeeze through the interendothelial slits in the endothelial-lined sinuses of the red pulp. The inclusions, which are not deformable, cannot pass through the slits and are simply nipped off; the red cells pass through and return to the circulation while the pitted material is ingested by local macrophages.

Effects of stasis

During the period of sequestration in the spleen, the red cells are subjected to another hazard. The stasis, combined with the presence of metabolically activated macrophages, results in oxygen and glucose deprivation, which stresses susceptible red cells, increasing their membrane rigidity and reducing their natural deformability. The cells are thus unable to pass through the sinus endothelium cells to enter the splenic sinus lumen, and thus will become trapped. This occurs in red cells that react excessively to stress due to an intrinsic metabolic abnormality, or because the cells are spherical, misshapen in some other way, or antibody-coated. The trapped cells undergo phagocytosis. The spleen also plays a minor role in the process of elimination of senescent red cells. The mononuclear phagocyte system, especially in the marrow, playing the major role in this respect.

Immunological functions of the spleen

Loss of the spleen, especially in young patients, is attended with additional risk of infection (see below). The spleen therefore makes a significant contribution to the immune integrity of the host. The immune functions operative in the spleen are as follows.

Immune surveillance

- Delivery of antigenic information
- Focus for lymphocyte traffic

Immune clearance

- Opsinization: initiation of specific antibody promotion recruitment of non-specific opsonins (e.g. complement)
- Phagocytosis: intravascular pathogens uptake of immune complexes disposal of senescent cells

Immune regulation

- Development of B- and T-memory cells
- Maturation of T-suppressor cells
- Control of autoimmunity

Blood pool

The normal red cell content of the spleen is 20–60 ml, or less than 5 per cent of the total red cell mass.

When the spleen is enlarged, and especially in myelo- and lymphoproliferative disorders, it is capable of developing a remarkably large pool with a high haematocrit and a slow exchange of red cells with those of the general circulation. This pooling will exclude a relatively large volume of red cells from the main arterial and venous circulation and thus will cause functional anaemia. There is no normal pool of granulocytes in the normal spleen, but there is sequestration of granulocytes, causing neutropenia, in splenomegaly. Platelets have a significant reservoir in the normal spleen (up to 30 per cent of normal platelet mass) rapidly interchangeable with the circulation. Cells may be held up temporarily in the spleen before returning to the circulation, a process known as sequestration.

Haemopoiesis and its regulation

Haemopoiesis is seen in the fetal spleen from 12 weeks of gestation to birth, after which it normally ceases. The potential for haemopoiesis remains in the spleen and it is regularly seen under conditions of severe anaemia. The microenvironment of the spleen imposes a different pattern of haemopoiesis as compared to the bone marrow. In the marrow the dominant proliferating elements are the myeloid series, while the splenic pulp favours erythropoiesis. In the marrow, haemopoiesis takes place exclusively in the tissues, but in the spleen haemopoiesis occurs both in the cords and in the sinus. This so-called reactive haemopoiesis has to be distinguished from myeloid metaplasia that occurs as part of myelosclerosis (the myeloproliferative condition). The latter is a neoplastic condition and the extramedullary haemopoiesis perhaps reflects the lack of fastidiousness of these cells for a normal microenvironemnt.

24.7.4   Hypersplenism and hyposplenism

The terms hypersplenism and hyposplenism were introduced at the beginning of the century when splenic function was thought to be analogous to the recently recognized disorders resulting from either excessive or inadequate endocrine activity. Subsequently it has been recognized that this is an oversimplistic approach to splenic function, bearing in mind that, although splenectomy does have consequences, the spleen is not essential to life. Nevertheless, the two terms do serve a purpose in outlining a series of syndromes associated with excess or absent splenic activity.

Splenomegaly: causes and effects

Splenomegaly occurs in a large number of aetiologically very different disorders, as summarized in Table 24.6.

The spleen responds to systemic inflammatory and necrotic processes by increasing the cellularity and the vascularity of the organ. This, in large measure, is a response of the constituents of the recticuloendothelial system to products from these

---

Table 24.6   Disorders accompanied by splenomegaly

Inflammatory conditions
1. *Infections*
   Bacterial
      splenic abscess, septicaemias, salmonellosis, relapsing fever, SBE, tuberculosis, brucellosis, syphilis
   Viral
      hepatitis, infectious mononucleosis, AIDS, cytomegalovirus infection
   Fungal   especially histoplasmosis
   Protozoal
      toxoplasmosis, malaria (major cause), leishmaniasis (major cause), trypanosomiasis
2. *Autoimmune disorders*
      Felty's syndrome, SLE, rheumatic fever, serum sickness, sarcoidosis and berylliosis, Graves' disease (hyperthyroidism)

Congestive splenomegaly
1. Intra-hepatic: cirrhosis, Wilson's disease, haemachromatosis, veno-occlusive disease, congenital fibrosis, bilharzia
2. Portal vein obstruction
      cavernous malformation, thrombosis, stenosis, or atresia
3. Splenic vein obstruction
      angiomatous malformation, thrombosis, atresia, or stenosis, obstruction by pancreatic disease or splenic arterial aneurysm
4. Hepatic venous occlusion, Budd–Chiari syndrome
5. Cardiac, especially chronic or recurrent congestive cardiac failure

Haematological disorders
1. Haemolytic disorders: red cell membrane disorders, e.g. hereditary sperocytosis; AIHA; thalassaemia, sickle cell, haemoglobinopatheis (Hb-SC)
2. Myeloproliferative disorders: myelosclerosis (major cause), polycythaemia vera (variable), essential thrombocythaemia (variable)
3. Miscellaneous: megaloblastic anaemia, iron deficiency

Malignancy
1. Haematological: acute leukaemia, chronic CGL (major cause), hairy-cell leukaemia, lymphoma, e.g. CLL, malignant histiocytosis, myelomatosis
2. Intrinsic angiosarcoma
      secondary carcinoma, melanoma
      Benign hamartoma, fibroma, haemagioma, lymphangioma
   Histiocytosis X, mastocytosis

Storage diseases
   Gaucher's disease (major cause), Niemann–Pick disease, Tangier's disease, Hurler's syndrome

Miscellaneous
   Cysts: parasitic, pseudocyst, epidermoid
   Amyloidosis, hereditary haemorrhagic telangiectasia
   Tropical and idiopathic splenomegaly

---

reactions. It manifests with hyperplasia of the macrophages located predominantly in the red pulp and the lymphoid cells and there is a concomitant response of the underlying stromal elements of the spleen. In the process of filtration, the splenic macrophages phagocytose a variety of particles, cells, and debris; this in turn can lead to significant and long-lasting hyperplasia. In experimental animals it has been shown that the injection of the non-digestible polymer, methyl cellulose, results in marked hyperplasia of red pulp macrophages and consequently splenic hyperplasia. Similar stimulation of macrophage proliferation occurs in many of the haemolytic anaemias. In congestive syndromes, such as in cirrhosis, the increased portal pressure results in pooling of blood in the cords and this, in turn, leads to secondary hyperplasia in the cordal macrophages.

The spleen is infiltrated in a variety of leukaemias, and in certain of these splenomegaly may be massive. Notable among these are chronic granulocytic leukaemia, the myeloproliferative disorders, hairy-cell leukaemia, and prolymphocytic leukaemia.

Hypersplenism, or the splenomegaly syndrome, is a disease complex characterized by enlargement of the spleen; deficits of one or more of the cell lines in the peripheral blood; normal or hyperplastic cellularity of the bone marrow, with at least normal representation of the cell line deficient in the circulation and correction of the defects by splenectomy.

The peripheral blood in the splenomegaly syndrome is dominated either by anaemia, granulocytopenia, or thrombocytopenia. The hyperplasia of the bone marrow is a strong indication that there is no lack of cell production, rather there is a loss of cells. Strenuous efforts have been made to determine whether or not the enlarged spleen causes marrow suppression. To date none has been found. Splenomegaly causes anaemia by splenic pooling, haemolysis, and haemodilution.

Splenic pooling As has been mentioned previously, the spleen has the ability to condition viable cells (culling, etc.) and to phagocytose effete cells. This may become harmful.

Sequestration and pooling refer to the temporary process whereby cells are held up in the sinuses before returning to the circulation, and the presence in the spleen of an increased amount of blood. In contrast to sequestration, pooled cells are in continuous exchange with the circulation.

The normal red cell content of the spleen is 20–60 ml, or less than 5 per cent of the total red cell mass, and there is no significant red cell pool. When the spleen is enlarged it is capable of developing a remarkably large pool of blood with a high haematocrit (the mechanism for concentrating red cells in the spleen was referred to earlier) which slowly exchanges with the red cells of the circulation. This pooling process will exclude a relatively large volume of red cells (20–60 per cent of the total) from the main circulation and thus will cause functional anaemia (Fig. 24.69).

Haemolysis Where splenomegaly coexists with immune haemolysis and major erythrocyte defects, e.g. hereditary haemolytic disease, red cell survival is greatly reduced. In

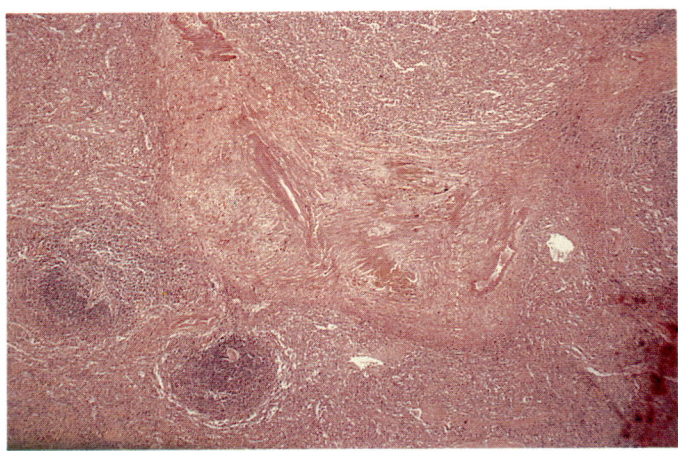

Fig. 24.69 A Gamna–Gandy body in the spleen from a case of portal hypertension. There is scarring with focal deposition of haemosiderin, giving a brown appearance macroscopically.

patients without major red cell defects there is only a moderate degree of haemolysis, i.e. red cell survival is modestly reduced. This can be attributed to increased splenic erythrocyte destruction. The rate of destruction is directly proportional to the size of the spleen.

Haemodilution Patients with splenomegaly, from whatever cause, invariably have increased plasma volume. This plasma volume expansion usually makes up about 30–60 per cent of normal values and, in some instances, the plasma volume may double. Plasma volume diminishes after splenectomy, the failure to do so implies that there are pathological changes in other organs, e.g. the liver. The expended plasma volume may be due to increased pressure in the portal vein resulting in an increase in the size of the total splanchnic bed, or possible effects on plasma proteins.

Platelets and the enlarged spleen

Thrombocytopenia is a common feature of splenomegaly, this has been shown to be due to pooling in the spleen. The normal spleen has 30 per cent of the total body platelet mass in an exchangeable pool. In massive splenomegaly this proportion may rise as high as 95 per cent. Rarely is the level of thrombocytopenia great enough to cause bleeding.

The degree of platelet pooling in the spleen is compensated for by increased marrow platelet production and consequently a danger of splenectomy is thrombocytosis, which may result in thrombosis in various organs.

Hyposplenism

The term hyposplenism was introduced by Eppinger to describe the condition that develops after splenectomy, and was adopted subsequently to describe the effects of impaired splenic function whatever the aetiology. The causes of hyposplenism are listed in Table 24.7. The hallmark of the gross hyposplenic state is the presence in the peripheral blood film of Howell–Jolly bodies (intra-erythrocyte inclusions consisting of nuclear remnants).

Table 24.7 Diseases in which hyposplenism may occur

Congenital
    Congenital asplenia
        1. Ivemark's syndrome
        2. isolated anomaly
    Congenital cyanotic heart-disease
Haematological
    Sickle-cell disease
    Essential thrombocythaemia
    Fanconi's syndrome
Autoimmune
    SLE
    Glomerulonephritis/vasculitis
    Rheumatoid arthritis
    Hashimoto's disease
    Graves' disease
Intestinal
    Coeliac disease
    Dermatitis herpetiformis
    Ulcerative colitis
    Crohn's disease
    Tropical sprue
    Whipple's disease
    Intestinal lymphangiectasia
    Chronic ulcerative jejunitis
Miscellaneous
    Splenic irradiation
        1. external
        2. thorotrast
    Amyloidosis
    Sarcoidosis
    Sezary's syndrome
    Chronic active hepatitis
    Thrombosis
        1. splenic artery
        2. splenic vein
    Graft versus host disease
    Immunodeficiency
    Hypopituitarism

Hyposplenism is most commonly due to splenectomy, but destruction of the spleen can result from a variety of other causes, such as sickle-cell disease, where repeated infarction leads to atrophy of the spleen and essential thrombocythaemia, where therapeutic irradiation results in destruction of the spleen. The concept of functional hyposplenism arose from the observations that Howell–Jolly bodies can occur in the peripheral blood of patients whose spleens are of normal size or enlarged and that in some conditions the haematological features are transient, suggesting that hyposplenism may be reversible. In systemic lupus erythematosus (SLE) and rheumatoid arthritis, the high levels of circulating immune complexes are associated with hyposplenism. It is thought that these complexes block macrophage function. The mechanism leading to hyposplenism in coeliac disease is not understood.

Sequelae of hyposplenism

Haematological Hyposplenism is frequently first diagnosed from peripheral blood films. Red blood cells often show a target appearance and nuclear remnants in the form of Howell–Jolly bodies appear in red cells.

Infection Overwhelming infection is now a well-known complication of splenectomy and, although the risk is greatest in children and within the first few years following operation, there is no doubt that patients of any age are at risk throughout their lives. The risk is least following splenectomy for trauma, probably because spilled splenic contents establish splenunculi in the peritoneal cavity, and increases when the spleen is removed because of disease such as idiopathic thrombocytopenic purpura (ITP) and hereditary spherocytosis. Hyposplenism is characteristically associated with pneumococcal infections. The illness is usually abrupt in onset and follows a fulminant course. Severe infections with other bacteria, in particular *Haemophilus influenzae* and meningococcus, are well documented, and overwhelming infection with organisms not usually pathogenic in man has been seen. In addition to bacterial infections, malaria and babesiosis appear to be more common in asplenic subjects. The spleen is important in clearing bacteria from the circulation and particularly important for encapsulated organisms, such as pneumococci, where the liver macrophages are inefficient in the absence of specific opsonizing antibody. There is also evidence that the functions of Kupffer's cells and the alveolar macrophages are impaired after splenectomy.

Hyposplenism results in defective antibody responses, particularly to antigens administered intravenously and to polysaccharide antigens. Both primary and secondary responses are abnormal and absence of the spleen causes a long-lasting B-cell defect characterized by a limited capacity of circulating B-cells to differentiate into antibody-secreting cells.

Autoimmune phenomena Splenic atrophy is associated with a high incidence of autoimmune disease, this may possibly be due to the fact that the spleen contains suppressor T-cells.

Thrombosis There is an increased incidence of myocardial infarction, probably due to thrombocytosis and increased blood viscosity that occur after splenectomy. Splenectomy itself can result in local thrombosis of the portal veins, and subsequent atrophy of the left lobe of the liver is a well-recognized complication of splenectomy.

24.7.5 Diseases of the red pulp

Congestive splenomegaly

This is caused by venous hypertension in the portal and splenic veins. This may be due to intrahepatic obstructive portal hypertension, extrahepatic portal obstruction, or chronic passive congestion of cardiac origin. The commonest cause is cirrhosis of the liver, in which 70 per cent of cases develop splenomegaly. The duration appears to be more important than the height of venous pressure. The spleen may become very enlarged and may necessitate splenectomy.

The spleen becomes hard due to fibroblastic and macrophage

proliferation resulting in thickening of the capsule and trabecular skeleton, and widening of the splenic cords. There is also dilation of the venous sinuses with collagenization of their walls. A further consequence of the sustained pressure is intraparenchymal haemorrhage. This is concentrated in the marginal zone and around the trabeculae. These undergo organization, producing focal scars encrusted with iron and calcium. Macroscopically these appear as small brownish spots throughout the pulp, known either as tobacco flecks or Gamna–Gandy bodies (Fig. 24.69). Since intrasplenic haemorrhage can arise from diverse causes, Gamna–Gandy bodies are not restricted to congestive diseases of the spleen. Lymphoid atrophy is a common feature in congestive splenomegaly.

Other circulatory abnormalities of the spleen

Infarction of the spleen

Infarction of the spleen can result from a variety of causes including embolism, torsion, thrombosis of the splenic artery, vasculitis, and sickle-cell disease. Splenic infarction may occur in splenomegaly of any cause.

Diseases of red blood cells

These are described in detail in Chapter 12.

Hereditary spherocytosis (HS)

Spleens from patients with HS are seen to have congested cords and fairly empty sinuses, which supports the theory that reduced deformability leads to entrapment of the spherocytes. Although the sinuses may appear empty by light microscopy, ultrastructural studies have demonstrated that the sinuses are filled with the ghosts of red cells. As a consequence of this trapping process there is hyperplasia of pulp macrophages and sinus littoral cells.

Haemaglobinopathies

Sickle-cell disease Sickle cells are extremely rigid and this is decisive in explaining the pathogenesis of the underlying disease and its effect on the spleen. Sickling in a capillary area compromises blood flow and thereby reduces oxygen tension. This may initiate further sickling and interference with local circulation.

During periods of acute sickling, often precipitated by hypoxia, red cells accumulate in the spleen and this accounts for periods of splenomegaly. The acuteness of the accumulation of cells in the spleen results in distension of the spleen and this causes pain, a condition often erroneously thought of as infarction. On the other hand, the accumulation of the cells in the spleen compromises the microcirculation and this results in infarction and progressive fibrosis. Ultimately this leads to hyposplenism.

Thalassaemia is not strictly a haemoglobinopathy, but an inherited defect of haemoglobin synthesis. The defective haemoglobin synthesis results in erythrocytes which are short-lived, and significant intra- and extramedullary haemolysis. The spleen is enlarged due, in part, to hyperplasia of the phagocytic cells and, in some cases, to extramedullary haemopoiesis.

Auto-immune diseases

Auto-immune haemolytic anaemia (AIHA)

The spleen may have an important role in the genesis of anaemia in auto-immune haemolytic processes. However, unlike auto-immune idiopathic thrombocytopenia, splenectomy is rarely curative. The red pulp shows well-marked macrophage activity with prominent erythrophagocytosis. The venous sinuses have prominent littoral cells and usually contain numerous red cells, often with poorly staining red cell stromata. There is commonly considerable haemosiderosis. Haemosiderin is found predominantly in macrophages, usually in the cords but also in the white pulp. In severe forms of the disease, haemosiderin is also found in sinus littoral cells. Extramedullary haemopoiesis, presumably in response to the anaemia, is frequently seen.

Idiopathic thrombocytopenic purpura (ITP)

In only 5 per cent of cases of ITP is there splenomegaly, yet splenectomy cures the disease in 80 per cent of cases. ITP is thus unique as a disease process which is cured by splenectomy, but does not manifest with splenomegaly.

This improvement may be the result of elimination of the specially required site for the removal of sensitized platelets, or removal of the source of anti-platelet antibody formation.

Histological appearances of the spleen may vary from being normal, to varying degrees of hyperplasia of the malpighian corpuscle with marked germinal centre formation. In the red pulp there may be foamy macrophages. This appearance results from the vacuole-like cytoplasmic inclusions, which are residual fragments of platelet membranes. When foamy macrophages are numerous there may be concomitant extramedullary haemopoiesis. The splenic histology does not discriminate between those cases that respond to splenectomy and those that do not.

Diseases associated with macrophage proliferation or accumulation

Lipid storage

The commonest form of lipid storage occurs in focal collections in the perifollicular zone (Fig. 24.70). This is commonly seen after lymphangiogram examinations and is due to the injected 'Lipiodol'. It may also be seen in individuals who have not received any form of lipid injection. Studies have often shown that this is mineral oil, probably derived from the diet or from the oral use of purgatives.

Storage disorders

These are inherited disorders of metabolism with enzyme defects. As a consequence various material accumulates in pulp macrophages.

Gaucher's disease Macrophages are filled with accumulated

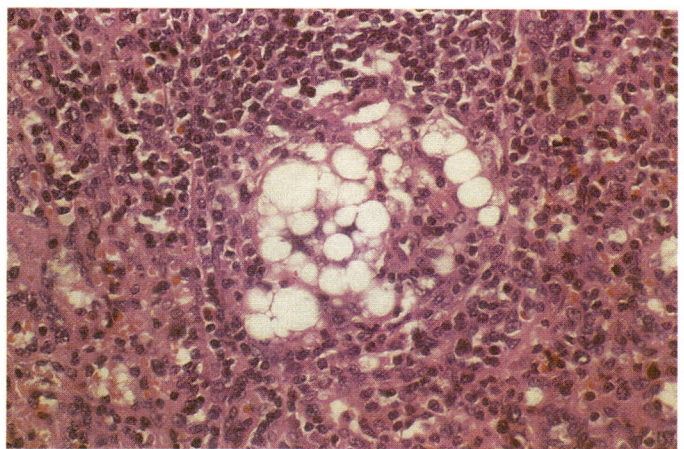

Fig. 24.70 A focal accumulation of lipid-filled macrophages. This is a very common finding in the spleen and is due to the accumulation of inorganic lipid, mostly dietary in origin, in macrophages.

glucocerebrosides. It affects especially the spleen, liver, and bone marrow. In the chronic type of the disease the spleen is most commonly very large, being the main storage place for the lipids, while hepatomegaly appears later in the course of the disease. The spleen (Fig. 24.71) is filled with large macrophages having cytoplasm of a ground-glass and streaky appearance.

Niemann–Pick disease This is rarer than Gaucher's disease. The spleen is once again the main storage site for sphingolipids; in contrast to Gaucher's disease, hepatomegaly occurs early in the disease.

Hurler's disease This is a rare childhood disorder due to increased acid mucopolysaccharides in the macrophages, accompanied by pronounced hepatosplenomegaly.

Wolman disease Deposition of cholesterol causes foam cells in

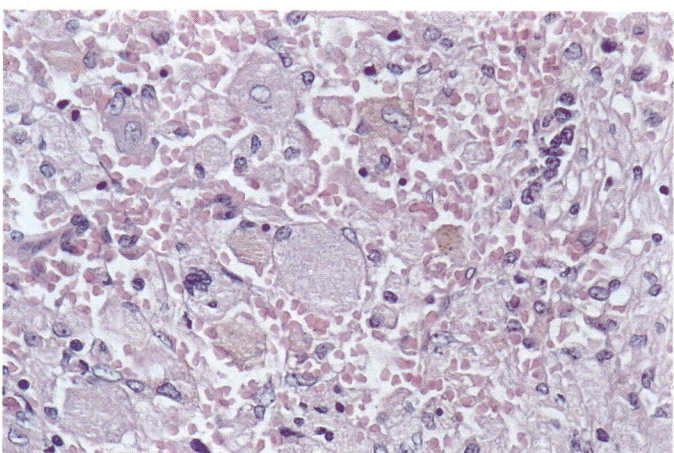

Fig. 24.71 Gaucher's disease. Cordal macrophages are filled with gluco-cerebroside, resulting in swollen macrophages with a ground-glass appearance and faint linear streaking.

many sites, but hepatosplenomegaly is the outstanding feature of this disease.

Gangliosiderosis This resembles Hurler's disease, with numerous foam cells due to the progressive deposition leading to splenomegaly.

Tangier's disease This is a serious familial cholesterol storage disease, sometimes associated with severe splenomegaly. The splenomegaly is probably due to phagocytosis of plasma high-density lipoproteins, splenectomy has been followed by a marked increase in serum lipid and its deposition in the skin.

Ceroid histiocytoses (sea-blue histiocytosis) Ceroid means wax-like and the term refers to a group of conditions in which there is an accumulation of macrophages with abundant foamy cytoplasm. The foamy nature is due to the accumulation of a variety of phospholipids. When stained with the Giemsa stain, the cells stain uniformly blue, hence the term sea-blue histiocytosis.

Histiocytosis X (Langerhans cell granulomatosis)

The histiocytosis X cells have the characteristic bland features of Langerhans cells with extremely folded nuclear membranes and small nucleoli. Splenic involvement is usually seen in the acute disseminated syndrome often seen in childhood as part of Letterer–Siwe disease.

Leukaemic infiltrates in the spleen

Most leukaemia patients show involvement of the spleen during the course of their disease, irrespective of the type of leukaemia. Splenomegaly, except in certain disease, is rarely the leading symptom, although it may contribute to anaemia and thrombocytopenia due to functional hypersplenism.

Leukaemic infiltration of the spleen carries with it the risk of spontaneous rupture, brought about as in the case of infectious mononucleosis, either by capsular infiltration, or possibly due to infarction. Although splenic rupture occurs in only about 1 per cent of leukaemic patients, leukaemia is the single most important cause for spontaneous rupture of the spleen, accounting for 40 per cent of cases. Rupture occurs most frequently in the acute leukaemias, particularly acute myeloid leukaemia and acute lymphocytic leukaemia, but also in hairy-cell leukaemia.

When malignancies of the lymphohaemopoietic system involve the spleen, their pattern of involement follows the migratory pathway of their normal benign counterparts. In line with the normal migratory location in the spleen, leukaemias of the myeloid, monocytic and erythroid, and megakaryocytic forms of differentiation are confined to the red pulp.

Chronic myeloid leukaemia Splenomegaly, often of appreciable degree, is present in more than 90 pr cent of untreated cases. The enlarged spleen is populated predominantly by cells of the myeloid system. However, megakaryocytes, often hypolobated in morphology, can be seen as well as a variable degree of erythropoiesis (Figs 24.72 and 24.73).

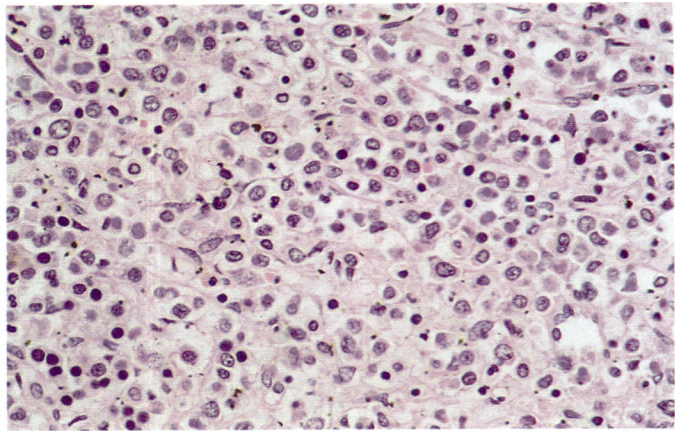

Fig. 24.72 Spleen in chronic myeloid leukaemia showing replacement of red pulp by a variety of cells, those with large open nuclei being myeloblasts. The scattered cells with dense small nuclei are erythropoietic elements.

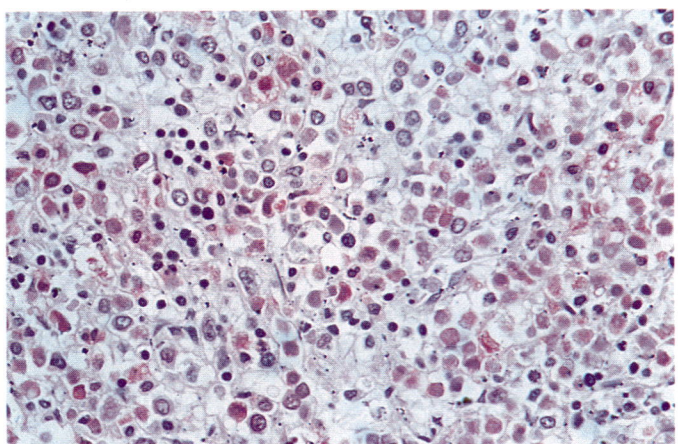

Fig. 24.73 Same case as shown in Fig. 24.72 stained for the enzyme chloracetate-esterase, which is found in myeloid cells. Note the pink (positive) staining of myeloid cells while erythroid precursors are unstained.

Myeloproliferative disorders In polycythaemia vera, although there is splenomegaly, there is minimal extramedullary haemopoiesis, although there is considerable trapping of mature red blood cells in the spleen. Commonly there are foamy macrophages in the red pulp, similar to those seen in ITP. In myelofibrosis there is considerable extramedullary haemopoiesis in the spleen, involving all three elements, i.e. myeloid, erythroid, and megakaryocytic. Splenic weight can be enormous, up to several kilograms (Fig. 24.74).

Hairy-cell leukaemia This is a malignant proliferation of B-lymphocytes. In contrast to other B-cell malignancies, the cells of hairy-cell leukaemia are confined to the red pulp. It produces a homogeneous infiltration of the cords, causing atrophy of the white pulp. Pools of red cells, the so-called red cell lakes, are

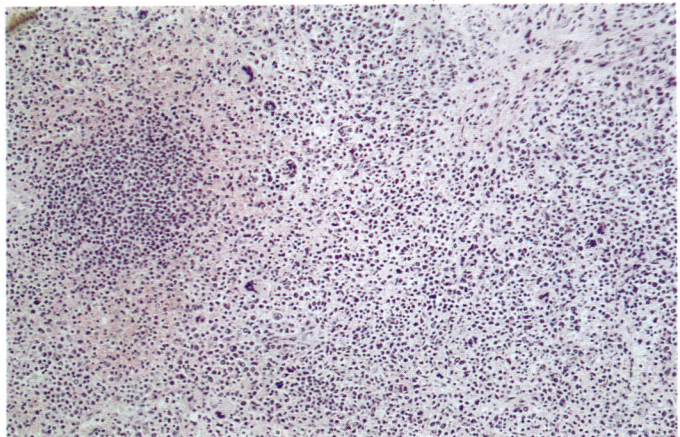

Fig. 24.74 The spleen in myelofibrosis showing infiltration of the red pulp, which includes numerous large megakaryocytes.

lined by hairy cells (pseudosinuses) (Fig. 24.75). The hairy cells are relatively small with bland round to oval nuclei, relatively open chromatin, and a paucity of mitotic figures. The cytoplasm is frequently abundant and clear. As a consequence the cells have a uniform, well-spaced arrangement. Hairy cells are frequently associated with numerous reactive plasma cells.

Hypersplenism is a regular feature of hairy-cell leukaemia and splenectomy is of considerable therapeutic benefit.

Splenomegaly due to infections

The filter-like function of the spleen in relation to the blood circulating through it commonly results in its involvement in generalized infections.

Acute suppurative diseases

In these diseases, with or without demonstrable septicaemia, the spleen may be 2–3 times larger than normal. In these conditions it is seldom palpable, because it is unusually soft. This type

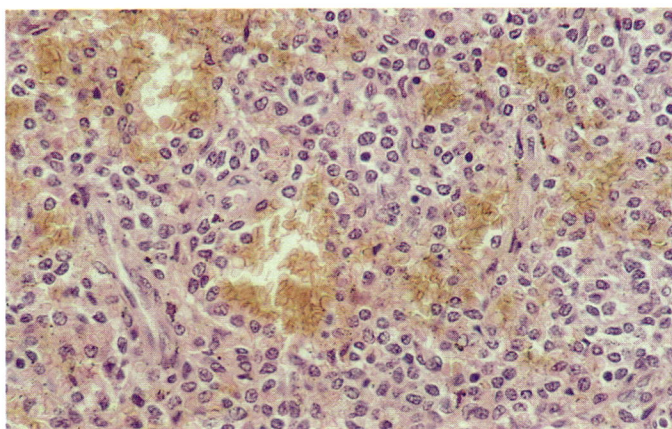

Fig. 24.75 Spleen from a case of hairy-cell leukaemia showing the morphology of the hairy cells and the formation of blood-filled pseudosinuses lined by these cells.

of splenomegaly used to be known as acute splenic tumour. The spleen is soft with a dull creamy red appearance. This appearance is due to the presence of numerous polymorphs and their products in the red pulp. The nature of the cell infiltrate is, to a certain extent, determined by the nature of the infectious agent, thus in typhoid and paratyphoid the spleen is packed with mononuclear cells instead of polymorphs. Chronic septicaemia illnesses, such as bacterial endocarditis, show the consequences of chronic stimulation, i.e. splenomegaly and hyperplasia of both the red pulp and the lymphoid tissue.

Granulomatous splenitis

There are numerous infectious causes for this, but in many instances the cause in unknown and sarcoidosis has to be always borne in mind. The spleen is regularly involved in cases of generalized miliary tuberculosis. Granulomas are seen in the secondary and tertiary stages of syphilis and in septicaemic forms of *Yersinia enterocolitica*, where lesions similar to those seen in the lymph nodes are visible. Granulomas are also seen in tularaemia and brucellosis. The spleen may contain granulomas in malignancies, particularly in Hodgkin's disease and non-Hodgkin's lymphoma.

Infectious mononucleosis

Cases of infectious mononucleosis may present as splenomegaly and sometimes with splenic rupture. The pulp cords and sinuses are filled with immunoblasts similar to those seen elsewhere in lymph nodes (see Section 24.3.11). In addition, there is infiltration of the capsule and the trabeculae by these same cells. In these cases the white pulp is usually atrophic.

Protozoal infections

Malaria There is enlargement of the red pulp of the spleen due to the increase in thickness of the red pulp cords primarily as a consequence of the proliferation of pulp-cord macrophages. In endemic areas the spleen may reach huge sizes and may be slate-grey in colour due to the accumulation of malarial pigment, which is altered haemoglobin.

The spleen is thought to play an important role in the attrition of the malarial infestation. Erythrocytes infected with plasmodia loose deformability and are therefore susceptible to filtration in the spleen by the mechanisms referred to previously. Splenectomy has therefore a deleterious affect in antimalarial host defence.

Leishmaniasis There is diffuse hyperplasia of the reticuloendothelial cells, especially of macrophages in the red pulp. This is one of the conditions which can manifest with massive splenomegaly. The infectious agent, *Leishmania donovani*, may be seen as an intracellular parasite in the macrophages.

Tropical splenomegaly syndrome (TSS) This is the term for the presence of a very large spleen of undetermined aetiology in an endemic malarious environment. Alternative terms are 'big spleen disease' or 'idiopathic splenomegaly'. TSS has been reported in Africa as well as in Vietnam and New Guinea. The syndrome is seen most often in young adults. Together with the splenomegaly there is enlargement of the liver, with a degree of portal hypertension. The patients show anaemia, leucopenia and thrombocytopenia. The IgM level is high and this is almost always associated with a high malaria antibody titre. The liver shows lymphocytic infiltration in the sinusoids and periportal fibrosis. The spleen shows little structural alteration. The white pulp is usually reduced, the sinuses are dilated and the pulp cords contain lymphocytes and plasma cells. The features are in no way diagnostic.

24.7.6 White pulp diseases

Lymphoproliferative diseases

Splenomegaly is frequently associated with malignant lymphoproliferative diseases and, in certain diseases such as pro-lymphocytic cell leukaemia, hairy-cell leukaemia, and the so-called pseudo-hairy-cell or villous-cell leukaemia, splenomegaly may be a dominant feature of the disease.

Lymphocytes traffic both in the red pulp and the white pulp and it is not surprising that these diseases may affect both sites. In general, however, the lymphomas and lymphoproliferative diseases affect particularly the white pulp. Hairy-cell leukaemia and large granular lymphocytic leukaemia are notable exceptions.

While normal lymphocytes traffic between the blood and the white pulp, it is unclear whether such trafficking occurs with neoplastic lymphocytes. Splenectomy of patients with chronic lymphocytic leukaemia is usually followed by increased lymphocytosis, suggesting that the spleen provides a pool for blood lymphocytes. It does not, however, prove that the cells of the white pulp exchange with the circulating pool. In a few patients splenectomy is followed by decreased lymphocyte counts, indicating that the spleen is a focus of tumour cell generation.

While most lymphomas tend to pick out the white pulp and follow the architecture of the spleen, large-cell anaplastic lymphomas, such as immunoblastic lymphoma, present as large tumour masses in the spleen.

Hodgkin's disease

The spleen may be involved either directly by tumour tissue in Hodgkin's disease, or show secondary effects. Early deposits of tumour tissue occur either in the peri-arteriolar zone or in the marginal zone (Figs. 24.76, 24.77). The tumour tissue shows similar components to that seen elsewhere. Involvement of the spleen may either consist of multiple nodules involving numerous white pulp areas, some of which coalesce, or there may be only a single tumour nodule.

In addition to infiltration of the spleen, epithelioid granulomas may be found in both the white and red pulp of the spleen in the absence of tumour tissue.

Non-Hodgkin's lymphomas

Although 40–50 per cent of non-Hodgkin's lymphomas involve the spleen, primary lymphoma of the spleen is very rare and is

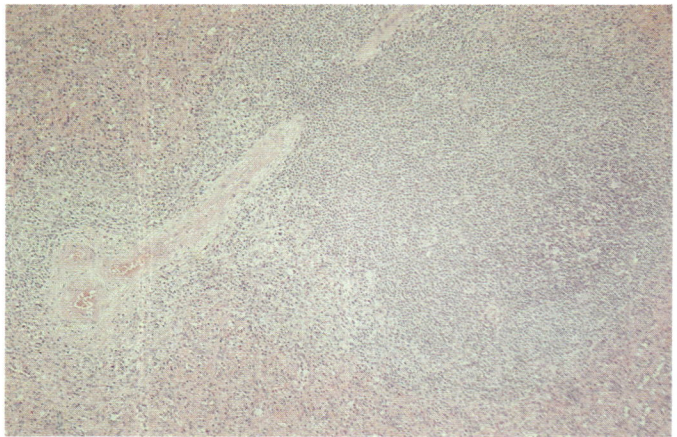

Fig. 24.76 Spleen from a case of Hodgkin's disease. The B cell follicle is hyperplastic and infiltration along the peri-arteriolar lymphocyte sheath by Hodgkin's disease is evident.

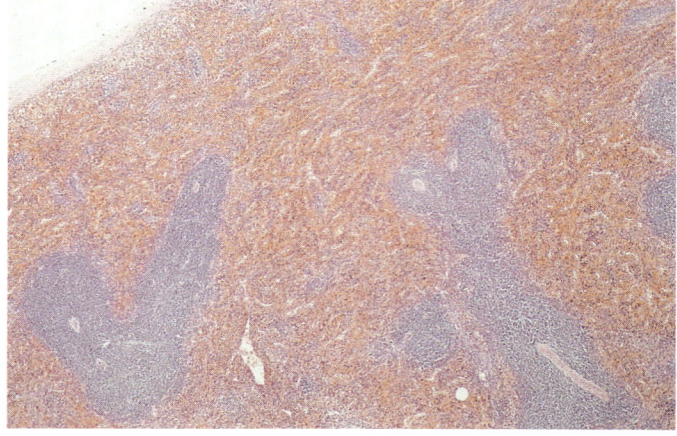

Fig. 24.78 Spleen in malignant lymphoma lymhocytic (chronic lymphocytic leukaemia) showing infiltration of the white pulp together with small infiltrates in the red pulp.

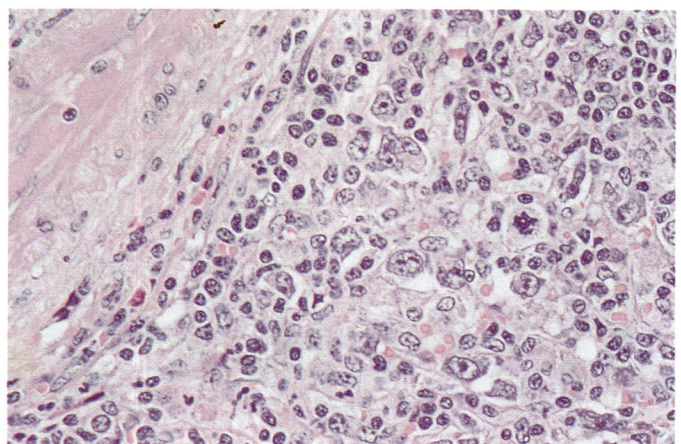

Fig. 24.77 Details of the infiltrate seen in Fig. 24.76. Reed–Sternberg and Hodgkin's cells are evident in a background of lymphocytes; plasma cells, and macrophages.

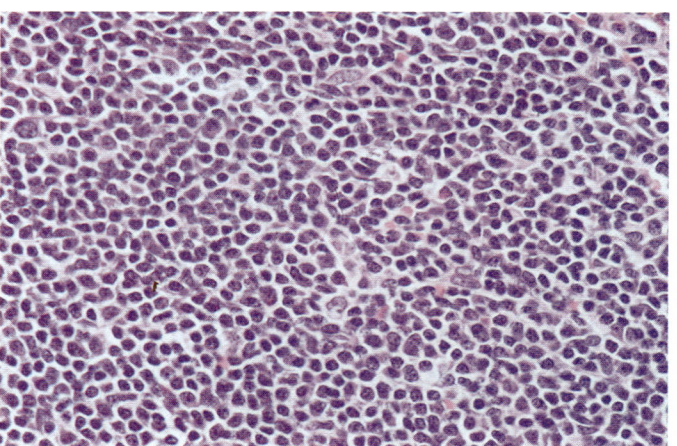

Fig. 24.79 Detail of infiltrate seen in Fig. 24.78, showing that it consists of small lymphocytes.

thought to occur in fewer than 1 per cent of all patients with lymphoma.

When splenic involvement by non-Hodgkin's lymphoma is early it may occur in a normal or slightly enlarged spleen showing no gross changes, or with only focal involvement on microscopic examination.

Lymphocytic lymphoma (chronic lymphocytic leukaemia (CCL)) In the majority of cases with B-CLL, splenomegaly is a late complication. However, in less than 5 per cent of patients there is a progressive enlargement of the spleen without significant enlargement of lymph nodes. There is a diffuse involvement of the spleen affecting both the red and white pulp. In general, the density of the lymphoid infiltrate in the red pulp reflects the severity of the peripheral blood lymphocyte count (Figs. 24.78, 24.79).

The usual range of cells seen in lymph nodes in CLL are found

in the spleen, i.e. small lymphocytes, prolymphocytes, and 'para-immunoblasts'. While these cell types are found both in the red and white pulp, they are differentially distributed between them. Thus there is a greater proportion of the prolymphocytes and 'para-immunoblasts' in the white pulp than in the red. In effect, the white pulp resembles the proliferation centres seen in the lymph nodes. In the 'accelerated phase' of the disease or 'prolymphocytoid change', there is considerable tumorous enlargement of the white pulp composed predominantly of para-immunoblasts and prolymphocytes.

In lymphocytic lymphoma, despite the absence of lymphocytosis in the peripheral blood, the histological findings in the spleen are similar to those in CLL.

Lymphoplasmacytic lymphoma Lymphoplasmacytic malignancies have a similar tissue distribution to CLL. There is a tendency for the prolymphocytic forms to accumulate on the periphery of the white pulp, producing a marginating effect, and this can cause difficulties if the obliteration of the marginal zone is relied upon as a diagnostic criterion. Plasma cells and plasmacytoid lymphocytes are to be found both in the white and red pulp. In a number of cases there is a concomitant leukaemia. Some of these have villous processes on their cell surface such that the cells superficially resemble hairy-cell leukaemia.

Prolymphocytic cell leukaemia Splenic enlargement occurs early on in this disorder in which there are high lymphocyte counts. Cytologically the disorder differs from CLL in having a prominent nucleolus in the presence of dense clumped chromatin. Unlike CLL, Ig is at a high density on the cell surface. The disease pursues an aggressive course. The pattern of infiltration in the spleen is similar to other lymphoproliferative disorders, with involvement of the red and white pulp. Margination of cells in the white pulp is striking.

Centroblastic/centrocytic lymphoma Splenic involvement is common and may be the presenting feature. The white pulp is predominantly involved. There is a broad marginal zone surrounding a central white pulp area consisting of centroblasts and centrocytes.

Centrocytic lymphoma This disease predominantly affects the white pulp, and the Malpighian corpuscle is diffusely affected. Frequently, the white pulp is surrounded by epithelioid macrophages.

Immunoblastic lymphoma This may take the form of proliferation of immunoblastic cells in the white pulp, resulting in a considerable expansion of lymphoid tissue in the spleen. In the most severe forms the disease presents with large round tumour masses in the red pulp.

T-cell lymphomas The histological features seen in the white pulp are a reflection of the features in the lymph nodes, i.e. lymphocytes with epithelioid cells in Lennert's lymphoma, a pronounced proliferation of vessels in angioimmunoblastic lymphadenopathy-like lymphoma, etc.

24.7.7 Primary non-lymphoreticular tumours of the spleen

The spleen is composed of tissues with a mesenchymal derivation, thus neoplasms of fibroblasts, vasoformative elements, arise in this organ. In addition, a variety of cysts are found in the spleen, in all likelihood originating from infoldings of the mesothelial lining. Benign lesions include haemangiomas, lymphangiomas, epidermoid cysts, mesothelial cysts, lipomas, and splenic hamartoma.

Comparatively few primary malignant tumours have been documented in the spleen, these include angiosarcoma, haemangioendothelioma, and fibrosarcoma.

24.7.8 Further reading

Burke, J. S. (1981a). Surgical pathology of the spleen: an approach to the differential diagnosis of splenic lymphomas and leukaemias. Part I. Diseases of the white pulp. *American Journal of Surgical Pathology* **5**, 551–63.

Burke, J. S. (1981b). Surgical pathology of the spleen: an approach to the differential diagnosis of splenic lymphomsa and leukaemias. Part II. Diseases of the red pulp. *American Journal of Surgical Pathology* **5**, 681–94.

Krieken, J. H. J. M. van and Te Velde, J. (1986). Immunohistology of the human spleen: an inventory of the localization of lymphocyte subpopulations. *Histopathology* **10**, 285–94.

Krieken, J. H. J. M. van, Te Velde, J., Hermans, J., Cornelisse, C. J., Welvaart, C., and Ferari, M. (1983). The amount of white pulp in the spleen: a morphometrical study done in methacrylate-embedded splenectomy specimens. *Histopathology* **7**, 767–82.

Lampert, I. A. and Thompson, I. (1988). The spleen in chronic lymphocytic leukaemia and related disorders. In *Chronic lymphocytic leukaemia* (ed. A. Polliack and D. Catovsky), pp. 193–208. Harwood Academic Publishers, London.

Lewis, S. M. (ed.)(1983). The spleen. *Clinics in haematology* **12** (2). W. B. Saunders, London.

Rappaport, H. (1970). The pathological anatomy of the splenic red pulp. In *Die Milz/The spleen* (ed. K. Lennert and D. Harms), pp. 24–40. Springer-Verlag, Berlin.

Videbaek, A., Christenson, B. J., and Jønsson, V. (1982). *The spleen in health and disease*. FADL's Forlag, Copenhagen.

Weiss, L. and Tavassoli, L. (1970). Anatomical hazards to the passage of erythrocytes through the spleen. *Seminars in Haematology* **7**, 372–9.

24.8 The thymus

M. A. Ritter and I. A. Lampert

24.8.1 Introduction

The thymus is a bilobed organ that lies in a mediastinal position just above the heart. It reaches its greatest size in childhood, and shows progressive involution following puberty. As early as 1777 the anatomist Magnus Falconer described the thymus as a gland that was filled with white corpuscles and whose external duct was the thoracic duct. However, little progress was made in the following 200 years, and in textbooks published as recently as 1956 it was considered to be an organ of unknown function. The true significance of the thymus remained a mystery until the early 1960s when J. F. A. P. Miller and R. A. Good demonstrated its vital role in the production of those lymphocytes that are responsible for mounting cell-mediated immune responses (e.g. graft rejection). Such lymphocytes were termed T-lymphocytes after their organ of origin.

24.8.2 Structure

The thymus is predominantly a lymphoepithelial organ surrounded by a connective tissue capsule (Fig. 24.80). The latter

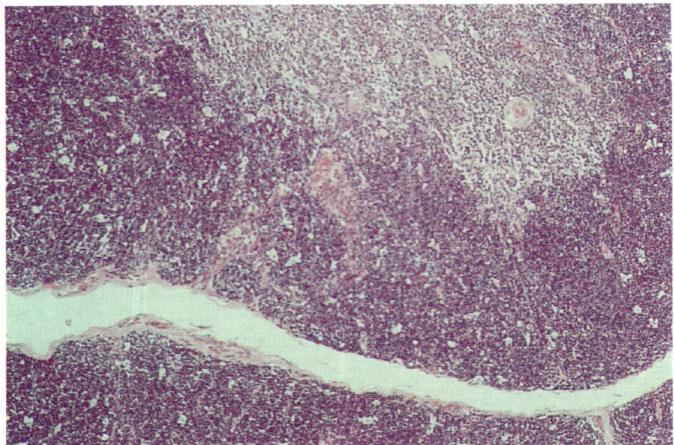

Fig. 24.80 Low-power view of paediatric thymus stained with haematoxylin to show lobular structure separated by septa.

extends deeply into the structure, forming septae (trabeculae) that divide each lobe into many pseudolobules. These septae carry vascular and neuronal supplies into the organ. A basement membrane lies immediately under the capsule and also surrounds the many blood vessels within the thymus. Reticulin fibres form a meshwork throughout the organ. In histological section, three main areas of the thymus can be recognized: the subcapsular zone, the cortex, and the central medulla—each characterized by distinctive cellular components (Fig. 24.81).

The main blood vessels enter the thymic lobules from the septa at the level of the cortical–medullary junction; these arterioles give rise to three sets of thymic blood vessels:

1. capillaries in the cortex which loop back to venules at the cortical–medullary junction and exit via the septa;

2. capillary loops in the medulla which also return to venules at the cortical–medullary junction and leave via the septa; and

3. cortical capillaries which do not form loops but which continue out through the cortex and drain into the surface venous plexus that lies external to the thymic capsule.

Short lengths of the venules in the cortical–medullary region are lined with high endothelium and it is in this area that cells probably enter and leave the organ via the vascular system. The capsule, septa, and perivascular spaces are also drained by lymphatics; however, unlike the vessels of the vascular system these do not arise from the thymus parenchyma itself.

The thymus is well innervated. Noradrenergic fibres enter the organ with the vasculature and form plexuses under the capsule and in septal regions. From the subcapsule, fibres branch and spread throughout the thymic cortex, while the septal-derived fibres extend to form venous and arterial plexuses at the cortical–medullary junction. Small fibres branch from these vascular plexuses and enter the medulla. Peptidergic innervation may also be important. VIP-like immunoreactive profiles that resemble nerve fibres have been detected, and epithelial cells (e.g. cortical thymic nurse cells) are known to contain, and presumably secrete, both oxytocin and vasopressin. The extent of thymic cholinergic innervation is unclear.

24.8.3 Cellular composition

Many cell types are found within the thymus: lymphocytes, epithelial cells, macrophages, and dendritic cells comprise the major populations; however, B-lymphocytes, neutrophils, eosinophils, and occasional myoid and erythroid cells are also seen within the organ.

The epithelial cells form a framework into which the other cell types are packed; this framework can be visualized with immunostaining for keratin intermediate filaments (Fig. 24.82), and has been analysed in detail by both light and electron microscopy. In the subcapsular regions they form a

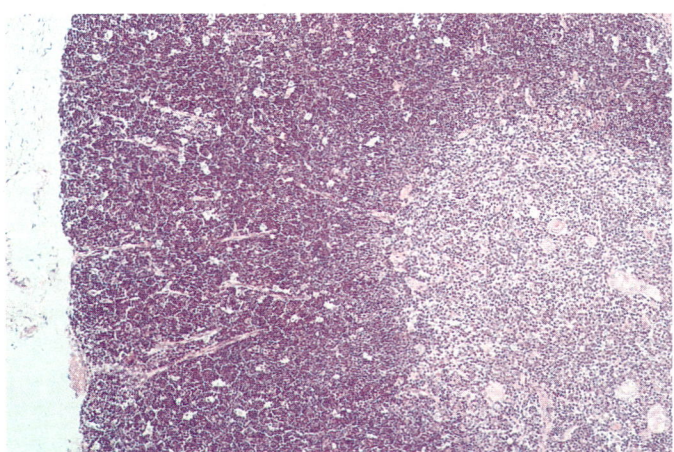

Fig. 24.81 Low-power view of paediatric thymus showing division into cortical (outer) and medullary (inner) regions.

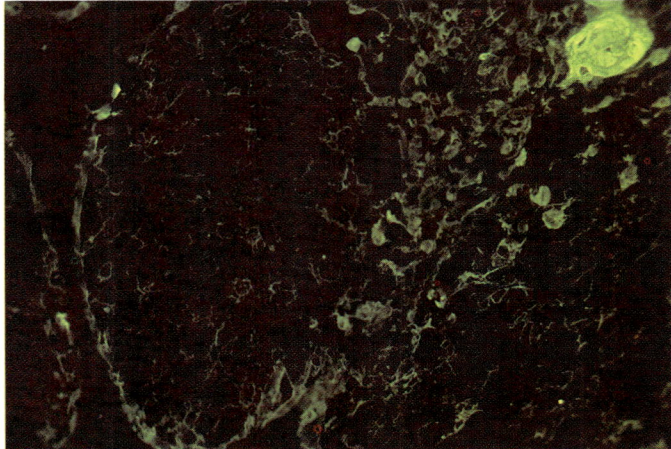

Fig. 24.82 Epithelial cells of subcapsular, cortical, and medullary zones of paediatric human thymus visualized by immunofluorescent (fluorescein) staining of keratin filaments. A highly keratinized Hassall's corpuscle can be seen in the upper right-hand corner of the photograph.

layer 1–2 cells deep, with the outermost layer lying on the base-ment membrane, just under the capsule. Similar cells line the septal invaginations and perivascular spaces. In contrast, the cortical epithelial cells are irregularly shaped with long pro-cesses that form a network within the cortex. These epithelial processes are in close contact with each other and are thought to form a syncytium. In the medulla, the epithelial cells do not interconnect; they are more oval in shape and have shorter, spatulate processes. Finally, whorls of epithelial cells, the 'Has-sall's corpuscles' are seen in the medulla (Fig. 24.83). These structures vary considerably in size: the smaller ones are com-posed of living epithelial cells arranged in concentric circles; in the larger ones the outer layers of living cells surround a cen-tral, non-living, highly keratinized core.

The thymus lymphocytes (thymocytes) also show character-istic differences according to their position within the organ (Figs 24.84, 24.85). Large lymphoblasts, which represent approximately 5 per cent of all thymocytes, lie in the sub-capsular region. The majority of the population (85 per cent)

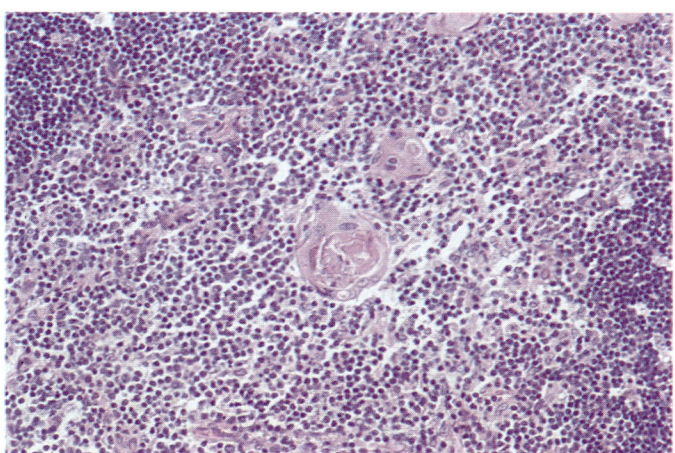

Fig. 24.83 Haematoxylin staining of human paediatric thymus show-ing Hassall's corpuscle (epithelial whorl) in the medullary region.

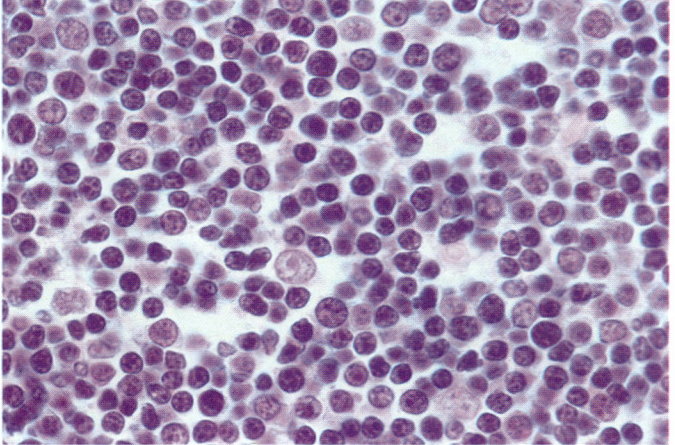

Fig. 24.84 Haematoxylin stain of human thymus to show closely packed small lymphocytes in the cortical zone.

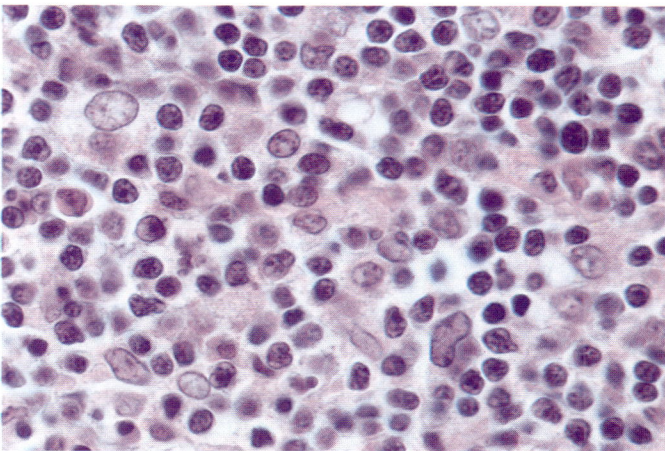

Fig. 24.85 Haematoxylin stain of human thymus to show loosely packed small lymphocytes in the medullary region.

comprises the cortical thymocytes. These are the smallest lymphocytes within the thymus and are found tightly packed in between the epithelial cells, forming lymphoid islands that are surrounded by epithelial cell processes. The final 10 per cent of thymocytes are situated in the medulla; these cells are slightly larger than those of the cortex and are essentially indistinguish-able from mature recirculating peripheral T-lymphocytes.

Macrophages are found scattered throughout all regions of the thymus; although morphologically relatively homo-geneous, enzyme, and immunohistochemical data indicate that different subpopulations of these cells occupy different sites within the organ. Dendritic cells, which are probably related to similar cells in many other organs, are found only in the medulla. Of the remaining cell types found within the thymus, neutrophils and eosinophils are fairly rare within the actual thymic lobules (although frequently present in the septa); they are seen as occasional scattered cells in both cortex and medulla, and are sometimes found within the Hassall's cor-puscles. In contrast, significant numbers of B-lymphocytes have been observed only in the medulla. Although originally thought to enter the thymus as mature cells, recent data suggest that these non-T-lymphoid haemopoietic cells may develop *in situ* under the inductive influence of intrathymic local micro-environmental niches.

Myoid cells form a relatively rare thymic population. They are found mainly in the medulla, often close to Hassall's cor-puscles. Myoid cells can be identified by immunostaining with antibodies to striated muscle. They are usually rounded, although some have fusiform tails which can be seen by elec-tron microscopy to contain striations characteristic of skeletal muscle. The cells are thought to be the source of auto-antigen in myasthenia gravis.

24.8.4 Ontogeny

The thymus develops from the third and fourth pharyngeal pouches early in embryogenesis. It is not clear whether both ectoderm and endoderm make a physical contribution to the final organ or whether the ectoderm plays only a inductive role in the organ's formation; a requirement for a mesenchymal inductive influence has been clearly demonstrated. During development, the thymus migrates from a cervical position to its final location above the heart. As migration proceeds, the two lobes come progressively closer together until in their final position above the heart they lie next to each other, linked by surrounding connective tissue.

Initially, the thymic anlagen is composed entirely of epithelial cells. During the 9th week of gestation large lymphoblastic haemopoietic stem cells and subsequently lymphocytes can be seen in the developing rudiment. The number of lymphocytes throughout the organ increases rapidly, and by the 14th week of gestation the distinction between cortex and medulla has become clear. Also at this time, macrophages appear throughout the thymus, and dendritic cells are seen entering the medulla from the mesenchymal septa and perivascular spaces. Myoid cells are first seen in the thymus in the 8th week of gestation, and can later be found as scattered clusters of round/elongated cells in the thymic medulla. By week 14, distinct subcapsular, cortical, and medullary zones can be distinguished. This regional differentiation is accompanied by development of the septal tissue. During the 9th–12th weeks the thymus becomes indented by mesenchymal septa. These push progressively further and further into the expanding thymic tissue, until by the 17th week the septa have reached the cortical–medullary junction, dividing the thymus into pseudolobules. Branches of these septa push into the thymus to form perivascular spaces in the cortical–medullary region. Blood vessels and nerves are brought into the organ via the septa and the thymus thus acquires its mature architecture. During subsequent fetal development there is a considerable increase in thymic size that involves all regions of the organ. Age-associated involution of the thymus is discussed in a later section.

24.8.5   Lymphopoiesis

The thymus is regarded as a primary lymphoid organ responsible for the production of T-lymphocytes. Haemopoietic stem cells (generated in the adult bone marrow and fetal liver) migrate via the bloodstream to the thymus. In the early fetal thymus, stem cells enter via the connective tissue capsule and lining basement membrane; after vascularization, stem cells leave the blood and enter the thymus at the level of the high endothelial venules and other vessels at the cortico–medullary junction. The T-lymphocyte progenitors (prothymocytes) then migrate out to the subcapsular region where they proliferate—hence their blastic appearance—and give rise to the large population of lymphocytes in the thymic cortex. The majority of these cortical thymocytes are thought to die *in situ* rather than to leave the organ. Evidence of such large-scale death and resultant phagocytosis is not obvious within the thymus. However it has been shown that the process of apoptosis (active programmed cell death via DNA cleavage by endogenous endo-

nuclease activity) is responsible for thymocyte deletion, giving rise to smaller and less conspicuous fragments of cell debris. The surviving minority of thymocytes, estimated to represent between only 5 and 20 per cent of the total lymphocytes produced within the thymus are thought to migrate to the medulla before leaving to enter the recirculating pool of mature peripheral T-lymphocytes.

24.8.6   Lymphocyte subpopulation—phenotypic analysis

The process of T-lymphocyte maturation within the thymus has been analysed by monoclonal antibody and molecular genetics techniques, making it possible to identify lymphocyte populations according to their surface antigenic phenotype and the rearrangement and expression of the genes encoding their surface receptors for antigen. As prothymocytes mature to cortical lymphocytes they sequentially acquire a number of cell surface protein/glycoprotein molecules (Fig. 24.86). Each molecule has been given a 'cluster of differentiation' number, according to World Health Organization nomenclature. CD1 is present only on the surface of cortical thymocytes, while CD2 and CD5 are expressed on essentially all cortical and medullary thymocytes. CD8 appears early in T-lymphocyte development; CD8$^+$ immature cells give rise to double-positive CD4$^+$CD8$^+$ cortical thymocytes. A minority of these double-positive cells give rise to the functionally mature, single-positive CD4$^+$ or CD8$^+$ lymphocytes of the thymic medulla, while the majority form the population that is thought to die *in situ*. It is during the development of thymocytes in the cortex that T-cell receptor expression first occurs. Rearrangement of the T-cell receptor genes takes place within the CD4$^+$CD8$^+$ population to generate the repertoire of functional T-cell receptor molecules. For the majority of T-cells the receptor is a heterodimeric structure composed of an α and a β polypeptide chain. The β gene locus is rearranged before the α, yielding cortical thymocytes that contain free cytoplasmic β

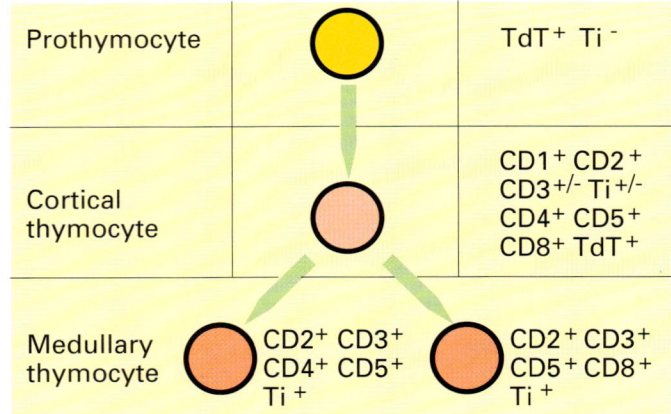

Fig. 24.86 Diagrammatic summary of the surface molecules present on subpopulations of thymocytes in man. TdT, Enzyme terminal deoxyribonucleotidyl transferase—adds nucleotides to DNA without a template; CD1, CD2, CD3, CD4, CD5, CD8, cell surface molecules detected by specific monoclonal antibodies; Ti, T-cell receptor.

chains. Only when the α locus has also been rearranged to give a functional α gene and α protein product does the fully assembled α–β heterodimer appear on the lymphocyte surface. As with all other T-cell receptor bearing lymphocytes, there is co-expression of the CD3 molecule. An alternative T-cell receptor, a heterodimer composed of γ and δ chains encoded by separate genes, is expressed during ontogeny and in approximately 5 per cent of adult T-cells. The enzyme terminal deoxyribonucleotidyl transferase (TdT) is present within the nucleus of all pro-thymocytes and cortical lymphocytes and is involved in the generation of T-cell receptor diversity (Fig. 24.87).

24.8.7 Functional aspects of cell surface molecules

The T-cell receptor can only recognize antigen when it is presented on the surface of a target cell in association with a molecule encoded by the major histocompatibility complex (MHC). CD4$^+$ T-cells recognize antigen in the context of MHC class II antigens (HLA-DP, DQ, or DR), while CD8$^+$ T-cells see antigen only when associated with MHC class I antigens (HLA-A, B, or C)—a phenomenon termed 'MHC restriction'. The CD4 and CD8 molecules are thought to bind to their respective MHC molecules in such a way as to increase the overall affinity of binding between the T-cell and its target. The co-expression of CD4 and CD8 on cortical thymocytes may provide a strong bond between developing T-lymphocytes and self MHC molecules on the cortical epithelium, and might by important in the processes of MHC restriction and tolerance to self. The CD3 molecule is very closely associated with the T-cell receptor, and monoclonal antibodies to CD3 are mitogenic, indicating that this molecule is involved in the proliferative response of the T-cell to antigen. Certain combinations of anti-CD2 monoclonal antibodies are also mitogenic; however, since this molecule appears earlier in development and is not tightly linked to the T-cell receptor it is likely that CD2 functions in a separate, anti-

gen non-specific expansion of lymphocytes within the thymus. The stimulus for this pathway is thought to be the LFA3 molecule that is present on thymic epithelial cells and is known to be a ligand for CD2.

24.8.8 Phenotypic heterogeneity of thymus microenvironmental cells

Monoclonal antibodies have also been used to identify subpopulations of cells within the thymic epithelium (Figs 24.88, 24.89), although no officially recognized clusters of differentiation have yet been established.

Epithelial cells of the subcapsular, perivascular, and medullary zones share many characteristics. Most monoclonal antibodies give identical labelling patterns of all these cell types (e.g. MR19, MR10, RFD4), while a few show staining of the subcapsular region alone (Thy-1, Leu7). Thymic hormone production has been demonstrated in all these areas and this, together with the fact that these cells bind the anti-ganglioside monoclonal antibody A2B5, has led to the use of the term 'neuro-endocrine' epithelium.

The epithelium of the cortex forms a distinct zone characterized by the expression of MHC class II molecules and labelling with monoclonal antibody MR6. The fine processes of these cells provides good contact between epithelium and lymphocytes, an interaction that culminates in the thymic nurse cell (an epithelial cell that appears to totally enclose a number of cortical lymphocytes).

The Hassall's corpuscles form an antigenically distinct and highly keratinized compartment within the thymic medulla. Less is known of the other thymic microenvironmental cell types. Dendritic cells are found only in the medulla. They are CD1$^+$, MR6$^+$ and constitutively express MHC class II molecules. Thymic macrophages are probably phenotypically heterogeneous, with different populations occupying different positions in the thymus. They can be induced to express MHC class II antigens when exposed to T-cell products (approximately 50 per cent are positive at any one time).

24.8.9 Function of the thymic microenvironment

Collectively, the cells of the thymic microenvironment are thought to be responsible for: the induction of T-lymphocyte maturation, including the generation of diversity of the T-cell receptor repertoire; the induction of tolerance to self, such that autoreactive T-cells are either eliminated or inactivated; and the induction of MHC restriction. However, the exact part played by the individual components of the microenvironment is not clear. Thymic epithelial cells are known to secrete a variety of soluble molecules (thymic hormones, e.g. thymulin, thymopoietins, thymosins) that can induce phenotyic changes in early lymphoid cells and hence may act as maturation signals during intrathymic T-cell development. Thymulin is present in the serum and is probably involved in some post-thymic T-lymphocyte maturation. Macrophage and epithelial cell-derived

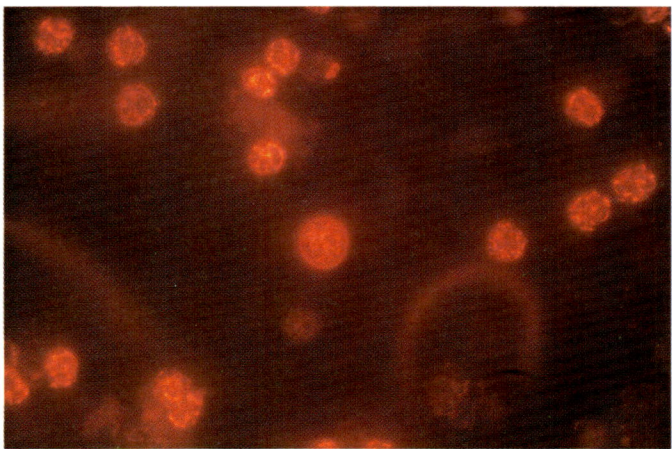

Fig. 24.87 Immunofluorescent (rhodamine) labelling to show the presence of the enzyme TdT in the nucleus of a prothymocyte (large cell in the centre of the field) and several cortical thymocytes.

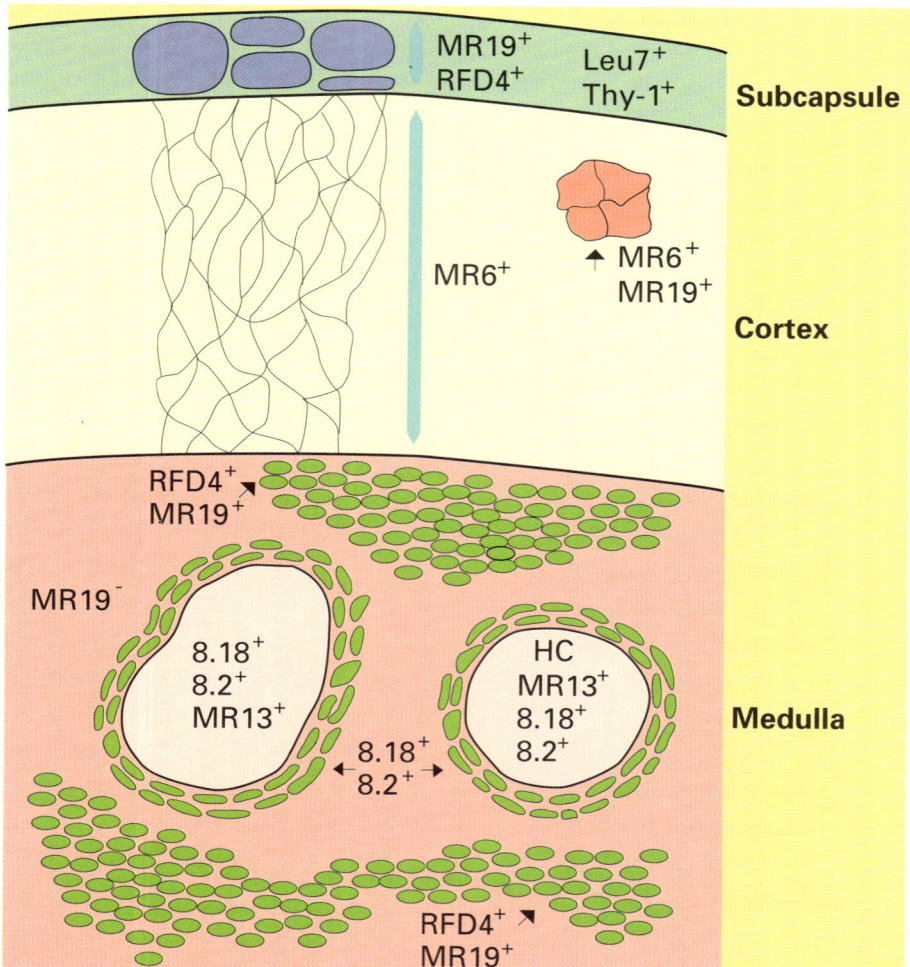

Fig. 24.88 Diagrammatic representation of epithelial subpopulations present in the human thymus, as defined by some monoclonal anti-epithelial cell antibodies (details of these are given in Ritter and Haynes 1987). HC, Hassall's corpuscles.

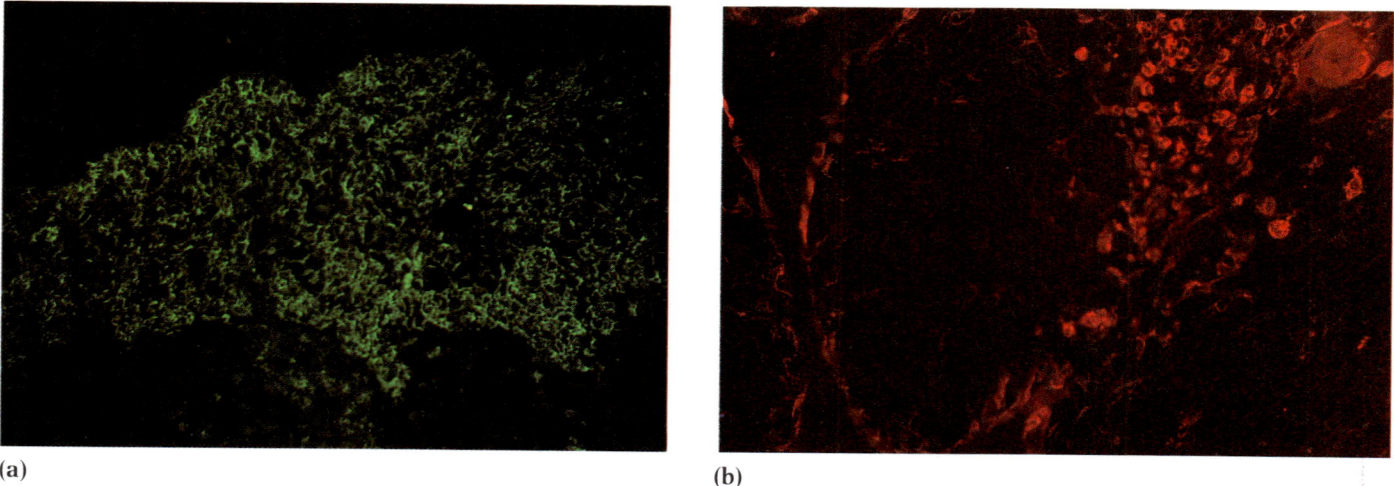

(a)   (b)

Fig. 24.89 Immunofluorescent staining of human paediatric thymus with (a) anti-cortical (MR6) and (b) anti-subcapsular/medullary (MR19) epithelial monoclonal antibodies.

interleukin 1, 6, and 7, and lymphocyte-derived interleukin 2 and 4 will interact with lymphocyte cell surface receptors to induce proliferation and expansion of the appropriate thymocyte populations, while cortical epithelial and medullary dendritic cells are thought to be the sites, respectively, of induction of MHC restriction and tolerance to self. In addition, it is likely that maturation signals required for other haemopoietic lineages may also be generated within the thymic microenvironment. B-lymphopoiesis is known to occur in the medulla, while macrophages, dendritic cells, and the scattered neutrophils and eosinophils may also develop *in situ*.

24.8.10 Factors affecting the thymus

Ageing

A progressive decrease in thymic size and weight is observed throughout life, with the fastest rate of involution occurring during the first 10 years. Involution involves all components of the thymus. The total amount of thymic tissue (lymphocytes, epithelium, and other non-lymphoid cells) declines progressively with age, from year 1 onwards, while the cellular content of the remaining tissue stays essentially normal and mitoses can still be seen. The total volume of the perivascular spaces increases up to the age of 20 years, after which it declines. The total amount of connective tissue continues to increase up to 30 years of age, after which it is progressively replaced with adipose tissue, which itself forms a progressively greater and greater proportion of the total organ. For example, the approximate adipose content of the thymus is 10 per cent at 20 years, 60 per cent at 35 years, and 80 per cent from 55 years onwards. The capsule becomes much thicker with age, such that the thymus in old age is small, fibrous, and fatty (Fig. 24.90). It is commonly, and probably erroneously, assumed that the adult thymus has no function. However, the fact that lymphocytes are still produced within the residual organ and that thymulin can be detected in the serum indicates that functional lymphopoiesis continues throughout life, albeit at a reduced level. Such low-level lymphopoiesis is probably necessary and sufficient to maintain the peripheral T-lymphocyte pool. It should be noted that the effects of ageing on the human thymus have been studied mainly from post-mortem material; this is unsatisfactory since stress (due to disease and/or hospitalization) can cause rapid weight loss in the thymus, thus exaggerating the age-associated involution.

Stress

The thymus is very sensitive to stress-induced involution. The effect is mediated via steroid hormones and results in the intrathymic death of the majority of cortical lymphocytes, probably by apoptosis (Fig. 24.91). This cell loss is reflected in a rapid loss in thymic weight. Regeneration occurs after the stress stimulus has been removed.

Hormones

Androgenic, oestrogenic, and adrenocortical steroid hormones (e.g. testosterone, oestrogen, ACTH) all cause thymic involution. Such hormones are responsible for the reduction in thymic size in ageing and during late pregnancy and lactation. Thymic involution is reversible. The organ recovers its pre-pregnancy size after lactation is stopped, and thymic involution in old male rats can be reversed by either surgical or chemical castration.

Chemicals

Toxic compounds such as Dioxin and organometals both cause rapid loss of cortical lymphocytes; however, the mechanisms of involution differ since organometals directly affect the lymphocytes while Dioxin exerts its primary toxic effect via the cortical epithelium. As before, the effects appear to be reversible.

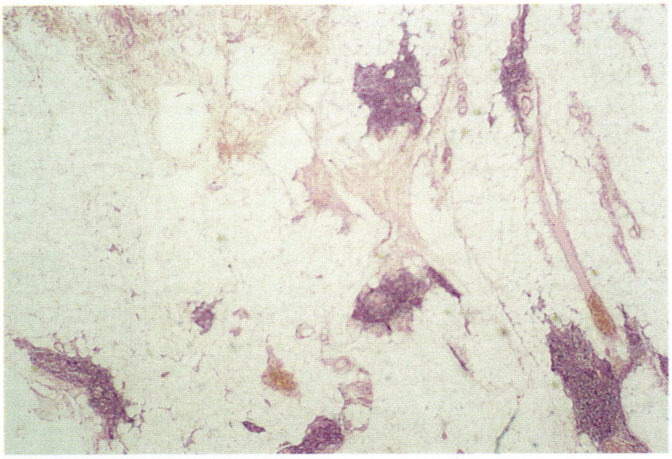

Fig. 24.90 The thymus involutes with age. Haematoxylin staining of thymus from a 60-year-old female, showing reduction in the lympho-epithelial elements and replacement of septa by expanded adipose tissue.

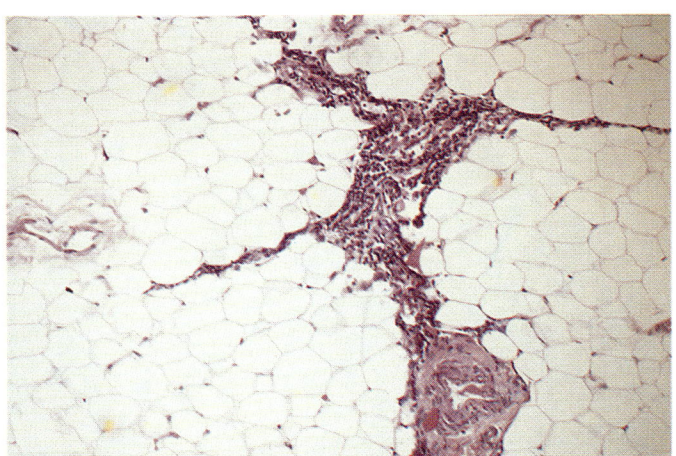

Fig. 24.91 Stress involution of the thymus. The thymus is dramatically reduced in size due to the loss of cortical thymocytes.

Immunosuppression

Steroid-mediated depletion of the cortex has been described above. In contrast, cyclosporin A (CSA) and the recently developed drug FK-506 have been shown experimentally to have the opposite effect, causing medullary depletion while sparing the cortex (Fig. 24.92). With CSA all medullary elements (lymphocytes, epithelium, dendritic cells, and macrophages) are equally affected, leading to a medullary remnant that, even after prolonged CSA treatment, is never entirely lost. After cessation of CSA immunosuppression the appearance of the medulla quickly returns to normal, but whether it is functionally normal is not known. The drug therefore appears to block the maturation step from cortical to medullary thymocyte, in addition to its well-documented immunosuppressive effects on mature peripheral T-lymphocytes.

Malnutrition

This leads to thymic atrophy, involving first the cortex and ultimately the whole organ. The degree of atrophy depends upon the duration and severity of the malnutrition. Both protein and calorie starvation cause thymic atrophy and the resultant deficiencies in immune responses. Since the levels of serum glucocorticoids increase considerably during periods of starvation it is possible that the thymic effects of malnutrition may be mediated by these hormones.

24.8.11   Immunodeficiency diseases that involve the thymus

Di George's syndrome

In this condition the congenital thymic and parathyroid aplasia probably results from an embryological failure of these organs to develop from the third and fourth pharyngeal pouches. The thymic remnant is often found ectopically in the neck region. In

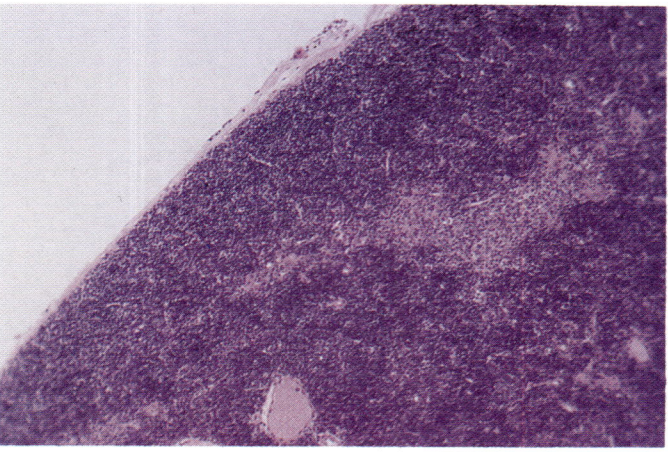

Fig. 24.92 Immunosuppression with Cyclosporin A drastically reduces the thymic medulla, but has no morphological effects on the cortex. Thymus from mouse treated intraperitoneally for 14 days with 10 mg/kg/day CSA.

the absence of a functional epithelial microenvironment, T-cells fail to develop and patients lack all T-cell-mediated immune responses. The deficit has, in some cases, been ameliorated by grafts of fetal thymic epithelium.

Hereditary ataxia telangiectasia

Patients exibit reduced T-cell immunity; thymic hypoplasia may involve the epithelium, leading to defects in the induction of T-cell differentiation. Many other, non-immune, defects are observed in this syndrome.

Severe combined immunodeficiency (SCID)

This group of diseases results from various defects of the haemopoietic stem cell rather than from a fault within the thymus itself, and as such is beyond the scope of this chapter. Interestingly, however, in the murine SCID model the defect is now known to lie in the recombinase enzyme that is required for rearrangement of both immunoglobulin and T-cell receptor gene loci necessary for the generation of lymphocyte receptor diversity.

MHC deficiency syndrome

Previously known as bare lymphocyte syndrome, the disease is characterized by the absence or reduction of expression of MHC class I and/or II antigens. This deficiency affects all cell types within the thymus, although the expression of other thymic molecules and the general thymic architecture appear normal Despite the presence of T- and B-lymphocytes and antigen-presenting cells (monocytes) in the periphery, antigen-specific responses are either absent or severely deficient.

24.8.12   Thymic tumours

A variety of tumours occur in the anterior mediastinum (Table 24.8), although the origin of these tumours is sometimes in doubt. Some, such as the thymomas and thymic carcinomas, clearly arise from the epithelial stroma of the organ, and it is likely that the carcinoids also come from this tissue. The origin of others, such as the germ-cell tumours, is not certain. Some lymphomas may originate in local lymph nodes with secondary spread to the thymus, whereas others clearly originate within the thymic tissue. Since the precise origin of these tumours in the anterior mediastinum (i.e. thymus versus surrounding tissue) is not always clear, they are best considered together. The term *thymoma* is restricted to those tumours known to arise out of thymic epithelial cells. The relative incidence of primary mediastinal tumours differs in childhood and in adult life (Table 24.9).

Thymomas

These are mainly tumours of middle to later life; mean age at diagnosis is approximately 50 years and there is no sex predilection. There are rare reports of thymomas (five cases) in children. Thymoma is the commonest of the neoplasms that occur in the anterior mediastinum, and the majority of thymomas

Table 24.8 Thymic tumours

Thymolipoma

Thymoma

Thymic carcinomas (malignant
thymomas—cytologically malignant)

Thymic sarcomas

Thymic carcinoids and other neuro-
endocrine tumours

Germinoma

Teratoma

Malignant lymphoma
  Hodgkin's disease
  Lymphoblastic lymphoma
    (Sternberg tumour)
  Mediastinal diffuse large-cell
    lymphoma with sclerosis
  Other lymphomas

Thymic cysts

Thymic hyperplasia

Castleman's disease

Other lesions of the mediastinum
(notably parathyroid adenomas occurring
within the thymus)

Table 24.9 Relative incidence of primary mediastinal tumours

	Percentage incidence
Adult tumours	
Thymic lesions (vast majority thymomas)	47
Lymphoma	23
Germ-cell tumours	15
Endocrine tumours (mainly thyroid and parathyroid)	16
Childhood tumours	
Lymphomas	45
Germ-cell tumours	24
Thymic lesions (primarily hyperplasia and cysts, only five cases of thymoma reported)	17
Messenchymal tumour	15

(75 per cent) occur in this site. The remainder occur largely elsewhere in the mediastinum, while rare cases are found in the neck.

Clinical presentation of thymoma is variable. Approximately half present with myasthenia gravis with or without tumour symptoms. Of all cases of thymoma, approximately 40 per cent present with symptoms related to the presence of the tumour mass. Non-myasthenic paraneoplastic syndromes are present in 10 per cent of cases.

Morphological and immunophenotypic studies have indicated that the neoplastic population in thymomas is the epithelium and that the lymphocytes are benign components responding to epithelium-derived proliferative signals. Studies of T-cell receptor genes in thymomas have not demonstrated any form of clonal proliferation and thus have confirmed the non-neoplastic nature of these lymphocytes.

Macroscopic appearance

The majority of thymomas present as well-circumscribed, firm, tan-pink to green masses totally enclosed by a fibrous capsule. Invasive thymomas are less well defined and tend to encase adjacent organs and blood vessels. The invasive nature of the tumour is best assessed at the time of surgery, together with the radiological appearances of the tumour. There is considerable variation in size, with the smallest being recognized incidentally at autopsy. The resected lesions measure from 2 to 20 cm in diameter and can weigh up to several kilograms; the median weight is approximately 150 g. The cut surface reveals fibrous trabecula creating a lobular appearance. Many tumours show areas of cystic degeneration filled with fluid or cellular debris. There may be calcification both of the capsule and within the tumour.

Histological appearances

By definition, all tumours included as thymomas are neoplasms consisting of thymic epithelial cells (Fig. 24.93). Since thymic epithelium creates a specialized microenvironment conducive to the proliferation and differentiation of T-cell precursors, it is not surprising that the neoplastic cells recreate this micro-environment and consequently the same proliferation and differentiation of T-cell precursors takes place here. This means that there is a variable density of lymphocytes accompanying the neoplastic epithelium, these are not regarded as intrinsic to the neoplastic tissue. Previously, when the nature and function of the thymus was unknown, pathologists thought that the lymphocytes were also neoplastic, hence the now outmoded term lymphoepithelial thymoma. The term, however, does serve to indicate that the density of lymphocytes is variable, such that at one extreme it is difficult to distinguish the tumours from lymphomas and at the other from epithelial and, indeed, connective tissue neoplasms. Where there is uncertainty as to the nature of the lesion, staining for cytokeratin and desmosomal junctions confirms the epithelial nature of the lesion. This is of help in the form of thymoma which is dominated by spindle medullary type cells that can simulate a connective tissue lesion. Additional helpful features are:

1. The fibrous bands which divide up the tumour giving it a lobulated appearance.

2. At the edge of the lesion there is a sharp palisaded border which marks the end of the epithelial sheet. In a similar fashion there is a connective tissue space between the vessels and the surrounding tumour, the so-called perivascular space. These are often filled with proteinaceous fluid and lymphocytes, red cells, and foam cells (macrophages).

3. Occasional foci of differentiation into Hassall's corpuscles (epithelial whorls).

4. Foci of cystic degeneration are frequent.

5. Occasionally there are glandular spaces lined by cuboidal epithelial cells.

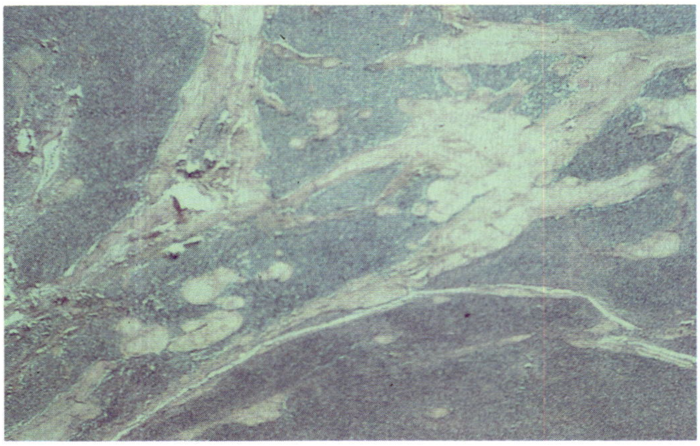

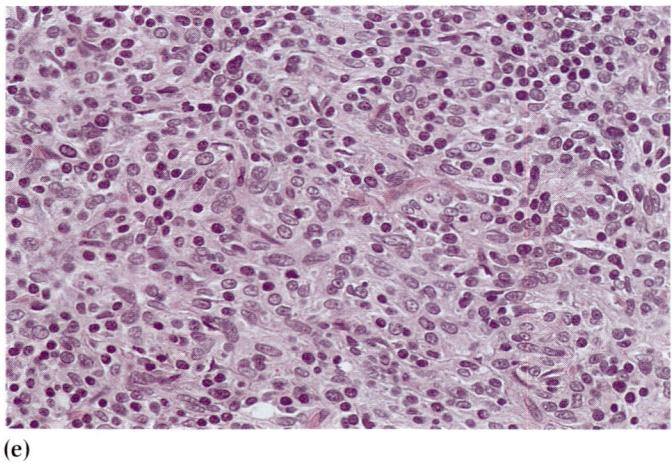

(a)

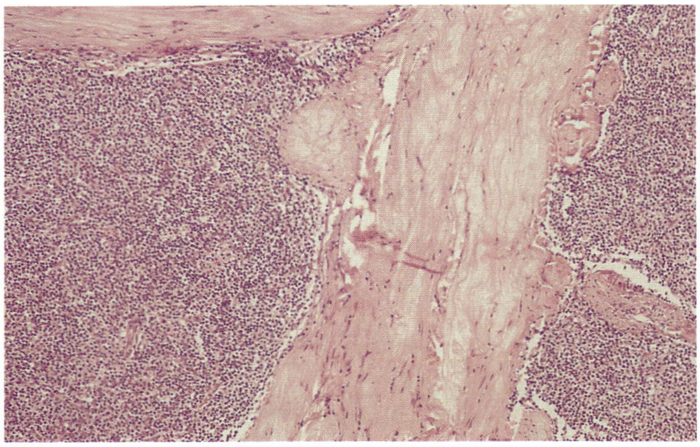

(b)

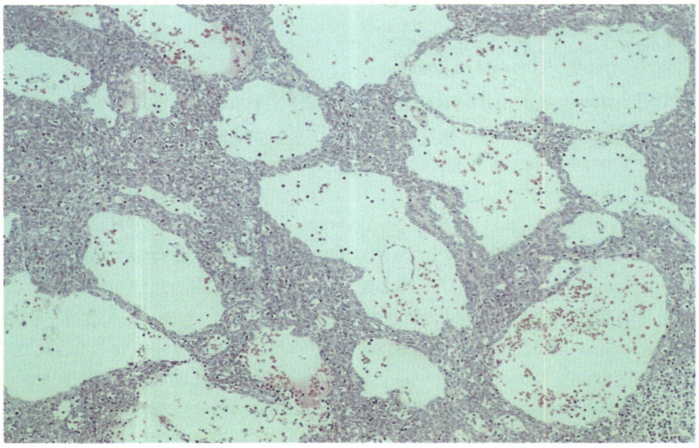

(c)

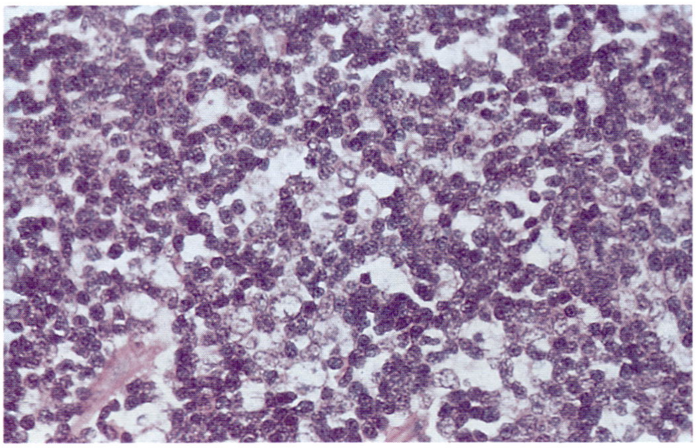

(d)

(e)

Fig. 24.93 Thymoma. (a) Thymomas are typically lobulated tumours. In this photograph the epithelial islands containing lymphocytes ('lymphoepithelial' thymoma) are separated by thick collagen bands. (b) The epithelial nature of the lesion may not be immediately apparent, due to the dense infiltrate of lymphocytes. The sharp margin of the epithelial sheet helps to distinguish it from a lymphoid neoplasm. (c) Perivascular formation. The apparent cystic spaces in this tumour are perivascular areas. Lymphocytes are seen frequently in these areas. Perivascular spaces are useful in distinguishing thymoma from a lymphoid neoplasm. (d) Thymoma resembling thymic cortex. The large pale cells with vesicular nuclei are the thymic cortical epithelial cells. (e) Thymoma in which the epithelial cells have a spindle shape, similar to medullary epithelial cells.

Classification

Histological and immunohistochemical techniques have been used to identify distinct subpopulations of thymic epithelial cells and lymphocytes (described earlier in this chapter). These techniques have been used to analyse thymomas and to classify

them according to the phenotype of the neoplastic epithelium; although it is too early to assess the clinical usefulness of this classification. The classification is as follows:

1. Cortical

2. Mixed
   Common
   Cortical predominant
   Medullary predominant
3. Medullary

Some thymomas are composed entirely of either 'cortical' or 'medullary' type epithelium, while others contain mixtures of these cells. These 'mixed' type thymomas vary in the relative proportions of the different epithelial cell populations. In some, one cell type predominates over the other (>75 per cent of cells), while in others the two cell types are more equally represented ('common' mixed thymoma). Double immunostaining of these thymomas has shown that many contain neoplastic epithelial cells that simultaneously express markers of both cortex and medulla. It has been suggested that the normal counterpart of these epithelial cells is the relatively rare, double-positive cortical epithelial cell, and that this cell represents an intrathymic epithelial stem cell (Fig. 24.94).

Paraneoplastic syndromes

A number of thymomas are associated with paraneoplastic syndromes. The most frequent of these are: myasthenia gravis, aplastic anaemia, pernicious anaemia, polymyositis, keratoconjunctivitis sicca, alopecia areata, mixed collagen vascular disease, Graves' disease.

The incidence of myasthenia gravis with thymoma ranges in different series from 7 to 54 per cent with a mean of 35 per cent. Conversely, approximately 10–15 per cent of people with myasthenia gravis are found to have thymomas. In general, myasthenics without thymomas tend to be younger than those with thymomas. Paraneoplastic syndromes other than myasthenia gravis occur in 10 per cent of patients with thymomas, the commonest of these are hypogammaglobulinaemia, pure red cell aplasia and aplastic anaemia. Myasthenia gravis is associated with cortical and mixed-type thymoma, whereas pure red cell aplasia and hypogammaglobulinaemia occur in spindle-cell (medullary) thymoma.

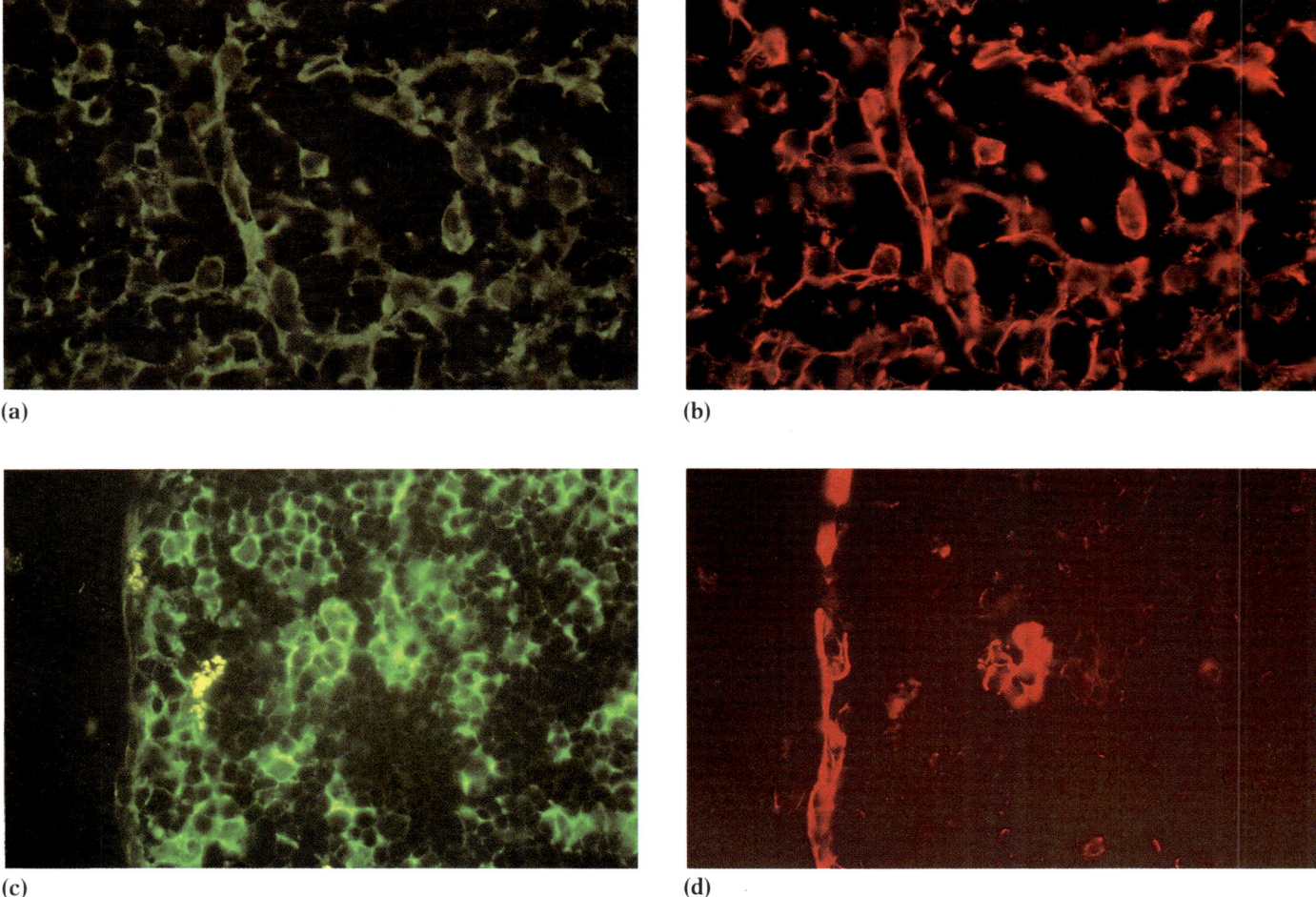

(a)

(b)

(c)

(d)

Fig. 24.94 Dual immunolabelling of thymoma from a patient with myasthenia gravis, (a) and (b), and normal paediatric thymus, (c) and (d), to demonstrate 'double-positive' epithelial cells that carry markers for both cortical and subcapsular/medullary epithelium. (a) and (c) MR6 (anti-cortical), (b) and (d) MR19 (anti-subcapsular/medullary).

Prognostic factors

Well-circumscribed tumours remain stationary in their growth and their prognosis is largely a function of the accompanying paraneoplastic syndrome, particularly in myasthenia gravis. Invasion is the most important factor affecting prognosis. This relates to tumour size, since most large tumours are invasive. Staging therefore provides a good indication of prognosis:

- *Stage I* intracapsular growth with the capsule intact, this is generally referred to as benign thymoma;
- *Stage II* disease is indicated by growth into surrounding organs particularly the mediastinal fat, pleura, or pericardium;
- *Stage III* intrathoracic metastasis;
- *Stage IV* extrathoracic metastasis.

Benign thymoma (Stage I) has an excellent prognosis (in the absence of a paraneoplastic syndrome). Malignant thymomas have a 5-year survival rate of between 20 and 50 per cent. Malignant behaviour is seen in some of the cases with cortical-type morphology, whereas the medullary lesions are, in general, benign.

Thymic carcinomas

These tumours are distinguished from the above on the basis of the presence of cytological atypia, i.e. nuclear hyperchromatism, prominent nucleoli, and mitotic figures (Fig. 24.95). The majority are squamous carcinomas, but lymphoepithelial carcinomas resembling those from the nasopharynx, oat cell carcinomas, and sarcomatoid carcinomas are also found. These are rare tumours with the prognosis being worst for squamous cell thymic tumours.

Germ cell tumours

Mediastinal germinal tumours are thought to arise in the thymus from primordial germinal crests that do not complete their migration from the urogenital ridge to the gonads during embryogenesis. The rarity of these tumours and their histological similarity to gonadal tumours have led some people to doubt the fact that they originated in this location. However, they are now accepted as primary tumours because of the extreme rarity with which germinal gonadal neoplasms metastasize solely to the anterior mediastinum. These tumours are classified as follows:

- Benign teratomas;
- Malignant teratomas (including choriocarcinoma, yolk sac carcinoma, embryonal carcinoma, and teratocarcinoma);
- Seminomas (germinomas).

Approximately 80 per cent of all mediastinal germ cell tumours are benign teratomas. They exhibit a variety of mature tissues from the three germ cell layers. They usually present in the second or third decade of life.

Malignant teratoma

Primary malignant teratoma is a disease virtually restricted to young men. As with the disease elsewhere it is associated with raised HCG and α-fetal protein levels in the blood. Despite their similarity to gonadal teratomas to date they have demonstrated a poor response to standardized therapy.

Seminomas (germinomas)

This is the commonest germ cell tumour in the anterior mediastinum, affecting males (exclusively) in the third decade of life. The lesions are similar in histological appearance to those seen elsewhere in the body (Fig. 24.96).

Thymic carcinoids

Carcinoids arise in the mediastinum and are presumed to be of thymic origin, because of the normal presence of Kulschitsky cells in the thymus. These tumours used to be referred to as

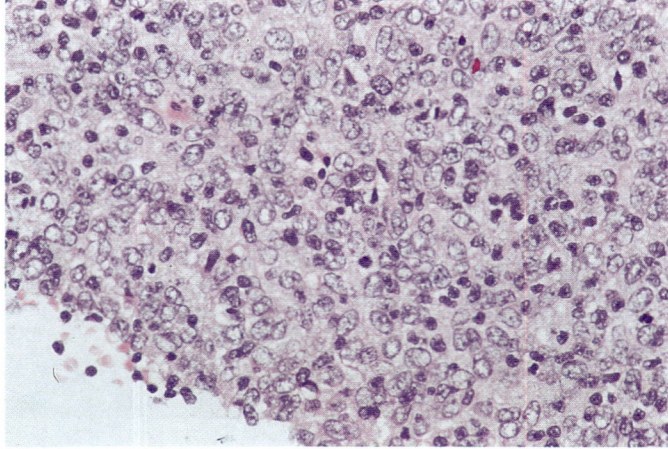

Fig. 24.95 Thymic carcinoma. The cytological atypia is evident in the large nuclei with prominent nucleoli, considerable pleomorphism, and mitoses (not shown); these features are characteristic of all carcinomas.

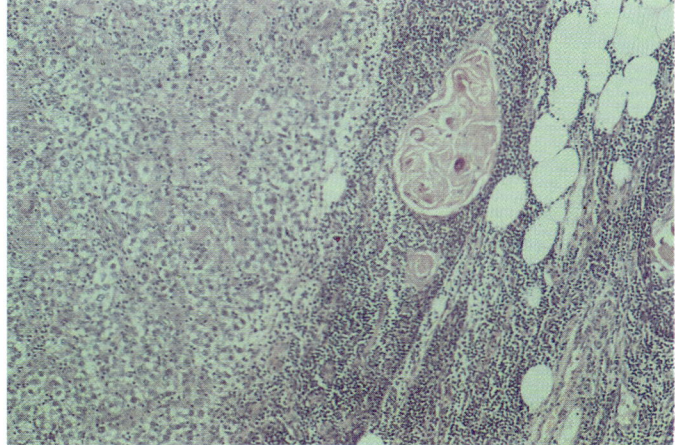

Fig. 24.96 Thymic seminoma. Low-power view of a seminoma developing within the thymus. This is similar to seminomas that develop elsewhere in the body.

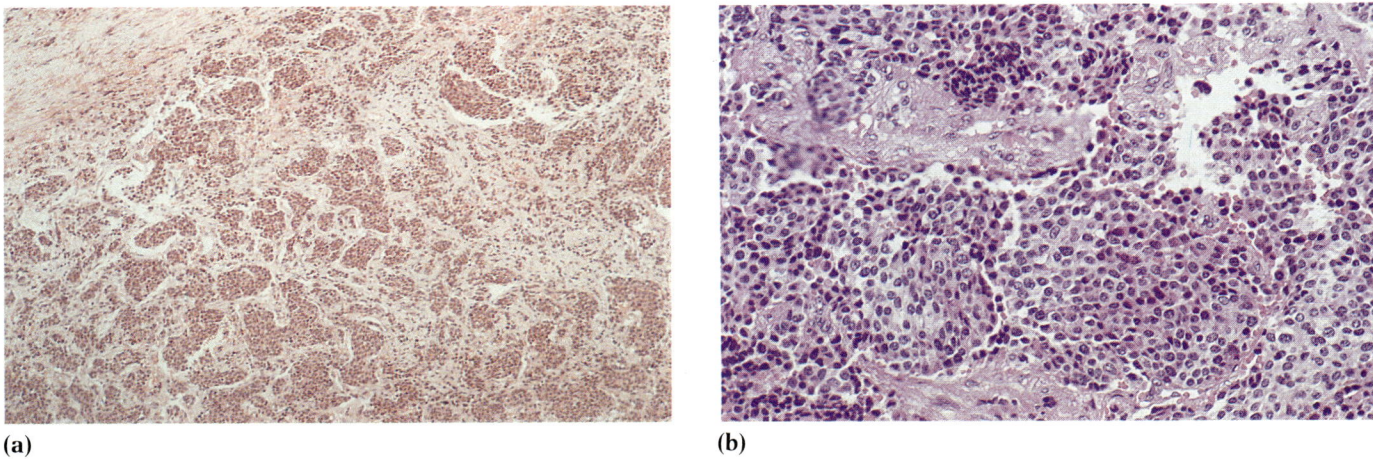

(a)   **(b)**

Fig. 24.97   Thymic carcinoid (a) low-power, (b) high-power view. Note the epithelial islands that contain no lymphocytes.

'pure' epithelial thymomas because they are not accompanied by any lymphoid element. The tumours have the typical features of carcinoids elsewhere, exhibiting anastomosing cords of epithelial cells, ribbons, festoons and, in places, a rosette-like arrangement (Fig. 24.97). Lymphocytes are notable by their absence. These are biologically aggressive tumours and metastases occur in a substantial proportion (up to 70 per cent). Some of these cases (up to 30 per cent) show the Cushing's syndrome, which is due to the ectopic production of ACTH. The disease is also associated with a familial endocrine neoplasia (MEN) syndrome.

Lymphomas

All types of leukaemias and lymphomas may involve the thymus.

Hodgkin's disease

Mediastinal involvement may be a prominent sign in Hodgkin's disease, especially of the nodular sclerosis (NS) type, in which it has been reported in as many as 60–70 per cent of cases. This type of lymphoma has for several years been misconceived as a form of thymoma, being referred to as 'thymoma of granulomatous type'. The features of NS Hodgkin's are similar to that seen elsewhere. A frequent feature of the thymic involvement is the presence of thymic cysts, these may be lined either with columnar or squamous epithelium. There is a tendency for invasion of the lung.

Non-Hodgkin's lymphoma

In non-Hodgkin's lymphoma mediastinal involvement is less often present (18–24 per cent) and is predominantly related to the lymphoblastic convoluted T-cell lymphoma (Sternberg sarcoma).

Mediastinal diffuse large-cell lymphoma of B-cell type with sclerosis

This is a recently described large-cell lymphoma of B-cell type which occurs in the mediastinum in young adults. The tumour cells are predominantly large with occasional multinucleated forms with abundant cytoplasm. They are often arranged in an alveolar pattern and the considerable sclerosis produces confusion with other tumours in the thymus, notably germinomas, nodular sclerosing Hodgkin's disease, and thymoma. Isaacson has recently described a unique population of B-cells in the thymic medulla that may be the benign counterparts of these tumours.

Thymic cysts

The majority of thymic cysts are probably developmental in origin: they are often asymptomatic and found incidentally on radiological examination. Most are lined by columnar or stratified squamous epithelium (Fig. 24.98). Secondary alterations may result from haemorrhage or rupture. Necrosis in thymic tumours has to be distinguished from true thymic cysts. It must be borne in mind that cystic change is a common phenomenon

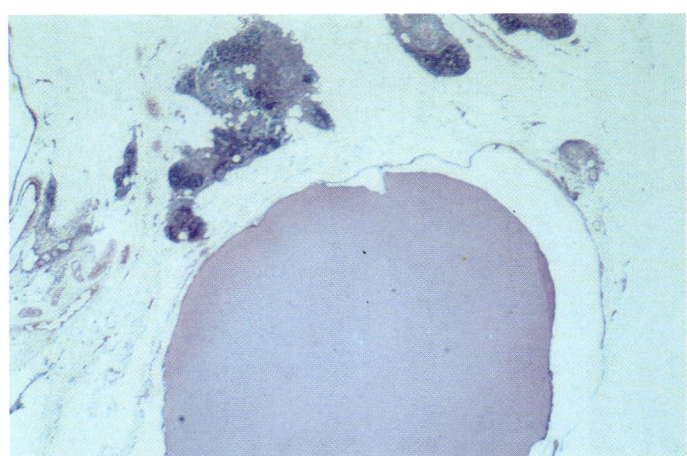

Fig. 24.98   Thymic cyst. This is an example of one of the many types of cyst. The cyst appears to be associated with glandular elements, illustrating the range of epithelial elements that can be involved in these structures.

in normal Hassall's corpuscles. The squamous pearl-like structure can show the development of mucous glandular epithelium which can enlarge to a millimetre or so.

Mesenchymal tumours

A wide variety of mesenchymal tumours occur in the thymus, both benign and malignant. Lipoma (thymolioma) is the commonest of these, accounting for 2 per cent of all primary mediastinal neoplasms (Fig. 24.99). Microscopically, lipoma consists of adult adipose tissue with varying numbers of lymphocytes in the stroma, and presents entirely within the thymus. Despite their essential benignity, these tumours are clinically very important because they tend to grow to enormous proportions. Total extirpation is essential because they have a tendency to recur.

Thymic hyperplasia

Hyperplasia of the thymus is a rare lesion occurring in childhood and is characterized by an increase in all the elements of the thymus. It is said to be a normal response of infants during recovery from serious illness, in particular recovery from burns, and after the recovery from chemotherapy for malignancy. Occasional cases occur without such antecedent history. This phenomenon is not associated with immunological abnormality or malignancy. Spontaneous involution occurs in the vast majority of these enlargements; occasionally surgical removal is required. Thymic enlargement may also occur as part of endocrine abnormalities, in particular acromegaly, Addison's disease, and thyrotoxicosis.

Castleman's disease

In 1956 Castleman and associates described a group of patients with benign mediastinal lymphoid masses that they entitled 'mediastinal lymph node hyperplasia', now referred to as Castleman's disease. These lesions can occur in any part of the

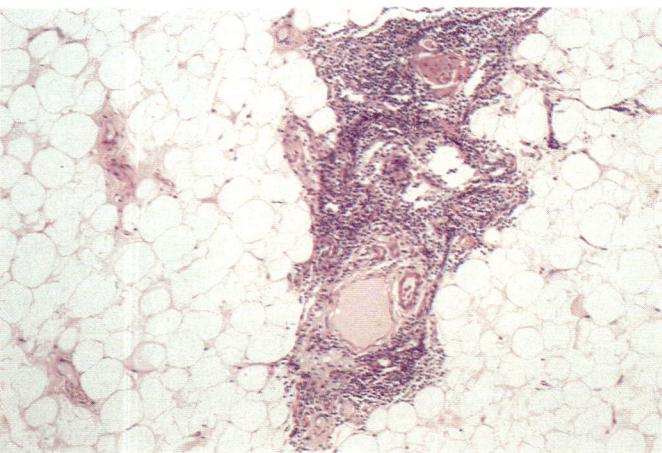

Fig. 24.99 Thymic lipoma. Note the normal thymic areas surrounded by considerably expanded adipose tissue.

body that contains lymphoid tissue, although 70 per cent are found in the anterior mediastinum. Two specific types of Castleman's disease have been identified. The most common is the hyaline vascular type accounting for 90 per cent of all lesions. Most patients are young (70 per cent less than 30 years) and asymptomatic (occasionally there may be pressure symptoms). Microscopically the paracortical lymphoid architecture is affected by a proliferation of post-capillary venules associated with lymphocytes, immunoblasts, and a variable number of plasma cells. The germinal centres are considerably changed. The centre of the germinal centre, which normally consists of proliferating centroblasts and centrocytes, is replaced by hyaline vascular proliferations. At the same time the mantle of the follicle is enormously thickened and surrounds these hyaline vascular structures. This form is benign and usually is cured after extirpation.

The second form, or plasma cell variety, is associated with enormous germinal centre hyperplasia and a diffuse infiltration of the tissue with sheet of plasma cells. In 50 per cent of cases this form is associated with fever, anaemia, and hypergammaglobulinaemia.

24.8.13   The thymus and myasthenia gravis

Myasthenia gravis (MG) is a disorder of the neuromusclar junction, characterized by muscular weakness which increases with effort. Auto-antibodies to the acetylcholine receptor of skeletal muscle lead to a reduction in receptor numbers, causing the clinical weakness. The frequent association of this disease with thymic abnormality has long been recognized. About 10–15 per cent of MG cases have a thymoma (see above), while in non-thymomatous myasthenics 75–84 per cent of patients have abnormalities in the thymus, mostly involving follicular hyperplasia in the medulla and associated anti-AChR antibody synthesis (Fig. 24.100). In these cases thymectomy improves the clinical myasthenia. In the hyperplastic MG thymus lymph-node-like elements have been brought into the thymic medulla via perivascular tissue. Electron microscopic and immunohistochemical studies have shown that these germinal centres are located in the connective tissue between the thymic epithelium and the vasculature, with a well-developed basement membrane separating the thymic epithelium and the germinal centre, although this may be perforated in some areas. In extreme cases the germinal centres are surrounded by T-cell zones and the medullary epithelium is reduced to thin bands, giving an 'onion skin' appearance (Fig. 24.99). Thus the term 'hyperplasia' is a rather poor one as the changes in myasthenia show features which are more akin to an inflammatory reaction. The term thymitis has been proposed for these changes, which are not unique as they are also seen in the thymus of patients with Addison's disease, Graves' disease, rheumatoid arthritis, and systemic lupus erythematosus.

A further interesting immune phenomenon in MG has been the detection of antibodies to the 'A' band of striated muscle, present in 50 per cent of patients with MG and in more than

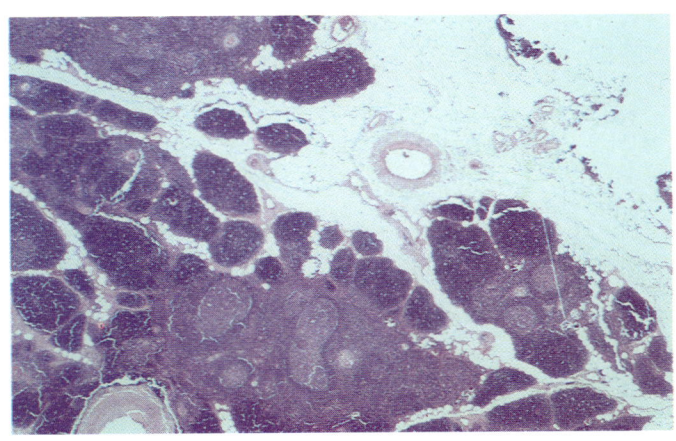

(a)

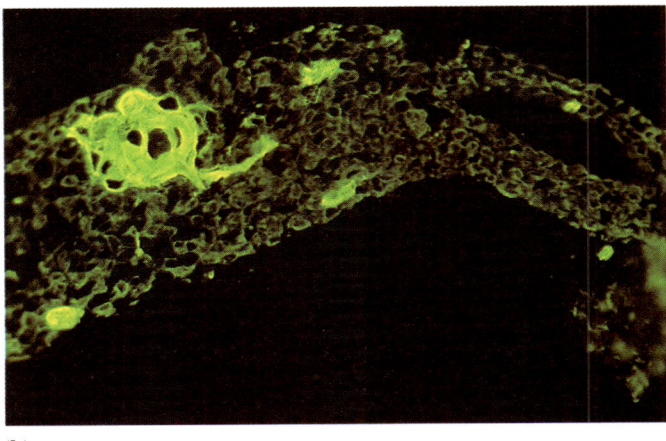

(b)

Fig. 24.100 Thymic hyperplasia (thymitis) in myasthenia gravis. (a) Low-power view, haematoxylin staining. The tissue thymic consists of small cortical islands surrounding medullary regions that have become expanded by the invasion of peripheral lymphoid tissue (germinal centres and associated T-cell zones). (b) High-power view of compressed band of medullary epithelium ('onion skin'), visualized by immunofluorescent staining for keratin, surrounding a germinal centre (not stained).

90 per cent of myasthenics with thymoma; curiously 30 per cent of patients with thymoma but without MG have these antibodies.

24.8.14 Further reading

Henry, K. and Farrer-Brown, G. (1981). *A colour atlas of thymus and lymph node histopathology with ultrastructure*. Wolf Medical Publications, London.

Janossy, G., Bofil, M., Trejdosiewicz, L. K., Willcox, H. N. A., and Chilosi, M. (1986). Cellular differentiation of lymphoid subpopulations and their microenvironments in the human thymus. *Current Topics in Pathology* **75**, 89–125.

Kendall, M. D. (ed.) (1981). *The thymus gland*. Academic Press, London.

Kendall, M. D. and Ritter, M. A. (eds) (1988). *Thymus update 1: The microenvironment of the human thymus*. Harwood Academic, London.

Kendall, M. D. and Ritter, M. A. (eds) (1989). *Thymus update 2: T-lymphocyte differentiation in the human thymus*. Harwood Academic, London.

Kendall, M. D. and Ritter, M. A. (1990). *Thymus update 3: The role of the thymus in tolerance induction*. Harwood Academic, London.

Kendall, M. D. and Ritter, M. A. (1991) *Thymus update 4: The thymus in immunotoxicology*. Harwood Academic, London.

Muller-Hermelink, H. K. (ed.) (1986). *Current Topics in Pathology*. Vol. 75: *The human thymus*. Springer-Verlag, Berlin.

Muller-Hermelink, H. K., Marino, M., and Palestro, G. (1986). Pathology of thymic epithelial tumours. *Current Topics in Pathology* **75**, 207–68.

Ritter, M. A. and Crispe, I. N. (1991). *The thymus. IRL in focus series*. Oxford University Press.

Ritter, M. A. and Haynes, B. F. (1987). Summary of thymic epithelium workshop. In *Leucocyte typing III* (ed. McMichael *et al.*) pp. 247–8. Oxford University Press.

Rosai, J. and Levine, G. D. (1975). Tumours of the thymus. In *Atlas of tumour pathology*, 2nd series, Fascicle 13. The Armed Forces Institute of Pathology, Washington.

Schluep, M., Willcox, N., Ritter, M. A., Newsom-Davis, J., Larche, M., and Brown, A. N. (1988). Myasthenia gravis thymus: clinical, histological and culture correlations. *Journal of Autoimmunity* **1**, 445–67.

25

The nervous system

25

The nervous system

25.1 Structure and function of cells in the nervous system

E. L. Rees and M. Berry

25.1.1 Introduction

The structure and function of cells as classically described using neuroanatomical methods is being superseded by molecular biological and immunocytological techniques. These new methods describe neurones and their pathways on the basis of the neuromediators they contain and the receptors they engage; whereas glial cells are being reclassified according to new ideas relating to immunologically defined phenotypes. This article breaks with the traditional approach to introduce the new descriptions.

25.1.2 Neurons

The conventional anatomy of the nervous system is well documented in standard neuroanatomical texts. We have attempted to summarize the recent works describing cell groups and their axonal projections according to the transmitter used. This neurochemical approach to the anatomy of neurones has great advantages in the understanding of both normal and deranged function, and also in devising a rational approach to neuropharmacology. The chemoarchitecture of the brain has been reviewed recently by Nieuwenhuys (1985) and this summary is an attempt to simplify a complex discipline, at present in its infancy, which will undoubtedly assume an increasing importance in neuropathology.

Cholinergic cell groups and pathways

Cholinergic (Ch) cells and their processes are specifically identified by an immunohistochemical method using an antibody raised against *choline acetyltransferase* (ChAT), an enzyme responsible for the synthesis of acetylcholine (ACh). All choliner-gic neurones are associated with *acetylcholinesterase* (AChE), an enzyme that degrades ACh. However, all AChE-associated neurones are not necessarily cholinergic.

In the central nervous system most Ch neurones are found in the brainstem and spinal cord, the rest mainly in the telencephalon. Ch cell groups are designated Ch1 to Ch6. Some are 'undesignated' because they form well-known cell groups which include α and γ motor neurones of the cranial and spinal nerves, and also preganglionic autonomic neurones of the brainstem and spinal cord. Certain intrinsic neurones of the neostriatum also form another 'undesignated' cholinergic group.

The Ch cell groups in the basal forebrain are probably involved in memory, affective behaviour, and mood. This system is affected in certain neurodegenerative disorders, such as *Alzheimer's disease*, *parkinsonism* associated with dementia, and also *Huntingdon's disease*. The cholinergic reticular formation is concerned with arousal and REM sleep.

Cholinergic cell groups of the basal forebrain

This population of large cholinergic neurones forms groups Ch1 to Ch4, and extends from the septal region rostrally to the sub-thalamus caudally (Fig. 25.1).

The Ch1 group forms 10 per cent of the neurones of the medial septal nucleus. The Ch2 and Ch3 groups are located in the nucleus of the diagonal band of Broca. Efferent fibres from all these groups pass via the stria medullaris to the habenula and to the base of the midbrain. They end in the medial habenular nucleus, the interpeduncular nucleus, and the ventral tegmental area of Tsai.

Other efferent fibres (septo-hippocampal) leave cell groups Ch1 and Ch2, and travel in the fornix to synapse on cells of the hippocampus and dentate gyrus. Fibres from Ch2 also terminate in the lateral hypothalamus; and some axons, mainly from Ch3, project to the olfactory bulb.

The Ch4 group of cells corresponds to the basal nucleus of Meynert, about 90 per cent of the neurones of this nucleus are cholinergic. The nucleus lies within the substantia innominata, a poorly defined area situated ventral to the globus pallidus.

Some of the efferent fibres from Ch4 project to the amygdala, but the bulk of the fibres are distributed to all areas of the cerebral neocortex.

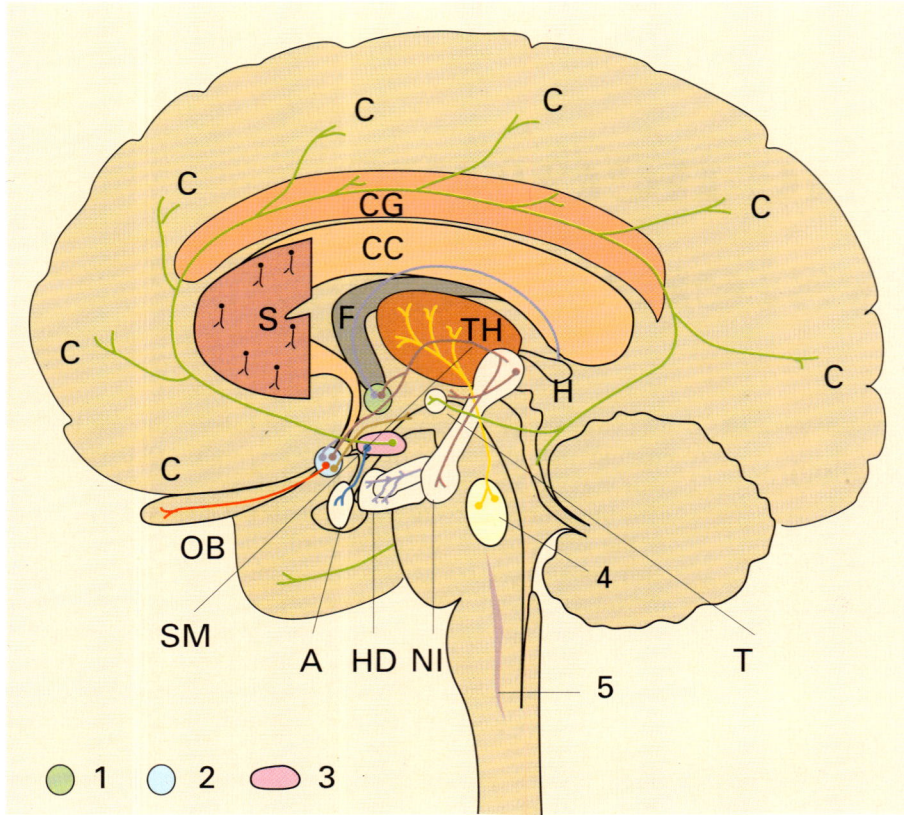

Fig. 25.1 Cholinergic cell groups and pathways. 1, Medial septal nucleus (Ch1); 2, nucleus of the diagonal band (Ch2, Ch3); 3, basal nucleus of Meynert (Ch4); 4, cholinergic cell groups (Ch5, Ch6); 5, cholinergic cells of the reticular formation; A, amygdala; C, cerebral neocortex; CG, cingulate gyrus; F, fornix (septo-hippocampal fibres); H, habenula; HD, hippocampus and dentate gyrus; NI, interpeduncular nucleus; OB, olfactory bulb; S, striatum; SM, stria medullaris; T, ventral tegmental area of Tsai; TH, thalamus. (Drawn after Nieuwenhuys 1985, with permission.)

The cholinergic reticular formation

Cholinergic neurones form lateral and medial columns in the brainstem tegmentum. Cholinergic cells of the lateral region are designated as the Ch5 group; and those of the rostral part of the medial region belong to the Ch6 group (Fig. 25.1). Both groups are functionally regarded as part of the 'ascending reticular activating system'.

The axons of dorsally situated, Ch reticular neurones form the dorsal tegmental cholinergic pathway which terminates in the tectum of the midbrain, the lateral and medial geniculate bodies, and the thalamus (anterior, midline, and intralaminar nuclei, especially the centromedian nucleus).

The ventral tegmental cholinergic pathway, formed of ascending fibres from ventrally sited, reticular neurones, is distributed to the thalamus (anterior and ventral nuclear groups), and to the hypothalamus, particularly the mamillary, supraoptic, and preoptic regions.

Noradrenergic cell groups and pathways

Neurones that synthesize noradrenaline are confined to the pontine and medullary tegmental regions. They have profuse, extensively branched projections which run the length of the neuraxis and are distributed to diverse regions of the central nervous system.

In rodents, seven noradrenergic (NA) cell groups are recog-

nized and designated A1–A7: all except A3 are present in primates. Groups A1 and A2 are situated in the lower part of the medulla oblongata, group A2 cells lying in and around the nucleus of the solitary tract and the dorsal motor vagal nucleus. Cells of group A4 lie subependymally along the superior cerebellar peduncle. Situated in the region of the facial nucleus are the cells forming group A5. Group A6 is a densely packed aggregation of neuromelanin-pigmented cells which forms the nucleus coeruleus, found in the floor of the fourth ventricle along the line of the sulcus limitans, in the rostral pons. Here, the nucleus may be seen macroscopically as a blue streak, known as the *locus coeruleus*. The nucleus has three extensions, one of which lies in the subcoeruleus area (A6sc), another is group A4 (already mentioned). Groups A4 and A6 (with its other extensions) are usually known as the locus coeruleus complex. Group A7 cells lie medial to the lateral lemniscus in the rostral part of the pons.

For descriptive convenience, the projections of the NA groups can be divided into two systems, the *locus coeruleus complex* (A4 and A6), which contains about 50 per cent of the total NA cells, and the '*lateral tegmental*' complex, composed of the rest of the NA cell groups.

The NA system regulates the fear and anxiety reactions, focuses attention, and maintains vigilance. The nucleus coeruleus also regulates the wake–sleep cycle, and may also regulate the cerebral blood flow. Noradrenaline mediates these effects as a typical neurotransmitter at synapses or as a neurohormone from along the nerves. Malfunction of the system has been implicated in depressive illness, Alzheimer's disease, schizophrenia, and parkinsonism.

The locus coeruleus complex system

Cells of this complex give rise to (1) descending and intrinsic brainstem; (2) cerebellar; and (3) ascending efferent fibres (see Fig. 25.2).

1. Some descending fibres travel in the dorsal longitudinal bundle of Schütz to end in the dorsal vagal nucleus. However, the majority descend in the central tegmental fasciculus of the pons to supply directly, or by collaterals, the chief and spinal nuclei of the trigeminal nerve, the cochlear nuclei, and the entire hindbrain reticular formation. Fibres whose collaterals innervate the above-mentioned structures descend in the ventrolateral funiculus of the spinal cord, as the coeruleospinal and subcoeruleospinal tracts, to innervate bilaterally cells in the base of the dorsal column (laminae IV, V, VI), the intermediate grey matter, and the ventral column of all cord segments. An extensive input passes to preganglionic parasympathetic neurones (S2, 3, 4) but none to the preganglionic sympathetic cells.

2. Coeruleocerebellar fibres enter the superior cerebellar peduncle to end in the roof nuclei and cortex of the cerebellum.

3. Ascending fibres are distributed through two routes: a large dorsal NA bundle, and a much smaller dorsal periventricular pathway.

The dorsal NA bundle, or dorsal tegmental bundle (Fig. 25.2), ascends in the midbrain, ventrolateral to the periaqueductal grey matter. It reaches the hypothalamus and then becomes a major constituent of the medial forebrain bundle. In the septal region, NA fibres are distributed to various forebrain structures via the rostral part of the forebrain bundle, the cingulum, stria medullaris, the fornix, and the diagonal band of Broca.

In the midbrain, branches of the dorsal NA bundle supply the periaqueductal grey matter, the tectum, and the dorsal raphe nucleus. Farther rostrally, fibres are distributed to the lateral and medial geniculate nuclei, and all the other thalamic nuclei except those of the medial and midline groups. The habenular nuclei are also supplied, largely by fibres leaving the medial forebrain bundle which then run caudally in the stria medullaris.

In the telencephalon, structures innervated by the dorsal NA bundle include:

1. the amygdala;

2. the hippocampal formation;

3. the septal area, the bed nucleus of the stria terminalis, and the nucleus of the diagonal band;

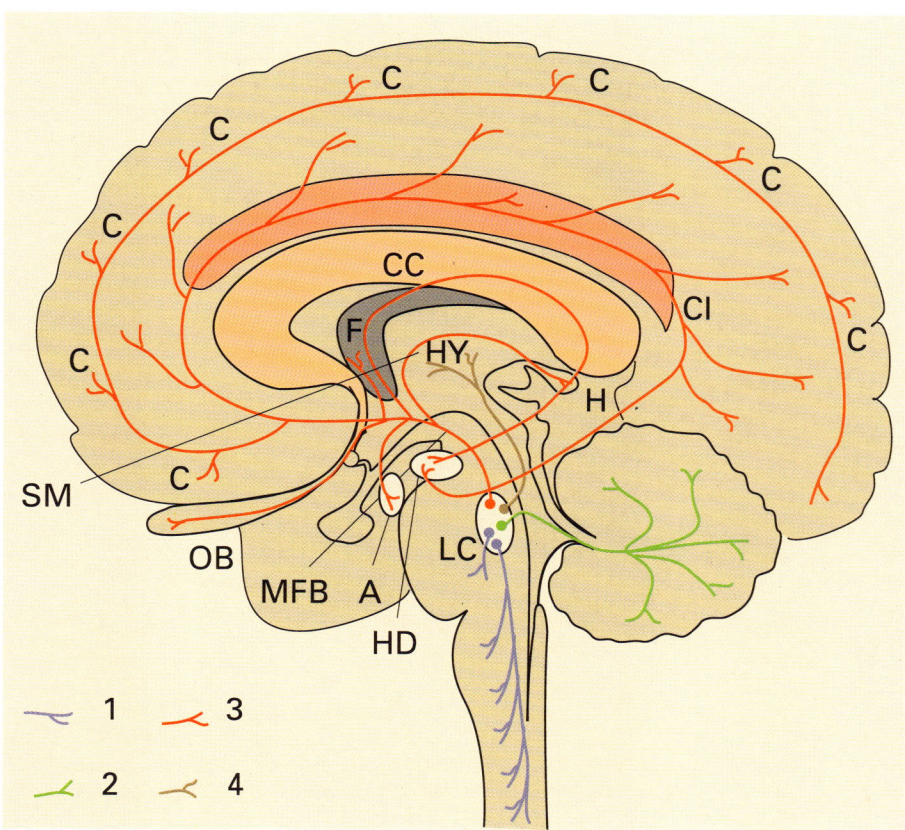

Fig. 25.2 The locus coeruleus and its pathways. 1, Descending pathway; 2, coeruleocerebellar pathway; 3, dorsal tegmental noradrenergic bundle; 4, dorsal longitudinal bundle of Schütz; A, amygdala; C, cerebral neocortex; CC, corpus callosum; CI, cingulum; F, fornix; H, habenula; HD, hippocampus; HY, hypothalamus; LC, locus coeruleus complex (A4 and A6); MFB, medial forebrain bundle; OB, olfactory bulb; SM, stria medullaris. (Drawn after Nieuwenhuys 1985, with permission.)

4. various olfactory centres, including the bulb and tubercle; and

5. the entire neocortex.

The smaller dorsal periventricular pathway is formed of axons arising from cells of the locus coeruleus complex. These axons enter the ventromedial part of the periaqueductal grey matter of the midbrain and form a component of the dorsal longitudinal bundle of Schütz (Fig. 25.2). The pathway continues as the diencephalic periventricular plexus which innervates certain parts of the hypothalamus. These include the paraventricular nucleus, the supraoptic nucleus, and the dorsomedial nucleus. However, the major hypothalamic NA projection comes from the lateral tegmental system (see below), so that the above-mentioned nuclei have a dual innervation from the two systems. Note that several structures receive NA coerulean fibres from more than one route, e.g. the amygdala (through the stria terminalis and a more direct path from the medial forebrain bundle), and the hippocampus (via the fornix and cingulum).

The lateral tegmental system

Noradrenergic fibres of this system arise from cell groups A1, A2, A5, and A7. They form (1) descending; (2) intrinsic brainstem; and (3) ascending pathways (Fig. 25.3).

1. Descending fibres form the dorsolateral NA bulbospinal tract which ends in the substantia gelatinosa (laminae I, II, III) and the thoracic intermediate columns, the latter having particularly profuse projections.

2. Intrinsic brainstem fibres project to mostly motor nuclei, namely: the dorsal vagal, facial, and trigeminal; but also to the solitary nucleus and the 'caudal' raphe nuclei.

3. Ascending fibres constitute the ventral NA pathway which is located in the central tegmental tract. This pathway passes rostrally, mainly continuing in the medial forebrain bundle (Fig. 25.3). *En route* the fibres supply the midbrain reticular formation, the entire hypothalamus, especially the supraoptic and paraventricular nuclei, the dorsomedial nucleus, and the tuberal nuclei. In the telencephalon they innervate the amygdala, the bed nucleus of the stria terminalis, and the septal area.

Adrenergic cell groups and pathways

Adrenergic neurones may be specifically identified by using an antibody raised against *phenylethanolamine-N-methyltransferase* (PNMT), an enzyme involved in the catecholamine biosynthetic chain, which finally converts noradrenaline into adrenaline (AD).

Out of all the major monoaminergic systems, the adrenergic one is the least understood anatomically, and the complete picture of its distribution is still to emerge. The PNMT technique has a low sensitivity. Biochemical methods have shown the presence of adrenaline in areas of the brain, such as the basal ganglia, the septal nuclei, and the amygdala, in which the PNMT technique failed to demonstrate any adrenergic terminals.

The adrenergic system may influence the secretion of oxytocin and vasopressin, and may also regulate respiration and blood pressure.

All PNMT-containing cell groups are situated in the caudal part of the hindbrain, and have been designated C1, C2, and C3 (Fig. 25.4). The largest is cell group C1, situated in the ventrolateral part of the medulla oblongata just dorsal to the inferior

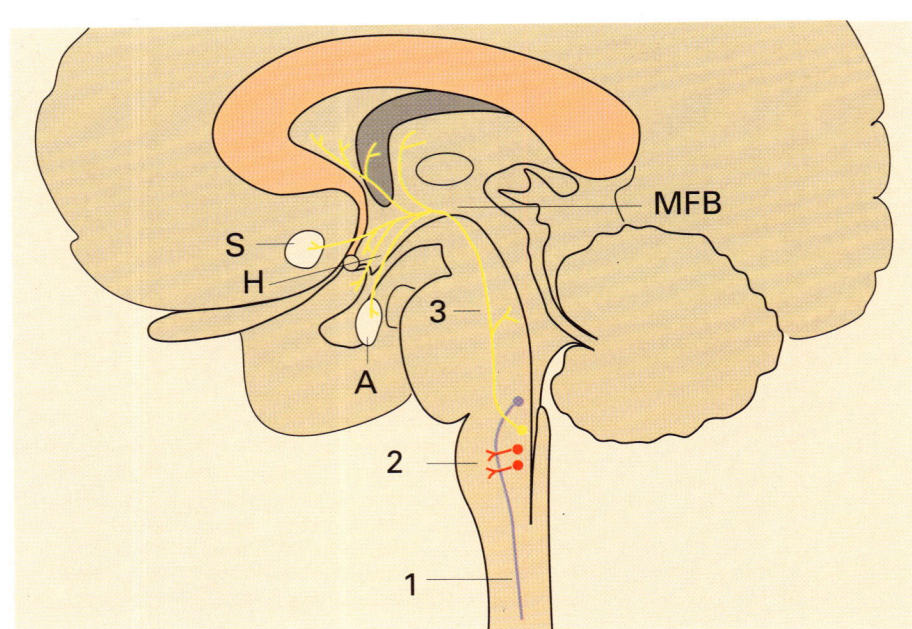

Fig. 25.3 The remaining noradrenergic pathways. 1, Descending pathways; 2, intrinsic brainstem fibres; 3, ascending pathway (ventral noradrenergic bundle); A, amygdala; F, fornix; H, hypothalamus; MFB, medial forebrain bundle; S, septal area. (Drawn after Nieuwenhuys 1985, with permission.)

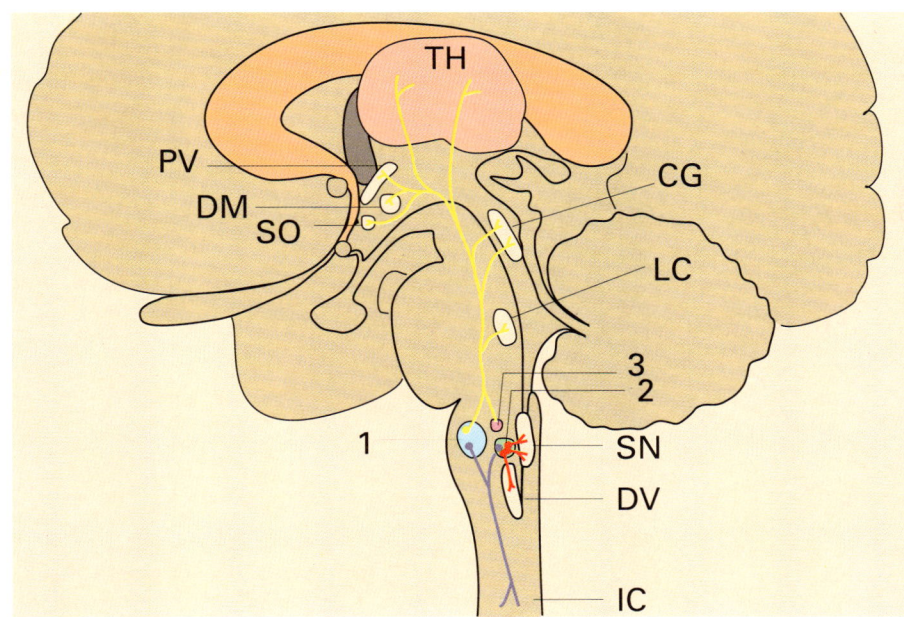

Fig. 25.4 Adrenergic cell groups and pathways. 1, Cell group C1; 2, cell group C2; 3, cell group C3; CG, central grey matter of the midbrain; DM, dorsomedial nucleus; DV, dorsal vagal nucleus; IC, intermediolateral column; LC, locus coeruleus; PV, paraventricular nucleus; SN, solitary nucleus; SO, supraoptic nucleus; TH, thalamus. (Drawn after Nieuwenhuys 1985, with permission.)

olivary nucleus. Cell group C2 lies within and around the solitary nucleus. The smallest, cell group C3, is found close to the midline at the level of the hypoglossal nucleus where it lies amongst the fibres of the medial longitudinal bundle.

From cell groups C1 to C3 axons ascend through the reticular formation, closely associated with the ventral noradrenergic bundle, to reach the lateral hypothalamus (Fig. 25.4). In the medulla, axons terminate in the solitary nucleus and the dorsal vagal nucleus, while in the pons they end in the locus coeruleus—the former two structures showing a particularly high density of adrenergic terminals. *En route* to the diencephalon, the ascending bundle distributes fibres to the periaqueductal grey matter, and finally supplies the thalamic midline nuclei, the dorsomedial, supraoptic, and paraventricular hypothalamic nuclei. Descending PNMT-containing axons have also been traced into the spinal cord where they end in high density in the intermediolateral column (part of lamina VII).

Serotonergic cell groups and pathways

Serotonergic (S) neurones are found throughout the brainstem, lying in or near the midline, in association with the rapheal nuclei. They are designated B1–B9 cell groups; and their projections are similar to those of the noradrenergic system, although less prolific. They are (1) descending; (2) intrinsic brainstem; (3) cerebellar; and (4) ascending projections (see Fig. 25.5). S axons also form the supra-ependymal plexus (5).

1. Medullary S cells from the 'caudal' raphe nuclei, specifically the nucleus pallidus (B1), the nucleus obscura (B2), and the nucleus magnus (B3), give rise to two descending bundles:
   (a) The lateral raphespinal bundle from B3 descends close to the lateral corticospinal tract, its fibres ending in the

dorsal grey columns including the substantia gelatinosa, and the intermediate grey matter (laminae I, II, and V). They prevent the transmission of noxious and thermal stimuli by activating enkephalinergic interneurones which inhibit spinothalamic projection neurones and certain primary afferent fibres.
   (b) The ventral raphespinal bundle travels in the medial part of the ventral white coumn, its axons terminating in the ventral grey column (laminae VIII and IX). Both sets of fibres form a diffuse projection system which runs the length of the cord, their collaterals influencing entire cell columns by projecting to extensor and flexor motor neurone pools, activating α- as well as γ-neurones, and thus increasing motor responsiveness. This is a gain-setting mechanism which is also facilitated by coeruleospinal fibres of the NA system.

2. Intrinsic projections arising from pontine and midbrain S neurones and by synapsing on cells of the nucleus coeruleus, the tegmental nuclei, and also the pontine and medullary reticular formation. They are probably concerned with the central control of cardiovascular function.

3. Cerebellar projections arise from pontine cell groups (B2, B5) and pass through the ipsilateral middle cerebellar peduncle to end in the roof nuclei and cells of the cerebellar cortex.

4. Ascending fibres from the 'rostral' raphe nuclei—the central superior (B6 and B8) and the dorsal raphe (B7) nuclei—form two bundles.
   (a) The dorsal ascending serotonergic bundle (Fig. 25.5), a small projection, arises from pontine S cells and enters the dorsal longitudinal bundle of Schütz which lies within the periaqueductal grey matter of the midbrain. These fibres end in the midbrain reticular nuclei, the

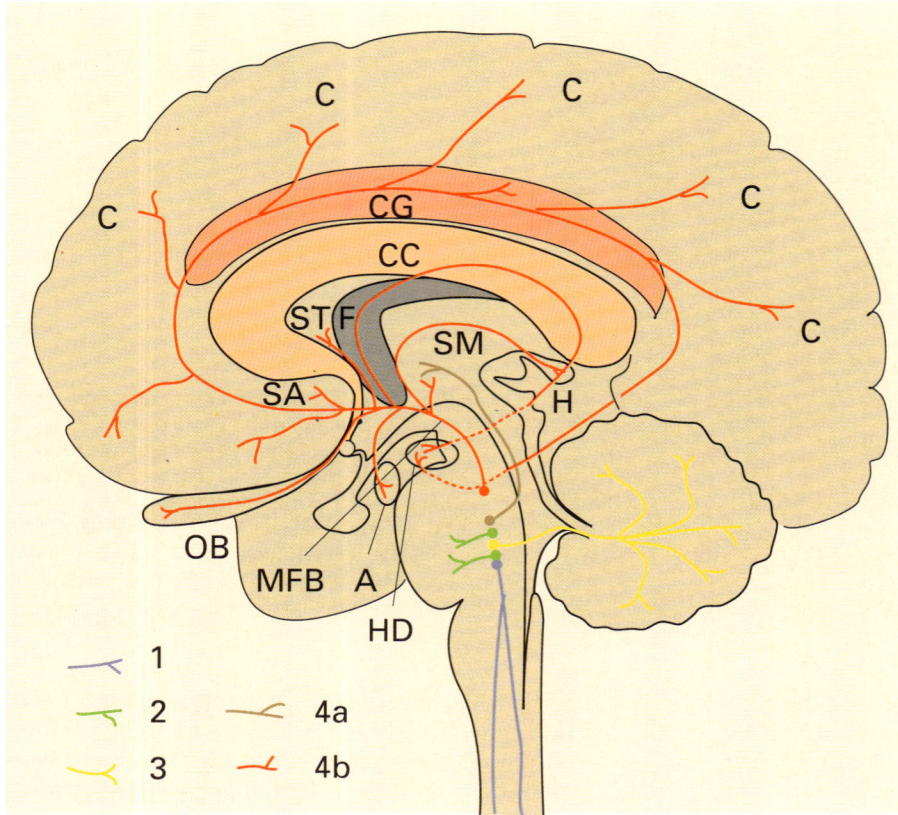

Fig. 25.5 The serotonergic pathways. 1, Descending pathways; 2, intrinsic brainstem projections; 3, cerebellar projections; 4a, dorsal ascending serotonergic bundle; 4b, ventral ascending serotonergic bundle; A, amygdala; C, cerebral neocortex; CC, corpus callosum; CG, cingulate gyrus; F, fornix; H, habenula; HD, hippocampus; MFB, medial forebrain bundle; OB, olfactory bulb; SA, septal area; SM, stria medularis; ST, striatum. (Drawn after Nieuwenhuys 1985, with permission.)

periaqueductal grey matter, and caudal regions of the hypothalamus.

(b) The ventral ascending serotonergic bundle (Fig. 25.5) is large and is a component of the central tegmental fasciculus of the midbrain. It then courses through the lateral part of the hypothalamus, where it joins the medial forebrain bundle. In the midbrain it supplies the substantia nigra and the interpeduncular nucleus. In the diencephalon it projects to the habenula, the thalamus (medial, midline, and parafascicular nuclei), and to the lateral hypothalamus and mamillary body. In the telencephalon it innervates the striatum and limbic system. In the latter, some fibres pass to the hippocampus via the fornix and also by way of the cingulum (dual innervation); others go to the amygdaloid nucleus, the septal areas, entorhinal cortex, and other olfactory areas, including the olfactory bulbs. The neocortex, especially the medial frontal, is also supplied. Ascending fibres from the 'rostral' raphe nuclei are involved in the regulation of sleep, possibly by blocking the NA (locus coeruleus) arousal mechanism. It is suggested that the serotonergic system is concerned with slow wave or deep sleep, whereas the NA system tends to govern REM sleep.

5. The supra-ependymal plexus extends throughout the ventricular surface, except for the ventral part of the third ventricle—the zone adjoining the hypothalamus. Its terminals make synapse-like contacts with ependymal cells.

Serotonin is released into the cerebrospinal fluid (CSF) for dissemination over the entire ventricular surface. The transmitter then re-enters the brain substance by transcellular routes through certain ependymal cells, where it is free to act at serotonergic receptors. The plexus is also concerned with modulating the motility of the cilia of ependymal cells, thus influencing the flow of CSF. It also controls the production of CSF and certain hormones produced by ependymal cells.

The concentration of serotonin and that of its major metabolite (5-hydroxyindoleacetic acid) in the CSF is reduced in some patients suffering from exogenous depression. Whether the entire serotonergic cell population is malfunctioning, or only cells of B6, B7, and B8 groups whose axons project to form the supra-ependymal plexus, remains to be seen.

Serotonergic fibres from mesencephalic raphe nuclei project to intracerebral arteries and arterioles. They regulate the cerebral blood flow, and may well be involved in the aetiology of serotonergic-related cerebrovascular disorders, e.g. migraine, ischaemia, and stroke.

The dopaminergic cell groups and pathways

Dopaminergic (DA) cell groups of the CNS (A8–A14) are situated in the mesencephalon and the hypothalamus. They give rise to two principal projections: the mesotelencephalic and hypothalamic systems, both of which are further subdivided.

The mesotelencephalic DA systems

1. The mesostriatal system (Fig. 25.6) arises from cells of the substantia nigra, pars compacta (A9), the ventral tegmental area of Tsai (A10), and the lateral tegmental area (A8), cell groups which are located in the rostral part of the midbrain. Their axons ascend through the medial tegmentum of the midbrain entering the dorsal part of the lateral hypothalamus, before diverging laterally and dorsally into the striatum.

   (a) Axons of cells of A9 (substantia nigra), A8, and A10 groups project to the caudate–putamen complex.
   (b) Axons of cells of A10 (ventral tegmental area of Tsai) and part of the A9 groups project to the nucleus accumbens (the ventral striatum).

This system regulates complex behaviour, and is concerned with the ability to switch motor programmes arbitrarily. In parkinsonian patients there is a progressive loss of DA neurones in the substantia nigra, with the consequent destruction of the nigrostriatal pathway. This results in muscular rigidity (*hypertonia*) and also paucity of movement (*akinesis*). The ventral tegmental area (A10) also shows loss of DA cells in parkinsonism, which results in patients being unable to change their behaviour arbitrarily; and thus they show a shifting aptitude disorder at both motor and cognitive levels.

2. The mesolimbocortical system (Fig. 25.6) arises from neurones of the ventral tegmental area (A10) and the medial part of the substantia nigra (A9). Axons from these cells ascend medial to the mesostriatal projection in the medial forebrain bundle to be distributed to:

   (a) the medial frontal, anterior cingulate, piriform, and entorhinal cortices; and
   (b) the olfactory bulb, olfactory area, anterior perforated substance, the lateral septal nucleus, and amygdala.

Activation of A10 with its projection to the nucleus accumbens enhances locomotor activity. Hyperactivity of A10, which projects to limbic structures, may play a role in the pathophysiology of schizophrenia. Post-mortem examinations of brains of some schizophrenic patients show an increase in the concentration of DA in the nucleus accumbens and the anterior perforated substance. There is also gross asymmetry of the dopamine concentration in the amygdalae (left greater than right). Overenthusiatic treatment of parkinsonian patients with L-dopa, a DA agonist, can result in schizophrenic behaviour. This is probably due to enhancement of activity either in the ventral area of Tsai (A10) or, more probably, in the dopamine receptor sites of the limbic system.

The hypothalamic DA systems

1. Hypothalamo-spinal projections arise from cells of the A11 group, situated in the caudal part of the hypothalamus

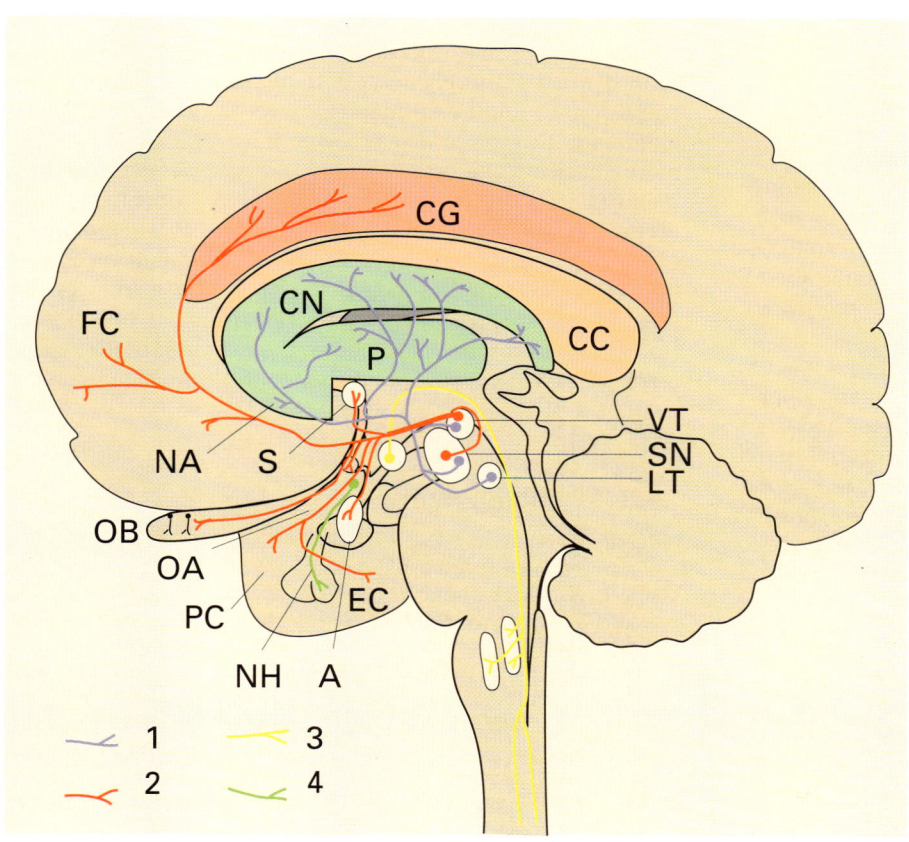

Fig. 25.6 The dopaminergic pathways. 1, Mesostriatal system, from A8, A9, and A10; 2, mesolimbocortical system, from A10 and part of A9; 3, hypothalamo-spinal system, from A11; 4, tubero-infundibular projections, from A12; A, amygdala; CC, corpus callosum; CG, cingulate gyrus (anterior part); CN, caudate nucleus; EC, entorhinal cortex; FC, frontal cortex; LT, lateral tegmental area; NA, nucleus accumbens; NH, neurohypophysis; OA, olfactory area and anterior perforated substance; OB, olfactory bulb, contains dopaminergic interneurones, A15; P, putamen; PC, prepyriform cortex; S, septal area; SN, substantia nigra; VT, ventral tegmental area. (Drawn after Nieuwenhuys 1985, with permission.)

(Fig. 25.6). Their axons descend in the brainstem through the dorsal longitudinal bundle of Schütz. In the spinal cord they form two bundles. One bundle continues in the postero-lateral tract and lamina I to supply neurones in the dorsal grey columns, the other descends close to the spinal canal to innervate preganglionic neurones of intermediolateral column in segments Th1 to L2 (the sympathetic outflow).

2. Hypothalamo-septal projections arise from cell groups A11, A13, and A14, situated in the rostral and caudal parts of the hypothalamus, and end by synapsing on cells of the lateral septal nucleus.

3. Tubero-infundibular projections (Fig. 25.6) arise from cells of the A12 group and synapse on cells of the median eminence. Functionally they are concerned with the inhibition of prolactin release.

Other monoaminergic neurones

γ-Aminobutyric acid (GABA), aspartate, glycine, and taurine are all recognized as CNS transmitters localized in specific neuronal groups. For example, GABA is a major inhibitory transmitter found in most inhibitory interneurones throughout the CNS, but also in the Purkinje cells of the cerebellum and other projection neurones such as those of the extra-pyramidal system. Glutamate and aspartate are excitatory transmitters in many systems, including the corticospinal, corticostriate, and corticothalamic pathways.

Peptidergic neurones

Aside from substance P-containing sensory terminals and certain enkephalin-containing neurones which are involved in pain perception, other peptidergic systems like those containing vasoactive intestinal polypeptide (VIP), cholecystokinin (CKK), and neurotensin (NT), although well described neuroanatomically, have poorly documented functions. Some act as neuromodulators, where they coexist with other neurotransmitters in the same cell, and may regulate the amount and duration of transmitter release as well as the sensitivity of the receptors in the post-synaptic membrane.

Receptor mapping of most transmitters is now well advanced, and a good example is that of the anatomy of μ, δ, and κ opiate receptors (Mansour et al. 1988). Matching receptor and transmitter distributions in the CNS is clearly a means of understanding regulatory mechanisms of, for example, opioid–peptide receptor interactions. Genetic regulation of receptor expression and transmitter production using in situ hybridization histochemical techniques is clearly a future direction with tremendous potential for understanding brain function.

25.1.3 Glia

Immunological markers are now used routinely to define the phenotypes of cells in the central nervous system in vitro. For example, antibodies to the surface glycoprotein THY-1, the ganglioside GM1, and the A2B5 ligand, together with those directed against the neurofilament triplet, are used to define neurones; anti-galactocerebroside (Gal-C) antibody for oligodendrocytes, and anti-glial fibrillar acid protein (GFAP) antibody for astrocytes. Working with the optic nerve of the rat, Raff and his colleagues have defined a migratory bipotential glial progenitor cell (A2B5+) which can differentiate into either oligodendrocytes (Gal-C+ cells) or astrocytes of a specific phenotype, GFAP+ and A2B5+, which have been called type 2 astrocytes (Raff and Miller 1984). All these latter cells are of the same lineage designated the O2A lineage. Another sort of astrocyte, designated type 1 astrocyte (GFAP+, A2B5−) is formed from a different population of stem cells resident in the optic nerve. Raff has also been able to identify the nature and source of the growth-promoting and inducer factors which control the proliferation and differentiation of O2A bipotential progenitor cells into either oligodendrocytes or type 2 astrocytes in vitro. However, the crucial step of demonstrating the existence of both bipotential progenitor cells and type 2 astrocytes in vivo is proving difficult, mainly because the cell surface antigens A2B5 and Gal-C are difficult to use on tissue sections. Moreover, attempts to discover whether gliogenesis elsewhere in the CNS follows a similar pattern to that inferred for the optic nerve from tissue culture experiments is also proving problematic. Thus, although bipotential progenitor cells appear to have the same phenotype in the developing cerebral hemisphere as those derived from the optic nerve, the A2B5 marker poorly discriminates type 1 from type 2 astrocytes.

Throughout the brain one important source of glia is the subependymal plate, a periventricular layer of cells characteristically made up of cells with darkly and lightly cresyl-fast-violet-stained nuclei. The phenotypic status of these cells vis-à-vis A2B5, Gal-C, and GFAP markers is yet to be determined. In mammals, two types of astrocytes have been described on morphological criteria, as fibrous and protoplasmic astrocytes (Penfield 1932; Fedoroff and Vernadakis 1986) which mainly occupy white and grey matter, respectively. It is tempting to equate type 1 cells with protoplasmic astrocytes and type 2 with fibrous; indeed Raff has suggested that type 2 astrocytes are cells with a specific function of servicing nodes of Ranvier. However, for reasons stated above, the existence of the type 2 astrocyte in vivo has yet to be demonstrated convincingly.

25.1.4 Bibliography

Fedoroff, S. and Vernadakis, A. (1986). Cellular neurobiology: a series: astrocyte, Vol. 1. Academic Press, New York.

Mansour, A., Khachaturian, H., Lewis, M. E., Akil, H., and Wilson, S. J. (1988). Anatomy of CNS opioid receptors. Trends in Neurosciences 11, 308–14.

Nieuwenhuys, R. (1985). Chemoarchitecture of the brain. Springer-Verlag, Berlin.

Penfield, W. (1932). Neuroglia, normal and pathological. M. Cytology and cellular pathology of the nervous system, Vol. II, pp. 423–79. Hoeber, New York.

Raff, M. C. and Miller, R. H. (1984). Glial cell development in the rat optic nerve. Trends in Neurosciences 7, 469–72.

25.2 Hypoxia

G. Cole

25.2.1 Brain hypoxia

Hypoxia is defined as a deficiency of oxygen, and, basically, hypoxic brain damage is brought about by either a reduction of oxygen in the blood, or inability of the brain to utilize oxygen at the cellular level. There is considerable evidence to show that a period of severe hypoxia of more than 3 or 4 minutes will cause irreversible brain damage. In an adult the average cerebral blood flow (CBF) is about 50 ml/100 g/min, and the brain normally consumes oxygen at the rate of about 3.3 ml/100 g/min.

Autoregulation

Autoregulation is the vital mechanism by which a relatively constant CBF is maintained over a wide range of perfusion pressures. The cerebral perfusion pressure represents the difference between the mean arterial blood pressure and the intracranial pressure, but under normal circumstances the arterial blood pressure can be viewed as the effective cerebral perfusion pressure. Autoregulation is affected by changes in the cerebrovascular resistance; thus when the arterial blood pressure falls, the cerebral arterioles dilate, and a rise in blood pressure will result in arteriolar constriction. Autoregulation usually fails when the blood pressure drops below 50 mmHg, and the cerebral blood flow falls rapidly. Any factor interfering with the ability of cerebral vessels to dilate or constrict interferes with autoregulation, and it may be impaired under a variety of conditions including *hypoxic or hypercapnic states*, *chronic hypertension*, and in a wide range of acute conditions such as *head injury*, *cerebral tumour*, and *stroke*.

25.2.2 Classification of brain hypoxia

Brain hypoxia is classified according to the underlying physiological factors, and very often in any particular case more than one factor may be active. The views of earlier workers have been incorporated in the widely used classification of hypoxia, which is outlined below.

1. Stagnant hypoxia (ischaemic and oligaemic).
   (a) *Ischaemic*: the brain or some portion of it is deprived of its blood supply.
   (b) *Oligaemic*: the brain or some portion of it receives a reduced supply of blood.
2. Anoxic and hypoxic hypoxia.
   (a) *Anoxic*: an absence of oxygen in the pulmonary alveoli leads to anoxaemia and brain anoxia.
   (b) *Hypoxic*: reduced oxygen in the pulmonary alveoli leads to brain hypoxia.

3. Anaemic hypoxia. In uncomplicated anaemias the oxygen content of the blood is reduced, but the oxygen saturation and tension may be normal. Carbon monoxide poisoning reduces the amount of circulating haemoglobin available to combine with oxygen, and is the only example of anaemic hypoxia that leads to brain damage.
4. Histotoxic hypoxia. In the presence of poisons such as cyanide there is an inhibition of brain respiratory enzymes, and oxygen canot be utilized.
5. Hypoglycaemia. Energy in the brain is derived almost exclusively from oxidative metabolism of glucose, and the effect of glucose deprivation is therefore very similar to that of oxygen deprivation.

It is clear that hypoxic damage to the brain may occur in a variety of medical emergencies, which include cardiac arrest, severe hypotension, respiratory obstruction, brainstem damage, hypoglycaemia, carbon monoxide poisoning, and drug overdose.

25.2.3 Neuropathological changes in hypoxia

In spite of the large variety of causes of hypoxic brain damage, the neuropathological changes are very similar. The extent and distribution of the lesions in the brain depend largely on the duration and severity of the hypoxia, and the length of survival of the patient. The neurones are most vulnerable to oxygen deprivation, but if a hypoxic episode is of sufficient severity, the nerve processes, glial cells, and blood-vessels will be affected to a variable degree.

Ischaemic cell change

The neurone affected by hypoxia undergoes ischaemic change, and this phenomenon may be seen at the microscopic level after survival of about 4–12 h. The earliest change in the cell is that of *microvacuolation*, but this is a transient event often obscured by autolytic changes and rarely identified in man. Typically, the affected neurone assumes a shrunken appearance with deeply eosinophilic cytoplasm, and finely dispersed Nissl substance. The nucleus is also shrunken, often triangular in shape, and stains darkly. This is followed by homogenization, in which the cytoplasm is structureless and the Nissl substance can no longer be discerned. The dead neurone eventually disappears.

25.2.4 Selective vulnerability

It has long been recognized that neurones in different anatomical sites vary in their susceptibility to hypoxia. The most vulnerable neurones are those of the hippocampus, the Purkinje and granule cells of the cerebellum, and the 3rd, 5th, and 6th layers of the cerebral cortex. Within the cerebral cortex, neuronal necrosis is usually most pronounced in the occipital and parietal lobes, and decreased towards temporal and frontal lobes. Brain damage may be restricted to *arterial boundary zones* in the cortex and cerebellum, and this pattern of damage is mostly encountered when there is a profound episode of hypotension and consequent fall in cerebral perfusion pressure. Because of their anastomotic blood supply, arterial boundary zones are particularly susceptible to hypoxia.

Hypoxic damage may occur in certain nuclei of the thalamus, particularly the anterior nuclear complex, and dorsomedial nuclei, and also the basal ganglia, especially the caudate nucleus and the putamen.

Within the adult brainstem, the reticular zones of the substantia nigra, the inferior colliculi, and inferior olives are relatively vulnerable. In young children, the brainstem is more vulnerable than in the adult, and hypoxic damage may include the nuclei of the 5th, 8th, and 10th cranial nerves. The hypothalamus is rarely affected in the adult, but the mamillary bodies in young children are more vulnerable to hypoxia.

25.2.5 Prolonged survival after hypoxia

After a severe hypoxic episode such as cardiac arrest, the majority of patients die within a few hours or days. However, there are an increasing number of patients who survive for months or even years. The brains of such patients demonstrate the patterns of selective vulnerability, and the secondary changes associated with widespread neuronal necrosis.

Macroscopic appearance

After prolonged survival the brain may be markedly reduced in weight, with atrophy of the cortical gyri and the cerebellar folia. On coronal sectioning of the brain, the ventricles may appear slightly enlarged after a few weeks, but may be grossly enlarged after months or years. The cortical layer may be thinned and show focal or widespread necrosis. With increasing length of survival there may be obvious shrinkage and discoloration of the basal ganglia and thalamus, and the white matter may show evidence of destruction, with areas of discoloration, pallor, or cystic necrosis (Fig. 25.7).

Microscopic appearance

The deeper cortical layers, or occasionally the whole width of the cortex, shows varying loss of neurones and cystic necrosis, which is accompanied by an often intense gliomesodermal reaction (Fig. 25.8), with reactive astrocytes producing glial fibres, thickened blood vessels, and often prominent macrophages in the perivascular spaces. Necrosis of the basal ganglia and thalamic nuclei is similarly represented, by varying neuronal loss and cystic gliosis. *Wallerian-type degeneration* within the white matter tracts is a consequence of neuronal destruction, in particular areas of the cortex and deeper grey nuclei. The affected white matter may show pallor or destruction of myelin with subsequent gliosis and an invasion of varying numbers of macrophages. Affected areas of the cerebellum show a varying loss of Purkinje cells and granule cells (Fig. 25.9) accompanied by marked gliosis.

Perinatal hypoxia

Hypoxic brain damage incurred during or after birth results in a variety of neurological disorders such as cerebral palsy, epilepsy, and mental retardation. Neuropathological lesions may affect the cortex, basal ganglia, cerebellum, and brainstem.

Primitive neural tissue has little reactive capacity and injured tissue tends to disappear without gliosis or scarring. Thus malformations or large cystic cavities may be produced if hypoxic damage occurs in early embryonic development.

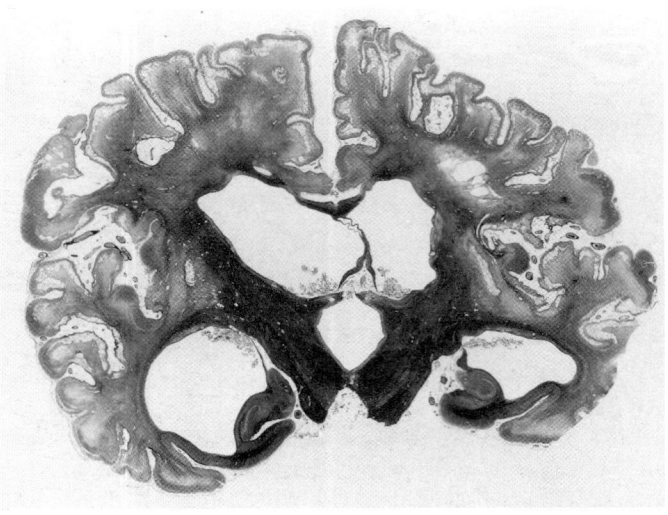

Fig. 25.7 Coronal section of the fronto-temporal region. Note the enlarged ventricles, cystic necrosis of the putamen and white matter, and necrosis of the cortex.

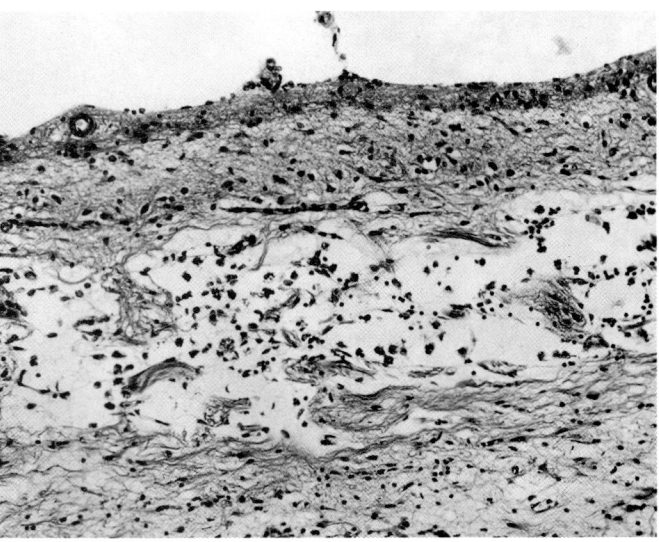

Fig. 25.8 Section of frontal cortex showing loss of neurones, cystic necrosis, and a gliomesodermal reaction.

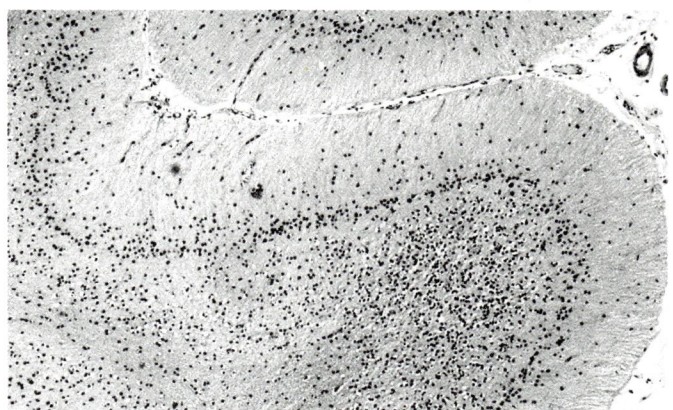

Fig. 25.9 Section of cerebellum with total loss of Purkinje cells and thinning of the granule cell layer.

25.2.6 Further reading

Brierley, J. B. and Graham, D. I. (1984). Hypoxia in vascular disorders of the central nervous system. In *Greenfield's neuropathology* (ed. J. Hume-Adams, J. A. N. Corsellis, and L. W. Duchen) (4th edn), pp. 125–207. Edward Arnold, London.

Brierley, J. B., Adams, J. H., Graham, D. I., and Simpson, J. A. (1971). Neocortical death after cardiac arrest. *Lancet* **ii**, 560–5.

Raichle, M. E. and De Vivo, D. C. (1974). Disorders of cerebral circulation. In *Neurological pathophysiology* (ed. S. G. Eliasson, A. L. Prensky, and W. B. Harder) (1st edn), pp. 242–67. Oxford University Press, New York.

25.3 Infections

Margaret M. Esiri

25.3.1 Bacterial and fungal infections

Despite its protected site inside the skull, many organisms are capable of reaching the brain and surrounding meninges to cause inflammatory diseases which are important causes of mortality and morbidity, and which are reviewed below. For an account of the bacterial disease, leprosy, which affects peripheral nerves, the reader is referred to Section 25.9.3.

Bacteria and fungi reach the central nervous system (CNS) in the blood or spread directly from a nearby focus of infection in bones, middle ears, or air sinuses of the skull. Bacterial invasion may also complicate *skull fractures*, insertion of a *ventricular shunt*, or occur in subjects with *malformations* that allow exposure of the CNS to the environment, for example, a *meningomyelocoele*. For the most part, bacterial and fungal organisms that are capable of growing well in cerebrospinal fluid (CSF) produce acute or chronic inflammation of the leptomeninges. If highly virulent organisms infect the brain, they give rise to an abscess, while organisms of lower virulence may produce granulomas in the brain as well as in the leptomeninges. Infections with the less virulent organisms are particularly liable to occur in immunodeficient subjects.

When a clinical diagnosis of a bacterial or fungal infection of the CNS or its coverings is made, it is usually possible to obtain confirmation of this by examination of the CSF from which the causative organism may be cultured, provided the sample is obtained before antibiotic treatment is started. Repeated cultures may be necessary to demonstrate the presence of some of the fungi, and in certain cases serological tests on CSF and serum provide a diagnosis more readily than culture. Frequently definitive isolation of the responsible organisms can be obtained, similarly, from the pus of an abscess or subdural empyema. Occasionally, it is necessary to resort to a tissue biopsy of the brain or meninges in order to diagnose bacterial or fungal granulomatous disease.

Acute bacterial leptomeningitis

Acute bacterial meningitis causes considerable mortality. Recent figures of nearly 20 per cent for pneumococcal and 5–10 per cent for meningococcal meningitis have been recorded. These are the two organisms most frequently responsible for adult cases (Table 25.1). In children under 5 years, *Haemophilus influenzae* accounts for the majority of cases and has a mortality of 5–10 per cent, in infants *Escherichia coli* is responsible for most cases, the remainder of paediatric cases being due, as in adults, principally to meningococcus and pneumococcus. Patients who have undergone splenectomy are at particular risk of pneumococcal septicaemia and meningitis.

In acute, fatal bacterial meningitis there is usually a purulent exudate readily visible in the subarachnoid space covering the surface of the brain (Fig. 25.10). The superficial vessels of the brain appear congested and there may be some generalized cerebral swelling. In occasional fulminating cases, there may be

Table 25.1 Bacterial and fungal organisms causing meningitis and/or brain granulomas

Bacteria	Fungi and yeasts
Actinomyces	*Aspergillus*
Arachnia	*Blastomyces*
Bacillus anthracis	*Candida albicans*
Borrelia burgdorfii	*Cladosporidium*
Brucella	*Coccidioides*
Coliforms	*Cryptococcus*
Haemophilus influenzae	*Histoplasma*
Leptospira	*Pseudoallescheria*
Listeria monocytogenes	*Sporothrix*
Meningococcus	Zygomycetes
Mycobacteria (tuberculosis and atypical)	
Nocardia	
Pneumococcus	
Serratia	
Staphylococci	
Streptococci	
Treponema pallidum	

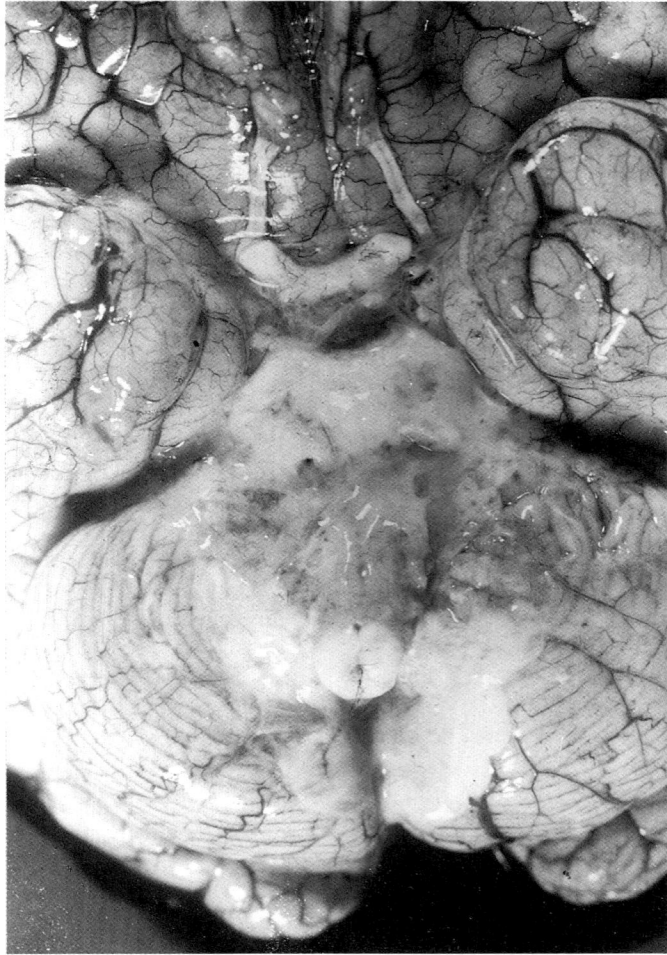

Fig. 25.10 Appearance of the base of the brain in acute meningitis, with collections of pus around the base of the pons and in the cisterna magna.

no obvious subarachnoid pus, but the meninges and surface vessels are acutely congested and show a few petechial haemorrhages and there is more severe cerebral swelling Microscopically, the subarachnoid space and leptomeninges contain a predominantly neutrophil polymorph infiltrate with some admixed mononuclear cells and strands of fibrin. Inflammation may extend as short cuffs of cells around the most superficial parenchymal vessels. Organisms should be demonstrable with appropriate stains unless antibiotic treatment has eradicated them. Outside the CNS, there may be adrenal haemorrhages or more widespread evidence of intravascular coagulation.

Chronic meningitis

Chronic meningitis occurs if infection in the subarachnoid space is due to less virulent organisms than pyogenic bacteria, or if pyogenic infection is inadequately treated. An inflammatory reaction that persists in the leptomeninges for more than 2 or 3 weeks is liable to lead to two important pathological com-

plications. The first of these is *hydrocephalus*, which is caused by impairment of the circulation of CSF due to collagen deposition in the subarachnoid space or at the outlet foramina of the fourth ventricle (Fig. 25.11). Obstruction at these sites results in a *communicating hydrocephalus* in which the third, fourth, and lateral ventricles are all dilated and contain CSF under increased pressure. The extent of the hydrocephalus varies from mild and clinically trivial to gross and life threatening. Obstruction to CSF flow through the aqueduct can also occur as a result of gliosis complicating *infective or non-infective ventriculitis*. This gives rise to a *non-communicating hydrocephalus* in which the lateral and third ventricles only are dilated.

The second important complication seen in chronic meningitis is the development of *endarteritis obliterans*, which can affect both major cerebral arteries that lie in the subarachnoid space, and the smaller leptomeningeal arteries. This produces narrowing of the arterial lumen with intimal thickening and chiefly adventitial inflammation (Fig. 25.12). It also predisposes to local thrombosis of affected vessels and infarction in their

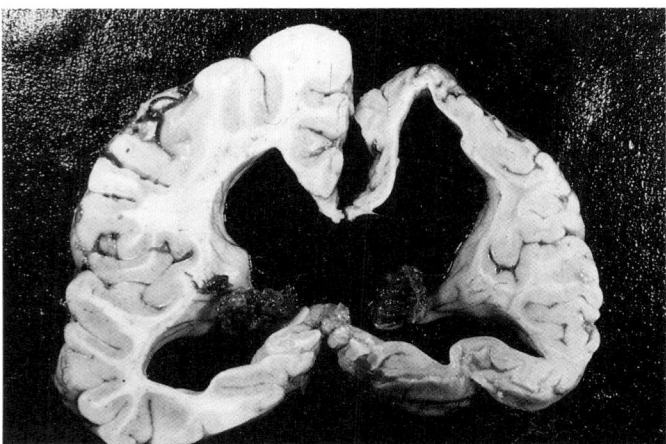

Fig. 25.11 Massive hydrocephalus due to tuberculous meningitis which developed and was treated many years before death.

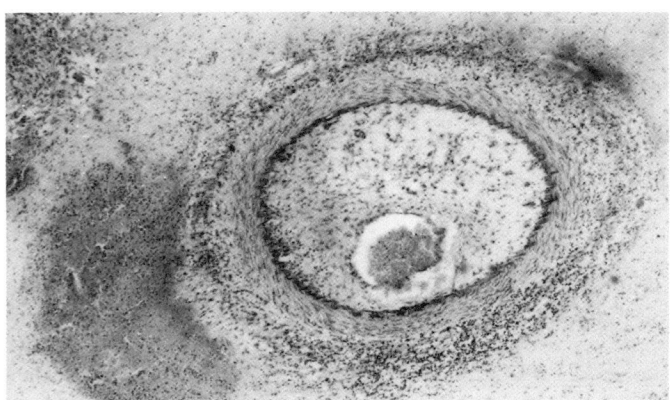

Fig. 25.12 Endarteritis obliterans affecting leptomeningeal vessels from a case of tuberculous meningitis. (Luxol fast blue/cresyl violet stain.)

territories of supply (Fig. 25.13). These infarcts are an important cause of persistent morbidity in survivors. Cerebral infarction is particularly liable to occur in forms of fungal meningitis, in which the organisms tend to invade the vessel wall (Fig. 25.14).

In chronic meningitis, due to *tuberculosis, cryptococcosis*, and some other *yeast or fungal infections*, there are likely to be granulomas present in the leptomeninges, choroid plexus, and superficial brain parenchyma. These contain the same cellular components as are found in similar granulomas elsewhere in the body, with multinucleate giant cells, epithelioid cells, macrophages, and lymphocytes present (Fig. 25.15). Caseation is seen in some of the tuberculous granulomas, and the organisms should be demonstrable with appropriate stains. Some other infections produce no well-defined granulomas, but a predominantly neutrophil polymorph reaction close to the organism.

The inflammatory process in chronic meningitis invariably extends to the ventricular surfaces where raised foci of inflammatory and reactive glial cells form nodules that protrude through the disrupted ependymal layer (*granular ependymitis*).

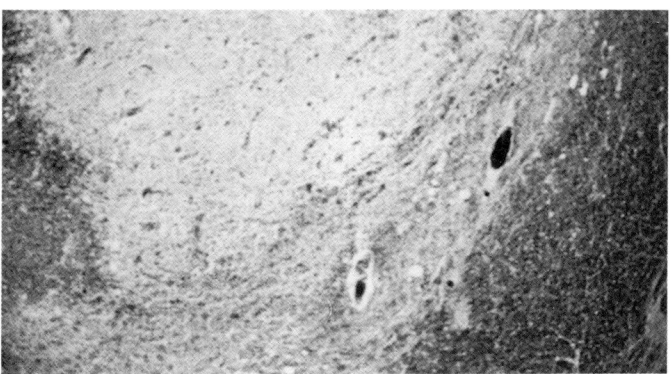

Fig. 25.13 Small pontine infarct associated with the development of endarteritis obliterans. (Luxol fast blue/cresyl violet stain.)

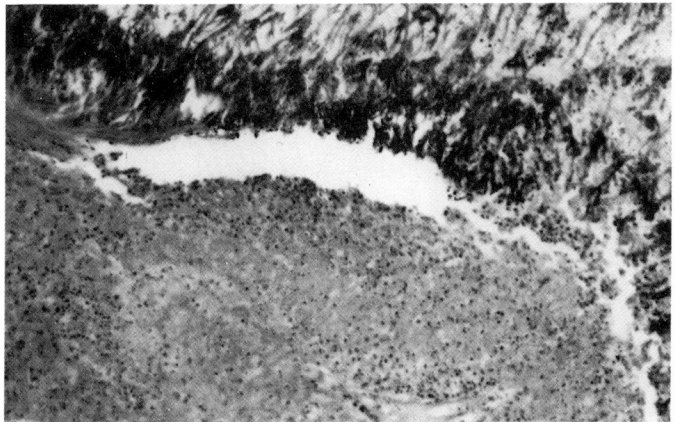

Fig. 25.14 *Aspergillus* organisms (top) invading the wall of a recently thrombosed leptomeningeal artery from a case of chronic aspergillus meningitis. (PAS stain.)

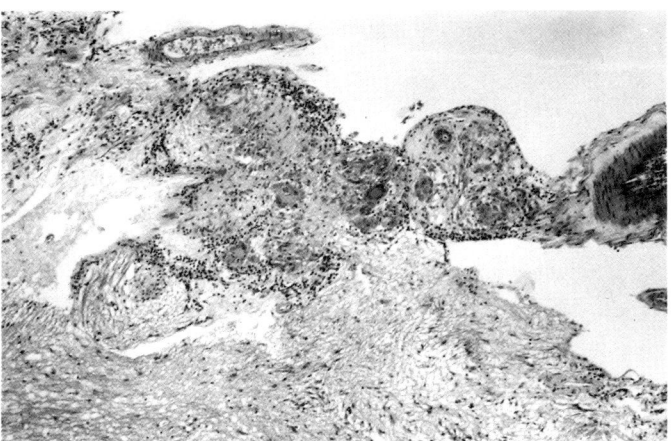

Fig. 25.15 Low-power view of the subarachnoid space in chronic tuberculous meningitis. Note the presence of coalescing multinucleate giant-cell granulomas.

These eventually form acellular fibrillary glial scars over which the ependyma is rarely fully restored.

Cranial and spinal nerve roots frequently become inflamed and damaged in chronic meningitis. After the inflammation has subsided, there is fibrosis and axonal loss. In *tertiary syphilis*, there is a *radiculitis* that particularly affects dorsal spinal roots, destroying some of the central axons of the sensory ganglion cells and resulting in Wallerian degeneration in the posterior columns of the spinal cord. Residual inflammation following treatment is sparse or absent. These are the characteristic findings in cases of *tabes dorsalis* (Fig. 25.16). The other manifestation of tertiary syphilis (*general paralysis of the insane*), rarely seen now, is a form of encephalitis chiefly affecting the frontal poles and producing marked frontal cortical atrophy. Microscopically, the condition is characterized by mononuclear inflammatory cell infiltrates, the presence of activated microglia, reactive astrocytosis, and neurone loss, chiefly in frontal lobe cortex. Iron deposits are found in the microglia. In untreated cases, spirochaetes can be demonstrated in affected cortex.

Occasionally, the spinal arachnoid membrane becomes involved in a chronic inflammatory process which results in painful, fibrotic tethering of the spinal nerve roots—*chronic spinal arachnoiditis*. This is most commonly seen at the lumbosacral or thoracic levels. It may be accompanied by calcification. Some cases have resulted from previous myelography when the introduction of radio-opaque contrast medium into the subarachnoid space has apparently been the precipitating cause. *Myodil*, an oily liquid, was particularly prone to produce such a reaction. Organisms are not usually identifiable in such cases. Another rare cause of chemical meningitis is release of the fluid contained in a craniopharyngioma into the subarachnoid space.

Subdural empyema

Subdural empyema usually results from spread of pyogenic infection from a local focus of *osteomyelitis* or *paranasal sinusitis*.

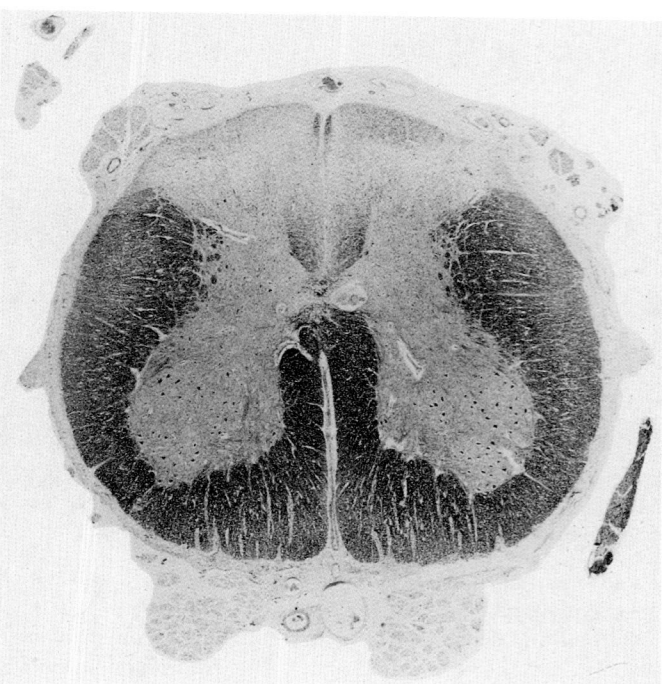

Fig. 25.16 Sacral spinal cord from a case of tabes dorsalis. There is pallor of myelin staining in the posterior columns and leptomeningeal fibrosis. (Luxol fast blue/cresyl violet stain.)

Because of the poor blood supply to the dura, it rarely develops from blood-borne spread of organisms and, for the same reason, the infection is difficult to eradicate once established. Pus in the subdural space is diffusely spread over the surface of the arachnoid, from which it can easily be removed. It may also loculate in pockets alongside the falx. There is a danger of *venous sinus thrombosis* and *venous infarction* of the brain developing as potentially fatal complications of subdural empyema.

Spinal epidural abscess

Pyogenic infection of the spinal epidural space is usually due to *Staphylococcus aureus* and results from local spread of the organism from infected bones of the vertebral column. The commonest site is at the thoracic level. Pus is liable to become loculated in pockets which may extend over several segments of the cord. Thrombosis of spinal vessels may occur as a complication of the infection.

Chronic infection of the epidural space occurs with spread of less virulent organisms from neighbouring bones, most notably with tuberculous infection. The granulation tissue formed shows the typical appearance of caseating granulomas, and organisms are detectable with the Ziehl–Neelsen stain.

Brain abscess

Abscesses may develop in any part of the brain but they are more common in white than grey matter. Those that occur as the result of local spread of organisms have particular sites of predilection. Thus, infection spreading from the middle ear tends to produce an ipsilateral *temporal lobe or cerebellar abscess*, while infection spreading from a frontal sinus produces an abscess in the adjacent frontal pole. If organisms are blood-borne, there may be multiple abscesses. The infection commences as a focus of *purulent encephalitis*. The softened and inflamed brain tissue rapidly breaks down to form a cavity filled with pus and surrounded by an abscess wall composed of glial fibrils and scanty collagen. The wall is fragile to start with, even barely existent in the presence of a highly virulent organism such as the pneumococcus, and may be insufficient to prevent rupture of the abscess into a ventricle. When well-established, the wall may appear laminated and contain fibrin, mononuclear inflammatory cells, neutrophil polymorphs and, more peripherally, reactive astrocytes, fibroblasts, collagen, and congested blood-vessels. Almost invariably, the surrounding brain is oedematous and the oedema may give rise to potentially fatal herniation (Fig. 25.17). Bacterial abscesses, by far the commonest type, frequently contain a mixed flora which includes anaerobic organisms. Rarely, abscesses are due to other organisms, such as amoebae.

Septic emboli arising from infected heart valves may give rise to solitary or multiple brain abscesses. Such emboli are also liable to cause cerebral infarction by blocking small arteries, or they may produce a *mycotic cerebral aneurysm* by lodging against, and weakening, the wall of an artery. The resulting infarct or haemorrhage can become secondarily infected by organisms contained in the embolus, or the organisms may reach the subarachnoid space to cause a complicating meningitis.

Brain granulomas

Granulomas in the brain vary in size from microscopic nodules to large, space-occupying lesions. They may be single or multiple, occur anywhere in the brain, and may be associated with

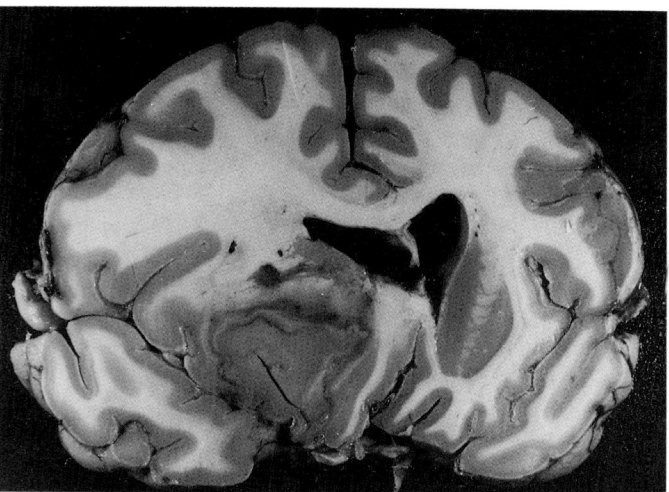

Fig. 25.17 Cerebral abscess situated in the left basal ganglia and inferior frontal lobe. Note the surrounding white matter oedema and shift of midline structures to the right.

localized or generalized chronic meningitis. They occur at all ages. In Western countries, macroscopic brain granulomas are not common and are seen more often in immunosuppressed than in immunocompetent individuals. In other parts of the world, the tubercle bacillus is responsible for many such brain granulomas and protozoal organisms for many more.

To the naked eye, macroscopic granulomas appear as ill-defined regions of granular, partially necrotic tissue, in some cases with patchy calcification (Fig. 25.18). They may abut on the ventricular system and give rise to *obstructive hydrocephalus*. Microscopically, the granulomas contain granulation tissue in which there are mixed mononuclear inflammatory cells, reactive astrocytes, a few fibroblasts, and many small blood vessels. Small, well-defined giant-cell granulomas are sometimes present. Plasma cells may also be a prominent component. In immunosuppressed subjects the inflammatory infiltrate is liable to be sparse or absent. The organisms responsible should be identifiable with appropriate stains.

Some cases of granulomatous disease of the meninges and CNS parenchyma are due to *sarcoidosis*. No organisms can be detected in these lesions which, apart from the absence of caseation, otherwise resemble those seen in tuberculosis. The diagnosis of sarcoidosis is supported if a positive Kveim test is obtained, and if granulomas are found elsewhere in the body at characteristic sites. However, some cases have lesions that are apparently confined to the CNS and its coverings.

Histiocytosis X

In this disease, foci of granulomatous inflammation develop in the bones of the skull and around the brain and pituitary gland. The spinal cord and cauda equina are also occasionally involved. The inflammatory cells include epithelioid cells, atypical macrophages with foamy cytoplasm, multinucleate cells,

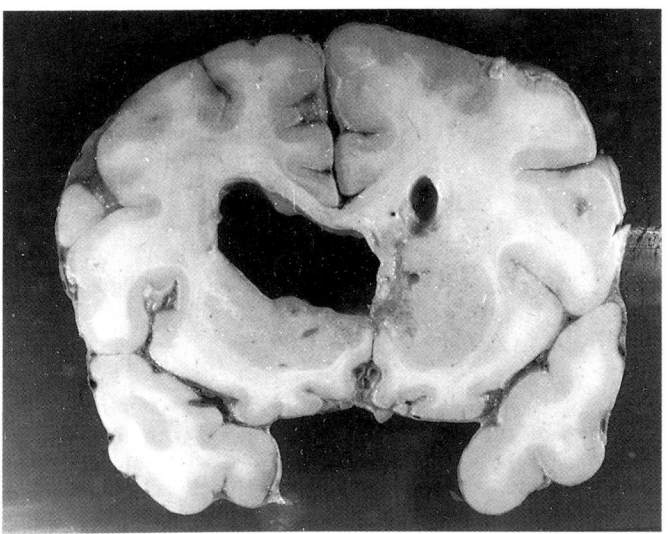

Fig. 25.18 Cerebral sarcoidosis producing granulomatous inflammation in the septum and structures surrounding the lateral ventricles, with the development of an obstructive hydrocephalus on the left.

lymphocytes, and plasma cells. In one form, *eosinophilic granuloma*, eosinophils also accumulate in the lesions.

Whipple's disease

The brain is occasionally a site of involvement in Whipple's disease, a condition in which bacteria accumulate in macrophages at various sites, most commonly in the walls of the intestine. The affected macrophages are strongly reactive with the PAS stain. Sites in the brain that are occasionally involved include the thalamus, hypothalamus, and other subcortical nuclei.

25.3.2 Viral and rickettsial infections

Viral and rickettsial infections may be localized to the meninges, brain, or spinal cord. Viruses reach the central nervous system (CNS) and its coverings via the blood or along nerves, while rickettsial infections are invariably blood-borne.

Viral meningitis

Viral meningitis is common and rarely fatal. It is a diagnosis that is often inferred when there are clinical features of meningitis, a predominantly mononuclear pleocytosis is found in the cerebrospinal fluid (CSF), and microscopy and culture of CSF for bacteria and fungi are negative ('aseptic meningitis'). Occasionally, virus can be cultured from CSF. Rare fatalities occur if viral meningitis is complicated by an encephalitic component to the infection. In such cases, the meninges show congestion and a predominantly mononuclear inflammatory cell infiltrate around leptomeningeal veins.

Viral encephalitis and myelitis

Diagosis of viral encephalitis depends on demonstrating the virus by culture, immunocytochemistry, or electron microscopy in cerebrospinal fluid or brain. Alternatively, immunological evidence of CNS infection may be sought by examining acute and convalescent pairs of sera and CSF for specific virus antibody. In many clinically diagnosed cases (about 70 per cent), no definitive virological diagnosis is achieved.

A great many different viruses may infect the brain or spinal cord and produce diseases that vary greatly in their tempo and severity (Table 25.2). Nevertheless, there are certain characteristic pathological features that many forms of viral encephalitis share in common. These are the following:

1. *cell death*, which varies enormously in its severity and selectivity, depending on the lytic capacities of the virus and its range of host cells;

2. *neuronophagia*, the clustering around the remnant of a dead neurone of a group of macrophages (Fig. 25.19);

3. *microglial nodules*, consisting of clusters of microglial cells admixed with a few lymphocytes (Fig. 25.20);

4. the presence of *inclusion bodies* in infected cells; these may be intranuclear, as in *herpes simplex* (HSV) or *cytomegalovirus*

Table 25.2   Viruses and rickettsiae causing human encephalitis, meningitis, or meningoencephalitis

Viruses

Herpes simplex types 1 and 2	Rabies
Herpes zoster	Lymphocytic choriomeningitis virus
Cytomegalovirus	
Herpes B	JC papova virus
Epstein–Barr virus	Arthropod-borne viruses (see Table 25.3)
Enteroviruses (polio, coxsackie, ECHO)	
	Rubella
Adenoviruses	Human immunodeficiency virus-1
Paramyxoviruses, especially measles virus; mumps virus	
	Human T-cell lymphotropic virus type I

Rickettsiae

Typhus and typhus-like fevers
Q fever

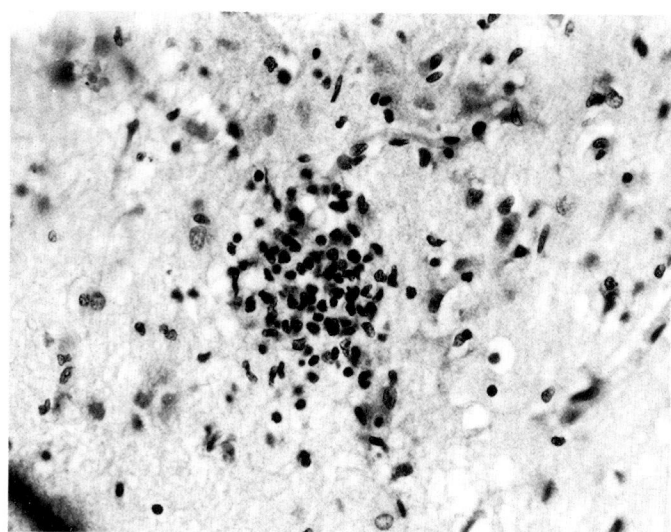

Fig. 25.20   Microglial nodules composed of mononuclear inflammatory cells in the cerebral cortex from a case of 'glial nodule' encephalitis in a renal transplant recipient.

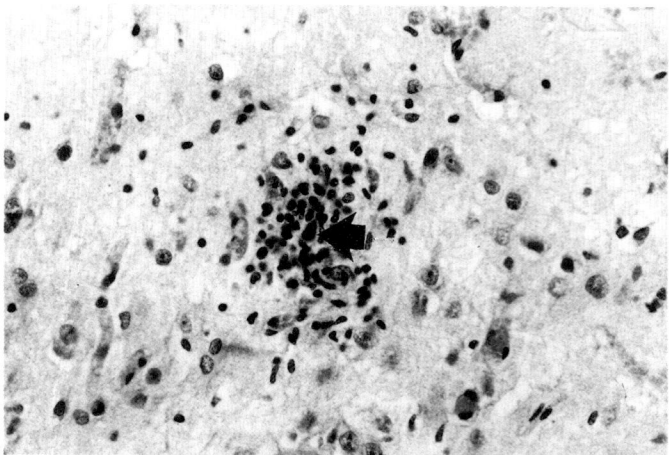

Fig. 25.19   Focus of neuronophagia surrounding the remnant of a cortical neurone (arrow) from the cerebral cortex of a case of subacute sclerosing panencephalitis.

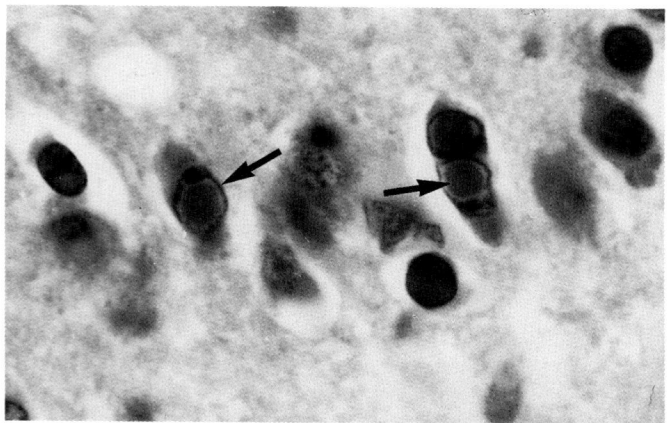

Fig. 25.21   Intranuclear inclusion bodies (arrows) in cerebral cortical neurones from a case of subacute sclerosing panencephalitis.

(CMV) *encephalitis*, and *subacute sclerosing panencephalitis* (SSPE) (Fig. 25.21), or intracytoplasmic, as with the *Negri body* characteristic of *rabies* (Fig. 25.22);

5. *inflammatory cell cuffing* in the Virchow–Robin spaces around small veins and venules, with infiltration of inflammatory cells in the CNS parenchyma, and frequently also in neighbouring leptomeninges (Fig. 25.23);

6. additional, less specific, reactive features of *astrocytosis* and *diffuse microglial activation*.

An important distinguishing feature of the pathology of different forms of viral encephalitis is its topographic localization. Different viruses have different sites of predilection for damage to the CNS. In some cases, this may reflect the route by which the virus reaches the CNS. Thus, *HSV* produces damage that is predominantly localized to the temporal lobes and a few other regions anatomically connected with them, while the *arboviruses* produce widespread focal changes maximal in the deep grey matter. These sites of damage may reflect access of the former virus along the olfactory pathways and the latter viruses from the blood, with entry to the CNS occurring at widely distributed sites. Differing selectivity with respect to host cell type also plays a part in determining the distribution of the pathology in different forms of viral encephalitis. Thus, *poliomyelitis virus*, which has a relative (but not absolute) predilection for infecting motor neurones, produces its main focus of pathology in spinal cord anterior horns, while the *JC papova virus* responsible for *progressive multifocal leukoencephalopathy* (PML) lytically infects oligodendrocytes and produces its main damage to cerebral white matter.

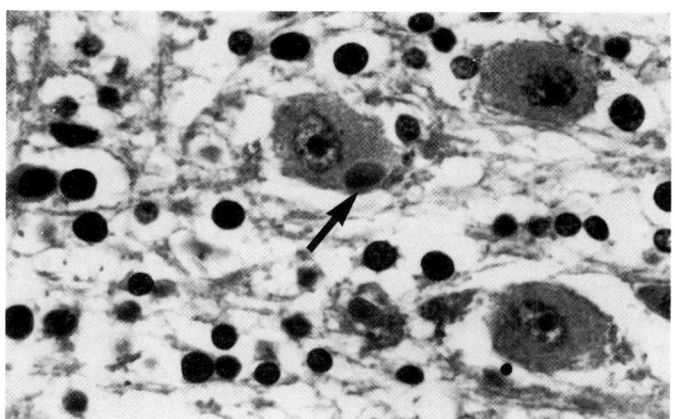

Fig. 25.22 Intracytoplasmic inclusion (Negri body) (arrow) in a Purkinje cell from a case of rabies.

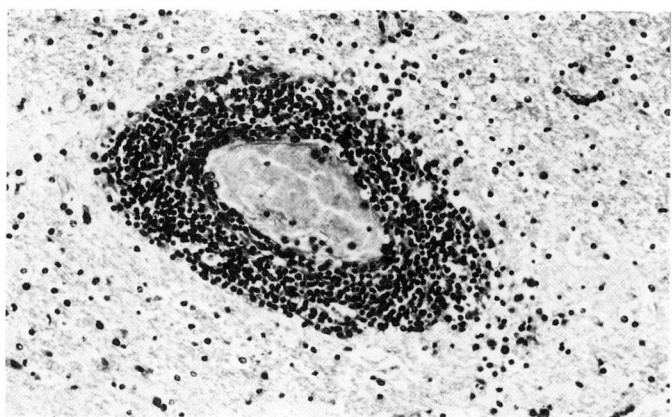

Fig. 25.23 Intense perivenous collection of mononuclear inflammatory cells from a case of subacute poliomyelitis.

Summarized below are the chief pathological findings in the main forms of viral encephalitis and myelitis.

Acute viral encephalitis and myelitis

HSV (type 1) is the commonest identified cause of sporadic viral encephalitis. It produces an acute encephalitis with onset of headache, fever, epilepsy, abnormal behaviour with confusion and memory loss progressing to drowsiness, hemiparesis, and coma within a few days. Before the advent of specific antiviral therapy (acyclovir), the mortality was as high as 70 per cent and there was serious residual neurological damage in many of the survivors. Treatment with acyclovir has reduced the mortality to around 20 per cent. The most reliable means of confirming the clinical diagnosis in the acute stage is by brain biopsy. CT scan appearances strongly suggest the diagnosis in some cases. Diagnosis by biopsy depends on viral culture or demonstration of specific viral antigen using the immunoperoxidase technique on smears or paraffin sections (Fig. 25.24). Herpes virions are detectable in infected cells by electron microscopy. It is also possible to detect specific HSV nuclei acid

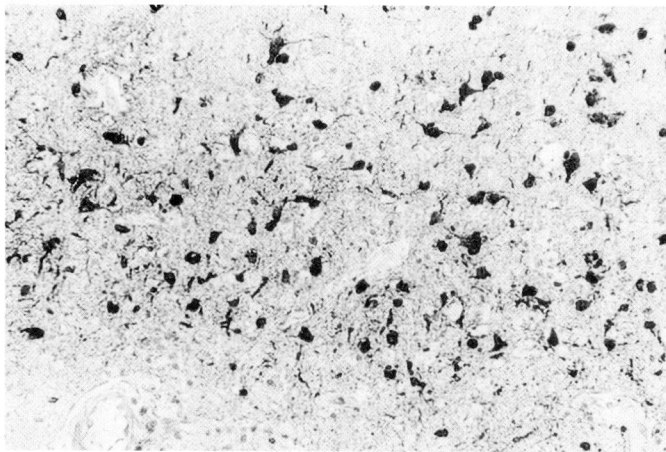

Fig. 25.24 Immunoperoxidase reaction for herpes simplex virus in cerebral cortical neurones from a case of acute herpes simplex encephalitis.

sequences by *in situ* hybridization techniques. Some clinicians prefer to avoid brain biopsy and base the diagnosis on the demonstration of a rise in titre of anti-HSV antibody in serum and CSF during the first 2 weeks of the disease, and on the demonstration of an antibody titre in CSF indicative of intrathecal antibody synthesis. Treatment with acyclovir is started in such cases on the basis of the clinical diagnosis, and the definitive diagnosis is made retrospectively.

In cases of HSV encephalitis dying during the acute stage of the disease, there is asymmetrical swelling, softening, congestion, and petechial cortical haemorrhages in the temporal lobes and adjacent insula, hippocampus, and amygdala (Fig. 25.25). The cingulate gyrus and orbital frontal cortex on one or both

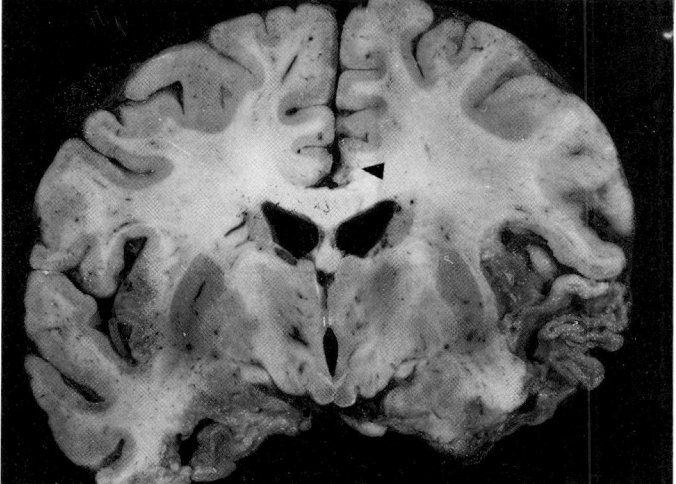

Fig. 25.25 Coronal slice through the cerebral hemispheres from a case of herpes simplex encephalitis. Death occurred about 6 months after the acute illness. There is extensive necrosis of the right temporal lobe and insula with less severe damage to the same structures on the left. Slight necrosis is also evident in the right cingulate gyrus (arrowhead).

sides may also be necrotic. Cerebral swelling is severe, particularly in the worst-affected hemisphere, with shift of midline structures to the opposite side and herniation of the uncus on the same or both sides. Microscopically, in the affected cortex, neurones, if still present, show acute homogenizing, eosinophilic change and there is intense mononuclear inflammatory cell infiltration and perivascular cuffing with lymphocytes, macrophages, and plasma cells (Fig. 25.26). In the first few days, *intranuclear inclusion bodies* may be seen in neurones. *Reactive astrocytosis* is present around the margins of necrosis. The leptomeninges are also inflamed and congested. The white matter is affected but to a lesser extent than the cortex. The inflammation persists for many more weeks and only slowly subsides thereafter. In subjects dying months or years later, the

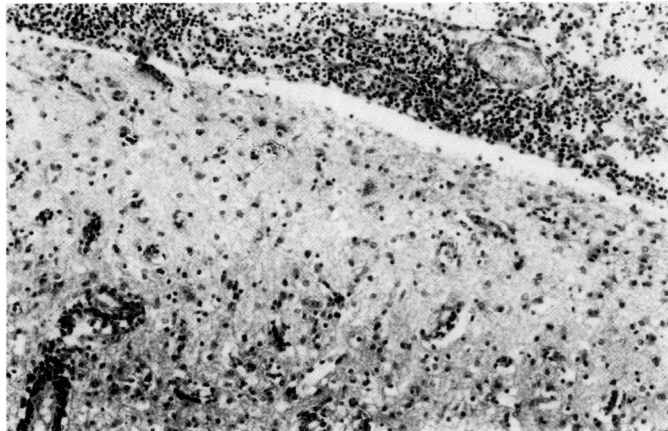

Fig. 25.26 Microscopical appearance of affected cerebral cortex in herpes simplex encephalitis, with necrosis and mononuclear inflammation in parenchyma, leptomeninges, and perivascular spaces.

softened temporal lobes are collapsed and the overlying leptomeninges thickened. The collapsed tissue is largely devoid of neurones and contains only a few vascular and glial elements, together with slight residual inflammation.

HSV type 1 encephalitis is thought to be a manifestation of secondary infection with the virus. Most subjects have serum antibody at the start of the illness, indicating earlier exposure to it. In some cases, it has been shown that the trigeminal ganglion harbours virus of identical genetic type to that found in the brain, but in other cases the viruses at these two sites are genetically distinct. The pathogenesis of the disease is not known for certain, but the virus is known to travel along nerves, and the anatomical distribution of the pathology is suggestive of entry of virus into the brain by the olfactory route, with possible reactivation from a site of latency close to or in the medial temporal lobes or hippocampus. Others have argued in favour of the virus gaining entry to the brain from the trigeminal ganglion, where it is known frequently to establish a latent infection, along branches of the trigeminal nerve that innervate the basal leptomeninges. Very rarely, HSV type 1 causes a primary brainstem encephalitis.

HSV type 2 occasionally causes a generalized encephalitis in neonates who acquire the infection at birth from an infected maternal genital tract. In these cases, the virus is blood-borne and there is usually evidence of infection of other organs, such as the liver and adrenal glands, as well as the brain.

Arbovirus encephalitis

Several different arthropod-borne viruses can give rise to epidemic forms of encephalitis (Table 25.3). The viruses are acquired from the bite of an infected insect. Each virus has specific mammalian hosts and insect vectors, the geographical distribution and seasonal availability of which determine the patterns of epidemic infection produced. Encephalitis only

Table 25.3 Summary of major arbovirus encephalitides

	Vector	Animal reservoir	Mortality	Geographical distribution
Togaviruses				
Alphavirus				
Eastern encephalitis	Mosquitoes	Birds	High (c.50%)	Eastern USA; Caribbean
Western encephalitis	Mosquitoes	Birds	Low (less than 3%)	West and South-western USA
Venezuelan encephalitis	Mosquitoes	Horses and small mammals	Variable (with different strains)	South and Central America; South-western USA
Flaviviruses				
St Louis encephalitis	Mosquitoes	Birds	Low (c. 10%)	USA
Japanese encephalitis	Mosquitoes	Birds	Variable (5—50%)	Japan; China; South-East Asia; India
Murray Valley encephalitis	Mosquitoes	Birds	Variable (18—42%)	Australia; New Guinea
West Nile virus	Mosquitoes	Birds	Low	Africa; Middle East
Tick-borne viruses				
	Ticks	Small mammals and birds	Variable (with different strains)	Different strains: Eastern central and northern Europe; USSR; Canada; Japan; India
Bunyaviruses				
California encephalitis	Mosquitoes	Small mammals	Low (less than 1%)	USA

occurs in a very small proportion of individuals infected with these viruses. The initial infection is manifested by a 'flu-like' systemic illness or is subclinical. Encephalitis follows as a second phase of illness, usually 10–14 days after the initial illness. Mortality and morbidity vary with the different viruses (Table 25.3). Diagnosis is usually based on clinical and epidemiological features and is confirmed by demonstrating a rising titre of specific antibody in serum and CSF during the course of the disease, and evidence of antibody synthesis in the CNS. In the acute stage of the disease, in fatal cases, the brain shows generalized congestion and swelling, sometimes with petechial haemorrhages. Microscopically, there are mononuclear inflammatory cell infiltrates, neuronophagia, microglial nodules, and reactive astrocytosis in many areas of grey matter, but particularly concentrated in the basal ganglia, thalamus, hypothalamus, midbrain, and upper pons. The cerebral cortex may also be affected. In some cases the cervical spinal cord grey matter is involved and motor neurones destroyed, with resulting upper limb weakness and muscle wasting. An unusual additional feature of the pathology in some forms of arbovirus encephalitis is the presence of multiple, well-circumscribed microscopic foci of *acellular necrosis* in grey matter (Fig. 25.27). Occasionally, larger lesions with cystic necrosis occur. In later stages, after the inflammation has subsided, there may be calcification associated with these foci. They are thought to have a probable ischaemic basis. Inclusion bodies are not found in arbovirus encephalitis. In a few acute cases, the virus has been demonstrated by electron microscopy.

Rabies

Rabies is a form of acute encephalitis which occurs in many parts of the world and is due to infection of the brain by a *rhabdovirus* which frequently infects dogs, foxes, and some other mammals including bats. Only a few islands, including the United Kingdom, are free of the infection. Humans acquire the infection usually by being bitten or licked by an infected dog,

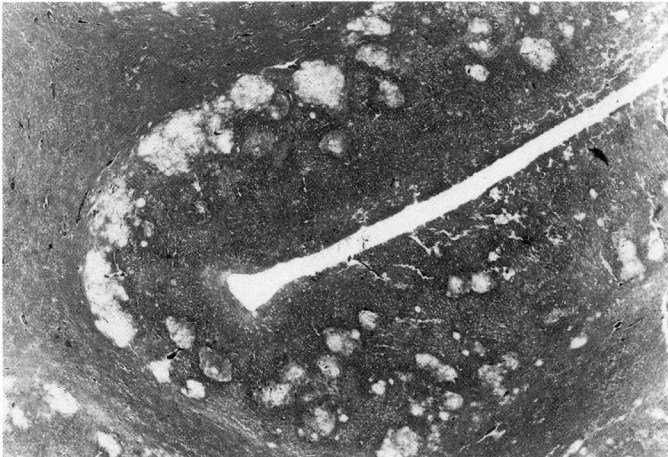

Fig. 25.27 Late effects of arbovirus encephalitis. Pale, acellular foci of necrosis scattered in the cerebral cortex. (Courtesy of Professor R. Iizuka.)

whose behaviour may have been rendered unusually aggressive by the infection of its brain, and whose saliva contains the virus. Occasionally infection is acquired from bites by other animals or from inhalation of the virus in infected bat-infested caves. The incubation period for the disease is usually long, varying from a few weeks to several months, but occasionally extending to over 2 years. Exceptionally, the incubation period is shorter, lasting only a few days. Not infrequently, there is no clear history of exposure to the virus. Symptoms frequently commence with itching or pain at the site of the bite and this is followed by fever; headache; sudden, paroxysmal inspiratory spasms; and the pathognomonic symptom of *hydrophobia*—painful pharyngeal spasms set off by the sight or taste of water. These are followed within a few days by autonomic disturbances, coma, and death. The mortality is virtually 100 per cent, recovery after onset of symptoms being documented but extremely rare.

The disease is prevented in most cases that receive pre- or rapid post-exposure immunization. Diagnosis can be confirmed by demonstrating the virus antigen immunocytochemically in intradermal nerves of a neck skin biopsy.

At post-mortem examination the brain appears congested and may be slightly swollen, but is not otherwise remarkable macroscopically. Histological sections show modest inflammatory changes and neuronophagia in the brainstem reticular formation and, to a lesser extent, in grey matter of the hypothalamus, thalamus, basal ganglia, cerebral cortex, and hippocampus. Spinal sensory ganglia are also characteristically inflamed. *Acute homogenizing, eosinophilic change* is usually present in neurones of the brainstem reticular formation, and the characteristic intracytoplasmic inclusion bodies, *Negri bodies*, can be found in large neurones at many sites (see Fig. 25.22). They are particularly conspicuous in hippocampal pyramidal neurones, Purkinje cells of the cerebellum, and large neurones of the hypothalamus and brainstem. Viral antigen can be demonstrated immunocytochemically in a wide distribution. It is not confined to cells containing Negri bodies and is predominantly present in neurones, but has also been described in oligodendrocytes. Virus with a typical rhabdovirus (bullet-shaped) structure can be found in infected neurones by electron microscopy.

In a few cases of rabies, clinically distinguished by the early onset of motor paralysis and sensory deficits (*paralytic rabies*), the spinal cord is severely affected and shows inflammation and necrosis. Inflammation and neuronophagia are also found in sensory spinal ganglia.

Some aspects of rabies infection are not yet satisfactorily explained. It is uncertain why the incubation period is frequently prolonged. During this time the virus is thought to be present in skeletal muscle and it appears to gain access to the nervous system by entering nerve endings in muscle. Thence, it travels to the spinal cord, and probably also within the CNS, by axonal transport. The cause of selective damage to the brainstem neurones is not clear since the virus appears to infect other neurones without obviously damaging them, and in tissue culture the infection is non-lytic. There are some suggestions from experimental studies of infected neuroblastoma cells that the virus may inhibit certain key reactions that control intermediary metabolism in cells with opioid receptors on their surface, and this is a possible mechanism of damage *in vivo*.

Poliomyelitis

Acute poliomyelitis is now rarely seen in countries that have instituted effective immunization regimes, but still occurs elsewhere. Occasionally, other *enteroviruses* are responsible for producing an acute or subacute poliomyelitis. *Enterovirus 70* infection has been associated with outbreaks of conjunctivitis with paralytic poliomyelitis, and *ECHO virus* infections in hypogammaglobulinaemic children occasionally cause a poliomyelitis-like illness.

Paralytic symptoms develop in only a very small proportion of those infected with poliomyelitis virus. The primary infection occurs in the gastrointestinal tract and may provoke symptoms of pharyngitis, diarrhoea, and fever. Otherwise, it is subclinical. It is followed, a few days later, by rapidly progressive weakness of one or more limbs and, in severe cases, of bulbar musculature. Meningitic symptoms may also be prominent. Paralysis tends to be particularly severe in muscle that have been vigorously exercised in the few days preceding the illness. There is a *viraemic phase* to the illness, before the onset of paralysis, and some authorities consider that the virus reaches the CNS in the blood. However, experimental studies clearly indicate that the virus is capable of being transported along axons, and it remains possible that, as a result of the viraemia, the virus enters muscle and is transported from the muscle to the spinal cord along axons.

In acute, fatal poliomyelitis, the brain and spinal cord are congested and petechial haemorrhages may be visible in the spinal cord grey matter. In microscopic sections, there is intense inflammation with neuronophagia of motor neurones in anterior horns and some inflammation also in dorsal grey matter, leptomeninges, and spinal sensory ganglia. In the brainstem, in cases with bulbar symptoms, the reticular formation of the medulla, pons, and midbrain show inflammation with lymphocytes, macrophages, and plasma cells, neuronophagia, and numerous activated microglial cells. Other regions of the brain that may also be affected are the substantia nigra, hypothalamus, thalamus, dentate nuclei of the cerebellum, and occasionally the motor cortex. In patients dying many years after the acute illness, the anterior roots of the affected spinal cord segments appear wasted and motor neurones in the cord depleted. Skeletal muscles involved show denervation atrophy and some fibre-type grouping due to compensatory re-innervation.

Subacute and chronic viral encephalitis or encephalopathy

Subacute sclerosing panencephalitis (SSPE)

SSPE is a rare subacute or chronic, progressive neurological disease of children. It has a duration of several months to several years and is eventually invariably fatal. Symptoms usually commence with deterioration in mental function, ac-companied by epilepsy, motor weakness and spasticity, ataxia and myoclonus, in varying combinations. It is due to infection of the brain by an incomplete form of *measles virus*. Most of those affected have been noted to suffer from acute measles infection at an unusually early age, usually when less than 2 years. It is almost unknown after measles immunization. The disease can be diagnosed by demonstrating a high titre of measles antibody in serum and CSF, with a titre in CSF that is indicative of intrathecal synthesis of measles antibody.

In SSPE, the appearance of the brain, post-mortem, varies according to the duration of the disease. There is usually a considerable degree of cerebral atrophy with narrowing of cortical gyri, widening of sulci, and dilatation of the lateral ventricles (Fig. 25.28). Atrophy is particularly severe in cases of long duration. The cerebral white matter appears abnormally granular and discoloured and feels firm and gliotic. In histological sections, there are inflammatory cells present in grey and white matter. These consist of lymphocytes, plasma cells, macrophages, and activated microglia. In grey matter, particularly in the cerebral cortex, neurones are depleted and there are inclusion bodies in the nuclei of some of those that remain. In white matter there is loss of myelin and axons, with inclusion bodies in some oligodendrocyte nuclei, and a marked reactive astrocytosis. Measles virus antigen can be demonstrated in neurones and oligodendrocytes using immunocytochemical techniques, and *paramyxovirus-like nucleo-capsids* can be found by electron microscopy in nuclei of cells bearing inclusion bodies. Complete virus particles are, however, not present. Measles virus can sometimes be cultured from explant cultures of the brain using co-cultivation techniques. Differential analysis for the various measles protein antigens shows that there is a deficiency of the *M protein* which is required for assembly of complete virus particles. There is also an absence of antibody to the M protein. Lack of the M protein explains the chronic and limited nature of the infection in the brain, but it is uncertain how it arises. The fact that fully infectious measles can be retrieved eventually from explant brain cultures from some cases suggests that there

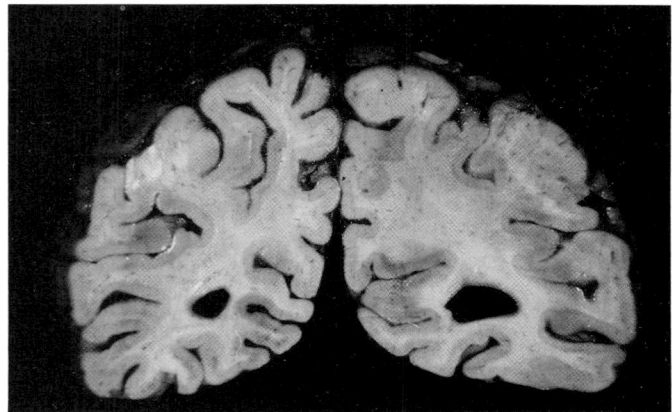

Fig. 25.28 Coronal slice through the cerebral hemispheres from a case of subacute sclerosing panencephalitis. There is generalized cortical atrophy, moderate ventricular dilatation, and discoloration of the white matter.

is no deficiency of the viral gene coding for the M protein, but rather a failure of its transcription.

Immunosuppressive measles encephalitis

This is a form of fatal, subacute measles infection of the brain seen in some children who suffer acute measles infection when immunodeficient, usually as a result of treatment for acute leukaemia. In this disease, there is sparse mononuclear inflammation in grey matter of the brain, reactive gliosis, neuronophagia, and inclusion bodies containing measles antigen in some remaining neurones.

Progressive rubella encephalitis

A few cases have been described of a chronic, progressive encephalitis in children suffering from intra-uterine infection with rubella virus. Antibody titres to rubella are elevated in serum and CSF. In such cases, there is usually atrophy of the brain, particularly of the cerebellum, with thickening of the overlying leptomeninges. Microscopically, there is widespread perivascular cuffing of small veins with lymphocytes and plasma cells, scattered microglial nodules, and reactive astrocytosis. A noteworthy feature is the presence of *basophilic amorphous deposits*, sometimes with calcification, in affected parenchyma and in the walls of small blood vessels. No inclusion bodies are seen.

Progressive multifocal leukoencephalopathy (PML)

This is a fatal subacute or chronic disease predominantly affecting white matter of the brain and caused by infection with *JC papova virus*. This is a virus to which the majority of the population has been exposed without it resulting in any detectable illness. Those who develop PML usually do so in the context of suffering from some form of immunosuppression, most commonly associated with Hodgkin's disease, chronic lymphatic leukaemia, sarcoidosis, prolonged steroid treatment, or AIDS. The disease presents with progressive neurological symptoms and signs, including mental deterioration and confusion, motor and sensory deficits, and ataxia. Low-density lesions in cerebral, and sometimes cerebellar, white matter are demonstrable on CT scans. A definitive diagnosis can only be made in many cases by brain biopsy, but in some cases a high titre of antibody to JC virus is present in CSF and this enables the diagnosis to be confirmed.

The characteristic lesions of PML are found in the white matter of the brain or at the junction between white matter and cortex. They consist of discrete foci of grey or yellowish discoloration of white matter, sometimes with necrotic softening. The lesions are usually numerous and vary from under 1 mm in diameter to several centimetres. The larger lesions are probably formed by coalescence of smaller ones. Similar foci may be present in the brainstem, where they are hard to detect with the naked eye, and in the cerebellum. In microscopic sections stained for myelin, the lesions appear as sharply defined regions of myelin pallor (Fig. 25.29). Axons are relatively preserved. There are macrophages containing neutral fat in the more recently formed foci, but other inflammatory cells are generally scarce. There is a noticeable absence of oligodendrocytes from

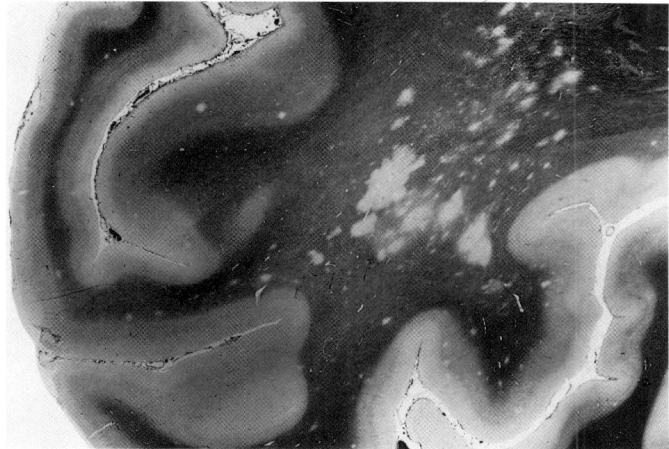

Fig. 25.29 Low-power view of a myelin-stained section from the cerebrum of a case of progresive multifocal leukoencephalopathy. Several sharply defined foci of myelin loss are evident in the white matter.

the centre of the larger lesions, but an astrocytic reaction is prominent. Oligodendrocytes at the margins of the lesions contain enlarged nuclei with effaced chromatin and basophilic inclusion bodies (Fig. 25.30). These can be shown by electron microscopy to contain numerous papova virus particles. JC virus antigens can be demonstrated in such nuclei by immunocytochemistry, and specific JC virus nucleic acid sequences by *in situ* hybridization. The other characteristic microscopic feature is the presence of enlarged, pleomorphic astrocyte nuclei, in some of which JC virus antigen can be demonstrated (Fig. 25.31). The JC virus infection of astrocytes, unlike that of oligodendrocytes, is non-lytic, but the pleomorphism it engenders in the nuclei may reflect the capacity of the virus to transform some glial cells. Inoculated in the brain of small laboratory animals, JC virus can cause the development of gliomas and some cases have been described of gliomas developing in human subjects with PML.

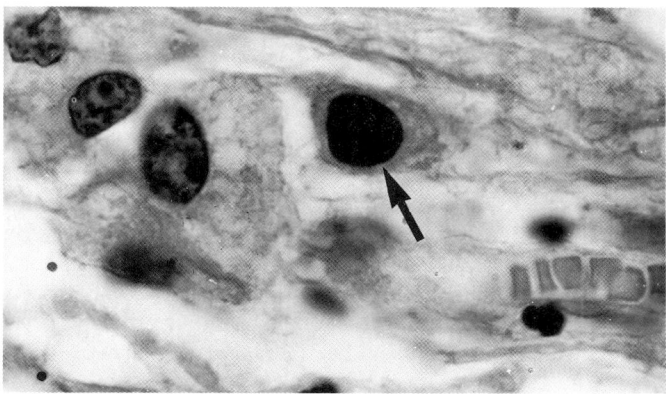

Fig. 25.30 Basophilic oligodendrocyte inclusion (arrow) at the margin of a demyelinated focus from a case of progressive multifocal leukoencephalopathy.

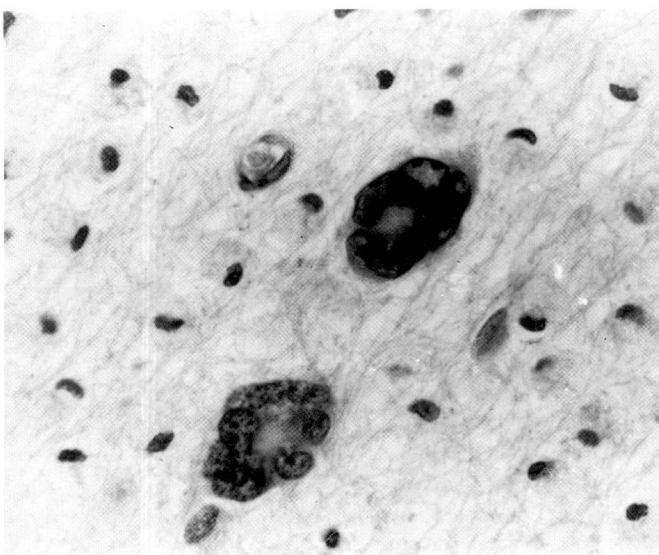

Fig. 25.31 Multinucleated astrocytes with bizarre nuclear morphology in a demyelinated lesion from a case of progressive multifocal leukoencephalopathy.

Cytomegalovirus (CMV) encephalitis

CMV is capable of producing a mild form of encephalitis in immunosuppressed adults, a more severe necrotizing encephalitis in some patients with severe prolonged immunosuppression, particularly in AIDS, and a severe encephalitis in fetuses infected *in utero*. Initially, the mild form of encephalitis was referred to as '*glial nodule*' encephalitis because it is characterized by the presence of scattered microglial nodules throughout the grey matter. Occasionally, at the centre of such nodules, there may be a neurone containing an intranuclear inclusion body. This form of encephalitis was noted particularly frequently in patients with evidence of CMV infection elsewhere in the body. It does not always give rise to any clinically detectable neurological disease.

Macroscopically, the brain appears normal or minimally atrophic. The glial nodules are not usually accompanied by any significant lymphocytic infiltrate but there may be mild astrocytosis. CMV antigens can be demonstrated immunocytochemically in the rare inclusion bodies.

Intra-uterine infection with CMV can result in severe encephalitis. Other organs besides the brain are usually also involved, particularly the liver. The infant may be premature or stillborn. The brain shows hydrocephalus, and sometimes microencephaly, indicating arrested development. There is patchy inflammatory change in foci of necrosis and astrocytosis. Calcification in the lesions is common. The periventricular regions are particularly susceptible to damage. A careful search shows typical intranuclear inclusion bodies in glial cells or neurones.

Human immunodeficiency virus (HIV) encephalopathy

About 40 per cent of those with AIDS develop neurological symptoms, and in as many as 80 per cent of cases in some autopsy series the brain is reported to be abnormal. In some of these cases, there are opportunistic infections of the brain or spinal cord, most commonly due to CMV or toxoplasmosis. A few have lymphomas. About 28 per cent have evidence of an HIV-associated encephalopathy, with or without additional pathology. HIV infection, detected immunocytochemically or by *in situ* hybridization, occurs in the brain chiefly in monocyte-derived cells: microglial cells, perivascular macrophages, and multinucleated cells which express macrophage antigens. The virus is thought to enter the brain in infected monocytes which then differentiate *in situ*. A few glial cells may also be infected, but infection of neurones has rarely been reported.

The pathology associated with the presence of HIV in the brain chiefly affects the white matter and basal ganglia. The main cerebral white matter shows diffuse pallor in myelin-stained sections and foci of rarefaction, with vacuolation and destruction of myelin sheaths and disruption of some axons. In these regions, and elsewhere, there are groups of macrophages and a few multinucleated cells with nuclei distributed around the periphery of the cell (Fig. 25.32). Similar mononuclear and multinucleate cells may also be found in perivascular spaces in the basal ganglia. A sparse lymphocytic infiltrate may also be present around small veins in grey and white matter and in the leptomeninges. Abnormal groups of glial nuclei, some possibly the slightly enlarged nuclei of oligodendrocytes, may be found in white matter, and mild diffuse astrocytosis and microglial activation commonly occur.

In the spinal cord of a few AIDS sufferers, a *myelopathy* is described which has also been attributed to HIV infection. Clinically, this is manifest as a spastic paraparesis with disturbance of bladder control. Pathologically, there is vacuolation and rarefaction of white matter in lateral and posterior white columns, particularly at the thoracic and cervical levels. HIV can be detected in some of these lesions.

A progressive encephalopathy occurs in 30–50 per cent of infants and children infected with HIV. Mental retardation and motor dysfunction are the commonest clinical features. There is less frequent infection of the brain with opportunistic organisms

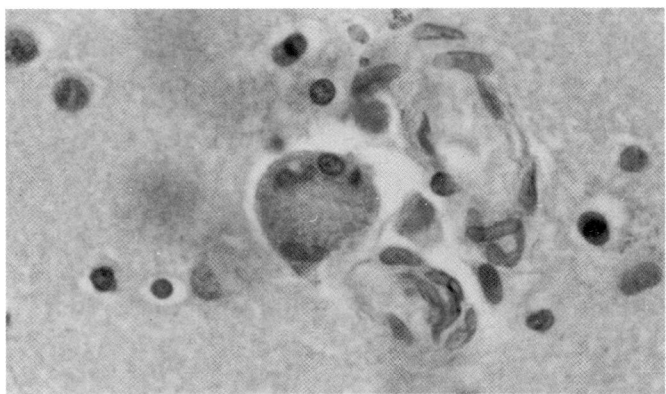

Fig. 25.32 Multinucleated perivascular cell of probable macrophage origin from a case of human immunodeficiency virus-associated encephalopathy.

than in adults with AIDS, though this occurs in some cases. HIV has been detected in infant brains by electron microscopy, culture, and immunocytochemistry. Its presence is associated, as in adults, with the presence of perivascular macrophages and multinucleate cells in basal ganglia and white matter, and a sparse lymphocytic infiltrate. Pallor of myelin staining and rarefaction of white matter also occur.

Herpes zoster encephalomyelitis and encephalopathy

Herpes zoster is an inflammatory disease of sensory ganglia (usually spinal or trigeminal) and nerves, caused by local reactivation of the varicella-zoster virus. Occasionally, there is an extension of the inflammatory process to the neuraxis at the level at which the inflammation arises. Thus, a necrotic myelopathy of the cord may complicate spinal zoster and a brainstem encephalitis ipsilateral to infection of the geniculate ganglion may complicate the *Ramsay–Hunt syndrome* (zoster affecting the ear-drum and surrounding skin). This is usually associated with immunodeficiency and, in the same circumstances, exceptionally, a generalized infection of the brain with varicella-zoster virus may ensue. A complication of zoster affecting the trigeminal ganglion is *ipsilateral cerebral infarction* associated with *middle cerebral or internal carotid artery thrombosis*. A further complication of herpes zoster, in which multifocal white matter lesions resembling those of PML occur in periventricular regions, has been described in immunosuppressed subjects, particularly those with AIDS. This demyelinating condition is associated with the presence of intranuclear inclusion bodies in oligodendrocytes which, in a few cases, have been shown to contain varicella-zoster virus antigen.

Human T-cell lymphotropic virus type I (HTLV-I) and tropical spastic paraparesis

Infection with the retrovirus HTLV-I, which was originally shown to be associated with adult T-cell leukaemia in parts of Japan, has recently been linked serologically with the occurrence of a *chronic progressive myelopathy* in several tropical countries (*tropical spastic paraparesis* (TSP)). This presents clinically with spastic weakness of the lower limbs and disturbance of bladder control. Antibodies to HTLV-I are found in sera from a much higher proportion of those with TSP, and at higher titre, than in control subjects from the same geographical area. Antibodies to HTLV-I have also been found in CSF from cases of TSP and a clinically similar form of myelopathy in Japan, termed *HTLV-I-associated myelopathy*. Some cases of the latter disease also contain abnormal lymphocytes in the CSF. The pathology of TSP, which is not usually fatal and has therefore only infrequently been studied in the early phase of its development, consists of degeneration of axons and myelin in the lateral and posterior white columns of the spinal cord, with fibrosis and sparse inflammation in the leptomeninges, spinal sensory roots, and spinal cord. Occasionally, the inflammation in the leptomeninges extends as far as the brainstem, but higher levels of the neuraxis are not usually affected.

Rickettsial encephalitis

Rickettsial infections caused by bacterium-like organisms, usually transmitted to man by insect vectors, produce systemic diseases involving multiple organs. The organisms multiply preferentially in endothelial cells of small blood vessels and neurological involvement results if vessels of the nervous system or leptomeninges are colonized. The lesions produced consist of small vasculitic foci, often accompanied by small cerebral infarcts. The diagnosis usually depends on demonstrating a rise in antibody to one of the rickettsiae at the time of the systemic illness.

25.3.3 Protozoal and metazoal infections

P. D. Lewis

Parasitic disease of tropical or subtropical zones may today be found in almost any part of the world, thanks to the ease and speed of air transport. Some protozoal infections of the nervous system are also of world-wide distribution, occurring in immunocompromised patients, including those with AIDS.

Protozoal infections

Malaria

Cerebral malaria is a lethal complication of infection with *Plasmodium falciparum*, the causal organism of *malignant tertian malaria*. The incubation period may be between 1 and 3 weeks. Malarial coma is usually fully reversible, but ischaemic brain lesions may result from cerebral oedema and capillary blockage by parasite-containing red blood cells. At autopsy, brain swelling and congestion are evident, while on dissection the cut surface has a dull grey appearance, sometimes with petechiae at the junction of cortex and white matter. Microscopically, oedema, necrosis of vein walls, parasites in red blood cells, and pigment granules are seen. *Plasmodium falciparum* antigens and IgG have been reported as occurring on capillary basement membranes, implicating immune mechanisms in vascular damage and blockage. In protracted cases, proliferation and aggregation of astrocytes together with pigment-laden macrophages, producing the *malarial nodules (granulomas) of Dürck*, may be seen. Hypoxic changes in nerve cells and myelin damage may also be present.

Amoebae

Primary amoebic meningoencephalitis Free-living amoebae of the *Naegleria* genus, which normally live in the soil and multiply in warm water, may cause meningoencephalitis. Those affected are generally children or young adults, previously healthy, who have a history of swimming or playing in stagnant fresh water. The incubation period lasts from a few days to 2 weeks, and the brain disease is almost always rapidly fatal. Autopsy appearances resemble acute suppurative meningitis. Olfactory bulbs and inferior frontal cortex are particularly severely affected, with extensive necrosis and haemorrhage in many cases. The pattern of lesions may reflect the pathway of infection, since it is believed that the organisms may enter through the nasal mucosa and invade the brain from the olfactory bulbs. The amoebae are smaller than *Entamoeba histolytica*, measuring up to 20 μm in diameter, and are numerous in perivascular spaces, where they may be mistaken for macrophages. Inflammatory cells are relatively sparse. Brain infection by *Acanthamoeba culbertsoni* occurs opportunistically in immune-deficient and chronically ill patients, of any age, and is not related to swimming in stagnant water. Infection with this organism is fatal, but courses of 4 months are recorded, in contrast to death generally within 7 days for *Naegleria*. At autopsy, meningitis and focal necrosis are seen, while chronic inflammatory changes with vasculitis are present, together with amoebae, 15–45 μm long, in vessel walls.

African trypanosomiasis

Trypanosoma rhodesiense and *T. gambiense* infect a variety of wild and domestic animals as well as man, transmission occurring by the bite of the *tsetse fly*. Parasitaemia develops several days after the bite and produces systemic febrile symptoms. *T. rhodesiense* causes acute or subacute meningoencephalitis, often fatal within weeks, some patients dying at a relatively early stage if there is severe cardiac involvement. Organisms are readily found in the CSF, and are thin flagellates, 10–30 μm long. *T. rhodesiense* has a natural reservoir in game, while *T. gambiense* is primarily a human disease, being spread from man to man by river tsetse flies. This causes a more chronic and progressive neurological disease (*West African sleeping sickness*) with somnolence and restlessness, fits, abnormal movements, and paralysis. Trypanosomiasis of either type produces chronic meningoencephalitis, with chronic inflammatory thickening of the pia-arachnoid and morular bodies, up to 20 μm in diameter, thought to be derived from plasma cells, and present in perivascular spaces as well as in leptomeninges.

American trypanosomiasis (Chagas' disease)

Infection with *Trypanosoma cruzi* is frequent in tropical South America and also occurs in Central and North America. It is spread by triatome bugs of the Reduviid family, which convey the infection to man from mammalian reservoirs, including rats, dogs, bats, and armadillos. Encephalitis may occur in the acute form of the disease, in which systemic features are prominent. Chronic disease affects older children and adults and is rarely associated with encephalitis. In contrast, it produces severe damage to nerves in the heart and gastrointestinal tract, resulting in cardiac dysfunction and dilatation of oesophagus, stomach, or colon.

Toxoplasmosis

Toxoplasmosis occurs world-wide and the rate of infection rises through adult life. Infection during pregnancy may lead to pla-

cental involvement and transmission of infection to the fetus, with resultant hydrocephalus, microcephaly, or choroidoretinitis. Lesions in the cerebral hemispheres are concentrated around the ventricles, where there is focal necrosis and calcification with chronic inflammation. Organisms may be seen both free and as cysts. Free trophozoites are 6–7 μm long and up to 2 μm wide, while cysts are rounded collections of organisms, measuring 15–30 μm. Periaqueductal lesions are the cause of hydrocephalus.

Systemic infection is often asymptomatic, and the development of host resistance does not always destroy parasites, which can encyst and remain dormant for years in a variety of tissues, including brain. The reactivation of previous infection in immunocompromised patients may be the mechanism underlying *fulminant cerebral toxoplasmosis* in AIDS sufferers. At least 10 per cent of patients with AIDS develop cerebral toxoplasmosis. Lesions are abscess-like and may measure from a few millimetres to several centimetres in diameter. Necrotizing, organizing, or chronic abscesses may be seen. Vascular proliferation and inflammation at their periphery cause ring contrast enhancement in CT scans; prompt treatment may produce clinical remission and evidence of healing on serial scanning.

Other protozoa

Metastatic cerebral abscesses in patients with *Entamoeba histolytica* abscesses of liver and lung occur rarely. *Babesia* may also produce neurological symptoms due to intravascular aggregation of parasitized red blood cells.

Metazoal infections

Cysticercosis

Cysticercosis is the outcome of eating the ova of *Taenia solium*, the cestode for which man is the only definitive host and the pig a common intermediate host. Cysticercosis is common in South and East Asia, Central and South America, and South Africa. Involvement of the central nervous system by cysticerci, which are the larval forms of the tapeworm, may produce focal neurological manifestations, including epilepsy. The lesions most commonly involve the cerebral hemispheres, where they are often situated subcortically like tumour metastases. They may also expand within the ventricles causing hydrocephalus. Spinal cord compression may occur. In young lesions, parasites are readily identifiable by the presence of suckers and hooklets on the rostellum of the scolex. A granulomatous zone surrounds parasites, which in the course of time may be obliterated in dense scar tissue, sometimes calcified.

Hydatid disease

Two dog tapeworms (*Echinococcus granulosus* and *E. multilocularis*) may cause hydatid disease in man. Man may be an intermediate host, and the ova, after hatching, penetrate the venules of the intestinal wall as embryos and become established in the liver. If they can get beyond the hepatic circulation, they lodge in the lungs. A small proportion may reach other tissues, including the brain. Cerebral hydatids occur in only a few per cent of all cases of hydatidosis. They may cause local pressure effects, including hydrocephalus, or may rupture, producing seeding and a local inflammatory response, resembling that of cysticercosis.

Schistosomiasis

The ova of three blood flukes may be carried in the bloodstream to the meninges, brain, and spinal cord, where they excite a granulomatous reaction. *Schistosoma japonicum* has been found in the central nervous system more often than *S. mansoni* and *S. haematobium*. This may be because it has the smallest eggs and an inconspicuous terminal spine, which could favour venous spread. A non-specific chronic inflammatory response with giant cells is seen in nervous parenchyma around the parasites, and fibrosis and calcification develop in long-standing lesions.

Paragonimiasis

Lung flukes *Paragonimus westermani* and *P. skryabini* are endemic in the Far East, the latter only in China. Adult worms are mainly parasites of the lungs, but can invade other organs, of which the brain is the most frequently involved. Infection occurs from eating uncooked Crustacea, the second intermediate host (snails are the first). Any part of the brain may be affected, though involvement of brainstem, cerebellum, and cord is rare. A granulomatous mass develops, generally superficial and with meningeal adhesion. Intact mature worms are rarely seen, even in apparently recent lesions.

Eosinophilic meningitis due to Angiostrongylus infection

The nematode *Angiostrongylus cantonensis*, a parasite of the rat lung, may invade human brain, meninges, and eyes. Infection is a result of eating uncooked terrestrial snails and slugs, and occurs in parts of South-East Asia. A severe meningitis with encephalopathy occurs and lumbar puncture shows gross CSF pleocytosis, almost entirely eosinophilic. Occasionally adult‧ nematodes may be found. *Angiostrongylus* infection is benign and self-limiting, with a mortality of less than 1 per cent.

Gnathostomiasis

Gnathostoma spinigerum, found in South-East Asia and especially in Thailand, is also capable of causing eosinophilic meningitis, and may involve the spinal cord and, less commonly, the brain. The adult worm is harboured by cats and dogs, and human infestation occurs when raw or undercooked fish is eaten. The organisms may migrate through the central nervous system, producing parenchymal foci of haemorrhage and necrosis. Sometimes multiple haemorrhagic tracks are seen.

Toxocariasis

Toxocara cati and *T. canis* are nematodes, 7–12 cm long, normally resident in the intestine of cats and dogs. Excreted ova may be ingested by other mammals, including man. The larvae can migrate to a variety of organs, including brain and eye, as well as liver and lungs. In children, intra-ocular granulomata can be mistaken clinically for retinoblastoma. Toxocaral brain lesions

are granulomatous and may include larval remnants. Clinical neurological disorders are minor.

Filariasis

Several species of filariae, including *Loa loa*, widespread in equatorial West Africa, are capable of invading brain and meninges. Parasitaemia occurs after insect bites, and occlusion of brain capillaries by organisms may produce petechiae and oedema. Granulomatous nodules, often centrally necrotic and sometimes containing identifiable *microfilariae*, can be found throughout the brain. Microfilariae may be present in lumbar CSF.

Other Metazoa

Cerebral involvement is sometimes seen in *sparganosis*, infection by larvae of diphyllobothriid tapeworms of the *Spirometra* genus. Brain lesions causing raised intracranial pressure, focal neurological features, and haemorrhage have been described.

Hyperinfestation with *Strongyloides stercoralis* may be associated with meningitis, cerebral microinfarcts, and brain abscesses.

The free-living nematode, *Micronema deletrix*, may cause fatal meningoencephalitis.

Muscle involvement by parasites

Clinically important involvement of human muscles is seen in the protozoal disorders *sarcosporidiosis*, *toxoplasmosis*, and both *African* and *American trypanosomiasis*; with the cestode infestations *cysticercosis*, *coenurosis*, *hydatidosis*, and *sparganosis*; and with the nematode diseases *trichinosis* and *toxocariasis*.

25.3.4 Further reading

Bacterial and fungal infections

Harriman, D. G. F. (1984) Bacterial infections of the central nervous system. In *Greenfield's neuropathology* (ed. J. H. Adams, J. A. N. Corsellis, and L. W. Duchen) (4th edn), pp. 236–59. Edward Arnold, London.

Scaravilli, F. (1984) Parasitic and fungal infections of the nervous system. In *Greenfield's neuropathology* (ed. J. H. Adams, J. A. N. Corsellis, and L. W. Duchen) (4th edn) pp. 304–37. Edward Arnold, London.

Viral and rickettsial infections

Booss, J. and Esiri, M. M. (1986). *Viral encephalitis: pathology, diagnosis and management*. Blackwell Scientific, Oxford.

Brownell, B. and Tomlinson, A. H. (1984). Virus diseases of the central nervous system. In *Greenfield's neuropathology* (ed. J. H. Adams, J. A. N. Corsellis, and L. W. Duchen) (4th edn), pp. 260–303. Edward Arnold, London.

Price, T. R., Wisseman, C. L., and Woodward, T. E. (1977). Rickettsial diseases. In *Scientific approaches to clinical neurology* (ed. E. S. Goldensohn and S. H. Appel), pp. 515–26. Lea and Febiger, Philadelphia.

Protozoal and metazoal infections

Lewis, P. D. (1990). Protozoal infections and metazoal infestation. In *Systemic pathology*, Vol. 4 (ed. R. O. Weller) (3rd edn), pp. 180–93. Churchill Livingstone, Edinburgh.

Pallis, C. A. and Lewis, P. D. (1988). Involvement of human muscle by parasites. In *Disorders of voluntary muscle* (ed. J. Walton) (5th edn), pp. 611–27. Churchill Livingstone, Edinburgh.

25.4   Cerebrovascular disease

G. Cole

The two major manifestations of cerebrovascular disease are *cerebral infarction* and *intracranial haemorrhage*, both of which are commonly referred to as *stroke*. About 85 per cent of strokes are due to cerebral infarction, and about 15 per cent are due to haemorrhage. It has been estimated that about 10 per cent of all deaths are caused by strokes, and of those that survive about half are severely disabled. The incidence of stroke rises rapidly with increasing age and the majority occur in subjects over the age of 65 years. The risk of stroke is considerably increased in the presence of *hypertension*, *diabetes mellitus*, and *heart disease*. Other factors that increase the risk of stroke include *hyperlipoproteinaemia*, *increased coaguability of the blood*, *diet*, and *cigarette smoking*.

25.4.1   Cerebral infarction

A cerebral infarct may be defined as an area of tissue necrosis which is the result of a critical reduction in the blood supply to the brain. Blood is supplied to the brain via the internal carotid and vertebral arteries, which anastomose at the base of the brain to form the circle of Willis (Fig. 25.33). The circle of Willis produces a potential collateral circulation which may be effective if one of the main arteries contributing to it is blocked before it reaches the circle.

The major causes of cerebral infarction are *arterial thrombus* or *embolus*. A cerebral infarct may measure only a few millimetres or involve an entire arterial territory. Occlusion of certain vessels, such as the *middle cerebral, anterior cerebral*, or *posterior inferior cerebellar artery*, often lead to a defined area of necrosis and classical neurological signs. However, the extent of the infarct may show poor correlation with the anatomical area of supply of a particular vessel. A vessel may be totally occluded without any corresponding area of infarction or lead to only a small area of necrosis. A number of factors contribute to such discrepancies. Variation of the vessels which contribute to the circle of Willis is a fairly common incidental finding in autopsy studies: for instance, one vertebral or posterior communicating artery may be much smaller than the other; in such circumstances occlusion of the smaller vessel may result in little damage, and occlusion of the larger vessel may produce more

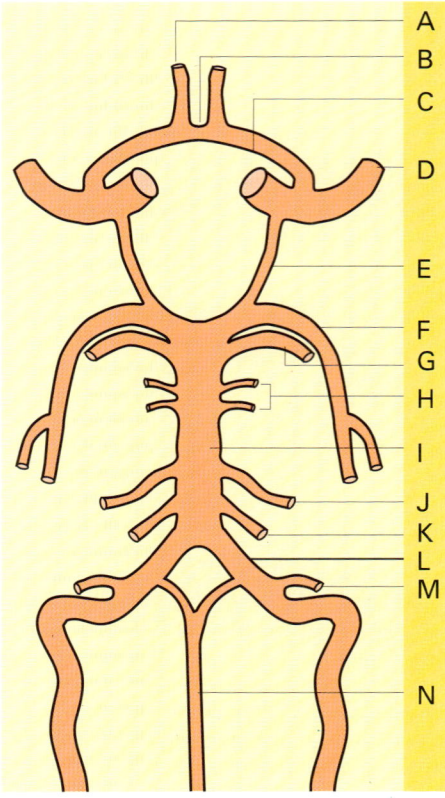

Fig. 25.33   The circle of Willis. A, Anterior cerebral artery; B, anterior communicating artery; C, internal carotid artery; D, middle cerebral artery; E, posterior communicating artery; F, posterior cerebral artery; G, superior cerebellar artery; H, pontine branches; I, basilar artery; J, labyrinthine artery; K, anterior inferior cerebellar artery; L. vertebral artery; M, posterior inferior cereballar artery; N, anterior spinal artery.

widespread infarction than is usual. The occurrence and extent of infarction also depends on available anastomoses. In addition to the circle of Willis itself there are other important anastomoses, such as between the middle and anterior, or middle and posterior cerebral arteries, and also between the larger arteries supplying the cerebellum. If one of these arteries is occluded, the infarcted area may be smaller than the area supplied by the vessel, since the periphery may be adequately supplied by the collateral circulation. Anastomoses also occur between the meningeal branches of the external carotid artery and the cortical branches of the internal carotid artery. A superficial shell of cortex may thus remain intact at the meningeal surface. Haemodynamic factors are also of importance: a severe episode of hypotension from whatever cause may produce infarction in the absence of vascular occlusion, and this usually occurs in the boundary zones between the territories supplied by the middle and anterior cerebral, or middle and posterior cerebral arteries. This is more likely to occur when the cerebral circulation is already compromised by pre-existing arterial disease.

An infarct may be *pale (ischaemic)* or *red (haemorrhagic)*. In the white matter there is a relatively poor anastomotic circulation and an infarct is usually pale, while there are abundant anastomoses within the grey matter and an infarct is likely to be haemorrhagic. Slow occlusion of a vessel by thrombosis tends to result in a pale infarct, while rapid occlusion by embolus often causes vascular spasm which, when it subsides or the embolus breaks up, may be followed by haemorrhage into the necrotic area.

25.4.2 Pathology of infarction

As indicated above, the location and extent of the infarct depends mainly on the vessel involved, the available anastomoses, pre-existing vascular disease, and the patient's haemodynamic balance. The gross and microscopic appearance of the infarct depends on the presence or absence of haemorrhage and the length of survival of the patient.

Macroscopic appearance

A recent infarct involving the cortex or grey matter is usually haemorrhagic and dark red in colour. Haemorrhage within the area of infarction is due to the leakage of blood from damaged capillaries. Blood re-entering these capillaries is thought to come from the collateral circulation or through the originally occluded vessel. Infarction involving the white matter is frequently pale and difficult to visualize within the first few days. The infarct is soft to the touch and slightly darker than the surrounding brain.

After about 3 days the whole area of infarction becomes oedematous and the red coloration of the cortex or deep grey matter begins to diminish. Affected white matter is now obviously swollen and soft. The oedema surrounding an infarct may be extensive, and in large infarcts such severe brain swelling may be fatal in itself.

By about the tenth day the oedema has decreased and the area of infarction is very soft and necrotic. Eventually the area becomes cystic as the necrotic tissue is removed. This process may take months or even years, depending on the size of the infarct, but finally the infarcted area is replaced by a thin-walled cyst with yellowish-brown pigmentation produced by altered blood pigments (Figs 25.34, 25.35).

Microscopic appearance

Within 8–12 hours, neurones in the infarcted zone show ischaemic cell change. The cytoplasm becomes densely eosinophilic and the nucleus is shrunken and pyknotic. If the infarct is haemorrhagic, there are varying numbers of petechial haemorrhages in the vicinity, and swollen capillary endothelium may be detectable. Another early manifestation is a brisk inflammatory cell response with polymorphonuclear leucocytes, which may be quite abundant around the vessels and at the edge of the infarct. The leucocytes tend to disappear within 3–6 days. By about the fourth day, lipid-filled macrophages increase in number and at this stage are the predominant cells. As the necrotic tissue is phagocytosed, the macrophages gradually decrease, but are often still present for some months in a large infarct. Swollen astrocytes make their appearance at the stage

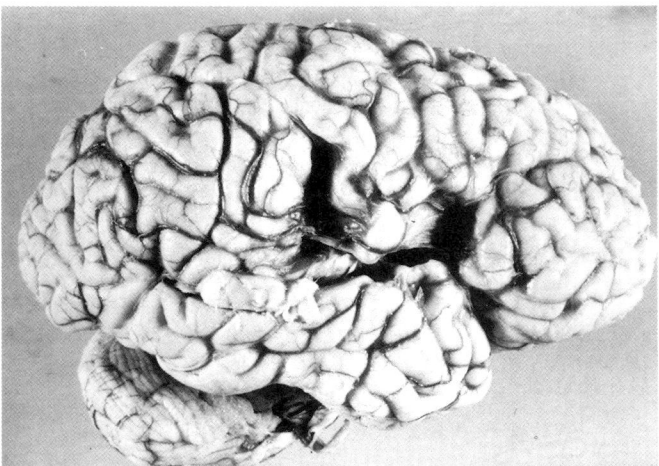

Fig. 25.34 Brain, showing cystic scar of old infarct within the territory of the right middle cerebral artery. (Reproduced from Pathy 1985, by permission of John Wiley and Son, Ltd.)

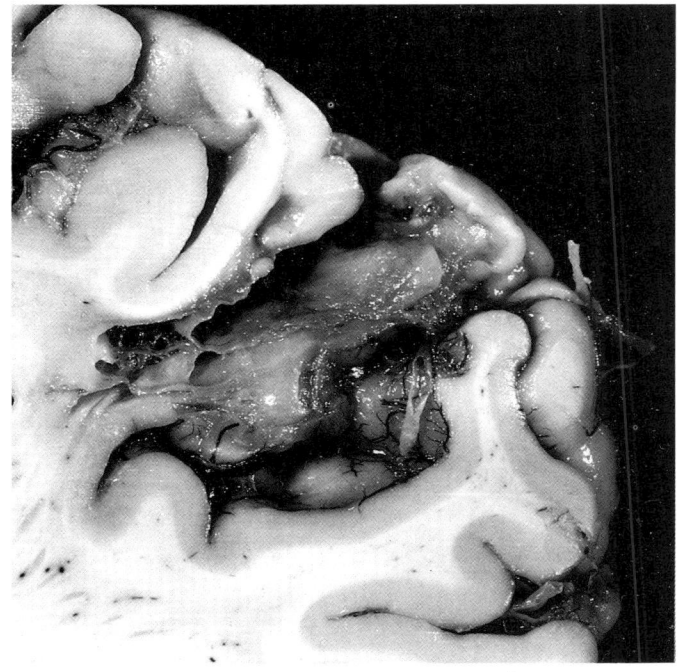

Fig. 25.35 Cystic scarring involving the right frontal region.

of oedema (Fig. 25.36) and, in time, numerous glial fibres dominate the area. Scattered blood vessels with thickened walls and occasional newly formed capillaries may be evident. Eventually, the whole area is transformed into a cyst surrounded and traversed by glial fibres (Fig. 25.37), and macrophages containing altered blood pigments often persist within it.

Infarction of the spinal cord

Spinal cord infarction is rare except as a complication of trauma or cord compression.

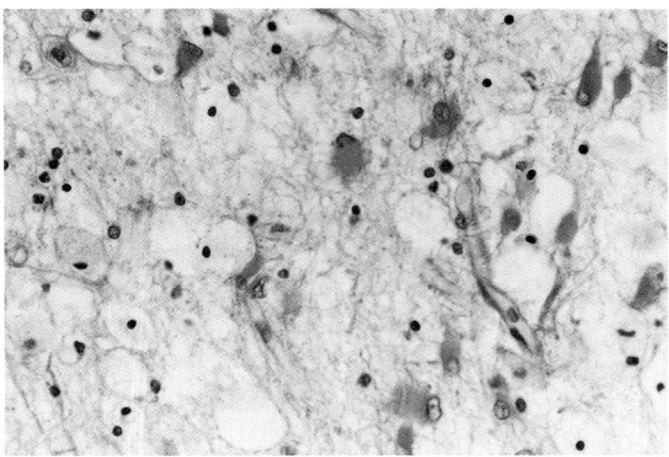

Fig. 25.36 Section showing an area of recent cerebral infarction with prominent foamy macrophages and reactive astrocytes.

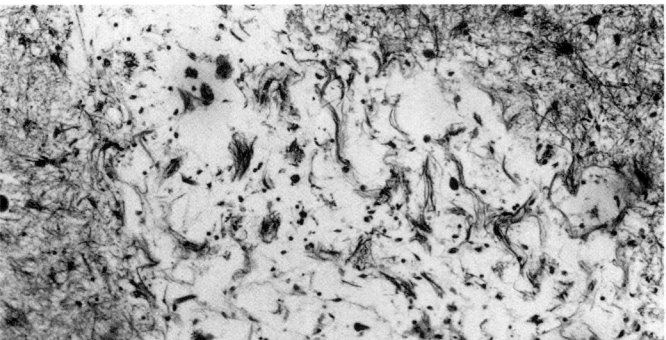

Fig. 25.37 Section of an old cerebral infarct, showing a cystic area traversed and surrounded by glial fibres.

25.4.3   Vascular disease associated with cerebral infarction

Atherosclerosis

Atheroma is the commonest disease to affect the arteries, and a major cause of cerebral infarction. Atherosclerosis generally affects the large muscular arteries, such as the extracranial parts of the common carotid and vertebral arteries and, within the cranium, the internal carotid, anterior, middle, and posterior cerebral arteries, and the basilar artery.

An atheromatous plaque is characterized by intimal thickening, which is largely contributed to by proliferating smooth muscle cells. Lipids, especially cholesterol, accumulate within the muscle cells and within macrophages. Fibrous thickening of the vessel wall and destruction and splitting of the elastic lamina occurs (Fig. 25.38) and, in a complicated plaque, there is calcification and ulceration of the surface. Atheromatous debris may form emboli, or thrombus deposition may reduce the lumen considerably, but rarely totally occludes it. Circulation through the vessel is further compromised by superimposed thrombus or haemorrhage into the plaque. The affected vessel

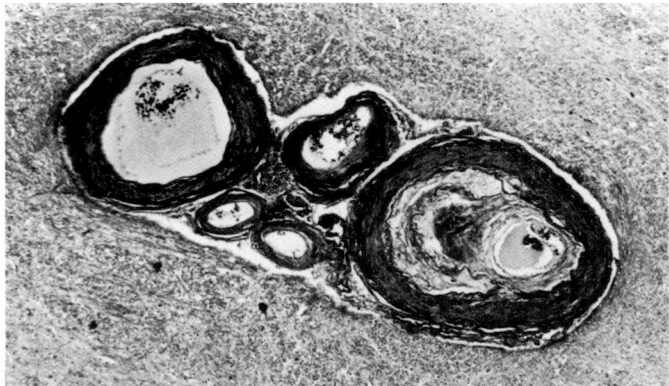

Fig. 25.38 Atherosclerotic vessels in brain showing thickening of media, and splitting of elastic lamina. An atheromatous plaque is evident in one artery, resulting in a marked reduction of the lumen. (Reproduced from Pathy 1985, by permission of John Wiley and Son, Ltd.)

shows a yellowish opacity of its wall, and in severe cases the whole artery may be elongated and tortuous. Furthermore, weakening of the vessel wall may lead to aneurysmal dilatation.

Hypertension

Within the large and medium-sized vessels sustained hypertension produces hypertrophy of the media, and thickening and reduplication of the elastic lamina. This eventually results in fibrous replacement of the media and breaking up of the elastic layer. In smaller arteries and arterioles the media is hypertrophied and the intima becomes thickened by connective tissue. The incidence and severity of atheroma affecting large muscular arteries is considerably increased in hypertension.

Lacunae

These small lesions are commonly found in the brains of patients with atherosclerosis, and particularly in those with hypertension. Lacunae occur in the brainstem, basal ganglia, and central white matter, and are represented by small cavities measuring from 2 to 20 mm in diameter. On microscopic examination they are found to consist of irregular areas of perivascular rarefaction, sometimes with scattered haemosiderin-laden phagocytes, and demarcated by a thin rim of gliosis. They are generally thought to be due to atheromatous change, hyalinization, or occlusion of small arteries.

Hypertensive encephalopathy

A severe and acute rise in blood pressure may occur in normotensive individuals with such conditions as *eclampsia* or *acute nephritis*, and in patients with *malignant hypertension*. Clinically, hypertensive encephalopathy is characterized by severe headache, followed by convulsions or coma. If death occurs, the main changes found within the brain are fibrinoid necrosis of small arteries, petechial haemorrhages, and oedema of the white matter.

Other types of vascular disease

Other forms of vascular disease affecting the brain are rare in comparison with atherosclerosis and hypertension. However, a variety of systemic diseases may affect the vasculature of the central nervous system and cause infarction or haemorrhage. Such diseases include polyarteritis nodosa, systemic lupus erythematosus, giant-cell arteritis, granulomatous arteritis, amyloid angiopathy, and syphilitic arteritis.

25.4.4   Cerebral embolism

Embolism is an important cause of cerebral infarction. Cerebral emboli are most commonly a result of cardiac disease, or atheromatous disease of the large arteries in the neck.

Emboli may originate within the heart, especially in patients with mural thrombus as a result of endomyocardial infarction, and in patients with prolonged atrial fibrillation. Formation of thrombus from vegetations on damaged valves is most commonly associated with rheumatic heart disease.

Emboli consisting of atheromatous debris or thrombus may arise from atheromatous plaques. Atheroma commonly affects the aorta, carotid, vertebral, or basilar arteries.

Large emboli from the aorta may impact in the carotid, basilar, or middle cerebral arteries. Emboli reaching the brain via the internal carotid arteries usually impact within the distribution of the middle cerebral artery.

Transient ischaemic attacks

These occur suddenly and are characterized by various neurological signs, which usually clear within about 24 hours. Such attacks are thought to be caused by microemboli, which are generally considered to have the same pathogenesis as small cerebral infarcts. Clinically they are a warning of impending complete cerebral infarction. Estimates of the risk of subsequent permanent strokes vary from 13 to 50 per cent.

Fat embolism

This may occur after bone fractures, when fat from the marrow enters damaged veins. If numerous emboli are formed, they may escape from the lungs where they usually lodge into the systemic circulation and thus reach the brain. In fatal cases the brains of patients who have survived 3 or 4 days show diffuse perivascular petechial haemorrhages within the white matter, and stains for fat will show strong positivity.

Air embolism

Air may enter the circulation in a variety of situations, such as abortion, trauma, or cardiac and lung surgery. A large amount of air is needed to cause symptoms, and it has been estimated that the amount required is between 300 and 500 ml. Death is due to pulmonary and cardiac dysfunction, and in such cases the brain may show ischaemic damage due to reduced cerebral blood flow and hypoxaemia.

25.4.5   Venous thrombosis

Aseptic thrombosis of the cerebral veins and dural sinuses may occur as a complication of a variety of conditions, including severe dehydration and malnutrition especially in children, pregnancy, abortion, blood disorders associated with increased blood coagulability, and trauma. The commonest site of thrombosis is the *superior sagittal sinus*. Localized thrombus formation rarely leads to permanent damage because of an adequate collateral circulation, but total obstruction of a sinus and its tributaries leads to severe impairment of venous drainage. Intense engorgement of the superficial veins will follow, and there may be subarachnoid haemorrhage within their vicinity. The affected areas of cortex and white matter show the features of haemorrhagic infarction. Extension of thrombus into the transverse and lateral sinuses may occur.

Thrombosis may also occur as a complication of pyogenic infections, and is usually the result of direct spread. Infection of the frontal air sinuses may cause superior sagittal sinus thrombosis. *Lateral sinus thrombosis* is most often a complication of otitis media or mastoiditis, and *thrombosis of the cavernous sinus* is frequently secondary to infected lesions of the central part of the face through the facial and ophthalmic veins. Thrombosis of the internal cerebral veins occurs most commonly in young children with or without infection, and may be secondary to thrombosis of the dural sinuses, or may occur primarily in the veins. Haemorrhagic infarction in the field of venous drainage is variable in its severity.

25.4.6   Intracerebral haemorrhage

The most important cause of spontaneous intracerebral haemorrhage is hypertension. The most common site of haemorrhage is the *basal ganglia* in the region of supply of the *lenticulostriate artery* (Fig. 25.39). The haemorrhage may remain circumscribed or progressively enlarge with diffusion into the white matter, rupture into the ventricles, or extension to the surface of the brain. A large haemorrhage is usually rapidly fatal and results in destruction of brain tissue. A steep rise in intracranial pressure follows with *transtentorial herniation* and *brain stem compression*.

Other sites in which haemorrhage may arise are the cerebellum and the brainstem. Within the cerebellum, circumscribed lesions may form in the white matter, and possible complications include *rupture into the fourth ventricle, tonsillar herniation*, or *medullary compression*. Haemorrhage into the brainstem usually involves the pons (Fig. 25.40) and may rupture into the fourth ventricle. Death occurs rapidly from cardiorespiratory arrest due to interference with vital brainstem functions.

The appearances of the haematoma will vary according to the severity of the bleeding and the length of survival of the patient. If the haemorrhage was large and rapidly fatal, the blood clot is semi-fluid in consistency. A smaller circumscribed haematoma, which has been survived, is gradually absorbed by macrophages, and the residual lesion is eventually represented by a cavity filled with yellowish fluid, and lined by a glial

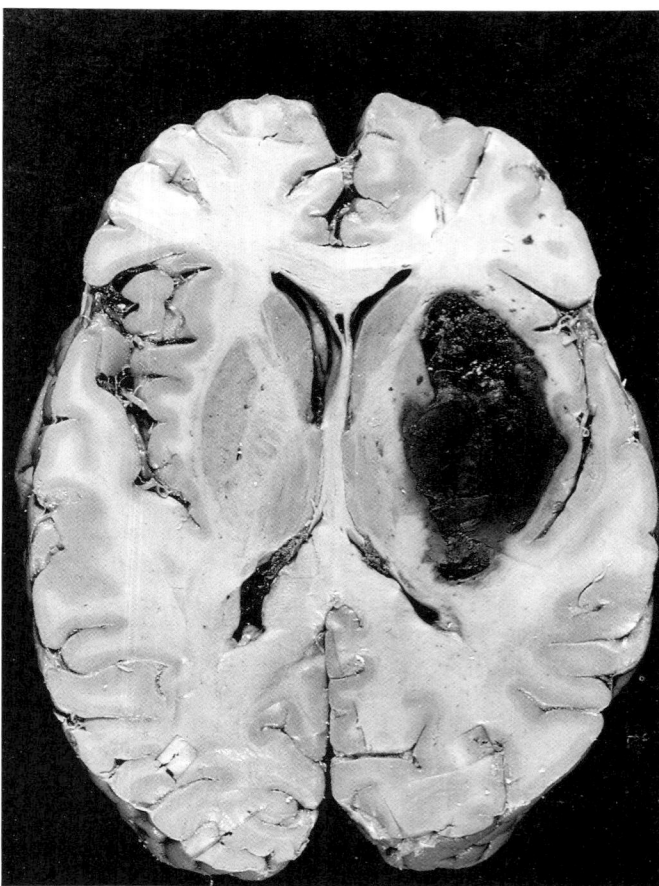

Fig. 25.39 Circumscribed haemorrhage in the region of the right basal ganglia, with narrowing of the right ventricle.

membrane. The brown colour of the lesion is imparted by altered blood pigments.

Pathogenesis

Miliary or microaneurysms that occur on small cerebral vessels were first described by Charcot. Haemorrhage was attributed to their rupture, and since that time a number of workers have confirmed this observation. Post-mortem studies have demonstrated microaneurysms on small, perforating arteries within the brain. They are usually multiple and measure up to 2 mm in diameter. They occur most commonly in hypertensive subjects and their incidence increases with age. Microaneurysms have been observed in the brains of normotensive individuals, but are rare compared with their incidence in cases with hypertension.

25.4.7 Subarachnoid haemorrhage

Haemorrhage into the subarachnoid space is most frequently caused by rupture of a saccular aneurysm arising from one of the vessels forming the circle of Willis at the base of the brain (Fig. 25.41).

Saccular (Berry) aneurysm

These aneurysms may be single or multiple, and are represented by thin-walled sacs varying in size from 2 to 10 mm. Giant aneurysms measuring around 2.5 cm occur in about 5 per cent of cases and may present as mass lesions. Saccular aneurysms usually arise at or close to points of branching of the arteries. About 40 per cent of aneurysms are related to the junction of the internal carotid and posterior communicating arteries, about 30 per cent found in the region of the anterior communicating artery, and about 20 per cent arise on a middle cerebral artery, usually at its proximal point of branching. Aneurysms in the posterior part of the circle of Willis are less common, and it is

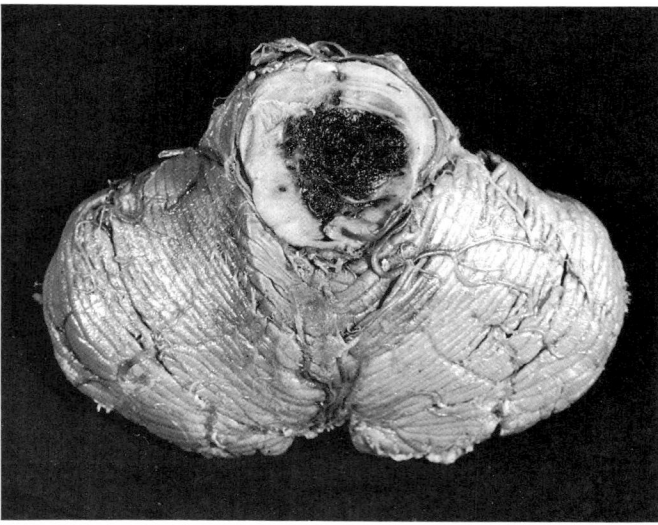

Fig. 25.40 Mid-pontine haemorrhage in a case of hypertension.

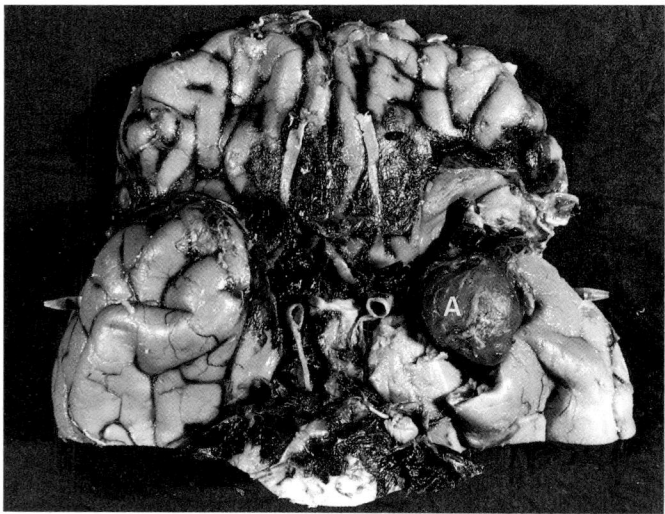

Fig. 25.41 A giant saccular aneurysm (A) is arising from the left middle cerebral artery. Subarachnoid haemorrhage is evident at the base of the brain.

estimated that about 5–10 per cent are associated with the posterior cerebral arteries, the vertebral arteries, and the basilar artery. Saccular aneurysms occur in 1–2 per cent of the population, and are multiple in about 20–30 per cent of individuals with aneurysms. Subarachnoid haemorrhage due to rupture of the aneurysm has a peak incidence in the 40–60 year age-group. Fewer than 10 per cent are encountered under the age of 30 years, and it is rare under the age of 20 years. There is a male predominance in patients under the age of 20 years, and a 2 : 1 female preponderance in patients over the age of 60 years.

Pathogenesis

Histological studies have shown that in the normal cerebral vessels of the circle of Willis, there is frequently a gap in the medial coat at the point of bifurcation. It is generally considered that most aneurysms form within this structurally weakened area, which is composed of the intimal layer, the elastic lamina, and adventitial tissue. Subsequent degenerative changes within the aneurysm, such as atherosclerosis, may further weaken the wall and predispose to rupture. This offers a reasonable explanation for the increased incidence of rupture in older age-groups. However, it is not known why aneurysms form in only about 2 per cent of the population, and other haemodynamic and inherited factors may be important. There is evidence to show that rupture of an aneurysm is more likely to occur in hypertensive subjects, particularly with a sudden rise in blood pressure, although rupture is by no means restricted to this group.

Pathology

Haemorrhage from a ruptured aneurysm is sometimes limited to that site, but more frequently there is extensive haemorrhage into the subarachnoid space. This may be complicated by blood ploughing into the brain to produce intracerebral haemorrhage, which may then rupture into the ventricles. Such an event is accompanied by acute brain swelling and herniation, and is invariably fatal. Another complication is infarction of the region of the brain supplied by the affected artery. Infarction is thought to be caused by arterial spasm which, in subarachnoid haemorrhage, frequently occurs in the vessel bearing the aneurysm, and may also affect those vessels surrounded by blood clot.

In some fatal cases, evidence of previous small subarachnoid haemorrhages may be demonstrated. In such cases the leptomeninges in the vicinity of the aneurysm are discoloured by altered blood pigments.

Prognosis

Rupture of an aneurysm carries a high mortality rate. About 25 per cent of cases die immediately or within hours of the first haemorrhage. If not treated surgically, there is a high risk of recurrent bleeding within the next few months. The success of neurosurgical intervention in uncomplicated subarachnoid haemorrhage is dependent upon a number of factors, including the condition of the patient at the time of surgery, the age, and the presence of hypertension.

It should be noted that not all aneurysms rupture, and they may be asymptomatic unless they are of sufficient size to cause local neurological symptoms.

Atherosclerotic fusiform aneurysm

Patients with severe atherosclerosis commonly develop fusiform dilatations of the basilar or internal carotid artery. Atherosclerotic plaques develop in the affected artery and the media is replaced by fibrous tissue. The wall of the artery stretches, the lumen is increased in size, and the vessel assumes a kinked or 'S'-shaped appearance. If the dilatation becomes excessive, a fusiform aneurysm develops. There may be no symptoms, but large aneurysms may compress and distort cerebral tissue and nerve roots, giving rise to local neurological signs. Thrombosis or embolus may result in infarction of the brain, but rupture of these aneurysms rarely occur.

Mycotic aneurysm

Infected thrombus may lead to secondary inflammation in the wall of an artery. Less commonly direct spread of an infection may involve the vessel wall. The inflammatory response in the wall of the artery leads to damage of the internal elastic lamina and the media, with subsequent aneurysmal dilatation. These aneurysms are usually small because of the acute nature of the process. The most common complication is cerebral infarction, but rupture of the aneurysm leading to subarachnoid or intracerebral haemorrhage may occur.

Dissecting aneurysm

Intracranial arteries are rarely affected by dissecting aneurysms. The plane of dissection is subintimal, and the cause has been attributed to trauma, syphilitic arteritis, or a congenital defect of the media. The middle cerebral artery is usually affected and cerebral infarction may occur, but haemorrhage has not been reported.

Vascular malformations

Three main types of vascular malformation affect the central nervous system, and may lead to haemorrhage or infarction:

1. arteriovenous malformation (AVM);
2. cavernous angioma;
3. capillary telangiectasis.

Arteriovenous malformation

These vascular anomalies are usually situated on the surface of the brain or spinal cord, but may extend into the brain to a varying degree. They vary in size from a small localized lesion to a large mass involving most of a hemisphere. An AVM is characterized by a mass of tangled, tortuous vessels, which are usually dilated. The main arteries and veins leading to and from the vascular mass are often enlarged. The arachnoid membrane covering the vessels is thickened and there may be a brown pigmentation indicating previous bleeding. Microscopic examination reveals large numbers of enlarged blood-vessels in the affected area. Within the arteries the internal elastic lamina may be reduplicated and distorted, and the media varies greatly in thickness in segments of the same vessel. The veins are thickened and hyalinized. The vessels may show secondary degenerative changes and thrombosis.

Rupture of an AVM produces a subarachnoid haemorrhage or, less commonly, an intracerebral haemorrhage. Haemorrhage may be slight and self-limiting, recurrent, or massive. Cerebral infarction may occur as a result of ischaemia or thrombus formation.

Spinal AVMs usually occur on the dorsal surface of the spinal cord, but may penetrate into the cord itself. Histologically they resemble the cerebral AVM and are subject to the same complications.

Cavernous angioma

These malformations occur most commonly in the white matter of the brain, then the pons, and rarely in the spinal cord. Multiple lesions may occur. Histologically, cavernous angiomas are composed of multiple abnormal vascular spaces which vary in size, and are closely opposed to each other. Gliosis is usually evident in the surrounding brain, and there may be evidence of previous haemorrhage.

Patients with this lesion usually present between the third and sixth decades, with epilepsy, focal neurological symptoms, or intracerebral bleeding.

Capillary telangiectasis

These lesions are usually an incidental finding at autopsy, and are rarely of clinical significance. They are most commonly situated in the pons but may also occur in the cerebral cortex or white matter. Microscopically these small lesions consist of groups of dilated capillaries which vary in size. The intervening brain tissue is normal. Spontaneous haemorrhage is a rare occurrence.

Sturge–Weber syndrome

This rare disease is characterized by an AVM involving the leptomeninges covering part or the whole of one cerebral hemisphere, with linear calcification and gliosis of the underlying cortex. In the complete syndrome there is a facial naevus involving the supraocular region, epilepsy, mental retardation, and often hemiparesis. Haemorrhage rarely occurs.

Other causes of intracranial haemorrhage

Spontaneous haemorrhage may occur as a complication of anticoagulant therapy, or of blood disorders such as haemophilia and leukaemia. Metastatic tumours are quite often vascular and liable to haemorrhage. Primary cerebral tumours such as haemangioblastomas and gliomas, especially the oligodendroglioma may also bleed spontaneously, and in such cases intracranial haemorrhage may be the first clinical manifestation of a cerebral tumour.

25.4.8 Further reading

Graham, D. I. and Brierley, J. B. (1984) Vascular disorders of the central nervous system. In *Greenfield's neuropathology* (ed. J. Hume-Adams, J. A. N. Corsellis, and L. W. Duchen) (4th edn), pp. 157–207. Edward Arnold, London.

Gresham, G. E., Phillips, T. F., Wolf, P. A., McNamara, P. M., Kannel, W. B., and Dawber, T. R. (1979). Epidemiological profile of long term stroke disability: The Framingham Study. *Archives of Physical Medicine and Rehabilitation* **60**, 487–91.

Pathy, M. A. (ed.) (1985). *Principles and practice of geriatric medicine*. John Wiley & Son, Chichester.

Weller, R. O. and Pickard, J. D. (1983). Cerebral vascular disease. In *Clinical neuropathology* (ed. R. O. Weller, M. Swash, D. L. McLellan, and C. L. Scholtz), pp. 57–84. Springer-Verlag, Berlin.

Yates, P. O. (1976). The pathogenesis of transient ischaemic attacks. In *Stroke* (ed. F. J. Gullingham, C. Mawdley, and A. E. Williams), pp. 178–87. Churchill Livingstone, Edinburgh.

25.5 Metabolic disorders

P. J. Gallagher

Neurological symptoms and neuropathological changes are well recognized in a wide variety of systemic and metabolic disorders, including malignant neoplasms, in chronic alcoholism, and some vitamin deficiencies. Furthermore, a number of therapeutic and recreational drugs, heavy metals, and industrial and agrochemicals have defined toxic effects on the central, and particularly the peripheral, nervous systems. Unfortunately, there is very little information on how neuropathological damage is produced in the majority of these instances. Even when there is a clearly defined histological or ultrastructural change, the underlying pathogenesis is often uncertain. It is also important to recognize that the neurological changes in many of these disorders are less important than those in other systems, particularly the liver, kidney, heart, and lung.

25.5.1 The neuropathology of alcoholism

The true incidence of alcohol dependence is uncertain but there may be as many as 750 000 'alcoholics' in the United Kingdom. In a large community hospital in Oslo, where the autopsy rate is between 70 and 80 per cent, evidence of alcohol-related disease was found in 713 of 8735 post-mortems (8.2 per cent) over a five-year period. The major neuro-psychiatric symptoms and neuropathological features of alcoholism are summarized in Table 25.4.

The exact ways in which alcohol induces damage in the central and peripheral nervous systems are unknown, but it is very probable that more than one mechanism is involved (Table 25.5). There is good evidence that long-term alcohol administration induces neuronal changes in the hippocampus in well-nourished experimental animals. Whether this is the direct result of alcohol toxicity, or the result of an alcohol breakdown

Table 25.4 Clinical and pathological features of alcohol-related neurological disease

Neuro-psychiatric features
  recurrent alcoholic intoxication
  alcohol withdrawal syndromes (including delirium tremens)
  psychoses (including Korsakoff's)
  depression
  reversible and irreversible dementia
  epilepsy

Neuropathological changes
  cerebral atrophy
  cerebellar degeneration
  Wernicke's encephalopathy
  peripheral neuropathy
  hepatic encephalopathy
  uncommon changes:
    central pontine myelinosis
    Marchiafava–Bignami disease
    tobacco–alcohol amblyopia
    fetal alcohol syndromes

Table 25.5 Pathophysiological changes related to alcoholic brain disease

Direct toxicity of alcohol, or its metabolites
Vitamin deficiencies secondary to malnutrition, especially thiamine
Hepatic encephalopathy due to alcoholic liver disease
Heart failure secondary to 'alcoholic cardiomyopathy'
Methyl alcohol toxicity
Traumatic head injuries

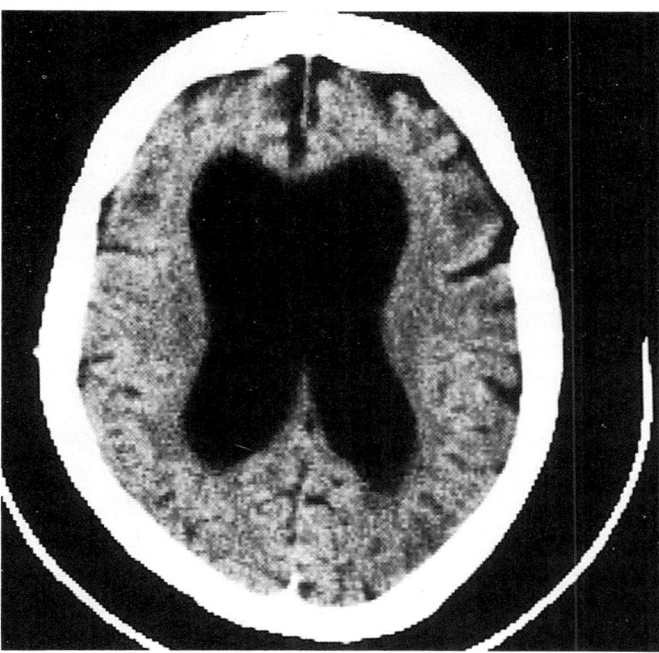

Fig. 25.42 Computerized tomographic scan in a patient with a long history of alcoholism. There is a marked cerebral atrophy, particularly in the frontal areas and dilatation of the ventricular system.

product such as acetaldehyde, is uncertain. Trauma, methyl alcohol poisoning, hepatic and cardiac failure also play some part in the neurological disease seen in long-standing alcoholics.

Pathological features

Both post-mortem studies and clinical investigations using computerized tomography indicate that cerebral atrophy is one of the commonest cerebral abnormalities in alcoholics. Ventricular dilatation, widening of the cerebral and cerebellar sulci, and enlargement of the Sylvian and interhemispheric fissures are the usual radiological changes. Brain weights are 30–70 g less than 'non-alcoholic controls'. No specific cerebral cortical changes have been described in these patients, although a number of non-quantitative studies have suggested that there may be a reduction in the number of cortical neurones. The structural basis for alcoholic dementia is uncertain and neither the classical changes of multi-infarct dementia or senile dementia of the Alzheimer type are particularly prominent in heavy drinkers.

Histological changes of *Wernicke's encephalopathy* are seen in between 1 and 3 per cent post-mortems. Macroscopic changes include shrinkage and brown discoloration of the mamillary bodies and ventricular dilatation. Unless the subependymal regions of the third and fourth ventricles are examined histo-

logically, many cases will be missed. In active Wernicke's encephalopathy there is pronounced swelling of the capillary endothelium, perivascular oedema, and patchy gliosis. It has been suggested that the changes in the thalamus and inferior olives are rather different to those in the mamillary bodies and resemble those of anoxia. Cerebellar atrophy is seen in over a quarter of long-standing alcoholics at post-mortem and is particularly common in the anterior vermis.

Central pontine myelinolysis presents with a rapidly evolving para- or quadriparesis with prominent pseudobulbar symptoms such as dysarthria or dysphagia. There is usually a history of alcoholism and the condition is often associated with severe electrolyte disturbances, particularly hyponatraemia. The lesion is uncommon, even in chronic alcoholics, and there is often extensive histological evidence of pontine demyelination.

Necrosis of the corpus callosum in heavy wine-drinkers was noted by Marchiafava and Bignami at the turn of the century. The clinical pattern of the disease is rather unlike other forms of alcoholic neurological disease. Initially there is a loss of emotional control and reasoning power, but upper motor neurone signs, tremor, and coma then develop rapidly and death usually occurs within months of the initial presentation. Although most of the changes are found in the corpus callosum, some areas of axonal loss and vascular proliferation may be found in the central white matter. The precise cause of these curious lesions is uncertain, but a toxic factor, other than alcohol or methyl alcohol, in cheap red wine has been suggested. As in most of the uncommon forms of alcoholic brain disease, other clinical and pathological features of alcoholism may also be present.

In the common forms of alcoholic neurological disease there are only limited ocular signs, as *pupillary miosis*, *slow pupil reflexes*, and *third, fourth, or sixth nerve palsies*. In 'tobacco–alcohol' or *nutritional amblyopia*, necrosis of retinal ganglion cells and structural changes in the optic nerves lead to deteriorating visual acuity and central scotomas. Most patients with this also smoke heavily and the precise mechanism of the ocular damage is uncertain. A similar condition has been reported from tropical Africa and related to cassava root consumption. Cyanide, as contaminants of these roots, and of some tobaccos, may impair vitamin B_{12} metabolism and some patients appear to respond to vitamin B_{12} therapy.

A symmetrical and distal peripheral neuropathy is a well-recognized feature of chronic alcoholism and may be the result of vitamin B_1 deficiency. Foot drop and weakness of the thigh and hand muscles are the most prominent clinical features. Autonomic neuropathy is rare in alcoholism, but both acute and subacute myopathies can develop.

25.5.2 Fetal alcohol syndrome

Neurological and pathological changes have been described in the children of mothers who consistently drink more than 30 g of alcohol per day during pregnancy (Table 25.6). The original descriptions of this so-called 'fetal alcohol syndrome' were from France, Scandinavia, and the USA, but it is now well recognized in the United Kingdom, and in Liverpool is seen in at least 1 in 2500 births. The toxic effects of alcohol, and more especially acetaldehyde, are compounded by poor maternal nutrition, vitamin deficiencies, and smoking. *Microencephaly* is the most prominent macroscopic, and *cerebellar dysplasia* the most frequent microscopic, change. Children who are severely affected are retarded, but there is some evidence that this is less obvious as they age. Experimental studies have reproduced most of the changes seen in humans and suggest that even the third trimester is a risk period. Alcohol impairs both cell migration and nerve cell maturation, particularly in the cerebellum.

25.5.3 Methyl alcohol poisoning

Methyl alcohol (methanol) is present in a variety of household solvents, cosmetics, and cleansing lotions but these are seldom responsible for poisoning. Illicitly prepared spirits can be contaminated with methanol and this is the usual cause of acute toxicity. There is an early phase of cerebral depression, followed 8–48 hours later by a severe metabolic acidosis. An alcohol dehydrogenase in the liver and kidney is responsible for the metabolism of methyl alcohol to formaldehyde and then to formic acid. This is responsible for the severe metabolic acidosis which is such a characteristic feature of methanol, though not ethanol, poisoning.

The earliest signs of ocular toxicity are blurring of vision, and papilloedema may develop. Demyelination of the optic nerve is now accepted as the major mechanism of ocular damage, but necrosis of retinal ganglion cells has also been observed.

Table 25.6 Clinical and pathological features of the fetal alcohol syndrome

Neurological changes
  Prenatal and postnatal growth retardation
  Acute neurological symptoms in the neonatal period
  Diminished IQ, behavioural and learning problems, occasionally mental retardation, speech disorders

Pathological features
  Microencephaly
  Micro-ophthalmia and short palpebral fissures
  Flat upper lip, small jaw, broad nasal bridge
  Increased incidence of cardial septal defects
  Minor skeletal abnormalities, especially of upper limbs

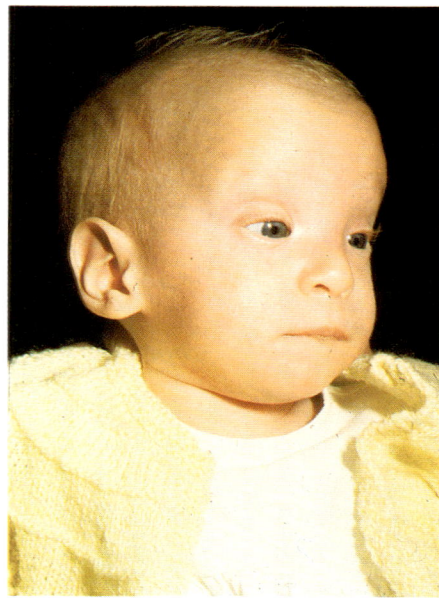

Fig. 25.43 Fetal alcohol syndrome. One of twins born to a mother with a history of heavy alcohol consumption throughout pregnancy. The head is smaller than usual, the eyes are small, and there is a broad nasal bridge.

Cerebral changes have also been identified in methyl alcohol poisoning, but whether these are primarily the result of methanol toxicity or the secondary effects of anoxia are uncertain. Areas of necrosis have also been described in the white matter of the frontal lobes and in the cerebellum. It may be that these lesions and the demyelinating process in the optic nerves are the result of formate toxicity. Necrosis of anterior horn cells in the spinal cord is probably the result of anoxia.

25.5.4 Deficiency disorders

Neurological disease follows deficiencies of a number of the B group of vitamins (Table 25.7). In contrast there are few, if any, characteristic neuropathological features associated with other vitamin deficiencies, lack of folic acid, or the various forms of protein or calorie malnutrition.

Table 25.7 Neuropathological changes associated with vitamin deficiencies

Vitamin deficiency	Underlying causes	Clinical features	Neurological and neuropathological changes
A	Protein-calorie malnutrition (usually in the tropics)	Dry eyes; keratitis; night blindness	*Occasionally*: myopathies, polyneuropathies
B Group			
B_1 (thiamine)	Malnutrition; alcoholism; anorexia nervosa; hyperemesis; G-1 disorders	Beri beri; Wernicke's encephalopathy (see text)	Haemorrhage, congestion and capillary proliferation in periventricular areas and mamillary bodies; polyneuropathies
B_2 (nicotinic acid)	Alcoholism; G-1 disorders; severe malnutrition	Pellagra (diarrhoea, dry skin, glossitis)	Mania, depression, dementia; loss of cortical and pontine neurones; degeneration of posterior, corticospinal, and spinocerebellar tracts
B_6 (pyridoxine)	Drug therapy (isoniazid, hydralazine, penicillamine)	Anaemia; convulsions	Polyneuropathy; optic atrophy
B_{12} (cobalamin)	Pernicious anaemia; total gastrectomy	Megaloblastic anaemia	Subacute combined degeneration of spinal cord (posterior columns, corticospinal tracts) causing ataxia, spasticity, and paraplegia; peripheral neuropathy, dementia, and psychoses
C	Dietary imbalances, especially in elderly	Scurvy	*Occasionally*: cerebral or retinal haemorrhage

In Western societies, vitamin B_1 deficiency (thiamine) is now almost restricted to alcoholics. Thiamine is not stored in the body and signs of deficiency can appear within a month. This is particularly true of beer-drinkers whose high carbohydrate intake increases the demand for thiamine. The characteristic *psychotic symptoms* described by Wernicke, and later by Korsakoff, are often the most dramatic feature of each patient's presentation. Other neurological symptoms include memory loss, peripheral neuropathies, ataxia, nystagmus, and extra-ocular palsies. Cerebral symptoms and peripheral neuropathy are said to be rare in tropical beri beri, but have been identified in detailed studies of European prisoners of war. Although a variety of cardiovascular disorders are seen in alcoholics, the severe 'high output' congestive cardiac failure with peripheral oedema and vasodilatation, so characteristic of beri beri, does not generally occur in alcoholics. In the West, left heart failure with dyspnoea, rales, and impaired left ventricular function is more common. The precise patterns of deficiencies in separate communities may be subtly different and it is very probable that nicotinic acid deficiency also contributes to the neurological disease seen in alcoholics. A large number of experimental studies have confirmed that thiamine deficiency induces areas of cerebral necrosis and haemorrhage. As in humans, neurological symptoms can develop after 3–4 weeks of dietary deficiency. Nicotinic acid deficiency produces *pellagra* (diarrhoea, dry skin, and glossitis). Abnormalities have been reported in the cerebral cortex, the pons, and the spinal cord.

The major neurological changes associated with *vitamin B_{12} (cobalamin) deficiency* are peripheral neuropathy, demyelination, and degeneration of the posterior and lateral columns of the spinal cord and a variety of confusional, amnestic, and psychotic alterations. In classical pernicious anaemia, the underlying pathology is a failure of gastric secretion of the glycoprotein, intrinsic factor. This complexes with dietary vitamin B_{12} and is absorbed in the terminal ileum. Vitamin B_{12} is involved in at least three enzymic reactions and, if deficient, affects the haemopoietic and nervous systems, epithelial surfaces, and osteoblast function. Methylcobalamin participates in a methyltransferase reaction involving a tetrahydrofolate, and therefore affects DNA synthesis and, ultimately, haemopoiesis. This might be important in the neurological disease but a cobalamine is also involved in a methylmalonyl-CoA mutase reaction. A deficiency leads to abnormal fatty-acid synthesis ('funny fatty acids') and this could affect the biochemical structure of myelin.

A fully developed neurological disease is now rare in pernicious anaemia but the changes were described in great detail at the turn of the century. There is some evidence that the thoracic cord is preferentially affected and symptoms appear in the lower, before the upper, limbs. Paraesthesia and ataxia are the first symptoms of spinal cord disease but can progress within weeks to complete paraplegia. Recovery in patients treated in the early stages of the disease is often excellent.

A peripheral neuropathy may be the presenting feature of pernicious anaemia and occasionally patients with cobalamin deficiency have neurological signs but no evidence of megaloblastic anaemia. The changes of subacute combined degeneration have been produced in monkeys fed a vitamin B_{12}-deficient diet. The earliest changes are in myelin sheaths, which show separation of lamellae, vacuolation, and ultimately full demyelination. Some axonal loss also occurs, but the exact cellular mechanism underlying these changes is uncertain. No unequivocal neuropathological changes have been described in association with folic acid deficiency.

25.5.5   Neurological changes in systemic disorders

Liver disease

Hepatic encephalopathy develops in both fulminant *acute hepatitis* and in *chronic liver failure*. There may be subtle differences in the clinical patterns of presentation in these two instances but the underlying neuropathological changes are probably similar. Encephalopathy can be precipitated by a rise in blood urea, often secondary to diuretic therapy, the use of sedatives or tranquillizers, and as a result of gastrointestinal haemorrhage.

The pathogenesis of hepatic encephalopathy is uncertain. Raised circulating levels of ammonia, mercaptans, phenols, short-chain fatty acids, and a number of essential and non-essential amino acids have been described. However, there is no conclusive proof that any of these alterations are directly responsible for the encephalopathy. Plasma levels of the inhibitory neurotransmitter aminobutyric acid (GABA) are increased in both patients and animals with hepatic encephalopathy. This is probably the result of increased absorption of bacterial GABA from an abnormally permeable large intestine and diminished plasma extraction by a diseased liver. The blood–brain barrier normally excludes GABA but may function abnormally in hepatic encephalopathy.

In some patients dying in liver failure there is undoubted cerebral oedema, but in most cases the brain weight is within normal limits. The chief histological changes are *neuronal necrosis* with associated *astrocytic gliosis*, particularly in the deep layers of the cerebral cortex, the basal ganglia, and the dentate nucleus of the cerebellum. Characteristic changes are observed in the astrocytes and these were first described by Von Hosslin and Alzheimer in 1912 in a case that was probably an example of Wilson's disease. Later authors divided the astrocytic changes into two groups and these are now named *Alzheimer type 1* and *type 2 change*. Type 1 astrocytes are enlarged and typically have a multilobed hyperchromatic nucleus. In contrast, Alzheimer type 2 astrocytes are also enlarged but have vacuolated and chromatin-poor nuclei which often appear in pairs. Although these changes are generally considered to be 'degenerative', it is not known whether they are reversible in man.

Many different experimental models of hepatic encephalopathy have been devised. Alzheimer type 2 astrocytes can be identified in rats within weeks of porto-caval shunting, particularly if ammoniated ion-exchange rhythms are also administered. The astrocytic enlargement is the result of hyperplasia of both mitochondria and rough endoplasmic reticulum. In the later stages, pronounced hydropic degeneration is identified. From the results of experiments such as these it has been suggested that hepatic encephalopathy is an 'ammonia-induced gliopathy'.

Although liver disease is a prominent feature of *Reye's syndrome*, the cerebral changes that have been reported are not

Table 25.8   Neurological changes in common systemic disorders

Disorder	Clinical features	Neuropathology
Hepatic encephalopathy	Early: anorexia, sleep disturbances, loss of judgement	Cerebral oedema (some cases only), astrocytic swelling, and degeneration
	Late: depression, confusion, flapping tremor (asterixis), coma	Some evidence of neuronal necrosis (cerebral cortex, basal ganglia, cerebellum)
Uraemic encephalopathy	Early: episodic loss of concentration, headache, vomiting	No consistent macroscopic changes
	Late: disorientation, dysarthria, confusion, dyspnoea, dementia (elderly especially), symmetrical distal peripheral neuropathy	Degeneration of cerebral cortical neurones with astrocytic and microglial reaction
Cardiovascular disorders		
Cardiac dysrhythmias	Light-headedness, syncope, Stokes–Adams attacks	No characteristic changes
Cardiac failure	Confusion, lethargy, depression	No characteristic changes
Hypertensive encephalopathy	Increasing headache, vomiting, convulsions, cortical vision loss, papilloedema	Cerebral oedema, petechial haemorrhages, multiple microinfarcts, necrosis of vessel walls
Infective endocarditis	Localizing signs due to emboli, encephalopathy	Cerebral infarction, meningitis, haemorrhage from mycotic aneurysms
Diabetes mellitus	Complex patterns of cranial, peripheral, and autonomic neuropathy; pseudotabes	Axonal degeneration, demyelination, microangiopathic changes, cerebral atherosclerosis
Connective tissue disorders		
Systemic lupus erythematosus	Fits, meningism, ataxia, extra-pyramidal syndromes Psychiatric symptoms	Multiple microinfarcts, occasionally vasculitis of medium-sized arteries
Polyarteritis nodosa	Symmetrical sensory polyneuropathy Mononeuritis multiplex Cerebral symptoms (especially memory loss)	Focal necrotizing vasculitis ? (cerebral vasculitis rare)
Rheumatoid disease	Cord signs due to atlanto-axial subluxation but no generalized symptoms	No primary CNS changes

obviously those of hepatic encephalopathy. The most prominent feature is *cerebral oedema*, which is often severe and occasionally requires decompressive surgery. The pattern of neuronal necrosis strongly suggests ischaemic damage, and in some acute cases there may be evidence of patchy microinfarction throughout the cerebral cortex. As in hepatic encephalopathy, substantially raised levels of blood ammonia are usually recorded but, paradoxically, Alzheimer type 2 change is not a prominent feature.

The cause of Reye's syndrome is uncertain, but salicylates may provoke the disorder. The incidence of Reye's syndrome appears to be declining, as is the use of aspirin preparations in children. There is an epidemiological association with outbreaks of influenza, but the histological appearances in the brain and liver are not especially suggestive of viral disease.

Renal failure

Many neurological symptoms occur during the course of both acute and chronic renal failure. The earliest are loss of concentration, headache, and vomiting. Myoclonic seizures, convulsions, and coma are later changes. Electroencephalographic abnormalities may be present before these clinical signs appear. As with most other extrarenal manifestations of uraemia, the cause of the cerebral alterations in renal failure are unknown. The clinical picture is often complicated by additional changes such as hypertension, congestive cardiac failure, metabolic acidosis, and hyperkalaemia. There is no evidence that raised blood urea, *per se*, is responsible for any of the pathological alterations. No characteristic macroscopic abnormalities have been detected in the central nervous system in patients dying in renal failure. There is evidence of degenerative changes in cerebral cortical neurones, with an associated astrocytic and microglial reaction. The occipital cortex is relatively spared and changes in the cerebellum are less pronounced.

In retrospect, it is clear that the severe pattern of encephalopathy seen in patients on prolonged dialysis was restricted to a comparatively small number of units, albeit in separate countries. In these patients there was a characteristic pattern of stuttering speech with *dysarthria*, *dyspraxia*, and *myoclonus*; some developed *dementia*. It is very likely that these patients absorbed *aluminium* from dialysis fluids. The full-blown syndrome is now rare and the aluminium content of dialysis fluids and its concentration in the water supply to dialysis units is now carefully monitored. Nevertheless, a rapid reduction of blood urea levels can be associated with headache, muscular twitching, and transient confusional states—the so called '*dialysis disequilibrium syndrome*'. These, and a variety of psychological symptoms, are most common when patients first enter a dialysis programme.

There are no specific neuropathological changes directly associated with renal transplantation. However, immunosuppressive treatment predisposes these patients to a variety of bacterial, viral, fungal, and protozoal infections. Cytomegalovirus and herpes simplex are particularly common and may produce small focal inflammatory lesions. Central pontine myelinolysis may unusually occur after renal transplantation, but the cause of this is uncertain. There is some evidence that in other clinical settings this may follow correction of severe electrolyte abnormalities, particularly profound hyponatraemia.

Cardiovascular disease

Cerebral symptoms can occur in patients with severe heart failure, particularly in the elderly. Confusion, insomnia, headache, and depression are the most common features. Some patients with ventricular dysrhythmias can complain of lightheadedness, may faint, or have typical Stokes–Adams attacks. No consistent neuropathological changes have been described in these patients.

Headache is a frequent but non-specific symptom in mild or moderate systemic hypertension. Cerebral atherosclerosis is accelerated in these patients and many will develop capillary microaneurysms of branches of the middle cerebral artery. In contrast, in typical cases of malignant hypertension there is severe and increasing headache, vomiting, convulsions, and retinal changes, including papilloedema. In patients who die in the acute stage, cerebral oedema is a frequent finding, and there are diffuse petechial haemorrhages throughout the white matter, areas of microinfarction with fibrinoid necrosis of the walls of small arterioles.

The most common neurological complication of endocarditis is cerebral infarction, secondary to embolization of mitral or aortic valvular vegetations. Dilatation or rupture of arteries follows bacterial or fungal infection of the wall ('mycotic aneurysms'). Although cerebral arteries are most often affected, pulmonary mycotic aneurysms and fungal ophthalmitis are increasingly seen in drug addicts. A non-specific encephalopathy with evidence of meningism is another feature of infective endocarditis.

Some patients develop neurological symptoms after *cardiopulmonary bypass*. Intra-operative hypotension may induce ischaemic changes with postoperative confusion or behavioural changes. Focal signs such as transient hemiplegia or visual-field deficits are probably the result of air embolism. Thromboembolism is uncommon but can occur after removal of a left ventricular aneurysm with mural thromus, or excision of a thrombosed atrial appendage. Calcified debris may be released into the systemic circulation when stenotic aortic or mitral valves are replaced.

Diabetes mellitus

The commonest and most important neurological lesion in diabetes is peripheral neuropathy, and while not directly influencing mortality, is a substantial cause of morbidity. Some sign or symptom of peripheral neuropathy is almost inevitable in any elderly insulin-dependent diabetics with long-standing disease. There is no entirely satisfactory classification of this disorder but a *symmetrical sensory and motor polyneuropathy*, a *mononeuritis* involving both cranial and peripheral nerves, and an *autonomic neuropathy* are well-recognized features (see p. 1897). The primary pathology appears as *axonal degeneration* but the cause of this is not known. It is strongly suspected that microangio-pathic changes are responsible for at least some of the neuro-logical lesions. The extensive and symmetrical peripheral nerve lesions are unlikely to have a purely vascular basis but, despite a number of recent detailed biochemical studies of human sural nerve biopsies, the exact underlying abnormalities have not been determined.

Diabetes is an important risk factor for atherosclerosis, not only in the aorta and coronary arteries, but also in the cerebral circulation. Recurrent attacks of insulin-induced hypogly-caemia may induce necrosis of cerebral cortical or anterior horn neurones, but this rarely produces substantial clinical prob-lems. Occasional diabetics develop posterior column signs, sometimes described as 'pseudotabes'.

Connective tissue disease

There is no universally agreed definition of a 'connective tissue disease'. Many are clearly multisystem disorders and in some there is good evidence of an underlying *diffuse vasculitis*. In most there are immunological abnormalities, with clearly defined patterns of circulating auto-antibodies and/or evidence of immune complex deposition (see Chapter 4). In some of these disorders, a primary pathological process in a joint such as the spine induces secondary neurological change. This is particu-larly important in rheumatoid disease, where dislocation of the atlanto-axial joint can produce cervical cord signs.

Cerebral signs are well described in systemic lupus eryth-ematosus. Over 25 per cent of patients have psychotic changes at some stage in the course of their illness, and up to 20 per cent have fits or convulsions. Migraine, hemiplegia, papilloedema, ataxia, and extrapyramidal syndromes are other well-described features. Multiple areas of microinfarction in the white matter have been described, but cerebral vasculitis is uncommon. Recurrent transient ischaemic attacks and cere-bral infarcts are features of the 'anti-phospholipid antibody' syn-drome. These patients have many of the usual signs of systemic lupus but are particularly liable to recurrent arterial and venous

thromboses and mid-pregnancy abortions. Circulating anti-bodies to *phospholipids* are characteristic, but the exact cause of the coagulopathy has not been determined.

In *polyarteritis nodosa* a focal vasculitis may lead to isolated peripheral nerve lesions or a *mononeuritis multiplex*. Occasion-ally a symmetrical sensory polyneuropathy develops. Focal neurological defects, transient ischaemic attacks, dementia, and hemiplegias have all been recorded with systemic vasculitis. *Cranial (giant cell or temporal) arteritis* has a particular predilec-tion for the ciliary and ophthalmic arteries and may produce substantial ocular signs. Granulomatous angiitis of the central nervous system has superficial histological similarities to cra-nial arteritis. It affects meningeal or intracerebral arteries and arterioles, and usually presents with increasing confusion or headache. Angiography may demonstrate a beaded appear-ance, and the diagnosis can be confirmed by meningeal or stereotactic cerebral biopsy. There are no extracranial features, and the disease may respond to steroids or cyclophosphamide therapy. In some patients there is associated cerebral amyloid angiopathy (see Section 5.5). Primary neurological abnormal-ities are uncommon in conditions such as rheumatoid disease, ankylosing spondylitis, scleroderma, polymyositis, or poly-myalgia rheumatica.

25.5.6   Neurological syndromes associated with malignant disease

A variety of 'non-metastatic' neurological complications have been described in association with malignant neoplasms (Table 25.9). Both clinically and pathologically these form a hetero-geneous group and the underlying pathological mechanisms are poorly understood. The early clinical features include anxiety, depression, and loss of recent memory. Dementia, a common presenting symptom of primary tumours of the central nervous system, may also occur as a 'non-metastatic' effect.

Most patients with malignant neoplasms who develop cere-bellar signs have evidence of metastatic deposits. However,

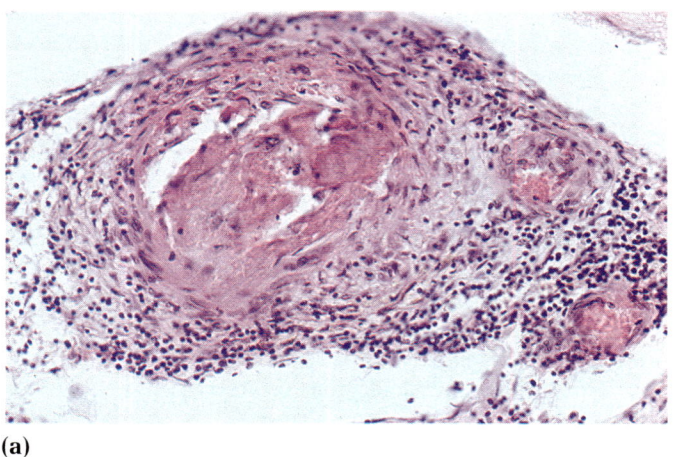

(a)

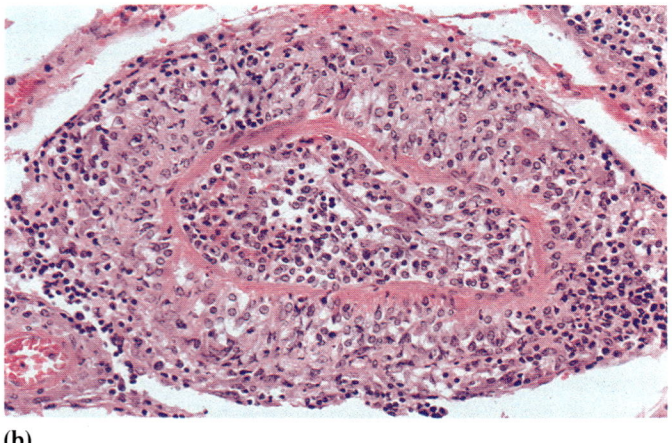

(b)

Fig. 25.44   (a) Subacute vasculitis in small cerebral arteries from a patient with systemic lupus erythematosus. (b) Florid chronic inflammatory and giant cell infiltrates in meningeal arteries of a patients with granulomatous angiitis of the central nervous system.

Table 25.9 Non-metastatic complications of malignant neoplasms in the nervous system

Complication	Clinical or pathological features
Cerebellar degeneration	Acute or subacute onset cerebellar signs, especially dysarthria and ataxia; Purkinje and some granular cell loss
Encephalitis and myelitis	Wide pattern of clinical symptoms, e.g. limbic encephalitis, brainstem signs (ophthalmoplegias, bulbar palsies, pyramidal weakness, or spinal symptoms resembling motor neurone disease); pathology—patchy perivascular inflammation with oedema and gliosis
Neuromuscular syndromes Peripheral neuropathy	Motor, sensory, or mixed; distal weakness, wasting, sensory loss, and paraesthesia; axonal loss with secondary demyelination
Myopathy (myastenic or Eaton–Lambert syndrome)	Proximal weakness; usually minimal histological abnormalities; occasionally polymyositis or dermatomyositis
Iatrogenic and infectious disease Drug-induced encephalopathies	Steroids, cytotoxic drugs, especially vincristine
Radiation necrosis Opportunistic infections	Herpes simplex encephalitis, papova virus infection (progressive multifocal encephalitis), bacteria (e.g. *Listeria*), fungi, toxoplasmosis

some patients with carcinoma of the bronchus, and less commonly the ovary or the breast, develop *acute or subacute cerebellar degeneration*. The Purkinje cells are particularly affected but other cortical neurones and the dentate nuclei can be involved. There may be associated gliosis and in some cases perivascular lymphocytic infiltration has been described. Ataxia and dysarthria are the most frequent symptoms but nystagmus, vertigo, and diplopia also occur. There are now several reports of antibodies that react with Purkinje cells in the serum of patients with this form of cerebellar degeneration. These antibodies sometimes cross-react with T-lymphocytes, and severe cerebellar degeneration is associated with T-cell lymphoma.

The *encephalomyelitic syndromes* associated with neoplastic disease produce a wide variety of clinical symptoms, largely dependent on the pattern of anatomical involvement. The underlying pathological changes include perivascular lymphocytic infiltration and oedema and neuronal necrosis. Recent memory loss, dementia, and mood disorders may be presenting cerebral signs. Changes are most frequent in the temporal lobe. Brainstem lesions also occur but cerebellar changes are rare. Spinal cord involvement may produce symptoms that mimic motor neurone disease—'carcinomatous amyotrophic lateral sclerosis'. However, it appears that classical motor neurone disease and carcinomatous myelitis are distinct pathological entities, even if there is some overlap of clinical symptoms. The cause of these forms of encephalitis and myelitis are unknown. The pathological changes are somewhat similar to viral encephalitis

but there is no direct or indirect evidence that a particular virus is implicated.

The *neuromuscular syndromes* are the commonest, but the least specific, complications of malignant tumours. Peripheral neuropathies may be motor, sensory, or mixed. The chief symptoms are distal weakness, wasting, sensory loss, and paraesthesiae (see p. 1900). Myopathic and myasthenic syndromes are well recognized in advanced malignancies but there are few, if any, histological alterations. Only the occasional patients develop classical dermatomyositis/polymyositis, with the characteristic cutaneous changes and dense inflammatory infiltrates (see p. 2158). Opportunistic infective agents in the central nervous system include *herpes simplex*, *papova virus* (progressive multifocal leukoencephalopathy), a variety of fungi, and toxoplasmosis (p. 1839).

25.5.7 Drug-induced neurotoxicity

There are comparatively few drugs that cause substantial neurological changes, at least in comparison with the wide range of toxic affects seen in the hepatic, renal, and cardiovascular systems. Although the blood–brain barrier excludes many therapeutic agents, the barrier effect is lost when tumours develop or there is diffuse meningitis.

It is notoriously difficult to study the precise neuropathological changes associated with many drug reactions. Liver, renal, or even cardiac biopsy can be justified on clinical grounds in many situations but this is seldom possible in the central nervous system. Post-mortem autolysis may obscure some of the underlying pathological changes in patients who die, and it can be difficult to distinguish drug-induced alterations from those caused by systemic disease. Many drugs induce a peripheral neuropathy (see p. 1900) and, as nerve biopsy is a relatively innocuous procedure, detailed histological and electron microscopic studies are possible.

Relatively few drugs induce changes that are restricted to the central nervous system (Table 25.10). The neurotoxic effects of cytostatic preparations are of growing importance and severe nausea and vomiting are common acute side-effects. *Intrathecal methotrexate* may cause more severe neurological symptoms and occasionally a *necrotizing leucoencephalopathy* with associated vascular changes. Early reports suggested that focal demyelination with ventricular dilatation occurred in a substantial proportion of leukaemic children treated prophylactically with cranial radiation and methotrexate. This has not been confirmed but it is very likely that some intellectual impairment does occur in young children treated in this way. *Vincristine* induces axonal abnormalities, and the clinical signs of neurotoxicity include motor weakness and loss of reflexes, parasthaesiae, peripheral, autonomic, and cranial nerve palsies. In most patients the neurotoxicity is dose related, but occasionally an acute reaction can develop shortly after treatment has commenced. Ultrastructural studies suggest that the drug, or one of its metabolites, combines with a protein associated with microtubular structures within axons, forming large abnormal crystalline masses.

Table 25.10   Neurotoxic drugs

Drug	Clinical effects	Neuropathology
Therapeutic agents		
Bismuth	Mood alterations, confusion, dysarthria, coma	Neuronal necrosis of hippocampus and cerebellum
Clioquinol	Subacute myelo-opticoneuritis (SMON)	Clinical and experimental evidence of degeneration in optic pathways and posterior columns, especially cervical cord
Cytotoxic agents		
Methotrexate	Confusion, ataxia, fits, meningitis	Necrotizing leucoencephalopathy, fibrinoid necrosis of vessels, synergistic effect of cranial irradiation
Vincristine	Peripheral neuropathy and myopathy	Axonal abnormalities—combines with microtubular protein to form crystalline masses; neuronal and axonal degeneration after intrathecal injection
Gold	Renal disease, peripheral neuropathy, encephalopathy	Few detailed descriptions
Hexachlorophane	Percutaneous absorption, especially in premature infants; irritability, convulsions	Swelling of myelin sheaths, especially in brainstem
Isoniazid	Peripheral neuropathy	Inhibition of pyridoxal phosphate kinase; axonal damage; experimental evidence of myelin swelling in central nervous system
Metronidazole	Ataxia, convulsions, peripheral neuropathy	Multiple focal spongiform lesions, especially vestibular and cochlear areas
Oral contraceptives	Migraine, involuntary movement	Cerebrovascular thrombosis
Addictive drugs		
Amphetamines and cocaine	Hypertension, convulsions, sudden death	Haemorrhage from berry aneurysm; occasionally intracerebral haemorrhage
Barbiturates	Drowsiness, coma	No characteristic pathology
Opiates	Coma, convulsions, sudden death	Ischaemic necrosis of neurones; infectious encephalitis and ophthalmitis, especially *Candida*
Solvents (especially hexanes)	Distal weakness, loss of ankle reflexes, paraesthesiae	Clinical and experimental evidence of axonal swelling due to accumulation of neurofilaments

Because of its activity against anaerobic bacteria, *metronidazole* is increasingly used in patients with postoperative infections, particularly abdominal sepsis. It can penetrate the blood–brain barrier and should not be used in patients with active neurological disorders. Side-effects are uncommon, but prolonged treatment can induce a *peripheral neuropathy*. Dizziness, ataxia, and transient convulsions have been reported in occasional patients treated with high doses. Older *bismuth* preparations occasionally caused encephalopathies, sometimes with dysarthria and coma, and there was some evidence of neuronal necrosis in the few patients examined post-mortem. Bismuth chelates are now popular for the treatment of peptic ulcers but as yet no definite neurological symptoms have been observed. Nausea, vomiting, headache, and migraine are side-effects of *combined oral contraceptives*. Occasional patients develop involuntary movements and there is an increased incidence of cerebral arterial thrombosis, especially in smokers, at age 35 years or older.

Subarachnoid and intracerebral haemorrhage are rare complications of both *amphetamine and cocaine abuse*. In most fatal cases, berry aneurysms have been detected at post-mortem and it is presumed that acute hypertension precipitates their rupture. Coronary arterial intimal thickening and ischaemic heart disease are other complications of prolonged cocaine use. There are no primary neuropathological changes that can be ascribed to either *barbiturates or opiates*. Careful post-mortem studies of

heroin addicts have identified areas of ischaemic necrosis within the cerebrum. Meningitis and ophthalmitis are increasingly seen in addicts who inject intravenously. Septicaemia may follow directly from injection of contaminated material, from septic thrombophlebitis or bacterial endocarditis. A particular pattern of peripheral neuropathy has been identified in gluesniffers and is ascribed to the solvent n-*hexane*. The primary abnormality is in axons, where focal accumulations of abnormal neurofilaments can be identified.

25.5.8   Metallic and industrial neurotoxins

Greek and Roman physicians recognized the neurological symptoms associated with the mining of lead or the use of mercury in the purification of silver. Some of these syndromes were described in detail in the seventeenth century by Ramazzini—the founding father of occupational medicine. Many industrial and agrochemicals have neurotoxic effects (Table 25.11). The agents responsible for these are generally well defined and, as voluntary and statutory safety measures are instituted, these disorders are becoming less common. However, safety regulations are of variable stringency in different countries and from time to time an unusual sequence of events may lead to unexpected clusters of new cases. Furthermore, although many novel industrial agents are carefully screened by toxicologists, it

Table 25.11 Metallic and industrial neurotoxins

Agent	Route of exposure	Clinical effects	Neuropathology
Aluminium	Renal dialysis fluids	Speech disorder, epilepsy, progressive dementia	Few detailed reports; glial reaction with some evidence of neuronal loss in the cerebral cortex
Arsenic	Pesticides	Acutely: GI disturbances Chronically: peripheral neuropathy, encephalopathy, hyperkeratosis, pigmentation	Few detailed reports
Lead (organic)	Petrol (tetraethyl lead)	Sleep disturbances, psychoses	Cerebral oedema and congestion; ?experimental evidence of neuronal necrosis
Lead (inorganic)	Paints, battery manufacturing, etc.	Children: encephalopathy, ataxia, fits Adults: anaemia and colic, peripheral motor neuropathy	Cerebral oedema and congestion axonal degeneration and demyelination
Mercury (organic)	Seed fungicides; methylation of inorganic mercury in food chain	Paraesthesiae, ataxia, concentric constriction of visual fields	Neuronal necrosis probably secondary to inhibition of neuronal protein synthesis
Mercury (inorganic)	Industrial exposure—historically in purification of silver and hat felting; now chloralkali plants	Psychological symptoms, coarse tremor, gingivitis	Less extensive neuronal changes but underlying mechanism as in organic mercury
Organophosphates	Insecticides, contaminated cooking oil	Acutely: anti-cholinesterase effects Chronically: few changes apart from peripheral neuropathy	Experimental evidence of 'distal degeneration of axons'

is more difficult to demonstrate more toxic effects in the nervous system than in other organs.

Lead and *mercury* are the metals that have the strongest neurotoxic effects in man. The many sources of inorganic lead poisoning include paints and lead-based pigments, battery and solder manufacturing, home-brewed alcohols, and the production of fuel additives. When lead is absorbed it is distributed widely through the body and in children is laid down in the metaphysis of long bones. In cases of acute poisoning, there may be marked cerebral oedema and congestion with associated areas of haemorrhage both in the grey and white matter. It is strongly suspected that lead is in some way toxic to endothelium, particularly in children or young animals. The patterns of inorganic lead poisoning in adults and in children are rather different. Adults develop abdominal colic and an anaemia with basophilic stippling of red cells. A peripheral motor neuropathy is characteristic and is most prominent in muscles that are used frequently. In contrast, children develop cerebral signs with ataxia and convulsions.

Tetraethyl lead is added to petrol as an 'anti-knock' agent and ensures a smoother pattern of combustion. Occasional workers engaged in its manufacture or storage have developed reactions varying from sleep disturbances to psychoses and acute cerebral oedema. Tetraethyl lead is also responsible for the psychological symptoms seen in habitual petrol syphoners! Cases such as these demonstrated that tetraethyl lead was toxic and, as it is emitted in vehicle exhaust fumes, raised the possibility of more widespread environmental contamination. The lead content in the atmosphere around lead smelting plants or close to major highways is significantly higher than in rural areas. Because lead appears to damage the developing nervous system selectively, surveys have been conducted in Australia, Germany, the United States, and in Great Britain to determine whether children in urban areas are at risk from lead-induced neurotoxicity. The results that have been published to date have not demonstrated any significant neurological disabilities that can be ascribed to lead exposure. However, when correction is made for a variety of sociological variables, intellectual development is inversely related to postnatal blood lead concentrations.

Mercury is a potent neurotoxin, both in the organic and inorganic form. It combines avidly with disulphide bonds, particularly in cell membranes, to form stable compounds known as mercaptans. There is also good experimental evidence that mercury impairs ribosomal protein synthesis in neurones. Organic compounds such as *methyl mercury* are lipid-soluble and enter the central nervous system more easily than inorganic mercury. Although the precise patterns of toxicity with organic and inorganic mercury are rather different, the underlying biochemical mechanisms are probably similar.

Historically, mercury was used to purify precious metals such as gold and silver. Fur treated with mercury was ideal for the manufacture of hats, and the symptoms seen in these workers—coarse tremor, emotional lability, and paranoia—prompted the expression 'mad as a hatter'. Mercury is still used in chloralkali plants during the production of sodium hydroxide. In a celebrated outbreak of mercury poisoning in Minamata Bay in Japan inorganic mercury was discharged into a land-locked sea basin, methylated by bacteria, and passed in the food chain to edible fish. Local fishermen developed organic mercury poisoning with prominent cerebellar signs and concentric constriction of the visual field. A larger outbreak of methyl mercury poisoning in Iraq resulted from the consumption of bread made from seed corn treated with an organic mercurial fungicide.

Organophosphorous compounds are used extensively in the

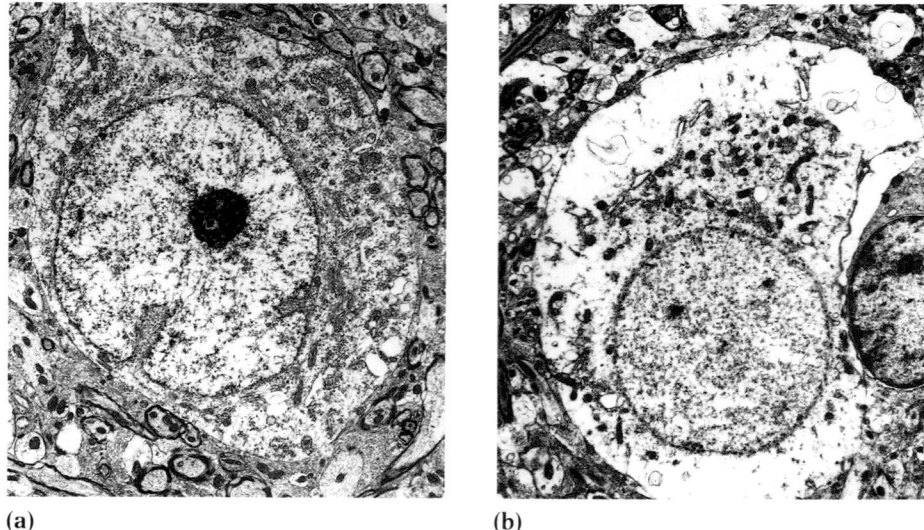

(a)   **(b)**

Fig. 25.45 Inorganic mercury toxicity. (a) There is a slight swelling of the cytoplasm of a neurone suggesting impairment of the sodium pump mechanism at the cell membrane. (b) Advanced cytoplasmic swelling and necrosis secondary to cell membrane damage.

manufacture of insecticides. These compounds have a strong anti-cholinesterase effect and acute toxicity is associated with headache, abdominal cramps, vomiting, and constriction of the pupils. Fortunately, these can be rapidly corrected with atropine-like compounds and there are no long-term effects. Chronic exposure to these compounds may produce peripheral neuropathy.

Arsenic is now rarely used therapeutically but it is incorporated into some pesticides. Some patients treated for syphilis with organic arsenic compounds developed a florid encephalopathy with a high mortality rate. This is extremely rare in occupational exposure, where a troublesome peripheral neuropathy is the major problem.

25.5.9 Further reading

Asbury, A. K. (1988). Understanding diabetic neuropathy. *New England Journal of Medicine* **319**, 577–8.

Cavanagh, J. B. (1979). Metallic toxicity and the nervous system. In *Recent advances in neuropathology* (ed. W. T. Smith and J. B. Cavanagh), pp. 247–75. Churchill Livingstone, Edinburgh.

Charness, M. E., Simon, R. P., and Greenberg, D. A. (1989). Ethanol and the nervous system. *New England Journal of Medicine* **321**, 442–54.

Cregler, L. L. and Mark, H. (1986). Medical complications of cocaine abuse. *New England Journal of Medicine* **315**, 1495–1500.

Duchen, L. W. and Jacobs, J. M. (1984). Nutritional deficiencies and metabolic disorders. In *Greenfield's neuropathology* (ed. J. Hume-Adams, J. A. N. Corsellis, and L. W. Duchen) (4th edn), pp. 573–95. Edward Arnold, London.

Fischer, J. E. (1985). Portal systemic encephalopathy. In *Liver and biliary disease* (ed. R. Wright, G. H. Millward Sadler, K. G. M. M. Alberti, and S. Karran), pp. 1245–82. Baillière Tindall, London.

Harper, C. (1983). The incidence of Wernicke's encephalopathy in Australia—a neuropathological study of 131 cases. *Journal of Neurology, Neurosurgery and Psychiatry* **46**, 593–8.

Harris, E. N., Gharavi, A. E., Asherson, R. A., Boly, M. L., and Hughes, G. R. (1984). Cerebral infarction in systemic lupus: association with cardiolipin antibodies. *Clinical and Experimental Rheumatology* **2**, 47–51.

Henson, R. A. and Urich, H. (1982). *Cancer and the nervous system: the neurological manifestations of systemic malignant disease*. Blackwell Scientific Publications, Oxford.

Lewis, P. D. (1985). Neuropathological effects of alcohol on the developing nervous system. *Alcohol and Alcoholism* **20**, 195–200.

Malpas, J. S. and Whitehouse, J. M. A. (1980). Cytostatic and immunosuppressive drugs. In *Meyer's side effects of drugs* (ed. M. N. G. Dukes) (9th edn), p. 738. Excerpta Medica, Amsterdam.

McMichael, A. J., Baghurst, P. A., Wigg, N. R., Vimpani, G. V., Robertson, E. F., and Roberts, R. J. (1988). Port Pirie Cohort study: environmental exposure to lead and childrens ability at the age of four years. *New England Journal of Medicine* **319**, 468–75.

Moore, P. M. and Fauci, A. S. (1981). Neurologic manifestations of systemic vasculitis. *American Journal of Medicine* **71**, 517–24.

Norenberg, M. D. (1981). The astrocyte in liver disease. In *Advances in cellular neurobiology* (ed. S. Federoff and L. Hertz), pp. 304–52. Academic Press, London.

Poskitt, E. M. E. (1984). Foetal alcohol syndrome. *Alcohol and Alcoholism* **19**, 159–65.

Torvik, A., Lindboe, C. F., and Rogde, S. (1982). Brain lesions in alcoholics: a neuropathological study with clinical correlations. *Journal of the Neurological Sciences* **56**, 233–48.

Walton, J. (1985). Paraneoplastic neurological syndromes. In *Brain's disease of the nervous system* (6th edn), pp. 486–9. Oxford University Press.

25.6 Demyelinating diseases

R. O. Weller

By definition, the term demyelination implies selective destruction of myelin sheaths with preservation of the axons. Demyelination is a feature of a number of different diseases of the central nervous system (Table 25.12) and of the peripheral nervous system (see Section 25.9). Of these diseases, *multiple sclerosis* is the most important in Britain, North America, much of Europe, and Australasia. Because of its chronic, progressive disabling course, with many patients living more than 20 years with the disease, multiple sclerosis is a significant medical and sociological problem, particularly in areas of high prevalence. In other diseases, such as *post-infectious encephalomyelitis* or *progressive multifocal leukoencephalopathy*, demyelination is related to *virus infections*. These disorders are not as common as multiple sclerosis and the clinical course does not show the relapsing and remitting features of multiple sclerosis. Demyelination can also be related to *toxic disorders* and to defects of lipid metabolism in the *leucodystrophies* (Table 25.12).

Demyelinating diseases affect mainly the white matter of the cerebral hemispheres, brainstem, cerebellum, and spinal cord. Those demyelinating diseases which affect the central nervous system do not involve the myelin of the peripheral nervous system, and similarly central nervous system myelin is virtually unaffected by demyelinating diseases of peripheral nerves. Part of the reason may be the chemical differences between central and peripheral nervous system myelin, particularly with regard to the proteins.

25.6.1 Normal myelin

Myelination begins in the spinal cord and brainstem during the second half of gestation, and at birth the cerebral hemispheres are still virtually free of myelin. Soon after birth, however, the internal capsules become myelinated, and myelin forms in the rest of the cerebral hemispheres and cerebellum during the first 6 months of postnatal life. Although by the age of 6 years myelination is almost complete, it continues slowly into the second decade.

Oligodendrocytes are the myelin-forming cells in the central nervous system. Each oligodendrocyte myelinates short segments of several axons by compaction of cell membranes derived from processes wrapped around the axons. Segments of

Table 25.12 Demyelinating diseases affecting the central nervous system

Multiple sclerosis
Post-infectious or post-vaccinial encephalomyelitis
Progressive multifocal leucoencephalopathy
Intoxications
Leucodystrophies

myelin formed by each oligodendrocyte are separated by *nodes of Ranvier* along the length of the axon. Conduction in myelinated fibres proceeds by *saltatory conduction* similar to that in the peripheral nervous system.

In histological preparations, myelin in the brain can be visualized in frozen sections by polarized light, as it is birefringent. Several stains, such as *luxol fast blue* and *haematoxylin-based myelin stains*, are used to identify myelin in paraffin sections (Weller 1984). The axons encompassed by the myelin can be stained by silver stains such a *Palmgren or Bodian*, or depicted by immunocytochemical techniques for *neurofilament proteins*. Electron microscopically, myelin has typical 12 nm periodicity with osmiophilic major and minor dense lines separated by unstained regions.

Some 40 per cent of myelin is water and 70 per cent of its dry weight is lipid, consisting mainly of cholesterol, phospholipids, and galactolipids in the proportions $4:4:2$ (Cuzner 1980). The other 30 per cent of dry weight is protein, of which proteolipid protein and myelin basic protein form 60–80 per cent. Proteolipid protein is a 30 000 Da hydrophobic protein residing mainly in the lipid layers of myelin. Myelin basic protein, on the other hand, is an 18 000 Da hydrophilic protein which forms part of the inner, or cytoplasmic, aspect of the compacted cell membrane (the major dense line). A small amount of the *Wolfgram protein*, 45 000–47 000 Da, is also present in mature myelin. Experimental studies have shown that an *allergic encephalomyelitis* (EAE) can be caused by the injection of myelin basic protein; this encephalogenic protein induces cell-mediated immunity to central nervous system myelin. Injection of *galactocerebroside*, on the other hand, results in the production of demyelinating antibodies (Hallpike *et al.* 1983).

When myelin breakdown occurs, lamellated myelin debris is ingested by invading macrophages, the proteins are degraded, and cholesterol within the myelin is esterified to form sudanophilic globules of cholesterol ester. Such lipid droplets can be stained in frozen sections by Sudan dyes or Oil Red O and this is a useful technique for detecting recent (i.e. 1 week to 3–4 months) myelin breakdown. Gradually the lipid debris is removed and macrophages disappear from the site of myelin damage. Remyelination in the central nervous system is not as effective as in the peripheral nervous system, and although it occurs in experimental systems, remyelination in multiple sclerosis and other human demyelinating diseases probably occurs to only a minor degree.

25.6.2 Multiple sclerosis

Age, incidence, and epidemiology

The peak onset of multiple sclerosis is from early adolescence until 30 years of age; its incidence thereafter declines and onset of the disease is uncommon after 60 years of age. In areas of high incidence, multiple sclerosis has a female:male incidence of $1:1$ but this rises to $2.8:1$ in regions of low incidence.

There is a distinct geographical distribution of multiple sclerosis (Matthews *et al.* 1985) (Fig. 25.46). It is a disease of temperate climates and is most prevalent in northern Europe,

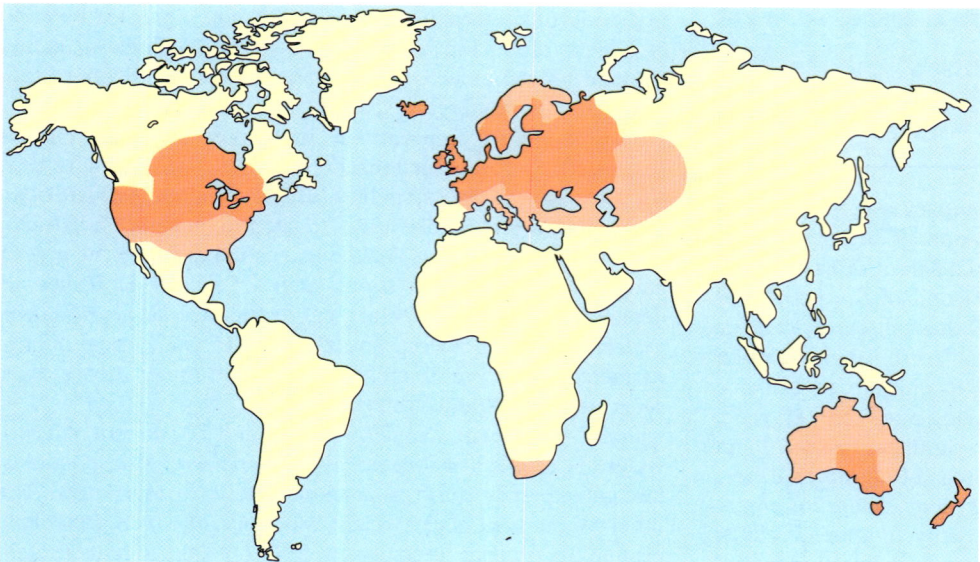

Fig. 25.46 Geographical distribution of multiple sclerosis. Red areas are of high incidence, orange areas are of intermediate incidence, and yellow areas are of low incidence or areas for which there are no figures available. (Drawn after Weller 1990, with permission).

the northern United States, southern Australia and New Zealand. The highest annual incidence, of 9.3 per 100 000, is in the Orkney Islands north of Scotland. A distinct north–south decline in incidence has been recorded in Europe and in the United States. Rochester, Minnesota has an annual incidence of multiple sclerosis of 3.2 per 100 000 whereas in New Orleans it is only 0.4 per 100 000. This difference in annual incidence (new cases occurring per year) is also reflected in the prevalance rates (the number of cases living on a particular date) of 144 per 100 000 in north-east Scotland and 10 per 100 000 in New Orleans. In the southern hemisphere, multiple sclerosis is more common in Tasmania than in Sydney. Individuals moving from high-risk to low-risk areas before the age of 15 adopt the low risk of multiple sclerosis. There is a marked racial difference in susceptibility to multiple sclerosis; the disease is rare in Bantu, Eskimos, and Oriental races. In northern Europe, most cases of multiple sclerosis are associated with *HLA DW2* suggesting some genetic basis for the disease.

Clinical features and investigations

The clinical features of multiple sclerosis are very varied (Matthews *et al.* 1985). Most patients present with a single neurological deficit which then remits. In 50 per cent of cases the neurological deficit involves limb weakness, whereas visual disturbances such as blurring of vision, blindness, or diplopia herald the onset of multiple sclerosis in 30 per cent of cases. The signs and symptoms remit, but relapses occur at varying intervals following the initial attack. Despite the remissions, patients are left with residual neurological deficits which accumulate following repeated episodes. Thus, in long-standing multiple sclerosis, patients exhibit ataxia, spasticity, motor weakness, sensory disturbances, and bladder dysfunction. Occasionally,

severe cases with an onset in early adult life run a progressive course from the onset and patients die without remission. More indolent chronic cases occur in middle age and may also run a progressive course. A number of distinct patterns of onset are recognized, for example *Devic's disease* in which there is *retrobulbar neuritis* and *severe spinal cord involvement*.

In the rare cases of multiple sclerosis dying in the acute stage, death may be due to respiratory paralysis and bronchopneumonia. In long-standing cases of multiple sclerosis, patients may die from causes unrelated to multiple sclerosis but they may also die from the effects of the disease, with pneumonia, or septicaemia from pyelonephritis and sepsis from bed sores.

There is no clinical investigation that is 100 per cent reliable for the diagnosis of multiple sclerosis. *Oligoclonal bands of immunoglobulin* are found in the cerebrospinal fluid in some 90 per cent cases of multiple sclerosis (Hallpike *et al.* 1983). *Plaques of demyelination* in the optic nerve may be detected by swelling and inflammation of the disc (*retrobulbar neuritis*) or by optic atrophy. Such plaques can also be detected electrophysiologically through abnormalities in visual evoked potentials. Although many of the axons may be preserved in multiple sclerosis plaques, loss of myelin causes slowing of conduction velocities. The measurement of visual evoked potentials from retina to occipital cortex will detect the slowing caused by multiple sclerosis plaques in the optic nerve. Measurement of auditory evoked potentials can be used to detect plaques in the brainstem.

Acute and chronic multiple sclerosis plaques can be detected by *CT scan* or, more reliably, by *magnetic resonance imaging* (MRI) (Fig. 25.47) (Huber *et al.* 1988). However, it is not possible on these images alone to be certain that the lesions are multiple sclerosis plaques; they may be confused with small infarcts.

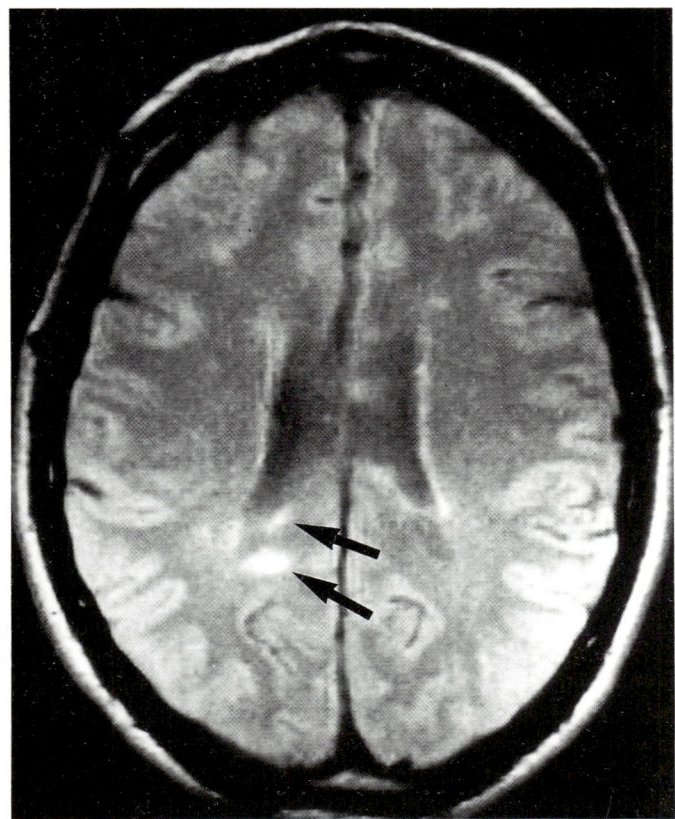

Fig. 25.47 Magnetic resonance imaging of multiple sclerosis plaques in the periventricular white matter (arrows). (Kindly supplied by Dr P. Cook.)

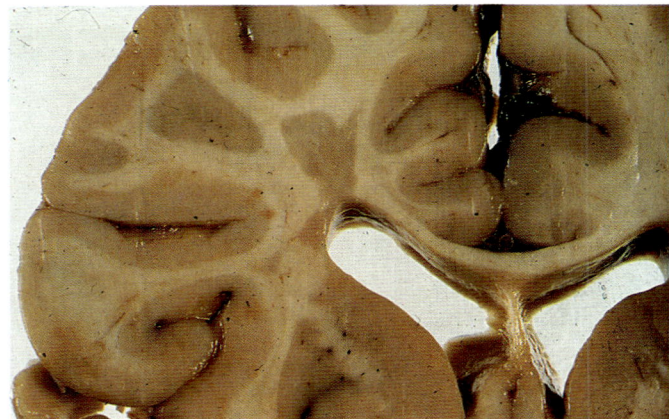

Fig. 25.48 Chronic multiple sclerosis plaque seen as a sharply defined grey area in the white matter just above the lateral ventricle in a coronal slice of cerebral hemisphere.

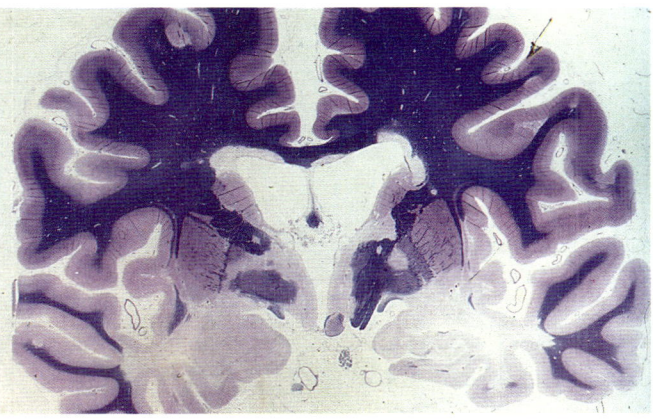

Fig. 25.49 Coronal slice of brain stained for myelin (dark blue). Multiple unstained demyelinated plaques are seen especially around the lateral ventricles, in both temporal lobes, scattered through central grey matter, and in the cortex (upper left). (Klüver–Barrera stain.)

Pathology

Most of the information regarding the pathology of multiple sclerosis is derived from the study of post-mortem brains. As most patients with the disease survive for many years, the commonest finding at post-mortem is *multiple sclerotic grey gliotic plaques* (Fig. 25.48) distributed throughout the cerebral hemispheres, brainstem, cerebellum, and spinal cord. It is from this appearance, described more than 100 years ago, that the disease derives its name. The distribution of plaques is a historical record of the previous episodes of the disease.

Occasionally, patients die within a few months of the onset of multiple sclerosis and acute active multiple sclerosis plaques are seen.

Examination of a fixed brain from a patient with multiple sclerosis may reveal some cerebral atrophy, but in many cases the external aspects of the cerebral hemispheres appear to be normal. Shrunken grey plaques may be seen on the surface of the optic nerves, the chiasma, or on the surface of the pons, medulla, and spinal cord, particularly if the leptomeninges are stripped away. When the brain is sectioned, it is seen that the majority of multiple sclerosis plaques are deep within the substance of the brain (Figs 25.48, 25.49). Distribution of the plaques is asymmetrical, with the optic nerves, chiasma,

periventricular regions, and the spinal cord most commonly involved. In one survey (Brownell and Hughes 1962), 40 per cent of plaques in the cerebral hemispheres were around the lateral ventricles; 22 per cent were in the frontal regions, 15 per cent parietal, 12 per cent temporal, and only 1 per cent in the occipital lobes. The majority of plaques (74 per cent) involved the white matter, 17 per cent involved the cortex and white matter, 5 per cent were small plaques restricted to the cerebral cortex, and 4 per cent were seen in the central grey matter areas of the cerebral hemispheres. Plaques of demyelination are frequently present in the periaqueductal regions of the midbrain and small plaques (3–4 mm diameter) are often found in the anterior parts of the pons and in the white matter of the middle cerebellar peduncles. In the spinal cord, the plaques may be circular or wedge-shaped and sited laterally in the white matter of the cord.

In the majority of cases, the multiple sclerosis plaques have

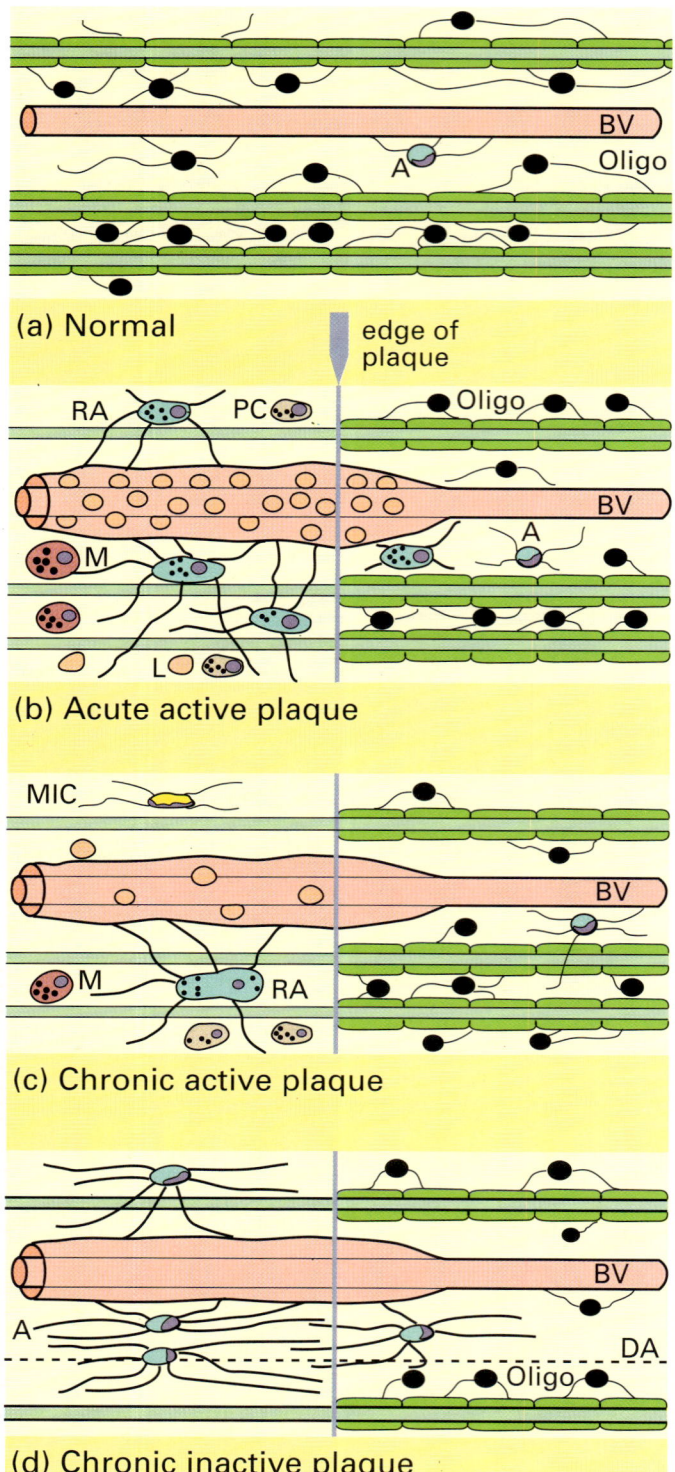

(a) Normal

(b) Acute active plaque

(c) Chronic active plaque

(d) Chronic inactive plaque

sharply defined borders but in some patients, often those who exhibit dementia, the whole of the cerebral white matter is involved and appears shrunken, grey, and almost translucent and gelatinous. This is the *Schilder's type* of multiple sclerosis.

Ballo's concentric sclerosis (Vinken and Bruyn 1970) is a rare type of multiple sclerosis in which bands of demyelination alternate with bands of preserved myelin.

Acute multiple sclerosis plaques are much less common than the old grey chronic sclerotic plaques. The acute plaques are soft, yellow, and granular due to the high content of disrupted myelin lipid within them.

Histology

It is from the histological and cytological study of multiple sclerosis plaques that most information has been gained regarding the pathogenesis of the lesions. The appearances range from the acute active plaques to chronic inactive (burnt-out) plaques. The acute active plaques are characterized by active myelin breakdown and infiltration by lymphocytes, plasma cells, and macrophages. Chronic, inactive (burnt-out) plaques, on the other hand, are sharply defined from the surrounding white matter and are composed of compacted astrocyte processes and reduced numbers of axons; the plaque is devoid of myelin and oligodendrocytes. Intermediate, chronic active plaques have a rim of lymphocyte, plasma cell, and macrophage infiltration in an area of active myelin breakdown at the periphery of the plaque. The histological appearances in the different phases of multiple sclerosis are summarized in Fig. 25.50.

Acute active plaques

In common with most multiple sclerosis plaques, these are sharply defined areas of demyelination seen best in sections stained by myelin techniques such as *Klüver–Barrera*. As axons enter the plaque from the surrounding myelinated white matter, they lose their myelin sheaths. Evidence of active myelin breakdown is present, with large numbers of foamy macrophages containing globular droplets of cholesterol ester. Intense perivascular lymphocyte and plasma cell accumulation may be seen at the edges and in the central regions of the plaque (Fig. 25.51). The lymphocytes are mainly T-cells with T-suppressor–cytotoxic cells in the perivascular regions and T-helper cells

Fig. 25.50 A diagrammatic summary of the different phases of multiple sclerosis. (a) Normal brain. (b) Acute active plaque showing perivascular lymphocyte and macrophage accumulation with reactive astrocytosis accompanying the demyelination. The plaque is on the left. (c) Chronic active plaque showing residual lymphocytes, macrophages, and reactive astrocytes in the demyelinated plaque (left). (d) Chronic inactive plaque showing fibrosis around the vessel, and gliosis with thickened astrocyte processes surrounding the demyelinated axons. Loss of axons in the plaque is represented by an interrupted line. Oligodendrocytes, present in the white matter surrounding the plaque (right), are lost from the plaque itself. Abbreviations: Oligo, oligodendrocyte; BV, blood vessel; A, astrocyte; RA, reactive astrocyte; PC, plasma cell; M, macrophage; L, lymphocyte; MIC, microglia cell; DA, degenerated axon.

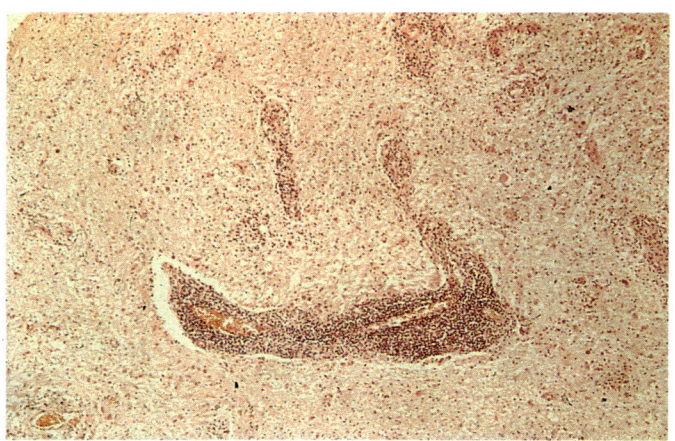

Fig. 25.51 Acute multiple sclerosis. There is perivascular cuffing by lymphocytes and macrophages in the centre of the plaque. Inflammatory cells have also invaded the tissue away from the vessel.

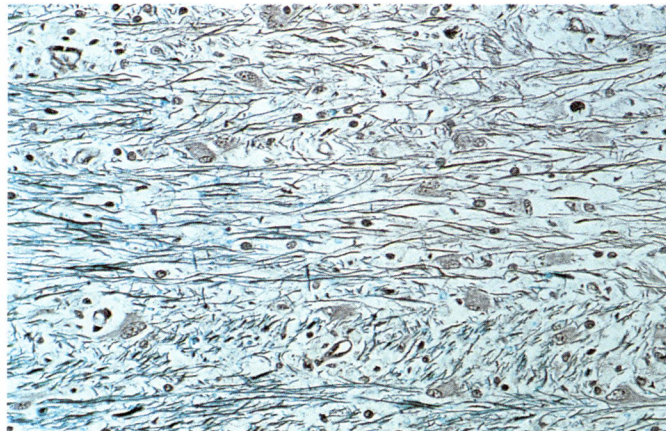

Fig. 25.52 The edge of a chronic multiple sclerosis plaque showing axons (stained black) passing from left to right. On the left side they are coated by green-blue myelin, but within the plaque (right) they have lost their myelin sheaths. (Palmgren luxol fast blue stain.)

away from the vessels towards the edges of the plaques, and in the adjacent white matter (Traugott *et al.* 1983). Many of the plasma cells secrete IgG but some produce IgA (Esiri 1980). The perivascular accumulation of inflammatory cells is mainly around veins but is sometimes also seen around arteries. In addition to the myelin breakdown and inflammation, large numbers of plump, reactive astrocytes are seen, with many thick processes extending from their cell bodies. Such astrocytes interweave among the axons that traverse the plaque (Weller 1984). Oligodendrocytes are difficult to identify in these active lesions but many, if not the majority, are probably destroyed at this stage (Fig. 25.50b).

Chronic inactive (burnt-out) plaques

These plaques (Fig. 25.50) are the most common lesions seen at post-mortem in patients dying with multiple sclerosis. They are again areas of demyelination sharply defined from the surrounding white matter (Fig. 25.48). As axons pass from normal white matter into the plaque, they completely lose their myelin sheaths (Fig. 25.52) and become surrounded by compacted astrocyte processes. There is almost a complete lack of oligodendrocytes within the chronic plaques and, although macrophages and lymphocytes may also be absent, the evidence of past inflammation is seen in the fibrosis of perivascular tissues around arteries and veins.

Chronic active plaques

Chronic active plaques (Fig. 25.50) are macroscopically very similar in appearance to chronic inactive plaques (Fig. 25.48). Histologically, however, they are characterized by continuing myelin breakdown at the edges with foamy macrophages, lymphocytes, microglial cells, and reactive astrocytes accompanying the breakdown of myelin at the periphery of the plaque.

Some loss of axons inevitably occurs from chronic multiple

sclerosis plaques, but many axons are still preserved; they can be stained by axon techniques, such as Bodian and Palmgren stains (Fig. 25.52), or by the use of antibodies to neurofilament proteins in immunocytochemical techniques. Although the plaques themselves do not respect the boundaries of the long tracts in the spinal cord, such as the corticospinal tracts and the dorsal columns, some degeneration in these tracts is often seen due to axon loss from plaques up and down the cord.

Pathophysiological correlations

There are many problems associated with correlation of the clinical features, physiological findings, and pathological observations in multiple sclerosis (Matthews *et al.* 1985). Although the plaques of demyelination can be mapped throughout the brain at post-mortem, the distribution may bear little relationship to the clinical course of the disease. Some patients may show significant disability with few plaques and others no disability with large numbers of plaques. The other major problem is that it is impossible to reconcile many of the clinical features of multiple sclerosis with the view that brain function is initially disturbed by demyelination and later by loss of axons by degeneration. Part of the difficulty is due to the inability to investigate the physiological function of patients during life and the even greater problem of correlating any physiological findings directly with the pathology, as the patient may live for many years following investigation.

Much of the research on the physiological effects of demyelination has been carried out on peripheral nerves and the results extrapolated to the central nervous system. Thus, it is assumed that demyelination causes slowing of conduction or failure of impulse conduction as axons cross the demyelination plaque. Demyelination obviously occurs in multiple sclerosis, and there is evidence from visual evoked potentials that slowing of conduction occurs in optic nerve plaques. This does not explain, however, why the neurological defects in the acute stages of the onset or relapse of multiple sclerosis partially, or almost completely, recover subsequently.

There is no evidence for significant remyelination in multiple sclerosis, so re-establishment of the myelin sheath cannot explain the return of function. However, it may be that the central nervous system adapts to the altered conduction patterns induced by the plaque and that, following this adaptation, function returns.

Pathogenesis of multiple sclerosis

Many experimental models of demyelination have been devised although none can be exactly equated with multiple sclerosis. Perhaps the nearest model is that of *experimental allergic encephalomyelitis* (EAE) induced by the injection of central nervous system myelin (Hallpike *et al.* 1983). Plaques of demyelination occur in the central nervous system in chronic relapsing EAE and are accompanied by lymphocyte and plasma cell infiltration, similar, in many ways, to multiple sclerosis. However, although the histological features of multiple sclerosis suggest that myelin breakdown is due to an immune mechanism, no aetiological agent has so far been identified. Genetic data indicate that multiple sclerosis may be due to an auto-immune process and the epidemiological findings suggest that the triggering agent may be environmental and geographically restricted.

Remyelination is a feature of many of the experimental models of demyelination such as EAE, but remyelination in multiple sclerosis does not occur to any significant degree. In experimental demyelination induced by the injection of toxins such as *cuprizone* (Ludwin 1980), remyelination proceeds once the toxin has been withdrawn and is preceded by multiplication of oligodendrocytes. This emphasizes the possibility that the lack of remyelination in multiple sclerosis may be due to the destruction of oligodendrocytes within the plaques.

The role of astrocytes within multiple sclerosis plaques and the part they play in the return of function are unclear.

25.6.3   Other demyelinating diseases

Demyelination occurs in a number of disorders of the human central nervous system but, unlike multiple sclerosis, the cause of the demyelination is known or the lesions are associated with known metabolic, toxic, or infective disorders. Much of the interest of these diseases stems from the desire to elucidate the mechanisms of demyelination in multiple sclerosis and to use other demyelinating diseases of known cause as models.

Acute post-infectious or post-vaccinial encephalomyelitis

This disease develops several days or up to 3 weeks after a viral infection or vaccination. Patients show the clinical signs of encephalitis with fever, seizures, and focal neurological disturbances. The illness occurs particularly after infection with measles, varicella zoster, and influenza virus or other respiratory tract infections. It may also follow vaccination for smallpox

or rabies. Most patients recover but in those who die, widespread perivascular infiltration by lymphocytes, monocytes, and plasma cells is seen around blood vessels in the grey and white matter of the brain. Perivascular zones of myelin destruction, 1–2 mm in diameter, are seen, in which the axons are relatively well preserved (Weller 1990). A fulminating acute haemorrhagic leucoencephalitis may also occur.

Progressive multifocal leucoencephalopathy (PML)

This term very adequately describes the pathology in this disease. On CT scan, patients with PML show multiple areas of decreased tissue density in the white matter of the cerebral hemispheres and sometimes in the brainstem. The disease presents with progressive dementia or neurological deficit and is usually seen in patients with Hodgkin's disease or other lymphomas, in patients with acquired immunodeficiency syndrome (AIDS), or in elderly people. Lesions in the brain appear at postmortem as soft, granular, yellow areas in the white matter, which histologically show extensive loss of myelin sheaths and relative preservation of axons (Weller 1990). Many macrophages are present within the demyelinated lesions and they contain sudenophilic lipid derived from the breakdown of myelin. A characteristic feature of this disease is the presence of bizarre astrocytes and oligodendrocytes, with large hyperchromatic nuclei, containing inclusions of *papova virus*.

The virus can be identified and localized in tissue sections by electron microscopy, by immunocytochemistry using antiviral antibodies, or by *in situ* hybridization using appropriate DNA probes. Specific strains of papova virus associated with this disease have been identified and the commonest is JC. The disease is thought to be an opportunistic virus infection by an organism which is widespread throughout the population and only becomes pathogenic in the brain in immunosuppressed individuals. PML is usually fatal.

Toxins

Triethyltin and hexachlorophene, in particular, can cause oedema and vacuolation of myelin sheaths. The myelin recovers unless the intoxication is prolonged, in which case there may be destruction of myelin and demyelination. A rare disorder—*central pontine myelinolysis*—has been described in alcoholics and other patients in which there is demyelination in the central regions of the pons. This disorder may be related to severe electrolyte disturbances.

Leucodystrophies

A variety of diseases in which there is demyelination in the central, and in some cases the peripheral, nervous system (Lake 1984) occur under this heading. Some show an X-linked inheritance pattern; this group includes *adrenoleucodystrophy* in which there is a defect in the degradation of very-long-chain fatty acids due to a deficiency in enzymes of the peroxisomal β-oxidation system. *Pelizaeus–Merzbacher* is also an X-linked inherited leucodystrophy but the cause is unknown. Other leucodystrophies include *metachromatic leucodystrophy* (MLD) (sulphatide lipidosis) and *Krabbe's globoid leucodystrophy*. Both these disorders affect the central and the peripheral nervous system (see Section 25.9), and are due to deficiencies of lysosomal enzymes. In the case of MLD it is an *arylsulphatase* which is deficient, allowing the accumulation of *sulphatide lipid* in the white matter and peripheral nerves. In Krabbe's disease, there is a deficiency of *galactocerebroside β-galactosidase* with the accumulation of *galactocerebroside* and related lipids in the brain and peripheral nerves.

A variety of other leucodystrophies occur, including *Alexander's disease* in which there is an accumulation of thickened astrocyte processes—*Rosenthal fibres*—in the white matter. Sporadic and familial cases of white matter demyelination, with no significant inflammation and no known enzyme defect, occur and usually present in childhood. When an enzyme defect is present, its detection in blood leucocytes may be used as a diagnostic test.

Acknowledgements

I would like to thank the staff of the Wessex Regional Neuropathology Laboratory, Southampton General Hospital for their technical assistance and Margaret Harris for typing the manuscript.

25.6.4   Bibliography

Brownell, B. and Hughes, J. T. (1962). The distribution of plaques in the cerebrum in multiple sclerosis. *Journal of Neurology, Neurosurgery and Psychiatry* 25, 315–20.

Cuzner, M. L. (1980). Recent biochemical and immunological observations in multiple sclerosis. *Neuropathology and Applied Neurobiology* 6, 405–14.

Esiri, M. M. (1980). Multiple sclerosis: a quantitative and qualitative study of immunoglobulin-containing cells in the central nervous system. *Neuropathology and Applied Neurobiology* 6, 9–21.

Hallpike, J. F., Adams, C. W. M., and Tourtellotte, W. W. (eds) (1983). *Multiple sclerosis*. Chapman & Hall, London.

Huber, S. J., *et al.* (1988) Magnetic resonance imaging and clinical correlations in multiple sclerosis. *Journal of the Neurological Sciences* 86, 1–12.

Lake, B. D. (1984). Lysosomal enzyme deficiencies. In *Greenfield's neuropathology*, (ed. J. H. Adams, J. A. N. Corsellis, and L. W. Duchen) (4th edn), pp. 491–572. Edward Arnold, London.

Ludwin, S. K. (1980). Chronic demyelination inhibits remyelination in the central nervous system. An analysis of contributing factors. *Laboratory Investigation* 43, 382–7.

Matthews, W. B., Acheson, E. D., Batchelor, J. R., and Weller, R. O. (1985). *McAlpine's multiple sclerosis*. Churchill Livingstone, Edinburgh.

Traugott, U., Reinherz, E. L., and Raine, C. S. (1983). Multiple sclerosis; distribution of T-cell subsets with an active chronic lesion. *Science* 219, 308–10.

Vinken, P. J. and Bruyn, G. W. (eds) (1970). *Multiple sclerosis. Handbook of clinical neurology*, Vol. 9. North Holland, Amsterdam.

Weller, R. O. (1984). *Colour atlas of neuropathology*. Harvey Miller and Oxford University Press.

Weller, R. O. (ed.) (1990). *Systemic pathology* (3rd edn), Vol. 4: *Nervous system, muscle and eyes*. Churchill Livingstone, Edinburgh.

25.7   Degenerative diseases

Margaret M. Esiri

The degenerative diseases of the nervous system that are discussed below are diseases in which nerve cells from selective populations die in a progressive and relentless fashion. The process occurs at a varying rate and is accompanied by *astrocytic gliosis, a minimal microglial reaction,* and *little other cellular response*. A characteristic feature is the *systemic* nature of the neurone loss, which corresponds to neuroanatomically discrete and, in some cases, interconnected functional groups of neurones, but is independent of their regional position or vascular supply. This results in a selective dismantling of parts of the nervous system concerned with particular functions; for example, of the upper and lower motor neurones in motor neurone disease and certain interconnected cortical pyramidal neurones in *Alzheimer's disease*. The pathology is usually, but not invariably, symmetrical. The age of onset of these diseases is variable; several commence in late middle or old age, but others commence in infancy or childhood. Some are familial, others usually sporadic. In some of the diseases, structural changes are found in those neurones surviving in the affected populations, while in others the neurones concerned simply disappear, sometimes after undergoing atrophy. Frequently, it is the distal ends of long neurones that are affected before the cell body shows pathological changes ('*dying back*' of neurones). Thus, loss of axons in the corticospinal tracts in motor neurone disease may be readily apparent at the lower spinal level when loss of motor neurones in the primary motor cortex is undetectable. In most of these diseases, the pathology is confined to the nervous system but, in a few, other organs are also affected. For example, the heart regularly shows pathological changes in *Friedreich's ataxia*, and the lymphoreticular tissue is abnormal in *ataxia telangiectasia*.

The causes of these diseases are, for the most part, unknown. The exception is *Creutzfeldt–Jacob disease*, which was shown 20 years ago to be transmissible (see below). The agent responsible for this disease has been only partially characterized and had several atypical properties which had led to it being classed as an 'unconventional' transmissible agent. Following the discovery of the transmissibility of Creutzfeldt–Jacob disease, attempts have been made to transmit other degenerative diseases of the nervous system, all without success. Further comments on the aetiology of these diseases are provided in the concluding remarks to this section.

25.7.1   Motor neurone diseases

The classical form of *motor neurone disease* presents most commonly in late middle or old age with progressive weakness of the limbs or bulbar musculature. Initially its effects may be limited to only one limb but as the disease advances virtually all muscle groups become involved. The mean duration of the disease is

3 years but some cases survive 10 years or more. Death is usually due to respiratory failure or aspiration pneumonia attributable to involvement of the muscles of respiration and deglutition. The disease accounts for about 1 in 1000 adult deaths. There is some epidemiological evidence to suggest that the incidence is higher in some parts of the world than others. For example, there is a remarkably high incidence of motor neurone disease, and of parkinsonism and dementia, on the Pacific island of Guam. The condition is only rarely familial.

The most obvious naked-eye changes to be found in motor neurone disease are marked wasting of the striated muscles, which results from denervation atrophy (see Section 25.9.2), and wasting of the anterior nerve roots as they emerge from the spinal cord (Fig. 25.53). In sections of the cord, the motor neurones in the anterior horns are clearly reduced in number, particularly at the cervical and lumbo-sacral levels (Fig. 25.54). Lower motor neurone loss occurs also in motor nuclei of the lower brainstem, particularly in the hypoglossal nuclei in the medulla. The facial nucleus is less regularly affected, and the motor nuclei of the cranial nerves innervating the extra-ocular eye muscles are spared both clinically and pathologically. In myelin preparations of the cord, a loss of axons, reflected in pallor of myelin staining, is usually evident in the crossed and uncrossed corticospinal tracts, and to a lesser extent in the rest of the white matter of the lateral and anterior columns. The posterior columns, in contrast, are well preserved (Fig. 25.55). (It is from the crossed corticospinal tract degeneration that the alternative name for motor neurone disease, *amyotrophic lateral sclerosis*, is derived.)

In addition to classical motor neurone disease, there are various uncommon inherited motor neurone diseases. These have an age of onset that ranges from early infancy, or even fetal life, through childhood to early adulthood. In general, the later the onset of these diseases the more benign is the course. They show an *autosomal recessive inheritance*. The earliest and most grave of these diseases is *Werdnig–Hoffmann disease*, which presents in infancy with hypotonia, weakness, and failure to thrive owing to an inability to suck strongly. The mother may have noticed that fetal movements were feeble. The striated muscles in the limbs are pale and wasted. Muscle fibres are, for the most part, unduly small and denervated. The few surviving groups of innervated fibres are, in contrast, hypertrophic (Fig. 25.56). In the central nervous system, there is loss of motor neurones in the spinal cord, with wasting of anterior roots, but the pyramidal and other long tracts are not affected.

The more chronic inherited motor neurone diseases, sometimes referred to as *spinal muscular atrophies*, show essentially the same distribution and type of pathology as Werdnig–Hoffmann disease, but at a later age and with more compensatory changes. Thus, as the disease progresses, in the skeletal

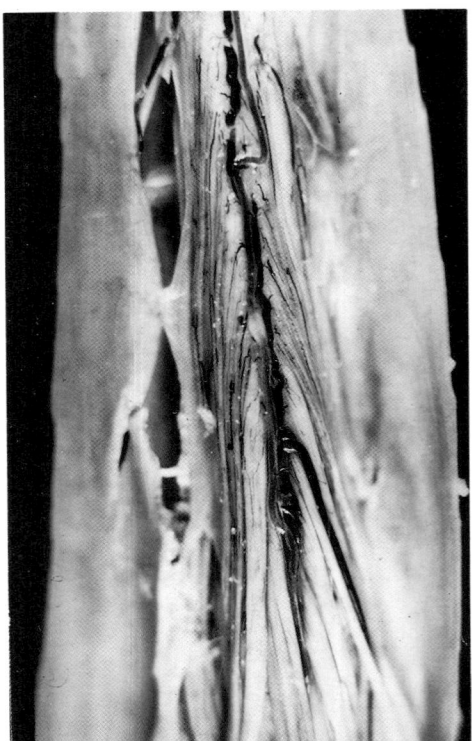 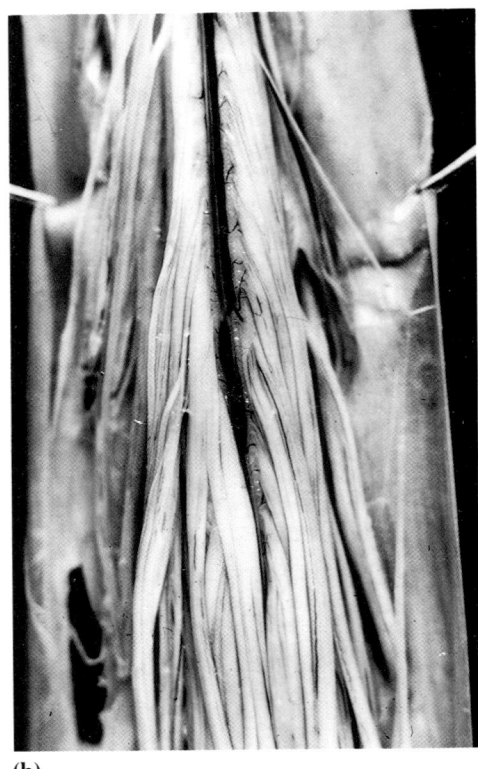

(a)   (b)

Fig. 25.53 Anterior aspect of the lower spinal cord and cauda equina from a case of motor neurone disease (a) and control (b). There is gross wasting of the anterior (motor) nerve roots in motor neurone disease.

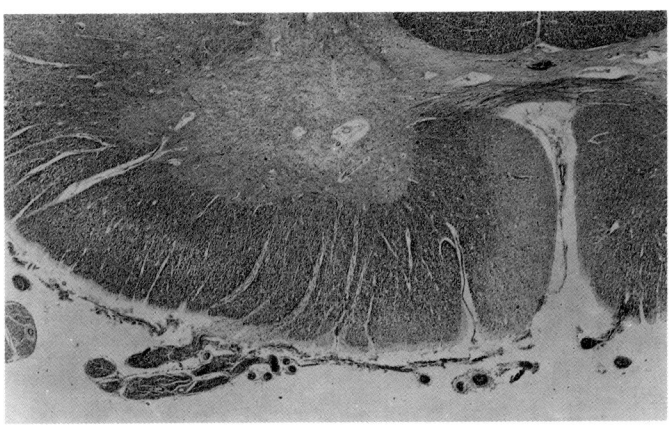

(a)

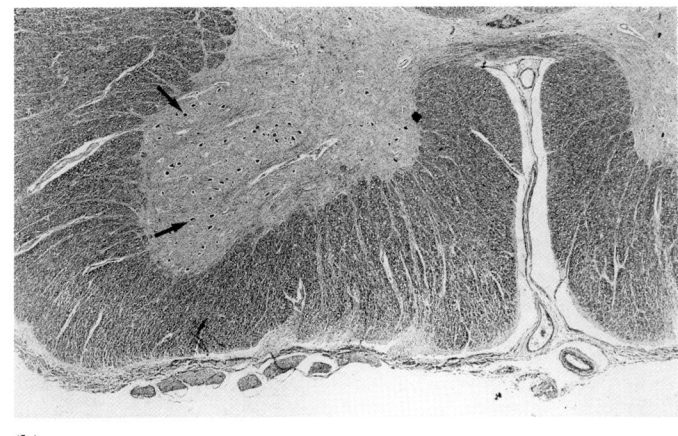

(b)

Fig. 25.54 Low-power view of sections of the cervical spinal cord to show the anterior horn from a case of motor neurone disease (a) and control (b). Motor neurones are readily visible in the right photograph (arrows) but are almost completely absent in the left one. (Luxol fast blue/cresyl violet stain.)

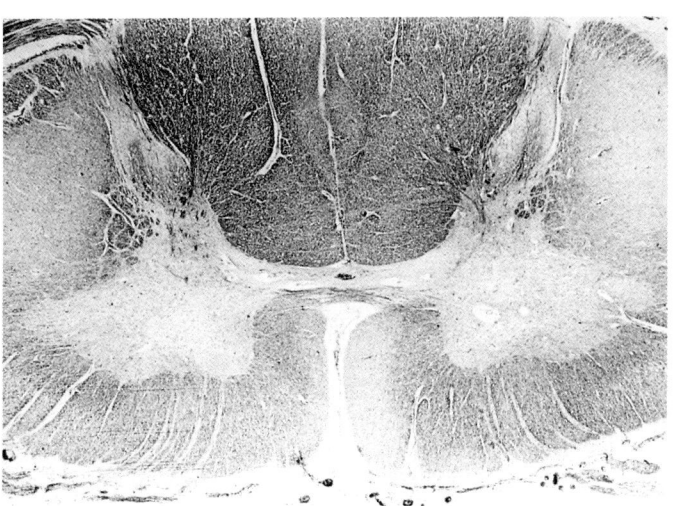

Fig. 25.55 Low-power view of a myelin-stained section of the cervical spinal cord from a case of motor neurone disease. There is pallor of myelin staining in the anterior (uncrossed) and lateral (crossed) corticospinal tracts.

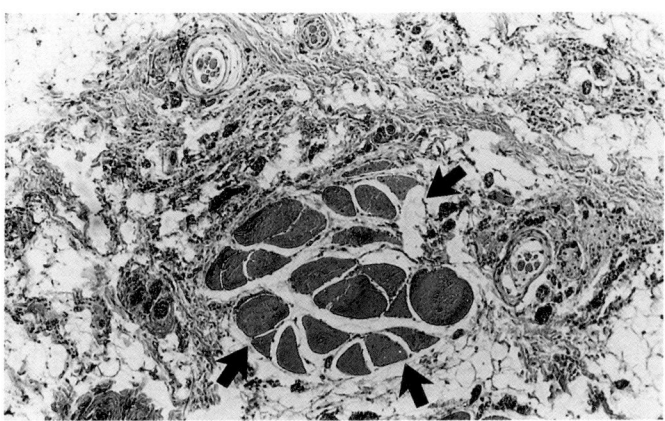

Fig. 25.56 Low-power view of a transverse section of skeletal muscle from a case of Werdnig–Hoffmann disease. In the centre there is a group of hypertrophied muscle fibres (arrow) surrounded by very atrophic muscle fibres, muscle spindles, and adipose tissue and collagen.

muscles there is usually extensive re-innervation of denervated fibres by terminal sprouting of the remaining intact pool of motor neurones. Skeletal muscles therefore frequently show *fibre type grouping*, as well as group atrophy due to denervation. Secondary skeletal changes such as scoliosis, resulting from the unequal pull of partially weak muscles on the vertebral column, are also liable to occur.

25.7.2 Parkinson's disease and parkinsonism

Parkinson's disease is a common disorder, principally of late middle and old age. Its main effects are seen as an interference in normal motor activity, with bradykinesia, resting tremor, and rigidity in the limbs, and poverty of facial expression. They were first clearly described by James Parkinson in 1817. It is a chronic disease which progresses gradually over several years. Treatment with *L-dopa* ameliorates the effects of the disease to some extent.

The characteristic naked-eye pathology in Parkinson's disease is loss of pigment from the pigmented nuclei of the brainstem, particularly the *pars compacta of the substantia nigra* and the *locus coeruleus* (Fig. 25.57). Microscopically, the same sites show loss of nerve cells, incontinence of melanin pigment, and the presence, in some of the surviving pigmented neurones, of characteristic intracytoplasmic inclusion bodies known as *Lewy bodies* (Fig. 25.58). The cell loss is most severe in the middle third of the substantia nigra. Lewy bodies are spherical structures, 5–25 μm in diameter, with a laminated appearance and a

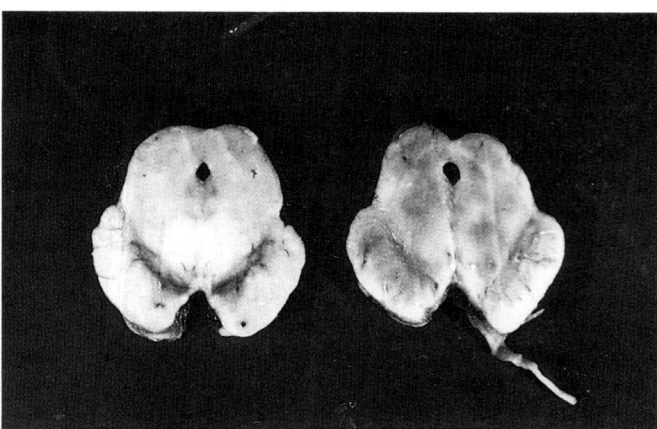

Fig. 25.57 Naked-eye appearance of the midbrain from a case of Parkinson's disease (right) and control (left). Note that there is a readily visible band of pigment in the substantia nigra normally and that this has almost entirely disappeared in the case of Parkinson's disease.

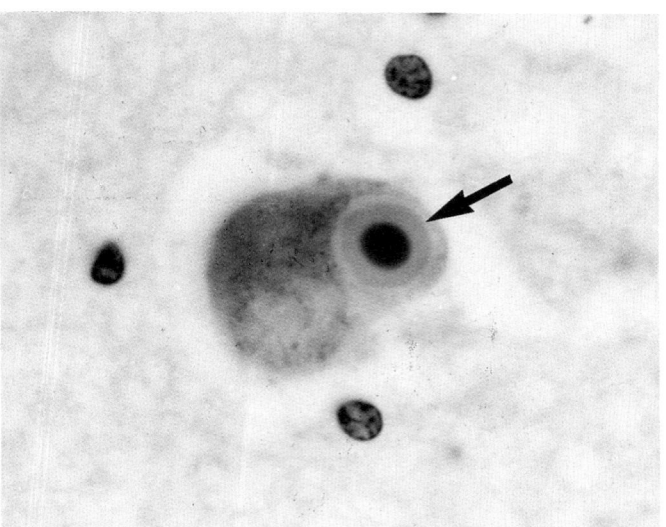

Fig. 25.58 High-power view of a pigmented neurone in the pars compacta of the substantia nigra from a case of Parkinson disease. A laminated, spherical inclusion body (Lewy body) occupies the cytoplasm (arrow). (Lendrum's stain.)

pale halo. They are readily visible in sections stained with haematoxylin and eosin or Lendrum's phloxine-tartrazine method. They react immunocytochemically with neurofilament antibodies, and ultrastructurally they are composed of aggregated filamentous and granular material. Lewy bodies are found in small numbers in about 5 per cent of non-parkinsonian subjects, particularly in old age. Possibly their presence in this context signifies a preclinical phase of Parkinson's disease. Neurone loss and Lewy bodies are not confined to melanin-containing neurones in Parkinson's disease, but are found also in non-pigmented cells of the nucleus basalis, hypothalamus, and upper brainstem. Rarely, they can be found widespread in the cerebral cortex.

The pigmented cells lost from the substantia nigra are dopaminergic, and in Parkinson's disease there is loss of dopamine in the striatum to which cells project. This dopamine deficit is thought to be responsible for many of the symptoms of Parkinson's disease. Cells lost from the locus coeruleus are *noradrenergic*, and in Parkinson's disease there is a corresponding loss of noradrenaline in the cerebral cortex and various subcortical nuclei to which they project. The nucleus basalis, from which cells are also lost in Parkinson's disease, contains neurones supplying a cholinergic projection at the cerebral cortex. Markers of cholinergic activity in the cortex, such as the activity of the enzyme *choline acetyltransferase* are likewise reduced in Parkinson's disease. It is thought possible that this deficit, and the deficit in noradrenaline in the cortex, may contribute to the development of dementia, which occurs in about 10–15 per cent of Parkinson's disease sufferers.

Other causes of parkinsonism

Elderly subjects with some of the clinical features of Parkinson's disease, particularly bradykinesia and rigidity, are sometimes found after death to lack the pathological features of Parkinson's disease but to have small areas of softening in the striatum. Small arteries in the striatum in such cases usually show considerable intimal thickening and hyaline degeneration. The term *arteriosclerotic parkinsonism* is sometimes used to refer to this condition.

A process responsible for many cases of severe parkinsonism in the past, and probably for a few sporadic cases still, is *post-encephalitic degeneration* of neurones, chiefly in the upper brainstem. Clinically, such patients suffer from severe parkinsonism with the added symptom of *oculogyric crises*. The condition was a common sequel in survivors of *acute encephalitis lethargica*, which was seen in epidemic form during and in the decade after the First World War. The pathological features of the condition are severe cell loss from all parts of the substantia nigra, scattered gliotic scars and variable cell loss in the upper brainstem and basal nuclei, and neurofibrillary tangles in remaining neurones in the same locations. Another condition in which neurofibrillary change and nerve cell loss occur predominantly in the substantia nigra in association with parkinsonian symptoms is *post-traumatic brain damage*, which is chiefly confined to some professional boxers. *Manganese poisoning* is another rare cause of parkinsonian symptoms afflicting a few miners of the element.

A rare disease with symptoms almost indistinguishable from Parkinson's disease is *striato-nigral degeneration*, one form of multiple system atrophy discussed below. This produces shrinkage and brown discoloration of the putamen and loss of pigment from all parts of the substantia nigra. Microscopically, these nuclei show neurone loss and gliosis, but no Lewy bodies.

25.7.3 Multiple system atrophy

There is a spectrum of disease subsumed under this heading, which has in common the occurrence of progressive loss of function in, and neurone loss and gliosis affecting, a number of different nuclei of the brain, several of them anatomically connected. No structural abnormalities are seen in the remaining neurones. Some cases are familial. In an individual case of multiple system atrophy, only a selection of the structures at risk are affected, and certain combinations of lesions occur characteristically together and have acquired their own name. The nuclei chiefly at risk are: *putamen, substantia nigra, locus coeruleus, intermediolateral column nuclei of the spinal cord, pontine nuclei, Purkinje cells of the cerebellum*, and *the inferior medullary olives; upper and lower motor neurones* and *sensory ganglia* may be mildly affected in some cases. One named variant of multiple system atrophy is striato-nigral degeneration, mentioned above. The other is *olivo-ponto-cerebellar atrophy*, in which the principal structures affected are the pontine nuclei, with their efferent tracts in the middle cerebellar peduncles; the inferior olives, with their efferent tracts in the inferior cerebellar peduncles; and Purkinje cells of the cerebellar cortex. The base of the pons, olives, cerebellar cortex, and inferior and middle cerebellar peduncles are all shrunken and the fourth ventricle is enlarged. The main clinical symptom is ataxia. In some cases, the lesions of striato-nigral degeneration and olivo-ponto-cerebellar atrophy are combined.

Progressive autonomic failure (Shy–Drager syndrome)

This syndrome may complicate cases of multiple system atrophy in which the pigmented nuclei are affected. A few cases of Parkinson's disease also show the same complication. The condition presents with orthostatic hypotension, loss of sweating, loss of bladder control, nocturnal stridor, and, in men, sexual impotence. The lesions responsible for this syndrome are found in the intermediolateral column nuclei of the thoracic and sacral spinal cord, where there is loss of neurones and gliosis. In Parkinson's disease there may also be a few Lewy bodies in these nuclei. The features of either multiple system atrophy or Parkinson's disease are found in the brain.

25.7.4 Friedreich's ataxia

This is an uncommon, progressive, familial disease, with the chief clinical symptom of ataxia. It has an onset in the first two decades of life, and runs a course lasting several years. In the later stages, the heart becomes affected and death is usually due to heart failure. Cerebrovascular accidents are also common, and result from emboli originating in the heart.

The most striking naked-eye changes in the nervous system are to be found in the *cauda equina, spinal cord*, and *brainstem*. The posterior nerve roots are severely wasted and the whole cord shrunken. Histological sections of the spinal cord and sensory ganglia show the following: loss of sensory ganglion cells and of their axons in the posterior columns of the cord (this change is most severe at the lower levels of the cord, and the gracile tract is correspondingly more affected than the cuneate tract in the posterior columns); loss of cells in the dorsal (Clarke's column) nuclei and loss of axons in the spinocerebellar tracts; loss of axons in the pyramidal tracts (Fig. 25.59). In the

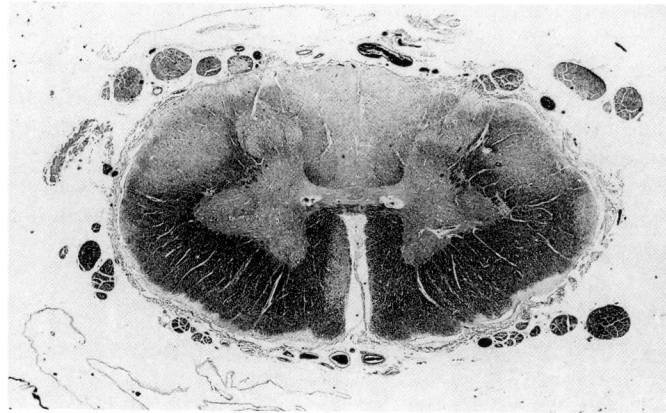

Fig. 25.59 Low-power view of a myelin-stained section of the cervical spinal cord from a case of Friedreich's ataxia. Note the pallor of the posterior nerve roots, crossed and uncrossed corticospinal tracts, posterior columns, and anterior and posterior spinocerebellar tracts.

brainstem, there is loss of neurones in the accessory cuneate nuclei (cephalic homologue of the spinal cord dorsal nuclei) and, in long-standing cases, in gracile nuclei. In the cerebellum, neurones in the dentate nuclei, and their axons in the superior cerebellar peduncles, are depleted. In the basal ganglia, some cases show cell loss in the globus pallidus and subthalamic nucleus. The optic nerve and tracts are also shrunken and depleted of axons. The pathological change in the heart consists of diffuse fibrosis and hypertrophy.

25.7.5 Cerebellar cortical degeneration

This is a rare, recessively inherited condition that produces slowly progressive ataxia from middle age. The pathology is found in the cerebellar cortex and inferior medullary olives. Purkinje cells are lost from the cerebellum, particularly from the superior aspects of the hemispheres and vermis. Neurone loss also occurs in the inferior olives in those parts that project to the affected cerebellar cortex. This olivary cell loss probably represents secondary retrograde change since it is also seen after traumatic, ischaemic, and other lesions affecting Purkinje cells.

25.7.6 Ataxia telangiectasia

This is a rare, familial disease with autosomal recessive inheritance, producing ataxia in childhood. This symptom is followed by the development of telangiectasis in the skin and conjunctiva. There is also a tendency to develop repeated respiratory tract infections. Growth is retarded and mental deterioration may occur in the later stages of the disease. Lymphomas are liable to develop terminally. IgA and IgE levels in serum and other body fluids are very low. Raised levels of α-fetoprotein are detectable in serum. Lymphocyte proliferation in response to phytohaemagglutinin is defective, and there may be a lymphopenia. At post-mortem examination, the thymus and lymph nodes are found to be markedly hypoplastic and the viscera infiltrated with large cells with bizarre nuclei. The telangiectases consist of dilated, tortuous venules. In the nervous system, the cerebellum is atrophic, showing loss in the cortex of Purkinje and granule cells. The inferior olives show secondary retrograde cell loss. In spinal sensory ganglia (Fig. 25.60) there is a deficiency of satellite cells and of the larger sensory neurones, whose central axons are also lost from the posterior columns, particularly in the gracile tracts.

25.7.7 Progressive supranuclear palsy

This sporadic disease was first described in 1964. It is uncommon, has an onset in late middle or old age, and affects males twice as often as females. It produces muscular rigidy, particularly of neck muscles, dysarthria, and an inability to move the eyes upwards. Mental function is also affected, probably mainly through a slowing of appropriate responses rather than by producing marked dementia.

   Pathological changes are found in the *globus pallidus*, *subthalamic nucleus*, *brainstem*, and *cerebellum*. Brainstem structures affected include the substantia nigra, tectum of the pons and midbrain, and the red nuclei. In these regions, in addition to loss of neurones and gliosis, there are neurofibrillary tangles present in remaining neurones (Fig. 25.61). Ultrastructurally, these tangles are composed of filaments, some of which are paired, helically wound, 11 nm diameter filaments, resembling those found in Alzheimer's disease (see below), while others are straight, unpaired 11 nm diameter filaments. The dentate nuclei in the cerebellum show neurone loss but no tangles. The superior cerebellar peduncles, containing the efferent outflow from the dentate nuclei, and the medial longitudinal fasciculus in the brainstem show loss of axons.

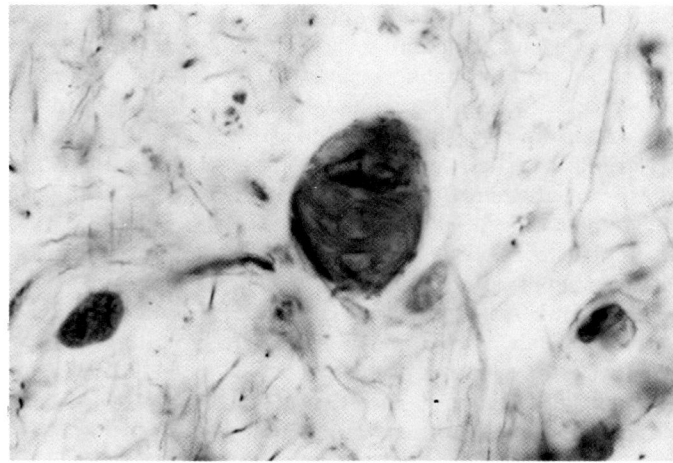

Fig. 25.61 Progressive supranuclear palsy. High-power view of a neurone from the substantia nigra, containing an intracytoplasmic neurofibrillary tangle.

25.7.8 Huntington's disease

This is a dominantly inherited condition presenting with movement disorders or progressive mental impairment usually in middle age. Both motor and mental facets of the disease eventually appear in most cases. The movement disorder commences as a pronounced fidgetiness and may progress to frank chorea.

   The main site of pathology is in the *striatum*. The caudate nuclei, in particular, are usually grossly atrophic and the frontal horns of the lateral ventricles compensatorily dilated (Fig. 25.62). Cerebral cortical atrophy is described in some

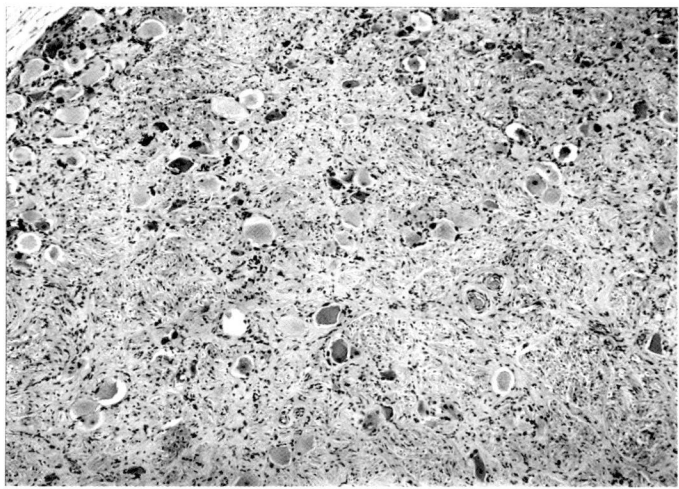

Fig. 25.60 Ataxia telangiectasia. Low-power view of spinal sensory ganglia, showing a shortage of both ganglion cells and satellite cells.

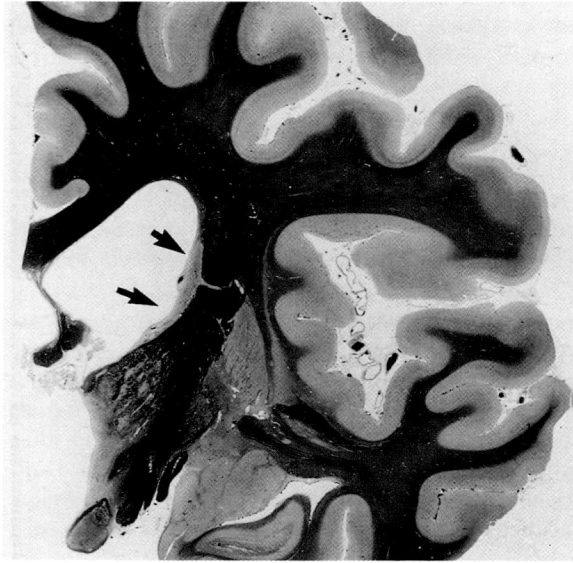

Fig. 25.62 Myelin-stained section of a coronal section through one cerebral hemisphere at the level of the mamillary body from a case of Huntington's disease. The caudate nucleus (arrows) is atrophied and the lateral ventricle dilated.

cases but not others. Histological sections of the striatum show a severe loss of small neurones with preservation of large ones, and there is striking reactive gliosis. Axonal loss is seen in the bundles of myelinated axons that pass from the putamen to the globus pallidus. Neurone loss may also be evident at other sites, including the cerebral cortex, thalamus, hypothalamus, substantia nigra, cerebellar cortex, dentate nuclei, and inferior olives. None of these sites show such severe cell loss as the striatum, however.

The small neurones that are lost from the striatum in Huntington's disease are neurones that release the neurotransmitter γ-aminobutyric acid (GABA). Striatal GABA content is markedly reduced in Huntington's disease. In contrast, neurones containing *somatostatin* and *neuropeptide Y* are selectively spared in the disease, as are the larger cholinergic neurones. A combination of diminished GABA release and excess dopaminergic activity resulting from loss of GABA control, with a relative excess of somatostatin in surviving neurones, is thought to cause *chorea*. At present, the pathological basis of the dementia in Huntington's disease is not clear. Most cortical neurotransmitters are preserved, and the extent of the neurone loss in the cortex is unclear and has not been correlated with the extent of the dementia.

25.7.9 Alzheimer's disease

Alzheimer's disease is the commonest cause of progressive dementia in late middle and old age. The first symptoms are usually of memory loss, but in the later stages all aspects of mental function and personality are affected. The incidence of the disease is estimated at 5 per cent of those over 65 years and 20 per cent of those over 80 years. Most cases are sporadic but about 10 per cent are familial. The pathological changes of Alzheimer's disease occur almost universally in subjects with *Down's syndrome* who survive to middle age or longer.

Death in cases of Alzheimer's disease is usually due to bronchopneumonia.

The pathological changes of Alzheimer's disease affect selected sites in the *cerebral cortex* and *subcortical nuclei*. There is usually some atrophy of the cortical gyri evident macroscopically. The bodies and inferior horns of the lateral ventricles usually show a modest degree of dilatation. The most characteristic pathology is seen in histological sections of the cerebral cortex, particularly medial temporal lobe cortex and hippocampus, and in the amygdala and certain other subcortical nuclei. It consists of the presence of numerous argyrophilic *plaques* and *neurofibrillary tangles* (Figs 25.63, 25.64). Sites that contain neurofibrillary tangles also show considerable neuronal loss. *Argyrophilic plaques* are rounded, shrub-like collections of degenerate nerve processes which react with silver stains and measure 50–200 μm across. In severe cases of Alzheimer's disease they may partially coalesce. Some plaques have a central core which also reacts with stains for *amyloid*. Plaques are most numerous in the outer half of the cerebral cortical ribbon. Ultrastructurally, they consist of abnormal neuritic processes containing excess lipofuscin, abnormal mitochondria, and a few paired, helical filaments, 11 nm in diameter. These are interspersed with astrocytes and microglial cell processes, and at the core are found collections of amyloid fibrils. Neurofibrillary tangles are abnormal argyrophilic, fibrillary structures whose appearance with silver stains resembles a twist or flame-shaped skein of wire (Fig. 25.64). They occupy the cell bodies of certain cortical and hippocampal pyramidal neurones, and react both with silver and amyloid stains. Ultrastructurally, they are composed of bundles of paired, helically wound filaments, each 11 nm in diameter. Both neurofibrillary tangles and argyrophilic plaques react with monoclonal antibodies to *neurofilament antigens*. The numbers of both neurofibrillary tangles and argyrophilic plaques in the brain in Alzheimer's disease is directly correlated with the severity of dementia. In

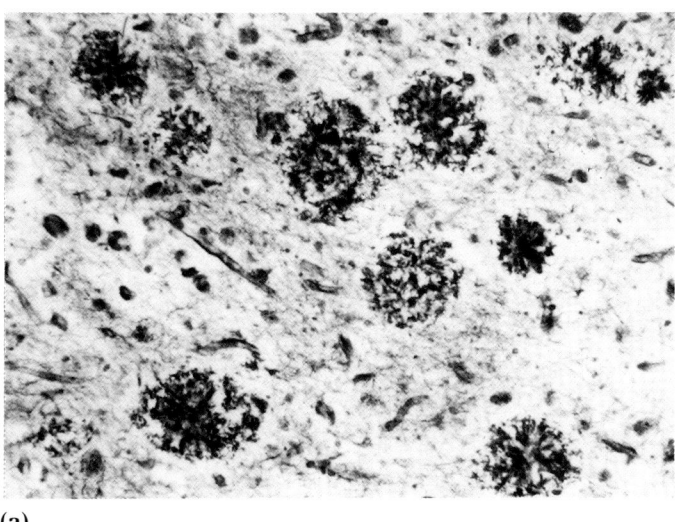

(a)

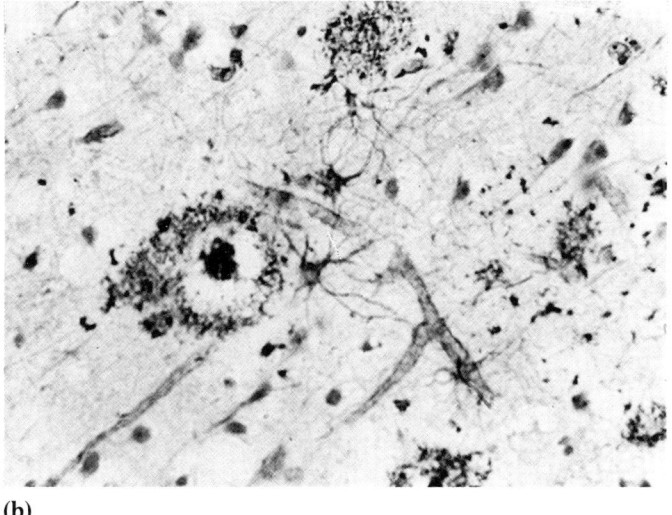

(b)

Fig. 25.63 Cortical argyrophilic plaques from a case of Alzheimer's disease. Those illustrated in (a) lack well-defined central cores, while that seen in (b) contains such a core. Also visible closely adjacent to this plaque are a few reactive astrocytes and nearby capillaries. (von Braunmühl's stain.)

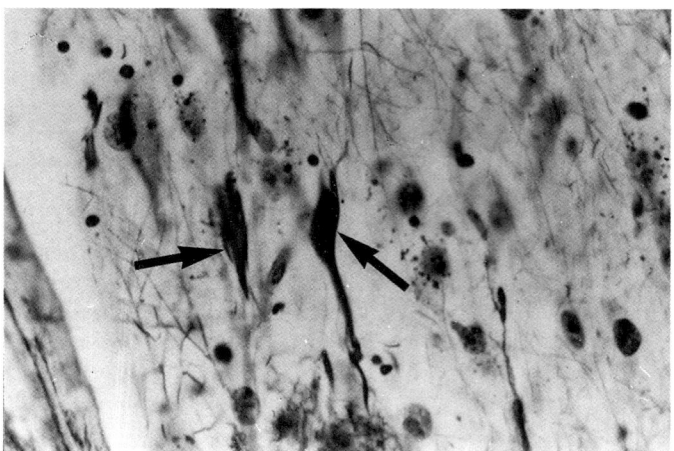

Fig. 25.64 Neurofibrillary tangles in the cerebral cortex in Alzheimer's disease (arrows).

the hippocampus, the pyramidal neurones, in addition to harbouring neurofibrillary tangles, may also contain *Hirano bodies*, eosinophilic rod-like cytoplasmic structures, and show *granulovacuolar degeneration* (Fig. 25.65).

Leptomeningeal and cortical blood vessels in Alzheimer's disease show a variable degree of *amyloid deposition* in their walls. This is not accompanied by vascular amyloid deposition elsewhere in the body. Protein extracted from the cerebrovascular amyloid in Alzheimer's disease has had its amino-acid sequence determined, a mutation of the gene encoding the amyloid precursor protein has been found in some familial cases. It has a molecular weight of about 4000 and is thought to be derived from a larger precursor membrane protein.

The most striking neurochemical change that has been detected in the cerebral cortex in Alzheimer's disease is loss of marker enzymes of cholinergic nerve endings, particularly the biosynthetic enzyme, *choline acetyltransferase*. This is thought to

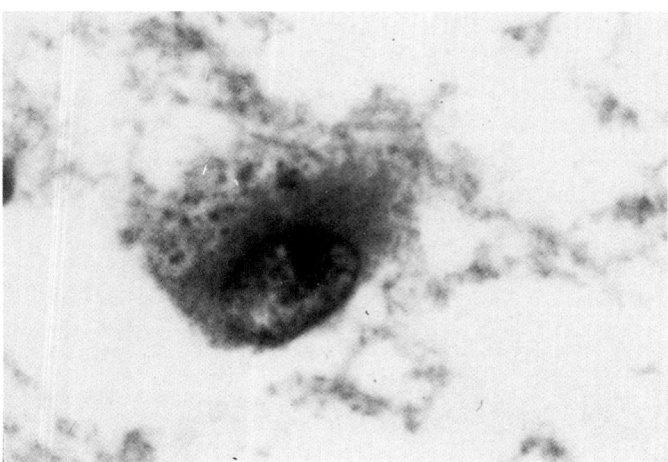

Fig. 25.65 Granulovacuolar degeneration in a hippocampal pyramidal neurone from a case of Alzheimer's disease.

be a consequence of loss of neurones in the nucleus basalis, which are the major source of acetylcholine in the cortex. There are lesser deficiencies of several other neurotransmitters in the cortex, notably of somatostatin, serotonin, and noradrenaline. The latter two transmitters are released at endings of projections from the raphé nuclei and locus coeruleus, respectively, both of which are involved pathologically in Alzheimer's disease. There are also probable deficiencies of the excitatory neurotransmitter, *glutamic acid*, which is thought to be the transmitter released at endings of the depleted cortical pyramidal neurones.

Alzheimer's-type changes seen in normal ageing

The pathological changes of Alzheimer's disease are seen, to a mild extent, and in more restricted locations, in elderly subjects known to have been undemented before death. In such subjects, argyrophilic plaques may be found in the hippocampus, amygdala, and association cortex in small or moderate numbers. Neurofibrillary tangles are few in number and virtually entirely restricted to the hippocampus, amygdala, and medial temporal cortex. Likewise, a slight degree of granulovacuolar degeneration may be found in the hippocampus in elderly, undemented subjects. The incidence of these features in such subjects rises with every decade beyond the fifth.

25.7.10   Pick's disease

This is another disease producing slowly progressive dementia. It is much less common than Alzheimer's disease. Many cases are familial. Symptoms of dementia and personality disorder develop from middle age.

The naked-eye appearance of the brain is very abnormal in Pick's disease. There is severe cortical atrophy which is characteristically lobar in its distribution. In most cases, the atrophy is maximal at the frontal and temporal poles. The posterior half of the superior temporal convolution is usually spared. Occasionally, the cortical atrophy is generalized. The caudate nuclei are atrophic in most cases, and the cerebral white matter also depleted. Lateral ventricles are correspondingly dilated (Fig. 25.66). In histological sections of the affected cerebral cortex, loss of neurones is severe. Among the remaining neurones are some Pick cells, neurones that are abnormally swollen, with pale cytoplasm and nucleus displaced to the cell margin, an appearance reminiscent of chromatolysis (Fig. 25.67). Some other neurone cell bodies are not swollen but contain spherical argyrophilic inclusions in the cytoplasm (Pick bodies). Pick cells and Pick bodies have been shown ultrastructurally to contain aggregates of neurofilaments. The cerebral white matter frequently shows pallor of myelin staining due to axonal loss.

25.7.11   Creutzfeldt–Jacob disease

Rare cases of fatal encephalopathy with rapidly progressive dementia and spongy change in the grey matter of the brain have been described since the 1920s and are now known as

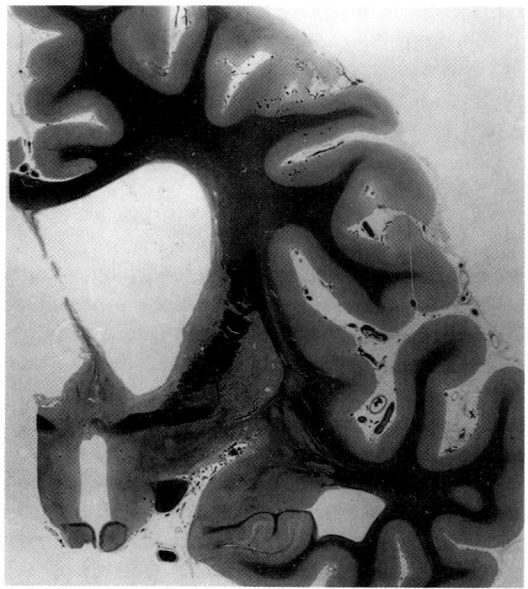

Fig. 25.66 Myelin-stained section of a coronal section of the cerebral hemisphere from a case of Pick's disease. The cortical ribbon is narrow, the sulci are widened, the caudate nucleus is atrophic, and the frontal and inferior horns of the ventricle are dilated.

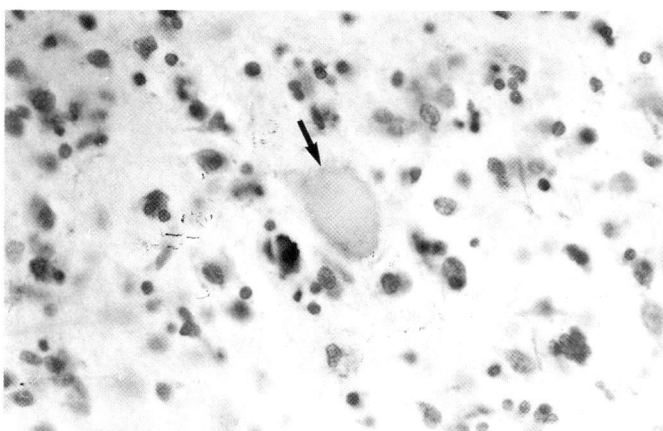

Fig. 25.67 High-power view of the cerebral cortex in Pick's disease. There is a swollen Pick cell at the centre of the field (arrow). Nissl stain.

Creutzfeldt–Jacob disease. In 1957, a disease, 'kuru', was described with similar clinical features and even more similar pathology. Kuru occurred in the restricted population of a remote tribe of the Pacific island of New Guinea. It was pointed out that the pathology of kuru closely resembled that of a degenerative neurological disease of sheep known as *scrapie*, a disease that had been shown to be transmissible many years previously. This observation led to successful attempts to transmit kuru and Creutzfeldt–Jacob disease to chimpanzees by means of intracerebral inoculation of affected brain homogenates. Scrapie and Creutzfeldt–Jacob disease were also subse-

quently shown to be transmissible to small laboratory animals. The incubation period for the transmitted disease is 12–18 months or more, and the disease produced resembles the natural diseases clinically and pathologically. The transmissible agents of scrapie, Creutzfeldt–Jacob disease, and kuru are now considered to be very similar and the conditions themselves are frequently classified together as the *spongiform encephalopathies*. Most cases of Creutzfeldt–Jacob disease are sporadic but about 10 per cent are familial. A small number of cases have occurred by iatrogenic transmission through the use of contaminated electrodes inserted into the brain, by corneal grafting and, most recently, by injection of human growth hormone to growth hormone-deficient children. The manner in which the disease is acquired in the majority of cases is not known. Kuru, which has now largely disappeared from New Guinea, was thought to have been formerly transmitted by the practice of cannibalism.

The brain usually appears grossly normal in Creutzfeldt–Jacob disease. In histological sections, the abnormal microscopic features of spongy change, consisting of *empty vacuoles in grey matter*, 5–50 µm diameter (Fig. 25.68), *neurone loss*, and *reactive astrocytosis*, are found in the cerebral cortex, basal ganglia, thalamus, and cerebellar cortex. Reactive astrocytosis without spongy change or neurone loss may occur at some sites from which efferent terminations have been lost. In the cerebellum, the spongy change is most clearly seen in the molecular layer of the cortex. Rarely, there may be small plaques of amyloid in cerebellar and cerebral cortex. These are much commoner in kuru than in Creutzfeldt–Jacob disease. A few cases of Creutzfeldt–Jacob disease show unusually severe atrophy of the cerebral or cerebellar cortex. These cases tend to have had an

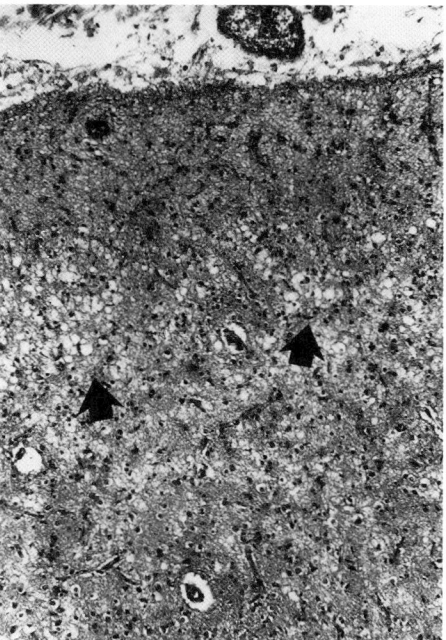

Fig. 25.68 Low-power view of the cerebral cortex in a case of Creutzfeldt–Jacob disease, showing foci of spongy change in layers 2 and 3 (arrows).

unusually long duration of disease. Another unusual feature seen in a few cases, and described mainly, but not exclusively from Japan, is spongy change in cerebral white matter.

A condition that has recently been recognized to be a probable variant of Creutzfeldt–Jacob disease is the *Gerstmann–Sträussler syndrome*. This is a familial condition in which progressive ataxia and dementia develop in middle age. In contrast to Creutzfeldt–Jacob disease, which rarely has a disease duration of more than 1 year, the condition progresses over several years before death occurs. Brain homogenates from cases of Gerstmann–Sträussler syndrome have been shown to produce an encephalopathy in animals after a prolonged incubation period, the pathology of which resembles that of transmitted Creutzfeldt–Jacob disease, kuru, and scrapie. A particularly prominent feature of the pathology is the presence of numerous plaques in the molecular layer of the cortex (Fig. 25.69). The spinal cord shows degeneration of dorsal nuclei (Clarke's column nuclei), neurones and loss of axons in the spinocerebellar tracts. These changes are accompanied by gliosis, but there is no spongy change.

Experimental studies aimed at characterizing the agents associated with the spongiform encephalopathies have been carried out chiefly with the scrapie agent, but many of the findings have been confirmed for the agent of Creutzfeldt–Jacob disease. The spongiform encephalopathies are remarkable in several respects: the long incubation periods for the transmitted diseases, the absence of any immune response to the agents, and the fact that in a minority of cases of Creutzfeldt–Jacob disease and in all cases of Gerstmann–Sträussler syndrome, the diseases can apparently be inherited. The agents themselves are also exceptional in their high resistance to inactivation, for example, by UV light, formalin, and other microbicidal agents; the absence of a clearly demonstrable nucleic acid component; and the lack of a well-defined ultrastructural form. After intravenous administration, the scrapie agent has been found to proliferate in lymphoreticular tissue before becoming detectable in the brain. Recent studies have demonstrated that the high-infectivity

fraction of scrapie brain contains a protein, termed *prion protein*, which has been partially sequenced. On extraction, this protein forms amyloid fibrils. Nucleic acid coding for the normal prion protein isotype has been shown to be present in normal human and mouse neurones, but the function of the protein is not known.

25.7.12   Concluding remarks

It seems certain that the degenerative neurological diseases discussed above will eventually be found to have different aetiologies. Some clues to what these might be are already to hand. It is known that large neurones are exceptional in the high metabolic demands made by their need to maintain the integrity of uniquely large surface membranes and long processes. Such large neurones are known to undergo degeneration of the 'dying back' type, not dissimilar to that shown in some of the degenerative diseases discussed above, under conditions of vitamin deficiency, certain intoxications, and the influence of some drugs. Inherited metabolic defects that limit the energy available to the cell can also produce diseases that resemble these degenerative diseases. Particularly pertinent to Parkinson's disease is the recent demonstration that a chemical, *1-methyl-4-phenyl-1,2,3,6-tetra-hydropyridine* (MPTP), produces selective death of pigmented neurones in the substantia nigra and locus coeruleus. It is not thought that most cases of Parkinson's disease are due to MPTP intoxication, though there is recognized to be a small group of parkinsonian patients who inadvertently poisoned themselves with this substance when it was produced as a contaminant of self-administered illicitly prepared opioids. Rather, the demonstration of the selective neurotoxicity of MPTP is acting as a stimulus for a search for other such neurotoxins, which may be more widely dispersed in the environment.

Further insights into toxic mechanisms that may be relevant to these human diseases are provided by experiments on the effects of certain excitatory amino acids, which are thought to mimic the effects of endogenous excitatory neurotransmitters, particularly glutamate. One such, *quinolinic acid*, exerts a neurotoxic action by binding locally to, and excessively activating, receptors for glutamate. The consequence of this action is death of the cell on which the receptors are situated. It has been found that injection of quinolinic acid into the striatum of rats results in a pattern of cell death that is closely similar to that occurring in Huntington's disease. This finding raises the possibility that Huntington's disease itself may be due to a genetically determined abnormal handling of endogenous excitatory transmitters in the striatum. Other excitatory amino acids are present in some naturally occurring food substances. Thus, *β-N-methylamino-1-allaline* (BMAA), a component of the cycad seed, which is used as a source of food in some parts of the world, particularly under famine conditions, has been shown to produce degeneration of upper and lower motor neurones when administered to monkeys. The high incidence of motor neurone disease on the island of Guam has recently been attributed to the use of this seed in the diet. Whether the observation of the

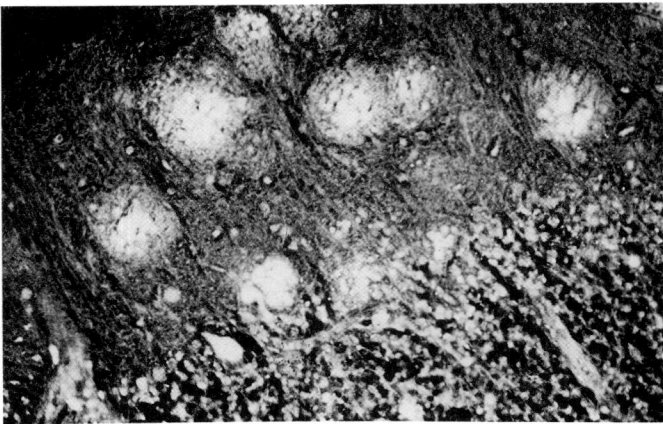

Fig. 25.69 Multiple amyloid plaques in the molecular layer of the cerebellar cortex from a case of Gerstmann–Sträussler syndrome. (Thioflavine T stain photographed under fluorescence illumination.)

neurotoxicity of BMAA in animals has relevance to other human motor neurone diseases is not yet known. Regarding the aetiology of Alzheimer's disease, there is some speculation that excitotoxic effects of endogenous cortical glutamate may be involved. However, others consider that potential environmental factors, such as *aluminium* and *viruses*, also deserve careful scrutiny as possible aetiological agents in Alzheimer's disease. In addition, the discovery of the amyloidogenic properties of the scrapie-associated prion protein has possible relevance to Alzheimer's disease, in view of the prominent congophilic elements in its pathology. Finally, the possibility has been raised that some of the degenerative diseases of the nervous system may be due to inherited or acquired deficiencies in the production and transport between neurones of trophic factors, such as *nerve growth factor*. However, until such factors are identified and their roles in the maintenance of normal central nervous system neurones clarified, such suggestions must remain speculative.

25.7.13 Further reading

Bridges, B. A. and Harnden, D. G. (eds) (1982). *Ataxia-telangiectasia.* John Wiley, New York.

Fahn, M. D. and Bergmann, K. J. (eds) (1986). *Advances in neurology,* Vol. 45: *Parkinson's disease.* Raven Press, New York.

Manuelidis, L. and Manuelidis, E. E. (1986). Recent developments in scrapie and Creutzfeldt–Jacob disease. *Progress in Medical Virology* **33**, 78–98.

Martin, J. B. and Gusella, J. F. (1986). Huntington's disease. *New England Journal of Medicine* **315**, 1267–76.

Oppenheimer, D. R. (1984). Diseases of the basal ganglia, cerebellum and motor neurons. In *Greenfield's neuropathology* (ed. J. H. Adams, J. A. N. Corsellis, and L. W. Duchen) (4th edn), pp. 699–747. Edward Arnold, London.

Prusiner, S. B., Gabizon, R., and McKinley, M. P. (1987). On the biology of prions. *Acta Neuropathologica* **72**, 299–314.

Roth, M. and Iversen, L. L. (eds) (1986). Alzheimer's disease. *British Medical Bulletin* **42**.

Rowland, L. P. (1987). Motor neuron diseases and amyotrophic lateral sclerosis: research progress. *Trends in Neurosciences* **10**, 393–8.

Tomlinson, B. E. and Corsellis, J. A. N. (1984). Ageing and the dementias. In *Greenfield's neuropathology* (ed. J. H. Adams, J. A. N. Corsellis, and L. W. Duchen) (4th edn), pp. 951–1025. Edward Arnold, London.

25.8 Tumours of the nervous system

P. L. Lantos

25.8.1 Introduction

Epidemiology

Incidence rates of tumours of the nervous system vary from one country to another and comparison is made difficult by different systems of data collection, reporting, standard of accuracy, and diagnostic criteria. Post-mortem statistics indicate that brain tumours are found in between 1 and 2 per cent of all necropsies. Data from four European centres, Vienna, Heidelberg, Tübingen, and Freiburg, reported an overall incidence of primary and metastatic neoplasms of 1.81 per cent. Primary tumours alone accounted for 1.4 per cent and half of these were gliomas (Weil 1946).

Age-adjusted mortality rated in 27 countries reveal an average incidence of 5/100 000, varying from 1.1/100 000 in Mexico to 6.8/100 000 in Israel (Goldberg and Kurland 1962). In England and Wales malignant brain tumours alone killed 2743 individuals in 1989, with a death rate of 6.4/100 000 for men and 4.6/100 000 for women (HMSO 1989). The incidence of brain tumours is higher in smaller populations in which errors inherent in data obtained from different countries can be eliminated. For example, in the Faroes the incidence rate is 9.9/100 000 and in Rochester, Minnesota it exceeds 14/100 000 (Codd and Kurland 1985; Zülch 1986).

The incidence of primary brain tumours shows little difference between sexes, although gliomas are somewhat more frequent in men and meningiomas in women (Codd and Kurland 1985). Zülch (1986), however, observed male preponderance in all but two types of tumours: only meningiomas and intracranial schwannomas occur more often in women.

Brain tumours constitute only 2 per cent of all malignancies, but they are disproportionately more common in children, in whom they rank second after neoplasms of the haemopoietic system (Willis 1962).

Aetiology and pathogenesis

The cause of neoplasia of the nervous system is not known, although modern investigative techniques, particularly molecular biology of human tumours and experimental induction of neural tumours, have considerably contributed to our knowledge in recent years. Since these tumours originate from different tissues, it is likely that the tumorigenic stimuli differ for various tumour types. The cause of a malignant glioma may differ from that of a meningioma or neuroblastoma.

Very little is known about early, preneoplastic changes which precede the appearance of overt neoplasia. This is particularly true of the tumours of the central nervous system: the brain and spinal cord, being both surrounded by bony coverings and fibrous membranes, are not readily accessible to repeated biopsies like the exposed epithelial surfaces of the skin, lung, or cervix. Moreover, tumours of the nervous system cause signs and symptoms after they have reached a considerable size, at a stage when secondary changes, haemorrhage, necrosis, and anaplasia have interfered with, or even obliterated, the original cytoarchitecture.

Chemicals

Carcinogens that have been shown to induce tumours in the nervous system are widely distributed in the environment. *Polycyclic aromatic hydrocarbons*, being formed during incomplete combustion of fossil fuels, are present in the air, water, and soil. The possible carcinogenic action of a particular polycyclic aromatic hydrocarbon is, however, impossible to assess accurately, since these compounds occur in complex mixtures of organic material contaminated with other carcinogens.

Carcinogenic nitroso compounds are also ubiquitous in the environment, and they occur in various foods, alcoholic drinks, and tobacco smoke. Moreover, these compounds can be formed from secondary amines and nitrites in the acidic milieu of the mammalian stomach. Although a wide variety of species is susceptible, evidence that man responds in the same way, in the absence of experimental exposure, could only be obtained from an epidemiological study. Even if man were susceptible, the effects of the small amounts present in the environment are not known (reviewed by Lantos 1986).

The possibility that environmental factors, particularly chemical carcinogens, may play a role in the causation of neural tumours should be seriously considered. Occupational risks have been reported for individuals employed in the rubber, oil and petrochemical, pharmaceutical, and electrical industries, for farmers, and for workers exposed to vinyl chloride. Professional groups, white- and blue-collar occupations, which apparently carry a higher risk of intracranial gliomas, have been reviewed recently (McLaughlin *et al.* 1987).

Viruses

Both DNA and RNA viruses induce neural neoplasms in experimental animals, but there is no direct evidence of viral aetiology of any of these tumours in man. Infection by human immunodeficiency virus is associated with primary lymphomas and Kaposi's sarcomas of the brain, but these arise in patients whose immunological state has been severely compromised by the virus. In acquired immunodeficiency syndrome (AIDS), there is also an increased incidence of *progressive multifocal leukoencephalopathy*. This degenerative, demyelinating disorder, which also occurs as a complication of malignancy, is caused by an oncogenic papova virus. One of its histological hallmarks is the presence of bizarre, but apparently non-neoplastic, astrocytes.

Irradiation

The high susceptibility of fetal and neonatal nervous system to irradiation has been well recognized. Although high doses can cause malformations, the effects of single or repeated diagnostic doses are disputed. Irradiation of pregnant mothers increased the incidence of neoplasms of the progeny, including tumours of the nervous system (McMahon 1962).

Therapeutic irradiation of the nervous system for benign and malignant tumours or for non-neoplastic lesions is known to induce new growths. Radiation-induced neoplasms should fulfil certain criteria: they should arise in the field of irradiation, have had a long latency, and should be histologically verified. A recent review of the literature revealed 96 such cases, of which 50 were meningiomas, 24 gliomas, and 22 sarcomas (Liwnicz *et al.* 1985).

Trauma

The role of trauma in the pathogenesis of neural tumours remains controversial. Careful examination of individual cases, statistical analysis of large series of human material, and observations in experimental animals using trauma as co-carcinogen have yielded controversial results. Trauma has been considered to be a possible cause of convexity meningiomas, and a few possible tumours associated with injury have been reviewed (Zülch 1986). The relationship between trauma and neuroepithelial tumours is even more tenuous: the likelihood that a glial response elicited by direct damage to the brain will become neoplastic is remote.

Hormonal and immunological factors

Most tumour types of the nervous system are more common in males, the two exceptions being meningiomas and schwannomas. These sexual predilections have raised the possibility of hormonal influences, but here is no evidence that endocrine imbalances cause neural neoplasms. That the growth of meningiomas is influenced by hormones is well known, and both the *oestrogen and progesterone receptors* in these tumours have been studied. The presence of specific progesterone receptors opens the possibility of hormonal manipulations in their treatment (Ironside *et al.* 1986). The results of animal experiments, in which various endocrine organs were removed and hormones administered, are controversial, but they do not exclude the possibility that hormones may act as co-carcinogens and promoters (Jänisch and Schreiber 1977).

Suppression of the immune system appears to be associated with a higher incidence of brain tumours. A nearly sixtyfold increase of non-Hodgkin lymphomas and an excess of squamous cell carcinomas of the skin and mesenchymal tumours were observed in patients who had been treated with immunosuppressive drugs for kidney transplantation. These tumours developed after a short latency and had a striking predilection for the brain, which was involved in 15 cases out of 34. The possible mechanisms thought to be responsible for this increased incidence include the *impairment of immune surveillance*, *prolonged antigenic stimulation*, *graft versus host reaction*, and the activation of *oncogenic viruses* (Kinlen *et al.* 1979). A cerebellar 'reticulum-cell sarcoma–microglioma' associated with similar lesions in the lung developed in a patient after cardiac transplantation (Schober and Herman 1973). The association of primary malignant lymphomas with AIDS has been considered previously. It is of interest to note that in all these cases, irrespective of the underlying cause of immunosuppression, the resulting cerebral tumours are lymphomas and not neuro-epithelial malignancies.

Embryonal rests and congenital tumours

Various tumour types have their peak incidence in childhood. Moreover, several neuro-epithelial, mesenchymal, and maldevelopmental tumours are discovered at birth or during the neonatal period. These include primitive neuro-epithelial neoplasms such as medulloblastomas, neuroblastomas, and retinoblastomas. Of the gliomas, some pilocytic astrocytomas and ependymomas fall into this category. The possible relationship of these tumours to embryonal cell rests lends support to, and has revived interest in, *Cohnheim's theory of carcinogenesis*.

This assumes that neoplasms could arise from primitive vestiges of ontogenesis. Similarities, both morphological and biological, exist between malignant and differentiating cells, and cells of primitive neuro-epithelial tumours have a propensity for differentiating into more mature forms. Although it is difficult to prove unequivocally the relationship in man between embryonal cell rests and neural neuroplasms, in experimental animals *ethylnitrosourea-induced malignant gliomas* were shown to originate from the *primitive cells of the subependymal plate* (Lantos 1985; Pilkington and Lantos 1990)

Genetic factors and familial tumours

Systemic, so-called *dysgenetic syndromes* often involve the nervous system. Three of these, *neurofibromatosis* (von Recklinghausen's disease), *tuberous sclerosis* (Bourneville's disease), and *angiomatosis of the central nervous system* (von Hippel–Lindau disease) are associated with neural neuroplasia: neurofibromas develop in the first, subependymal giant-cell astrocytomas in the second, and haemangioblastomas in the third. In von Recklinghausen's disease, schwannomas, gliomas, and meningiomas also occur. These syndromes have a familial background and the underlying genetic mechanism is the subject of intense investigations. They have been particularly fruitful in elucidating the molecular genetic abnormalities of von Recklinghausen's disease (Rouleau *et al.* 1987; Jadayel *et al.* 1990). Other familial tumours in the nervous system are rare and their occurrence in the brain has been reviewed (Tijssen *et al.* 1982).

Oncogenes

It has been long realized that chromosome abnormalities in brain tumours abound, but only recent research on oncogenes has started to shed light on the molecular basis of malignancy. Acoustic schwannomas and meningiomas are associated with loss of genes on human *chromosome 22*, indicating that a common event may underlie the development of these tumours (Seizinger *et al.* 1986). Qualitative and quantitative abnormalities of oncogene expression have been reported in a variety of cerebral neoplasms. The best-characterized oncogene is N-*myc*, which has been found to be amplified in neuroblastomas, astrocytomas, and retinoblastomas. Moreover, a relationship between the amplification of N-*myc* and tumour progression was observed in neuroblastomas: the level of amplification was directly related to higher degrees of malignancy as expressed by clinical staging. Conversely, *retinoic acid*, known to induce cellular differentiation, caused a decrease of N-*myc* expression in a neuroblastoma cell line before cell cycle changes and morphological differentiation (Thiele *et al.* 1985). Other oncogenes, including *erb B*, *fos*, *neu*, *n-ras*, *src*, *sis*, and *ros* have also been demonstrated in tumours of the nervous system, and their presumptive mode of action has been reviewed (Schmidek 1987; Whittle 1989). The cause and mechanism of gene amplification in mammalian cells remain largely unknown, but this phenomenon is associated with neoplastic growth, most likely with progression of neoplastic phenotype (Bishop 1987).

Oncogenes could play a role in cell differentiation and divi-

sion: they are closely related to growth factors. The oncogene c-*erb B* encodes a truncated epidermal growth factor receptor and c-*sis* encodes one of the polypeptides of the platelet-derived growth factor. Both these growth factors are known to stimulate mitotic activity in normal glial cells. Thus, the molecular manipulation of tumour differentiation and malignancy through oncogene expression and growth factors is relevant not only to the understanding of the molecular basis of tumorigenesis, but also to future approaches to therapy.

25.8.2 General features

Tumours of the nervous system have several unique features. First, most originate and grow in a limited space: the brain and spinal cord are encased in unyielding fibrous and bony structures. This is particularly important in the case of brain tumours: there is a conflict between the expanding tumour mass and the rigid dura and skull. The results are the signs and symptoms of increased intracranial pressure, and brain tumours may often present with the classical triad of headache, nausea and vomiting, and double vision. Intrinsic growths often cause distortion of normal anatomy and lead to dislocation and herniation of structures (Fig. 25.70). The cingulate gyrus may be forced towards the contralateral hemisphere under the free edge of the falx (*cingulate or supracallosal herniation*), the uncus and the medial part of the parahippocampal gyrus may shift medially and downward through the tentorial opening (*uncal or tentorial herniation*), and the cerebellar tonsils could be displaced caudally through the foramen occipitale magnum (*tonsillar herniation*). The herniated structure in severe cases may suffer haemorrhage and become necrotic. Interference with the CSF may cause hydrocephalus. Disturbance of the cerebral circulation leads to haemorrhages; those occurring in the brainstem are often lethal complication of space-occupying lesions. Another serious and potentially life-threatening complication is *cerebral oedema*. Thus, brain tumours can initiate a

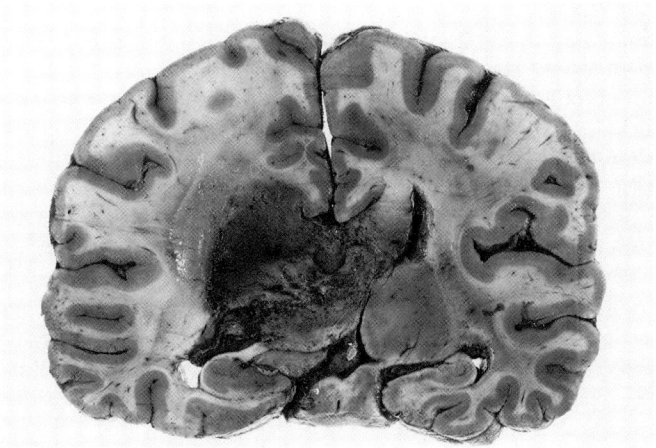

Fig. 25.70 A glioblastoma multiforme spreading to the contralateral hemisphere via the corpus callosum and causing distortion of normal anatomy.

sequence of events which lead to a serious disturbance of the haemodynamics of the central nervous system (reviewed by Miller and Adams 1984).

Secondly, the usual histological and cytological criteria of malignancy cannot be automatically applied to the intrinsic, neuro-epithelial neoplasms of the brain. These tumours are not encapsulated and invade the surrounding brain. Consequently, their surgical extirpation is fraught with difficulty: since their complete removal is hardly ever achieved, they tend to recur and carry a poor prognosis. Even histologically low-grade gliomas may prove fatal, particularly if they develop in areas which contain important functional centres. A low-grade astrocytoma of the brainstem, for example, is biologically a malignant tumour: it allows very little surgical intervention and interferes with vital centres of the brainstem.

Thirdly, neoplasms with mixed cell populations and cellular pleomorphism are common: the histological pattern may vary within the same tumour. More than one cell type may form the tumour: gliomatous and sarcomatous components, glial and neuronal cells, and various glial types may occur within a single neoplasm. Cellular pleomorphism results from differentiation and anaplasia: neuro-epithelial tumours often contain cells at various stages of differentiation, primitive precursors, and bizarre or anaplastic forms.

25.8.3 Grading and classification

A system of grading of neuro-epithelial tumours was introduced to indicate prognosis: four grades of increasing malignancy were distinguished from *grade I to IV* (Kernohan *et al.* 1949). The concept of grading, although useful in histological studies, particularly in assessing tumour progression, and essential in prognosis, presents considerable practical difficulties and hazards. Since many neuro-epithelial tumours display varied histological patterns even within the same tumour, and since anaplasia is often focal, grading of small biopsies is of limited value and can be misleading. Moreover, the site of the tumour, particularly its relationship to CSF pathways and to vital centres, is an important clinical factor which histological grading does not take into account.

Tumours of the nervous system presents a great variety of histological appearances and cytological derivations. Neoplasms can originate from neuro-epithelial cells (neuronal, glial, pineal, and retinal cells), from the meninges, from the components of the peripheral nerves and blood vessels, and from endocrine cells of the adenohypophysis. The nervous system is liable to harbour teratomas and hamartomas, may be involved in neoplasms of adjacent structures and prone to host secondary deposits. Thus, attempts to achieve a universally accepted classification have previously been doomed to failure. The classification by the World Health Organization (Zülch 1979), although far from being perfect, has provided a reasonable framework and eliminated some of the more controversial and confusing entities. This system has now been revised and the following description of pathology has adopted this classification (Kleihues *et al.* 1991).

25.8.4 Tumours of neuro-epithelial tissue

These are intrinsic neoplasms of the nervous system system originating from astrocytes, oligodendrocytes, ependymal and choroid plexus cells, neurones, and pineal cells. Although the term 'glioma' has assumed a wider application, occasionally denoting any primary brain tumour, the name should be reserved for neoplasms of neuroglial tissue.

Astrocytic tumours

Astrocytic neoplasms constituting 20 per cent of neuro-epithelial tumours (Russell and Rubinstein 1989) can develop at any age, the peak of frequency is in the fourth and fifth decades, and affect men more frequently than women, the ratio being 3:2. Astrocytomas can occur anywhere along the neuro-axis, but they are found most commonly in the white matter of the cerebral hemisphere in adults and may extend to the cortex or the basal ganglia. The histology, evolution, and prognosis of astrocytomas greatly depend upon the site of origin: the cerebellar astrocytomas of children, the brainstem gliomas of young adults, and the astrocytomas of the cerebral hemispheres in adults are neoplasms which differ in all these aspects. In the spinal cord they are the second commonest intrinsic tumours after ependymonas. Astrocytomas, like other tumours of neuro-epithelial origin, are single lesions in the overwhelming majority of cases, but microscopical statellite foci and large, widely separated growths are found occasionally.

Astrocytomas

Histologically three different subgroups can be distinguished: *fibrillary*, *protoplasmic*, and *gemistocytic astrocytomas*.

1. *Fibrillary astrocytomas* are relatively slow-growing neoplasms composed of fibrillary astrocytes. The border of the tumour is poorly defined: under the microscope the neoplastic cells diffusely invade the apparently normal-looking, surrounding brain tissue. The fibrillary astrocytes show little pleomorphism: the fusiform cells, frequently arranged in bundles, contain oval or elongated nuclei, and the cytoplasm extends into tapering processes. Other cells are, however, rendered stellate by many cytoplasmic processes. The most important cytoplasmic organelles are fibres, the amount of which depends upon the degree of cellular differentiation. They can be demonstrated by special histological stains, including Mallory's phosphotungstic acid haematoxylin (PTAH) and by the more complicated metallic impregnation techniques. Electron microscopy reveals the fibres to consist of astrocytic filaments of 10 nm in diameter. These intermediate filaments of the cytoskeleton are composed of the *glial fibrillary acidic protein* (GFAP) which was originally extracted from gliotic tissue (Eng *et al.* 1971). The immunohistochemical demonstration of GFAP using anti-GFAP antibodies has provided an invaluable method in the diagnosis of astrocytic tumours. *Glutamine synthetase* (GS) offers a practical alternative to GFAP as an astrocytic marker, particularly in the diagnosis of poorly differentiated astrocytic tumours (Pilkington and Lantos 1982).

2. *Protoplasmic astrocytomas* are rare in pure form and the temporal lobe is the commonest supratentorial site. They tend to be superficial and expand the cortex by ill-defined growth of soft, greyish tissue, which involves the underlying white matter and occasionally the leptomeninges. The neoplastic cells contain few or no astrocytic filaments and resemble normal protoplasmic astrocytes, but are larger with fewer processes. The swollen cytoplasm frequently undergoes degeneration, resulting in microcysts.

3. *Gemistocytic astrocytomas* are restricted to the cerebral hemispheres and, like protoplasmic astrocytomas, are rare in pure forms. The histological appearances are distinctive and unmistakable: the cells are large and polygonal, and the oval or round, relatively small nuclei are eccentric in the abundant, uniformly eosinophilic cytoplasm. Cellular pleomorphism, including binucleate cells, is not uncommon. Electron microscopy shows the cells to be distended by masses of astrocytic filaments and other organelles, including rough endoplasmic reticulum and mitochondria.

Anaplastic (malignant) astrocytomas

Most astrocytic gliomas have a propensity to undergo anaplastic changes and up to 80 per cent show anaplastic areas; astrocytomas of the cerebral hemispheres in adults are particularly prone to become malignant. Anaplastic astrocytomas are large, poorly demarcated, and their cut surface displays a variegated appearance of greyish-white viable tumour tissue alternating with areas of necrosis and haemorrhage. Histologically the entire spectrum of malignancy can be seen: cellular pleomorphism, nuclear hyperchromasia, high mitotic activity, vascular abnormalities, necrosis, and haemorrhage. The cell types vary; in addition to fibrillary, protoplasmic, or gemistocytic astrocytes, poorly differentiated cells and giant forms may also be present. The tumour is richly vascularized and newly formed capillaries with hyperplastic endothelium, particularly at the infiltrating edge, abound.

To distinguish an anaplastic astrocytoma from a glioblastoma multiforme on histological grounds in biopsy specimens may present considerable difficulties, and a clear-cut distinction, however desirable, may not be possible. These tumours invariably carry a poor prognosis, but the survival rate is somewhat better than for glioblastoma multiforme.

Glioblastomas

The incidence of these highly malignant tumours is difficult to establish, for their definition as a separate entity from malignant astrocytomas has been the subject of long controversy. They constitute some 50 per cent of all gliomas and therefore represent the single, most important group of brain tumours. The peak incidence is between 45 and 55 years of age and there is a slight preponderance of males. The deep white matter of the cerebral hemispheres is the common site of occurrence; the tumour develops most frequently in the frontal lobes and the incidence decreases in the posterior parts of the brain. The involvement of more than one lobe is not unusual and the

neoplasms, spreading across the corpus callosum to the contralateral hemisphere, can produce the characteristic 'butterfly' configuration (Fig. 25.70). The relatively well-defined appearances of the growth are deceptive, for diffuse invasion of surrounding tissues is the rule.

Histology reveals a highly cellular neoplasm with endless structural variations, not only in different patients but also within the same tumour. This architectural pleomorphism is ensured by the different constituent cell types and the supervening secondary changes. Spindle-shaped, round, or polygonal cells without any particular features of differentiation are intermingled with bizarre and often multinucleate giant cells. Astrocytic areas are not uncommonly found, whereas oligodendroglial foci are rare and ependymomatous features exceptional. Mitoses are plentiful and frequently abnormal. Pseudopalisading by primitive cells around serpiginous areas of microscopic necrosis is prominent (Fig. 25.71), while massive necroses can devastate all but the peripheral rim of the tumour. The variability of blood vessels is another striking feature and newly formed capillaries with hyperplastic endothelium are plentiful: this can be demonstrated by antibodies to factor VIII-related antigen and to the lectin, *Ulex europaeus* in immunocytochemical reaction. The exuberant vascular proliferation may occasionally become malignant and the resulting tumour is a mixed glioblastoma and sarcoma.

Another variety is the *giant-celled glioblastoma*, in which multinucleated monstrous cells predominate and the abundant stroma is rich in reticulin. Despite the ominous histology, these neoplasms have a slightly better prognosis after surgery and irradiation than typical glioblastomas. All glioblastomas are, however, of grade IV malignancy.

The pathogenesis of glioblastomas has been the subject of controversy between two schools of thought. One regards glioblastomas to represent an end-state in the evolution of gliomas, predominantly of astrocytomas, which have undergone anaplasia, widespread and severe enough to eradicate any distinctive features of glial differentiation. The opposite view maintains

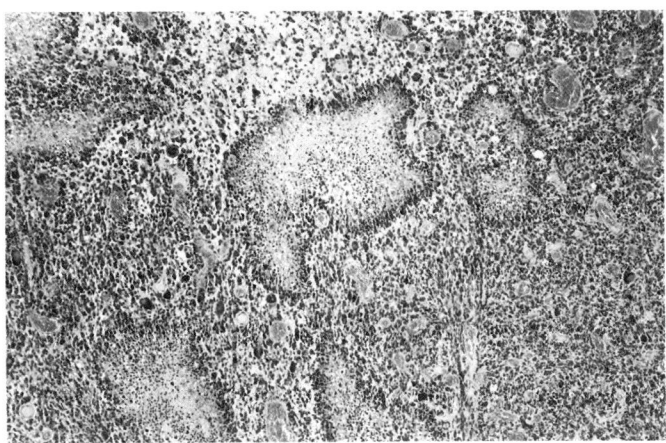

Fig. 25.71 Necrotic areas surrounded by neoplastic cells (pseudopalisading) in a glioblastoma multiforme.

that glioblastomas arise *de novo* from primitive cells and not from pre-existing astrocytomas by anaplasia. The controversy, however exciting, is of academic importance and unlikely to be unequivocally decided, since the earliest changes of tumour development cannot be studied in man. Although well-documented cases with successive biopsies have gone a long way to shed some light on tumour progression, the factors initiating and governing anaplasia have remained largely unknown.

Pilocytic astrocytomas

This category comprises a variety of astrocytic tumours, including cerebellar astrocytomas, and many of the brain stem gliomas. Gliomas of the neurohypophyseal region, inappropriately called 'infundibulomas', also belong to this group.

The predominant cell is the *pilocytic astrocyte*: a bipolar cell with fusiform nucleus and attenuated fibrillary processes, forming parallel bundles (Fig. 25.72). Astrocytomas can assume a pilocytic growth pattern when they invade the corpus callosum or the long fibre tracts of the brainstem and adapt themselves to their environment: this structural plasticity is a salient astrocytic feature. Stellate astrocytes are also commonly encountered. Some pilocytic astrocytomas, particularly those of the cerebellum, have a biphasic architecture: solid, pilocytic tissue alternates with loose, microcystic areas. Exaggerated microcystic degeneration may lead to the formation of large cysts at the expense of solid tumour tissue which survives as a mural nodule. Pilocytic astrocytomas often display *Rosenthal fibres* and *intracytoplasmic droplets*. The Rosenthal fibres are eosinophilic, PTAH-positive, irregular carrot-shaped structures, which in the electron microscope appear to be composed of osmiophilic bodies associated with dense feltwork of thickened glial filaments. Accordingly, they show a varying pattern of reaction for GFAP: larger fibres are entirely negative or have a narrow peripheral positive ring, whereas occasional smaller fibres are

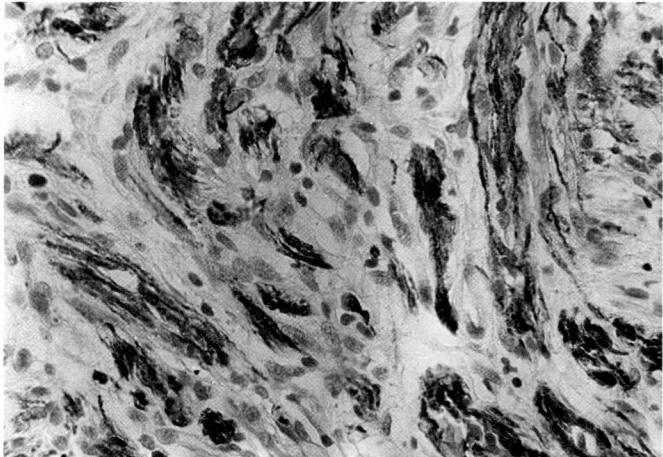

Fig. 25.72 A cerebellar astrocytoma shows GFAP-positive cell processes, some arranged in bundles. (Biotin–streptavidin immunoperoxidase reaction.)

positive. The intracytoplasmic droplets or granules may be formed by the fusion of autophagic vacuoles, and thus represent an advanced stage of cellular degeneration.

Pilocytic astrocytomas are slow growing and, although locally invasive, anaplasia is of rare occurrence. Moreover, *optic gliomas*, a rare variety, are thought to be hamartoma-like growths, on the basis of both biological and clinical behaviour.

Pleomorphic xanthoastrocytomas

These tumours have been recently identified by their distinctive site, morphology, and prognosis as a new entity within the group of astrocytic gliomas (Kepes *et al.* 1979). Pleomorphic astrocytomas usually develop in children and adults as supratentorial, superficial growths which may reach a considerable size, involving the leptomeninges. The histology is strikingly pleomorphic with many bizarre and multinucleate giant forms, and tumour cells are often heavily lipidized. There is an abundant reticulin network which, in the electron microscope, corresponds to basal lamina around tumour cells. This suggests that pleomorphic xanthoastrocytomas originate from subpial astrocytes which are known to be partly covered by basal lamina. GFAP positivity further supports the astrocytic derivation of these neoplasms. Despite the pleomorphic histology, these gliomas carry a good prognosis, and for this reason it is important to distinguish them from glioblastomas.

Subependymal giant cell astrocytomas

These are ventricular tumours of the *tuberous sclerosis complex*; frequently multiple nodules forming the classical appearance of candle gutterings of the ventricular wall. They may also occur in the absence of tuberous sclerosis. Tumours, developing at strategic points, e.g. occluding the foramen of Monro, can interfere with the flow of the CFS and cause hydrocephalus. Histologically, the tumours are composed of large, often fusiform and pyramidal cells, which are embedded in a dense fibrillary and frequently calcified matrix. They are circumscribed, slow growing, and carry a good prognosis. However, immunohistochemical evidence challenged the purely astrocytic nature of these tumours: variable staining for GFAP and neurone-specific enolase suggests that some cells may have unique, neither astrocytic, nor neuronal phenotypes.

Oligodendroglial tumours

These constitute only 5 per cent of all intracranial gliomas and their peak incidence is in the fourth and fifth decades of life. They occur most frequently in the cerebral hemispheres, while other sites, including the region of the third ventricle, the cerebellum, and the spinal cord, are rarely affected. Oligodendrogliomas involve the subcortical white matter and cortex, spreading to the leptomeninges, or develop in the deep white matter, reaching the ventricles. The soft, sometimes well-defined tumour displays occasional cystic degeneration and frequent calcification: the latter feature is of diagnostic importance in neuro-imaging.

The tumour is composed of a uniform population of oligodendrocytes. The round or oval nuclei are embedded in clear

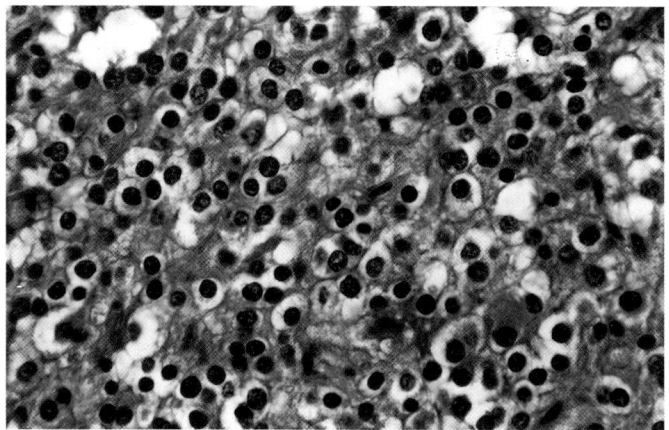

Fig. 25.73 The typical honeycomb appearance of an oligodendroglioma: regular round nuclei are embedded in the clear cytoplasm, demarcated by well-defined cell membranes.

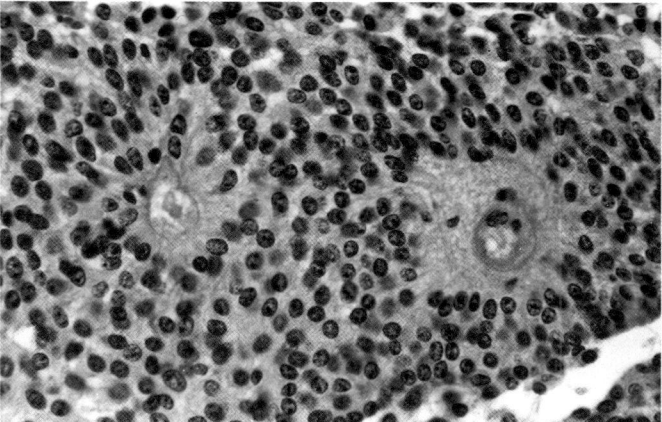

Fig. 25.74 Cells of an ependymoma forming a rosette and a perivascular pseudorosette.

cytoplasm demarcated by a well-defined cell membrane: this imparts the characterstic honeycomb appearance to the tissue (Fig. 25.73). A delicate supporting fibrovascular stroma breaks up the uniform mass of tumour cells. The thin-walled blood vessels are liable to become encrusted with calcium, and spontaneous haemorrhage, causing sudden coma and death, is not uncommon.

The view that oligodendrogliomas are always benign and of slow evolution had to be revised, for it was recognized that some tumours contain an astrocytic component, while others are prone to become anaplastic. Mixed oligo-astrocytomas and anaplastic oligodendrogliomas have a worse prognosis, but even the classical oligodendroglioma may run an unpredictable course.

Ependymal and choroid plexus tumours

Ependymomas

These tumours constitute only about 6 per cent of intracranial gliomas, but they are the commonest intraspinal neoplasms. Although ependymomas can occur in adults, they are predominantly tumours of childhood and adolescence; the maximal incidence is well below the age of 10 years. The fourth ventricle in children is the most frequent site: 60 per cent of intracranial ependymomas are subtentorial, whereas 40 per cent are situated above the tentorium. The neoplasms can reach a considerable size, occasionally obliterating the ventricles and causing hydrocephalus. The growths appear to be well defined and their consistency varies from firm, solid mass to soft, gelatinous tissue. In the spinal cord they distend the affected segments, whereas in the region of the cauda equina, a preferential site, lobulated, gelatinous masses are common.

Histologically the ependymal cells form rosettes, canals, perivascular pseudorosettes, and groups of various sizes (Fig. 25.74). In rosettes, the cells surround a central lumen: these structures are diagnostic hallmarks of better differentiated ependymomas. A more common configuration is the *perivascular pseudorosette*, in which the cells are orientated towards a blood vessel.

Electron microscopy reveals features resembling normal ependyma: vestiges of *bipolar cytoarchitecture*, elaborate *intercellular junctions*, *cytoplasmic filaments*, and *basal bodies*. These latter are the structures, the shaft of cilia, which correspond to the rod-shaped, PTAH-positive *blepharoplasts* seen after meticulous search in the light microscope. Ependymomas show GFAP positivity, particularly the processes of cells forming pseudorosettes.

Ependymomas are usually slowly growing tumours, but occasional anaplastic forms are recognized. These are malignant cellular neoplasms which, although containing areas of anaplasia, show recognizable ependymomatous features. A rapidly growing and diffusely invading rare variety is the *ependymoblastoma*; this tumour is composed of primitive cells resembling spongioblasts, but areas of ependymal differentiation are also present. Other histological variants include the *myxopapillary ependymomas*, occurring nearly always in the region of the cauda equina; the *papillary ependymomas*, resembling occasionally choroid plexus papillomas; and *subependymomas*. In these last tumours, frequently incidental findings at post-mortem examinations in the fourth or lateral ventricles, groups of ependymal cells are embedded in a dense matrix of glial fibres. Large, infiltrating tumours of the fourth ventricle with a poor prognosis have also been reported. The process of proliferation appears to be maintained by fibrillary astrocytes and not by the more inert ependymal cells.

Choroid plexus tumours

Papillomas of the choroid plexus are rare. They occur in adults, but a considerable proportion is found in children and even congenital forms have been recorded. The fourth, lateral, and third ventricles are involved, in this order of frequency, nearly

50 per cent being subtentorial. The tumours form reddish, cauliflower-like growths, which often become heavily calcified. The histology simulates the normal architecture of the choroid plexus: the papillary fronds are composed of a single layer of columnar or cuboidal epithelium which is mounted on a well-vascularized connective tissue stroma. This feature helps to distinguish choroid plexus papillomas from papillary ependymomas: the stroma of this latter contains chiefly neuroglial tissue. However, this distinction is not so clear-cut: a large proportion of choroid plexus papillomas contain GFAP, suggesting focal ependymal differentiation. Choroid plexus papillomas are benign, although seedlings may be carried by the CSF to distant parts of the neuroaxis. The tumour is liable to spontaneous haemorrhage, resulting in blood-stained or xanthochromic CSF. Hydrocephalus is a common complication: the papillomas may expend the ventricles locally, may cause obstruction, or may produce an excessive amount of CSF.

Malignant forms, *choroid plexus carcinomas*, are very rare and occur mainly in children; when they develop in adults, secondary deposits from a distant carcinoma should be excluded before the diagnosis is made. Choroid plexus carcinomas diffusely invade the brain and in doing so lose their regular papillary architecture.

Pineal cell tumours

Tumours originating from pineal cells are rare and can be divided into two groups according to their degree of differentiation; *pineocytomas* and *pineoblastomas*. The term 'pinealoma', frequently used to denote any tumour of the pineal region, should be reserved for these neoplasms. Other tumours of this area, but not of the pineal parenchyma, are teratomas, gliomas, and cysts.

Pineocytomas and pineoblastomas

These tumours represent various stages of differentiation of the pineal cells and transitional forms between the two groups exist. The more primitive pineoblastomas afflict younger age-groups, mainly children, whereas the better differentiated pineocytomas can occur at any age from childhood to senescence.

Pineocytomas are usually well-defined growths composed of relatively uniform cells resembling their normal counterparts. Rosettes, perivascular pseudorosettes, and linear palisades may all be seen within the framework of a fine fibrovascular stroma. The scanty cytoplasm may extend into a single polar process which can be best appreciated in silver impregnation. The biological behaviour of pineocytomas is unpredictable and depends upon their potential to differentiate into glial or ganglionic lines, or both. 'Pure' pineocytomas are malignant, while those with neuronal or neuronal and astrocytic differentiation are relatively benign. Pineocytomas with astrocytic maturation may be slowly growing or malignant.

Pineoblastomas are malignant tumours similar to medulloblastomas: invasion of surrounding tissues and formation of widespread cerebrospinal metastases are common. Histology shows a cellular growth composed of undifferentiated cells with hyperchromatic nuclei surrounded by a narrow rim of cytoplasm. Differentiation is evidenced by occasional rosettes of the *Homer–Wright type* and, in rare instances, retinoblastomatous features testify the role of the pineal gland as a photoreceptive organ at earlier stages of phylogenesis. The survival time for patients with pineoblastomas or pineocytomas without any evidence of differentiation is less than 2 years (Rubinstein 1981).

Neuronal and mixed neuronal-glial tumours

This group includes a variety of neoplasms originating from nerve cells and their precursors.

Gangliocytomas are rare tumours and occur most often around the third ventricle or in the temporal lobe of young adults. Mature neurones are the constituent cells with conspicuous Nissl substance and well-formed, argyrophilic processes. These slowly growing, benign neoplasms should be distinguished from occasional cases of gliomas in which entrapped neurones at the infiltrating edge may lead to the false diagnosis of gangliocytoma.

Gangliogliomas are mixed tumours of both nerve and glial cells; the presence of the latter component carries a less favourable prognosis, for it invests the tumour with a potential for malignant transformation. Occasional nerve cell tumours may contain pleomorphic cells at various stages of differentiation from mature neurones to neuroblasts; in these cases the diagnosis of *ganglioneuroblastoma* is warranted. These tumours are more malignant than the previous varieties and it may be difficult to distinguish them from neuroblastomas with foci of neuronal differentiation.

Desmoplastic infantile gangliogliomas are supratentorial tumours composed of neuroepithelial cells with divergent astrocytic and neuronal lines and an extensive desmoplastic tissue elicited by the leptomeninges. They present as large, superficial cystic masses during infancy and have a relatively favourable prognosis after surgical removal (VandenBerg et al. 1987). A recently defined entity in children and young adults is the *dysembryoplastic neuroepithelial tumour* which is associated with intractable epilepsy. These lesions are multicentric, forming well-demarcated nodules in the cortex and underlying white matter, and occurring most often in the temporal lobes. Histologically, they are composed of astrocytes, oligodendrocytes, and neurons. The prognosis is excellent following surgical removal (Daumas-Duport et al. 1988).

Central neurocytomas develop in association with the ventricular system of young adults. Although their histology superficially resembles that of oligodendrogliomas, they are predominantly composed of neuronal cells as demonstrated by electron microscopy and positive reaction with antibodies to neuron specific enolase and synaptophysin. The neoplastic cells may also express GFAP, indicating bipotential differentiation and probably an origin from the primitive cells of the subependymal plate (von Deimling et al. 1990).

Embryonal tumours

This group includes medulloepitheliomas, ependymoblastomas, retinoblastomas, neuroblastomas and primitive neuroectodermal tumours. *Medulloepitheliomas* are rare, primitive tumours composed of epithelial cells which form tubular or papillary patterns, and may differentiate into neuronal and glial lines. *Ependymoblastomas* has been described under ependymomas, and *retinoblastomas* will not be considered here.

Neuroblastomas

Neuroblastomas, while rare in the brain, are common tumours of the peripheral nervous system. Cerebral neuroblastomas occur most frequently in children during the first few years of life and are malignant tumours with a high recurrence rate and a metastatic spread in the cerebrospinal pathways in 40 per cent of cases. Histologically three variants have been distinguished: *classical* (similar to peripheral neuroblastomas), *desmoplastic* (characterized by prominent connective tissue stroma), and *transitional* (containing an admixture of the features of the two previous types).

The peripheral tumours develop in the adrenals and sympathetic ganglia, and are composed of small primitive cells with round or oval, hyperchromatic nuclei and sparse, ill-defined cytoplasm. However, the cells have a tendency to form Homer–Wright rosettes in which the central space is filled with cell processes, and to grow neurofibrillary processes. These features and the presence of mature ganglionic cells testify that the undifferentiated cells of neuroblastomas have a potential to achieve some degree of maturation. Neuroblasts metabolize, store, and secrete *catecholamines*. The breakdown products of these neurotransmitters, including *vanillylmandelic acid* and *homovanillic acid*, are to be found in the urine and serum: the quantitative assessment of these compounds is important not only in prognosis, but also in monitoring the efficacy of chemotherapy. Ultrastructural investigation reveals secretory granules (which are dense-cored vesicles of 100 nm), bundles of neurofilaments, microtubules, and synapse-like structures—features all in support of neuronal derivation. A positive correlation exists between the number of secretory granules, the urinary excretory patterns, and the clinical course: plentiful neurosecretory granules hold the promise of a better prognosis. Antibodies against *neurone-specific enolase* and *neurofilament proteins* are used in immunohistochemical reactions to demonstrate nerve cells and their precursors in this group of neoplasms.

Primitive neuroectodermal tumours

The term primitive neuroectodermal tumour (PNET), was introduced by Rorke (1983) who originally intended to group all the embryonal tumours under this name. This view has not been universally accepted and now PNET is applied to medulloblastomas of the cerebellum and to similar tumours which rarely may develop in the cerebral hemispheres or in the spinal cord.

Medulloblastomas

These tumours occur most frequently in the midline of the cerebellum in children and the incidence gradually decreases with increasing age. A second peak is found in young adults in whom the tumour may be laterally situated. In the differential diagnosis of posterior fossa tumours of children and young adults, medulloblastomas should always be considered: astrocytomas, medulloblastomas, and ependymomas are the commonest neuro-epithelial tumours in children, in this order of frequency, and the cerebellum is the site most frequently involved. Medulloblastomas form 7–8 per cent of intracranial tumours of neuro-epithelial derivation. Their site of origin has been attributed to the *fetal granular layer of Obersteiner*, although primitive cell nests in the posterior medullary velum and the neurones in the internal granular layer have also been considered as alternative sources.

The tumours often occupy the fourth ventricle, occluding the cavity and invading the floor. The cerebellar peduncles may be involved and the cisterna magna obliterated. The laterally located neoplasms are usually well-defined masses over the dorsal surface of the cerebellar lobes, with involvement of the leptomeninges. This access both to the ventricle and to the leptomeninges promotes distant metastases by the CSF pathway. The tumours are extremely cellular: diffuse sheets of primitive cells display hyperchromatic nuclei and sparse cytoplasm (Fig. 25.75). In many meduloblastomas, this cellular monotony is not relieved by any special architectural patterns, whereas in others the cells have a propensity for differentiation towards neuronal or glial cells. This maturation can be demonstrated by immunocytochemical markers of glial, chiefly astrocytic, cells and neurones. Medulloblastomas are highly malignant, but the survival rate depends upon age, sex, and site. Adults and females have longer survival than children and males, and lateral tumours are associated with a better prognosis.

Desmoplastic medulloblastoma is a histological variant with an abundant fibrous stroma rich in reticulin fibres. These tumours are usually laterally situated, develop in adults rather than in children, and carry a marginally better prognosis.

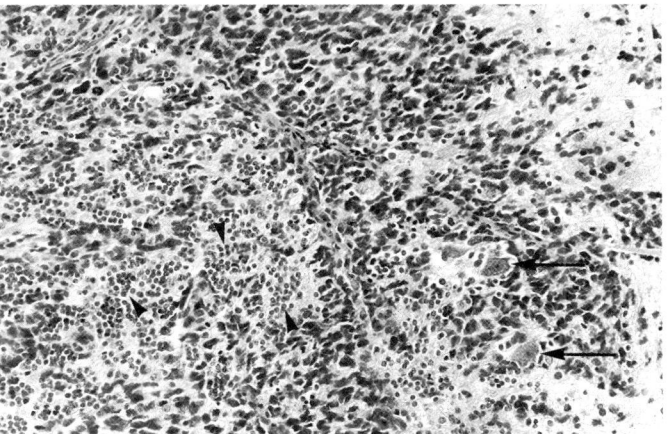

Fig. 25.75 Primitive cells of a medulloblastoma invading the cerebellum. Note surviving Purkinje cells (arrows) and groups of granule cells (arrowheads).

Neuroepithelial tumours of uncertain origin

Three tumour types, astroblastoma, polar spongioblastoma and gliomatosis cerebri, are grouped together, since their histogenesis has not been clarified. *Pure astroblastomas* are rare, and usually occur in the cerebral hemispheres of children and young adults, although an astroblastic pattern may be occasionally found in astrocytomas and glioblastomas. Histology reveals a loose-textured tumour with the characteristic perivascular pattern: the stout processes of neoplastic cells radiate towards the central blood vessel. *Polar spongioblastomas* develop in the vicinity of the ventricular system in children and adolescents. The uni- and bipolar cells are arranged in parallel arrays with conspicuous palisading of the elongated nuclei. Although these neoplasm are undifferentiated, astrocytic maturation may be evidenced by the formation of fine neuroglial fibrils. *Gliomatosis cerebri* is a diffuse malignant growth involving the brain extensively. The neoplastic cells are by no means always undifferentiated, and astrocytic cells are usually present, together with occasional foci of glioblastoma.

25.8.5   Tumours of nerve sheath cells

Schwannomas (neurilemmomas)

These tumours involve the cranial and spinal nerve roots and the peripheral nerves. Intracranial schwannomas constitute 8 per cent of all primary tumours in this region. The tumour has a striking affinity to involve sensory nerves; of these the auditory nerves are far the most frequent site, whereas the trigeminal, vagal, and glossopharyngeal nerves are seldom affected. Schwannomas manifest themselves in middle-aged patients and there is a female preponderance. They tend to be single, while multiple lesions are often associated with von Recklinghausen's disease. Bilaterial acoustic schwannomas are regarded as a manifestation of central von Recklinghausen's disease, even in the absence of cutaneous lesions: these tumours develop earlier, grow faster, attain larger size, and form more cellular growths. The tumours are usually well circumscribed, encapsulated, and firm, with occasional cystic degeneration in the larger examples.

Schwannomas of the spinal nerve roots arise selectively in the posterior roots and, although they can develop anywhere in the cord including the cauda equina, the lumbar segments are most frequently involved. Occasionally they extend through the intervertebral foramen to form the so-called *hour-glass tumour*, the peripheral part of which can reach a considerable size. Schwannomas of the peripheral nerves usually occur in major nerve trunks, frequently on the flexor aspects of the limbs. They are not uncommon in the posterior mediastinum, a region often involved by neural neoplasms, and in the intercostal nerves.

Histological examination reveals, in the overwhelming majority of cases, the classical appearance of two patterns. The dense *Antoni A-type tissue* consists of interlacing bundles of spindle-shaped cells; the elongated nuclei are frequently arranged to form palisades (Fig. 25.76). This pattern alternates with the loosely structured *Antoni B-type tissue*, in which a more

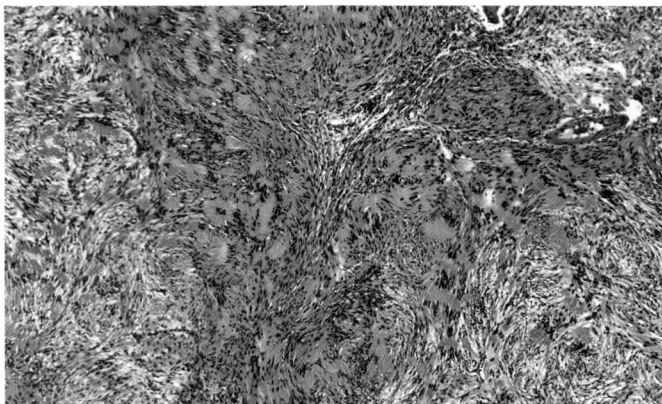

Fig. 25.76 The fusiform cells of a schwannoma form interlacing bundles and show typical palisading of nuclei.

pleomorphic cell population is haphazardly distributed. The loose, eosinophilic matrix lends itself to mucinous degeneration, microcyst formation, and xanthomatous change. There is a rich network of reticulin fibres, particularly in the Antoni A-type tissue. Electron microscopy reveals basement membrane around the tumour cells, the material responsible for the reticulin staining, and so-called *Luse bodies*, extracellular fibrillary structures with a regularly repeated cross-banding at 120–150 nm. Schwannomas contain *S100*, a highly acidic protein present in, but not restricted to, tumours derived from the neural crest. Moreover, most schwannomas (80 per cent) also give a positive immunocytochemical reaction with an antibody against *Leu-7*.

The principal cell of origin of schwannomas has been ascribed to the *endoneurial fibroblast*, perineurial cell, and *Schwann cell*. Electron microscope investigations have eliminated the endoneurial fibroblasts, and the current view favours the schwannian derivation of these tumours. The histological evolution of schwannomas has been reconstructed in neoplasms of various sizes. Small tumours are solid cellular nodules with few blood vessels and without degenerative changes. Antoni B-type tissue appears in large growths in which irregular vascular spaces and extensive secondary changes develop.

Schwannomas are benign tumours of slow growth. Larger intracranial examples, by compressing adjacent structures, particularly the brainstem, undoubtedly represent a serious hazard and the solution lies in surgical removal. Very rare cases may show malignant, anaplastic changes with loss of architectural pattern, high mitotic activity, and invasion of surrounding structures.

Neurofibromas

Neurofibromas are benign, solitary, or multiple, the latter examples are associated with von Recklinghausen's disease. In this condition, in addition to neurofibromas, there is an increased incidence of schwannomas, gliomas (including optic gliomas, astrocytomas, ependymomas, and diffuse glial tumours), meningiomas, and phaeochromocytomas.

The affected nerves display fusiform cylindrical or even spherical enlargements. Neurofibromas consist of a mixture of Schwann cells and fibroblasts. When compared with schwannomas, they are less cellular, looser in texture, and without the characteristic pattern of alternating Antoni A- and B-type tissue. The rich reticulin network of schwannomas is absent, but collagen is plentiful and nerve fibres can be encountered without difficulty.

A malignant counterpart of the benign neurofibroma exists: neurofibromas, usually those associated with von Recklinghausen's disease, may undergo anaplasia resulting in neurofibrosarcoma.

25.8.6 Tumours of meningeal and related tissues

Meningiomas are common tumours, constituting 14 per cent of all primary intracranial neoplasms and 12 per cent of those arising within the spinal canal (Russell and Rubinstein 1989). Although they can afflict any age-group, the maximal incidence is during the middle decades of life and there is a female preponderance. Meningiomas are usually attached to the dura and it is generally accepted that most arise from the arachnoid villi enclosed in the dura, yet others may originate in the perivascular mesenchymal cells within the Virchow–Robin spaces. The source of origin of the intraventricular examples has been ascribed to the tela choroidea or the stroma of the choroid plexus. The tumours can grow to a considerable size, and compress, but do not invade, underlying neural tissues. Many are found incidentally at necropsy.

Half of the intracranial meningiomas over the convexity of the brain are related to the sagittal sinus (parasagittal meningiomas), usually over the middle third. Laterally, the Sylvian fissures and at the base the sphenoidal ridges, olfactory grooves, and the pituitary region are frequent sites. In the spinal canal meningiomas are the commonest primary neoplasms, exceeding the incidence of schwannomas. Although they may occur along the entire length of the spinal canal, the thoracic segments are most often involved. Intraventricular meningiomas also occur, and rare sites include the orbital cavity and the petrous bone.

The histological picture reveals a striking variety of patterns; and the new classification lists no fewer than 11 types (Kleihues et al. 1991). Of these the four commonest forms are the meningothelial, fibrous, transitional, and psammomatous variants. However, quite often more than one pattern may be encountered within the same tumour. Meningothelial meningiomas are composed of sheets of cells with round or oval nuclei and indistinct cell membranes; hence the alternative name of syncytial meningiomas. Bipolar, fibroblast-like cells with elongated nuclei form parallel or interlacing bundles in the fibrous or fibroblastic type. The transitional or mixed variety combines features of the previous two, but the most obvious hallmark is the presence of concentric cellular whorls (Fig. 25.77). In psammomatous meningiomas mineralized structures, the psammoma bodies predominate. This type is most common in

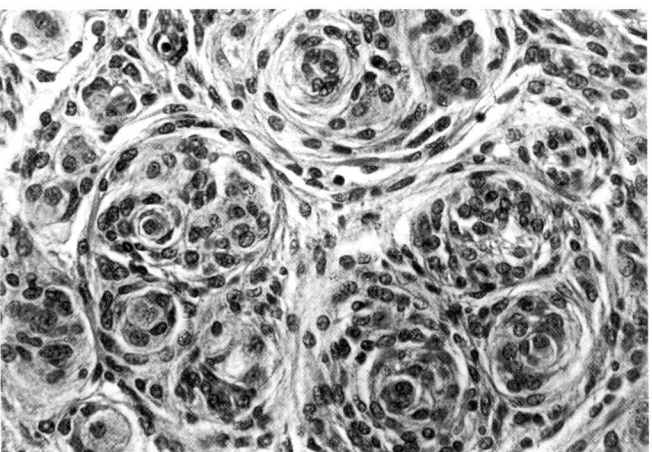

Fig. 25.77 Whorl formation in a meningioma. (van Gieson's stain.)

the spinal canal. They tend to permeate venous sinuses and bones, but only the invasion of the adjacent brain or spinal cord is an ominous sign. Malignant meningiomas fall short of being classified as sarcomas; although anaplastic changes may supervene, some original features of the meningioma are still retained. Papillary meningiomas also pursue a biologically aggressive course. These malignant meningiomas not only invade the brain, but also may give rise to distant secondary deposits. Although most meningiomas can be diagnosed without 'special' stains, an intriguing immunohistochemical feature of these tumours is their expression of both mesenchymal and epithelial antigens: they give positive reactions with antibodies to epithelial membrane antigen, vimentin, and S100 protein.

Primary sarcomas of the meninges are rare and the variants include the *spindle-celled fibrosarcoma*, *polymorphic cell sarcoma*, and *primary meningeal sarcomatosis*. The meninges may also harbour a variety of benign and malignant growths, including xanthomatous tumours and primary melanotic neoplasms.

25.8.7 Primary malignant lymphomas

Amongst the various lymphomatous proliferations which involve primarily the nervous system, malignant lymphomas are the most important. These tumours, previously known as *microgliomas*, were thought to originate from primitive reticulum cells which then could differentiate into metallophilic microglia. Immunohistochemical investigations have convincingly demonstrated the lymphoid derivation of these tumours. Recent evidence indicates the involvement of Epstein–Barr virus in the causation of these lymphomas (Hochberg and Miller 1988). They may be solitary, multifocal, or diffuse, involving more than one lobe. The maximum incidence is in the fifth and sixth decades, and both sexes are equally affected. Histology reveals a cellular, pleomorphic tumour in which the predominant cell type belongs to the lymphoid series: they are B-type lymphocytes at various stages of maturation. Perivascular cuffing is a constant and prominent feature and the neoplastic cells infiltrate not only the distended Virchow–Robin spaces, but also

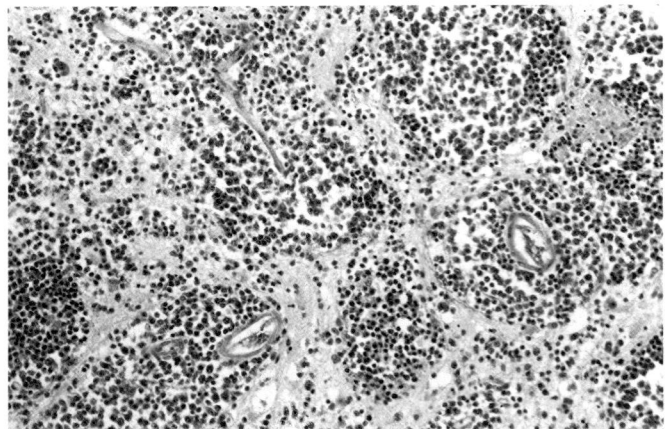

Fig. 25.78 Malignant non-Hodgkin lymphoma in a patient with AIDS, showing a typical multicentric, often perivascular arrangement of cells.

the vascular wall, splaying its layers apart (Fig. 25.78). The presence of macrophages and reactive astrocytes also contributes to the cellular pleomorphism. Immunohistochemistry is essential in the accurate diagnosis: staining for κ and λ light chains reveals monoclonal immunoglobulin production in most cases, although a few lymphomas may synthesize both. The macrophage constituent, including microglial cells, can be demonstrated by staining for *muramidase*, *α-1-antitrypsin*, and *α-1-antichymotrypsin*. For these cells and for the lymphocytes a range of other antibodies are available (Adams and Howatson 1990). These tumours are frequently associated with naturally occurring and artifically induced abnormalities of immunological mechanisms: patients with AIDS and those who received immunosuppressive therapy for organ transplantation are particularly at risk. AIDS-associated lymphomas tend to be extensive, multicentric, and of B-cell origin. With the spreading epidemic, their frequency is likely to increase. There is a tendency to apply the classification of non-Hodgkin lymphomas to these tumours, but until a universally accepted classification is agreed upon this may prove to be more confusing than helpful.

25.8.8   Tumours of blood-vessel origin

Of these tumours, *capillary haemangioblastomas* are common: they constitute between 1.1 and 2.4 per cent of all intracranial tumours. They involve most frequently the cerebellum where the paramedian site is preferred, but the spinal cord, medulla, and supratentorial regions may also harbour these neoplasms. Most examples are solitary, but multiple lesions are not uncommon, suggesting *Lindau's syndrome*. This is a familial, inherited condition frequently associated with angiomatosis of the retina (*von Hippel's disease*), benign cysts of the pancreas and kidneys, and neoplasms of the adrenals and kidneys. The association of haemangioblastomas with erythrocythaemia has been well established. The tumours are well defined, although not encapsulated, and tend to become cystic. They may be found outside

the parenchyma of the central nervous system, particularly in the spinal canal. The most conspicuous histological feature is the presence of vascular channels of various sizes: capillary structures and dilated sinusoidal vessels intermingle with polygonal, frequently foamy, stromal cells. The endothelial cells lining the vessels may be hypertrophied, but without any evidence of pleomorphism or crowding. Electron microscopy reveals three cell types: *endothelial cells, pericytes,* and *stromal cells*. The origin of stromal cells and their role in the formation of haemangioblastomas have been disputed. Opinions are divided as to whether they have an exclusively supporting function or are endowed with angiogenic potential. It has been suggested that stromal cells are, in fact, stem cells which differentiate into the 'vasoformative' elements of endothelial cells and pericytes. The possibility that some of the stromal cells may be of astrocytic origin has been considered on the basis of their GFAP content, but this finding could result from the uptake of this protein by non-glial cells in the vicinity of fibrillary gliosis.

Reflecting this uncertainty of histogenesis, the new classification places capillary haemangioblastomas, together with haemangiopericytomas, into a subgroup within the large group of mesenchymal, non-meningothelial tumours. Haemangiopericytomas of the meninges, previously regarded as a variant of meningiomas, have been shown to be identical with those which occur elsewhere in the body. In the meninges, they are cellular, mitotically active, and liable to recur.

The vascular malformations include *capillary telangiectasias, cavernous angiomas, arteriovenous malformations, venous malformations,* and *Sturge–Weber disease. Arteriovenous malformations,* frequently referred to as *angiomas,* are relatively common; the incidence varies from 0.5 per cent to 3.7 per cent of intracranial tumours in the material of different neurosurgical clinics, but 1 per cent appears to be a realistic figure. There is a clear male preponderance of 2:1. The preferential site is the territory of the middle cerebral artery, while the cerebellum, midbrain, and spinal cord may also be involved. Their size varies from the large examples which become embedded into the substance of the brain, causing atrophy and degeneration, to small cryptic cases which, being prone to cause fatal intracerebral haemorrhage, may be difficult to recover in the haematoma. These malformamations are composed of a collection of abnormal blood-vessels; the size and configuration of the vascular channels, and the thickness and histological composition of their walls vary considerably.

25.8.9   Germ cell tumours

Germinomas, embryonal carcinomas, choriocarcinomas, and *teratomas* belong to this group, tumours which most often occur in the pineal region. *Germinomas,* or *atypical teratomas,* are the commonest growths in this area: they may develop adjacent to the pineal gland or in a suprasellar position, involving the third ventricle. Males are more often affected and the tumours are usually discovered between the ages of 15 and 26 years.

Germinomas, particularly the larger ones, extensively invade surrounding tissues, and access to the ventricular system promotes distant metastasis. Histologically, the tumour is indistinguishable from testicular seminomas and ovarian dysgerminomas and is composed of two cell types. Large polygonal cells (which are the cardinal neoplastic elements with high mitotic rates) and small lymphoid cells are intermingled in a lobular pattern maintained by the fibrovascular stroma.

25.8.10 Malformative tumours and tumour-like lesions

This mixed group includes various *cystic and hamartomatous lesions: craniopharyngiomas* and *Rathke's cleft cysts, epidermoid* and *dermoid cysts, colloid cysts of the third ventricle,* and *enterogenous cysts. Lipomas, choristomas (granular cell myoblastomas), hypothalamic neuronal hamartomas,* and *nasal gliomas* complete the full list. All these conditions are entirely benign. Of these malformations, craniopharyngiomas and epidermoid cysts will be considered.

Craniopharyngiomas, or suprasellar cysts, are thought to originate from the remnants of the Rathke's pouch, which is an evagination of the primitive stomatodeum. They are common, constituting 3 per cent of all intracranial tumours, and more than half are detected in childhood and adolescence. Craniopharyngiomas are partly solid and partly cystic, or may be entirely cystic. Larger examples may compress the optic chiasma in front, the floor of the third ventricle above, and the pituitary gland below. The solid part of the tumour is composed of trabeculae and islands of epithelial cells supported by a connective tissue stroma. Degeneration of epithelium with formation of keratin masses and secondary changes in the stroma, including inflammatory exudate and microcyst formation, commonly occur. The lining of the cystic part is stratified squamous epithelium mounted on a collagenous basement membrane.

Epidermoid cysts or *cholesteatomas* are rarer than craniopharyngiomas and usually are detected later in life. They favour the cerebello-pontine angle, but the pituitary region, rhomboid fossa, and the diploe are well-recognized sites. The cysts vary in size and their capsule, displaying a mother-of-pearl sheen, has warranted the name of *pearly tumour.* The cyst lining is composed of simple squamous epithelium which continuously sheds keratinous material into the cavity. The keratin lamellae gradually expand the cyst and, escaping into the CSF, may cause *granulomatous meningitis.*

25.8.11 Tumours of the anterior pituitary

The incidence of pituitary adenoma varies from 7 to 17.8 per cent in various material, the former figure being the more realistic. The real incidence, however, is more difficult to assess, since apparently normal glands may contain, on thorough histological examination, one or more areas of adenomatous proliferation, so-called *microadenomas.* The distinction between hyperplasia and neoplasia in endocrine organs is often blurred, but these microadenomas will increase the overall incidence.

The classification of these tumours, based on the tinctorial propensities of cells, into chromophobe, acidophil, and basophil adenomas is convenient, but in the light of recent ultrastructural and immunohistochemical investigations can hardly be maintained. There is a tendency to classify adenomas on the basis of functional criteria, whether they are endocrinologically active or not, and the former group is then subdivided according to the hormones produced: growth hormone, prolactin, corticotroph, thyrotroph, gonadotroph, etc. cell adenomas. The recent classification, based on morphogenesis, ultrastructure, clinical features, and structure–function relationship is discussed in Section 26.1.

Pituitary adenomas are usually detected between 30 and 50 years of age, although earlier manifestations of those associated with growth hormone production do occur. On the whole, the tumours are benign, but they may encroach upon the brain and, by occupying the cavity of the third ventricle, can cause hydrocephalus. Compression of the optic chiasma, erosion of bones, particularly the floor of the sella, and involvement of the cavernous sinus are not unusual. The capsule may be breached with consequent permeation of adjacent structures, but this complication is not an unequivocal evidence of malignancy. Only when there is considerable mitotic activity, nuclear pleomorphism with hyperchromasia, and permeation of vessel walls by tumour cells should the diagnosis of malignant adenoma be entertained.

25.8.12 Local extension from regional tumours

This mixed group includes tumours which spread to the nervous system from adjacent structures: they are chiefly, but not exclusively, neoplasms of bones and other mesodermal elements. Amongst the various entities *chordomas* merit a special comment, because they are not only relatively common, but also of interest to pathologists and clinicians alike. Chordomas originate from the embryonic vestiges of notochord represented by the nucleus pulposus of the intervertebral discs. They are detected during the third and fourth decades of life, although the sacrococcygeal examples cause clinical signs and symptoms earlier. There is a male predominance. They develop at the base of the skull and in the vertebral column: of the 600 cases reviewed, 50 per cent originated in the sacrum, 35 per cent in the spheno-occipital region, and the rest in the vertebrae. Macroscopically, chordomas are soft, almost translucent, and gelatinous. Histology reveals the characteristic *physaliphorous cells*: the vacuolated cytoplasm contains hyperchromatic nuclei. They are locally invasive, tend to recur after surgical removal, and are resistant to radiotherapy: thus they carry a poor prognosis, despite the benign histological appearances.

25.8.13 Metastatic tumours

Secondary neoplasms of the nervous system, being common, constitute an important group. Although the incidence ranges from 3.2 per cent to 36.81 per cent; a figure of 20 per cent of all intracranial tumours seems realistic. Carcinoma are far the commonest source of secondary deposits: undisputedly, *bronchial cancer* leads the list, followed by *carcinoma of the breast, kidney, alimentary tract*, and *thyroid*. Choriocarcinomas, testicular tumours, and malignant melanomas are also liable to involve the central nervous system. Bronchial carcinomas not uncommonly manifest with a brain metastasis, and in these cases the clinical diagnosis of a primary brain tumour is likely to be made. Occasionally, the primary bronchogenic tumour is small and may prove difficult to detect at autopsy. Sarcomas can also give rise to metastasis in the brain, but the incidence is relatively low, for every patient with a sarcoma metastasis there are 10 cases of secondary carcinoma. Lymphomas and leukaemias can also spread to the nervous system and the involvement may be more diffuse than in carcinomas. The neurological manifestations of systemic malignant disease have been comprehensively reviewed (Henson and Urich 1982).

Secondary deposits tend to be well defined and frequently spherical, surrounded by oedematous brain. Multiple secondary growths are frequent and, even when there is a single solitary deposit, histology may reveal many minute seedlings. Microscopical examination also shows extensive invasion of the surrounding brain, the circumscribed appearance of secondary deposits is therefore deceptive. The distribution appears to be haphazard, but small metastases are frequently discovered at the border of the cortex and white matter, at a site where emboli tend to be lodged. This suggests that haemodynamic factors, the difference between the well-vascularized cortex and the less well-supplied white matter, may play an important role in determining the site.

The leptomeninges may become involved by direct spread from metastases reaching the surface of the brain, but the more *diffuse* 'carcinomatous meningitis' may occur after the secondary deposit has gained entry into the ventricular system. Malignant cells may reach the neural tissue not only directly by the bloodstream, but also by spreading from an established metastasis in the adjacent bone.

25.8.14   Bibliography

Adams, J. H. and Howatson, A. G. (1990). Cerebral lymphomas: review of 70 cases. *Journal of Clinical Pathology* **43**, 544–7.

Bishop, J. M. (1987). The molecular genetics of cancer. *Science* **235**, 305–11.

Codd, M. B. and Kurland, L. T. (1985). Descriptive epidemiology of primary intracranial neoplasms. *Progress in Experimental Tumor Research* **29**, 1–11.

Daumas-Duport, C., *et al.* (1988). Dysembryoplastic neuroepithelial tumour: a surgically curable tumor of young patients with intractable partial seizures. *Neurosurgery* **23**, 545–56.

von Deimling, A., Janzer, R., Kleihues, P., and Wiestler, O. D. (1990). Patterns of differentiation in central neurocytoma: an immunohistochemical study of eleven biopsies. *Acta Neuropathologica* **79**, 473–9.

Eng, L. F., Vanderhaeghen, J. J., Bignami, A., and Gerstl, B., (1971). An acidic protein isolated from fibrous astrocytes. *Brain Research* **28**, 351–4.

Goldberg, I. D. and Kurland, L. T. (1962). Mortality in 33 countries from diseases of the nervous system. *World Neurology* **3**, 444–65.

Henson, R. A. and Urich, H. (1982). *Cancer and the nervous system*. Blackwell, Oxford.

HMSO Mortality Statistics (1989) *Cause*. Office of Population Censuses and Surveys, Series DH2, no. 16. HMSO, London.

Hochberg, F. H. and Miller, D. C. (1988). Primary central nervous system lymphoma. *Journal of Neurosurgery* **68**, 835–53.

Ironside, J. W., Battersby, R. D. E., Dangerfield, V. J. M., Parsons, M. A., Timperley, W. R., and Underwood, J. C. E. (1986). Cryostat section assay of oestrogen and progesterone receptors in meningiomas: a clinicopathological study. *Journal of Clinical Pathology* **39**, 44–50.

Jadayel, D. *et al.* (1990). Paternal origin of new mutations in von Recklinghausen neurofibromatosis. *Nature* **343**, 558–9.

Jänisch, W. and Schreiber, D. (1977). *Experimental tumours of the central nervous system*. Upjohn, Kalamazoo.

Kepes, J. J., Rubinstein, L. J., and Eng, L. F. (1979). Pleomorphic xanthoastrocytoma: a distinctive meningocerebral glioma of young subjects with relatively favourable prognosis—a study of 12 cases. *Cancer* **44**, 1839–52.

Kernohan, J. W., Habon, R. F., Svien, H. J., and Adson, A. W. (1949). A simplified classification of the gliomas. *Proceedings of the Mayo Clinic* **24**, 71–5.

Kinlen, L. J., Sheil, A. G. R., Peto, J., and Doll, R. (1979). Collaborative United Kingdom–Australasian study of cancer in patients treated with immunosuppressive drugs. *British Medical Journal* **2**, 1461–6.

Kleihues, P., Burger, P. C., and Scheithauer, B. W. (1991). *Histological typing of tumours of the central nervous system* (2nd edn). Springer-Verlag, Berlin, in press.

Lantos, P. L. (1985). Cerebral neoplasia. In *Scientific basis of clinical neurology* (ed. M. Swash and C. Kennard), pp. 557–82. Churchill Livingstone, Edinburgh.

Lantos, P. L. (1986). Development of nitrosourea-induced brain tumours—with a special note on changes occurring during latency. *Food and Chemical Toxicology* **24**, 121–7.

Liwnicz, B. H., Berger, T. S., Liwnicz, R. G., and Aron, B. S. (1985). Radiation-associated gliomas: a report of four cases and analysis of postradiation tumors of the central nervous system. *Neurosurgery* **17**, 436–45.

McLaughlin, J. K., *et al.* (1987). Occupational risks for intracranial gliomas in Sweden. *Journal of the National Cancer Institute* **78**, 253–7.

McMahon, B. (1962). Prenatal X-ray exposure and childhood cancer. *Journal of the National Cancer Institute* **28**, 1173–91.

Miller, D. J. and Adams, J. H. (1984). The pathophysiology of raised intracranial pressure. In *Greenfield's neuropathology* (ed. J. H. Adams, J. A. N. Corsellis, and L. W. Duchen) (4th edn), pp. 53–84. Edward Arnold, London.

Pilkington, G. J. and Lantos, P. L. (1982). The role of glutamine synthetase in the diagnosis of cerebral tumours. *Neuropathology and Applied Neurobiology* **8**, 227–36.

Pilkington, G. J. and Lantos, P. L. (1990). Pathology of experimental brain tumours. In *Neuro-oncology: primary malignant brain tumours* (ed. D. G. T. Thomas), pp. 51–76. Edward Arnold, London.

Rorke, B. R. (1983). The cerebellar medulloblastoma and its relationship to primitive neuroectodermal tumors. *Journal of Neuropathology and Experimental Neurology* **42**, 1–15.

Rouleau, G. A., *et al.* (1987). Genetic linkage of bilateral acoustic neurofibromatosis to a DNA marker on chromosome 22. *Nature* **329**, 246–8.

Rubinstein, L. J. (1981) Cytogenesis and differentiation of pineal neoplasms. *Human Pathology* **12**, 441–8.

Russell, D. S. and Rubinstein, L. J. (1989). *Pathology of tumours of the nervous system* (5th edn). Edward Arnold, London.

Schmidek, H. H. (1987). The molecular genetics of nervous system tumours. *Journal of Neurosurgery* **67**, 1–16.

Schober, R. and Herman, M. M. (1973). Neuropathology of cardiac transplantation. Survey of 31 cases. *Lancet* **i**, 962–7.

Seizinger, B. R., Martuza, R. L., and Gusella, J. F. (1986). Loss of genes on chromosome 22 in tumorigenesis of human acoustic neuroma. *Nature* **322**, 644–7.

Thiele, C. J., Reynolds, C. P., and Israel, M. A. (1985) Decreased expression of N-*myc* precedes retinoic acid-induced morphological differentiation of human neuroblastoma. *Nature* **313**, 404–6.

Tijssen, C. C., Halprin, M. R., and Endtz, L. T. (1982). *Familial brain tumours. A commented register.* Martinus Nijhoff, The Hague.

VandenBerg, S. R., *et al.* (1987). Desmosplastic supratentorial neuroepithelial tumors of infancy with divergent differentiation potential ('desmoplastic infantile gangliogliomas'). *Journal of Neurosurgery* **66**, 58–71.

Weil, A. (1946). *Textbook of neuropathology* (2nd edn). Heinemann, London.

Whittle, I. R. (1989). Oncogenes and neuro-oncology. *British Journal of Neurosurgery* **3**, 3–12.

Willis, R. A. (1962) *The pathology of the tumours of children.* Oliver and Boyd, Edinburgh.

Zülch, K. J. (ed.) (1979). *Histological typing of tumours of the central nervous system*, International histological classification of tumours, No. 21. World Health Organization, Geneva.

Zülch, K. J. (1986). *Brain tumors. Their biology and pathology.* Springer-Verlag, Berlin.

25.9 Peripheral nerves

R. O. Weller

Peripheral nerve diseases present clinically with various combinations of sensory disturbance, muscle weakness and wasting, and defects of autonomic function. The sensory and motor disorders predominantly affect the distal parts of the limbs; this distribution helps to distinguish peripheral nerve diseases from primary muscle disease in which the proximal muscles of the limbs are mainly affected. Different patterns of *peripheral neuropathy* are seen; in some, many nerves are affected in a symmetrical pattern (*polyneuropathy*, or *polyneuritis*); alternatively a single nerve may be affected (*mononeuritis*) or several individual nerves may be affected in an asymmetrical pattern (*mononeuritis multiplex*). Neuropathies are often characterized by the time scale of their onset; thus, they may be acute, subacute, chronic, progressive, or relapsing.

Despite the wide range of clinical presentation seen with neuropathies, peripheral nerves exhibit only two major pathological reactions, viz. *axonal degeneration* and *segmental demyelination*. The clinical signs, symptoms, and progression of peripheral nerve diseases depend upon the anatomical location of the disease process and the predominant pathological reaction.

25.9.1 Normal peripheral nerves

The majority of cranial and spinal peripheral nerves are *mixed motor* and *sensory nerves*. Motor nerves arise from anterior horn

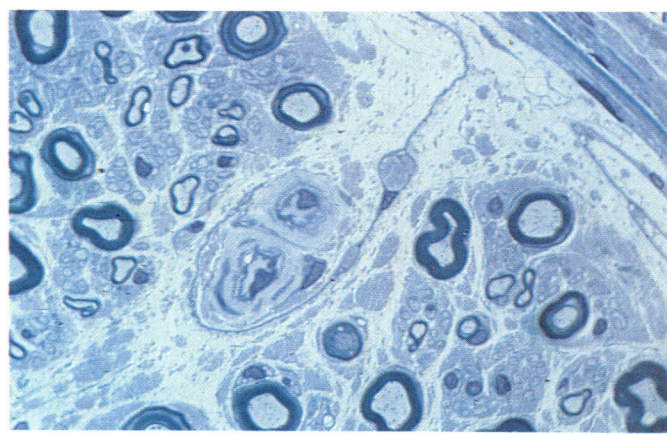

Fig. 25.79 Normal peripheral nerve. The perineurium (top right) encloses the fascicle and, within the endoneurium, there are blood-vessels (centre) and large and small myelinated fibres, seen here cut in cross-section. (1 μm resin section stained with toluidine blue.)

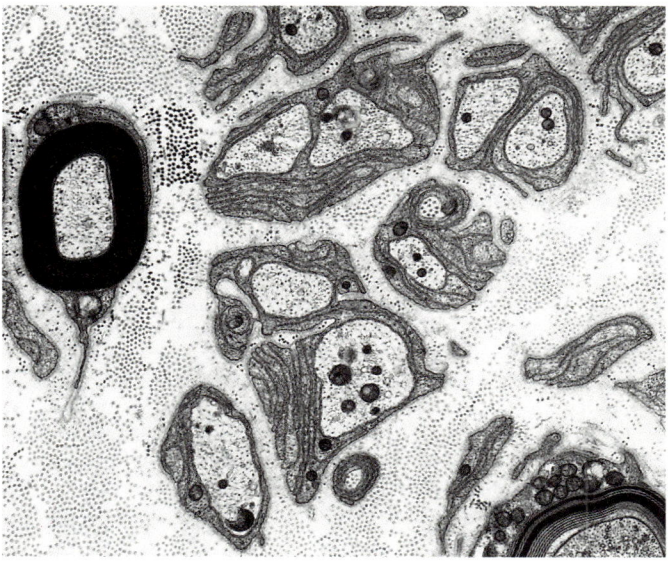

Fig. 25.80 Electron micrograph of normal peripheral nerve, showing a myelinated fibre (left) and number of non-myelinated axons, represented here as circular or eliptical profiles surrounded by Schwann cell cytoplasm. Longitudinally orientated endoneurial collagen (cut transversely) is seen as black dots between the cells.

cells in the spinal cord or from motor neurones in the brainstem. The cell bodies of sensory nerves are in the dorsal root ganglia or in the ganglia of sensory cranial nerves. Each sensory ganglion cell has a peripheral axonal process and a central process which enters the dorsal columns or spino-thalamic tracts, etc. of the spinal cord and ascends towards the brain.

In transverse section, a typical spinal nerve is composed of a connective tissue sheath—*the epineurium*—containing a major muscular artery and a vein (see Fig. 25.86). The epineurium surrounds several fascicles of nerve fibres, each encompassed by a perineurium composed of layers of flattened cells (Figs 25.79,

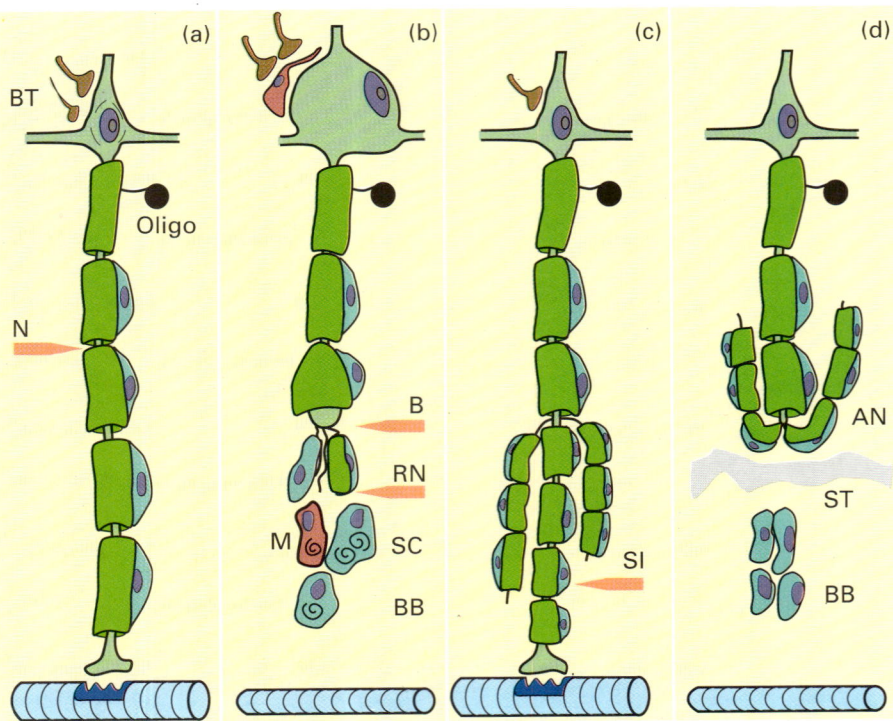

Fig. 25.81 Axonal degeneration and regeneration. (a) Normal nerves showing an anterior horn cell (top) with boutons termineaux (BT) on its surface. The axon extends to innervate striated muscle (bottom). An oligodendrocyte (oligo) myelinates the axon within the spinal cord, whereas Schwann cells myelinate the peripheral part of the axon and are separated by nodes of Ranvier (N). (b) 3–8 days after axonal injury. The neurone is swollen and chromatolytic and the boutons have been lifted from the surface by a microglial cell. The proximal stump of the axon has formed a swelling—axon balloon (B)—and from this, regenerating neurites (RN) extend into Schwann cells, forming bands of Büngner (BB). Schwann cells (SC) and macrophages (M) contain myelin debris. The muscle fibre has undergone neurogenic atrophy. (c) Axonal regeneration. One of the three regenerating neurites has re-innervated the muscle. The neurite has become remyelinated and is recognized by short internodes of myelin (SI) formed during regeneration. (d) Amputation neuroma. Axonal regeneration and re-innervation of the muscle has been blocked by scar tissue (ST). Regenerating neurites have curled back to form a swelling or amputation neuroma (AN). Schwann cells devoid of axons remain in the distal part of the nerve as bands of Büngner (BB).

25.86). Within the *perineurium* is the *endoneurium*, in which the nerve fibres lie surrounded by a mucopolysaccharide matrix and longitudinally orientated collagen fibres. There is a blood–nerve barrier which is maintained by the endothelial cells of the endoneurial capillaries and by the perineurium; this barrier prevents many substances, including proteins and drugs, from entering the normal peripheral nerve. It is broken down when the nerve is injured and fluid and inflammatory cells flow into the endoneurium, resulting in oedema and inflammation of the nerve.

Large myelinated fibres (Fig. 25.79) within the nerve have a total diameter of 10–20 μm; they conduct at up to 100 m/s and subserve motor functions and sensory modalities such as light touch. Small myelinated fibres (mean diameter 5 μm) conduct impulses more slowly (12–30 m/s) and subserve pain and temperature sensation. The non-myelinated fibres (Fig. 25.80) are 0.5–3 μm in diameter and are invaginated into the surface of Schwann cells and their processes; they conduct slowly, at 0.3–1.6 m/s and are referred to as *C fibres* by electrophysiologists. Such fibres subserve pain sensation and are the postganglionic autonomic axons.

Each myelinated nerve fibre is surrounded by a *myelin sheath* of a thickness proportional to the axon diameter. The myelin is formed from the compaction of Schwann cell membranes with one Schwann cell myelinating a single segment (Fig. 25.81). Nodes of Ranvier separate sequential segments along the nerve fibre. Biochemical analyses have shown that myelin is composed of 50 per cent protein and 50 per cent lipid—predominantly cholesterol and phospholipids.

25.9.2 General pathology of peripheral nerves

Peripheral nerve disorders result either from damage to motor or sensory neurones (*neuronopathies*), damage to axons [*axonopathies*—axon (Wallerian) degeneration], or from selective damage to myelin sheaths (*demyelination*).

Axonal degeneration and regeneration

Following destruction of a neurone or damage to its axon, the distal part of the axon dies and degenerates. Within the first 24 hours, the distal part of the injured axon fragments and the surrounding myelin sheath becomes distorted as it retracts from the nodes of Ranvier. Globules of myelin sheath and axon debris are initially contained within the parent Schwann cells, and breakdown of the myelin is initiated by lysosomal enzymes. Although there may be loss of myelin basic protein from the degenerating nerve as early as 24 hours after damage, changes in the myelin lipids may not be seen for 6–7 days. *Sudanophilic cholesterol esters* are formed from the cholesterol within the myelin and the sheath loses its lamellated birefringent structure to form amorphous *osmiophilic globules*. At the time of nerve damage, blood monocytes invade the nerve from the blood, and become the macrophages which play an active role in the degradation of myelin and axon debris.

Within the first 2–3 days after injury, the proximal stump of the damaged axon swells (Fig. 25.81) due to the accumulation of cytoplasm and cytoplasmic organelles, including neurofilaments and mitochondria. Such swellings may be several hundred microns in length and 50–100 μm in diameter. They form because the axoplasmic flow of cytoplasmic elements from the neurone cell body still continues along the axon but is impeded at the point of axon injury.

Axonal regeneration may start within 6 or 7 days of axonal damage. Several axon sprouts grow from the terminal axon balloon towards the distal part of the nerve (Fig. 25.81b). Changes may be seen in the neuronal cell body at this stage, with an axon reaction characterized by swelling of the neurone cell body (Fig. 25.81b), peripheral displacement of the nucleus, and disappearance of the granular endoplasmic reticulum (Nissl substance) from the cell cytoplasm (*chromatolysis*). An increase in the amount of ribosomal RNA within the neurone and an increase in protein synthesis accompanies axonal regeneration.

If continuity of the nerve fascicle is maintained at the time of the injury, clusters of fine regenerating nerve sprouts (Fig. 25.82) will grow distally at 2–5 mm/day along columns of proliferating Schwann cells (*bands of Büngner*) in the distal part of the nerve. As the axons regenerate, they become myelinated and, if they reach the appropriate end-organ, they may attain normal diameter and normal sheath thickness (Fig. 25.81c). Non-myelinated axons regenerate in a similar way to myelinated axons, except that they do not become myelinated.

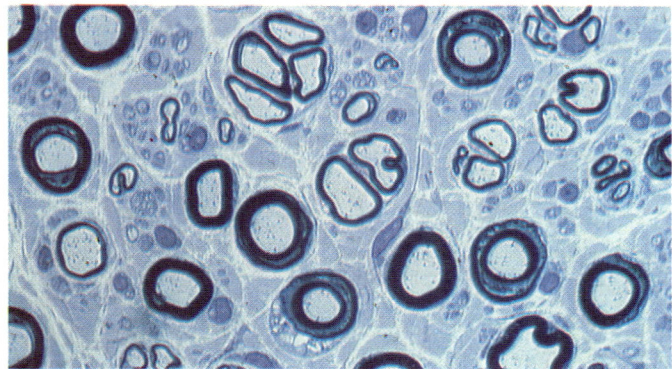

Fig. 25.82 Regeneration following axonal degeneration. The nerve is cut in cross-section and clusters of small axons with thin myelin sheaths are seen (top centre). These are regenerating fibres. They can be compared with the normal large- and small-diameter myelinated fibres, which are also seen in the nerve. (1 μm resin section stained with toluidine blue.)

Regeneration of axons is more successful if damage has occurred at the extreme distal end of the nerve such that distances for regrowth are short and free of obstruction. Severe damage to a large peripheral nerve trunk by ischaemia or trauma, however, may result in little effective regeneration and poor return of function. When a nerve is transected or disrupted by trauma, scar tissue may intervene between the proximal stump of the nerve and the distal end. Regenerating axons may, therefore, be unable to enter the distal end of the nerve and may spread out in a random distribution and even curl back to form an amputation neuroma (Fig. 25.81d).

Secondary effects of axonal degeneration and unsuccessful regeneration include muscle wasting and skin denervation with loss of sensation.

Demyelination and remyelination

If injury to a peripheral nerve primarily affects the myelin sheath or the metabolism of the Schwann cell, demyelination occurs with selective destruction of the myelin sheath and preservation of the axon. Because each Schwann cell myelinates one segment of an axon, demyelination may occur in a segmental pattern along the nerve, as in *Guillain–Barré syndrome*, *diphtheritic neuropathy*, *mild ischaemia*, and some cases of *diabetes*.

The first signs of myelin damage in segmental demyelination are seen as the myelin retracts from the node of Ranvier (Fig. 25.83b). In some cases, only part of the internodal myelin may break down but in other fibres there is destruction of the myelin throughout the whole length of the internode. The myelin may be primarily destroyed by the Schwann cell or by invading macrophages, as in allergic peripheral neuropathies (e.g. Guillain–Barré syndrome). Myelin debris is broken down in lysosomal vacuoles and sudanophilic cholesterol ester droplets are formed within Schwann cells.

The Schwann cells undergo mitosis following the breakdown of the myelin sheath and remyelination of the preserved axons

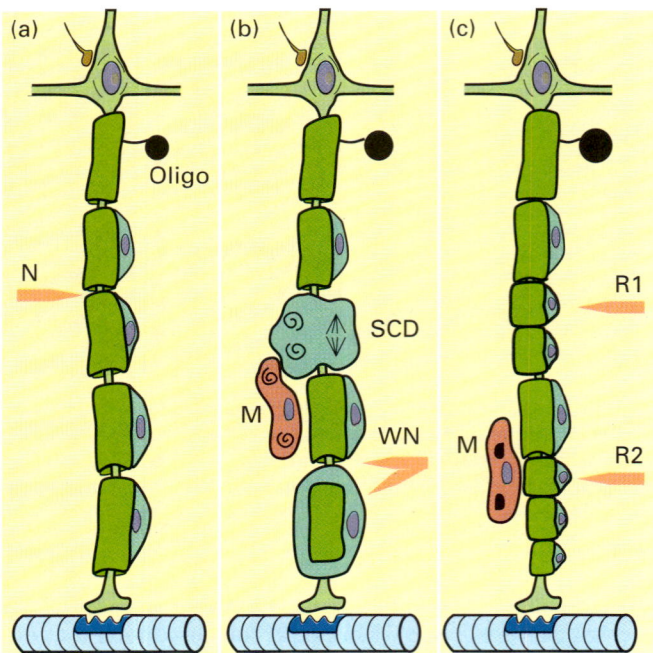

Fig. 25.83 Segmental demyelination and remyelination. (a) Normal nerve innervation striated muscle. Node of Ranvier, N; oligodendrocyte, Oligo. (b) Early segmental demyeliation (3–5 days). Retraction of the myelin sheath from the node of Ranvier, producing a widened nodal gap (WN), is the earliest change. Later, myelin is broken down with Schwann cells and taken up by macrophages (M). Schwann cells divide (SCD). The muscle remains innervated. (c) Remyelination. Although the myelin sheaths have regained their normal thickness, the internodes are short (R1 and R2). Macrophages containing myelin debris (M) may remain for some time.

begins. Initially, therefore, a demyelinated segment of axon is surrounded only by a layer of Schwann cell (Fig. 25.83b) but, within 3–5 days, a thin myelin sheath forms and progressively increases in thickness, to regain its original thickness within a few weeks of demyelination (Fig. 25.83c). In some hereditary and severe metabolic disorders remyelination is inhibited and demyelinated or thinly myelinated axons persist within the nerve (Fig. 25.84).

When significant segmental demyelination occurs in a peripheral nerve, there is functional impairment with muscle weakness and sensory disturbances. As the axons remain intact, however, they still conduct impulses but with a significant slowing of conduction velocity (by more than 50 per cent) which can be detected by electrophysiological techniques. As remyelination proceeds, conduction velocities return towards normal values and, as the axons remain intact, function recovery following remyelination may be virtually complete.

Hypertrophic neuropathies

One of the most striking pathological changes in peripheral nerves is that of *hypertrophic neuropathy*. It is associated in most cases with recurrent segmental demyelination and remyelination and is characterized by the formation of whorls of Schwann

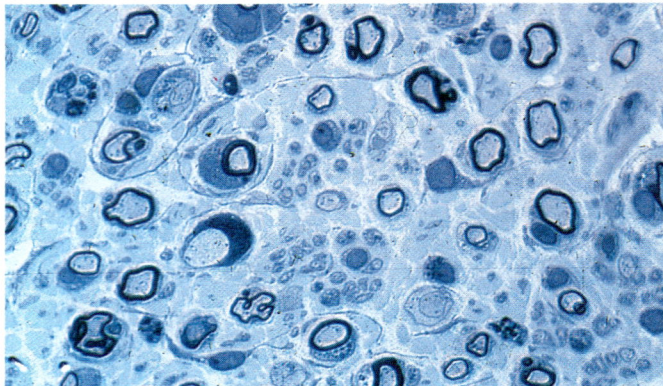

Fig. 25.84 Segmental demyelination and remyelination. Biopsy from a patient with metachromatic leukodystrophy, showing extensive loss of myelin with some demyelinated axons and other thinly myelinated remyelinating axons. (1 μm resin section stained with toluidine blue.)

cells containing a central demyelinated or myelinated axon (Fig. 25.85); such whorls have been likened to '*onion bulbs*'. Hypertrophic neuropathy is seen in a number of *hereditary neuropathies* and in *sporadic relapsing segmental demyelinating neuropathies*.

25.9.3   Pathology of peripheral nerve diseases

Many peripheral nerve axons are very long; they may, for example, extend from neurone cell bodies in the anterior horns of the grey matter in the lumbar spinal cord to supply small muscles of the feet. Axons arising from sensory neurones in the dorsal root ganglia may be even longer, with a peripheral axon supplying the skin of the foot and the central axon from the same cell extending up a gracile tract in the dorsal columns of the spinal cord to the gracile nucleus at the lower end of the medulla. Neurones and their axons may, therefore, be exposed to injury from disorders affecting the spinal cord or brainstem,

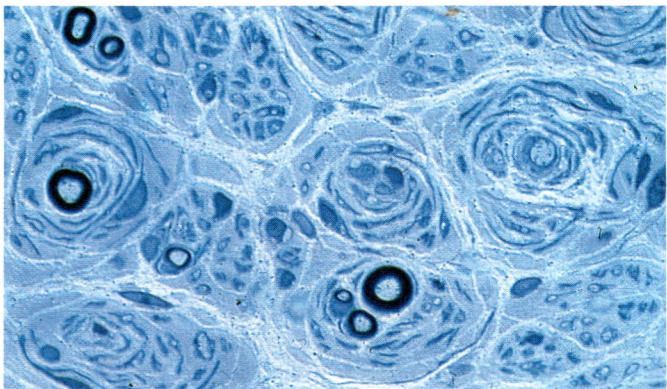

Fig. 25.85 Hypertrophic neuropathy (Charcot–Marie–Tooth disease) showing 'onion-bulb' whorls of Schwann cells around myelinated and demyelinated (top right) axons. Non-myelinated axons are not involved in this process and can be seen separate from the whorls. (1 μm section toluidine blue stained.)

nerve roots, nerve trunks, and the fine terminal branches which may be some 1 metre or more distant from the cell body of the neurone.

Table 25.13 is a summary of peripheral nerve diseases. It is constructed partly on an anatomical basis and partly on a pathological basis, depending upon the site of damage and whether the disease process destroys neurones, axons, or myelin sheaths.

Neuropathies (Table 25.13) are characterized by neuronal cell death. In *motor neurone disease* (amyotrophic lateral sclerosis), for example, cortical motor neurones and anterior horn cells die and the motor axons degenerate. As a consequence, patients present with a combination of upper and lower motor neurone signs. In *spinal muscular atrophy*, on the other hand, only the lower motor neurones in the anterior horns of the spinal cord are affected. In both these conditions, denervation of affected muscles is seen but in the early stages there is re-innervation of muscle fibres by surviving axons. *Shy–Drager syndrome* is characterized by postural hypotension, incontinence, sweating, muscle rigidity and tremor, and by the loss of neurones from the thoracic nuclei (Clarke's column) in the spinal cord from which sympathetic fibres originate. There is also degeneration of neurones in the caudate nucleus and the substantia nigra of the brain. Destructive lesions of the spinal cord result in the loss of anterior horn cells. This is seen in *myelomeningocele* and in *syringomyelia*, in which a large fluid-filled cyst forms in the centre of the cervical spinal cord. *Poliomyelitis virus infection* also destroys anterior horn cells. Spinal cord tumours may locally damage anterior horn cells either by growth within the cord (gliomas) or by compression of the spinal cord from the outside (meningiomas, schwannomas, metastatic carcinoma, lymphomas).

Dorsal root ganglion cells may be damaged by *herpes simplex* and *varicella-zoster* viruses. Such infections are associated with a vesicular rash in the skin regions supplied by those neurones. Hereditary sensory neuropathies are rare and associated with loss of neurones from sensory ganglia. A similar loss is seen in *ataxia telangiectasia*, a disorder associated with *progressive cerebellar ataxia* and symmetrical telangiectases of the skin and conjunctiva. Neuronal loss from autonomic ganglia is seen in amyloid and diabetes.

Axonopathies are characterized by axonal degeneration. Long motor and sensory axons are susceptible to various disease processes along their course; the majority of these diseases cause axonal degeneration which may be followed by varying degrees of regeneration.

Spinal nerve roots may be compressed within the spinal canal or intervertebral foramina by prolapsed intervertebral discs or by vertebral collapse. Tumours within the theca and in the extradural tissues may also damage nerve roots. Isolated or multiple cranial or spinal nerve root lesions may occur in *tuberculous meningitis* or *carcinomatous meningitis* due to vascular occlusion or invasion of the nerve roots by carcinoma cells.

Major peripheral nerves and their terminal branches may be affected by a large number of disease processes (Table 25.13). Nerves may be damaged by trauma or compressed around

Table 25.13   Pathology of peripheral nerve diseases

Neuronopathies (neuronal cell death)
  Spinal cord disorders:
    loss of anterior horn cells
    motor neurone disease (amyotrophic lateral sclerosis)
    spinal muscular atrophy
    Shy–Drager syndrome
    dysraphism—myelomeningocele
    syringomyelia
    poliomyelitis
    spinal cord tumours
    paraneoplastic encephalomyelitis
  Diseases of posterior root sensory ganglion cells
    virus infections: varicella-zoster (herpes zoster) and herpes simplex
    hereditary sensory neuropathies
    ataxia telangiectasia
  Autonomic neuropathies
    diabetes
    amyloid neuropathies

Axonopathies [axonal (Wallerian) degeneration]
  Damage to spinal and cranial nerve roots
    spinal osteoarthritis and prolapsed intervertebral disc: nerve root compression
    trauma to spine, vertebral collapse
    tumours: schwannoma, neurofibroma, meningioma, carcinomatous and leukaemic involvement of meninges with root invasion, extradural metastases
    bacterial meningitis: tuberculous
    arachnoid adhesions
  Diseases involving peripheral nerve trunks
    trauma: direct injury, traumatic (amputation) neuromas
    compression: disordered joints (e.g. rheumatoid arthritis); ulna nerve at the elbow, carpal tunnel (median nerve), posterior interosseous nerve
    vascular disease: peripheral vascular disease—arteriosclerosis; vasculitis in rheumatoid arthritis, polyarteritis nodosa, and other immunological disorders
  metabolic disorders: diabetes
  amyloid neuropathy: hereditary and Ig related
  hereditary neuropathies, e.g. Charcot–Marie–Tooth disease—neuronal type; giant axonal neuropathy
  distal axonopathies
    nutritional deficiencies, e.g. vitamins B_1, B_6, B_{12}
    toxins, e.g. acrylamide organophosphorus compounds
    drugs, e.g. isoniazid
    infections—leprosy

Demyelinating peripheral neuropathies
  Guillain–Barré syndrome: idiopathic (or post-infectious) polyradiculoneuropathy
  diphtheria
  mild trauma and compression
  diabetes
  IgM paraproteinaemia
  disorders of lipid metabolism
    metachromatic leukodystrophy (sulphatide lipidosis)
    Krabbe's globoid leukodystrophy
  hypertrophic neuropathies
    hereditary sensorimotor neuropathies
      Type I, peroneal muscular atrophy (Charcot–Marie–Tooth disease)
      Type 3, Dejerine–Sottas disease
      Type 4, Refsum's disease (disorder of phytanic acid metabolism)
    hereditary pressure-sensitive neuropathy

Tumours
  schwannoma (neurilemmoma)
  malignant schwannoma
  neurofibroma
  malignant neurofibroma
  neuroblastoma
  ganglioneuroblastoma
  ganglioneuroma
  granular cell tumour
  tumour-like lesions
    nerve sheath myoxomas, amputation neuroma

damaged joints. Ischaemia is a common cause of peripheral nerve damage, often presenting clinically with mononeuritis multiplex. In Fig. 25.86, a major epineurial artery in a case of *polyarteritis nodosa* shows fibrinoid necrosis and inflammation of its wall and thrombotic occlusion of the lumen. Because of the anastomotic blood supply of peripheral nerves, complete infarction of a nerve is rarely seen, but extensive axonal degeneration occurs. Patients with severe atherosclerosis in lower limb arteries also suffer ischaemic damage to their peripheral nerves and axonal degeneration.

In general, when axonal damage occurs, it is usually the large axons that are the most susceptible and degenerate first, then the smaller myelinated fibres, and the non-myelinated fibres are most resistant to damage. Notable exceptions to this rule, however, are *amyloid neuropathy*, in which the small myelinated and non-myelinated fibres are typically the first to be affected, and *porphyria*, in which small myelinated fibres selectively degenerate. If damage has occurred sporadically along the nerves, as in *ischaemic neuropathies*, it is the long nerves that are most severely affected and the patient presents with distal limb weakness and sensory loss.

In a few axonopathies, there are characteristic histopathological findings. Amyloid is seen within the endoneurium in amyloid neuropathy, and *giant axonal swellings* may be seen in the rare *familial giant axonal neuropathy*.

Large peripheral nerves such as the sural nerve, a nerve that is often biopsied for diagnosis, may be normal in the distal axonopathies caused by nutritional deficiencies, toxins, and drugs. It is the smaller, intramuscular and sensory branches in the skin that are most severely affected in these disorders. Similarly, the distal parts of the nerves are initially the most severely affected in leprosy, particularly in lepromatous leprosy. In this disorder, the lepra bacilli (*Mycobacterium leprae*) may be detected within Schwann cells and even within axons.

Demylinating peripheral neuropathies are not as commonly

seen in their pure form as axonopathies. In mild *ischaemic* and mild *diabetic neuropathies*, segmental demyelination may be detected in addition to axonal degeneration.

Clinically, the segmental demyelination in a neuropathy may be detected by showing a significant slowing of nerve conduction velocities by electrophysiological techniques. *Guillain–Barré syndrome* is the commonest acute peripheral neuropathy. It usually occurs some days after a viral infection and is characterized by extensive segmental demyelination with invasion of macrophages and lymphocytes into the nerve. It is thought to be due to cell-mediated immune attack on peripheral nerve myelin.

Many of the other segmental demyelinating neuropathies are uncommon, but they may have pathological features which are useful in the diagnosis of the disorder. In patients with *IgM paraproteinaemia*, for example, the paraprotein binds to glycoproteins associated with peripheral nerve myelin. Bound IgM can be detected by immunocytochemistry in the myelin of peripheral nerve biopsies from such patients, and this is associated not only with segmental demyelination but also with widening of myelin sheath periodicity in surviving fibres. Symptoms improve following plasmaphoresis. Pathognomonic appearances in peripheral nerve biopsies are also seen in disorders of lipid metabolism. In *metachromatic leukodystrophy*, for example, there is an accumulation of sulphatide within the Schwann cells, due to a deficiency of *arylsulphatase A*. The sulphatide shows brown metachromasia when stained with cresyl violet.

Hypertrophic neuropathy is a feature of a number of hereditary diseases. In some of the hereditary sensory motor neuropathies, such as *Type 1 peroneal muscular atrophy (Charcot–Marie–Tooth disease)*, there is recurrent segmental demyelination due to a basic defect in the Schwann cells themselves. In *Refsum's disease*, there is a disorder of long-chain fatty-acid metabolism. Hypertrophic changes are also seen in sporadic disorders in which there is relapsing and recurrent segmental demyelination.

A distinctive histological picture is present in the hereditary pressure-sensitive neuropathies, in which the myelin sheaths become very thick in sausage-shaped ovoids along the axons; this is seen particularly at points of compression near joints.

25.9.4   Tumours of peripheral nerves

Schwannomas and neurofibromas are the commonest tumours of the peripheral nervous system and they arise on cranial and spinal nerve roots and on more peripheral parts of nerves (see Section 25.8).

von Recklinghausen's neurofibromatosis is now recognized as two major diseases. The peripheral form is the most common inherited disorder affecting the human nervous system. It is characterized by *café-au-lait spots* on the skin in childhood and neurofibromatosis of the skin developing in adults. The disorder is complicated by mental retardation, epilepsy, spinal deformities, and other tumours such as gliomas and phaeochromocytomas. Sarcomatous change may occur in the neurofibromas of

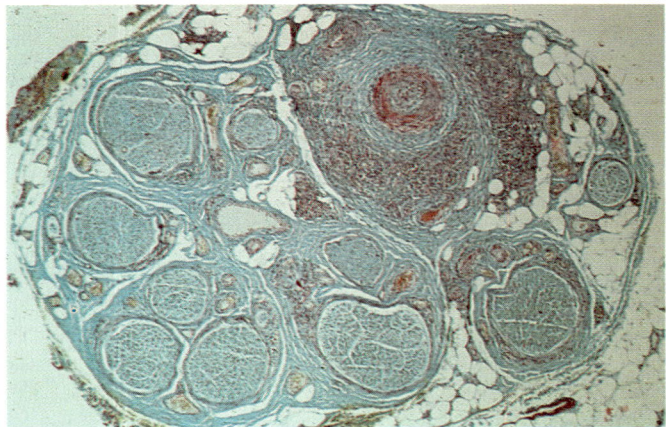

Fig. 25.86 Polyarteritis nodosa. The nerve has been cut in cross-section and shows multiple fascicles surrounded by perineurium. The epineurial artery (top) is surrounded by inflammatory cells and shows fibrinoid necrosis (red) within its wall. (Masson trichrome stain.) (Reproduced with permission from Weller 1984.)

the skin or elsewhere in the body. There is an autosomal dominant pattern of inheritance with a high penetrance, but half the cases may be spontaneous mutations. The gene defect for this disorder is linked to the locus encoding *nerve growth factor receptor* located on the *long arm of chromosome 17*. It is thought that a mutation in the nerve growth factor receptor gene is unlikely to be the main defect in the peripheral form of von Recklinghausen's neurofibromatosis.

A much less common type of von Recklinghausen's neurofibromatosis is the central form, or bilateral acoustic neurofibromatosis. It is an autosomal dominant disorder, genetically and clinically distinct from the peripheral form. It is characterized by multiple intracranial and spinal tumours which are mainly schwannomas and meningiomas. There is a specific loss of alleles from *chromosome 22* in several of the different tumour types examined, although it is possible that chromosome 17 may be involved.

Acknowledgements

I would like to thank the staff of the Wessex Regional Neuropathology Laboratory, Southampton General Hospital for their technical assistance and Margaret Harris for typing the manuscript.

25.9.5   Further reading

Dyck, P. J., Thomas, P. K., Lambert, E. H., and Bunge, R. (eds) (1984). *Peripheral neuropathy* (2nd edn). Saunders, Philadelphia.

Seizinger, B. R., *et al.* (1987). Genetic linkage of von Recklinghausen neurofibromatosis to the nerve growth factor receptor. *Cell* 49, 589–94.

Swash, M. and Schwartz, M. S. (1988). *Neuromuscular diseases. A practical approach to diagnosis and management* (2nd edn). Springer-Verlag, London.

Thomas, P. K., Landon, D. N., and King, R. H. M. (1984). Diseases of the peripheral nerves. In *Greenfield's neuropathology* (ed. J. H. Adams, J. A. N. Corsellis, and L. W. Duchen) (4th edn). Edward Arnold, London.

Walton, N. N. (1985). *Brain's diseases of the nervous system* (9th edn). Oxford University Press.

Weller, R. O. (1984). *Colour atlas of neuropathology*. Harvey Miller and Oxford University Press.

Weller, R. O. (ed.) (1990). *Systemic pathology* (3rd edn), Vol. 4: *Nervous system, muscle and eyes*. Churchill Livingstone, Edinburgh.

Weller, R. O., Swash, M., McLellan, D. L., and Scholtz, C. L. (eds) (1983). *Clinical neuropathology*. Springer-Verlag, Heidelberg.

25.10   Eye

D. R. Lucas

The eye and its adnexa are affected by many of the pathological processes to which similar tissues elsewhere are susceptible. However, the eye itself has various specialized structural and functional features which govern its response to such processes and also make it subject to a number of unique disorders. The present section necessarily concentrates on these special features and some of the most important unique disorders.

25.10.1   Applied anatomy and physiology

The anatomy of the human eye is illustrated diagrammatically in Fig. 25.87. The arrangement of the principal intra-ocular structures within the corneoscleral shell effectively divides the interior of the globe into three chambers. The anterior and posterior chambers contain aqueous fluid. The vitreous chamber is separated from the posterior chamber by the 'lens–iris-diaphragm'. For convenience, the eye is often roughly divided into anterior and posterior segments. The former comprising structures anterior to the ora serrata.

Sclera and cornea

The sclera and cornea provide a tough collagenous envelope which protects the delicate intra-ocular structures. In the sclera, the collagen fibres are obliquely arranged in interlacing bundles and there is an admixture of elastic fibres. In the corneal stroma, the collagen fibres are uniform in diameter and regularly spaced in a proteoglycan matrix. This arrangement *inter alia* enables transparency to be achieved. The limbus is the boundary line observed clinically between the cornea and sclera. Histologically there is a transitional zone extending from the margin of *Bowman's* and *Bruch's membranes* anteriorly to the posterior margin of the *scleral spur* posteriorly.

The adult sclera is generally resistant to stretching when intra-ocular pressure is raised, but local areas of thinning may occur, particularly in the limbal area. In childhood, the sclera expands in response to sustained increased intra-ocular pressure, with the result that the globe may be enormously increased in size (buphthalmos).

The fibres of the optic nerve pass through a sieve-like aperture in the sclera, the *lamina cribrosa*. This is an area of potential weakness which stretches as a result of chronically increased intra-ocular pressure.

Progressive gradual expansion of the sclera also occurs in pathological myopia (myopia of more than 8 dioptres), though the factors responsible are not known at present.

The ciliary vessels and nerves enter the eye through emissary canals in the sclera. These are important because they also provide routes through which choroidal melanomas may escape.

The cornea is covered by a layer of non-keratinizing squamous epithelium. In the limbal zone it becomes continuous with the bulbar conjunctiva, which is a mucous membrane. The surface of the cornea and conjunctiva is covered by a film, derived from lacrimal and mucous secretions, which contains the protective agents lysozyme and lactoferrin as well as immunoglobulins. Deep to the epithelium is a layer of acellular collagen, of between 10 and 16 μm in thickness, known as *Bowman's membrane*. The collagen fibres of the stroma are embedded in a matrix of complex saccharides, including keratan and chondroitin sulphates, and there is a sparse population of keratocytes

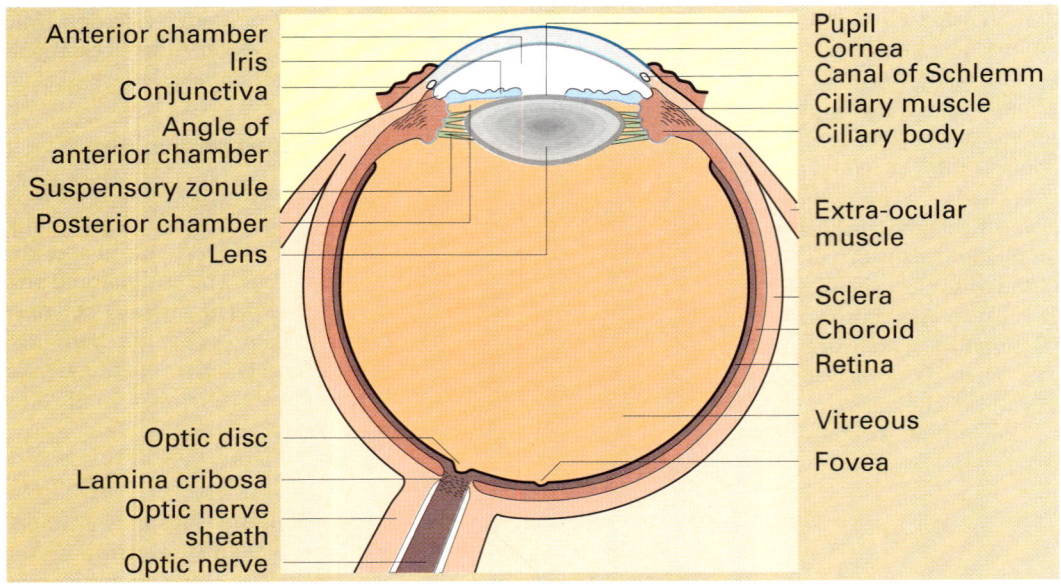

(a)

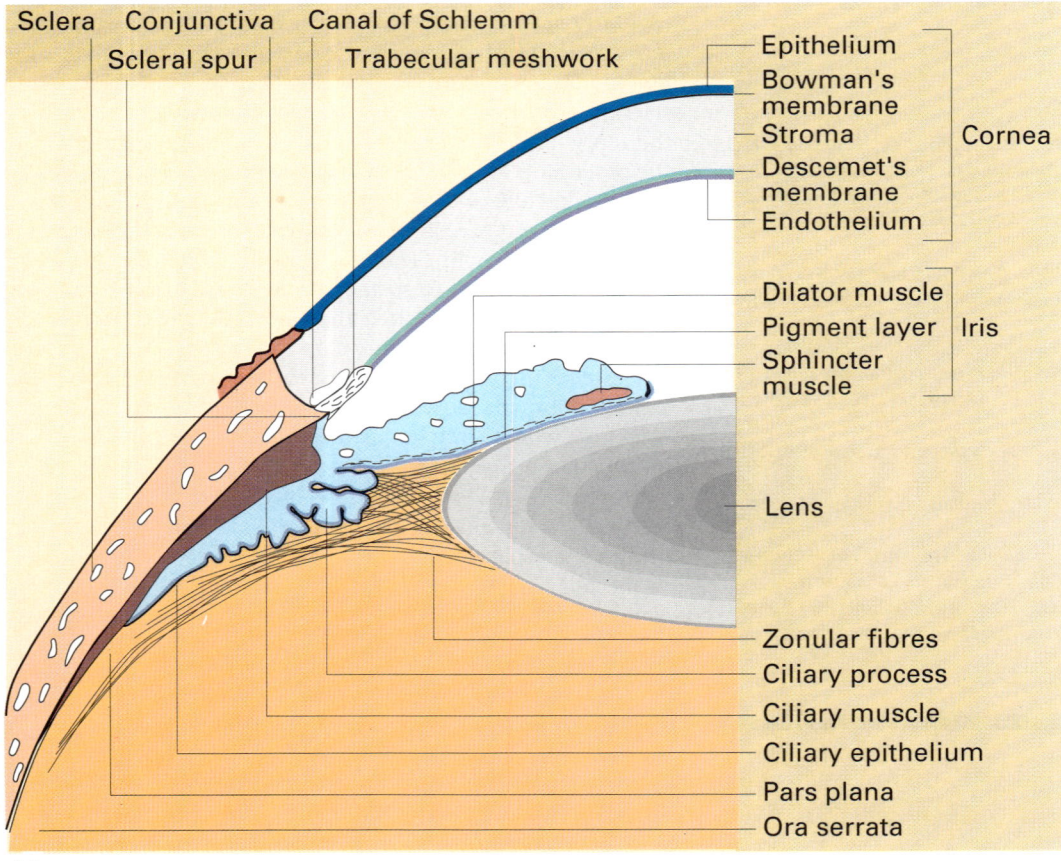

(b)

Fig. 25.87   Basic structure of the eye. (a) Diagram of right eye seen from above; (b) anterior segment in more detail. [(a) Drawn after Parr, J. (1982). *Introduction to ophthalmology* (2nd edn), Oxford University Press.]

which are fibrocytic in character. The posterior surface of the cornea is lined by *Desçemet's membrane,* which is effectively the basement membrane of the corneal endothelium. The endothelium is a single layer of hexagonal cells which have the vital function of maintaining corneal hydration. It is not a true endothelium and there is evidence that the cells may be of neural crest origin. In man, at least, its powers of replication are very limited and loss of cells is compensated for by enlargement of residual cells.

Blood–ocular barriers

Two blood–ocular barriers regulate exchanges between the blood and the eye. The blood–aqueous barrier resides in the ciliary body and iris. Cells of the ciliary epithelium are linked by tight junctions which limit the passage of macromolecules, and iris capillaries are not fenestrated.

The blood–retina barrier exists at two levels. The retinal capillaries that supply the inner layers of the retina are non-fenestrated and do not allow the passage of macromolecules such as horseradish peroxidase or substances such as fluorescein. The latter property is exploited clinically in the procedure of clinical angiography. The outer layers of the retina are supplied by the choriocapillaris, the capillaries of which are freely permeable. However, Bruch's membrane acts as a diffusion barrier to molecules of large size and the cells of the pigmented epithelium are joined by *zonulae occludentes,* which have similar permeability characteristics to those of the retinal capillary endothelium.

Breakdown of the blood–ocular barriers is common in intra-ocular disease. In the anterior chamber this leads to an increase in the protein content of the aqueous, which is observed clinically as 'flare' under the slit lamp. It is commonly seen as a result of inflammatory processes affecting the anterior part of the globe.

Breakdown of the blood-retina barrier at the level of the retinal capillaries may occur for many reasons, of which the most important are inflammatory conditions such as uveitis, venous occlusions, diabetic retinopathy, and surgical trauma. The result is retinal oedema. Because of the arrangement of the retinal capillaries around the macula, the pools of fluid show a petaloid appearance by fluorescein angiography. The histological appearance is illustrated in Fig. 25.88. The fluid is at first low in protein, but if it does not resolve, the protein content gradually increases.

Breakdown of the blood–retina barrier at the level of Bruch's membrane and the pigmented epithelium results in accumulation of fluid between the pigmented epithelium and the neuroretina, which thus becomes detached. This occasionally occurs spontaneously in the macular region, but is more often secondary to inflammation or tumours involving the choroid.

Maintenance of intra-ocular pressure

Pressure within the globe is regulated by the rate at which aqueous secreted by the ciliary epithelium passes through the outflow pathways. The most important pathway is via the tra-

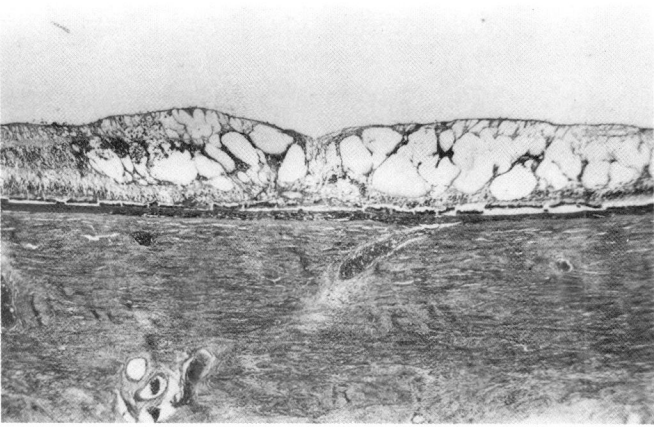

Fig. 25.88 Cystoid macular oedema; F, fovea. (Masson trichrome.)

becular meshwork into the canal of Schlemm (Fig. 25.89) and thence into the venous drainage system of the eye. Aqueous resembles protein-free plasma in composition.

25.10.2 Raised intra-ocular pressure— glaucoma

In glaucoma, obstruction of aqueous drainage results in intra-ocular pressure being sustained at a level sufficient to damage ocular tissues, especially the retina and optic nerve. The common causes of obstruction are:

1. increased outflow resistance at the level of the trabecular meshwork—'*open-angle*' *glaucoma;*

2. occlusion of the trabecular meshwork by the root of the iris—'*angle-closure*' *glaucoma;*

3. *pupillary block.* This may occur acutely from impaction of the lens in the pupil as a concomitant of angle-closure glaucoma. Blockage of more gradual onset results from adhesions binding the pupillary border to the lens (Fig. 25.90).

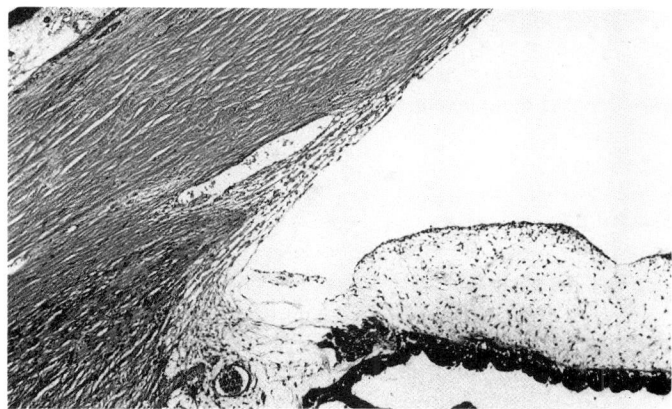

Fig. 25.89 Normal drainage angle. Asterisk indicates canal of Schlemm; S, scleral spur. (Masson trichrome.) (From Lucas 1989, by courtesy of Blackwell Scientific Publications Ltd.)

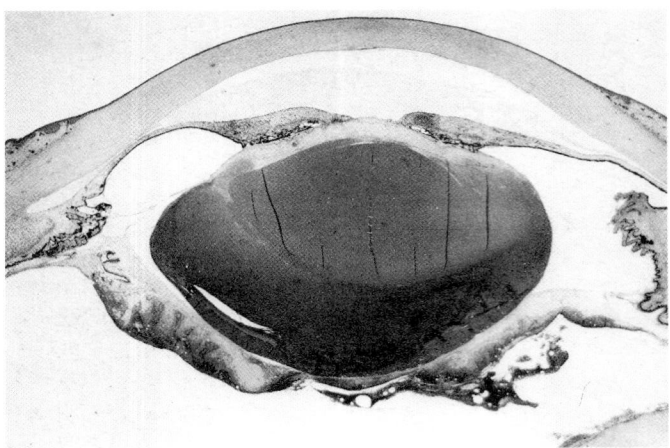

Fig. 25.90 Secondary glaucoma due to occlusion of the pupil. The pupillary border of the iris is firmly bound to the anterior surface of the lens, causing complete blockage of aqueous flow through the pupil and ballooning forwards of the iris (iris bombé). Case of long-standing retinal detachment. The detached retina can be seen posterior to the lens. (From Lucas 1989, by courtesy of Blackwell Scientific Publications Ltd.)

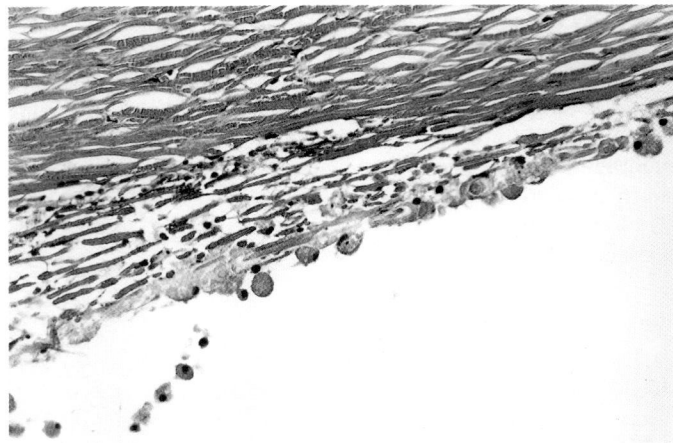

Fig. 25.91 Phacolytic glaucoma. Note the macrophages adhering to the surface of the trabecular meshwork and in the pores. (From Lucas 1989, by courtesy of Blackwell Scientific Publications Ltd.)

This is usually a consequence of inflammation in the anterior segment.

While all glaucoma is, like vascular hypertension, strictly speaking secondary, some categories are commonly described as 'primary' because their precise pathogenesis is obscure. This is partly because satisfactory material from early cases is not readily available.

Open-angle glaucomas

Primary

Chronic simple glaucoma is a common 'primary' form of open-angle glaucoma which has an insidious onset and occurs in the middle-aged and elderly. The disease is familial, but the mode of inheritance is imprecise. Both eyes are affected, though not necessarily synchronously. There is an increased resistance to aqueous outflow through the trabecular meshwork. The pathological basis is uncertain. The changes described in the meshwork, such as sclerosis, depletion of endothelial cell population, and deposition of amorphous plaques, are of a non-specific character and may be secondary to the raised pressure. Similar, but less marked changes also occur with ageing.

Secondary

1. Various forms of particulate matter may lodge in the meshwork. Of these, the most important are:
   (a) red cells or red cell debris after trauma resulting in intraocular haemorrhage;
   (b) macrophages crammed with lens protein from a ruptured hypermature cataract (see below)—this is termed phacolytic glaucoma (Fig. 25.91);
   (c) pigment derived from the iris, though this is rarely heavy enough to cause obstruction (pigmentary glaucoma);

   (d) 'exfoliative material'. In the 'exfoliation (pseudoexfoliation) syndrome', which is often associated with 'open angle' glaucoma, flakes of PAS–positive material are deposited on the trabecular meshwork, the zonular fibres, the ciliary processes, the posterior surface of the iris, and on the anterior surface of the lens where the material is brushed towards the equator by the action of the iris. By electron microscopy, the material has a fibrillary structure. It is thought to originate from basement membrane. Unlike pigment, it is not taken up by macrophages;
   (e) inflammatory exudates (v.i.).

2. Prolonged administration of corticosteroids may result in glaucoma, but the pathological basis has not been established for certain.

Angle-closure glaucomas

Primary

Primary angle-closure glaucoma occurs in the middle-aged and elderly, but is much less common than chronic simple glaucoma. Small (hypermetropic) eyes with a large lens and narrow angle are predisposed. Onset is sudden and usually unilateral, although the contralateral eye is usually also at risk. Dilatation of the pupil in subdued light may precipitate an attack, as may the application of mydriatics. The root of the iris covers the trabecular meshwork. At the same time, the lens may become impacted in the pupil. The condition is reversible, but permanent adhesions may develop between the iris and cornea if the eye is not treated.

Secondary

Secondary angle-closure is due to fibrovascular adhesions between the root of the iris and the peripheral cornea—anterior peripheral synechiae (Fig. 25.92). These are commonly seen in

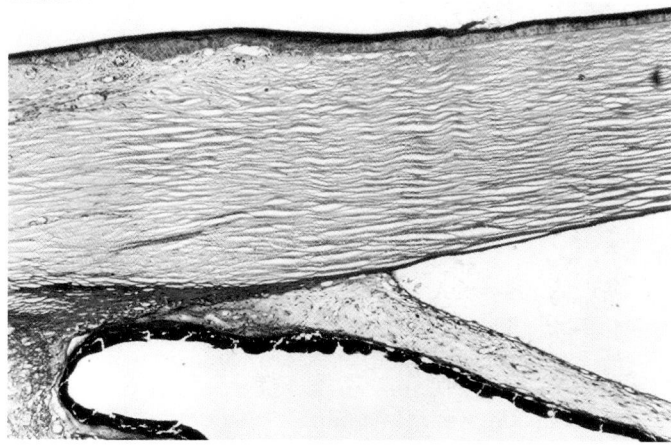

Fig. 25.92 Anterior peripheral synechia. Note capillaries (new vessels) on anterior surface of iris with attachment of the root of the iris to the posterior surface of the cornea (Desçemet's membrane is indicated by arrows). The trabecular meshwork is collapsed and no canal of Schlemm is seen. (PAS–Tartrazine.) (From Lucas 1989, by courtesy of Blackwell Scientific Publications Ltd.)

post-thrombotic glaucoma (see below), but also occur following inflammation and trauma.

Congenital glaucomas

Glaucoma occasionally occurs in infancy, commonly as a result of failure of development of the outflow apparatus. The condition has a familial tendency and one or both eyes may be affected. The drainage angle retains a fetal appearance and the affected eye becomes enlarged (q.v.).

Effects of raised intra-ocular pressure

Cornea

An acute rise in pressure leads to corneal oedema and may result in irreversible endothelial damage. Chronically raised

pressure is associated with the ingrowth from the limbus of a thin layer of fibrovascular tissue between Bowman's membrane and the epithelium, which is referred to clinically as degenerative 'pannus'.

Retina

Ganglion cells are lost from the retina, probably as a result of ischaemia (Fig. 25.93a).

Optic nerve

The loss of ganglion cells from the retina is associated with atrophy of their axons in the optic nerve. The increased pressure within the eye also causes outward displacement of the cribriform plate through which the nerve fibres pass, and results in the familiar 'cupping' of the optic nerve head seen in long-standing glaucoma (Fig. 25.93b). It is possible that interference with axonal transport by distortion of the fibres as they pass through the cribriform plate is a contributory factor in glaucomatous optic atrophy.

25.10.3   Diseases due to infective agents

The eye may be involved incidentally in many systemic diseases due to infective agents, especially in the immunologically compromised. In this section, only those in which ocular involvement is of primary interest can be covered.

Bacterial infections

Acute bacterial conjunctivitis

Acute bacterial conjunctivitis is characterized by hyperaemia, oedema, and infiltration by neutrophils and mononuclear cells. A fibrino-purulent exudate is formed in the conjunctival sac. The most important causes are *Staphylococcus aureus*, *Streptococcus pneumoniae*, and *Haemophilus aeqyptius*. Infants appear to be especially susceptible to infection by *Neisseria gonorrhoeae*, which is a cause of *ophthalmia neonatorum*.

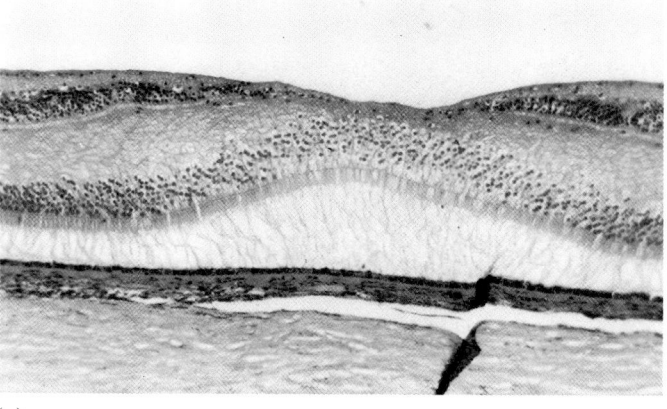

(a)

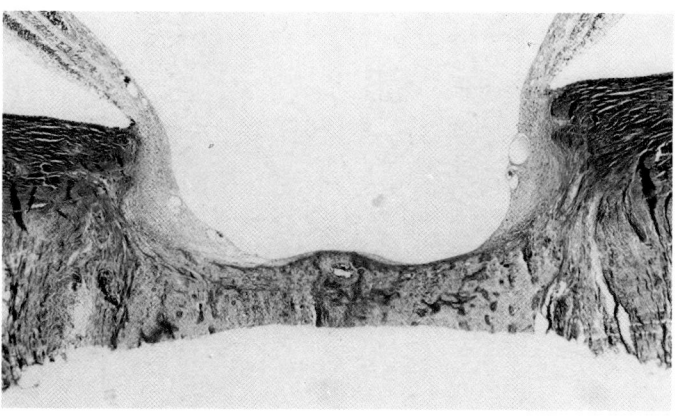

(b)

Fig. 25.93 Effects of long-standing glaucoma. (a) Foveal retina in glaucoma showing complete loss of ganglion cells (cf. Fig. 25.94). (From Lucas 1989, by courtesy of Blackwell Scientific Publications Ltd.) (b) Cupping of the optic nerve head. The retinal detachment at the margins of the cup is factitious. (Masson trichrome.)

Chronic bacterial conjunctivitis

Chronic bacterial conjunctivitis is usually associated with infection of the lid margin. *S. aureus* is the commonest cause, but certain coliforms, especially *Proteus* may be implicated.

Bacterial ulceration of the cornea

Bacterial ulceration of the cornea is usually slightly subcentral. Infection may follow an apparently trivial injury and corneas affected by chronic oedema are particularly vulnerable. It is thus a common terminal event in chronically diseased eyes. Of the causative organisms, apart from *S. aureus*, *S. pneumoniae*, and *Proteus mirabilis*, *Pseudomonas aeruginosa* deserves special mention because it is a contaminant of contact lens solutions.

The formation of the ulcer is characterized by oedema, necrosis, and infiltration by neutrophils. Severe destruction of the stroma sometimes exposes Desçemet's membrane, which then bulges forwards (Desçemetocoele) and may perforate. Neutrophils from vessels in the iris and ciliary body are attracted chemotactically into the anterior chamber where they form a sediment (hypopyon) (Fig. 25.94). Dilatation of the capillaries of the limbal conjunctiva, and oedema and infiltration by inflammatory cells of the *substantia propria* result in what is described clinically as 'inflammatory pannus'.

If the infection is resolved, the residual scarring will depend on the amount of tissue destroyed. Bowman's membrane does not regenerate. Thus, even minimal destruction in the optical axis is serious.

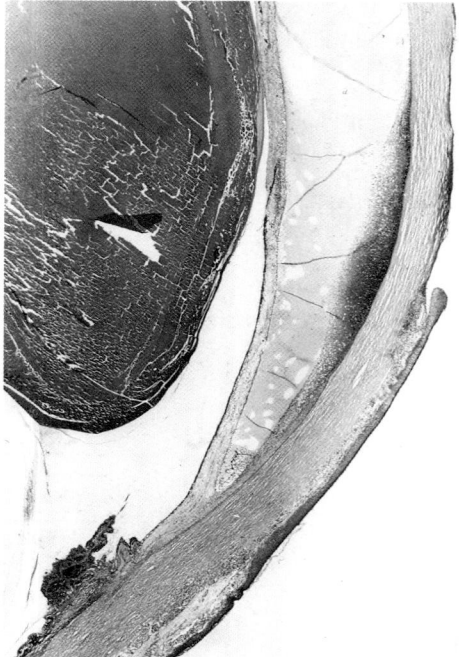

Fig. 25.94 Hypopyon ulcer. Mass of polymorphs (P) adherent to posterior surface of the cornea deep to the inferior margin of the ulcer. (From Lucas 1989, by courtesy of Blackwell Scientific Publications Ltd.)

Mycotic infections

Mycotic infections are uncommon in temperate climates, but various species, of which the most important are *Aspergillus* and *Candida*, may cause indolent and intractable corneal ulceration or endophthalmitis. The latter is particularly liable to affect patients on prolonged immunosuppressive and steroid therapy. Candidial infection of the vitreous also occurs in intravenous drug-abusers.

Chlamydial infections

Local infection by *TRIC* (*trachoma inclusion conjunctivitis*) agent, an intracellular bacterium, causes trachoma in developing countries, where it is the single most important cause of blindness. In Westernized countries, it is primarily a sexually transmitted disease, occasionally causing conjunctivitis in the new-born and in sexually active young adults.

Trachomas

Infection is mainly by serotypes A, B, and C, and eye-to-eye transmission by eye-seeking flies is common. Seasonal epidemics of conjunctivitis by bacteria such as *Haemophilus* may be contributory. The disease progresses through four stages:

1. *Incipient.* Lymphocytic follicles appear in the conjunctiva of the upper tarsus, fornix, and limbus, which becomes hyperaemic and oedematous. Cytoplasmic inclusions can be found in conjunctival epithelial cells.

2. (a) *Follicular hypertrophy.* The lymphoid follicles enlarge, develop germinal centres, and undergo necrosis; infiltration of the stroma by plasma cells and macrophages is conspicuous.

    (b) *Papillary hypertrophy.* Intense stromal cellular infiltration causes papillary folding.

3. *Cicatrization.* As the inflammation subsides, the infiltrate is gradually replaced by granulation tissue and later by more dense collagenous tissue. The epithelium becomes stratified squamous and goblet cells are lost. The scarring causes obstruction of the lacrimal ducts, inturning of the lashes (trichiasis) and lids (entropion), and fusion of lid margins (symblepharon).

4. *Healed.* The inflammation has subsided and the follicles and papillae are replaced by scar tissue. Small surface dimples, which are scars derived from limbal follicles, are known as Herbert's pits and are characteristic of old trachoma.

Conjunctivitis (paratrachoma)

Infection is mainly by subgroups D–I. In infants, infection by TRIC agent contracted in the birth canal is now the commonest form of *ophthalmia neonatorum* (inclusion blenorrhoea).

In adults, infection causes a subacute follicular conjunctivitis with associated punctate keratitis.

The cytoplasmic inclusions may be found in epithelial cells in Giemsa-stained conjunctival scrapings, typically in the form of perinuclear caps.

Viral infections

Adenovirus

Infection by adenovirus is the commonest infectious cause of acute follicular conjunctivitis, which may occur as isolated cases, or in small local outbreaks, usually in children or young adults. The follicles consist of aggregates of lymphocytes, together with a few macrophages. Intranuclear inclusions can rarely be demonstrated in conjunctival scrapings, but the virus may be isolated from conjunctival swabs. The serotypes commonly identified are 1, 3, 4, and 7. When there is an associated infection of the upper respiratory tract and pyrexia, it is known as pharyngoconjunctival fever.

Certain serotypes, notably type 8, may produce explosive epidemics, usually based in eye departments. The conjunctivitis is generally more severe and may be pseudomembranous. There is an associated punctate keratitis. The spots are small subepithelial aggregates of lymphocytes and fibroblasts which may take years to resolve.

Herpes simplex

Primary herpetic keratoconjunctivitis affects only the ocular surface, and healing without scarring is usual. Recurrent infections are more common due to the virus residing in a dormant state in the trigeminal ganglia. Normally, only one eye is affected, and to a variable extent:

1. *Dendritic ulcer.* The infection is largely confined to the epithelium, which shows branching ulceration. This recognized clinically by staining with fluorescein which stains Bowman's membrane where the epithelium is defective. Healing without scarring takes place if Bowman's membrane is not damaged. However, the branches of the ulcer may widen to assume a geographic configuration, and treatment by steroids may result in rapid and catastrophic progress.

2. *Stromal keratitis.* The features include epithelial and stromal oedema with local granular degeneration of Bowman's membrane and focal infiltration by lymphocytes and polymorphs. Intranuclear inclusions may be found in the epithelial cells. These are PAS-positive and also stain brilliantly red by Masson's trichrome (Fig. 25.95). Local oedema in the deeper stroma may be well circumscribed and is responsible for the disciform opacification observed clinically. A characteristic feature is the presence of giant cells along Desçemet's membrane. Recurrent attacks lead to thinning, scarring, and vascularization of the stroma. Post-herpetic scarring is a serious cause of visual disability, for which a corneal transplant is necessary. Unfortunately, the disease may recur in the graft. Rejection is a further hazard, especially if the cornea is vacularized.

3. *Anterior uveitis.* Herpetic iridocyclitis may complicate herpetic keratitis.

4. *Vitreo-retinitis.* Some cases of necrotizing vitreoretinitis (acute retinal necrosis syndrome) have been shown to be due to HSV. Both immunosuppressed and immunocompet-

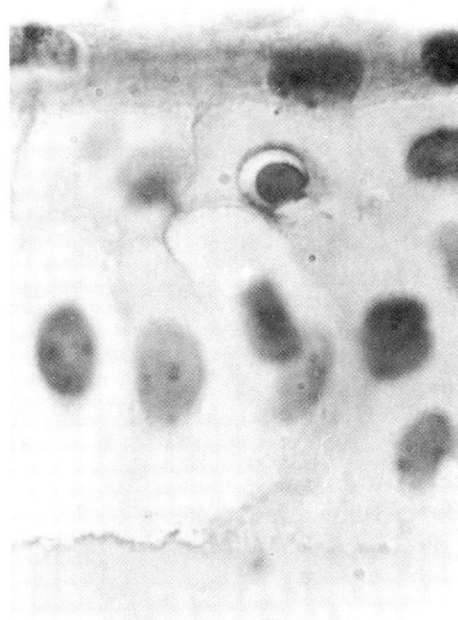

Fig. 25.95 Herpetic keratitis. Intranuclear inclusion (arrow) in corneal epithelium. (Masson trichrome.) (From Lucas 1989, by courtesy of Blackwell Scientific Publications Ltd.)

ent subjects may be affected (Duker and Blumenkranz 1991).

Cytomegalovirus

Retinitis due to cytomegalovirus is seen in the majority of patients dying from HIV infection and sometimes also in immunosuppressed renal transplant cases. All layers of the retina are affected by a patchy necrosis and the typical 'owl-eye' inclusions may be found.

Herpes zoster

The eye is usually affected when the nasociliary branch of the ophthalmic division of the trigeminal nerve is involved in shingles. The corneal lesions vary in severity from discrete superficial stromal opacities or vesicular lesions which heal without scarring, to neurotrophic keratitis and severe ulceration which results in serious scarring.

There may also be an associated iritis.

Measles

Acute catarrhal conjunctivitis is part of the prodromal phase of measles and Koplik's spots may be seen on the caruncle. Punctate fluorescein-staining opacities appear in the corneal and conjunctival epithelium and are accompanied by severe photophobia.

It is noteworthy that in sub-Saharan Africa acute corneal ulceration following measles is the commonest cause of childhood blindness. Malnutrition, vitamin A deficiency, and secondary herpes simplex infection may be local contributory factors.

Protozoa

Toxoplasma

Ocular involvement is well recognized in congenital toxoplasmosis. There is usually a choroidoretinitis which is localized posteriorly and ultimately leads to retinal detachment, secondary cataract, and shrinkage of the eye as the inflammation subsides and internal fibrosis progresses. Parasitic cysts can be demonstrated in histological sections. Free forms are more difficult to recognize if there is much pyknotic debris.

Ocular involvement may also occur in acquired toxoplasmosis, but is uncommon. However, a fulminating retinochoroiditis has been observed in immunocompromised patients.

Acanthamoeba

That an intractable ulcerative keratitis, which may progress to a hypopyon uveitis, can be caused by acanthamoeba is being recognized with increasing frequency. The organism is normally found in brackish or sea water and in the soil but may contaminate contact lenses or lens solution. There is usually a history of minor corneal trauma or contact lens wear. Two species, *A. castellani* and *A. polyphaga*, have been isolated. The parasites may be difficult to see in histological sections or corneal scrapings, but can be grown in culture.

Helminths

Toxocara

Circulating larvae of *Toxocara canis* may lodge in the eye, usually in children. The commonest sites are in the anterior vitreous or intraretinally, either near the posterior pole or at the *ora serrata*. A local eosinophilic granuloma is set up. When the larva is located anteriorly, the associated fibrosis in the anterior vitreous usually results in a traction detachment of the retina.

25.10.4   Other inflammatory diseases

Allergic conjunctivitis

Some cases are clearly related to pollens, animal dander, etc., but often a specific cause is not identified. Contact lens wearers may suffer from giant papillary conjunctivitis.

Vernal conjunctivitis

Vernal conjunctivitis is a chronic recurrent bilateral inflammation usually showing seasonal exacerbations. Flat-topped 'papillae' are formed on the upper tarsal conjunctiva. The conjunctival epithelium is fixed at intervals to the tarsal plate, and oedema and exudation in the *substantia propria* elevates the epithelium between these points (Fig. 25.96). A light cellular infiltrate rich in eosinophils is found in the *substantia propria*, and eosinophils may be found in conjunctival scrapings. In long-standing cases considerable scarring may occur.

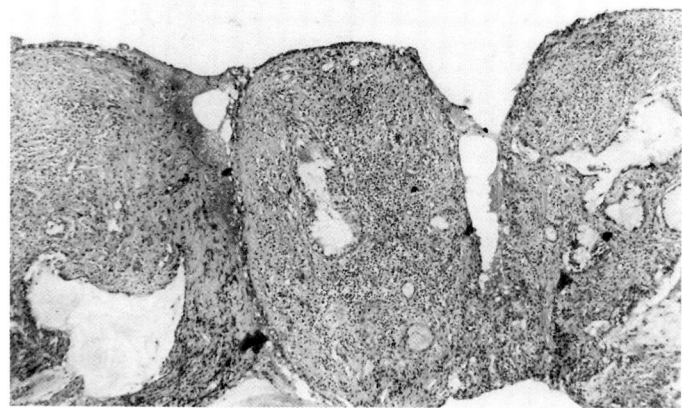

Fig. 25.96   Vernal conjunctivitis. Swelling and inflammatory infiltration of the conjunctiva has resulted in a pseudopapillary appearance. (From Lucas 1989, by courtesy of Blackwell Scientific Publications Ltd.)

Uveitis

The term uveitis is used to describe various diseases in which the inflammation is largely localized to the uveal tract. The diseases considered in this section comprise a somewhat heterogeneous mixture. In some, the ocular involvement is part of a systemic disease.

Anterior uveitis

The inflammation is usually of a non-specific character and localized in the anterior segment. If the process is not controlled, serious sequelae ensue, such as glaucoma due to interference with aqueous drainage by adhesions.

Anterior uveitis may occur:

1. for no demonstrable cause, though there is an increased incidence in carriers of HLA-B27;

2. in association with a variety of systemic diseases, including *Reiter's syndrome, ankylosing spondylitis, juvenile rheumatoid arthritis, ulcerative colitis*, and *Behçet's disease*.

The HLA antigens associated with these diseases are well known and dealt with elsewhere.

The microscopic features are infiltration of the iris and ciliary body with lymphocytes and plasma cells, and leakage of plasma proteins and inflammatory cells into the aqueous. Onset is often acute and the condition tends to recur.

Fuchs heterochromic iridocyclitis

Fuchs' heterochromic iridocyclitis is a common and well-defined entity in which there is a unilateral mild iridocyclitis of unknown aetiology. Atrophy of the iris stroma and pigmented epithelium result in the affected eye becoming paler in colour. The condition tends to be mild and few cases have been examined pathologically. Inflammatory infiltration is light and new vessels which form on the iris rarely progress to form adhesions.

Sympathetic ophthalmitis

Sympathetic ophthalmitis is now an extremely rare but potentially blinding complication of penetrating ocular injuries, in which there is prolapse of uveal tissue (Fig. 25.97a). The essential features of the condition are:

1. There is an interval usually of 4–6 weeks, but sometimes of months or years, before inflammation begins to affect not only the injured eye, but later also the other (sympathizing) eye.

2. Removal of the injured eye before the second eye is affected effectively protects it. However, once the second eye has become involved, removal of the injured eye does not influence the progress of the inflammation of the other eye.

3. The inflammation in both eyes is granulomatous and affects the choroid (Fig. 25.97b) and tends to track out along emissary channels in the sclera.

Aetiology

The disease has long been regarded as an auto-immune reaction to uveal tissue or choroidal pigment, but more recent work has suggested that the reaction is to retinal S-antigen. In injuries complicated by uveal prolapse, the antigen, which is normally confined to an intra-ocular compartment lacking lymphatic drainage, probably gains access to the conjunctival lymphatics, and can thus provoke an immune response.

Lens-induced endophthalmitis

Disorganized lens matter released into the ocular cavities following injury or spontaneous rupture of a hypermature cataract (see below) is usually disposed of by macrophages with minimal disturbance. Reference has already been made to phacolytic glaucoma. Occasionally, however, the release excites an inflammatory reaction, which is thought to be auto-immune. The reaction may occur within 48 hours or may take several days to develop, and is confined to the anterior segment and focused on the lens. Initially, the infiltrate is predominantly composed of neutrophils and eosinophils, but macrophages and giant cells soon appear. The neutrophils are probably attracted by complexes resulting from the reaction of complement-fixing anti-lens antibodies with the released lens antigen. The reaction subsides with evacuation of residual lens matter.

Sometimes lens-induced endophthalmitis occurs in association with sympathetic ophthalmitis.

25.10.5 Disease of the retina

General considerations

Basic structure

The neural retina (Fig. 25.98) comprises the layer of photoreceptors and the neurones which relay the signals generated in the former to the brain. In man there are both 'rods', which respond to low levels of illumination, and 'cones', which are stimulated at normal 'daylight' levels and can discriminate colour. In the foveal region the cones are slender and resolution is at its most critical. The region is also avascular, but is surrounded by a rich capillary bed derived from the superior and inferior temporal branches of the central retinal artery. The photoreceptors are linked to the bipolar neurones in the inner nuclear layer by synapses (outer fibre layer of Henle). It is now recognized that there are complex cross-connections, particularly between cones, and that considerable image processing occurs in the retina. The bipolar neurones form synapses with the ganglion cells in the middle fibre layer. The axons of the ganglion cells form the nerve fibre layer whose fibres converge to form the optic nerve. The Müller fibres are large glial cells which extend perpendicularly through the retina. Their footplates form the inner limiting membrane. The outer limiting membrane is formed by a series of terminal bars between the Müller fibres and the photoreceptors. The outer segments of the photoreceptors are invested by fine cytoplasmic processes from the cells of the pigmented epithelium. By electron microscopy,

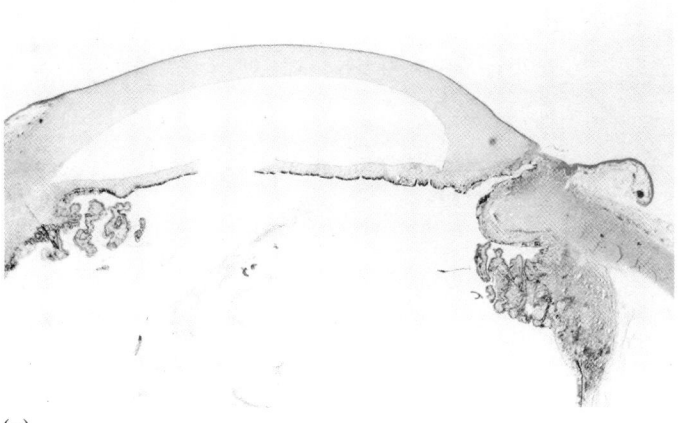

(a)

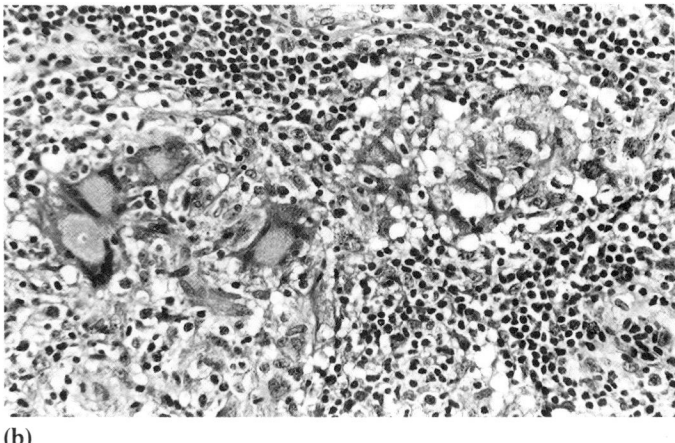

(b)

Fig. 25.97 Sympathetic ophthalmitis following extraction of a traumatic cataract. (a) Low-power view of anterior segment, showing prolapse of the iris into the cataract section (arrow). Note the absence of an infiltrate in the iris and ciliary body. (Masson trichrome.) (b) Typical granulomatous exudate in the choroid. (Both figures are from Lucas 1989, by courtesy of Blackwell Scientific Publications Ltd.)

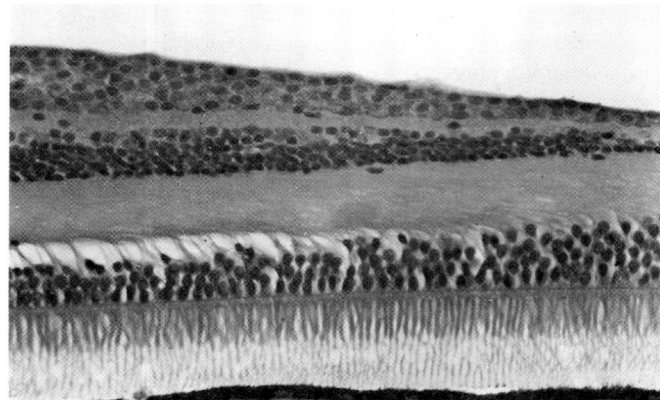

Fig. 25.98 Normal foveal retina. GC, ganglion cells; INL, inner nuclear layer; F, Henle's fibre layer; PR, photoreceptors; PE, pigmented epithelium. The nerve fibre layer (axons of the ganglion cells) cannot be distinguished in this area. (From Lucas 1989, by courtesy of Blackwell Scientific Publications Ltd.)

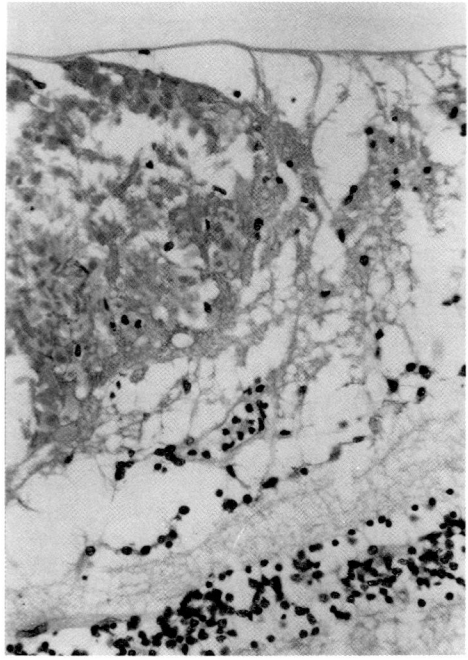

Fig. 25.99 Edge of a microinfarct, showing cytoid bodies (arrows) in the nerve fibre layer. (Specimen by courtesy of Dr M. Filipic.)

the outer segments of the photoreceptors are composed of membrane stacks, which are renewed from the base as their tips are phagocytosed by the pigmented epithelium. Adhesion between the neural retina and the pigmented epithelium depends on the visco-elastic properties of a glycosaminoglycan ground-substance between the outer segments and active transport of fluid by the pigmented epithelium, which maintains a negative pressure and prevents dilution of the ground-substance.

Non-specific pathological changes

Intra-retinal haemorrhages Haemorrhages in the superficial nerve fibre layer track along the line of the fibres, they are thus linear or 'flame-shaped'. Deeper ('dot and blot') haemorrhages are contained by the Müller fibres.

Cotton-wool spots are microinfarcts in the superficial nerve fibre layer due to arteriolar occlusion. Microscopically they consist of swollen axons crammed with mitochondria and other intracellular organelles, which in cross-section superficially resemble large cells and are thus known as 'cytoid bodies' (Fig. 25.99).

Hard exudates are pools of proteinaceous and fatty material in Henle's layer (Fig. 25.100) which, due to the arrangement of the capillary network from which they are derived, tend to be laid down in an arc or circle around the macula.

Microaneurysms occur in conditions in which there is retinal ischaemia. Though best seen in flat preparations, they may be recognized in histological sections because they intrude into the outer fibre (plexiform) layer (Fig. 25.101), because the wall of the microaneurysm tends to be permeable, they are often associated with exudates.

Drüsen are seen in sections as hemispherical excrescences of Bruch's membrane, thought to be formed by the pigmented epithelium. They are hyaline and strongly PAS-positive (Fig.

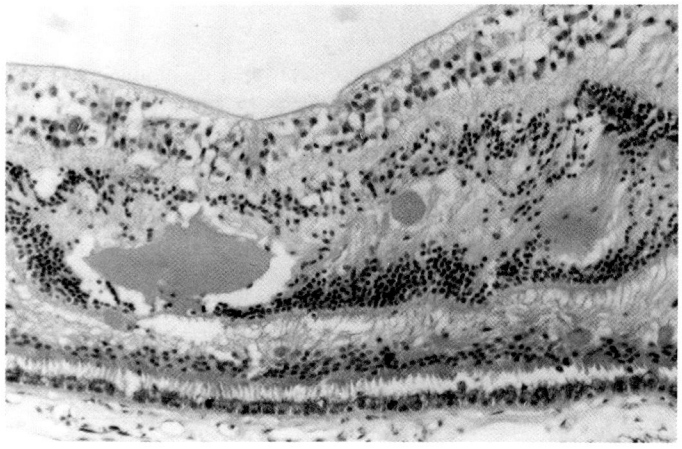

Fig. 25.100 Serous (hard) exudates in the layer of bipolar cells in diabetic retinopathy. (From Lucas 1989, by courtesy of Blackwell Scientific Publications Ltd.)

25.102a) and increase in number with age. As they increase in number, they become more granular (Fig. 25.102b) and this probably heralds the onset of macular degeneration (see below).

Vascular disease

Occlusion of the central retinal artery

Occlusion of the central retinal artery is most commonly due to atheroma or embolism, but cranial arteritis accounts for about

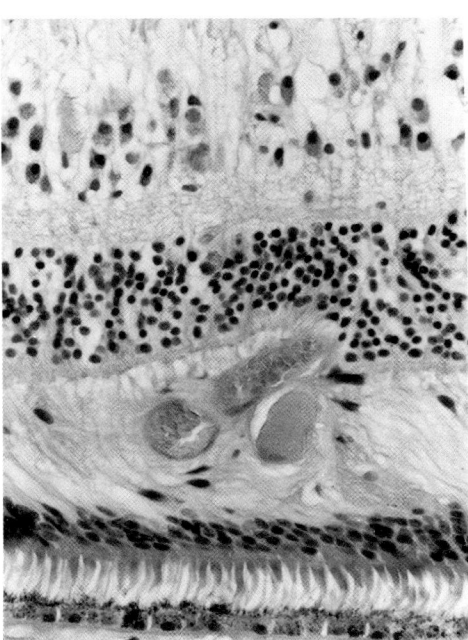

Fig. 25.101 Microaneurysm in diabetic retinopathy. The aneurysmal capillary (asterisks) has intruded into Henle's fibre layer and there is an adjacent pool of exudate (E) which has presumably leaked from it. (From Lucas 1989, by courtesy of Blackwell Scientific Publications Ltd.)

10 per cent of cases. The site of occlusion is usually just posterior to the cribriform plate. The inner retinal layers are affected, since the photoreceptors are maintained through the pigmented epithelium. After removal of the necrotic debris derived from these layers by phagocytosis, there is not much gliosis because the Müller fibres are destroyed.

Occlusion of the central retinal vein

Occlusion of the central retinal vein is a common event in hypertensive and elderly arteriosclerotic patients. Raised intra-ocular pressure is also a predisposing factor. The consequences are serious, as recovery of much useful vision seldom occurs. The site of the occlusion is usually, as in the case of the artery, just posterior to the cribriform plate. The immediate effect of such an occlusion is retinal oedema and intra-retinal haemorrhages. These spread from the optic nerve head along the fibres as described above. The deeper haemorrhages may rupture into the subretinal space or through the internal limiting membrane. Later, hard exudates and cotton-wool spots appear.

In about 20 per cent of cases, new vessels spread over the anterior surface of the iris and retina (see below). Those on the iris form anterior peripheral synechia with occlusion of the drainage angle and intractable glaucoma (q.v.). This type of glaucoma is often called 'thrombotic', though it is strictly 'post-thrombotic' and perhaps best referred to as neovascular.

New vessels on the anterior surface of the retina usually arise at the margin of the optic nerve head. They may spread on the retina and form fronds posterior to the vitreous. The latter are prone to bleed, and organization of such haemorrhages eventually leads to a traction detachment.

'Painful blind eyes' following thrombosis of the central retinal vein are amongst the commonest specimens seen by an ophthalmic pathologist. In such eyes, special study is necessary to demonstrate the site of the venous thrombosis and, because of the lapse of time, may not actually be possible. The central vein in sections of the optic nerve often appears collapsed and shows cuffing by lymphocytes. The retinal vessels usually show a conspicuous degree of hyaline sclerosis (Fig. 25.103). Thick-walled vessels in which new capillary channels are forming are also characteristic.

Occlusion of a major retinal branch vein

Branch veins are commonly occluded by thrombosis at the sites of arteriovenous crossings. The predisposing factors are the same as for occlusion of the central vein. The effects are also similar, but confined to the quadrant involved. There is usually useful residual vision and post-thrombotic glaucoma is much less likely to supervene.

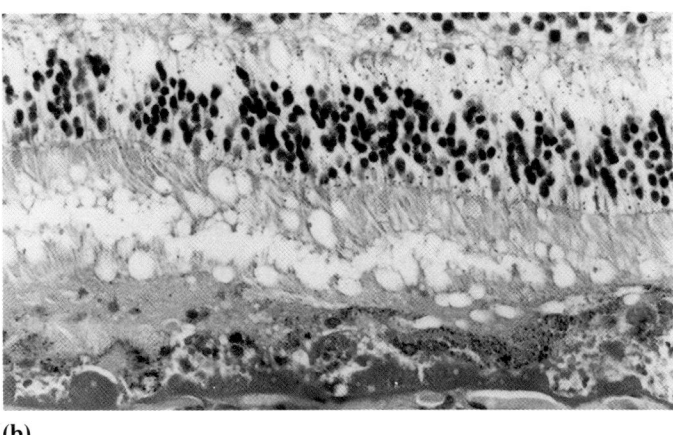

(a)   (b)

Fig. 25.102 Drüsen: (a) solitary drüse; (b) multiple granular drüsen. (PAS-tartrazine.) (From Lucas 1989, by courtesy of Blackwell Scientific Publications Ltd.)

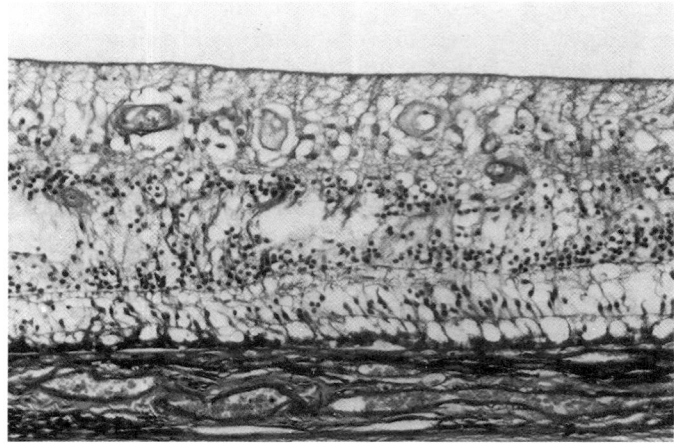

Fig. 25.103 End-stage post-thrombotic glaucoma. Typical hyalinized small retinal vessels (arrows).

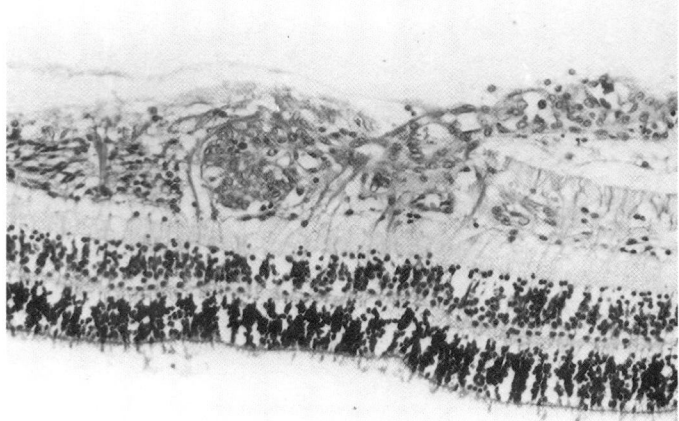

Fig. 25.104 Retinopathy of prematurity. Capillary knot (K) in the nerve fibre layer, with adjacent spindle cells (S) (orientated parallel to the retinal surface) from which capillaries (C) are seen proliferating on to the retinal surface. (PAS-tartrazine.) (From Lucas 1989, by courtesy of Blackwell Scientific Publications Ltd.)

Diabetic eye disease

The vascular changes in diabetic retinopathy are *hyaline arteriolosclerosis, thickening of the capillary basement membrane, degeneration of pericytes, capillary closure, microaneurysm formation,* and *increased tortuosity of venules.* Most of these changes are not unique to the retinal vasculature. Shunt vessels showing endothelial proliferation appear in the areas of capillary closure and, as the retinopathy progresses, cotton-wool spots, hard exudates, and cystoid macular oedema may all complicate the picture.

A serious complication of diabetic retinopathy is the growth of new capillaries on the retina and iris as has already been described following occlusion of the central retinal vein. The release of an angiogenic factor by ischaemic retina has long been thought to account for the proliferation of these new vessels. Angiogenic factors with properties similar to those isolated from certain tumours have been isolated from the retinae of several species.

A further feature, unrelated to vascular disease, seen in some diabetic eyes is the occurrence of deposits of glycogen in the pigmented epithelium of the iris. If the glycogen is lost during processing, the iris epithelium has a vacuolated appearance.

Retinopathy of prematurity

Retinopathy of prematurity (*retrolental fibroplasia*) occurs in premature infants who have usually been subjected to sustained hyperoxia. Under normal conditions, the retinal vessels develop from mesenchymal spindle cells, which migrate anteriorly from the optic nerve head. Under hyperoxia, capillary closure occurs and the migration is inhibited. The spindle cells proliferate and subsequently form arteriovenous shunts. At this stage, arrest and partial regression is possible. Further progress leads to capillary proliferation on the retinal surface (Fig. 25.104) with exudation, haemorrhage, and secondary detachment of the retina. Hyaline membranes may be found in the pulmonary alveoli of affected infants.

Inherited retinal degenerations

The retina is subject to a large number of inherited degenerative conditions, some of which are part of wider syndromes. Even in the more common, such as retinitis pigmentosa, the pathology is often not well known because few examples have been seen, particularly in the early stages. Of these conditions, retinitis pigmentosa is a significant cause of visual disability in the young and merits a brief account.

Retinitis pigmentosa

Retinitis pigmentosa is usually inherited as an autosomal recessive, although autosomal dominant and X-linked transmission have also been demonstrated and several clinical and pathological variants have been described. The disease is not inflammatory, but retention of the technically incorrect name was recommended at a recent symposium of experts (Marmor *et al.* 1983). Atrophy of the pigmented epithelium in the post-equatorial region, with migration of pigment along attenuated blood vessels (Fig. 25.105a) gives the 'bone corpuscular' pattern seen ophthalmoscopically. Initially, the rods in the post-equatorial region are most severely affected by the degenerative process, hence the 'night-blindness'. Eventually, the process affects the photoreceptors more widely and, in the typical late case, stumpy remnants of cones and a single layer of cone nuclei are all that remain in the foveal area (Fig. 25.105b).

In *Usher's syndrome*, retinitis pigmentosa is associated with neurosensory deafness. Other conditions associated with eye disease clinically resembling retinitis pigmentosa are the Bardet–Biedl (Laurence–Moon) syndrome, Refsum's and Cockayne's syndromes, and the Bassen–Kornzweig syndrome.

Finally, it may be added that contusion of the retina may lead to late changes clinically and histologically resembling retinitis pigmentosa.

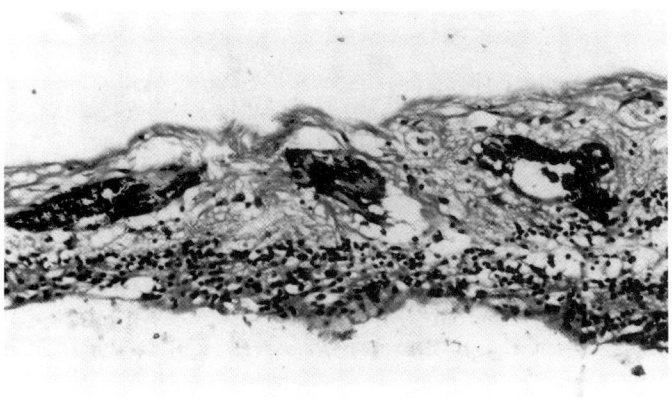
(a)

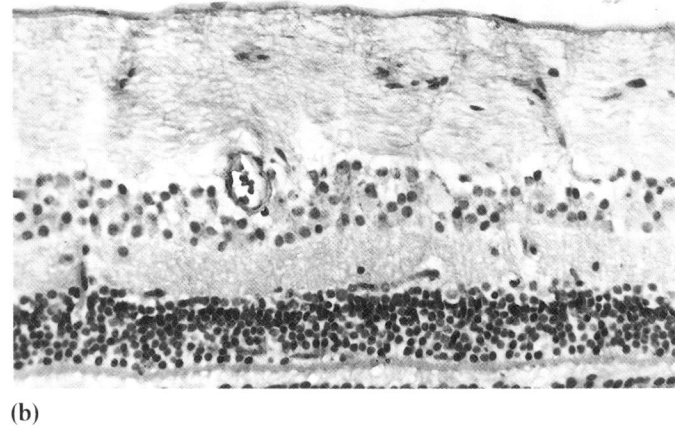
(b)

Fig. 25.105 Retinitis pigmentosa: (a) pigment migrating along retinal vessels in the peripheral retina (Masson trichrome); (b) single layer of cone nuclei (CN) with stumpy cones in the central retina. (Both figures are from Lucas 1989, by courtesy of Blackwell Scientific Publications Ltd.)

Age-related macular degeneration

In this category are included interrelated conditions that affect predominantly the macular region in elderly subjects, although a 'juvenile' variant also occurs. They are a common cause of visual disability and often affect both eyes, though not necessarily synchronously. Because the peripheral retina is usually spared, some vision is retained long after central vision has been lost.

Senile macular degeneration

The pathological features of this condition are:

1. thickening of Bruch's membrane with increasing basophilia and deposition of lipids;

2. flattening, depigmentation, and fragmentation of the pigmented epithelium and proliferation of small heaps of cells;

3. the appearance of drüsen and a PAS-positive 'basal linear deposit' between Bruch's membrane and the pigmented epithelium (Fig. 25.106);

4. distortion and loss of photoreceptors.

Pathogenesis Senile macular degeneration may be regarded as a functional failure of the pigmented epithelium, due perhaps to accelerated senescence. The accumulation of incompletely degraded material in the cells of the pigmented epithelium through failure of the cellular digestive system compromises the maintenance of the photoreceptors and leads to extrusion of aberrant material (drüsen and linear deposit) on Bruch's membrane (Young 1987).

Some accumulation of lipid in Bruch's membrane is normal with increasing age. When excessive, the membrane probably becomes hydrophobic so that transport of fluid and metabolites between the choriocapillaries and the pigmented epithelium is impeded. Plasticizers such as phthalates, adipates, and tributyl acetyl citrate, which are lipid soluble, have been found in the

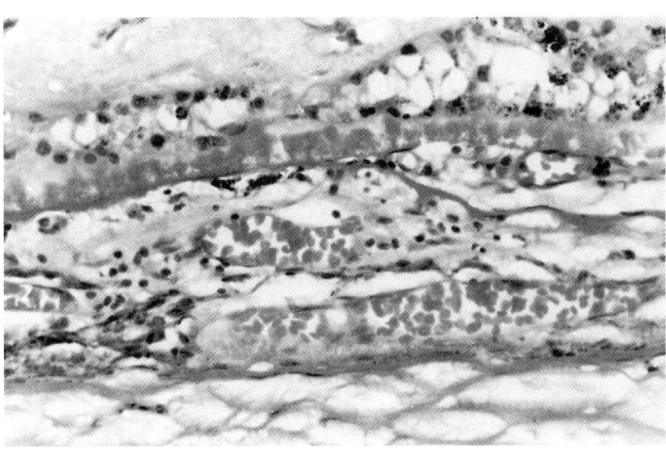

Fig. 25.106 Senile macular degeneration. Basal linear deposit (D) along Bruch's membrane (BM) with a capillary (asterisk) on the retinal side of Bruch's membrane. (PAS-tartrazine.) (From Lucas 1989, by courtesy of Blackwell Scientific Publications Ltd.)

lipid deposits. Their role in the pathogenesis is unknown, but they may stabilize the deposits (Bird 1991).

Disciform degeneration

In addition to the changes already described, breaks are found in Bruch's membrane. The other essential features are:

1. Invasion of the subretinal space by new capillaries (Fig. 25.106). These enter through the breaks in Bruch's membrane and sometimes from the margins of the nerve head. The retinal vasculature may also contribute.

2. Exudation and haemorrhage from the new vessels result in a subretinal haematoma.

3. Organization of the haematoma leaves a flat, disc-shaped scar over which there is usually no functional retina.

4. Secondary haemorrhages and exudation may occasionally be large enough to simulate a choroidal melanoma or even break through the retina into the vitreous chamber.

Other retinal degenerations

Peripheral cystoid degeneration

Typical cystoid degeneration affects the peripheral retina in all eyes from childhood onwards. Expanding lacunae are seen in the outer nerve fibre layer, bridged by pillars composed mainly of Müller fibres. The condition rarely, if ever, leads to detachment.

Lattice degeneration

Lattice degeneration has been found in 10 per cent of cases in large autopsy series. It is a localized degenerative change in which first the neurones of the inner layers and later the photoreceptors are replaced by proliferating glia and associated with pigment hyperplasia. The overlying vitreous becomes condensed and glial filaments extend into it to form traction bands. This may result in a retinal break and subsequent detachment.

Retinal detachment

Retinal detachment implies the breakdown of adhesion between the neural retina and the pigmented epithelium. This may occur for various reasons and detachments fall into three main categories.

Rhegmatogenous detachment

By definition this type of detachment is associated with a hole or break in the retina. However, for a detachment to occur there must also be vitreous traction. This arises because the vitreous is firmly attached anteriorly at the *pars ciliaris* and peripheral neural retina (the vitreous base) and retracts forwards if degenerative changes occur or as a result of trauma. Factors that predispose to rhegmatogenous detachment are:

1. myopia (retinal breaks are 10 times more common in high myopes);
2. lattice degeneration;
3. cataract surgery;
4. accidental trauma.

The subretinal fluid, which is derived from vitreous, initially has a low protein content in this type of detachment.

Exudative detachment

Exudative detachments are due to a leakage of fluids from blood vessels and are seen in association with uveal inflammation, choroidal neoplasms, and retinoblastoma. The subretinal fluid has a high protein content approximating to that of plasma.

Coats' disease is a rare, usually unilateral, vascular retinopathy affecting male infants, in which massive leakage occurs from dilated peripheral retinal capillaries.

Tractional detachment

Tractional detachments are associated with fibrovascular proliferation within the vitreous chamber, such as has already been described in diabetic retinopathy, post-thrombotic glaucoma, retinopathy of prematurity, or organization of the vitreous following inflammatory conditions such as vitreous abscess, toxocara, or toxoplasma.

Effects on retina

The outer retinal layers are dependent on contact with the pigmented epithelium and detachment results in fragmentation of the outer segments. These are phagocytosed by pigment-laden macrophages, probably derived at least in part from the pigmented epithelium. There is also a diffuse oedema of the inner layers of the retina.

If the retina is restored to its normal position within a few days, the changes are reversible. This can normally be accomplished in rhegmatogenous detachments by sealing the hole surgically.

25.10.6   Diseases of the conjunctiva and cornea

Degenerations

Pannus

Pannus is the clinical term used to describe the ingrowth from the limbus of a thin layer of fibrovascular tissue between the epithelium and Bowman's membrane. It is seen in conditions associated with chronic corneal oedema such as *chronic glaucoma* and *Fuch's endothelial dystrophy*.

Pinguecula

A pinguecula is a yellowish elevated spot at the limbus in the interpalpebral fissure. Degenerative changes in the *collagen substantia propria* result in the appearance of coarse basophilic curlicues which stain for elastin. Calcific granules may be deposited.

Pterygium

Pterygia occur in the interpalpebral fissure and are found more often on the nasal side. They consist of a triangular (wing-shaped) growth of fibrovascular tissue covered by conjunctival epithelium, the apex of which extends into the cornea, eroding Bowman's membrane as it progresses. Degenerative changes similar to those seen in pingueculae are usually present and there may be dysplastic changes in the overlying epithelium.

The pathogenesis is unknown, but they are commoner in hot, dry climates.

Band keratopathy

Band keratopathy is a form of dystrophic calcification seen in long-standing eye diseases such as chronic iridocyclitis or glaucoma. The calcium is deposited in the epithelial basement membrane and Bowman's membrane (Fig. 25.107). Eventually, Bowman's membrane may fragment and scarring of the superficial stroma may ensue.

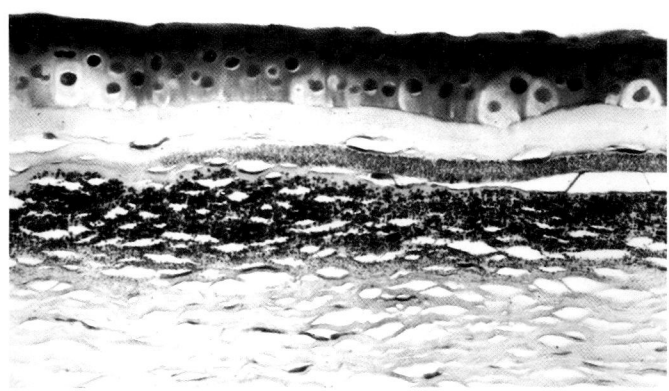

Fig. 25.107 Band keratopathy. Calcific stippling of Bowman's membrane (BM) and the anterior stroma. A hyaline fibrous pannus is present between Bowman's membrane and the epithelium. Masson trichrome.) (From Lucas 1989, by courtesy of Blackwell Sci(entific Publications Ltd.)

Fuch's endothelial dystrophy

Fuch's endothelial dystrophy is an age-related degenerative condition, primarily affecting Descemet's membrane and the endothelium. The former becomes thickened and develops excrescences on its posterior surface (Fig. 25.108), while the latter becomes depleted. This eventually results in chronic epithelial oedema. The latter may commonly be precipitated by cataract surgery.

Keratoconus

Keratoconus affects young adults and is associated with atopy. It also occurs in Down syndrome. Ectasia of the axial part of the cornea results in gross astigmatism. Microscopically, there are breaks in the epithelial basement membrane and Bowman's

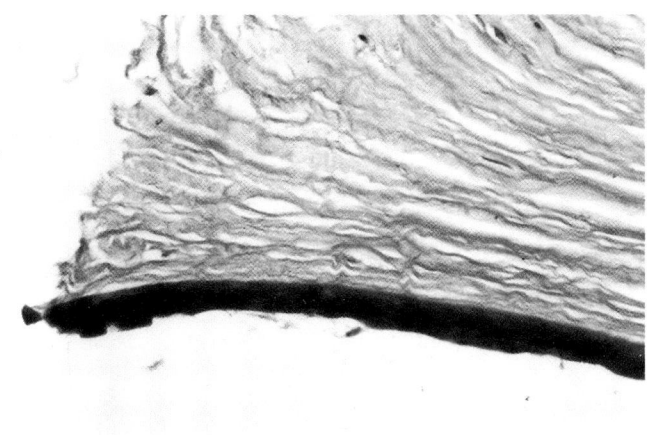

Fig. 25.108 Fuch's endothelial dystrophy. Thickening of Desçemet's membrane with irregularities of its posterior surface. (PAS-tartrazine.) (From Lucas 1989, by courtesy of Blackwell Scientific Publications Ltd.)

membrane and the number of stromal lamellae is reduced in the axial region. Occasionally, Descemet's membrane ruptures spontaneously with resulting gross oedema (hydrops) of the cornea. The pathogenesis of keratoconus is unknown.

Inherited corneal dystrophies

The cornea is subject to a number of rare familial dystrophies. They are characterized by deposition of abnormal material. This is presumably derived from an accumulated metabolite for which the appropriate enzyme system is defective. They tend to recur gradually after grafting. The three major types are described here.

Lattice dystrophy

Lattice dystrophy is the most commonly encountered of the group. It is inherited as an autosomal dominant. The abnormal material deposited in the stroma has the properties of amyloid. There is also marked fibrosis affecting the anterior stroma and Bowman's membrane, which is probably responsible for much of the visual impairment. This may be serious by age 40. No associated deposition of amyloid elsewhere has been identified in these cases.

Granular dystrophy

Granular dystrophy is inherited as an autosomal dominant. Proteinaceous material, which stains brilliantly by the red counterstain in Masson's trichrome, is deposited mainly deep to Bowman's membrane in the central cornea. Under the electron microscope, the deposit consists of masses of electron-dense rods or plates, 100–500 nm in length, which are protein crystals. Associated fibrosis is minimal and serious visual impairment usually occurs late.

Macular dystrophy

Macular dystrophy is inherited as an autosomal recessive. There is a diffuse cloudiness of the central stroma which spreads peripherally. The abnormal material is a glycosaminoglycan, rich in keratan sulphate, which stains brilliantly by the PAS method, Alcian blue, etc. It is usually most abundant in the superficial stroma, but deposits are spread throughout the stroma and also in the endothelium. Electron microscopy shows the deposits to be membrane-bound aggregates of fibrillary material. Some associated fibrosis is usually seen and visual impairment may be serious by age 30.

25.10.7 Cataract

The lens is derived from surface epithelium which continues to generate new fibres at the equator throughout life, where there is thus a thin layer of nucleated fibres. The weight of the lens actually trebles between birth and age 80. The content of a yellowish pigment, hydroxykynurenin glucoside, which is present in the lens, also increases with age. Cataracts may be described in terms of age, the location of the opacities, or the clinical situation in which they have appeared.

Many factors that may cause or contribute to the risk of developing cataract have been identifed. The most important are:

1. *Genetic.* There may be a clear inheritance or familial prevalence, or the cataract may be part of a systemic syndrome, e.g. Lowe's, Alport's, Marfan's.

2. *Radiations.* Ionizing (X-rays etc.) and non-ionizing (infra-red and microwaves) radiation have clearly been implicated. Sunlight and ultraviolet radiation are under suspicion.

3. *Drugs.* Corticosteroids are the most important. They cause posterior lens opacities.

4. *Trauma.*

5. *Diabetes mellitus.*

6. *High blood pressure.*

7. *Chronic intra-ocular disease.*

It is difficult to classify cataracts satisfactorily on a pathological basis, but the following pathological changes are observed in cataractous lenses:

1. *Disappearance of the lens epithelium and nucleated equatorial fibres.* At the same time, nucleated fibres appear along the posterior capsule.

2. *Swelling and vacuolation of the superficial cortical fibres.* The deeper fibres fragment and liquefy, and eosinophilic (Morgagnian) globules are deposited between the fragmented fibres (Fig. 25.109a). At the cataract 'matures', the cortex liquefies and the nucleus becomes smaller and smaller, and eventually a small nuclear remnant is left floating in a sac of fluid ('hypermature' or Morgagnian cataract). It is at this stage that phacolytic glaucoma or lens-induced endophthalmitis may be caused by escape of the liquefied lens matter through capsular breaks or pores.

Osmotic imbibition of fluid during the process of liquefaction may cause swelling of the lens and pupillary block. In diabetics, saturation of the hexokinase pathway by the high levels of glucose results in increased production of sorbitol by aldose reductase. Intracellular accumulation of sorbitol also causes intake of water.

Brown discoloration, probably due to the accumulation of products of tryptophan degradation, is a conspicuous feature of cataractous lenses.

3. *Nuclear sclerosis.* The nucleus has a 'glassy' look in conventional sections, though this can be difficult to detect. Electron microscopically, there is increasing density of the lens fibres, associated with an increase in the number and complexity of the interdigitations between the fibres. These appear to be age-related changes, although 'senile' cataracts are not necessarily nuclear.

4. *Anterior subcapsular fibrosis.* The subcapsular epithelium undergoes metaplasia into fibrocyte-like cells which lay down a plaque consisting of layers of collagen and basement membrane material deep to the capsule, which becomes wrinkled (Fig. 25.109b).

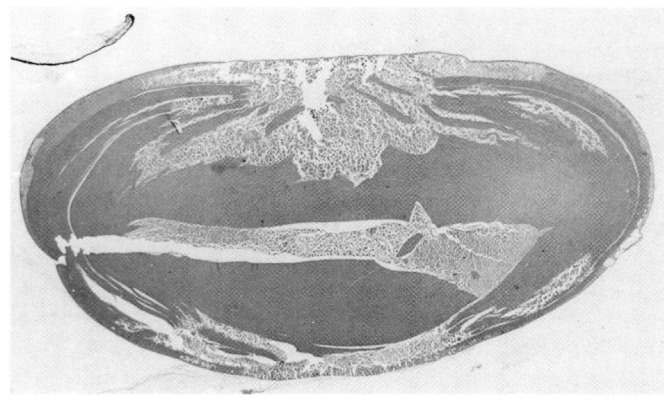

(a)

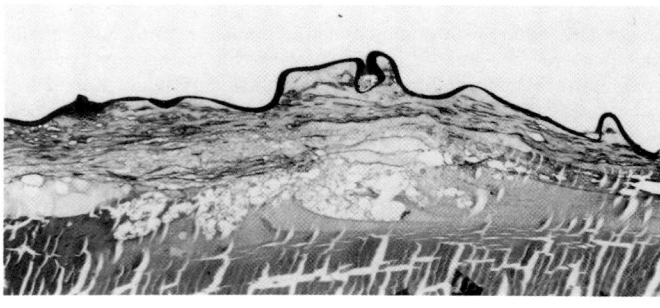

(b)

Fig. 25.109 Cataract: (a) showing breakdown of lens fibres into globules; (b) subcapsular fibrosis with convolution of anterior lens-capsule (PAS-tartrazine). (From Lucas 1989, by courtesy of Blackwell Scientific Publications Ltd.)

25.10.8   Peri-ocular tumours

Most of the tumours that arise on the lids and within the orbit are similar to those that arise in corresponding tissues elsewhere. However, several benign conjunctival tumours have special features that deserve mention.

Choristomas of the conjunctiva

Dermolipoma

These are common malformations that occur in the fornices, especially at the outer canthus. They consist mainly of fatty tissue in which may be found pilary adnexal structures and sweat gland coils. Occasionally, more complex examples contain lacrimal gland, cartilage, smooth muscle, and nerve fibres.

Dermoid tumours

These are essentially plaques of ectopic skin, often complete with pilosebaceous follicles and sweat glands, which commonly lie across the limbus, but occasionally replace the entire cornea.

Conjunctival papillomas

These are typical papillary growths arising on the lid margin, limbus, or caruncle in young adults. They often contain koilocytes and are probably virus-induced. Although they are prone to recur, they do not become malignant. Carcinoma of the conjunctiva is, indeed, extremely rare.

Conjunctival naevi

Naevi are not uncommon on the conjunctiva and are usually located at the limbus, although they also occur on the lid margin and caruncle. Cryptic downgrowths of bulbar conjunctiva are a constant feature of limbal naevi (Fig. 25.110) and junctional activity may persist in their epithelium after it is no longer seen in the surface epithelium. Accumulation of mucus in the crypts can lead to cyst formation, which simulates growth. Naevi of the lid margin may show extensive ramifications around adnexal structures and the meibomian glands, which can be confused with malignant infiltration. Conjunctival melanomas are extremely rare.

25.10.9   Intra-ocular tumours

Naevi

Naevi may be observed incidentally in the choroid, usually in adult life. Microscopically, they are composed of varying proportions of spindly, polyhedral, or dendritic cells. The polyhedral cells are often heavily pigmented. Naevi are usually symptomless and rarely show measurable growth. However, some may occasionally become large enough to expand the choroid locally. The choriocapillaris then becomes compressed and drüsen form on Bruch's membrane. Because naevus-like cells are found in the base of many choroidal melanomas (v.i.), it has been claimed that most or all such tumours arise in naevi.

Malignant melanomas

Malignant melanoma is the commonest primary intra-ocular tumour, but it is, nevertheless, a rare tumour. The incidence in Causcasians is approximately 15 times greater than that in coloured races. The majority of melanomas arise in the choroid

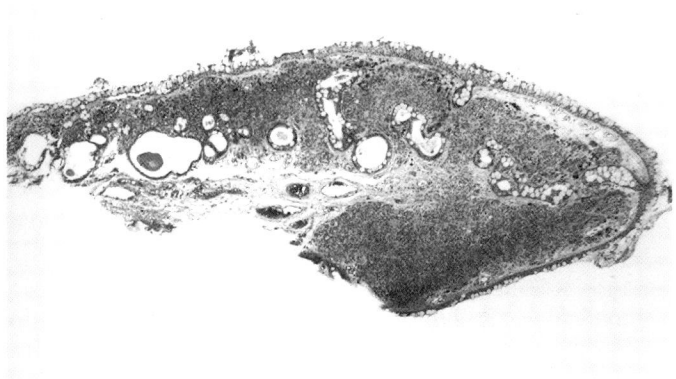

Fig. 25.110 Cystic naevus of bulbar conjunctiva. Dilated epithelial crypts are seen in the large mass of naevus cells in the substantia propria.

and the posterior supratemporal quadrant is the commonest subsite.

The growth initially expands the choroid, but as it enlarges Bruch's membrane may be ruptured and a head of tumour then forms in the subretinal space, to give the characteristic mushroom or collar-stud shape (Fig. 25.111a).

General structure

The tumours are composed of spindle or epithelioid cells, resembling those seen in melanomas elsewhere. Tumours in which the so-called *spindle B-type cells* (Fig. 25.111b) predominate are the commonest. Pigment content is variable and often quite light. The cells are often arranged in interlacing bundles. Lymphocytic infiltration in the tumour or adjacent choroid is unusual.

Local complications

Detachment of the retina is usual even with small, posteriorly located tumours (q.v.), and is responsible for the common presenting symptom of painless, progressive unilateral loss of vision. Other complications include massive necrosis which may simulate spontaneous endophthalmitis, vitreous haemorrhage, and secondary glaucoma.

Spread and metastasis

Within the globe, the tumour spread locally in the choroid and may infiltrate between the adjacent scleral lamellae. Anteriorly located ciliochoroidal tumours may invade the anterior chamber through the root of the iris and the trabecular meshwork. More serious still is the propensity to spread along scleral emissary channels through which vessels and nerves enter the eye (Fig. 25.111c). Posteriorly this leads to extension into the orbit, and anteriorly on to the surface of the globe under the limbal conjunctiva.

Intra-ocular melanomas differ from melanomas elsewhere in not having direct access to lymphatics until extra-ocular extension has occurred, but, as with other melanomas, the liver is the prime site for haematogenous metastases.

Mortality

The mortality after enucleation has been estimated in many different series. The figures range from 16 to 86 per cent after 5 years and from 27 to 64 per cent after 10 years. There has been some controversy in the literature recently as to the value of enucleation in the management of choroidal melanomas. It has been claimed that choroidal melanomas in general metastasize late, and that the peak mortality rate, seen 2–3 years after enucleation, may actually be the result of metastases promoted by handling the tumour at the time of enucleation. This implies that there is no urgency to remove a tumour-containing eye which retains useful vision. The contrary view is that any eye diagnosed as containing a malignant melanoma should be enucleated forthwith to minimize the risk of metastasis (the topic is reviewed in depth in Nicholson 1980, Chapters 11–13).

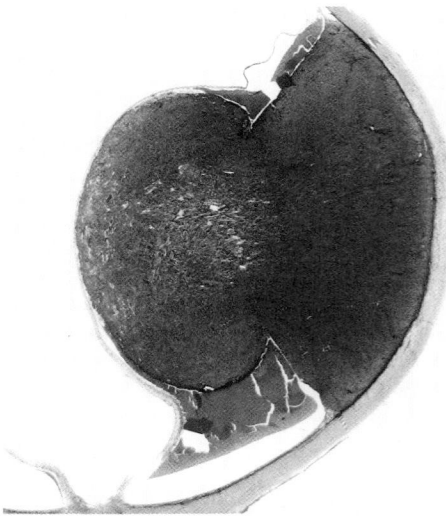

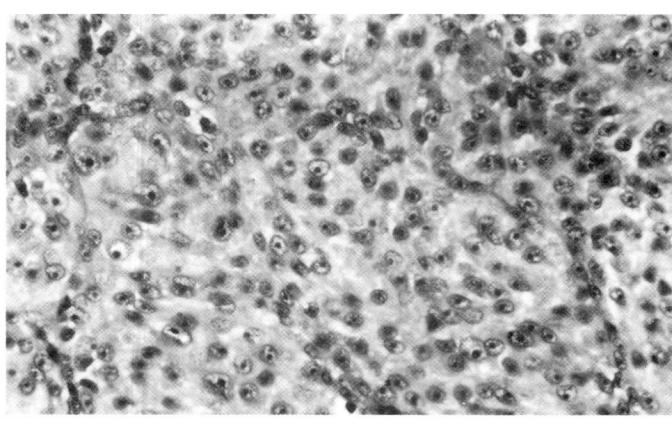

(b)

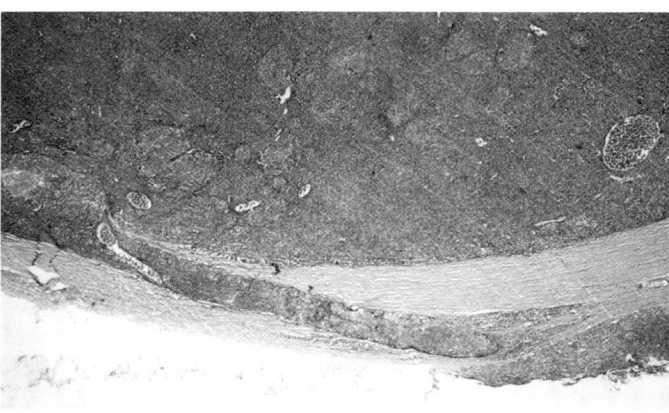

(c)

Fig. 25.111　Malignant melanoma: (a) Low-power view of a large equatorial melanoma, showing the typical mushroom-profile; (b) typical spindle B-cells with conspicuous nuceoli; (c) extension of an intra-ocular melanoma through a scleral canal to form an extrascleral deposit (S, sclera). [Both (a) and (b) are from Lucas 1989, by courtesy of Blackwell Scientific Publications Ltd.]

Prognostic factors

Many factors have been claimed to be of prognostic value:

1. *Cell type.* Contrary to experience with cutaneous melanomas, there is ample evidence that cell type influences prognosis. Tumours composed predominantly of small spindle cells with nuclei lacking nucleoli (spindle A) have a much better prognosis that epithelioid cell tumours.

2. *Size.* Small melanomas (< 1 cm in cross-sectional area) have a favourable prognosis.

3. *Location.* Anteriorly located tumours have a less favourable prognosis than posteriorly located tumours, but they usually cause symptoms later and thus tend to be larger when the eye is enucleated.

4. *Rupture of Bruch's membrane.* This is an unfavourable sign, probably because it reflects rapid growth.

5. *Reticulin content.* It has long been thought that slowly growing tumours lay down more reticulin. In practice this is rarely useful because reticulin content tends to be high in the oldest part of the tumour and low in the part which is actively growing, such as the head after rupture through Bruch's membrane.

6. *Pigment content.* Heavy pigmentation appears to be an adverse prognostic factor.

7. *Necrosis.* Necrosis is common and, although it has been claimed to be immunologically based, it probably more often results from failure of vascular supply and is not a favourable prognostic indicator.

8. *Extrascleral extension.* The presence of tumour outside the globe at the time of enucleation indicates a very poor prognosis.

Haemangiomas

The choroid is the occasional site for a cavernous-type haemangioma. Adults are usually affected. Haemangiomas are usually located posteriorly and may cause visual loss through interference with the retinal vascular supply via the choriocapillaris. Retinal detachment may also occur. Choroidal haemangiomas are occasionally misdiagnosed clinically as melanomas, but this has become less common with the introduction of fluorescein angiography and ultrasonography.

Retinoblastomas

Retinoblastoma is a rare malignant neoplasm derived from embryonic neuronal cells. It is estimated to occur in 1 in 15 000–20 000 live births and comprises about 3 per cent of childhood malignancies. The sexes are equally affected. Presentation is usually within the first 3 years of life, and often within the first 3 months.

Genetic retinoblastomas

Genetic retinoblastomas result from a mutation in the parents of the child or their antecedents. The gene is an autosomal dominant and has a penetrance of approximately 80 per cent. Of all cases of retinoblastoma, some 25–30 per cent are bilateral and genetic, and 10–20 per cent are unilateral and genetic.

Non-genetic retinoblastomas

Non-genetic retinoblastomas result from somatic mutations in the retina of the affected child and are thus always unilateral, but indistinguishable clinically and pathologically from unilateral genetic retinoblastomas.

Chromosomal abnormalities

The karyotype is normal in most cases of retinoblastoma, but 20 per cent of patients with partial deletion of the long arm of chromosome 13 (13q-syndrome) develop retinoblastoma. The mutation appears to occur at the D gene locus at 13q14.

General structure

Macroscopically the tumour is seen to arise from retina and usually expands posterior to the retina (exophytum type),

which is thus detached (Fig. 25.112a). Less commonly, growth is forwards within the vitreous space (endophytum type). The cut surface of the tumour often shows white flecks of calcium.

Microscopically, the tumour is composed of masses of small hyperchromatic cells. In undifferentiated retinoblastoma, many cells in mitosis are present and there are areas of necrosis in which calcium is precipitated (Fig. 25.112b). Blood-vessels may be stained by calcium–DNA complexes, as in other rapidly growing, necrotizing, malignant tumours such as oat-cell carcinoma of the lung.

Some tumours exhibit more differentiation and form rosettes. The so-called *Flexner–Wintersteiner rosettes*, which are characteristic of retinoblastoma, are composed of 15–40 tapering cells in a radial arrangement around a central lumen (Fig. 25.112c). Electron microscopy shows the cells to be connected by terminal bars, thus mimicking normal retinal structure. Microvilli, and sometimes cilia, showing primitive photoreceptor differentiation may be demonstrated projecting into the lumen.

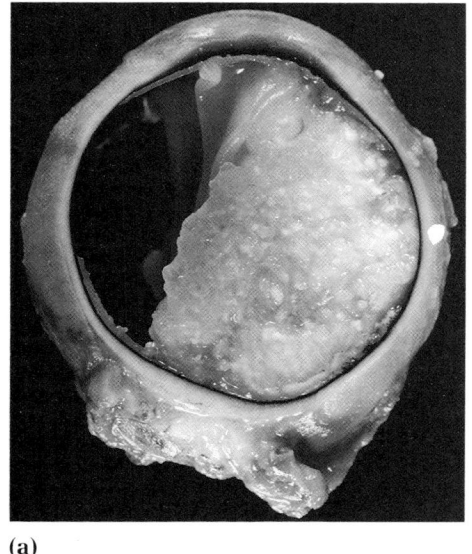

(a)

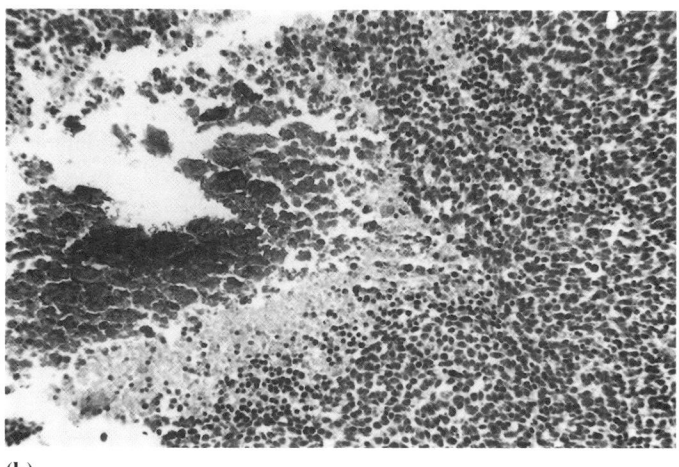

(b)

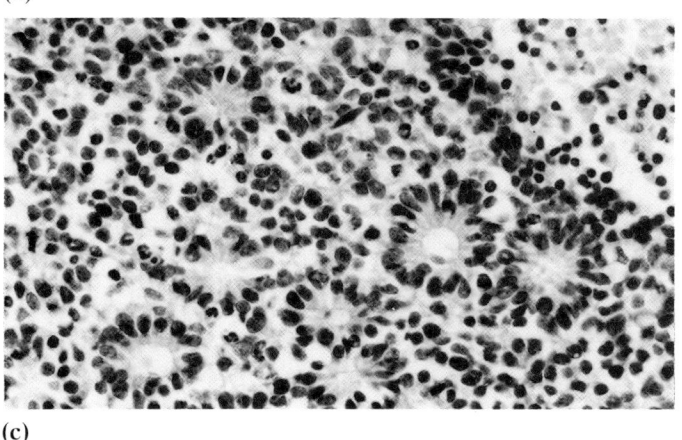

(c)

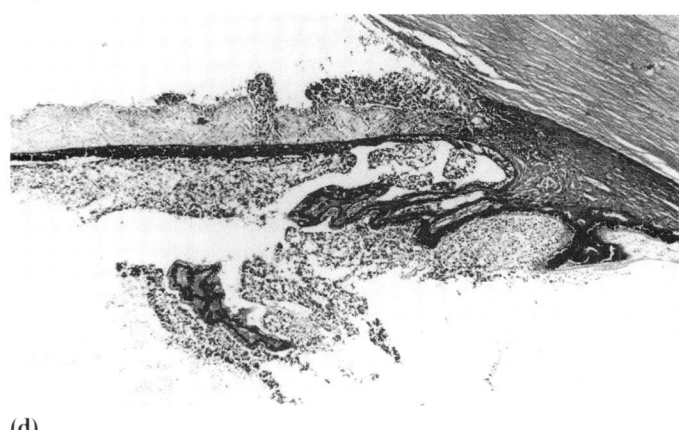

(d)

Fig. 25.112 Retinoblastoma. (a) Macroscopic picture of exophytum type with retinal detachment. The retina is just visible (R). (b) Area of necrosis, with deposition of calcium, in an undifferentiated retinoblastoma. (c) Retinoblastoma rosettes. (d) Intra-ocular spread of retinoblastoma in anterior segment. Deposits of growth can be seen around the ciliary processes, in the drainage angle, and on both surfaces of the iris. [Figures (c) and (d) are from Lucas 1989, by courtesy of Blackwell Scientific Publications Ltd.]

Spread and metastasis

Local seeding with the globe is characteristic of retinoblastoma. With the exophytum type it is within the subretinal space, while the endophytum type seeds in the vitreous chamber, on the posterior surface of the lens, and eventually into the anterior chamber (Fig. 25.112d) where the cells may sediment and simulate a hypopyon.

Invasion of the optic nerve head is common, and spread along the optic nerve to the brain eventually occurs. Careful examination of the optic nerve is important in globes enucleated for retinoblastoma. Spread beyond the cribriform plate is an unfavourable prognostic sign. Spread to the cut end of the nerve is an indication for radiotherapy.

Extension into the choroid occurs at the optic nerve head, around the margin of Bruch's membrane, and from there the orbit may be invaded. Choroidal extension is an unfavourable feature because it foreshadows haematogenous dissemination, particularly to bones such as skull, ribs, and humerus. From the orbit the tumour may invade the orbital bones and spread by lymphatic channels to local lymph nodes.

Prognosis

Cure by enucleation is estimated to be from 50 to 90 per cent in the absence of any of the unfavourable indications noted above.

The tumour is radiosensitive and cure is possible by radiotherapy. Such treatment is obviously advantageous in bilateral cases.

Spontaneous regression and arrest

Between 1952 and 1983, regressed retinoblastomas had been reported in 85 eyes (Aaby *et al.* 1983). These eyes are of two types:

1. *Phthisical globes.* Calcified remnants of tumour have been demonstrated in phthisical globes, usually from close relatives of cases of retinoblastoma. Necrosis of the tumour had presumably occurred because of failure of vascular supply. Islands of viable tumour cells may indeed persist.

2. *Functional globes.* Flat, partially calcified tumours have been observed in the parents of cases of retinoblastoma. In the few cases that have been examined histologically, they were composed of 'benign-looking' cells with evidence of photoreceptor differentiation. They may represent 'arrested' or 'regressed' tumours. They have been variously called 'retinomas', 'retinoblastoma group 0', and retinocytoma. They carry the same genetic risk as retinoblastomas.

Second malignancies in retinoblastoma survivors

Second malignancies are rare in cases of unilateral retinoblastoma, but with bilateral cases there is a 20 per cent chance that the patient will develop a second non-ocular malignancy up to over 40 years later, especially if radiotherapy has been given. Most examples have been osteogenic sarcomas, which may arise not only in the orbit within the field of irradiation, but also in the lower limbs.

25.10.10   Secondary carcinomas

Carcinomas commonly metastasize to the eye during the natural history of the malignancy, but, in about half the eyes found to contain secondary carcinoma, the primary growth has not been diagnosed at the time of enucleation.

Approximately 40 per cent of secondaries originate from the breast and about 40 per cent from the lung. The remainder come from gut, pancreas, thyroid, prostate, and kidney.

Most metastatic tumours are located in the choroid, where they form a grey-white saucer-shaped plaque. Retinal detachment occurs, but it is exceptional for Bruch's membrane to be ruptured.

25.10.11   Further reading

Aaby, A. A., Price, R. L., and Zakov, Z. N. (1983). Spontaneously regressing retinoblastomas, retinoma or retinoblastoma group 0. *American Journal of Ophthalmology* **96**, 315–20.

Albert, D. M. and Puliafilo, C. A (1979). *Foundations of ophthalmic pathology.* Appleton-Century-Crofts, New York.

Apple, D. J. and Rabb, M. F. (1985). *Ocular pathology. Clinical applications and self-assessment* (3rd edn). C. V. Mosby Co., St Louis.

Bird, A. C. (1991). Pathogenesis of retinal pigment epithelial detachment in the elderly: the relevance of Bruch's membrane change (Doyne lecture). *Eye* **5**, 1–12.

Boniuk, M. (ed.) (1964). *Ocular and adnexal tumours, new and controversial aspects.* C. V. Mosby Co., St Louis.

Duker, J. S. and Blumenkranz, M. S. (1991). Diagnosis and management of the acute retinal necrosis (ARN) syndrome. *Survey of Ophthalmology* **35**, 327–43.

Easty, D. L. (1985). *Virus diseases of the eye.* Lloyd Luke (Medical Books), London.

Fine, B. S. and Yanoff, M. (1979). *Ocular histology, a text and atlas* (2nd edn). Harper & Row, New York.

Garner, A. and Klintworth, G. K. (eds) (1982). *Pathobiology of ocular disease. A dynamic approach*, Parts A and B. Dekker, New York.

Jakobiec, F. A. (ed.) (1978). *Ocular and adnexal tumours.* Aesculapius, Birmingham, AL.

Jensen, O. A. (1986). *Human ophthalmic pathology.* Munksgaard, Copenhagen.

Kaufman, J. E., Barron, B. A., McDonald, M. B., and Waltman, S. R. (eds) (1988). *The cornea.* Churchill Livingstone, New York.

Kraus-Mackiw, E. and O'Connor, G. R. (eds) (1983). *Uveitis. Pathophysiology and therapy.* Thieme-Stratton, New York.

Lucas, D. R. (1989). *Greer's ocular pathology.* Blackwell Scientific Publications, Oxford.

Marmor, M. F., *et al.* (1983). Retinitis pigmentosa. A symposium on terminology and methods of examination. *Ophthalmology* **90**, 126–31.

Naumann, G. O. H. and Rabb, D. J. (1986). *Pathology of the eye.* Springer-Verlag, New York. (Translation and update of Naumann, G. O. H. (1980). *Pathologie des Auges.* Springer-Verlag, Berlin.)

Newsome, D. A. (ed.) (1988). *Retinal dystrophies and degenerations.* Raven Press, New York.

Nicholson, D. H. (ed.) (1980). *Ocular pathology update.* Masson Publishing, New York.

Rahi, A. H. S. and Garner, A., (1976). *Immunopathology of the eye.* Blackwell Scientific Publications, Oxford.

Reese, A. B. (ed.) (1976). *Tumours of the eye* (3rd edn). Harper & Row, New York.

Ritch, R., Shields, M. B., and Krupin, T. (eds) (1989). *The glaucomas*, Vols 1 and 2. C. V. Mosby Company, St Louis.

Spencer, W. H. (ed.) (1985–6). *Ophthalmic pathology. An atlas and text* (3rd edn), 3 volumes. W. B. Saunders, Philadelphia.

Yanoff, M. and Fine, B. S. (1989). *Ocular pathology. A text and atlas* (3rd edn). J. B. Lippincott Company, Philadelphia.

Young, R. W. (1987). Pathophysiology of age-related macular degeneration. *Survey of Ophthalmology* **31**, 291–306.

Zimmerman, L. E. and Sobin, L. H. (1980). *Histological typing of tumours of the eye and its adnexa*, International Histological Classification of Tumours, No. 24. World Health Organization, Geneva.

25.11 Developmental abnormalities of the brain

J. S. Wigglesworth

25.11.1 Introduction

Developmental abnormalities of the brain, as described in this section, cover a wide spectrum of pathological processes ranging from faults of organogenesis to a variety of forms of cerebral damage or disease process arising later in the course of prenatal or perinatal development. The latter include infective, toxic, and anoxic-ischaemic forms of injury.

25.11.2 Congenital anomalies

As stated in Chapter 11, the CNS is one of the most frequent sites of major congenital anomalies. The common lesions are due to abnormalities of closure of the primitive neural tube at 24–26 days post ovulation.

Anencephaly

Anencephaly, the most severe anomaly, is due to lack of closure, or secondary breakdown, of the anterior end of the neural tube. The affected fetus has a distinctive appearance with lack of cerebral hemispheres or cranial vault bones. The crown of the head comprises a mass of vascular tissue without covering skin. The fetus has bulging eyes, a broad nose, and malformed ears.

Myelocele and meningomyelocele

A similar lesion involving the posterior end of the neural tube leads to one of the forms of spina bifida comprising lack of formation of the vertebral arches and an exposed bulging mass of meninges or granulation tissue over a segment of abnormal spinal cord in the lumbar or sacral region. The severe lesion may be termed a *myelocele* or *meningomyelocele* according to whether the cord tissue is open or covered by a sac of meninges. The spinal cord lesion is associated with an elongation of the 4th ventricle and medulla extending through the foramen magnum into the upper cervical canal along with a tongue of cerebellar vermis. This condition, the *Arnold–Chiari malformation*, appears to result from the tethering of the spinal cord tissue by the skin attachment and leads in turn to the development of hydrocephalus, although the precise mechanism remains in dispute. A less severe form, *meningocele*, has a normal covering of skin over the lesion and is not associated with the Arnold–Chiari malformation. Both spina bifida and anencephaly are now commonly diagnosed antenatally by ultrasound techniques allowing therapeutic termination of pregnancy early in the second trimester. Consequently the abnormalities are seen less seldom in the mature fetus than previously. In addition there is some indication that spina bifida may be related to maternal nutrition and the frequency of the condition has been falling for a number of years.

Hydrocephalus

Hydrocephalus, expansion of the cerebral hemispheres by excessive CSF, occurs in association with a number of cerebral anomalies including *agenesis of the corpus callosum* and the *Dandy–Walker malformation* (cyst of the 4th ventricle with hypoplasia of the vermis) in addition to the association with spina bifida. It may also be due to congenital obstruction of the aqueduct of Sylvius. One form of hydrocephalus due to aqueduct stenosis has been linked to the X chromosome as a dominantly inherited disorder presenting in boys. Hydrocephalus also occurs as a result of obstruction to the aqueduct or to CSF outflow at the foramina of the 4th ventricle due to infections or haemorrhage in fetal or early neonatal life. An extensive ischaemic destruction of the brain *in utero* may cause an apparent hydrocephalus (i.e. dilatation of the ventricular system without expansion of the hemispheres).

Other gross cerebral anomalies

Failure of formation of separate cerebral hemispheres in the second month of development leads to a single, rather simple, hollow mass of cerebral tissue, *holoprosencephaly* (Fig. 25.113). This is often associated with trisomy of chromosome 13. The cerebral lesion is often accompanied by defects of the nose and eyes, of which the most severe is a fused central eye, *cyclopia*. Herniation of part of the brain, encephalocele, occurs with defects of the cranial vault, most often in the occipital region. The combination of a small occipital encephalocele with cystic kidneys, ductal plate malformation in the liver and polydactyly, Meckel syndrome, is of autosomal recessive inheritance.

Other grossly recognizable anomalies include abnormalities of cerebral size, microencephaly and megalencephaly, agenesis of the cerebellum, and a number of vascular malformations.

Abnormalities of cerebral architecture

Variations in brain size and in gyral appearance such as a smooth brain (*agyria*), or increase in gyral folding (*micropolygyria*), are consequences of a whole range of conditions involving failure of development of the normal microarchitecture of the brain. Subtle abnormalities of this type may result in severe functional consequences such as intractable epilepsy.

Brain malformation due to exogenous causes

Gross exposure to ionizing radiation causes microcephaly and mental retardation and a number of chemicals and drugs have been shown to cause abnormalities of cerebral architecture.

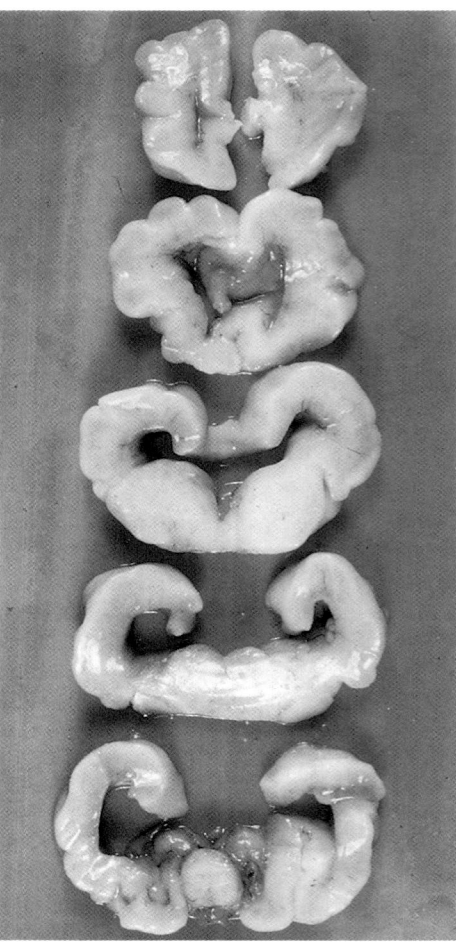

Fig. 25.113 Slices through a fetal brain showing incomplete formation of separate cerebral hemispheres, a form of holoprosencephaly.

25.11.3   Infections

Prenatal infections

The *Rubella* virus, *cytomegalovirus*, and *Toxoplasma gondii* are the three major infections known to damage the fetal brain following transplacental transmission from the mother. Rubella causes microcephaly following infection in the first trimester and is often considered teratogenic. The infections due to cyto-megalovirus and toxoplasmosis cause destructive inflammatory lesions around the ventricle and may result in microcephaly or hydrocephaly.

Perinatal bacterial infections

Infection with *Listeria monocytogenes*, β-haemolytic streptococci of Lancefield's Group B, and a range of Gram-negative organisms can cause *meningitis* or *meningoencephalitis* in the early neonatal period. Obstruction of the foramina of the 4th ventricle by organizing inflammatory exudate can lead to secondary hydrocephalus.

25.11.4   Haemorrhagic lesions

These include bleeding into the subdural and subarachnoid spaces and into the ventricular system.

Subdural and subarachnoid haemorrhage

Subdural haemorrhage is mainly due to rupture of small veins passing between the cerebral veins and the dural venous sinuses during traumatic deliveries, but occasionally forms part of a generalized haemorrhagic disorder in the newborn. Subarachnoid haemorrhage usually results from coalescence of hypoxic petechiae emanating from leptomeningeal vessels or from blood in the ventricular system which has entered the subarachnoid space through the foramina of the 4th ventricle. Subarachnoid haemorrhage of either origin is most frequent in preterm infants.

Subependymal and intraventricular haemorrhage

This condition is common and important in the small preterm infant. It is related to the presence of a thick zone of proliferating neural cells, the *subependymal matrix*, on the lateral aspect of the lateral ventricles during the latter part of the second and early third trimesters. Bleeding into this immature tissue develops as a result of a fluctuating haemodynamic state in hypoxic preterm infants. Animal experiments and human observations suggest that the likely sequence is hypotension with hypoperfusion of the periventricular region, followed by restoration of flow and capillary rupture. The inability of the preterm infant to maintain an appropriate cerebral circulation in conditions of asphyxia is partly due to the relative size of the brain. In the newborn infant the brain represents some 12 per cent of body mass, whereas in the adult it represents only 2 per cent. It is easy to imagine any of us as having difficulty in maintaining an appropriate circulation to a 9 kg brain while running for a bus! The subependymal haemorrhage secondarily ruptures into the ventricular system, which may become dilated by liquid blood and blood clot (Fig. 25.114). Organization of blood that has leaked into the subarachnoid space may result in *posthaemorrhagic hydrocephalus*. Large haemorrhages can prove fatal and posthaemorrhagic hydrocephalus often results in death or severe handicap. However, many preterm infants in whom significant intraventricular haemorrhage is recognized on imaging studies in the neonatal period are now known to survive with little evidence of handicap.

25.11.5   Anoxic–ischaemic lesions

These comprise a large and important range of related conditions which may develop in fetal life, during labour or in the neonatal period.

Major destructive cerebral lesions

These are usually central lesions involving cerebral white matter, *cystic encephalomalacia*, but may also spread out to the cerebral cortex in the more extreme forms such as *hydranencephaly*, in which most of the cerebrum has necrosed and been replaced

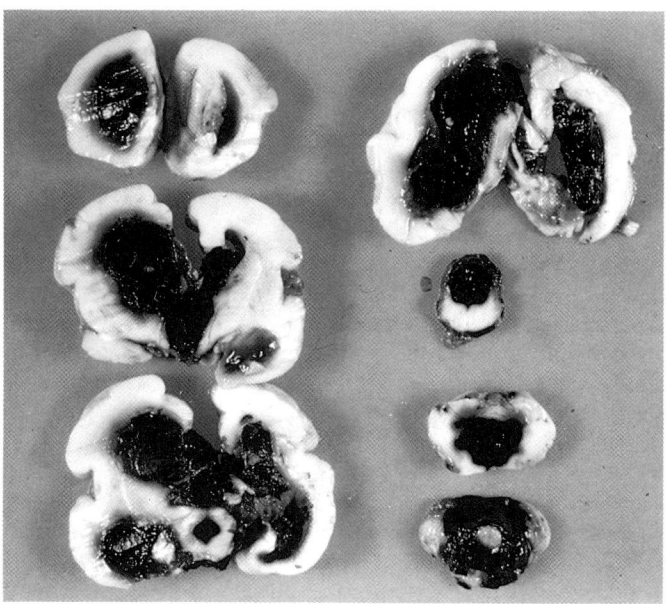

Fig. 25.114 Slices through a preterm infant brain shown massive intraventricular haemorrhage.

by fluid in the early fetal period. In general, the lesions of early onset tend to be more severe. Sometimes there is a history of some form of maternal shock, such as a respiratory arrest, which might be expected to cause an episode of fetal anoxia and hypotension. One specific example of prenatal brain damage resulting in cystic encephalomalacia is the cerebral injury sometimes seen in a survivor of a monochorial twin pair after the co-twin has died *in utero*. The lesion has usually been attributed to the transfer of thromboplastins or emboli from the dead twin via the placenta but recent observations suggest that in many cases the problem is due to an acute transfusion of blood across placental vascular anastomoses from the surviving twin into the dying or dead twin as its blood pressure drops. In addition, classic forms of cerebral infarction due to arterial occlusion sometimes develop in the perinatal period.

Periventricular leukomalacia

This comprises foci of ischaemic necrosis in the future white matter area of the hemispheres round the trigone of the lateral ventricle and in the deep white matter near the dorsolateral angle of the lateral ventricle. Small necrotic foci become infiltrated with lipid-filled macrophages: larger ones may break down to form cysts. The lesions are spatially related to the boundary between arterial branches passing in from the cortex and arteries supplying the basal ganglia, as well as the boundaries between the anterior and middle, and middle and posterior, cerebral arteries. The anatomical location and the production of similar lesions by induction of hypotension in experimental animals have caused the condition to be ascribed to episodes of hypotension. There is a gradation between the small necrotic and cystic lesions of periventricular leukomalacia and the mas-

sive destructive lesions of cystic encephalomalacia. Periventricular leucomalacia develops in preterm infants in the first month or so of life, but is now also recognized to occur before birth in many cases. The condition is of major importance in neonatology as the lesions occupy the site of the future internal capsule and optic and auditory radiations. Surviving infants may suffer multiple handicaps including cerebral palsy, blindness, and mental deficiency.

Anoxic-ischaemic neuronal necrosis

Selective necrosis affecting neurons throughout the brain is the characteristic anoxic lesion of the mature infant as periventricular leucomalacia is of the preterm infant. There are a number of patterns of damage to the brain according to the nature and severity of the anoxic stress. Thus a slowly progressive asphyxial process, due, for instance, to abnormal uterine contractions, will allow some attempt at compensation for fetal hypoxia by increasing cerebral circulation. When the process finally breaks down there may be onset of cerebral oedema with widespread death of neurons of the cortex and basal ganglia and some sensitive sites in the pons and cerebellum. If the fetus or neonate suffers an acute episode of almost total anoxia, due to an event such as umbilical cord obstruction or cardiac arrest, there is no scope for compensation and the neurons die off in sequence according to their metabolic requirements. The most vulnerable neurons are those of the deep nuclei of thalamus, midbrain, medulla, and spinal cord. The immature neurons of the cerebral cortex are relatively resistant to anoxia, in contrast to those of the adult brain. Thus a fetus or newborn infant who has suffered a catastrophic anoxic-ischaemic event may have a relatively normal cortex but almost total loss of neurons from deep nuclei in thalamus, midbrain, and brainstem. The same range of lesions may occur in the late stages of pregnancy, during labour, or in the early neonatal period. Fragmentation of the nucleus (*karyorrhexis*), is one of the most frequent histological appearances in acute neuronal necrosis at this time of life. Following widespread neuronal death there may be marked proliferation of astrocytes.

25.11.6 Metabolic brain damage

Bilirubin encephalopathy (*kernicterus*) is the most important form of metabolic brain damage in the newborn. It is now relatively infrequent due to prevention of Rhesus isoimmunization and treatment of jaundiced preterm infants by phototherapy. Preterm newborn infants have immature hepatic enzyme systems and may be unable to conjugate and excrete bilirubin due to poor activity of glucuronyl transferase. Unconjugated bilirubin is lipid soluble and in high concentration may enter the deep nuclei and cause neuronal death. At post-mortem examination in the acute stage the affected nuclei may be bright yellow in colour. Other forms of metabolic brain damage seen in the newborn include those due to hypoglycaemia and amino acidopathies.

25.11.7 Further reading

More detailed descriptions of perinatal neuropathology are found in current texts on perinatal pathology including:

Harding, B. N. (1989). The brain. In *Diseases of the fetus and newborn* (ed. G. B. Reed, A. E. Claireaux and A. D. Bain). Chapman and Hall, London.

Larroche, J.-C. (1991). The central nervous system. In *Textbook of fetal and perinatal pathology* (ed. J. S. Wigglesworth and D. B. Singer). Blackwell Scientific Publications, Oxford.

Laurence, K. M. (1987) Hydrocephalus and malformations of the central nervous system. In *Fetal and neonatal pathology* (ed. J. W. Keeling). Springer-Verlag, London.

Laurini, R. N. (1987). Acquired disorders of the central nervous system. In *Fetal and neonatal pathology* (ed. J. W. Keeling). Springer-Verlag, London.

Wigglesworth, J. S. (1984). *Perinatal pathology*. Major Problems in Pathology No. 15, W. B. Saunders, Philadelphia.

25.12 The pathology of cerebral trauma

P. D. Lewis

Head injuries are responsible for 1 per cent of all deaths in the United Kingdom, about half of the deaths caused by road traffic accidents and a quarter of deaths from all forms of physical trauma. Disability in survivors of head injury is substantial, even in those cases sustaining only concussion.

25.12.1 Mechanisms of brain damage in closed head injury

Non-penetrating head injury may produce severe parenchymal damage in the brain. Cortical contusions and lacerations are seen, together with evidence of tearing of nerve fibres within the substance of the brain. In closed head injuries, the cortical areas particularly affected include frontal poles, orbital gyri, para-Sylvian cortex (i.e. the brain close to the lesser wings of the sphenoid), temporal poles, particularly their under-surface, and sometimes the under-surface of the occipital poles. Small lesions of the uncus of the temporal lobe are common. Involvement of under-surface of frontal and temporal lobes is so frequent, wherever the site of primary injury may be, as to demand a physical explanation. It was first recognized nearly 50 years ago that when the head was free to move following blunt trauma, rotational movements of the brain occurred within the skull. These are considered likely to account for the commonly observed 'contre-coup' pattern of damage. Brain movement is restricted by the brainstem, tentorium, and falx, leaving the frontal and temporal poles most at risk to external physical forces. It has been shown experimentally that all the major types of parenchymal pathology seen in closed head injury can be produced by acceleration forces alone, a direct blow to the skull not being necessary.

Patterns of injury

Cortical contusions and lacerations

The pia covering contusions is intact, but that over lacerations is torn. The cerebral lesions are identical in the two types of damage. In the early stages, haemorrhage is seen. In the course of time, healing occurs with the formation of depressed orange/brown scars which erode the cerebral cortex over the crests of gyri, contrasting with the lesions of focal ischaemia which are typically in the depths of cortical sulci. In the course of time, these *plaques jaunes* lose their colour, but they are nevertheless identifiable for very many years after head injury has occurred. Cortical contusions and lacerations are not commonly seen in infants, where blunt injury more often produces white matter tears.

Nerve fibre tears

Tears in nerve fibres are a major feature in patients who are unconscious from the moment of injury. Initially, small haemorrhages may indicate where tears have occurred. Survival for more than two to three months permits degeneration of myelin to occur, and in patients who have survived for longer than this extensive changes may be seen in the white matter. Grossly, lesions may be visible at the lateral extremities of the corpous callosum and in the cerebellar peduncles, while extensive loss of white matter may result in enlargement of the cerebral ventricles. Microscopic evidence of white matter degeneration can be found years after injury. Nerve fibre tearing damages axons, as well as myelin, producing retraction balls, a consequence of accumulation of axoplasm in the proximal end of the torn nerve fibre. Retraction balls are seen scattered throughout the white matter, sometimes adjacent to blood-vessels, and are concentrated in sites of macroscopic white matter damage. Small nerve fibre tears heal as *microglial stars*, clusters of reactive brain macrophages which are characteristic of head injury. Microglial clusters may be the only evident pathological abnormality in patients with a history of concussion.

Brain swelling

Cerebral oedema is sometimes seen as a delayed consequence of head trauma, and may be the cause of clinical deterioration occurring 24–48 hours after injury. Swelling adjacent to cortical lesions is commonplace, minor, and due to blood–brain barrier damage. In contrast, diffuse swelling of both cerebral hemispheres may occur in the absence of contusions or other focal traumatic lesions. The causal mechanism is unclear, though in some cases there has been prior cerebral hypoxia from cardio-respiratory arrest. Diffuse brain swelling occurs almost exclusively in children; adults with a similar pattern of post-traumatic neurological deterioration have usually developed an *intracranial haematoma*.

Intracranial haematomas

Traumatic haematomas usually produce a delayed effect, and manifest themselves clinically as more or less rapidly expanding space-occupying lesions. The three principal varieties are *extra-dural*, *subdural*, and *intracerebral*.

Extradural haematoma

Extra-dural haemotoma usually results from tearing of a meningeal artery. Typically they are caused by an injury which produces fracture of the squamous temporal bone and laceration of branches of the middle meningeal artery. Arterial laceration cannot always be identified and, in about a third of cases of acute extra-dural haematoma, the source of bleeding may appear to be torn veins, dural sinuses, or bone itself. As the haematoma enlarges it strips the dura from the skull, ultimately forming a large rounded mass that indents the underlying brain. Although the temporal region is the most common site, frontal, parietal, and posterior fossa extradural haematomas are sometimes seen. About a third of cases show evidence of injury to the underlying brain, with cortical contusion or subdural bleeding. Classically, the injury that causes extradural haematoma produces initial concussion, which is followed by a lucid interval of hours, following which the patient shows rapid deterioration into coma.

Subdural haematoma

This form of intracranial bleeding is due to rupture of bridging veins in the subdural space. The accelerational forces on the brain produced in closed head injury cause a shearing of these drainage vessels. Subdural haematoma is often bilateral, and in contrast to the localized nature of extradural haematoma, it tends to spread diffusely over the cerebral hemispheres. A thin, *acute subdural haematoma* is often seen in severe head injury with contusion. A larger or more extensive acute haematoma may be seen in the type of severe head injury that produces a 'burst lobe' (see below). *Subacute subdural haematomas* present within ten days to a fortnight of head injury and are also commonly associated with contusion of the underlying brain. *Chronic subdural haematoma*, presenting weeks or months after an often trivial head injury, is the variety which may cause great clinical and forensic pathological problems. A slow ooze of blood into the subdural space starts to undergo fibrous organization at its edges after about two weeks, and eventually an *encysted hygroma* is formed. The slow enlargement displaces cerebrospinal fluid and brain tissue (and may in an old person with cerebral atrophy take months to produce clinical effects). Without treatment severe neurological compressive problems, ultimately affecting vital centres in the brainstem, will occur. From the medico-legal standpoint, grading the early chronic subdural haematoma may be difficult because fresh blood sometimes continues to ooze for many weeks, and the rate of fibrous capsule formation is very variable. Landmarks in the histological dating of subdural haematoma include the appearance of a fibroblastic layer on the dural side of the haematoma at four to five days, the layer thickening to one half the width of the dura by two weeks. At this stage there is also a fibroblastic membrane on the pia-arachnoid side of the haematoma, while vascular sinusoids are apparent within the clot. By four weeks the haematoma is surrounded by a well-formed relatively avascular fibrous membrane as thick as the dura, and contains a liquified clot. By three months the investing membranes have become hyalinized. Ultimately, calcification or even ossification may occur.

Intracerebral haematoma

Intracerebral haematoma occurs in a minority of fatal head injuries. Intracerebral haematomas can be single or multiple and behave as rapidly expanding lesions. Most are associated with contusions or lacerations, and if the surface is breached by the injury and the intracerebral haematoma, the latter is found in continuity with an acute subdural haematoma, constituting the *burst lobe*. Such lesions usually occur in the inferior frontal or temporal regions. Intracerebral haematomas may be found deep in the cerebral hemispheres, presumably resulting from shearing of small arteries. A single intracerebral haematoma in a head injured patient may be the cause rather than the consequence of the head injury; the patient may have had a stroke and then fallen, injuring his head. Traumatic intracerebral haematomas sometimes develop after a delay, which may be two weeks or more, and are then amenable to treatment.

25.12.2 Other types of injury

Head-injured patients may develop neuropathological changes secondary to raised intracranial pressure and comparable to those found in patients with brain tumours. These result from internal herniations, and include occipital infarction, due to compromise of posterior cerebral arteries in the edge of the tentorium, secondary haemorrhage in midbrain and pons, due to interference with basilar arterial flow, and uncal haemorrhage, due to compression against the edge of the tentorium. Such changes are likely to be terminal events in already critically injured patients. Severely head-injured patients may additionally show focal or diffuse ischaemic/hypoxic changes, principally in the boundary zones between cerebral arterial territories. Some cranial nerves are frequently traumatized in closed head injury. Damage to the olfactory bulbs is often seen in association with inferior frontal contusion, and sometimes with fracture of the orbital plate. Optic nerves commonly sustain direct injury; occasionally brainstem swelling may produce infarction of an optic tract. Ocular motor nerves are much more commonly damaged consequent to brain swelling and herniation than directly. Basal skull fracture may produce direct injury of the trigeminal nerve, while petrous temporal fracture may produce injury of facial and auditory nerves. Head injury may damage intracranial vessels, carotico-cavernous fistula, traumatic aneurysm formation, and carotid artery occlusion being the most frequently encountered lesions.

Cerebral fat embolism

Patients with multiple injuries may show delayed neurological deterioration due to cerebral fat embolism consequent to bony fractures. The white matter shows numerous perivascular foci of necrosis in which walls of blood vessels may appear necrotic. There are few fat emboli in the white matter, but many in the grey, which is less obviously affected macroscopically. White matter lesions heal with scarring, and survivors show little long-term neurological deficit.

Boxing injury

The chronic repetitive head trauma of boxing may produce a clinical 'punch drunk' syndrome with dementia, cerebellar, and extrapyramidal features. The main neuropathological findings are a degree of cerebral cortical atrophy, perforation of the septum pellucidum, variable depigmentation of the substantia nigra in the midbrain, and neurofibrillary degeneration but no senile plaques in grey matter.

Infection

Basal skull fracture may result in dural tearing and CSF leakage. Purulent meningitis or rarely abscess formation may result.

Intracranial infection is more frequently seen after penetrating head injury and may develop months to years later.

Non-accidental injury in children

Violent shaking of infants may produce acute subdural haemorrhage. Inter-hemispheric and intracerebral haemorrhage may also be seen. White matter tears may be visible macroscopically, and there may be evidence of diffuse axonal injury. Brain swelling is often seen. Retinal haemorrhage is a frequent consequence of violent shaking of infants. As noted earlier, head-injured infants rarely show cortical contusions.

Decompression sickness

Any part of the nervous system may be affected, but involvement of dorsal and lumbar spinal cord is especially important. Focal necrosis of white matter has been shown in this region.

26

The endocrine system

26

The endocrine system

In this chapter we meet the several organs that go together to make up a very large system; that of a series of glands which secrete their potent products directly into the blood and co-ordinate a large number of integrated physiological activities.

Moreover, there is a large diffuse endocrine system, largely confined to the gut, where, in addition to blood-borne products, there are important local or paracrine effects.

26.1 The pituitary gland

Margaret M. Esiri

26.1.1 Introduction

The pituitary gland, weighing a mere 1 g or so and measuring approximately 1.5 cm across, has an endocrinological and pathological importance out of all proportion to its size. Although subject to a number of different pathological processes, by far the most common of these is tumour formation, which occurs almost exclusively in the anterior lobe and has important clinical consequences in many cases. In some neurosurgical centres, pituitary adenomas comprise almost 25 per cent of surgical intracranial neoplasms. The classification of pituitary adenomas has undergone considerable development in the past 20 years, following the introduction of radio-immunoassay for accurate measurement of hormone levels in blood, and the application of immunocytochemistry and electron microscopy as routine techniques for the analysis of tumour tissue removed surgically or studied at autopsy. Apart from the tumours that originate in the pituitary gland, the most important pathological changes are those related to vascular or inflammatory disease.

The pituitary gland is divided anatomically into two distinct parts, *anterior and posterior lobes*; the latter is continuous with the pituitary stalk linking it with the hypothalmus above. An *intermediate lobe*, readily identifiable in animals, is not distinctly demarcated in humans. In *anencephalic fetuses*, which lack a forebrain, the pituitary gland is hypoplastic or absent.

In the mature anterior pituitary lobe there are distinct epithelial cell types responsible for producing *growth hormone* (GH), *prolactin* (PRL), *adrenocorticotropin* (ACTH), *thyroid stimulating hormone* (TSH), and the *gonadotropins* (LH, FSH). The cells are arranged in acini in which the cells producing the different hormones are intermingled. The acini are separated by delicate strands of collagenous vascular connective tissue, adjacent to which are found scattered non-epithelial *folliculo-stellate cells*. These react immunocytochemically for *glial fibrillary acidic protein* (GFAP).

26.1.2 Tumours arising in the anterior lobe of the pituitary gland

Tumours arising in the anterior lobe of the pituitary gland are generally *benign adenomas* of limited growth potential. Although they may exhibit a relatively invasive local growth pattern, and may recur following incomplete removal, they only very rarely metastasize in the central nervous system and even more rarely outside it. Histological features such as frequency of mitoses, presence or absence of necrosis, and pleomophism of nuclei, which might be expected to signify a tumour's growth potential, are, surprisingly, of no value in predicting the biological behaviour of the pituitary adenomas. Accordingly, the term *carcinoma* is only appropriate when it is applied to a pituitary tumour that has already metastasized outside the central nervous system.

Pituitary adenomas produce clinical symptoms in two ways. In some patients these may combine. First, if the adenoma secretes a functionally active hormone, attention will be drawn to its presence by the development of symptoms due to excess hormone secretion; *gigantism or acromegaly* with excess GH secretion; *Cushing's disease* with excess ACTH secretion; and combinations of menstrual irregularities, galactorrhea, and infertility in women of child-bearing age, and impotence or loss of libido in men, with excess PRL secretion. Secondly, if the tumour has enlarged sufficiently, whether or not it secretes an active hormone, it will produce symptoms due to compression of surrounding structures. Most frequently, these consist of *visual symptoms* related to suprasellar extension of the tumour with compression of the optic nerves and chiasm, and *headache*. There may also be *cranial nerve palsies*, due to encroachment on the cavernous sinuses; symptoms of *hypothalamic compression or hydrocephalus*, due to compression of the third ventricle; or *cerebrospinal fluid rhinorrhoea*, due to erosion of the floor of the pituitary fossa. In addition, if there has been sufficient local compression of the pituitary gland to destroy at least three-quarters of the functioning tissue, there may be symptoms of *hypopituitarism*. Spontaneous haemorrhage or infarction in a pituitary tumour, if extensive, produces symptoms of *pituitary apoplexy*. More often haemorrhage is slight and asymptomatic.

Microadenomas confined within the pituitary fossa are a common incidental finding at autopsy. Larger adenomas that extend to the suprasellar compartment are also occasionally found incidentally (Fig. 26.1). About half of such incidentally discovered adenomas contain PRL, and most of the remainder contain small groups of cells containing gonadotropins or no detectable hormones.

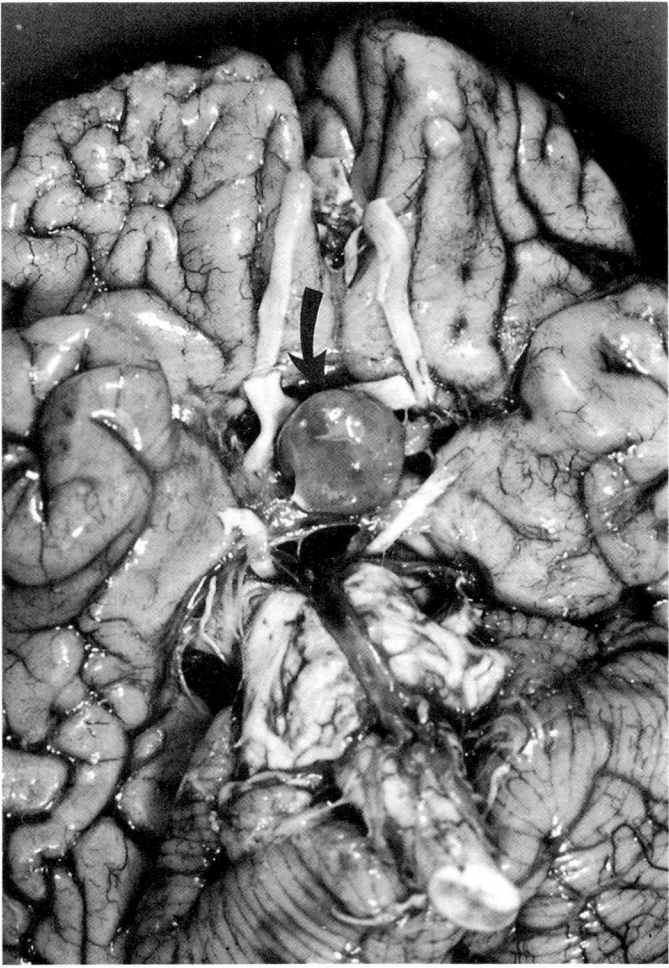

Fig. 26.1 Pituitary adenoma with suprasellar extension (arrow) found incidentally at autopsy.

Most pituitary adenomas apparently arise spontaneously. They occur over a wide age-range from childhood to old age but present most commonly in middle-age. Exceptionally, they may arise under conditions of hyposecretion of the target gland; for example, rare TSH producing tumours have arisen in patients with long-standing hypothyroidism. Adenomas may also be exceptionally associated with the presence of a *hypothalamic hamartoma* or *intracellular ganglioneuroma* capable of stimulating adenoma formation by neurosecretion.

Although many adenomas produce one hormone, consistent with a derivation from one transformed cell, it is also quite common for adenomas to be composed of cells of more than one morphological type, each producing a different hormone; or to be composed of one cell type which itself produces more than one hormone (see below). These *pluri-hormonal adenomas* raise questions about their mode of origin to which there is no simple answer at present. Most such tumours contain GH-producing cells and are associated with acromegaly. PRL is the most frequent additional hormone detectable in these tumours. It is thought possible that such mixed tumours may arise from hypothetical *bipotential* or *multipotential precursor cells*. It is also possible that differentiated pituitary epithelial cells and their progeny are capable of producing multiple, biochemically unrelated hormones. Recently recognized gonadotropin-producing tumours may produce FSH alone, FSH and LH, or (rarely) LH alone. In these tumours, production of more than one hormone is unremarkable since normal gonadotropin-producing cells are known to be capable of synthesizing both hormones. Similarly, the presence in ACTH-producing tumours of *β-lipotropin*, *α-MSH*, *endophins*, and *enkephalins* is not surprising, since these peptides are all derived normally from a common precursor molecule, *proopiomelanocortin*.

A puzzling feature of some pituitary adenomas is the lack of correlation between their hormonal content as detected immunocytochemically, by radioimmunoassay of tumour fragments, or by their cell perfusates derived from *in vitro* perfusion and the presence of physiological effects of excess hormone or, indeed, evidence of elevated blood levels of their contained hormones. Thus, in acromegalics whose adenomas can be demonstrated to contain PRL and/or a glycoprotein as well as GH, there may be no elevation of PRL or glycoprotein hormone levels in the blood. Similarly, not all gonadotropin-containing adenomas are associated with elevated blood levels of gonadotropins. There are several possible explanations for these discrepancies. There may be production of the hormone but failure of secretion, either because the hormone remains stored in the tumour cell cytoplasm, or is broken down in the cell before it is released. Alternatively, the hormone may be secreted in a form that is immunologically and biologically inactive; or insufficient amounts may be secreted to raise blood levels and produce physiological effects. The latter seems to be the case with some gonadotropin-containing tumours since it has been found that it is only those tumours that contain the highest percentages of immunoreactive cells which are associated with elevated levels of the appropriate gonadotropin hormone in the blood. An additional complication that further confounds clear-cut correlation of tumour hormone content with blood hormone levels is the frequent moderate elevation of blood PRL level that occurs if any type of pituitary tumour enlarges sufficiently to compress the pituitary stalk, thus interfering with normal inhibitory mechanisms for the control of PRL secretion from the pituitary gland.

Classification of pituitary adenomas

The classification of pituitary adenomas can be approached from the endocrinological, surgical, or pathological standpoints. Enocrinologically, they are classified as *functional* or *nonfunctional*, with the functional tumours further subclassified according to the clinical symptoms and elevated blood hormone levels that are present. At surgery (or autopsy) the tumours can be classified according to their size and growth pattern. Thus, tumours may be confined within the sella as *microadenomas* (less than 10 mm diameter) or *macroadenomas* (more than 10 mm diameter) ('enclosed' tumours); extend through the dura to form a *suprasellar extension*; and/or extend downwards through the bone of the sella floor to reach the sphenoid sinus (*locally invasive tumours*); or grow extensively in all directions to invade the *cavernous sinuses* laterally, the *subarachnoid space* superiorly, and the *sphenoid sinus* inferiorly (*diffuse invasive tumours*). Here, however, we are primarily concerned with the pathological classification of these tumours. Formerly, this was based on their tinctorial properties; there were *acidophil, basophil*, and *chromophobe adenomas*. Acidophil tumours were generally found in acromegalics, basophil tumours in patients with Cushing's disease, and chromophobe tumours in endocrinologically silent or non-functioning tumours. With the more recent recognition that a wider range of functioning tumours occurs (PRL-producing, TSH-producing, and gonadotropin-producing), and particularly since the advent of immunocytochemistry, which enables the hormone content of the tumour to be revealed, the inadequacy of this classification has become clear. For example, some GH-producing tumours are chromophobe or contain a mixture of acidophil and chromophobe cells, some acidophil or chromophobe tumours produce PRL, and some non-functioning tumours are acidophil (Table 26.1c).

The most satisfactory basis for the pathological classification of pituitary adenomas now is that based on the hormone content of the tumours as demonstrated by the use of immunocytochemistry (Table 26.1a). With the routine use of electron microscopy, further subclassification of these tumours can be achieved (Table 26.1b). To provide a complete diagnostic classification, it is necessary to perform immunocytochemistry with antisera to all the major anterior pituitary hormones, and electron microscopy. Immunocytochemistry can be performed on formalin-fixed, paraffin-embedded material using the indirect immunoperoxidase, PAP, or avidin–biotin detection systems with appropriate controls. The tinctorial properties of the tumours are satisfactorily displayed with *a combined orange G and PAS stain*, with which acidophils stain orange and basophils pink. Also of value in the assessment of pituitary surgical tissue is a reticulin stain, which is particularly useful for distinguishing anterior lobe from microadenoma by the manner in which it demonstrates the effacement of the normal reticulin pattern in microadenomas.

Pituitary adenomas composed solely of GH-containing cells

Most adenomas containing GH arise in one of the lateral wings of the pituitary gland where many of the GH cells are located. Most form tumours that are confined to the pituitary fossa but they may extend locally beyond it. Rarely, these tumours may occupy an *ectopic site* in the sphenoid sinus or parapharyngeal region, sites that are thought to reflect the path of developmental migration of cells from *Rathke's pouch*. Also, rarely, a GH-producing adenoma in the pituitary fossa may be closely associated with a ganglioneuroma capable of stimulating GH-cell proliferation.

Adenomas composed solely of GH-containing cells comprise about 12–15 per cent of all surgically removed pituitary adenomas. They are removed most frequently from middle-aged subjects who may have a long history of acromegaly extending back several years. Males and females are equally commonly affected. The adenomas are composed of epithelial cells, usually arranged in a diffuse pattern, and immunostaining shows a positive reaction for GH and negative reactions for all other pituitary hormones (Fig. 26.2). Ultrastructurally, the tumours fall into two groups: one in which the tumours are composed of *densely granulated cells*, the granules being relatively large in size (Fig. 26.3); these tumours appear acidophil by light microscopy. The other group consists of tumours composed of cells with fewer, smaller granules and possessing characteristic *intracytoplasmic inclusions* ('fibrous bodies') containing aggregates of intermediate filaments, diameter 11 nm, and microtubules (Fig. 26.4). Cilia and centrioles are also frequently found in these cells. These tumours are predominantly chromophobe by light microscopy. The two types of tumour occur with about the same frequency, and one or other of them is found in the majority of cases of acromegaly. The sparsely granulated

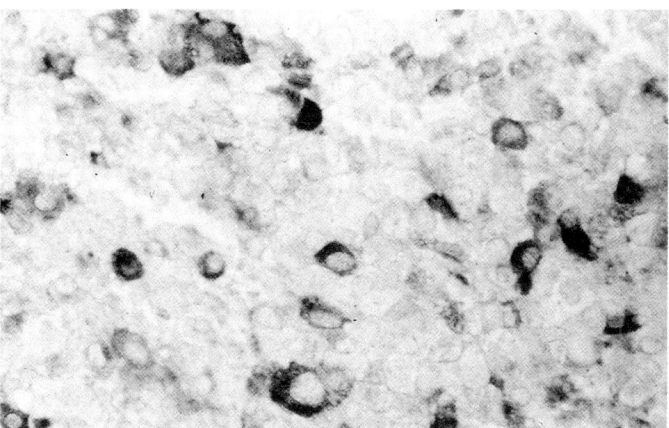

Fig. 26.2 Immunoperoxidase reaction for growth hormone (GH) in the cytoplasm of the tumour cells of a pituitary adenoma associated with acromegaly. (Weakly counterstained with haematoxylin.)

Table 26.1 Pathological classification of pituitary adenomas

(a) Immunocytochemistry (common clinical presentation)	(b) Electron microscopic features	(c) Tinctorial properties
GH only (Usually acromegaly or gigantism)	Two subdivisions:	
	Densely granulated: granules 300–600 nm diam., prominent RER and Golgi complex	Acidophil
	Sparsely granulated: granules 100–300 nm diam.; cells contain cytoplasmic fibrous bodies composed of 11 nm diam. filaments, frequent centrioles and some cilia	Chromophobe or weakly acidophilic
Only PRL (Hyperprolactinaemia or SOL*)	Two subdivisions:	Acidophil
	Densely granulated: large granules, 400–700 nm diam; spherical, oval, or pleomorphic; misplaced exocytosis	
	Sparsely granulated: granules variable in size; abundant RER; misplaced exocytosis	Chromophobe
GH and PRL in different cells (Acromegaly; sometimes with hyperprolactinaemia)	Two distinct cell types present, one resembling densely or sparsely granulated GH cells (see above), the other densely or sparsely granulated PRL cells (see above)	Acidophil, chromophobe, or mixture of the two
GH and PRL in the same cells (Usually hyperprolactinaemia; less often acromegaly)	Cells with combined features of sparsely granulated GH cells and sparsely granulated PRL cells (see above). Some oncocytic change may be present (excess mitochondria with some abnormal forms)	Chromophobe or weakly eosinophil
GH and PRL with some cells containing both hormones and extracellular material reactive for GH (Usually acromegaly)	Cells with combined features of densely granulated GH cells and densely granulated PRL cells (see above)	Acidophilic
ACTH (Usually Cushing's or Nelson's syndrome)	Cells with granules of variable size and number; usual diam. 300–500 nm; perinuclear bundles of filaments 7 nm diam.	Basophilic, occasionally chromophobe
TSH (Usually hyperthyroidism, rarely long-standing hypothyroidism)	Large cells with variable numbers of small granules 60–150 nm diam., large Golgi complex; some cells may contain short microfilaments	Slightly basophilic
Gonadotrophins (FSH, LH, or both) (Usually a SOL)	Cells with generally sparse, small granules 50–250 nm diam., of variable electron density and sometimes with clear haloes; oncocytic change common	Usually chromophobe, sometimes acidophil, rarely weakly basophilic
No detectable hormones (SOL)	Cells with sparse, small secretory granules resembling those of gonadotropin-secreting tumours (see above)	Chromophobe, less often acidophil
More than two hormones Usually GH, PRL, and a glycoprotein (TSH, FSH, LH, or α-subunit of these) (Usually acromegaly)	May show one, two, or three distinct cell types. In most tumours these include cells of densely or sparsely granulated GH type (see above), may also include cells showing misplaced exocytosis (PRL cells) and cells with small granules resembling those of gonadotropin cells (see above)	Variable; usually mixed acidophil and chromophobe

* SOL, space-occupying lesion.

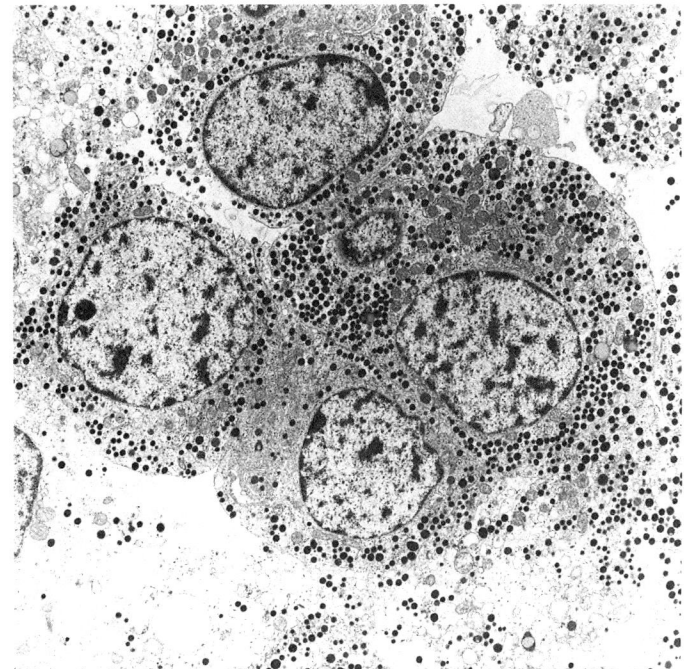

Fig. 26.3 Electron micrograph of tumour cells from a GH-producing pituitary adenoma. The cytoplasm contains many medium- and large-sized, electron-dense secretory granules. (Uranyl acetate and lead citrate.)

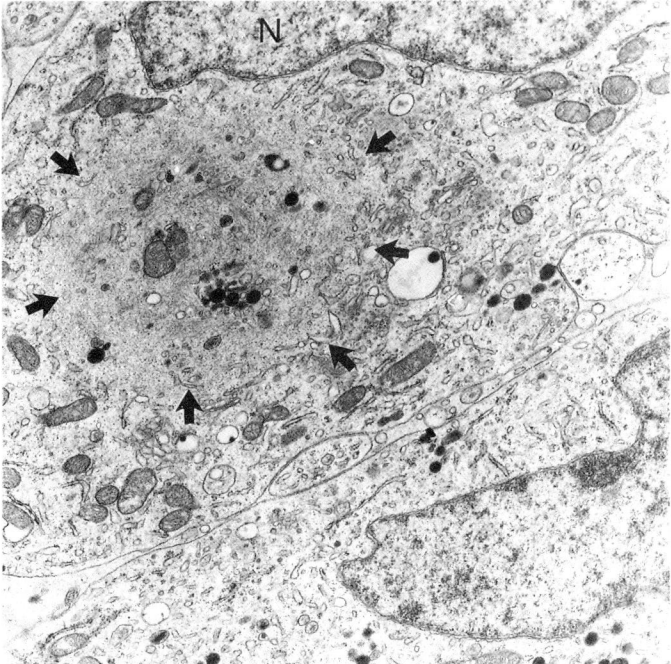

Fig. 26.4 Electron micrograph of the cytoplasm of a tumour cell from a pituitary adenoma associated with acromegaly. In the perinuclear region, there is a fibrous body (arrows) containing filaments, micro-tubules, and admixed dense granules and mitochondria. N, nucleus. (Uranyl acetate and lead citrate.)

tumours are considered by some authorities to have a higher growth rate, a more invasive pattern of growth, and a greater rate of recurrence than the densely granulated tumours.

Pituitary adenomas composed solely of PRL-containing cells

PRL-containing adenomas account for around 25 per cent of all surgically removed pituitary adenomas. These tumours tend to come to medical attention earlier in women than in men because they produce *amenorrhoea*, *infertility*, and sometimes *galactorrhoea* in women of child-bearing age, whereas their endocrine effects in men are less well defined, consisting of *loss of libido*, *depression, or impotence*. Most women are aged between 20 and 35 years when operated upon and the adenomas are *microadenomas* or *intrasellar macroadenomas*. Men are operated on generally at a later age and frequently have tumours that extend outside the sella, where they are likely to have produced local symptoms of space occupation. Space occupation is also the principal means of presentation of PRL tumours in post-menopausal women, who consequently also tend to have large adenomas. Occasionally, PRL adenomas occur in adolescence of both sexes. Overall, their sex incidence is about equal.

Most PRL-cell adenomas are chromophobe or weakly acido-phil. They have a variable histological pattern, either papillary, sinusoidal, or diffuse. Calcification in the form of *calcospherites* is fairly common (Fig. 26.5). Occasionally, amyloid deposition is present. Immunocytocehmistry shows PRL in all tumour cells. Ultrastructurally, most PRL tumours are composed of cells with sparse, medium-sized granules scattered throughout the cyto-plasm. Some granules can be found outside cell membranes, a feature that is characteristic only of PRL-containing cells in adenomas (Fig. 26.6). A further characteristic feature is the abundance of rough endoplasmic reticulum which sometimes forms concentric arrays. Rarely, PRL adenomas are composed of cells with numerous large secretory granules. Such tumours are acidophil by light microscopy.

Recently, there has been a tendency to treat PRL adenomas

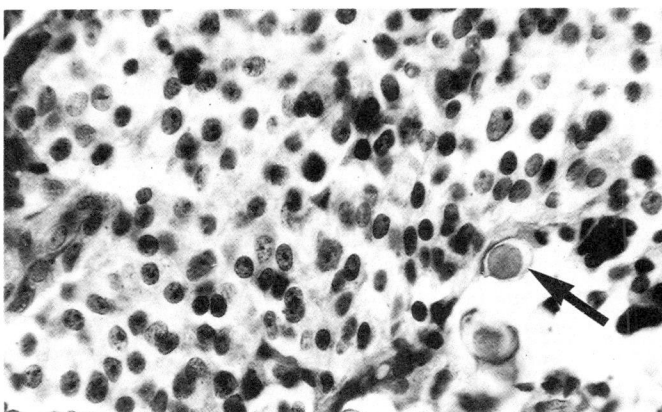

Fig. 26.5 Light microscopical appearance of a prolactin (PRL)-containing chromophobe adenoma in which there are scattered calco-spherites (arrow).

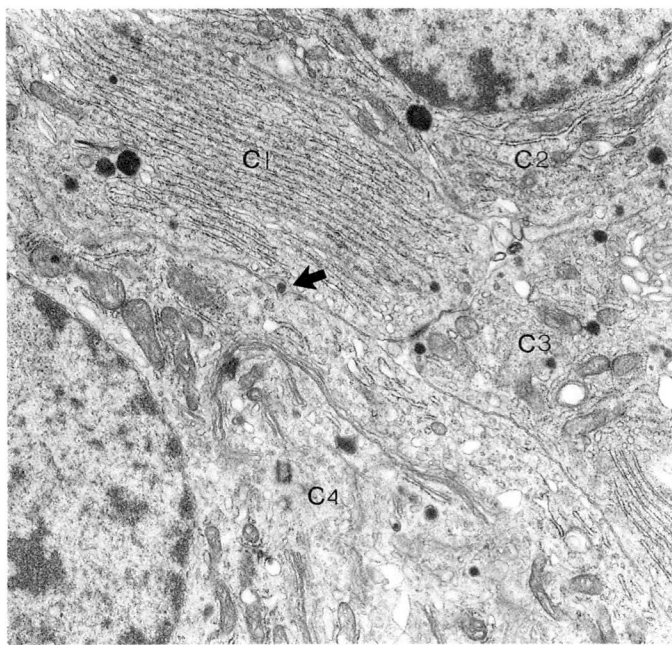

Fig. 26.6 Electron micrograph of the cell membranes of four adjacent tumour cells (C1–C4) from a PRL-containing pituitary adenoma. There are scanty secretory granules and abundant rough endoplasmic reticulum (especially in C1). A misplaced exocytotic granule lies between the cell membranes of C1 and C4 (arrow). (Uranyl acetate and lead citrate.)

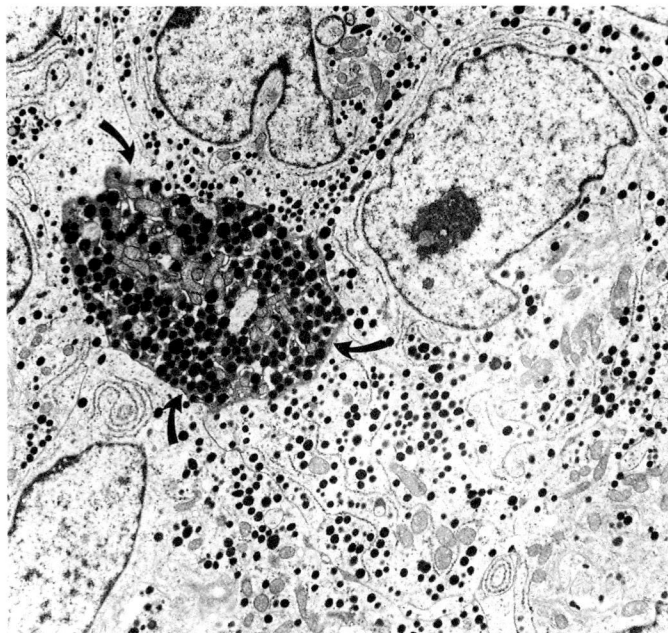

Fig. 26.7 Electron micrograph of a pituitary adenoma containing many GH-immuno-reactive and a few PRL-reactive cells. One cytoplasmic process (arrows) contains abundant, large secretory granules (probably a PRL-containing cell, as some misplaced exocytosis was found associated with such processes) while the surrounding cells (probably GH-containing) show more dispersed and slightly smaller secretory granules. (Uranyl acetate and lead citrate.)

with *bromocriptine*, a dopamine agonist. This, and related substances, have been found to reduce the size of PRL adenomas, as assessed by scanning techniques, to lower blood PRL levels, and restore fertility to young, infertile women. PRL adenomas removed from patients who have been treated with bromocriptine show marked changes in morphology compared with tumours of patients not so treated. The cells are reduced in size, with particular reduction in cytoplasmic volume, and contain very few secretory granules. Little or no PRL is demonstrable immunocytochemically. In some areas, the cells may appear necrotic. After long periods of treatment with bromocriptine, markedly increased reticulin and collagen deposition is liable to occur and may render surgery very difficult to perform.

Pituitary adenomas containing GH and PRL in different cells

These are uncommon adenomas usually presenting with *acromegaly*, in some cases with additional features of *hyperprolactinaemia*. They contain a mixture of GH- and PRL-containing cells. By light microscopy, they are acidophil, chromophobe, or a mixture of the two. By immunocytochemistry, it can be shown that the cells containing one hormone are different from those containing the other, and two different cell types can be found ultrastructurally, containing granules of differing size and abundance (Fig. 26.7). Both the GH- and the PRL-containing cells may be densely or sparsely granulated. Extruded granules are found in association with the PRL cells.

Pituitary adenomas containing GH and PRL in the same cells

These adenomas are regarded as probably arising from a stem cell common to both GH- and PRL-producing cells of the pituitary gland. They are uncommon and usually present with symptoms of *hyperprolactinaemia*. By light microscopy, they appear chromophobe or weakly acidophil, and immunocytochemistry shows GH and PRL in the same cells. Ultrastructurally, the cells are all similar and combine features found in cells of sparsely granulated GH adenomas and sparsely granulated PRL adenomas (Table 26.1). Some cells may contain excess mitochondria (*oncocytic change*).

Pituitary adenomas containing GH and PRL in the same cells and with the presence of extracellular GH-reactive material

These uncommon tumours are slow growing, generally acidophil, and usually present with *acromegaly*. Both hormones are detectable in the same cells by immunocytochemistry. Secretory granules are numerous and large, and some extruded granules can be found. *Extracellular material reactive for GH* forms a prominent feature at the light microscopic level (Fig. 26.8).

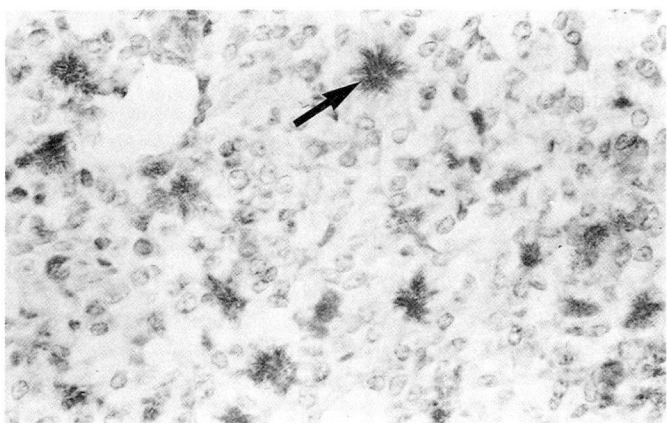

Fig. 26.8 Light microscopical appearance of a pituitary adenoma associated with acromegaly in which there are extracellular deposits of material which are reactive for GH (arrow). (Immunoperoxidase reaction for GH, with weak haematoxylin counterstain.)

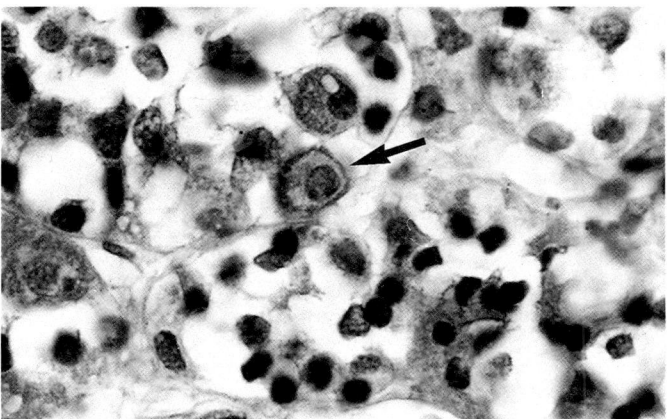

Fig. 26.9 Crooke's hyaline change in a pituitary gland basophil (arrow) close to an ACTH-containing adenoma from a patient with Cushing's disease. (Orange G/PAS stain.)

Pituitary adenomas containing ACTH

Adenomas containing ACTH present clinically as *Cushing's disease* or, in those who have had a previous bilateral adrenalectomy, *as Nelson's syndrome*. They account for 9–15 per cent of pituitary adenomas removed surgically. Adenomas associated with Cushing's disease occur over a wide age-range with a peak incidence in middle age, and with a female:male preponderance of 2:1. A few ACTH-containing adenomas that are endocrinologically silent have been described. These present as space-occupying lesions. The much commoner, endocrinologically active tumours are frequently small, sometimes only 1 mm across. In some cases of pituitary-dependent Cushing's disease, it is not possible to demonstrate an adenoma. Some cases of this type have been attributed to *hyperplasia of ACTH-producing basophils*. Adenomas in Cushing's disease are basophil or, rarely, chromophobe. Some cells show a clear, hyaline, perinuclear region with the granules displaced to the margins of the cell. The appearance of such cells, and a similar appearance seen in ACTH cells in the pituitary gland in conditions of high circulating glucocorticoids, is known as *Crooke's hyaline change* (Fig. 26.9). Ultrastructurally, the tumour cells are found to contain variable numbers of medium-sized or large secretory granules, which may show varying electron density and be aligned close to the cell membrane (Fig. 26.10). A distinctive ultrastructural feature of these tumours is the presence of bundles of *fine intracytoplasmic filaments* (7 nm in diameter) which lie close to the nucleus (Fig. 26.11). These are the ultrastructural equivalent of Crooke's hyaline change.

Adenomas containing TSH

These are rare tumours accounting for no more than 1 per cent of pituitary adenomas. They are associated with elevated blood levels of TSH and usually with clinical hyperthyroidism. The tumours tend to be large, extending beyond the sella turcica. They are composed of large, irregular-shaped cells, some showing pleomorphism of their nuclei (Fig. 26.12). Their cytoplasm

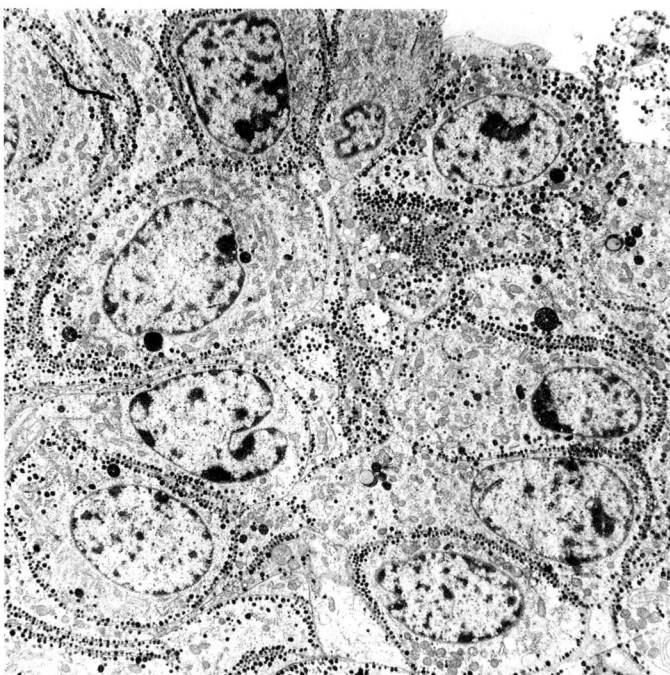

Fig. 26.10 Low-power electron micrograph of an ACTH-containing pituitary adenoma from a case of Cushing's disease. Tumour cells contain secretory granules aligned adjacent to cell membranes. (Uranyl acetate and lead citrate.)

is weakly basophil and contains weakly argyrophilic granules. TSH can be demonstrated in the cytoplasm of some tumour cells. Other hormones, particularly GH, may be present in other cells. Small secretory granules, 60–110 nm in diameter, can be seen with electron microscopy in the TSH cells. They tend to be aligned adjacent to the cell membrane. The cell cytoplasm also contains a large Golgi complex and may contain short microfilaments.

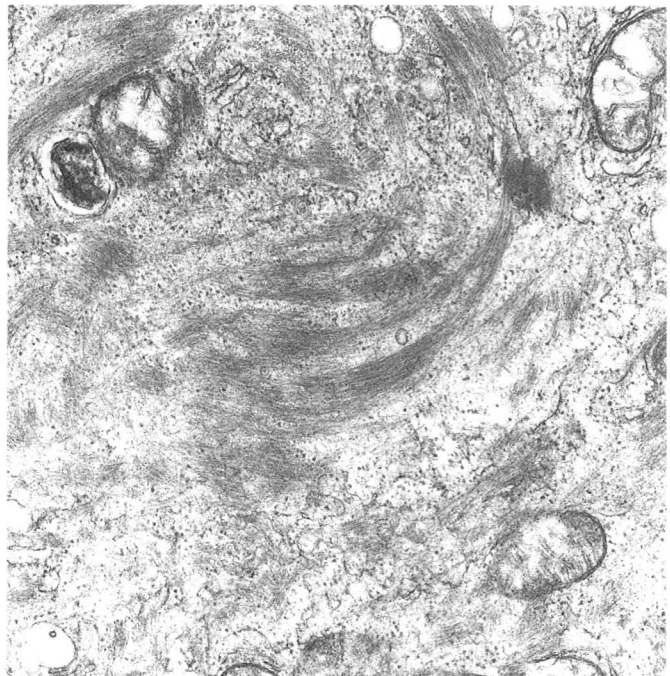

Fig. 26.11 Fine cytoplasmic filaments in the cytoplasm of tumour cells from an ACTH-containing pituitary adenoma associated with Cushing's disease. (Uranyl acetate and lead citrate.)

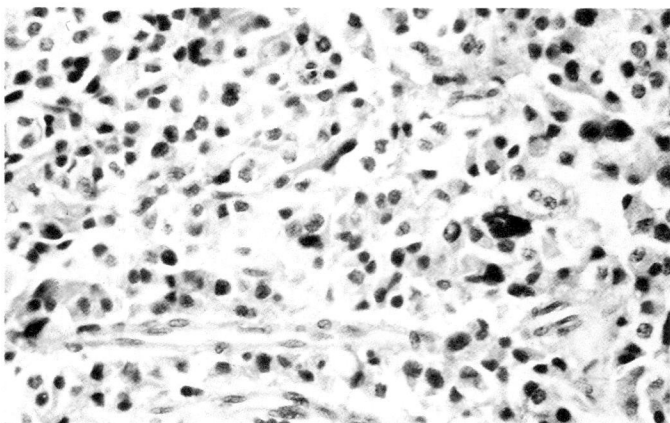

Fig. 26.12 Light microscopical appearance of a tumour containing thyroid stimulating hormone. There is considerable pleomorphism of nuclei.

Adenomas containing gonadotropins

Since immunocytochemistry has come into routine use for the diagnosis of pituitary adenomas, it has been recognized that a considerable proportion of endocrinologically 'silent' tumours presenting as space-occupying lesions, contain a few gonadotropin-reactive cells. Most such cases show no elevation of blood gonadotropins. However, there are a few tumours that contain frequent gonadotropin-reactive cells by immunocyto-chemistry, some of which are associated with elevated blood

gonadotropin levels before surgery and reduction in these levels after surgery. Although symptoms related to local space occupation predominate in the clinical presentation, there are also reports of *loss of libido* in men and *galactorrhoea* or *amenorrhoea* in some women with tumours of this sort. In most of their histological and ultrastructural appearances, these tumours are indistinguishable from non-functioning tumours (see below).

Adenomas containing no detectable hormones

Endocrinologically silent adenomas, in which the great majority of tumour cells contain no detectable pituitary hormones, constitute one of the largest groups of pituitary tumours, 50 per cent in some series. Most of these tumours are large with supra-sellar extensions, and present as space-occupying lesions. They occur most frequently in middle- and old age and show no clear sex preponderance. They are *chromophobe* or weakly acidophil by light microscopy and the cells show a variable arrangement in diffuse sheets or with a sinusoidal or papillary orientation. Fibrosis or haemorrhage, the latter occasionally extensive and giving rise to *pituitary apoplexy*, may be found in some tumours. Immunocytochemically, these tumours show entirely negative reactions for pituitary hormones, or contain small foci of cells reactive for various hormones, most frequently gonadotropins in varying combinations, as in the gonadotropin-containing tumours (Fig. 26.13). Some contain only the α-subunit of the glycoproteins. The cells that contain gonadotropins appear slightly argyrophilic. Ultrastructurally, they show a uniform appearance of polygonal cells, with well-defined apposed cell membranes, and generally small, sparse secretory granules 100–250 nm in diameter (Fig. 26.14). Many of the tumours contain some cells showing oncocytic change (Fig. 26.15).

26.1.3 Other pituitary tumours

The posterior pituitary lobe may be the site of origin of two uncommon, slowly growing tumours: *granular cell tumour* and

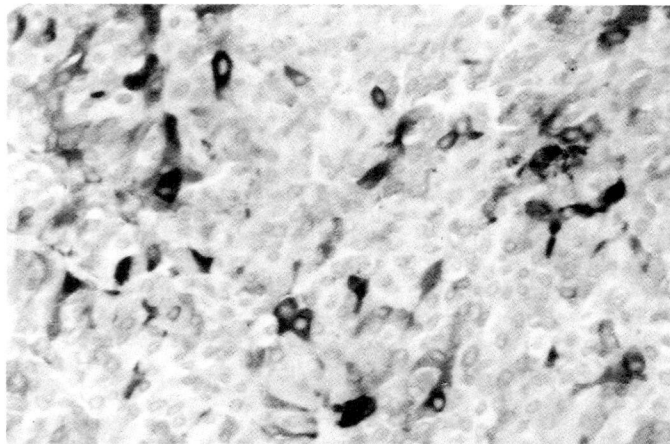

Fig. 26.13 Scattered tumour cells showing immunoreactivity for FSH in a clinically non-functioning pituitary adenoma. (Weak haematoxylin counterstain.)

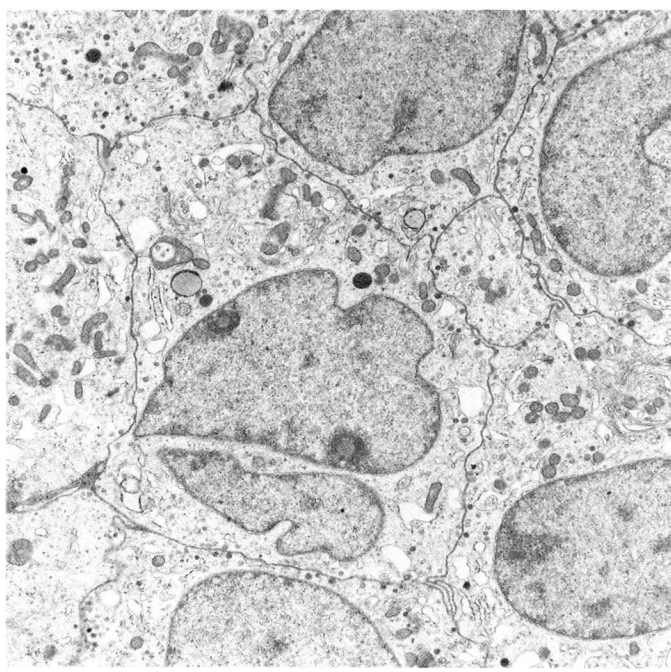

Fig. 26.14 Electron micrograph of the tumour cells in a clinically non-functioning pituitary adenoma. There are very small secretory granules aligned near cell membranes and scattered in the cytoplasm. (Uranyl acetate and lead citrate.)

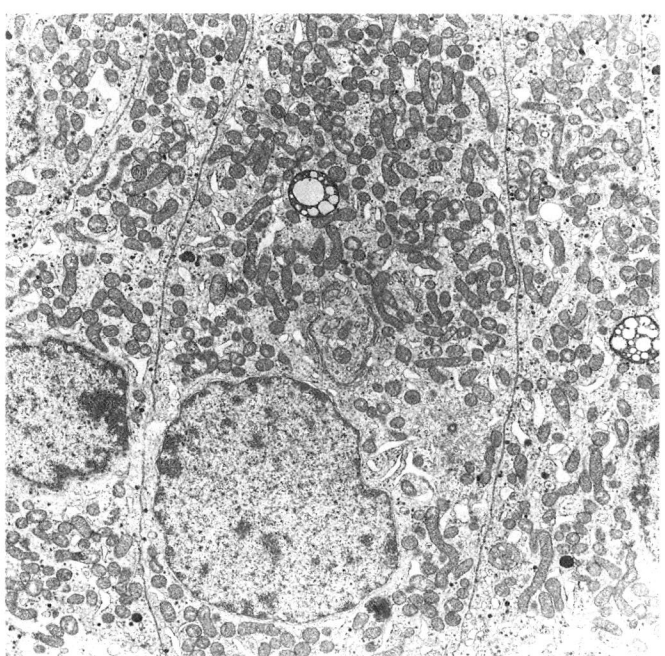

Fig. 26.15 Electron micrograph of tumour cells in a clinically non-functioning pituitary adenoma. The most abundant cytoplasmic constituents are mitochondria. In addition, there are small secretory granules and a few multivesicular bodies. (Uranyl acetate and lead citrate.)

a tumour of the *glial-derived pituicytes* (*pituicytoma*). The *granular cell tumour* is composed of medium-sized, diffusely arranged, uniform cells with abundant granular cytoplasm and small central nuclei. Its cell of origin is uncertain but in their immunocytochemical reactions, the tumour cells resemble Schwann cells (S100-positive, vimentin-positive). The *pituicytoma* is composed of elongated spindle cells arranged around blood vessels (Fig. 26.16). The tumour cells resemble normal pituicytes of the posterior pituitary and are reactive for glial fibrillary acidic protein (GFAP). Other tumours may extend into the posterior lobe from above, most frequently *gliomas* or *hamartomas* of the hypothalamus. There are a number of tumours that may arise close to the pituitary fossa and extend locally to involve the gland. These include *craniopharyngioma*, *meningioma*, *atypical teratoma* (*germinoma*), *lymphomas*, *chordoma* or *chondrosarcoma* arising in the bone of the clivus, and *nasopharyngeal carcinoma*. The pituitary gland may also, rarely, be the site of a *metastatic tumour deposit*.

26.1.4 Pituitary cysts

Simple cysts of the pituitary gland give rise to clinical symptoms infrequently through progressive space occupation. They are lined by cuboidal epithelium and most are thought to be derived from remnants of the epithelium lining Rathke's cleft, which can be seen as microscopic epithelial-lined cysts in most normal glands, lying between anterior and posterior lobes. *Epidermoid cysts* occasionally occur also in the parasellar region.

26.1.5 Infarction and haemorrhage of the pituitary gland

The anterior lobe of the pituitary gland is at risk of infarction in circumstances that produce a severe drop in pressure in the *hypothalamo-hypophysial portal blood vessels*. The risk is enhanced during *pregnancy* and in the *puerperium* because of the increased size and metabolic activity of the gland. At this time, the most common event predisposing to pituitary infarction is

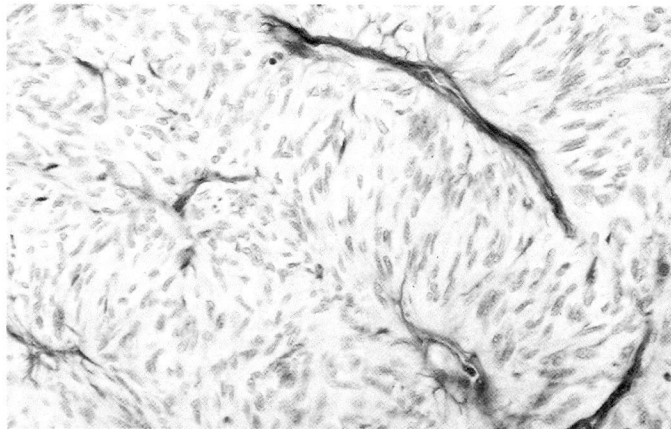

Fig. 26.16 Light microscopical appearance of pituicytoma arising in the posterior pituitary gland. (Orange G/PAS stain.)

massive haemorrhage related to childbirth. This produced the formerly well-recognized *Sheehan's syndrome*, now infrequently seen because such haemorrhage is promptly treated and pituitary infarction avoided. Another circumstance in which pituitary infarction or haemorrhage occurs is as a consequence of severe head injury in which the delicate vessels supplying the gland may be torn. Large *aneurysms of the intracavernous sinus* portions of the internal carotid arteries occasionally produce hypopituitarism by exerting pressure on the pituitary gland.

26.1.6   Inflammatory diseases of the pituitary gland

The pituitary gland can be the site of infection by a number of organisms, chiefly those that produce a chronic inflammatory process. Organisms can spread to the pituitary fossa from neighbouring air sinuses. *Aspergillus* can, in this way, become established as a chronic infection in the pituitary fossa and result in *panhypopituitarism. Tuberculosis* may do likewise, causing production of caseating granulomas. *Pyogenic infections*, when they affect the pituitary, tend to do so by extention from air sinuses and the subdural space.

Inflammatory reactions of uncertain aetiology may also affect the pituitary gland and cause distinct destructive effects. Thus, *sarcoidosis* may produce non-caseating granulomas and cause *hypopituitarism*. Occasionally, the pituitary gland is the site of a *lymphocytic hypophysitis* in which a mononuclear inflammatory cell infiltrate extends throughout the gland. Even less common is a *granulomatous inflammation* confined to the pituitary gland with the presence of many multinucleate giant cells. These conditions are thought to have an auto-immune aetiology. *Histiocytosis X* is another chronic inflammatory disease in which pituitary function may be compromised and both lobes of the gland infiltrated by atypical foamy histiocytes.

26.1.7   Metabolic diseases

The pituitary gland may be affected by a number of metabolic diseases. Chief among these are the *inherited mucopolysaccharidoses* or *haemochromatosis*.

26.1.8   Radiation necrosis of the pituitary gland

Although relatively resistent to radiation damage, the pituitary gland undergoes necrosis when subjected to large doses of irradiation. Occasionally, *sarcomas* have arisen in the parasellar region following irradiation.

26.1.9   The empty sella syndrome

The empty sella syndrome refers to the radiological finding of an *air-filled sella turcica* in patients presenting with symptoms of *hypopituitarism*. The pituitary gland is shrunken, occupying only the rim of the sella. The causes are probably variable and include vascular and inflammatory processes mentioned above.

26.1.10   Further reading

Robert, F. and Martinez, A. J. (eds) (1986). Pituitary adenomas. *Seminars in Diagnostic Pathology* **3**, (1).

Scheithauer, B. W. (1984). Surgical pathology of the pituitary: the adenoma. In *Pathology annual*, Vol. 19 (ed. S. C. Sommers and P. P. Rosen), Pt. 1, pp. 317–74 and Pt. 2, pp. 269–329.

Scheithauer, B. W. (1985). Surgical pathology of the pituitary and sellar region: exclusive of pituitary adenomas. In *Pathology annual*, Vol. 20 (ed. S. C. Sommers, P. P. Rosen, and R. E. Fechner), Pt. 1, pp. 67–155.

Treip, C. S. (1984). The hypothalamus and pituitary gland. In *Greenfield's neuropathology* (ed. J. H. Adams, J. A. N. Corselis, and L. W. Duchen) (4th edn), pp. 748–78. Arnold, London.

26.2   The thyroid gland

R. B. Goudie

26.2.1   Introduction

Diseases of the thyroid gland are among the most common endocrine disorders encountered in clinical practice. Thyroid enlargement (goitre) and mental retardation, the effects of impaired thyroid hormone production, are endemic in many parts of the world where there are inadequate amounts of iodine in the diet. Indeed, the prevention of iodine deficiency in affected communities by the use of iodized foods ranks among the greatest triumphs of medical science. Auto-immunity to organ-specific antigens in the thyroid is another major factor in the pathogenesis of several thyroid diseases. It is of historical interest that hypothyroidism was the first endocrine deficiency to be successfully treated, the missing hormone being replaced by subcutaneous injection of thyroid juice.

26.2.2   Anatomy

The thyroid is the largest single endocrine gland in the body. Normally it weighs 15–25 g and it is slightly heavier in females, especially at puberty, menstruation, and during pregnancy. It consists of two pear-shaped *lateral lobes* about 5 cm long, 3 cm wide, and 2 cm deep. These lie on either side of the lower part of the larynx and upper part of the trachea and are usually joined in front of the second, third, and fourth rings of the trachea by a narrow *isthmus* from which a small pyramidal lobe sometimes projects upwards towards the larynx, slightly to the left of the midline.

The gland is separated from the skin of the front of the neck only by subcutaneous tissue and the thin, strap-like sternothyroid and sternocricoid muscles, and by the sternomastoids laterally. It is therefore readily visible and palpable when even slightly enlarged and it moves on swallowing because the pretracheal fascia which invests it is also attached to the larynx and trachea.

Clinically its most important anatomical relations are the trachea and oesophagus (Fig. 26.17). Stridor and difficulty in swallowing may result from compression of these structures by a greatly enlarged thyroid, particularly when it extends downwards behind the sternum into the mediastinum or when the swelling is asymmetrical and markedly displaces the trachea and oesophagus to the opposite side. Other neighbouring structures include the carotid arteries laterally and the recurrent laryngeal nerves and parathyroid glands which lie posterior to the thyroid.

Structure

The thyroid is surrounded by a vascular fibrous capsule from which fibrous septa extend inwards dividing the parenchyma into irregularly shaped lobules which are most readily apparent when the gland is enlarged. The parenchyma itself has a brown glistening appearance due to the presence of gelatinous *colloid* stored within tiny cyst-like follicles, the largest of which are just visible to the naked eye. Each follicle is surrounded by a rich plexus of capillaries and lymphatics which are separated from the folliclar epithelium by a thin basement membrane. When the gland is inactive, the follicles are lined by a layer of flat or cubical epithelium but under the influence of *thyroid stimulating hormone* (TSH) from the anterior pituitary the epithelial cells become larger and more numerous and assume a columnar shape (Fig. 26.18). The colloid within the follicles secreted by the epithelium and its main constituent, the 660 kDa glycoprotein *thyroglobulin*, is the site where the iodinated amino acids *thyroxine* and *3,5,3'-tiiodothyronine*, the principal thyroid hormones, are formed and stored.

Somewhat less than 1 per cent of the epithelium in the thyroid is composed of parafollicular neuro-endocrine cells, which may lie singly or in small clusters on either side of the follicular basement membrane. Because of their clear cytoplasm in histological sections, the *parafollicular cells* are often referred to as *C-cells* but their most characteristic feature is the presence in their cytoplasm of secretory granules containing the polypeptide hormone *calcitonin*, which can readily be demonstrated by immunohistochemical staining.

Development

The thyroid develops from the endoderm of the floor of the pharynx as a midline tubular diverticulum, the *thyroglossal duct*, which grows downwards in front of the laryngeal cartilages then bifurcates to form the isthmus and most of the

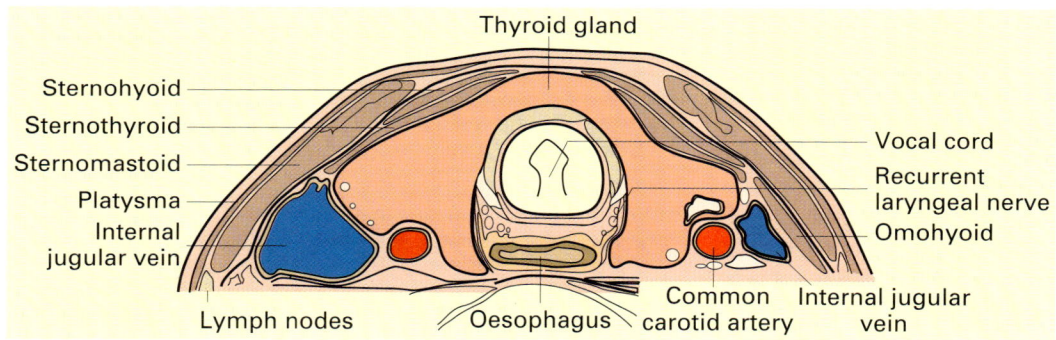

Fig. 26.17   Anatomical relationships of the thyroid gland at the level of the isthmus.

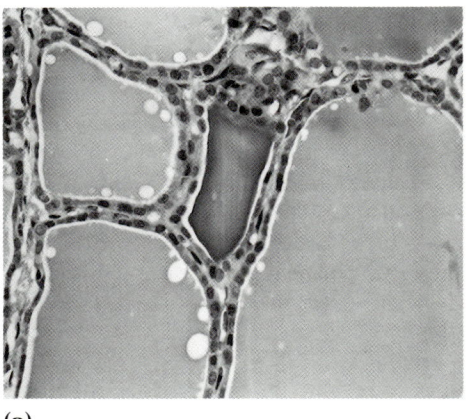 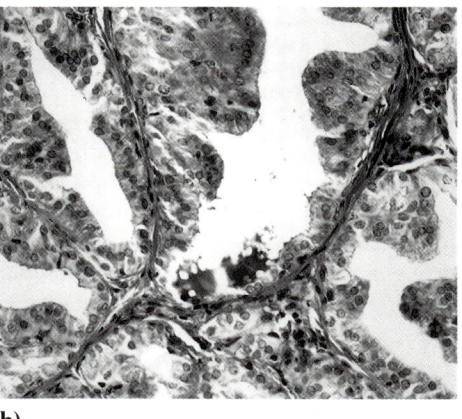

(a)   (b)

Fig. 26.18   (a) Normal resting thyroid: the follicles are lined by cubical epithelium and are full of colloid. (b) Thyroid epithelial hypertrophy and hyperplasia; the epithelium is columnar and heaped up to form papillary projections. The follicles are small and depleted of colloid.

lateral lobes. It is probable that the *ultimobranchial bodies* derived from the ectoderm of the fourth branchial clefts also contribute to the developing lateral lobes, and there is some evidence that they give rise to the parafollicular cells which are thought to originate, at an earlier stage of development, from the neural crest.

In the adult, remnants of the thyroglossal duct may be found in the line extending between the foramen caecum near the back of the tongue to the pyramidal lobe of the thyroid. These remnants may take the form of masses of *ectopic thyroid tissue* (*lingual thyroid*, for example), *thyroglossal sinuses* opening on the midline of the neck, or *thyroglossal cysts* lined with squamous or respiratory-type epithelium, which may form fistulae with the overlying skin. Sometimes the thyroid fails to descend and the lingual thyroid may then be accompanied, lower in the neck, with isolated small bilateral masses of follicles and C-cells, which are possibly derived from the ultimobranchial bodies. Interestingly, thyroglobulin has recently been found in epithelial cells lining occasional branchial cysts. Ectopic follicles are found in skeletal muscle surrounding the thyroid in infants and are sometimes present in cervical lymph nodes in adults where they may be difficult to distinguish from deposits of well-differentiated metastatic thyroid carcinoma.

26.2.3 The thyroid hormones

Thyroxine (T4) and *3,5,3′-triiodothyronine* (T3), are iodinated forms of the amino acid thyronine (Fig. 26.19) and chemically quite unlike the hormones produced by other endocrine glands. Their unusual chemical composition is reflected in the unusual way they are synthesized and secreted into the bloodstream by the follicular epithelium, and in their storage in large reservoirs of extracellular colloid which can provide a continuing supply of hormones for about 3 months if iodine is absent from the diet.

Iodine for thyroid hormone synthesis is provided partly by recycling within the thyroid and partly by dietary intake, an average of 150 μg a day being absorbed in the form of *iodide* from the small intestine. Depending on the amount of TSH stimulation, some of the absorbed iodide is actively removed from the bloodstream by the thyroid epithelium, the remainder being excreted by the kidney. Within the follicular epithelial cells the iodide is rapidly oxidized by a *peroxidase–H_2O_2 system* and bound to tyrosyl residues in thyroglobulin to form *monoiodotyrosine* (MIT) and *diiodotyrosine* (DIT). Coupling of two neighbouring DITs within the thyroglobulin molecule leads to the formation of T4 while one DIT and one MIT couple to form T3, the ratio of T3:T4 formed being greater when the supply of iodine is limited or when the time available for iodination is decreased due to rapid turnover of thyroglobulin. After iodination, thyroglobulin is discharged from the epithelium into the colloid in the follicular lumen.

The secretion of T4 and T3 into the bloodstream is also controlled by TSH, which promotes endocytosis of stored colloid by the follicular epithelium. Within the epithelial cells the colloid droplets fuse with primary lysosomes, whose proteolytic enzymes digest the thyroglobulin, releasing T4 and T3 which then pass out of the cells into the perifollicular capillaries and lymphatics. Normally about 80 μg of T4 and 5 μg of T3 are secreted per day. Physiologically, T3 may be the main thyroid hormone, having four times the metabolic effect of T4 which can, however, be converted to the more active T3 by a specific *deiodinase*. Uncoupled MIT and DIT are also released when thyroglobulin is digested, but these molecules are nearly all retained within the epithelial cells where their iodine is removed by deiodinase enzymes and recycled for iodination of newly synthesized thyroglobulin.

Because of their poor solubility in water, most of the circulating thyroid hormones are transported bound to plasma proteins, mainly a *specific thyroxine-binding globulin* (one of the alpha globulins) but also to prealbumin and albumin for which they have much lower affinity. The concentrations of unbound T4 and T3 thus depend on the total amount of hormone in the plasma and on the concentrations of the various binding proteins. Only 0.03 per cent of total plasma T4 and 0.3 per cent of T3 are unbound or 'free' and available to enter target cells and exert their hormonal effects. Since the concentration of thyroxine-binding globulin in the plasma varies markedly, depending on genetic factors, pregnancy, and disease, measurements of free T4 and T3 are preferable to total plasma assays in the diagnosis of borderline cases of thyroid hormone excess or deficiency.

Unbound T3 and T4 are lipid soluble and are thought to enter cells by diffusion across the cell membrane. Inside the cell they combine with a specific receptor, which probably functions as a transport protein and conveys them to the nucleus where they have a direct action at specific hormone-binding sites. It is of interest that the *thyroid-hormone receptor* is the product of the *proto-oncogene c-erb A* and is a member of the same family of proteins as the various steroid-hormone receptors.

Effects of thyroid hormones

The functions of the primary targets to which T3 and T4 bind in the nucleus are unknown, but directly or indirectly they lead to profound changes in protein, carbohydrate, and fat metabolism. Thyroid hormones also have important effects on development, particularly on the nervous and skeletal systems. Deficiency during fetal life and in infancy leads to *cretinism*. In severe cases the appearance is characteristic—a mentally retarded dwarf with coarse skin and hair, large tongue, and a pot-belly with an umbilical hernia (Fig. 26.20). Sometimes most of these features are absent apart from neurological abnormalities, which include deaf mutism, spastic paralysis, and ataxia. Most of the effects of cretinism can be prevented or corrected by timely hormone replacement but some impairment of intellectual function is liable to persist.

Hypothyroidism

Hypothyroidism developing later in life is insidious in onset and easily overlooked. By definition, the concentrations of (free) T4 and T3 in the blood are subnormal. Unless secondary to hypopituitarism, the circulating level of TSH is increased. The basal metabolic rate is subnormal. The patient complains of feeling

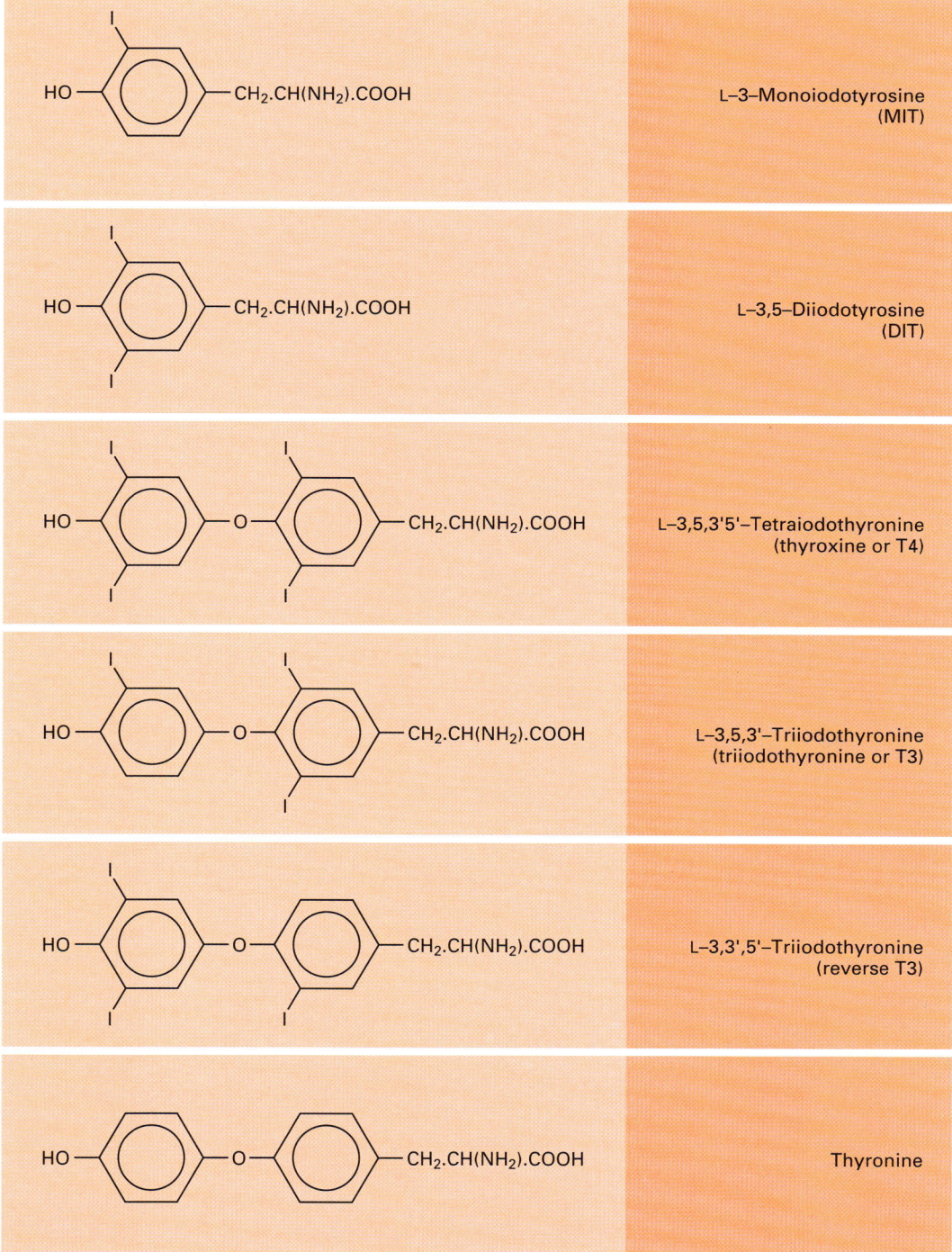

Fig. 26.19 Some thyroid amino acids derived from tyrosine. Only T3 and T4 are hormonally active.

the cold and gradually becomes apathetic and slow in thought and movement. Some cases become frankly psychotic. Lassitude, constipation, weight gain, and anaemia are common. The hair is sparse, dry, and unkempt. Swelling of the connective tissues due to increase in the mucoid ground substance (the origin of the term 'myxoedema') is responsible for the swelling of the face (Fig. 26.21) and croaking voice which are typical of the disease, and for the development of deafness and carpal tunnel syndrome which are sometimes encountered. Hypercholesterolaemia is often present and predisposes to atheroma

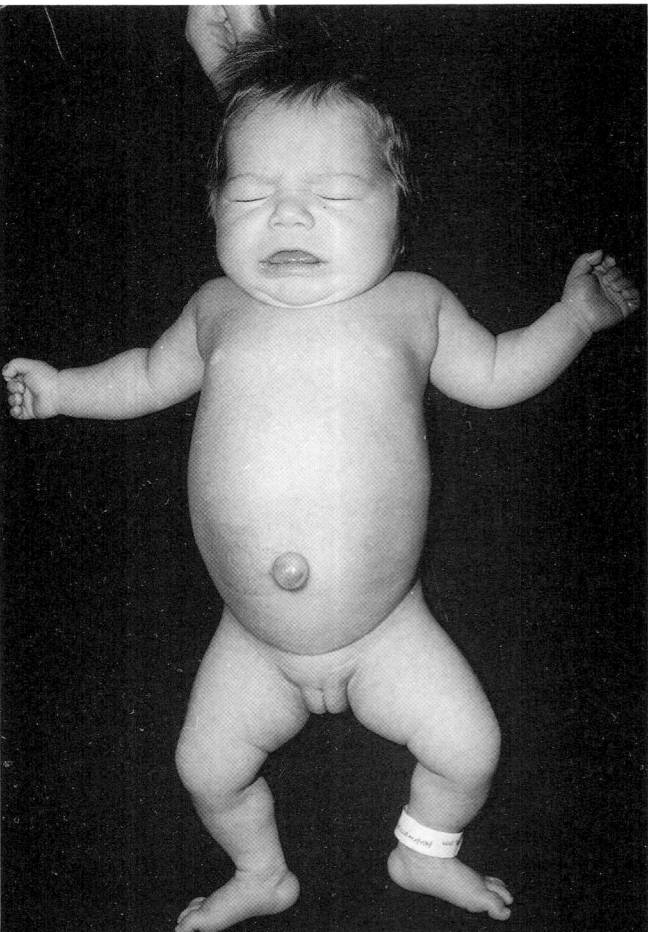

Fig. 26.20 Cretinism. Note the large protruding tongue, pot-belly and umbilical hernia. By the time such changes are present there is already irreversible intellectual impairment.

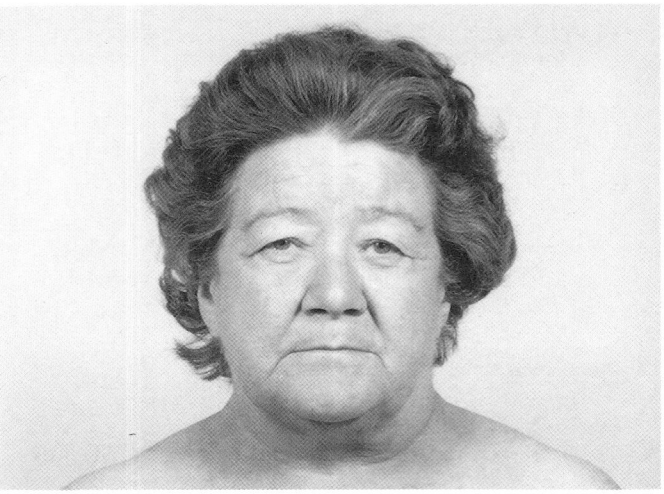

Fig. 26.21 Hypothyroidism. There is puffiness of the face and supra-clavicular fossae and the hair is lacklustre in this patient who had raised TSH and subnormal T4 blood levels.

and its complications, particularly ischaemic heart disease. With the exception of atheroma and its effects, all these changes can be reversed with thyroxine therapy. Table 26.2 lists the main causes of hypothyroidism.

Table 26.2 Causes of hypothyroidism (after Hoffenberg 1987)

TSH deficiency
    Hypopituitarism
Developmental abnormality
    Thyroid agenesis
Impaired synthesis or release of T3 and T4
    Iodine deficiency
    Dyshormonogenesis
    Antithyroid drugs
    Hashimoto's disease
Destruction of thyroid
    Thyroidectomy
    Irradiation
    Auto-immune atrophic thyroiditis
Blocking of TSH receptor
    Auto-immune atrophic thyroiditis
    Neonatal hypothyroidism
Peripheral resistance to thyroid hormone

Hyperthyroidism

This is usually characterized by thyroid enlargement and elevated levels of free T3 and T4 in the circulation, but in mild cases only T3 may be increased. Pituitary TSH production is totally suppressed except in cases due to thyrotroph tumours of the pituitary. The effects of hyperthyroidism are the converse of those found in hypothyroidism. Those directly due to hypersecretion of T3 and T4 include hypermetabolism, resulting in weight loss, increased appetite, heat intolerance, and physical and mental overactivity. Skeletal myopathy gives rise to weakness, while cardiac myopathy is associated with tachycardia and arrhythmias, including atrial fibrillation and cardiac failure. Osteoporosis and amenorrhoea may also be present. A second group of effects, based on potentiation of sympathetic receptor effects by the thyroid hormones, include tachycardia, sweating, intestinal hypermotility, and a staring expression due to retraction of the eyelids by contraction of Müller's muscle. The principal causes of hyperthyroidism are shown in Table 26.3.

Control of thyroid function

Thyroid hormone production is, for the most part, controlled by the level of circulating thyroid stimulating hormone (TSH), a 28 kDa glycoprotein produced by the thyrotroph cells of the anterior pituitary. A negative feedback mechanism (Fig. 26.22) is involved. When the concentrations of T3 and T4 in the blood are too low there is increased production of TSH, while excessive formation of thyroid hormone leads to a fall in circulating TSH. The secretion of TSH is also influenced by *thyrotrophin releasing hormone* (TRH), a tripeptide that is produced under

Table 26.3 Causes of hyperthyroidism (after Hoffenberg 1987)

Auto-antibody induced
  Graves' disease
  Toxic nodular goitre
  Neonatal

Autonomous tumour
  Toxic adenoma
  Well-differentiated thyroid carcinoma

Leakage of iodoprotein from damaged follicles
  Diffuse lymphocytic thyroiditis
  de Quervain's disease

Excessive TSH secretion
  Tumour of pituitary thyrotrophs
  Hydatidiform mole
  Choriocarcinoma
  Embryonal carcinoma of testis

Administration of thyroid hormone
  Intentional (factitious)
  Overenthusiastic therapy

Iodide induced
  Jod Basedow
  Radiographic contrast media

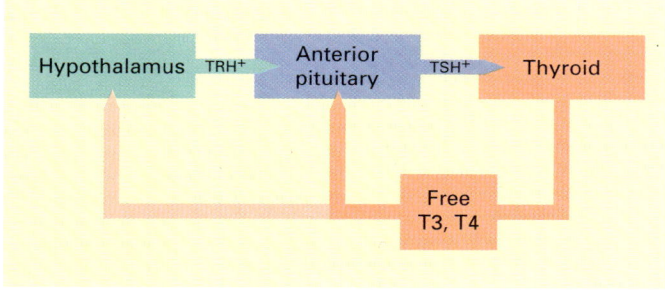

Fig. 26.22 Negative feedback control of thyroid hormone secretion.

neural and perhaps feedback control in the median eminence of the hypothalamus, whence it reaches the pituitary by way of the hypophyseal–portal vascular system. TSH consists of two polypeptide chains linked by sulphydryl bonds. The α-chain is identical to the α-chain of the pituitary and chorionic gonado-trophins but the β-chain is peculiar to TSH and forms the basis of sensitive immunological assays which are of great value as screening tests for hypothyroidism, especially in neonates. Receptors specific for TSH are found on the surface of follicular epithelial cells and also on adipocytes. Combination of TSH with its receptor leads to an increase in intracellular adenyl cyclase and cyclic AMP (cAMP), which in turn stimulates the produc-tion of T3 and T4 and their secretion into the circulation.

Control of thyroid growth

By acting through adenyl cyclase and cAMP, TSH stimulates not only thyroid function but also thyroid growth. Blockade of thyroid hormone synthesis in rats by prolonged administration of goitrogen leads to sustained elevations in plasma TSH level

and uptake of iodide by follicular epithelium. The growth re-sponse shows three distinct phases:

1. A self-limiting period of thyroid growth during which the epithelial cells become columnar and their number increases by a factor of 10 as a result of a thirtyfold mitotic burst which lasts for 1 or 2 months.

2. A plateau in which TSH, iodide uptake, and cell number remain elevated and constant although mitotic activity has almost returned to normal. If goitrogen treatment is inter-rupted for several weeks during the plateau phase, the number of epithelial cells scarcely falls and resumption of goitrogen does not cause a second mitotic burst. If, however, an incision is made in the gland a marked rise in follicular cell mitotic activity occurs in the neighbourhood of the wound, equal to that seen in the normal non-goitrous thy-roid. These findings point to the existence of a growth-desensitizing mechanism which specifically turns off the growth, but not the function-stimulating effects of TSH.

3. Following goitrogen administration for 6 months to 1 year focal TSH-dependent follicle cell tumours appear, apparently derived from cells which have circumvented the TSH-specific growth-desensitizing mechanism of the plateau phase.

In vitro experiments with isolated thyroid follicles have shown that the growth-desensitizing mechanism is intrinsic to the follicular epithelium itself, independent of the surrounding stroma. The molecular basis is unknown but it seems unlikely to be due to *down-regulation* of TSH receptors. The mitotic re-sponse of plateau epithelium to surgical trauma points to stimu-lation of a receptor responding to some growth factor other than TSH, possibly *insulin-like growth factor* (IGF-I).

The dissociation of growth and functional responses during TSH stimulation may have some parallel in the existence of distinct populations of thyroid auto-antibodies which stimulate follicle cell function and growth. However, it is not yet fully established that thyroid growth-stimulating immunoglobulins act through the TSH receptor.

26.2.4   Thyroid epithelial hyperplasia

By far the most prevalent diseases of the thyroid gland are those associated with hyperplasia of the follicular epithelium. This usually results from increased TSH stimulation in response to inadequate formation of T3 and T4 due to deficiency of dietary iodine which is endemic in many parts of the world, but other cases are due to blocking of some essential function of the fol-licular cells in thyroid hormone production. The thyroid may be uniformly enlarged, as would be expected in hyperplasia induced by a trophic hormone, but in most cases of long stand-ing the goitre is composed of multiple nodules whose patho-genesis is not yet fully understood. Affected patients are euthyroid or hypothyroid. In yet other cases, thyroid epithelial hyperplasia is stimulated not by TSH but by auto-antibodies directed against the TSH receptors. Such auto-antibodies often cause hyperthyroidism which in turn leads to suppression of pituitary TSH.

In practice, three important questions should be considered in a case of thyroid hyperplasia:

1. Is there an avoidable cause, such as iodine deficiency, genetic abnormality, or exposure to a goitrogen?

2. Does the patient require treatment for hypo- or hyper-thyroidism?

3. Is surgery required to relieve pressure symptoms, remove an unsightly goitre, or exclude the diagnosis of neoplasia?

Iodine-deficiency goitre

Seafood is the main source of dietary iodine. Endemic iodine deficiency affecting man and animals thus tends to occur in mountainous regions far from the sea, such as Switzerland, the Himalayas, and Andes; and inland areas, such as those surrounding the Great Lakes in North America. Liability to iodine deficiency is greatest when there is an increased physiological requirement for the element during childhood, puberty, pregnancy, and lactation. After puberty, females are more often affected than males. In pregnancy, extra iodine is required not only to meet the needs of the growing fetus but also because the maternal blood volume and thyroxine-binding globulin levels are increased, and additional T3 and T4 must be produced to provide an adequate concentration of free hormone for the tissues of the mother. Minor inborn defects of thyroid hormone synthesis or the ingestion of goitrogenic foods such as cabbage, kale, and turnip may further exaggerate the effects of iodine deficiency. Dietary fads are a possible cause of sporadic iodine deficiency. The development of the condition can be completely prevented in communities that are at risk by the addition of iodide to salt, flour, or milk products.

The pathological appearance of the thyroid varies considerably from case to case and three forms of iodine-deficiency goitre are recognized.

Diffuse hyperplastic goitre

The gland shows slight to moderate enlargement and is usually firm and symmetrical. On section it is composed of uniform fleshly lobules consisting of small follicles lined by columnar epithelium and containing little colloid. This variant is seldom encountered in biopsy or thyroidectomy specimens but, on the basis of animal experiments, it is presumed to be the normal response of a thyroid that has recently been exposed to iodine deficiency for the first time.

Diffuse colloid goitre

This form is found mainly in adolescents and pregnant females. The gland is uniformly affected, soft and only moderately enlarged. On section the follicles are seen to be greatly distended with gelatinous colloid. Histologically they are lined with flat epithelial cells (Fig. 26.23). These changes may be a stage in the involution of diffuse hyperplastic goitre when iodine deficiency has become less severe. Withdrawal of TSH stimulation during the plateau phase of thyroid growth in the rat rapidly leads to increased colloid storage and shrinkage of the hypertrophied columnar epithelium lining the follicles to flat cuboidal cells. Interestingly, the decline in total number of epithelial cells is slight and gradual.

Nodular goitre

This is the most common type of goitre in areas of endemic iodine deficiency. There is irregular bossing of the surface of the thyroid due to the presence within the substance of the gland of nodules, which range in size from a few millimetres to several centimetres in diameter. The gland may be very large and obviously multinodular (Fig. 26.24) or almost normal in size with an apparently single localized asymmetrical swelling, but on section the nodules are invariably found to be multiple. Each nodule has a poorly formed fibrous capsule surounding a spherical mass of gelatinous thyroid tissue, which may be dis-

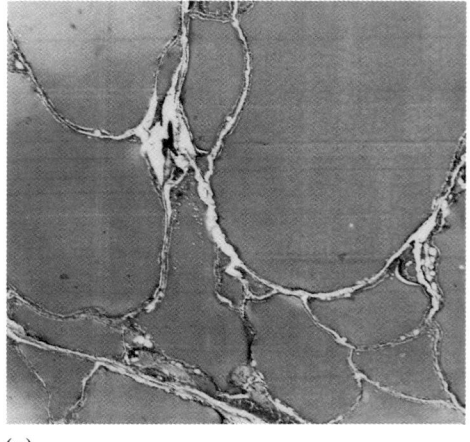 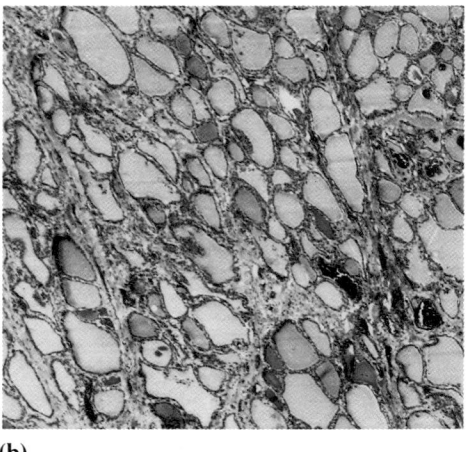

(a)   (b)

Fig. 26.23 (a) Colloid goitre showing greatly distended follicles lined by flat epithelial cells; (b) normal thyroid at the same magnification for comparison.

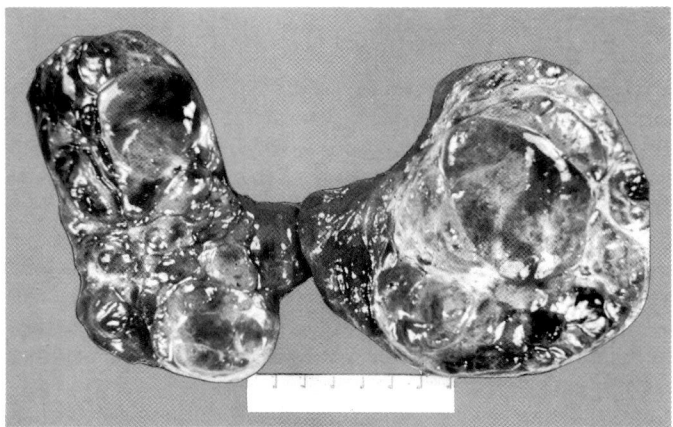

Fig. 26.24 A large non-toxic nodular goitre. The lateral lobes have been sectioned to show multiple, poorly encapsulated nodules of various sizes.

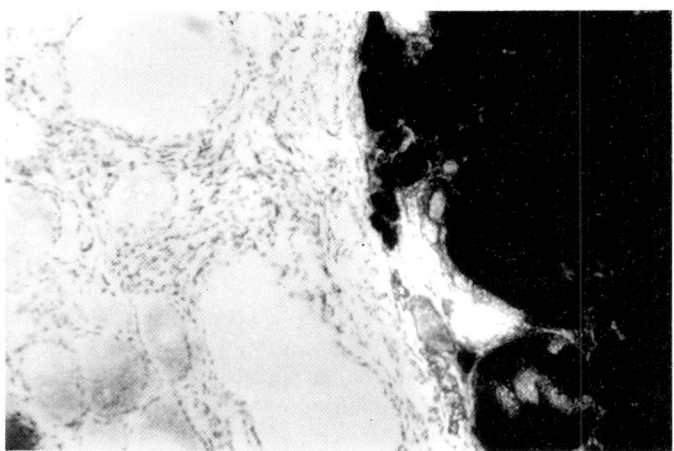

Fig. 26.26 Non-toxic nodular goitre. Autoradiograph following administration of radioiodine. Part of a hot nodule is shown (right) in which the isotope (black) is concentrated.

coloured due to old or recent haemorrhage and show cyst formation, fibrosis, and calcification. Microscopically, the follicles within individual nodules characteristically vary considerably in size from 2 mm or so in diameter to abnormally small microfollicles (Fig. 26.25). The epithelial lining is usually cubical and in some of the larger follicles it may form papillary ingrowths with thin fibrovascular cores. The fibrous stroma is often oedematous and, in areas of previous haemorrhage, haemosiderin and cholesterol crystals may be abundant. The irregular structure of the gland is reflected in patchy functional activity, as revealed by autoradiography. Radioiodine may be taken up from the blood by clusters of follicles lying between cold nodules, and sometimes a hot nodule is found (Fig. 26.26).

Mechanism of nodule formation There is no satisfactory animal model of nodular goitre. According to one theory the development of nodules in man is secondary to local factors such as

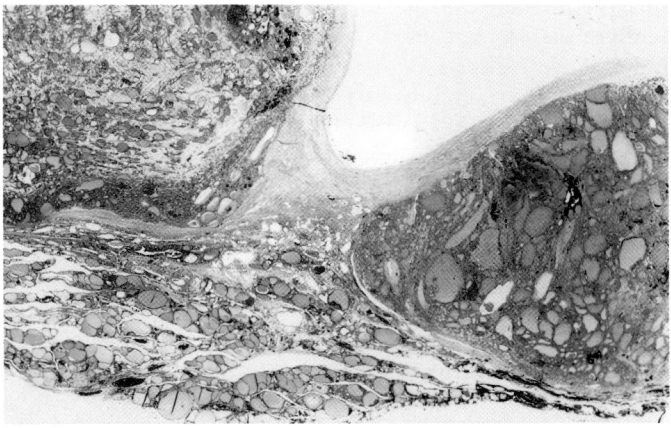

Fig. 26.25 Non-toxic nodular goitre. Two nodules are shown, the right with an incomplete fibrous capsule and marked variation in follicle size, the left with stromal oedema. Above is part of a cyst surrounded by dense collagen. The follicles in the lower part of the photograph are not involved in nodule formation.

ischaemia, which could lead to focal necrosis followed by nodular regeneration of the follicular epithelium. A second explanation is based on detailed studies of normal thyroids which show marked heterogeneity of function and growth potential of individual cells and follicles. It has therefore been proposed that nodule formation is based on *clonal proliferation of epithelial cells* responsive to slightly increased TSH acting over a long period of time. No suitable clonal markers are available to test this hypothesis in man, but in strains of mice in which this can be done most TSH-induced nodules with a structural resemblance to those in human nodular goitre are shown not to be derived from single cells but to be *polyclonal* in origin. A third possibility, still to be explored, is regulation of epithelial growth and function by *heterogeneous clones of stromal cells*.

Clinical effects

During phases of iodine deficiency, blood levels of T4 and T3 are low normal or within the hypothyroid range and TSH is increased. Characteristically, iodide uptake by the thyroid is raised relative to the amount excreted in the urine. Clinically, by far the most serious effect is *hypothyroidism*, especially when it gives rise to cretinism in children born to iodine-deficient mothers. Large goitres, besides being unsightly, are liable to cause difficulty in breathing and congestion of neck veins, particularly when the gland extends behind the sternum. The risk of carcinoma is said to be increased but the evidence is questionable. Pain and swelling of a lobe may suddenly develop due to haemorrhage into a cyst. Treatment with thyroxine or resumption of adequate iodine intake may lead to shrinkage of the goitre, but the swelling is unlikely to disappear if the gland is large and nodular.

Other causes of non-toxic goitre

Dyshormonogenesis

This term implies defective synthesis of thyroid hormone due to an inborn error of metabolism. Such errors show a *Mendelian recessive mode of inheritance*. Phenotypically normal parents may have one or more affected children and the risk is increased when the parents are consanguineous. Goitre may be present at birth or develop shortly thereafter and cretinism is commonly, but not invariably, present. As in iodine deficiency, there is excessive TSH stimulation of the thyroid and this leads to nodular goitre. In dyshormonogenesis the follicular epithelium tends to be more hyperplastic and there may be epithelial atypia sugestive of carcinoma, although frank malignancy with metastasis is extremely rare. The diagnosis of dyshormonogenesis mainly rests, however, on the familial occurence of congenital goitre or goitrous cretinism in a community with adequate dietary iodide. The genetic defects responsible represent errors in the various stages of thyroid hormone synthesis. Thus failure of *iodide trapping, thyroglobulin synthesis, iodination of thyroglobulin, coupling of MIT and DIT to form iodothyronines*, and *release of T3 and T4* into the circulation have all been recognized, and various structural abnormalities have been observed in thyroglobulin. Two other conditions are also included in the group—the *dehalogenase defect*, in which MIT and DIT are excreted in the urine, leading to secondary iodine deficiency, and *target organ unresponsiveness*, in which hypothyroidism is present despite raised plasma concentrations of T3 and T4. Much remains to be discovered about the molecular aspects of these uncommon disorders but failure of iodination of thyroglobulin depends on defects of peroxidase activity or production of H_2O_2, while coupling defects are associated, as a rule, with structural abnormalities of thyroglobulin. In *Pendred's syndrome* a mild defect of iodination of thyroglobulin, giving rise to familial goitre with or without hypothyroidism, is associated with eighth nerve deafness. In general, the various forms of dyshormonogenesis are identified by *in vivo* tests with radioiodine or by *in vitro* metabolic studies on excised samples of thyroid tissue.

Goitrogens

Thyroid hyperplasia and nodular goitre may develop following ingestion of many different substances that interfere with one or other of the steps in thyroid hormone synthesis, as in the various forms of dyshormonogenesis. For example, *perchlorate* and *thiocyanate* inhibit the iodide-trapping mechanism while many drugs, including *thiouracil, resorcinol*, para-*amino-salicyclic acid, colbalt*, and some *sulphonamides*, prevent iodination of thyroglobulin, probably by blocking the enzyme *peroxidase*. Plants of the *Brassica* family, such as cabbage, kale, and turnip, have the same effect, but the quantities required to produce goitre are very large. In normal individuals large doses of *iodide* block the secretion of the thyroid hormones, and the amount of iodide present in certain cough mixtures, asthma remedies, and even the normal diets of some districts of Japan where *seaweed* is eaten in large amounts, can cause nodular goitre and hypothyroidism in susceptible individuals. *Lithium*, used for the treatment of manic depressive states, has similar effects in a small proportion of cases.

When pregnant women are treated for hypothyroidism with *iodide* or *methimazole*, these substances cross the placenta and may lead to congenital goitre in the fetus, with or without hypothyroidism. It is noteworthy that neither TSH nor T3 and T4 cross the placenta.

Thyroid-growth-stimulating immunoglobulins When all the above causes have been excluded there still remains a substantial number of sporadic cases of non-toxic goitre which are unexplained. In about two-thirds of such cases, thyroid-growth-stimulating immunoglobulin has been found in the blood. This is capable of inducing DNA synthesis, as measured by tritiated thymidine uptake in human or rat thyroid cell cultures, but much more effectively demonstrated by ultrasensitive techniques such as nucleic acid cytophotomety in organ culture of guinea-pig thyroid or assay of glucose-6-phosphate dehydrogenase activity, which is the rate-controlling enzymatic step in the pentose shunt, the major source of ribose sugars needed for DNA synthesis. Positive results are found most often in diffuse goitres and in nodular goitres that recur after thyroidectomy. In non-toxic goitre the concentration of thyroid-growth-stimulating immunoglobulin is relatively low and it has been suggested that only some of the thyroid cells respond, as possible explanation for unequal cell proliferation and nodule formation. Thyroid-growth-stimulating immunoglobulin may react with the TSH receptor in such a way that thyroid cell function is not increased, but another possibility is that some growth factor receptor other than the TSH receptor may be involved.

26.2.5   Hyperthyroidism

Most cases of hyperthyroidism are due to *thyroid-stimulating* auto-antibodies, which induce hyperplasia of the follicular epithelium and excess thyroid hormone production, which in turn suppresses pituitary TSH. Graves' disease and many cases of toxic nodular goitre come into this category. Other rare causes, which together account for little more than 1 per cent of cases, include *thyroid tumours* (nearly always benign adenomas), follicular damage in some forms of *thyroiditis*, and administration of large doses of *thyroid hormones*, intentionally or due to overenthusiastic therapy. In these conditions pituitary TSH is suppressed and thyroid epithelial hyperplasia is absent, but on rare occasions hyperthyroidism occurs due to excessive production of TSH by tumours, or hyperplasia of pituitary thyrotrophs or of chorionic epithelium. Hyperthyroidism sometimes develops when a patient with non-toxic goitre is given iodide.

Graves' disease

Graves' disease (also known as primary thyrotoxicosis or eponymously as Parry's or von Basedow's disease) is characterized clinically by hyperthyroidism; diffuse goitre, often with a bruit; and ocular abnormalities, of which exophthalmos is most common (Fig. 26.27). In some cases there is mucoid swelling of the dermis and subcutaneous tissue of the legs (*pretibial myxoedema*).

Either sex may be affected and the disease may occur at any

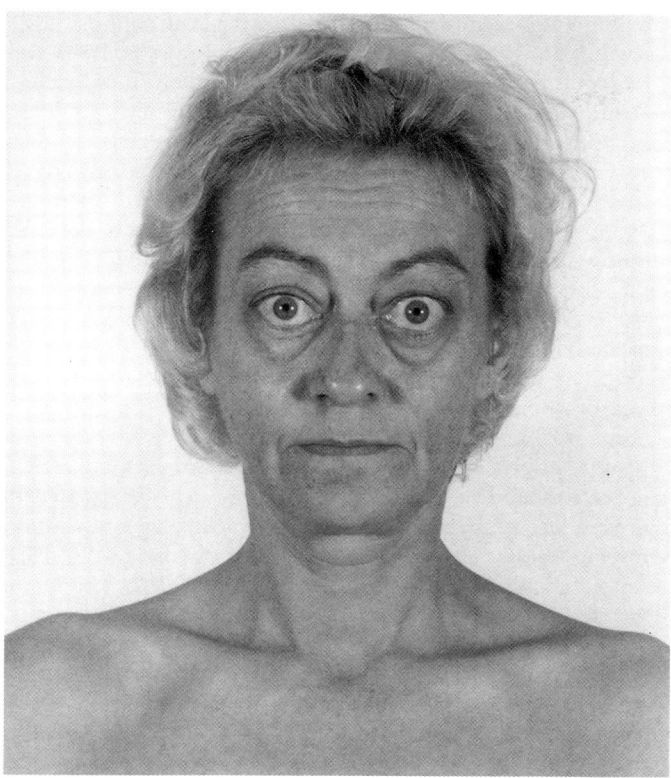

Fig. 26.27 Appearance of a patient with Graves' disease. Note the presence of goitre and exophthalmos.

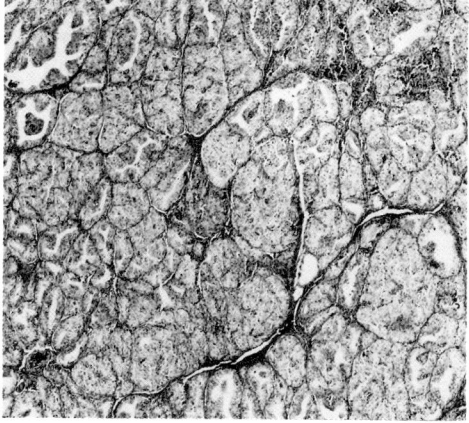

Fig. 26.28 Untreated Graves' disease. Note the diffuse uniform epithelial hypertrophy and hyperplasia. The dark areas of stroma are infiltrated with lymphocytes.

age, but it is most common in women in the third and fourth decades.

Diagnosis rests on the clinical findings and the demonstration of raised serum levels of T3 and usually of T4. Following a tracer dose of radioactive iodine or technetium there is rapid diffuse uptake by the thyroid which cannot be suppressed by T3, since the gland is not under the control of the pituitary. The increase of iodide uptake by the thyroid normally seen after injection of TRH is diminished or absent, presumably due to feedback suppression of the pituitary by high circulating levels of thyroid hormone.

In untreated cases the thyroid is highly vascular, uniformly enlarged, and fleshy in appearance due to reduced colloid storage. There is *diffuse epithelial hyperplasia and hypertrophy* (Fig. 26.28), the cells being tall and columnar and forming papillary projections which increase the surface area of the follicles. Mitotic figures and large hyperchromatic polyploid nuclei may be found. In paraffin sections the colloid is weakly stained and reduced in amount, and it contains numerous vacuoles at the edge of the follicular lumina where it is in contact with the epithelium ('marginal scalloping'). There is usually an increased number of stromal lymphocytes and plasma cells distributed singly and in clusters, and in some cases there is marked lymphoid infiltration with germinal centre formation. Thyroidectomy specimens are usually obtained after the disease has been controlled by drugs which modify the histological

appearance of the gland. Antithyroid drugs, such as *methimazole*, which block iodination of thyroglobulin and so diminish thyroid hormone production, also appear to have an immunosuppressive effect and diminish the lymphoid infiltrate. Iodides are often used pre-operatively because they markedly reduce the vascularity of the gland and block hormone secretion; they profoundly affect thyroid morphology, reducing the degree of epithelial hyperplasia and increasing the storage and staining intensity of the colloid (Fig. 26.29). The appearance of the gland is little affected by β-adrenoreceptor blockers. As in most other thyroid disorders, and particularly in view of the effects of pre-operative drug therapy, the histological appearance is a poor indicator of hormone production.

Pathological changes are not confined to the thyroid. There may be lymphoid hyperplasia of thymus, spleen, and cervical lymph nodes. The primary changes in the orbit responsible for exophthalmos appear to be oedema and lymphoid infiltration of the extra-ocular muscles with subsequent fibrosis which

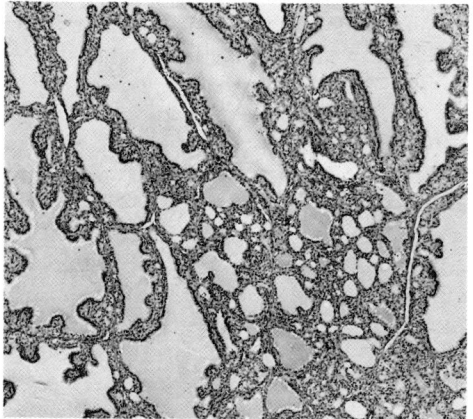

Fig. 26.29 Graves' disease treated with iodide. Epithelial hypertrophy and hyperplasia are still evident but greatly reduced. There is a marked increase in colloid storage.

spreads to the orbital fat. In addition to proptosis, there may be limitation of eye movements, diplopia, ulceration of the cornea due to inability to close the eyes, and loss of sight due to compression of the optic nerve.

Aetiology

There is now good evidence that Graves' disease is one of the organ-specific auto-immune diseases, and that its occurrence is, in part, genetically determined.

The serum in approximately 90 per cent of thyrotoxic patients contains abnormal auto-antibodies against the *TSH receptor*. In the sensitive *in vitro* bioassays some of these antibodies behave as thyroid-stimulating immunoglobulins. Further evidence of their pathological significance is their association with congenital thyrotoxicosis, which results from transplacental transfer to the babies of thyrotoxic mothers. Thyroid-stimulating auto-antibodies also cause transient hyperthyroidism when injected into guinea-pigs or mice. Relapse or remission of thyrotoxicosis is related to the presence or absence of thyroid-stimulating immunoglobulin at the time antithyroid drug therapy is stopped. Thyroid-growth-promoting immunoglobulin is found in two-thirds of thyrotoxic patients, especially those with large goitres, but not in cases without thyroid enlargement. Auto-antibodies are frequently found against other thyroid-specific auto-antigens such as thyroglobulin and thyroid microsomes. There is also an increased incidence of antibodies against organ-specific antigens in other tissues, such as the stomach and adrenal glands, and of the corresponding organ-specific auto-immune diseases, atrophic gastritis and chronic adrenocortical insufficiency.

It is uncertain in Graves' disease whether the basic defect leading to auto-antibody formation against the TSH receptor and other thyroid auto-antigens resides in the thyroid gland, the immune system, or both. As explained elsewhere, antibody formation by B-cells is regulated by the opposing effects of helper and suppressor T-lymphocytes. Abnormalities reported in peripheral blood lymphocytes in Graves' disease include the presence of T-helper cells specifically sensitized against the TSH receptor and a reduction in the amount of thyroid-specific suppressor T-cell activity compared with normal.

Approximately 50 per cent of thyrotoxic patients have a family history of the disease, and more than a third of apparently healthy first-degree relatives have thyroid auto-antibodies. Comparison of concordance rates in monozygotic (50 per cent) and dizygotic twins (5 per cent) points to the importance of genetic factors in the causation of the disease, while the discordant monozygotic twin pairs indicate that environmental factors also have a role. Inheritance appears to be polygenic. There is general agreement that Caucasian patients with Graves' disease inherit the HLA antigens DR3 and B8 with undue frequency, DR3 being associated with an early onset and greater risk of relapse following treatment. In Japanese and Chinese patients, other DR antigens are implicated. Involvement of the DR locus is especially interesting in an immunological disorder since helper T-cells can recognize a potential antigen only if they encounter it in the context of DR molecules on the surface of antigen-presenting cells. DR is the homologue of the *Ir (immune-reactivity) genes* of the major histocompatibility complex of the mouse, which determine antibody formation against certain thymus-dependent antigens. Studies using immunoglobulin allotypes (Gm) as genetic markers have shown that in certain families thyroid-stimulating immunoglobulin formation is associated with inheritance of the immunoglobulin heavy-chain genes on one particular chromosome 14, possibly because rearrangement of the immunoglobulin gene on this chromosome has an increased likelihood of producing antibody complementary to the TSH receptor. A preponderance of λ light chains in thyroid-stimulating immunoglobulin may have a similar explanation.

In normal individuals the expression of DR molecules is found only on antigen-presenting cells, such as macrophages, B-lymphocytes, and vascular endothelium. In Graves' disease DR molecules are present on the surface of follicular epithelium, rendering these cells capable of presenting their own TSH receptors as potential auto-antigens. The reason for the inappropriate DR expression is unknown. It could be a genetically programmed primary defect in the thyroid epithelium, or a secondary consequence of the release of lymphokines such as *γ-interferon* by activated T-cells in the neighbourhood.

Environmental factors that have been suspected include *Yersinia* infections. *Yersinia* cross-reacts with thyroid-specific antigens and could thus favour the development of thyroid auto-immunity by abolishing self-tolerance. Emotional stress is another factor suspected of precipitating the disease.

No discussion of the aetiology of Graves' disease can be complete without considering the associated eye changes, which are clinically apparent in about two-thirds of patients. The presence of ophthalmopathy does not correlate with circulating levels of thyroid-stimulating immunoglobulin or with the severity of the hyperthyroidism. Eye changes other than lid retraction and lid lag cannot be produced experimentally by administration of thyroid homone. It thus appears possible that the thyroid and ocular manifestations are two different diseases, which develop at about the same time in the same individual. Attempts to demonstrate a separate auto-immune basis for the ophthalmopathy have so far been unsuccessful. Various immunological abnormalities, ranging from auto-antibodies or cell-mediated immunity directed against the extrinsic eye muscles to the deposition of immune complexes containing thyroglobulin in the orbital tissues, have been reported, but none of the findings have been adequately confirmed.

Toxic nodular goitre

This condition (Plummer's disease) differs clinically from Graves' disease in several respects. It affects older patients, eye signs are unusual, and cardiac arrhythmia or cardiac failure may be the presenting feature. Auto-antibodies stimulating hormone production and thyroid growth are, however, frequently present. The patient often has a history of non-toxic nodular goitre for a decade or more before hyperthyroidism develops. Many sporadic cases of non-toxic goitre attributed to growth-stimulating immunoglobulins show a diminished or absent response to TRH, as in Graves' disease, and in such cases hyperthyrodism may supervene when hormone production by autonomous functioning nodules exceeds a critical level. Alternatively, some cases may simply be examples of Graves' disease superimposed on non-toxic goitre of whatever cause, following the onset of thyroid-stimulating antibody production. It has long been recognized in iodine-deficient areas that the introduction of iodized salt sometimes leads to the development of hyperthyroidism (Jod Basedow). The mechanism is unknown, but it is possible that pre-existing latent hyperthyroidism has been masked by iodine deficiency. The gross and microscopic appearances of the thyroid in toxic nodular goitre are indistinguishable from those of non-toxic goitre.

Toxic adenoma

Most thyroid tumours have little functional activity but occasionally hyperthyroidism is due to a simple adenoma which appears as a solitary hot nodule in a cold, but otherwise normal thyroid gland. Significant hormone production by thyroid carcinoma is exceptional, but a few examples of hyperthyroidism have been recorded in well-differentiated follicular tumours with extensive metastases.

26.2.6   Thyroiditis

Acute suppurative thyroiditis may result from local or haematogenous spread of pyogenic bacteria to the thyroid, but it is rare. Chronic inflammation due to *tuberculosis, syphilis, actinomycosis,* or *fungal infection* is also occasionally encountered. Non-infective thyroid granulomata may be found in *sarcoidosis, rheumatoid arthritis,* and perhaps as a result of *trauma—palpation thyroiditis.* By far the most common chronic inflammatory condition of the thyroid, *auto-immune thyroiditis,* is characterized by infiltration of the gland with autoreactive lymphoid cells and various epithelial abnormalities. Depending on the extent and nature of the lymphoid infiltrate and epithelial abnormality, three main forms of auto-immune thyroiditis are recognized; *Hashimoto's disease, atrophic thyroiditis,* and *focal thyroiditis.* Two other forms of thyroiditis are recognized clinically and pathologically and are usually referred to eponymously as *de Quervain's disease* and *Riedel's disease.*

Hashimoto's disease (lymphadenoid goitre)

This disease characteristically occurs in middle-aged women, although men are occasionally affected. Clinically the thyroid is enlarged, firm, and usually painless. Half of the patients are hypothyroid and the remainder are liable to become so, particularly if partial thyroidectomy is performed. The level of circulating TSH is often increased.

The thyroid is not adherent to the surrounding tissues. On section it presents a pale, solid, lobulated appearance, similar to normal pancreas. There is no necrosis. The local lymph nodes may be enlarged. The cardinal histological features are the diffuse nature of the lymphoid infiltrate and epithelial changes,

and some degree of thickening of the fibrous interlobular septa (Fig. 26.30). The lymphoid infiltrate consists of mature lymphocytes and many plasma cells which crowd round individual thyroid follicles and groups of follicles. Lymphoid follicles with germinal centres are nearly always present. Mitotic figures are seldom encountered, except in the follicle centres. The thyroid follicles are small and the colloid sparse and often densely stained; some contain a few macrophages, plasma cells, and an occasional multinucleated giant cell. Often the epithelial clusters have no visible lumen. The epithelial cells themselves are large and cubical (Fig. 26.31). The cytoplasm has a characteristic granular eosinophilic appearance due to the presence of greatly increased numbers of mitochondria. The nuclei may be large, hyperchromatic, and irregular in shape but mitoses are uncommon. These metaplastic mitochondrion-rich epithelial

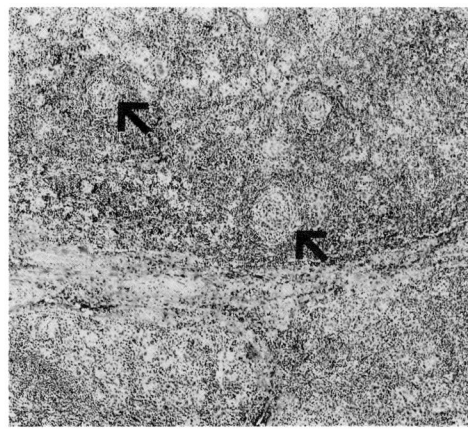

Fig. 26.30 Hashimoto's disease. Diffuse infiltration with lymphoid cells and lymphoid follicles with germinal centre (arrows). Note the absence of normal thyroid follicles.

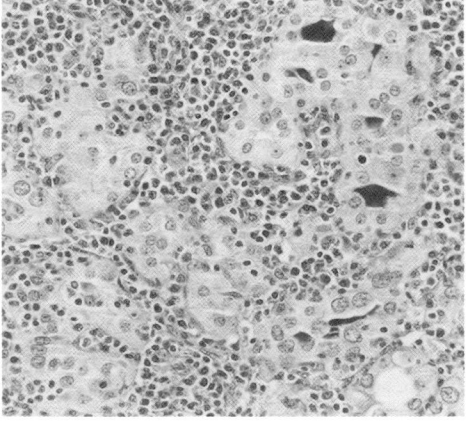

Fig. 26.31 Hashimoto's disease. Numerous small follicles, a few of which contain dark colloid. The epithelial cells are abnormally large (compare with Fig. 26.18a) with abundant eosinophilic granular cytoplasm (Askanazy cells). Note the large number of plasma cells in the infiltrate.

cells are variously described as *Hürthle cells*, *Askanazy cells*, *oxyphil cells*, or *oncocytes*. Despite their increased content of mitochondria and respiratory enzymes, their ability to iodinate thyroglobulin and produce thyroid hormone is impaired. Sometimes squamous metaplasia is also present. In most cases of Hashimoto's disease there is an increase in the total volume of epithelium, which thus contributes to the overall thyroid enlargement. In the fibrous variant of Hashimoto's disease much of the gland may be replaced by dense, relatively acellular collagen but the surviving areas of parenchyma show the typical epithelial and lymphoid abnormalities.

The features described above are mainly encountered in middle-aged and elderly patients. The corresponding auto-immune disorder in adolescents and young adults appears to be a diffuse lymphocytic thyroiditis with fewer plasma cells in the infiltrate and conspicuous epithelial hyperplasia, the follicles being larger, devoid of colloid, and lined by pale cubical epithelium lacking the eosinophilic granular cytoplasm of Askanazy cells. Clinically, there is painless goitre and the patient may be hyperthyroid, due to release of iodoprotein from damaged follicles, euthyroid, or hypothyroid. The hyperthyroidism and hypothyrodism may be transient, especially in cases developing after pregancy, and hypothyroidism may follow a hyperthyroid phase.

Occasionally Hashimoto's disease is complicated by a *primary malignant lymphoma* or *plasmacytoma* of the thyroid. The diagnosis can be made readily by histological or cytological examination of a needle biopsy. There is no increased risk of carcinoma.

Atrophic thyroiditis

This condition is responsible for *non-goitrous hypothyroidism* ('primary myxoedema') which is common in the elderly. Either sex may be affected, but there is a slight predominance of females. The thyroid gland is reduced to a fibrous remnant, weighing as little as 3 g. Histologically no normal thyroid tissue is seen. Within the fibrous tissue there are scattered islands of lymphoid cells surrounding small follicles lined by Askanazy cells or solid or cystic masses of squamous epithelium (Fig. 26.32). The fibrous component may include a few adipocytes.

Focal auto-immune thyroiditis

Unlike Hashimoto's disease and atrophic thyroiditis, in which there is diffuse lymphoid infiltration, in focal auto-immune thyroiditis the lymphoid infiltrate is patchy (Fig. 26.33) and may remain so over a period of many years. In some parts of the world, including the United Kingdom, clinically latent focal thyroiditis is present in about 10 per cent of middle-aged and elderly women. Patchy Askanazy cell change is often present. There may be subclinical hypothyroidism with raised plasma TSH levels, and some cases may represent an early stage of atrophic thyroiditis. Focal auto-immune thyroiditis is an almost invariable accompaniment of Graves' disease and, when severe ('Hashitoxicosis'), increases the risk of hypothyroidism following partial thyroidectomy.

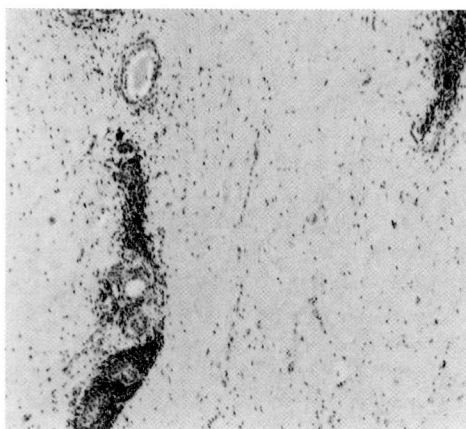

Fig. 26.32 Atrophic thyroiditis. The thyroid consists mainly of fibrous connective tissue with small islands of abnormal epithelium surrounded by lymphocytes and plasma cells.

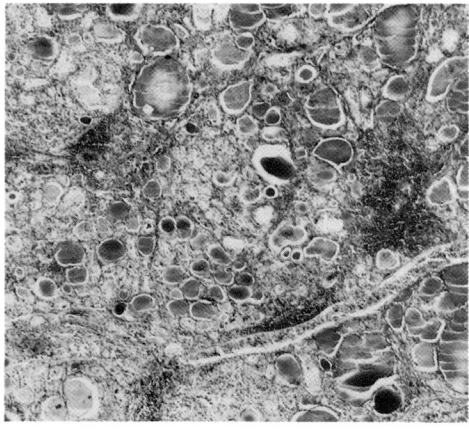

Fig. 26.33 Focal auto-immune thyroiditis. From an elderly woman whose blood contained antithyroid microsomal antibody but with no clinical evidence of thyroid disease. Patchy lymphoid infiltrate and small thyroid follicles lined with Askanazy cells.

Evidence of auto-immunity

Many, but not all, patients with the above morphologically defined conditions have circulating antibodies directed against one or more organ-specific auto-antigens present in the normal human thyroid. These include *thyroglobulin* and a *microsomal antigen* closely associated with thyroid peroxidase. These antibodies can be demonstrated by conventional serological techniques, are polyclonal, mainly IgG, and react *in vitro* with the patient's own thyroid antigens, i.e. they are *organ-specific auto-antibodies*. Auto-antibodies, especially in high titres, are found most often in typical Hashimoto's disease and least often in focal lymphocytic thyroiditis, presumably reflecting the number of antibody-secreting plasma cells in the gland. In some cases of Hashimoto's disease the concentration of antithyroglobulin antibody exceeds twice the total level of IgG normally present in the serum.

Pathogenesis of auto-immune thyroiditis

Antithyroglobulin antibody is demonstrable in some of the plasma cells infiltrating the thyroid, and thyroid auto-antibodies tend to disappear following thyroidectomy or when antigenic stimulation declines in advanced cases of atrophic thyroiditis, further evidence of their local production in the thyroid. It is thus certain that an immune response to thyroid antigen is at least in part responsible for the lymphoid infiltration encountered in this group of diseases. However, the possibility of other sources of antigenic stimulation, for example virus infection, cannot be ruled out.

Unlike Graves' disease, in which passive transmission experiments have shown convincingly that thyroid-stimulating immunoglobulin directed against the TSH receptor is responsible for the epithelial hyperplasia and hyperthyroidism in that condition, it is by no means clear that any of the antibodies demonstrable by serological methods are responsible for the abnormalities of the follicular epithelium in auto-immune thyroiditis. *Transitory neonatal hypothyroidism* has been observed in the babies of some women with atrophic thyroiditis, and it is possible that epithelial atrophy may be due to antibody that blocks the TSH receptor. It has been proposed that the epithelial damage in Hashimoto's disease is mediated by antibody together with *K-cells* or *complement*, or by *cytotoxic T-cells*, but none of these studies are based on *in vivo* transmission experiments and none have addressed the problem of the genesis of the peculiar metaplasia of the follicular epithelium to mitochondrion-rich Askanazy cells.

Aetiology

The peripheral blood of normal individuals contains both measurable amounts of thyroglobulin and B-lymphocytes with specific receptors for thyroglobulin. The same is probably true for other potential thyroid auto-antigens. The mechanisms that normally hold the clonal expansion of these lymphocytes in check are not known, nor are the defects that lead to a major auto-immune response with infiltration of the target organ. As in Graves' disease, *inappropriate expression of HLA DR molecules* on the surface of follicular epithelial cells has been observed in Hashimoto's disease and in the neighbourhood of lymphoid infiltrates in focal thyroiditis, suggesting that abnormal auto-antigen presentation to T-helper cells may be a factor. There are also reports of deficiency of thyroid-specific T-suppressor cells. The various forms of auto-immune thyroiditis tend to run in families, along with other organ-specific auto-immune diseases such as Graves' disease, pernicious anaemia, juvenile diabetes, and vitiligo. Affected individuals may have clinical or serological evidence of more than one of these conditions. Atrophic thyroiditis, like Graves' disease, is in linkage disequilibrium with HLA DR3, whereas Hashimoto's disease is associated with DR5.

Normal pregnancy is known to be accompanied by mild immunosuppression, and lymphocytic thyroiditis has been observed to remit during pregnancy and to relapse after childbirth, sometimes producing transient hyperthyroidism followed by temporary or permanent hypothyroidism. Administration of iodide is another factor with an adverse effect on Hashimoto's disease.

Spontaneous auto-immune thyroiditis with thyroid auto-antibodies and hypothyroidism are encountered in obese-strain chickens. The disease develops shortly after hatching and thyroid epithelial abnormalities appear to precede the development of auto-immunity. Experimental thyroiditis and thyroglobulin autoantibody can be induced by injection of autologous thyroglobulin in Freund's complete adjuvant in genetically susceptible animals possessing appropriate MHC-linked immune response genes homologous to HLA DR in man. Similar lesions can be produced without injection of antigen by neonatal thymectomy to reduce the number of suppressor T-cells.

de Quervain's thyroiditis

Also known as *granulomatous, giant-cell, pseudotuberculous,* or *subacute thyroiditis,* this condition is characterized by sudden onset of painful enlargement of one or both lobes of the thyroid, fever, leucocytosis, diminished thyroidal uptake of radioiodine, and transient hyperthyroidism due to release of iodoprotein from damaged thyroid follicles. At an early stage affected follicles are invaded by neutrophils, but later these are replaced by epithelioid granulomas with one or more multinucleated giant cells centred on the follicular lumina and giving the disease its characteristic histological appearance (Fig. 26.34). Interstitial fibrosis and infiltration with lymphocytes, plasma cells, and macrophages are also features. As a rule, thyroid function returns to normal following recovery. The cause of de Quervain's disease is unknown. Though not familial, there is a strong genetic predisposition associated with HLA Bw35. One outbreak was associated with mumps infection, and more recently de Quervain's disease has been linked with human syncytial virus, a foamy retrovirus. Following the illness there may be transitory production of thyroid auto-antibody but the condition is quite distinct from the thyroid-specific auto-immune diseases.

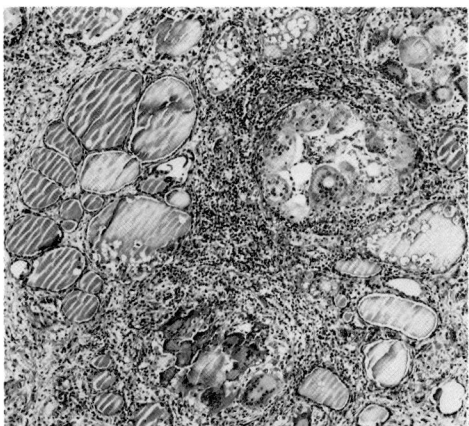

Fig. 26.34 de Quervain's disease. Some of the follicles contain large multinucleated giant cells but others appear normal. There is also stromal fibrosis and lymphoid infiltration.

Riedel's disease

This is an extremely rare form of chronic thyroiditis of unknown aetiology, characterized by a focus of dense fibrosis that completely replaces the affected part of the thyroid and invades the adjacent strap muscles of the neck, to form a hard adherent mass. Obliterative vasculitis affecting both veins and arteries is usually prominent in the fibrotic area and there are chronic non-specific inflammatory changes in the thyroid bordering the lesion (Fig. 26.35). Clinically the lesion simulates a locally invasive tumour. Hypothyroidism does not occur since only part of the gland is involved. The disease is sometimes associated with retroperitoneal or mediastinal fibrosis.

26.2.7   Tumours of the thyroid gland

Thyroid neoplasia is relatively uncommon, having been responsible for only 120 deaths in England and Wales in 1985. A tumour of the thyroid may present clinically as a solitary thyroid nodule, as a rapidly enlarging diffuse goitre (often giving rise to symptoms due to pressure on adjacent structures in the neck), or, in cases with a small primary, as metastatic disease, especially in bone or cervical lymph nodes. Tumours rarely cause hyperthyroidism. In clinical practice it is desirable to exclude other disorders with which thyroid cancer may be confused, and in many cases a positive diagnosis can be established by needle biopsy. However, solitary thyroid nodules sometimes give rise to management problems since, in a minority of cases, the lesion is a well-differentiated follicular carcinoma, which can be diagnosed with confidence only by histological examination of an excision biopsy.

Thyroid tumours form a very heterogeneous group and are generally categorized as shown in Table 26.4. The biological behaviour and prognosis of individual tumours can be predicted largely from their histogenesis and, in the case of those arising from follicular epithelium, the pattern of differentiation

Table 26.4   Classification of thyroid tumours

Benign
  Thyroid adenoma
  Embryonal
  Fetal
  Follicular (including Hürthle cell)
  Atypical
Malignant
  Derived from follicular epithelium
    Well differentiated
      Follicular adenocarcinoma ⎫ (including Hürthle cell and clear
      Papillary adenocarcinoma   ⎭ cell variants)
    Anaplastic
      Small-cell carcinoma
      Giant-cell carcinoma
      Spindle-cell carcinoma
    Others (including squamous carcinoma)
  Derived from parafollicular (C) cells
    Medullary carcinoma
  Others
    Secondary carcinoma
    Malignant lymphoma, including plasmacytoma
    Sarcoma
    Teratoma

(Fig. 26.36). Furthermore, different causal factors can be recognized in the different histogenetic categories.

Thyroid adenoma

Thyroid adenomas are benign tumours derived from follicular epithelium. They are usually solitary, measuring up to 10 cm or more in diameter, and are sharply demarcated from the surrounding gland by a fibrous capsule. On section they may have the brown gelatinous appearance of thyroid colloid or be pink and fleshy if there is little colloid storage. Patchy haemorrhage, cyst formation, fibrosis, and calcification may be present. Under the microscope the epithelial cells are usually uniform in appearance with pale, regularly sized nuclei, inconspicuous nucleoli, and scant mitoses. The cells may be arranged as solid trabeculae (*embryonal adenoma*), minute follicles (*fetal adenoma*), or masses of small follicles containing colloid (*follicular adenoma*). These variations are of no clinical significance, nor is the presence of epithelial cells with the granular oxyphilic cytoplasm characteristic of mitochondrion-rich Askanazy or Hürthle cells (*Hürthle cell adenoma*), or of cellular pleomorphism provided the fibrous capsule is intact (*atypical adenoma*). Adenomas composed of follicles that are lined by columnar epithelium and contain little colloid are sometimes associated with hyperthyroidism (*toxic adenoma*). The fibrous capsule of many adenomas includes whorls of smooth muscle derived from obliterated blood vessels. Some compression of adjacent normal thyroid parenchyma is invariably present.

Most thyroid adenomas take up less radioiodine than the surrounding normal thyroid and, on scanning, appear as 'cold nodules'. In toxic adenoma the scan shows a hot nodule, the rest of the thyroid being cold due to feedback suppression of pituitary TSH. In clinical practice, small nodular goitres are by far the most common cause of apparently solitary hot or cold

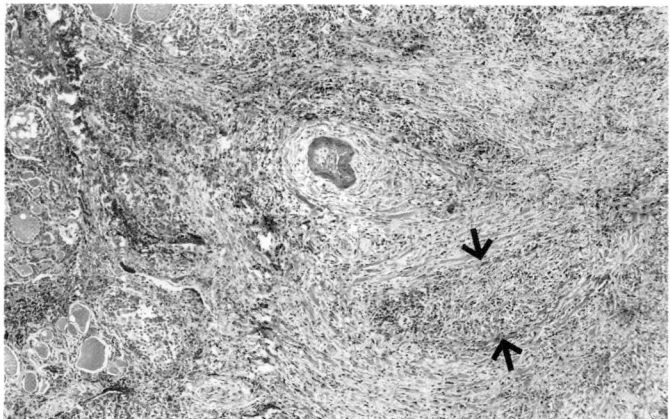

Fig. 26.35   Riedel's disease. Part of a massive area of fibrosis is shown with obliterative vasculitis of a small vein (between arrows) and artery. The adjacent thyroid (left) shows non-specific chronic inflammation.

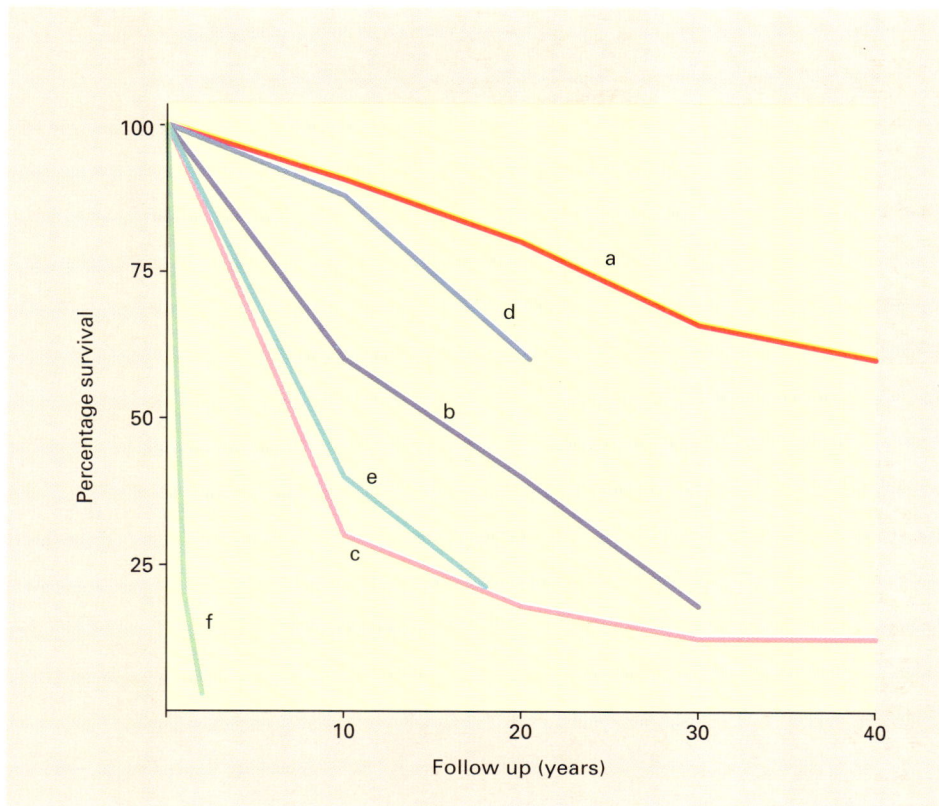

Fig. 26.36 Survival curves in thyroid cancer (after Woolner *et al.* 1968). (a) Occult or intrathyroid papillary carcinoma with or without nodal metastases; (b) papillary carcinoma directly invading perithyroid tissues; (c) follicular carcinoma with moderate or marked invasive growth; (d) medullary carcinoma, negative nodes; (e) medullary carcinoma, positive nodes; (f) anaplastic carcinoma.

thyroid nodules. Pathologically these differ from thyroid adenomas; on section they are seen to be poorly encapsulated and to consist of multiple, closely packed nodules, which are particularly prone to haemorrhage, cyst formation, and calcification; histologically, the presence of large and small follicles irregularly distributed within a single nodule is also distinctive. The differential diagnosis between adenoma and follicular carcinoma of thyroid is considered below.

Follicular carcinoma of thyroid

This tumour is the malignant counterpart of thyroid adenoma, which it sometimes closely resembles clinically and on naked-eye examination (Fig. 26.37). In other cases the tumour is non-encapsulated and infiltrates the surrounding tissues. The neoplastic follicles are usually smaller than normal and solid areas may be present. The tumour often closely resembles normal thyroid (Fig. 26.38) but varying degrees of atypia may be present. In non-encapsulated tumours *invasion of neighbouring normal thyroid* is an important criterion of malignancy. In encapsulated tumours the demonstration of neoplastic follicles *invading thin-walled vascular channels* within the fibrous capsule indicates malignant potential (Fig. 26.39), especially if many vessels are involved. The above diagnostic criteria also apply to *Hürthle-cell* and *clear-cell variants* of follicular carcinoma. It thus follows that unless a thyroglobulin-containing metastatic adenocarcinoma has already been shown to be present, for

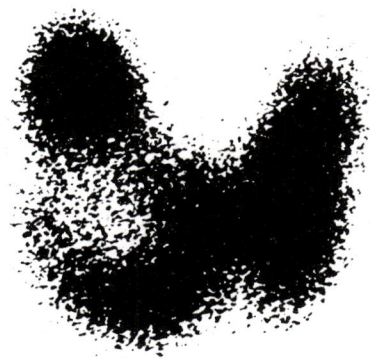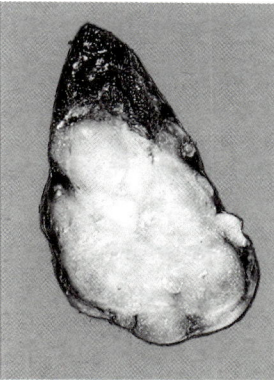

Fig. 26.37 Follicular carcinoma of the thyroid. The tumour presented as a thyroid nodule which appeared as a cold area in the thyroid scan (left). Right lobectomy was carried out and a section (right) showed a pale encapsulated mass replacing the lower part of the specimen.

example by needle biopsy (Fig. 26.40), the diagnosis of well-differentiated follicular carcinoma of the thyroid depends on histological examination of multiple sections taken from the surgically excised tumour to establish the presence of invasive growth. Poorly differentiated follicular carcinoma, such as that shown in Fig. 26.41, can readily be diagnosed by needle biopsy.

Follicular carcinoma may occur at any age but predominantly affects patients in their forties, particularly females. It

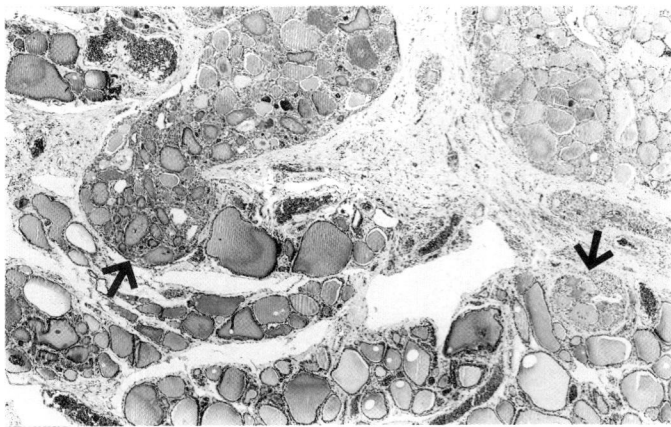

Fig. 26.38 Follicular carcinoma of the thyroid (same case as Fig. 26.37). The tumour (top right) is well differentiated and composed of follicles which closely resemble those of the normal thyroid (below and left). Note that the tumour penetrates the fibrous capsule at two points (arrows).

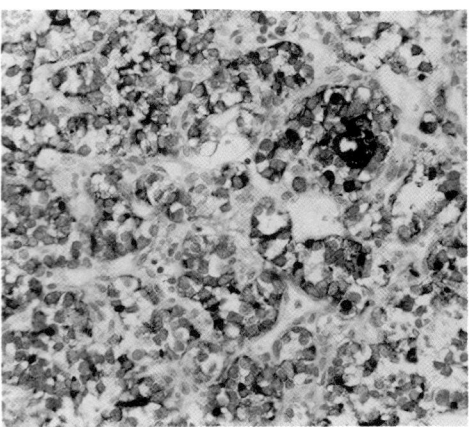

Fig. 26.40 Metastatic follicular carcinoma of the thyroid. The patient presented with an intracranial tumour and biopsy revealed a follicular adenocarcinoma which was shown to originate in the thyroid by the presence of thyroglobulin (black) in tumour cells and follicles. (Indirect immunoperoxidase.)

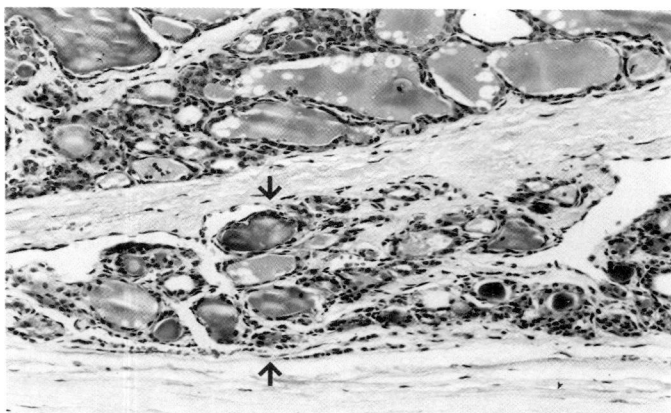

Fig. 26.39 Follicular carcinoma of thyroid (same case as Figs. 26.37 and 26.38). A thin-walled vascular channel (arrowed) in the fibrous capsule contains neoplastic follicles covered with endothelium. Part of the main tumour is seen above. Capsular vascular invasion is an important sign of malignancy in a well-differentiated encapsulated follicular carcinoma.

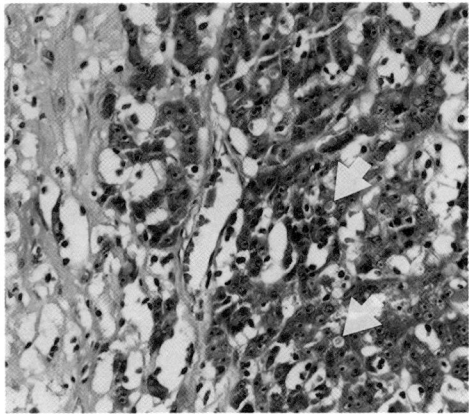

Fig. 26.41 Poorly differentiated follicular carcinoma. The tumour is composed of sheets of atypical cells with the formation of occasional microfollicles (white arrows). Note the prominent nucleoli and area of old necrosis.

tends to metastasize by the bloodstream to lung and bone, involvement of regional lymph nodes being uncommon. Patients with metastases, particularly from well-differentiated tumours, may survive for many years.

Papillary carcinoma

The gross appearance of this interesting tumour varies considerably from case to case. Most are irregular in outline, non-encapsulated, and hard and white with cystic spaces. A few are well encapsulated and closely resemble follicular tumours, but thin-walled cysts containing colloid and papillary projections may be visible to the naked eye. In about one-third of the cases the primary is a clinically inapparent, predominantly fibrous nodule less than 1.5 cm in diameter (*occult sclerosing carcinoma*

of the thyroid) and the disease presents with metastatic deposits in the cervical lymph nodes.

Histological diagnosis is usually straightforward and is based on the presence of cystic follicles with characteristic papillary ingrowths composed of a fibrous core covered with epithelial cells (Fig. 26.42). The epithelium is usually cuboidal or columnar and may be several layers thick. Occasionally there is extensive *squamous metaplasia* and some tumours are composed of Hürthle cells. Often the tumour is multicentric with microscopic papillary lesions in the surrounding normal thyroid and sometimes in the contralateral lobe, appearances that are probably the result of intrathyroidal spread. When even a few typical papillae are present in a predominantly follicular tumour, the lesion is likely to behave as a papillary carcinoma and should be diagnosed as such. In such cases the diagnosis is sometimes first

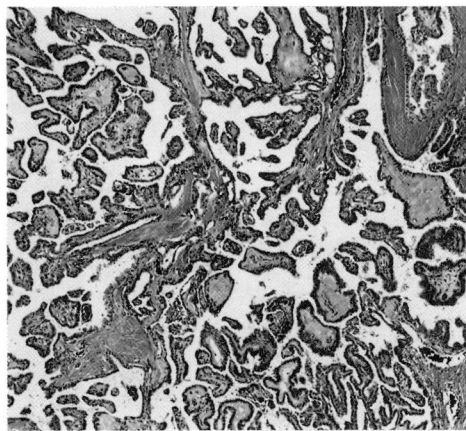

Fig. 26.42 Papillary adenocarcinoma of the thyroid. Typical appearance of cystic spaces containing papillae with fibrovascular cores covered with neoplastic epithelial cells.

suspected from the findings of laminated basophilic *psammoma bodies* in the stroma, or a peculiar 'ground-glass' or 'empty' appearance of the nuclei of the tumour cells ('Orphan Annie') (Fig. 26.43), features which, when present, are highly suggestive of papillary rather than follicular carcinoma. There is little point in attempting to distinguish papillary carcinoma from benign papillary adenoma.

Papillary carcinoma of thyroid is a most remarkable tumour. Affected patients, commonly young women, have a virtually normal expectation of life, even when lymph node metastases are present and left untreated (Fig. 26.36). The tumour is hormone sensitive and suppression of pituitary TSH with thyroxine can lead to shrinkage of lesions. Spontaneous regression also occurs, as shown by the presence of psammoma bodies in tumour-free lymph nodes of individuals with the disease. Small, clinically inapparent tumours are found at post-mortem in

several per cent of the population. Local invasion of extra-thyroidal tissue from the primary is uncommon but may lead to death from laryngeal involvement. Other unfavourable prognostic factors include: advanced age at onset and progression of the tumour to anaplastic cacinoma. Metastasis to lymph nodes is common but haematogenous spread to lung or bone is exceptional.

Anaplastic carcinoma of thyroid

This rare tumour usually causes rapid unilateral thyroid enlargement and often gives rise to stridor and difficulty in swallowing. The tumour is ill-defined, necrotic, and adherent to adjacent tissues. *Small-cell*, *giant-cell* (Fig. 26.44), and *spindle-cell varieties* are encountered. The tumour cells synthesize little or no thyroglobulin. Death is usually due to local invasion and compression of surrounding structures in the neck, but widespread metastases may also be present.

Causation of tumours of follicular epithelium

There is good epidemiological evidence that *ionizing radiation* is a significant cause of thyroid tumours. The frequency of adenoma and follicular and papillary carcinoma is increased in survivors of atomic explosions. External X-ray irradiation to the neck for the treatment of birthmarks or supposed thymic enlargement in childhood leads to the same group of tumours. Thyroid tumours can be induced in experimental animals by moderate doses of *radioiodine* and the number is greatly increased if goitrogens are administered to promote thyroid growth. It is noteworthy that doses of radioactive iodine that are large enough to reduce thyroid function (for example, in the treatment of hyperthyroidism) do not lead to clinically apparent tumour formation.

There is considerable geographical variation in the incidence of papillary and follicular tumours. The frequency of follicular carcinoma is said to be increased in nodular goitre associated with low dietary iodine, but the risk is very small. Evidence of

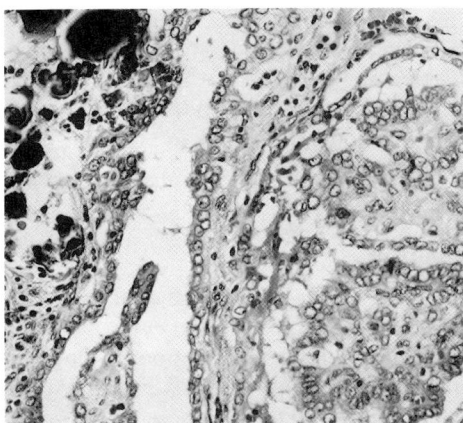

Fig. 26.43 Papillary adenocarcinoma of the thyroid, with typical 'ground-glass' nuclei and laminated calcified psammoma bodies. If present, these features can be of value in distinguishing between papillary and follicular carcinoma when the diagnosis is in doubt.

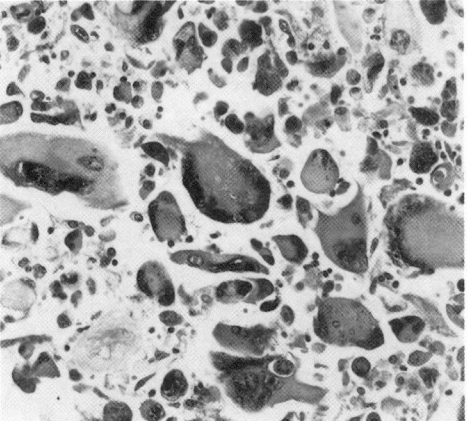

Fig. 26.44 Anaplastic carcinoma of the thyroid, giant-cell type. Compared with normal follicular epithelium (Fig. 26.18a) the multinucleated tumour cells are very large.

pre-existing low-grade follicular or papillary tumours is found in most cases of anaplastic carcinoma.

Activation of ras oncogenes by point mutation occurs at an early stage in the development of follicular tumours with increased expression of transforming growth factor beta in the malignant phase. Such changes are less common in papillary carcinomas, some of which have rearrangements to the tyrosine kinase domain of the ret proto-oncogene.

Medullary carcinoma

This tumour is derived from *parafollicular* (*C*) cells and occurs in two forms. In *sporadic cases* there is usually a single, sharply defined and sometimes ecapsulated mass up to 10 cm in diameter. The *familial form* of the disease is symmetrical, with tumours affecting both lateral lobes. When diagnosed early the lesions may be only 1–2 mm in diameter. Histologically the tumour cells are polyhedral or spindle shaped and are characteristically arranged in solid nests (Fig. 26.45). The cytoplasm is granular, argyrophilic, and it contains *calcitonin* which can be demonstrated by immunocytochemistry (Fig. 26.46). Electron microscopy shows the presence of *neurosecretory granules*. Mitoses are usually scanty. Some tumours contain entrapped follicles of normal thyroid but in a small proportion of cases neoplastic follicles are formed by tumour cells which may contain both thyroglobulin and calcitonin, a finding which raises interesting questions about the supposed neuroectodermal origin of the C-cells. In familial cases, the tumour may be preceded or accompanied by C-cell hyperplasia. An important, though not invariable, diagnostic feature is the presence in the stroma of deposits of endocrine amyloid which incorporate calcitonin and often show patchy calcification. When the disease is restricted to the thyroid the prognosis is very good, but lymph-node metastasis is associated with a 40 per cent ten-year survival (Fig. 26.36). Sometimes there is a rapid downhill course with extensive metastases.

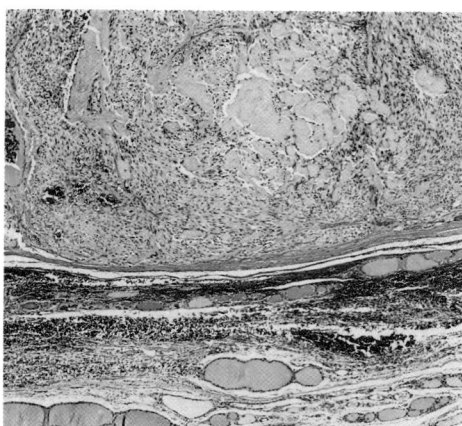

Fig. 26.45   Medullary carcinoma of the thyroid. The tumour (above) is separated from normal thyroid (below) by a fibrous capsule. Note the solid nests of spindle-shaped C-cells and hyaline masses of amyloid within the tumour.

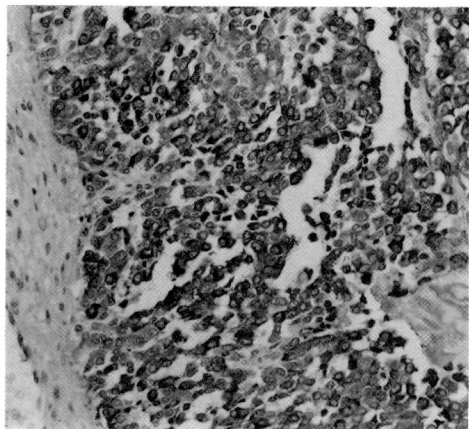

Fig. 26.46   Medullary carcinoma of the thyroid. Calcitonin (black) is seen in the cytoplasm of the tumour cells but not in the stromal cells (left). (Indirect immunoperoxidase.)

Medullary carcinoma has interesting endocrine and genetic aspects. Calcitonin is secreted with no ill-effects but it provides an excellent marker for the early detection of affected family members. For the diagnosis of small tumours, *pentagastrin* may be administered to increase the level of calcitonin in the blood. Sometimes Cushing's syndrome results from ectopic ACTH production by the tumour, while diarrhoea, which is troublesome in a third of patients, has been variously attributed to secretion of serotonin, bradykinin, and prostaglandins.

In the familial forms, medullary carcinoma is inherited as a Mendelian dominant. In some families it is accompanied by *bilateral phaeochromocytomas* and *parathyroid hyperplasia* or *adenoma* (*multiple endocrine neoplasia, type IIA*). The abnormal gene is inherited on chromosome 10 but a second (somatic) mutation often occurs in chromosome 1 before the tumours develop. In *Sipple's syndrome* (*multiple endocrine neoplasia type IIB*), medullary carcinoma is associated with phaeochromocytoma, mucosal neuromas (Fig. 26.47), and long, thin limbs.

Histologically, *endocrine amyloid* in medullary carcinoma is quite unlike AA amyloidosis secondary to rheumatoid arthritis, chronic infection, etc., which may affect the thyroid and cause firm diffuse enlargement of the gland. The typical appearance of amyloid goitre is shown in Fig. 26.48, the follicles being lined by flat epithelium and separated by hyaline stroma containing numerous adipocytes.

Thyroid lymphomas

Before the advent of immunocytochemical methods of distinguishing anaplastic lymphoid and epithelial tumours, most primary thyroid lymphomas were wrongly diagnosed as anaplastic small-cell carcinomas. Now it is clear that *plasmacytomas* and malignant lymphomas like those of mucosa-associated lymphoid tissues arise in Hashimoto's disease, presumably from lymphoid cells participating in the auto-immune reaction. There is sometimes difficulty in distinguishing morphologically between florid examples of lymphoid hyperplasia in auto-

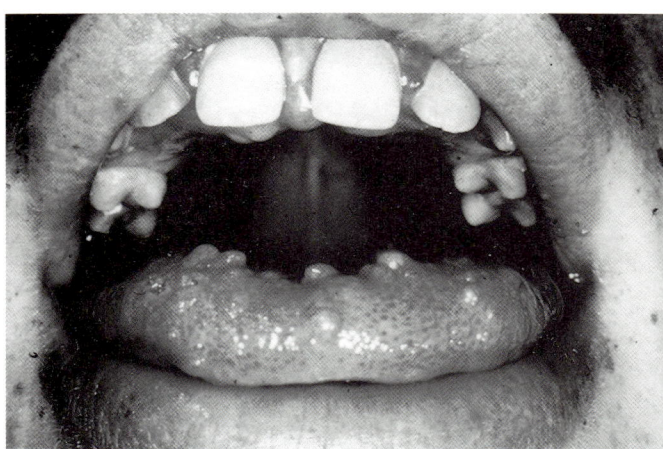

Fig. 26.47 Mucosal neuromas in Sipple's syndrome. A young man was noted by his dentist to have swellings of his tongue and conjunctivae. Biopsy showed mucosal neuromas which led to the discovery of medullary carcinoma and bilateral phaeochromocytomas.

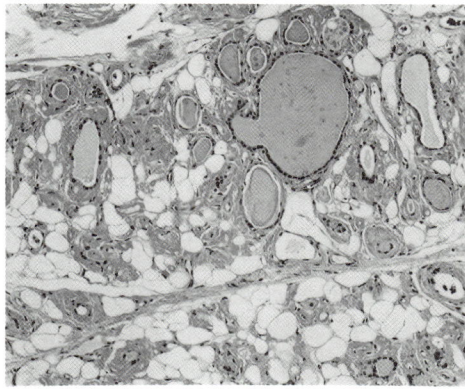

Fig. 26.48 Amyloid goitre. Follicles lined by flat epithelium are separated by hyaline (amyloid) stroma containing numerous adipocytes.

immune thyroiditis and well-differentiated thyroid follicular lymphoma, a problem that can be resolved by tests for monotypic immunoglobulin or immunoglobulin gene rearrangements. Thyroid lymphoma commonly infiltrates the surrounding tissues and spread sometimes takes place to gut-associated lymphoid tissue in the small intestine. Elderly females are usually affected and often give a history of recent rapid growth of a long-standing goitre. Large-cell lymphomas usually lead to death in a few months, but there are some long survivals.

26.2.8 Further reading

General

Hoffenberg, R. (1987). Thyroid disorders. In *Oxford textbook of medicine* (2nd edn) (ed. D. J. Weatherall, J. G. G. Ledingham, and D. A. Warrell). Oxford University Press.

Johnson, R. L. and Hartmann, W. H. (1983). The thyroid. In *Principles and practice of surgical pathology* (ed. S. G. Silverberg). John Wiley and Sons, New York.

McGregor, A. M. (1986). *Immunology of endocrine diseases*. MTP Press, Lancaster.

Rosai, J. (1981). Thyroid gland. In *Ackerman's surgical pathology* (6th edn). C. V. Mosby, St. Louis.

Sommers, S. C. (1982). Thyroid gland, In *Endocrine pathology, general and surgical* (2nd edn) (ed. J. M. B. Bloodworth). Williams and Wilkins, Baltimore.

Recent developments

Burt, A. D., Kerr, D. J., Brown, I. L., and Bolye, P. (1985). Lymphoid and epithelial markers in small cell anaplastic lymphoid tumours. *Journal of Clinical Pathology* **39**, 893.

Knight, J., Laing, P., Knight, A., Adams, D., and Ling, N. (1986). Thyroid-stimulating autoantibodies usually contain only lambda light chains: evidence for the 'Forbidden Clone' theory. *Journal of Clinical Endocrinology and Metabolism* **62**, 342.

Londei, M., Lamb, J. R., Bottazzo, G. F., and Feldmann, M. (1984). Epithelial cells expressing aberrant MHC class II determinants can present antigen to cloned human T cells. *Nature* **312**, 639.

Mathew C. G. P., Smith, B. A., Thorpe, K., Wong, Z., Royle, N. J., Jeffries, A. J., and Ponder, B. A. J. (1987). Deletion of genes on chromosome 1 in endocrine neoplasia. *Nature* **328**, 524.

Perrone, T. (1986). Mixed medullary–follicular thyroid carcinoma. *American Journal of Surgical Pathology* **10**, 362.

Peters, H. J., Gerber, H., Studer, H., and Smeds, H. (1985). Pathogenesis of heterogeneity in human multinodular goitre: a study on growth and function of thyroid tissue transplanted onto nude mice. *Journal of Clinical Investigation* **76**, 1992.

Ramsay, I. (1986). Postpartum thyroiditis—an underdiagnosed disease. *British Journal of Obstetrics and Gynaecology* **93**, 1121.

Sap, J., Munoz, A., Damm, K., Goldberg, Y., Ghysdael, J., Leutz, A., Beug, H., and Vennstrom, B. (1986). The c-erbA protein is a high affinity receptor for thyroid hormone. *Nature* **324**, 635.

Smith, P., Williams, E. D., and Wynford-Thomas, D. (1987). *In vitro* demonstration of a TSH-specific growth desensitising mechanism in rat thyroid epithelium. *Molecular and Cellular Endocrinology* **51**, 51.

Werner, J. and Gelderblom, H. (1979). Isolation of foamy virus from patients with deQuervain thyroiditis. *Lancet* **ii**, 258.

Woolner, L. B., Bearhs, O. H., McConahey, W. M., Keating, F. R., and Black, B. M. (1968). Thyroid carcinoma: general considerations and follow up data on 1181 cases. In *Thyroid neoplasia* (ed. S. Young and D. R. Inman). Academic Press, London.

26.3 Parathyroid glands

H. A. Ellis

26.3.1 Introduction

Ivar Sandström (1879) is credited with the first detailed description of the human parathyroid glands. He began his studies in 1877 while still a medical student at Uppsala University. The glands are found in all terrestrial vertebrates. Although small and frequently overlooked in the anatomical dissecting room and by pathologists at necropsy, the parathyroids are of paramount importance in the regulation of calcium and phosphorus homeostasis.

In man there are generally four parathyroid glands, with five glands being present in about 6 per cent and six glands in 0.4 per cent of the population. The two upper glands, derived from the *fourth pharyngeal pouch*, undergo a short embryonic migration and are relatively constant in position on the dorso-medial aspect of the thyroid lobes, about half-way between the upper and lower poles. The two lower glands, derived from the *third pharyngeal pouch*, are located at or near the posterior surfaces of the lower poles of the thyroid. Parathyroid development is closely related to that of the thymus and one or more glands may be embedded in thymic tissue. The lower glands may be 'carried' with thymic tissue during development well below the level of the thyroid, sometimes as far as the anterior mediastinum. Occasionally the glands lie just beneath the capsule of the thyroid or are deeply embedded in its substance. These variations in the number and location of the parathyroid glands are of more than academic interest to the surgeon when undertaking operations to remove diseased parathyroid glands.

A knowledge of the structure and functions of the normal parathyroid glands is essential for an understanding of the histopathology and pathophysiology of parathyroid disease.

26.3.2   The normal parathyroid

Each parathyroid is a pale yellow or light to dark tan coloured, more-or-less flattened ovoid, measuring about 6 × 3 × 1.5 mm in the adult, but glands may be moulded by adjacent structures to become elongated or compressed. Individual glands weigh from as little as 7.5 mg up to 75 mg, but average about 20–40 mg. In one subject, individual glands can vary in weight by as much as 100 per cent, but the combined weight of four glands is about 130 mg for normal women and 120 mg for normal men. Parathyroid parenchymal tissue accounts for about 70 per cent of these weights.

Parathyroid gland structure

The histology of the parathyroid glands changes from infancy to old age. Glands of the new-born comprise sheets and cords of uniform parenchymal chief cells, are richly vascularized, and do not include interstitial fat cells or oxyphil cells. The glands of older children and adults (Fig. 26.49) include a variable amount of interstitial fat (from almost nil up to 50 per cent or more of the gland) and there are two main types of parenchymal cells present—the *chief (principal) cells* and the *oxyphil cells*. Light microscopy reveals principal cells with a uniform, dark-staining cytoplasm (dark chief cells) or cells with some degree of vacuolization due to the presence of glycogen and lipid. These are known as *transitional and clear chief cells*. Oxyphil cells appear first near puberty as isolated cells amongst the chief cells, and their numbers increase with age to form aggregates or even micronodules up to 1–2 mm in diameter in the aged. The

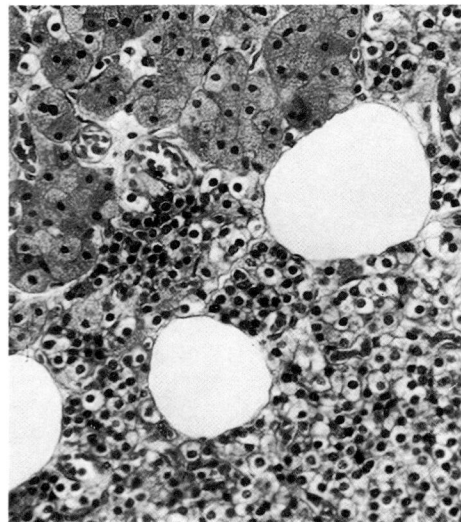

Fig. 26.49   Normal adult (male, 67 years) parathyroid tissue, comprising chief cells (mainly clear type), oxyphil cells with granular cytoplasm, (top left), and fat cells.

oxyphil cell cytoplasm is rich in eosinophilic granules. Electron microscopy (Nilson 1977), reveals that these granules are large mitochondria which pack the cytoplasm leaving little space for other organelles (Fig. 26.50). The cytoplasm of chief cells includes rough endoplasmic reticulum (RER), a Golgi complex, smaller and fewer mitochondria, and membrane-bound secretory granules. There are varying amounts of lipid complexes and glycogen. The oxyphil cells are derived from chief cells, and intermediate forms known as *transitional oxyphils* occur with increased numbers of mitochondria, although they also contain RER, a Golgi complex, and secretory granules.

Cellular pathways of biosynthesis, secretion, and degradation of parathormone

Although all varieties of parathyroid cells are capable of synthesizing parathormone, the oxyphil cells play little or no part in this process in the normal gland. Individual chief cells undergo a cycle of hormone synthesis and secretion with an intervening resting phase, and there are corresponding appearances on electron microscopy. Resting cells have abundant lipid and glycogen and the RER, Golgi complex, and secretory granules are inconspicuous. During hormone synthesis intracellular glycogen and lipid are diminished and the RER becomes prominent and aggregated into parallel arrays, the Golgi complex enlarges, and secretory granules appear on its surface.

Nature and biosynthesis of parathormone

Parathormone is a single-chain polypeptide comprising 84 amino acids (MW 9600) but the hormone has several precursors (Fig. 26.51). The first formed is *preproparathormone*, a polypeptide comprising 115 amino acids which is synthesized on ribosomes attached to the cisternae of the RER, the specific

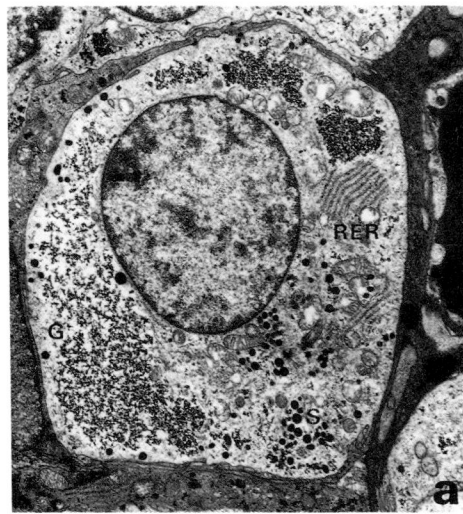

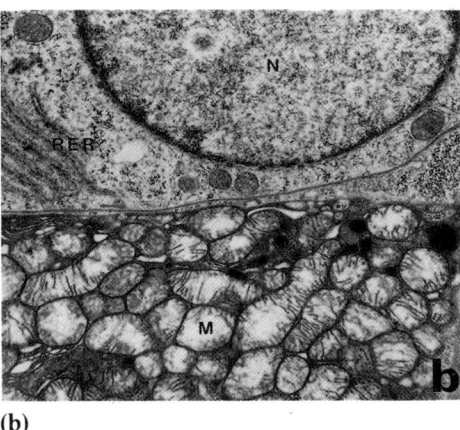

(b)

Fig. 26.50 Ultrastructure of (a) a chief cell with stacked rough endoplasmic reticulum (RER), mitochondria, secretory granules (S) and glycogen (G); (b) parts of adjacent chief and oxyphil cells with numerous closely packed large mitochondria (M) in the latter (lower half).

amino-acid sequence being determined by mRNA-encoded information. Preproparathormone comprises an 'initiator' peptide (-30, -31), a signal or 'leader' sequence (-29, to -7) and the proparathormone component. The 'leader' component facilitates transport of the hormone peptide chain into the lumen of the RER and during this process the preproparathormone is immediately converted by proteolytic cleavage to *proparathormone*, comprising a chain of 90 amino acids which is now enclosed in the cisternal lumen of the RER. Proparathormone is transferred within minutes to the Golgi complex where it is converted by further proteolytic cleavage into *parathormone*. This is then packaged into secretory granules for transport to the cell surface where the membranes of the granules fuse with the cell membrane and discharge their contents (exocytosis) into the extracellular space. Parathormone may be secreted from the cell shortly after synthesis, or stored in membrane-bound secretory granules within the cell. Some 'unwanted' parathormone passes to the cytoplasm where it is cleaved and degraded by lysosomal activity. Fragments of hormone as well as intact parathormone are secreted.

Circulating parathormone

Peripheral metabolism of intact secreted parathormone occurs primarily in the Kupffer cells of the liver, the hormone being cleaved into a biologically active amino-terminal fragment (1 to 34) and a carboxy-terminal fragment which appears to be biologically inactive (Fig. 26.51). The latter fragment constitutes the major form of circulating parathormone. The parathyroid glands secrete carboxy-terminal fragments, and possibly amino-terminal fragments, as well as intact parathormone and the kidney is responsible for clearance of carboxy-terminal fragments, however derived. Proteolytic metabolism of parathormone in the glands, liver, kidney, and bone result in a short-lived amino-terminal fragment. The heterogeneity of hormone fragments in the circulation has led to the development of a wide variety of assays.

Assay of parathormone An ideal assay should measure the biologically active molecule. In clinical practice, levels of circulating parathormone are commonly determined by means of *radioimmunoassay* (Armitage 1986) using antibodies directed against one or more of the hormone fragments (*immunoreactive parathormone, iPTH*). The alternative cytochemical bioassays for parathormone give values suggesting that only about 10 per cent of circulating hormone as detected by radioimmunoassay is biologically active. The bioassay technique is complicated and not a practical alternative to radioimmunoassay in routine clinical practice. In hypoparathyroidism the serum iPTH is diminished or undetectable; in hyperparathyroidism, serum iPTH (both intact parathormone and carboxy-terminal fragments) is increased or inappropriately normal in the presence of hypercalcaemia. Since the major circulating component is the carboxy-terminal fragment, this is more readily detectable by radioimmunoassay and, although not biologically active, determination of this fragment has proved useful clinically in the diagnosis of parathyroid disorders.

Functions of parathormone

The level of serum ionized calcium plays a major role in the control of parathyroid gland activity. A fall causes increased parathormone secretion whereas a rise inhibits release of parathormone and accelerates intraglandular hormone degradation, the inactive carboxy-terminal fragment being the major secretory product. Changes in calcium ion concentration also regulate the biosynthesis of new hormone, probably by controlling the number of mRNA molecules that are synthesized.

Parathormone controls serum calcium and phosphorus in three ways:

1. by mobilizing calcium from bone;
2. by *stimulating reabsorption of calcium* and *inhibiting reabsorption of phosphate by the renal tubules*; and

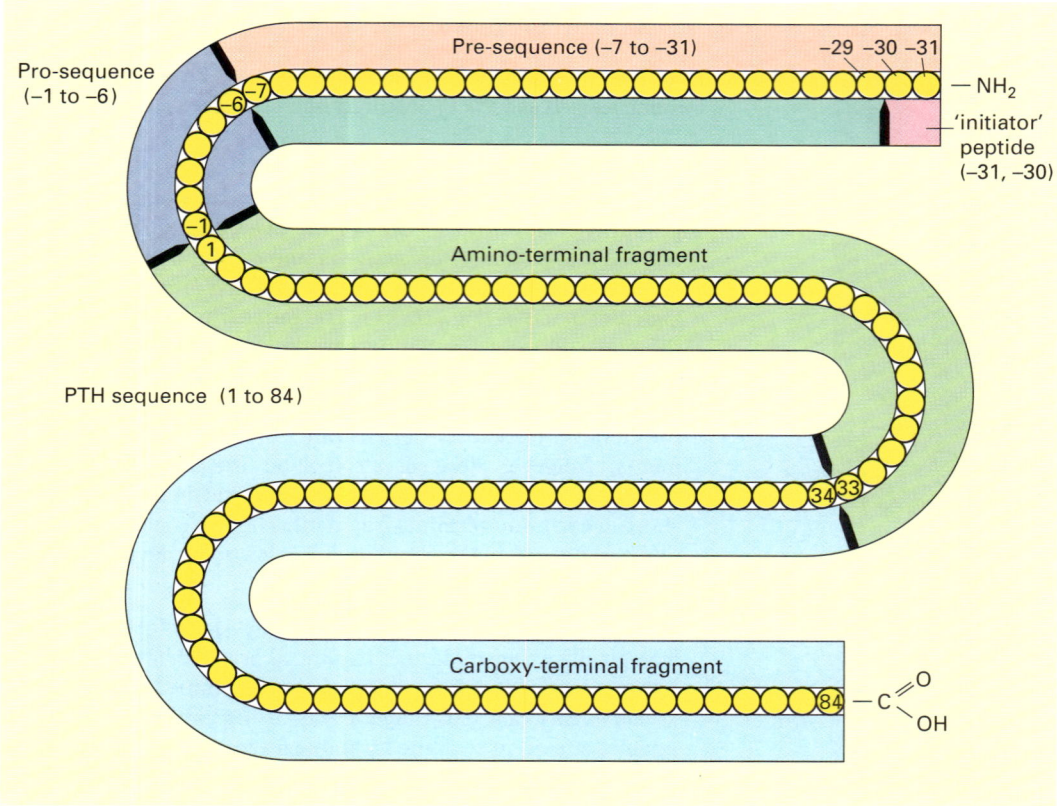

Fig. 26.51   Diagram of the nature of parathormone and its precursors.

3. indirectly by *increasing the activity of renal tubular 25(OH)D₃ 1α-hydroxylase to stimulate the conversion of 1,25(OH)D₃ to the active vitamin D metabolite 1,25(OH)₂D₃*. This in turn increases small intestinal absorption of calcium and phosphorus. There are receptors for $1,25(OH)_2D_3$ in the parathyroid cells and a *negative feedback mechanism* exists by which $1,25(OH)_2D_3$ inhibits synthesis of parathormone by the glands.

Mechanism of parathormone action
Parathormone binds to specific cell-membrane receptors in the target organs (kidney and bone) to activate adenylate cyclase, resulting in an increased intracellular formation of cyclic AMP from adenosine triphosphate. In turn, cyclic AMP activates a sequence of intracellular events that are responsible for the effects of parathormone in bone and kidney.

Calcitonin
Although we are here concerned with disturbances of metabolism brought about by diseases of the parathyroid glands, it should be appreciated that the calcitonins, which are secreted by the *C-cells* (*parafollicular cells*) of the thyroid (see Section 26.2), also play a role in the regulation of mineral homeostasis (Martin 1985). Calcitonin inhibits osteoclastic resorption of bone and retards the transfer of calcium from bone to the extra-

cellular fluid and blood. Secretion (release) of calcitonin is suppressed by hypocalcaemia and stimulated by hypercalcaemia. Calcitonin secretion is partly meal-related, release of calcitonin being produced by gastrin and enteroglucagon secreted during digestion, as well as by the intake of calcium-rich food. Patients with chronic hypercalcaemia due to vitamin D intoxication or hyperparathyroidism often have C-cell hyperplasia and increased levels of circulating calcitonin.

26.3.3   Disturbances of parathyroid structure and function
Diseases of the parathyroid glands will be considered in relation to whether they are associated with hyper- or hypofunction.

Parathyroid hyperfunction
Hyperfunction of the parathyroid may be (1) *primary* or (2) *secondary* in type. In *primary hyperparathyroidism* there is excessive secretion of parathormone by the diseased gland(s) in the absence of any known extraglandular stimulus. The primary parathyroid abnormality may be *hyperplasia*, *adenoma*, or *carcinoma*. In contrast, *secondary hyperparathyroidism* develops as a result of compensatory hyperplasia in response to increased stimulation mediated by hypocalcaemia. The hypocalcaemia

may be the result, for example, of nutritional vitamin D deficiency, intestinal malabsorption, or from the disordered vitamin D metabolism in patients with chronic renal failure. In some patients with prolonged secondary hyperparathyroidism, the glands eventually appear to become 'autonomous' with regard to both their growth and hyperfunction, and troublesome hypercalcaemia develops simulating the effects of primary hyperparathyroidism. St Goar suggested that the term 'tertiary' hyperparathyroidism was appropriate for such cases.

Primary hyperparathyroidism

Incidence and modes of presentation

Primary hyperparathyroidism occurs in 1–2 per 1000 of the population. Although no age is exempt, middle-aged adults are most commonly affected. Excess parathormone causes hypercalcaemia and hypophosphataemia from its action on bone (increased mobilization) and the kidneys (increased tubular reabsorption of calcium and diminished reabsorption of phosphate, with hyperphosphaturia). Although parathormone reduces tubular clearance of calcium, the hypercalcaemia still results in hypercalciuria.

The symptoms may be many and varied (Potts 1987). The relatively recent practice of determining the serum calcium as part of routine medical examinations has led to an increase in the detection of asymptomatic patients with hypercalcaemia due to hyperparathyroidism, and in some centres as many as half the patients are asymptomatic at the time of diagnosis. Renal stones of calcium phosphate or calcium oxalate, especially when recurrent, often provide the first indication that there is hyperparathyroidism. Before the introduction of biochemical screening tests about 60–70 per cent of patients presented with renal complications but the incidence is now lower. The calcium-rich calculi are visible on X-radiography. There may be parenchymal calcification and fibrosis of the kidneys (nephrosclerosis) with loss of nephrons and eventually chronic renal failure. Metastatic calcification may also be found in the elastic lamellae and tunica media of arteries, in the lungs in bronchial and alveolar walls, and in the gastric mucosa or myocardium.

Symptoms relating to the effects of excess parathormone on bone (osteitis fibrosa), such as bone pain and fractures, are relatively uncommon. Von Recklinghausen in 1891, when giving his classical account of generalized osteitis fibrosa cystica, was unaware of the parathyroid origin of the disease, and although Askanazy in 1903 had observed a case of von Recklinghausen's disease of bone associated with a parathyroid tumour, it was not fully accepted that the bone changes were the result of hyperparathyroidism until 1926 when Mandl, the Viennese surgeon, successfully treated a case by parathyroidectomy (Mandl 1947). Only about 15 per cent of patients have X-radiographic evidence of bone disease, such as subperiosteal resorptions of the phalanges, and even fewer have so-called 'brown cysts' (osteitis fibrosa cystica). A transiliac bone biopsy is a much more sensitive means of detecting hyperparathyroidism, many patients showing some degree of histological osteitis fibrosa. There is increased bone turnover with excess osteoclastic resorption,

and increased bone formation by prominent surface osteoblasts. The plasma alkaline phosphatase activity (bone isoenzyeme) is then increased. In spite of the increased bone turnover, in most patients the balance between bone formation and resorption is sustained, although in some patients there is a negative balance eventually leading to clinically significant osteoporosis. The more severe symptoms of bone disease tend to occur in patients with rapidly growing large adenomas or carcinoma of the parathyroids.

Hypercalcaemia may be associated with general lassitude, polyuria, thirst, muscular weakness, anorexia, and vague gastrointestinal symptoms. Nervous manifestations from mild personality disorders to severe psychosis may occur. Duodenal ulceration is commoner than in the general population.

Parathyroids in primary hyperparathyroidism

It is usually stated that about 80 per cent of cases of primary hyperparathyroidism are the result of an adenoma, with primary hyperplasia of all glands accounting for 16 per cent and parathyroid carcinoma for 4 per cent of cases. In practice it may be difficult to distinguish between an adenoma and primary hyperplasia, particularly when only one diseased gland is available for microscopic examination, and some so-called 'adenomas' are undoubtedly examples of hyperplasia masquerading as adenomas.

Primary hyperplasia

There are two distinct types of primary parathyroid hyperplasia: (1) water-clear ('Wasserhelle') cell hyperplasia; and (2) chief-cell hyperplasia.

Primary water-clear cell hyperplasia This was the first to be recognized, in the early 1930s. All the glands are markedly enlarged, mahogany brown, and lobulated, and in 80 per cent of cases weigh 5–10 g or more. The upper glands are often larger than the lower glands. Microscopically there is a uniform hyperplasia with characteristic large cells, up to 40 μm in diameter, more-or-less filled by intracytoplasmic vacuoles, giving a 'clear cell' appearance. A tubular architecture may give rise to an appearance reminiscent of that of a renal tubular clear-cell carcinoma. On electron microscopy the membrane-bound vacuoles appear empty and are presumed to be derived from the RER or the Golgi complex, and the cells may contain the usual secretory granules in addition. It should be stressed that these clear cells of primary hyperplasia are quite distinct from the transitional and clear-cell varieties of chief cells which occur in normal and diseased glands and in which the vacuolation results from the presence of intracytoplasmic glycogen (see above).

For some unexplained reason, primary water-clear cell hyperplasia is much less common now than it was in the past, and currently probably accounts for only 1–2 per cent of cases of primary hyperplasia.

Primary chief-cell hyperplasia Chief-cell hyperplasia was not fully accepted as a cause of primary hyperparathyroidism until the late 1950s (Castleman *et al.* 1976). Previously it had been thought that primary hyperplasia was always of the water-clear cell variety and chief-cell hyperplasia was considered to occur only in secondary parathyroid disease. The glands are all enlarged, but generally less so than in water-clear cell hyperplasia, and are pale to dark tan. Although the combined weight may be between 5 and 10 g, larger glands are uncommon, and in about 55 per cent of patients the combined glands weigh less than 1 g. In about half the patients the glands are more-or-less equally enlarged, but in the others one gland may be much enlarged while the rest are slightly affected and may even appear more-or-less normal to the surgeon. In such cases the single large gland may be mistaken at operation for an adenoma.

Microscopically, in primary hyperplasia there are initially multiple islands of hyperplastic tissue within otherwise relatively normal tissue, which often includes interstitial fat cells. Later, the whole gland becomes diffusely hyperplastic or there are discrete areas of nodularly hyperplastic tissue. Relatively unaffected parts of a gland may be pushed aside and compressed by hyperplastic nodule(s) and the appearance may then closely resemble that of an adenoma. The hyperplastic tissue comprises uniform chief cells or a mixture of chief cells, transitional oxyphil cells, and oxyphil cells. There is some cellular and nuclear enlargement, and careful search reveals very occasional normal mitoses (which are never found in normal glands) in about 60 per cent of cases. Electron microscopy reveals parathyroid cells in various stages of the secretory cycle, and active cells show conspicuous plasmalemmal convolutions.

Parathyroid adenoma

An adenoma is a benign neoplasm with an expansile growth which compresses surrounding parathyroid tissue from which it is clearly demarcated, often with a thick fibrous capsule which may be patchily calcified. Most are small and are not clinically palpable. They measure from as little as 10 mm in maximum dimension to 50 mm and weigh from less than 1 g to 20 g or more. Generally, there is one adenoma only but multiple adenomas occur occasionally. The displaced normal parathyroid tissue, with its adipose interstitium and located at the pole or to one side of the adenoma, contrasts sharply with the cellular adenoma, which lacks adipose tissue (Fig. 26.52). The adenoma may be a single homogeneous mass or composed of nodules with fibrous septa. Commonly, one cell type predominates in the adenoma but there may be various mixtures of chief cells, including transitional and clear chief cells, transitional oxyphil cells, and oxyphil cells. Occasional cases of primary hyperparathyroidism are due to a *pure hyperfunctioning oxyphil cell adenoma*. The architectural arrangement of cells is variable and may cause diagnostic confusion when examining intra-operative frozen sections. This is particularly likely when there are numerous acinar formations with eosinophilic colloid, and the tissue is mistaken for a *microfollicular area of thyroid*. The parathyroid cells and their nuclei are generally slightly enlarged and, as in hyperplasia, occasional normal mitoses may be found in 60–70 per cent of cases. In addition, there may be scattered

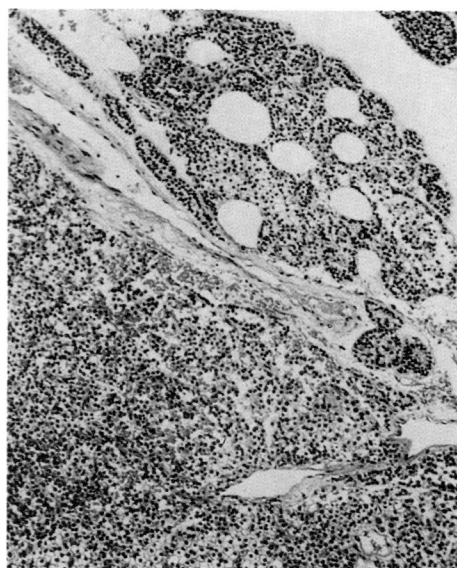

Fig. 26.52 Parathyroid adenoma; margin contrasting unaffected parathyroid tissue with fat cells (top right) and compact structure of the cellular adenoma.

individual parathyroid cells with enlarged hyperchromatic nuclei. The presence of such cells does not indicate malignancy.

Parathyroid carcinoma

Parathyroid carcinoma may be associated with severe bone disease—osteitis fibrosa cystica—and accounts for about 4 per cent of cases of primary hyperparathyroidism. Diagnosis may be difficult and the true nature of the parathyroid disease may not be revealed for many years when local invasion and metastasis occur.

Most parathyroid carcinomas are hard and greyish-white in comparison with the softer, tan-coloured adenomas, and there may have been adherence to surrounding tissues at operation. Typically there is a dense hyaline capsule with fibrous septa dividing up the tumour, which is not explicable on the basis of organization of old haemorrhage or necrosis that may occur in benign adenomas. The cells are generally large, with enlarged uniform nuclei, and may be columnar in outline and palisaded around blood vessels. As mentioned already, mitoses may be found in adenomas and hyperplastic glands as well as in carcinomas and are of little diagnostic value, although the presence of numerous mitoses, including abnormal forms, is suggestive of carcinoma. Local invasion of thyroid and nerves or the finding of metastases confirms a diagnosis of carcinoma. In metastatic tumours of doubtful origin it may be possible to demonstrate a parathyroid origin by the immunoperoxidase staining technique, using an antiserum to parathormone.

In addition to the foregoing types of patathyroid disease, there is a special group of patients in which there is involvement of several endocrine organs in addition to the parathyroids. These will be mentioned briefly.

Multiple endocrine neoplasia (MEN)

This term relates to a collection of uncommon syndromes in which there is familial hyperplasia or neoplasia of several endocrine organs. In *MEN type I* (*Wermer's syndrome*) there may be hyperplasia or *adenomas* of the *pancreatic islet cells, anterior pituitary, adrenal cortex,* and the *parathyroid glands,* and *peptic ulceration.* In *MEN type II* (*Sipple's syndrome*) there is *phaeochromocytoma* of the *adrenal medulla* (which may be bilateral) and *medullary carcinoma* of the *thyroid.* The pancreas is uninvolved, but there may be *parathyroid hyperplasia.* In some MEN type II patients, there are *multiple mucosal neuromas of lips and tongue, skin pigmentation,* and *ganglioneuromas of the bowel.*

Secondary hyperparathyroidism

Modes of presentation

Frequently, symptoms related to the underlying disorder causing hypocalcaemia, such as malabsorption or chronic renal failure, overshadow those of hyperparathyroidism, which is revealed only by biochemical investigations including estimation of the serum iPTH. In end-stage renal failure, for example, the majority of patients have some degree of raised levels of circulating iPTH and histological osteitis fibrosa in bone biopsies, but few have related symptoms such as bone pain or fractures. With the introduction of various forms of renal replacement therapy, many more patients now survive and eventually develop severe uncontrollable hyperparathyroidism with hypercalcaemia, simulating primary hyperparathyroidism, sometimes with clinically significant bone disease and metastatic calcification.

Serum iPTH in renal failure. In comparison with primary hyperparathyroidism, the serum iPTH, measured as the carboxy-terminal fragment, is markedly increased in renal secondary hyperparathyroidism. In both situations the liver degrades intact hormone with formation of carboxy-terminal fragments, but the kidneys in the patient with renal failure are unable to remove these and they accumulate in the circulation. Following successful renal transplantation, the excess fragments are rapidly taken up by the kidney and serum iPTH returns to normal within a day or so, whereas after parathyroidectomy the carboxy-terminal fragments may persist in the circulation for several weeks.

Parathyroid glands in secondary hyperparathyroidism

It is more-or-less impossible, solely on histological grounds, to distinguish between primary chief-cell hyperplasia and secondary hyperplasia of the parathyroid glands. Glands in the early stages may be little enlarged but the amount of parenchyma is increased at the expense of interstitial fat. Later, the glands become obviously enlarged, together weighing up to 5 g or more. The enlargement may affect all glands about equally, or one or more may be particularly enlarged. The larger glands often appear nodular and individual nodules are pale grey to white, compared with the usual tan colour of parathyroid tissue (Fig. 26.53). Microscopically there is diffuse hyperplasia, nodu-

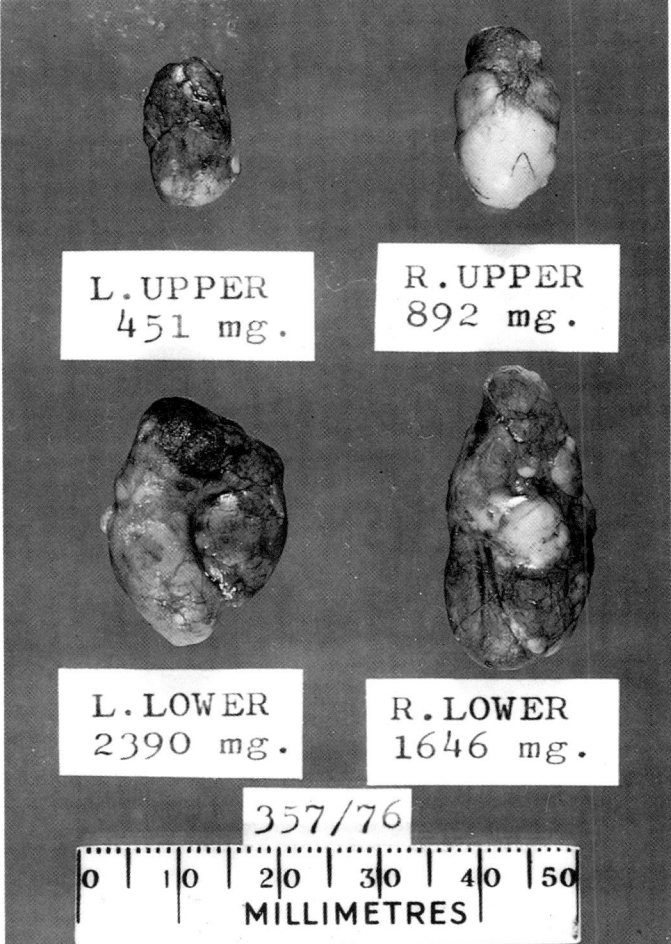

Fig. 26.53 Nodular secondary hyperplasia of parathyroid glands in long-standing renal failure; combined weight of glands 5379 mg (i.e. 40 × normal). There was severe osteitis fibrosa.

lar hyperplasia, or an admixture of these. Diffusely hyperplastic glands are usually not as enlarged as are nodular glands, and often show a predominance of one cell type, such as transitional chief cells. In nodular glands the nodules may comprise one or more cell types and in long-standing cases of chronic renal failure aggregates and nodules of oxyphil cells may be a conspicuous feature. Individual expansile nodules may become encapsulated by fibrous tissue and appear adenomatous. There is some nuclear enlargement, especially in nodular and adenomatous areas, and occasional normal mitoses may be present in chief cells and in transitional oxyphils. Larger glands are sometimes subject to episodes of localized ischaemic necrosis and haemorrhage. Very rarely this is sufficiently extensive as to cause spontaneous remission of severe hyperparathyroidism. Electron microscopy reveals a variable cytology, with cells in different phases of the secretory cycle, but it is not possible ultrastructurally to distinguish clearly between adenomatous and non-adenomatous areas.

26.3.4 Hypercalcaemia of malignancy

Hypercalcaemia may be discovered during the investigation of patients with malignant disease. Rarely, the discovery of hypercalcaemia is the first indication that a patient is suffering from some malignancy. The hypercalcaemia may either occur in association with skeletal metastases, or be due to the secretion of a parathyroid hormone-like substance by the tumour cells in the absence of skeletal metastases or parathyroid disease. The latter is known as *humoral hypercalcaemia of malignancy* or *ectopic hyperparathyroidism*. Ectopic hyperparathyroidism is most commonly associated with squamous carcinoma of the lung, being found in 10–15 per cent of such cases, and the prognosis is very poor. The hypercalcaemia results from the action of parathormone-like tumour products on bone to increase resorption, and on the kidneys, increasing reabsorption of calcium. *Hypophosphataemia* results from the increased urinary phosphate secretion. The use of immunoassays against various parathormone fragments in the serum and tumours gives inconsistent and sometimes conflicting results, and commonly serum iPTH is not increased. Furthermore, parathormone mRNA has not been demonstrated in the tumours; and for these reasons the existence of the mechanism has been challenged. However, the tumour cells react positively when stained by the Immunoperoxidase technique for parathormone and have secretory granules similar to those in parathyroid tumour cells on electron microscopy. Recently (Suva *et al.* 1987) further credence has been given to the concept of ectopic hyperparathyroidism with the isolation from lung cancer cells of a *parathryoid-hormone-related protein*, comprising 151 amino acids, that has homology with parathormone. This homology explains the interaction with normal parathormone receptors in bone and kidney, while differences in the remainder of the molecule explain the frequent failure to demonstrate increased circulating iPTH in patients with the hypercalcaemic malignant syndrome.

26.3.5 Parathyroid hypofunction

Parathyroid deficiency causes a reduction in plasma ionized calcium and an increase in plasma phosphate. Clinical hypoparathyroidism may be the result of either (1) an *inadequate output of parathormone* or (2) a *failure of the target organs to respond to parathormone* (so-called *pseudohypoparathyroidism*).

Clinical manifestations of hypoparathyroidism

Apart from the skeletal and developmental defects which may be associated with certain types of hypoparathyroidism (to be mentioned later), the main symptoms relate to the hypocalcaemia.

Tetany

The abnormally low levels of calcium in the blood and extracellular fluid cause increased neuromuscular excitability. In mild cases there are '*pins and needles*' (paraesthesiae), otherwise there is spasm of voluntary muscle with characteristic *carpo-pedal involvement, spasm of the larynx (laryngismus stridulus), and convulsions* that may resemble epilepsy. In less severe cases, latent tetany may be induced by tapping over the facial nerve, which causes twitching of facial muscles (*Chvostek's sign*), or by compressing the upper arm with a sphygmomanometer cuff, which precipitates carpo-pedal spasm (*Trousseau's sign*).

Other clinical features

These include various mental disorders, such as *anxiety*, attacks of *inexplicable panic* and, most commonly, *depression*. *Parkinsonism* is sometimes present and can result from the soft tissue calcification of the basal ganglia, which is common in 'idiopathic' hypoparathyroidism and in pseudohypoparathyroidism but not in post-operative hypoparathyroidism. *Loss of hair, brittleness of the nails*, and *subcapsular cataracts* may complicate any form of hypoparathyroidism. The lens is not calcified and the precise pathogenesis is unclear.

Candidiasis

Patients with 'idiopathic' hypoparathyroidism have a predisposition to suffer from *chronic mucocutaneous candidiasis* and this may be a presenting symptom preceding other manifestations by several years.

Hypoparathyroidism as a result of inadequate parathormone secretion

Lack of parathormone may result from several causes, which will be considered in turn.

Removal of parathyroid glands

Probably the commonest cause of hypoparathyroidism is the inadvertent removal of the glands or damage to their blood supply during thyroid surgery, but this occurs less frequently than in the past. Hypoparathyroidism may follow removal of a hyperfunctioning parathyroid adenoma, but the hypocalcaemia is generally transient and largely simply the result of bone 'hunger' for calcium as the hyperparathyroid bone disease resolves. Repeated cervical operations for recurrent hyperparathyroidism sometimes result in hypoparathyroidism.

Congenital hypoparathyroidism

This is rare. Abnormalities related to the development of the third and fourth pharyngeal pouches may lead to *congenital absence* of the parathyroid glands associated with *thymic aplasia, mandibular hypoplasia, and abnormalities of the great blood vessels* (*Di George's syndrome*). There is hypocalcaemia with tetany, and repeated infections due to abnormalities in cell-mediated immunity frequently cause death in infancy.

Suppression of parathormone secretion

Neonatal tetany may result from hypoparathyroidism when developmentally normal parathyroid glands in the unborn infant have been suppressed by hypercalcaemia in the mother who is suffering from hyperparathyroidism. This may be the presenting clinical manifestation of the mother's parathyroid disease.

Acquired parathyroid diseases

Miscellaneous disorders are known to be the cause of very occasional cases of hypoparathyroidism. These include *post-irradiation damage* and fibrosis of the glands following ^{131}I therapy of thyrotoxicosis and fibrosis associated with *haemochromatosis*. Deposition of *amyloid or malignant tumour* in the parathyroid glands are sometimes mentioned as possible causes of hypoparathyroidism. Amyloid is commonly deposited in the glands of patients with either AL or AA types of systemic amyloidosis but seldom causes hypoparathyroidism. Often the presence of even large amounts of amyloid in the glands does not appear to interfere with their function and the parathyroid glands are still capable of undergoing secondary hyperplasia should renal failure develop. Leukaemic infiltrates and metastatic deposits of carcinoma may be found in the parathyroid glands, but again seldom, if ever, are the cause of parathyroid hypofunction.

'Idiopathic' hypoparathyroidism

In the past when the cause of hypoparathyroidism could not be determined the term 'idiopathic' was used. This term is now often inappropriate since it is known that many of these rare cases of acquired hypoparathyroidism result from an organ-specific auto-immune disorder, and in about one-third of patients there are *circulating antiparathyroid antibodies*, demonstrable by immunofluorescence. Radioimmunoassay fails to reveal circulating parathormone, although very low levels may be detected by cytochemical bioassay. Clinically unaffected members of the family may also have circulating antiparathyroid antibodies. Patients may have other auto-immune manifestations, such as *pernicious anaemia, adrenal cortical insufficiency (Addison's disease), chronic thyroiditis,* and *testicular atrophy,* and it may be possible to demonstrate antibodies to these organs.

There are very few adequate descriptions of the pathology of the parathyroid glands in cases of 'idiopathic' hypoparathyroidism. Features that have been described include chronic inflammatory cell infiltration, fibrosis, and atrophy. Sometimes the glands have been found to be fatty, or no glandular tissue at all could be identified at necropsy.

Hypoparathyroidism as a result of failure of target organ response (pseudohypoparathyroidism)

Failure of end-organ response to normal parathormone causes:

1. *deficient renal phosphate excretion and hyperphosphataemia;*
2. *reduced flow of calcium from bone into the extracellular fluid, with hypocacaemia;* and
3. *reduced blood levels of the active vitamin D metabolite* $1,25(OH)_2D_3$, since the renal resistance to parathormone interferes with the normal stimulatory effect the hormone has on *renal* $25(OH)D_3$-1α-*hydroxylase activity.* This lack of $1,25(OH)_2D_3$ in turn *reduces intestinal absorption of calcium* and contributes to the hypocalcaemia.

Injection of parathormone does not induce the usual increases in urinary cyclic AMP and phosphate.

Paradoxically, since the parathyroid glands are perfectly normal they respond to the chronic hypocalcaemia and undergo *secondary (compensatory) hyperplasia*. Circulating parathormone levels are increased and in about a third of patients this results in osteitis fibrosa.

The disease is accompanied by features of *Albright's hereditary osteodystrophy,* such as short stature, rounded facies, brachydactyly, soft-tissue calcification, enamel hypoplasia with 'pitted' teeth, and mental retardation. The age of onset of symptoms is usually between 1 and 10 years but unrecognized cases may be encountered clinically in adults. Pseudohypoparathyroidism is a heritable disease with a complex mode of inheritance, involving autosomal dominance and not an X-linked dominant mechanism as was originally thought to be the case.

The term *pseudo-pseudohypoparathyroidism* has been applied when the above same skeletal and other stigmata are present but the biochemical abnormalities are absent and the patient is normocalcaemic.

Subtypes of pseudohypoparathyroidism have been recognized according to the particular biochemical abnormality present (Drezner and Neelon 1983). *Pseudohypoparathyroidism type I* results from an abnormality in the *parathormone-receptor–adenylate-cyclase moiety* in the kidney tubule cell membrane, causing deficient cyclic AMP production which in turn retards the sequence of intracellular events that normally bring about the effects of parathormone. In *pseudohypoparathyroidism type II* there is an inability of intracellular cyclic AMP to initiate these parathormone-directed metabolic events. The hypocalcaemia of pseudohypoparathyroidism results from defective mobilization of bone calcium, due to an abnormality in bone corresponding to that in the kidney and to the diminished production of $1,25(OH)_2D_3$ by the renal tubules.

26.3.6 Principles of treatment related to pathology

In primary hyperparathyroidism an attempt should be made to identify all glands at operation to distinguish between primary hyperplasia and adenoma. When only one gland appears enlarged this, together with the whole of one other gland, should be examined intra-operatively by the pathologist, using the frozen-section technique. This is to exclude the possibility that there is multigland hyperplasia which is marked in one masquerading as an adenoma. If the smaller gland is considered to be normal, then the case is one of adenoma and no further excision is required; if mildly hyperplastic then there is multi-glandular disease (hyperplasia) and subtotal parathyroidectomy is indicated. When all four glands are enlarged at operation and hyperplastic on frozen-section examination, again subtotal parathyroidectomy is carried out.

In secondary hyperparathyroidism there is a need to treat the underlying cause as well as the hyperparathyroidism. In renal failure treatment with the *active vitamin D metabolite* $1,25(OH)_2D_3$ short-circuits the inability of the renal tubules to produce active vitamin D, improving intestinal absorption of calcium and correcting the hypocalcaemic stimulus to hyperparathyroidism. Also, $1,25(OH)_2D_3$ binds to receptors in the parathyroid cells and directly reduces parathormone secretion by interference with parathormone gene transcription. In those patients with secondary hyperparathyroidism uncontrolled by medical means (that is, the hyperparathyroidism has become 'autonomous') then subtotal or total parathyroidectomy may be necessary.

Recently a new procedure, *total parathyroidectomy combined with autografting* of selected fragments into the forearm muscle, has proved a useful means of achieving an optimal parathyroidectomy (Saxe 1984).

Hypocalcaemia of hypoparathyroidism responds to treatment with *calcium supplements* and *vitamin D* or *the active metabolite*, $1,25(OH)_2D_3$. In pseudohypoparathyroidism, use of $1,25(OH)_2D_3$ bypasses the defective renal hydroxylation stage of vitamin D metabolism. Attempts have been made to treat a few cases of Di George syndrome by allo-grafting of parathyroid tissue. This procedure, with appropriate immunosuppression, has also been used to treat some patients with 'idiopathic' hypoparathyroidism who have developed severe complications attributable to prolonged treatment with vitamin D (Duarte *et al.* 1985).

26.3.7   Bibliography

Armitage, E. K. (1986). Parathyrin (parathyroid hormone): metabolism and methods for assay. *Clinical Chemistry* **32**, 418–24.

Castleman, B., Schantz, A., and Roth, S. I. (1976). Parathyroid hyperplasia in primary hyperparathyroidism. A review of 85 cases. *Cancer* **38**, 1668–75.

Drezner, M. K. and Neelon, F. A. (1983). Pseudohypoparathyroidism. In *The metabolic basis of inherited disease* (5th edn), (ed. J. B. Stanbury, J. B. Wyngaarden, D. S. Fredrickson, J. L. Goldstein, and M. S. Brown), pp. 1508–27. McGraw-Hill, New York.

Duarte, B., Mozes, M. F., John, E., Aronson, I., Pollak, R., and Jonasson, O. (1985). Parathyroid allotransplantation in the treatment of complicated idiopathic primary hypoparathyroidism. *Surgery* **98**, 1072–6.

Mandl, F. (1947). Hyperparathyroidism. A review of historical developments and the present state of knowledge on the subject. *Surgery* **21**, 394–440.

Martin, C. R. (1985). Parathyroid hormone, calcitonin, and other regulators of calcium and phosphorus metabolism. In *Endocrine physiology*, pp. 463–96. Oxford University Press.

Nilson, O. (1977). Studies on the ultrastructure of the human parathyroid glands in various pathological conditions. *Acta Pathologica et Microbiologica Scandinavica, Section A* Suppl. **263**, 1–88.

Potts, J. R. (1987). Diseases of the parathyroid gland and other hyper- and hypocalcaemic disorders. In *Harrison's principles of internal medicine* (11th edn) (ed. E. Braunwald, K. J. Isselbacher, R. G. Petersdorf, J. D. Wilson, J. B. Martin, and A. S. Fauci), pp. 1870–89. McGraw-Hill, New York.

Sandström, I. (1879–1880). On a new gland in Man and several mammals. *Upsala Läkareförenings Forhandlingar* **15**, 441–71. See: Seipel, C. M. (1938). An English translation of Sandström's 'Glandulae Parathyroideae'. *Bulletin of the Institute of the History of Medicine* **6**, 179–222.

Saxe, A. (1984). Parathyroid transplantation. A review. *Surgery* **95**, 507–26.

Suva, L. J., Winslow, G. A., Wettenhall, R. E. H., Hammonds, R. G., Moseley, J. M., Diefenbach-Jagger, H., Rodda, C. P., Kemp, B. E., Rodriguez, H., Chen, E. Y., Hudson, P. J., Martin, T. J., and Wood, W. I. (1987). A parathyroid hormone-related protein implicated in malignant hypercalcaemia: cloning and expression. *Science* **237**, 893–6.

26.4   The adrenal cortex

A. Munro Neville

26.4.1   Introduction

The adrenal gland consists of two structurally and functionally distinct components. The inner part, called the medulla, produces catecholamines and certain peptide hormones; its pathology is discussed elsewhere (p. 1987). The outer part is referred to as the *cortex*; it produces *steroid hormones*. Disorders of the human adrenal cortex are uncommon but are important as they are associated with a series of protean and fascinating endocrine disturbances, many of which are curable by either medical or surgical intervention.

In general, the important disorders of the human adrenal cortex are due to either increased or decreased secretion of one or more of its hormones. The principle pathological changes in these disorders are *hyperplasia, neoplasia,* or *atrophy*. In addition, nodular changes can affect the gland, particularly as a facet of the ageing process. The purpose of this section is to discuss and highlight those disorders which serve to illustrate the value of correlating structure and function in the study of pathology.

26.4.2   The normal adult adrenal cortex

In fetal life, the adrenal cortex consists of two components: an *inner fetal zone* and an *outer adult (definitive) zone*. It is from the outer definitive zone that the cortex of the adult develops; the fetal zone undergoes regression postnatally.

The adrenal glands sit atop either kidney. The right gland is pyramidal, and the left, crescentic in shape (Fig. 26.54). The cut surface reveals a grey inner medulla occupying the head and body of the gland, i.e. its more medial parts, but absent from the tail and the alae.

The weight of the normal adrenal gland removed at surgery or at the autopsy of someone who has died suddenly, e.g. in a traffic accident, is 4 g. The cut surface of the adrenal cortex in these circumstances presents an inner brown and an outer yellow zone.

The autopsy weight of the gland is 6 g, in those who have died as a result of stress, e.g. following a prolonged illness. The cortical cut surface of such glands is often diffusely brown in colour. This difference is due to the effect of adrenocorticotropin

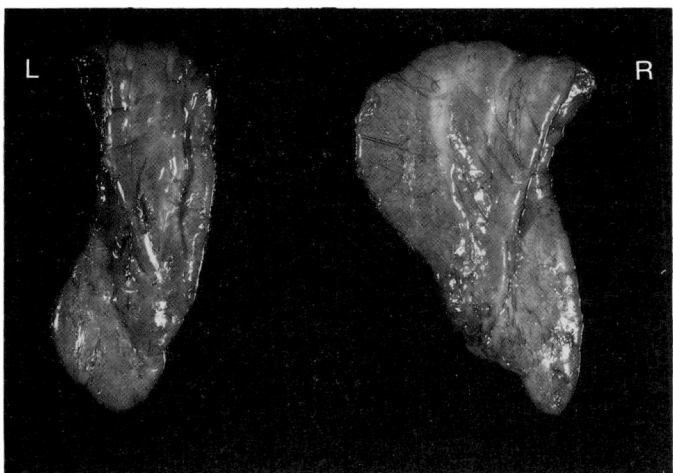

Fig. 26.54 The gross appearance of the adult adrenal gland is shown from the anterior aspect.

(ACTH) (see below) (Symington 1969). With increasing age, and particularly in patients with hypertension, *nodules* of varying size and frequency may be detected (see below).

The adrenal cortex comprises three distinct morphological zones contained within the outer gland capsule. They comprise the outer, but focally present, *zona glomerulosa*, the inner *zona reticularis*, and, in between, the *zona fasciculata*. Structural differences between those three zones are due to their different cell types, arrangement, cytoplasmic constituents, and vascular framework (Fig. 26.55).

The zona glomerulosa forms an ill-defined zone immediately below the capsule where it is present only in a focal manner. It is the sole source of *aldosterone*, the important mineralocorticoid. This zone consists of rounded collections of small cells with a high nuclear:cytoplasmic ratio. Their cytoplasm contains sparse amounts of lipid. The cell nests are surrounded by a delicate capillary network.

The zona reticularis comprises the inner one-third to one-quarter of the cortex. Its cut surface has a brown colour due to the cells having a low lipid content. In conventionally prepared histological material, the cells have eosinophilic lipid-sparse cytoplasm and are referred to as *compact cells*. They are arranged in a series of nests and short cords separated by an anastomosing sinusoidal network.

The zona fasciculata lies between the zona glomerulosa and the zona reticularis and comprises the remainder of the cortex. It extends to the capsule where the zona glomerulosa is deficient. The cells of the zona fascuculata are arranged in radially dispersed columns. The cells are large with prominent cell membranes, a low nuclear:cytoplasmic ratio and a high content of lipid, predominantly cholesterol and cholesterol esters. In conventionally prepared histological material, the lipids are dissolved out during processing, so that the cells take on a vacuolated appearance. They are referred to as *clear cells*.

The adrenal cortex receives its blood supply from a myriad of arteries which form an anastamosing network on the capsular

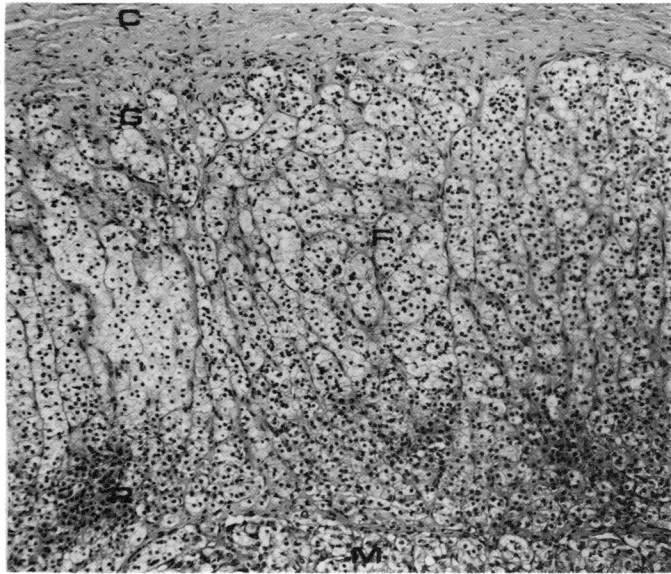

(a)

(b)

Fig. 26.55 The normal human adrenal cortex. A 4.0 g gland removed at surgery from a patient with metastatic breast cancer is shown (a). The zona glomerulosa (G) is only focally present while the zona reticularis (R) is present on the inner aspect. The clear cell zona fasciculata (F) comprises the rest. A small part of the medulla (M) is also present. The effect of ACTH administration for 4 days is shown in (b) with compact lipid-sparse cells extending out almost to reach the capsule. This gland weighed 6.8 g.

surface. Small arteries penetrate the capsule to reach the capillaries of the zona glomerulosa, from whence the blood flows centripetally through the cortex.

The cortical vascular effluent feeds into the central vein of the adrenal gland, either directly or after passing through the medulla. Around the central vein and its main tributaries is a small collar of cortical cells, known as the 'cortical cuff'. It separates the medulla from the central vein and, like the main cortex, is divisible into the three zones. It receives its blood supply from arteries accompanying the central vein, an important point in relation to the genesis of adrenal nodules (p. 1972).

Functional properties

Understanding the pathological changes in adrenocortical disorders requires a knowledge of both the functional zonation of the cortex, i.e. which zones produce the several types of hormones, and the effect of ACTH on its structure and function.

Zonation

The cortex produces three broad categories of steroid hormones, namely *mineralocorticoids*, as typified by aldosterone and 18-hydroxycorticosterone; *glucocorticoids*, such as cortisol and corticosterone; and *sex steroids*, including the androgens, testosterone and DHA, and oestrogens, including oestradiol (Fig. 26.56). The adrenal cortex does not store significant con-

centrations of steroid hormones. All the hormones are derived from a common precursor, *cholesterol*, which is converted, under the agency of ACTH, first to the key intermediate, *pregnenolone* (Fig. 26.57). The subsequent conversion of pregnenolone to the various different metabolically active steroid hormones involves the sequential action of a series of highly specific enzymes. Depending upon which enzymes are involved, structurally different compounds with different effects will be produced (Figs 26.56, 26.57), e.g. aldosterone lacks a hydroxyl group at position 17, whereas this is present in cortisol. While mineralo- and glucocorticoids have 21 carbon atoms, the sex steroid hormones do not have a side-chain and contain only 19 carbon atoms if they are androgens and 18 carbon atoms when oestrogens. Knowledge of these different enzymes and their sequence of action is important: inherited enzyme defects occur in *congenital adrenocortical hyperplasia* with dramatic results.

Aldosterone, as stated before, is produced only by the zona glomerulosa. The control of aldosterone secretion is multifactorial and complex. It involves both *electrolyte levels* as well as polypeptide hormones, such as *angiotensin II*.

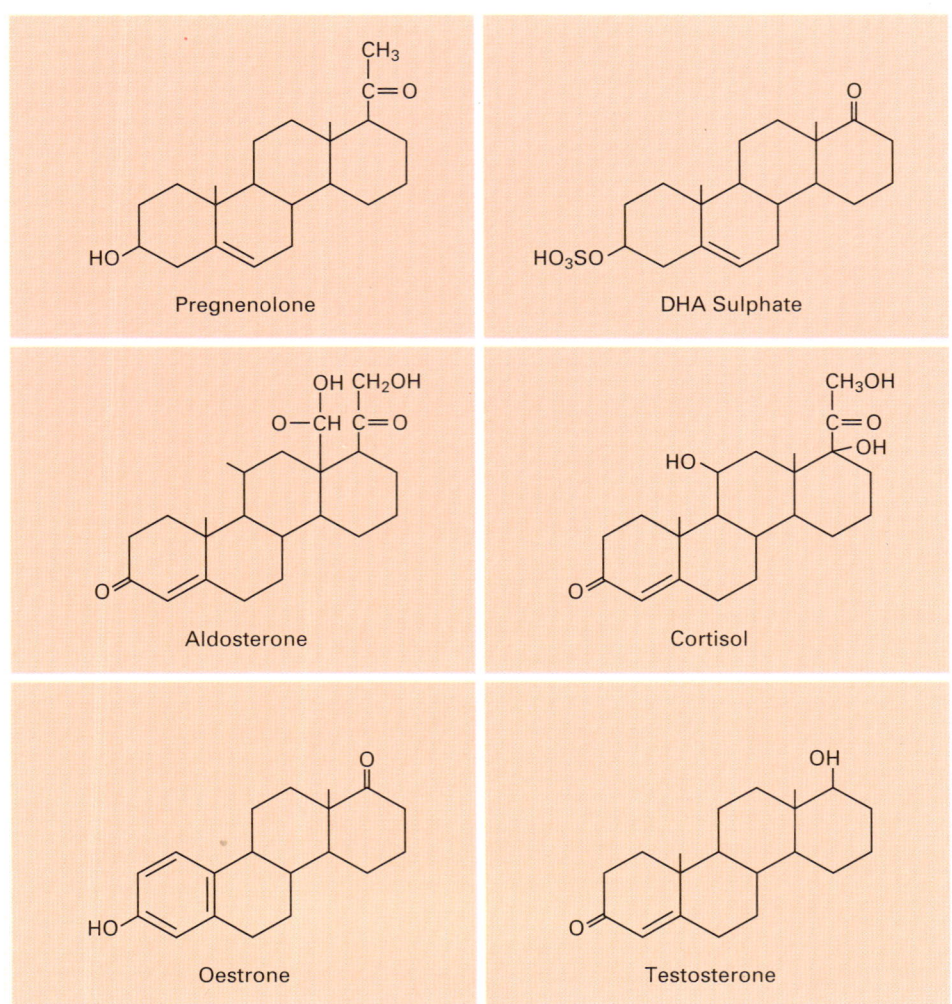

Fig. 26.56 Structures of the quantitatively predominant steroid hormones of different classes secreted by the human adrenal cortex.

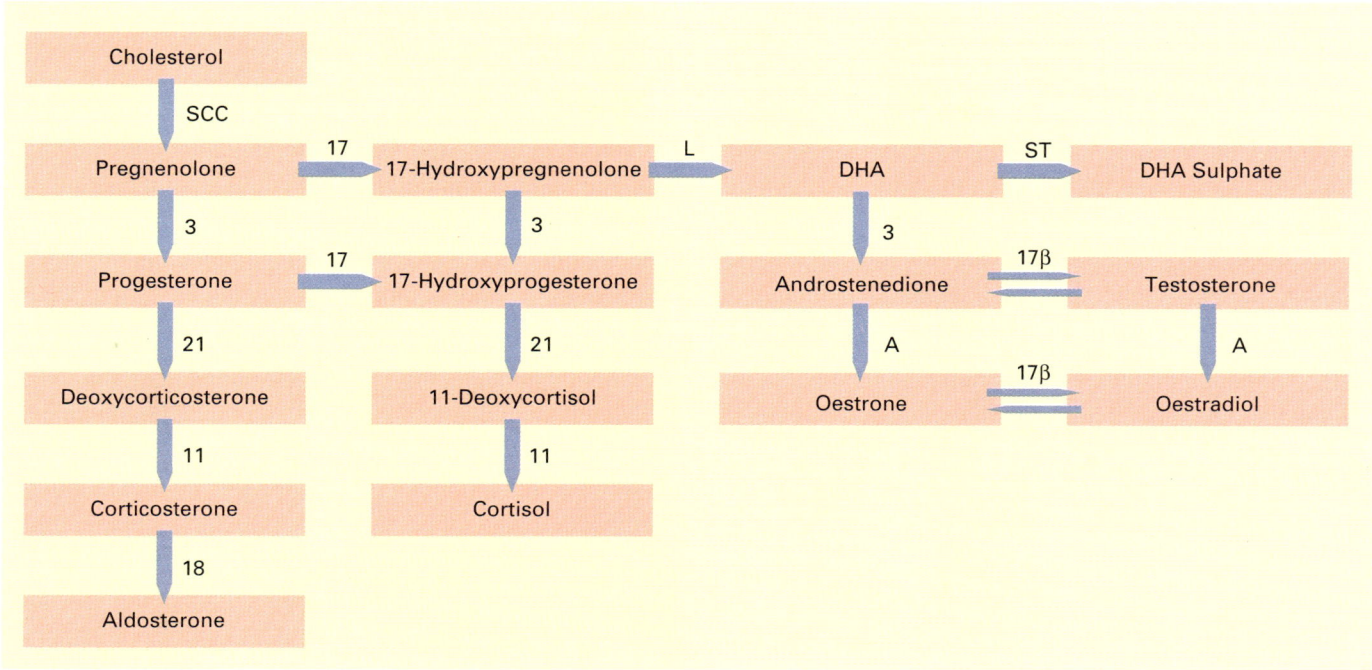

Fig. 26.57 Major pathways of steroidogenesis in the human adult cortex. SCC, Cholesterol side-chain cleavage system; 3, 3β-hydroxysteroid dehydrogenase-5-en-4-en-isomerase system; 17, 17α-hydroxylase; 21, 21-hydroxylase; 11, 11β-hydroxylase; L, C_{17-20} lyase (desmolase); ST, steroid sulphotransferase; 17β, 17β-hydroxysteroid dehydrogenase; A, Aromatase; 18, 18-hydroxylase.

While there are subtle differences in the steroids produced, the zona fasciculata and zona reticularis are best viewed as functioning as a *single unit* producing both glucocorticoid and sex steroid hormones. The zona fasciculata and zona reticularis together produce such steroids required on a day-to-day basis but, the clear cells, with their high content of cholesterol and its esters, function additionally as a reserve zone to provide increased amounts of steroids such as cortisol, in times of stress, infection, and in response to increased ACTH levels.

It would appear that both androgen and oestrogen production by the adrenal, like cortisol, are under the control of ACTH.

Effects of ACTH

The *in vivo* administration of ACTH results in an almost immediate rise in adrenal blood flow and steroid hormone output, in particular, cortisol, as a result of its stimulating the conversion of cholesterol to pregnenolene (Fig. 26.57). Continued administration may well result in the steroid hormone output rising tenfold. After approximately 48 h, the effects of increased ACTH administration will be such that there is an increase in adrenal weight. This is due to cellular hyperplasia which assists in maintaining the continued high steroid output. At the same time as the weight begins to rise, it is possible to begin to discern morphologically that the clear cells of the zona fasciculata at the border with the zona reticularis lose their cholesterol and cholesterol ester content and are converted into lipid-sparse *compact cells*. With continuing ACTH administration, this pro-

cess will gradually extend outwards to involve all the clear cells and reach the zona glomerulosa or the capsule where the zona glomerulosa is deficient (Fig. 26.55).

In response to the stress of dying, with its increased circulating ACTH levels, similar changes occur in the cortex and will be seen in most autopsy glands. As before, there is conversion of the clear cells of the zona fasciculata into lipid-sparse compact cells but this occurs in a focal manner and is referred to as *focal lipid depletion* (Fig. 26.58). With continued, prolonged stress, however, the entire gland can be depleted of its lipid; the process is then called *complete lipid depletion*, and is frequently associated with some pseudotubule or lumina formation which separates the cortical cell columns (Symington 1969).

When the ACTH levels have returned to normal, the gland also will revert to its normal weight, size, and zonation. The first morphological evidence of this process is a change from compact to clear cells, occurring first where the border between the original zona fasciculata and the zona reticularis used to exist. This change then extends progressively out towards the capsule. This process is known as *reversion*.

If ACTH levels fall below normal, the weight of the gland will be reduced. The cortex will be significantly narrowed and contain only clear lipid-laden cells of the zona fasciculata type (see Fig. 26.63b). This is one form of *atrophy*; its commonest cause will arise from the administration of pharmacological amounts of glucocorticoids for disorders responding to such steroid therapy. It is also associated with cortisol-producing tumours causing *Cushing's syndrome* (p. 1976).

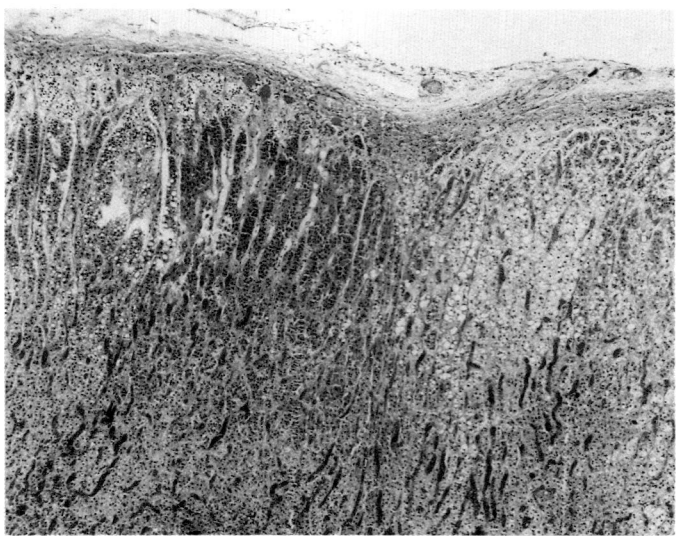

Fig. 26.58 The human adult cortex. Response to stress. Focal lipid depletion. The broadened cortex consists of segments with inner compact cells and outer clear cells together with areas where the compact cells extend out to reach the capsule, or zona glomerulosa.

Adrenocortical nodules

Nodules are common adrenal lesions. Their frequency increases with age and they are especially prone to occur in subjects with 'essential' hypertension.

Nodules, formerly referred to as 'non-functioning adenomas', are generally rounded, localized overgrowths of adrenocortical cells varying from microscopic dimensions to 2–3 cm in diameter (Fig. 26.59). They arise within the substance of the gland, gradually enlarge and may come to protrude through the capsule, forming mushroom-like lesions. Nodules are not true tumours, but need to be distinguished from such in certain forms of hypercorticalism (see below). Nodules are generally detected either at autopsy or, during life, as an incidental finding as a result of a CT or NMR scan of the abdomen for general abdominal complaints. Nodules, generally, are not associated with evidence of adrenal dysfunction. However, they can occur with disorders associated with adrenocortical hyperfunction. In particular, nodules occurring in essential hypertension require to be distinguished from the true benign tumour associated with hyperaldosteronism with low plasma renin (*Conn's syndrome*) and which produces hypertension.

Nodules have a yellow cut surface and are composed of clear lipid-laden cells similar in size and appearance to those of the zona fasciculata. The cells are arranged in small cords or groups separated by prominent fibrovascular trabeculae (Fig. 26.59). Rarely, and particularly at autopsy, a nodule may have a black cut surface and be composed of compact lipid-sparse zona reticularis-type cells; *lipofuscin*, and possibly *neuromelanin*, in the cell cytoplasm account for the dark colour. While nodules may increase the total adrenal cellular mass, they are apparently not associated with increased adrenocortical hormone secretion *in vivo*. They are, however, capable of steroid synthesis

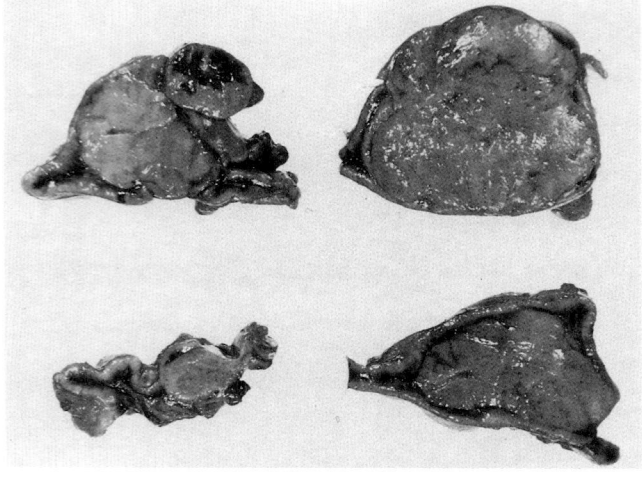

(a)

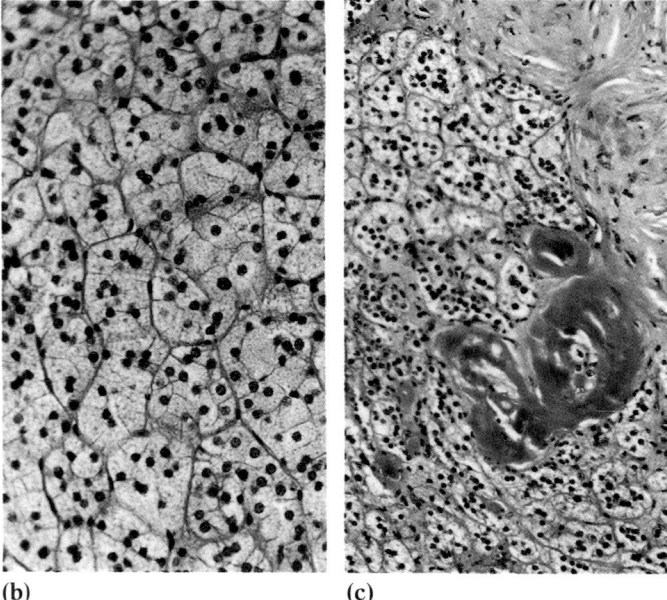

(b)   **(c)**

Fig. 26.59 The nodular adrenal gland. In (a) several typical nodules of varying size and distribution are shown. They consist of nests of lipid-laden zona fasciculata-type cells (b). The arteriopathic changes noted in relation to nodules are illustrated in (c).

in vitro. Nodules are a favoured site for metastatic carcinomatous foci and for certain infections, such as tuberculosis.

The rationale for their development and existence is unknown; one theory believes that they represent focal areas of cellular hyperplasia which come to fill ischaemic defects in the cortex resulting from a related arteriopathy (Fig. 26.59). In agreement with this thesis is the observation that many nodules arise from cortical tissue around the central vein. This part of the cortex receives its blood supply from a different source (the *arteriae comitantes* that accompany the central vein) from that to the main cortex. These arteries accompanying the central vein are less compromised by arteriopathy.

Table 26.5 Adrenocortical hyperfunction: the pathology of the adrenal cortex in 401 patients*

Disease	Number of patients	Adrenal lesion		
		Bilateral hyperplasia	Adenoma	Carcinoma
Cushing's syndrome	202 (50%)	157	26	19
Hyperaldosteronism with low plasma renin (Conn's syndrome)	153 (38%)	28	120	5
Adrenogenital syndrome				
Virilism	41 ⎱ (12%)	20	8	13
Feminization	5 ⎰	—	—	5
Total	401 (100%)	205	154	42

* Neville and O'Hare (1982).

26.4.3 Hypercorticalism

Increased functional activity of the adrenal cortex (hypercorticalism) takes one of three forms:

1. *Cushing's syndrome*, excess production of glucocorticoids, such as cortisol;

2. *hyperaldosteronism with low plasma renin* (*Conn's syndrome*), excess production of salt-retaining hormones, typically aldosterone; or

3. the *adrenogenital syndrome*, virilism or feminization, due to increased androgen or oestrogen production.

In pathological practice, Cushing's syndrome is the most commonly encountered disorder (Table 26.5); all, however, are *uncommon*. Each syndrome may be due to either bilateral adrenocortical hyperplasia or adrenal neoplasms, benign or malignant. Tumours are usually unilateral. While each syndrome is a distinct entity, admixtures, e.g. virilism and Cushing's syndrome, may occur, particularly with carcinomas.

Cushing's syndrome

Cushing's syndrome is due to a chronic increased level of circulating glucocorticoid hormone which leads *inter alia* to *truncal obesity, abdominal striae, amenorrhoea, hirsutism, and hypertension*. It should be remembered that a more frequent cause of the same clinical features, than their being of endogenous adrenocortical origin, is due to the administration of pharmacological levels of *glucocorticoid steroid hormones* for the treatment of other disorders responding to such therapy. Similar signs can also be associated with an excessive *alcohol intake* (Kapcala 1987).

Cushing's syndrome, and its associated adrenal changes, occurs at all ages but is commoner in adult females; most commonly, it is due to *bilateral adrenocortical hyperplasia* (Table 26.6). In children, carcinomas are the most frequent cause; when due to bilateral hyperplasia, it tends to occur around puberty (Neville and Symington 1966; Neville and O'Hare 1982; Page *et al*. 1986).

Bilateral hyperplasia of the adrenal cortex is associated with an increased effective stimulation of the adrenocortical cells by

Table 26.6 Incidence of adrenal lesions in Cushing's syndrome as a function of age*

Adrenal lesion	Incidence (%)	
	Adults	Children
Hyperplasia	78	42
Adenoma	13	12
Carcinoma	9	46

* Neville and O'Hare (1982).

ACTH. This may have as its basis a *microadenoma, basophil adenoma, chromophobe adenoma*, or rarely, *a carcinoma of the pituitary gland* (Gabrilove *et al*. 1986). *In many cases, such lesions are not found.*

Increased ACTH levels in these circumstances may result from increased corticotrophin-releasing factor (CRF) production by the hypothalamus. Frequently, the periodic or *nycterohemeral rhythmicity of ACTH* levels is lost. Increased levels may also arise from so-called 'non-endocrine tumours', e.g. *small cell carcinomas of the lung*, which can produce ACTH. This is the so-called 'ectopic ACTH' syndrome. ACTH levels are reduced in the blood when Cushing's syndrome is caused by the autonomous production of glucocorticoid hormones by an adrenal tumour. In adults, benign and malignant adrenal lesions occur with about equal frequency (Table 26.6).

Bilateral adrenocortical hyperplasia

On the basis of size, weight, gross and histological features, it is possible to subdivide bilateral adrenocortical hyperplasia into one of three forms:

1. *simple* (or *diffuse*) *hyperplasia*;

2. *nodular hyperplasia*; and

3. *hyperplasia with 'non-endocrine' tumours* (the 'ectopic ACTH' syndrome).

The relative incidences are given in Table 26.7.

Table 26.7 The relative incidence of different pathologies in bilateral adrenocortical hyperplasia in Cushing's syndrome*

Pathology	Adults			Children		
	%	Age (yr)	Sex (F:M)	%	Age (yr)	Sex (F:M)
Simple hyperplasia	62	20–40	3:1	62	9–15	2:3
Nodular hyperplasia	20	40–50	3:1	23	<1	3:1
Hyperplasia with the 'ectopic ACTH' syndrome	18	40–60	1:3	15	Any	1:1

* Neville and O'Hare (1982).

Simple (or diffuse) hyperplasia This entity afflicts females more often than males, especially between the ages of 20 and 40 years (Table 26.7). The adrenal appearances are totally accounted for by an effective chronic increase in ACTH stimulation.

Both glands are enlarged with rounded contours (Fig. 26.60) and usually weigh more than normal when surgically removed, between 6 and 12 g. The cortex, which is broadened, presents a dark-brown cut surface on its inner one-third to one-half; the outer part is yellow (Fig. 26.60). Small nodules (<0.25 cm) may be seen.

Morphologically, the appearances accord with the known long-term effects of ACTH on the cortex. In conventionally prepared histological material, the brown inner cortical zone corresponds to a broadened compact-cell lipid-sparse zona reticularis separated by an undulating boarder from the outer zone fasciculata which is also broader than normal (Fig. 26.61). The zona glomerulosa remains focal with gener-

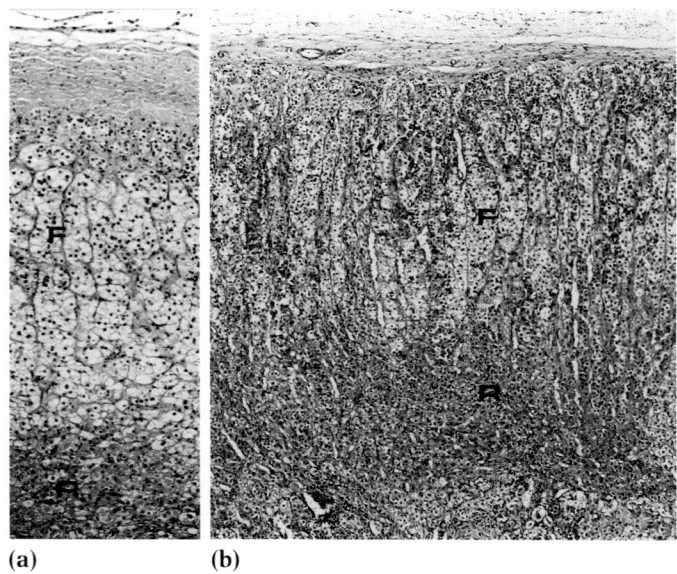

(a)   **(b)**

Fig. 26.61 Cushing's syndrome. Bilateral diffuse hyperplasia (operation specimen; 6.6 g). On the right (b) is the Cushing's gland where the cortex is wider than normal and has a broadened zona retcularis (R), which has an undulating border with the zona fasciculata (F). On the left (a), a normal gland removed at operation is shown for comparison.

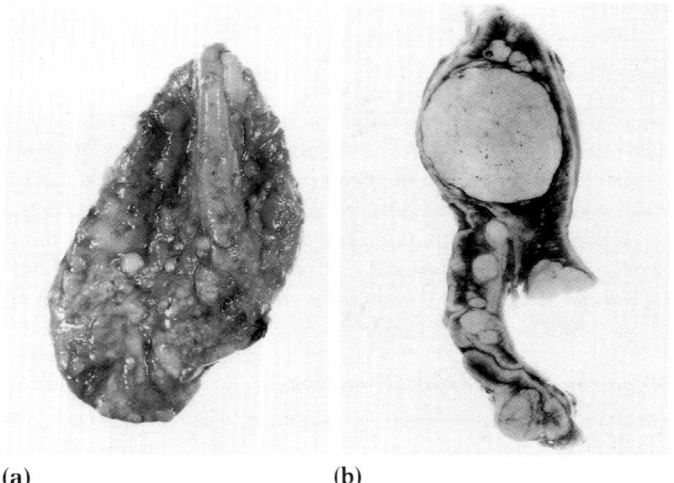

(a)   **(b)**

Fig. 26.60 Cushing's syndrome. (a) Bilateral diffuse hyperplasia. A gland of 6.0 g in weight, removed at surgery, is shown with its characteristic rounded contours. (b) Bilateral nodular hyperplasia. The gland weighed 12 g and contained numerous yellow nodules, the largest being 2.5 × 1.5 cm in size. The attached cortex shows the typical gross features associated with bilateral hyperplasia, with its inner brown and outer yellow layers.

ally a normal distribution. In both the zona reticularis and zona fasciculata, the cells are normal in size and appearance. Ultrastructurally, the cells are also normal in appearance. As stated above, small yellow nodules with their clear, lipid-laden zona fasciculata-type cells situated in the cortex or near the central vein may be present.

From time to time, hypertrophy of the adrenocortical cells may be noted. This tends to be associated with an overt pituitary tumour or the 'ectopic ACTH' syndrome. When present, such aetiologies require to be excluded. If the adrenal glands are examined at autopsy in a case of untreated Cushing's syndrome, the effects of stress will be superimposed on the above features.

Nodular hyperplasia Bilateral nodular hyperplasia accounts for 20 per cent of all examples of adrenocortical hyperplasia (Table 26.7). It also is an ACTH-dependent disorder occurring in an older age-group (40–50 years of age) than those with bilateral hyperplasia. However, again it is commoner in females (Table 26.7). When it occurs in children, it tends to be in infancy and can even be congenital.

The term nodular hyperplasia is reserved for glands containing one or more prominent yellow nodules from 0.5 cm upwards, often measuring 2.0–2.5 cm in diameter (Fig. 26.60). Such nodules are almost always *bilateral*. The glands attached to such nodules have the same gross appearance as those of diffuse hyperplasia but are usually heavier, often showing a significant weight disparity due to different numbers and sizes of nodules on either side.

The cut surface of the nodules is yellow, often with small brown foci. Microscopically, the nodules consist predominantly of clear lipid-laden zona fasciculata-type cells of normal size and appearance, which correspond to the yellow areas seen on gross examination, while the brown foci consist of compact lipid-sparse zona reticularis-type cells (Fig. 26.62). The attached gland always shows bilateral hyperplasia with microscopic features identical to those of diffuse hyperplasia (Figs 26.61, 26.62).

Accordingly, nodular hyperplasia is simply an extension of diffuse hyperplasia where, given more time as the disease occurs mostly in older people, there has been further growth of the small nodules seen in diffuse hyperplasia.

This entity requires to be clearly distinguished from an *adenoma* causing Cushing's syndrome. However, such benign tumours, whose microscopic appearances are similar to those of a nodule, are almost always unilateral and the attached and contralateral glands always show cortical atrophy (see below).

A particular form, called *micronodular hyperplasia*, has been reported recently. It may be congenital and is most frequent in children. The nodules may be pigmented. Moreover, it is said that it can occur unilaterally on occasion and that it is not ACTH-dependent. While opinions vary as to its aetiology (Aiba

et al. 1990), this condition may be, in part, an auto-immune disorder; *serum immunoglobulins* from affected patients have been shown to stimulate adrenal cell growth (Oelkers *et al.* 1986).

Hyperplasia and the 'ectopic ACTH' syndrome This is a rare cause of Cushing's syndrome, most frequent in men, as one of the commonest sources of non-endocrine tumour-derived ACTH is small cell lung carcinoma (Table 26.7). Some tumours produce, in addition, CRF and ACTH precursor forms, including proopiomelanocortin (Gabrilove *et al.* 1986). Other neoplasms, including those of pancreatic islets, thymus, adrenal medulla, and ovary, as well as carcinoid tumours, can be associated with this syndrome. Blood levels of ACTH are often very high and probably account for such glands weighing between 14 and 16 g or more each. Morphologically, the effects of high ACTH levels are manifest. The cortex is much broadened and consists solely of compact lipid-sparse cells extending outwards in columns to the capsule or, where present, the zona glomerulosa (Fig. 26.62). The cells are frequently hypertrophied with enlarged nuclei. Significant cell and nuclear pleomorphism is often noted. Metastatic carcinomatous foci may be present.

Adrenocortical tumours

Approximately 25 per cent of all examples of Cushing's syndrome are due to an adrenal tumour (Tables 26.5, 26.6). Carcinomas, whose incidence is higher in children, may simultaneously cause other forms of hypercorticalism, in particular, *virilism*.

Adenoma These benign tumours occur at all ages, but especially between 30 and 50 years and in females (Table 26.8). They are almost always unilateral, do not exhibit a side predilection and are circumscribed, rounded, and encapsulated. Most weigh less than 50 g. Their cut surface is bright yellow with small red–brown foci.

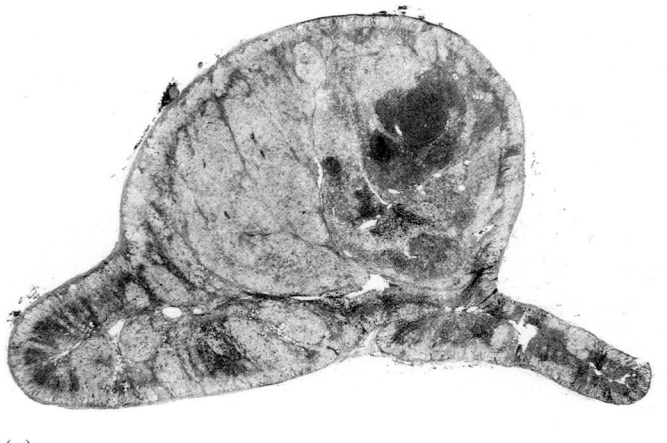

(a)

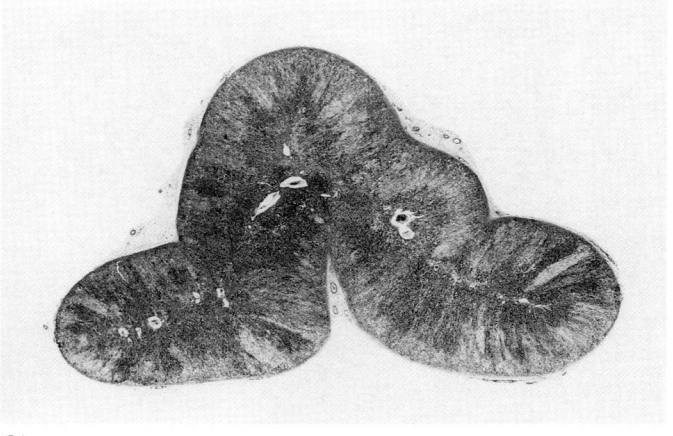

(b)

Fig. 26.62 Cushing's syndrome. (a) Bilateral nodular hyperplasia. This gland weighed 18 g. The nodule (1.5 cm diameter) on the superior surface of the gland is seen to be composed mainly of clear cells with foci of compact cells. The attached cortex shows diffuse hyperplasia and contains numerous clear-celled micronodules. (b) Ectopic ACTH syndrome. This gland weighed 12.1 g. The broadened cortex consists of a prominent inner zona reticularis with compact-cell columns extending out to reach the capsule or be capped by residual clear cells.

Table 26.8   Age, sex, and site of incidence of forty personally studied* adrenocortical tumours causing Cushing's syndrome*

Age (yr)	Adenoma	Carcinoma
0–10	1	2
11–30	2	3
31–50	17	9
51–60	1	4
>60	1	—
Sex (M:F)	1:3	1:8
Site (L:R adrenal)	4:3	1:1

* Neville and O'Hare (1982).

Microscopically, within a tenuous capsule, the yellow areas, noted on gross examination, correspond to lipid-laden zona fasciculata-type cells while the red–brown foci consist of compact lipid-sparse zone reticularis-type cells (Fig. 26.63). The cells and their nuclei are normal in appearance and size; seldom is there nuclear or cellular pleomorphism. The cells are arranged in nests and short cords; generally, clear cells predominate. Ultrastructurally, the cell appearances are similar to those of their normal counterparts. Rarely, compact cells with lipofuscin-laden and possible also neuromelanin-containing cytoplasm comprise the entire lesion, when it has a dark, cut surface and may be referred to as a 'black adenoma'.

The attached and contralateral adrenal glands *always* show *cortical atrophy* (Fig. 26.63).

Carcinoma Adrenocortical carcinomas causing Cushing's syndrome tend to be large lesions weighing over 100 g and often in excess of 1000 g. Such a size may be related to a long gestation phase as, on a per cell basis, carcinomas are inefficient hormone producers. Carcinomas occur more often in females than in males, and especially between 30 and 50 years. Cushing's

tumours in children are most likely to be malignant (Table 26.8).

Carcinomas are unilateral, encapsulated, and soft in consistency. Occasionally, tumour spread through the capsule is seen. The cut surface is red–brown with areas of manifest haemorrhage and necrosis. Calcification and cystic change may be observed. Metastases, when they develop, tend to occur in the related lymph glands, the liver, lungs, bone marrow, and contralateral adrenal gland.

Microscopically, such tumours consist of compact lipid-sparse cells with their typical eosinophilic cytoplasm arranged in cords, alveoli, and sheets, separated by fine fibrovascular trabeculae (Figs 26.64, 26.65). The tumour cells are enlarged, exhibit cellular and nuclear pleomorphism, and pronounced nuclear vesicularity with one or more prominent nucleoli, features that are the hallmark of adrenal carcinoma cells. Mitotic figures are often most difficult to detect. Giant and bizarre cellular forms may be present. Large areas of necrosis with or without haemorrhage are typical. Vascular invasion, even when overt metastases have developed, is often difficult to note within or around the tumour.

Electron microscopy shows few features not seen in cells of the normal cortex and does not aid in the morphological discrimination of difficult cases as to whether they are benign or malignant.

These morphological features are similar to those of other carcinomas causing the other forms of hypercorticalism, as well as the so-called 'non-functioning' carcinomas (Figs 26.65, 26.73). The attached adrenal gland, which shows steroid-induced atrophy (Fig. 26.63), is the morphological clue that one is dealing with a Cushing's syndrome-associated lesion.

The attached and contralateral gland In association with benign and malignant adrenal tumours causing Cushing's syndrome, the associated adrenal cortex shows *steroid-induced atrophy*. The hormonal function of these tumours produces

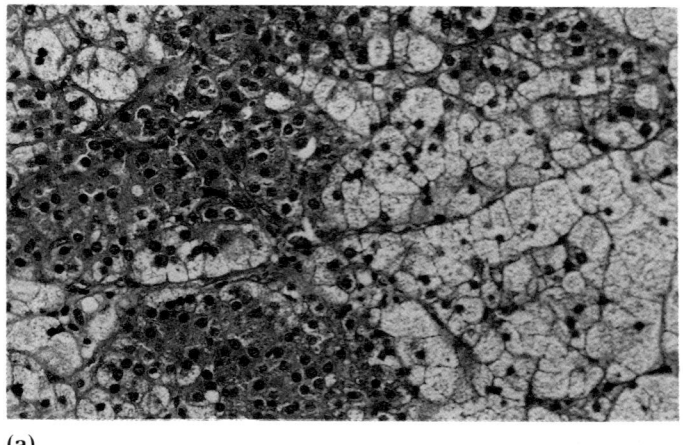

(a)

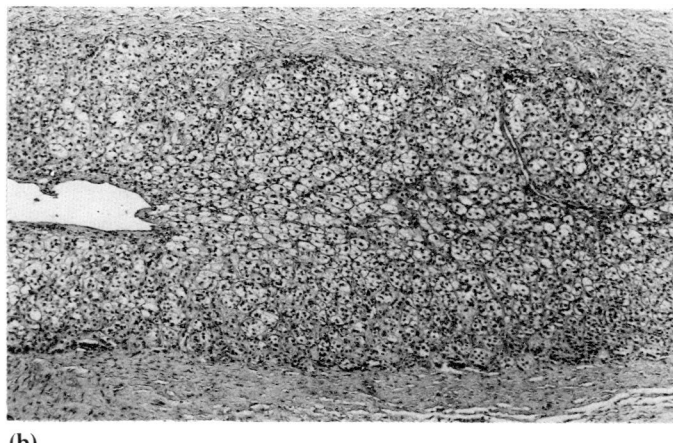

(b)

Fig. 26.63 Cushing's syndrome. Adrenocortical adenoma and attached atrophic gland. The tumour shown in (a) weighs 6.0 g and consists predominantly of cords of clear lipid-laden cells with foci of compact cells interspersed between them. The cells are of normal size and show little pleomorphism. The attached (and contralateral) adrenal cortex (b) is atrophic, narrower than normal, and is surrounded by a thickened oedematous capsule. The cortex is composed solely of clear cells of the zona fasciculata type.

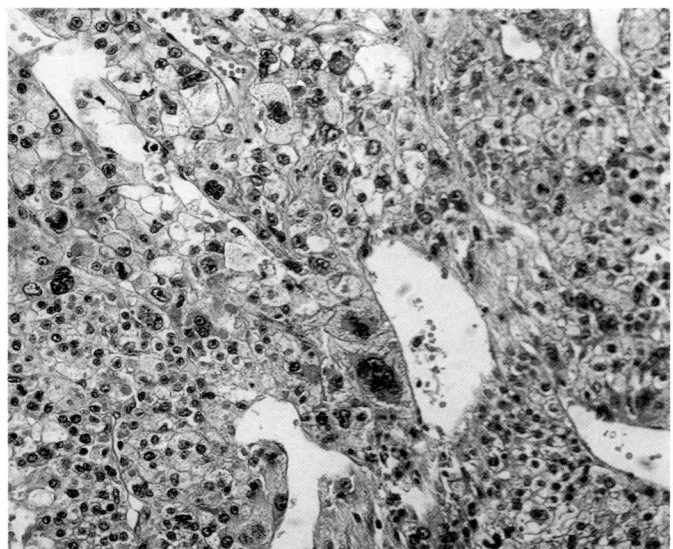

Fig. 26.64 Cushing's syndrome. Adrenocortical carcinoma, 125 g. The carcinoma, from which overt metastases developed 8 months after operation, consists of nests of cells showing marked cellular and nuclear pleomorphism. The enlarged nuclei are vesicular with prominent nucleoli.

increased blood levels of cortisol and, hence, suppression of ACTH production by the pituitary.

Accordingly, on the basis of knowledge of the effect of ACTH on the cortex, its paucity will result in a gland of reduced size, decreased cortical width, and composed solely of clear lipid-laden zona fasciculata-type cells (Fig. 26.63). The capsule, which is often oedematous, appears thickened.

Prognosis

Spontaneous remissions of Cushing's syndrome, due to bilateral hyperplasia or an adenoma, have been recorded but are rare. Untreated, Cushing's syndrome carries a high mortality. However, surgery will cure the disorder due to an adenoma or bilateral hyperplasia, except in the case of patients with the 'ectopic ACTH' syndrome. More recently, medical adrenalectomies have been employed to treat patients with bilateral hyperplasia. Surgical adrenalectomy can result in the subsequent development of ACTH-producing pituitary tumours (*Nelson's syndrome*). Adrenal carcinomas are associated with a very poor prognosis, with patients dying within 3 years, although some long-term (> 5 years) survivors have been recorded. The recent introduction of adjuvant chemotherapy with *o'p-DDD* may be advantageous. *Streptozotocin* may also have a cytotoxic role to play in therapy (Oberg *et al.* 1988).

The adrenogenital syndrome

The adrenogenital syndrome encompasses those disorders of sexual differentiation due to adrenocortical dysfunction. It is associated with abnormal levels of circulating sex steroid hormones.

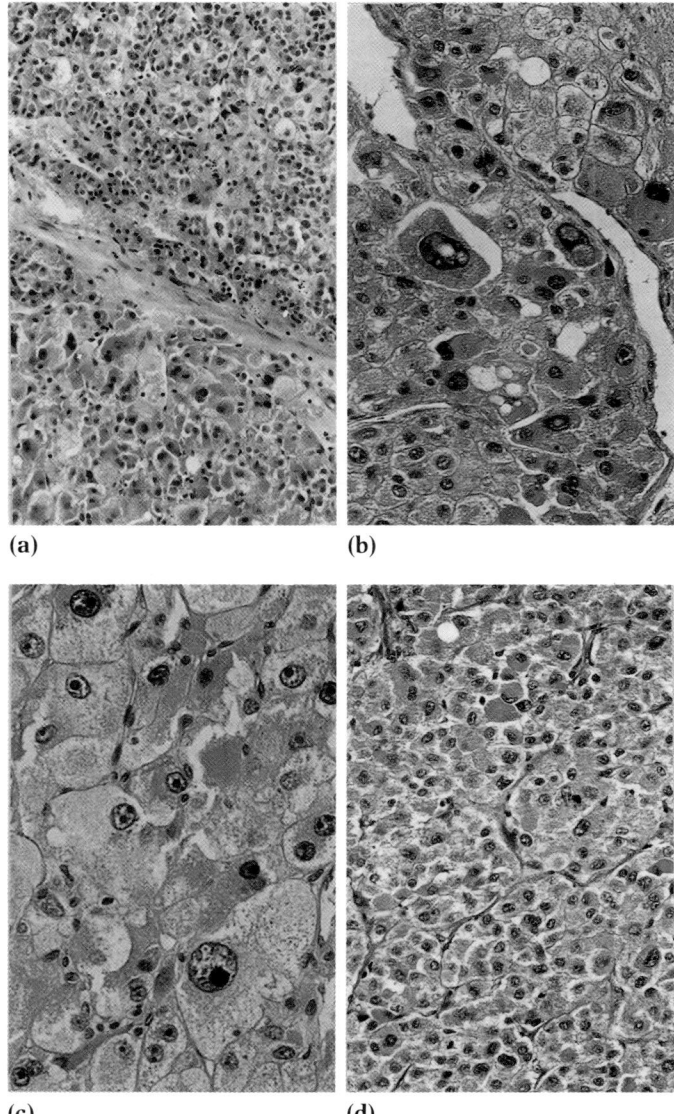

(a) (b)

(c) (d)

Fig. 26.65 Adrenocortical carcinomas. (a) and (b) are two proved carcinomas, weighing 71 g and 1143 g respectively, causing Cushing's syndrome; (c) (1500 g) and (d) (1250 g) are from the adrenogenital syndrome, virilism and feminization respectively. The cells are compact in type in each lesion and show the nuclear features associated with malignancy (pleomorphism, marked vesicularity, and prominent enlarged nucleoli). The lesions are indistinguishable morphologically. It is not possible to predict their functional properties. Attention to the appearance of the attached adrenal gland as well as steroid biochemical analyses are required to distinguish the syndromes with which such lesions are associated (see text).

The commonest cause of this syndrome is *congenital adrenocortical hyperplasia* due to a genetic deficiency of one of the cortisol-synthesizing enzymes. Tumours, both benign and malignant, may also cause this syndrome. They occur at all ages; benign lesions tend to occur, however, before the age of 12 years (Heinebecker *et al.* 1957).

Congenital adrenocortical hyperplasia

Congenital adrenocortical hyperplasia is the most important cause of the adrenogenital syndrome, a fascinating condition or series of related conditions. It affects both sexes equally and manifests itself during infancy or childhood, although delay until adult life has been reported.

All of the cortisol-synthesizing enzymes have been reported as being genetically deficient in the syndrome. However, *in any one patient, only one enzyme is affected*. All the defects cause a decline in cortisol synthesis which leads to increased ACTH production by the pituitary with the end result of increased weight and size of both adrenal glands.

As examples of this condition, two enzyme defects will be presented, namely the *21-hydroxylase defect* (Fig. 26.66) and the enzyme involved in the degradation of *cholesterol to pregnenolone* (Fig. 26.57). Only the former is associated with virilization.

Congenital adrenal hyperplasia with virilization: 21-hydroxylase defect

This enzyme defect is the commonest abnormality, causing 90 per cent of all examples of congenital adrenal hyperplasia. The 21-hydroxylase defect results in lowered cortisol production leading to increased pituitary ACTH secretion with the end result of bilateral adrenocortical hyperplasia (enlarged and heavier glands). The increased ACTH production results in an increased conversion of cholesterol to pregnenolone and thereafter to an accumulation of cortisol precursors (Fig. 26.66), such as *17-hydroxyprogesterone* and *17-hydroxypregnenolone*, which are then converted into DHA and, thence, to the potent androgen, *testosterone*. Hence, virilization results.

There are two forms of this disorder, *classic* and *non-classic* (Table 26.9). In the classic form, virilization commences *in utero* so females are born as *pseudohermaphrodites* with clitoral enlargement, labioscrotal fusion, and, in extreme cases, a penile urethra. Such females still have a uterus and Fallopian tubes. Males, by contrast, appear normal at birth, but sexual precocity develops and, if untreated, gives rise to early epiphyseal fusion and a small final stature.

In many with the classic form, the 21-hydroxylation of progesterone is also affected so that aldosterone synthesis is also compromised (Fig. 26.66) with the development of a *salt-losing syndrome*. In this variant, an acute adrenal crisis may develop 10–15 days after birth and be life-threatening, particularly for males, in whom no other symptoms or signs are yet visible.

In the non-classic form, the defect is milder and evidence of excess androgens only develops after birth so that such female subjects have normal external genitalia at birth.

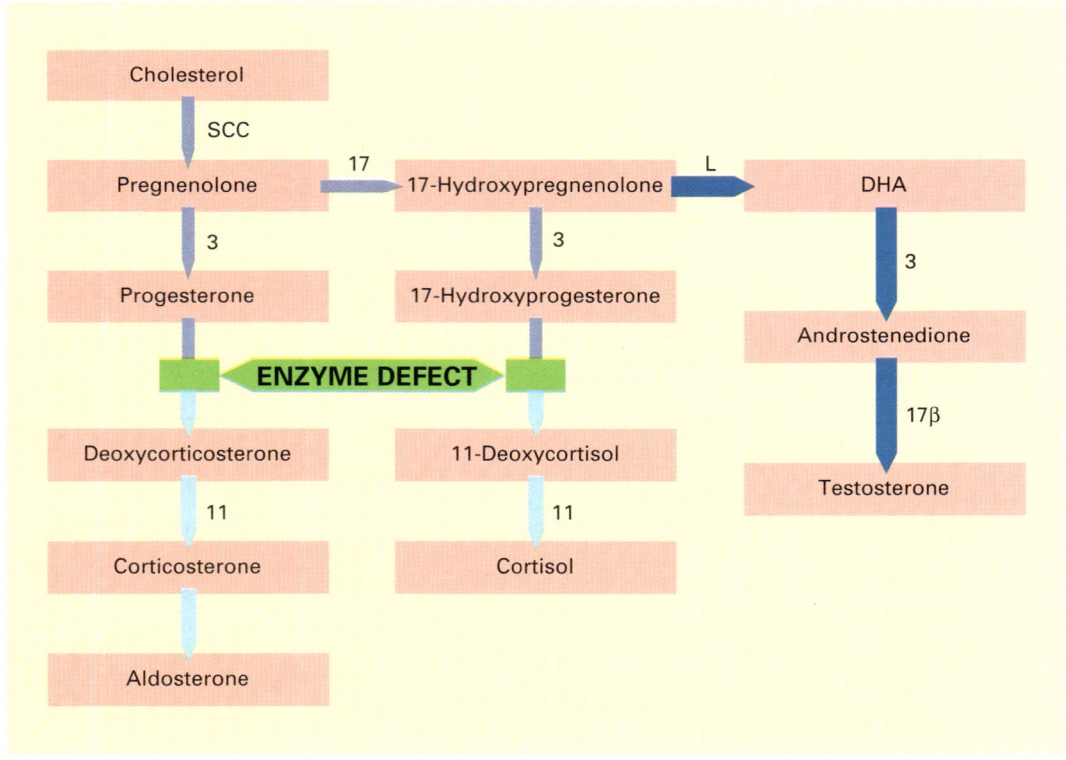

Fig. 26.66 Congenital adrenocortical hyperplasia. Pathways of steroidogenesis in the classic 21-hydroxylase deficiency syndrome. The enzyme defect results in less cortisol production (from 17 hydroxprogesterone) and less aldosterone from progesterone (blue arrows). Hence, ACTH levels rise producing more precursor steroids that are channelled to produce excess DHA and testosterone (purple arrows) and, thus, virilization.

Table 26.9 A résumé of some of the features of the 21-hydroxylase form of congenital adrenocortical hyperplasia*

Feature	Classic form	Non-classic form
Disease frequency	1:12 000	1:100 all whites: 1:30 Ashkenazic Jews
Prenatal virilization	Females	No
Postnatal virilization	60–75% of cases	No
Genotype of CYP21B	Severely affected allele/severely affected allele	Mildly affected allele/mildly affected allele or severely affected allele/mildly affected allele
Associated HLA haplotype	B47, DR7	B14, DR1
Mutation	Deletion, frameshift, nonsense: Ile to Asn-172	Val to Leu-281

* Data culled from Speiser *et al.* (1988).

On examination, the adrenal glands exhibit the end result of significant and prolonged exposure to excessive ACTH levels. The glands can weigh as much as 15 times the weight anticipated for the age of the subject, e.g. 15 g instead of 1 g in neonates and 30–35 g in adults. Macroscopically, such glands have a cerebriform outline with a diffuse brown-coloured cut surface (Fig. 26.67). Histologically, the cortex is markedly broadened and, in conventionally prepared material, consists exclusively of compact lipid-sparse zona reticularis-type cells. Small compact-cell nodules are often present. In neonates, the fetal cortex will also be present showing varying degrees of involution depending on the subject's age (Fig. 26.68a). In cases with defective aldosterone production, bilateral hyperplasia of the zona glomerulosa will also be present.

These histological features are also noted in patients with defects of the *11β-hydroxylase* or *3β-hydroxysteroid dehydrogenase-isomerase enzymes* (Fig. 26.57). Zona glomerulosa hyperplasia does not occur with the 11β-hydroxylase defect as excess *deoxycorticosterone* (DOC) is also produced (Fig. 26.57). This steroid, while preventing salt loss, does cause hypertension.

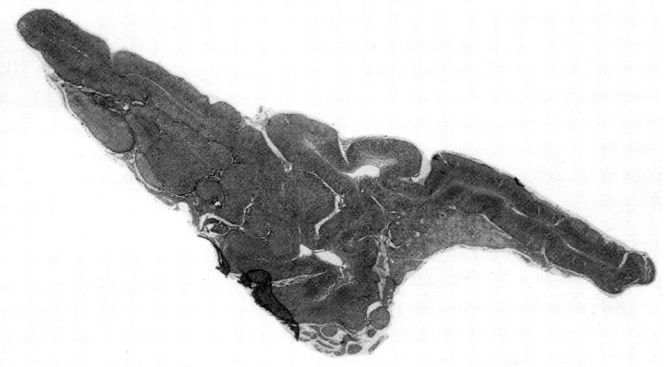

Fig. 26.67 Congenital adrenocortical hyperplasia. 21-Hydroxylase defect. This gland, from a 2½-year-old girl, weighed 6.5 g. It has a typical convoluted cerebriform outline. The cortex, brown in colour on its cut surface, consists solely of compact lipid-sparse cells.

Non-virilizing congenital adrenal hyperplasia syndromes All enzyme defects causing this syndrome are extraordinarily rare, and are still documented in the world literature when recognized. Of the several enzyme defects which can be a cause of this aspect of the syndrome, only the one associated with *defective cholesterol utilization* will be discussed.

Defective cholesterol utilization In this disorder, there is a congenital deficiency of the *side-chain cleavage enzyme* so that cholesterol fails to be converted to pregnenolone. This is the first step leading to the formation of cortisol and aldosterone (Fig. 26.57). Such neonates exhibit salt loss due to inadequate aldosterone production (Fig. 26.57). In males, there is *incomplete masculinization* due to the enzyme defect also affecting the fetal testis and its production of testosterone.

Accordingly, cholesterol and its esterified forms accumulate in the cells of the adrenal cortex. The lack or relative lack of cortisol results in increased ACTH production and bilateral cortical hyperplasia; this time, the cortical cells with their high cholesterol content in conventionally prepared, paraffin-embedded material morphologically will resemble clear lipid-laden zona fasciculata-type cells and occupy the entire broadened cortex, extending out to the capsule (Fig. 26.68b). Foci of cholesterol clefts also occur. The term *congenital 'lipoid' hyperplasia* is given to this entity. In children dying shortly after birth, similar 'lipoid' features will be seen in the fetal cortex.

Genetics

The study of families with the 21-hydroxylase defect has shown that the abnormal genetic locus is situated in the *HLA major histocompatibility complex of chromosome 6* (Speiser *et al.* 1988). Both the classic and non-classic forms are inherited in a recessive manner as allelic variants. Different HLA alleles are associated with the different forms (Table 26.9). Molecular studies have shown that the 21-hydroxylase gene (CYP 21B) is in the HLA complex. Different point mutations of the gene cause the various syndromes (Table 26.9).

The defect, due possibly in some instances to an absence of the enzyme which converts cholesterol to pregnenolone, has

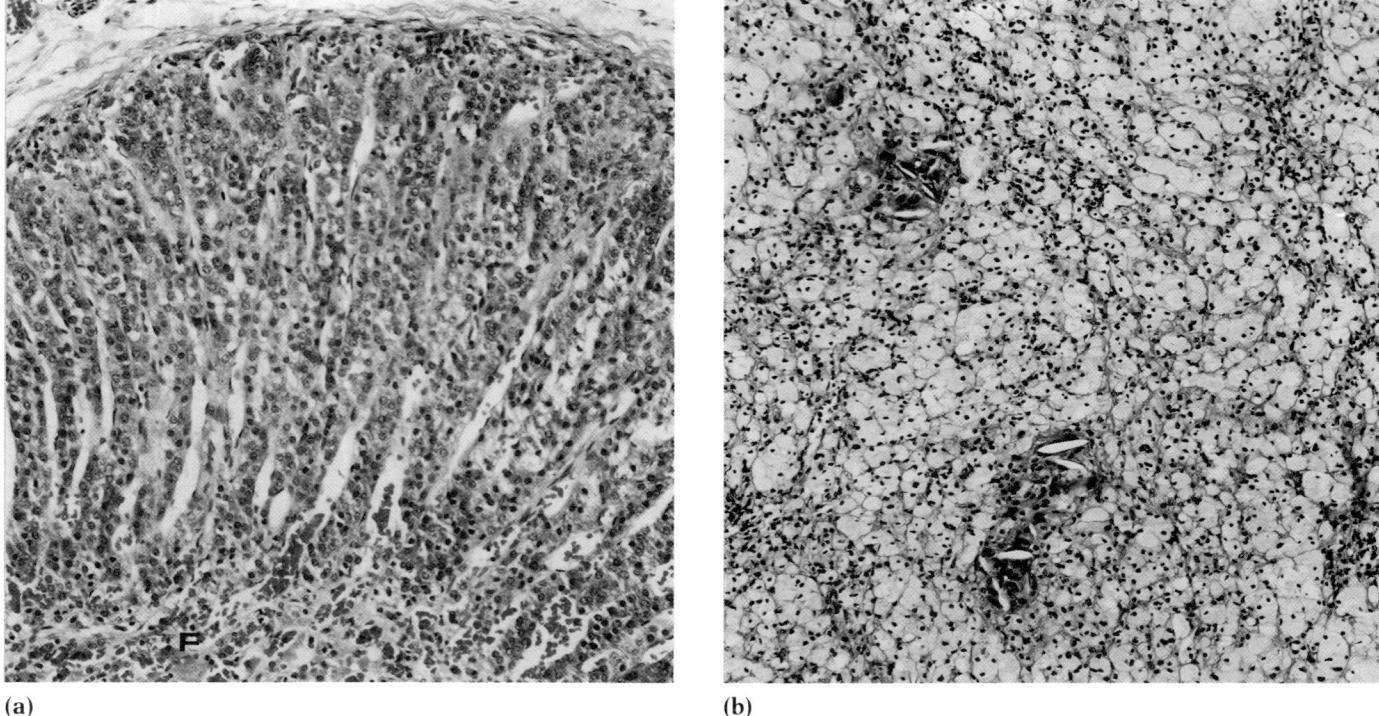

(a)

(b)

Fig. 26.68 Congenital adrenocortical hyperplasia. (a) 21-Hydroxylase defect. This neonatal example shows a broadened outer cortex composed solely of compact-cell columns separated by prominent simusoids. The fetal cortex, on the innermost aspect, is congested and undergoing degeneration. (b) Defective cholesterol utilization (congenital lipoid hyperplasia). The cortex consists exclusively of lipid-laden clear cells. Numerous cholesterol clefts, together with associated foreign-body giant cells, are also present.

been shown by DNA hybridization studies not to be associated with gene deletions (Matteson *et al.* 1986).

Prognosis

The prognosis for children presenting with the adrenogenital syndrome is now good provided diagnosis is made early and therapy instituted promptly. Growth and development can be normal and the cosmetic results of plastic reconstructive surgery, when needed, are also most satisfactory.

Virilizing adrenocortical tumours

Little or nothing is known regarding the causation of such lesions, which tend to occur in children, females more than males, although no age is exempt. In female children, such lesions cause *clitiromegaly* and *hirsutism*, while in female adults, *oligomenorrhoea* develops with *increased musculature* and *hirsutism*. In male children, *precocious isosexual pseudopuberty* develops; in adult males, there may be no overt evidence. Occasionally, and especially with carcinomas, mixed syndromes may be found, e.g. virilism with Cushing's syndrome.

All these adrenocortical tumours, whether benign or malignant, have enzyme defects or changes, often multiple, which channel steroid production towards male sex hormone production, and hence are the basis of the presenting features.

In general, the smaller tumours, especially in young people, are benign, while larger lesions, in excess of 100 g, are gener-

ally carcinomas. However, unlike Cushing's syndrome (p. 1976), the distinction between benign and malignant tumours in this syndrome is not clear cut (Neville and O'Hare 1982; Page *et al.* 1986).

Virilizing tumours, like most adrenocortical tumours, are usually well encapsulated and discrete. Their cut surface usually has a uniform brown–red colour although, in smaller tumours, small yellow-coloured foci may be present. With increasing size, areas of haemorrhage, necrosis, and calcification become frequent. Rarely, cyst formation may be noted.

Small adenomas consist exclusively, or almost so, of compact lipid-sparse cells similar in size and appearance to those of the normal zona reticularis. Occasional foci of clear cells may be present. The tumour cells are arranged in short cords, trabeculae, or strands, with a fine interweaving fibrovascular network (Fig. 26.69a). Nuclear and cellular pleomorphism are not marked. Individual cell necrosis, but not large areas of necrosis, may be present.

In proved carcinomas, the morphological picture is identical to that of the malignant tumours causing Cushing's syndrome (Fig. 26.65), with the lesions consisting of compact-type cells with their typical eosinophilic lipid-sparse cytoplasm arranged in large trabeculae, alveoli, and solid cords. The nuclei are pleomorphic and enlarged, vesicular, with one or more enlarged nucleoli, so typical of the features of adrenocortical carcinomas.

The distinction between the functional activity of Cushing's

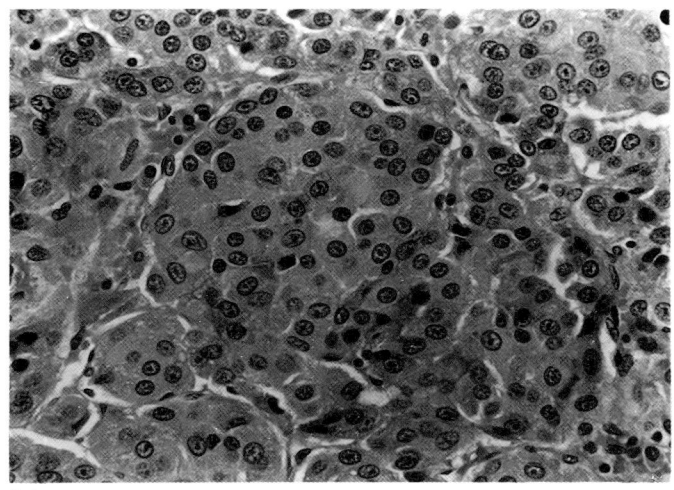

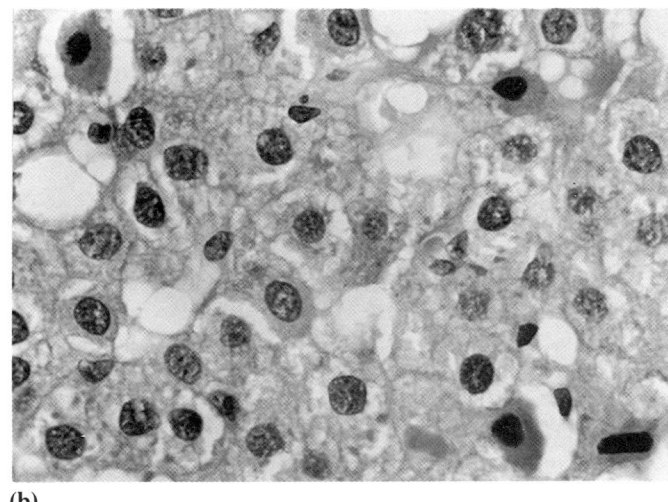

(a)   (b)

Fig. 26.69 Adrenogenital syndrome. Virilizing adrenocortical adenoma. (a) A 25 g lesion, consisting of uniform, normal-sized, compact lipid-sparse cells arranged in nests and strands separated by fine fibrovascular trabeculae. (b) A 228 g adenoma, removed from a 8-year-old boy. The tumour cells, compact in type, are larger than normal and show pleomorphism. This lesion caused great diagnostic difficulty in deciding whether it was benign or malignant. Nucleoli, while present, are not prominent and the nuclei, although enlarged, are not markedly vesicular. The patient is alive and well 20 years later.

and adrenogenital tumours lies in the appearance of the associated adrenal cortex. In Cushing's syndrome, the attached and contralateral adrenal glands exhibit *steroid-induced atrophy* (Fig. 26.63) due to the increased production of cortisol by the tumour. In the pure adrenogenital syndrome, the appearances of the glands are within normal limits.

It is important to remember that, in many virilizing lesions, the light morphological distinction between a benign and malignant tumour is often far from easy, at least by current morphological and related methods. Ultrastructural analysis has no part to play in this context. Such difficulties tend to be encountered when tumours weigh between 100 and 400 g. They consist of large lipid-sparse zona reticularis-type cells forming trabeculae and sheets with intervening sinusoids (Fig. 26.69b). The cells and nuclei are larger than normal and may show pleomorphism, even with giant forms. This type of lesion is difficult or impossible to classify as benign or malignant.

Recently, several studies involving flow cytometric analysis of nuclear DNA from adrenal tumours have revealed that such an approach may assist in predicting the outcome. The presence of *aneuploidy* was seen to correlate with recurrence or metastases (Amberson *et al.* 1987). *In vitro* biochemical and cell culture methods can also assist in this context (Neville and O'Hare 1982).

Prognosis Benign lesions may be cured by surgery; as a group, carcinomas of the virilizing type metastasize more slowly than those found in Cushing's syndrome. The prognosis, however, is poor.

Feminizing adrenocortical tumours

Less than 100 oestrogen-producing adrenocortical tumours causing feminization have been recorded (Gabrilove *et al.* 1965; Neville and O'Hare 1982).

Males are most often affected when the presenting sign is *bilateral gynaecomastia*. However, pre-pubertal females and post-menopausal women may also exhibit feminization. Hyper-oestrogenism is, naturally, difficult to detect clinically in adult females.

The size of such tumours is very variable and many weigh over 1 kg. Their morphological features are similar to those of virilizing tumours and consist of compact cells of the zona reticularis-type (Fig. 26.65). In many reported cases, the morphological appearance of the cells has often seemed benign and yet they have been found subsequently to metastasize. Accordingly, all, irrespective of their histology, should be regarded as carcinomas.

Rare examples of feminization with raised oestrogen levels, which decline in response to dexamethasone administration and are associated in men with spermatogenic arrest, have been described. The adrenal abnormalities in those cases remain to be reported, but a non-neoplastic aetiology is suspected.

Hyperaldosteronism with low plasma renin (primary aldosteronism; Conn's syndrome)

This syndrome of hyperaldosteronism and low plasma renin (so-called primary aldosteronism), epitomized by *hypertension and hypokalaemic alkalosis*, was first described by Conn in 1955. It is due to the increased production of *aldosterone*, although similar features can develop when adrenal corticosteroids, other than aldosterone, but with mineralocorticoid effects, are produced in excess. It is thought that between 1 and 2 per cent of unselected hypertensive subjects may have this disorder, but the precise incidence is difficult to gauge.

Unlike Cushing's and the adrenogenital syndromes, *adrenocortical tumours*, almost all benign, are the commonest cause of Conn's syndrome. Rarely, a carcinoma or bilateral hyperplasia of the zona glomerulosa is the precipitating lesion (Neville and Symington 1966; Neville and O'Hare 1982; Page *et al.* 1986).

Adenomas

Adrenal tumours causing hyperaldosteronism with low plasma renin are almost always benign, single, and occur in females more often than males, especially between the ages of 30 and 50 years (Table 26.10). Most tumours weigh less than 4 g and are unilateral, involving the left more often than the right gland.

While larger benign lesions may project from one pole of the adrenal gland, many are of such small size that they are contained wholly within the gland. Typically, the tumours are encapsulated and circumscribed with a distinctive golden-yellow cut surface.

Microscopically, their appearance is very characteristic and unexpected. Most adenomas consist of clear lipid-laden cells similar in size and appearance to those of the zona fasciculata. Such cells may comprise all the lesion or be the dominant type admixed with other lipid-laden cells whose size lies between that of zona fasciculata and the smaller zona glomerulosa cells. They are known as *intermediate cells* (Fig. 26.70). Zona glomerulosa cells may or may not be found; when present they tend to surround the periphery of the lesion in a subcapsular location dipping into the tumour in a tongue-like manner, or they are found in the immediate vicinity of fibrovascular septae which permeate and punctuate the whole tumour (Fig. 26.71). Compact zona reticularis cells may also be present. Varying degrees of admixtures of these cell occur in any one lesion, but usually the large clear cells predominate together with intermediate cells; rarely, a tumour has been found to consist only of zona glomerulosa-type cells.

The tumour cells are arranged in short cords or nests separated by a fine fibrovascular stroma (Figs 26.70, 26.71). The nuclei often contain vacuolated inclusions and are more vesicular than normal. Nuclear and cellular pleomorphism is often present although not marked; giant and bizarre forms can occur but do not indicate malignancy. Ultrastructurally, the

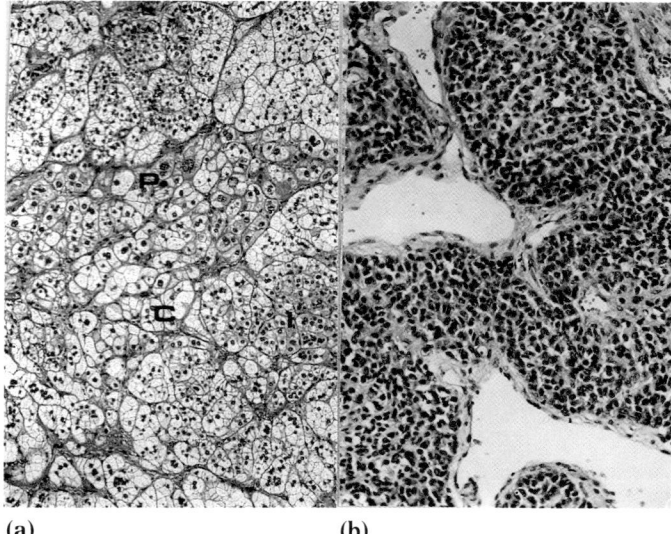

(a)   **(b)**

Fig. 26.70 Hyperaldosteronism with low plasma renin. (a) Adrenocortical adenoma. The typical appearance of a 2.5 g adenoma is presented with its composition of large clear (C) and intermediate (I) cells. They are arranged in nests separated by prominent fibrovascular trabeculae. Nuclear pleomorphism is readily apparent (P). (b) Adrenocortical carcinoma. This lesion weighed 2000 g and is composed of zona glomerulosa-type cells arranged in characteristic large trabeculae with intervening prominent sinusoids and fibrovascular trabeculae.

component cells, both large and intermediate clear-cell types, have features, such as mitochondria and RER, that resemble those of normal zona glomerulosa cells or are intermediate between this cell type and those of the normal, typical lipid-laden zona fasciculata cell.

Why do such aldosterone-producing adenomas not follow the expected morphological appearance and be composed of zona glomerulosa cells only? This is, after all, the cell type that produces aldosterone. There is no doubt but that such lesions are the source of the excess aldosterone production. The answer to this quandary may lie in the glucocorticoid levels of the arterial blood entering and flowing through the adrenal cortex. High glucocorticoid levels *in vitro* are known to inhibit aldosterone production.

The normal zona glomerulosa is situated immediately below the adrenal capsule and is the first zone to receive arterial blood, which is relatively low in glucocorticoid levels compared to the adrenal venous effluent. From experimental data, it would appear that the normal zona glomerulosa may produce both aldosterone and glucocorticoids. In the effluent from this zone, therefore, the level of glucocorticoids becomes high. Such high levels may suppress aldosterone secretion elsewhere deeper in the cortex. Hence, this mineralocorticoid is only produced in the outermost zone of the cortex. If similar constraints exist in adrenocortical adenomas associated with hyperaldosteronism, it is not unreasonable to find 'true' zona glomerulosa-type cells in relation only to the periphery of the tumour and with the permeating fibrovascular trabeculae where afferent arterial

Table 26.10 Primary aldosteronism: analysis of 240 patients with benign tumours of the adrenal cortex*

	Male	Female
Sex incidence	30%	70%
Modal age incidence (years)	30–50	30–50
Site of tumours (left:right)		
Single	1:1	7:4
Multiple	1:4	4:1
Weight of tumours (g)		
<2		34%
<4		58%

* Neville and O'Hare (1982).

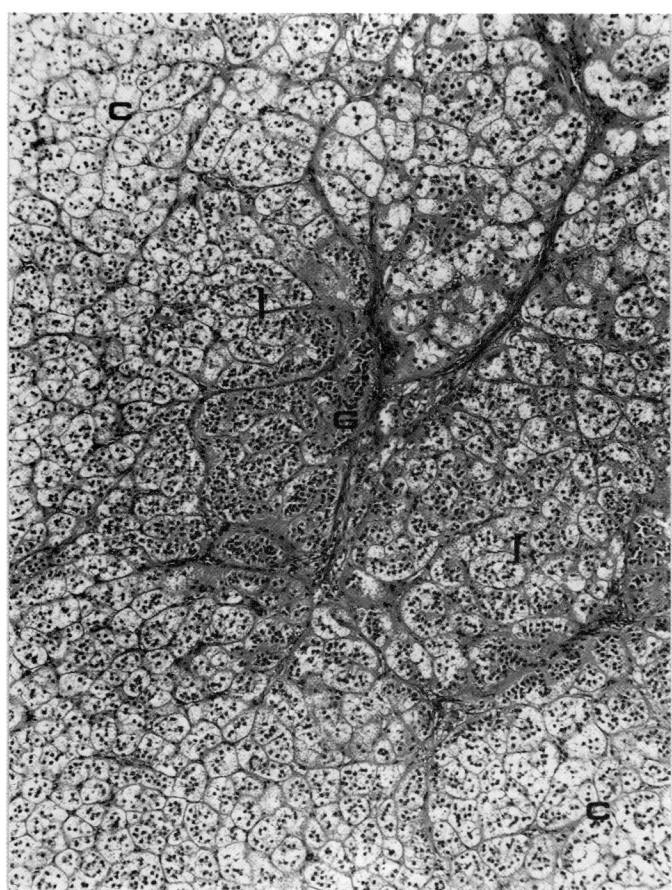

Fig. 26.71 Hyperaldosteronism with low plasma renin. Adrenocortical adenoma (1.0 g). Cells of the large clear type (C) are the main constituents of this tumour. Toward the periphery of the lesion, numerous fibrovascular trabeculae dip into the tumour and appear to carry with them zona glomerulosa-type cells (G). Intermediate cells (I) are present between the zona glomerulosa-type and large clear cells.

blood vessels also exist. In other areas, the influence of cortisol secretion will result in intermediate-type cells and eventually large clear zona fasciculata-type cells (Neville and O'Hare 1982; Sasano *et al.* 1989).

In a preceding section, it was mentioned that adrenocortical nodules were frequently associated with so-called '*essential*' *hypertension*. Is it possible that such nodules represent the end result of '*cortisol-differentiation*' of an aldosterone-producing adenoma which was the original cause of the hypertension? Subsequently, despite normal aldosterone levels being reached eventually, the hypertension has become permanent due to the established vascular changes.

The attached and contralateral cortex The adrenal cortex associated with hyperaldosterone-producing adenomas exhibits a degree of narrowing of the cortex, resulting in an apparently increased width of the zona glomerulosa. Such changes are consistent with some cortisol production by the tumour causing a degree of cortical atrophy. Many of the glands also exhibit

nodules of varying size. Their features have already been described (Fig. 26.59) (p. 1972).

Other adrenal changes

Adrenocortical carcinomas, often large, may cause hypertension. They are extremely rare. Those producing aldosterone have a typical microscopic appearance (Fig. 26.70); others secreting alternative hypertension-inducing steroids such as deoxycorticosterone (Fig. 26.57) are more typical of zona fasciculata and zona reticularis functions and are morphologically indistinguishable from those causing Cushing's and the adrenogenital syndromes (Fig. 26.65).

In some subjects with primary aldosteronism, no tumours are found. These subjects who tend to be older than those with adenomas, are found to have bilateral hyperplasia of the zona glomerulosa, with or without associated adrenocortical nodules (Fig. 26.72).

An even rarer cause of hyperaldosteronism is a disorder called *dexamethasone-suppressible hyperaldosteronism*. It is familial and may be a form of congenital hyperplasia involving a partial defect in the action of the *17α*-hydroxylase enzyme (Fig. 26.57). Morphologically, 17α-hydroxylase deficiencies result, however, in enlarged glands with appearances similar to those of the 21-hydroxylase defect and quite different from the hyperplasia of Conn's syndrome (Sasano *et al.* 1987).

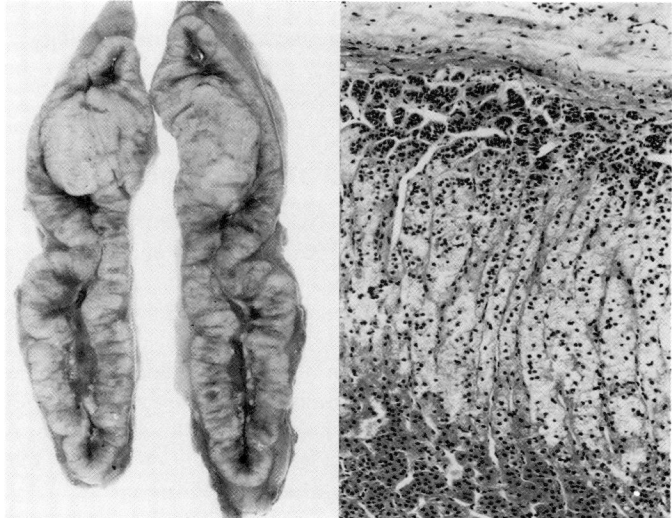

Fig. 26.72 Hyperaldosteronism with low plasma renin. Bilateral nodular hyperplasia. The appearances of the gland, illustrated here, were similar on both sides. This gland (4.89 g) is opened to show a small 0.6 cm yellow intraglandular nodule with numerous further micronodules in the rest of the cortex. The nodules were typical morphologically (see Fig. 26.59). The cortex showed bilateral hyperplasia of the zona glomerulosa with broad sinusoids between the nests of glomerulosa cells. These features may occur alone to cause hyperaldosteronism or be present in the attached and contralateral glands in cases of adenomas causing the syndrome. In this latter case, the cortex may be slightly reduced in width (see text).

Prognosis

The outlook following surgical extirpation of an adenoma is good, often with complete reversal of the hypertension. However, the hypertension in patients with non-tumourous hyperaldosteronism due to bilateral zona glomerulosa hyperplasia seldom abates following surgery to remove the glands. The prognosis for subjects with carcinomas is poor, such lesions pursuing a very aggressive course.

Hyperaldosteronism with high plasma renin (secondary aldosteronism)

Elevated aldosterone levels, in response to an increase in renin and angiotensin circulating levels, occur in association with numerous extra-adrenal disorders. They are usually associated with oedema of renal, cardiac, or hepatic origin. Such cases exhibit bilateral hyperplasia of the zona glomerulosa (Fig. 26.72). Consequently, careful history and adequate biochemical analyses are essential in the diagnosis of the different forms of non-tumourous aldosteronism.

Mineralocorticoid excess without hyperaldosteronism

Hypertension may be induced by adrenal lesions producing steroids such as *deoxycorticosterone* (DOC). These include congenital adrenocortical hyperplasia due to 11β-hydroxylase or 17α-hydroxylase defects.

Some adrenocortical carcinomas produce significant amounts of deoxycorticosterone and cause hypertension. Rarely, increased deoxycorticosterone levels are raised due to bilateral hyperplasia of the zona glomerulosa. The aetiology of this last anomaly is unknown; the hypertension may be reversed with the drug *spironolactone*.

26.4.4   Non-functioning (non-hormonal) adrenocortical carcinomas

From time to time, patients will present with an abnormal mass located by clinical and/or radiographic means in one or other adrenal gland. No overt evidence of hormonal imbalance will be noted clinically.

However, detailed chemical analyses of the blood or urinary steroid profiles will reveal that such tumours are not inert, but are producing a wide variety of non-hormonally active precursor steroids, e.g. *pregnenolone* (Fig. 26.57). Such lesions are, thus, not non-functioning, but rather non-hormonal.

These tumours are rare, and invariably malignant. They tend to afflict men more than women, especially between the ages of 40 and 60 years, although no age is exempt (Lewinsky *et al.* 1974). Because they do not cause hormonal symptoms and signs, these lesions are often late in recognition and frequently large, weighing over 1 kg. Many have metastasized at the time of initial diagnosis. Morphologically, they display features identical to those of carcinomas causing Cushing's syndrome (Figs 26.65, 26.73). The attached and contralateral glands are normal in appearance, consistent with the fact that cortisol and ACTH production are not affected in this disorder.

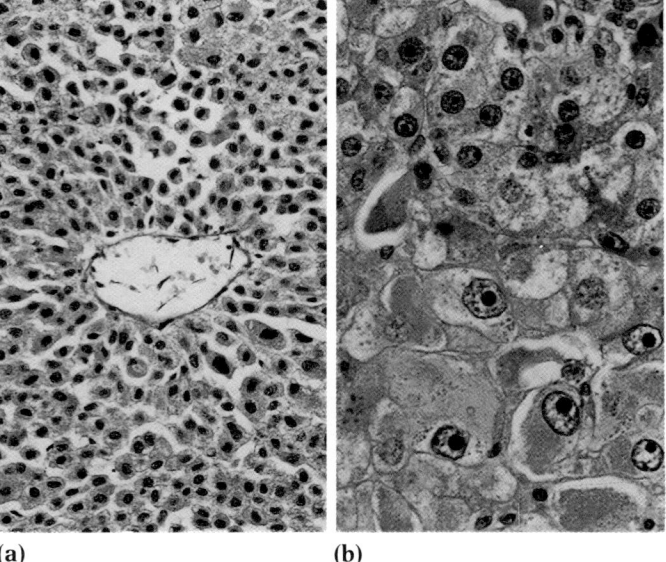

(a)   **(b)**

Fig. 26.73   Non-hormonal adrenocortical carcinoma. The tumour cells in both examples are of the compact type arranged in trabeculae punctuated by vascular sinusoids (a). While pleomorphism is present, it is more marked in (b), where the nuclei are enlarged and vesicular with prominent nucleioli, so typical of adrenal carcinomas.

The prognosis for patients with these lesions is poor; most patients succumb with metastases within 1 year of diagnosis, although about one-third survive beyond 3 years (Oberg *et al.* 1988). In the follow-up of these patients, it is essential to characterize the nature of the precursor steroids being released and to use them as index substances to monitor the clinical course.

26.4.5   Hypocorticalism

The several causes of decreased adrenocortical function are shown in Table 26.11. The term *adrenoprivic* implies that the origin of the hypocorticalism lies within the cortex itself, while *tropoprivic* infers that reduced ACTH stimulation of the cortex is the basic aetiology.

All forms of hypocorticalism are extremely rare and the reader is referred to detailed texts for further information as only the least uncommon conditions will be discussed in this section (Neville and O'Hare 1982).

Acute acquired adrenoprivic hypocorticalism

This term implies that the hypocorticalism is of acute onset, of adrenal origin, and due to causes affecting the gland as opposed to an inherent adrenal defect.

Formerly, *bilateral adrenal haemorrhage* was considered a prime cause of this condition. However, most, but not all, recent studies negate its importance in this context. The commonest cause of acute adrenocortical insufficiency is, therefore, probably that which can occur in patients who are receiving *substitution steroid therapy* following bilateral adrenalectomy, or in patients with *chronic acquired adrenoprivic hypocorticalism*

Table 26.11 Aetiological classification of hypocorticalism

Adrenoprivic hypocorticalism

1. Congenital
  (a) Idiopathic congenital adrenocortical hypoplasia and the syndrome of ACTH unresponsiveness
  (b) Congenital adrenocortical hyperplasia (adrenogenital syndrome)

2. Acquired
  (a) Acute
    (i) Withdrawal of glucocorticoid substitution therapy
    (ii) Bilateral adrenal haemorrhage
  (b) Chronic
    (i) Addison's disease (see Table 26.12)

Tropoprivic hypocorticalism

1. Congenital
  (i) Adrenal hypoplasia in anencephalia

2. Acquired
  (i) Iatrogenic—exogenous glucocorticoid therapy
  (ii) Cortisol-producing adrenal tumours
  (iii) Sheehan's syndrome
  (iv) Simmond's disease
  (v) Idiopathic ACTH deficiency disease

Table 26.12 Aetiology of chronic acquired adrenoprivic hypocorticalism (Addison's disease)

Idiopathic
  Organ-specific auto-immune adrenalitis
Inflammatory
  Granulomata
  Tuberculosis
  Sarcoidosis
  Protozoa and fungi
  Histoplasmosis
  Blastomycosis
  Coccidiomycosis
  Candidiasis (moniliasis)
  Torulosis (cryptococcosis)
  Viruses
  Cytomegalovirus
  Herpes simplex
Metabolic
  Amyloidosis
Neoplastic
  Metastatic carcinoma
  Lymphoma
Iatrogenic
  Ketoconazole therapy

(*Addison's disease*). When such treatment is withdrawn or these patients are further stressed as, for example, by an operation or infection, then minor or even major degrees of insufficiency may rapidly evolve if replacement therapy is not augmented.

Chronic acquired adrenoprivic hypocorticalism (Addison's disease)

Patients with chronic acquired adrenoprovic hypocorticalism present clinically with the symptoms and signs of Addison's disease, which include *weakness, fatigue, hyperpigmentation, hypotension, and weight loss.* Of the many causes (Table 26.12), *idiopathic organ-specific auto-immune adrenalitis* (*idiopathic Addison's disease*) is the commonest, followed by *tuberculosis* of the adrenal gland. It was formerly considered that bilateral involvement of the adrenal glands by *metastatic carcinomas* did not cause, or was a rare cause, of adrenal insufficiency. However, the use of more esoteric and sophisticated tests has shown biochemical evidence of adrenal insufficiency in such patients, although overt clinical manifestations seldom are detectable or develop.

Organ-specific auto-immune adrenalitis (idiopathic Addison's disease)

Addison's disease is the least uncommon of the group of disorders causing hypocorticalism. It occurs most commonly between the third and fifth decades and tends to afflict women. It is often associated with other auto-immune disorders involving the thyroid and parathyroid glands, ovary and stomach, e.g. the *auto-immune polyglandular disease type I.* It is associated with an increase in the level of circulating ACTH.

The adrenal glands are smaller than normal. For individual glands, weights of 0.2 g are not uncommon. Adrenocortical tissue may not be detectable macroscopically at autopsy, and only be found by microscopic examination of the adrenal bed.

Histologically, the whole cortex exhibits *diffuse atrophy.* The capsule is thickened. When cortical tissue is definable, the cells exist in isolation, as small clusters or short cords (Fig. 26.74a). The adrenal cells are compact in type with lipid-sparse cytoplasm and are similar in size to those of the normal zona reticularis. Abundant lipofuscin may be seen in the cytoplasm. An

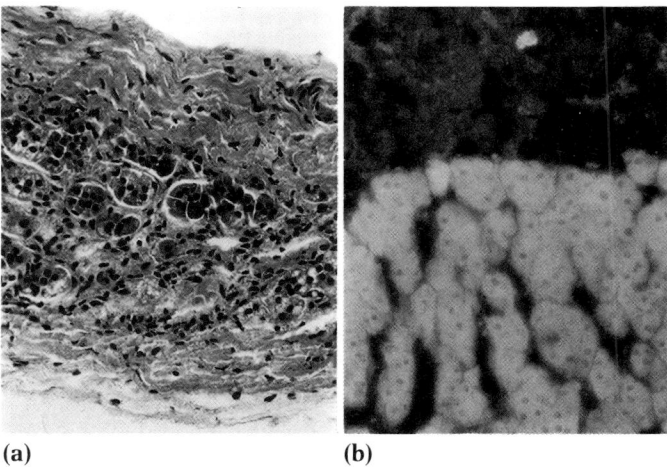

(a)   **(b)**

Fig. 26.74 Idiopathic Addison's disease. The atrophic gland (a) has a thickened capsule and contains islands of surviving compact-type cells. A chronic inflammatory infiltrate is present. An immunofluorescent illustration of auto-antibodies to adrenocortical cells in a subject with hypocorticalism is presented in (b). (Courtesy of Professor J. Anderson, Glasgow.)

extensive and diffuse infiltration of lymphocytes, together with plasma cells and macrophages, is always present. The adrenal medulla is normal in appearance. These appearances require to be distinguished from the atrophy due to increased levels of glucocorticoid hormones (steroid-induced atrophy) (Fig. 26.63) or with other inflammatory infiltrates (Table 26.12)

The cause of organ-specific auto-immune adrenalitis is unknown, but there is a higher risk of its occurring in patients with a *HLA DR3 constitution*. Many of these patients also have auto-antibodies directed against the thyroid, stomach, para-thyroid gland, and the ovary, as well as having type I diabetes mellitus. Most of the auto-antibodies are organ specific and occur in about 70 per cent of patients (Fig. 26.74b). Antibodies reacting with steroid-producing cells may also be found. Auto-antibodies to cell surface antigens of the cortical cells have recently been detected, and some believe that they are the most relevant ones in causing the atrophy and cell death in this dis-order, and that the other auto-antibodies develop subsequently. However, there are reports that infer that the organ-specific and steroid-cell auto-antibodies are present prior to biochemical and overt clinical manifestation of hypofunction (Ahonen *et al.* 1987). The adrenocortical cells show an increased expression of *class II MHC antigens*, but this may well be due to their induc-tion by the lymphokines produced by the inflammatory cells rather than their being related to the basic aetiology.

Adrenoleukodystrophy

A variant form, referred to as *Schilder–Addison's disease*, or bet-ter *adrenoleukodystrophy* (ALD), has been described in recent years. Here, Addison's disease is associated with diffuse demy-elination of the central and peripheral nervous systems. ALD is a fatal disorder that belongs to the genetic peroxisomal group of diseases. It takes one of three forms:

1. *neonatal ALD*, an autosomal recessive disorder;

2. *childhood ALD*, an X-linked recessive disease; or

3. *adrenomyeloneuropathy*, an X-linked recessive disease which, however, does not present until early adulthood. In it, tes-ticular failure also occurs.

Generally, the neurological aspects supersede evidence of adrenal hypofunction. Steroid replacement therapy does not halt the progress of these diseases.

The adrenal cortex shows progressive cytolysis, atrophy with decreasing cell numbers, and often consists solely of clusters of swollen 'ballooned' cells with granular eosinophilic cytoplasm, occasionally with a unique striated appearance quite typical of the disorder. This latter change is best seen by electron micro-scopy. Eventually, only the medulla remains (Powers *et al.* 1980).

The cause is due to a defect in the oxidation of *very-long-chain fatty acids*. An accumulation of C_{26} relative to C_{22} fatty acids occurs and, once esterified to cholesterol, interferes with intra-cellular enzyme functions, to create cell toxicity. Other defects involving *plasmalogen* and *β-galactosidase* have been described. Determination of the $C_{26}:C_{20}$ fatty acid levels in blood or fibro-blasts allows diagnosis and, by using amniotic cells, prenatal diagnosis is possible.

26.4.6   Other anomalies

While this chapter has concentrated upon functioning lesions of the adrenal cortex, it is important to remember that other con-ditions, including benign and malignant tumours, not unique to the adrenal gland, may be detected from time to time, the more since the introduction of CT scanning. Reference to the incidental detection of adrenocortical nodules has already been made (p. 1972). Other lesions include *myelolipoma*, *cysts*, *pseudocysts*, and *neonatal haemorrhage*. Clinical acumen and histological examination serve to identify such conditions.

Neoplasms of the adrenal stroma will occur from time to time, arising from connective, vascular, or adipose tissues. Their appearances and therapy are the same as when they occur at commoner sites.

26.4.7   Bibliography

Alba, M., Hirayama, A., Iri, H., Kodama, T., Fujimoto, Y., Kusakabe, K., *et al.* (1990). Primary adrenocortical micronodular dysplasia: Enzyme histochemical and ultrastructural studies of two cases with a review of the literature. *Human Pathology* **21**, 503–11.

Ahonen, P., Miettinen, A., and Perheentupa, J. (1987). Adrenal and steroidal cell antibodies in patients with autoimmune poly-glandular disease type I and risk of adrenocortical and ovarian failure. *Journal of Clinical Endocinology and Metabolism* **64**, 494–500.

Amberson, J. B., Vaughan, E. D., Gray, G. F., and Naus, G. J. (1987). Flow cytometric analysis of nuclear DNA from adrenocortical neo-plasms. *Cancer* **59**, 2091–5.

Gabrilove, J. L., Sharma, D. C., Wotiz, H. H., and Dorfman, R. I. (1965). Feminizing adrenocortical tumors in the male. A review of 52 cases including a case report. *Medicine* **44**, 37–79.

Gabrilove, J. L., Anderson, P. J., and Halmi, N. S. (1986). Pituitary proopiomelanocortin-cell carcinoma occuring in conjunction with a glioblastoma in a patient with Cushing's disease and subsequent Nelson's syndrome. *Clinical Endocrinology* **25**, 117–26.

Heinbecker, P., O'Neal, O., and Ackerman, L. V. (1957). Functioning and non-functioning adrenal cortical tumors. *Surgery, Gynecology and Obstetrics* **105**, 21–33.

Kapcala, L. P. (1987). Alcohol-induced pseudo-Cushing's syndrome mimicking Cushing's disease in a patient with an adrenal mass. *American Journal of Medicine* **82**, 849–56.

Lewinsky, B. S., Grigor, K. M., Symington, T., and Neville, A. M. (1974). The clinical and pathologic features of 'non-hormonal' adrenocortical tumors. *Cancer* **33**, 778–90.

Matteson, K. J., Chung, B.-C., Urdea, M. S., and Miller, W. L. (1986). Study of cholesterol side-chain cleavage (20, 22 desmolase) defi-ciency causing congenital lipoid adrenal hyperplasia using bovine-sequence P450scc oligodeoxyribonucleotide probes. *Endocrinology* **118**, 1296–1305.

Neville, A. M. and O'Hare, M. J. (1982). *The human adrenal cortex*. Springer-Verlag, Berlin.

Neville, A. M. and Symington, T. (1966). Pathology of primary aldo-steronism. *Cancer* **12**, 1854–64.

Oberg, K., Goldhirsch, A., and Neville, A. M. (1988). In *Textbook of uncommon cancer*, (ed. C. J. Williams, J. G. Krikorisin, M. R. Green, and D. Raghavon), pp. 731–62. John Wiley and Sons, Chichester.

Oelkers, W., Bähr, V., Hensen, J., and Pickartz, H. (1986). Primary adrenocortical micronodular adenomatosis causing Cushing's syndrome. Effects of ketoconazole on steroid production and *in vitro* performance of adrenal cells. *Acta Endocrinologica* **113**, 370–7.

Page, D. L., DeLellis, R. A., and Hough, A. J. (1986). *Tumors of the adrenal.* Armed Forces Institute of Pathology, Washington, DC.

Powers, J. M., Schaumburg, H. H., Johnson, A. B., and Raine, C. S. (1980). A correlative study of the adrenal cortex in adreno-leukodystophy: evidence for a fatal intoxication with very long chain saturated fatty acids. Enzyme histochemistry, fine structure, tissue culture, proposed molecular model and cellular pathogenesis. *Investigative and Cell Pathology* **3**, 353–62.

Sasano, H., Mason, J. I., and Sasano, N. (1989). Immunohistochemical study of cytochrome P-450$_{17a}$ in human adrenocortical disorders. *Human Pathology* **20**, 113–17.

Sasano, H., Masuda, T., Ojima, M., Fukuchi, S., and Sasano, N. (1987). Congenital 17α-hydroxylase deficiency: a clinico-pathologic study. *Human Pathology* **18**, 1002–7.

Speiser, P. W., New, M. I., and White, P. C. (1988). Molecular genetic analysis of nonclassic steroid 21-hydroxylase deficiency associated with HLA-B12, DR1. *New England Journal of Medicine* **319**, 19–23.

Symington, T. (1969). *Functional pathology of the human adrenal gland.* Livingstone, Edinburgh.

26.5 The adrenal medulla

A. Gallimore

26.5.1 Introduction

The adrenal medulla forms a specialized adjunct to the sympathetic nervous system. The constituent chromaffin cells are functionally similar to postganglionic neurones of the sympathetic system and secrete either adrenaline or noradrenaline. In addition to adrenal chromaffin cells, aggregates of similar cells are found associated with the sympathetic nervous system, distributed symmetrically and segmentally in the paraxial regions of the trunk and neck. These form the *extra-adrenal paraganglionic system*. Less commonly, *ectopic chromaffin rests* are found in the wall of the urinary bladder, the gut, gonads, and elsewhere.

26.5.2 Embryology

Chromaffin cells are derived from the neural crest and are so named because their stored catecholamine granules turn brown when fixed in dichromate salts. *Sympathoblasts* invade the primitive adrenal cortex at about seven weeks' gestation and subsequently migrate centrally. Similar cells migrate to areas where sympathetic nervous tissue is found to form, subsequently, the extra-adrenal paraganglionic system. Up until birth the development of the adrenal medulla is relatively slow,

after which it accelerates. Indeed, prenatally the only source of adrenaline, in the fetus, is the *organ of Zuckerkandl*, and the medulla lacks the necessary enzyme for converting noradrenaline to adrenaline until after birth. Postnatally extra-adrenal chromaffin tissue regresses as the adrenal medulla develops.

26.5.3 Physiology

Chromaffin cells elaborate, store, and secrete *catecholamines*. These are hydroxylated aromatic amino acids synthesized from tyrosine. The predominant adrenal catecholamines are *adrenaline* and *noradrenaline*, but very small amounts of tyramine and dopamine are produced also. The relative proportion of adrenaline and noradrenaline found in the adrenal medulla is 9:1. The important metabolites of medullary catecholamines are *metanephrine, normetanephrine, vaniyll mandelic acid, and 3-methoxy-4-hydroxyphenoglycol*. The principal effects of adrenaline, which evokes both *alpha* and *beta responses*, are positive inotropic and chronotropic cardiac effects, vascular and bronchial smooth muscle relaxation, and enhancement of glycogenolysis and lipolysis. Noradrenaline has chiefly *alphaadrenergic effects*, causing contraction of vascular smooth muscle, producing an elevation of peripheral resistance.

Chromaffin cells receive input from preganglionic sympathetic innervation, and their hormones act as neurochemical transducers, producing a physiological response from electrical activity. Unlike most hormones, there is rapid onset of effect with equally rapid dissipation, commensurate with the role of the adrenal medulla in response to emotional or physical stress.

The CNS areas regulating sympathoadrenal activity are not fully identified, but there are specific centres in the medulla, pons, and hypothalamus. Neurotransmitters involved in CNS connections include adrenaline, noradrenaline, dopamine, serotonin, and oxytocin. Impulses arrive at the receptors of the adrenal medulla via preganglionic fibres arising form levels T1 to L2 of the spinal cord. These nerves synapse with postganglionic neurones of the paravertebral sympathetic ganglia or pass through the ganglia at level T5 to L2, to form the splanchnic nerves. These neurones synapse later with receptors of the adrenal medulla. The CNS centres themselves receive input from the cerebral cortex, hypothalamus, and limbic system. Afferent impulses also form reflex arcs and elicit changes in sympathetic discharge at the level of the brain stem. In addition, the composition of the extracellular fluid with regard to tonicity, hormone concentration, and pH also influences discharge of brain stem centres.

26.5.4 Morphology

The combined weight of the adrenal medullae is about 1.0 g and this represents 10 per cent of total adrenal mass. The arterial supply to the adrenal is through branches of the inferior phrenic artery (superior adrenal artery), the aorta (middle adrenal artery), and the renal artery (inferior adrenal artery). These vessels form an anastomosing plexus within the capsule of the gland. The medulla is supplied both directly from tributaries of this system and via venous channels, forming a portal system, from the cortex. The portal blood is rich in corticosteroid hormones, which play an important part in the functioning of the adrenal medulla. Capillaries ultimately coalesce to form a single adrenal vein which drains into the vena cava on the right side and into the renal vein on the left.

The adrenal medulla is composed of densely packed groups of chromaffin cells, in cords or clumps, set within a stroma consisting of a fine capillary network together with nervous and connective tissue. Chromaffin cells are irregular, polyhedral cells with strongly basophilic cytoplasm, containing *secretory granules*. The granules are seen ultrastructurally as dense core granules 100–300 nm. Adrenaline-secreting granules occur in 85 per cent; most of the remainder contain noradrenaline granules.

26.5.5   Phaeochromocytoma

The name phaeochromocytoma is derived from the dusky (*phaeo*) colour (*chromo*) of its cut surface. Although uncommon, its great clinical importance stems from the hypertensive effects of catecholamine release from the tumour, along with its association with multiple endocrine neoplasia and other familiar syndromes. Phaeochromocytomas occur in only 0.1 per cent of hypertensives, although in autopsy series its incidence in the general population reaches up to 0.3 per cent. The peak incidence occurs in the fourth decade and it arises only rarely after 60 years of age. In adults there is a slight female preponderance, but in children it is twice as common in males. Ninety per cent of tumours are *intra-adrenal*, most of the remainder occur along the *sympathetic chain*, especially at the aortic bifurcation. Infrequently, paragangliomas occur in the intrathoracic paravertebral ganglia, in the bladder or other rare ectopic sites, such as the spermatic cord. Extra-adrenal tumours are relatively more common in children. In non-familial cases 10–20 per cent of tumours are bilateral, rising to 70 per cent in familial cases. Only 5–10 per cent of intra-adrenal phaeochromocytomas are malignant but in some series up to 30 per cent of extra-adrenal tumours are malignant.

Clinical course

Phaeochromocytomas in adults produce *sustained hypertension* with additional *paroxysmal elevations* in one-third of cases. The remaining two-thirds divide evenly between those which produce intermittent hypertension only and those producing sustained hypertension without paroxysms. In children 90 per cent of cases have sustained hypertension. Paroxysms may be triggered by several stimuli, including emotional stress, physical exertion, postural changes, or palpation of the tumour mass. Some small tumours produce no hypertension.

Presenting symptoms of phaeochromocytoma include headache, which occurs in 90 per cent of patients with paroxysmal hypertension, along with nausea and vomiting. Headache occurs in 70 per cent of patients with sustained hypertension. Night sweats, palpitation, tachycardia, anxiety, and tremor are more common in patients with paroxysms, and weakness, fatigue, even prostration may be severe at the end of a paroxysm. Less common presenting symptoms include chest pains, abdominal pain, dyspnoea, visual disturbance, constipation, and weight loss. Mild glucose intolerance occurs in 50 per cent of patients.

The main complications of tumour-associated hypertension involve the cardiovascular and cerebrovascular systems and include *myocardial infarction, cardiac arrhythmias, cardiac failure, and cerebral haemorrhage*. The characteristic myocardial lesion, which may be induced in animals by long-term administration of catecholamine, is *multifocal myofibrillar degeneration* together with *interstitial fibrosis* and *chronic inflammation*. This is found predominantly subendocardially in the left ventricle and may have secondary hypertensive changes superimposed.

Approximately 30 per cent of tumours secrete only noradrenaline; 15 per cent secrete mainly adrenaline but the majority secrete predominantly noradrenaline with some adrenaline also. A biochemical diagnosis of phaeochromocytoma is based on demonstrating excessive secretion of catecholamines or metabolites in urine or blood. Elevated levels of catecholamine and metabolites are shown in a 24 h urine collection in 95 per cent of patients. Estimation of urinary metanephrine levels is the most reliable single screening test. Plasma catecholamine levels may be used but are more open to interference by diet or drug intake and also give a false negative rate of 30 per cent in those patients with paroxysmal hypertension only.

Various imaging techniques may be employed to localize tumours, including plain X-ray, intravenous urography, ultrasound, computerized tomography, and angiography. Full alpha- and beta-adrenergic blockade is required before invasive procedures are used such as angiography, but this latter procedure has the advantage of allowing selective venous sampling of vessels draining the tumour.

Morphology

Adrenal phaeochromocytoma may weigh up to 4 kg, but the average weight is about 100 g. Most measure between 3 and 5 cm diameter. Tumours are well demarcated by compressed adrenal cortex or connective tissue (Fig. 26.75). The cut surface is pale grey or brown with slight lobulation produced by fibrovascular trabeculae. There is variable necrosis and haemorrhage, and larger tumours may be markedly calcified.

The cellular appearance is variable but most resemble normal adrenal medulla. The predominant growth pattern is as cords or alveolae, although trabecular and diffuse appearances may occur. Typically, adjacent groups of cells are separated by fibrovascular stroma rich in reticulin. In a minority there is an angiomatous growth pattern. In the majority the tumour is clearly demarcated from the adrenal cortex by a connective tissue rim, but in some there is invasion of the cortex. This and vascular invasion are *not* indicative of malignancy. Myxomatous change, haemorrhage, and necrosis occur more often in large tumours. Tumour cells are larger than normal phaeochromocytes and they contain abundant basophilic, granular

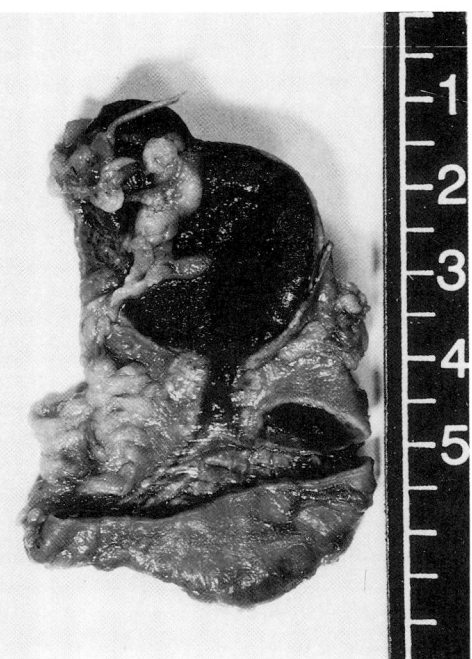

Fig. 26.75 A typical phaeochromocytoma; well-demarcated from adjacent adrenal tissue.

cytoplasm (Fig. 26.76). Nuclei are vesicular, round to oval with coarsely clumped chromatin and a distinct nucleolus. Pleomorphism is marked and mitoses may be present but are not common. Neither pleomorphism nor mitotic activity correlate with malignancy. Less common cytological variants include a small-cell form, cells with small, hyperchromatic nuclei and little cytoplasm. A spindle-cell variant accounts for less than 5 per cent of histological subtypes. Fibrovascular stroma surrounding nests of tumour cells may contain amyloid. A rim of *sustentacular cells*, strongly positive for S100 protein, may be

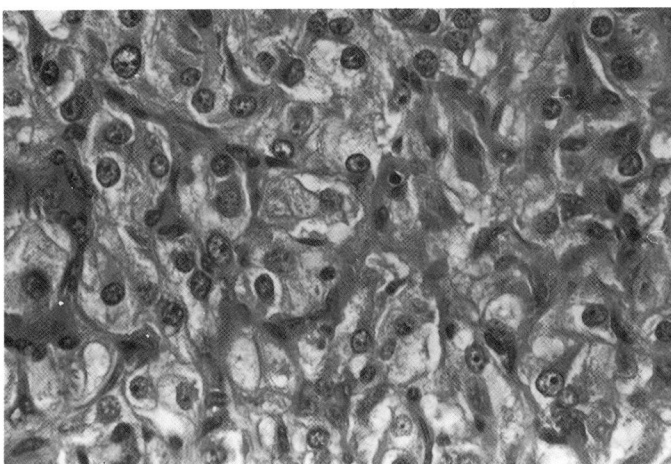

Fig. 26.76 Phaeochromocytoma. Large tumour cells with granular cytoplasm, surrounded by fibrovascular stroma.

present around groups of tumour cells. A diagnosis of malignancy is not made on histological grounds in the tumour alone. The only absolute criterion of malignancy is *the presence of metastases*. Malignant phaeochromocytomas do, however, tend to show less pleomorphism than benign tumours. Tumours with large numbers of mitoses are more likely to be malignant. Metastases occur most commonly in related lymph nodes, liver, lungs, and bones.

Familial patterns of phaeochromocytoma

A familial predisposition to phaeochromocytoma is transmitted as an *autosomal dominant trait*, with incomplete penetrance. Tumours arise in childhood and are multiple or bilateral in more than 50 per cent of cases.

Multiple endocrine neoplasia syndrome (MEN) type IIA (*Sipple's syndrome*) consists of the association of phaeochromocytoma, *medullary carcinoma of the thyroid*, and *parathyroid adenoma* or hyperplasia. This syndrome is also transmitted as an autosomal dominant, but with a high degree of penetrance. Tumours occur later in life, most often in the fourth decade. Tumours are bilateral or multifocal in more than 50 per cent of cases and probably arise from *adrenal medullary hyperplasia*. They are mostly adrenaline secreting and paroxysmal hypertension is the rule, fewer than 50 per cent of patients suffer sustained hypertension. Phaeochromocytoma occurs in 50 per cent of patients with kindred affected by Sipple's syndrome.

MEN type IIB is the association of phaeochromocytoma, medullary carcinoma of the thyroid, and *mucosal neuromas*. Parathyroid hyperplasia or adenoma is rare. This is an autosomal dominant syndrome and may be associated with *Marfanoid habitus*.

One per cent of patients with neurofibromatosis also have phaeochromocytoma, and 5 per cent of patients with a phaeochromocytoma have neurofibromatosis. If expressed only partially, the neurofibromatous aspect of the syndrome may be missed. Partial forms may include patients with only 5–6 *café-au-lait* spots, vertebral deformity, or kyphoscoliosis.

Phaeochromocytoma may occur in up to 10 per cent of patients with *von Hippel–Lindau disease*, but probably only certain kindreds are at risk; as many as 25 per cent may have clinically silent phaeochromocytoma.

MEN type I (*Wermer's syndrome*) *consists of hyperparathyroidism, pituitary adenoma, and pancreatic islet cell tumour.* Phaeochromocytoma is not usually a feature of this syndrome, but the familial occurrence of phaeochromocytoma and pancreatic islet cell tumour has been described.

Patients of kindreds with familiar phaeochromocytoma have been described who exhibit *cross-over syndromes*, that is they show features of other related syndromes, such as MEN I, MEN II, neurofibromatosis, or von Hippel–Lindau disease.

26.5.6 Neuroblastoma

Neuroblastoma is a tumour of *neuroblasts*, which are cells of neural crest origin. Most, 25 per cent, arise in the adrenal medulla, but they are also found at sites of extra-adrenal chromaffin tissue, along the sympathetic chain. The second commonest location is in a paravertebral position in the posterior mediastinum. Other sites include the pelvis, neck, lower abdomen, and, rarely, the posterior cranial fossa. It is the third commonest solid tumour of childhood and infancy, behind only cerebral tumours and lymphoma. The overall incidence of neuroblastoma in children is 9.6 per million, although autopsy series on infants less than three months of age show an incidence of *in situ* neuroblastoma of up to 1 : 39. Sixty per cent of patients are less than 1 year old, and 26 per cent between 1 and 2 years. In contrast to the common location in the abdomen or mediastinum in children, neuroblastomas are found most frequently in peripheral sites such as the leg, buttocks, head, and neck in adults.

Clinical course

In children younger than 2 years old, the commonest presenting complaint is of abdominal mass. Fever, bone pains, and weight loss are also prevalent. Some cases of neuroblastoma may undergo spontaneous maturation or regression. This phenomenon is rare in children over 1 year of age and often occurs in patients with remote disease confined to either the liver, skin, or bone marrow, without radiological evidence of bone involvement. This tumour regression may explain why some patients with apparently late-stage disease often do remarkably well, even without treatment. Pulmonary metastases are, however, a sign of widespread dissemination and indicate a poor prognosis. Diagnosis of neuroblastoma may be aided by imaging techniques such as intravenous pyelography and computerized tomography. Radionuclide studies are of use in detection of metastatic disease, and the presence of urinary catecholamines or metabolites, secreted by tumour cells, may be helpful in monitoring disease progress following therapy. Vanillylmandelic acid (VMA) and homovanillic acid (HVA) secretion occurs in combination in 80 per cent of patients and high VMA : HVA ratios indicate a better prognosis.

The single most important variable in the determination of prognosis is the age of the patient at presentation. The two-year survival for patients less than 1 year old at presentation is 74 per cent, falling to 12 per cent for those over 2 years old at diagnosis. The site of tumour is also important: patients with mediastinal tumours have a better prognosis than those with subdiaphragmatic lesions. Aggressive lesions have been found to be associated with amplification of the N-myc oncogene.

Morphology

Neuroblastoma may vary in size from a microscopic lesion to tumours that fill the abdominal cavity. Tumours are well delineated and may be encapsulated. They are friable, soft grey–pink masses which often show cystic degeneration, haemorrhage, or calcification. Medullary tumours often grow towards midline structures and may envelope the great vessels and other retroperitoneal structures. Direct invasion of the inferior vena cava or renal vein may occur, or there may be infiltration of the adjacent kidney. Occasionally, large tumours cross the midline

and involve the contralateral adrenal gland. Neuroblastomas in the sympathetic chain may permeate the vertebral foramina in a dumb-bell fashion and mediastinal tumours may involve vertebral bodies and ribs. The lungs are rarely involved by direct extension.

Neuroblastoma has a variable microscopic appearance. The least well-differentiated forms grow as sheets of cells with small hyperchromatic round/oval nuclei and little cytoplasm. Cell borders are ill-defined and cohesion is minimal. Mitotic activity varies but may be plentiful, especially in younger patients.

Fibrovascular bands may give the appearance of lobulation. The background fibrillary, eosinophilic matrix, representing tangles of unmyelinated nerve fibres, is a characteristic feature. Lymphatic or vascular invasion is commonly seen, as are foci of necrosis, haemorrhage, and calcification. True *Homer–Wright rosettes* are seen in only one-third of cases (Fig. 26.77), but rosettes are more commonly present, and may indeed be a predominant feature.

In more-differentiated tumours, amongst the small cells, there are clusters or single cells with large vesicular neuclei and a prominent single nucleolus. These cells contain more cytoplasm and may have cytoplasmic processes. In some tumours, cells resembling immature ganglion cells may be present.

In situ neuroblastoma

These lesions, most often seen in infants younger than 3 months of age, are discrete nodules of neural crest elements found within the adrenal gland. No tumour is present elsewhere. Most tumours show degenerative changes. In 70 per cent of cases there are associated severe congenital anomalies. The relatively high incidence of *in situ* neuroblastoma compared to that of clinically apparent lesions in later life could be explained by an absence of a second 'hit' in *Knudson's two 'hit' hypothesis* of carcinogenesis, with subsequent regression of the neuroblastoma.

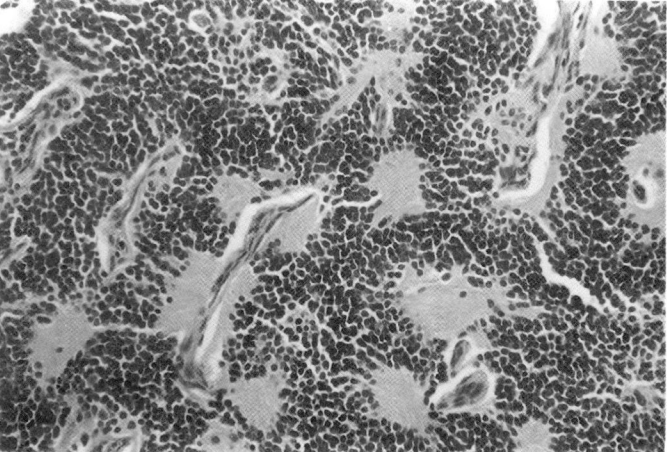

Fig. 26.77 Neuroblastoma, showing Homer–Wright rosettes, composed of collections of tumour cells around a central core of fibrillary tissue.

Familial syndromes and associated lesions

Neuroblastoma is rarely a familial tumour, but several kindreds have been reported in which more than one family member is affected. Pattern of inheritance in these cases suggests an autosomal dominant mode of inheritance. These are a small number of conditions in which neuroblastoma may be associated. They include von Recklinghausen's syndrome, colonic aganglionosis, and a variety of developmental defects, mainly congenital heart defects. Neuroblastoma has developed in patients treated with radiotherapy for a number of tumours, including osteosarcoma, fibrosarcoma, thyroid carcinoma, and renal cell carcinoma. There are also reported associations with some other tumours in the absence of treatment. These include soft-tissue sarcomas, ependymomas, and Hodgkin's disease. In 70 per cent of cases, structural chromosomal abnormalities have been found in tumour cells, including deletions of the short arm of chomosome 1.

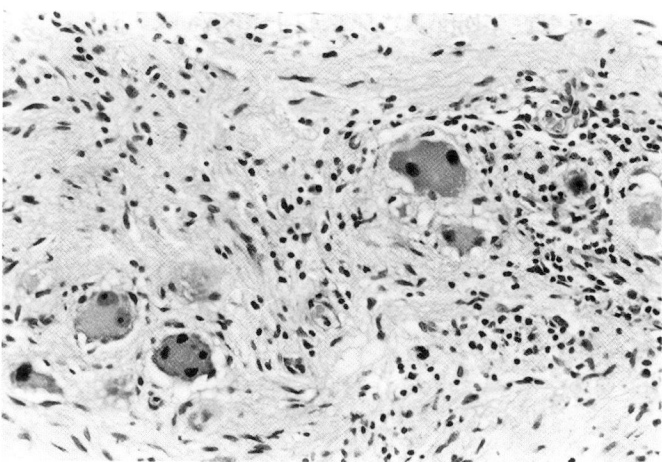

Fig. 26.78 Ganglioneuroma. Ganglion cells admixed with other neural elements.

26.5.7 Ganglioneuroma

Ganglioneuroma is a benign neoplasma. They occur at all ages, but adrenal tumours tend to occur at an older age (30–50 yr) than extra-adrenal lesions. They arise in the adrenal gland and along the sympathetic chain, particularly at the base of the skull and neck, posterior mediastinum, and the retroperitoneum. Uncommon, miscellaneous sites include the gut, uterus, ovary, and skin. In one series, 56 per cent were found in the mediastinum or retroperitoneum and 30 per cent within the adrenal, with 14 per cent arising from several other sites.

Clinical course

Intra-adrenal tumours are most often asymptomatic and only rarely present with abdominal pain. They may calcify and be discovered after X-ray. Very uncommonly they are associated with hypertension and even less commonly they may produce watery diarrhoea, hypochlorhydria, and alkalosis from vasoactive intestinal polypeptide (VIP) secretion. Growth of tumours is slow and due to proliferation of the Schwann cell population. Adequate excision is curative.

Morphology

Adrenal tumours are unencapsulated, but well delineated, and usually weigh less than 50 g. Extra-adrenal tumours often reach greater size and are often encapsulated. In both the cut surface is firm and grey-white. Tumours may be bilateral.

Tumours are composed of mature ganglion cells, sheathed neurites, Schwann cells, and collagen in varying proportions (Fig. 26.78). Ganglion cells may be distributed diffusely or, more commonly, in clusters. The ganglion cells have an eccentrically placed vesicular nucleus with large nucleolus, and abundant cytoplasm with well-developed Nissl substance. They often have associated satellite cells. The stroma may be either compact or oedematous and there may be a lymphocytic infiltration. The predominant cell type is the *spindle-shaped Schwann*

cell, these are often in interlacing bundles with variable intercellular collagen. Cystic degeneration is a prominent feature.

26.5.8 Ganglioneuroblastomas

Ganglioneuroblastomas are composed of variable proportions of mature sympathetic ganglion cells, immature neuroblastic cells, intermediate cells, and Schwann cells. The majority arise in the retroperitoneum with the remainder found in the mediastinum, neck, and adrenal gland. They have an equal incidence in males and females and usually occur below the age of 10 years.

Clinical course

Usually the tumour presents due to some local effect of a mass. Only rarely is hypertension or intractable diarrhoea with VIP secretion manifest clinically. Behaviour of these tumours is unpredictable. Well-encapsulated lesions may be cured by adequate excision. Some tumours, however, show local or distant spread.

Morphology

Tumours are often encapsulated, but this is not invariable. The better-differentiated tumours have a glistening, tan, fibrous cut surface. The less-differentiated tumours have foci of necrosis or haemorrhage. Calcification is often found.

Cellular appearances range from immature neuroblast populations to mature sympathetic ganglion cells. The ganglion cells have a similar appearance to those in the benign ganglioneuromas, with vesicular nuclei and abundant eosinophilic cytoplasm with prominent Nissl substance. Satellite cells often surround ganglion cells. Tumours may be composed of a mixture of cells showing varying degrees of differentiation (imperfect/diffuse pattern) or they may resemble a benign ganglioneuroma but for the presence in discrete foci of nodular collections of immature neuroblastic elements (immature/composite type). In both patterns some ganglion cells may be multinucleate and appear immature. Lymphocytic infiltration, haemorrhage, and necrosis are common features. Despite encapsulation, extension of tumour beyond the capsule is a common finding. Metastatic deposits are more likely to occur in primary tumours of composite type (65 per cent) than in those with diffuse pattern (18 per cent).

26.5.9   Further reading

Phaeochromocytoma

Alpert, L. I., Pai, S. H., Zak, F. G, and Werthamer, S. (1972). Cardiomyopathy associated with a phaeochromocytoma. *Archives of Pathology* **93**, 544–8.

Carmon, C. T. and Brashear, R. E. (1960). Phaeochromocytoma as an inherited abnormality. *New England Journal of Medicine* **263**, 419–23.

Carney, J. A., Sizemore, G. W., and Sheps, S. G. (1976). Adrenal medullary disease in multiple endocrine neoplasia type II; phaeochromocytoma and its precursors. *American Journal of Clinical Pathology* **66**, 279–90.

Carney *et al.* (1980). Familial phaeochromocytoma and islet cell tumour of the pancreas. *American Journal of Medicine* **68**, 515–21.

Das Gupta, T. K. and Brasfield, R. D. (1971). Von Recklinghausen's disease. *Cancer Journal for Clinicians* **21**, 174–83.

Horton, W. A., Wang, V., and Eldridge, R. (1976). Von Hippel-Lindau disease: clinical and pathological manifestations in nine families with fifty affected members. *Archives of Internal Medicine* **136**, 769–77.

Lips, K. J. M., Veer, J. S., Struyuenberg, A., Alleman, A., Leo, J. R., Wittebol, P., *et al.* (1981). Bilateral occurence of phaeochromocytoma in patients with the multiple endocrine neoplasia syndrome type 2a (Sipple syndrome). *American Journal of Medicine* **70**, 1051–9.

Manger, W. M. and Gifford, R. W., Jr. (1977). *Phaeochromocytoma*. Springer-Verlag, New York.

Melicow, M. M. (1977). One hundred cases of phaeochromocytoma (107 tumours) at the Columbia Presbyterian Medical Centre 1926–1976. *Cancer* **40**, 1987.

Neville, A. M. (1969). The adrenal medulla. In *Function pathology of the human adrenal gland* (ed. T. Symington), pp. 217–324. Williams and Wilkins, Baltimore.

Saad, M. F., Frazier, O. H., Hickey, R. C., and Samaan, N. A. (1983). Intrapericardial phaeochromocytoma. *American Journal of Medicine* **75**, 371–5.

St John Sutton, M. G., Sheps, S. G., and Lie, J. T. (1981). Prevalence of clinically unsuspected phaeochromocytoma: A review of a 50-year autopsy series. *Mayo Clinic Proceedings* **56**, 354–60.

Samaan, N. A. and Hickey, R. C. (1987). Phaeochromocytoma. *Seminars in Oncology* **14** (3), 297–305.

Stackpole, R. H., Melicow, M. M., and Uson, A. C. (1963). Phaeochromocytoma in children. *Journal of Pediatrics* **63**, 315–30.

Neuroblastoma and ganglioneuroma

Beckwith, J. B. and Perrin, E. V. (1963). *In situ* neuroblastomas: A contribution to the natural history of neural crest tumours. *American Journal of Pathology* **43**, 1089–104.

Bill, A. H. (1968). The regression of neuroblastoma. *Journal of Pediatric Surgery* **3**, 103–6.

Bolande, R. P. (1979). Developmental pathology. *American Journal of Pathology* **94**, 627–84.

Breslow, N. and McCann, B. (1971). Statistical estimation of prognosis for children with neuroblastoma. *Cancer Research* **31**, 2098–103.

Cloyoma, C., Qualman, S. J., Shimada, H., and Newton, W. A. (1988). Composite ganglioneuroblastoma (C-GNB). Immunohistochemical distinction of stromal components correlates with prognosis. *Laboratory Investigation* **58**, 5A.

D'Angio, G. J., Evans, A. E., and Koop, C. E. (1971). Special pattern of widespread neuroblastoma with favourable prognosis. *Lancet* **i**, 1046–9.

Evans, A. E. (1982). Staging and treatment of neuroblastoma. *American Journal of Roentology* **138**, 75–8.

Jaffe, N. (1976). Neuroblastoma: review of the literature and an examination of factors contributing to its enigmatic character. *Cancer Treatment Reviews* **3**, 61–82.

Jansen-Goemans, A. and Engelhardt, J. (1977). Intractable diarrhoea in a boy with vass active intestinal polypeptide-producing ganglioneuroblastoma. *Pediatrics* **59**, 710–16.

Knudson, A. G. and Meadows, A. T. (1976). Developmental genetics of neuroblastoma. *Journal of the National Cancer Institute* **57**, 675–82.

Rosenthal, I. M., Greenberg, R., Kathan, R., Falk, G. S., and Wang, R. (1969). Catecholamine metabolism of a ganglioneuroma. *Pediatric Research* **3**, 413–24.

Someren, A. and Karcoiglu, Z. (1977). Malignant vagal paraganglioma. Report of a case and review of the literature. *American Journal of Clinical Pathology* **68**, 400.

Staley, N. A., Polesky, H. F., and Bensch, K. G. (1967). Fine structural and biochemical studies on the malignant ganglioneuroma. *Journal of Neuropathology and Experimental Neurology* **26**, 634–53.

Stowens, D. (1957). Neuroblastoma and related tumours. *Archives of Pathology* **63**, 451–59.

Witzelben, C. L. and Landy, R. A. (1974). Disseminated neuroblastoma in a child with von Recklinghausen's disease. *Cancer* **34**, 786–90.

Young, J. L. and Miller, R. W. (1975). Incidence of malignant tumours in children. *Journal of Pediatrics* **86**, 254–8.

26.6   The carotid body, chemodectomas, and the non-chromaffin system

D. Heath

26.6.1   The non-chromaffin paraganglionic system

Scattered throughout the body are tissues that constitute the so-called non-chromaffin paraganglionic system. This is an inaccurate term since the chromaffinity of their chief cells is very faint rather than absent. Furthermore, these collections of tissue do not meet the strict criteria for non-chromaffin paraganglia, which should be homologous to postganglionic parasympathetic ganglion cells and have their main innervation in parasympathetic efferent nerve fibres. Nevertheless, they share common histological features and form a well-defined system throughout the body. These tissues tend to assume the form of a spherical conglomeration of cells and small blood vessels, or *glomus*.

The groups of glomera

There are four groups of non-chromaffin glomera. The first is *branchiomeric*, that is laid down at the site of branchial arches in contrast to the older concept of branchiogenic glomera thought to be actually derived from cells of the arches. This group includes the *carotid bodies* and the *aortico-pulmonary bodies*, one of which is found on the bifurcation of the pulmonary trunk where it has acquired the spurious designation of the 'glomus pulmonale' in spite of receiving its blood supply from the coronary rather than the pulmonary arteries. This group also includes the glomus jugulare, and glomera in the orbit and larynx; their tumours are described below.

Intravagal groups of glomic cells are found interior to the perineurium just beneath the nerve sheath or between nerve fibres within the ganglion nodosum of the vagus nerve. This 'glomus intravagale' is not related to an artery but cannot be distinguished from other glomic tissue on grounds of histology, ultrastructure, or cytochemistry.

Aortico-sympathetic glomera are associated with segmental ganglia of the sympathetic chain. A specially prominent member of this group in the fetus and new-born is the *organ of Zuckerkandl*.

Visceral–autonomic glomera associated with blood vessels of the respective organs are found in the interatrial septum of the heart, the hilus of the liver, the wall of the urinary bladder, and the wall of the duodenum.

Neoplasms may arise from glomera in any of these four groups and reactions to generalized disease may occur in some of the branchiomeric glomera.

The basic histological unit

Each glomus has a very similar histological appearance but the account given here applies specifically to the carotid body, which has been studied in detail (Heath and Smith 1985). It is composed of lobules, some 400 μm in diameter, embedded in a fibrous stroma which contains elastic interlobular branches of the glomic arteries, derived from the common or external carotid arteries. Also running in the interlobular fibrous tissue are branches of the glossopharyngeal (ninth cranial) nerve, which appear to be sensory for chemoreception, and of the ganglioglomerular nerve from the superior cervical sympathetic ganglion, which innervates the blood vessels of the carotid body.

The lobules are composed of clusters, some 80 μm in diameter, which are made of *chief* (or *type 1*) cells and *sustentacular* (or *type 2*) cells. In man three variants of chief cells can be recognized, *the light*, *the dark*, and *the progenitor*, thought to give rise to the other two variants. Chief and especially dark cells contain cytoplasmic dense core-vesicles which are typical of 'APUD' cells and comprise a central osmophilic core and a surrounding clear halo. Concentrations of six peptides as determined by radioimmunoassay and expressed as picomoles per gram of wet tissue were found in the human carotid body to be methionine–enkephalin 612, leucine–enkephalin 162, bombesin 73, neurotensin 67, substance P16, and vasoactive intestinal peptide 9 (Heath *et al.* 1988). Met- and leu-enkephalins occur predominantly in the dark variant of chief cells and to lesser extent in progenitor cells while bombesin is found in close approximation to the smooth muscle cells of the walls of the glomic arties (Smith *et al.* 1990). The function of the peptides in the human carotid body is unknown. The clear surrounding halo contains biogenic amines such as dopamine, adrenaline, noradrenaline, and serotonin. These amines are thought to be associated with chemoreception, but the mechanisms involved are at present obscure. In light cells the cytoplasm stains faintly with haematoxylin, contains vacuoles, and has an irregular outline forming a syncytium with adjacent cells. The nucleus is round or ovoid, some 7 μm in diameter, and has a characteristic open vesicular appearance. In dark cells the nucleus is smaller and shows numerous small clumps of chromatin giving a coarsely granular appearance. The cytoplasm is darker and has a more clearly defined border. In progenitor cells the nucleus is small and intensely haematoxyphilic.

In each cluster the central spherule of chief cells is surrounded by a covering of elongated sustentacular cells whose average nuclear dimensions are 13×4 μm. These cells are closely akin to Schwann cells. They enfold non-myelinated nerves and their cytoplasmic extensions extend deeply into the centres of the clusters, where the nerves come into contact with chief cells. On the outer surface of the clusters the sustentacular cells merge almost imperceptibly into Schwann cells which lie closely around larger myelinated nerves in the stroma. The sharing of the same histological features by the carotid body and the other glomera should not be taken to imply that they share the same function. Only the carotid and aortico-pulmonary bodies are known to be chemoreceptors.

26.6.2 Enlargement of the carotid bodies

The carotid bodies enlarge and show histological changes in *chronic hypoxaemia and systemic hypertension*. This important aspect of the pathology of the carotid bodies has been largely ignored by morbid anatomists who usually do not examine the carotid bodies at post-mortem and thus remain unaware of the involvement of the non-chromaffin paraganglionic system in generalized disease. It is important for the pathologist to be able to distinguish between carotid body hyperplasia and normal anatomical variation which involves up to 10 per cent of carotid bodies. On either side of the neck these organs may be double, bilobed, or leaf-shaped (Khan *et al.* 1988).

The carotid bodies of Quechua Indians living at high altitude in the Peruvian Andes are larger and heavier than those of mestizos living at sea level (Arias-Stella and Valcarcel 1973). The enlargement is progressive throughout life, in contrast to what occurs in lowlanders, and was subsequently reported by these authors as being associated with a prominence of the chief cells so that the clusters of parenchymal cells grow larger. The same enlargement of clusters and lobules was found in Andean cattle to such an extent that the histological appearances were thought to resemble the tumour of the carotid body described below. In the native highlanders there was a pronounced fall in formalin-induced fluorescence in their carotid bodies indicating a loss of catecholamines. The stimulus for the progressive enlargement of the human and bovine carotid bodies was thought to be chronic exposure to the hypobaric hypoxia of the mountains.

Subsequent studies revealed that the carotid bodies also increase in size and weight in some patients with chronic bronchitis and emphysema (Heath *et al.* 1970). The enlargement is not related to the type of emphysema present or its severity, but rather to the accompanying degree of hypoxaemia. Thus big carotid bodies are found in subjects who exhibit the clinical manifestations of the *blue and bloated syndrome* with hypoxaemia, hypercarbia, frequently associated systemic oedema, and right ventricular hypertrophy with some increase in pulmonary vascular resistance. In subjects with chronic obstructive lung disease of this type, the histological appearances of the carotid bodies are different from those reported in the enlarged glomera of native highlanders. There is proliferation of the sustentacular cells, which form thick shells around the chief cells forming the cores of the clusters. This pressure and encroachment upon the chief cells may be associated with the loss of hypoxic respiratory drive which characterizes subjects chronically exposed to hypoxia, such as native highlanders and patients with either chronic obstructive lung disease or cyanotic congenital heart disease.

There is a relation between the weight of the carotid bodies and that of the left ventricle as well as that of the right (Edwards *et al.* 1971). This is because enlargement of the carotid bodies occurs in systemic hypertension as well as in states of chronic alveolar hypoxia. The histological changes found in the two conditions are identical, with proliferation of sustentacular cells and associated nerve axons. It is as though the glomera are unable to distinguish between the stimuli of chronic hypoxaemia and raised intravascular pressure and this may be because the systemic hypertension induces occlusive changes in the radicles of the glomic arteries which render the parenchyma of the carotid bodies ischaemic. In carotid body hyperplasia the combined carotid body weight increases from a mean of 18 mg to one exceeding 30 mg (Heath *et al.* 1982). While the cell clusters remain at the same diameter of some 80 μm, the lobules increase in size from 400 μm to 600 μm. In normal carotid bodies the differential cell count of sustentacular cells is about 45 per cent but in cases of hypoxaemia secondary to pulmonary emphysema, it may exceed 60 per cent. In a case of coarctation of the aorta associated with systemic hypertension and severe left ventricular hypertrophy, the proliferation of sustentacular cells was gross, with extensive compression and ablation of the clusters of chief cells (Heath *et al.* 1986). Young subjects with systemic hypertension may show disturbances of hypoxic drive indicating the connection between the carotid bodies and raised systemic pressure. The carotid bodies also appear to be involved in sodium metabolism so that their stimulation in rats leads to a natriuresis, which is independent of nerve control in the kidney and appears to be endocrine in nature. Systemic blood pressure in man and rats is lowered by exposure to the hypobaric hypoxia of high altitude. In rats this amelioration is associated with a natriuresis and it is prevented by their free access to salt.

Spontaneously hypertensive rats develop enlargement of their carotid bodies which may be genetic, rather than related to raised vascular pressure.

Characteristic age changes occur in the carotid bodies (Hurst *et al.* 1985). In youth, considerable numbers of the dark variant of chief cell are to be found. In middle age there is concentric proliferation of sustentacular cells around the clusters of chief cells. The carotid bodies of the elderly show progressive fibrosis which becomes acellular and hyalinized and tends to encroach on the clusters of chief cells. At the same time there is age-change intimal fibrosis in the radicles of the glomic arteries. Over the age of 50 years, a diffuse infiltrate of lymphocytes appears amongst the glomic tissue. In up to 29 per cent of subjects over the age of 70 years, the lymphocytes from aggregates in the substance of the carotid body with streamers extending between the glomic tissue (Khan *et al.* 1989). T-cells account for virtually all the diffuse lymphocytes and for about half to three-quarters of the aggregates. The appearances are reminiscent of focal chronic thyroiditis or other autoimmune conditions. In a few cases of glomitis, plasma cells appear in abundance especially around ageing nerve fibrils (Heath *et al.* 1989). Similar aggregates of lymphocytes are also to be found in the glomus pulmonale of elderly subjects, suggesting that chronic glomitis may be a feature of the non-chromaffin paraganglionis system, rather than be confined to the carotid bodies (Khan and Heath 1990).

Dark cell proliferation

When rabbits are subjected to hypoxia for a period of about three months, their carotid bodies show initially a proliferation of dark cells but when they are left exposed to hypoxia for a period of six months, there is only a hyperplasia of the light variant of chief cells. The same chain of events seems to take place in man. In a woman with a ventricular septal defect and pulmonary hypertension, reversal of the intracardiac shunt occurred a few months before her death, thus exposing the carotid bodies to a stimulus of hypoxaemia for that short period. Histological examination revealed a prominence of dark cells suggesting that this represented the first cellular response to hypoxaemia. Patients with chronic bronchitis and emphysema or long-standing systemic hypertension who have established carotid body hyperplasia with proliferation of sustentacular cells sometimes show superimposed focal accumulations of the dark variant of chief cells (Heath and Smith 1985). It seems likely that this may represent a subacute tissue response to an exaggeration of the hypoxic or hypertensive stimulus. This might occur, for example, during an acute pulmonary infection complicating the condition of chronic obstructive lung disease and leading to an acute, sudden worsening of hypoxaemia. Focal accumulations of progenitor dark cells are also found in such situations. The carotid bodies of cattle in transit through the hypoxic atmosphere of the Andes also show focal collections of dark cells. In the rat, dark variants of chief cells are hard to make out and have been dismissed as an artefact produced by autolysis. In man they appear to be a distinct entity of pathological significance. The carotid bodies may swell and become engorged with blood on acute exposure to hypoxia without any cellular involvement. This may be readily demonstrated experimentally in animals but it is likely that it occurs in acute episodes of hypoxia induced by respiratory infection in the course of chronic respiratory disease.

26.6.3   Non-chromaffin parangliomas

Tumours may develop in the carotid bodies and the other glomera throughout the body. Although these tissues do not meet the strict criteria for designation as non-chromaffin paraganglia, some authorities (Glenner and Grimley 1974) accept tumours arising from them as 'non-chromaffin paragangliomas'. The histological features of tumours arising from the various glomera are very similar.

Chemodectomas

Early researchers used the non-committal term of 'carotid body tumour', and there is much to recommend it, but in 1950 Mulligan coined the term 'chemodectoma' in recognition of the function of chemoreception exhibited by this glomus. Chemodectomas form fairly smooth globular or ovoid tumours, between 2 and 4 cm diameter, but rarely tumours up to 15 cm in diameter have been reported. On section, they present a firm, resilient cut surface, which varies in colour from pink–grey to red–brown. There is a fibrous capsule, which may be wide or ill-defined. When a chemodectoma is received as a surgical specimen, it will commonly show the grooving produced by the closely adjacent and adherent arteries at the site of the carotid bifurcation where it was growing (Pryse-Davies et al. 1964). Its surface will show tags and adhesions of fibrous tissue binding chemodectoma and adventitia of the carotid arteries.

Chemodectomas may present at any age and there is no sex preponderance. In a large series from the Mayo Clinic, the age of presentation ranged from 12 to 63 years (Shamblin et al. 1971). The usual complaint is one of a mass growing very slowly in the neck. Usually the tumour is present for over 5 years before the patient presents for surgery, but in one celebrated case it was present for 47 years. It is worthy of note that, in one large series, 19 of the 90 patients reported that there had been a noticeable increase in size of the tumour in the 6 months before examination. Since the chemodectoma is fixed to the adventitia of the carotid arteries, it commonly does not move with swallowing and will move laterally but not vertically. Usually the swelling is not tender on palpation and pain from the tumour is exceptional. Traditionally the chemodectoma has been regarded as hard and on this account designated a 'potato-like tumour' but this was a historical blunder for this term was originally applied to cervical lymphosarcomas. In fact, when carotid body tumours have a significant angiomatous component, they may feel soft.

The carotid body is a highly vascular structure and in a minority of cases this high blood flow causes the tumour to pulsate and develop a murmur and bruit. This high blood flow is utilized in the diagnosis of chemodectomas by angiography although computerized tomography and magnetic resonance imaging have now assumed greater importance in this respect. Headache is a common but non-specific symptom, which could have a pyschological basis. Hoarseness, or vocal cord or hypoglossal paralysis are occasionally seen, but care must be taken that any cranial nerve involvement noted is not ascribed to the tumour when, in fact, it may be due to previous surgery. Dizziness, tinnitus, and loss of hearing have also been recorded.

Chemodectomas tend to show a familial incidence and the genetic transmission is most consistent with autosomal dominance. As a group, non-chromaffin paragangliomas frequently have a multicentric origin. Carotid body tumours do not usually show endocrine activity, but noradrenaline secreting examples have been described and they are usually intimately attached to the cervical sympathetic chain near the superior cervical ganglion.

Most chemodectomas tend to reproduce the histological features of the normal carotid body. In particular they show cell clusters or 'zellballen' (Fig. 26.79). Not infrequently the clusters are large and well-defined and are delineated by fine reticulin fibres, which are easily picked out by silver stains to present a characteristic pattern of a network of boxes. The reticulin fibres do not penetrate between individual tumour cells. The tumour cells appear to be derived from chief cells and have typical open, round, or oval nuclei, 5–12 μm in diameter, with occasional prominent nucleoli. The margins of the cells cannot be distinguished clearly and present a syncytial appearance; the cytoplasm is palely eosinophilic and often contains small vacuoles. Electron microscopy of these closely applied cells may reveal intercellular adhesions which, in fact, correspond to the *puncta adherentia* of normal chief cells and which resemble the *desmosomes* in tight junctions of epithelial tissues. Hence the presence of desmosomes in a tumour queried as a chemodectoma should not be taken as proof that it is, in fact, a tumour of epithelial origin. A characteristic feature of the chemodectoma is the presence of broad bands of relatively acellular fibrous tissue.

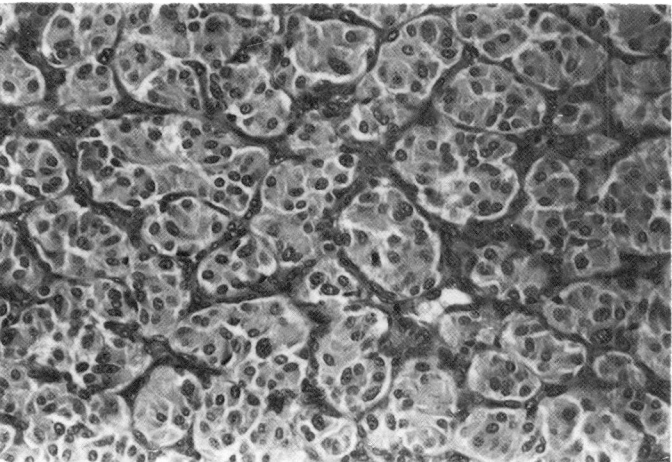

Fig. 26.79 Carotid body paraganglioma (chemodectoma). Nests of tumour cells ('*zellballen*') surrounded by fibrovascular stroma including sustentacular cells.

Not all chemodectomas have this classical appearance. In some the neoplastic cell clusters are very small and, if their organization into these separate units is not recognized, could be interpreted as sheets of epithelial cells. *Zellballen* may occur within these expanses of neoplastic mini-clusters. Dilated sinusoid-like vascular channels are sometimes seen and these may isolate individual cell clusters into discrete bands. Glenner and Grimley (1974) believe that there are differences in the cytoplasmic density in the cells of a chemodectoma, which correspond to that of light and dark variants of chief cells described above. This is easier to make out in thin, plastic sections of tumour fixed well in glutaraldehyde. It is difficult to distinguish in routine paraffin sections. Sometimes the clusters of chief cells are surrounded by a rim of more elongated cells, which might represent sustentacular cells. Some chemodectomas are composed entirely of spindle-shaped cells, but such an appearance should raise the possibility of malignancy.

The chemodectoma tends to show nuclear pleomorphism, even in tumours which are unequivocally benign on clinical grounds. There may be considerable variation in the size and shape of the chief cells. Hyperchromatic nuclei, and even bi- and tri-nucleate cells, may be found but mitotic figures are exceedingly rare. Even a large giant cell with a single nucleus may be discovered, although this may represent a surviving ganglion cell. Such appearances may be disturbing but the histopathologist must be on his guard against accepting such appearances as indicators of malignancy. Nevertheless, undoubted malignant change with local or distant spread does occur in the chemodectoma.

Local invasion of the wall of the carotid arterial bifurcation occurs in about 5 per cent of cases, and metastasis to regional lymph nodes and distant viscera also takes place. Shamblin and his colleagues (1971) found that in the 500 cases of chemodectomas reported up to that year, 3 per cent showed local infiltration of the carotid arteries and 3 per cent showed distant metastasis. The lungs and skeleton are especially susceptible to metastasis. Prediction of the behaviour of a chemodectoma from its histological appearance is difficult, if not impossible. Cellular and nuclear pleomorphism are not uncommon features of benign tumours but are also commonly found with malignant changes. Even multinucleated giant cells are not reliable indices of malignancy. A series of cases from the Mayo Clinic included two that had metastasized; in neither was there any histological evidence of malignancy. Romanksi (1954) carefully compared two clinically malignant chemodectomas with five benign tumours and was unable to detect histological differences from which the differing biological behaviour could have been predicted. Sometimes chemodectomas or their metastases in lymph nodes show unequivocal features of malignancy, such as gross pleomorphism.

A suspected diagnosis of chemodectoma can usually be confirmed by electron microscopy, since the neoplastic cells retain many of the ultrastructural features of normal glomic cells, such as dense core-vesicles. However, the technique will not distinguish between a carotid body tumour and a vagal paraganglioma, since both have an identical fine structure. Sustentacular cells and nerve axons are not ultrastructural features of chemodectoma.

Chemodectomas occur more frequently in man and cattle living at high altitude, where the chronic stimulus of hypobaric hypoxia may be responsible. All but two of 25 Peruvians with chemodectomas of the head and neck studied by Saldaña and his colleagues (1973) had been born and lived at altitudes between 2105 and 4350 m above sea level. There is also some association with chronic hypoxia induced by lung disease. Chedid and Jao (1974) reported the occurrence of 11 tumours of the carotid body and one of the ganglion nodosum of the vagus nerve in six members of two consecutive generations of a family. Four of these six patients had chronic obstructive lung disease with hypoxaemia and hypercarbia. An association of chemodectoma with thyroid carcinoma of papillary or follicular type has been reported in Mexico City, at an altitude of 2380 m.

Tumours of other glomera in the non-chromaffin paranganglionic system

The other glomera in the body may give rise to tumours that have a similar histological picture to that of the chemodectoma, in being composed of chief cells without incorporating a significant number of sustentacular cells or nerve endings, thus pointing to their true neoplastic nature.

The *glomus jugulare tumour* is more common in women and is located along the course of the tympanic branch of the glossopharyngeal nerve or the circular branch of the vagus nerve. The tumour of the middle ear forms a reddish mass which bleeds easily and appears initially as an aural polyp. Occasionally it arises in the adventitia of the jugular bulb immediately beneath the bony floor of the middle ear and presents as a lesion at the base of the skull with enlargement of the jugular foramen, and may extend as finger-like projections into the lumen of the jugular vein.

The *laryngeal paraganglioma* arises on either side of the midline above the anterior end of the vocal cords. It may also arise between the thyroid and cricoid cartilages, or from glomera within the recurrent branch of the vagus nerve. It commonly leads to pain in the throat, hoarseness, and bleeding, and has a tendency to become malignant. An *aortic body tumour* may arise from glomera situated in the adventitia of the pulmonary trunk, ascending aorta, and subclavian artery. Usually it is attached to, or lies within, the pericardium surrounding the left auricle, or intimately associated with the ascending aorta. The so-called *orbital chemodectoma* may develop any time between childhood and middle age. It is red–brown to tan in colour, is lobulated, and is rubbery on section. It may be as much as 4 cm in diameter and occurs in the retrobulbar area or may involve the rectus muscles. The usual presentation is visual loss with orbital throbbing. If the optic nerve is involved, there is also macular degeneration. Glaucoma may be present. There is no sex preponderance. The *vagal body tumour* arises from nests of glomic cells within the perineurium of the vagus nerve just below or at the ganglion nodosum. Like the glomus jugulare tumour, it is commoner in women. It usually presents as a mass in the anterolateral aspect of the neck, leading to hoarseness and difficulty in swallowing. The histological features are as in all the non-chromaffin paragangliomas and, as in them, it may metastasize, especially to lymph nodes or bones. A tumour may arise from the *organ of Zuckerkandl* or one of the other retroperitoneal glomera associated with the sympathetic chain at the bifurcation of the abdominal aorta. It is ovoid or lobulated and is tan, grey, or red in colour, and may present as an adbominal mass up to 15 cm in diameter. These tumours occur in a younger age-group. Metastases to regional lymph nodes and the skeleton are not uncommon. A high proportion of them show functional activity due to secretion of catecholamines, producing the signs and symptoms of a phaeochromocytoma. Finally, nests of *glomic tissue within the trigone* or about the ureteric orifices may give rise to a paraganglioma. They may bulge into the urinary bladder to produce painless haematuria.

26.6.4   Bibliography

Arias-Stella, J. and Valcarcel, J. (1973). The human carotid body at high altitudes. *Pathologia et Microbiologia* **39**, 292–7.

Arias-Stella, J. and Valcarcel, J. (1976). Chief cell hyperplasia in the human carotid body at high altitudes. Physiologic and pathologic significance. *Human Pathology* **7**, 361–73.

Chedid, A. and Jao, W. (1974). Hereditary tumours of the carotid bodies and chronic obstructive pulmonary disease. *Cancer* **33**, 1635–41.

Edwards, C., Heath, D., and Harris, P. (1971). The carotid body in emphysema and left ventricular hypertrophy. *Journal of Pathology* **104**, 1–13.

Glenner, G. G. and Grimley, P. M. (1974). *Tumors of the extra-adrenal paraganglion system (including chemoreceptors)*. Armed Forces Institute of Pathology, Washington, DC.

Heath, D. and Smith, P. (1985). *The pathology of the carotid body and sinus*. Edward Arnold, London.

Heath, D., Edwards, C., and Harris, P. (1970). Post-mortem size and structure of the human carotid body. *Thorax* **25**, 129–40.

Heath, D., Khan, Q., Nash, J., *et al.* (1989). Carotid body disease and the physician—chronic carotid glomitis. *Postgraduate Medical Journal* **65**, 353–7.

Heath, S., Quinzanini, M., Rodella, A., *et al.* (1988). Immunoreactivity to various peptides in the human carotid body. *Research Communications in Chemical Pathology and Pharmacology* **62**, 289–93.

Heath, D., Smith, D., and Hurst, G. (1986). The carotid bodies in coarctation of the aorta. *British Journal of Diseases of the Chest* **80**, 122–30.

Heath, D., Smith, P., and Jago, R. (1982). Hyperplasia of the carotid body. *Journal of Pathology* **138**, 115–27.

Hurst, G., Heath, D., and Smith, P. (1985). Histological changes associated with ageing of the human carotid body. *Journal of Pathology* **147**, 181–7.

Khan, Q. and Heath, D. (1990). Chronic carotid glomitis and the glomus pulmonale. *Journal of Clinical Pathology* **43**, 39–42.

Khan, Q., Heath, D., Nash, J., *et al.* (1989). Chronic carotid glomitis. *Histopathology* **14**, 471–81.

Khan, Q., Heath, D., and Smith, P. (1988). Anatomical variations in human carotid bodies. *Journal of Clinical Pathology* **41**, 1196–9.

Mulligan, R. M. (1950). Chemodectoma in the dog. *American Journal of Pathology* **26**, 680–1.

Pryse-Davis, J., Dawson, I. M. P., and Westbury, G. (1964). Some morphologic, histochemical, and chemical observations on chemodectomas and the normal carotid body, including a study of the chromaffin reaction and possible ganglion cell elements. *Cancer* **17**, 185–202.

Romanski, R. (1954). Chemodectoma (non-chromaffin paraganglioma) of the carotid body with distant metastases. With illustrative case. *American Journal of Pathology* **30**, 1–13.

Saldaña, M. J., Salem, L. E., and Travezan, R. (1973). High altitude hypoxia and chemodectomas. *Human Pathology* **41**, 251–63.

Shamblin, W. R., ReMine, W. H., Sheps, S. G., and Harrison, E. G. (1971). Carotid body tumor (chemodectoma). Clinicopathologic analysis of ninety cases. *American Journal of Surgery* **122**, 732–9.

Smith, P., Gosney, J. R., Heath, D., *et al.* (1990). The occurrence and distribution of certain polypeptides within the human carotid body. *Cell Tissue Research* **261**, 565–71.

26.7   The endocrine pancreas

J. M. Polack and S. R. Bloom

26.7.1   Introduction

The role of the pancreas as an endocrine as well as exocrine gland was recognized almost 100 years ago, 20 years after the discovery in 1869 of the pancreatic islets. Paul Langerhans described the islets as clusters of clear cells in the pancreatic gland (Fig. 26.80). With the application of special histological stains, it was soon realized that this conglomerate of endocrine cells is highly heterogeneous. Thus, the endocrine cells of the islets were first subclassified as *β and non-β (A)* types, using techniques like *aldehyde fuchsin* and *pthalaldehyde acid haematoxylin*. Nowadays, using immunocytochemistry and specific peptide antibodies, at least four endocrine cell types, with a distinct distribution, are recognized within the pancreatic islets (see Fig. 26.81a–d) (Ferri *et al.* 1987). These light microscopical

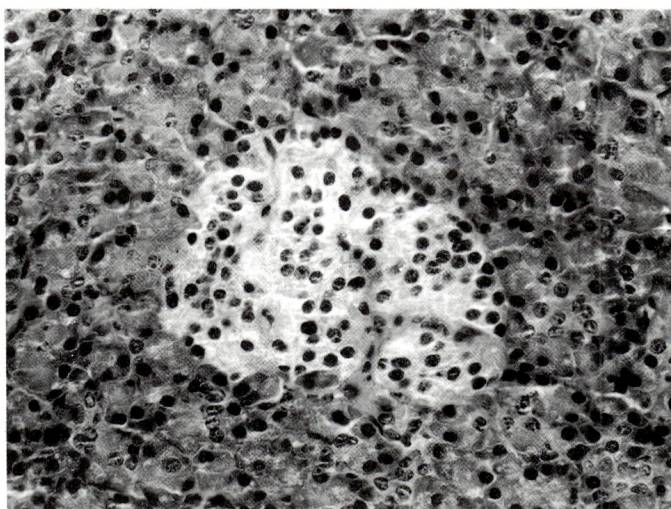

Fig. 26.80 Haematoxylin and eosin stain of an islet from normal human pancreas.

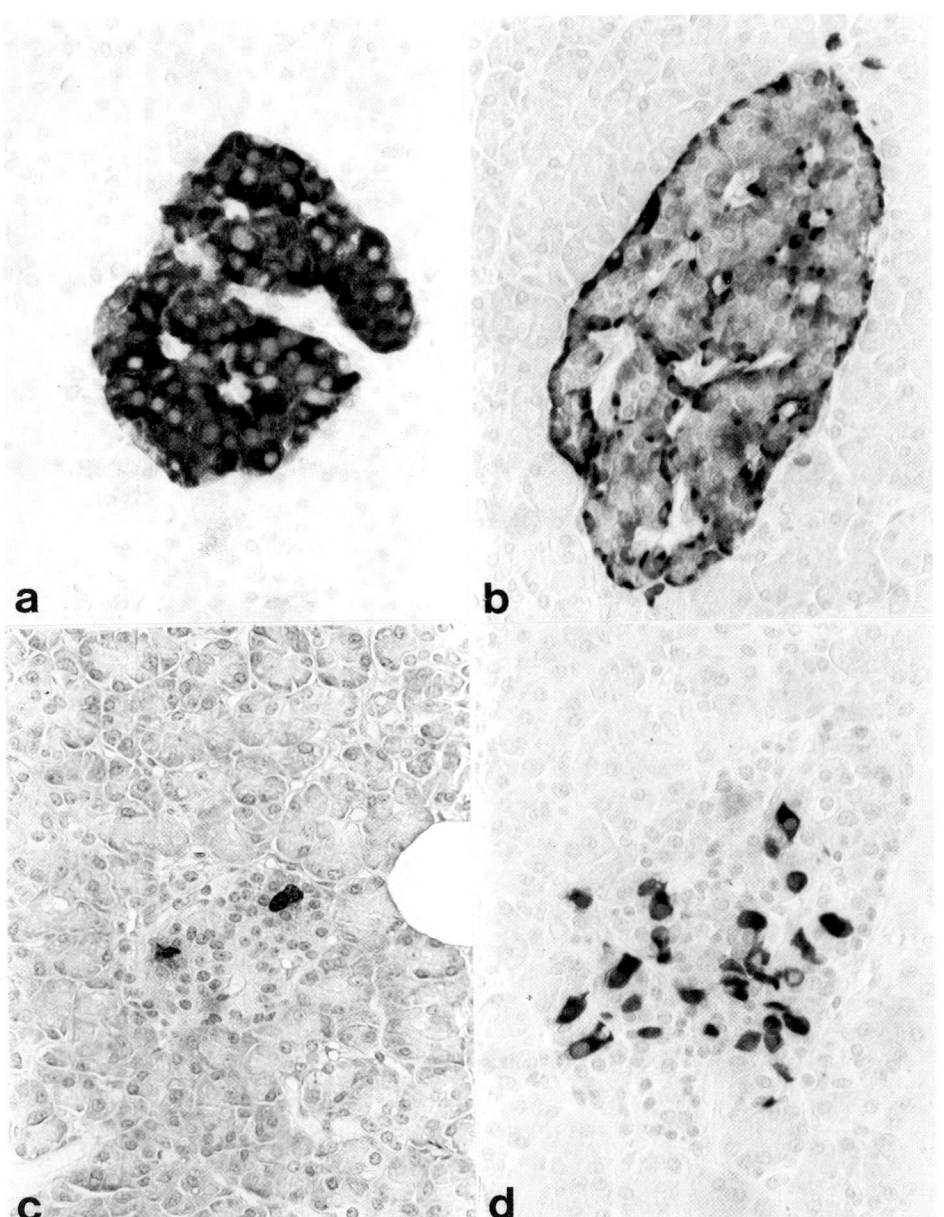

Fig. 26.81 Sections of normal human pancreas immunostained for (a) insulin—β cells form the majority cell population of the islet; (b) glucagon—α cells lie at the periphery of the islet; (c) pancreatic polypeptide—PP cells are few in islets other than those of the ventral head region; and (d) somatostatin—D cells are scattered in the islet. Peroxidase anti-peroxidase immunostains with weak haematoxylin counterstain.

findings correlate well with ultrastructural features, which also distinguish at least four separate endocrine cell types by the morphology of the electron-dense secretory granules (Fig. 26.82). Additional cell types have been described on the basis of their electron-dense secretory granules but no peptide hormones have been attributed to them as yet. The main staining properties, distribution characteristics, and ultrastructural features of the endocrine cell types of the pancreatic islets are summarized in Table 26.13. The islets of Langerhans contain most of the endocrine cells of the pancreas. In the adult, only scattered single cells are found outside the islets. The islets are evenly distributed in the gland, except for the posterior portion of the head of the adult pancreas, where they are more numerous and irregularly scattered. Two types of islets can be recog-

nized in the pancreas according to their anatomical location and endocrine cell composition: *β-cell-rich and PP-cell-rich islets*. β-cell rich islets are round to oval in shape and sharply outlined. In contrast, PP-rich islets, described over 70 years ago, are of irregular size and outline and may show a conspicuous trabecular architecture. While the occurrence of PP-rich islets is restricted to the posterior part of the pancreatic head, the β-cell-rich islets are scattered throughout the gland. The posterior lobe may be separated from the anterior portion by a band of connective tissue, thus allowing, on occasions, a blunt dissection of the lobe. It has been suggested that the PP-rich lobe derives from the ventral pancreatic primordium during embryogenesis.

The islets are embedded in collagen and reticulum fibres, but

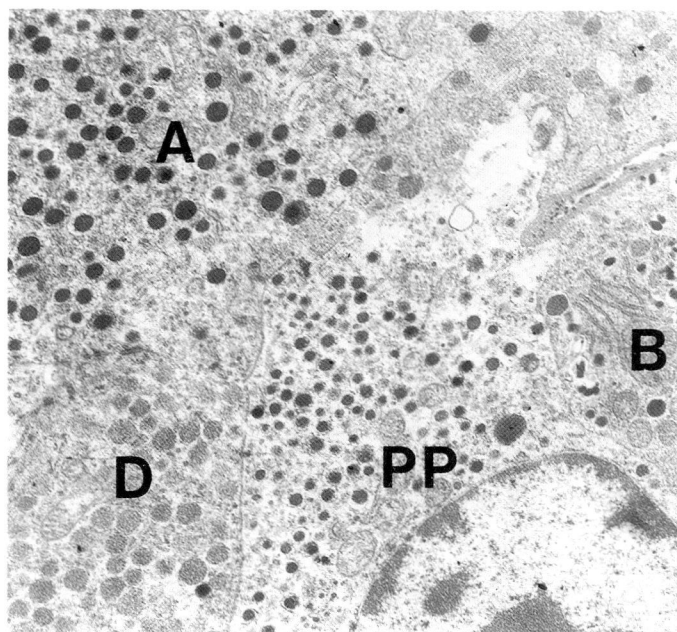

pancreas is the presence of *vasoactive intestinal polypeptide* (VIP) in parasympathetic neurones (Bishop *et al.* 1980) (Fig. 26.83a,b), *neuropeptide tyrosine* (NPY) in sympathetic neurones, and *calcitonin gene-related peptide* (CGRP) in sensory neurones (Su *et al.* 1987).

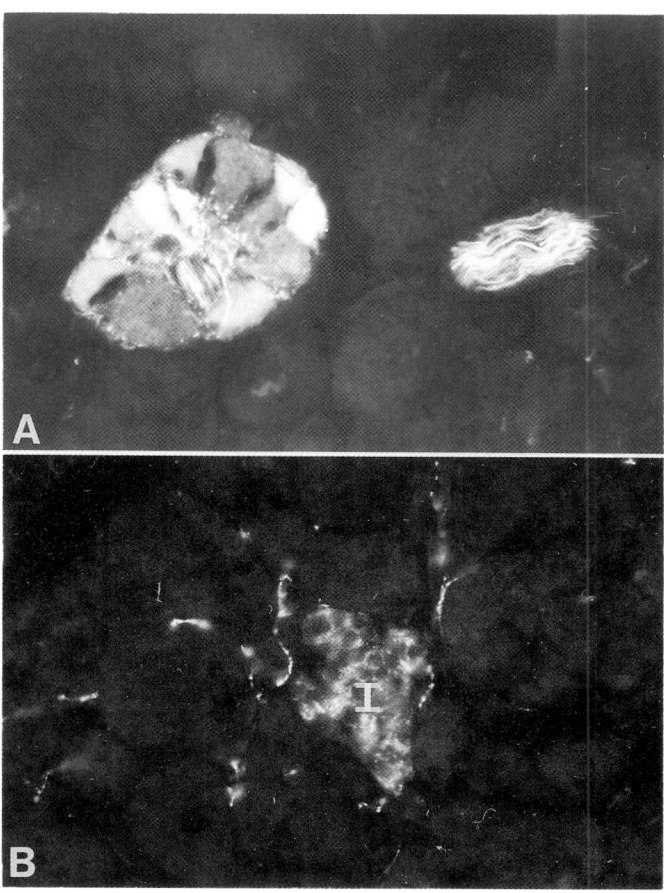

Fig. 26.82 An electron micrograph of a normal human pancreatic islet, showing secretory granules typical of the four endocrine cell types; A cell (granule diameter 200–300 nm), B cell (250–400 nm), D cell (150–400 nm), PP (100–200 nm).

lack any true capsule. They have one or two afferent arterioles which terminate in capillaries. These form a glomerulus-like network between the endocrine cells, and are lined by *fenestrated endothelial* cells. Although the islets receive parasympathetic, sympathetic, and sensory inputs, nerve terminals adjacent to islets (neuro-insular complexes) are seen only rarely and synaptic clefts are lacking (Ferri *et al.* 1987). Parasympathetic nerve fibres originate locally from cell bodies found scattered in the pancreatic parenchyma. By contrast, the adrenergic and sensory innervation originates from neurones outside the gland, from the superior mesenteric ganglion (sympathetic) and from primary sensory neurones located mainly in the dorsal root ganglia. Neuropeptides are found in cholinergic, adrenergic, and sensory nerves. Particularly noticeable in the

Fig. 26.83 VIP immunoreactivity in nerves of the human pancreas demonstrated using the technique of indirect immunofluorescence. (A) Ganglion cells and a nerve bundle showing dense VIP immunoreactivity; (B) fine, varicose VIP-immunoreactive fibres in close association with an islet (I). The islet has been made visible by double immunostaining with insulin.

Table 26.13 Main morphological features of endocrine pancreatic cells

Cell types	A (A2 or α)	B (β)	D (A1 or δ)	PP (F)
Hormones	Glucagon immunoreactants	Insulin/proinsulin, C peptide	Somatostatin/RSCP (rat somatostatin cryptic peptide)	Pancreatic polypeptide
Actions	Metabolism (amino acid)	Sugar	Suppresses exocrine and endocrine secretion	? Suppresses enzyme secretion and gall-bladder contraction
Localization	Islet periphery	Islet centre	Paracentral in association with A cells	Islet periphery, extra-insular (in tail of pancreas)
Granule structure	Eccentric electron-dense core, grey halo, tightly fitting membrane	Polymorphic (bar shape, crystalline shape) electron-dense with wide clear halo	Large, round core of flocculent appearance, tightly fitting membrane	Small, round, electro-dense core, narrow clear halo
Granule size (nm)	200–300	250–400	150–400	100–200

26.7.2　Embryology and development

The origin of the endocrine cells of the pancreas has been much debated (Pearse 1984). Basically, there are two main trends of opinion; the one that predominates is the concept that endocrine cells differentiate from *multipotential (endodermal)* stem cells. The other, less favoured, opinion is that the endocrine cells are of *neuro-ectodermal origin*. Thus, the latter theory states that pancreatic endocrine cells are irrevocably programmed as neuro-endocrine in the early embryo, whereas the former indicates that neuro-endocrine differentiation is the result of a much later differentiation. In man, the first islet bud appears in the outer layer of the primitive tubules from 9 weeks of gestation onwards. At 10–11 weeks, the endocrine cells form small clusters within the tubular formations. Primitive islet cell clusters are found at around the 12th week of gestation. At about 15 weeks, the islets are surrounded by exocrine acini and they often maintain an intimate relationship with ductules. By electron microscopy, the first identifiable cell type is the *A cell*. It appears at 9 weeks and is followed by the *D cell* and *β cell* at 10.5 weeks. The *PP cell* is the last to occur.

While A, D, and PP cells show a constant nuclear size, *β* cells may occasionally have large, polyploid nuclei (? B cell hyperfunction). This phenomenon of hypertrophy is observed frequently in the pancreas of new-born babies of diabetic mothers.

26.7.3　Diabetes mellitus

Although early investigators described much of the wide spectrum of islet alterations in diabetes mellitus, the recognition of diabetes-specific lesions and their relationship with the natural course of the disease was possible only after the development of advanced methodological approaches (Klöppel 1984). In 1980, the WHO expert committee on diabetes mellitus defined this disease as '*a state of chronic hyperglycaemia*' (i.e. the state of having an excessive concentration of glucose in the blood, which may result from many environmental and genetic factors, often acting jointly). The causes of hyperglycaemia are either an absolute or a relative insulin deficiency, which leads to defective carbohydrate metabolism. The various clinical and pathogenetic types of sustained hyperglycaemia, i.e. diabetes mellitus, are classified in Table 26.14.

Diabetes mellitus is one of the most common chronic diseases. Throughout the world, about 30 million people are thought to be affected by the disease and it is one of the leading causes of death in developed countries. The prevalence of discovered and undiscovered diabetes in the adult population is estimated to be 5–6 per cent. This rate appears to increase in populations which are older and obese. In *insulin-dependent diabetes mellitus* (IDDM), the peak incidence is between 10 and 14 years of age. There is no sex preponderance in IDDM. The female:male ratio in non-insulin-dependent diabetes mellitus (NIDDM) is about 1:4. The greatest risk factor for NIDDM in the Western countries is adiposity, the risk being directly related to duration and degree of obesity. In IDDM, in contrast, obesity plays no role. Other major factors concerning both IDDM and NIDDM are of

Table 26.14　WHO classification of diabetes mellitus (1980) (from Klöppel and Heitz 1984)

Diabetes mellitus
　Insulin-dependent type—type I
　Non-insulin-dependent type—type II
　　(a)　non-obese
　　(b)　obese
Diabetes mellitus associated with
　Pancreatic diseases
　Diseases of hormonal aetiology
　Drug- or chemical-induced conditions
　Insulin receptor abnormalities
　Genetic syndromes
　Miscellaneous
Impaired glucose tolerance
　(a)　non-obese
　(b)　obese
　(c)　associated with certain conditions or syndromes
Gestational diabetes

genetic origin. It has been suggested that a polygenetic, multi-factorial inheritance underlies diabetes mellitus. Evidence for inheritance of diabetes mellitus comes from studies on HLA-typing in diabetes, from the frequent familiar aggregation of NIDDM, and from studies of identical twins with diabetes.

Insulin-dependent diabetes mellitus (IDDM)—type I diabetes

Since the classical publication by Gepts on the pathology of the pancreas in recent onset (duration less than one year) type I (insulin-dependent) diabetes mellitus, it has been widely accepted there is a dramatic reduction in the number of insulin-secreting *β* cells and that *insulitis*, a chronic inflammatory cell infiltrate affecting a proportion of the islets, is frequently present (Foulis 1987). Gepts proposed this pathology to be characteristic of IDDM and suggested that an *auto-immune reaction* to *β* cells or a viral infection could explain these morphological features. Indeed this seems to be the case as there is evidence of both mediated and humoral immunity to islet antigens in the majority of patients. Furthermore, there seems to be serological evidence of viral infection in some patients, in particular with coxsackie B virus. Indeed, coxsackie B virus was demonstrated in the pancreata of two patients (albeit clinically atypical) who died at clinical presentation of type I diabetes. The major contribution to the understanding of the pathogenesis of type I diabetes has come from studies of the role of hereditary factors in the disease, mainly the association of this disease with *major histocompatibility complex (MHC) genes (especially class II)*. The seminal work of Foulis clarified the pathology of type I diabetes mellitus since he was able to examine suitable samples of pancreas from 75 patients who died within a year of the onset of diabetic symptoms. In 'classical' cases, there are essentially three populations of islets. The majority of islets are insulin-deficient but contain a normal complement of the remaining pancreatic endocrine cells, including glucagon-, somatostatin-, and PP-producing cells. Furthermore, a proportion of islets are affected by insulitis. The inflammatory process, mainly lymphocytic, affects in particular those islets that still contain β cells, thus suggesting that insulitis represents an immunologically mediated destruction of β cells. A proportion of islets remain totally unaffected and show a normal array of the four endocrine cell types. Thus, within one pancreas and even within one microscopic section of the pancreas, heterogeneous features are noticed; insulin-deficient islets (characteristic of a pancreas with long-standing type I diabetes), islets where β cells are being destroyed selectively by chronic inflammation, and islets where this process has not yet started. There is, therefore, a full spectrum of lesions (Fig. 26.84a–d). According to a recent hypothesis, aberrant expression of class II major histocompatability complex (MHC) products on a target cell may allow presentation of organ-specific surface antigen(s) to potentially autoreactive T-helper lymphocytes and thus lead to auto-immunity. Aberrant expression of class II MHC was demonstrated immunohistochemically by Foulis (1987) on β cells in 21 out of 23 patients with recent onset diabetes. No such expression was seen on the other pancreatic endocrine cells. These abnormalities of MHC expression appear to precede insulitis within a given islet and were found to be unique to type I diabetes.

Non-insulin-dependent diabetes mellitus (NIDDM)-type II diabetes

The histological features of the islets in NIDDM are either indistinguishable from those of non-diabetics or are characterized by *islet amyloidosis*. The identification of deposits of a 'hyaline' material (which was later shown to be amyloid) in the islets of Langerhans of a diabetic subject was first made in 1901 (Opie 1901). Islet amyloid is present in 59–72 per cent of tye II diabetic subjects over the age of 40 and the extent of the deposits increases with the severity of diabetes, judged by the need for insulin therapy (Schneider *et al.* 1980). Islet amyloid is also present in older, spontaneously diabetic domestic cats (Johnson and Stevens 1973) and in some insulinomas (Westermark *et al.* 1987b) but is absent in type I diabetes. Amyloid lies between the islet capillaries and the endocrine cells and may totally replace the islet cells in severe disease (Westermark and Wilander 1978). Its insolubility and low concentration in the pancreas has, until now, prevented the identification of the component peptide. All islets with and without amyloidosis contain normal numbers of β cells and degranulation of the β cells is rare. The frequency and degree of islet amyloidosis is related to the age of the patient; the older the patient, the more marked the amyloidosis. Islet amyloid shows birefringence after staining with Congo red and non-branching, irregularly arranged fibrils (100 Å) at the ultrastructural level. It is located in the perisinusoidal spaces, where it forms nodular to cord-like deposits. Based on its immunocytochemical, biochemical, and clinicopathological characteristics, *insular amyloid*, or as it is now called, *amyloid of endocrine origin*, is distinctly different from systemic amyloid of L or A type. Endocrine amyloid, a form of organ-limited amyloid, can also be found in islet cell tumours. This protein has been characterized and found to have strong sequence homologies with a novel neuropeptide termed *calcitonin gene-related peptide* (Westermark *et al.* 1987a). In addition to amyloidosis, insular fibrosis is a frequent finding in NIDDM. Islet regeneration may be observed occasionally in areas where ductules proliferate. A general trend towards a reduction of endocrine cell mass in NIDDM is mainly due to the reduced numbers of β cells; other cell types may remain unchanged or are increased.

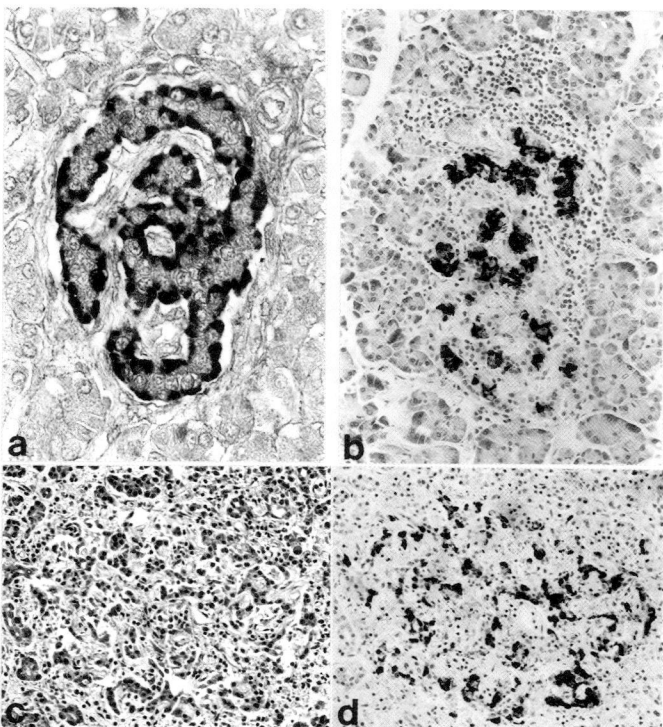

Fig. 26.84 Sections of human pancreas showing damage to islets in diabetes mellitus (type I). (Courtesy of Dr A. Foulis.) (a) A section of an insulin-deficient islet which has been immunostained simultaneously for somatostatin, glucagon, and pancreatic polypeptide. All of the endocrine cells are stained. (b) An islet with marked insulitis immunostained for insulin. (c) Haematoxylin and eosin stain showing extensive β cell necrosis. (d) Adjacent section to (c) immunostained for glucagon. Although no β cells remain in this islet, the α cells are preserved. The fact that the α cells are separate indicates recent β cell destruction. Later, the islet would have collapsed in on itself and resembled the islet shown in (a). (Immunoperoxidase stain with haematoxylin counterstain.)

26.7.4 Persistent hyperinsulinaemic hypoglycaemia in infancy

While the clinical features of persistent hyperinsulinaemic hypoglycaemia are uniform, the pathology of the endocrine pancreas is heterogeneous and has received a most diverse terminology including: *diffused or generalized islet hyperplasia, β cell nesidioblastosis, microadenomatosis, focal adenomatosis, congenital insulinomas (nesidioblastoma), multifocal and focal ductulo-insular proliferation (nesidioblastosis), endocrine dysplasia*, and *nesidiodysplasia* (Heitz *et al.* 1980; Bishop *et al.* 1981; Klöppel and

Heitz 1984). The term *nesidioblastosis* was introduced by Laidlaw to indicate a proliferation of cells that differentiate out of the duct epithelium to build islets. It is now known that the clinical syndrome may include a variety of lesions of the pancreas, ranging from a normal pancreas to a marked diffuse or focal β-cell hyperplasia, on many occasions with derangements of the normal islet cell architecture, leading to lack of paracrine (from the D cells) control of insulin release from the β cells (Fig. 26.85a–c).

26.7.5   Islet-cell tumours

Various terms have been used to describe this class of tumours. Oberndorfer proposed the term 'carcinoid' to describe tumours with a 'carcinoma-like' structure. Laidlaw (1938) introduced the term 'nesidioblastoma' for tumours of the endocrine pancreas and 'nesidioblasts' for cells that differentiate from the epithelium of secretory ducts to form islets. Islet cell tumours of the pancreas were, prior to immunocytochemistry, also termed β- and non-β-cell tumours. The term APUDoma (Sziij *et al.* 1969), meaning tumours derived from APUD (amine precursor uptake decarboxylation) (Pearse 1969) cells, has also been proposed. However, islet-cell tumours or peptide-producing endocrine tumours are now the favoured names. The advent of modern technology, such as immunocytochemistry and radio-immunoassay, has allowed further characterization of these tumours in terms of their function (see Polak and Bloom, 1985). In spite of the fact that these tumours frequently produce more than one peptide (*mixed endocrine tumours*), often one circulating peptide is responsible for the associated clinical syndrome. Thus, in clinical terms, endocrine tumours are often named after their major active secretory product, e.g. *gastrinoma* and *insulinoma*.

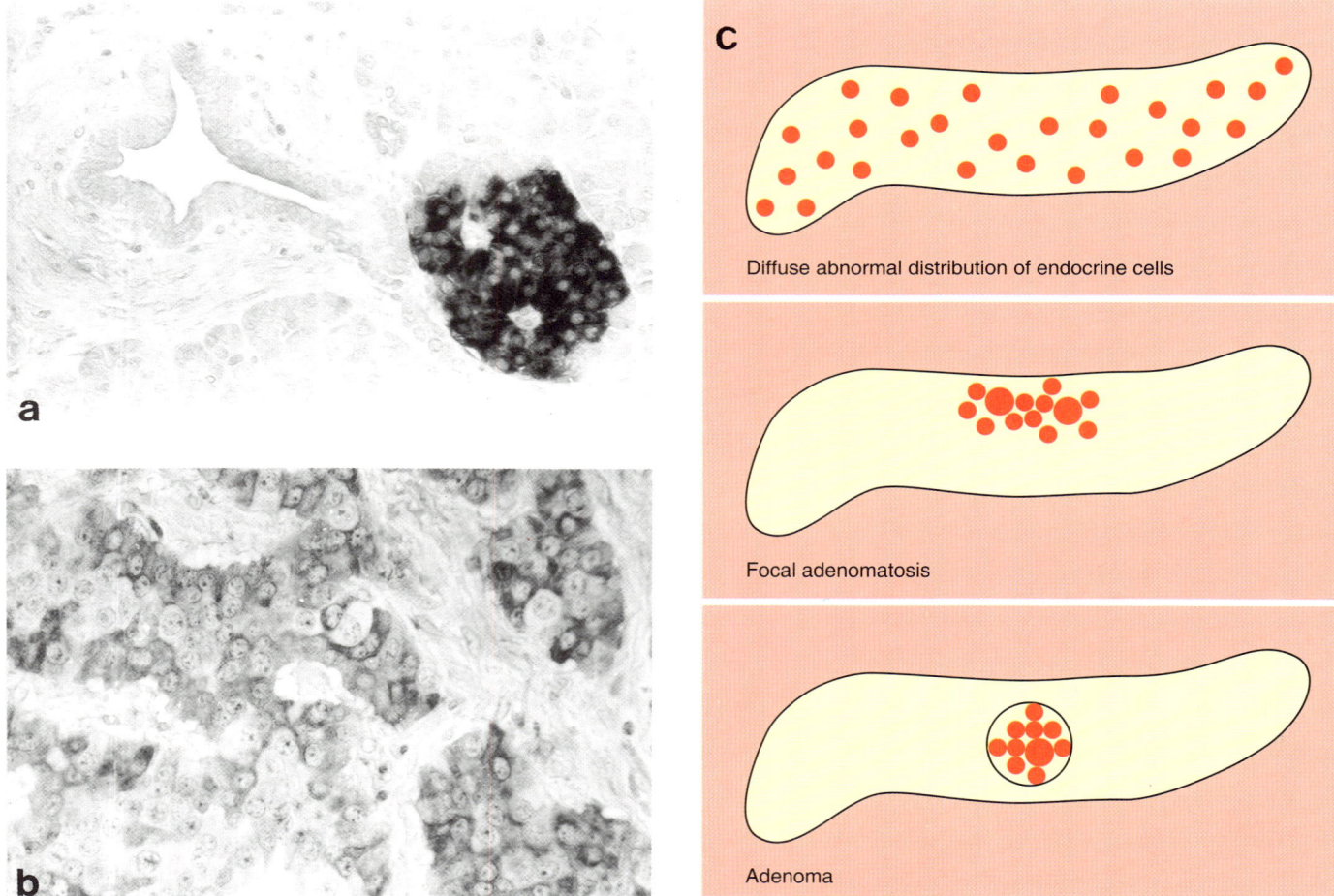

Fig. 26.85   (a) Focal ductulo-insular proliferation (nesidioblastosis) in pancreas taken from a child with persistent hyperinsulinaemic hypoglycaemia. An islet, immunostained for insulin, can be seen budding off a duct. Peroxidase anti-peroxidase immunostain with haematoxylin counterstain. (b) Insulin immunostained in numerous cells of a pancreatic microadenoma removed from a child with persistent hyperinsulinaemic hypoglycaemia. Peroxidase anti-peroxidase immunostain with haematoxylin counterstain. (c) Diagrammatic representation of the pancreatic lesions associated with the clinical syndrome of persistent hyperinsulinaemic hypoglycaemia. (Reproduced by permission from *Pancreatic pathology* (ed. G. Klöppel and Ph. Heitz), Churchill Livingstone, Edinburgh, 1984.)

Clinical features

It is difficult to assess the true incidence of islet-cell tumours, but well recognized, functioning tumours are clearly uncommon. Islet-cell tumours are often characterized by the hypersecretion of active regulatory peptides which are responsible for their clinical manifestation. However, clinical features of some functioning tumours may be obscured or altered by the presence in the circulation of more than one regulatory peptide with counteracting effects. In addition to hormonal effects, nonspecific manifestations depending on site, size, and invasion may be present. Clinical suspicion is usually aroused when more common diseases have been excluded. This sometimes delays diagnosis, with resultant adverse effects on the prognosis. Many pre-operative, non-invasive techniques are also used widely, including a series of stimulation and suppression tests for the particular hormone. Further, a series of tumour localization methods are applied, in particular angiography, ultrasound, or isotope scanning and high resolution computerized tomography. Percutaneous, trans-hepatic portal, and pancreatic veno-sampling, with parallel measurement in systemic blood, may also be useful. Other localization techniques include radioisotope-tagged specific antibodies and nuclear magnetic resonance.

Histology

Peptide-producing endocrine cells are often distributed unevenly within a tumour. It is therefore very important to sample a large number of specimens, taken randomly throughout the tumour mass. The growth pattern of endocrine tumours is quite characteristic. These tumours are composed of uniform cells with little atypia and few mitoses arranged in irregular masses, ribbons, or glandular structures. In the past, it has been claimed that a specific growth pattern may have some diagnostic significance in the typing of endocrine tumours. However, this view is not uniformly accepted and, in our experience and that of others, the criterion of growth pattern has proved unreliable for precise diagnosis. The use of antibodies to *neurone-specific enolase* and to *chromogranin*, as well as *silver impregnation methods* (see Chapter 30), in particular *Grimelius' silver impregnation technique*, are of good diagnostic value (Fig. 26.86). Hyalinization of the tumour stroma is common and sometimes extensive. It is seen especially in some classes of tumours, such as insulinomas and medullary carcinomas. It has been claimed that this substance is related to the hormone produced by the tumours. Classical histochemical stains for amyloid (e.g. tryptophan and tyrosine) are negative and therefore it is possible that this amyloid is chemically different from classical amyloid. Specific names have been proposed such as *APUDamyloid* (Pearse *et al.* 1972) or *endocrine or tissue-associated amyloid*. Assessment of malignancy may be difficult histologically. This class of tumours is slow growing, and unless there is clear-cut evidence of massive infiltration into neighbouring tissue or the presence of metastases, it may be impossible to predict behaviour. A more functional criterion of malignancy has been proposed recently (Heitz *et al.* 1983). This is the production, and release of α *human chorionic hormone* (HCG) by many malignant endocrine tumours, in particular pancreatic endocrine tumours, although 30 per cent of those which behave malignantly show no reactivity for HCG.

Electron microscopy

On electron microscopy, pancreatic endocrine tumours can be seen to contain variable numbers of secretory granules, but often peptide-producing tumour cells store less peptide than their normal counterparts. This suggests that one of the metabolic defects in endocrine tumour cells resides in the control of hormone secretion. Partial or complete loss of control of secretion by the tumour cells results in inappropriate production and secretion of peptide. At present, the process behind this defective conversion remains unknown.

Biochemistry

Highly sensitive and specific radioimmunoassays for the measurement of regulatory peptides in blood and tissue are readily available (Bloom and Long 1982), allowing early diagnosis of functioning tumours. Thus, very small tumours may be diagnosed clinically and biochemically, presenting a challenge both to specialists in localization techniques and to surgeons. However, it must be remembered that circulating levels of active peptides can be elevated in diseases other than tumours, for example *gastrin in atrophic gastritis*. Such cases must be excluded before making the diagnosis of endocrine tumour.

Ectopic hormone production

Liddle and co-workers in 1965 (Liddle *et al.* 1965) coined the term 'ectopic hormone' for tumour cell products that cause remote effects resembling non-biological actions of hormones. By definition, ectopic hormones are produced by a tumour arising in an organ which does not secrete the substance under normal conditions. Synthesis, and sometimes secretion, of a number of peptides by endocrine and non-endocrine tumours may be much more common than is realized presently. Strictly speaking, gastrin and VIP are hormones ectopic to the pancreas, since there is substantial evidence against the production of these peptides by endocrine cells of the normal adult organ. However, gastrin is found in endocrine cells of the fetal pancreas and VIP in neurones of fetal and adult pancreas.

Proof of ectopic hormone production is difficult and requires clinical and biochemical methods, as well as morphological techniques and cell culture. On the other hand, symptoms of ectopic hormone secretion may precede other signs of tumour growth. A knowledge of potential tumour markers is therefore important. For instance, pancreatic endocrine tumours are the cause of approximately 10 per cent of ectopic cases of Cushing's syndrome and are thus second in frequency only to bronchogenic tumours, the commonest site for ectopic ACTH production.

Multihormonal tumours

Multiple hormone production may be caused by single or multiple endocrine tumours [for example those of multi endocrine

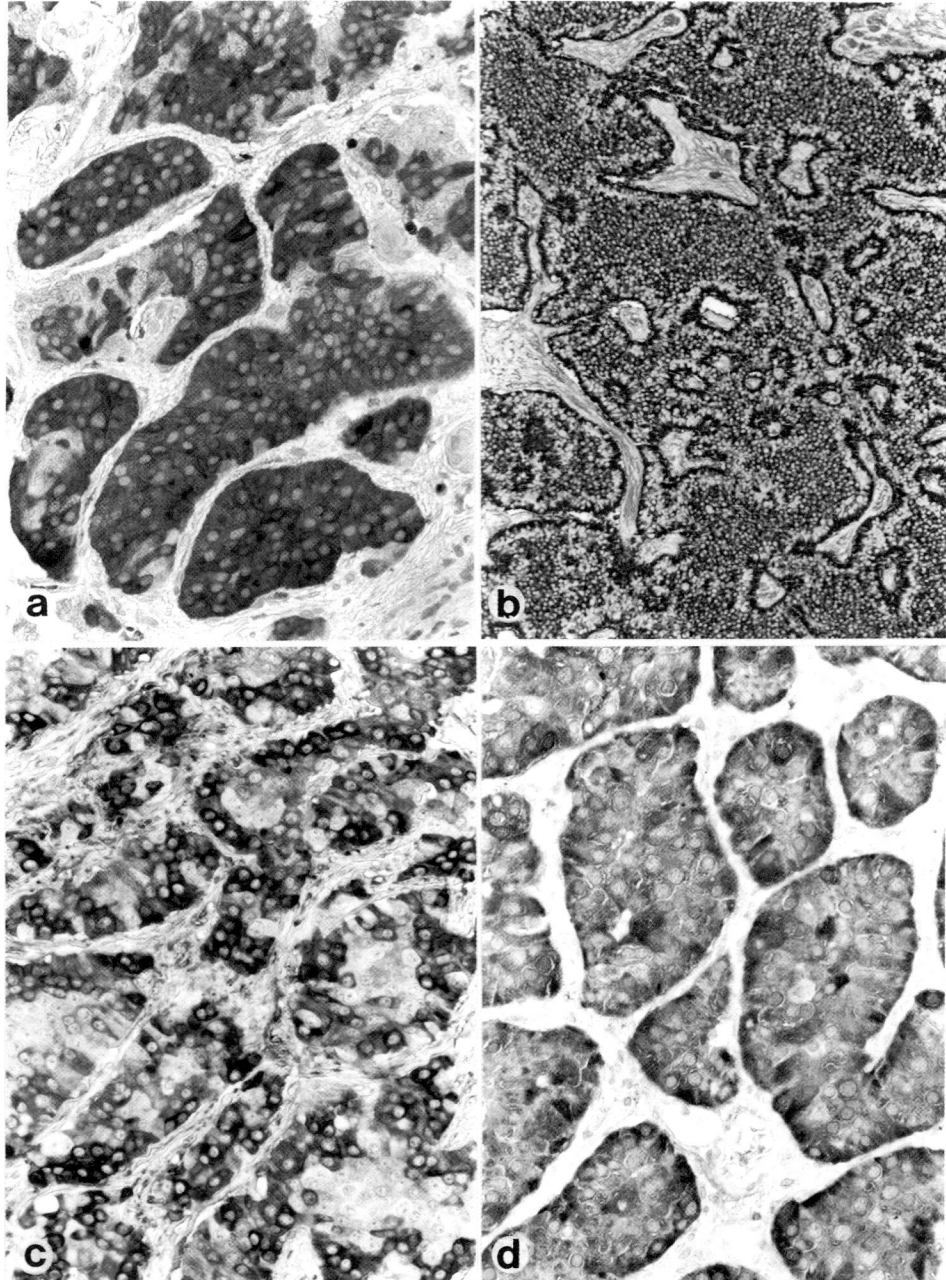

Fig. 26.86   Sections of the same β-cell (insulin-producing) tumour stained in different ways. (a) NSE immunostain. All endocrine cells show some degree of immunoreactivity. (b) Grimelius' silver impregnation method demonstrates argyrophil cells. (c) immunoreactivity for chromogranin can be seen in a proportion of tumour cells. Unlike NSE, which is a cytosolic marker for even poorly granulated endocrine cells, chromogranin immunoreactivity indicates granulated cells. (d) C-peptide immunoreactivity is present in numerous cells, mainly towards the edge of cell nests (a), (c), and (d) peroxidase stain with haematoxylin counterstain.

adenomatosis type I syndrome (MEA-1)]. However, until recently the production of more than one hormone by a single endocrine tumour was considered uncommon. This was due mainly to the fact that the effects of one secreted hormone were clinically predominant and thus obscured the presence of other

less active peptide(s). It is now recognized that some patients have symptoms attributable to the simultaneous secretion of more than one hormone. Furthermore, patients have been reported with symptoms derived from the combination of two syndromes and have even shown transition from one to another, sometimes due to treatment (chemotherapy). In most instances the appropriate hormones have been shown to be produced by separate cell types by both light and electron microscopy.

26.7.6   Tumours associated with characteristic clinical syndromes (Cohen and Soloway 1985)

Gastrinomas (Zollinger–Ellison syndrome)

The discovery by Zollinger and Ellison in 1955 of a potent gastric secretogue being produced and released by a pancreatic tumour challenged and the existing view that the only functioning pancreatic endocrine tumours were insulinomas. Gastrin was characterized fully by Gregory *et al.* in 1960, who extracted it from tumours associated with the Zollinger–Ellison syndrome and showed that it caused the symptoms associated with the syndrome. Subsequently, plasma gastrin was shown to be elevated in this disease. Nowadays, the *Zollinger–Ellison syndrome* is associated with the word gastrinoma.

Gastrinomas represent 20–25 per cent of pancreatic endocrine tumours. They occur most often between 30 and 50 years of age (age-range 20–92 years) and there is a slight male preponderance (60 per cent). The clinical features include *intractable gastric, duodenal*, and *jejunal ulceration, bleeding, and greatly increased gastric acid secretion*. These features are found rarely nowadays since the tumours are usually diagnosed at an early stage due to the increasing awareness of the condition and availability of gastrin assays. Basal plasma gastrin levels are usually extremely elevated, but *calcium stimulation of gastrin levels* is a commonly employed diagnostic test, permitting the distinction between a gastrinoma and other hypergastrinaemic conditions associated with recurrent peptic ulcer (e.g. retained or excluded antrum). Suspicion of a gastrinoma should be aroused if a patient with duodenal ulcer has very high levels of gastric acid secretion and the symptoms do not remit after modern therapy. In view of the association of gastrinomas with parathyroid adenomas in multiple endocrine adenomatosis type I syndrome, all patients with gastrinomas should be investigated for *parathyroid hormone and calcium levels*. Approximately 50 per cent of gastrinoma patients also have chemical evidence of hyperparathyroidism, and temporary improvement of peptide ulcer disease, as well as a fall in gastrin, may occur after parathyroidectomy.

Eighty-five per cent of gastrinomas are found in the pancreas. Extrapancreatic gastrinomas are found, for instance, in the duodenum (13 per cent) and in other areas (1 per cent), including the stomach, upper jejunum, and biliary tree. Solitary intrapancreatic gastrinomas are most often localized in the head and tail of the pancreas, but some occur in the body. This distribution in frequency of anatomical sites for gastrinomas does not fit with the distribution of gastrin-containing cells in normal tissue. G cells are most prominent in the antrum and less frequent in the duodenum, jejunum, and fundus (in this order). At least 60 per cent of gastrinomas are malignant and they frequently metastatize, especially to the liver. This percentage is possibly underestimated and might well be as high as 70–90 per cent.

Histologically, these tumours have the typical appearance of endocrine tumours; frequently duodenal gastrinomas are diagnosed as intestinal carcinoids. Neurone-specific enolase immunostaining, although always positive, is sometimes variable, possibly reflecting the metabolic state of each individual cell. Chromogranin immunostaining and Grimelius' silver impregnation depend on the density of secretory granules. Peptide immunocytochemistry using region-specific antibodies recognizing various segments of the gastrin and preprogastrin molecules, is of good diagnostic value. Furthermore, tumours producing gastrin frequently produce other regulatory peptides, in particular pancreatic polypeptide. Thus, double immunostaining, using a variety of separate peptide antibodies, can aid the diagnosis of the 'mixed' nature of these tumours. By electron microscopy, electron-dense secretory granules can be found in variable quantities. Morphologically distinguishable separate types of electron-dense secretory granules further confirm the 'mixed' nature of some of the gastrin-producing tumours. Secretory granules could resemble the normal antral gastrin type of granule (electron-lucent and with a mean diameter of 240 nm). Other tumours contain predominantly small, electron-dense secretory granules. The features attributed to the Zollinger–Ellison syndrome can sometimes be seen in the so-called *G-cell* hyperplasia/hyperfunction syndrome.

Insulinomas

Insulinomas represent one of the many causes of hypoglycaemia. They constitute 70–75 per cent of all pancreatic endocrine tumours and are about equally common in both sexes. All patients with insulinomas should also be checked for other endocrine disturbances, since β- or non-β-cell adenoma can be associated with other inherited endocrine neoplasms of the MEA-1 syndrome. Clinical features are almost always present, even with small tumours. Hypoglycaemia manifests as headaches, blurred vision, sweating, hunger, and palpitations. Symptoms are usually intermittent and thus a patient can be misdiagnosed as psychiatric, cardiac, or neurological. Other causes of hypoglycaemia must be excluded, including factitious hypoglycaemia, retroperitoneal tumours (producing insulin-like substances), alcohol-induced hypoglycaemia, and Addison's disease. The highest incidence of insulinomas is found between the ages 30 and 60 years old and infants with nesidioblastosis may present with β-cell hyperplasia, focal adenomatosis, and/or a clear-cut β-cell adenoma. Virtually all insulinomas are localized in the pancreas. Approximately 90 per cent of them are solitary and can be excised.

The diameter of the tumours is generally less than 3 cm and they weigh less than 10 g, but the size of the tumours varies considerably and is unrelated to the severity of the symptoms. Most insulinomas are benign; the ratio of malignant tumours varies between 4 and 16 per cent. Histologically, a solid or trabecular growth pattern is most often found. This pattern varies from region to region of the same tumour. Amyloid

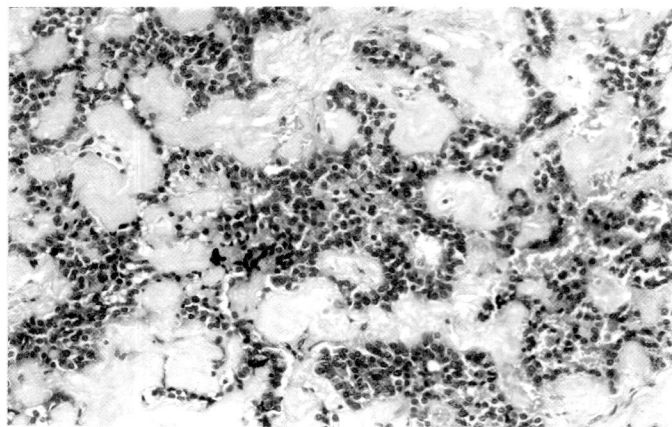

Fig. 26.87 A β-cell tumour with abundant amyloid between tumour cells.

(Fig. 26.87), with a characteristic fibrillary appearance at the electron microscopical level, is frequently found in insulinomas. Insulinomas can be characterized by special histological stains, including aldehyde fuchsin. Silver impregnation methods are only helpful in some cases, but peptide immunostaining and electron microscopy result in the most accurate diagnosis. Antibodies to insulin, C-peptide, and proinsulin reveal a pattern of different staining intensity as insulinomas, like most other endocrine tumours, produce different molecular forms in variable proportions. Electron microscopy and electron immunocytochemistry are also of value. Secretory granules may sometimes resemble the classical β cells of the pancreas, with a crystalline core, but frequently the granules are round and small, many of them have been demonstrated to be immunostained by antibodies to *proinsulin*. Insulinomas are also frequently mixed and, again, pancreatic polypeptide is one of the frequent contaminants of this class of tumours. Sometimes the variable staining intensity pattern correlates with the differing granularity of the tumour and the presence or absence of features of active biosynthesis, e.g. RER, Golgi, etc.

Glucagonomas

The first description of *diabetes* and *necrolytic migratory erythema* associated with a glucagon-secreting tumour was published in 1966 (McGavran *et al.* 1966). The syndrome, however, was recognized as a clear-cut clinical entity by Mallinson and co-workers in 1974 (Mallinson *et al.* 1974), on the basis of the findings made in nine patients. The typical clinical picture shows the following symptoms:

1. a skin rash, *necrolytic migratory erythema*, characterized by superficial epidermal destruction, erythema, a tendency to migrate, and a localization in the lower abdomen, perineum, and legs;

2. an abnormal glucose tolerance test;

3. normocytic, normochromic anaemia;

4. a sore, red tongue;

5. an angular stomatitis;

6. severe weight loss;

7. depression;

8. a tendency to develop overwhelming infection;

9. venous thrombosis (in about one-third of patients).

Many of the symptoms have been ascribed to high gluconeogenesis due to *excess of circulating (normal and/or abnormal) glucagon* and to *low levels of circulating amino acids*. After removal of the glucagonoma, the serum concentration of amino acids may rise to normal or supranormal levels and symptoms may disappear very quickly. In addition, administration of *zinc* induces a fast remission of the skin rash. This led to the postulate that this condition may be partly due to zinc deficiency. The disease occurs most often between 40 and 70 years of age and appears to be slightly more common in women than in men. More than 60 per cent of glucagonomas causing the symptoms are malignant. This percentage is even higher if tumours inducing hyperglucagonaemia but not causing the complete syndrome are included. Glucagonomas are a frequent autopsy finding (about 0.8 per cent).

Histologically, glucagonomas show no remarkable features other than general endocrine morphology. Grimelius' silver impregnation method, neurone-specific enolase, and chromogranin immunostaining are good neuro-endocrine markers. Peptide immunocytochemistry, in particular if antibodies to the preproglucagon molecule are available (Fig. 26.88), is of an excellent diagnostic value (Hamid *et al.* 1986). The 'mixed' nature or multiple hormone production by glucagonomas, also quite a common feature, is further validated by peptide immunocytochemistry. *Pancreatic polypeptide-producing cells* are frequently present, but also *insulin-, somatostatin, and gastrin-producing cells* may be found. Glucagon-producing pancreatic adenomas constitute part of a multiple endocrine adenomatosis type I (MEA-1) syndrome, some cases even presenting with a

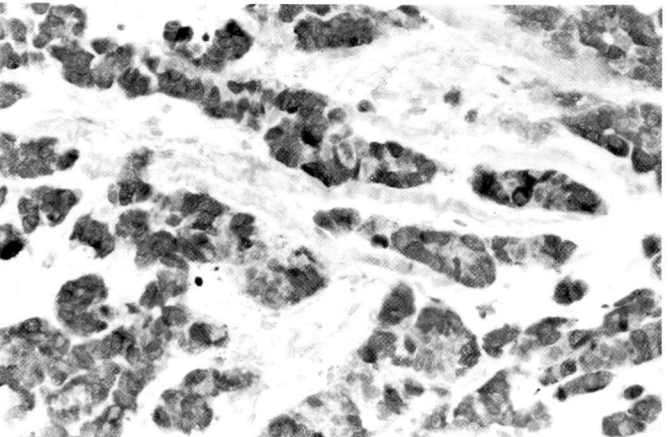

Fig. 26.88 An α-cell (glucagon-producing) tumour immunostained with antibodies to GLP-2 (glucagon-like peptide-2) a peptide derived from the preproglucagon molecule. (Peroxidase anti-peroxidase immunostain with haematoxylin counterstain.)

full glucagonoma syndrome; thus, if a diagnosis of glucagonoma is reached, the search for a possible MEA-1 syndrome is obligatory. By electron microscopy, a variable number of secretory granules can be seen. In general, 'benign' glucagonomas are fully granulated; malignant ones are not and show features of high peptide synthesis and secretion. Secretory granules, in particular in adenomas, may frequently resemble A-cell granules of the pancreas, but malignant tumours or highly active tumours generally show an atypical type of secretory granules.

VIPoma/PHMoma, diarrhoegenic (WDHA) tumour syndrome

VIPomas represent 3–5 per cent of all pancreatic endocrine tumours (Long *et al.* 1981). The syndrome consists of *diarrhoea of a highly fluid consistency*, free of blood and mucus, and with a volume of 4–20 ml/kg/day, of *hypokalaemia and hypo- or achlorhydria*. Approximately two-thirds of patients complain of *abdominal colic* and some have *intermittent high faecal fat output*. There is often a significant weight loss. At operation, a large amount of alkaline secretion from the pancreas is found. Some patients may also suffer from occasional flushing attacks. The rate of tumour malignancy is 50–75 per cent.

The tumours are often quite large (2–7 cm). Histologically, the tumours show either the classical features of islet-cell tumours or features of *ganglioneuroblastomas* (Fig. 26.89). Grimelius' silver impregnation method, neurone-specific enolase, and chromogranin immunostaining give variable results, depending on the granularity of the tumour. Equally, peptide immunostaining is also variable, but nowadays the availability of region-specific antibodies, recognizing various parts of the preproVIP molecule (Fig. 26.90), permits a much better evaluation of these tumours. Ultrastructurally, tumours associated with the VIPoma syndrome, being either islet-cell tumours or ganglioneuroblastomas, are generally poorly granulated. The secretory granules are small and round (Fig. 26.91). These tumours are frequently mixed, the most common additional peptide produced by them being *pancreatic polypeptide*.

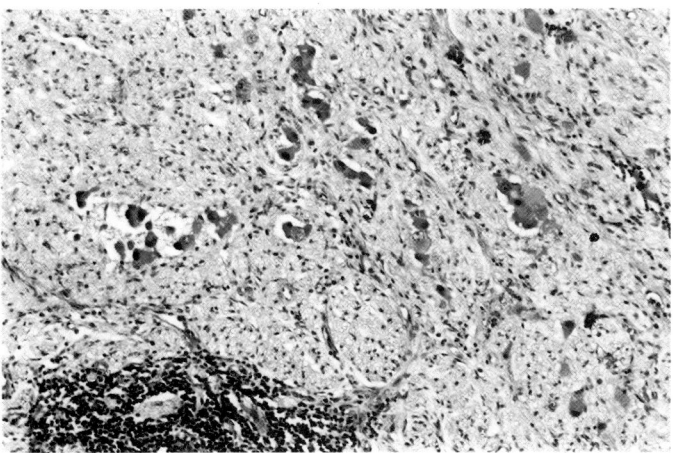

Fig. 26.89 A haematoxylin and eosin stain of a ganglioneuroblastoma showing neuroblasts and fully differentiated nerve cell bodies.

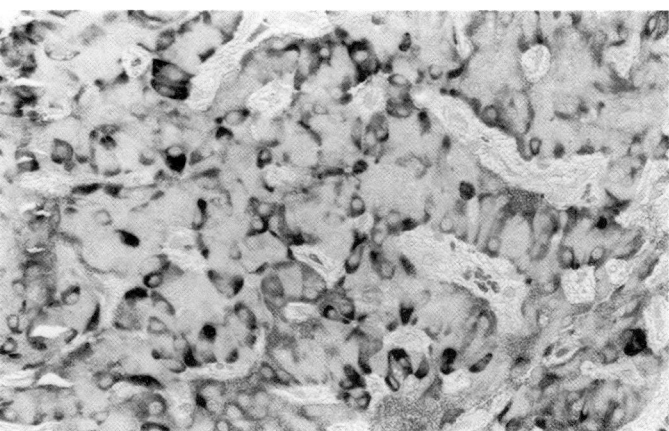

Fig. 26.90 A pancreatic endocrine tumour with a predominantly trabecular structure immunostained for VIP. Many immunoreactive cells can be seen scattered in the tumour. (Peroxidase anti-peroxidase stain with haematoxylin counterstain.)

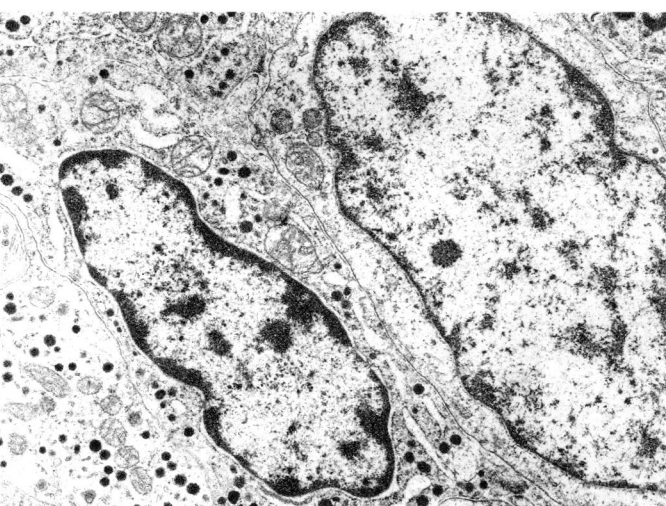

Fig. 26.91 An electron micrograph of two cells from a pancreatic VIP-producing tumour. Typically small, electron-dense secretory granules can be seen.

Somatostatinomas

The association of somatostatin production by endocrine tumours and a clinical syndrome of *diabetes mellitus, steatorrhoea, hyperchlorhydria* and, in some cases, *gallstones*, was described some time ago. However, the entity of the somatostatinoma syndrome is still being discussed (Cohen and Soloway 1985). Most somatostatinomas are solitary and localized in the pancreas. Fewer tumours have been described in the gut and tumours with the features of duodenal 'carcinoids' with psammomatous bodies have been shown to react to somatostatin antibodies. These tumours have been described in association with neurofibromatosis and phaeochromocytomas.

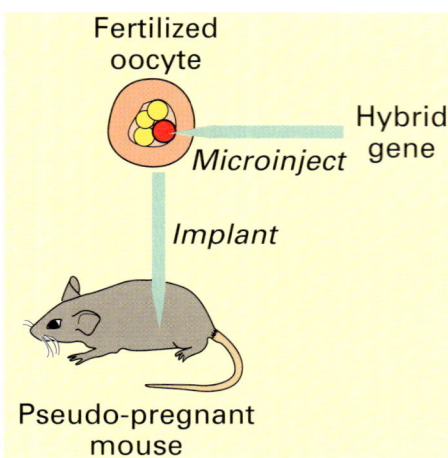

Fig. 26.92 Diagrammatic representation of the production of transgenic mice. A hybrid gene is constructed, e.g. from the promoter region of SV40 and the regulatory region of the insulin gene, and microinjected into a fertilized oocyte. This is implanted into a pseudo-pregnant mouse. The progeny show β-cell pathology, including formation of neoplasms.

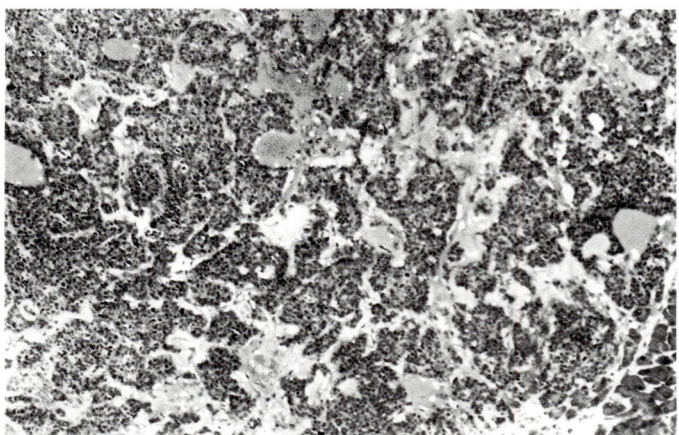

Fig. 26.93 Haematoxylin and eosin stain of a β-cell tumour removed from an SV40–insulin transgenic mouse.

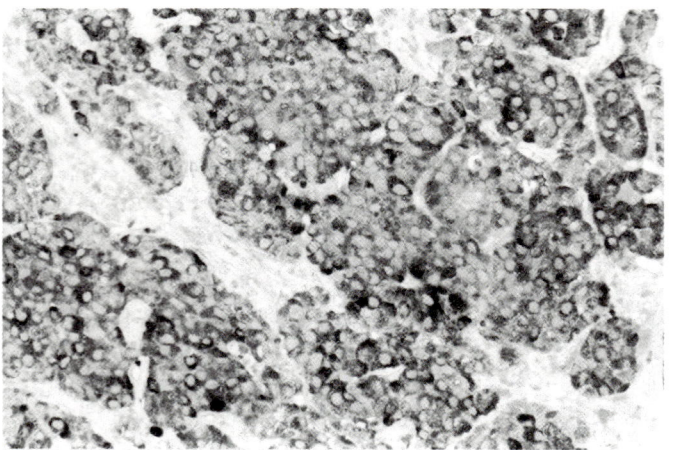

Fig. 26.94 A similar tumour to that shown in Fig. 26.93 immunostained for insulin. Peroxidase anti-peroxidase stain with no counterstain.

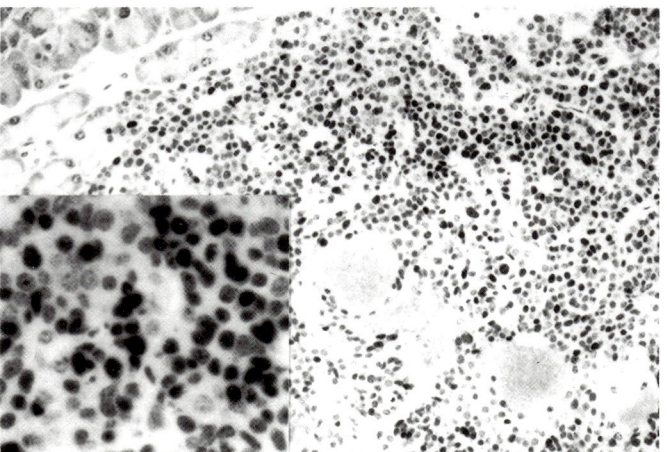

Fig. 26.95 A similar tumour to that shown in Fig. 26.93 immunostained for large T-antigen, an antigenic marker for SV40. Peroxidase anti-peroxidase stain with no counterstain.

Somatostatin-containing tumours are frequently malignant and their growth pattern is similar to those described for endocrine tumours. The immunocytochemical demonstration of somatostatin is easy, as tumour cells react strongly to antibodies. Silver impregnation methods, in particular Davenport's (Helleström–Hellman) method, are useful and by electron microscopy the tumours are, in general, well granulated, many of them presenting granules similar to their normal counterparts. Other hormones have been found to be present in somatostatinomas, including pancreatic polypeptide.

Tumours producing pancreatic polypeptide: PPomas

Oversecretion of PP is one of the most frequent associations noted with well-defined, functioning endocrine tumours (Cohen and Soloway 1985). Tumours most frequently containing PP cells include VIPomas, glucagonomas, and insulinomas. Gastrinomas show less frequent PP production. PP is rarely present in other classes of endocrine tumours (ileal or lung carcinoids may occasionally also produce PP). Therefore, PP-positive immunostaining in a metastasis of an endocrine tumour of unknown origin points to the possibility of the primary being in the pancreas. Frequent PP immunostaining has also been noted in *duodenal paragangliomas* and 'pure' PPomas have also been described. In the described cases of so-called 'pure' PPomas, none of the patients presented with specific symptoms that could be ascribed to high secretion of PP. Most 'PPomas' are benign.

Growth hormone-releasing factor-producing tumours, GRFomas, or acromegalic tumours

Tumours of the pancreas associated with acromegaly have frequently been described in the literature and GRF has now been found to be produced by pancreatic endocrine neoplasms.

Experimental production of endocrine tumours

Until recently the experimental production of endocrine tumours was difficult. Advances in gene transfer technology has allowed the production of pancreatic endocrine tumours in mice (Hanahan 1985). This is achieved by microinjection of a hybrid gene into an oocyte. The hybrid gene consists of the coding sequence of the *oncogene virus SV40* (*promoter region*) and the *regulatory region of hormone gene*. Thus, successful production of insulinomas has recently been achieved using transgenic mice (Figs 26.92–26.95).

26.7.7   Bibliography

Bishop, A. E., Polak, J. M., Green, I. C., Bryant, M. G., and Bloom, S. R. (1980). The location of VIP in the pancreas of man and rat. *Diabetologia* 18, 73–78.

Bishop, A. E., Polak, J. M., Garin Chesa, P., Timson, C. M., Bryant, M. G., and Bloom, S. R. (1981). Decrease of pancreatic somatostatin in neonatal nesidioblastosis. *Diabetes* 30, 122–6.

Bloom, S. R. and Long, R. G. (eds) (1982). *Radioimmunoassay of gut regulatory peptides*. W. B. Saunders, London.

Cohen, S. and Soloway, R. D. (eds). (1985). *Hormone-producing tumours of the gastrointestinal tract*. Churchill Livingstone, New York.

Ferri, G.-L., Bloom, S. R., and Polak, J. M. (1987). Morphology of the islets of Langerhans. In *Surgical diseases of the pancreas* (ed. J. M. Howard, G. L. Jordan, Jr., and H. A. Reber), pp. 779–87. Lea & Febiger, Philadelphia.

Foulis, A. K. (1987). The pathogenesis of beta cell destruction in type 1 (insulin-dependent) diabetes mellitus. *Journal of Pathology* 152, 141–8.

Hamid, Q. A., Bishop, A. E., Sikri, K. L., Varndell, I. M., Bloom, S. R., and Polak, J. M. (1986). Immunocytochemical characterization of 10 pancreatic tumours, associated with the glucagonoma syndrome, using antibodies to separate regions of the pro-glucagon molecule and other neuroendocrine markers. *Histopathology* 10, 119–33.

Hanahan, D. (1985). Heritable formation of pancreatic B-cell tumours in transgenic mice expressing recombinant insulin/simian virus 40 oncogenes. *Nature* 315, 115–22.

Heitz, Ph. U., Klöppel, G., and Polak, J. M. (1980). Morphology of the endocrine pancreas in persistent hypoglycaemia in infants. In *Current views on hypoglycemia and glucagon* (ed. D. Andreani, P. J. Lefebvre, and V. Marks), pp. 355–65. Academic Press, London.

Heitz, Ph. U., Kasper, M., Klöppel, G., Polak, J. M., and Vaitukaitis, J. L. (1983). Glycoprotein-hormone alpha-chain production by pancreatic endocrine tumours: a specific marker of malignancy. Immunocytochemical analysis of tumors of 155 patients. *Cancer* 51, 277–82.

Johnson, K. H. and Stevens, J. B. (1973). Light and electron microscopic studies of islet amyloid in diabetic cats. *Diabetes* 22, 81–90.

Klöppel, G. (1984). Islet histopathology in diabetes mellitus. In *Pancreatic pathology* (ed. G. Klöppel and P. U. Heitz), pp. 154–92. Churchill Livingstone, Edinburgh.

Klöppel, G. and Heitz, P. U. (eds) (1984). Persistent hyperinsulinaemic hypoglycaemia in infancy. In *Pancreatic pathology*, pp. 193–205. Churchill Livingstone, Edinburgh.

Laidlaw, G. F. (1938). Nesidioblastoma, the islet tumor of the pancreas. *American Journal of Pathology* 14, 125–34.

Liddle, G. W., Givens, J. R., Nicholson, W. E., and Island, D. P. (1965). The ectopic ACTH syndrome. *Cancer Research* 25, 1057–61.

Long, R. G., Bryant, M. G., Mitchell, S. J., Adrian, T. E., Polak, J. M., and Bloom, S. R. (1981). Clinicopathological study of pancreatic and ganglioneuroblastoma tumours secreting vasoactive intestinal polypeptide (vipomas). *British Medical Journal* 282, 1769–71.

McGavran, M. H., Unger, R. H., Recant, L., Polk, H. C., Kilo, C. H., and Levin, M. E. (1966). A glucagon secreting alpha-cell carcinoma of the pancreas. *New England Journal of Medicine* 274, 1408–13.

Opie, E. (1901). The relation of diabetes mellitus to lesions of the pancreas. Hyaline degeneration of the islands of Langerhans. *Journal of Experimental Medicine* 5, 527–40.

Pearse, A. G. E. (1969). The cytochemistry and ultrastructure of polypeptide producing cells of the APUD series and the embryologic, physiologic and pathologic implication of the concept. *Journal of Histochemistry and Cytochemistry* 17, 303–13.

Pearse, A. G. E. (1984). Islet development and the APUD concept. In *Pancreatic pathology* (ed. G. Klöppel and P. U. Heitz), pp. 125–32. Churchill Livingstone, Edinburgh.

Pearse, A. G. E., Ewen, S. W. B., and Polak, J. M. (1972). The genesis of apudamyloid in endocrine polypeptide tumours. Histochemial distinction from immunamyloid. *Virchows Archiv B—Cell Pathology* 10, 93–107.

Polak, J. M. and Bloom, S. R. (eds) (1985). *Endocrine tumours*. Churchill Livingstone, Edinburgh.

Schneider, H. M., Storkel, S., and Will, W. (1980). Das amyloid der Langerhansschen inseln und seine beziehung zum diabetes mellius. *Deutsche Medizinische Wochenscrift* 105, 1143–7.

Su, H. C., Bishop, A. E., Power, R. F., Hamada, Y., and Polak, J. M. (1987). Dual intrinsic and extrinsic origins of CGRP- and NPY-immunoreactive nerves of rat gut and pancreas. *Journal of Neuroscience* 7, 2674–87.

Sziij, I., Csapo, Z., Laszlo, F., and Kovacs, K. (1969). Medullary cancer of the thyroid gland associated with hypercorticism. *Cancer* 24, 167–73.

Westermark, P. and Wilander, E. (1978). The influence of amyloid deposits on the islet volume of maturity onset diabetes mellitus. *Diabetologia* 15, 417–21.

Westermark, P., Wernstedt, C., O'Brien, T. D., Hayden, D. W., and Johnson, K. H. (1987a). Islet amyloid in Type 2 human diabetes mellitus and adult diabetic cats contain a novel putative polypeptide hormone. *American Journal of Pathology* 127, 414–17.

Westermark, P., Wernstedt, C., Wilander, E., Hayden, D. W., O'Brien, T. D., and Johnson, K. H. (1987b). Amyloid fibrils in human insulinoma and islets of Langerhans of the diabetic cat are derived from a neuropeptide-like protein also present in normal islet cells. *Proceedings of the National Academy of Sciences, USA* 84, 3881–5.

26.8   Pathophysiology of the diffuse neuro-endocrine system

J. M. Polak and S. R. Bloom

26.8.1   Introduction

Recognition that the cells of the endocrine system do not exist solely in endocrine glands came from the work of Feyrter and his alumni (cf. Ratzenhofer *et al.* 1984). Feyrter described the existence of characteristic '*endocrine/paracrine*' cells widely distributed throughout the body, often as single cells interspersed with non-endocrine cells. These '*clear*' *cells*, or *Helle Zellen*, as Feyrter called them, took up conventional stains only poorly but could be demonstrated by the application of silver impregnation methods. Later on, the presence of *dense-cored secretory granules* was demonstrated in Feyrter's endocrine cells by electron microscopy (Creutzfeldt *et al.* 1970). Since the discovery of potently active regulatory peptides in almost every tissue of the body, it has been possible to demonstrate by immunocyto-chemistry that these substances, often termed '*regulatory peptides*', are present both in endocrine cells and the organ innervation, forming together the so-called '*diffuse neuro-endocrine system*'. Details of the 'diffuse neuro-endocrine system' of the gastrointestinal tract and pancreas and the involvement of this system in tumour and non-tumour pathology are given in Sections 26.7 and 16.17. In this section, the nature, distribution, and pathophysiology of the 'diffuse neuro-endocrine system' of non-gastroenteropancreatic tissues richly provided with regulatory peptides will be described.

26.8.2   Respiratory tract

The respiratory tract contains a rich variety of regulatory peptides (Table 26.15) present both in mucosal endocrine cells and in autonomic/sensory nerves (Polak and Bloom 1986). The finding of numerous *bombesin/GRP* (*gastrin-releasing peptide*) immunoreactive mucosal endocrine cells in the fetal and neonatal developing human lung (Fig. 26.96) led, in the early

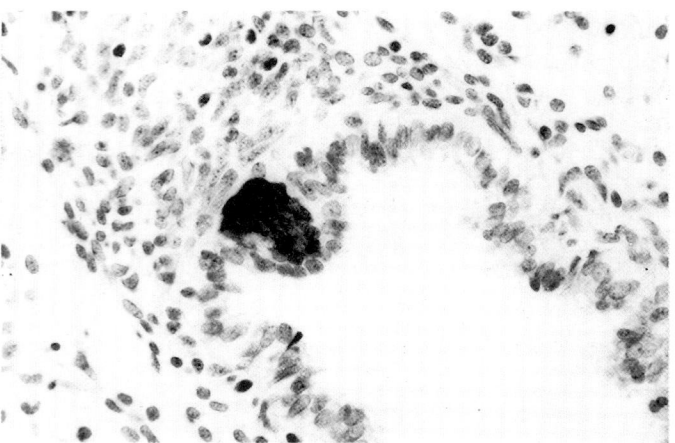

Fig. 26.96   Bombesin-immunoreactive cells in lung of 18 week human fetus. Bouin's fluid-fixed, wax-embedded tissue. Peroxidase anti-peroxidase method.

days, to the postulate that this peptide may exert growth-promoting properties. This was further substantiated by the later finding that hypoplastic lungs of babies with respiratory distress syndrome have a marked deficiency of bombesin-containing cells (Ghatei *et al.* 1983). However, the firmest evidence for bombesin being a growth-promoting factor comes from the study of tumour pathology: bombesin/GRP is frequently produced by one of the most malignant and rapidly growing neuro-endocrine tumours of pulmonary and non-pulmonary origin, the small cell carcinoma (Fig. 26.97) (Ghatei *et al.* 1983; Springall *et al.* 1986; Hamid *et al.* 1987*a*). If

Table 26.15   Distribution and characteristics of the major regulatory peptides of the respiratory system

Peptides	Number of amino acids of main molecular form*	Location	Cell bodies	Coexistence	Distribution
Bobesin (GRP)	27 (in man)	Endocrine cells (mainly developing lung)	NA	Serotonin	Trachea, bronchi
VIP	28	Nerves	Local cell bodies	Acetylcholine, galanin, PHI (M)	Around seromucous glands, blood vessels, smooth muscle
PHI (M)	27	Nerves	Local cell bodies	Acetylcholine, galanin, VIP	Around seromucous glands, blood vessels, smooth muscle
Galanin	29	Nerves	Local cell bodies	Acetylcholine, VIP, PHI (M)	Around seromucous glands, blood vessels, smooth muscle
CGRP	37	Endocrine cells and nerves	Extrinsic (sensory) neurones	? Substance P in nerves, cells NK	Bronchial and vascular smooth muscle, intra-epithelial nerve endings
Calcitonin	37	Endocrine cells	Very scattered, only in adults	Serotonin	Main bronchi
Enkephalin	5	Endocrine cells	Very scattered, unconfirmed reports	? Bombesin, ? serotonin	Main bronchi
Tachykinins (substance P/ neurokinin A)	11	Nerves	Extrinsic (sensory) neurones	? With CGRP	Bronchial and vascular smooth muscle, intra-epithelial nerve endings
NPY	36	Nerves	Extrinsic (sympathetic) neurones	Catecholamines	Around blood vessels mainly

GRP, gastrin-releasing peptide; VIP, vasoactive intestinal polypeptide; PHI (M), peptide histidine isoleucine (methionine); CGRP, calcitonin gene-related peptide; NPY, neuropeptide Y; NA, not applicable; NK not known.
* All these regulatory peptides are present in multiple molecular forms.

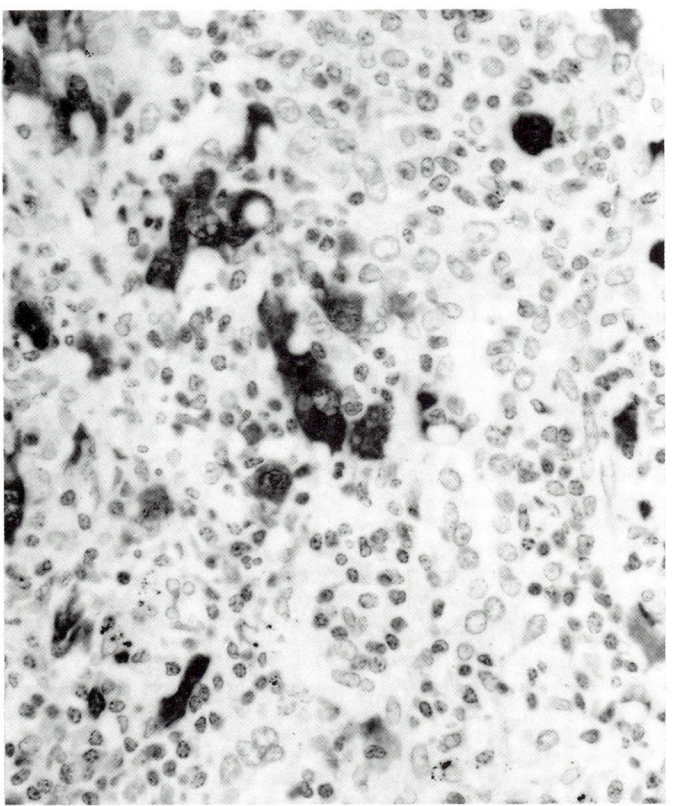

Fig. 26.97 Bombesin immunoreactivity in a small cell carcinoma of the lung (intermediate type). (Formalin-fixed, wax-embedded tissue. PAP method.)

this tumour is grown in culture or in nude mice, the growth is markedly impeded by the addition of specific monoclonal antibodies to bombesin/GRP. Furthermore, addition of pure bombesin enhances growth, both in nude mice and in tumour cell lines (Cuttitta *et al.* 1985). This observation led to the postulate that bombesin-producing malignant tumour cells have on their surface bombesin receptors and thus, once this growth-promoting factor is released from the malignant cell, it activates its own receptors and this in turn stimulates cell growth (*autocrine effect*) (Cuttitta *et al.* 1985). Indeed, the existence of binding sites for bombesin has been demonstrated both biochemically, on isolated cell membranes, and morphologically, using dimeric forms of bombesin which bind on one side to the receptor on the surface of the bombesin-producing malignant cells and on the other to specific bombesin antibodies (Lackie *et al.* 1985). The final reaction product can be visualized at the electron microscopical level by the use of gold-labelled antibodies (Fig. 26.98).

Calcitonin gene-related peptide (CGRP) is present in innervated mucosal endocrine cells (Fig. 26.99), the position of which within the bronchial epithelium suggests a possible role in sensing oxygen concentrations in airways (Cadieux *et al.* 1986). This postulate is substantiated by the changes observed in CGRP-containing endocrine cells after chronic hypoxia (Springall *et al.* 1987).

Vasoactive intestinal polypeptide (VIP), and possibly peptide histidine isoleucine (PHI), modulate airway diameter and bronchial secretions, and VIP/PHI-containing nerve fibres abundantly innervate bronchial smooth muscle and seromucous glands (Power *et al.* 1987). It is therefore possible to postulate

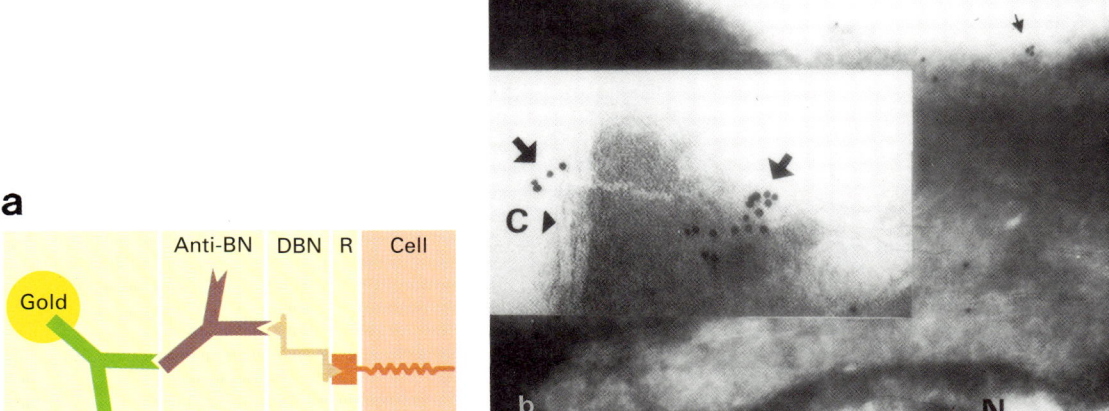

Fig. 26.98 (a) Diagram showing the localization of bombesin receptor (R) on the cell surface using a divalent bombesin ligand (DBN) and the immunogold staining method with an anti-bombesin serum (Anti-BN). (b) An electron micrograph showing bombesin receptors (arrows) on the surface (C) of cultured pulmonary small cell carcinoma cells, using the method described in (a). N, nucleus.

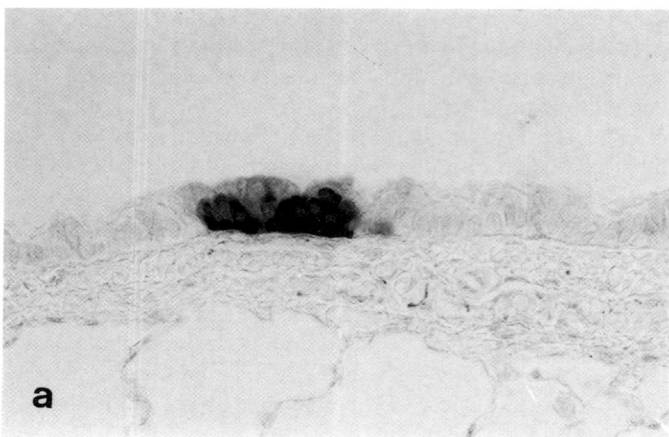 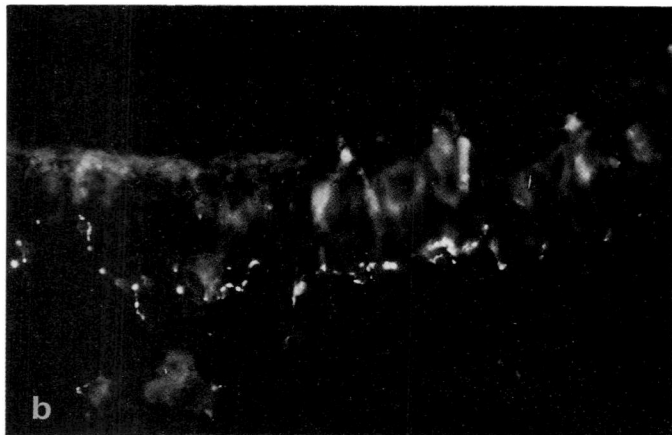

Fig. 26.99 Cells immunoreactive for CGRP in intrapulmonary bronchus of rat. (Wax-embedded, Bouin's fluid-fixed tissue. PAP method.) (b) Nerve fibres immunoreactive for CGRP running below and within the epithelium of rat trachea. (Benzoquinone-fixed tissue, immunofluorescence method.)

that patients with bronchial hyper-reactivity (asthma) or cystic fibrosis may show a depletion of the VIP/PHIergic nervous system. This has been shown recently. Changes in the VIPergic system have also been demonstrated in the nasal mucosa of patients with *uncontrollable vasomotor rhinitis* (Kurian *et al.* 1983).

26.8.3   Cardiovascular system

The majority of peptides present in the cardiovascular system (Table 26.16) are found in nerves, with the exception of *atrial natriuretic peptide* (ANP) which is present in *specialized myoendocrine cells*, present in particular in the atrium of heart (Fig. 26.100) (Wharton and Gulbenkian 1987). The entirety of the innervation of the cardiovascular system can be revealed easily by the use of antibodies *to protein gene product 9.5* (PGP)

(Fig. 26.101) and to *synaptophysin*. The former is a protein originally extracted from the brain and thought to be present in the cytoskeleton, whereas the latter, also termed *P38* is a *Ca^{2+}-regulating glycoprotein* present, in particular, in the membrane of small neurosecretory vesicles. Antibodies to PGP immunostain all classes of nerves (autonomic/sensory) and large nerve trunks, whereas immunostaining of synaptophysin is particularly useful for axon terminals. PGP immunostaining reveals with clarity the conduction system. *Neuropeptide tyrosine* (NPY) is the most abundant neuropeptide in nerves of the human conduction system (Fig. 26.102).

In man, abundant ANP can be produced by the ventricles in disease states (e.g. cardiac insufficiency). Gene expression in ventricular myocytes can be investigated by the use *in situ* hybridization which demonstrates the mRNA directing the synthesis of a given peptide (Hamid *et al.* 1987*b*) (Fig. 26.103).

Table 26.16   Distribution and characteristics of the major regulatory peptides of the cardiovascular system

Peptides	Number of amino acids in main molecular form*	Species abundance	Distribution	Nature
NPY	36	Man	Coronary blood vessels, myocardium, conduction system	Sympathetic
CGRP	37	Rat and guinea-pig	Coronary and other blood vessels, myocardium	Sensory
Substance P	11	Rat and guinea-pig	Coronary and other blood vessels, myocardium	Sensory
Somatostatin	28	Man	Conduction system, myocardium	NK
VIP	28	Cat and man	Blood vessels	? Parasympathetic
ANP	36	Most species	Myoendocrine cells of atrium and in ventricular branches of the conduction system	NA

VIP, Vasoactive intestinal polypeptide; ANP, atrial natriuretic peptide; CGRP, Calcitonin gene-related peptide; NPY, neuropeptide Y; NA, not applicable; NK not known.
* All these regulatory peptides are present in multiple molecular forms.

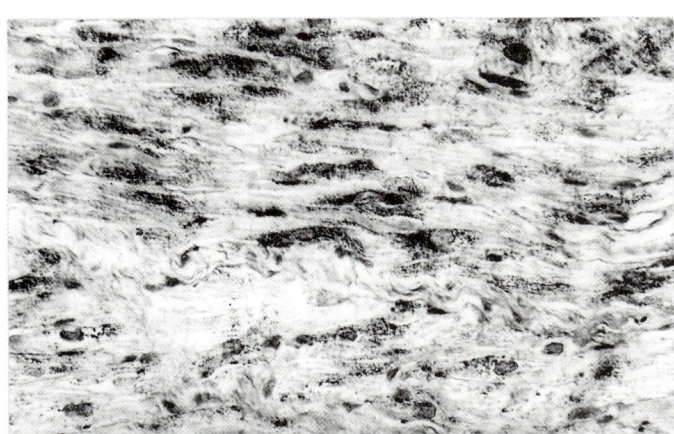

Fig. 26.100 Section of human atrial appendage immunostained for ANP with PAP method. ANP immunoreactivity is concentrated around the nuclei and nuclear poles of myocardial cells. Normaski optics.

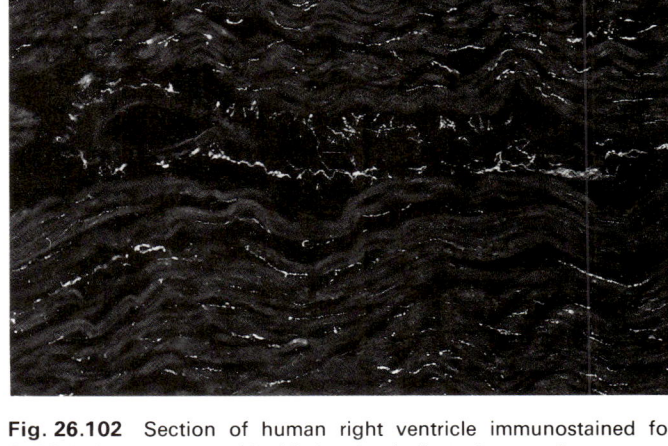

Fig. 26.102 Section of human right ventricle immunostained for C-PON (pro-neuropeptide Y) by the indirect immunofluorescence technique. C-PON immunoreactive nerve fibres concentrated around a coronary artery branch and in the myocardium.

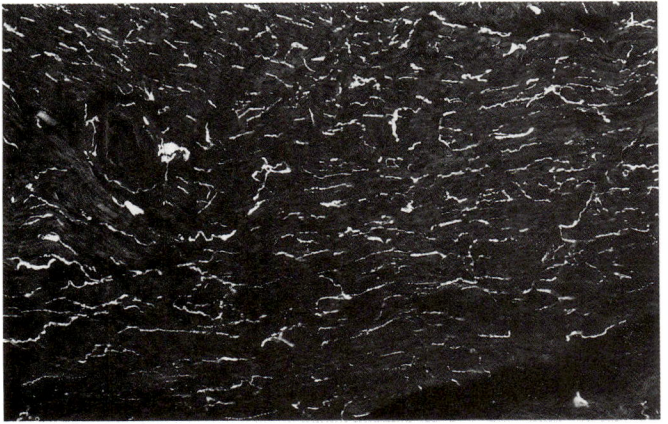

Fig. 26.101 Section of human left atrium immunostained for PGP. A dense network of nerve fibres and fasicles can be seen associated with the atrial myocardium and around a coronary artery branch.

26.8.4 Genital tract

The male and female genital tracts contain numerous regulatory peptides (Table 26.17), in particular in their innervation. Scattered endocrine cells have been described but the peptide production of these cells remains to be elucidated, although *serotonin* has been shown to be present in endocrine cells (Fetissof *et al.* 1986). In the female, one of the most abundant neuropeptides in the genital tract is *VIP*. VIP-containing nerves innervate vascular and non-vascular smooth muscle, seromucous glands as well as endometrial, cervical, and Fallopian tube epithelium. VIP-containing nerves are present throughout the male genital tract and are concentrated particularly around blood vessels of the erectile tissue of the penis (Fig. 26.104a) (Polak *et al.* 1981). These nerves are markedly depleted in various forms of impotence (Fig. 26.104b) (Gu *et al.* 1984).

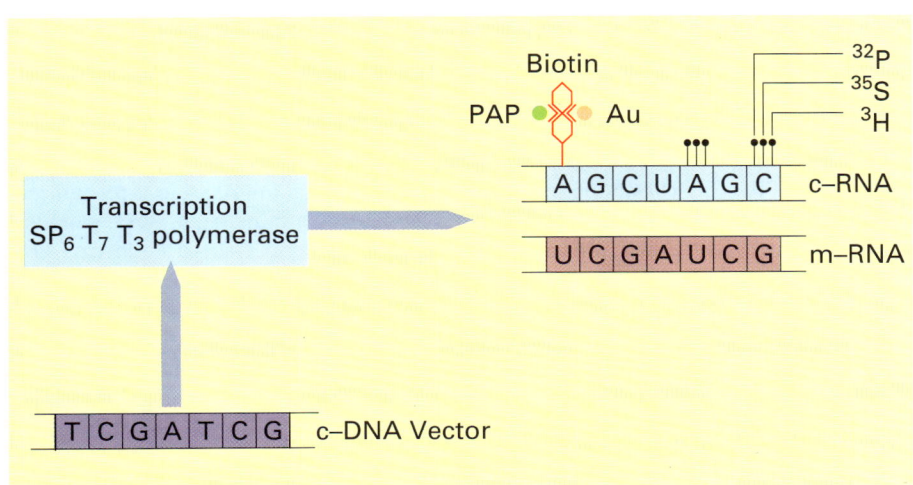

Fig. 26.103 A diagrammatic representation of the production of cRNA probes for *in situ* hybridization showing the various methods that can be used to label the probes.

Table 26.17   Distribution and characteristics of the major regulatory peptides of the genitourinary system

Peptides	Main actions	Main distribution	Origin of nerves
VIP	Vasodilation, smooth muscle relaxation, secretion	Nerve fibres in lamina propria, muscle layers, and close to blood vessels	Pelvic plexus
PHI	Smooth muscle relaxation, secretion	Nerve fibre distribution closely mimics that for VIP	Pelvic plexus
NPY	Vasoconstriction, smooth muscle contraction	Nerve fibres in muscle layers and around blood vessels	Pelvic plexus, inferior mesenteric ganglion, aortico-renal plexus, sympathetic chain
Sub P	Sensory neurotransmission, vasodilation, smooth muscle contraction	Nerve fibres in subepithelial locations and around blood vessels and muscle	Dorsal root ganglia: T_{11}-L_3-hypogastric nerve, L_6-S_1-pelvic nerve
CGRP		Similar to substance P	

VIP, Vasoactive intestinal polypeptide; PHI, peptide histidine isoleucine; NPY, neuropeptide Y; Sub P, substance P; CGRP, calcitonin gene-related peptide.

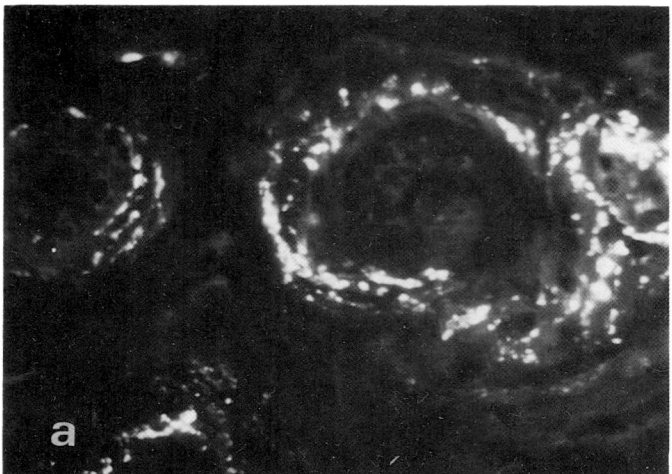 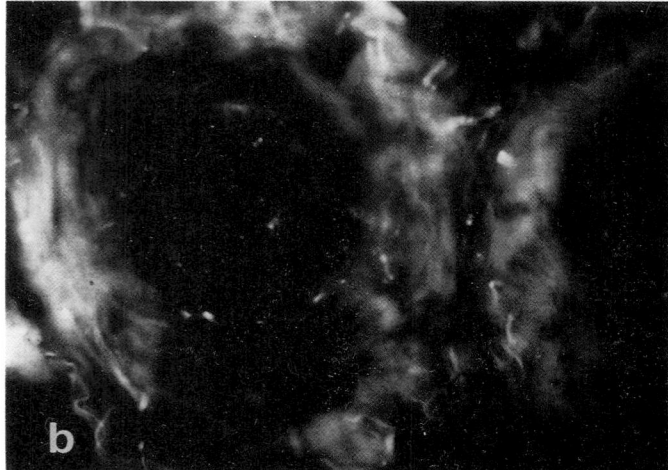

Fig. 26.104   Sections of human penis immunostained for VIP. (a) Numerous immunoreactive nerve fibres can be seen surrounding blood vessels in normal penis. (b) A penile biopsy from a diabetic patient with impotence. Extensive fibrosis can be seen with a lack of VIP-immunoreactive nerve fibres. Benzoquinone-fixed tissue, immunofluorescence method.

26.8.5   Urinary system

Like the genital tract, the urinary system contains a variety of neuropeptides and scattered epithelial serotonin-containing endocrine cells (Table 26.17). VIP is one of the most abundantly found neuropeptides, particularly in humans (Polak and Bloom 1984). The bladder is richly innervated by VIP-containing nerves present in the smooth muscle, lamina propria, and beneath the epithelium. Local cell bodies can be found, albeit scattered in the wall of the bladder. VIP exerts potent muscle relaxant properties and is markedly depleted in patients with unstable bladders (Gu *et al.* 1983*a*). The ureter, in particular that of rat and guinea-pig, is richly innervated by CGRP- and substance P-containing nerve fibres whose cell bodies originate from primary sensory neurones located in the dorsal root ganglion. The network of nerves innervating the urinary system and their links with the spinal cord can be mapped by the use of *retrograde tracing methods combined with immunocytochemistry* (Fig. 26.105) (Su *et al.* 1986).

26.8.6   Skin

The endocrine cell type of human and animal skin is recognized as the *Merkel cell* and possibly contains regulatory peptides (Table 26.18). The Merkel cell is a specialized endocrine cell with putative pressor receptor functions and is found in certain areas of the skin in the basal epidermis. Ultrastructurally, the cell contains neurosecretory granules. Numerous nerve terminals can be distinguished, at both the light and electron microscopical levels, in close opposition to Merkel cells and, although these cells can be stained by the so-called 'general neuro-endocrine markers' (Fig. 26.106), the presence of peptides in Merkel cells remains controversial. Merkel cell tumours

Table 26.18 Distribution and characteristics of the major regulatory peptides of the skin

Peptides	Species	Actions	Distribution	Coexistence
CGRP	Most species	Sensory, vasodilation—potently causes long-lasting flare	Intra- and sub-epithelial nerves, smooth muscle, touch receptors, hair follicles, blood vessels	? SP
SP/NKA	Most species	Sensory, vasodilation—wheal flare	As for CGRP but also around sweat glands	? CGRP
VIP/PHI (M)	Most species	Autonomic and sensory, vasodilation—wheal and flare, secretomotion	Free nerve endings—dermis, epidermis, blood vessels, sweat glands	? Cholinergic
NPY	Most species	Autonomic, vasoconstriction, sensory and autonomic	Blood vessels, sweat glands, subepidermal nerves, touch receptors	? Catecholamines

CGRP, Calcitonin gene-related peptide; SP, substance P; NKA, neurokinin A; VIP, vasoactive intestinal polypeptide; PHI (M), peptide histidine isoleucine (methionine); NPY, neuropeptide Y.

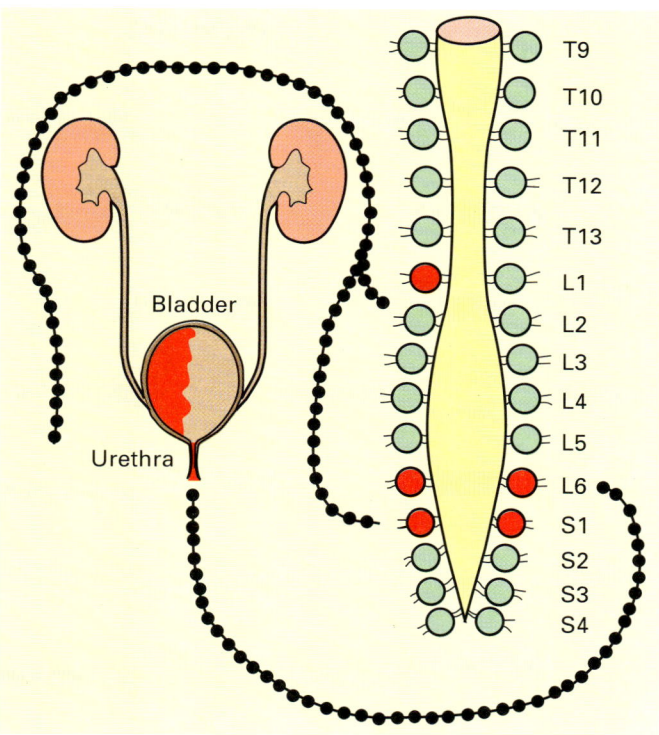

Fig. 26.105 Diagram showing the origin in dorsal root ganglia of the CGRP-immunoreactive innervation of the rat urinary tract obtained by the use of combined retrograde tracing and immunocytochemistry.

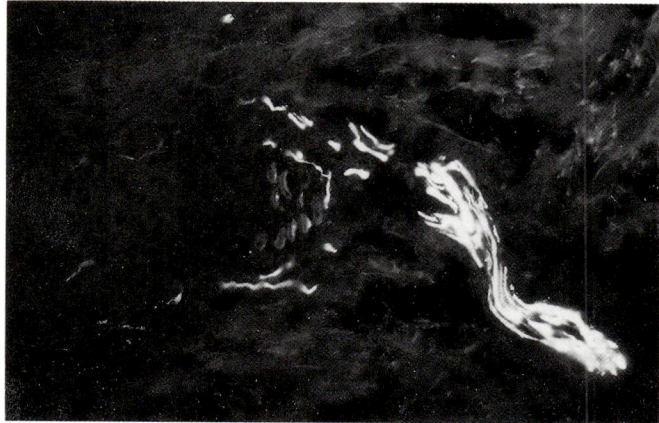

Fig. 26.106 Human nose skin immunostained with antiserum to neurofilaments, showing a Merkel disc with associated nerves. Benzoquinone-fixed tissue, immunofluorescence method.

(Gu *et al.* 1983*b*), one of the types of neuro-endocrine tumours found in the skin, can be immunostained and thereby characterized using antibodies to the so-called 'general neuro-endocrine' markers. Neuropeptides have been found to be abnormal in skin diseases, including eczema, 'painful' skin, psoriasis, and leprosy. The entire innervation of the skin can be demonstrated by the use of antibodies to *protein gene product 9.5*, (PGP) *neurofilament triplet proteins*, or *neurone-specific enolase*.

26.8.7 Bibliography

Cadieux, A., *et al.* (1986). Occurrence, distribution and ontogeny of CGRP immunoreactivity in the rat lower respiratory tract: effect of capsaicin treatment and surgical denervations. *Neuroscience* **19**, 605–27.

Creutzfeldt, W., Gregory, R. A., Grossman, M. I., and Pearse, A. G. E. (eds) (1970). *Origin, chemistry, physiology and pathophysiology of the gastrointestinal hormones.* F. K. Schattauer Verlag, Stuttgart.

Cuttitta, F., Carney, D. N., Mulshine, J., Moody, T. W., Fedorko, J., Fischler, A., and Minna, J. D. (1985). Bombesin-like peptides can function as autocrine growth factors in human small-cell lung cancer. *Nature* **316**, 823–6.

Fetissof, F., Dubois, M. P., Heitz, P. U., Lansac, J., Arbeille-Brassart, B., and Jobard, P. (1986). Endocrine cells in the female genital tract. *International Journal of Gynecological Pathology* **5**, 75–87.

Ghatei, M. A., Sheppard, M. N., Henzen-Logman, S., Blank, M. A., Polak, J. M., and Bloom, S. R. (1983). Bombesin and VIP in the developing lung: marked changes in acute respiratory distress syndrome. *Journal of Clinical Endocrinology and Metabolism* **57**, 1226–32.

Gu, J., *et al.* (1983*a*). Vasoactive intestinal polypeptide in the normal and unstable bladder. *British Journal of Urology* **55**, 645–7.

Gu, J., Polak, J. M., Van Noorden, S., Pearse, A. G. E., Marangos, P. J., and Azzopardi, J. G. (1983*b*). Immunostaining of neuron-specific enolase as a diagnostic tool for Merkel cell tumours. *Cancer* **52**, 1039–43.

Gu, J., *et al.* (1984). Decrease of vasoactive intestinal polypeptide (VIP) in the penises from impotent men. *Lancet* **ii**, 315–18.

Hamid, Q. A., *et al.* (1987*a*). Expression of the C-terminal peptide of human pro-bombesin in 361 lung endocrine tumours, a reliable marker and possible prognostic indicator for small cell carcinoma. *Virchows Archiv A—Pathological Anatomy and Histopathology* **411**, 185–92.

Hamid, Q., *et al.* (1987*b*). Localization of atrial natriuretic peptide mRNA and immunoreactivity in the rat heart and human atrial appendage. *Proceedings of the National Academy of Sciences, USA* **84**, 6760–4.

Kurian, S. S., *et al.* (1983). Vasoactive intestinal polypeptide (VIP) in vasomotor rhinitis. *IRCS Medical Science* **II**, 425–6.

Lackie, P. M., Cuttitta, F., Minna, J. D., Bloom, S. R., and Polak, J. M. (1985). Localisation of receptors using a dimeric ligand and electron immunocytochemistry. *Histochemistry* **83**, 57–9.

Polak, J. M. and Bloom, S. R. (1984). Localisation and measurement of VIP in the genitourinary system of man and animals. *Peptides* **5**, 225–30.

Polak, J. M. and Bloom, S. R. (1986). Regulatory peptides of the gastro-intestinal and respiratory tracts. *Archives Internationales de Pharmacodynamie* **280**, 16–49.

Polak, J. M., Gu, J., Mina, S., and Bloom, S. R. (1981). VIPergic nerves in the penis. *Lancet* **ii**, 217–19.

Power, R. F., *et al.* (1987). Anatomical distribution of VIP binding sites in peripheral tissues investigated *in vitro* autoradiography. *Annals of the New York Academy of Sciences*, **527**, 314–25.

Ratzenhofer, M., Höfler, H., and Walter, G. F. (eds) (1984). Frontiers of hormone research. In *Interdisciplinary neuroendocrinology*, Vol. 12. S. Karger, Basel.

Springall, D. R., Ibrahim, N. B. N., Rode, J., Sharpe, M. S., Bloom, S. R., and Polak, J. M. (1986). Endocrine differentiation of extra-pulmonary small cell carcinoma demonstrated by immunohistochemistry using antibodies to PGP 9.5, neuron-specific enolase and the C-flanking peptide of human pro-bombesin. *Journal of Pathology* **150**, 151–62.

Springall, D. R., Collina, G., Barer, G., Suggett, A. J., Bee, D., and Polak, J. M. (1987). Increased intracellular levels of calcitonin gene-related peptide-like immunoreactivity in pulmonary cells of hypoxic rats. *Journal of Pathology* **151**, 33–4A.

Su, H. C., *et al.* (1986). Calcitonin gene-related peptide immunoreactivity in afferent neurons supplying the urinary tract: Combined retrograde tracing and immunohistochemistry. *Neuroscience* **18**, 727–47.

Wharton, J. and Gulbenkian, S. (1987). Peptides in the mammalian cardiovascular system. *Experientia* **43**, 821–32.

27

The locomotor system

Locomotor system

27.1 Bone

N. A. Athanasou and C. G. Woods

27.1.1 Normal structure and function

A knowledge of the normal structure and function of bone is essential for an understanding of the pathological changes that can occur in bone.

Gross organization of a long bone

The gross structure and regions of a long bone are illustrated in Fig. 27.1. Bone is anatomically composed of a periosteum, cortex, and medulla. The periosteum consists of a thick adherent fibrous membrane covering the outer surface of the bone. The cortex is the thick outer sheath of hard compact bone. The medulla (marrow cavity) is the inner central part of the bone and consists of numerous thin cancellous (spongy) bone trabeculae which surround haemopoietic marrow and adipose tissue. The regions described in a long bone are:

1. Diaphysis or bony shaft;
2. Epiphysis, the expanded end of a long bone which includes the articular surface;
3. Metaphysis, the junctional zone between the epiphysis and the shaft;

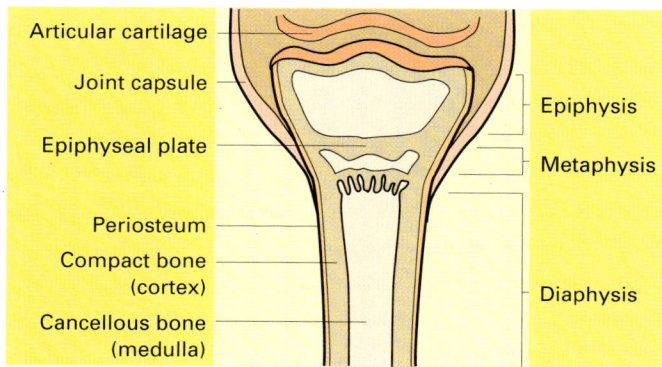

Fig. 27.1 Schematic diagram of the main compartments and structures in a long bone.

Labels in figure:
Articular cartilage
Joint capsule
Epiphyseal plate
Periosteum
Compact bone (cortex)
Cancellous bone (medulla)
Epiphysis
Metaphysis
Diaphysis

4. Epiphyseal plate, a cartilaginous line that separates the epiphysis from the metaphysis; this is the zone of endochondral ossification in actively growing bone.

Microscopic structure of bone

Bone exists in two main forms in the human skeleton: lamellar bone and woven bone.

In the mature skeleton, both compact and cancellous bone is of the lamellar type, i.e. the osteoid contains collagen fibres which are arranged in parallel sheets or lamellae. Collagen fibres in each of these sheets lie parallel to each other but their orientation differs from that of collagen fibres in adjacent lamellae; this is best seen by polarization microscopy (Fig. 27.2a). In cortical bone, the lamellae are concentrically arranged around a central channel containing blood and lymphatic vessels and nerves. These cylindrical columns (Haversian systems or osteons) are oriented in the long axis of the bone. Spaces between individual osteons are filled with iregularly arranged interstitial lamellae. In addition, several parallel non-Haversian circumferential lamellae of dense compact bone are found at the periosteal and, less regularly, at the endosteal surface. Cancellous bone is also composed of non-Haversian lamellar bone separated by cement lines. Cement lines, which are also present in cortical bone, are found where there is a discontinuity or change in orientation of the collagen lamellae.

Woven (or immature) bone is the type of bone found in the developing skeleton, fracture callus, and a variety of pathological bone conditions where there is rapid bone formation. It is characterized by random orientation of the collagen fibres and a matrix rich in ground substance (Fig. 27.2b). The cells in woven bone are larger and more closely packed than in lamellar bone (Fig. 27.3a). Woven bone is mechanically weaker than lamellar bone and is usually replaced by the latter in the normal skeleton.

Bone cells

Three main types of cell are found in bone: osteoblasts, osteocytes, and osteoclasts (Fig. 27.3).

Osteoblasts

These are mononuclear cells which line the external surfaces of bone trabeculae (the endosteum), the inner layer of the periosteum and the surface of bone lining Haversian canals (Fig. 27.3b). They are derived from the marrow stromal cell

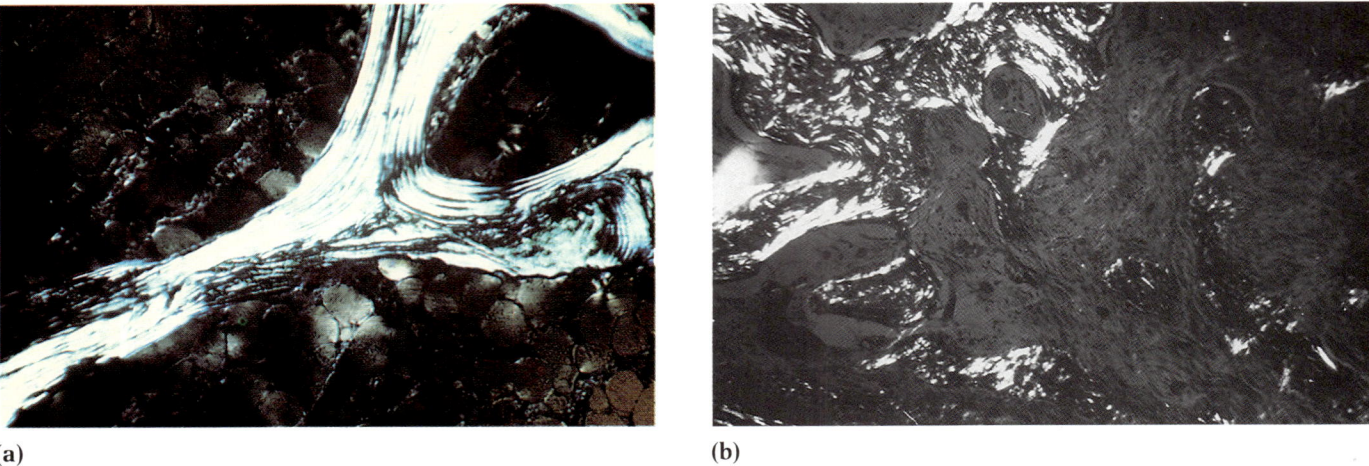

(a)   **(b)**

Fig. 27.2 (a) Lamellar bone trabeculae viewed by polarization microscopy. Parallel arrangement of collagen fibres. (b) Woven bone trabeculae viewed by polarization microscopy. Random orientation of short collagen fibres.

system and are responsible for producing collagen and other proteins that make up the organic bone matrix. They are also implicated in the deposition and exchange of calcium and other ions. In areas of active bone formation, osteoblasts form a continuous layer of plump cells with polygonal outline, basophilic and pyroninophilic cytoplasm, and a large ovoid nucleus. In areas of mature or resting bone, they appear as a layer of flattened elongated 'lining cells' with little cytoplasm and a central basophilic nucleus. Osteoblasts display alkaline phosphatase and phosphorylase activity.

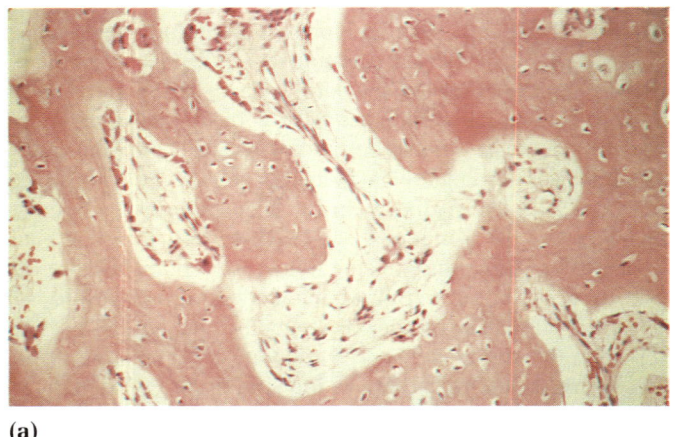

(a)

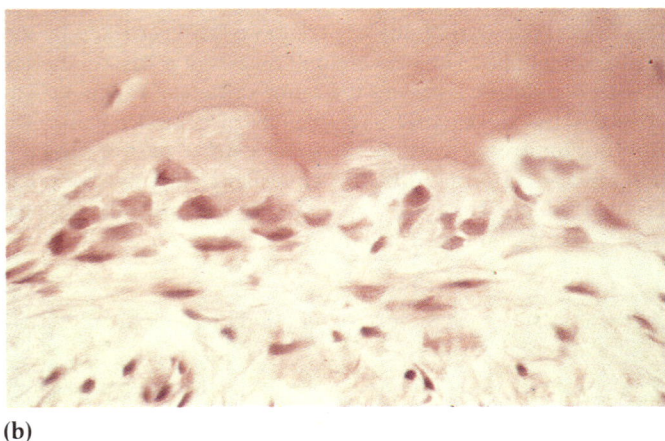

(b)

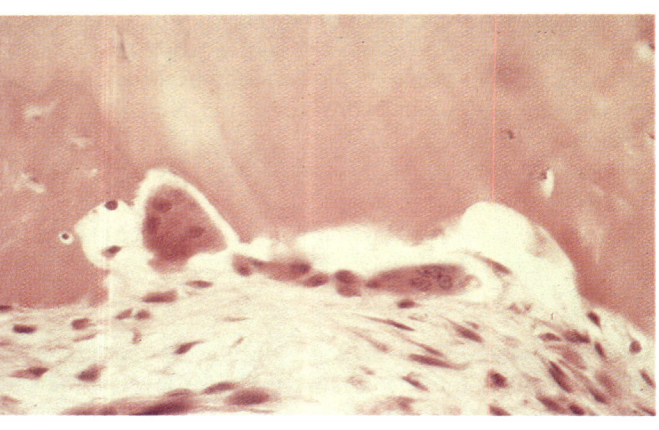

(c)

Fig. 27.3 (a) Woven bone with mononuclear osteoblasts lining bone trabeculae, multinucleated osteoclasts, and numerous osteocytes in lacunae. (b) Osteoblasts forming a thin layer of pale-staining osteoid over a bone trabecula. (c) Multinucleated osteoclasts lying in Howship's lacunae.

Osteocytes

When osteoblasts become entrapped within forming bone, they stop secreting bone matrix and lose many of their protein-synthesizing organelles. They are now called osteocytes (Fig. 27.3a) and lie in lacunae completely surrounded by bone, but they retain continuity with each other and the exterior by means of fine protoplasmic processes which lie in hollow channels called canaliculi. The function of the osteocyte is uncertain but is most likely concerned with preservation of the bone matrix and maintenance of its mineral content.

Osteoclasts

These are multinucleate cells which are responsible for bone resorption. They are uncommonly seen in normal mature bone but are prominent in areas of active bone resorption where they lie in depressions on the bone surface called resorption or Howship's lacunae (Fig. 27.3c). They have abundant pale-staining cytoplasm, which is strongly acid-phosphatase positive, and a variable number of round or oval nuclei, each of which contains little chromatin and a prominent nucleolus. Osteoclasts are formed by fusion of mononuclear precursors which are derived from the haemopoietic stem cell and are most likely members of the mononuclear phagocyte system.

Bone matrix

Bone differs from other connective tissues (except dentine) in that, in addition to an organic extracellular matrix or osteoid, it contains a mineral matrix of calcium salt. This is largely in the form of hydroxyapatites and is deposited on the organic matrix of bone. This provides bone with structural rigidity and is the major store of body calcium. The mechanisms underlying bone mineralization are poorly understood. There are sufficient amounts of calcium and phosphorus in the extracellular fluid of bone to initiate and maintain bone mineralization. This may be prevented by the action of naturally occurring inhibitors, such as pyrophosphate. Osteoblasts could control mineralization by the production of an alkaline phosphatase and a pyrophosphatase which may locally remove pyrophosphate. These enzymes have been found in membrane-bound matrix vesicles which are present in mineralizing bone and cartilage.

Collagen forms 90 per cent of the organic matrix of bone. The collagen molecule is a triple-stranded polymer of three polypeptide α-chains (see Chapter 1). At least 10 genetically different collagens have been described. Bone collagen is largely type I and is produced by the osteoblast. The synthesis of each type of α-chain of collagen is controlled by specific genes with different chromosomal locations. Several important post-translational modification steps follow and the large precursor molecule is secreted from the osteoblasts. This procollagen molecule is modified before molecular self-assembly and formation of the collagen fibre. Mineralization commences in areas between the collagen molecules. Both inherited (e.g. osteogenesis imperfecta) and acquired (e.g. scurvy) disorders of bone may result from defects in collagen synthesis.

There are numerous other non-collagenous proteins in bone, such as osteocalcin (bone Gla protein), matrix Gla protein, osteonectin, bone morphogenic protein, bone sialoproteins (including osteopontin), and bone proteoglycans. Bone matrix also contains phosphoproteins, lipids, and bone-derived growth factors. The proteoglycans are large branching molecules with a protein core and polysaccharide side-chains; they are of less structural importance than collagen but may affect its synthesis and fibre formation. In the mucopolysaccharidoses, inherited enzyme defects lead to accumulation of incompletely degraded proteoglycans and consequent skeletal abnormalities.

Bone development, growth, and remodelling

In the fetus, bone development involves ossification of pre-existing connective tissue, either by the process of intramembranous or endochondral ossification. Most bones are, in fact, composite structures formed partly by intramembranous or endochondral ossification. These processes result in the formation of a woven type of bone which is then remodelled by osteoclastic resorption and appositional growth to form the lamellar bone of the mature skeleton.

Intramembranous ossification

This is seen in the development of the calvarium and the clavicle and is the process whereby bone is directly formed from primitive mesenchymal connective tissue. In centres of ossification, mesenchymal cells proliferate and differentiate into osteoblasts which synthesize and secrete osteoid that is rapidly mineralized (Fig. 27.4a). Each centre of ossification enlarges and fuses with adjacent centres to form ultimately a continuous mass of woven bone.

Endochondral ossification

This process is seen in the development of the tubular long bones, vertebrae, pelvis, and bones of the base of the skull. It involves progressive ossification of a continuously enlarging cartilage model and is the process whereby most bones grow in length. Endochondral ossification is seen initially in the diaphyseal primary ossification centre but later becomes localized to the epiphyseal growth plate. In this process, the cartilage cells essentially undergo a sequence of changes including proliferation, growth, hypertrophy, and degeneration (Fig. 27.4b). The cell walls of the degenerate hypertrophic chondrocytes and the surrounding matrix become calcified and the resultant lacunae of calcified matrix are invaded by capillaries from the marrow cavity and remodelled by osteoblasts and osteoclasts. The osteoblasts lay down osteoid on the spicules of calcified cartilage matrix. This is rapidly mineralized to form the immature bone found in the metaphysis, and is termed the primary spongiosa. This is selectively resorbed by osteoclasts. A lamellar type of bone is laid down in its place (the secondary spongiosa) and this extends into the diaphysis of the bone. Endochondral ossification is not seen in the normal mature skeleton but may be seen in pathological conditions such as tumours of cartilage-forming cells, fracture repair, or osteoarthrosis.

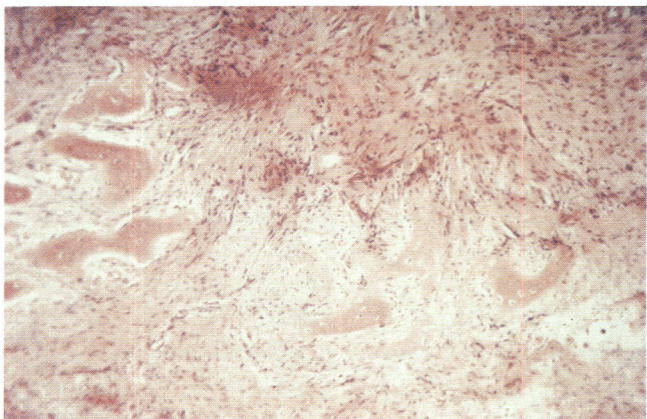

(a)

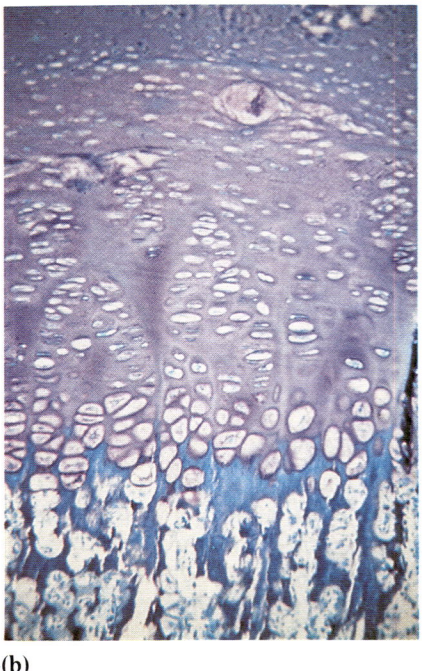

(b)

Fig. 27.4 (a) Intramembranous ossification. Irregular bone trabeculae are formed directly from cellular fibrous tissue. (b) Endochondral ossification in growth plate.

Appositional bone growth

This is the deposition of bone matrix by osteoblasts on pre-existing bone (either of woven or lamellar type) and its subsequent mineralization. It is seen as part of endochondral and intramembranous ossification and is the means by which new bone is formed in the normal continuous turnover of bone in the mature skeleton. During the growth period, enlargement of the diameter of the shaft of a long bone occurs by appositional growth at the periosteal surface with production of lamellar bone which has a predominantly circumferential arrangement. These circumferential lamellae are removed at a later stage and replaced by Haversian bone. Interstitial lamellar bone is composed partly of residual circumferential lamellar bone.

Remodelling occurs continually throughout life and all bones in the body are in a dynamic state of formation and resorption in response to constantly changing mechanical stresses and the demands of mineral homeostasis. The anatomical basis for this activity has been termed the bone multicellular unit (BMU), wherein there is coupling of bone resorption and formation. In each BMU, remodelling is initiated by osteoclastic bone resorption; this is followed by a phase of reversal and osteoblastic bone formation in the same location. Several coupling factors are thought to link bone resorption and formation and it has been shown that several known stimulators of bone resorption do not act directly on osteoclasts but on osteoblasts which, in turn, may control osteoclast function.

Physiological control of bone composition

The factors controlling bone composition are not completely understood. They are related to overall calcium and phosphorus metabolism and include not only systemic hormones and vitamins, e.g. vitamin D, vitamin C, parathyroid hormone (PTH), and calcitonin, but also locally acting substances, such as growth factors and prostaglandins.

Vitamin D

Although vitamin D is known to be an important factor in the prevention of rickets, it is best regarded as a hormone rather than a vitamin (i.e. an essential dietary requirement). Only a small amount of the natural form of vitamin D, vitamin D_3 (cholecalciferol) comes from dietary sources such as fish, liver oils, and dairy products. Most vitamin D_3 is, in fact, produced in the skin by the action of ultraviolet light on the precursor 7-dehydrocholesterol. A synthetic form, vitamin D_2 (ergocalciferol) is prepared artificially by the ultraviolet radiation of ergosterol, a plant sterol; vitamin D_2 is added to foods and is the form used in treatment.

Both vitamin D_2 and vitamin D_3 undergo a 25 hydroxylation in the liver. 25 hydroxy-vitamin D_3 ($25(OH)D_3$) is the major circulating metabolite of vitamin D_3, and its plasma concentration closely reflects the vitamin D status of a patient. The next step occurs in the kidney where there is further specific hydroxylation of $25(OH)D_3$ to either $1,25(OH)_2D_3$ or $24,25(OH)_2D_3$. $1,25(OH)_2D_3$ is the most active metabolite of vitamin D, and its production is stimulated by low calcium concentration and suppressed by high calcium concentration. The activity of the renal 1 α-hydroxylase is also affected by plasma phosphate, parathyroid hormone, calcitonin, oestrogen, prolactin, and somatomedins. The production of $1,25(OH)_2D_3$ is closely controlled by a negative feedback system. PTH stimulates 1 α-hydroxylation of $25(OH)D_3$ to $1,25(OH)_2D_3$. As more $1,25(OH)_2D_3$ is synthesized, it raises plasma calcium which, in turn, reduces secretion of PTH. This effectively removes the stimulus for further $1,25(OH)_2D_3$ production.

Vitamin D_3 increases plasma calcium mainly by increasing calcium absorption across the small intestine and stimulating bone resorption. Vitamin D_3 promotes mineralization of bone but its mechanism of action is uncertain. It is suspected that this is due to the direct effect of vitamin D_3 metabolites rather than an indirect consequence of increasing the concentration of calcium in the extracellular fluid by its effect on intestinal calcium absorption and bone resorption. Receptors for vitamin D_3 are not confined to intestine and bone but have been found in a large number of other organs and cells. Macrophages express the vitamin D_3 receptor protein and are also capable of 1 α-hydroxylation of $25(OH)D_3$. This may be associated with an autocrine effect on macrophage function and could account for the hypercalcaemia seen in sarcoidosis. $1,25(OH)_2D_3$ also has a role in controlling cellular proliferation and differentiation, including that of myeloid cell lines amongst which the osteoclast can be included. The involvement of vitamin D_3 in so many important and diverse cellular processes suggests that it has a fundamental role in cellular metabolism, possibly the regulation of intracellular calcium.

Parathyroid hormone (PTH)

PTH, secreted by the parathyroid glands, is a single-chain, 84 amino-acid hormone produced from a large precursor molecule. Specific cleavage of PTH between residues 33 and 34 occurs mainly in the liver to produce two major circulating fragments: an amino-terminal, biologically active portion with a short half-life, and a carboxy-terminal portion which is biologically inactive and has a long half-life.

Secretion of PTH is mainly in response to a fall in the plasma calcium concentration, particularly the ionized fraction of blood calcium. Other factors, such as plasma magnesium concentration, prostaglandins, catecholamines, and vitamin D metabolites, also influence PTH secretion. The overall effects of PTH are to raise plasma calcium and increase phosphate excretion. This is achieved by its action on the kidneys, the intestine, and bone. The main renal effects of PTH are an increase in the renal tubular reabsorption of calcium and an increase in phosphate excretion. PTH also stimulates the renal 1 α-hydroxylase to produce $1,25(OH)_2D$, the active metabolite of vitamin D. This effect on vitamin D metabolism partly accounts for the PTH stimulation of calcium absorption by the small intestine and its effect on bone resorption. In vitro, PTH also directly inhibits osteoblast synthesis of collagen and other matrix proteins, and stimulates osteoclastic bone resorption. PTH and vitamin D_3 do not stimulate osteoclasts directly but acts indirectly via osteoblast mediation.

PTH-related peptide This has been discovered recently. It is secreted by some neoplastic cells and is a 177 amino-acid protein with an amino-terminal sequence very similar to human PTH. PTH-related peptide mobilizes calcium from bone both in vitro and in vivo and is likely to be an important factor in the production of the humoral hypercalcaemia of malignancy.

Calcitonin

Calcitonin (thyrocalcitonin) is a calcium-lowering hormone produced by the parafollicular (C-cells) of the thyroid. It is a short (32 amino-acid) polypeptide which acts in many ways as the physiological antagonist of PTH. Its secretion is stimulated by a rise in plasma calcium and it acts to lower plasma calcium and phosphate. It acts directly on osteoclasts to reduce bone resorption and increases renal calcium (and phosphate) clearance by the kidney. It also has a number of non-skeletal effects, including those on sodium metabolism. The importance of calcitonin in the control of calcium and phosphate metabolism in the normal individual is unclear as neither calcitonin excess (e.g. medullary carcinoma of the thyroid) nor calcitonin deficiency alone produces an effect on blood calcium or phosphate. Calcitonin secretion is increased at times of physiological stress, such as growth and pregnancy, and is decreased in post-menopausal women. Calcitonin is particularly effective as a therapeutic agent in the suppression of osteoclastic bone resorption in conditions associated with rapid bone turnover, e.g. Paget disease. Katacalcin and calcitonin-gene-related peptide are also products of the gene that produces calcitonin; their precise function and importance in bone physiology is uncertain.

Other endocrine hormones and vitamins

The hormones secreted by other endocrine organs also affect bone growth and composition.

Growth hormone This promotes long bone and cartilage growth through the mediation of somatomedin which is synthesized in liver. Somatomedin stimulates the incorporation of amino acids into mucoproteins of cartilage and promotes RNA and DNA synthesis. Amongst other changes, growth hormone excess results in overgrowth of long bones before epiphyseal closure in childhood (gigantism), and in periosteal new bone formation with enlargement of the acral parts of the skeleton in adults (acromegaly).

Thyroid hormone This accelerates bone turnover and is important in skeletal maturation. Hyperthyroidism results in excessive bone resorption compared with bone formation and is a cause of osteoporosis. It can also reduce intestinal absorption of calcium and increase urinary excretion of calcium, leading to a negative calcium balance. A deficiency of thyroid hormone retards skeletal growth and development, particularly in infancy and early childhood (cretinism).

Adrenal corticosteroids These inhibit the formation and activity of osteoblasts and are associated with increased osteoclastic bone resorption. In conditions of corticosteroid excess osteoporosis can be severe.

Androgens These accelerate growth and somatic development, including skeletal maturation. Whether androgens act directly on bone cells to exert this effect is uncertain. Excessive androgen secretion is associated with rapid growth but premature closure of the epiphysis. Male hypogonadism, however, is associated with osteoporosis.

Oestrogens These have been shown to prevent PTH-mediated bone resorption and to stimulate renal 1 α-hydroxylase activity. However, the precise biological effect of oestrogens on bone composition is unknown and their mechanistic relevance to post-menopausal osteoporosis is uncertain.

Insulin This is also necessary for normal skeletal growth and bone composition and diabetes mellitus is associated with osteoporosis.

Vitamin C Ascorbic acid is essential for the maintenance of the integrity of all connective tissues, including bone. It is a necessary cofactor for the hydroxylation of proline and lysine in collagen synthesis, and is also important in the synthesis of matrix glycosaminoglycans. Deficiency of vitamin C results in impaired formation of the organic bone matrix, with disturbances of endochondral growth and abnormal bone repair due to the failure of osteoblasts to lay down osteoid. In addition, formation of defective intercellular cement substance results in weakening of capillary walls, with consequent haemorrhage.

Vitamin A This stimulates osteoclastic bone resorption and has an effect on epiphyseal cartilage growth *in vitro*. *In vivo* hypervitaminosis A is associated with hypercalcaemia, excessive bone resorption, and periosteal calcification.

Local regulatory factors

A number of local factors influence bone cell function and bone composition. These include not only physical factors, such as mechanical stress or pressure, but also paracrine or autocrine factors produced and secreted by cells in bone. Of these, the cytokines, growth factors, and prostaglandins are best known.

Cytokines These are short-range soluble mediators which are important in cell-to-cell communication. Osteoclast activating factor (OAF) was the first cytokine identified to affect bone cell function. OAF is produced by myeloma and other cell lines. It stimulates bone resorption and inhibits collagen synthesis *in vitro*. Recently, OAF was purified and found to be identical to the macrophage-derived cytokine, interleukin-1 (IL-1). It is likely that IL-1 and related cytokines, tumour necrosis factor-α (TNF-α) and TNF-β, are important factors in the bone destruction and hypercalcaemia associated with malignant haematological neoplasms and solid tumours. With other cytokines, e.g. γ-interferon, which inhibits osteoclastic bone resorption, TNF, IL-1, and transforming growth factor may also have a role in normal bone remodelling and bone resorption associated with age and inflammation.

Growth factors These are glycoproteins that have the ability to stimulate either progenitor (colony-stimulating factors) or normal cells (transforming growth factors) to form colonies *in vitro*. Transforming growth factor-β (TGF-β) induces cartilage formation and stimulates bone resorption *in vitro*. TGF-α, which is synthesized and secreted by a variety of tumour cells, increases the production of osteoclast progenitors in the bone marrow and also stimulates osteoclastic bone resorption. TGF-α and β have both been implicated in tumour osteolysis and the humoral hypercalcaemia of malignancy. Other bone-derived growth factors have also been identified but their precise significance is not yet understood.

Prostaglandins These are a widely distributed family of local hormones of 20-carbon fatty acid structure, which act near their tissue or cell of production. Several prostaglandins are produced in bone. Prostaglandins of the E series are particularly associated with bone resorption and their production is affected by mechanical stress, pressure changes, and electric fields. They have been implicated in the bone resorption seen with inflammation and the osteolysis and hypercalcaemia of malignancy. Both prostaglandins and cytokines have been postulated as coupling factors, linking bone resorption and formation.

27.1.2 Abnormal development of the skeleton

Skeletal development is dependent upon the formation of growth cartilage and subsequent endochondral ossification, the activity of osteoblasts and osteoclasts, the development of extraosseous connective tissues, and the composition of extracellular fluid. There are, therefore, a large number of abnormalities which lead to maldevelopment of the skeleton. Some of these are tabulated in Table 27.1. Those disorders in which the skeletal abnormality is but part of the overall effect are discussed in other chapters. Some are considered more appropriately in later sections of this chapter.

Osteochondrodysplasias

These heritable disorders of skeletal connective tissue form a heterogeneous group composed of a large number (80 or more) of apparently distinct conditions identified by radiographic, clinical, and genetic characteristics. With increasing information the terminology has changed over the years.

Reports of the microscopic appearances in the growth plates of chondrodysplasia have been reasonably consistent in some of the named conditions, but have been conflicting in others. This is, to some extent, due to the different degrees of severity of the abnormality in the growth plates of an affected individual and even within a single growth plate. Hopefully, identification of the basic molecular biological defect will bring some order to what is a confusing area of pathology.

The most important investigation that a pathologist can arrange when confronted with a case showing evidence of skeletal malformation is a comprehensive radiological survey from vertex to phalanges. Without that evidence, a satisfactory diagnosis may not be possible. The radiographs should dictate the specimens to be removed for histopathological study.

It is not possible to describe here more than a selection of the skeletal dysplasias, and Sillence *et al.* (1979) should be consulted for more information regarding the chondrodysplasias.

Achondroplasia

This is the commonest form of chondrodysplasia. Most of the patients appear to have developed the disease as the result of a new mutation. Family histories indicate that transmission is by

Table 27.1 Some causes of abnormal skeletal development

1. Osteochondrodysplasias
   (a) Disorder primarily in growth cartilage
       (i) general, e.g. achondroplasia
       (ii) local, e.g. enchondroma
   (b) Disorder primarily affecting bone
       (i) general, e.g. osteogenesis imperfecta, osteosclerosis
       (ii) local, e.g. Englemann disease

2. Chromosomal abnormality
   e.g. Turner syndrome

3. Inborn errors of metabolism
   Mucopolysaccharidoses
   Lipidoses
   Cystinosis
   Oxalosis
   Hypophosphatasia?

4. Endocrinological abnormalities
   Growth hormone
   Corticosteroid excess, endogenous or iatrogenic
   Hypothyroidism

5. Secondary metabolic disorders
   Renal disease
   Liver disease
   Diabetes

6. Nutritional disorders
   Coeliac disease
   Malnutrition

7. Familial tall or short stature

8. Extraosseous connective tissue abnormalities
   (a) general, e.g. Marfan, Ehlers–Danlos syndromes
   (b) local, e.g. congenital hip dislocation and club foot

9. Fluorosis

an autosomal dominant trait. It is a condition known for thousands of years; the Ancient Egyptians have left records of the characteristic appearance. The disease can be recognized at birth. There is short limb rhizomelic (proximal segment) dwarfism, normal trunk, large head with bulging forehead and depressed bridge of nose. It is uncommon for the infant to die, unless it has acquired paired abnormal genes from parents both of whom are achondroplastic. The condition does not change significantly as the child develops. There are numerous causes of short-limbed dwarfism and many patients have been thought to be achondroplastic who have some other skeletal abnormality, either primary or secondary.

Contrary to the name of the disorder, the growth plates are generally well organized and undergo endochondral ossification (Fig. 27.5). There may be greater separation of the cell columns by cartilage matrix, and clusters of proliferative zone chondrocytes surrounded by a fibrous matrix with shortening of the related columns. Endochondral ossification appears remarkably little altered. Periosteal bone formation may be increased and partly surround the growth plate. Electron-dense granules and threads within membrane-bound inclusions are described in the chondrocytes. In the homozygous form of the disease there is more obvious abnormality of the growth cartilage hypertrophic zone and of endochondral ossification.

Of the skeletal dysplasias affecting bone formation primarily both osteogenesis imperfecta and osteopetrosis are described here.

Osteogenesis imperfecta (OI; brittle bone syndrome)

This is a rare, genetic disorder of bone collagen synthesis which is manifest principally, but not exclusively, in the effect on bone formation, which is, in essence, failure to produce an adequate amount of mature, lamellar-type bone. The severity of bone formation failure varies widely and the extent to which other collagen-containing tissues, teeth, sclera, skin, ligaments, are affected also differs. Some forms of the disease are inherited as a dominant characteristic and a small proportion show a recessive pattern of transmission. New dominant mutations cause some of the severe lethal cases. Combinations of skeletal abnormality with other manifestations of defective collagen production produce a number of recognizable patterns which have formed the basis for a classification of the syndrome which currently comprises four major categories (see Smith 1986).

Opportunities to examine bone from patients are uncommon; cadaveric tissue from lethal perinatal disease has been more extensively studied. Bone obtained from patients is often taken from sites of fracture and may be mainly reactive bone rather

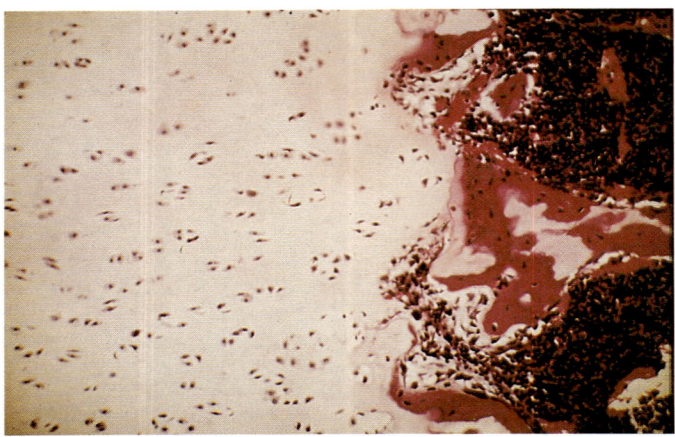

Fig. 27.5 Achondroplasia, growth plate. Poorly organized columns of cells, paucity of hypertrophic cells, and abnormal arrangement of metaphyseal bone.

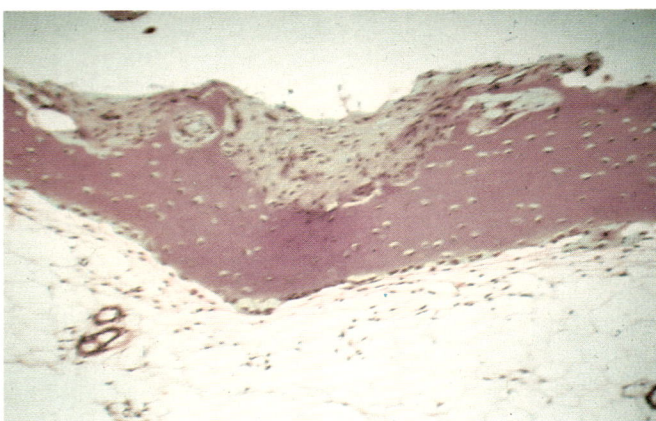

Fig. 27.6 Osteogenesis imperfecta type II. Bone cortex composed of immature bone forming a thin shell without Haversian canals.

than the primarily abnormal tissue. This may lead to confusion of interpretation of the true abnormality.

Studies of biopsies removed from non-traumatized parts of the skeleton indicate that there are differences in the histological abnormalities corresponding to the type of osteogenesis imperfecta.

Type I OI

The lamellar bone is formed and is organized into compact and cancellous structure. There is less bone than normal, i.e. the patient is osteoporotic, and the density of osteocytes per unit area of bone tissue is greater than normal. The latter feature is best appreciated in sections of compact bone. A simplistic interpretation of these findings is that each osteoblast produces less collagen matrix than normal. These findings equate with a disorder that is characterized by a susceptibility to fracture that is not sufficient to be life-threatening and does not lead to either marked deformity of the skeleton nor diminution of stature. The abnormality is transmitted as a dominant trait.

Type II OI

The patient with type II disease has a very restricted ability to form lamellar bone and has a skeleton that is deficient in quantity of bone, mainly of woven type (Fig. 27.6). As a consequence the bone is extremely fragile and multiple fractures are usually present at or shortly after birth. Many affected subjects are stillborn or die shortly after birth. Those who survive into childhood have severe deformities of bones and are, as a result, of short stature. The inheritance pattern of this type of the disorder indicates a recessive gene.

Type III OI

This disease presents, in some of those affected, a distinctive radiographic feature described as 'popcorn bone'. This is due to the formation of spherical masses of cartilage in both the metaphyseal and epiphyseal areas of the bone (Fig. 27.7). In the

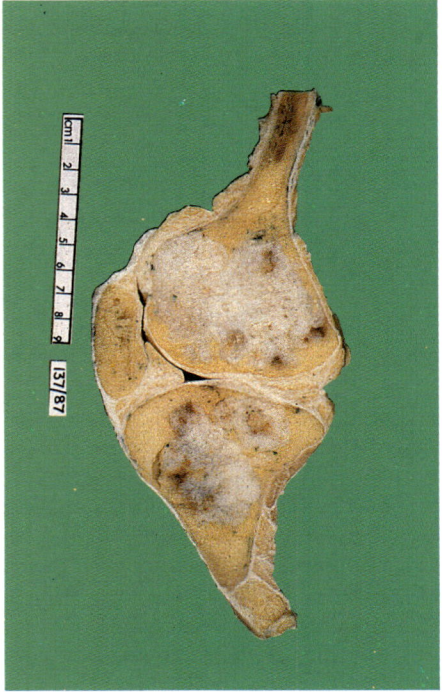

Fig. 27.7 Osteogenesis imperfecta type III. Bisected femur and tibia showing nodular masses of cartilage in epiphyses and metaphyses ('popcorn' bones).

immature skeleton some of these masses are directly continuous with the growth plate and are presumably derived from that structure.

Bones with the popcorn appearance are enlarged in those areas which contain the abnormal cartilage. The mode of formation of the cartilage nodules is unknown: it is unlikely that it is simply a consequence of abnormal structure and fragility of the bone. Bone formation in this type of disease leads to a lamellar-type of tissue but with the persistence of woven bone, and both types can usually be found in any area of the skeleton.

The quantity of bone is markedly reduced. It is inherited as a recessive trait.

Type IV OI

The skeletal tissue in type IV is composed of lamellar bone but appears to have been organized abnormally in that the cement lines are arranged irregularly and there are small segments of bone rather than the long continuous strands of collagenous matrix as in normal bone. This arrangement reduces the mechanical stability and augments the fragility of the bone resulting from the reduced amount of tissue formed. These patients suffer more fractures than the type I patients, have a deformed skeleton, and are of short stature. The associated gene is dominant.

With the possible exception of the bones that show the popcorn change, the cartilage growth plates are inherently normal in osteogenesis imperfecta.

Osteopetrosis (marble bone disease)

This is one of a group of conditions characterized by excessive amounts of mineralized bone, termed the osteoscleroses or sclerosing bone dysplasias. The extent and distribution of skeletal involvement varies within the group. Some appear to be the result of failure of bone resorption and remodelling whereas others are probably the result of increased bone deposition.

Osteopetrosis is a generalized skeletal abnormality in which the major abnormality is a reduction in bone resorption during bone modelling. There are two genetically distinct forms, recessively and dominantly inherited. The former is the more severe.

The severe form causes problems from early infancy resulting from the marked restriction of the medullary cavities by the excessive bone tissue. Bruising and bleeding occur, liver and spleen are enlarged. There is a leucoerythroblastic anaemia and extramedullary haematopoiesis occurs. Neurological complications include blindness, deafness, and facial nerve palsy. Osteomyelitis, notably of the jaw, is common. The bones fracture more easily. Radiographs show the increased mineralized bone, sometimes with a striking 'os-in-os' appearance. Descriptions of the histological appearances vary somewhat, but there is general agreement that there has been failure to resorb bone, although the number of osteoclasts seems normal. This suggests a functional abnormality, an impression supported by the observation that the ruffled borders of the osteoclasts are not so well developed in osteopetrotic bone as in normal bone.

Patients with the mild form of the disease may suffer more fractures than normal, and from neurological problems. As in the severe form, growth may be impaired. The radiographic features are of the same type, but less striking than in the severe form and may be difficult to distinguish from other types of myelosclerosis.

An elevated serum alkaline phosphatase level has been found in all patients in whom it has been estimated, presumably another indication of abnormal function of osteoclasts or their precursor cells.

Hypophosphatasia

In the table of causes of skeletal maldevelopment this condition is tentatively included with the inborn errors of metabolism. The uncertainty arises because the related abnormalities occur only in cartilage and bone, but there is another biochemical abnormality, an increased output of phosphoethanolamine in the urine. Neither the cause, nor the effect of the second abnormality is known.

This is a very rare disease, presumably inherited as a recessive characteristic, with marked variation in severity of clinical expression. The most severe form is apparent in the neonatal period, with undermineralization of the skeleton and apparently widened skull sutures, and symptoms suggesting generalized ill health. Radiographic changes may be mistaken for osteogenesis imperfecta. When the disease becomes apparent in later childhood, there are changes in the growth plates and metaphyses like those of rickets, the limbs are bowed, and growth is retarded. Cranial synostosis may occur.

It is rare for the condition to present in adult life; at that time pathological fracture is the principal problem.

The skeletal changes are due to a failure of mineralization of both growth cartilage and bone and the histological appearances are indistinguishable from those of rickets and osteomalacia. Secondary hyperparathyroidism is not a feature.

Spontaneous fluctuations occur and phases of normal mineralization are interspersed with calcification failure. This may account for the reports of normal serum alkaline phosphatase levels in patients who have phosphoethanolamine in their urine. Hypercalcaemia has also been recorded. Chondrocalcinosis, which may be the result of either hypercalcaemia or abnormal pyrophosphatase activity, is a further problem for some patients.

Fluorosis

Ingestion of fluoride in sufficient quantity and over a prolonged period can produce marked changes in the composition of bone. Naturally occurring high-fluoride-containing drinking water in parts of India, and exposure of workers in aluminium plants to fluoride contamination have resulted in endemic fluorosis. Elderly patients with idiopathic osteoporosis have been treated with fluoride. There is no evidence that fluoridation of water as a prophylactic against dental caries, or the normal use of fluoride-containing toothpaste leads to significant changes in the skeleton.

The effect of fluoride is to promote osteoblastic differentiation and bone formation. Additional bone is laid down in the medullary cavity, on the subperiosteal surface, and at ligamentous insertions. The bones appear more dense in radiographs, may be wider than normal, and have exosteophytes, including bridges of bone between vertebral bodies.

An abnormal bone is formed. The matrix is not of either typical lamellar or woven type but a mixture of both, and mineralization is irregular or, in some areas, fails completely. Mineralization failure is probably due to the formation of fluorapatite crystals which inhibit further crystal deposition at the site. The pattern of tissue deposition is disordered. Osteoclastic activity also increases, particularly in the cortical bone where the endosteal zone becomes cancellized.

A small, but significant proportion of patients with endemic fluorosis have been reported as developing hyperparathyroidism. It is presumed that skeletal calcium is less accessible for homeostasis because of fluorapatite deposition and that the parathyroid overactivity is secondary. Bone cell activity will be additionally stimulated in this situation.

Localized skeletal changes due to soft-tissue abnormalities

Talipes equinovarus

If ligaments or tendons fail to elongate at a normal rate they serve as a 'tether' which inhibits endochondral ossification. In the talipes equinovarus (club foot) deformity, for example, there is retardation of growth of the tarsals, especially on the medial side. When the condition is unilateral, the smaller size of the ossific nuclei on the affected side is easily recognized in radiographs. If the abnormal soft tissues can be effectively detached from the bones, ossification will proceed and the foot may be restored virtually to normal.

Femoral head dislocation

The secondary centre of ossification in the femoral head which is dislocated at birth is also underdeveloped and will revert to normal if the femoral head can be relocated in the acetabulum.

Other causes

Local overgrowth in bone length occurs if there is paralysis of muscle in childhood, and patients with anterior poliomyelitis show this effect. The other well-recognized cause of local bone overgrowth is the presence of a large soft-tissue vascular hamartoma, and in these cases it is assumed that increased blood flow through the metaphysis of the bone increases cartilage cell proliferation and endochondral ossification.

27.1.3 Fracture repair, bone necrosis, and miscellaneous bone conditions

Fracture repair

A fracture is a disruption in the continuity of the bone. It may be caused by a single violent mechanical injury or by repeated injuries or stress (fatigue or stress fracture). A fracture through a bone area weakened by disease is termed a pathological fracture, and may occur after trivial injury or even spontaneously. Causes of pathological fracture are shown in Table 27.2. Fractures may be simple (closed) when there is no communication between the fractured bone and the body surface, or open (compound) when there is a wound of the body surface communicating with the site of fracture. Fractures are also described grossly on the basis of their shape or pattern, e.g. transverse, oblique, spiral, comminuted, crush, greenstick.

The sequence of events following fracture of a previously normal bone begins with disruption of blood vessels in the medulla, cortex, periosteum, and surrounding soft tissues. A haematoma forms between the bone ends and extends beneath the periosteum around the fracture site. Organization and granulation tissue formation follow rapidly with growth of immature fibroblasts and capillaries into the haematoma. The area also shows evidence of traumatic inflammation with early infiltration by polymorphonuclear leucocytes and later by macrophages which remove necrotic bone and marrow debris.

Fracture healing is characterized by the formation of callus; this is a hard mass of repair tissue which unites the bone ends and is composed of new vessels, fibrous tissue, cartilage, and bone. Callus is derived largely from osteoprogenitor cells of the periosteum and endosteum. Although fracture callus describes a single mass of tissue, it is customarily divided into three zones by its location. Internal callus is formed in the original medullary cavity, intermediate callus is adjacent to the ends of cortical bone, and external callus is the hard fusiform swelling on the external surface of the bone.

Formation of external callus begins by the end of the first

Table 27.2 Causes of pathological fracture

1. Inherited and congenital diseases
   Osteogenesis imperfecta
   Osteopetrosis
   Neurofibromatosis
   Gaucher disease
   Enchondromatosis

2. Metabolic bone disease and endocrine disturbances
   Hyperparathyroidism
   Osteoporosis (localized or generalized)
   Osteomalacia
   Vitamin C deficiency
   Cushing disease
   Hyperthyroidism

3. Paget disease

4. Bone infections

5. Tumours and tumour-like conditions of bone—benign and malignant

week with proliferation of cells of the inner layer of the peri-osteum along the entire shaft but especially in the region of the fracture. Here, they form a distinct cuff around the bone ends and show signs of differentiation to bone- or cartilage-producing cells. The osteoblasts lay down osteoid which is later mineralized to form immature woven bone trabeculae. Differen-tiation into chondroblasts and the formation of cartilage is seen where callus develops rapidly and has a poor blood supply (Fig. 27.8). This is particularly evident in the outer, more superficial part of the external callus where the formation of new capillar-ies cannot keep up with the proliferation of osteoprogenitor cells. Mechanical stress, e.g. a poorly immobilized fracture, also favours cartilage formation in the callus. The two enlarging collars of external callus form around each bone end and grow towards each other, finally uniting to form a bridge of woven bone around the fracture site.

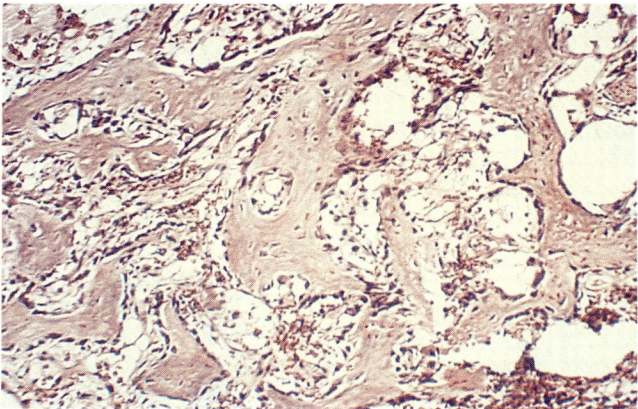

Fig. 27.9 Fracture callus. Interlocking trabeculae of reactive bone in medullary cavity (internal callus).

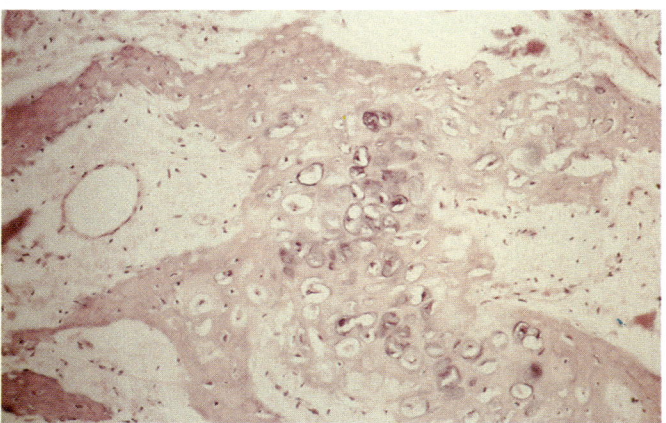

Fig. 27.8 Fracture callus. External callus composed of trabeculae of reactive bone and a central mass of reactive cartilage.

At the same time as subperiosteal proliferation and external callus formation, osteoprogenitor cells covering the endosteal surface of the cortex and medullary trabeculae also proliferate and differentiate into cells that produce internal callus (Fig. 27.9). Cartilage formation is less common in internal cal-lus as the medullary cavity is a more vascular location and less subject to mechanical forces. Osteoblasts lay down osteoid and woven bone in the medullary cavity partly on the surface of necrotic bone trabeculae. Resorption of necrotic bone and tissue debris by osteoclasts and macrophages also continues during this period. The woven bone trabeculae of internal callus de-velop from each bone end and finally bridge the fracture gap in the medullary cavity. Similarly, intermediate callus forms between the fractured cortical bone ends.

The external, intermediate, and internal calluses that are first formed make up what is termed provisional callus. This mass of woven bone unites and stabilizes the fracture, and reaches its maximal size by about the end of the second or third week in an uncomplicated fracture. With progressive ossification and mineralization of new osteoid, the reparative process becomes visible radiographically.

In the subsequent and longest stage of fracture repair, there is active bone remodelling with reconstitution of the strength and normal contour of the bone. Cartilaginous callus becomes mineralized and is replaced by woven bone trabeculae in a pro-cess resembling endochondral ossification. Intramembranous bone formation also occurs. Osteoclasts, which are more prominent at this stage, resorb mineral, dead bone, and un-necessary trabecular bone that formed in the fracture callus. At the same time, new bone trabeculae are laid down in an arrangement largely determined by the stresses and strains to which the callus is subjected. In this way, the woven bone of provisional callus is gradually removed and replaced by lamel-lar bone. The external callus almost entirely disappears and the intermediate callus is slowly converted to compact bone, with its usual osteon structure, and the medullary cavity reforms and contains normal cancellous bone. This process of gradual remodelling occurs relatively slowly over a variable period of time (generally months or years) and is more rapid in children.

Primary union of fracture

Fracture healing, particularly of cortical bone, may occur with-out formation of significant amounts of fracture callus if there is accurate and close apposition of the bone surfaces and rigid fixation of the fracture. This is sometimes described as an ex-ample of fracture repair by primary union. It is more likely, however, that the mechanical factors limit the amount of callus production and that this phenomenon does not differ qualitat-ively from normal fracture repair.

Abnormalities of fracture repair

Several complications may occur if fracture healing does not occur normally. These include a complete failure of union to occur (non-union). This may be associated with the interposi-tion of soft tissue, such as muscle or fascia, between the fractured bone ends, wide separation of the fractured ends, pathological fracture, and lack of immobilization. In non-union, the fragments are united by scar tissue and the bone ends are covered by dense hyaline fibrous tissue which may undergo a metaplastic change to fibrocartilage. An area of fibrinoid necrosis may develop in this cartilage; this may enlarge and develop a lining of synovial cells with production of a false joint or pseudoarthrosis. This is a well-recognized complication of fractures of the tibia.

Delayed union of the fracture may be due to a number of local and general considerations. These include the presence of foreign body material or abundant necrotic bone fragments in the fracture, infection, and inadequate immobilization. A poor blood supply will also delay healing and is a particularly well-recognized sequel of fractures of the femoral neck or carpal scaphoid. Abnormalities of the general nutritional and metabolic status of the patient, including hypoproteinaemia, vitamin D and vitamin C deficiencies, may also delay fracture healing.

Avascular necrosis of bone

Bone necrosis may occur as part of a number of disease processes, not all of which are primarily vascular in origin (Table 27.3).

In adults, trauma, in particular fracture of the femoral neck or dislocation of the femoral head, with consequent interruption of the blood supply, is the most common cause of avascular necrosis and infarction. There are numerous other non-traumatic conditions associated with bone necrosis and these, too, most commonly affect the femoral head, although other bones, especially long bones, may be affected. The mechanism whereby osteonecrosis is brought about by these non-traumatic conditions is unknown. Factors that may contribute include: embolism (fat, nitrogen, or vascular); infiltration with abnormal cells (as in Gaucher disease) leading to compression of small blood vessels in bone; clotting abnormalities leading to sludging, thrombosis, or haemorrhage; or repeated mechanical stress on bone which is abnormal (e.g. osteoporotic) leading to microfractures with impaired bone remodelling and rupture of small intratrabecular vessels and consequent vascular insufficiency at the capillary level.

Radiological features in avascular necrosis can vary depending on the age of the lesion. Although, initially, no abnormality may be seen, the earliest sign is often a subchondral crescentic radiolucent zone which represents a subchondral fracture between infarcted bone trabeculae inserting into subchondral bone. Later, an irregular area of increased radiodensity due to dystrophic calcification or reparative new bone formation is seen. The articular surface may be collapsed or appear irregular (Fig. 27.10). Disuse osteoporosis in surviving bone can complicate the radiological appearances.

Histologically, necrosis of bone is recognized by death of osteocytes and empty osteocyte lacunae (Fig. 27.11). However, the earliest change is seen in the bone marrow where there is necrosis of fat and haemopoietic cells with haemorrhage and exudation of serum in fatty marrow and formation of large 'fat cysts'. Dystrophic calcification may also be seen in necrotic

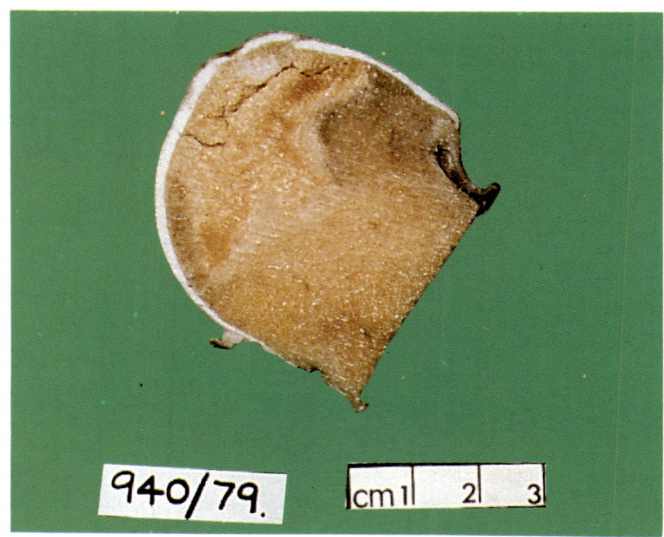

Fig. 27.10 Avascular necrosis. Bisected femoral head. Necrosis of bone in most of the superior segment of the head extending to the subchondral zone.

Table 27.3 Conditions associated with bone necrosis

1. Trauma—fractures (especially of femoral neck); dislocations
2. Non-traumatic
   (a) Decompression states and Caisson disease
   (b) Haemoglobinopathies (sickle-cell disease)
   (c) Corticosteroid therapy; Cushing disease
   (d) Gaucher disease
   (e) Alcoholism
   (f) Pancreatitis
   (g) Renal transplant
   (h) Metabolic abnormalities—gout and hyperuricaemia, hyperlipidaemia, iron overload
   (i) Immunosuppressive therapy
   (j) Non-steroidal anti-inflammatory drugs
   (k) Small vessel disease in polyarteritis, rheumatoid arthritis, systemic lupus erythematosus, giant-cell arthritis, diabetes mellitus
   (l) Radiation

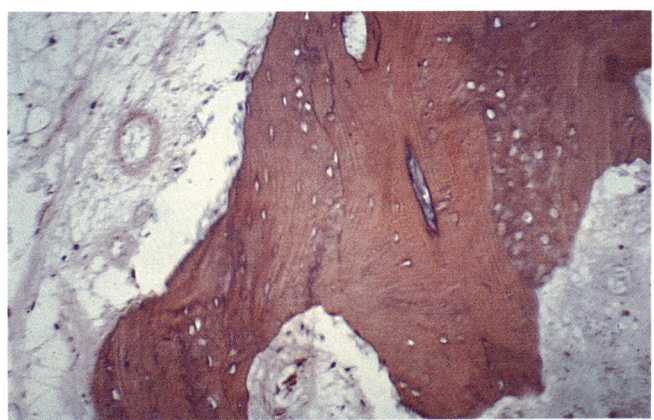

Fig. 27.11 Avascular necrosis. Compact bone in which all the osteocyte lacunae are empty. The inferior surface is undergoing osteoclastic resorption.

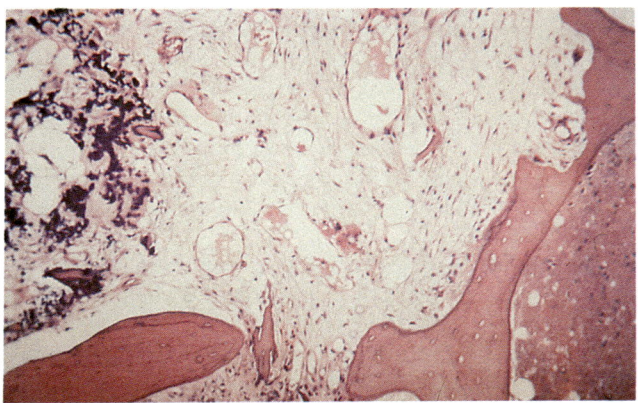

Fig. 27.12 Avascular necrosis. Dead bone trabeculae with osteoclastic resorption of part of the surface and osteoblasts on other parts. Amorphous debris on the right, dystrophic calcification on the left, and revascularized marrow in the centre.

intertrabecular tissue, particularly in large infarcts (Fig. 27.12). Reparative granulation tissue, including new blood vessels and marrow fibroblasts, is present at the peripheral margin of necrotic areas. The marrow fibroblasts differentiate into osteoblasts and form woven bone in apposition to dead bone trabeculae ('creeping substitution') as well as by intramembranous ossification. In uncomplicated infarcts, the articular cartilage remains viable as it receives its nutrition from the synovial fluid.

Some infarcts heal without sequelae but many are complicated by collapse of the necrotic segment and consequent flattening and distortion of the articular surface. Avascular necrosis of bone is now recognized as a significant cause of secondary degenerative arthritis in the hip and other joints.

Osteochondritis juvenilis

This is a general term used to describe a large number of ep-onymous conditions occurring in the epiphyses and apophyses of children and adolescents. Although primary avascular necrosis of epiphyseal bone prior to closure of the growth plate was thought to be the common pathology underlying these various conditions, other mechanisms are now known to be involved. True avascular necrosis is still widely regarded as the cause of Legg–Calve–Perthes (Perthes) disease, the most common and important of these conditions. Perthes disease results in partial or total necrosis of the femoral capital epiphysis. It is more common in male children and the age of onset is usually between 5 and 11 years. There is a family history in 30 per cent of cases and, in many, radiological evidence of skeletal immaturity. The condition is bilateral in about 10 per cent of cases. The clinical and pathological changes and sequelae are those of adult avascular necrosis. Radiologically, there is widening of the joint space, deformity and widening of the epiphysis, and often lytic lesions in the metaphysis. Subchondral collapse following avascular necrosis results in fragmentation and a mushroom-shaped flattening of the femoral head with widening of the metaphysis. Secondary degenerative arthritis is a common sequel in later life. Other common sites in which osteochondritis due to true avascular necrosis occurs include the carpal lunate bone (Kienbock disease), the tarsal navicular bone (Kohler disease), and the head of the metatarsal bone (Frieberg disease). A partial or total avulsion of the tendon insertion which removes a flake of bone which only then becomes necrotic is thought to underlie Osgood–Schlatter disease of the tibial tubercle, Sever disease of the calcaneal apophysis, and Sinding–Larsen disease of the lower pole of the patella. Bone necrosis is not involved in Calve disease of the vertebral body epiphysis, which is thought to be due to eosinophilic granuloma; nor is Scheuermann disease of the ring-shaped vertebral epiphysis, which is now known to be due to herniation of disc material through the weakened bony end plate.

Transplantation of bone

Bone transplants (or grafts) are commonly used to promote fracture healing in non-union, or to fill a space within a bone that has been destroyed by accident or disease. It is also used in reconstructive plastic surgery and to bring about the union of bones separated by a diseased joint (arthrodesis).

Following transplantation of autologous compact or cancellous bone (autograft), most of the grafted bone becomes necrotic as it is cut off from its blood supply; only a few superficial osteocytes and lining osteoblasts may survive. Transplants of homologous bone (homografts), which have been sterilized and stored, consist entirely of non-viable bone. In both cases the graft acts as a framework for the ingrowth of granulation tissue and formation of new bone.

Osteogenic cells from the surrounding host periosteum, endosteum, and marrow proliferate and accompany capillaries which grow into the transplant area. These osteogeneic cells lay down osteoid and bone while necrotic bone of the graft is removed and replaced by new bone (creeping substitution). In an autograft, surviving superficial osteogenic cells of the periosteum and endosteum may also contribute to bone formation.

Woven bone is formed initially and fills the grafted area. This is later remodelled to form normal lamellar cancellous or cortical bone. The process thus resembles repair following fracture or bone necrosis.

The effect of radiation on bone

Bone cells are less sensitive to radiation than haemopoietic marrow cells. Nevertheless, heavy doses of radiation, whether from an external or internal source (e.g. ingested radium), do produce pathological changes in bone. These include general tissue effects of radiation, such as thickening of the walls and obliteration of small blood vessels. There is consequent bone necrosis and scarring with fibrous repair tissue containing abnormal stellate fibroblasts. There is also loss of osteoblasts and osteocytes with abnormal bone resorption by osteoclasts. The bone structure is weakened and pathological fracture may ensue. Osteomyelitis is more likely to develop in ischaemic or necrotic irradiated bone, particularly in the jaw. Cartilage cells of the epiphyseal growth plate may also be directly damaged, leading to growth retardation or sometimes growth arrest with premature closure of the epiphysis.

Focal areas of proliferating abnormal osteogenic tissue may also develop following radiation. Development of bone sarcoma following external radiation, however, is rare; as a rule, the risk is directly proportional to the dosage employed. Sarcoma development is a more common complication of internal radiation. The latent interval before sarcoma development may range from 3 to 30 or more years. It is most often an osteosarcoma or fibrosarcoma. Leukaemia may develop following therapeutic external radiation of the skeleton (e.g. in the treatment of ankylosing spondylitis), and carcinoma of the nose and nasal sinuses following radium ingestion is also well recognized. The dosage of radiation required to induce leukaemia is generally much smaller than that which induces sarcoma or carcinoma. High dose accidental radiation causes leukaemia, as in the recent Chernobyl disaster.

The effects of bone damage and the small risk of neoplasia are generally too great for the treatment of non-neoplastic or benign lesions of bone and joint but are acceptable in the treatment of malignancy, when the lowest dose calculated to be effective should be used.

Hypertrophic pulmonary osteoarthropathy

In this condition there is subperiosteal new bone formation usually affecting the shafts of long bones, often symmetrically. Digital clubbing as well as painful swelling of the joints are also seen. The condition is most commonly associated with pleural mesothelioma or lung carcinoma but has also been seen with malignancies of other organs and in non-neoplastic lung and liver disease, amongst other conditions. The aetiology is unknown. In the bone, several layers of subperiosteal bone are laid down and there is a mild lymphocytic infiltrate in the periosteal tissues. Oedema and a mild lymphocytic infiltration is also seen in the soft tissues beneath clubbed fingers and the affected joints show a mild non-specific synovitis. Hypertrophic osteoarthropathy may predate other manifestations of bronchial carcinoma and may disappear after removal of the diseased lung. Similar subperiosteal new bone formation on shafts of large tubular bones can also accompany vascular disturbances, such as severe varicose veins with ulceration; it also occurs with polyarteritis nodosa.

27.1.4   Infection of bone (osteomyelitis)

Infection of bone may affect the periosteum, the cortex, or the medullary cavity alone, and the resulting reaction designated periostitis, osteitis, and osteomyelitis, respectively. In practice, the infective process involves more than one tissue plane and the term osteomyelitis is now in common usage to describe all bone infections regardless of localization.

Bone becomes infected by haematogenous spread from another lesion, by direct implantation via an open wound, or by spread from an infected organ or subcutaneous tissue. A wide variety of organisms has been cultured from bone infections. The commonest cause of pyogenic infection is *Staphylococcus aureus* and of granulomatous osteomyelitis, *Mycobacterium tuberculosis*. Other bacteria are recognized as an important cause in certain circumstances. Neonates, for example, may be infected by *E. coli*, *H. influenzae*, and group B streptococci. The elderly or debilitated patient may have a coliform osteomyelitis. Patients with sickle-cell disease are more likely to have a *Salmonella* infection.

Compound fractures and surgical operations may be complicated by infection by more than one organism, including anaerobic bacteria, at the time of trauma; or may become infected during the healing phase by haematogenous dissemination from urinary- or respiratory-tract infections or during tooth extraction.

Fungal infections may occur by any of the same routes followed by bacteria. *Candida*-induced osteomyelitis occurs by haematogenous spread in neonates and intravenous drug abusers and by direct implantation. Blastomycosis and maduromycosis extend from soft-tissue foci. Bone infections by *Coccidioides* and *Cryptococcus* are always blood-borne.

Parasitic infestations are blood-borne. Echinococcosis (hydatid disease) of bone is uncommon. Cysticercosis has been described.

The only described cases of viral infection of bone have been due to variola or vaccinia. Finding the infective agent is the problem when attempts are made to establish a connection between inflammatory reactions and viruses.

Types of inflammatory response

Tissue reactions to infection fall into three major patterns, pyogenic, chronic non-specific, and granulomatous. To designate osteomyelitis as simply acute or chronic is not adequate. Osteomyelitis may be chronic, in the clinical sense, either because it is an inadequately treated pyogenic infection or because it is caused by an organism that provokes a slowly progressing reaction. The implications in both cases are different.

Pyogenic infections

An acute polymorphonuclear response is the usual reaction to bacterial infection by any of the organisms previously mentioned, except *M. tuberculosis*, *Coccidioides* and, sometimes, blastomycosis. Brucellosis may also cause pyogenic osteomyelitis.

In general, the cellular reactions following pyogenic infection of bone are the same as those that occur in other tissues (see Chapter 4). The differences are due to the effects on bone tissue. In the early phase a combination of vascular stasis, products of tissue cell death, and bacterial toxins cause death of bone tissue (Fig. 27.13). This is followed, in the phase of resolution, by a phagocytic response directed at the necrotic bone, and osteoclasts appear in the affected area (Fig. 27.14). The dead bone may be either completely resorbed or separated from the viable bone and persist as a sequestrated fragment within the inflammatory tissue (Fig. 27.15). Viable organisms may be contained within the marrow spaces of the dead bone and be a cause of recurrence of active infection.

When cortical bone dies and is resorbed, a communication

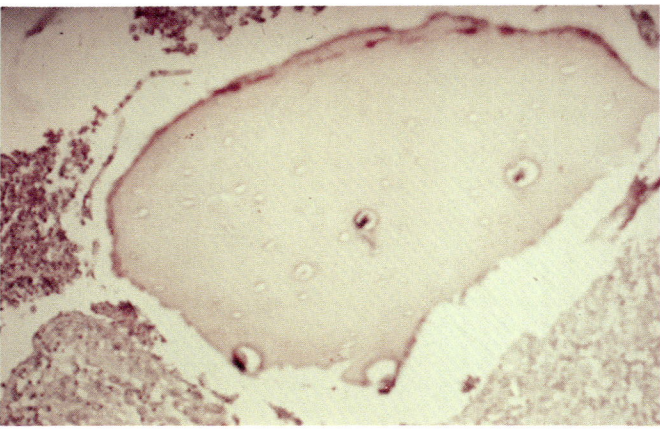

Fig. 27.15 Pyogenic osteomyelitis. An isolated fragment of necrotic bone (sequestrum) surrounded by purulent exudate.

between the medullary cavity and extraosseous tissue is established. This is called a cloaca and from it the inflammatory tissue may extend to the skin surface and discharge. The sinus offers a portal for other organisms to colonize the bone. The periosteum covering an area of infected bone is commonly lifted away from the bone surface by exudate, but is not affected by the infection and remains viable. Bone of reactive type is formed between the periosteum and the bone and, if it is extensive and encloses the original bone in a sleeve, is called an involucrum (Fig. 27.16). Reactive bone formation occurs also within the bone during the repair phase of the reaction (Fig. 27.17). The intramedullary bone may be of lamellar type opposed to preexisting trabeculae; or of woven type usually in the form of trabeculae within reactive fibrous tissue.

Very little is known about the factors that influence bone resorption and formation related to pyogenic infection. It is postulated that cytokines such as interleukin-1 activate osteoclasts, but it is not clear how important this is for the resorption of necrotic bone.

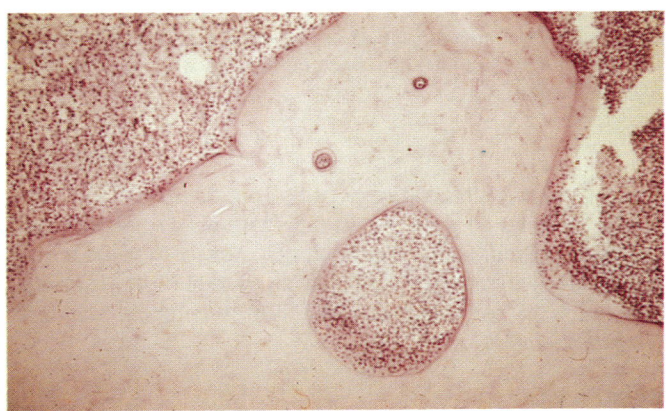

Fig. 27.13 Acute pyogenic osteomyelitis. Necrotic compact bone and purulent exudate in Haversian canal and marrow space.

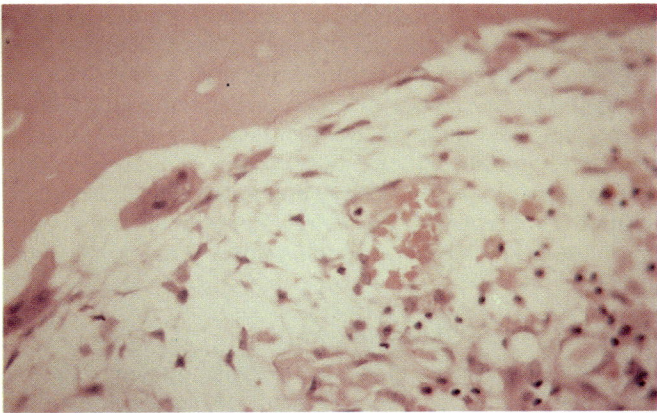

Fig. 27.14 Pyogenic osteomyelitis. Necrotic bone (top left) undergoing osteoclastic resorption.

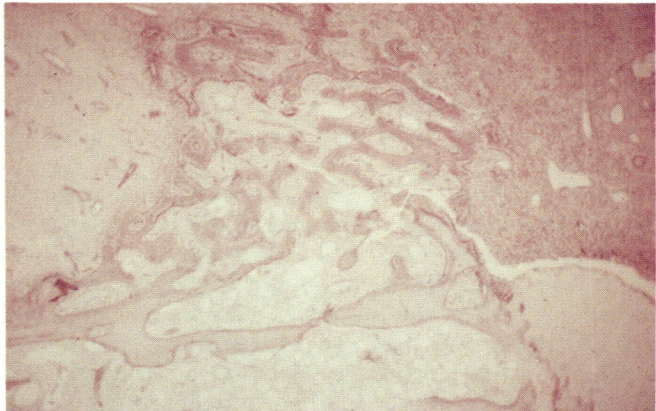

Fig. 27.16 Pyogenic osteomyelitis. Involucrum. Trabeculae of reactive bone (centre) on periosteal surface of juxta-articular cortex (articular cartilage lower right).

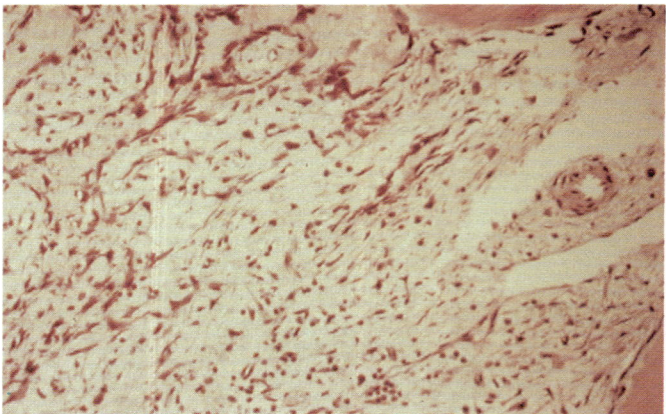

Fig. 27.17 Pyogenic osteomyelitis. Reactive bone formation in medullary cavity.

Collagenase in the purulent exudate may also contribute to bone resorption as it contributes to the dissolution of cartilage that becomes involved in a pyogenic reaction. Bone formation is initiated and regulated by mechanisms that are not understood or are guessed at. Involucrum formation appears to be only a particular example of the general observation that new bone will be deposited whenever the periosteum is separated from the bone cortex and remains viable. Formation of bone within and around the infected area can occur only when the inflammatory cells have been replaced by fixed connective tissue cells. Substances released by macrophages may promote recruitment and proliferation of fibroblasts, but no stimulus to intramembranous bone formation or bone apposition is known to come from inflammatory cells. (See Chapter 4 for discussion of molecular mechanisms of the inflammatory response.) It may be that new bone is formed in response to mechanical stresses which are abnormal because of bone resorption.

Blood-borne infection of bone in children is located most commonly in the metaphyseal region; the upper tibia and lower femur are sites most likely to be affected. The blood vessels in the metaphyses are at the end of the nutrient-artery-derived system and capillaries are most numerous in these areas. Common involvement of bone around the knee is possibly merely a reflection of the relative size of those metaphyses. Trauma is said to precede blood-borne infection in a substantial minority of children, and this may be an additional factor in the pattern of involvement.

From the initial area of infection extension to involve medullary cavity, cortical bone, and sometimes the extraosseous soft tissues occurs quickly (Fig. 27.18). Changes in the texture of the bone may be visible within 3 days of the first symptoms. Metaphyseal lesions will invariably come to impinge on the growth cartilage, which may be partially destroyed. Extension to the soft tissues around the metaphysis may lead to synovial involvement, septic arthritis, and destruction of articular cartilage. From the joint space, infection may gain access to the epiphyseal region of the bone.

Complications of pyogenic osteomyelitis include: patho-

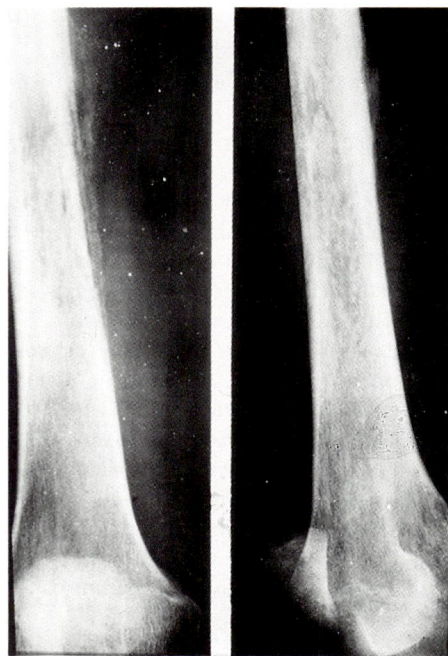

Fig. 27.18 Pyogenic osteomyelitis. Radiograph of lower femur. Diffuse loss of bone from medulla and cortex. Involucrum on medial and posterior diaphysis.

logical fracture; metastatic infection from recurrences of active disease; damage to growth cartilage with growth disturbance; damage to articular cartilage leading to ankylosis of the joint or premature degenerative arthritis; amyloid disease; squamous carcinoma in recurrent sinuses; and sarcoma in the intraosseous scar tissue.

Brodie's abscess
This is a relatively small and well-defined focus of osteomyelitis which appears on a radiograph as an area of complete bone loss, surrounded by a zone of increased bone density (Fig. 27.19).

In some lesions the osteolytic area contains pus or pyogenic granulation tissue and viable staphylococci. Some of these lesions contain predominantly reparative tissue with few inflammatory cells, while others contain encysted fluid which is almost cell-free. Bacterial examination does not reveal the causative organism in the majority of cases. While some of these lesions appear to be the result of inadequate chemotherapeutic treatment of a pyogenic infection, it seems probable that many are the result of infection by an organism of low-grade pathogenicity.

Chronic non-specific osteomyelitis
Inadequate treatment of acute pyogenic osteomyelitis may cause the disease to become chronic and change the composition of the inflammatory cell reaction to one in which lymphocytes, plasma cells, and macrophages dominate the

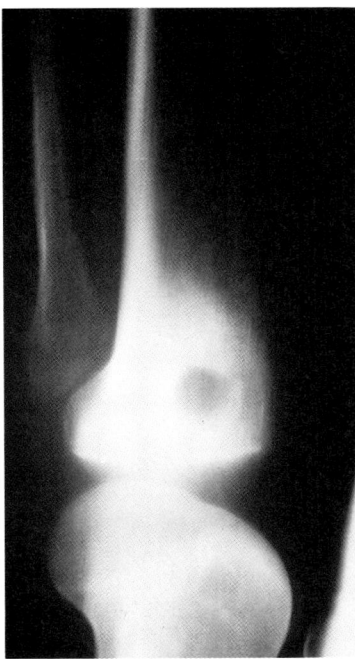

Fig. 27.19 Brodie's abscess; radiograph (tomogram). Well-defined lytic focus surrounded by sclerotic bone.

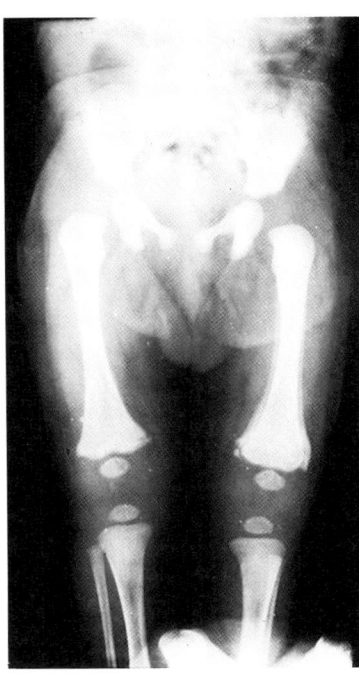

Fig. 27.20 Congenital syphilis; radiograph. Asymmetry of lower femoral growth plates and periosteal new bone formation, right femur.

histopathological appearances; this should not be confused with an inflammatory response which is characterized by a mixture of inflammatory cells without evidence of suppuration, in the absence of any treatment. The former condition commonly retains small foci of pus cells and a very large proportion of plasma cells, features not found in the latter. Some bacteria produce a chronic non-specific response quite often, especially *Salmonella* and *Brucella*. There is also a very rare form of bone inflammation, affecting children and young adults, designated transitory, migratory osteomyelitis in which the cellular infiltrate may be almost purely lymphocytic. The cause of this disease is not known.

Congenital syphilitic infection of bone affects the metaphyses, which are infiltrated by chronic inflammatory cells at the expense of normal connective tissue cells. Endochondral ossification is impeded, the metaphysis is mechanically unstable, and incomplete fracture may occur. In addition, the periosteum of the long bones may be displaced and a layer of reactive bone formed on the cortical surface. Periosteal displacement might be the result of inflammatory cell infiltration (periostitis) or of slipping of the epiphysis (Fig. 27.20). Bone resorption and reactive formation occur in association with this type of inflammation as in pyogenic osteomyelitis.

Brucellosis of the spine leads to ossification of the annulus of the intervertebral disc and the spinal ligaments, producing a radiographic appearance termed 'bamboo spine; this is similar to the effect of ankylosing spondylitis. Sequestrum formation is not a feature of this type of inflammation, nor do sinuses occur spontaneously. Pathological fracture may occur, particularly of

vertebral bodies. Extension of infection to a joint does not usually cause the severe cartilage damage seen in septic arthritis, but can lead to premature osteoarthritis. Amyloid disease and malignant changes are not known complications.

Granulomatous osteomyelitis

As previously indicated the most common cause of this type of chronic bone infection is *M. tuberculosis*. Before considering that disease, other types of granulomatous inflammation require brief consideration.

Brucellosis may induce a granulomatous type of reaction. There is no caseation and the granulomata resemble those of sarcoid reactions rather than tuberculosis.

Acquired syphilis and yaws also cause osseous lesions. Syphilitic gummata may lead to bone destruction with very little reactive bone formation and, in the case of thin flat bones, for example skull vault and palate, perforations are produced (Fig. 27.21). In contrast, there may be very active bone formation related to a gumma and the radiographic appearances can resemble those of an osteosarcoma. All degrees of bone destruction and formation, between these extremes, occur. The osseous lesions of framboesia (yaws) are characteristically more osteoblastic than osteolytic and produce irregular subperiosteal deposits, usually over the diaphysis of a long bone (Fig. 27.22).

Mycotic infections which may induce a granulomatous reaction include maduromycosis, blastomycosis, and coccidioidomycosis. The first two affect bone by direct extension from soft-tissue infections and the reaction may be either purulent or granulomatous. Coccidioidomycotic bone lesions are the result

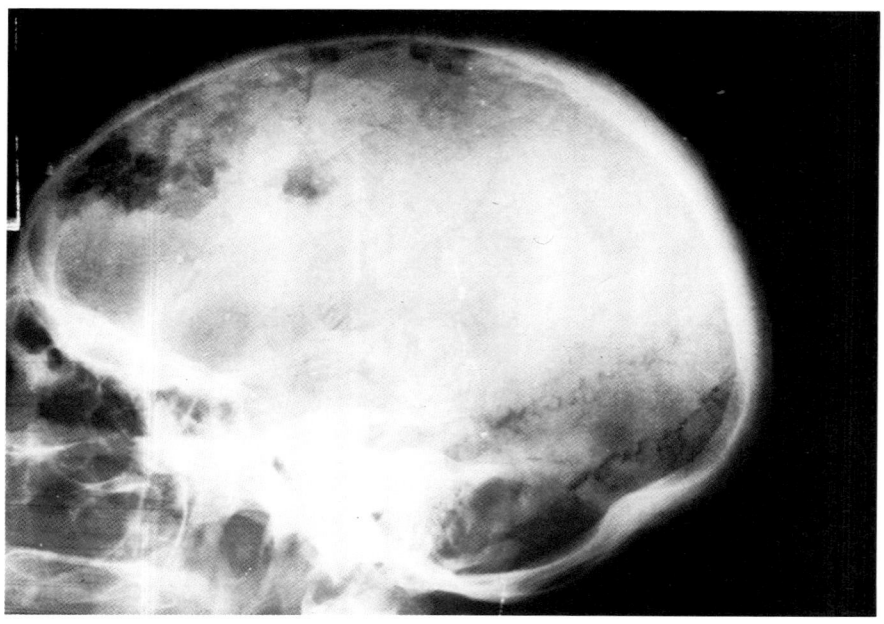

Fig. 27.21   Tertiary syphilis; radiograph. Skull with perforating lesions and a sclerotic reaction.

of haematogenous spread, may be multiple, and can very closely resemble tuberculous osteomyelitis.

Tuberculous osteomyelitis

With the rare exception of infection resulting from penetrating injury, bone infection by *Mycobacterium tuberculosis* is by haematogenous dissemination from a primary infection, usually of the lung and by the human variety of this organism. At the time of presentation with the osseous lesion, the primary

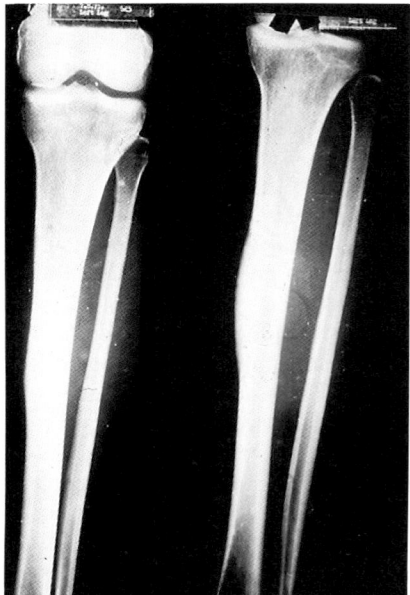

Fig. 27.22   Yaws; radiograph. Fusiform thickening in central diaphysis of tibia.

focus may be inactive. The patient will usually demonstrate a hypersensitivity reaction (positive Mantoux test). Any bone in the body may be affected, the vertebral bodies most frequently. Infection in long bones is frequently accompanied by arthritis.

The cellular reaction is composed of macrophages and lymphocytes in which there are epithelioid and giant-cell granulomata with necrotic centres. There is also diffuse necrosis of the inflammatory tissue and bone, especially in the centre of the reaction (Fig. 27.23). The relative amount of necrosis varies widely. Proliferation of the inflammatory reaction leads to bone resorption and the lesion appears osteolytic in a radiograph. Residual bone may be seen in the centre of the lesion, corresponding with an area of caseous necrosis in which all cellular activity has ceased. Caseous material does not contain collagenase.

Tubercle bacilli may be observed in histopathological sections, usually after a long search. If acid-fast bacilli are present in large numbers the possibility of infection by 'atypical' mycobacteria should be considered (see below).

Reactive new bone formation is not a significant feature of tuberculous osteomyelitis. Continuing bone resorption will eventually cause pathological fracture. This complication is most serious when it occurs in tuberculous osteomyelitis of the spine (Pott disease), especially when thoracic vertebral bodies are involved. When the vertebral body fractures it also collapses and tends to break into several fragments. Thoracic vertebral body collapse always produces a kyphotic deformity and bone fragments, together with the contents of the lesion, are driven posteriorly, encroach on the spinal canal, and may compress the spinal cord, causing paraplegia. Infection of the spine is commonly multifocal, often affecting consecutive bodies and leading to severe angular kyphosis. Marginal, subligamentous foci also occur (Fig. 27.24) and extension of these lesions under

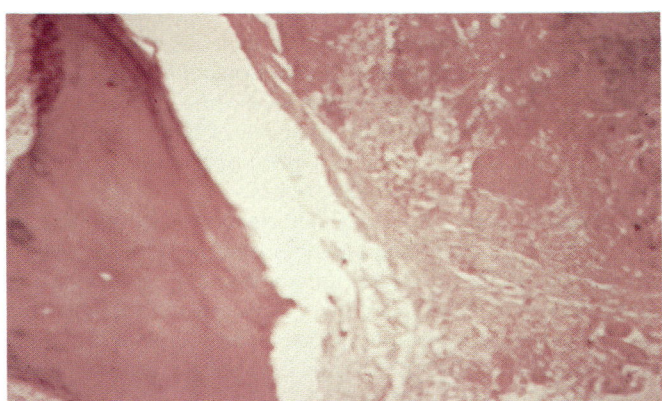

Fig. 27.23 Tuberculous osteomyelitis. Necrosis of bone and caseous debris in marrow.

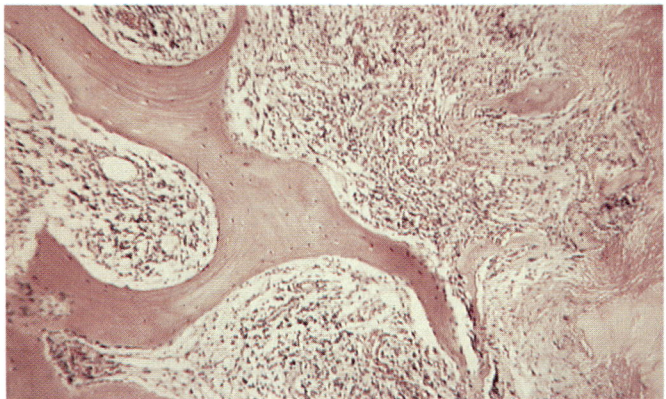

Fig. 27.25 Tuberculous osteomyelitis. Proliferative reaction beneath articular cartilage (right). The subchondral plate and calcified zone of cartilage have been destroyed but the hyaline cartilage remains.

the spinal ligament may obstruct the blood-supply to the cord, producing a paraplegia that cannot be relieved by removal of the tuberculous material.

Intraosseous lesions frequently extend and make contact with cartilaginous tissue, which the advancing edge of macrophages resorbs (Fig. 27.25). In the spine this produces a discrete perforation in the intervertebral disc, with residual disc material separating the vertebral bodies. Hyaline cartilage is similarly destroyed, separates from the subchondral bone, and

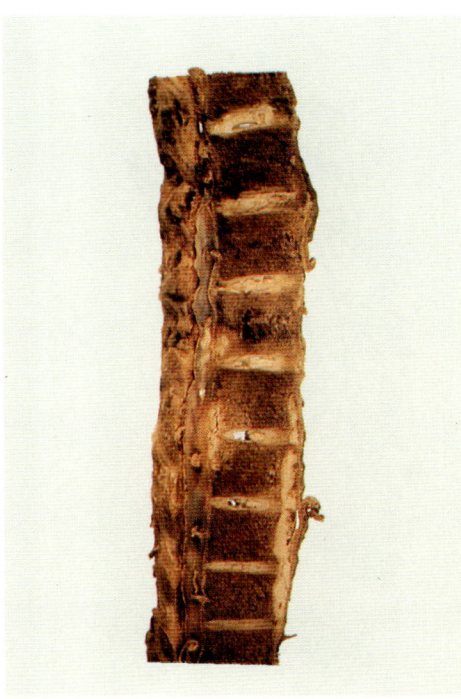

Fig. 27.24 Tuberculous osteomyelitis of spine (Pott disease). Sagittal section of thoracic spine. There are two lesions. The upper has eroded through the posterior part of the intervertebral disc. Note that the residual disc is of normal thickness.

lies free in the joint space, which is often, at that stage, filled with granulomatous tissue and caseous debris.

Sinus formation occurs most frequently from long-bone lesions, and secondary bacterial infection with pyogenic organisms occurs. The tissue reactions in the bone can then become more like those of a primary pyogenic osteomyelitis.

The patient with tuberculous osteomyelitis often has metastatic lesions in other organs and tissues, especially the kidney.

Complications of the osseous lesions, other than those already mentioned, are rare. Joint involvement leads to disintegration of the articular surfaces and fibrous ankylosis during the healing phase. Malignant change in bone or skin is not to be expected unless secondary pyogenic infection is superadded. The same is true of amyloid deposition.

Bone is occasionally infected by 'atypical' mycobacteria, either by direct implantation or via the bloodstream. Organisms may be seen in large numbers in macrophages; the latter cell dominates the cellular reaction. Although granuloma may not be evident, there is usually necrosis of the inflammatory tissue.

Ecchinococcal infestation (hydatid disease)

Only a small proportion of patients with hydatid disease have osseous lesions. In bone there is usually a number of small thinwalled cysts, formed in the medullary marrow and inducing bone resorption as they enlarge (Fig. 27.26). The radiographic appearances indicate the presence of several cysts with surviving septae of bone between. As the cysts encroach on the endosteal surface of the cortex, new bone may be formed on the periosteal surface and the bone enlarges in diameter. Pathological fracture may occur. While the cysts are intact and contained within the bone they do not provoke an inflammatory response. Cysts ruptured by pathological fracture or incomplete excision are surrounded by a giant-cell reaction of foreign-body type (Fig. 27.27). Spinal involvement may cause cord compression and paraplegia. Infestations of all long tubular and flat bones, including the skull, have been described.

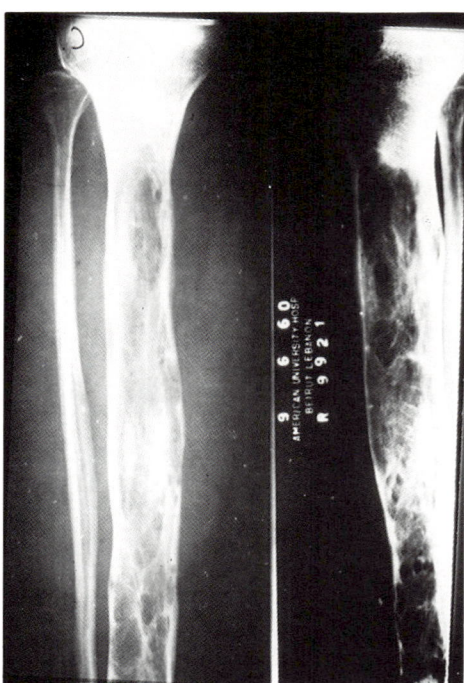

Fig. 27.26 Hydatid disease of bone; radiograph of tibia.

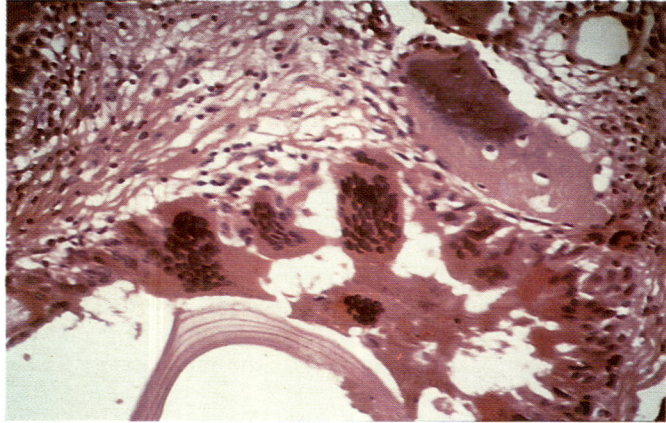

Fig. 27.27 Hydatid disease. Foreign-body reaction to chytinous cyst wall after fracture of affected bone.

27.1.5 Metabolic bone disease

This general title encompasses those disorders of the skeleton that result from disordered function of bone cells. It excludes those conditions that are genetically inherited.

Osteoporosis

The skeleton is said to be osteoporotic when it contains a reduced mass of bone tissue per unit area, which has a normal ratio of mineral to organic content. It results from an imbalance in the activity of osteoblasts and osteoclasts. Either type of cell

may be increased or decreased in number and/or functional activity; the only requirement is that bone resorption exceeds the amount of bone deposited. Some forms of osteoporosis are described as generalized, alhough it is very uncommon for every bone in the skeleton to show evidence of bone loss and extremely rare for the reduction in bone mass to be equal in every bone. Localized osteoporosis also occurs.

Osteoporosis is an important abnormality because it predisposes to fracture. The consequences may be fatal, especially those which render the elderly immobile and predispose to pulmonary infection. Apart from the serious complications of fractures of the femoral neck and ribs, osteoporosis-related fractures of vertebral bodies (Fig. 27.28) and limb bones may be followed by deformity and chronic invalidity.

The causes of generalized osteoporosis are numerous, as Table 27.4, which is certainly incomplete, indicates. Heritable causes of osteoporosis are included in Table 27.4 in order to indicate the range of differential diagnosis.

Some patients with generalized osteoporosis will have more than one factor contributing to skeletal loss. For example, the elderly female patient will be post-menopausal, may be very restricted in her activities, and could also have a diet grossly deficient in calcium. Hormone-related osteoporosis may be due to a direct effect of the hormone on bone cell activity, or be an indirect influence. Cortisone depresses bone formation; thyroxine stimulates bone cell activity, with excess osteoclasis; androgens affect the skeleton by their influence on muscle bulk and the effect that has on the forces applied to the skeleton. Liver disease, partial gastrectomy, coeliac disease, and chronic renal

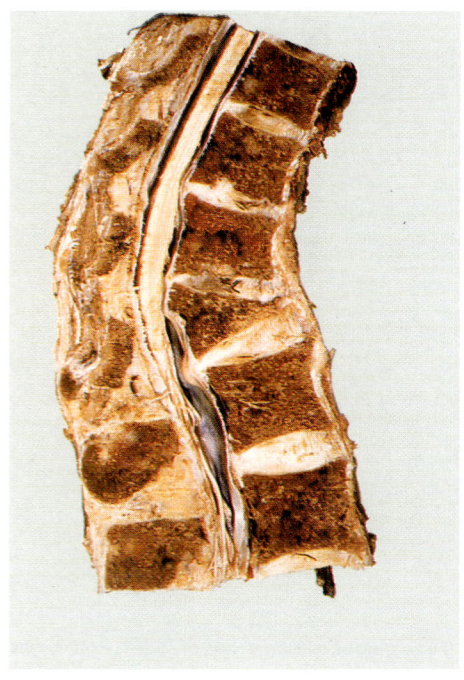

Fig. 27.28 Osteoporosis. Sagittal section of the lumbo-sacral spine showing collapse and anterior wedging of the T12 vertebral body.

Table 27.4 Causes of generalized osteoporosis

1. Idiopathic osteoporosis
   (a) Of the elderly
   (b) Of young adults
   (c) Juvenile
   (d) Pregnancy-related (may occur postpartum)
2. Hormone-related
   (a) Oestrogen deficiency
       (i) menopause and oophorectomy
       (ii) Turner syndrome (? due to lack of sex hormones)
   (b) Hypercortisonism
       (i) adrenal tumour
       (ii) iatrogenic
   (c) Thyrotoxicosis
   (d) Androgen deficiency
   (e) Hypopituitarism
   (f) Hyperparathyroidism
3. Vitamin C deficiency
4. Liver disease
5. Partial gastrectomy
6. Coeliac disease
7. Chronic renal failure
8. Cytotoxic drugs
9. Diffuse infiltration of marrow by malignant cells
10. Mastocytosis; heparinization
11. Osteogenesis imperfecta
12. Marfan syndrome
13. Fibrogenesis imperfecta
14. Immobility
15. Calcium dietary deficiency

failure may also lead to failure of mineralization. The skeleton consequently has both a decrease in bone mass and an excessive amount of unmineralized osteoid, i.e. a combination of osteoporosis and osteomalacia.

The causes of localized osteoporosis are fewer (Table 27.5). Pregnancy-related and juvenile osteoporosis may involve restricted areas of the skeleton, e.g. vertebral bodies or metaphyses of lower-limb long-bones, respectively.

The histopathological diagnosis is based on the recognition that there is less bone per unit area of section than normal. Provided that one knows the normal value for the piece of bone under examination and that there are no artefacts that make the method invalid, the ratio of bone tissue area to section area can be determined by very simple histomorphometric methods.

Table 27.5 Causes of localized osteoporosis

1. Immobility
   (a) Fracture
   (b) Rheumatoid disease
   (c) Septic arthritis
   (d) Sudek's atrophy
2. Tumour infiltration
3. Paget disease

There is wide biological variation in normal values and measurement of bone tissue content at one point in time may not identify osteoporosis unless it is marked. With experience it is often possible to recognize that the bone is porotic without formal measurements. Loss of bone from the cortical area results in enlargement of the Haversian canals, especially those in the deep, endosteal, zone. So much bone may be lost that the inner cortex assumes a more cancellous-like arrangement. Porosis of cancellous bone may be manifest as thinning of trabeculae or as total removal of some trabeculae with residual trabeculae of normal thickness, or as a combination of thinning and total loss (Fig. 27.29). The diameter of fat cells in the marrow is a useful comparison for trabecular width and the number of trabeculae visible in the field of the $10 \times$ objective can be used to assess total loss of trabeculae. This method of judging cancellous bone area is again dependent on knowing what is normal for that particular area.

Added to the features of osteoporosis may be abnormalities of the bone cell population or of the marrow contents, which will suggest the primary cause and indicate whether there is active bone loss. When bone is being lost very quickly as, for example, in Sudek's atrophy, osteoclasts may be very numerous and osteoblasts with an associated marrow fibrosis a prominent feature. The appearances may resemble hyperparathyroid bone disease, except that the cement lines will not be grossly

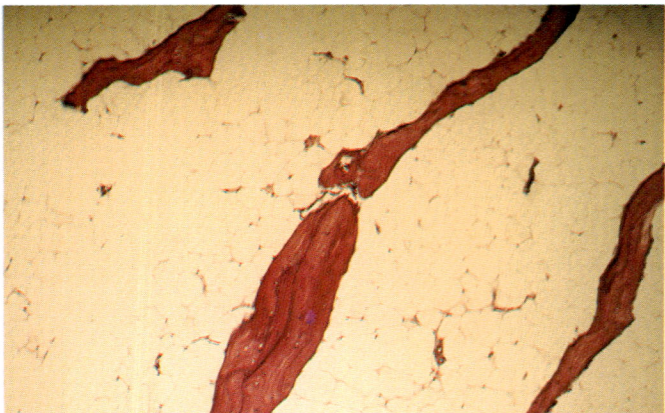

Fig. 27.29 Osteoporosis; cancellous bone. The lower central trabecula is of normal thickness. All other trabeculae are thin.

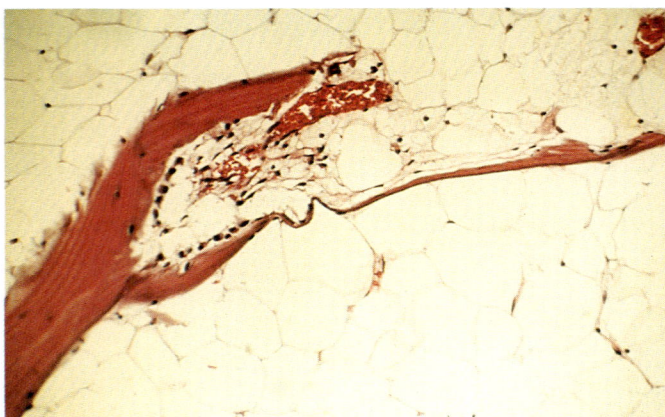

Fig. 27.30 Osteoporosis. Cancellous bone undergoing active resorption, leaving a thinned strut of bone (right centre). Rapid bone loss following immobilization.

abnormal (Fig. 27.30). In some biopsies there may be no evidence of active resorption, rather the appearances will indicate an increase in bone apposition. This may be a purely local phenomenon, perhaps as a response to stress, or a more extensive change when the cause of the osteoporosis has been removed and the skeleton is being restored to normal. An explanation for some of these incongruous appearances may be found in the clinical history and the radiographic appearances.

Rickets and osteomalacia

In both conditions there is failure of mineralization of bone matrix. The difference is related to skeletal maturity, rickets being a disorder that affects both bone and growth cartilage and leads to enlargement and distortion of epiphyseal plates. Causes of rickets and osteomalacia are tabulated in Table 27.6.

Rickets is characterized by widening of epiphyses and lateral bowing deformity of long bones (Fig. 27.31). The broad costochondral junctions are responsible for the chest wall swellings described as the 'rachitic rosary'. Bowing of long bones occurs in the metaphyseal region and commonly affects the tibia. Failure of growth plate calcification prevents endochondral ossification (Fig. 27.32), impedes growth in length of bone, and is a cause of short stature.

Table 27.6   Causes of rickets and osteomalacia

1. Vitamin D deficiency
   - (a) Inadequate intake
   - (b) Deficient synthesis
   - (c) Malabsorption
       - (i) gluten-sensitive enteropathy
       - (ii) gastric operations
       - (iii) bowel resection
       - (iv) biliary cirrhosis

2. Renal disorders
   - (a) Glomerular disease (failure of vitamin D metabolism)
   - (b) Tubular disease (phosphate loss)
       - (i) familial hypophosphataemic rickets
       - (ii) adult onset hypophosphataemic osteomalacia
       - (iii) inherited tubular acidosis
       - (iv) ureterocolic anastomosis (acquired tubular acidosis)
       - (v) cystinosis
       - (vi) oculo-cerebro-renal syndrome
       - (vii) Wilson disease
       - (viii) cadmium poisoning

3. Anticonvulsant therapy (failure of vitamin D absorption and/or of hydroxylation in liver)

4. Tumour-related rickets and osteomalacia (hypophosphataemia, pathogenesis uncertain)

5. Diphosphonate therapy (blocks hydroxyapatite crystal formation)

6. Aluminium hydroxide (lowers phosphate)

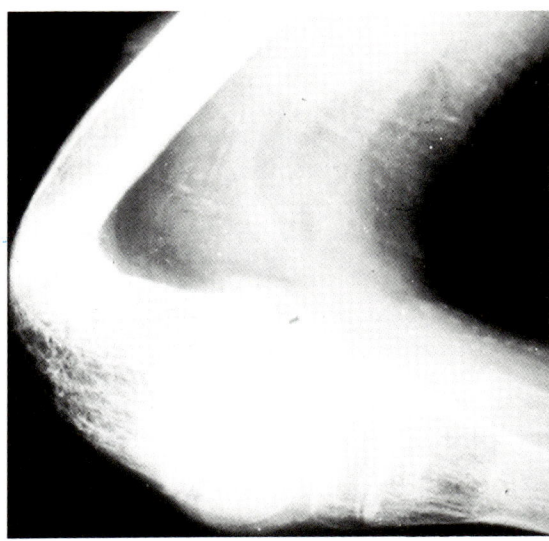

Fig. 27.31   Rickets; radiograph. Broad irregular growth plates. Severely bowed femoral diaphysis with incomplete fracture at apex of curve.

Osteomalacia is associated with bowing deformity of limbs, distortion of the pelvis, and pathological fractures which are often incomplete (Looser's zones) and do not unite by bone formation unless the primary disorder is corrected (Fig. 27.33). Patients with rickets and osteomalacia resulting from vitamin D deficiency may also experience severe weakness of muscles, especially around the pelvis and shoulder.

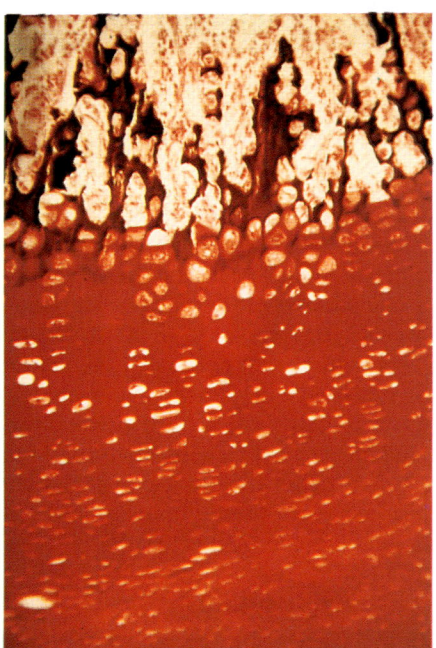

Fig. 27.32   Rickets; growth plate. Incomplete mineralization of hypertrophic zone of cartilage and of metaphyseal bone. (Undecalcified section; v. Kossa stain.)

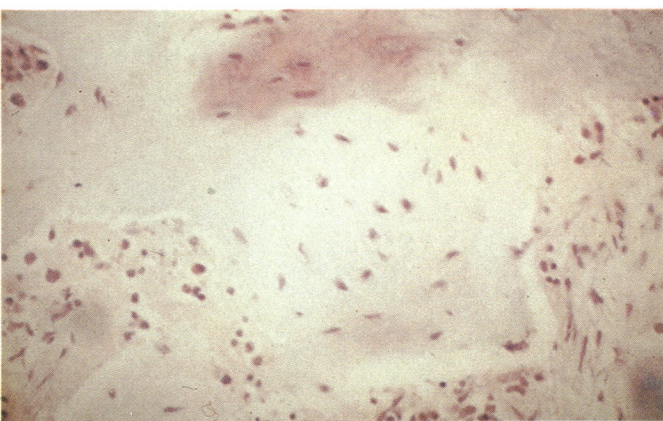

Fig. 27.33   Osteomalacia; Looser's zone. Unmineralized cartilage occupies the lucent zone.

Rickets and osteomalacia can be identified reliably only on microscopic sections prepared from undecalcified tissue which have been stained by the v. Kossa technique. Failure of calcification in the hypertrophic zone of growth cartilage is usually gross and easily identified.

What constitutes osteomalacia as an histopathological entity is a question that has been answered in several different ways and has generated a lot of debate. While all are agreed that the answer depends on a quantitative analysis, the disagreements are over the methods of quantitation and the features that should be enumerated. Recognition of failure of osteoid mineralization is relatively easy, if the v. Kossa-stained section is examined in polarized light using a 20 × or 40 × microscope objective. This will reveal the lamellar osteoid as being composed of layers of alternating birefringent and non-birefringent collagen (except the thinnest layer which will be a single sheet). Osteoid which is being mineralized normally will not have more than four birefringent layers in any seam. If there are five or more birefringent lamellae in even one osteoid seam, that is histological osteomalacia (Fig. 27.34). Other methods, which involve measurement of length, thickness, area, volume, rate of apposition, the amount of calcification front, and other parameters, may be of value for comparative studies or the elucidation of pathogenesis, but are not needed to establish the basic diagnosis.

The histological appearances may be modified by parathyroid overactivity in those patients who have vitamin D (or metabolite) deficiency (see p. 2022). Features of hyperparathyroid bone disease are added to those of osteomalacia (secondary hyperparathyroidism) (Fig. 27.35). A similar increase in osteoblastic and osteoclastic activity may be observed after the establishment of adequate treatment of vitamin D deficiency. When osteomalacia is due to phosphate deficiency, secondary hyperparathyroidism does not occur (Fig. 27.36). Diphosphonates are compounds in which the oxygen in a phosphate bond is replaced by nitrogen. When the ethanehydroxy form is administered the production of hydroxyapatite is inhibited and can be totally halted. This compound may be used in the treatment of

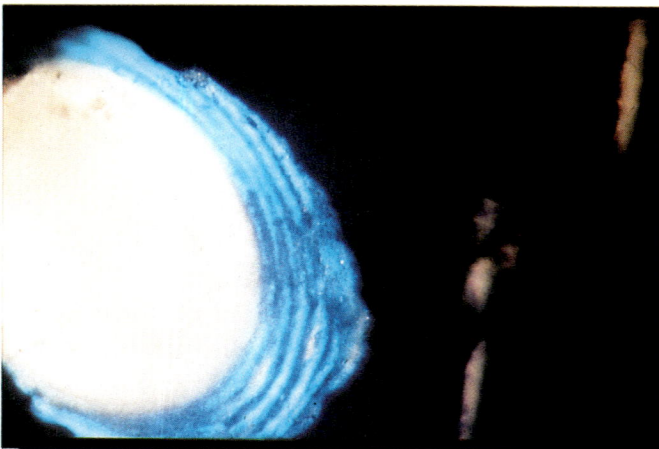

Fig. 27.34 Osteomalacia. Undecalcified section of bone stained by v. Kossa method with toluidine blue. There are five birefringent lamellae in the osteoid seam.

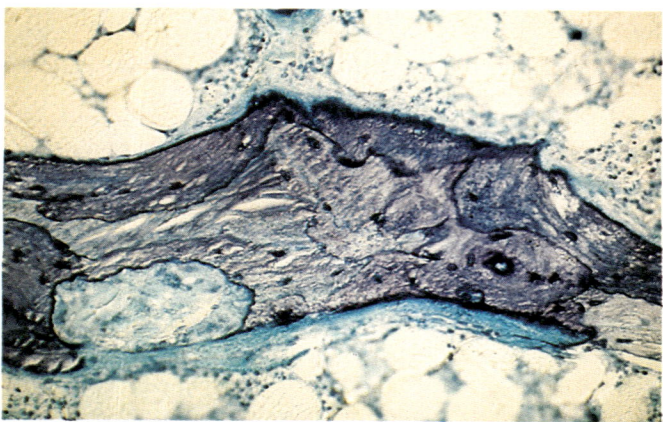

Fig. 27.35 Secondary hyperparathyroidism. Undecalcified section of bone stained with toluidine blue. Bone surface is covered by osteoid (turquoise blue) and bone resorption is occurring beneath an osteoid seam (lower parts of bone trabecula, left and right).

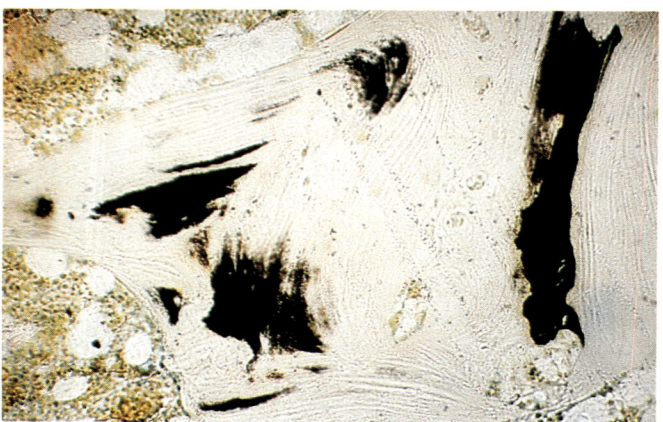

Fig. 27.36 Hypophosphataemic osteomalacia. Undecalcified bone section stained v. Kossa/neutral red. There is a larger area of osteoid than of bone, but no evidence of osteoclastic resorption.

Paget disease because the accumulation of unmineralized osteoid prevents osteoclastic resorption and osteoblastic activity is also suppressed (Fig. 27.37). Growth plate mineralization is also inhibited by diphosphonate.

The relationship between aluminium and bone disease is not clear, despite claims to the contrary. There is no doubt that if aluminium hydroxide (in the form of Aludrox) is ingested, the serum phosphate level can be lowered to a degree that causes osteomalacia. It is also true that aluminium can be demonstrated in the bone and osteoid of some patients with osteomalacia. The uncertainty is because aluminium can also be seen in the bone of patients who do not have osteomalacia, and aluminium may not be present in all areas where osteoid mineralization is inhibited. In these circumstances the presence of aluminium in bone might be a clue to the cause of the osteomalacia (Aludrox ingestion) but cannot be assumed to be the mechanism responsible for failure of mineralization.

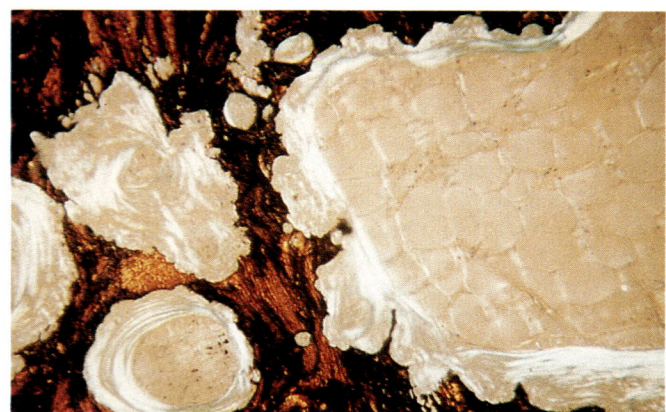

Fig. 27.37 'Osteomalacia' following treatment of Paget disease with diphosphonate. Undecalcified section. v. Kossa/toluidine blue (polarized light).

From the list of causes of histopathological osteomalacia, it is clear that the bone abnormality might be the result of interference with the activity of osteoblasts or due to a change in the availability or composition of the calcium and phosphate ions required to make hydroxyapatite. In most cases, the histopathological appearances will not reveal the proximate cause and, in many, not even the primary abnormality. The terms osteomalacia and rickets were applied originally to patients, radiographs, and histological sections that showed the effects of vitamin D deficiency. While the number of recognized causes of 'soft bones' has increased, the terminology has remained the same and no longer has precision.

Hyperparathyroid bone disease

The skeleton may be affected by increased parathormone production from an adenoma or carcinoma of the parathyroid, or by hyperplasia of the glands. What proportion of patients with hyperparathyroidism have skeletal abnormalities is not known, but examination of biopsies taken from patients who have neither radiographic nor clinical features of overt bone disease have shown histopathological changes indicative of increased bone cell activity.

These histological changes are of two types: generalized and focal; and the latter may not be present. The general change consists basically of an increase in both osteoclastic and osteo-blastic activity (Fig. 27.38). Other abnormalities are usually present whicn are related to, or consequent on, the increased cellular activity.

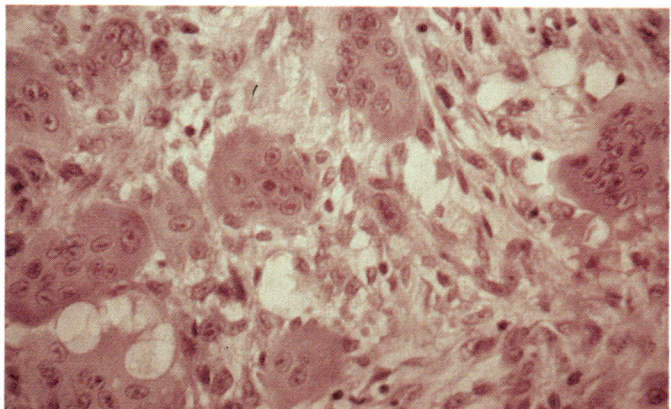

Fig. 27.39 Hyperparathyroidism; 'brown tumour'. Osteoclast-like giant cells interspersed amongst spindle cells. Central part of lesion.

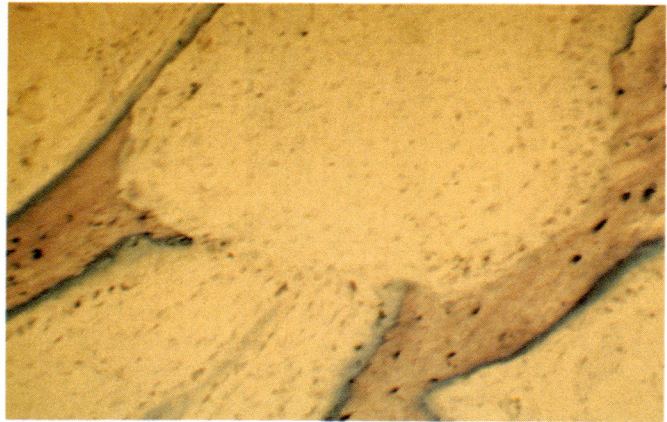

Fig. 27.38 Primary hyperparathyroidism. Osteoclastic bone resorption has produced a large Howship's lacuna in each of the bone trabeculae. The remaining bone surfaces are the site of osteoid deposition. Undecalcified section stained with toluidine blue.

Secondary hyperparathyroidism can usually be distinguished from primary, in the untreated patient, because there is also evidence of osteomalacia in the former, together with a mode of osteoclastic activity which leads to 'dissecting' or 'tunnelling' resorption.

Increased osteoclastic activity is recognized by the presence of an increased number of osteoclasts per unit length of bone surface and of Howship's lacunae cut into the surfaces of bone trabeculae. Tunnelling resorption results from osteoclasts resorbing the central part of a trabecula along the long axis of the bone struts. Undecalcified sections will show that this occurs usually when the trabecular surfaces are covered by a thick layer of osteoid. Osteoblasts are usually also increased in number and the proportion of bone surface covered by osteoid is correspondingly increased. Some of the osteoblasts may be found in Howship's lacunae, replacing bone which has been resorbed.

Where bone resorption is followed by new bone apposition, the limit of the bone removal is marked by a cement line (in this situation sometimes called a 'reversal' line). When the hyperparathyroid condition has been present for more than a few months the increased number of cement lines and their abnormal configuration can be appreciated. It is unusual for the distribution of the cement lines to be so abnormal as in Paget disease of bone (the 'mosaic' appearance), but it has been de-

scribed as 'pseudo-mosaic', reflecting the close similarity. After successful treatment of hyperparathyroidism, the abnormal cement lines remain for many years after the other indications of bone disease have disappeared.

When osteoblasts and osteoclasts are active, the marrow tissue adjacent to the active cells usually contains fibrous tissue. In hyperparathyroid bone disease this fibrous tissue usually forms a thin sheet covering the active cells and normal fatty and haematopoietic tissue remains in the centre of the inter-trabecular space. This contrasts with the appearance of active Paget's disease, when the whole marrow space is occupied by vascularized fibrous tissue.

In the fibrous tissue, trabeculae of immature bone may form—intramembranous ossification—and this appears to be more common in areas where bone resorption has greatly exceeded the apposition of lamellar bone and is a constant feature of the focal lesions.

As mentioned above, primary and secondary hyperparathyroidism can usually be distinguished in the abnormal bone. In primary disease the total amount of osteoid will be increased because there are more osteoblasts, but the matrix mineralizes correctly, so no osteoid layer contains more than four brightly birefringent lamellae. There is a delay in, or complete failure of, mineralization of the osteoid in secondary hyperparathyroidism and many of the osteoid seams contain five or more brightly birefringent lamellae. Sometimes the primary abnormality producing the hyperparathyroid state can be suggested on the basis of the thickness of the osteoid. In renal failure, the osteoid seldom consists of more than 11 lamellae, whereas in D-deficiency forms of osteomalacia there are often 12 or more lamellae in some of the osteoid deposits.

Although hyperparathyroid bone disease affects the whole skeleton, the changes are not of uniform intensity throughout. In particular, there may be focal areas in which bone is totally removed and replaced by fibrous tissue in which there are numerous giant cells of osteoclast type and sufficient haemosiderin pigment to give the lesion a distinctive colour, which has earned the lesion the description of 'brown' tumour

(Fig. 27.39). This lesion may be confused histologically with giant-cell tumour (osteoclastoma) of bone. The histo-pathological features which distinguish a 'brown' tumour are the spindle cell nature of the tissue between the giant cells, the large amount of haemosiderin pigment, the presence of reactive bone trabeculae around the periphery of the soft-tissue mass, and the changes of hyperparathyroidism in the surrounding bone (Fig. 27.40). Brown tumours are often multiple and are commonly diaphyseal in location (Fig. 27.41). There may be radiological evidence of hyperparathyroidism and there will be biochemical abnormalities. The serum calcium, phosphorus, and alkaline phosphatase must always be checked before a diagnosis of osteoclastoma can be firmly established.

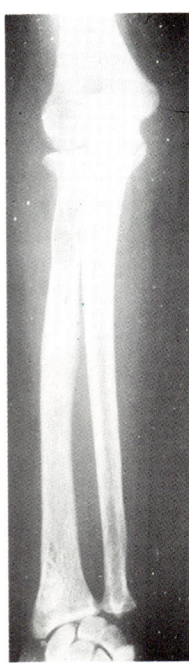

Fig. 27.41　Hyperparathyroidism; radiograph of forearm. Three 'brown tumours' in radius and general abnormality of bone texture.

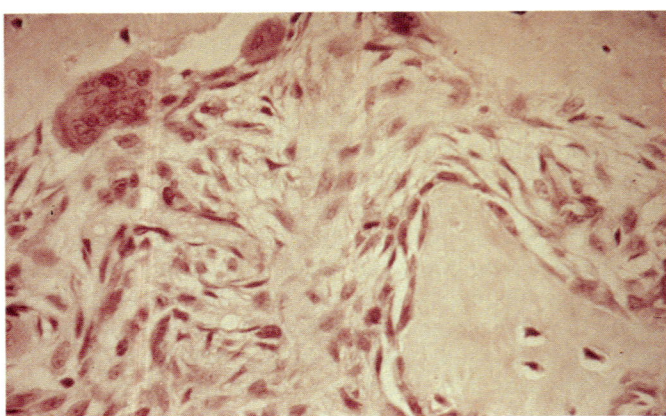

Fig. 27.40　Hyperparathyroidism; 'brown tumour'. Peripheral part of lesion showing predominantly spindle cell tissue, part of a trabecula of reactive bone, and osteoclastic resorption of enclosing bone.

When a patient with vitamin-D-deficiency osteomalacia is established on adequate therapy there will be a phase in the skeletal response when osteoblasts and osteoclasts are increased in number and the appearances will resemble secondary hyperparathyroidism. This phase begins at about the second week of treatment and is indicated by a rise in the level of the patient's serum alkaline phosphatase.

Paget disease

The inclusion of Paget disease with metabolic bone disorders is a matter of convenience and is justified only on the tenuous grounds that the disease process is the result of greatly increased ostoclastic and osteoblastic activity. It is never a truly generalized disorder, and in many patients appears to be monostotic.

There have been, in recent years, suggestions that the disease is due to the presence of viral bodies in the nuclei of osteoclasts. The original interpretation of the nuclear inclusions was that they were derived from the measles virus and this was followed by the suggestion that the respiratory syncytial virus was responsible. There is as yet no evidence, other than the morphological appearances, that the disease is viral induced.

The condition appears to occur only in the mature skeleton and patients are usually over 40 years of age when they present for treatment. Many people have asymptomatic lesions and the true incidence of the disease is not known. Different races have different disease incidence and there are local geographical variations. The indigenous population of the United Kingdom and their descendants in Commonwealth countries have a relatively high incidence (about 2.5 per cent of the population at risk) and there is a higher incidence in parts of north-west England than in any other area of the UK. The incidence decreases from northern to southern Europe. Arabic and Asiatic people are rarely affected. These observations suggest a genetic factor, the mode of action of which is not known.

Skeletal involvement is mainly in those bones that normally contain haematopoietic tissue in adult life, a useful aid to remembering the distribution of lesions, but of no other known significance. Peripheral long bones and the hands and feet are also susceptible.

The disorder appears to start with excessive bone resorption and the appearance of a large number of osteoclasts on bone surfaces. This is an assumption based on the observation that lesions which are actively enlarging are osteolytic at the advancing edge. Increased osteoblastic activity follows and active lesions usually have bone surfaces on which Howship's lacunae containing osteoclasts alternate with smooth bone surfaces with a covering of osteoid and plump osteoblasts. This cellular activity is disordered. Bone trabeculae become very irregular in thickness and Haversian canals irregularly enlarged. Bone is laid down on the periosteal surface. The result is a bone which is enlarged overall and has a grossly disordered trabecular structure, which is no longer orientated by mechanical considerations (Fig. 27.42). Long bones becomes bowed. Microscopic structure of the bone is also abnormal, the collagenous matrix being disposed as relatively short bundles at differing angles one block to another. These blocks of matrix are separated by cement lines and the resultant histological appearances is described as a mosaic (Fig. 27.43). While the cells are active the marrow tissue is replaced by fibrous tissue in which there are numerous thin-walled vascular channels (Fig. 27.44).

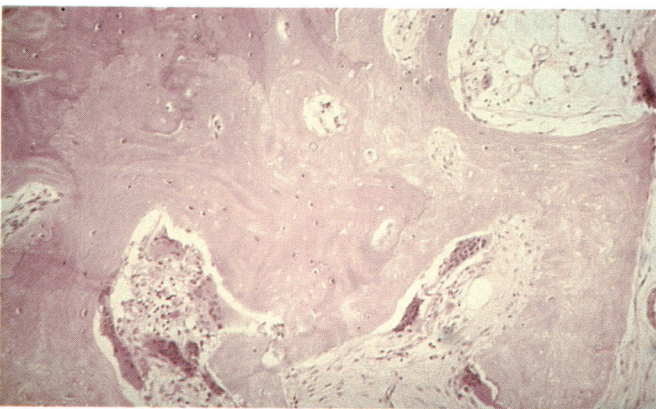

Fig. 27.44 Paget disease. Irregularly shaped bone surfaces on which there are numerous osteoclasts and osteoblasts. The marrow contains fibrous tissue in which there are dilated, thin-walled vascular channels.

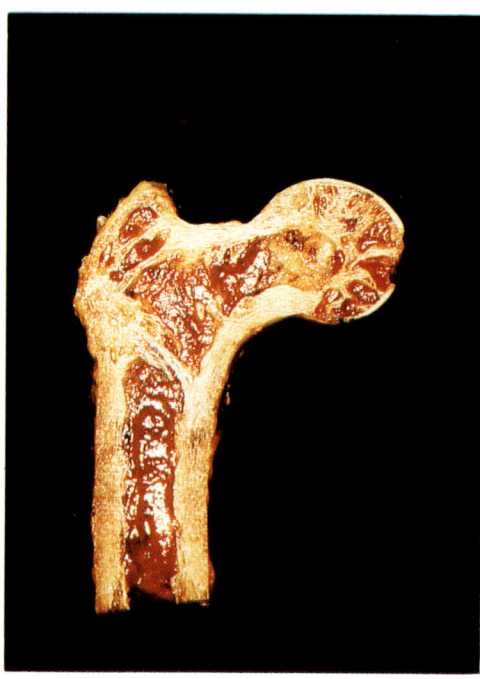

Fig. 27.42 Paget's disease. Proximal femur bisected to show irregular shape of compact and cancellous bone tissue.

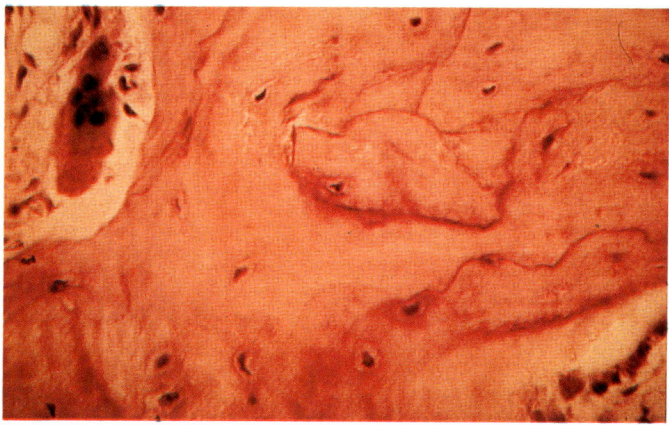

Fig. 27.43 Paget disease. Abnormal arrangement of cement lines producing the mosaic feature.

Spontaneous remission of the disease occurs. Usually only part of the abnormal tissue becomes totally quiescent, relatively large areas may contain a few scattered osteoclasts and active osteoblasts on a small proportion of the bone surface. In these areas, fatty and haematopoietic tissue return to the marrow. Evidence of previous active disease remains in the abnormally shaped trabeculae and the mosaic appearance of the bone matrix. There is no predictable pattern to the activity of the disease. Because of this, the effects of drug treatment on the disease cannot be reliably assessed solely on the basis of bone biopsy appearances.

Active Paget disease causes an elevation in serum alkaline phosphatase and hydroxyproline levels and an increased urinary excretion of hydroxyproline. Although these also fluctuate independently of treatment, they are more reliable indicators of disease activity than a small, random bone biopsy.

Pagetic bone is more fragile because it is both grossly and microscopically mechanically unstable. The affected bone is liable to fracture at both the microscopic and gross levels (Fig. 27.45). Microfractures induce reactive bone formation within the lesion and both trabeculae and compact masses of woven bone are abundant in parts of Pagetic lesions. Complete fractures unite, with the usual pattern of callus formation, if treated appropriately.

Deformity of subarticular bone leads to degenerative arthritis and is a particular problem when the pelvis or proximal femur is involved. The pain due to the arthritis may be the presenting symptom, the patient being unaware of the primary disease. Enlargement of bone may encroach on foramina or the spinal canal. Deafness and spinal nerve deficits occur, and cord compression. The highly vascularized marrow tissue may produce what is effectively an arterio-venous anastomosis and lead to cardiac failure.

Malignant change occurs in a small proportion of cases. The exact incidence cannot be calculated, but is estimated at about 1 per cent of clinical cases. Sarcomatous transformation produces a predominantly radiolucent lesion, which erodes the

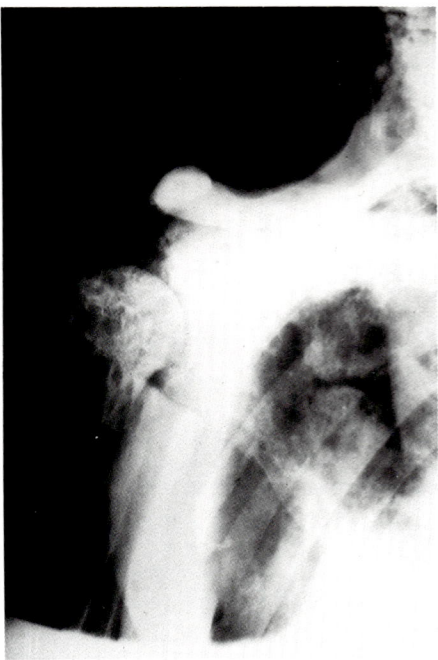

Fig. 27.45 Paget's disease; radiograph. There is a pathological fracture in the proximal diaphysis of the humerus. Both head and shaft of humerus are involved by Paget disease.

bone cortex and infiltrates the extraosseous tissues. The patient may experience severe local pain or present because of pathological fracture. There are a variety of histological patterns presented by the tumour. Some are predominantly osteoblastic, others fibroblastic or giant-cell containing lesions resembling malignant fibrous histiocytoma. Sarcomata showing all these appearances within the same tumour also occur. Predominantly chondroblastic lesions are uncommon, and lesions which could be properly called chondrosarcoma are rare.

Very occasionally a purely osteolytic, sometimes expansile, area will be seen in a Pagetic lesion and will be found to contain a large number of osteoclast-like giant cells separated by vascularized spindle cell tissue of benign appearance. These should not be confused with osteoclast-rich sarcoma; they do not have a sinister significance. Nor should they be confused with true giant-cell tumours, the 'brown' tumours of hyperparathyroidism, or giant-cell reparative granuloma.

Disordered bone modelling and remodelling producing histopathological appearances very similar to those of Paget disease occurs in hyperparathyroid disease; as a developmental abnormality; and as a localized reaction.

Idiopathic hyperphosphatasia

This is one of the sclerosing bone dysplasias and is the result of disordered and excessive activity of both osteoblasts and osteoclasts. The bone is architecturally abnormal and, in some cases, a mosaic arrangement of the bone matrix makes the appearances indistinguishable from Paget disease. The alkaline phosphatase level in the serum is greatly increased. What distinguishes this condition from Paget disease is that it is an inherited condition, manifest in childhood.

Localized disordered bone remodelling

A Paget-like change may be induced in bone in proximity to another lesion, usually one that causes significant changes in the stress pattern in bone. The most common site for this change is in the subchondral bone, beneath an area from which the articular cartilage has been eroded in an osteoarthritic joint, and the femoral head affords frequent opportunities to observe this phenomenon. Bone tumours and tumour-like conditions also lead to disordered remodelling, and fibrous dysplasia is a frequent association. This can be a particularly difficult differential diagnosis to resolve if the patient is adult and the material available for study is a small biopsy.

Fibrogenesis imperfecta ossium

This is a rare disorder of the skeleton characterized by the production of a collagen matrix of abnormal fibre diameter and spacing which does not mineralize correctly. As a result the skeleton becomes extremely fragile, pathological fractures are frequent, and the patient becomes progressively more disabled. Most patients die as an indirect result of their immobility within a few years of the first symptom. Not only is there abnormal collagen formation but the distribution of the tissue is disorganized, resulting in abnormally shaped trabeculae which vary greatly in width. Overall there is loss of mineralized bone. The bones do not increase in diameter, but otherwise appear in radiographs somewhat similar to bone affected by Paget disease. In every patient who has been examined there is an abnormal globulin of myeloma type circulating in the plasma. The significance of this finding has yet to be explained as there is no evidence that the patients have myelomatosis.

The histological appearances are distinctive, provided that the sections are examined in polarized light (Fig. 27.46). There are trabeculae of widely variable thickness, the central parts of

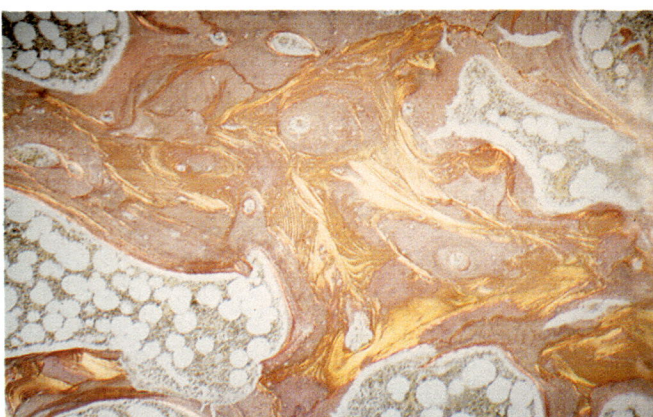

Fig. 27.46 Fibrogenesis imperfecta ossium; decalcified section; polarized light. Parts of the bone show a normal lamellar pattern whereas others appear non-birefringent.

which are composed of lamellar mineralized bone. On the surface there is some birefringent, lamellar osteoid mixed with areas of eosinophilic material, which is very poorly and only patchily birefringent, in which there are small collections of basophilic granules (Fig. 27.47). This basophilic material is calcified and is probably hydroxyapatite. Both osteoclasts and osteoblasts may be present and increased in number but there is no fibrosis of the marrow, nor have abnormal cells been described in the marrow.

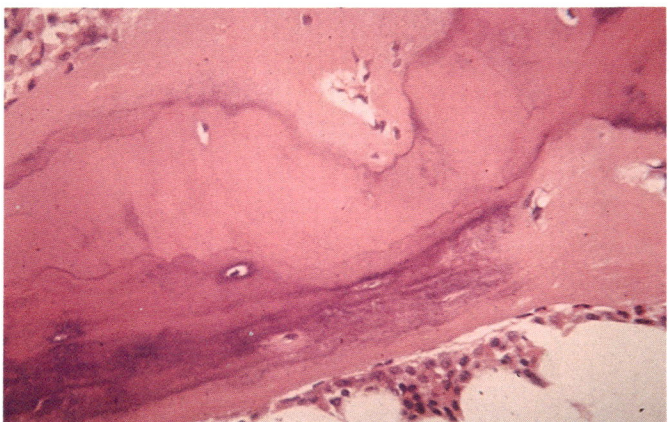

Fig. 27.47 Fibrogenesis imperfecta ossium; decalcified section. There are thick, irregular layers of abnormal pale-staining matrix on both upper and lower surfaces of normal bone. In the lower layer of matrix there is basophilic staining, indicating the site of abnormal calcification.

There is no known treatment for the condition, which runs a relentless course. Because the histological changes are not quantitatively homogeneous throughout the skeleton, claims that treatment has produced some alleviation of the condition on the basis of comparative histological studies must be regarded with caution.

27.1.6 Bone tumours and tumour-like conditions of bone

Primary bone tumours

Introduction and classification

Primary bone tumours are relatively uncommon and malignant primary tumours of bone are distinctly rare; the latter account for less than 1 per cent of all deaths from neoplastic disease. Despite their rarity, a large number of types has been described and classification has proved difficult, largely due to the uncertainty that exists regarding their histogenesis. The classification presented in this chapter is shown in Table 27.7. Essentially, this is based on the path of differentiation that the tumour cells follow and not on the tissue or cell type from which the tumour is thought to have arisen, e.g. osteosarcoma probably does not arise from transformed normal osteoblasts but most likely from multipotential mesenchymal cells or tissue that differentiate predominantly towards osteoblasts in the process of neoplastic transformation. This is evidenced by the production of osteoid or bone by the tumour cells. Not all the tumour cells, however, differentiate towards osteoblasts, as is shown by the phenomenon of cartilage production in osteosarcomas.

Aetiology and predisposing factors

The aetiology of most spontaneously occurring bone tumours is unknown. However, several aetiological factors, including some benign bone conditions, are significantly associated with an increased risk of bone tumour development. Viruses, ionizing radiation, and chemical carcinogens, including beryllium salts and carcinogenic hydrocarbons, can cause malignant bone tumours in experimental animals. Ionizing radiation is also known to cause malignant bone tumours in man. Large bone infarcts of long bones have been associated with an increased incidence of primary malignant bone tumours, particularly osteosarcoma, fibrosarcoma, and malignant fibrous histiocytoma. Trauma has not been shown to be a significant aetiological factor. Paget disease predisposes to the development of malignant bone tumours, but the overall incidence of this occurrence is probably less than 1 per cent. Fibrous dysplasia, particularly the polyostotic type, has also uncommonly been complicated by the development of a bone sarcoma. Both enchondromatosis and hereditary osteochondromatosis (hereditary multiple exostoses) are associated with an increased risk of chondrosarcoma development. It should also be recalled that chronic suppurative osteomyelitis with recurrent or persistent sinus formation can rarely be complicated by the development of squamous cell carcinoma in the lining of the sinus epithelium.

Clinical features and diagnosis of bone tumours

Bone tumours present clinically in a limited number of ways. Patients may complain of pain, swelling, or limitation of movement in a bone containing a benign or malignant lesion. Examination may reveal local tenderness or a palpable swelling. Both benign and malignant tumours can also present as a pathological fracture consequent upon replacement of bone by abnormal tissue. There are thus few specific clinical features that reveal whether a bone lesion is benign or malignant, and virtually none that allow accurate classification of a bone tumour. Further investigation is thus always necessary for accurate diagnosis of a suspected bone tumour. For this reason, bone tumour diagnosis is generally a multidisciplinary effort based on all available clinical, biochemical, haematological, and radiological information, as well as the gross and microscopic pathology of the lesion.

Diagnostically, the most important clinical details are the age of the patient and the bone involved by the suspected tumour. In children, a bone tumour is more likely to be primary than metastatic. In adults, however, metastatic bone tumours are far more common than primary malignant tumours. Certain bone tumours or tumour-like conditions also show a strong tendency to occur within a given age-range and are more common at certain sites. A history of factors known to predispose to bone malignancy (ionizing radiation, Paget disease, etc.) should

Table 27.7   Classification of primary bone tumours

1. Bone-forming tumours
    Benign
        (i)   osteoma; enostosis
        (ii) osteoid osteoma; osteoblastoma
    Malignant
        (i)   osteosarcoma
        (ii) parosteal osteosarcoma

2. Cartilage-forming tumours
    Benign
        (i)   chondroma (enchondroma; periosteal chondroma)
        (ii) osteochondroma
        (iii) benign chondroblastoma
        (iv) chondromyxoid fibroma
    Malignant
        (i)   chondrosarcoma
        (ii) mesenchymal chondrosarcoma
        (iii) clear-cell chondrosarcoma

3. Giant-cell tumour of bone

4. Tumours of marrow origin
    (a) Plasma cell myeloma
    (b) Malignant lymphoma

5. Other connective-tissue/neural tumours
    Benign
        (i)   desmoplastic fibroma
        (ii) lipoma
        (iii) neurilemmoma
        (iv) neurofibroma
    Malignant
        (i)   fibrosarcoma
        (ii) malignant fibrous histiocytoma
        (iii) liposarcoma

6. Vascular tumours
    Benign
        (i)   haemangioma
        (ii) lymphangioma
        (iii) glomus tumour
    Intermediate/malignant
        (i)   haemangioendothelioma
        (ii) haemangiopericytoma
        (iii) angiosarcoma

7. Other tumours
    (a) Chordoma
    (b) Adamantinoma of long bones
    (c) Ewing tumour

8. Tumour-like lesions of bone
    (a) Metaphyseal fibrous defect/non-ossifying fibroma
    (b) Fibrous dysplasia
    (c) Histiocytosis X
    (d) Myositis ossificans
    (e) Solitary bone cyst
    (f) Aneurysmal bone cyst
    (g) Other cysts of bone (ganglion, subchondral, epidermal inclusion)

also be sought. A general medical examination should also be carried out if involvement of bone by metastatic tumour is suspected or to search for metastasis from a primary bone tumour.

Useful biochemical investigations include determination of serum calcium, phosphate, alkaline phosphatase, and acid phosphatase, to exclude metabolic bone disease, Paget's disease, or metastatic carcinoma of the prostate respectively. Myelomatosis may also be evidenced by proteinuria, hypercalcaemia, hyperuricaemia, and raised serum globulins with a monoclonal M band. Measurement of serum and urine catecholamines can also confirm the diagnosis of metastatic neuroblastoma in bone. Haematological investigations are essential where there is a suspicion of myeloma, lymphoma, or leukaemia involving bone.

Radiological investigation is essential for the diagnosis of a suspected bone tumour. X-rays indicate the precise location of the lesion within a given bone (i.e. whether diaphyseal, metaphyseal, epiphyseal, cortical, or medullary) as well as the extent of the lesion within bone and soft tissue. Other features such as the size, shape, outline, and content (e.g. areas of calcification or ossification), as well as the reaction of the bone surrounding the lesion, also provide useful diagnostic information. Accurate localization of the lesion in bone can also be achieved using computerized transverse axial tomography. Radioisotope bone scans, most commonly with [99]TC-labelled polyphosphate, indicate areas of active bone formation and are also useful in the diagnosis of a suspected bone tumour, especially of skeletal metastases.

Biopsy, whether by blind-needle aspiration or through an open surgical incision, is always required to establish the correct diagnosis and treatment of a suspected bone tumour. Histopathological diagnosis of bone tumours is difficult and requires an adequate biopsy from a representative part of the lesion. Frozen section can be performed on softer areas of the lesion to immediately determine the above, as well as to allow rapid diagnosis. Frozen sections, as well as cytological imprints of the tumour, can also be used for enzyme histochemistry and immunohistochemistry. The latter can also be performed on fixed decalcified material. It is also possible for tissue received fresh to be optimally fixed for electron microscopy.

Bone-forming tumours

Osteoma

This term includes a group of slow-growing, possibly hamartomatous benign lesions composed of mature bone with a predominantly lamellar structure.

The classical 'ivory' osteoma is found in the skull and facial bones near the external surface of the bone. Most are tiny and asymptomatic but the lesion can grow into the orbit and paranasal sinuses and cause obstructive symptoms in the cranial cavity or a neighbouring air sinus. They may also be seen as part of Gardner syndrome (intestinal polyposis, osteoma, and soft tissue tumours, see Chapter 16). Osteomas are radio-opaque, well-defined lesions. They are usually composed of dense lamellar bone with Haversian systems but may also contain immature bone (Fig. 27.48). Excision is indicated if the lesions are symptomatic.

An enostosis (bone island) is an osteoma found in medullary cancellous bone. They are most commonly found in the femur or tibia and are generally less than 1 cm in diameter. They are clinically insignificant and are not uncommonly seen in bone radiographs as round, distinct radio-opacities. Rarely, they can increase in size and it is then necessary to distinguish them from osteoid osteoma or an osteosclerotic bone metastasis. Histologically, they are composed of mature lamellar compact bone which merges with surrounding cancellous bone. Unlike 'ivory' osteomas, they do not protrude from the bone surface or alter the bone contour.

Osteoid osteoma and osteoblastoma

Osteoid osteoma is a relatively common benign lesion found usually in the diaphysis or metaphysis of any bone but especially in the long bones of the lower limbs of children or young adults. Males are more commonly affected than females. Characteristically, the patient complains of severe, well-localized pain and tenderness, often worse at night and relieved by salicylates. Swelling and redness may accompany superficial lesions and there may be focal muscle atrophy. Joint effusion with reactive synovitis may occur if the lesion is intracapsular. Vertebral lesions may be accompanied by muscle spasm and a consequent painful scoliosis. Radiologically, there is a localized central area of bone density (the nidus) surrounded by a thin lucent zone and a prominent but variable surrounding bone sclerosis (Fig. 27.49). Grossly, it is a well-defined, soft, fleshy, pink tumour, one centimetre or less in diameter, surrounded by a zone of dense sclerotic bone (Fig. 27.50). Microscopically, the lesion has a cellular and highly vascular stroma in which there are plump osteoblast-like cells forming osteoid and immature bone in a disorganized fashion (Fig. 27.51). Osteoclastic resorption is seen on the surface of the bone trabeculae. Cartilage is never produced in this lesion and the bone-forming cells show no atypical features. The surrounding bone appears sclerotic.

Osteoblastoma (synonyms: ossifying fibroma, giant osteoid

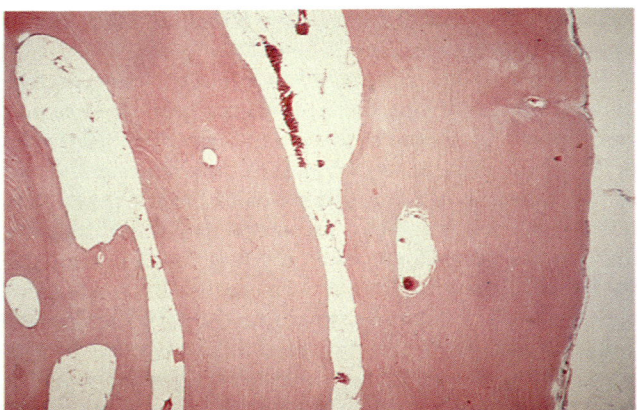

Fig. 27.48 Osteoma; compact or 'ivory' type. A mass of compact lamellar bone with Haversian canals of different diameters.

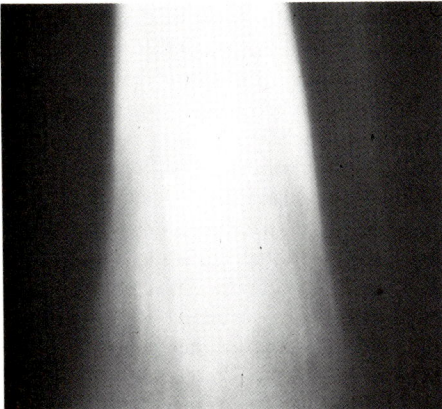

Fig. 27.49 Osteoid osteoma; radiograph (tomogram). Osteolytic area with central calcified nidus. Sclerosis of bone around the osteolytic focus.

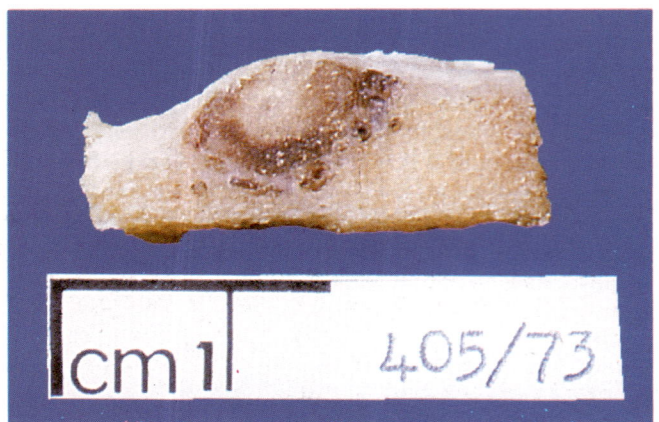

Fig. 27.50 Osteoid osteoma; bisected resection specimen. Osseous 'nidus' surrounded by vascularized tissue.

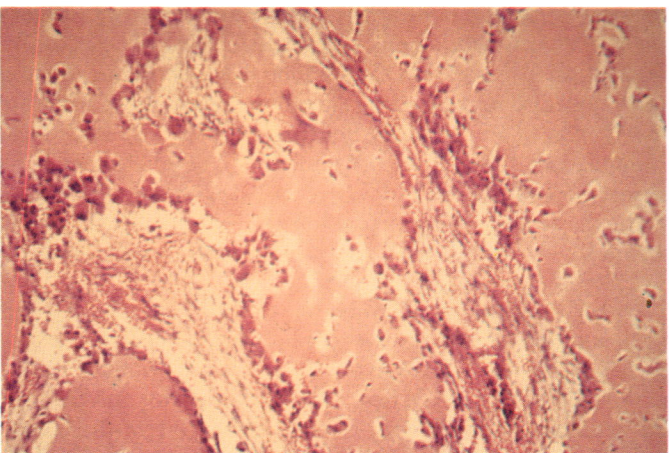

Fig. 27.52 Benign osteoblastoma. Large irregular masses of osteoid with included osteocytes. Plump osteoblasts cover most of the osteoid surfaces.

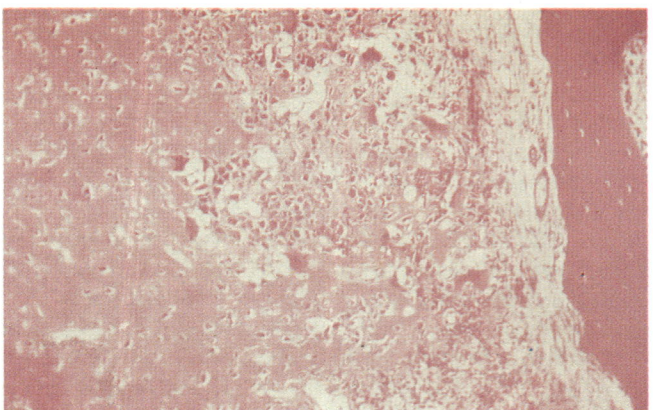

Fig. 27.51 Osteoid osteoma. The lesion consists of irregular trabeculae of bone with osteoclasts and osteoblasts on the bone surfaces. Vascularized fibrous tissue, also part of the lesion, abuts on normal bone (right).

but do not metastasize, are termed aggressive osteoblastomas. These lesions are often more cellular and osteoblasts show nuclear and cellular pleomorphism with increased mitotic activity.

Both osteoid osteoma and osteoblastoma are cured by total excision. Incomplete removal may be followed by recurrence. The above lesions must not only be differentiated from each other but also other bone-forming lesions, particularly osteosarcoma. A solitary enostosis or chronic bone abscess may resemble osteoid osteoma radiologically but these are easily distinguished histopathologically.

Osteosarcoma

Osteosarcoma is a malignant primary tumour of bone characterized by the formation of osteoid or bone by tumour cells. Although an uncommon neoplasm, it is nevertheless the most common of all primary malignant bone tumours (if myeloma is excluded).

Osteosarcomas arise most often in adolescents and young adults. In older patients it may be associated with Paget disease of bone or local irradiation therapy. Males are affected more commonly than females, by a ratio of 2:1.

Osteosarcomas most commonly arise in the medullary cavity of the metaphysis of long bones, particularly the lower end of femur, upper end of tibia or femur, and upper humerus. They may, however, arise in any bone, including bones of the axial skeleton, especially when associated with Paget disease. Paget disease is also most commonly associated with the development of multifocal osteosarcoma. Rarely, synchronous development of multifocal osteosarcomas has been reported in the absence of Paget disease; this typically occurs in childhood and adolescence and has a poor prognosis. Multifocal metachronous osteosarcomas also occur and, unlike the synchronous type, are found predominantly in older patients and have a better prognosis. Osteosarcoma also occurs in patients who have survived retinoblastoma removal. In these osteosarcomas, as in retino-

osteoma) closely resembles osteoid osteoma histologically but is distinguished largely on the basis of clinical and radiological features. These include its larger size (more than 1 cm), equal sex incidence, and preferential involvement of flat and short bones, especially the vertebrae and bones of the hands and feet. Other affected sites include the long bones of upper and lower limbs and skull and jaw bones. Clinically, bone pain is usually dull and poorly localized, and there is often a detectable swelling. Radiological features are non-specific but there is usually expansion of the affected bone. The lesion is radiolucent or variably sclerotic and radiolucent. The normal bone reaction around an osteoblastoma is variable but does not usually show dense sclerosis. Histologically, the lesion closely resembles osteoid osteoma (Fig. 27.52). The pattern of osteoid and bone production, as well as the amount of cellularity and vascular stroma, is variable throughout the lesion. Rarely, mitotic figures are seen but frankly atypical mitoses are never seen. Osteoblastomas which exhibit local invasion and tend to recur, blastoma there is reduction to hemizygosity of the RB locus on the long arm of chromosome 13 (see Chapter 9).

Clinically, there is a relatively short history of pain or limitation of movement associated with a tender swelling and increase in local heat. Pathological fractures are relatively uncommon. Serum alkaline phosphatase is elevated in about 50 per cent of patients.

Radiologically, there is evidence of bone destruction and tumour expansion with subperiosteal extension, cortical perforation, and invasion of surrounding soft tissues (Fig. 27.53). A characteristic radiological sign (Codman's triangle) is produced when the tumour breaks through the periosteum and a triangle is formed by the remaining bone cortex, the elevated periosteum, and the advancing tumour mass. In addition, long fine spicules of bone are laid down at right angles to the elevated periosteum, producing a pattern of radiating 'sun-burst' spiculation. These signs are not specific for osteosarcoma and may be seen with any aggressive tumour or even in benign conditions.

By the time of diagnosis, most osteosarcomas are large tumours which extensively involve the medulla and have penetrated through the cortex into surrounding soft tissue. The tumour tissue is generally grey-white and often contains areas of necrosis, haemorrhage, and cystic degeneration (Fig. 27.54a, b). The appearance and consistency depends largely on the relative amount of bone, osteoid, cartilage, or fibrous tissue produced by the tumour cells. Sclerosing tumours show abundant bone and osteoid production; they are hard and obviously contain calcified material. Osteolytic tumours,

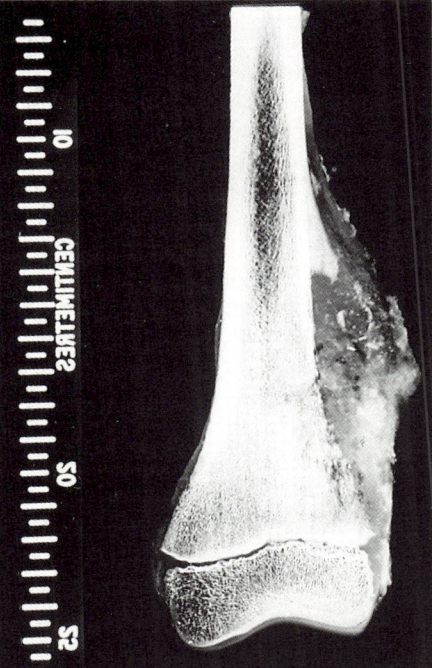

(a)

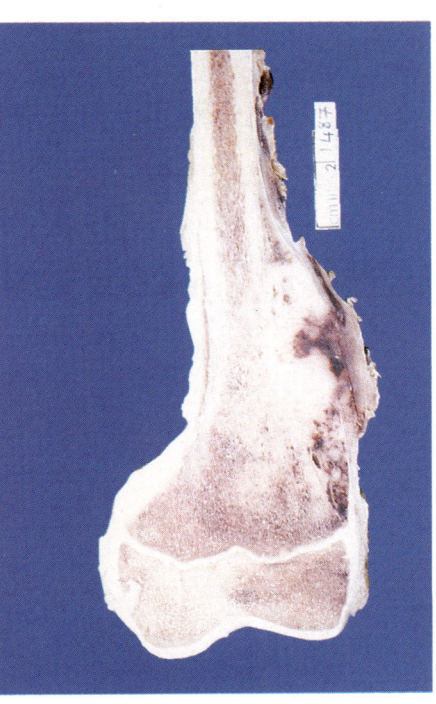

(b)

Fig. 27.54 (a) Osteosarcoma; radiograph of a coronal slice through the distal femur. A tumour in the metaphysis is extending through and destroying the cortex on the lateral side (right). At the proximal end of the soft-tissue extension of the lesion there is a triangular-shaped area of bone projecting from the cortical surface—a 'Codman's triangle'. (b) Photograph of same specimen as (a).

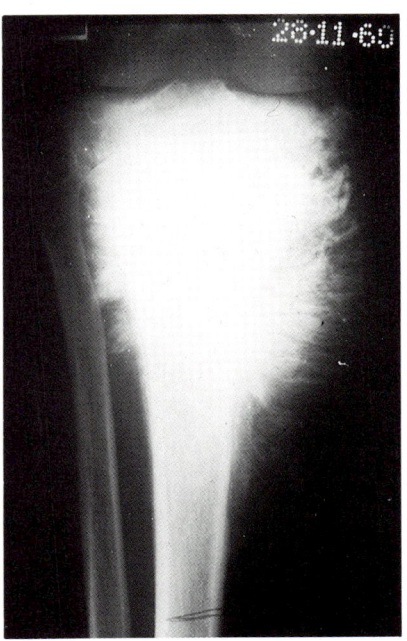

Fig. 27.53 Osteosarcoma; radiograph upper tibia. Osteoblastic lesion in metaphysis and diaphysis extending into soft tissues and producing a 'sun-ray' spicular appearance.

however, contain little ossified tumour tissue and are softer. Most osteosarcomas usually contain areas of both sclerosing and osteolytic tumour tissue. Areas of chondroid differentiation within the tumour appear glistening white or blue-grey. Highly vascular tumours with little evidence of tumour bone formation appear as haemorrhagic, often multicystic tumours. Osteosarcomas rarely involve the joint space. Extension through the cartilaginous growth plate is also uncommon but can occur, particularly in older adolescents reaching skeletal maturity.

Histopathologically, the essential feature that distinguishes an osteosarcoma is the production of bone or osteoid by malignant tumour cells (Fig. 27.55). Within this context, however, the microscopic pattern is highly variable. Poorly differentiated tumours are composed of highly pleomorphic cells with large, abnormal, hyperchromatic nuclei showing increased mitotic activity (Fig. 27.56). Tumour giant cells are occasionally seen. Well-differentiated tumours contain relatively well-organized bone, with a few tumour cells often in the intertrabecular tis-

sue. The tumour may contain a variable amount of cartilage, fibrous, or myxoid tissue. Such low grade tumours may superficially resemble fibrous dysplasia, desmoplastic fibroma, osteoblastoma, or chondromyxoid fibroma. Osteoid or bone formation and evidence of invasion is, however, invariably present. Osteosarcomas are often described histopathologically as osteoblastic, chondroblastic, or fibroblastic, depending on which tissue element predominates. Osteosarcomas may also be highly vascular and contain large vascular spaces surrounded by pleomorphic tumour cells and scattered osteoclast-like giant cells. This 'telangiectatic' variant of osteosarcoma may show little osteoid or bone formation and must be distinguished from aneurysmal bone cyst and other giant-cell lesions of bone (Fig. 27.57).

The many different tissues that may be present in an osteosarcoma may lead to difficulty in histopathological diagnosis. It is especially important to distinguish tumour bone formation from reactive bone formation, e.g. in exuberant fracture callus or Paget disease. Cartilaginous tumours may also show evidence of endochondral ossification and this may be confused with tumour bone formation. Benign bone-forming lesions and lesions of tumours showing reactive bone formation in their stroma, e.g. fibrous dysplasia, giant-cell tumour of bone, must also be distinguished from osteosarcoma.

Osteosarcomas are aggressive tumours with poor prognosis (5–20 per cent five-year survival rate). Metastases occur early via the bloodstream to the lung, viscera, and other bones. Osteosarcomas of the jaw and distal skeleton have a better prognosis. Treatment usually involves surgery and chemotherapy.

Periosteal or peripheral osteosarcoma is a rare distinct entity, which arises on the surfaces of long bones, especially the tibia and femur of children. They are characterized radiologically by an ill-defined radiolucent soft-tissue swelling with periosteal new bone formation at right angles to the underlying bone cortex. Histopathologically, they are osteosarcomas with prominent malignant cartilage formation. The prognosis is better

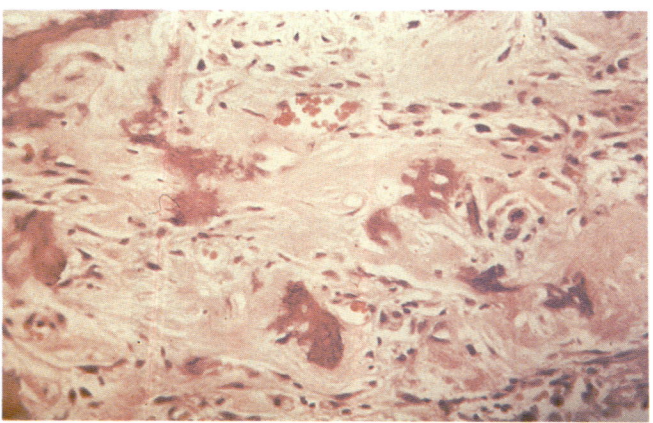

Fig. 27.55 Osteosarcoma. Amongst the neoplastic cells there are irregularly shaped deposits of matrix, part osteoid (pink-staining) and part mineralized (basophilic-staining).

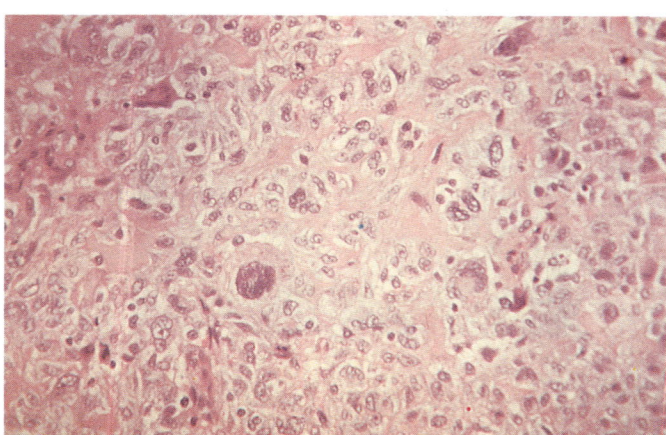

Fig. 27.56 Osteosarcoma. Highly cellular, pleomorphic tumour in which there are irregular thin strands of eosinophilic matrix between malignant cells.

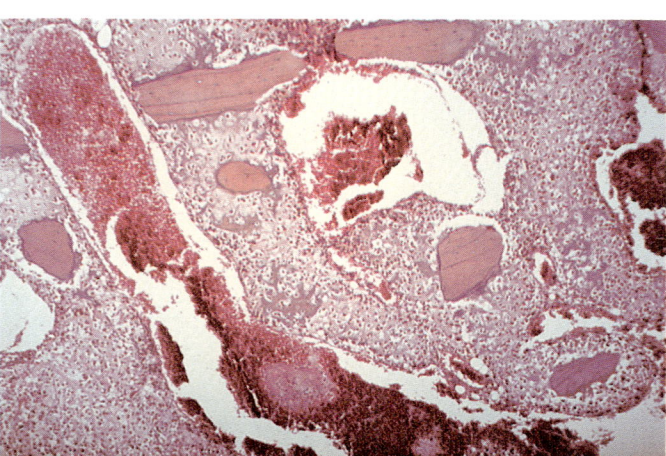

Fig. 27.57 Osteosarcoma. Within the tumour there are numerous dilated blood-filled channels. The 'telangiectatic' form of osteosarcoma.

than for typical osteosarcomas. This entity closely resembles juxtacortical chondrosarcoma.

Parosteal (juxtacortical) osteosarcoma

This is a rare type of osteosarcoma which arises in the subperiosteal region. It is distinguished from medullary osteosarcoma on the basis of its occurrence in an older age-group (young to middle-aged adults), equal sex incidence, its site of origin, well-differentiated microscopic appearance, and better prognosis. The tumour most commonly arises in the metaphysis of a long bone (most commonly the lower femur) and is a hard, lobulated mass which grows towards the periosteum and soft tissues and tends to encircle the shaft (Fig. 27.58). Medullary involvement occurs later and is usually associated with a worse prognosis. Radiological and clinical features are important in the diagnosis of this lesion and its distinction from the benign condition of myositis ossificans. Histopathologically, the tumour is composed of relatively well-ordered bone trabeculae separated by intertrabecular fibrous spindle-cell stroma (Fig. 27.59). Malignant tumour cells or evidence of tumour bone formation may be difficult to find. Foci of cartilage formation are often seen (Fig. 27.60). In distinguishing parosteal osteosarcoma from myositis ossificans it is important to note that peripheral parts of a sarcoma are less well differentiated than more central parts of the tumour. This is the reverse of what is seen in benign lesions, especially those due to trauma, where the most mature tissue is at the periphery. The tumour grows slowly and the prognosis is good provided that the tumour is completely excised.

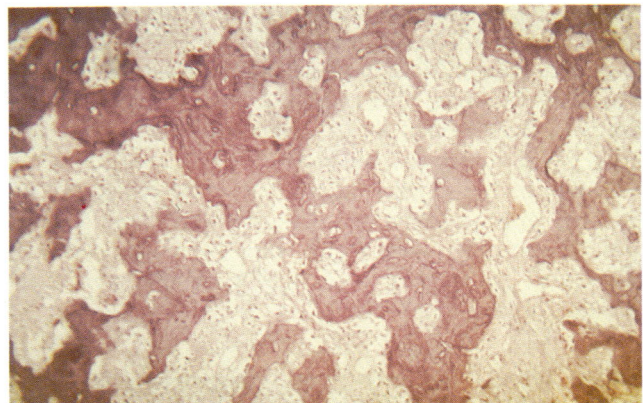

Fig. 27.59 Parosteal osteosarcoma. The lesion consists of relatively well-organized trabeculae and compact masses of bone. Moderately cellular and differentiated spindle-cell tumour fills the intertrabecular spaces.

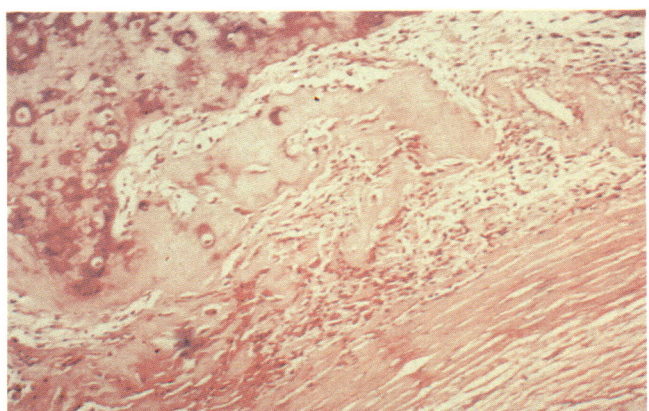

Fig. 27.60 Parosteal osteosarcoma. The lesion abuts on normal fibrous connective tissue (bottom right). In addition to bone, cartilage is also being formed by this tumour (top left).

Cartilage-forming tumours

Chondroma (synonym: enchondroma)

This is a relatively common benign tumour, characterized by the formation of abundant mature hyaline cartilage. Children, adolescents, and young adults are predominantly affected; the sex incidence is equal. Chondromas affect all bones that develop in cartilage and are most commonly found in the medullary cavity of the diaphysis of small bones of the hands and feet, but are also seen less commonly in the ribs and long bones. Chondromas may be single or multiple. If multiple, tumours are present in one or several bones and the condition is called enchondromatosis. If the multiple enchondromas have a predominantly unilateral distribution, the condition is referred to as Ollier disease, and, when multiple chondromas are associated with multiple soft-tissue haemangiomas, as Mafucci syndrome. The above conditions are neither hereditary nor familial. Chondromas arise initially in the metaphysis but

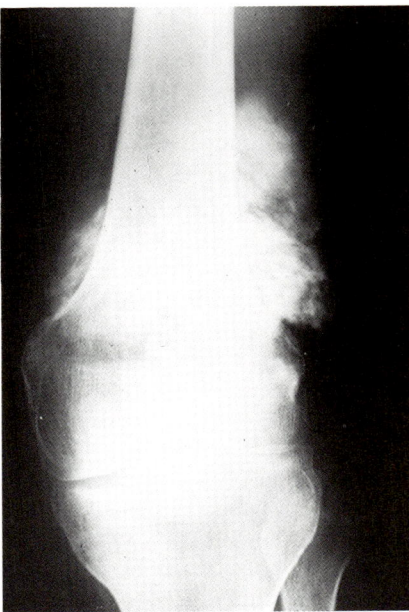

Fig. 27.58 Parosteal osteosarcoma. Radiograph of lower femur and knee joint. The lesion is producing an irregularly and densely ossified mass projecting from the periosteal surface of the femoral diaphysis. An adult patient; the epiphyseal growth plates have closed.

usually enlarge into the diaphysis. They may originate in heterotopic nests of cartilage cells that have been demonstrated in the metaphyseal area of normal bone, and become left behind as growth continues. Clinically, the lesion may be asymptomatic or produce pain, local tenderness, swelling, or pathological fracture. Grossly, the lesion is well circumscribed and composed of bluish translucent cartilage, which is often lobulated and contains focal areas of calcification. These features are also seen radiologically, when the lesion appears as a well-defined radiolucent lesion which expands and slightly thins the cortex (Fig. 27.61).

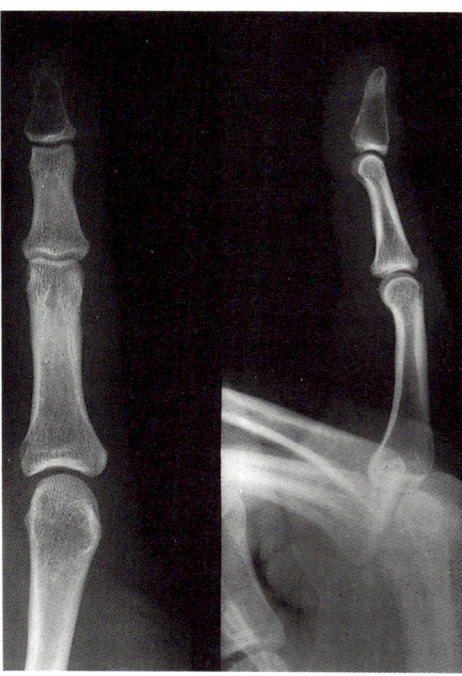

Fig. 27.61 Enchondroma; radiograph of finger. In the centre of the terminal phalanx there is a sharply demarcated translucent lesion. There is bone enclosing the tumour and the diameter of the diaphysis is slightly increased.

Microscopically, mature hyaline cartilage is present with abundant matrix and irregularly scattered cartilage cells (Fig. 27.62). A lobular pattern may be evident. The lesion may be unusually cellular and may contain smaller cells with dark irregular nuclei and occasional binucleate cells; these are particularly evident in peripheral chondromas in children, or in adults with enchondromatosis. Unless the clinical and radiological features indicate otherwise, these features alone are not evidence of malignancy. However, in an adult patient with a cartilaginous tumour showing the same histological features in a more proximally located bone, these features should be regarded as suspicious of malignancy. Focal areas of calcification, necrosis, or myxoid change may also be present, but mitoses are never seen in chondromas. Endochondral ossification is commonly seen.

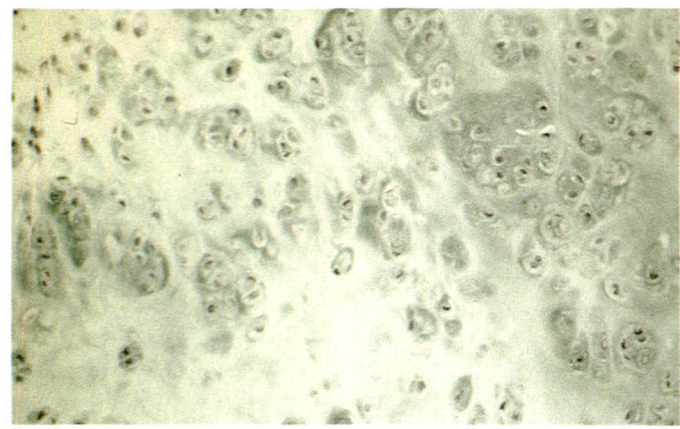

Fig. 27.62 Enchondroma. There is a moderate number of chondrocytes of uniform morphology scattered in the cartilage matrix.

Solitary chondromas rarely undergo malignant change; this occurs almost exclusively in tumours located in flat bones or proximal limb bones and is rare in peripheral locations. A significant percentage of patients with multiple enchondromatosis, however, do develop chondrosarcoma, again mostly in lesions located in flat and proximal limb bones.

Periosteal (juxtacortical) chondroma This is a rare benign cartilaginous tumour lying against the external surface of the bone cortex. The tumour is usually seen in young adults who complain of a slowly enlarging swelling. Grossly, the cartilaginous tumour is well circumscribed and the base may extend into cortical bone (Fig. 27.63). Histological features resemble those of enchondroma but the tumour is covered by fibrous tissue which is continuous with that of the periosteum. As with solitary chondromas, the main differential diagnosis is chondrosarcoma and other cartilage-forming tumours.

Osteochondroma (synonym: cartilage-capped/ osteocartilaginous exostosis)

This is a cartilage-capped bony projection from the external surface of the metaphyseal part of a long tubular bone. This is the most common benign tumour of bone and may be a solitary lesion or occur as part of the generalized autosomal dominantly inherited condition of hereditary multiple exostosis. The pathogenesis of osteochondroma is uncertain but possible origins are from a displaced fragment of growth cartilage which has rotated through 90° and grows transversely to the long axis of the shaft; or from subperiosteal cartilage rests; or herniation of growth cartilage through periosteal defects. The lesion most commonly presents in childhood and adolescence, and may be asymptomatic or present with pain, swelling, and deformity. Osteochondromas may arise in any bone that is formed from cartilage but are most commonly found in the femur, tibia, and humerus.

Macroscopically, the tumour is a sessile or pedunculated bony protuberance, which is covered by periosteum and a cartilage cap not usually more than 1 cm in thickness; generally,

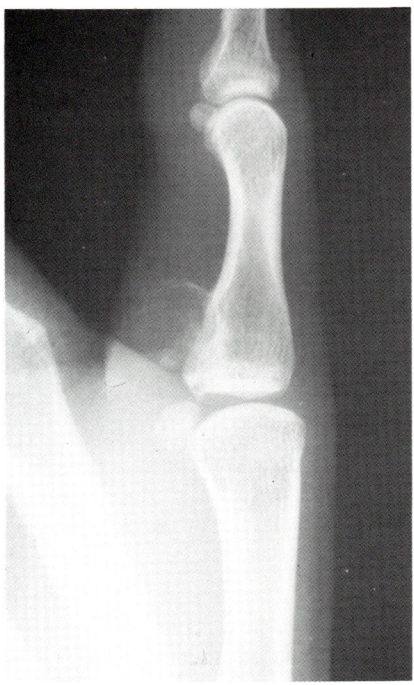

Fig. 27.63 Periosteal chondroma; radiograph of thumb. On palmar surface of proximal end of proximal phalanx, there is a predominantly translucent lesion outlined by a thin shell of calcified tissue. A small, saucer-shaped erosion is present in the cortical bone on the deep surface of the tumour.

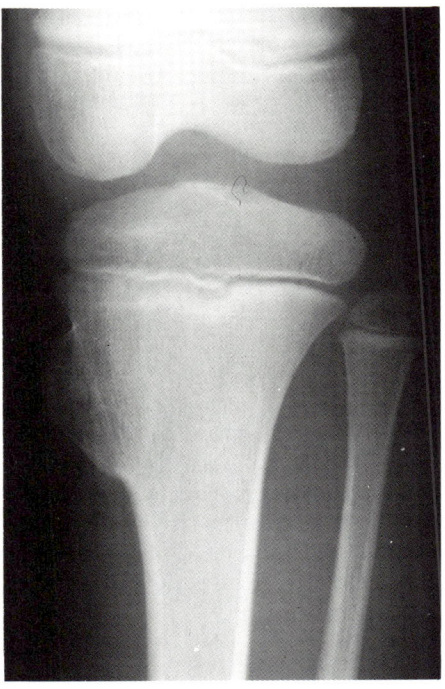

Fig. 27.64 Osteochondroma; radiograph of upper tibia. There is a bony projection from the medial side of the proximal metaphysis. The lesion has a broad base which appears to extend to the growth plate. The cartilage covering the lesion is not visible.

the younger the patient the thicker the cartilaginous cap (Figs 27.64, 27.65). An adventitious bursa may overlie the cartilage cap in the extraskeletal connective tissue. Radiologically, the sessile or pedunculated lesion is of variable size and often points away from the epiphysis. Histopathologically, beneath the fibrous periochondrium, the superficial part of the cartilage cap is composed of a zone of randomly arranged chondrocytes. Beneath this there is a zone of chondrocytes which have a columnar arrangement and undergo irregular endochondral ossification in a manner similar to a growth plate (Figs 27.66, 27.67). The cellularity of the cartilage cap and the extent of endochondral ossification occurring in the lesion is age-related. As with enchondromas, the interpretation of features indicating chondrocyte multiplication, such as binucleate cells, depends on the age of the patient and other clinical and radiological details.

Malignant change (usually chondrosarcoma) is rare in solitary osteochondromas (less than 1 per cent) and is usually first seen in the outer zone of randomly arranged chondrocytes. Malignant change is, however, more common in patients with hereditary multiple exostoses. Surgical removal is only undertaken if the lesion is symptomatic but lesions should be followed radiographically to determine whether there is any increase in size. Differential diagnosis includes not only chondrosarcoma but other cartilage-forming tumours and tumours which contain cartilage elements, such as parosteal osteosarcoma.

Subungual exostosis This is a painful lesion which projects from the distal portion of the terminal phalanx, usually of the great toe. It is thought to arise from osseous or cartilaginous metaplasia in fibrous tissue or the cambium layer of the periosteum following infection or trauma. However, some lesions do have a zonal callus-like arrangement of bone and cartilage,

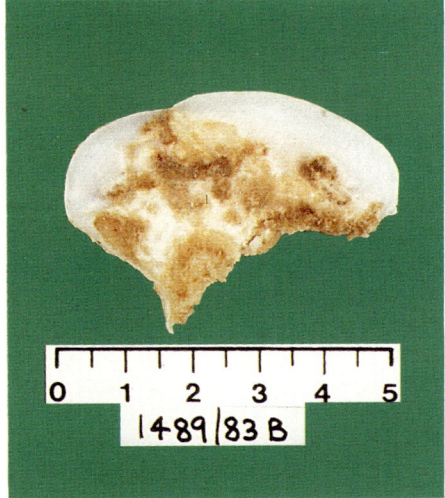

Fig. 27.65 Osteochondroma; bisected excised lesion.

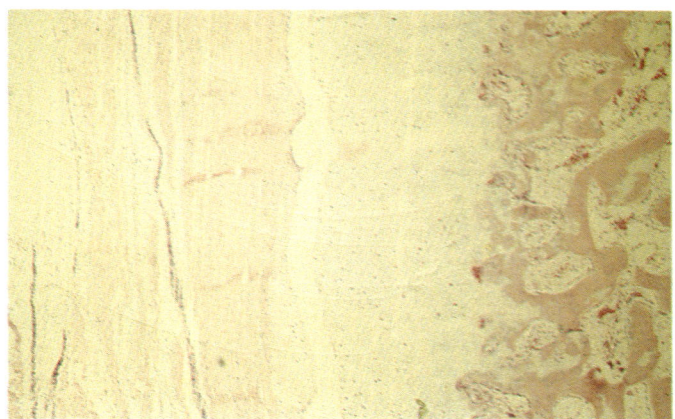

Fig. 27.66 Osteochondroma. Section to show, from the left, loose connective tissue, the fibrous perichondrium sharply demarcated from the cartilage cap, and the bone produced by endochondral ossification at the base of the cartilage.

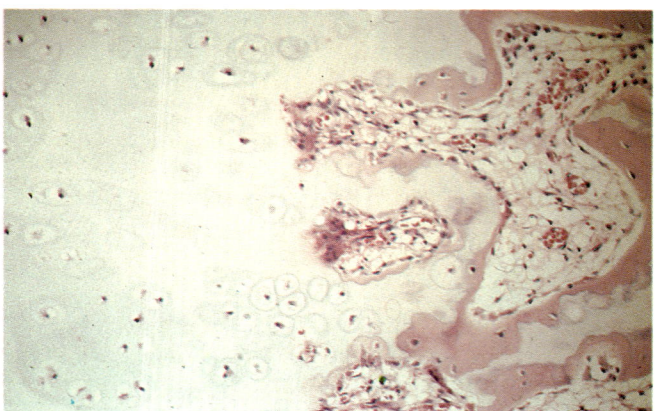

Fig. 27.67 Osteochondroma. The zone of endochondral ossification at the base of the cartilage cap.

with the external surface of the fibrous cartilaginous cap merging with the dermis. Unlike conventional osteochondromas, they grow relatively quickly and are found more often in the mature patient.

Benign chondroblastoma

This is a rare, benign cartilaginous tumour which occurs predominantly in adolescents and young adults; males are more commonly affected than females. The lesion almost always involves the epiphysis and the epiphyseal growth plate, and is found chiefly around the knee joint and upper humerus. Clinically, there may be pain, local tenderness, swelling, or limited joint movement. Radiologically, the tumour is usually a well-demarcated radiolucent lesion, lying entirely within the epiphysis or extending across the epiphyseal line into the metaphysis. (Fig. 27.68). Grossly, the tumour is a well-defined, firm, round or ovoid grey tumour containing calcific material and small nodules of cartilage. Microscopically, the lesion is highly cellular and consists largely of small, round or polyhedral cells

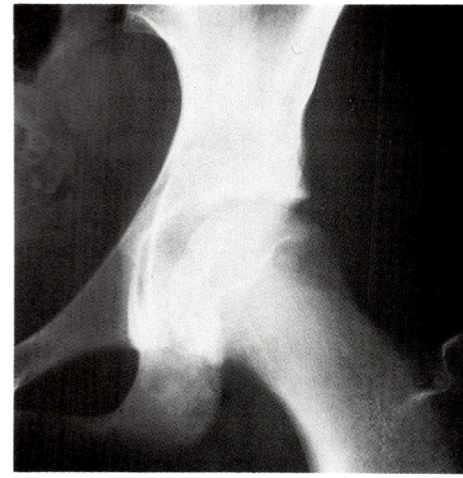

Fig. 27.68 Benign chondroblastoma; radiograph of hip joint. The lesion is situated in the lateral part of the femoral head and neck and extends across the growth plate.

with a thick, well-defined cell membrane and hyperchromatic and variably shaped nuclei. There is a variable amount of amorphous chondroid matrix, which may contain irregular areas of calcification, particularly in areas where the cells appear necrotic and in septa separating the tumour cells. A characteristically delicate 'lacy' pattern of calcification is often seen around individual tumour cells (Fig. 27.69). A moderate number of osteoclast-like giant cells are scattered amongst the tumour cells, usually in relation to calcified cartilage or small areas of haemorrhage within the tumour (Fig. 27.70).

Chondroblastomas must be distinguished from other cartilage-forming tumours and giant-cell-containing bone lesions. The tumour is benign and is usually cured by curettage, although recurrence may follow incomplete removal.

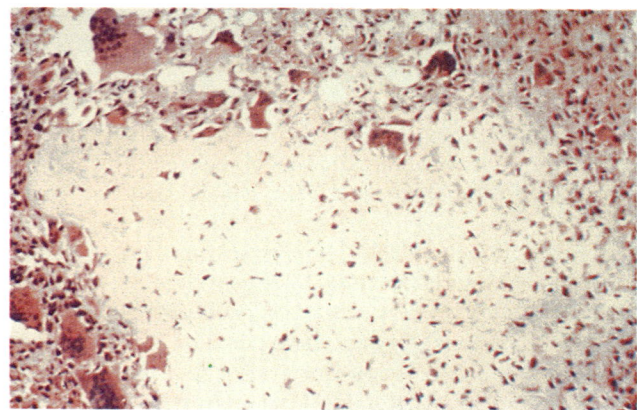

Fig. 27.69 Benign chondroblastoma. The chondroid matrix in the centre contains a moderate number of chondrocytes and merges into more densely cellular tissue on the right. At top and left osteoclast-like giant cells and mononuclear cells abut on to the cartilage matrix.

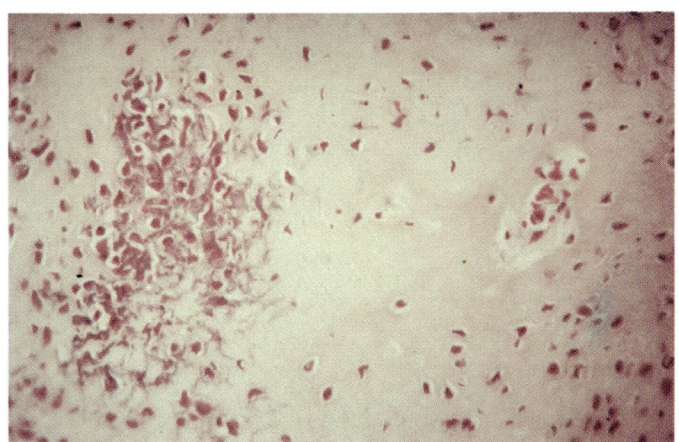

Fig. 27.70 Benign chondroblastoma. In the cellular area (left of centre) there is a fine lace-like deposition of basophilic matrix.

Chondromyxoid fibroma

This is a rare benign cartilaginous tumour arising chiefly in the metaphysis of long bones in young adults and adolescents. Sex incidence is equal. The upper end of the tibia is most commonly involved but other long bones and small bones of the hands and feet may be affected. Clinically, there may be pain, local tenderness, swelling, or limitation of movement. Radiologically, it is an eccentric, well-defined radiolucent lesion producing expansion of the overlying cortex; the epiphysis is usually spared and, even if the lesion is large, does not extend into extraskeletal soft tissue. Grossly, the tumour is firm, lobulated, whitish, large, and well defined. Microscopically, there is a lobular pattern with the lobules composed of abundant, partly vacuolated myxoid or chondroid matrix and scattered spindle-shaped or stellate cells (Fig. 27.71). The lobules are separated by bands of fibrous tissue which contain similar mononuclear cells and a few osteoclast-like giant cells. Mitoses are unusual.

The tumour is benign but local recurrence is quite common after currettage, so wide exicision or block resection is often the treatment of choice. Metastases do not occur. Differential diagnosis includes other cartilage-forming tumours, particularly chondrosarcoma, and other giant-cell containing lesions.

Chondrosarcoma

This is a malignant tumour of cartilage-forming cells and is the second most common primary malignant bone tumour. About 10 per cent arise from known pre-existing benign cartilaginous lesions, particularly osteochondromas, and are often termed 'secondary' chondrosarcomas. Chondrosarcomas occur more commonly in males than females. In contrast to osteosarcoma, chondrosarcomas are extremely rare before skeletal maturity and are seen most often in those older than 30 years. Patients usually complain of pain and swelling. In contrast to the distribution of enchondroma, chondrosarcomas are most common in the more proximal parts of the skeleton, particularly the pelvis, ribs, and proximal long bones.

Chondrosarcomas may be divided grossly by their location in the bone into central (i.e. situated in the medullary cavity) or peripheral types (i.e. attached to the external surface of the bone). Central chondrosarcomas are the more common type. They arise in the metaphysis or diaphysis and are slow-growing, obviously cartilaginous tumours which are firm, translucent or blue-white, and have a lobulated outline (Fig. 27.72). Areas of calcification, ossification, cystic degeneration, and haemorrhage may also be present within the tumour. The tumour expands the bony shaft and invades the cortex, finally extending into soft tissues. Peripheral chondrosarcomas may arise *de novo* in subperiosteal tissue or from malignant change in the cartilage cap of an osteochondroma. These tumours are often large and show extensive calcification

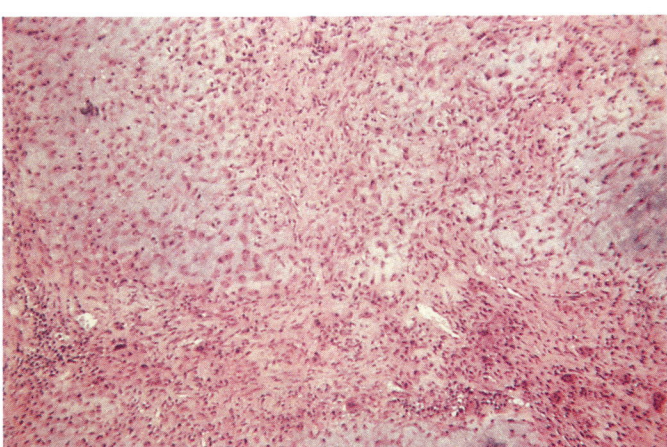

Fig. 27.71 Chondromyxoid fibroma. Round, spindle, and stellate cells in a basophilic, chondroid matrix.

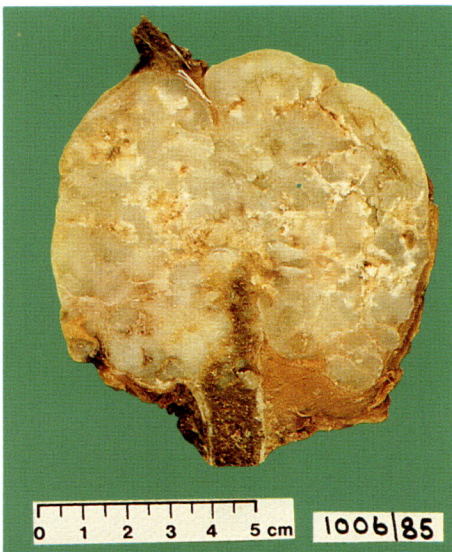

Fig. 27.72 Chondrosarcoma; bisected tumour arising from rib. Nodular pattern of proliferation into muscle (lower right). The irregular streaks of opaque white within the lesion are areas of calcification of cartilage.

and myxoid degeneration. Radiological features mirror the gross changes with irregular destruction and fusiform expansion of the bony shaft, and cortical perforation by a lobulated radiolucent tumour containing focal, large or small, areas of calcification (Fig. 27.73).

Microscopically, slow-growing, well-differentiated chondrosarcomas are often difficult to distinguish from benign cartilage tumours. They consist of an abundant cartilaginous matrix containing scattered, small, round cartilage cells, which may show slight cellular pleomorphism or nuclear variation (Figs 27.74, 27.75). Mitoses are rarely seen in cartilage tumours but occasional binucleate cells are present. None of these histological features is absolutely diagnostic of malignancy, and such minor changes may be acceptable in the small bones of the hands and feet of a child; they are, however, highly suspicious of malignancy if found in the skeleton of an adult. It is therefore important to consider all the available clinical and radiological information, and to closely examine the tumour, particularly the growing edge, for evidence of invasion. Poorly differentiated tumours are highly cellular with numerous pleomorphic and binucleate cells, occasional mitotic figures, and evidence of invasion. Focal calcification and endochondral ossification may be seen in neoplastic cartilage but the direct formation of osteoid or bone by malignant cells, as in osteosarcoma, is never seen.

Chondrosarcomas must especially be differentiated from benign cartilage tumours but, on occasion, may be confused with chordomas or metastatic tumours with an abundant mucinous or myxoid matrix.

Chondrosarcomas grow more slowly and are less malignant than osteosarcomas. Metastasis is generally a late feature, and

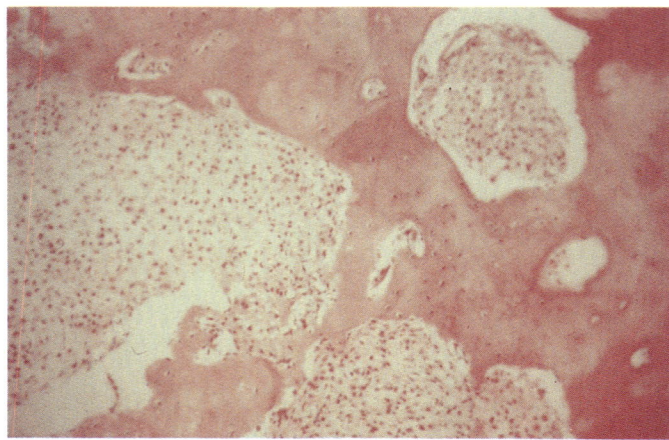

Fig. 27.74 Chondrosarcoma. A highly cellular cartilaginous tumour is infiltrating compact bone.

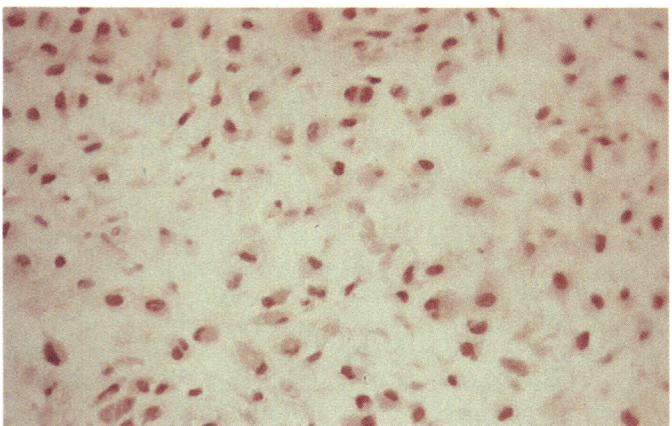

Fig. 27.75 Chondrosarcoma. A moderately cellular lesion with several binucleate chondroblasts indicative of active cellular proliferation.

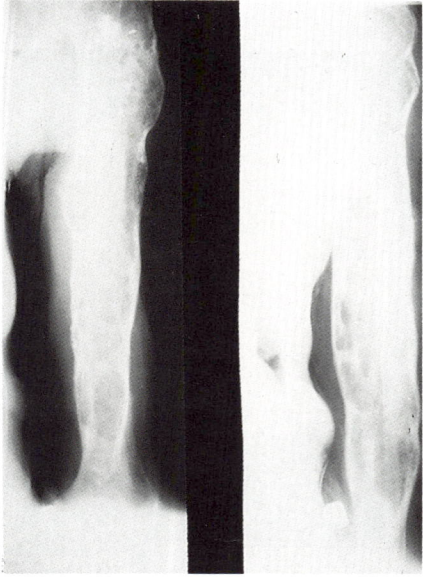

Fig. 27.73 Chondrosarcoma; radiograph of humerus. Virtually the whole bone is expanded by tumour in which there are focal opacities, best seen at the proximal end. Erosion of cortex and extension of tumour into soft tissue is evident on the medial side of the diaphysis.

the prognosis following adequate surgical therapy is better than for other types of malignant bone tumour. In contrast to osteosarcoma, the microscopic degree of differentiation has prognostic value. Low-grade (well-differentiated) chondrosarcomas are slow-growing and uncommonly metastasize, whereas high-grade (poorly differentiated) tumours are rapidly growing and metastasize early via the bloodstream, especially to the lungs. Chondrosarcomas have a marked tendency to directly invade and grow along regional veins. In addition, after biopsy or other surgical manipulation, tumour cells can implant and grow in soft tissues. For this reason, radical excision is often considered in the initial surgical treatment of chondrosarcoma.

Rarely, a poorly differentiated spindle-cell sarcoma component resembling a fibrosarcoma may develop in a primary or, more commonly, recurrent chondrosarcoma previously classified as well differentiated. This change to a 'dedifferentiated' chondrosarcoma considerably worsens the prognosis.

A rare clear-cell variant of chondrosarcoma is also described, characterized by numerous cells with abundant clear, vacuolated cytoplasm and scattered chondroid matrix (Fig. 27.76). There are also stromal cells and benign giant cells similar to those seen in chondroblastoma, of which this may be an aggressive or malignant form. Areas of typical chondrosarcoma may also be present. This variant is a low-grade tumour, usually located in the epiphysis of long bones, particularly the femoral head and upper humerus of adults.

Mesenchymal chondrosarcoma is a specific variant of chondrosarcoma. It can arise in either bone or soft tissues and is often multicentric. It is characterized by areas of well-differentiated cartilage scattered amongst a highly cellular undifferentiated spindle- or round-cell stroma which forms the bulk of the tumour (Fig. 27.77). This variant is a highly aggressive tumour.

Juxtacortical (periosteal) chondrosarcoma This is a rare malignant cartilage-forming tumour arising from the external surface of the shaft of a long bone, most commonly the femur. Grossly, the tumour is lobulated, well defined, and contains areas of spotty calcification and production of bone at right angles to the shaft. Histopathologically, the tumour is a well-differentiated malignant cartilaginous tumour with a lobular pattern; it seldom infiltrates the cortex and contains scattered areas of calcification and endochondral ossification. It resembles closely the entity known as periosteal osteosarcoma but no malignant osteoid production is seen. It must also be distinguished from a periosteal chondroma, and a chondrosarcoma arising in a pre-existing osteochondroma. Prognosis is relatively better than with central chondrosarcomas of a similar grade of malignancy.

Giant-cell tumour of bone (synonym: osteoclastoma)

This is an uncommon osteolytic tumour with characteristic clinical, radiological and histopathological features. It is seen most commonly between the ages of 20 and 50 years, and is rare in patients with open epiphyses. Females are more frequently affected than males. The tumour arises in the epiphysis of a long bone where it usually spreads to involve the metaphysis. It is most common in the lower femur, upper tibia, and lower radius but any bone can be affected. The jaw, pelvis, and vertebral column above the sacrum are rarely involved. Clinically, pain, swelling, and tenderness are most commonly encountered.

Grossly, the tumour is usually an eccentric osteolytic lesion which expands the end of a long bone. The tumour is red or brown, fleshy, and partly friable (Fig. 27.78). There is bone destruction with thinning and expansion of the cortex. Areas of necrosis, haemorrhage, and cyst formation are common. In most cases, the tumour does not penetrate the periosteum and

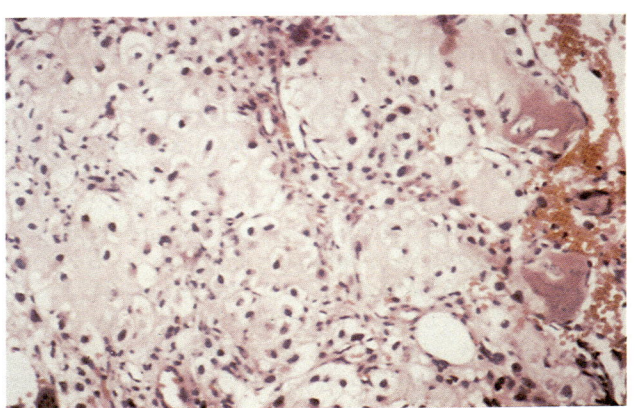

Fig. 27.76 Clear-cell chondrosarcoma. Small nodules of cartilage in which some of the chondrocytes have abundant clear cytoplasm. At the edge of the cartilage (right) there are small foci of bone-like matrix which are in continuity with the cartilage.

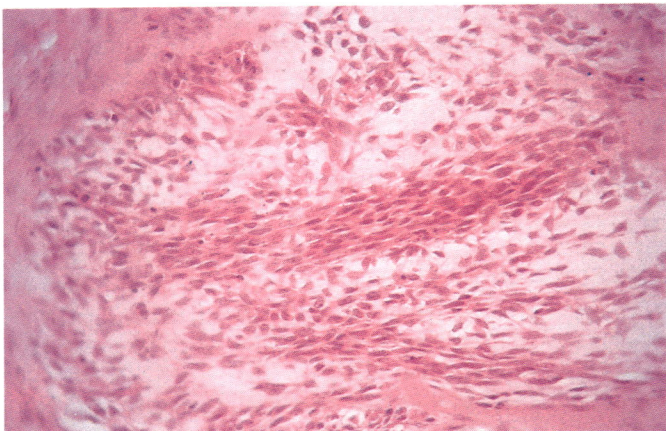

Fig. 27.77 Mesenchymal chondrosarcoma in which there are undifferentiated pleomorphic tumour cells.

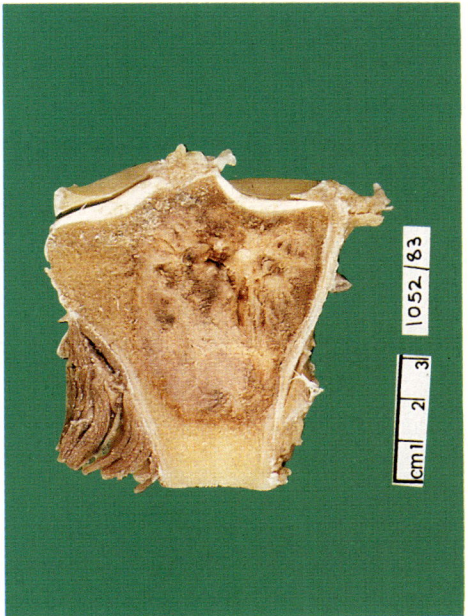

Fig. 27.78 Giant-cell tumour at upper end of tibia.

does not involve the joint. Radiologically, the tumour is a lobu-lated, translucent lesion involving the epiphysis and metaphysis (Fig. 27.79). Generally, there is no sclerotic border or periosteal reaction.

Histopathologically, abundant osteoclast-like giant cells are scattered amongst mononuclear round or spindle-shaped mononuclear stromal cells (Fig. 27.80). The giant cells contain a variable, occasionally huge, number of nuclei; no mitoses or nuclear atypia is seen in these cells. The mononuclear stromal cells alone show mitotic figures and nuclear pleomorphism. The tumour is highly vascular and may contain focal areas of

necrosis, haemorrhage, and osteoid or reactive bone formation. Microscopic grading of these tumours is usually not helpful in predicting behaviour.

All giant-cell tumours are locally aggressive lesions which frequently recur after curettage. For this reason, *en bloc* excision is often the treatment of choice. The concept of malignant giant-cell tumour is controversial. Primary malignant giant-cell tumour is very rare and most reported cases probably represent mistakenly diagnosed cases of telangiectatic osteosarcoma, malignant fibrous histiocytoma, or other sarcomas rich in giant cells. Reported sarcomatous transformation of giant-cell tumours, mostly to fibrosarcoma or less commonly to osteo-sarcoma, is almost always associated with radiation therapy. There is also a small number of reported cases which showed pulmonary metastases from giant-cell tumours that showed no histological evidence of malignancy; these deposits usually remain static or regress.

Giant-cell tumour of bone needs to be distinguished from several other lesions that contain numerous osteoclast-like giant cells (giant-cell variants). The 'brown' tumour of hyper-parathyroidism can so closely resemble giant-cell tumour of bone histologically that serum calcium, phosphorus, and alkal-ine phosphatase should always be determined; a radiological search for subperiosteal erosions should also be carried out if this diagnosis is considered. Many giant-cell variants, including chondroblastoma, aneurysmal bone cyst, simple bone cyst, and non-ossifying fibroma, occur almost exclusively in young patients below the age of 20. Other lesions that should also be considered are giant-cell reparative granuloma (particularly in the jaw and in small tubular bones), chondromyxoid fibroma, eosinophil granuloma, fibrous dysplasia of bone, and increased osteoclast numbers and activity associated with any rarefying bone lesion, e.g. Paget disease, trauma, infection, osteolytic tumours.

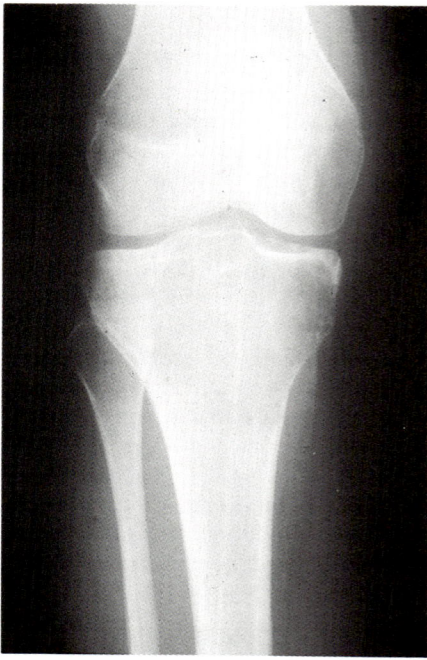

Fig. 27.79   Radiograph of the tumour in Fig. 27.78, showing a well-defined, radiolucent, eccentric lesion.

Tumours of marrow origin

Plasma cell myeloma

This is a neoplastic proliferation of plasma cells in the bone marrow which may be localized (solitary plasmacytoma) or more commonly disseminated (myelomatosis or multiple myel-oma). Plasma cell myeloma is associated wih the monoclonal production of immunoglobulin or immunoglobulin compon-ents and is often accompanied by systemic disease (see also Chapter 23).

Multiple myeloma is the most common of all primary bone tumours. It is rarely seen below 40 years of age and is more common in males. Bones where there is active haemopoiesis (e.g. spine, skull, pelvis, ribs, and upper femur and humerus) are most commonly involved. These contain multiple focal osteolytic lesions; or areas of diffuse marrow replacement pro-ducing bony rarefaction.

Clinically, there may be pain referable to an osteolytic lesion that has caused pathological fracture or pressure effects on the spinal cord or spinal nerves. There are also numerous systemic effects, including weakness, anaemia, a predisposition to infec-

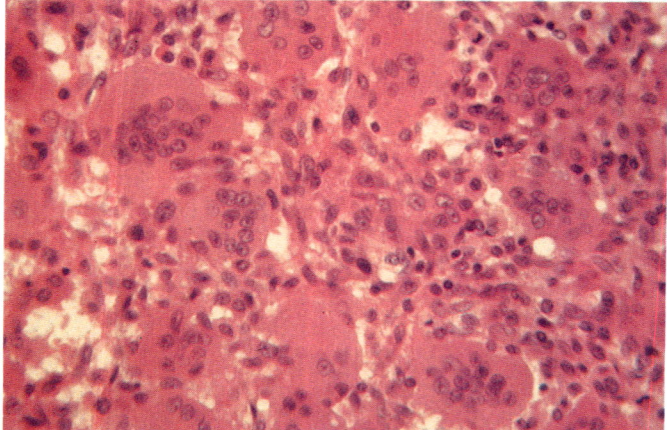

Fig. 27.80   Giant-cell tumour of bone. Large multinucleated giant cells are evenly scattered throughout the lesion and are separated by mononuclear stromal cells.

tions, raised erythrocyte sedimentation rate, clinical effects of hypercalcaemia and amyloid deposition, and numerous renal complications. There may also be extraskeletal spread of myeloma and, rarely, plasma cell leukaemia.

Grossly, myeloma deposits are soft and pink, often with areas of haemorrhage (Fig. 27.81). Focal osteolytic lesions are usually well defined and do not alter the bone shape. Radiologically, the lesions are usually multiple and punched out, with no surrounding bone reaction (Fig. 27.82).

Microscopically, the tumour is composed of sheets of plasma cells of varying degrees of differentiation; there is cellular and nuclear pleomorphism and occasional multinucleate plasma cells may be seen (Fig. 27.83). The cells are pyroninophilic and immunohistochemistry shows the production of immuno-globulin proteins of a single light-chain type. There is usually little stromal connective tissue. Small deposits of amyloid often

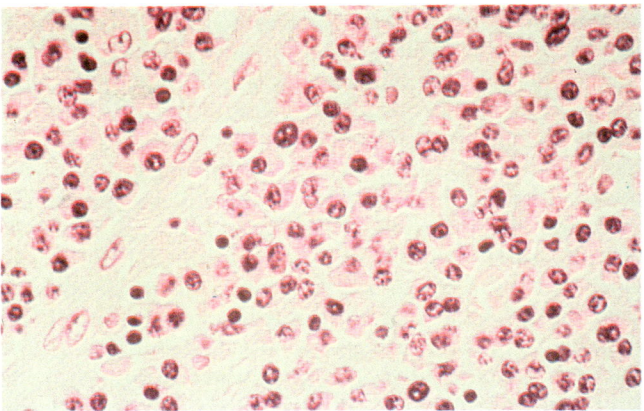

Fig. 27.83 Multiple myeloma cells resemble mature plasma cells but show cellular and nuclear pleomorphism.

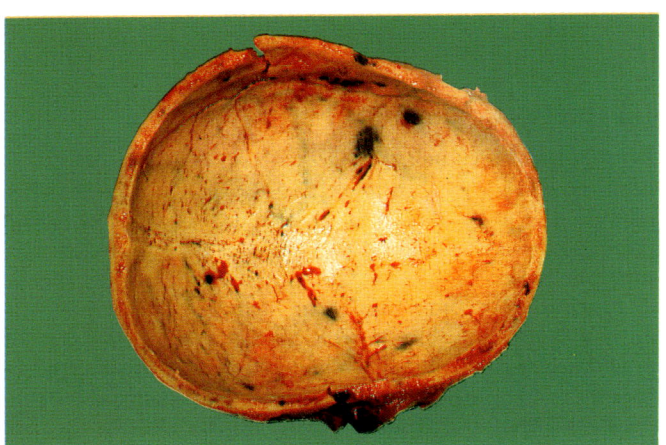

Fig. 27.81 Multiple myeloma deposits in the skull.

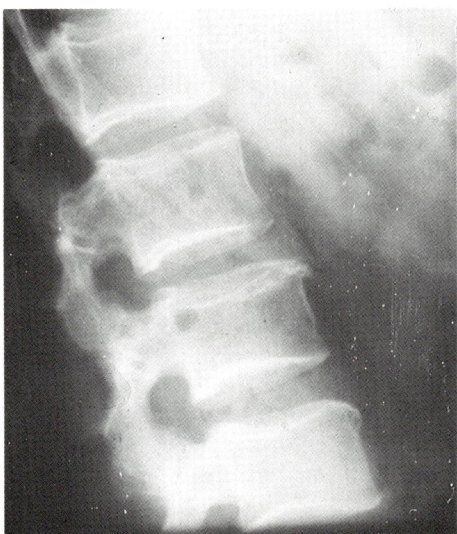

Fig. 27.82 Multiple osteolytic areas of myeloma in the vertebral bodies.

surounded by foreign-body giant cells may be found in myelomas. These should be distinguished from those associated with uraemic patients who have received long-term haemodialysis where the amyloid protein is β_2 microglobulin and not of immunoglobulin light-chain type.

The histopathological differential diagnosis includes malignant lymphoma, metastatic small cell carcinoma, and chronic inflammatory lesions rich in plasma cells. The diagnosis of multiple myeloma is usually made by haematologists via bone marrow aspiration (see Chapter 23). It is confirmed by serum or urine immunoelectrophoresis which shows a dense M band corresponding to the immunoglobulin component produced; this is usually IgG, less commonly IgA or light-chain components alone (Bence–Jones protein), and rarely IgD. Prognosis for patients with multiple myeloma is poor, with median survival 25–50 months.

Solitary plasmacytoma or localized myeloma is seen in younger patients than multiple myeloma. It consists of a single deposit of myeloma, usually in a long bone or vertebral body or, less commonly, in soft tissue. Systemic features of multiple myeloma are not usually present at the time of diagnosis and the condition has a better prognosis. However, the majority eventually progress to multiple myeloma.

Malignant lymphoma of bone (synonyms: reticulosarcoma, reticulum cell sarcoma of bone)

Malignant lymphoma is a rare primary tumour of bone and is more commonly encountered secondary to generalized malignant lymphoma arising in lymph nodes or spleen (see Chapter 23). Primary non-Hodgkin malignant lymphoma is seen most commonly in patients older than 30 and is rare in childhood. Males are affected more frequently than females. It commonly arises in the metaphysis or diaphysis of a long bone, but also involves flat bones and the axial skeleton.

Clinically, pain, local tenderness, and swelling of insidious onset are most common. Systemic symptoms, in contrast to multiple myeloma or secondary lymphoma, are uncommon. Radiologically, there is irregular osteolysis of the cortex and medulla with little periosteal new bone formation (Fig. 27.84). The tumour is grey-white or pink and often extensive.

Microscopically, the tumour is usually a high-grade, diffuse B-cell lymphoma and consists of a mixtue of lymphoid cell types, including lymphocytes, lymphoblasts, centroblasts, and centro-cytes (Fig. 27.85). In contrast to the tumour cells of Ewing tumour, these cells have well-defined cell outlines and complex nuclei containing prominent nucleoli. Glycogen is usually absent from the tumour cells which are separated by a dense reticulin network. Immunohistochemical staining for immuno-globulin components and B-cell markers are also useful. The usual treatment involves surgery and radiotherapy, sometimes combined with chemotherapy. The prognosis of primary malig-nant lymphoma in bone is relatively good compared with that of secondary lymphoma in bone, which is invariably fatal within 2 years. Metastases in other organs, including lymph nodes, can occur. The lungs and other bones are less commonly involved than in Ewing sarcoma.

Systemic Hodgkin disease (particularly of the lymphocyte-depleted or mixed-cellularity types) can also quite commonly produce multifocal osteolytic or osteoblastic secondary deposits which are commonly asymptomatic. Hodgkin disease rarely presents as a 'primary' bone tumour.

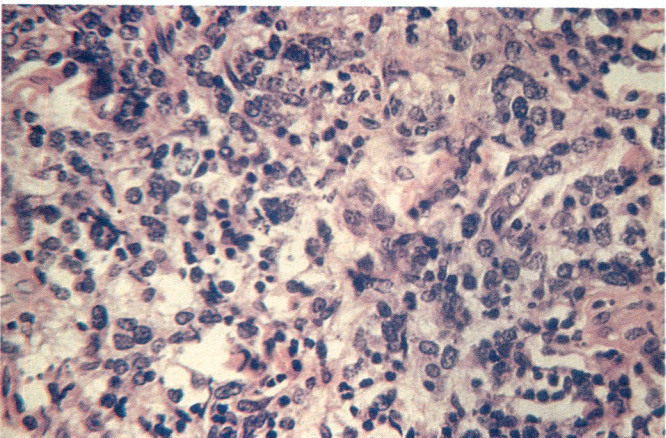

Fig. 27.85 High-grade malignant lymphoma of bone: highly pleo-morphic, rounded lymphoid cells with irregular nuclei and prominent nucleoli.

Connective-tissue tumours

Desmoplastic fibroma

This is a rare, locally aggressive, fibrous-tissue tumour which is probably the intraosseous counterpart of soft-tissue fibro-matosis or desmoid tumour. The lesion occurs over a wide age-range but is seen most commonly in the first three decades of life. It arises most commonly in the metaphysis or diaphysis of long bones or in the pelvis. Clinical features include pain or pathological fracture. Radiologically, there is a translucent cen-tral area in the diaphysis or metaphysis with cortical destruc-tion from the endosteal side. Grossly, it is an infiltrative, firm, white tumour. Histopathologically, it is composed of mature fibroblasts and abundant collagen fibres (Fig. 27.86). There is no cellular pleomorphism, mitotic activity, necrosis, or bone production, and the degree of cellularity is not high. The lesion is slow growing and locally aggressive and recurrence is com-mon after curettage. It should be distinguished from fibro-sarcoma, fibrous histiocytoma, metaphyseal fibrous defect, and fibrous dysplasia.

Fibrosarcoma

This is a rare tumour of fibroblasts in which collagen is present but bone and cartilage are absent. The tumour may arise in the medullary cavity (endosteal) or beneath the periosteum (perios-teal). It usually occurs at the metaphyseal end of long bones, particularly around the knee joint. It has a wide age-range but generally affects older patients than does osteosarcoma. Clini-cally, there is usually pain, swelling, or pathological fracture. Grossly, the tumour is firm grey-white, often with areas of necrosis or haemorrhage. Radiologically, there is usually a poorly defined translucent lesion with 'moth-eaten' destruction of involved bone. Histopathologically, it is a highly cellular spindle-cell tumour, producing variable amounts of collagen (Fig. 27.87). Cellular and nuclear pleomorphism, mitoses, and tumour giant cells with bizarre, atypical nuclei are common. A

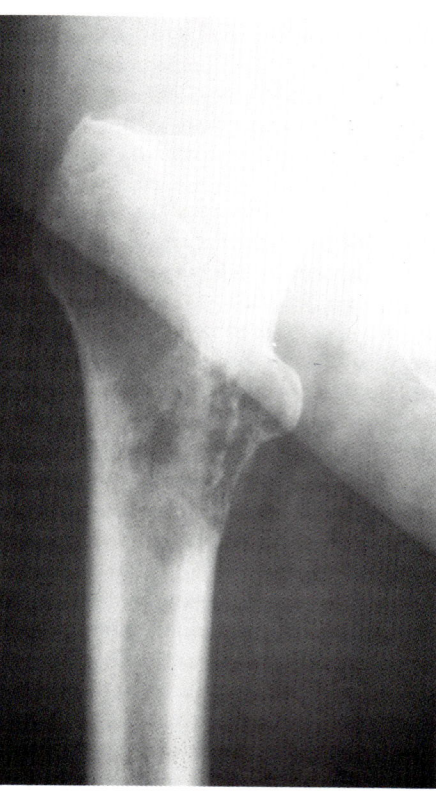

Fig. 27.84 Malignant lymphoma of bone: an infiltrative lesion with poorly defined margins.

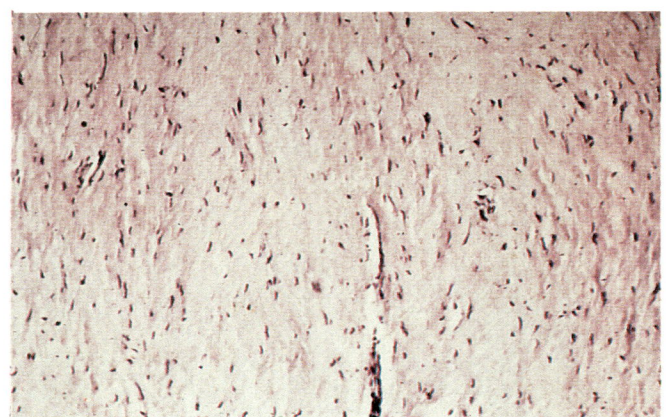

Fig. 27.86 Desmoplastic fibroma. Hyalinized bands of collagen fibres with scattered fibroblasts.

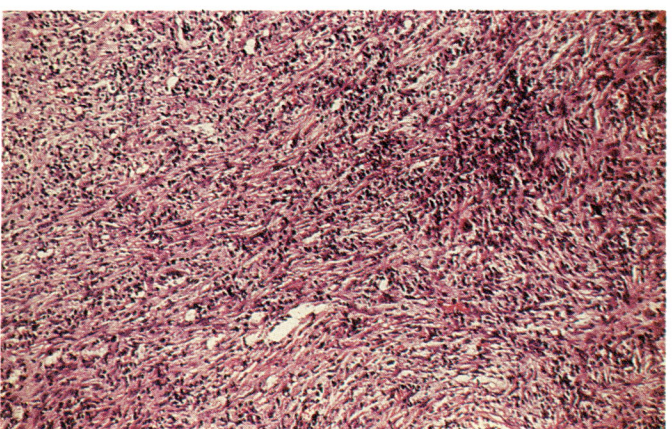

Fig. 27.87 Fibrosarcoma. Interlacing bundles of spindle-shaped tumour cells.

herring-bone pattern may be present. The tumour matrix contains collagen but no cartilage or bone.

Fibrosarcoma should be distinguished from other connective-tissue tumours and metastatic carcinomas or melanomas that show a spindle-cell pattern. The tumour inevitably metastasizes but the prognosis is better than for osteosarcoma. There is some correlation between the prognosis and the degree of tumour cell differentiation.

Malignant fibrous histiocytoma

This is a rare malignant bone tumour, which shares many similar clinical, radiological, and gross features with fibrosarcoma. Histopathologically, it is composed of spindle-shaped pleomorphic cells in bundles and whorls, with a prominent cartwheel or storiform arrangement (Fig. 27.88). Occasional foamy or vacuolated cells and multinucleate giant cells are seen and they commonly contain phagocytosed material. Cellular pleomorphism and mitotic activity is variable but usually prominent. Prognosis is generally poor.

Both benign and malignant fat and smooth muscle tumours

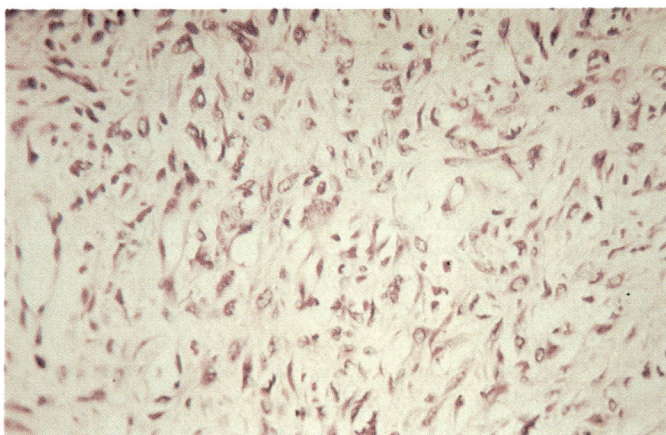

Fig. 27.88 Malignant fibrous histiocytoma. Rounded and spindle-shaped tumour cells and occasional giant cells.

have rarely been described in bone. Neurogenic tumours are also very rare, with intraosseous neurilemmoma most commonly seen.

Vascular tumours

Benign haemangioma is the commonest vascular tumour in bone; it probably represents a vascular hamartomatous malformation and not a true neoplasm. It is most commonly found in the vertebral bodies, skull, or jaw bone. It is usually a small, solitary, red, cyst-like lesion but can be of varying size. Larger tumours can expand the bone and induce periosteal new bone formation. Histopathologically, it consists of thin-walled cavernous blood spaces and capillaries lined by endothelium (Fig. 27.89).

Hemangiomas are usually asymptomatic and are common incidental radiological or post-mortem findings. Larger lesions may be complicated by pathological fracture of extraosseous extension. Skeletal haemangiomas are occasionally multiple and are then usually associated with cutaneous, visceral, or

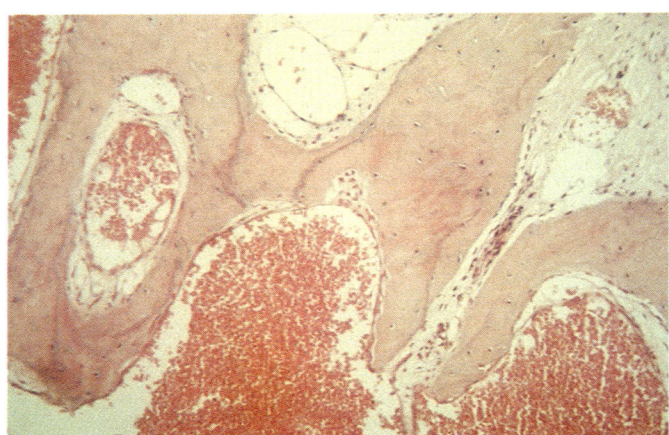

Fig. 27.89 Haemangioma composed of dilated blood-filled vascular channels.

soft-tissue haemangiomas. The condition is not familial and is usually seen in children or young adults.

Massive osteolysis (Gorham disease) is a rare skeletal condition of unknown aetiology, characterized by extensive progressive replacement of bone by fibrous tissue containing numerous thin-walled vascular spaces and channels. One or more bones may be involved, usually around the hip or shoulders, and the condition usually affects children or young adults. Recurrence is common after resection.

Other rare benign vascular tumours, including lymphangioma (solitary or multiple), glomus tumour, and benign haemangioendothelioma, have also rarely been reported in bone. Malignant vascular tumours are also rare and include malignant haemangioendothelioma, haemangiopericytoma, and angiosarcoma. These are discussed later (Chapter 12).

Other tumours of bone

Chordoma

This is a rare, slow-growing tumour, which arises from remnants of the notochord, the embryonic axial skeleton. Notochord is normally found in the nucleus pulposus of the intervertebral discs, but occasionally is found in the sacrum, coccyx, spheno-occipital region, and, less commonly, other vertebral bodies or the tissues surrounding them. Most, if not all, chordomas arise in the bone substance rather than the nucleus pulposus. Chordomas are most commonly found in the sacral region with the spheno-occipital region the next most common site. It is more common in males than females, and uncommon below the age of 30 years. Clinically, sacral and other vertebral chordomas cause pain and neurological dysfunction, often associated with compression of the spinal cord or nerve roots. Spheno-occipital tumours present with the effects of a slowly enlarging intracranial neoplasm. Grossly, the tumour is lobulated and superficially well encapsulated. It is usually blue-grey, gelatinous, and contains areas of cystic degeneration and haemorrhage (Figs 27.90, 27.91).

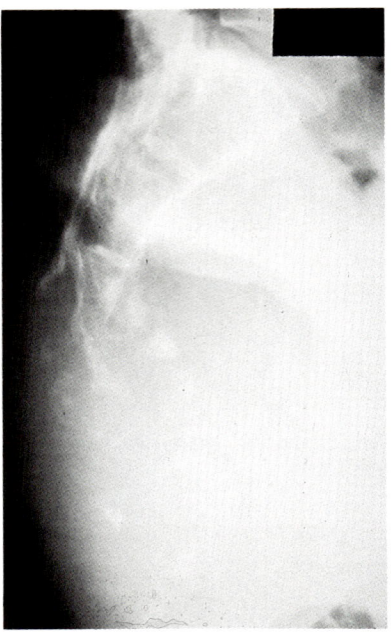

Fig. 27.91 Chordoma. Lateral radiograph of sacrum and coccyx, which has been partly replaced by a large, ill-defined mass in which there are several irregularly shaped calcified foci.

Histopathologically, the tumour has an abundant mucoid stroma which contains clumps and cords of round or polyhedral cells (Fig. 27.92); these cells have a characteristically vacuolated appearance (physaliphorous cells), prominent vesicular nuclei, and are positive for epithelial cytokeratins on immunohistochemistry. Foci of cartilage, fat, bone, and calcification may be present within the tumour. Some spheno-occipital chordomas contain a significant cartilaginous component; they are called chondroid chordomas and have a relatively good prognosis.

Chordomas must be differentiated from mucus-secreting adenocarcinoma, chondrosarcoma, and myxopapillary ependy-

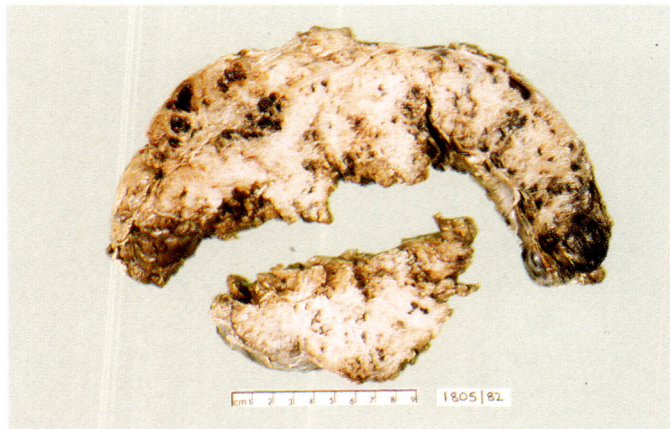

Fig. 27.90 Chordoma. Bisected specimen of sacro-coccygeal chordoma removed piecemeal. The lesion is not encapsulated and is composed of gelatinous tissue in which there are small areas of haemorrhage.

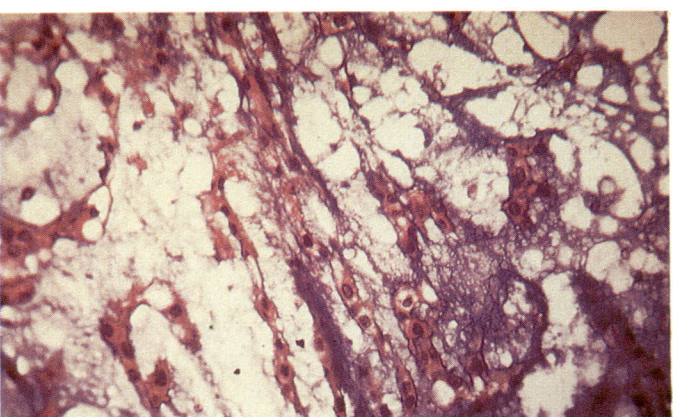

Fig. 27.92 Chordoma. Short chains of cells and isolated physaliferous cells are embedded in a basophilic matrix.

moma. Chordomas are slow-growing malignant tumours which extensively infiltrate adjacent structures. The tumour does not commonly metastasize but is invariably fatal.

Adamantinoma of long bones

This is a rare, slow-growing, malignant tumour of uncertain histogenesis with a histological appearance resembling that of adamantinoma (ameloblastoma) of the jaw. It occurs in the shaft of long bones, particularly the tibia, and is seen most commonly in young and middle-aged adults. It usually presents with pain of insidious onset, and is a well-circumscribed, rubbery, firm white or grey tumour with a characteristically multicystic translucent radiographic appearance (Figs 27.93, 27.94).

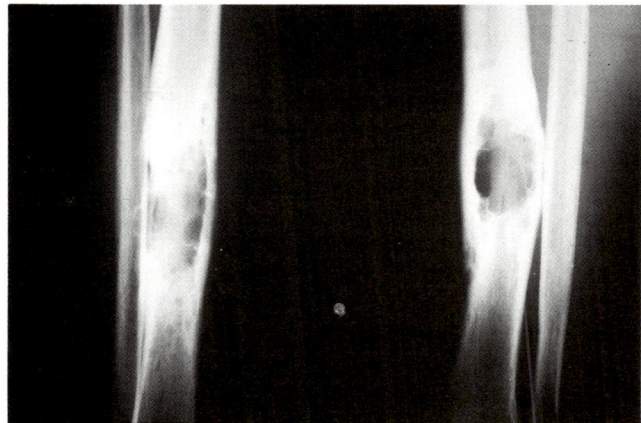

Fig. 27.94 Adamantinoma of long bone; radiograph of tibia. The diaphysis is expanded by an osteolytic lesion which is fairly sharply defined and appears lobulated.

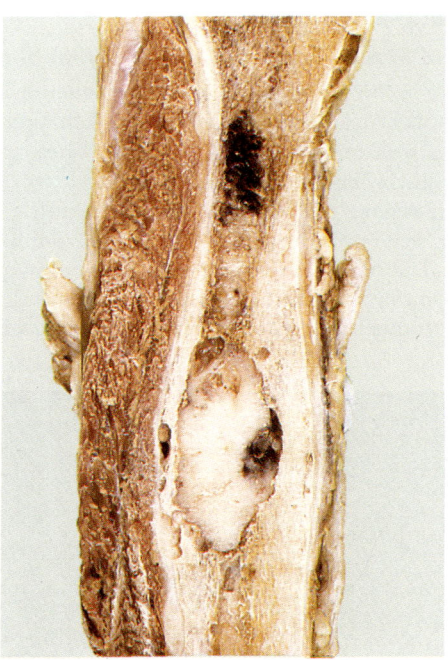

Fig. 27.93 Adamantinoma of long bone; part of tibia bisected. An ovoid mass of pale tumour extends across the medullary cavity and is inducing cortical erosion. The haemorrhagic areas in the tumour and in the medullary cavity are sites of pre-amputation biopsies.

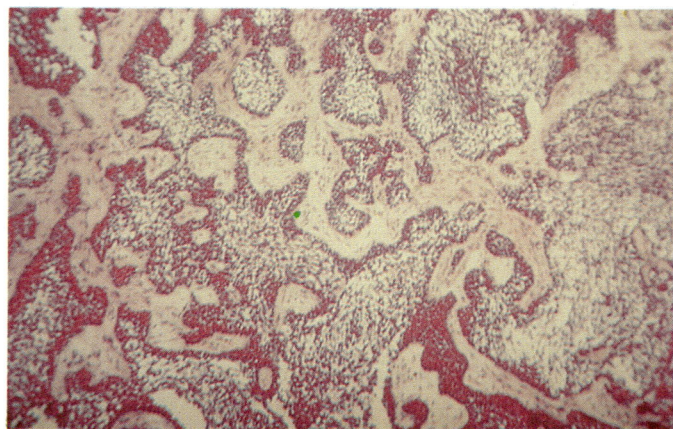

Fig. 27.95 Adamantinoma of long bone. Irregular cords and islands of spindle and ovoid cells, randomly distributed in the centre and radially arranged at the periphery. Strands of poorly cellular fibrous tissue enclose the tumour masses.

Histopathologically, it usually consists of nests or groups of cells separated by a cellular fibrous stroma (Fig. 27.95). Larger nests may exhibit peripheral palisading of the cells or show squamous metaplasia of the tumour cells or cystic change resembling the stellate reticulum of the ameloblastoma of the jaw.

Origin from epithelium either displaced traumatically or in early embryonic development is favoured, but origin from synovial or vascular tissue have also been proposed. The tumour is slow growing and should be completely excised as recurrence is common and metastasis can occur.

Ewing tumour

This is a rare, highly malignant tumour of uncertain histogenesis. It usually involves the long bone of a child or adolescent; it is most common between the ages of 5 and 20 and is rare in patients younger than 2 years or older than 30 years. The tumour arises in the medullary canal in the diaphysis or metaphysis of long bones, but occasionally occurs in flat bones. Typical clinical features include pain and swelling. There are also systemic effects such as pyrexia, anaemia, leukocytosis, and a raised erythrocyte sedimentation rate; thus, Ewing tumour can clinically mimic as osteomyelitis.

Radiologically, there is extensive irregular osteolysis of the medullary shaft, often with patchy subperiosteal bone formation which may be in layers, resembling an onion skin (Fig. 27.96). Grossly, it is a soft, white tumour containing areas of necrosis and haemorrhage. Extensive involvement of the

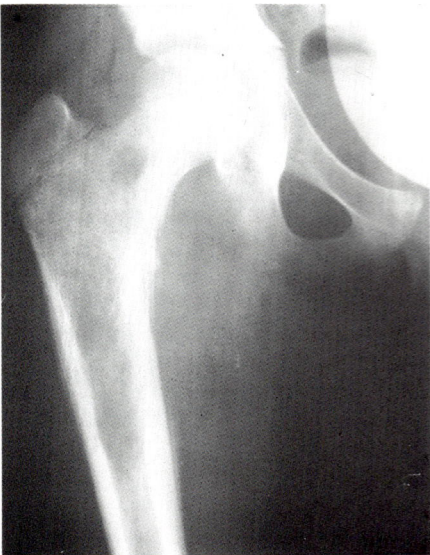

Fig. 27.96 Ewing tumour; radiograph of hip joint and proximal femur. There is irregular destruction of bone from the femoral neck down the diaphysis and a small layer of subperiosteal reactive bone on both lateral and medial surfaces of the diaphysis enclosing the tumour.

medullary shaft, cortical bone and surrounding soft tissue is often seen.

Microscopically, the tumour is composed of densely packed small cells with relatively large, pale, round or oval nuclei, scanty cytoplasm, and poorly defined cytoplasmic outline (Fig. 27.97). Occasional mitoses are seen. The sheets of tumour cells are irregularly divided into lobules by fibrous strands. Large areas of necrotic tumour separate surviving masses of tumour cells, which are commonly centred around a blood vessel in pseudorosette fashion. The reticulin network is scanty and

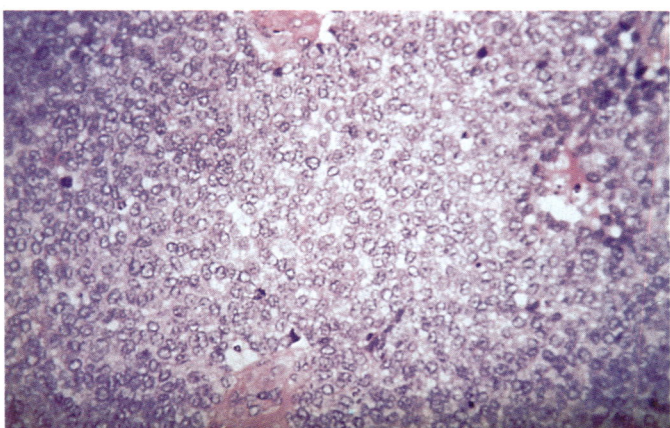

Fig. 27.97 Ewing tumour. A compact mass of cells with poorly defined cytoplasm and round or slightly ovoid nuclei. The cells are of fairly uniform morphology. Mitotic figures are not commonly so numerous as in this field.

the tumour cell cytoplasm contains abundant PAS-positive diastase-resistant glycogen. Necrosis and haemorrhage are common.

Untreated, the tumour is highly aggressive with early metastatic spread, particularly to the lungs, liver, and other bones. Surgery with combination chemotherapy and radiotherapy has greatly improved the prognosis for these patients. The differential diagnosis is essentially that of other round-cell tumours of bone, and includes metastatic neuroblastoma, malignant lymphoma, leukaemia, and osteosarcoma.

The histogenesis of Ewing tumour is unknown. Undifferentiated mesenchymal or myeloid cells, endothelial cells or 'reticulum' cells have all been proposed as the cell of origin. Origin from an undifferentiated or primitive pluripotential cell, which may differentiate into various different cell lines, has also been proposed.

Tumour-like lesions of bone

Metaphyseal fibrous defect and non-ossifying fibroma

This is a rare lesion of unknown aetiology which usually presents in the subcortical metaphyseal region of children and adolescents. It is seen most commonly in long bones, particularly the tibia or lower femur. Radiologically, the lesion lies in the metaphyseal region and is well-defined, eccentric osteolytic lesion with scalloped margins (Fig. 27.98). Smaller lesions (metaphyseal fibrous defects) are usually asymptomatic and found incidentally in radiographs, but larger lesions (non-ossifying fibromas) can present with pathological fracture.

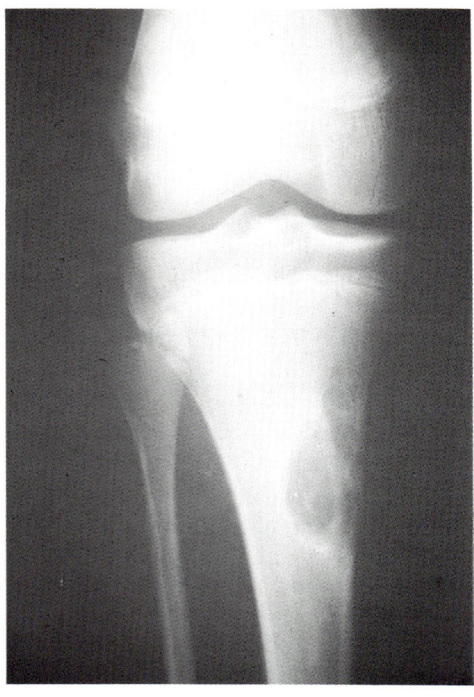

Fig. 27.98 Non-ossifying fibroma; radiograph. Well-defined osteolytic lesion in the metaphyseal/diaphyseal region on the medial side of the tibia. The growth plates are open.

Grossly, the lesion is composed of firm tissue of yellow or brown colour. Histopathologically, the lesion resembles a benign fibrous histiocytoma of soft tissue and is composed of a whorled pattern of mature cellular fibrous tissue containing occasional foamy or haemosiderin-laden histiocytes and giant cells (Fig. 27.99). Smaller lesions tend to regress spontaneously but larger lesions will require curettage. The lesion should be distinguished from fibrous dysplasia, fibrous tumours of bone, and bone lesions containing giant cells.

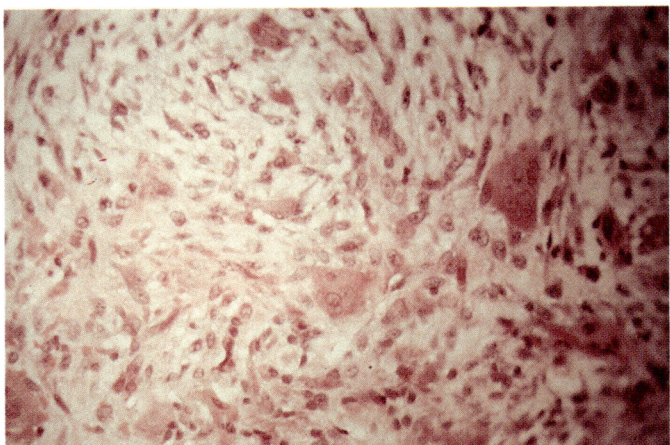

Fig. 27.99 Non-ossifying fibroma. The lesion is composed of spindle-shaped cells with small amounts of intercellular collagen and osteoclast-like giant cells interspersed amongst the spindle cells. 'Foamy' histiocytes and macrophages containing haemosiderin pigment may also be present but are not essential components.

Fibrous dysplasia

This is a relatively common benign lesion composed of bone and fibrous tissue. The aetiology is unknown but it is thought to be a development abnormality. It usually presents as a solitary (monostotic) bony lesion and multiple (polyostotic) bone involvement is less common. Rarely, mostly in females, poly-ostotic fibrous dysplasia is associated with patchy skin pigmentation and precocious puberty (Albright syndrome). The condition is not familial. The monostotic form most commonly involves the ribs, jaw, skull, or long bones, but any bone may be affected. Polyostotic fibrous dysplasia may affect one region predominantly or have a unilateral distribution. Monostotic fibrous dysplasia usually presents in children or young adults in whom it is often asymptomatic and found incidentally on radiological examination. Pain, localized swelling or deformity, and pathological fracture may also be noted; these are more common in the polyostotic form which, in addition, usually presents at an earlier age. There is an equal incidence in males and females. Some cases show a moderate rise in serum alkaline phosphatase but the serum calcium and phosphorus are usually normal.

Radiologically, the lesion is well defined and has a 'ground-glass' translucent appearance (Fig. 27.100). Grossly, it is com-

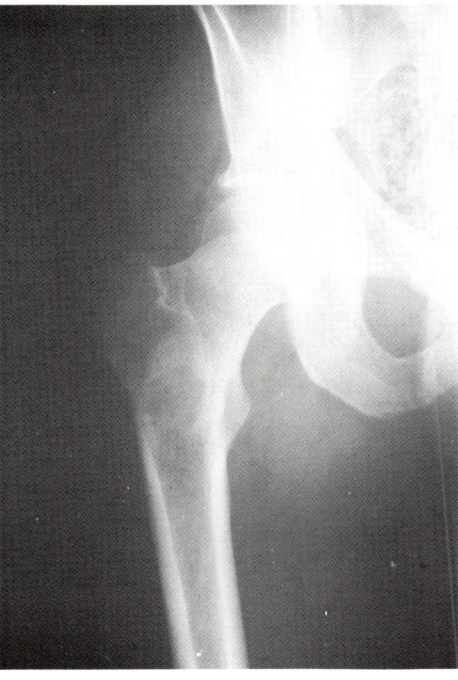

Fig. 27.100 Fibrous dysplasia; radiograph. In the distal femoral neck and proximal diaphysis there is a poorly defined lytic area in the medullary cavity producing irregular erosion of the endosteal surface of the cortex. The lesion produces a hazy radiographic shadow because of the bone formed within it.

posed of a well-demarcated mass of firm, white, fibrous tissue containing small amounts of recognizable bone or cartilage and cysts. This expands the bone, filling the medulla and thinning the cortex. Histopathologically, it consists of small, thin, irregular trabeculae of woven bone, many of which have a characteristic 'fish-hook' appearance and are not usually lined by osteoblasts (Fig. 27.101). A few trabeculae may show osteoblastic bone formation and osteoclastic resorption. These bony spicules lie in a relatively avascular and abundant fibrous spindle-cell stroma. Nodules of cartilage and mucinous cystic degeneration may also be present in the stroma.

Fibrous dysplasia should be distinguished from both benign and malignant lesions that contain woven bone, such as hyperparathyroidism, osteoid osteoma, osteosarcoma, and lesions containing abundant cellular fibrous tissue, such as non-ossifying fibroma or desmoplastic fibroma.

The lesion is benign and grows slowly, often ceasing to enlarge at the time of skeletal maturation. Some lesions, however, continue to grow in adult life or are reactivated after a period of quiescence. Rapid increase in size may be associated with haemorrhage or cyst formation. Rarely, sarcomatous change (usually a fibrosarcoma) has arisen in an area of fibrous dysplasia; this is usually associated with the polyostotic form and in patients who have had previous radiotherapy.

Histiocytosis X (synonym: Langerhans cell histiocytosis)

The term 'histiocytosis X' designates a group of conditions

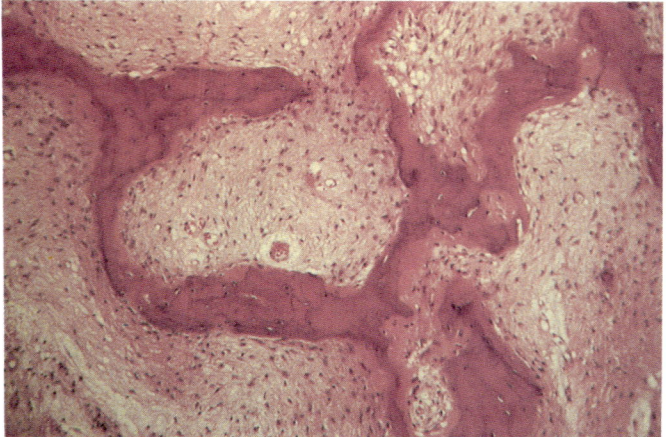

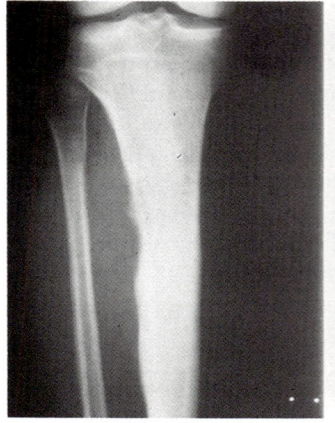
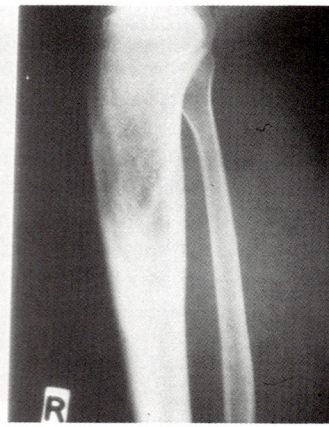

Fig. 27.101 Fibrous dysplasia. The lesion is composed of fibrous tissue which is poorly to moderately cellular. Within this fibrous tissue irregularly shaped trabeculae of bone are formed by intramembranous ossification. The amount of bone varies considerably in different areas of each lesion.

Fig. 27.102 Eosinophilic granuloma (histiocytosis X); radiograph. A poorly defined osteolytic lesion in the proximal diaphysis of an immature tibia. The lesion has caused destruction of both medullary and cortical bone and there is subperiosteal reactive bone formation.

characterized by the presence of a polymorphic inflammatory infiltrate containing Langerhans cells. The latter are normally present in skin, and similar cells have been reported in lymph nodes and elsewhere; Langerhans cells are characterized ultra-structurally by intracytoplasmic racket-shaped inclusion bodies called Birbeck granules. Histiocytosis X is often categorized as one of three conditions on the basis of the type and extent of organ involvement: eosinophilic granuloma, Hand–Schüller–Christian disease and Letterer–Siwe disease.

Eosinophilic granuloma is usually seen as solitary- or multiple-focal bone lesions affecting children or young adults. The skull bones, jaw, ribs, vertebrae, and proximal long bones are most commonly affected. There is no systemic involvement. Patients may present with pain, local tenderness, or pathological fracture. Radiologically, it is generally an osteolytic, well-defined, round or ovoid lesion, with or without a sclerotic margin. The radiographic appearances are not characteristic and mimic those of many other conditions, both benign and malignant (Fig. 27.102). Grossly, the lesion is reddish-grey and contains flecks of yellow material. In developing lesions there is a polymorphic cellular infiltrate composed of numerous histiocytes, eosinophils, lymphocytes, plasma cells, giant cells, and fibroblasts (Figs 27.103, 27.104).

Langerhans cells may be identified in the infiltrate as large cells with indented or lobulated nuclei, which may have a longitudinal groove. Areas of necrosis may also be present. In later stages, there is fibrosis and scattered eosinophils. Differential diagnosis includes pyogenic granulation tissue, non-ossifying fibroma and other giant-cell lesions of bone, as well as small round-cell tumours of bone. The lesions may regress spontaneously and are usually cured by local treatment; occasionally, other lesions may develop in the same or other bones. Cases of multiple osseous lesions without organ involvement are less

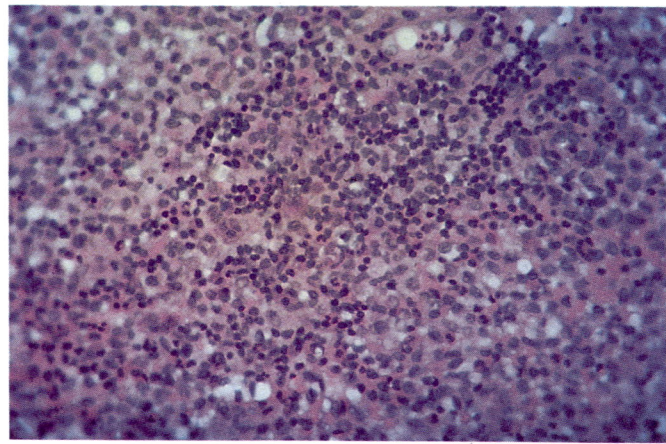

Fig. 27.103 Eosinophilic granuloma (histiocytosis X). Large mononuclear cells of histiocytic types, eosinophilic leucocytes, and lymphocytes are randomly admixed. The proportion of each cell type varies from area to area.

common and characterized by a more prolonged clinical course. Prognosis is usually favourable.

In Hand–Schüller–Christian disease, adolescents and young adults are predominantly affected, and may develop hypopituitarism, diabetes insipidus, exophthalmos, hepatosplenomegaly, lymphadenopathy, and multiple osteolytic bone lesions. The prognosis is difficult to predict but poor prognostic features include bone marrow and liver involvement and young age at the time of diagnosis.

Letterer–Siwe disease is seen most commonly in infancy and very young children and is the most aggressive form of histiocytosis X. It is characterized by extensive multiple organ infiltration, including skin, with little or no bone involvement. This is discussed more fully in Chapter 28.

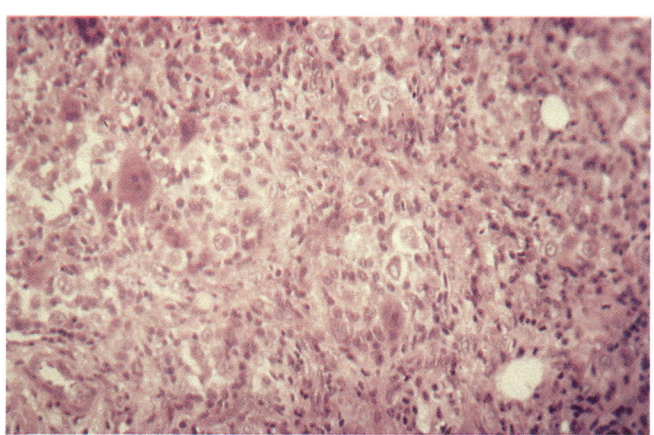

Fig. 27.104 Eosinophilic granuloma (histiocytosis X). In this field fibrous tissue and osteoclast-like giant cells are a prominent feature, and leucocytes and histiocytes are less conspicuous.

Myositis ossificans

Myositis ossificans (circumscripta) is a benign, solitary, reactive, ossifying condition which must be distinguished from osteosarcoma. It most commonly occurs in adolescents or young adults who present with a painful lump, usually in the upper arm or thigh, of several weeks' duration. A history of trauma is often, but not always, elicited. Radiologically, there is initially a poorly defined radio-opaque lesion; later, a well-defined bony lesion is evident (Fig. 27.105). Grossly, the fully developed lesion consists of a gritty, red-brown mass surrounded by bone. Histopathologically, the centre of the lesion shows granulation tissue with proliferating fibroblasts and

small areas of haemorrhage in early lesions, and with more mature fibrous tissue in older lesions. Reactive formation of bone can be seen at the periphery of the lesion and shows a characteristic maturation pattern (Fig. 27.106). The most peripheral areas consist of well-organized woven or lamellar bone trabeculae and the intermediate zone shows poorly organized woven bone, osteoid production, or small areas of cartilage undergoing endochondral ossification. This zonal maturation pattern is important in histologically distinguishing the lesion from a parosteal osteosarcoma and should be correlated with the clinical and radiological findings.

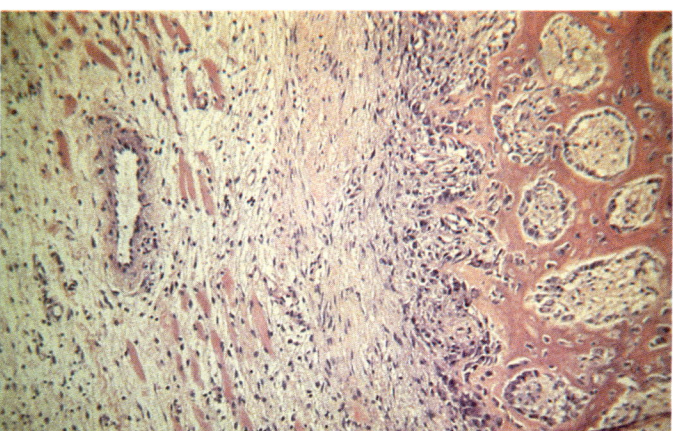

Fig. 27.106 Myositis ossificans. On the left there are atrophic muscle fibres with fibrosis of the interstitial tissue. This merges with fibrous tissue which defines the lesion. The lesion (right) consists of interlocking trabeculae of immature bone with active osteoblasts on the surfaces. The intertrabecular tissue is poorly cellular fibrous tissue.

Myositis ossificans progressiva (MOP) is a rare muscle condition in which there is a progressive ossification of muscle groups, ligaments, and tendons, as well as characteristic skeletal abnormalities (phalangeal abnormalities including short big toe or thumb, abnormalities of long bones and exotases, fusion of the cervical vertebrae). Symptoms usually begin in childhood and most often affect muscles around the neck, upper back, and major joints including the hip. Affected muscles become painful, red, and hard, and progressively ossify with consequent limitation of movement and functional disability including severe loss of pulmonary function. Histologically, the lesion contains fibrous scar tissue, cartilage, and poorly organized woven or lamellar bone. MOP is thought to be inherited as an autosomal dominant condition with variable penetrance. Plasma alkaline phosphatase may be elevated during active myositis but other biochemical measurements are usually normal.

Solitary (simple, unicameral) bone cyst

This is a benign, non-neoplastic, solitary cystic defect, most commonly found in the metaphyseal region of the humerus, femur, and other long bones. Solitary cysts form and most commonly present in children and adolescents. They are more

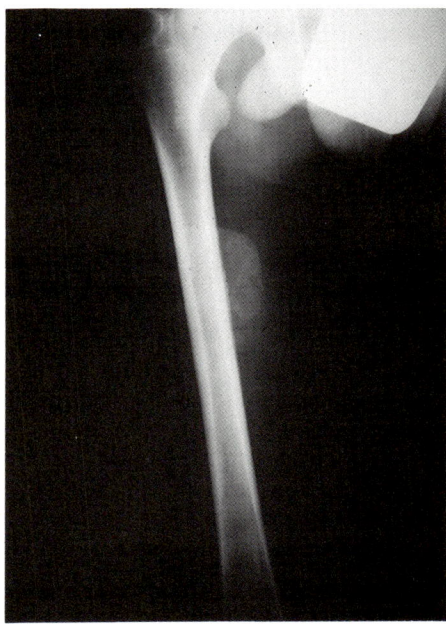

Fig. 27.105 Myositis ossificans; radiograph of thigh. Calcified ovoid mass in soft tissue in close proximity to, but separate from, the femur.

common in males. Radiologically, there is a well-defined radio-lucent lesion expanding the bone and thinning the cortex (Fig. 27.107). In serial radiographs, the lesion appears to migrate away from the epiphyseal plate.

Grossly, it is a cyst lined by fibrous tissue containing clear fluid. Secondary changes, particularly pathological fracture are common. The fluid in the cyst may then become bloody or brownish and the fibrous lining brownish with areas of haemorrhage. Histologically, the uncomplicated cyst is lined by simple fibrous tissue (Fig. 27.108). Most cysts, however, also show evidence of secondary haemorrhage with reparative granulation tissue, calcification, cholesterol clefts, osteoclasts, macrophages, and other inflammatory cells.

The usual treatment is curettage of the contents but the lesion has a tendency to recur, especially if it lies close to the epiphyseal plate.

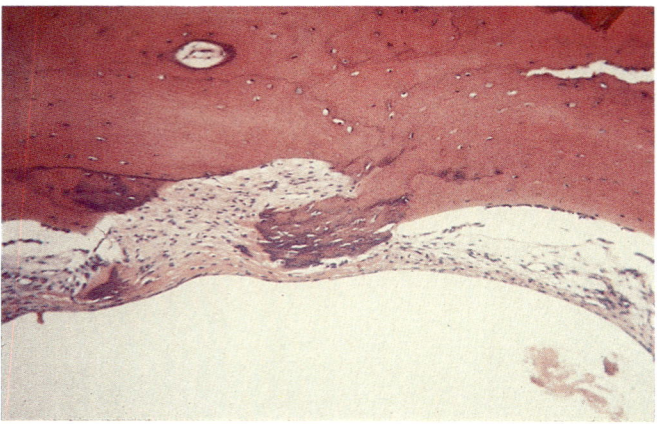

Fig. 27.108 Unicameral bone cyst. The cyst is lined by a thin layer of loose, textured, poorly cellular fibrous tissue, which is apposed to the internal surface of the cortical bone (above) which is undergoing resorption.

Aneurysmal bone cyst

This is a solitary, large, rapidly expanding lesion of unknown aetiology, most commonly involving the shaft of long bones or the vertebrae of children or adolescents. It presents with pain and swelling, or with neurological defects if the spine is involved. The rapid growth raises the clinical suspicion of malignancy. Grossly, it is often an eccentric, highly vascular multiloculated lesion, covered by a thin shell of reactive bone. Radiologically, the multilocular structure of the osteolytic cyst is usually obvious (Fig. 27.109). Histopathologically, the lesion contains cystic spaces that are filled with blood (Fig. 27.110). These are separated by cellular fibrous tissue septae containing unevenly scattered osteoclast-like giant cells, foci of haemorrhage and haemosiderin-laden macrophages, and occasionally foci of osteoid or immature bone formation. The vascular spaces are not lined by endothelium but by mononuclear cells and giant cells. No cytological atypia is seen in any of the cellular components.

Aneurysmal bone cyst should be distinguished histologically from giant-cell tumour of bone and other giant-cell-containing lesions, telangiectatic osteosarcoma simple bone cyst, and vascular tumours of bone. The lesion is usually cured by curettage.

Other cysts of bone

Rarely, an intraosseous ganglion cyst is found in the epiphyseal end of long bones, particularly the medial malleolus of the tibia. It rarely involves the joint, and morphologically resembles a soft-tissue ganglion. Subchondral bone cysts are simple cysts lined by fibrous tissue, characterized by their location in bone beneath the articular cartilage; they are, by definition, not associated with degenerative joint disease. Epidermal inclusion cysts have also rarely been described in bone.

Metastatic tumours in bone

This is the most common of all malignant tumours that involve bone and is much more common than primary bone tumours.

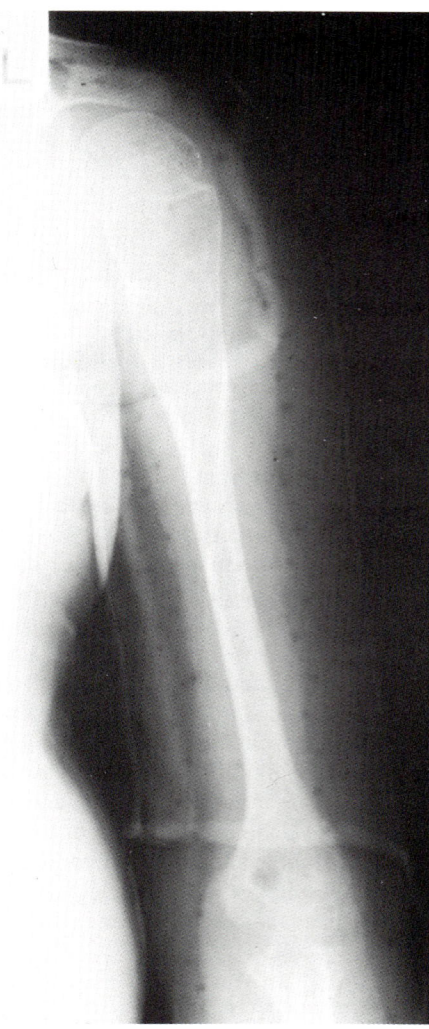

Fig. 27.107 Unicameral bone cyst. Radiograph of lesion affecting the proximal metaphysis and diaphysis of humerus. The lesion is osteolytic and has caused expansion of the bone diameter. Note that the growth plate is open.

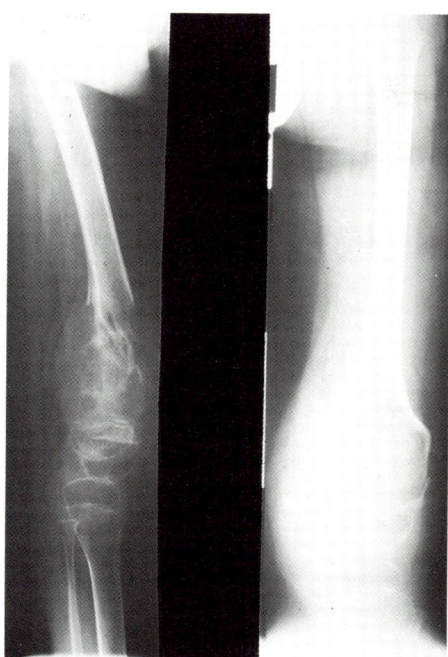

Fig. 27.109 Aneurysmal bone cyst. Radiograph of lesion in distal femoral metaphysis and diaphysis. There is an osteolytic lesion which appears multilocular and has produced an expansion of the bone, seen most clearly in the lateral view.

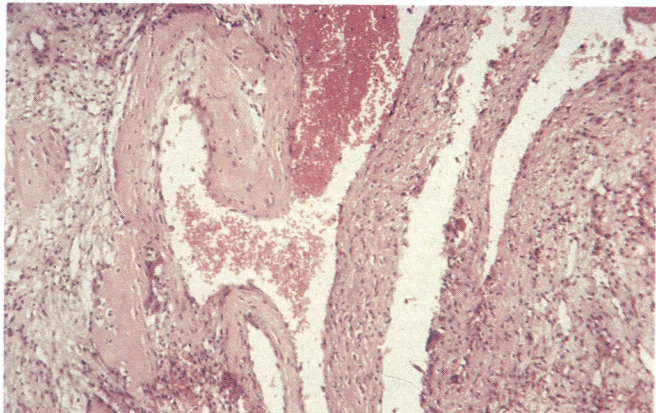

Fig. 27.110 Aneurysmal bone cyst. The cystic spaces contain blood. The spaces are separated by cellular fibrous tissue containing haemosiderin-laden macrophages.

A few present as pain, local tenderness, swelling, pathological fracture, or neurological complications consequent upon involvement of the vertebral column, but most secondary tumours are clinically silent. Radiological studies, including skeletal surveys and isotope bone scans, are useful but still do not reveal the full extent of bone involvement by tumour. Even the reported incidence of bony secondaries is difficult to evalu-

ate as this depends largely on the thoroughness of post-mortem examination. Suffice it to say that only the lungs and the liver are more frequent sites of secondary spread.

In adults, the most common primary tumours that metastasize to bone are carcinomas of the breast, prostate, lung, thyroid, kidney, gastrointestinal tract, malignant melanoma, and lymphoma. Neuroblastoma is the commonest in young children. Nevertheless, almost any malignant tumour can metastasize to bone, and no primary site should be eliminated on the grounds of probability alone.

Metastatic tumour usually involves the haemopoietic marrow and is thus most common in the axial skeleton, particularly the vertebral column, innominate bones, ribs, and skull bones. The proximal ends of the femur and the humerus are also commonly affected but skeletal secondaries are uncommon below the knees or elbows. The tumour deposits may be well circumscribed or diffusely involve the marrow. They arise largely from arterial tumour cell emboli, although retrograde spread along the vertebral venous plexus of veins has also been suggested as a possible route of metastasis from tumours of pelvic organs.

Bone destruction is the usual consequence of skeletal metastases and secondary tumours causing this commonly termed osteolytic (Figs 27.111, 27.112). Tumour cells are known to produce or stimulate the production of prostaglandins and cytokines, which are capable of stimulating osteoclastic bone resorption. It is unlikely that they resorb the bone directly. Hypercalcaemia may be a consequence of this bone destruction but this is not the sole means by which hypercalcaemia develops in malignancy. Some secondaries stimulate local bone

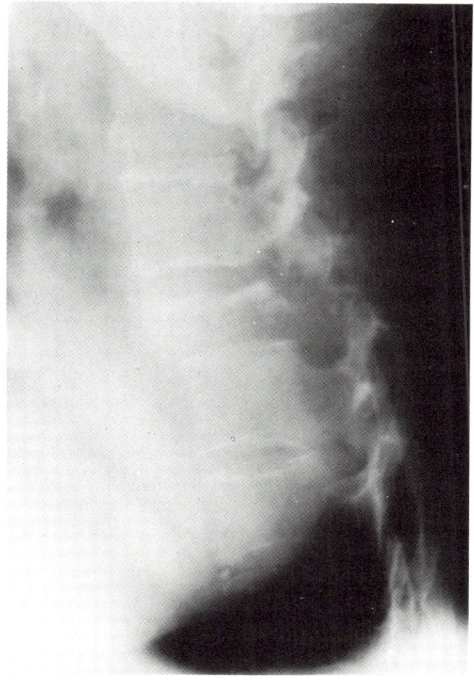

Fig. 27.111 Metastatic carcinoma; radiograph of thoracic spine. One vertebral body has been extensively destroyed and has collapsed.

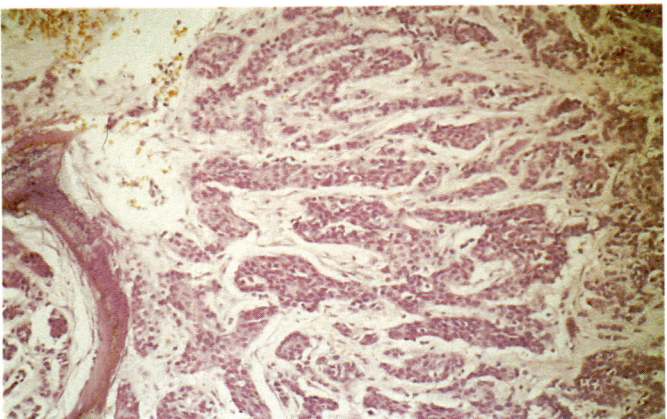

Fig. 27.112 Metastatic carcinoma. Cords of tumour cells and reactive fibrous tissue have replaced both bone and marrow tissue. Variable amounts of immature bone form in the fibrous tissue.

formation by osteoblasts and are termed osteosclerotic; these are most commonly associated with prostatic carcinoma but can be seen in metastases from any primary site, as can mixed osteolytic and osteoblastic tumour secondaries. The serum alkaline phosphatase activity may be increased with osteoblastic secondaries or if pathological fracture has occurred.

Metastatic tumour deposits are usually multiple, although clinically they may appear to be solitary. Surgical resection of apparently solitary skeletal metastases is thus rarely undertaken. However, in some cases of renal carcinoma, which has a tendency to metastasize to only one bone, this may be considered. Palliative radiotherapy is otherwise the most common treatment.

27.1.7   Further reading

Bone—normal structure and function

Caplan, A. L. and Pechak, D. G. (1987). The cellular and molecular embryology of bone formation. In *Bone and mineral research* (ed. W. A. Peck), pp. 117–83. Elsevier, Amsterdam.

Marks, S. C. and Popoff, S. N. (1988). Bone cell biology: The regulation of development, structure and function in the skeleton. *American Journal of Anatomy* **183**, 1–44.

Mundy, G. R. and Roodman, G. D. (1987). Osteoclast ontogeny and function. In *Bone and mineral research*, Vol. 5 (ed. W. A. Peck), pp. 209–79. Elsevier, Amsterdam.

Smith, R. (1984). Recent advances in the metabolism and physiology of bone. In *Recent advances in physiology*, Vol. 10 (ed. P. F. Baker), pp. 317–48. Churchill Livingstone, Edinburgh.

Vaughan, J. (1981). *The physiology of bone* (3rd edn). Oxford University Press, Oxford.

Abnormal development of the skeleton

Sillence, D. O. *et al.* (1979). Morphologic studies in the skeletal dysplasias. *American Journal of Pathology* **96**, 813–60.

Smith, R. (1979). *Biochemical disorders of the skeleton*. Butterworth, London.

Smith, R. (1986). Osteogenesis imperfecta. *Clinics in Rheumatic Diseases* **12**, 655–89.

Wynne-Davies, R. *et al.* (1985). *Atlas of skeletal dysplasias*. Churchill Livingstone, Edinburgh.

Fracture repair, bone necrosis, and miscellaneous bone conditions

Glimcher, M. J. and Kenzora, J. E. (1979). The biology of osteonecrosis of the human femoral head and its clinical implications III. Discussion of the aetiology and genesis of the pathological sequelae: comments on treatment. *Clinical Orthopaedics and Related Research* **140**, 273–312.

Ham, A. W. and Harris, W. R. (1971). Repair and transplantation of bone. In *The biochemistry and physiology of bone* (ed. G. H. Bourne), Vol. 3 (2nd edn), pp. 338–400. Academic Press, New York.

Inove, A. and Ono, K. (1979). A histological study of idiopathic avascular necrosis of the head of the femur. *Journal of Bone and Joint Surgery* **61B**, 138.

Woods, C. G. (1972). *Diagnostic orthopaedic pathology*. Blackwells, Oxford.

Infection of bone

Revel, P. A. (1986). *Pathology of bone*, pp. 235–55. Springer-Verlag, Berlin.

Smith, R. (1985). Recovery and tissue repair. *British Medical Bulletin* **41**, 295–301.

Metabolic bone disease

Ellis, H. A. and Macwhinney, W. H. B. (1982). Aluminum induced dialysis osteomalacia. *Journal of Clinical Pathology* **35**, 792–3.

Revel, P. A. (1986). *Pathology of bone*, pp. 86–167. Springer-Verlag, Berlin.

Smith, R. (1979). *Biochemical disorders of the skeleton*. Butterworth, London.

Swan, C. H. J. *et al.* (1976). Fibrogenesis imperfecta ossium. *Quarterly Journal of Medicine* **45**, 233–53.

Woods, C. G. (1982). Pathology of endocrine bone disease. In *Current endocrine concepts* (ed. E. D. Williams), pp. 165–70. Praeger, Eastbourne, New York.

Bone tumours

Dahlin, D. C. (1987). *Bone tumors* (3rd edn). Thomas, Springfield, Illinois.

Jaffe, H. L. (1958). *Tumors and tumorous conditions of the bones and joints*. Lea and Febiger, Philadelphia.

Lane, J. M. (1986). Ten most common bone and joint tumors: symposium. *Clinical Orthapaedics and Related Research* **204**, 2–142.

Mirra, J. M. (1989). *Bone tumours: clinical, radiologic and pathologic correlations*. Lea and Febiger, Philadelphia.

Schajowicz, F. (1981). *Tumors and tumor-like lesions of bone and joints*. Springer-Verlag, New York.

Schajowicz, F. (1983). Current trends in the diagnosis and treatment of malignant bone tumors. *Clinical Orthopaedics and Related Research* **180**, 220–52.

Schajowicz, F., Ackerman, L. V., and Sissons, H. A. (1972). *Histological typing of bone tumours*. International histological classification of tumours, No. 6. World Health Organization, Geneva.

Spjut, H. J., Dorfman, H. D., Fechner, R. E., and Ackerman, L. V. (1970). *Tumors of bone and cartilage*, 2nd series, Fascicle 5. Armed Forces Institute of Pathology, Washington, DC.

27.2 Joint disease

P. A. Revell

27.2.1 Normal structure and function

The connections between different parts of the skeleton are brought about in a variety of ways, all of which are generally termed joints or articulations. Classifications of joints are based either on the extent to which movement is allowed or on their histological features. Thus, there are:

1. diarthroses, which are freely mobile joints (e.g. knee joint);
2. amphiarthroses, in which slight movement is permitted (e.g. intervertebral joints); and
3. synarthroses, where there are fixed and rigid junctions (e.g. skull sutures).

Consideration of the type of tissue forming joints leads to their division into:

1. synovial types (e.g. knee);
2. cartilaginous (symphyses, synchondroses); and
3. fibrous (skull sutures, syndesmoses, gomphoses).

A brief description of diarthrodial or synovial joints and spinal joints (which are symphyses) will be given here.

Synovial joints

The synovial joints are mostly situated in the limbs. The opposing ends of the bones are covered by a layer of hyaline cartilage and there is a surrounding fibrous capsule, lined on its inner aspect by synovial membrane. The potential space delineated by these structures contains synovial fluid. Ligaments may reinforce the capsule, and other structures, such as the fibro-cartilaginous menisci in the knee or discs in the sternoclavicular and temporomandibular joints, are peripherally attached to the capsule. Tendons pass in close proximity to joints where they may be attached to the capsule. Tendons may have sesamoid bones embedded in them.

Articular cartilage

Articular cartilage is glistening bluish-white in children and young adults; duller yellowish-white in middle age; and yellowish-brown in elderly individuals. It varies in thickness from one joint to another and in different areas over the same joint surface. The variations are related to the size of joint, load-bearing and other mechanical factors, joint congruity, and age.

Detailed descriptions of the biochemistry, histology, and ultrastructure of hyaline cartilage are available elsewhere. Essentially cartilage is composed of chondrocytes in a matrix of collagen fibres with proteoglycan and water, the last of which makes up 70–75 per cent of its weight. The collagen fibres are arranged in 'arcades'. They are closely packed and orientated parallel to the surface in the uppermost zone. In the deepest part of the cartilage, they are perpendicular to the surface, while in the intermediate zone they cross over in various directions to form a lattice-like arrangement. Recently, a different arrangement of the collagen fibres has been proposed, in which there is a three-dimensional collagen lattice-work within which are trapped large hydrophilic molecules of proteoglycan. According to this theory, there are no arcades of collagen fibres. The deepest collagen fibres are embedded in a calcified zone of the cartilage and the junction between this and the overlying cartilage is called the 'tidemark' (Fig. 27.113).

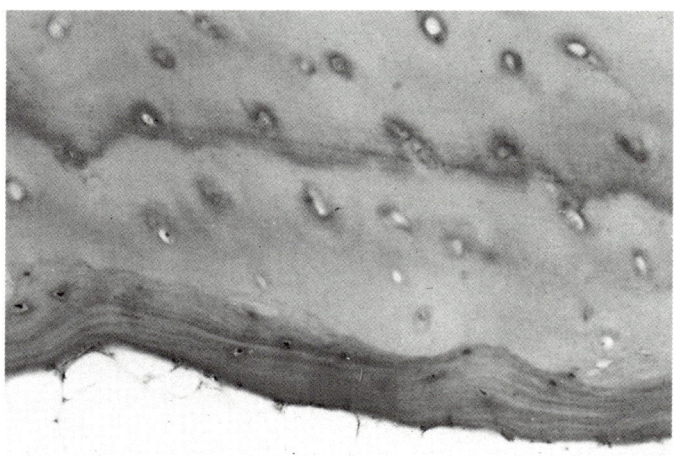

Fig. 27.113 Deeper zones of articular cartilage to show calcified cartilage and subchondral bone (bottom). Note linear calcification at interface between calcified and non-calcified cartilage at the tidemark.

The calcified cartilage is supported by subchondral bone which is formed by horizontal bridging between the trabeculae of the underlying cancellous bone to form a more or less complete layer beneath the cartilage, through which small vessels pass to supply the deepest, calcified cartilage region.

Between the cartilage collagen fibres there are massive molecules formed by the aggregation of hyaluronic acid with proteoglycans; the latter comprise chondroitin sulphate and keratan sulphate glycosaminoglycans linked to a core protein. These hyaluronic acid–proteoglycan aggregates are retained immobile within the collagen framework. They possess numerous fixed negative charges and hydroxyl groups which hold large amounts of water so that they are responsible for the swelling pressure of cartilage, giving resilience and turgidity.

Chondrocytes vary in appearance, being smaller and flattened with their long axes parallel to the surface in the superficial zone; larger and rounded in the deeper regions where they are often arranged in pairs or small groups (Fig. 27.114). As well as confirming the arrangement of collagen fibres, ultrastructural studies show that the chondrocytes contain those organelles normally associated with active protein synthesis and secretion, such as rough endoplasmic reticulum, free

Fig. 27.114 Surface and middle zone of normal articular cartilage, showing flattened chondrocytes near the surface and more randomly arranged cells, some of which are in pairs, in the middle zone.

ribosomes, Golgi apparatus, and mitochondria. The collagen immediately around the chondrocytes is different both ultra-structurally and biochemically (type IX collagen) from that else-where in the cartilage matrix, viz. type II collagen, which is the major cartilage collagen. The movement of fluid into and out of cartilage is necessary for load bearing, lubrication, and the nutrition of chondrocytes. Opinions differ as to the exact mech-anisms but repetitive loading and unloading during normal joint function appears to be an important factor in cartilage nutrition, which is obtained almost exclusively from the syn-ovial fluid.

Synovial membrane

The fibrous capsule of a joint is firmly attached to the peri-osteum at or near the joint margins. Within this dense fibrous tissue is a combination of looser vascular fibrous tissue and fat, which may vary in proportion from site to site even within a particular joint. The surface of this tissue is covered by a layer of cells, variously termed synovial cells, synoviocytes, synovial lining cells, or intimal cells. The synovial membrane (syno-vium) so constituted is sometimes referred to as being divisible into an 'intima' (surface cells) and 'subintima' (vascular con-nective tissue). Normal synovial membrane often has small finger-like villous projects at its synoviocyte surface; these are developed to an excessive extent in certain pathological states (e.g. rheumatoid arthritis).

In the normal joint, the synovial intima comprises a thin layer of cells, usually no more than one or two cells deep, over the surface of the fibrofatty tissue (Fig. 27.115). There is no basement membrane. Synoviocytes have been subdivided into type A and type B cells, mainly on the basis of electron micro-scopical appearances, and have been considered by many to belong to a single population, which differentiates according to functional demands. Recent evidence from monoclonal anti-body and experimental studies shows that type A cells are members of the macrophage series and that type B cells are fibroblastic. The subintima mainly contains fat, fibroblasts, and macrophages, with other cells present in small numbers. Numerous small vessels are present and there is vascular pro-liferation together with cellular infiltration of this region in joint disease.

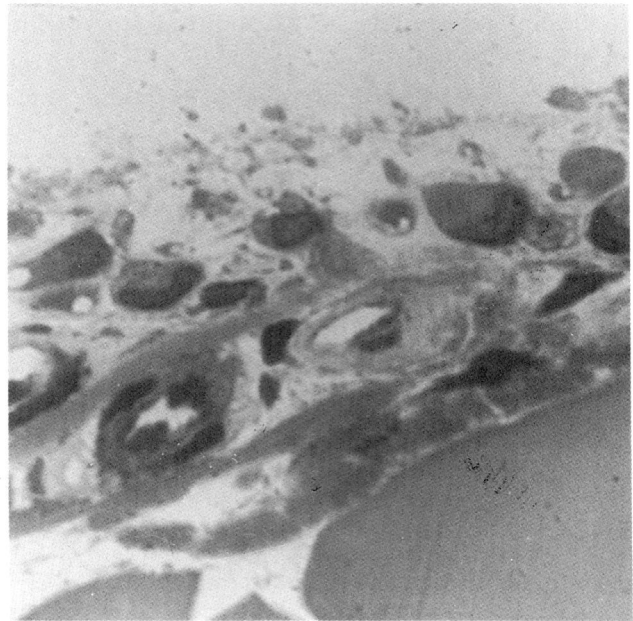

Fig. 27.115 Resin-embedded section of normal synovium, showing fatty tissue (bottom), small vessels and a thin layer of surface cells with no basement membrane (thionin stain).

Synovial fluid and intra-articular pressure

Normal joints contain only small amounts of synovial fluid, which is a dialysate of plasma to which hyaluronic acid–proteo glycan has been added. The high viscosity of normal synovial fluid is dependent on the content of hyaluronic acid, which is produced by the synovial intimal cells. Normal synovial fluid is yellow and transparent with a pH from 7.2 to 7.4. Large pro-teins do not enter synovial fluid because they do not pass through the walls of normal vessels, and therefore synovial fluid does not clot since it contains no fibrinogen or clotting factors. Immunoglobulins are normally absent, but smaller molecules, such as uric acid, bilirubin, and glucose, pass more readily into the synovial fluid. The normal glucose level, for example, is similar to that in the blood. Values for the normal white cell count vary from series to series, but there are usually fewer than 0.5×10^9–1×10^9 cells/dl, with mononuclear (lymphocytes and macrophages) cells predominating over polymorphonuclear leucocytes. The exact way in which synovial fluid lubricates the joint surfaces is still under discussion; concepts include boundary lubrication and weeping lubrication.

Synovial fluid volume and pressure have been measured in disease states but little information about the normal intraarticular pressure is available and this applies almost exclusively to the knee. The pressure of synovial fluid is normally just below atmospheric pressure in extended joints and is raised by only a small amount in full flexion. Increased synovial fluid volume may result in an increase in pressure to levels of the same order as those in the arteries, which will impair blood flow or even result in joint rupture.

Menisci and intra-articular discs

Intra-articular fibrocartilaginous structures are found in the knee (menisci) and at other sites, such as the wrist, temporomandibular and sternoclavicular joints (discs). The periphery of each disc is attached to the joint capsule; so also are the menisci, but these crescenteric structures are also anchored to the upper tibia in the intercondylar region. Elastic fibres are intermingled with the collagen of the fibrocartilage of these structures. While there is little information about their function, it is likely that the menisci alter in shape in order to provide contiguity of the joint surfaces through the full range of movement at the knee. They are in contact with both joint surfaces, but whether or not they are weight bearing is controversial. They transmit most of the force under light loads and as the weight is increased more underlying cartilaginous surface is exposed, up to a point where the menisci will still transmit up to half the load.

Ligaments, tendons, synovial sheaths, and bursae

Ligaments and tendons are made of dense collagenous tissue and, although collagen fibres are not elastic, they can be arranged in such a way as to allow some elastic deformation. Elastic fibres enable deformation under applied force with later return of the fibres to their original state. Collagen and elastic fibres are intermingled in ligaments while collagen fibres are predominant in tendons. Synovial sheaths are present around many tendons, for example at the wrist. They have an outer (parietal) and inner (visceral) layer which are separated by synovial fluid. Microscopically, the tendon sheath resembles synovial membrane.

Bursae are flattened, sac-like structures containing synovial fluid and lined by synovial membrane. Subcutaneous bursae are present between skin and bony prominences, for example at the olecranon and patella. Bursae near joints may be in continuity with the joint cavity.

Biomechanics of joints

Since mechanics is about forces, motions, and the effects that they have, its study in relation to joint function is appropriate.

Mechanical properties of materials describe their elasticity, their strength in tension and compression, and their resistance to wear. There will be frictional resistance between any two surfaces moving relative to one another and wear of the surfaces will result. Lubricants reduce friction and therefore decrease wear as well. An unfortunate difficulty in the biomechanics of joints is that the materials being evaluated are not homogeneous.

A joint like the knee has 'materials'—bone, hyaline cartilage, fibrocartilage, fibrofatty tissue, synovial fluid—all with different properties. Furthermore, each individual component shows variation; for example, the orientation of the collagen fibres in cartilage, as well as differing from the surface to the deep aspect (see above), also varies across the joint surface, the superficial fibres being arrayed along definite (Hultkrantz) lines, analogous to Langer's lines in the skin. Joint structures are subjected to compressive, tensile, and shearing forces. Friction at loaded surfaces is expressed as the friction coefficient. This is between 100 and 1000 times smaller in a healthy synovial joint than for metal or plastic; and 10–20 times smaller compared to polished metal and polyethylene in the presence of synovial fluid, as in an artificial joint. Wear is the removal of material from surfaces and is low in prostheses lubricated by synovial fluid.

The spine

The spine has two kinds of joint. The small apophyseal joints are situated posteriorly and are diarthrodial joints linking the pedicles. The articulations between the vertebral bodies are formed by fibrocartilaginous discs having an outer, multilayered 'annulus fibrosis' and an inner, softer 'nucleus pulposus'. The turgidity and resilience of the intervertebral discs results from the high water content, retained within the nucleus pulposus by hyaluronic acid–proteoglycan aggregates similar to those in hyaline articular cartilage. The discs are delineated above and below by a layer of hyaline cartilage and beneath this there is subchondral bone forming an 'end plate'. The spine at any one level must be considered as a unit, taking the apophyseal joints and disc together. Impaired or increased mobility at one joint has effects on the other joints at the same level, so that, for example, subluxation of one vertebra on another (spondylolisthesis in the lumbar spine) requires changes to be present in both the discs and posterior joints. Severe disc disease in the absence of apophyseal involvement does not give rise to displacement of vertebrae.

27.2.2 Congenital abnormalities and developmental defects

Details of congenital abnormalities of the skeleton and developmental defects as they relate to the joints are available elsewhere (Revell 1986 and Section 27.1). A number of conditions are summarized here.

Dwarfism and the chondrodysplasias

Shortness of stature may be present at birth or develop during childhood. It may be due to one of the group of unrelated disorders called the chondrodysplasias, many of which result in short-limbed dwarfism and some of which show spinal involvement. The commonest of the chondrodysplasias is achondroplasia in which there is a characteristic skull shape and facies, limb shortening, lordosis, dorsolumbar kyphosis, and abnormalities of the ribs and pelvis. There may be coxa vara and genu varum. The ends of the shortened limb bones are enlarged.

Cleidocranial dysostosis

Cleidocranial dysostosis is inherited as an autosomal dominant. The clavicles and calvaria are the principal sites of abnormality but deficient ossification or absence of parts of the pelvis, hip joint deformities, spina bifida occulta, and dental abnormalities have also been reported. The clavicles are not completely formed. The fragmentary clavicles articulate normally with the sternum but have non-articulating lateral ends which are either freely mobile or joined by fibrous bands to the choranoid process, acromion, first rib, or glenoid cavity.

Congenital dislocation of the hip

Congenital dislocation of the hip with bilateral femoral head displacement is rare. By comparison, the condition more usually called congenital dislocation of the hip (which does not actually exist at birth) in most cases is the result of hip-joint anomalies which predispose to subsequent dislocation (see also Section 27.1). In the true form (present at birth), the acetabular socket is decreased in size and flattened while the femoral neck is shortened. The commonest form of hip dysplasia, not true congenital dislocation, occurs more frequently in some families. There is hypoplasia of the osseous nuclei, the acetabular roof is more oblique, the socket flattened, and the femoral head anteverted at the stage before subluxation (dislocation) occurs.

After subluxation, the femoral head protrudes from the acetabulum, though much of the original articular surfaces remain in contact. The femoral head flattens and later moves out of the acetabular socket, the displacement being always upwards (Fig. 27.116) but sometimes anteriorly, posteriorly, or laterally. A second socket becomes formed adjacent to this displaced femoral head.

Talipes equino varus (club foot) and talipes calcaneovalgus

A deformity of the foot in which there is involvement of the talus is called talipes. One of the commonest skeletal malformations at birth is talipes equino varus (club foot), a composite deformity in which the sole is turned medially so that the lateral side of the foot touches the ground in varus, while the toes are lower than the heel in equinus. Talipes equino varus occurs as part of the constellation of abnormalities in the chondrodystrophies such as the campomelic, diastrophic, spondyloepiphyseal, and Kniest dysplasias.

In congenital talipes calcaneovalgus, the foot is dorsiflexed and everted so that its dorsum easily touches the antero-lateral aspect of the leg.

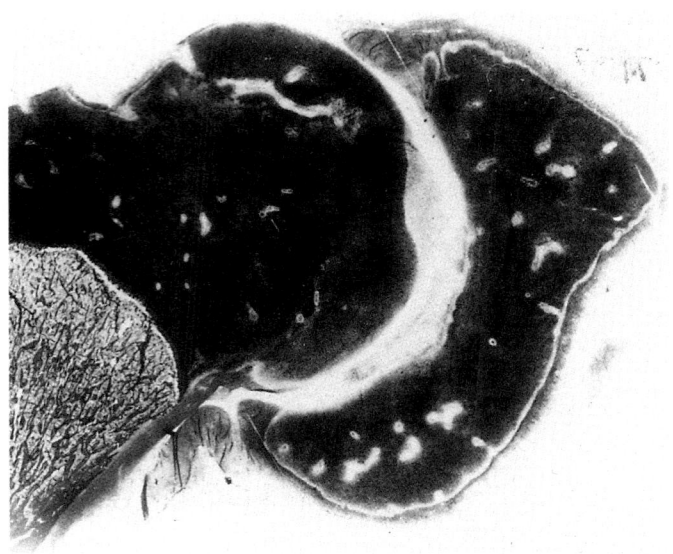

Fig. 27.116 Upward displacement of the femoral head in a case of hip dysplasia (thionin stain).

Perthes disease

The ossification centre of the femoral head undergoes partial or complete aseptic necrosis in Perthes disease and alterations in the femoral neck and acetabulum accompany this change almost from its outset (see Section 27.1). Boys are affected more often than girls, and in nearly all cases the disease is unilateral. There is segmental necrosis of the bone and this results eventually in alteration in the shape of the femoral head due to collapse. The overlying articular cartilage remains viable. There is revascularization of the dead bone of the epiphysis with appositional new bone formation. The femoral head is flattened and the femoral neck shortened as viewed later when this remodelling is complete. This deformity of the femoral head predisposes the hip joint to the subsequent development of osteoarthritis.

Slipped capital femoral epiphysis

Slipping of the epiphysis of the femoral head off the neck may be unilateral or bilateral and affects boys more than girls, in the first half of the second decade of life. The epiphyseal cartilage plate is fragmented, reduplicated, and folded, but the epiphysis itself is not usually directly affected. Vascular fibrous tissue is seen in the region of the epiphyseal plate and reunion eventually occurs with the femoral head frequently malaligned to the neck. Ischaemic necrosis of the slipped femoral capital epiphysis may occur. There may be secondary osteoarthritis later in life.

Congenital pseudoarthrosis of the tibia

Pseudoarthrosis of the tibia is noted at birth or in childhood. It is characterized by a thinning of the tibial cortical bone with subsequent fracture, fibrous union, and development of the pseudoarthrosis. Nearly half the cases reported have a history of cutaneous lesions or manifestations of von Recklinghausen's disease (neurofibromatosis; see Chapter 20).

Osteochondritis dissecans

Osteochondritis dissecans is a condition in which a small piece of detached cartilage with related subchondral bone is found free in the joint. These loose bodies or 'joint mice' are round or ovoid with viable cartilage covering necrotic bone. Males of 15–20 years are most commonly affected and the knee joint is usually involved, especially the medial condyle. A small groove on the articular surface indicates the site from which the loose body has arisen. Other joints sometimes affected are the hip, shoulder, and elbow.

27.2.3 Infective arthritis

Infection of joints occurs in one of two ways: by direct involvement, as in open wounds and extension of infection from adjacent structures; or by the haematogenous route. Involvement is usually monoarticular and the larger joints of the lower limb (knee, hip) are those mostly affected. Infection in the spine may spread from a vertebral body to affect the adjacent disc. It may occur at any level, but most frequently happens in the lumbar region of adults. Predisposing factors in the development of infective arthritis of peripheral joints include corticosteroid treatment, diabetes mellitus, and rheumatoid arthritis. Infection of joints may be due to a variety of bacteria (including *Mycobacterium tuberculosis*), viruses, treponemes, and fungi.

Bacterial arthritis

Septic arthritis is most commonly caused by *Staphylococcus aureus*, haemolytic streptococci, *Neisseria gonorrhoeae*, and *Haemophilus influenzae* in adults. A similar spectrum is seen in children, although staphylococcal infections are more usual in the very young and gonococcal infection in teenagers. Other organisms include *N. pneumoniae*, *Pseudomonas*, *Proteus*, *Salmonella*, *Enterobacter*, *Escherichia coli*, and *Bacteroides*. An important function of the histopathologist in relation to joint replacement surgery is the recognition of infection in cases undergoing revision surgery.

Since involvement is usually monoarticular, the pathologist is faced with the problem of differentiating septic arthritis from the effects of trauma, crystal deposition, and a chronic synovitis such as rheumatoid arthritis presenting in a single joint. The joint is clinically inflamed and enlarged due to increased synovial fluid as well as synovial membrane swelling and proliferation. The synovial fluid shows a high white cell count with numerous polymorphonuclear leucocytes, and may contain abundant fibrin and organisms (Fig. 27.117). The synovial membrane is also heavily infiltrated with polymorphonuclears and macrophages, with increased vascularity and variable numbers of lymphocytes and plasma cells. Abundant surface fibrin may be seen and the causative organisms may be distinguished in a Gram stain. The patient may sometimes receive

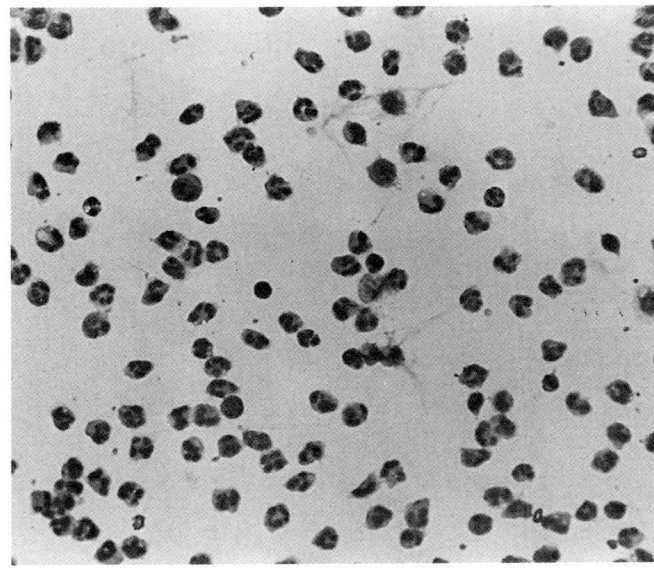

Fig. 27.117 Numerous polymorphonuclear leucocytes and occasional streaks of fibrin in the synovial fluid from a joint with septic arthritis (May–Grunwald Giemsa).

several days of antibiotic treatment before biopsy is performed, so that the histopathological appearances may be modified. The differential diagnosis of synovitis containing plentiful polymorphonuclear leucocytes includes crystal synovitis and Behcet syndrome. If untreated for any significant length of time, septic arthritis can give rise to severe damage to the joint surfaces. Cartilage involvement may be both by direct action of inflammatory cells and by alteration of its nutrition, so that chondrocyte degeneration occurs. Eventually, erosion of the cartilage and extension of the infective process into adjacent bone may occur.

Tuberculous arthritis

Tuberculosis of joints usually results from haematogenous spread of organisms, although spread from an adjacent focus of osteomyelitis may occur. Disc involvement may accompany tuberculous osteomyelitis of the spine, which occurs most frequently in the lumbar, followed by the cervical, region. The hips and knees are the joints most affected, though other sites are involved. The synovial membrane becomes inflamed and may show the presence of a creamy-coloured surface exudate or occasionally small whitish tubercles. The cartilage may merely have a 'lack-lustre' appearance due to a surface covering of tuberculous fibrous tissue, while at an advanced stage, there may be detachment of fragments of cartilage to expose the underlying bone.

The synovial membrane shows the presence of tuberculoid granulomata containing Langhans giant cells (Fig. 27.118). These granulomata may be caseating but this is by no means common. Organisms may be identified with Ziehl–Nielson or other stains. Elsewhere in the synovial membrane there may

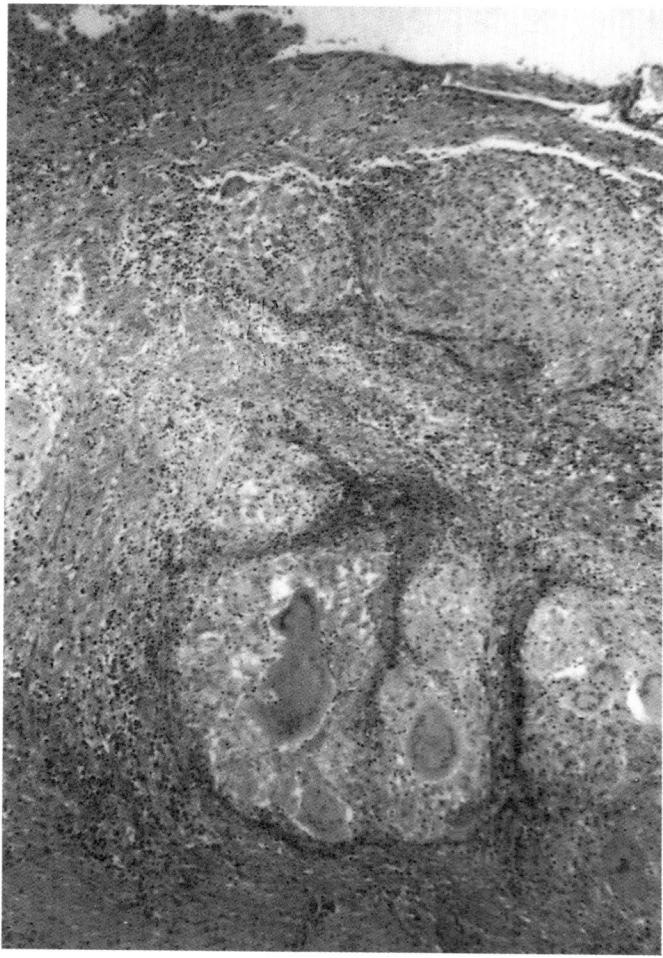

Fig. 27.118 Synovial membrane showing the presence of several epithelioid granulomata containing Langhans giant cells in tuberculous synovitis.

be lymphoid follicles and a plasma cell infiltrate, resembling rheumatoid arthritis. A careful and thorough examination of multiple levels of the tissue for the presence of granulomata is essential when there is a suspicion of tuberculosis, but the histopathological picture is apparently of a non-specific chronic synovitis.

Other conditions should be borne in mind when granulomata are seen in a synovial biopsy. These include atypical mycobacterial infection, sarcoidosis, foreign body reactions, fungal arthritis, and Crohn disease. Organisms such as *M. kansasii*, *M. marinum*, *M. avium*, and *M. fortuitum* may be responsible for a 'sausage digit' or diffuse swelling of the palm or other parts of the hand. The condition typically remains unrecognized for a considerable period of time, being treated conservatively or with corticosteroid injections before there is resource to biopsy and/or microbiological examination. Sarcoidosis of joints undoubtedly occurs, but attention to the exclusion of other causes of granulomatous synovitis is essential before reaching this diagnosis.

Syphilis of joints

Joints are only rarely involved by syphilis of either congenital or acquired type. Large joints are those affected, the knee being the most frequent, followed by the elbow, ankle, shoulder, and wrists. Involvement may be bilateral and symmetrical.

Joint involvement occurs relatively late in congenital syphilis with erosion of cartilage and bone together with periostitis. There is a lymphocyte and plasma cell infiltrate in the synovial membrane. Older children have increased joint laxity and excessive amounts of synovial fluid in 'Clutton's joints'. Gummata may be present in the synovial membrane. In the secondary stage of acquired syphilis details are sparse. In established cases there may be gummata in the synovial membrane and adjacent bone, cartilage, and ligaments, all of which are destroyed. The synovial membrane shows a non-specific chronic synovitis. Loss of nerve supply to the knee joint in tabes dorsalis results in the severe disruption seen in neuropathic joint disease, which is described later in this chapter.

Brucellosis and joints

Arthritis occurs in a small proportion of those having *Brucella* infections. Peripheral joint and spinal involvement both occur, with chronic synovitis in the former and osteomyelitis spreading to the intervertebral discs in the latter. Granulomata may be present. The knees and other large peripheral joints are those usually affected.

Fungal arthritis

The fungal infections that may affect joints are candidiasis, coccidioidomycosis, sporotrichosis, blastomycosis, histoplasmosis, and cryptococcosis, all of which are rare. Patients are likely to be immunosuppressed with haematological malignancy, steroid treatment, or a severe debilitating systemic illness such as carcinomatosis; the exceptions are coccidioidomycosis, sporotrichosis, and blastomycosis. Coccidiomycosis and blastomycosis are endemic in parts of the USA. Most fungal infections of joints are monoarticular and they usually involve large joints, particularly the knee. Granulomata are seen in coccidioidomycosis, sporotrichosis, blastomycosis, and cryptococcosis, but not in candidiasis, in which there is a non-specific mononuclear cell infiltrate.

Lyme arthritis

Lyme disease is a multisystem disorder affecting children or adults, and was first described in a small area of Connecticut. The condition, at first thought to be a childhood complaint, has a characteristic skin lesion called erythema chronicum migrans. Cardiac, neurological changes, and an arthritis are also present. The latter is oligoarticular and typically intermittent, but may proceed to a chronic erosive and destructive joint disease. The histopathological appearances are those of a non-specific chronic synovitis with thickening of the intimal cell layer, and a lymphoplasmacytic infiltrate, sometimes with lymphoid follicle formation. Lyme disease is caused by a recently recognized spirochaete belonging to the genus *Borrelia* and this is transmitted to man by *Ixodes dammini* or related ixodid ticks. Cases have been described in other parts of the USA, in Europe, and in Australia.

Viral diseases and the joints

Rubella, mumps, lymphogranuloma venereum, variola, infectious mononucleosis, hepatitis B, chicken-pox, varicella, influenza, and smallpox may all be accompanied by joint disease. Involvement is transient and acute with arthralgia predominating. Little detailed information is available about histopathological features in the synovium in these conditions because biopsy material is very rarely submitted for examination. A non-specific lymphocytic synovial infiltration with thickening of the intimal cell layer has been noted in mumps-associated arthritis and similar changes are seen with rubella. It seems likely that this is the appearance in the other viral arthritides. Virus has been demonstrated by immunohistochemical methods in the synovial membrane following smallpox and rubella vaccination.

Rheumatic fever

The arthritis occurring in association with rheumatic fever is typically a transient, acute, and migratory disorder which follows a group A haemolytic streptococcal infection. It is not an infective arthritis but reactive. Large joints, such as the knee, ankle, and elbow, are affected but the small joints of the wrist may also be involved. The synovial membrane contains polymorphonuclear leucocytes and macrophages at first, though there may later be a lymphocyte and plasma cell infiltrate. Subcutaneous 'rheumatic' nodules may develop adjacent to the affected joints. These nodules have a central eosinophilic zone surrounded by a rim of lymphocytes, macrophages, and giant cells. There may be vasculitis in nearby vessels. The nodules disappear after a few weeks, unlike those of rheumatoid arthritis which persist and occur in particular anatomical sites (see Section 27.2.5).

27.2.4   Joint involvement in generalized diseases

Ochronosis

Ochronosis is due to an inborn error of metabolism in which homogentisic acid oxidase is deficient. A brown pigment, the polymerized oxidation product of homogentisic acid, is deposited in cartilage. The pigment becomes deposited in cartilage everywhere; in the peripheral joints, the intevertebral discs, and other sites, such as the ears. Cartilage degeneration takes place so that there is development of polyarticular osteoarthritis and spondylosis, both of which are severe. The knee joint is particularly liable to severe damage. The heavily pigmented articular cartilage becomes fibrillated and large fragments

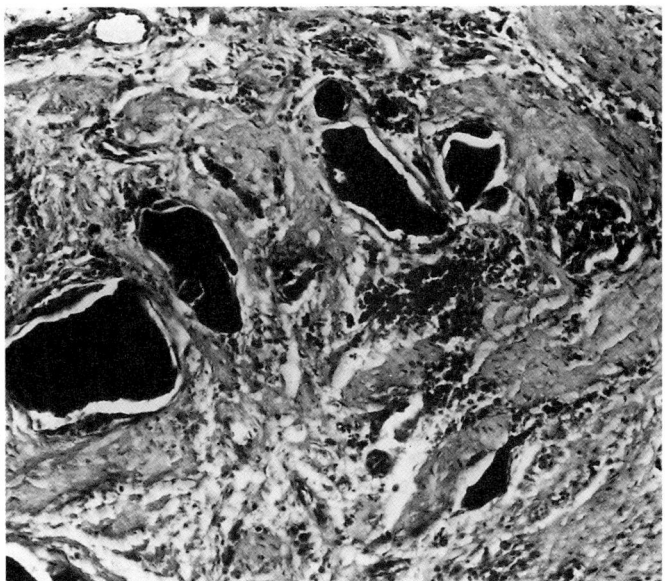

Fig. 27.119 Synovial membrane in ochronosis, showing the presence of fragments of pigmented cartilage (shards) with some chronic inflammatory cells.

(shards) of pigmented cartilage are shed from the joint surface. They are readily distinguished histologically in the synovial membrane (Fig. 27.119). Calcium pyrophosphate dihydrate crystal deposition may be associated with ochronosis.

Haemochromatosis

Joint involvement occurs in a significant proportion of patients with haemochromatosis, the sites affected being the fingers, knees, hips, and wrists, together with the spine. Haemochromatosis is one of those conditions in which calcium pyrophosphate dihydrate (CPPD) crystal deposition also occurs, so that there may be fine, chalky, white deposits, both on the articular cartilage and in the synovial membrane which is otherwise discoloured brown because of iron deposition. Histopathological examination of the synovial membrane shows the presence of iron (haemosiderin) deposits in the cells of the thickened intimal layer and in the underlying synovial macrophage infiltrate. No other evidence of significant inflammation is seen apart from occasional fibrin deposits. The articular cartilage undergoes changes similar to osteoarthritis (see Section 27.2.6); CPPD crystals may be demonstrable in both cartilage and synovial membrane by compensated polarization microscopy (see Section 27.2.7). Recent evidence suggests that there may be a defect in the calcified zone of cartilage with iron deposition in the tidemark region. Separation of cartilage from subchrondral bone occurs at this level.

Other conditions in which there is iron deposited in the synovial membrane are transfusional haemosiderosis, haemophilia, haemarthrosis due to trauma, vascular tumours, and pigmented villonodular synovitis. Local bleeding into the joint is responsible for the heavy iron load in these patients, except in haemosiderosis, which resembles haemochromatosis in the synovial appearances produced.

Haemophilia and similar disorders

Haemorrhage into the joints is a common occurrence in haemophilia and in Christmas disease. Recurrent haemarthroses are responsible for the changes seen. The synovial membrane is discoloured brown and, on histopathological examination, shows the presence of numerous iron-laden intimal cells and subintimal macrophages. There may be erosion of the articular cartilage, subchondral bone sclerosis, and the development of other features of osteoarthritis, including pseudocyst formation.

Haemarthrosis

Trauma is an important cause of bleeding into the joint and phagocytosis of red blood cells ultimately leads to accumulation of iron deposits in the synovial intimal cells and macrophages. Not only may obviously significant episodes of trauma lead to this picture, but it may also occur with joint derangements, such as damaged menisci and similar mechanical problems. Moderate amounts of iron may be seen in various other disorders—notably rheumatoid arthritis—and, while there have been suggestions that this may play a role in the aetiopathogenesis of the disease, it is likely that iron deposition is a reflection of past haemorrhage into the inflamed rheumatoid tissues.

Haemophiliac arthropathy

Recurrent episodes of haemarthrosis occur in haemophilia so that there is heavy haemosiderin deposition in the synovial tissues. There is thickening of the intimal cell layer and the synovial membrane may assume a more villous appearance. There is vascular proliferation and fibrosis may also occur. The cellular infiltrate usually contains significant numbers of lymphocytes as well as pigment-laden macrophages. Secondary degenerative changes occur in the cartilage with the development of osteoarthritis.

Sickle-cell disease

Sickle-cell disease (see Chapter 23) results in the blockage of small vessels by sickled red blood cells and platelets in various sites in the body, including the joints. Areas of necrosis of subchondral bone with subsequent loss of overlying cartilage may lead to 'degenerative' joint disease. Ischaemic necrosis of the femoral head may also occur, and in the affected child may resemble Perthes disease, though the latter occurs at a younger age and rarely affects Negroes. The synovium may show reactive changes related to the presence of cartilage and bone fragments from the joint surface, or there may be low-grade inflammation with a mononuclear cell infiltrate and focal areas of soft-tissue necrosis. Infection may spread to joints from nearby bone or soft tissue or there may be haematogenous spread of organisms. *Salmonella* is the usual infective agent.

Acromegaly

As well as stimulating bone growth with lengthening of limb bones, enlargement of the hands and feet, and the facial (skull) changes, cartilage production is increased in acromegaly. This results in changes at sites of endochondral ossification, such as the costochondral junctions, but also involves articular cartilage, which becomes thickened and then is the site of secondary degenerative changes similar to those of osteoarthritis. The vertebral bodies become increased in diameter and there is a commensurate increase in intervertebral disc size. The changes may resemble spondylosis deformans.

Amyloid deposition in joints

Amyloid can be deposited in joints in one of two different ways; as part of age-related changes and in association with generalized amyloidosis. The formation of amyloid occurs in many ageing tissues, and small deposits of amyloid have been described in the cartilage of osteoarthritic joints and in degenerating intervertebral discs. The term 'amyloid arthropathy' is used to describe a polyarthritis due to the deposition of amyloid in and around joints in association with multiple myeloma. The shoulder joints are particularly affected and may become swollen to the size of a football, but elbows, hands, knees, hips, temporomandibular, and sternoclavicular joints are also commonly involved. The synovial membrane has a stiffened appearance and there may be a greyish waxy deposition of amyloid in the joint space, though free amyloid in the synovial fluid may require electron microscopy of a spun sediment for its detection. Amyloid may be detected with appropriate stains, such as Congo red, as a thin layer at or just below the surface of the articular cartilage and as deposits in the synovium and para-articular soft tissues. Localized masses of amyloid may be present in the bone marrow space of the subchondral bone. The optical properties of amyloid may not be demonstrable in the free synovial fluid deposits which are nevertheless stained with Congo red. By electron microscopy, typical amyloid fibrils of 7.5–10 nm diameter and a periodicity of two or three bands per 10 nm length are found extracellularly in the synovial membrane and synovial fluid.

Amyloid is also present around small vessels in the synovium of patients on long-term dialysis. The amyloid is composed partially of β_2 microglobulin.

Pulmonary hypertrophic osteoarthropathy

Hypertrophic osteoarthropathy occurs predominantly in association with severe lung disease, such as bronchogenic carcinoma, but is also seen in association with congenital heart disease and with some gastrointestinal and liver diseases. Clubbing of the fingers and toes, due to thickening of subungual soft tissues, periosteal new bone formation with widening of the bone ends in the peripheries, and painful swelling of joints are the important features. The radius and ulna, the tibia and fibula, are more often affected than the humerus or the femur, and the metacarpals or metatarsals more than the phalanges. Enlargement of joints is mainly due to periosteal new bone formation but thickening of the synovial membrane and the presence of synovial effusions may also occur. Histological examination may show a focal lymphocyte infiltrate and increased vascularity.

27.2.5 Chronic inflammatory joint disease

Rheumatoid arthritis

Rheumatoid arthritis (RA) is a chronic non-suppurative inflammatory polyarthritis, mainly affecting peripheral synovial joints and usually in a symmetrical pattern. The wrists and small joints of the hands, for example, are frequently involved. The arthritis is part of a generalized disease of unknown aetiology, characterized by a prolonged course with exacerbations and remissions. Onset may be at any age, but is most frequent in those from 35 to 50 years old. Women are affected around three times more often than men. There are no absolute features for the clinical diagnosis but the American Rheumatism Association (ARA), now called the American College of Rheumatology, has provided criteria that are normally used to assess whether patients have probable, definite, or classical RA. There is no certain diagnostic laboratory test for the disease, though patients with severe involvement frequently show rheumatoid factor activity (IgM anti-IgG) in the serum although IgG and IgA antiglobulins (rheumatoid factors) also occur. The following description will be confined to the changes in the joints. Pathological changes in other systems are described in the appropriate chapter.

The joints in early rheumatoid arthritis show redness, pain, heat, and localized swelling. The small joints of the fingers and toes, the knees, elbows, wrists, and hips are usually affected, though any of the synovial joints may be involved. There is a synovial effusion containing increased numbers of polymorphonuclear leucocytes. The synovial membrane is congested and swollen with a pronounced villous pattern. Histological examination may show the presence of increased numbers of polymorphonuclears and fibrin, giving rise to the suspicion of an infective process, but, more often, there is a chronic inflammatory appearance with abundant lymphocytes and plasma cells, polymorphonuclears, and fibrin, together with an increase in numbers of synovial lining cells (erroneously called synovial hyperplasia), even in the early stage of the disease.

Vascular fibrous tissue (granulation tissue) grows from the margins of the joint across the articular surface and comprises the 'pannus' (Latin: a cloth) which becomes increasingly adherent to the cartilage. Adhesions between villous processes of the synovium and this granulation tissue also occur, and later there may be fibrous or even bony ankylosis, though the latter is more common in other diseases, such as destructive infective arthritis or ankylosing spondylitis. When the disease process is well established, villous processes of synovial membrane are yellowish-brown in colour due to iron deposition; the articular surface shows patchy areas of cartilage loss, mainly extending inwards from the joint margins; and there is destruc-

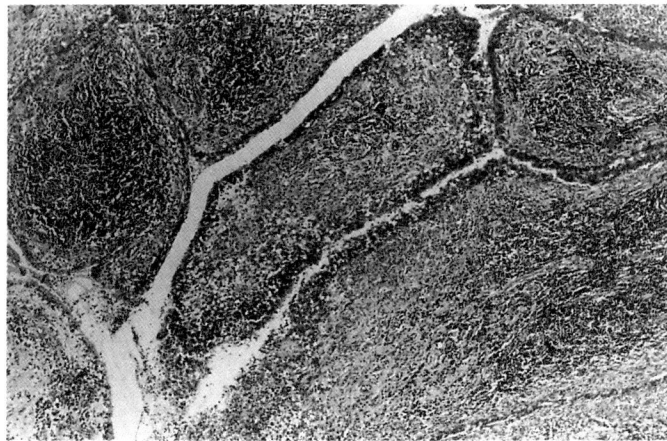

Fig. 27.120 Rheumatoid synovial membrane, showing an increase in surface cells and heavy chronic inflammatory cell infiltration with formation of lymphoid follicles.

tion of the bone at the sides of the joint, which is the morphological counterpart of 'erosions' in clinical radiographs.

Light microscopy of the synovial membrane in established rheumatoid arthritis shows marked infiltration with inflammatory cells, comprising diffuse lymphocytes and plasma cells but with lymphocytes also arranged in follicles, some of which may contain germinal centres (Fig. 27.120). There is increased vascularity and there may be diffuse fibrosis and perivascular fibrosis. The surface of the synovial membrane is covered by a layer of intimal cells which is considerably increased in thickness. There may be surface fibrin deposition, and fibrin is also incorporated into the superficial part of the heavily inflamed underlying synovial connective tissue. Polymorphonuclear leucocytes are not a prominent feature of routinely stained sections, and where present they are usually most numerous in relation to fibrin.

These features in combination have in the past been considered typical of rheumatoid arthritis but careful comparative studies have shown that the appearances of the rheumatoid synovial membrane cannot be distinguished from those of other chronic inflammatory joint diseases, including ankylosing spondylitis, Reiter syndrome, psoriatic arthritis, enteropathic arthritis, and even some cases of osteoarthritis. True rheumatoid nodules sometimes occur in synovial tissues and are the only feature characteristic of rheumatoid arthritis. Structures resembling rheumatoid nodules which have partly discharged their contents into the joint space are sometimes also seen, and they have been called 'hemigranulomas'. Care is required in separating these from true rheumatoid nodules since they have been found occasionally in other joint diseases, such as psoriatic arthritis, ankylosing spondylitis, and osteoarthritis. Large focal collections of fibrin which have become incorporated into the synovial membrane, organized, and surrounded by macrophages are the probable explanation for these hemigranulomas.

Immunohistochemical methods have been used to study the

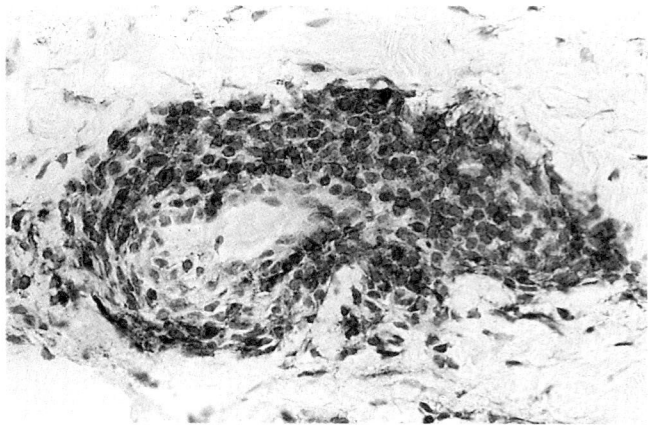

Fig. 27.121   Perivascular collection of T-helper lymphocytes (CD4⁺) in synovial membrane (indirect immunoperoxidase).

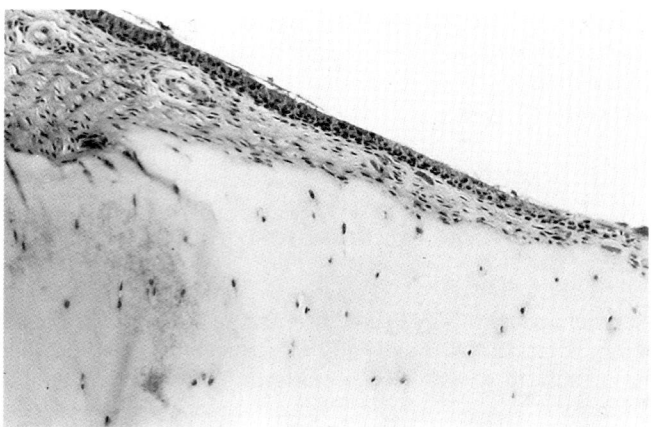

Fig. 27.122   Cartilage–pannus junction in rheumatoid arthritis, showing vascular fibrous tissue (pannus) with a surface layer of cells resembling synoviocytes.

rheumatoid synovial membrane. Most of the plasma cells contain IgG immunoglobulin, followed in frequency by IgA, then IgM. Synovial membranes from seropositive rheumatoid arthritis patients show significantly more IgM-containing plasma cells than those from seronegative rheumatoid or the other chronic synovitides. Rheumatoid factor (antiglobulin) activity has been demonstrated *in situ* in a proportion of synovial plasma cells, using several different techniques. Although classical rheumatoid factor is an IgM antibody and IgM-rheumatoid factor is found in these plasma cells, double-labelling experiments show that most plasma cells contain IgG-rheumatoid factor. Immunoperoxidase light microscopic and immunogold electron microscopic studies have shown that the synovial intimal cells (type A synoviocytes) are labelled with monoclonal antibodies for HLA-Dr, lysozyme, α_1-antitrypsin, and a number of macrophage markers, while others (type B synoviocytes) contain and produce fibronectin. These cells have recently been shown to be surrounded by type IV collagen and laminin. The cellular infiltrate has also been further examined and the cell populations present have been identified. Macrophages are extremely numerous, both in the diffuse infiltrate and in lymphoid follicles. Staining with monoclonal antibodies also shows the presence of many more polymorphonuclear leucocytes than are detectable in routine sections. Characterization of synovial lymphocytes shows a preponderance of T-cells with CD4⁺ cells much more numerous than CD8⁺ cells both in lymphoid follicles and perivascular lymphocyte collections (Fig. 27.121). There are also B-lymphocytes present in follicles and these follicles may contain germinal centres.

The margin of the joint affected by progressive rheumatoid arthritis invariably shows the presence of granulation tissue, forming pannus, and it is this which accounts for the destruction of the cartilage. Pannus extends inwards from the edge of the joint to replace the cartilage. The cartilage adjacent to pannus shows decreased basophilia, a reflection of proteoglycan loss, a finding that may be confirmed using dyes such as toluidine blue or alcian blue. There are differences of opinion as to the nature of the process occurring at the cartilage–pannus junction. While it may be that the granulation tissue containing inflammatory cells (polymorphonuclear leucocytes, lymphocytes, plasma cells, macrophages, mast cells) is actively destroying the cartilage, an alternative explanation is that cartilage damage and loss may be due to some other mechanism (for example, failure of cartilage nutrition) and that pannus represents a healing reaction. Although there are variations, the interface between pannus and cartilage is usually clearly demarcated, and the cells close to the margin may be polymorphonuclears, mast cells, or macrophages (Fig. 27.122). Similar vascular fibrous tissue containing inflammatory cells is seen sometimes undermining the cartilage through the subchondral bone, but this is a poorly understood lesion. Cartilage loss gives rise to the so-called loss of joint space seen in clinical radiographs. The encroachment of inflammatory fibrous tissue inwards into the subchondral bone from the joint margin gives rise to the erosions. Cyst-like defects (pseudocysts) are also formed in the bone immediately deep to the articular surface where it has lost its cartilage covering. The bone adjoining affected joints in rheumatoid arthritis is often osteoporotic and it is thought that synovial fluid or granulation tissue is forced into this weakened bone under pressure to form these flask-shaped pseudocysts, which histologically come to contain fibrous tissue. Degenerative changes in the abnormal cartilage lead to secondary osteoarthritis in rheumatoid joints. Altered joint mechanics contribute to this and these in turn are related to the instability caused by damage to soft tissues. Progressive damage to the joint capsule, ligaments, and tendons occurs as the rheumatoid inflammatory process extends to adjacent structures. Subluxation of unstable joints results and subsequent healing with fibrosis gives rise to the well-known and characteristic fixed deformities of rheumatoid joints, for example in the hand.

Seronegative arthropathies

Various forms of chronic synovitis are known to occur as part of, or in association with, other diseases. The affected patients have no evidence of rheumatoid factor in their blood and the disorders are often put together into a seronegative group. Ankylosing spondylitis (AS) is one of these disorders and 90 per cent of such affected people have the histocompatibility antigen HLA-B27, compared to 8 per cent of healthy Caucasians. There are also associations between HLA-B27 and other seronegative arthropathies, e.g. Reiter's syndrome and psoriatics, with spinal and peripheral joint involvement.

Ankylosing spondylitis

This is a disease, predominantly of young men, which starts in the lumbar spine and sacro-iliac joints. There is inflammation at the attachment of ligaments to bone, mainly consisting of a lymphocytic infiltrate. Subsequent healing with fibrosis and ossification gives rise to early bony ankylosis across the margins of the intervertebral discs. Ultimately, the whole spine may become completely fused to form a rigid 'bamboo spine'. Peripheral joint involvement occurs in around one-quarter of all cases and there is usually a monoarticular (sometimes pauci-articular) arthritis affecting mainly the hip, knee, ankle, or shoulder. Histopathologically, the affected synovial membrane shows features similar to those of rheumatoid arthritis, with a villous pattern, intimal layer thickening, fibrin deposition, increased vascularity, and a diffuse lymphoplasmacellular infiltrate with development of lymphoid follicles.

Psoriatic arthritis

Although the combination of psoriasis and arthritis is more than coincidental, arthritis is present in only around 5 per cent of psoriatics. The arthritis may be pauciarticular, with a mild or moderately progressive course; symmetrical and polyarticular, with a slowly destructive course; or show the presence of sacro-iliitis and spondylitis, with or without peripheral arthritis. The last group are mostly HLA-B27 positive. Involvement of the distal interphalangeal joints of the hands is peculiar to psoriatic arthritis, and occurs more frequently in those with pauci-articular than those with symmetrical disease, being least often seen in those with spondylitis. While there have been considered to be differences in the histological appearances in the synovial membrane in the past, the picture is actually similar to that of rheumatoid arthritis, as demonstrated in recent careful comparative studies. Severely destructive osteolytic changes occur in relation to the distal phalanx, and these are associated with osteoblastic remodelling activity to give rise to a broadened mushroom-shaped distal phalanx.

Reiter syndrome

Reiter syndrome originally included the combination of conjunctivitis, urethritis, and arthritis. Mucosal ulceration, keratoderma blenorrhagica, and cardiovascular abnormalities are now also sometimes included. Reiter syndrome is an example of a 'reactive' arthritis, in that prior infection with *Chlamydia trachomatis* is followed by development of the syndrome after a short interval. The organisms are not present drome after a short interval. The organisms are not present within the joint. Most affected are males, and 80 per cent of patients are HLA-B27 positive. The arthritis is asymmetrical and pauciarticular, usually affecting the ankle or knee. The synovial membrane is hyperaemic, with some granulocytes but mostly lymphocytes and plasma cells, so that the picture resembles that of rheumatoid arthritis and the other chronic synovitides. Occasionally, the arthritis becomes more destructive, with pannus formation and loss of cartilage. Spondylitis, when it occurs, resembles that seen in the other seronegative arthropathies.

Enteropathic arthritis

A 'reactive' arthritis may occur one or two weeks after enteritis caused by *Salmonella*, *Shigella*, *Yersinia*, or *Campylobacter* infection, particularly in those who are HLA-B27 positive. This acute sterile synovitis, associated with infection localized elsewhere in the body (hence reactive), shows histological features like those of Reiter syndrome. Involvement is usually mono-articular or pauciarticular. A small proportion of those with ulcerative colitis or Crohn disease develop a similar reactive type of arthritis. Sarcoid-like granulomata have occasionally been seen, and the differential diagnosis of other granulomatous synovitides (tuberculosis, sarcoidosis) has to be considered in these circumstances. A transient migratory arthritis also occurs sometimes in Whipple disease. The synovitis is non-specific but periodic acid–Schiff positive macrophages may be present (see Chapter 16).

Behcet syndrome

Behcet syndrome is a multisystem disorder affecting the skin, eyes, oral and genital mucous membranes, cardiovascular and nervous systems, as well as joints. Behcet syndrome is relatively uncommon in Britain and is seen mostly in Japan, the eastern Mediterranean, and Turkey. Arthritis occurs at some time in a large proportion of cases and has an intermittent pauciarticular pattern affecting the knees, ankles, wrists, and shoulders. The microscopic appearances are unlike those of rheumatoid arthritis or the other chronic synovitides. Lymphoid follicles and plasma cells are uncommon. There is usually abundant granulation tissue, with a mixed polymorphonuclear leucocyte, lymphocyte, and macrophage infiltrate. The surface lacks intimal cells over large areas and there may be abundant fibrin deposition. The presence of numerous polymorphonuclear leucocytes suggests the differential diagnosis of infection or acute gout.

Systemic lupus erythematosus

The general features of systemic lupus erythematosus are dealt with elsewhere in this book (Chapter 4). Polyarticular joint disease is a frequent but not very prominent feature, lasting for a short period and only occasionally progressing to deforming chronic disease. Wrists, knees, and fingers are mostly affected. The synovial membrane shows increased vascularity, a low-grade lymphoplasmacellular infiltrate with perivascular lymphocytic cuffing and surface fibrin deposition. Haematoxy-lin bodies are the only specific feature and they are rarely seen.

Scleroderma

Arthritis is an occasional accompaniment of scleroderma. The synovial membrane shows surface fibrin deposition and the in-timal cell layer is attenuated or absent. Occasional collections of lymphocytes and plasma cells are present, and fibrosis occurs in the later stages of synovial involvement.

Familial Mediterranean fever

Familial Mediterranean fever is an inherited disorder, having its onset in childhood and characterized by brief attacks of fever, arthritis, and serositis (pleural, peritoneal) lasting up to a week. A more chronic arthritis occurs sometimes and then affects a single joint. The synovial membrane shows a mixed inflammat-ory cell infiltrate with granulocytes, macrophages, lympho-cytes, and plasma cells. Lymphoid follicles are not a feature.

27.2.6   Osteoarthritis

Osteoarthritis (OA) is a non-inflammatory disorder of diar-throdial joints characterized by progressive loss of cartilage; sclerosis of the underlying bone; and proliferation of bone and cartilage at the joint margins. Changes similar to those seen in modern man can be detected in the bones of prehistoric animals and in ancient human populations. There is potential confusion over the use of terms in osteoarthritis, which is frequently classified as being primary or secondary. The latter occurs after some other insult to the joint, such as rheumatoid arthritis, other synovitis, gout, calcium pyrophosphate dihydrate (CPPD) arthropathy, hip dysplasia, acromegaly, haemochromatosis, and even neuropathic joint (see Section 27.2.4). Osteoarthritis of this secondary type could be considered to represent 'end-stage' joint disease, and thus parallel cirrhosis of the liver and granular contracted kidney.

The naked-eye appearances of osteoarthritic joints vary in detail from site to site. Most studies have been performed on the hip, followed by the knee. Large areas of the articular cartilage are lost with exposure of the underlying bone, which becomes grooved and/or polished, depending on the joint. Around the joint margin there is outgrowth of bone (covered by cartilage on its articular surface) to form osteophytes. The North American tendency is to call this type of involvement degenerative joint disease and, while osteoarthritis occurs with increasing fre-quency with increasing age from the fourth decade onwards, it is becoming clear that individuals vary in their capacity for regrowth and remodelling of cartilage and bone so that con-tinuing deterioration of ageing joints is by no means a certainty. Thus degenerative joint disease may not be an entirely appro-priate alternative name.

The way in which these changes come about is best under-stood by consideration of the biochemistry of cartilage and the histological appearances. A large amount of specialist biochem-istry has been performed in primary osteoarthritis, but the

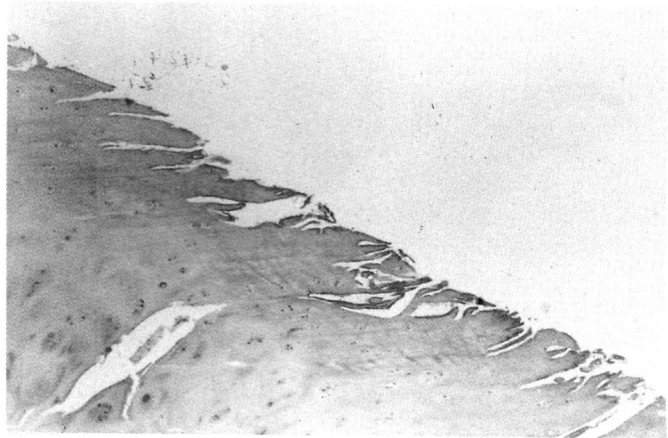

Fig. 27.123   Osteoarthritic cartilage showing the presence of numer-ous splits in the surface in the process of fibrillation.

cause of this condition remains unknown and it is likely that no single factor is responsible. Early changes in the proteoglycan content and collagen of articular cartilage are subtle, as are alterations in subchondral bone. Which of these various factors is most important is unknown. Cartilage depends for its resi-lience (and turgidity) on the presence of large hydrophilic aggregates of hyaluronic acid with chondroitin sulphate- and keratan sulphate-containing proteoglycans held between a tightly packed network of collagen fibrils (see Section 27.2.1). In older cartilage, the chondroitin sulphate content decreases and that of keratan sulphate increases. Proteoglycan loss in osteoarthritis, which may be related to collagen damage, means loss of water, so that the cartilage undergoes splitting at its surface; the process is known as fibrillation (Fig. 27.123). There is a question about whether fine splitting is part of the ageing process and does not progress to OA. Evidence of prolifer-ative activity by chondrocytes is seen with the development of large clusters, or chondrocyte clones, in the fibrillated cartilage of OA. Pieces of fibrillated cartilage become broken off and even-tually there is progressive thinning as the cartilage shelves to bare bone in a process known as eburnation (Fig. 27.124).

These changes occur at predictable sites in affected joints and these correspond to the main mechanical load-bearing areas of the articular surfaces. Thus the medial compartment of the tibio-femoral joint and the zenith region of the femoral head next to the fovea are early sites of cartilage loss. The loading of the bone beneath the articular surface depends on the type of surface covering it. Thus normal cartilage has different load-bearing properties from thinned fibrillated cartilage, which again is different from direct load transmission by the bone itself. Appositional new bone formation occurs in the sub-chondral bone in response to this altered loading, so that in the area where cartilage has been lost there is sclerotic bone. On naked-eye examination this thickened bone of the eburnated part of the joint surface has a polished, shiny appearance, like ivory, due to the abrasive effects of movement. Radiologically,

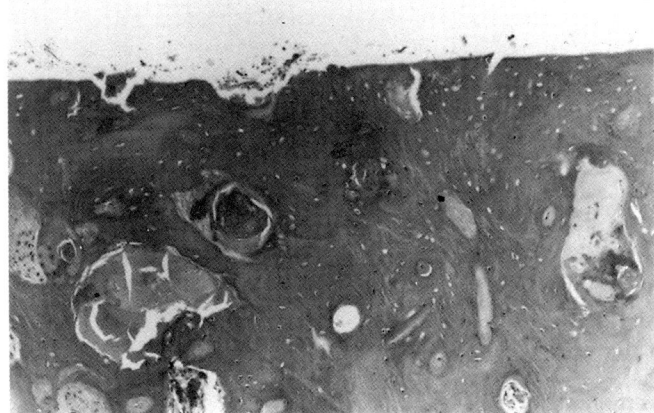

Fig. 27.124 Osteoarthritic joint showing exposed bone which is greatly increased in density in the process of eburnation.

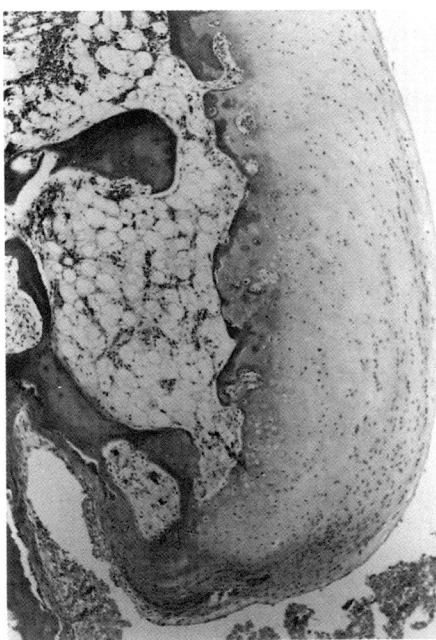

Fig. 27.125 Osteophyte, in osteoarthritis, showing fibrocartilaginous covering of the bone outgrowth from the joint margin. The original bone is to the extreme left. The trabeculae and intertrabecular fatty and haemopoietic tissue are in continuity with this. The growing tip of the osteophyte is seen at the bottom of the picture.

cyst-like spaces are seen immediately beneath the bony articular surface and histological examination reveals these to be either completely circular/oval defects or flask-like areas opening on to the surface. The exact mode of formation of these lesions is obscure. While it has been suggested that they may be due to localized necrosis of subchondral bone, a more likely suggestion is that they represent the effects of the injection of synovial fluid under pressure during normal joint function through a point of weakness in the articular surface, with subsequent expansion within the interosseous soft tissues to achieve the cyst-like space. Fractures of the subchondral bone plate can be seen in OA and could form the basis for this transmission of synovial fluid pressure to the marrow space. These lesions are more correctly called pseudocysts since they do not contain fluid. They may contain either proteinaceous material or fibrovascular tissue. This fibrous tissue may undergo metaplasia to fibrocartilage in the flask-like areas. The pseudocysts become surrounded by bone through endochondral ossification of the margin of the fibrocartilage and direct new bone formation in the fibrous tissue (intramembranous ossification).

Altered distribution of load due to cartilage loss over the load-bearing area results in mechanical stimulation of structures towards the periphery of the joint. Proliferation of fibrocartilage occurs at the joint margin where the fibrous tissue of the capsule is inserted. This fibrocartilage becomes vascularized and converted to bone at its base by endochondral ossification. This process continues with progressive growth of fibrocartilage undergoing ossification outwards away from the joint margin to form an osteophyte (Fig. 27.125). The osseous tissue of the osteophytic process becomes populated by fatty or haemopoietic tissue in continuity with the trabecular bone of the original bone. There is remodelling with more or less pronounced loss of the original marginal subchondral bone and adjacent cortex at the side of the bone.

The synovial membrane in osteoarthritis may show only minor changes, with increased vascularity and fibrosis. There may, however, be increased numbers of intimal cells, fibrin deposition, and a lymphocyte and plasma cell infiltrate, even with lymphoid follicle formation, so that the appearances resemble those of chronic inflammatory joint disease. Fragments of cartilage and bone debris are often incorporated into the synovial membrane and calcium pyrophosphate crystals are sometimes seen. There is no evidence that either detritus or crystals are the reason for this chronic lymphocytic infiltration, although, of course, both may themselves excite a macrophage response.

Primary generalized hypertrophic osteoarthritis

Osteoarthritis frequently involves one or just a few joints, the knee, hip, shoulder, fingers and thumb, and ankle being common sites. Recent clinical studies suggest that there may be particular distribution patterns of osteoarthritic joint involvement but no information exists as to whether there are pathological correlates. A well-recognized form of osteoarthritis, known as primary generalized hypertrophic or nodular osteoarthritis, may be distinguished, and occurs particularly in post-menopausal women. Various joints are involved, but in particular the distal and proximal interphalangeal joints of the fingers. Small, hard nodules, known as Heberden's nodes, are a characteristic feature adjacent to the terminal phalangeal joints, and these are small marginal osteophytes on histopathological examination. The features of osteoarthritis are seen at the affected joint surfaces, with cartilage and bone changes as described above.

Endemic osteoarthritis

There are several forms of polyarticular osteoarthritis which have a high frequency of occurrence in certain parts of the world, namely the USSR, China, South Africa, and India. All show onset in the first or second decades of life; are acquired rather than inherited; affect impoverished rural communities; and cause variable growth restriction. Kashin–Beck disease, an example of this type of osteoarthritis, will be described briefly. It is a condition that occurs in the region of south-eastern Siberia, northern China, and North Korea. The prevalence of the disease is unknown, but may be as high as 80 per cent in some villages.

There is initially swelling, pain, and stiffness of the interphalangeal joints, with metacarpophalangeal and wrist joints sometimes affected. This phase is followed by generalized osteoarthritis affecting the elbows, knees, and ankles, although hip involvement is uncommon. Early Kashin–Beck disease is characterized by zonal necrosis of chondrocytes in the growth plate and articular cartilage. Later, deformity develops due to disintegration of the cartilage. Osteochondral loose bodies and osteophyte formation are both seen. The aetiopathogenesis of the condition is unknown, but two possibilities that have been suggested are:

1. an abnormality in the trace element content of soil or water; and

2. toxins produced by moulds and local grain crops.

Neuropathic joints

Severe damage results when joints are subjected to loss of their nerve supply, as first pointed out by Charcot in tabes dorsalis. The lower limb is usually affected in tabes, but an analogous change occurs in the upper limb in syringomyelia. Diabetic neuropathy may occasionally give rise to severe arthropathy; and other rarer, but recognized, causes include congenital insensitivity to pain, transverse myelitis, and even peripheral nerve trauma or neuritis.

In tabes dorsalis, the knee is most commonly affected, followed by the hip, ankle, and shoulder. Usually a single joint is involved, but sometimes several may be affected. Clinically and radiologically there may be fracture(s) of the shaft of the bone adjacent to the joint, which may extend up to the articular surface, though there may be few or no clinical complaints. Recurrent swellings and effusions occur with mechanical derangement, loosening of the capsule and ligaments, and subsequent subluxation. In the early stages, a Charcot's joint may be mistaken for osteoarthritis, but at a more advanced stage there is gross abnormality with destruction of the articular surfaces and the subchondral bone. Macroscopic examination shows severe disruption of the joint surfaces, often with loose osteochondral fragments in the joint space and osteophytes at the joint margins. The synovial membrane is thickened and villous, containing incorporated detritic fragments. Microscopy

shows fibrous thickening of the synovial membrane with embedded fragments of bone and cartilage and a variable low-grade inflammatory infiltrate, sometimes with surface fibrin deposition if there has been a recent episode of trauma. Continued growth of detached cartilage may be evident in the loose bodies, and incorporated osteochondral fragments in the synovial membrane.

The articular surfaces show no evidence of original cartilage, and comprise either bare bone, with or without a covering layer of fibrous tissue, or fibrocartilage. There may be areas of marked osteosclerosis in abnormally loaded parts of the joint and marked bone atrophy in unloaded parts as a result of altered mechanics due to reunion of malaligned fractures.

The changes in syringomelia are similar except that fractures of the shafts of the upper limb long bones are much more common than they are in tabes dorsalis.

Neuropathic involvement of joints in diabetes mellitus is mainly in the lower limb, although the upper limb is sometimes affected. The bones and joints of the foot are involved and, since infection is a common complication of diabetes, the changes may not be merely related to the presence of neuropathy. The changes include osteoporosis of the affected bones and juxta-articular erosive changes. Later, there may be marked destruction of the ends of the bones of the phalanges and distal ends of the metatarsals, which become tapered and subluxed. The ankle may show radiological changes like those of a true Charcot's joint.

Loose bodies (osteochondral bodies)

Loose bodies in joints usually comprise fragments of cartilage or cartilage with related subchondral bone (Fig. 27.126). Such osteochondral bodies may become incorporated in the synovial membrane, where the cartilage can continue to grow (see synovial chondromatosis).

Loose bodies may be secondary to osteochondral fractures in joint trauma, degenerative and destructive disease of the articular surfaces (e.g. neuropathic joints), or separation of fragments in osteochondritis dissecans. The origins of many loose bodies

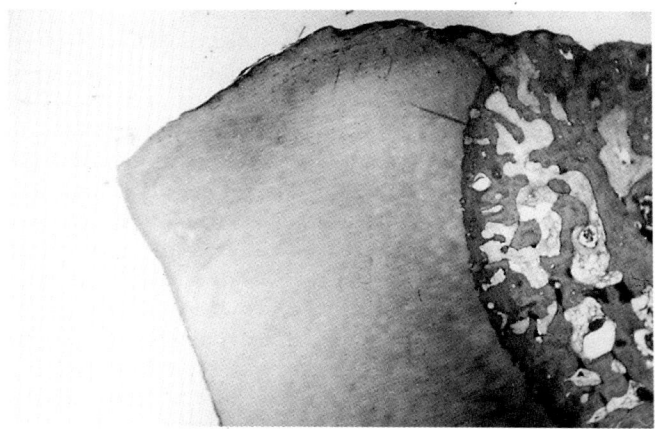

Fig. 27.126 Osteochondral body, showing viable cartilage (left) and necrotic subchondral bone (right).

are, however, frequently unknown. Radiological examination may reveal the presence of one or more radio-opaque loose bodies, and macroscopically there are small nodules which are sometimes composed of obvious bone and cartilage, or have a nobbly cartilaginous mulberry-like structure. Histological examination shows a variety of appearances, depending on the duration of time that the osteochondral fragment has been separated. There may be viable cartilage covering the bone which still shows the presence of osteocytes in its lacunae. The bone may be dead, lacking osteocytes, osteoblasts, or osteoclasts (Fig. 27.126) while viable cartilage may have proliferated to replace the tissue in the intertrabecular space. Fibrous tissue and cartilage may grow from the edge of the original hyaline cartilage along the sides of the attached bone to surround the whole loose body. Finally, the original bone may be encased in multiple layers of fibrous tissue and cartilage.

27.2.7 Crystal-induced diseases

Gout

Gout is a condition in which crystals of monosodium urate are deposited in the joints and other tissues, where they cause inflammation. Hyperuricaemia is present and there is a disturbance of purine metabolism. The high serum uric acid levels result from either increased uric acid production with normal excretion, or from reduced excretion in the presence of normal production. One example of the former is the predisposition to urate crystal deposition of patients with lymphoma and leukaemia undergoing treatment for their malignancy; these patients are treated prophylactically to avoid the effects of increased purine breakdown products arising from the tumour. Dietary factors are also important, as evidenced by the virtual disappearance of gout in Germany during the Second World War but the subsequent rise to the present incidence of 2 per cent of males in the western part of Germany. Reduced excretion is shown by the consistent presence of hyperuricaemia in patients with renal failure and uraemia, although a personal autopsy study of over 60 first metatarsal heads from such cases failed to show a single example of even subclinical crystal deposition in cartilage. Clearly, hyperuricaemia does not automatically lead to gout, and local tissue conditions such as pH, low temperature, and the presence of sulphated glycosaminoglycans are among other important factors.

The classical clinical picture is of acute attacks of severely painful arthritis with some joints, such as the metatarsophalangeal of the great toe, particularly affected. Apart from joints, urate crystals may also be precipitated in the ear cartilages, the soft tissues, and in the interstitial tissue of the kidney, where urate stones also form in the tubules.

Gout affects males overwhelmingly more often than females (95 per cent of cases), although cases in post-menopausal females do occur. It appears from the second to the sixth decades. While arthritis of the toes, knees, ankles, elbows, and fingers is usual, joint involvement does not occur in all patients suffering from gout. Lesions may be confined to periarticular tissues and extraskeletal sites, such as the outer ear, eyelids, and kidneys.

Gout can be diagnosed rapidly by the recognition of negatively birefringent needle-shaped crystals on polarization light microscopy of synovial fluid, or in a scraping from a chalky white deposit which may be present over the ear cartilages or a gouty tophus which has ulcerated the skin surface. For microscopical examination, care is needed to avoid aqueous solutions in the preparation of all materials likely to contain water-soluble urate crystals. Alcohol and formal–alcohol are best used as fixatives whenever gout is suspected. Examination of the synovial fluid in an acute gouty arthritis reveals a high white cell count (over 10×10^9 cells/dl) with a predominance of polymorphonuclear leucocytes. The crystals are seen in polymorphonuclears and macrophages as well as in free suspension. It is rare for synovial membrane to be biopsied during acute gout because the diagnosis is usually reached without recourse to this procedure. The synovial membrane, however, shows the presence of an acute inflammatory infiltrate with abundant polymorphonuclears and fibrin deposition at this stage. The important differential diagnosis is from septic arthritis, though Behcet syndrome can also show a similar picture (see Section 27.2.5). Urate crystals and organisms should be sought when this acute inflammatory picture is seen. The histopathologist is more likely to see tissue from the established lesions of gout in the joints, soft tissues, and kidney. Urate crystals are deposited as a chalky white precipitate on the surface of affected cartilage. Polarization microscopy shows the deposition of crystals in the superficial part of the articular cartilage and there is accompanying loss of staining of the matrix due to secondary changes in chondrocyte metabolism with proteoglycan loss (Fig. 27.127). This damage to cartilage predisposes the joint to development of secondary osteoarthritis.

Collections of urate crystals in the synovial tissues and nearby juxta-articular soft tissues are surrounded predominantly by macrophages with some giant cells (Fig. 27.128). No cells are present in the centre of the deposit, which may be because the crystals are cytotoxic, or merely because the crystals are closely packed together allowing cellular access only at the periphery of the mass. A vascular fibrous layer surrounds these granuloma-like collections of crystals and cells. These extra-articular collections of urate crystals and accompanying granulomatous reaction form white masses which are called tophi. They occur particularly adjacent to an affected joint, and the macrophage response to crystals at the joint margin may itself result in destruction of adjacent cartilage and bone. The inflammatory process then extends into the subchondral bone and across the joint surface with erosive damage. Calcification or secondary infection may occur in tophi, and fistulae may develop from deeper lesions to the skin surface.

The renal effects of uric acid deposition are described elsewhere in this book (see Chapter 19).

Lesch–Nyhan syndrome

A severe familial, X-linked form of gout, the Lesch–Nyhan syndrome, presents in childhood and is due to deficiency of the enzyme hypoxanthine-guanidine phosphoribosyl transferase (HGPRT). The affected children show hyperuricaemia, renal damage, mental retardation, choreoathetosis, convulsions, spasticity, aggressive behaviour, and self-mutilation.

Calcium pyrophosphate dihydrate (CPPD) deposition

Calcium pyrophosphate dihydrate (CPPD) crystals are deposited in the hyaline cartilage of diarthrodial joints and the fibrocartilage of the menisci and intervertebral discs. Clinically, the presence of CPPD crystals may be an incidental radiological finding in the menisci and discs, and this condition is then called chondrocalcinosis. There may be a fairly severe and acute synovitis, known as pseudogout. Sometimes there is more chronic joint involvement, resembling chronic synovitis of rheumatoid

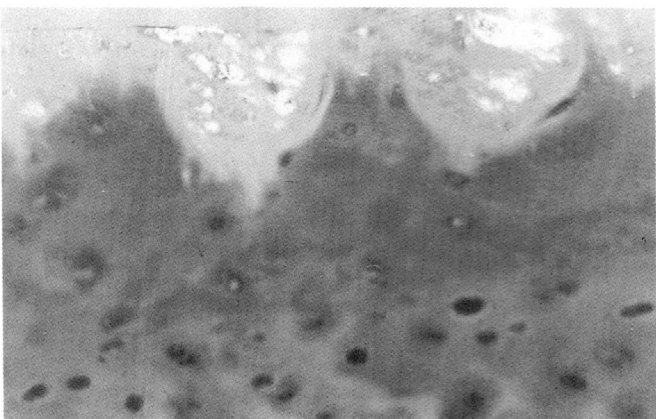

Fig. 27.127 Surface of articular cartilage in gout showing deposition of crystals (top) of monosodium urate with loss of staining in the related cartilage matrix (polarization microscopy).

type in clinical presentations and features. There is an association between osteoarthritis and CPPD deposition in joints, but this is likely to be because both conditions occur at increasing frequency with increasing age. Finally, some patients develop a severely destructive form of osteoarthritis resembling a neuropathic joint, but CPPD and apatite crystals are both deposited in the joint tissues. At the shoulder, this is known as Milwaukee shoulder, but similar changes have also been observed at the hip and knee.

Inorganic pyrophosphate (PPi) is produced in a wide variety of biochemical pathways; for example, the biosynthesis of proteins, lipids and phospholipids, nucleotides and nucleic acids, steroids, polysaccharides, and glycogen. Inorganic pyrophosphatases catalyse the hydrolysis of PPi. These comprise the better-known glucose-6-phosphatase and alkaline phosphatases, as well as specific pyrophosphatases.

Certain other conditions predispose to the precipitation of CPPD in the tissues, namely hypothyroidism, hyperparathyroidism, haemochromatosis, haemosiderosis, hypophosphatasia, hypomagnesaemia, and Wilson disease. CPPD deposition and gout also sometimes coexist. The possible mechanisms for CPPD crystal deposition in these other diseases may be related to the effect they have on local conditions in the joint. For example, other joint disease, such as gout, may give rise to a focus for epitaxy of crystals, or result in lowering of pH because of inflammation. Not all forms of joint inflammation predispose to CPPD deposition. It is rare, for example, in rheumatoid arthritis. Raised levels of Ca^{2+} and/or PPi may be responsible for precipitation in hyperparathyroidism; while raised PPi levels are responsible in hypophosphatasia. Iron and copper may act as nucleating agents for crystal growth or inhibitors of pyrophosphatase in haemachromatosis and Wilson disease, respectively.

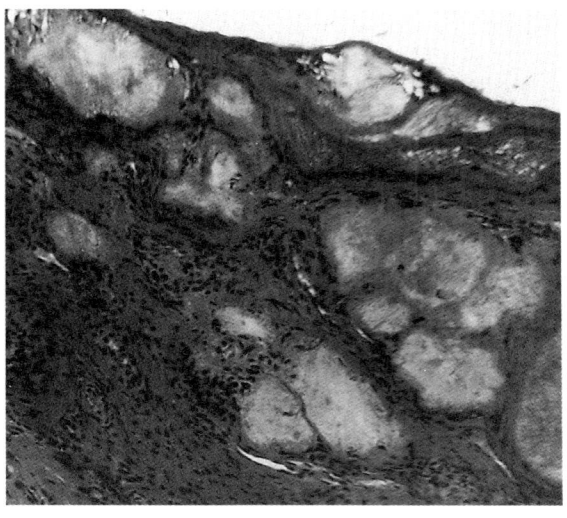

(a)

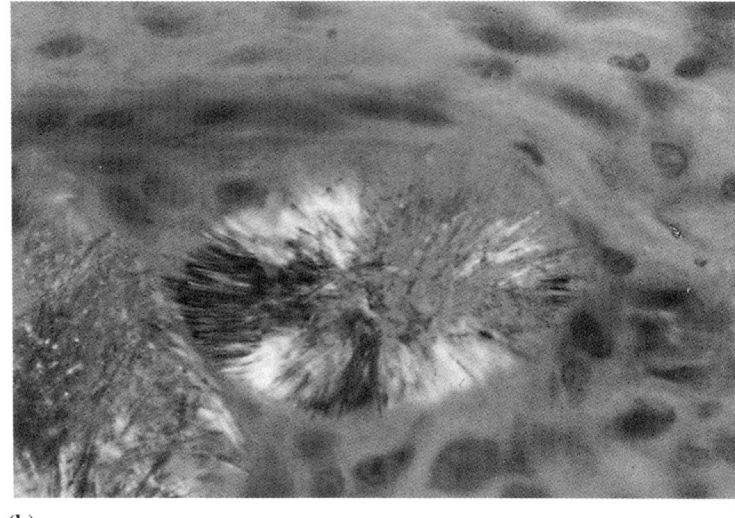

(b)

Fig. 27.128 (a) Synovial soft tissues from a case of tophaceous gout, showing numerous collections of monosodium urate crystals with macrophage and giant-cell reaction (polarization microscopy). (b) High-power view of a collection of needle-shaped urate crystals, with macrophage reaction (polarization microscopy).

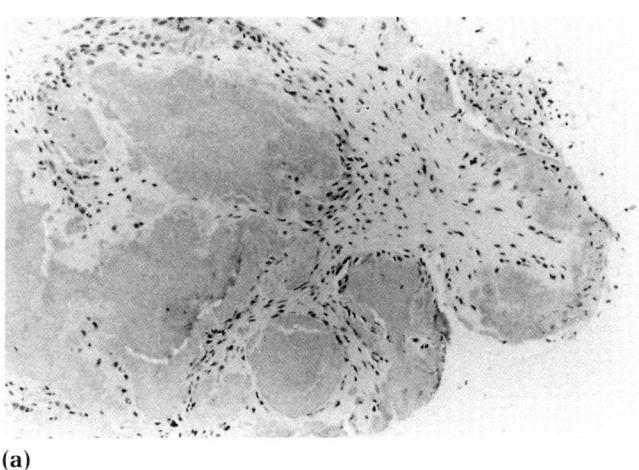
(a)

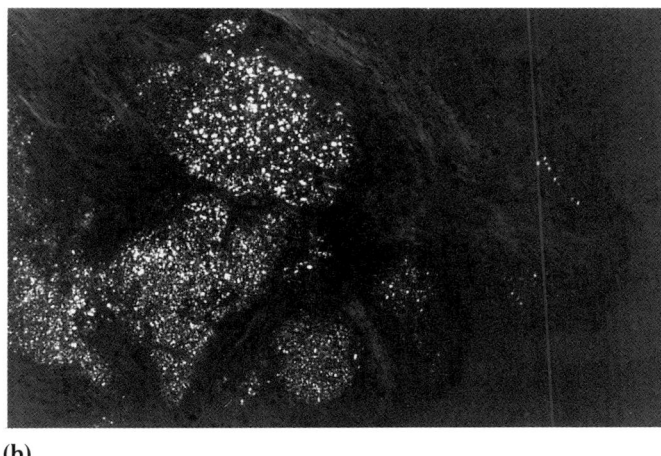
(b)

Fig. 27.129 (a) Synovial membrane containing several collections of haematoxyphil calcified deposits. (b) Polarization microscopy of the same field, showing the presence of numerous small calcium pyrophosphate dihydrate crystals.

CPPD crystal deposition disease occurs in the knee, ankle, shoulder, wrist, metacarpophalangeal, hip, and elbow joints, and also in the intervertebral discs. Linear calcification is seen on radiological examination of the intervertebral discs and the menisci of the knee in chondrocalcinosis. Histopathological examination shows the presence of deeply located crystals in these sites, usually in the absence of a significant cellular reaction. CPPD crystals are weakly positive birefringent on compensated polarization microscopy. They may be detected in synovial fluid as free crystals and within phagocytic cells. In the synovial membrane, there may be a diffuse deposition of crystals in the intimal cell layer, sometimes only detected by careful polarization microscopy; or there may be large, sharply delineated deep deposits which are a fairly characteristic purple-grey colour in haematoxylin- and eosin-stained sections and are surrounded by more or less numerous macrophages and giant cells (Fig. 27.129a). Polarization may show relatively few preserved birefringent crystals in these masses in routinely processed material (Fig. 27.129b).

Deposits of CPPD crystals in cartilage, and to a lesser extent in the synovial surface, are seen as a milky white material on naked-eye examination. Microscopy reveals collections of crystals in the superficial and mid zones of the articular cartilage close to, but never within, the chondrocyte lacunae. There is loss of metachromasia in the adjacent matrix, due to changes in proteoglycan content, and the cartilage is frequently fibrillated. The question of the association between pyrophosphate deposition and osteoarthritis has already been mentioned. Severe degenerative joint disease with marked destruction of the joint surfaces and nearby bone occurs in Milwaukee shoulder; CPPD and apatite crystals are seen in the tissues. Small crystals, identified as apatite, have also been identified in the synovial fluid of some patients with acute arthritis. It is possible that calcium phosphates other than apatite and CPPD might also give rise to crystal-induced arthropathy.

27.2.8 Joint replacement

Most prosthetic joint implants are made of metal (cobalt–chrome alloy, stainless steel, titanium–aluminium–vanadium alloy) and plastic (usually high-density polyethylene, HDP). Ceramics and other materials, for example, carbon fibre, are used in some designs. The components are either fixed to the skeleton by bone cement (polymethyl methacrylate) or by various procedures that allow cementless fixation. The histological appearances in the tissues adjacent to a prosthetic joint (at the implant bed) will depend on the materials used, the type of fixation, and the extent to which there is wear and failure of the prosthesis.

For a short period of time after implantation, there is evidence of bone and bone marrow death immediately adjacent to the prosthesis. This results partly from the trauma of preparing the implantation site by reaming or sawing. In the case of a cemented component, the changes extend for up to 3 mm into the osseous tissues and are considered to result from the heat of polymerization of the bone cement as it cures *in situ*, as well as local toxic effects of unincorporated (excess) methyl methacrylate monomer. There is gradual healing of tissues near the prosthesis by fibrosis, with woven bone and appositional new bone formation, which is followed by remodelling of this bone adjacent to the implant so that it becomes orientated parallel to the prosthesis surface. Exact changes vary with the type of implant. The stem of a femoral component at the hip, for example, becomes surrounded by a cylinder of bone linked to the related trabeculae. There is always a layer of fibrous tissue between bone and implant or cement and this undergoes chondroid metaplasia where there has been compressive loading.

Loosening of prostheses may occur for a variety of reasons, including mechanical and surgical factors (e.g. malalignment of components, overloading), infection, excessive wear, failure of components, and so-called aseptic loosening, the mechanism of

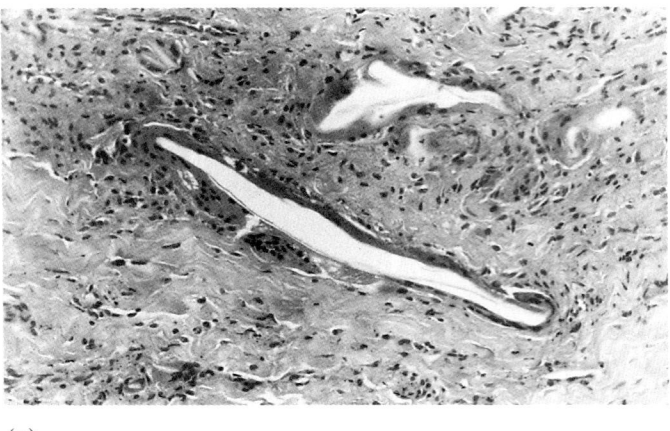

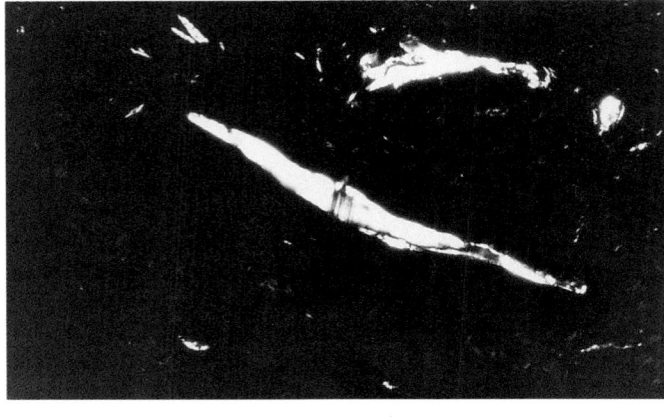

(a)   (b)

Fig. 27.130   (a) Macrophages and multinucleate giant cells in synovial tissue adjacent to a failed joint prosthesis. (b) Polarization microscopy of the same field, showing the presence of birefringent flakes and fragments of high-density polyethylene.

which is poorly understood. Infection is far less of a problem than in the early days of prosthetic surgery but adequate examination of tissues to exclude infection remains vital in the pathological study of loosened prostheses. Usually, polymorphonuclear leucocytes are present where there is active infection, but infection with organisms such as *Bacteroides* may show only a low-grade, predominantly lymphocytic, infiltrate on histological examination. Proper microbiological study of tissue from prostheses is important where infection is suspected.

Inevitably, prosthetic components wear and generate debris which is shed into the joint. Elevated metal levels can be detected in the synovial fluid and synovial membrane related to prostheses. The highest levels occur where metal articulates against metal, followed by metal against bone, then metal and plastic articulations. Metal, polyethylene, and cement debris all provoke a macrophage and giant-cell response in the synovial membrane and implant bed. The size of particle mainly determines the cell type, so that fine black granules of metal debris are found in a predominantly macrophage infiltrate; while small particles and larger flakes of birefringent polyethylene debris are present in macrophages and giant cells (Fig. 27.130). Bone cement is soluble in the solvents used in routine tissue processing so that the sites which contained this material are seen as spaces which are surrounded by macrophages and giant cells. Many bone cements contain radiographic contrast material so that a residual fine grey-green granular material in such spaces is a useful clue to the fact that they contained bone cement. Low levels of wear debris in the joint are removed by phagocytic cells, and foreign material can be detected in draining lymph nodes. However, excess wear overloads the defence mechanisms and large amounts of debris accumulate. Not only are they present in the synovial membrane but they also find their way into the interface between prosthesis and bone. Phagocytic cells at this site are thought to contribute to the loosening of the prosthesis by causing resorption of bone. Macrophages have recently been observed adjacent to the bone cement in well-fixed prostheses in the absence of wear debris.

Other foreign materials are used in prosthetic joint replacement, including ceramics and carbon fibre, the latter to reinforce polyethylene. Ceramics are seen as fine grey granules in macrophages, while carbon fibre occurs in short lengths with accompanying macrophages and giant cells. Carbon fibre is also used in tendon and other soft-tissue repair operations.

27.2.9   Tumours and tumour-like conditions

Pigmented villonodular synovitis

Pigmented villonodular synovitis (PVNS), which may be nodular or diffuse, has been given a variety of other names—giant-cell tumour of tendon sheath and synovium, benign synovioma, xanthoma of tendon sheath, and xanthogranuloma—none of which is satisfactory. The aetiology of the process is unknown, although similarities of the histopathological appearances in the nodular and diffuse processes suggest that they may have a common histogenesis.

PVNS is a localized monoarticular proliferative process, most often affecting the knee joint or the tendon sheaths of the fingers. It also occurs in the hip, toes, ankle, wrist, elbow, and shoulder. Localized nodular lesions of tendon sheath and synovium are seen in the hands, while diffuse PVNS mostly occurs in the knee, though nodular lesions may also be present in this site. All ages from young adulthood onwards may be affected and there is no difference in the sex incidence. There may be no, or only mild, symptoms with lesions of the hand. Moderate pain, swelling, and tenderness may occur in knee involvement. Aspiration of a swollen knee due to PVNS characteristically yields a brown or blood-stained synovial fluid. Suspicion that a particular lesion is a destructive, even malignant, tumour may arise from radiological examination of the affected part, both in large joints, such as the knee and hip, and in the fingers, since there may be local erosive damage to the joint surface and bone.

Macroscopically, the synovium of the affected knee in diffuse PVNS is thickened, with a villous or 'mossy' appearance and a

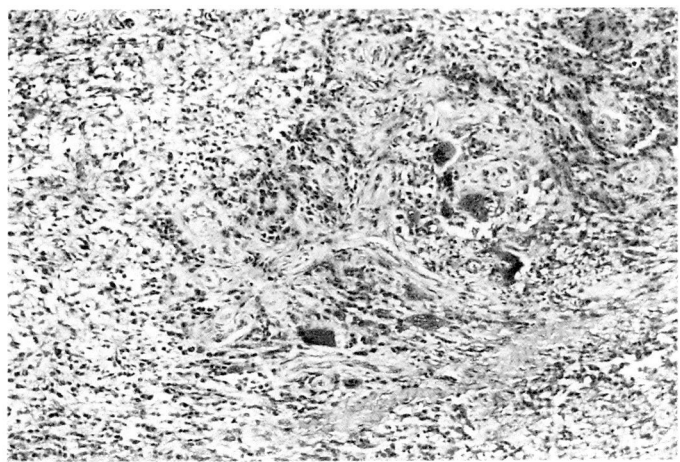

Fig. 27.131 Nodular pigmented villonodular synovitis, showing the presence of giant cells, macrophages, and collagen formation. Note the presence of numerous foamy macrophages (left).

rusty brown and/or yellow colour due to the presence of iron or lipid. Nodular areas may coexist in this thickened synovium. Histopathology shows a predominance of macrophages with finely vacuolated cytoplasm. Synovial cells and macrophages are variably laden with haemosiderin, which may also lie free in the tissues. Spindle-shaped and lipid-laden cells are also present, together with multinucleate giant cells. Variable numbers of lymphocytes may be seen. Diffuse PVNS is easily overdiagnosed if a heavily iron-loaded synovium is not examined carefully. The implications to the patient are important since true PVNS is known to recur in up to 45 per cent of cases. Other conditions in which there is significant iron present include haemophilia, haemosiderosis and haemochromatosis, haemangioma of the synovium, trauma, and rhematoid arthritis. The presence of all the histological features together with clinical and macroscopical corroboration should be sought in diagnosing PVNS.

The nodular form of pigment synovitis occurs either in a joint or tendon sheath and comprises circumscribed lobulated masses with a greyish cut surface containing yellow or brown areas. Nodular tenosynovitis occurs particularly near the phalanges of the hands, but also elsewhere in the hand, foot, ankle, and wrists. The lesion contains two main types of cell; spindle-shaped fibroblastic cells, and oval/polygonal macrophages. Masses of foamy macrophages may be present and there are multinucleate giant cells (Fig. 27.131). Variable amounts of collagen are present between these cells, and some lesions may have a predominance of dense fibrous tissue with only small areas of cellular infiltrate revealing their true nature. Haemosiderin pigment is usually present and there may be a mild lymphocyte and plasma cell infiltrate. Some lesions bear a strong resemblance to benign fibrous histiocytomas seen in soft tissues (see Section 27.4.5).

Synovial chondromatosis

The presence of islands of metaplastic cartilaginous tissue

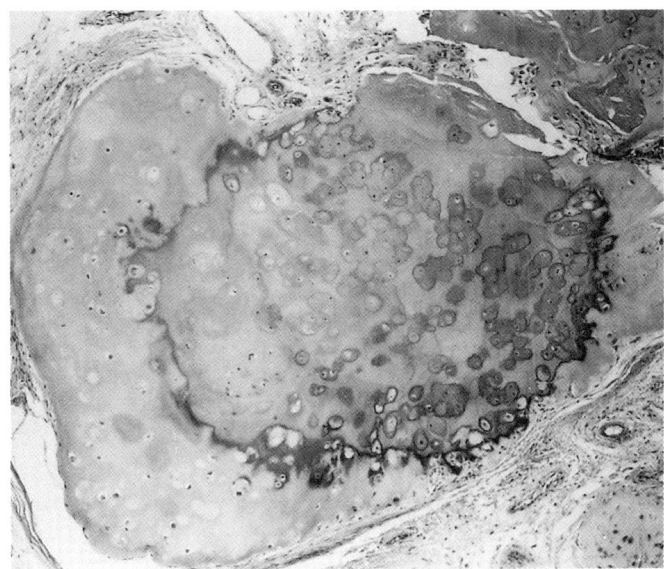

Fig. 27.132 Synovial chondromatosis, showing a nodule of chondroid tissue undergoing calcification and situated in the synovial membrane.

within the synovium may be due to two distinctly different processes, both of which are often referred to as synovial chondromatosis. In osteochondritis dissecans, trauma, inflammatory, and non-inflammatory degenerative joint diseases, cartilaginous and osteocartilaginous fragments may become detached and embedded in the synovial membrane. These cartilage fragments may then continue to grow (as described under loose bodies, Section 27.2.6; this process is sometimes referred to as secondary chondrometaplasia (secondary chondromatosis)).

Primary synovial chondromatosis is a benign, slowly progressive condition affeting the hip and knee, although other joints (wrist, ankle, digits, elbow) may be involved. Presentation is with pain, stiffness, or swelling, at any time from teenage to the seventh decade. Since the lesions are sometimes radiolucent, radiological detection may not always be easy. Radio-opaque lesions may be seen in and around a joint and frankly erosive damage to adjacent bone may cause suspicion of a malignant neoplasm. Small cartilaginous masses are seen in the synovial soft tissues on macroscopical examination and histological sections show foci of chondroid tissue in the synovium. These have a markedly disorganized appearance, with clusters of chondrocytes, considerable cellular atypia, and occasional mitoses present. Calcification and endochondral ossification may be seen (Fig. 27.132).

Considerable care is required in differentiating this lesion from chondrosarcoma, particularly where the radiograph shows a destructive lesion. Evidence for a synovial origin may be available within the sections. A clear idea of the site of origin of the lesion should be obtained from the referring clinician. True synovial chondrosarcoma is extremely rare and this diagnosis must be made taking great care to differentiate it from chondromatosis. Synovial chondromatosis may recur locally.

Synovial haemangioma

Haemangiomas in joints may be diffuse or localized; the latter may be sessile or pedunculated. Haemangioma may lead to repeated haemorrhage into the joint cavity, which often starts in childhood and may go on for many years. Histological examination shows capillary, cavernous, mixed capillary and cavernous, or venous patterns. Massive amounts of iron may accumulate in synovial macrophages and there may also be lipid-laden cells present. Care is required over the erroneous diagnosis of pigmented villonodular synovitis.

Other benign tumours

Lipoma and neurofibroma have been reported in joints. Other lesions, called xanthofibroma and xanthoma, are probably variants of nodular pigmented villonodular synovitis.

Malignant tumours of joints

Synovial sarcomas are malignant soft-tissue tumours which occur at any time in life from early adulthood to old age but mostly under 40 years of age. They present as a mass and sometimes with pain or tenderness. The lower limb is affected in a little over half the cases. Other sites are the upper limb and trunk. The percentage of cases occurring in or near joints or tendon sheaths varies from 10 to 58 per cent in different studies. Most of these are likely to be para-articular rather than truly within the joint. Those occurring in sites such as the abdominal wall have no apparent connection with any synovial structures.

Radiological examination shows a round or oval lobulated mass or masses of moderate density. There may be evidence of focal calcification or ossification and periosteal reaction; bone erosion or invasion are sometimes seen. Macroscopically slowly growing lesions are well circumscribed with a yellowish-grey cut surface, while higher-grade lesions are, not surprisingly, poorly defined at the margins and have a variegated appearance with areas of haemorrhage and necrosis on sectioning. By light microscopy, the tumour contains two different elements, epithelial cells resembling carcinoma and spindle cells resembling fibrosarcoma, giving a typical 'biphasic' appearance. The spindle cells are usually predominant. Monophasic forms have been reported, mostly of spindle-cell type; monophasic–epithelial synovial sarcoma may also occur. Immunohistochemical studies show that the carcinoma-like cells react with epithelial markers. Mitoses are seen in both elements, but are frequent only in poorly differentiated tumours. Focal calcification is present in about 40 per cent of synovial sarcomas.

Little is known of the tissue of origin of synovial sarcoma. There is no convincing evidence that it is related to any benign synovial lesion, or that it is even derived from the synovial membrane on histochemical, immunohistochemical, and ultrastructural grounds.

Synovial sarcoma is liable to recur. The recurrence rate probably depends on the degree of malignancy and adequacy of treatment as much as anything else. Metastases develop in over 50 per cent of cases, mainly in the lungs, followed by lymph nodes and bone marrow. Metastasis may occur after a long interval. Reported five-year survival rates vary between 25 and 63 per cent.

Other tumours and joints

Rare examples of metastases to joints, and leukaemia and lymphoma in the synovium, have been described. Amyloid deposition occurs in multiple myeloma (see Section 27.1.6). A mild non-specific chronic synovitis with lymphoid follicles is sometimes seen in the joint adjacent to benign and malignant tumours in bone, especially osteoid osteoma.

Multicentric reticulohistiocytosis (lipoid dermatoarthritis)

Multicentric 'reticulohistiocytosis' is a rare disease of unknown aetiology and histogenesis, affecting women more than men and usually occurring over the age of 40 years. Reddish nodules up to 1 cm in diameter appear on the skin of the hands and face. The mucous membranes are involved and there is a polyarthritis which runs an apisodic course of remissions and exacerbations leading to joint deformity. The synovial membrane shows the presence of large foamy macrophages and multinucleate giant cells with finely granular cytoplasm. Small numbers of lymphocytes may be present.

27.2.10   The menisci

Menisci that have been lacerated or have undergone degenerative changes may be submitted for pathological diagnosis. This subject is often omitted from pathology texts.

Lacerated/torn meniscus

Traumatic injury to menisci occurs under various conditions, particularly in some sports. A rotational force in a partially flexed knee is the usual mode of injury. Extensive injury leads to a bucket-handle tear, while lesser types of laceration also may be seen. Longitudinal tears are the commonest, and the medial meniscus is affected much more often than the lateral. The meniscus is best sectioned vertically across the plane of the laceration. Microscopic examination shows fraying of the collagenous tissue of the fibrocartilage, sometimes with focal new capillary formation. There may be some fibrin deposition. The appearances are unremarkable but should be readily distinguishable from an incision made at the time of surgery.

Meniscal cysts

Cysts of the menisci are usually situated in the antero-medial part of the lateral meniscus and occur as a result of focal 'myxoid degeneration' and softening of the fibrocartilaginous tissue. Multifocal cystic areas become coalescent. Microscopical examination shows separation and fraying of the fibrocartilage and the cystic cavity may be lined by cells resembling the synovial intimal cells.

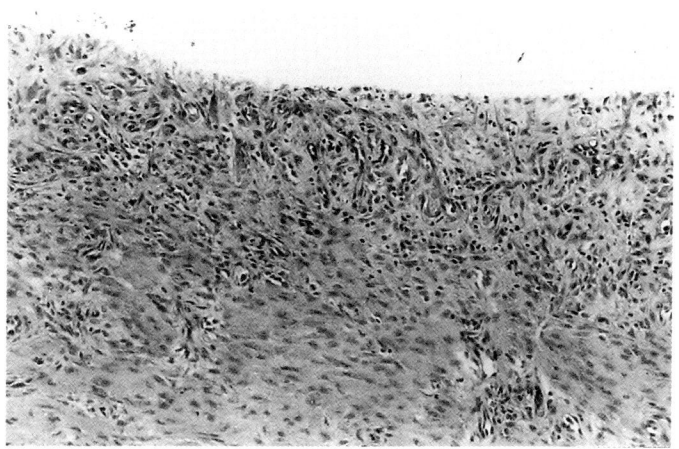

Fig. 27.133 Wall of a bursa with a low-grade chronic inflammatory cell infiltrate and small vessels. A synovial cell layer is present over part of the surface (left and right), although the central area shows no such cells.

Meniscal calcification

Calcium pyrophosphate dihydrate (CPPD) crystals become deposited in the menisci in chondrocalcinosis. Typically, no cellular reaction is seen in relation to these crystals in this site. The effects of crystals on joints, including CPPD, are discussed in Section 27.2.7.

Discoid meniscus

The lateral meniscus may have a discoid shape rather than semilunar. Medial discoid meniscus has been described. This anomaly of development is prone to horizontal splitting and degenerative changes.

27.2.11   Bursae, cysts, and ganglia

Bursae arise after birth in response to mechanical stimuli and comprise fluid-filled cystic spaces lined by synovial membrane at sites where there is movement of tendon, fascia, or skin and subcutaneous tissue across a bony surface. While a blow to the elbow may result in an olecranon bursa and a prepatellar bursa may similarly form at the knee, bursae are more usually the result of repeated injury such as excessive pressure. A good example of this is housemaid's knee, which is an enlarged and painful prepatellar bursa. In general, bursae develop where there is friction in gliding surfaces or over bony prominences. The bursal sac has an irregular yellowish discoloured surface; there may be strands of fibrin in the lumen and attached to the surface. Inflammation is relatively uncommon, even though these lesions are frequently called 'bursitis' (Fig. 27.133). There may, however, be changes of acute inflammation with pus formation where a bursa has become infected.

A cyst-like structure in the popliteal region is frequently called a 'Baker's cyst'; this term is now used to encompass all simple cysts at this site, rather than its original meaning of a cystic extension arising posteriorly from a rheumatoid knee joint. Sometimes such a popliteal cyst represents a herniation of the posterior capsule of the knee joint, which is thin walled with a synovial lining, but bursae also occur in this site.

Bursae are involved by the rheumatoid process in at least 5 per cent of cases, most commonly the popliteal, olecranon, subacromial, supradeltoid, and Achilles bursae. Baker's cysts are connected to the knee joint by a valvular mechanism, and increased intra-articular pressure due to the presence of a rheumatoid synovial effusion can lead to the development of a large swelling. All the histological features of rheumatoid synovitis are seen in the synovial lining of such bursae.

Ganglia are thin-walled cysts, containing viscous mucoid fluid, found usually on the hand and wrist. They also occur on the dorsum of the foot, near the ankle or knee, or occasionally near almost any other joint. A ganglion develops as an area of degeneration and softening in the collagenous tissue of a tendon sheath. It may be lined by cells resembling synovial lining cells but these are frequently absent.

Whether bursae, cysts, and ganglia are clearly distinct from each other, apart from the site at which they occur, is a matter of personal belief rather than scientific fact. It is likely that cystic change in the menisci of the knee is also a closely related phenomenon.

27.2.12   Further reading

Enzinger, F. M. and Weiss, S. W. (1983). *Soft tissue tumors.* C. V. Mosby, St. Louis.

Eulderink, F. (1982). The synovial biopsy. In *Bone and joint disease* (ed. C. L. Berry), Current Topics in Pathology, Vol. 71, pp. 26–72. Springer, Berlin.

Fassbender, H. G. (1975). *Pathology of rheumatic diseases.* Springer, Berlin.

Gardner, D. L. (1972). *The pathology of rheumatoid arthritis.* Arnold, London.

Ghadially, F. N. (1983). *Fine structure of synovial joints.* Butterworths, London.

Jaffe, H. L. (1972). *Metabolic, degenerative and inflammatory diseases of bones and joints.* Lea and Febiger, Philadelphia.

Levick, J. R. (1983). Joint pressure-volume studies: their importance, design and interpretation. *Journal of Rheumatology* **10**, 353–7.

Rao, A. S. and Vigorita, V. J. (1984). Pigmented villonodular synovitis (giant cell tumor of the tendon sheath and synovial membrane). *Journal of Bone and Joint Surgery* **66A**, 76–94.

Resnick, D. and Niwayama, G. (1981). *Diagnosis of bone and joint disorders*, Vol. 1. W. B. Saunders, Philadephia.

Revell, P. A. (1982). Examination of synovial fluid. In *Bone and joint disease* (ed. C. L. Berry), Current Topics in Pathology, Vol. 71, pp. 1–24. Springer, Berlin.

Revell, P. A. (1982). Tissue reactions to joint prostheses and the products of wear and corrosion. In *Bone and joint disease* (ed. C. L. Berry). Current Topics in Pathology, Vol. 71, pp. 73–101. Springer, Berlin.

Revell, P. A. (1986). *Pathology of bone.* Springer, Berlin.

Revell, P. A. (1987). The synovial biopsy. In *Recent advances in histopathology*, No. 13 (ed. P. P. Anthony and R. N. M. MacSween), pp. 79–93. Churchill Livingstone, Edinburgh.

Revell, P. A. (1989). Diseases of bones and joints. In *Paediatric pathology* (ed. C. L. Berry) (2nd edn), pp. 451–85. Springer-Verlag, Berlin.

Spjut, H. J., Dorfman, H. D., Fechner, R. E., and Ackerman, L. V. (1971). Tumors of bone and cartilage. In *Atlas of tumor pathology*, 2nd series, fascicle 5. Armed Forces Institute of Pathology, Washington, DC.

Villacin, A. B., Brigham, L. N., and Bullough, P. G. (1979). Primary and secondary synovial chondrometaplasia. *Human Pathology* **10**, 439–51.

27.3 Muscle

A. J. Franks

27.3.1 The structure of muscle and its reactions to disease

Human skeletal muscle consists of specialized contractile elements aligned longitudinally within a fibrovascular framework with attachments (usually by tendons) at each end to fixed structures (usually skeletal elements). Non-neoplastic diseases affecting muscle can be broadly grouped into neuropathies (resulting from disturbances of innervation), myasthenic disorders of the motor end plate, and myopathies (resulting from primary disturbances of muscle structure).

Innervation

The contractile cells are a heterogeneous mixture which broadly correspond to the physiologically defined fast- and slow-twitch muscle fibres. The nature of an individual fibre is determined by its innervation and, in consequence, all the fibres supplied by an individual neurone are of the same type. A motor unit consists of a neurone and the fibres (up to 2000) it supplies, which randomly intermingle in a muscle. It is possible to identify fibres of different types (type I, slow/oxidative; type II, fast/glycolytic) by the application of a histochemical method for myosin ATPase to cryostat sections of muscle. This results in a random mosaic pattern of fibres (Fig. 27.134).

Since the type of a fibre, and the maintenance of its structure, is dependent on its innervation, alterations in the pattern of innervation will result in alterations in fibre size and the distribution of fibre type. If the neurone supplying a motor unit dies, the muscle fibres supplied by that neurone will atrophy (Fig. 27.135), typically taking on a compressed angular profile which may show enhanced staining for oxidative enzymes (see Fig. 27.143). Surviving intramuscular axons form collateral branches which connect with the denervated fibres and these fibres will display the characteristics of the type determined by their new innervation (Fig. 27.136). This process can be detected by methods, such as supravital staining with methylene blue, that demonstrate the terminal innervation; its continuation will result in greater numbers of fibres of the same

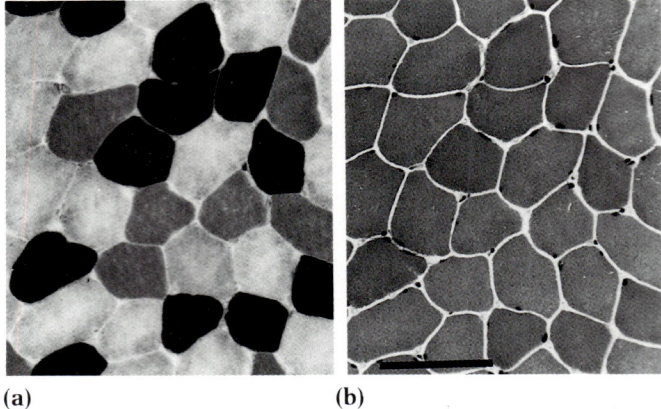

(a)   **(b)**

Fig. 27.134 (a) Apparently homogeneous muscle fibres, (b) can be separated into subgroups (type I, black; type IIA, white; type IIB, grey) by the myosin ATPase reaction with preincubation at pH 4.63. (bar = 100 μm).

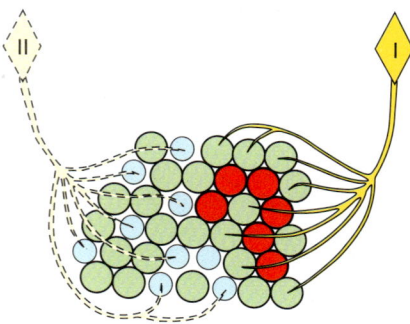

Fig. 27.135 Degeneration of type II neurone results in atrophy (blue) of the fibres it innervates (green). See text for explanation.

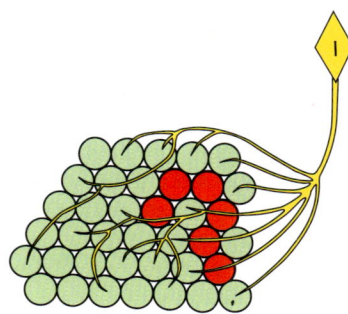

Fig. 27.136 Collateral branches from surviving type I intramuscular nerves reinnervate denervated (previously type II) fibres, which then become type I.

type occurring in a particular area. This fibre-type grouping is characteristic of the reinnervated state and is thus indicative of a neuropathic disorder (Fig. 27.137).

Another consequence of this process is that motor units enlarge. If the neurone supplying such a motor unit degenerates, a larger number of fibres will atrophy and these will also be

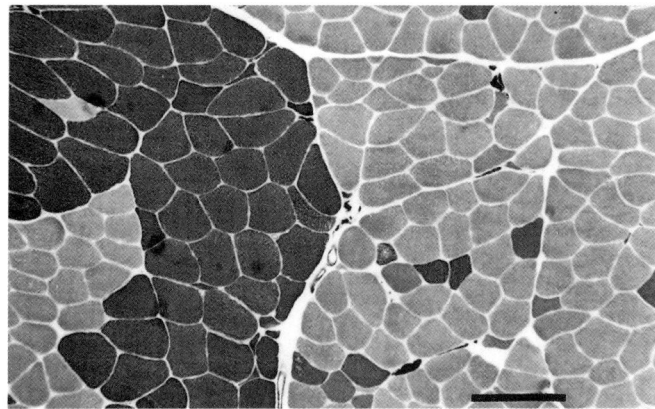

Fig. 27.137 Clustering of fibres of the same type following re-innervation results in fibre-type grouping (bar = 200 μm).

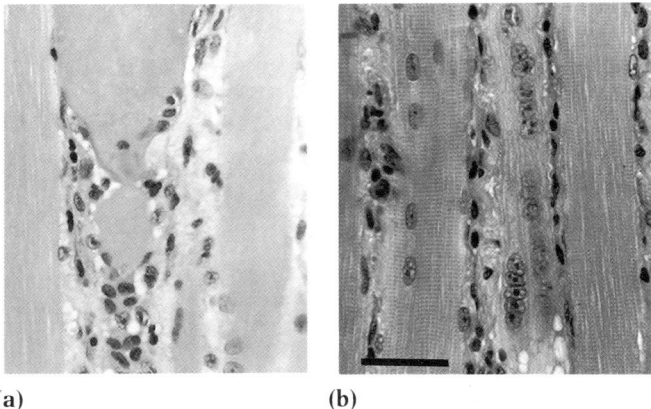

(a)   (b)

Fig. 27.139 (a) Necrotic debris is removed by infiltrating macrophages. (b) Regenerating myocytes align longitudinally and fuse to form new fibres (bar = 50 μm).

more likely to be grouped together; similarly, surviving fibres that may undergo compensatory hypertrophy will also be more likely to be in a group. The result is a pattern of atrophy and hypertrophy of large and small groups of fibres (see Fig. 27.141) which is typical of neurogenic disease.

In addition to disturbances of fibre size and type distribution, a characteristic change is often found in the structure of individual fibres in response to denervation (or possibly reinnervation). The centre of the fibre shows disruption of myofilaments with loss of mitochondria and other subcellular elements, resulting in a central zone that stains differently from the remaining cytoplasm and may resemble an archery target (Fig. 27.138). Such disruptions may be difficult to distinguish from the central cores that are a feature of a specific congenital myopathy (see central core disease, below). Although the two structures do differ (true cores extend the entire length of a fibre while targets are discontinuous), this distinction cannot usually be made on a transverse section and the term core–targetoid fibre is applied.

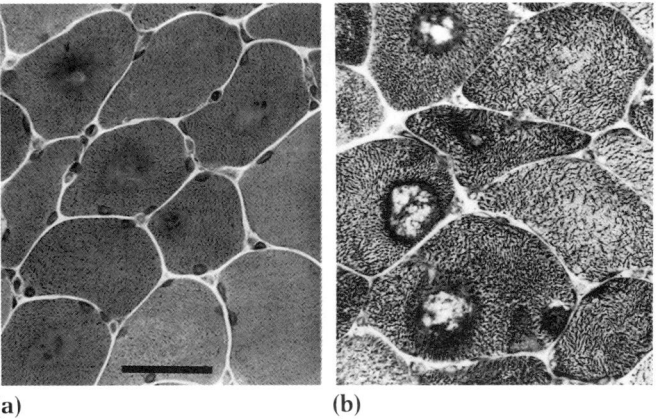

(a)   (b)

Fig. 27.138 (a) The disruption of structure in core–targetoid fibres is ill-defined with routine stains (Gomori Trichrome), but (b) is easy to see in oxidative enzyme preparations (NADH diaphorase) (bar = 50 μm).

Reactions of the muscle cell

Necrosis of muscle cells is a central process in many myopathies and may result in elevated serum levels of the muscle isoenzyme of creatine phosphokinase (CPK). Although the basic cause is often unknown, necrosis in X-linked muscular dystrophies and idiopathic myositis has been linked with the inappropriate expression of surface class I histocompatability antigens. When a muscle fibre dies the cell debris is typically removed by phagocytic cells (Fig. 27.139a). Within the basement membrane sheath that encloses individual muscle fibres resides a population of quiescent stem cells (satellite cells). On appropriate stimulation these enter the cell cycle and, by a combination of proliferation, contractile protein synthesis, and fusion (Fig. 27.139b) form new muscle fibres to replace those lost through disease.

This regenerative capacity delays the onset of symptoms in progressive degenerative diseases (muscular dystrophies) and allows full recovery from episodes of muscle fibre necrosis.

The dependence of muscle fibres on their innervation may relate in part to the stimulus the latter provides for contraction. If muscle fibres are not used they atrophy, although this is far more obvious among type II (fast) fibres. In consequence, atrophy of type II fibres (specifically subtype B) is a common finding in the context of disuse and systemic illness, and as a response to steroid therapy. Atrophy of muscle fibres is basic to many myopathic and neurogenic disorders and distinction from the non-specific atrophy of disuse is an important diagnostic step.

Individual muscle fibres are capable of hypertrophy by increasing their complement of contractile proteins and thus increasing their functional capacity. Increased fibre diameter is often associated with a tendency for myocyte nuclei to migrate from their normal subsarcolemmal location to the internal areas of the muscle cell (see Fig. 27.145b). In the face of continued fibre hypertrophy, longitudinal infoldings of the cell membrane may occur, resulting in the splitting of a single fibre into several fibres of smaller diameter. Hypertrophy may provide compensation for weakness in other fibres due to either denervation or primary disease and is a feature of many chronic

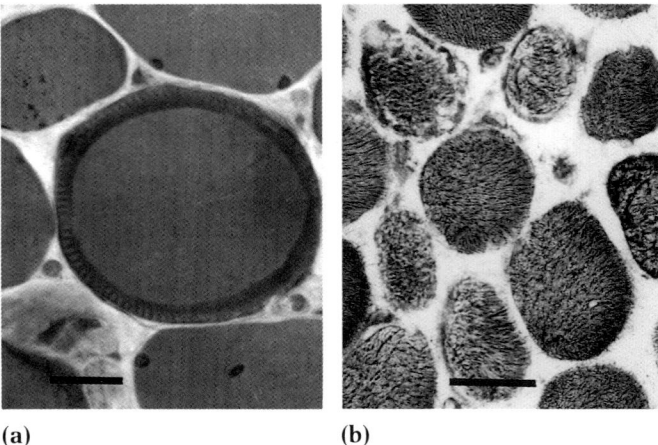

(a)   **(b)**

Fig. 27.140 (a) Malaligned myofibrils form recognizable cross-striations in a ring fibre. (b) The normally regular distribution of mitochondria (centre) contrasts with the moth-eaten appearance of surrounding fibres. (bars = 50 μm).

muscle disorders, although internal migration of nuclei and fibre splitting tend to be commoner in myopathic states.

Other architectural changes are encountered in which the normal components of the cell show various degrees of disorganization. None of these is specific to any one condition but their presence may assist diagnosis. Ring fibres (Fig. 27.140a) show a peripheral band of myofibres arranged at right angles to the normal longitudinal bundles and a similar but less-organized tendency results in whorled fibres. Patchy loss of mitochondria results in a 'moth-eaten' appearance (Fig. 27.140b) in preparations stained for oxidative enzymes (which are located in mitochondria), and is seen in many myopathic disorders.

With progressive loss of muscle fibres, an increase in the relative volume of the interstitial connective tissue will be apparent and fibrosis is a common feature of many chronic disorders of muscle.

Although most of the changes described in this section are more typical of myopathic disorders, they may be found in advanced states of neurogenic atrophy. First recognized in muscle from victims of poliomyelitis, these 'pseudomyopathic' changes may be an important source of confusion in some chronic progressive neurogenic diseases in which the clinical picture of proximal weakness may suggest a myopathic condition.

The role of muscle biopsy in diagnosis

Although histological changes in the muscle may occasionally prove absolutely diagnostic, in most circumstances account has to be taken of the clinical context so that a full clinicopathological synthesis can be arrived at. Thus it is essential that the pathologist has access to full clinical information or (ideally) has personally examined the patient and advised on the biopsy site most likely to yield useful information. Since prior needling of muscle (for EMG) may produce focal changes of necrosis, regeneration, and inflammation, such sites should be avoided.

27.3.2   Neurogenic disease

Diseases of the motor neurone

Spinal muscular atrophy (SMA)

These are a group of inherited (usually autosomal recessive) disorders resulting from degeneration of anterior horn cells. Four major clinical groups are recognized, each distinguished by the age of onset and speed of progression (Table 27.8).

All forms are characterized by neurogenic changes in muscle, although these are modified by muscle immaturity in types 1 and 2 and by chronicity in type 4 and, to a lesser extent, type 3.

Types 1 and 2 show large groups of atrophic fibres which (apparently because of fibre immaturity) retain a circular profile rather than the angular shape of other neurogenic states (Fig. 27.141). Hypertrophic fibres (which are usually type I) are also present in groups and singly. These two groups have identical biopsy appearances and distinction is made on clinical grounds. Anterior-horn cells show shrinkage or ballooning change, and in some cases neuronal loss is found in non-motor areas, such as the thalamus.

Types 3 and 4 SMA have a more typically neurogenic appearance, with angular fibres, extremely atrophic fibres (in the form of clumps of pyknotic nuclei), and hypertrophied fibres. Because of chronicity, pseudomyopathic features may be prominent, and in type 4 SMA may be so marked that a mis-diagnosis of a primary myopathic state may be made, especially if there is a 'limb-girdle' distribution (see limb-girdle dystrophy).

Table 27.8   Clinical subgroups of spinal muscular atrophy

Type	Onset	Progression
1. Acute infantile (Wernnig–Hoffmann)	<6 months	Rapidly fatal
2. (a) Severe chronic (b) Intermediate chronic	<3 yr	Inexorably progressive; usually severely disabled by age 10 yr; incapacity earlier in (a) than in (b)
3. Mild/juvenile (Kugelberg–Welander)	3–14 yr	Usually able to walk; life-span may be normal
4. Adult onset	15–50 yr	Frequently presents as limb-girdle syndrome

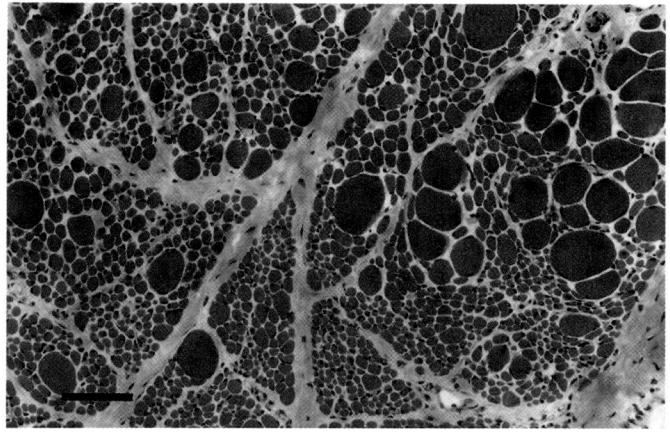

Fig. 27.141 In this typical picture of type 1 spinal muscular atrophy, groups of atrophic fibres contrast with the hypertrophic fibres, although all retain a circular profile (bar = 100 μm).

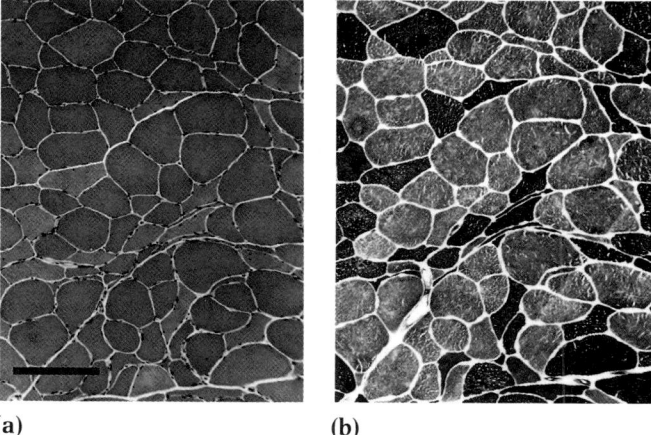

(a) (b)

Fig. 27.142 In early motor neurone disease, clusters of atrophic angular fibres are recognizable in routine H & E preparations (a), but ATPase pH 9.4 (b) reveals that both major fibre types are involved (bar = 200 μm).

Motor neurone disease

This is a group of sporadic conditions in which both upper and lower motor neurones degenerate. They are usually of late adult onset but rare familial examples have an earlier onset. High local incidences in some geographical locations, such as the Pacific island of Guam, have raised the possibility that environmental agents (viruses, toxins, or heavy metals) are involved in causation (see Chapter 25). An increase in incidence over the past 20 years in the UK, USA, and Scandinavia also supports an environmentally determined causal factor or factors. Motor neurones in the cortex, brain stem, and anterior horns are involved, and different clinical patterns result from predominant involvement of one or more of these groups (Table 27.9) although intermediate or 'mixed' forms are not uncommon. All variants are progressive and death usually results from an intercurrent chest infection.

The muscle shows changes of denervation (Fig. 27.142) with fewer core–targetoid fibres than in peripheral neuropathies but no consistent changes are attributable to upper motor neurone involvement. Typically, both fibre types are involved in both the atrophic and hypertrophic processes. Because of its more rapid progression, motor neurone disease differs from adult SMA in that pseudomyopathic change is less likely to be present.

Table 27.9 Clinical subgroups of motor neurone disease

Type	Upper motor neurones	Lower motor neurones	Brainstem nuclei
Bulbar palsy	−	−	+ +
Amyotrophic lateral sclerosis	+ +	+ +	−
Progressive muscular atrophy	−	+ +	−

Peripheral neuropathies

Diseases of the peripheral nerve may be acute, chronic, or hereditary; may affect sensory, motor, or both types of nerve; and may result from damage to the axon, the Schwann cell, or both. The details of the pathology of the nerve changes are dealt with in Section 25.9.3. When the motor innervation is affected by peripheral nerve disease, whether axonal degeneration or demyelination, the muscle shows characteristic changes of denervation (Fig. 27.143). These consist of atrophy and hypertrophy of both fibre types, fibre-type grouping, group atrophy, and collateral branching (the latter three indicative of reinnervation). Core–targetoid fibres are often numerous, although they become less common with time. With chronicity, pseudomyopathic features may be very severe but the clinical picture will usually allow distinction from genuine myopathic states.

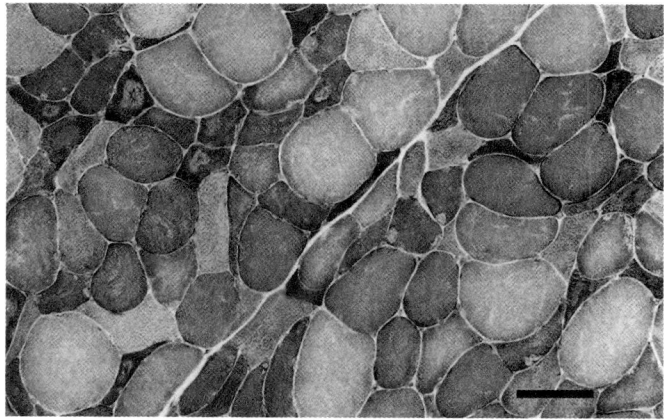

Fig. 27.143 In neurogenic atrophy, core–targetoid fibres are common and atrophic fibres often show intense staining (centre) in oxidative enzyme preparations (NADH diaphorase) (bar = 100 μm).

27.3.3 Diseases of the motor end plate

Myasthenia gravis

This disease is associated with the presence of circulating antibodies to skeletal muscle and the acetylcholine receptor. These antibodies bind in the region of the motor end plate. They are associated with structural simplification of the normally complex membrane infoldings of this structure, resulting in reduced availability of post-synaptic receptors for acetylcholine and thus muscle weakness. Antibody production may be associated with disease of the thymus, and three main clinical groups have been defined by Compston *et al.* (1980) (Table 27.10).

Thymectomy is generally more successful when hyperplasia is present, since it removes the source of antibody. In contrast, removal of a thymoma may remove the initiating antigen (inappropriately expressed on tumour-cell surfaces) but antibodies may continue to be produced in peripheral lymphoid tissue. Consistent muscle changes are usually limited to attenuation of the motor end plate and thus biopsy is of little value in diagnosis. Collections of lymphocytes (lymphorrhages) may be found but, although characteristic, they are not specific.

Myasthenic/Eaton–Lambert syndrome

This is a rare syndrome associated with malignancy, usually an oat cell carcinoma, in which defective release of acetylcholine due to a defect (probably antibody-mediated) in the pre-synaptic membrane results in a clinically myasthenic syndrome. No specific morphological changes occur and the post-synaptic membrane does not show the simplification of myasthenia gravis.

27.3.4 Diseases of muscle

Muscular dystrophies

These are inherited, progressive primary degenerations of muscle, although in some of the milder later-onset forms (especially limb-girdle distribution) there have been suggestions of an underlying chronic neurogenic process. The diseases are broadly grouped on the basis of age of onset, severity, and clinical pattern of muscle involvement. The severer forms are X-linked and therefore restricted to males, although very rare autosomal recessive severe forms do occur which can affect either sex.

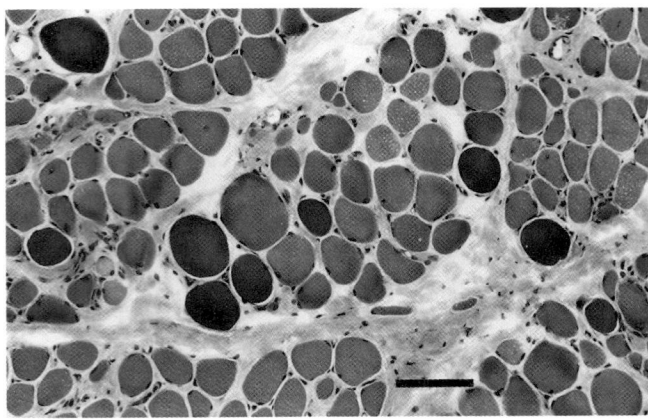

Fig. 27.144 Fibrosis and enlarged hyaline fibres (dark in this photograph) are typical features of Duchenne dystrophy (bar = 100 μm).

Duchenne muscular dystrophy

This, the severest form of dystrophy, has an X-linked recessive inheritance with onset usually before 5 years; survival beyond the end of the second decade is rare. Muscle weakness is commonly associated with mental retardation. A frequent finding is calf hypertrophy which is, at first, compensatory but eventually reflects extensive fatty replacement.

The defective gene on the X-chromosome can now be detected with DNA probes, and carrier detection and antenatal diagnosis are now being done. A deletion (not necessarily a constant one) on the short arm of the X-chromosome is the usual abnormality.

The muscle shows fibre necrosis and regeneration and frequent hyaline fibres (Fig. 27.144), which are thought to be hypercontracted due to a basic membrane defect. A similar basic defect may explain the fact that the distinction between fibre types is less clear than normal. Associated secondary changes include fibrosis (which causes contractures) and a focal chronic inflammatory cell infiltrate which may be quite intense.

The continuing fibre necrosis results in extremely high serum levels of CPK and the eventual inability of regeneration to compensate results in progressive weakness. There is an associated cardiomyopathy which is responsible for the frequent finding of ECG abnormalities.

Table 27.10 Clinical subgroups of myasthenia gravis

Sex	Age	AChR* Abs	Skeletal muscle Abs	HLA Type	Thymic pathology	Response to thymectomy
1. M = F	not specific	high	present	none	thymoma	variable
2. F > M	<40 yr	present	low	A1, B8, DRW3	hyperplasia	good
3. M = F	>40 yr	low	other auto-antibodies present	A3, B7, DRW2	—	—

* AChR, acetylcholine receptor; Abs, antibodies.

Becker muscular dystrophy

This is a milder X-linked dystrophy than Duchenne, with a later onset and slower progression. It is not associated with mental retardation, cardiac changes are less common, and death may be delayed until after the age of 40. Histologically the muscle shows appearances qualitatively similar to Duchenne dystrophy, although less severe for the patient's age; there is generally less fibrosis and fibre types are more clearly distinguished.

The same gene is involved in both Duchenne and Becker dystrophies but different sites of deletion may determine the severity and rate of progression and thus the clinical grouping. The normal product of the defective gene, dystrophin, has now been identified and abnormalities of its structure in both diseases are thought to result in its defective integration into the sarcolemma with consequent defects in muscle function. Characterization of dystrophin abnormalities is likely to prove of considerable value in both diagnosis and prognostication.

Congenital muscular dystrophy

Presentation of this disease ranges from simple hypotonia to contractures present at birth. Despite similar histological appearances these may represent distinct nosologic entities. One inherited form (Fukuyama) is associated with abnormalities of cerebral cortical development.

The diagnosis is based on the presence of dystrophic features in an appropriate clinical setting. These consist of fibre atrophy and hypertrophy, necrosis and regeneration, and fibrosis, although the hyaline fibres of the severe X-linked dystrophies are not usually present. Progression is variable from patient to patient and prediction of behaviour on biopsy appearances is unreliable.

Facio-scapulo-humeral dystrophy

This has an autosomal dominant inheritance with characteristic involvement of facial and upper limb girdle muscle. It may be mimicked by other disorders, including inflammatory myopathies and some neurogenic disorders (especially SMA).

The muscle shows myopathic features, although degeneration and regeneration are less frequent than in other dystrophies. In addition, lobulated fibres (due to peripheral aggregates of mitochondria) and small angular fibres (similar to those seen in neurogenic states) may be present. As with Duchenne and Becker muscular dystrophies, focal inflammation may be present and, in some cases, may make distinction from polymyositis so difficult that a trial of steroid therapy may be required.

Oculopharyngeal dystrophy

This late-onset, autosomal dominant condition combines involvement of external ocular, oropharyngeal and, to a variable extent, upper limb girdle muscles. Even though the latter may only be mildly involved, clinically they will usually show sufficient abnormality for biopsy to be diagnostically valuable. The changes in the muscle are broadly myopathic and, characteristically, intrafibre autophagic vacuoles (Fig. 27.145a) will be present, although these are neither inevitable nor specific.

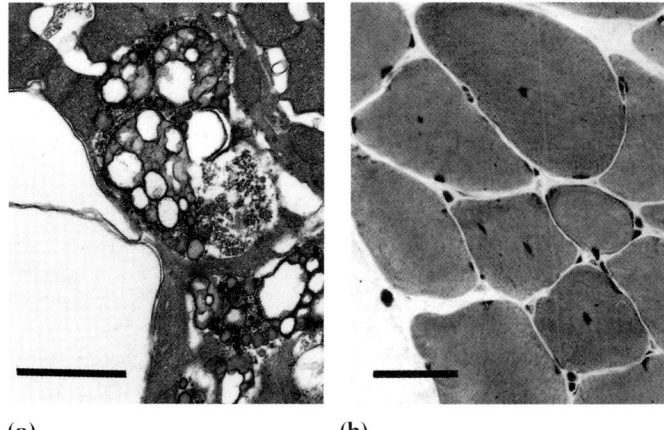

(a)   **(b)**

Fig. 27.145 (a) Autophagic vacuoles, usually membrane-bound, are typical of oculopharyngeal dystrophy, but are only identifiable with the electron microscope (bar = 1 μm). (b) Fibre calibre variation, internal nuclei and scattered ring fibres typify adult myotonic dystrophy (bar = 75 μm).

Limb-girdle dystrophy

In its genuine form this is an uncommon, autosomal recessive, proximal dystrophy with progressive upper and lower limb involvement. Many cases labelled as limb-girdle dystrophy are, in reality, examples of late-onset SMA in which low-grade chronic denervation is masked by gross pseudomyopathic features.

Myopathic features typically dominate with fibrosis, fibre hypertrophy and atrophy, and ring and whorled fibres. Small-group atrophy and collateral branching of motor innervation will identify an underlying neurogenic state, even if CPK levels are elevated.

Myotonic dystrophy

This is a progressive autosomal dominant condition of adult onset in which there is muscle wasting, especially of the face; premature balding; cataracts; testicular atrophy in affected males; and cardiac conduction defects. The muscle wasting is associated with a membrane abnormality which results in the clinical sign of myotonia: an inability of muscle to relax after cessation of voluntary or stimulated contraction. The muscle shows numerous internal nuclei (Fig. 27.145b) and type I fibre atrophy. Ring fibres and subsarcolemmal masses are both characteristic and may reflect the fundamental abnormality of the cell membrane, which also results in disordered cytoarchitecture.

Occasionally the disease may present as hypotonia in infancy (congenital myotonic dystrophy), but is always associated with maternal disease, suggesting an additional circulating 'factor' acting on the heterozygote infant. Clinical myotonia is usually absent, although EMG may show characteristic changes. The muscle shows features interpreted as immaturity and many fibres show peripheral zones (haloes) that lack myofibrils.

Myotonia congenita This is a rare autosomal dominant disease in which myotonia is not associated with progressive muscle degeneration. The muscle may be structurally normal or show fibre hypertrophy.

Congenital myopathies

A wide range of disorders of muscle structure and function presenting in early life (usually as hypotonia) have been described. These vary in their severity, progression, and heredity but many are distinguished by characteristic structural features on which the diagnosis is based. Clear distinction between these types is not always easy, and the occurrence of mixed patterns must be recognized. Inheritance patterns are variable in most groups and need to be assessed for each individual pedigree in which milder cases may present in adult life although with a characteristic histology. Many cases may be non-progressive, but the hypotonia that results may be sufficiently severe to be life threatening due to involvement of respiratory muscles. These conditions are all rare, and only a selected few are described here.

Congenital fibre-type disproportion

Type I fibre smallness is associated with a usually nonprogressive weakness, which may improve with increasing age. Type I smallness may also occur in conjunction with other architectural abnormalities in the context of other congenital myopathies and these must be excluded before the diagnosis is certain.

Nemaline/rod-body myopathy

This myopathy is characterized by the presence in most (but not necessarily all) fibres of numerous thread-like structures (Fig. 27.146a), which are aggregates of Z-band material. These structures are often difficult to identify in routine sections but they are well stained by trichrome or phosphotungstic acid haematoxylin (PTAH). Clinical states range from severe (with neonatal death) to mild (with a late onset).

Central-core disease

This is an autosomal dominant condition which may present as hypotonia, or be associated with little motor abnormality. Life expectancy is not usually significantly shortened. There is a definite association with susceptibility to malignant hyperthermia (see below) and diagnosis should lead to investigation of the entire family for this latter trait. The muscles show central cores (see above for distinction from core–targetoid fibres) in most, if not all, type I fibres (Fig. 27.146b), which are usually increased in number relative to type II fibres.

Centronuclear/myotubular myopathy

In this condition muscle fibres retain central nuclei and thus resemble fetal myotubes. The centres of the fibres lack myofibrils, and satellite cells are scarce. Both a severe X-linked and a less severe form with an inconstant inheritance pattern are described.

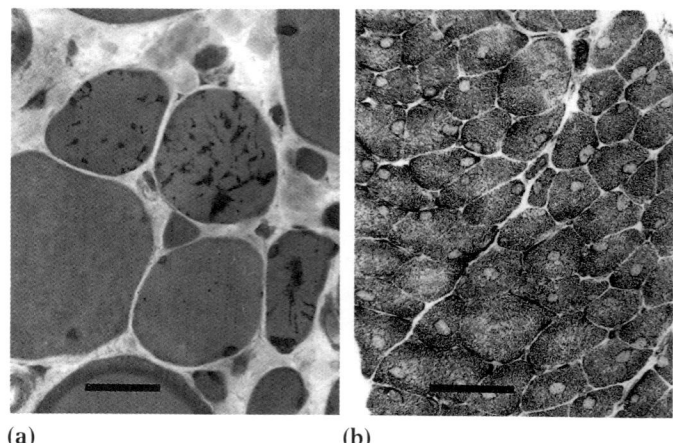

(a)   **(b)**

Fig. 27.146 (a) Darkly stained rod bodies fill many fibres in rod-body myopathy but require trichrome·stains for best visualization (Gomori trichrome; bar = 25 μm). (b) The presence in most fibres of pale-staining cores in this oxidative enzyme preparation (NADH diaphorase) identifies central-core disease (bar = 75 μm).

Multicore disease

In this condition there is predominance of type I fibres, many of which contain small areas of myofibrillar disruption sometimes described as minicores. Clinically it usually causes a nonprogressive hypotonia.

Benign congenital hypotonia

This is a heterogeneous category in which other defined entities and central nervous system causes have been excluded. Progression is not usual and the muscle shows only mild defects of maturation.

Metabolic myopathies
Mitochondrial myopathies

A wide range of disorders of mitochondrial function may result in symptoms of muscle disease. In some of these a defined mitochondrial defect is known, while in others the mitochondria may be structurally abnormal allowing the diagnosis to be made (Fig. 27.147a). Where the defect involves lipid metabolism (i.e. carnitine deficiency) abnormally large lipid droplets will also be evident, but in other cases the only abnormality will be aggregates of mitochondria within fibres (Fig. 27.147b) which are termed 'ragged-red' because of their appearance on trichrome preparations.

Some of these conditions are associated with defined clinical syndromes, often involving extra-ocular muscles, but no clear pattern of enzyme deficiency has been delineated for these cases.

Glycogen disorders

Myophosphorylase deficiency/McArdle disease (glycogenosis V) Lack of myophosphorylase results in exercise-induced cramps without a rise in serum lactate but sometimes with myoglobinuria. Myophosphorylase can be shown to be absent histochemically (and biochemically) and glycogen aggregates

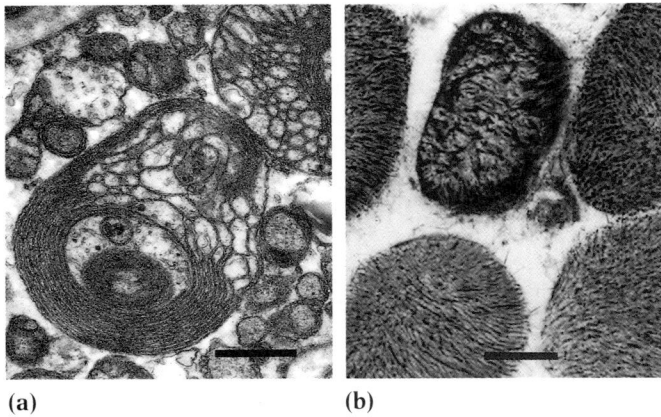

(a)   **(b)**

Fig. 27.147 (a) Ultrastructural abnormalities in mitochondria are rarely specific or consistent but abnormal collections can be recognized (b) as subsarcolemmal densities in trichrome or (as here) oxidative enzyme preparations. (Bars: (a) 0.1 μm; (b) 25 μm.)

(not membrane bound) form beneath the sarcolemma and give rise to a vacuolar appearance.

A very similar syndrome is found with phosphofructokinase deficiency (glycogenosis VI), which can also be detected histochemically.

Acid maltase deficiency (glycogenosis II) Lack of the lysosomal enzyme, acid maltase, results in the accumulation of undegraded excess glycogen within lysosomes which form vacuoles. The infantile form (Pompe disease) has an early mortality due to multi-system involvement but later- and adult-onset forms are milder and muscle symptoms may predominate.

Periodic paralyses

These are a rare group of disorders in which episodes of weakness are usually associated with changes in serum potassium levels. Although usually hereditary, sporadic cases may be seen in the context of thyrotoxicosis. During attacks (and sometimes between them) the muscle may show a vacuolar change due to sarcoplasmic reticulum distension.

Malignant hyperthermia (MH)

In this autosomal dominant condition certain general anaesthetic agents (especially halothane) trigger prolonged muscular contraction resulting in hyperthermia that may be fatal. In such cases the muscle shows evidence of hypercontraction, but in susceptible (but unexposed) individuals may show little. Myopathic changes do occur, but these are not an inevitable feature of the disease and probably represent acquired abnormalities in susceptible muscle. Diagnosis at present depends on *in vitro* testing of an open biopsy specimen. Central-core disease has a recognized association with this trait but underlies very few cases of MH.

Inflammatory disorders

Infective diseases

Viral, bacterial, fungal, protozoal, and metazoal infection and infestation of muscle all occur. Viral infection (notably coxsackie) may result in acute rhabdomyolysis; while bacteria and fungi cause lesions with local destruction and abscess formation. Metazoal parasites (notably *Taenia solium* and *Trichinella spiralis*) may involve muscle as part of their life cycle but the biopsy picture is usually dominated by the organism and the muscle shows only local reaction to this.

Polymyositis and dermatomyositis

These conditions may occur together, separately, or in association with multisystem disorders which may or may not conform to a definable syndrome, such as systemic lupus erythematosus or rheumatoid arthritis. They have an immunological basis, with muscle necrosis and inflammation (polymyositis) and, in dermatomyositis, a superficial dermatitis with characteristic facial oedema and swelling. The fibre necrosis that is central to this condition results in the usual finding of high serum levels of CPK. Typically the proximal limb-girdle muscles are involved but a facio-scapulo-humeral distribution may occur. An identical syndrome may occur in association with neoplastic disease (breast, ovary, lung, or stomach) and as many as 20 per cent of cases over 50 years of age may be in this category. The basis for the apparent auto-immune cellular reaction is unknown but there is some evidence to implicate previous viral infection, or, in the case of tumour-associated disease, cross-reacting antigens.

The muscle shows a mixed picture of individual fibre necrosis and phagocytosis, regeneration, and an interstitial lymphocytic (mostly T-cell) and monocytic infiltrate (Fig. 27.148). Although the inflammatory infiltrate is frequently perivascular, a true vasculitis is not usual in adult cases. This contrasts with the disease in children where vascular involvement is much commoner, and confluent areas of necrosis amounting to micro-infarcts may be found. Vascular compromise is also thought to underlie the perifascicular atrophy that is characteristic of childhood polymyositis (Fig. 27.149a).

The changes, especially in adult disease, may be focal, and a

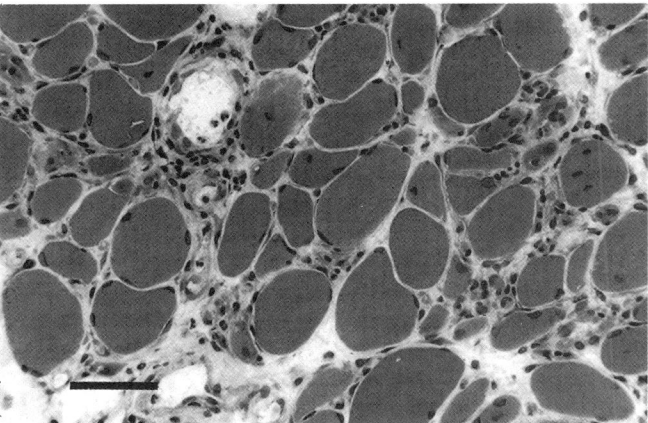

Fig. 27.148 Fibre degeneration and regeneration accompany the inflammatory infiltrate of typical adult polymyositis (bar = 75 μm).

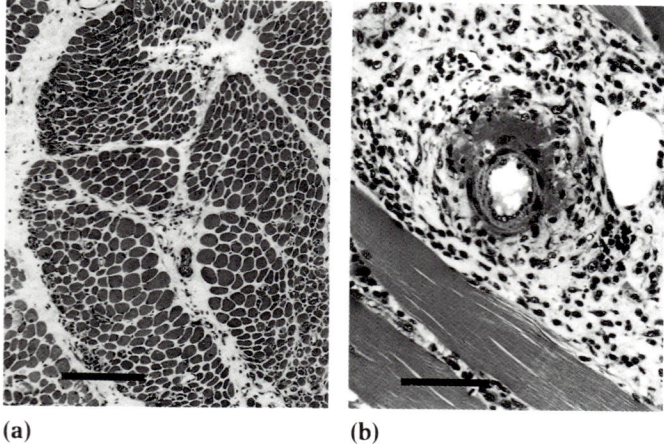

(a)   **(b)**

Fig. 27.149 (a) The tendency for atrophic fibres to be perifascicular in childhood polymyositis is best appreciated at low magnification (bar = 200 μm). (b) Segmental necrosis of the wall of a small interstitial artery with fibrin exudation distinguishes the true vasculitis of polyarteritis nodosa from simple perivascular inflammation (bar = 75 μm).

variant is encountered in which fibre necrosis and regeneration occur without an accompanying inflammatory infiltrate. It is not clear whether these 'necrotizing myopathies' are variants of polymyositis, the result of sampling error, or a heterogeneous group of conditions of unrecognized aetiology.

Localized nodular myositis is an acute, painful, localized necrotizing myopathy which may progress to a generalized myositis identical to polymyositis.

Muscle involvement in systemic disease

The muscle may show evidence of focal inflammatory cell infiltrates in many connective tissue disorders, but unless these are accompanied by active fibre breakdown and regeneration the diagnosis of polymyositis is not justified. Granulomatous inflammation occurs in the context of systemic sarcoidosis, which may occasionally be diagnosed by muscle biopsy.

Polyarteritis nodosa is most likely to produce clinical weakness due to involvement of peripheral nerves, but sometimes muscle symptoms are prominent and biopsy may reveal typical necrotizing lesions in affected vessels (Fig. 27.149b). Random biopsy is only likely to be positive in one-third of cases.

27.3.5   Interstitial fibroproliferative disorders

Although skeletal muscle has a capacity for true regeneration at a cellular/myofibre level, this requires an intact basement membrane tube within which satellite cells can proliferate and form new myofibres. Although this may be the case in minor injury, most traumatic and ischaemic damage to muscle will heal by fibrous repair. Reactions of muscle, or more importantly its connective tissue, to injury may result in tumour-like lesions whose importance lies in their distinction from true neoplasms (see also Section 27.4).

Myositis ossificans

This is probably an abnormal response to local haemorrhage which results in a proliferating mesenchymal mass with marked, inappropriate, osteoblastic differentiation with the formation of both woven and lamellar bone. In its early stages the condition may be mistaken for osteogenic sarcoma but, in distinction to the latter, myositis ossificans shows an organized architecture with more advanced maturation at the periphery and a central, less differentiated zone of mesenchyme. Not surprisingly, there is usually (but not inevitably) a history of trauma preceding the onset of symptoms (see also Section 27.1.6).

Proliferative myositis and musculoaponeurotic fibromatosis (desmoid tumour)

These both represent non-neoplastic fibroblastic proliferations. Proliferative myositis is distinguished by the presence of large, sometimes bizarre, myofibroblastic cells which may resemble ganglion cells, although there is no evidence to support such a relationship.

Musculoaponeurotic fibromatosis typically affects the anterior abdominal wall but may be found at other sites. It is a locally infiltrative fibroblastic proliferation which, despite its tendency to recur locally after excision, rarely, if ever, metastasizes.

27.3.6   Further reading

Anderson, J. R. (1985). *Atlas of skeletal muscle pathology. Current histopathology*, Vol. 9. MTP Press, Lancaster.

Compston, D. A. S., Vincent, A., Newsom-Davis, J., and Batchelor, J. R. (1980). Clinical, pathological, HLA antigen and immunological evidence for disease heterogeneity in myasthenia gravis. *Brain* **103**, 567–601.

Dubowitz, V. (1985). *Muscle biopsy. A practical approach* (2nd edn). Baillière Tindall, London.

Hoffman, E. P., Brown, R. H., and Kunkel, L. (1987). Dystrophin: the protein product of the Duchenne muscular dystrophy locus. *Cell* **51**, 919–28.

Mastaglia, F. L. and Ojeda, V. J. (1985). Inflammatory myopathies. Parts 1 & 2. *Annals of Neurology* **17**, 215–27 and 317–23.

Weller, R. O. (1984). Muscle biopsy and the diagnosis of muscle disease. In *Recent advances in pathology*, Vol. 12 (ed. P. P. Anthony and R. N. M. MacSween). Churchill Livingstone, Edinburgh.

27.4   Soft tissue tumours

C. D. M. Fletcher and P. H. McKee

27.4.1   Introduction

Soft tissue tumours are notorious for the diagnostic problems that they cause to histopathologists, largely because so many of the entities in this category are relatively uncommon, with the obvious exceptions of the ubiquitous lipoma and benign fibrous histiocytoma. Furthermore, massive recategorization and subclassification of soft tissue tumours has occurred over the past 30 years, with the recognition of many new histological entities, making it rather difficult for the non-specialist to keep up with the clinicopathologically important literature. It should be remembered, however, that malignant connective tissue tumours, known collectively as sarcomas, are outnumbered in frequency by both carcinomas and benign soft tissue neoplasms by about 100 to 1 in each instance.

One of the principal difficulties in categorizing soft tissue tumours lies in the fact that the histogenetic origin of the majority of cases is entirely unknown and many lesions are therefore diagnosed solely on their pattern of differentiation. Indeed, many cases originate in tissues lacking the mature (fully differentiated) counterpart of the tumour itself. For example, most embryonal rhabdomyosarcomas arise at sites totally devoid of skeletal muscle and both extraskeletal osteosarcomas and chondrosarcomas develop, by definition, at sites unrelated to any osteoarticular structure. Sadly, at the present time, one can only ascribe such phenomena to the remarkable plasticity of differentiation of mesenchymally derived tumours. To make matters worse, a significant number of these neoplasms show no evidence of differentiation which is at all comparable to normal tissues, for example fibrous histiocytomas (both benign and malignant), epithelioid sarcoma, and alveolar soft-part sarcoma.

Against this seemingly depressing background, more than 95 per cent of all soft tissue tumours (benign and malignant combined) can, in fact, be classified into recognizable histopathological categories with reasonably predictable clinical implications. Admittedly, however, between 10 and 15 per cent of sarcomas (i.e. malignant lesions) are unclassifiable, even in specialist centres. To give a general ideal of relative importance, approximate proportional frequencies of the identifiable histological types of sarcoma are given in Table 27.11. It is important, when examining this frequency distribution, to be aware that more than 90 per cent of rhabdomyosarcomas occur in childhood or adolescence, at which ages this tumour accounts for the majority of sarcomas. Conversely, it is exceedingly uncommon in adulthood. Similarly, malignant fibrous histiocytoma and liposarcoma are virtually confined to adult life and are very rare in children.

Table 27.11 Frequency distribution (%) of histologically classifiable soft-tissue sarcomas* (St. Thomas's Hospital data, 1989)

Liposarcoma	17
Leiomyosarcoma	14
Rhabdomyosarcoma	12
Malignant fibrous histiocytoma (all types)	11
Malignant nerve sheath tumour	9.5
Synovial sarcoma	6

* No other single histological type accounts for more than 4 per cent of all soft-tissue sarcomas, and it should be remembered that between 10 per cent and 15 per cent are unclassifiable.

27.4.2 Tumours of fat

Lipoma

Clinical features

Lipomas are the single commonest soft tissue tumour. The overwhelming majority present as a slowly growing, soft subcutaneous mass on the trunk or limbs of middle-aged adults of either sex, but almost any site may be affected on occasion. They are usually mobile, painless, and may measure from 1 to 20 cm or more in diameter. Local recurrence is uncommon and malignant transformation, for all practical purposes, never occurs.

Histopathology

These lesions are typically lobulated and have a thin capsule. They are composed of a well-circumscribed mass of mature, univacuolated adipocytes with small monomorphic nuclei and no mitoses. Some cases contain irregular bands of dense fibrous tissue (fibrolipoma) and, more rarely, osseous or chondroid metaplasia may be a feature. Areas of fat necrosis or myxoid degeneration are not infrequently present.

Variants

Approximately 2 per cent of lipomas are deeply located and are predominantly found within or between skeletal muscles (Fletcher and Martin-Bates 1988). Such lesions tend to be larger and often have infiltrative margins, suggestive of a sarcoma. These tumours recur locally in up to 15 per cent of cases unless widely excised. Deeply located lipomas may also rarely be seen within joints or tendons.

Angiolipoma

Clinical features

Angiolipomas are outnumbered by ordinary lipomas by about 10 to 1, are commonest in young or middle-aged adults, particularly males, and most often arise in the arm, although up to 30 per cent may develop on the trunk or leg. Up to 75 per cent of patients have multiple lesions, which are invariably located in subcutaneous fat, are typically mobile and encapsulated and are painful or tender in 50 per cent or more of cases. Local recurrence is very unusual and malignant transformation does not occur. It is noteworthy that there is no deeply located equivalent of angiolipoma, and cases reported as intramuscular angiolipoma appear to represent intramuscular haemangiomas with a prominent fatty component (see Section 12.5).

Histopathology

Angiolipomas differ from ordinary lipomas by the presence of variable numbers of small, thin-walled vascular channels (Fig. 27.150), which are usually most prominent at the periphery of the lesion and form a complex anastomosing meshwork which may occupy from 5 to 90 per cent of the tissue examined. Occasional cases may contain large, thick-walled vessels, sometimes with associated fibrosis. There is no endothelial atypia or multilayering.

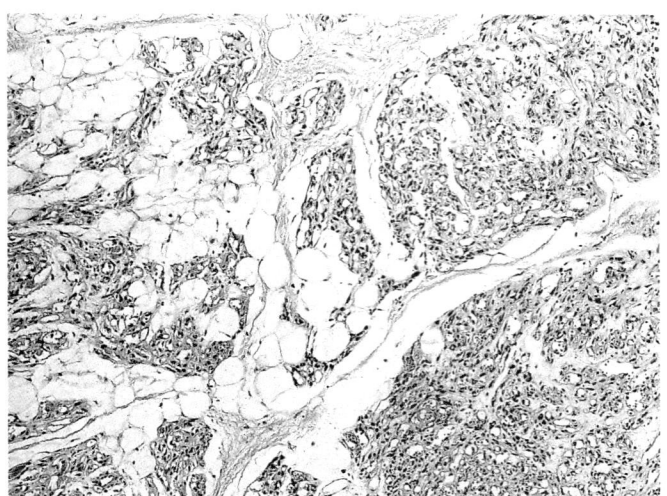

Fig. 27.150 Angiolipoma. Note the prominent proliferation of small vascular channels within mature adipose tissue.

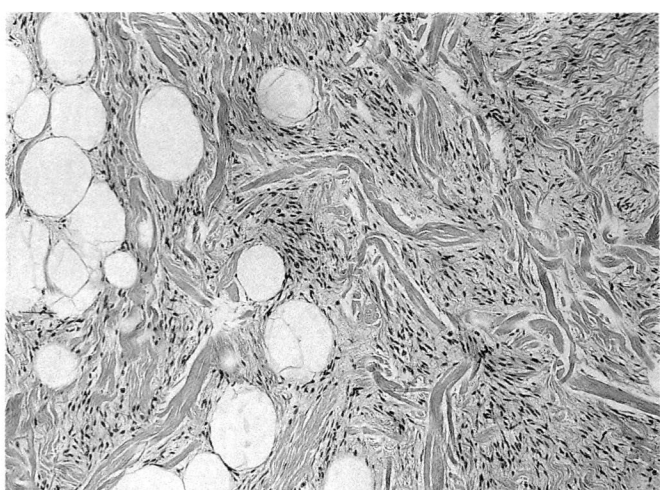

Fig. 27.151 Spindle cell lipoma. Short fascicles of spindle cells are orientated between collagen bundles and mature adipocytes.

Angiomyolipoma

These hamartomatous lesions may rarely be seen outside the kidney, but are histologically identical to their renal counterparts (see Chapter 19). Such examples only seem to occur in the retroperitoneum, often close to the kidney, and appear to be less often associated with tuberous sclerosis.

Spindle cell lipoma

Clinical features

Spindle cell lipomas (Fletcher and Martin-Bates 1987) are outnumbered by ordinary lipomas by about 60 to 1, present most often in the fifth to eighth decades, and show a striking predilection for males. The majority of cases arise on the back of the neck, upper back, or the posterior aspect of the shoulder but, occasionally, almost any site may be affected. They are typically slowly growing and painless, almost always develop in subcutaneous fat and only very rarely recur locally.

Histopathology

These tumours are characterized by very variable proportions of three principal components: mature adipocytes; small monomorphic basophilic spindle cells; and short bundles of eosinophilic, rather hyalinized collagen (Fig. 27.151). Mitoses and lipoblasts are absent, enabling ready distinction from liposarcoma. There is often a striking infiltrate of mast cells, but blood vessels are generally inconspicuous. Nuclear palisading of the spindle cells is not uncommon and may be sufficiently pronounced as to resemble a schwannoma (see below). The precise nature of the spindle cells remains uncertain, but they seem likely to represent either primitive fat cells (prelipoblasts) or uncommitted mesenchymal cells.

Pleomorphic lipoma

Pleomorphic lipoma (Shmookler and Enzinger 1981) is clinic-

ally indistinguishable from spindle cell lipoma, but is much less common. It is also histologically similar, except for the additional presence of bizarre, hyperchromatic giant cells, which often have multiple nuclei arranged in a floret pattern. A further difference is the presence of very occasional multivacuolated lipoblasts. Chronic inflammatory cells may be prominent in the stroma. These lesions are differentiated from liposarcoma by their generally small, encapsulated, superficial nature and the usual absence of necrosis or mitotic activity.

Lipoblastoma

Clinical features

Lipoblastoma (Chung and Enzinger 1973) is a rare tumour of infancy which most often arises in the subcutaneous tissue of a limb and may be either encapsulated or diffuse and deeply infiltrative, the latter type being known as lipoblastomatosis. It presents as a slowly growing painless mass, sometimes noticeable from birth. Local recurrence is very uncommon and usually reflects incomplete excision of a diffuse lesion.

Histopathology

Both forms of lipoblastoma are histologically similar and are composed of lobules of fat cells showing very variable differentiation, ranging from spindle-shaped prelipoblasts through multivacuolated and univacuolated (signet-ring) lipoblasts to mature adipocytes. There often appears to be a zoned pattern, with the most primitive cells at the periphery of the lobules and mature fat cells centrally. An arborizing network of thin-walled blood vessels, similar to that in myxoid liposarcoma, is frequently prominent. Distinction from liposarcoma is largely aided by the fact that liposarcoma is virtually unheard of in infancy. Furthermore, the nuclei in lipoblastoma are not pleomorphic or hyperchromatic and never show abnormal mitotic figures. The pronounced lobular pattern and almost invariable absence of necrosis also argue against liposarcoma.

Lipomatosis

This is a rare condition, characterized by diffuse overgrowth of mature adipose tissue, which may take several forms, of which the best known is probably symmetrical involvement of the neck and shoulders (sometimes known as Madelung's disease). This is commonest in middle-aged males and may be associated with alcohol abuse or various endocrine disorders. Another form, also affecting middle-aged males, although with no known clinical associations, involves the pelvis and often leads to ureteric compression. Possibly the rarest type is that seen in infants or young children, which most often diffusely affects a large part of a limb and is extremely difficult to excise.

Fibrolipomatous hamartoma of nerve

Clinical features

Fibrolipomatous hamartoma of nerve (Silverman and Enzinger 1985) is a very rare lesion which is probably hamartomatous in nature and is characterized by a rather fusiform swelling, usually located in the hand or wrist of adolescents or young adults. In the majority of cases, the median nerve or one of its branches is affected and symptoms of a compression neuropathy are not uncommon. Frequently the mass has been noted since birth or early childhood, and about 25 per cent of patients have associated macrodactyly. Attempts at excision invariably lead to a severe neurological deficit, therefore surgical intervention should be confined to a diagnostic biopsy and nerve decompression if necessary.

Histopathology

The nerve bundles are widely separated by copious adipose tissue and mature fibrous tissue laid down within the epineurium. Individual bundles show striking perineural and endoneural fibrosis.

Hibernoma

This is the only tumour that shows pure differentiation into brown fat, although liposarcomas may occasionally contain hibernoma-like foci. Brown fat, under normal circumstances, is principally found in fetuses and young infants and is mainly located between the scapulae, in the axillae and groins, and around retroperitoneal viscera. Small amounts may persist into adult life. Brown fat, which is characterized by large numbers of mitochondria and less actual lipid than ordinary adipocytes, is thought to be important in heat production.

Clinical features

Hibernomas are, surprisingly, commonest in middle-aged adults of either sex and arise most often between the scapulae, in the axilla, or the neck. They have also been recorded at many other sites and may be subcutaneous or intramuscular. They are slowly growing, often attain a considerable size, and never recur. There is no malignant equivalent.

Histopathology

These lesions are well circumscribed and encapsulated and typ-

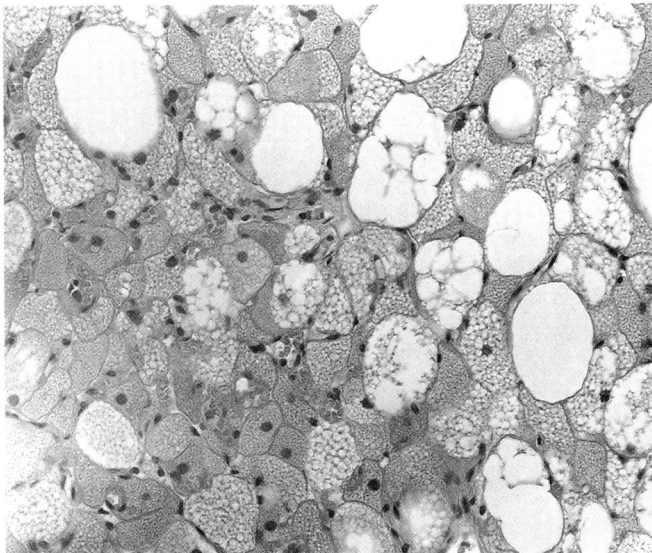

Fig. 27.152 Hibernoma. Note the granular eosinophilic and multi-vacuolated cells typical of brown fat.

ically have a tan-brown colour. They are composed of three principal cell types: multivacuolated cells with variably eosinophilic cytoplasm and small central nuclei; smaller granular, eosinophilic cells containing little or no lipid; and ordinary univacuolated adipocytes (Fig. 27.152). Mitoses and nuclear pleomorphism are absent. Numerous small capillaries are often present in the stroma.

Liposarcoma

Liposarcoma (Kindblom et al. 1975, Hashimoto and Enjoji 1982, Azumi et al. 1987) is one of the commonest malignant connective tissue tumours of adult life but is exceedingly rare in children. Other than very occasional radiation-induced cases, the aetiology is unknown. Histologically, liposarcoma is divided into four subtypes: well-differentiated; myxoid; round cell; and pleomorphic. These subtypes have prognostic relevance. The well-differentiated group can be further subclassified (see below). An absolute prerequisite for the diagnosis of liposarcoma is the presence of multivacuolated lipoblasts, characterized by two or usually more intracytoplasmic lipid droplets of variable size associated with a large hyperchromatic, often pleomorphic, nucleus which is indented or 'scalloped' by the lipid droplets. Univacuolated (signet-ring) forms are also quite common but are hard to recognize in the absence of their multivacuolated counterparts.

Clinical features

Liposarcoma may present at any time during adult life but is commonest in the fifth and sixth decades and shows a slight male predominance. The most frequently affected sites are the lower limb and retroperitoneum. Patients complain of a painless mass of variable duration and growth rate, which is usually much larger than most lipomas and averages 10–15 cm in diameter. Overall, around 50 per cent of cases recur locally, about 25 per cent metastasize, and the median five-year survival is 60 per cent. The prognosis is heavily dependent upon site and histological subtype. Tumours in the retroperitoneum, irrespective of microscopic appearance, have a five-year survival of about 35 per cent owing to their usual incomplete excision and repeated local recurrence with involvement of vital structures. In contrast, limb lesions of the pure well-differentiated or myxoid types do extremely well and only rarely metastasize, whereas round cell and pleomorphic tumours, irrespective of site, commonly metastasize and have a five-year survival of around 20 per cent.

Histopathology

Well-differentiated liposarcoma This tumour may be divided into four types: lipoma-like; sclerosing; inflammatory; and dedifferentiated, of which the first is the commonest. The lipoma-like variant, as it sounds, is composed mainly of univacuolated adipocytes showing some variation in size and shape, associated with only scattered multivacuolated lipoblasts and occasional hyperchromatic spindle or stellate cells, which are often found within dense fibrous septa. The sclerosing variant is typified by large, hyperchromatic, pleomorphic cells set in an abundant, variably fibrillary or dense collagenous stroma, associated with occasional lipoblasts and areas of relatively mature adipose tissue. The inflammatory variant resembles the lipoma-like type except for the addition of a dense, often rather nodular infiltrate of lymphocytes and plasma cells. Patchy fibrosis is a common feature and lipoblasts may be hard to find. The dedifferentiated variant may resemble any of the above types but, in addition, contains variably sized foci of pleomorphic or undifferentiated tumour, often resembling malignant fibrous histiocytoma and usually showing no discernible adipocytic differentiation.

It is important that all well-differentiated examples are extensively sampled, both to ensure identification of lipoblasts (hence avoiding confusion with, for example, intramuscular lipoma) and secondly to exclude the presence of a dedifferentiated element, which confers a much worse prognosis with up to 50 per cent metastasizing. The current trend is to classify all *pure* well-differentiated cases arising in a *limb* as atypical lipoma, since they never metastasize and therefore wide excision should be curative. However, it must be remembered that local recurrence may be associated with the development of a more aggressive-type histology, hence altering the prognosis.

Myxoid liposarcoma This is the single commonest histological type of liposarcoma and is characterized by small, undifferentiated mesenchymal cells and variable numbers of lipoblasts, set in an abundant myxoid matrix composed predominantly of hyaluronic acid (Fig. 27.153). A typical feature is the presence of a prominent anastomosing network of thin-walled capillaries, having a so-called 'chicken-wire' or 'crow's feet' appearance. Pooling of mucin to give a multicystic appearance is not uncommon. All myxoid liposarcomas should be carefully sampled to exclude the presence of a round cell element (see below).

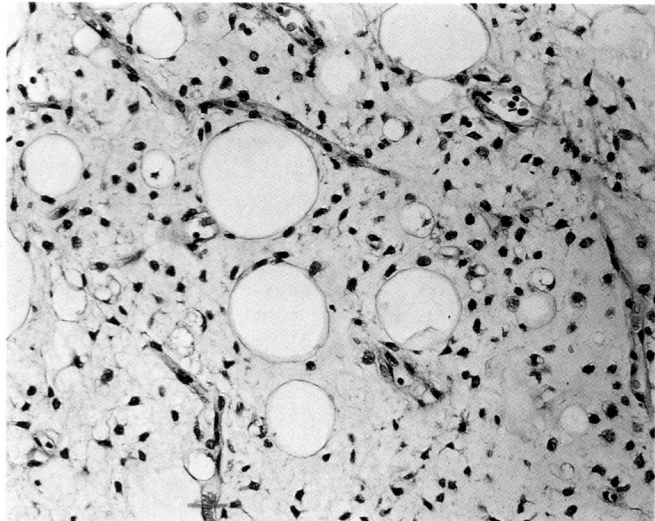

Fig. 27.153 Myxoid liposarcoma. Note the scattered small lipoblasts and prominent capillary network.

Round cell liposarcoma This relatively uncommon type of liposarcoma is widely regarded as the poorly differentiated counterpart of the myxoid variant and frequently contains typical areas of myxoid liposarcoma. The bulk of the tumour, however, is composed of solid sheets of uniform, small to medium-sized, round basophilic cells with little discernible cytoplasm. Lipoblasts may be quite hard to find within these areas and, similarly, the plexiform vascular network (described above) may be largely obscured by the dense cellularity.

Pleomorphic liposarcoma As the name would suggest, these tumours have a very pleomorphic appearance characterized by spindle cells and numerous giant cells, and are only distinguishable from other types of sarcoma by the presence of variable, usually small, numbers of multivacuolated lipoblasts (Fig. 27.154). This is the only variant of liposarcoma in which mitoses are usually numerous.

The differential diagnosis of liposarcoma typically presents no great problem if careful attention is paid to the accurate identification of lipoblasts. The only cells that bear any great resemblance to lipoblasts are lipid or mucin-laden macrophages, seen in areas of fat necrosis or a variety of tumours, particularly myxoid malignant fibrous histiocytoma. These cells tend to have much smaller, less well-defined, rather bubbly vacuoles, with a smaller, euchromatic, and often centrally placed nucleus which is not indented by the vacuoles.

27.4.3   Reactive lesions of fibrous tissue

The group of tumours considered under this heading are generally believed to be reactive, rather than neoplastic, in nature, although the initiating stimulus is often unknown. Trauma is, however, the most popularly implicated aetiological agent. Despite their general clinical insignificance, they may cause great

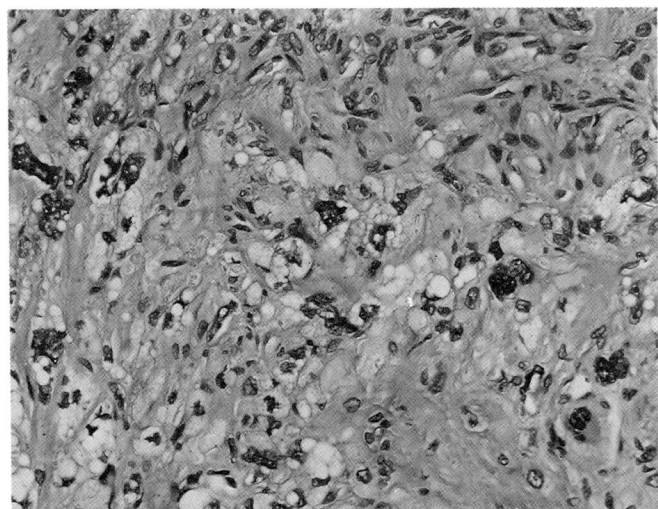

Fig. 27.154 Pleomorphic liposarcoma. Multivacuolated lipoblasts are readily identified in this pleomorphic neoplasm.

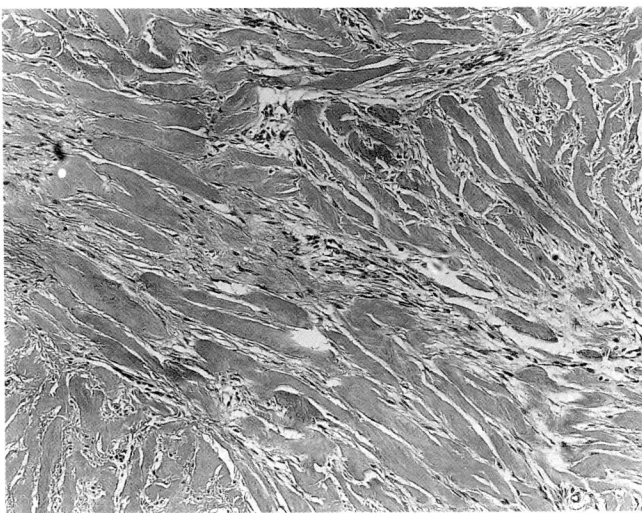

Fig. 27.155 Keloid. Note the characteristic thick, hyalinized collagen bundles.

difficulties in diagnosis, particularly in the case of nodular fasciitis (and its variants) which seems to be frequently mistaken for a sarcoma.

Keloid

Clinical features

Keloids are best regarded as exuberant variants of a scar and are, for practical purposes, always related to preceding trauma, be it mechanical, inflammatory, or otherwise. They are commonest in adolescents and young adults, show a marked predilection for negroid races and affect females rather more often than males. They present most often around the face, neck, earlobes, sternum, and forearms as raised, smooth nodules or plaques, which are frequently itchy or tender and characteristically extend beyond the site of the initiating injury. They are extremely prone to local recurrence following excision and are generally rather difficult to treat.

Histopathology

The microscopic appearance of a keloid is dependent upon its duration. Early lesions are characterized by a partly nodular, partly fascicular intradermal mass of cellular fibrous tissue, often showing mitotic activity. The more typical long-standing cases show very striking brightly eosinophilic hyalinization of collagen with a marked reduction in cellularity (Fig. 27.155).

Hypertrophic scar

Hypertrophic scars are less common than keloids but show some similarities. They, too, are related to previous trauma but show no predilection for Negro patients and do not extend beyond the boundaries of the initial tissue damage. They are less often symptomatic and only occasionally recur after excision. Histologically, while distinction from a keloid may be very difficult in the early stages, hypertrophic scars do not go on to show striking hyalinization but, rather, persist as an intradermal nodule of moderately cellular, mature fibrous tissue.

Nodular fasciitis

Clinical features

Nodular fasciitis (Bernstein and Lattes 1982, Shimizu et al. 1984) is a relatively common condition which presents most often as a tender nodule, typically of less than three months' duration, in patients of almost any age but most frequently in young adults. The forearm is by far the single commonest site, followed by the leg and trunk. Cases in children frequently affect the head and neck. The majority of lesions are located in subcutaneous fat, but up to 10 per cent involve skeletal muscle. Following local excision only about 1 per cent of cases recur locally and, in fact, a small proportion of untreated examples regress spontaneously.

Histopathology

Most tumours measure less than 3 cm in diameter and superficially appear quite well circumscribed, although infiltrative margins are often evident microscopically. To some extent the appearances seem dependent on the duration of the lesion. The classical picture (Fig. 27.156) is one of rather plump, uniform fibroblasts, randomly arranged in fascicles or whorls and showing moderate numbers of normal mitotic figures. These cells are set in a loose myxoid matrix, giving rise to the so-called feathery appearance. Within the myxoid stroma, numerous small blood vessels lined by plump endothelium, extravasated red cells, and lymphocytes are usually prominent. Very early examples are often particularly myxoid, whereas long-standing lesions tend to hyalinize, with a concomitant reduction in vascularity and inflammation. Notably, however, at no stage is there nuclear pleomorphism or hyperchromasia.

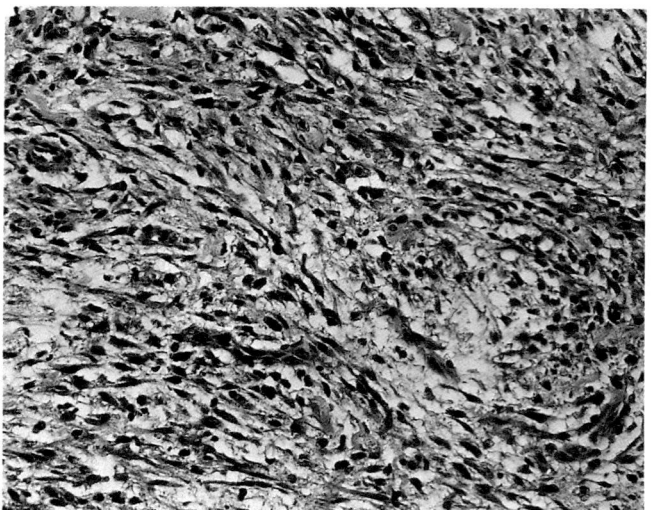

Fig. 27.156 Nodular fasciitis. A typical disorderly proliferation of plump fibroblasts, associated with extravasated red cells and lymphocytes.

Variants

Intravascular fasciitis This lesion (Patchefsky and Enzinger 1981) is uncommon, most often presenting as one or more nodules in the arm of children or young adults. While histologically similar to conventional nodular fasciitis, it also involves the full thickness of blood vessel walls and shows prominent intraluminal growth, simulating a sarcoma. Up to 20 per cent of cases may recur locally.

Cranial fasciitis (Lauer and Enzinger 1980) is a very rare entity, which almost always occurs in young infants and is only distinguishable from conventional nodular fasciitis by the presence of invasion into (and sometimes through) the underlying skull bone. Local excision is curative.

Parosteal fasciitis This is also an extremely rare lesion, of which cranial fasciitis is best regarded as a variant, which, while histologically unremarkable, arises from the periosteum and may or may not be associated with destruction of bone. There are insufficient data upon which to base a clear clinical picture.

While the differential diagnosis of nodular fasciitis often seems to cause great problems, the typical clinical history and lack of pleomorphism or atypical mitoses allows ready distinction from most types of sarcoma. Fibromatoses are distinguished by their more orderly fasciculated and collagenous appearance and their relative paucity of blood vessels and inflammatory cells.

Proliferative fasciitis

Clinical features

Proliferative fasciitis (Chung and Enzinger 1975) is clinically and macroscopically indistinguishable from nodular fasciitis (see above), but for the fact that it appears confined to later adult life (predominantly the fifth and seventh decades) and does not occur in childhood. As in nodular fasciitis, local recurrence is unusual.

Histopathology

This lesion has many microscopic similarities to nodular fasciitis but is more often truly located around superficial fascia and tends to have more extensively infiltrative margins. The cardinal and distinctive feature is the presence of numerous basophilic, ganglion-like giant cells, which seem never to have more than two nuclei and which may contain eosinophilic 'collagenous' inclusions. These cells are often aggregated in clusters and may show scattered normal mitoses. They are thought to represent an unusual type of 'activated' fibroblast.

Proliferative myositis

Clinical features

Proliferative myositis (Enzinger and Dulcey 1967) is the intramuscular equivalent of proliferative fasciitis and has a similar age distribution. It presents as a painless swelling, usually of less than one month's duration, and is most often located in the major muscles of the chest wall. As with these other reactive lesions, local recurrence is very uncommon.

Histopathology

This lesion is characterized by diffuse proliferation of plump fibroblasts both between and within muscle bundles, associated with large numbers of basophilic ganglion-like cells, as described above. Mitotic activity is often prominent both in the fibroblasts and giant cells. A striking feature is the remarkable preservation of muscle fibres which, despite this infiltrative process, tend not to show either atrophic or reactive features.

Elastofibroma

Clinical features

Elastofibroma (Jarvi et al. 1969) has a very typical clinical picture, almost always presenting as an ill-defined subscapular mass of prolonged duration in an elderly patient, most often a female. Up to 10 per cent of cases are bilateral. Despite claims to the contrary, there is no consistent relationship with a history of heavy manual labour, although repeated trauma between the lower border of the scapula and the chest wall is probably aetiologically important. Local excision is curative and recurrence is not a feature.

Histopathology

The microscopic appearances are characteristic and consist of irregular bundles of dense collagen located within adipose tissue and associated with a very marked proliferation of elastic fibres, which have a beaded, rod-like, or globular appearance (Fig. 27.157). The lesion is generally hypocellular and has very ill-defined margins.

There has been much controversy over the nature and origin of these diagnostic elastic fibres but current evidence would suggest that they are truly composed of elastin (as opposed to

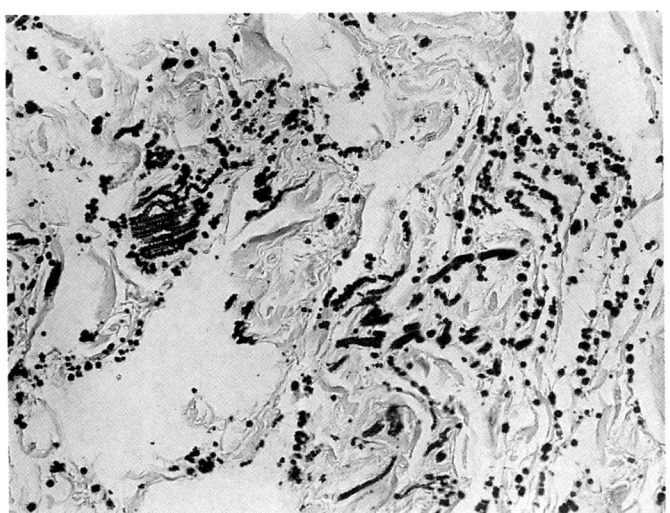

Fig. 27.157 Elastofibroma. Using a special stain for elastin (elastic van Gieson), the abnormal fibres show a typical beaded or globular appearance.

degenerate 'elastotic' collagen) and that they reflect abnormal elastogenesis with increased cross-linkages.

27.4.4 Tumours of fibrous tissue

In this section the hamartomatous, and truly neoplastic, lesions of fibrous tissue are described. It is worth noting that many of these tumours are composed largely, and sometimes entirely, of myofibroblasts, which appear (under most circumstances) to represent a relatively immature stage of fibroblastic differentiation. These cells are characterized by the presence of intracytoplasmic contractile filaments (hence the resemblance to smooth muscle cells). The proportion of such cells within a given tumour usually seems to diminish in parallel with increasing duration and decreasing cellularity; eventually, mature fibroblasts become the predominant cell type.

Fibrous hamartoma of infancy

Clinical features

Fibrous hamartoma of infancy (Enzinger 1965, Fletcher *et al.* 1988a) almost invariably presents within the first two years of life, is not infrequently congenital, and shows a marked predilection for males. It usually arises as a solitary mobile subcutaneous mass, most often in the region of the shoulder girdle (predominantly the axilla), but has been described at a wide variety of sites. Very rarely, patients may present with multiple lesions. Local recurrence is uncommon following excision but spontaneous regression seems not to occur.

Histopathology

This lesion may involve subcutaneous fat or the deep dermis and has ill-defined, infiltrative margins. There are four principal histological components: small foci of primitive, often rather stellate mesenchymal cells set in a myxoid matrix; fascicles of uniform, rather wavy spindle cells arranged in a fibrillary collagenous background; islands of mature adipose tissue; and areas showing disorderly fibrosis. The relative proportions of these components varies markedly between cases. There is no pleomorphism and mitoses are scarce. Despite the rather neural appearance of some cases, the histogenesis of these tumours remains unknown although there are features to suggest disorderly recapitulation of primitive mesenchymal differentiation.

Calcifying aponeurotic fibroma

Clinical features

Calcifying aponeurotic fibroma (Allen and Enzinger 1970) almost always presents in the first two decades of life, shows a very marked male predominance, and usually arises in the hand or foot (typically the palm or sole). Patients complain of a solitary, slowly growing, diffuse mass. Local recurrence occurs very frequently, particularly in younger patients, but radical surgery is not indicated since these tumours seem to become quiescent and cause little problem with increasing age.

Histopathology

The earliest lesions, typically seen in infants, are characterized by an infiltrative cellular mass composed of plump fibroblasts with scattered small foci of calcification. With increasing age, calcification becomes more prominent, cellularity diminishes and, not infrequently, cartilaginous metaplasia is evident in calcified areas. Multinucleate giant cells are quite often found around calcified foci.

Fibroma of tendon sheath

Clinical features

Fibroma of tendon sheath (Chung and Enzinger 1979, Pulitzer *et al.* 1989) is a common neoplasm which presents most often in middle-aged adults, predominantly males, as a solitary, well-circumscribed nodule typically attached to a tendon on a finger or hand. It may also arise in the foot or around the knee. Up to 20 per cent of cases recur locally, usually reflecting incomplete primary excision.

Histopathology

The tumour is characteristically encapsulated and lobulated. It is usually composed of dense, rather hyalinized fibrous tissue, within which are characteristic long, slit-like vascular channels lined by normal endothelium. Occasional cases have a much more cellular appearance with scattered mitoses, but distinction from other tumours, such as fibrous histiocytoma, is facilitated by the characteristic lobulation and vascular pattern.

Infantile digital fibromatosis

Clinical features

Infantile digital fibromatosis (Allen 1972) is a relatively uncommon tumour which, as the name would suggest, usually arises on the finger or toe of children of either sex, usually before the age of 3 years. Multiple nodules on the same or different digits are frequently seen and may develop simultaneously or over a period of years. Confusingly, identical cases have now been recognized both in adulthood and outside the digits. Irrespective of the clinical background, around 50 per cent of cases recur following local excision. However, once the initial diagnosis has been made, there is often no need to treat recurrences or separate new lesions since the majority will regress spontaneously with time.

Histopathology

These lesions are predominantly intradermal but may extend right down to periosteum. While superficially appearing to be composed of a rather non-specific infiltrative mass of moderately cellular fibrous tissue showing occasional mitoses, they have one absolutely characteristic feature. Variable numbers of the spindle cells contain a brightly eosinophilic, rounded intracytoplasmic inclusion, often located close to the nucleus. These inclusions are now known to represent abnormal aggregates of close-packed actin filaments, the cause of which remains unknown.

Infantile myofibromatosis

Clinical features

Infantile myofibromatosis (Chung and Enzinger 1981) is an uncommon disorder which usually presents in the first 2 years of life and is more frequent in males. Most often it arises as a solitary dermal, subcutaneous, or intramuscular nodule, but about 25 per cent of patients have multiple lesions which may affect soft tissue, bone, or visceral organs, particularly the lung and gastrointestinal tract. Up to 5 per cent of cases seem to have an inherited basis, being either autosomal recessive or autosomal dominant with incomplete penetrance. Local recurrence is uncommon and the majority of lesions in soft tissue or bone regress spontaneously. In contrast, multiple visceral lesions often lead to respiratory failure or severe intestinal symptoms and such cases often pursue a fatal course.

Histopathology

This lesion tends to have a rather zoned appearance, being composed of small, round, rather primitive cells centrally and of eosinophilic spindle cells, resembling smooth muscle cells, peripherally. In the central areas there is often a prominent branching, haemangiopericytoma-like (see Section 12.5) vascular pattern. Extensive necrosis is not uncommon and irregular calcification may be evident in the spindle-cell areas. The relative proportions of the two cell types varies considerably between cases. The presence of necrosis and mitotic activity may suggest the diagnosis of leiomyosarcoma, but this tumour is very rare in infants and typically lacks either a small cell component or an arborizing vascular pattern. Whether infantile myofibromatosis is truly derived from myofibroblasts or is, in fact, a primitive smooth muscle tumour remains undecided.

Juvenile hyaline fibromatosis

Clinical features

Juvenile hyaline fibromatosis (Remberger et al. 1985) is a very rare condition characterized by the development of multiple, often disfiguring, dermal and subcutaneous masses, predominantly in male children under the age of 5 years. The head and neck region is particularly affected. There may be associated flexural contractures, gingival hyperplasia, and similar masses within bone. A proportion of cases appear to be autosomal recessive in origin and the underlying abnormality seems likely to be a defect in collagen synthesis. While individual lesions tend not to recur, new masses may continue to develop into early adult life.

Histopathology

Most lesions are composed of relatively hypocellular masses of eosinophilic hyaline material, within which spindle cells and blood vessels are distributed in artefactual cleft-like spaces. While the hyaline matrix resembles dense collagen, it lacks the typical staining characteristics of the latter and contains very little connective tissue mucin.

Fibromatosis colli

Clinical features

Fibromatosis colli, often referred to as a sternomastoid tumour, is not uncommon and is typified by the development of a firm mass in the sternocleidomastoid muscle of a neonate. Males are affected more frequently than females and, despite popular suggestions to the contrary, there is no evidence that these lesions are related to birth trauma or intrauterine position. While most cases regress spontaneously, up to 10 per cent go on to develop torticollis (wry neck deformity).

Histopathology

The only feature that distinguishes this tumour from a typical desmoid fibromatosis (see below) is the fact that the proliferating fibroblasts are diffusely and extensively distributed between individual muscle fibres, the latter often showing marked atrophy or reactive changes. The cellularity of the lesion is directly proportional to its duration.

Palmar fibromatosis (Dupuytren's contracture)

Clinical features

Palmar fibromatosis is a very common condition, characterized in its early stages by the development of nodules in the palmar fascia and later by the appearance of dense fibrous bands, leading to the typical flexion deformity at the metacarpophalangeal joints known as Dupuytren's contracture. The ring finger is most often affected, and up to 25 per cent of cases are bilateral. Patients, who are usually in their fifth or sixth decade, show a marked male predominance, a probable genetic predisposition, and an increased incidence of alcohol abuse, epilepsy, and diabetes mellitus. They may also develop plantar fibromatosis, knuckle pads, and Peyronie's disease. Treatment is rendered very difficult by the fact that local recurrence is almost inevitable unless total palmar fasciectomy is performed.

Histopathology

The nodular stage of palmar fibromatosis is typified by a markedly cellular proliferation of plump spindle cells, showing normal mitotic figures and frequent nucleoli. There is no pleomorphism and minimal collagen deposition. In the later stages, once a contracture has been established, the lesions are far less cellular and are composed mainly of slender mature fibroblasts set in a dense collagenous matrix which is often rather hyalinized.

Plantar fibromatosis

Plantar fibromatosis (also known as Ledderhose disease) is less common than its palmar equivalent and differs clinically from the latter by the absence of any contraction deformity and by the fact that it not infrequently presents in young adults or adolescents. It shows the same tendencies to bilaterality and local recurrence and is histologically almost identical to palmar fibromatosis, but for the occasional presence of haemosiderin or chronic inflammatory cells, which probably reflect the secondary effects of local trauma.

Peyronie's disease

Clinical features

Peyronie's disease (penile fibromatosis) is a relatively uncommon condition which presents in the fourth to sixth decades with abnormal curvature and pain on erection. Palpable nodules or a fibrous cord are usually evident in the dorsal aspect of the penile shaft. The aetiology is unknown, although a primary vasculitic process has been proposed. A small proportion of cases regress spontaneously but, in all other cases, there is no reliable treatment.

Histopathology

Early lesions are said to be typified by chronic inflammation in and around the corpus cavernosum. However, by the time of presentation, most examples show only dense, variably cellular fibrous tissue, quite often with marked hyalinization.

Desmoid fibromatoses

The group of lesions that fall under this heading are characterized by a deep, typically intramuscular location, an infiltrative growth pattern, and a marked tendency to local recurrence. They often attain a considerable size, averaging 10–15 cm in diameter. These are therefore locally aggressive tumours, which may be hard to eradicate and often necessitate radical surgery. They do not metastasize and are only occasionally fatal due to locally destructive effects.

Clinical features

Extra-abdominal desmoid fibromatosis This tumour arises most often around the shoulder girdle, the trunk, or in the lower limb and has a peak incidence in the third and fourth decades. There is a slight female predominance. Patients complain of a deeply seated, poorly defined mass of variable duration. The aetiology is uncertain, although some cases may arise in a surgical scar and others appear to have a genetic predisposition, particularly those associated with familial polyposis coli (Gardner syndrome).

Desmoid fibromatosis of the anterior abdominal wall This is perhaps the best-known type of 'desmoid tumour', although it is rather less common than the extra-abdominal variant. It arises most frequently in the rectus abdominis muscle of young adults and shows a marked predilection for females, most of whom have borne children (often in the recent past). It may also arise in an abdominal scar or may be a feature of Gardner syndrome. Aetiologically there is some evidence to suggest that 'trauma' to the abdominal wall during pregnancy, combined with the promoting effects of oestrogens, may be important.

Intra-abdominal desmoid fibromatosis This relatively uncommon variant, which usually arises in the mesentery but may also develop in the retroperitoneum, affects mainly young adults and is associated with Gardner syndrome in the majority of cases. Intra-abdominal desmoid tumours seem often to be particularly aggressive but this may reflect their usually greater size and the fact that adequate excision often necessitates resection of a considerable length of bowel.

Infantile desmoid fibromatosis This is the least common member of the group of desmoid fibromatoses. It usually presents in the first five years of life as a mass in the head and neck region or around the shoulder girdle. There is a male predominance, as is the case with most fibroblastic tumours of childhood. The aetiology is unknown. The anatomical site, combined with the age of the patient, often render complete excision impossible, therefore local recurrence is particularly common and may be very destructive.

Histopathology

Desmoid fibromatoses arising in adulthood are histologically similar irrespective of site, and are composed of irregularly interlacing bundles of uniform, slender spindle cells set in a prominent collagenous stroma (Fig. 27.158). The cellularity is variable and is inversely proportional to the amount of collagen laid down. The spindle cells have palely eosinophilic cytoplasm and typically have euchromatic thin, tapered nuclei, although more cellular foci may show plump, rounded nuclei with prominent nucleoli. Scattered normal mitoses are a common finding, but there is no pleomorphism or significant hyperchromasia. The tumour infiltrates surrounding skeletal muscle and, at the advancing edge, bizarre, reactive muscle cells and a lymphocytic infiltrate are frequently present. Mesenteric examples often have a rather more myxoid stroma in which blood vessels may be prominent. While infantile cases may closely resemble the adult form, they are often characterized by a more cellular, primitive appearance with a very myxoid, rather fibrillary stroma (largely lacking in collagen) and are often associated with fatty replacement of adjacent muscle.

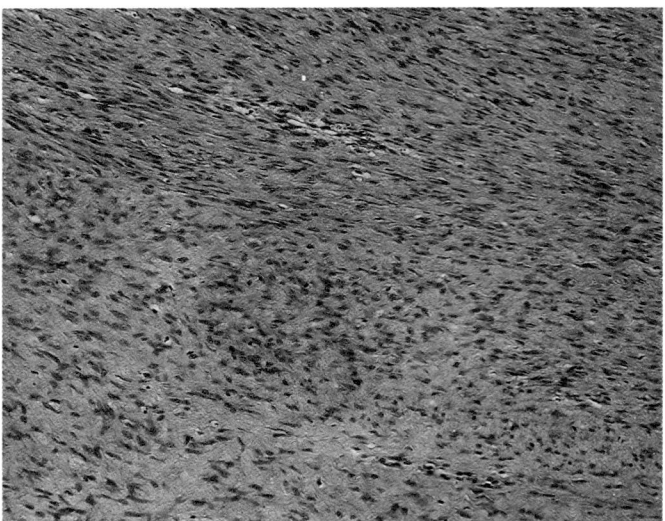

Fig. 27.158 Desmoid fibromatosis. Note the dense collagenous background and uniformity of the spindle cells.

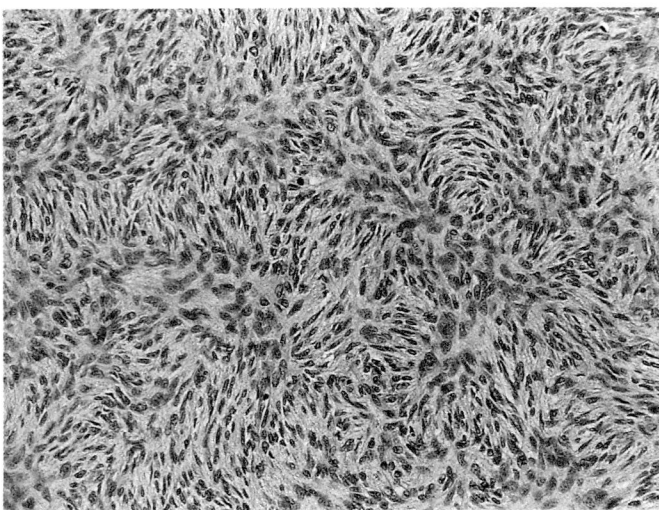

Fig. 27.159 Dermatofibrosarcoma protuberans. Uniform spindle cells arranged in a typical storiform or cartwheel pattern.

Dermatofibrosarcoma protuberans

Clinical features

Dermatofibrosarcoma protuberans (Fletcher *et al*. 1985) presents most often between the ages of 20 and 50 as a slowly growing, multinodular or plaque-like intradermal mass, usually located on the trunk or lower limb. There is a slight predilection for males. The aetiology is generally unknown. Between 30 and 50 per cent of cases recur locally unless widely excised at the outset, but metastasis is exceedingly rare (amounting to less than 0.3 per cent of reported cases). This fact has led some authors to classify this entity as a soft-tissue tumour of borderline malignancy.

Histopathology

Dermatofibrosarcoma has a characteristic, reproducible histological appearance in the majority of cases, being composed of uniform, palely eosinophilic spindle cells with elongated nuclei, arranged in a storiform (Latin *storia*, a rush mat) or whorled pattern (Fig. 27.159). Moderate mitotic activity is usually evident but there is little, if any, pleomorphism, and giant cells are rare. The tumour cells are arranged in a variable collagenous matrix, which may be very sparse or may show marked hyalinization. Small foci of necrosis or haemorrhage are only occasionally present. A typical feature is the infiltrative nature of the lesion, which often extends widely into subcutaneous fat and may involve skeletal muscle at certain anatomical sites. Occasional cases, particularly recurrences, may show a fascicular appearance reminiscent of fibrosarcoma (see below). The nature of the spindle cells in these tumours is disputed, but most evidence would favour fibroblastic or perineural fibroblastic origin. The previous designation as a fibrohistocytic tumour is no longer tenable.

Variants

Pigmented dermatofibrosarcoma protuberans This is also known as a Bednar tumour (Fletcher *et al*. 1988b). Approximately 2 per cent of histologically otherwise typical cases show a variable number of dendritic or delicate spindle-shaped cells which contain copious melanin pigment. These lesions seem to be more common in coloured patients but are otherwise clinicopathologically indistinguishable from the conventional variant.

Myxoid dermatofibrosarcoma protuberans While focal myxoid degeneration is a relatively frequent occurrence, rare cases have a very prominent myxoid stroma, which may largely obscure the storiform pattern. Such examples have to be distinguished from myxoid liposarcoma by the identification of more typical foci (using careful sampling) and by the absence of lipoblasts.

Fibrosarcoma

While fibrosarcoma was formerly regarded as one of the commonest types of soft-tissue sarcoma, modern methods of classification have transferred many such cases to the categories of either malignant fibrous histiocytoma, monophasic synovial sarcoma, or malignant peripheral nerve sheath tumour, leaving less than 5 per cent of soft-tissue malignancies with this designation.

Clinical features

Fibrosarcoma falls into two distinct groups—those arising in adults and those arising in children, of which the former are more common.

Adult fibrosarcoma Adult fibrosarcoma (Scott *et al*. 1989) presents most often as a deeply located, painless mass in the lower limb (particularly the thigh) or trunk in middle-aged adults of either sex. Occasional cases are associated with previous irradiation; a chronic sinus or ulcer; or arise in a scar, often due to burns. Following excision, local recurrence occurs in about 50 per cent of cases and the overall five-year survival is approximately 40 per cent.

Infantile fibrosarcoma (Chung and Enzinger 1976) typically arises within the first two years of life and, in fact, is often congenital. It shows a predilection for males and may develop either within muscle or deep subcutis, typically in the distal area of a limb. Importantly, in contrast to adult cases, only about 20 per cent recur locally and only between 10 and 15 per cent metastasize and pursue a fatal course. No clear reason has been identified for this striking difference in behaviour.

Histopathology

Adult fibrosarcoma is typified by angulated fascicles of spindle cells arranged in a so-called herring-bone pattern (Fig. 27.160). These cells have hyperchromatic, elongated, tapered nuclei with a straight contour and show prominent, often abnormal mitotic activity (Fig. 27.161). The amount of stromal collagen is much less than that in a desmoid fibromatosis, but increasing amounts correlate with greater differentiation and a better prognosis. In contrast to malignant fibrous histiocytoma, marked nuclear pleomorphism and multinucleate giant cells are not features of fibrosarcoma.

Infantile fibrosarcoma This tends to show a less orderly fascicular pattern than its adult counterpart, and is usually composed of rather smaller, more primitive spindle cells. These cells are, however, very uniform in appearance and collagen deposition is relatively sparse in most cases. Mitoses are frequent and an irregularly branching vascular pattern, resembling an haemangiopericytoma, is often seen.

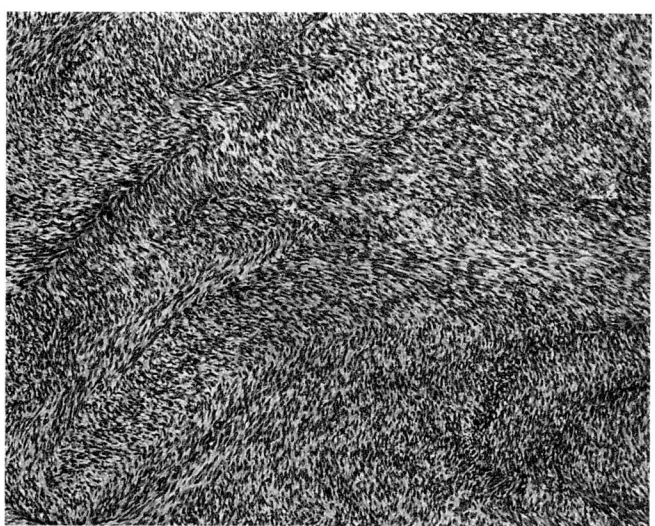

Fig. 27.160 Fibrosarcoma. Note the typical herring-bone pattern of the fascicles.

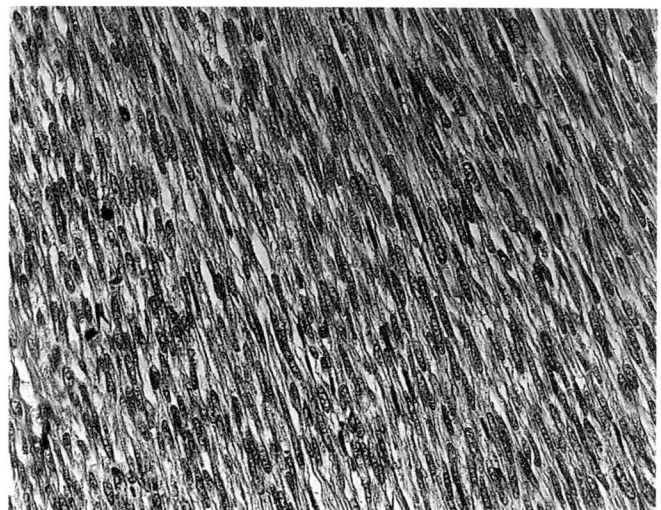

Fig. 27.161 Fibrosarcoma. The nuclei are elongated with tapering ends, are very monomorphic, and show marked mitotic activity.

27.4.5 Tumours showing fibrohistiocytic differentiation

The concept of a fibrohistiocytic group of soft-tissue tumours has been a source of controversy ever since its inception almost 30 years ago and, to this day, remains a very mixed and poorly understood diagnostic 'rag-bag', particularly with regard to malignant fibrous histiocytoma. Perhaps the most important fact to come to light in recent years is that these tumours *are not* derived from histiocytes, nor do they bear any direct relationship to cells of monocyte/macrophage lineage. Rather, they appear to arise from either a fibroblast or primitive mesenchymal stem cell, which then manifests the ability to express histiocytic features to a varying degree (Fletcher 1987). Since, however, the precise histogenesis and the extent to which these tumours are truly interrelated remains uncertain, they are still classified as fibrohistiocytic by their apparent patterns of differentiation. This category is likely to be the subject of refinement and change in the coming decades and has already lost one of its founder members, dermatofibrosarcoma protuberans (see above).

Benign fibrous histiocytoma

Clinical features

The majority of benign fibrous histiocytomas are located in the skin and these represent one of the commonest soft-tissue tumours. They present most often in young or middle-aged adults of either sex as a raised cutaneous nodule, usually situated on a limb although almost any site may be affected. Most are white or red in colour, but some may show brownish pigmentation, resembling a malignant melanoma, due to the deposition of haemosiderin. Approximately 20 per cent of patients have multiple lesions. Occasional cases recur locally if incompletely excised but malignant transformation does not occur.

A small proportion of cases present as a larger, encapsulated subcutaneous, intramuscular, or intra-abdominal mass (Fletcher 1990). The age and sex distribution is similar to that of the cutaneous lesions. Local recurrence is rather more common.

Histopathology

The light-microscopic appearance of these lesions is variable, hence the wide range of names used in the past. Nearly all, however, are typified by a poorly circumscribed, purely intradermal mass. The commonest form comprises an admixture of uniform spindle cells, arranged in a vaguely whorled or curlicue pattern, scattered foamy macrophages and variable numbers of chronic inflammatory cells (Fig. 27.162). Small numbers of multinucleate giant cells may be present and mitoses are scarce. Some cases are composed almost solely of spindle cells set in a hyalinized collagenous stroma (syn. 'dermatofibroma'). Others contain numerous small blood vessels (often with hyalinized walls), associated with extravasation of red cells and marked haemosiderin deposition (syn. 'sclerosing haemangioma'). Least commonly, there is predominance of the foamy, lipid-laden macrophages (syn. 'histiocytoma cutis'). Distinction from dermatofibrosarcoma is afforded by the latter's greater mitotic activity, more conspicuous storiform pattern, deeper infiltration, and relative paucity of foamy histiocytes or giant cells. Atypical fibroxanthoma is readily distinguished by its far greater pleomorphism (see below). Interestingly, the epidermis overlying cutaneous fibrous histiocytomas may show a wide variety of reactive changes, the commonest of which are acanthosis or pseudoepitheliomatous hyperplasia. Basal cell carcinomas may also sometimes be seen.

Deeply located examples are histologically similar to their cutaneous counterparts, but for the facts that foamy histiocytes and giant cells are generally sparse and that there is often, at least focally, an obvious haemangiopericytoma-like vascular pattern. Large areas closely resembling dermatofibrosarcoma are common.

Giant cell tumour of tendon sheath

Clinical features

Giant cell tumour of tendon sheath may be either localized or diffuse, of which the former is much more common (Myers *et al.* 1980). The localized type presents usually as a circumscribed mass on either the extensor or flexor aspect of a digit (most often a finger) in young or middle-aged adults. Females are affected more frequently than males. The lesion is typically slowly growing and, on examination, is fixed to deep articular structures, characteristically a tendon. The aetiology is unknown. Approximately 10 per cent of cases recur locally, usually as a result of inadequate primary excision.

The diffuse type (sometimes referred to as pigmented villonodular tenosynovitis) tends to arise around the knee or ankle joint in a similar age-group but with an equal sex incidence. The tumour is usually larger than the localized form, is often painful, and is frequently associated with an intra-articular component. Radiologically there may be cortical erosion or even invasion of adjacent bone. Up to 50 per cent recur locally but truly malignant behaviour with metastatic spread is exceedingly rare.

Histopathology

Localized giant cell tumours are characterized by an encapsulated, often lobulated mass, composed of plump eosinophilic, histiocyte-like cells, bland spindle cells, foamy macrophages, chronic inflammatory cells, and varying numbers of osteoclast-like multinucleate giant cells (Fig. 27.163). The cells are set in a

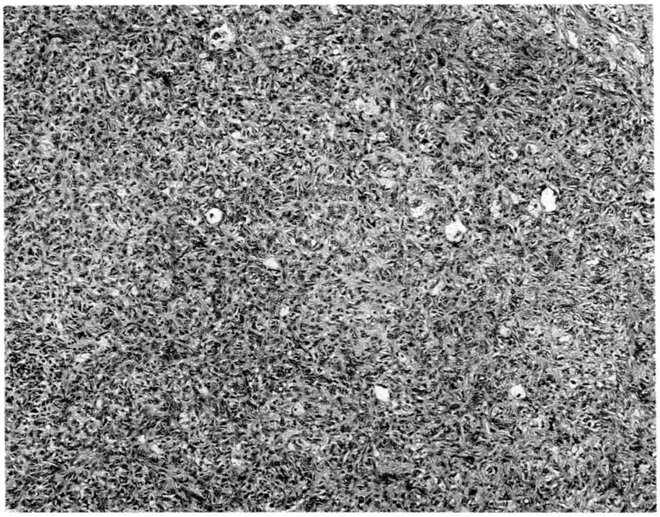

Fig. 27.162 Benign fibrous histiocytoma. Spindle cells, lymphocytes, and histiocytes in a whorled arrangement, along with scattered foamy macrophages.

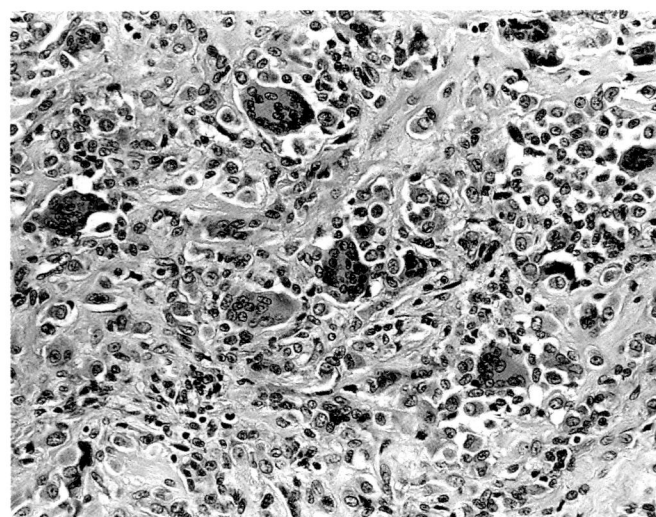

Fig. 27.163 Giant cell tumour of tendon sheath. The tumour consists mainly of histiocytes and osteoclast-like giant cells in a collagenous matrix containing lymphocytes.

variably dense collagenous stroma in which haemosiderin deposition is usually prominent. Mitotic figures of normal configuration are quite frequent. The diffuse type is histologically very similar, although less clearly encapsulated, and is often covered by synovium. Cleft-like spaces lined by polygonal or spindle-shaped cells are a common feature, but are readily distinguished from the glandular spaces of synovial sarcoma by the lack of an epithelial lining. Multinucleate giant cells are often less prominent in the diffuse type than the localized form.

Although both types of giant cell tumour show morphological evidence of fibrohistiocytic differentiation, there is much evidence to suggest that they are actually derived from synovium, of which type A cells have histiocytic features even under normal circumstances.

This lesion is also referred to in the section on Joint Disorders (Section 27.2).

Juvenile xanthogranuloma

Clinical features

Juvenile xanthogranuloma (Sonoda *et al.* 1985) is a relatively uncommon lesion which presents most often by the age of 5 years as one, or more, yellow, cutaneous papules or nodules, which are typically located in the head and neck region or trunk of either sex. Infants with multiple lesions occasionally also have visceral nodules, particularly in the iris but occasionally in the lungs or pericardium. Despite the name, up to 20 per cent of cases arise in adolescents or young adults, in which circumstance they are usually cutaneous and solitary. Very rarely, lesions may develop in deep soft tissue (including skeletal muscle) in either age-group. At whatever site, most examples tend to regress spontaneously and aggressive behaviour is never a feature. These features would suggest that this may, in fact, be a reactive, rather than neoplastic entity, although the cause is entirely unknown. There is certainly no convincing evidence of an underlying metabolic defect.

Histopathology

The microscopic appearances appear to be related to the duration of a given lesion. Early examples are typified by an ill-defined, intradermal mass of monomorphic, eosinophilic histiocytes associated with a mild, mixed inflammatory infiltrate. More typical cases of rather longer standing show, in addition, collections of lipid-laden macrophages (xanthoma cells) and variable numbers of multinucleate giant cells, usually of the Touton type (Fig. 27.164). Regression is characterized by the development of progressive stromal fibrosis. At all stages the epidermis and epidermal appendages remain uninvolved, an important distinguishing feature from histiocytosis X (see Section 27.1.6).

Reticulohistiocytoma

Clinical features

Reticulohistiocytoma is a rare lesion which may take two forms. In the more common, purely cutaneous variant (Purvis and Helwig 1954), the lesion usually presents as a solitary nodule in

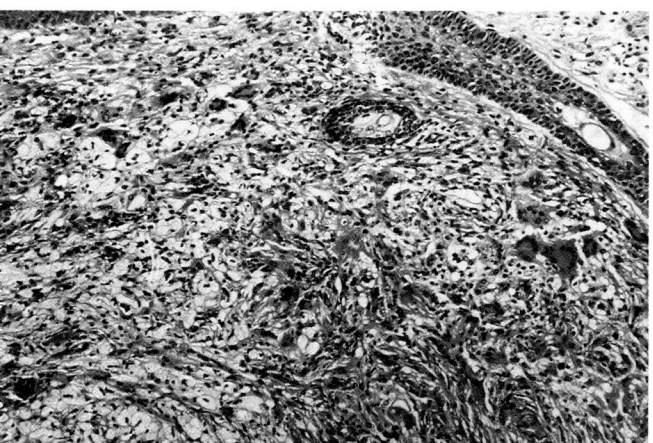

Fig. 27.164 Juvenile xanthogranuloma. Typical, ill-defined mass of foamy histiocytes, Touton giant cells, and inflammatory cells within the dermis.

the head and neck region or trunk of an adult. Multiple lesions are rare. The biological behaviour varies from spontaneous regression through to local recurrence in occasional cases. In the classical systemic form, known as multicentric reticulohistiocytosis (Barrow and Holubar 1969), identical lesions develop in large numbers in the skin, subcutaneous tissue, mucosal surfaces, and joints (particularly interphalangeal). Patients are typically middle-aged, predominantly female, and often present with weight loss, malaise, and pyrexia. Joint involvement is of particular importance since it often leads to a rapidly progressive, destructive arthropathy. In these patients, the cutaneous and muscosal nodules eventually regress spontaneously but the residual joint deformities are irreversible. Both variants are regarded as reactive conditions of uncertain aetiology.

Histopathology

Both forms of the disease have similar histological appearances at whatever site. They are characterized by a well-circumscribed collection of eosinophilic histiocytes, associated with scattered chronic inflammatory cells and large numbers of diagnostic multinucleate giant cells with peripherally located nuclei and ground-glass, eosinophilic cytoplasm. In the absence of a typical clinical history, distinction from juvenile xanthogranuloma may be achieved in difficult cases by the demonstration of both mucopolysaccharide and lipid in the cells of reticulohistiocytoma, as opposed to just lipid in xanthogranuloma.

Plexiform fibrohistiocytic tumour

Clinical features

Plexiform fibrohistiocytic tumour (Enzinger and Zhang 1988) is a recently described, uncommon neoplasm which arises most often in the distal extremities (particularly the forearm) and usually presents as a subcutaneous nodule or plaque in children or adolescents, predominantly in females. Owing to its infiltrative growth pattern, around one-third of cases recur locally and very occasional, non-fatal, lymph node metastases have been described.

Histopathology

This tumour is typically poorly defined and tends to affect the subcutis and deep dermis. It consists of a variable admixture of ramifying fibroblastic fascicles and discrete, small nodules, composed of plump, histiocyte-like cells and scattered osteoclast-like giant cells. Extravasation of red blood cells and haemosiderin deposition are sometimes prominent. There is no significant pleomorphism and mitoses are sparse.

Atypical fibroxanthoma

Clinical features

Atypical fibroxanthoma (Fretzin and Helwig 1973) arises most often on the sun-exposed areas of the head and neck region in elderly patients, predominantly males. Up to 10 per cent, however, are said to present on the limbs or trunk of young or middle-aged adults. Occasionally there is a history of previous irradiation to the affected site. The lesion usually presents as a cutaneous nodule, up to 3 cm in diameter, which is frequently ulcerated and has only been noticed for a few weeks or months. Less than 10 per cent of cases recur locally and, if strict diagnostic criteria are adopted (see below), metastasis is exceedingly rare—there being fewer than ten acceptable cases in the world literature.

Histopathology

These lesions are well circumscribed and should be almost entirely confined to the dermis. Microscopically they are very similar to pleomorphic malignant fibrous histiocytoma, being composed of hyperchromatic spindle cells, bizarre multinucleate giant cells, and occasional foamy histiocytes. Mitoses are very frequent and often abnormal. While focal haemorrhage is occasionally seen, the presence of marked necrosis, vascular or perineural invasion, or infiltration of deeper tissues generally warrants the more sinister diagnosis of malignant fibrous histiocytoma with all that this implies. Signs of actinic damage in the adjacent skin are common but, importantly, there is no evidence of either an epidermal origin or junctional activity, allowing distinction from spindle-cell variants of squamous cell carcinoma or malignant melanoma. In ulcerated or otherwise difficult cases, this differential diagnosis may also be achieved by the use of immunohistochemistry, the former showing epithelial markers (such as keratin) and the latter expressing neuroectodermal markers (such as S-100 protein).

Malignant fibrous histiocytoma

No single soft-tissue tumour has caused more dissent or confusion in terms of diagnostic criteria or classification than has malignant fibrous histiocytoma (MFH) in recent years. These problems stem largely from the facts that the histogenesis is uncertain; that the name MFH is often inappropriately used for any unclassifiable pleomorphic sarcoma; and that almost any identifiable type of sarcoma may 'dedifferentiate' either within foci of the primary neoplasm or in recurrences to produce a picture indistinguishable from MFH. It must, however, be remembered that the pattern known as MFH is one of the commonest soft tissue sarcomas of adulthood and, with careful application of this diagnosis, may be subclassified into five clinically and prognostically relevant histological types: pleomorphic/storiform (60–70 per cent of cases); myxoid (10–20 per cent); giant cell (5–15 per cent); inflammatory (5–10 per cent); and angiomatoid (1–3 per cent) (Weiss 1982).

Clinical features

Pleomorphic MFH (Weiss and Enzinger 1979) is the commonest variant, and classically presents in the sixth or seventh decades as an enlarging, painless mass, which is most often deeply located in a limb (particularly the thigh). The retroperitoneum is much less often affected and, at all sites, males predominate slightly over females. In the majority of cases the aetiology is unknown, although a small proportion appear to be radiation-induced. Local recurrence and/or metastasis occurs in up to 60 per cent of patients and the overall five-year survival is about 50 per cent.

Myxoid MFH (Weiss and Enzinger 1977) has a similar age distribution but is much more commonly located in subcutaneous tissue and is virtually confined to the limbs. Clinically it often has a discontinuous, multinodular configuration. About 40 per cent recur locally, but less than 25 per cent are associated with metastasis and a fatal outcome.

Giant-cell MFH (Guccion and Enzinger 1972) also presents in middle to late adult life, most often as a deep-seated mass in a limb, particularly the leg. However, up to a third of cases arise in subcutaneous tissue. This is of prognostic significance since, although 30 per cent recur at any site, only about 20 per cent of superficial tumours metastasize, in contrast to 75 per cent of deep lesions.

Inflammatory MFH (Kyriakos and Kempson 1976) presents in middle to late adulthood and shows a striking predilection for the retroperitoneum, followed in frequency by the limbs. Patients not infrequently have systemic symptoms such as pyrexia. Owing to the preferential site of origin, local recurrence is much more common than metastasis but overall five-year survival is only about 30 per cent.

Angiomatoid MFH (Enzinger 1979) is clinically very different from the other variants, being commonest in children and adolescents and usually presenting as a slowly growing, subcutaneous mass in a limb, most often the arm. Although up to 50 per cent recur locally, metastatic spread is extremely rare (Costa and Weiss 1990).

Histopathology

Pleomorphic MFH This is typified by a large, infiltrative mass, often showing areas of haemorrhage and necrosis. Cytologically it is composed of irregularly arranged, rather eosinophilic

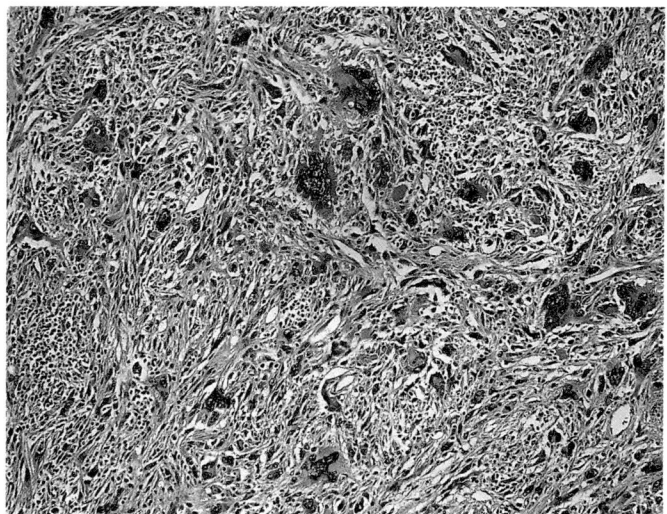

Fig. 27.165 Malignant fibrous histiocytoma. Note the very striking pleomorphism and vague storiform pattern.

spindle cells with hyperchromatic nuclei, bizarre giant cells, foamy histiocytes, and a variable number of chronic inflammatory cells (Fig. 27.165). A focal storiform pattern is often evident and there is usually prominent, abnormal mitotic activity. The amount of collagenous stroma is inversely proportional to the cellularity. Vascular or perineural invasion are frequently identified.

Exclusion of any other type of pleomorphic sarcoma requires a careful search for lipoblasts or rhabdomyoblasts and the use of both immunohistochemistry and electron microscopy. The latter should also be useful in distinguishing a metastatic pleomorphic carcinoma, for example, from the kidney or lung. Although currently a very controversial topic, there is increasing evidence (Fletcher 1991a) that pleomorphic MFH may, in fact, represent the shared morphology of a wide range of heterogeneous neoplasms, the true nature of which can often only be identified by ancillary diagnostic techniques. It is therefore possible that, in the coming years, this tumour may cease to exist as a discrete entity.

Myxoid MFH This usually shows foci very similar to pleomorphic MFH, but for the most part shows a very pronounced myxoid matrix composed of hyaluronic acid. As a result the tumour cells are widely dispersed but still tend to show similar pleomorphism to that described above. A proportion of cases are cytologically much more bland, consisting almost solely of more widely dispersed spindle- or stellate-shaped cells: such tumours are sometimes referred to as myxofibrosarcomas. Distinction from myxoid liposarcoma is achieved by the absence of lipoblasts or a characteristic plexiform vascular pattern, and by the presence of even minimal pleomorphism.

Giant-cell MFH This is also histologically very similar to pleomorphic MFH but for the presence of numerous osteoclast-like multinucleate giant cells and a frequently multinodular growth

pattern. These lesions, therefore often resemble the better-known osteoclastoma (see Section 27.1.6). Foci of metaplastic benign-looking osteoid or bone are often present, typically towards the periphery of the tumour. Not infrequently, however, the cytology of the associated stromal cells warrants a diagnosis of extraskeletal osteosarcoma.

Inflammatory MFH This is usually microscopically very different from the preceding variants, although typically pleomorphic foci may be present. Most often the bulk of the lesion is composed of sheets of relatively uniform, foamy histiocytes (similar to those seen in xanthogranulomatous inflammation). Admixed with these histiocytes are large numbers of inflammatory cells (classically polymorphs), which are unassociated with necrosis. Cytological features of malignancy may be hard to find, unless the tumour is thoroughly sampled.

Angiomatoid MFH This is histologically very dissimilar, being typified by a well-circumscribed mass, composed of sheets or nodules of rather bland eosinophilic histiocytes, which are often arranged around large, blood-filled cystic spaces. A dense lymphocytic infiltrate is also a characteristic feature, notably towards the periphery of the lesion, producing a superficial resemblance to a lymph node. It is highly likely that this tumour will be removed from the fibrohistiocytic category in the future, and there is some evidence to suggest myogenic differentiation (Fletcher 1991b).

27.4.6 Tumours of smooth muscle

Pilar leiomyoma

Clinical features

Pilar leiomyoma is a relatively uncommon cutaneous neoplasm, which most often presents as multiple, discrete papular or nodular lesions in the skin of the limbs or trunk of young adults. These are small, slowly growing, and are often tender or painful, particularly if compressed or exposed to cold. Solitary examples are much less frequent. Up to 15 per cent of cases appear to have an autosomal dominant inheritance and all examples are thought to be derived from arrector pili muscles. Local recurrence is quite common, although it is sometimes unclear wheather this represents the development of a separate new lesion. Malignant transformation does not occur.

Histopathology

These lesions are characterized by an infiltrative, poorly circumscribed intradermal mass, composed of interlacing fascicles of spindle-shaped, bland, smooth muscle cells. The latter are typified by brightly eosinophilic cytoplasm and blunt-ended or cigar-shaped nuclei. Histochemically useful features by which to demonstrate smooth muscle cells are the presence of intracytoplasmic glycogen (if suitably fixed) and longitudinal striations on a trichrome or phosphotungstic acid haematoxylin stain. Pilar leiomyomas show no pleomorphism and no mitoses.

Genital leiomyoma

Clinical features

Genital leiomyomas (Newman and Fletcher 1991a) are rare lesions that arise from the superficial muscle of the scrotum, vulva, or nipple. They are typically solitary and tend to affect middle-aged adults. They are painless and only very rarely recur after excision.

Histopathology

Other than their generally slightly larger size, these tumours are histologically similar to pilar leiomyoma.

Angioleiomyoma

Clinical features

Angioleiomyoma is a common subcutaneous or deep dermal tumour, which arises from vascular smooth muscle (most probably a vein). It is typically solitary, mainly affects middle-aged adults, with a marked predominance of females, and almost always develops in a limb, most especially the leg. Approximately 50 per cent are painful when compressed. Local recurrence is very rare and malignant transformation has never been reported.

Histopathology

In contrast to pilar leiomyoma, angioleiomyoma is characteristically well circumscribed and encapsulated. It is composed of bundles of mature smooth muscle cells (as described above), orientated around variable numbers of generally thick-walled blood vessels with narrow lumina (Fig. 27.166). Hyalinization or myxoid degeneration are common findings and, occasionally, the vascular component may show marked dilatation. The smooth muscle cells show no mitoses and pleomorphism is absent.

Leiomyoma of deep soft tissue

Clinical features

This is an uncommon and poorly documented tumour, which seems to present most often in young or middle-aged adults as a slowly growing, often quite large mass, either within limb musculature, mesentery, or retroperitoneum. In our experience, local recurrence is very uncommon.

Histopathology

Deep leiomyomas are well circumscribed and encapsulated and are very similar in appearance to angioleiomyomas but for the relative dearth of vascular channels. These lesions frequently seem to show marked degenerative changes in the form of hyalinization, myxoid change, cyst formation, or calcification. The smooth muscle cells, however, are uniform in appearance and mitoses are only very rarely identified. If mitotic activity amounts to as much as one per 10 high-power fields in number, then the lesion is best regarded as a leiomyosarcoma.

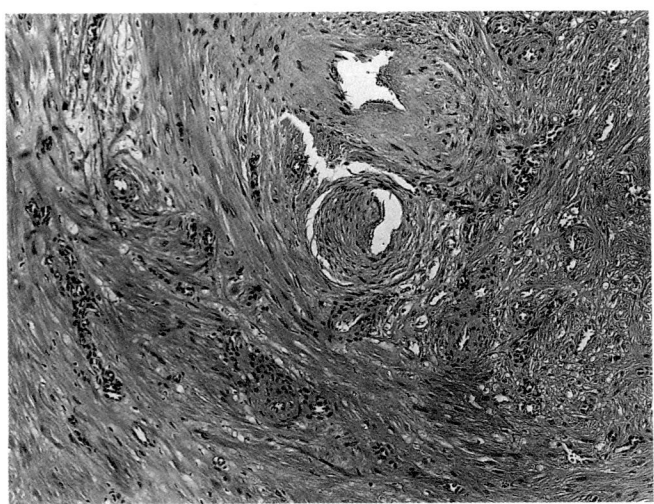

Fig. 27.166 Angioleiomyoma. Fascicles of mature smooth muscle cells arranged around thick-walled blood vessels.

Epithelioid smooth muscle tumours

These lesions, which are well recognized in the stomach or uterus, are extremely rare in soft tissue but may occasionally be seen in the mesentery. Readers are referred to the Alimentary or Female Reproductive sections for a histological description. Most such tumours arising in soft tissue appear to pursue a malignant course.

Leiomyosarcoma

Clinical features

Leiomyosarcoma arising in non-visceral soft tissue may be divided into four principal types: cutaneous; subcutaneous or intramuscular; vascular; and intra-abdominal (Fields and Helwig 1981, Berlin *et al.* 1984, Hashimoto *et al.* 1985).

Cutaneous leiomyosarcoma This arises typically in the limbs (particularly the leg) of middle-aged adults, with a slight predominance of males. It is thought to originate usually from pilar smooth muscle. The tumour is frequently fairly small (averaging less than 3 cm in diameter) and is often painful. While about 50 per cent of cases recur locally, usually as a result of inadequate excision, metastatic spread is very uncommon and fatalities are rare.

Subcutaneous and intramuscular leiomyosarcomas These have a very similar age, sex, and anatomical distribution to their cutaneous counterparts, but tend to be larger at presentation. They are thought to be derived from the muscle coat of small, unapparent blood vessels. Most importantly, although the recurrence rate is similar, up to 40 per cent metastasize and have a fatal outcome.

Vascular leiomyosarcoma This is relatively uncommon and is characterized by both intramural and luminal involvement of a large blood vessel, almost always a vein, in addition to the usually more obvious soft-tissue component. These tumours arise most often from the inferior vena cava, femoral, or saphenous veins. The vast majority occur in females between the ages of 40 and 60. The prognosis is generally very poor, most patients dying either with the Budd–Chiari syndrome or early and widespread blood-borne metastases.

Intra-abdominal leiomyosarcomas These are probably the single commonest group and mainly arise in either the retroperitoneum or mesentery in late adult life and show a moderate predilection for females. Irrespective of size or histological appearance, such tumours are generally very hard to remove adequately (particularly if retroperitoneal), and up to 80 per cent of patients succumb to recurrent or metastatic disease within five years.

Histopathology

Leiomyosarcoma has a similar histological appearance at whatever site; therefore, all the above clinical subgroups are described as one. The tumour is composed of interlacing fascicles of eosinophilic spindle cells with plump, blunt-ended nuclei (Fig. 27.167). The latter are much more hyperchromatic and pleomorphic than those seen in benign smooth muscle tumours, and mitoses, which are often abnormal, tend to be prominent (Fig. 27.168). It is worth noting, however, that, in contrast to gastrointestinal or uterine smooth muscle tumours, *any* mitotic activity in a smooth muscle tumour of soft tissue should be viewed with concern, and if one or more mitoses are identified per 10 high-power fields then the lesion is best regarded (and treated) as a leiomyosarcoma.

Stromal hyalinization or myxoid degeneration are quite common, as is the presence of nuclear palisading, which may simulate a neural neoplasm. A focal storiform pattern may also be evident and a small number of cases may show very marked

cytological pleomorphism, hence resembling malignant fibrous histiocytoma. Distinction from other types of sarcoma, particularly of the predominantly spindle-cell type, is facilitated by the characteristic nuclear morphology, the identification of intracytoplasmic glycogen and longitudinal striations, and, in about 60–70 per cent of cases, by the immunohistochemical demonstration of the intermediate filament, desmin.

27.4.7 Tumours of striated muscle

Rhabdomyoma

Clinical features

Rhabdomyomas are rare benign tumours of striated muscle which may be divided into three types: adult, fetal, and genital.

Adult rhabdomyomas These generally arise in the head and neck region of middle-aged or elderly males. They often arise beneath a mucosal surface and are sometimes multicentric. Up to 10 per cent recur locally.

Fetal rhabdomyomas These are the least common of the three types; they tend to arise in the head and neck region of young male infants, particularly in the retroauricular region. Local recurrence is not a feature.

Genital rhabdomyomas These arise in the vulvovaginal region or cervix of middle-aged females and also do not seem to recur.

Histopathology

Rhabdomyomas of the adult type are well circumscribed and are composed of a solid mass of large, polygonal eosinophilic or vacuolated cells with small bland nuclei. Cross-striations and bizarre filamentous inclusions are readily demonstrated by the phosphotungstic acid haematoxylin (PTAH) technique. Fetal examples have a much more primitive cellular appearance, resembling embryonal rhabdomyosarcoma (see below), but are

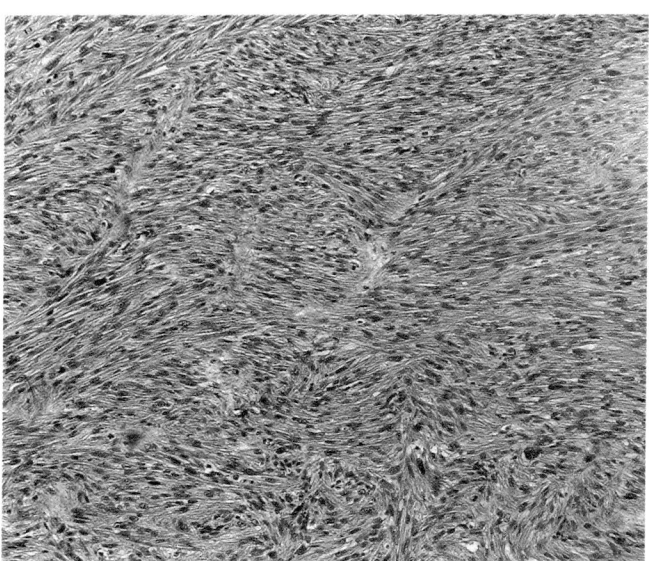

Fig. 27.167 Leiomyosarcoma. Irregularly interlacing fascicles of spindle cells with copious eosinophilic cytoplasm.

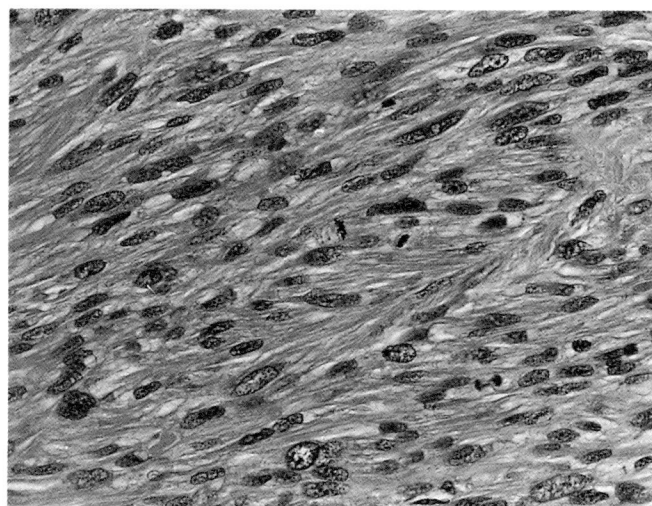

Fig. 27.168 Leiomyosarcoma. The tumour cells have plump, blunt-ended nuclei and mitoses are obvious.

well circumscribed, non-necrotic, show no pleomorphism, and only rare mitoses. Obvious differentiation into strap-like rhabdomyoblasts may only be evident towards the periphery of the lesion. Genital lesions are ill-defined and consist of numerous, eosinophilic strap-shaped rhabdomyoblasts (totally lacking in pleomorphism or mitoses) set in a prominent fibro-collagenous stroma.

Rhabdomyosarcoma

Rhabdomyosarcoma is by far the commonest malignant soft-tissue neoplasm in infants and children but is rare in adults. Criteria for its diagnosis have varied over the years and have often been a source of disagreement. It is essential, however, that there be demonstrable skeletal muscle differentiation. In some cases, morphologically typical rhabdomyoblasts are readily identified but, often, ancillary techniques are necessary to prove the nature of the tumour. These include demonstration of cytoplasmic cross-striations by the phosphotungstic acid haematoxylin technique, a feature that is only present in 50 per cent of cases at most; immunohistochemical positivity with markers such as desmin, creatine kinase-MM, β-enolase, or myoglobin; or ultrastructural identification of sarcomeric features, such as bundles of alternating thick and thin filaments and Z-bands. Rhabdomyosarcoma is traditionally subdivided into embryonal, alveolar, and pleomorphic subtypes; the botryoid form is simply a variant of embryonal (see below).

Clinical features

Embryonal rhabdomyosarcoma This is the commonest subtype and presents most often in the first six years of life, showing a predilection for males. It classically arises, in descending order of frequency, in the head and neck region (especially the orbit, nasopharynx, or middle ear), the genito-urinary tract (particularly the paratesticular region or bladder), the limbs, or the retroperitoneum. Those developing beneath a mucosal surface and presenting as a protuberant mass resembling a bunch of grapes are known as *botryoid*. The aetiology is generally unknown and it is worth noting that most cases are thought to originate from primitive mesenchymal cells, since the majority arise at sites normally devoid of striated muscle. With the advent of modern multimodal therapy, three-year survival rates of 60–80 per cent are becoming the norm, representing a dramatic improvement over the past 20 years. Poor prognostic factors are site, and hence operability (parameningeal cases do particularly badly), and extent of the disease at presentation.

Alveolar rhabdomyosarcoma (Enzinger and Shiraki 1969) accounts for about 25 per cent of cases and typically presents between the ages of 10 and 20 years in either sex as a deep-seated intramuscular mass in the limbs, especially the arm, or trunk. Many patients have either lymph node or distant metastases at the time of presentation and this is one of the major reasons why the average five-year survival in this group is only 10–20 per cent.

Pleomorphic rhabdomyosarcoma (De Jong *et al.* 1987) is much

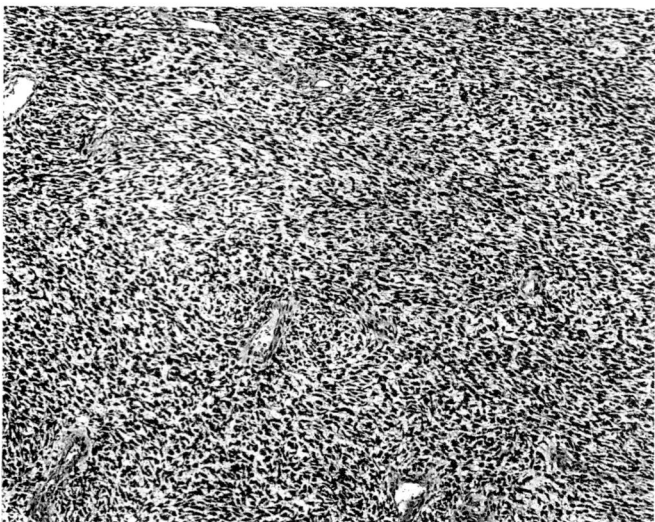

Fig. 27.169 Embryonal rhabdomyosarcoma. A typically very cellular, rather undifferentiated example with a variably prominent myxoid stroma.

the rarest subtype and tends to arise in the limbs of either adults or children. The majority of tumours classified as pleomorphic rhabdomyosarcoma of adulthood in the past tend nowadays to be recategorized as pleomorphic MFH. There is insufficient data available on accurately diagnosed cases by which to create a clear clinical or prognostic picture.

A small proportion of rhabdomyosarcomas show a *mixed pattern*, most often being predominantly embryonal in type but with foci showing an alveolar or pleomorphic pattern. Cases with even only small areas of alveolar differentiation behave as (and should be treated as) full-blown alveolar rhabdomyosarcoma.

Histopathology

Embryonal rhabdomyosarcoma This most often shows relatively little in the way of obvious skeletal muscle differentiation, being mainly composed of small, basophilic, round or spindle-shaped cells with hyperchromatic nuclei, set in a variably prominent myxoid matrix (Fig. 27.169). The degree of pleomorphism is variable but generally only of moderate degree, although mitotic activity is typically marked. Rhabdomyoblasts, which vary greatly in number, have deeply eosinophilic cytoplasm and may be round, strap-shaped, tadpole-shaped, or very vacuolated (the so-called spider cell) (Fig. 27.170). A significant number of cases show no recognizable rhabdomyoblasts on ordinary haematoxylin and eosin sections, but are diagnosed solely on the basis of immunohistochemistry or electron microscopy. The botryoid variant is often fairly well differentiated and tends to show both a very myxoid stroma and a characteristic submucosal zone of dense cellularity, known as the cambium layer.

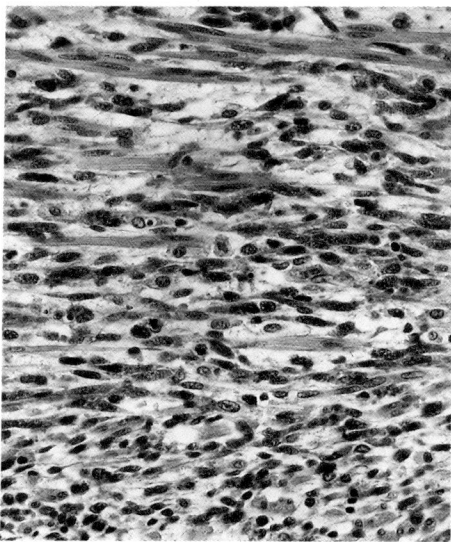

Fig. 27.170 Embryonal rhabdomyosarcoma. Strap- and tadpole-shaped eosinophilic rhabdomyoblasts are clearly evident in this field.

Alveolar rhabdomyosarcoma This is distinguished from the embryonal type firstly by the fact that it almost invariably arises within voluntary muscle. It is characterized by small, round basophilic cells arranged in nests or sheets, separated by variably prominent dense fibrous septa. Many of these nests show loss of cellular cohesion centrally, producing an appearance reminiscent of pulmonary alveoli (Fig. 27.171). Within these central looser areas, larger eosinophilic or polygonal rhabdomyoblasts are usually evident after careful searching. An additional diagnostic feature is the frequent presence of large, palely eosinophilic giant cells with multiple, peripherally located nuclei (giving a so-called wreath-like appearance). A

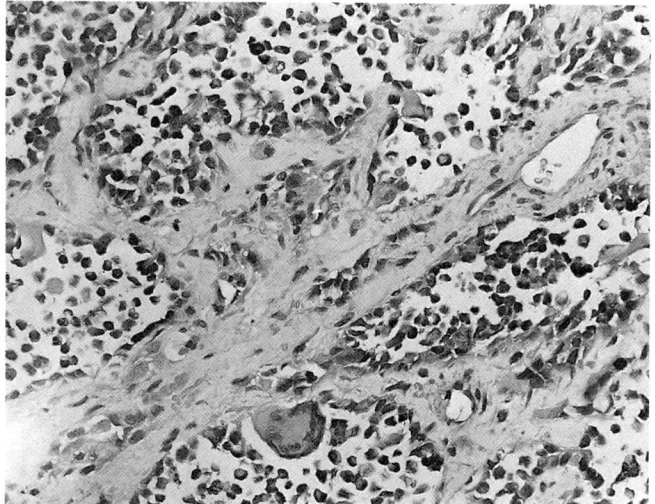

Fig. 27.171 Alveolar rhabdomyosarcoma. Note the striking alveolar pattern, the small, round rhabdomyoblasts and the multinucleate giant cell.

small proportion of cases are composed almost entirely of solid sheets of tumour cells with very few identifiable rhabdomyoblasts: these lesions are said to carry a particularly poor prognosis.

Pleomorphic rhabdomyosarcoma In many ways this is the best differentiated of the three types, being characterized by a proliferation of very large, polygonal eosinophilic cells with pleomorphic nuclei. Markedly vacuolated rhabdomyoblasts are often prominent. In addition to the techniques mentioned earlier, these rare lesions may also be distinguished from MFH by the presence of large amounts of intracytoplasmic glycogen.

Ectomesenchymoma

This is a very rare neoplasm (Kawamoto *et al.* 1987) which may present at a variety of sites, usually in early infancy, and carries about a 50 per cent overall mortality. Histologically it is characterized predominantly by embryonal rhabdomyosarcomatous tissue but shows, in addition, areas of ganglion cell, neuroblastic, or Schwannian differentiation.

27.4.8 Tumours of neuroectodermal origin

Traumatic neuroma

Clinical features

Traumatic neuroma is a reactive lesion that results from severe trauma to, or complete severance of, a peripheral nerve of almost any size. As a consequence, a wide variety of sites may be affected at any age and the lesion typically presents as a solitary nodule which is often painful. Perhaps the single commonest site is a limb amputation stump, in which a large nerve (or nerves) is affected. Local recurrence is not a feature.

Histopathology

Adjacent to the transected end of the nerve, if identifiable, is a poorly circumscribed mass composed of an irregular proliferation of small axons, Schwann cells, and fibroblasts (Fig. 27.172). There is no pleomorphism or hyperchromasia. The various components of the lesion are embedded in a collagenous stroma, which becomes progressively hyalinized with time.

Morton's metatarsalgia

Clinical features

Morton's metatarsalgia is also a reactive lesion, which presents in adulthood with paroxysmal pain in the region of the metatarsophalangeal joints, which is worse on walking and relieved by rest. Usually there is no palpable mass but, at operation, there is characteristic fibrous thickening around a plantar digital nerve. Up to 25 per cent of patients have bilateral involvement. The aetiology is uncertain but is probably related to repeated trauma in the region of the balls of the feet. Local recurrence following excision does not occur.

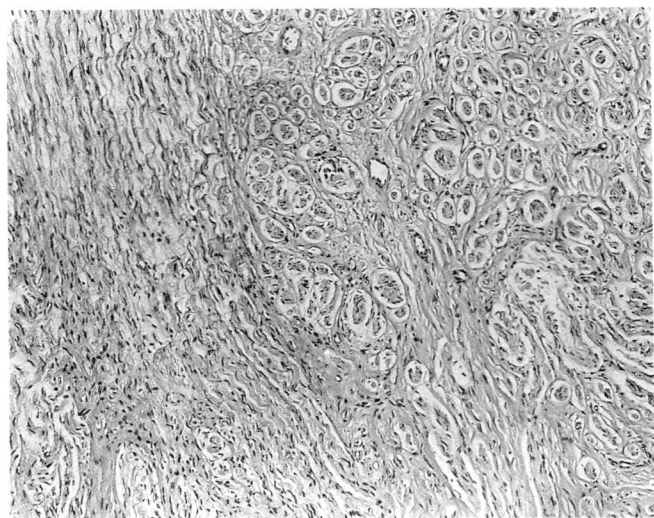

Fig. 27.172 Traumatic neuroma. Arising from the cut end of a nerve (top left) is a mass of small axons and hyalinized fibrous tissue.

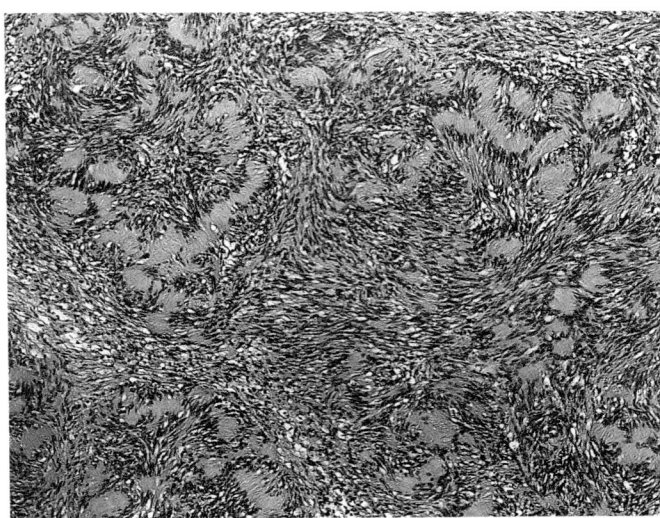

Fig. 27.173 Schwannoma. A typical Antoni A area, consisting of spindle cells showing prominent Verocay bodies.

Histopathology

The characteristic features are the presence of marked endoneural and perineural fibrosis, often with hyalinization and sometimes adjacent myxoid change. Adjacent vessels also show adventitial scarring, hyalinization, and fibrointimal proliferation.

Nasal glioma

Clinical features

Nasal glioma (Fletcher *et al.* 1986a) is a developmental anomaly, which typically presents at birth or in early infancy as a mass either on the bridge of the nose (60 per cent of cases), within the nasal cavity (30 per cent), or with both components (10 per cent). The lesion represents a frontal encephalocoele which has become partially, or more often completely, separated from the frontal lobes by closure of the cranial sutures. Up to 20 per cent may retain some sort of communication with the underlying cerebrum and may therefore be complicated by CSF rhinorrhoea or meningitis, particularly after incautious surgery. Local recurrence following excision is very rare.

Histopathology

The lesion is typically poorly circumscribed and involves predominantly the subcutaneous tissues. It consists of multiple nodules of mature astrocytes arranged in a neurofibrillary stroma. Oligodendroglia are present in smaller numbers, but neurons are almost always absent.

Schwannoma (neurilemmoma)

Clinical features

Benign Schwannomas, also known as neurilemmomas, are common tumours which predominantly present during adult life in either sex as a well-circumscribed, slowly growing mass most often situated in the head and neck region or flexor aspect of a limb. The vast majority are solitary and usually arise in subcutaneous tissue, although a proportion develop deeply in skeletal muscle, retroperitoneum or mediastinum, or superficially in the dermis. They are only rarely associated with von Recklinghausen neurofibromatosis and are very seldom painful. Surgically, those lesions arising in an identifiable nerve are located eccentrically within the nerve sheath and are readily removed without damage to the nerve. Local recurrence is not a feature and malignant change has only been acceptably documented in less than ten cases.

Histopathology

These lesions are well circumscribed and encapsulated. They generally have an instantly recognizable appearance, with a biphasic appearance composed of two types of tissue known as Antoni A and B. Antoni A areas are cellular and consists of rather eosinophilic spindle cells with ill-defined cell margins, arranged in random fascicles or whorls. In these areas, nuclear palisading is a common feature and parallel rows of nuclei with intervening cell processes, known as Verocay bodies, are frequently seen (Fig. 27.173). Mitoses of normal type are occasionally identified. In contrast, Antoni B tissue comprises small, round, or spindle-shaped cells set in a copious myxoid matrix, often showing microcystic degeneration. In these areas, blood vessels with thick hyalinized walls are a characteristic feature (Fig. 27.174). Ultrastructurally these tumours are composed predominantly of Schwann cells, the myelin-producing cells of peripheral nerve sheath.

Variants

Ancient Schwannoma This is the term used to describe Schwannomas showing severe degenerative change, most often

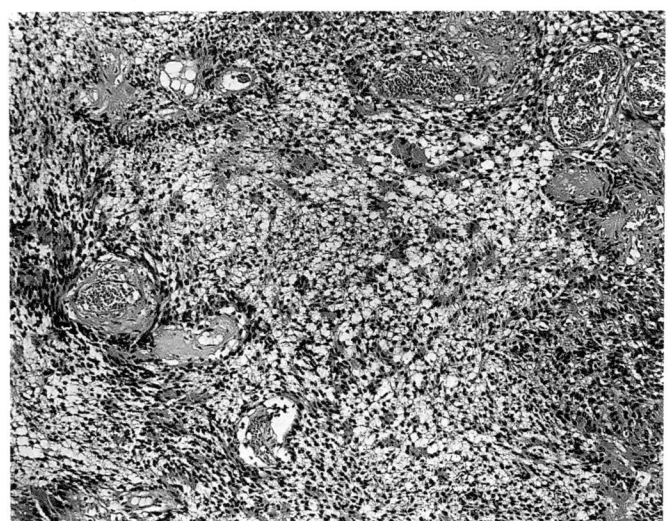

Fig. 27.174 Schwannoma. Antoni B areas are much more hypocellular and myxoid. Note the hyalinized blood vessel walls.

typified by relative loss of Antoni A tissue, marked hyalinization, cystic change, vascular thrombosis and patchy haemosiderin deposition. Such lesions often show moderate nuclear pleomorphism, suggestive of malignancy, but mitoses are absent. Most cases are deeply located and often present in the elderly, suggesting that the changes are simply a reflection of prolonged duration.

Cellular Schwannoma (Fletcher *et al.* 1987) is much less common but typically arises in the mediastinum or retroperitoneum of middle-aged adults. Although benign, it is often mistaken for a sarcoma since it is composed largely of eosinophilic spindle cells, generally lacking in palisading or Verocay bodies, which may show up to five normal mitoses per 20 high-power fields. The cellular areas are, however, not pleomorphic; the lesion is encapsulated; typical hyalinized vessels are usually present; and S100 protein, an immunohistochemical marker of neuroectodermal differentiation, is always positive, allowing ready distinction from leiomyosarcoma, the most frequent misdiagnosis.

Plexiform Schwannoma (Iwashita and Enjoji 1987) is a rare entity that usually develops in the dermis or superficial subcutis of children or young adults and shows a predilection for the trunk or head and neck region. Histologically it consists of multiple (up to 50) discontinuous nodules of typical Schwannomatous tissue. Its importance lies in that, in contrast to plexiform neurofibroma, it is only rarely associated with neurofibromatosis and never undergoes malignant change.

Melanotic Schwannoma (Font and Truong 1984) is a rare neoplasm that typically seems to arise as a pedunculated mass from either the sympathetic chain or a spinal nerve root in middle-aged adults. Histologically it is composed mainly of Antoni A-type tissue combined with numerous polygonal cells showing heavy melanin pigmentation, reflecting dual neural crest differ-

entiation. About 20 per cent of cases behave in a malignant fashion, but there are no reliable means of predicting such behaviour.

Neurofibroma

Clinical features

Neurofibromas are usually solitary, but up to 10 per cent of patients have multiple lesions and, within this latter group, a large proportion have von Recklinghausen neurofibromatosis. Solitary lesions are commonest in young or middle-aged adults of either sex and typically arise in the dermis or superficial subcutis at almost any site as a painless nodule. Less frequently they may arise more deeply from an identifiable nerve, in which circumstance they are usually inextricably tangled with the nerve bundles. The lesions in neurofibromatosis also have a very wide anatomical distribution and often develop at an earlier age. Local recurrence is very rare but a small percentage, particularly those associated with neurofibromatosis or deeply situated, undergo transformation to a malignant peripheral nerve sheath tumour (see below).

Histopathology

In contrast to Schwannomas, these lesions are poorly circumscribed with ill-defined margins. They are typified by a relatively hypocellular proliferation of bland, palely eosinophilic spindle cells with rather wavy, S-shaped or buckled nuclei set in a copious fibrillary or rather myxoid background (Fig. 27.175). Blood vessels are generally scanty and significant pleomorphism or mitoses are not seen and should raise the possibility of malignancy. Small nerve fibres are usually readily identified within the tumour, a feature which is entirely absent from Schwannomas. The stroma of these lesions occasionally undergoes marked myxoid or hyaline change. Ultrastructurally these neoplasms are composed of an admixture of Schwann cells and perineural fibroblasts.

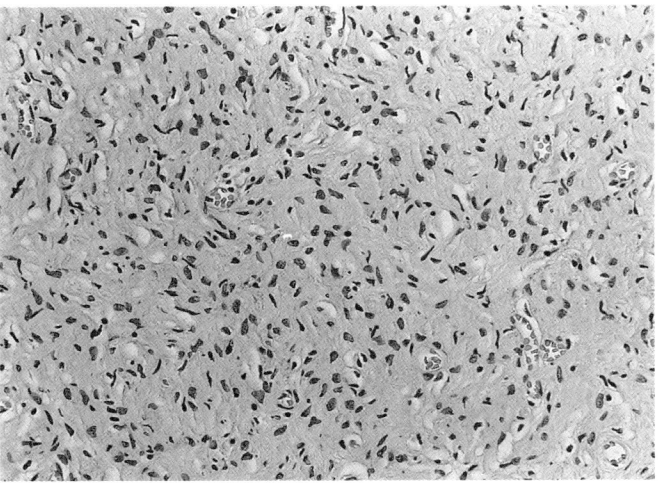

Fig. 27.175 Neurofibroma. Small, ill-defined spindle cells with wavy or comma-shaped nuclei in a collagenous stroma.

Variants

Plexiform neurofibroma This is much less common than the ubiquitous conventional neurofibroma and takes two principal forms: a relatively small type seen in the dermis or superficial subcutis; and a larger, usually deeply situated type, which often involves voluntary muscle or visceral structures. It is an important lesion for two reasons: first, at whatever site, it is pathognomonic of neurofibromatosis; secondly, it runs a small but significant risk of undergoing malignant change, particularly if deeply located. Histologically it is composed of multiple, discrete nodules of often rather myxoid neurofibromatous tissue, associated with hypertrophic nerve bundles both within and adjacent to the nodules (Fig. 27.176).

Diffuse neurofibroma This is also relatively uncommon but presents as a variably sized, often large, area of marked dermal and subcutaneous thickening, most often on the trunk or head and neck region of adolescents or young adults. At least 70 per cent of cases are associated with neurofibromatosis, but malignant change is exceedingly rare. Microscopically the lesion consists of an extensively infiltrative mass of neurofibromatous tissue, containing hypertrophic nerve trunks. Foci of Meissnerian differentiation are common and occasional cases contain melanin pigment.

Other variants These include the very rare epithelioid neurofibroma, typified by focal differentiation into plump, rather eosinophilic cells; Pacinian neurofibroma, in which rudimentary Pacinian corpuscles are seen; and granular cell neurofibroma, in which the spindle cells have periodic acid-Schiff (PAS)-positive, granular eosinophilic cytoplasm.

Solitary circumscribed neuroma

Clinical features

Solitary circumscribed neuroma (Fletcher 1989) is not uncom-

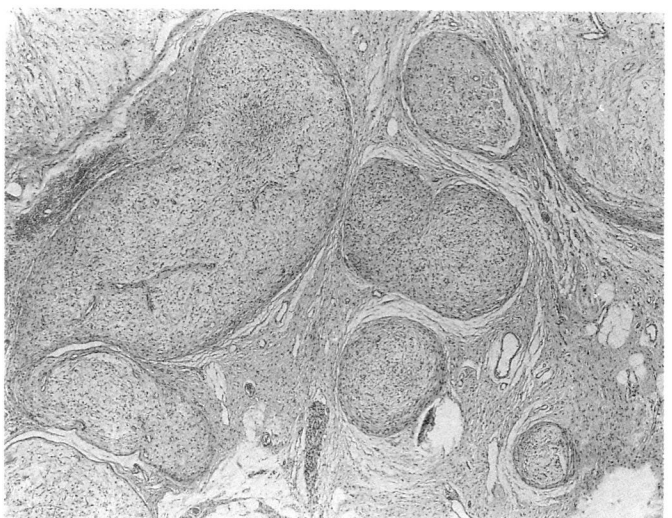

Fig. 27.176 Plexiform neurofibroma. Typical, large discrete nodules of neurofibromatous tissue.

mon but is a little-known benign lesion, which typically presents as a painless, solitary, cutaneous nodule on the face. Other sites may more rarely be affected. Affected patients are most often middle-aged adults of either sex and there is no association with either von Recklinghausen disease or the type II multiple endocrine neoplasia syndrome. These lesions are entirely benign and do not recur.

Histopathology

The tumour is generally small (< 1 cm), is situated in the dermis and is subtotally encapsulated. It consists of short interlacing fascicles of bland, monomorphic Schwann cells, scattered between which are innumerable tiny axons which can usually only be identified by special stains. It is this latter feature which clearly distinguishes this entity from a simple benign Schwannoma. A nerve of origin is often evident at the base of the lesion.

Granular cell tumour

Clinical features

Granular cell tumour, formerly known as granular cell myoblastoma, is a not uncommon benign lesion of probable Schwann cell origin. It presents most often in young or middle-aged adults, with a marked predominance of females, as a solitary, dermal or subcutaneous nodule. Up to 10 per cent of patients have multiple lesions. While almost any site may be affected, the tongue, chest wall (including breast), and upper limbs are favoured locations. The aetiology is unknown. Local recurrence is very uncommon. A very small number of cases have been reported to pursue a malignant course, but this is exceedingly rare and very difficult to predict on histological grounds.

Histopathology

Granular cell tumours have a very characteristic, uniform appearance, typified by a poorly circumscribed, ill-defined mass composed of a diffuse sheet of large, palely eosinophilic polygonal cells with granular cytoplasm and a small, often central, nucleus (Fig. 27.177). The cells characteristically contain small amounts of PAS-positive, diastase-resistant material, thought to represent glycolipid. A frequent and striking feature is the presence of perineural and endoneural tumour cells both within, and at the periphery of, the lesion. In up to 20 per cent of cases, particularly if located in the oral cavity, the overlying epidermis (or mucosa) shows striking pseudoepitheliomatous hyperplasia (Fig. 27.177) which is easily mistaken for squamous cell carcinoma. The differential diagnosis of granular cell tumours is rarely a problem.

Dermal nerve sheath myxoma

Clinical features

Dermal nerve sheath myxoma, sometimes known as neurothekeoma (Gallager and Helwig 1980), is an uncommon benign tumour, which typically presents as a small, solitary

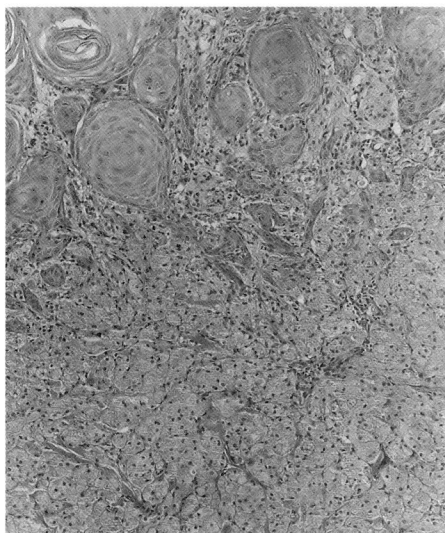

Fig. 27.177 Granular cell tumour. Note the sheet of large, uniform cells with granular cytoplasm and the overlying pseudoepitheliomatous hyperplasia.

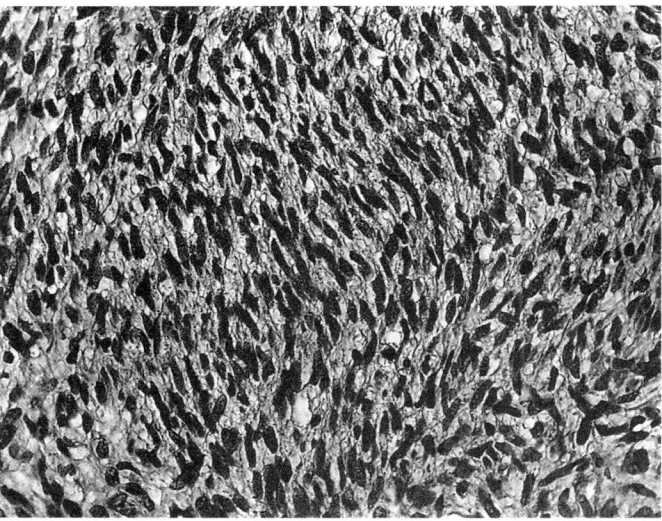

Fig. 27.178 Malignant peripheral nerve sheath tumour. The nuclei are hyperchromatic, tapering, and have a wavy configuration reminiscent of neurofibroma.

nodule on the face or upper limb of adolescents or young adults, predominantly females. Whether it is derived from Schwann cells or perineural fibroblasts remains unknown. Local recurrence is rare and probably reflects inadequate excision.

Histopathology

The tumour has a poorly circumscribed, multinodular appearance and is usually confined to the deep dermis and superficial subcutis. The nodules have a variable pattern, mainly being composed of spindle- or stellate-shaped cells in an abundant myxoid matrix, but focally consisting of plump, eosinophilic rather epithelioid cells. Occasional multinucleate giant cells are usually identified and scattered normal mitoses are to be expected. There is no nuclear pleomorphism or hyperchromasia. Tiny amounts of tissue identical to the tumour itself are often found within small nerve bundles adjacent to the lesion.

Malignant peripheral nerve sheath tumour

Criteria for the diagnosis of malignant peripheral nerve sheath tumour (MPNST) have varied over the years, largely because many cases have a non-specific spindle-cell pattern similar to fibrosarcoma or monophasic synovial sarcoma. These lesions should, however, either demonstrably arise from a nerve, be contiguous with a recognizable neurofibromatous element, or show ultrastructural or immunohistochemical evidence of Schwann cell differentiation. Even so, there is no doubt that a small proportion of cases that fail to fulfil one of these criteria, have, to some extent, a characteristic histological appearance identical to proven MPNSTs and probably also belong in this category.

Clinical features

MPNST (Ghosh *et al.* 1973, Ducatman *et al.* 1986) presents most often in middle-aged adults as an enlarging, deep-seated mass in the limbs or trunk, which is sometimes associated with pain or other neurological symptoms. Between 30 and 40 per cent of cases arise in patients with neurofibromatosis, in which cirumstance affected individuals are usually aged between 20 and 40 years. Up to 10 per cent in either clinical group develop at the site of previous irradiation. Approximately 40 per cent of tumours recur locally and the overall five-year survival is 40–60 per cent, although patients with von Recklinghausen's disease do significantly worse and have a five-year survival of about 15 per cent. These latter patients also run the risk of developing a separate, asynchronous MPNST.

Histopathology

Typically the tumour measures more than 5 cm in diameter, has infiltrative margins, and shows widespread haemorrhage or necrosis. It is composed of pale spindle cells with ill-defined cytoplasmic borders and tapering, often wavy nuclei showing prominent mitotic activity (Fig. 27.178). These cells are arranged in parallel interlacing fascicles and tend to show alternating hypercellular and rather myxoid areas, associated with striking perivascular whorling and infiltration of vessel walls (Fig. 27.179). Focal hyalinization, which is sometimes nodular in configuration, is quite common, but nuclear palisading, so typical of benign Schwannomas, is rare. Heterologous differentiation, most often in the form of rhabdomyoblasts, osteoid or cartilage, occurs in about 10–15 per cent of cases (see also below). Contiguous areas with the typical features of a neurofibroma are found in about 30 per cent of lesions and are particularly frequent in patients with neurofibromatosis.

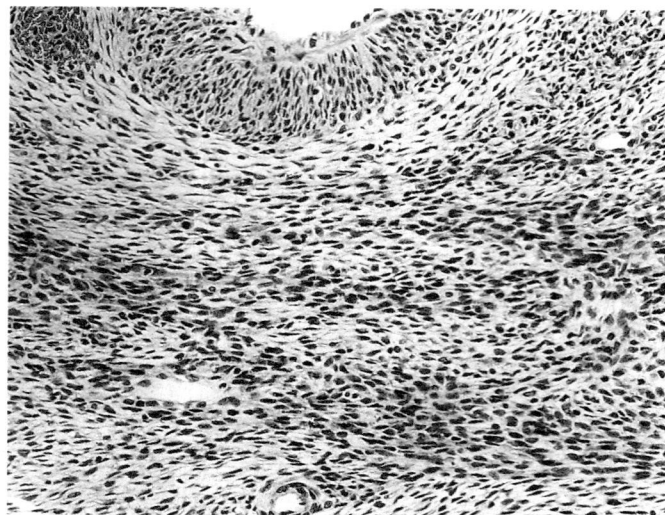

Fig. 27.179 Malignant peripheral nerve sheath tumour. Note the focally myxoid background and the striking perivascular whorling (top).

Variants

MPNST with rhabdomyoblastic differentiation Also known as the malignant Triton tumour (Brooks *et al.* 1985), this occurs mainly in patients with neurofibromatosis and has a very poor prognosis. It is usually characterized by variably prominent areas of tissue resembling well-differentiated embryonal rhabdomyosarcoma within an otherwise typical MPNST.

Epithelioid MPNST This is a rare variant typified by the presence of nodules or cords of large, often rather basophilic epithelioid cells. If these cells occupy a large proportion of the tumour, then distinction from a metastatic melanoma or carcinoma may be very difficult, although origin from a nerve or immunohistochemistry may be helpful. The prognosis appears no different from conventional MPNST.

Malignant melanotic Schwannoma (see p. 2123).

Pigmented neuroectodermal tumour of infancy

Clinical features

Pigmented neuroectodermal tumour of infancy (Young and Gonzalez-Crussi 1985), formerly known as a retinal anlage tumour, arises classically in the maxilla of young infants but may also present in the soft tissues of the head and neck or at a variety of other sites, such as the epididymis. In the vast majority of cases it is a benign tumour which is not usually associated with elevated urinary levels of catecholamine metabolites.

Histopathology

The tumour has infiltrative margins and consists of sheets of small basophilic neuroblast-like cells and clusters of larger, more epithelioid cells, many of which contain melanin pigment and closely resemble melanocytes. The pigmented cells are frequently arranged in a pseudoacinar pattern around the smaller primitive cells. Both cell types are set in a relatively hypocellular

fibrocollagenous stroma. It is presumed, therefore, that these tumours are derived from a primitive neuroectodermal cell, which then manifests dual differentiation.

Peripheral neuroepithelioma

Peripheral neuroepithelioma, or malignant primitive neuro-ectodermal tumour of soft tissues, has only become widely recognized in recent years as a consequence of careful ultrastructural and immunohistochemical studies. In a very simplistic sense, it is best regarded as the peripherally located equivalent of neuroblastoma (see Chapter 26).

Clinical features

This rare tumour (Hashimoto *et al.* 1983) most often presents in adolescents or young adults, with a slight predominance in females, but may occur at any age. It usually arises in a limb, is often rapidly growing and painful, and may show demonstrable origin from a major nerve. Urinary catecholamine metabolites are not usually raised in concentration. A specific clinical subgroup, formerly known as the Askin tumour, arises in the chest wall, pleura, or peripheral lung of younger patients, again mainly in females (Askin *et al.* 1979). Both types usually carry a poor prognosis, with 75 per cent or more patients dying within two years of diagnosis, although survival is improving with modern chemotherapeutic regimes.

Histopathology

The histological features in both clinical groups are relatively similar. The tumours are composed of small basophilic cells, with little or no cytoplasm and hyperchromatic nuclei, arranged in diffuse sheets or nests (Fig. 27.180). Rosettes or pseudorosettes can often be found after thorough sampling, and a proportion of cases contain small amounts of intracytoplasmic glycogen. Proof of their neuroectodermal nature can be obtained by immunohistochemistry (for example, positivity for

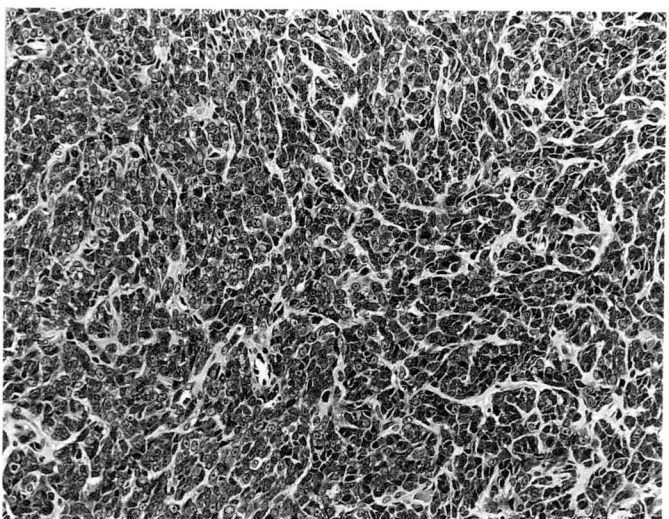

Fig. 27.180 Peripheral neuroepithelioma. Nests and trabeculae of small basophilic cells with ovoid nuclei and prominent nucleoli.

neurone-specific enolase or neurofilaments) or electron microscopy (interdigitating cell processes, microtubules, and neurosecretory granules).

Clearly with these appearances, the possibility of metastatic spread from an underlying neuroblastoma (particularly in childhood cases) should always be excluded.

Malignant melanoma of soft tissues

Clinical features

Malignant melanoma of soft tissues (Chung and Enzinger 1983), which was formerly known as clear cell sarcoma of tendons and aponeuroses, is a fairly uncommon tumour which shows a predilection for adolescents or young adults of either sex. It presents most often as a deeply situated, slowly growing mass in a limb, most especially in the region of the foot. It is generally fairly small (less than 5 cm in diameter) and, at operation, classically involves tendo-aponeurotic structures. Up to 50 per cent recur locally and a similar number eventually metastasize and pursue a fatal course, often after a very prolonged interval (even 10 years or more).

Histopathology

This neoplasm typically has a lobulated appearance and infiltrative margins. It is composed of ovoid or polygonal cells, with clear cytoplasm and vesicular nuclei, arranged in nests or fascicles which are separated by fibrous septa. The majority of cases contain histochemically demonstrable melanin in a variable proportion of the clear cells; another cardinal feature is the presence of multinucleate giant cells in the fibrous septa (Fig. 27.181).

Occasional cases have a more eosinophilic, spindle-celled appearance with a fascicular pattern. The immunohistochemical demonstration of S100 protein in these tumours, combined with ultrastructural evidence of melanogenesis within tumour cells, has effectively proved their neuroectodermal nature. However, the precise cell of origin remains uncertain; it is postulated that these lesions may arise from melanocytes which have shown aberrant migration during embryogenesis.

Extracranial meningioma

Meningiomas may very rarely present in soft tissue (Lopez et al. 1974) as a primary phenomenon or occasionally as a secondary event due to direct extension of an intracranial neoplasm (see Chapter 25). The latter occurrence has often been preceded by craniotomy. Primary meningiomas (Theaker et al. 1990) in soft tissue usually present in the head and neck region, but may be paravertebral, and are thought to arise from developmentally ectopic arachnoid cell nests. These primary lesions are histologically similar to their intracranial counterparts and behave in a benign fashion.

Extraspinal ependymoma

Ependymomas presenting in soft tissue (Anderson 1966) are extremely uncommon but may develop either from a neural

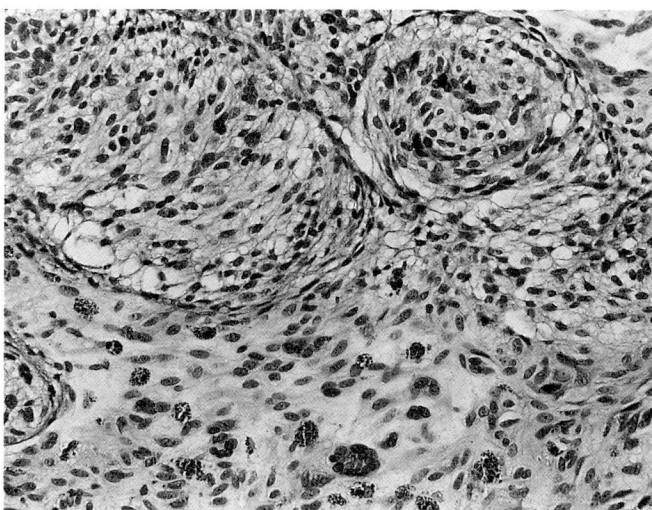

Fig. 27.181 Malignant melanoma of soft tissues. Nests of clear cells along with granular pigmented cells and a multinucleate giant cell (bottom centre).

tube remnant or from ectopic ependymal cells, sometimes associated with spina bifida. They present as a subcutaneous mass located over the sacrococcyx and, histologically, usually resemble the conventional myxopapillary ependymomas which arise from the cauda equina (see Chapter 25). Up to 20 per cent of cases metastasize, often after a very prolonged latent period.

27.4.9 Cartilaginous and osseous tumours

Soft tissue chondroma

Clinical features

Soft tissue chondroma (Chung and Enzinger 1978) is not uncommon and presents, in the vast majority of cases, as a slowly growing, well circumscribed subcutaneous mass on a finger or toe. Middle-aged adults, predominantly males, are most often affected. Radiologically there is no evidence of bone involvement and, at operation, the lesion quite often seems to arise from a tendon sheath or joint capsule. Up to 10 per cent of cases recur locally but malignant transformation has never been reported (cf. chondromas of bone, Section 27.1).

Histopathology

The tumour is typically composed of an encapsulated, lobulated mass of mature hyaline cartilage which may show striking hypercellularity and nuclear pleomorphism (Fig. 27.182). Lacunae containing multiple nuclei are a frequent finding but mitoses are scarce. Dystrophic calcification or osseous metaplasia are common. Some cases contain multinucleate giant cells, typically distributed around the edges of the cartilaginous lobules, while occasional examples may have a very myxoid stroma.

Distinction from extraskeletal chondrosarcoma (q.v.) is usually simple, since, for practical purposes, well-differentiated

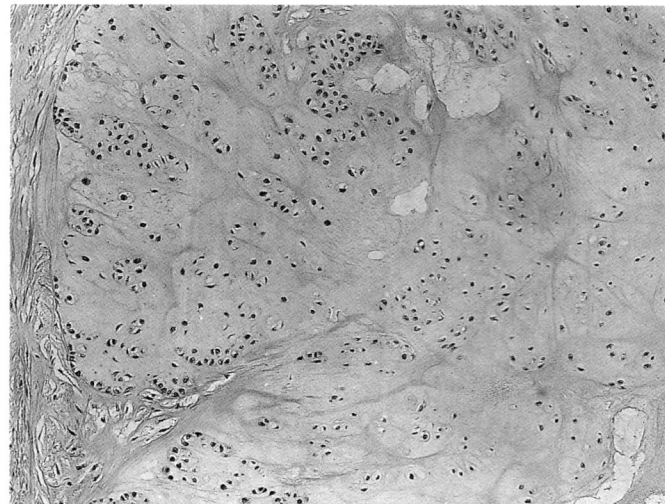

Fig. 27.182 Soft tissue chondroma. A lobulated, encapsulated mass of hypercellular mature cartilage.

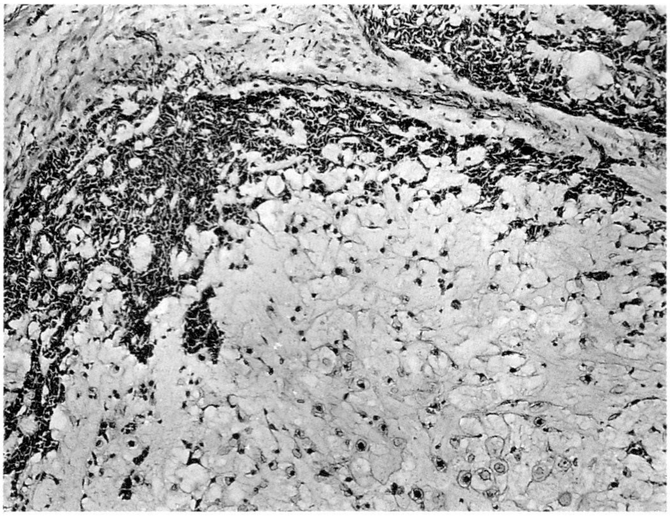

chondrosarcoma arising in soft tissue is almost unheard of. In view of the cytologically worrying features described above, it is obviously mandatory to exclude an underlying bone lesion but it is also reassuring to realize that metastasizing chondrosarcomas of phalangeal bones are vanishingly rare.

Extraskeletal chondrosarcoma

Chondrosarcomas arising primarily in soft tissue are uncommon and are almost always divisible into one of two types: myxoid or mesenchymal. Tumours resembling the better-known, well- or moderately differentiated chondrosarcomas of bone are exceedingly infrequent in soft tissues and have never been properly documented.

Clinical features

Extraskeletal myxoid chondrosarcoma (Fletcher *et al.* 1986b) presents most often in early to middle adult life as a slowly growing, deeply located mass in a limb (particularly the leg). It is usually totally unrelated to any osteoarticular structure, although it has been described within a joint. Up to 20 per cent of cases recur locally and the overall five-year survival is about 85 per cent.

Extraskeletal mesenchymal chondrosarcoma This chondrosarcoma (Guccion *et al.* 1973) is rarer than the myxoid variant and tends to show a predilection for the head and neck region of adolescents and young adults. It is generally a larger, more aggressive tumour than myxoid chondrosarcoma, with up to 60 per cent of cases metastasizing and pursuing a fatal course.

Histopathology

Extraskeletal myxoid chondrosarcoma This has a characteristically lobulated appearance, the periphery of the lobules being composed of a rim of small, basophilic, rather primitive

Fig. 27.183 Extraskeletal myxoid chondrosarcoma. Note the zoned appearance, with peripheral hypercellularity and a myxoid core.

cells and the remainder consisting of uniform, round, palely eosinophilic cells set in a copious myxoid matrix (Fig. 27.183). Only about 50 per cent of cases show obvious chondroblastic differentiation, typically in small foci. There is usually little pleomorphism and mitoses are very scanty.

Extraskeletal mesenchymal chondrosarcoma By contrast, this is largely composed of sheets of small, basophilic, polygonal, or spindle-shaped cells with little discernible cytoplasm, dispersed within which are occasional small islands of well-differentiated cartilage (Fig. 27.184). Within the primitive basophilic areas there is often a striking network of arborizing vascular channels

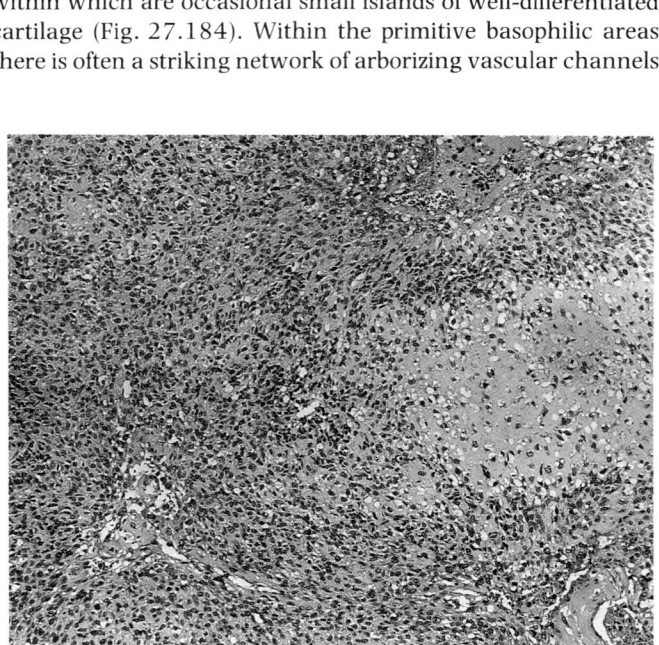

Fig. 27.184 Extraskeletal mesenchymal chondrosarcoma. A mass of small undifferentiated cells within which is a nodule of cartilage (right).

resembling an haemangiopericytoma (see Section 12.5). Accurate diagnosis of this variant is very much dependent upon thorough sampling to allow identification of cartilaginous foci.

Osteoma

For practical purposes there appears to be no such lesion as a soft-tissue osteoma. A variety of dermal lesions have been labelled osteoma cutis in the past but, on the whole, these seem to represent extensive metaplastic ossification within other entities such as melanocytic naevi, pilomatrixomas, calcinosis cutis, or scars.

Myositis ossificans

Clinical features

Myositis ossificans (Sumiyoshi *et al.* 1985) is a relatively uncommon reactive lesion which may present at any age but shows a predilection for young adults of either sex. It typically arises within a major limb muscle, most often in the thigh, as a painful swelling that has rapidly enlarged over a period of a few weeks. Only about 40 per cent of cases have a convincing history of recent trauma to the affected site. Radiologically the lesion appears well circumscribed with a peripheral rim of calcification. Excision is almost never complicated by local recurrence and, if no treatment is employed, most examples soon cease to grow and eventually regress spontaneously. In those cases lacking a history of trauma, the aetiology remains unknown.

Histopathology

By the time most lesions are excised, they have a characteristically zoned appearance, being composed of a central core of cellular proliferating fibrous tissue (closely resembling nodular fasciitis, see p. 2107); a middle zone in which plump osteoblasts are seen laying down unmineralized osteoid; and an outer zone consisting of trabeculae of fairly mature bone (Fig. 27.185).

Foci of cartilaginous differentiation may also be evident between the osteoid layer and the bone. Identification of the zoned pattern is of paramount importance in the diagnosis; small biopsies are therefore contraindicated since tissue taken from the central cellular area, along with fragments of osteoid, may be very difficult to distinguish from osteosarcoma. The clinical history and X-ray appearances should also be helpful.

Fibro-osseous pseudotumour of the digits

Clinical features

Fibro-osseous pseudotumour of the digits (Dupree and Enzinger 1986) basically represents an anatomically and histologically distinct variant of myositis ossificans. It is a rare entity with a similar age-distribution to myositis ossificans, which usually presents as a painful localized swelling on a finger. The history is typically short and is often related to trauma. Local recurrence is rare.

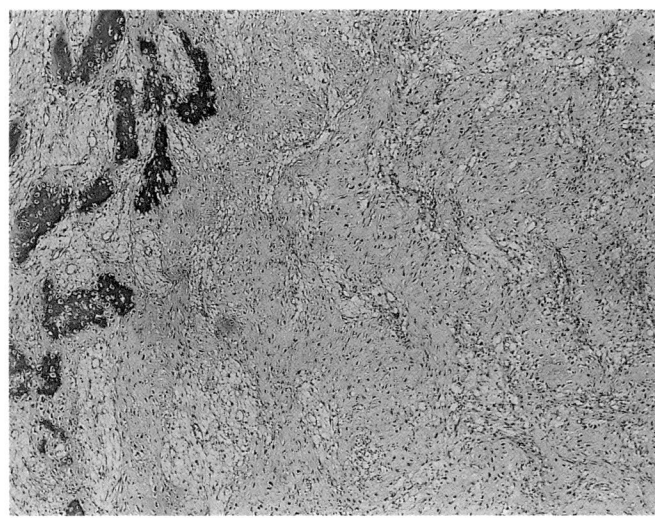

Fig. 27.185 Myositis ossificans. Note the typical zoning with peripheral bone (left), an intermediate layer of primitive osteoid, and central loose fibrous tissue (right).

Histopathology

The microscopic appearances are very similar to those of myositis ossificans in terms of content but the zoning pattern is generally absent. These lesions may therefore be misdiagnosed as extraskeletal osteosarcoma (q.v.) unless the age, site, and relatively bland appearance of the osteoblasts are taken into account.

Fibrodysplasia ossificans progressiva

Clinical features

Fibrodysplasia ossificans progressiva (Cramer *et al.* 1981) is a very rare condition which classically presents in infancy as a progressively enlarging mass in the trunk or neck region. The lesion extends to involve more and more of the musculature, meanwhile progressively ossifying and thus giving rise to increasing rigidity of such structures as the spine and rib cage. A characteristic feature is the associated presence of congenital phalangeal anomalies, most often in the form of hypoplasia or aplasia of two or more digits. The aetiology is unknown, although some cases are familial, and most patients eventually die after 15 years or more with respiratory failure.

Histopathology

The features are quite similar to those of an infantile desmoid fibromatosis (q.v.) but for the vital fact that the infiltrative fibroblastic mass gradually and relentlessly ossifies in an irregular fashion. One eventually sees irregular masses of mature bone distributed throughout the dermis, subcutis, and musculature.

Extraskeletal osteosarcoma

Clinical features

Extraskeletal osteosarcoma (Chung and Enzinger 1987) is uncommon but typically presents in late adult life as an

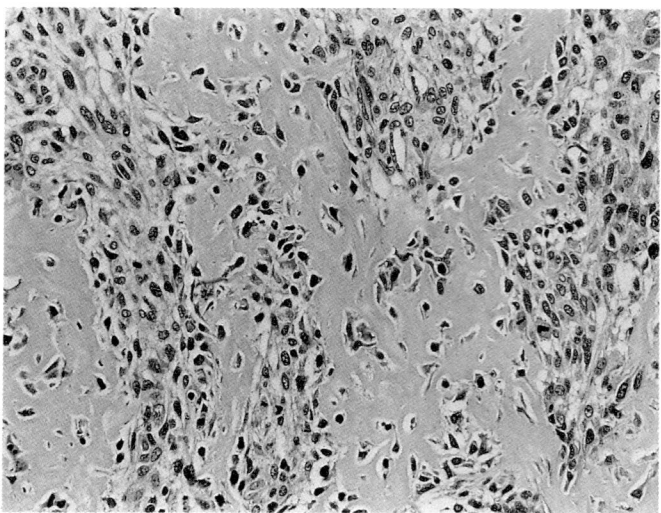

Fig. 27.186 Extraskeletal osteosarcoma. Typical pleomorphic, hyperchromatic spindle cells in an osteoid matrix.

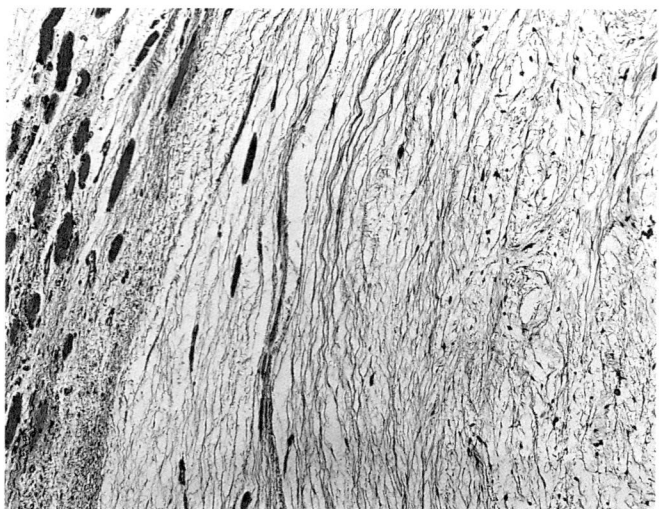

Fig. 27.187 Intramuscular myxoma. Note the typical hypocellularity and paucity of blood vessels.

enlarging, deeply seated mass in a limb, particularly the thigh. A wide variety of sites may be affected on occasion, including quite often the retroperitoneum, but lesions in the hand or foot are exceedingly rare (cf. fibro-osseous pseudotumour). There is a slight predominance of males and some patients have a history of irradiation or significant trauma. This is generally an aggressive neoplasm and the five-year survival is only about 30 per cent.

Histopathology

The microscopic appearances parallel exactly those of osteosarcomas arising in bone (see Section 27.1) and are therefore not repeated in detail here. The osteoblastic (Fig. 27.186) or MFH-like variants are the most frequently encountered. In contrast to myositis ossificans, osteoid is laid down in an irregular, patternless manner and the tumour cells nearly always show far greater anaplasia.

27.4.10   Tumours of uncertain histogenesis

Intramuscular myxoma

Clinical features

Intramuscular myxoma (Miettinen *et al.* 1985) is a not infrequent benign tumour that typically presents in middle-aged adults, predominantly females, as a slowly growing, rather soft painless mass, which is most often located within a thigh or buttock muscle. Occasional patients have multiple lesions or may have an underlying bony abnormality such as fibrous dysplasia. The aetiology is unknown but an inherent metabolic abnormality of connective tissue has been suggested. Local recurrence is very uncommon and usually results from significantly incomplete excision.

Histopathology

These tumours have an extremely bland appearance, being composed of a relatively scanty population of bland spindle- or stellate-shaped cells set in an abundant myxoid matrix consisting of hyaluronic acid (Fig. 27.187). There is no nuclear pleomorphism and mitoses are generally absent. In contrast to myxoid liposarcoma, blood vessels are very scarce and do not have a plexiform pattern. While many cases are well circumscribed, about 50 per cent show irregular infiltration of adjacent skeletal muscle or fascia. These lesions are currently thought to be derived from primitive mesenchymal cells which may show fibroblastic or myofibroblastic differentiation.

Giant cell fibroblastoma

Clinical features

Giant cell fibroblastoma (Fletcher 1988) is an uncommon, recently recognized benign entity which predominantly affects male infants under the age of 5 years and presents as a solitary, slowly growing subcutaneous mass. While the trunk is the commonest site, almost any superficial location may be involved. Although the lesion is usually fairly small (less than 4 cm in diameter), up to 50 per cent of cases recur locally.

Histopathology

The histological features are very distinctive and show two main components. The predominant element is an infiltrative mass of bland, elongated spindle cells with wavy nuclei, set in a variably myxoid or hyalinized stroma in which scattered bizarre multinucleate cells are often found. The other component, found within the spindle-cell areas, consists of large, irregular sinusoid-like spaces, which are lined by either hyperchromatic mononuclear cells or large, multinucleate cells showing nuclear pleomorphism. These spaces give the tumour a vascular appearance but lack an endothelial lining and usually contain pale mucin. Currently available data would suggest that these lesions are composed of fibroblasts having an unusual morphology, but this is to some extent controversial.

Parachordoma

Clinical features

Parachordoma (Dabska 1977) is a very rare benign tumour, which usually presents as a deeply located mass in a limb of an adolescent or adult. It is often closely related to osteoarticular structures and may have been noticed for many years. A small proportion of cases recur locally but metastatic spread has never been reported.

Histopathology

The tumour is typically well circumscribed and lobulated and consists mainly of large vacuolated or eosinophilic cells arranged in cords or alveoli. These cells are set in a copious myxoid matrix, which may have a rather hyaline chondroid appearance. The tumour lobules are dispersed in a dense fibrocollagenous stroma. The histogenesis remains unknown; despite the resemblance to notochordal tissue, there is no evidence that any such tissue is ever found in a limb.

Congenital granular cell tumour

Clinical features

Congenital granular cell tumours (Lack et al. 1982) are rare lesions, which are present at birth in all cases, always arise in the gingivae, and are virtually confined to female infants. They are not associated with any other congenital abnormality and do not recur after excision, in fact some cases appear to regress spontaneously.

Histopathology

The features are basically very similar to those of ordinary granular-cell tumours (see p. 2133), but for the additional presence of a prominent network of capillaries and small islands of odontogenic epithelium. Overlying pseudoepitheliomatous hyperplasia is never a feature. These lesions lack any immunohistochemical or ultrastructural features of neuroectodermal differentiation. Their origin remains undecided but possibilities include odontogenic epithelium or a reactive histiocytic lesion.

Ossifying fibromyxoid tumour

Clinical features

Ossifying fibromyxoid tumour (Enzinger et al. 1989) is a very recently described, rare neoplasm which typically presents as a deep subcutaneous mass in the limbs of adults, predominantly males. Up to 30 per cent of cases recur locally but metastasis is exceedingly uncommon.

Histopathology

This lesion is most often encapsulated and frequently exhibits a subcapsular shell of lamellar bone. The tumour itself consists of lobules or nests of small, bland, palely eosinophilic cells with pale vesicular nuclei, in which mitoses are infrequent. These tumour cells are set in a variably prominent myxoid or collagenous matrix and are often S100-protein positive. Cartilaginous or neural origins have been proposed but the histogenesis remains undecided.

Synovial sarcoma

Despite the well-known name of this tumour, there is little or no evidence to suggest that this tumour actually arises from synovial lining cells, furthermore, anatomical origin within a joint is very uncommon. It is highly likely that this sarcoma will be renamed in the coming years. (See also Section 27.3).

Clinical features

Synovial sarcoma (Wright et al. 1982) most often presents in adolescents or young adults, with a slight predominance of males, as a deep-seated painful mass of very variable duration. The majority of cases arise in the limbs, particularly around the thigh or knee, but occasionally such sites as the abdominal wall or head and neck region may be affected. The tumour is frequently large and in most cases pursues an aggressive course, often over a prolonged period, such that the overall ten-year survival rate is only about 30 per cent. The aetiology is entirely unknown.

Histopathology

Classically, synovial sarcoma has a biphasic appearance, being composed of an admixture of elongated basophilic spindle cells and nests or glandular structures made up of plump or columnar epithelial cells (Fig. 27.188). The spindle-celled areas often closely resemble conventional fibrosarcoma (q.v.), but, in addition, usually show (at least focally) an haemangiopericytoma-like vascular pattern, a notable infiltrate of mast cells, and quite

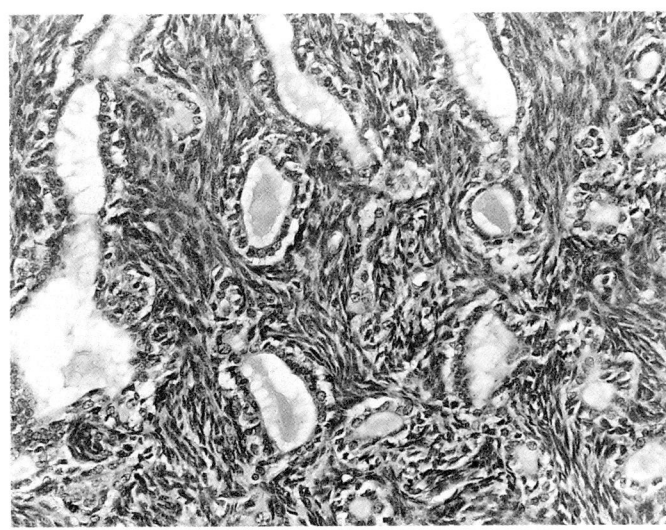

Fig. 27.188 Synovial sarcoma. A classical biphasic example consisting of spindle cells and gland-like spaces.

often also show small areas of calcification or metaplastic bone. The epithelial cells are usually large, with pale cytoplasm and vesicular nuclei, and contain acid mucopolysaccharide, which is also evident within the glandular spaces.

Up to one-third of cases have a purely monophasic spindle-cell appearance, even after extensive searching for an epithelial element, in which circumstances the diagnosis is based on the features described above combined with either immunohistochemical demonstration of epithelial differentiation or ultrastructural studies. The fact that virtually all biphasic cases express epithelial markers (cytokeratin or epithelial membrane antigen) has been one of the key pieces of evidence both in excluding origin from synovium (which never bears these antigens) and in supporting the existence of a monophasic variant on the basis of immunohistochemical similarities.

A small proportion of biphasic tumours show very heavy and extensive calcification, often with ossification, both in the spindle-cell areas and glands and this variant seems to carry a much better prognosis (Varela-Duran and Enzinger 1982).

Epithelioid sarcoma

Clinical features

Epithelioid sarcoma (Chase and Enzinger 1985) is a relatively uncommon neoplasm, which typically arises in adolescents or young adults and shows a predilection for males. The vast majority present in the subcutis or dermis of the limbs, particularly around the hand or forearm, as a multinodular mass which has often been noticed for several years. Around 75 per cent of cases recur locally, often repeatedly, and about 40 per cent metastasize with fatal results, frequently after a very prolonged latent interval.

Histopathology

Although, in the past, this tumour has been confused with a carcinoma or granulomatous process, the histological features are usually distinctive. The tumour is typically composed of multiple nodules, made up of eosinophilic cells which are both plump and epithelioid in nature and also spindle shaped. The two cell types merge imperceptibly and the centre of the nodules quite often shows so-called geographic necrosis, within which dystrophic calcification may be seen. The tumour cells are set in a very dense collagenous stroma. There is usually only minimal cytological pleomorphism, although mitoses may be prominent. Interestingly, the epithelioid cells (and to a lesser extent the spindle cells) also express immunohistochemical markers of epithelial differentiation in the same way as synovial sarcoma. Whether the two entities are related remains undecided but seems unlikely.

Alveolar soft-part sarcoma

Clinical features

Alveolar soft-part sarcoma (Auerbach and Brooks 1987, Lieberman et al. 1989) is a rare neoplasm, which predominantly presents in young adults of either sex as a deeply located mass in the leg or around the limb girdles. The tumour is often large

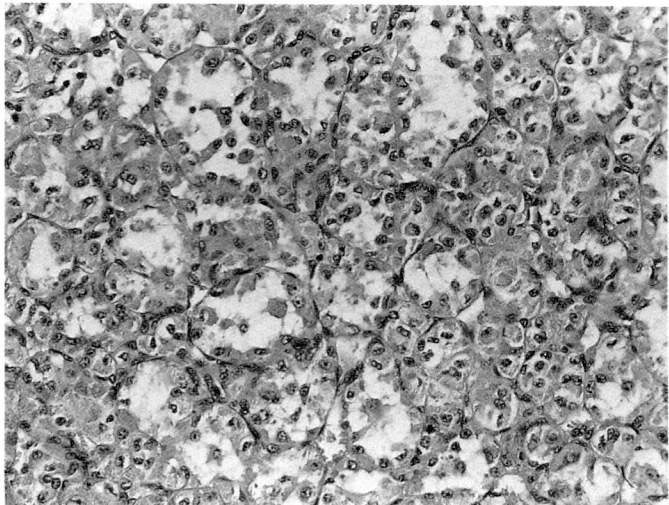

Fig. 27.189 Alveolar soft-part sarcoma. Nests of granular eosinophilic cells showing loss of cohesion centrally, hence the alveolar pattern.

(almost always more than 5 cm in diameter) and has frequently grown slowly over a period of several years. No aetiological factors have been identified. Around 25 per cent recur locally but, more significantly, up to 70 per cent metastasize, often over a very long period.

Histopathology

This tumour has a classical and instantly recognizable appearance, being composed of large round or polygonal cells, with eosinophilic granular cytoplasm, arranged in nests or alveolar structures which often show loss of cohesion centrally (Fig. 27.189). The nuclei are hyperchromatic but tend to be fairly uniform in shape and size. The diagnostic feature is the presence of intracytoplasmic crystalline material or granules which are uniformly PAS positive after diastase digestion. These 'crystals' appear to be composed of filamentous proteins, the nature of which is still undecided. The histogenesis remains unknown despite a wide range of published hypotheses, but increasing evidence favours rhabdomyoblastic differentiation.

Extraskeletal Ewing sarcoma

Clinical features

Extraskeletal Ewing sarcoma (Angervall and Enzinger 1975) is a rare tumour, which typically affects adolescents or young adults and most often presents as a rapidly enlarging, deeply located mass in the trunk or limbs. Approximately 60 per cent of patients die with widely disseminated disease, frequently within a very short period of time.

Histopathology

The microscopic appearances are, for practical purposes, the same as those of Ewing sarcoma arising in bone (see Section 27.1). Although the histogenesis of these tumours has been disputed for many years, compelling evidence has accumulated in recent years to suggest that extraskeletal Ewing's sarcoma is probably a primitive neuroectodermal tumour, based largely on cytogenetic and immunohistochemical findings (Dehner 1986; Fletcher 1991a).

Extrarenal rhabdoid tumour

Clinical features

This recently described, very rare neoplasm (Sotelo-Avila *et al.* 1986) typically presents in early infancy or childhood (although young adults may be affected). It may be located at a very wide variety of sites, predominantly in deep soft tissue, although lesions in various viscera or the brain have been described. The aetiology is unknown but patients are at increased risk of developing a separate, often asynchronous intracranial malignancy. The prognosis is generally appalling, most patients dying with widespread metastases within two years of presentation.

Histopathology

Extrarenal rhabdoid tumours are characterized by an often large, infiltrative mass showing extensive necrosis. They are very cellular lesions composed of sheets of small, round cells with brightly eosinophilic cytoplasm (hence the resemblance to rhabdomyosarcoma), many of which contain large hyaline paranuclear inclusions made up of intermediate filaments. Areas showing a more basophilic spindle-celled appearance are often present. There is very little pleomorphism but mitoses are usually prominent. The histogenesis is unknown but immuno-histochemical studies to date have shown very heterogeneous results, suggesting that this histological appearance may represent a pattern shared in common by a range of both mesenchymal and epithelial neoplasms showing almost complete loss of differentiation.

Malignant mesenchymoma

Malignant mesenchymoma is a very uncommon neoplasm, which is only rarely described in the literature, but which is characterized by two or more separate differentiated sarcomatous elements (other than fibrosarcoma) within the same tumour. By convention, malignant peripheral nerve sheath tumours showing heterologous differentiation do not fall into this category and, clearly, nor do sarcomas containing foci of benign metaplastic bone or cartilage. Most cases seem to arise in either the retroperitoneum or limbs of adults and the commonest combinations seen are rhabdomyosarcoma with liposarcoma, osteosarcoma, or chondrosarcoma. The prognosis is very variable but seems to be surprisingly good (Newman and Fletcher 1991b).

27.4.11 Bibliography

Allen, P. W. (1972). Recurring digital fibrous tumours of childhood. *Pathology* **4**, 215–23.

Allen, P. W. and Enzinger, F. M. (1970). Juvenile aponeurotic fibroma. *Cancer* **26**, 857–67.

Anderson, M. S. (1966). Myxopapillary ependymoma presenting in the soft tissue over the sacrococcygeal region. *Cancer* **19**, 585–90.

Angervall, L. and Enzinger, F. M. (1975). Extraskeletal neoplasm resembling Ewing's sarcoma. *Cancer* **36**, 240–51.

Askin, F. B., Rosai, J., Sibley, R. K., Dehner, L. P., and McAllister, W. H. (1979). Malignant small cell tumor of the thoracopulmonary region in childhood. A distinctive clinicopathologic entity of uncertain histogenesis. *Cancer* **43**, 2438–51.

Auerbach, H. E. and Brooks, J. J. (1987). Alveolar soft part sarcoma. A clinicopathologic and immunohistochemical study. *Cancer* **60**, 66–73.

Azumi, N., Curtis, J., Kempson, R. L., and Hendrickson, M. R. (1987). Atypical and malignant neoplasms showing lipomatous differentiation. A study of 111 cases. *American Journal of Surgical Pathology* **11**, 161–83.

Barrow, M. V. and Holubar, K. (1969). Multicentric reticulohistiocytosis. A review of 33 patients. *Medicine* **48**, 287–305.

Berlin, O., Stener, B., Kindblom, L.-G., and Angervall, L. (1984). Leiomyosarcomas of venous origin in the extremities. A correlated clinical, roentgenologic and morphologic study with diagnostic and surgical implications. *Cancer* **54**, 2147–59.

Bernstein, K. E. and Lattes, R. (1982). Nodular (pseudosarcomatous) fasciitis, a nonrecurrent lesion: clinicopathologic study of 134 cases. *Cancer* **49**, 1668–78.

Brooks, J. S. J., Freeman, M., and Enterline, H. T. (1985). Malignant Triton tumors. Natural history and immunohistochemistry of nine new cases with literature review. *Cancer* **55**, 2543–9.

Chase, D. R. and Enzinger, F. M. (1985). Epithelioid sarcoma. Diagnosis, prognostic indicators and treatment. *American Journal of Surgical Pathology* **9**, 241–63.

Chung, E. B. and Enzinger, F. M. (1973). Benign lipoblastomatosis. An analysis of 35 cases. *Cancer* **32**, 482–92.

Chung, E. B. and Enzinger, F. M. (1975). Proliferative fasciitis. *Cancer* **36**, 1450–8.

Chung, E. B. and Enzinger, F. M. (1976). Infantile fibrosarcoma. *Cancer* **38**, 729–39.

Chung, E. B. and Enzinger, F. M. (1978). Chondroma of soft parts. *Cancer* **41**, 1414–24.

Chung, E. B. and Enzinger, F. M. (1979). Fibroma of tendon sheath. *Cancer* **44**, 1945–54.

Chung, E. B. and Enzinger, F. M. (1981). Infantile myofibromatosis. *Cancer* **48**, 1807–18.

Chung, E. B. and Enzinger, F. M. (1983). Malignant melanoma of soft parts. A reassessment of clear cell sarcoma. *American Journal of Surgical Pathology* **7**, 405–13.

Chung, E. B. and Enzinger, F. M. (1987). Extraskeletal osteosarcoma. *Cancer* **60**, 1132–42.

Costa, M. J. and Weiss, S. W. (1990). Angiomatoid malignant fibrous histiocytoma. A follow-up study of 108 cases with evaluation of histologic predictors of outcome. *American Journal of Surgical Pathology* **14**, 1126–32.

Cramer, S. F., Ruehl, A., and Mandel, M. A. (1981). Fibrodysplasia ossificans progressiva: a distinctive bone-forming lesion of the soft tissue. *Cancer* **48**, 1016–21.

Dabska, M. (1977). Parachordoma. A new clinicopathologic entity. *Cancer* **40**, 1586–92.

Dehner, L. P. (1986). Peripheral and central primitive neuroectodermal tumors. A nosologic concept seeking a concensus. *Archives of Pathology and Laboratory Medicine* **110**, 997–1005.

De Jong, A. S. H., Van Kessel-van-Vark, M., and Albus-Lutter, C. E. (1987). Pleomorphic rhabdomyosarcoma in adults: immunohistochemistry as a tool for its diagnosis. *Human Pathology* **18**, 298–303.

Ducatman, B. S., Scheithauer, B. W., Piepgras, D. G., Reiman, H. M., and Ilstrup, D. M. (1986). Malignant peripheral nerve sheath tumors. A clinicopathologic study of 120 cases. *Cancer* **57**, 2006–21.

Dupree, W. B. and Enzinger, F. M. (1986). Fibro-osseous pseudotumor of the digits. *Cancer* **58**, 2103–9.

Enzinger, F. M. (1965). Fibrous hamartoma of infancy. *Cancer* **18**, 241–8.

Enzinger, F. M. (1979). Angiomatoid malignant fibrous histiocytoma. A distinct fibrohistiocytic tumor of children and young adults simulating a vascular neoplasm. *Cancer* **44**, 2147–57.

Enzinger, F. M. and Dulcey, F. (1967). Proliferative myositis. Report of thirty three cases. *Cancer* **20**, 2213–23.

Enzinger, F. M. and Shiraki, M. (1969). Alveolar rhabdomyosarcoma. An analysis of 110 cases. *Cancer* **24**, 18–31.

Enzinger, F. M. and Zhang, R. (1988). Plexiform fibrohistiocytic tumor presenting in children and young adults. An analysis of 65 cases. *American Journal of Surgical Pathology* **12**, 818–26.

Enzinger, F. M., Weiss, S. W., and Liang, C. Y. (1989). Ossifying fibro-myxoid tumor of soft parts. A clinicopathological analysis of 59 cases. *American Journal of Surgical Pathology* **13**, 817–27.

Fields, J. P. and Helwig, E. B. (1981). Leiomyosarcoma of the skin and subcutaneous tissue. *Cancer* **47**, 156–69.

Fletcher, C. D. M. (1987). Malignant fibrous histiocytoma. *Histopathology* **11**, 433–7.

Fletcher, C. D. M. (1988). Giant cell fibroblastoma of soft tissue: a clinicopathological and immunohistochemical study. *Histopathology* **13**, 499–508.

Fletcher, C. D. M. (1989). Solitary circumscribed neuroma of the skin (so-called palisaded, encapsulated neuroma): a clinicopathologic and immunohistochemical study. *American Journal of Surgical Pathology* **13**, 574–80.

Fletcher, C. D. M. (1990). Benign fibrous histiocytoma of subcutaneous and deep soft tissue: a clinicopathologic analysis of 21 cases. *American Journal of Surgical Pathology* **14**, 801–9.

Fletcher, C. D. M. (1991a). Recent advances in the pathology of soft tissue tumours. *Diagnostic Oncology* **1**, 5–11.

Fletcher, C. D. M. (1991b). Angiomatoid 'malignant fibrous histiocytoma': an immunohistochemical study indicative of myoid differentiation. *Human Pathology* **22**, 563–8.

Fletcher, C. D. M. and Martin-Bates, E. (1987). Spindle cell lipoma: a clinicopathological study with some original observations. *Histopathology* **11**, 803–17.

Fletcher, C. D. M. and Martin-Bates, E. (1988). Intramuscular and intermuscular lipoma: neglected diagnoses. *Histopathology* **12**, 275–87.

Fletcher, C. D. M., Evans, B. J., Macartney, J. C., Smith, N., Wilson-Jones, E., and McKee, P. H. (1985). Dermatofibrosarcoma protuberans: a clinicopathological and immunohistochemical study with a review of the literature. *Histopathology* **9**, 921–38.

Fletcher, C. D. M., Carpenter, G., and McKee, P. H. (1986a). Nasal glioma: a rarity. *American Journal of Dermatopathology* **8**, 341–6.

Fletcher, C. D. M., Powell, G., and McKee, P. H. (1986b). Extraskeletal myxoid chondrosarcoma: a histochemical and immunohisto-chemical study. *Histopathology* **10**, 498–9.

Fletcher, C. D. M., Davies, S. E., and McKee, P. H. (1987). Cellular Schwannoma: a distinct pseudosarcomatous entity. *Histopathology* **11**, 21–35.

Fletcher, C. D. M., Powell, G., Van Noorden, S., and McKee, P. H. (1988a). Fibrous hamartoma of infancy: a histochemical and immunohistochemical study. *Histopathology* **12**, 65–74.

Fletcher, C. D. M., Theaker, J. M., Flanagan, A., and Krausz, T. (1988b). Pigmented dermatofibrosarcoma protuberans (Bednar tumour): Melanocytic colonisation or neuroectodermal differen-tiation? A clinicopathological and immunohistochemical study. *Histopathology* **13**, 631–43.

Font, R. L. and Truong, L. D. (1984). Melanotic schwannoma of soft tissues. Electron microscopic observations and review of literature. *American Journal of Surgical Pathology* **8**, 129–38.

Fretzin, D. F. and Helwig, E. B. (1973). Atypical fibroxanthoma of the skin. A clinicopathologic study of 140 cases. *Cancer* **31**, 1541–52.

Gallager, R. L. and Helwig, E. B. (1980). Neurothekeoma—a benign cutaneous tumor of neural origin. *American Journal of Clinical Pathology* **74**, 759–64.

Ghosh, B. C., Ghosh, L., Huvos, A. G., and Fortner, J. G. (1973). Malignant schwannoma. A clinicopathologic study. *Cancer* **31**, 184–90.

Guccion, J. G. and Enzinger, F. M. (1972). Malignant giant cell tumor of soft parts. An analysis of 32 cases. *Cancer* **29**, 1518–29.

Guccion, J. G., Font, R. L., Enzinger, F. M., and Zimmerman, L. E. (1973). Extraskeletal mesenchymal chondrosarcoma. *Archives of Pathology* **95**, 336–40.

Hashimoto, H. and Enjoji, M. (1982). Liposarcoma. A clinico-pathologic subtyping of 52 cases. *Acta Pathologica Japonica* **32**, 933–48.

Hashimoto, H., Enjoji, M., Nakajima, T., Kiryu, H., and Daimaru, Y. (1983). Malignant neuroepithelioma (peripheral neuroblastoma). A clinicopathologic study of 15 cases. *American Journal of Surgical Pathology* **7**, 309–18.

Hashimoto, H., Tsuneyoshi, M. and Enjoji, M. (1985). Malignant smooth muscle tumors of the retroperitoneum and mesentery: a clinicopathologic analysis of 44 cases. *Journal of Surgical Oncology* **28**, 177–86.

Iwashita, T. and Enjoji, M. (1987). Plexiform neurilemoma: a clinico-pathological and immunohistochemical analysis of 23 tumours from 20 patients. *Virchows Archiv A*, **441**, 305–9.

Jarvi, O. H., Saxen, A. E., Hopsu-Havu, V. K., Wartiovaara, J. J., and Vaissalo, V. T. (1969). Elastofibroma—a degenerative pseudo-tumor. *Cancer* **23**, 42–63.

Kawamoto, E. H., Weidner, N., Agostini, R. M., and Jaffe, R. (1987). Malignant ectomesenchymoma of soft tissue. Report of two cases and review of the literature. *Cancer* **59**, 1791–802.

Kindblom, L.-G., Angervall, L., and Svendsen, P. (1975). Liposarcoma. A clinicopathologic, radiographic and prognostic study. *Acta Pathologica Microbiologica Scandinavica A* Suppl. No. 253, 1–71.

Kyriakos, M. and Kempson, R. L. (1976). Inflammatory fibrous histiocytoma. An aggressive and lethal lesion. *Cancer* **37**, 1584–606.

Lack, E. E., Perez-Atayde, A. R., McGill, T. J., and Vawter, G. F. (1982). Gingival granular cell tumor of the newborn (congenital 'epulis'): Ultrastructural observations relating to histogenesis. *Human Pathology* **13**, 686–9.

Lauer, D. H. and Enzinger, F. M. (1980). Cranial fasciitis of childhood. *Cancer* **45**, 401–6.

Lieberman, P. H., Brennan, M. F., Kimmel, M., Erlandson, R. A., Garin-Chesa, P., and Flehinger, B. Y. (1989). Alveolar soft-part sarcoma. A clinico-pathologic study of half a century. *Cancer* **63**, 1–13.

Lopez, D. A., Silvers, D. N., and Helwig, E. B. (1974). Cutaneous meningiomas—a clinicopathologic study. *Cancer* **34**, 728–44.

Miettinen, M., Hockerstedt, K., Reitamo, J., and Totterman, S. (1985). Intramuscular myxoma—a clinicopathological study of twenty three cases. *American Journal of Clinical Pathology* **84**, 265–72.

Myers, B. W., Masi, A. T., and Feigenbaum, S. L. (1980). Pigmented villonodular synovitis and tenosynovitis: a clinical epidemiologic study of 166 cases and literature review. *Medicine* **59**, 223–38.

Newman, P. L. and Fletcher, C. D. M. (1991a). Smooth muscle tumours of the eternal genitalia: clinicopathological analysis of a series. *Histopathology* **18**, 523–9.

Newman, P. L. and Fletcher, C. D. M. (1991b). Malignant mesenchymoma: clinicopathologic analysis of a series with evidence of low grade behaviour. *American Journal of Surgical Pathology* **15**, 607–14.

Patchefsky, A. S. and Enzinger, F. M. (1981). Intravascular fasciitis. A report of 17 cases. *American Journal of Surgical Pathology* **5**, 29–36.

Pulitzer, D. R., Martin, P. C., and Reed, R. J. (1989). Fibroma of tendon sheath. A clinicopathologic study of 32 cases. *American Journal of Surgical Pathology* **13**, 472–9.

Purvis, W. E. and Helwig, E. B. (1954). Reticulohistiocytic granuloma ('reticulohistiocytoma') of the skin. *American Journal of Clinical Pathology* **24**, 1005–15.

Remberger, K., Krieg, T., Kunze, D., Weinmann, H.-M., and Hubner, G. (1985). Fibromatosis hyalinica multiplex (juvenile hyalin fibromatosis). Light microscopic, electron microscopic, immunohistochemical and biochemical findings. *Cancer* **56**, 614–24.

Scott, S. M., Reiman, H. M., Pritchard, D. J., and Ilstrup, D. M. (1989). Soft tissue fibrosarcoma. A clinicopathologic study of 132 cases. *Cancer* **64**, 925–31.

Shimizu, S., Hashimoto, H., and Enjoji, M. (1984). Nodular fasciitis: an analysis of 250 patients. *Pathology* **16**, 161–6.

Shmookler, B. M. and Enzinger, F. M. (1981). Pleomorphic lipoma: a benign tumor simulating liposarcoma. A clinicopathologic analysis of 48 cases. *Cancer* **47**, 126–33.

Silverman, T. A. and Enzinger, F. M. (1985). Fibrolipomatous hamartoma of nerve. A clinicopathologic analysis of 26 cases. *American Journal of Surgical Pathology* **9**, 7–14.

Sonoda, T., Hashimoto, H., and Enjoji, M. (1985). Juvenile xanthogranuloma. Clinicopathologic analysis and immunohistochemical study of 57 patients. *Cancer* **56**, 2280–6.

Sotelo-Avila, C., Gonzalez-Crussi, F., DeMello, D., Vogler, C., Gooch, W. M., Gale, G., and Pena, R. (1986). Renal and extra-renal rhabdoid tumors in children: a clinicopathologic study of 14 patients. *Seminars in Diagnostic Pathology* **3**, 151–63.

Sumiyoshi, K., Tsuneyoshi, M., and Enjoji, M. (1985). Myositis ossificans. A clinicopathologic study of 21 cases. *Acta Pathologica Japonica* **35**, 1109–22.

Theaker, J. M., Fletcher, C. D. M., and Tudway, A. J. (1990). Cutaneous heterotopic meningeal nodules: a light microscopic and immunohistochemical study. *Histopathology* **16**, 475–9.

Varela-Duran, J. and Enzinger, F. M. (1982). Calcifying synovial sarcoma. *Cancer* **50**, 345–52.

Weiss, S. W. (1982). Malignant fibrous histiocytoma. A reaffirmation. *American Journal of Surgical Pathology* **6**, 773–84.

Weiss, S. W. and Enzinger, F. M. (1977). Myxoid variant of malignant fibrous histiocytoma. *Cancer* **39**, 1672–85.

Weiss, S. W. and Enzinger, F. M. (1979). Malignant fibrous histiocytoma. An analysis of 200 cases. *Cancer* **41**, 2250–66.

Wright, P. H., Sim, F. H., Soule, E. H., and Taylor, W. F. (1982). Synovial sarcoma. *Journal of Bone and Joint Surgery* **64A**, 112–22.

Young, S. and Gonzalez-Crussi, F. (1985). Melanocytic neuroectodermal tumor of the foot. Report of a case with multicentric origin. *American Journal of Clinical Pathology* **84**, 371–8.

28

The skin

28

The skin

28.1 Normal skin, anatomical variations, and disease terminology

K. A. Fleming

It is a curious fact that despite the extreme ease in sampling and investigating skin lesions, progress towards understanding the cellular and molecular pathobiology has been relatively slow. Thus, a great many purely descriptive terms (often in dubious Latin), are still used in both the clinical and pathology literature, frequently with wild abandon, but often without contributing much insight. Accordingly, to try to minimize the confusion that this plethora of names can cause, this chapter presents skin diseases, classified in broad groups. Where relevant, it emphasizes the clinical features important in making the diagnosis and also discusses the aetiology or pathogenesis (where known). It includes a description of the important histopathological features, the differential diagnosis, and an indication of the clinical or pathological features that might support one or other diagnosis. Where relevant, an indication of what variation may occur, particularly as a result of duration, treatment, site, etc., is given.

This chapter is not intended to be a compendium of all skin diseases. The criteria for describing any lesion have included:

1. frequent occurrence;
2. important pathogenetic mechanism;
3. characteristic or unusual pathology;
4. difficult differential diagnosis;
5. treatment or management is greatly influenced by the pathology.

Since knowledge of the normal is essential before attempting to understand the abnormal, a short description of normal skin is included at the start. Also included is a description of abnormalities common to most skin diseases. Before starting on the specific disease groups, there is a brief discussion of the particular reasons why diagnosis of skin lesions can be amongst the most demanding in pathology and why clinical correlation is often paramount.

There are two layers: epidermis and dermis, beneath which is the subcutaneous fat. There are also two types of skin, hair-bearing and non-hair-bearing (glabrous), e.g. palms and soles.

28.1.1 Epidermis

This is derived from the ectoderm. It is conventionally divided into layers depending on the state of maturation (Fig. 28.1). The basal layer is that adjoining the dermis and consists of a single row of cells of columnar configuration with basal nuclei. This is the germinative cell of the epithelium. The basal cells attach to surrounding epidermal cells through desmosomes in their plasma membranes and to the dermis by hemidesmosomes (see Chapter 1.1). They contain fibrils of prekeratin tonofilaments which associate with the desmosomes. The junction zone between dermis and epidermis has three layers on electron microscopy—beneath the plasma membrane of the basal cell is the lamina lucida, then the basal lamina (lamina densa), and lastly the fibrillar zone.

Interspersed amongst the basal cells are melanocytes (derived from the neural crest), about one melanocyte for every 4–10 basal cells, depending on the site; melanocytes are more frequent on sun-exposed areas, such as the face. Melanocytes are recognized by being spherical/oval, with dendritic processes which interdigitate with surrounding epithelial cells. They have a central nucleus and clear cytoplasm, unlike the basal cells.

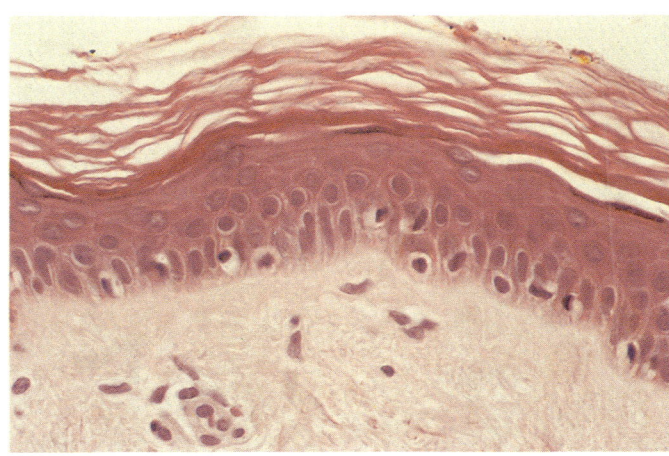

Fig. 28.1 Normal skin showing basal, prickle, and keratin layers. Note the occasional clear melanocyte scattered amongst the basal cells. The granular layer is inconspicuous in this section, which is from the arm.

Special stains, such as Masson–Fontana (a silver stain) will detect the melanin synthesized by melanocytes. Melanin is also normally found in epidermal cells, having been phagocytosed after secretion from the melanocytes. The degree of melanin pigmentation of epidermal cells varies according to race and ultraviolet exposure, amongst other factors. Ultrastructurally, melanocytes contain an almost unique cytoplasmic organelle where melanin is synthesized, the premelanosome and its derivative the melanosome.

Above the basal cells, the majority of the epidermis consists of prickle cells, so called from their tonofilamentous and desmosomal connections to surrounding cells. These are large polygonal cells with central nuclei and eosinophilic cytoplasm. Electron microscopically, the prickle cells contain many more prekeratin tonofilaments than basal cells, and they also contain a few membrane-coated granules (Odland bodies). The latter are thought to be related to the formation of the keratohyalin granules in the granular layer, where they are much more numerous. Normally, depending on the site, the prickle layer is about five cells thick. In pressure areas, e.g. elbows, palms, and soles, it is much thicker. In other areas—facial skin and forearms—it can be thinner. When the epidermal cells, particularly the prickle cells, increase in size and number compared to the normal for that site, the epidermis is said to be acanthotic (Fig. 28.2), and when they increase in number, hyperplastic. Intercellular oedema of the epidermis (spongiosis) (Fig. 28.3) is easily seen in the prickle cell layer by virtue of the residual desmosomal connections between the cells. Acantholysis (Fig. 28.4) is a rare form of disruption of the epithelium, where the desmosomal connections are destroyed as a primary event, resulting in individual separation and rounding up of the epithelial cells.

Above the prickle cells, as they further mature and begin to keratinize, the keratohyalin becomes visible as basophilic granules—hence the name granular layer. This is usually only one or two cells thick, but may be thicker (hypergranulosis) when

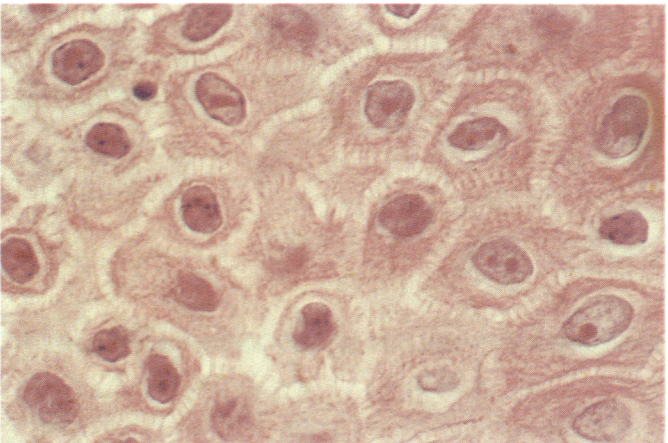

Fig. 28.3 Spongiosis. Subacute dermatitis with marked intercellular oedema (spongiosis). The intercellular connections (desmosomes) are largely intact, giving the appearance of prickle cells.

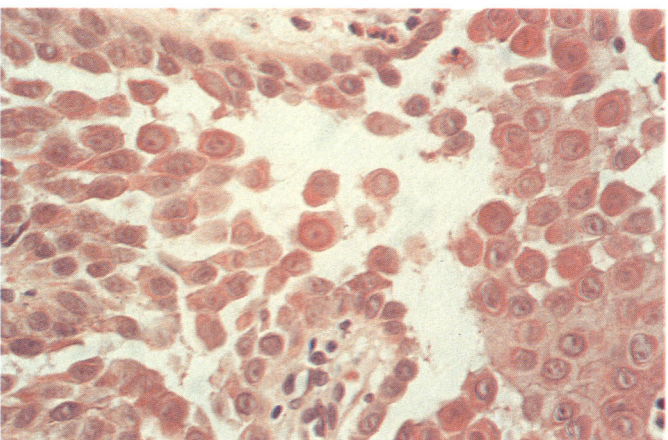

Fig. 28.4 Acantholysis. Pemphigus vulgaris with intra-epidermal blister formation due to acantholysis. In contrast to spongiosis, the cells are rounded up and dissociated from each other.

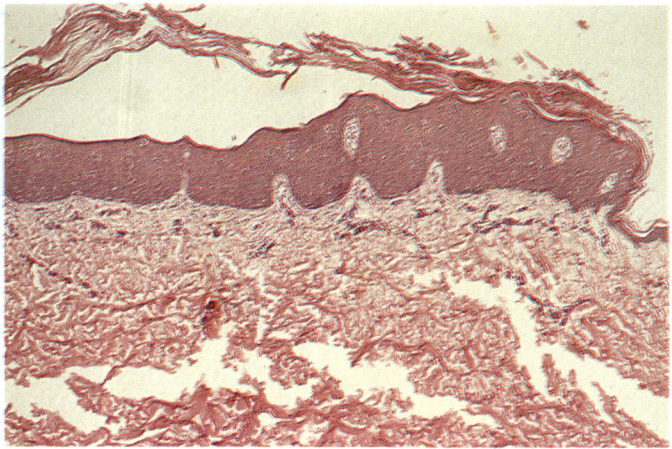

Fig. 28.2 Acanthosis. Bowen's disease of the skin, showing marked thickening (acanthosis) due to an increase in the number and size of epithelial cells. Normal epidermis is at the right-hand side.

the epithelium is hyperplastic or acanthotic. It is also normally particularly thick in areas of physiological stress, such as palms and soles, etc. The presence of a granular layer is one of the features that separates skin epithelium from mucosal epithelium, such as mouth and anus, where keratinohyalin is not formed. Keratinohyalin is also not present in the tricholemmal layer of hair follicles.

Above the granular layer is the stratum lucidum, where the nuclei have disappeared as part of normal maturation. This is only well seen in certain sites, particularly the palms and soles. The top layer of the epidermis is the keratin layer (stratum corneum) usually about the equivalent of 3–4 cells thick. This normally forms a 'basket weave' pattern since the keratin skeletal outline of the cells is all that is left. In regions of trauma and pressure the keratin layer is concentrated and thickened. In certain varieties of abnormal maturation, keratohyalin is not formed, the granular layer is absent and nuclei persist in the keratin layer—this is called parakeratosis. Hyperkeratosis is the name given to thickening of the keratin layer. If nuclei are absent, this is called orthokeratosis, as opposed to the parakeratotic epithelium, where nuclei persist.

The prickle layer also contains scattered dendritic Langerhans cells which are bone marrow derived and which probably function as antigen-presenting cells. They can be identified by a variety of histochemical and other stains, but staining for HLA class II antigens identifies them easily. They also have characteristic Birbeck (tennis-racquet) granules on ultrastructural examination. An infrequent cell found in and around the basal cells of the epithelium is the Merkel cell, recognized ultrastructurally by the presence of membrane-bound, dense-core granules. Its functional role is unclear but may be related to local neuronal interactions, particularly sensation. Its main importance is that, very rarely, it forms a tumour partially resembling, on conventional light microscopy, a basal cell carcinoma.

When maturation of the prickle cell layer is disordered (usually as part of a neoplastic process) the term dyskeratosis is used (Fig. 28.5). This is characterized by the presence of premature or abnormal keratinization of individual cells, often with mitotic figures, some of which can be abnormal. Ballooning (reticular) degeneration (Fig. 28.6) is the hallmark of viral infection of the skin and is recognized by swelling and disintegration of the cytoplasm of the infected prickle cells, the nuclei often containing inclusions. Liquefaction of the basal layer (Fig. 28.7) is characteristically seen in the lichenoid group of conditions. This term means clearing and swelling of the cytoplasm of the basal cells, with eventual loss, resulting in a clear zone between the prickle cell layer and the underlying dermis. Colloid or cytoid bodies are often associated with this lesion and probably represent apoptotic, dyskeratotic, basal cells. They are found in and around areas of basal cell liquefaction, especially in lichen planus, but are also seen in other conditions. Bullae are fluid-filled spaces in the skin greater than 1 cm diameter, vesicles being less than 1 cm in diameter. The precise site of a blister in the skin layer is of paramount diagnostic importance.

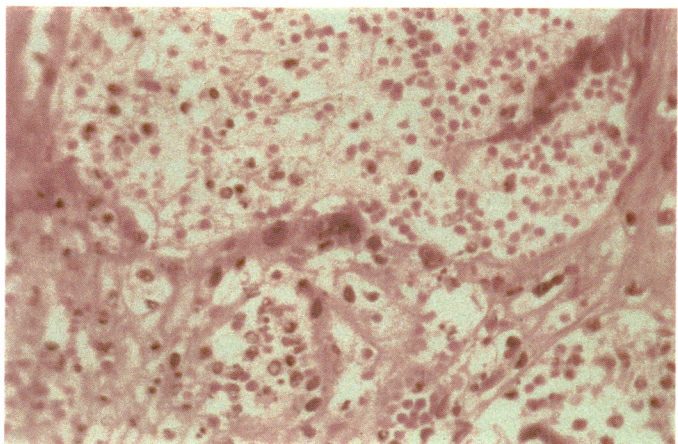

Fig. 28.6 Reticular degeneration. An intra-epidermal blister formed by the ballooning degeneration of herpes simplex infected cells. There is considerable inflammation and haemorrhage.

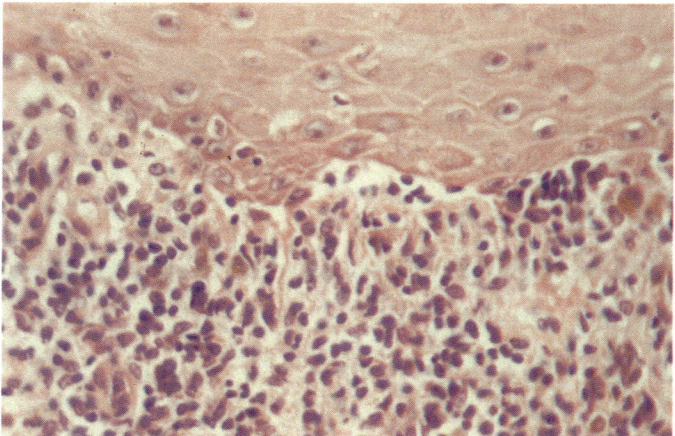

Fig. 28.7 Basal cell liquefaction. Lichen planus with liquefaction of the basal cells forming a cleft at the junction between the epidermis and the dermis. There is a dense mononuclear inflammatory infiltrate.

Microabscesses of the epidermis are seen in a variety of conditions, including the psoriasiform lesions and in mycosis fungoides. The basic lesion is a localized collection of leucocytes in the epidermis, the site and type of leucocyte being important in differentiating the causative disease.

The histology of the hair and nail is highly specialized and is dealt with in other texts.

28.1.2 Dermis

The dermis has two parts: the papillary dermis, just beneath the epithelium; and the reticular dermis, lying between the papillary dermis and the subcutaneous fat. The epithelium has downward prolongations into the dermis, called rete ridges which, by demarcating papillae in the dermal connective tissue, give the papillary dermis its name. These papillae contain loops

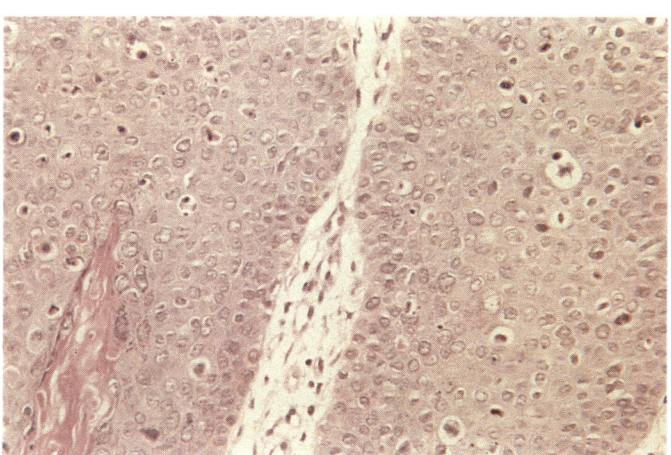

Fig. 28.5 Dyskeratosis. Note the loss of polarity of the epithelium.

of thin-walled blood vessels, nerve endings, and loose connective tissue, including elastin fibres, all of which are orientated, in general, upwards towards the epithelium. In certain diseases, the papillae are elongated and often broadened, the lesion being called papillomatosis.

Just beneath a line drawn along the tips of the rete ridges, the dermal collagen changes in orientation and structure. It becomes thicker and coarser and lies in an interweaving pattern roughly parallel to the surface epithelium. This is the reticular dermis. Scattered through this are the adnexal structures, namely hair follicles and their associated sebaceous and apocrine glands and arrectores pilorum muscles. The eccrine sweat glands are separate. Hair follicles are not found in certain sites (palms and soles), but are numerous elsewhere, being particularly numerous and large in the scalp. The sebaceous glands are also most numerous and large in the head region. In addition to the sweat glands of eccrine type, in certain areas—scalp, neck, axillae, and groins—apocrine glands become numerous. The epidermis through which the hair follicles and sweat glands pass, is called the follicular and poral epidermis, respectively. These epidermal cells do not have the same physiology as the surrounding epidermal cells and thus can sometimes be identified. The best example of this is in actinic (ultraviolet) damaged epithelium, where the intervening epidermis shows dysplastic changes early in the process; the epidermal cells of the sweat glands and hair follicles are only affected later.

28.2   Problems particular to the histopathology of skin

Histopathology of skin lesions, particularly inflammatory conditions, differs from that of other organs for several reasons.

1. Clinical observation of lesions is obviously easier, resulting in detection and biopsy of a wider range of lesions (and their stages) than might be the case elsewhere.

2. The response of the skin to a wide variety of insults is relatively limited, such that differentiation of different diseases on purely histopathological grounds may be impossible.

3. It is a very unusual patient who, having a skin lesion of sufficient concern to warrant biopsy, has not applied some medicament, either self or medically prescribed. These applications can considerably modify the appearances in a variety of ways.

4. The time between onset of the lesion and biopsy is also of importance. Many conditions only show characteristic features at a particular stage in the illness. Sampling outwith that stage can result in a non-diagnostic biopsy.

5. Trauma, either accidental or deliberate (as in scratching), can also considerably modify the appearances, due to the addition of reactive inflammatory changes.

6. The site involved can also modify the features. Unlike some internal organs, which are relatively homogenous, skin shows considerable variation in appearance, e.g. the thickness and content of adnexal structures vary with site.

7. The age of the patient and the degree of ultraviolet exposure also modify the skin. With increasing age and sun exposure, the epidermis and dermis can show marked atrophy and degenerative changes.

8. Mainly because of the ease of observation, most dermatologists do not biopsy lesions with a clinically obvious diagnosis! Therefore, biopsy tends to be carried out on lesions which are unusual in some way.

In addition to these factors, certain technical aspects of skin biopsy are important. This results from the small size of most skin biopsies, and relates to handling, preparation, and sampling. Crush artefact is as destructive to diagnostic histopathology in skin biopsies as in any tissue. However, as the tiny nature of many biopsies makes handling difficult, it is therefore more likely to be traumatized during removal, especially by inexperienced operators. Injection of local anaesthetic close to the lesion can markedly alter the histopathology and must be avoided. Accurate vertical orientation of the specimen in the laboratory is absolutely vital. It is only too easy to embed small biopsies incorrectly and a diagnosis cannot be made (Fig. 28.8). Although occasionally sectioning the biopsy at levels may retrieve the situation, more frequently no improvement is obtained. Even re-embedding the block is often unhelpful, as by the time the tissue has been refaced, no diagnostic material is left. Lastly, cutting of multiple levels is a useful routine in skin biopsies. It is surprising how frequently a non-diagnostic biopsy is converted to a diagnostic one, simply by examining multiple levels of the tissue. In our experience, skin is almost unique in this respect.

In view of all the potential problems outlined above, successful diagnosis of skin lesions demands as close clinico-histopathological collaboration as possible and optimal use of the material obtained. Even then, it may be impossible to arrive

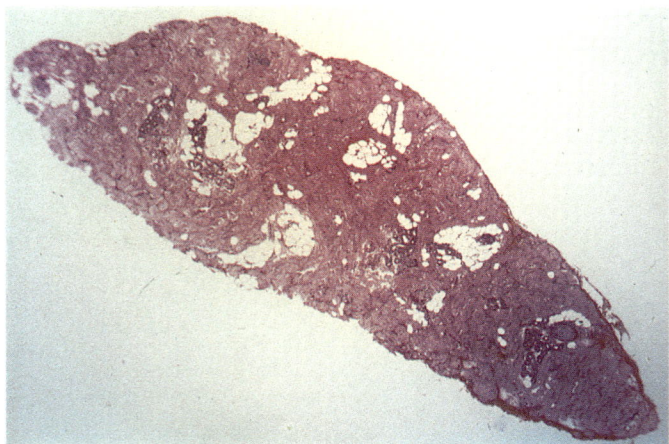

Fig. 28.8 Skin biopsy that has been poorly orientated. No epithelium is present, preventing accurate assessment of the material.

at a precise diagnosis and a differential diagnosis is all that can be given.

28.3   Hereditary lesions

There are a number of hereditary conditions which predominantly affect the skin.

28.3.1   Ichthyosis ('fish skin' disease)

This is a complex group of conditions, all characterized by generalized, non-inflammatory flaky and scaly skin. One of the major difficulties in diagnosing and understanding the group has been the many names applied to the many clinical variants, some of which, however, may not be truly separate entities. Classification on the basis of genetic linkage has imposed some order (Table 28.1). The role of the pathologist in diagnosis is limited, being restricted predominantly to excluding other conditions and occasionally confirming those few variants with distinctive histopathology.

The aetiopathogenesis of the ichthyosiform lesions is unknown. It appears to be a disorder of keratinization, although some variants are probably an abnormality of desquamation. Given the variety of clinical appearances that can be produced by different molecular defects of the same gene, e.g. the thalassaemias (see Chapter 2), it may be that there are surprisingly few genes involved in the ichthyosis complex, and that the large number of clinical and pathological variants reflects differing lesions of the same gene(s). In view of the current capabilities of molecular biology, significant insights into the pathogenesis of the ichthyosiform dermatoses may appear soon.

Bullous ichthyosiform erythrodema

Occasionally, solitary or localized lesions identical to epidermo-

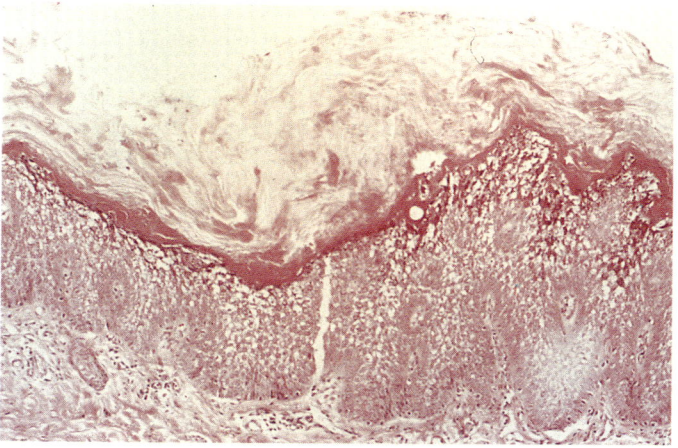

Fig. 28.9   Epidermolytic hyperkeratosis. The epithelium shows widespread vacuolation due to perinuclear degeneration of the prickle cells in the mid and upper layers of the epithelium.

lytic hyperkeratosis (bullous ichthyosiform erythrodema) are present in the skin (Fig. 28.9). These are often classified as epidermal naevi. In addition, there are a number of systemic conditions in which the cutaneous ichthyosiform lesions are only part of a more generalized disorder of ectodermal development. There are also some acquired variants of ichthyosis associated with internal malignancy and drugs. Details of these two groups of ichthyosiform dermatoses can be found in specialized dermatology textbooks (see Further reading).

28.3.2   Darier disease (follicular keratosis)

This is an uncommon autosomal dominant condition, in which warty, 'greasy', dark-brown papules are present in the skin, particularly the hands, trunk, scalp, and folds in the groins, axillae, and neck. The pathogenesis is unknown, but electron microscopy suggests a disorder of the tonofilament–desmosome complex.

Table 28.1   Classification of some of the ichthyosiform dermatoses (ichthyosis)

Type	Clinical	Histopathology
Sex-linked X-linked recessive	Present at birth; males affected; large, dark scales, shed infrequently	Prominent granular layer; acanthosis; non-specific mononuclear inflammation
Ichthyosis vulgaris autosomal dominant	Appears about 3 months; small white scales, shed continuously; 45% have atopic state; relatively common	Faint to absent granular layer; no acanthosis; mild lamellar hyperkeratosis
Epidermolytic hyperkeratosis (bullous congenital ichthyosiform erythroderma) autosomal dominant	Presents around birth; large yellow/brown flakes; occasional bullae; rare	Granular layer shows perinuclear halo; ballooning degeneration; eventual intra-epidermal blister. Some lesions show only hyperkeratosis, acanthosis and parakeratosis; levels may reveal vacuolar degeneration of granular layer
Lamellar ichthyosis autosomal recessive	Varying severity from intra-uterine death to mild erythroderma; rare	Similar to sex-linked, although the granular layer may be normal

The most striking low-power histopathological features are of papillary down-budding and of discrete, small supra-basal splits, involving predominantly the epidermis around hair follicles and sweat ducts (Fig. 28.10). Occasionally, only a very small clump of cells is involved, requiring careful scrutiny and multiple levels for accurate assessment. The clefting is the result of supra-basal acantholysis (Fig. 28.11) and the acantholytic cells show premature keratinization (dyskeratosis), giving rise to basophilic 'corps ronds'. The epidermis above the clefts is hyperkeratotic and parakeratotic. These parakeratotic cells are

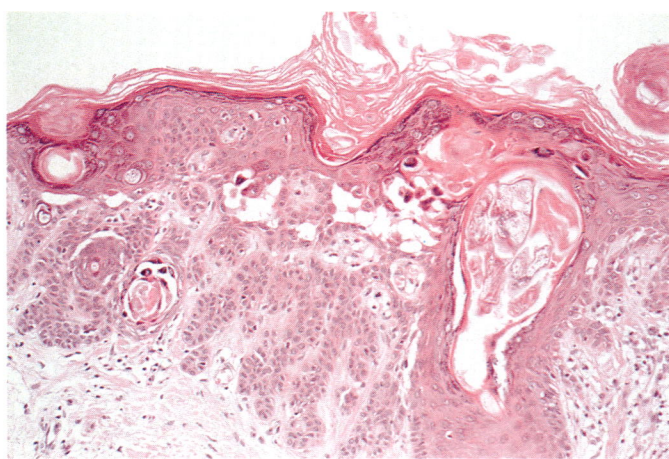

Fig. 28.10 Darier disease. There is marked hyperkeratosis, with the formation of intra-epidermal clefts.

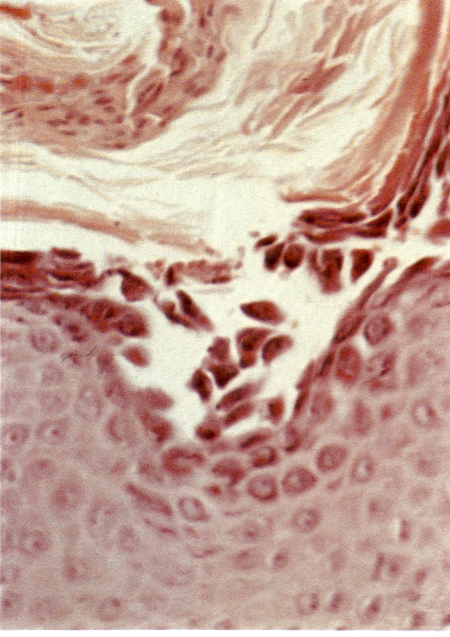

Fig. 28.11 Darier disease. The intra-epidermal cleft is formed by acantholytic basophilic cells called corps ronds. There is marked hyperkeratosis and parakeratosis (grains).

graced with the name 'grains' in Darier disease and probably represent maturing corps ronds. There may be a perivascular upper dermal mononuclear inflammatory infiltrate. Sometimes the basal down-budding becomes extremely complex and ramified and can simulate the acantholytic variants of actinic keratosis, even squamous cell carcinoma. Not infrequently, a similar picture is seen as a solitary lesion in sun-exposed skin of older patients. While it has been suggested that these may represent a 'forme fruste' of Darier disease, it is now generally held that these lesions represent abnormal keratinization resulting from actinic damage. The lesions are called warty dyskeratoma. Similarly, occasionally linear lesions, sometimes confined to one half of the body, are biopsied which show histopathological features of Darier. These probably represent epidermal naevi.

Differential diagnosis

The histopathological differential diagnosis of Darier disease is Hailey–Hailey disease, the acantholytic dermatoses, and the pemphigus group of disorders. Careful consideration of the histopathology (particularly the absence of dyskeratosis) and immunofluorescence, should provide easy delineation from the pemphigus group (see below).

Hailey–Hailey disease (benign familial chronic pemphigus)

Hailey–Hailey disease, also a hereditary condition, is more difficult to distinguish from Darier disease. The principle clue is the more extensive and uniform involvement of the epidermis in Hailey–Hailey. The upper layers of the epidermis are more often involved, giving rise to larger clefts (lacunae) in the affected epidermis (Fig. 28.12). There is much less tendency to show dyskeratotic changes and hair follicles are not involved. However, the histopathology of both conditions can be very similar. Fortunately, the clinical features of Hailey–Hailey are distinct from Darier disease, there being a recurrent vesicular and crusted eruption on the friction sites of neck, axillae, and groins. This is in contrast to Darier; there the lesions are hyperkeratotic, follicular, and predominantly affect the hands, trunk, and head region, as well as the folds. Hailey–Hailey usually develops in early adult life, unlike Darier which starts in the teens. The genesis of Hailey–Hailey is unknown, but it is an autosomal dominant condition and it may result from a defect in the tonofilament–desmosomal complex or in synthesis of intercellular matrix. Infection and trauma can precipitate and complicate lesions.

Grover disease (transient acantholytic dermatosis)

This was described in 1970. It presents as an acute eruption of discrete, flat-topped, pruritic papules, mainly on the trunk. The patients are mainly elderly, and males are more commonly affected than females. The condition normally lasts a few weeks to months, although rarely it can last over one year. This latter feature has given rise to the concept of a separate entity—persistent acantholytic dermatosis. This persistent variety has a

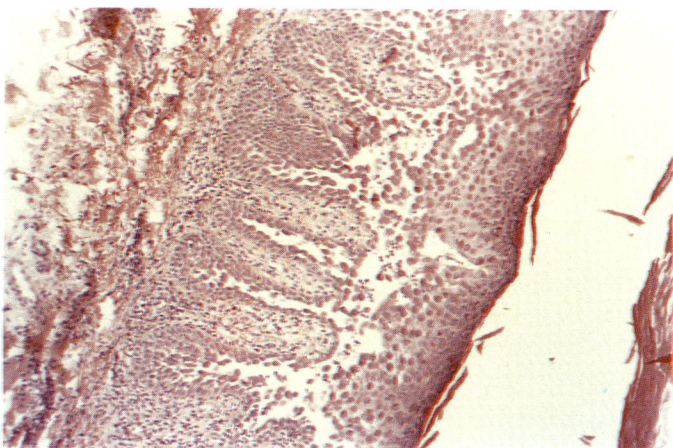

Fig. 28.12 Hailey–Hailey disease. There is a large intra-epidermal vesicle due to widespread acantholysis. This appearance is said to resemble a dilapidated brick wall.

strong association with actinic damaged skin, including skin showing actinic keratoses. Histopathologically, the lesions of acantholytic dermatoses vary and consist of a sharply demarcated intra-epidermal vesicle with features identical to either Darier and/or Hailey–Hailey and/or the pemphigus group. There is also a spongiotic variety, where intra-epidermal acantholysis and vesicle formation is associated with surrounding spongiosis. These various histopathological variants appear clinically similar, with no resemblance to the mimicked diseases. The genesis of Grover disease is unknown.

28.3.3 Epidermolysis bullosa (mechano-bullous diseases)

This is a rare and complex group of conditions, characterized by increased fragility of the skin and mucosae, with a tendency to form blisters either on relatively minor trauma or spontaneously. Like ichthyosis, there are different hereditary forms and also an acquired form. The acquired form appears to be immunologically mediated. To date, five main groups have been described, the differentiation depending on the site on the body and the site within the skin where blister formation takes place, the genetic mode of inheritance, the age of onset, and the resultant clinical picture. The features are summarized in Table 28.2. Within these groups, there are a considerable number of clinical variants, all of which have different eponyms.

On light microscopy, all the forms show blister formation at the dermo-epidermal junction, with little or no inflammation. An important characteristic of the dystrophic types is the scarring which accompanies the healing process. This can result in considerable deformity. In the simple forms, the lesion forms through the basal and supra-basal cells (cytolysis) and this feature can be identified on light microscopy (Fig. 28.13). The junctional form shows only a dermo-epidermal blister on light microscopy, while ultrastructurally the lesion is seen to form in the lamina lucida and may represent a defect of basal cell hemidesmosomes. The dystrophic variants show a blister forming in the upper papillary dermis, sometimes with dermal fragments remaining attached to the roof of the lesion. Electron microscopically, the lesion forms through the fibrillar zone of the dermo-epidermal junction. Antibodies to various components of the basement membrane zone on frozen sections (e.g. antilaminin, bullous pemphigoid sera) can help to define the site of the lesion.

28.4   Psoriasiform lesions

These are a group of conditions in which the pathological features are characterized by focal lamellar parakeratosis, regular

Table 28.2   Classification of epidermolysis bullosa

Disease	Clinical features	Site of lesion	Abnormality
Epidermolysis bullosa simplex	Autosomal dominant; whole body involvement from birth	Intrabasal cell split	Tonofilaments
Epidermolysis bullosa (hands and feet)	Autosomal dominant; delayed onset	Intrabasal cell split	Tonofilaments
Junctional epidermolysis bullosa	Autosomal recessive; present at birth	Lamina lucida of basement membrane	Hemidesmosomes
Dystrophic epidermolysis bullosa	Autosomal dominant; delayed onset. Recessive; onset from birth	Below lamina densa	Anchoring fibrils
Epidermolysis bullosa acquisita	Associated with inflammatory bowel disease, auto-immune disease, and internal malignancy	Below lamina densa	Immune-mediated disease of collagen VII in dermis, with deposition of IgG or IgM

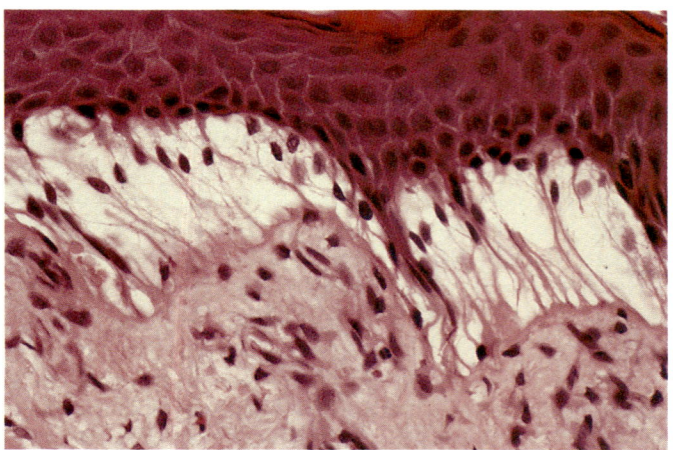

Fig. 28.13 Epidermolysis bullosa simplex. There is formation of a cleft through lysis of the basal cells. The residual basal cell nuclei are clearly visible.

acanthosis, prolongation of rete ridges, and 'squirting papillae'. The latter is a term coined by Pinkus to describe the exudation of neutrophil polymorphs and fluid from dilated thickened capillaries at the tip of papillae and emigration upwards of these polymorphs into the overlying epidermis. Often the epidermal polymorphs are few and degenerate, but occasionally they form rather larger collections amounting to microabscesses (of Munro). The differential diagnosis is of psoriasis, and its various clinical variants, of seborrhoeic dermatitis, asteatotic dermatitis, pustulosis palmaris et plantaris, Reiter's syndrome, and the rare pityriasis rubra pilaris and impetigo herpetiformis. Normally, these are easily distinguished clinically, while the histopathology is less distinct.

28.4.1 Psoriasis

Clinical features and aetiology

This is a common skin disease affecting the sexes equally and about 2 per cent of the population. It can affect children, but is predominant in adults, and typically produces pink/red, well-defined, slightly raised plaques covered by silvery scales. It is a chronic relapsing condition varying in intensity from occasional patches to involvement of all the body, including the nails, but only rarely (if at all) the mucosae. About 5 per cent of patients have an arthropathy, very similar to rheumatoid arthritis, but sero-negative. There is a well-established, but ill-defined, genetic component, with strong association with HLA-Cw6 and HLA-DR7.

There are several clinical varieties, e.g. guttate, pustular, flexural, erythrodermic. Histopathologically, the appearances of these variants, apart from pustular, are essentially similar. Psoriasis can occur at the site of trauma—Koebner phenomena.

The aetiology has been the subject of a vast amount of research, but is still unknown. There is undoubtedly a great disturbance in the growth kinetics of the epithelial cells; increased production of new epidermal cells, probably in excess of 20 times normal, increased mitotic index, and shortened epidermal transit time (56 days reduced to 7 days). There is also decreased cyclic AMP which regulates cell proliferation, and increased inflammatory mediators such as arachidonic acid. However, some of these features are found in uninvolved skin. Inevitably there are immunological abnormalities, such as increased numbers of cells expressing HLA class II antigens, with increased release of cytokines. However, the basic defect remains obscure.

Histopathology

There are changes in the epidermis and dermis. In the fully developed lesion (Fig. 28.14) the epidermis is thickened due to a combination of increased cell number and size (acanthosis). This acanthosis tends to be quite regular and principally manifests as elongated rete ridges with bulbous tips and with thinning of the suprapapillary epithelium. Not infrequently, these ridges fuse to give a more complex picture. The granular layer is lost with prominent parakeratosis, usually forming large, layered patches. In and around the thinned suprapapillary epithelium, there are often degenerate neutrophil polymorphs (PMLs) representing the squirting papillae (Fig. 28.15). The PMLs can be found in all layers of the epithelium and may occasionally form the microabscess of Munro (Fig. 28.16). Marked spongiosis is not a feature. The dermis characteristically contains a mild to moderate perivascular inflammatory infiltrate of lymphocytes and macrophages in the upper dermis, except in the squirting papillae, where occasional PMLs are seen. Excessive inflammation, or presence of large numbers of

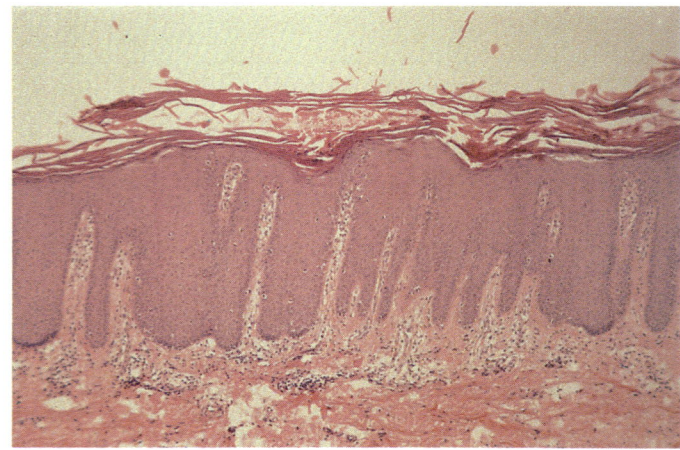

Fig. 28.14 Chronic psoriasis. There is lamellar hyper- and parakeratosis with marked acanthosis of the epithelium. This acanthosis has resulted in fusion of some of the rete ridges.

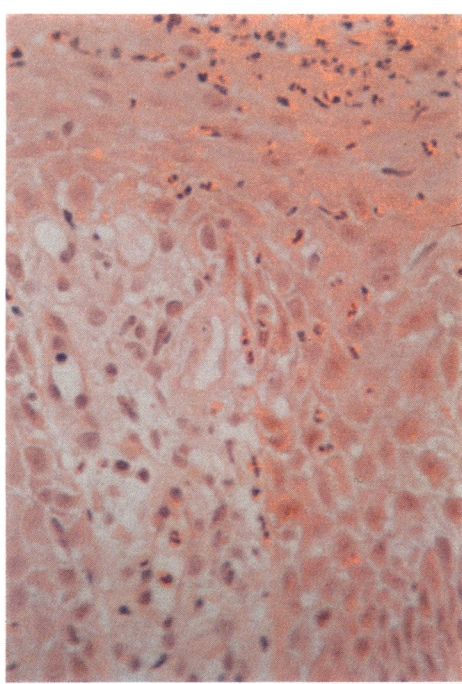

Fig. 28.15 Acute psoriasis. A dermal papilla showing dilation of capillaries and emigration of polymorphs upwards into the epithelium.

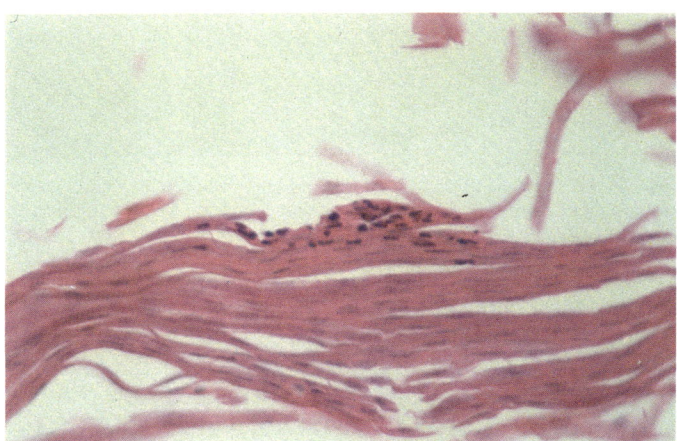

Fig. 28.16 Psoriasis. A localized collection of neutrophil polymorphs in an area of parakeratosis (microabscess of Munro).

plasma cells, should cast doubt on the diagnosis of psoriasis. In papillae, there is often a prominent capillary loop, the prominence being due to a combination of dilatation and apparent increased thickness of the wall.

In contrast to the fully developed lesion, the earliest change in psoriasis is in the dermis, namely oedema and mononuclear inflammation around dilated capillaries in the papillae. The mononuclear cells emigrate into the epidermis and are associated with loss of the granular layer and parakeratosis. PMLs

appear later to give the classic 'squirting' papillae. These changes typically are cyclical in nature, being repeated several times, and manifesting as the presence of multiple Munro's abscesses in the same area of epidermis.

Pustular psoriasis is a state where there appears to be more acute psoriasis with formation of sterile pustules. Clinically there are localized forms (confined mainly to the hands and feet) and generalized forms. Microscopy shows large collections of neutrophil PMLs in the upper epithelium, with the residual epithelium having a spongiform appearance (spongiform pustule of Kogoj). The surrounding epithelium will show some or all of the other features of psoriasis. Lesions confined to the palms and soles of feet without other signs of psoriasis, either clinically or microscopically, are called palmoplantar pustulosis, a condition of unknown aetiology. Acute pustular psoriasis occurring in pregnancy is called impetigo herpetiformis.

Differential diagnosis

Seborrhoeic dermatitis is a condition of scaly skin which affects predominately the scalp, axillae, and groins. It is very common, affecting either infants or adults. The aetiology is unknown and it runs a chronic relapsing and remitting course. Microscopy shows a combination of psoriasiform and dermatitic features, e.g. spongiosis. The latter is not found in psoriasis except where some topical application has caused a dermatitic reaction, a not uncommon event. Reiter syndrome (urethritis, conjunctivitis, and arthritis) can affect the skin and mimic psoriasis on microscopy. However, it is clinically distinct and rare. Occasionally patients present with a clinically and microscopically atypical psoriasis. In these cases, the possibility of drug-induced psoriasis or a psoriasiform drug reaction must be considered. There are no diagnostic features, but an unusually dense inflammatory component is a suggestive feature. Drugs that produce these reactions include methyldopa and beta-blockers, such as practolol. The latter produces marked fibrosis, a feature not found in conventional psoriasis. Occasionally, lichen simplex chronicus (chronic dermatitis) resembles psoriasis clinically, but the histopathology is distinct (see Section 28.6). The differential diagnosis of the pustular psoriasis lesions is of impetigo infectiosum and subcorneal pustular dermatosis (see below).

28.5　Lichenoid lesions

The prototype of this group of conditions is lichen planus. The hallmark is basal cell liquefaction and a 'band-like' chronic inflammatory infiltrate in the papillary dermis. There are other conditions that can show these features. These include lichen nitidus, graft versus host disease (GVHD), poikilodermatous lesions, lupus erythematosus (LE), dermatomyositis, some actinic keratoses, and lichen sclerosus (balanitis xerotica). Occasionally resolving melanocytic lesions can show basal cell liquefaction, which can cause diagnostic problems. Certain drug eruptions can mimic lichen planus. Lichen amyloid and erythema dyschromicum are unusual lesions that also occasionally show basal cell liquefaction.

28.5.1   Lichen planus

Clinical features and aetiology

The classical clinical features of lichen planus are of an intensely itching, papular rash which persists for months to a couple of years, before healing spontaneously to leave deeply pigmented patches. The rash is papular, often very small, and typically is violaceous in colour. Wickham's striae are white lines or dots on the surface of the shiny flat papule. Papules can appear along scratch marks (Koebner phenomenon) and occasionally an annular rash is found (especially on the penis). Spiny lesions, arising around hair follicles, are occasionally seen.

The disease is world-wide and relatively common. It typically affects young to middle-aged adults and the sexes equally. Any part of the body can be involved, including any mucous membrane (70 per cent of cases), nails, and hair, but the flexor surfaces (front of the wrists and around the ankles), lumbar region, and mouth are commonest.

There are several clinical varieties which have histopathological counterparts. These include hypertrophic, atrophic, bullous, follicular (lichen planopilaris), and annular lichen planus.

The cause of lichen planus is unknown. While a viral aetiology has been suggested, current speculation centres on immune mechanisms. Immunofluorescence reveals IgM deposits in spotty patches in the basal layer, often in degenerate eosinophilic cells called colloid or Civatte bodies. There are also increased Langerhans cells in the epidermis early in the lesions, and T-cells in the inflammatory infiltrate. One possible pathogenesis is that antigen is presented to the epidermis, processed by Langerhans cells, resulting in some way in T-cell cytotoxicity against epidermal cells, similar to GVHD.

Histopathology

The histopathology is characteristic. The diagnostic feature is basal cell liquefaction (see Fig. 28.7). In addition, the keratin layer is thickened, there being orthokeratosis, and rarely parakeratosis. Indeed, the presence of parakeratosis should cast doubt on the diagnosis. However, occasionally parakeratosis is seen if there is superimposed infection or scratching. The epithelium is thickened, this acanthosis typically being irregular, giving rise to a 'saw-tooth' appearance (Fig. 28.17). The granular layer is also more prominent in an irregular fashion, like the irregular acanthosis. As mentioned above, the most characteristic finding is of basal cell liquefaction, often of considerable length and prominence in contrast to the basal cell liquefaction found in other conditions, such as LE. These are also occasional

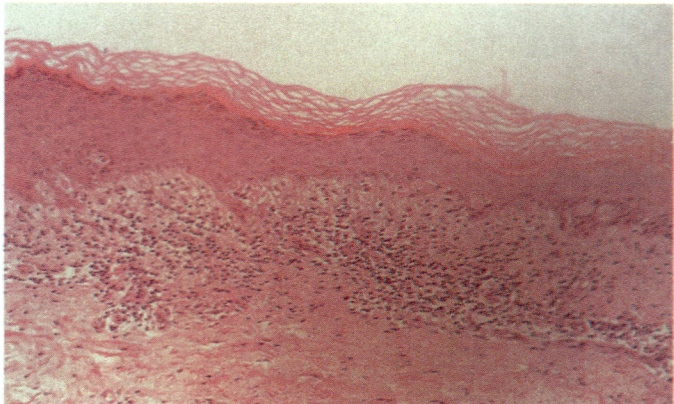

Fig. 28.17   Lichen planus. The epithelium shows focal hypergranularity and acanthosis (saw-toothed epithelium). There is a chronic inflammatory infiltrate occupying the papillary and upper reticular dermis.

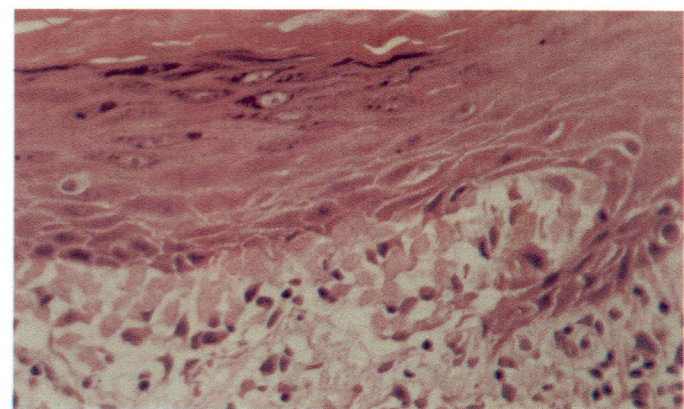

Fig. 28.18   Lichen planus. Marked basal cell liquefaction with localized collections of colloid (Civatte) bodies. Note the focal hypergranularity of the epithelium.

apoptotic basal/prickle cells (Fig. 28.18) which are eosinophilic (colloid or Civatte bodies). Colloid bodies are normally infrequent, but occasionally clumps (sometimes in the papillary dermis) are seen. Another characteristic feature is a dense mononuclear inflammatory infiltrate confined essentially to the papillary dermis, usually in a continuous band beneath the abnormal epidermis. Plasma cells are very infrequent, as are polymorphs. The presence of any substantial inflammatory infiltrate in the reticular dermis should cast doubt on the diagnosis.

The picture can be modified in a variety of ways. As the age of the lesion increases, the inflammatory infiltrate decreases and becomes patchy in the papillary dermis. Released melanin from damaged basal cells is ingested by macrophages to form melanophages. This incontinence of pigment can occasionally become very prominent. The epidermis also tends to thin, as opposed to the acanthosis of the acute lesion.

The clinical variants show associated histopathological variation. In the bullous variety, the basal cell liquefaction becomes sufficiently marked and continuous to allow the epidermis to separate from the dermis. In the hypertrophic variant, there is an unusual degree of thickening of the epidermis, often with relatively little inflammation. This is often clinically a solitary lesion. As mentioned above, atrophy is seen in older lesions, and in lichen planopilaris the changes are predominant in and around hair follicles, resulting in follicular plugging with keratin. Destruction of hair follicles leads to scarring alopecia (see below).

Differential diagnosis

The differential microscopic diagnosis is that given at the beginning of this section. Lupus erythematosus does not normally show the irregular acanthosis and the relatively prominent and continuous basal cell liquefaction of lichen planus. Also, in lupus erythematosus, there is prominent follicular plugging and characteristic patchy, solid, mononuclear inflammatory infiltrate scattered through the dermis, often quite deep. In actinic keratosis, the presence of dysplasia and basal cell down-budding is usually enough to separate the two conditions. In dermatomyositis and poikilodermatous reactions, the epithelium is often atrophic, inflammation is sparse and colloid bodies are not seen. Drug-induced lichenoid reactions can mimic lichen planus exactly, but occasionally the presence of parakeratosis, spongiosis, and patchy inflammation suggest the possibility of a drug-induced lesion. The commonest drugs include gold, and mepacrine. Colour-film developers can cause a similar reaction.

Lichen nitidus

This is a rare condition which is histopathologically similar to lichen planus. In addition, clinically the lesions show some overlap, except that the lesions of lichen nitidus remain as papules, with little or no tendency to coalesce. The main differential features are the extremely small size of the lesion, the sharply demarcated configuration, the frequent presence of parakeratosis, and the granulomatous nature of the inflammatory infiltrate, none of which are found in lichen planus.

Graft versus host disease

This occurs in two variants—acute and chronic. In the acute phase, there is focal basal cell liquefaction and associated sparse mononuclear inflammation at the dermo-epidermal junction. Colloid bodies can be seen. The chronic variant of GVHD can mimic lichen planus very closely, except the changes are more focal and less dense. Eosinophils may be prominent, while fibrosis is a late manifestation. This can result in a systemic sclerosis-like picture.

Poikilodermatous reactions

This is not a disease, but a group of conditions characterized clinically by atrophy, depigmentation, and telangiectasia. The histological features are of epidermal atrophy, focal (often insignificant) basal cell liquefaction, melanin incontinence, and patchy, sparse mononuclear inflammation. This inflammation is not solely confined to the papillary dermis and there is associated vascular dilation. The main differential diagnosis in adults is dermatomyositis, lupus erythematosus, systemic sclerosis, the pre-mycotic phase of mycosis fungoides, drug reactions, and radiation dermatis. The rarer congenital and/or hereditary forms show similar features.

28.6 Dermatitic (eczematous) lesions

The term dermatitis is one of the most misused in dermatopathology, for a variety of reasons. The name is often used by pathologists to describe any inflammation in the skin. However, this is incorrect and the term should be restricted to a specific type of epidermal reaction characterized by a mixture of focal parakeratosis, hyperkeratosis, acanthosis, and, most importantly, spongiosis. Part of the histopathologist's confusion also arises from the large number of clinical entities that include 'dermatitis' in their names. These range from atopic and endogenous dermatites, through primary irritant and sensitization forms, to exfoliatitive dermatitis, seborrhoeic dermatitis, stasis dermatitis, radiodermatitis, and dermatitis herpetiformis. Restricting the definition of a dermatitic reaction to the strict histopathological criteria above, allows simple classification into acute, subacute, and chronic varieties. Having done this, unfortunately, it is impossible and fruitless to attempt to identify histopathologically the specific clinical entities underlying the reaction. Furthermore, dermatitic reactions are not infrequently complicated by superimposed features of scratching and/or infection, and can also be modified by therapy. This, again, can lead to confusion and difficulty in diagnosis. Thus, the correct diagnosis of dermatitis reactions is yet another example of the absolute necessity of clinico-pathological correlation in dermatopathology. Dermatitis is synonymous with eczema.

28.6.1 Acute and subacute reactions

Clinical features

The two major types of acute and subacute dermatitic reactions are endogenous dermatites, particularly atopic dermatitis and all its variants (asteatotic and nummular dermatitis), and exogenous dermatites, particularly primary irritant and allergic contact dermatitis and all their variants. The clinical features of these extremely common conditions are protean and can be complex. They are illustrated in dermatology textbooks.

The prevalence of dermatitis and its variants is extremely difficult to estimate, but it undoubtedly accounts for a large amount of skin disease. For instance, it has been estimated that around 2 per cent of the population suffer from some form of dermatitis at any one time. Clinically, an acute dermatitic reaction shows erythema and vesiculation of the skin. The vesicles rupture easily or are scratched and a weeping phase occurs. As the lesion subsides, the vesicular phase starts to settle, the exudate reduces, and crusting occurs. This is the subacute phase.

With further resolution, the damaged epithelium flakes off to give a scaly phase. If the lesion persists, either due to inadequate treatment, continued exposure to the aetiological agent, or as a result of habitual rubbing or scratching, the epidermis thickens, resulting in a clinical appearance of exaggerated skin markings. This is chronic dermatitis, and as the skin is said to resemble the bark of a tree overgrown with lichens, it is described as lichenification. Note that this has nothing to do with lichenoid reactions, e.g. lichen planus, which is another source of confusion.

Histopathology

It is extremely rare to see a pure acute dermatitic reaction unless a patch test is biopsied. Normally the appearances are a mixture of acute and subacute dermatitis with parakeratosis, spongiosis, acanthosis, and mononuclear inflammation. All of these features are focal (Fig. 28.19). This focality is characteristic of a dermatitic reaction, and in its absence, the diagnosis should be reconsidered.

The first abnormality seen in an acute dermatitic reaction is inter- and intracellular oedema of the prickle cell layer. As this develops, the intercellular oedema enlarges to form intra-epidermal vesicles (Fig. 28.20), in which the damaged epithelial cells often line up vertically. The desmosomes are the last part of the cells to disassociate, so allowing visualization of the characteristic prickles. As the maturation of the epithelium is eventually disturbed by the damage to the prickle cells, keratinization becomes abnormal, resulting in parakeratosis. From experiments with patch tests (allergic contact dermatitis), it is clear that this lesion is generated by Langerhans cells interacting with antigen, releasing cytokines causing vasodilation, and recruiting mononuclear inflammatory cells into the epidermis. However, these epidermal inflammatory cells can be strikingly few in number, considering the extent of the epidermal disorder. They include lymphocytes and macrophages, with variable numbers of eosinophils. Plasma cells are very infrequent. The infiltrate in the dermis is characteristically perivascular. It is often confined to the papillary and upper reticular dermis.

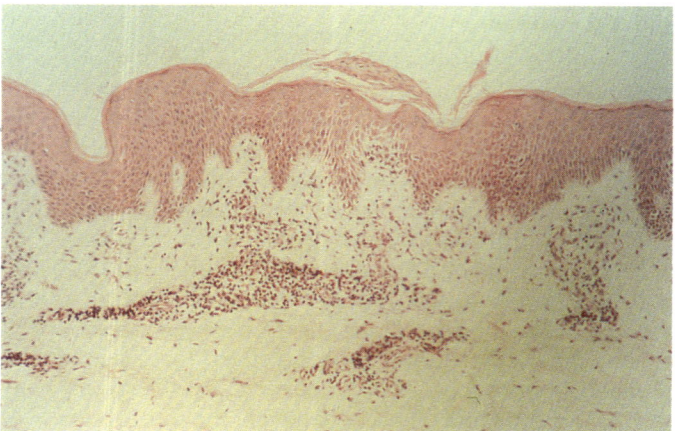

Fig. 28.19 Subacute dermatitis. There is focal parakeratosis overlying an area of intra-epidermal vesicle formation. The epithelium is acanthotic and there is a perivascular inflammatory infiltrate in the upper dermis.

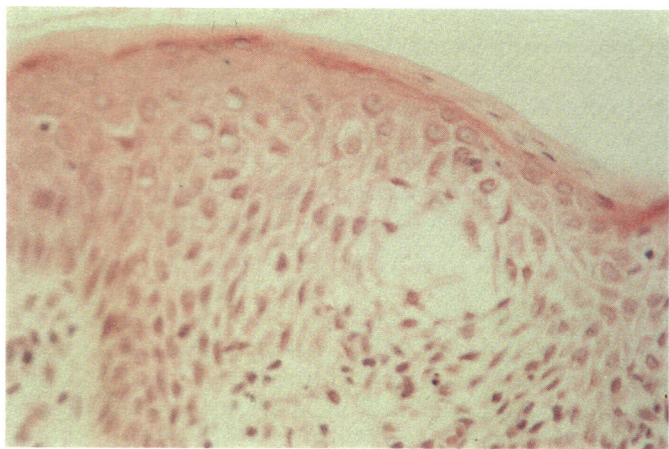

Fig. 28.20 Subacute dermatitis. An intra-epidermal blister formed by spongiosis. There is a small amount of parakeratosis present, but only occasional mononuclear inflammatory cells.

The mechanism by which a dermatitic reaction is generated in other types of dermatitis is unclear. In acute lesions, vesicles form under the keratin layer, but eventually rupture on to the surface. This produces the clinical weeping lesion. As the lesion ages, parakeratosis and acanthosis become prominent and clinically a crusting lesion appears where serum coagulates on the epithelium. This has a characteristic appearance, being a mixture of eosinophilic plasma protein, parakeratosis, and degenerate epidermal inflammatory cells. It is strikingly focal and has residual spongiosis in the surrounding epidermis. As the dermatitis itches, scratch marks are often superimposed. These can have an identical appearance to the crusted lesion. Not infrequently there is infection. This is suggested by a larger than usual inflammatory component, often with neutrophil polymorphs.

Differential diagnosis

The histopathological differential diagnosis of an acute/subacute dermatitic reaction, apart from the endogenous and exogenous dermatites, is pityriasis rosea, superficial fungal infections, pre-mycosis fungoides, pityriasis lichenoides, seborrhoeic dermatitis, papular urticaria, and drug reactions, especially photosensitization reactions. In addition, any skin condition that causes itching can have scratch marks and/or infection superimposed. If the biopsy is taken from an area including such scratch changes, with little or no features of the underlying condition, this can result in misdiagnosis of a dermatitic reaction. Furthermore, it must be remembered that any skin condition is liable to have been subjected to a large variety of medicaments, so that superimposed sensitization to these not infrequently appears. This can lead to a histopathological diagnosis of dermatitis, if the pre-existing lesion is missed or not adequately represented in the biopsy.

Pityriasis rosea is essentially identical to a dermatitic reaction and requires clinical differentiation. A superficial fungal infection usually has minimal epidermal involvement; thus, in any mild dermatitic lesion, relevant stains for fungus can be helpful. Pre-mycosis fungoides should only be diagnosed in the appropriate clinical situation and when there are 'suspicious' mononuclear cells present. Pityriasis lichenoides usually has a more florid dermal inflammatory component and clinical information should be helpful. Seborrhoeic dermatitis can occasionally cause confusion, but it will normally show squirting papillae and Munro's microabscess, as in psoriasis. Clinically it is distinct. The papular urticarias will only cause problems in later lesions where scratching and/or infection can cause spongiosis and parakeratosis. Unfortunately, drug reactions can often cause a dermatitic reaction which is not distinguishable from other forms of dermatitis. Accordingly, this cause should always be considered, if only for exclusion.

28.6.2 Chronic dermatitic reactions

The major clinical entities of a chronic dermatitic histopathological picture are the chronic phases of acute/subacute lesions, any chronic rubbing, as in prurigo nodularis, Picker's nodule, lichen simplex chronicus, and chronic neurodermatitis. The appearances of chronic dermatitis or lichenification are in striking contrast to the acute/subacute dermatites. The characteristic and principal feature is of parakeratosis and acanthosis, with little spongiosis. Focality is also less striking. The acanthosis can be either irregular or regular, and is often marked (Fig. 28.21). There is a variable inflammatory infiltrate of similar nature to that of the acute dermatitis. Occasionally the papillary dermis shows some fibrosis, particularly in severe and prolonged chronic dermatitis.

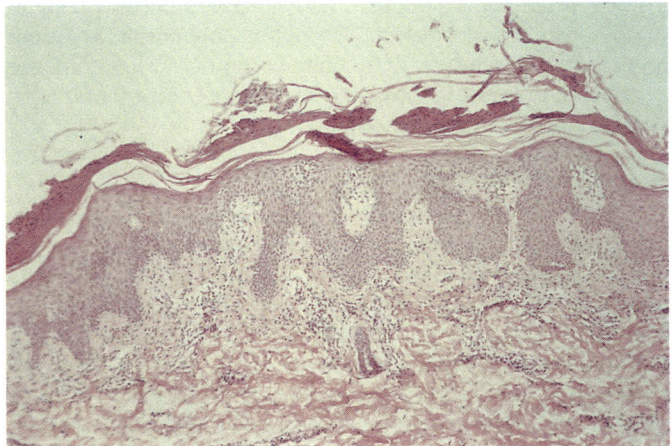

Fig. 28.21 Chronic dermatitis. The epithelium shows marked thickening (acanthosis) with associated hyperkeratosis.

The differential diagnosis is of psoriasis, epidermal naevi, and some variants of ichthyosis. The cause of a chronic dermatitic reaction is impossible to determine on histological examination alone and requires clinical information.

28.7 Blistering eruptions/pemphigus disorders

Blistering occurs not uncommonly in acute dermatitic reactions and as a complication of a variety of conditions, such as impetigo, drug reactions, and insect bites. However, primary blistering disorders are relatively uncommon.

For classification, it is convenient to group the lesions according to the microanatomical site in the skin involved, i.e. intraepidermal, subepidermal. Several of the blistering diseases have an auto-immune component and, indeed, the principle use of immunofluorescence in the skin is in the investigation of blisters. Of all skin diseases, biopsy of an early lesion is paramount in diagnosis of blisters. If necessary, the patient should be admitted to permit biopsy of a lesion within 12 hours of its appearance. After this, regenerative and secondary inflammatory changes lead to loss of the diagnostic features.

The pemphigus disorders are an interrelated group of lesions in which blisters involve the epidermis and are characterized by acantholysis, i.e. separation of epithelial cells from each other, through loss of intercellular substances and disruption of the desmosomes. This results in individually separated, smooth-surfaced epidermal cells.

Two types of pemphigus are recognized. Pemphigus foliaceus with its variant, Fogo Selvagem, and pemphigus vulgaris with its variant, pemphigus vegetans. They have in common the presence of an antibody in the serum to squamous epithelial intercellular substance, which is also found *in situ*.

28.7.1 Pemphigus foliaceus

Clinical features

This is uncommon in the UK, but a variant called Fogo Selvagem is seen in epidemic and endemic form in South America (Brazil) and is thought to be due to an infectious agent. The patients are usually young to middle-aged, but it can affect children. The rash is usually localized, predominantly on the face, scalp, and upper trunk, especially the seborrhoeic areas. Small flaccid bullae may be found, but often only scaly, crusting lesions are present. The lesions may spread slowly to involve the whole body, giving an erythroderma with the appearance of exfoliative dermatitis. The disease is relatively benign with a remitting course.

A condition with similarities, called Senear–Usher syndrome or pemphigus erythematosus, has clinical features both of pemphigus foliaceus and lupus erythematosus, namely an erythematous rash, with butterfly distribution in the face, and presence of antinuclear antibodies in the serum. While this disease was originally classified as a variant of pemphigus foliaceus, it is now regarded as a separate entity. Interestingly, the patient's serum contains antibodies both to the intercellular antigen of the pemphigus group of diseases and to the basement membrane antigen of lupus erythematosus.

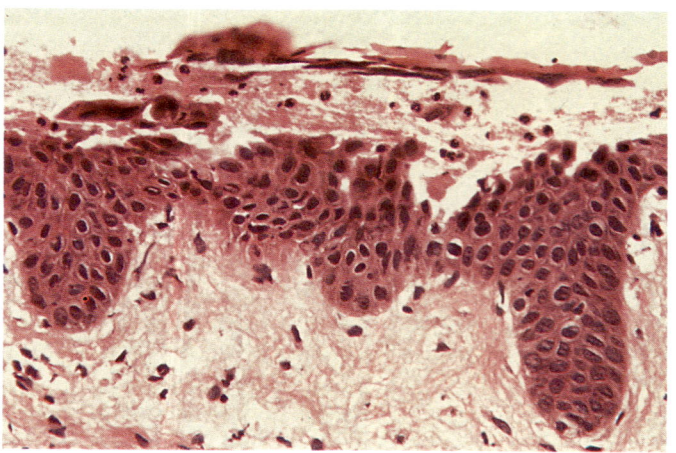

Fig. 28.22 Pemphigus foliaceus. An upper epidermal cleft due to acantholysis.

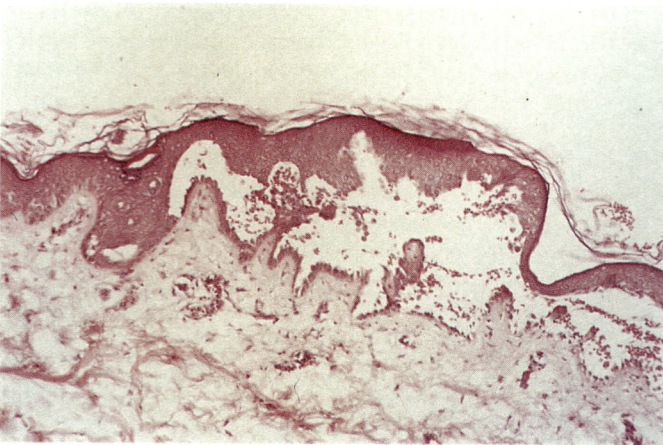

Fig. 28.23 Pemphigus vulgaris. There is a large intra-epidermal cleft formed in the supra-basal region. The rest of the epidermis and dermis appears remarkably normal.

Histopathology

All of these disorders are characterized by acantholysis in the upper epidermis just within the stratum granulosum or corneum (Fig. 28.22). Usually there is only a small blister or, indeed, often no discrete blister and the only visible change is an irregular, ill-defined cleft formed by occasional acantholytic cells in the stratum corneum. There may be parakeratosis and dyskeratosis. The lesions are usually very small and rather easy to miss. The dermis is uninvolved and there is no inflammation of note.

28.7.2 Pemphigus vulgaris

Clinical features

This is a relatively uncommon disease of world-wide distribution. It is a disease of the middle-aged, equally distributed amongst the sexes, with an apparent increased susceptibility amongst Jews. The disease often starts with oral mucosal lesions some months before skin lesions. These are characteristically painful and often denuded; the latter presumably because of trauma. In the skin, the early appearances are somewhat similar with flaccid, fragile, blisters which tear easily leaving bleeding, denuded, painful erosions. This gives a crusted, impetiginous appearance. Some months after onset, the lesions spread with generalized eruption of flaccid blisters. Nikolsky's sign on unaffected skin is positive, i.e. sliding pressure applied by a finger leads to separation of the epidermis. Before the advent of corticosteroids, this disease was virtually always fatal in a year or so.

Histopathology

There is acantholysis (see Fig. 28.4) of the supra-basal region of the epidermis. This leads to blister formation. This is in contrast to the lesions of pemphigus foliaceus and erythematosus which affect the upper epidermis. The lesions usually form a distinct, large gap in the epidermis, the roof of which is formed by the

ragged edges of the unaffected overlying epithelium (Fig. 28.23). The basal cells are left in place as a relatively regular row, but occasionally the basal cells lift off into the blister. If denudation occurs, then serum crusting, parakeratosis, and even secondary infection are present. There is normally little or no inflammation, either in the blister or the dermis. The blister can extend into the surrounding epidermis as a supra-basal cleft.

Eosinophilic spongiosis

An unusual variant is eosinophilic spongiosis. This appears to arise as a preclefting lesion in some cases of pemphigus vulgaris. There is prominent spongiosis, with a dense infiltrate of inflammatory cells in the epidermis. Eosinophil polymorphs are prominent, but not exclusive, with other mononuclear inflammatory cells being present. Eosinophilic spongiosis is also found as an early lesion in bullous pemphigoid.

Pemphigus vegetans

This is a variant of pemphigus vulgaris in which the epidermis shows hyperkeratosis and marked papillary prolongation, particularly down hair shafts and sweat glands, with often a dense localized collection of eosinophils and mononuclear inflammatory cells. The dermis becomes involved in the same type of inflammatory infiltrate. Lesions arise particularly in the groins, axillae, and flexures and are often seen in patients with pemphigus vulgaris on steroid treatment. It has been suggested that it represents pemphigus vulgaris in a patient with a greater resistance to the disease. Clinically the lesions are granular, raw-looking, and have a warty appearance on progression.

Differential diagnosis

There are several other diseases that must be considered in the differential diagnosis of intra-epithelial blisters. Hereditary conditions, including Darier and Hailey–Hailey disease (benign familial chronic pemphigus), infections such as impetigo and certain viruses, dermatitic reactions, drug reactions, pustular psoriasis, Reiter syndrome, and subcorneal pustular dermatosis (Sneddon–Wilkinson disease). One of the variants of Grover disease is identical to pemphigus (see earlier). Most of these (except Sneddon–Wilkinson disease) are dealt with in other parts of this chapter.

Pathogenesis of pemphigus disorders

One of the major advances in the understanding of aetiology and pathogenesis of skin conditions in the past 20 years has been the recognition of auto-antibodies in a variety of skin conditions, particularly the blistering eruptions.

In pemphigus, there is a circulating IgG antibody to intercellular substances of squamous epithelia. This antibody can be detected by applying patient's serum to frozen sections of mucosal squamous epithelia, e.g. guinea-pig lip mucosa, and detecting bound human antibody with fluorescent- (Fig. 28.24) or perioxidase-labelled antibodies to human immunoglobulins. Direct testing of frozen sections of the patient's skin taken from within or beside a blister, show bound immunoglobulin and complement (C3) in the intercellular areas.

In pemphigus vulgaris and vegetans, bound antibody is localized predominantly in the basal layers, while the upper layers are involved in pemphigus foliaceus and erythematosus. The titre of the serum auto-antibody reflects clinical activity. These features suggest strongly that the auto-antibody is causative in the genesis of blisters, probably in conjunction with complement or protease activation. The target antigen has not been identified, but it appears to be in the intercellular material, per-

haps an intercellular adhesion molecule, rather than tonofilaments or desmosomes. By election microscopy, the intercellular substance shows the first changes of degradation and vacuolation, while the tonofilaments and desmosomes are affected later. Development of the antibody is not unique to pemphigus as it can be detected in D-penicillamine-induced pemphigus foliaceus.

28.7.3 Subcorneal pustular dermatosis (Sneddon–Wilkinson dermatosis)

Clinical features and pathogenesis

This is a rare disease of middle-aged women. It runs a chronic relapsing, but eventually benign, course. The disease presents as a pustular rash of acute onset with a mild surrounding erythema, often in the axillae and groins, but sparing mucosae. These lesions occur in groups and the patients are afebrile. After a few days, the pustules dry up to leave a flaky crust. There is then a quiescent phase, followed by another wave of pustules. No organisms have been isolated and no auto-antibodies have been detected. At present, the genesis is unknown. After some years, spontaneous resolution occurs.

Histopathology

There is formation of a pustule of neutrophil polymorphs in a subcorneal location. No spongiosis or acantholysis is seen in typical cases. The roof is quite sturdy and not often lost. The blisters are often large and, curiously, despite the quite dense accumulation of polymorphs in the pustule, the underlying and surrounding epidermis shows relatively little inflammation. However, the dermis is quite often inflamed with neutrophil polymorphs and mononuclear inflammatory cells.

Differential diagnosis

The histopathological differential diagnosis is of impetigo infectiosum, pustular psoriasis, Reiter syndrome, impetigo herpetiformis, and seborrhoeic dermatitis. Impetigo infectiosum can be identical, but the clinical features and microbiological culture should prevent confusion. Of the others, a combination of the clinical and histopathological features should allow differentiation. These features are described elsewhere in this chapter. As acantholysis can occur in late lesions, this can cause confusion with pemphigus foliaceus.

28.7.4 Toxic epidermal necrolysis— scalded-skin syndrome

There has been some confusion in the classification of this condition. There appear to be two types of processes that give rise to the clinical appearance of scalded skin.

Lyell/Ritter disease

This is a disease of infants and young children who suddenly develop sloughing skin in the fold regions. It usually follows

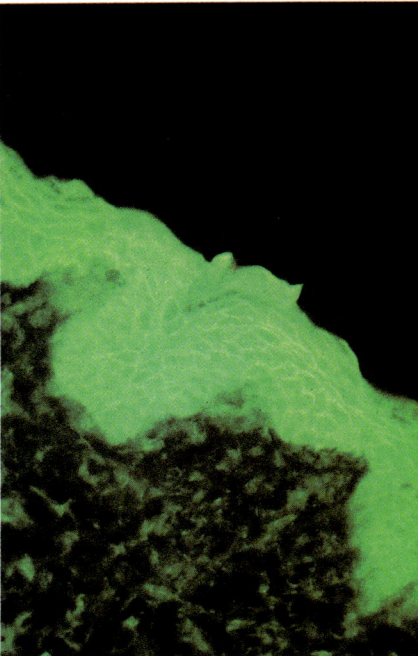

Fig. 28.24 Pemphigus vulgaris. Indirect immunofluorescence showing localization of pemphigus auto-antibody to the intercellular regions.

impetigo or skin infection and is associated with staphylococcal infection, usually of phage type 71. It resolves spontaneously after antibiotics. Histologically there is an intra-epidermal blister formed by necrosis of the squamous cells just beneath the granular layer. With ageing of the blister, sloughing and inflammation supervene.

Drug-induced erythema multiforme

This is the other major cause of the clinical appearance of the scalded-skin syndrome. The major drugs are phenylbutazones, sulphonamides, and barbiturates. The clinical picture often affects the mucosae first, particularly eyes and mouth, before involving the skin, and there is considerable overlap with Stevens–Johnson syndrome, i.e. another clinical variant of erythema multiforme. Unlike Lyell disease, the histopathology is of erythema multiforme, there being a subepidermal blister with epidermal necrosis (see below).

28.7.5 Pemphigoid—bullous and cicatricial

Clinical features and pathogenesis

This is a disease of middle-aged and elderly people, although it can occur in children. There is a tendency for female preponderance in younger sufferers, with reversal of this sex predominance in older patients. While an uncommon condition, it is more frequent than pemphigus. As in pemphigus, auto-antibody is found in the serum, but in this condition it is directed against antigens in the basement membrane junction zone of the epidermis and dermis (Fig. 28.25). The location of

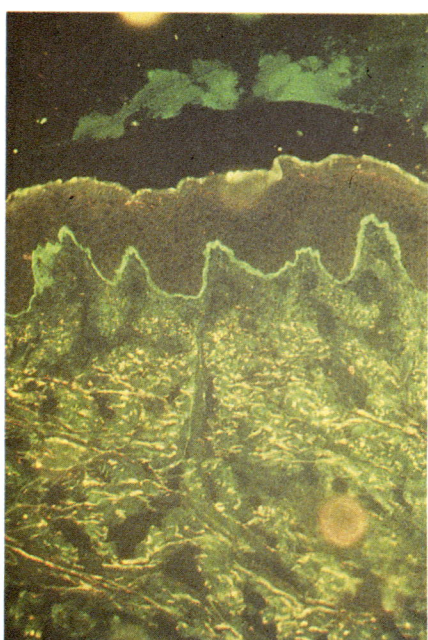

Fig. 28.25 Bullous pemphigoid. Direct immunofluorescence, showing linear deposition of IgG in the basement membrane zone.

the antigens can be determined by split-skin biopsies or by chemical separation of the skin. This shows that the antigen site varies between patients, some showing a location in the upper part of the basement membrane lamina lucida, others in the lower part, and others as a combination. The antibody is predominantly IgG in type (although occasionally IgM, IgA, or IgE), and usually is deposited in a linear configuration in the skin. Direct immunofluorescence shows it in the basement membrane of the blister and perilesional skin, with accompanying complement components of both classical and alternate pathways. A small proportion of bullous pemphigoid patients are negative for auto-antibodies at the time of biopsy. It is thought that activation of the complement pathways after binding of antibody to pemphigoid antigen (a glycoprotein of 29 kDa) results in release of proteases and inflammatory mediators, thus producing the patient's lesion.

Typically, the patient suffers large, tense, haemorrhagic, tough blisters anywhere on the skin, but often on the abdomen and flexor aspects of limbs. There is often a prodromal non-specific rash of some weeks' duration. The oral mucosa is occasionally involved and the blisters heal with minimal residual pigmentation. In contrast to bullous pemphigoid, cicatricial pemphigoid (benign mucous membrane pemphigoid) predominantly affects the mucosae of the mouth, eyes, and genitals, although it can involve the skin, particularly around mucosal orifices. Unlike bullous pemphigoid, there is usually healing by scarring which can cause considerable deformity, particularly of the conjunctivae. Despite these marked clinical differences, cases occur in which there is much overlap, and indeed there is essentially no difference in the features of early blisters by light microscopy and immunohistology.

Histopathology

Both forms of pemphigoid show a subepidermal blister, usually quite large (Fig. 28.26). The epidermis lifts off in a clean separation with tapering off at the edges. Often there is no inflammation or only a few scattered non-specific mononuclear inflammatory cells. The base of the blister is formed by the dermis.

Occasionally there is quite dense inflammation, of lymphocytes, macrophages, and eosinophil polymorphs. Much is made of this division into cell-rich and cell-poor pemphigoid, but in our experience this is unimportant. The controlling factors for the presence or absence of inflammation are unclear. As the blister ages, the epithelium often becomes necrotic, inflammation increases, and regenerative epithelial cells grow out from hair follicles and sweat duct openings to form the floor of the blister. Occasionally eosinophilic spongiosis can be seen as a manifestation of bullous pemphigoid (Fig. 28.27). In cicatricial pemphigoid, as the lesions heal, fibrosis of the dermis becomes prominent. Whether bullous pemphigoid is associated with an increased occurrence of internal malignancy has been debated for many years. Recent evidence suggests that there is no such association.

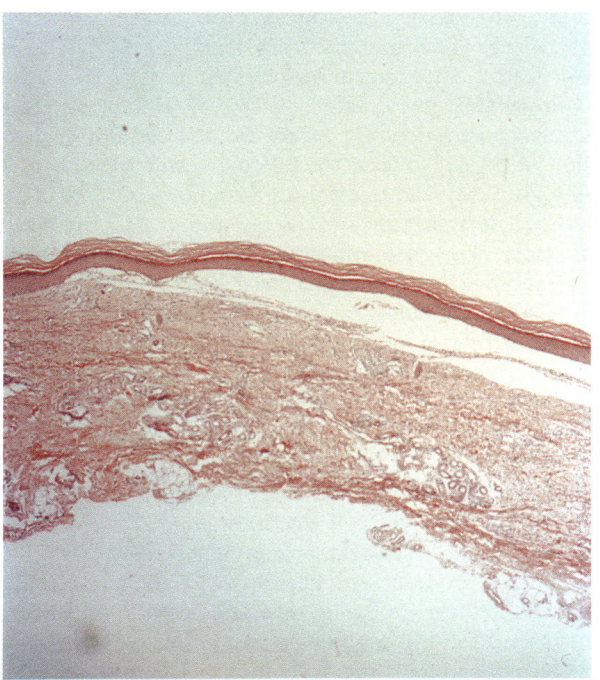

Fig. 28.26 Bullous pemphigoid. There is formation of a large sub-epidermal blister with only a sparse inflammatory infiltrate.

28.7.6 Dermatitis herpetiformis

Clinical features and pathogenesis

Another major differential diagnosis of subepidermal blisters is dermatitis herpetiformis (DH). Clinically, this disease is rare and affects predominantly middle-aged males. There is an intensely itching, urticarial rash, usually distributed symmetrically over the extensor surfaces of the limbs and over the buttocks and natal cleft. The blisters are usually small and often excoriated. The disease runs a relapsing and remitting course over years.

Most patients have a gluten enteropathy indistinguishable from coeliac disease. The skin lesions are gluten dependent and there is a high incidence of HLAB8 and HLADRw3 in dermatitis herpetiformis, similar to the association seen in coeliac disease without DH. The mechanism by which gluten damages the skin and causes the lesions is unknown, but gluten withdrawal from the diet can reduce or prevent lesions. Characteristically, by immunofluorescence, the skin contains granular deposits of IgA (plus infrequent IgM or IgG) and complement (particularly C3) in dermal papillae in the lesional and perilesional skin (Fig. 28.28). Occasionally there may be linear deposits of IgA. The antigen is unknown but is probably related to the dermal microfibrillary bundles. Unlike pemphigus, there is no direct relationship with clinical activity. There is no circulating antibody, and complement activation is by the alternate pathway.

Histopathology

The earliest lesion consists of collections of neutrophil polymorphs forming microabscesses in the tips of the dermal papillae (Figs 28.29, 28.30). Instead of microabscess, one sometimes finds a long, single cell layer of degenerate neutrophil polymorphs lined up just below the epidermis. As the lesion progresses, the microabscesses coalesce and the epidermis lifts off the dermis to form a sub-epidermal blister in which there are many neutrophil polymorphs; a few eosinophil polymorphs are present. If an early blister is biopsied, the features are characteristic, but multiple levels may need to be examined to detect the papillary microabscesses.

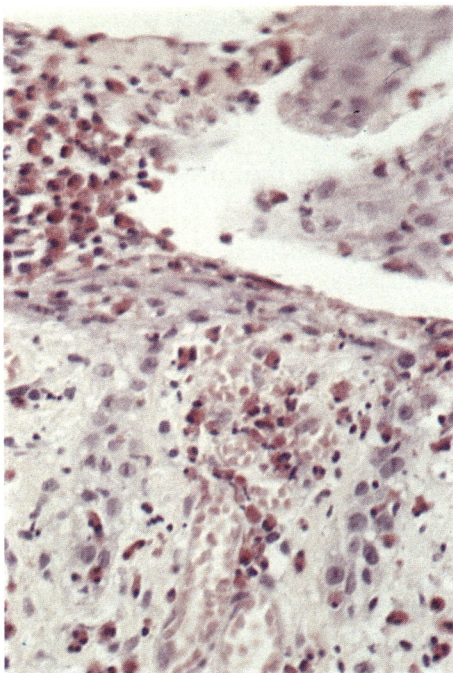

Fig. 28.27 Bullous pemphigoid. Intra-epidermal spongiosis with numerous eosinophil polymorphs and formation of a blister (eosinophilic spongiosis).

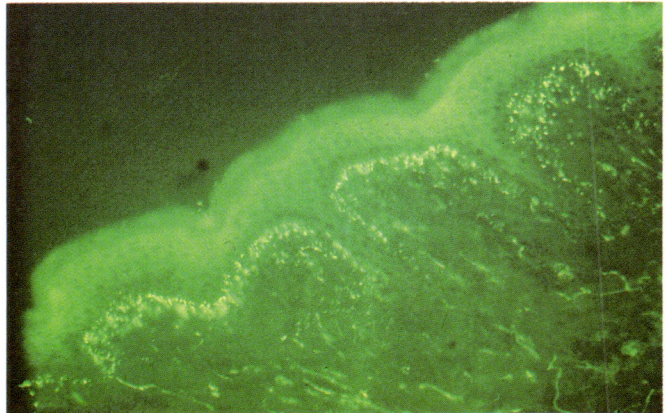

Fig. 28.28 Dermatitis herpetiformis. Direct immunofluorescence showing granular deposits of IgA in upper regions of the papillae.

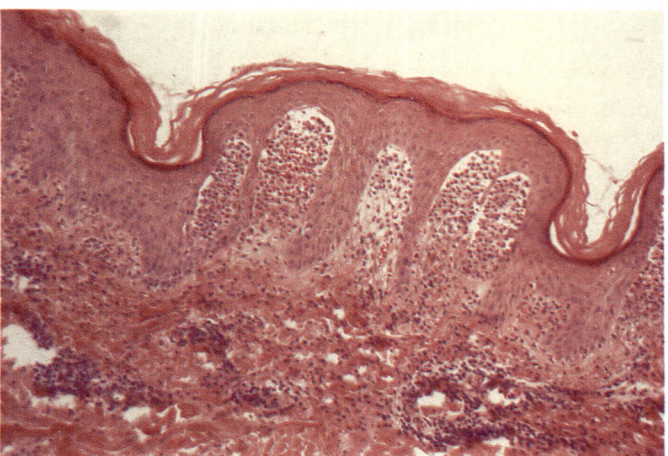

Fig. 28.29 Dermatitis herpetiformis. Numerous papillary micro-abscesses with early subepidermal vesicle formation.

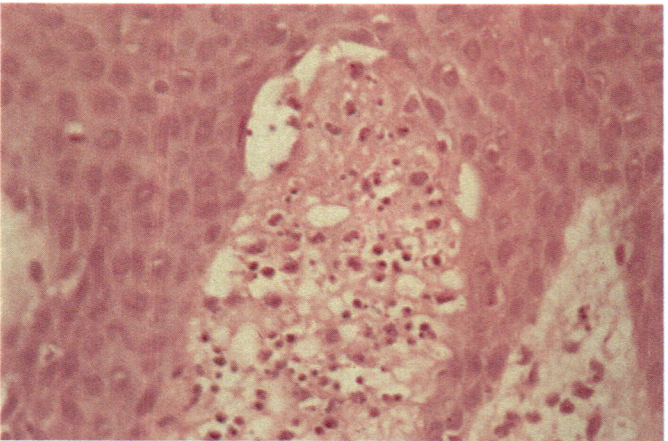

Fig. 28.30 Dermatitis herpetiformis. Papillary microabscess of neutrophil polymorphs.

Linear IgA dermatoses of adults and childhood

This is a rare group of conditions in which subepidermal blisters are found in association with continuous linear basement membrane IgA deposits. Clinically, linear IgA of childhood is usually different from that of adults and both are different from DH. However, occasionally the presentations merge towards one another and immunofluorescence is necessary to differentiate the disorders. Another major differential feature is that the childhood or adult linear IgA disease is associated with gluten sensitivity in only a few patients and is often a very mild form.

28.7.7   Erythema multiforme

Clinical features and pathogenesis

This is a relatively common condition usually affecting young adults. It has a variety of clinical manifestations and can be recurrent. The classic appearance is the 'target' lesion where there is a large erythematous urticarial oval/round lesion with central clearing. The central region often blisters. The rash can occur anywhere and is often pruritic. The Stevens–Johnson syndrome is a particularly severe form, often due to a drug reaction. It typically affects the mucous membranes, as well as the skin, and can lead to death in a small percentage of cases. Often the blisters ulcerate and can become secondarily infected.

The cause of erythema multiforme is often unknown but it may be preceded by a viral or bacterial infection. Drugs, particularly the sulphonamides, can cause the disease, and it is rarely associated with internal malignancy. It probably represents an immune-complex-mediated entity.

Histopathology

The hallmark is epidermal necrosis. This takes the form of either individual keratinocyte cell death, manifest as eosinophilic apoptotic cells, or confluent epidermal necrosis (Fig. 28.31). These changes are associated with an acute and chronic inflammatory cell infiltrate in the dermis. The necrotic epidermis lifts off the dermis to form a subepidermal blister. In some lesions, the epidermis is initially relatively intact and the major lesion is extensive papillary oedema and dermal inflammation, with both acute and chronic inflammatory cells and sometimes dermal necrosis. Confluent epidermal necrosis (Fig. 28.32) quickly occurs (less than 12 hours). Fibrinoid necrosis of blood vessels can be seen, raising the suspicion of a vasculitic component. However, this may be a secondary event. In accordance with the recurrent nature of the lesions, one sometimes sees lesions with alternating horizontal layers of necrotic and viable epidermis, reflecting the recurrent necrosis and healing.

28.7.8   Differential diagnosis of subepidermal blisters

There are a variety of conditions that cause subepidermal blisters on light microscopy. These include bullous pemphigoid, cicatricial pemphigoid, dermatitis herpetiformis, and erythema multiforme. More unusual lesions are the epidermolysis bullosa group of conditions (mechano-bullous disorders), blisters of coma, the bullous itching rashes of pregnancy (herpes gestationis), and systemic conditions in which blisters occasionally occur, e.g. porphyria and amyloidosis.

If a subepidermal blister is biopsied later than 12 hours after development, secondary changes of inflammation, necrosis, crusting, and regrowth of epithelium from sweat ducts and hair follicles can totally preclude accurate assessment. Again, it is essential to obtain fresh blisters for examination.

The differential diagnosis of the individual epidermal cell death in erythema multiforme is of GVHD, lichen striatus, lichen planus, and regressing melanocytic lesions; that of the subepidermal blister is bullous pemphigoid and dermatitis herpetiformis—particularly late lesions. Early lesions of bullous

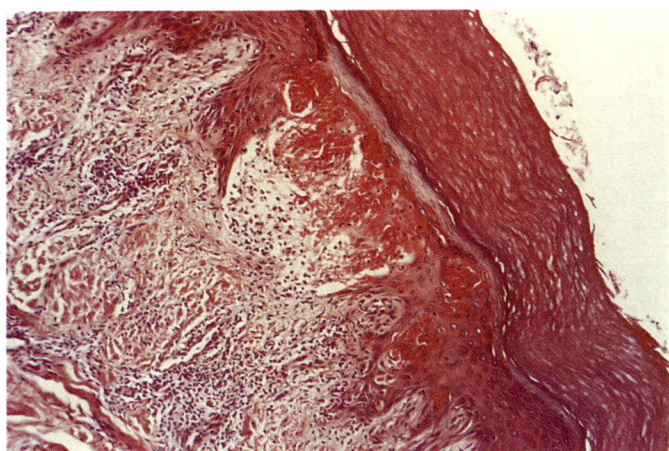

Fig. 28.31 Erythema multiforme. Early formation of a subepidermal blister with confluent eosinophilic necrosis of overlying epidermal cells.

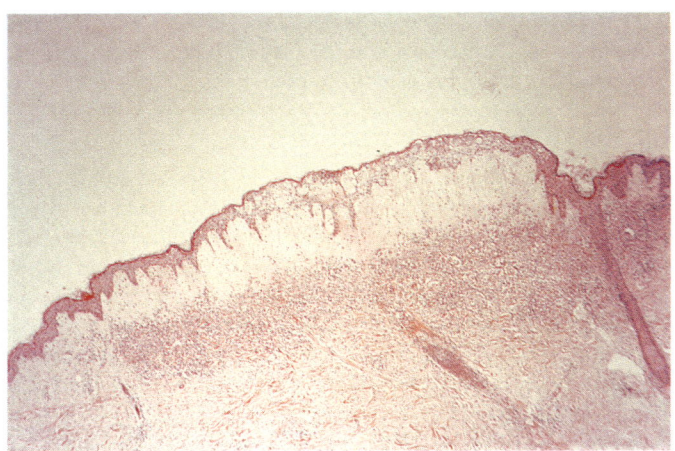

Fig. 28.32 Erythema multiforme. Formation of a subepidermal blister due to severe papillary oedema. The epidermis overlying the blister is necrotic and there is a dense inflammatory infiltrate in the upper dermis.

pemphigoid and dermatitis herpetiformis do not show epidermal necrosis, and immunofluorescence of both late and early lesions is diagnostic: dermatitis herpetiformis shows papillary granular IgA deposits; bullous pemphigoid shows linear basement membrane IgG; and erythema multiforme shows vascular IgM and C3.

The other rarer causes of subepidermal blisters normally produce acellular lesions. The diagnosis is reached by a combination of clinical details and, where appropriate, specific changes, e.g. amyloid. Herpes gestationis is a very rare blistering eruption of pregnancy which has many features in common with bullous pemphigoid and is probably a variant.

28.8 Connective tissue diseases

28.8.1 Lupus erythematosus

Clinical features and pathogenesis

The two major forms of lupus erythematosus (LE) both affect the skin. In the systemic illness, there are a multiplicity of types of skin rashes. In the cutaneous form (discoid), the skin only is involved, and typically as scaly, variable-sized erythematous patches, which often affect the sun-exposed areas and heal by scarring and atrophy. Within these two extremes, there are patients who have a greater or lesser mixture of cutaneous and systemic manifestations. There is a female preponderance and it affects the middle-aged. There is also a genetic predisposition and a well-recognized immunological component of immune complex deposition and auto-antibodies (see Chapter 4). The role of stress, sunlight, and cold in precipitating or exacerbating the illness is well recognized in many patients.

Histopathology

Although the clinical lesions may be variable in cutaneous LE, the histopathological appearance is relatively restricted. The major features are hyperkeratosis and (in the more long-standing lesions), epidermal atrophy (Fig. 28.33). There is focal and often insignificant basal cell liquefaction (Fig. 28.34) and atrophy of pilosebaceous units. There is often thickening of the basement membrane (Fig. 28.35), best seen with a PAS

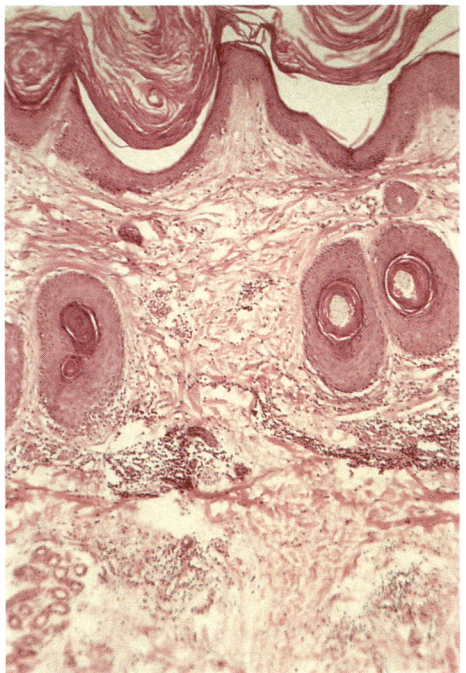

Fig. 28.33 Discoid lupus erythematosus. Marked hyperkeratosis with focal atrophy of the epidermis. There is also follicular plugging and a focal mononuclear inflammatory infiltrate within the dermis.

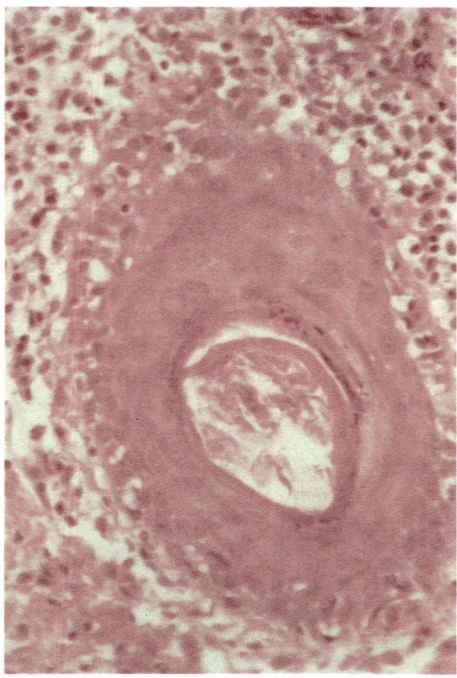

Fig. 28.34 Discoid lupus erythematosus. Basal cell liquefaction and dense mononuclear inflammatory infiltrate around hair follicle.

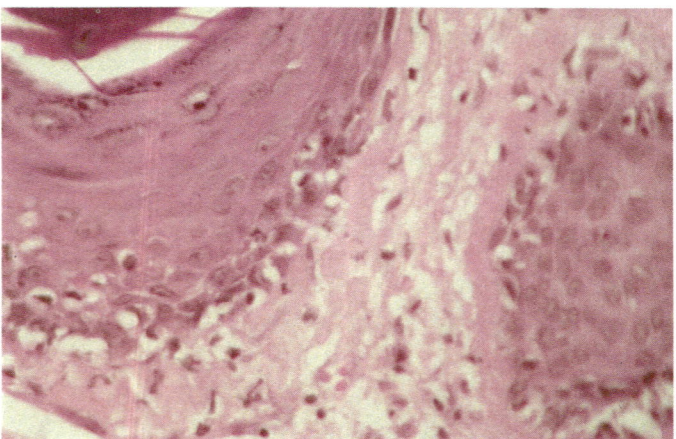

Fig. 28.35 Discoid lupus erythematosus. Basal cell liquefaction of hair follicle with thickened basement membrane.

stain, and a strikingly dense, patchy, lymphocytic infiltrate predominately located in the upper half of the dermis (Fig. 28.36). All these features are very often restricted to the periphery of the hair follicles and, indeed, if LE is suspected, the most reliable place to find the basal cell liquefaction is in the basal cells of the pilosebaceous units. Unlike lichen planus, the basal cell liquefaction is quite often very indistinct and difficult to see, and, of course, may result in pigment incontinence.

Another feature of LE that may be helpful is the presence of an ill-defined change to the connective tissue of the papillary dermis. This appears as a mixture of vague sclerosis and oedema

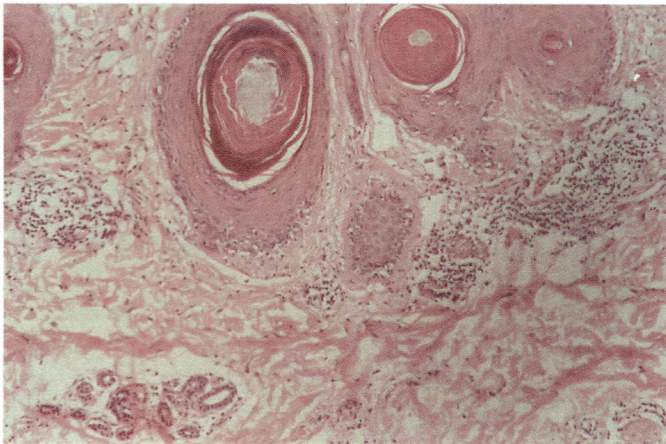

Fig. 28.36 Discoid lupus erythematosus. Follicular plugging and focal inflammation in relation to the hair follicles.

and, while not invariable, is useful when present. Overall, the characteristic of LE is the spotty nature of the changes, particularly centred on hair follicles, and the peculiarly dense nature of the lymphocytic infiltrate. LE is one of the diseases which causes dilatation and plugging of hair follicles with keratin. Others are lichen planus and pityriasis rubra pilaris.

Differential diagnosis

The differential diagnosis is of the lesions associated with basal cell liquefaction (lichen planus, poikiloderma, actinic keratosis, etc.) and those associated with lymphocytic infiltrates, particularly lymphoma, toxic erythema, and Jessner's eruption. Occasionally the lymphoid infiltrate of LE lies particularly deep in the dermis and can extend into the subcutaneous fat. This variant is known as LE profundus and can be recognized by the dermal changes described above; these may be difficult to find and require multiple levels.

In systemic LE, the microscopic changes in the skin are usually non-specific, consisting of sparse perivascular mononuclear inflammation in the upper dermis and occasional hyperkeratosis or atrophy. In some cases, there is the more diagnostic feature of basal cell liquefaction, but in our experience this is not often seen. In such instances, the appearances are of poikiloderma (see below). In other cases, the features are those of a vasculitis.

The best way to check the diagnosis of either systemic or cutaneous LE is by use of immunohistology. In both conditions, immunoglobulins, particularly IgG, are deposited in a linear form along the basement membrane in the histopathologically abnormal skin. Complement components (C3, C1q) are also present. In systemic LE, in contrast to cutaneous LE, this material may also be deposited in the clinically uninvolved non-sun-exposed skin (60–80 per cent), an extremely useful feature.

28.8.2 Dermatomyositis and systemic sclerosis

Other connective tissue disorders that often involve the skin are

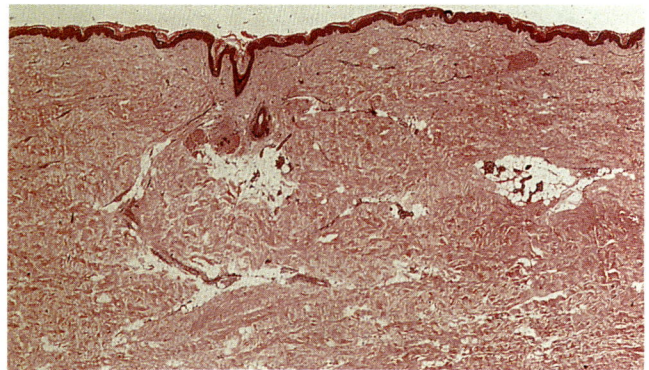

Fig. 28.37 Systemic sclerosis. Thickening of the dermis with sweat glands, hair follicles, and subcutaneous fat apparently situated in the mid- to upper dermis.

dermatomyositis and systemic sclerosis. The changes in dermatomyositis are similar to those of systemic LE (as in poikiloderma), while in systemic sclerosis the major abnormality is apparent increased thickness of the dermis, as judged by the presence of sweat coils and fat in the mid-dermis, as opposed to the dermo-subcutaneous junction (Fig. 28.37). There is often surprisingly little to see, particularly in early lesions. In late lesions the collagen bundles can be thickened, with loss of the distinction between the papillary and reticular dermis. Whether there is an increase in collagen synthesis in systemic sclerosis is unresolved, as is the role of small vessel disease. In early lesions, a sparse perivascular mononuclear inflammatory infiltrate can be found. The localized form of scleroderma (morphea) shows thickening of the collagen bundles and loss of the interstitial space, similar to late systemic sclerosis, but, in my experience, there is loss of adnexal structures, unlike systemic sclerosis. To that extent, morphea resembles scarring (particularly keloid), but the elastic pattern is usually preserved, unlike scarring.

28.9 Granulomatous inflammation

There are two types of granulomatous inflammation in the skin. First, there are those composed of epithelioid or mixed cell granulomas. The major differential diagnoses are: tuberculosis, sarcoid, fungal and protozoal infection, foreign body reaction, syphilis, leprosy, and drug reactions. Often there are no specific diagnostic features of these conditions (although occasionally special stains or polarized light can help) and diagnosis rests on a combination of clinical and other laboratory investigations, e.g. serology and culture. In general, however, the presence of granulomas with polymorphs shoud lead one to suspect a fungal infection or halogen drug eruption, while the presence of numerous plasma cells should raise the possibility of syphilis. A history of foreign travel would obviously direct attention towards certain organisms, as would a history of AIDS.

Secondly, in contrast, certain specific skin conditions cause palisading granulomatous inflammation. These are granuloma annulare, necrobiosis lipoidica, and rheumatoid nodules (see Chapter 27).

28.9.1 Granuloma annulare

This is not uncommon in children and young adults. It involves the skin of the hands or trunk. The lesions are annular and self-limiting, lasting a few months to years.

Histopathologically the diagnostic feature is focal degeneration of the dermal collagen of a peculiarly ill-defined nature, called necrobiosis (Fig. 28.38). The dermal connective tissue is sometimes obviously necrotic with loss of nucleic and amorphous debris, but often the main abnormality is a faint loss of collagen eosinophilia with some basophilia, a slight fragmentation of collagen, and loss of fibroblast nuclei. This change is best recognized in low power and is usually noticed because of the surrounding palisade of inflammation (Fig. 28.39). This is composed of a few ill-defined, epithelioid cells and multinucleate giant cells with scattered mononuclear inflammatory cells. The lesion is small and situated in the upper reticular dermis. Occasionally the palisade is almost non-existent and levels may help to confirm the changes. The epidermis is uninvolved but, occasionally, the lesion can be very high in the dermis and ulcerate through the epidermis. Conversely, it can be found in the deep dermis and/or subcutaneous fat. The aetiology is unknown, although a cell-mediated, delayed hypersensitivity reaction has resemblances.

28.9.2 Necrobiosis lipoidica

This shows similar changes to granuloma annulare but with

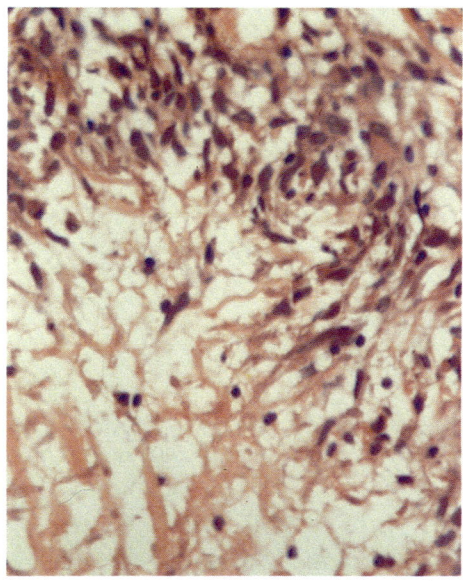

Fig. 28.38 Granuloma annulare. Palisade of epithelioid cells surrounding an area of eosinophilic necrotic collagen.

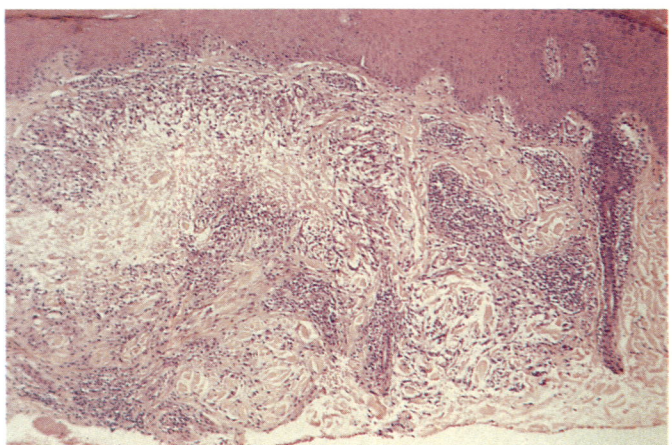

Fig. 28.39 Granuloma annulare. Formation of an ill-defined area of necrobiosis with surrounding palisade of inflammation.

some differences. The necrosis is usually larger and more obvious, the inflammation is more marked and intense, and the lesion is found in the mid to lower half of the reticular dermis. It is said that the necrotic material contains a heavy deposit of lipid, in contrast to that of granuloma annulare and rheumatoid disease. Necrobiosis lipoidica is associated with diabetes mellitus in about 40 per cent of cases. It typically affects the legs of middle-aged females and forms large, round/oval, symmetrical, raised, yellow plaques which heal by scarring. A few other conditions can show changes similar to those described above, namely rheumatic disease and rheumatoid nodules. Differentiation requires clinical correlation (see also Chapter 27).

28.10   Vasculitides

A large variety of conditions can cause inflammation of the vessels of the skin. Clinically there are two main groups: those systemic diseases that involve the skin as well as other organs, and conditions that involve the skin only. However, there are no histopathological differences. Vasculitis in the skin shows three main histological patterns:

1. leukoclastic vasculitis;
2. mononuclear vasculitis; and
3. granulomatous vasculitis.

All are characterized by damage to the vessel wall, either in the form of necrosis and/or endothelial swelling, with associated inflammation.

28.10.1   Leukoclastic vasculitis

This is characterized by vascular wall necrosis, often fibrinoid in nature, and inflammation of small endothelial channels, either capillaries or post-capillary venules. The diagnostic feature is necrosis of the vessel wall and neutrophil polymorphs, often with marked nuclear dusting (Fig. 28.40). However, there may be occasional mononuclear inflammatory cells. Extravasation of red blood cells is inevitable. The vessels involved can be found anywhere in the dermis (Fig. 28.41), although usually the changes are found in one zone, e.g. papillary dermis or papillary–reticular junction. The degree of inflammation can vary from sparse to dense. If a large number of vessels are involved, there is often necrosis of the epidermis and superficial dermis, on which there may be superimposed infection. Fibrin thrombi are not infrequent.

There are many causes of a leukoclastic vasculitis. The predominant causes are immune complex diseases (e.g. LE, Henoch–Schönlein purpura), erythema multiforme, drug reactions, and septicaemia. If larger vessels are involved, particularly in the subcutaneous fat, the possibility of polyarteritis nodosa must be considered.

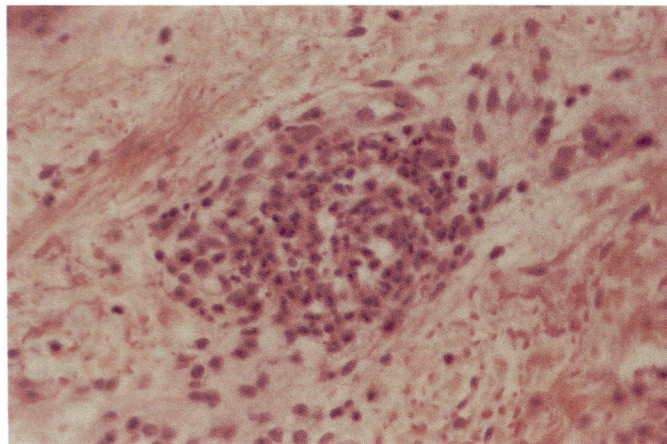

Fig. 28.40 Leukoclastic vasculitis. Small blood vessel in the papillary dermis with a dense circumferential neutrophil polymorph infiltrate. The lumen and vessel wall are obscured by the inflammation.

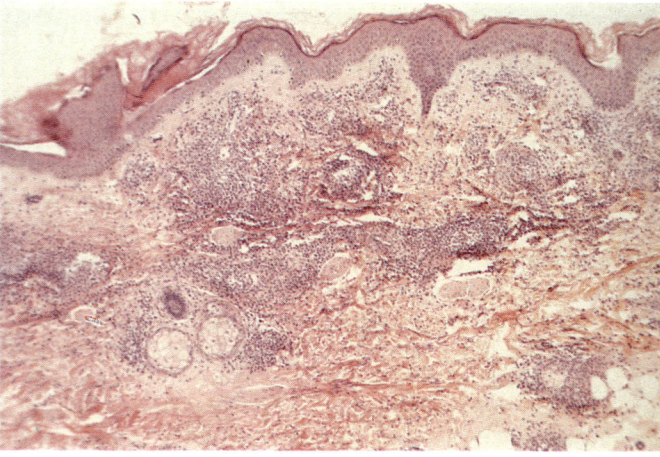

Fig. 28.41 Leukoclastic vasculitis. A widespread, dense perivascular infiltrate is spread throughout the full thickness of the dermis. Note that the epidermis is normal.

28.10.2 Mononuclear vasculitis

This must be differentiated from perivascular inflammation; both are often confused. Mononuclear vasculitis is uncommon. The features are similar to those of leukoclastic vasculitis, except that the inflammation does not contain neutrophil polymorphs, and necrosis of vessel walls is infrequent. Most often the endothelial cells only show swelling. The most frequent cause is a drug reaction, but a chronic urticarial reaction can produce similar appearances. Pityriasis lichenoides also shows a mononuclear vasculitis (see below). Chilblain (pernio) is an infrequently biopsied mononuclear vasculitis.

28.10.3 Granulomatous vasculitis

The best known example is Wegener disease, a rare condition. The changes are characterized by the presence of epithelioid granulomatous inflammation and multinucleate giant cells in and around the damaged blood vessels.

Differential diagnosis

In all vasculitides, while the skin biopsy can support or suggest the diagnosis, the results of clinical and other investigations need to be considered to establish the diagnosis. In addition to those conditions outlined above, two rare specific skin lesions are of interest—erythema elevatum diutinum (EED) and granuloma faciale. Both show essentially a leukoclastic vasculitis. Although much is made in the literature of the presence of toxic hyaline in EED and is contrasted with the fibrinoid necrosis in other forms of leukoclastic vasculitis, in our experience this is unjustified. These diagnoses are made by consideration of the clinical story.

28.10.4 Other vascular lesions

Gravitational changes

Venous 'stasis' of the lower limbs is often associated with discoloration and thickening of the skin as well as ulceration and scarring. Stasis may be a misnomer, as some investigations have shown an increased venous blood flow, not stasis.

Histopathologically the most striking lesion is proliferation of capillaries in the boundary between papillary and reticular dermis and in the reticular dermis (Fig. 28.42). These can form regular nodules, rather like microscopic pyogenic granulomata, and can be mistaken for Kaposi sarcoma. These nodules are associated with haemosiderin deposition in the tissues. There is often atrophy of adnexal structures, chronic inflammation, and fibrosis, presumably reflecting ischaemia. In addition, in cases of stasis dermatitis, there is superimposed on these dermal vascular changes an epithelial picture of a dermatitic reaction, the mechanism of which is unknown.

Progressive pigmented purpuric dermatoses

These represent a group of clinical conditions in which annular or patchy purpuric lesions appear, usually on the legs, which

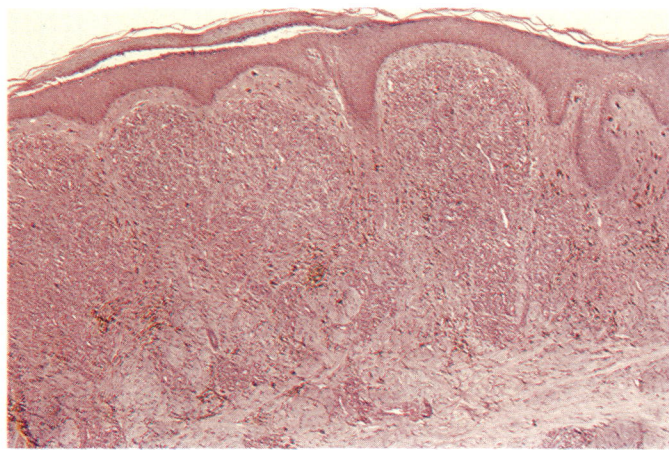

Fig. 28.42 Stasis dermatitis. There are large nodules of proliferating capillaries occupying most of the papillary and upper reticular dermis. Haemosiderin pigment is widespread, indicating previous haemorrhage.

progress into hyperpigmented plaques. There are a variety of different clinical names, depending on the stage of the lesion—Majocchi disease, Schamberg disease, lichenoid dermatitis of Gougerot and Blum, and lichen aureus.

The common denominator is the presence of extrasavated red blood corpuscles (RBCs) in the upper reticular and papillary dermis, with associated mononuclear inflammatory infiltrate (Fig. 28.43). There is also oedema, with increased numbers of

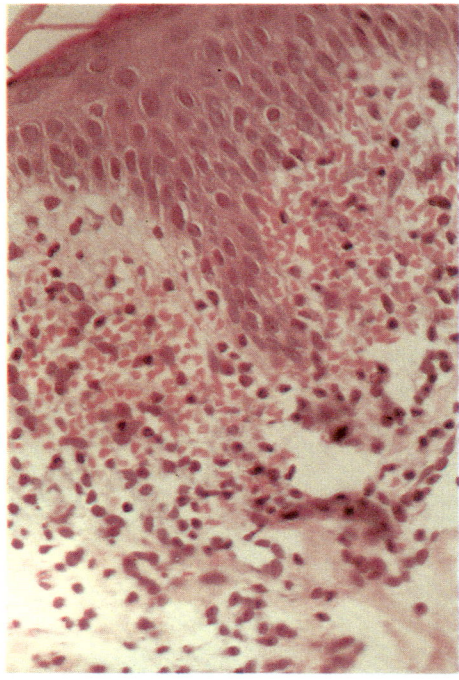

Fig. 28.43 Pigmented purpuric dermatosis. Widespread free blood cells in the papillary dermis indicating haemorrhage. There is also a moderate mononuclear inflammatory infiltrate. There is some prominence of the endothelium of the small vessels.

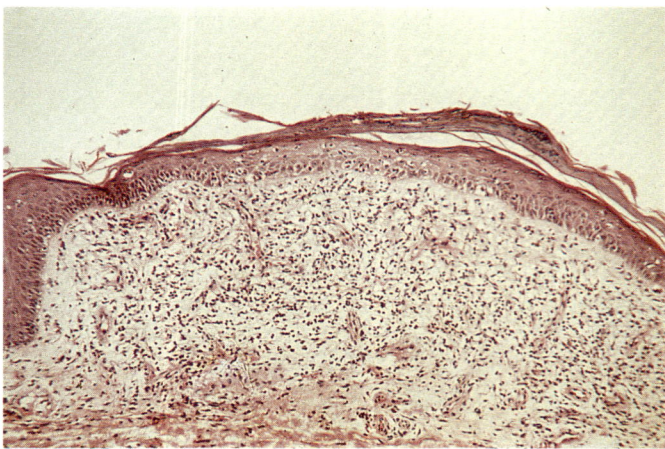

Fig. 28.44 Pigmented purpuric dermatosis. This lichenoid form shows lamellar hyper- and parakeratosis. There is some epidermotropism of mononuclear inflammatory cells. The papillary and upper reticular dermis show a widespread mononuclear inflammatory infiltrate, with some prominence of the small blood vessels.

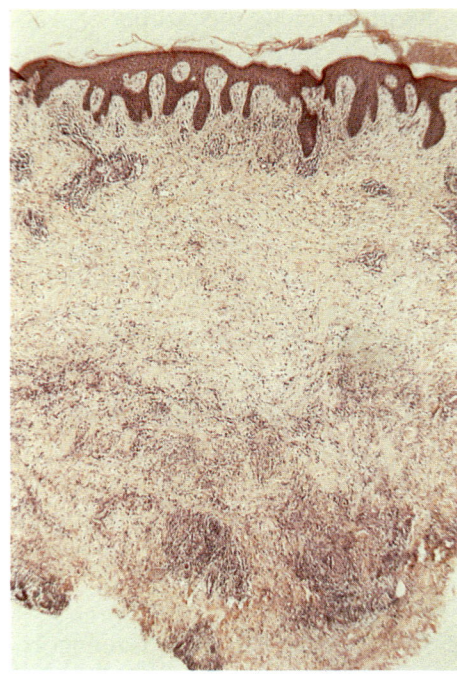

Fig. 28.45 Pityriasis lichenoides. There is focal hyperkeratosis and irregular acanthosis. There is a dense perivascular mononuclear inflammatory infiltrate spread throughout the full thickness of the dermis.

capillaries in the papillary dermis. This abnormality of the vessels appears to be the prime lesion and is associated with increased amounts of haemosiderin in macrophages, resulting from breakdown of free RBCs. The epidermis can also become involved with focal parakeratosis.

In the lichenoid purpuras, the epidermal changes are more marked, with acanthosis producing the lichenoid clinical appearance (Fig. 28.44). Lichen aureus is relatively uncommon and presents as a few grouped, golden-coloured papules anywhere on the body. The histological changes are similar to those of the other progressive purpuric dermatoses (PPD), but epidermal involvement is not seen.

It should be noted that, on biopsy, all these conditions can be confused with stasis changes and those of trauma, so that clinical information is necessary for differentiation. The aetiology is unknown.

Pityriasis lichenoides

In this condition there appears to be a vascular abnormality in the papillary dermis, although it is not usually considered a variant of PPD. Typically it affects young adult males, but there is a spectrum of clinical forms, from acute and varioliform to chronic varieties, all of which are uncommon and have, as usual, their own eponyms. Most cases of lymphomatoid papulosis are probably examples of pityriasis lichenoides. The chronic varieties show a prominent epidermal scale formed by orthokeratosis and parakeratosis (Fig. 28.45). There is some epidermotropism of mononuclear inflammatory cells and a mild mononuclear inflammatory reaction in the papillary dermis. Some of these lymphoid cells can be rather hyperchromatic and pleomorphic.

The appearances are rather non-specific, apart from the epidermal change, and suggest a large differential diagnosis: the chronic dermatites, the psoriasiform lesions, the pigmented purpuric dermatoses, and occasionally pre-mycosis fungoides.

In the more acute forms, the degree of inflammation increases, with papillary oedema, free RBCs, and scattered mononuclear inflammatory cells; this is sometimes associated with microscopic subepidermal blister formation. The epidermis shows increasing damage, with oedema and crusting. Eventually necrosis can occur with ulceration; the necrosis involves the underlying papillary dermis. The endothelium of the papillary dermal capillaries is often prominent and the changes suggest a vasculitis (lymphocytic) with ischaemic necrosis.

28.11   Panniculitis

Inflammation of the subcutaneous fat is yet another source of considerable confusion for pathologists. This is partly bcause of the relative infrequency of such lesions, and hence unfamiliarity, but also because the subcutaneous fat has essentially only one reaction, no matter what the stimulus. Furthermore, a deep biopsy, including a considerable depth of subcutaneous fat, is usually necessary for diagnosis, a criterion which is frequently absent. The response of subcutaneous fat to inflammation invariably involves similar changes to those found in inflammation of fat anywhere in the body. These are necrosis, foamy macrophages, multinucleate giant-cell formation, and result-ant fibrosis. The inflammation is predominantly mononuclear, but epithelioid granulomatous inflammation is almost invari-able, if sufficient necrosis has occurred. Polymorphs are found in some lesions. Furthermore, vessels are often damaged in pan-niculitis, but whether this is primary (as in polyarteritis nodosa) or secondary is unclear. However, the most helpful diagnostic feature is the location of the inflammatory changes. There are two patterns, septal and lobular panniculitis. In septal pannicu-litis, the inflammation is largely confined to the fibrous tissue septae which divide the fat into lobules. The changes extend into the lobule to a varying extent, but low-power examination clearly shows the septal predominance of the inflammation. Lobular panniculitis is quite different, with uniform density of inflammation affecting the fat lobules. The clinical manifest-ations of panniculitis are usually of swollen, painful, eryth-ematous nodules of the legs.

Differential diagnosis

The diseases that are associated with septal panniculitis are erythema nodosum, nodular vasculitis (with its clinical vari-ants, including nodular migratory thrombophlebitis), and polyarteritis nodosa. The differential diagnosis rests primarily on clinical correlation, but a search should be made for a damaged large vessel. These vessels are most commonly detected in the interlobular septa at the junction of dermis and subcutaneous fat, but may require multiple sections and special stains, e.g. EVG, for delineation of the damaged vessel. Demon-stration of such a vessel suggests a diagnosis of nodular vasculi-tis or polyarteritis nodosa.

Occasionally lupus erythematosus profundus and angio-immunoblastic lymphadenopathy can involve the subcuta-neous fat, causing a septal panniculitis. Erythema induratum is another lesion presenting as septal panniculitis, but should be regarded as a variant of TB of the skin (Bazin's disease).

Very rarely, pancreatic disease (inflammatory or neoplastic) can be associated with a septal or lobular panniculitis. This lesion has a peculiarly amorphous calcification, superimposed on 'ghost-like' necrotic cells.

Lobular panniculitis is classically associated with Weber–Christian disease and frequently shows necrosis and neutrophil polymorph infiltrate, in addition to the other features of fat damage. Subcutaneous sarcoid (Darier–Roussy) may also present in this way, as can α-1-antitrypsin deficiency and cold panniculitis.

28.12 Non-specific erythemas (toxic erythema) and urticaria

There are a group of conditions that present clinically as an erythematous and/or whealing rash, with essentially no

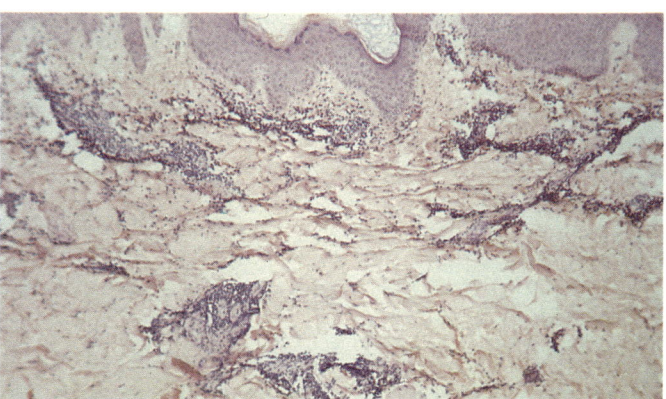

Fig. 28.46 Toxic erythema. The striking feature is the presence of a dense perivascular infiltrate scattered through the dermis. There is mild papillary oedema. The epidermis is essentially normal.

epidermal involvement. The distribution and subsequent pro-gress of these rashes allows separation into clinical entities, but histopathologically the appearances are similar and usually non-specific. There is usually variable oedema of the papillary dermis and around blood vessels in the reticular dermis, but the predominant feature is a perivascular mononuclear infiltrate of varying intensity (Fig. 28.46). The degree of oedema and inflammation seen is in direct proportion to the degree of urti-caria and erythema seen clinically. When pruritic, there is often superimposed scratch damage and reaction in the epidermis, recognized by the strictly focal serum-crusting and parakerato-sis, sometimes with ulceration of the epidermis.

Differential diagnosis

This is extensive and includes acute and chronic urticaria, insect bite and its variant erythema chronicum migrans (Lyme disease), erythema marginatum rheumaticum, erythema annulare centrifugum, drug reaction, erythema gyratum repens, papular eruptions of pregnancy, Jessner's lymphocytic infiltration, lupus erythematosus profundus, vasculitis, photo-sensitivity, pigmented purpuric dematoses, and even lymphoid neoplasms. As can be seen from this list, the need for clinical correlation is mandatory and almost invariably all that can be said histopathologically is that the appearances are consistent or otherwise with the suggested clinical diagnosis.

28.13 Miscellaneous scaly lesions

These include pityriasis rosea and superficial fungal infections.

Clinically, pityriasis rosea is a papulo-squamous rash, usually in young female adults. There is typically a solitary, early lesion (herald patch) followed some days to a week later by a self-limiting, generalized rash lasting for weeks to months. It may represent a peculiar reaction to a systemic viral illness.

Microscopically, the skin is largely normal. However, there is focal parakeratosis, often mild and quite insignificant. Related to this focus of parakeratosis, the epidermis shows mild spongiosis, often with a tiny intra-epidermal vesicle, with a mild perivascular mononuclear infiltrate in the underlying papillary dermis. The appearances are similar to focal subacute dermatitis.

The differential diagnosis is of dermatitis, superficial fungal infection, and drug reactions.

Fungal infections can be identified by a periodic acid-Schiff stain (PAS).

28.14   Follicular lesions

A variety of conditions predominantly affect the pilosebaceous follicle. The commonest is probably simple folliculitis, which shows varying inflammation within and around the hair follicle, often with abscess formation.

28.14.1   Acne vulgaris

This disease is associated with parakeratotic plugging of the follicle, simulating an epidermoid cyst, which ruptures stimulating a foreign-body giant-cell response, dense inflammation, and scarring. Acne vulgaris is thought to be a result of the pilosebaceous unit responding inappropriately to the circulating androgens of puberty and thereafter.

28.14.2   Keratosis pilaris and lichen spinulosus

Keratotic plugging of hair follicles is typical of a variety of diseases, some of which are discussed elsewhere, e.g. lichen planus, lupus erythematosus, lichen sclerosis, and Darier disease. Keratosis pilaris and lichen spinulosus are characterized by the presence of a simple keratotic plug in the hair follicle with variable surrounding inflammation and fibrosis, and are essentially clinical diagnoses. Keratosis pilaris may be a variant of ichthyosis vulgaris.

28.14.3   Rosacea

This is a common condition with a variable clinical appearance including facial flushing, erythema, papules, and pustules. Histopathologically the papular and pustular lesions consist of a folliculitis, with acute and chronic inflammation in the pilosebaceous unit, associated with variable epidermal changes of seborrhoeic dermatitis. In addition, a characteristic feature is the presence of small epithelioid granulomata, usually located in the upper and mid-reticular dermis, often juxtaposed to pilosebaceous units. Depending on the clinical appearance, this latter change can be the only histological feature and raises the differential diagnosis of all granulomata (TB, sarcoid, etc.). *Demodex folliculorum* within hair follicles are particularly

numerous and common in rosacea, suggesting a pathogenic role. Rhinophyma (a clinical variant of rosacea) shows excessive enlargement of sebaceous glands and dilatation of the pilosebaceous units, but usually there are few or none of the associated inflammatory changes of rosacea.

28.14.4   Pityriasis rubra pilaris

This is a rare disease in which it is said that there is abnormal metabolism of vitamin A. Histopathologically, early lesions resemble psoriasis, but, in later lesions, there is follicular plugging with chronic dermatitic changes in the surrounding epidermis.

28.14.5   Alopecia

For the pathologist, alopecia may cause difficulty because biopsy changes may be insignificant. There are two main histopathological groups: one with little or no change; and the other with scarring and hair follicle destruction. The major clinical management decisions are to determine:

1. if there is a hair follicle disorder; and
2. if this is likely to lead to permanent hair loss.

Alopecia areata

This disease and its variants are relatively common and occasionally biopsied. The skin often shows very minor and subtle changes: apparently normal empty, or catagen/telogen follicles interspersed with occasional anagen follicles, which have a peribulbar inflammatory reaction. The increased number of catagen or telogen follicles is abnormal. Recognition of these minor changes requires both a good biopsy (i.e. from the affected area) and familiarity with the pattern of normal hair in the region biopsied. Accordingly, often the biopsy looks normal! The aetiology of alopecia areata is unknown, but there is an association with organ-specific auto-immune diseases in about 10 per cent of cases, a history of atopy in a further 10 per cent, and a family history of alopecia areata in up to 50 per cent.

Scarring alopecias

The scarring alopecias can result in permanent hair loss and include diseases such as lupus erythematosus and lichen planus (lichen planopilaris), which can involve hair follicles as part of a more general skin lesion. In addition, there are patients who develop scarring alopecia, for which, currently, no cause can be identified (pseudopelade of Brocq).

If the biopsy is from a suitable area, the major abnormality is loss of recognizable hair follicles with replacement by a fibrous shadow, often recognizable on H & E, but highlighted by connective tissue stains (EVG). The intervening epidermis is normal and, even in areas of scarring, hair follicles are often remarkably little disturbed. However, some follicles may show perifollicular mononuclear inflammation and variable scarring and loss of the outer root sheath; the inflammatory reaction gradually appears to extend into and replace the hair follicle. While this scarring replacement of hair follicles may be recognized by special stains, occasionally the only sign of loss of hair follicles in the biopsy may be the presence of residual normal arrectores pilorum muscles, in the abscence of associated hair follicles. This appearance should stimulate the careful search (special stains and levels) for evidence of scarred or inflamed hair follicles.

28.15 Infection

Infections of the skin are common and are given a variety of names, depending on the clinical appearances and circumstances (e.g. ecthyma, impetigo). The majority show no significant histopathological differences from their counterparts in other organs and will not be dealt with in detail here. Thus, staphylococcal lesions form abscesses, while streptococcal lesions have a more diffuse, acute inflammatory reaction (cellulitis, erysipelas). However, the differential diagnosis of an acute inflammatory infection in the skin includes the specific skin diseases of subcorneal pustular dermatosis (see above) and Sweet syndrome (acute febrile neutrophilic dermatosis). In the latter rare condition, the patient, often female and middle-aged, develops multiple oedematous erythematous plaques in association with fever and leucocytosis. Histopathologically it consists of a diffuse or perivascular infiltrate of neutrophil polymorphs of varying density in the dermis. The aetiology is unknown, but it is said that 10 per cent are associated with leukaemia.

28.15.1 Viral infections

Epidermal infections are common. These are usually either viruses of the herpes family (simplex, zoster, cytomegalovirus), or molluscum contagiosum. Other viral infections (e.g. adenovirus) are much rarer.

Herpes

The principle clue to herpes infection is the presence of syncytial multinucleate epidermal cells, necrosis and ballooning of epidermal cells, leading to formation of intra- or subepidermal blisters (Fig. 28.47) and eventually ulceration. There is a dense, mainly mononuclear, inflammatory infiltrate in the dermis. Eosinophilic, viral, intranuclear inclusions are visible, but precise delineation of the various virus types is only possible at present by use of either immunohistochemistry for antigen or *in situ* hybridization for nucleic acid.

Molluscum contagiosum

This is a disease of children, with clusters of papular white/pink spots which extrude white 'pus' on pressure from the central punctum. Typically there is a crateriform lesion with marked

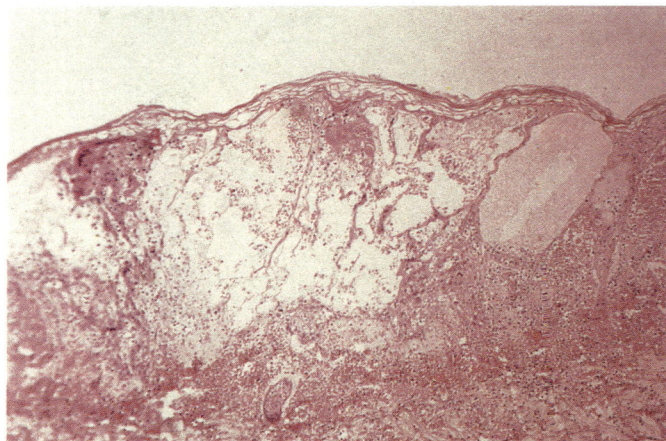

Fig. 28.47 Herpes simplex infection. There is a large intra-epidermal and subepidermal blister. This has been formed by ballooning and reticular degeneration of the infected epithelial cells. At one edge, the infected epithelial cells are forming a syncytium of multinucleated giant cells. There is a considerable amount of haemorrhage.

epithelial hyperplasia, a pattern not dissimilar to keratoacanthoma. However, the cells contain large eosinophilic, cytoplasmic inclusions which become basophilic as they approach the surface.

Human papilloma virus (HPV)

This is a common viral infection of the skin. It is not usually biopsied, except in the anogenital region (Chapter 21) and in immunocompromised patients (Chapter 4) where HPV infection has a premalignant connotation. There are a large number of clinical varieties which show some association with the 60 or so HPV types. The characteristic feature of all HPV infections is hyperplasia of the epidermis, which can range from a focus of a few hundred cells to large pedunculated verrucous lesions (Fig. 28.48). There is a curious absence of inflammation. The

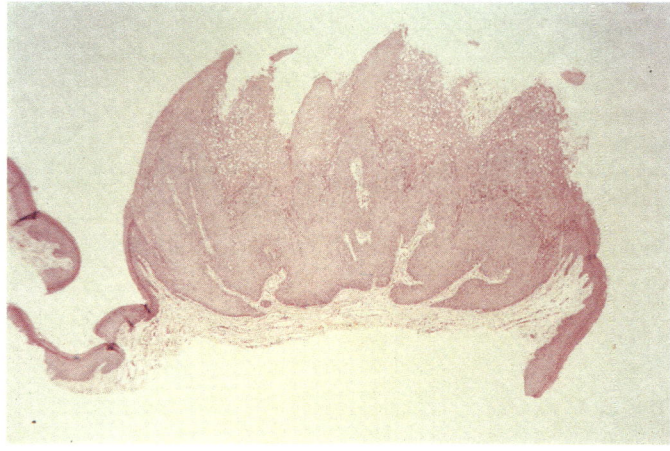

Fig. 28.48 Verruca vulgaris. There is a localized proliferation of the epithelium. The lateral edges of the proliferated epithelium point in towards the centre of the lesion.

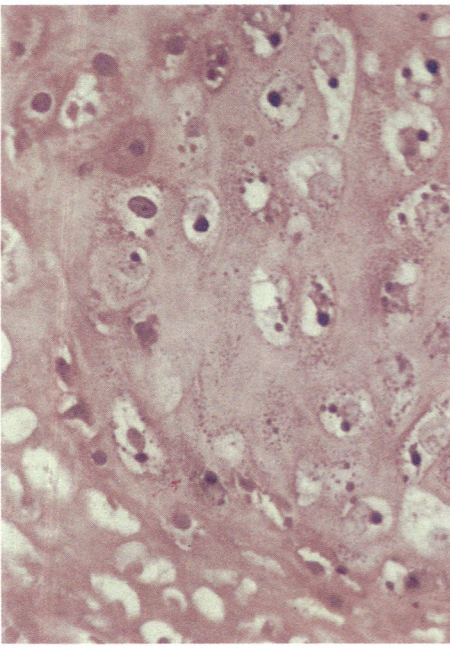

Fig. 28.49 Human papilloma virus infection of skin. Numerous 'koilo-cytic' cells with clearing of cytoplasm and basophilic granules.

presence of intranuclear eosinophilic inclusions is rare, but should raise the possibility of HPV in an otherwise non-inflamed acanthotic and hyperplastic epidermis. More typically, intra-cytoplasmic basophilic inclusions are seen. Both types of inclusion may be associated with 'koilocytic' change (Fig. 28.49) and occasional syncytial multinucleated appearances.

28.16 Pigmentary disorders

A variety of skin conditions can result in either increased or decreased pigmentation. A few of the commoner causes are listed in Table 28.3. In the majority of cases, the diagnosis is straightforward, as is the mechanism of increased or decreased pigmentation.

Table 28.3 Pigmentary disorders

Pigment	Epithelium	Dermis
Increased melanin	Sun-tan, freckles, lentigines, chloasma, naevi, melanoma	Post-inflammatory, blue naevi, incontinentia pigmenti
Decreased melanin	Vitiligo, albinism, naevi	Scarring
Others	Hyperkeratosis	Blood/haemosiderin, tattoos

28.16.1 Incontinentia pigmenti (Bloch–Sulzberger disease)

This rare, specific condition occurs in neonates. It should not be confused with the much commoner pigment incontinence which occurs in many epithelial inflammatory conditions, par-ticularly those with destruction of basal cells, e.g. lichen planus, lupus erythematosus. In these inflammatory conditions, the destroyed epithelial cells appear to release their melanin, which is then taken up and concentrated in the papillary dermal macrophages. In contrast, incontinentia pigmenti presents in neonates as blisters and is much commoner in females. The epithelium contains small vesicles (in the prickle cell layer) which characteristically contain eosinophil polymorphs. The blisters subside, to be replaced by a pseudo-epitheliomatous change, which again subsides to leave a depigmented, other-wise normal, epithelium. The papillary dermis contains hyper-pigmented macrophages. The aetiopathogenesis is totally obscure, but it may be an X-linked dominant condition which is lethal in male fetuses.

28.16.2 Vitiligo

Vitiligo is a common lesion (around 0.5 per cent of the popula-tion) which appears to have an auto-immune mechanism. Antibodies to melanocytes have been identified in the serum, and the lesions are associated with other organ-specific auto-immune disorders. The skin shows a mixture of changes, depending on the stage of progression of the lesion. At the early stage, there is a scattered, mild mononuclear inflammatory reaction which is focal in the lower epidermis and related papil-lary dermis. In the late stages, there is no inflammation and the only abnormality visible is decreased melanocyte numbers and epithelial depigmentation.

28.17 Tumours of the skin

Beryl Crossley and K. A. Fleming

This section includes not only lesions that are benign and malig-nant, but also a variety of hamartomata and hyperplasias. Included here is the term naevus (naevi). This name has caused difficulty for several reasons. There is no generally accepted de-finition, but normally a naevus is a benign proliferation of one or several components of the skin, causing discoloration and arising at or around birth or infancy. However, while many are congenital, and present at birth, not all are: some arise quite late in life. Also, some authors (particularly pathologists) have used the term in a very restricted sense to encompass only melanocytic naevi, while others (particularly clinicians) have used the term widely and applied it to almost any discoloration of the skin. Furthermore, while some have used naevus and hamartoma synonymously, this can cause problems, since so-called 'minus naevi' consist of a reduction or absence of components of the skin, quite the opposite of hamartoma. Thus, it would be preferable to abandon the name naevus completely. However, as it is deeply entrenched, this will probably be impossible. Accordingly, if the name is to be used, it should be done realizing that a naevus does not imply a specific pathology and is applied to a variety of different processes.

For ease of classification, the lesions will be described according to the skin region primarily involved, i.e. epidermis, pilosebaceous follicle, etc.

28.17.1 Benign epidermal lesions

Naevi

Epidermal naevi have a variety of clinical forms, but all basically show a roughened warty skin, sometimes with hyperpigmentation. Linear epidermal naevi are arranged in a linear fashion, while naevus unius lateris is a more extensive unilateral lesion. Bilateral extensive lesions are called ichthyosis hystrix, while solitary isolated lesions are called acrokeratosis of Kopf, or hard naevus of Unna. The degree of keratinization can vary, resulting in a hard or soft clinical appearance.

Histopathologically all lesions consist of hyperkeratotic, acanthotic, papillomatous epithelium, the quantity of each being variable and accounting for the clinical impression of hardness or softness. Inflammation can be extensive, particularly in inflammatory linear verrucous epidermal naevi (ILVEN).

Several points are worthy of note.

1. Ichthyosis hystrix can often show epidermolytic hyperkeratosis, as is found in some forms of ichthyosis.

2. The microscopic differential diagnosis of most epidermal naevi is of viral wart, simple squamous papilloma, seborrhoeic keratosis, and acanthosis nigricans. These require clinical differentiation.

3. Occasionally the clinical diagnosis is of a dermatitic or psoriatic plaque which is not responding to treatment and is therefore biopsied.

4. Often epidermal naevi are associated with malformation of adnexal components and are thus part of an organoid naevus (see below).

Organoid naevus (naevus sebaceous of Jadassohn)

These are developmental lesions that have both epidermal and dermal components in the malformation. The epidermal component is usually a hyperkeratotic, acanthotic epidermis, showing variable papillomatosis. The dermal component is of malformed, small pilosebaceous units, often with multiple sebaceous glands. There are frequently apocrine sweat glands present.

Clinically the lesions present in early life (often at birth) as a roughened yellow area. It is frequently found in the scalp. Hair growth is reduced. At puberty, the sebaceous elements enlarge, causing clinical presentation. In later life, there is an increased risk of tumour development, particularly basal cell carcinoma. However, syringocystadenoma papilliferum is the commonest tumour to develop in organoid naevi. Other tumours, such as malignant melanoma, squamous cell carcinoma, syringoma, sebaceous epithelioma, and nodular hidradrenoma can also develop.

Seborrhoeic keratosis (basal cell papilloma)

This common lesion typically arises in middle to old age and appears to be 'stuck on to' the skin. It is usually dark brown in colour due to melanin hyperpigmentation and is warty and greasy in appearance. It is slowly growing and can occur anywhere in the body. It is entirely benign.

Histopathologically it is comprised of a mixture of immature small basaloid cells and squamous cells keratinizing through a granular layer. The latter frequently form keratinous microcysts (horn cysts). The epithelium is papillomatous, acanthotic, and hyperkeratotic. The major diagnostic feature is the architectural structure of the lesion (Fig. 28.50).

Several variants are recognized, including solid, reticular, and papillomatous. More importantly, many lesions show reactive changes that are accompanied by more widespread maturation and keratinization. Often this keratinized squamous epithelium forms distinct nodules within the epithelium, called squamous eddies (Fig. 28.51). This 'activated' seborrhoeic keratosis may be accompanied by inflammation. It can mimic a well-differentiated squamous cell carcinoma. Differentiation is by recognition of the 'stuck-on' architecture.

Melanoacanthoma

In this variant there is melanocyte proliferation in addition to the normal epithelial cells of seborrhoeic keratosis.

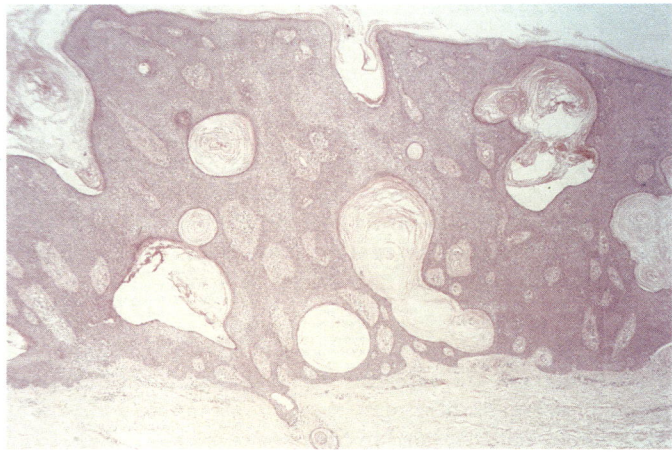

Fig. 28.50 Basal cell papilloma. Classic pattern with horn cysts and large islands of proliferating basaloid epithelial cells. This epithelium is raised above the rest of the skin to give a 'stuck on' appearance.

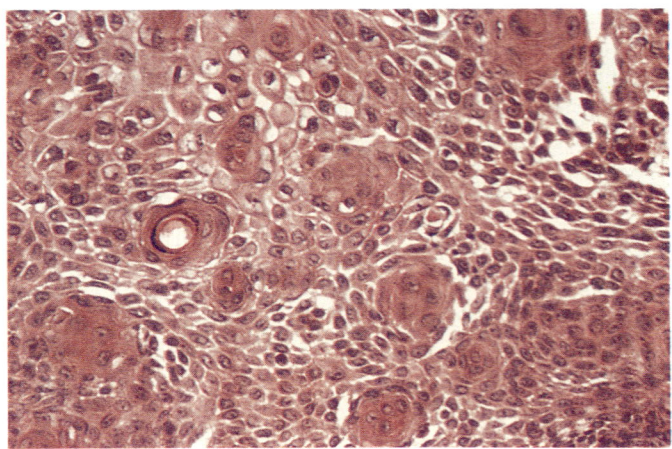

Fig. 28.51 Activated basal cell papilloma. Focal squamous differentiation and marked intercellular oedema resulting in the appearance of 'squamous eddies'. These appearances can mimic a well-differentiated squamous cell carcinoma.

Inverted follicular keratosis

This is similar to an activated seborrhoeic keratosis, but appears to arise in the follicular infundibulum—hence the alternate name of follicular poroma. This intradermal location can lead to difficulty in differentiation from squamous cell carcinoma. The main tool in making the diagnosis is considering whether the lesion could be an inverted follicular keratosis.

Squamous cell papilloma

This is a purely descriptive diagnosis, depending on the presence of papillomatous proliferation of squamous epithelium, often with hyperkeratosis. These lesions probably represent a collection of different entities, including reactive hyperplasia, human papilloma virus induced hyperplasia, naevoid lesions, and even actinic keratosis.

Clear cell acanthoma

This is an uncommon lesion found in the lower limbs of the middle-aged or elderly. It is usually solitary, but can be multiple. It presents as a raised plaque-like lesion with a sharply demarcated edge. There is often a scale around the edge. Histopathologically there is characteristic acanthosis of pale, clear keratinocytes, which contain abundant glycogen. The demarcation from non-involved epidermis is strikingly abrupt. Whether it is a benign tumour, reactive hyperplasia, or a naevoid lesion is unclear. It is entirely benign.

Epidermal cysts

Many lesions in the skin can be cystic, but a very common lesion is a keratin-filled cyst lined by squamous epithelium. These are usually situated in the upper reticular dermis. They are of two types: those in which there is keratinization through formation of keratohyalin (epidermal cysts) and those in which the keratinization is of tricholemmal type (tricholemmal cysts).

Both are entirely benign and often rupture to produce a foreign body granulomatous inflammatory reaction. Occasionally multiple tricholemmal cysts are seen in the scalp, forming a large and discrete lesion. These proliferating tricholemmal cysts (pilar tumour) (Fig. 28.52) are characterized by marked squamous proliferation and widespread rupture and reactive inflammation. This appearance mimics an invasive squamous cell carcinoma. Recognition of the tricholemmal nature of this lesion should permit diagnosis. It is benign.

28.17.2   Premalignant epithelial disease

Solar keratosis

Solar keratoses present as keratotic, raised or atrophic plaques on the sun-exposed skin of the middle-aged and elderly. They are a consequence of cumulative sun exposure. Histopathologically the epidermis may be either acanthotic with papillomatosis (Fig. 28.53) or, more rarely, it is atrophic. There is always a variable degree of epithelial dysplasia, which may be focal, ranging from mild atypia of basal cells to full thickness epithelial dysplasia. If large or multinucleated giant cells are present, the lesion can resemble Bowen disease (Bowenoid solar keratosis). There is often striking basal down-budding. The surface of the lesion shows alternating hyperkeratosis and parakeratosis. This alternating hyper- and parakeratosis is the hallmark of actinic keratoses. It arises because of the variable biology of different parts of the epithelium. The epithelial cells formed by the sweat ducts and hair follicles are apparently slower to become dysplastic than the intervening epithelium (Fig. 28.54). Accordingly, while the stratum corneum above the dysplastic epithelium shows abnormal keratinization with retention of nuclei (parakeratosis), that above the intra-epithelial sweat ducts/ pilosebaceous follicles keratinizes more normally, resulting in orthokeratotic hyperkeratosis. Another result of this relative resistance of intra-epithelial duct cells to UV light is that the

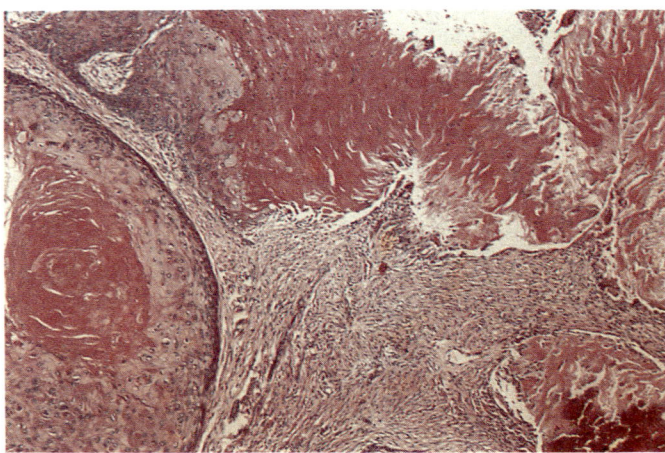

Fig. 28.52 Pilar tumour. Numerous keratin-filled cysts, some of which have ruptured and have evoked a focal inflammatory infiltrate. There is no granular layer at the junction of the keratin and the squamous epithelium, indicating the tricholemmal origin of the cells.

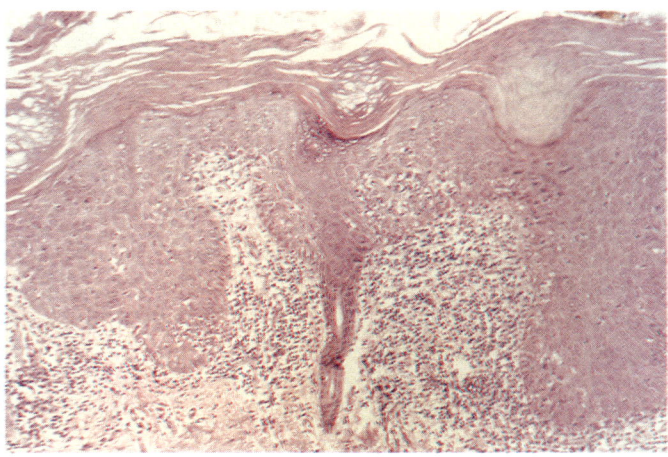

Fig. 28.53 Actinic keratosis. Note the thickening of the keratin layer which shows alternating parakeratosis and orthokeratosis. The orthokeratosis is situated above the intra-epidermal portion of a sweat duct. The surrounding epidermis shows dysplasia, evidenced by different staining characteristics.

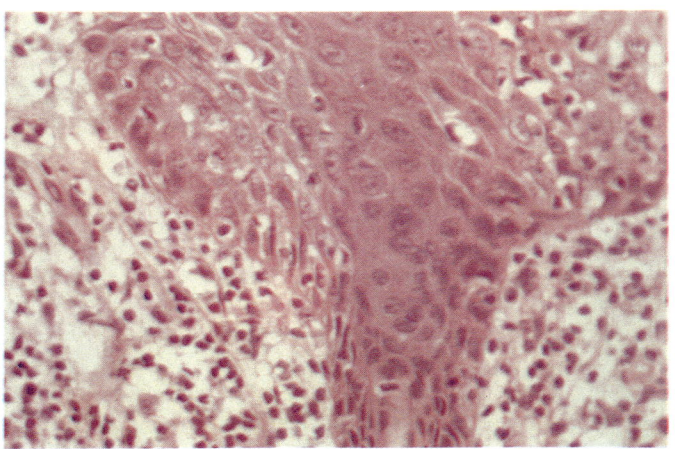

Fig. 28.54 Actinic keratosis. Higher-power view of Fig. 28.53. This shows the relatively normal epithelium of the intra-epidermal sweat duct, while the surrounding basal epithelium shows loss of polarity and pleomorphism of the cells. Note that this dysplastic epithelium is growing down the outside of the sweat duct.

intervening dysplastic epithelial cells grow down the outside of the sweat ducts and pilosebaceous units in a characteristic 'cuffing' fashion. Another relatively common feature in actinic keratoses is acantholysis. This affects the supra-basal cells particularly and can sometimes form significant clefting. It can mimic pemphigus, Darier disease, and warty dyskeratoma. In all of these variants the superficial dermis shows solar elastosis, a basophilic homogeneous change caused by accumulation of abnormal elastic tissue. A chronic inflammatory infiltrate surrounds the lesion.

A small proportion of solar keratoses will develop into infiltrating squamous carcinoma, but the prognosis for this tumour is good, with only a minority resulting in metastasis. Indeed, it is claimed by some that metastases never occur.

Bowen disease

This is characterized by slightly raised, gradually expanding plaques in areas that are not normally exposed to the sun. Histopathologically, these lesions show full-thickness epithelial dysplasia with overlying hyper- and parakeratosis (Fig. 28.55). Flow cytometric studies of the amount of cellular DNA shows aneuploidy within all lesions of Bowen disease studied, even though the proportion that will develop into squamous carcinoma is low (5 per cent). Occasionally Bowen disease occurs on the vulva and when it appears on the glans penis it is graced with the name erythroplasia of Queyrat.

Bowen disease is said to herald or predate an internal malignancy in a proportion of patients. There is no explanation for this association.

28.17.3 Squamous cell carcinoma

This tumour of the keratinocytes is most frequently found in sun-exposed areas of the fair-skinned. It is probably the second most common cancer of the skin after basal cell carcinoma. Typically the lesion presents as an ulcerating indurated nodule on a sun-exposed site in an elderly male. There is often preexisting actinic damage in the skin, with actinic keratosis and elastosis. Squamous cell carcinoma can also arise in a site of pre-existing ulceration, such as stasis ulcers of the leg.

Most squamous cell carcinomas (SCC) are well-differentiated tumours which show keratinization (Fig. 28.56). The malignant squamous cells invade into the dermis, extension beyond the sweat ducts being diagnostic (Fig. 28.57). This is in contrast to keratoacanthoma, where the infiltrating epithelium does not penetrate beyond the sweat gland level. Occasionally the tumour shows widespread acantholysis reminiscent of pemphigus. Infrequently a poorly differentiated pattern is present

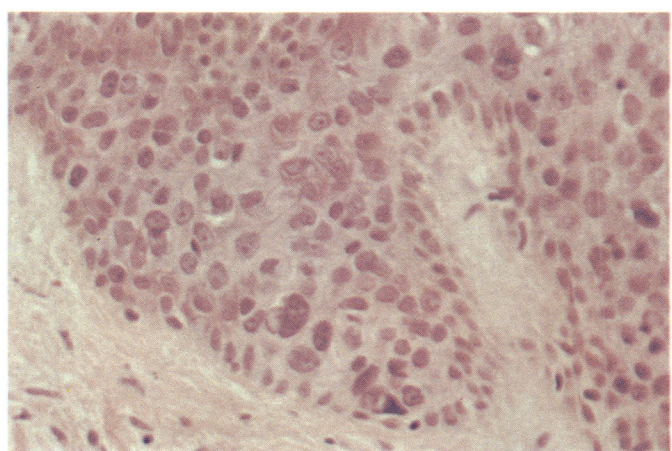

Fig. 28.55 Bowen disease. Marked dysplasia of the squamous epithelium with numerous pleomorphic, hyperchromatic, squamous cells.

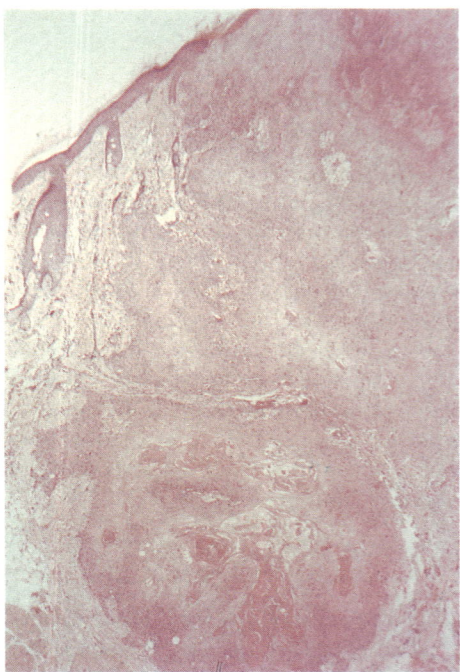

Fig. 28.56 Squamous cel carcinoma of the skin. A large, well-differentiated squamous cell carcinoma extending deeply into the subcutaneous fat. The tumour is originating from the surface epithelium.

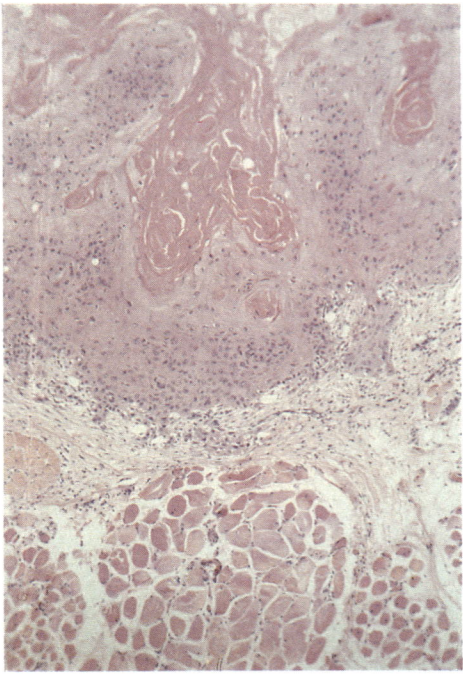

Fig. 28.57 Squamous cell carcinoma. A higher-power view of the tumour seen in Fig. 28.56. Note that the tumour is very well differentiated, showing marked keratinization. Its lower edge infiltratēs the deep structures and has almost reached voluntary muscle.

with spindle cells. This unusual variant occurs in the head and neck region of the elderly. Metastasis of all variants is normally to the local and regional lymph nodes. The prognosis of all the tumours is good with conventional treatment (surgery, radiation, etc.), the five-year survival rate being about 90 per cent. The rare variant, verrucous carcinoma, rarely metastasizes unless treated inadequately by radiation. This lesion arises on oral and genital mucosa and appears as a large, well-differentiated, bulbous tumour. A wart virus-induced lesion of similar appearance is the giant condyloma of Buschke–Loewenstein, which is found on the genitals. Another well-differentiated variant of SCC is found occasionally on the skin of the foot (epithelioma cuniculatum).

The differential diagnosis is normally not difficult since most are well-differentiated lesions. However, the spindle-cell variant needs to be delineated from spindle-cell malignant melanoma and atypical fibroxanthoma. This is most easily achieved by examination of multiple levels and by immunohistochemistry (cytokeratins, melanoma-associated antigens, and connective tissue markers).

Pathogenesis of squamous cell dysplasia and cancer

Besides ultraviolet light, a number of agents have been proposed as promoters or initiators of epithelial dysplasia. Arsenic is known to induce an atypical epithelial proliferation following prolonged topical exposure or ingestion. In renal transplant patients there is a higher incidence of skin cancers and their precursor lesions, especially in sunny climates and on sun-exposed skin. This is related to the presence of human papilloma virus, often of relatively uncommon types. It has also been related to azathioprine therapy given to reduce transplant rejection. Azathioprine is metabolized to 6-thioguanine which is incorporated into DNA. Thiopurines are known to be unstable in the presence of ultraviolet light of wavelength between 320 and 360 nm, so exacerbating the damaging effects of sunlight. Therapeutic X-irradiation slightly increases the probability of later development of skin cancer in the area of irradiation after a latency period of over 20 years. This effect is seen more often in females, and resultant basal cell carcinomas outnumber squamous tumours or their precursors. Polycyclic aromatic hydrocarbons have been long recognized as a cause of squamous carcinoma (Potts carcinoma of the scrotum in chimney sweeps) and, indeed, much of the theory of initiation and promotion of chemical and viral carcinogens has been devised from the results of work done on induction of squamous carcinomas on the skin of animals.

Epidermodysplasia verruciformis and HPV infection

The association between wart virus infection and squamous epithelial dysplasia has recently become topical. One example of this is the disease epidermodysplasia verruciformis (EV), which is a generalized cutaneous viral infection caused by human papilloma virus (HPV) of many types. There are now over 60 types of human papilloma virus identified. Most common skin warts (verruca vulgaris) are due to HPV type 2 while the plantar warts of the feet are often due to HPV-1. Other types of HPV are found infrequently in skin lesions, unless there is some systemic abnormality, e.g. immunosuppression (as in renal transplant) or EV. In EV there is a familial predisposition which may have autosomal recessive inheritance. It appears that there is genetic immunodeficiency of T-cell responses. When the lesions of EV are caused by HPV-5 there is a very high incidence of cutaneous malignancy. Most of these lesions occur on sun-exposed sites.

There is also good evidence for a causative role for wart virus in some dysplastic lesions of the genitals. One such condition, known as Bowenoid papulosis, presents in the anogenital region of younger adults as multiple pigmented papules. Histopathologically, the papules show irregular acanthosis with vacuolation of cells of the granular layer and overlying hyper- and parakeratosis. Throughout the lesion there is epithelial dysplasia, often with individual atypical cells at all levels of the epidermis superimposed upon otherwise normal maturation. Electron microscopy and immunohistology using a polyclonal rabbit anti-HPV antibody suggest the presence of wart virus within the lesions of Bowenoid papulosis. Also DNA hybridization using labelled cloned sequences from HPV-16 shows the presence of closely related sequences in a majority of cases. The precise role of human papilloma viruses in carcinogenesis is the subject of intense investigation, but no definitive mechanism has been identified. The function of the E7 gene (7th early gene) is currently the most promising candidate (see also Chapter 21).

28.17.4 Keratoacanthoma

A keratoacanthoma is a rapidly growing lesion of the elderly, often confused both clinically and histologically with a squamous carcinoma. It presents as an enlarging, keratotic mass, and microscopy shows a cup-shaped lesion filled with keratin and surrounded by proliferating epithelium (Fig. 28.58). The latter is thickened and often papillomatous and composed of large epithelial cells with pale, homogeneous, eosinophilic cytoplasm. Characteristically, the lesion is very well defined, showing shoulders of normal surface epidermis. The base of the lesion, though also defined and delineated by a chronic inflammatory infiltrate, often shows proliferating tongues of epithelial cells, and there may be significant dysplasia. The epithelium never extends beyond the level of the sweat glands. Spontaneous resolution occurs within 3–6 months and persistence beyond this should cast doubt on the diagnosis. Often these lesions are curetted or badly oriented in section, which makes appreciation of the architecture difficult and sometimes impossible to distinguish from a squamous carcinoma.

28.17.5 Basal cell carcinoma

The most common malignant tumour of man, basal cell carcinoma presents usually after middle age on sun-exposed skin, initially as a small, slowly growing lesion with a depressed centre and raised edges. If left, these tumours continue to grow and to infiltrate and destroy surrounding tissues ('rodent'

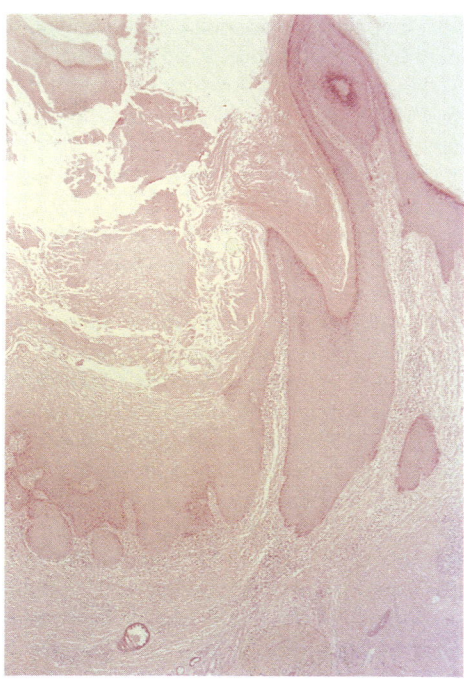

Fig. 28.58 Keratoacanthoma. The classic structure of a keratin-filled cup-shaped tumour is present. The shoulder of the keratoachanthoma is formed by relatively normal squamous epithelium. The proliferating squamous epithelium is well differentiated and shows pale eosinophilic cytoplasm. The lower edge is above the sweat gland present at the base of the figure.

ulcer). They have a very low metastatic potential (< 1 per cent).

Histopathologically, basal cell carcinoma (BCC) consists of irregular islands of epithelial cells within the dermis, sometimes clearly arising from the overlying epidermis (Fig. 28.59). The epithelial cells of the islands are relatively homogeneous, with oval, deeply basophilic nuclei and a little cytoplasm. Around the

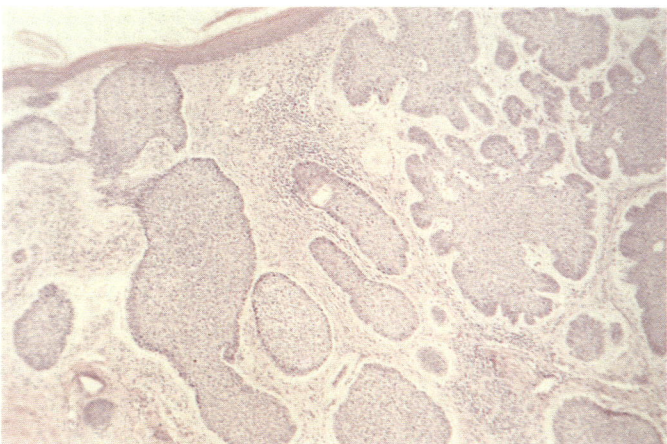

Fig. 28.59 Basal cell carcinoma. This is a typical basal cell carcinoma taking origin from the surface epithelium. There are islands of basaloid cells with surrounding pale eosinophilic stroma. Note the peripheral palisade of nuclei in tumour islands.

periphery of the tumour islands, the epithelial nuclei are arranged parallel to each other, lined up perpendicular to the edge of the island, a feature known as peripheral nuclear palisading (Fig. 28.60). The immediately surrounding stroma is characteristically loose. Indeed, the presence of such stroma is almost universal in BCC, such that it has been suggested that the growth and differentiation of the tumour is controlled by this stroma. The rest of the dermis may show solar elastosis and variable fibrosis, with a chronic inflammatory infiltrate. A common artefact seen is shrinkage of the stroma away from the tumour islands, leaving a gap or hole. The surrounding inflammation includes a high proportion of lymphocytes, especially T-suppressor cells, and immune cytotoxicity has been suggested to explain the slow growth and low metastatic rate of basal cell carcinomas despite a short cell-doubling time. It has been noticed that defects in cell-mediated immunity, including the acquired immune deficiency syndrome (AIDS), are associated with a higher rate of metastazing basal cell carcinomas.

BCCs show a huge variety of microscopic patterns. This represents differentiation of the basaloid cells towards various adnexal components of the epithelium. While these variations are of interest to the morphologist, with few exceptions they carry no prognostic implications (see below). Thus, islands of basal cell carcinoma occasionally show central cystic degeneration, and when this is a prominent feature the tumour is called an adenoid cystic basal cell carcinoma. However, this tumour behaves in exactly the same manner as a typical BCC. Similarly, tumour islands close to the epidermis may have a central area of

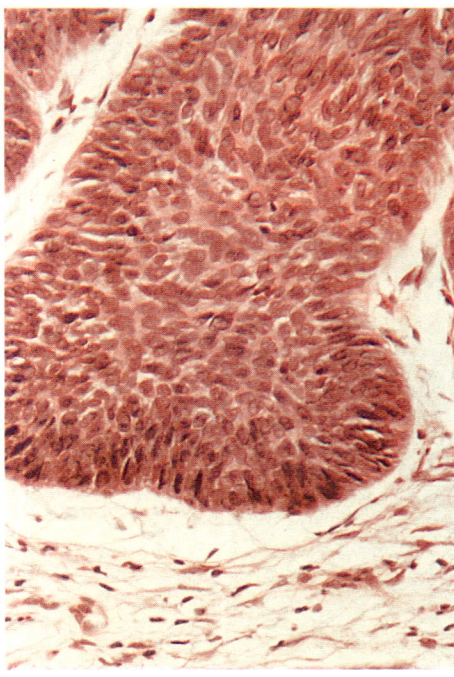

Fig. 28.60 Basal cell carcinoma. A nodule of tumour showing a poorly defined peripheral palisade. The tumour cells are small with large round/oval nuclei. Note that the stroma has shrunk away from the epithelium to form a cleft.

squamous differentiation, but the tumour will behave as a basal cell carcinoma.

Basosquamous cancer

In contrast, the term basosquamous carcinoma is reserved for that small percentage of tumours in which there is recognizable basal cell carcinoma and unequivocal squamous carcinoma, with a transition between. These rare tumours have an increased tendency to metastasize and, as such, should be specifically identified.

Aggressive BCC

In addition, a few basal cell carcinomas have a tendency to infiltrate particularly extensively. These 'aggressive' variants of BCC can be recognized by their peculiar tendency to infiltrate widely and deeply, often in very small clumps of cells and usually without any noticeable stroma, unlike all other variants. It is important to recognize the aggressive BCC early, since adequate excision requires wider and deeper surgery than normal. Failure to do so results in extensive deep infiltration, often into and through bone, which in the head and neck then becomes virtually inoperable. Very occasionally they show lymphatic and perineural invasion.

The recurrence or re-emergence rate of a basal cell cancer is dependent on the adequacy of the original excision, though an apparent recurrence may be another tumour arising in an area of 'field change' of sun-damaged skin.

Solar exposure is unequivocally associated with the development of basal cell carcinoma. A number of genetically determined conditions exacerbate the effects of ultraviolet light and result in multiple basal cell carcinomas at an earlier age than normal. These diseases include xeroderma pigmentosum and Gorlin syndrome. In both these conditions a defect in cellular DNA repair following damage by ultraviolet light has been proposed.

28.17.6   Benign melanocytic lesions

The normal melanocyte

Melanocytes are melanin-producing cells characterized by their intracytoplasmic development of melanosomes. They originate in the neural crest during early fetal life and migrate to the periphery from as early as 6 weeks' gestation, along developing nerves and vessels. Within the skin, they are found between basal epidermal cells and communicate with 30–40 keratinocytes, transferring melanin to the epidermal cells. All human races possess a similar number of peripheral melanocytes, but the cells vary in their melanin-producing activity and in the state of maturation of their melanosomes. Normal melanocytes are present as singly disposed cells along the dermo-epidermal junction.

Melanocytic proliferations: lentigo

A lentigo simplex is clinically a flat, pigmented lesion consisting of a localized proliferation of single melanocytes at the dermo-epidermal junction. In a senile lentigo there may also be irregular acanthosis and solar elastosis. A gradually expanding flat pigmented lesion of the face of the elderly may include some atypical melanocytic cells and this lesion is known as a lentigo maligna, carrying a risk of future development of melanoma (see below).

Melanocytic naevus

This is a raised, pigmented lesion which may be present at birth or acquired during life. In the acquired form, small groups of melanocyte nests proliferate at the dermo-epidermal junction and are then released as packets into the underlying dermis (Fig. 28.61). As the melanocytes descend into the deeper dermis, the packeted arrangement may become obscured and the cells apparent as sheets. At these deeper levels, the melanocyte nuclei become smaller and more hyperchromatic, with no nucleolus visible, a process that is known as maturation and is said to be characteristic of a benign lesion. Sometimes, the deeper cells of a benign naevus become spindle-shaped, with wavy cytoplasm, and this is known as neuroid change. Occasionally they can mimic neurofibroma. The whole lesion is typically a nodule in the skin.

The congenital lesions, in contrast, are much more diffuse than the acquired variant, involve predominantly the mid–lower dermis and show extensive infiltration of the melanocytes in and around the dermal appendages (sweat glands etc.). There is only a little lentigenous proliferation of melanocytes at the dermo-epidermal junction. Clinically there are three types, depending on the size: small naevi are less than 1.5 cm diameter, giant naevi are greater than 20 cm diameter, and intermediate naevi lie between. The importance of differentiating the two forms of melanocytic naevi (congenital versus acquired) lies in the recognition that giant (and possibly smaller) congenital naevi have an increased risk of malignant transformation. Un-

fortunately, however, the histopathological differences between the two are not as clear-cut as indicated above. Undoubtedly, some naevi presenting at birth show features of the acquired type. Thus, confident diagnosis of a congenital melanocytic naevus requires close clinical and histopathological cooperation.

A benign naevus follows a well-documented pattern of development. A junctional naevus consists of groups of cells at the dermo-epidermal junction only, with no involvement of the dermis. In a compound naevus, there is proliferative activity at the dermo-epidermal junction and naevus cells present within the dermis. An intradermal naevus no longer shows evidence of junctional activity.

Unusual variants of melanocytic naevi

Spitz naevus

An uncommon compound melanocytic naevus occurring in children and occasionally in adults, Spitz naevus presents as a well-defined, often only lightly pigmented, raised pink or red lesion. The histopathological appearance may be mistaken for malignant melanoma because the melanocytes are large and sometimes atypical, with epithelioid, multinucleated giant and spindle forms. There may be mitotic activity. Vessels are telangiectatic and there is often a lymphohistiocytic infiltrate. Frequently, the epidermis shows pseudo-epitheliomatous change. Differentiation from malignant melanoma is possible because of the clinical and microscopic appearance and also because there is no significant epidermal invasion by melanocytes although occasional single innocuous cells may be present. Furthermore, there is maturation of cells within the dermis. Typically the lesion is symmetrical around the centre.

Pigmented spindle-cell naevus (Reed)

In this variant of compound naevus most, or all, of the melanocytes have a spindle-cell configuration. There is often an impressively large amount of melanin present, both within the melanocytes and the melanophages. There is no significant epidermal involvement although occasional single innocuous cells may be present, and recognition largely depends on awareness. It is common on the thigh of females, presenting as a dark nodule.

Blue naevus

A blue naevus is a discrete, often flat, blue-coloured lesion which consists of collections of small, regular, often spindle, melanocytic cells within the deep dermis. Melanin pigmentation is variable and there may be much coarse pigmentation within melanophages, tending to obscure the melanocytic cells. A cellular variant usually shows a lesser degree of pigmentation. The naevus is thought to be the result of arrested migration melanocytes during fetal life, with their subsequent proliferation.

Dysplastic naevus

A dysplastic naevus differs clinically from a typical benign naevus in showing either large size (greater than 5 mm

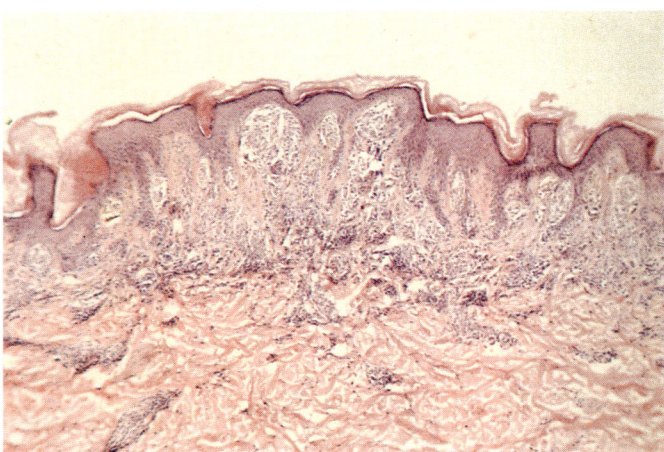

Fig. 28.61 Compound melanocytic naevus. There are nests of melanocytic cells present at the dermo-epidermal junction. These melanocytic cells are extending down into the papillary and upper reticular dermis. There is no spread of the melanocytes into the overlying epithelium.

diameter), irregularity of the margin, nodularity, erythema or variable pigmentation, and accentuated skin markings. Histopathologically, the features of a dysplastic naevus are either melanocytic nuclear atypia, a lymphocytic infiltrate, or some evidence of dermal response to the naevus (for example lamellar fibrosis). In addition, there may be architectural changes, such as epithelial hyperplasia and prominent junctional activity at the tips of the dermal papillae, with bridging of junctional nests across a dermal papilla. Dysplastic naevi may be sporadic or part of an inherited condition (see below). Whether the sporadic forms carry an increased risk of *in situ* development of melanoma is controversial. Furthermore, many clinically typical melanocytic naevi show these features and identification is not possible purely on histopathological grounds. Absence of pagetoid spread of melanocytes is an important feature allowing distinction from malignant melanoma.

28.17.7   Malignant melanoma

Incidence and risk factors

World-wide, the reported incidence of malignant melanoma has increased dramatically over the past 30 years. The rise is seen particularly amongst persons of pale complexion with fair or red hair who expose themselves to periodic intense sunshine. In general, patients with melanoma report more past episodes of painful sunburn than controls. Melanins within keratinocytes absorb and therefore protect against the harmful effects of ultraviolet-B light (see Chapter 10). Such light is certainly a promoter and may act as an initiator for malignant melanoma.

All common malignant skin tumours show a seasonal variation in presentation, with a peak incidence from mid-August to mid-September. For basal cell and squamous carcinomas, total cumulative sunlight exposure over many years is of importance, suggesting a prolonged induction period with multiple stages. In contrast, for malignant melanoma (with the exception of lentigo maligna), several studies support a short induction period; the tumours developing during the summer months and presenting towards the end. Such a theory would explain the wide age-range of presentation of melanoma.

Other risk factors for malignant melanoma include preexisting melanocytic naevi, particularly the giant congenital type, the presence of one or more atypical or dysplastic naevi, and a family history of malignant melanoma. The latter ranges from a polygenic trait to an autosomal dominant condition in which the lifetime incidence of melanoma approaches 100 per cent; these melanomas often arise within a dysplastic naevus (familial dysplastic naevus or B-K mole syndromes).

There is no good evidence that oral contraceptives or exposure to fluorescent light are significant risk factors for the development of melanoma. A proportion of melanomas possess tumour cells that exhibit oestrogen receptors, and there is some evidence that women who have a large number of children have a slightly lower incidence. However, exogenously administered oestrogens have not been found to have a significant effect. Though multiple individual case reports propose a role for

trauma in the aetiology of melanoma, careful review fails to link trauma with the great majority of tumours.

Pathogenesis of malignant melanoma

Melanoma is a malignant tumour of melanocytes, cells that are derived from the neural crest and migrate to the periphery during fetal life. Primary cutaneous melanomas usually arise from malignant cells proliferating at the dermo-epidermal junction which then infiltrate the epidermis and often the dermis. In a proportion of cases, the lesion consists only of malignant tumour, while in others there is clinical and/or histopathological evidence of a pre-existing benign naevus. The proportion of melanomas apparently arising within a benign naevus ranges from 18 per cent to 83 per cent, depending on the investigator. As described above, benign naevi may be either present at birth or acquired during life. A small proportion of neonates (1 in 500 000) possess a giant, or bathing-trunk, congenital naevus and it has been estimated that their lifetime risk of melanoma is greater than 6.3 per cent. In contrast, it has not yet been convincingly demonstrated that acquired or smaller congenital melanocytic naevi carry an increased risk of developing melanoma.

Between 0.4 per cent and 12 per cent of melanomas occur in patients with an inherited susceptibility. Some of these have the dysplasic naevus (or B-K mole) syndrome, which often has autosomal dominant inheritance and may be due to a mutation in a gene on the short arm of chromosome 1, close to the rhesus gene. Abnormal-appearing naevi are noticed from late childhood and the median age of development of melanoma is 35 years, some 16 years earlier than the general population. Cultured fibroblasts and lymphoblasts from affected patients are mutated or killed more readily by ultraviolet light of wavelength 254 nm than those of controls. Dysplastic naevi also occur sporadically with no known family history but with a tendency to develop melanoma, and a small number of melanoma patients have diffuse melanocytic dysplasia which appears clinically as a mottling or freckling of the skin.

Classification of melanoma

Clinically, one of the hallmarks of a developing melanoma is a changing lesion. This change may be apparent as an increase in size, pigmentation, erythema, or irregularity of a mole, or the mole may become symptomatic with parasthetic 'awareness', itching, irritation, or ulceration.

Clincally and histopathologically, four subtypes of melanoma are recognized:

1. superficial spreading melanoma, accounting for over 70 per cent;
2. nodular melanoma, comprising 14.7 per cent;
3. lentigo maligna melanoma, 4.9 per cent;
4. acral lentiginous melanoma, relatively rare in the Caucasian population, but the most common form of melanoma amongst Negroes.

Superficial spreading melanomas

This is the most common and microscopically shows a prominent radial growth pattern along the dermo-epidermal junction and into the epidermis (Fig. 28.62). This is accompanied by a variable dermal component. The presence of spread of individual dysplastic melanocytes into and along the epidermis (pagetoid spread) is by far the most helpful diagnostic sign of malignant melanoma. The tumour cells are present singly or in nests, are often epithelioid in appearance and, in common with all melanomas, are atypical with finely dispersed cytoplasmic melanin pigmentation and a variable mitotic rate. A chronic inflammatory infiltrate within the dermis may be band-like beneath the tumour.

Nodular melanomas

These have a predominantly downward growth pattern into the dermis and do not spread laterally for more than three rete ridges beyond the bulk of the tumour (Fig. 28.63). The tumour cells show invasion of the epidermis and the dermis singly, as sheets, or as nests, and may be epithelioid or spindle cell. Unlike benign naevi, the cells in the dermis do not become smaller with regular hyperchromatic nuclei at increasing depth (a change often referred to as 'maturation' in a naevus), but remain atypical throughout the lesion (Fig. 28.64). Pigmentation, inflammation, and mitotic activity vary with the individual tumour.

Lentigo maligna melanoma

This is the development of malignancy in a slowly growing atypical lesion of sun-exposed areas in the elderly. Lentigo maligna presents clinically as a pigmented patch with an irregular margin, usually on the face, and is characterized by slow growth and changes in pigmentation. Histopathologically, atypical melanocytes proliferate singly along the dermo-epidermal junction and there is associated solar elastosis, a variable dermal inflammatory infiltrate, and often a degree of epidermal and dermal atrophy (Fig. 28.65). The onset of malignancy is

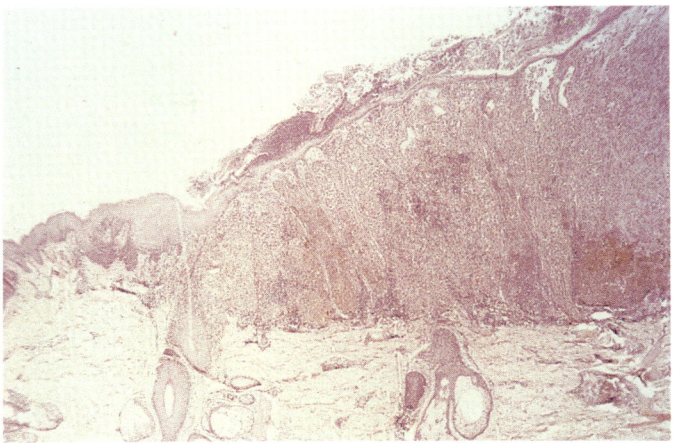

Fig. 28.63 Nodular malignant melanoma. There is a large tumour forming a discrete nodule in the skin. This tumour has extended halfway into the reticular dermis. There is focal melanin pigmentation. Note the relatively abrupt transition of the melanoma into normal skin.

heralded clinically by a recent change in the lesion—increasing nodularity or pigmentation. Histopathologically this is associated with invasion of the dermis or epidermis by malignant cells.

Acral lentiginous melanoma

Subungual regions, the palms and soles, are favoured sites. A prolonged lentiginous phase is characteristic, with proliferation of abnormal melanocytes at the dermo-epidermal junction, either singly or in nests, often accompanied by acanthosis. Melanoma is seen as invasion of the dermis and epidermis, the dermis often being invaded by spindle tumour cells.

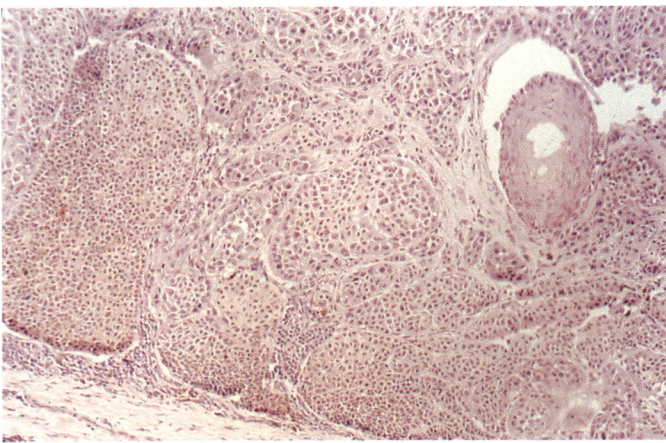

Fig. 28.64 Nodular malignant melanoma. A higher-power view of the tumour shown in Fig. 28.63. The melanoma cells are of variable size and are surrounding a hair follicle. There is marked variation in the pigmentation of the melanocytes. There is only a sparse mononuclear inflammatory infiltrate present at the edge of the tumour. The majority of these tumour cells are polygonal with abundant eosinophilic cytoplasm.

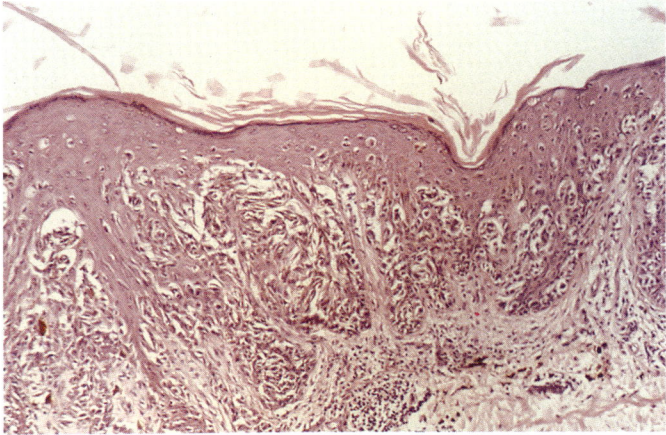

Fig. 28.62 Superficial spreading malignant melanoma. The epidermis shows extensive pagetoid spread of dysplastic melanocytes. At one side, there is invasion into the upper part of the papillary dermis.

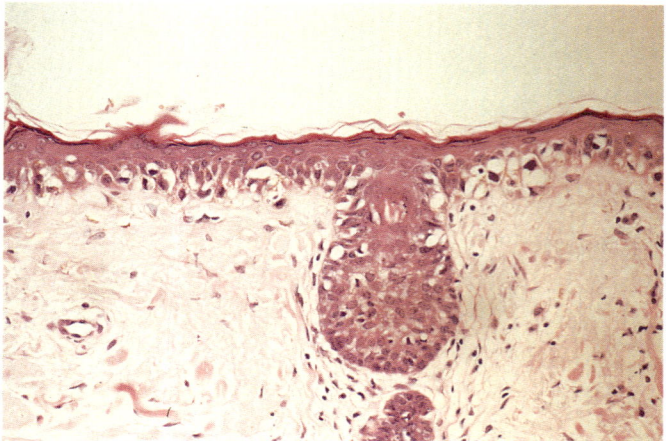

Fig. 28.65 Lentigo maligna. This is a portion of skin from a sun-damaged area showing increased numbers of melanocytes at the basal layer. These melanocytes show considerable nuclear hyperchromatism and pleomorphism. There is also cytoplasmic pleomorphism. The tumour cells are increased in number along the side of the hair follicle. Note that there is no significant pagetoid spread into the upper epidermis.

Differential diagnosis

Clinically, malignant melanoma must be distinguished from seborrhoeic keratosis, vascular lesions such as angiokeratoma and pyogenic granuloma, pigmented basal cell carcinoma, and benign or dysplastic naevi. Histopathologically it can be difficult to differentiate between a melanoma and a Spitz, spindle-cell, or a dysplastic naevus. Also amelanotic melanomas, especially if metastatic, may be difficult to distinguish from undifferentiated tumour of other histogenetic origin. Melanoma cells are often large, epithelioid, polygonal or spindle in shape, with pleomorphic nuclei, many of which possess a large eosinophilic nucleolus. The cytoplasm may be clearly defined, eosinophilic or occasionally clear ('balloon' cells), and melanin pigment may be apparent following a Masson–Fontana stain. Electron microscopic examination reveals melanosomes present within the cell cytoplasm. Immunohistological studies show S100 protein in melanocytes and their tumours, both benign and malignant. Also, several recently developed antibodies (e.g. NKI/C3) may be able to distinguish between malignant melanocytic and non-melanocytic lesions. As mentioned above, pagetoid spread of dysplastic melanocytes is almost universal in malignant melanoma, but is not found in benign lesions.

Prognostic indicators

A number of clinical parameters influence prognosis. With the exception of lentigo maligna melanoma, the greater the age of the patient at presentation, in general the worse the prognosis. Females have a better survival than males. An ulcerated lesion carries a worse prognosis than one with intact overlying epidermis. Melanomas arising on the trunk show worse survival figures than those arising elsewhere.

Histopathologically, two parameters are used regularly as prognostic indicators; the thickness of the lesion (Breslow thickness) and the depth of invasion (Clark's level). The tumour thickness is measured in millimetres from the granular layer of the epidermis to the deepest tumour cell. A tumour thickness of less than 0.76 mm confers almost 100 per cent survival; between 0.76 mm and 1.5 mm the five-year survival falls to 66 per cent; and is only 44 per cent for lesions greater than 1.5 mm. Clark's level refers to the anatomical structures involved by the tumour:

Level 1 Tumour confined to epidermis;

Level 2 Invasion into papillary dermis;

Level 3 The tumour reaches the junction between papillary and reticular dermis;

Level 4 There is extension into the reticular dermis;

Level 5 Melanoma extends to the subcutis.

A recent additional parameter is the Prognostic Index (PI). This is obtained by multiplying the Breslow thickness in mm by the number of tumour cell mitoses per square millimetre. A PI of less than 19 may be useful in predicting a better survival in those patients with tumours of medium thickness. Evidence of vascular invasion is a poor prognostic sign.

Regressing melanocytic lesions

Not infrequently, melanocytic naevi undergo changes including itching, erythema, and tenderness. These raise clinical suspicion of malignancy. However, these changes can be associated with apparent spontaneous destruction of the melanocytes. This is manifest histopathologically as increased mononuclear inflammation in and around the melanocytes, with swelling and necrosis of the same melanocytes (Fig. 28.66). Often there is a collection of residual eosinophilic debris in which the pattern of a melanocyte nest can be detected. These changes suggest an immune-mediated destruction of the melanocytes, but whether this is correct is currently

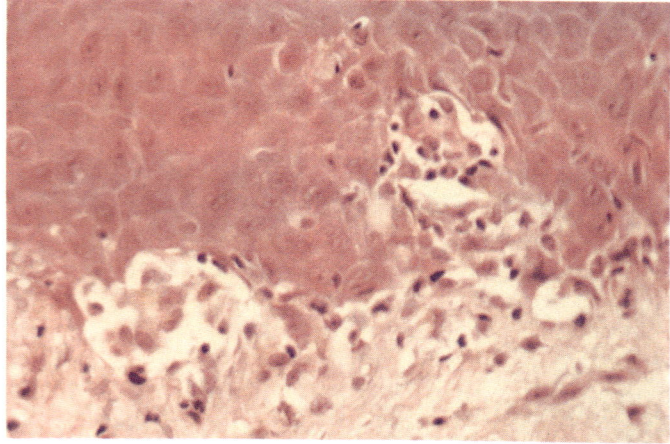

Fig. 28.66 Regressing melanocytic naevus. There are nests of residual melanocytes at the dermo-epidermal junction. These show considerable degenerative changes and have a sparse mononuclear inflammatory infiltrate around them.

unclear. It may be that the melanocytes become apoptotic for other reasons and the inflammatory response is reactive. The changes can be seen at times in all melanocytic lesions, ranging from melanocytic naevi (Sutton's halo naevus) to malignant melanomas.

28.17.8   Eccrine gland tumours

The normal eccrine gland

Eccrine sweat glands are present over most of the body surface. They consist of:

1. A secretory coil situated within the deep reticular dermis and composed of small gland lumina bounded by two cell layers, an inner epithelial and outer myoepithelial layer. Differentiation towards secretory coil is suggested by the detection of eccrine enzymes; by the presence of cytoplastic granules, cell-surface microvilli, and intercellular canaliculi on electron microscopy; and by the detection of S100 protein by immunohistology.

2. A sweat duct which connects the secretory coil to the surface. The duct is lined by two layers of epithelial cells which contain glycogen. The duct has an intra-epidermal and an intradermal component and the deeper part of the latter is coiled. Duct differentiation is suggested by glycogen within the cells, luminal microvilli covered by an amorphous layer, and keratohyalin granules within the cells of the intra-epidermal portion.

Eccrine gland tumours (Table 28.4) derive from these normal sweat gland components.

Eccrine poroma

Poromas usually occur as single pedunculated growths on the distal extremities at any age. Histopathologically, interconnecting bands of very homogeneous basaloid epithelial cells grow from the epidermis (Fig. 28.67) with a sharp distinction

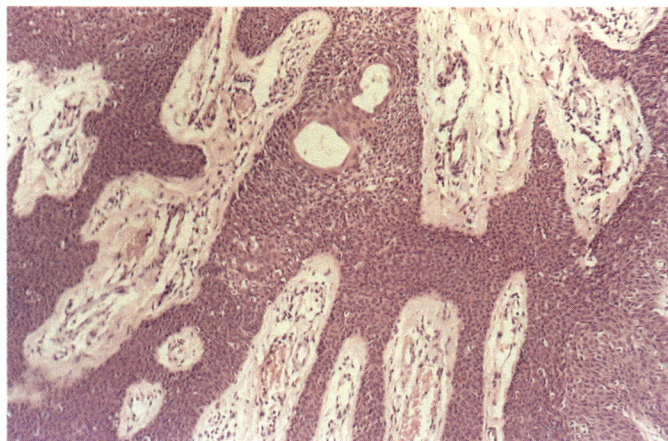

Fig. 28.67   Eccrine poroma. There are interlacing bundles of basaloid cells, scattered through which there are occasional ductal structures. These tumour cells are extending down from the surface epithelium.

between tumour and epidermal cells. The tumour cell bands show no peripheral nuclear palisading. Occasional lumina may be seen within the tumour. The cells contain glycogen. Electron microscopy and histochemistry support an origin from the intra-epidermal part of the eccrine duct. A rare malignant variant occurs on the upper thighs and buttocks of elderly people and is usually slow growing and locally invasive with metastases in a small proportion.

Syringoma

These small tumours usually occur as groups of yellow papules on the lower eyelids but may present as crops on the extremities. Light microscopy shows small nests and islands of epithelial cells within a fibrous dermis (Fig. 28.68). Some of the nests contain lumina and a few have a characteristic comma shape. The tumour cells sometimes contain glycogen and the nests

Table 28.4   Tumours of the eccrine gland

Name	Site	Malignant variant	Age/sex	Histogenesis	Single/multiple
Eccrine poroma	Feet and hands	Occasional	Middle age	Intra-epidermal sweat duct	Usually solitary
Syringoma	Eyelids	Occasional	Young; females	Intradermal sweat duct	Often multiple
Cylindroma	Scalp and face	Occasional; may arise in old benign tumour	F > M	Intradermal sweat duct	Sporadic single; genetic multiple
Eccrine hidrocystoma	Face	No	—	Intradermal sweat duct	Often multiple
Eccrine spiradenoma	Anywhere	Rare; may arise in benign tumour	Young	?Secretory coil; ?eccrine duct	Usually solitary
Hidradenoma	Head	Occasional; aggressive	F > M; middle age	Eccrine gland and duct	Usually solitary
Eccrine carcinoma	—	—	Rare	—	Solitary

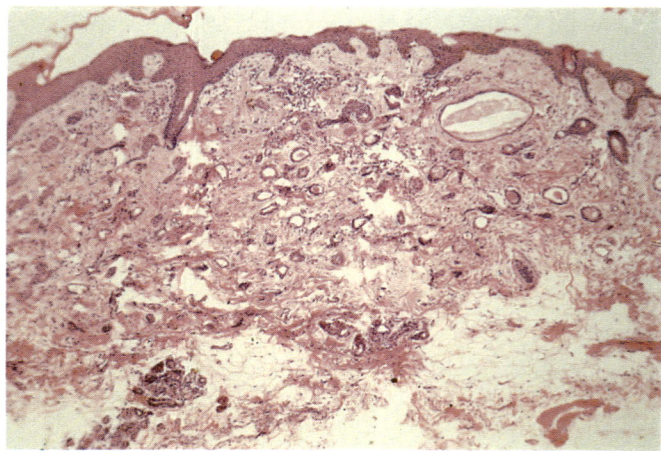

Fig. 28.68 Syringoma. A classic appearance of a syringoma with small tubular structures scattered through the dermis. The tubules towards the skin surface show cystic dilatation and keratinization.

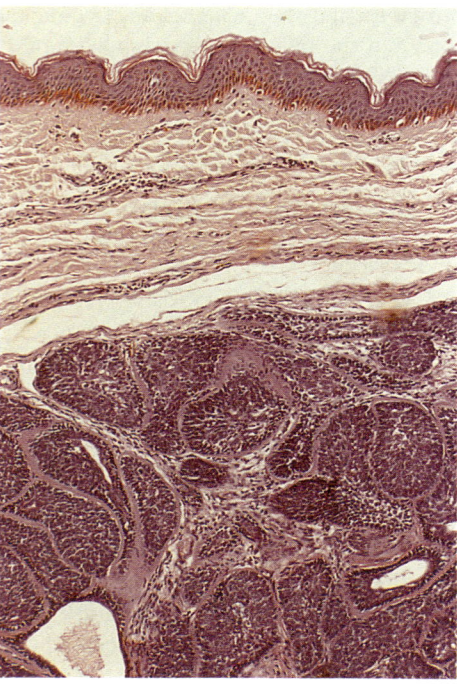

Fig. 28.69 Cylindroma. There is a discrete nodule in the dermis which is formed by interlacing islands of epithelial cells. The striking appearance is a thick layer of eosinophilic basement membrane material around each of the islands. There are scattered ductular structures.

may keratinize close to the surface. Syringomas are thought to arise from the intradermal sweat duct.

Cylindroma

Dermal cylindromas occur sporadically and also as multiple scalp tumours in those with an autosomal dominant genetic predisposition. The tumours are often circumscribed and consist of multiple islands of epithelial cells closely arranged in the dermis like a jigsaw Fig. 28.69). The islands are each encased by a hyaline sheath and similar hyaline droplets are often seen between tumour cells. Occasional lumina may be present. Electron microscopy and immunohistology suggest an origin from the intradermal eccrine duct, but an apocrine glandular origin has also been proposed.

Eccrine hidrocystoma

A small cystic lesion occurring on the face, this consists of a single cyst with papillary infoldings and lined by eccrine duct-like epithelium. A similar apocrine variant is recognized.

Eccrine spiradenoma

Presenting as a painful, very well-circumscribed dermal nodule, eccrine spiradenomas can occur at any age and site. Lobules of closely packed epithelial cells are separated by thin connective tissue bands which may contain telangiectatic vessels. A rare, highly vascular type may be mistaken for a vascular tumour. The tumour cells appear to be of two types; at the periphery of the lobules are cells with small dark nuclei, while more centrally are cells with larger, pale nuclei. A few lumina are observed. Rarely, malignant transformation of a benign lesion is seen. The histogenesis of eccrine spiradenoma is controversial, some favouring an origin from the duct while the reported presence of myoepithelial cells and S100 protein favours the secretory coil.

Hidradenoma

This tumour has a variety of patterns, each of which has been given a selection of names—nodular, tubular, clear cell myoepithelioma, chondroid syringoma, mixed tumour, and acrospiroma. Basically all are tumours of the eccrine coil and ducts. They tend to be encapsulated and form distinct dermal nodules in the skin. The most common regions in which they are found are the head and neck, usually in older people. They show a variety of differentiation patterns, hence the different names. There are two cell types present: a small cuboidal basophilic cell and a larger, rounder cell, often with clearer cytoplasm. These tend to form lobules, sheets, or clumps of cells, interspersed with cystic spaces sometimes containing eosinophilic material. There is a variable amount of connective tissue present. The cystic spaces have a duct lining, composed of the two cell types, the smaller cells forming the luminal border. This double-layered duct pattern is characteristic of all hidradenomas. Sometimes the ducts or tubules are predominant and hence the designation tubular hidradenoma. At other times, there is a striking increase in stroma, which shows chondroid features like a pleomorphic adenoma of salivary gland—this is called a chondroid syringoma or mixed tumour. All of these lesions are benign, although there are a few reports of malignant variants.

Sweat gland carcinoma

Some sweat gland carcinomas are malignant variants of benign tumours and, occasionally, malignancy arises in a long-standing benign lesion (e.g. eccrine spiradenoma, cylindroma). In addition, there are some malignancies that do not appear to have a benign counterpart. These include: mucinous sweat gland carcinoma, in which tumour cells are present within pools of mucin, the tumour possibly arising from the secretory coil; classical eccrine carcinoma, in which obviously malignant tissue lies adjacent to normal eccrine glands; and adenoid cystic carcinoma, which closely resembles the tumour of salivary gland and has a disputed histogenesis in the skin.

28.17.9 Tumours of apocrine glands and the pilosebaceous unit

The normal apocrine gland and pilosebaceous unit

Apocrine glands are found in the axilla and anogenital regions, and in a modified form in the eyelids, breasts, and external ear canal. A few glands are present on the scalp and face. They consist of a secretory coil composed of glands of wide lumen lined by large eosinophilic cells showing decapitation secretion, surrounded by a layer of myoepithelial cells. Apocrine glandular differentiation is indicated by the presence of secretory granules, by the presence of apocrine enzymes, and by the characteristic decapitation secretion. For most apocrine glands, the secretory coil communicates with the infundibular region of a hair follicle by means of a straight duct lined by two layers of epithelial cells. It is suggested that apocrine and eccrine glandular differentiation can be distinguished by the presence of carcino-embryonic antigen (CEA). This can be detected immunohistologically in the coil and duct of the former but not of the latter.

The hair follicle has a central hair matrix surrounded by bands of epithelial cells known as the inner and outer root sheaths. At the base of the follicle is a fibrovascular core known as the papilla. The infundibulum of the follicle is delineated by the duct of the associated sebaceous gland.

Tumours arise from all of these microscopic elements (Table 28.5).

Hidradenoma papilliferum

A small encapsulated dermal tumour arising principally on the labia majora of adults, this lesion is composed of cystic glandular structures with papillary infoldings. Enzyme histochemistry and electron microscopy support an origin from the apocrine secretory coil.

Syringocystadenoma papilliferum

Seen on the face or scalp of children and adolescents, often in association with organoid naevus (naevus sebaceous of Jadassohn), this tumour consists of cysts and duct-like structures with papillary projections, often communicating with the epidermis. The cysts and ducts are lined by a double epithelial cell layer. Characteristically, within the associated stroma are numbers of chronic inflammatory cells, principally plasma cells. Studies favour an origin from the apocrine duct.

Apocrine carcinoma

A very rare malignant tumour, which usually presents as an axillary growth in adults. Malignancy may also arise within the modified apocrine glands of the eyelid and external ear canal. Histopathologically, there is an apparent transition between recognizable apocrine gland and malignant tumour.

Extramammary Paget disease

Extramammary Paget disease is the intra-epidermal spread of malignant glandular cells in sites other than the nipple (Fig. 28.70). It is most often seen in the vulval and perianal

Table 28.5 Tumours of the apocrine gland and pilosebaceous unit

Name	Site	Age/sex	Malignant	Histogenesis
Hidradenoma papilliferum	Labia majora	F	Rare	Apocrine secretory coil
Syringocystadenoma papilliferum	Scalp, face	Child; may be associated with organoid naevus	No	Apocrine duct
Apocrine carcinoma	Axilla	F = M	Yes	Apocrine gland
Extramammary Paget disease	Vulva, anus, axilla	F > M; middle-aged, elderly	Yes	Apocrine secretory cells
Trichofolliculoma	Face	—	No	Pilosebaceous unit
Trichoepithelioma	Face	—	No	Pilosebaceous unit
Pilomatrixoma	Face, upper extremities	Child; young adult	Rare	Hair matrix
Trichilemmoma	Face	All ages; M > F	No	Outer root sheath
Tumour of follicular infundibulum	Face	Mid–old; F > M	No	Outer root sheath

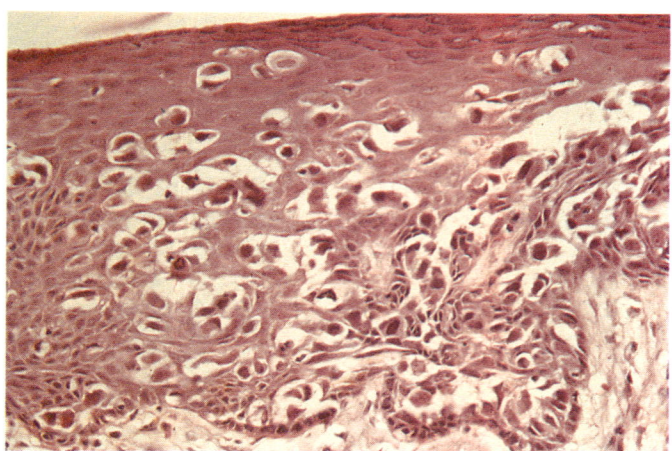

Fig. 28.70 Extramammary Paget disease. There are numerous dysplastic cells spreading throughout the epithelium, either as small clumps or as individual cells. The tumour cells have abundant cytoplasm and markedly aberrant nuclei.

regions and is occasionally associated with an underlying adenocarcinoma, for example of the anal canal. Where no underlying malignancy is discovered, it is suggested that the tumour cells are derived from cutaneous apocrine glands. Such a conclusion is based on immunohistochemistry, using anti-CEA and an antibody raised to a glycoprotein of breast cystic disease fluid, which was found to stain apocrine glands and their derivative lesions. The malignant cells of extramammary Paget disease are often Alcian blue/PAS positive. They are also frequently positive for Masson–Fontana silver stain, consistent with the presence of melanin. This should not be taken to indicate a deposit of malignant melanoma.

Trichofolliculoma

A single nodule arising on the face of an adult, the trichofolliculoma may possess a central tuft of hairs on clinical examination, and histopathologically these can be seen to be arising from an abnormal central hair channel. Multiple secondary hair follicles grow radially from this primary channel.

Trichoepithelioma

These tumours occur on the face, singly as a sporadic event or as multiple lesions when inherited as an autosomal dominant condition. Situated within the dermis are multiple small collections of basal cells and horn cysts. The islands of basal cells may be indistinguishable from those of a basal cell carcinoma. A rare variant has a surrounding fibrous stroma (desmoplastic trichoepithelioma).

Pilomatrixoma

Hard lesions arising within the dermis of the face and upper extremities of children and young adults, pilomatrixomas are thought to originate from the hair matrix. They consist of a mixture of proliferating basaloid cells and masses of ghost cells

derived from the former. This matrix excites a foreign body reaction in the surrounding stroma and in time may calcify. The lesion is sometimes known by the alternative name of calcifying epithelioma of Malherbe.

Trichilemmoma, tumour of follicular infundibulum

The common trichilemmoma is an overgrowth of the outer root sheath of the hair follicle infundibulum and consists of lobules of clear (glycogen-rich) cells connecting with the epidermis. The tumour of hair follicle infundibulum is thought to have a similar origin and presents as a plate of clear epithelial cells growing in the dermis and showing multiple connections to the epidermis.

Sebaceous gland neoplasms

Tumours of sebaceous glands range from completely benign adenomas to aggressive carcinomas, the latter often arising from the specialized glands of the eyelid. In a variety of dominantly inherited conditions there is an association of multiple sebaceous neoplasms with a high incidence of visceral malignancy, most often gastrointestinal (Torre, Muir–Torre syndromes).

Sebaceous adenomas occur on the face and neck and are circumscribed collections of sebaceous gland lobules consisting mainly of mature sebocytes, with a few peripheral basophilic germinative cells. The sebaceous 'epithelioma' has a greater proportion of germinative cells, and in places may resemble a basal cell carcinoma. The sebaceous carcinoma grows as sheets and lobules of malignant cells in which there is a variable degree of recognizable sebaceous differentiation. In the eyelid the tumours tend to be more aggressive and may sometimes invade the epidermis in a pagetoid manner.

Sebaceous hyperplasia

This is a lesion which is commonly mistaken clinically for a basal cell carcinoma. It presents as a raised pearly/white nodule on the face, often on the nose, in elderly people. Histopathologically there is a central hair follicle, usually dilated and enlarged, containing keratin. There is a proliferation of sebaceous glands around this hair follicle, like the flower heads in a vase. Occasionally more than one hair follicle is present. It is entirely benign.

28.17.10 Dermal connective tissue

Tumours of the dermal components of the skin are not infrequent and can involve any structure. Many are similar in both clinical and pathological details to their counterparts in the rest of the body (e.g. lipoma, neurofibroma) and will not be discussed here (see Sections 12.18 and 27.4).

28.17.11 Vascular growths

Pyogenic granuloma (capillary haemangioma)

This is a common lesion, presenting as a rapidly growing moist nodule which is friable and haemorrhagic. It often occurs after minor injury. Pathologically it has a characteristic nodular polypoid configuration, the epithelium being normal or ulcerated and the lesion consisting of a solid nodule of proliferating capillaries. The epithelium grows in at the sides of the nodule to form a collarette. It is benign and spontaneously regresses.

Angiokeratoma

This is a relatively uncommon lesion in which angiomatous elements extend into the epidermis. There are four clinical varieties: angiokeratoma of Fabry, in which there is a genetic defect in ceramide trihexosidase; angiokeratoma of Fordyce (a lesion of the scrotum); angiokeratoma of Mibelli (a lesion of the finger); and isolated angiokeratoma. The epidermis is often ulcerated. The vascular component consists of thin-walled, dilated vacular channels. The overlying epidermis is hyperkeratotic.

Glomus tumour

This is a lesion of the Sequet–Hoyer canal, which forms the arteriovenous anastomosis in the skin. There are two types: the solitary lesion, which often occurs in the subungual region; and multiple lesions, which are hereditary and often occur in the thigh. The lesions are exquisitely tender, although the hereditary entity is said to be less so. Histopathologically the lesion forms a nodule of vascular channels in the reticular dermis, the characteristic appearance being the cuffing of compact regular clear cells around the blood vessel (Fig. 28.71). These can form large clumps of cells, particularly in the solitary variety, in which the vascular element is often of capillaries. The multiple lesions have much larger vascular channels and relatively few glomus cells. Indeed, it is sometimes easy to miss them. The solitary variety has a capsule, unlike the hereditary form.

Kaposi sarcoma

This is an uncommon lesion, which until recently was largely confined to Africa. However, Kaposi sarcoma is frequently found in AIDS patients and forms part of the diagnostic criteria. There has been controversy over the nature of the lesion; namely whether it is a neoplasm or whether it represents reactive hyperplasia. Each view has its supporters, although the majority opinion is that it is neoplastic. The lesions show foci of proliferating capillaries, spindle and lymphoid cells in the mid- to upper dermis. Characteristically the capillaries have no intervening stroma (back to back). There is often haemosiderin deposition, indicating previous haemorrhage. The early lesions are often very inconspicuous, being scattered, small foci in the dermal collagen. They may be noticed by the curious vertical orientation of the capillaries. As the lesions develop, the capillaries form nodules (Fig. 28.72) and spindle cells become more numerous. There may also be larger vascular channels with pooled red blood cells. These nodules can occupy much of the dermis. The histogenesis of the lesion has been controversial, but the current consensus is that the origin is from endothelium (see also Section 12.18). The differential diagnosis is of stasis dermatitis and reactive granulation tissue.

28.17.12   Fibro-histiocytic lesions

Dermatofibroma

This is a common lesion, often found on the limbs. It arises in young adults and forms a firm, often small, nodule in the skin. The colour varies from yellow/white to red/brown.

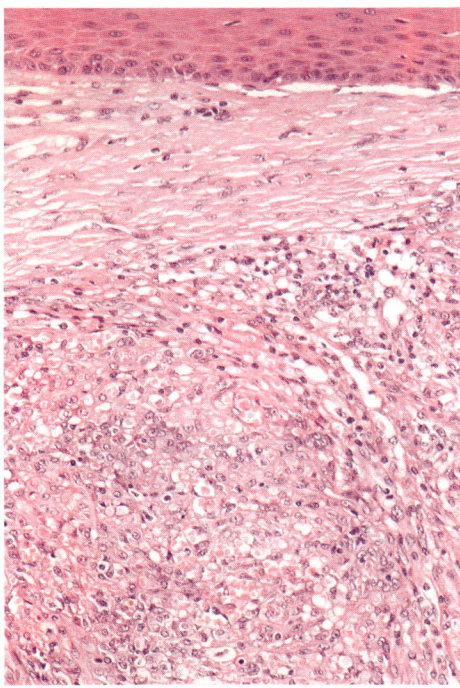

Fig. 28.72 Kaposi sarcoma. A high power view of a nodule of tumour cells within the epidermis. The tumour is composed of densely packed spindle cells between which there are vascular spaces, some of which contain red blood cells (see also Chapter 12).

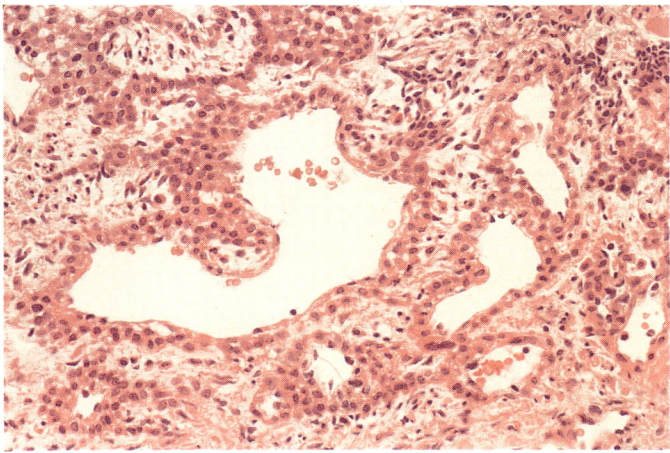

Fig. 28.71 Glomangioma. The tumour is formed by numerous blood vessels which are surrounded by a cuff of eosinophilic small cuboidal (glomus) cells.

Histopathologically the lesion consists of a nodule of spindle cells in the reticular dermis, often extending down to the subcutaneous fat (Fig. 28.73). The spindle cells have a characteristic pattern in which they encircle collagen bundles, particularly well seen at the periphery of the lesion (Fig. 28.74). The lesion does not have a storiform pattern. There is often a mixture of histiocytic cells and multinucleated giant cells of Touton type. These histiocytic cells often contain haemosiderin and fat. Sometimes the lesion appears to be formed by proliferating capillaries. Typically, the epidermis is acanthotic above the dermal lesion. Mitotic figures can be present in the dermal mass, but there is no significant atypia. Occasionally the lesions can be extremely large, but despite this, they are benign.

The aetiology is unknown, and it is not clear whether they are a reactive hyperplasia or a benign tumour. The cell of genesis is also unclear, suggestions ranging from fibroblasts to endothelial cells or histiocytes.

Dermatofibrosarcoma protuberans

This is a rare tumour of the dermis. It presents usually as a slowly enlarging lesion of the skin, frequently in the upper leg or around the shoulders. The overlying epidermis is often thinned or ulcerated (Fig. 28.75), in contrast to dermatofibroma, and the lesion characteristically extends widely on to either side of the central nodule to form a shelf. It can merge imperceptibly with the normal dermis. It is composed of spindle cells and the diagnostic feature is a storiform pattern (Fig. 28.76), although other areas resemble a low-grade fibrosarcoma. There is only mild cytological atypia, but mitoses are not infrequent. The lesion has a high local recurrence rate (50 per cent), particu-

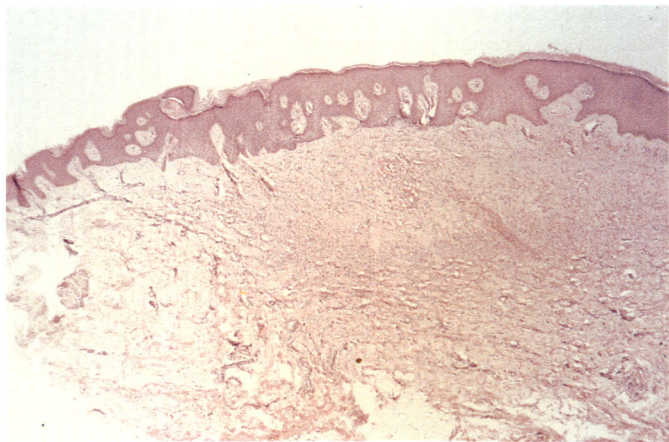

Fig. 28.73 Dermatofibroma. A typical lesion, with acanthosis of the surface epithelium and an oval-shaped circular tumour located in the centre of the dermis. The lesion is extending out on either side and down towards the subcutaneous fat.

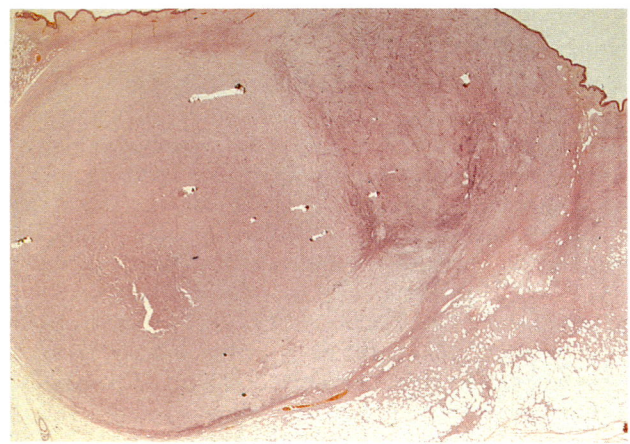

Fig. 28.75 Dermatofibrosarcoma protuberans. There is a large nodular protuberant tumour invading down into the subcutaneous fat. There are two patterns, of high and low cellularity.

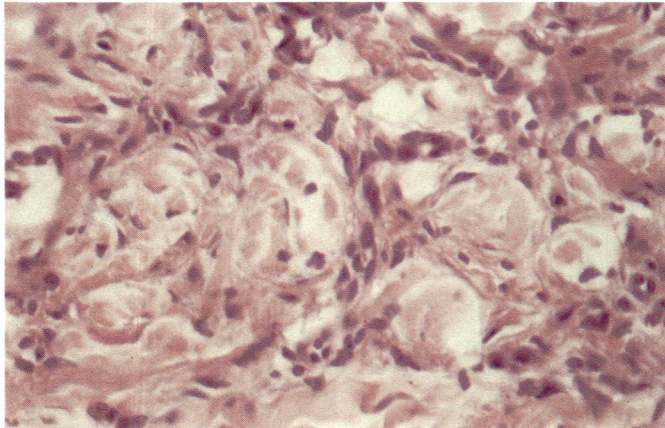

Fig. 28.74 Dermatofibroma. A view from the periphery of a dermatofibroma. This shows individual collagen bundles being surrounded and delineated by the spindle-shaped tumour cells.

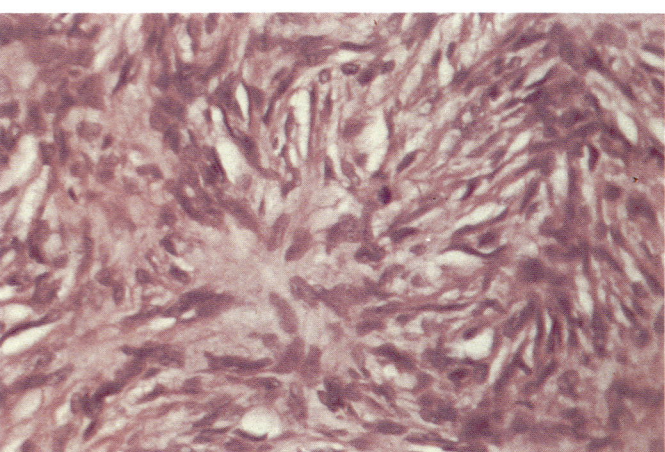

Fig. 28.76 Dermatofibrosarcoma protuberans. A high-power view from the centre of the tumour presented in Fig. 28.74, showing a storiform pattern. This is a highly cellular tumour showing considerable cytological and nuclear atypia. There is a mitotic figure in the centre of the field.

larly if excision is incomplete. Wide excision is necessary, but metastases are rare.

Atypical fibroxanthoma

This is a rare benign tumour of the sun-exposed skin, most often seen in the head and neck region of elderly patients. It may follow X-radiation. It often presents as a rapidly growing nodule, sometimes with ulceration. It is a highly cellular tumour involving the dermis, up to the epidermis. There is a characteristic mixture of highly pleomorphic cells, often multinucleate, and many dysplastic spindle cells. Mitotic figures are numerous. The overall impression is of a highly malignant spindle-cell tumour, frequently forming a large nodule and extending down to the subcutaneous fat. However, its clinical course is essentially benign. The diagnosis rests in the clinical presentation, age, and site. The differentiation is from spindle-cell squamous carcinoma, malignant melanoma, or malignant fibrous histiocytoma (see also Chapter 27). Cytokeratin and melanoma-associated antigen staining can help to resolve the first two, while the last is often less malignant-looking and has a storiform pattern, not seen in atypical fibroxanthoma.

28.17.13 Lymphoma of the skin

There are a variety of lymphoproliferative lesions of the skin, some of which are listed in Table 28.6. In addition, many of the non-cutaneous lymphoproliferative conditions, such as Hodgkin disease, non-Hodgkin lymphoma (T- and B-cell), and leukaemias, can involve the skin in the course of the systemic disease. These will not be considered here further (see Chapter 24).

Intermediate lesions

Lymphomatous proliferations of the skin fall into two broad groups. The intermediate lymphoproliferative lesions are a source of great confusion and controversy. Some of these lesions can behave in a benign fashion but have histopathological appearances that suggest malignant lymphoma. Some have a non-specific or benign appearance, but ultimately can develop a

Table 28.6 Cutaneous lymphoproliferative conditions

Behaviour	Designation
Intermediate	Spiegler–Fendt sarcoid; Jessner lymphocytic infiltrate (insect bite, drug reaction)
	Actinic reticuloid; pityriasis lichenoides (lymphomatoid papulosis)
	Angiolymphoid hyperplasia with eosinophils; lymphomatoid granulomatosis
	Pre-mycosis fungoides—large plaque parapsoriasis, poikiloderma
Malignant	Mycosis fungoides—Sézary syndrome, Worlinger–Kolopp disease, follicular mucinosis
	Hodgkin and non-Hodgkin lymphoma
	Leukaemia

malignant lymphoma. Currently there is no way of accurately determining which will behave in which fashion. This includes investigation by cytogenetics, immunophenotyping, and assessment of T-cell receptor and light-chain gene rearrangements. Essentially all these procedures are directed at showing the presence of a monoclonal proliferation of T- or B-cells, on the assumption that such monoclonality denotes malignancy. However, this has not proved to be the case, with many examples of monoclonal lesions behaving in a benign fashion. In the absence of an obvious benign cause, e.g. insect bite, the best that can be done it to regard all lymphoproliferative lesions of the skin as having potential for malignancy and advising follow-up accordingly. This is especially important in monoclonal lesions.

Bearing in mind the preceding comments, several entities can be identified. Spiegler–Fendt sarcoid is characterized by the presence of dermal lymphoid proliferation, either in a perivascular distribution or as more diffuse masses and with germinal follicles. Jessner lymphocytic infiltrate is similar, but does not have germinal follicles. Sometimes a definite cause for either of these lesions can be identified (insect bite, drug reaction, photosensitization) and they can be confidently called benign. In other cases, there is no obvious cause and circumspection is advised. Actinic reticuloid is a disease of the elderly in which an acute, persistent, generalized, red, photosensitive rash covers the body. Histopathologically there are atypical lymphoid cells present, which raises the suspicion of malignancy. However, few, if any, of these patients develop malignant lymphoma. Pityriasis lichenoides and its variant lymphomatoid papulosis have been discussed earlier. Again, the presence of atypical lymphoid cells suggests malignancy, but the clinical behaviour is of a benign lesion. Angiolymphoid hyperplasia with eosinophils and lymphomatoid granulomatosis occasionally affect the skin. As in the lymph nodes (see Chapter 24) and lungs, the ultimate outcome and course of these lesions is variable.

The pre-mycosis fungoides conditions of large plaque parapsoriasis, poikiloderma variegata, and poikiloderma vasculare atrophicans are notoriously difficult to diagnose. Large plaque parapsoriasis is characterized by scaly red patches of many years' duration. The histopathology is non-specific, there being focal parakeratoses, acanthosis, some epidermotropism of lymphoid cells, and a perivascular mononuclear inflammatory infiltrate. Very occasionally, atypical cells may be present. The differential diagnosis, apart from pre-mycosis fungoides, is of chronic dermatitis, the psoriasiform lesions, the pigmented purpuric dermatoses, and pityriasis lichenoides. Poikiloderma variegata and poikiloderma vasculare atrophicans show essentially identical features to the other types of poikiloderma (see earlier). The differential diagnosis is of pre-mycoses fungoides, lupus erythematosus, dermatomyositis, systemic sclerosis, drug reaction, and radiation.

It is impossible to determine on histopathological grounds the precise diagnosis of all the preceding conditions. Clinical information is necessary. Indeed, in many cases, even then all that can be said is that the appearances are consistent with the clinical diagnosis, e.g. pre-mycosis fungoides, but that other lesions (e.g. chronic dermatitis) cannot be excluded. It is wise to suggest follow-up, with repeat biopsy to monitor the development of malignancy.

T-cell neoplasms: mycosis fungoides and Sézary syndrome

Clinically, mycosis fungoides (MF) usually evolves gradually through three stages, beginning as an erythematous rash, progressing to multiple indurated plaques, and finally presenting with unequivocal tumours. The malignancy occasionally makes a first presentation in the tumour stage, or may manifest as generalized erythroderma, and these presenting indices of advanced disease carry a worse prognosis.

Sézary syndrome is mycosis fungoides with the presence of abnormal hyperconvoluted cells in the peripheral blood (more than 5 per cent of total white cell count). Pathogenetically, as will be described later, mycosis fungoides and Sézary syndrome represent the same disease.

A biopsy of the erythematous or patch stage shows a superficial mild perivascular and sometimes band-like chronic inflammatory infiltrate in the dermis. Occasional abnormal (see below) lymphoid cells are also present within the epidermis and the epithelium of the adnexae, either singly, or collected into small groups known as Darier–Pautrier microabscesses. If these cells are very sparse, distinction from a benign inflammatory process may be very difficult at this stage (see pre-mycosis fungoides). Histopathology of the plaque form (Fig. 28.77) shows a more profound dermal infiltrate, usually mixed and polymorphous and often inclusive of atypical large cells (Fig. 28.78)

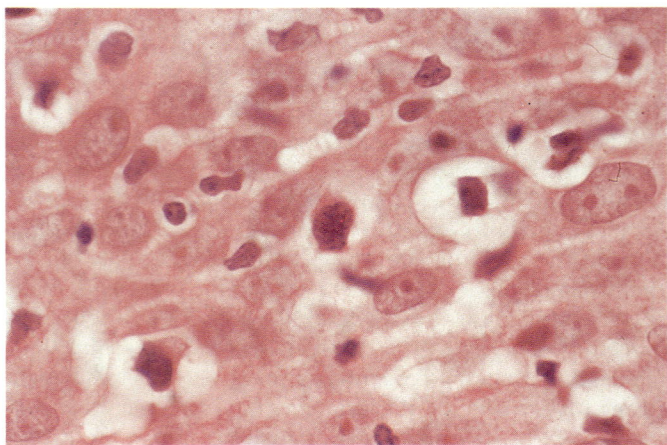

Fig. 28.78 Mycosis fungoides. High-power view of Lutzner cells in epithelium in the plaque stage of mycosis fungoides. The nuclei are hyperchromatic and lobulated. Compare with normal, small, regular, round lymphocytes.

with hyperconvoluted nuclei (Sézary or Lutzner cells, sometimes called 'cerebriform'). There are typically more of these cells within the epidermis and within adnexae compared to the patch stage. Microabscesses may be easy to find, though they are not an invariable feature. The epidermis is sometimes acanthotic and there may be dermal fibrosis and loss of elastic tissue. When there is dense pagetoid spread of Lutzner cells through the epidermis, this variant of MF is called Worlinger–Kolopp disease. Occasionally the pilosebaceous units show mucinous degeneration, this being the malignant variant of follicular mucinosis—the benign variant occurs earlier in life and does not show a lymphomatous infiltrate.

The tumour stage consists of a dense and deep dermal infiltrate, which includes atypical cells and sometimes bizarre forms. There may be epidermal ulceration.

Pathogenesis of mycosis fungoides

Immunological and immunohistochemical studies on the infiltrate of mycosis fungoides suggest that this is a tumour of T-lymphocyte origin with differentiation towards T-helper cells (more than six times the number of T-suppressor cells). Current research suggests that this may be a disease of antigen persistence, in which a foreign antigen is introduced to the Langerhans cells of the epidermis and is carried by them to regional lymph nodes. Here clones of sensitized T-helper cells are induced and these cells migrate back to the skin via the bloodstream. Eventually one clone becomes malignant. Because there is a haematogenous phase during the development of the disease, mycosis fungoides and Sézary syndrome are, for practical purposes, the same entity.

The antigen that initiates the process is unknown, though a type C retrovirus has been isolated from mycosis cells. This retrovirus is very similar to that which has been linked to adult T-cell leukaemia/lymphoma in Japan (HTLV-I) and it is interesting that classical mycosis fungoides is extremely rare amongst the Japanese (see also Chapter 24).

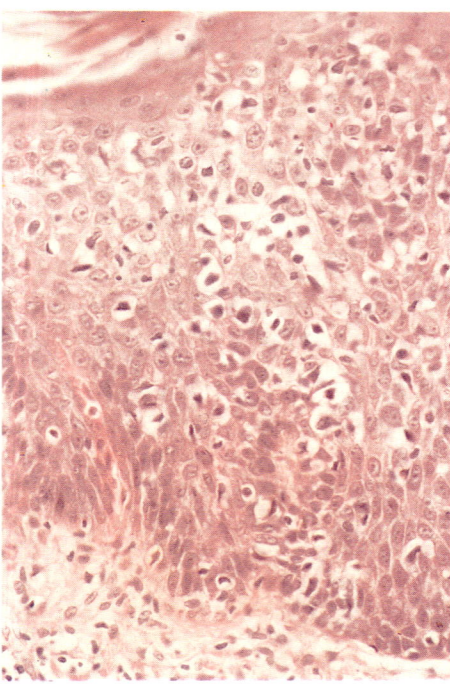

Fig. 28.77 Mycosis fungoides. The epithelium is thickened. There is widespread infiltration of epidermis by pleomorphic lymphoid cells (epidermotropism), but no Pautrier abscesses.

Prognosis of mycosis fungoides

When fatal, mycosis fungoides terminates as immunoblastic T-cell lymphoma. Presentation with visceral dissemination is usually fatal within 6 months. In the tumour stage, or if there is generalized erythroderma, the five-year survival is 40 per cent, and this rises to 90 per cent if the patient has a limited number of plaques. A patient with an erythematous rash may survive many years with limited progression.

Other cutaneous T-cell malignancies

Adult T-cell leukaemia/lymphoma is a systemic malignancy with cutaneous infiltration and is seen amongst the Japanese and the indigent Negro population of the Caribbean. The malignant cell is usually a T-helper cell and the disease is thought to be related to infection with a retrovirus similar to that which has been identified in mycosis fungoides. Adult T-cell leukaemia/lymphoma may therefore be a variation of a host response to this virus in particular racial groups.

T-cell chronic lymphatic leukaemia often has a cutaneous tumour infiltrate, manifest clinically as erythroderma. The phenotype may be either T-suppressor or T-helper cell, with the former more common.

Cutaneous B-cell lymphomas

When a B-cell lymphoma has a cutaneous phase, in a quarter of cases this is a first manifestation. Typically, the tumour infiltrate within the dermis spares the epidermis, in contrast to T-cell tumours which predominantly infiltrate the epidermis, and thus there is a Grenz zone of uninvolved papillary dermis (Fig. 28.79). However, this is not invariable and cannot be used as a feature to distinguish B-cell from T-cell cutaneous lymphoma.

The commonest patterns of cutaneous B-cell lymphoma are lymphoplasmacytoid and immunoblastic. Separation of a benign from a malignant lymphohistiocytic infiltrate may be very difficult in the skin. Immunohistology may be of some use,

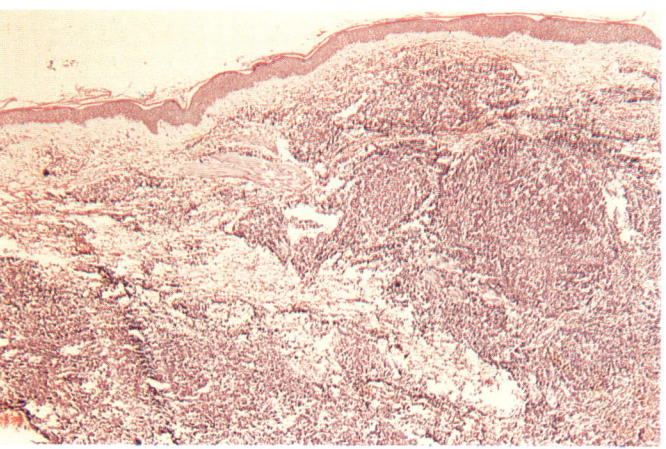

Fig. 28.79 Non-Hodgkin lymphoma. There are numerous widespread clumps of lymphoid cells present throughout the dermis. Note the relative sparing of the upper dermis (Grenz zone).

as a benign infiltrate will often show compartmentalization of T- and B-lymphocytes, similar to that seen in a reactive lymph node.

28.17.14   Further reading

Ackerman, A. B. (1978). *Histological diagnosis of inflammatory skin diseases. A method by pattern analysis.* Lea and Febiger, Philadelphia.

Fry, L., Wojnarowska, F. T., and Shahrad, P. (1985). *Illustrated encyclopaedia of dermatology* (2nd edn). MTP Press, Lancaster.

McGovern, V. J. (1983). *Melanoma: histological diagnosis and prognosis.* Biopsy Interpretation Series (ed. A. Blaustein). Raven Press, New York.

McKee, P. H. (1989). *Pathology of the skin.* Gower Medical, London.

MacKie, R. M. (ed.) (1984). *Milne's dermatopathology* (2nd edn). Edward Arnold, London.

MacKie, R. M. (1989). *Skin cancer.* Martin Dunitz, London.

Pinkus, H. and Mehregan, A. H. (1981). *A guide to dermatohistopathology* (3rd edn). Appleton-Century-Crofts, New York.

Rook, A., Wilkinson, D. S., Ebling, F. J. G., Champion, R. H. and Burton, J. L. (eds) (1986). *Textbook of dermatology* (4th edn). Blackwell Scientific Publications, Oxford.

29

Pathology of tropical infections

S. Lucas

29

Pathology of tropical infections

S. Lucas

29.1   Introduction

Medicine in the tropics is not limited to parasitic disease. But it is convenient to group and summarize in one section the range of pathologies caused by parasites globally. Rapid international travel means that virtually any parasitic infection may now present in any country, imported albeit uninvited.

Parasitism

Parasitism is a process whereby one organism derives energy and subsistence at the expense of another (the host). This ranges from *mutualism* whereby both parasite and host benefit, through *commensalism* where they share nutrients without harm to the host, to *pathogenic parasitism* where the host suffers, sometimes to death. In the human host, there are no examples of mutualism.

Parasitic infections of man theoretically include all infective agents—from prions to tapeworms—that live on or in the human body for part or all of their life cycles. In practice, the term 'parasite' is restricted to the unicellular protozoa, metazoan helminths (worms), and arthropods. The 1987 International Nomenclature of Diseases lists 14 non-invasive species and 34 tissue-invasive, pathogenic species of protozoa. Of helminths, some 90 species are non-invasive (mostly in the intestinal lumen) and about 180 species are invasive.

Parasite life cycles

These range in complexity from simple man-to-man transmission, to those utilizing a series of different intermediate hosts, including insect vectors. If there is sexual reproduction in the life cycle, the term *definitive host* indicates that in which it occurs. Many infections are *zoonotic*, i.e. are transmitted from an animal reservoir host, man being an 'accidental' recipient. A few parasites such as *Clonorchis* and *Schistosoma japonicum* use man or animals equally.

Pathogenic parasites usually mature or multiply in man, but a few (e.g. *Toxocara*) do not develop despite remaining and moving in the host tissues for long periods. This is termed *paratenesis*.

Susceptibility to infection

Host susceptibility is complicated. For any parasite, the prevalence of infection (the proportion of a community infected) and intensity of infection (the quantity of organisms in peoples' bodies) are often positively correlated. In any community, there will be some people who have apparent immunity to a given endemic infection. The extent to which this is due to lack of exposure versus genuine immunity following exposure is often unclear. Conversely, there will be a small proportion of those infected who have very intense infections. They present a disproportionate amount of the clinical burden of pathology.

Pathogenesis of disease

Infection is not equivalent to disease. The variables that determine the sequelae of parasitic infection include:

1. the number of parasites in the body or organ;
2. which organ(s) or cells are infected;
3. the size of the parasite;
4. the age at which infection is acquired;
5. the life-span of the parasite;
6. the secretion of toxic substances by the parasite;
7. the type and intensity of host inflammatory and immune reaction (i.e. immunopathology).

As a result of these interacting factors, there are four patterns of disease versus infection intensity (Fig. 29.1).

Opportunistic parasitic infections

Most pathogenic parasites of man are *principal pathogens*; they cause disease in people with apparently normal host defence

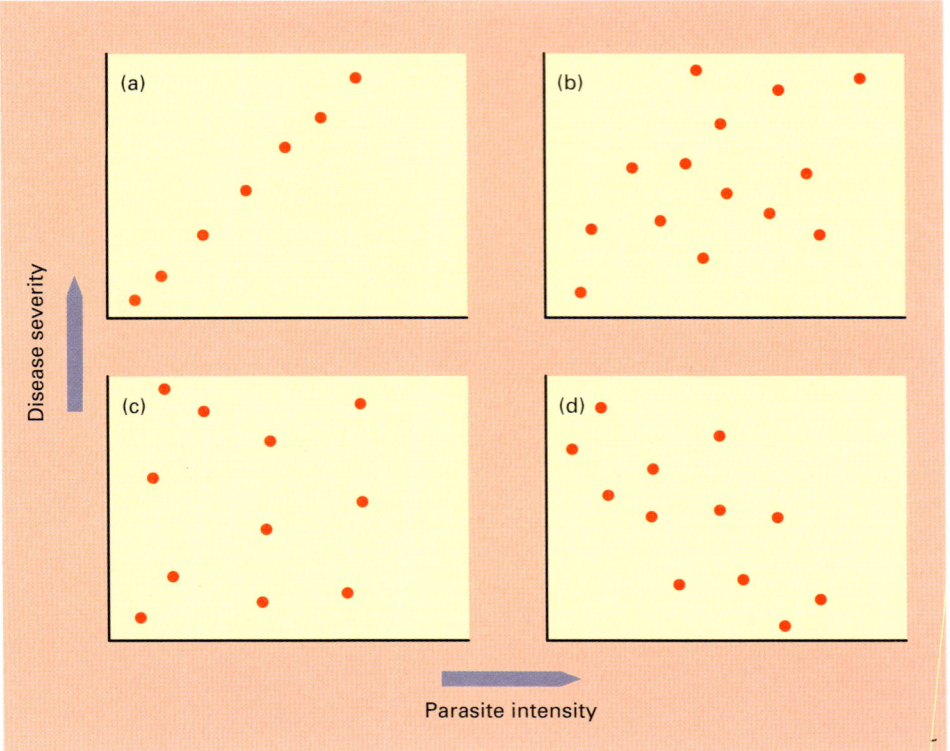

Fig. 29.1 General relationships between the intensity of parasite infection and the severity of disease. (a) Monotonic: each parasite inflicts a unit amount of damage, e.g. hookworm infection; (b) general positive correlation, e.g. schistosomiasis, malaria; (c) no overall correlation, where the site of infection may be more important than the numbers of parasites, e.g. cysticercosis; (d) negative correlation, where the host reaction simultaneously eliminates parasites and causes tissue damage, e.g. the filariases.

systems. Some of these parasites are also *opportunists*; they produce more severe disease in people with damaged specific and non-specific defences. A very few are purely opportunistic (*Pneumocystis carinii* and *Enterocytozoon*); they cause disease only in immunocompromised people.

Many opportunist parasites are normally controlled by cell-mediated immunity. Despite latent infection or constant reinfection, they cause little or no disease in immunocompetent people. Thus the advent of human immunodeficiency virus infections (HIV-1 and HIV-2) has irreversibly altered the geographical and clinical pathology of several parasitic infections. Previously uncommon infections such as *Cryptosporidium*, *Pneumocystis*, and adult cerebral toxoplasmosis are now common because of HIV.

This chapter discusses the major protozoan and helminth parasites. Details of epidemiology, life cycles, morphology, serology, and other diagnostic techniques are not given. They are available in numerous medical parasitology texts (see Further reading). Classical taxonomies are followed, which are based on both parasite morphology and on patterns of disease. However, with the new techniques of molecular biology, the definitions of what constitutes a species or strain of parasite are changing. Emphasis here is placed on the descriptive pathology and pathogenesis of parasitic disease: to explain why people do (or do not) become ill following infection.

29.1.1   Further reading

General reference books on parasitic pathology

Garcia, L. S. and Bruckner, D. A. (1988). *Diagnostic medical parasitology*. Elsevier, New York. [Good for parasitology and diagnostics.]

Gutierrez, Y. (1990). *Diagnostic pathology of parasitic infections with clinical correlations*. Lea & Febiger, Philadelphia. [Good on morbid anatomy.]

General accounts of parasitic disease

Weatherall, D. J., Ledingham, J. G. G., and Warrell, D. A. (eds) (1987). *Oxford textbook of medicine* (2nd edn), Chapter 5, pp. 446–594. Oxford University Press.

Regular updates on parasitic diseases and their pathogenesis

Parasitology Today, published monthly by Elsevier Trends Journals, Cambridge, UK.

Protozoan infections

These unicellular parasites range in size from 2 μm (e.g. microsporidia) to 200 μm (e.g. *Balantidium*). They include intracellular organisms that induce disease through immunopathology, i.e. by eliciting a tissue-destructive host reaction (e.g. *Leishmania*); and extracellular organisms that are directly toxic to host cells (e.g. *Entamoeba*).

Asexual reproduction is by binary fission or by multiple fission (*schizogony*). The latter is subtyped *merogony* if it produces *merozoites*, and *sporogony* if *sporozoites* result. Sexual reproduction is by *gamogony* to produce *gametes*. The term *trophozoite* (or *zoite*) is used generally to indicate protozoan forms that are not multiplying (= mature merozoite). Many protozoa form *cysts* (or *oocysts*), with more than one nucleus, during their life cycles.

29.2 Intra-erythrocytic protozoa

Two genera infect human erythrocytes: *Plasmodium* and *Babesia*. *Plasmodium* is the cause of one of the most important human diseases—malaria.

29.2.1 *Plasmodium*

Four species of *Plasmodium* cause malaria in man: *P. falciparum*, *P. vivax*, *P. malariae*, and *P. ovale*. The major burden of morbidity and virtually all the mortality come from *P. falciparum*.

Epidemiology

As an infection of the tropics and subtropics, 2.1 billion people are at risk for malaria. Some 270 million are infected, 250 million in Africa, the rest in Asia and the Americas. Over 4500 cases are imported annually into Europe. Susceptible groups are children, and adults who have lost or never acquired immunity. In Africa, about one million children die of malaria each year.

Life cycle and morphology (Fig. 29.2)

Malaria is transmitted by anopheline mosquitoes taking a blood meal. Sporozoites are injected into the bloodstream and rapidly enter hepatocytes. In all *Plasmodium* species, merogony then occurs with release of merozoites that enter erythrocytes. This pre-erythrocytic phase causes no liver damage. Schizogony takes place in the erythrocytes, releasing more merozoites (and rupturing the host cell) to enter further erythrocytes. Gamogony forms gametes which are taken up by a mosquito, in which they fuse and develop eventually into sporozoites. With *P. vivax* and *P. ovale*, some sporozoites entering hepatocytes become latent forms, *hypnozoites*, which can undergo schizogony months or years later. This explains late post-treatment relapses with those malarias.

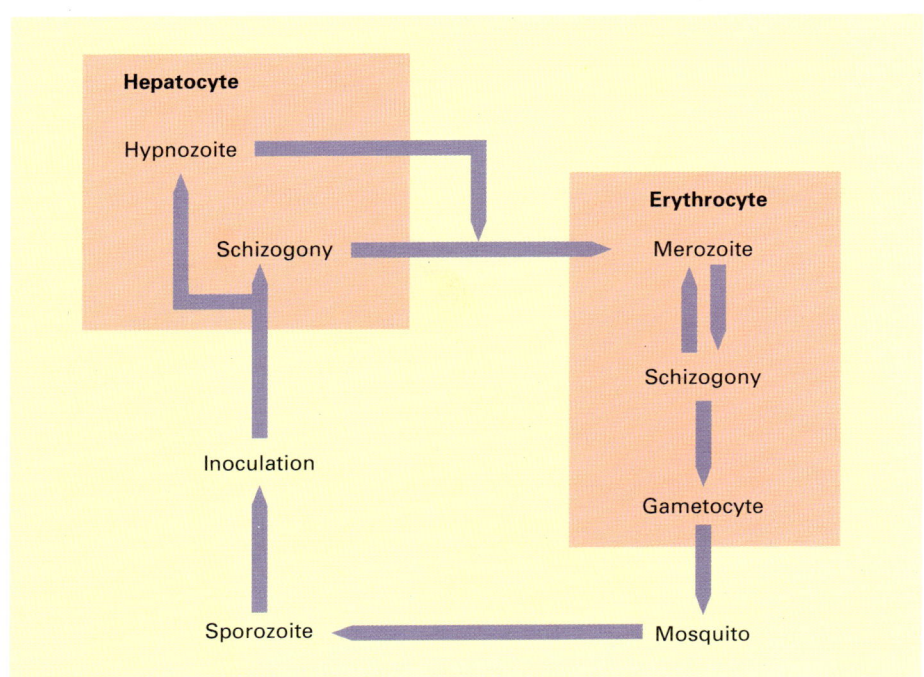

Fig. 29.2 The life cycle of malaria parasites. The hypnozoite (latent) form only occurs in *P. vivax* and *P. ovale* infections.

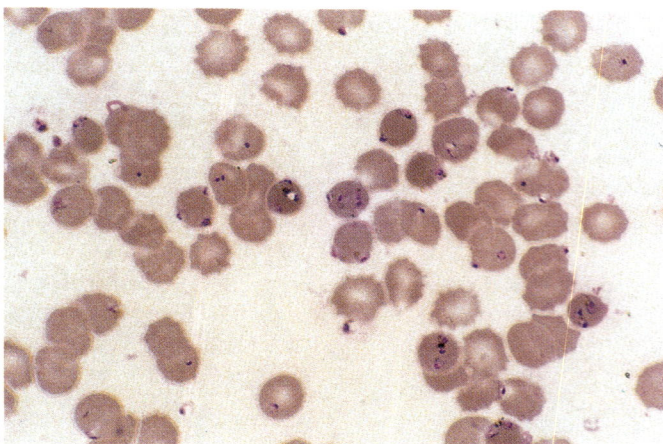

Fig. 29.3 Peripheral blood smear with ring-form trophozoites of *Plasmodium falciparum* in erythrocytes. (Giemsa stain.)

The parasites inside erythrocytes have characteristic forms according to species. In falciparum malaria, only ring-form trophozoites are seen in peripheral blood (Fig. 29.3). Malaria parasites produce a brown pigment (haemozoin) as a product of haemoglobin breakdown.

Clinical features and pathology

Common to all malarias are periodic fevers, headache, nausea, and splenomegaly. The periodicity of fever depends on the time taken for merogony and erythrocte rupture; for *P. malariae* it is 72 hours ('quartan' fever), for the others it is 48 hours ('tertian' fevers). The non-falciparum malarias are benign, and the anaemia they cause is mild. Their main contribution to mortality is rupture of an enlarged spleen following trauma.

P. falciparum infection is often severe and fatal. This is the result of:

1. rapid replication: with *P. falciparum*, 40 000 merozoites are released after merogony in an erythrocyte, far more than with the other species;

2. the phenomenon of sequestration (cytoadherence), whereby parasitized erythrocytes adhere to the endothelium of deep vessels.

Apart from the *P. malariae* nephrotic syndrome, only falciparum malaria is discussed hereon. This may be divided into the features of acute and chronic infection. HIV infection does not influence the course of malaria.

The acute effects of falciparum malaria

Anaemia, hepatosplenomegaly, and diarrhoea are common features of acute infection. Severe and complicated falciparum malaria comprises the following:

1. severe normocytic anaemia, with haemoglobin < 5 g/dl and parasitaemia of > 10 000 per microlitre of blood; more than 50 per cent of erythrocytes may be parasitized, with counts of > 10^6 per microlitre;

2. pulmonary oedema;

3. renal failure with or without haemoglobinuria ('blackwater fever');

4. shock ('algid' malaria);

5. hypoglycaemia;

6. cerebral malaria.

The overall mortality of falciparum malaria is 1–2 per cent per episode. Immunity is acquired by survivors of childhood malaria, so that adults in endemic zones are infrequently ill, although they may manifest low-grade parasitaemias. An exception to this is in pregnancy, when acquired immunity is lost and severe malaria is common.

Anaemia

The anaemia of falciparum malaria is multifactorial. The major cause is haemolysis when meronts rupture the erythrocytes. The bone marrow is dark red. It is hyperplastic, with accumulations of pigmented macrophages containing haemozoin, but there is some dyserythropoiesis hindering the compensatory release of new erythrocytes. This may be an effect of local cytokine secretion. Antibody-mediated immune haemolysis plays little part in ordinary malaria. However, in blackwater fever it may contribute to the massive intravascular haemolysis.

Lymphoreticular system

In acute falciparum malaria, the liver and spleen are enlarged. In fatal cases, they weigh up to 2 500 and 500 gm, respectively. They are congested and pigmented dark-brown (Fig. 29.4). Histologically, the liver shows no parenchymal damage or cholestasis unless there has been shock and ischaemic necrosis. The portal tracts have a chronic inflammatory infiltrate; the sinusoids are dilated with parasitized red blood cells (PRBC), and the Kupffer cells are hypertrophied. They contain haemozoin, so giving the liver its macroscopic colour (Fig. 29.5). Lymphadenopathy is not a feature of acute malaria.

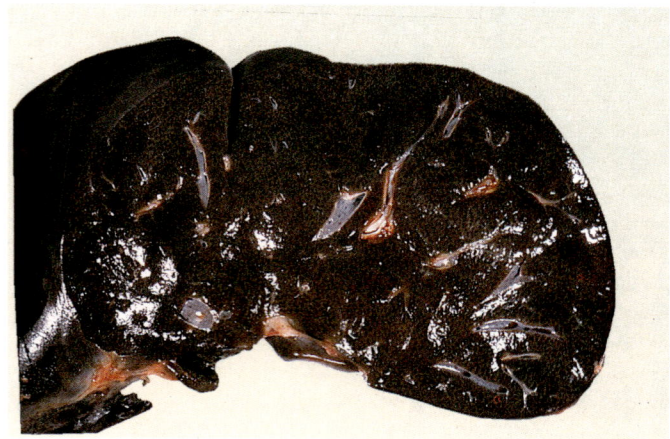

Fig. 29.4 Liver in fatal falciparum malaria. It is congested and dark-brown from accumulated haemozoin pigment.

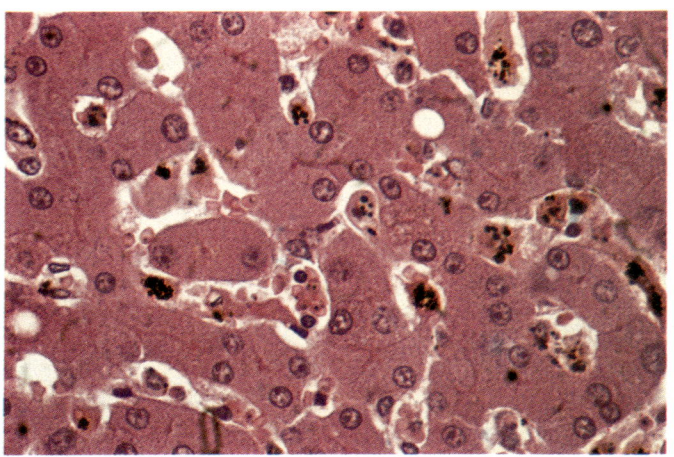

Fig. 29.5 Liver in falciparum malaria. Dark-brown granules of haemozoin pigment in Kupffer cells.

Lung

Pulmonary oedema developing in falciparum malaria has a high mortality. Histologically, numerous PRBC are seen in the interstitial capillaries. In addition to alveolar oedema, there may also be hyaline membrane disease (shock lung). Oedema may follow iatrogenic overhydration. In other cases, it is possible that cytokine secretion (e.g. tumour necrosis factor) induces the capillary wall damage.

Kidney and shock

In autopsied cases of malaria, the vessels and glomeruli appear congested, and there is haemozoin pigment in mesangial cells. In acute falciparum malaria, acute nephritis is uncommonly seen. Histologically it is an acute proliferative glomerulonephritis and has an excellent prognosis on antimalarial chemotherapy. Immune complexes with *P. falciparum* antigens can be demonstrated in glomeruli.

Acute tubular necrosis associated with circulatory collapse occurs in some adult cases. The pathogenesis is probably not cytoadherence of PRBC and obstruction of renal vessels. Nor is it usually the consequence of disseminated intravascular coagulation, which occurs infrequently in adult patients with severe malaria. The shock state of malaria is clinically similar to that of Gram-negative septicaemia. Cytoadherence probably impairs the perfusion of the gut mucosa, with consequent absorption of endotoxins and release of tumour necrosis factor to induce systemic shock.

Historically, a syndrome of acute severe haemolysis, haemoglobinuria, renal failure, shock, and high mortality was seen in expatriates with falciparum malaria. It was often associated with quinine therapy. This 'blackwater fever' is rarely encountered now. Its pathogenesis is uncertain, but an auto-immune haemolytic anaemia triggered by quinine may have been causative. Currently, severe haemoglobulinuria in malaria usually occurs in those with glucose-6-phosphate dehydrogenase deficiency who have been treated with oxidizing antimalarial drugs. Histologically, there are the features of acute tubular necrosis, accompanied by haemoglobin casts in the tubules.

Placenta

Pregnancy is adversely affected by malaria. Maternal death, increased abortion and still-birth rates, premature delivery, and low fetal birth weight are all complications, particularly in the first pregnancy. Pathologically, there is heavy parasitism of red cells in the maternal sinuses, accompanied by monocytosis containing haemozoin pigment (Fig. 29.6).

Fetal nutrition is impaired by maternal sinus parasitism. Transplacental infection (congenital malaria) is uncommon. It presents with anaemia and splenomegaly in the early neonatal period.

Hypoglycaemia

Low blood glucose (< 2.2 mmol/l) occurs in children and adults (particularly pregnant women) in association with other features of severe malaria. Hypoglycaemia may be symptomatic or asymptomatic, and can be obscured by cerebral malaria. In some cases, it is attributable to the direct hyperinsulinaemic effect of quinine therapy. In others with high parasitaemia loads, glycolysis by the parasite is probably important. Further, gluconeogenesis in the liver is impaired both by endotoxaemia (see above) and the reduced blood flow through the liver from cytoadherence. Histologically, post-mortem liver samples from children dying of malaria with hypoglycaemia are depleted of glycogen.

Cerebral malaria (CM)

This is the major cause of death in falciparum malaria. A wide range of neurological disorders is seen, up to coma: changes in behaviour, drowsiness, fits, cerebellar ataxia, hemiplegia, spasticity, decerebrate rigidity, and flaccidity. In children, the onset of CM is rapid, with progress from mild drowsiness to full coma in 1–2 days. Spontaneous recovery from CM without specific chemotherapy is rare. On specific chemotherapy, recovery is

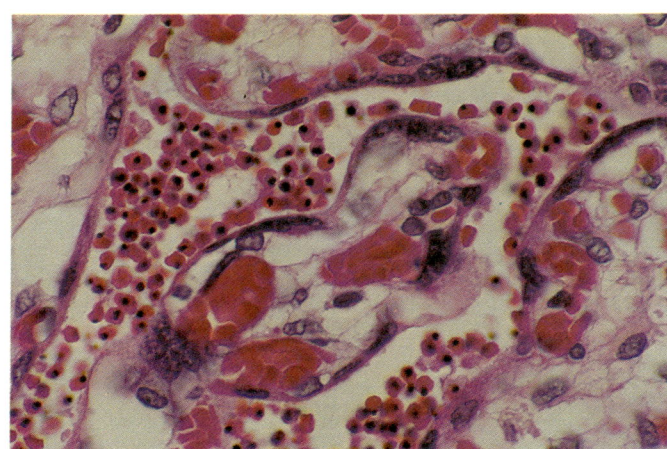

Fig. 29.6 Placenta in falciparum malaria: all the erythrocytes in the maternal sinuses contain parasites; the fetal erythrocytes do not.

rapid (2–6 days) in those who survive. In general, those who recover from CM are neurologically and intellectually normal, indicating that there is little significant damage to the brain tissue. However, neurological deficits such as hemiparesis are observed after recovery in up to 10 per cent of children. The morbid anatomical basis of these residual lesions is not described, but it is likely that they follow cerebral haemorrhages (see below) or hypoglycaemia.

Externally, the brain in CM has meningeal congestion, and may show some swelling. On slicing, the brain may be normal. Usually there is congestion and slight grey discoloration of the cortex from the haemozoin pigment. In about half of fatal autopsied cases, the brain shows petechial haemorrhages, 1–2 mm diameter, mainly in the white matter from frontal lobes to brain stem (Fig. 29.7).

Histologically, all zones of the brain show congested small vessels, with most red cells containing haematoxyphilic dots (parasites) and granules of haemozoin pigment. If there are macroscopic haemorrhages, microscopy shows ruptured capillaries and post-capillary venules with surrounding haemorrhage, often seen as a ring haemorrhage (Fig. 29.8). Around these lesions the myelin is often pale and degenerate. Parasitized vessels, with or without haemorrhage, have no surrounding inflammatory reaction, i.e. there is no morphological evidence of an immunopathological process. Thrombosis in cerebral small vessels is unusual. If a small piece of brain from a fatal case of CM is smeared on a slide, stained with Giemsa, and the arcades of small vessels examined microscopically, they are

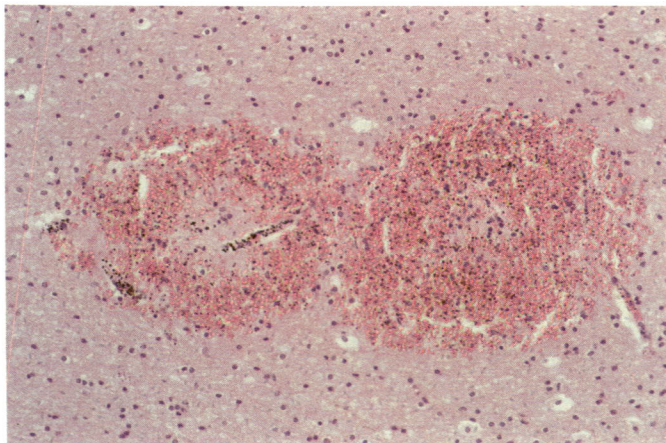

Fig. 29.8 Brain in falciparum malaria. Two ring haemorrhages in the white matter, around obstructed small vessels.

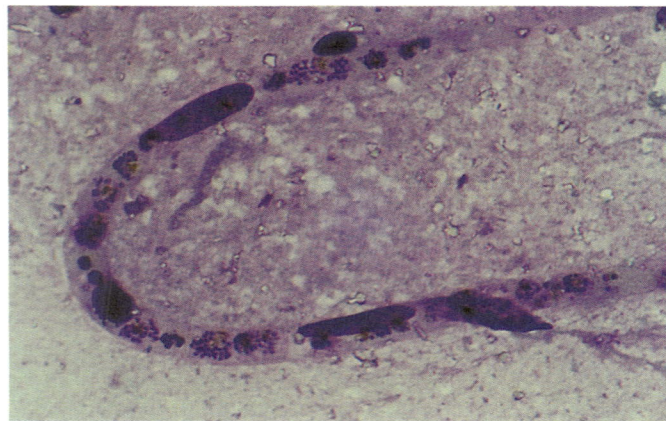

Fig. 29.9 Squash smear of a falciparum malaria brain showing a capillary. There are numerous erythrocytes containing meronts (with haemozoin pigment dots), adhering to the endothelial cells. (Giemsa stain.)

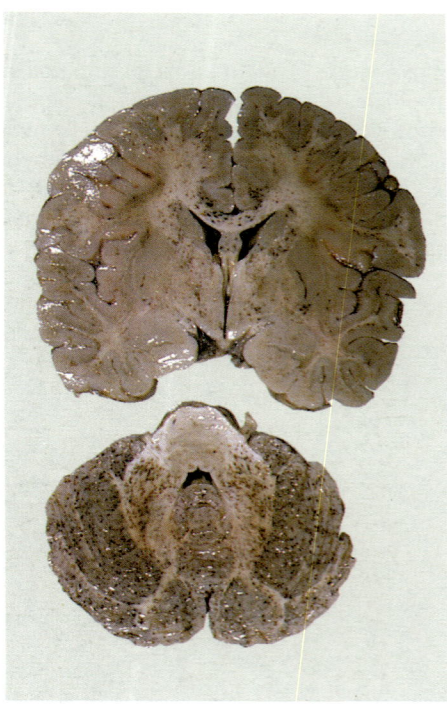

Fig. 29.7 Cerebrum and cerebellum in falciparum malaria. Widespread small haemorrhages, mainly in the white matter. (Photograph courtesy of the late Dr F. MacDonald and Professor M. S. R. Hutt.)

seen to contain closely packed PRBC, the parasites being ring forms or schizonts (Fig. 29.9).

Patients who live for a week or more after lapsing into coma, but then die, manifest a repair reaction in the brain to the petechial haemorrhages and demyelination. Microglial nodules ('Durck granulomas') phagocytose the haemorrhage and degenerate neuropil.

Cytoadherence and the pathogenesis of cerebral malaria. The pathogenesis of falciparum malaria and cerebral malaria in particular have been much debated. Earlier concepts stressed disseminated intravascular coagulation (which is uncommon in malaria), or an increased permeability of parasitized brain capillaries with accompanying cerebral oedema. However, *in vivo* studies using CT scans show that cerebral oedema in CM is uncommon, though it may develop at the time of death as an agonal event. The contribution of hypoglycaemia towards CM is limited. Correction of the blood sugar does not result in rapid recovery. However, some of the post-recovery deficits seen in children may follow hypoglycaemic damage.

Erythrocytes parasitized by *P. falciparum* adhere to the surface of endothelial cells. This sequestration occurs preferentially in the internal visceral capillaries and post-capillary venules, so that patients with severe clinical malaria may have few or, uncommonly, no PRBC in a peripheral blood sample. The proposed endothelial cell receptors for adherence include the glyco-proteins thrombospondin, CD36, and ICAM 1 (intercellular adhesion molecule). Parasitized adhering cells have numerous tiny surface protrusions termed 'knobs' (Fig. 29.10), sites of adhesion to endothelial cells. Transmission electron microscopy shows knobs to be electron-dense deposits just under the surface membrane. They are complexes of parasite-derived material with components of the host red cell cytoskeleton.

The current explanation of CM proposes that PRBC adhere to endothelium, the blood flow through capillaries slows, and there is reduced metabolic activity through impaired delivery of oxygen and nutrients to the brain cells. *In vivo* studies demonstrate reduced cerebral blood flow, which returns to normal after successful therapy, and CSF analysis shows increased lactate concentration as an indication of anaerobic glycolysis. In other organs, such as the intestine, similar cytoadherence and ischaemia probably takes place (Fig. 29.11).

Haemorrhages in CM occur when the blood flow through small vessels is so sluggish that they undergo ischaemic necrosis. Since they are not always seen in fatal cases, haemorrhages are not the initial cause of cerebral dysfunction and coma; but they may represent a pathological 'point of no return'.

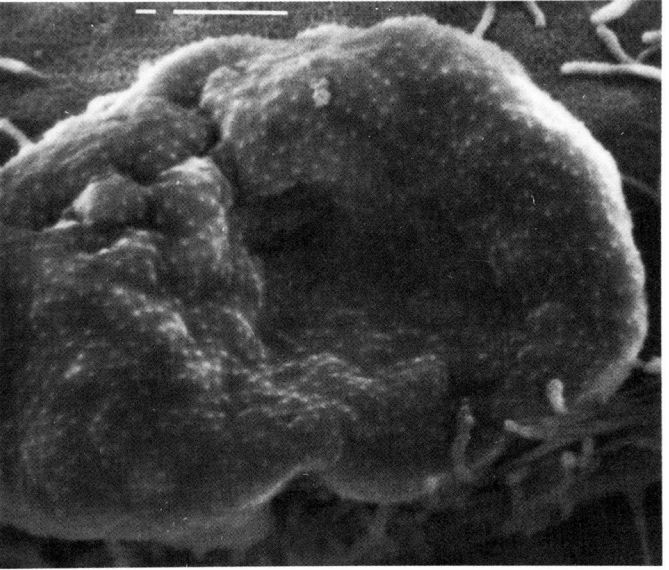

Fig. 29.10 Scanning electron micrograph of an erythrocyte parasitized with *P. falciparum*. There are abundant small 'knobs' on the cell surface; these facilitate cytoadherence to endothelial cells. (Photograph courtesy of Professor M. Hommel.)

The rupturing meront releases substances which stimulate macrophages to release cytokines such as tumour necrosis factor (TNF). This has been proposed as the pathogenesis for many aspects of severe malaria, such as pulmonary oedema, algid malaria, and CM. TNF can induce expression of endothelial receptors for cytoadherence. However, the correlation of circulating TNF levels with symptoms is not close. Variable secretion of TNF and other undetermined cytokines might explain why only some infected people suffer from severe malaria.

The chronic effects of malaria

'Tropical splenomegaly syndrome' (TSS)

Some young adults in zones endemic for *P. falciparum* malaria develop marked chronic splenomegaly. The spleen may enlarge over years to a weight of 3–4 kg, resulting in severe hypersplenism. Occasionally, Caucasian expatriates develop the same syndrome. Significant portal hypertension is not a feature, and variceal bleeding is rare. This 'tropical splenomegaly syndrome' is differentiated from other causes of large spleens in the tropics, such as schistosomiasis, visceral leishmaniasis, and leukaemia. Patients have characteristically very high blood IgM concentrations. Mortality is high, with 90 per cent of those with massive splenomegaly dead within 15 years of onset.

The enlarged spleen is congested and firm. There is no haemozoin pigment accumulation, for there is minimal or no detectable parasitaemia. The lymphoid pulp is hyperplastic, but most of the hyperplasia is of the red pulp. The liver is of normal size, but has a characteristic histological appearance. The Kupffer cells are hypertrophied but not pigmented. There is an infiltration of T-lymphocytes throughout the sinusoids, which may be very marked (Fig. 29.12). Immunostaining shows deposition of IgG and IgM along the sinusoids.

There is consensus that TSS is caused by a chronic, very low-intensity infection by *P. falciparum*:

1. TSS is confined to endemic malarious zones;
2. it is rare in HbAS heterozygous individuals, who are relatively protected against malaria;
3. TSS patients have high serum titres of antimalaria antibodies;
4. the condition regresses on long-term antimalarial chemotherapy.

The syndrome most commonly occurs in members of population groups whose exposure to malaria is recent. HLA studies indicate a genetic immune response link to TSS. In susceptibles, malaria infection induces both specific IgG and IgM antibodies and a polyclonal B-cell activation with formation of IgG and IgM auto-antibodies. These induce the hypersplenism and impair primary immune responses. Impaired T-suppressor cell control of antibody production is thought to be the fundamental defect. Recently, the syndrome has been more precisely renamed 'hyperreactive chronic malarial splenomegaly'.

Quartan malaria nephrotic syndrome

The patterns of nephrotic syndrome in children in sub-Saharan

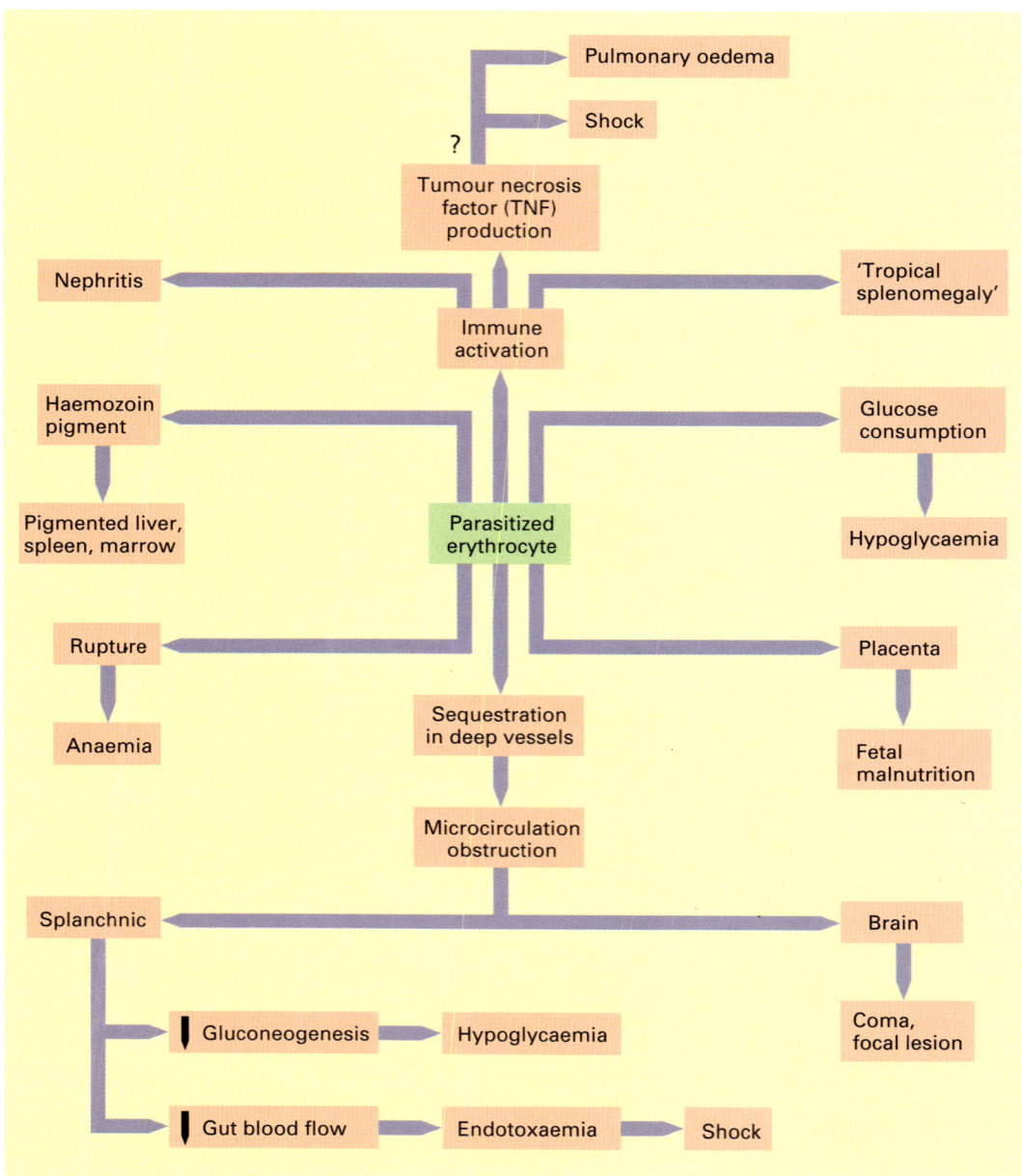

Fig. 29.11 Schematic flow diagram of the major pathophysiological sequelae of *Plasmodium falciparum* infection.

Africa are not the same as those found in European countries where minimal change disease (MCD) is the commonest diagnosis. In Africa, MCD underlies only 10–20 per cent of nephrosis cases; most cases have proliferative or sclerosing glomerulonephritis. A characteristic histological type is associated with endemic *P. malariae* infection, and immunofluorescence shows *P. malariae* antigen in the glomeruli. This 'quartan malaria nephrotic syndrome' has a poor prognosis, with chronic renal failure as the usual outcome, irrespective of antimalarial treatment.

Histopathologically, the early lesion is focal and segmental glomerulitis, capillary wall thickening, and mesangial accumulation of PAS-positive material (Fig. 29.13). Later the lesion becomes diffuse with progressive glomerular sclerosis; there is no endothelial cell proliferation.

Malaria and malignant lymphoma

In Africa, South America, and Papua New Guinea, high endemicity for *P. falciparum* is geographically associated with a high-grade B-cell lymphoma in children, Burkitt's lymphoma (BL)

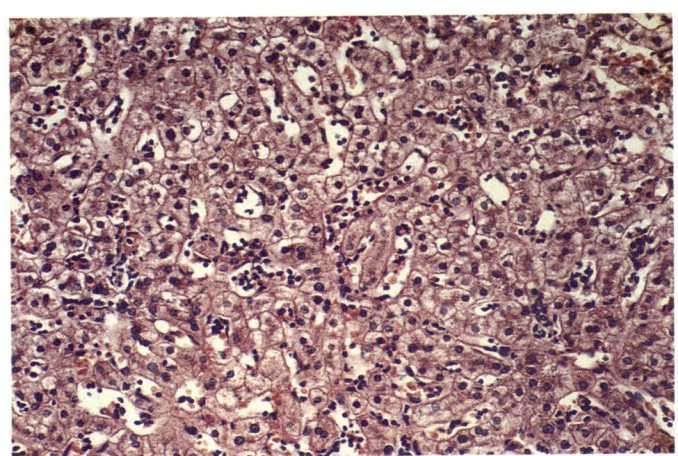

Fig. 29.12 Malaria. Liver in tropical splenomegaly syndrome (TSS), showing sinusoidal lymphocytosis. There is no parasitaemia.

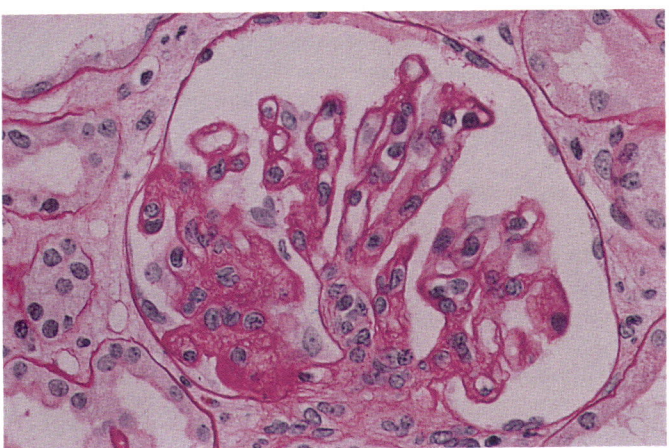

Fig. 29.13 Glomerulus in quartan malaria nephrotic syndrome (QMNS). There is segmental sclerosis. (Periodic acid-Schiff stain.)

(see Chapter 24). Pathogenetically, BL is also associated with early infection by Epstein–Barr virus (EBV). EBV is oncogenic for B-cells and BL tumour cells have chromosomal translocations near the c-*myc* oncogene. The precise role of malaria in oncogenesis is uncertain. During acute falciparum malaria, peripheral blood T-helper cell counts are reduced, which could remove a modulating effect on EBV replication and increase the chance of a mutation. However, in people who are both HIV and EBV seropositive, the incidences of EBV-expressing lymphomas are relatively low. Malaria probably has a specific but undetermined pathogenetic role in endemic Burkitt's lymphoma.

There is epidemiological evidence that high-grade non-Burkitt non-Hodgkin's malignant lymphomas are over-represented in areas of Africa where falciparum malaria is holoendemic. Again, this argues for an aetiological role for malaria in lymphoma-genesis.

Diagnosis and treatment

Examination of thick and thin blood smears diagnoses malaria and the *Plasmodium* species. Tissue biopsies may reveal parasitized erythrocytes in previously unsuspected cases. Antimalarial chemotherapy is complex and under constant reappraisal.

29.2.2 *Babesia*

Babesiosis in man is a zoonosis, all infections being accidental intrusions on the natural transmission cycles.

Life cycle and morphology

Ticks are the vectors of *Babesia*, transmitting to a wide variety of mammals, including rodents, dogs, and cattle (the vectors include the same tick species that transmit Lyme disease). In the mammal erythrocytes, only merogony occurs; the cycle in the tick is complex and unlike that of *Plasmodium* in mosquitoes. The parasites resemble *P. falciparum* ring-form trophozoites, although they are often flame-shaped (hence also known as 'piroplasms'—Fig. 29.14). Unlike *Plasmodium*, there is no haemozoin pigment production.

Epidemiology and clinical features

These are global infections of animals. Of particular economic importance is *B. divergens* infection of cattle, which causes red-water fever. For man, there are two clinico-pathological patterns of babesiosis.

B. microti infection occurs in the USA (normal hosts are rodents). It may be asymptomatic, or produce haemolytic anaemia with fever, myalgia, and splenomegaly. The illness is self-limiting and recovery takes place after a month.

Conversely, bovine *B. divergens* infection is usually fatal in man. It is sporadic in Europe, and only occurs in splenectomized people. There is profound haemolytic anaemia, shock with renal failure and haemoglobinuria, and jaundice.

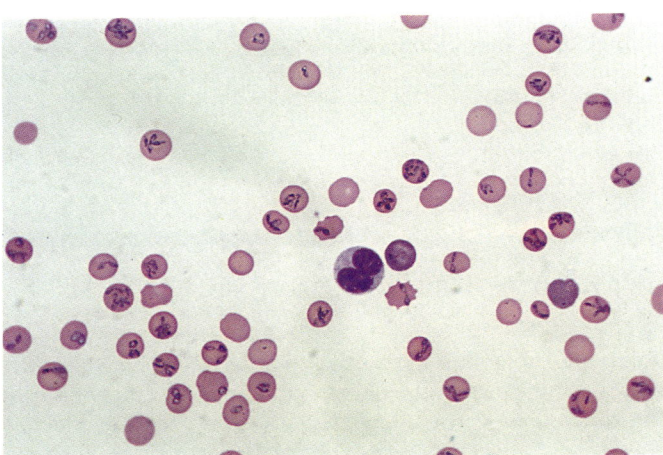

Fig. 29.14 Peripheral blood smear of a patient infected with *Babesia divergens*. The erythrocytes contain merozoites, some arranged in the shape of a Maltese cross. (Giemsa stain.)

Pathology

Benign *B. microti* infection causes parasitaemia without known specific tissue morphological changes. In fatal *B. divergens* infection, the kidneys show congestion and oedema, the lungs are oedematous with the appearances of shock lung, the liver is enlarged, and the brain is hyperaemic but not haemorrhagic. There is no dark pigmentation as in malaria. The peripheral blood has a high parasitaemia. Histologically, there is pulmonary oedema and hepatic centrilobular necrosis. The kidneys show acute tubular necrosis with abundant casts of haemoglobin. In the few cases studied at autopsy, small vessels of the brain contain numerous parasitized erythrocytes, as well as leuko-erythroblasts, but there is not the adherence of parasitized red cell to the endothelium typical of *P. falciparum* infection.

Pathogenesis

Haemolysis is the major factor in babesiosis, caused by rupture of erythrocytes as the parasites emerge to infect other red cells. In *B. divergens* infection, where the absence of a spleen renders the host unable to control the parasitaemia, systemic shock follows. The cytoadherence characteristic of severe falciparum malaria is not evident in human infections. Experimental models suggest that tumour necrosis factor is important in producing the organ damage; but whether this may be a direct consequence of infection (an interaction between parasite and macrophages), or whether it follows from haemolytic shock with intestinal hypoperfusion and leakage of endotoxins, is unclear.

Diagnosis and treatment

Diagnosis is by observing the erythrocytic parasites in thin or thick blood films, with careful distinction from malaria infection. Serology is available for epidemiological studies. There are no generally effective drugs for treating babesiosis.

29.2.3   Further reading

Warrell, D. A., Molyneux, M. E., and Beales, P. F. (1990). Severe and complicated malaria (2nd edn). *Transactions of the Royal Society of Tropical Medicine and Hygiene* **84** (Suppl. 2), 1–65.

29.3   Intestinal protozoa

There are numerous species of protozoa that have vegetative reproductive cycles in the human gut lumen, but do not invade the mucosa or cause significant disease. They include *Entamoeba coli*, *Endolimax nana*, *Iodamoeba buetschlii*, and *Blastocystis hominis*—all globally distributed.

The three clinically significant intestinal infections in man are *Giardia*, *Entamoeba histolytica*, and *Balantidium*.

29.3.1   *Giardia*

Giardia lamblia (*G. duodenalis*) is a common cause of enteritis—giardiasis.

Epidemiology, life cycle, and morphology

The infection is cosmopolitan. Whether it is purely anthroponotic is disputed, since animals such as monkeys, pigs, and beavers carry the parasite and could be a zoonotic reservoir. In some communities, more than 10 per cent of people are infected. The life cycle is simple vegetative, with binary fission and cyst production in the small bowel lumen. There is no mucosal invasion. Transmission of infection is by faecal–oral passage of cysts. Giardiasis is common in the gay population. Water supplies may become contaminated, causing epidemics of giardiasis. The trophozoites measure 20×15 μm, with characteristic flagella. Cysts are 10×8 μm in size.

Clinical features

Only a minority of those with *Giardia* in the gut are symptomatic. They have abdominal pains and diarrhoea of varying severity, which in a smaller proportion may be associated with malabsorption and weight loss. Children and people with hypogammaglobulinaemia are at particular risk of symptomatic infection.

Pathology

The correlation of pathology with clinical features is not close, although there is a trend for those with malabsorption to have more severe intestinal damage. *Giardia* parasites attach to the enterocytes' brush border by their suction disk. The duodenal and jejunal villi may be otherwise nearly normal; or show degrees of villous blunting that can even mimic that seen in tropical sprue and coeliac disease (Figs 29.15, 29.16). The lamina propria has a plasma cell infiltrate and intra-epithelial lymphocytes are increased. Small polymorph accumulations in the surface epithelium are common. Patients with hypo-

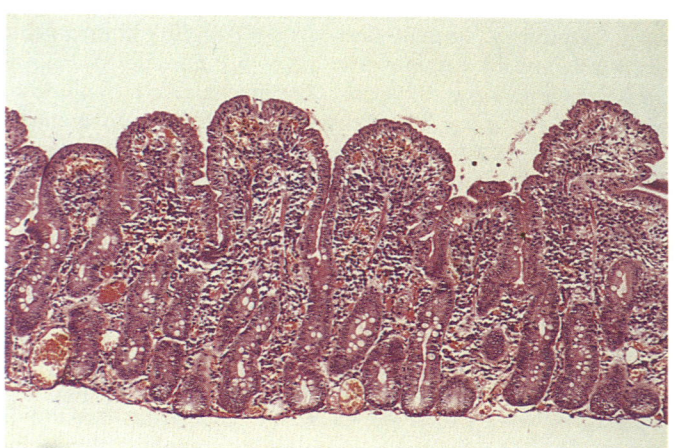

Fig. 29.15 Jejunal biopsy in giardiasis. There is partial villous atrophy.

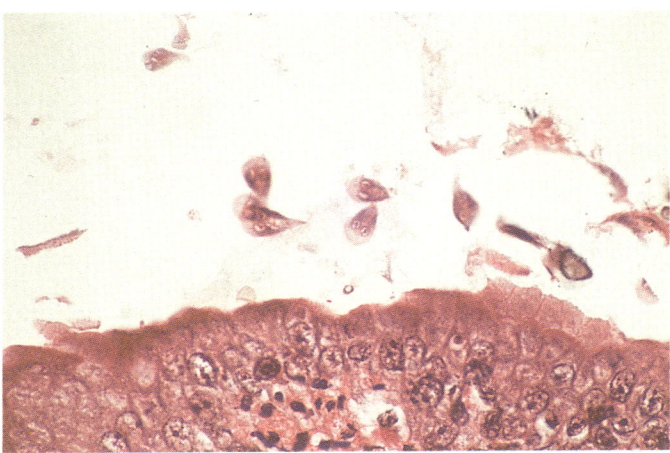

Fig. 29.16 Giardiasis. The pear-shaped trophozoites are seen above the enterocytes.

gammaglobulinaemia may have nodular lymphoid hyperplasia of Peyer's patches.

Pathogenesis

Only a minority of those infected are symptomatic. Variation in virulence between different strains of *Giardia* is possible but not proven. The postulated pathogenetic mechanisms of disease include:

1. mechanical blockade of the villi by parasites;
2. toxin production by *Giardia*;
3. immune injury to the mucosa: antibody and/or T-cell mediated;
4. co-infection with bacteria.

There is evidence that bacterial co-infection is common in symptomatic *Giardia* infection. Thus the pathogenesis may be similar to that of 'tropical sprue' (see Chapter 16).

Diagnosis and treatment

Aspiration of duodenal or jejunal juices are the most sensitive techniques. Identification of cysts in the faeces is unreliable. Small bowel biopsy may identify the infection, or provide alternative diagnoses for the symptoms. Treatment is with metronidazole.

29.3.2 *Entamoeba histolytica*

Amoebiasis produces a wide range of pathological sequelae (Fig. 29.17), and is a leading parasitic cause of death after malaria and schistosomiasis.

Epidemiology

Infection is global. Approximately 10 per cent of the world's population have *Entamoeba histolytica* in the colorectum. Clinical disease ('amoebiasis' proper) occurs in 0.1–20 per cent of those infected (see 'Pathogenesis'), with most cases in the tropics. Gay communities have asymptomatic *E. histolytica* prevalences of up to 25 per cent.

Life cycle and morphology

Only man is infected. Following ingestion of faecal cysts, from food, water, or sexual practices, the parasites exist and reside in the large bowel lumen. Vegetative asexual multiplication and cyst production take place. The trophozoites are 20–30 μm in diameter, with a single nucleus (Fig. 29.18). Cysts are 12–14 μm in size and contain four nuclei.

Clinical features

Disease results from invasion of the mucosa by *Entamoeba*. This occurs from caecum to rectum (and occasionally the appendix), and may be focal or diffuse. Painful diarrhoea with blood (dysentery) is typical. This may resolve spontaneously, persist, or progress to more extensive ulceration. In up to 4 per cent of cases there is perforation and amoebic peritonitis. Pregnant women and people on steroids are more susceptible to severe amoebiasis. Uncommonly, a florid inflammatory mass forms around a site of invasion (mimicking a carcinoma), known as an *amoeboma*.

Extra-intestinal amoebiasis is most commonly to the liver, following invasion by amoebae of the mesenteric veins and transport there. There is tender hepatomegaly, fever, leucocytosis, and, sometimes, cholestatic jaundice. Untreated amoebic liver abscess is fatal. It perforates through the capsule into the peritoneal cavity, or (less commonly) across the diaphragm to produce empyema, lung abscess, and pericarditis. Amoebic peritonitis has a very high mortality. Direct spread of amoebae from rectum to anus produces an ulcerating proliferative lesion, as may a fistula from colon to abdominal wall. Venereal infections of the penis and cervix also occur. These epithelial lesions may resemble squamous carcinoma. From the liver, haematogenous spread to the brain is rare.

Pathology

Intestinal amoebiasis

The disease commences as mucosal oedema, proceeding through small erosions to ulcers (Fig. 29.19). These may become confluent, to produce massive shaggy necrosis with thickening of the bowel wall. Histologically, the early colitis is similar to bacterial colitis, with oedema and polymorph infiltration of crypts; amoebae are seen adherent to the surface epithelium. Epithelial necrosis follows, often with much slough. Amoebae invade vertically through the mucosa and laterally in the submucosa, so producing the undermined ('flask-shaped') ulcers (Figs 29.20, 29.21). The amoebae are seen in greatest numbers at the advancing edges of ulcers; characteristically, they phagocytose erythrocytes (Fig. 29.18). Attendant inflammation includes polymorphs and plasma cells, but is not granulomatous. Invasion by amoebae of arteries in the bowel wall and their subsequent thrombosis contributes to the necrosis in severe cases.

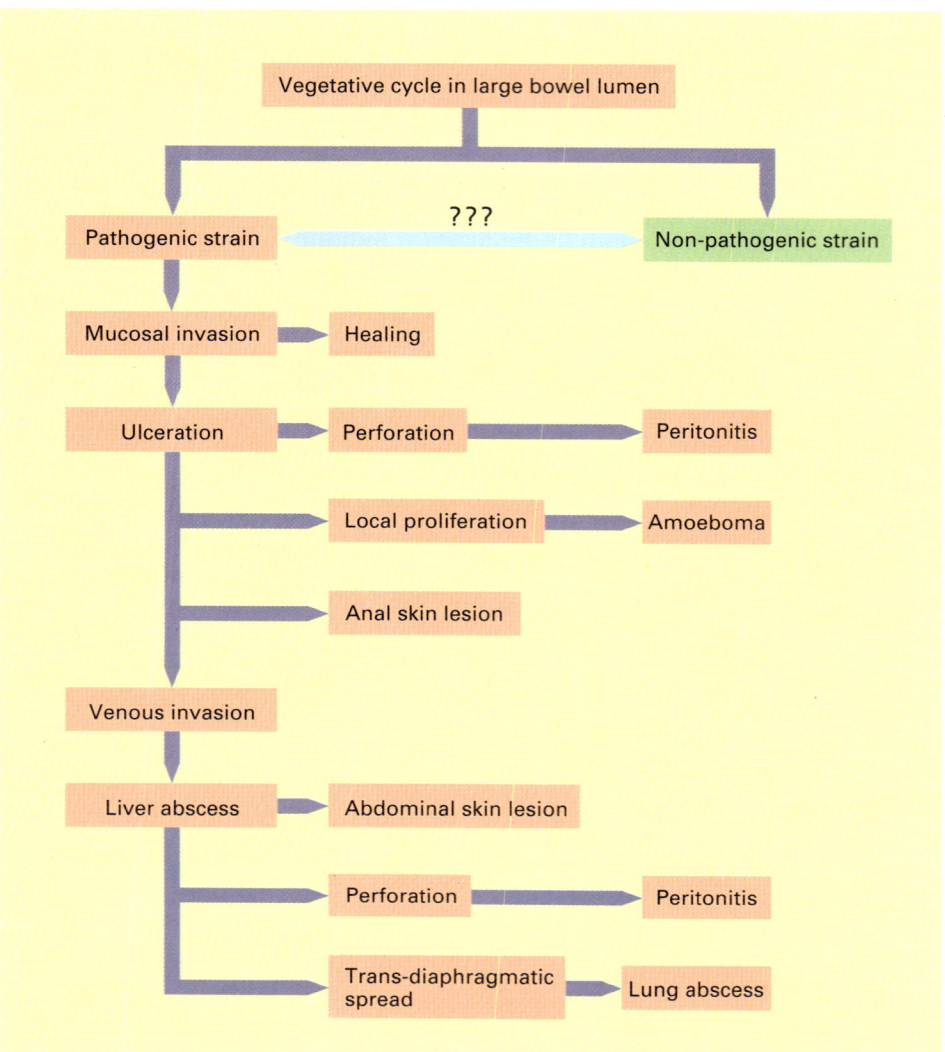

Fig. 29.17 Sequelae of infection with *Entamoeba histolytica*.

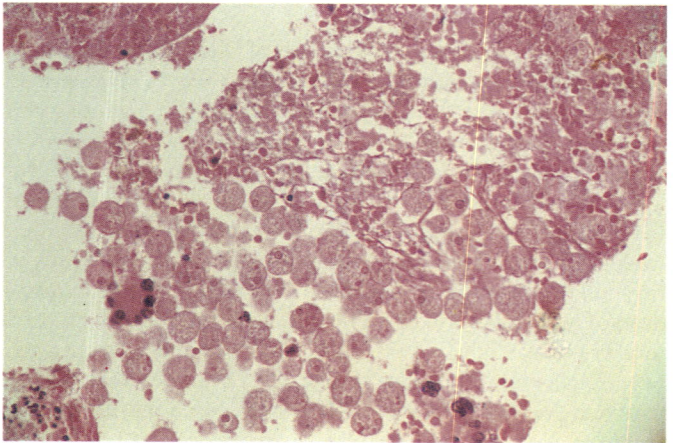

Fig. 29.18 *Entamoeba histolytica* trophozoites. They have a single nucleus and many contain phagocytosed erythrocytes.

An amoeboma (Fig. 29.22) comprises a parasitized central necrotic zone with surrounding granulation tissue and fibrosis, replacing the colon wall. Trophozoites are not numerous. This degree of fibrosis is unusual in amoebiasis; usually the ulceration heals well on treatment, without significant scarring.

In parasitization by non-pathogenic *E. histolytica* (see below), trophozoites without phagocytosed erythrocytes proliferate near the mucosal surface, but do not invade or elicit significant inflammation.

Extra-intestinal amoebiasis

Early foci of hepatic infection are small, white necrotic zones. These expand and the centres liquefy, producing the characteristic brownish material resembling anchovy sauce (it comprises necrotic liver tissue, blood, and plasma exudate). Amoebic abscesses are usually multiple, and the right lobe is more affected than the left (Fig. 29.23). Their size at presentation ranges from

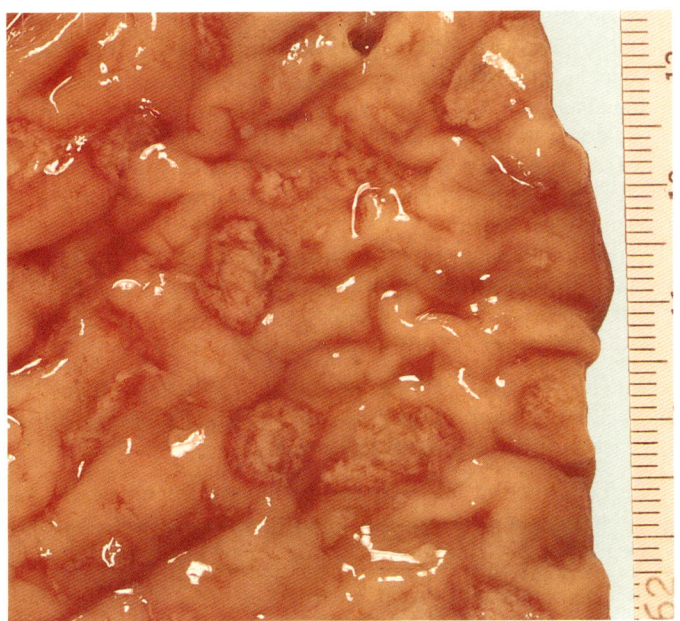

Fig. 29.19 Colon mucosa with several amoebic ulcers. The intervening mucosa is oedematous.

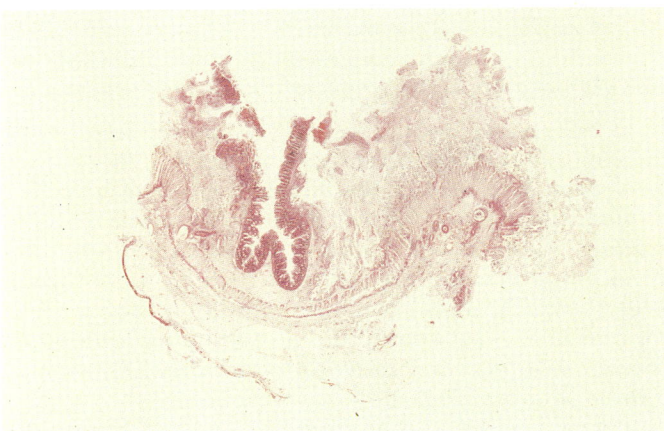

Fig. 29.20 Colonic amoebiasis. The mucosa is undermined by invading amoebae.

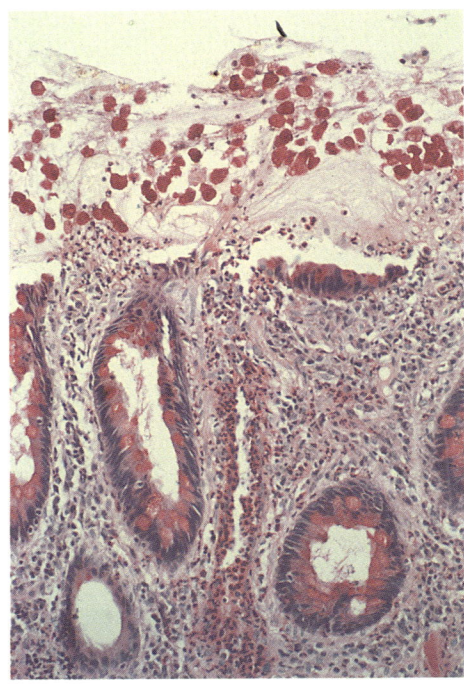

Fig. 29.21 Colonic amoebiasis. The *Entamoeba* trophozoites (stained red) cause necrosis of the enterocytes following cell contact. (Periodic acid-Schiff stain.)

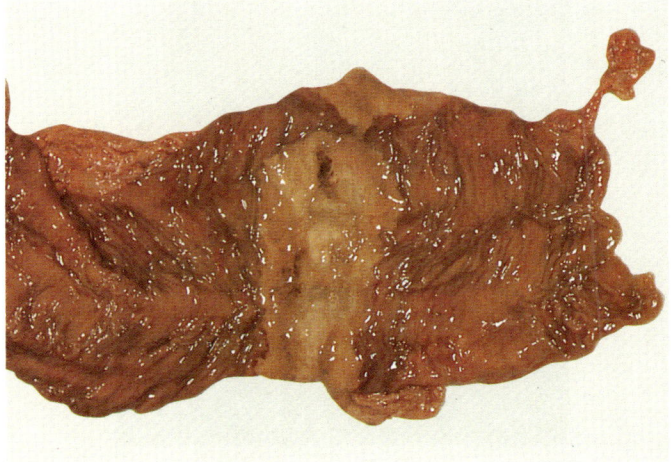

Fig. 29.22 Colonic amoeboma. There is a focal inflammatory and fibrotic mass protruding into the lumen; this caused intestinal obstruction. (Photograph courtesy of the late Dr F. MacDonald and Professor M. S. R. Hutt.)

4 to 12 cm in diameter. The inner lining is irregular, and in long-standing cases there is a fibrous rim around the abscess. Histologically, the trophozoites invade from portal veins into the liver, destroying and phagocytosing hepatocytes, eliciting oedema and a mild chronic inflammatory reaction. The clinical condition of 'amoebic hepatitis'—indicating liver damage without parasitization—does not, in fact, exist. In established abscesses, parasites are variable in number, but are only visualized around the edge of the abscess next to the granulation tissue lining. Similar histopathology is found in other infected viscera, such as lung and brain, although there is less fibrosis.

On therapy, amoebic liver abscesses resolve over 2–20 months (as visualized ultrasonographically). Despite the fibrosis, resolution of liver lesions is nearly complete, with little residual scarring.

Infected squamous epithelium is chronically inflamed around the ulceration, often with pseudo-epitheliomatous hyperplasia (Fig. 29.24). Amoebic trophozoites are seen in large numbers at the epithelial surface.

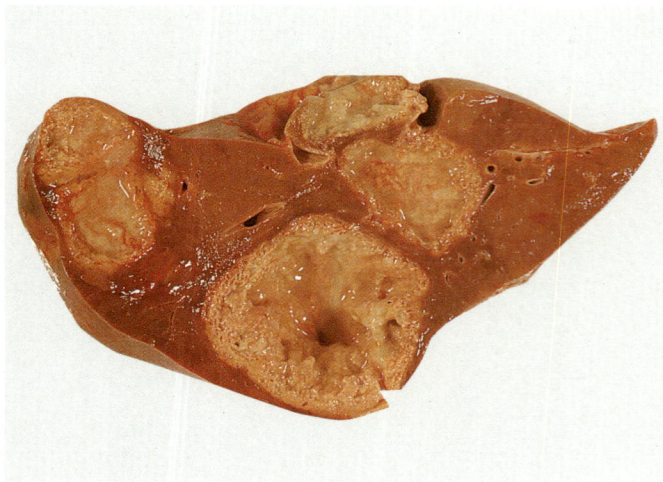

Fig. 29.23   Liver with multiple amoebic abscesses. (Photograph courtesy of the late Dr F. MacDonald and Professor M. S. R. Hutt.)

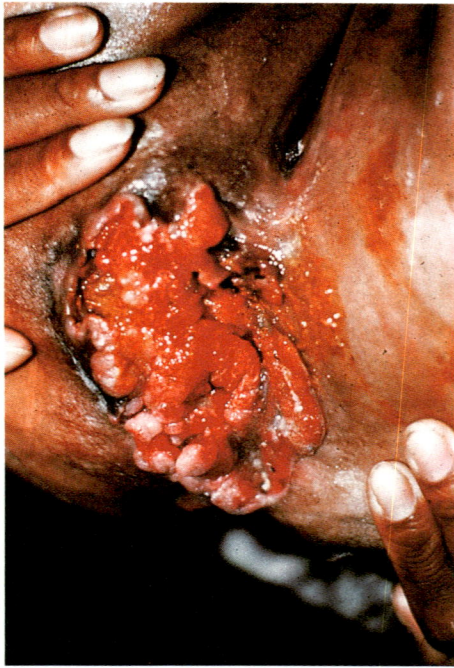

Fig. 29.24   Anal amoebiasis (spread from the rectum). The hyperplastic overgrowth resembles carcinoma.

Pathogenesis

Morphologically, *E. histolytica* from asymptomatic cyst passers are identical to those from patients with invasive disease. But there are numerous different strains of *E. histolytica*, which can be identified by enzyme electrophoresis of cultured amoebae and, more recently, by DNA probes. All strains isolated from patients with invasive amoebic colitis or liver abscess share the characteristic of an absent α-band and a present β-band in electrophoresis of the enzyme phosphoglucomutase. These are pathogenic zymodemes (PZs). Non-pathogenic zymodeme (NPZ) strains, which have never been associated with invasive disease, lack this feature.

Claims that NPZs can switch to PZs by incubation with irradiated gut bacteria from invasive colitis patients (and vice versa) have not been substantiated. DNA probe analysis further supports the firm division of *E. histolytica* into pathogenic and non-pathogenic strains.

There may be a genetic susceptibility to invasive disease, as revealed by different HLA-DR types in amoebiasis patients compared with controls. Given a pathogenic strain and a susceptible host, four processes follow during invasion:

1. The amoebae adhere to colonic epithelial mucins. Of several candidate proteins, one characterized amoebic adherence lectin is a 260 kDa galactosamine.

2. The amoebae disrupt the epithelium. PZ *Entamoeba* secretes proteinases *in vitro*, which may dissolve epithelial barriers by degrading fibronectin, laminin, and type I collagen.

3. The trophozoites lyse epithelial cells and the responding host inflammatory cells. Direct contact between the parasite and host epithelial cell initiates the secretion of a pore-forming protein (PFP) termed 'amoebapore', a 28 kDa protein which creates a 2 nm hole in the host cell membrane. This ion channel collapses the transmembrane electric potential, water enters the cell which then swells and bursts. The host cell can then be phagocytosed. *In vitro*, and presumably *in vivo*, amoebae can also kill host polymorphs, lymphocytes, and macrophages.

4. The parasite resists host defences during deeper tissue invasion and in distant organs such as the liver. The nature of host resistance is unclear. Specific anti-trophozoite antibody is formed following invasion, but has no protective role. That cell-mediated immunity is important is surmised from the fact that pregnant women and patients on steroids are more likely to suffer severe invasive amoebiasis. Further, patients treated for colonic or hepatic amoebiasis do not usually get a second invasive infection. And delayed hypersensitivity skin tests to *Entamoeba* antigens become positive after recovery.

In vitro, amoebae can be killed by stimulated lymphocytes and macrophages (but they can also resist lysis by complement). It is possible that antibodies to the adherence lectin may be important in post-infection resistance. However, people with HIV infection are not more likely to acquire invasive amoebiasis, indicating that our explanations of host resistance to *Entamoeba* are incomplete.

Diagnosis and treatment

E. histolytica cysts and trophozoites in the faeces are distinguishable by morphological criteria from the numerous non-*histolytica* non-pathogenic species. Distinction of PZs from NPZs requires culture in reference centres; but the presence of many trophozoites with phagocytosed erythrocytes indicates a pathogenic strain. For enteric infection, biopsy is less sensitive than scraping a mucosal ulcer and direct microscopy. Amoebic serology is very useful since it is positive in invasive amoebiasis, but not in non-invasive cyst passage.

Liver abscess is usually diagnosed on clinical and ultrasonographic criteria, supported by positive amoebic serology. Aspiration does not always yield parasites, which may be scanty even at the edge of an abscess. For skin lesions, surface scrapes and biopsy are diagnostic.

Metronidazole effectively treats invasive amoebiasis, but diloxanide is often required to eliminate parasites from the bowel lumen.

29.3.3 *Balantidium*

Epidemiology, life cycle, and morphology

Balantidium coli is the largest protozoon to infect man, and is also the only invasive pathogenic ciliate. It is widely distributed in hogs in the tropics and subtropics as an intestinal infection. The life cycle, like that of *Entamoeba histolytica*, has trophozoites and cysts. Human infection is accidental, by the ingestion of cysts. The trophozoite is ovoid, cilated, and up to 200 μm long. It has two elongated nuclei.

Clinical features and pathology

Gastrointestinal upset, often with severe dysentery, occurs. The colon is affected. Since the parasite is invasive, perforation of the bowel and peritonitis may follow.

Mucosal ulceration may be focal or extensive. The undermining typical of *Entamoeba* is not found, but deep penetration into

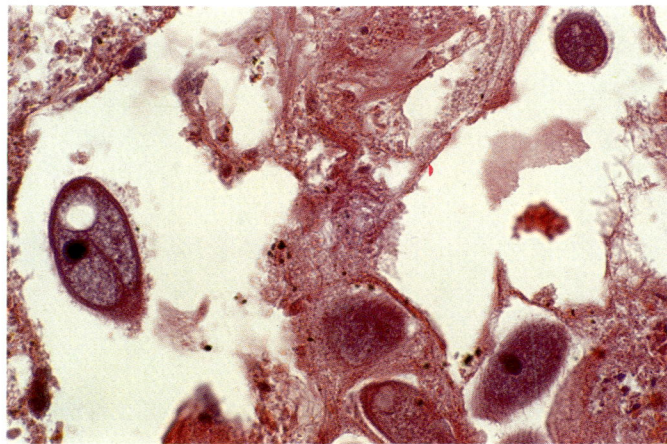

Fig. 29.26 Balantidiasis. The trophozoites are larger than *Entamoeba*, and are ciliated.

the muscularis and serosa is common (Fig. 29.25). The *Balantidium* trophozoites are seen at the advancing ulcer edges (Fig. 29.26), accompanied by a mixed acute and chronic inflammatory reaction.

29.3.4 Further reading

Ravdin, J. I. (1989). Amebiasis now. *American Journal of Tropical Medicine and Hygiene* **41** (Suppl. 3), 40–8.

29.4 Free-living amoebae

Two genera of amoebae that live entirely in soil or water can accidentally infect man. *Acanthamoeba* and *Naegleria* cause meningoencephalitis; *Acanthamoeba* also infects the eye.

29.4.1 *Acanthamoeba*

Epidemiology, life cycle, and morphology

Acanthamoeba species are common organisms in water and soil globally. On morphological and immunostaining criteria, four species affect man: *A. castellani*, *A. polyphaga*, *A. culbertsoni*, and *A. astronyxis*. (*Hartmanella*, often bracketed with *Acanthamoeba*, are distinct, non-pathogenic free-living amoebae.) Only trophozoite and cyst stages form the life cycle. Cysts survive for years in dry soil, and can be found in air samples. Man is infected either by inhalation and infection of the nasopharynx with cysts or by their inoculation into the skin (Fig. 29.27). Although *Acanthamoeba* disease is uncommon in man, asymptomatic carriage of amoebae occurs in the nasopharynx of healthy people. Acanthamoebiasis is predominantly an opportunistic infection, most cases occurring because of a breach in

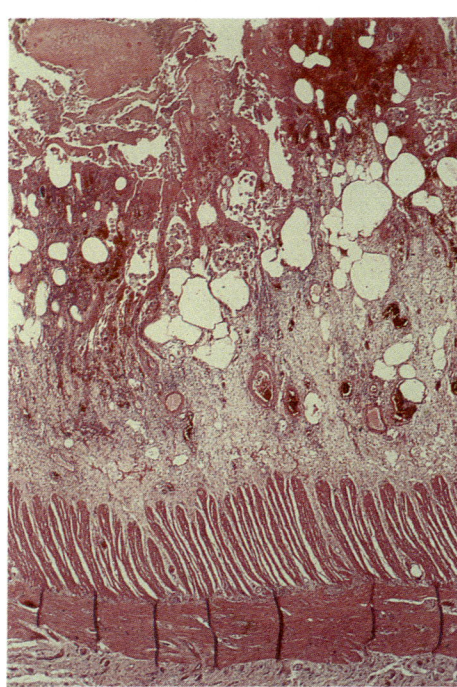

Fig. 29.25 Balantidiasis of the colon. Low-power view showing mucosal necrosis and invasion of the submucosa.

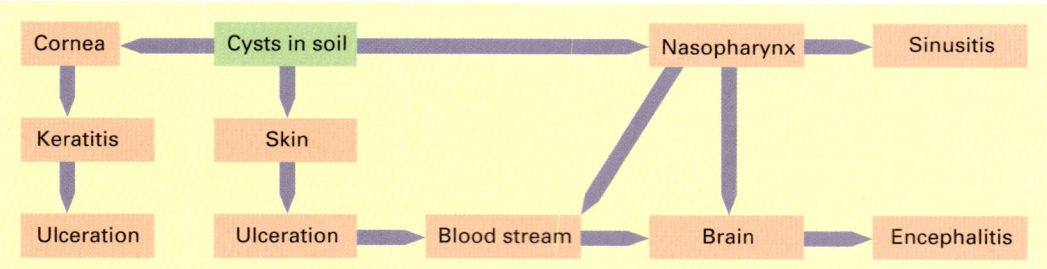

Fig. 29.27 Sequelae of infection with *Acanthamoeba*.

host defences, either local (in the eye) or systemic. The trophozoites measure 20–45 μm; the cysts 10–25 μm.

Clinical features

Two distinct clinico-pathological patterns of disease occur in man. *Acanthamoeba* keratitis (predominantly *A. castellani*) is associated with the use of soft contact lenses; non-sterile lens cleaning solutions become contaminated. The eye shows conjunctival infection and a white infiltrate of the cornea. It thins, ulcerates, and may perforate.

The second pattern is visceral disease, which occurs in those immunocompromised by diabetes, alcoholism, cancer, or HIV infection. Cerebral involvement is the most common, with a course lasting weeks or months. Focal neurological signs, dementia, and coma occur, fatal unless treated. Some patients have a simultaneous *Acanthamoeba* skin ulcer, and a few have nasal infection with purulent discharge, or pneumonia.

Pathology

In *Acanthamoeba* keratitis, the corneal stroma is necrotic, with an intense underlying polymorph infiltrate. The trophozoites and cysts are seen in the superficial layers (Fig. 29.28).

The cerebral disease is a multifocal haemorrhagic necrotizing meningoencephalitis, with brownish lesions several centimetres in diameter. There tends to be centrifugal spread from the deeper to the superficial parts of the brain. The olfactory bulbs are often involved. Histologically, the amoebae are most dense around vessels that are necrotic and thrombosed, accompanied by a polymorph reaction. There is much surrounding oedema, gliosis, and, in older lesions, a granulomatous reaction to necrotic material and to the trophozoites and cysts (Figs 29.29, 29.30). This disease is often termed 'granulomatous amoebic encephalitis'.

Skin lesions are deep ulcers with a granulomatous reaction to trophozoites. It is postulated that, in some cases, the amoebae spread via the olfactory nerves into the brain (like *Naegleria*, see below) as well as via the bloodstream after skin or respiratory tract infection.

The mechanism of host tissue necrosis is unclear, but a toxin released from the parasite—as with *Entamoeba histolytica*—is postulated.

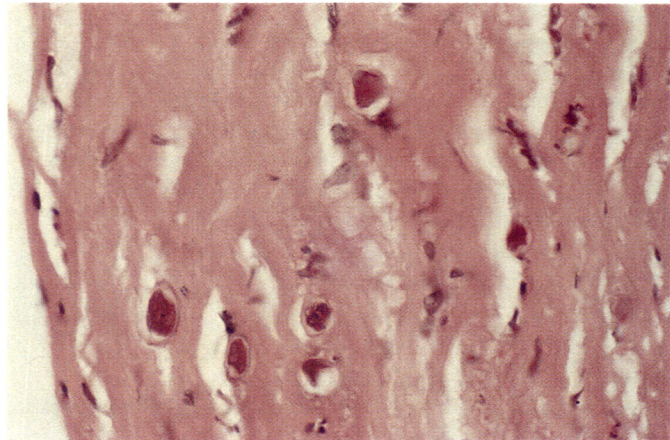

Fig. 29.28 Cornea in *Acanthamoeba* keratitis. There are trophozoites and cysts in the degenerate stroma.

Diagnosis and treatment

Diagnosis is by identification of *Acanthamoeba* from scrapings from the cornea and in the CSF, respectively. Culture and immunostaining with specific antisera confirm the morphological diagnosis, and aid the distinction from *Naegleria*. Anti-

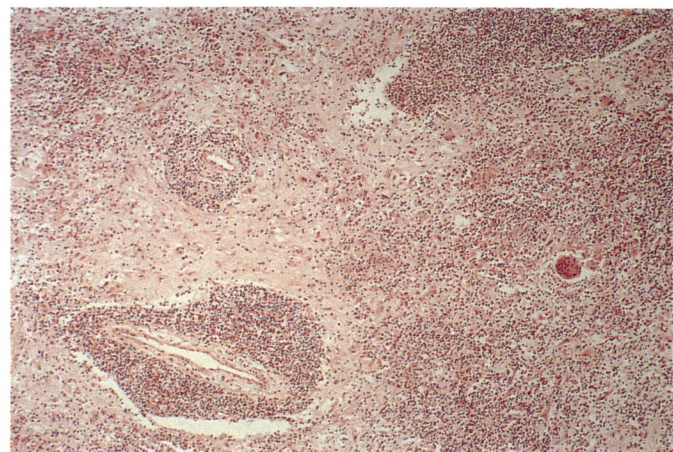

Fig. 29.29 *Acanthamoeba* encephalitis. Oedema, perivascular inflammation, and a giant cell granuloma (to the left).

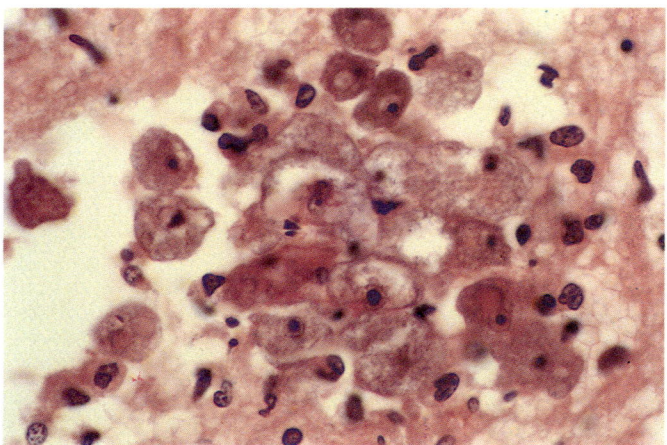

Fig. 29.30 *Acanthamoeba* trophozoites in brain. They are larger than *Entamoeba*.

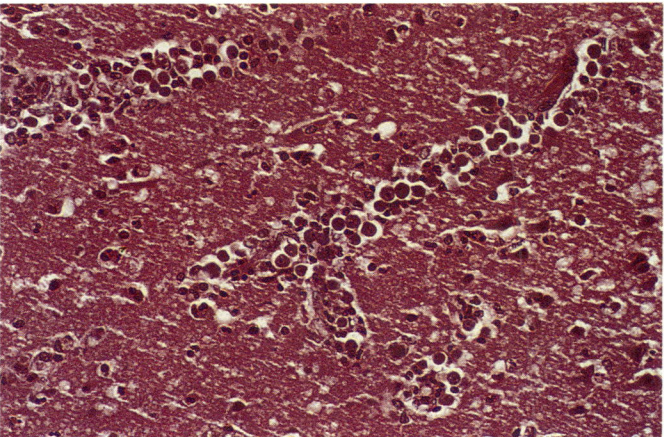

Fig. 29.31 *Naegleria* meningoencephalitis. Trophozoites infiltrating along vessels in the grey matter.

fungal agents may be effective if used early in cerebral acanthamoebiasis. Corneal transplantation is usually required for keratitis.

29.4.2 *Naegleria*

Epidemiology, life cycle, and morphology

These protozoa live in hot springs and waters (heated naturally or by power plants) all round the world. Human infection is with *N. fowleri*, following swimming in contaminated water. The amoeba penetrates the olfactory epithelium and the cribriform plate of the skull, infects the olfactory bulb, and then invades the brain along the Virchow–Robin spaces. Only the trophozoites are seen in human infection; they are smaller than *Acanthamoeba*, at 10–35 μm in diameter.

Clinical features

Immunocompetent people are susceptible. The incubation period after exposure is short, usually 2–10 days. Fulminant meningitis ('primary amoebic meningoencephalitis') develops, with rapid deterioration to coma and death unless treated.

Pathology

The meninges are hyperaemic, the brain swollen, and on section there are cortical haemorrhages affecting the frontal and basal parts predominantly. The olactory bulbs are necrotic, and the nasal cavity inflamed. Histologically, the amoebae penetrate along small vessels into the brain, causing vascular and surrounding necrosis. There is a mixed mononuclear and polymorph reaction (Fig. 29.31). *N. fowleri* secretes a 54 kDa poreforming protein and causes tissue necrosis in a similar manner in *Entamoeba*.

Diagnosis and treatment

Naegleria can be identified in cerebrospinal fluid (CSF) (which is often haemorrhagic), and early treatment with amphotericin B has been successful.

29.5 Blood and tissue flagellate protozoa

Trypanosoma and *Leishmania* species are grouped together. They share a flagellate morphology at some stage during their life cycle; they are mostly zoonotic with animal reservoir hosts, and have complex man–vector–reservoir cycles (Fig. 29.32).

29.5.1 *Trypanosoma brucei*

Two closely related subspecies of *Trypanosoma brucei*—*T. brucei gambiense* and *T. brucei rhodesiense*—cause human African trypanosomiasis (HAT; sleeping sickness) in West and Central Africa (Fig. 29.33).

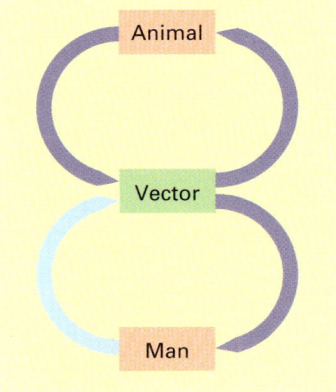

Fig. 29.32 Outline of the life cycles of *Trypanosoma* and *Leishmania* species infecting man. Transmission is from animal to vector to man, with the exceptions of *T. b. gambiense*, and *L. donovani* in India, where it is man–vector–man.

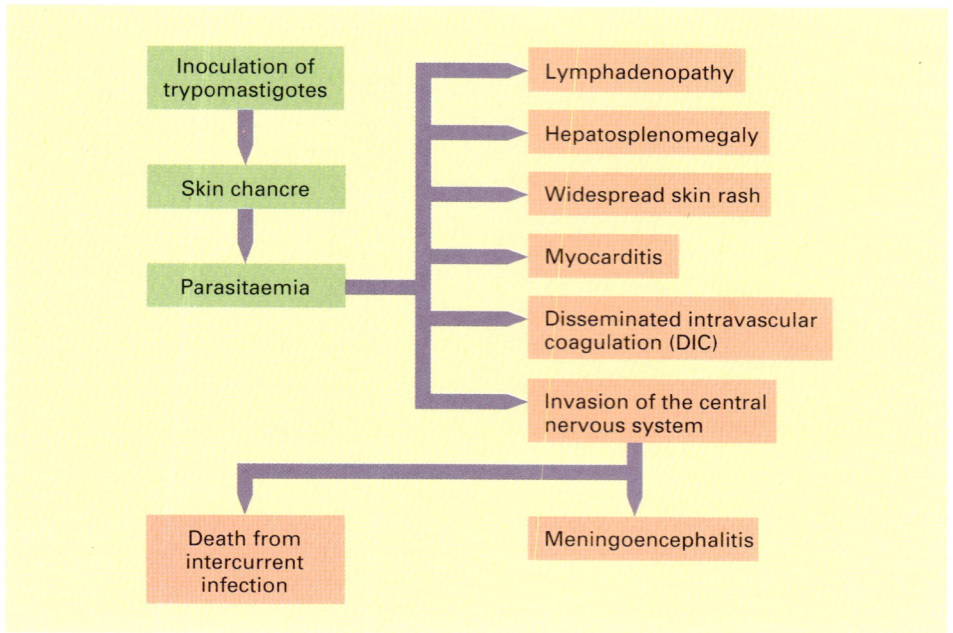

Fig. 29.33 Sequelae of infection with African *Trypanosoma* species.

Epidemiology

Trypanosoma brucei parasites infect many animal species in Africa. In West Africa, the parasite is *T. b. gambiense* and man is the main host; domestic animals are reservoir hosts. In Central Africa, *T. b. rhodesiense* is primarily a parasite of game animals. The highest incidences of HAT are in Uganda and Zaïre. Currently some 25 000 cases are reported annually, with periodic epidemics.

Life cycle and morphology

The tsetse fly is the vector. Trypanosomes are sucked from the host during a blood meal, develop into infective forms, and are transmitted from the tsetse salivary glands by biting. The trypomastigote blood forms are 10–30 μm long (Fig. 29.34).

Clinical features

The cadence of HAT differs according to geography and parasite, with *rhodesiense* disease being more acute than *gambiense*. In both, there are three stages:

1. the local skin lesion;
2. blood and lymphatic infection but before cerebral invasion;
3. cerebral invasion by trypanosomes (this is usually stated to occur about a month after infection, but on little direct evidence).

The skin lesion is the trypanosomal chancre, a large inflamed zone at the site of infection. Weeks or months later, there are waves of trypomastigote parasitaemia accompanied by fever. Lymphadenopathy (particularly the posterior cervical nodes), hepatosplenomegaly, and sometimes a petechial skin rash de-

velop. Anaemia is common. Disseminated intravascular coagulation and urine changes indicative of glomerulonephritis are uncommon. In *T. rhodesiense* infection, a pancarditis may cause death from heart failure before severe CNS disease occurs.

The later encephalitis produces personality changed, heaache, abnormal sleep patterns, focal neurological signs, and finally stupor and cachexia. Spontaneous recovery is rare, and death is from an intercurrent infection such as bacterial pneumonia. Very high IgM antibody levels (mostly non-specific and not anti-trypanosomal) are found in the blood. There is no apparent interaction between African trypanosomiasis and HIV infection.

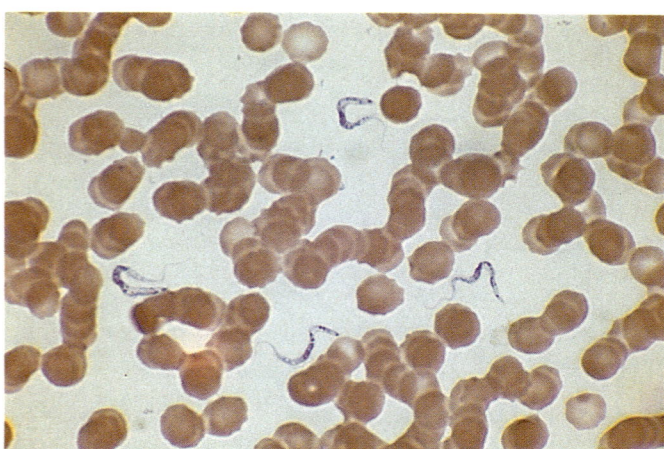

Fig. 29.34 Peripheral blood smear with trypomastigotes of *Trypanosoma rhodesiense*.

Pathology

The trypanosomal chancre is a mixed acute and chronic inflammatory reaction with oedema; the parasites lie in the interstitium. The lymphadenopathy of HAT shows follicular hyperplasia, medullary plasmacytosis, and sinus histiocytosis, but parasites are not frequently seen in the nodes.

The heart is usually of normal size and macroscopic appearance. Unlike Chagas' disease (see below), aneurysms do not form. But histologically there is a pancarditis. The endocardium and epicardium are inflamed and fibrosed. The myocardium and valves show patchy lymphocytic and plasmacytic inflammation, muscle fibre degeneration, oedema, and fibrosis. The conducting system has similar lesions. Trypanosomes are not found in the tissues (Fig. 29.35).

The brain in autopsied cases has opaque meninges. On section it is normal or swollen (Fig. 29.36). The diencephalon and mesencephalon are most severely affected by encephalitis, but the cerebral cortex, cerebellum, and brain stem are also involved. Histologically there is a chronic meningoencephalitis, with small lymphocytes and plasma cells densely cuffing the arachnoid and penetrating vessels. Necrotizing vasculitis does not occur in untreated patients. Many plasma cells are in the form of Russell bodies with intracytoplasmic IgM globules, which in HAT are then termed the 'morular cells of Mott'. In the white and grey matter, there may be widespread oedema, demyelination, and gliosis (Figs 29.37, 29.38). But neurone necrosis is uncommon and trypanosomes are virtually never seen in brain tissues. Chronic inflammation of the choroid plexus occurs.

About 10 per cent of patients treated with melarsoprol (see below) develop arsenical encephalopathy. Some die of epilepsy, and the brain shows anoxic changes in addition to the trypanosomal encephalitis. Others have an acute haemorrhagic encephalopathy, with fibrinoid necrosis of vessels, thrombi, and perivascular haemorrhages.

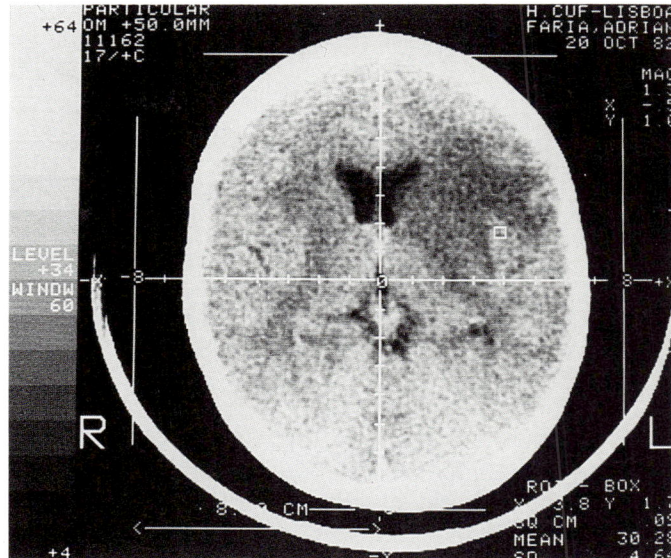

Fig. 29.36 CT scan of a child with African trypanosomiasis. There is irregular oedema, seen as more radiolucent zones. (Scan courtesy of Dr H. Ree.)

Pathogenesis

The successive waves of parasitaemia are due to antigenic variation at the parasite surface. As antibodies are produced, they eliminate the current clone, but successive new patterns of surface antigens are produced to evade this host response.

The high levels of immunoglobulin and immune complexes in the blood also result from the chronic polyclonal B-cell stimulation. A putative B-cell mitogen secreted by the parasite is now unlikely; deranged T/B-cell interactions are more important. The organ lesions are characterized by proliferating B-cells (and in the lymph nodes and spleen, reduced T-cell zones). This immune paralysis accounts for the terminal intercurrent

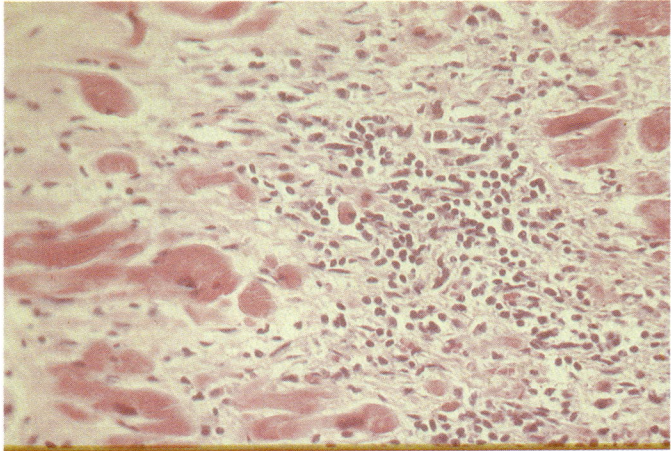

Fig. 29.35 Myocarditis in African trypanosomiasis. Degeneration of muscle fibres and chronic inflammation. (Photograph courtesy of Dr A. Poltera.)

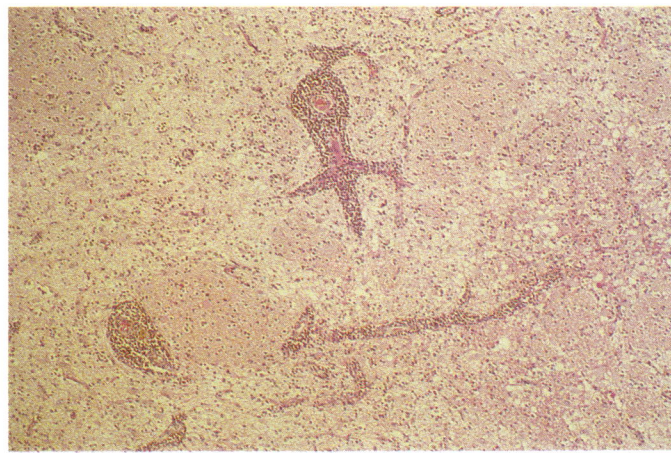

Fig. 29.37 African trypanosomal encephalitis. Perivascular inflammation and oedema.

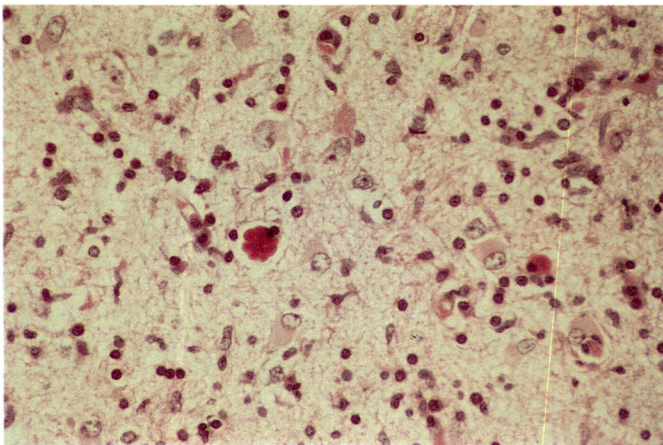

Fig. 29.38 African trypanosomal encephalitis. Gliosis, oedema, and Mott cells plasma cells with intracytoplasmic globules of immunoglobulin (Russel bodies).

infections. Antibody production may be relevant in the causation of anaemia, presumed nephritis, and the skin rash.

The mechanisms underlying heart and brain damage are still mysterious. Although trypanosomes enter the CSF, associated with a progressively leaky blood–brain barrier, they are not seen in the neuropil. The cerebral lesions are not classical Gell and Coombs' immunological reactions. There is no polymorph reaction to indicate activation of deposited immune complexes; there is no macrophage or granulomatous reaction. Despite the pathological meningoencephalitis, there is no direct neuronal damage. The current hypotheses depict interactions at the cerebral vasculature between trypanosomal antigens, B-cells, T-cells, and astrocytes. The latter control permeability of vessels via their end-feet, and can act as both antigen-presenting cells and secretors of cytokines (such as interleukin-1). The neurological disorders could follow from local production of cytokines affecting neurotransmitters and the structural integrity of brain cells.

Diagnosis and treatment

Finding trypanosomes in blood, lymph node aspirate, and CSF are the standard methods of diagnosis. The criteria that indicate cerebral invasion are:

1. trypanosomes in the CSF;
2. CSF white cell counts of > 5 per mm^3;
3. CSF protein > 25 mg%;
4. the presence in the CSF of IgM antibody.

The standard treatment for early infection (blood only) has been suramin, and that for cerebral involvement is the arsenical melarsoprol. Because the latter is toxic (see above), it is restricted to cases of definite or presumed cerebral involvement. Recently, difluoromethylornithine has been introduced as a successful non-toxic chemotherapy for all stages of HAT.

29.5.2 *Trypanosoma cruzi*

Symptomatic infection with *Trypanosoma cruzi* is also known as Chagas' disease (South American trypanosomiasis).

Epidemiology

The infection is endemic in 21 Central and South American countries (particularly Brazil), with 90 million people at risk and about 18 million people infected. Trypanosomiasis is predominantly a rural disease, the vectors living in the mud and thatch roofs of households and biting at night.

Life cycle and morphology

The vectors are reduviid bugs (kissing bugs). They take up parasites from man and other reservoir mammal hosts during a blood meal. After development within the bug intestine, the trypomastigote forms are deposited on the skin when the bug defaecates after feeding; and scratching the skin or eye completes the inoculation. Within the host, the parasite circulates in the blood as a 20 μm long trypomastigote (resembling *Trypanosoma brucei*), but on entering host cells it converts to the smaller non-flagellate amastigote form (resembling *Leishmania*), 2 μm in diameter. The amastigotes possess a kinetoplast rod of DNA. There are periodic episodes of parasitaemia as amastigotes leave tissues and reinvade the blood, but over time the intensity of blood infection declines markedly. In addition to vector-borne infection, many cases follow infection by blood transfusion.

Clinical features

Acute infection is predominantly in children. A week after infection, the site of infection becomes swollen (a chagoma) due to parasite multiplication and host inflammation, and the draining lymph nodes enlarge. If the conjunctiva is involved, there is conjunctivitis with palpebral oedema, known as Romaña's sign. Fever, mild hepatosplenomegaly, and a myocarditis of varying severity follow. Of those infected, 5–10 per cent die in the acute episode from heart failure. Encephalitis is also common, and transplacental infection occurs (Fig. 29.39).

The survivors enter the latent infective stage, which may last up to 30 years. Some 30–40 per cent then develop chronic Chagas' disease, which also happens to many who had no clinically evident acute infection. Predominantly, this affects the heart and the gastrointestinal tract. The heart enlarges, suffers from arrythmias, and is the site of thrombi which embolize to cause, for example, strokes. Death is from chronic congestive heart failure, or an acute fatal arrythmia. Segments of the gut, from oesophagus to rectum, dilate massively, producing the 'mega' syndromes that cause difficulty in swallowing (like achalasia), and constipation (like Hirschsprung's disease).

Pathology

In the acute infection, parasites disseminate haematogenously to all organs and parasitize many host cells, including endothe-

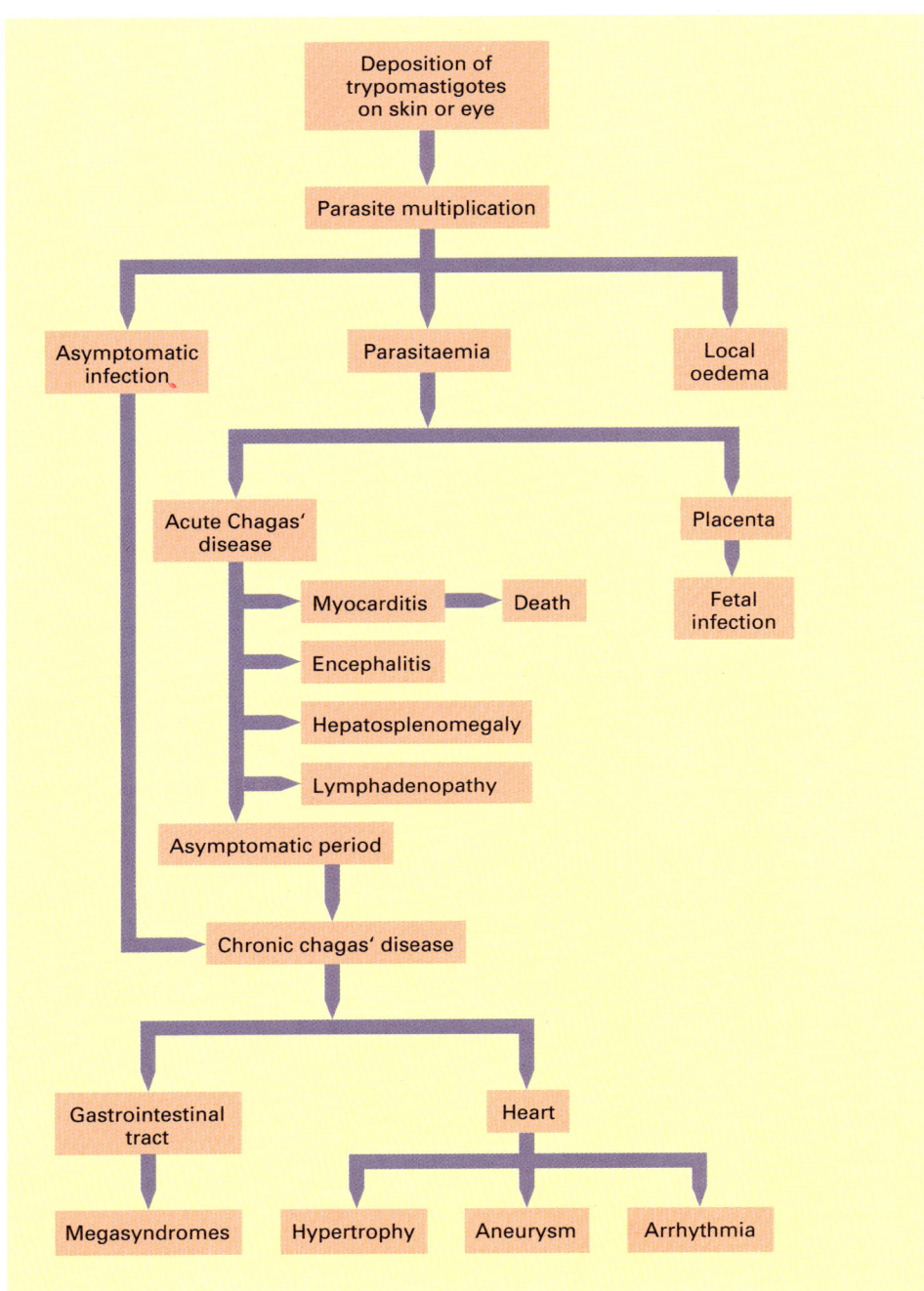

Fig. 29.39 Sequelae of infection with *Trypanosoma cruzi* (South American trypanosomiasis; Chagas' disease).

lial cells, cardiac fibres, cerebral and spinal neurones and glial cells, autonomic ganglia, macrophages, and placental stroma. The heart in fatal acute carditis is flabby and oedematous. Histologically, muscle fibres are degenerate or necrotic, separated by a massive infiltrate of mononuclear cells and fewer polymorphs or eosinophils. The fibres contain clusters of parasite amastigotes (Fig. 29.40). The brain shows meningoencephalitis with foci of lymphocytes and macrophages around parasitized neurones and astrocytes. Visceral autonomic ganglion cells contain parasites with surrounding lymphocytes.

Congenital Chagas' disease manifests as inflammatory foci of cells with amastigotes and necrosis in numerous organs, including the heart, brain, and gut. Similar lesions are also seen in the placenta.

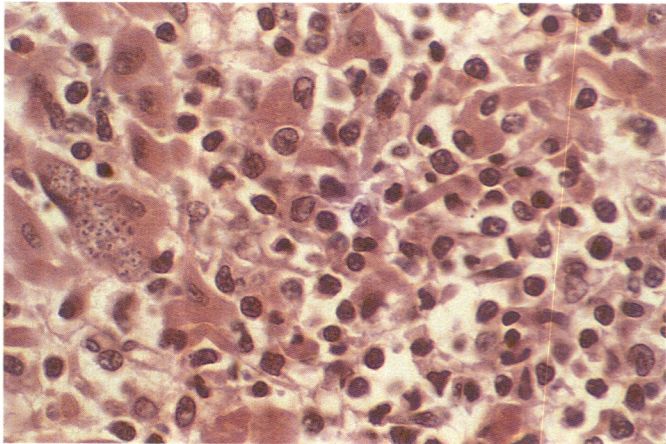

Fig. 29.40 Acute Chagasic myocarditis. Oedema, muscle fibre degeneration, and chronic inflammation. The fibre at top left contains *Trypanosoma cruzi* amastigotes.

Chronic Chagasic heart disease shows enlargement, due to biventricular hypertrophy and dilatation. The valves are not directly affected. Mural thrombi and left ventricle apical aneurysms are common (Fig. 29.41). Histologically, there is diffuse fibrosis, chronic inflammation, and residual myofibre hypertrophy. The apical aneurysms have thin fibrous walls. The condition system is fibrosed, and counts of atrial wall ganglion cells show reduced numbers. Parasites are found, with difficulty, in less than half of hearts at autopsy.

The intestinal segments affected are most commonly the oesophagus and colon (Fig. 29.42). They are thinned, with

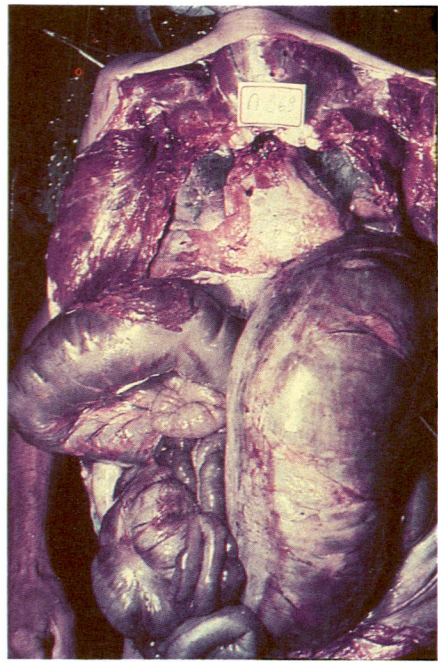

Fig. 29.42 Chronic Chagas' disease. Autopsy showing megacolon.

fibrosed walls and reduced or absent ganglion cells in the myenteric plexi. Parasites are very rarely identified in the gut wall at this stage.

Pathogenesis

In the acute illness, the necrosis in all organs is due partly to a direct toxic effect of the intracellular multiplying parasites (which escape from phagosomes and lie free in the cytoplasm) and partly to the florid host inflammatory reaction. Acute Chagas' disease thus has some resemblance to severe toxoplasmosis; and, in both infections, the parasites persist in small numbers in the tissues for life.

In chronic Chagas' disease, the intestinal dilatation is considered a consequence of myenteric ganglion cells' destruction by parasites, commencing during the acute phase and proceeding during the long latent period. However, the pathogenesis of the heart disease is the subject of much controversy. Classically, the damage to the parasympathetic nervous innervation of the heart is held to be primary, with the hypertrophy and dilatation due to chronic unopposed sympathetic action. Alternatively, there is a chronic parasite-driven myofibre necrosis; this could be a direct process, or it might involve cross-reacting humoral and cell-mediated immunological reactions, as there is evidence for common antigens between heart cells and *T. cruzi*. Physiological studies indicate that myocardial damage precedes the functional parasympathetic abnormalities, and the denervation could be a non-specific consequence of chronic myocarditis and ventricular dilatation. Finally, experimental models also suggest a role for platelet adherence to parasitized heart endothelial cells. Vascular spasm and occlusion in the acute phase, with

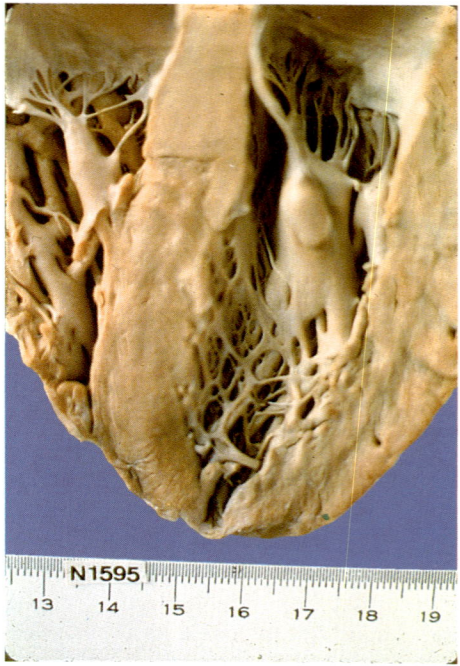

Fig. 29.41 Chronic Chagas' heart disease. Left ventricular hypertrophy and an apical aneurysm.

progressive intimal proliferation, could produce myocytolysis and fibrosis.

Diagnosis and treatment

In acute disease, blood smears show the trypomastigotes. In the latent and chronic disease, parasitaemia is low or apparently absent, and blood cultures or xenodiagnosis are used. In the latter, a previously uninfected reduviid bug feeds on the patient's skin, and its intestine is later examined for evidence of *T. cruzi* infection. Serodiagnostic tests remain positive after infection.

Treatment of trypanosomiasis is difficult. The trypanocidal drug, nifurtimox, is used in the acute stage but does not always prevent the development of chronic disease (the intracellular parasites being more resistant). Once chronic intestinal or car-diac signs have developed, anti-parasitic chemotherapy has no effect.

29.5.3   *Leishmania*

Infection with *Leishmania* produces a complex and wide range of clinico-pathological patterns of leishmaniasis (Fig. 29.43).

Epidemiology

Leishmania are widely distributed through tropical and temperate zones. Some 350 million people are at risk of infection, and about 12 million have the disease (6 million in the Middle East and Asia, 5 million in Central and South America, 1 million in Africa, and 10 000 in Mediterranean Europe).

Most *Leishmania* species are strictly zoonotic; the reservoirs

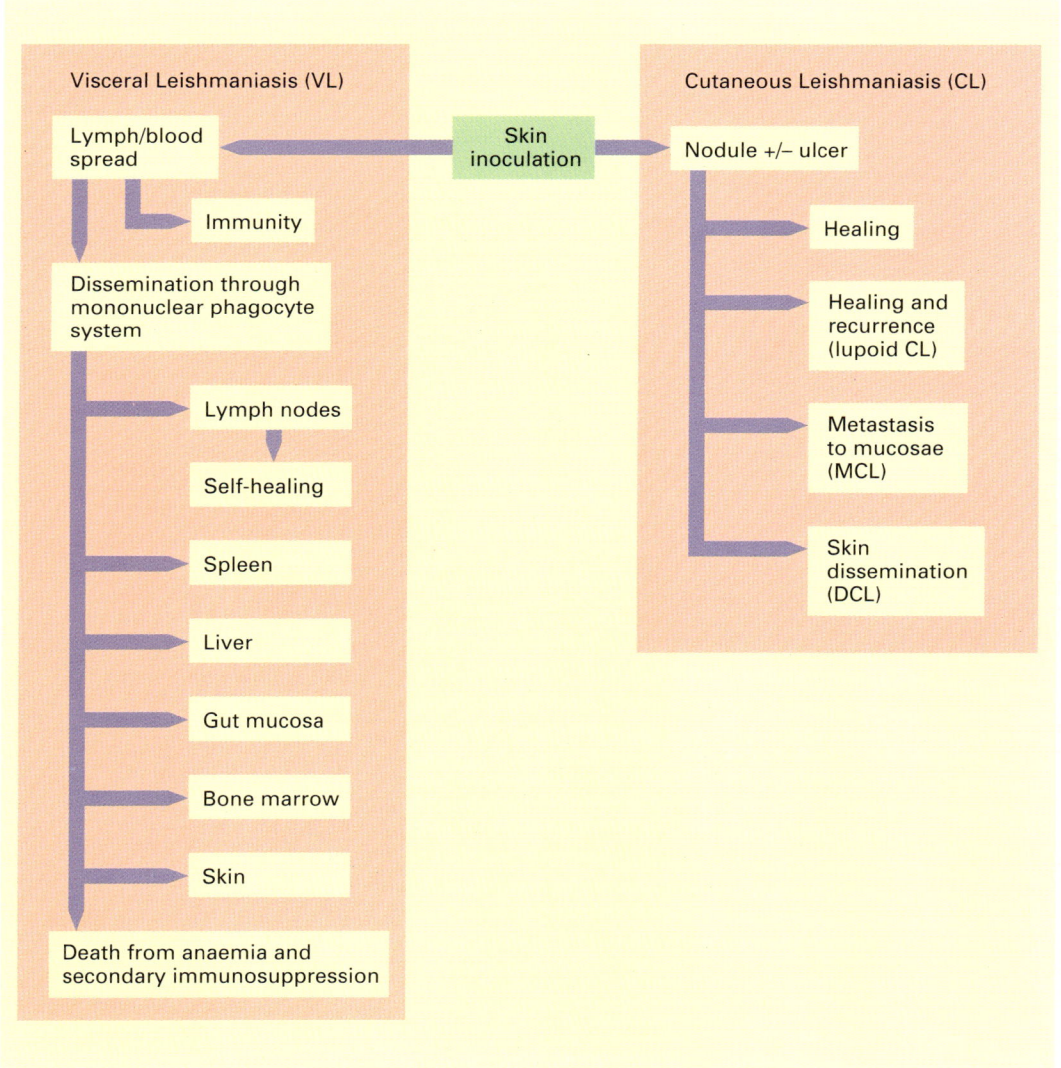

Fig. 29.43 Sequelae of infection with *Leishmania* species. MCL, mucocutaneous leishmaniasis; DCL, disseminated cutaneous leishmaniasis.

are canines or rodents, and the vectors are sandflies. Man is accidentally infected (Fig. 29.32). The speciation of *Leishmania* (which morphologically are similar) is highly complex, and utilizes DNA probes and isoenzyme analysis. The main groups, their geography and disease associations, are indicated in Table 29.1.

Table 29.1 The main species groups of *Leishmania*, their geography, and the clinical diseases they cause

Species	Geography	Disease
L. major	North and sub-Saharan Africa, Middle East, south USSR	ZCL
L. tropica	Mediterranean Basin east to Pakistan	ACL; rarely AVL
L. aethiopica	Ethiopia, Kenya	ZCL, DCL
L. donovani	East Africa, India, China	ZVL, PKDL; AVL in Asia
L. infantum	Mediterranean basin, S. America	ZVL, ZCL
L. mexicana	Central and South America	ZCL, DCL
L. brasiliensis	Central and South America	ZCL, MCL

ZCL, zoonotic cutaneous leishmaniasis; ACL, zoonotic cutaneous leishmaniasis; ACL, anthroponotic cutaneous leishmaniasis; DCL, diffuse cutaneous leishmaniasis; AVL, anthroponotic visceral leishmaniasis; ZVL, zoonotic visceral leishmaniasis; PKDL, post-kala-azar dermal leishmaniasis; MCL, mucocutaneous leishmaniasis.

Life cycle and morphology

After inoculation into man by sandflies, the leishmanias lose their flagella to become amastigotes. These are 2–4 μm in diameter, with a kinetoplast rod of DNA, and are known as Leishman–Donovan (LD) bodies (Fig. 29.44). They are obligate intracellular parasites, mainly of macrophages. Sandflies take up amastigotes from the skin during a blood meal (Fig. 29.32).

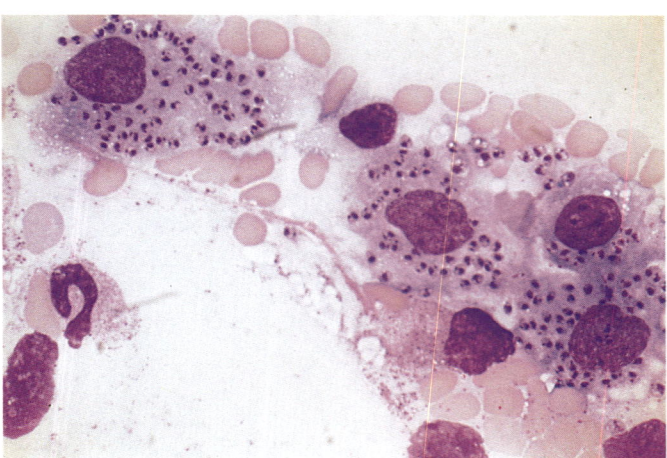

Fig. 29.44 Leishmaniasis. Aspirate from spleen in visceral leishmaniasis showing Leishman–Donovan (LD) bodies in macrophages. The small rod-shaped bodies next to the nuclei are the kinetoplast. (Giemsa strain.)

Clinical and pathological features

These depend on the species of *Leishmania* and on the host response. Classically, leishmaniasis is described as cutaneous (CL), visceral (VL; kala-azar), or mucocutaneous (MCL), with clear associations between parasite species and disease. Modern speciation techniques have revealed more complex patterns (Table 29.1). For example, similar zymodemes of *L. infantum* (a subgroup of *L. donovani*, the classical cause of VL) can cause both CL and VL. But from *in vitro* cultural characteristics, the dermatotropic parasites are genetically distinct from the viscerotropic strains.

Cutaneous leishmaniasis

The different dermatotropic *Leishmania* species produce characteristic lesions at the sites of sandfly bites, with varying numbers of lesions, incubation periods, tendencies to exude and ulcerate, rates of healing, and degrees of late scarring. In general, lesions develop over several months, usually ulcerate, and usually heal spontaneously over a year or more (Fig. 29.45). Chemotherapy accelerates the healing process and reduces subsequent scar-

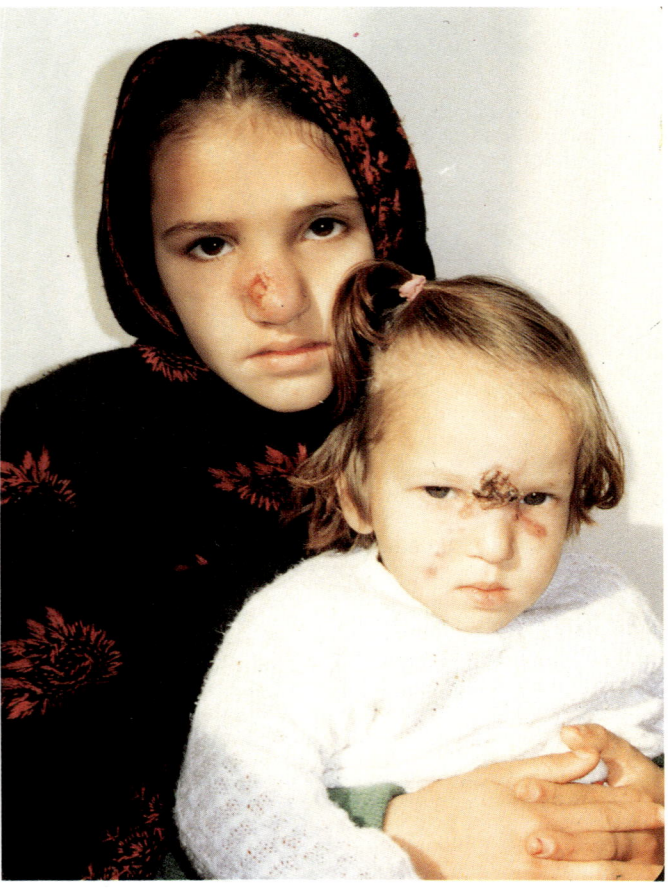

Fig. 29.45 Cutaneous leishmaniasis. Two sisters with multiple nodules and ulcers on the face. (Photograph courtesy of Sister A. Nestele.)

ring. After healing, there is immunity to infection from homologous species.

Skin biopsy in the early stages shows a diffuse macrophage infiltrate in the dermis, accompanied by plasma cells and some lymphocytes. The macrophages contain numerous LD bodies (Fig. 29.46). At this stage, delayed hypersensitivity skin tests to leishmanin antigen (the Montenegro test) are unreactive. Some cases heal without ulceration (e.g. with *L. aethiopica*): the infiltrate becomes granulomatous and the parasite load decreases. More commonly, there is focal or diffuse necrosis within the macrophage mass, associated with an influx of neutrophil polymorphs and of plasma cells. The overlying epithelium ulcerates and often shows a marked pseudo-epitheliomatous hyperplasia (but CL is not associated with the development of skin cancer). Epithelioid cell and giant cell granulomas form, often with central fibrinoid necrosis. The parasite density declines, and the skin heals with scarring. The differential diagnosis from mycobacterial and other granulomatous diseases of the skin may be impossible histologically (Fig. 29.47).

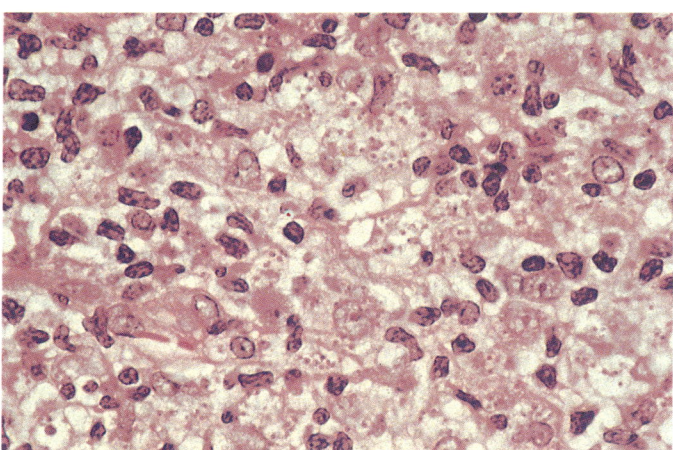

Fig. 29.46 Acute cutaneous leishmaniasis. Abundant LD bodies in dermal macrophages; no granuloma formation.

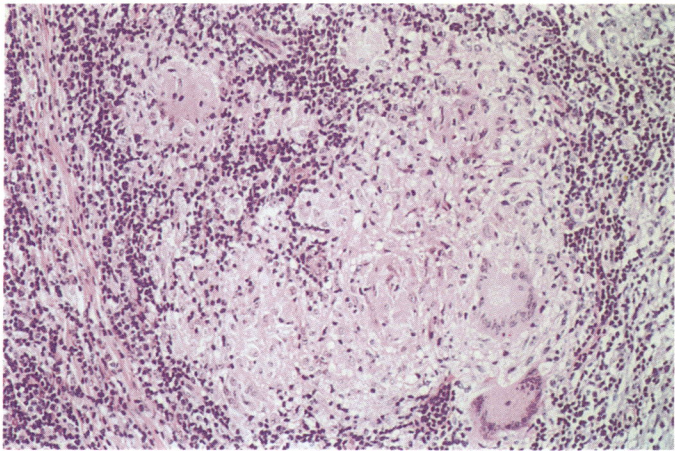

Fig. 29.47 Chronic cutaneous leishmaniasis. Tuberculoid granulomas and lymphoplasmacytic infiltration, but no LD bodies.

In some patients with *L. tropica* infection, the lesion may heal and then recrudesce at the same site with ulceration. This is called *lupoid (recidivans) leishmaniasis*. Histologically it is granulomatous, with many Langhans giant cells, and no LD bodies evident. Characteristically ther is no plasmacytic infiltrate. It heals with chemotherapy.

In most CL infections, there is a minor degree of dermatopathic lymphadenitis, which does not represent nodal infection. Ascending lymphatic spread of parasites ('sporotrichoid' spread) may occur. Lymph nodes then show granulomas and necrosis, with scanty LD bodies in macrophages. Such nodes may discharge through a sinus on to the skin, like scrofuloderma.

In a few individuals, infection with *L. aethiopica* and *L. mexicana* does not ulcerate or heal, but progressively spreads over the skin. It does not visceralize. This *diffuse cutaneous leishmaniasis* (DCL) has some resemblances to lepromatous leprosy (Fig. 29.48). Histopathologically, the epidermis is flattened, there is a clear subepidermal zone, and the dermis is filled with vacuolated macrophages that are heavily parasitized. Although unable to control *Leishmania*, patients with DCL are immunocompetent for other infections. Chemotherapy reduces the lesions, but relapse is usual.

Leishmaniasis is also an opportunistic infection, as the parasites can remain latent. Reactivation with skin lesions can occur up to four decades later if an immunosuppresssive state intervenes.

Mucocutaneous leishmaniasis ('espundia')

With *L. brasiliensis* infections, up to 40 per cent of people develop mucocutaneous leishmaniasis (MCL) after the initial skin

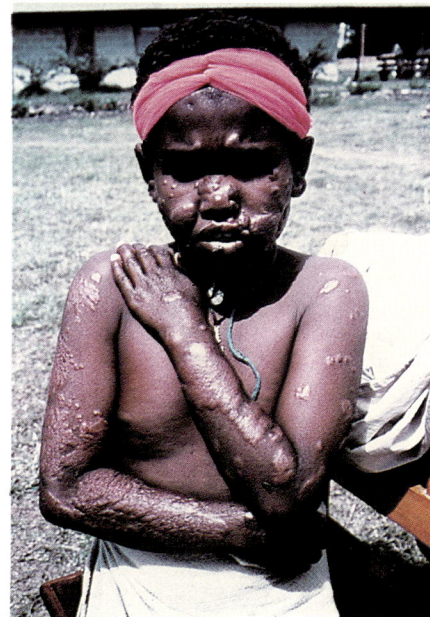

Fig. 29.48 Disseminated cutaneous leishmaniasis (DCL) in a child. Multiple non-ulcerating papules over the body. (Photograph courtesy of Dr A. Bryceson.)

lesion has healed. This presentation may be delayed for up to 10 years. At junctions of mucosa and skin—usually the nasopharyngeal area, but also the perineum—progressively destructive ulceration takes place (Fig. 29.49). Soft tissues, cartilage and bone are destroyed, and the ulceration extends down the pharynx to the larynx. Clinically it can resemble lymphoma. Spontaneous resolution does not occur and, even with therapy, death from bacterial infection of the respiratory tract is common. Histologically, there is ulceration and a mixed inflammatory reaction, with granulomas, acute inflammation, vasculitis, and much granulation tissue. LD bodies are usually scanty or undetectable.

Visceral leishmaniasis

In the classic VL disease there is no significant skin lesion, and after an incubation period of some months, patients develop fever, hepatosplenomegaly, and anaemia. Children are disproportionately affected (Fig. 29.50). Liver function tests are normal. The spleen may be massive (up to 4 kg in adults). The skin becomes darkened (hence the name 'kala-azar'). Untreated, the infection persists until death from a secondary bacterial infection, such as pneumonia or septicaemia. Leishmanin skin tests are negative. There are high blood antibody titres of both IgG and IgM, much of it non-specific, but including auto-antibodies.

Effective chemotherapy for VL reduces the parasite density (as recorded by splenic aspirates) 1000-fold over the first week, and to zero by 4 weeks.

In fatal cases, the spleen is congested and the liver is pale. Macrophages throughout the lymphoreticular system are hyperplastic, hypertrophied, and heavily parasitized by LD

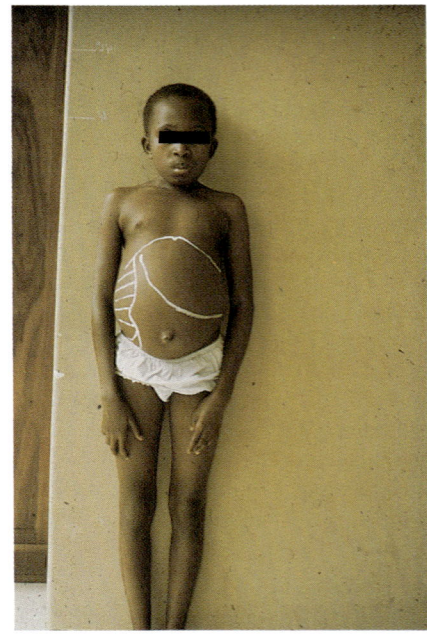

Fig. 29.50 Visceral leishmaniasis (kala-azar) in a child. Gross hepatosplenomegaly.

bodies. A plasma cell infiltrate accompanies. In the liver, the Kupffer cells contain numerous LD bodies, with portal tract plasmacytosis. The lymphoid follicles of the spleen are reduced, but the red pulp sinuses are packed with parasitized macrophages. Similarly, lymph nodes have a parasitized sinus histiocytosis. The small bowel lamina propria macrophages may also be parasitized, which may explain the mild malabsorption that can occur in VL. Bone marrow is hyperplastic and heavily parasitized (Fig. 29.51). LD bodies are found in circulating monocytes in half the patients, and in skin smears of many patients, although clinical skin lesions are rare.

Autopsied cases often show an interstitial pneumonitis with

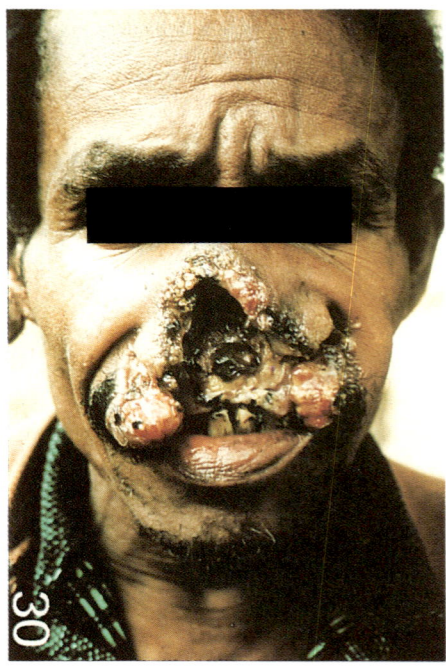

Fig. 29.49 Mucocutaneous leishmaniasis (MCL). Gross destruction of the upper lip and nose.

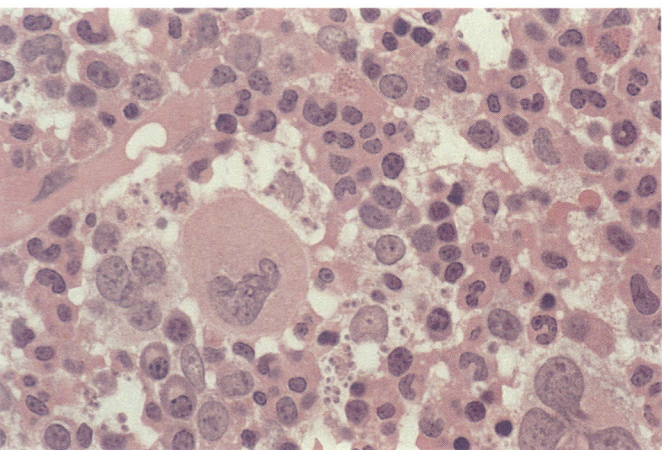

Fig. 29.51 Bone marrow in visceral leishmaniasis. Numerous LD bodies in macrophages, associated with plasmacytosis.

infiltrates of lymphocytes, plasma cells, and parasitized macrophages. In VL in South America, a form of diffuse intralobular hepatic fibrosis is described (rather similar to that seen in congenital syphilis). This results from chronic sinusoidal inflammation and is not a true cirrhosis.

This simple picture of VL has necessarily become modified by detailed epidemiological studies. Skin test surveys show that for each case of classical VL there are 10–30 cases of subclinical infection (Fig. 29.43). Many have complete immunity, with the infection being stopped at the skin inoculation site. Some infections have a localized dissemination to lymph nodes. Epithelioid cell granulomas in paracortex and germinal centres are seen (as in toxoplasmosis); necrosis is frequent, mimicking tuberculosis. The parasites are killed and further disease progression does not take place.

Another subset of infected people manifest a mild chronic non-specific malaise with slight hepatosplenomegaly. They have LD bodies on bone marrow aspirate and positive leishmanial serology. Liver biopsy shows a granulomatous reaction with fewer LD bodies compared with classic VL. If untreated, one-quarter go on to develop severe VL and the others resolve spontaneously.

After chemotherapy for VL, some patients develop a maculopapular skin rash or skin nodules. This occurs in 10 per cent of Indian patients, and <5 per cent of African patients, and is called *post-kala-azar dermal leishmaniasis* (PKDL). Leishmania skin tests are usually positive. Pathologically, the lesions range from dense lymphocytic infiltrates and tuberculoid granulomas with few parasites (typical of Asian cases; Fig. 29.52) to a diffuse, heavily parasitized macrophage infiltrate (typical of African cases). PKDL patients do not get a recurrence of VL.

HIV infection and leishmaniasis

Viscerotropic parasites may reside in the host for years without causing disease. Steroids may permit amastigote replication, producing VL with hepatosplenomegaly. In HIV-seropositive

people, *L. infantum* infection causes VL with parasitism of the spleen, liver, and marrow.

Not all such patients have splenomegaly, and not all have anti-leishmania antibodies. Some cases have been diagnosed by finding parasitized macrophages in the skin on biopsy for Kaposi's sarcoma lesions. Relapse after standard chemotherapy is common.

Pathogenesis

From these pathological descriptions, there is a form of immunopathological spectrum in leishmaniasis. Unactivated macrophages are unable to kill parasites (as in DCL and VL). In the more granulomatous pathological types, parasite densities are low or absent (e.g. in CL, recidivans CL, and self-healing VL). The healing of CL lesions is due, in part, to the activation of macrophages through cell-mediated immunity. Initially, parasites inside phagolysosomes resist attack. More activated macrophages kill *Leishmania* through oxygen radicals and tumour necrosis factor (TNF). In CL, the role of antibody in parasite elimination is uncertain. In VL, death follows from secondary immune paralysis: the macrophage functions of antigen presentation and phagocytosis are inhibited by the heavy *Leishmania* load.

Experimental models of leishmaniasis show that susceptibility to infection is inherited. Some mice resist *L. donovani* inoculation, whereas others develop visceral infection. Such host differences may be relevant to human infection, and explain why some develop DCL rather than healing CL lesions. The wide variations in response to *Leishmania* that can cause visceral disease may also have a basis in innate host cell-mediated responses. These interactions with specific parasite characteristics are being investigated intensively.

Diagnosis and treatment

Direct identification of the parasite is usual. With samples from CL skin lesions, the current diagnostic sensitivities are: immunocytochemical staining or DNA probe > *in vitro* culture > Giemsa staining of a smear > histological identification in a biopsy. The Montenegro skin test and serology are not reliable for individual cases, although useful epidemiologically.

For VL, needle aspiration of the spleen is highly sensitive (Fig. 29.44). Liver and bone marrow biopsy also contribute. Serology is useful epidemiologically. Pentavelent antimonials are the mainstay of therapy for all types of leishmaniasis. Pentostam is the standard compound.

29.5.4 Further reading

Poltera, A. A. (1985). Pathology of human African trypanosomiasis. *British Medical Bulletin* 41, 169–74.

Ridley, D. S. (1988). *Pathogenesis of leprosy and related diseases*. Wright, London.

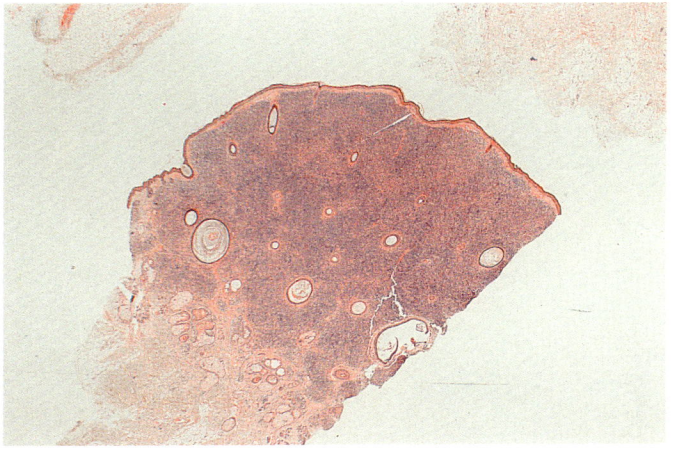

Fig. 29.52 Skin biopsy of post-kala-azar dermal leishmaniasis (PKDL). Flat epidermis and dense lymphoplasmacytic infiltration (mimicking lymphoma).

29.6   *Pneumocystis carinii*

This organism is the cause of *Pneumocystis carini* pneumonia (PCP; pneumocystosis).

Epidemiology

The infection is global. In developed and developing countries, serological studies show that more than 70 per cent of children have been infected by the age of 8 years. However, the clinical disease shows marked variations in prevalence, since only immunocompromised people develop the disease (Fig. 29.53). The states that induce susceptibility to PCP include congenital and acquired diseases:

1. primary immune deficiencies—humoral, cell-mediated, and combined forms;
2. secondary immune deficiencies—prematurity and malnutrition; cancer (especially lymphoma and lymphocytic leukaemia); cytotoxic chemotherapy for organ transplantation, cancer, and connective tissue diseases; HIV infection.

Life cycle and morphology

The taxonomic position of *Pneumocystis* is uncertain. Until recently it has been classified as a protozoan. Ultrastructural evidence and analysis of ribosomal RNA suggest that it is a fungus. However, its biochemical characteristics are unlike those of fungi. A case may be made for placing it as a new class of organism.

Pneumocystis affects both man and lower mammals, such as

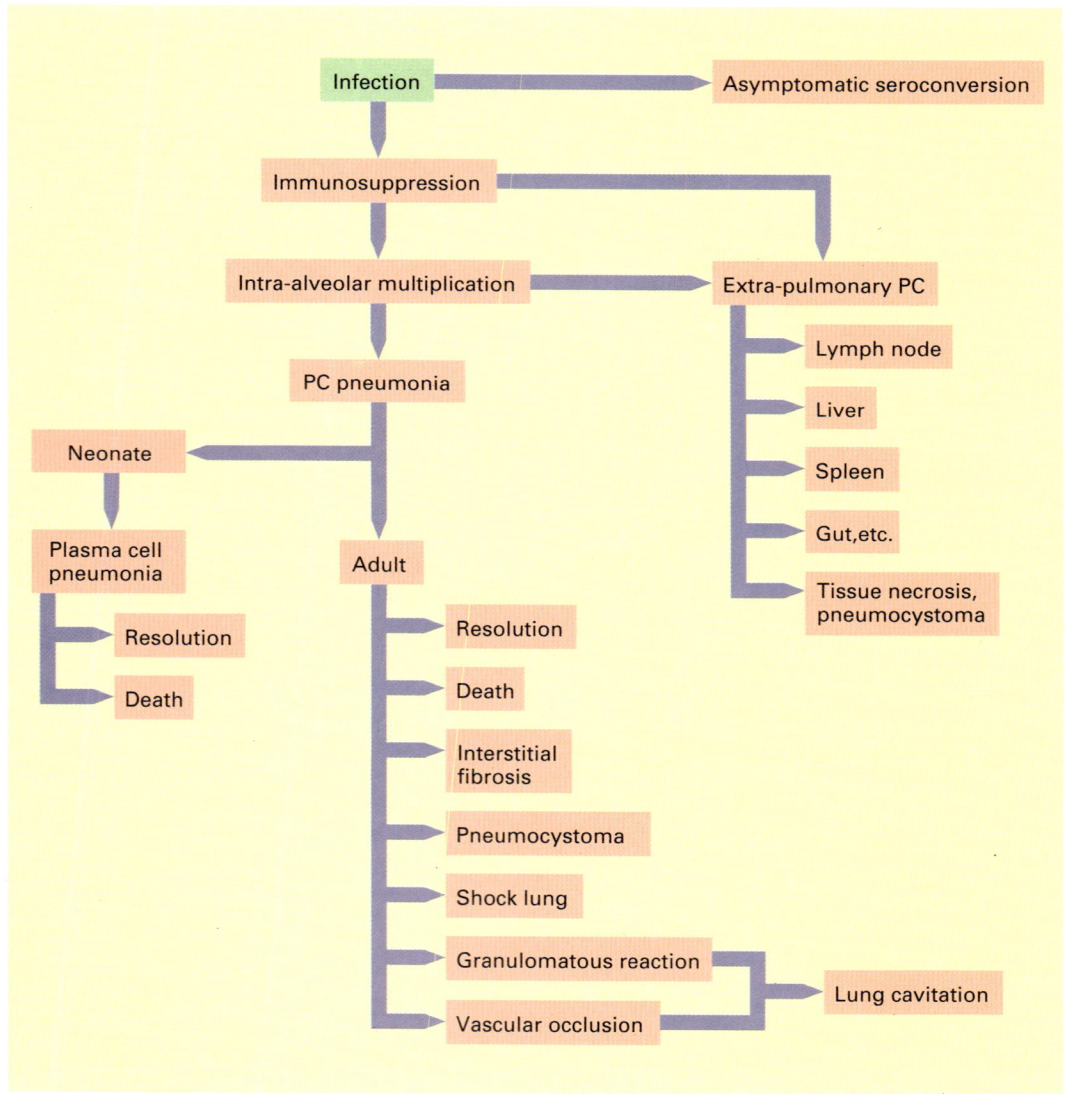

Fig. 29.53 Sequelae of infection with *Pneumocystis carinii* (PC).

rats. The mode of transmission is presumed to be by inhalation. The organism must be ubiquitous in air or soil but its state outside the hosts is unknown. Outbreaks of PCP within hospital units of immunocompromised patients show that nosocomial transmission also occurs. The cysts are 4–6 μm diameter, circular or distorted in shape. The trophozoites within are seen as tiny dots.

Clinical features

PCP has two basic forms, that in malnourished infants ('epidemic' PCP) and that in immunocompromised older children and adults ('sporadic' PCP). The infantile form of PCP occurs in premature and marasmic children aged 10–24 weeks. The progression of cyanosis, cough, and dyspnoea is rapid; death within 24–48 hours is common. Without treatment, mortality is nearly 100 per cent, but survivors recover completely.

In adults the disease has a more insidious course. Breathlessness and cough develop over weeks. Without treatment, mortality is 100 per cent. Therapy reduces the first episode mortality to 25 per cent. Recent advances in chemotherapy and prophylaxis delay the first presentation of PCP during the course of HIV-related immunosuppression but (in developed countries) approximately 80 per cent of HIV seropositives will have PCP at some time, and many will die of it. Pneumothorax is a common sequel to PCP.

Pneumocystis can infiltrate organs outside the lungs. This phenomenon is increasingly seen in HIV-seropositive people (in up to 10 per cent of autopsied cases), especially those inhaling pentamidine chemotherapy into the lungs. Although extrapulmonary pneumocystosis (EPPC) infection usually occurs in association with present or past lung infection, EPPC may sometimes be the first presentation.

The commonest location of EPPC is in hilar lymph nodes. Infiltration of abdominal and inguinal nodes, liver, spleen, bone marrow, gut wall, kidney, adrenals, thyroid, heart muscle, choroid of the eye, Virchow–Robin space of the brain, skin dermis, and peripheral arteries have all been observed. Symptoms depend on the site and extent of infiltration: gut perforation and peritonitis, goitre and hypothyroidism, skin nodules, digital gangrene, and visual deficit are examples.

Pathology

The classical appearance of infantile PCP at autopsy is of multilobar red consolidation (red hepatization). In adults, acute fatal PCP is a paler consolidation; the combined weight of the lungs can exceed 2.5 kg (Fig. 29.54).

Infantile PCP is also known as interstitial plasma cell pneumonia. The alveoli are filled with eosinophilic exudate, including clusters of organisms. *Pneumocystis* does not invade host cells. The alveolar walls are greatly thickened by an infiltrate of plasma cells and lymphocytes (Fig. 29.55, 29.56). Resolution occurs by phagocytosis of PC organisms by alveolar macrophages.

In immunosuppressed adults, the degree of interstitial inflammation is less than in infants. Following successful therapy, the

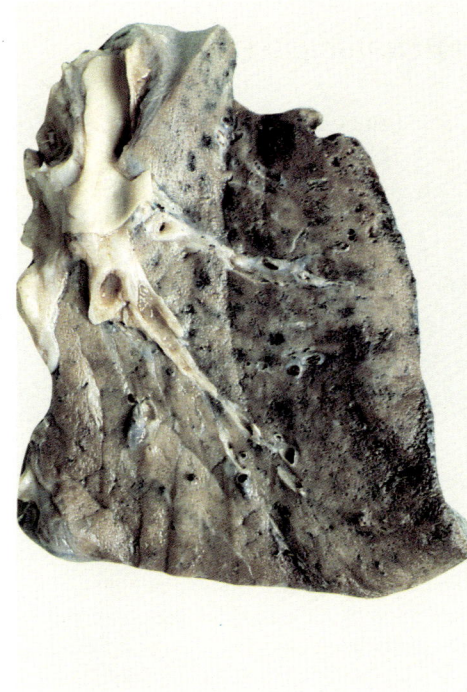

Fig. 29.54 *Pneumocystis carinii* pneumonia in an adult with T-cell lymphoma. The consolidation is pale; in neonates the lung is more red.

lung may return to normal. Pathological complications include diffuse fibrosis and shock lung (adult hyaline membrane disease). Parasites also invade and occlude pulmonary vessels. There may be cavities of 2–3 cm diameter, resembling tuberculosis. A granulomatous reaction to *Pneumocystis* may be found in such cases. Cavities underneath the pleura present as emphysematous bullae. Less frequently, PCP is multinodular, resembling metastatic deposits with eosinophilic exudate infiltrating and destroying alveoli. A bronchiectatic pattern is

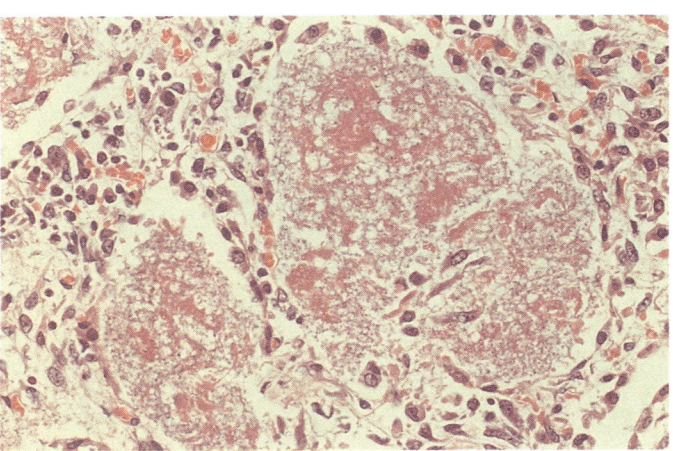

Fig. 29.55 *Pneumocystis* pneumonia in a neonate. In the alveoli, eosinophilic exudate, pale cysts, and small dots (trophozoites); in the interstitium, lymphocytes and plasma cells.

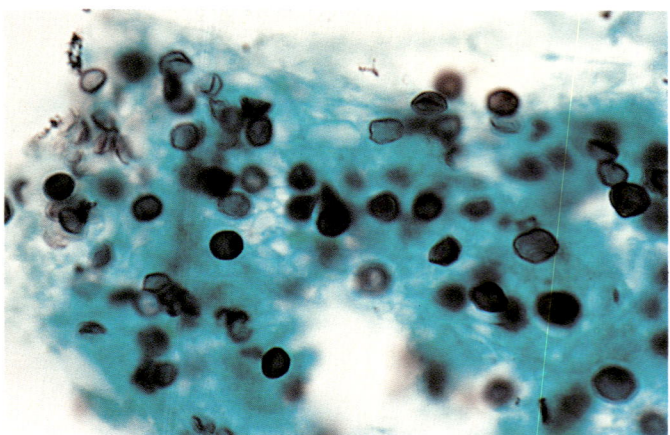

Fig. 29.56 *Pneumcystis* pneumonia. Smear of broncho-alveolar lavage, showing cysts. (Silver stain.)

seen where there is bronchial destruction. In long-standing infection, dystrophic calcification is frequent.

Extrapulmonary PC infection appears as yellow granular masses, often gritty from calcification, replacing the host tissue. Histologically, it infiltrates tissue similarly to a tumour (Fig. 29.57) and obstructs arteries.

Pathogenesis

It is likely that the organism is continually inhaled and that disease follows multiplication of *Pneumocystis* in the lungs, released from the normal (but unknown) control processes. In infantile PCP, defective macrophage function and low IgG production are considered important (the alveolar plasmacytic infiltrate secretes IgM). Adult PCP is nearly always related to defective cell-mediated immunity. In HIV-positive people, PCP is uncommon until the peripheral blood count of CD4 (T-helper) lymphocytes drops from the normal 1000 per mm³ to below 200 per mm³.

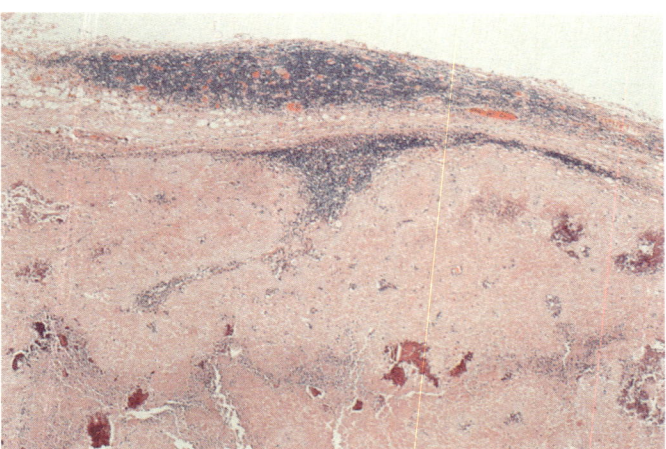

Fig. 29.57 Extrapulmonary pneumocystosis. Hilar lymph node infiltrated by eosinophilic deposits of *Pneumocystis*.

The destructive lung disease found in AIDS patients may result both from granulomatous inflammation (with macrophage enzymes dissolving alveolar walls), and from ischaemia. The latter follows widespread occlusion of pulmonary vessels.

Pneumocystis evidently visceralizes to all parts of the body by bloodstream dissemination. That it does not normally proliferate outside the lung is shown by the rarity of extrapulmonary disease until large numbers of HIV-positive patients were given inhalation chemotherapy (nebulized pentamidine) for treatment and prophylaxis of PCP. This inhibits proliferation in the lung but does not give systemically effective drug concentrations.

Diagnosis and treatment

Examination of smears prepared from broncho-alveolar lavage is the method for diagnosing PCP. Transbronchial biopsy is also used but carries the risk of pneumothorax. Therapy includes systemic trimethoprim-sulphamethoxazole and inhaled pentamidine.

29.6.1　Further reading

Santa Cruz, D. J. (ed.) (1989). *Pneumocystis carinii* infection. *Seminars in Diagnostic Pathology* **6** (3). Saunders, Philadelphia.

29.7　Coccidian protozoa

The class Coccidea includes four genera that are widely distributed among animals and man: *Toxoplasma*, *Sarcocystis*, *Cryptosporidium*, and *Isospora*. Their reproductive cycles include asexual and sexual phases in host enterocytes (Fig. 29.58). *Toxoplasma*, *Cryptosporidium*, and *Isospora* depend on cell-mediated immunity for control of infection, and have thus assumed great clinical importance because of the HIV epidemic.

29.7.1　*Toxoplasma gondii*

Toxoplasmosis is characterized by a high infectivity but low symptomatology. Neonates and immunocompromised adults are the most severely affected groups (Fig. 29.59).

Epidemiology

The proportions of peoples infected by *T. gondii* are estimated by serology. Prevalence increases with age. There are wide variations globally, depending on the intensity of exposure to domestic cats, social habits of eating raw or undercooked meat, and on climate (dry soils favour low prevalence). The highest seroprevalence is in Paris, France, where 90 per cent of people are infected. In the USA and UK, about 50 per cent of adults are infected. In Africa, the rates vary from 5 to 60 per cent in adults.

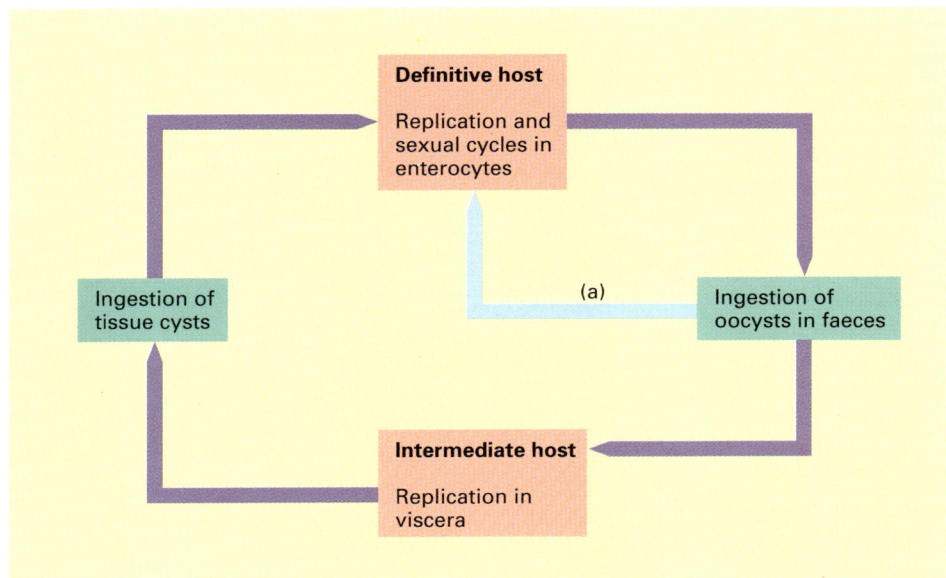

Fig. 29.58 Life cycles of coccidian parasites. *Toxoplasma gondii* and *Sarcocystis* follow the full cycle. *Cryptosporidium* and *Isospora* have no intermediate hosts and follow cycle (a).

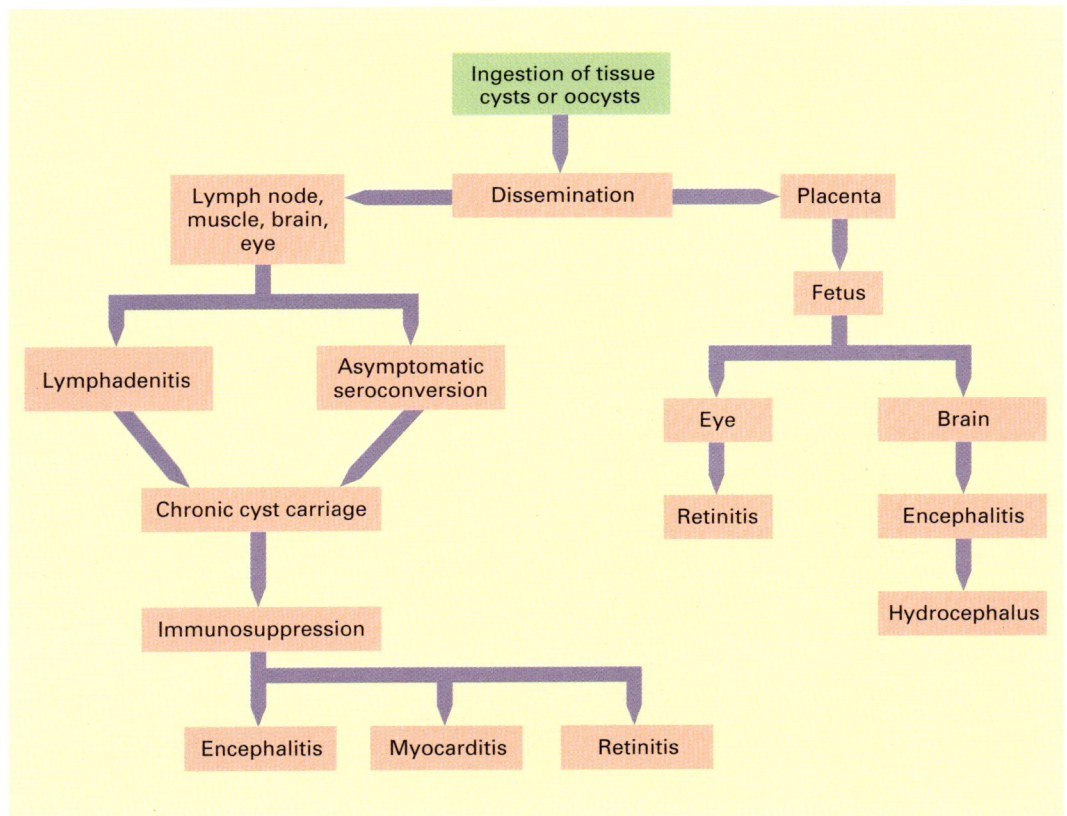

Fig. 29.59 Sequelae of infection with *Toxoplasma gondii*.

Life cycle and morphology

The definitive host is the cat, in whose intestine sexual reproduction occurs with excretion of oocysts in the faeces. Mammals and birds are intermediate hosts. After ingestion of oocysts, parasites disseminate through the body to infect a wide range of cells: macrophages, neurones, muscle, and placenta (Fig. 29.59; similar to *Trypanosoma cruzi*). Multiplication forms zoites which cluster together as intracellular bradycysts (the more latent form), or free tachyzoites which signify active infection and pathology. The cat eats infected tissues to continue the cycle. Man is infected by ingesting oocysts from domestic cats, or by eating undercooked meat containing tissue bradycysts. Occasionally transmission is via a transplanted heart with latent infection. Once infected, *Toxoplasma* remains in the body for life; brain neurones and muscle cells are common sites of latent infection. Tachyzoites are 2–4 μm in diameter and do not possess a kinetoplast. The bradycysts are about 30 μm across (Fig. 29.61).

Clinical features and pathology

Acquired toxoplasmosis

Primary infection in adolescence and adulthood is usually asymptomatic, but a febrile illness with cervical lymphadenopathy may occur. Histologically, the lymph nodes show follicular and paracortical hyperplasia. The characteristic feature is multiple small, non-necrotic epithelioid cell granulomas, both within and without the follicle germinal centres (Fig. 29.60). Parasites are very rarely identified in nodes.

More common is toxoplasmosis in immunosuppressed people. Conditions such as lymphoma, cancer chemotherapy, transplantation, and HIV infection permit reactivation of latent infection (Fig. 29.61). About 30 per cent of HIV-infected people who are seropositive for *T. gondii* will develop cerebral toxoplasmosis.

Cerebral lesions present with headache, focal neurological signs, and coma. Despite modern imaging methods, distinction

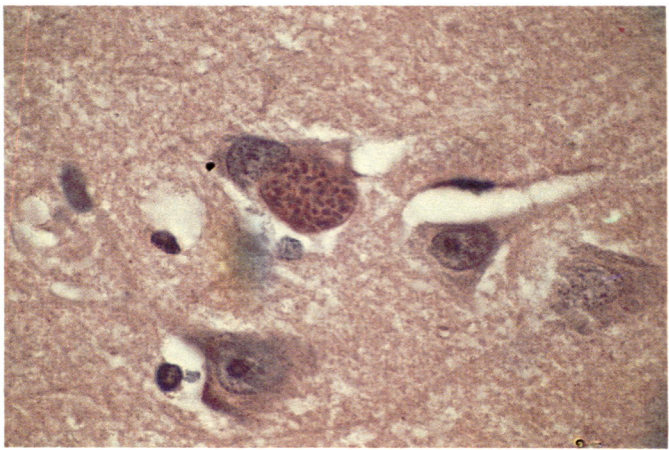

Fig. 29.61 *Toxoplasma* bradycyst in brain, neurone containing numerous zoites.

from cerebral lymphoma is often impossible without biopsy. Ophthalmitis and myocarditis are frequent in toxoplasmosis in immunosuppressed patients. Other organs involved include the intestine (focal myositis), lung (focal or lobar pneumonic changes), and skin (producing a papular rash).

Grossly, cerebral toxoplasmosis usually shows swelling with multiple necrotic and haemorrhagic foci in white and grey matter throughout the brain (Fig. 29.62). Sometimes, despite widespread infection on histology, the brain appears normal. The necrotizing abscess has haemorrhage, polymorphs, and mononuclear cells. Tachyzoites are extracellular, and encysted bradyzoites are seen in neurones (Fig. 29.63). Arteries have panmural inflammation with or without necrosis, endothelial parasitization and hyperplasia; the lumina are greatly narrowed (Fig. 29.64). Another pattern is central coagulative necrosis with surrounding macrophages and few parasites. This may become cystic. Such changes are common after chemo-

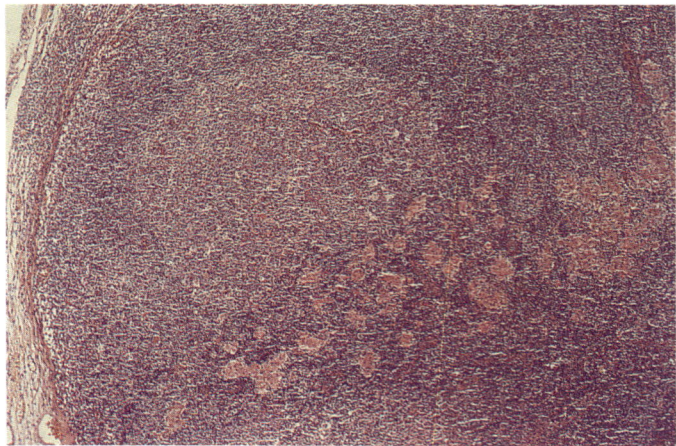

Fig. 29.60 Toxoplasmosis. Lymph node with hyperplastic follicles and small, pink-staining epithelioid cell granulomas.

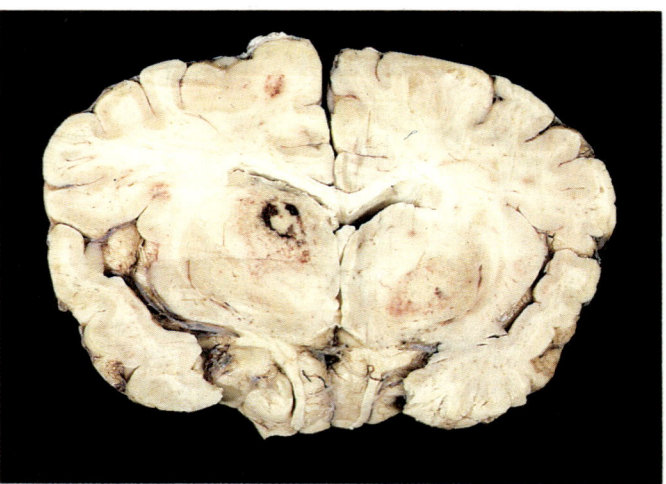

Fig. 29.62 *Toxoplasma* encephalitis. Multiple foci of haemorrhagic necrosis, and cerebral swelling.

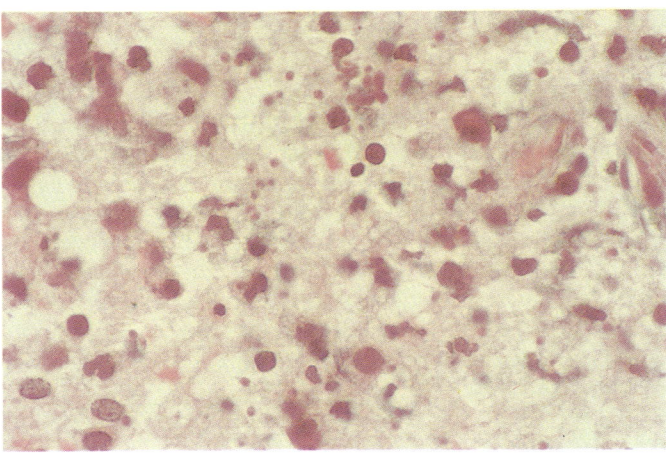

Fig. 29.63 *Toxoplasma* encephalitis. Inflammation, oedema, and numerous small unicellular tachyzoites.

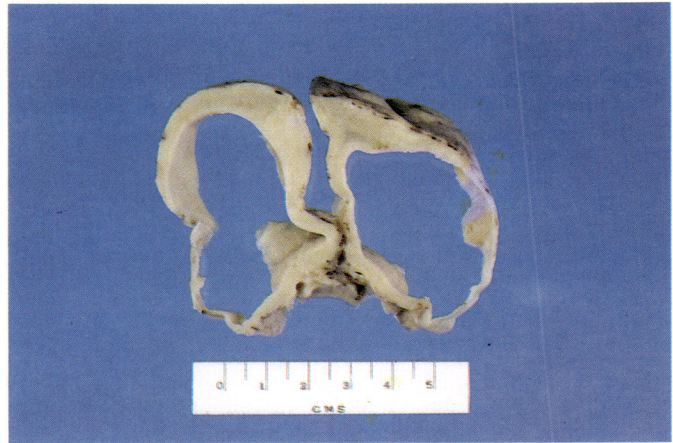

Fig. 29.65 Congenital *Toxoplasma* infection. Gross ventricular dilation following earlier necrotizing encephalitis. (Photograph courtesy of the late Dr F. MacDonald and Professor M. S. R. Hutt.)

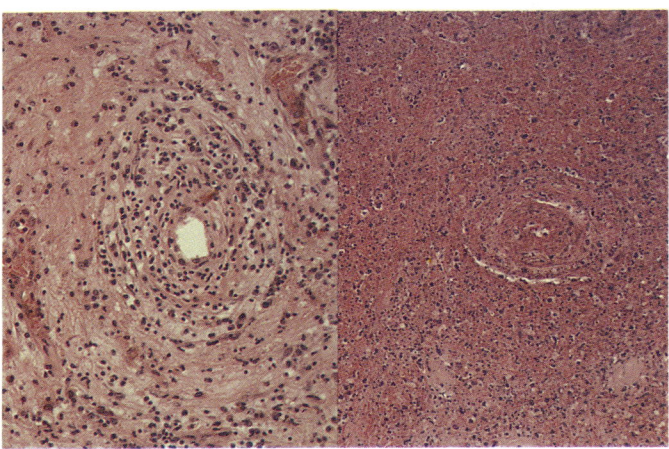

Fig. 29.64 *Toxoplasma* encephalitis. Vasculitis and severe narrowing of the lumen; in the left picture, the surrounding brain is necrotic (infarcted).

therapy, and parasites may be identified only with immunocytochemical staining for antigen.

Toxoplasma myocarditis is grossly normal, or pale and flabby. Histologically, myofibres contain parasites and there are foci of inflammation around degenerate fibres. Toxoplasma lung infection is an interstitial pneumonia with alveolar exudate, parasites, and often multiple foci of necrosis.

Ophthalmic disease is a single or multifocal choroidoretinitis. In immunosuppressed patients there is retinal necrosis and haemorrhage associated with tachyzoites. Immunocompetent people also develop eye disease, but the reaction is more granulomatous.

Congenital toxoplasmosis

The tetrad of choroidoretinitis, hydrocephalus, epilepsy, and intracranial calcification typifies severe congenital infection.

Milder forms can become evident in later childhood. Ophthalmitis is also frequent.

Autopsied children show an encephalitis that is particularly severe in the periventricular zones, and hydrocephalus (Fig. 29.65). The necrosis is histologically similar to that seen in immunocompromised adults, and there is dystrophic calcification. The placenta in congenital infection has a chronic villitis with foci of necrosis, calcification, and scanty parasites.

Pathogenesis

The host is unable to eliminate *T. gondii* infection. In macrophages, the parasites are in a phagosome but resist fusion with a lysosome, so inhibiting killing. The fetus and immunocompromised patients both lack intact cell-mediated immunity (CMI). Control of parasite proliferation is T-cell-mediated, so latent bradycysts release zoites which multiply and induce lesions. The necrosis of toxoplasmosis results from direct cytotoxicity of the parasite, antigen–antibody reactions, and from cell-mediated immunopathology. In those with some CMI, disintegrating cysts induce death of surrounding cells via the secretion of macrophage products. In the granulomatous ophthalmitis, sensitization to retinal antigens (sympathetic ophthalmitis) also plays a role. In immunosuppressed patients, some of the cerebral necrosis is infarction, due to the vasculitis and subsequent ischaemia.

The periaqueductal and periventricular necrosis of congenital cerebral toxoplasmosis has a unique pathogenesis. Parasitized ependymal cells leak antigen into the CSF and antibody diffuses into subependymal tissues. Through a type III hypersensitivity reaction, vasculitis occurs, obstructs the aqueduct of Sylvius, and results in hydrocephalus. Dystrophic calcification follows the necrosis.

Diagnosis and treatment

The parasites may be identified on tissue biopsy or cytology. If these are negative, tissue inoculation into mice (which are highly susceptible) is a bioassay. Serology for *T. gondii* infection is complex. IgG antibodies denote latent or active infection; IgM titres indicate active infection. Chemotherapy is with pyrimethamine and sulphonamides.

29.7.2   Sarcocystis

Two distinct conditions result from infection by *Sarcocystis* (Fig. 29.58).

Intestinal sarcocystosis

Man is a definitive host for *S. hominis* and *S. suihominis* as an enteric infection. The intermediate hosts are cattle and pigs, respectively; their muscle contains encysted merozoites. Such veterinary infection is global but symptomatic disease in man is rare. Transmission is from eating infected meat.

Clinically there is vomiting, diarrhoea, and abdominal pain. The few resected specimens show ileitis with focally ulcerated villi and an eosinophil reaction. Lamina propria cells under the epithelium are infected with zoites similar in morphology to *Isospora*.

Muscle sarcocystosis (sarcosporidiosis)

More common than the intestinal infection is an asymptomatic infection of skeletal and heart muscle. Here, man is the intermediate host, infected by oocysts. The parasite is group-named *S. lindemanni*, although there are morphologically several subspecies. The cysts are within muscle cells, and may be over 1 mm long. They contain thousands of small zoites, and excite no inflammatory reaction (Fig. 29.66). Cysts are detected as incidental findings at autopsy or in a biopsy containing muscle.

29.7.3   Cryptosporidium

There are numerous *Cryptosporidium* species affecting the gut and respiratory tract of mammals (particularly calves) and birds. *C. parvum* is the cause of human illness—cryptosporidiosis.

Epidemiology

Undescribed in man until 20 years ago, *Cryptosporidium* is a cause of diarrhoea globally. Up to 14 per cent of episodes of childhood diarrhoea are associated with *Cryptosporidium* oocysts in the stools. Cattle workers are frequently infected from contact with calf faeces. In the USA and Europe, about 10 per cent of HIV-positive patients with diarrhoea have cryptosporidiosis. In Africa, the proportion is often nearer 50 per cent. Other predisposing host defects are hypogammaglobulinaemia and low IgA states.

Life cycle and morphology

The oocyst is ingested from water, invades gut enterocytes, and undergoes cycles of merogony; merozoites invade adjacent cells. Oocysts are passed in the faeces. The organism occupies an intracellular but extracytoplasmic location. It is seen as 1–4 μm haemotoxyphilic dots (Fig. 29.67). A thin membrane from the brush border covers the parasite (Fig. 29.68).

Clinical features

In the immunocompetent, the watery diarrhoea is self-limiting and infection ceases, with subsequent immunity. The incubation period is 1 week, and the duration of diarrhoea about 2 weeks. In HIV-seropositive patients, the infection continues indefinitely with persistent diarrhoea, sometimes producing up to 17 litres of faeces daily. It is associated with profound wasting (a cause of the HIV-associated 'slim' syndrome), and is a major cause of death in AIDS. A second clinical form of cryptosporidiosis is cholangitis, with high alkaline phosphatase enzyme levels. Bronchiolitis and pneumonitis are occasionally associated with cryptosporidial lung infection in HIV-seropositive people.

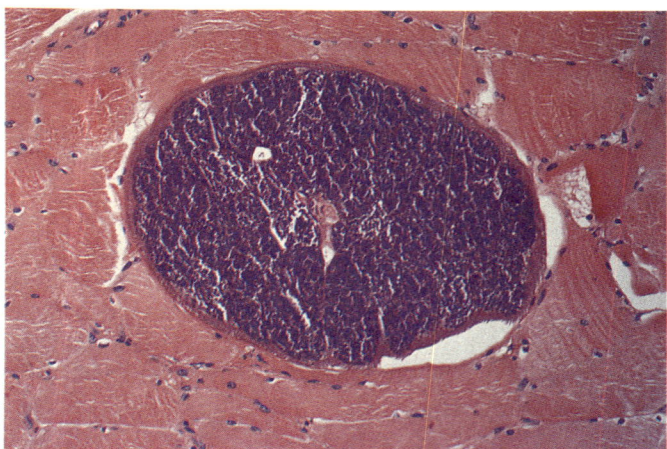

Fig. 29.66 Sarcocystosis. The cyst in the skeletal muscle contains numerous zoites, and is exciting no inflammatory reaction.

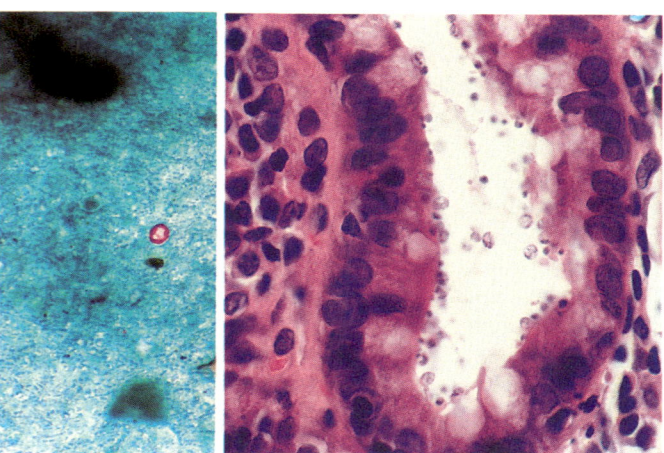

Fig. 29.67 *Cryptosporidium* enteritis. Left picture: faecal smear with an oocyst (Ziehl–Neelsen stain). Right picture: duodenal crypt with numerous parasites near the surface of enterocytes.

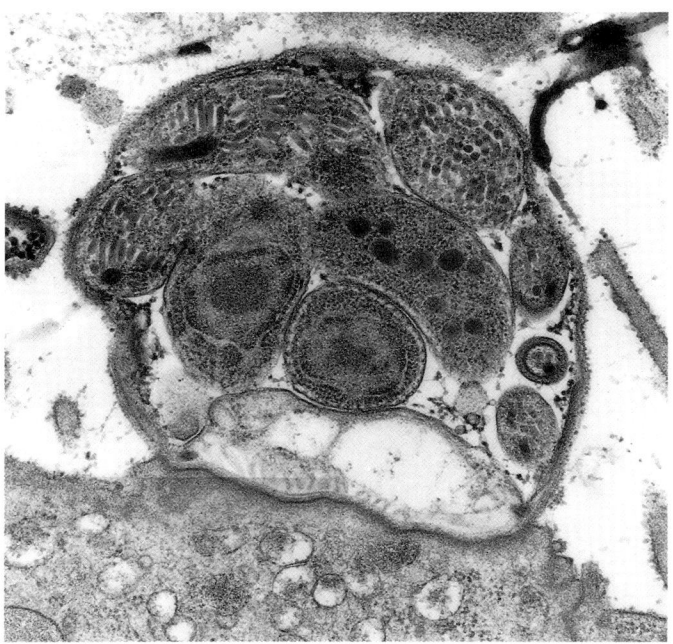

Fig. 29.68 *Cryptosporidium* in an enterocyte. Electron micrograph of a meront containing numerous merozoites. The whole structure is extracytoplasmic but still intracellular, being covered by a thin rim of host cell membrane. (Photograph courtesy of Dr A. Curry.)

Pathology

Although most often found in the small and large bowel, *Cryptosporidium* can parasitize oesophagus, trachea and bronchi, and the biliary tree. The bowel appears enteritic; the mucosa is oedematous, but not ulcerated in the absence of other pathogens. Histologically, the small bowel mucosa ranges from virtually normal to partial villous atrophy, with plasmacytic infiltrate of the lamina propria and a variable increase in intra-epithelial lymphocytes. Often, in HIV-seropositive people the pathology is complicated by co-infection with cytomegalovirus. In colorectal infection, focal crypt abscesses and hyperplasia are common.

The cholangitis affects the whole biliary tree, from common bile-duct and gall-bladder to large intrahepatic ducts. Chronic inflammation is usual and fibrosis (sclerosing cholangitis) may develop. Where there is ulceration of the mucosa, it is due to co-infection with cytomegalovirus. The parasite are located at the surface of the biliary epithelium.

Pathogenesis

This is obscure. The host inflammatory response is variable. For the watery diarrhoea, it is possible that a cholera-like toxin is secreted by the parasites in the small bowel. Intact humoral and cell-mediated immunity are required to eliminate the infection, but the mechanisms are unknown.

Diagnosis and treatment

Most cases of gut infection are identified by finding oocysts in the faeces. Ziehl–Neelsen methods stain the cysts red (Fig. 29.67). Immunocytochemical methods can also be used. Biopsy is required to identify the site of bowel infection, and the presence of biliary or lung infection. No specific therapy is available for the persistent infections in immunocompromised patients.

29.7.4 *Isospora*

Before the HIV epidemic *Isospora belli* was a rare cause of enteritis, but isosporiasis (sometimes referred to as 'human coccidiosis') is now increasingly common.

Epidemiology

Most infections are acquired in the tropics or subtropics; it is much less common in temperate zones. Infants, children, and adults—immunocompetent as well as immunocompromised—may be infected. In African HIV-seropositive patients, up to 16 per cent of those with chronic diarrhoea have isosporiasis. The disease may be latent for months following infection.

Life cycle and morphology

The parasite multiplies by merogony and gamogony entirely within the enterocytes of the small bowel. As far as is known, there is no animal reservoir host for *I. belli*. Transmission is human to human via faecal–oral contamination by oocysts. The oocyst is 25×15 μm in size.

Clinical features

These range from moderate diarrhoea, through abdominal pain and steatorrhoea, to severe watery diarrhoea. This may last a few days before spontaneous cure, or persist for months until death from malabsorption and wasting. The latter pattern is common in immunocompromised patients. Blood eosinophilia of > 500 per mm^3 is seen in about half the cases (an unusual phenomenon in protozoan infections).

Pathology

The entire small bowel is involved. There is inflammation of the lamina propria, often with marked eosinophilia. The villi are blunted through crypt hyperplastic atrophy, which may be as severe as that seen in coeliac disease. The parasites are seen in their various life stages in the villous enterocytes, but not in crypts or the lamina propria (Fig. 29.69). Dissemination of *Isospora* to mesenteric lymph nodes has been recorded in association with HIV infection.

The pathogenesis of the diarrhoea and the immune processes relevant to immunity and recovery from infection are unknown.

Diagnosis and treatment

Finding the characteristic oocysts in faeces is the main method. Small bowel biopsy is less sensitive since the

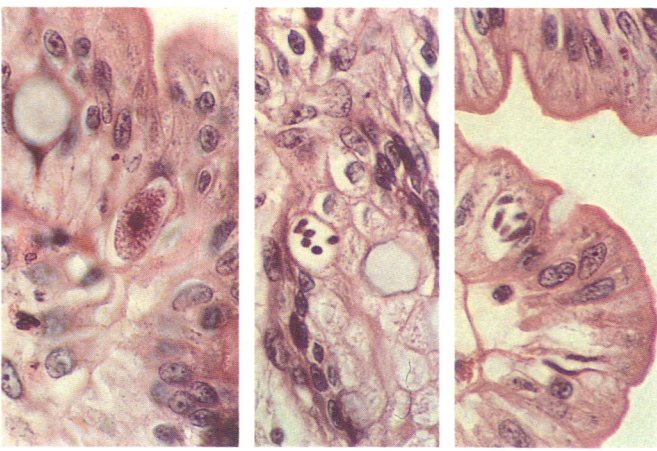

Fig. 29.69 Isosporiasis. Jejunal biopsy. Sickle-shaped merozoites in enterocytes (left and middle photographs); uninucleate early meront in the right photograph. (Slide courtesy of Dr M. Mathan.)

parasites may be relatively scanty. Treatment with trimethoprimsulphamethoxazole clears the infection and symptoms in some patients.

29.8　Microsporidian protozoa

Members of this large phylum are obligate intracellular parasites of vertebrates and invertebrates. Three genera infect man: *Nosema*, *Encephalitozoon*, and *Enterocytozoon*; only the last two are at all common. They are mainly associated with host immunosuppression. The means of transmission are not known. The life cycle is unique. Within the spore forms, there is a coiled filament; this uncoils and injects the infective sporoplasm directly into host cells.

29.8.1　*Encephalitozoon cuniculi*

This is a definite cause of keratoconjunctivitis. All the documented cases have been in patients with AIDS. There is conjunctival irritation and photophobia, often with a history of ocular trauma or contact-lens wearing. Examination reveals minimal hyperaemia but granular opacity of the cornea. In time, the cornea may ulcerate and perforate. There is no specific treatment for this infection.

Biopsy or scrapes of conjunctiva show minimal inflammation, but the epithelial cells contain 2 μm ovoid spores and meronts that stain with Giemsa and Gram methods. Electron microscopy confirms the diagnosis by identifying the polar filaments in spores.

Serological evidence links *Encephalitozoon* infection with neurological diseases in man, but there has been no direct visualization of parasites in human brain.

29.8.2　*Enterocytozoon bieneusi*

Unlike encephalitozoonosis, this is not a zoonotic infection. It has only been observed in the small bowel enterocytes of HIV-seropositive people with chronic diarrhoea; in some series, 7 per cent of such patients are infected. The parasites are found in the superficial parts of surface enterocytes (Fig. 29.70).

Inflammation is slight or absent. Electron microscopy provides the definitive diagnosis (Fig. 29.71). It is presumed that these organisms are pathogenic rather than passengers, but proof is awaited. There is no specific therapy.

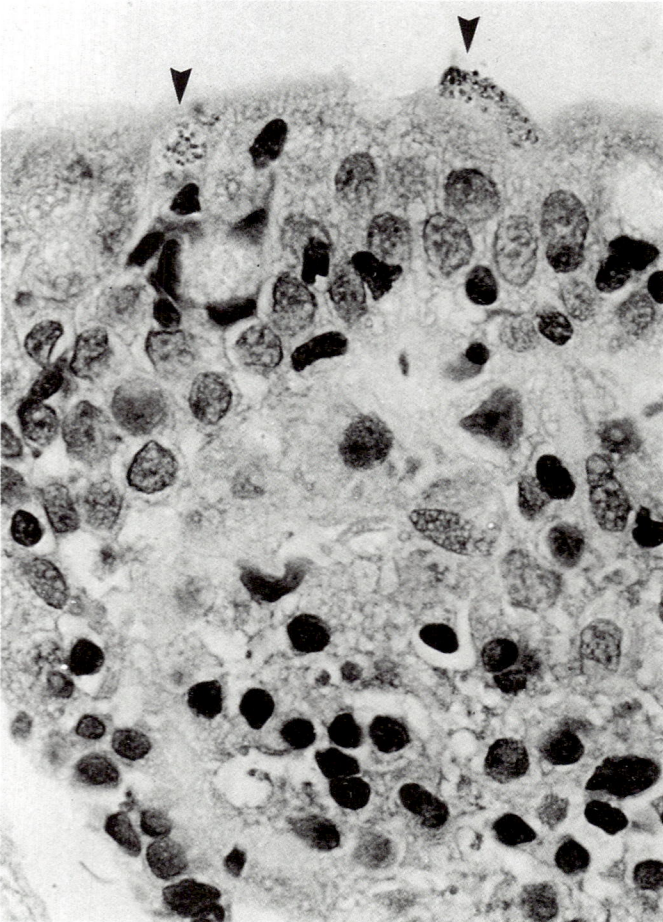

Fig. 29.70 Microsporidiosis. Spores of *Enterocytozoon bieneusi* in the apical parts of two enterocytes (arrowed).

Helminth infections

Helminths (worms) are divided into Nematodes (roundworms) and Platyhelminths (flatworms). The flatworms are subdivided

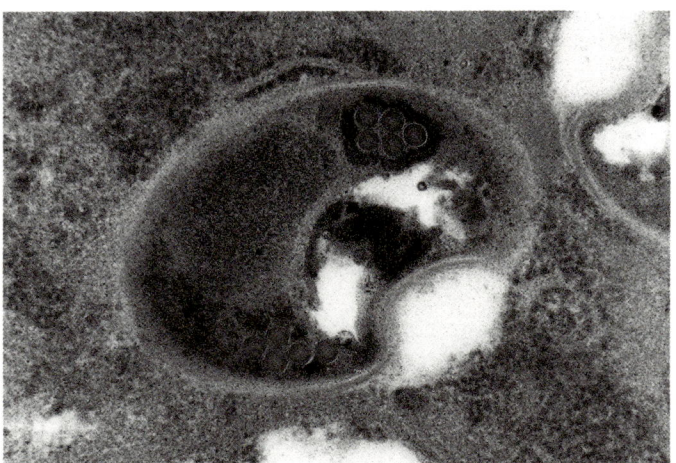

Fig. 29.71 Microsporidiosis. Electron photomicrograph of an *E. bieneusi* spore. Either side of the nucleus are cross-sections of the coiled polar filament that elongates to eject the nuclear material and infect a nearby cell. (Photograph courtesy of Dr A. Curry.)

into cestodes and trematodes. The human parasites in these three groups range in size from the barely visible to 10 m in length.

Nematodes are unsegmented, have an intestine, have separate sexes, and moult four times between the egg stage and adulthood. Their life cycles range from direct man-to-man transmission to complex cycles with one or more intermediate host.

Cestodes are composed of a chain of similar segments (proglottids) which contain both male and female sexual organs. The adults all live in the host intestine and the head segment has a scolex for attachment to the mucosa, often with hooklets. Eggs develop into larvae, which are mostly cystic, in intermediate hosts.

Trematodes are unsegmented, have an intestine, are hermaphrodite (except *Schistosoma*), and require a snail as the first intermediate host.

In human parasitology, nematodes are grouped into the intestinal nematodes, filarial worms, and other non-filarial nematodes.

29.9 Intestinal nematodes

The major infections by adult worms are by *Enterobius*, *Trichuris*, the hookworms (*Necator* and *Ankylostoma*), *Ascaris*, and *Strongyloides*. Their sequelae are often regarded, wrongly, as being of little clinical importance unless there is massive infection. Hookworms, *Ascaris*, and *Trichuris* commonly co-infect the same people. The life cycles of intestinal nematodes are given in Fig. 29.72.

29.9.1 *Enterobius vermicularis*

Enterobiasis (also known as oxyuriasis and pin-worm infection) is very common in children. It causes pruritus ani, but only rarely more severe pathology.

Epidemiology

In temperate zones, infection in childhood is near universal, but declines in adolescence. In institutionalized children, 96 per cent may be infected. In the tropics, it is reportedly less common, perhaps because the eggs survive best in a cool, moist environment. Globally, 300–500 million people are affected.

Life cycle and morphology

The worms live free in large numbers in the caecum, colon, and appendix, unattached to mucosa. At night, females emerge through the anus to deposit eggs on the perianal skin, before (usually) retreating back into the intestine. The adult worm lifespan is 5–8 weeks. Eggs are transferred from anus to fingernails, bed-linen, walls, floor surfaces, and other furniture, to the hands and thence to the mouth to complete an infection cycle. The incubation period is 4 weeks.

Adult female worms are 10×0.4 mm. Along their length there are bilateral pointed ridges (alae) on the cuticle which aid identification (Fig. 29.73). The eggs measure 55×25 μm and are oval with a characteristic flattening on one side.

Clinical features

Most infections are unnoticed. Symptoms are a mild to severe perianal pruritus. In childhood infections, parents may observe the white worms wriggling around the perineum of children at night. Infection appears to be associated with bacterial cystitis in females.

Uncommonly, an intra-abdominal helminthoma or abscess results from migrating worms—*invasive enterobiasis*. This almost always occurs in women and presents as general abdominal discomfort, salpingitis, peritonitis, perirectal mass, or hepatic tenderness. Although people with the common intestinal infestation do not have a peripheral blood eosinophilia, patients with invasive enterobiasis can have eosinophil counts from normal to 3000 per mm³.

Pathology

The pruritus ani as a typical eczematous rash. *Enterobius* is not considered to be a cause of acute appendicitis, though it is often seen in resected specimens with or without inflammation. The intra-abdominal lesions vary according to site, the commonest being within the bowel wall. There, and in the liver and peritoneum, they are greenish-white solid nodules up to 2 cm in diameter. They mimic carcinoma deposits. Salpingo-oophoritis is usually unilateral and may be part solid inflammation, part cystic abscess, green in colour.

The pathologist most commonly observes *Enterobius* lying in the lumen of an appendix removed for appendicitis (Fig. 29.73). The invasive solid intra-abdominal lesions centre around adult

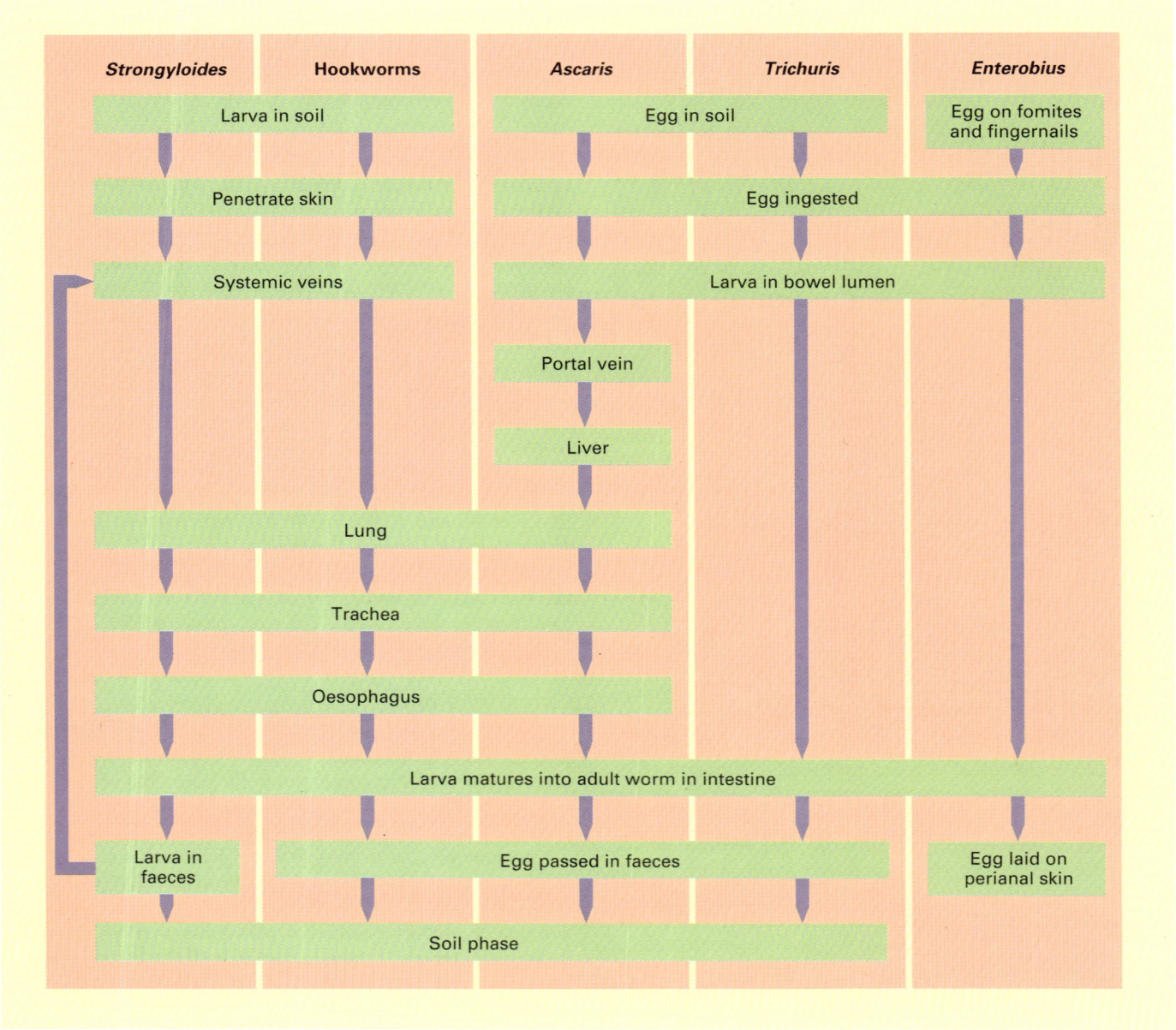

Fig. 29.72 Life cycles of intestinal nematodes: *Strongyloides*, hookworms, *Ascaris*, *Trichuris*, and *Enterobius*. *Strongyloides* also has an auto-infection cycle.

worms and eggs. The worms may be degenerate or unidentifiable by the time of sampling (Fig. 29.74). There is surrounding eosinophilic necrosis, including numerous eosinophils and their granules. There is a peripheral granulomatous rim with epithelioid cells and giant cells. Bowel wall lesions are solid necrotic areas usually in the submucosa or serosa. In a tubal abscess, the predominant cell is the eosinophil, hence the green coloration. Worm fragments and eggs lie in the lumen.

Pathogenesis

The pruritus ani is a hypersensitivity contact dermatitis to egg antigens on the skin. The invasive lesions can follows from worms (both male and female) penetrating through the large bowel wall. This implies a breach in the mucosa, such as inflammatory bowel disease or carcinoma. Occasional cases of intramural rectal helminthoma occur without an evident predisposing lesion. More commonly, an adult worm migrates up the female genital tract after depositing eggs. Depending on where it becomes arrested, the host inflammatory reaction to adult and/or eggs produces an endometritis, salpingo-oophoritis, or peritonitis. The worm can penetrate the liver capsule, and may enter an ovary via a recently ruptured Graafian follicle.

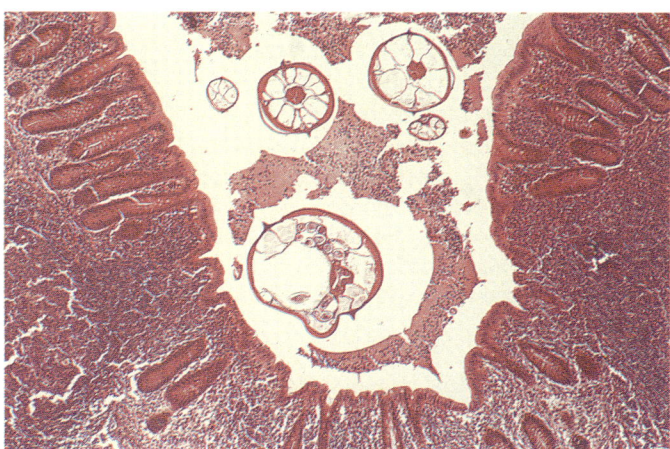

Fig. 29.73 Enterobiasis. Appendix lumen containing cross-sections of several female worms; note the lateral spine-like alae. There is no inflammation.

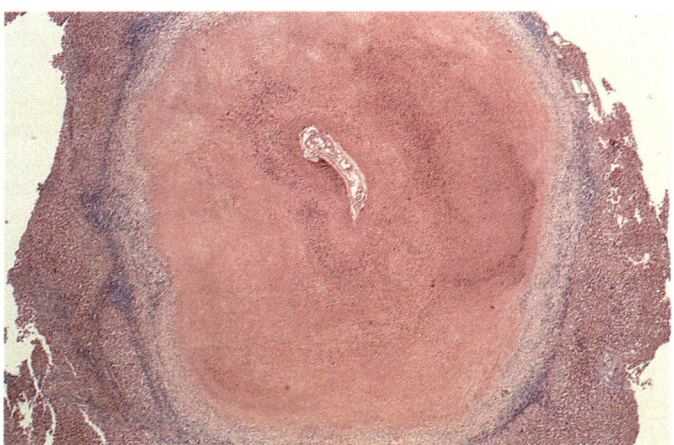

Fig. 29.74 Invasive enterobiasis. Necrotic liver nodule with a central degenerate worm. At operation, this was thought to be metastatic carcinoma.

Diagnosis and treatment

Faecal preparations are not suitable diagnostic samples. Worms are seen at the anus at night and eggs may be found on the perineal skin. The invasive lesions are only diagnosed histopathologically following resection. The shape of the eggs, the size and the characteristic lateral alae on the female worm provide identification. Antihelminthic chemotherapy cures the lumenal infection. Surgery is required for the invasive disease.

29.9.2   *Trichuris trichiura*

Epidemiology

About 800 million people in the tropics, mainly children, are infected by this worm. In some communities, 90 per cent of children have *Trichuris*, often with the other soil-transmitted helminths—hookworms and ascarid worms.

Life cycle and morphology

As with *Enterobius*, the cycle is simple and direct (Fig. 29.72). Adult worms pass eggs into the faeces. Ingested eggs hatch into larvae in the intestine and the adults attach to the colorectal mucosa but do not invade into the lamina propria. Adults are 30–50 mm long, and live for 3 years. The eggs have characteristic bipolar plugs and measure $50 \times 22 \ \mu m$.

Clinical features

Most infections are asymptomatic apart from minor abdominal discomfort. The severe clinical trichuriasis syndrome occurs when >200 worms are present; this affects 5 per cent of children in an infected community. The main features are chronic dysentery with blood loss, anaemia (haemoglobin <10 g/dl), and growth retardation. Rectal prolapse occurs in a third of heavily infected children. Blood eosinophilia is mild.

Pathology

Grossly, worms are seen attached to the large bowel mucosa (Fig. 29.75). In heavy infections, the mucosa is congested and friable. The head of the worm is buried within the superficial mucosa but is surrounded by epithelium. The lamina propria has dilated capillaries and a moderate eosinophilia.

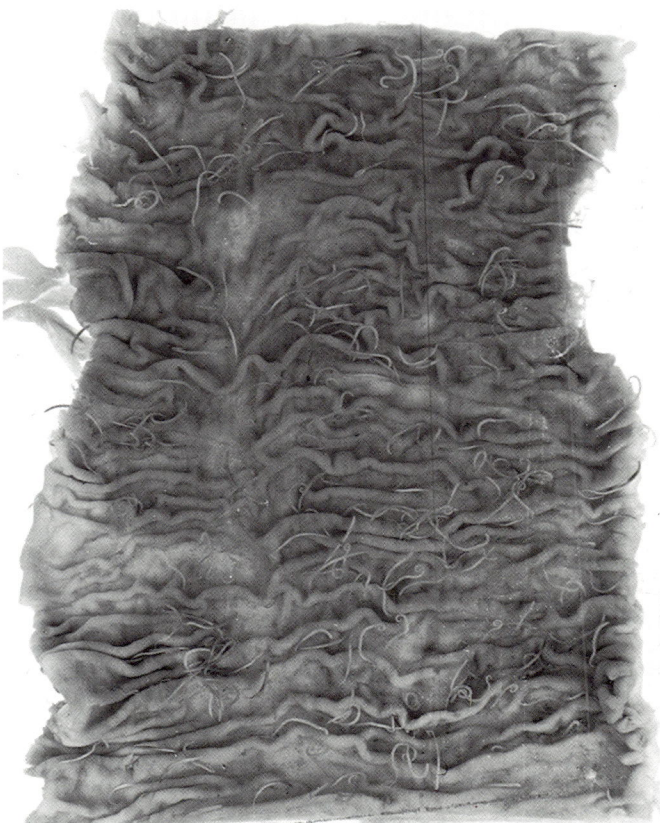

Fig. 29.75 Trichuriasis. Massive colon infection with *Trichuris* worms attached to the mucosa. (Photograph courtesy of the Wellcome Museum of Medical Science.)

The aetiology of the trichuriasis syndrome is unclear. There is not a diffuse proctocolitis, but focal inflammation where the worms are embedded. Separately, and also in conjunction with hookworms and ascarids, *Trichuris* affects child growth by aggravating protein–energy malnutrition. Mass treatment of children significantly aids growth in heavily infected populations. The mechanism is not diarrhoea *per se*, but a combination of decreased nutrient intake and disturbed efficiency of nutrient metabolism.

29.9.3   Hookworms

Two species, *Necator americanus* and *Ankylostoma duodenale*, mature in man and produce chronic intestinal infection ('ankylostomiasis'). Several animal hookworms infect man but remain paratenic (i.e. do not mature) and cause cutaneous larva migrans.

Epidemiology

Hookworms are widely distributed through the tropics, subtropics, and southern temperate zones such as the Mediterrranean basin and southern USA. About 1000 million people have intestinal hookworms, and in many poor areas the prevalence is virtually 100 per cent.

Life cycle and morphology

Eggs excreted in faeces have a larval phase in the soil. Larvae invade the skin, migrate to the lung, penetrate into alveoli, migrate up the trachea and into the oesophagus (Fig. 29.72). They mature in the upper small bowel and attach to the mucosa (Fig. 29.76). *Ankylostoma* larvae are also infective by mouth, with direct maturation in the gut. Adults may live for 14 years, but usually die sooner. There is no apparent immunity to re-infection. The adults are 9–11 mm long. The characteristic eggs measure $60 \times 40 \ \mu m$.

Clinical features

There are three phases:

'Ground itch' and cutaneous larva migrans

A transient itchy papular and vesicular rash may develop at the site of skin infection, shortly after penetration ('ground itch'). If the hookworm species is zoonotic (e.g. *Ankylostoma caninum*), the larva may wander for several centimetres, leaving an erythematous raised track (Fig. 29.77). This cutaneous larva migrans also occurs with *Strongyloides* and *Gnathostoma*.

Pneumonitis

Several larval intestinal nematodes pass through the lungs during maturation: hookworms, *Strongyloides*, and *Ascaris*. In heavy synchronous infections, particularly in those sensitized by previous infection, a pulmonary syndrome often known as Loeffler's pneumonitis occurs 2 weeks after infection. Clinically, dyspnoea with cough and bronchospasm last for about 10 days. The chest X-ray shows miliary mottling. Blood eosinophilia is marked.

Chronic gut infection

Iron deficiency anaemia (microcytic, hypochromic) is the major manifestation of hookworm infection. Globally, hookworms remove 2×10^6 litres of blood daily, equivalent to the total exsanguination of 400 000 people. Once chronic infection is established, there is little or no blood eosinophilia. Heavy hookworm infection also aggravates protein–energy malnutrition (see under *Trichuris* above).

Pathology

Penetrating larvae induce an eosinophilic reaction in the skin, with much oedema. Biopsies of cutaneous larva migrans show the larvae burrowing in the lower epidermis, associated with dermal perivascular inflammation, including eosinophils (Fig. 29.78). Human studies of Loeffler's pneumonitis are

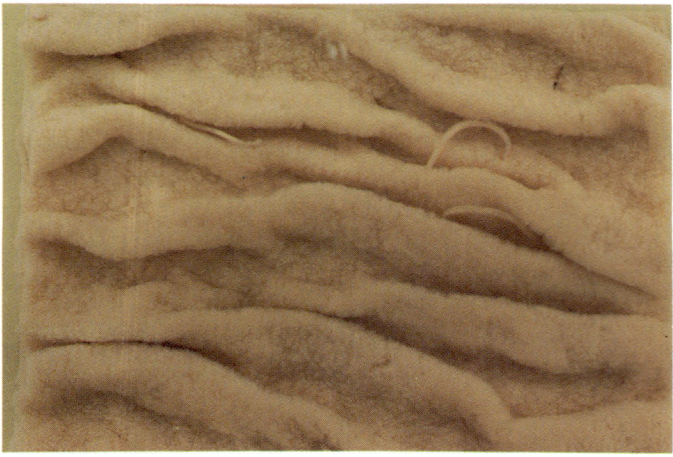

Fig. 29.76 Hookworm infection. Jejunum with several small *Ankylostoma* worms attached to the mucosa. (Photograph courtesy of the late Dr F. MacDonald and Professor M. S. R. Hutt.)

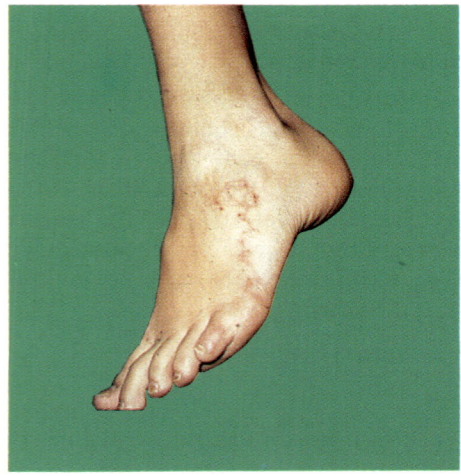

Fig. 29.77 Cutaneous larva migrans (canine *Ankylostoma*). Serpiginous track of inflammation from larva migrating through the skin.

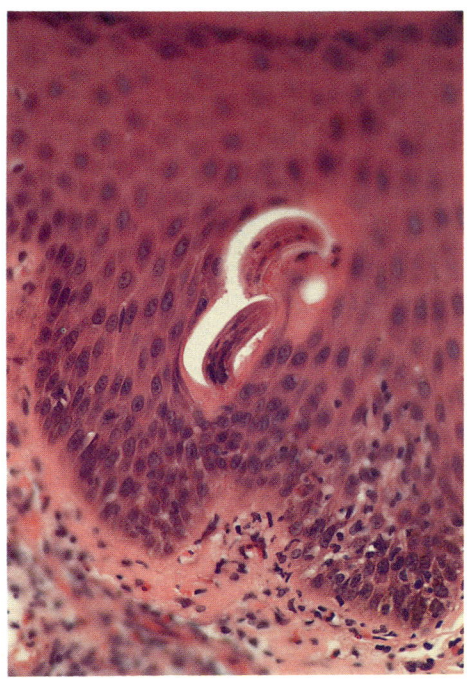

Fig. 29.78 Cutaneous larva migrans. Larva invading through the epidermis.

scanty. There is haemorrhage, fibrinous exudate and an eosinophilic infiltrate in alveoli. Larvae, intact and degenerating, are seen in the alveolar walls and spaces and in small blood vessels.

In the small bowel, hookworms wriggle continuously, bite off fragments of small bowel villi with their mouthparts, and attack a new mucosal site every 10 minutes. This results in constant

bleeding. Each *Necator* worm causes the loss 0.03 ml of blood per day, and each *Ankylostoma* 0.5 ml/day. There is little host inflammatory reaction in the few human biopsy observations. The critical level of infection for significant anaemia is > 200 worms. Rarely, hookworms can invade the mucosa to form haemorrhagic submucosal nodules.

Diagnosis and treatment

Hookworm infection is diagnosed by identifying the eggs in faeces. Standard antihelminthics kill the adult worms, but do not prevent re-infection.

29.9.4   *Ascaris lumbricoides*

Ascariasis illustrates the principle that, usually, helminths become clinically important when infection is heavy, but also that a single worm in an unusual site may prove fatal (Fig. 29.79).

Epidemiology

Ascaris is widespread in the tropics and subtropics. One-quarter of the world's population has ascarids in the intestine, i.e. 1–1.3 billion people. Children are more affected than adults, and have prevalences at up to 98 per cent in some communities. It is calculated that there are about 10^{10} ascarids in the world, shedding 100 tons of eggs daily into the environment.

Life cycle and morphology

Eggs are passed out in faeces. When ingested, they hatch into larvae in the small bowel. These penetrate the gut and are carried haematogenously to the liver and then the lungs. Larvae

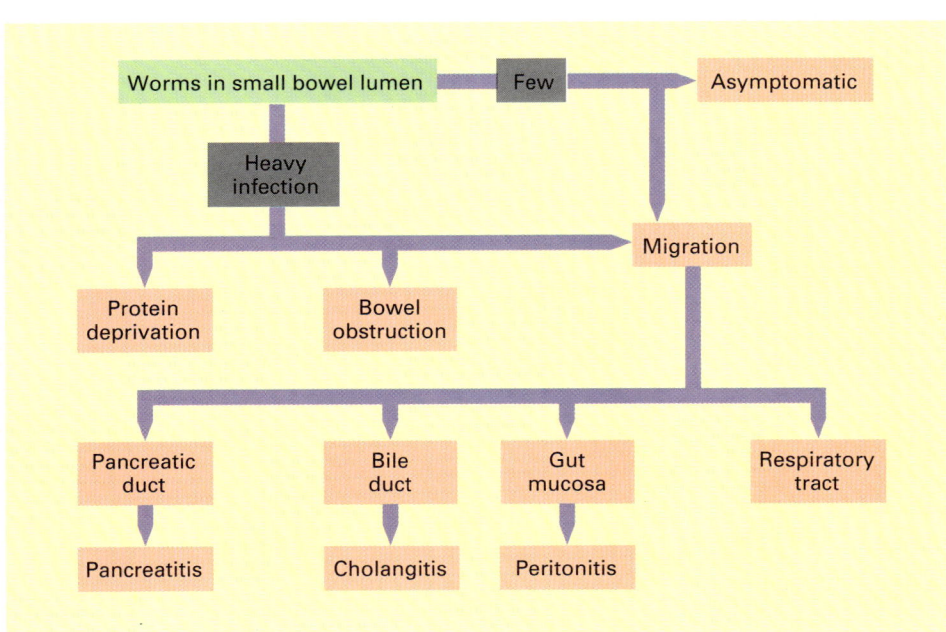

Fig. 29.79 Sequelae of infection with *Ascaris*.

then follow the same path as hookworms and *Strongyloides*, via alveoli, trachea, and oesophagus, to mature in the small bowel (Fig. 29.72). Worms lie in the lumen but rarely invade the mucosa. The prepatent period (infection to egg production) is 70 days. Adult worms live for 1–2 years, and there is no apparent immunity to re-infection. Female ascarids are up to 400 × 8 mm in size. The eggs are 60 × 40 μm.

Clinical features and pathology

The early larval phases in the intestine and liver are asymptomatic, although perilarval granulomas are occasionally found in liver samples. Heavy synchronous infections induce Loeffler's pneumonitis when the larvae moult in and traverse the lung (see above).

The major features of ascariasis are due to chronic intestinal infection and the wanderlust tendency of adult worms. In children, ascarids contribute to protein–energy malnutrition; it is calculated that 26 worms consume one-tenth of the total daily intake of protein. Heavy infections cause intestinal obstruction (a 'bolus' effect) and can precipitate small bowel volvulus (Fig. 29.80). It is estimated that up to 100 000 children die from obstructive ascariasis each year.

Ascaris worms migrate. This is seen pre-mortem and post-mortem, when worms can emerge from the mouth and nares. General anaesthesia can have the same effect. In life, they can migrate into the common and intrahepatic bile ducts (Fig. 29.81). Obstructive cholangitis may lead to liver abscess. Worms also predispose to cholelithiasis, degenerate fragments forming the nidus. Worm migration into the pancreatic duct can initiate acute haemorrhagic pancreatitis.

Occasionally, ascarids can penetrate intact bowel mucosa, or follow a pre-existing defect. The worm disintegrates in the peritoneal cavity, causing peritonitis. A granulomatous reaction with eosinophils forms around the released eggs (Fig. 29.82).

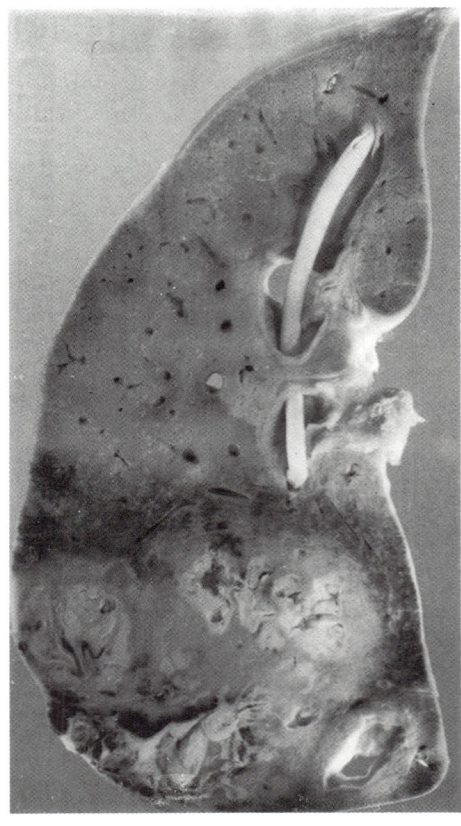

Fig. 29.81   Ascariasis. Worm in the bile duct causing cholangitis and abscesses. (Photograph courtesy of the Wellcome Museum of Medical Science.)

Diagnosis and treatment

Ascariasis is diagnosed by finding the eggs in faeces. Antihelminthic drugs kill the adult worms. Surgery is often needed for the sequelae of heavy infections in children.

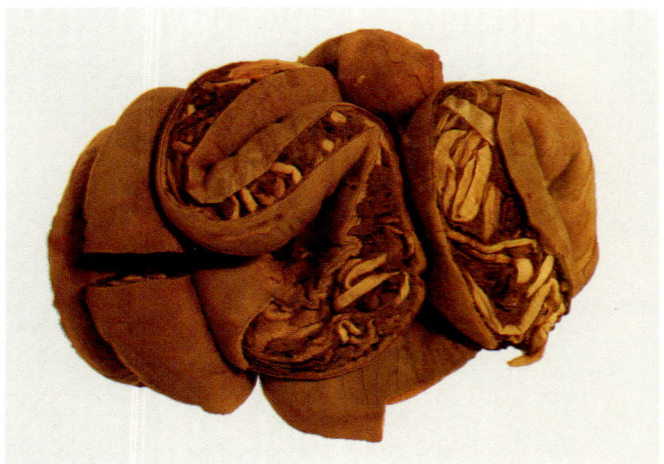

Fig. 29.80   Ascariasis. Ileum resected for obstruction, and opened to show massive infection with worms. (Courtesy of St Thomas's Hospital pathology museum.)

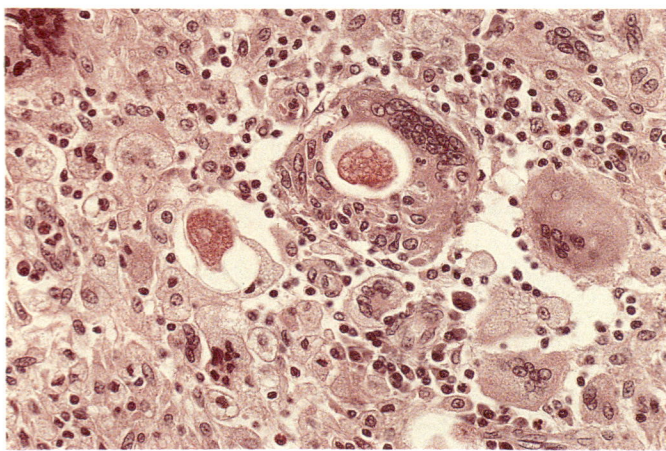

Fig. 29.82   Peritoneal ascariasis. Granulomatous reaction around *Ascaris* eggs.

29.9.5 *Strongyloides*

Strongyloides stercoralis results in clinical pathology that ranges from asymptomatic to fatal systemic disease, due to its almost unique auto-infection life cycle (Fig. 29.83).

Epidemiology

Some 50–100 million people carry *Strongyloides* in their gut. All the tropical and subtropical zones are affected, including southern Europe and the USA. Surveys show infection prevalence rates of 3 per cent in the USA and up to 45 per cent in some parts of central Africa. Because infection is potentially lifelong, cases are encountered in people who have not visited endemic zones for decades.

Life cycle and morphology

The adult female worm measures 2.5 mm in length by 40 μm in diameter and lives in the crypts (non-invasive) of the small bowel. The eggs are rarely encountered in faecal specimens since they hatch in the bowel lumen into rhabditiform larvae (350 × 20 μm). These moult into filariform larvae (630 × 20 μm) both inside and outside the bowel. The infection is acquired from skin contact with soil that harbours larvae. The life cycle is complex because it includes a free-living soil phase and, more importantly, an auto-infective cycle whereby filariform larvae may directly invade the gut mucosa, reach the lungs and thence the intestine to perpetuate the infection (Fig. 29.72). This auto-infection may result in chronic infection for 40 years or more after exposure. In man, only female worms are found; egg production is by parthenogenesis.

Clinical features

The great majority of infections with *S. stercoralis* are asymptomatic. Disease affects the intestine and the skin in those with moderate symptoms. Intermittent diarrhoea and abdominal pain feature.

Strongyloides is a cause of cutaneous larva migrans (CLM), along with hookworm infections and gnathostomiasis. An itchy serpiginous erythematous rash with urticaria moves under the skin of the perineum, trunk, and limbs. Wandering filariform larvae are the cause. CLM due to *Strongyloides* can move particularly rapidly (5 cm/hour is documented) and is also named 'larva currens'.

A special group of patients with strongyloidiasis has been Far-Eastern prisoners of war (FEPOWs) who were interned in Burma during the Second World War. Nearly fifty years later, up to one-third of them have had recurrent cutaneous larva migrans every few months. Mild intestinal symptoms have been less common.

In immunocompromised people (see below), the numbers of parasites can increase rapidly to cause an intestinal hyperinfection syndrome, and then disseminated infection which can

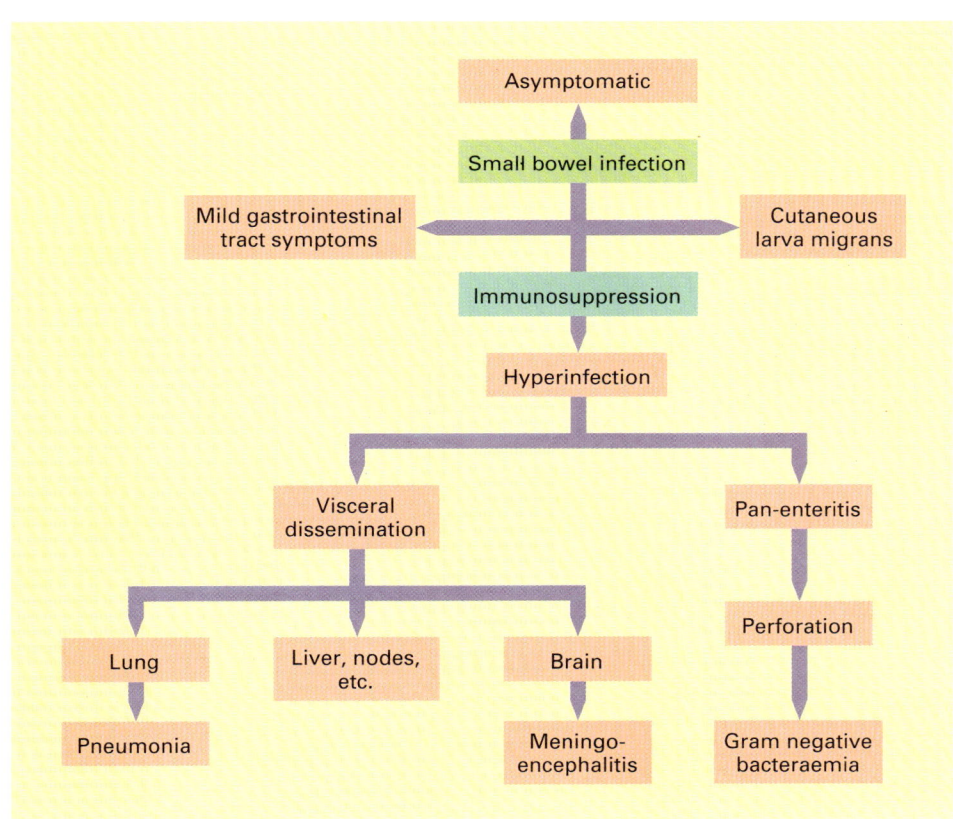

Fig. 29.83 Sequelae of infection with *Strongyloides*.

involve all organs of the body. Pneumonia is common and the brain is particularly affected, with focal neurological signs and reduced consciousness. Hyperinfection strongyloidiasis has a 100 per cent mortality if untreated.

Blood eosinophilia is common in all forms of strongyloidiasis. It can reach 2000 per mm^3, and may be the reason for identifying the infection in a previously unsuspected case. In the disseminated hyperinfection syndrome, the patients with the lower or normal eosinophil counts have the higher mortality.

Pathology

In the common asymptomatic infection, the bowel is macroscopically normal. Traditionally, the small bowel in symptomatic disease is classified as catarrhal, oedematous, or ulcerative enteritis. In the mildest form, there is mucosal congestion and increased mucus. Mucosal oedema and a rubbery thickening of the small bowel characterize the second pattern. In the hyperinfection state, there are numerous small erosions and ulcers up to 5 mm across. Serosal congestion and fibrinous exudate are common. The disease is often segmental, with relatively normal sections of bowel intervening, reminiscent of Crohn's disease. In the severest forms, the colorectum is also similarly involved.

Disseminated strongyloidiasis can affect all organs, but there are no specific gross appearances. In fatal cases, there may be purulent meningitis and cerebral petechiae. The lungs show consolidation with haemorrhages and pleural effusions.

Because the CLM rash moves so fast, biopsy misses it. The histopathology is presumably similar to that of hookworm CLM. The duodenum and jejunum in the asymptomatic person are structurally normal, apart from scanty female worms lying in the crypts, along with eggs and larvae. There is no significant inflammation of the lamina propria and no eosinophilia. In heavier infections, villous blunting is found, and filariform larvae throughout the bowel wall (Figs 29.84, 29.85). Inflammation is variable and mononuclear in type, but eosinophils are not frequent. Mucosal ulcers in small and large bowel may penetrate to the muscularis externa; they are filled with

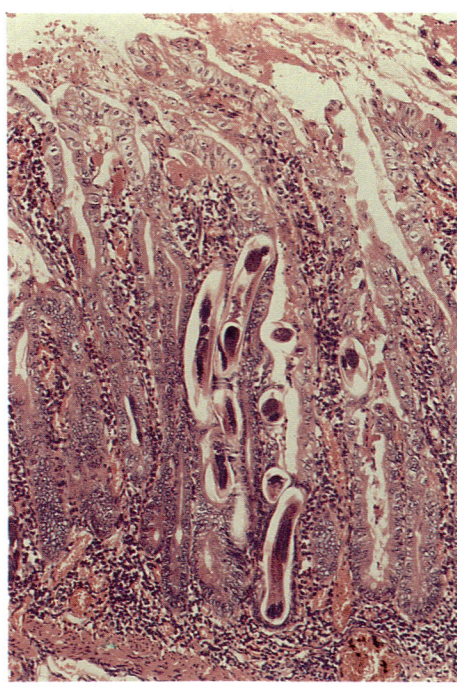

Fig. 29.85 Strongyloidiasis. Hyperinfection of ileum; long- and cross-sections of adult worms in crypts. There is no tissue eosinophilia.

exudate, dead cells, and parasites, and the adjacent villous mucosa is atrophic.

In disseminated infection, there are larvae in bronchi and alveoli associated with interstitial inflammation, necrosis, and alveolar polymorphs (Fig. 29.86). The liver in disseminated infection has larvae in portal veins and sinusoids, associated with acute inflammation or granulomas. In the brain, larvae may be seen in vessels unaccompanied by any inflammation, or they are surrounded by polymorphs and macrophages with haemorrhages. In the small vessels of any organ (e.g. skin, glomeruli, spleen), larvae can be found.

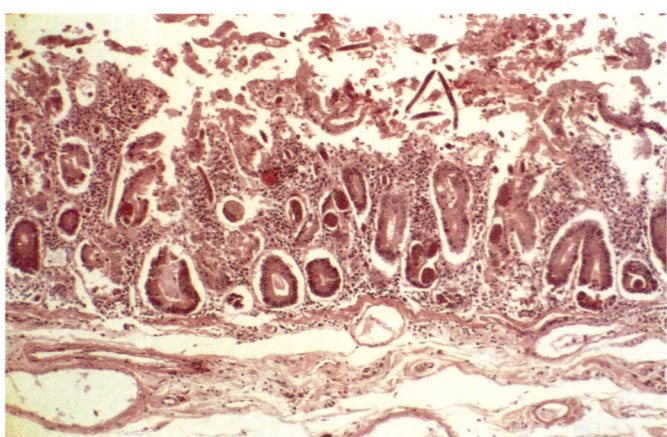

Fig. 29.84 Strongyloidiasis. Hyperinfection of ileum showing disrupted mucosa, adult worms in crypts, and larvae on the surface.

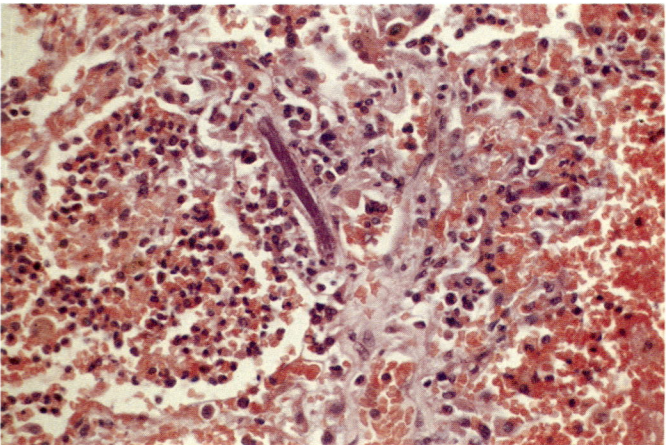

Fig. 29.86 Strongyloidiasis. Disemination to lung; a larva in an alveolus associated with acute inflammation.

Pathogenesis

The inflammation of larva currens is presumably a host allergic response, perhaps mediated by IgE; its frequency is notably variable in different countries. Although the life cycle of *Strongyloides* involves maturation in the lung, immunocompetent people do not get pulmonary syndromes as frequently as occurs with ascariasis or hookworm infections (Loeffler's pneumonitis). As reflected in the scanty intestinal infection load in most people, the challenge to the lungs is low following initial infection or the usual auto-infection rate.

The extent to which damage is induced by mechanical factors (including invasion) and by host immune mechanisms is unclear. Disseminated disease shows filariform larvae invading tissues with associated inflammation that may range from pure pyrogenic to granulomatous. *Escherichia coli* septicaemia is very frequent in disseminated strongyloidiasis, and is the common cause of the meningitis. The bacilli enter the blood through the intestinal ulceration, or by carriage on the larvae themselves.

The circumstances in which the hyperinfection and dissemination syndromes develop usually involve immunosuppression, endogenous or iatrogenic. The commonest group are those patients receiving organ transplants (20 per cent), followed by those with leukaemia or lymphoma (16 per cent). T-cell leukaemia/lymphoma associated with human T-cell lymphotrophic virus (HTLV-1) may present clinically with diarrhoea caused by strongyloidiasis. The majority of all these patients have received steroid therapy, which itself is a predisposing factor. Malnutrition and tuberculosis are also associated with hyperinfection. This suggests that cell-mediated immune defences, probably at the mucosal interface, are crucial to the normal containment of *S. stercoralis* infection. When the host defences fail, more larvae are permitted to invade, pass to the lungs, re-enter the bowel to produce more larvae, and thus rapidly build up a hyperinfection state.

However, some 15 per cent of cases of hyperinfection have no definable defect in cell-mediated immunity. And, most significantly, people with both intestinal *S. strongyloides* and HIV infection do not show an increased risk of hyperinfection, despite their lowered blood CD4 lymphocyte counts and inverted CD4 : CD8 lymphocyte ratio in the intestinal lamina propria.

Various other factors may be critical in controlling *S. stercoralis* infection in the intestine. Mast-cell function is a candidate, based on analogies with other nematode intestinal infections in experimental animals. The roles of mucus, of enterocyte turnover, and of mucosal antibodies are unexplored—but they could be affected by drugs and other diseases. Once hyperinfection has commenced, there is often intermittent ileus, and the increased intestinal transit time could permit more larvae to moult and invade the bowel wall. Finally, a change in the rate at which rhabditiform larvae moult and transform into the potentally invasive filariform larvae could be a major variable, and may be altered by the known predisposing factors.

Diagnosis and treatment

Identification of larvae in faeces, aspirates, and biopsies is the main mode of diagnosis. In low-intensity infections, faecal examination has low sensitivity, whereas duodenal aspiration and the string test have a higher success (the latter involves swallowing a length of string which is then pulled back and examined microscopically for larvae sticking to it). In heavy infections, larvae may be found in gastric aspirate, sputum, bronchial lavage, pleural and peritoneal fluid, and urine, as well as in faeces. Duodenal or rectal biopsy reveals abundant parasites, and the only helminthic differential diagnosis is *Capillaria philippinensis* (see Section 29.10.5).

Enzyme-linked immunosorbent assay (ELISA) serology for strongyloidiasis is available in reference centres, and has sensitivity and specificity of over 90 per cent. High specific IgE levels are common in strongyloidiasis. Thiabendazole is the main drug for *Strongyloides*, but the worm is often difficult to eradicate and recurrences are common.

29.9.6 Further reading

Genta, R. M. (1986). *Strongyloides stercoralis*: immunobiological considerations on an unusual worm. *Parasitology Today* 2, 241–6.

29.10 Other non-filarial nematodes

The following are a group of seven non-filarial nematode infections that are zoonoses, man being an accidental host. Some of the worms migrate through the tissue (larva migrans), but most do not mature to produce infective eggs.

29.10.1 *Anisakis*

Anisakiasis is a zoonotic larval infection of the gastrointestinal tract.

Epidemiology

Human anisakiasis is found wherever people eat undercooked sea fish and squid. Proportions of fish infected vary over time and place (in the North Sea, the proportion of whiting with musculature containing anisakine larvae varied from 1.5 to 60 per cent over a decade). Japan, the USA, and Europe have reported the most cases; the current fashion of eating *sushi* (raw fish) is relevant. The larvae can survive in fish for long periods, even in vinegar, but freezing ($-20°C$ for >3 days) or cooking ($>60°C$) kills them. Countries that have introduced appropriate treatment of fish have eliminated anisakiasis.

Life cycle and morphology

Many morphologically similar nematodes parasitize the intestines of marine mammals, such as dolphins, seals, and sea lions. Eggs excreted in their faeces develop into first-stage larvae which infect small crustaceans such as krill. These are eaten by squid and fish (cod, herring, whiting, etc.) and larvae parasitize these intermediate host's viscera. This is eaten by the definitive mammalian host, the worms maturing and inducing an inflammatory mass in the bowel wall.

Anisakis species (the 'herringworm') and *Pseudoterranova* species (the 'codworm') are the commonest to affect man, producing similar clinico-pathological features collectively called 'anisakiasis'. The larvae measure 20×0.5 mm.

Clinical features

Disease occurs when the parasite invades the mucosa of the gastrointestinal tract. Symptoms can start within hours of eating infected fish. In Japan, most cases affect the stomach, with abdominal pain and haematemesis, mimicking peptic ulcer. In the USA and Europe, the small bowel is equally affected; a few days after ingestion there is colicky pain, appendicitis-like symptoms, and peritonitis. A minority of patients have had months of gastrointestinal symptoms before presentation.

The worm may burrow further to cause an omental mass. Rarely, it may reach the liver and pancreas. Pleural effusions have been attributed to anisakiasis, but the worm has not been shown to invade lung.

Radiology may show a filling defect in the stomach, or a segmental narrowing of the ileum; Crohn's disease is a common diagnosis prior to laparotomy. Marked leucocytosis with eosinophilia is common. In gastric anisakiasis, endoscopy is diagnostic when the tail of the larva is visualized poking out of the mucosa.

Pathology

In the stomach, mucosal oedema is usual and in half the endoscoped cases a tumour, 1–8 cm across, forms within the wall. It has a soft, indurated centre. The serosa is congested or exudative. Although ulceration is uncommon, the worm may be seen penetrating the mucosa or submucosa. The intestinal form can involve any part of the ileum, and occasionally the proximal colon. It shows segmental oedematous mural thickening, often with one or more small abscesses on section, and serositis. If there is a mucosal ulcer, the tail of the worm may be seen sticking out. Some cases are described where the worm has not penetrated the bowel mucosa but lies on it. In the bowel wall, the omentum, or other extra-intestinal organs an abscess has greenish contents due to the high eosinophil infiltrate. Mesenteric lymph nodes are enlarged.

The histological appearances depend on the duration of infection. The degree of oedema is out of proportion to the small size of the larva. Early, the larva is intact, surrounded by an oedematous, predominantly eosinophil infiltrate; these cells degranulate, depositing much eosinophilic material around the cuticle (Fig. 29.87). Away from the worm, the whole bowel wall may be infiltrated by eosinophils. Later, the worm degenerates and an abscess forms with persistent eosinophils. Granulation tissue with granulomas form at the edge. The healed lesion is fibrotic.

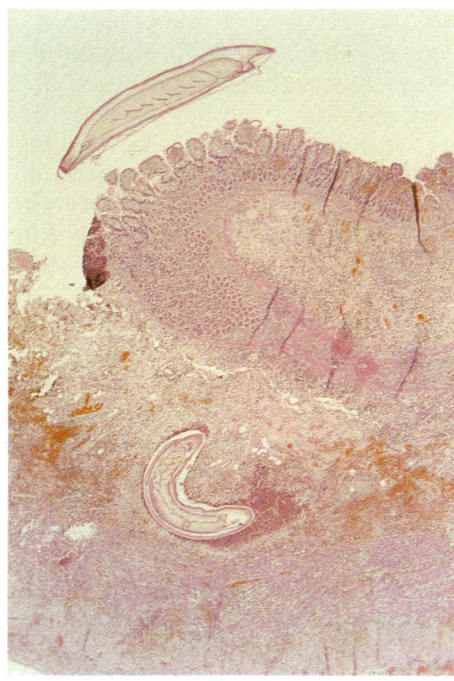

Fig. 29.87 Anisakiasis. Ileum with a larva penetrating into the submucosa, associated with eosinophilia.

Pathogenesis

Larvae of anisakine worms cannot mature in man. They secrete proteinases that lyse the gut mucosa, enabling the worm to burrow into the gut wall and occasionally beyond. The invasion induces a florid eosinophilic and granulomatous response in the bowel wall. Secretory products are chemotactic for eosinophils which degranulate on the worm surface. The eosinophil cytotoxic components (include MBP and eosinophil cationic protein) do not damage the worm cuticle, but may contribute to the host tissue destruction. Ultimately, the larva dies and degenerates within the abscess.

Given the presumed frequency of ingestion of viable larvae, invasive disease is relatively uncommon. How often the mere passage of larvae through the gut lumen is sufficient to precipitate an allergic enteritis is uncertain. It would be termed 'idiopathic eosinophilic enteritis' unless a worm was identified.

Diagnosis and treatment

Endoscopy, radiology, and histology contribute diagnostically. Serology is currently not completely sensitive nor specific. Treatment is by endoscopic removal of the larvae when in the stomach, or surgical excision of the inflamed bowel or omental mass.

29.10.2 *Toxocara*

Certain ascarid intestinal worms of dogs (*Toxocara canis*) and cats (*T. cati*) are able to parasitize virtually any host, including man, paratenically; the larvae can live for years, migrating through tissues but not developing. Most cases of toxocariasis in man come from canines, and the term *visceral larva migrans* (VLM), when used unqualified, is taken to indicate *T. canis* infection.

Epidemiology

Toxocariasis is global. Up to 80 per cent of puppy dogs are infected, declining to 20 per cent of dogs after one year of age. In cats, the prevalence is 10–75 per cent. Soil sample surveys of public parks in north America and Europe found eggs of *T. canis* in 10–66 per cent. The pica syndrome of indiscriminate eating of soil and dirt is closely associated with VLM in young children. Human sero-prevalences for *T. canis* infection vary from 6 per cent in the USA and Europe to 80 per cent in some Caribbean islands. Most infections are asymptomatic. The annual incidence of ocular larva migrans in the USA is estimated at 1 per 100 000 people.

Life cycle and morphology

Toxocara has complex cycles. The normal canine cycle is the same as for *Ascaris* in man: ingestion of eggs, larval migration via the lungs to the small intestine, and egg-laying. There is also transplacental infection to fetal pups. Deposition of eggs in dog faeces provides the source of human disease. The ingested eggs hatch in the gut, penetrate the bowel wall, pass to the liver, and then can migrate to any organ in the body. The larva in man measures $300 \times 20\ \mu m$.

Clinical features and pathology

Toxocariasis comprises two syndromes, which relate to the intensity of infection (Fig. 29.88).

Visceral larva migrans

This results from heavy infection. Overt VLM comprises cough and asthma, fever, hepatomegaly, and eosinophilia (usually over 20 000 per mm^3 of blood). It mainly affects children with the pica habit, aged 18 months to 3 years. There may be focal neurological signs, but, epidemiologically, epilepsy is not specifically associated with toxocariasis despite invasion of the brain.

The pathology of VLM varies. The liver has the highest infection intensity, with 60 larvae/g recorded in one autopsied case (the brain and skeletal muscle had 5 larvae/g). In heavy infection, white spots are visible grossly in the parenchyma. Histologically, often there is only eosinophilic debris in the wake of a migrating larvae (Fig. 29.89). A larva in tissues without any host reaction may be seen; or a granulomatous reaction around a larva, but not usually killing it (Fig. 29.90). Granulomas without larvae are also often encountered. Serologically, patients with VLM have high titres of anti-*Toxocara* antibodies.

A milder syndrome of 'covert' toxocariasis is now recognized in children with raised antibodies. It comprises non-specific symptoms such as cough, anorexia, abdominal pain, pharyngitis, cervical lymphadenitis, and headache. Epidemiologically, it may reasonably be attributed to toxocariasis. Eosinophilia may be absent in one-quarter of cases.

Ocular larva migrans (OLM)

OLM presents as visual deficit, squint, and leukocoria. It mimics retinoblastoma, for which presumed diagnosis surgical excision of the eye has often been done. Older children (mean age 8 years) and even young adults are the usual patients. The symptoms may be episodic as the larva migrates within the eye. Pathologically, there is necrotizing retinitis and usually retinal detachment; uveitis is less common. One larva is found surrounded by necrosis, granulomas, and eosinophils.

People rarely have both overt VLM and OLM. It is postulated that heavy infections (in pica children) induce immune responses against larvae, most of which are destroyed as they migrate, so producing symptoms. A light infection induces much less immune reaction. Larval migration continues

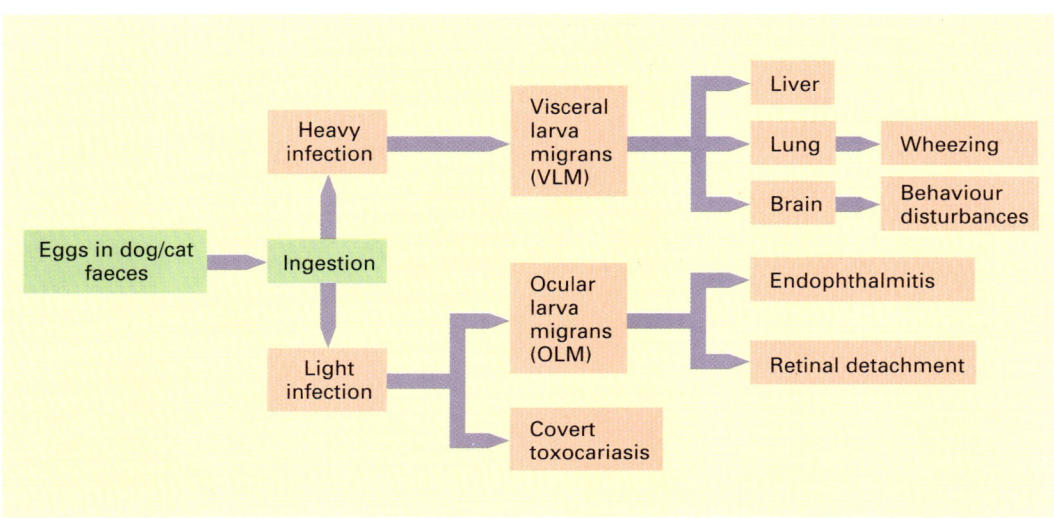

Fig. 29.88　Sequelae of infection with *Toxocara* species.

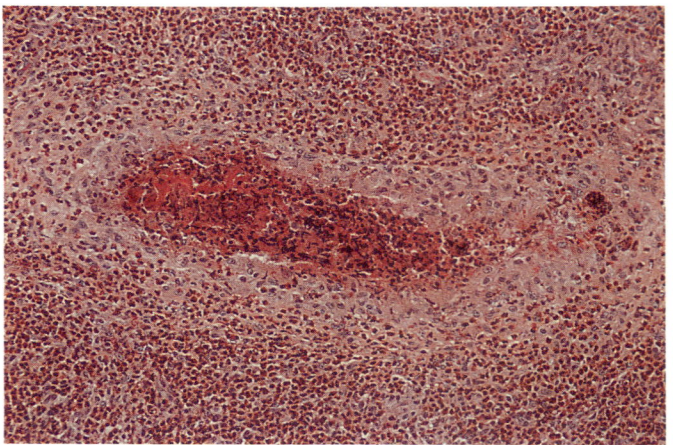

Fig. 29.89 Toxocariasis of the orbit. An eosinophil abscess marking the track of a migrating larva.

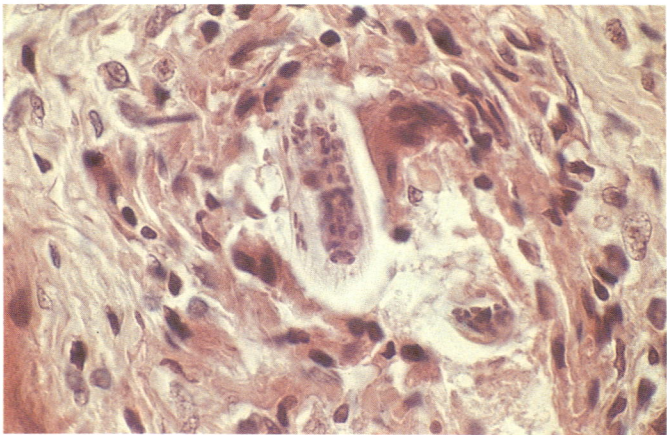

Fig. 29.90 Cerebral toxocariasis. Granulomatous reaction around a larva. (Slide courtesy of Dr C. Scholtz.)

out clinical manifestation until a larva reaches the eye and draws attention by causing retinitis.

Diagnosis and treatment

Clinical features and serology are the means of diagnosing toxocariasis. Diagnostic biopsy is rarely performed since the likelihood of finding a larva is small. Treatment with antihelminthics ameliorates symptoms, but recurrences are common.

Further reading

Schantz, P. M. (1989). *Toxocara* larva migrans now. *American Journal of Tropical Medicine and Hygiene* **41** (Suppl. 3), 21–34.

29.10.3 *Trichinella*

Consumption of meat that is infected with *Trichinella spiralis* causes trichinosis.

Epidemiology

Several species or strains of *Trichinella* affect numerous animals in all parts of the world. Pigs, hogs, boars, and bears are the main hosts, but rats may also be intermediate hosts. Human disease is of declining frequency. Sixty years ago, 16 per cent of autopsied diaphragms in the USA contained *Trichinella* larvae; by 1970 it was only 4 per cent. Nevertheless, epidemics still occur where improperly cooked pork is consumed.

Life cycle and morphology

The life cycles are complicated and vary according to climate. Essentially, the pig/hog/bear is the definitive host. It eats food scraps infected with intramuscular larvae. The latter mature in the duodenum, and begin releasing larvae after 5 days. The larvae invade the bowel and disseminate haematogenously, eventually reaching skeletal muscle. There the larva penetrates a myofibre and converts it into a 'nurse cell' (Fig. 29.91); this is eaten, so continuing the cycle. This cycle has similarities to that of *Toxoplasma gondii*. Man is infected by eating infected pig meat.

The nurse cell–parasite unit contains the largest intracellular parasite in man. It develops, over 5 weeks, by replacing the muscle components with whorls of smooth membranes and mitochondria, a thick outer collagen coat, and by acquiring a rich plexus of surrounding capillaries to sustain it. The cyst within the nurse cell measures up to $400 \times 250\ \mu m$; the larva is $35\ \mu m$ in diameter. In man, the nurse cell and parasite eventually die and calcify.

Clinical features

Light infections are often asymptomatic. The enteric phase may induce pain, diarrhoea, and vomiting. Dissemination to muscle causes myalgia, fever, oedema (often peri-orbital); heavy infections are associated with abnormalities of eye movements and swallowing. Cardiac invasion by larvae results in a myocarditis. Cerebral invasion may lead to encephalitis and meningitis. High blood eosinophil counts up to 4000 per mm^3 are characteristic of trichinosis. Deaths are now rare.

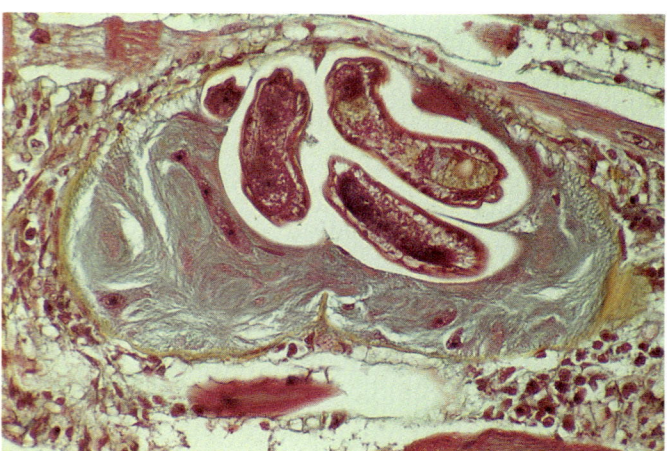

Fig. 29.91 Trichinosis. Larva in skeletal muscle 'nurse cell', with associated chronic inflammation. (Movat stain.)

Pathology

The enteric phase of trichinosis has not been studied in man. All skeletal muscles can be affected. Grossly, the foci of inflammation form small white spots in muscle. During the development of the nurse cell, there is myositis, with eosinophils and oedema separating the fibres. When the nurse cell unit has matured, inflammation ceases; eventually there is dystrophic calcification.

In severe cases of myocarditis—which is the principle cause of death—the heart is enlarged and flabby. There is myocarditis with focal necrosis and eosinophilia. Larvae are rarely seen and are not encysted. The pathogenesis of the myocarditis is not clear, but it may be a bystander effect of larval destruction by macrophages and eosinophils.

Brain invasion by larvae causes some meningeal exudation and cerebral swelling. Histologically, there are focal necroses with eosinophils and glial nodules, but larvae are infrequently found.

Most human infections have 1–10 larvae/g of skeletal muscle and many are asymptomatic. Moderately severe infections occur, with 50–100 larvae/g, and >5000 larvae/g has been recorded in a fatal case.

Diagnosis and treatment

In suspected cases, serology is sensitive but remains positive long after infection. A skeletal muscle biopsy can be taken during the symptomatic phase. It is crushed and directly examined for larval cysts, or the muscle digested first. Thiabendazole kills the larvae, and steroids may be used to reduce symptoms.

29.10.4   Oesophagostomum

Species of *Oesophagostomum* parasitize the intestines of many mammals and pass eggs via the faeces. Human infection occurs in Africa, Brazil, and Indonesia. Larvae in the soil are ingested and invade the bowel wall. Maturation is usually incomplete and egg production is rare in man. The worm measures 10–30 mm × 0.7 mm.

Clinical features and pathology

Oesophagostomiasis is a cause of helminthoma in and around the intestines. Hence there is abdominal pain, sometimes with a palpable mass. Peripheral blood eosinophilia is present. Intestinal obstruction does not usually occur unless the lesion has initiated an intussusception. At laparotomy, there is focal peritonitis and a nodular lesion inside or outside the bowel wall with adherent omentum. Clinically and radiologically oesophagostomiasis may simulate carcinoma or tuberculosis.

Multiple nodules may be present in the wall of small and large intestine. Or there is a single nodule, usually at the ileo-caecal junction. Uncommonly, the lesion is within the anterior abdominal wall.

Macroscopically, the helminthoma is up to 6 cm in diameter and usually located in the submucosa. The overlying mucosa is usually intact. There is yellowish pus in the centre and a solid

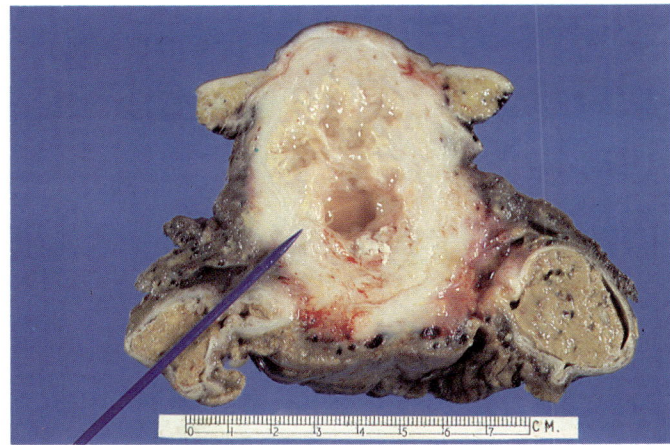

Fig. 29.92 *Oesophagostomum* abscess (helminthoma) of the mesentery. Thick fibrous wall around the cavity; the pointer indicates a small worm. (Photograph courtesy of the late Dr F. MacDonald and Professor M. S. R. Hutt.)

necrotic surround. The worm may be visible in the centre (Fig. 29.92). Histologically, around the worm is an eosinophil abscess, caseation necrosis, granulomas, and granulation tissue.

The diagnosis is made histopathologically or by examination of the whole worm. Similar inflammatory lesions containing no evident worm on resection are often presumed to represent helminthomas—of *Oesophagostomum* or other zoonotic nematodes such as *Gnathostoma*—in which the worm has degenerated.

29.10.5   Capillaria

Two species of *Capillaria* cause zoonotic disease in man. *Capillaria hepatica* results in liver disease; *C. philippinensis* causes enteritis.

Capillaria hepatica

This is a parasite in the liver parenchyma of many mammals, widely distributed throughout the world. Human cases are rare, but are reported from all continents except Australasia. In animals, the worm lays eggs in the liver, and after the death and decay of the host, the eggs develop further in the soil. Man is infected by eating eggs in contaminated dirt.

Clinical feature and pathology

Infection presents as a hepatitis with enlarged liver. There is prominent blood eosinophilia. Mortality is low. The liver has numerous small white spots through the parenchyma. Microscopy reveals a granulomatous and eosinophilic reaction to *Capillaria* larvae, adult worms, and eggs (Fig. 29.93). With older infections, there is more fibrosis. Adult worms are 20 × 0.1 mm, and eggs measure 60 × 30 μm. The diagnosis is made on liver biopsy or at post-mortem (no eggs are excreted).

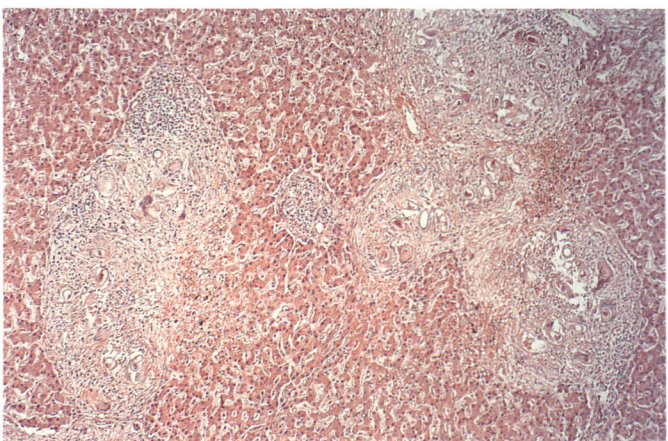

Fig. 29.93 *Capillaria hepatica* infection in liver. Granulomas around eggs, and fibrosis.

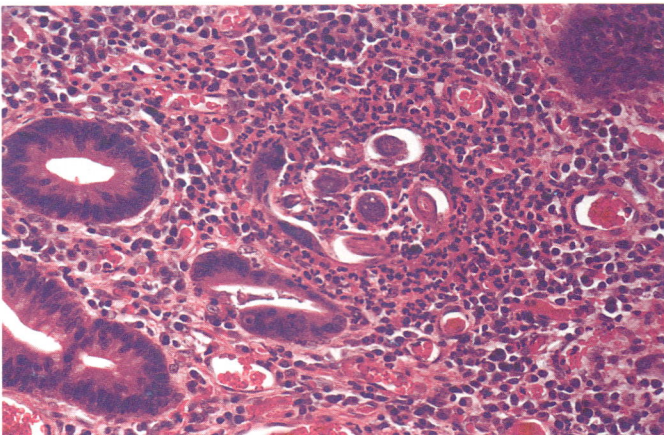

Fig. 29.94 *Capillaria philippinensis* infection in small bowel. Adult worms in a crypt, associated with acute inflammation.

Capillaria philippinensis

Epidemiology

The disease was first described in the 1960s. Most cases have been documented in the Philippines; many are now reported from Thailand. Sporadic cases have been seen in Japan, Iran, and Egypt. The natural definitive hosts are probably fish-eating birds.

Life cycle and morphology

Man acquires this zoonosis by eating larvae in uncooked fresh-water fish. The adult worms reside in the jejunum and upper ileum in large numbers; at autopsy up to 200 000 worms have been found per litre of bowel fluid. Eggs may embryonate into larvae within the human bowel and invade the mucosa. This auto-infection cycle (similar in principle to that of *Strongyloides*) permits the build-up of heavy infection loads. Female worms are up to 4.3 mm long × 40 μm in diameter. Eggs are elongated, measuring 40 × 20 μm.

Clinical features

Intestinal capillariasis is mainly a disease of young adults. The features are of a small bowel severe enteritis with abdominal pain, vomiting, and watery diarrhoea. Prolonged enteritis leads to wasting, hypokalaemia, and protein-losing enteropathy. The case fatality was initially up to 10 per cent but, with treatment, deaths are now rare. Unlike strongyloidiasis, which causes a pathologically similar enteritis, *C. philippinensis* larvae do not invade beyond the intestinal mucosa and disseminate.

Pathology

The jejunal and upper ileal mucosa are inflamed and oedematous in fatal cases. The other systemic morbid features are those of prolonged enteritis.

The adult worms and eggs are seen within the crypts. The lamina mucosa is inflamed with cells, lymphocytes, and some eosinophils (Fig. 29.94). Partial villous atrophy and mucosal erosions follow heavy infection. Eggs, adult worms, and larvae are seen in the faecal stream. The extent to which mucosal inflammation and disruption is a consequence of mechanical damage by intra-crypt worms, of toxic worm secretions, or of a host immunological reaction to worm antigens is not known.

Diagnosis and treatment

Intestinal capillariasis is diagnosed by identifying adult worms, worms, and eggs in the faeces. Histologically, the infection resembles strongyloidiasis. Serodiagnostic tests are still being evaluated. Antihelminthic drugs such as thiabendazole eliminate the infection, but long courses are needed to prevent relapse.

29.10.6   Gnathostoma

This worm is another cause of visceral larva migrans.

Epidemiology

Gnathostoma spinigerum is endemic in South-East Asia, particularly Thailand, and India. A prevalence of gnathostomiasis of 4 per 1000 people in Thailand has been claimed.

Life cycle and morphology

The main hosts are carnivores such as dogs and cats. Eggs are excreted in faeces in water. Hatched larvae penetrate *Cyclops* crustacea, which are eaten by the second intermediate hosts—fish or rodents. Ingestion of infected muscle from these second hosts transmits the infection to the definitive host and man. The larva burrows through the gut wall, passes to the liver, and then—in animals—migrates back to the intestine where it forms a helminthoma and excretes eggs. In man, the infection is paratenic. The larva found in man measures up to 13 × 1 mm. It has a characteristic head bulb with eight rows of spines which, mechanically, aid tissue invasion by the worm.

Clinical features and pathology

The larva migrates through the subcutis to cause migratory oedematous swellings on the extremities (similar to loiasis) and face. Loss of vision follows invasion of the eye. Pulmonary invasion produces cough and focal infiltrates on chest X-ray. A helminthoma in the intestine can develop, causing intestinal obstruction. The most severe manifestations follow invasion of the central nervous system. Radiculitis, paraplegia, meningitis, cerebellar and cerebral focal lesions may all occur. The larva can survive for several years to produce recurrent symptoms. Blood eosinophilia is marked.

The cerebral lesions at autopsy comprise subarachnoid haemorrhage and multiple parenchymal haemorrhages up to 4 cm in diameter. The moving worm may be found near a haemorrhage. Histologically, larvae are found on biopsy material only rarely. Haemorrhage, granulation tissue, and local eosinophilia are the typical constituents of the track of a migrating *Gnathostoma*.

Diagnosis and treatment

Most cases are diagnosed on clinical grounds, supported by specific serology. Surgical removal of the parasite is rarely possible. Antihelminthics do not appear to kill the worm.

29.10.7 *Angiostrongylus*

Two species of *Angiostrongylus*, which live in blood vessels, affect man. In both, the normal definitive hosts are rodents, and the intermediate hosts are snails or slugs. After eating such infected gastropods or eating vegetables coated with larvae, the latter migrate in the body. *A. costaricensis* is endemic in Latin America and Costa Rica. *A. cantonensis* is distributed through the Far East, Central America, and Africa.

Angiostrongylus costaricensis

The larvae invade the bowel wall and mature in mesenteric arteries, where the adult worms lay eggs. The females are 40×0.35 mm, the eggs 90 μm long.

Children are most often affected. Clinically, there is abdominal pain and a palpable mass, usually in the right lower quadrant, with fever and blood eosinophilia. Pathologically there is an inflammatory pseudotumour in and around the caecum and appendix. The worms are seen in vessels, but the main reaction is to eggs and hatched larvae. There is a granulomatous response with marked eosinophilia (Fig. 29.95).

Angiostrongylus cantonensis

In the normal rat host, ingested larvae move rapidly to the meningeal arteries, and thence via the heart to the pulmonary arteries where the adults mature and lay eggs. In man, the migration is arrested at the brain, causing an eosinophilic meningoencephalitis. Meningism, cranial nerve palsies, and other focal neurological signs develop over the month following exposure. There is blood eosinophilia. Recovery is usual,

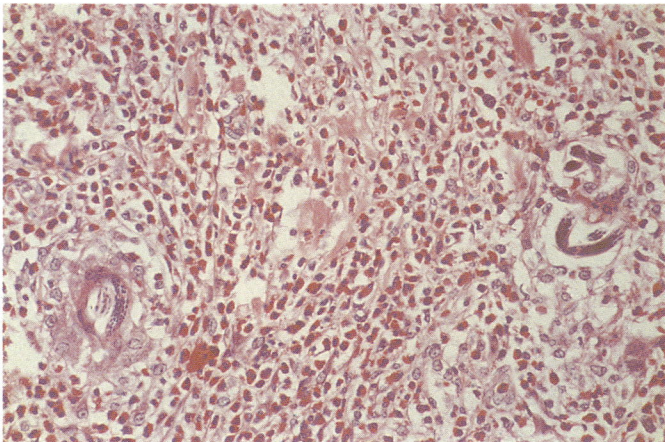

Fig. 29.95 *Angiostrongylus costaricensis* infection of the mesentery. Eosinophilia and granulomas around larvae.

though with some residual deficits. Mortality is about 1 per cent, due to massive infection.

Pathologically the meninges are hyperaemic and there are small grey and white matter haemorrhages. Worms (up to 12 mm long and 0.4 mm in diameter) may be seen in subarachnoid vessels. Intact worms elicit little reaction but degenerate worms in vessels and those that have migrated through brain tissue induce an eosinophilic and sometimes granulomatous reaction.

As well as this parasite, eosinophilic meningitis is also caused by *Gnathostoma*, *Trichinella*, cysticercosis, *Schistosoma*, and *Paragonimus*.

29.11   Filarial nematodes

This group of nematodes is characterized by having a *microfilaria* stage of development, between the egg and the fully developed larva. The microfilariae migrate in blood and lymph, or through tissues. All filariases require an insect vector (Fig. 29.96). The major filariases—lymphatic filariasis, loiasis, and onchocerciasis—are solely human infections, but dirofilariasis is zoonotic.

29.11.1   Lymphatic filariasis—*Wuchereria* and *Brugia*

These cause a very wide range of clinical pathology depending on the degree of host immune reaction to adults and microfilariae (Fig. 29.97).

Epidemiology

Wuchereria bancrofti is widely distributed in the tropics, in Africa, South America, the West indies, Asia, and the Far East.

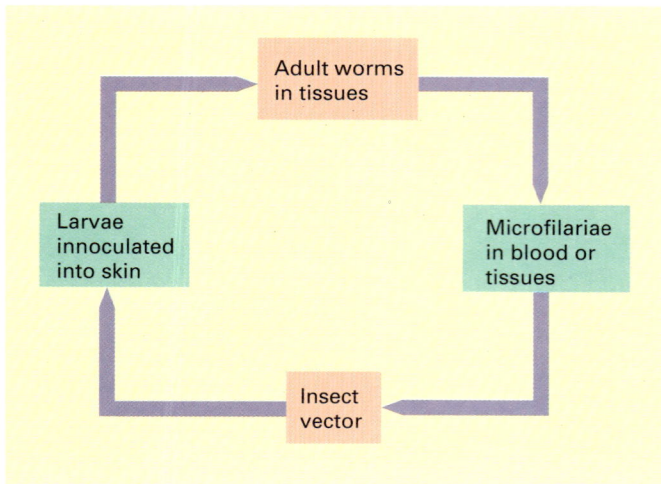

Fig. 29.96 General life cycle of filarial infections.

Brugia malayi is confined to Asia. Altogether 900 million people are at risk in 76 countries. An estimated 90 million are infected: 28 million in Africa, 60 million in Asia, and 0.9 million in South America.

Life cycle and morphology

The adult worms live in lymph sinuses and release microfilariae into the lymph. These circulate in the bloodstream, showing periodicity: the highest densities occur around midnight (nocturnal periodicity), coinciding with the likeliest times for the mosquito vector to bite. During the day, microfilariae are sequestered in the pulmonary circulation; this elicits no host reaction except in patients with tropical eosinophilia (see below). The microfilariae develop into infective larvae within the mosquito. After inoculation into man during a blood meal, the larvae migrate to lymph nodes and mature into adults over

a year. The commonest sites for adult worms are in the pelvic and inguinal nodes.

Adult lymphatic filariae live for up to 17 years. *Wuchereria* female adults measure 100×0.3 mm (Fig. 29.98); *Bruga* measure 50×0.15 mm. The microfilariae live for up to 6 months and measure 300×10 μm (Fig. 29.99).

Clinical features and pathology

There are five distinct patterns of infection with *Wuchereria* and human *Brugia*, depending on the age of first infection and the host immune response (Fig. 29.97).

1. In endemic zones, exposure to infection is universal. Yet the majority of people are asymptomatic, have antibodies against filaria, but no microfilaraemia ('endemic normals'). They could be either immune or have cryptic filariasis with no clinical manifestations from adult worms or microfilariae. From experimental evidence, the latter is thought to be more likely.

2. Another common pattern is for people to be asymptomatic, antibody-positive, and have circulating microfilaraemia. There is no host reaction to the occult adults.

3. Patients with acute lymphatic filariasis present with recurring malaise, fever, lymphadenitis, and perilymphadenitis. This may start in childhood, and episodes last up to 2 weeks. The inguinal lymph nodes and the scrotal contents are the most commonly affected, with axillary node disease also frequent. The nodes are enlarged and tender, and there is usually microfilaraemia.

Histologically, an intact filarial adult worm may be seen (usually as an incidental finding) in a node sinus without any host reaction: this corresponds to clinical group 2 above (Fig. 29.98). When symptomatic nodes are resected, there is acute inflammation around the worm, with eosinophils, distorting the sinuses. In time, the reaction becomes more granulomatous and the worm is destroyed, with obliteration of

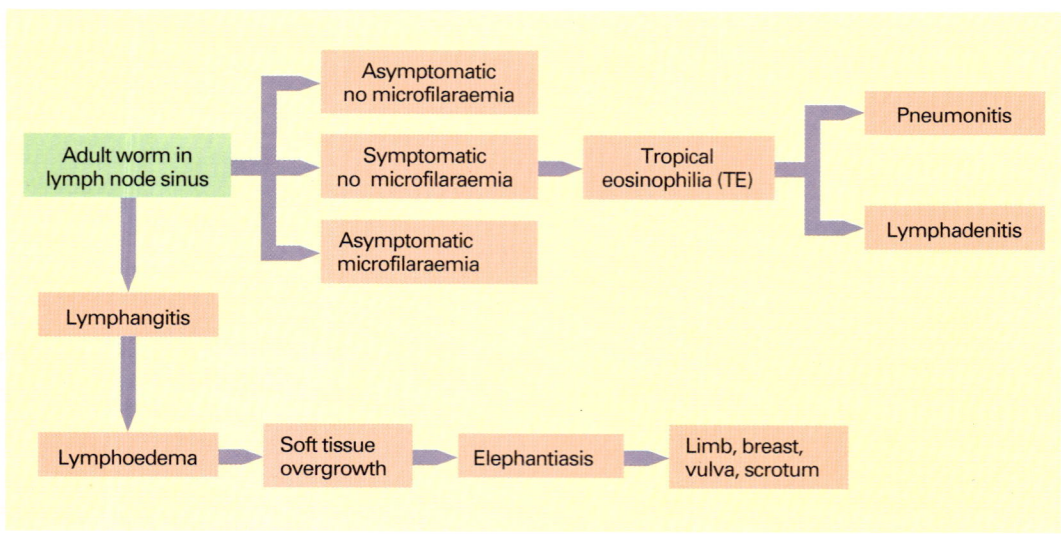

Fig. 29.97 Lymphatic filariasis—sequelae of infection.

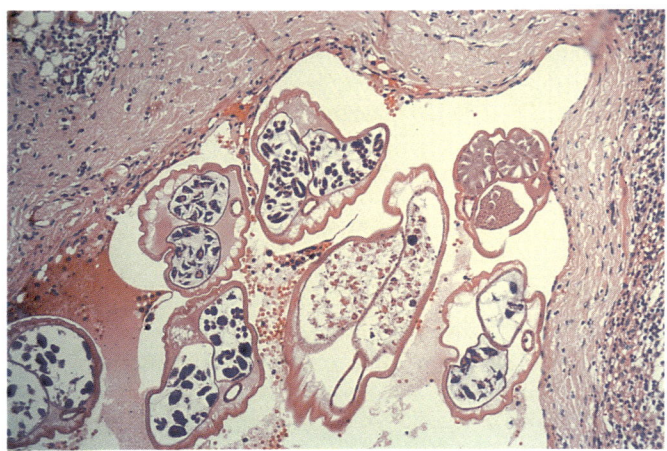

Fig. 29.98 Lymphatic filariasis. Adult female *Wuchereria bancrofti* worm in a lymph node sinus. Note the lack of inflammation.

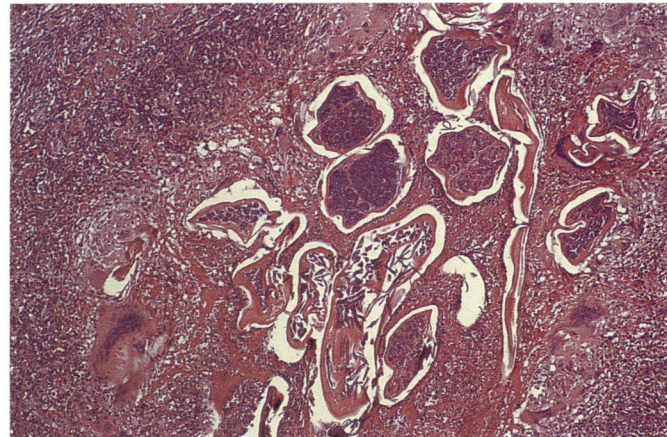

Fig. 29.100 Lymphatic filariasis. Granulomatous inflammation around degenerate worm, with surrounding fibrosis.

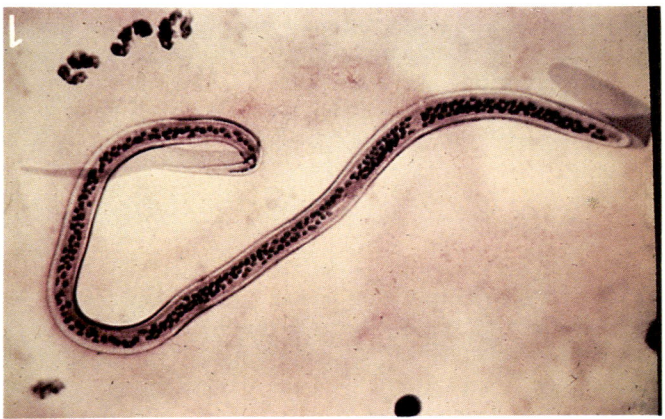

Fig. 29.99 Peripheral blood smear with a microfilaria (sheathed) of *W. bancrofti*.

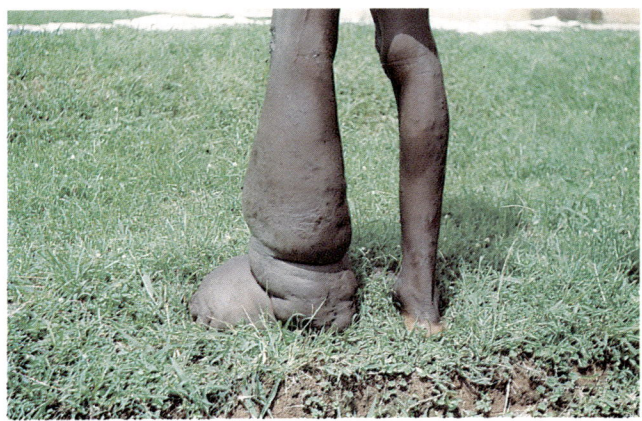

Fig. 29.101 Lymphatic filariasis. Elephantiasis of the leg. (Photograph courtesy of the late Dr F. MacDonald and Professor M. S. R. Hutt.)

the node and fibrosis which extends into the surrounding tissues. The same occurs in the epididymis if a worm is located there (Fig. 29.100).

People who are exposed to lymphatic filariasis for the first time when adults, for example servicemen, may develop acute filariasis. But unlike the endemic population, this is self-limiting, does not proceed to chronic pathology, and micro-filaraemia is virtually never detected.

4. Patients with chronic lymphatic obstructive pathology present later, after at least a decade of infection and episodes of acute filariasis. Hydrocoele is the commonest manifestation. Chronic lymphoedema causes soft-tissue proliferation in the extremities, usually the leg—*elephantiasis* (Fig. 29.101). There is often verrucous skin proliferation as well, termed 'mossy foot'. The arm, breast, scrotum, and vulva may be similarly involved by elephantiasis, although brugian filariasis never causes scrotal elephantiasis. If lymphatics are obstructed proximal to the bladder by pelvic nodal filariasis, there may be chyluria. Microfilaraemia is rare by this stage of the disease.

Histologically, the skin shows dilatation and proliferation of the dermal lymphatics, perilymphatic and perivenular fibrous rims, diffuse dermal fibrosis, and pseudo-carcinomatous epidermal hyperplasia. These are the effects of persistent protein-rich oedema. The cause of the lymph obstruction cannot be identified from skin biopsies.

The lymph nodes at this stage are sclerotic. Residual worm fragments may be calcified. The pathogenesis is bystander destruction of the lymph node and afferent sinuses when the adult worms within are attacked.

5. A smaller proportion of patients of any age have 'tropical eosinophilia' (TE). The commonest pattern is of pulmonary disease with nocturnal cough and wheezing. There is blood eosinophilia, often $> 10\,000$ per mm^3. On chest X-ray there is diffuse mottling. Hepatomegaly, splenomegaly, and lymphadenopathy may also be present, sometimes in the absence of lung symptoms. Neither adult worms nor microfilariae are found, but antibody titres to filaria are very high.

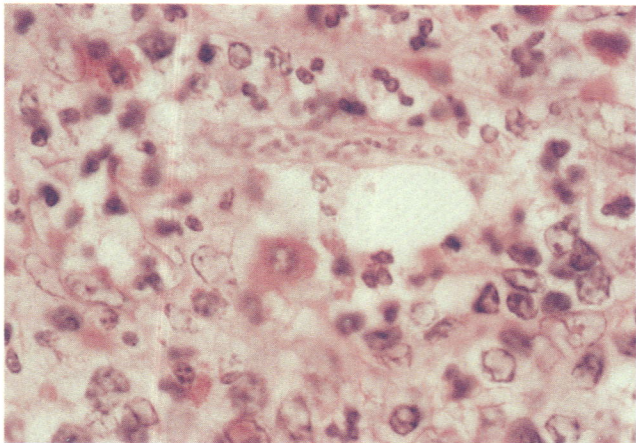

Fig. 29.102 Lymphatic filariasis. Eosinophil and macrophage reaction around a microfilaria in a lymph node.

Lung biopsies in TE show interstitial pneumonitis and alveolitis: eosinophils surround degenerating microfilariae. Later, the reaction becomes granulomatous with fibrosis. Lymph node and liver biopsies show a similar histopathology (Fig. 29.102). The extrapulmonary TE is known as the Meyers–Kouwenaar syndrome. TE is the only pattern of lymphatic filariasis where pathology results from a host response to microfilariae.

A rare pattern of *Brugia* infection occurs in the Americas following transmission of a zoonotic species. These do not produce microfilaraemia, but cause subcutaneous inflammatory masses, similar to subcutaneous dirofilariasis (see Section 29.11.4).

Pathogenesis

Studies of cellular and humoral immunity in zones endemic for lymphatic filariasis show near universal seropositivity, indicating infection at some time. Specific IgE titres are highest in those with TE, lower in those with chronic lymphoedema, and lowest in endemic normals and those with asymptomatic microfilaraemia. Measures of lymphocyte reactivity are increased in patients with elephantiasis compared with asymptomatics with microfilaraemia. Conversely, asymptomatics have higher titres of IgG blocking (neutralizing) antibodies to filarial antigen than symptomatic patients.

It is clear that the degree of host reactivity to adult and microfilarial antigens determines the clinical pathology. The reason why so many people in endemic zones are asymptomatic probably reflects tolerance induced *in utero*. Cord blood sera from babies of seropositive mothers commonly have IgE antifilarial antibodies. Since IgE does not cross the placenta, this indicates prenatal sensitization. Subsequent production of neutralizing antibodies is then a critical factor in determining the pattern of filarial infection later. Expatriates infected in adulthood are evidently very intolerant and rapidly eliminate the infection (see above).

Diagnosis and treatment

Blood samples for microfilaria are the main means of confirming lymphatic filariasis, supported by serology and tissue biopsies. Treatment is problematic. Diethylcarbamazine and ivermectin clear microfilariae from the blood temporarily, and have variable effects on the adult worm.

29.11.2   *Loa loa*

Epidemiology

This infection is limited to West and Central Africa. In hyperendemic regions, infection is universal and > 95 per cent of people have antibodies to *Loa* antigens by the age of 2 years. But only one-third have microfilaraemia or symptoms of loiasis. The amicrofilaraemic majority have *cryptic loiasis*, and have higher specific IgG antibody levels.

Life cycle and morphology

The adult worm migrates through the subcutaneous tissues. Microfilariae circulate in the blood, and are picked up by tabanid flies during a blood meal. Infective larvae are inoculated into the skin and develop into adults over a year. Adults live for up to 17 years, and measure 70×0.5 mm. The microfilariae measure 250×7 μm.

Clinical features

Most infections are asymptomatic. The major clinical manifestations are cutaneous and ocular. The adult worms move freely under the skin. Periodically they induce local allergic oedematous reactions—'fugitive' or 'Calabar' swellings. These may develop on any part of the body, and last for several days. Worms deeper in the fascial planes produce a shifting ache. A worm migrating under the conjuctival epithelium may be seen moving at about 1 cm/min (Fig. 29.103). Periorbital oedema is common. Microfilaraemia of up to 40 per ml is found.

A high blood eosinophilia is characteristic of loiasis, often

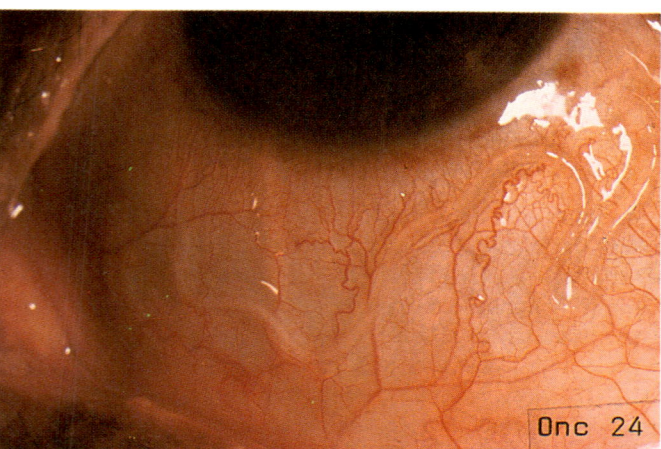

Fig. 29.103 Loiasis. Adult worm wandering under the conjunctiva. (Photograph courtesy of TALC.)

over 20 000 per mm³. Endomyocardial fibrosis (EMF) is associated with persistent eosinophilia; speculation on whether there is a true association between EMF and loiasis in Africa continues.

Expatriates infected with *Loa* as adults often show a hyperreactive states, with Calabar swellings but no microfilaraemia. This is similar, pathogenetically, to lymphatic filariasis in expatriates. Occasional cases of encephalitis are associated with loiasis. Enlarged inguinal lymph nodes have been attributed to *Loa* infection.

Pathology

Calabar swellings are rarely biopsied. The adult worm migrates through dermis or subcutis and elicits a surrounding eosinophil reaction and much oedema. There is also some dermal fibrosis.

Patients with *Loa* encephalitis have microfilariae in the CSF, and histology shows granulomas throughout the brain around microfilariae in small vessels. In lymph nodes, microfilariae may be seen in capillaries; whether nodal fibrosis results from this (as it certainly follows *Onchocerca* microfilarial infection in nodes) is uncertain.

Diagnosis and treatment

Loiasis is diagnosed by the very typical clinical appearances, and by finding microfilariae in the blood. Worms, particularly in the conjuctiva, may be removed surgically. Diethylcarbamazine is effective against adult *Loa*, but can induce adverse allergic reactions. Ivermectin kills microfilariae without side-effects.

29.11.3 *Onchocerca*

Onchocerciasis, from infection with *Onchocerca volvulus*, is an important cause of dermatitis and ophthalmitis in the tropics (Fig. 29.104).

Epidemiology

O. volvulus currently infects about 17 million people out of 90 million at risk by living in endemic zones. These are sub-Saharan Africa (where >90 per cent of infected people are), central and northern South America, and the Yemen. The American foci follow the transport of infected slaves from Africa.

In endemic areas, infection occurs throughout life from infancy. There is no definite evidence of acquired immunity, although infection intensities do plateau after childhood. The patterns of disease in different countries are broadly similar. However, in Africa, people who live in the savannah zones tend to suffer significantly more blindness from onchocerciasis compared with those living in rain-forest regions: 15 per cent versus

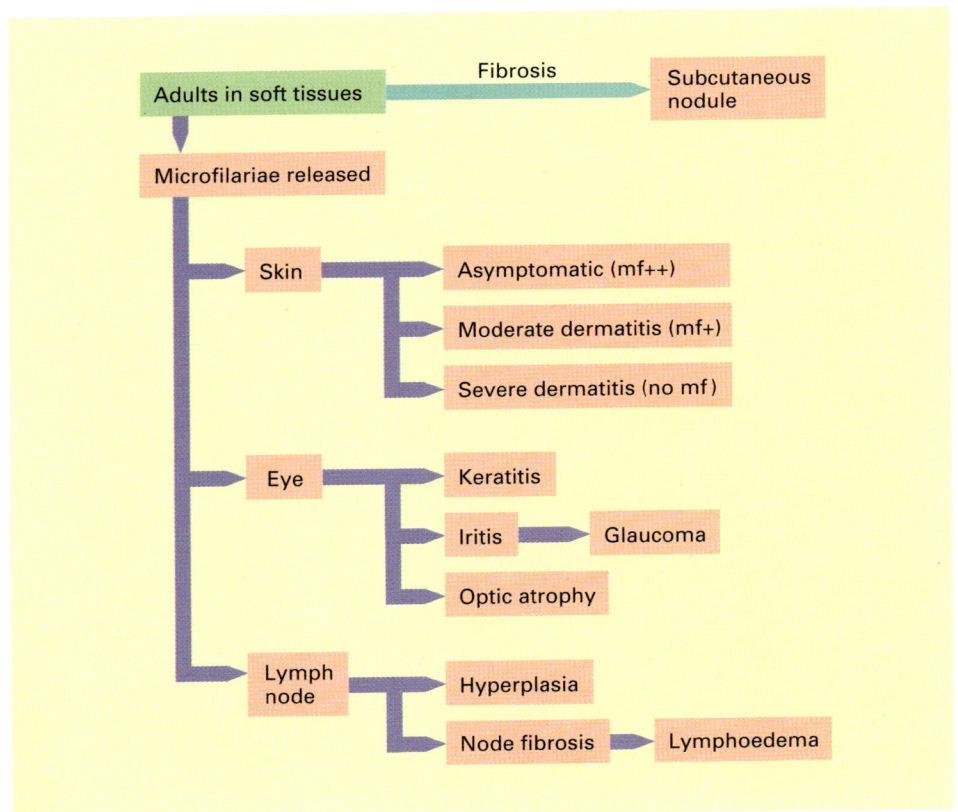

Fig. 29.104 Sequelae of infection with *Onchocerca*. mf, Microfilaria.

2 per cent prevalences of blindness. Expatriates may acquire the infection and present with dermatitis back home.

Life cycle and morphology

Simulium blackflies transmit the infection by injecting larvae in the dermis while taking a blood meal. The larvae develop into adult males and females, which pair and copulate in the sub-cutis and fascial planes. Many, but not all, worm pairs are located within palpable fibrous nodules. Autopsy studies have found occasional adult worm pairs in the retroperitoneum. A female adult may release one million microfilariae per year. The microfilariae move away through the dermal connective tissue, whence they may infect a biting blackfly. Microfilariae are not usually found circulating in the blood. Adult worms can live for more than a decade. It is not certain how long microfilariae may survive: possibly up to 2 years. In a heavily infected person, there may be 50–200 million microfilariae within the body. Adult female worms measure 500 × 0.4 mm. The microfilariae measure 300 × 8 µm.

Clinical features and pathology

Subcutaneous nodules, skin lesions, eye disease, and lymph-adenopathy are the major clinical features of onchocerciasis. As in lymphatic filariasis, there is a wide range of severity of infection, depending on the host immune reaction to *Onchocerca* (Fig. 29.104). The incubation period ranges from 7 to 24 months.

Nodules

Onchocercal nodules are subcutaneous, palpable, fibrotic reactions around adult worms. They are found in 15–50 per cent of infected people, and are typically over bony prominences. These include the head, hip bones, and ribs (Fig. 29.105). Nodules are 2–5 cm in diameter, but are not painful. Ultrasound studies detect more subcutaneous worms, which have not induced such fibrosis, than clinical palpation.

A nodule has an ill-defined outer fibrous capsule and contains coiled worms, usually two, but the range is 1–7 (Fig. 29.106). Nodules have a vascular pedicle, and the worms are presumed to feed from the host blood supply by eroding small vessels. They are seen histologically as multiple cross-sections of female and male worms, the former containing abundant microfilariae in the uterus. The worms lie in a matrix that may be granulation tissue (Fig. 29.107), or an abscess with giant-cell granulomas. Microfilariae are seen in the surrounding collagen, migrating away from the worms. In a given nodule, part of the worms may be degenerating or dead. Dead worms are phagocytosed, leaving fibrous scars and sometimes dystrophic calcification.

Why some *Onchocerca* worm aggregates should induce more fibrosis than others is unclear, but external trauma may play a role and would account for the presence of palpable nodules over bony surfaces. The differential diagnosis of an onchocercal nodule includes tumoral calcinosis and soft-tissue neoplasms.

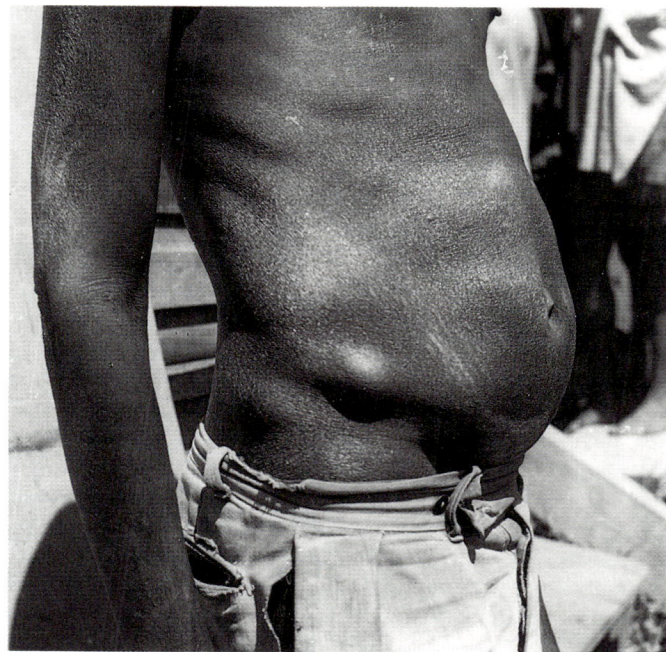

Fig. 29.105 Onchocerciasis. A nodule (onchocercoma) over the iliac crest. Scratch marks and lichenification on the arm and trunk illustrate the pruritic dermatitis.

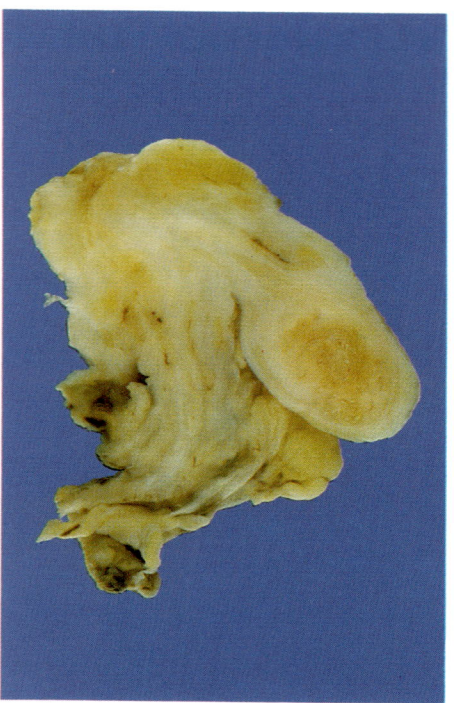

Fig. 29.106 An onchocercal nodule bisected showing a coiled worm and the vascular pedicle.

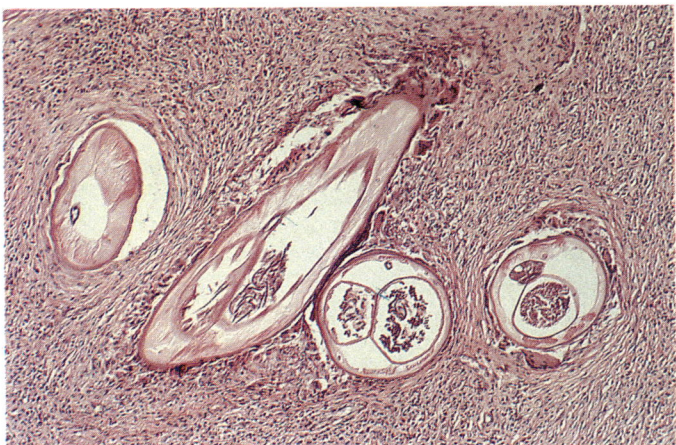

Fig. 29.107 Onchocercal nodule. Cross-sections of adult female worms containing microfilariae, and surrounding fibrosis.

Skin lesions (onchodermatitis)

Despite high densities of microfilariae in the skin, some infected people are asymptomatic. In symptomatic people, the early skin lesions are pruritic macules and papules. Hyper- and hypopigmentation may develop. Scratching induces lichenification (Fig. 29.105), and secondary bacterial infection may supervene. Any part of the body may be affected.

Chronic onchodermatitis has many facets. Atrophic, parchment-like skin ('lizard skin') is frequent. In the inguinal region, it may hang loose ('hanging groin', see below). A spotty depigmentation ('leopard skin') may develop; it is most probably an end-result of prolonged itchy dermatitis, although it has been postulated to be a host reaction to *Simulium* bites *per se*.

In the Yemen, and sometimes in Africans, a localized chronic hyper-reactive dermatitis occurs, called *sowda*. It is asymmetrical, intensely itchy, with papules and crusts, and is accompanied by regional lymphadenopathy.

The pathology of onchodermatitis is due entirely to the host reaction to microfilariae in the dermis. There is a wide spectrum with a general inverse relationship between the degree of inflammation (which correlates with symptoms) and the density of microfilariae (Fig. 29.1). Density is usually measured from skin-snips: a small fragment of superficial skin is sliced off with a scalpel, weighed, and immersed in saline. Microfilariae present in the dermis emerge into the saline, can be counted under the microscope, and the infection load expressed as microfilariae per mg of skin. More than 250 microfilariae per mg may be encountered, although the modal count in symptomatics is around 50 per mg.

In asymptomatic people, microfilariae are seen in the upper dermis without attendant inflammation (Fig. 29.108). Those with acute or chronic papular dermatitis have variable numbers of intact microfilariae, dermal oedema, and a perivascular infiltrate of lymphocytes and plasma cells, but few eosinophils. Dermal mast cells are increased.

In sowda, the dermal perivascular infiltrate is more marked. There is acanthosis and melanin incontinence, but microfilariae

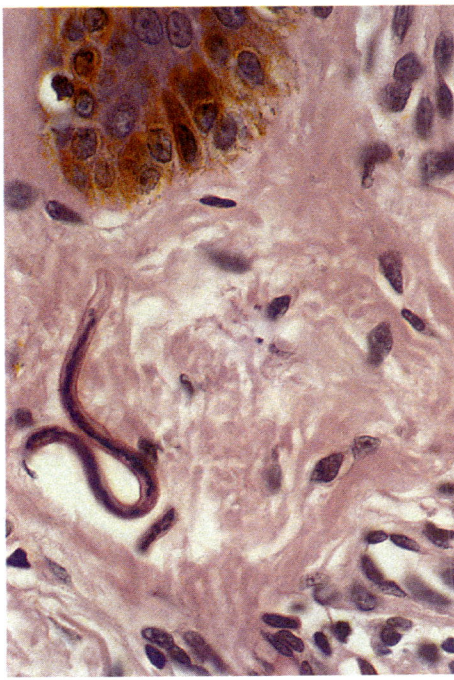

Fig. 29.108 Skin in onchocerciasis. A microfilaria under the epidermis, but no inflammation.

are rarely found. Expatriates infected for the first time in adulthood tend to be more reactive, with active dermatitis and rare or no detectable microfilariae.

The late sequelae of onchodermatitis are not histopathologically specific. There is epidermal acanthosis, hyperkeratosis, melanin depletion, and reduced dermal elastic tissue. Around the dermal vessels, the fibrous tissue is often concentrically arranged, as it is in chronic onchocercal lymph nodes (see below).

The effects of *treatment* are important in the clinical pathology of onchocerciasis. Until recently, the mainstay of chemotherapy has been diethylcarbamazine (DEC). This does not kill adult worms, or microfilariae *in vitro*. But *in vivo* it renders the microfilariae susceptible to immune-mediated destruction. This occurs in all patients, whether they were symptomatic or not from their infection. The resulting reactions are called the *Mazzotti reaction*. In the skin there are itchy oedematous papules developing within 24 hours, sometimes associated with fever, in sites where microfilariae are present.

Histopathologically, the Mazzotti reaction shows increased dermal oedema and perivascular inflammation. Specifically, there are small eosinophil abscesses at the dermo-epidermal junction, around a degenerating microfilaria (Fig. 29.109). Although this feature is not seen in biopsies of untreated onchodermatitis, it reinforces the accepted dogma that live microfilariae induce little or no host reaction, whereas damaged and degenerating ones are associated with pathology.

In summary, onchodermatitis shows an immunopathological spectrum comparable to that seen in lymphatic filariasis

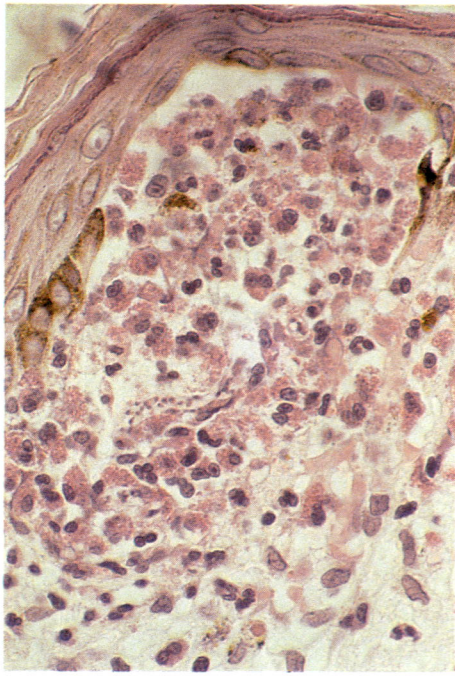

Fig. 29.109 Mazzotti skin reaction in onchocerciasis, after diethylcarbamazine treatment. At the dermo-epidermal junction is an eosinophil abscess around a degenerating microfilaria.

(see Section 29.11.1). Those people with absolute or relative tolerance to microfilarial antigens have less clinical disease than those who react to microfilariae.

Eye disease

Eye lesions are due to microfilariae migrating from adjacent facial skin. There are five ocular lesions:

1. punctate keratitis, fluffy opacities mainly at the periphery of the cornea, which leads to

2. sclerosing keratitis;

3. iridocyclitis, which produces synechiae and secondary glaucoma;

4. choroidoretinitis, with depigmentation of areas of retina;

5. optic neuritis and atrophy.

Slit-lamp examination reveals microfilariae floating in the anterior chamber of the eye, the modal densities being 10–30 microfilariae per eye. Histology of the cornea shows a process similar to onchodermatitis. Under the epithelium, microfilariae elicit oedema and a perivascular infiltrate of plasma cells and some eosinophils. The iritis is similar. Following DEC therapy, there is a more florid reaction to degenerating microfilariae; this Mazzotti reaction can produce acute irreversible inflammatory damage in the eye.

Lymph nodes

Enlarged lymph nodes, particularly inguinal, are common in patients with onchocerciasis. In Africa, it is associated with 'hanging groin', where a fold of lax inguinal skin containing a large node hangs down over the thigh. Elephantiasis of the scrotum may occasionally be associated with onchocerciasis, but chronic leg elephantiasis is not (any leg oedema usually resolves when the onchodermatitis resolves). In patients with hyperreactive skin lesions (sowda), node biopsy shows follicular hyperplasia and few or no microfilariae. More commonly, in Africa, the lymphadenopathy shows a progression. Early, there is follicular hyperplasia with numerous microfilaria in the nodal connective tissue, and surrounding eosinophils. Later, fibrosis replaces much of the node and the follicles atrophy. Blood vessels acquire a striking hyaline perivascular onion-skin-like proliferation; immunostaining shows local deposition of complement and immunoglobulin.

Pathogenesis

The major pathogenetic factor in onchocerciasis is the host reaction to microfilariae. It is probable that live migrating microfilariae cause no reaction; when they degenerate, either spontaneously or following chemotherapy, an inflammatory reaction results.

Immunocytochemical studies of onchodermatitis show that live microfilariae that are not involved in an inflammatory response are coated with IgE. In a Mazzotti reaction, specific IgG is found on microfilariae. IgG is known to mediate antibody-dependent cytotoxicity to microfilariae *in vitro*. Eosinophil degranulation and macrophage adherence result in death of the microflariae. Eosinophil MBP is an important toxic factor. Thus the current hypothesis is that non-reactive infected people have microfilariae coated with IgE, and no inflammation and no clinical dermatitis. In those people with dermatitis, IgG binds to the microfilariae and initiates cell-mediated killing. A correlation between severity of dermatitis and both serum antibody responses and delayed hypersensitivity skin reactions to onchocercal antigens supports this concept. All infected people produce a Mazzotti reaction when given DEC, indicating that everyone has the potential to react to onchocercal antigens.

One marked geographical difference in onchocerciasis is the higher incidence of blindness in people living in savannah zones compared with rain-forest. This may correlate with the proportion of adult worm nodules found on the head, which increases the likelihood of microfilariae migrating into the eye. But isoenzyme analysis also points to strain differences within *O. vulvulus*. These might also become important in explaining the different severities of onchodermatitis between people. None the less, as with lymphatic filariasis, the degree of intra-uterine or early postnatal exposure to onchocercal antigens may be relevant in determining the later outcome of infection.

Diagnosis and treatment

The diagnosis is made definitively by identifying adult worms or microfilariae. Biopsy of nodules, skin, or lymph nodes reveal the parasite. In the field, skin-snips are standard (see above). For ocular infection, a slip-lamp is needed.

Serodiagnosis, using crude *Onchocerca* worms as antigen, is sensitive, although the current systems lack specificity by cross-reacting with antibodies to other nematodes.

Treatment of onchocerciasis includes surgery (nodulectomy) and chemotherapy. Suramin kills adult worms, but is too toxic for general use. Diethylcarbamazine (DEC) removes microfilariae but in so doing causes the Mazzotti reaction (see above). The new drug, ivermectin, is promising. It does not kill adults but reduces microfilarial density in the skin to near zero within a week by an unknown process. The host reaction accompanying ivermectin therapy is not so severe as that seen with DEC. It also reduces microfilarial output from adult females by paralysing microfilariae in the uterus. However, microfilarial densities in skin-snips rise again to 30 per cent of pretreatment levels by 12 months.

29.11.4 *Dirofilaria*

Epidemiology

Dirofilaria species are parasites of dogs, cats, and wild mammals in all continents. *D. immitis* is distributed globally; *D. repens* is found in Europe, Africa, and Asia; *D. tenuis* occurs in North America. When man is accidentally infected with these zoonoses the worms do not mature to fertility, but die sterile.

Life cycle and morphology

In animals, *D. immitis* adults live in the right heart lumen; adults of other *Dirofilaria* species are in subcutaneous tissues. All have microfilariae circulating in the blood. The vector is a mosquito, when it takes a blood meal. After infection in man, the developing larva migrates. Microfilaraemia virtually never occurs in human infection. The adult worms are from 5 to 30 cm in length and have a diameter of 200–800 µm.

There are two clinico-pathological syndromes of human dirofilariasis, *D. immitis*, affecting the lungs, and *D. tenuis* and *D. repens* causing subcutaneous and orbital tumour-like swellings.

Pulmonary dirofilariasis

Clinical features and pathology

Adults are affected. Usually, the disease is picked up on chest X-ray as a coin-lesion, and resected as a presumed tumour. Symptoms such as cough and haemoptysis are unusual. Blood eosinophilia is not usually found.

Whereas in dogs the worm elicits no reaction within the right heart and pulmonary arteries, in man it causes pulmonary infarction. Probably the worms die in the right heart, are carried into the pulmonary arteries and impact. Grossly, the resected portion of lung has a peripheral necrotic nodule 1–4 cm in diameter. Histologically, the degenerate worm is embedded in thrombus within an artery. Early, the surrounding lung is pneumonic, with eosinophils and giant cells. Later, it becomes an organized infarct, with the worm barely dis-

tinguishable. Most cases have had a single worm. Virtually all the female *D. immitis* worms in man have been sterile. Only rarely, in an immunocompromised patient, have microfilariae been seen in the worm's uterus, indicating a fertile infection.

Subcutaneous dirofilariasis

Clinical features and pathology

The initial infective bite is not usually recalled. Where a migrating worm has become trapped by inflammation in subcutaneous tissues, a nodule forms, 1–3 cm in diameter, becoming tender. Arms, groin, breast, and salivary gland are typical sites. Conjunctival lesions occur when the worm can be seen migrating under the epithelium. Orbital infection results in proptosis. The nodules are usually solitary. Blood eosinophilia is mild.

The diagnosis is only made by surgical resection, which reveals a solid inflammatory mass or an abscess. Histologically, there is granulation tissue or an abscess containing longitudinal and cross-sections of a live or degenerate worm. In addition there is a fibrous capsule, variable tissue eosinophilia and often a granulomatous reaction. The worm is seen as several cross- and long-sections with a cuticle 10 µm thick. If a female, there may be unfertilized eggs in the uterus, but no microfilariae (Fig. 29.110). The lesions heal with scarring if not excised.

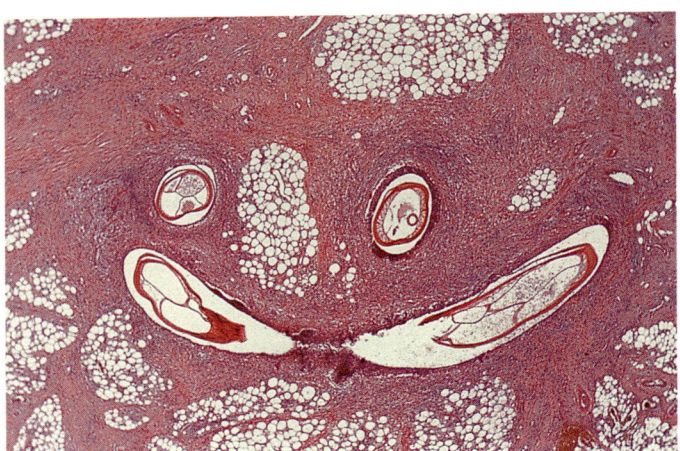

Fig. 29.110 Dirofilariasis. An inflammatory pseudotumour of the orbit; cross-sections of an adult *D. repens* worm.

The differential diagnosis is from a nodule containing *Onchocerca volvulus*. The latter occur particularly over bony prominences and contain more than one worm. Adult females are fertile, and microfilariae are seen in the uterus and migrating through the host tissues. The cuticle of the adult *O. volvulus* is thinner than that of *Dirofilaria*.

29.11.5 Further reading

Lichtenburg, F. von (1987). Inflammatory responses to connective tissue parasites. *Parasitology* **94**, S101–S122.

29.12   *Dracunculus*

Infection with the guinea-worm, *Dracunculus medinensis*, causes dracunculiasis. Although the adult resembles a filarial worm, it is not; it does not produce microfilariae.

Epidemiology

Infection occurs in many African countries, India, and Pakistan. Some 130 million rural inhabitants are at risk but recent estimates are of about 1 million cases per year (mainly in Africa) as eradication projects take effect. The global programme for eradication aims at breaking transmission at water sites (see 'Life cycle') by providing clean water. It is therefore hoped that a second edition of this textbook will require no reference to dracunculiasis.

Life cycle and morphology

Larvae freed from the host during contact with water enter a *Cyclops* crustacean intermediate host. Man is infected by drinking such contaminated water. The larvae burrows through the small bowel into the retroperitoneal connective tissues. Males and females mate, and the female migrates along muscle planes towards the skin surface. A skin blister forms through which the adult deposits larvae (of which she contains over 1 million). This cycle takes about 1 year. The adult female worm is up to 120 cm long and 1 mm wide. The larvae are 500×15 μm.

Clinical features

The intestinal phase is asymptomatic. The migrating adult may die before reaching the skin and form, for example, a paravertebral abscess. A tortuous subcutaneous worm track may be seen under the skin prior to the blister. The blister develops on the legs in 85 per cent of cases (Fig. 29.111), and less commonly on the groin, genitals, and back. The blister is preceded by fever, urticaria, and an itchy oedematous papule. The tip of

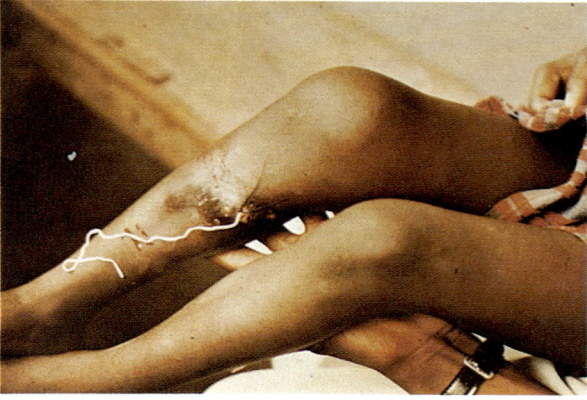

Fig. 29.111   Dracunculiasis (guinea-worm infection). A worm emerging from a sinus track below the knee, with associated soft-tissue swelling.

the worm protrudes through the subsequent ulcer and releases the larvae.

Secondary bacterial infection of the blister and subcutaneous tissues contributes to the morbidity. Such infection may involve joints, to cause septic arthritis and subsequent ankylosis. Arthritis may also follow migration of the worm into the joint space. Another complication is tetanus, which is the cause of death in this disease.

Apart from pain, the major effect of dracunculiasis is economic. The lack of mobility while the worm is discharging impairs the agricultural activity of infected farmers.

Pathology

Degenerate worms in the deep tissues calcify and may be found on X-ray. The main pathology commences once the female ruptures its uterus at the anterior end and larvae emerge. These induce an acute inflammatory reaction with polymorphs (but relatively few eosinophils) and make the blister, which then ulcerates. Following uterine rupture, a chronic inflammation develops along the length of the adult, which impedes its mechanical removal. Release of larvae into the synovial cavity causes an acute arthritis. If a worm ruptures prematurely in deeper tissues, such as muscle, an abscess containing up to 0.5 l of pus may form. Later there is a peripheral granulomatous reaction around the necrotic material.

Diagnosis and treatment

Diagnosis is usually obvious from the clinical appearances. No chemotherapeutic treatment is available; antihelminthics may reduce inflammation but apparently do not kill the worm. Careful removal of the intact worm through the blister—classically wound on to a stick—is still the mainstay.

29.13   Cestode infections

The taxonomy of cestode parasites is very complex, with new DNA studies altering the established concepts based on morphology, life cycles, and hosts. However, pathologically, cestode infections of man are categorized according to whether man is the definitive or the intermediate host. As definitive host, with adult tapeworms in the gut lumen, man is host to *Taenia saginata*, *T. solium*, and *Diphyllobothrium latum*. Much more important are the infections by larvae of *T. solium*, *Multiceps*, *Spirometra*, and, especially, *Echinococcus* species, where man is an intermediate host.

Cestode life cycles are essentially similar (Fig. 29.112). Adult worms live in the gut lumen, cause minimal damage, and release eggs which are eaten by an intermediate host. There the larvae forms a cyst containing a *scolex*, which is the head of a future adult worm. The definitive host eats this cyst and acquires a tapeworm in the bowel. With *Diphyllobothrium* and

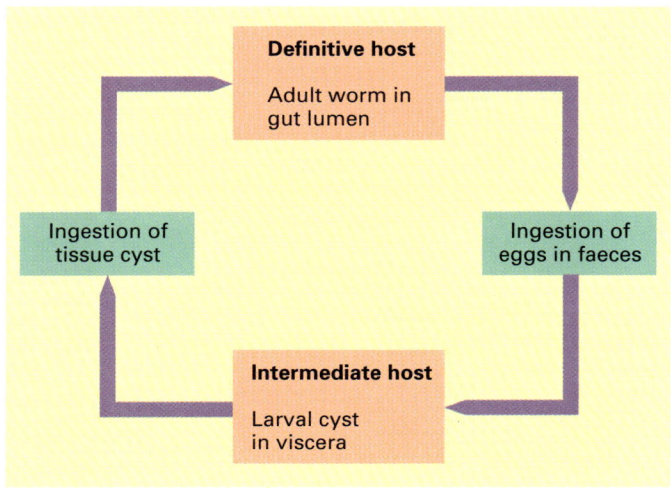

Fig. 29.112 General life cycle of the common human cestode infections.

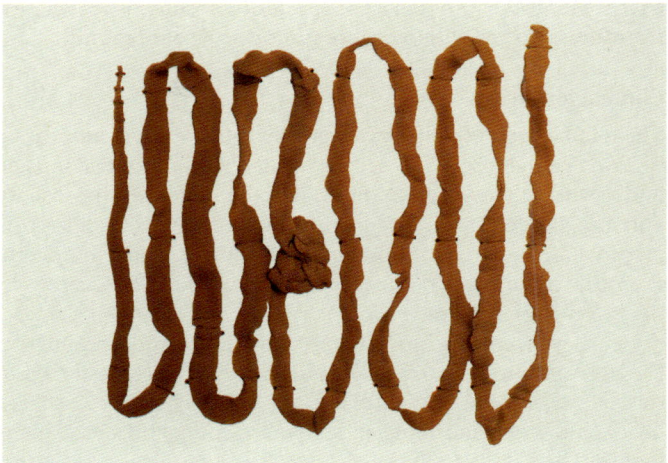

Fig. 29.113 A *Taenia saginata* worm, with head at the left. (Courtesy of St Thomas's Hospital Medical School Pathology Museum.)

Spirometra, there is a more complex sequence of intermediate hosts without formation of larval cysts.

29.13.1 Intestinal tapeworms—*Taenia* and *Diphyllobothrium*

Taenia saginata

Taenia saginata (the 'beef tapeworm') is cosmopolitan in distribution. It is acquired by eating undercooked cattle meat that contains larval cysts. The prevalence depends on the vigilance of veterinary inspection of meat in abattoirs (it has been eradicated from Britain). Some communities may have infection rates of up to 20 per cent.

The scolex (head) attaches to the small bowel mucosa, and the worm grows to a length of 5 m or more. There is usually only one worm at a time. The 1000–2000 proglottids that comprise the worm each measure 12×10 mm (Fig. 29.113). They contain eggs which measure 43×31 μm. Distal gravid proglottids are shed from the worm into the faeces.

The worm causes no clinical or pathological lesion by its presence in the intestine. But there may be psychological upset when shed segments are felt crawling about the anus or are seen in faeces. Unlike *T. solium*, *T. saginata* cannot produce a larval infection in man.

Taenia solium

Taenia solium (the 'pork tapeworm') is also cosmopolitan, and is acquired by eating undercooked pig meat that contains larval cysts. The adult worm is similar to *T. saginata* morphologically; the eggs are identical. Distinction between the species is made on the morphology of the uterus in a proglottid.

Like *T. saginata*, *T. solium* does not cause any clinical disease as an intestinal infection. However as a larval infection, cysticercosis (see below), *T. solium* is highly pathological.

Diphyllobothrium latum

Diphyllobothrium latum is the third and longest (up to 10 m) intestinal tapeworm infection of man. *D. latum* is widespread in temperate and Arctic zones, acquired from eating fish. The tapeworm is generally listed as a cause of vitamin B_{12} deficiency because it can consume the vitamin in the diet. However, the incidence of this complication is vanishingly rare.

29.13.2 *Taenia solium* cysticercosis

Man may be both definitive and intermediate host to *T. solium*. As the latter host, the disease caused by larval cysts is called *cysticercosis*. The larvae migrate via the bloodstream to the viscera.

Epidemiology

Cysticercosis is cosmopolitan. To acquire the disease requires ingestion of eggs (Fig. 29.112). Seventy-five per cent of patients do not have the adult *T. solium* tapeworm in their intestine. Despite the oft-quoted notion of auto-infection, by swallowing regurgitated eggs from a worm in their own bowel, most patients probably ingest eggs from another person's worm.

The most serious form of cysticercosis is intracranial disease, *neurocysticercosis*. In areas of high prevalence, such as Mexico and South-East Asia, neurocysticercosis is a commoner cause of intracranial space-occupying lesions than neoplasms.

Morphology

The classical cysticercus is a 0.5–1.5 cm diameter, translucent, white, fluid-filled vesicle. It contains one invaginated scolex (the head of a future adult worm) that has four suckers and two rows of hooks. In the brain, there is also an uncommon variant form called a *racemose* cyst. This is larger, at 10–20 cm diameter, rounded or forming a lobulated bladder resembling a cluster of grapes. It contains no scolex. It has been proposed that such cysts are of different species or strains of *Taenia*, but transitional forms with a disintegrating scolex are found.

Clinical features

The incubation period for cysticercosis may be a few months or several years. Most cysticerci are located within skeletal muscle and are usually asymptomatic. When the cysts die, they calcify and may be identified on radiology. Subcutaneous cysticercosis presents as one or more soft small tumours. Cardiac cysticerci are found at autopsy, but are not symptomatic. A cysticercus in the eye causes impaired vision.

Neurocysticercosis has several presentations, depending on the site and number of cysts within the brain: focal lesions and raised intracranial pressure are the main features, causing headache, focal neurological signs, epilepsy, and basal meningitis. The CSF usually has a raised protein level. Peripheral blood eosinophilia is absent or slight.

The majority of patients with neurocysticercosis do not have identifiable cysts elsewhere in the body. The precise mortality of neurocysticercosis is difficult to assess, but is significant.

Pathology

The cysts grow slowly and live for an uncertain length of time (though estimates are 6 months to 2 years). In muscle or subcutis, they appear grossly as small bladders within a capsule. In the brain, they may be located in the meninges, parenchyma, and in or around the ventricles (Fig. 29.114). Those around the ventricles and in the meninges produce symptoms by disturbing the flow of CSF and causing intracranial hypertension.

The host reaction to a viable cyst is often minimal, particularly in the brain: a thin rim of fibrous tissue, slight chronic inflammation without granulomas, and no eosinophilia (Fig. 29.115). In the subcutis, the fibrous capsule may be thicker. When a cyst dies spontaneously or following chemotherapy, there is usually more inflammation. Local eosinophilia, granulation tissue, sometimes a polymorph abscess,

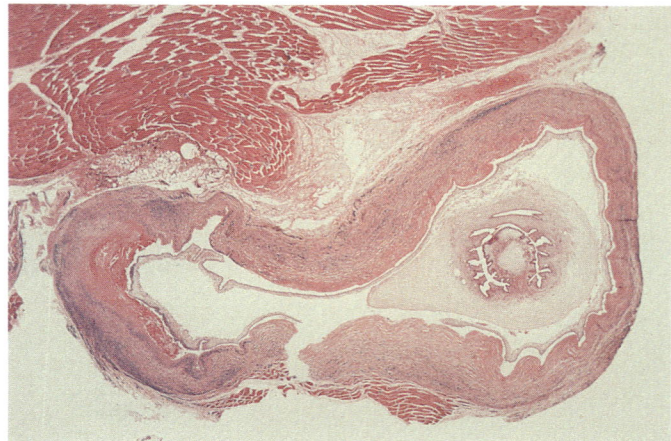

Fig. 29.115   Cysticercus in muscle. The fibrous capsule and the scolex are seen.

and a granulomatous reaction follow. Thus, the size of the cysticercus, and its space-occupying effect, increase. With neurocysticercosis, this is seen as oedema around the cysts on CT scans, and increased protein and cell content in the CSF. In all tissues, the parasite disintegrates and often calcifies within a residual fibrous scar.

This host reaction follows release of antigenic material from the degenerating larval cyst. Initial clinical presentation is often due to this. In patients with neurocysticercosis, chemotherapy often exacerbates symptoms and signs as the inflammation enlarges the lesions. If there has been meningitis, fibrosis, and subsequent raised intracranial pressure, then anticysticercal chemotherapy will not necessarily ameliorate the condition.

Diagnosis and treatment

The diagnosis is made on clinical features, CT scanning, biopsy, and serology. Serology is not totally sensitive, since only 80 per cent of those with neurocysticercosis are positive. The current chemotherapy is praziquantel, which kills cysts. To reduce the subsequent inflammation, steroids are often administered. Praziquantel reduces the number and size of intracranial cysts as indicated on follow-up CT scans.

29.13.3   *Multiceps*

Several species of carnivore taeniid tapeworms can parasitize man accidentally, with visceral larval cysts similar to cysticercosis. But the cysts (in man and natural intermediate hosts) contain numerous scolices, not one as in *T. solium* cysticercosis; hence the genus term *Multiceps*. The disease is called *coenurosis*. It is widespread, if uncommon, in temperate and tropical countries.

Infection is by eating eggs, which hatch, penetrate the bowel, and disseminate. In Africa, most cases present as subcutaneous or intramuscular tumours on the chest wall or trunk. Outside Africa, the brain and eye are more commonly parasitized, the

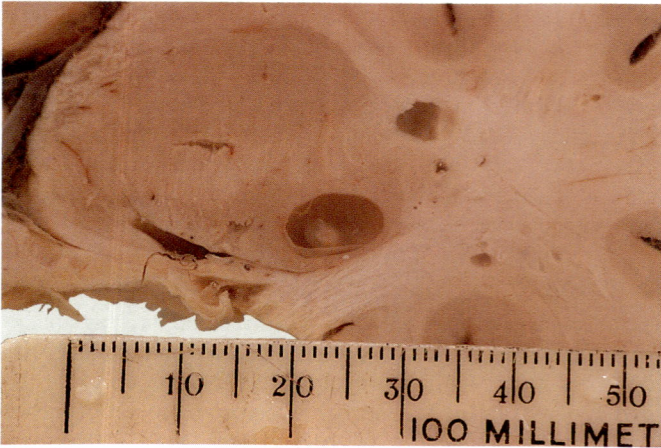

Fig. 29.114   Brain with cysticercosis. In the basal ganglia is a cyst containing a solid scolex.

coenurus cysts forming space-occupying lesions. These clinical differences probably represent different species of *Multiceps*.

Pathologically, the inflammatory lesion is 1–10 cm in diameter. The coenurus cyst is rounded or branching. The host reaction includes granulomas, fibrosis, and eosinophilia. Within the parasite cyst wall, dozens of scolices with hooks may be seen.

29.13.4 *Spirometra* (sparganosis)

Infection by the larva of *Spirometra* species is known as *sparganosis*, 'sparganum' being the taxonomic term for the larva. *Spirometra mansoni* is the usual parasite in man.

Epidemiology, life cycle, and morphology

Human sparganosis is uncommon, but distributed throughout the tropics and subtropics. The normal hosts for the adult tapeworm are carnivores. From eggs deposited in water, larval stages pass along the food chain from *Cyclops* crustacea, to amphibians and reptiles, to carnivorous mammals. Many vertebrates, including man, can be paratenic hosts. Human infection is usually by drinking water containing infected *Cyclops*, or by eating meat containing a sparganum.

The sparganum is a non-segmented, solid white worm, 20–40 cm long and 2–3 mm wide. It has no hooks or sucker.

Clinical features and pathology

The larva penetrates the bowel wall and migrates through the tissues to virtually any site of the body. It may cause peritonitis by perforating the intestine, but more commonly presents as a migratory subcutaneous swelling or as a localized inflammatory mass. This may be in the subcutis, for example in the groin and breast, or the orbit (causing proptosis), and even within the brain.

The infection is diagnosed by resection. A viable sparganum elicits little host reaction, but a degenerating larva produces an encapsulated inflammatory mass with surrounding fibrosis (Fig. 29.116). There is an intense eosinophilic response, with Charcot–Leyden crystals and variable numbers of granulomas (Fig. 29.117).

29.13.5 *Echinococcus*

Dogs and other carnivores, such as wolves and foxes, in all parts of the world may harbour various *Echinococcus* tapeworms in the bowel. These are small, all less than 1 cm long. The natural intermediate hosts that eat eggs and acquire larval cysts (Fig. 29.112) are in two categories:

1. domestic animals such as sheep, cattle, horses, and camels—the 'domestic' or 'pastoral' life cycle; and

2. wild herbivores such as deer, elk, and field rodents—the 'feral' or 'sylvatic' life cycle.

Man may acquire larval cysts, called *hydatids*. The subsequent

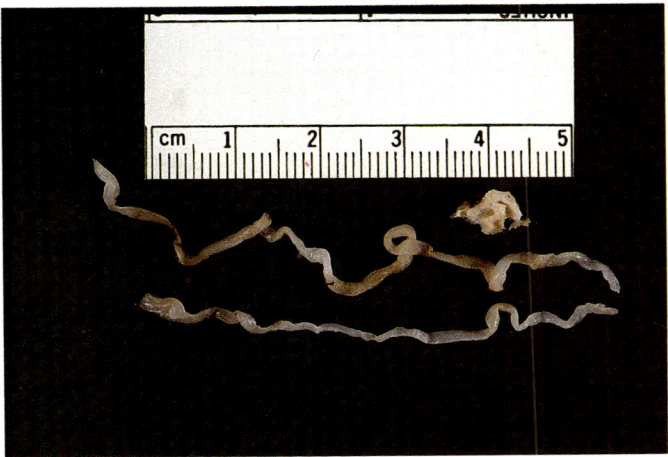

Fig. 29.116 Sparganosis. A sparganum resected from an inguinal mass.

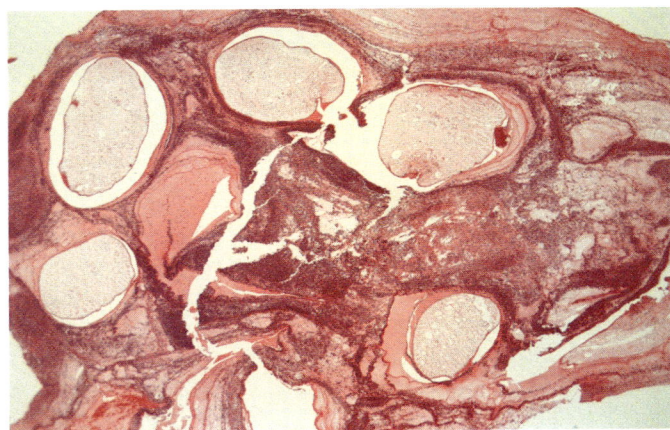

Fig. 29.117 Sparganosis. Cross-sections of a coiled sparganum in an eosinophil abscess.

disease, *echinococcosis*, is the most important of human cestode infections.

The commonest *Echinococcus* species to affect man is *E. granulosus*. It causes disease as a space-occupying lesion (Fig. 29.118). Less common, but more morbid, is *E. multilocularis*.

Echinococcus granulosus

Epidemiology

Although global in distribution (Iceland used to have a high prevalence until dog control was introduced), the highest prevalences of hydatid cyst in men are in north and east Africa, and the Middle East. Ultrasound surveys in Kenya show that, in some areas, up to 10 per cent of people have one or more intra-abdominal cysts. The proportion increases with age. Most infections are acquired through the domestic life cycle, there being close contact with dogs that harbour worms.

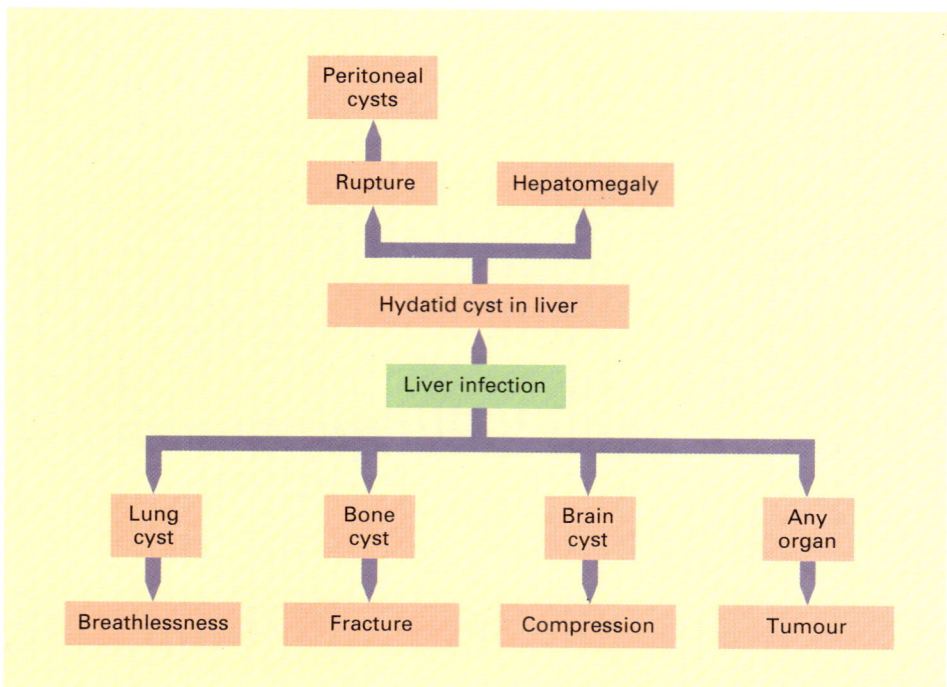

Fig. 29.118 Sequelae of infection with *Echinococcus granulosus*.

Although 'E. granulosus' is a species, it is evident that there are significant strain variations. In the UK, the dog/horse cycle is common (50 per cent of horses are affected), but man is nearly always infected via the dog/sheep life cycle, which is a genetically distinct strain.

Morphology

The larva that hatches from an egg in the bowel travels to the liver, and may then pass via the bloodstream to any part of the body. Hydatid cysts grow slowly, up to 2 cm per year. At presentation they may be up to 50 cm across, but 8–10 cm is more usual, depending on the organ involved. The parasite has an outer 1–2 mm thick white, soft, smooth membrane ('laminated' membrane). On its inner surface is the single-layer germinal epithelium, from which bud the scolices (the heads of future tapeworms). A scolex is ovoid and 100 μm long. It has four suckers, and hooks; these mouth-parts are often seen invaginated. The cyst is filled with clear fluid—'hydatid fluid'. Loose scolices in the fluid may be seen as tiny refractile dots with the naked eye—'hydatid sand'.

In about half the cases, the hydatid cyst is unilocular. The rest contain one or more 'daughter cysts', which are smaller internal cysts that have developed off the germinal membrane (Figs 29.119–29.121). Not all hydatid cysts are alive and fertile. Degenerate ones collapse and fold up (through not secreting hydatid fluid).

Clinical features

Many hydatid cysts are asymptomatic. The sites most commonly affected are liver (80 per cent of all cysts), upper abdominal peritoneal cavity, lung, spleen, and bone. However, in highly endemic zones, a tumour at any site may be presumed to be a hydatid cyst until proved otherwise. Multiple cysts, in several organs, are common.

Clinical presentation depends on the size and site of cysts. They act as space-occupying lesions. Within the liver, they cause hepatomegaly, but do not usually compress the biliary tree to produce jaundice. Occasionally, a liver hydatid cyst becomes secondarily infected with bacteria, and fills with pus.

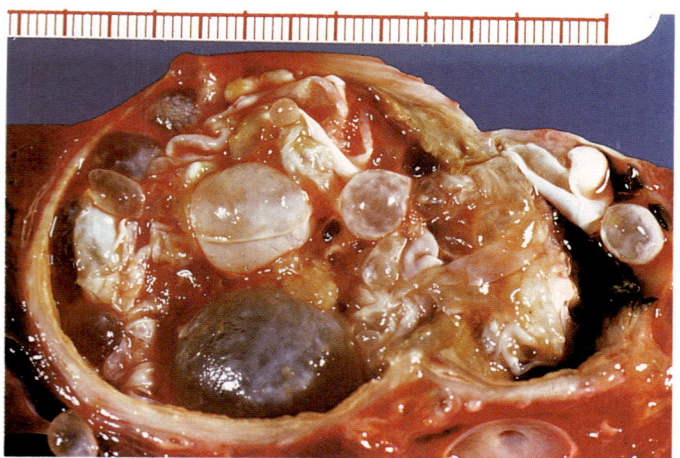

Fig. 29.119 Liver hydatid cyst with several smaller daughter cysts. The cyst is encapsulated by fibrous tissue.

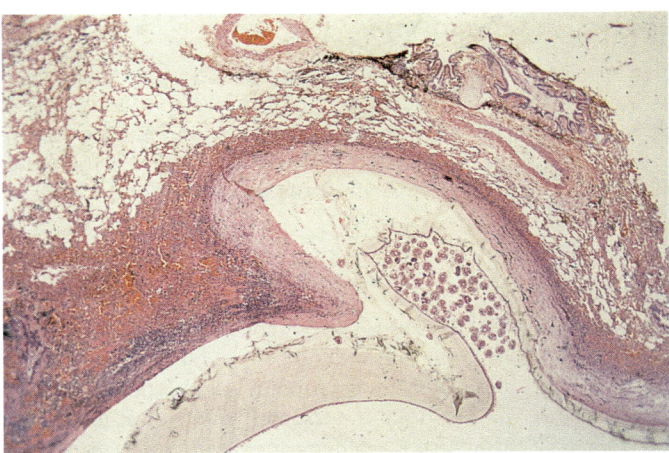

Fig. 29.120 Hydatid cyst in lung, showing thin fibrous capsule, the pale laminated membrane, and several scolices.

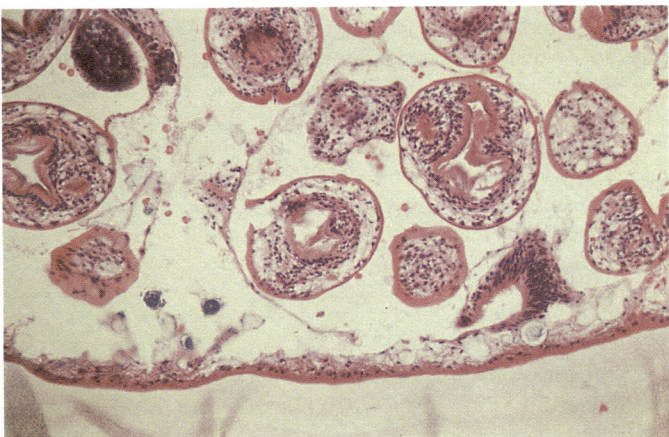

Fig. 29.121 Hydatid cyst. Numerous scolices that are budding off the germinal layer.

Loops of bowel may adhere to peritoneal cysts and cause intestinal obstruction. A splenic hydatid is the commonest aetiology of a cyst in that organ. Pulmonary cysts cause cough and dyspnoea and are seen on chest X-ray as rounded opacities. Hydatid cysts within bone produce pathological fractures; if in the vertebrae they compress the spinal cord. Intracranial hydatids may obstruct the flow of CSF and dilate ventricles. Hydatid cysts may rupture: this can discharge the contents into the pleural cavity, bronchus, biliary tree, or peritoneum, depending on the site of the original cyst. Secondly, such rupture disseminates the disease by spreading germinal membrane and scolices which can seed and initiate another cyst.

If hydatid fluid (containing antigen) leaks into the bloodstream of a sensitized individual, there may be an immediate anaphylactic reaction with respiratory and circulatory distress. This can happen after inadvertent liver biopsy of a cyst; but curiously, anaphylaxis does not occur if such leakage takes place under general anaesthesia.

Pathology

The intact hydatid cyst induces a small host reaction: a thin fibrous wall, slight non-granulomatous inflammation, and no significant eosinophil infiltrate (Fig. 29.120). This pattern is seen in all affected organs. When part or all of a cyst degenerates, the laminated membrane collapses and fragments. Then a giant-cell granulomatous reaction develops with phagocytosis of membranes. In degenerate cysts, scolices are not usually found on histology. In chronic cases of hydatid cyst there may be persistent discharge through a skin sinus of fragments of degenerate membrane, accompanied by a mixed inflammatory infiltrate.

Diagnosis and treatment

The diagnosis of hydatid cyst includes clinical features, ultrasound, surgical resection, and serology. Fine-needle aspiration cytology is often diagnostic, finding scolices or only hooks (which stain red with the Ziehl–Neelsen method).

Treatment is difficult. Cysts in some sites may be readily resected, but care not to spill hydatid material and thus disseminate the disease is essential. Silver nitrate or formalin is instilled into an opened cyst prior to resection to sterilize the contents. There is no satisfactory chemotherapeutic agent that is certain to kill the germinal membrane and treat inoperable hydatids (which comprise the majority of presentations). Albendazole and related compounds do reduce the size of cysts in many patients.

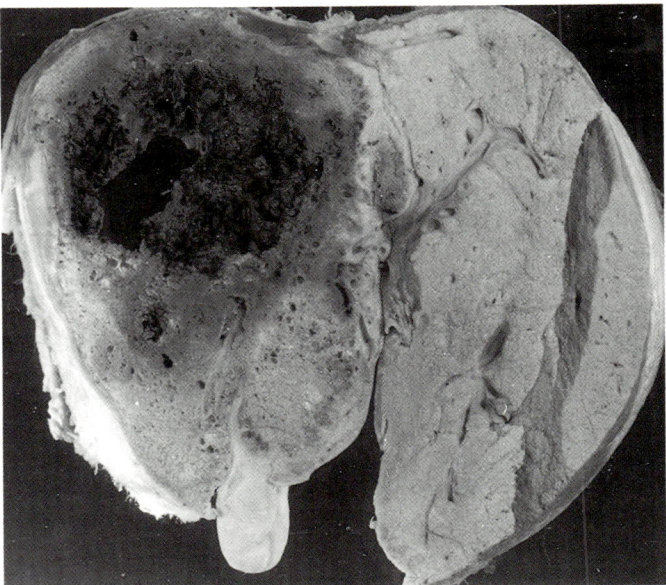

Fig. 29.122 *Echinococcus multilocularis* cyst in liver (alveolar hydatid). In contrast with an *E. granulosus* cyst, this is not contained within a capsule but invades the liver like a malignant tumour, causing massive necrosis. (Photograph courtesy of the Wellcome Museum of Medical Science.)

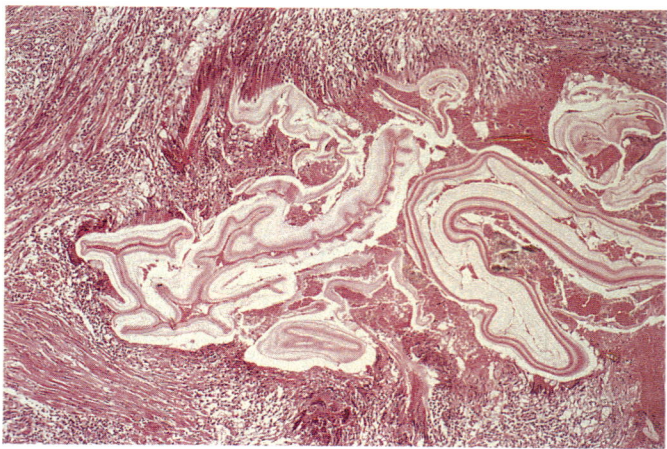

Fig. 29.123 *E. multilocularis* cyst. It is infiltrating the liver with much necrosis, and there are no scolices.

Echinococcus multilocularis

Epidemiology and morphology

E. multilocularis infection in man is called 'alveolar hydatid'. It is restricted to the temperate and Arctic regions of mainland Europe, Asia, and North America.

In natural intermediate hosts, the larval cyst grows more rapidly than does *E. granulosus*. In man the same applies, but *E. multilocularis* infection is so unnatural that scolices do not form within the proliferating cyst.

Clinical features and pathology

The infection commences in the liver. It presents as a rapidly growing tumour, simulating a cancer, with anorexia and wasting. Metastasis of the infection to lung and brain are common. Death is usually rapid, although recently chemotherapy with albendazole appears to be successful in some cases.

In the liver at autopsy *E. multilocularis* is a part-solid part-multicystic, expanding, and destructive lesion (Fig. 29.122). Histologically, the cyst wall is acellular and irregular. It invades into the parenchyma and produces a wide rim of peripheral necrosis. There is no host fibrotic reaction to encapsulate (and restrict) the growing cyst (Fig. 29.123). Surrounding inflammation may be absent or granulomatous. Scolices are not found within the cysts.

29.14   Trematode infections

Five genera of flukes are important as invasive human infections: *Schistosoma*, *Fasciola*, *Clonorchis*, *Opisthorcis*, and *Paragonimus* (Fig. 29.124). There are several intestinal trematodes (e.g. *Fasciolopsis*) which do not invade tissues and cause relatively little disease.

29.14.1   *Schistosoma*

Five species of *Schistosoma* flukes produce the visceral disease in man called *schistosomiasis*, or *bilharzia* (Fig. 29.125). The three most important are *S. mansoni*, *S. haematobium*, and *S. japonicum*. Small numbers of people have *S. intercalatum* and *S. mekongi*. Various animal schistosomes can cause a transient skin infection.

Epidemology

Globally some 600 million people living in the tropics are at risk of schistosomiasis, with 200 million people infected, the majority in Africa. *S. haematobium* is found in Africa and the Middle East; *S. japonicum* in China and the Philippines (but no longer infects people in Japan); *S. mansoni* in Africa, South America, and the West Indies; *S. intercalatum* in West and Central Africa; and *S. mekongi* along the Mekong River in South-East Asia.

In zones of intense transmission, infection is constant and the peak prevalence and intensity of infection occur, between the ages of 10 and 20 years. Nearly 100 per cent of children may be infected. Prevalence of infection then declines to about 50 per cent by the age of 65 years. This is partly due to decreased water contact and hence reduced reinfection. But there is also evidence that acquired immunity to reinfection develops in time. As with many worm infections, the burden of infection is skewed, the majority having light and mild or asymptomatic infection. However, a light infection may prove clinically serious if it is in an unusual organ (e.g. spinal cord).

Life cycle and morphology

The transmission of schistosomiasis is by contact with fresh water (Fig. 29.124). A *cercaria* burrows through the skin and sheds its tail to become a *schistosomulum* (immature worm). This migrates via veins to the pulmonary vasculature to mature for about 4 weeks (it is at this skin/lung stage that attrition of worms through immunity occurs). Then the worm migrates with the cardiac output arterial flow to a final location. For *S. mansoni*, *S. japonicum*, *S. mekongi*, and *S. intercalatum* this is usually the mesenteric veins, reached via the intestinal capillaries. For *S. haematobium*, the perivesical and perirectal veins are the preferred sites. However, worms may end up within any veins in the body and produce local disease ('ectopic' schistosomiasis).

In veins, male and female worms copulate and release eggs into the bloodstream (Figs 29.126, 29.127). Although worms may live for more than 30 years and cause disease long after infection, this is unusual and the average life-span for *Schistosoma* adults is 3–5 years. *S. japonicum* is estimated to release 3000 eggs per worm pair per day; the other species about 300 per day. About half the eggs exit the body (*S. haematobium* via the urine or faeces; the other species via the faeces). The remainder are retained in the body.

On contacting fresh water, an egg hatches into a miracidium, which penetrates a water snail of the appropriate species. Within the snail hepatopancreas, further multiplication takes

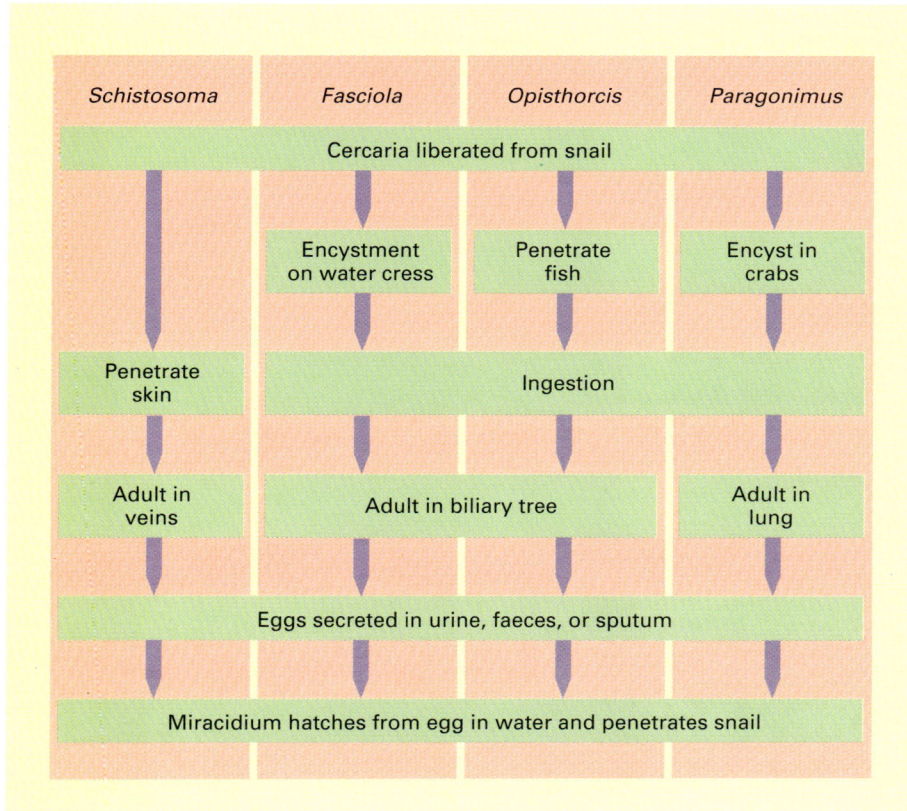

Fig. 29.124 Life cycles of trematode infections: *Schistosoma*, *Fasciola*, *Opisthorcis/Clonorchis*, and *Paragonimus*.

place and cercariae are released into the water. As well as man, *S. japonicum* infects animals, ranging from rodents to dogs and cattle. The other *Schistosoma* species are anthropophilic only.

Adult male schistosome worms are 10–20 mm long and females are up to 30 mm long; they are 0.3 mm wide. The eggs are characteristic of the species. *S. mansoni* has a lateral spine and measures 140×60 μm (Fig. 29.127); *S. haematobium* and *S. intercalatum* have a terminal spine and measure 160×60 and 180×60 μm respectively; *S. japonicum* and *S. mekongi* eggs possess tiny lateral spines and are rounder, measuring 85×60 and 60×45 μm, respectively. The function of the spine is unknown.

Clinical features and pathology

Schistosomiasis may be divided into two phases: early disease, comprising cercarial dermatitis and acute schistosomiasis (Katayama syndrome); and chronic infection, which is by far the most important aspect.

Cercarial dermatitis (swimmer's itch)

Usually cercarial penetration is asymptomatic. But in heavy infections, especially those infected for the first time, a local itchy papular rash develops within a few hours and lasts for a week. A similar rash follows infection with purely zoonotic schistosomes (usually parasites of birds), which are not restricted to the tropics; these infections do not mature beyond the skin stage in man. Histologically, the schistosomulum in the upper dermis elicits an eosinophil-rich perivascular infiltrate and granulomas, which kill the worm in zoonotic infections.

Acute schistosomiasis

Often known as the *Katayama syndrome*, acute schistosomiasis is a systemic disease seen mainly in people acquiring any *Schistosome* infection for the first time. It is most severe in schistosomiasis japonicum, and least common and serious in *S. haematobium* infection. The interval between infection and symptoms is generally 30–40 days. The major manifestations are fever, abdominal pain, diarrhoea, cough, urticaria, lymphadenopathy, mild hepatosplenomegaly, and (in *S. japonicum* infection) meningoencephalitis. Eosinophilia, raised IgM and IgG levels, and high titres of species-specific antischistosomal antibodies are found in blood samples. The syndrome lasts up to several weeks; death is uncommon.

Pathogenetically, several processes operate in Katayama syndrome. The pulmonary lesions, sometimes accompanied by diffuse fine infiltrates on chest X-ray, may reflect host reaction to maturing worms. Many cases commence at the onset of egg-laying, and the intestinal and hepatic disturbances could be due to local anti-egg inflammation. However, the syndrome is also noted within 1–2 weeks of infection, long before eggs are laid. Circulating schistosomal antigen and immune complexes have been identified in the blood. This suggests a humoral

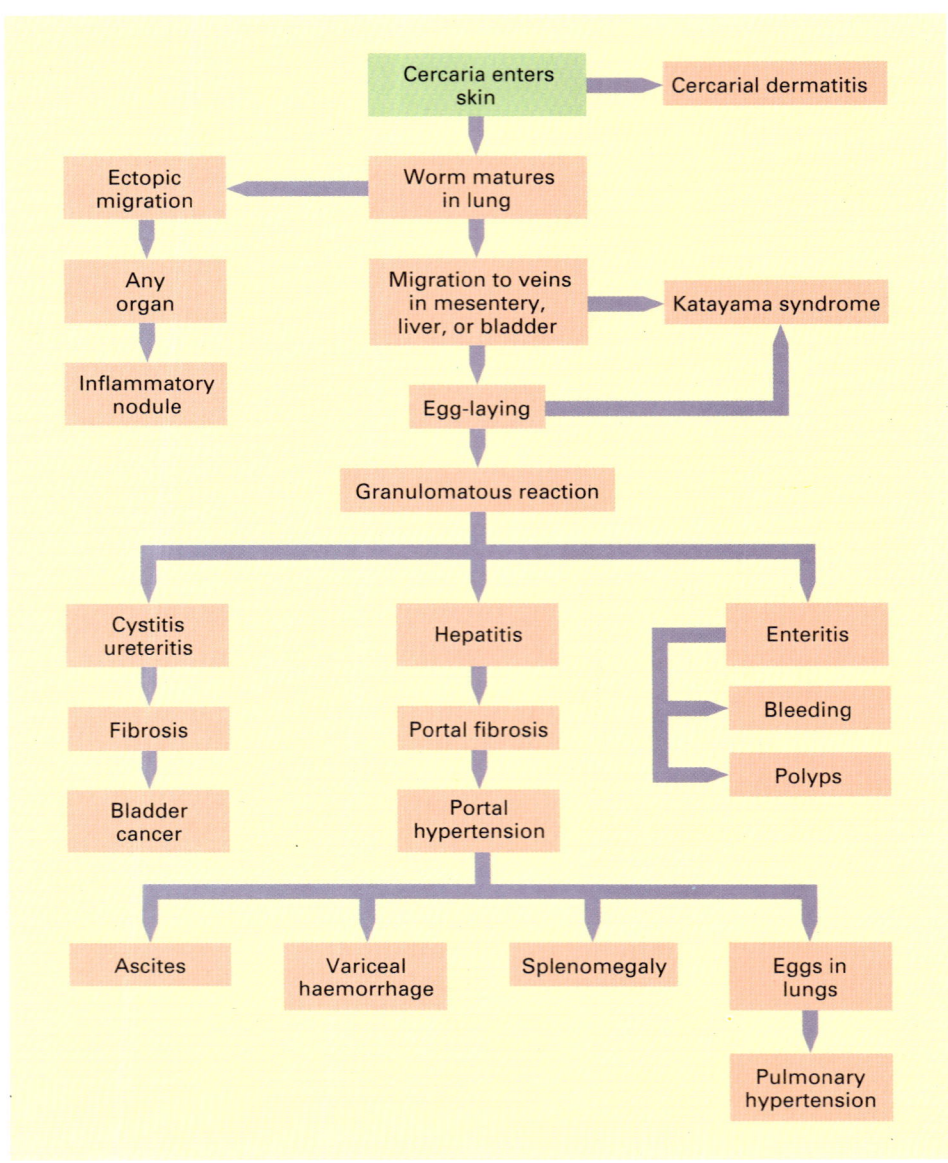

Fig. 29.125 Sequelae of infection with *Schistosoma* species.

immunological process affecting small blood vessels around the body, analogous to serum sickness (although nephritis does not occur).

Chronic schistosomiasis

Schistosome worms do not multiply in the host. The eggs released from the female induce an inflammatory host reaction where they impact in vessels, and this produces disease. Peripheral blood eosinophilia is usual in patients with schistosomiasis.

Schistosoma mansoni

The main pathologies of schistosomiasis mansoni are in the

liver and intestine. Schistosomiasis is the commonest cause of significant portal hypertension in the world.

Liver disease

Liver disease is the major clinical pathology due to infection with *S. mansoni* (and *S. japonicum*). A large proportion of eggs retained in the body are carried to the liver in the portal vein. In the early stages of heavy infection, there is mild hepatomegaly. The syndrome of *hepatosplenic schistosomiasis* (HSS) occurs when there is significant periportal fibrosis and portal hypertension. The liver is then usually small or of normal size. The spleen is enlarged (up to 1 kg or more), there is porto-systemic venous shunting, and, in the late stages, ascites. Clinical presentation is

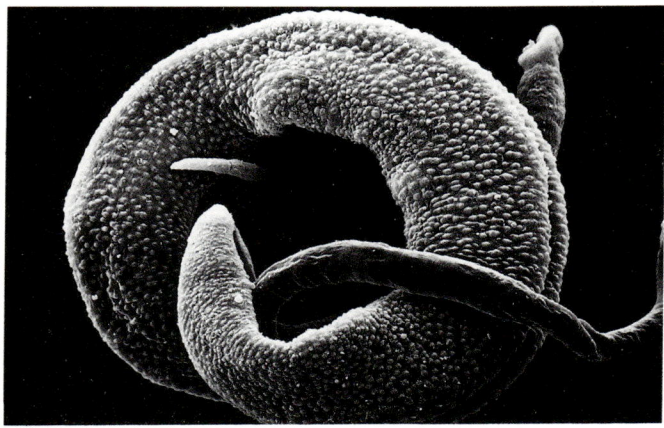

Fig. 29.126 Scanning electron micrograph of *Schistosoma mansoni* worms. The thinner female is wrapped within the larger male. (Photograph courtesy of Dr V. Zaman.)

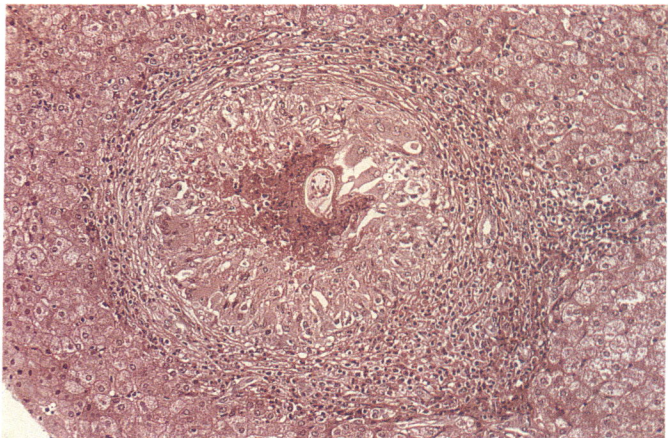

Fig. 29.128 Hepatic schistosomiasis. An egg in a portal tract is surrounded by a fibrinoid deposit and a tuberculoid granuloma.

veins of about 50 μm diameter. Secreted egg antigens induce a mixed tuberculoid granuloma and eosinophil reaction in portal triads (Fig. 29.128). The diameter of the egg granuloma is about 230 μm (one hundred times the volume of the egg itself). In some cases, there may be a rim of fibrinoid material around an egg, composed of antibody, fibrin, and eosinophil granules. This is termed a Hoeppli–Splendore reaction (and may also be found around other infectious agents). In older granulomas the eggs are phagocytosed and healing is with fibrous scars. Grossly, this is the miliary pattern of liver schistosomiasis. In Kupffer cells and portal tract macrophages, a haemozoin pigment similar to that of malaria infection accumulates. This is a metabolic product of the *Schistosoma* worm as it feeds on haemoglobin.

In HSS, the major portal tracts are grossly thickened with fibrous tissue, often termed *Symmers' clay pipestem fibrosis* (Figs 29.129–29.131). The external appearance of the liver is irregular and nodular. However, this is not true cirrhosis; the architecture of the hepatic lobules is intact. The periportal fibrosis comprises dense collagen and blood vessels, and, typically, few

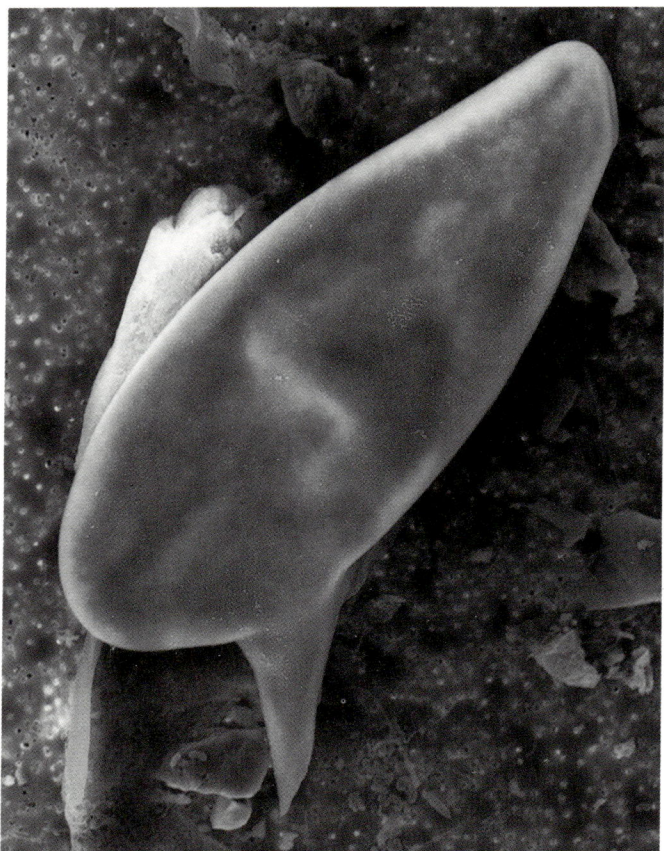

Fig. 29.127 Scanning electron micrograph of a *S. mansoni* egg. The lateral spine is distinctive for this species but of no obvious function.

commonly with bleeding oesophageal varices. Ultrasound epidemiological studies confirm that HSS can develop within a decade of chronic infection, with 5 per cent of adolescents in endemic zones having severe periportal fibrosis.

The eggs that are carried into the liver are entrapped in portal

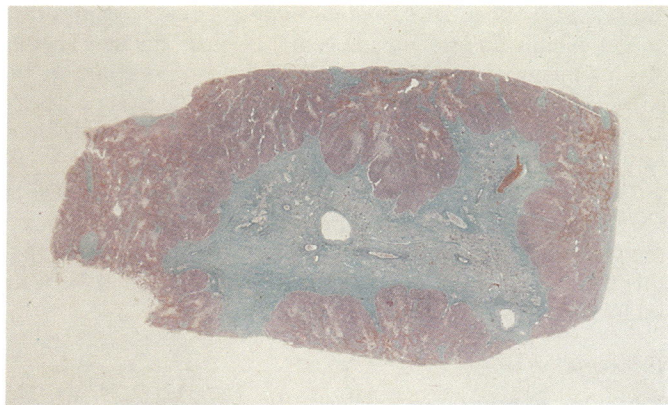

Fig. 29.129 Hepatic schistosomiasis. A whole mount showing severe portal fibrosis (green = collagen; trichrome stain).

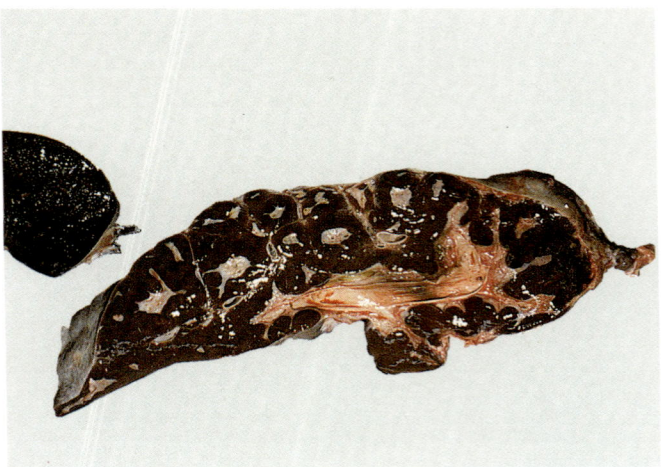

Fig. 29.130 Symmers' clay pipestem fibrosis of the liver. Around the portal tracts is dense, white fibrous tissue.

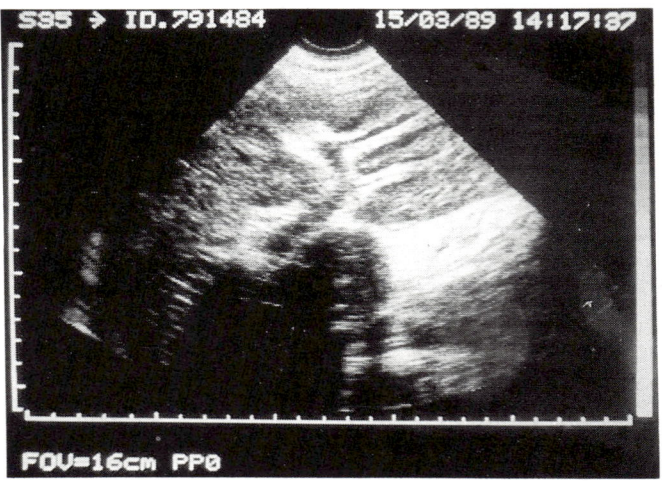

Fig. 29.131 Hepatic schistosomiasis. An ultrasound scan showing thickened fibrotic portal veins. (Photograph courtesy of Dr S. Houston.)

granulomas. When HSS patients suffer variceal bleeding, they do not usually go into hepatic coma. Because the liver lobules are relatively normal, the metabolic load from blood in the bowel can be processed by the hepatocytes. There is no association between hepatic schistosomiasis and primary liver carcinoma.

The spleen in HSS has a thickened capsule. Pathologically, it shows sinusoidal congestion and lymphoid hyperplasia. Part of the splenomegaly is the immunological reactive hyperplasia to this intravascular infection. There is no association between schistosomiasis and lymphoma of the spleen.

Intestinal disease

Intestinal schistosomiasis affects the large bowel with diarrhoea, pain, and bleeding per rectum. The bleeding is caused by the eggs breaking out of vessels in the submucosa and

mucosa, and penetrating through the mucosal crypt epithelium. Grossly, the mucosa has small petechial haemorrhages. In heavy infection, the bowel wall may be thickened and there are inflammatory polyps (Fig. 29.132). Histologically, live eggs induce an eosinophilic and granulomatous reaction (Fig. 29.133). It is very likely that the host inflammation facilitates excretion of eggs from the bowel. Degenerate eggs retained in the bowel wall may have no apparent host reaction.

In patients without hepatosplenic schistosomiasis, the intensity of infection in the intestine, as measured by counting tissue eggs, declines linearly from rectum to small bowel. In those with hepatosplenic disease, the main load is shifted proximally to the transverse colon. Tissue digestion studies show that in grossly normal bowel, the mean egg density ranges from 500 to 2000 eggs per gram of tissue. In polyps, there may be > 20 000 eggs/g.

Schistosomal granulomas (of all species) are found in the appendix, usually in the submucosa. However, there is no evidence that it predisposes to acute obstructive appendicitis.

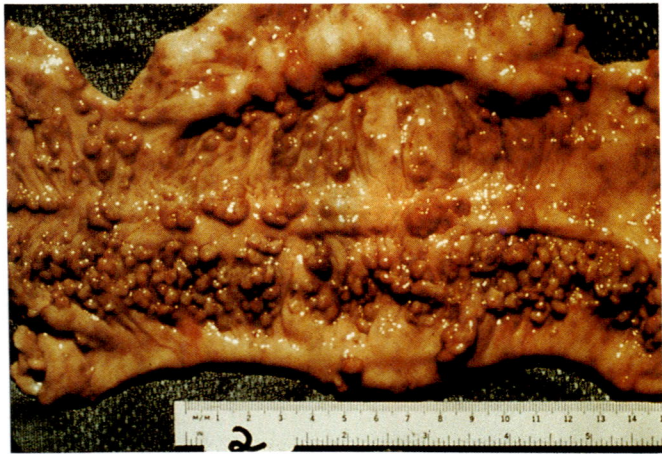

Fig. 29.132 Intestinal schistosomiasis. Numerous inflammatory polyps on the colonic mucosa.

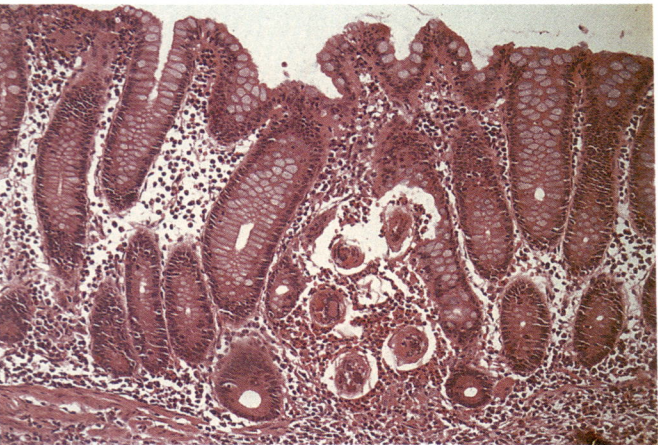

Fig. 29.133 Schistosomal colitis. Eggs in the mucosa, breaking into crypts.

Pulmonary disease

Schistosomal eggs are commonly found in the lungs of patients with hepatosplenic schistosomiasis. The porto-systemic collateral circulation permits eggs to be carried to the lungs. However, significant pathology with pulmonary hypertension is uncommon: in patients with *S. mansoni*, cor pulmonale is the cause of death in only 2 per cent. The eggs impact in small pulmonary arteries and induce a granulomatous reaction. This causes obliterative pulmonary arteriolitis; egg granulomas are also seen outside the vessels (Fig. 29.134). In heavy infections, plexiform dilatation lesions develop as in other types of pulmonary hypertension.

'Ectopic' and unusual disease

Worm pairs within the mesenteric venous system may deliver eggs constantly to a localized area, so building up over time a huge focal egg load. The accompanying host reaction forms a tumour-like mass—a *bilharzioma*. These are commonly found on the serosal surface of the large bowel, the mesentery, and on the retroperitoneum. Grossly, they are white, firm masses, often resembling a sarcoma. Histologically, eggs of all ages are seen within granulomas and surrounding fibrosis.

During maturation, worms can become trapped in unusual sites, i.e. outside the portal venous system, and mate. The granulomatous reaction to the eggs causes local inflammation and a space-occupying lesion. Any part of the body can be affected, such as skin, testis, and outer ear (a rare cause of aural polyp). A schistosoma anal polyp, although usually due to *S. haematobium*, may also be caused by *S. mansoni*. It presents as a skin nodule, and shows eggs, granulomas, and fibrosis within the dermis.

Central nervous system (CNS) schistosomiasis This is the most severe form of 'ectopic' schisitosomiasis. *S. mansoni* and *S. haematobium* usually affect the spinal cord, and *S. japonicum* usually affects the brain. Presentation is with focal neurological signs, epilepsy, and, in the case of spinal disease, paraplegia.

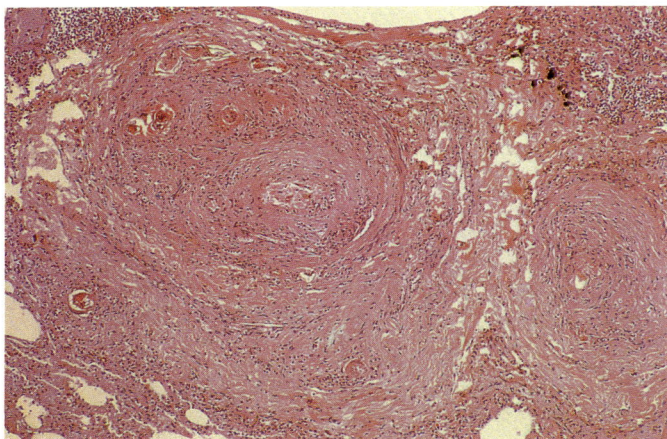

Fig. 29.134 Schistosomal pulmonary hypertension. Lung tissue showing eggs with granulomatous reaction around vessels and marked fibrosis.

Without biopsy the diagnosis is difficult to make. The histology is of neuropil with aggregated eggs, surrounding necrosis, eosinophils, and a granulomatous reaction. In some cases, adult worms are identified in vessels near the inflammation. Patients with CNS schistosomiasis may have no other evidence of the disease. It is an example of how a parasitic disease which normally requires heavy and chronic infection to produce significant morbidity, may be severe if the parasite is in a critical site.

Renal disease

In South America, up to 15 per cent of patients with hepatosplenic schistosomiasis have significant progressive glomerulonephritis, and it is generally agreed that *S. mansoni* is a major aetiological factor. The pattern is usually of membrano-proliferative glomerulonephritis, with electron-dense deposits seen in the mesangium and along the basement membrane. Immunofluorescence shows immune complexes in glomeruli. Eluates of affcted kidney contain antibodies that bind to the adult *Schistosoma* worm tegument and gut, indicating that the adult, and not the egg, provides the relevant antigen. Through the development of a collateral circulation, hepatosplenic schistosomiasis reduces the clearance of immune complexes by the liver, which may then be deposited in the glomeruli.

Despite being a chronic infection, there is no association between any of the schistosomiases and amyloidosis in man.

Schistosoma japonicum

The clinical and pathological effects are similar to those of *S. mansoni* infection. Hepatosplenic and intestinal disease predominate. However, pulmonary hypertension is very uncommon, and there is no association with glomerulonephritis. *S. japonicum* egg granulomas are smaller than those of *S. mansoni*.

There is controversy over whether *S. japonicum* intestinal schistosomiasis is aetiologically associated with colorectal carcinoma. In South America and Africa, no such claim has been made for *S. mansoni*. In China, there is some evidence for an increased incidence of carcinoma in those provinces endemic for *S. japonicum* infection. In particular, case control studies support an association with rectal adenocarcinoma but not with colonic carcinoma. Patients without overt carcinoma are reported to have epithelial dysplasia of the large bowel, raising an analogy with chronic ulcerative colitis and dysplasia. Further epidemiological studies are needed to resolve this issue.

Schistosoma haematobium

The bladder, lower ureters, and large bowel are main sites of pathology in schistosomiasis haematobium.

Urological disease

The worms in the perivesical venous plexi lay eggs that pass through or become trapped in the bladder wall: about half the eggs escape in urine. Clinically, this produces haematuria and dysuria. There is a sequence of changes of schistosomal cystitis as the infection passes from active (with heavy deposition of new eggs) to inactive (after most worms have died). Early, there are erythematous polypoid patches which bleed easily. Later, they become fibrous and then flat sandy patches, which may ulcerate. The polyps can be several centimetres in size and are analogous to the inflammatory polyps of intestinal schistosomiasis. Histologically, the eggs induce eosinophilia and granulomas. The urothelium is often hyperplastic and may show cystitis cystica (Fig. 29.135).

Ureteric infection is a common cause of hydro-ureter and may lead to hydronephrosis and permanent renal damage (Fig. 29.136). The eggs in the ureteric wall induce granulomas which act as a space-occupying lesion and obstruct the lumen (Fig. 29.137). If treated early, before significant fibrosis has supervened, this obstruction is reversed.

In heavy infections of the bladder, over time there is progressive fibrosis from the granulomatous reaction. This involves the subepithelial layers and bladder muscle and compromises the function of the bladder, with incomplete emptying. Bacterial cystitis may follow; this, as well as the chronic schistosomiasis, can result in squamous metaplasia of the urothelium.

S. haematobium eggs often remain in tissues in large numbers and become calcified. By this time there may be no host reaction, and the eggs are embedded in fibrous tissue. Egg loads of 250 000 per gram of bladder tissue are common in older people. This is often visible on X-ray, as a calcified ring in the pelvis. The seminal vesicles also accumulate huge numbers of eggs (Fig. 29.138).

Epidemiologically, there is no association between urolithiasis and schistosomiasis haematobium.

Bladder cancer There is no doubt that schistosomiasis haematobium is aetiologically associated with bladder carcinoma. In Egypt, 20 per cent of all cancers in males are of the bladder, and in southern Malawi the male incidence rate for bladder carcinoma is high, at 55/100 000/year: in both countries, schistosomiasis haematobium is highly prevalent. The peak age at presentation in such people is 35–45 years. The tumour is exo-

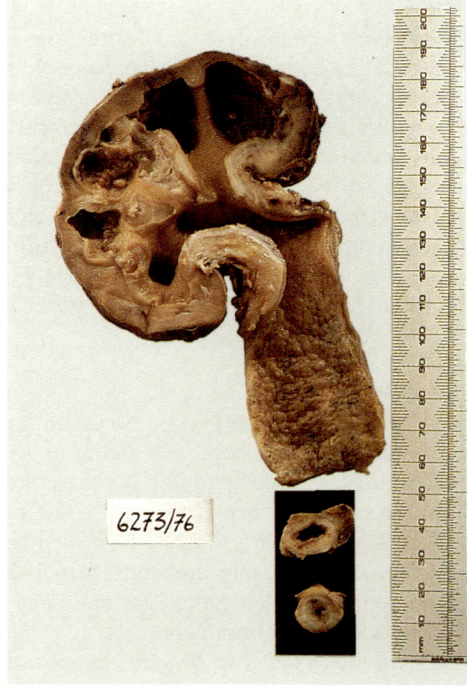

Fig. 29.136 Hydronephrosis and hydro-ureter due to schistosomiasis thickening the lower ureter and stenosing the lumen (inset).

phytic, originating on the posterior or lateral walls of the bladder, and may fill the bladder (Fig. 29.139). It invades through the bladder wall to obstruct the ureters, and metastasizes to local lymph nodes and lung. It is the major cause of death attributable to *S. haematobium*.

Histologically, the majority of bilharzial bladder cancers are squamous cell carcinoma, usually well differentiated. The adjacent bladder is fibrosed, has calcified schistosome eggs, and often shows squamous metaplasia of the urothelium.

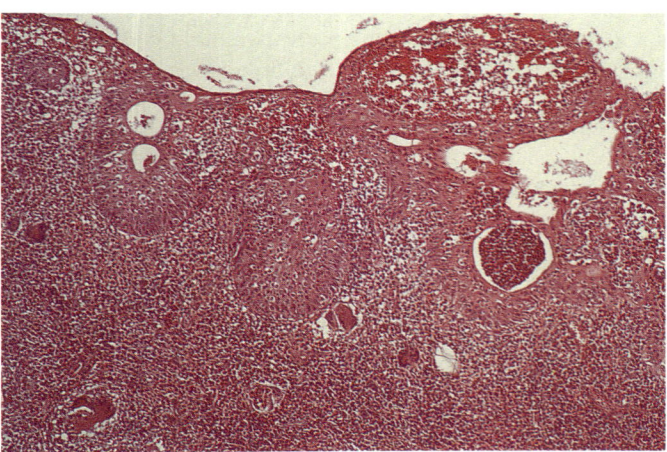

Fig. 29.135 Schistosomal cystitis. The reaction to the eggs is eosinophilic inflammation, vascular congestion, and epithelial hyperplasia.

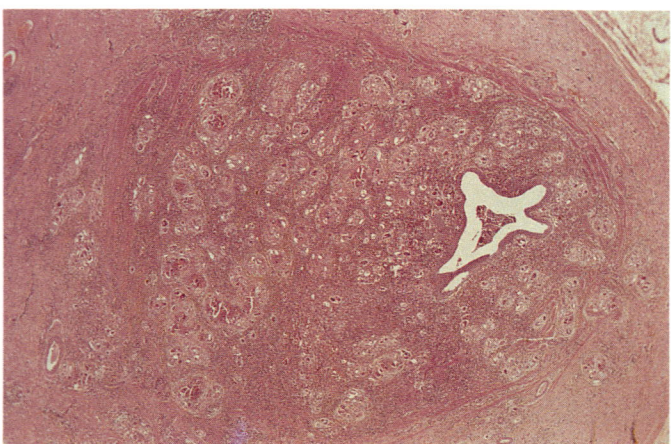

Fig. 29.137 Cross-section of schistosomal ureter, illustrating the obstructive effect of numerous egg granulomas.

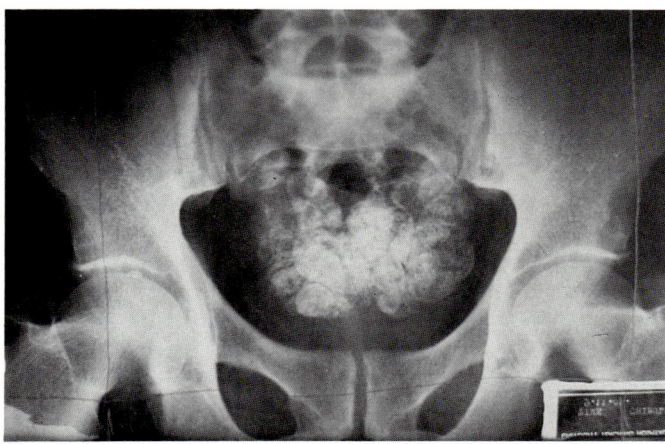

Fig. 29.138 Plain X-ray of pelvis. Both seminal vesicles are radio-opaque through massive deposition of calcified *S. haematobium* eggs (X-ray courtesy of Mr B. Elem).

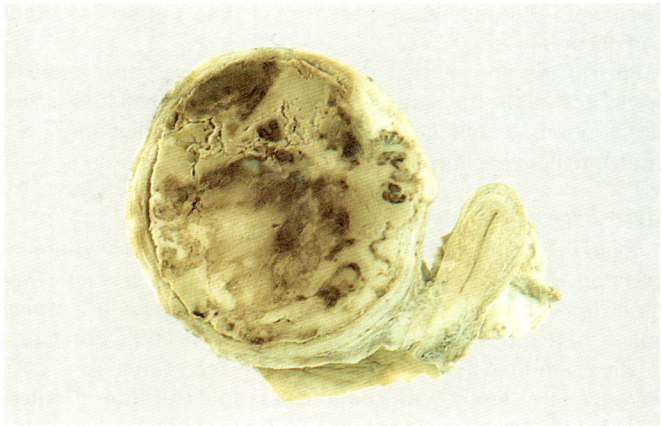

Fig. 29.139 Large exophytic bladder cancer in a 30-year-old woman with schistosomiasis. Histology showed a squamous cell carcinoma.

Intestinal and other organ disease

Worms lie in the mesenteric and systemic veins around the rectum and colon. Schistosomiasis haematobium is an important cause of large bowel disease, similar clinically and pathologically to *S. mansoni* infection. Although *S. haematobium* eggs are carried directly to the lungs via the inferior vena cava, significant pathology with pulmonary hypertension is uncommon. *S. haematobium* does not cause significant liver disease, although some hepatic egg granulomas may be found. Central nervous system disease is discussed above.

Within the pelvis, the genital tract is commonly affected by *S. haematobium*. Seminal vesicles, prostate, testis, ovary, Fallopian tube, and endometrium may all have schistosomal granulomas, and heavy infections may produce bilharziomas in those sites. The skin, vulva, vagina, and cervix may have schistosomal nodules which bleed.

Salmonella *bacteraemia*

Schistosoma haematobium infection is associated with persistent *Salmonella* bacteraemia which may cause recurrent symptoms. The bladder may be a site of such latent infection. Although *S. haematobium per se* is not associated with membranoproliferative glomerulonephritis, an immune complex nephritis—acute proliferative glomerulonephritis—may be found in children who have persistent *Salmonella* bacteraemia. This is associated with *Salmonella* antigen in the glomeruli, and it resolves with appropriate antibiotics.

Schistosoma intercalatum

This infection is common in endemic areas, as measured by rectal samples; however, clinical disease is mild. Diarrhoea with blood, from egg deposition in the rectum, is the main feature. Although liver biopsies show *S. intercalatum* egg granulomas in portal tracts—and with granuloma diameters comparable to

those of *S. mansoni*—hepatosplenic schistosomiasis has not been recorded.

Schistosoma mekongi

Few clinico-pathological studies of *S. mekongi* infection are available. Only a small proportion of these infected are symptomatic. Hepatosplenic schistosomiasis due to periportal fibrosis is the major feature. The pathology is thus similar to *S. japonicum* infection.

Pathogenesis

Three particular aspects of schistosomiasis pathogenesis require discussion:

Host inflammatory response

The adult worms in veins elicit no host reaction: they coat themselves with host glycoproteins (such as blood-group substances) to become non-antigenic, and also secrete anticoagulants. The pathology comes from the host reaction to eggs. Eggs live for only 3 weeks before degenerating, and there is constant removal of eggs by the macrophage system. None the less in, for example, *S. haematobium* infection, around 100 eggs per female worm accumulate in the tissue each day, so building up massive egg loads over time. The histopathological reaction around eggs may appear polymorphic: it includes eosinophil abscess, tuberculoid granuloma, the Hoeppli–Splendore phenomenon, fibrinoid necrosis, varying numbers of plasma cells and neutrophil polymorphs, fibrosis, and (particularly around dead eggs) no reaction at all. However, the experimental evidence shows that a T-cell-mediated macrophage activation (cell-mediated immunity) is the dominant process in all schistosomal granulomas. In experimental animals with chronic infection, there is a modulation of granulomatous reaction, i.e. the granulomas become smaller and less pathogenic. This is a cell-mediated process with *S. mansoni* infection, but may also be influenced by antibody in *S. japonicum* infection. However, in human disease, there is no morphological evidence yet that immune modulation occurs.

Part of the fibrosis that dominates chronic schistosomiasis originates in the healing of granulomas with residual scars. Numerous macrophage products, such as interleukin-1, are known to activate fibroblasts to secrete collagen.

Liver disease

A major determinant of liver disease is intensity and duration of infection. Autopsy studies on *S. mansoni* infection show that clinically significant hepatic fibrosis does not usually develop unless there has been chronic infection from > 160 worm pairs. However, in heavily infected people, the degree of fibrosis does not correlate closely with the intensity and duration of infection. It is evident that some people have a greater fibrogenic potential than others to given stimuli. Hepatosplenic schistosomiasis (HSS) is strongly associated with HLA types A1 and B5, which may influence the degree of fibrosis. Whether variations in parasite strain are also important is not yet clear.

The precise pathogenesis of the periportal fibrosis is also not certain. It is not only the accumulation of units of fibrous scarring from healing granulomas. In the fibrous bands, granulomas are often scanty. The portal hypertension is presinusoidal in type, but it is probably not due to the macroscopic pipestem fibrosis. With the inflammatory disruption of portal triads, arteriovenous anastomoses open up and raise portal pressure. Secondly, ultrastructural studies show that the space of Disse between sinusoids and hepatocytes becomes collagenized, providing a barrier between hepatocytes and the circulation.

Hepatitis B virus (HBV) infection is common in those areas where schistosomiasis is endemic. However, there is no epidemiological association between the prevalences of HSS and HBV. HBV co-infection may be important in determining the prognosis in individual patients with HSS.

Bladder cancer

Schistosome worms and eggs are not themselves carcinogenic. The current aetiological hypothesis links the poor functioning of a schistosomal bladder due to fibrosis, urine retention, secondary bacterial urinary superinfection, and squamous metaplasia. This sequence also occurs in the bladders of non-schistosomal patients with paraplegia. The bacteria form nitrosamines from dietary nitrates and nitrites that are excreted in urine. The carcinogenic nitrosamines act on the metaplastic urothelium and induce squamous carcinoma.

Diagnosis and treatment

Schistosomiasis is usually diagnosed by finding the eggs. Urine and faeces may be sampled; a more sensitive technique is to biopsy bladder or rectum and examine the crushed tissue directly for eggs. Tissue histopathology contributes to the diagnosis of liver, bladder, intestinal, pulmonary, ectopic, and tumoural schistosomiasis. With the exception of *S. haematobium*, the shells of all human schistosomes retain the red colour of the Ziehl–Neelsen stain. Serology can be helpful in diagnosis, but does not distinguish an active from a past infection.

Treatment with praziquantel is effective for all species of *Schistosoma*. It kills the adult worms, which then cease producing eggs, but does not suppress the host reaction to previously laid eggs.

29.14.2   *Fasciola*

Fascioliasis is a zoonosis caused by the fluke *Fasciola hepatica*. The major pathology is in the liver.

Epidemiology

Fascioliasis is primarily a disease of herbivores: sheep, goats, and cattle. Human infection is not common; 2600 cases have been documented over the past two decades, in all continents except Australasia. But the number of subclinical cases is unknown. The countries reporting the most cases are France, Portugal, and Cuba.

Life cycle and morphology

After leaving a snail, the cercaria encysts on water-plants and loses its tail; for man the main plant thus infected is watercress. After ingestion on cress, the metacercaria penetrates the duodenum into the abdominal cavity, develops into an immature fluke, and by 6 days after ingestion has begun to penetrate the liver. Within the parenchyma the fluke feeds on the liver tissue, and reaches a bile duct by 5–6 weeks, where it matures, resides, and commences egg-laying some 2 months later (Fig. 29.124). Adult flukes live in man for several years (13 years is the maximum documented). Egg production depends inversely on intensity of infection, and is about 5000 per fluke per day. Adult *Fasciola* flukes are hermaphrodite, flat, leaf-shaped worms, 30×13 mm when full-grown. The eggs are 140×80 μm. The flukes live in the bilary tree and gall bladder, attached to the biliary epithelium.

Clinical features

The first symptoms are fever, abdominal pain, and urticaria—the acute phase of liver invasion. The liver is enlarged and tender. Eosinophilic ascites may occur, but there is no jaundice. Most patients have leucocytosis with eosinophilia. The latent phase, when mature flukes have entered the bile ducts and commenced egg-laying, is asymptomatic. It may last months or years, and only peripheral blood eosinophilia may mark the infection. The chronic obstructive phase of fascioliasis is characterized by biliary colic, cholangitis, and cholecystitis. The proportion of those infected who develop these clinical features is not certain. Fascioliasis is not associated with bile duct carcinoma, in contrast to clonorchiasis (see below).

Pathology

The acute phase of fascioliasis shows yellowish nodules on the surface and on section. These lesions, which may resemble metastatic carcinoma deposits, are the necrosis and inflammatory reactions around migrating flukes. Histologically, there are granulomas and eosinophilia around the necrosis. Some scarring remains after these tracks heal.

Established bile duct parasitism dilates the ducts in which the flukes are seen (Fig. 29.140); up to 40 flukes have been noted in post-mortem livers. There is ductal fibrosis, and hyperplasia of the epithelium, with moderate eosinophilia. Granulomas around eggs in the bile duct walls may occasionally be seen. Secondary obstructive cholangitis and cholelithiasis develop in some patients. Cholecystitis also occurs, and the gall bladder may contain blood from flukes eroding the epithelium.

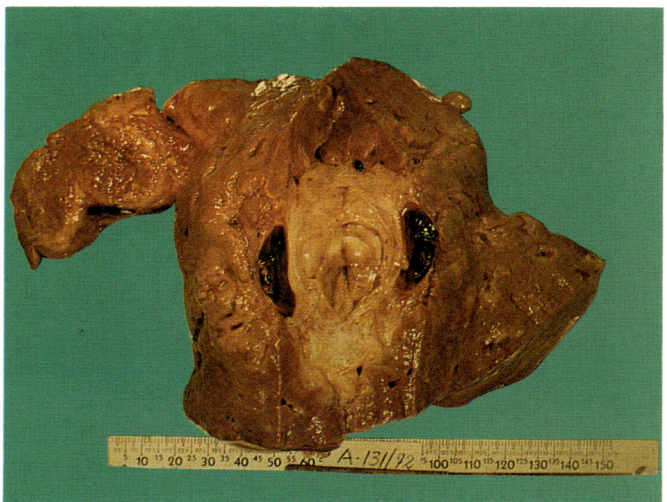

Fig. 29.140 Fascioliasis. Post-mortem liver cut to show portal fibrosis and two brown *Fasciola* flukes.

Ectopic fascioliasis

Occasionally the juvenile flukes migrate to non-liver sites. They die and induce an inflammatory mass. Such ectopic disease has been recorded in the intestinal serosa, the pancreas, the epididymis, and abdominal subcutis. An abscess-like cavity forms around the degenerating worm, lined histologically by an eosinophilic granulomatous reaction. At one time, the parasite causing the syndrome of 'halzoun'—acute dysphagia and laryngeal obstruction after eating raw sheep liver, with a worm attaching to the posterior pharynx—was thought to be *Fasciola*. Now it is attributed to the pentastome *Linguatula*.

Diagnosis and treatment

Cholangiography and CT scan of liver may suggest fascioliasis. Definitive diagnosis depends on finding eggs in the faeces, or by liver biopsy. Many cases are now diagnosed serologically without identifying the parasite. The effective drug for fascioliasis is praziquantel.

29.14.3   *Clonorchis* and *Opisthorcis*

There are three similar species of bile duct flukes: *Clonorchis*

sinensis, *Opisthorcis viverrini*, and *O. felineus*. Geography apart, the diseases they cause are similar, and are hereon termed 'clonorchiasis'.

Epidemiology

Clonorchis sinensis is prevalent in China, Vietnam, and Korea. *Opisthorcis viverrini* is endemic in north-east Thailand (with > 7 million people infected, and overall prevalences of 90 per cent in some foci) and along the Mekong river. *Opisthorcis felineus* is found in eastern Europe and the USSR. In endemic zones, acquisition of worms starts in childhood, infection loads becoming stable by the age of 20 years.

Life cycle and morphology

The adult worms are slenderer than *Fasciola hepatica*. They reside in the small bile-ducts. Eggs pass in bile to the faeces, and are ingested by aquatic snails in which they develop into cercariae (Fig. 29.124). These penetrate the second intermediate host, fish, and encyst in the muscle. Eating uncooked, pickled, or smoked fish transmits the infection; the metacercariae excyst in the upper gut and the larvae migrate through the ampulla of Vater into the biliary tract. These infections are not solely anthroponotic. Dogs, cats, and other fish-eating mammals are reservoir hosts. *Clonorchis* measures 25×5 mm and *Opisthorcis* 20×4 mm; the eggs of all three species measure 25×15 μm.

Clinical features

The acute infection in previously unexposed individuals comprises fever, malaise, slight jaundice, tender enlarged liver, and blood eosinophilia. In endemic zones re-infection is constant (protective immunity appears to be non-existent), and infection loads accumulate. Only about 5–10 per cent of those with chronic clonorchiasis experience symptoms: flatulence, weakness, and abdominal pain. Hepatomegaly attributable to clonorchiasis occurs in 5 per cent, and jaundice in 2 per cent of those infected.

Cholangiocarcinoma is unquestionably associated with clonorchiasis, with an incidence of up to 50/100 000/year in north-east Thailand (the usual incidence globally is about 2/100 000/year). In endemic areas, the ratio of cholangiocarcinoma to the ubiquitous and more common hepatocarcinoma is 1 : 5. The peak incidence is in the fifth to seventh decades, and the survival rate is < 6 per cent at 4 years post-diagnosis.

Pathology

In mild infections, the liver is externally normal. Heavier infections cause hepatomegaly and cholestasis. There is irregular dilatation and fibrous thickening of the walls of second-order, smaller bile ducts, 2–6 mm in diameter. The ducts contain visible worms, thick bile, and often stones. The common bile duct often contains worms that have migrated down. Generalized bile duct dilatation is uncommon. The gall bladder is often thickened and fibrotic, and contains mainly dead worms (they do not live long there).

Bile stones are seen in about 10 per cent of infected people.

They form around dead worms and epithelial debris, and are the main cause of obstruction that leads to septic cholangitis (usually an *E. coli* infection) and liver abscesses, which are found in 5 per cent of autopsied cases. In some autopsied cases, the pancreatic duct is parasitized and dilated, but pancreatitis is a rare complication. Clonorchiasis is not associated with cirrhosis of the liver. The spleen size is variable and there is no significant portal hypertension.

Cholangiocarcinoma is multifocal, affecting the second-order bile-ducts. It appears as numerous well-circumscribed grey nodules, 1–14 cm in diameter, attached to ducts, and also as annular thickenings of ducts. Many of the deposits are intra-hepatic metastases. The common bile duct and gall bladder are not commonly the sites of primary carcinoma. Extrahepatic metastasis is to periportal lymph nodes and lung.

Histologically, the predominant change in the parasitized bile ducts is epithelial hyperplasia and goblet-cell metaplasia. Periductal fibrosis to a thickness of 1 mm is frequent, but inflammation is not prominent unless there is acute cholangitis. A mild eosinophil infiltration is common. Parasitized gall bladder has hyperplastic epithelium and mural fibrosis (Figs 29.141, 29.142). The intra-ductal worms are viable unless there is acute cholangitis, in which case they degenerate. Free eggs are not seen in ducts unless there is obstruction. A parasitized pancreatic duct is dilated and shows squamous metaplasia.

The cholangiocarcinoma is a mucin-secreting adenocarcinoma. In autopsied cases, the multiple tumours show all stages from *in situ* to invasive carcinoma.

Pathogenesis

Disease from clonorchiasis is directly related to intensity of infection. Asymptomatic people harbour about 10 worms, as judged by counting worms recovered from the faeces after chemotherapy. Those people with cholecystitis and hepatic disease have 100–300 worms. There is a trend for higher infection loads to correlate with more severe bile duct hyperplasia and cholangiocarcinoma.

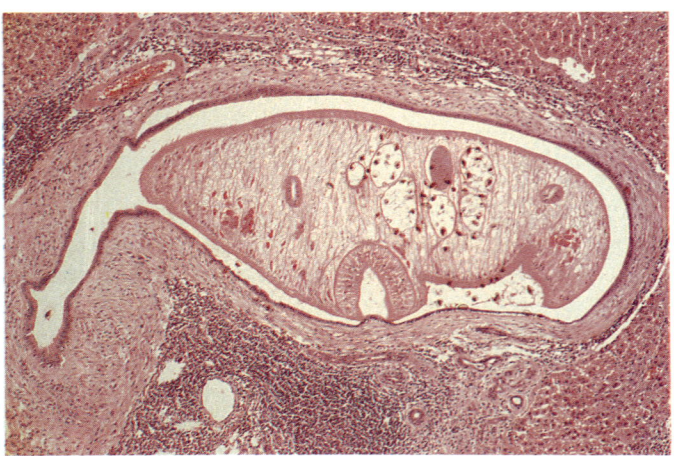

Fig. 29.141 Opisthorciasis of the liver. An *Opisthorcis* fluke attached by a sucker to the bile duct epithelium.

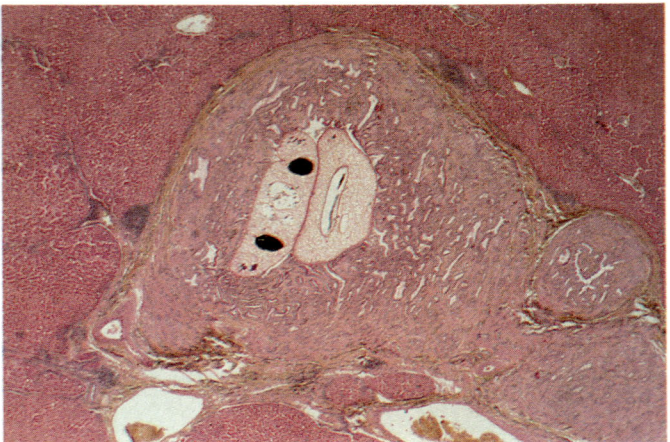

Fig. 29.142 Two *Opisthorcis* flukes in a bile-duct, exciting biliary epithelial hyperplasia.

The worms live for up to 25 years, providing constant irritation of the biliary epithelium by the fluke, which has a spiny cuticle and attaches by its suckers to epithelium. Worm secretory products may also stimulate the epithelium to undergo hyperplasia. The severe obstructive complications of clonorchiasis are caused not by worms but by stones, post-inflammatory stricture, or the development of cholangiocarcinoma.

The worms are not themselves carcinogenic. The host response is the hyperplasia of bile ducts, which could increase the likelihood of malignant change given the existence of carcinogens in the bile. Dietary nitrosamines and aflatoxins are considered candidate factors. In experimental rodent models of clonorchiasis, dimethylnitrosamine induces cholangiocarcinoma more readily in those previously infected with *O. viverrini* compared with controls. A protein-deficient diet increases the degree of bile duct hyperplasia in rodents with opisthorciasis. Given the poverty of people in those areas most endemic for clonorchiasis, this may be relevant in the genesis of cholangiocarcinoma.

Diagnosis and treatment

The main diagnostic method is finding eggs in the faeces. The stage of disease induced by clonorchiasis can be evaluated by ultrasonography of the liver and biliary tree, estimating gall bladder thickening, cholelithiasis, and dilatation of intrahepatic bile ducts. Endoscopic retrograde cholangiography demonstrates the biliary abnormalities as well as enabling removal of worms and drainage of the common bile duct. The standard chemotherapy for clonorchiasis is praziquantel, which kills the worms.

29.14.4 *Paragonimus*

Several *Paragonimus* species infect the lungs of carnivores. When man accidentally contracts the zoonosis, the disease is called *paragonimiasis*.

Epidemiology

There are foci of paragonimiasis in South America, China and South-East Asia, and Africa. Infection prevalence may reach 2 per cent. These are all usually ascribed to *P. westermani*, but other species are certainly involved.

Life cycle and morphology

Infection is by eating crabs or crayfish that contain cercariae. These hatch and penetrate the bowel wall, then burrow through the diaphragm into the pleural cavity and lung parenchyma. The flukes mature over 6 weeks. Although hermaphrodite, they usually pair up, and release eggs into the bronchial tree. Eggs are coughed up and spat out or swallowed and passed in the faeces. The eggs infect water-snails, so completing the life cycle (Fig. 29.124). Adult *Paragonimus* is a brown 15×6 mm fluke. The eggs measure 100×50 μm, with a characteristic operculum. The flukes live for about 10 years.

Clinical features

Paragonimiasis affects young adults. The major features are chronic cough and haemoptysis: this closely simulates post-primary pulmonary tuberculosis, and the chest X-ray may also suggest tuberculosis. But, unlike tuberculosis, pulmonary paragonimiasis is rarely fatal.

Paragonimus worms may remain within the abdominal cavity, or migrate to ectopic sites, outside the lung. Brain, intra-abdominal lymph nodes, liver, and subcutaneous tissues are typical sites. There the fluke produces an inflammatory tumour. In the brain, it causes focal neurological signs, meningitis, and epilepsy. A moderate blood eosinophilia is usual.

Pathology

The subpleural zones of the lung are most affected. The flukes produce abscesses and cavities in the lung by eroding the alveoli (Fig. 29.143). There is usually communication of cavities with the bronchial tree. The lesions are 1–5 cm in diameter and produce collapse of surrounding lung tissue. Most patients have fewer than 20 cavities in the lungs.

Around the fluke is an inflammatory reaction which increases with time (Fig. 29.144). Early, there is an eosinophil polymorph infiltrate. Later, there is more necrotic slough, granulation tissue, and fibrosis, and the fluke degenerates. Eggs embedded in the host tissue induce granulomas. Old lesions may become calcified.

In other sites, the host reaction is similar with an eosinophil abscess, fibrosis, and granulomatous reaction to *Paragonimus* eggs.

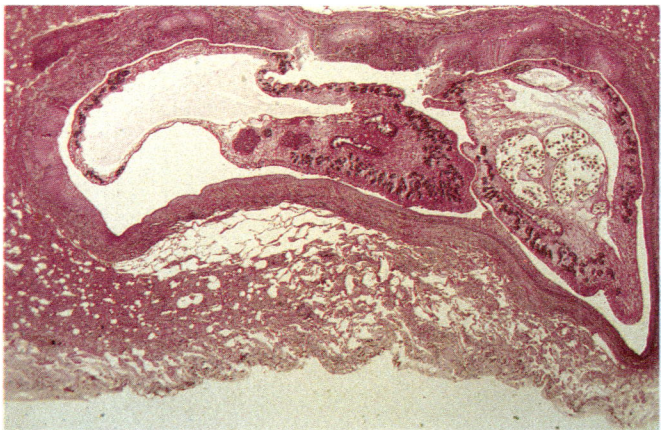

Fig. 29.144 Adult *Paragonimus* fluke in lung, with a thin capsule.

Diagnosis and treatment

Pulmonary paragonimiasis is diagnosed by finding eggs in sputum or faeces. Surgical excision of a segment of lung or of an ectopic infection site shows eggs and fluke on histology. Chemotherapy with praziquantel kills the worms.

29.14.5 Further reading

Chen, M. G. and Mott, K. E. (1988). Progress in assessment of morbidity due to schistosomiasis. *Tropical Diseases Bulletin* **85** (6), R2–R45. [*S. japonicum*.]

Chen, M. G. and Mott, K. E. (1988). Progress in assessment of morbidity due to schistosomiasis. *Tropical Diseases Bulletin* **85** (10), R2–R56. [*S. mansoni*.]

Chen, M. G. and Mott, K. E. (1989). Progress in assessment of morbidity due to schistosomiasis. *Tropical Diseases Bulletin* **86** (4), R2–R36. [*S. haematobium*.]

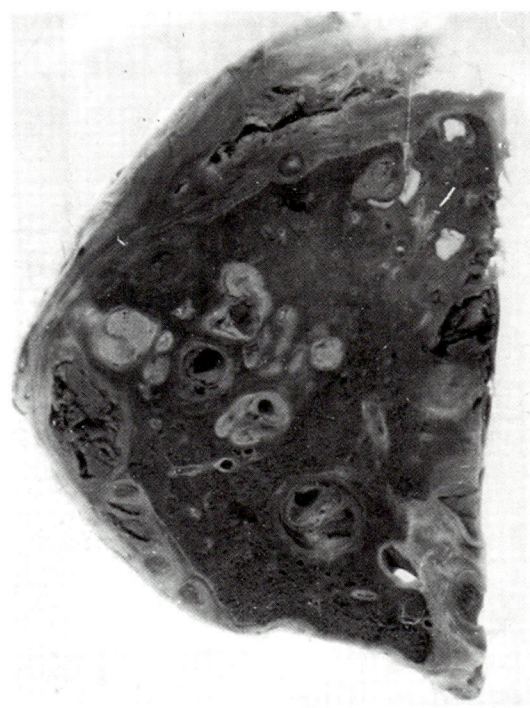

Fig. 29.143 Paragonimiasis of the lung, showing several cavities and abscesses in the parenchyma. (Photograph courtesy of the Wellcome Museum of Medical Science.)

30

Diagnostic and investigative techniques

30

Diagnostic and investigative techniques

30.1 Diagnostic biopsy preparation

A. J. Chaplin

30.1.1 Introduction

The differential coloration of cells and tissues remains fundamental to histopathological diagnosis. In recent years, the manner in which this can be achieved has been supplemented quite dramatically as more sophisticated techniques facilitate the specific demonstration and localization of individual cells and subcellular components. The gamut of methodology now includes not only the traditional and often empirical light microscopical staining procedures, but also a range of immunocytochemical protocols, utilizing an apparently endless spectrum of monoclonal antibodies, and the most recent addition to the histopathologist's repertoire, *in situ* hybridization and other molecular techniques (see Section 30.3).

In spite of these alternatives, some of which are discussed in greater detail later in this chapter, the majority of histopathological diagnoses are still made with the aid of the time-honoured haematoxylin and eosin stain, together with application of the considerable array of 'special' stains that have become well established over many years. It is to the preparation of tissues for these traditional methods that the greater part of this section is devoted.

30.1.2 Utilization of material

For many years histopathology departments functioned on the premise that best results were obtained when samples were immersed in a large bulk of fixing fluid, usually formalin, at the earliest possible moment. Although providing good basic morphological information, such a policy inevitably limited the number of investigations that could be performed. Certain recent innovations have demanded a reassessment of this approach such that, in contemporary times, various questions must be posed before tissue is committed to a fixative:

1. Are non-histopathological procedures required? The polypeptide hormone content of a tumour may need to be assessed by radioimmunoassay. Bizarre organisms in opportunistic infection may only be identified reliably by microbiological culture.

2. Are enzyme histochemical, fluorescent, monoclonal antibody, or molecular pathology studies likely to be relevant? A significant proportion of techniques in such categories are prohibited by primary fixation.

3. Is a fixative other than formalin preferable? Gluteraldehyde for ultrastructural studies, or a chromate fixative for the chromaffin reaction, for example.

4. What type of procedure is most appropriate to satisfy the diagnostic requirements? Touch preparations and smears, frozen or fixed sections, freeze-dried preparations, paraffin, celloidin- or resin-embedded material are all legitimate pathways, and many will be alluded to in the account that follows.

30.1.3 Preparatory techniques

Fixation

A prerequisite for the majority of histopathological techniques is that tissue, cells, and extracellular substances be preserved in as near life-like a manner as possible, with minimal alteration not only to the physical and morphological structure but also the chemical composition of the living tissue. Ideally, tissue components should be rendered insoluble in all of the reagents to which they may be subsequently exposed, without suffering any spatial displacement. Not surprisingly, a fixative capable of achieving this ideal is in reality an impossibility and, in practice, all fixative solutions are a compromise.

Many of the most important components of tissue are composed wholly or in part of protein. Consequently, fixation is normally directed primarily towards the preservation of simple proteins, lipoproteins, glycoproteins, etc. by rendering them insoluble. Occasionally it may be necessary to demonstrate some specific tissue component, not normally preserved by conventional fixation. Its preservation may be achieved only at the expense of the general morphology by using one of a number of obscure fixatives introduced for a particular purpose, such as cyanuric chloride, benzoquinone, and tannic acid.

Apart from these unusual fixatives there are only a small number of substances useful as fixatives. Traditionally they are divided into two groups according to their visible reaction with protein, namely coagulant or non-coagulant. They may be further classified as additive or non-additive, depending on whether the fixative is chemically incorporated into some part of the protein (Table 30.1).

Although most fixatives harden tissues to a greater or lesser extent, some may also cause either shrinkage or swelling. Consequently, many of the fixative mixtures in common use comprise a balance of several primary fixatives (and therefore also a mixture of coagulant and non-coagulant compounds), formulated to obviate these undesirable effects. In addition, aqueous fixing solutions may also contain 'indifferent' substances such as sodium chloride, sucrose, and buffer salts in order to maintain tonicity, pH, etc.

Just as there is no single fixative which will satisfy all the needs of even a routine diagnostic laboratory, so it is not expedient to have more than a few solutions readily available for routine use. As a compromise, most tissues can be satisfactorily fixed in the formalin-based solution of choice, and special requirements met by utilizing one or other of a limited range of alternative solutions.

General fixative solutions

Formaldehyde (HCHO), a gas, is available for diagnostic laboratories as a saturated solution known as formalin, which contains 37–40 per cent of the gas in water. Commercial solutions also contain about 10 per cent methanol, added to inhibit polymerization of formaldehyde to a solid white polymer, paraformaldehyde. The standard concentration of formaldehyde in working solutions is about 4 per cent—this is commonly designated 10 per cent formalin, i.e. a 10 per cent (v/v) solution of 40 per cent commercial formaldehyde.

Formaldehyde fixes by cross-linking protein molecules, a relatively slow process which is reversible in the early stages. It also preserves most lipids, but does not react significantly with carbohydrates and appreciable quantities of glycogen, for example, may be lost.

Prolonged storage of tissue in formaldehyde solutions may sometimes lead to excessive hardening, loss of staining potential and, particularly in acid solutions and with bloody tissues, the formation of a haemoglobin degradation product known as formalin pigment. This may be prevented, or at least minimized, by using a neutral buffered solution of formalin. For convenience, many laboratories use a formal saline solution as a routine fixative, though with this, pigment formation is frequently evident.

Mercuric chloride–formalin (Formal sublimate) A useful solution, suitable for most purposes, including post-fixation of routinely (formalin) fixed material. It enhances nuclear staining and improves subsequent staining of connective tissue with trichrome procedures, but tends to impair silver impregnation methods. It is both corrosive and toxic, and the latter in particular prohibits more widespread use.

Bouin's fluid A fairly rapid fixative for small biopsies which preserves the morphology well, especially of connective tissue. Although prolonged fixation impairs nuclear staining, Bouin's fluid is recommended for testicular biopsies, since the particularly clear nuclear detail obtained with optimal fixation is useful for assessing abnormalities of spermatogenesis.

Carnoy's fluid This is particularly useful as a rapid fixative (2–4 h for a small biopsy) providing good nuclear preservation. Tissue may suffer considerable shrinkage and become excessively hard. Carnoy's fluid extracts lipids, and so may be detrimental to subsequent staining for acid-fast bacilli, for example, but is useful for histochemical studies on proteins and carbohydrates. This fixative is preferred in this department for rapid routine biopsy fixation.

Helly's fluid This variant of Zenker's fixative gives good cellular detail and so is often used for bone marrow, spleen, etc., as well as for cytoplasmic organelles such as mitochondria. It is only suitable for small pieces of tissue, which must be washed thoroughly after fixation and prior to processing in order to prevent dichromate fixation precipitate. Characteristic mercuric chloride fixation artefact is frequently produced.

Orth's fluid One of many similar formulae, having limited application, but recommended for the demonstration of chromaffin tissue, and therefore for phaeochromocytomas. Again, tissue should be washed thoroughly after fixation (before processing) to remove excess dichromate.

Microwave fixation

The application of microwave technology provides a rather different approach to fixation, offering a rapid, non-chemical alternative to traditional methods. Although presently at an early stage of development in histopathological techniques, the

---

Table 30.1 Types of fixative

Coagulant	Non-coagulant
Additive	Additive
Picric acid	Formaldehyde
Mercuric chloride	Potassium dichromate
Chromic acid	(Osmium tetroxide)
Non-additive	Non-additive
Ethanol	Acetic acid
Trichloracetic acid	

use of microwaves for fixation, and also for conventional as well as immunocytochemical staining, is clearly an area of some considerable potential.

Fixation for special components

Proteins Neutral buffered formalin or Carnoy fixation is compatible with most histochemical methods for amino acids. Mercury-containing fixative should be avoided.

Nucleic acids For routine work, standard formaldehyde fixation is generally adequate. Carnoy's fluid is preferable for more precise study. Note that acid hydrolysis in the Feulgen method (for DNA demonstration) varies in time according to the fixative used.

Carbohydrates There is no single ideal fixative. Various substances, such as cetylpyridinium chloride, have been added to routine fixatives to try to improve the preservation of glycosaminoglycans and proteoglycans. For glycogen, alcoholic fixatives are generally preferred.

Lipids Most procedures require frozen sections of unfixed or formalin-fixed tissue. Mercury- or dichromate-containing fixatives are sometimes more effective for preserving lipids in cryostat sections.

Enzymes There is remarkable variation in the ability of different enzymes to remain active after fixation. For example, dehydrogenases are sensitive to even the briefest fixation, whereas chloracetate esterase is well preserved in routinely fixed paraffin-embedded tissues. This is exceptional, however, and most enzymes are shown to best effect using minimal fixation of frozen sections.

Biogenic amines Apart from immunocytochemical techniques applied to frozen or formalin-fixed material, most commonly used is the so-called chromaffin reaction, particularly for adrenal medullary cells and their tumours. The chromaffin reaction is normally accomplished using dichromate fixatives, but can be effected using other strong oxidizing agents.

Inorganic substances, crystals The need to demonstrate iron, calcium, and, to a lesser extent, copper is commonplace in diagnostic material. There is undoubtedly some loss of all of these elements into aqueous, particularly acid fixatives, and this is more pronounced if fixation is prolonged. Many crystals, such as urates and cystine, are water soluble, and tissues in which such substances may be present should be alcohol fixed.

Decalcification

Normally mineralized or pathologically calcified tissues cannot satisfactorily be sectioned by conventional procedures and need to be softened by chemically removing the insoluble calcium salts present. This is achieved by treating the specimen with a suitable acid decalcification or a chelating agent.

Common decalcifying agents

As with fixation, there is no single ideal decalcificant. For example, methods which are suitable for the study of dense cortical bone may be totally unsuited for the study of fine detail in bone marrow. All decalcifying fluids cause some loss of histological detail, if only in terms of staining quality. This loss is most conspicuous following rapid decalcification with strong mineral acids and is compounded by prolonged treatment and inadequacy of initial fixation. For diagnostic purposes it is useful to have available a selected strong acid formula, a weak acid, and EDTA for special purposes.

Nitric acid A reliable and rapid agent which can be used from 5 to 10 per cent without undue tissue maceration. It tends to harden tissue and may impair staining. It is a major component of Perenyi's fluid, slower acting than the parent acid but causing less swelling and useful for softening hard tissues and for surface decalcification.

Hydrochloric acid This is almost as rapid in action as nitric acid but causes too much swelling to be used alone, and is invariably used in conjunction with other balancing components. Nuclear staining is likely to be poor.

Trichloroacetic acid Used at 5 per cent trichloroacetic acid is vigorous in action, but does not cause undue damage and facilitates good subsequent staining because it precipitates protein and nucleic acids.

Formic acid This is slower than the other acids mentioned, but less disruptive and compatible with reasonable staining. It can be used alone or in conjunction with alcohol, buffers, etc.

Citric acid—citrate buffer Citric acid is much slower than the other agents mentioned previously, but causes no perceptible damage to tissue components and so may be useful if histochemistry is required.

EDTA Again a much slower decalcificant (EDTA is a chelating agent) but not injurious to tissues, and so is useful for delicate tissues or where histochemical methods are to be applied.

Proprietary solutions Although the precise formulation of these decalcifying fluids is unknown, they must be regarded as strong acid solutions. They have a tendency to macerate tissues, and subsequent nuclear staining may be impossible if decalcification is prolonged.

Processing and embedding procedures

The aim of these techniques is to thoroughly impregnate and embed the tissue in a solid medium which is sufficiently soft to allow sections to be cut with a microtome blade but, at the same time, sufficiently hard to give rigidity to the tissue in order to preserve morphology and facilitate the cutting of thin, even sections. A number of embedding media are available, each offering particular advantages for certain types of investigation.

Common embedding media

Paraffin wax is used almost universally for routine diagnostic work in one of its formulations, either alone or with various additives such as ceresin or synthetic polymers. Tissues need to be dehydrated, usually in graded alcohols, and 'cleared' in a suitable 'ante-medium' such as xylene, toluene, chloroform, or trichloroethane before impregnation in molten wax. Many laboratories now enjoy the improved safety and versatility of enclosed tissue processors to achieve this operation. Most also utilize some form of labelled cassette in which tissue may be securely processed and later embedded. Particularly small or friable tissues may need special containment, and may usefully be embedded in an agar block prior to conventional processing.

Resins The principal use of resins in histopathology is as embedding media for electron microscopy. There are, in addition, several well-defined applications in light microscopy, particularly the preparation of sections of undecalcified bone, and the preparation of particularly thin sections (0.5–2.0 μm) for studying glomerular or lymphoid morphology where high resolution is often required.

Epoxy resins are used mostly for ultrastructural work and may be aromatic, e.g. araldite, or aliphatic, e.g. Epon, Spurr. The number of conventional tinctorial stains that can be satisfactorily performed on epoxy-embedded material is limited and so, for light microscopy, the acrylic resins, particularly methacrylates, have achieved greater popularity.

Celloidin and LVN Although now less popular than in previous years, celloidin (cellulose tetranitrate), and LVN (low-viscosity nitrocellulose) share a unique role as embedding media for tissues of the central nervous system. They are particularly useful for large blocks of brain which may undergo considerable gross and cellular distortion if processed to paraffin wax. The rubbery consistency of these media also makes them useful in supporting hard tissues or tissue comprising a mixture of adjacent hard and soft constituents.

Frozen sections

There are some techniques, such as lipid and enzyme histochemistry and some monoclonal immunocytochemistry, for which the use of frozen sections is frequently a prerequisite. Frozen sections cannot be matched for speed and so remain important for rapid diagnostic reporting, and many metal impregnation techniques, particularly those used in neuropathology, rely heavily on frozen sections. Sections may be produced with a freezing microtome or with a cryostat. The former is more suited to the production of sections of fixed material, and the cryostat to the preparation of sections of fresh tissues.

30.1.4 Staining methods

Haematoxylin stains

The combination of haematoxylin and eosin, now over 100 years old, remains the basis of the majority of histopathological diagnoses, and many laboratories continue to use some of the oldest formulae devised, for example the solutions first described by Ehrlich, Mayer, and Harris. Haematoxylin is a natural product, and with few exceptions requires oxidation to haematein

Table 30.2 Some applications of haematoxylin staining

Stain type	Mordant	Component stained
Ehrlich	Potassium alum	Nuclei, mucin
Heidenhain	Iron	Muscle striations, mitochondria, etc.
Verhoeff	Iron	Elastic
Mallory	Tungsten	Fibrin, glial fibres, muscle striations
Solcia	Lead	Endocrine cell granules
Mallory	—	Iron, copper, lead

and 'mordanting' with certain cations before it has any value as a histological dye. Used in this way, however, it displays considerable versatility by demonstrating not only nuclei, and thence general morphology, but also a remarkable number of quite different tissue components (Table 30.2). Eosin is the most frequently used partner stain because of its ease of use, and its red colour contrasts well with blue haematoxylin.

Special stains

Whereas haematoxylin and eosin staining is invaluable as a general staining procedure, it is frequently necessary to revert to alternative staining techniques in order to demonstrate more selectively a particular tissue component. A small selection of methods suitable for general use is discussed briefly below. For convenience, methods are arranged in groups according to the component demonstrated, but it should be remembered that few techniques are entirely specific and the rationale may be only incompletely understood. It should be remembered too that many components may be revealed to good effect by means of immunocytochemical procedures.

Connective tissue and muscle fibres

Collagen Van Gieson's stain and trichromes may be used to demonstrate most collagens. At least 13 types of collagen have been characterized by chemical composition, distribution, and function, and may be distinguished by immunocytochemical methods.

Reticulin, a main component being type III collagen, is invariably demonstrated by one of the silver impregnation techniques.

Basement membrane This material, rich in type IV collagen, is well demonstrated with the periodic acid-Schiff method or by silver impregnation. Jones's methanamine silver method is recommended for revealing abnormalities of the glomerular basement membrane.

Elastin Elastic fibres display considerable variation in composition and structure according to age and site, and therefore a corresponding variety of staining characteristics. None the less, they are well demonstrated by Verhoeff's haematoxylin method, by one of the polyaromatic solutions such as resorcin fuchsin, or by orcein.

Muscle Muscle fibres are well shown using trichrome methods or phloxine tartrazine. Striations are best demonstrated with phosphotungstic acid haematoxylin (PTAH) or Heidenhain's haematoxylin, but may also be seen to good advantage in preparations using a silver impregnation method for peripheral nerves.

Bone

The inherent nature of bone and metabolic bone disease dictates the need for special procedures, particularly methods for producing sections of undecalcified material to assess osteoid, etc. Thus in bone pathology, frozen, paraffin, and LVN sections of decalcified material, as well as undecalcified resin or ground sections, all have an important role. An alternative to von Kossa staining of undecalcified sections is the Tripp and MacKay silver impregnation method, a technique which requires neither resin embedding nor specialized microtomy and is thus within the scope of all diagnostic laboratories.

Bone marrow In order to study the cell populations accurately, thin sections are necessary and so resin embedding is preferable in many instances. The periodic acid-Schiff method, Perl's reaction, reticulin stains, and the methyl green pyronin technique may all prove useful adjuncts to haematoxylin and eosin (H & E) or Giemsa stains; most laboratories routinely stain bone marrows with H & E and Giemsa stains.

Central nervous system

A considerable range of techniques is available. Many of these are applicable only to tissues from the nervous system and may require frozen, paraffin-, or celloidin-embedded sections. Gold and silver impregnation methods exist for both neurones and their fibres, and for glial cells and their processes. Myelin can be stained by one of the special haematoxylin methods or with luxol fast blue, whereas degenerate myelin and its products are shown by Marchi-type methods and lipid stains. Many of these procedures require particular expertise in order to achieve consistent results, and frequently methods suitable for brain or spinal cord are not recommended for peripheral nerve tissues.

Nucleic acids and proteins

Nucleic acids Both DNA and RNA may be localized in tissue by virtue of the mutual affinity of their phosphate groups for basic dyes. Haematoxylin, suitably prepared, is taken up strongly by nuclear DNA but less so by cytoplasmic RNA. Methyl green and pyronin are two basic dyes which stain DNA and RNA respectively when used in appropriate combination. Nuclear DNA can be stained by the Feulgen method; this is based on hydrolysis of the deoxyribose sugar, and visualization of the engendered aldehyde groups with Schiff's reagent. Specific nucleic acids (DNA and mRNA) are demonstrable by *in situ* hybridization (see Section 30.3).

Proteins Although histochemical methods exist for the demonstration of many individual amino acids and side-chain or terminal groups, they are rarely used in routine histopathology.

Some structures, such as Paneth cell granules, may be stained by visualizing their high concentration of basic protein with acid dyes. Others, such as fibrin, may be demonstrated by physico-chemical methods which may be selective but by no means specific. Many individual proteins are now regularly, and indeed more satisfactorily, demonstrated by immunocytochemical techniques.

Carbohydrates

Complex carbohydrate-containing substances form an important group of structural or metabolically active tissue components. Their demonstration depends on reaction of vicinal glycol groups, various anionic groupings or residues, and specific sugars. The most widely used technique is the periodic acid-Schiff method for vicinal glycol groups. This can be performed with or without predigestion with diastase and in sequence with alcian blue, a basic phthalocyanin dye with potential to discriminate between acid and sulphated glycosaminoglycans and glycoproteins. The specificity of some mucin stains can be increased by staining parallel sections after treatment with mucin-degrading enzymes such as hyaluronidase or sialidase, and by utilizing other modifying reactions such as methylation and saponification. The wider application of sugar-specific lectins may prove useful in diagnosis.

Amyloid The β-pleated sheet configuration of amyloid glycoprotein confers characteristic tinctorial properties on this curious material. Affinity for Congo red, combined with birefringent and dichroic properties is highly typical of amyloid, which may be further characterized by its sensitivity to treatment with potassium permanganate; its reaction with dimethylaminobenzaldehyde; staining with basic dyes; and immunocytochemical procedures.

Lipids

A considerable range of selective methods is available by which tissue lipids may be identified. Apart from the positive demonstration of simple lipids in tumours etc. such methods may be helpful in the diagnosis of disorders of lipid metabolism. In practical terms it is usually sufficient to identify three main classes of lipid. Oil red O or the Sudan dyes stain most lipids, Nile blue sulphate selectively distinguishes acidic and neutral lipids; and Schultz's method reveals cholesterol and its esters.

Enzymes

The normal activity of some enzymes in particular cells or organelles may be exploited by utilizing such activity as a marker of the cell or a particular subcellular function. Although a multitude of techniques exist for the histochemical demonstration of enzymes, few have achieved widespread acceptance in diagnostic work. None the less, the demonstration of acetylcholinesterase (Hirschsprung disease), acid phosphatase (metastatic adenocarcinoma of the prostate), chloracetate esterase (myeloid cell marker), DOPA oxidase (amelanotic melanoma), and non-specific esterase (classification of leukaemias) may provide useful information in diagnostic situations.

Biogenic amines

Although accurate identification of biogenic amines and neuroendocrine cells requires immunocytochemical and ultrastructural studies in addition to simple staining procedures, there is a small range of methods which may contribute useful information in studies of these components and related tumours. The most useful are the masked metachromasia and lead haematoxylin methods, and agyrophil (e.g. Grimelius), argentaffin (e.g. Masson Fontana), and alkaline diazo techniques.

Pigments

Endogenous pigments are frequently useful indicators of pathological processes. Their natural colour and situation generally permit confident identification, but in some instances it may be necessary to utilize more selective histochemical procedures.

Fixation artefacts These may confuse the identification of genuine endogenous pigments. Formalin pigment, and the closely related malaria pigment, can be removed by treatment of sections with saturated alcoholic picric acid, whilst mercury fixation deposit is eliminated by treatment of sections with an iodine-hypo sequence.

Haemosiderin Derived from haemoglobin, haemosiderin is normally a bright yellow-gold colour, stainable with Perl's method for ferric iron. It may be deposited locally at sites of trauma, haemorrhage, or inflammation, or diffusely in haemachromatosis.

Bile pigments A group of pigments, also derived from haemoglobin, but lacking iron, display a range of chemical and physical properties. All forms give a positive reaction with Gmelin's method, whilst Fouchet's method is simple, but little more informative than van Gieson's stain used alone.

Melanins A group of yellow to brown to black pigments whose physical and chemical properties may vary according to location. Melanins are generally identified by the Masson Fontana silver method in conjunction with solubility and bleaching characteristics. The DOPA reaction for tyrosinase should be positive in any cell capable of synthesizing melanin.

Chromaffin The brown pigment seen characteristically in adrenal medullary cells and their tumours after suitable fixation is derived from adrenaline and noradrenaline. It can be effectively demonstrated by Giemsa's stain or Schmorl's ferric ferricyanide method.

Lipofuscins A heterogenous group of yellow-brown pigments derived from the oxidation of lipids and lipoproteins and found most commonly as perinuclear granules in ageing or atrophic tissues. Staining characteristics are not uniform and it is advisable to use several methods, such as Sudan black, periodic acid-Schiff, a long Ziehl–Neelsen stain, and Schmorl's method.

Inorganic and miscellaneous components

Calcium Different techniques are required for demonstrating the varying physico-chemical states in which calcium may occur in tissues. In practice, most commonly used are von Kossa's method (which, in fact, demonstrates the anion rather than calcium itself) and the alizarin-type chelation methods.

Copper Of the various methods available, the rhodanine and rubeanic acid techniques give the best results with the deposits of copper found in Wilson's disease, primary biliary cirrhosis, etc. Even though the copper deposited in such diseases may be lost in fixation, characteristic copper-associated protein can be usefully demonstrated by Shikata's orcein stain.

Barium Identification of residual barium from radiographic use, particularly pertinent if the procedure has been invasive, is best achieved using the sodium rhodizonate method.

Others A host of exogenous and endogenous substances may be seen in sections from time to time, many of which may be recognized by tinctorial procedures or by using polarized light, e.g. starch (periodic acid-Schiff method), urates (alkaline methanamine silver after alcoholic fixation), and asbestos (ferruginous) bodies (Perl's method).

Micro-organisms

Although histology is far from ideal as a means of identifying micro-organisms, it may in some cases be the only option. The range of organisms found incidentally in tissues is becoming increasingly bizarre as unusual infections occur in immunosuppressed or immunodepressed patients. Many may be identified with a reasonable degree of confidence using the classic Gram and Ziehl–Neelsen stains; the Wade–Fite method for leprosy; Grocott's silver method for fungi and *Pneumocystis*; periodic acid-Schiff and Giemsa's stain for protozoa, helminths, etc; and the Dieterle or Warthin and Starry methods for spirochaetes and *Legionella*. The surface antigen of hepatitis B virus can be detected using Shikata's orcein stain, and many organisms can now be specifically identified by immunocytochemical staining.

30.1.5 Further reading

Bancroft, J. D. and Stevens, A. (1990). *Theory and practice of histological techniques* (3rd edn). Churchill Livingstone, Edinburgh.

Filipe, M. I. and Lake, B. D. (1983). *Histochemistry in pathology.* Churchill Livingstone, Edinburgh.

Horobin, R. W. (1982). *Outline of histochemistry and biophysical staining.* Gustav Fischer Verlag, Stuttgart.

Lillie, R. D. and Fullmer, H. M. (1976). *Histopathologic technique and practical histochemistry* (4th edn). McGraw-Hill, New York.

Pearse, A. G. E. (1980). *Histochemistry. Theoretical and applied* (4th edn), Vol. 1, *Preparative and optical technology.* Churchill Livingstone, Edinburgh.

Pearse, A. G. E. (1985). *Histochemistry. Theoretical and applied* (4th edn), Vol. 2, *Analytical technology.* Churchill Livingstone, Edinburgh.

Underwood, J. C. E. (1981). *Introduction to biopsy interpretation and surgical pathology.* Springer-Verlag, Berlin.

30.2 Immunocytochemical analysis of human tissue

D. Y. Mason

Immunocytochemical techniques allow antigenic molecules to be detected *in situ* in human cell and tissue samples, and have been used widely in recent years both in diagnostic pathology and in research into human disease. This section outlines the technical aspects of these techniques and also considers the way in which immunocytochemical reactions should be interpreted by the pathologist.

30.2.1 Methodology

Handling samples

Techniques for processing human tissue prior to immunocyto-chemical labelling can be divided into two categories:

1. routine histological fixation and paraffin embedding;
2. specialized fixation and embedding procedures.

Routine tissue processing

The traditional means of handling human tissues for diagnostic purposes are detailed in the preceding section (30.1). The most widely used histopathological fixatives are based upon formalin, and fixatives also contain additional chemicals, such as picric acid and dichromate. Although traditional fixatives and embedding procedures ensure good preservation of tissue morphology, they tend to denature or mask antigenic molecules present in tissues, and thereby restrict the scope of immunohistological analysis. Antigenic reactivity can in some instances be restored by treating sections with proteolytic enzymes (e.g. trypsin, pronase, etc.), but this is not always effective and some antigens are irretrievably lost.

Specialized tissue processing procedures

The problem of antigenic denaturation in routine fixatives has led many laboratories to explore alternative processing procedures. One of the simplest and most effective methods is to perform immunocytochemical staining on cryostat sections prepared from a frozen block of tissue. Cryostat sections are usually fixed in acetone prior to staining, since this improves the final cellular morphology and causes minimal antigenic denaturation.

The preservation of morphological detail in frozen sections is not as good, however, as that in wax-embedded tissue, and for this reason, and also to avoid the inconvenience of storing frozen tissue, a number of laboratories have explored wax-embedding procedures in which non-denaturating fixatives are used. A mixture of periodate, lysine, and paraformaldehyde (PLP) is the most popular of these fixatives, combining good immunohistochemical reactions with acceptable morphology.

Another approach is to freeze-dry rather than to fix tissues before wax embedding. Specialized tissue-processing methods are of limited use in the context of diagnostic immunocyto-chemistry, however, since they can only be used when fresh tissue is available.

Antibodies

Polyclonal antisera

Prior to the introduction of monoclonal antibodies, all immuno-histochemical studies were performed using polyclonal reagents raised by immunizing animals with purified antigen. Reagents prepared in this way suffer from a number of disadvantages; they have tended increasingly to be superseded by monoclonal reagents. One major drawback of polyclonal antisera is that, even when they have been raised against highly purified anti-gens they may contain unwanted antibodies against other constituents present in human tissue. The possibility of unwanted reactivity due to such contaminating antibodies can be reduced by absorbing the serum before use with an insolubilized prep-aration of antigen(s). However, since the specificity of these unwanted antibodies is usually unknown, this procedure offers, at best, only a probability that the performance of the antiserum will be improved.

An alternative means of increasing the specificity of a poly-clonal antiserum is to affinity purify the specific antibodies on an immunoadsorbent prepared by immobilizing the immuniz-ing antigen on a matrix such as Sepharose. Use of antibody eluted from such an immunoadsorbent reduces the risk of con-taminating antibodies but cannot guarantee their specificity (since impurities present in the antigen used for immunization are likely also to be present in the immunoadsorbent). Further-more, the method is only feasible when a substantial supply of purified antigen is available.

A further drawback of polyclonal antibodies is that, although a particular batch of antiserum may be of high specificity, the maintenance of the same quality in subsequent batches may be difficult to ensure. This problem of quality control may pose an obstacle to the use of any individual polyclonal antiserum in more than a few laboratories.

Monoclonal antibodies

The technique, first reported by Köhler and Milstein in 1975, for the production of antibodies from hybridomas prepared by the fusion of immune spleen cells and a myeloma cell line, has been widely used in immunocytochemistry. Since the antigen-combining site in all the molecules in a given monoclonal anti-body preparation will be of identical specificity, the risk of unwanted reactions is minimized. The problem of quality con-trol, referred to above in the context of polyclonal antisera, is also easily overcome when monoclonal reagents are used, since a hybridoma cell line can produce an unlimited amount of identical antibody. In consequence, it has been possible to distribute many monoclonal antibodies on a wide scale inter-nationally.

The first monoclonal antibodies to be produced were directed against white cell-associated antigens, and by the early 1980s a large number of these reagents had been reported in the literature. It was far from clear how many of them were of identical specificity, and this uncertainty led to the organization of the first of a series of international workshops on leucocyte antigens in Paris in 1982. Monoclonal antibodies produced in many different laboratories around the world were analysed by indirect immunofluorescent staining of white cell suspensions, by biochemical analysis of the target antigen(s) for the antibodies, and by immunohistological staining of tissue sections. Subsequent workshops have been held in Boston (1984), Oxford (1986), and Vienna (1989) and the fifth is being organized at the time of writing (1991).

As a result of these collaborative studies, much new information has been gathered on the nature of human leucocyte antigens and on the monoclonal antibodies which detect them. A system for the nomenclature of white cell antigens was established at the first workshop, in which antigens are referred to by a number, prefixed by the letters 'CD'. A total of 78 such designations were established in the first four workshops, as summarized in Table 30.3; readers should consult the proceedings of these workshops for further details.

Monoclonal antibodies against other human antigens have not been studied in the same depth, but nevertheless the range of molecules which can now be detected using monoclonal reagents is extensive, and includes intermediate filaments, growth factor receptors, and microbial and viral antigens.

Labelling techniques

All immunocytochemical techniques depend upon the linkage of a marker, which can be detected by microscopy, to a specific antibody. There are two major types of procedure, one based upon the use of a fluorescent marker molecule, and the other upon an enzyme which yields a visible reaction product. More recently, colloidal gold has been used, but this labelling system, although it has major advantages for ultrastructural visualization of antigens (the application for which it was first introduced), is not used on a wide scale in histopathology.

Immunofluorescent techniques

In the 1940s Coons reported experiments in which he had coupled fluorescein to crude antibody fractions of antisera raised against bacterial antigens, e.g. streptococci. He was able to show that micro-organisms in tissue sections could be visualized under the microscope using these reagents, and he is thus justly considered the originator of the science of immunocytochemistry.

The principle behind immunofluorescent labelling is that a fluorescent marker molecule is excited at one wavelength and then emits light at a different wavelength. Selective filters are used to prevent the excitation light being visible to the observer, with the result that the fluorescent signal is viewed against a dark background (Fig. 30.1). This is necessary because the small amount of light emitted by the excited fluorochrome would be swamped by conventional bright-field illumination.

Fluorescein, the label used in the pioneering experiments of

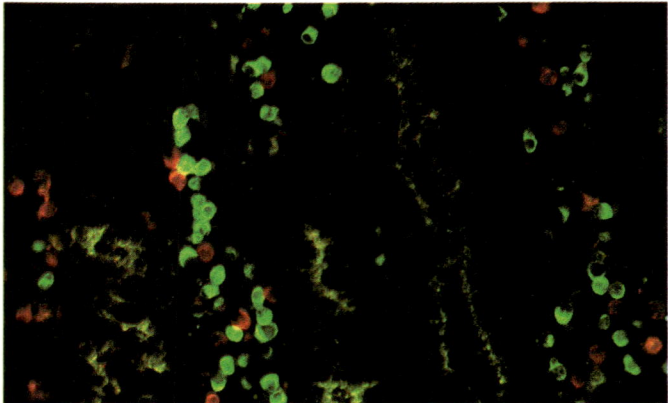

Fig. 30.1 Section of human jejunum from a case of coeliac disease double stained by an immunofluorescent technique using fluorescein to detect IgA (in green) and rhodamine to detect IgM (in red). Numerous IgA-positive plasma cells are seen in the lamina propria, together with smaller numbers of IgM-positive plasma cells. The yellow cytoplasmic staining in the glandular crypt epithelium represents the presence of the two fluorescent labels at the same site and indicates that both IgM and IgA are taken up and transported to the intestinal lumen. (No counterstain: photomicrograph kindly provided by Professor P. Brandtzaeg.)

Coons, continues to be the most widely used fluorochrome, but it has been joined more recently by rhodamine and Texas Red™ (both of which emit red light when illuminated with green excitation). A fluorochrome that has been used in recent years is phycoerythrin, an algal pigment that accounts for the red colour of some seaweeds and which increases the efficiency of photosynthesis by absorbing light of wavelengths which cannot directly stimulate chlorophyll. However, the major use of this fluorochrome has been in flow cytometry, since it has the advantage that both it and fluorescein can be excited by the same laser beam, and it is not widely used for the localization of antigens in tissue sections.

Regardless of the fluorochrome used, there are basically two major techniques for fluorescent immunocytochemistry, as illustrated in Fig. 30.2. In the direct procedure the fluoro-

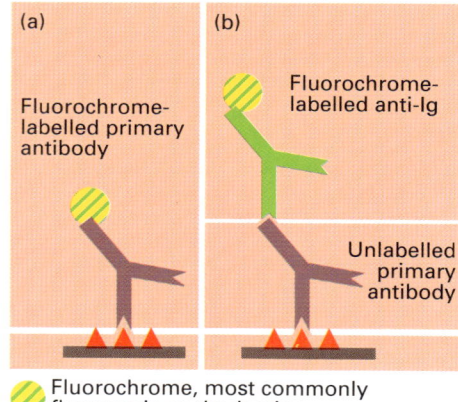

Fig. 30.2 Techniques for immunofluorescent staining of human tissues: (a) direct immunofluorescence; (b) indirect immunofluorescence.

chrome is coupled directly to the primary antibody, whereas in the indirect method a secondary reagent (directed against the species in which the first antibody is raised) is labelled with the fluorochrome. Direct techniques offer the advantage of rapidity, since only a single reagent need be applied, but they are of lower sensitivity than indirect techniques and depend on the availability of labelled primary antibodies. In contrast, the indirect method can be used with any primary antibody, provided that a fluorescently labelled second-stage reagent is available.

Immunoenzymatic techniques

These procedures first began to be used in the 1960s, the pioneers in the field being Avrameas, Sternberger, and Nakane. The most widely used enzyme in these procedures is horseradish peroxidase. This molecule is small (molecular weight approximately 40 kDa) by comparison to an antibody molecule, relatively easy and inexpensive to purify, and enzymatically stable. It can be detected by a number of different cytochemical reactions which yield sharply localized insoluble reaction products, but the commonest substrate contains diaminobenzidine and hydrogen peroxide (Fig. 30.3). In some laboratories aminoethylcarbazole and hydrogen peroxide is used as an alternative substrate, since the possibility has been raised that diaminobenzidine may be carcinogenic.

More recently a number of laboratories have utilized calf intestinal alkaline phosphatase as an alternative enzyme to peroxidase. Although this enzyme is of larger molecular weight and less easily purified than peroxidase, in practice it produces results which are equal to, if not better than, those obtained using peroxidase. Commonly used substrates contain naphthol phosphate together with hexazotized New Fuchsin or Fast Red; the bright red colour of these reaction products contrasts well in tissue sections with haematoxylin counterstain (Fig. 30.4). Immuno-alkaline phosphatase methods offer the advantage that endogenous tissue enzymatic activity (see below) poses less of a problem than in immunoperoxidase techniques. It is also

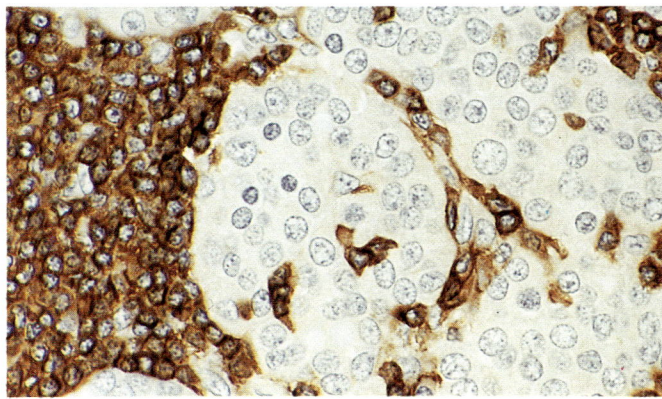

Fig. 30.3 Immunoperoxidase labelling of a human lymph node with a monoclonal antibody against leucocyte common antigen using the diaminobenzidine/H_2O_2 substrate. Lymphoid cells are strongly stained; metastatic carcinoma cells are negative. (Haematoxylin counterstain.)

possible to use immunoalkaline phosphatase and immunoperoxidase techniques together for double labelling procedures, since the two enzymes can be revealed in sharply contrasting colours (Fig. 30.5).

As in the case of immunofluorescent procedures, immunoenzymatic techniques may be performed by direct or indirect methods, as illustrated in Fig. 30.6. In choosing between these two techniques the same considerations apply as for immunofluorescent procedures. Many laboratories favour the three-stage indirect technique (Fig. 30.6c) since it is of higher sensitivity than the two-stage technique. In all of these procedures the enzyme must be covalently coupled to antibody, and a variety of techniques are well established for this purpose, most frequently using either a bifunctional reagent, such as glutaraldehyde, or alternatively a procedure in which carbohydrate on the enzyme is oxidized with periodate so that these groups can react with amino groups on the antibody molecule.

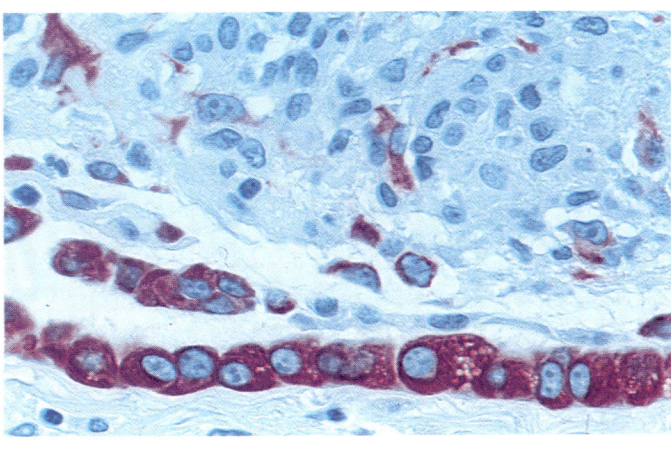

(a)

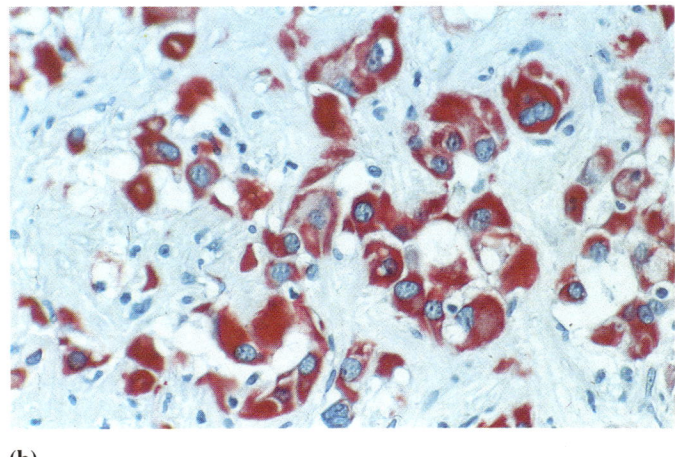

(b)

Fig. 30.4 Immuno-alkaline phosphatase labelling of cytokeratins in human lung showing the characteristic red reaction product. (Haematoxylin counterstain.) (a) Normal mesothelium, showing an orderly array of pleural lining cells; (b) mesothelioma showing cytokeratin-positive malignant cells with atypical morphological features.

Table 30.3   CD classification of leucocyte antigens

Antigens	Other title	Mol. weight	Main cellular distribution	Comments
CD1a, b, c	T6	49, 45, 43	Cortical thymocytes, Langerhans cells	Similar to HLA Class I (associated with $\beta2$ microglobulin)
CD2	T11	50	T-cells	Receptor for sheep erythrocytes and LFA-3
CD2R		50	Activated T-cells	CD2R epitope associated with T-cell activation
CD3	T3	16–29	T-cells	Five chains (γ–η), associated with T-cell receptor
CD4	T4	59	T-cells subset, monocytes/macrophages	Receptor for HLA-Class II and AIDS virus (HIV)
CD5	T1	67	T-cells, B-cell subset (weak)	
CD6	T12	100	T-cells, B-cell subset (weak)	
CD7		40	Most T-cells	
CD8	T8	32	T-cell subset, splenic sinusoidal cells	HLA-Class I receptor. Associated with $pp56^{lck}$ kinase
CD9	p24	24	Platelets, monocytes, pre-B-cells, many non-leucocytes (e.g. brain)	? Protein kinase. Anti-CD9 aggregates platelets
CD10	CALLA	100	Stem cells, renal epithelium, etc.	Neutral endopeptidase
CD11a	LFA-1	180	Many white cells	α-chain of LFA-1 integrin. Binds ICAM-1. Mediates T-cell cytoxicity and cell:cell adhesion (see CD18)
CD11b	Mac-1, CR3	165	Granulocytes, monocytes	α-chain of Mac-1. Receptor for C3bi, fibrinogen, Factor X (see CD18)
CD11c	p150, 95	150	Macrophages, granulocytes, NK cells, hairy cell leukaemia	α-chain of p150,95. ? C3bi receptor (see CD18)
CD12		No data	Myeloid cells	Little data available
CD13	My7, gp150	150	Granulocytes, monocytes, non-leucocytes (e.g. bile canaliculi, connective tissue)	Aminopeptidase N
CD14	gp55	55	Monocytes, Kupffer cells, granulocytes, FDC	Good monocyte/macrophage marker
CD15	Hapten X	50–180	Granulocytes, epithelium, RS cells	Gal 1-4 (Fuc1-3) GlcNac
CD16	FcRγIII	50–65	Granulocytes, some macrophages, NK cells	Low-affinity IgG receptor
CDw17	Lactosyl-ceramide	No data	Granulocytes, monocytes, platelets	Cer Glc, β1-4 Gal
CD18	LFA-1	95	Many white cells (see CD11a, b and c)	β-chain of LFA/Mac-1 integrin family (see CD11)
CD19	B4	90	B-cells	Belongs to Ig supergene family
CD20	B1	35/37	B-cells	? Involved in membrane ion transport
CD21	CR2	140	B-cells, FDC	Receptor for C3d and EBV
CD22		135	B-cells	Intracytoplasmic in early B-cells. Belongs to Ig supergene family. Homologous to myelin-associated glycoprotein, CD33, and N-CAM
CD23	FC$_\varepsilon$RII	45–50	Activated B-cells, some FDC	Low affinity receptor for IgE. ? Soluble form has growth factor activity
CD24	BA1	41/38	Some B-cells, granulocytes	
CD25	Tac	55	Activated cells, macrophages	Low affinity Interleukin-2 receptor
CD26		120	Activated T- and B-cells, macrophages	Dipeptidylpeptidase IV
CD27		55	T-cells, plasma cells	Present on cell surface as a homodimer (110 kDa)
CD28		44	T-cell subset	Present on cell surface as a homodimer (88 kDa)
CD29	GPIIa, VLA-β chain	130	T-cell subset, many non-leucocytes	Forms heterodimer with at least six different VLA-α chains (see CDw49)
CD30	Ki-1	105	Activated lymphocytes, R–S cells, anaplastic large cell lymphoma	
CD31	GPIIa'	140	Granulocytes, monocytes, platelets, B-cells, endothelium	CEA-like molecule
CDw32	FcγRII	40	Granulocytes, B-cells, monocytes, macrophages, platelets, endothelium	IgG receptor. Several isoforms with differing distributions have been identified
CD33	My9	67	Myeloid progenitors, monocytes	
CD34		105–120	Haemopoietic progenitors, endothelium	
CD35	CR1	160, 190 220 or 250	FDC, B-cells, red cells, granulocytes, glomeruli, some NK-cells	C3b receptor. Four allotypes differ in MW
CD36	GPIV	90	Monocytes/macrophages, platelets	Receptor for falciparum infected RBC and (?) thrombospondin
CD37		40–52	B-cells, also macrophages, T-cells (both weak)	
CD38	T10	45	Germinal centre cells, plasma cells, activated T-cells, thymocytes	
CD39		79–100	B-cells, macrophages, endothelium, other cells	
CD40		44–48, 50	B-cells, interdigitating reticulum cells, carcinomas, other cells	? Receptor for growth factor

Table 30.3 CD classification of leucocyte antigens—*continued*

Antigens	Other title	Mol. weight	Main cellular distribution	Comments
CD41	GPIIb/IIIa	155+110	Megakaryocytes, platelets	Ca^{2+} dependent complex of gpIIb and gpIIIa (CD61, 110 kDa), (120 kDa α-chain+33 kDa β-chain). Deficient in Glanzmann's thrombasthenia. Binds fibrinogen, fibronectin and VWf
CD42a	GPIX	23	Megakaryocytes, platelets	Complexes with GPIb (CD42b) to form receptor for VWf. Deficient in Bernard–Soulier syndrome
CD42b	GpIb	135+25	Megakaryocytes, platelets	Two chain molecule comprising 135 kDa α-chain and 25 kDa β-chain
CD43	Leucosialin, sialophorin	95	White cells, red blood cells, brain	Defective in Wiskett Aldrich syndrome
CD44	HERMES	80–95	White cells, brain	Cell homing receptor
CD45	LCA	180–220	Most white cells	Tyrosine phosphatase. Different isoforms (see below) produced via alternative splicing
CD45RA		220	B-cells, T-cell subset, monocytes/macrophages	Epitope encoded by exon A
CD45RB		190/205/220	B-cells, T-cell subset, monocytes/macrophages, granulocytes	Epitope encoded by exon B, detected by antibody PD7/26
CD45RO		180	T-cells, B-cell subset, monocytes/macrophages	Epitope not encoded by exon A, B, or C, detected by antibody UCHL1
CD46	MCP	56/66	Many cell types	Co-factor for cleavage of C3b/C4b
CD47		47–52	Pan-reactive	? Associated with Rhesus blood group
CD48		? 41	Monocytes and neutrophils (weak)	Can be used in diagnosis of PNH
CDw49	VLA-α chain	120–170	Platelets, lymphocytes, monocytes	Three chains (β, δ, φ) which complex to CD29 (VLAβ-chains) to produce, respectively, GP1a/IIa, a lymphocyte homing receptor, and laminin receptor
CDw50		108/14) (?)	Luecocytes	
CD51	VNR α-chain	125+25	Platelets, non-leucocytes	Complexes with VNR β-chain (CD61/CPIIIa) to form vitronectin receptor
CDw52	Campath-1	21–28 (?)	Leucocytes	Antibody used in preventing GVH disease
CD53		32–40	Leucocytes	
CD54	ICAM-1	90	Endothelial cells, activated lymphocytes, epithelial cells	Ligand for LFA-1. Receptor for rhinovirus
CD55	DAF	70	Many cells types	Limits complement activation. Absent from PNH red cells
CD56	NKH1	135/220	NK cells, neuroectodermal cells	Isoform of neural cell adhesion molecule (N-CAM)
CD57	HNK1	110	NK cells, T-cell subset	
CD58	LFA-3	40–65	Many cell types	Ligand for CD2 (SRBC-receptor)
CD59	MAC inhibitor	18–20	Many cell types	Inhibits complement mediated lysis
CDw60		Carbohydrate	T-cell subset, platelets	NeuAc-NeuAc-Gal sequence on gangliosides
CD61	GPIIIa, VNR β-chain	110	Platelets, megakaryocytes	Associates with GPIIb (in CD41) or with VNR α-chain (CD51) to form receptors for fibrinogen, vitronectin, VWf
CD62	PADGEN, GMP-140	140	Activated platelets, endothelium	Present in platelet α-granules. Expressed on surface after activation
CD63		53	Activated platelets, monocytes/macrophages	
CD64	FcγRI	75	Monocytes	High affinity receptor for IgG
CDw65		Carbohydrate	Granulocytes, monocytes	Type II chain fucoganglioside
CD66		180–200	Granulocytes	
CD67		100	Granulocytes	
CD68		110	Monocytes/macrophages, myeloid cells	Good cytoplasmic pan-macrophage marker
CD69	AIM	28–34	Activated cells, NK cells	Involved in early lymphocyte activation events
CDw70	Ki-24	??	Activated lymphocytes, R-S cells, anaplastic large cell lymphoma	
CD71	T9	95	Activated cells, macrophages, proliferating cells	Homodimer. Transferrin receptor
CD72		39/43	B-cells, some macrophages, epithelium	
CD73		69	B-cells and T-cell subset	Ector-5′ nucleotidase
CD74	LN2	35/33/41	B-cells, monocytes/macrophages, epithelial cells	Invariant chain of HLA-Class II
CDw75	LN1	53	Mature B-cells, epithelial cells	
CD76		67–85	Mature B-cells, T-cell subset, epithelial cells	
CD77	BLA	Carbohydrate	Follicle centre B-cells	Neutral glycosphingolipid. Equivalent to P^k blood group
CD78	Ba	??	B-cells	

AIM = Activation inducer molecule. CEA = Carcinoembryonic antigen. DAF = Decay accelerating factor. FDC = Follicular dendritic cells. GVH = Graft versus host. I-CAM = Intracellular adhesion molecule. LCA = Leucocyte common antigen. LFA = Leucocyte function antigen. MCP = Membrane co-factor protein. PNH = Paroxysomal nocturnal haemoglobinuria. R–S = Reed–Sternberg. VLA = Very late activation. VWf = Von Willebrand factor.

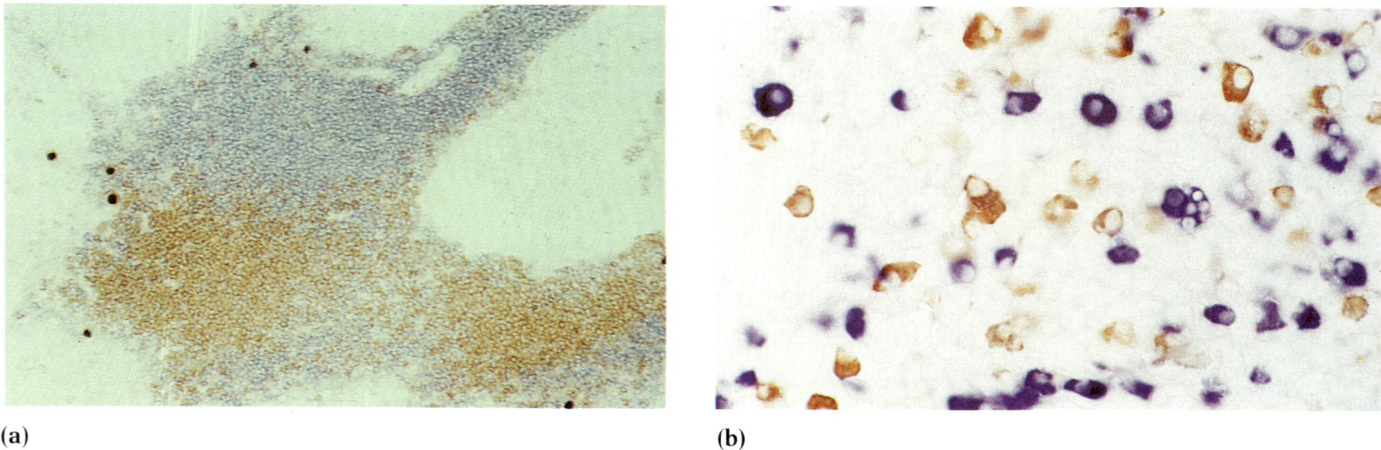

(a)   **(b)**

Fig. 30.5   Double staining of pairs of antigens in human tissue using alkaline phosphatase (blue reaction product) and peroxidase (brown reaction product) as enzyme labels (no counterstain). (a) Human thymoma stained for B- and T-lymphoid cells (brown and blue, respectively); (b) double labelling of plasma cells in a lymphoid tissue biopsy for κ and λ light chains (brown and blue, respectively).

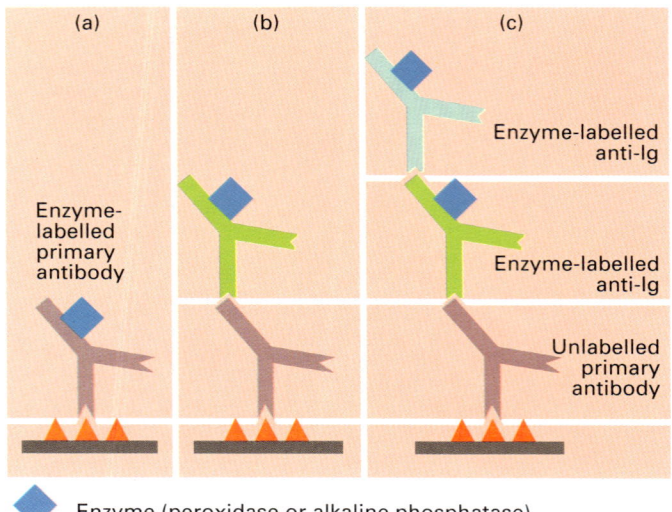

Fig. 30.6   Techniques for immunoenzymatic staining of human tissue based on covalent enzyme : antibody conjugates. (a) Direct immunoenzymatic staining; (b) indirect immunoenzymatic staining (two-stage); (c) indirect immunoenzymatic staining (three-stage).

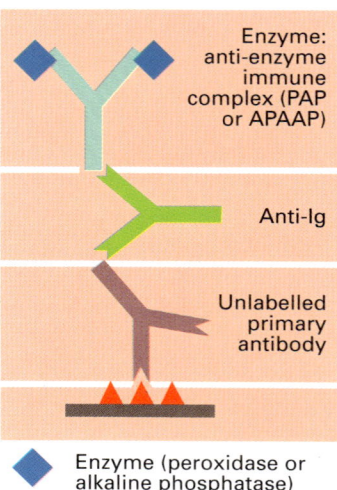

Fig. 30.7   Unlabelled antibody techniques for staining human tissues. The unlabelled antibody in the second stage acts as a bridging antibody, one of its antigen-binding sites reacting with the primary antibody and the other with immunoglobulin in the enzyme/antibody immune complexes. For this reason, the anti-enzyme antibody and the primary antibody must be raised in the same species.

An alternative to these covalent conjugate-based techniques is the 'unlabelled antibody' method. This was first developed in the laboratories of Spicer and of Sternberger in the late 1960s, and its principle is that the enzyme, rather than being coupled covalently to antibody, is bound by antibody which has been raised against the enzyme. These immune complexes of enzyme and antibody can be linked to the primary antibody by a bridging antibody, provided that the anti-enzyme antibody has been raised in the same species as the primary antibody. The most widely used of these techniques is the peroxidase : anti-peroxidase technique (PAP), as illustrated in Fig. 30.7. More recently an 'unlabelled antibody' procedure, based on alkaline

phosphatase, known as the alkaline phosphatase : anti-alkaline phosphatase (APAAP) technique, has been used widely (Fig. 30.7).

One of the attractions of unlabelled antibody techniques is that they do not necessitate the covalent coupling of antibody to enzyme, a process which has to be carefully monitored to avoid the formation of under- or over-conjugated material, or the production of high molecular aggregates which might bind to tissues non-specifically. Unlabelled antibody techniques tend to give low background and are of comparable or better sensitivity than indirect procedures. Furthermore, their sensitivity may be further increased by repeating the bridging anti-Ig antibody and PAP and APAAP steps.

A further important category of immunoenzymatic procedure exploits the high affinity of the reaction between the protein avidin and the vitamin biotin. A variety of procedures based upon this principle have been used, of which the most widely used is the ABC technique (Fig. 30.8). The rationale behind all of these procedures is that avidin has a very high affinity for its ligand, and this is thought to ensure strong binding of the final enzyme label to the tissue. It might be argued, on the principle that a chain is only as strong as its weakest link, that the very high affinity of this binding is less important for the intensity of the final reaction than the affinity of the second stage antibody for the primary antibody, or of the primary antibody for tissue antigen. In practice, avidin:biotin techniques are not clearly more sensitive than the other procedures described above, but they are nevertheless widely used for the immunocytochemical staining of pathological tissue.

Many human tissues contain endogenous peroxidase activity, principally myeloperoxidase and eosinophil peroxidase in white cells and haemoglobin in red cells. This may cause problems when staining tissues by immunoperoxidase techniques since the substrate will reveal both the endogenous enzyme and the horseradish peroxidase immunoenzymatic label. In consequence, a blocking step (e.g. incubation in methanol and hydrogen peroxide) is sometimes performed prior to immunoenzymatic labelling, with the aim of inhibiting endogenous enzyme activity. A potential complication is that this may denature antigens present in the tissue, and in these circumstances immuno-alkaline phosphatase procedures may be preferable. Alkaline phosphatase is present in some human tissues

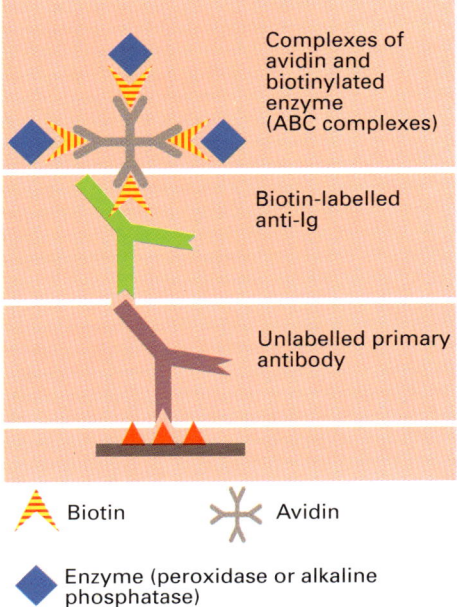

Complexes of avidin and biotinylated enzyme (ABC complexes)

Biotin-labelled anti-Ig

Unlabelled primary antibody

Biotin   Avidin

Enzyme (peroxidase or alkaline phosphatase)

Fig. 30.8 The ABC avidin:biotin technique. The complexes of avidin and biotinylated enzyme are usually pre-formed, so that the procedure involves only three incubation stages prior to addition of substrate.

but most of its activity can be blocked by an inhibitor (levamisole) which does not affect the calf intestinal alkaline phosphatase immunoenzymatic label.

30.2.2   Interpretation of results

Specific and non-specific staining

The aim of immunocytochemical labelling of human tissue is to reveal the 'antigenic content, the whole antigenic content and nothing but the antigenic content'; in other words it is desirable to avoid non-specific staining which does not reflect the presence of antigen, and equally well to ensure that any antigen which is present is revealed. The factors that may thwart this goal by causing either non-specific or false negative stainings are considered below.

Non-specific staining

As mentioned above, polyclonal antisera carry a risk of non-specific staining in that they may contain unwanted antibodies against antigens other than those to which they are primarily directed. However, the increasing use of monoclonal antibodies has tended to make this type of non-specific staining a thing of the past. Immunologists with experience of working with living cells are well aware that immunoglobulin may bind via its Fc portion to specific receptors on the surface of human cells. However, when staining tissue sections, this appears not to present a major problem, probably because fixation destroys receptor activity. It has sometimes been claimed in the past that monoclonal antibodies of IgM class tend to bind non-specifically to human tissues, but this has not been borne out by practical experience. Antibody may also bind to tissue sections as a result of other, poorly characterized mechanisms (e.g. collagen sometimes picks up antibody non-specifically, especially in polyclonal antisera) and this may cause some diffuse background labelling. A preliminary blocking step, in which the tissue is first incubated with non-immune serum, is therefore sometimes used. In practice, however, particularly with the use of monoclonal antibodies, this procedure is unnecessary, although it still survives in many laboratories for reasons related more to tradition than to necessity.

The possibility that a monoclonal antibody will detect a conformational epitope present on two unrelated molecules is a theoretical risk which in practice has turned out to be a very rare event. A much commoner situation is that a molecule which is believed initially to be specific for a particular cell type proves, on further study, to be more widely distributed. One widely studied example is in the field of intermediate filament immunocytochemistry: it was initially believed that different categories of intermediate filaments were highly specific for different cell types (e.g. cytokeratins for epithelium, desmin for muscle, vimentin for mesenchymal tissues, etc.). However, more detailed analysis has shown that these rules are far from absolute, particularly when malignancies are studied, and co-expression of more than one class of intermediate filament by a cell type is now well documented. Thus, carcinoma cells may express not only cytokeratins, as expected on the basis of their epithelial origin, but also vimentin, and both normal muscle and rhabdomyosarcomas can co-express desmin and cytokeratin (Fig. 30.9).

This phenomenon of antigens showing a wider cellular distribution than was initially thought is also commonly seen in the case of white cell-associated antigens. Examples of this phenomenon include CD1 antigen, shared between cortical thymocytes and Langerhans cells; CD4 antigen, present on helper-inducer T-cells and macrophages; CALLA antigen (CD10), which is found not only on haemopoietic stem cells but also on renal epithelium, fibroblasts, granulocytes, and several other cell types; and CD25 (the Tac antigen or interleukin-2 receptor), which was initially thought to be specific for activated T-cells but subsequently turned out to be present on macrophages and B-cells. This sharing of antigens between unrelated cell types, which often receives the emotive designation of lineage 'infidelity' or 'promiscuity', should be borne in mind when interpreting the reactions of antibodies on tissue sections.

It is frequently assumed, when a cell gives a positive immunocytochemical reaction in a tissue section, that it must have synthesized the antigen which it contains. However, it is now clear that diffusion and artefactual uptake of extracellular antigens may occur, probably during tissue processing, with the result that the cytoplasm of a cell may contain an antigen which it has acquired from its environment. Proteins which are normally present in the serum in high concentration, e.g. immunoglobulin and transferrin (Fig. 30.10), are particularly likely to cause this artefact.

False-negative staining

When a cell in a tissue section gives a negative immunocytochemical reaction, the obvious interpretation is that it does not contain the antigen in question. However, a variety of different mechanisms may account for a cell which does contain an antigen failing to give a positive immunocytochemical reaction.

Denaturation of antigens has already been referred to in the context of tissue-processing techniques. The recognition of this phenomenon is made easier when cells known to be positive for the antigen are present in the section as a positive control. For example, if a biopsy of lymphoid tissue containing metastatic tumour is stained for leucocyte common antigen (CD45), normal lymphoid cells expressing this antigen will always be present (Fig. 30.3), and negative staining of the tumour would be discounted as artefactual if these normal lymphoid cells were unstained. In contrast, staining of the same section for cytokeratin might be more difficult to interpret, given that non-lymphoid tissue normally contains no cytokeratin-positive cells as a positive control, and in these circumstances staining of a different tissue (e.g. normal human breast) known to contain cytokeratin might be performed as a positive control in the same experiment.

There are at least two other reasons why cells that synthesize an antigen may fail to stain by immunocytochemical methods. First, the level of antigen in the cell may be too low to be

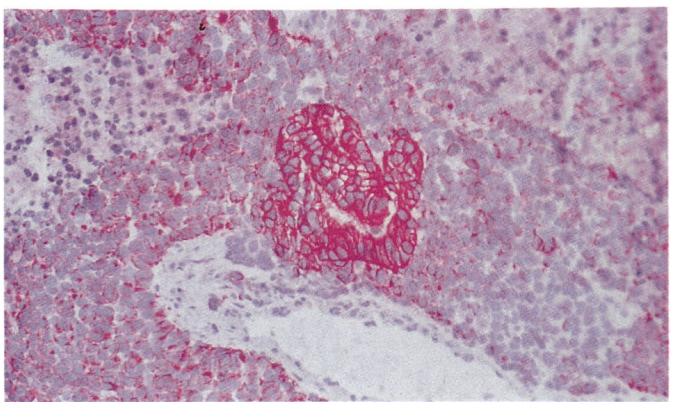

(a)

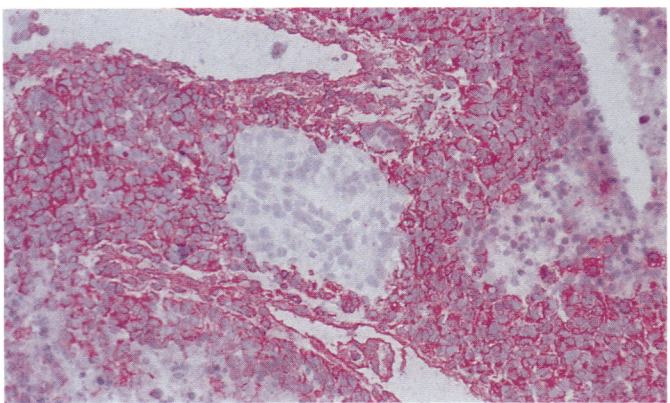

(b)

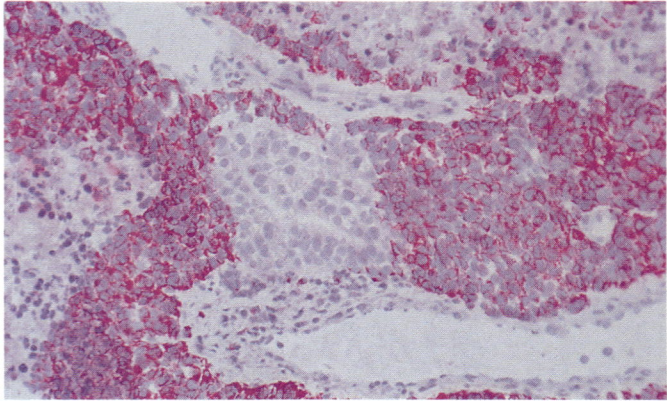

(c)

Fig. 30.9 Biopsy of human lung carcinoma stained for three different classes of intermediate filament. (Immuno-alkaline phosphatase technique, haematoxylin counterstain.) (a) A small area of normal bronchial epithelium is strongly positive for cytokeratin. It is surrounded by carcinoma cells which express lower levels of this antigen. (b) An adjacent section stained for vimentin shows that the normal epithelium is vimentin-negative but that the malignant cells aberrantly express this intermediate filament. (c) An adjacent section shows that the malignant cells also aberrantly express desmin, a class of intermediate filament which is normally confined to muscle. The normal epithelium is desmin-negative.

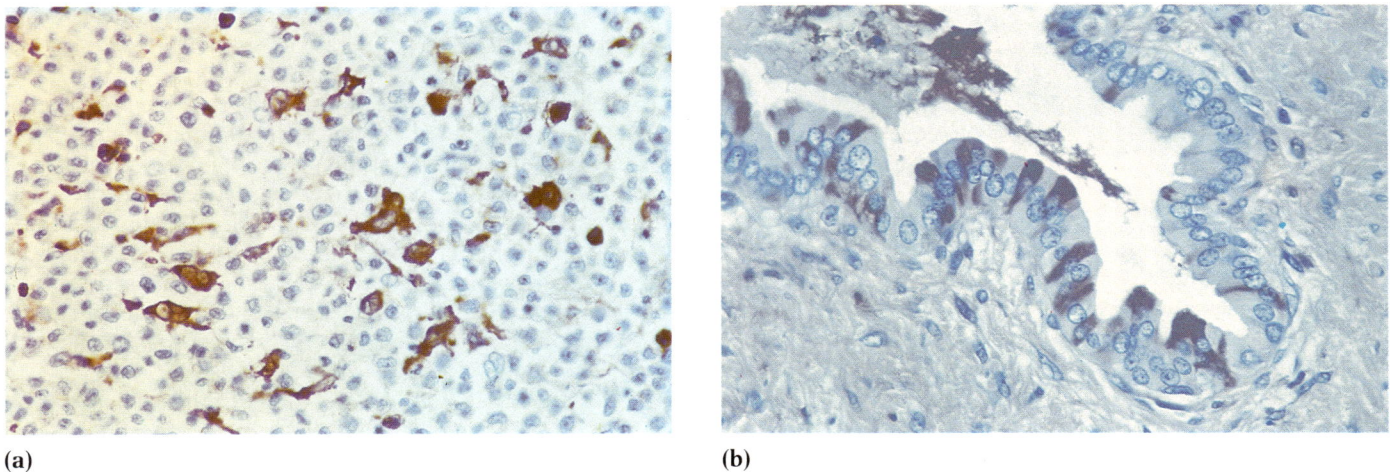

(a)　　　　　　　　　　　　　　　　　　　　　　　　　(b)

Fig. 30.10 Misleading staining patterns suggestive of cellular synthesis, which in reality, reflect passive uptake of extracellular protein. (Immunoperoxiclase technique, haematoxylin counterstain.) (a) A human lymphoma biopsy containing scattered cells, strongly stained for immunoglobulin which was absorbed from their environment. Staining for other serum proteins, e.g. albumin and transferrin, showed identical labelling patterns. (b) Scattered cells in human bile duct epithelium are strongly positive for serum albumin, which was also acquired through passive diffusion rather than by synthesis.

detected. This might be because only small amounts of antigen are synthesized by the cell; an example would be a growth factor receptor present at low density on the cell surface. Alternatively, a molecule may be synthesized in large amounts but be exported rapidly from the cell, and hence never accumulate at detectable concentration. The handling of an individual antigen may vary between two different cell types, e.g. lysozyme is synthesized and stored within intracytoplasmic granules in myeloid cells, where it is easily detectable by immunocytochemical staining, whereas when the same enzyme is produced by mono-

cytes and macrophages it tends to be liberated rapidly into the cells' environment and hence may not be detectable.

Controls

Two principal types of control reactions are performed in order to detect both false-positive and false-negative staining. These consist of either using the same antibody to stain different tissue, or else staining the same tissue with a different antibody, and their interpretation is summarized in Fig. 30.11. Techniques are available for more detailed analysis of the specificity

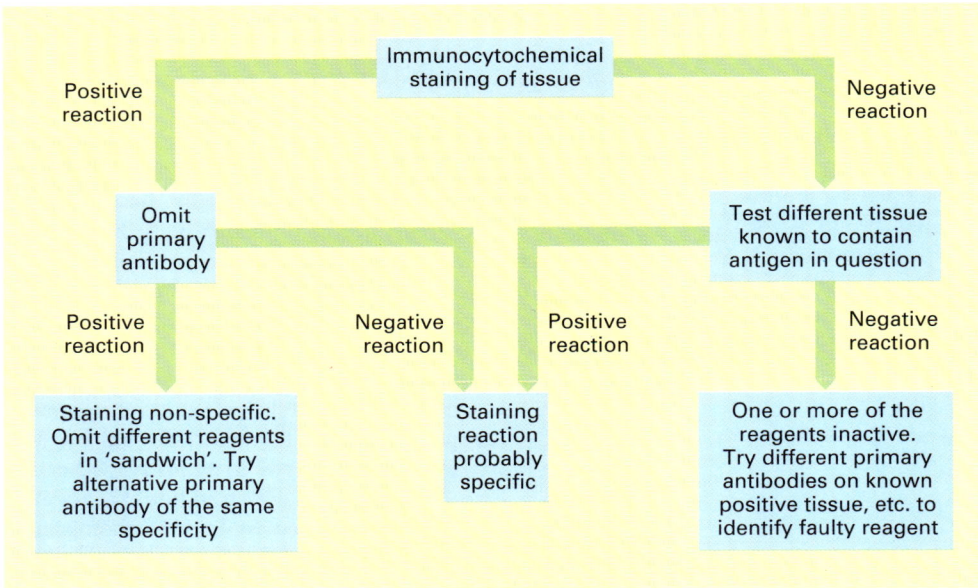

Fig. 30.11 Flow chart showing how simple controls may be used to investigate the cause of positive- and negative-staining reactions.

of antibodies used for immunocytochemical staining of human tissues (e.g. analysis by biochemical techniques which yield information on the molecular weight of the constituent recognized by an antibody), but these procedures are usually not suitable for use in diagnostic pathology laboratories.

30.2.3   Conclusions

Immunocytochemical procedures have developed in the past 20 years from techniques used primarily for research into methods which are indispensable for histopathological diagnosis. Applications, as detailed elsewhere in this book, include the differential diagnosis of tumours, the classification of lymphomas, and the evaluation of white cell reactions in a variety of different disease states (see Chapters 9 and 24). This field will continue to expand as the range of antibodies available to the pathologist grows; in contrast, the basic techniques and the principles behind them, as outlined in this section, are likely to remain substantially unchanged for the foreseeable future.

30.2.4   Further reading

DeLellis, R. A. (ed.) 1988). *Advances in immunohistochemistry*. Raven Press, New York.

Polak, J. and van Noorden, S. (eds) (1986). *Immunocytochemistry. Practical applications in pathology and biology* (2nd edn). Wright PSG, Bristol.

Proceedings of fourth workshop on human leucocyte differentiation antigens. (1990). Oxford University Press.

30.3   Tissue nucleic acid analysis

J. Burns and James O'D. McGee

30.3.1   Introduction

This section is concerned with the principles and applications of *in situ* nucleic acid analytical procedures in pathology. The previous section (*in situ* antigenic analysis) described the immunocytochemical localization of certain cellular products (antigens). Production of the latter and other cellular products is mediated by translation of appropriate messenger ribonucleic acid (mRNA) which in turn is derived by transcription of genomic deoxyribonucleic acid (DNA) (see Chapter 2.3). Both forms of nucleic acid are demonstrable within cells and tissue sections by a process known as *in situ* hybridization. Other techniques applicable to nucleic acid analysis are also included in this section.

30.3.2   *In situ* hybridization

Definition and general description

In situ hybridization uses the knowledge that DNA is a duplex molecule composed of two complementary polynucleotide strands which can be reversibly separated by denaturation with acid, base, or heat. The reassociation reaction is highly specific and is dependent on the high complementarity of the two separated polynucleotide strands. By introducing an exogenous but complementary labelled polynucleotide strand (probe) to the milieu of denatured DNA, during reassociation (hybridization) it will combine with one of the disassociated polynucleotide strands (target) to form a labelled hybrid DNA duplex *in situ*. Although the mRNA molecule, unlike DNA, is single stranded it may fold back on itself and base pair internally, forming short complementary double-stranded segments which may require mild heat and aldehyde denaturation in order to hybridize with complementary labelled nucleic acid probes.

In situ hybridization, therefore, results in the formation of an intracellular nucleic acid hybrid between single-standed (denatured) endogenous DNA or mRNA and an exogenous labelled complementary single-stranded nucleic acid sequence. The hybrid and, hence, the nucleic sequence of interest (target) is detected *in situ* by autoradiography if the probe is labelled with a radioisotope, or by regular light or fluorescence microscopy when the label is biotin, digoxigenin, or a fluorescent reporter (Fig. 30.12).

Type of probe and label

The probe may be produced in several ways. It may be double-stranded DNA derived from an isolated and cloned segment of genomic DNA; cDNA made from mRNA using reverse transcriptase; single-stranded, sense or anti-sense RNA; or chemically synthesized oligonucleotides. The reporter molecule used to label the probe may be either isotopic (^{3}H, ^{32}P, ^{35}S, or ^{125}I) or non-isotopic [acetylaminofluorene (AAF), dioxigenin, biotin: see below for alternative labels]. These labels are incorporated into the probe by enzymatic or chemical means without significantly affecting the base sequence or binding capacity of the probe.

Isotopic v. non-isotopic labelled probe   Isotopically labelled probes are highly sensitive; single genes may be detected on metaphase chromosome spreads, and 1–20 copies of specific mRNA per interphase cell (Fig. 30.13). They possess intrinsic disadvantages, however, which although acceptable in research and allied areas, are incompatible with routine diagnostic laboratories. Radioisotopes have a short half-life. Autoradiography of isotopically labelled probes, such as ^{32}P-labelled probes, typically require at least 12 h exposure; while tritium-labelled probes require several weeks, in order to obtain a positive signal. Due to these long exposure times, background noise invariably occurs with concomitant difficulties in interpretation of results. This is especially true of tissue sections but less so of mononuclear preparations (e.g. cells in culture). Other disadvantages include incompatibility with traditional histopathological staining methods, the need to handle photographic emulsions, and the ever present hazard of radioactivity.

Alternative non-isotopic labels such as AAF, fluorochromes, enzymes, mercuric cyanide, sulphone, 5-bromodeoxyuridine, biotin, and digoxigenin have been extensively investigated in

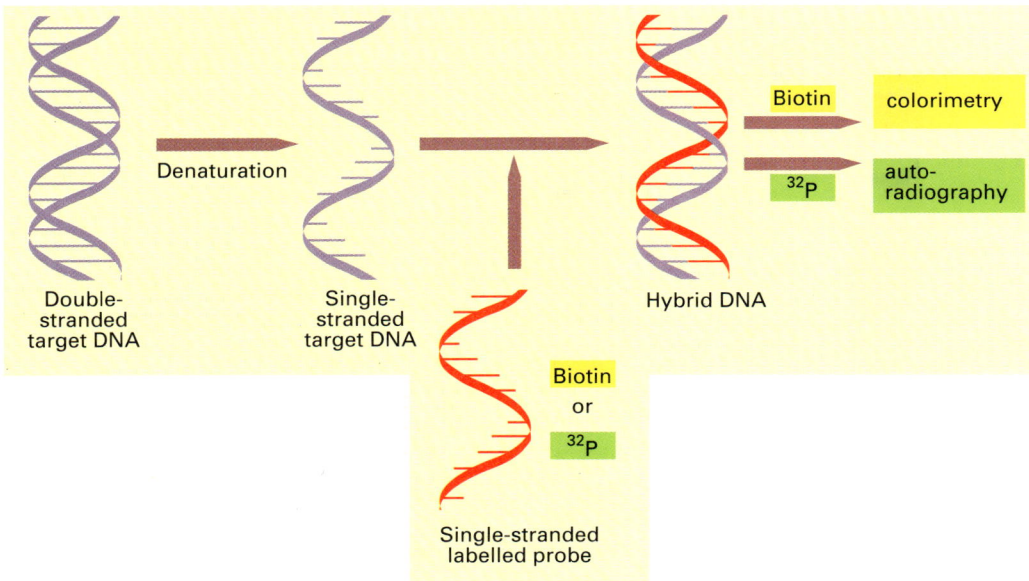

Fig. 30.12 Schematic outline of *in situ* hybridization protocol for DNA targets and modes of detection.

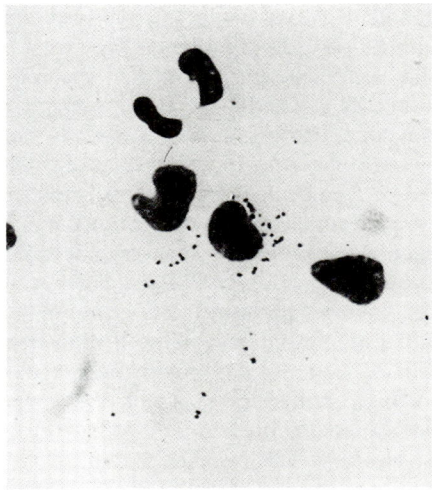

Fig. 30.13 AIDS patient, peripheral blood mononuclear cells hybridized with ^{35}S-labelled HIV-specific RNA probe showing HIV mRNA expression (perinuclear silver grains). Detection, autoradiography. See also Fig. 30.20 illustrating ^{32}P-labelled probe detection. (Reproduced from Harper *et al*. 1986.)

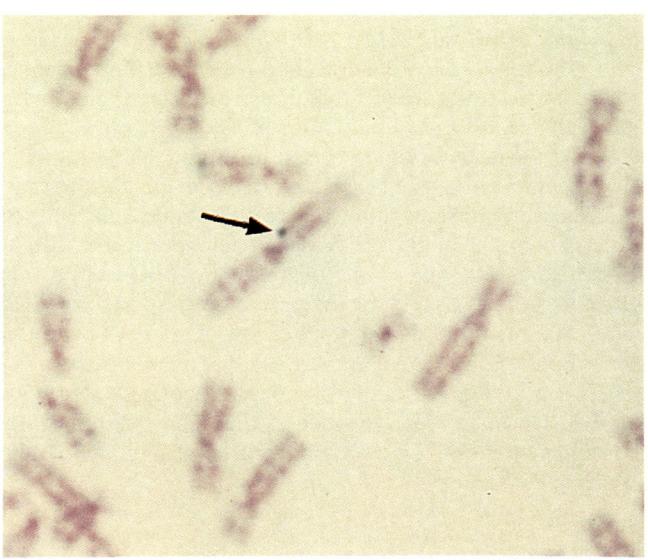

Fig. 30.14 Conventional metaphase chromosome spread hybridized with biotinylated N-*ras* probe. The location of the N-*ras* gene is detected as a single black dot on chromosome 1p13. Detection, immunogold-silver immunocytochemistry. Giemsa banded.

an effort to resolve the problems associated with radioactivity. Biotin and digoxigenin are preferred in this laboratory; these reporters overcome most of the disadvantages of isotopically labelled probes. Biotinylated probes are sensitive enough to locate single genes in chromosomes (Fig. 30.14) and less than 10 copies of HPV/cell in cervical lesions. Biotinylated and digoxigenin-labelled probes have a storage life of many months at 4°C, are easy to use, and are detectable within a short period of hybridization. The whole procedure, including hybridization and detection, takes less than 12 h.

30.3.3 Preparation of material for *in situ* hybridization

Type of material

Material used for *in situ* DNA analysis is derived from several sources and includes cellular preparations from tissue culture, cytological and cytogenetic origin, and tissue sections from cryostat and routine paraffin-embedded biopsy specimens.

Archival histopathological material is also suitable. The analysis is not confined to human nucleic acids but is also applicable to nucleic acids of infective agents such as bacteria, fungi, parasites, or viruses which play an important role in certain disease states. Nucleic acids 'in situ' are prepared in quite a different manner to those used for Southern, Northern, or dot blot or polymerase chain reaction (PCR) nucleic acid analysis. Nucleic acid for any of these analyses (except PCR) needs to be purified from other cellular elements beforehand. Intracellular nucleic acids for in situ analysis are 'fixed' in situ in the milieu of other cellular constituents.

Fixation

Nucleic acids are fixed in situ in intact cells in association with other cellular proteins, lipids, and carbohydrates with routine fixatives. Alcohol:acetic acid-based fixatives (Carnoy or Clarke's fluid) and 10 per cent aqueous formol–saline (formalin) are most commonly used for this purpose. All three fixatives preserve both DNA and mRNA but the latter may be better preserved with formalin alone or with paraformaldehyde and/or glutaraldehyde. Reagents used for processing fixed material to paraffin wax do not appear to affect the 'unmasking' of nucleic acids for analysis.

Unmasking of nucleic acids Aldehyde-fixed cells or cryostat sections and sections from formalin-fixed paraffin-embedded material may require mild proteolysis to render their nucleic acids available for in situ study. This procedure was established previously for unmasking antigens, in similar material, for in situ antigenic analysis. The enzymes used for this purpose include pepsin, pronase, or proteinase K. Formalin–paraffin sections are mounted on glass microscope slides precoated with an adhesive such as aminosilane or photo-flow-600 so that they withstand proteolysis and the manipulations required for in situ hybridization without detachment or loss of microscopic detail. Paraffin sections are baked on these slides at temperatures ranging between 60 and 80 °C in order to reinforce these objectives. Multiwell slides are recommended as they allow simultaneous in situ hybridization of test and control probes on parallel sections of the same material.

30.3.4 *In situ* hybridization (ISH) protocol

The major steps used for in situ hybridization are denaturation, hybridization, stringency washings, and detection.

Denaturation

Denaturation from a double-stranded to a single-stranded state is essential for in situ location of genomic nucleic acid sequences. Under appropriate conditions of temperature, ionic strength, and pH, it makes the target genomic base sequences available for hydrogen bonding with the complementary base sequences of the labelled probe. Denaturation can be performed with acid, base, or heat. Elevated temperatures ($\sim 95\,°C$), however, are invariably used for this purpose. Thereafter, preparations are cooled rapidly on ice to keep the nucleic acid

strands apart before subjecting them to hybridization, at appropriate temperatures, with nucleic acid probes. Double-stranded nucleic acid probes are heat denatured, either alone or together with the target DNA. It is important to remember that since mRNA in fixed material is probably only minimally damaged by heat it may hybridize with a probe used for targeting a heat-denatured genomic sequence. Difficulties in interpretation of results are resolved, to some extent, by using nuclease (DNase or RNase) digestion controls. Such controls are not always satisfactory. Synthetic oligonucleotide probes are often found to be more discriminatory.

Hybridization and stringency

Hybridization is the term used to describe the bonding between target nucleic acid sequences and that of the probe. The degree of stability exhibited by the newly formed hybrid is a function of the amount of base sequence homology between the two hybridizing strands of nucleic acid. It increases with increasing G + C content of the complementary regions. The stability of the hybrid is not only affected by base content but also by probe size, hybridization and wash temperatures, salt, dextran sulphate, and formamide concentrations. Formamide reduces the working temperatures required for the formation of stable hybrids. Dextran sulphate increases the rate of hybridization and sensitivity by forming networks of probe on the target. The hybridization buffer may contain denatured sheared salmon or herring sperm DNA, tRNA, ficoll, polyvinylpyrollidone, or bovine serum albumin to reduce non-specific binding of the probe to other cellular constituents or tissue elements.

The degree of complementary binding between target and probe is not only dependent on hybridization conditions but also on the stringency washing conditions employed prior to detection (visualization) of the hybrid. Hybridization and washing conditions of low temperature, low formamide, and high ionic strength (low stringency) allow a high degree of non-homologous base-sequence binding in the hybrid. Conversely, conditions of high stringency in which the temperature and formamide are raised and the ionic strength of the hybridization and/or washing buffer is lowered, facilitates dissociation of hybrid nucleic acid strands which contain imperfectly matched base sequences.

Detection

The method used to detect the intracellular hybrid is dependent on the type of label incorporated in the probe. As mentioned earlier, isotopic labels like ^{32}P are detected by autoradiography, and non-isotopic labels such as biotin by colorimetric methods. The technique of autoradiography is dealt with adequately elsewhere. Only the principles of visualizing non-isotopic labels (e.g. biotin) will be outlined here.

Two principle methods are available: immunocytochemistry or affinity cytochemistry. With immunocytochemistry, the biotin label incorporated in the hybrid is treated as a tissue antigen. High copy numbers of DNA or mRNA are readily detected 'in situ' by the majority of currently available immunocyto-chemical methods (including those used for detecting antigens '*in situ*' as described in the previous section). The simplest and most effective are the indirect or ABC immunoperoxidase/gold/ alkaline phosphatase of fluorochrome procedures, where the first antibody is directed against biotin. Silver amplification of the end-product of the immunoperoxidase or gold procedure is helpful for detecting unique sequences such as single genes in chromosome spreads. Affinity cytochemistry is based on the highly specific and strong non-covalent interaction between biotin (vitamin H) and the egg-white glycoprotein, avidin (MW 68 000), or the non-glycosylated protein, streptavidin (MW 60 000), produced by *Streptomyces ovidinii*, which leads to the formation of a high-affinity complex (KD 10^{-15}M). Avidin has four binding sites for biotin. This unique binding capacity of avidin for biotin has been utilized in the development of simple conjugates, e.g. avidin–peroxidase; avidin–colloidal gold; avidin–alkaline phosphatase, or avidin–fluorochrome for detecting both low and high copy numbers of nucleic acid sequences hybridized *in situ* with biotinylated probes. Simple histochemical substrates or fluorescence microscopy are used to visualize these affinity-bound cytochemical reagents, the immune complexes of immunocytochemistry and non-isotopically labelled oligonucleotides.

30.3.5   ISH in cytogenetics

Material used for routine cytogenetic investigation is suitable for *in situ* DNA analysis. This type of cellular material ranges from routine metaphase spreads to cellular explants from tumour tissue. It includes fresh and cultured amniotic and chorionic villi cells and cells from most body sources.

Introduction

In situ nucleic acid analysis was first used for cytogenetic studies by Pardue and Gall in the late 1960s. In these studies DNA was isolated from toad (*Xenopus laevis*) or mouse cells cultured in medium containing radiolabelled thymidine. DNA isolated from each cell type contained incorporated radioactive [³H]thymidine which acted as a label or reporter molecule. These labelled DNA extracts or probes were applied to toad oocytes or cultured mouse cells and formed DNA–DNA duplex molecules located by autoradiography. Although each probe located specifically to its cell (DNA) type of origin, in both interphase nuclei or metaphase chromosomes the technology available at that time was too insensitive to detect single genes in chromosomes. Such technology had to await developments in recombinant DNA technique in the mid 1970s, gene cloning in particular.

Gene assignment and chromosome banding

Recombinant DNA technology allows the production of large quantities of gene-specific probes from a variety of vectors. Probes of high specificity can be prepared and labelled with radioisotopes. Using this technology, the first single genes (unique sequences) were located on chromosomes by Harper and Saunders in the early 1980s. Since then gene mapping on chromosomes (gene assignment) of new genes with either isotopic, or non-isotopic, labelled probes is a relatively common event. Staining such preparations with the dye Giemsa induces a characteristic banding pattern peculiar to each chromosome type and is an essential accompaniment to *in situ* hybridization when mapping genes. The banding facilitates regional and sub-band-location of genes and direct visualization of chromosomal translocations, deletions, and break points in defined sequences (see Section 2.1).

Clinical application

In situ hybridization in cytogenetics enables the molecular and routine cytogeneticist to localize specific genes in mitotic (metaphase spreads) and meiotic chromosomes, assign translocations, deletions, and other chromosomal aberrations in human cancer and make more accurate diagnosis of genetic disorders. Detection of specific chromosomal numerical aberrations in interphase nuclei, called interphase cytogenetics, can be made with non-isotopic hybridization technology (see Chapter 9). This allows combined flow cytometry (Section 30.6) and fluorescence-activated cell sorting with *in situ* hybridization. In fact, 95 per cent of all chromosomal abnormalities would be covered if all interphase chorionic and amniotic cell preparations were hybridized with X, Y, and 21 (Down syndrome) chromosome-specific probes (Burns *et al.* 1985; Julien *et al.* 1986) Figs 30.15, 30.16). Location of point mutations, i.e. single base changes in mutant genes, is necessary for delineating molecular pathology of some inherited and acquired human diseases. Standard recombinant DNA-produced probes are invariably too large for this purpose. Short synthetic DNA fragments (oligonucleotides) can be made to detect single base changes in mutant genes. They are particularly valuable in prenatal diagnosis.

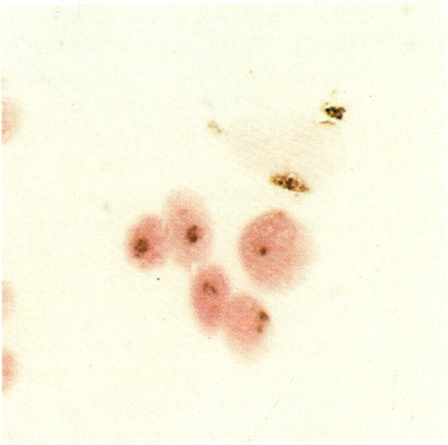

Fig. 30.15 Conventional cultured chorionic villous (male) cells hybridized with biotinylated Y-chromosome 'specific' probe (Y-chromosomes black). Detection, immunoperoxidase/silver immunocytochemistry. (Pyronin counterstained.)

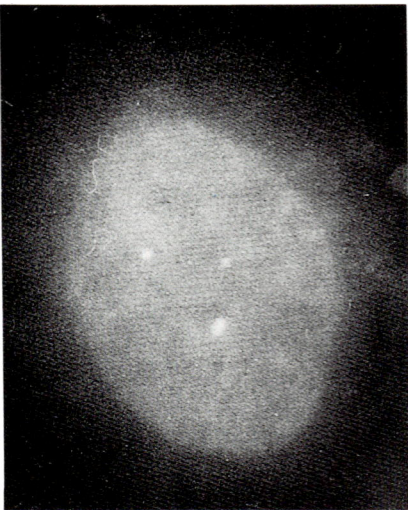

Fig. 30.16 Three intranuclear fluorescent dots from hybridization of biotinylated chromosome 21-DNA probe with an uncultured amniotic fluid cell from a trisomy-21 affected pregnancy. Detection (combined immuno- and affinity cytochemistry), fluorescein isothiocyanate (FIT-C)–avidin conjugate, biotin-labelled anti-avidin antibody, FITC–avidin conjugate. Fluorescence microscopy. (Reproduced from Julien *et al.* 1986, with permission.)

30.3.6   Viral detection

K. Cooper and James O'D. McGee

Introduction

One out of every two cancers in some parts of the world may be virus associated (Marx 1986). The cancers in question include adult T-cell leukaemia, which is associated with human T-cell lymphotrophic virus m(HTLV-1); liver carcinoma, which is associated with hepatitis B virus; Burkitt lymphoma and naso-pharangeal carcinoma, both associated with Epstein–Barr virus; cervical cancer, associated with various forms of human papilloma virus (Figs 30.17, 30.18). *In situ* hybridization, besides confirming the association of viruses with certain cancers, helps in the diagnosis of herpes simplex viral encephal-itis and other viral-induced diseases of the central nervous system (CNS). It also provides a better understanding of the less acute CNS diseases, such as progressive multifocal leuko-encephalopathy or subacute sclerosing encephalitis, in which human papovavirus, JC virus, and measles virus are associated respectively. As a consequences of these findings, *in situ* hybridization is being used to determine whether chronic neurological diseases of unknown aetiology are induced by viruses, and to what extent viruses exist in the CNS of clinically normal indi-viduals. The casual or causal role of viruses in myocarditis, artherosclerosis, type II diabetes, various connective tissue dis-

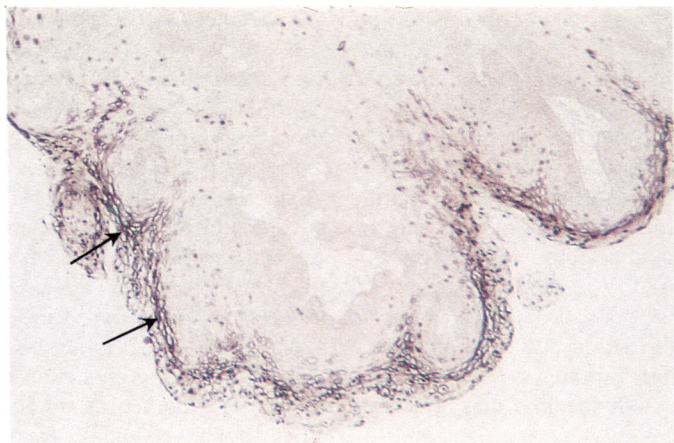

Fig. 30.17 Conventional formalin–paraffin section of a cervical biopsy of condyloma acuminatum hybridized with a biotinylated HPV6 probe. Nucleic acids unmasked with pepsin/HCl before hybridization. Koilo-cytes and many suprabasal cells are labelled. The cytoplasmic (mRNA) reaction is indicated with arrows (see also Fig. 30.18). Detection, avidin (modified)–alkaline phosphatase. A similar nucleic acid unmasking and detection system was used in Figs 30.18a and 30.19a,b.

orders, and many other disease processes is being conducted in a similar manner.

In situ hybridization (ISH) is useful for identification of viruses, fungi, bacteria, or parasites which are difficult or im-possible to culture *in vitro*, e.g. HPV (Figs 30.17, 30.18) and *Pneumocystis carinii* (Fig. 30.19).

Before the introduction of ISH, the detection of viruses in histological sections was always an enigma to the histopatholo-gist. The identification of characteristic intranuclear and intra-cytoplasmic inclusions facilitated the diagnosis of viral diseases on surgical and autopsy tissue sections for many years. Electron microscopy was an adjunct to detecting viruses with specific structural characteristics. More recently, the use of immuno-cytochemistry has allowed the histopathologist grappling with this problem an additional investigative technique in his quest for diagnostic accuracy.

However, with the advent of 'state-of-the-art' molecular techniques it soon became evident that even with the above methods viral detection still remained elusive to the histopatho-logist in certain instances. For example, latent/subclinical viral infections often do not display typical inclusion bodies, nor express structural capsid proteins for detection by immunocyto-chemical methods. Further, electron microscopy is only capable of detecting intact virions and does not distinguish between certain viral types that resemble each other.

Hence it is imperative for the histopathologist to explore some of the available molecular techniques in order to improve diag-nostic accuracy. These methods involve nucleic acid probes with diagnosis being made at the genetic level. It is the aim of this section to illustrate that it is not necessary for the histo-pathologist to become a molecular scientist in order to apply and benefit from the ever-expanding field of molecular patho-logy. Since viruses are typed according to their nucleic acid

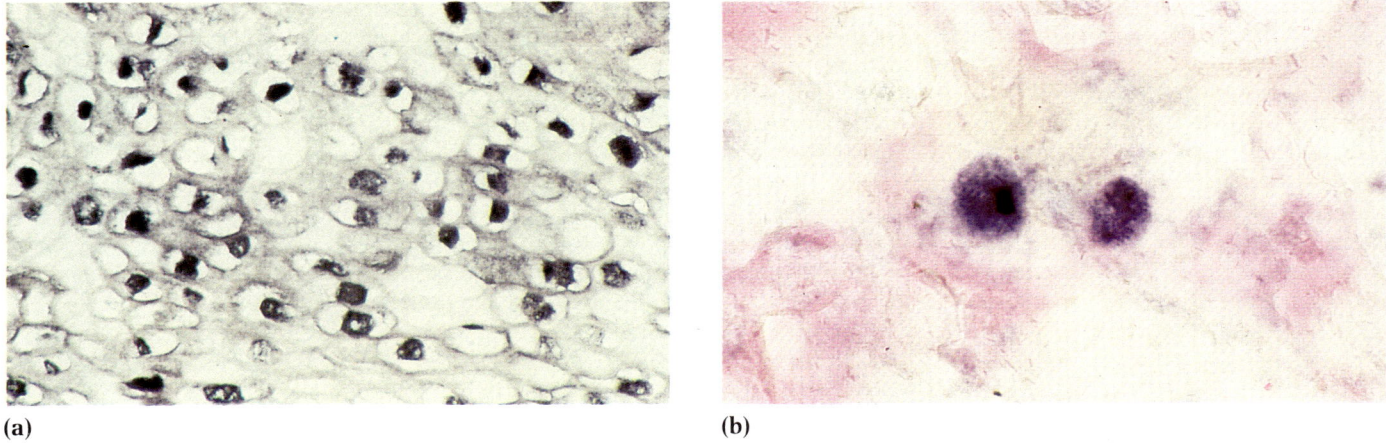

Fig. 30.18 (a) High-power view of an upper epithelial area of Fig. 30.17. Hybridization reaction for HPV in both koilocyte nuclei and cytoplasm; some of the cytoplasmic signal is HPV RNA. (b) Routine cervical smear from a case of CINIII probed with biotinylated HPV16. Detection as for Fig. 30.17 but *no* protease treatment. (Pyronin counterstained.)

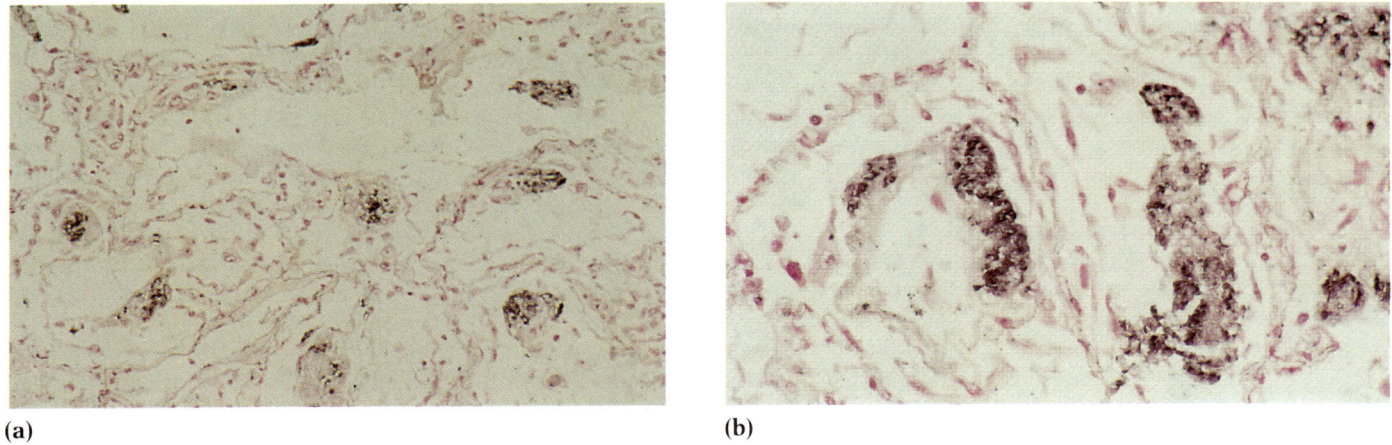

Fig. 30.19 Conventional formalin–paraffin section of an AIDS patient's lung, hybridized with biotinylated genomic *Pneumocystis carinii* probe. The hybridization signal is evident in alveoli in both (a) and (b). Characteristic beaded nuclear ring structures of pneumocystis are clearly shown, at a higher magnification, in (b). (Pyronin counterstained.)

content, the detection of nucleic acid in clinical material is therefore the most appropriate way of achieving a clinical diagnosis and of investigating the epidemiology and natural history of viral infections.

Nucleic acid hybridization is based on the unique ability of nucleic acid molecules to hybridize. Quite simply, a probe of known sequence is allowed to mix with a sample nucleic acid under conditions which allow specific complementary base pairing to occur. Subsequent detection of hybridization would then indicate the presence of a particular virus in the sample. The 'gold standard' technique for such a procedure is Southern blot hybridization. However, this time-consuming procedure of DNA extraction and analysis by restriction digestion is often only available in specialized centres and hence not applicable to routine diagnostic laboratories (see Section 30.3.9). In contrast, ISH is within access to the histopathologist for two reasons. Firstly, the technique can be performed on formalin-

fixed, routinely processed, paraffin-embedded material, thus allowing the pathologist to utilize a constantly expanding source of archival material. Secondly, detection of viral sequences is conducted with the maintenance of morphologic integrity of the sample tissue section on light microscope slides. An additional feature is that ISH is also performed using non-isotopic labelled probes, thus avoiding the problems associated with the use of radioactive isotopes. Non-isotopic *in situ* hybridization (NISH) is the only form of nucleic acid hybridization that combines the art of morphological analysis with a powerful non-isotopic genetic analysis, thus permitting definite localization of viral particles.

Human papilloma virus (HPV) in cervical disease

HPV detection by NISH is used in this section as an example of the facility of NISH to provide clinically and biologically relevant data.

Over 60 HPVs have been detected in lesions of squamous epithelia with specific types being implicated in the aetiology of cervical squamous cell cancers. HPV comprise circular double-stranded DNA that replicate within the cell nucleus. The nucleic acids may remain extra-chromosomal, i.e. episomal, or may integrate into one or more chromosomes. It has been postulated that this difference may be discernible with NISH by analysing the signal type. Episomal viruses are replicating and present in large numbers which facilitates their detection by NISH. Integrated virus, on the other hand, may be present in low numbers requiring sensitive procedures for their detection.

Integrated HPV have been detected in both CIN and SCC. This physical state of the virus is thought to play a role in the multi-step process of cervial carcinogenesis. It is probably the basal cells of squamous epithelium that first become infected by HPV, with viral replication and capsid production being related to squamous differentiation in the upper layers. It has also been noted that the morphological characteristics of episomal virus (koilocytes) disappear with progression of squamous epithelial morphology from benign to malignant. This may imply integration of the viral genome. Further, there is also an urgent need to detect those cervical HPV lesions that will progress to higher grades of CIN and invasive cancer. In an attempt to answer some of these questions the detction of HPV in cervical biopsies of CIN and SCC has been investigated extensively (see also Chapter 21).

Non-isotopic in situ hybridization protocol

Ideally, 6 μm paraffin sections are fixed on to multispot slides coated with aminopropyltriethoxysilane (section adhesive) to prevent detachment of sections from slides during the procedure. The adherence of sections is enhanced by overnight baking at 60°C. Dewaxing of sections by plunging in xylene and alcohol, is followed by enzymatic proteolysis to remove both viral and cellular proteins that impede diffusion and access of probe to target viral DNA sequences. This process has been termed *unmasking* and has been performed with 500 μg/ml proteinase K diluted in phosphate buffer at 37°C for 15 minutes in this laboratory. The object of this process is to make target nucleic acid available for hybridization while ensuring that the cytoskeletal structure is preserved to be identified by routine haematoxylin staining. The slides are then washed thoroughly in distilled water and dried at 75°C.

Hybridization is preceded by simultaneous *denaturation* of both double-stranded target viral nucleic acid and probe, at 95°C for 15 minutes on a solid steel plate in a hot oven into single-stranded DNA. Simultaneous heat denaturation of sample and digoxigenin or biotin labelled probes may favour penetrance and minimize the native nucleic acid from reannealing with its endogenous homologue. The hybridization mix/cocktail comprising labelled probe, formamide, salt, and dextran sulphate is added to multispot slides covered with 14 mm coverslips and placed in a moist Terasaki plate.

Following simultaneous *denaturation* of probe and target nucleic acids at 95°C, the conditions are then slowly reversed so that the *annealing* reaction can occur between labelled probe

and target nucleic acids with complementary base-pair sequences. Thus a 'hybrid' double stranded molecule is formed. A period of 2 hours in a 42°C oven is sufficient for this reaction to occur.

A series of salt washes is then performed to remove unhybridized probe and mismatched or heterologous duplexes. Prior to detection of the reporter molecule, non-specific binding of antibody and other proteins is reduced by preincubation with bovine serum albumin. Non-fat dry milk is also useful for the inhibition of non-specific nuclear staining and in this laboratory is incorporated into the detection system.

The presence of hybrids between labelled probes and target DNA is then visualized using an *amplified three-step detection* method. Thus, the combination of monoclonal antibody to the reporter molecule (in this instance monoclonal anti-digoxin) linked via a biotinylated linker antibody to an avidin conjugate produces high specificity (monoclonal antibody) and sensitivity (avidin conjugate). The latter depends on the high affinity of avidin for biotin which is approximately 1000 times greater than that of antibodies for antigen. This amplified detection procedure increases the sensitivity of detection up to tenfold and hence enhances potential detection of low-copy-number infections.

Briefly, slides are incubated in monoclonal anti-digoxin for 30 minutes at 22°C. Second incubation is in biotinylated rabbit anti-mouse [F(ab')$_2$ fragment] and third in avidin-peroxidase containing 5 per cent non-fat milk. Signal is then developed using amino-ethylcarbazole (AEC) and hydrogen peroxide. After probe detection, slides are air-dried at 42°C, counterstained progressively in haematoxylin and mounted in glycerol jelly.

During the investigation of the comparative prevalence of HPV in CIN and SCC in the UK and South Africa it soon became evident that there were three distinct morphological types of NISH signal patterns. Type 1 signal was characterized by a diffuse staining of the nuclei in the upper half of the epithelium in CIN lesions showing typical morphological features of wart virus infection (WVI) (Fig. 30.20). Type 2 signal comprised a punctate red dot within a clean background of haemtoxylin stained nuclei. This type of signal was generally confined to undifferentiated and dysplastic nuclei in a random distribution (Fig. 30.21). The third signal, type 3, was a combination of type 1 and type 2 signals either in the same or adjacent nuclei (Fig. 30.22). Examination of the SCC showed a punctate signal in all the tumours that were positive (68 per cent) for HPV DNA although a few tumours did have a superimposed diffuse signal (type 3). This latter feature was present particularly in tumours which showed keratin differentiation. Taken in conjunction with the type 1 signal in koilocytic cells showing squamous differentiation in CIN lesions, this feature bears testimony to the theory that viral replication is related to keratin production. It was this statement that led to the postulate that type 1 signal represents episomal viral particles. The punctate type 2 signal in contrast was present predominantly in atypical cells in CIN lesions and undifferentiated tumour cells in SCC. Hence this morphological transformation of signal type from 1 to 2 with

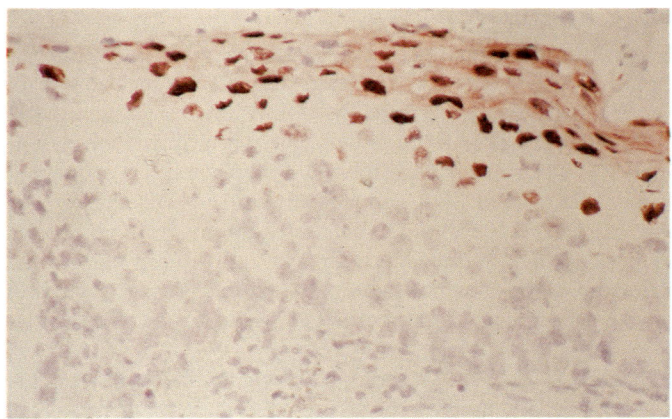

Fig. 30.20 Type 1 pattern of NISH signal confined to the upper half of the squamous epithelium. Diffuse red intranuclear signal present predominantly in cells showing morphological evidence of wart virus infection.

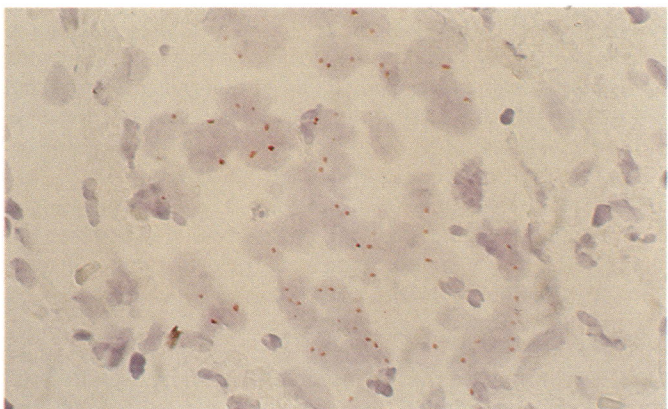

Fig. 30.21 Red punctate signal (dots) on a clean background of haematoxylin stained collection of squamous cancer cells within a vascular space (Type 2 NISH signal).

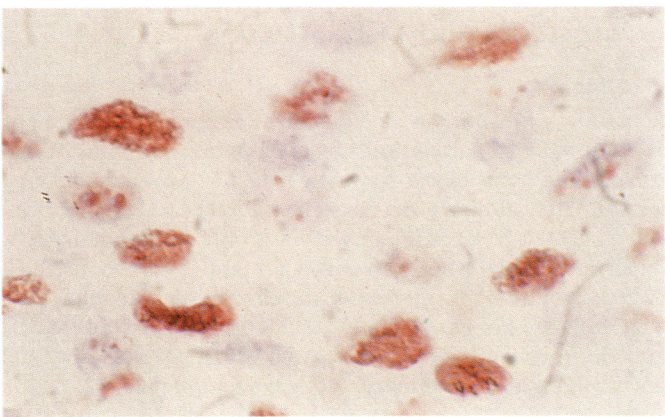

Fig. 30.22 Type 3 NISH signal comprising diffuse/granular (Type 1) intranuclear staining and punctate (Type 2) signal in cervical intraepithelial neoplasia.

progression of squamous epithelial cells from benign to malignant gave rise to the hypothesis that the punctate/dot signal may indicate integration of the viral genome into the host gene. In support of this is the additional observation of an identical signal type in CaSki and HeLa cells lines derived from cervical tumours known to contain HPV 16 and 18 in an integrated physical state. There is mounting evidence that integration of HPV into host genome may play a major role in the multi-step process of cervical carcinogenesis. If this proves to be true then the detection of a type 2 signal in a WVI with associated CIN may indicate those HPV lesions that are likely to progress to high-grade dysplasias and invasive cancers. Further, it has been estimated that about 14 per cent of cervical HPV infections will progress, indicating the need to have a morphological indicator of the onset of this progression. The type 2 punctate/dot NISH signal may help satisfy this void in determining clinical management in these instances.

30.3.7 *In situ* mRNA analysis

Eric P. H. Yap and James O'D. McGee

Introduction

Messenger ribonucleic acid (mRNA) constitutes only about 3 per cent (1 pg/cell) of total mammalian cellular RNA, but it plays an important role as an intermediary molecule in the transfer of genetic information between DNA (Section 2.4) and functional polypeptides. The regulation of gene expression through transcriptional control within a cell, and hence its functional state, is reflected in the cellular content and distribution of specific message and proteins. The fact that RNA forms duplexes with complementary nucleic acid sequences and that RNA and DNA are interconvertible *in vitro*, enables many of the techniques for DNA analysis and manipulation to be adapted for RNA work. The presence of protein as detected by immunohistochemistry (Section 30.2) or Western blotting, usually but not necessarily implies synthesis, as endocytosis and adsorption can account for its intracellular presence. Conversely, mRNA is subject to post-transcriptional control and is not always translated into a functional protein. mRNA and protein assays therefore complement each other in the analysis of gene products.

There are several aims of mRNA characterization. First, structural information regarding the base sequence and presence of introns, extrons, and untranslated regions can be derived by comparing the sequences of complementary (cDNA) and genomic DNA. Mutations causing base substitutions, deletions, insertions, and frame shifts, as well as alternative and abnormal RNA splicing may be found in a variety of diseases (Section 2.3). It is often more feasible to sequence the RNA of genes that have a large number of introns than to sequence the genomic DNA. Secondly, mRNA analysis allows the study of gene activation and inactivation, under various disease (*in vivo*) and experimental (*in vivo* and *in vitro*) conditions. A particular mRNA can be quantitated in absolute terms or relative to a constitutionally expressed gene. Spatial distribution can be studied in intact histological sections or by microdissection of tissues followed by *in vitro* amplification. The accumulation of mRNA can be localized to histological, cellular, or subcellular sites. Finally, the temporal pattern of mRNA distribution can also be studied with respect to various external stimuli or intrinsic development and disease processes.

Tools

Several enzymes are useful tools for molecular RNA work. DNA-dependent RNA polymerases transcribe double-stranded DNA into RNA. RNA polymerases encoded by bacteriophages of *E. coli* (T3, T7) and *Salmonella typhimurium* (SP6) are used with expression vectors (e.g. Bluescript, Gemini plasmids) that contain the relevant promoter sequences to synthesize single-stranded transcripts of specific cDNA inserts that have been cloned into the vector. Reverse transcriptase (RNA-dependent DNA polymerase), an enzyme isolated and cloned from avian myeloblastosis and murine leukaemia retroviruses, is used to synthesize single- and double-stranded cDNA from RNA. Ribonucleases which specifically digest and degrade single-stranded RNA or the RNA strand of RNA-DNA hybrids, are useful in removing RNA from DNA preparations, for reducing background due to unbound RNA probes in hybridization experiments, and for mapping regions of DNA/RNA homology.

Since ribonucleases are thermoresistant and are not destroyed by autoclaving, special precautions are required to prevent extrinsic contamination during handling of RNA and reagents. RNAse inhibitors used include diethyl pyrocarbonate (DEPC), a protein inhibitor derived from the human placenta and vanadyl-ribonucleoside complexes. Degradation by intrinsic RNAses can be limited by rapid fixation of tissue specimens, and this is underscored by the decreasing yields of RNA obtained from freshly fixed endoscopic biopsy, laparotomy, and post-mortem gut specimens.

There are several methods for studying mRNA in clinical samples. Poly(A) RNA can be extracted and purified from large samples, and run on Northern blots as described in Section 30.3.8. Smaller biopsies (e.g. from punch biopsies, needle aspirations), microdissection of tissue (e.g. individual renal tubules), or single cells (e.g. ovum) can be analysed for RNA content by *in vitro* amplification. A limited extraction procedure is performed to lyse cells and inactivate RNAses. Reverse transcription in the presence of oligo(T) or specific oligonucleotide primers results in cDNA-RNA hybrids. The polymerase chain reaction (PCR) is then used to amplify a specific cDNA, and this amplified fragment can subsequently be fractionated by electrophoresis, restricted by endonucleases, sequenced, or cloned into vectors (Section 30.3.9). If a poly(G) tail is added to the cDNA by terminal transferase after reverse transcripton, the whole cDNA library can be amplified by anchored PCR using poly(T) and poly(C) primers, and this library is useful for subtractive hybridization or cloning.

In situ hybridization

In contrast to the methods alluded to above, RNA *in situ* hybridization (ISH) allows the detection and precise localization of specific RNA sequences directly within intact cells and tissue sections. It is based on the principle of hybridizing labelled fragments of DNA or RNA containing complementary sequences (probes) to cellular RNA and detecting the labelled hybrids (see Fig. 30.12). This technique facilitates the investigation of the expression of a single gene within an individual cell, and the detection of specific viral sequences (e.g. measles, retroviruses) within cells and tissues for pathological diagnosis or for elucidation of disease aetiology.

Detection of RNA *in situ* requires very small quantities of tissues and cells. It enables the study of highly heterogeneous cell populations, since there is no need for extraction and homogenization of cell contents. Detection sensitivity may also be higher because there is no dilutional effect. Limits of detection of less than 10 copies per cell have been claimed, and this enables the detection of very rare mRNA species. Moreover, it is possible to determine simultaneously the biochemical, morphological, and immunocytochemical properties of the cells containing specific messages. Two or more nucleic acid sequences may be studied at the same time using different reporter molecules and detection systems. By using non-isotopic labels, detection time is reduced considerably, and the whole procedure can be performed within one working day. With automation of the pretreatment and detection steps, it may soon be feasible to employ ISH for routine diagnosis and prognostication. Further developments in the future include improving the detection sensitivity, standardization of protocols, and computer-aided analysis.

Biopsy preparation

A variety of samples may be used: cell cultures, aspirates and lavages, smears, cells mechanically disaggregated from tissues, and frozen or paraffin-embedded tissue sections. Cells are deposited on glass microscope slides by smearing or cytocentrifugation, or adherence of cells in monolayer culture. Pre-treatment of washed slides with poly-L-lysine or aminoalkylsilane improves adherence of cells and sections to slides and prevents loss during hybridization and washing steps.

Fixation

Generally, cross-linking aldehyde fixatives are preferred. Four per cent buffered paraformaldehyde is optimal in many circumstances, but tissue blocks routinely fixed in 10 per cent buffered formalin may also be used. Abundant mRNA species have been demonstrated in paraffin-embedded archival specimens. It is important to fix clinical samples promptly and to use pH-buffered solutions to minimize nucleic acid degradation. Precipitating alcohol-based fixatives such as methanol/acetic acid and Carnoy's solution may be used but RNA retention and preservation of cellular morphology is sub-optimal.

Permeabilization

The aims of permeabilization are to expose target mRNA to probes while preserving good tissue morphology and minimizing RNA loss. This step is often the single most critical factor to good hybridization results, and the treatment duration and concentration of permeabilizing agent should be empirically established for each experimental set-up. The optimum conditions for these conflicting goals depends on the type of tissue, section thickness, type and extent of fixation, and the type and length of probe used. Tissue extensively cross-linked (e.g. after glutaraldehyde fixation) requires more permeabilization, while precipitant-fixed tissue may not require further treatment. Proteases such as proteinase K, pepsin, and trypsin are most commonly used, and a further post-fixation step may be used to promote tissue adherence.

Prehybridization

Non-specific background signal arises from a variety of sources: hybridization with non-homologous nucleic acids, electrostatic attraction and physical entrapment of probe, and intrinsic cellular substances interacting with detection system (e.g. endogenous biotin and peroxidase). Several steps are employed to reduce this background and hence improve signal:noise ratio. Acetic anhydride is used to remove basic groups in proteins by acetylation. Post-hybridization RNase digestion to remove probe not bound to nucleic acid markedly decreases non-specific signal. Inactivation of endogenous peroxidase and blocking of tissue biotin can also be performed if necessary. The non-specific binding of probe to cell components can be blocked by saturating these sites during a pre-hybridization step. Blocking agents commonly used are ficoll, polyvinyl pyrolidone, Triton detergent, herring sperm DNA, and yeast-transfer RNA. Additionally, heat pre-treatment of samples may denature the secondary structure of mRNA and facilitate probe binding.

Probes

There are several types of probes available for RNA ISH. Double-stranded genomic DNA or cDNA probes labelled by nick-translation or random-primed labelling may be used for both DNA and RNA hybridzation. While they theoretically enable networking of hybrids and hence signal enhancement, they suffer from the disadvantage that they reanneal in solution and this reaction competes with the diffusion and hybridizing to target mRNA. Single-stranded probes are hence preferable in mRNA analysis, and also offer strand-specific controls. Single-stranded DNA probes cloned in M13 bacteriophage vectors have been difficult to produce, but this can be overcome by the use of asymmetric PCR to produce and label ssDNA. Synthetic oligonucleotides can be prepared conveniently and are end-labelled either by T4 polynucleotide transferase at the 5′ end or by terminal deoxynucleotidyl transferase at the 3′ end. They can be very useful in cases where closely homologous sequences need to be discriminated or where the entire cDNA sequence is not known or has not been cloned. Cocktails of several oligomers are required to compensate for the low specific activity of these probes. Complementary single-stranded 'antisense' RNA (cRNA) probes seem to be the most useful for mRNA ISH. Produced and labelled by *in vitro* transcription, they can be densely labelled, have a high binding stability, do not contain vector sequences that may cross-hybridize with cellular sequences, and are amenable to post-hybridization digestion of unbound (single-stranded) probe. These advantages result in high sensitivity and low background.

^{32}P-labelled probes were first used in ISH to demonstrate abundant ribosomal RNA in 1969. Since then, marked improvements of sensitivity and resolution were achieved using isotopes with shorter β-emission track lengths (^{35}S, ^{125}I, ^{3}H), and better emulsion detection methods. Non-isotopic ISH developed over the last decade has superseded the use of radioisotopes in ease of use, routine availability, environmental and personal safety, and cellular resolution, and is of comparable detection sensitivity. Many different compounds have been used as reporter molecules, but biotin, which binds to the naturally occurring avidin with an extremely high affinity, and digoxigenin, which is detected with specific monoclonal antibodies, are now the labels of choice.

Hybridization

Hybridization of probe-to-tissue mRNA is performed by incubating slides with hybridization solution under cover slips for 2–16 hours. Hybridization solutions comprise the probe, blocking reagent used in prehybridization, RNAse inhibitors, formamide, and salt. The hybridization temperature, formamide content, and salt concentrations affect the annealing rate and thermal stability (T_m) of RNA-probe duplexes. High temperatures, high formamide, and low salt concentrations allow only perfectly matched duplexes to anneal, and constitute conditions of high stringency. The level of stringency chosen for hybridization depends on the degree of homology allowed, the type and length of probe, and the guanine-cytosine content of short probes. Due to the greater stability of RNA–RNA hybrids, hybridization with cRNA probes is carried out 10–15°C higher than for DNA probes.

Other variable factors to be considered are probe length and concentration. The optimum lengths for probe diffusion and penetration vary, but long probes greater than 1 kb in length can be hydrolysed by heating. The optimal concentration is the minimum required to saturate target binding sites and give maximum signal to noise ratio, since background increases linearly with probe concentration. Economy of probe can be achieved by the addition of the polymer, dextran sulphate to increase the effective probe concentration, presumably by a volume exclusion effect.

Post-hybridization washes at increasing stringencies ensure dissociation of poorly matched hybrids, leaving only probe binding to specific complementary nucleic acid sequences. RNA probes in particular tend to bind non-specifically, and such background can be greatly diminished by incubation with RNAses which selectively degrade unbound single-stranded RNA.

Probe detection

Isotopic probes are detected by autoradiography. Exposure times are determined empirically, depending on abundance of mRNA species being detected and the isotope used, but typical durations range from days to weeks (Fig. 30.23).

A variety of detection systems exist for non-isotopic reporter molecules, including both immunocytochemical (specific antibody) and affinity cytochemical (e.g. avidin, streptavidin) methods. The addition of multiple layers of antibodies can be used to enhance and amplify the signal, though background is also increased in the process. Finally, the labelled duplex-detection complex is visualized either by enzyme-chromogenic substrate combinations, immunofluorescence, or more recently, by chemiluminescence. Several nucleic acid sequences can be visualized by using different chromogenes or fluorescent indicators of contrasting colours, or a combination. The slide can also be counterstained with histochemical stains to identify features of morphological interest.

Methods are available to quantify the signal. The signal density from tritium-labelled probes can be measured by counting the grains per cell or per unit area on emulsion autoradiograms. At lower resolutions, comparison can be made between tissue signal and known standard controls on autoradiograms, using computer-assisted densitometry. Computer-aided image analysis and scintillators are being developed for non-isotopic labels detected by chemiluminescence.

Interpretation

Appropriate controls are necessary for the interpretation of ISH results, since specific signal may easily be confused with non-specific binding to non-homologous mRNA, DNA, or other cellular and extracellular components. Negative controls should include probe-free hybridization, use of sense-strand RNA, vector and irrelevant probes, and RNAse pre-treatment of

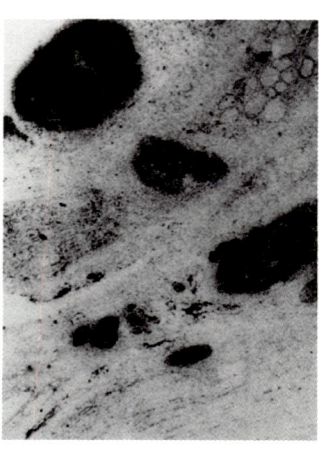 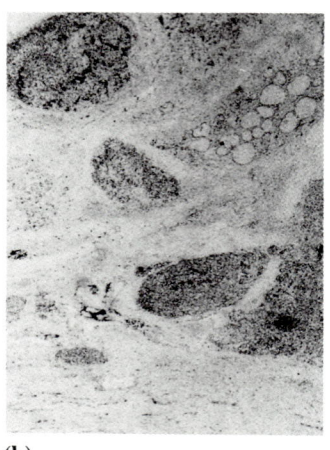

(a)   **(b)**

Fig. 30.23 Parallel formalin–paraffin sections of human medullary carcinoma of thyroid. Proteinase K was used to unmask nucleic acids. (a) Hybridized with an anti-sense (cRNA) probe for N-*myc*, (b) with the sense strand of the same probe [(b) acts as an internal control for (a)]. Both probes were labelled with ^{32}P. Note the intense hybridization signal given by nests of tumour cells in (a) compared with that given in (b). Detection, autoradiography (10 days). (Figures and data kindly supplied by D. Wynford-Thomas, University of Wales College of Medicine, Cardiff.) (Haematoxylin counterstained.)

samples. Positive controls may include using a cell line which expresses the gene being studied and using abundant constitutionally expressed gene probes. Using multiple probes for the same target, competitive inhibition with unlabelled probe, melting point analysis of *in situ* formed hybrids, and comparing signal localization to known anatomic or immunocytochemical distribution will all provide a strong indication of specificity.

In situ transcription

A new technique, a modification of *in situ* hybridization, developed recently is *in situ* transcription (IST). Briefly, it involves *in situ* hybridization of mRNA with specific oligonucleotide primers, followed by reverse transcription in the presence of labelled nucleotides and synthesis of a labelled cDNA *in situ*. This transcript can then be detected visually, or eluted into solution for further analysis by PCR or blotting. This method allows the localization of specific mRNA, and is particularly useful where only part of the sequence is known or where they may be alternate splicing. It enables allele or mutation-specific message detection since short discriminatory primers are used, and can also be used for tissue quantitation of mRNA.

30.3.8 DNA and messenger RNA extraction and analysis by Southern and Northern blotting

Julia E. Stickland and James O'D. McGee

The application of molecular biology techniques to the analysis of the human genome is highly relevant to many problems in human disease. Efficient extraction of pure, high-molecular-weight DNA and undegraded mRNA from biopsy samples taken for diagnostic purposes is essential, since samples are frequently small and cannot be repeated at will. It is often desirable to identify an individual fragment in a complex mixture that has been resolved by gel electrophoresis. For DNA samples, this is accomplished by Southern blotting, in which the fragments are transferred from the gel to a filter and the fragment of interest is identified by hybridization with a labelled nucleic acid probe. This approach has been applied in the diagnosis of genetic diseases (see Chapter 2). Linkage analysis using restriction fragment length polymorphisms (RFLPs) have helped to locate candidate genes for several diseases (Section 2.3) and to identify the location of putative tumour-suppressor genes in informative patients by loss of heterozygosity of a specific allele (Section 9.6). In addition, Southern blotting is used to detect T-cell receptor and immunoglobulin gene rearrangements, and the presence of viruses in cells. These two applications are essential for diagnostic accuracy in cases where routine methods have given an equivocal answer.

Resolution of single-stranded RNA and its subsequent transfer from the gel to a solid filter support has 'playfully' become known as the Northern blot. The presence, size, and amount of specific mRNA molecules in preparations of total RNA or polyadenosine triphosphate RNA (poly(A)$^+$ RNA) are determined by hybridization with labelled DNA or RNA probes.

The principles of DNA and RNA extraction from clinical specimens, cultured cells, peripheral blood, and paraffin embedded tissue will be discussed together with their analysis by Southern and Northern blotting respectively.

DNA extraction

There are a number of different protocols for the preparation of genomic DNA. These protocols consist of two parts: a technique which gently lyses the cells and solubilizes the DNA, followed by one of several enzymatic or chemical methods to remove contaminating proteins, RNA, and other macromolecules. Human genomic DNA is usually isolated by digesting cells with the powerful proteolytic enzyme proteinase K combined with the protein denaturing ionic detergent sodium dodecyl sulphate (SDS) in the presence of EDTA. Protein is subsequently extracted with phenol, which efficiently denatures proteins and probably dissolves denatured protein. Low-molecular-weight contaminants are removed by ethanol precipitation. All material should be processed as quickly as possible to avoid action by nucleases. Tissue samples can be stored in liquid nitrogen until required or placed directly into extraction buffer. Tissue culture cells should be cooled and washed quickly several times in ice-cold phosphate-buffered-saline (PBS). As soon as the tissue is frozen, or extraction buffer is added to the samples, the DNA is protected from action of nucleases. Subsequently the tissue must be cut into small pieces and ground up to permit rapid and efficient access to proteinase K and SDS. The presence of EDTA in the digestion buffer chelates divalent cations which could otherwise mediate aggregation of nucleic acids to each other and may act as cofactors for endogenous nucleases.

For blood samples, fresh blood is collected in tubes containing an anticoagulant (acid citrate dextrose solution is superior to EDTA in preserving high-molecular-weight DNA during storage of blood). The blood may be stored at $0\,^{\circ}$C for several days, or at $-70\,^{\circ}$C indefinitely, before the DNA is prepared. Whole blood is washed extensively in a hypotonic saline solution, which lyses the red blood cells. Complete lysis is essential since red blood cell products are potent inhibitors of restriction endonucleases. Extraction buffer is then added directly to the white blood cells. Samples derived from whole tissue, cultured cells, or blood are incubated in proteinase K extraction buffer for several hours. The now highly viscous samples are extracted with an equal volume of phenol equilibrated with Tris-HCl pH 8.0. If the pH of the phenol is lower than 7.5, the DNA becomes trapped at the interface between the organic and aqueous phases. The viscous aqueous DNA-containing phase is transferred to a clean tube using a wide-bore pipette (0.3 cm) to minimize DNA shearing and the extraction is repeated twice more with a mixture of phenol:chloroform:isoamyl alcohol. Chloroform stabilizes the boundary between the aqueous phase and the phenol layer, and isoamyl alcohol prevents foaming of the mixture and also aids in the separation of the organic and aqueous phases.

To isolate very high-molecular-weight DNA (~ 200 kb) for the construction of cosmid libraries, the aqueous phase is dialysed at $4\,^{\circ}$C. For DNA in the size range 100–150 kb (adequate for the construction of phage λ libraries and Southern blots) the DNA is ethanol precipitated.

DNA can also be extracted from paraffin-embedded sections by dewaxing in xylene and rehydration by passage through graded alcohols. A five-day incubation with proteinase K extraction buffer is required to produce good yields of DNA. Unfortunately the DNA is frequently partially degraded and whilst suitable for PCR analysis (see Section 3.3.9), probably only 1 in 50 blocks would provide DNA of a quality suitable for restriction enzyme analysis and Southern blotting.

RNA extraction

The isolation of undegraded preparations of eukaryotic mRNA from cells and tissues involves four steps: (1) inhibition of endogenous nucleases, by using inhibitors of RNases or methods that disrupt cells and inactive RNases simultaneously; (2) deproteinization of the RNA; (3) physical separation of the RNA from the other components of the homogenate; and (4) the selection of poly(A)$^+$ RNA by affinity chromatography on oligo (dT)-cellulose. It is important to avoid the accidental introduction of trace amounts of RNase from other potential sources in the laboratory, e.g. glassware, plasticware, contamination by workers, and contaminated solutions. Wherever possible solutions should be treated with 0.1 per cent diethyl-pyrocarbonate (DEPC). DEPC is a potent ribonuclease inhibitor.

Procedures using strong protein denaturants such as guanidinium thiocyanate and guanidine hydrochloride effectively combine the first two steps. Denaturation by guanidinium thiocyanate is enhanced by including a reductant, such as 2-mercaptoethanol or dithiothreitol which breaks intramolecular disulphide bonds which are essential for RNase activity. For precious samples with unknown RNase content guanidinium thiocyanate solution should be used since both cation (guanidinium) and anion (thiocyanate) are chaotropic agents.

Freshly removed tissue should be cut into small pieces and frozen in liquid nitrogen, or placed directly into the guanidinium solution and homogenized immediately using a polytron blender. Failure to treat the sample immediately results in nucleolytic damage to the RNA. Cultured cell lines grown in suspension may be recovered by centrifugation, washed once with PBS, and resuspended in guanidinium solution. Adherent cells, washed once in PBS, are lysed directly in the tissue culture dish. Normal human lymphocytes isolated from peripheral blood by Ficoll Hypaque are resuspended by vortexing in guanidinium solution. Once the RNA is dispersed in the guanidinium solution steps (1) and (2) have been completed and only steps (3) and (4) remain. These include the physical separation of the RNA from the other macromolecular components of the homogenate and selection of the poly(A)$^+$ RNA. A number of separation methods have been documented, which can be divided into two main categories: selective precipitation based on solubility, and selective sedimentation (by ultracentrifugation) based on buoyant density. Selective precipitation based on solubility works well for many tissues. A protocol combining acid guanidinium thiocyanate-phenol-chloroform extraction (AGPC) followed by ethanol precipitation gives comparable yields of equally pure RNA (Chomczynski and Sacchi 1987) to that obtained by guanidinium thiocyanate and cesium chloride centrifugation (Chirgwin *et al.* 1979).

Briefly, the AGPC method combines the action of a strong protein denaturant (guanidinium thiocyanate) with an acid phenol protein extraction. At pH 5–6 DNA is selectively retained in the organic phase and interface, leaving RNA in the aqueous phase. The centrifugation method uses guanidinium thiocyanate to disrupt the cells and the resulting homogenate is then layered on to a cushion of dense cesium chloride solution. The buoyant density of RNA in cesium chloride is much greater than that of the other cellular components. During centrifugation, the RNA forms a pellet on the bottom of the tube, while the DNA and protein float in the supernatant. Polytron homogenization of all cell lysates, whether derived from tissue or cultured cells, is a prerequisite for this protocol as this shears nuclear DNA which would otherwise form an impenetrable mat on top of the cushion of cesium chloride, which might block sedimentation of the RNA to the bottom of the centrifuge tube. In both the AGPC and the ultracentrifugation method, the RNA is normally reprecipitated at least twice with ethanol to eliminate already denatured ribonuclease from the nucleic acid pellets.

Due to its simplicity and the elimination of ultracentrifugation, the AGPC method allows simultaneous processing of a large number of samples and the degradation and loss of RNA is minimized by the limited handling in this technique.

The methods outlined above permit independent extraction of DNA or RNA from cultured cells and solid tissue. More recently, a procedure for the simultaneous extraction of high-molecular-weight DNA and RNA using frozen-phenol followed by two-step cesium chloride centrifugation has been described (Chan *et al.* 1988). This method may be the one of choice where both the DNA and RNA warrant investigation, especially in small biopsy samples. Procedures for RNA extrction from paraffin embedded material are not well documented. A technique identical to that employed to extract DNA from such tissue involves proteinase K digestion. This method yields a considerable amount of RNA which is suitable for PCR analysis, but not for Northern blotting.

Messenger RNA can be readily purified from total RNA preparations by affinity chromatography on oligo-(dT) cellulose. The vast majority of mRNAs of mammalian cells carry lengths of poly(A) at their 3′ terminus making it possible to purify mRNA by virtue of its base pairing with immobilized oligo-(dT). Heat denatured RNA, which removes any secondary structure, is normally applied to a column of oligo-(dT) in high salt buffer. High salt aids the binding of the poly(A)$^+$ fraction to the oligo-(dT) column, whilst poly(A)$^-$ RNA flows through the column. Poly(A)$^+$ RNA is eluted from the oligo-(dT) cellulose in low salt buffer, ethanol precipitated, and resuspended in DEPC treated water. Usually between 1 and 2 per cent of the total RNA applied to the column is recovered as poly(A)$^+$ RNA. Poly(A)$^+$

RNA usually yields better results than total RNA when analysed by Northern hybridization.

Southern blotting of genomic DNA

Genomic DNA is digested to completion with one or more restriction enzymes, and the resulting fragments are separated according to size by electrophoresis through an agarose gel containing ethidium bromide. Ethidium bromide binds to DNA by intercalating between the bases. The DNA can then be detected as ethidium bromide fluoresces under ultraviolet light. Molecular-weight standards are also electrophoresed on the gel (e.g. phage λ cleaved with *Hind*III), which is run slowly for several hours. After electrophoresis is completed the gels are photographed with a transparent ruler alongside the marker lanes, so that the distance that any band of DNA has migrated can be read directly from the photographic image. Prior to transfer of the restricted genomic DNA the gel is incubated in weak acid to partially depurinate the DNA which assists in the transfer of larger fragments (15 kb) from the gel. The DNA is then denatured in the gel with strong alkali rendering it single stranded so that it may bind to the solid support (nitrocellulose filter or nylon membrane). Before transfer of the DNA to nitrocellulose filters it must be neutralized to pH 7.5 by incubation in a Tris-HCl buffered solution, otherwise the filters become very fragile and crack easily. DNA fragments are normally transferred from agarose gels to solid supports by capillary transfer. The fragments are transferred from the gel by capillary flow of buffer and deposited on the surface of the solid support. Capillary action is aided by a stack of absorbent paper towels. Vacuum transfer is a viable alternative for the transfer of DNA or RNA to filters. Electrophoretic transfer requires large electric currents and it is difficult to maintain the elctrophoresis buffer at a temperature compatible with efficient transfer of DNA, so this is not recommended.

Transfer of nucleic acids

High ionic strength buffers are used for transfer, particularly for binding DNA to nitrocellulose filters. Transfer is allowed to proceed for 8–24 hours. Nitrocellulose filters are baked at 80°C for 2 hours to fix the nucleic acids to the filter by hydrophobic interactions. Nucleic acids become covalently attached to nylon membranes if they are exposed to low doses of ultraviolet irradiation when dry. The amount of irradiation required to produce the maximum hybridization signal must be determined empirically. Over-irradiation leads to a decrease in hybridization signal. Nylon membranes bind nucleic acids irreversibly and are more durable than nitrocellulose filters. They can therefore be hybridized sequentially. Filters may be stored wrapped loosely in aluminium foil or in a sealed bag at room temperature until required for hybridization.

Northern blotting of RNA

RNA agarose gels are either run under denaturing conditions, e.g. formaldehyde or methylmecuric hydroxide gels, or the RNA is denatured by treatment with glyoxal prior to electrophoresis. Ease of handling and lack of toxicity recommend use of either the glyoxal or the formaldehyde methods for the fractionation of RNA prior to transfer to hybridization membranes. Gels containing glyoxal/dimethyl sulphoxide (DMSO) treated samples are run slowly for several hours and the electrophoresis buffer must be circulated. This avoids unacceptable hydrogen ion gradients during electrophoresis. Glyoxal readily dissociates from RNA at pH >8.0, allowing formation of secondary structures within the RNA molecule which may affect migration through the gel. Glyoxylated molecular-weight markers removed from the gel following electrophoresis are stained with ethidium bromide and a photograph is taken as described for DNA gels. RNA is transferred from the gel to a nitrocellulose filter or nylon membrane directly, as no subsequent denaturation is necessary. However, before hybridization to a labelled probe, the glyoxal must be removed from the RNA by washing the filter in Tris-HCl buffer, pH 8.0 at 65 °C.

Formaldehyde-agarose gels are denaturing gels which do not require constant circulation of buffer during electrophoresis. However, after 1–2 hours, buffer should be collected, mixed, and returned to the gel apparatus. Prior to loading, RNA samples are denatured in a mixture of both formaldehyde and formamide, then loaded immediately, and electrophoresed as for glyoxal gels. At the end of the run, marker lanes are stained in ethidium bromide and photographed as previously described for DNA. The formaldehyde-containing gel requires pretreatment before RNA transfer. The gel must be rinsed in several changes of DEPC-treated water to remove the formaldehyde and equilibrated in transfer buffer before placing in contact with the transfer membrane. Capillary transfer is carried out as described for Southern blotting.

Hybridization

The conditions for prehybridization, hybridization, and washing of RNA/DNA immobilized on filters are essentially the same. These conditions are applicable whether the nucleic acid is bound to a nitrocellulose filter or a nylon membrane. A wide variety of probes may be used to detect DNA or RNA transferred to filters. These include: double-stranded DNA labelled by nick-translation or random priming, single-stranded DNA prepared by primer extension, labelled synthetic oligonucleotides, and RNA synthesized in vitro with prokaryotic DNA-dependent RNA polymerases. A choice between $[\alpha^{32}P]dNTP$ radioactively labelled probes or non-radioactive probes such as the haptens biotin or digoxygenin is available. The disadvantages of using radioisotopes—safety, disposal, short half-life, and duration of autoradiographic exposure—must be balanced against its higher sensitivity and generally greater reproducibility than nonradioactive probing methods. To obtain maximum sensitivity with nonradioactive probes, published protocols should be followed exactly. For detecting biotinylated DNA probes, readers are referred to Chan et al. (1985) and for digoxygenin labelled probes to Holtke and Kessler (1990).

There are many methods available to hybridize radioactive probes in solution; the choice depends to a large extent on personal preference. Prehydbridization of filters is normally carried out in a solution identical to the hybridization solution (without the probe). Compounds such as dextran sulphate or polyethylene glycol increase the rate of hybridization of probe to bound nucleic acid by approximately tenfold. The prehybridization solutions contain agents such as Denhardts reagent, SDS and denatured fragmented DNA which block the non-specific attachment of the probe to the surface of the filter. Hybridizations are usually carried out in solutions of high ionic strength to maximize the rate of annealing of the probe with its target in either 50 per cent formamide at 42 °C or at 68 °C in aqueous solution. To minimize background problems, filters are prehybridized for a minimum of 2 hours in at least 0.2 ml of solution per cm^2 of filter. Hybridization is carried out for the shortest possible time using the minimum amount of probe in a small volume of solution. Doube-stranded probes should be denatured by boiling for 5 minutes and chilled on ice. Approximately 10 ng/ml of radiolabelled probe (specific activity of 10^8 cpm/μg or greater) should be added to fresh hybridization solution and hybridization is carried out for 16–40 hours. The washing conditions should be as stringent as possible. A combination of temperature and salt concentration should be chosen that is approximately 12–20 °C below the calculated Tm of the hybrid. These conditions should be determined empirically for the probe of interest. It is important not to let the filter dry out as this increases non-specific background hybridization. Damp filters covered in plastic cling film should be exposed to X-ray film at -70 °C with an intensifying screen. Single copy sequences in genomic DNA can usually be detected after 16–24 hours of exposure, however rare mRNAs may require up to 1 week autoradiography.

30.3.9   The polymerase chain reaction

David Flannery and James O'D. McGee

Since its invention in 1985, the use of the polymerase chain reaction (PCR) has been in exponential growth in research and clinical departments. This method (in seven years) has progressed from the molecular biologist's laboratory to become an indispensable diagnostic tool for the future pathologist.

At a time when the genetic bases for several common and previously poorly understood conditions (e.g. cystic fibrosis, Duchenne's muscular dystrophy), and the significance of viruses in disease (e.g. HTLV1 in adult T-cell leukaemia, HIV in AIDS, and HPV in cervical cancer) are being uncovered, the process of detection of the endogenous or exogenous sequence has shortened from a matter of weeks to days. Theoretically the nightmare of pinpointing a single aberrant gene amongst thousands of cells has been circumvented by the amplification of a portion of this gene by up to 10^8-fold, in effect overshadowing the genetic haystack with a mountain built of needles.

Methodology

The automated process of PCR amplification involves the binding of two artificially synthesized oligonucleotide primers, typically 20 bases long (statistically, the length of a unique sequence within the human genome is 16 bases), to opposite strands of the double helix flanking the target DNA. The orientation of these primers is such that, by repeated cycles of heat denaturation (92–95°C), annealing of primers (37–60°C) and extension of the primers by a heat-stable DNA polymerase, Taq1 (around 72°C), DNA synthesis proceeds across the target sequence. The incorporation of the primer into an extension product which can itself act as a template for its partner primer essentially means the doubling, in each cycle, of a DNA fragment of size defined by the distance between the 5′ termini of the primers on the target DNA. As each copy gives rise to two new copies, this approximately exponential amplification means theoretically that one target sequence among 10^6 cells can now be visualized after 30–40 cycles by size differentiation using gel electrophoresis, although in practice most investigators would claim sensitivity of 10–50 copies. Sequences of up to 10 kilobases have been amplified, but the optimum length for amplification is 100–500 bases.

Applications

The ability of this technique to pull out a short sequence against seemingly insurmountable odds has enabled the study of DNA from a diversity of materials: million-year-old archaeological specimens, embryos, hair roots, buccal washes, smears, Guthrie spots, urine, cerebral spinal fluid, pleural and peritoneal effusions, and even single sperm. The commonest source for the pathologist is the paraffin block, and the DNA can be extracted from a dewaxed section simply by boiling for 10 minutes, or removing protein with proteinase K followed by heat denaturation of the enzyme. Alongside the morphological examination of contiguous haemotoxylin and eosin stained sections, this method has opened the door to a wealth of material available for restrospective study.

Prenatal diagnosis

On the other end of the spectrum, a single cell can be removed from *in vitro*-fertilized embryos prior to implantation and analysed for genetic defects or the presence of the Y-chromosome in the case of a sex-linked disease. However, the high error rate in Taq1 polymerase nucleotide incorporation (as high as 1 in 400 bases) could conceivably give rise to a 'false' mutation in the early cycles, which would later be emphasized. This reaction should therefore be ideally repeated on a second cell to reduce the possibility of an erroneous interpretation. Chorionic villous biopsies can be carried out after 6–8 weeks of gestation with low fetal loss and provide ample material for PCR. Fetal cells that have crossed the placental barrier during early pregnancy can also be amplified from the expectant mother's blood for the Y-chromosome, potentially obviating the necessity for invasive techniques in the detection of sex-linked disease. The creation of monoclonal antibodies to fetal cells will enable their removal

from maternal cells and their consequent (confident) analysis for single genetic disorders.

Viral diagnosis

The immediately obvious use of PCR analysis is to produce a discrete band by judicial use of primers and optimization of, principally, the annealing temperature and Mg^{2+} ionic concentration, but also the extension time for that reaction. A simple choice of primers would include those composed of viral sequences which would not amplify normal human DNA. The PCR reaction is very useful in the study of the role of HPV in cervical cancer, and for the detection of latent HIV in, as yet, sero-negative patients and babies born to sero-positive mothers.

Lymphoma diagnosis

Most B-cell follicular lymphomas contain a t(14; 18) chromosomal translocation. PCR can act as a diagnostic marker in the detection of residual disease using a primer from chromosome 14 and another from 18, since the breakpoints occur in a very small area, and the primers would only produce a discrete band if the translocation brings the primers into juxtaposition. The problem with detection of the Philadelphia chromosome in chronic myeloid leukaemia is that the breakpoints are too far apart to be easily amplified. This can be circumvented by translating the uniquely leukaemic 'fusion' mRNA, bcr-abl, into cDNA using the retroviral enzyme, reverse transcriptase. The cDNA produced, being shorter than the original gene (since mRNA is processed to remove non-coding information), can now act as a substrate for the PCR reaction. Again, a fragment is produced that would not result from normal DNA since the primers are derived from separate genes on separate chromosomes.

Point mutations

Along with gross chromosomal alterations, the reaction can bring to light single base mutations. Since the polymerase will only function properly if the 3′ end of the primer (the end to which it attaches) is annealed to its target, two reactions can be carried out: one with a pair of normal (wild type) primers, and the other with one wild type primer and one containing the base mutation at its 3′ end, as in the detection of sickle cell anaemia and α-1-antitrypsin deficiency. The inherent problem with this technique is that conditions for the reaction have to be stringently optimized and heterogeneous single base mutations cannot be detected.

An extension of this basic idea is the marrying of PCR with restriction enzyme analysis. Restriction enzymes each recognize a certain DNA sequence and cut the DNA at that site. Since mismatches of the primer sequence other than at the 3′ end do not significantly affect the PCR reaction, partial restriction sites can be engineered into the primers, so that if the mutation is present a complete restriction site is produced and amplified. Production of this site and its subsequent digestion with an appropriate restriction enzyme gives a smaller PCR product which can be visualized by size using polyacrylamide gel electrophoresis. Alternatively, the primers could be perfectly matched to the target and changes in the internal amplified sequence detected with the same technology. Mutations or rearrangements that alter or create a restriction site will change the number of fragments after digestion, whereas insertions or deletions will change the size of fragments. This is a rapid method of analysis, as the restriction enzyme can occasionally be directly added to the PCR reaction mix after amplification with no need for product purification, and is also useful in verification of a specific PCR reaction. However, other methods are also required for the verification of PCR products, since single base mutations can only be detected if they abolish or create a restriction site, and some insertions or deletions will be too small to be detected.

Another widely used method is hybridization of the PCR product with a labelled internal allele-specific oligonucleotide probe using blotting techniques, with either the product or the probe immobilized on a filter. This was initially used for detection of the sickle cell anaemia mutation; a probe containing the mutation hybridized to the homozygote's product, an unmutated probe only hybridized to normal DNA, and both probes hybridized to the product from heterozygotes. Here, stringency conditions for hybridization have to be optimized.

The 'gold standard' of PCR product verification and analysis is DNA sequencing, since any mutation can be detected, and sequencing can be carried out directly using one of the PCR primers. In this way, heterogeneous mutations have been discovered in α-1-antitrypsin and β-thalassaemia. The method, however, is laborious and time-consuming in comparison with the others.

Controls

Why this constant need for product verification? The answer is that non-specific amplification can occur when the primers anneal to sites other than the target. Although this non-specific amplification usually results in a different sized product, this may not be the case if a closely related virus or gene is amplified.

Another problem with PCR is that of 'false negatives', when the reaction simply fails to occur for technical reasons (inactive Taq1, or an incorrectly prepared reaction mix, etc.). For this reason a positive control should be included. Alternatively an additional pair of primers to another DNA region, that produce a differently-sized fragment, can be included in the same reaction.

The great strength of the PCR reaction is also its greatest weakness: its sensitivity. A single contaminant molecule could theoretically be amplified to produce a 'false positive'. This problem is magnified if a large number of cycles is carried out, so the number of PCR cycles should be reduced to the minimum necessary. Negative controls containing no DNA, or preferably a related negative DNA, should be included. The principal source of contamination is that from the amplified PCR product. As a consequence, the preparation of reaction mixes and their subsequent analysis should be carried out in separate rooms with separate pipettes (preferably positive displacement), ideally in a laminar flow hood. Other safeguards include aliquoting re-

agents to minimize handling, or carrying out a second round of amplification on the product using 'nested primers', sequences internal to the original primers. Novel methods used by some laboratories to minimize contamination include employing only female staff to assay for the Y-chromosome, and, where plasmids containing the target sequence are used in the same laboratory, to design primers for the target DNA that are separated by the vector DNA, thus producing a much larger fragment if the plasmid contaminates the reaction mix.

Summary

In this section we have concentrated on the clinical relevance to the pathologist of this new technology, but novel uses for this method are continually being found. The site of insertion of, for example, a virus within the genome can be located by selecting primers that extend away from each other, copying the DNA outside the primer pair. The template DNA is digested with a restriction enzyme and the two ends joined into a circle. This undergoes a PCR reaction in both directions across the join to give a linear product copied from DNA flanking the primers, which can then be labelled easily for use as a probe.

The ability of PCR to detect and amplify any nucleic acid, even a single molecule, from almost any material in a day (provided some of the sequence is known) has revolutionized molecular biology in just seven years. So what of the future? The Human Genome Project will unravel more of the genetic basis for disease whilst providing the necessary sequence information for detection. By using conserved sequences within viral families, e.g. HPV, novel but related viruses will be discovered. The whole process should become even more automated; DNA sequences being tapped into a machine, the primers synthesized and the PCR reaction carried out completely in a closed environment, making the technology more readily usable outside the research laboratory.

The most promising future prospect of the technology for the pathologist could be *in situ* PCR, since the amplified product would be directly correlated with morphology, and the margin for error (i.e. false positives) reduced. The primer or nucleotides could be labelled, or the product could be probed for with a labelled internal oligomer. The problem with this method at the moment is the difficulty of anchoring the PCR product in the cell.

30.3.10   Summary

In situ hybridization bridges the gap between molecular biology (recombinant DNA technology) and the morphological disciplines of cytogenetics, cytology, and histopathology. It allows direct investigative study into chromosomal gene location (translocation and other aberrational assignments) and single gene expression (mRNA) in normal, abnormal, and neoplastic cellular material. These studies are conducted in conjunction with Southern, Northern, dot blot, or PCR nucleic acid analyses and immunocytochemistry, if enough material is available. By such measures a better understanding of the molecular biology, aetiology, or pathogenesis of viral and other infectious diseases, neoplastic, and hereditary processes in man may be obtained.

30.3.11 Further reading

Alitalo, K. and Peltonen, L. (eds) (1986). Recombinant DNA in clinical medicine. *Annals of Clinical Research* 18, 217–343.

Bhatt, B., Burns, J., Flannery, D., and McGee, J. O'D. (1988). Direct visualisation of single copy genes on banded metaphase chromosomes by nonisotopic *in situ* hybridization. *Nucleic Acids Research* 16, 3951–61.

Biberfeld, P., Chayt, K. J., Marselle, L. M., Biberfeld, G., Gallo, R. C., and Harper, M. E. (1986). HTLV-III expression in infected lymph nodes and relevance to pathogenesis of lymphadenopathy. *American Journal of Pathology* 125, 436–42.

Bresser, J. and Evinger-Hodges, M. J. (1987). Comparison and optimization of *in situ* hybridisation procedures yielding rapid, sensitive mRNA detections. *Gene Analysis Techniques* 4, 89–104.

Burns, J., Chan, F. T.-W., Jonasson, J. A., Flemming, K. A., Taylor, S., and McGee, J. O'D. (1985). Sensitive system for visualising biotinylated DNA probes hybrised *in situ* rapid sex determination of intact cells. *Journal of Clinical Pathology* 38, 1085–92.

Burns, J., Graham, A. K. Frank, C., Fleming, K. A., Evans, M. F., and McGee, J. O'D. (1987). Detection of low copy human papillomavirus DNA and mRNA in routine paraffin sections of cervix by non-isotopic *in situ* hybridisation. *Journal of Clinical Pathology* 40, 858–64.

Chan, V.T.-W., Fleming, K. A., and McGee, J. O'D. (1985). Detection of subpicogram quantities of specific DNA sequences on blot hybridisation with biotinylated probes. *Nucleic Acids Research* 13, 8083–91.

Chan, V. T.-W., Fleming, K. A., and McGee, J. O'D. (1988). Simultaneous extraction from clinical biopsies of high-molecular-weight DNA and RNA: comparative characterisation of biotinylated and 32-P labelled probes on Southern and Northern blots. *Analytical Biochemistry* 168, 16–24.

Chan, F. T.-W. and McGee, J. O'D. (1987). Cellular oncogenes in neoplasia. *Journal of Clinical Pathology* 40, 1055–63.

Chirgwin, J. M., Przbyla, A. E., MacDonald, R. J., and Rutter, W. J. (1979). Isolation of biologically active ribonucleic acid from sources enriched in ribonuclease. *Biochemistry* 18, 5294–9.

Chomczynski, P. and Sacchi, N. (1987). Single step method of RNA isolation by acid guanidinium thiocyanate-phenol-chloroform extraction. *Analytical Biochemistry* 162, 156–9.

Cooper, K., Herrington, C. S., Graham, A. K., Evans, M. F., and McGee, J. O'D. (1991). *In situ* HPV genotyping of cervical intraepithelial neoplasia in South African and UK patients: evidence for putative HPV integration *in vivo*. *Journal of Clinical Pathology* 44, 400–5.

Cooper, K., Herrington, C. S., Graham, A. K., Evans, M. F., and McGee, J. O'D. (1991). *In situ* evidence for HPV 16,18,33 integration in cervical squamous cell cancer in the UK and South Africa. *Journal of Clinical Pathology* 44, 406–9.

Cooper, K., Herrington, C. S., Stickland, J. E., Evans, M. F., and McGee, J. O'D. (1991). Episomal and integrated HPV16 in cervial neoplasia demonstrated by non-isotopic *in situ* hybridisation. *Journal of Clinical Pathology* (in press).

Davies, K. E. (ed.) (1986). *Human genetic diseases: a practical approach.* IRL Press, Oxford.

DeLellis, R. A. and Wolfe, H. J. (1987). New techniques in gene product analysis. *Archives of Pathology and Laboratory Medicine* 111, 620–7.

Fenoglio-Preiser, C. M. and Willman, C. L. (1987). Molecular biology

and the pathologist. General principles and applications. *Archives of Pathology and Laboratory Medicine* 111, 601–19.

Glover, D. M. (1986). *DNA cloning. A practical approach*, Vols I and II. IRL Press, Oxford.

Grody, W. W., Cheng, L., and Lewin, K. J. (1987). Application of *in situ* DNA hybridization technology to diagnostic surgical pathology. In *Pathology annual* (ed. P. P. Rosen and R. Fechner), Part 2, pp. 151–75. Appleton-Lange, USA.

Hames, B. D. and Higgins, S. J. (eds) (1985). *Nucleic acid hybridisation: a practical approach.* IRL Press, Oxford.

Harper, M. E., Marselle, L. M., Gallo, R. C., and Wong-Staal, F. (1986). Detection of lymphocytes expressing human T-lymphotropic virus type III in lymph nodes and peripheral blood from infected individuals by *in situ* hybridization. *Proceedings of the National Academy of Sciences, USA* 83, 772–6.

Herrington, C. S., Graham, A. K., and McGee, J. O'D. (1991). Interphase cytogenetics III: Increased sensitivity and flexibility of digoxigenin-labelled DNA probes for HPV detection in cervical biopsies and cell lines. *Journal of Clinical Pathology* 44, 33–8.

Holtke, H.-J. and Kessler, C. (1990). Non-radioactive labelling of RNA transcripts *in vitro* with the hapten digoxygenin (DIG); hybridisation and ELISA-based detection. *Nucleic Acids Research* 18, 5843–57.

Julien, C., Bazin, A., Guyot, B., Forestier, F., and Daffos, F. (1986). Rapid prenatal diagnosis of Down's syndrome with *in situ* hybridisation of fluorescent DNA probes. *Lancet* ii, 863–4.

Larsson, L-I., Christensen, T., and Dalboge, H. (1988). Detection of proopiomelanocortin mRNA by *in situ* hybridization, using a biotinylated oligodeoxynucleotide probe and avidin-alkaline phosphatase histochemistry. *Histochemistry* 89, 109–16.

Lloyd, R. V. (1987). Use of molecular probes in the study of endocrine diseases. *Human Pathology* 18, 1199–211.

Martinez-Montero, J. C., *et al.* (1991). Model system for optimising mRNA non-isotopic in situ hybridisation: riboprobe detection of lysozyme mRNA in archival gut biopsy specimens. *Journal of Clinical Pathology* 44, 835–9.

Marx, J. L. (1986). Viruses and cancers. *Science* 231, 919–20.

Matthews, J. A. and Kricka, L. J. (1988). Review. Analytical strategies for the use of DNA probes. *Analytical Biochemistry* 169, 1–25.

Moyzis, R. K., Albright, K. L., Bartholdi, M. F., Cram, L. S., Deaven, L. L., Hildebrand, C. E., Joste, N. E., Longmire, J. L., Meyne, J., and Schwarzacher-Robinson, T. (1987). Human chromosome-specific repetitive DNA sequences: Novel markers for genetic analysis. *Chromosoma (Berl)* 95, 375–86.

Pardue, M. L. and Gall, J. G. (1969). Molecular hybridisation of radioactive DNA to the DNA of cytological preparations. *Proceedings of the National Academy of Sciences, USA* 64, 600–4.

Penschow, J. D., Haralambidis, J., Aldred, P., Tregear, G. W., and Coghlan, J. P. (1986). Location of gene expression in CNS using hybridisation histochemistry. *Methods in Enzymology* 124, 534–48.

Pfeifer-Ohlsson, S., Goustin, A. S., Rydnert, J., Wahlstrom, T., Bjersing, L., Stehelin, D., and Ohlsson, R. (1984). Spatial and temporal pattern of cellular myc oncogene expression in developing human placenta: implications for embryonic cell proliferation. *Cell* 38, 585–96.

Piper, M. A. and Unger, E. R. (1989). *Nucleic acid probes. A primer for pathologits.* American Society of Clinical Pathologists Press, Chicago.

Shapshak, P., Tourtellotte, W. W., Wolman, M., Verity, N., Verity, M. A., Schmid, P., Syndulko, K., Bedows, E., Boostanfar, R., Darvish, M., Nakamura, S., Tomiyasu, U., Steiner, R. C., Hawkins, S., Hoffman, D., Adhami, F., and Martinez, S. (1986). Search for virus nucleic acid sequences in postmortem human brain tissue using *in situ* hybridization technology with cloned probes: some solutions and results on progressive multifocal leukoencephalopathy and subacute sclerosing panencephalitis tissue. *Journal of Neuroscience Research* 16, 281–301.

Tecott, L. H., Barchas, J. D., and Eberwine, J. H. (1988). *In situ* transcription: specific synthesis of complementary DNA in fixed tissue sections. *Science* 240, 1661–4.

Trask, B., van den Engh, G., Pinkel, D., Mullikin, J., Waldman, F., van Dekken, H., and Gray, J. (1988). Fluorescence *in situ* hybridization to interphase cell nuclei in suspension allows flow cytometric analysis of chromosome content and microscopic analysis of nuclear organization. *Human Genetics* 78, 251–9.

Uhl, G. R. (ed.) (1986). In situ *hybridisation in brain*. Plenum Press, London.

Valentino, K. L., Eberwine, J. H., and Barchas, J. D. (eds) (1987). In situ *hybridization. Applications to neurobiology*. Oxford University Press, Oxford.

General reviews

Herrington, C. . and McGee, J. O'D. (eds) (1992). *Diagnostic molecular pathology: a practical approach*, Vols 1 and 2. IRL Press at Oxford University Press.

Maniatis, T., Fritsch, E. F., and Sambrook, J. (1989). *Molecular cloning: a laboratory manual*. Cold Spring Harbor Laboratory, New York.

Polak, J. M. and McGee, J. O'D. (1990). In situ *hybridisation: principles and practice*. Oxford University Press.

30.4   Exfoliative cytopathology

Dulcie Coleman

30.4.1   Introduction

One of the most remarkable changes to occur in clinical practice in the past 10 years has been the increased demand for cytopathology services. This change in medical practice stems from an increased awareness of the value of cytological investigation as a diagnostic tool; and a changing attitude to cancer prevention and primary health care.

The aim of this section is to provide the reader with information about the collection, preparation, and interpretation of cytology specimens so that he/she can report with confidence on cervical smears, sputum, effusions, and other specimens which constitute the majority of the samples submitted for cytopathological diagnosis.

30.4.2   Principles of cytological investigation

The success of cytological methods of investigation stems from the fact that the presence of malignancy in a tissue or organ can be accurately predicted by the examination of a small sample of cells in the light microscope. The sample may contain cells that have been exfoliated spontaneously (e.g. sputum, urine, effu-sions, or cyst aspirates) or cells that have been forcibly detached (e.g. endoscopic brushing or fine-needle aspiration biopsy specimens), or a mixture of both (e.g. cervical scrapes).

In every case where an adequate sample has been obtained, the analysis of fixed and stained smears by light microscopy will reveal information about the organ or tissue from which the cells were harvested.

30.4.3   Advantages and limitations of cytopathology

Cytological investigation has several advantages over surgical biopsy. The samples can be taken from the conscious patient in an out-patient setting with the minimum of trauma; and anaesthesia is rarely required. The techniques are safe, simple, and inexpensive and the complications of haemorrhage and sepsis, which frequently accompany biopsy, are rare. Moreover, if samples are of insufficient size or of poor quality, repeat samples can be taken, with minimum inconvenience to the patient. The development of a range of sampling techniques in the past 30 years has meant that cytological samples can be obtained from almost every site in the body.

The main use of cytology is in the diagnosis of malignancy. Since malignant cells lack the cohesiveness of normal cells, the smallest and earliest neoplastic lesions can be detected by these methods of sampling. Another advantage of cytology is that diseases other than neoplasia can be diagnosed from the samples, e.g. virus infection, hormonal inbalance, granulomatous change.

One of the important limitations of cytology is that it is not always possible to precisely localize the malignant lesion, even though tumour cells are present in the sample. This is a particular limitation of exfoliative cytology (cervical cytology, urine cytology, sputum cytology) so that endoscopy may be required to ascertain the site of a pre-invasive or early invasive cancer which may be inapparent clinically or radiologically. Another disadvantage is that invasive cancer cannot always be distinguished from pre-invasive disease and tumour type cannot always be predicted. Biopsy will also be required in cases where there is any doubt about the nature of the malignant lesion.

30.4.4   Accuracy of cytopathology

The presence of neoplastic cells can be diagnosed with a high degree of accuracy by cytopathologists and cytotechnologists who make an effort to build up their experience by careful scrutiny of a wide range of cytological samples and by comparative analysis of histopathological and cytopathological material.

The accuracy of a cytopathological diagnosis depends on several factors besides the interpretative skill of the cytopathologist. As cytopathology is essentially a 'sampling' technique, the accuracy of diagnosis will depend on the quantity and quality of the sample. It follows therefore that the larger the sample of cells available for analysis, the greater the chances of making an accurate diagnosis. This, of course, only holds true if the sample is appropriate to the area under investigation. For example, a sample composed mainly of saliva would be inappropriate for the investigation of a patient suspected of having carcinoma of the lung. A good quality sample in such an instance would be a deep cough sample of sputum.

To ensure accurate diagnosis, collection methods must be designed to ensure that the sample taken from the tissue or organ under investigation is as large as possible; and preparatory techniques must be modified to ensure that as many cells as possible are displayed for light microscopic examination. A range of instruments, e.g. spatulae, brushes, and aspirators, have been developed to optimize specimen collection and many preparatory techniques involve cell concentration by centrifugation, membrane filtration, or the use of mucolytic agents. It is often advantageous to eliminate red blood cells from a heavily bloodstained sample by gradient separation techniques as the RBCs may obscure the cells of interest.

Accuracy of cytodiagnosis can be assessed in terms of its sensitivity and specificity and the predictive value of a report. These vary from laboratory to laboratory, depending upon collection methods, preparatory technique, and diagnostic skill of the cytopathologists. In experienced hands the specificity of cytodiagnosis is very high (99 per cent) and a confirmatory biopsy is rarely indicated in those patients with clinical or radiological evidence suggestive of malignant disease. Similarly, clinicians should be advised to investigate fully those patients for whom a confident cytodiagnosis of malignancy has been given in the absence of clinically or radiologically obvious disease. On the other hand, the sensitivity of the technique can vary considerably (70–85 per cent) and a negative cytodiagnosis in the presence of clinical symptoms or signs suggestive of malignant disease should be ignored. In a laboratory where sensitivity is low it can often be improved by repeated sampling and review of methods of specimen collection and preparatory techniques.

30.4.5   The Papanicolaou smear

The alcohol-fixed Papanicolaou-stained smear is the trademark of modern cytotechnology. This elegant stain reveals details of cytoplasmic and nuclear structure that are inapparent in a formalin-fixed, paraffin-embedded section and is particularly appropriate for the evaluation of epithelial cells. The key to satisfactory staining with the Papanicolaou stain is rapid fixation of the smear. The smear must not be allowed to air-dry as this impairs the quality of the stain and renders the smear unsuitable for analysis. Of course, most of the staining techniques used for histopathological diagnosis can be applied to cytological samples and should be used freely where clinically indicated: for example, periodic acid–Schiff stain should be used routinely for the distinction between mesothelial cells and adenocarcinoma in effusions, and leucocyte common antigen is a useful marker when there is a problem of discriminating between poorly differentiated carcinoma and lymphoma. The use of May–Grunwald Giemsa stain has a particular advantage in those samples where analysis of the non-epithelial element is significant, e.g. serous effusions, cerebrospinal fluid; or where

the smears are thin and devoid of mucus so that air drying cannot be avoided—fine-needle aspirates and touch biopsies. Electron microscopic techniques and immunocytochemical techniques (Section 30.2) can be applied to cytological samples with minor modifications.

30.4.6   Principles of reporting

It is not always appreciated that the preparation of a cytopathology report requires just as much care as the preparation of a histopathology report. The report should be written in narrative form and classification systems such as that described by Papanicolaou (Papanicolaou 1954) should be avoided as they are open to misinterpretation. The report should answer the following questions:

1. Is the sample adequate for a reliable diagnosis to be made? Are there sufficient cells in the sample? Is there evidence that the tissue or organ under investigation has been properly sampled—the presence of alveolar macrophages in a sputum sample, or the presence of endocervical cells in a cervical smear?

2. Are there abnormal cells present? If so what type of neoplastic lesion is suspected?

3. Are there other features of the sample which indicate the presence of some other pathological process, e.g. *Trichomonas vaginalis* infection in cervical smears, asbestos bodies in sputum?

4. Can useful advice on further investigation or management of the patient be given to the clinician on the basis of the cytological findings? For example, if the cytopathologist is uncertain of tumour type this should be clearly stated and a biopsy requested.

In the majority of cases, a cytopathology report of 'No evidence of malignancy' or 'Malignant cells seen' can be given with confidence. There will, however always be a few cases where a confident diagnosis cannot be given and this should be made clear in the report. Such cases should be few and far between. Two types of sample fall into this category:

1. those cases where the number of cells in the sample are scanty or not representative of the organ or tissue being sampled (unsatisfactory smears); and

2. those cases where only a few atypical cells (borderline changes) are present in the smear and the cytopathologist is suspicious but not confident of malignancy.

The number of cases that fall into these two categories must not exceed 10 per cent of the workload, otherwise the cytopathology service becomes valueless to the clinician.

The principles of reporting cervical smears provide the basis for a document prepared by the British Society of Clinical Cytology on *Terminology in gynaecological cytopathology*, and the reader is referred to this document for further information on the subject (Evans *et al.* 1986).

30.4.7 Cytopathology in clinical practice

Cytopathology has many uses in clinical practice and these are discussed below.

1. *Screening of well women for precancerous changes in the cervix.* Cytology has a major role to play in the prevention of cervical cancer and as such the cytopathologist becomes involved in a programme of community care beyond the boundaries of the pathology laboratory. This is a relatively new role for the pathologist and unless he or she is equipped to participate in the planning and implementation of the screening service at every stage, the effectiveness of the screening programme suffers. The principles of screening strategy are described in the section on cervical cytopathology.

2. *Diagnosis of the patient with symptoms and signs suggestive of malignant disease.* This is the main role of cytological investigation in a hospital setting, and the laboratory can expect to receive specimens from almost every hospital department. For example, sputum samples and bronchial aspirates will be sent from patients attending the chest clinic and urine samples are the predominant specimen received from genitourinary clinics. Rapid diagnosis can be offered to patients attending dermatology clinics or breast clinics as analysis of skin scrapes or fine-needle aspiration samples takes a matter of minutes. Serous effusions and endoscopy samples also form a major part of the workload of hospital cytopathology laboratories. Sputum cytology, urine cytology, and the cytology of serous fluids are discussed in this section. Fine-needle aspiration cytology is discussed in Section 30.5.

3. *Evaluation of response to treatment.* Cytological investigation after tumour excision, radiotherapy, or cytotoxic drug therapy will indicate whether the tumour has been completely excised or eliminated.

4. *Long-term follow up of treated patients.* Regular cytological investigation will detect recurrence of a lesion at the earliest stages or metastatic spread of the disease.

5. *Selective screening of high-risk individuals.* Workers in the rubber and dye industry exposed to chemical carcinogens and women receiving hormone replacement therapy are screened at regular intervals for evidence of disease.

6. *Diagnosis of specific non-malignant diseases.* Pneumocystis carinii in bronchial lavage samples, herpes simplex in cervical smears, and inappropriate hormone secretion are examples of non-malignant disease which can be diagnosed by cytopathology.

30.4.8 Cervical cytopathology

The majority of specimens submitted for cytopathological investigation in most pathology departments offering a cytodiagnostic service are cervical smears taken from well women as part of national programmes for the prevention of cervical cancer. The concept of screening for pre-invasive lesions in the cervix stems from the work of Dr George Papanicolaou over 50 years ago (Carmichael 1973). He was the first to describe the various types of cells seen in smears prepared from the healthy and diseased cervix and he also developed a nomenclature to describe the cell types, which is in use today. The classification of the epithelial cells in the smear depends on careful examination of nuclear structure and the quality of the cytoplasm as well as observation of the nuclear cytoplasmic ratio. The appearance of the cytoplasm seen with the Papanicolaou stain can be of value in deciding whether a cell is of glandular or squamous origin.

Specimen collection: the cervical scrape

The collection of the cell sample and the preparation of the cervical smear is not usually in the hands of the cytopathologist. However, it is essential for him or her to be familiar with the techniques of sampling so that advice can be given in the event of the sample being improperly taken.

Detection of neoplastic lesions in the uterine cervix depends on adequate sampling of the cervical epithelial cells in the transformation zone as it is at this site that the pre-malignant changes occur. This can be achieved most efficiently by scraping the cervix at the site of the squamo-columnar junction with a wooden or plastic spatula. The ideal spatula should have a pointed end which can be inserted into the narrow endocervical canal of a nulliparous woman and a rounded end so that the patulous os of a multiparous female can be sampled. There are many spatula designs to choose from (Fig. 30.24) but those which have been most widely tested are the Ayre spatula and the Aylesbury spatula. An excellent account of the technique of sampling is contained in a booklet published by the British Society for Clinical Cytology (1989).

The cervix must be clearly visualized and the spatula inserted into the cervical os and rotated through 360°. The cervical mucus and cells adhering to the spatula are spread across a glass microscope slide which has been previously labelled with the patient's name in pencil or diamond pen (Fig. 30.25). The slide must be fixed immediately by immersion in 95 per cent ethanol, and left in fixative for a minimum of 30 min, after

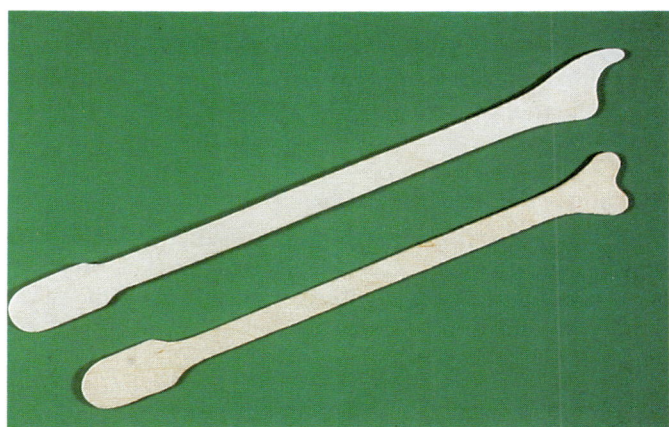

Fig. 30.24 Cervical spatulae. The Ayre spatula (top) and the Aylesbury spatula (bottom) have been most thoroughly tested and are most widely used.

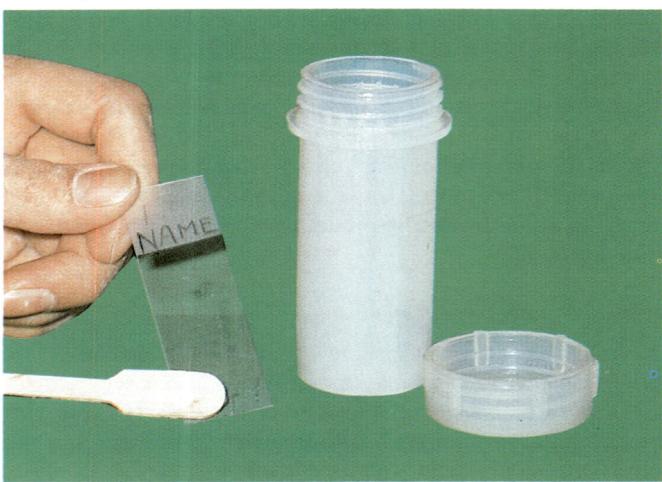

Fig. 30.25 Preparation of a cervical smear. The cervical sample is spread across a glass microscope slide and fixed immediately in alcohol.

which it may be safely removed and stored dry at room temperature. Spray fixatives or carbowax fixatives may be used as an alternative to ethanol fixation. On no account should the smear be allowed to dry before fixation as this impairs the staining quality.

Other methods of sampling the cervix

Cytological examination of material aspirated from the posterior vaginal fornix will reveal cells exfoliated from the portio vaginalis of the cervix and endocervical canal. Abnormal cells from an area of neoplasia in the cervix or uterine cavity can also be detected in these samples. However, several studies have shown that aspiration of the posterior fornix is a less sensitive method of detecting pre-invasive and invasive cervical cancer than the cervical scrape, and this method should be reserved for those cases where the cervix cannot be visualized.

Another method of sampling the cervix involves the use of the endocervical brush. This is particularly appropriate in those cases where the squamo-columnar junction is high in the endocervical canal or the cervix is stenosed. The former is most likely to occur in post-menopausal women, while the latter may be a complication of cone biopsy. It should be remembered that a scrape of the ectocervix should be taken at the same time.

The components of a cervical smear

A cervical smear taken with an Ayre spatula contains cells forcibly detached from the cervical mucosa as well as exfoliated cells trapped in the cervical mucus. The contents of the smear can be conveniently categorized as follows:

1. epithelial cells derived from the surface layers of the original squamous epithelium of the cervix and vagina;
2. columnar epithelial cells from the endocervical canal;
3. metaplastic cells from the transformation zone;
4. cells from the endometrial lining and stroma;

5. leucocytes and erythrocytes;
6. commonsal organisms;
7. mucous strands;
8. contaminants, e.g. spermatozoa.

Cells shed from the original (native) squamous epithelium

Three types of squamous cell can be recognized in cervical smears. According to convention they are designated superficial cells, intermediate cells, and parabasal cells. The three different cell types reflect the response of the epithelium to ovarian hormones at the time the smear was taken.

Superficial cells These appear as large polygonal squames with transparent cytoplasm and angular borders measuring 40–50 μm in diameter (Fig. 30.26). They are shed from the surface of fully mature squamous epithelium and are usually found in large sheets and stain a delicate pink colour with the Papanicoloau stain. They have a single pyknotic nucleus 5 μm or less in diameter. Karyorrhexis is sometimes seen.

Intermediate cells These are shed from the surface of squamous epithelium which is showing a diminished response to oestrogen or the effect of progesterone. These squames are only slightly smaller than superficial cells but can be recognized by the fact that the cytoplasmic borders may be slightly rounded and the nucleus is larger and has a vesicular structure (Fig. 30.27). They usually assume an azure hue with the Papanicolaou stain, but this is not an invariable finding. In pregnancy, intermediate cells assume an elliptical, boat-shaped appearance and are often described as *navicular cells* (Fig. 30.28). The cytoplasmic borders appear to be thickened and the nucleus eccentrically placed. Electron microscopy reveals that the cytoplasm contains abundant glycogen granules, which may account for the change in shape.

Parabasal cells These are small, rounded cells approximately 15–30 μm in diameter with cyanophilic cytoplasm and a centrally placed nucleus occupying one-third of the volume of the

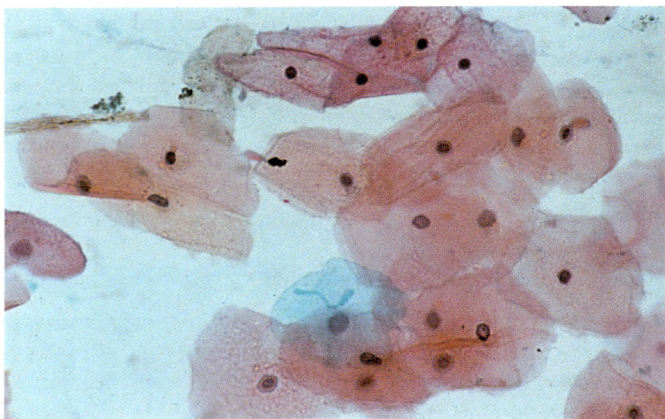

Fig. 30.26 Superficial squamous cells in a cervical smear. The scrape was taken mid-cycle. (Papanicolaou stain.) All samples shown in Figs 30.27–95 are stained with Papanicolaou stain unless otherwise stated.

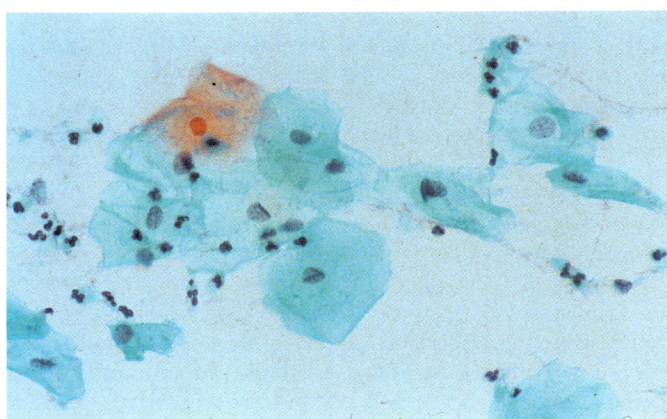

Fig. 30.27 Intermediate squamous cells in a cervical smear taken on the eighth day of the cycle.

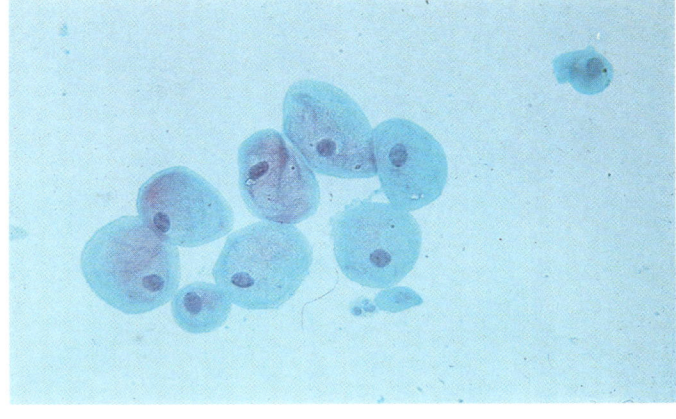

Fig. 30.29 Parabasal cells in a cervical smear. Note the rounded appearance, indicating that they have been shed spontaneously.

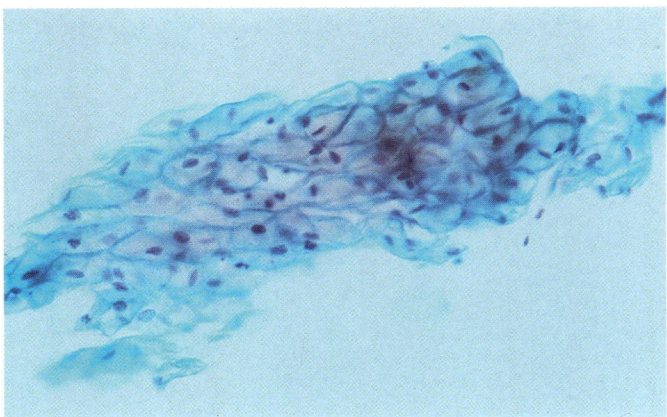

Fig. 30.28 Navicular cells in a cervical smear. Note the thickened cellular borders and eccentric nucleus.

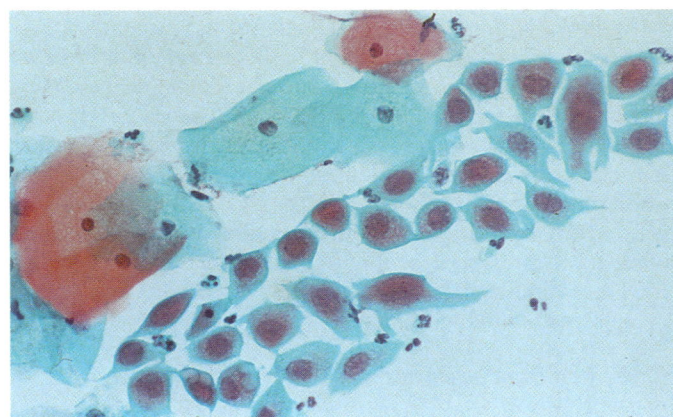

Fig. 30.30 Parabasal cells in a cervical smear. Note the cytoplasmic processes, indicating that they have been forcibly detached. Superficial cells and intermediate cells are also present in this field, indicating that this specimen has been taken from the transitional zone.

cell (Fig. 30.29). The cells may be found singly or in sheets. Single cells appear rounded if they have been exfoliated (Fig. 30.29). If they have been forcibly detached by the spatula they may have long cytoplasmic processes (Fig. 30.30). The cytoplasm is particularly fragile and may fragment so that sometimes only the free nuclei are seen.

Parabasal cells are found in smears taken from pre-pubertal and post-menopausal women, as well as smears taken from an area of immature metaplasia. Although the morphology of the parabasal cells in the smear is very similar, the overall smear patterns differ considerably. Smears taken from an atrophic cervix present a uniform appearance, as they will be composed entirely of parabasal cells (Fig. 30.31). The number of parabasal cells in the smear is often scanty and leucocytes abundant, reflecting a senile vaginitis. Mucous strands may be seen. In contrast, smears from an area of immature metaplasia will contain mature squames as well as parabasal cells, reflecting the patchy nature of metaplastic change in the transformation zone (Figs 30.30 and 30.32).

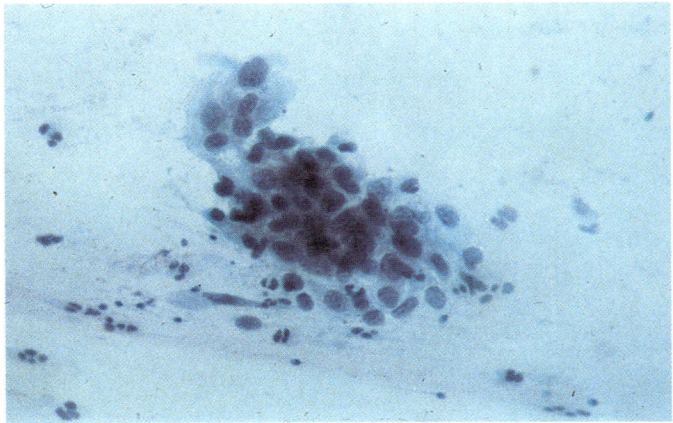

Fig. 30.31 Parabasal cells in a post-menopausal smear. Note the monomorphic pattern.

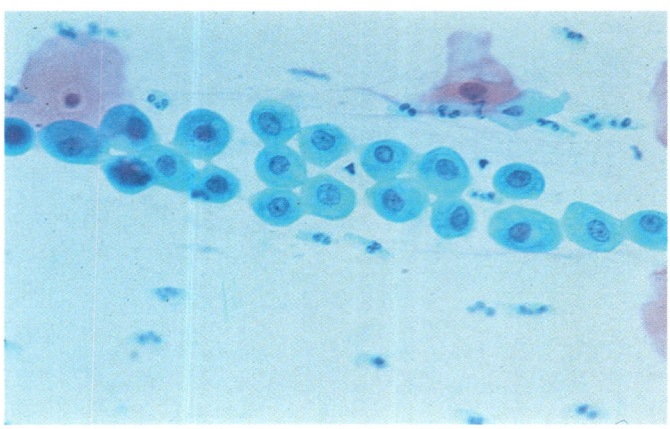

Fig. 30.32 Mature squamous cells and parabasal cells in a cervical smear taken from an area of immature metaplastic epithelium at transformation zone.

Cells shed from the endocervical canal

Endocervical cells appear singly or in sheets. Individual cells can be readily recognized by their columnar shape, delicate vacuolated cytoplasm, and basal nucleus. Cilia are rarely seen. Single cells seen 'en face' may be difficult to distinguish from parabasal cells. Sheets of columnar cells may appear in palisade or present a honeycomb appearance (Fig. 30.33). Endocervical cells which have been exfoliated into the cervical mucus are often poorly preserved, so that the outline of the cytoplasm and nucleus is indistinct. Occasionally free nuclei and fragments of cytoplasm are all that remain.

Cells shed from other parts of the genital tract

Cells of endometrial origin may be trapped in the cervical mucous plug and appear in cervical smears. They are frequently seen in smears taken at the time of menstruation and are also found in smears from women fitted with an intrauterine contraceptive device. Exfoliated endometrial cells can be distinguished from endocervical cells by their size (they are rarely larger than

20 μm) and by the structure of their nucleus which contains both coarse and fine chromatin granules (Fig. 30.34). They are often poorly preserved and characteristically appear in rounded, berry-like clusters (Fig. 30.35) or as a dense core of stromal cells surrounded by an outer rim of glandular cells.

Commensal organisms

A variety of organisms is present in the vagina in the absence of disease. They include lactobacilli (Doderlein bacilli), streptococci, staphylococci, micrococci, *Gardnerella vaginalis*, *Neisseria*, *Pseudomonas*, *Mycoplasma*, *Leptothrix*, and *Candida* species. Apart from the Doderlein bacilli and *Leptothrix*, the bacteria cannot be reliably identified with the Papanicolaou stain. Doderlein bacilli appear as pale-blue-staining rods, 1–2 μm in length (Fig. 30.36). They are particularly abundant in the genital tract during the secretory phase of the menstrual cycle and in pregnancy, at which time they metabolize the glycogen in the intermediate cells, destroying the cytoplasm of the cells in the process. Thus smears taken at these times will contain many broken cells and have a characteristic cytolytic pattern.

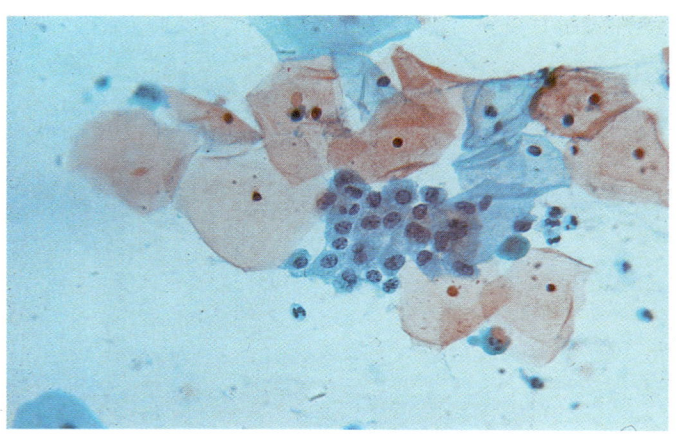

Fig. 30.34 Discrete endometrial cells in a cervical smear.

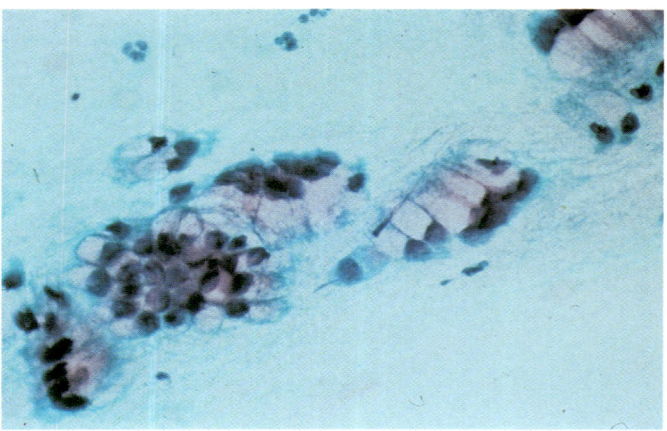

Fig. 30.33 Endocervical cells in a cervical smear. Note the honeycomb pattern.

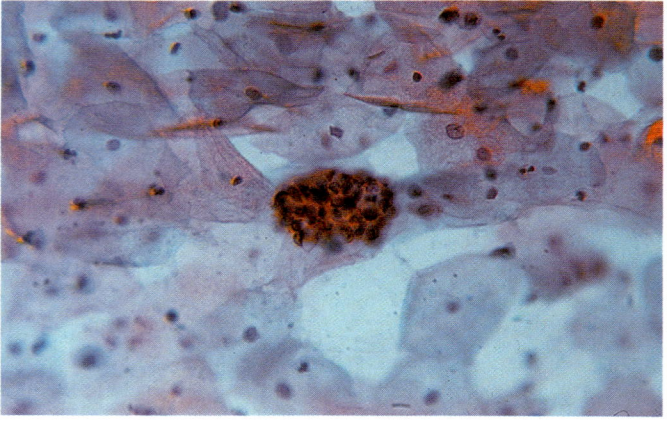

Fig. 30.35 Berry-like cluster of endometrial cells in a cervical smear.

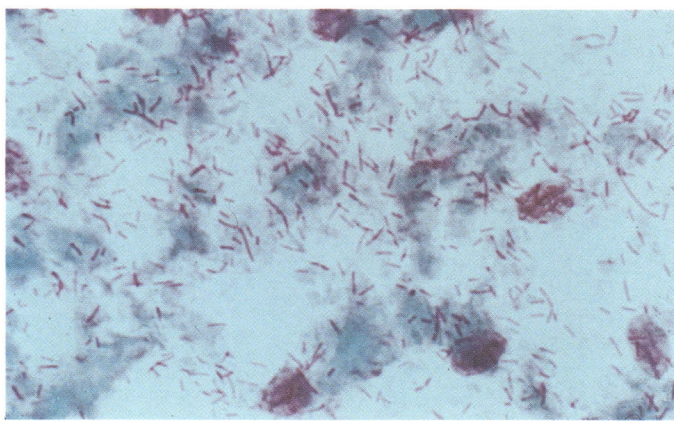

Fig. 30.36 Doderlein bacilli in a cervical smear taken during the secretory phase of the menstrual cycle. Note the marked cytolysis.

Other components of the smear

Some leucocytes and erythrocytes are present in almost every smear. The leucocytes are present in cervical mucous and reflect the response of the cervix to local trauma. In acute cervicitis, they may be so abundant as to render the smear unsuitable for a reliable cytological assessment. Heavily blood-stained smears taken during menstruation also fall into this category. Post-coital smears may contain numerous spermatozoa (Fig. 30.37) or seminiferous cells which may be mistaken for malignant cells. Mucin strands are transparent with the Papanicoloau stain and rarely interfere with the interpretation of the smear. However, in atrophic smears, mucus may form into dense inspissated basophilic masses which may be mistaken for malignant nuclei. Their amorphous structure should permit a correct diagnosis to be made.

Histiocytes are a common finding in smears taken at the time of menstrual flow and can be recognized by their rounded, oval, or reniform nuclei, and delicate vacuolated cytoplasm. They are particularly abundant immediately after the menopause and appear as a dense sheet of cells with foamy cytoplasm. This

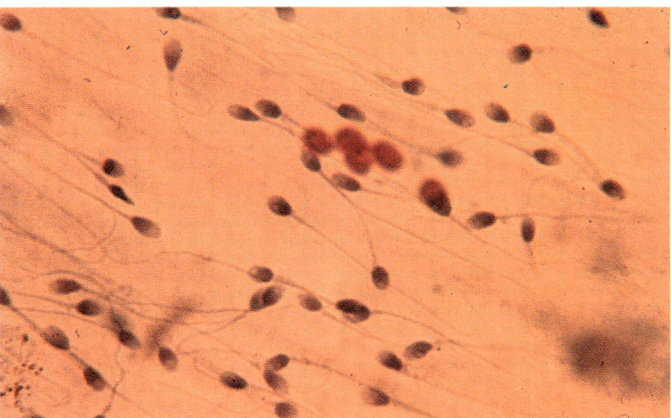

Fig. 30.37 Post-coital smear contains numerous spermatozoa.

cytological pattern was designated 'the exodus' by Papanicolaou.

Factors influencing the cell content of smears

The types of epithelial cells found in cervical smears taken by an experienced clinician in the absence of local disease are determined by two factors:

1. the hormonal status of the woman at the time the smear is taken; and

2. the position of the squamo-columnar junction.

Effect of hormonal status As mentioned in Chapter 21 the squamous epithelium of the cervix and vagina is sensitive to ovarian hormones and responds to oestrogen by becoming thicker and by maturation of the surface cells. Thus a smear taken mid-cycle will contain the large flat, mature squames designated by Papanicolaou as superficial cells. As oestrogen levels decline, intermediate cells predominate. In the secretory phase and in pregnancy a progesterone effect is seen and navicular cells may be found. Doderlein bacilli proliferate, causing extensive cytolysis. In the absence of hormones in the pre-pubertal female, or the postpartum or post-menopausal woman, the epithelium of the cervix is atrophic and the smear is composed of scanty parabasal cells (see Fig. 30.31). An intermediate pattern is usually found in smears from women on oral contraceptive therapy.

Location of the squamo-columnar junction Fundamental research has shown that pre-invasive and invasive cervical cancer arise in the transformation zone (TZ), hence the importance of sampling this area. The cytopathologist may infer that this area has been adequately sampled if endocervical cells and/or immature metaplastic cells, together with more mature squamous cells, are present in the smear (see Figs 30.30, 30.32). The TZ is most readily sampled when it is at the external os. The squamo-columnar junction may be high in the endocervical canal in post-menopausal women and an endocervical brush specimen may improve sampling in these cases.

Inflammation, infection, and repair

Acute cervicitis is usually associated with an inflammatory exudate. Bacterial culture may reveal the presence of pathogenic streptococci or staphylococci or *Neisseria gonorrhoea*. Coliform bacilli and *Gardnerella vaginalis* may also be isolated. Alternatively the cervicitis may be due to fungal or viral infection.

The presence of acute inflammation in the cervix is reflected in the smear by the presence of polymorphs which may be so numerous that they obscure any other elements in the smear. Bacteria may be seen in the background of the smear, although the individual bacterial species cannot be reliably identified by the Papanicolaou stain (Fig. 30.38). Acute cervicitis is also associated with degenerative changes in the cytoplasm and nucleus of the epithelial cells in the smear. Degenerative cytoplasmic changes include vacuolation, fragmentation, phagocytosis of polymorphs or red blood cells. Variation in the staining reaction of the cytoplasm is also seen (Fig. 30.39).

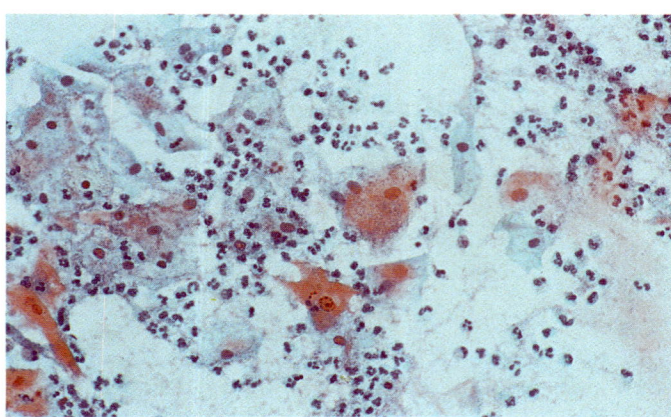

Fig. 30.38 Acute cervicitis. There is a heavy bacterial background and many polymorphs are present in the smear.

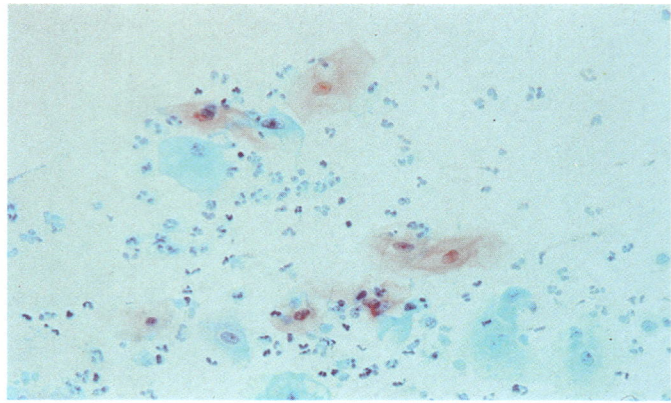

Fig. 30.39 Acute cervicitis. Note the degenerative changes in the cytoplasm of the epithelial cells. Numerous polymorphs are also present.

Degenerative nuclear changes include swelling of the nucleus and loss of chromatin structure, pyknosis, karyorrhexis, intra-nuclear vacuolation, irregularity of nuclear outline, and thickening of the nuclear membrane (Fig. 30.40). These changes are most likely to be seen in endocervical cells and metaplastic cells as these are the cells which are most vulnerable to the destructive effects of bacterial toxins. Shrinkage of the nucleus may result in the formation of perinuclear haloes. The degenerative changes seen in cervical smears in acute cervicitis are much more marked than those seen in histological section—possibly a reflection of the superior fixation of the nucleus and cytoplasm achieved with ethanol compared with formalin.

In smears from those cervices where infection is indolent and long standing (chronic cervicitis), lymphocytes and macrophages (and multinucleate giant cells) may be found in significant numbers among the polymorphs. Thus the distinction between acute and chronic cervicitis from the appearance of a cervical smear is arbitrary. However, chronic cervicitis is often associated with hyperkeratosis, parakeratosis, and squamous metaplasia and these changes may well be reflected in the smear (Fig. 30.41).

Certain specific infections produce a smear pattern which can be diagnostic for the organism involved. Specific infections that can be readily recognized include those due to *Candida* species, *Trichomonas vaginalis*, actinomycosis, herpes simplex, and wart virus infection. Senile vaginitis and follicular cervicitis also produce a characteristic smear pattern and these are described in the following paragraphs. The validity of a cytodiagnosis of *Chlamydia trachomatis* and *Gardnerella vaginalis* is discussed briefly for completeness.

Trichomas vaginalis *Trichomonas* infection of the vagina is very common. It has been estimated that it can be demonstrated in 20 per cent of women. Infection may be asymptomatic, but is more usually associated with vaginal discharge. Examination of the smear will reveal the presence of trichomonads which appear in Papanicolaou-stained smears as pyriform, slate-grey bodies with an ill-defined elliptical nucleus (Fig. 30.42). They

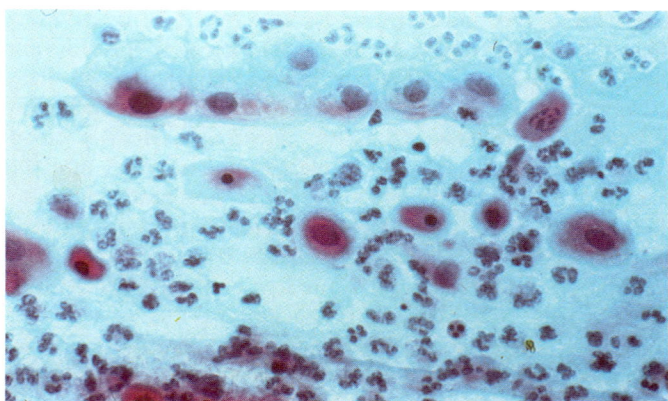

Fig. 30.40 Acute cervitis. Note the degenerative changes in the nuclei of the epithelial cells. Pyknosis and karyorrhexis can be seen together with numerous polymorphs.

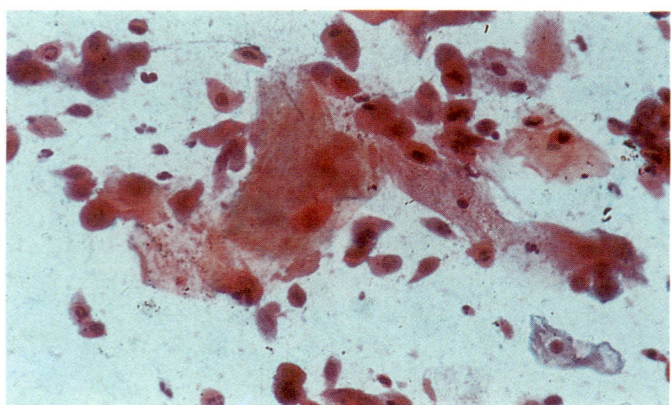

Fig. 30.41 Evidence of hyperkeratosis in a smear from a case of chronic cervicitis. Note the highly keratinized anucleate squames.

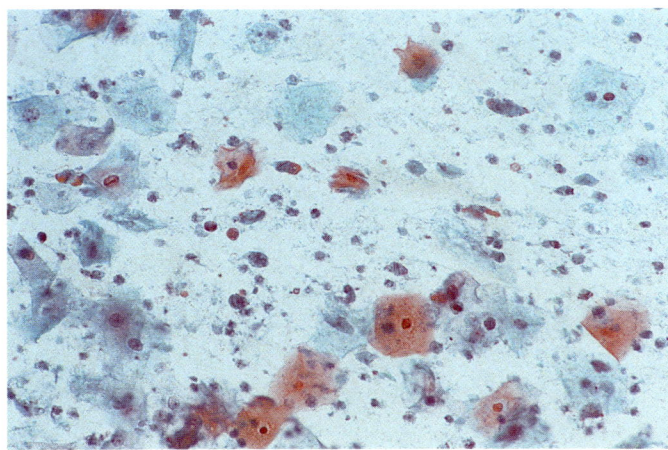

Fig. 30.42 Trichomonas vaginalis in a cervical smear. The organisms appear as pear-shaped slatey-grey bodies, 10–15 μm in diameter.

vary in size from 10 to 30 μm and pink-staining granules may be seen in the cytoplasm. The whip-like flagellae are rarely seen. The epithelial cells in the smear often assume a violet hue and develop perinuclear vacuolation.

Trichomonas infection of the vagina is occasionally associated with *Leptothrix* infection and the long filamentous strands of these bacilli may be found in the smear.

Candida albicans *Candida* infection is common in pregnancy, in women using a high-progesterone contraceptive pill, in patients taking broad-spectrum antibiotics, and in diabetic patients and patients receiving immunosuppressive therapy. The branching hyphae and tiny elliptical spores are closely applied to the cell surface and may appear bright pink with the Papanicolaou stain (Fig. 30.43). Cytolysis is a frequent feature of these smears.

Actinomyces israeli *Actinomyces* are filamentous micro-organisms that are related to bacteria. Infection is almost always associated with the presence of an intra-uterine contra-

ceptive device although it may occasionally follow surgical instrumentation or septic abortion. In the absence of trauma, progression to pelvic inflammatory disease is rare. In Papanicolaou smears the organisms can be recognized as dark, dense balls with an indistinct central core. Branched filamentous structures may be seen at the periphery of the mass (Fig. 30.44).

Herpes simplex The diagnosis of herpes genitalis can be made from a cervical smear with a high degree of accuracy. Approximately half the cases of genital infection with the herpes virus can be detected by this method. The large multinucleate cell shown in Fig. 30.45 is pathognomonic for this infection. These cells may measure up to 100 μm in diameter and are formed as a result of cell fusion induced by the virus. They contain up to 50 nuclei which show a characteristic moulding without overlapping, which helps to distinguish these cells from multinucleate foreign-body giant cells. The individual nuclei are devoid of chromatin which has been pushed to the margin of the nucleus. The marginated chromatin confers on the nucleus an empty, ballooned, ground-glass appearance. Occasionally, intranuclear inclusions may be seen which appear as large, round, centrally placed acidophilic bodies surrounded by

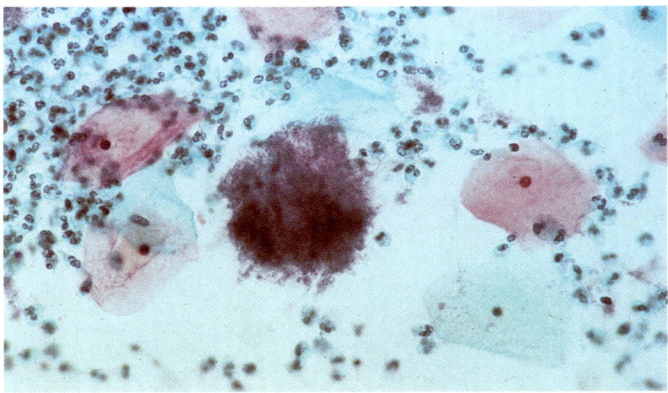

Fig. 30.44 Actinomyces-like organism in a cervical smear from a patient fitted with an intra-uterine contraceptive device.

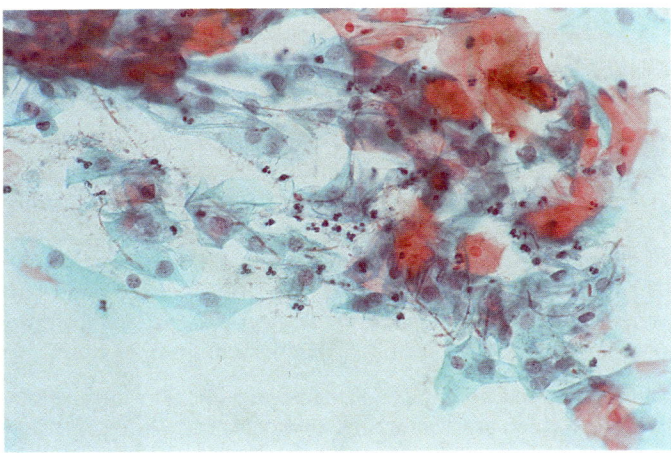

Fig. 30.43 *Candida* in a cervical smear.

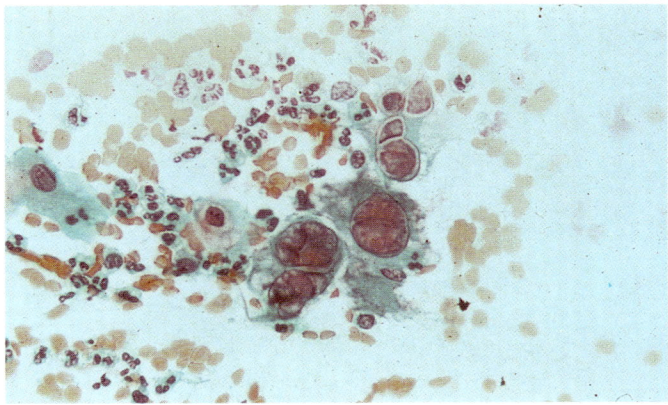

Fig. 30.45 Herpes simplex in a cervical smear. Note the multinucleate giant cells with 'ground-glass' nuclei.

a clear area or halo (Fig. 30.46). Both squamous and columnar epithelium may show these changes.

Human papilloma virus infection The presence of human papilloma virus (HPV) infection in the cervix is manifest in the cervical smear by koilocytotic atypia. Koilocytes are large squamous cells in which the nucleus is surrounded by a clear or transparent zone, bordered by a dense rim of cytoplasm (Fig. 30.47). The nucleus may be only slightly enlarged or may show changes indistinguishable from those seen in dyskaryotic cells shed from an area of cervical intra-epithelial neoplasia (CIN). The latter are thought to reflect the presence of HPV infection in an area of CIN. Other features of HPV infection in the cervical epithelium, e.g. multinucleation (Fig. 30.48), parakeratosis (Fig. 30.49), and hyperkeratosis, may also be reflected in the smear. It should be remembered that the presence of koilocytes in the cervical smear is only presumptive evidence of HPV infection. Confirmation by objective methods of diagnosis, e.g. electron microscopy, immunocytochemical staining, and *in situ* hybridization, is essential for a definitive diagnosis. Indeed, cytology is a relatively insensitive method of detecting these viruses, which can be identified by hybridization techniques in

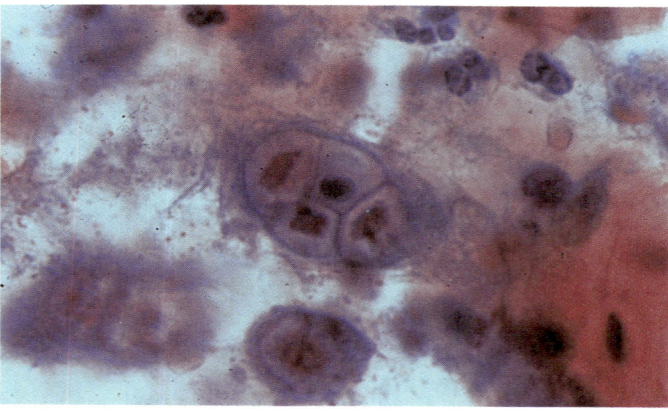

Fig. 30.46 Herpes simplex in a cervical smear. Note intranuclear (type-A) inclusions.

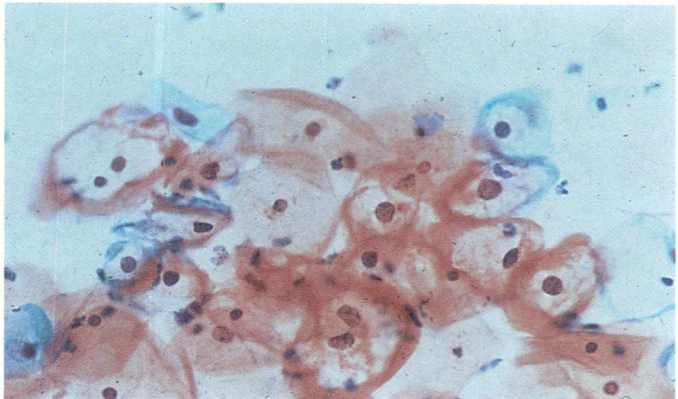

Fig. 30.47 Human papillomavirus infection. Note the koilocytes in the cervical smear.

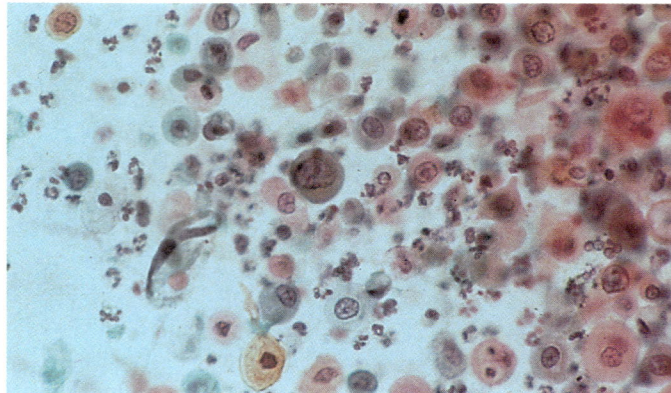

Fig. 30.48 Human papillomavirus infection. Note multinucleate cells and highly keratinized single cells typical of this infection. Koilocytes were also seen in another part of the smear.

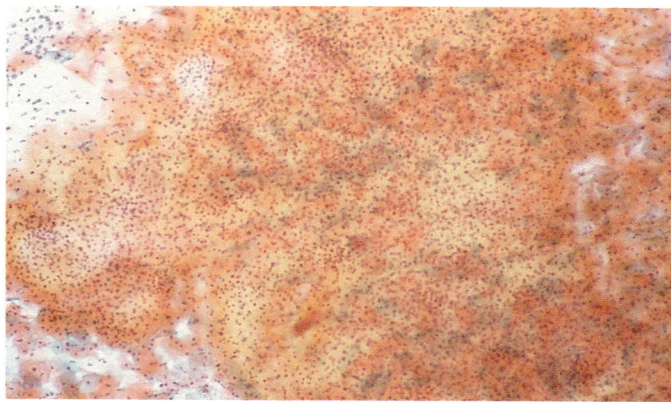

Fig. 30.49 Parakeratotic change in the cervical epithelium reflected in the smear. Note the sheets of small, highly keratinized squames with pyknotic nuclei. This pattern is frequently found in association with human papillomavirus infection.

5–40 per cent of normal and 60–80 per cent abnormal cervices. The variation in incidence of HPV detected by hybridization depends on the method of hybridization used to detect the viral DNA. The higher values have been derived from polymerase chain reaction (PCR) analysis. The 80 per cent value in the normal cervix derived from the latter may be artificially high.

Gardnerella vaginalis (syn. Haemophilus influenzae) This is a small pleomorphic coccobacillus which stains dark blue in Papanicolaou-stained smears. Infection may be suspected when large numbers of these bacteria are seen adhering to the surface of squamous cells, giving them a uniquely stippled appearance. These cells are called 'clue' cells (Fig. 30.50). Since other bacteria may produce a similar cytological pattern, confirmatory tests are advised for a definitive diagnosis of this infection.

Chlamydia trachomatis *Chlamydia* are obligate intracellular parasites which are a common cause of venereal infection. They have a complex developmental cycle which involves the formation of elementary bodies and initial bodies. There are several

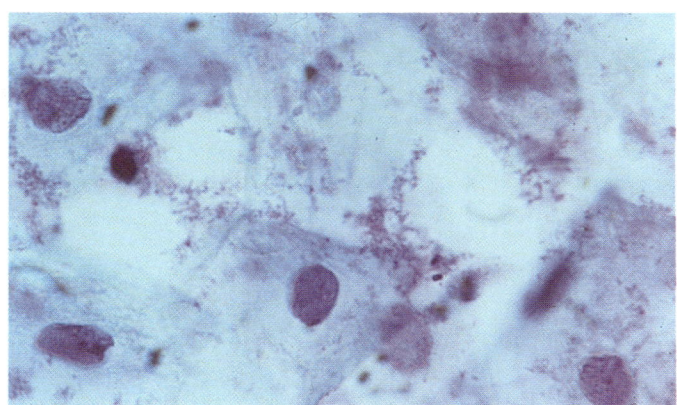

Fig. 30.50 'Clue cell' suggestive of *Gardnerella vaginalis*.

reports claiming that elementary bodies can be seen in the vacuolated cytoplasm of metaplastic cells in Papanicolaou-stained smears but recent comparative studies by the author using *Chlamydia* isolation and immunofluorescence techniques to identify the organisms indicate that cytology cannot be relied on for the accurate diagnosis of this infection.

Atrophic ('senile') vaginitis The thin, atrophic epithelium of the post-menopausal woman is particularly vulnerable to infection. This is manifest in the smear by a number of features (Fig. 30.51). Single, round parabasal cells showing remarkable variation in size and staining reaction dominate the smear. Some have abundant pale-staining cyanophilic cytoplasm and others have dense eosinophilic cytoplasm. The nuclei of the parabasal cells may be large and pale or small and irregular. Karyorrhexis and pyknosis are common and free nuclei are often seen. Leucocytes are abundant and mucous strands or blobs of densely staining basophilic mucus may be found. The bizarre changes may be mistaken for malignancy. In some instances the differential diagnosis can be extremely difficult. It has been suggested that in difficult cases local oestrogen therapy should be given and a repeat smear taken 2 or 3 days later, after which time, mature squamous cells will be seen.

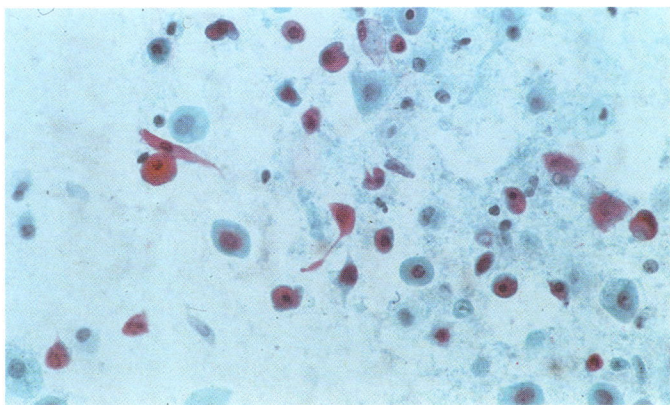

Fig. 30.51 Atrophic cervicitis manifest in the smear by numerous leucocytes and degenerative changes in the parabasal cells.

Follicular cervicitis This type of cervicitis is associated with the formation of lymphoid follicles in the cervix. During the taking of a cervical smear the fragile epithelium overlying the follicles may be scraped off and the lymphocytes released into the smear. Thus the smear will contain streaks of mature and immature lymphocytes, histiocytes, and plasma cells (Fig. 30.52). Errors of diagnosis are common in view of the relative rarity of detecting this condition in smears, and cases of follicular cervicitis are frequently misdiagnosed as endometrial cancer or CIN by the inexperienced cytopathologist. It should be remembered that lymphocytes do not form the cohesive cell sheets or cell clusters which are characterisitic of epithelial cells.

Regeneration and repair Studies of the cervix after laser therapy have shown that when an area of cervical epithelium is destroyed, the adjacent surviving epithelial cells proliferate to cover the defective surface. Similar changes occur in patients with acute ulcerating cervicitis. Thus regenerating epithelial cells often occur side by side with degenerating epithelial cells in a smear. In such cases, the smear will contain sheets of proliferating epithelial cells. They may appear undifferentiated with large nuclei and prominent nucleoli (Fig. 30.53). The chromatin pattern is regular and finely granular although several chromocentres may be found. Mitotic figures are occasionally seen.

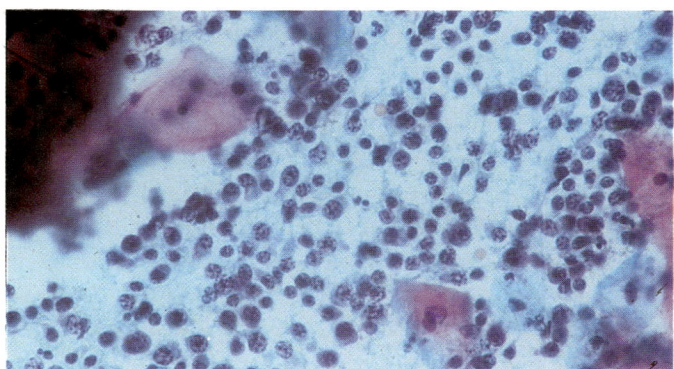

Fig. 30.52 Follicular cervicitis. Note the streaks of lymphoid cells and macrophages in the smear.

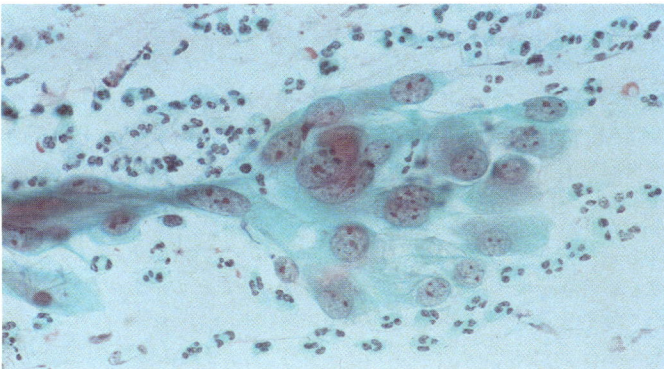

Fig. 30.53 Regenerating epithelial cells in a cervical smear. Note the prominent nucleoli and high nuclear/cytoplasmic ratio of the dividing cells.

Intra-epithelial neoplasia of the cervix

It is widely accepted that most cancers pass through a stage in which transformed cells are confined to the epithelium (intra-epithelial neoplasia) and that intra-epithelial neoplasia, if left untreated, will progress in a proportion of cases to invasive disease. Cervical screening provides an opportunity to diagnose pre-invasive disease in the cervix, thereby preventing invasive disease. The recognition of cells scraped or shed from an area of cervical intra-epithelial neoplasia is one of the most important tasks of the cytologist and one of the most difficult in view of the pleomorphism of the neoplastic cells.

Terminology

By convention, the term 'dyskariosis' (Greek, dys = abnormal; karyos = nucleus) is used to indicate the presence of abnormal epithelial cells in a cervical smear which are considered to be derived from an area of cervical intra-epithelial neoplasia (CIN). The number of dyskariotic cells in a smear is very variable—there may be many hundreds or just one or two. It should be remembered that the number of cells does not reflect the extent of the lesion.

Dyskariosis and the diagnosis of CIN

Dyskariotic cells are characterized by the following features.

1. Nuclear enlargement, hyperchromasia, and irregularity of outline. The nucleus is at least twice the size of a normal intermediate cell nucleus.

2. The chromatin content is increased and coarsely granular. Abnormal nucleoli and mitotic figures may be seen.

3. The cytoplasm may be very scanty indeed, or very abundant. Abnormal keratinization may be seen.

4. The cells are usually discrete, reflecting the loss of cohesion which is a feature of neoplastic change; or they may be present in small sheets.

Dyskariotic cells have been classified further into subgroups to enable the cytopathologist to more accurately identify the grade of the underlying neoplastic lesion. Three types of dyskariotic cells have been described—mild, moderate, and severe. In general, cells showing mild dyskariosis in a smear reflect a low-grade lesion (CIN-I); cells showing a degree of moderate dyskariosis reflect underlying CIN-II; and cells showing a severe dyskariosis reflect a high grade lesion (CIN-III).

Mild dyskariosis Cells showing mild dyskariosis have abundant cytoplasm with angular borders resembling superficial or intermediate cells (Fig. 30.54). The nucleus occupies less than half the total area of the cytoplasm. The cells may occur singly or in sheets or as highly keratinized plaques. The cells frequently show changes suggestive of human papilloma virus infection and koilocytotic atypia and multinucleation may be seen.

Moderate dyskariosis Cells showing a moderate dyskariosis are characterized by a greater degree of nuclear enlargement, so that the nucleus occupies one-half to two-thirds of the total area of the cytoplasm. The nuclei of cells showing moderate dys-

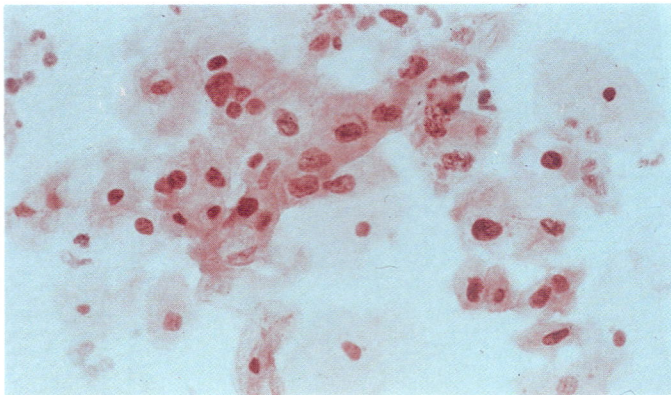

Fig. 30.54 Mild dyskariosis. Note the abundant cytoplasm. The nucleus occupies less than half the total area of the cytoplasm.

kariosis tend to show a greater degree of hyperchromasia and greater irregularity of nuclear outline than the nuclei of cells showing mild dyskariosis.

Severe dyskariosis Cells showing severe dyskariosis typically have a narrow rim of cytoplasm and a very abnormal nucleus which practically fills the cell or two-thirds of it (Fig. 30.55). Occasionally, they have the abundant cytoplasm which is characteristic of mild dyskariosis. However, the degree of dyskariosis can be determined on the basis of the large, irregular hyperchromatic nucleus.

The cytodiagnosis of invasive squamous carcinoma and adenocarcinoma of the cervix

Many of the features which are suggestive of CIN-III can also be found in smears from an area of invasive squamous carcinoma. Thus a definitive diagnosis of CIN-III cannot be made on a cervical smear report and confirmation by colposcopy and biopsy is mandatory. However, there are a number of features of a cervical smear which strongly suggest the presence of invasive

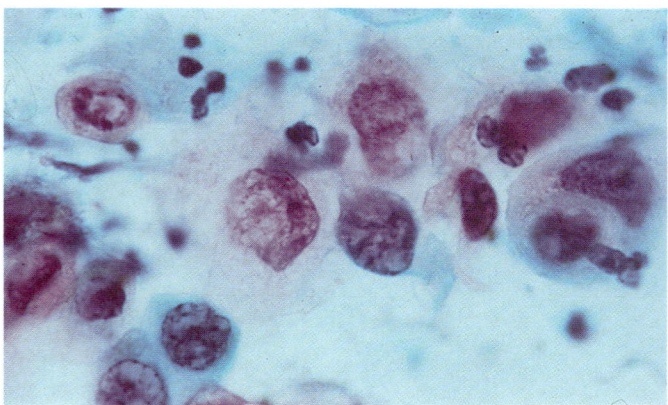

Fig. 30.55 Severe dyskariosis. Note the abundant cytoplasm, but the nucleus is greatly enlarged, irregular in outline, and has an abnormal chromatin content.

cancer rather than intra-epithelial cancer. The most striking feature is the presence of blood and polymorphs in the smear (sometimes called 'the malignant diathesis') which reflects the ulceration and infection usually associated with invasive disease. Keratinizing invasive squamous carcinoma of the cervix can be recognized by the presence of numerous highly keratinized orangeophilic squames in the smear. These may assume bizarre shapes (tadpole or fibre cells) and contain small irregular pyknotic nuclei (Fig. 30.56). Occasionally, keratinized plaques or anucleate squames or 'ghost cells' can be seen.

Primary adenocarcinoma of the cervix (or endometrial carcinoma involving the cervix) may be suspected by the presence of numerous atypical glandular epithelial cells in the smear. In a well-differentiated tumour of endocervical type the glandular cells appear remarkably uniform, although the nuclei are slightly enlarged and hyperchromatic. Rosettes and palisades may be found (Fig. 30.57). In mucin-producing lesions, the tumour cells may be discrete or in rounded clusters. The individual cells have vacuolated cytoplasm and large nucleoli.

Poorly differentiated carcinomas present cytologically as large, dense clusters of closely packed hyperchromatic nuclei (Fig. 30.58). The individual cell borders in the tissue fragments may be difficult to identify but examination of the clumps at high magnification will reveal a marked anisonucleosis and nuclear pleomorphism. It should be remembered that exfoliative cytopathology is an unreliable method for detecting advanced invasive cancers of the cervix. The erythrocytes and polymorphs in the smear may obscure any abnormal epithelial cells present, leading to a false negative report. For this reason, a clinical suspicion of cancer should always override a negative smear report.

Screening strategy

The importance attached to cervical cytopathology as a method of preventing invasive cervical cancer is reflected by the number of developed countries which offer a national or regional cervical cytology screening programme. In those countries or regions where coverage of the population has been complete (British Columbia, Iceland, Finland, Sweden, Scotland, and Holland) a significant fall in morbidity and mortality from cervical cancer has been observed. In other countries where cervical screening is offered on an *ad hoc* basis, the results of screening have been less satisfactory.

Several reasons for failure have been identified.

1. Women most at risk of cervical cancer have not been screened. These are older women (> 35 years) who have been sexually active for many years.

2. Follow-up of women with abnormal smears has not been rigorous, so that CIN lesions identified by cytology have not been treated.

3. Laboratory performance has been suboptimal due to a lack of trained staff and qualified screeners. The accuracy of reporting has also been impaired by poor standards of smear taking.

The resolution of some of these problems often, but not always, depends on an increase in resources put into the screening programme. For example, more money may need to be spent on

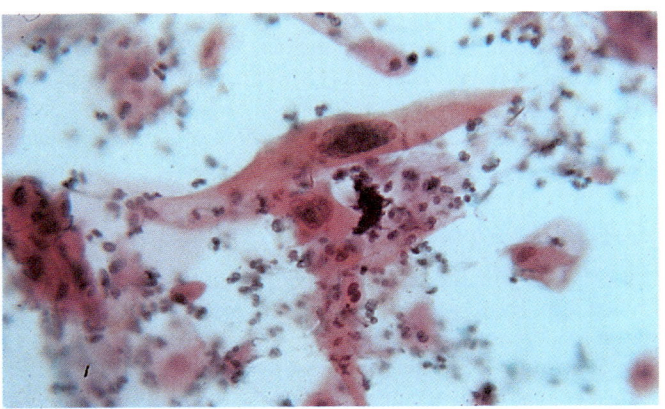

Fig. 30.56 Highly keratinized squame with abnormal nucleus suggestive of invasive squamous carcinoma. Notice the numerous red blood cells and polymorphs in the smear.

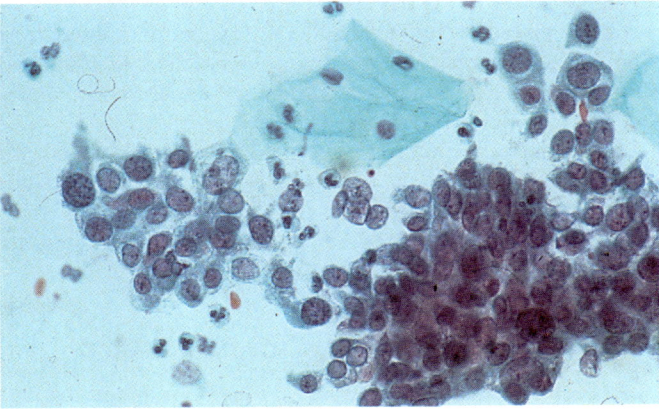

Fig. 30.57 Adenocarcinoma of the cervix. The smear contains numerous glandular epithelial cells with slightly enlarged hyperchromatic nuclei. The cells form small clusters and rosettes.

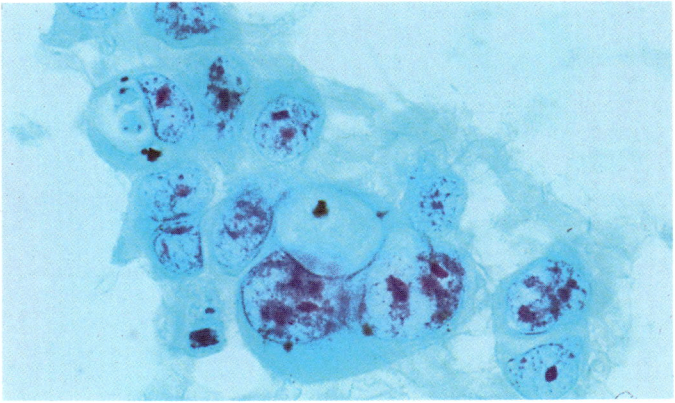

Fig. 30.58 Malignant cells from a poorly differentiated carcinoma in a cervical smear.

health education, or for salaries for cytoscreeners, or to establish a computerized record system for call and recall. In many cases, however, improvements can be effected by better use of resources already available. For example, restricting screening to high-risk groups (usually selected by age) or to women who have not had a smear within the past 5 years is a very effective way of limiting the cost of a screening programme without reducing its effectiveness.

One of the most important methods of making the cervical cancer prevention programme more effective is by improving laboratory standards and monitoring laboratory performance by a series of quality control measures. These may include obvious exercises, such as histopathological/cytopathological correlation of all cases that are referred for biopsy, or more complex exercises involving certification of laboratories on the basis of the performance of the laboratory personnel (medical and non-medical) confronted with a set of test slides. In order that these exercises are successful and the results comparable from one laboratory to another, terminology must be standardized and uniform reporting formats used.

The following reporting format has been used for many years in this laboratory in London and has been found to be very satisfactory (Table 30.4). The cytopathological findings are described and the underlying histopathological changes predicted. Thus, a normal smear predicts a normal cervix and mild dyskariosis is suggestive of an area of CIN-I in the cervix. It is not uncommon for a smear to contain mild, moderate, and severely dyskariotic cells reflecting areas of CIN-I, II, and III in the cervix. By convention, only the most severe changes are included in the report. The smear should always be interpreted in the light of the clinical data provided; otherwise errors of management may occur. For example, a well oestrogenized smear from a post-menopausal woman could be a significant

observation for the clinician as it may reflect the presence of an oestrogen-producing tumour. On the other hand, information that is irrelevant to the clinical management of the patient should not be included in the report. For example, the presence of inflammatory changes in the epithelial cells has no clinical relevance; in contrast, a note to the effect that specific infection with *Trichomonas vaginalis* is present may be most useful to the clinician in management of the patient.

Every smear report should include a statement on the quality of the specimen. A smear may be considered unsatisfactory if it contains scanty epithelial cells or if it is air-dried or heavily bloodstained. An adequate smear is defined as one which contains numerous squamous epithelial cells whose morphology is well preserved and whose structure is clearly displayed. Evidence that the smear has been taken from the transformation zone should be sought. The presence of endocervical cells or parabasal cells from an area of immature metaplasia is acceptable evidence of correct sampling procedure. However, the absence of these cell types does not necessarily mean that the smear is unsatisfactory.

Finally, many clinicians welcome a recommendation from the cytopathologist regarding the management of the patient with an abnormal smear. Guidelines for management have been set out by the British Society for Clinical Cytology (Evans *et al.* 1987). They may need updating as new information about the pathobiology of cervical cancer becomes available (especially the association with human papilloma virus infection).

30.4.9   Cytopathology of the vagina and vulva

The collection of smears from the vaginal vault is routinely advised after hysterectomy as a method of ensuring early detection of recurrence of a primary tumour. Occasionally, the presence of granulation tissue in the vault may result in fibroblasts being detected in the smear. These may be misdiagnosed as malignant cells. Similarly, the bizarre changes associated with radiotherapy may give rise to misdiagnosis unless the cytopathologist is aware of the clinical history (see Fig. 30.94).

Vaginal scrapes are recommended if information about the hormonal status of the patient is required and facilities for biochemical assay are not available. By convention the scrape should be taken from the upper two-thirds of the lateral vaginal walls. Two hormonal patterns can be recognized with confidence—an atrophic pattern and an oestrogen effect.

Vulval smears are useful for the investigation of patients with an ulcerated lesion of the vulva. Smears from benign lesions characteristically contain few cells, whereas smears from neoplastic lesions are often cellular and frequently contain abnormal highly keratinized squames.

30.4.10   Cytopathology of the corpus uteri

It has been known for many years that benign and malignant endometrial cells may be present as a coincidental finding in cervical smears taken primarily for the detection of cervical neoplasia. Benign endometrial cells (see Figs 30.34, 30.35) may be

---

Table 30.4 Cytopathological changes in cervical smears and predicted histopathology

Cytopathology report*	Predicted histopathology
Smear unsuitable for cytological assessment	
Findings essentially normal	Normal cervix; no evidence of malignancy
Borderline changes	Probably inflammatory changes not amounting to neoplasia
Mild, moderate dyskariosis, suggestive of CIN-I or II	CIN-I or II
Severe dyskariosis suggestive of CIN-III	CIN-III
Severely dyskariotic cells with features suggestive of invasive squamous carcinoma	Invasive squamous carcinoma
Abnormal glandular cells present	Endocervical adenocarcinoma; endometrial hyperplasia; or adenocarcinoma
Abnormal cells suggestive of other tumour types	Other tumour types

* Other findings of pathological significance, e.g. specific vaginal infection, endometrial cells in smears from post-menopausal women, or hormonal effects inconsistent with the clinical condition of the patient should also be described.

found in menstrual smears or in smears from women fitted with an intra-uterine contraceptive device (see Section 30.4.14 on iatrogenic changes). Endometrial carcinoma may be suspected when only a few abnormal glandular cells are found in the smear. The cells are often poorly preserved (indicating their origin from the fundus uteris) and usually have abundant vacuolated cytoplasm and large irregular nuclei (Fig. 30.59).

Although endometrial pathology can be diagnosed from a cervical smear, it should be remembered that endometrial exfoliation is capricious and the cervical smear is a most unreliable method of screening for endometrial cancer. A more reliable approach depends on direct sampling of the endometrium, and several cytological techniques have been developed which offer an alternative to curettage or Vabra suction in those cases where carcinoma of the corpus uteri is suspected on clinical grounds. These techniques have an advantage over classical curettage. They can be carried out in an out-patient setting and anaesthesia is not required; vacuum curettage, however, is now frequently performed without anaesthesia. Tissue for cytological studies can be obtained by washing out the endometrial cavity with saline (Gravlee jet wash) or abrading the endometrium (the Mi Mark or Accurette). The Isaacs endometrial sampler creates a negative pressure in the syringe so that endometrial cells from the uterine cavity are aspirated into the cannula.

Endometrial cells obtained by direct sampling differ in their appearance in the light microscope from endometrial cells shed spontaneously into the cervical canal and trapped in cervical mucus. They are better preserved so that cell morphology is clearly displayed. The cells appear in sheets rather than in rounded balls (Fig. 30.60). Tumour cells, if present, are usually abundant.

In some centres, endometrial sampling is used to monitor the response of the endometrium in women on hormone replacement therapy. Smears are taken every 3 months with a view to detecting endometrial hyperplasia at the earliest stage in its development.

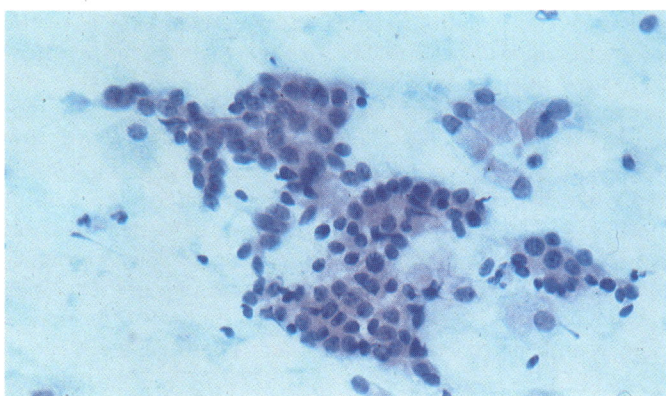

Fig. 30.60 Endometrial cells in a smear prepared from an endometrial aspirate obtained with an Isaacs aspirator.

30.4.11 Cytopathology of the respiratory tract

The value of cytology as a method of diagnosing malignant tumours of the respiratory tract has been appreciated by pathologists and clinicians for many years. The classical description of tumour cells in sputum by Dudgeon and Wrigley in 1935 did much to promote the use of sputum cytology for the investigation of patients suspected of bronchial cancer. Subsequent studies showed that a wide range of pulmonary lesions could be identified from a single sputum sample. Experience with bronchial secretions, bronchial washings, broncho-alveolar lavage, and bronchial brush samples collected through a rigid or fibre optic bronchoscope shows that these samples are also suitable for cytological studies. These techniques permit localization of the lesion (see Chapter 13), which is a major limitation of sputum cytology.

Specimen collection

Sputum

Sputum production in significant amounts is evidence of lung pathology. In the majority of cases the underlying disease process is benign but sputum cytology remains the simplest, quickest, and most cost-effective way of providing pathological evidence of lung cancer. The procedure involves no risk to the patient and can be repeated as often as necessary.

Research has shown that optimal results can be achieved if three separate samples are examined from each patient and three smears prepared from each sample. This will result in a cancer detection rate of 60–70 per cent, although the detection rate will, of course, depend on the size, location, and type of the tumour. For example, centrally located tumours will be detected more efficiently than peripheral ones; hence squamous carcinoma of the lung is more likely to be detected than adenocarcinoma. A small improvement in the detection rate can be achieved if additional specimens are examined or additional smears prepared, but the slight increase in sensitivity is out of proportion to the additional work involved in specimen preparation and analysis.

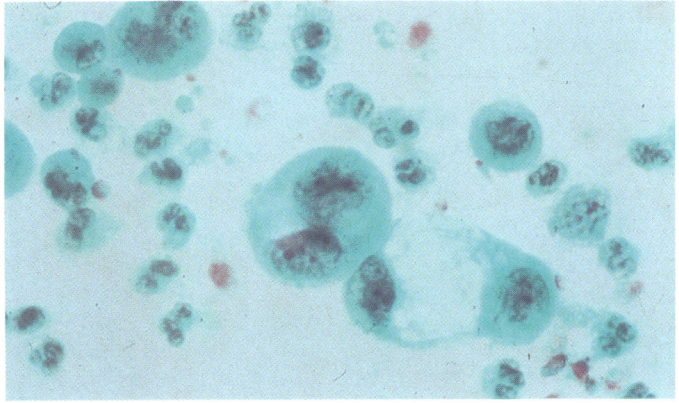

Fig. 30.59 Adenocarcinoma cells shed from an endometrial carcinoma in a cervical smear. Curettage is mandatory in such cases. Should it prove negative, carcinoma of the ovary or Fallopian tubes should be excluded.

A satisfactory sputum sample must contain cells from the lower respiratory tract and it is advisable to instruct the patient as to how this can be achieved. Sputum samples taken after physiotherapy are usually satisfactory, as are induced sputum samples following percutaneous injection of saline into the trachea. Specimens should be collected at the beginning of the day whenever possible, to avoid contamination with food or toothpaste. Heavily bloodstained samples or watery samples may require special processing in the cytopathology laboratory to optimize the chances of detecting tumour cells in the sample. Specimens should be processed within 4 hours of collection. If delay is anticipated the specimen should be stored at 4°C.

Bronchial secretions, bronchial washings, and lavage specimens

Bronchial secretions can be obtained by applying suction through a bronchoscope and collecting the aspirated mucus in a trap. Bronchial washing can be collected after a small amount of normal saline (10 ml) is instilled into the trachea and re-aspirated. Broncho-alveolar lavage was developed to facilitate the investigation of interstitial lung disease. Its use has been extended to the investigation of patients with peripherally sited lung tumours outside the field of bronchoscopic inspection. It is also used for the investigation of immunocompromised and HIV-positive patients with symptoms and signs suggestive of pulmonary infection with *Pneumocystis carinii*. Sampling is carried out by impacting the fibre-optic bronchoscope in the appropriate segmental bronchus and flushing 100 ml sterile saline through it. The saline is then aspirated into the trap. About half the sample can be recovered in this way. Specimen preparation in the cytopathology laboratory will involve concentration methods to ensure that the maximum number of cells in these samples are harvested for cytological studies.

Bronchial brush specimens

A disposable nylon brush is usually used. If reusable brushes are preferred, care must be taken to clean them thoroughly after use to avoid cross-contamination of specimens. Smears must be fixed immediately in 95 per cent ethanol before air-drying occurs, and stained by the Papanicolaou method. After the smears have been made, the brush can be washed in a small volume of normal saline to recover any remaining cells adhering to it and the saline suspension transferred to the laboratory where the cells can be harvested.

Cytopathological patterns in benign respiratory tract disease

A satisfactory sputum sample is characterized by the presence of carbon-laden macrophages (Fig. 30.61). These are large cells (30–40 μm in diameter) with round or oval nuclei and abundant foamy cytoplasm which contains variable numbers of carbon particles. The particles are brown/black in the Papanicolaou stain and range in size from fine granules to large angular masses. The macrophages may be multinucleate and their presence is evidence of the lower respiratory tract origin of the

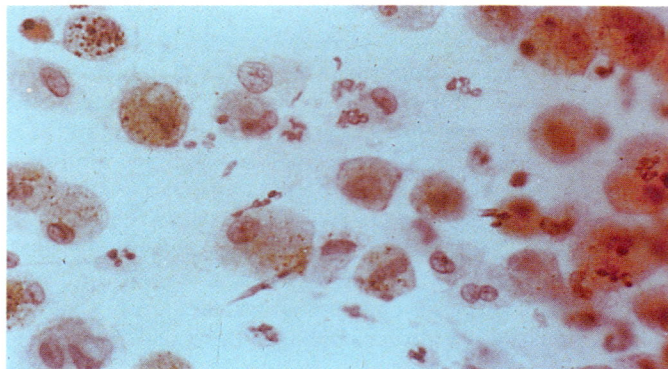

Fig. 30.61 Pulmonary macrophages in sputum. Two macrophages in top left corner contain carbon granules.

sample. A striking cytopathological pattern is seen in sputum from patients with pulmonary oedema. In these samples the macrophages are loaded with haemosiderin, and are sometimes called 'heart-failure cells'.

Sputum samples may also contain a few bronchial epithelial cells which may be ciliated or mucus secreting (Fig. 30.62). These cells may appear singly or in clumps and are recognized by their columnar or cuboidal shape and basal nuclei. Occasionally, large dense papillary clusters of bronchial epithelial cells may be seen which have been designated 'Creola bodies'. These reflect the hypertrophy of the bronchial epithelium seen in chronic bronchitis or bronchiectasis. Careful examination of the cluster will reveal a clear border of cytoplasm around the periphery of the cells, which is consistent with a benign origin for the cells (Fig. 30.63).

Squamous cells from the mouth are also present in sputum, often in considerable numbers. Polymorphs and lymphocytes are invariably present.

A proportion of samples submitted to the laboratory as sputum are composed of saliva only. They appear watery and do not contain macrophages and must be regarded as unsuitable for analysis.

Bronchial secretions, bronchial washings, and bronchial brushings are characterized by the large numbers of bronchial

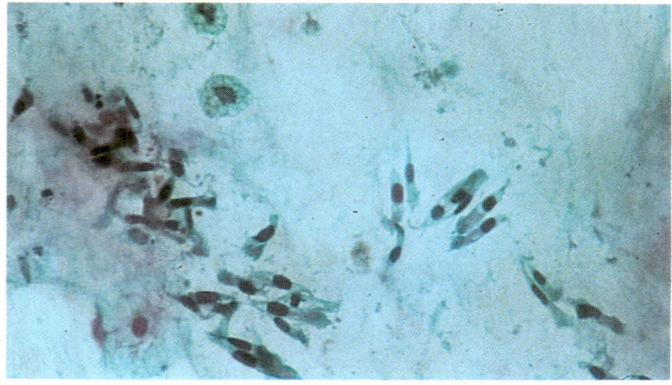

Fig. 30.62 Bronchial epithelial cells in sputum.

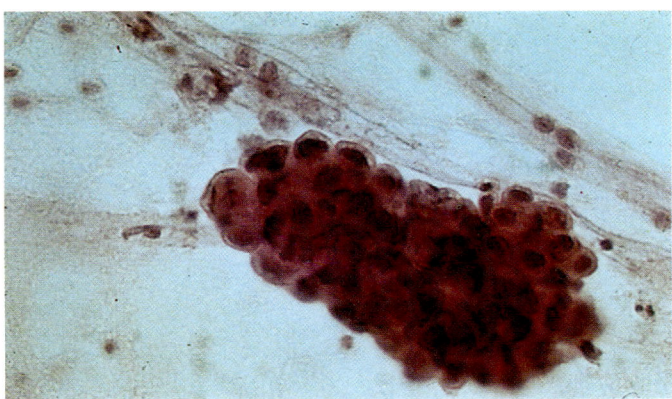

Fig. 30.63 Large papillary cluster of bronchial epithelial cells (Creola body) in sputum.

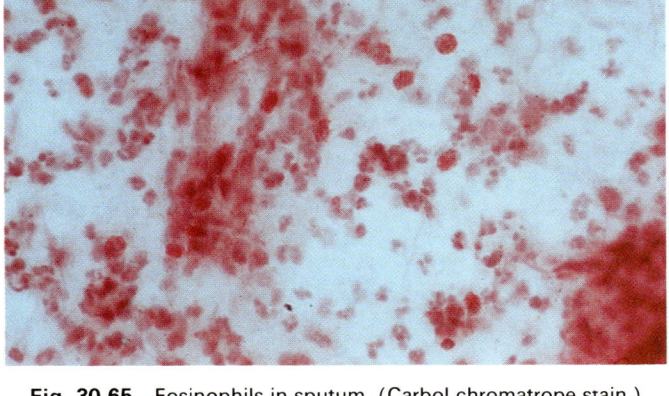

Fig. 30.65 Eosinophils in sputum. (Carbol chromatrope stain.)

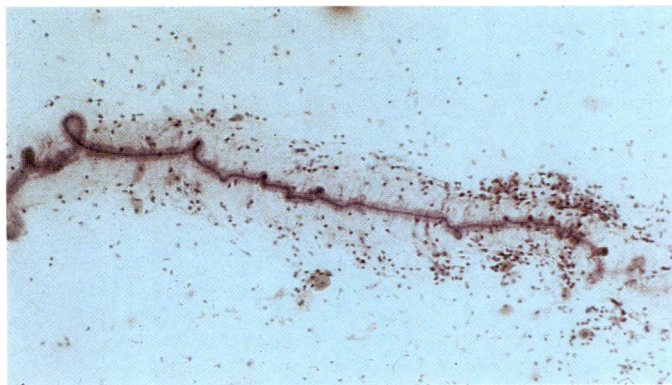

Fig. 30.64 Mucous cast of a small bronchiole in sputum (Curshmann spiral).

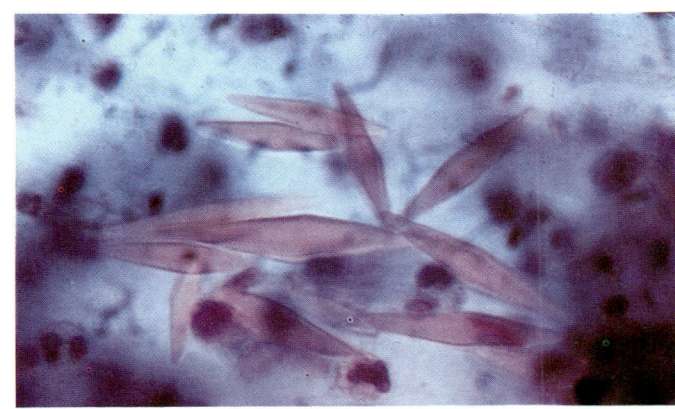

Fig. 30.66 Charcot–Leyden crystals in sputum.

epithelial cells they contain. The epithelial cells are often in a palisade or honeycomb arrangement. The nuclei of the bronchial cells may be distorted as a result of surgical manipulation of the specimen, and appear crowded and hyperchromatic and may be mistaken for anaplastic carcinoma. Careful examination will reveal that the nuclei are squashed together and do not show the moulding characteristic of carcinoma. Macrophages and polymorphs may also be found in these specimens, whereas buccal squames are rare.

The non-cellular elements of sputum are also of significance for the cytopathologist. Mucus is present in abundance in sputum, but is less prominent in lavage specimens or brushings. It generally forms an even cyanophilic background to the smear but may appear in dense strands which obscure the cells. Sputum from patients with asthma or other diseases causing chronic airway obstruction may contain mucous strands in the form of Curshmann spirals (Fig. 30.64). These represent inspissated casts of the small bronchioles. Sputum from these patients may also contain numerous eosinophils (Fig. 30.65). Other non-cellular elements of significance are asbestos bodies and Charcot–Leyden crystals derived from the eosinophil leucocytes (Fig. 30.66).

Care must be taken not to confuse contaminants, such as meat or vegetable fibres or pollen grains, with tumour cells in the sputum.

Infectious disease in immunosuppressed patients

Cytopathology has an important role to play in the diagnosis of specific infection of the respiratory tract in patients whose immune reactions are impaired by drugs or disease. These patients are susceptible to opportunistic infection with viruses, fungi, and protozoa, and cytology offers a non-invasive method of detecting these organisms. Induced sputum samples and broncho-alveolar lavage specimens are used routinely for the investigation of AIDS patients with impaired lung function, as they have proved to be particularly sensitive methods of detecting *Pneumocystis carinii* infection (Fig. 30.67). Other infections of the respiratory tract that can be diagnosed with confidence are herpes simplex (Figs 30.68, 30.69), cytomegalovirus infection, cryptococcus, *Candida albicans*, *Aspergillus fumigatus*, and *Histoplasma capsulatum*. We have also recognized the granulomatous changes of tuberculosis (Fig. 30.70) and the larval forms of *Strongyloides stercoralis* (Fig. 30.71) in sputum samples.

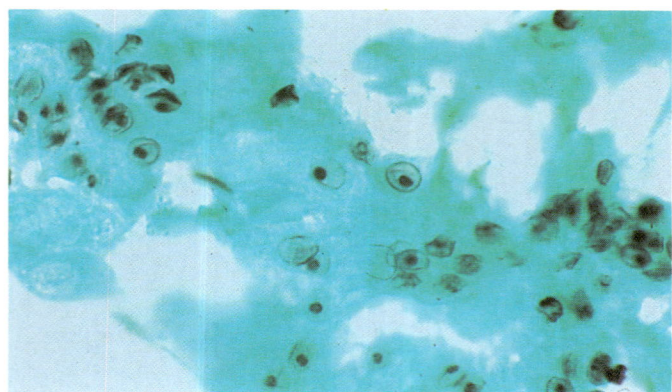

Fig. 30.67 Cysts of *Pneumocystis carinii* in sputum. (Grocott stain.)

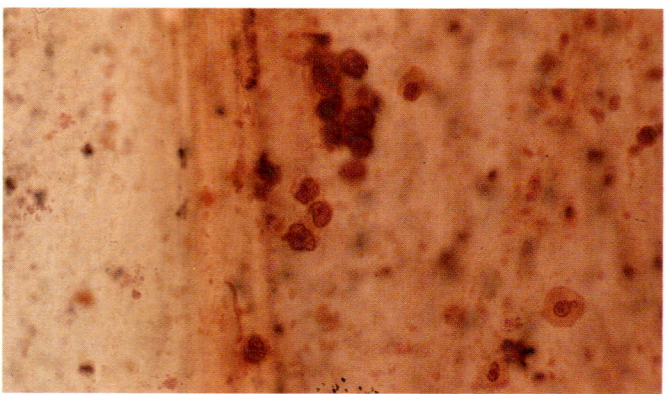

Fig. 30.70 Epithelioid cells in sputum from a case of bronchocentric granuloma.

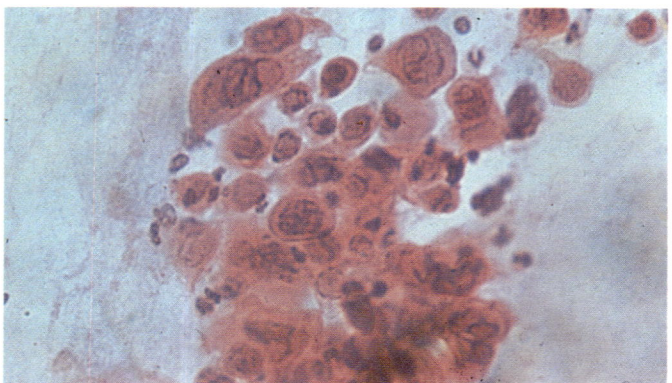

Fig. 30.68 Herpes virus-infected cells in sputum. Note the multinucleate cells with 'glassy' nuclei.

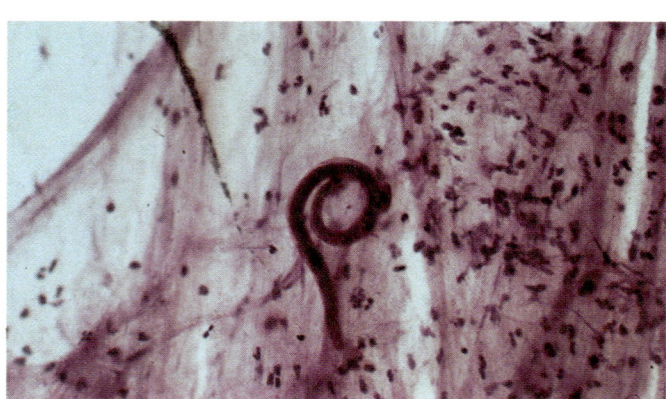

Fig. 30.71 *Strongyloides stercoralis* in sputum from an HIV-positive patient.

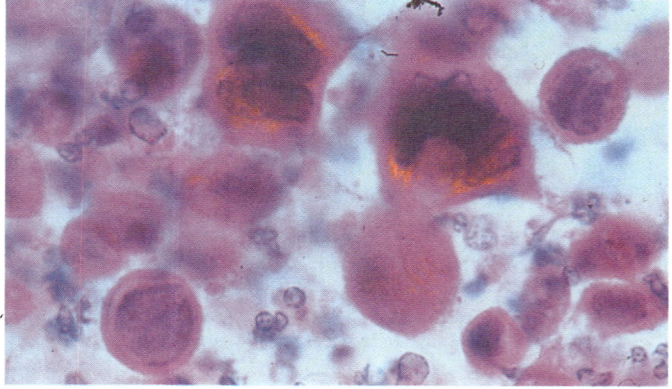

Fig. 30.69 Herpes virus-infected cells in sputum. Note the abnormal keratinization of cells. They may be misdiagnosed as squamous carcinoma. However, the 'glassy', structureless appearance of the nucleus is not consistent with malignant change.

Cytopathology of malignant disease of the respiratory tract

Cytopathology is a very successful method of identifying the majority of tumours which arise in the respiratory tract. Predictive typing is accurate in approximately 90 per cent of squamous carcinomas and small cell cytopathology carcinoma and in 70 per cent of adenocarcinomas. The correlation between the cytopathological findings and the histopathological classification is best for well-differentiated tumours. *In situ* carcinoma cannot reliably be distinguished from invasive carcinoma of the bronchus by cytopathological methods.

Squamous carcinoma

Keratinizing squamous carcinoma can be recognized in Papanicolaou-stained smears by the presence of irregularly shaped cells with dense, brightly eosinophilic cytoplasm, which has a refractile quality, and keratinized plaques may be seen (Fig. 30.72). The nuclei are usually small pyknotic and irregu-

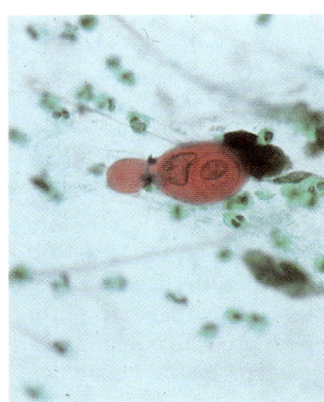 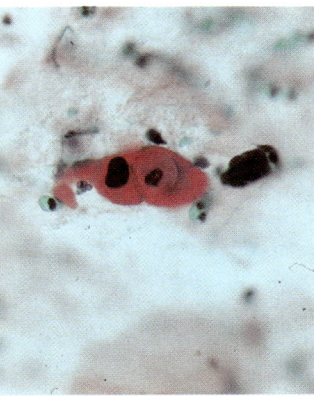

Fig. 30.72 Abnormal keratinized squames in sputum from a patient with a well-differentiated keratinizing squamous carcinoma of bronchus.

lar and show a marked pleomorphism. Anucleate cells or 'ghost cells' may be seen. The shapes of the cells may be quite bizarre; tadpole- or spindle-shaped cells are common.

Malignant cells from non-keratinizing squamous carcinoma have dense cyanophilic cytoplasm and large hyperchromatic nuclei with a coarse chromatin content and irregular nuclear outline (Fig. 30.73). They tend to occur singly or in loose groups or 'streaks' of cells. It has been noted that an individual squamous carcinoma may give rise to well-differentiated malignant cells in the sputum and poorly differentiated cells in the bronchial brushings or washings. Sputum samples from patients with squamous carcinomas often contain abundant cell debris, reflecting the extensive necrosis which is a feature of these tumours.

Adenocarcinoma

Tumour cells from well-differentiated adenocarcinoma of the lung can be recognized in sputum or bronchial material by their large size and foamy vacuolated cytoplasm. Nuclear pleomorphism and prominent nucleoli are features of these tumour cells, which may be found as discrete entities or in papillary clusters (Fig. 30.74). Broncho-alveolar carcinoma can be

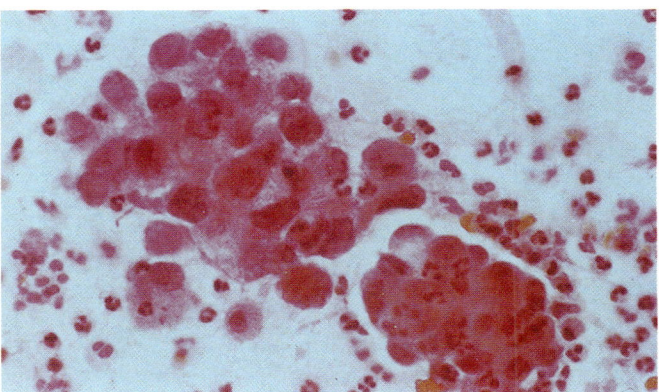

Fig. 30.74 Adenocarcinoma cells in a sputum sample.

recognized by the fact that the tumour cells occur in well-demarcated groups and the individual cells resemble normal columnar cells with slightly hyperchromatic and enlarged nuclei (Fig. 30.75).

Anaplastic carcinoma

Large cell anaplastic carcinomas exfoliate readily and present cytologically as large discrete epithelial cells with scanty cytoplasm. There is marked nuclear pleomorphism and adjacent nuclei may show moulding. Small cell anaplastic carcinoma (oat cell carcinoma) can be recognized by the presence of small cells barely 20 μm in diameter, with scanty cytoplasm and hyperchromatic nuclei which fill the cell (Fig. 30.76). The tumour cells tend to occur in clusters or in an elongated sheaf, which gives them their name. When the cells occur in tight clusters they mould each other and it is this feature, above all others, that enables them to be differentiated from lymphocytes (Fig. 30.77).

Other tumours

Metastatic deposits from adenocarcinoma of breast, prostate, and kidney may be found in the lung. Tumour cells from the

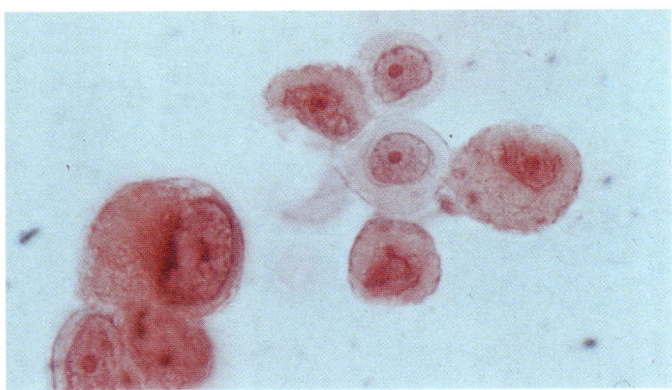

Fig. 30.73 Tumour cells from a non-keratinizing squamous carcinoma of bronchus.

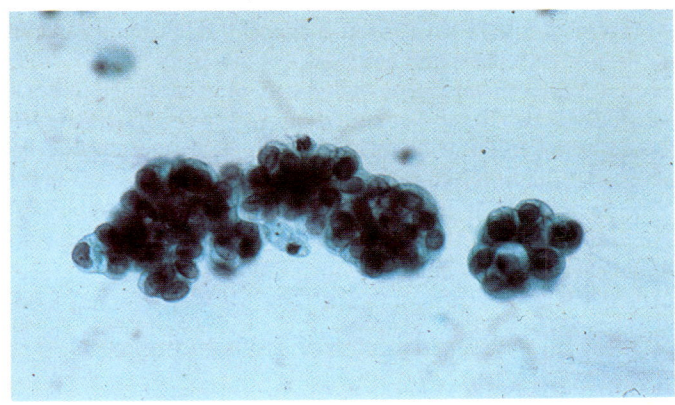

Fig. 30.75 Well-demarcated clusters of small glandular epithelial cells with hyperchromatic nuclei typical of broncho-alveolar carcinoma. Sputum sample.

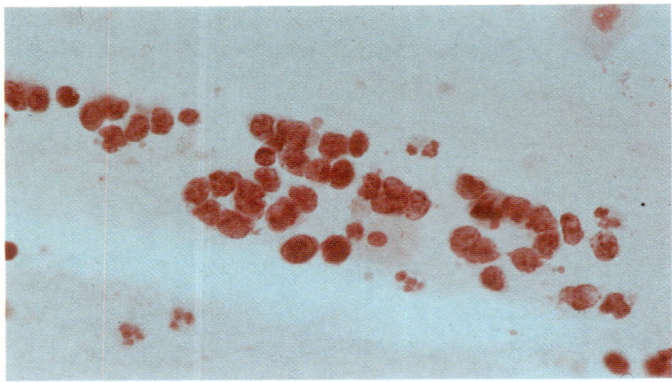

Fig. 30.76 Oat cell carcinoma in sputum. Note the elongated sheaf of cells and nuclear moulding.

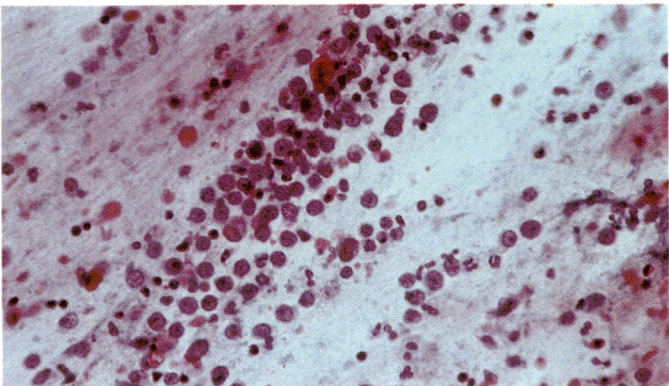

Fig. 30.77 Lymphoid cells in sputum.

deposits rarely appear in sputum as the metastases are usually peripherally sited. However, when cells from these tumours are exfoliated into the bronchial tree they can, rarely, be distinguished from primary adenocarcinoma of lung on the basis of their cytomorphology alone. Other metastatic tumours that can be recognized in sputum samples include melanoma, transitional cell carcinoma, and lymphoma.

Carcinoid tumours are rarely diagnosed cytologically as they lie deep to the epithelium and do not exfoliate unless ulceration occurs. When this happens the sputum may contain clusters of small cells (10–20 μm in diameter) which resemble histiocytes or respiratory epithelial cells rather than tumour cells. Diagnosis is much more likely to be made on a bronchial brush specimen than on a sputum sample. When a diagnosis of carcinoid is suspected, it can be confirmed by immunocytochemical staining or ultrastructural studies.

30.4.12   Cytopathology of serous effusions

Accumulation of fluid in the pleural or peritoneal cavities is an expression of local or systemic disease, and examination of the cells in the fluid can be of value in diagnosing the underlying disease process (see Chapters 14 and 16). Light microscopic analysis of smears can reveal whether the disease process is benign or malignant, inflammatory or reactive, and is one of the most useful tests for the patient with an effusion.

Effusions are usually classified clinically as transudates or exudates, according to the specific gravity or protein content of the fluid. Classically, exudates are distinguished by a high protein content (greater than 30 g protein/l) and a high cell count, whereas transudates contain few cells and have a low protein content. The value of making a distinction on the basis of the protein content of the sample is doubtful as the clinical correlation is poor. For example, it is not unusual to find that transudates due to cardiac failure have a high protein content and are very cellular, possibly due to associated pulmonary infarction.

Specimens should be collected into a sterile container and as much fluid as possible should be sent to the laboratory for cytological studies. Although a cytodiagnosis can occasionally be made on as little as 10 ml of fluid, it is advisable to routinely request 100 ml to ensure that an adequate number of cells are available for analysis. If delay in preparing the specimen for cytology is anticipated, the specimen should be stored at 4 °C. If the specimen is rich in protein and has a tendency to clot, 2 ml of 3.8 per cent sodium citrate should be added to every 50 ml of fluid. Bloodstained fluids that give a heavy deposit of red blood cells (RBCs) after centrifugation require special preparatory techniques to eliminate the red cells, which will otherwise obscure the cells of interest in the smear. At least two smears should be prepared for cytological studies—a wet fixed smear stained by the Papanicolaou method and an air-dried smear stained by the Giemsa method. The Papanicolaou stain is particularly appropriate for examination of mesothelial or cancer cells, whereas the Giemsa stain permits analysis of the nonepithelial cells in the fluid. Several spare smears should be made routinely for special stains (e.g. PAS immunocytochemistry), should these be needed.

Cell content of effusions

The cells found in effusions fall into four main categories: leucocytes, macrophages, mesothelial cells, and malignant cells.

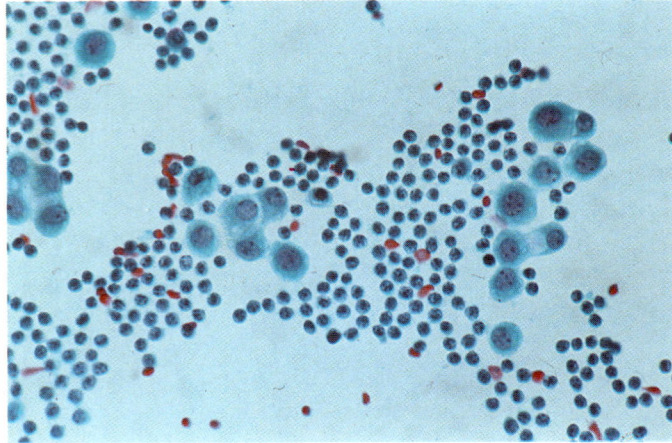

Fig. 30.78 Mesothelial cells and lymphocytes in pleural effusion fluid.

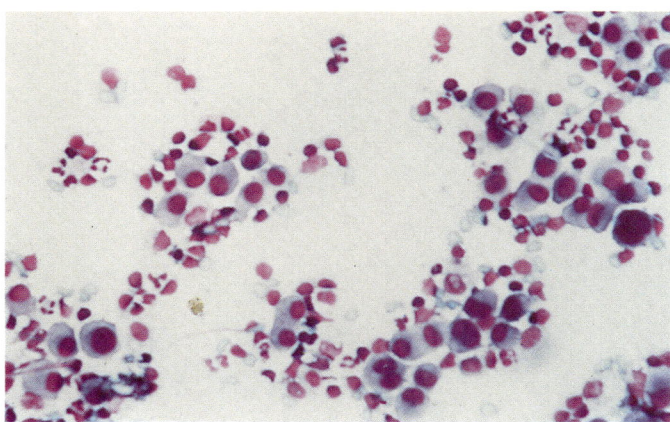

Fig. 30.79 Mesothelial cells and leucocytes in pleural fluid. (Giemsa stain.)

Leucocytes

In Giemsa-stained smears the leucocytes have exactly the same morphology as those found in blood films. Neutrophils predominate in effusions due to infection but lymphocytes and plasma cells are commonly seen in fluid due to cardiac failure or malignancy. Less frequently, primitive cells of the myeloid series may be encountered and care should be taken not to misinterpret them as malignant cells. Although eosinophils in effusions are classically associated with allergic disease, they are frequently found in effusions associated with pneumothorax.

Macrophages

A number of different cell types are included under this heading. Sometimes small mononuclear cells identical to blood monocytes are seen in the smears. A more usual finding is a large mononuclear cell with vacuolated cytoplasm and flattened nucleus. A range of cells with cytoplasm in varying stages of degeneration and 'signet-ring' cells are also seen. Many of the cells appear to have phagocytosed RBCs or cell debris. Some of these cells are believed to be derived from blood or tissue macrophages, but others appear to be altered forms of mesothelial cells which have been shed into the fluid.

Mesothelial cells

These are usually found in discrete cells or smears in small clusters (Figs 30.78, 30.79). They vary in size from 15 to 30 μm and binucleate and multinucleate forms may be seen. They assume a cuboidal shape and the nucleus is often eccentrically placed. In Papanicolaou-stained smears, the cytoplasm assumes a dense azure hue but degenerating forms indistinguishable from macrophages may be seen. When the mesothelium becomes multilayered, the number of mesothelial cells in the fluid may be very large. They may proliferate freely in the fluid and mitotic figures may be seen. It is this massive proliferation of mesothelial cells which makes the distinction between benign proliferation and mesothelioma so difficult. It is frequently seen in ascitic fluid in cirrhosis or in pleural effusions due to pulmonary infarction.

In certain conditions, e.g. effusions due to tuberculosis or rheumatoid arthritis, the mesothelium is covered by a fibrinous exudate. The effusions associated with these diseases are remarkable for the absence of mesothelial cells (Fig. 30.80).

Malignant cells

The presence of malignant cells in effusions usually represents metastatic spread of a tumour from a primary site elsewhere in the body. In the majority of cases the morphology of the tumour cells is so bizarre that a diagnosis of malignancy can be made without hesitation. However, a small proportion of effusions contain cells that present problems of diagnosis, and the use of special stains is indicated to ascertain the nature of the cells. Several different types of tumour can be recognized in the smears. These include adenocarcinoma, squamous carcinoma, anaplastic carcinoma, and lyphoma.

Adenocarcinoma Two distinct cytological patterns have been described:

1. a papillary or acinar form (Fig. 30.81); and
2. a free-cell form (Fig. 30.82).

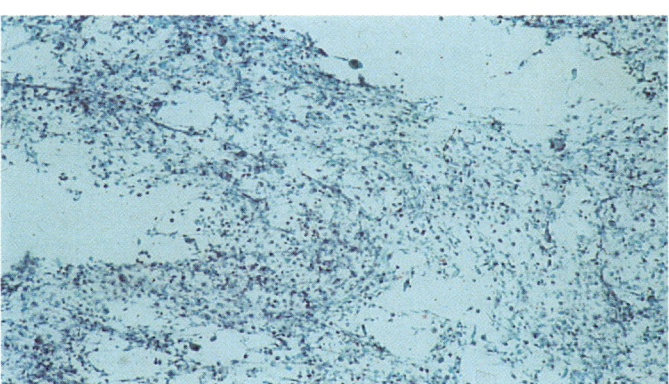

Fig. 30.80 Cytology of effusion due to rheumatoid arthritis. Note the background of proteinaceous debris and the absence of mesothelial cells. No multinucleate giant cells (typical of rheumatoid disease) were seen in this sample.

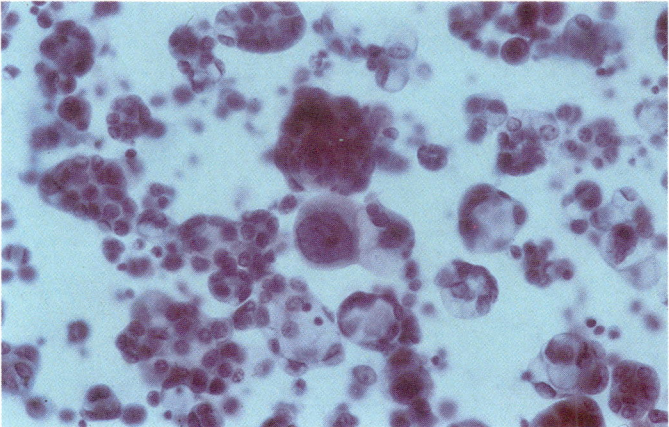

Fig. 30.81 Adenocarcinoma cells in effusion: papillary form.

The majority of adenocarcinoma cells in effusions form papillary clusters (Fig. 30.81a). The aggregates may be irregular or rounded and form hollow balls of cells. The balls may be composed of few tumour cells or reach enormous size containing thousands of cells. Such large aggregates are visible to the naked eye as cloudy shimmering particles in the fluid when it is held up to the light. Other features of the cells in the papillary clusters are their vacuolated cytoplasm and giant nucleoli.

A minority of effusions due to metastatic adenocarcinoma present cytologically in the free-cell form. In these cases the smears are composed almost entirely of discrete tumour cells (Fig. 30.81b). When the tumour cells are small these cases present problems of diagnosis. The presence of mucin can be demonstrated using the periodic acid-Schiff reaction to distinguish them from mesothelial cells. Carcinoembryonic antigen (CEA) is a useful marker of malignancy in these cases, as several large studies have shown that it is specific for epithelial tumours and false positive staining does not occur (Fig. 30.82). Occasionally, the discrete adenocarcinoma cells display a fringe of microvilli which stains pink with the Giemsa stain (Fig. 30.83).

One of the limitations of the cytological diagnosis of effusions is that the primary site of the adenocarcinoma cells cannot be deduced from their morphology in the smears. Immunocytochemical staining for thyroglobulin, prostatic-specific antigen, etc. may be helpful to identify the origin of the tumour in some cases.

Squamous carcinoma Abnormal keratinized squames from a keratinizing squamous carcinoma are rarely found in effusions. An exception occurs in malignant empyema due to direct invasion of the serosal surface by primary bronchial carcinoma (Fig. 30.84). In these cases the smears are composed of sheets of necrotic debris and fragments of highly keratinized cells. A more frequent finding is clusters of tumour cells with dense cyanophilic cytoplasm and large hyperchromatic irregular nuclei (Fig. 30.85).

Small cell anaplastic carcinoma At least half the effusions associated with small cell anaplastic carcinoma of the lung (oat

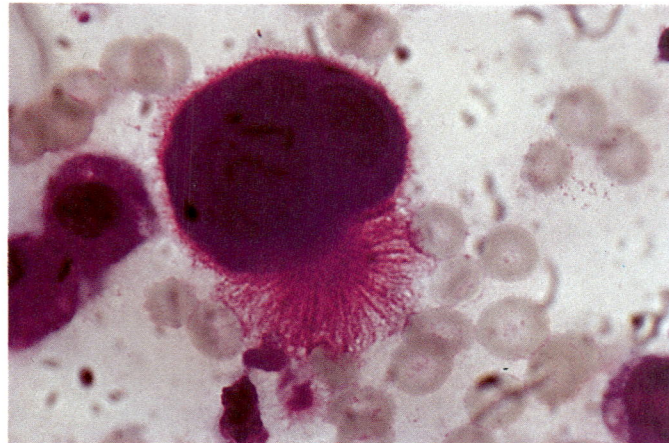

Fig. 30.83 Pseudociliated tumour cell in pleural effusion due to metastatic ovarian carcinoma. (Giemsa stain.)

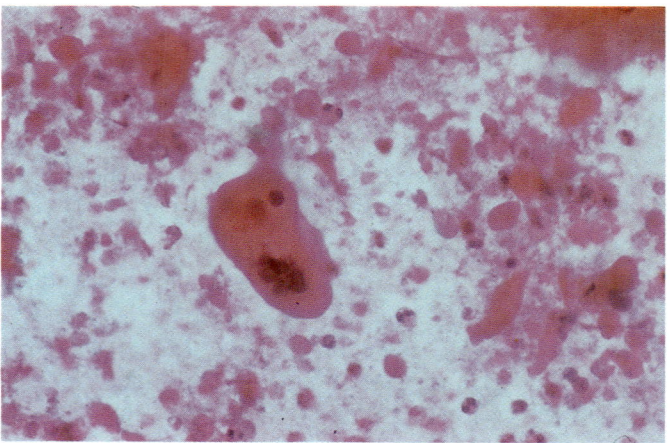

Fig. 30.84 Keratinized squames in effusion due to malignant empyema. Note the necrotic debris.

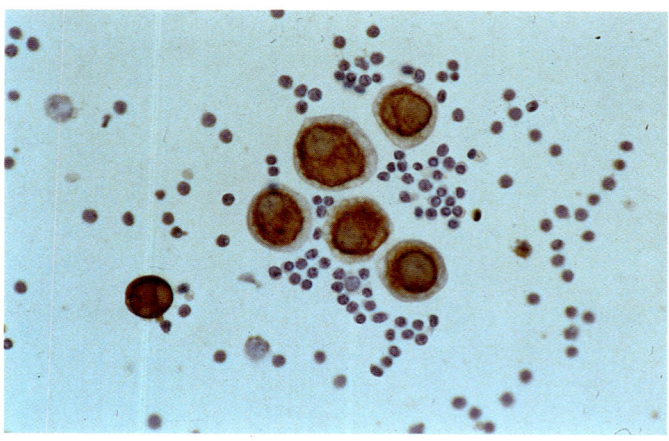

Fig. 30.82 Adenocarcinoma cells (free cell form) in pleural effusion stained for carcinoembryonic antigen. (Immunoperoxidase.)

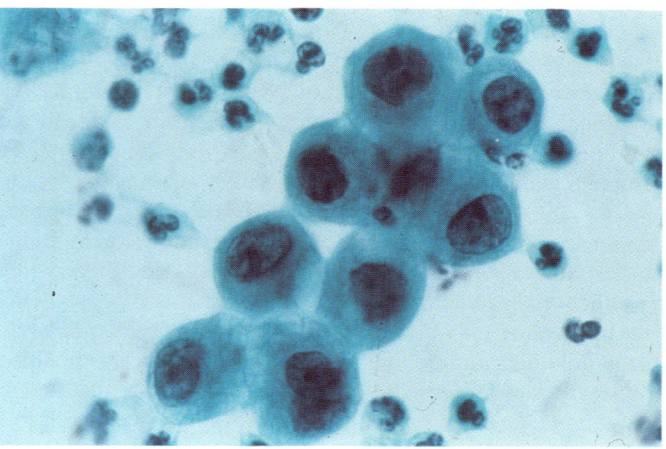

Fig. 30.85 Squamous carcinoma cells in effusion.

cell carcinoma) contain tumour cells. The tumour cells are small and appear to be devoid of cytoplasm. They are frequently mistaken for lymphocytes. Unlike lymphocytes, the oat cells form small clusters or occur in pairs. Careful examination of the cell clusters at high magnification will reveal the nuclear pleomorphism and moulding similar to that seen in sputum samples (Fig. 30.86). It is this characteristic which distinguishes them from lymphocytes.

Mesothelioma This primary mesothelial tumour presents cytologically in several different ways. It may closely resemble the papillary form of adenocarcinoma and special stains for mucin and hyaluronic acid (periodic acid-Schiff/diastase and Alcian blue/hyaluronidase) may be needed to make the distinction. Alternatively, the tumour may resemble anaplastic carcinoma or sarcoma. The most distinctive cytological picture is that of a smear composed of many large papillary clusters of mesothelial cells, together with many discrete mesothelial cells (Fig. 30.87). The papillary clusters are solid and angular, and in this respect they differ from those formed by adenocarcinoma cells, which are hollow and rounded. The clusters may appear crenated, rather like a blackberry, and individual mesothelial cells may be

binucleate or multinucleate and mitotic figures may be seen. Many of these features apply to a description of benign mesothelial proliferation but the changes seen in benign proliferation are never as marked as those associated with mesothelioma.

Lymphomas and other tumours The highly malignant group of non-Hodgkin lymphoma frequently metastasizes to the serous cavities. The tumour cells vary in size and are always discrete. It is this characteristic that makes it possible to distinguish them from metastatic anaplastic carcinoma (see Fig. 30.88). Lymphoma cells in effusions usually exhibit marked nuclear pleomorphism and cleaved cell forms can be readily identified. Immunocytochemical staining can be used to distinguish between T- and B-cell tumours.

Hodgkin lymphoma, when accompanied by an effusion, cannot be distinguished from other high-grade lymphomas. Reed–Sternberg cells are rarely seen.

The malignant cells of plasmacytoma are readily recognizable in Giemsa-stained smears (Fig. 30.89). They are large oval cells with deep cyanophilic cytoplasm with a clear zone adjacent to

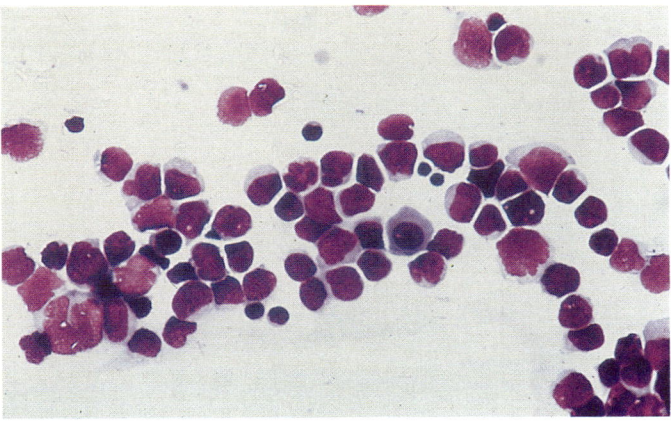

Fig. 30.86 Anaplastic tumour cells from oat cell carcinoma in pleural fluid.

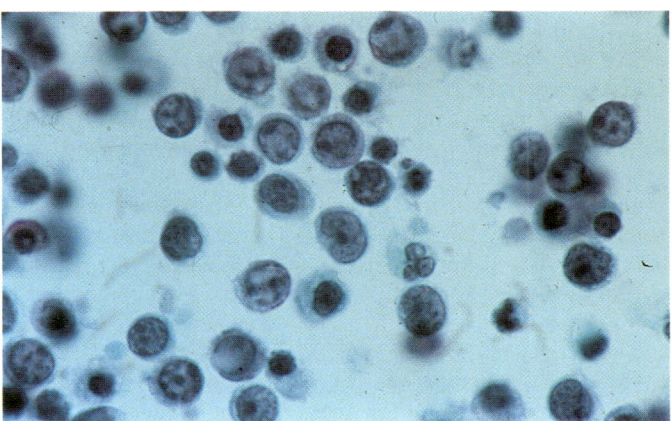

Fig. 30.88 Malignant cells from T-cell lymphoma in pleural fluid. Note that the tumour cells are always discrete.

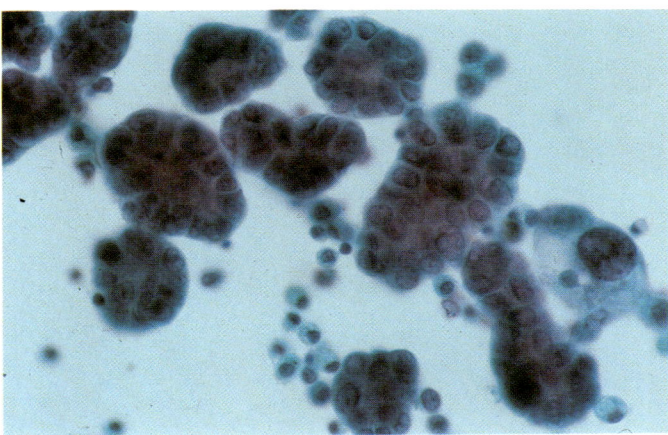

Fig. 30.87 Mesothelioma cells in pleural effusion.

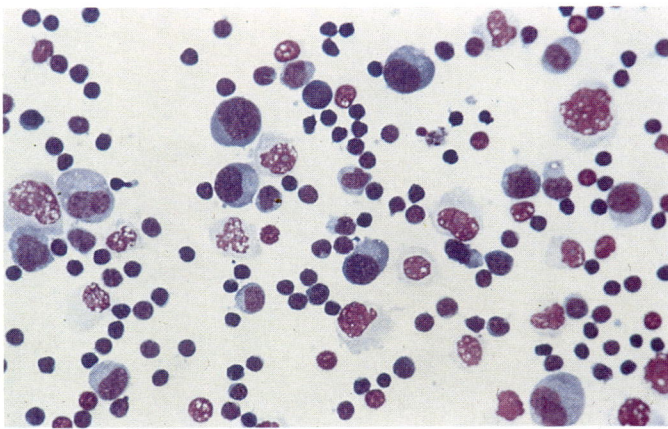

Fig. 30.89 Malignant cells in an effusion in a patient with multiple myelomatosis. Notice the clear zone adjacent to the nucleus and variation in nuclear sizes. (Giemsa stain.)

the nucleus. The nuclei of the malignant plasma cells are eccentrically placed and show marked variation in size. The diagnosis can be confirmed by immunocytochemical staining for κ or λ light chains.

The cells from metastatic melanoma, sarcoma, and germ cell tumours may occasionally be found in effusions.

30.4.13 Cytopathology of the urinary tract

There are four types of sample that are routinely sent for cytological studies: voided urine, catheter urine, ileal loop urine, and bladder washings. Samples should be sent to the laboratory within 3 h of collection. If delay is anticipated, 10 ml fixative (95 per cent alcohol plus normal saline in equal volumes) must be added to the sample.

Processing should proceed without delay if the specimen is received unfixed. Cell concentration techniques must be employed and many centres rely on centrifugation to concentrate the cells. Numerous studies have shown that membrane filtration is a much more effective method of recovering the cells from the sample.

In health, most cells found in voided urine are from the urothelial lining and are few in number. Under pathological conditions (see Chapter 19) transitional cells may be abundant (Fig. 30.90). Contaminating cells from the squamous epithelium of the vagina and vulva in the female and seminiferous fluid in the male may also be found. Leucocytes abound in the presence of infection. Light microscopy will also reveal the presence of tumour cells (Fig. 30.91), casts, and crystals. A number of specific infections (human polyomavirus infection (Fig. 30.92), cytomegalovirus infection, and schistosomiasis (Fig. 30.93), can also be diagnosed on the basis of the cytological findings.

The cytological investigation of urine has an important role to play in the investigation of haematuria as it permits detection of transitional cell tumours arising in the bladder, ureter, or renal pelvis at their earliest stage. It is less satisfactory for the diagnosis of carcinoma of the renal parenchyma, as the tumours are usually well advanced before malignant cells appear in the urine. Cytology is also used for screening workers

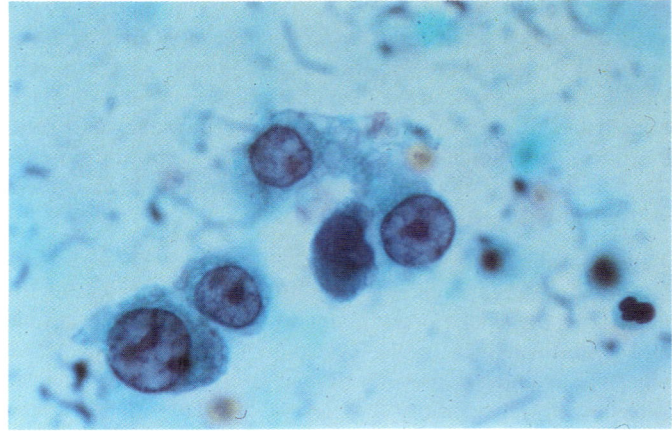

Fig. 30.91 Malignant cells from transitional cell carcinoma in voided urine.

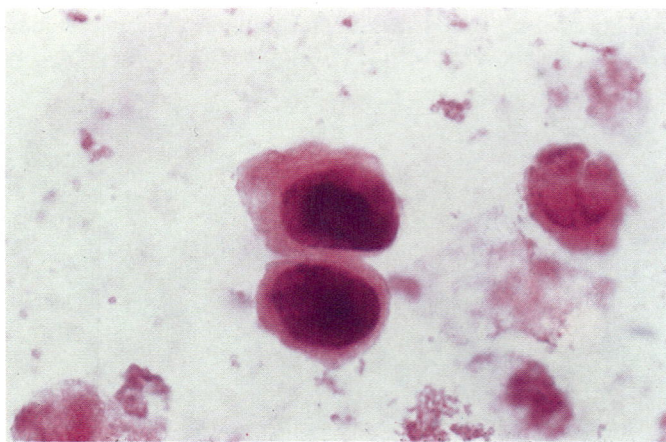

Fig. 30.92 Two inclusion-bearing cells in urine from renal allograft recipient. Electron microscopy revealed polyomavirus particles in the nuclei of the cells.

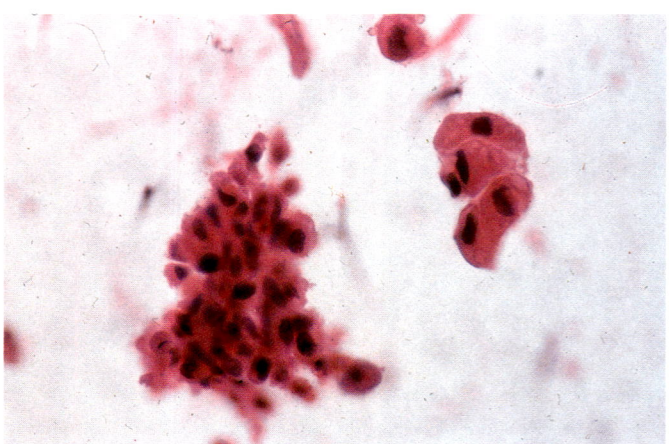

Fig. 30.90 Sheet of transitional cells in catheter specimen of urine.

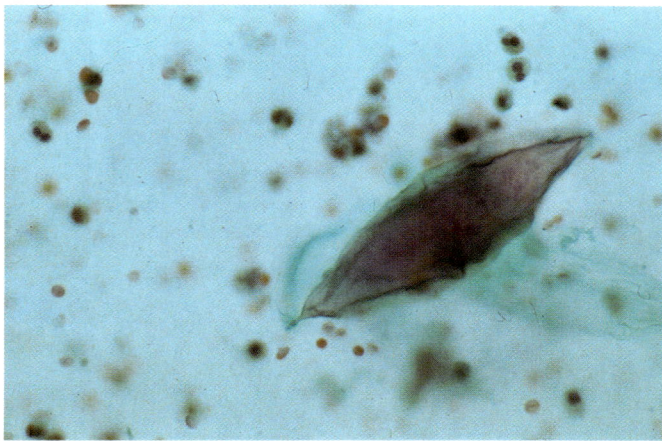

Fig. 30.93 Schistosoma haematobium in a smear of a urine sediment.

in the rubber and dye industry who are at high risk of transitional cell carcinoma. Regular examination of urine samples is a much more acceptable form of monitoring the health of these workers than twice yearly cystoscopy.

Urine cytology also offers a practical way of monitoring the progress of patients who have been treated for bladder cancer: the first evidence of recurrence may be detected by cytology.

The appearance of transitional cells in smears of urine sediment varies according to the method of collection of the sample. In voided urine in the absence of infection large superficial cells (umbrella cells) which have been exfoliated spontaneously are seen. These are flat polygonal cells, 30–50 μm in diameter. They may contain one or more nuclei and are almost always discrete. Single, deeper-layer transitional cells may also be found. These appear as rounded cells 20–30 μm in diameter with a single, round nucleus; a small nucleolus is often seen. In the presence of infection these cells may show degenerative changes; i.e. cytoplasmic vacuolation, nuclear pyknosis, or karyorrhexis. These features disappear after treatment.

Catheter specimens can be recognized by the fact that the urine will contain sheets of transitional cells which have been forcibly detached (see Fig. 30.90). They differ in shape from the spontaneously exfoliated cells and assume a cuboidal or columnar appearance. Large syncytial cells with multiple nuclei may also be seen in these samples. Their origin is uncertain but may be ureteric in origin.

Malignant cells shed from a high-grade transitional cell carcinoma can be readily recognized in smears of urine sediment by their pleomorphism and variation in nuclear size (see Fig. 30.91). The distinction between low-grade tumours and normal transitional epithelium can be difficult if the diagnosis is attempted on a catheter specimen of urine. However, in voided urine the presence of numerous transitional cells with hyperchromatic nuclei and some degree of anisonucleosis should raise the suspicion of malignancy, especially if this pattern is seen in a patient with painless haematuria in the absence of infection.

A cytopathology report of abnormal transitional cells in urine sediment should always be followed by cystoscopy. In the event of negative cystoscopic findings, efforts should be made to exclude carcinoma *in situ* or a lesion in the ureters or renal pelvis. The possibility of a lesion arising in a diverticulum should also be entertained. Errors of diagnosis are rare, but may occur if the cytopathologist is unaware that the patient has received treatment for a bladder carcinoma, as iatrogenic changes may mimic carcinoma (see below).

Occasionally, abnormal squamous cells or glandular cells will be found in urine sediment, reflecting squamous carcinoma or metastatic adenocarcinoma of the bladder. It is not unusual to find contaminating dyskariotic squamous cells in smears of urine sediment from females with CIN or invasive squamous carcinoma of the cervix or vagina.

A recent development in cytology has been the application of exfoliative cytopathology to renal transplantation and the identification of graft rejection. Rejection is manifest by the presence of red blood cells. lymphocytes, renal tubular cells, casts, and necrotic cell debris. The regular examination of urine samples from the post-transplantation patient will permit identification of acute rejection to be made on cytological grounds even before there is clinical evidence of impaired function of the graft. Renal allograft recipients are susceptible to fungal and viral infections and cytological changes characteristic of these infections can be seen in smears of urine sediment.

30.4.14 Iatrogenic pathology

One of the most perplexing problems in modern medical practice is the amount of damage and disease which is caused as a result of treatment. The pathological changes induced by therapy are frequently reflected in cytological smears and the cytopathologist must be alert to this problem as the changes frequently mimic malignancy. Therapeutic manœuvres which may cause problems of cytodiagnosis include cryotherapy, electrocautery and laser therapy, radiation therapy, cytotoxic drug therapy, and exogenous hormone therapy. The presence of an intra-uterine contraceptive device can also affect the cytological pattern, as can endoscopy and catheterization.

Ablative therapy to the cervix

Smears taken one week after carbon dioxide laser ablation contain abundant necrotic debris together with bizarre elongated cells of connective-tissue origin, probably reflecting a shearing action adjacent to the area of destruction. Within two weeks of treatment evidence of repair processes are visible in the smear. Smears taken at this time contain regenerating parabasal cells with enlarged hyperchromatic nuclei and large nucleoli. There may be slight anisonucleosis, which may make it difficult to distinguish the repair process from CIN. Epithelial regeneration is usually complete within a month but, in view of the difficulty in interpreting these post-laser smears, it is advisable to wait for two months after treatment before taking a follow-up smear to assess the effectiveness of therapy. Similar changes are found after cryotherapy and electrocautery.

Changes due to ionizing radiation

Unlike laser therapy, the effect of ionizing radiation on the cervix is long lived and may be seen many months or years after treatment. The immediate effect of radiotherapy is one of cell destruction with swelling of the epithelial cells and loss of morphological detail. Other early degenerative changes include vacuolation of the cytoplasm and nucleus, wrinkling of the nuclear membrane, and condensation of the nuclear chromatin, all of which are precursors of cell death. They may be seen in benign and malignant epithelial cells alike.

Six months later a different pattern is seen. Nuclei may be enlarged, hyperchromatic, and irregular, reflecting a post-radiation dysplasia which is difficult to distinguish cytologically from neoplastic change. Multinucleate, bizarre-shaped cells with abundant vacuolated cytoplasm may also be seen, compounding the problems of diagnosis (Fig. 30.94). However, smudging of the nuclear chromatin and loss of nuclear detail

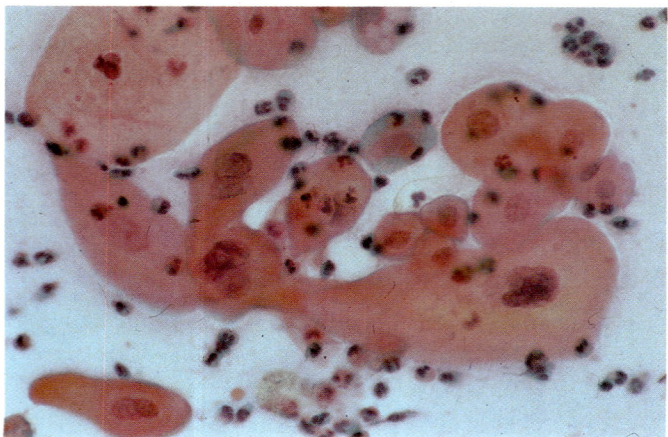

Fig. 30.94 Radiotherapy changes in epithelial cells in a cervical smear. Note the large size of cells and the lack of nuclear structure.

are features of radiation that are not found in neoplasia, and are useful markers for the cytopathologist faced with the differential diagnosis of tumour recurrence or radiation change. The presence of enlarged nucleoli, coarse chromatin, and mitotic figures in the cells supports a diagnosis of tumour recurrence.

Changes due to chemotherapy

The iatrogenic changes due to cytotoxic therapy are of two types: they promote dysplastic changes in epithelial cells and they predispose the patient to opportunistic infection. Both these are reflected in cytological material. Drug-induced dysplastic changes have been described in cells from cervix, bronchial epithelium, bladder, and gastric mucosa, as well as many other sites (Fig. 30.95). The changes mimic those found in frankly malignant epithelium and a complete clinical history must be taken if misdiagnosis is to be avoided. In some instances, especially when cytotoxic therapy is used for the

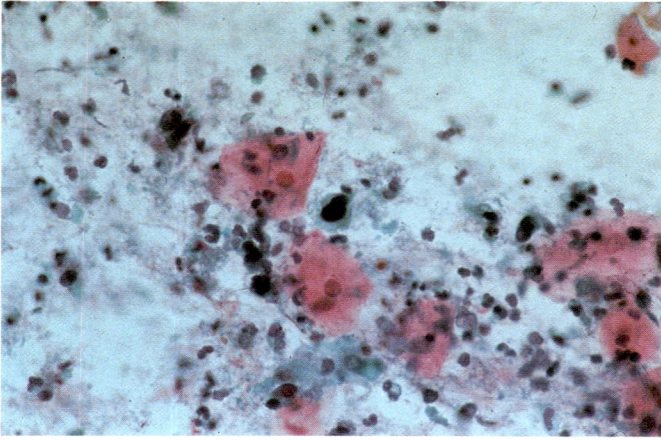

Fig. 30.95 Abnormal cells in sputum from a patient receiving busulphan for treatment of chronic myeloid leukaemia. Note their resemblance to the malignant cells shown in Fig. 30.72.

treatment of bladder carcinoma, it is impossible to distinguish cytologically between iatrogenic change and recurrence.

The impaired immune response induced by cytotoxic therapy results in increased susceptibility of the patient to opportunistic infection by viruses, fungi, and parasites. These can be recognized in cytological material.

The intra-uterine contraceptive device (IUCD)

Several different cytological patterns have been associated with the insertion of an IUCD. Macrophages and other inflammatory cells may abound in the smear, reflecting a foreign-body reaction in the uterus. Atypical endometrial cells may also be found reflecting a chronic endometritis. *Actinomyces* and *Entamoeba gingivalis*-like organisms are frequently seen in smears from women with an IUCD. These are non-pathogenic organisms and reflect the fact that the conditions in the vagina and cervix favour the growth of these organisms on the string of the IUCD.

Effect of hormone administration

Exogenous hormones are frequently given to counter the symptoms of the menopause. Thus a smear from a post-menopausal woman may appear unexpectedly well-oestrogenized if the clinical information provided with the specimen is incomplete. However, the possibility of a granulosa cell tumour should be borne in mind. Occasionally, hormone replacement therapy may result in endometrial hyperplasia, and the presence of endometrial cells in a post-menopausal woman is an indication for curettage.

30.4.15   Conclusions

Exfoliative cytopathology offers a method of diagnosing malignant disease which is quick, safe, inexpensive, and accurate, as well as being acceptable to the patient. Techniques have been developed to obtain samples from most epithelial surfaces and the body cavities. In this section we have discussed the collection and interpretation of specimens which are most commonly submitted for cytological examination, namely cervical and vaginal smears, endometrial aspirates, sputum samples, bronchial secretions and lavage specimens, urine samples, and serous effusions. Other specimens suitable for cytological examination include brushings from the oral mucosa and gastrointestinal tract, scrapings from skin lesions and the conjunctival mucosa, and samples of cerebrospinal fluid.

30.4.16   Bibliography

British Society for Clinical Cytology (1989). *Taking cervical smears.* Copies available from Dr K. J. Randall, Red Tree House, Pine Glade, Keston Park, Orpington, Kent BR6 8NT.

Carmichael, D. E. (1973). *The Papanicolaou smear: life of George N. Papanicolaou.* Charles C. Thomas, Springfield, Illinois.

Coleman, D. V. and Chapman, P. A. (eds) (1990). *Clinical cytotechnology.* Butterworth, London.

Coleman, D. V. and Evans, D. M. D. (eds) (1988). *Biopsy pathology and cytology of the cervix.* Chapman and Hall, London.

Dudgeon, L. S. and Wrigley, C. H. (1935). On the demonstration of particles of malignant growth in sputum by means of the wet film method. *Journal of Laryngology and Otology* **50**, 752–3.

Evans, D. M. D., Hudson, E. A., Brown, C. L., Boddington, M. M., Hughes, H. C., McKenzie, E. F. D., and Marshall, T. (1986). Terminology in gynaecological cytopathology: report of the working party of the British Society for Clinical Cytology. *Journal of Clinical Pathology* **39**, 933–4.

Evans, D. M. D., Hudson, A. E., Brown, C. L., Boddington, M. M., Hughes, H. C., and McKenzie, E. F. D. (1987). Management of women with abnormal cervical smears: supplement of terminology in gynaecological cytopathology. *Journal of Clinical Pathology* **40**, 530–1.

Papanicolaou, G. N. (1954). *Atlas of exfoliative cytology*. Harvard University Press, Cambridge, Massachusetts.

30.5 Fine-needle aspiration cytopathology

M. W. Stanley, L. Skooge, and T. Lowhagen

30.5.1 Historical perspective

Cytopathology has gradually assumed an important role in the diagnosis of malignancy. Its use in screening for diseases of the uterine cervix as well as its growing acceptance as a means to diagnose pulmonary, urologic, and haematopoietic neoplasia is well documented. These traditional techniques, which are based on analysis of exfoliated cells, have been extended to brushings, washings, and lavage of pulmonary, bladder, and gastrointestinal sites.

It is logical to extend tumour diagnosis by analysis of cellular samples to material obtained by fine-needle aspiration (FNA) of palpable masses. This technique is not new, having originated in the United States in the 1930s. Following its enthusiastic initial description as successfully applied to over 2500 cases, it was not widely disseminated, perhaps because it represents a very special type of practice for the pathologist. By contrast, this method is widely used in Scandinavia. At the Karolinska Hospital (Stockholm, Sweden), over 10 000 such FNA biopsies are performed annually and definitive therapy for malignancies of the breast, thyroid, prostate, and other sites is based on the results. This method is currently enjoying wide use in many countries.

Further application of this methodology has come with the use of aspirated material in the evaluation of deep-seated lesions, including metastases from known tumours. These techniques take full advantage of the radiologists' ability to delineate and sample these masses using modern imaging technology, and frequently eliminate the need to obtain such material with open surgical biopsy procedures.

A useful historical analogy can be drawn between current attitudes toward FNA and those expressed about frozen section histopathology when it was new. Although frozen section is now a routine procedure which frequently defines surgical therapy, it was once felt to be a 'fad or pose' and that 'the number of cases requiring it is very small'. Furthermore, it was felt 'that the diagnosis of malignancy, erroneously made . . . will lead to unnecessary radical operations' (Abele *et al.* 1983). In some areas, FNA biopsy is already achieving the status of a routine procedure for diagnosis and follow-up evaluation of palpable masses. This will become increasingly so with the public demand for relatively non-invasive investigative techniques.

30.5.2 Technique

The majority of samples are obtained with 25 gauge (0.6 mm) needles affixed to a 10 ml syringe. A pistol-like holder enables the physician to control the entire aspiration procedure with one hand, while the other hand is free to stabilize the mass being studied (see Figs 30.96, 30.97 for details of fine-needle aspiration).

The specimens obtained consist not of a few single cells widely dispersed over the relatively large surface of a microscope slide, but as numerous tissue fragments. These are, in many cases, as large as, and better preserved than, the fragments obtained by endoscopic biopsy of the bronchial or gastrointestinal linings, so that while requiring the use of expanded diagnostic criteria, they are more than adequate for the diagnosis of malignancy. This generous sampling is made possible by aspiration of tissue fragments excised by the needle tip as it is moved back and forth within the mass under continuous negative pressure from the syringe. In most cases, the stromal scaffold is left behind and only epithelial elements are aspirated, thus concentrating the diagnostic portion of the tissue.

30.5.3 Possible complications

Owing to the small size of the needle, complications are quite rare. The following have been discussed extensively in the literature on FNA.

Implantations of malignant cells in the needle tract

Fear of this possibility is the most frequently raised objection to FNA. This subject has been carefully addressed in the European and American literatures. Based on thousands of cases, there is strong evidence that this complication is very uncommon. Fifteen year follow-up of breast carcinomas diagnosed by FNA showed no difference in outcome from cases in which this technique was not employed (Berg and Robbins 1962). A Canadian series of 2500 transabdominal and transthoracic FNA biopsies revealed no instance of tumour seeding (Tao *et al.* 1980). Even aspiration of parotid mixed tumours, which are notorious for their ability to recur if surgically violated, is deemed safe (Frable 1983).

Infections

The best evidence for the rarity of FNA-associated infections comes from reports of transrectal prostatic aspiration, during

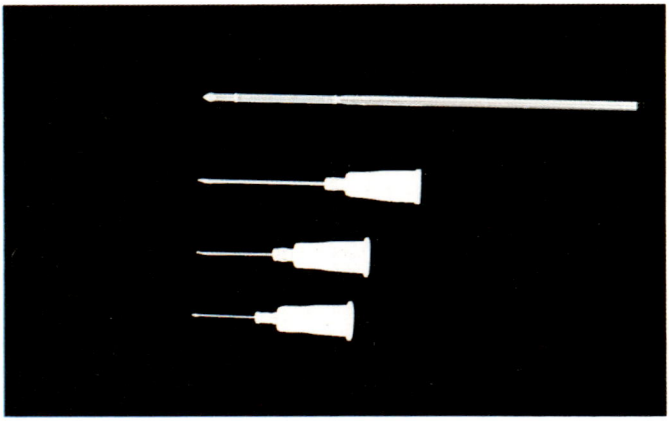

(a)

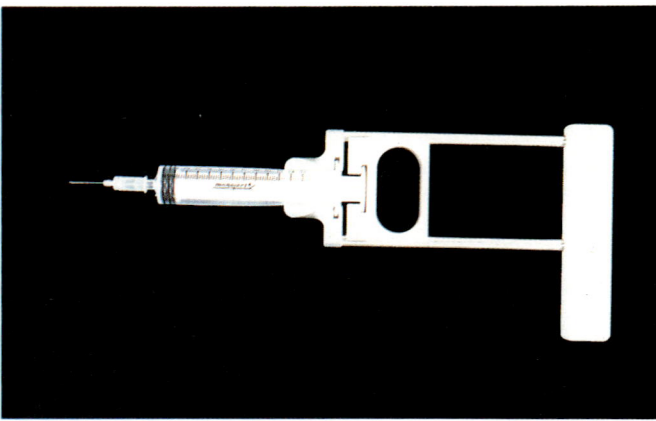

(b)

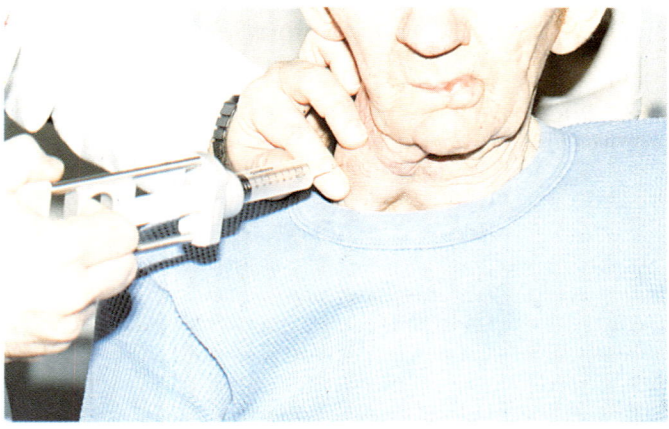

(c)

Fig. 30.96 FNA procedure and equipment. (a) A comparison of various sized needles is shown. A cutting core needle (for biopsy) is shown at the top of the picture and beneath this are needles generally used for fine-needle aspiration. These are of standard gauges 23, 25, and 27. (b) The assembled apparatus with needle, syringe, and syringe pistol is shown. The syringe pistol adds a great deal of control and makes the left hand completely free for stabilization of the mass or other attention required by the patient. (c) Aspirating a recurrent tonsillar carcinoma.

which rectal contents are often aspirated with prostatic epithelium. This is the principle method for diagnosis of prostatic carcinoma in Sweden, and large series are also reported in the American literature. Esposti found four cases of Gram-negative sepsis in 14 000 prostate FNA biopsies. This rate is much lower than seen with needle core biopsies (Esposti and Norlen 1985; Chodak *et al.* 1986).

Other complications

Experience with parotid aspiration also demonstrates the rarity of other complications; no instance of facial nerve damage or infection has been reported (Cohen *et al.* 1986).

30.5.4   Accuracy

The accuracy of FNA is well documented. More than 90 per cent of malignancies will be readily diagnosed by this technique. Table 30.5 shows representative accuracy figures for several frequently aspirated sites. Factors contributing to this success include the experience of the person performing the aspirate, the care used in preparing and staining the aspirated material, and the experience of the person interpreting the cytological findings.

Although the biopsy technique is simple, training in the best methods as well as frequent exercise of one's skill are needed to consistently obtain diagnostic material (Frable 1983; Barrows *et al.* 1986). Proper smear preparation and staining will convert a small amount of aspirated material to a highly diagnostic form. Persons performing FNA biopsies must use optimum smearing techniques. For the pathologist (whether or not he or she actually performs the biopsy), the examination of FNA smears requires an acquaintance with new patterns and diagnostic criteria. These are not mere extensions of those applied to traditional exfoliative cytopathology, but in many instances represent totally different criteria. Furthermore, the degree to which FNA diagnosis can be extrapolated from surgical pathology varies in different body sites, so that once again, new criteria must be embraced.

In exfoliative cytopathology, small numbers of cells are studied in great detail for evidence of malignancy. In FNA, more abundant material is examined for architectural features, the relation of cells to one another, and the nature of extracellular materials. Thus, details of nucleocytoplasmic ratio, chromatin clumping patterns, nucleolar numbers or morphology, and nuclear membrane contours are much less important in FNA than in exfoliative cytology. Instead, the critical features are often assessed at relatively low magnification and include smear cellularity, the degree of cellular dyshesion, and the types of extracellular material which may be present.

For example, smears from a typical infiltrating ductal breast carcinoma will show high cellularity and marked cellular dyshesion, as indicated by the presence of many single cells. That these cells are larger and more polymorphous than benign ductal epithelial cells will also be apparent at intermediate magnification (Fig. 30.98). While the previously noted nuclear features

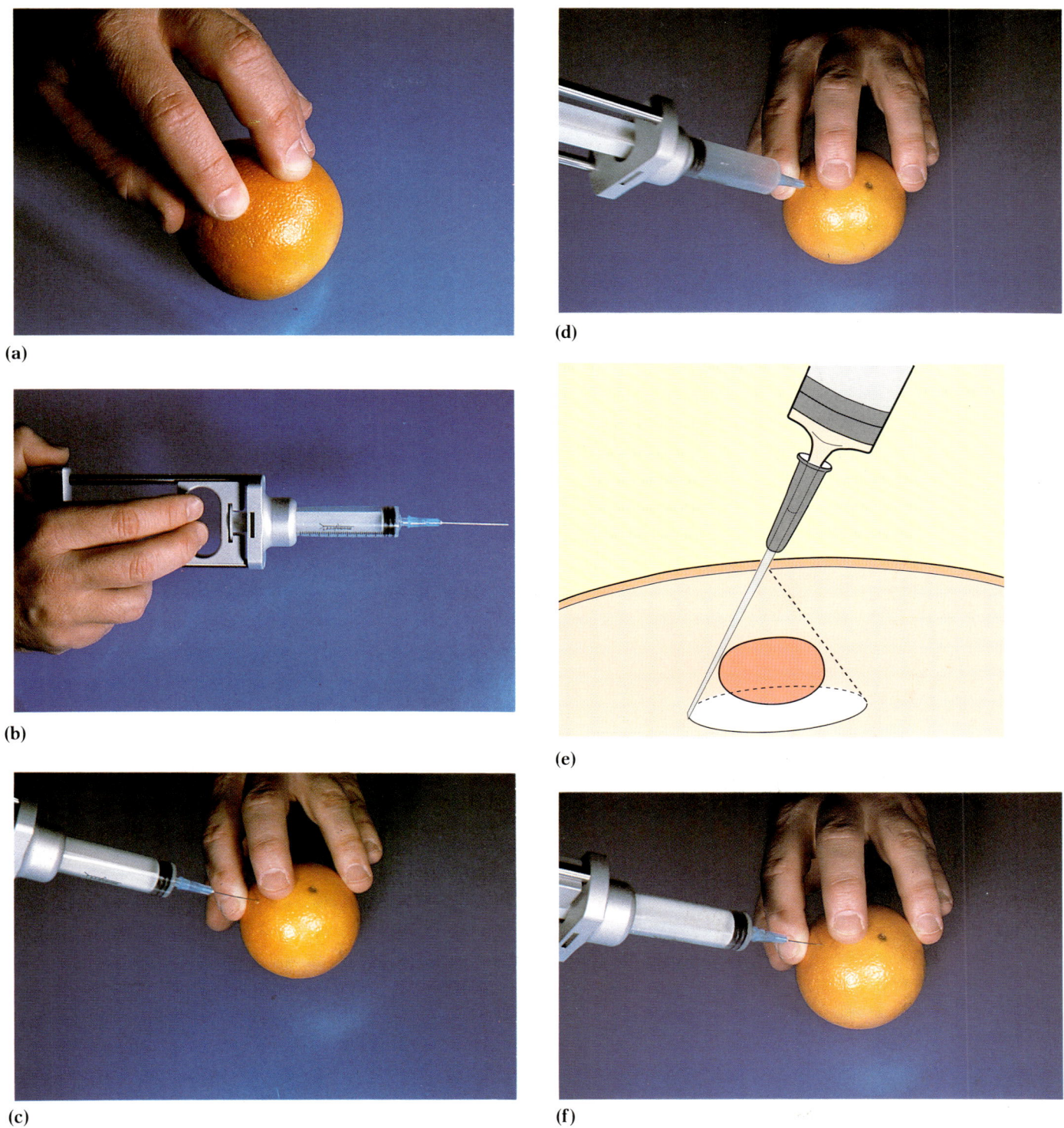

Fig. 30.97 Step-wise guide to FNA. This series of figures is a step-wise guide to fine-needle aspiration. An orange, representing the lump, is used to demonstrate the steps involved.

(a) The left hand is used to palpate the lump. By using a syringe pistol, the index and second fingers of the left hand can stabilize the lesion. (b) The syringe pistol apparatus is held in the right hand. (c) The needle is introduced to the lesion which is palpated beneath the index and second fingers. At this point the plunger of the syringe is still down. (d) The needle is advanced into the lesion and only at this time is the suction applied by withdrawing the plunger. (e) The needle is moved in and out in different directions with suction applied. The needle is moved through the cone-shaped area indicated. (f) While the needle remains in the lesion, suction is let off so that the plunger is now completely relaxed.

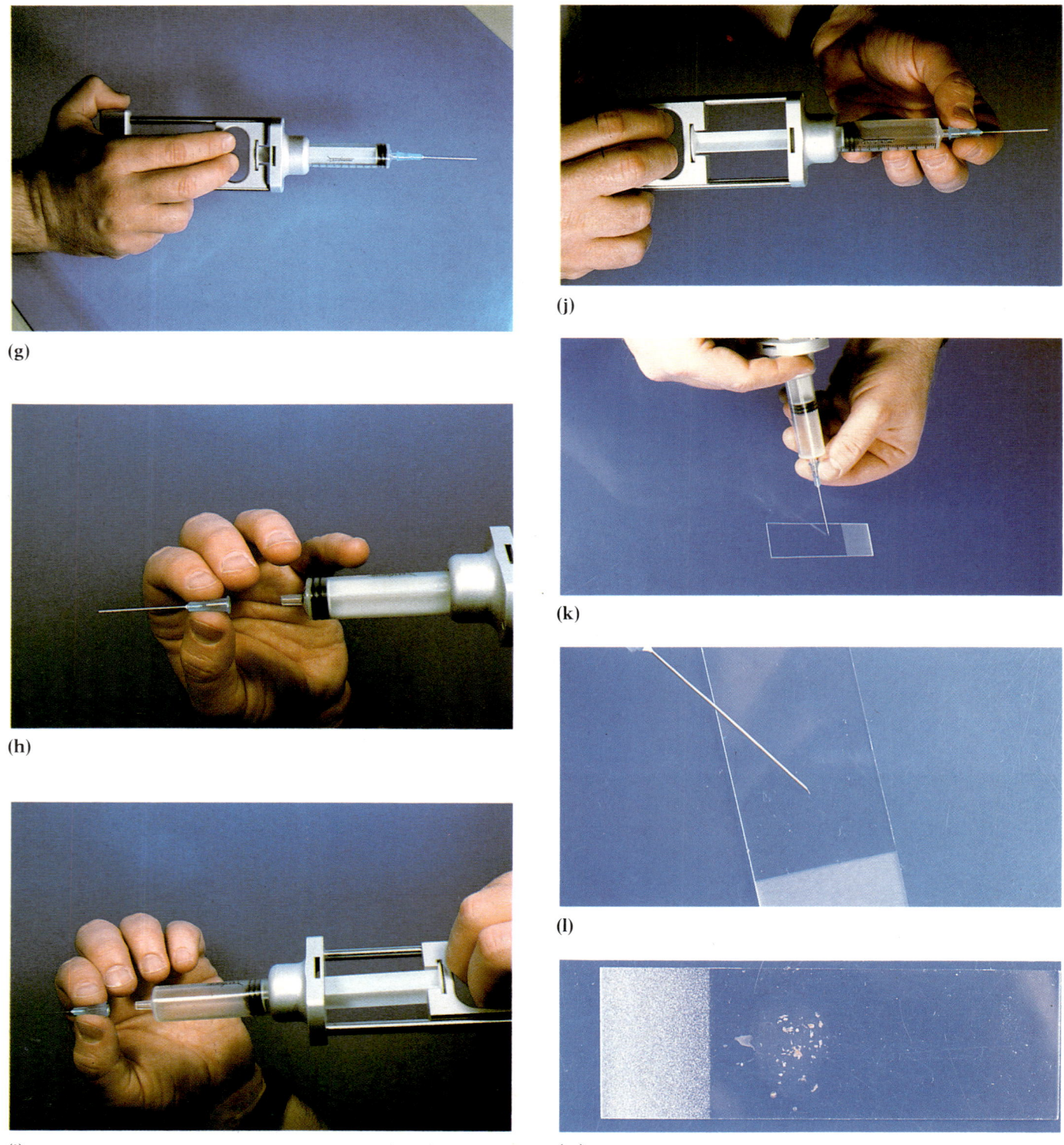

Fig. 30.97 (*cont.*)   (g) The entire apparatus is withdrawn from the lesion. (h) The needle is removed from the syringe. At this point, most of the sample is actually within the needle and not in the syringe. (i) With the needle still off the syringe, the plunger is withdrawn and the syringe barrel filled with air. (j) The needle is replaced on to the syringe. (k) The air now in the syringe is used to expel the specimen on to a clean, uncoated glass slide. (l) and (m) The contents of the needle, including fluid and tissue fragments, are expelled on to the glass slide near the label end. The bevel of the needle (l) is usually down or only slightly raised so that the specimen is very gently layered on to the slide.

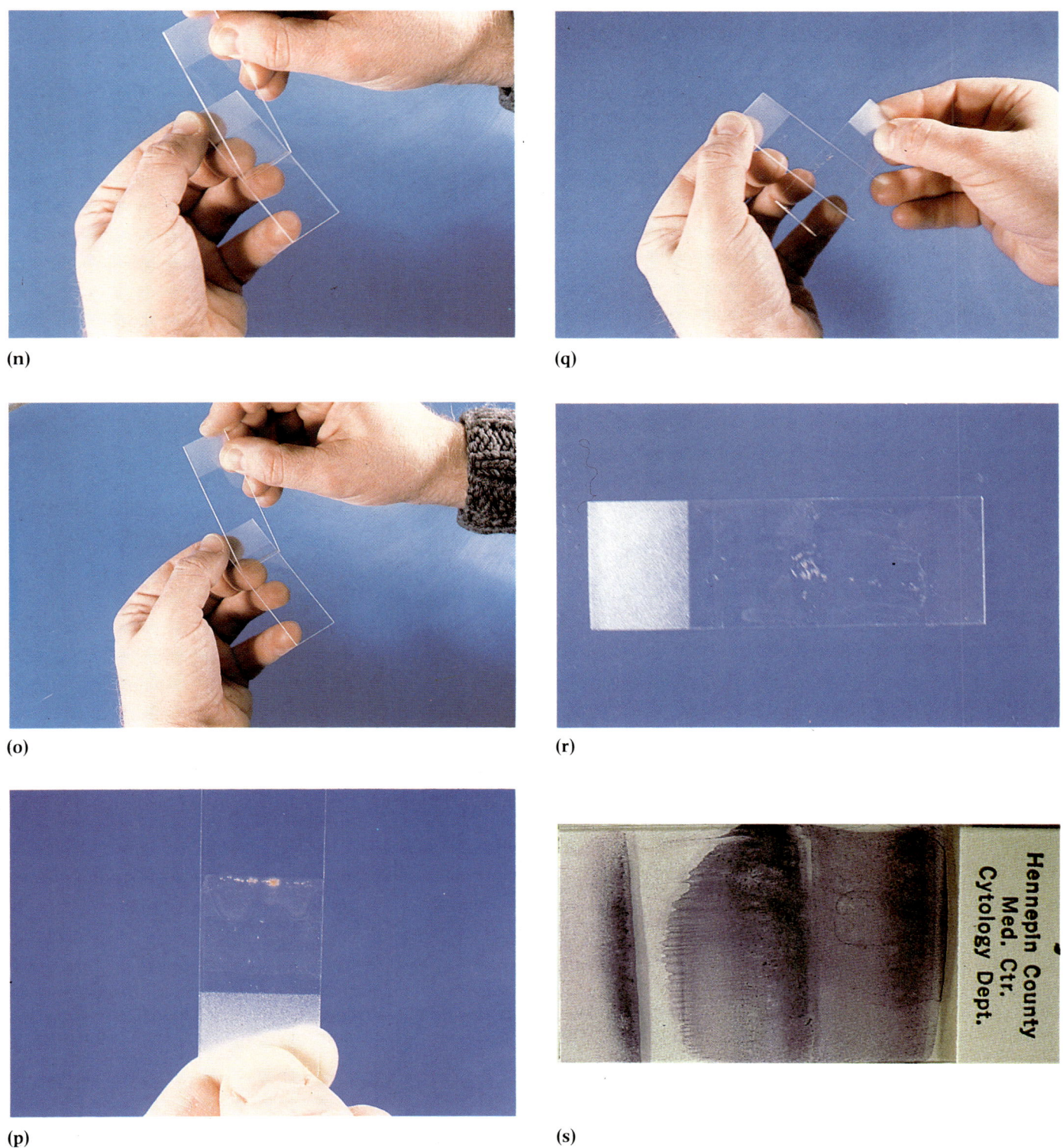

(n)

(q)

(o)

(r)

(p)

(s)

(n) The fluid and particles are collected into a line using surface tension in a manner very similar to that in which blood smears are made. (o) The smear is drawn to the labelled end with the particles still collected under the edge of the spreading slide by surface tension. (p) After this, the line of particles is brought back toward the centre of the slide, the spreader slide is lifted and the slide bearing the material to be smeared is inverted so that fluid drains from the tissue particles. (q) This line of particles is then smeared. (r) The smeared material is concentrated on a small area of the slide which is then either dried or fixed as required by the laboratory using the smears. (s) The finished product is stained by Romanovsky, Giemsa, or other stain and cover-slipped as shown in this photograph.

Table 30.5   Representative accuracy figures for fine-needle aspiration biopsy diagnosis of malignancy

Organ	Sensitivity (%)	Specificity (%)	False positive rate (%)	False negative rate (%)	Reference
Breast	—	—	0.17*	5–10	Feldman and Covell (1985) Silverman *et al.* (1987)
Prostate	—	—	0	7–10	Walsh (1986) Stanley *et al.* (1989)
Salivary gland	98	100	—	—	Frable and Frable (1982)
Lymph node†	92	99	—	—	Frable (1983)

     * Cumulative review of 25 180 cases in several series.
     † Series of 1000 cases assessed for malignancy (metastatic carcinoma or malignant lymphoma). Slightly lower accuracy is noted when specific types of malignant lymphoma are considered.

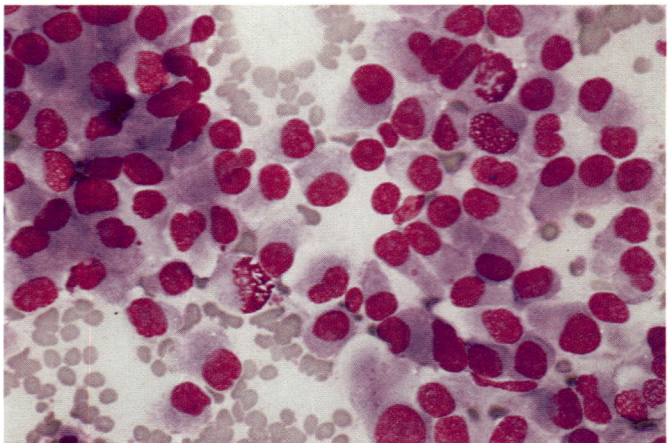

Fig. 30.98   Fine-needle aspiration smear of infiltrating ductal carcinoma of the breast. The smear is very cellular and shows enlarged, polymorphous, malignant-appearing epithelial cells lying singly and in three-dimensional groups.

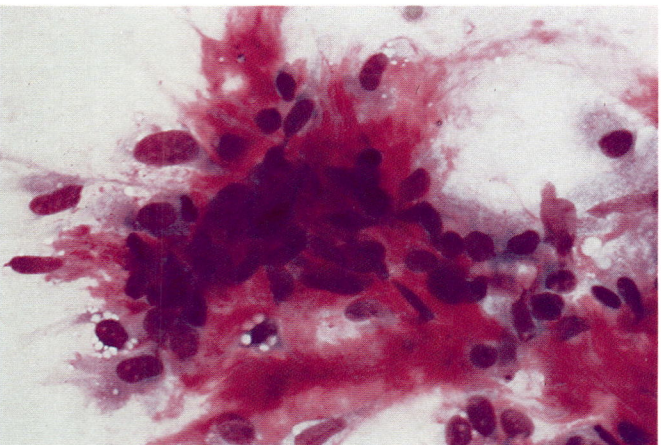

Fig. 30.99   Pleomorphic adenoma (benign mixed tumour) of the parotid gland. FNA smear showing abundant fibrillar metachromatic matrix. The small number of epithelial cells present are embedded within this matrix and are obscured by it so that they tend to take on a pale ghost-like appearance.

of malignancy will be present in many cases, they assume less importance than the overall smear pattern.

Extracellular material is of diagnostic importance in many tumours. A frequently studied example of this situation is the benign pleomorphic adenoma (mixed tumour) of salivary gland origin. The chondroid extracellular matrix which typifies this neoplasm has a very characteristic appearance in smears (Fig. 30.99). Even when present in very small amounts, it indicates pleomorphic adenoma. This finding outweighs the many other features which may be seen in these tumours (cystic change, mucin, squamous metaplasia, epithelial atypia, and sebaceous elements) and permits accurate diagnosis despite a wide range f cytological details which may be present.

30.5.5   Advantages

The advantages of diagnosis by FNA are numerous. It is a safe, reliable, rapid, accurate, and inexpensive means of diagnosing most malignancies and of following clinically benign masses. It can be performed as an office procedure and requires no anaesthesia, drapes, Betadine, or even gloves—only alcohol cleansing of the skin similar to that used in drawing blood for laboratory tests. It leaves no scars, is nearly painless, and is attended by minimal complications. These features suggest that its utility should not be compared with surgical procedures, but rather with the unaided physical examination. By extending the physician's examining finger tips with a very small-gauge needle, this technique permits rapid diagnosis of most palpable masses.

30.5.6   General guidelines for FNA

1. Most palpable masses, as well as those which are deep-seated but can be approached with radiographic guidance, can be sampled by FNA for diagnostic purposes.

2. For the highest diagnostic yield and greatest consistency, the aspirations should be performed and interpreted by the same individual. Only in this way can all available clinical and morphologic findings be synthesized into the most accurate possible diagnosis.

3. An FNA negative for malignancy, infection, or other specific benign diagnosis leaves the clinical problem unsolved. Such an aspiration should be followed by another diagnostic procedure, either repeat FNA or tissue biopsy by other means.

4. Radiographic or clinical evidence of malignancy should overrule a benign or inconclusive FNA report. This is especially true in the breast, where evidence of malignancy may be clinical, radiographic or cytological.

30.5.7 Bibliography

Abele, J. S., Miller, T. R., Goodson III, W. H., Hunt, T. K., and Hohn, D. C. (1983). Fine needle aspiration of palpable breast mass: a program for staged implementation. *Archives of Surgery* **118**, 859–63.

Barrows, G. H., Anderson, T. J., Lamb, J. L., and Dixon, J. M. (1986). Fine needle aspiration of breast carcinoma: relationship of clinical factors to cytology results in 689 primary malignancies. *Cancer* **58**, 1493–8.

Berg, J. W. and Robbins, G. F. (1962). A late look at the safety of aspiration biopsy. *Cancer* **15**, 826–7.

Chodak, G. W., Steinberg, G. D., Bibbo, M., Wied, G., Strauss II, F. S., Volgelzang, N. J., and Schoenberg, M. W. (1986). The role of transrectal aspiration biopsy in the diagnosis of prostatic carcinoma. *Journal of Urology* **135**, 299–302.

Cohen, M. B., Ljung, B.-M. E., and Boles, R. (1986). Salivary gland tumors: Fine needle aspiration vs. frozen section diagnosis. *Archives of Otolaryngology* **112**, 867–9.

Esposti, P. L. and Norlen, A. E. (1985). Complications of transrectal aspiration biopsy of the prostate. *Scandinavian Journal of Urology and Nephrology* **9**, 208–13.

Feldman, P. S. and Covell, J. L. (1985). *Breast and lung in fine needle aspiration cytology and its clinical application*, pp. 27–43. Chicago American Society of Clinical Pathologists Press.

Frable, W. J. (1983). *Thin-needle aspiration biopsy.* W. B. Saunders, Philadelphia.

Frable, M. A. and Frable, W. J. (1982). Fine-needle aspiration biopsy revisited. *Laryngoscope* **92**, 1414–18.

Silverman, J. F., Lannin, D. R., O'Brien, K., and Norris, H. T. (1987). The triage role of fine needle aspiration biopsy of palpable breast masses. Diagnostic accuracy and cost-effectiveness. *Acta Cytologica* **31** (6), 731–6.

Stanley, M. W., Hedlund, P. O., Ronstrom, L., and Lowhagen, T. (1989). Determination of the false negative rate in fine needle aspiration of the prostate: A study of sequential aspirations of 30 untreated carcinoma patients. *Urology* **34**, 73–5.

Tao, L. C., Pearson, F. G., DeLarue, N. C., Langer, B., and Sanders, D. E. (1980). Percutaneous fine needle aspiration biopsy: I. Its value to clinical practice. *Cancer* **45**, 1480–5.

Walsh, P. (1986). Fine needle aspiration of the prostate—why has it taken so long to accept? *Journal of Urology* **135**, 334–5.

Zajicek, J. (1974). *Aspiration biopsy cytology: Part I: Cytology of supradiaphragmatic organs.* S. Karger, Basle.

30.6 Flow cytometry

Phil Quirke

30.6.1 Introduction

The flow cytometer is an instrument offering a rapid, reproducible, and quantitative technique for the measurement of a variety of physical and fluorescence-associated parameters. Three major areas of use have emerged: first, measurement of cell-surface markers in immunology; secondly, as a method of quantitating DNA content and cell proliferation; and thirdly, as a cell sorter in research laboratories. Flow cytometry is not just restricted to cells but can be applied to a variety of small particulate structures, including bacteria and chromosomes.

30.6.2 Analysis

For analysis by flow cytometry, the cells under study must be in a single cell suspension. Athough this problem does not arise for blood or semen, all other tissues must be disaggregated by the use of enzymatic or physical methods. The cells are then stained with a fluorescent dye to demonstrate the substance to be quantitated. As shown in Fig. 30.100, upon insertion into the machine (1) cells are forced by gas pressure into an injection needle, from which on exit they are hydrodynamically focused by a faster flowing stream of sheath fluid (2). This process compresses the sample stream and controls the rate of ejection of the cells. Individual cells pass downwards from the flow chamber in single file under the influence of gravity into the path of a light source, which may be either a laser or a mercury arc lamp. The laser beam provides high intensity illumination with a restricted number of wavelengths of excitation, whereas a mercury arc lamp provides low intensity light of multiple wavelengths. Light is focused on to the stream (3) where it physically interacts with each cell and is scattered in all directions. Light scattered in the forward direction is detected as forward angle light scatter (4) and is proportional to the size of the cell. Light collected at 90° to the cell's trajectory is proportional to the internal granularity or density of the cell. Incoming light also excites the fluorochrome with which the cell has been stained, leading to the emission of light of a longer wavelength, which can be directed by means of optical filters to one of several photomultiplier tubes (PMT). More than one fluorochrome may be used, the limiting factors being the number of excitation sources that can be applied and the number of PMTs available for measurement of emissions. The PMT (5) converts light into an analogue electrical signal (6) which is changed into a digital signal (7) by an analogue to digital converter. The signals are processed by the computer and a frequency histogram generated (8). The greater the intensity of fluorescence or the ability of the cells to scatter light, the further along the X-axis the event is plotted. The signal from any one PMT may be correlated with up to two other PMTs,

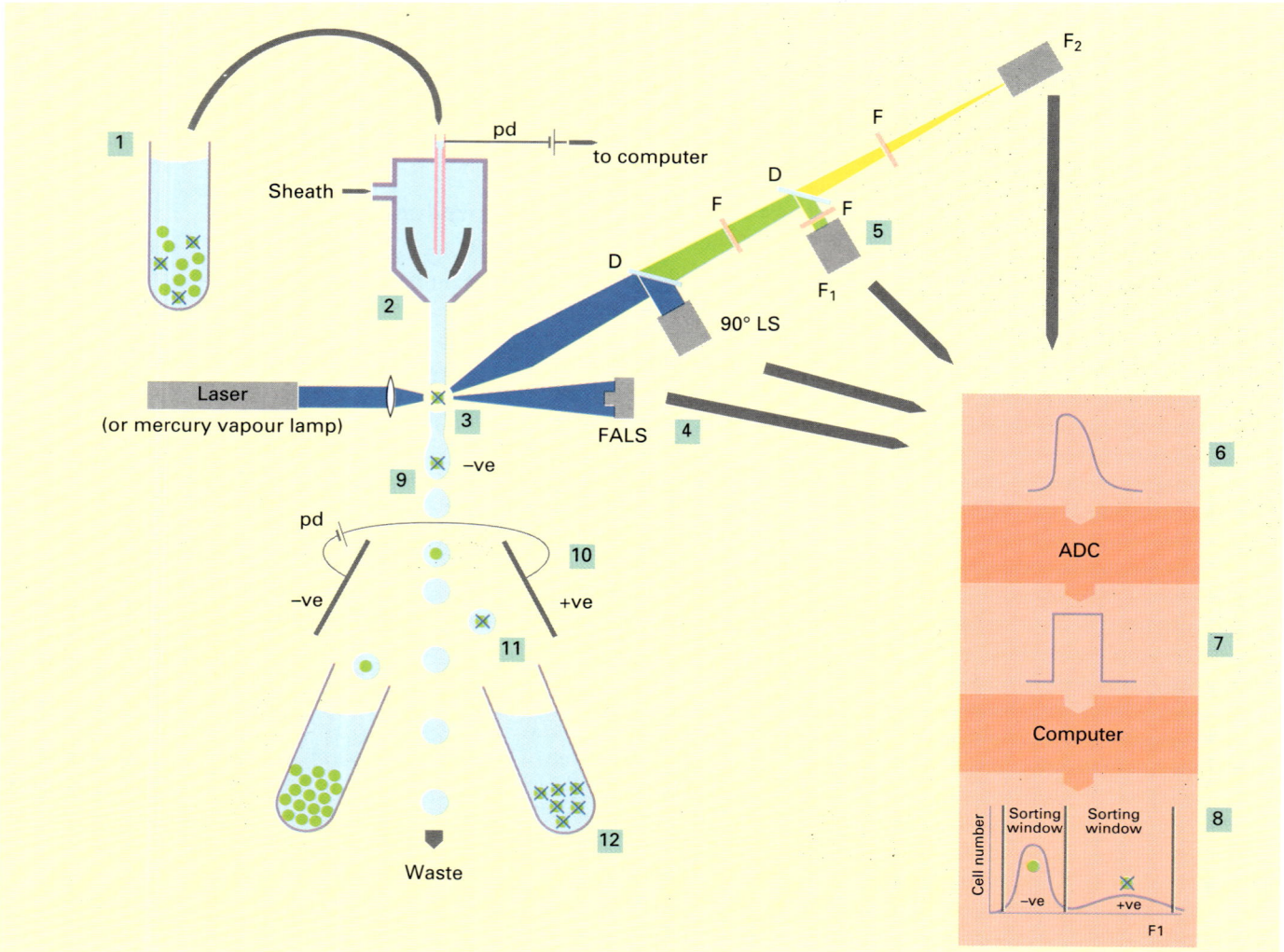

Fig. 30.100 Schematic diagram of a flow cytometer (see text for details). The crossed circles represent fluorescent cells and the circles fluorescent negative cells. Abbreviations used: FALS, forward angle light scatter; 90° LS, 90° light scatter; D, dichroic filter; F, filter; F1 F2, fluorescence signals 1 and 2; pd, potential difference; ADC, analogue to digital converter. (Drawn after the *Journal of Pathology*, with permission.)

allowing the identification of multiple phenotypic properties of an individual cell. Quantitation of the resultant populations is then performed using computer software.

30.6.3   Cell sorting

If cells are to be isolated from the sample then the fluorescent or physical properties of the required subpopulation are programmed into the computer (8). After passing through the light beam (3) the stream breaks up into individual droplets (9) caused by the vibrations of a piezo-electric crystal. If a cell of the required subpopulation (crossed circles) is identified by the computer from its electronic profile, then a transient negative potential difference is applied to the stream, charging the droplet containing the cell of interest. This breaks off, carrying the charge, and the stream reverts back to its non-charged state. The negatively charged droplet containing the cell falls under

gravity between two plates at a high constant potential difference (10). It is attracted towards the oppositely charged positive plate (11) and leaves the central stream to fall into a collecting vessel (12). By changing the charge applied to the stream at breakoff from negative to positive it is possible to sort a second population (uncrossed circles). These cells are attracted to the negatively charged plate, thereby leaving the central stream and falling into a second collection vessel. Further investigations are now possible on either population of cells. Sorting purity can vary between 95 per cent and 99.9 per cent, depending on the sort of conditions applied.

30.6.4   Applications of flow cytometry

Flow cytometry can be applied to the quantitation of any substance which will give a fluorescent emission, and can therefore provide important information in many fields.

Immunology

Since blood is a natural single-cell suspension, flow cytometry is a favoured tool of immunologists. Whole blood samples or purified subpopulations are labelled with cell-surface phenotypic markers (which may be either antibodies or lectins), by direct or indirect fluorescent techniques. Populations and subpopulations of T- or B-cells may be rapidly quantitated and used, for example, to derive CD4 : CD8 ratios in AIDS patients, determine the monoclonality of B-cell tumours, or assess the phenotypic expression of leukaemias. Flow cytometry has become a routine instrument in immunology laboratories.

DNA content

The application of flow cytometry currently of most interest to pathologists is the measurement of nuclear DNA content and cell-cycle analysis. This depends on the use of a fluorescent stain which has a stoichiometric reaction with DNA, i.e. where there is a linear relationship between the amount of DNA in the nucleus and the fluorescence emission intensity. Cells increase the amount of DNA they contain when passing through the cell cycle (see Fig. 30.101) and therefore the position of the cells on a DNA histogram moves to the right. The frequency histogram of fluorescence (DNA content) versus cell number has a characteristic pattern which allows the proportion of cell nuclei in G_0/G_1, S, and G_2/M phases to be calculated by computer software (see below). Measurements may be performed on nuclei extracted from fresh, fixed, or paraffin-embedded material, and can therefore be applied retrospectively to stored material from previous years.

Malignant and, to a lesser extent, premalignant conditions frequently show gross aberrations of DNA content, where the cell nuclei contain over 50 chromosomes. Such DNA aneuploid cell populations can be easily identified by flow cytometry since a second DNA peak becomes apparent which is separate from the first. An example of a diploid and a DNA aneuploid histogram are shown in Fig. 30.102. The presence of DNA aneuploidy in malignant tumours from sites such as the colorectum, lung, ovary, and prostate is associated with poor prognosis, and there is some evidence to suggest that flow cytometry predicts prognosis more accurately than histopathological assessment.

One valuable application of flow cytometry is in the differential diagnosis of hydatidiform molar pregnancy. Partial hydatidiform molar pregnancies contain 69 chromosomes and are therefore triploid, seen on the DNA histogram as a second peak halfway through S phase (Fig. 30.103a). Complete hydatidiform moles are diploid and reveal a high level of cell proliferation (Fig. 30.103b). Analysis by flow cytometry is important in helping to distinguish complete and partial moles, but it does not appear to predict those cases of complete molar pregnancy at risk of persistent trophoblastic disease (see Chapter 21).

Cell-cycle analysis

The DNA distribution of diploid tumours may be broken into their constituent G_0/G_1, S, and G_2/M phases by computer software to derive values for the percentage G_0/G_1, S-phase, and G_2/M populations (see Fig. 30.104). This is only an assessment of the relative distribution of the cell population and does not reveal how rapidly these cells are passing through the cell cycle. Such information can, however, be obtained by flow cytometry using bromodeoxyuridine labelling in a manner analogous to autoradiography. The presence of high cell proliferation has been found useful in the assessment of prognosis in a variety of tumours, such as rectal carcinoma, lung carcinoma, and non-Hodgkin lymphoma, with tumours demonstrating a high level of cell proliferation having a poorer prognosis.

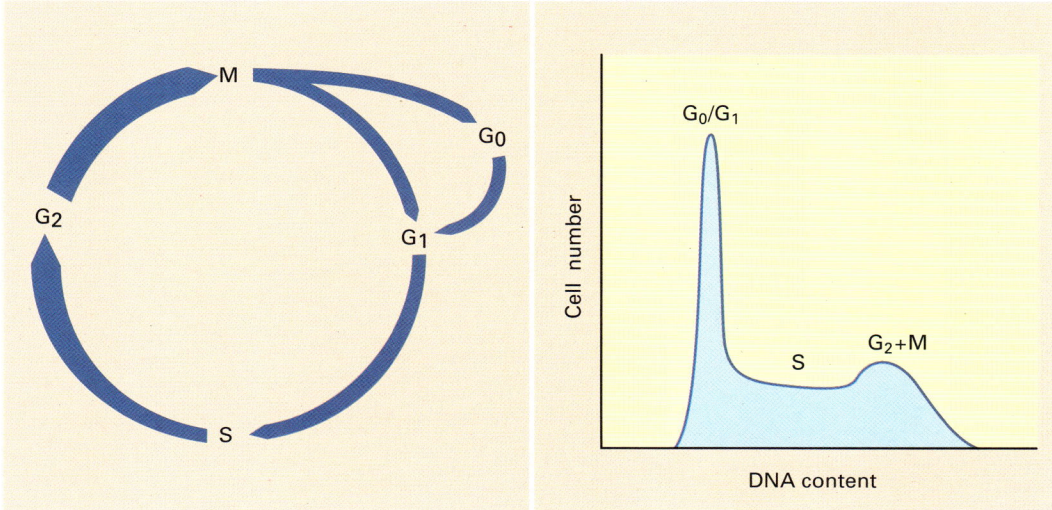

Fig. 30.101 Diagram to show the compartments of the cell cycle. DNA content increases progressively during S-phase until it reaches double the normal level at G_2; after mitosis it returns to normal levels. The flow cytometric histogram shows the fluorescence distribution of a normal cell population. The histogram represents cell number (Y-axis) versus fluorescence DNA content (X-axis).

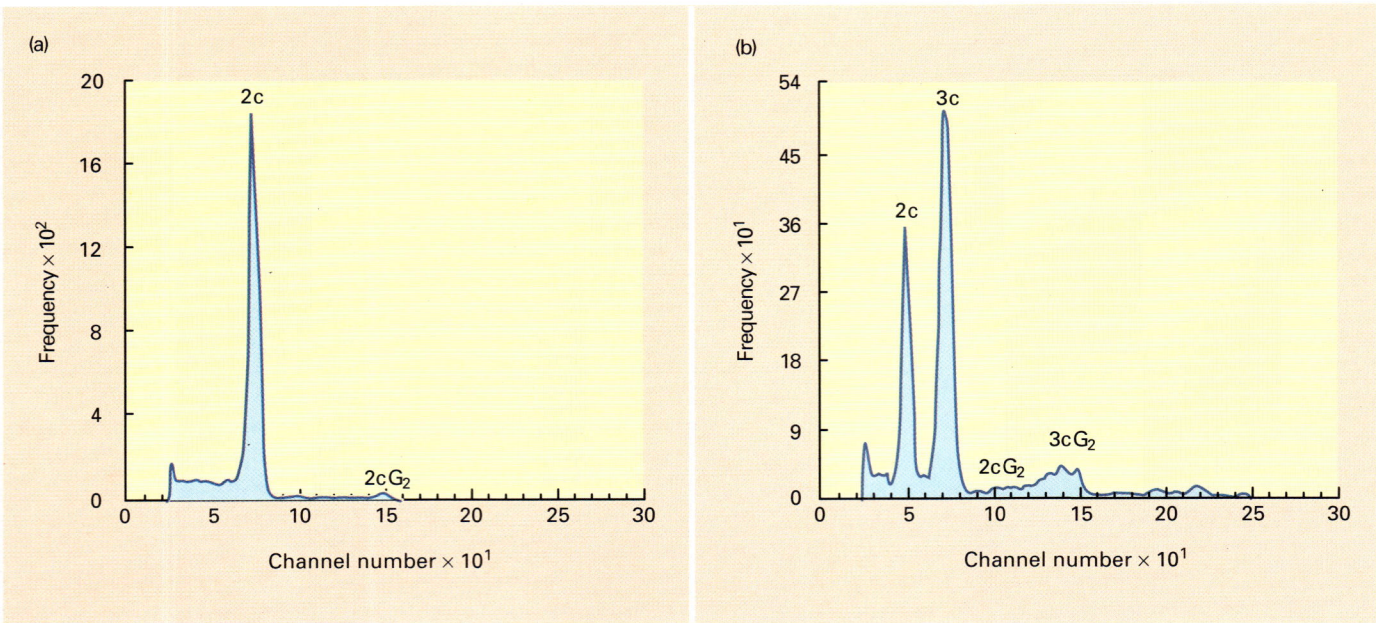

Fig. 30.102 Two DNA histograms: (a) of a diploid tumour with a single G_0/G_1 peak, and (b) a DNA aneuploid tumour with two G_0/G_1 peaks. (Drawn after the *Journal of Pathology*, with permission.)

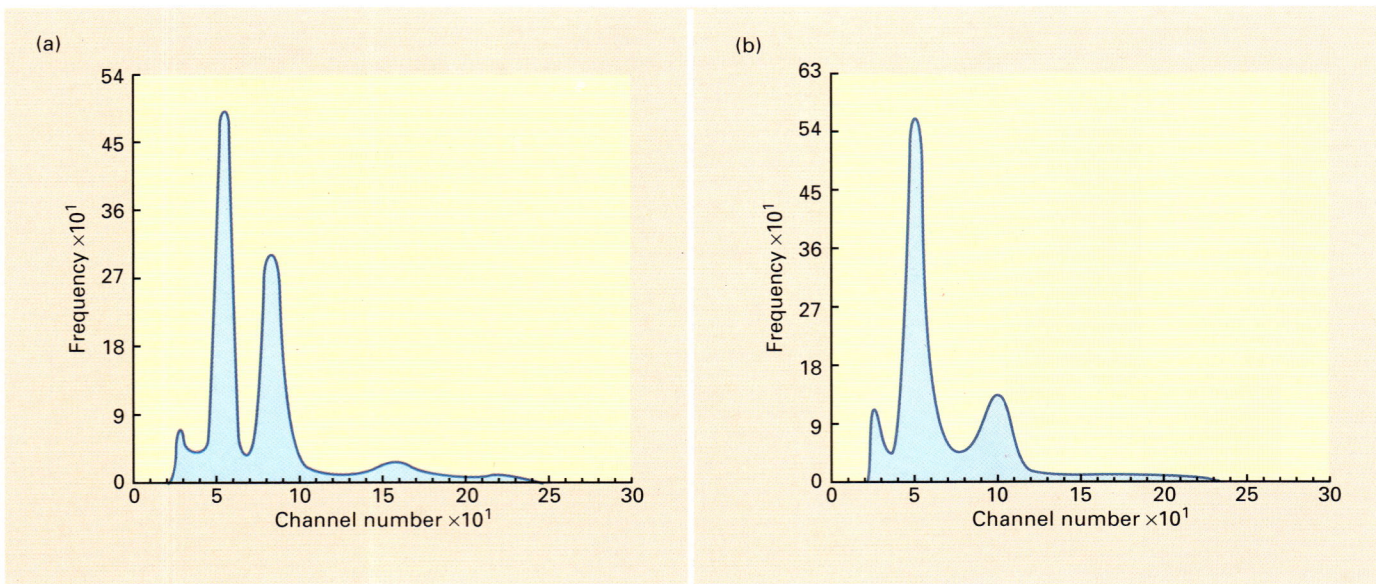

Fig. 30.103 DNA histograms from (a) partial hydatidiform mole and (b) a diploid complete mole. In (a) the first peak (diploid G_0/G_1: 46 chromosomes) represents normal maternal decidua with the second peak (triploid G_0/G_1: 69 chromosomes) derived from the abnormal placental tissue. In (b) the first peak represents the diploid G_0/G_1 (maternal and placental tissue). Accompanying this are elevated S and G_2/M phases, revealing the high degree of cell proliferation seen in this condition. A small polyploid population can be seen stretching out to the right of the DNA histogram. (Drawn after the *Journal of Clinical Pathology*, with permission.)

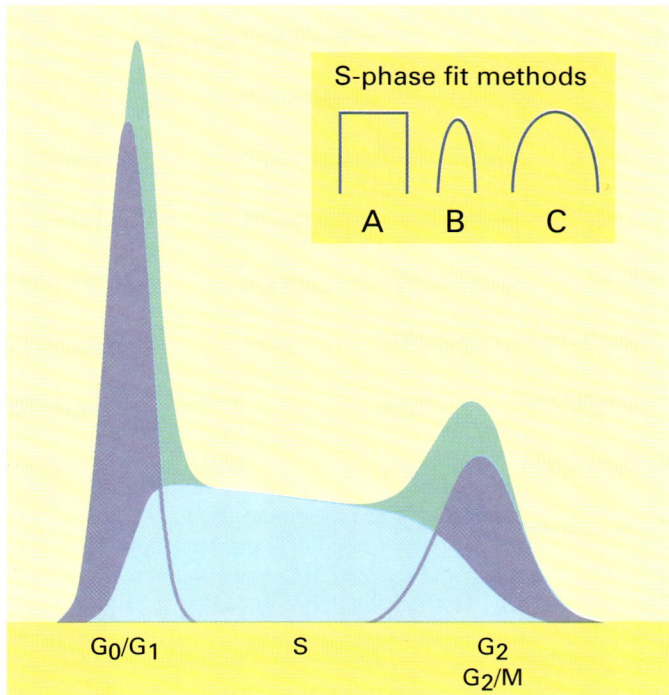

S-phase fit methods

A   B   C

G$_0$/G$_1$ S   G$_2$
G$_2$/M

Fig. 30.104 A DNA histogram broken down into its constituent parts of G_0/G_1, S, and G_2/M phases (or G_2 only if nuclear isolation techniques have been used because mitotic cells are destroyed using this method). S-phase can be calculated by removing the two Gaussian G_0/G_1 and G_2/M peaks from the histogram to give a residual S-phase value, or by integrating the area of S-phase using mathematical methods based on either rectangular (A), Gaussian (B), or polynomial (C) equations.

Treatment

It is known that the sensitivity of cells to radiotherapy is dependent on their DNA content; increasing DNA content suggesting an increased radiosensitivity in a variety of animal tumours with different nuclear DNA content. There is also evidence for increased radiosensitivity of DNA aneuploid cells in human tumours in cervical cancer, acute lymphoblastic leukaemia, and neuroblastoma. Such assessments may in future enable rational planning of the optimum type of therapy where choice exists.

Cytology and semenology

Flow cytometry has been relatively unsuccessful in attempts to automate cervical cytology owing to the relatively high false negative rates reported, but probably has an important role to play in semenology where it is able to assess sperm concentration, viability, and motility, possibly in combination with surface labelling when tests for antisperm antibodies are required.

Other methods

Flow cytometric methods have been developed for a variety of other applications such as the measurement of calcium levels, cytoplasmic pH, membrane potential, and enzymes within individual cells. The unique advantage of flow cytometry lies in the facility for the cross-correlation of results for each individual cell, thus enabling relative assessments to be made of the parameters under study.

30.6.5　Summary

Flow cytometry provides rapid quantitative information in immunology and tumour pathology combined with the ability to separate cell populations. Its use in other areas has been relatively limited owing to the cost of such machines, although with a continuing reduction in price, valuable new diagnostic techniques and applications will emerge in the next 5 years.

30.6.6　Further reading

Beisker, W., Dolbeare, F., and Gray, J. W. (1987). An improved immunocytochemical procedure for high sensitivity detection of incorporated bromodeoxyuridine. *Cytometry* **8**, 235–9.

Evenson, D. P., Darzynkiewicz, Z., and Melamed, M. R. (1982). Simultaneous measurement by flow cytometry of sperm cell viability and mitochondrial membrane potential related to cell motility. *Journal of Histochemistry and Cytochemistry* **30**, 279–80.

Hemming, J. D., Quirke, P., Womack, C., Wells, M., Elston, C. W., and Bird, C. C. (1987). Diagnosis of molar pregnancy and persistent trophoblastic disease by flow cytometry. *Journal of Clinical Pathology* **40**, 615–20.

Quirke, P. and Dyson, J. E. D. (1986). Flow cytometry: methodology and applications in pathology. *Journal of Pathology* **149**, 79–87.

30.7　Future directions in molecular biology

Eric P. H. Yap and James O'D. McGee

Clinical observation defines a disease/syndrome. Its cellular basis gives some insight into the general mechanisms likely to be involved in its pathogenesis. Some of the investigative techniques discussed in this chapter go some way towards elucidating the cellular and molecular events underlying these mechanisms. The aim of this section is to give an overview of two areas which will have an impact on the way pathology will evolve over the next few years—the Human Genome Project and gene sequence screening. These will be important not only in analysing disease processes at a molecular level but also in laboratory diagnosis of disease.

30.7.1　The Human Genome Project

The aim of the Human Genome Project is to determine the complete DNA sequence of the human genome. This does not merely mean elucidating the sequence of the 6 thousand million base pairs (bp) that comprise the human genome, of which only about 10 per cent code for proteins, but also knowing the relative positions (linkage map), structure (physical map), spatial and temporal expression, and functions of the estimated 50 000 genes present. One of the ultimate goals is for this comprehensive atlas of human genetic information to be meaningfully applied across biomedicine, including developmental biology and disease genetics, aetiology, and pathogenesis. At the moment, more than 2000 genes have been sequenced, though the number is expected to grow rapidly with the advent of new technology and intensified efforts.

The genomes of several other organisms are being studied concurrently as models. Ethical and scientific considerations preclude liberal experimental manipulation of humans. Smaller, simpler, and often better characterized genomes offer testing grounds for new strategies and technologies. Protein coding sequences are often conserved between various species and also often exhibit functional homology. The genome mapping project therefore includes study of the genomes of the bacterium *Escherichia coli* (4.7 Mbp), yeast *Saccharomyces cerevisiae* (15 Mbp), water cress *Arabidopsis thaliana* (100 Mbp), the nematode *Caenorhabditis elegans* (80 Mbp), fruit fly *Drosophila melanogaster* (150 Mbp), mouse, and pig. Other species of biotechnological interest such as maize, rice, disease-causing parasites, and domestic mammals may be added to this list in future. Complete DNA sequences of many viruses including phage ϕX174 (5 kbp), simian virus 40 (5 kbp), human papilloma-viruses (8 kbp), bacteriophages T7, and lambda (50 kbp), and the herpesviruses EBV (172 kbp) and CMV (230 kbp) have already been determined.

Mapping the human genome occurs at several levels. At the top of the hierarchy are individual chromosomes containing about 100 million bases, with bands about 10 centiMorgans (10 Mbp) apart. Linkage maps constructed from known polymorphic markers such as restriction fragment polymorphisms (RFLP), minisatellite repeats, variable number tandem repeats (VNTR), and microsatellite dinucleotide sequences (Weber and May 1989) will provide resolutions of 5–10 Mbp. Restriction maps of rare cutting endonucleases have been used to characterize 5 Mbp segments of DNA. Overlapping cloned DNA used as probes (contiguous mapping) are used in the final level, where the DNA in yeast artificial chromosomes (0.5 Mbp), cosmid (50 kbp), phage (20 kbp), and plasmid vectors (1–10 kbp) can be sequenced base by base. Each of these maps is important in the development of the next, and are themselves useful in establishing the location of disease genes.

Several strategies are being used in physically mapping the entire genome. In the 'genomic' approach, DNA segments are systematically analysed and mapped in a sequential manner. This may occur in a top-down fashion, where the entire genome or chromosome is gradually subdivided into regions of smaller and smaller size, or in a bottom-up method, where long range maps are assembled by arranging cloned DNA according to their overlapping regions. Chromosome walking and jumping are terms used to describe the incremental and quantum serial search for DNA of interest (Rommens *et al.* 1989). These methods are used in the isolation of disease genes on the basis of their approximate chromosomal positions ('positional cloning') (Wicking and Williamson 1991).

The 'cDNA' approach has recently been used with success to isolate expressed genes. The mRNA of a normal, developing, or abnormal cell is reverse transcribed to form a library of cDNA sequences, where each of them can subsequently be mapped physically on to chromosomes, sequences, and compared against known sequences for homology. Transcripts from different cells may be semi-quantitatively compared with each other through subtractive hybridization to yield genes uniquely expressed or suppressed in developing, specialized, or diseased cells.

Technological advances have made possible the increasingly rapid and economical sequencing of large tracts of DNA. Mechanical robotization and the use of fluorescent-labelled primers have enabled automated sequencing machines that perform the initial purification, sequencing reactions, electrophoresis, scanning, and data processing, with a potential ouput of 100 kbp of DNA per day (Endo *et al.* 1991). Innovations in DNA fractionation such as capillary and pulsed field gel electrophoresis have increased the speed and enabled the separation of megabases of DNA respectively. Methods have been adapted to sequence directly the products of the polymerase chain reaction, bypassing the cloning step. The use of sequence tagged sites (STS) means that any laboratory can synthesize or analyse mapped unique sequences based on published PCR primers without the need for physical exchange of DNA clones (Olson *et al.* 1989).

Another important aspect of the Human Genome Project is information storage, analysis, retrieval, and dissemination. Internationally accessible databases exist as repositories of DNA sequences (EMBL, Genbank), genes, chromosomal markers and maps (Genome Database), and protein sequences (PIR, Swiss-prot). Sophisticated computer programs enable searching, comparison, and anaysis of stored sequences. However, data verification, protocols of information exchange, and coordination of research plans remain to be fully worked out. While regional efforts are directed by the respective research funding agencies in individual countries (e.g. National Institutes of Health and Department of Energy in the US, the Medical Research Council and others in the UK, and other European and Japanese agencies), the Human Genome Organisation (HUGO) has been formed to co-ordinate international efforts and also investigate other issues such as bioethics and information dissemination.

30.7.2   Gene sequence screening

Introduction

While few of the 2500 Mendelian inherited diseases in man have been characterized at the molecular level, the emphasis and thrust of the Human Genome Project (Section 30.7.1) has been isolating and sequencing disease-associated genes, and the number of such genes known is increasing rapidly. There is, therefore, a growing need to identify perturbations of gene structure and expression in the clinical setting. Gross abnormalities in chromosome structure and gene expression have been detected by karyotyping, and DNA/RNA filter and *in situ* hybridization immunocytochemistry respectively. As many mutations are quite small (e.g. oligonucleotide or single base insertions, deletions, and substitutions), several methods have recently been developed to detect point differences in DNA sequence (Table 30.6). These avoid the need for costly and time-consuming definitive sequencing which may be unnecessary when the mutation–disease association is known. Rapid analysis of large numbers of samples for mutations is now feasible. Many of these techniques have been adapted for DNA amplified *in vitro* by the polymerase chain reaction (PCR) which offers advantages in speed and flexibility in small, impure, or degraded samples such as clinical samples.

Gross mutations

Gross deletions and rearrangements in genomic DNA can be detected by hybridization with cloned probes on filters (Southern, Northern, and dot blots) and *in situ* (see Section 30.3). Moderate-sized deletions or rearrangements can be easily detected by the absence of any PCR product due to absence of one or both primer annealing sites. Using multiple primer pairs, several fragments can be co-amplified in the same tube (multiplex PCR) to screen for deletions that may occur in a large gene with many introns. Insertions and deletions within the amplified segment will yield a product of abnormal size detectable by

Table 30.6 Rapid gene sequence screening and some applications

Method	Example	Reference
I. Gross mutations		
Filter Hybridization: Northern, Southern, dot blots		Section 30.3
In situ hybridization		Section 30.3
Polymerase Chain Reaction (PCR)		Section 30.3
product absence/presence		
product size anomaly		
multiplex PCR (simultaneous coamplification)	dystrophin	Chamberlain *et al.* 1988
II. Point mutations		
A. Known sequence variants		
Polymerase Chain Reaction (PCR)		
allele-specific oligo (ASO) probe hybridization of product		
Southern blot	β-globin	Saiki *et al.* 1988
direct dot blot	N-*ras*	Saiki *et al.* 1986
reverse dot blot	DQA, β-thalassaemia	Saiki *et al.* 1989
loss/gain of restriction site	HbS (β-globin)	Chehab *et al.* 1987
loss/gain of introduced restriction site	Ki-*ras*	Halliassos *et al.* 1989
allele-specific PCR using sequence variant-specific primers	HbS (β-globin)	Wu *et al.* 1989
amplification refractory mutation system (ARMS) using destabilized primers	α_1-anti-trypsin deficiency	Newton *et al.* 1989
colour PCR using fluorescent-labelled primers	HbS (β-globin)	Chehab and Kan 1990
B. Unknown sequence variants		
Nucleotide analogue mobility shift	insulin receptor gene	Kornher and Livak 1989
Heteroduplex electrophoresis		
Agarose		Wenger and Nielsen 1991
Polyacrylamide	Tay–Sachs disease (Hexosaminidase A)	Nagamine *et al.* 1989
Acrylamide-substitute (e.g. Hydrolink)	retinitis pigmentosa (rhodopsin)	Keen *et al.* 1991
Denaturing gradient gel electrophoresis		
Denaturant gradient (DGGE)		Myers *et al.* 1985a
	polymorphisms in Southern blots	Burmeister *et al.* 1991
with GC-clamping	HbS, HbC (β-globin)	Sheffield *et al.* 1989
Temperature gradients (TGGE)	cucumber mosaic virus RNA	Po *et al.* 1987
	quantitative PCR	Henco and Heibey 1990
Temperature-sweep (TGSE)	coliphage gene VIII	Yoshino *et al.* 1991
RNAse A cleavage	β-thalassaemia	Myers *et al.* 1985b
Chemical mismatch cleavage		
Hydroxylamine and osmium teteroxide	human factor IX	Cotton *et al.* 1988
Potassium permanganate	Drosophilia chorion gene	Gogos *et al.* 1990
Carbodiimide modification		
Gel retardation	H-*ras*	Novack *et al.* 1986
Immunoelectronmicroscopy	HbS (β-globin)	Ganguly *et al.* 1989
Primer extension	collagen	Ganguly and Prockop 1990
Single strand conformation polymorphism (SSCP)	*ras*	Orita *et al.* 1989b
Non-isotopic SSCP	Tay–Sachs B1 disease	Ainsworth *et al.* 1990
Two-dimensional SSCP	HRV virus	Kovar *et al.* 1991

electrophoresis on agarose, or polyacrylamide for greater resolution.

Screening for known point mutations

Hybridization of DNA with a labelled oligonucleotide (allele-specific oligonucleotide, ASO) probe is sufficiently discriminatory to detect single base differences if short probes and conditions of high stringency are used. A wide variety of formats have been used for PCR products, including Southern blot, solution hybridization followed by gel electrophoresis, direct dot blot, reverse dot blot, and sandwich capture assays exploiting biotin–avidin affinity binding to solid supports.

Where the base difference spans an endonuclease recognition site, restriction digestion of PCR products followed by agarose gel electrophoresis may be used to distinguish between alleles or between mutant and wild-type sequences. Restriction sites, when absent at the points of interest, may be created by introducing mismatches in the 3' end of PCR primers which are designed to abut the polymorphic/mutation site. Alternatively primers specific to the various expected alleles may be used to amplify selectively particular alleles or mutations at high annealing stringency (allele-specific PCR). In the amplification refractory mutation system (ARMS), a deliberate mismatch is introduced into the 3' end of a primer to increase its specificity. Amplification in the presence of allele/type-specific primers that have been prelabelled with different fluorochromes yields products of different colours.

Screening for small uncharacterized sequence changes

The methods described above are only useful where the site and nature of the sequence variants are known. Other methods are available for screening and discovery of mutations and polymorphisms in unsequenced DNA or sequences longer than those spanned by oligoprobes, primers, and restriction recognition sites. Most of these are based on the detection of heteroduplexes formed between sample DNA and a reference DNA of known sequence, or of known origin, i.e. wild-type. Some heteroduplexes, particularly if they involve deletions spanning at least several base pairs, may migrate with slower mobility in agarose or more obviously in non-denaturing polyacrylamide gels. Single base mismatched duplexes have been separated on Hydrolink gels. Differential electrophoretic mobilities due to varying base content in short DNA sequences can be enhanced by incorporating nucleotide analogs such as biotin-11-dUTP during PCR and detection on a sequencing gel.

The decreased thermal stability of a domain containing a base mismatch is utilized in denaturing gradient gel electrophoresis (DGGE) where the differential mobilities of partially denatured homoduplexes and heteroduplexes are detected on polyacrylamide gels with a gradient of increasing denaturant (formamide and urea), or increasing temperature (TGGE). While the efficacy for mutation detection is increased by the addition of a GC-rich sequence to the 5' end of a PCR primer (GC-clamping), the main disadvantages are the difficulty of pouring such gels and use of radioisotopes, and cost of the setup, respectively. A variant, called temperature sweep gel electrophoresis, whereby the temperature at which a uniform gel is run is gradually increased, may simplify the technique. TGGE has also been used to separate normal from point mutated internal standard product in competitive PCR for quantifying DNA templates. DGGE has been used as an alternative to restriction fragment length polymorphism (RFLP) analysis for identifying polymorphic sequence variation in genomic DNA by Southern blotting.

The differential susceptibility of single- and double-stranded DNA to enzymatic and chemical cleavage may be used to detect the mismatched areas in a heteroduplex. Single-strand nuclease S1 and more effectively, RNase A digestion of the single-stranded parts of a labelled reference RNA probe and target DNA duplex may be used to detect point mutations as well. However, this method requires RNA probe synthesis and is only sensitive for large segments of mismatch. Chemical mismatch cleavage operates on the same principle; piperidine is used to cleave mismatched thymine and cytosine bases that have been modified by osmium tetroxide and hydroxylamine respectively. This method also requires ^{32}P or ^{35}S labelling and the use of various highly toxic chemicals. Potassium permanganate in the presence of tetraalkylammonium salts may be used in place of the more noxious osmium tetroxide and the reactions performed with DNA immobilized on a solid support to simplify the method. A related method is to use carbodiimide to tag mismatched bases; the large molecule retards gel migration of the DNA fragment, can be detected by immunoelectronmicroscopy and also stearically prevents subsequent primer extension at that site.

Relative merits of methodologies

These methods of detecting mutations are simpler than sequencing each base and are useful for screening DNA samples prior to sequencing. The number of methods suggests that no one technique is ideal for all applications (Rossiter and Caskey 1990). Heteroduplex electrophoresis, while simple in principle and practice, does not seem efficacious enough for mutation screening, and so far has been reported for only a few specific mutations. GC-clamped denaturing gradient gel electrophoresis has been reported to be more efficacious in detecting β-glucosidase mutations compared to chemical cleavage and RNase A protection (Theophilus 1989) but is not without its technical difficulties. The same criticism may apply to chemical mismatch cleavage. One distinct advantage of the latter is that it localizes the site of sequence diversion, which is useful when subsequent sequencing of the mutation is performed.

The common disadvantages of the methods mentioned, with exception of heteroduplex electrophoresis, are that they are still relatively time-consuming and inconvenient compared to sample preparation and in vitro DNA amplification technology that is currently available. Furthermore most of these require the use of radioactivity. A reference or wild-type sequence DNA is also required in most of these methods, which precludes their use where such is unavailable, as in screening for genomic polymorphisms. Furthermore, they are only useful where sequences are relatively similar to the original reference sequence such that, firstly, the kinetics of heteroduplex annealing are favourable and secondly, there are one or only a few sites of base mismatches. This may not be so for many situations, such as type/subtype variations in viral sequences. The ideal method is one that is simple, robust, non-isotopic, and which can be routinely employed in most laboratories that are equipped to carry out DNA amplification of samples by PCR. Single strand conformation polymorphism was recently invented and in its modified form, fulfils some of these requirements.

Single strand conformation polymorphism

Single strand conformation polymorphism (SSCP) is based on the principle of denaturing native double-stranded DNA and fractionating the single strands on a non-denaturing polyacrylamide gel. Under the appropriate conditions, the electrophoretic mobility of the DNA is dependent not only on its length and molecular weight, but also on its overall conformation. This secondary structure is determined by the balance between destabilizing thermal forces and weak local stabilizing forces such as short intra-strand base pairings and stackings, which are in turn determined by the primary structure of the strand. In practice, not only do the complementary strands migrate as separate bands on the gel, but small differences in sequence can also be detected. This effect is used in the application of SSCP in mutation and polymorphism analysis (reviewed by Hayashi 1991).

Method

SSCP was first described using Southern blots. Total genomic DNA was restricted, alkali-denatured, electrophoresed on non-denaturing glycerol polyacrylamide gel, transferred to filter, and hybridized to ^{32}P-labelled probes. Polymorphic fragments varied from 100–700 bp, and were detected with *ras* and anonymous probes. Subsequently, SSCP was used to detect polymorphisms and mutations in small sized PCR-amplified genomic DNA or cDNA. ^{32}P is incorporated in the DNA either by 5′ end-labelling of one or both primers. The DNA is then heat or alkali denatured and loaded on to non-denaturing polyacrylamide gel with or without 10 per cent glycerol. Electrophoresis is performed at 4°C or room temperature for 1–6 hours, the gel is fixed and dried, and exposed to X-ray film for 0.5–72 hours.

Recent improvements have been made in the area of non-isotopic DNA detection. Silver-staining has been employed using a semi-automated gel running system. This adaptation avoids the need to prelabel PCR product/primers and is reported to take under 2 hours for electrophoresis and staining. Ethidium bromide staining of gels has recently been shown to be reproducible, sensitive, and rapid for routine analysis of PCR products. Asymmetric PCR can be used to produce only one of the strands, thus reducing overlapping and simplifying patterns obtained from heterozygous sources. The use of primers labelled with different fluorochromes may also be helpful in identifying separate strands.

Modifications of the procedure have been described to overcome the length limitation of 300–400 bp. Long PCR products may be digested with restriction enzymes, the resultant fragments separated on, excised, and eluted from non-denaturing acrylamide gels before SSCP analysis in the usual manner. In two-dimensional SSCP, the DNA is first restricted into smaller fragments which are separated by denaturing capillary electrophoresis, and then run under non-denaturing conditions in the second dimension in a conventional slab SSCP gel. Point mutations in the 2.7 kb long capsid encoding region of HRV14 genome were detected, and the method was claimed to be highly reproducible.

Physical variables While relatively little is known about the secondary structure or conformation of ssDNA under different physical or chemical conditions, several factors have been empirically determined to have an effect on the electrophoretic mobility of ssDNA under non-denaturing conditions.

Temperature destabilizes the weak van der Waals and hydrophilic/phobic forces that are thought to account for the folding of ssDNA, and at high temperatures these forces are overcome and the strands migrate according to the log of their molecular weights. SSCP is therefore usually performed at room temperature or at 4°C. Even at these two temperatures, the conformation of a DNA strand varies as demonstrated by the different relative mobilities of denatured DNA. However base differences can usually be demonstrated at either temperature.

Glycerol has also been found empirically to affect mobility. While bromophenol blue and xylene migrate more slowly in the presence of glycerol, in keeping with its role of increasing the density of the gel, ssDNA tends to migrate faster, though to an unpredictable extent. The mobility differences between variant strands may thus be enhanced or diminished by glycerol. In practice, both gels with and without 5 per cent glycerol are run to maximize the chance of detecting different conformers.

Buffer ionic strength is also a determinant of conformation, though this has not been systematically studied. It is not known if lower ionic concentration of the gel and buffer predisposes to denaturation of secondary structure as it does to interstrand base-pairing.

In a limited study of p53 and HPV mutations, it was determined empirically that optimum conditions for discriminating single base substitutions in SSCP gels on a sequencing gel apparatus were: $0.5 \times$ TBE without glycerol at 4°C and $0.5 \times$ TBE with 5 per cent glycerol at room temperature. There was no significant difference with polyacrylamide concentrations above 6 per cent.

Efficacy There has not been a systematic study of the efficacy of SSCP in detecting either point (base) or larger sequence differences. While the effect of sequence change on electrophoretic mobility is unpredictable, it is unlikely that all single base changes can be detected by SSCP. Occasionally, one of two strands shows a mobility difference while the complementary strand does not. Estimates of sensitivity of between 80 per cent and 99 per cent by empirical and theoretical methods have been quoted, and it is thought that point mutations in smaller (100–300 bp) fragments are more easily detected than in larger (300–400 bp) ones.

Applications

SSCP has been used for the rapid identification of sequence variants in DNA fragments, both for differentiating between known variants of known sequence as well as for identifying the presence of sequence variation between samples (see Table 30.7). These aberrations are termed polymorphisms or mutations depending primarily on the expressed phenotypic manifestation of the gene under investigation, and secondarily on the genetic frequencies of the variants in the general population.

SSCP was initially developed as an alternative for RFLPs of total genomic DNA. Known Mendelian-inherited polymorphisms have been demonstrated on Southern blots. The presence of unknown polymorphisms at particular loci may also be rapidly sought by SSCP. The technique is also useful for identifying known mutations at well characterized sites. Point mutations known to activate cellular proto-oncogenes (e.g. *ras*) can rapidy be detected by this technique. By far the most common application of SSCP is the screening for uncharacterized gene mutations. mRNA of putative tumour suppressor genes

may be analysed for mutations that may inactivate their normal cellular function. Many inborn errors of metabolism can be diagnosed on the basis of specific mutations in genes encoding enzymes and cell proteins.

SSCP has also been used to separate the variant sequences so that a particular variant or allele may be selected for further PCR and direct sequencing. The ability to distinguish single-base differences between target and exogenous control sequences has been used in competitive PCR for the quantification of DNA. In a similar manner, gene dosage can be measured against other genes, or the relative amount of two alleles in a heterozygous genome compared. Loss of heterozygosity implying gene deletion has been detected in this way.

Since it is rapid and convenient, SSCP may be used in many applications where PCR is performed. False positives due to contamination by exogenous cloned DNA can be identified if the plasmid clone contains a sequence that differs from the wild type. Similarly, the amplification of certain viruses (e.g. retroviruses) from different sources is expected to yield sequence

Table 30.7 Single strand conformation polymorphism (SSCP) and some applications in disease*

Application	DNA segment	Disease	Reference
Detection of polymorphisms			
Known			
	D13S2		Orita *et al.* 1989a
	p53	breast cancer	Yap and McGee 1992a
Unknown			
	Alu repeat		Orita *et al.* 1989b
	coding loci		Poduslo *et al.* 1991
	glucose transport gene		Muraoka *et al.* 1991
Detection of mutations			
Known			
	H-*ras*		Orita *et al.* 1989a
	N-*ras*, K-*ras*	cancer cell lines	Orita *et al.* 1989b
	ras	lung cancer	Suzuki *et al.* 1990
Unknown			
	retinoblastoma Rb	lung cancer	Murakami *et al.* 1991
	p53	acute lymphoid leukaemia	Sugimoto *et al.* 1991
		chronic lymphoid leukaemia	Gaidano *et al.* 1991
		cancer cell lines	Mohabeer *et al.* 1991, Murakami *et al.* 1991
		gastric cancer	Tamura *et al.* 1991
	translocation breakpoint region gene	neurofibromatosis NF1	Cawthon *et al.* 1990
	transmembrane conductance regulato gene	cystic fibrosis	Dean *et al.* 1990
	SRY/testis determining factor	XY female	Berta *et al.* 1990
	lipoprotein lipase	hereditary lipolytic deficiency	Hata *et al.* 1991, Hegele *et al.* 1991
	phenylalanine hydroxylase PAH gene	phenylketonuria	Labrune *et al.* 1990, Dockhorn *et al.* 1991
	factor IX	haemophilia B	Demers *et al.* 1990
	dopamine D2 receptor gene	?alcoholism	Bolos *et al.* 1990
	hexosaminidase A (Hex A)	Tay–Sachs disease	Ainsworth *et al.* 1991
	vitamin D receptor	rickets	Saijo *et al.* 1991
	human papillomavirus		Spinardi *et al.* 1991
Separation of variant sequences for further analysis			
	lipoprotein lipase	hereditary lipolytic deficiency	Hata *et al.* 1990, Suzuki *et al.* 1991
Quantification of gene dosage			
	p53	breast cancer	Yap and McGee 1992b

* See text for further applications.

variation; this can be detected by SSCP, and lack of heterogeneity may imply contamination by one DNA sequence. The fidelity of Taq polymerase extension may also be checked by SSCP in instances where *in vitro* mutation has to be excluded (e.g. indirect sequencing of PCR products). When combined with other allele detection methods (e.g. ARMS), SSCP may be effective in discriminating poly-allelic loci (e.g. HLA).

30.7.3   Further reading

General reading

Hayashi, K. (1991). PCR-SSCP: a simple and sensitive method for detection of mutations in the genomic DNA. *PCR Methods and Applications* 1, 34–8.

Herrington, C. S. and McGee, J. O'D. (1992). *Diagnostic molecular pathology*. Vols 1, 2. Oxford University Press.

Maddox, J. (1991). The case for the human genome. *Nature* 352, 11–14.

Rossiter, B. J. F. and Caskey, C. T. (1990). Molecular scanning methods of mutation detection. *Journal of Biological Chemistry* 265, 12753–6.

Watson, J. D. (1990). The human genome project: past, present and future. *Science* 248, 44–9.

Weatherall, D. J. (1991). *The new genetics and clinical practice* (3rd edn). Oxford University Press.

Human Genome Project

Endo, I., Soeda, E., Murakami, Y., and Nishi, K. (1991). Human genome analysis system. *Nature* 352, 89–90.

Little, P. F. R. (1990). Gene mapping and the human genome mapping project. *Current Opinion in Cell Biology* 2, 478–84.

Olson, M., Hood, L., Cantor, C., and Botstein, D. (1989). A common language for physical mapping of the human genome. Science 245, 1434–5.

Rommens, J. M., et al. (1989). Identification of the cystic fibrosis gene: chromosome walking and jumping. *Science* 245, 1059–65.

Weber, J. L. and May, P. E. (1989). Abundant class of human DNA polymorphisms which can be typed using the polymerase chain reaction. *American Journal of Human Genetics* 44, 388–96.

Wicking, C. and Williamson, R. (1991). From linked marker to gene. *Trends in Genetics* 7, 288–93.

Gene sequence screening

Burmeister, M. diSibio, G., Cox, D. R., and Myers, R. M. (1991). Identification of polymorphisms by genomic denaturing gradient gel electrophoresis: application to the proximal region of human chromosome 21. *Nucleic Acids Research* 19, 1475–81.

Chamberlain, J. S., Gibbs, R. A., Ranier, J. E., Nguyen, P. N., and Caskey, C. T. (1988). Deletion screening of the Duchenne muscular dystrophy locus via multiplex DNA amplification. *Nucleic Acids Research* 16, 11141–56.

Chehab, F. F., et al. (1987). Detection of sickle cell anaemia and thalassaemias. *Nature* 329, 293–4.

Chehab, F. F. and Kan, Y. W. (1990). Detection of sickle cell anaemia mutation by colour DNA amplification. *Lancet* 335, 15–7.

Cotton, R. G. H., Rodrigues, N. R., and Campbell, R. D. (1988). Reactivity of cytosine and thymine in single-base-pair mismatches with hydroxylamine and osmium textroxide and its application to the study of mutations. *Proceedings of the National Academy of Science USA* 85, 4397–401.

Ganguly, A., Rooney, J. E., Hosomi, S., Zeiger, A. R., and Prockop, D. J. (1989). Detection and location of single-base mutations in large DNA fragments by immunomicroscopy. *Genomics* 4, 530–8.

Ganguly, A. and Prockop, D. J. (1990). Detection of single-base mutations by reaction of DNA heteroduplexes with a water-soluble carbodiimide followed by primer extension: application to products from the polymerase chain rection. *Nucleic Acids Research* 18, 3933–9.

Gogos, J. A., Karayiorgou, M., Aburatani, H., and Kafatos, F. C. (1990). Detection of single base mismatches of thymine and cytosine residues by potassium permanganate and hydroxylamine in the presence of tetralkylammonium salts. *Nucleic Acids Research* 18, 6807–14.

Haliassos, A., et al. (1989). Modification of enzymatically amplified DNA for the detection of point mutations. *Nucleic Acids Research* 17, 3606.

Henco, K. and Heibey, M. (1990). Quantitative PCR: the determination of template copy number by temperature gradient gel electrophoresis. *Nucleic Acids Research* 18, 6733–4.

Keen, J., Lester, D., Inglehearn, C., Curtis, A., and Bhattacharya, S. (1991). Rapid detection of single base mismatches as heteroduplexes on Hydrolink gels. *Trends in Genetics* 7, 5.

Kornher, J. S. and Livak, K. J. (1989). Mutation detection using nucleotide analogs that alter electrophoretic mobility. *Nucleic Acids Research* 17, 7779–84.

Myers, R. M., Lumelsky, N., Lerman, L., and Maniatis, T. (1985a). Detection of single base substitutions in total genomic DNA. *Nature* 313, 495–8.

Myers, R. M., Larin, Z., and Maniatis, T. (1985b). Detection of single base substitutions by ribonuclease cleavage at mismatches in RNA:DNA duplexes. *Science* 230, 1242–6.

Nagamine, C. M., Chan, K., and Lau, Y.-F. C. (1989). A PCR artifact: generation of heteroduplexes. *American Journal of Human Genetics* 45, 337–9.

Newton, C. R., et al. (1989). Analysis of any point mutation in DNA: The amplification refractory mutation system. *Nucleic Acids Research* 17, 2503–16.

Novack, D. F., Casna, N. J., Fischer, S. G., and Ford, J. P. (1986). Detection of single base-pair mismatches in DNA by chemical modification followed by gel electrophoresis in 15% polyacrylamide gel. *Proceedings of the National Academy of Science USA* 83, 586–90.

Po, T., Steger, G., Rosenbaum, V., Kaper, J., and Riesner, D. (1987). Double-stranded cucumovirus associated RNA 5: experimental analysis of necrogenic and non-necrogenic variants by temperature-gradient gel electrophoresis. *Nucleic Acids Research* 15, 5069–83.

Saiki, R. K., Bugawan, T. L., Horn, G. T., Mullis, K. B., and Erlich, H. A. (1986). Analysis of enzymatically amplified β-globin and HLA-DQα DNA with allele-specific oligonucleotide probes. *Nature* 324, 163–6.

Saiki, R. K., et al. (1988). Primer-directed enzymatic amplification of DNA with a thermostable DNA polymerase. *Science* 239, 487–91.

Saiki, R. K., Walsh, P. S., Levenson, C. H., and Erlich, H. A. (1989). Genetic analysis of amplified DNA with immobilized sequence-specific oligonucleotide probes. *Proceedings of the National Academy of Science USA* 86, 6230–4.

Sheffield, V. C., Cox, D. R., Lerman, L. S., and Myers, R. M. (1989). Attachment of a 40-base-pair G + C rich sequence (GC-clamp) to genomic DNA fragments by the polymerase chain reaction results in improved detection of single-base changes. *Proceedings of the National Academy of Science USA* 86, 232–6.

Shenk, T. E., Rhodes, C., Rigby, P. W. J., and Berg, P. (1975). Biochemical method for mapping mutational alterations in DNA with S1 nuclease: the location of deletions and temperature-sensitive mutations in simian virus 40. *Proceedings of the National Academy of Science USA* **72**, 989–93.

Theophilus, B. D. M., Latham, T., Grabowski, G. A., and Smith, F. I. (1989). Comparison of RNAse A, a chemical cleavage and GC-clamped denaturing gradient gel electrophoresis for the detection of mutations in exon 9 of the human acid β-glucosidase gene. *Nucleic Acids Research* **17**, 7707–22.

Wenger, R. H. and Nielsen, P. J. (1991). Reannealing of artificial heteroduplexes generated during PCR-mediated genetic isotyping. *Trends in Genetics* **7**, 178.

Wu, D. Y., Ugozzoli, L., Pal, B. K., and Wallace, B. (1989). Allele-specific enzymatic amplification of β-globin genomic DNA for diagnosis of sickle cell anemia. *Proceedings of the National Academy of Science USA* **86**, 2757–60.

Yoshino, K., Nishigaki, K., and Husimi, Y. (1991). Temperature sweep gel electrophoresis: a simple method to detect point mutations. *Nucleic Acid Research* **19**, 3153.

Single-strand conformation polymorphism

Ainsworth, P. J., Surh, L. C., and Coulter-Mackie, M. B. (1991). Diagnostic single strand conformation polymorphism (SSCP): a simplified non-radioisotopic method as applied to a Tay–Sachs B1 variant. *Nucleic Acids Research* **19**, 405.

Berta, P., *et al.* (1990). Genetic evidence equating SRY and the testis-determining factor. *Nature* **348**, 448–50.

Bolos, A. M., *et al.* (1990). Population and pedigree studies reveal a lack of association between dopamine D2 receptor gene and alcoholism. *Journal of the American Medical Association* **264**, 3156–60.

Cawthon, R. M., *et al.* (1990). A major segment of the neurofibromatosis type I gene: cDNA sequence, genomic structure, and point mutations. *Cell* **62**, 193–201.

Dean, M., *et al.* (1990). Multiple mutations in highly conserved residues are found in mildly affected cystic fibrosis patients. *Cell* **61**, 863–70.

Dean, M. and Gerrard, B. (1991). Helpful hints for the detection of single-stranded conformation polymorphisms. *Biotechniques* **10**, 332–3.

Demers, D. B., Odelberg, S. J., and Fisher, L. McA. (1990). Identification of a factor IX point mutation using SSCP analysis and direct sequencing. *Nucleic Acids Research* **18**, 5575.

Dockhorn-Dworniczak, B., *et al.* (1991). Non-isotopic detection of single strand conformation polymorphism (PCR-SSCP): a rapid and sensitive technique in diagnosis of phenylketonuria. *Nucleic Acids Research* **19**, 2500.

Gaidano, G. L., *et al.* (1991). p53 mutations in Ph negative chronic myeloproliferative disorders: analysis by SSCP method and direct sequencing. *Experimental Haematology* **19**, 540.

Hata, A., Robertson, M., Emi, M., and Lalouel, J.-M. (1990). Direct detection and automated sequencing of individual alleles after electrophoretic strand and separation: identification of a common nonsense mutation in exon 9 of the human lipoprotein lipase gene. *Nucleic Acids Research* **18**, 5407–11.

Hegele, R. A., *et al.* (1991). A hepatic lipase gene mutation associated with heritable lipolytic deficiency. *Journal of Clinical Endocrinology and Metabolism* **72**, 730–2.

Kovar, H., Jug, G., Auer, H., Skem, T., and Blaas, D. (1991). Two dimensional single-strand conformation polymorphism analysis: a useful tool for the detection of mutations in long DNA fragments. *Nucleic Acids Research* **19**, 3507–10.

Labrune, P., *et al.* (1991). Single-strand conformation polymorphism for detection of mutations and base substitutions in phenylketonuria. *American Journal of Human Genetics* **38**, 1115–20.

Mohabeer, A. J., Hiti, A. L., and Martin, W. J. (1991). Non-radioactive single strand conformation polymorphism (SSCP) using the Pharmacia 'PhastSystem'. *Nucleic Acids Research* **19**, 3154.

Murakami, Y., Hayashi, K., and Sekiya, T. (1991). Detection of aberrations of the p53 alleles and the gene transcript in human tumor cells lines by single-strand conformation polymorphism analysis. *Cancer Research* **51**, 3356–61.

Murakami, Y., *et al.* (1991). Inactivation of the retinoblastoma gene in a human lung cancer carcinoma cell line detected by single-strand conformation analysis of the polymerase chain reaction product of cDNA. *Oncogene* **6**, 37–42.

Muraoka, A., Sakura, H., Kishimoto, M., Akanuma, Y., Buse, J. B., *et al.* (1991). Polymorphism in exon 4AA of the human GLUT4 muscle-fat facilitative glucose transport gene detected by SSCP. *Nucleic Acids Research* **19**, 4313.

Orita, M., Iwahana, H., Kanazawa, H., Hayashi, K., and Sekiya, T. (1989a). Detection of polymorphisms of human DNA by gel electrophoresis as single-strand conformation polymorphisms. *Proceedings of the National Academy of Science USA* **86**, 2766–70.

Orita, M., Suzuki, Y., Sekiya, T., and Hayashi, K. (1989b). Rapid and sensitive detection of point mutations and DNA polymorphisms using the polymerase chain reaction. *Genomics* **5**, 874–9.

Orita, M., Sekiya, T., and Hayashi, K. (1990). DNA sequence polymorphisms in Alu repeats. *Genomics* **8**, 271–8.

Poduslo, S. E., Dean, M., Kolch, U., and O'Brien, S. J. (1991). Detecting high-resolution polymorphisms in human coding loci by combining PCR and single-strand conformation polymorphism (SSCP) analysis. *American Journal of Human Genetics* **49**, 106–11.

Saijo, T., *et al.* (1991). A unique mutation in the vitamin-D receptor gene in 3 Japanese patients with vitamin-D dependent rickets type-II—utility of single-strand conformation polymorphism analysis for heterozygous carrier detection. *American Journal of Human Genetics* **49**, 668–73.

Spinardi, L., Mazars, R., and Theillet, C. (1991). Protocols for an improved detection of point mutations by SSCP. *Nucleic Acids Research* **19**, 4009.

Sugimoto, K., *et al.* (1991). Mutations of the p53 gene in lymphoid leukaemia. *Blood* **77**, 1153–6.

Suzuki, Y., Orita, M., Shiraishi, M., Hayashi, K., and Sekiya, T. (1990). Detection of ras gene mutations in human lung cancers by single-strand conformation analysis of polymerase chain reaction products. *Oncogene* **5**, 1037–43.

Suzuki, Y., Sekiya, T., and Hayashi, K. (1991). Allele-specific polymerase chain reaction: a method for amplification and sequence determination of a single component among a mixture of sequence variants. *Analytical Biochemistry* **192**, 82–4.

Tamura, G., *et al.* (1991). Detection of frequent p53 gene mutations in primary gastric cancer by cell sorting and polymerase chain reaction single-strand conformation polymorphism analysis. *Cancer Research* **51**, 3056–8.

Yap, E. P. H. and McGee, J. O'D. (1992a). Nonisotopic SSCP detection in PCR products by ethidium bromide staining. *Trends in Genetics* (in press).

Yap, E. P. H. and McGee, J. O'D. (1992b). Nonisotopic SSCP and competitive PCR for DNA quantification: p53 in breast cancer cells. *Nucleic Acids Research* (in press).

Index

The alphabetical arrangement is letter-by-letter.

Page numbers in **bold** indicate major discussions; those in *italics* indicate tables.

The following abbreviations have been used in sub-headings: ACTH, adrenocorticotrophic hormone; CNS, central nervous system; CSF, cerebrospinal fluid; G-CSF, granulocyte colony-stimulating factor; GH, growth hormone; HBV, hepatitis B virus; HCV, hepatitis C virus; HDL, high-density lipoprotein; HIV, human immunodeficiency virus; HPV, human papilloma virus; MHC, major histocompatibility complex; PRL, prolactin; RFLP, restriction fragment length polymorphisms; TSH, thyroid-stimulating hormone; UV, ultraviolet; VIP, vasoactive intestinal polypeptide.

Bruch's membrane (*cont.*)
 tumour-induced rupture 1919, 1920
Brugia malayi 928, 2240
 see also filariasis, lymphatic
Brugia timori 928
Brunner's glands 1177
Brunn's nests 566, 1516, 1520
brush-border cells, small intestine 35, 1176, 1177
brush cytology
 bronchi 2316
 oesophagus 1148
BSC-1 growth inhibitor *678*
buccal mucosa 1053, 1054
Budd–Chiari syndrome 921, **1344**, 1421
 chronic, hepatocellular carcinoma and 1392
 inferior vena cava webs 1292
 liver transplant recipients 1400
Buerger disease (thromboangiitis obliterans) 846, 919–20
bulbo-urethral (Cowper's) glands 1516
bullae, skin 2141
bullous ichthyosiform erythroderma 2143
bull's neck, diphtheria 954
Büngner, bands of 1898, 1899
bunyaviruses, entry into host cells 445
buphthalmos 1903
Burkitt-like lymphoma 1782
Burkitt lymphoma (BL) **1781–2**
 endemic 1781–2
 Epstein–Barr virus and 652, 691, 1765, 1782, 2197
 malaria and 652, 691, 1782, 2196–7
 non-endemic 1782
burns
 Curling ulcers 550
 hypovolaemic shock 541
 neutrophil function 328
 thrombosis 513
bursae 2075, **2093**
Bursa of Fabricius 1689
bursitis 2093
burst lobe, head injury 1927
Buschke–Loewenstein, giant condyloma of 1279, 2170
bush teas 1345
busulphan 692, 987
butazolidin, hepatotoxicity *1332*
butylated hydroxytoluene (BHT) 725
Byler disease *1352, 1365*

C1
 activation 260–1
 deficiency 265
C1 inhibitor 260–1
C1q
 deposits in glomerulonephritis 1459
 IgG binding 222–3
C2 200, 261
 deficiency 265, 278

C3 259, 261
 cleavage reaction 259, 260, 263
 deficiency 225, 265, 392
 deposits in glomerulonephritis 1459, 1462, 1463, 1464
 nephritic factor 1464, 1465
 receptors, *see* complement receptors
 serum levels in glomerulonephritis 1459, 1464, 1465
C3a 259
 functions 264, 363, 438
 type II hypersensitivity reaction 277
C3b 363, 438
 cleavage 260, 261, 263
 cofactors for cleavage 262, 264
 function 223, 225, 277
C3bi
 formation 259, 260, 263
 phagocytosis and 358, 363
 receptors 263, 264
C3d 207
C4 259, 261
 deficiency 265, 278
C4a 200, 261, 264
C4b 200, 261
C5 261
C5a 261
 functions 264, 277, 363, 438
 receptors 322
C5b6 261
C5bC789 261, 438
C6 261
C7 261, 481
C8 261, 481
C9 155, 261–2, 481
Ca-1 antigen 707
CA19-9 antigen, pancreatic carcinoma 1447
cachectin, *see* tumour necrosis factor
cachexia **715–17**
 animal models 715
 associated problems 717
 clinical and laboratory features 715–16
 management 717
 pathogenesis 716–17
cadmium
 aminoaciduria 1499
 pulmonary reaction *721*
caecocystoplasties, carcinomas in 1526
caecum 1178
 solitary diverticulum 1258
Caenorhabditis elegans, trans-splicing 94
caeruloplasmin 1290–1, 1363
café-au-lait spots 1902
caffeine/coffee
 analgesic nephropathy and 1483
 pancreatic carcinoma and 1444
caisson disease (decompression sickness) **523–4**, 1010, 1928
CAH, *see* hepatitis, chronic active
Calabar (fugitive) swellings 2242, 2243
calcification
 aortic valve 870, 904
 arterial 846

calcification (*cont.*)
 atherosclerotic plaques 801
 breast carcinoma 1676, 1678
 breast cysts 1672, 1673
 cardiac valves 868
 cytoplasmic deposits 172, 173, 174
 dystrophic 527
 endomyocardial, cardiac grafts 897
 menisci 2093
 metastatic 1963
 mitral ring 868, 874, 875
 mitral valve 872, 874
 renal 1489, 1490, 1511–12
calcifying aponeurotic fibroma 2109
calcitonin (CT)
 ectopic tumour-derived *695*, 696, **702**, 1041
 gene, splicing 97
 hepatocyte proliferation and 1385
 mineral homeostasis 1962, 2023
 thyroid medullary carcinoma *581*, 702, 1958
 thyroid secretion 1941
calcitonin gene-related peptide (CGRP) 97, 702, 1270, 2023
 cardiovascular system *2012*
 endocrine amyloid and 2001
 gastrointestinal tract *1184*
 genitourinary system 2014, 2015
 inflammatory activity 364
 pancreatic nerves 1999
 respiratory tract *2010*, 2011, 2012
 skin *2015*
calcium (Ca^{++})
 absorption 736, 740
 blood coagulation 505, 506, 507
 bone 2021
 cytosolic
  apoptosis and 146, 147
  epidermal growth factor receptor regulation 677
  injured cells 182
  mast cell/basophil activation 333
  mechanisms of cytotoxicity and **189–91**
  menadione toxicity and 193
  necrosis and **153**
  neutrophil activation and 325
  paracetamol toxicity and 192
  regulation 189
 dietary requirements *732*
 function 737
 gastrin stimulation 2005
 histochemistry 2274
 hormonal regulation of serum levels 1961–2, 2023
 mitochondrial overloading 163–4
 platelet contraction and 510, 511
 supplements 1968
 see also hypercalcaemia; hypocalcaemia

calcium bilirubinate 1404, 1406
calcium carbonate, gallstones 1404
calcium-containing renal stones 1494
calcium pyrophosphate dihydrate (CPPD) crystal deposition 2079, **2088–9**
 menisci 2093
 osteoarthritis 2085, 2088, 2089
calcospherites, pituitary adenoma cells 1935
calculus, dental 1097
 subgingival 1093
California encephalitis *1842*
CALLA, *see* CD10
Call–Exner bodies 1625
callus, fracture 2028–9
 external 2028–9
 intermediate 2029
 internal 2029
 provisional 2029
calorimetry 738
calpains 189
calpastatin 189, 190
Calve disease 2031
Calymmatobacterium granulomatis 1574
CAM 120/180 26
Campbell de Morgan spots (cherry angiomas) 931
Campylobacter coli 1223
Campylobacter infections 1209, 1210, 1222, **1223**
 reactive arthritis 2083
Campylobacter jejuni 467, 1223
Campylobacter pylori, see Helicobacter pylori
CAMs, *see* cell adhesion molecules
canalis reuniens 1106
canal of Schlemm 1904, 1905
cancer
 age-related incidence 679–80
 animals 571
 causes
  general 681–3
  specific cancers 683–94
 definitions *in vivo* 571–3
 epidemiology **679–94**
 genes 114–15, 124–5
  see also tumour suppressor genes
 gene therapy 630–1
 genetic/environmental interaction 644–5, 646
 genetic susceptibility 644–7
 history 571
 immunology **706–9**
 immunotherapy 629, 630, 708–9, 712
 infection susceptibility 441
 in vitro criteria of malignancy 573–7
 latent period 634, 680–1
 microscopic appearance 572–3
 nomenclature 572
 primary 572
 secondary 572
 sex-related incidence 680, *681*
 'suture-line' 375, 378–9
 virus-induced, *see* virus-induced cancer

cytokeratins (*cont.*)
cultured keratinocytes 40
immunocytochemistry *581*, 2282
malignant mesothelioma 1047, 1048
mesothelial cells 1042
oral mucosa cells 1053, 1061
oral squamous cell carcinoma 1061
pancreatic carcinoma 1446
thymic epithelial cells 1808–9
tumour classification *581*, 584–5
cytokines 556
antimicrobial activity 438
bone, effects on 2024
endothelial cell 498–9
hypercalcaemia of malignancy 698, 699
inflammatory activity 363–4
macrophages and 238–9, *240*
mediating T–B interaction 268–9
natural killer cells and 346–7
in neoplasia **709–15**
networks 711
polarized secretion 268
T-cell production 232
see also specific cytokines
cytology
cervical 1593–4, 2303–14
corpus uteri 2314–15
exfoliative **2301–27**
fine-needle aspiration, *see* fine-needle aspiration biopsy
flow cytometry in 2337
iatrogenic pathology 2325–6
pancreatic 1447
respiratory tract 2315–20
serous effusions 2320–4
urinary tract 2324–5
vagina 2314
vulva 2314
cytolysis, cervical smear cells 2306, 2307
cytomegalic inclusion disease 962
cytomegalovirus (CMV) 651
AIDS and HIV infection 288
cardiac graft recipients 897, 898
colitis 1230
encephalitis 1839–40, **1846**
eye infections 1909
fetal/neonatal infection 450, 787, 953
brain pathology 1846, 1924
parotid glands 1072–3
gastritis 1154
gastroenteritis 1214
liver involvement 1298
liver transplant recipients 1400
lymphadenopathy 1765
oesophageal lesions 1143
persistence 485
pneumonia 962–3
reactivation 485
renal graft recipients 315
respiratory tract cytology 2317
salivary glands 1072–3
skin lesions 2165
cytometry, flow, *see* flow cytometry
cytopathic effect (cpe), viral 450
cytopathology 1593

cytopathology (*cont.*)
exfoliative **2301–27**
accuracy 2301–2
advantages and limitations 2301
clinical applications 2303
Papanicolaou smear 2302
principles 2301
reporting principles 2302
viral 450
cytoplasm **8–25**
determinants in embryos 39–40
granules 20–4
membrane systems 11–13
cytoplasmic inclusions *149*, **172–5**
cytosine arabinoside (ara-C)
hepatotoxicity 1340
pulmonary oedema 989
small intestinal effects 380, 381
cytoskeleton **15–19**
calcium-mediated alterations **190**
injured cells 167
metastatic cells 619–20
tissue-specific variation **34–6**
cytosol 11
cytotoxic drugs
carcinogenicity 664, 1717
exfoliative cytopathology and 2326
intestinal crypt regeneration after 380, 381
intestinal toxicity 1200
leucopenia/neutropenia induction 1705–6
neurotoxicity 1863, *1864*
teratogenicity 783
wound healing and 374
cytotoxic T cells, *see* T-cytotoxic cells
cytotrophoblast cells,
choriocarcinoma 1558, 1560, 1629, 1638

D1-cells, gastric mucosa 1150
Dacron, vascular grafts 903
Dandy–Walker malformation 1923
Dane particle 1295, 1301
dantrolene, hepatotoxicity 1335
dapsone 1334, 1701
Darier–Pautrier microabscesses 2184
Darier–Roussy disease 2163
Darier disease (follicular keratosis) **2143–5**
differential diagnosis 2144–5
daunorubicin, adverse reactions 886
D-cells, gastric mucosa 1150
D cells (δ-cells), pancreatic 1998, 1999, 2000
DDT **726–7**, 728
debrisoquine 1331
decalcifying agents 2271
decamethrin 729
decay accelerating factor (DAF) 262
decidualization
endometrium 1595, 1596
Fallopian tube 1610
decompression sickness (caisson disease) **523–4**, 1010, 1928
dedifferentiation 40–1

defence mechanisms **197–347**, 415–16
impairments 435, **440–1**
non-specific 197, 415–16, *436*
deeper **438–9**
directional flow 437–8
impaired *440*
mechanical barriers 437
normal commensal flora 435–7
surface **435–8**
surface secretions 437
respiratory tract 197, 437, 947, 956
specific, *see* immune response
urinary tract 437–8, 1477–8
see also immunity
defensins 323
definitive host 2189
degenerative nervous system diseases 1873–83
dehydration 743
renal cortical necrosis 1490
renal vein thrombosis 1473
thirst in 731
dehydroepiandrosterone (DHA) 1971
dehydroepiandrosterone (DHA) sulphate 1970, 1971
deiodinase 1942
Del Castillo syndrome 1553
deletions, *see* chromosome deletions; chromosome microdeletions; gene deletions
delirium tremens 754
delta agent, *see* hepatitis D virus
δ-cells (D cells), pancreatic 1998, 1999, 2000
dementia
alcoholic 1857
Alzheimer disease 1879
dialysis 1861
malignant disease 1862
Parkinson disease 1876
Pick disease 1880
senile, amyloid deposits 411
Demodex folliculorum 2164
demolition phase
infarction 527
wound healing 367
demyelinating diseases
central nervous system **1867–73**
peripheral nervous system 1867, 190, 1902
demyelination 1867
multiple sclerosis 1871–2
peripheral nerves 1897, **1899–900**, 1899
denaturation, nucleic acids 2286, 2290
dendritic cells 242
antigen presentation 200, 267, 270
follicular (dendritic reticulum cells) 207, 208–9
antigen presentation 200, 267, 270
immunocytochemistry 1749
lymph nodes 1746–8
malignant lymphoma
centrocytic 1780–1

dendritic cells (*cont.*)
follicular (dendritic reticulum cells) (*cont.*)
Peyer's patches 1752–3
graft rejection and 308
interdigitating, *see* interdigitating dendritic/reticulum cells
Steinman–Cohn 237, 242, 251
thymus 1809, 1811, 1813
dendritic ulcer, herpes simplex 1909
dengue haemorrhagic fever 451
Dennovillier's fascia 1541
dense bodies, platelet 503
dense-body deficiency *1733*, 1734
dense tubular system, platelets 510, 511
dens invaginatus *1087*
dental abscess 473, **1083**
caries-associated 1099, 1101, 1102
paradontal 1083
periapical 1083
dental caries **1096–102**
aetiology 1097
dentine 1099–101
enamel 1097–9
epidemiology 1096–7
root 1096, 1097, 1099
xerostomia 1069
dental follicle 1081, 1082
dental infections, acute 473
dental lamina rests 1081, 1082
dental plaque 1091
microbiology 471, 1092–3
pathogenesis of periodontal disease and 1094–5
role in dental caries 1097
subgingival 1092, 1093
dental pulp, caries involvement 1099–101
dental work, infective endocarditis and 875
dentate line 1181
dentine
caries 1099–101
development 1082
dentinoma *1087*
dentures, ill-fitting 392
deoxycorticosterone (DOC) 1971, 1979
adrenal lesions producing 1984
adrenocortical carcinoma producing 1983
11-deoxycortisol 1971
deoxyribonuclease, *see* DNase
deoxyribonucleic acid, *see* DNA
depression
hypoparathyroidism 1966
manic 124
pituitary adenomas and 1935
serotonin and 1830
de Quervain thyroiditis 1951, **1953**
dermal nerve sheath myxoma 2124–5
dermatan sulphate *37*, 59, 60
dermatitis **2149–511**
acute and subacute 2149–51
clinical features 2149–50
differential diagnosis 2150–1
histopathology 2150

nephropathy (*cont.*)
  reflux 1480
nephrotic syndrome
  congenital **1455**
  glomerulonephritis 1456
  oedema **537–8**
  quartan malaria 2195–6, 2197
  renal vein thrombosis 1473
nephrotoxic nephritis 1469
nerve biopsy 1863, 1902
nerve conduction velocities,
    demyelinating disease 1900,
    1902
nerve fibres, *see* axons
nerve growth factor (NGF) *676*,
    1883
  receptor *676*, 1903
nerves, peripheral, *see* peripheral
    nerves
nerve sheath cell tumours **1892–3**
nerve sheath myxoma, peripheral
    2124–5
nerve sheath tumour, malignant
    peripheral (MPNST) 2125–6
nervous system **1825–928**
  cell structure and function
    1825–33
  degenerative diseases 1873–83
  healing and regeneration 385–6
  hypoxia **1833–5**
  infections 1835–50
  metabolic disorders 1856–66
  microglia, *see* microglia
  radiation-induced damage 775
  type I hypersensitivity reaction
    275
  vascular malformations 917,
    1855–6, 1894
  see also central nervous system;
    enteric nervous system
nesidioblastosis 2001–2, 2005
neu oncogene, *see* c-*erb B2* oncogene
neural cell adhesion molecule
    (NCAM) 26, 38, 222
neural-glial cell adhesion molecule
    (NgCAM) 26, 38
neural tube defects 783, 1923
neural tumours **1883–97**
  aetiology and pathogenesis
    1883–5
  anterior pituitary, *see* pituitary
    tumours
  congenital 1884–5
  epidemiology 693, 1883
  familial 1885
  gastrointestinal tract 1172,
    1268, 1274
  general features 1885–6
  germ cell tumours 1894–5
  grading and classification 1886
  immunocytochemistry *581*
  local extension from regional
    tumours 1895
  malformative tumours and
    tumour-like lesions 1895
  meningeal and related tissues
    1893
  metastatic 1895–6
  nerve sheath cells 1892–3
  neuro-epithelial 1886–92

neural tumours (*cont.*)
  primary malignant lymphomas
    1893–4
  vascular 1894
  see also brain tumours
neuraminidase (N) 445, 464, 513
neurilemmoma, *see* schwannoma
neuritis, retrobulbar 1868
neuroblastoma 572, 791, **1887**,
    1989–91
  cerebral 1887
  clinical course 1990, 2071
  familial syndromes and associated
    lesions 1991
  immunocytochemistry 580
  in situ 1990
  morphology 1990
  N-*myc* expression 1885, 1990
  olfactory **1117**
  origin 1884–5
  peripheral 1887
  recessive genes 114, 115
neuroblasts 1989, 1991, 1992
neurocysticercosis 1848, 2249,
    2250
neurocytoma, central 1891
neuroectodermal tumour(s)
  interphase cytogenetics 592
  pigmented, of infancy 1091,
    2126
  primitive 1887
  of soft tissue, malignant primitive
    2126–7
  soft tissues **2121–7**
neuroendocrine cells, *see* endocrine
    cells
neuroendocrine system
  cardiovascular system 2012,
    2013
  diffuse 1182, **2009–16**
  genital tract 2013, 2014
  gut **1182–7**
    non-neoplastic disorders
      1185–7
  respiratory tract 2010–12
  skin 2014–15
  urinary system 2014, 2015
neuroendocrine tumours (carcinoid
    tumours)
  ampulla of Vater 1273, 1448
  breast 1657
  ectopic hormones 695, 696,
    700, 1269, 2008
  gall bladder 1415
  gastrointestinal **1269–75**
    classification 1272
    clinical and biochemical
      features 1269–70
    foregut 1155, 1272, **1273–4**,
      1699
    hindgut 1272, **1274–5**
    histology 1270
    main features 1272–5
    midgut 1272, **1274**
    mixed exo/endocrine 1275
  hepatic 1395
  lung 696, **1041**, 1273, 2320
    atypical 1041
  middle ear 1111
  ovary 1631
  pancreas, *see* islet-cell tumours

neuroendocrine tumours (carcinoid
    tumours) (*cont.*)
  specialized techniques for
    demonstrating *581*, **1271–2**
  thymic 1273, 1814, **1818–19**
neuroepithelial tumours **1886–92**
  dysembryoplastic 1891
  uncertain origin 1891–2
neuroepithelioma, peripheral
    2126–7
neurofibrillary tangles *149*, 407,
    408, 411
  Alzheimer's disease 1879, 1880
  progressive supranuclear palsy
    1878
  undemented elderly 1880
neurofibroma **1892–3, 2123–4**
  clinical features 2123
  diffuse 2124
  histopathology 2123–4
  joints 2092
  multiple, *see* neurofibromatosis
  nose 1118
  oesophagus 1146
  plexiform 2124
  stomach 1172
  variants 2124
neurofibromatosis (von
    Recklinghausen disease)
    1885, 1892, 2123
  cancer susceptibility 647, 648,
    1893, 2125, 2126
  central form 1892, 1903
  intestinal neurofibromas 1268
  mutant locus *123*
  neuroblastoma 1991
  peripheral form 1902–3
  phaechromocytoma and 1989
  plexiform neurofibromas 2124
neurofibrosarcoma 1893
neurofilament proteins *581*, 1832,
    1867
  Alzheimer disease 1879
  multiple sclerosis 1871
  neuroblastomas 1887
  skin 2015
neurofilaments 19, *36*, 584
neurogenic bladder 1516
neurogenic muscle disease 562,
    2094–5, **2096–7**
neuro-insular complexes 1999
neurokinin A (NKA) *2010, 2015*
neurokinins, midgut carcinoid
    tumours 1274
neuroleptic drugs, tardive dyskinesia
    754
neuroleukin 147
neurological disorders
  AIDS and HIV infection 1846–7
  alcoholism 1856–8
  fetal alcohol syndrome 1858
  malaria 2193–4
  methyl alcohol poisoning 1858
  paraneoplastic **703–6**, 717,
    1862–3
  systemic diseases 1860–2
  vitamin deficiencies 1858–60
neuroma
  acoustic, *see* acoustic
    schwannoma
  amputation 1898, 1899, 2121

neuroma (*cont.*)
  solitary circumscribed 2124
  traumatic 2121, 2122
neuromedin U *1184*
neuromelanin, adrenocortical
    nodules 1972
neuromuscular syndromes,
    neoplastic disease 1863
neuronal dysplasia, intestinal 1191
neuronal-glial tumours, mixed
    1891
neuronal necrosis
  anoxic-ischaemic, perinatal 1925
  brain hypoxia 1833–4
  liver failure 1860
  shock 546
neuronal tumours **1891**
neurones
  apoptosis 147
  cerebral infarction 1851
  'dying back' 1873, 1882
  immunological markers 1832
  inflammatory response 364
  ischaemic change in hypoxia
    1833
  response to injury 385
  shock-induced lesions 545–6
  structure and function **1825–32**
  vulnerability to hypoxic injury
    1833–4
neurone-specific enolase (NSE)
  gut neuroendocrine tumours
    1270, **1271–2**
  islet-cell tumours 2003, 2004,
    2005, 2006
  jugulotympanic paraganglioma
    1111
  lung tumours 1041
  neuroblastomas 1887
  skin 2015
neuronopathies 1899, 1901
neuronophagia, viral encephalitis
    1839, 1840
neuropathic joints 2086
neuropathies
  hereditary 1900, 1901, 1902
  hereditary pressure-sensitive
    1902
  hypertrophic 1900, 1902
  peripheral, *see* peripheral
    neuropathies
  sporadic relapsing segmental
    demyelinating 1900
neuropeptides
  CNS neurones 1832
  enteric nerves 1184
  hypertension and 839
  inflammatory activity 364
  type I hypersensitivity reaction
    275
neuropeptide tyrosine (NPY) *1184*
  cardiovascular system 2012,
    2013
  enteric nerves 1187
  genitourinary system *2014*
  Huntington disease 1879
  pancreatic nerves 1999
  respiratory tract *2010*
  skin *2015*
neurophysin 701, 703
neurosyphilis 403, 1837, 1838

processus vaginalis 1552
procidentia 1586
procollagen 54, 55, 371, 372
proconvertin, *see* factor VII
proctitis
  allergic 1248
  follicular 1238, 1239
  herpes simplex virus 1230
  lymphogranuloma venereum 1228
  non-LGV *Chlamydia trachomatis* 1228
  schistosomiasis 1233
  syphilis 1227–8
  ulcerative 1236
proctocolectomy, ulcerative colitis 1240–1
pro-erythroblasts 1693
progesterone 1971
  breast development and 1645–6
  cervical effects 1584, 2307
  endometrial effects 1595, 1597–8
progesterone receptors (PR)
  breast carcinoma 1654, 1667
  endometrial adenocarcinoma 1605
  meningiomas 1884
progestogens, endometrial effects 1598
progressive multifocal leukoencephalopathy (PML) 1840, **1845**, 1846, **1872**
  AIDS 1884
  demyelination 1867
  Hodgkin disease 1770
progressive supranuclear palsy **1878**
progressive systemic sclerosis, *see* systemic sclerosis, progressive
proinsulin 107–8, *1999*, 2006
prolactin (PRL) 1931, 1933
  ectopic production 702
  pituitary adenomas secreting 1931, 1932, *1934*, **1935–6**
  regulation of expression 96
prolapse
  genital **1586**
  rectal 1253
proliferation centres, lymphocytic lymphoma 1777, 1778
prolyl hydroxylase 371, 1392
prolymphocytes 1712, 1713, 1714, 1806
prolymphocytic leukaemia (PLL) 1713, 1714, 1807
promoters 92, 94, 95
  GC-rich 95
  mutations *110*, 114
  TATA box 95
promoting agents, tumour 663, 666, 667
promotion, tumour 635–6
promyelocytes 1704, 1720–1
promyelocytic leukaemia, acute 1720–1
N-proopiocortin (N-POC) 699, 700
proopiomelanocortin (POMC) 99, 699, 1932
  N-terminal mitogenic factors 384
prooxyphysin 703

proparathormone 1961, 1962
properdin 259, 1464
  deficiency 265
Propionobacterium acnes 436
propressophysin 701, 703
prostacyclin (PGI$_2$) 361
  endothelial cells and 498, 796, 797
  heart failure 537
  hypovolaemic shock and 542
  inflammatory activity 357, 360–1
  smoking and 513
prostaglandin D$_2$ (PGD$_2$) 275, 332, 335, 361
  inflammatory activity 360
prostaglandin E$_1$ (PGE$_1$) 438
prostaglandin E$_2$ (PGE$_2$) 361, 1175
  ascites 1422
  heart failure 537
  inflammatory activity 360–1
prostaglandin F$_{2\alpha}$ (PGF$_{2\alpha}$) 360, 361
prostaglandins
  acute renal failure and 1508
  bone, effects on 2024
  duodenal ulcer disease 1175
  endothelial cells 796
  gastric mucus–bicarbonate barrier 1152
  heart failure 536, 537
  hypercalcaemia of malignancy 698
  hypertension and 839–40
  hypovolaemic shock and 541–2
  inflammatory reaction 360–1
  periodontal disease and 1096
  platelets and 511, 514–15
  synthesis 361
prostate gland 385, **1535–43**
  atrophy 142, 563
  congenital abnormalities 1536
  inflammatory conditions 1536–8
  macrophages 253
  structure and function 1535–6
  transrectal fine-needle aspiration 2327–8
prostate-specific antigen *581*, 1536
prostatic acid phosphatase *581*, 1536
prostatic adenocarcinoma 1539
  see also prostatic carcinoma
prostatic adenoma 1539
prostatic carcinoma 1535, 1536, **1539–43**
  aetiology and epidemiology 1539–40
  bone metastases 1541–2, 2071, 2072
  breast carcinoma in males vs. 1658
  clinical 1540
  cytology 1543, *2332*
  epidemiology **690**
  histogenesis 1540
  incidental (latent) 1540
    grading and staging 1542–3
  macroscopic appearances 1540–2
  microscopic appearances 1542
  mucoid 1543
  occult 1540

prostatic carcinoma (*cont.*)
  spread 1531, 1541–2, 1562
prostatic duct 1516
prostatic glandular epithelium 1535–6
  dysplasia/carcinoma *in situ* 1539, 1540
  squamous metaplasia 1538
prostatic hyperplasia
  benign nodular 561, 1535, **1538–9**
    atypical 1539
    gross appearances 1538–9
    prostatic carcinoma and 1540
    variants 1539
  post-sclerotic 1540
prostatic infarction 1538
prostatic intra-epithelial neoplasia (PIN) 1540
prostatic polyps, benign 1530
prostatic resection, transurethral 1522, 1537
prostatic tumours *581*, **1539–43**
prostatic utricle 1535
prostatitis **1536–7**
  acute 1536
  chronic 1536
  eosinophilic 1537
  gonorrhoea 1543
  granulomatous 1536–7
  tuberculous 1537, 1543
prostatodynia 1536
protamine sulphate 755
protease–anti-protease imbalance hypothesis, emphysema 979
protease inhibitors 152
proteases
  calcium-activated 153, **189**
  host cell, virus pathogenicity and 445
  macrophage 341
  mast cells/basophils 334
protective antigen (PA), *Bacillus anthracis* 461
protein(s)
  abnormal cytoplasmic inclusions 175
  abnormalities in single gene disorders 102–9
  absorption 740
  ascites fluid 1421
  biological value 733–4
  body
    excessive loss 716
    total 733
  cationic, neutrophils 323, 327
  dietary *732*, **733–4**
    allergies 1198, 1249
    deficiency, wound healing and 374
  fixatives 2271
  immunogenicity 199
  membrane 8
  metabolism in cancer patients 716–17
  molecular lesions causing reduced synthesis 109–15
  neutrophil specific granules 324
  peroxidation 151
  phosphorylation 99
  processing and trafficking **98–9**

protein(s) (*cont.*)
  serum/plasma
    adverse drug reactions and 750
    embryonic synthesis 601
    hepatic synthesis 1290
    leakage in acute inflammation 355–6
    nutritional status and 738
    vascular deposition 836
  signal sequence 108
  staining methods 2273
  ubiquitination 148–9
protein 4.1 1700
  deficiency 1700
β-protein (A4 protein) 408, *409*, 411
protein A, staphylococcal 464, 465
proteinase
  staphylococcal 465
  streptococcal 462, 465
α_1 proteinase inhibitor, *see* α-1-antitrypsin
protein C *506*, 508, 509
protein efficiency ratio (PER) 734
protein energy malnutrition **742–3**
  ascariasis and 2230
  hookworms aggravating 2228
  infection susceptibility 286, 441
  intestinal mucosal changes 1202
  pancreatic features 1435
  trichuriasis aggravating 2228
protein gene product 9.5 (PGP) **1272**, 2012, 2013, 2015
protein kinase A 333
protein kinase C 146–7, 325, 677
protein-losing enteropathy 1194
proteinosis, pulmonary alveolar **986–7**
protein synthesis 91, 98
  liver 1290–1
    effects of alcohol 1325
  regulation 93, 98
  sites 11–12, 158, 165
  virus-induced 450
protein-thiol modification 185–7, 192
proteinuria 175
  glomerulonephritis 1456
  pre-eclampsia 1496
  Waldenstrom macroglobinaemia 1497
proteoglycans 37, **58–60**
  basement membrane 59, 60
  bone 2021
  cell-surface 59, 60
  endothelial 60
  function 59–60
  interstitial 59, 60
  intracellular 59
  loss in osteoarthritis 2084
  structure 58–9
  wound healing 369
proteolipid protein 1867
proteolysis, *in situ* hybridization 2286, 2290
proteolytic enzymes, emphysema induction 979
Proteus 467
  conjunctivitis 1908
  hospital-acquired infections *493*

nu

struct.
vascula

N.J. Mitchell

Oxford Textbook
of Pathology

Oxford Textbook of Pathology

Volume 2a
Pathology of Systems

Edited by

James O'D. McGee
Nuffield Department of Pathology
and Bacteriology
University of Oxford

Peter G. Isaacson
University College and Middlesex
School of Medicine
University College, London

Nicholas A. Wright
Royal Postgraduate Medical School
Hammersmith Hospital

Associate editors
Heather M. Dick
Department of Medical Microbiology
University of Dundee

Mary P. E. Slack
Nuffield Department of Pathology
and Bacteriology
University of Oxford

OXFORD   NEW YORK   TOKYO
Oxford University Press
1992

Oxford University Press, Walton Street, Oxford OX2 6DP

Oxford   New York   Toronto
Delhi   Bombay   Calcutta   Madras   Karachi
Petaling Jaya   Singapore   Hong Kong   Tokyo
Nairobi   Dar es Salaam   Cape Town
Melbourne   Auckland

and associated companies in
Berlin   Ibadan

Oxford is a trade mark of Oxford University Press

Published in the United States
by Oxford University Press, New York

A catalogue record for this book is available from the British Library

Library of Congress Cataloging-in-Publication Data
(Cataloging data is available)
ISBN 0–19–261976–4 (hbk. : set)
ISBN 0–19–261973–X (hbk. Vol. 1)
ISBN 0–19–261975–6 (hbk. Vol. 2a)   } Available as part of set only
ISBN 0–19–262273–0 (hbk. Vol. 2b)
ISBN 0–19–261972–1 (pbk. Vol. 1)
ISBN 0–19–261974–8 (pbk. Vol. 2)
ISBN 0–19–262274–9 (pbk. Vol. 2a)   } Available as part of Vol. 2 'set' only
ISBN 0–19–262275–7 (pbk. Vol. 2b)

Typeset by
Cotswold Typesetting Ltd, Gloucester
Printed in Great Britain by
William Collins Sons and Company Ltd, Glasgow

Preface

Pathology has been revolutionized over the past 20 years by an explosion of new knowledge generated by extensive scientific investigation of the cellular and molecular biology of human tissues. This has resulted from the introduction of a plethora of new molecular techniques, and the use of endoscopic and fine-needle tissue sampling which provide tissues previously only seen after surgical excision or at autopsy. What students of pathology need to know and learn today, therefore, is very different from the requirements two decades ago. The speed and magnitude of changes in pathology and in the pathologist's role are such that there is now a need to redefine the science of pathology and its future directions. It is in this context that we have embarked on this book. No textbook can ever take the place of careful study of original papers but we trust that this book will constitute an authoritative text for trainee and established pathologists as they get to grips with the new pathology.

The science of pathology does not lend itself easily to an encapsulating definition. The definitions proposed are either too narrow (the morphological basis of disease) or too broad (the study of disease) to be useful. It is clear, however, that pathology as we know it today grew from the gross morphological description of diseased organs, and following Virchow's discovery of the cellular basis of disease in the last century, pathology established itself as the core of medicine. As tissue preparative techniques and light microscopes improved, pathologists described natural and experimentally induced diseases in ever greater detail, culminating in the ultrastructural descriptions of the late 1950s and early 1960s. At about that time, Sir Roy Cameron summed up the direction of pathology as follows: 'The main endeavour has been to resolve the fundamental problems of pathology—injury, recovery, death—into simpler cellular, subcellular and eventually chemical components.' This we can now do with considerable accuracy. For some, this descriptive approach is sufficient; the problem is defined and the challenge is to treat the patient.

There is, however, a radically different view. In 1892, Victor Horsley wrote 'What is currently thought of as pathology is nothing of the sort—it is morbid anatomy. The pathologist should be a student of disordered function.' We strongly endorse this view. The advent of *in situ* phenotyping and genotyping of cells in the 1970s and 1980s respectively made it possible to ascribe synthetic function and dysfunction to intact cells. This, together with diagnostic morphology, has led to a new understanding of disease mechanisms and with it more accurate diagnosis and improved patient management. Over the past six years, new analytical nucleic acid techniques have emerged almost monthly. Some, such as the polymerase chain reaction, have had an immediate and profound impact on laboratory medicine, while others are being assimilated more cautiously. As practising clinicians, we foresee that these new and future methodologies will advance our knowledge of disease aetiopathogenesis and hence patient care. As medical scientists, we are excited by the future prospects because pathology laboratories will provide the largest repositories of fully documented DNA and RNA.

Volume 1 of the Oxford Textbook of Pathology examines the Principles of Pathology linking basic science and clinical observation to explain disease processes. Here, concepts of normal cell and chromosome/gene structure and function are described as a prelude to an account of the cellular, subcellular, and molecular mechanisms involved in genetic disorders, cell death, defence mechanisms, inflammation, pathophysiology of infection, neoplasia, and vascular disorders. Environmental and developmental pathology are also included. Emphasis is placed on the application of cell and molecular biology and the impact that these have had in unravelling the origins of disease. Because it is clear that we are far from a complete understanding of any single general principle, the text highlights our areas of ignorance and suggests ways of thinking and future experimental approaches. We believe it will provide a sound basis from which pathologists and basic scientists can approach the latest literature.

In Volume 2 (2a and 2b), we present the Pathology of Systems. Because of our conviction that the practice of clinical medicine should be multidisciplinary in its approach, we have shown the structural basis of disease in a clinical context. Each chapter starts with an overview of the normal structure and function of the system. The description of each disease is preceded by a précis of its clinical presentation and is followed by an analysis of aetiopathogenesis where this is known. In putting together Volume 2, we have been comprehensive in our approach without necessarily being encyclopaedic. The relevance of molecular pathology to specific disease processes is stressed. However, the main emphasis in this volume remains the cellular basis of disease and the role of pathology in clinical diagnosis. The book ends with a chapter on diagnostic and molecular investigative techniques which we hope will encourage pathologists to look deeper than the images conveyed by visible light through a microscope tube. By combining traditional methods of observation with the new molecular pathology, medical and non-medical scientists will each grow in their appreciation and understanding of disease processes. The future of pathology lies not only in the refinement of diagnosis and aetiology of disease but also in analysis of the mechanistic networks which regulate cellular responses to tissue and cell injury.

Our aim in this book has been to make a definitive statement. Thus we have elected to invite contributions from many leading experts. What may have been lost in continuity of style will, we hope, be compensated for by the high quality of the content. We have endeavoured to give the authors the opportunity to present their subjects comprehensively and encouraged the liberal use of colour diagrams and gross and microscopic photographs. This has resulted in a substantial book—rather more substantial than we originally envisaged—but one which we trust is pleasing to read in depth whilst being accessible for brief consultation. Our thanks are due to all contributors for their patience and for the care and enthusiasm with which they have approached their task. We believe that the finished product will expunge the memories of inevitable irritations along the way. To readers, we hope you enjoy the text and share in the excitement of discovery and the satisfaction of solving some of the problems we have outlined. We encourage readers to write to us with suggestions for improvement, or for changes of emphasis, which we will be glad to consider when planning future editions.

University of Oxford,   J.O'D.M.
University College, London, and   P.G.I.
Royal Postgraduate Medical School,   N.A.W.
    Hammersmith Hospital
November 1991

Acknowledgements

We would like to thank Mrs Penny Messer, Miss Lesley Watts, Mrs Sue Slaymark, Mrs Jean Garnet, and Miss Susan Chandler, whose organizational and administrative skills and eye for detail have kept this project flowing smoothly. We would also like to thank the many staff at Oxford University Press who have been involved in the production of this book. It has been a particular pleasure working with them as they have been professionally competent, encouraging, and effectively persistent over what sometimes seemed major problems.

Without the patience and encouragement of our wives and families, this book would not have seen the light of day. We express our gratitude to them for what they have had to endure during the gestation of this book.

The illustrations were drawn by Jane Fallows, Jane Templeman, and Focal Image Ltd.

List of chapters

Contents

13   The respiratory system   941

14   The mouth, salivary glands, jaws, and teeth   1051

15   Ear, nose, and throat   1103

18 The exocrine pancreas 1429
J. Rode

20 The male generative system   1533

21 The female genital tract and ovaries   1563
H. Fox and C. H. Buckley

Contributors

M. Alison, Department of Histopathology, Royal Postgraduate Medical School, Hammersmith Hospital, Du Cane Road, London W12 0HS, UK

S. P. Allwork, British Heart Foundation Museum of Heart Diseases, Institute of Child Health, Guildford Street, London WC1N 1EH, UK

R. H. Anderson, National Heart and Lung Institute, Dove House Street, London SW3 6LY, UK

T. J. Anderson, University of Edinburgh, Department of Pathology, The Medical School, Teviot Place, Edinburgh EH8 9AG, UK

I. D. Ansell, Department of Pathology, City Hospital, Hucknall Road, Nottingham NG5 1PB, UK

P. P. Anthony, University of Exeter, Postgraduate Medical School, Area Department of Pathology, Church Lane, Heavitree, Exeter EX2 5DY, UK

J. P. Arbuthnott, Vice-Chancellor, University of Strathclyde, Glasgow, UK

J. K. Aronson, University of Oxford, Medical Research Council Clinical Pharmacology Unit, Department of Clinical Pharmacology, Radcliffe Infirmary, Woodstock Road, Oxford OX2 6HE, UK

N. A. Athanasou, Department of Histopathology, Nuffield Orthopaedic Centre, Headington, Oxford OX3 7LD, UK

F. Barker, Department of Histopathology, Royal Postgraduate Medical School, Hammersmith Hospital, Du Cane Road, London W12 0HS, UK

J. H. Baron, Department of Surgery, Royal Postgraduate Medical School, Hammersmith Hospital, Du Cane Road, London W12 0HS, UK

C. L. Berry, Department of Pathology, The London Hospital Medical College, The London Hospital, London E1 2AD, UK

M. Berry, Department of Anatomy, Guy's and St Thomas's Hospitals, London Bridge, London SE1 9RT, UK

E. Beutler, Department of Molecular and Experimental Medicine, The Scripps Research Institute, 10666 North Torrey Pines Road, La Jolla, CA 92037, USA

P. C. L. Beverley, Imperial Cancer Research Fund Human Tumour Immunology Group, The Courtauld Institute of Biochemistry, University College and Middlesex School of Medicine, 91 Riding House Street, London W10 8BT, UK

S. R. Bloom, Department of Medicine, Royal Postgraduate Medical School, Hammersmith Hospital, Du Cane Road, London W12 0HS, UK

L. G. Bobrow, Department of Histopathology, University College and Middlesex School of Medicine, University Street, London WC1E 6JJ, UK

A. R. Boobis, Department of Clinical Pharmacology, Royal Postgraduate Medical School, Hammersmith Hospital, Du Cane Road, London W12 0HS, UK

J. Bridger, Department of Histopathology, Royal Postgraduate Medical School, Hammersmith Hospital, Du Cane Road, London W12 0HS, UK

C. H. Buckley, Central Manchester Health Authority, Department of Pathology, St Mary's Hospital, Whitworth Park, Manchester M13 0JH, UK

J. Burns, University of Oxford, Nuffield Department of Pathology and Bacteriology, John Radcliffe Hospital, Headington, Oxford OX3 9DU, UK

K. A. Calman, Chief Medical Officer, Department of Health, Richmond House, 79 Whitehall, London SW1A 2NS, UK

S. Cameron, The Queen's University of Belfast, Department of Pathology, Grosvenor Road, Belfast B12 6BL, UK

R.L. Carter, Histopathology Department, Institute of Cancer Research, Royal Marsden Hospital, Sutton, Surrey SM2 5PX, UK

T.J. Chambers, Department of Histopathology, St George's Hospital Medical School, Cranmer Terrace, Tooting, London SW17 0RE, UK

I. Chanarin, Medical Research Council Clinical Research Centre, Watford Road, Harrow, Middlesex HA1 3UJ, UK

A. J. Chaplin, Department of Histopathology, John Radcliffe Hospital, Headington, Oxford OX3 9DU, UK

R. W. Chapman, Gastroenterology Unit, Level 2, John Radcliffe Hospital, Headington, Oxford OX3 9DU, UK

J. Cohen, Infectious Diseases Unit, Department of Bacteriology and Medicine, Royal Postgraduate Medical School, Hammersmith Hospital, London W12 0HS, UK

G. Cole, Department of Pathology, University of Wales College of Medicine, Heath Park, Cardiff CF4 4XN, UK

D. V. Coleman, Department of Cytopathology, St Mary's Hospital, London W2 1NY, UK

K. Cooper, University of Oxford, Nuffield Department of Pathology and Bacteriology, John Radcliffe Hospital, Headington, Oxford OX3 9DU, UK

T. Creagh, Department of Histopathology, Royal Postgraduate Medical School, Hammersmith Hospital, Du Cane Road, London W12 0HS, UK

J. Crocker, Department of Histopathology, East Birmingham Hospital, Bordesley Green East, Birmingham B9 5ST, UK

B. Crossley, 27422 La Cabra, Mission Viejo, CA 92691, USA

A. J. D'Ardenne, Histopathology Department, St Bartholomew's Hospital Medical College, West Smithfield, London EC1A 7BE, UK

D. S. Davies, Department of Clinical Pharmacology, Royal Postgraduate Medical School, Hammersmith Hospital, Du Cane Road, London W12 0HS, UK

M. J. Davies, St George's Hospital Medical School, Department of Cardiological Sciences, Cranmer Terrace, London SW17 0RE, UK

J. Denekamp, Cancer Research Campaign, Gray Laboratory, PO Box 100, Mount Vernon Hospital, Northwood, Middlesex HA6 2RN, UK

V. J. Desmet, Universitaire Ziekenhuizen Leuven, Dienst Pathologische Ontleedkunde II, Minderboredersstraat 12, B-3000 Leuven, Belgium

T. M. Dexter, Paterson Institute for Cancer Research, Christie Hospital (NHS) Trust, Wilmslow Road, Manchester M20 9BX, UK

H. M. Dick, Department of Medical Microbiology, University of Dundee Medical School, Ninewells Hospital, Dundee DD1 9SY, UK

R. Doll, University of Oxford, Imperial Cancer Research Fund, Cancer Epidemiology and Clinical Trials Unit, Gibson Building, Radcliffe Infirmary, Oxford OX2 6HE, UK

M. S. Dunnill, Department of Histopathology, Level 1, John Radcliffe Hospital, Headington, Oxford OX3 9DU, UK

E. Duvall, University of Edinburgh, Department of Pathology, The Medical School, Teviot Place, Edinburgh EH8 9AG, UK

M. Eastwood, University of Edinburgh, Wolfson Gastrointestinal Laboratories, Western General Hospital, Edinburgh EH4 2XU, UK

H. A. Ellis, 16 Southland, Tynemouth, Tyne and Wear, UK

M. M. Esiri, University of Oxford, Department of Neuropathology, Radcliffe Infirmary, Woodstock Road, Oxford OX2 6HE, UK

D. J. Evans, Department of Histopathology, St Mary's Hospital Medical School, Paddington, London W2 1PG, UK

D. J. Fawthrop, Department of Clinical Pharmacology, Royal Postgraduate Medical School, Hammersmith Hospital, Du Cane Road, London W12 0HS, UK

M. Feldmann, The Charing Cross Sunley Research Centre, Lurgan Avenue, Hammersmith, London W6 8SW, UK

M. A. Ferguson-Smith, University of Cambridge, Department of Pathology, Tennis Court Road, Cambridge CB2 1QP, UK

J. D. Firth, Nuffield Department of Clinical Medicine, John Radcliffe Hospital, Headington, Oxford OX3 9DU, UK

A. M. Flanagan, Department of Pathology, St George's Hospital, Cranmer Terrace, Tooting, London SW17 0RE, UK

D. M. J. Flannery, University of Oxford, Nuffield Department of Pathology and Bacteriology, John Radcliffe Hospital, Headington, Oxford OX3 9DU, UK

K. A. Fleming, University of Oxford, Nuffield Department of Pathology and Bacteriology, John Radcliffe Hospital, Headington, Oxford OX3 9DU, UK

C. D. M. Fletcher, Cancer Research Campaign Soft Tissue Tumour Unit, United Medical and Dental Schools, Guy's and St Thomas's Hospitals, Department of Histopathology, St Thomas's Hospital, London SE1 7EH, UK

H. Fox, University of Manchester, Department of Pathology, Stopford Building, Oxford Road, Manchester M13 9PT, UK

A. P. Fraise, Microbiology Department, Selly Oak Hospital, Raddle Barn Road, Birmingham B29 6JD, UK

A. J. Franks, University of Leeds, Department of Public Health Medicine, 32 Hyde Terrace, Leeds LS2 9LN, UK

P. J. Gallagher, Department of Pathology, Southampton University Hospitals, Southampton SO9 4XY, UK

A. Gallimore, Department of Histopathology, Royal Postgraduate Medical School, Hammersmith Hospital, Du Cane Road, London W12 0NN, UK

K. C. Gatter, University of Oxford, Nuffield Department of Pathology and Bacteriology, John Radcliffe Hospital, Headington, Oxford OX3 9DU, UK

A. R. Gibbs, Department of Pathology, Llandough Hospital, Penarth, Glamorgan CF6 1XN, UK

J. M. Goldman, Medical Research Council Leukaemia Research Unit, Department of Haematology, Royal Postgraduate Medical School, Hammersmith Hospital, Du Cane Road, London W12 0HS, UK

S. Gordon, University of Oxford, Sir William Dunn School of Pathology, South Parks Road, Oxford OX1 3RE, UK

R. B. Goudie, University of Glasgow, Department of Pathology, Royal Infirmary, Castle Street, Glasgow G4 0SF, UK

C. F. Graham, University of Oxford, Cancer Research Campaign Growth Factors Group, Department of Zoology, South Parks Road, Oxford OX1 3PS, UK

D. G. Grahame-Smith, University of Oxford, Clinical Pharmacology Department, Radcliffe Infirmary, Oxford OX2 6HE, UK

G. A. Gresham, University of Cambridge, Department of Morbid Anatomy and Histopathology, The John Bonnet Clinical Laboratories, Addenbrooke's Hospital, Hills Road, Cambridge, CB2 2QQ, UK

D. Griffiths, Department of Pathology, University of Wales College of Medicine, Heath Park, Cardiff CF4 4XN, UK

M. Griffiths, University College and Middlesex School of Medicine, Department of Histopathology, Bland Sutton Institute, The Middlesex Hospital, London W1P 7PN, UK

P. D. Griffiths, Department of Virology, Royal Free Hospital, Hampstead, London NW3 2QG, UK

N. R. Grist, University of Glasgow, Communicable Diseases (Scotland) Unit, Ruchill Hospital, Glasgow G20 9NB, UK

B. A. Gusterson, Institute of Cancer Research, Royal Cancer Hospital, Department of Histopathology, The Haddow Laboratories, Clifton Avenue, Sutton, Surrey SM2 5PX, UK

T. J. Hamblin, Southampton University, Faculty of Medicine, Medicine 1, Level D, Centre Block, Southampton General Hospital, Tremona Road, Southampton, SO9 4XY, UK

D. G. Harnden, Paterson Institute for Cancer Research, Christie Hospital (NHS) Trust, Wilmslow Road, Manchester M20 9BX, UK

G. Hart, University of Oxford, Department of Cardiovascular Medicine, John Radcliffe Hospital, Headington, Oxford OX3 9DU, UK

D. A. Heath, University of Liverpool, Department of Pathology, Duncan Building, Royal Liverpool Hospital, PO Box 147, Liverpool L39 3BX, UK

C. S. Herrington, University of Oxford, Nuffield Department of Pathology and Bacteriology, John Radcliffe Hospital, Headington, Oxford OX3 9DU, UK

S. T. Holgate, Faculty of Medicine, Medicine 1, Level D, Centre Block, Southampton General Hospital, Tremona Road, Southampton SO9 4XY, UK

E. R. Horak, University of Oxford, Nuffield Department of Pathology and Bacteriology, John Radcliffe Hospital, Headington, Oxford OX3 9DU, UK

W. J. Hume, University of Leeds, Department of Dental Surgery, School of Dentistry, Clarendon Way, Leeds LS2 9JT, UK

S. E. Humphries, The Charing Cross Sunley Research Centre, 1 Lurgan Avenue, Hammersmith, London W6 8LW, UK

H. R. Ingham, Newcastle Regional Public Health Laboratory, Institute of Pathology, General Hospital, Westgate Road, Newcastle upon Tyne, Tyne and Wear NE4 6BE, UK

P. G. Isaacson, Department of Histopathology, University College and Middlesex School of Medicine, University Street, London WC1E 6JJ, UK

J. R. Jass, University of Auckland, Department of Pathology, School of Medicine, Private Bag, Auckland, New Zealand

H. M. H. Kamel, The Queen's University of Belfast, Department of Pathology, Grosvenor Road, Belfast BT12 6BL, UK

J. W. Keeling, Paediatric Pathology Department, Royal Hospital for Sick Children, 2 Rillbank Crescent, Edinburgh EH9 1LF, UK

P. M. A. Kelly, Department of Pathology, Mater Misericordiae Hospital, Eccles Street, Dublin 7, Ireland

T. Krausz, Department of Histopathology, Royal Postgraduate Medical School, Hammersmith Hospital, Du Cane Road, London W12 0HS, UK

P. J. Lachmann, University of Cambridge, Department of Pathology, Medical Research Council Centre, Hills Road, Cambridge CB2 2QH, UK

I. A. Lampert, Department of Histopathology, Ealing Hospital, General Wing, Uxbridge Road, Southall, Middlesex UB1 3HW, UK

P. L. Lantos, Department of Neuropathology, Institute of Psychiatry, de Crespigny Park, Denmark Hill, London SE5 8AF, UK

J. G. G. Ledingham, University of Oxford, Nuffield Department of Clinical Medicine, John Radcliffe Hospital, Headington, Oxford OX3 9DU, UK

F. D. Lee, University of Glasgow, Department of Pathology, The Royal Infirmary, Castle Street, Glasgow G4 0SF, UK

C. E. Lewis, University of Oxford, Nuffield Department of Pathology and Bacteriology, John Radcliffe Hospital, Headington, Oxford OX3 9DU, UK

P. D. Lewis, Department of Histopathology, Royal Postgraduate Medical School, Hammersmith Hospital, Du Cane Road, London W12 0HS, UK

G. B. M. Lindop, University of Glasgow, Department of Pathology, Western Infirmary, Glasgow G11 6NT, UK

J. Lorenzen, Universitat zu Koln, Abteilung Pathologie, Joseph-Stelzmann- Strasse 9, 5000 Koln 4, Germany

T. Lowhagen, Division of Clinical Cytology, World Health Organization Collaborating Centre, Department of Pathology, Karolinska Institute and Hospital, S 104 01, Stockholm, Sweden

D. R. Lucas, Department of Ophthalmology, Manchester Royal Eye Hospital, Oxford Road, Manchester M13 9WH, UK

S. Lucas, Department of Histopathology, University College and Middlesex School of Medicine, University Street, London WC1E 6JJ, UK

D. C. Linch, Department of Haematology, University College and Middlesex School of Medicine, University Street, London WC1E 6JJ, UK

I. C. M. MacLennan, The University of Birmingham, Department of Immunology, The Medical School, Vincent Drive, Birmingham B15 2JT, UK

I. A. Magnus, Institute of Dermatology, Guy's and St Thomas's Hospitals Medical Schools, London SE1 7EH, UK

D. Y. Mason, Leukaemia Research Fund, Immunodiagnostics Unit, University of Oxford, Nuffield Department of Pathology and Bacteriology, Haematology Section, John Radcliffe Hospital, Headington, Oxford OX3 9DU, UK

D. F. W. McCormick, The Queen's University of Belfast, Department of Pathology, Grosvenor Road, Belfast BT12 6BL, UK

J. O'D. McGee, University of Oxford, Nuffield Department of Pathology and Bacteriology, John Radcliffe Hospital, Headington, Oxford OX3 9DU, UK

P. H. McKee, Department of Histopathology, Guy's and St Thomas's Hospitals Medical Schools, St Thomas's Hospital, London SE1 7EH, UK

A. E. M. McLean, Department of Clinical Pharmacology, University College and Middlesex School of Medicine, 5 University Street, London WC1E 6JJ, UK

A. J. McMichael, University of Oxford, Nuffield Department of Medicine, John Radcliffe Hospital, Headington, Oxford OX3 9DU, UK

L. Michaels, Department of Histopathology, University College and Middlesex School of Medicine, London WC1E 6JJ, UK

A. Michalowski, Onkologiska Kliniken, Lasaretet 1 Lund,, 221-85 Lund, Sweden

N. A. Mitchison, Forschungslaboratorium, Robert Koch Institut, Haus 11, Nordufer 20, D-1000 Berlin 65, Germany

J. Monjardino, Department of Medicine, Queen Elizabeth the Queen Mother Wing, St Mary's Hospital Medical School, London W2 1PE, UK

W. J. Mooi, Netherlands Cancer Institute, Plesmanlaan 121, 1066 CX Amsterdam, The Netherlands

P. R. Morgan, Department of Oral Medicine and Pathology, Floor 28, Guy's Tower, Guy's Hospital, London SE1 9RT, UK

A. Morley, Department of Pathology, Royal Victoria Infirmary, Newcastle upon Tyne, Tyne and Wear NE1 4LP, UK

P. J. Morris, University of Oxford, Nuffield Department of Surgery, John Radcliffe Hospital, Headington, Oxford OX3 9DU, UK

A. M. Neville, Ludwig Institute for Cancer Research, Hedges House, 153/5 Regent Street, London W1R 7FD, UK

D. C. Old, University of Dundee, Department of Medical Microbiology, Ninewells Hospital, Dundee DD1 9SY, UK

E. G. J. Olsen, Department of Histopathology, Royal Brompton National Heart and Lung Hospital, Sydney Street, London SW3 6ND, UK

D. L. Page, Department of Pathology, Vanderbilt University Medical School, Nashville, TN 37232, USA

J. Parr, Department of Opthalmology, Manchester Royal Eye Hospital, Oxford Road, Manchester M13 9WH, UK

D. V. Parums, University of Oxford, Nuffield Department of Pathology and Bacteriology, John Radcliffe Hospital, Headington, Oxford OX3 9DU, UK

K. Paterson, Department of Haematology, University College and Middlesex School of Medicine, University Street, London WC1E 6JJ, UK

R. S. Patrick, University Department of Pathology, Royal Infirmary, Castle Street, Glasgow G4 0SF, UK

A. J. Pinching, Department of Immunology, St Mary's Hospital Medical School, London W2 1PG, UK

J. M. Polak, Histochemistry Department, Royal Postgraduate Medical School, Hammersmith Hospital, Du Cane Road, London W12 0NN, UK

A. Pomerance, Histopathology and Cytopathology, Harefield and Mount Vernon Pathology Laboratories, Mount Vernon Hospital, Northwood, Middlesex HA6 2RN, UK

J. S. Porterfield, University of Oxford, Sir William Dunn School of Pathology, South Parks Road, Oxford OX1 3RE, UK

B. Portmann, Institute of Liver Studies, King's College School of Medicine and Dentistry, Denmark Hill, London SE5 8RX, UK

C. S. Potten, Cancer Research Campaign, Department of Epithelial Biology, Paterson Institute for Cancer Research, Christie Hospital (NHS) Trust, Wilmslow Road, Manchester M20 9BX, UK

A. B. Price, Department of Histopathology, Northwick Park Hospital, Watford Road, Harrow, Middlesex HA1 3UJ, UK

L. Pusztai, University of Oxford, Nuffield Department of Pathology and Bacteriology, John Radcliffe Hospital, Headington, Oxford OX3 9DU, UK

P. Quirke, The University of Leeds, Department of Pathology, Leeds, Yorkshire LS2 9JT, UK

A. D. Ramsay, University of Southampton, Department of Pathology, Faculty of Medicine, Level E, South Lab/Path Block, Southampton General Hospital, Tremona Road, Southampton SO9 4XY, UK

J. G. Ratcliffe, Wolfson Research Laboratories, Department of Clinical Chemistry, Queen Elizabeth Medical Centre, Edgbaston, Birmingham B15 2TH, UK

P. J. Ratcliffe, University of Oxford, Nuffield Department of Clinical Medicine, John Radcliffe Hospital, Headington, Oxford OX3 9DU, UK

E. L. Rees, Department of Anatomy, Guy's and St Thomas's Hospitals, London Bridge, London SE1 9RT, UK

H. C. Rees, Department of Histopathology, St Bartholomew's Hospital, West Smithfield, London EC1A 7BE, UK

P. A. Revell, Department of Morbid Anatomy, The London Hospital Medical College, The London Hospital, London E1 1BB, UK

M. D. Richardson, Department of Medical Mycology, Anderson Building, 56 Dumbarton Road, Glasgow G11 6NU, UK

P. W. J. Rigby, Laboratory of Eukaryotic Molecular Genetics, Medical Research Council National Institute for Medical Research, The Ridgeway, Mill Hill, London NW7 1AA, UK

M. A. Ritter, Department of Immunology, Royal Postgraduate Medical School, Hammersmith Hospital, Du Cane Road, London W12 0HS, UK

C. R. Rizza, Oxford Haemophilia Centre, Churchill Hospital, Headington, Oxford OX3 7LJ, UK

J. W. Rode, Department of Anatomical Pathology, St Vincent's Hospital and University of Melbourne, 41 Victoria Parade, Fitzroy, Melbourne, Victoria 3065, Australia

J. Rosai, Department of Pathology, Sloan Kettering Institute of Cancer Studies, New York, NY, USA

R. Ross, University of Washington, Department of Pathology, School of Medicine, Seattle, WA 98195, USA

T. J. Ryan, Department of Dermatology, Slade Hospital, Oxford OX3 7JH, UK

V. Sams, Department of Histopathology, University College and Middlesex School of Medicine, University Street, London WC1E 6JJ, UK

P. J. Scheuer, University of London, Department of Histopathology, Royal Free Hospital School of Medicine, The Royal Free Hospital, Pond Street, London NW3 2QG, UK

J. B. Schofield, Department of Histopathology, Royal Postgraduate Medical School, Hammersmith Hospital, Du Cane Road, London W12 0HS, UK

A. W. Segal, Department of Medicine, University College and Middlesex School of Medicine, The Rayne Institute, University Street, London WC1E 6JJ, UK

J. B. Selkon, Oxford Regional Public Health Laboratory, Level 6/7, John Radcliffe Hospital, Headington, Oxford OX3 9DU, UK

N. A. Shepherd, Department of Histopathology, Gloucestershire Royal Hospital, Great Western Road, Gloucester GL1 3NN, UK

B. J. Shepstone, University of Oxford, Department of Radiology, John Radcliffe Hospital, Headington, Oxford, OX3 9DU, UK

P. R. Sisson, Newcastle Regional Public Health Laboratory, Institute of Pathology, General Hospital, Westgate Road, Newcastle upon Tyne, Tyne and Wear, NE4 6BE, UK

L. Skooge, Division of Clinical Cytology, World Health Organization Collaborating Centre, Department of Pathology, Karolinska Institute and Hospital, S 104 01 Stockholm, Sweden

J. M. W. Slack, University of Oxford, Imperial Cancer Research Fund Developmental Biology Unit, Department of Zoology, South Parks Road, Oxford OX1 3PS, UK

M. P. E. Slack, University of Oxford, Nuffield Department of Pathology and Bacteriology, Microbiology Section, Level 7, John Radcliffe Hospital, Headington, Oxford OX3 9DU, UK

P. M. Speight, Joint Department of Oral Pathology, The London Hospital Medical College and Institute of Dental Surgery, Eastman Dental Hospital, 256 Gray's Inn Road, London WC1X 8LD, UK

J. Spencer, Department of Histopathology, University College and Middlesex School of Medicine, University Street, London WC1E 6JJ, UK

C. J. F. Spry, St George's Hospital Medical School, Cardiovascular Immunology Research Group, Department of Immunology, Jenner Wing, Cranmer Terrace, London SW17 0RE, UK

M. W. Stanley, Hennipin County Medical Center, Department of Pathology and Laboratory Medicine, 701 Park Avenue South, MN 55415, USA

A. G. Stansfeld, Department of Pathology, St Batholomew's Hospital, West Smithfield, London EC1A 7BE, UK

J. E. Stickland, University of Oxford, Nuffield Department of Pathology and Bacteriology, John Radcliffe Hospital, Headington, Oxford OX3 9DU, UK

B. C. Sykes, University of Oxford, Nuffield Department of Pathology and Bacteriology, John Radcliffe Hospital, Headington, Oxford OX3 9DU, UK

P. J. Talmud, The Charing Cross Hospital, Sunley Research Centre, 1 Lurgan Avenue, Hammersmith, London W6 8LW, UK

D. Tarin, University of Oxford, Nuffield Department of Pathology and Bacteriology, John Radcliffe Hospital, Headington, Oxford OX3 9DU, UK

J. M. Theaker, Department of Pathology, Level E, Southampton General Hospital, Tremona Road, Southampton SO9 4XY, UK

H. C. Thomas, Department of Medicine, Queen Elizabeth the Queen Mother Wing, St Mary's Hospital Medical School, Praed Street, Paddington, London W2 1NY, UK

H. Thompson, Department of Histopathology, The General Hospital, Steelhouse Lane, Birmingham B4 6NH, UK

S. Tinkler, 53 Mount View Road, London N4, UK

P. G. Toner, The Queen's University of Belfast, Department of Pathology, Grosvenor Road, Belfast BT12 6BL, UK

J. Trowell, University of Oxford, Department of General Medicine, John Radcliffe Hospital, Headington, Oxford, OX3 9DU, UK

D. True, Department of Pathology, Yale University, Connecticut, USA

J. L. Turk, Department of Pathology, Royal College of Surgeons of England, Hunterian Institute, 35/43 Lincoln's Inn Field, London WC2A 3PN, UK

D. R. Turner, University of Nottingham, Department of Pathology, University Hospital, Queen's Medical Centre, Nottingham, NG7 2UH, UK

M. W. Turner, University of London, Molecular Immunology Unit, Institute of Child Health, 30 Guildford Street, London WC1N 1EH, UK

N. C. Turner, Department of Clinical Pharmacology, Royal Postgraduate Medical School, Hammersmith Hospital, Du Cane Road, London W12 0NN, UK

C.A. Wagenwoort, Erasmus University, PO Box 1738, 3000 Rotterdam, The Netherlands

J. C. Wagner, Medical Research Council External Staff, Team on Occupational Lung Diseases, Llandough Hospital, Penarth, Glamorgan CF6 1XW, UK

J. S. Wainscoat, Department of Haematology, Level 4, John Radcliffe Hospital, Headington, Oxford, OX3 9DU, UK

M. J. Walport, Rheumatology Unit, Royal Postgraduate Medical School, Du Cane Road, London W12 0PP, UK

F. M. Watt, Imperial Cancer Research Fund Laboratories, PO Box 123, Lincoln's Inn Fields, London WC2A 3PX, UK

D. J. Weatherall, University of Oxford, Nuffield Department of Clinical Medicine, John Radcliffe Hospital, Headington, Oxford OX3 9DU, UK

A. D. B. Webster, Clinical Research Centre, Division of Immunological Medicine, Watford Road, Harrow, Middlesex HA1 3UJ, UK

H. K. Weinbren, Royal Postgraduate Medical School, Hammersmith Hospital, Du Cane Road, London W12 0HS, UK

R. O. Weller, Department of Neuropathology, Level E, South Lab/Path Block, Southampton General Hospital, Tremona Road, Southampton SO9 4XY, UK

J. S. Wigglesworth, Department of Histopathology, Neonatal and Child Health, Royal Postgraduate Medical School, Hammersmith Hospital, Du Cane Road, London W12 0HS, UK

D. G. D. Wight, Department of Morbid Anatomy and Histopathology, The John Bonnet Clinical Laboratories, Addenbrooke's Hospital, Hills Road, Cambridge CB2 2QQ, UK

M. J. Wilkins, Department of Pathology, St Mary's Hospital Medical School, Paddington, London W2 1PG, UK

D. M. Williams, Department of Oral Pathology, Dental School, The London Hospital Medical College, Turner Street, London E1 2AD, UK

G. T. Williams, Department of Pathology, University of Wales College of Medicine, Heath Park, Cardiff CF4 4XN, UK

S. P. Wolff, Department of Clinical Pharmacology, University College and Middlesex School of Medicine, 5 University Street, London WC1E 6JJ, UK

C. G. Woods, Department of Histopathology, Nuffield Orthopaedic Centre, Headington, Oxford, UK

N. Woolf, Department of Histopathology, University College and Middlesex School of Medicine, The Bland-Sutton Institute, The Middlesex Hospital, London W1P 7PN, UK

D. H. Wright, The University of Southampton, Faculty of Medicine, South Lab/Path Block, Southampton General Hospital, Tremona Road, Southampton SO9 4XY, UK

N. A. Wright, Department of Histopathology, Royal Postgraduate Medical School, Hammersmith Hospital, Du Cane Road, London W12 0HS, UK

A. H. Wyllie, University of Edinburgh, Department of Pathology, The Medical School, Teviot Place, Edinburgh EH8 9AG, UK

E. P. H. Yap, University of Oxford, Nuffield Department of Pathology and Bacteriology, John Radcliffe Hospital, Headington, Oxford OX3 9DU, UK

The circulatory system

12

The circulatory system

12.1 Normal arterial anatomy and function

R. Ross

12.1.1 Normal anatomy

Arteries characteristically consist of three layers: the intima, the media, and the adventitia. The intima is bounded on its inner aspect at the lumen of the vessel by a continuous monolayer of endothelial cells and on its outer aspect by the internal elastic lamina. The media is bounded by the internal elastic lamina on its inner aspect and by the external elastic lamina on its outer aspect. The adventitia is bounded by the external elastic lamina and the outer surface of the vessel (Fig. 12.1).

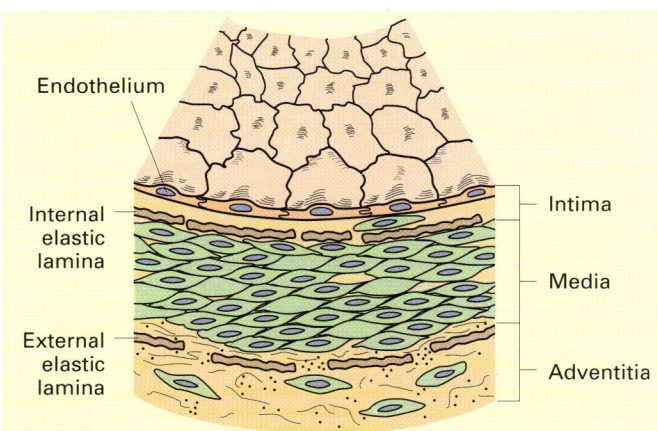

Fig. 12.1 Structure of a normal muscular artery. This diagram demonstrates the characteristic structure of most muscular arteries, which contain three layers: an intima, bounded by endothelium and the internal elastic lamina; a media, bounded by the internal and external elastic laminae; and the adventitia, representing the outermost layer of the artery. The medial smooth muscle cells form an interlocking spiral band of cells, surrounded by connective tissue, that are attached to each other by junctional complexes. (Drawn after Ross and Glomset 1976, with permission.)

At birth, the intima generally contains no cells other than the endothelium, although occasional single smooth muscle cells may be found. The endothelium rests on a relatively continuous layer of a specialized form of connective tissue, the basement membrane. The basement membrane may be separated from the internal elastic lamina by a space that contains other connective tissue elements, which have little apparent morphological structure and which consist principally of proteoglycans. Although the endothelial cells that line each vessel may appear to be similar morphologically, evidence is developing that there may be marked differences in the functional activities of endothelial cells from artery as well as between arteries, veins, capillaries, etc., which include the formation of vasoactive substances and growth factors, as well as differing permeability characteristics. These differences are poorly understood at present, but are under investigation. Of the functional characteristics that remain to be elucidated, some may be critical in explaining why some arteries become involved in the process of atherosclerosis, whereas others do not. For example, the characteristic anatomic sites where lesions of atherosclerosis form are at branches and bifurcations of the superficial femoral and iliac arteries, abdominal and thoracic aortas, coronary arteries, carotid arteries, and cerebral arteries. The remainder of the arterial system is, in general, spared from the atherosclerotic process, although exceptions have been observed. It has been suggested that one of the reasons these anatomic sites are involved is because of the effects of rheologic changes at branches and bifurcations that act synergistically with other causative agents affecting these specific arteries, but not others. It is also possible that functional differences in the endothelial cells at these sites may be important in these reactions.

The media of each artery consists of interconnected layers of smooth muscle cells that tend to spiral in a helical fashion in the wall of the artery. In muscular arteries, the media is delineated by the internal elastic lamina on the luminal aspect and by the external elastic lamina on its outer aspect. In large elastic arteries such as the aorta, there are varying numbers of lamellae of smooth muscle cells, each separated by an elastic lamina that is not as well developed as the internal elastic lamina, but which has a structure similar to that found in muscular arteries (Fig. 12.2). Vasa vasorum can be observed in very thick vessels, but

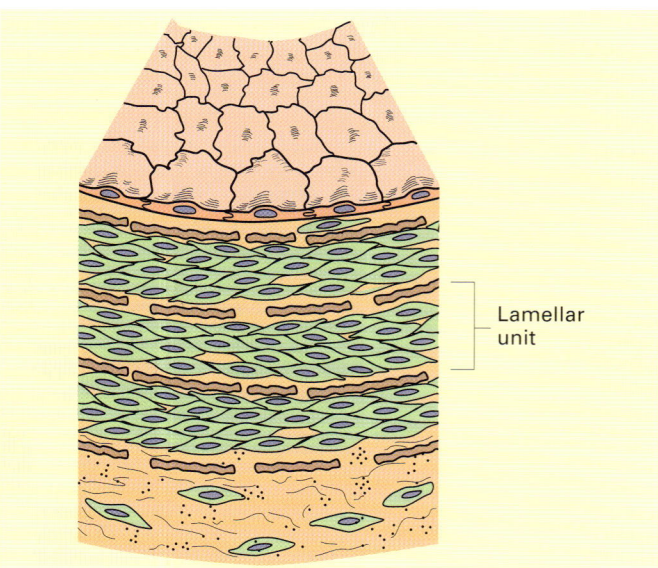

Fig. 12.2 Structure of a normal elastic artery. The normal elastic artery contains the same three regions as observed in the muscular artery; namely, intima, media, and adventitia. The principal difference in the elastic artery is in the media, which consists of numerous lamellae of smooth muscle cells, each of which is bounded by elastic laminae on both the luminal and adventitial aspects. Elastic arteries, such as the aorta, can have 20 or more lamellae. (Drawn after Ross and Glomset 1976, with permission.)

Lamellar unit

apparently are not observed until the artery contains at least 29 smooth muscle lamellae. It would appear that less than this number is sufficient to permit nutrients to reach the layers of the artery based on pressure filtration from the lumen. At thicknesses greater than 29 lamellae, vasa vasorum appear to be necessary to provide appropriate levels of oxygenation and nutrition to the outer layers of the artery.

Each elastic lamina consists of a fenestrated sheet of elastic fibres that criss-cross one another to form a structure that *en face* would appear something like a fisherman's net. The elastic fibres that are present in the lamina are mature in the sense that they consist of a mixture of homogeneous-appearing elastin together with embedded 100 Å microfibrils. The latter are known to consist of a glycoprotein that is different in amino-acid composition from elastin, which is a highly cross-linked protein with elastomeric properties. As one approaches the outer aspect of an elastic artery, each elastic lamina is less highly structured and less prominent than the internal elastic lamina.

12.1.2   Vascular cell function

Endothelial cells are one of the two known sources of factor VIII–von Willebrand factor, a protein that plays a critical role in platelet adherence. The dense, rod-shaped Weibel–Palade bodies found in many endothelial cells have been shown to be storage granules for von Willebrand factor. There is emerging data that other proteins, such as growth factors, may also be stored in these granules. Not all endothelia contain Weibel–Palade bodies. For example, although they are commonly found in human arterial endothelium, bovine arterial endothelium lacks these storage granules, suggesting that these substances may be stored differently in the bovine system.

Endothelial cells play a critical role in maintaining a balance in eicosanoid formation in the artery wall so that they normally form prostaglandin derivatives such as prostacyclin (PGI_2) that tend to prevent platelet and leucocyte adherence. When placed in culture, endothelial cells from most sources contain the enzyme cyclo-oxygenase, which utilizes arachidonic acid to synthesize PGI_2. PGI_2 is a potent vasodilator and one of the most potent antithrombotic substances that has been discovered. Its turnover is extremely rapid; consequently it has a very short half-life in the blood.

In contrast, platelets also use cyclo-oxygenase to form a different prostaglandin derivative, thromboxane A2 (TXA_2), which acts in opposition to PGI_2; namely, it promotes platelet adherence and aggregation, and thus thrombosis. Therefore, the same fatty acid substrate, arachidonic acid, can serve to provide opportunities for both prothrombotic and antithrombotic substances to be formed at a given site in the arterial tree, and the balance between these substances may play a critical role in determining whether platelet adherence, and thus thrombosis, may occur at a given site.

Endothelial cells also form a second substance that tends to counter platelet adherence, the anticoagulant proteoglycan, heparan sulphate. Endothelial cells in culture are capable of synthesizing heparan sulphate proteoglycan that bonds tightly to antithrombin due to the presence of an antithrombin-binding domain in the molecule. Such antithrombin-active proteoglycans have been located on the surface of arterial endothelial cells in culture, and thus may be partly responsible for some of the non-thrombogenic properties of arterial endothelium. Endothelial cells have relatively uniformly distributed, positively charged groups on their surfaces, as well as a heterogeneous pattern of negatively charged groups. The latter appear to be represented in part by sialic-acid-containing glycoproteins, which can be unmasked by neuraminidase treatment and which may play a role in the adhesion of leucocytes to the surface of the endothelium.

Bovine aortic endothelial cells have been shown to be capable of propagating procoagulant as well as anticoagulant activities. Aortic endothelial cells can bind factors IX and IXa. Factor IXa in the presence of factor VIII can activate factor X, which can lead to activation of prothrombin (see Chapter 7). In addition, when endothelial cells are injured or presented with substances such as endotoxin, they may release tissue factor activity. Thus there are several ways in which the endothelial cells can be involved in procoagulant activity as well as in anticoagulant activities. This procoagulant activity can be increased by interleukin-1 (IL-1), which is a potent inducer of such activity in human vascular endothelial cells. IL-1 appears to induce endothelial cells to produce tissue-factor-like activity. This can be demonstrated through the interaction of blood monocytes or macrophages, which induce procoagulant activity by endothe-

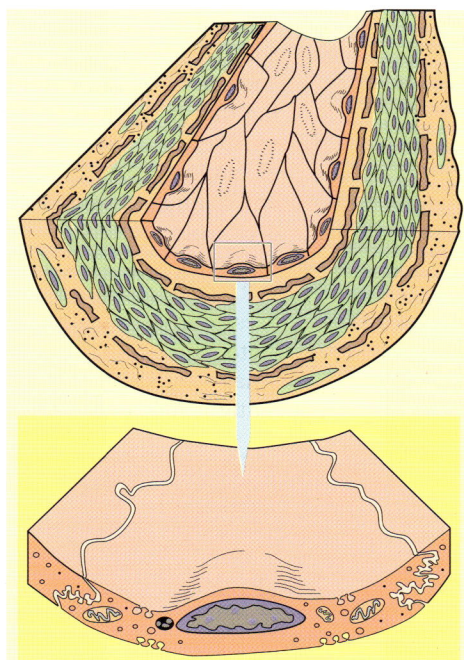

Endothelial cell function

1. Permeability barrier
2. Non-thrombogenic properties
   a. Cell surface
   b. PGI_2
3. Metabolism of vasoactive substances
4. Production of growth factors
5. Connective tissue formation

Fig. 12.3 This diagram shows the endothelial barrier present in the normal artery wall. In the higher magnification insert, the borders between the endothelial cells are irregular, allowing the cells to interdigitate. Vesicles and infoldings at either cell surface permit the cells to transport materials from the lumen of the artery to the tissue by endocytosis. Transport also occurs below the cell junctions, between the cells, and by vesicles that fuse with the membranes in these regions. In the artery, each endothelial cell rests on a connective tissue matrix that consists of a basement membrane intermixed with collagen fibrils. (Drawn after Ross and Glomset 1976, with permission.)

lial cells, some of which requires lymphocyte co-operation. Thus, cellular interactions that occur at sites of inflammation or in experimentally induced atherogenesis may aggravate this process by inducing such procoagulant activity.

Endothelial cells can induce vasodilation not only through PGI_2 formation, but also by their capacity to form endothelial-derived relaxing factor (EDRF). EDRF has been identified as nitric oxide (NO), which is also an inhibitor of platelet aggregation. By its capacity to produce PGI_2 and EDRF, endothelium can have a profound effect on smooth muscle relaxation and thus vasodilation. The combination of EDRF (NO) and PGI_2 would potentiate the anti-aggregating activity of PGI_2 alone, an activity that can be abolished with a cyclo-oxygenase inhibitor such as indomethacin. Counteracting the activity of these vasodilating agents is the capacity of endothelial cells to make angiotensin-converting enzyme, which could have a pivotal role in vasoconstriction and in blood pressure homeostasis. Endothelial cells in culture appear to be capable of forming angiotensin-converting enzyme (ACE) when they are confluent and have low turnover levels, as would be the case in normal intact vessels. Regenerating endothelial cells appear to be less capable of generating ACE, and thus the balance between these competing vasoconstricting and vasodilating activities may ultimately be important in vascular homeostasis (Fig. 12.3).

The smooth muscle cells of each artery provide a level of tonus that permits the artery to dampen each diastole and systole. In addition, the smooth muscle cells are capable of forming all of the connective tissue macromolecules, and are the principal connective tissue synthetic cells of the artery wall. These cells are capable of responding both chemotactically and mitogenically, and thus can serve as a reservoir of cells that can

migrate into the intima to form the lesions of atherosclerosis. In addition, there may be a 'stem cell' variety of smooth muscle in the media that provides numerous progeny that may also be important in atherogenesis.

The cells in the adventitia are poorly studied. They are said to consist of a mixture of fibroblasts and smooth muscle together with a relatively loose, poorly defined connective tissue. Nerves and small arterioles and venules are also embedded in this loose outer connective tissue layer.

12.1.3 Further reading

Bevilacqua, M. P., Pober, J. S., Majeau, G. R., Cotran, R. S., and Gimbrone, M. A. (1984). Interleukin 1 (IL-1) induces biosynthesis and cell surface expression of procoagulant activity in human vascular endothelial cells. *Journal of Experimental Medicine* **160**, 618–23.

Buchanan, M. R., Butt, R. W., Magas, Z., Van Ryn, J., Hirsh, J., and Nazir, D. J. (1985). Endothelial cells produce a lipoxygenase derived chemo-repellent which influences platelet/endothelial cell interactions—effect of aspirin and salicylate. *Thrombosis and Haemostasis* **53**, 306–11.

Del Vecchio, P. J. and Smith, J. R. (1981). Expression of angiotensin-converting enzyme activity in cultured pulmonary artery endothelial cells. *Journal of Cellular Physiology* **108**, 337–45.

Furchgott, R. F. and Zawadzki, J. V. (1980). The obligatory role of endothelial cells in the relaxation of arterial smooth muscle by acetylcholine. *Nature* **288**, 373–6.

Marcus, A. J., Weksler, B. B., Jaffe, E. A., and Broekman, M. J. (1980). Synthesis of prostacyclin from platelet-derived endoperoxides by cultured human endothelial cells. *Journal of Clinical Investigation* **66**, 979–86.

Moncada, S., Palmer, R. M. J., and Higgs, E. A. (1987). Prostacyclin and endothelium-derived relaxing factor: biological interactions and significance. *Thrombosis and Haemostasis* **58**, 597–618.

Nawroth, P. P. and Stern, D. M. (1986). Implication of thrombin formation on the endothelial cell surface. *Seminars in Thrombosis and Hemostasis* **12**, 197–9.

Ross, R. and Glomset, J. A. (1976). The pathogenesis of atherosclerosis. *New England Journal of Medicine* **295**, 369–77, 420–5.

Stern, D., Nawroth, P., Handley, D., and Kisiel, W. (1985). An endothelial cell-dependent pathway of coagulation. *Proceedings of the National Academy of Sciences USA* **82**, 2523–7.

12.2   Atherosclerosis

R. Ross

Atherosclerosis represents a series of cellular changes in the arterial system that take the form of different lesions, the composition of which may be dependent upon anatomic location, the age and sex of the individual, and the risk factors to which the individual has been exposed. These lesions range from fatty streaks to gelatinous lesions to various forms of fibrous plaques and complicated lesions. It is the fibrous plaque and the complicated lesion that may partially or fully obstruct the lumen of an artery and lead to the common clinical sequelae of infarction, gangrene, or reduced function of an organ or limb (see Chapter 7). For many years, the cellular content of the different lesions of atherosclerosis was poorly understood. Recent advances in immunology, cell and molecular biology now permit an unambiguous definition of the cellular content of the different lesions. Furthermore, appropriate animal models have provided insight into the cellular interactions that lead to lesion development. Thus we are beginning to understand how hypercholesterolaemia and hypertension lead to the development of atherosclerotic lesions. As a consequence, the future is bright for improved understanding of how diabetes and cigarette smoking result in a similar disease process. In some cases, there may be a continuum between the fatty streak and the advanced lesions of atherosclerosis, whereas in others this may not be the case. This section will attempt to put these ideas into perspective, to provide understanding and insight into the nature of the lesions and their cellular make-up, and how they occur.

The principal changes that take place in the artery wall during the development of the lesions of atherosclerosis occur largely within the intima of medium and large arteries. Thus the entry of substances from the plasma, as well as cells from the blood, into the artery depends upon alterations in the barrier presented by the endothelial cells; and upon the formation of substances within the intima which can attract cells from the blood, and smooth muscle cells from the media, to migrate into the intima. Cells from the blood are not normally present within the intima of the artery. Smooth muscle cells can be present in diffuse intimal thickenings which occur during development and which are commonly found in all human arteries, either as eccentric thickenings at bifurcations opposite the flow divider, or as concentric thickenings throughout the arterial tree. The thickness of these regions appears to increase gradually with age (see Section 7.11).

12.2.1   The lesions of atherosclerosis

The principal lesions of atherosclerosis are the fatty streak, the fibrous plaque, and the complicated lesion.

The fatty streak

The fatty streak is a ubiquitous lesion found throughout the arterial tree at all ages. It is present in children in early infancy and even at birth in some cultures, depending upon dietary habits and life-style. Fatty streaks are particularly prominent in those societies whose diets contain large amounts of milk and saturated fats. A series of monoclonal antibodies have been developed that are specific for smooth muscle cells, for macrophages, and for lymphocytes of varying subtypes. Using these monoclonal antibodies coupled with immunohistochemical methodology and examination by light and electron microscopy, the cellular content of the different lesions of human atherosclerosis can be unambiguously determined. The fatty streak consists largely of monocyte-derived macrophages that have entered into the intima. These monocyte/macrophages become foam cells due to the uptake and intracellular aggregation of large amounts of lipid in the form of lipid droplets, which principally contain cholesterol ester (Fig. 12.4). Advanced fatty streaks have been described that consist of variable numbers of lipid-filled smooth muscle cells and lipid-filled macrophages, each of which can take the form of foam cells. Based upon geographic pathology study, it has been assumed that some of these fatty streaks will progress to become fibrous plaques, that others will regress and disappear, while still others may remain unchanged during the individual's lifetime. This will be discussed in greater detail below.

Another lesion that may be an early or intermediate lesion of atherosclerosis is the so-called 'gelatinous lesion' that appears to contain a large amount of extracellular matrix. This matrix in the gelatinous lesion appears to be relatively rich in proteoglycan, and contains numerous cells embedded within the matrix. Most of these cells appear to be macrophages and smooth muscle. The relationship of the gelatinous lesion to the fatty streak and to the advanced lesions of atherosclerosis is not understood. It has been suggested that some gelatinous lesions may go on to become advanced fibrous plaques (Fig. 12.5).

The fibrous plaque and complicated lesion

The lesions that result in clinical sequelae are the fibrous plaque and the so-called complicated lesion (Fig. 12.6). The complicated lesion is probably a fibrous plaque that has become altered by calcification or that may develop cracks or fissures, or undergo ulceration. This could then lead to secondary haemorrhage within the plaque, which may be accompanied by thrombosis. It is this secondary involvement with thrombosis that

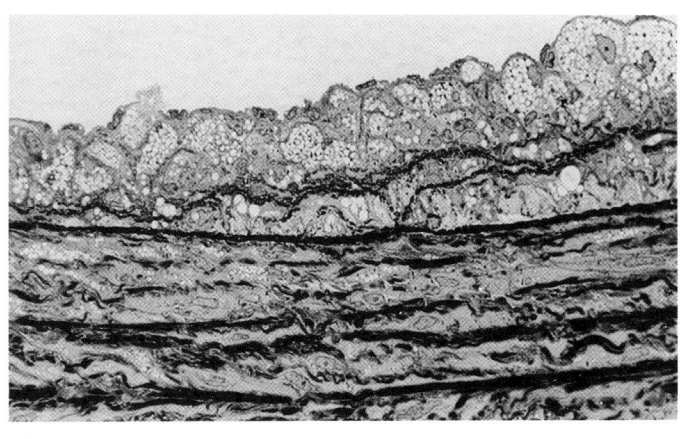

(a)

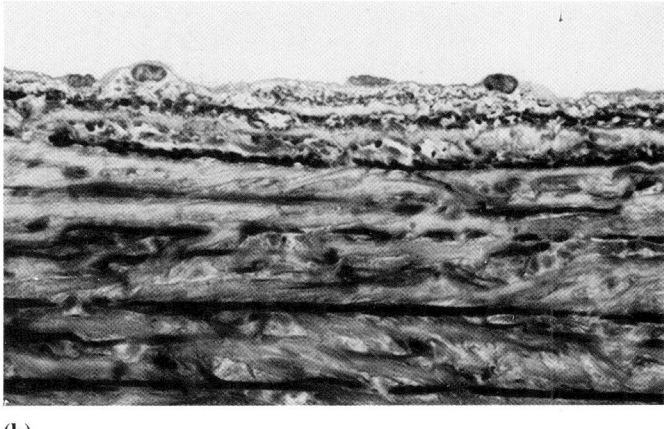

(b)

Fig. 12.4 (a) This is a light micrograph of a human fatty streak. This lesion from a coronary artery contains areas of vacuolation in the intima due to the presence of foam cells, which are principally lipid-filled macrophages together with lipid-filled smooth muscle cells that have migrated into this area and taken up lipid. The identity of these cells is difficult to appreciate in a light micrograph such as this one, which is routinely stained with haematoxylin and eosin. Note that one of the foam cells is exposed to the lumen through a break in an endothelial cell junction (upper right). (b) Contrast the artery containing the fatty streak (a) with this artery, which contains a relatively normal intima in which the endothelial cells lie close to the internal elastic lamina, with some elements of connective tissue between the endothelium and the elastic lamina, but few to no cells.

often leads to clinical sequelae such as myocardial or cerebral infarction, or gangrene. When advanced lesions are examined with the different monoclonal antibodies that are cell-type specific, each lesion can be subdivided into approximately three different regions. The region closest to the lumen generally consists of a dense fibrous cap. This fibrous cap contains thick bands of collagen-rich connective tissue matrix, which surround numerous smooth muscle cells, together with some macro-

phages, and is lined on the lumen by endothelium. These cells appear to be embedded in elliptical spaces that look somewhat like lacunae. Each smooth muscle cell in the fibrous cap has a relatively flat, pancake-shaped appearance under the electron

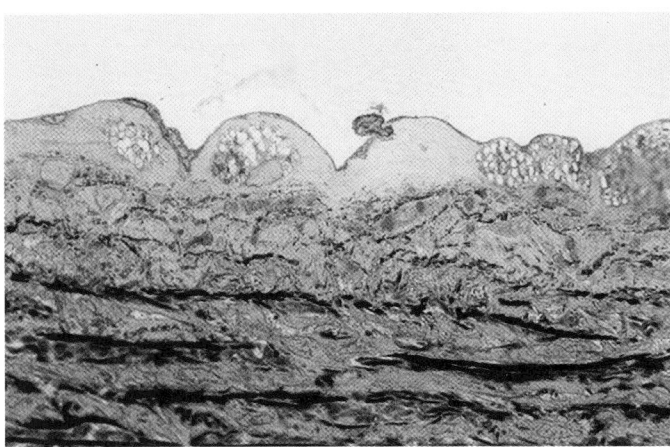

Fig. 12.5 This light micrograph demonstrates an early gelatinous lesion from a section of human aorta. This lesion contains a few foam cells, which appear to lie within relatively large areas that contain amorphous-appearing material that is probably proteoglycan in nature. A mononuclear cell can be seen in the process of either entering or exiting the intima in the centre of the micrograph. In a lesion such as this one, which contains foam cells as well as mononuclear cells, all of which are surrounded by amorphous material, it is difficult to know whether such a lesion will progress or remain in this state for a prolonged period.

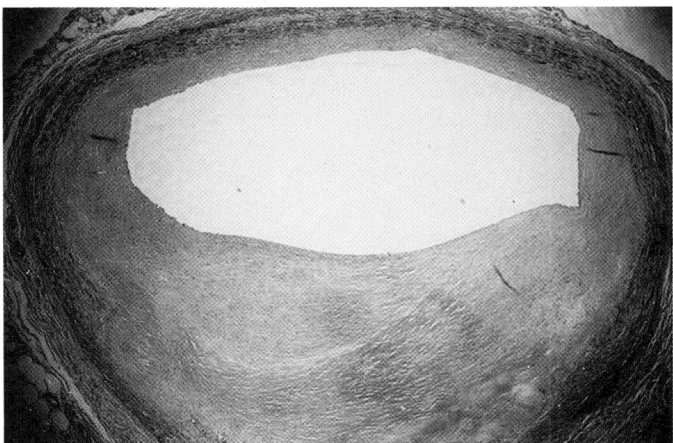

Fig. 12.6 This fibrous plaque in a human coronary artery demonstrates the asymmetric nature of the lesion, the occlusive potential of the lesion, and the marked intimal thickening that is visible in this low-power light micrograph. Characteristically, fibrous plaques are covered by a fibrous cap of dense connective tissue, which surrounds flattened smooth muscle cells together with varying numbers of intermixed macrophages. This layer covers a collection of smooth muscle cells, lymphocytes, and lipid-containing macrophages, the amount of which depends upon the state of hyperlipidaemia of the patient. In this particular case, the fibrous plaque is densely fibrous and contains relatively little lipid. The cellular detail described above is not apparent in arteries routinely prepared, such as this one, but is confirmed in studies such as those demonstrated in Figs 12.7 and 12.8. The appearance of such advanced lesions is very common.

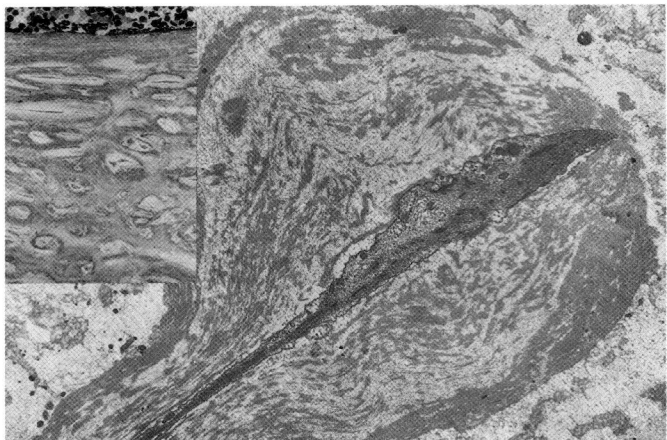

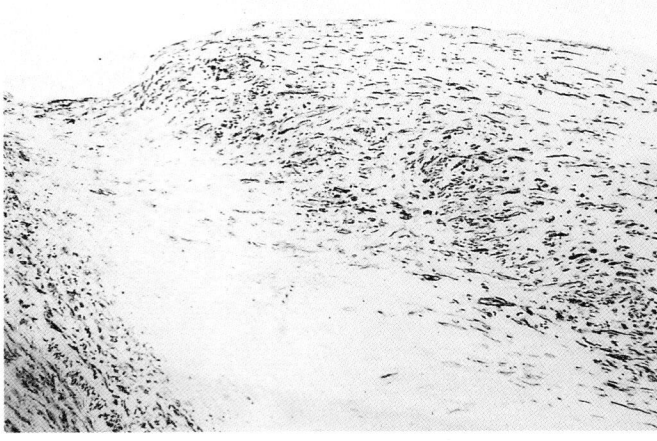

(a)

Fig. 12.7 An electron micrograph of a portion of one of the pancake-shaped cells similar to those shown in the inset. These cells can be identified as smooth muscle by their complement of myofilaments and because they are surrounded by concentric layers of amorphous material resembling basal lamina. Small dark-staining granules representing proteoglycan are interspersed among the basal-lamina-like material. Notice that the basal lamina covering follows the contours of the cell. (Reproduced from Ross *et al.* 1984.)

microscope (Fig. 12.7). This appears to be due, in part, to the formation by these cells of a large amount of dense connective tissue matrix, which then compresses the cells. Numerous macrophages are located around and between these smooth muscle cells. As a result, this layer is a dense, fibrous, smooth-muscle-rich region in which the smooth muscle cells are surrounded by variable numbers of macrophages (Fig. 12.8).

Beneath the fibrous cap lie varying numbers of smooth muscle cells and macrophages, each of which may contain deposits of lipid. Beneath this is a layer rich in macrophages that are often full of lipid and appear like foam cells, particularly in hypercholesterolaemic individuals. There may be numerous T-lymphocytes associated with this layer of macrophages as well (Fig. 12.8). These T-cells may be located in the region encompassing the fibrous cap and the luminal aspect of the foam-cell-rich zone. This foam cell layer may also be involved with necrotic changes and therefore some areas may contain few definable cells and have large amounts of extracellular lipid debris that has resulted from necrosis and breakdown of many of the foam cells. At the base of the fibrous plaque, there may be large numbers of proliferated smooth muscle cells surrounded

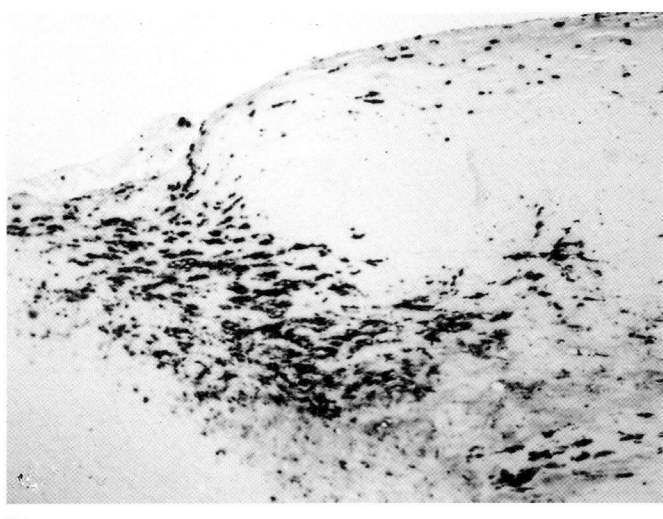

(b)

Fig. 12.8 These light micrographs represent a set of serial sections of a shoulder region of a fibrous plaque from a human carotid artery. (a) This section is stained with an anti-muscle cell antibody HHF-35 that, when used with an immunoperoxidase technique, stains only smooth muscle cells. (b) A serial section with an immunoperoxidase stain demonstrating an anti-macrophage antibody, HAM-56, an antibody specific for monocytes and macrophages only. (c) A serial section that has been stained with an antibody-T200 antibody that stains lymphocytes and some monocytes. Further study with these sections has shown that these cells are principally T-lymphocytes. (Reproduced from Gown *et al.* 1986.)

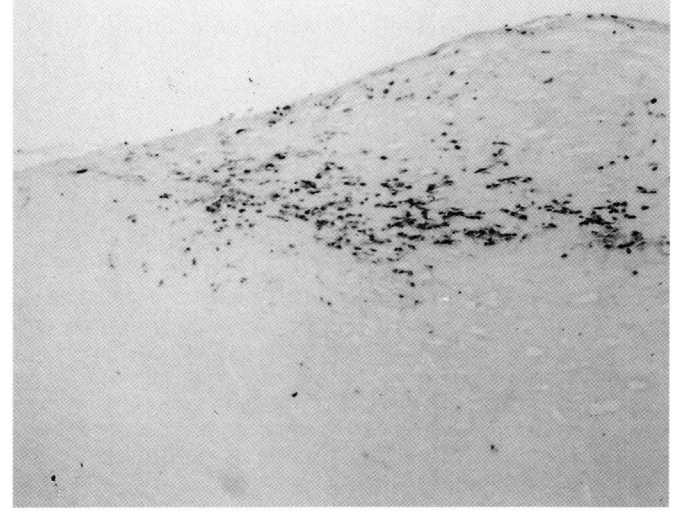

(c)

by varying amounts of connective tissue matrix (Fig. 12.8). This schema is a general one, and most lesions represent variations on this theme. When fibrous plaques become calcified, this usually occurs deep within the lesion, often associated with the areas of necrosis and cell debris. If the lesions undergo ulceration at their luminal surface, they may go on to develop cracks or fissures. These may subsequently become involved in secondary haemorrhage from vasa vasorum, or in thrombosis. If the thrombus does not occlude the vessel and lead to acute clinical sequelae, it will become organized. If this should occur, the lesion may become highly distorted in appearance, making it difficult to assign specific morphological characteristics to the lesion, which may become highly variable in appearance.

It has been assumed that the above description of the fibrous plaque is typical of the advanced lesions of atherosclerosis in different parts of the arterial tree; however, it is not clear that this is necessarily the case. Studies are underway to determine whether there are differences in the cellular content and in the distribution of cells, particularly in advanced lesions of atherosclerosis, in different parts of the arterial tree. It is also not clear whether there are differences in lesion morphology and location in association with each of the different risk factors with which the patient may be involved, including hypercholesterolaemia, hypertension, cigarette smoking, diabetes, or less common entities such as homocystinuria. The important demonstration that the fatty streak consists largely of monocyte-derived macrophages suggests that these cells must be derived from blood-borne monocytes since there is no evidence that macrophages in any tissue come from cells other than the blood monocyte at some time during their life-span.

It should be pointed out that although risk factors such as hypercholesterolaemia, cigarette smoking, hypertension, and diabetes have long been associated epidemiologically with an increase in the incidence of atherosclerosis, in some instances it has not been demonstrated that each of these individual factors is necessarily causally related. In some cases, such as hypercholesterolaemia, this may be true, whereas in others, such as hypertension, the relationship may be an indirect one. Furthermore, when the factors are causally related, it is not entirely clear in each case which specific factor is the causative agent. For example, although cigarette smoking is known to be one of the major risk factors associated epidemiologically with increased incidence of atherosclerosis, the specific agent or agents derived from smoking cigarettes that are aetiologic in this process have not, as yet, been defined. The risk factor concept therefore represents an epidemiological association and is thus a statistical concept. This is in contrast to specific agents or molecules that can be shown to be causally responsible in the aetiology and pathogenesis of the disease process.

12.2.2 Lipids and the lipoproteins in atherosclerosis

Since hypercholesterolaemia is the major risk factor associated with the increased incidence of atherosclerosis in the United States, Europe, and many other parts of the world, it is important to understand the role that lipids play in atherogenesis. Although many lesions of atherosclerosis are fibrous and contain relatively little lipid (as may be true from some cigarette-smokers), the effects of lipid on endothelium, on monocytes, and on smooth muscle, and the accumulation of lipid in the lesions of hypercholesterolaemic individuals, can be critical components of the process of atherogenesis. Consequently, it is important to understand specifically how elevated levels of cholesterol-bearing lipoproteins are related to the process of atherogenesis.

Thanks to the investigations of a series of patients with familial hypercholesterolaemia (FH disease), we know that the surfaces of normal hepatocytes, fibroblasts, and smooth muscle cells contain receptors for plasma low-density lipoproteins, and that these receptors are either physically absent or unable to function in patients with FH disease and, to varying degrees, in other individuals such as heterozygotes or individuals with various polygenic forms of hyperlipidaemia (see also Section 2.7).

The concentrations of cholesterol and triglycerides in the plasma are controlled by several metabolic processes and are influenced by a variety of factors. There are two sources of circulating plasma lipoproteins. These are exogenous dietary fat, which is absorbed through the intestinal tract and enters the plasma as chylomicrons, and endogenous fats of hepatic origin. Although cholesterol is ubiquitous as a constituent of the membranes of all mammalian cells, it also serves as a precursor for the formation of bile acids, adrenal and gonadal hormones, as well as other biologically active compounds. It can have disastrous effects when it is present in excess amounts in the plasma as constituents of the lipoproteins. On the other hand, triglycerides, many of which are derived from dietary carbohydrate, represent on average about 40 per cent of the total calories consumed in the United States on a daily basis. Triglycerides are stored in adipose tissue and can provide unesterified fatty acids that are also transported to distant sites by plasma lipoproteins and as fatty acid–albumin complexes.

Hyperlipoproteinaemia generally reflects a defect in the metabolism of lipoproteins, which represent a diverse species of particles containing cholesterol, triglycerides, and other lipids, together with a series of specific apoproteins. Although it is not possible to discuss lipoprotein metabolism in detail in this section, a brief review follows. For a more complete discussion, the reader is referred to reviews noted in Sections 12.2.11 and 2.7.9.

The different classes of lipoprotein have been separated, based upon the size of the particles and their density. Within each major class of lipoproteins, there is a fair amount of variation in size. This variation, and consequent hererogeneity, probably results not only from the synthesis of the lipoproteins, but from the catabolic processes that change the size of lipoproteins while they circulate in the plasma. The triglyceride-rich lipoproteins are the largest particles and include the chylomicrons and the very-low-density lipoproteins (VLDL), both of which are progressively reduced in size by the action of lipoprotein lipase in the capillary endothelium of adipose tissue after they come into the plasma from the gut and liver, respectively. As these

particles are reduced in size, there is a transfer, or reorganiza-
tion, of some of the apoproteins that are associated with each
particle. Consequently, each class of lipoprotein may consist of a
mixture of particles that are in various stages of conversion due
to metabolic alteration. These particles have generally been
classed as high-density (HDL), intermediate-density (IDL), and
low-density (LDL) lipoproteins. The major classes of apoproteins
and the particles they are associated with are presented in Table
12.1. The binding to cells of the different lipoprotein particles
occurs via their apoproteins, each of which binds to specific
receptors on cells such as endothelium, smooth muscle, and
macrophages. Just as the particles of a certain class of lipoproteins are heterogenous in size, they are also heterogeneous in
the content of their apoproteins, with the exception of LDL,
which contains only apoprotein-B. This also reflects the fact
that the lipoprotein particles are in different stages of metabolic
alteration or conversion.

Triglyceride-rich lipids are generally absorbed in the intestinal tract and are secreted by the cells of the intestine into the
lymph as chylomicrons. Apoprotein-B is synthesized and incorporated into the chylomicron prior to its secretion into the
lymph, as is apoprotein-A. Once the chylomicrons enter the
bloodstream from the lymph, apoprotein-A, together with some
phospholipids, is transferred to another class of particle that is
relatively rich in cholesterol, the HDL particle, and in so doing
the chylomicrons accept apoC and apoE proteins from the HDL
particles. Thus apoA proteins may be contributed from chylomicron particles to HDL particles in the plasma. One of the apoC
proteins, apoC-II, is a cofactor for the enzyme lipoprotein lipase,
generally thought to be derived from adipose cells, where it is
secreted and binds to the surface of capillary endothelial cells.
Individuals who are deficient in lipoprotein lipase activity or are
deficient in apoC-II generally have a markedly elevated concen-

tration of triglyceride-rich lipoproteins in their plasma. Because
they are deficient in lipoprotein lipase activity, these individuals
also accumulate chylomicrons, particularly after they have
eaten diets rich in triglyceride.

The intestine also secretes some VLDL in addition to chylomicrons. However, most of the plasma VLDL is derived from the
liver, which forms these particles from fatty acids derived from
adipose tissue and fatty acids that are synthesized in the liver.
Ingested cholesterol and cholesterol synthesized in the liver is
transported to the extrahepatic tissues in the form of VLDL particles. VLDL formation and secretion also involves apoprotein-B,
and when the VLDL particles enter the plasma, they pick up
other apoproteins, including apoC and apoE, from HDL. Thus
the VLDL particles present in the plasma can be derived from
both the liver and intestine. An additional class of particles are
also present. They are described as 'remnants' since they result
from the breakdown of VLDL and perhaps of chylomicrons, both
of which have lost their apoA and gained apoC and apoE. These
remnants then go on to be metabolized further to provide a class
of IDL that are rich in cholesterol esters, apoB, and apoE. IDL
particles are formed largely by the activity of lipoprotein lipase
and go on to be processed, probably in the liver, to form LDL,
which represents the final product in the plasma of the breakdown of VLDL. LDL particles are poor in triglycerides, rich in
cholesterol esters and free cholesterol, and contain apoB as their
only apoprotein.

The liver is the principal site where LDL is removed from the
plasma. This occurs via high-affinity cell-surface receptors in
the hepatocytes. The remainder of the LDL is bound to peripheral cells such as fibroblasts, smooth muscle, and endothelium, where it can also be removed. LDL can be modified by
malonation, by glycation, by oxidation, or by other chemical
changes. Such modified LDL can bind to 'modified LDL recep-

Table 12.1 Composition and properties of human plasma lipoproteins (after Beigel and Gotto 1986)

Lipoprotein	Density	Electrophoretic mobility	Major lipid constituents	Apoprotein constituents
Chylomicrons	0.95	Origin	Triglyceride	ApoA-I ApoA-II ApoA-IV ApoB-48
VLDL	0.95–1.006	Pre-beta	Triglyceride, phospholipid	ApoB-100 ApoC-I ApoC-II ApoC-III ApoE
IDL	1.006–1.019	Beta	Esterified cholesterol, phospholipid	ApoB-100 ApoE
LDL	1.019–1.063	Beta	Triglyceride, esterified cholesterol	ApoB-100
HDL	1.061–1.210	Alpha	Phospholipid, cholesterol	ApoA-I ApoA-II ApoC-II ApoE

VLDL, very-low-density lipoprotein; IDL, intermediate-density lipoprotein; LDL, low-density lipoprotein; HDL, high-density lipoprotein.

tors', sometimes called scavenger receptors, on cells such as macrophages (see also Section 12.3). These receptors have the capacity to take up large amounts of the modified form of the LDL particle. Some individuals who are both hyper-triglyceridaemic and hypercholesterolaemic have a particular form of VLDL called β-VLDL. This particle contains a high ratio of cholesterol ester to triglyceride and large quantities of apoE as well as apoB. β-VLDL appears to be particularly atherogenic in experimental animals and probably plays a similar role in humans.

Abnormal accumulation of lipoprotein in the plasma can occur from overproduction, from deficient removal, or from a combination of both abnormalities. There are a number of forms of genetic hyperlipidaemias that are either monogenic or polygenic (see also Section 2.7). The different forms of genetic hyperlipidaemias are presented in Table 12.2. Perhaps more common are forms of hyperlipoproteinaemia that are secondary to other diseases. The most common diseases resulting in eleva-tion of the different classes of lipoproteins include diabetes mel-litus, renal disease, alcoholism, treatment with corticosteroids or oestrogens, hypothyroidism, and the dysglobulinaemias.

One of the best demonstrations of the role of hyper-cholesterolaemia in atherogenesis can be seen in patients with FH disease. Although FH disease is much less common than the secondary hyperlipoproteinaemias or other genetic hyper-lipidaemias, we know a great deal about its course in both humans and animals. In these cases, the plasma cholesterol and LDL are inordinately high due to the fact that these individuals either lack LDL receptors or have receptors that are incapable of binding or responding to LDL. Investigations that examined patients with deficient or missing LDL receptors led to the dis-covery of the LDL receptor and to identification of the mech-anisms of control of cholesterol metabolism at the cellular level, and thus of events that lead to the development of hypercholes-terolaemia in such individuals. Under these circumstances, the LDL receptor normally acts by a feedback inhibitory mechanism so that when LDL is bound to its receptor, it suppresses the activity of the rate-limiting enzyme for cholesterol synthesis, HMG CoA reductase. Both the liver and the peripheral cells of individuals with FH disease continue to synthesize large amounts of cholesterol, and the liver secretes very large amounts due to the fact that absent or faulty receptors fail to generate a feedback inhibitory signal, and the cholesterol syn-thetic process goes on unabated. Under such conditions, these individuals have markedly elevated plasma LDL cholesterol levels, go on to develop rampant atherosclerosis with advanced lesions. As a consequence, myocardial infarcts have been des-cribed in young children with FH disease. Such individuals have been reported to have infarcts as early as 2 years of age and are often dead by the age of 20. The process of atherogenesis appears to occur at a slower rate in most hypercholesterolaemic individuals, presumably because their levels of LDL are lower. These observations and numerous studies suggest that reduc-tion of LDL should lead to a decrease in the incidence of atheros-clerosis.

Recent studies have been performed on large numbers of hypercholesterolaemic individuals who have been treated with pharmacological agents that reduce plasma cholesterol levels. These clinical trials have shown unequivocally that decreasing cholesterol levels over time will lead to a decrease in the incid-ence of clinical sequelae directly attributable to the advanced lesions of atherosclerosis in such individuals. Consequently, new guidelines have been recommended to physicians in the United States for both routine determination of cholesterol levels and for treatment (dietary, or dietary and pharmacolo-gical, dependent upon the level of plasma cholesterol) to reduce cholesterol levels to an accepted safe range. Plasma cholesterol levels are considered acceptable if they are below 200 mg/dl. Levels between 200 and 240 mg/dl should be treated by diet, and above 240 mg/dl by diet and, if necessary, cholesterol-lowering agents. These agents include inhibitors of HMG CoA reductase, bile acid sequestrants, and others. In addition, since elevations in HDL are as beneficial as reductions in LDL in relation to prevention of atherosclerosis, the ratio of these two lipoproteins is considered an important part of the diagnostic work-up of hypercholesterolaemic individuals. Such approaches will undoubtedly change the attitude toward diagnosis and treatment of diseases associated with hyper-cholesterolaemia, particularly atherosclerosis.

12.2.3 Hypertension

Hypertension has long been recognized as a risk factor associ-ated with increased incidence of coronary heart disease,

Table 12.2 Single-gene disorders that predispose to premature coronary artery disease (after Goldstein and Brown 1988)

Disorder	Typical age for myocardial infarction	Primary biochemical defect	Mechanism of inheritance	Estimated population frequency
Familial hypercholesterolaemia		Defective cell surface receptor for plasma LDL	Dominant	
heterozygous form	Adult			1 in 500
homozygous form	Childhood			1 in 1 000 000
Multiple lipoprotein hyperlipidaemia (familial combined hyperlipidaemia)	Adult	Not known	Dominant	1 in 200
Familial hypertriglyceridaemia	Adult	Not known	Dominant	1 in 300
Familial dysbetalipoproteinaemia	Adult	Abnormal apoE-II	Recessive	1 in 40 000
Cholesterol ester storage disease	Young adult	Deficiency of lysosomal acid lipase	Recessive	1 in 1 000 000

cerebrovascular disease, and accelerated atherogenesis (see also Section 12.5). Epidemiologically, the effects of hypertension appear to be unrelated to those of other risk factors; however, when coupled with risk factors such as hypercholesterolaemia, there appears to be a synergistic effect of these in increasing the incidence of atherosclerosis-induced disease.

The mechanisms by which hypertension causes the cellular changes that result in atherosclerosis are not clear. Experimentally induced hypertension in rabbits has demonstrated cellular interactions not too dissimilar from those observed in hypercholesterolaemia (discussed below), namely, increased monocyte adherence and intimal localization of monocyte-derived macrophages which, however, do not accumulate lipid but are localized as macrophages within the intima. The potential role of these cells in the subsequent cellular events that lead to proliferative lesions of atherosclerosis remains to be elucidated in these experimentally induced hypertensive animals. Humoral mediators of blood pressure may be important participants in the process, ranging from angiotensin and renin to substances that have not yet been defined. Altered haemodynamic properties have been suggested to be important in hypertensive individuals, and since it is clear that many lesions occur at branches and bifurcations opposite the flow divider, where it is known that the characteristics of the flow are strikingly different than they are in other parts of the arterial system, it is conceivable that in individuals with increased blood pressure, these rheologic properties may be further changed and may play important roles in inducing cellular interactions that result in proliferative intimal smooth muscle lesions.

12.2.4   Cigarette smoking

Perhaps one of the strongest epidemiological associations with the increased incidence of atherosclerosis is that of cigarette smoking. Substances released within the plasma in individuals who smoke cigarettes have not been identified as yet; however, a series of tobacco glycoproteins has been isolated which is said to somehow be associated with an immune response within the artery wall. Should this prove to be the case, cigarette smoking and immune injury to the endothelium, resulting in a series of cellular interactions culminating in proliferative lesions of atherosclerosis, may prove to be important in individuals who smoke and who mount an immune response to these tobacco-derived substances. Clearly, cessation of cigarette smoking decreases the risk for the development of the clinical sequelae of atherosclerosis; however, further research remains to be pursued to clearly determine which factors in cigarette smoking are important in this process.

A series of studies was performed to examine the nature of the lesions of atherosclerosis in middle-aged men who had a history of smoking and had occlusive lesions of the superficial femoral artery. These patients were normolipaemic or moderately hyperlipaemic. The lesions of the normolipaemic individuals were occlusive, densely fibrotic, and contained little to no demonstrable lipid. In contrast, the moderately hyperlipaemic individuals had lesions with deposits of lipid within them.

12.2.5   Diabetes

Diabetes represents an equally important risk factor for increased incidence of atherosclerosis. Individuals who have clinical diabetes mellitus have increased incidence of atherosclerosis and myocardial infarction. Many diabetic individuals are hypercholesterolaemic. However, for those who are normocholesterolaemic, the mechanisms by which diabetes results in increased lesions of atherosclerosis is poorly understood. Some diabetics demonstrate decreased levels of HDL and often are hypertensive in association with their hyperglycaemia. Nevertheless, specific substances in the plasma or changes in the artery wall that may be associated with this process have yet to be identified.

12.2.6   Experimental studies

A large number of morphological investigations have been performed using non-human primates, rabbits, swine, pigeons, and other species to determine the cellular changes and interactions that lead to the development of each of the different lesions of atherosclerosis. Studies in diet-induced hypercholesterolaemic non-human primates and hypercholesterolaemic swine, and in endogenously hypercholesterolaemic Watanabe heritable hyperlipidaemic rabbits (WHHL) compared to matched fat-fed rabbits have demonstrated similar types and chronology of cellular interactions that precede lesion development. The WHHL rabbit is the only hypercholesterolaemic animal model of FH disease, in which LDL receptors are non-functional. Thus each WHHL rabbit becomes hypercholesterolaemic regardless of diet. The cellular changes that have been described in all of the hypercholesterolaemic animals, regardless of the basis for the increase in cholesterol, appear to be the same. The anatomic sites at which they occur will vary with the species. They are as follows.

Within 7–12 days after inducing high levels of hypercholesterolaemia (500–1000 mg/dl) or within 6–8 months after lower levels (250–300 mg/dl), the first cellular response that can be observed occurs in the form of numerous clusters of leucocytes that are attached to the endothelium of the artery wall throughout the aorta, iliac, coronary, and carotid arteries (Fig. 12.9). The leucocytes consist principally of monocytes together with some lymphocytes. The attached cells migrate along the surface of the endothelium and are chemotactically attracted to probe between endothelial cells and migrate subendothelially (Fig. 12.10), where they localize within the intima. In hypercholesterolaemic animals, the monocytes take up lipid which has accumulated in the intima due to transendothelial transport from the hypercholesterolaemic plasma. The intimal lipid contains numerous particles of lipid as well as small membranous constituents presumably derived from lipoprotein, which may have been altered as they passed into the connective tissue space of the intima. Within a relatively short period of time, the monocytes take up the lipid and gradually expand to take on the appearance of macrophages full of lipid droplets, so that some of them eventually become foam cells (Fig. 12.11).

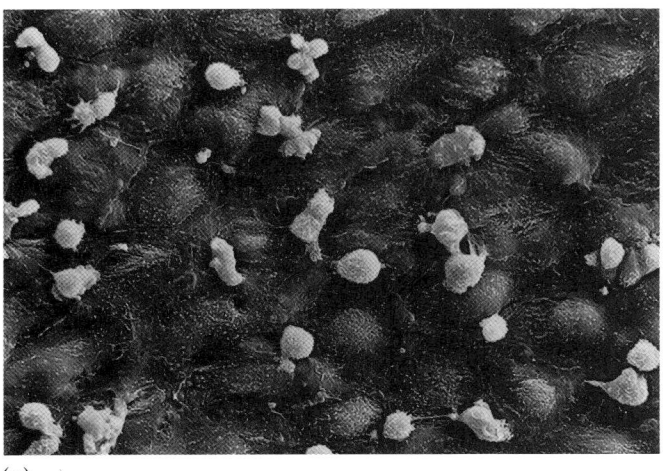

(a)

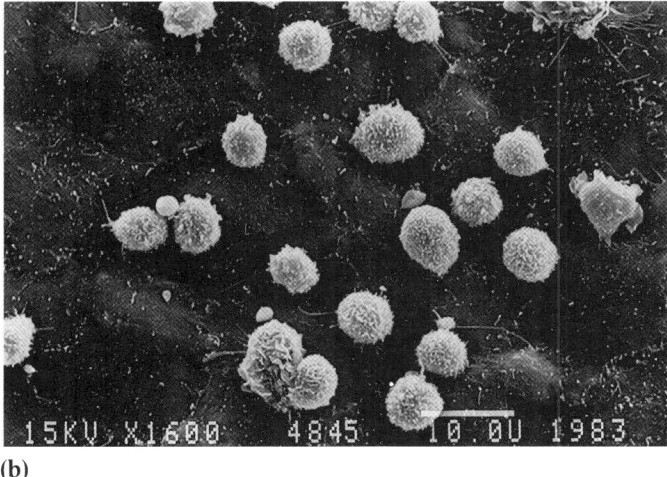

(b)

Fig. 12.9 (a), (b) These scanning electron micrographs demonstrate the endothelial surface of the thoracic aorta of a hypercholesterolaemic non-human primate 12 days after induction of a high level of hypercholesterolaemia (700–1000 mg/dl). Numerous mononuclear cells, principally monocytes, are attached to the surface of the endothelium. This attachment and the chemotactic activity of these monocytes occur due to substances, released in the plasma and within the artery wall, that cause the monocytes to adhere preferentially to endothelium at sites in the artery, to migrate on the endothelial surface, to probe between the endothelial cells, and to localize subendothelially, where they become converted to macrophages.

These collections of intimal foam cells, or fatty streaks, enlarge by the process of continued chemoattraction of additional monocytes to attach to the surface of the lesions and to enter into the lesion (Fig. 12.12).

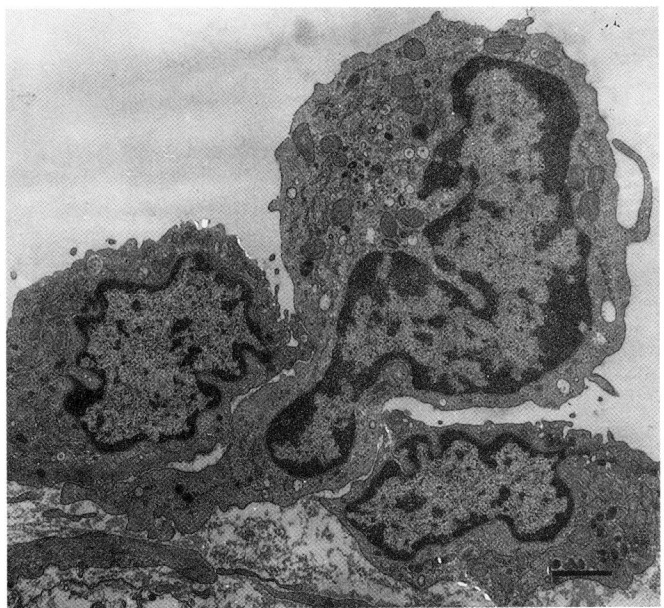

Fig. 12.10 In this transmission electron micrograph, this peripheral blood monocyte is half within the intima and half in the lumen of the artery. It is never possible to know the direction the cell is moving in any given micrograph. Since this cell contains no lipid and appears like a relatively inactive monocyte, it is probably a monocyte that is in the process of entering the artery prior to its development into a macrophage or a foam cell. (Reproduced from Faggiotto *et al.* 1984, by permission of the American Heart Association, Inc.)

With increasing duration of hypercholesterolaemia, a second cell type appears in the fatty streak. These are smooth muscle cells, which are attracted from the underlying media into the intima, where they also begin to take up lipid and become foam cells (Fig. 12.11). Observations in the hypercholesterolaemic animals suggest that the majority of the fatty streaks progress to fibrous plaques by a continuing process of attraction of smooth muscle cells and macrophages into the lesion. These sometimes form alternating layers of cells, but eventually the cells become intermixed, a fibrous cap of smooth muscle starts to form at the lumen, and the lesions then evolve into the shape and substructure of the human fibrous plaques described above. The period of time required for this may depend on many factors, including the degree and duration of hypercholesterolaemia, the artery and anatomic site involved, and the genetic susceptibility of the host.

At some branches and bifurcations opposite the flow divider of some arteries, a second set of changes has been observed in hypercholesterolaemic non-human primates, swine, and rabbits. Because these are, in general, only observed at branches and bifurcations, they are thought to be related in part to the haemodynamic characteristics of the blood flow at these particular sites. These changes consist of junctional separations between individual endothelial cells overlying the fatty streak, accompanied by retraction of these endothelial cells to uncover many of the lipid-filled macrophages in the lesion. In some cases, these macrophages appear to be swept into the bloodstream, where they can be found in the circulation. In other cases they appear to remain *in situ*. In either case, where endothelial retraction and/or macrophage exposure has occurred, platelets may be found adherent to exposed connective tissue or to some of the macrophages that have been exposed to the circulation. Platelet adhesion has also been observed at sites where

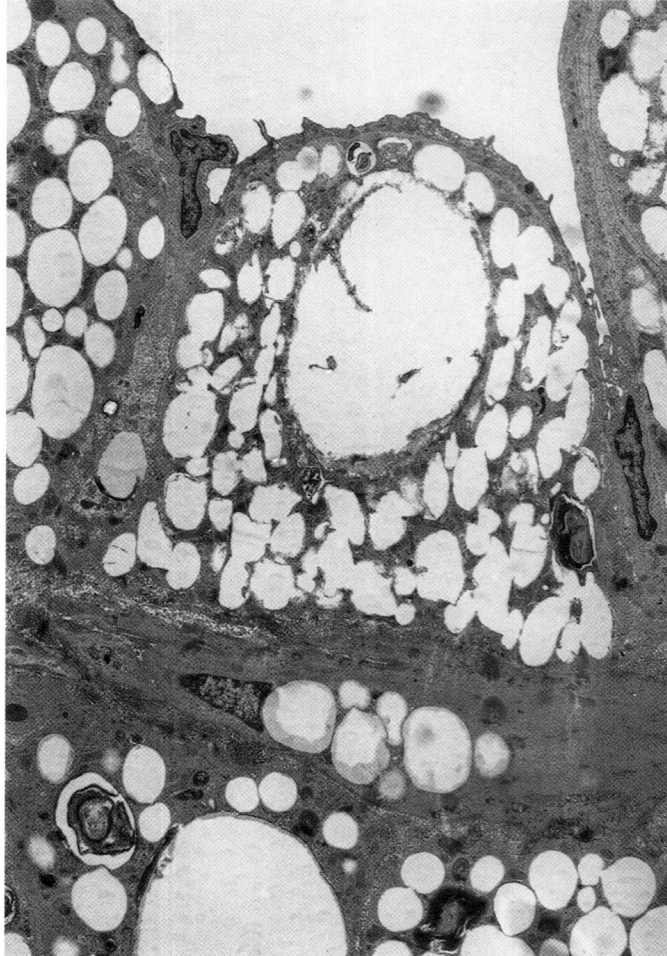

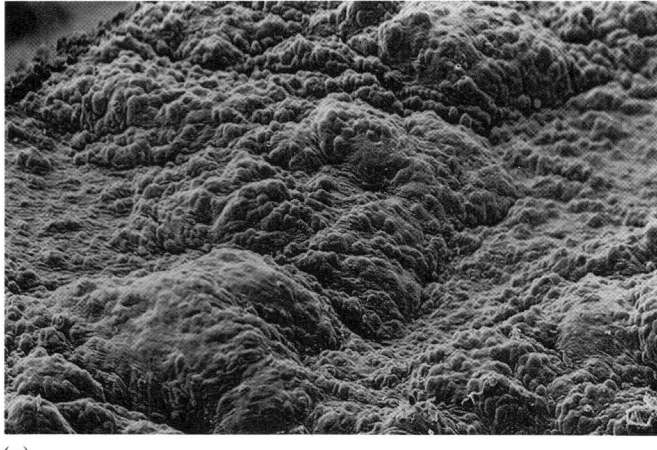

(a)

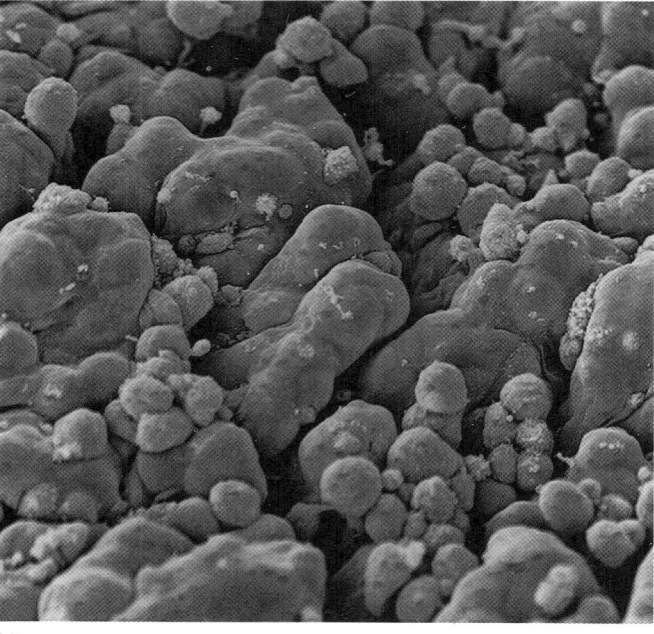

(b)

Fig. 12.11 In this transmission electron micrograph, several lipid-filled macrophages constitute the fatty streak. These were found in a monkey that had been hypercholesterolaemic for 2 months. Beneath the lipid-filled macrophages can be seen a lipid-filled smooth muscle cell that has migrated from the media into the intima, has taken up lipid, and will also become a foam cell. Thus fatty streaks can become mixed macrophage-smooth muscle lesions. (Reproduced from Faggiotto *et al.* 1984, by permission of the American Heart Association, Inc.)

Fig. 12.12 (a) This low-power scanning electron micrograph demonstrates the marked change in the surface contours of the lining of the artery in this hypercholesterolaemic non-human primate 2 months after being on a hypercholesterolaemic regimen. (b) At high magnification, a region of such a fatty streak can be seen to consist of numerous elevations and deep folds in the surface of the aorta. Attached to this fatty streak are large numbers of mononuclear cells that participate in expansion of the fatty streak as long as the animal is hypercholesterolaemic. Thus the fatty streak can continue to expand as long as factors responsible for its initiation and progression remain present within the artery.

individual macrophages are exposed to the circulation, possibly because they are in the process of exiting the lesion to return to the circulation (Fig. 12.13). At sites where such platelet adherence may have occurred, it would appear that, within relatively short periods of time, extensive proliferative smooth muscle lesions form at similar anatomic sites. This suggests that where platelet interactions occur, they may be associated with more rapid lesion formation, possibly due to substances released locally by platelets. It should be emphasized that, at most sites, the endothelium remains intact and the fatty streaks appear to be converted with time to proliferative smooth muscle lesions.

These observations have suggested a series of questions that require further investigation to determine the factors that are responsible for increased adhesion and attraction of monocytes

into the artery, as well as the factors that chemotactically induce migration of smooth muscle cells from the media into the intima. Establishing which factors are responsible for the proliferation of the smooth muscle cells and for the formation of connective tissue, and thus for the formation of the proliferative

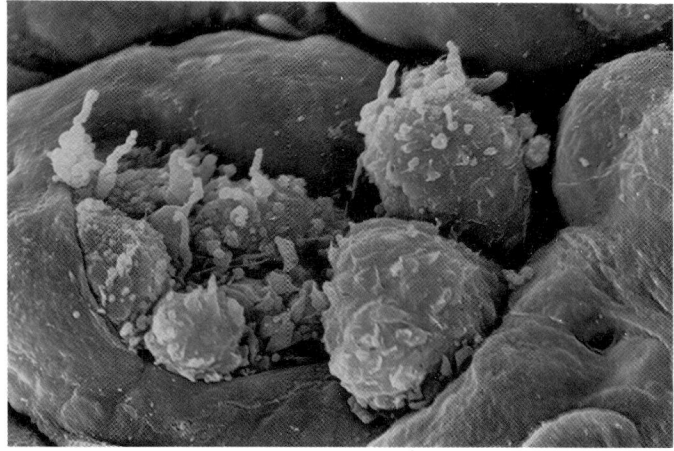

(a)

(b)

Fig. 12.13 (a) In this scanning electron micrograph, a section of a fatty streak has lost its endothelial cover by endothelial retraction. The retracted smooth edge of the endothelium has exposed several of the underlying lipid-filled macrophages, or foam cells, some of which can act as a nidus for platelet adherence and thrombus formation. (b) A scanning electron micrograph of a portion of a fatty streak in an artery from a chronically hypercholesterolaemic monkey. Numerous platelets can be seen adherent to these exposed macrophages in a part of this fatty streak. Changes such as these, when they occur, usually do so at branches and bifurcations. (Reproduced from Ross 1986.)

fibrous plaque, is of particular importance since it is the advanced lesion that results in clinical sequelae including thrombosis, myocardial infarction, cerebral infarction, peripheral vascular disease, and gangrene.

12.2.7 Cells involved in atherogenesis

If we are to understand the pathogenesis of the lesions of atherosclerosis, it is necessary to understand the functional roles of each cell and the alterations in each of the cells involved in lesion development. Therefore, not only is an understanding of arterial endothelium and smooth muscle paramount in this process, but the role of circulating blood cells, including platelets, monocyte/macrophages, and lymphocytes is equally critical. This is true, as indicated above, because each of these cells is involved either in different stages of formation of the lesions or, in the case of the monocyte/macrophage and the lymphocyte, are found to varying degrees in both the early and the advanced lesions of human atherosclerosis. Consequently, it is important to understand the roles each of these cells can play in both lesion induction and progression and, of particular import, the nature of the cellular interactions that occur in circumstances such as hypercholesterolaemia, hypertension, and the other risk factors associated with increased incidence of atherosclerosis.

Endothelium

The endothelial cells perform a large number of functions. Of particular interest in atherogenesis is the functional capacity of endothelium to modify and transport lipoproteins, to participate in the adherence of leucocytes, to form vasoactive substances, to participate in procoagulant and anticoagulant activity, and to form growth factors (see Section 12.1). When endothelial cells are presented with low-density lipoprotein, they will bind, internalize, and modify the lipoprotein and can oxidize it, making it available for macrophage uptake via the scavenger receptor on the surface of the macrophage. Endothelial cell turnover is reasonably low in most parts of the adult, fully developed arterial system, except at sites where rheologic changes have an influence on this property. Continuous tritiated thymidine administration to experimental animals suggests that an increase in endothelial turnover may be more common than previously suspected. Increased turnover and 'injury' to the endothelial cells at given anatomic sites, or exposure of the endothelium to cytokines such as tumour necrosis factor, can induce the endothelial cells to express the genes for mitogens such as platelet-derived growth factor (PDGF) and interleukin-1. Furthermore, exposure of endothelium to coagulant factors such as activated factor X or thrombin can also induce early secretion of stored PDGF and, later, gene expression and synthesis, and secretion of PDGF. Thus under appropriate conditions, the endothelium can become a rich and potentially important source of mitogens. This may be particularly important in the development and progression of fatty streaks to more advanced lesions, since in these cases the endothelium is positioned in close proximity to potentially activated macrophages.

Very advanced lesions of atherosclerosis often become vascularized by vasa vasorum, usually derived from the adventitia. When this occurs, the endothelium from the vasa could also serve as a source of growth factors, if appropriately stimulated.

Smooth muscle

As discussed earlier, smooth muscle cells are the principal source of connective tissue in the fibrous plaques and, in addition, have the capacity when appropriately stimulated to form growth factors; in particular, PDGF A-chain. Under normal circumstances in adult animals, there appears to be little or no gene expression for growth factors, and thus little to no mitogen formation by smooth muscle. It has been demonstrated, however, that in smooth muscle cells obtained from developing rat aorta and from experimentally induced proliferative lesions in rats, as well as from human fibrous plaques, some of the smooth muscle cells from these lesions express the genes for the A-chain of PDGF and have the capacity to secrete this mitogen when these cells are grown in culture. At what stage of lesion development this may occur and whether the mitogen is actually secreted *in vivo* remains to be determined.

It is important to emphasize that the most important aspect of the advanced lesions of atherosclerosis is the fact that they are intimal proliferative lesions. Consequently, smooth muscle multiplication accompanied by new connective tissue formation with variable amounts of lipid accumulation are the critical components of lesions that lead to clinical sequelae. The smooth muscle replication that occurs may take place either in a pre-existing region of diffuse intimal thickening that occurred during normal development and ageing, or in a region of the artery where the intima is very thin. In the former situation, the smooth muscle cells will have migrated and proliferated at a low level during an earlier interval. In the latter, acute migration into the intima associated with smooth muscle proliferation must occur. At present it is difficult to know which of these has occurred at any given lesion; however, the end result is probably the same—a fibrous plaque or complicated lesion.

Three other principal players in this process that must be considered are the monocyte/macrophage, the platelet, and the lymphocyte.

The monocyte/macrophage

The monocyte has been amply demonstrated to be the precursor cell of macrophages in all tissues. When it enters a tissue, it has a variable life-span and turnover, dependent upon the tissue and the stimulus for entry. Monocytes can be activated by numerous substances, and when this occurs can synthesize and secrete a wide panoply of biologically active agents, including growth factors. Thus the activated macrophage can secrete growth factors for connective tissue cells, such as fibroblasts and smooth muscle, in the form of both chains of PDGF. They can also form fibroblast growth factor (FGF), although it is not clear if FGF is secreted by these cells. FGF is also a potent angiogenic agent and thus can play a role in capillary formation as

well as in connective tissue proliferation. Activated macrophages can also secrete a mitogen that can induce epithelial migration and proliferation, namely, transforming growth factor-α (TGF-α), and substances that may modulate or moderate growth factor activity, such as transforming growth factor-β (TGF-β). TGF-β is the most potent inhibitor of cell proliferation that has thus far been discovered. TGF-β is also one of the most potent inducers of collagen synthesis and is undoubtedly important in this process in the artery wall. In addition, interleukin-1 (IL-1) can be formed by activated macrophages. This can have an indirect and profound effect on lymphocyte proliferation, and is also a modest mitogen for some connective tissue cells. Finally, activated macrophages may also form colony-stimulating factor-1 (CSF-1), which may in turn act in an autocrine fashion on macrophages or possibly on stem cell precursors of the macrophages that may be present in a given tissue.

An important cytokine, tumour necrosis factor (TNF-α or cachectin), is also one of the major factors formed and released by the activated macrophages. As described above, when TNF-α is exposed to endothelial cells, it will induce endothelial gene expression for PDGF, resulting in PDGF synthesis and secretion. Therefore in the fatty streak, where activated macrophages may find themselves in close juxtaposition to endothelial cells, TNFα secretion may be associated with activated macrophages, endothelial activation, and growth factor formation by both cell types associated with the progression of the fatty streak to a fibrous plaque.

Macrophages also act as scavenger cells and can induce free radical formation by oxidizing ingested lipids. If they secrete such oxidized material together with other agents such as hydrolytic enzymes, these could be injurious to neighbouring cells, including endothelium and smooth muscle. In this way, the macrophage could play a major role in inducing further tissue injury. Thus a complicated set of events combining cell–cell interactions, lipid accumulation, tissue injury, and mitogenesis surround the role of the macrophage in lesion formation and progression in atherosclerosis. The macrophage is probably the key cell responsible for mitogenic stimulation of smooth muscle, and thus is critical in lesion formation and progression in atherogenesis (also Section 12.3).

The platelet

Platelets are a rich source of multiple growth factors or mitogens. PDGF was first described because of its release from activated platelets; however, it did not take long to demonstrate that activated platelets also secrete relatively large amounts of an epidermal growth factor (EGF)-like substance, TGF-β, and a specific growth factor for arterial endothelial cells that is in the process of being characterized. In addition, platelets play a major role in the coagulation process and, of course, thrombosis. It is common to observe that thrombi readily organize by ingrowth and proliferation of smooth muscle cells, which are responsible for deposition of new connective tissue. This undoubtedly occurs because of the wealth of growth factors present in the thrombus that have been released from the aggregated degranulated platelets. It is also possible that platelets may be important as a source of mitogens during development of some lesions of atherosclerosis where mural thrombi may form at sites of altered endothelium. Such thrombi have been observed in experimental hypercholesterolaemic animals if, for several possible reasons, the endothelial cells have lost their capacity to provide a non-thrombogenic surface. In addition, complicated lesions may form by progression of fibrous plaques at sites where ulceration, fissuring, or cracking of the fibrous plaque may occur. This could lead to haemorrhage into the plaque and secondary thrombosis, followed by additional smooth muscle proliferation and connective tissue formation, and thus lesion progression.

The lymphocyte

More recently, it has been appreciated that T-cells are also a feature of many advanced lesions of atherosclerosis (see Fig. 12.8). The role of the T-cells in the process of atherogenesis is not understood, but their presence suggests that immune or auto-immune responses may be involved. Many of the T-cells observed in fibrous plaques were found to be activated, based upon their ability to express class II HLA surface antigens. A majority of the plaque cells were observed to be HLA-DR positive, and many of these were smooth muscle cells. It is assumed that T-cells are attracted into the artery wall by the formation of cytokines, or some form of chemotactic factor, and that they interact with cell-surface antigens on macrophages and/or smooth muscle cells or endothelium. On the assumption that appropriate antigens are present and that T-cell/macrophage/endothelial or smooth muscle interactions may occur, other cytokines may be generated, such as γ-interferon (IFN) or IL-1. These may lead to further intercellular reactions that culminate in the release of substances, including growth factors, that may play an important role in the cellular proliferative response. In addition, in situations where an immune response to antigens occurs in the vessel wall, as in rejection of cardiac transplants, it is common to find that the rejected transplants have rampant atherosclerotic involvement of the coronary arteries. This is probably similar to atherosclerosis induced in experimental animals by serum sickness. In these cases, immunological injury to associated cells in the artery walls may play a key role in generating the proliferative response due to the release of growth factors from these cells.

What risk-factor-associated phenomena could result in autoimmunity in atherosclerosis? Could substances such as organic tobacco glycoproteins released during cigarette smoking, or complement components associated with extracellular lipids in developing lesions be involved? Pharmacological agents, such as cyclosporin, that inhibit the immune response of T-helper cells have been observed to result in a decrease in the incidence and size of lesions formed in experimentally induced atherosclerosis. Thus, immunity and auto-immunity may be important in the genesis and progression of the lesions of atherosclerosis and their sequelae; this is discussed further in Section 12.3.

12.2.8 Growth factors

There are several putative candidates to consider when attempting to determine the nature of the mitogenic substances responsible for the intimal proliferative response that characterizes the fibrous plaque and complicated lesions of atherosclerosis. One mitogen that is potentially important in this process is PDGF, which is both a potent mitogen and a chemoattractant for smooth muscle cells. As discussed above, it can be formed by appropriately activated arterial endothelial cells, by activated monocyte/macrophages, and is released from platelets at sites where platelet adherence, aggregation, and degranulation occur. Furthermore, PDGF A-chain messenger RNA has been observed in some smooth muscle cells derived from proliferative lesions of human atherosclerosis when they are grown in cell culture, suggesting that under these conditions PDGF may act in an autocrine capacity. Stimuli that can induce endothelial cells to secrete and express the gene for PDGF include increased turnover of the endothelium, exposure to coagulation factors, such as factor Xa and thrombin, or platelet-derived factors, as well as exposure to IL-1 or TNF-α. The latter is of particular interest in view of the fact that one of the principal products of activated macrophages is TNF-α. Thus the fatty streak represents an ideal milieu in which activated macrophages could serve to stimulate overlying endothelial cells in the fatty streak to synthesize and secrete PDGF.

Activated macrophages express the genes for both A- and B-chains of PDGF, and appear to secrete homodimers of each of these chains after appropriate stimulation. If macrophages in the fatty streak are in such states of activation, and if they also produce TNF-α so that they have stimulated the overlying endothelial cells, then both of these cells could play critical roles in secreting PDGF as well as other growth factors, which might be important in chemotactically attracting smooth muscle cells to migrate from the media into the intima, to proliferate, and to secrete connective tissue proteins. Connective tissue synthesis can be induced by numerous factors, but in particular by transforming growth factor-β (TGF-β). Activated macrophages and endothelial cells can secrete TGF-β. TGF-β acts in a complicated fashion as both an inhibitor of proliferation and perhaps more importantly, as an inducer of cell differentiation and a stimulator of both collagen and proteoglycan formation. Thus, in the environment in which appropriate growth factors and modulators of proliferation and differentiation are present, smooth muscle cells may respond to these factors by proliferating and by laying down new connective tissue matrix, both of which are integral to the development of the fibroproliferative lesions that occur during atherogenesis. In addition, the formation of IL-1 by macrophages may serve to attract lymphocytes into the lesion. This would then present a complex picture in which lymphocytes and macrophages may interact with smooth muscle cells, resulting in alternating layers of smooth muscle and macrophages mixed with varying numbers of lymphocytes, characteristic of the morphology observed in the complex advanced lesions of atherosclerosis.

12.2.9   Response to injury hypothesis of atherosclerosis

The events described above in experimentally induced hypercholesterolaemia in primates, swine, and rabbits have also been described in some forms of experimentally induced hypertension, in baboons made homocysteinaemic, and in lesions induced by immune responses such as serum sickness or graft rejection of transplanted hearts. These observations have led to the formulation of a hypothesis that has been modified and refined during the past 16 years, termed the 'response to injury hypothesis' (Fig. 12.14).

This hypothesis suggests that some form of 'injury' to the endothelium lining that artery results in a sequence of events that lead to the development of the lesions of atherosclerosis. The 'injury' may be a subtle event and may result in functional but no observable morphological alterations in the endothelium. Some observations suggest that the 'injury' may alter cell surface glycoproteins of the endothelial cells as well as those on the circulating monocytes and lymphocytes. Such changes could lead to increased monocyte and lymphocyte adhesion to the endothelium and would be accompanied by chemotactic attraction of these cells into the subendothelial space.

Those forms of injury that lead to no phenotypic alterations in the endothelium may lead to increased endothelial turnover, although morphological observation of the vessel surface itself may provide no evidence for such increased turnover. Nevertheless, this may be sufficient to induce expression of genes for growth factors in the endothelium or, at the very least, generation of chemotactic factors for monocytes. When the monocytes have attached, migrated between the endothelium and entered into the subendothelial space, they may then become activated as macrophages, which are capable of expressing genes for numerous growth factors, including PDGF A- and B-chains, TGF-α, TGF-β, IL-1, TNF-α, CSF-1, PGE, and γ-IFN. There is also evidence that macrophages may form FGF, although FGF secretion has not yet been demonstrated. The observation that both macrophages and activated endothelial cells can form growth factors appropriate for activating and attracting smooth muscle cells into the intima from the media suggests that during atherogenesis these cells are the principal source of growth factors that initiate intimal smooth muscle migration, accumulation, and proliferation.

Furthermore, should endothelial integrity be lost at particular anatomic sites, such as branches or bifurcations, and should conditions develop such that platelet interactions occur, platelets are also a rich source of all the growth factors capable of attracting smooth muscle cells into the intima. Thus the presence of appropriate conditions to provide growth factors in the intima for cells of the artery are readily determined by a number of events, since all of the cells capable of interacting in the artery wall are also capable of forming the growth factors critical to the development of the intimal proliferative smooth muscle response. As a consequence, the varying forms of injury, including hypercholesterolaemia, hypertension (the basis of 'injury' is unknown unless it is mechanically associated with rheologic factors), toxins, viruses, substances such as homocysteine or substances from tobacco smoking (such as tobacco glycoproteins), or immune injury could be postulated to play a role in bringing about changes in endothelium, macrophages, and smooth muscle cells that can result in the development of intimal proliferative lesions that ultimately take the form of the advanced lesions of atherosclerosis.

Once the smooth muscle cells have been attracted into the intima in sufficient quantity, a complex series of cellular interactions could then occur (according to the response to injury hypothesis), in which lymphocytes and macrophages may interact to stimulate macrophages to secrete growth factors; macrophages and endothelium may continue to interact to induce the endothelium to do the same; and both endothelium and macrophages may stimulate smooth muscle cells to multiply and perhaps to induce gene expression for PDGF in the smooth muscle cells themselves. In this way, if PDGF genes are expressed in some of the smooth muscle cells in the proliferating lesion, they may represent a further basis for lesion progression in which the smooth muscle cells may play a role as well.

Observations derived from testing the 'response to injury hypothesis' permit one to postulate means of preventing lesion formation by finding ways of protecting the endothelium, or developing approaches to selectively prevent monocyte adherence and conversion to macrophages within the artery wall. Specific antagonists to the different growth factors and/or their

Fig. 12.14   The 'response to injury hypothesis'. Advanced intimal proliferative lesions of atherosclerosis may occur by at least two pathways. The pathway demonstrated by the clockwise (green) arrows to the right has been observed in experimentally induced hypercholesterolaemic in non-human primates, rabbits, and swine. Injury to the endothelium (A) may induce growth factor secretion (short arrow). Monocytes attach to endothelium (B), which may continue to secrete growth factors (short arrow). Subendothelial migration of monocytes (C) may lead to fatty streak formation and release of growth factors such as PDGF (light blue arrow) by these cells as they become activated macrophages. Fatty streaks may become directly converted to fibrous plaques (green arrow from C to F) through release of growth factors from macrophages, or endothelial cells, or both. Macrophages may also stimulate and/or injure the overlying endothelium. In some cases, macrophages may lose their endothelial cover and platelet attachment may occur (D), providing three possible sources of growth factors—platelets, macrophages, and endothelium (light blue arrows). Some of the smooth muscle cells in the proliferative lesion itself (F) may form and secrete growth factors such as PDGF (light blue arrows). An alternative pathway for development of advanced lesions of atherosclerosis is shown by the bright blue arrows from A to E to F. In this case, the endothelium may be injured but remain morphologically intact. Increased endothelial turnover may result in growth-factor formation by endothelial cells (A). This may stimulate migration of smooth muscle cells from the media into the intima, accompanied by endogenous production of PDGF by smooth muscle, as well as growth factor secretion from the 'injured' endothelial cells (E). These interactions could then lead to fibrous-plaque formation and further lesion progression (F). (Drawn after Ross 1986, with permission.)

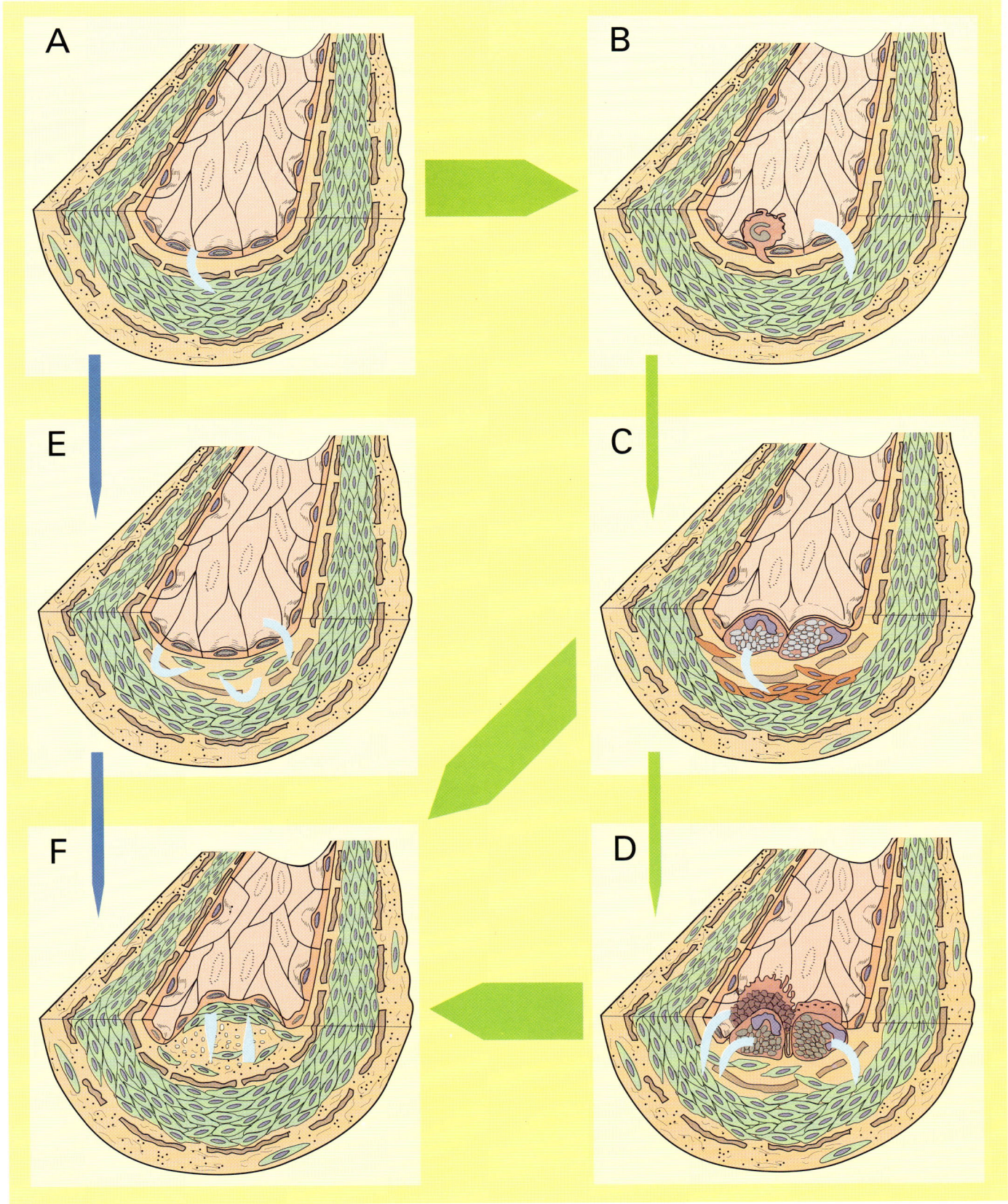

receptors should also provide opportunities to develop new diagnostic tools that might permit one to detect patients who are at risk on a genetic basis or on the basis of substances released by the altered cells in the artery.

This hypothesis suggests that it should be possible to find means of 'protecting' the endothelium from 'injury' and of developing antagonists to specific growth factors or to their receptors that would then inhibit the intimal migration as well as the proliferation of monocytes and/or smooth muscle cells, thus precluding lesion development.

12.2.10   Regression of atherosclerosis

Until recently, the question as to whether advanced lesions of atherosclerosis could regress was a controversial one. In experimentally induced atherosclerosis, fatty streaks are totally reversible, and it is presumed that this is also true for humans. There is also evidence in hypercholesterolaemic non-human primates containing advanced proliferative lesions that it is possible to induce regression of these lesions if the animals are placed on a normocholesterolaemic diet.

There is now evidence that it is also the case in humans. In a series of studies of hypercholesterolaemic patients with angiographically demonstrable advanced fibrous plaques, the plasma cholesterol of these patients was subsequently lowered by a combination of diet and hypercholesterolaemia-inducing drugs. Over a period of six months to several years, a significant proportion of these individuals showed statistically significant reductions in the size of their lesions, manifested by increase in the lumen of their arteries as seen in angiograms. Thus, there is good reason to believe that some advanced lesions in some individuals can regress. It is not yet understood what factors are important in permitting or preventing lesion progression and in which individuals these factors will be relevant. These data, however, suggest that the development of mechanisms to remove factors responsible for the formation of the lesions, or to impede substances that play a role in lesion formation, will be critical not only in preventing the formation of new lesions, but perhaps in inducing lesion regression as well.

12.2.11   Bibliography

Beigel, Y. and Gotto, A. (1986). *Lipoproteins in health and disease: diagnosis and management*. The Baylor College of Medicine, Cardiology Series 9–6, No. 1.

Faggiotto, A., Harker, L., and Ross, R. (1984). Studies of hypercholesterolaemia in the nonhuman primate. I. Changes that lead to fatty streak formation. *Arteriosclerosis* **4**, 323–40.

Goldstein, J. L. and Brown, M. S. (1988). Genetics and cardiovascular disease. In *Heart disease* (ed. E. Braunwald). W. B. Saunders, Philadelphia.

Gown, A. M., Tsukada, T., and Ross, R. (1986). Human atherosclerosis. II. Immunocytochemical analysis of the cellular composition of human atherosclerotic lesions. *American Journal of Pathology* **125**, 191–207.

Nathan, C. F., Murray, H. W., and Cohn, Z. A. (1980). The macrophage as an effector cell. *New England Journal of Medicine* **303**, 622–6.

Ross, R. (1986). The pathogenesis of atherosclerosis—an update. *New England Journal of Medicine* **314**, 488–500.

Ross, R. and Glomset, J. A. (1976). The pathogenesis of atherosclerosis. *New England Journal of Medicine* **295**, 369–77, 420–5.

Ross, R. and Harker, L. (1976). Hyperlipidemia and atherosclerosis. *Science* **193**, 1094–100.

Ross, R., Wight, T. N., Strandness, E., and Thiele, B. (1984). Human atherosclerosis. I. Cell constitution and characteristics of advanced lesions of the superficial femoral artery. *American Journal of Pathology* **114**, 79–93.

Ross, R., Raines, E. W., and Bowen-Pope, D. F. (1986). The biology of platelet-derived growth factor. *Cell* **46**, 155–69.

Unanue, E. R. (1980). Cooperation between mononuclear phagocytes and lymphocytes in immunity. *New England Journal of Medicine* **309**, 977–85.

12.3   Aortic atherosclerosis: pathogenesis and local complications

Dinah V. Parums

12.3.1   Introduction

This section will consider the role of macrophages in the pathogenesis of atherosclerosis in the human lesion and the local complications of aortic atherosclerosis. If the atherosclerotic plaque were an innocent intimal lesion without local complications or sequelae, it would not be the principal cause of death in Europe and the USA. It is the local complications of atherosclerosis which lead to its clinical sequelae. The local complications of the advanced 'complicated' atherosclerotic plaque include stenosis of the arterial lumen; plaque ulceration and fissuring ($\pm$ athero-emboli); thrombosis ($\pm$ thrombo-emboli); calcification; haemorrhage into the plaque; aneurysm formation ($\pm$ thrombosis, $\pm$ thrombo-emboli); and chronic inflammation. We see atherosclerosis in terms of its clinical horizon (Fig. 12.15), most commonly as ischaemia and infarction. At present, the only means of visualizing the extent and severity of an individual's atherosclerosis is at autopsy. There are no other laboratory, or clinical parameters, that estimate the generality of this diffuse arterial disease. *In vivo*, methodology to achieve this in patients is under development in this laboratory.

12.3.2   Macrophages in atherosclerosis

The atherosclerotic plaque consists of cells and non-cellular elements (Fig. 12.16). The 'response to injury hypothesis' (see Section 12.2.9) has been modified in recent years to incorporate the 'macrophage hypothesis'. The macrophage can be considered a major cellular component in atherogenesis and may be equally important in its clinical complications.

Over 50 years ago, Anitschkow and Duff realized that intimal

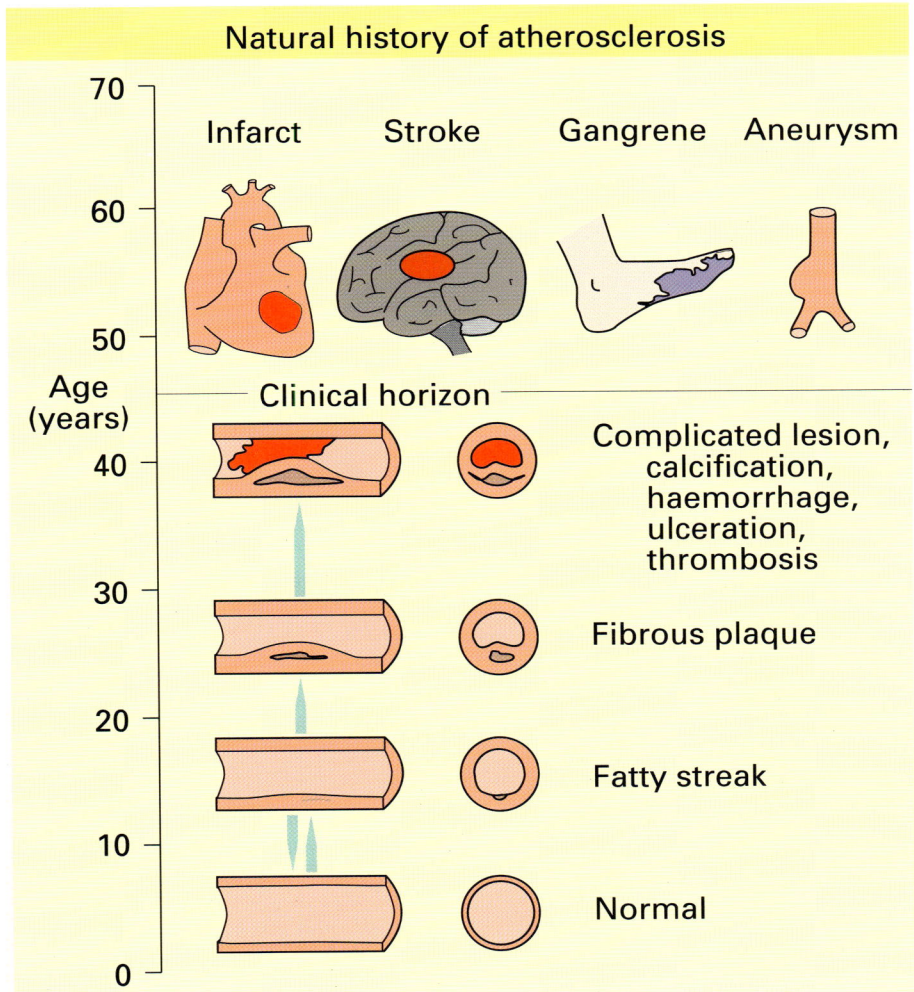

Natural history of atherosclerosis

Fig. 12.15 The clinical horizon of atherosclerosis.

foam cells were macrophages. It is now apparent that foam cells, present in fatty streaks and at the edges of most advanced plaques, are macrophages and that macrophages are found in the necrotic base of advanced atherosclerotic plaques. Smooth muscle cells are present in diffuse intimal thickening and are increased in number in larger lesions.

Ceroid is the insoluble yellowish pigment present in mammalian tissues, especially in vitamin E deficiency. It is associated with human atherosclerotic plaques and can be regarded as the hallmark of the advanced lesion. It is insoluble in lipid solvents and is recognizable in routinely processed tissue sections by lipid stains (Fig. 12.17); it is also auto-fluorescent. It has a characteristic laminated appearance on electron microscopy, with a periodicity to the laminae of 8 nm (Fig. 12.18). It probably consists of polymerized products of oxidized lipoproteins. It can be made artificially in the laboratory by oxidizing low-density lipoprotein (LDL).

The interaction with and uptake of lipoprotein by macrophages is summarized in Fig. 12.19. The macrophage hypothesis is a unifying concept of atherogenesis and permits some understanding of how atherosclerosis causes human disease.

The potential functions of macrophages in the pathogenesis of atherosclerosis include:

1. transport of LDL into the intima from blood-borne monocytes;

2. secretion of cytokines chemoattractant for monocytes and smooth muscle cells to the intima;

3. secretion of growth factors for smooth muscle and endothelial cells;

4. secretion of factors which induce phenotypic modulation of smooth muscle cells from a contractile to a secretory state;

5. secretion of angiogenic factors which stimulate new vessel formation at the base of the plaque;

6. secretion of neutral proteases (collagenases, elastases) which contribute to the formation of the necrotic 'gruel'-like content of the advanced plaque and may be involved in aneurysm formation; degraded collagen is thrombogenic and is also a common site for dystrophic calcification;

7. production of toxic oxygen radicals which contribute to (6)

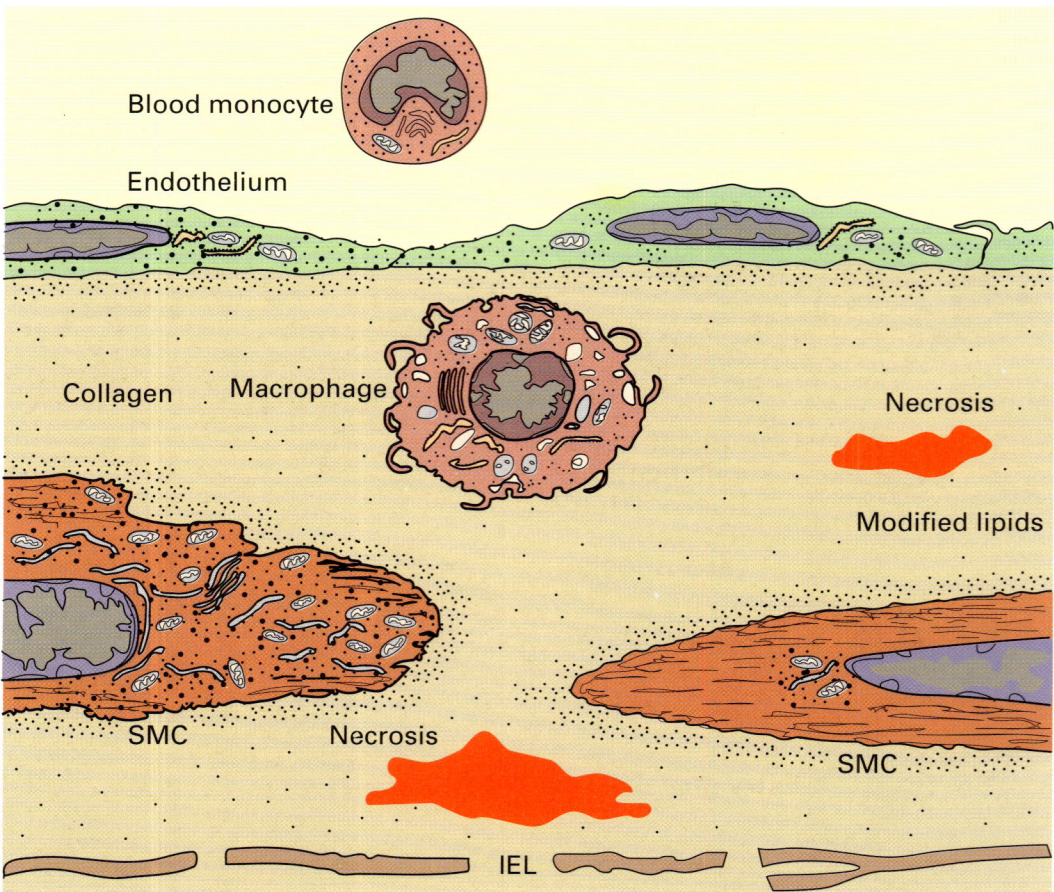

Fig. 12.16 This diagram represents the cellular and non-cellular constituents of the advanced or 'complicated' atherosclerotic plaque. (SML = smooth muscle cell; IEL = internal elastic lamina)

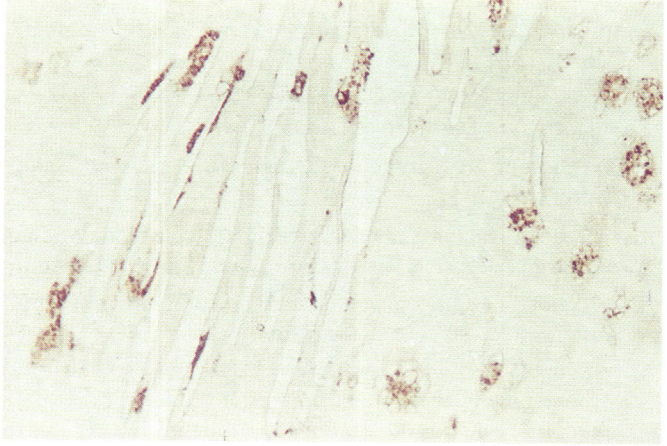

Fig. 12.17 This light micrograph shows ceroid rings and granules, both within macrophages and extracellularly in the base of the atheromatous plaque; stained with oil-red-O.

and further oxidize free LDL, enhancing its uptake by macrophages;

8. secretion of lipoprotein lipase by macrophages, leading to uptake and degradation of lipoproteins by macrophages;

9. re-emergence of lipid-laden intimal macrophages into the blood; although there is no evidence that this occurs in man, it could be the mechanism for the regression of early lesions;

10. oxidation of lipid within macrophages leading to the production of ceroid;

11. oxidation of LDL by macrophages is antigenic; this may be due to modification of lysyl residues in apolipoprotein B;

12. action of macrophages as antigen-presenting cells, secreting cytokines which recruit lymphocytes to the lesion.

In the development of the clinical complications of atherosclerosis, the most important roles of the macrophage include

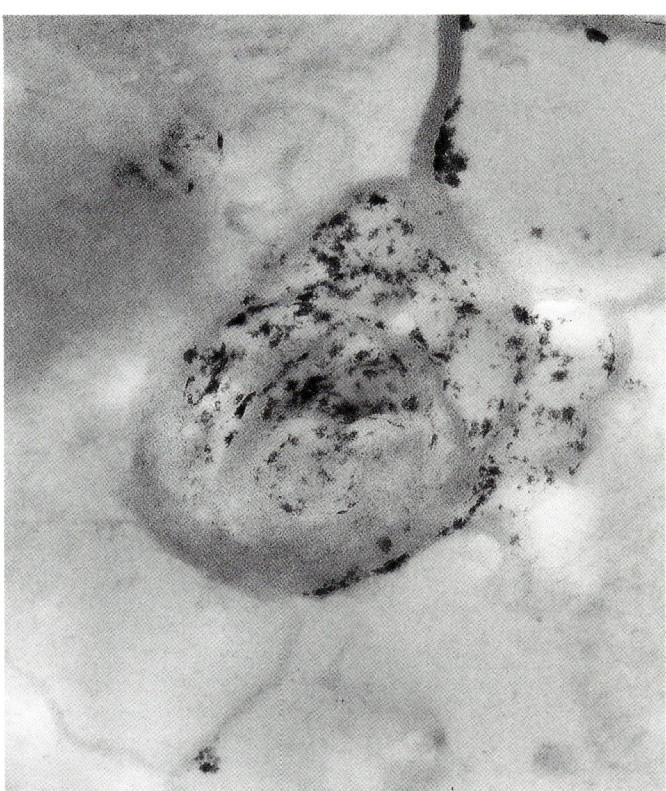

Fig. 12.18 This electron micrograph of the base of the atheromatous plaque shows ceroid lamellae of 8 nm periodicity and globular proteins of 50–100 nm diameter.

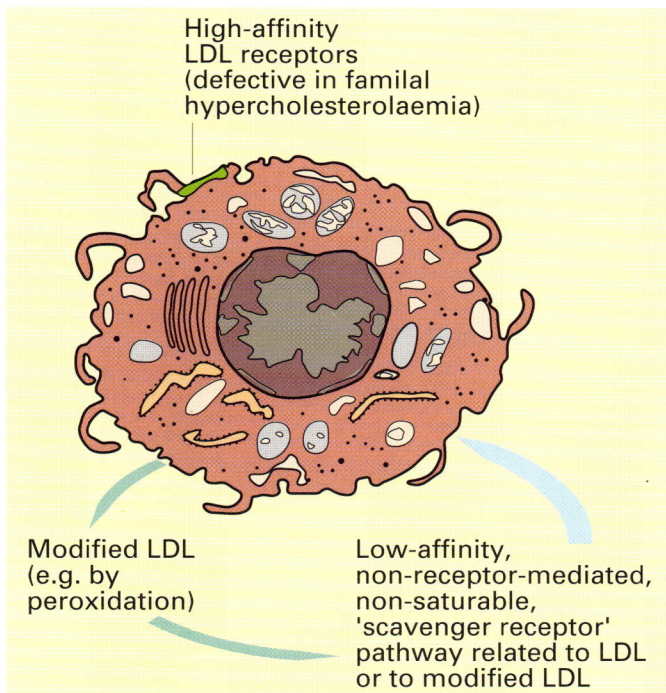

High-affinity LDL receptors (defective in familal hypercholesterolaemia)

Modified LDL (e.g. by peroxidation)

Low-affinity, non-receptor-mediated, non-saturable, 'scavenger receptor' pathway related to LDL or to modified LDL

Fig. 12.19 Handling of LDL by macrophages can occur by a receptor-mediated pathway which becomes downregulated when the cell has sufficient cholesterol. In familial hypercholesterolaemia, these receptors are defective and plasma LDL levels are abnormally high. Macrophages and endothelial cells possess a 'scavenger receptor pathway' which allows them to take up modified LDL. As the scavenger receptors for modified LDL are not downregulated by high cellular cholesterol levels, the macrophage continues to acquire lipid and eventually forms a bloated foam cell.

their interactions with lipoproteins; secretion of cytokines which recruit and modulate the behaviour of other cells; release of enzymes; release of oxygen radicals; and their ability to modify lipoprotein, rendering it toxic, immunogenic, and more amenable to the scavenger receptor pathway (Fig. 12.20).

12.3.3 Aneurysm formation

Aneurysms are permanent, irreversible, localized dilatations of arteries. Arterial medial thinning or degeneration associated with atherosclerosis was described by Sir James Paget in 1850 in the small arteries of the brain in a patient who died of cerebral haemorrhage. He wrote of a 'fatty degeneration' of the vessel wall with 'varicose enlargement'. The aorta is exceptional; unlike most other organs, its length and breadth increase inexorably throughout life. Since Erdheim's original description, in 1929, of fragmentation of the elastin in the aortic media with age, it has become apparent that these changes are instrumental in formation of aortic aneurysms.

Abdominal aortic aneurysms are primarily atheromatous in origin, but other factors may be involved. Medial degeneration that accompanies all but the earliest stages of atherosclerosis further damages a wall already weakened by ageing or by a presumptive defect in collagen. These aneurysms are most frequent below the renal orifices and around the aortic bifurca-

tion, where atheroma is usually most severe (Fig. 12.21). Other types of aneurysms occasionally encountered at this site, although commoner elsewhere, include dissecting aneurysms, traumatic aneurysms, mycotic aneurysms, and aneurysms due to Takayasu arteritis (see Section 12.6).

12.3.4 Chronic periaortitis

Introduction

In 1890, Hutchinson commented that 'in elderly patients, arteries are liable to a spreading inflammation which glues the artery to its sheath'. He regarded it as the hallmark of atheroma which differentiated it from 'senile change' or 'fatty degeneration'. Over the intervening years it has been suggested that arterial infiltrates of lymphocytes and plasma cells correlated with severity of the intimal atheromatous lesion and not with the anatomical site of the plaque nor with the patient's age or sex (Fig. 12.22). (The adventitial cellular changes in polyarteritis nodosa, giant cell arteritis, and disseminated lupus erythematosus are different to those associated with the advanced atherosclerotic plaque (see Section 12.6).) These changes may be involved in the pathogenesis rather than the

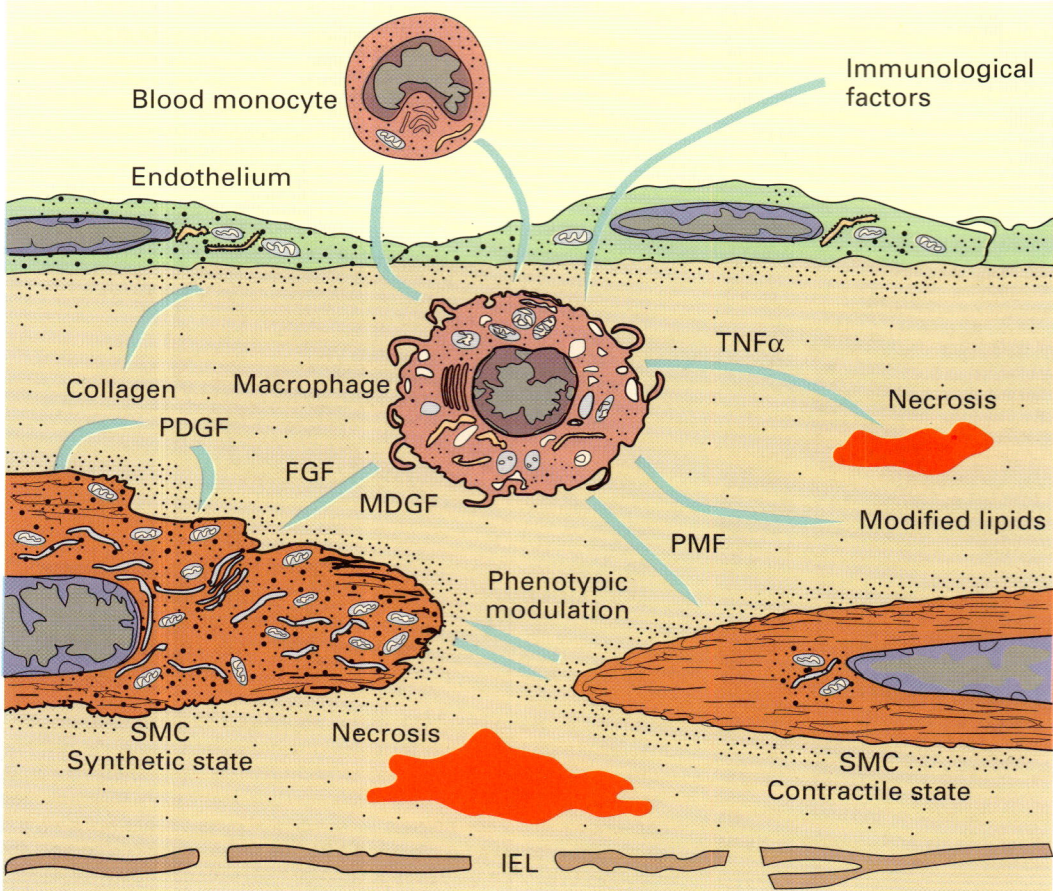

Fig. 12.20 The interaction between macrophages and the cellular and non-cellular constituents of the advanced ('complicated') atherosclerotic plaque. MDGF=macrophage-derived growth factor; SMC=smooth muscle cell; PDGF=platelet-derived growth factor; IEL=internal elastic lamina; PMF=platelet mitogenic factor; TNF=tumour necrosis factor; FGF=fibroblast growth factor. See also Section 12.2.8 for discussion of growth factors.

aetiology of atherosclerosis and may be due to some 'change in immunological tolerance' to a component of the plaque itself.

Lymphocytes and macrophages are present in the intima of atherosclerotic arteries. In the rat, it has been proposed that infiltration of blood-borne mononuclear cells into the intima is a response to a chemical message, perhaps an antigen, originating from the media. Adventitial inflammation in the atherosclerotic plaques is generally underestimated. Those who have studied immunological phenomena in human atherosclerosis, have done so with a view to elucidating the mechanism of atherogenesis and have largely ignored the adventitial inflammatory cells.

'Idiopathic retroperitoneal fibrosis'

'Idiopathic retroperitoneal fibrosis' (IRF), typically, is a disease of middle-aged to elderly males who develop chronic inflammation and fibrosis around the lower abdominal aorta. This inflammatory process tends to drag neighbouring hollow structures towards the midline. The disease usually presents as a

urological problem with obstruction of one or both ureters, often with hydronephrosis.

The peri-aortic distribution of the IRF first emerged from necropsy studies (Fig. 12.23) and has been confirmed by computed tomography (CT) (Fig. 12.24). It is associated with a raised erythrocyte sedimentation rate (ESR), often a dramatic response to steroids, and advanced aortic atherosclerosis with medial disruption and adventitial infiltrates of lymphocytes and plasma cells (Fig. 12.25).

A similar, chronic inflammatory process occurs, much less commonly, around the thoracic aorta. This is known as 'idiopathic mediastinal fibrosis' (IMF). The histopathological findings in IMF are identical to those in IRF and the two conditions may occur in continuity through the diaphragm.

Rarely, IRF can be associated with other fibrotic disorders, including Reidel thyroiditis, sclerosing cholangitis, and pseudotumour of the orbit. These fibrotic diseases have been grouped under the heading 'multifocal fibrosclerosis'.

Retroperitoneal fibrosis has been associated with the use of

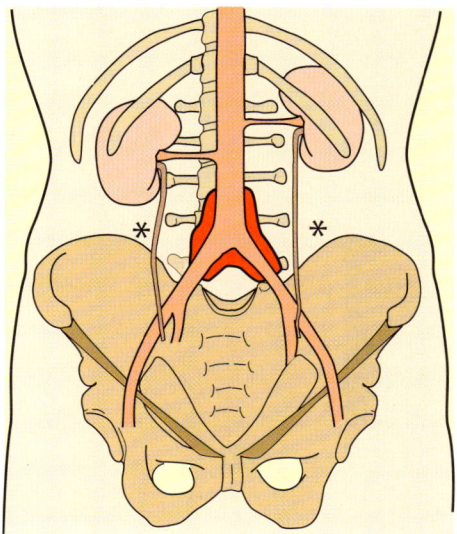

Fig. 12.21 This shows the classic peri-aortic distribution of both 'idiopathic retroperitoneal fibrosis' (IRF) and 'inflammatory aneurysm' at L3, L4, L5 where aortic atheroma is usually most severe. In dilated and undilated aortas, the peri-aortic inflammation and fibrosis may be so severe that neighbouring mobile structures, like the ureters (∗) are dragged medially.

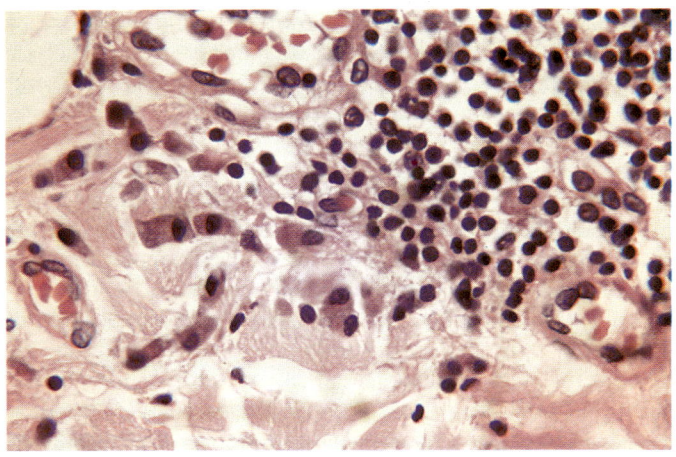

Fig. 12.22 Chronic inflammatory cells consisting of lymphocytes, plasma cells, and macrophages are clustered around the vasa vasorum in the adventitia. (Reproduced from Parums 1990.)

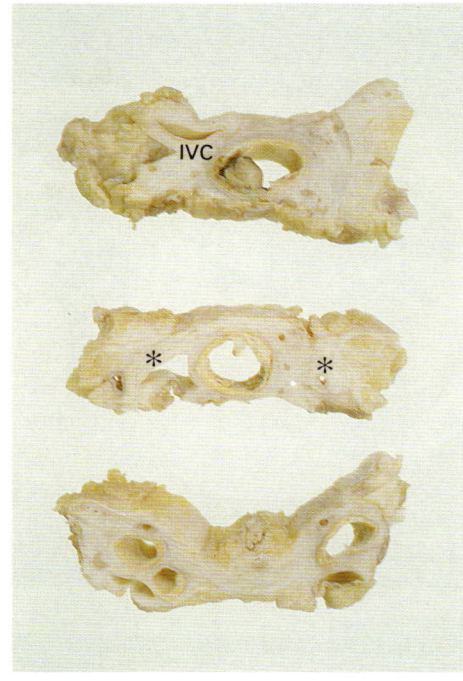

Fig. 12.23 The macroscopic appearance of the abdominal aorta, removed at necropsy and sectioned transversely down its length from a case of 'idiopathic retroperitoneal fibrosis'. The top section shows the area of maximal peri-aortic thickening (25 mm) just below the renal artery origin where the aortic diameter is 24 mm maximally. The middle section is at the aortic bifurcation and the bottom section shows the inflammation and fibrosis around the internal and external iliac vessels. The ureters (∗) are encased in fibrous tissue and the inferior vena cava (IVC) is also involved. (Reproduced from Parums 1990.)

methysergide, an indole derivative, with a structural similarity to serotonin. It is used in the treatment of migraine. Its mechanism of action is uncertain but in the context of IRF it may damage the vessel wall by provoking vasospasm, simulating the peripheral effects of serotonin. IRF in patients treated with methysergide is often accompanied by fibrosis at other sites.

The benefits of corticosteroid therapy for IRF was first suggested by Ross and Tinkler in 1958. The rapidity of response seen in patients with ureteric obstruction supports the view that the ureter is not blocked by fibrosis but rather by oedema and inflammation. This is confirmed histologically. It is not known whether oedema and inflammation obstruct the ureter directly or indirectly, by interfering with nerve or blood supply. Despite the value of steroid therapy, almost all surgeons still regard ureterolysis as the first line of management.

As early as 1972, Mitchinson proposed that the inflammation in IRF may be due to 'leakage of atherosclerotic material into the adventitia'. He suggested the examination of serum from these patients to search for circulating antibodies to components of the plaque, such as lipoproteins.

'Inflammatory aneurysm'

Occasionally, surgeons see an aneurysm encased in fibrous tissue which extends into the retroperitoneal tissues. 'Inflammatory aneurysms' form 2–10 per cent of all aortic aneurysms. The term 'inflammatory aneurysm' was first used to describe aneurysms which had a macroscopically thickened wall, and was considered a different clinical entity from the atheromatous variety. It has been supposed that it is due to an auto-immune response to a transudate of blood products through a weakened aneurysm wall. Review of the histopathology of atherosclerotic aortic aneurysms, have shown that all are accompanied by adventitial inflammation and fibrosis of varying degree.

It has been suggested that these 'inflammatory aneurysms'

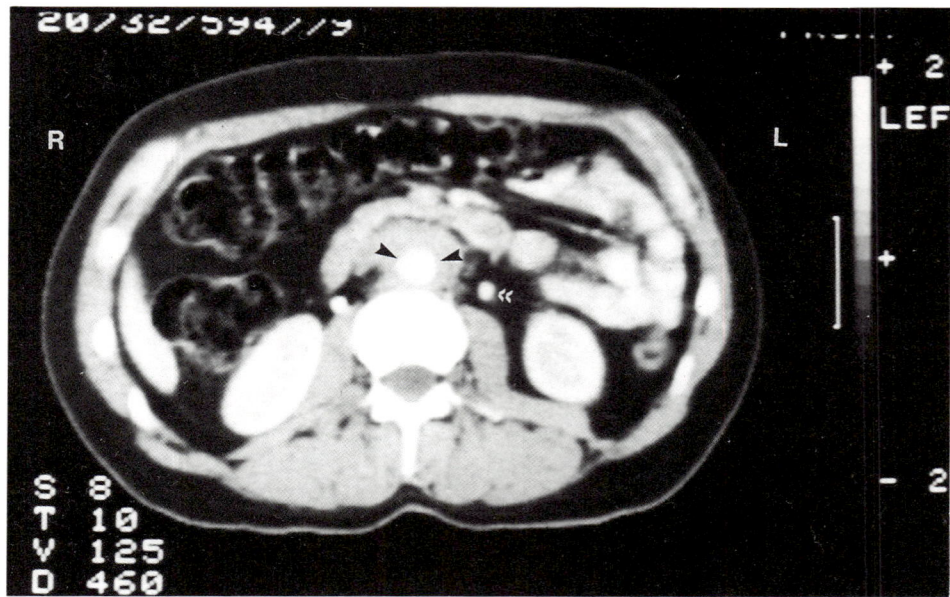

Fig. 12.24   CT scan showing a dense, peri-aortic mass measuring 25 mm in thickness (arrows). The aorta is 24 mm in diameter. There is an associated hydronephrosis due to obstruction of the right ureter by the inflammatory process.

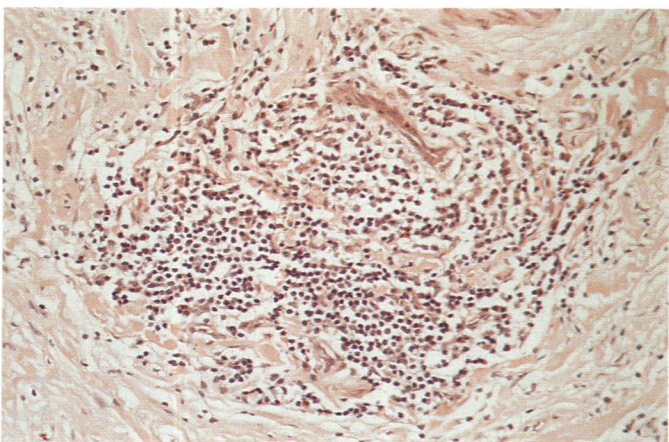

Fig. 12.25   This biopsy was taken during surgical ureterolysis. There is dense fibrous tissue and a mixture of lymphocytes, plasma cells, and macrophages.

are caused by inflammation rather than atherosclerosis. The other view is that the inflammation differs only in degree from that seen around atherosclerotic aneurysms and that they are, therefore, a consequence of atherosclerosis.

To add to the confusion, the term 'peri-aneurysmal retroperitoneal fibrosis' has been used to describe the condition in which ureteric blockage has occurred as a result of fibrosis around atherosclerotic aneurysms of the abdominal aorta. But, the inflammatory infiltrate is the same as that in both 'idiopathic retroperitoneal fibrosis' and 'inflammatory aneurysms'; there is a raised ESR; the disease is sensitive to corticosteroids; and ureteric involvement occurs in 23 per cent of patients with inflammatory aneurysms.

In a 30 year review of 2816 abdominal aortic aneurysms undergoing elective surgical repair, there was an incidence of 4.5 per cent of 'inflammatory aneurysms' (Pennell *et al*. 1985). The histopathology of medial degeneration, adventitial thickening, and infiltration with lymphocytes and plasma cells was identical to those of idiopathic retroperitoneal fibrosis, except that in IRF the aorta is undilated. This has been confirmed by direct comparison of 12 cases of 'inflammatory aneurysm' and eight cases of 'idiopathic retroperitoneal fibrosis' (Parums 1990).

Histopathology of atherosclerotic aneurysms has shown that all are accompanied by inflammation and fibrosis, which is usually slight. Severe degrees of this inflammation are visible macroscopically and give rise to the conditions variously named, 'inflammatory aneurysm' or 'peri-aneurysmal retroperitoneal fibrosis'. This condition appears to be identical to IRF except that in the latter, the aorta is undilated. Therefore, on histopathological grounds, the unifying term, 'chronic periaortitis' should be used to describe the association between advanced atherosclerosis, medial thinning, and chronic adventitial inflammation and fibrosis.

Chronic periarteritis

Inflammation and fibrosis frequently occur around coronary arteries in association with advanced atherosclerotic plaques and this has been reported in association with IRF. In this situation, the triad of atherosclerosis, medial thinning, and adventitial inflammation may be termed 'chronic periarteritis' (Fig. 12.26).

Pathogenesis of chronic periaortitis

A spectrum of chronic inflammation is commonly seen in association with advanced human atherosclerotic plaques when the media is thinned. The inflammatory infiltrate consists of lymphocytes, plasma cells, and occasional lymphoid follicles

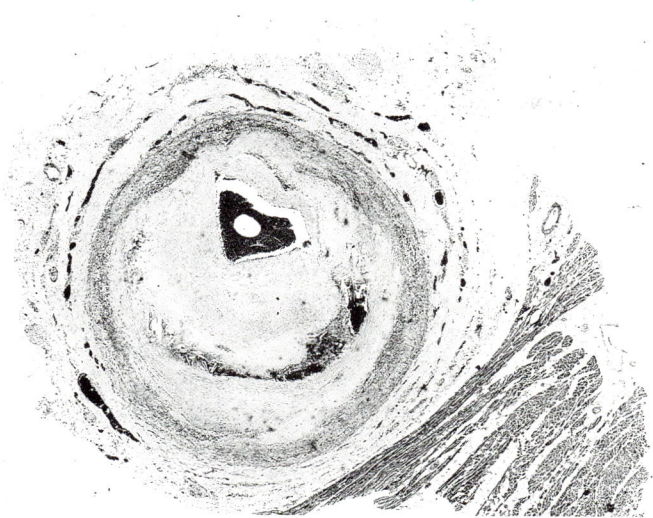

Fig. 12.26 Coronary artery with advanced atherosclerosis, medial thinning, and a mild chronic inflammatory cell infiltrate in the adventitia. This is sub-clinical chronic periarteritis.

(Fig. 12.27). Chronic periaortitis is usually not associated with clinical manifestations. In the most severe forms, however, this periaortic inflammation may present clinically in the form of 'inflammatory aneurysm' or 'idiopathic retroperitoneal fibrosis', depending upon whether or not the aorta is dilated. Pleomorphic adventitial cellular infiltrates are found in syphilis, mycotic arteritis, and Takayasu's arteritis, while non-lymphocytic coronary adventitial infiltration occurs in rheumatic heart disease (see Section 12.6). In none of these conditions do the aggregates resemble those of atheromatous arteries in type or distribution.

In the normal aorta, the media represents about 60–70 per cent of the total aortic wall thickness. The intima and adventitia occupy about 15–20 per cent each. The atherosclerotic aorta is

thickened 1.5–2 fold. In chronic periaortitis, there is similar intimal proliferation, but the media is markedly attenuated and there is profound thickening of the adventitia. The total aortic wall thickness may be increased several times (Figs 12.28, 12.29).

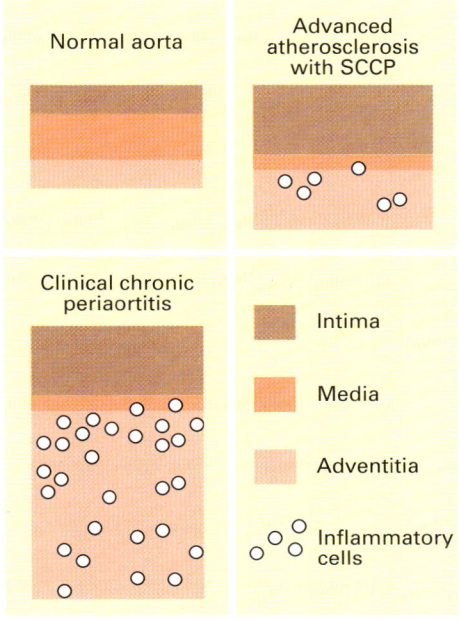

Fig. 12.28 Schematic comparison of the wall of a normal aorta, an atherosclerotic aorta with sub-clinical chronic periaortitis (SCCP), and an aorta with clinical chronic periaortitis ('idiopathic retroperitoneal fibrosis' or 'inflammatory aneurysm'). This highlights the differences in the contribution of the intima, media, and adventitia to wall thickness, and the presence of chronic inflammatory cells.

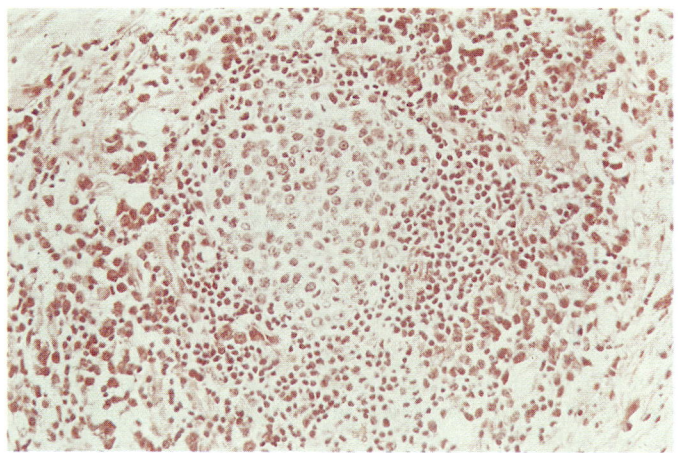

Fig. 12.27 The adventitia in clinical chronic periaortitis contains a dense chronic inflammatory cell infiltrate which may form lymphoid follicles.

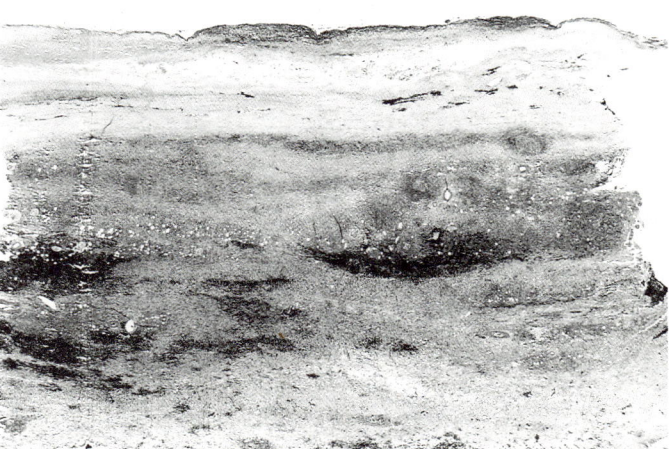

Fig. 12.29 This low-power scanning view of the aorta in a case of clinical chronic periaortitis shows the atheromatous intima, thinned media, and thickened adventitia (10 mm). The outer limit of the fibrosis extends below the lower edge of the photomicrograph. (Reproduced from Parums 1990.)

The inflammation could be the cause or a consequence of atheroma. It is likely that the latter is the case, for the following reasons. Inflammation is not seen in the adventitia of normal arteries and aortas. Advanced atherosclerotic plaques are seen which show no evidence of adventitial inflammation. The degree of inflammation, when present, is related to severity of the atheromatous plaque. The plaque itself appears to be the prerequisite for the inflammatory response and not vice versa. There is also a significant relationship between increased adventitial inflammation and increased number of macrophages/foam cells in the plaque.

Immunoglobulin-secreting plasma cells in the aortic adventitial infiltrate occur in chronic periaortitis; this has been interpreted as evidence that chronic periaortitis is due to an auto-allergic reaction to a component of the atherosclerotic plaque. Ceroid is found in all advanced atherosclerotic plaques. Immunoglobulin, predominantly IgG, is associated with ceroid in plaques in patients with severe chronic periaortitis. Ceroid can be manufactured *in vitro* by oxidizing LDL. Furthermore, antibodies to ceroid and oxidized LDL are always detectable in patients with severe chronic periaortitis.

The nature of the inflammatory cell population in chronic periaortitis has been investigated using immunohistochemistry. This confirmed the presence of IgG-containing plasma cells in the aortic adventitia, together with B-cells and T-helper cells. HLA-DR was displayed by the majority of lymphocytes, macrophages, and by some vascular endothelial cells and smooth muscle cells (Fig. 12.30). B-lymphocytes predominated in aortic adventitia (including within lymphoid follicles), but were not detected in atheromatous plaques. Plasma cells in chronic inflammation are thought to produce antibodies specific for antigens present locally. B-lymphocytes encountering antigen for which they have specific receptors, will be retained and stimulated to divide and differentiate. Lymphokine release from

locally activated T-cells may provide a further, stimulatory, amplifying signal to B-cell maturation.

A T-helper:T-cytotoxic-cell ratio of approximately 4:1 is seen in chronic periaortitis. These helper T-lymphocytes may be responsible for inducing cell-mediated reactions to antigens (e.g. oxidized lipids) which are elaborated in atheromatous plaques in chronic periaortitis. The paucity of T-suppressor/cytotoxic cells, which are involved in immunoregulatory activity, may allow the persistence of this ongoing chronic inflammatory process and lead to uncontrolled proliferation of antigen-reactive cells in some individuals.

These studies confirm findings reported by Hansson and colleagues (1989). They found T-lymphocytes and macrophages in atherosclerotic plaques, but B-lymphocytes were absent; T-cells, macrophages, and smooth muscle cells expressed HLA-DR. T-cells also expressed interleukin-2 (IL-2) receptor and were associated with γ-interferon secretion. They suggested that T-cell–smooth muscle cell interactions occur during atherogenesis. More recently, it was shown that lymphocyte populations in various stages of human atherosclerotic plaques consist of HLA-DR-positive T-helper and T-cytotoxic cells, which express IL-2 receptors, leading to the postulate that local immune-mediated reactions are associated with atherogenesis. Neither of these recent studies make mention of the cell populations in the aortic adventitia, possibly because some workers used surgical endarterectomy specimens which did not include adventitia, and possibly because the atherosclerotic plaques examined were not sufficiently advanced to cause medial thinning. The findings of these workers could reflect the initial stages of the immunologically based inflammation which is initially confined to the atheroma and is more cellular in its early stages. The atherosclerotic plaque may represent a site of relative immunological privilege until the media is breached or new vessels form in advanced or complicated plaques in which chronic periaortitis is common. Chronic periaortitis may be the end-stage of the immune response, directed at antigens elaborated in the atherosclerotic plaque during atherogenesis.

Chronic periaortitis is also characterized by peri-aortic fibrosis. What determines the degree of fibrosis is unknown. In its severest form, the fibrotic reaction leads to the clinical manifestations of the disease, such as ureteric obstruction. Cells of the immune system are sources of mediators regulating fibroblast function. The macrophage and T-lymphocytes synthesize fibroblast growth factor, and macrophages produce TGFβ which stimulates collagen production.

These recent data suggest that as well as circulating antibodies from locally stimulated B-cells, responses mediated by T-helper cells and directed at major histocompatibility complex (MHC) class II antigen-bearing cells may be of importance in the pathogenesis of chronic periaortitis (Fig. 12.31). Chronic periaortitis is a local complication of advanced atherosclerosis. It appears to be a consequence rather than a cause of human atherosclerosis and is likely to be relevant in disease progression.

Computed tomography (CT) has an established role in the preoperative diagnosis of chronic periaortitis, by demonstrating the

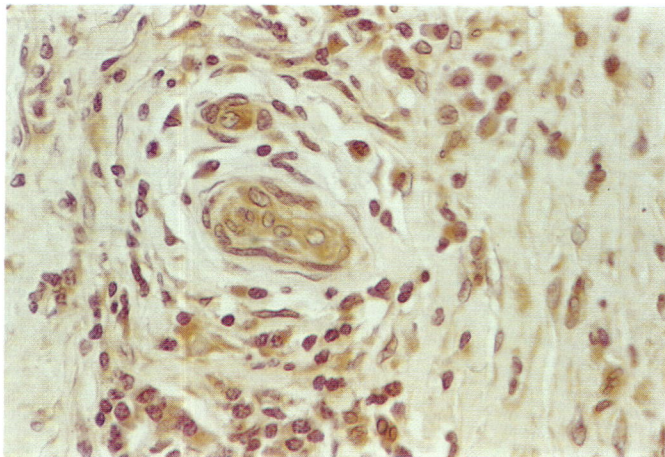

Fig. 12.30 Immunohistochemical labelling of a case of chronic periaortitis with monoclonal antibody TAL-1B5 (directed against MHC class II antigen). Many lymphocytes, macrophages, and endothelial cells in the adventitial inflammation are HLA-DR positive.

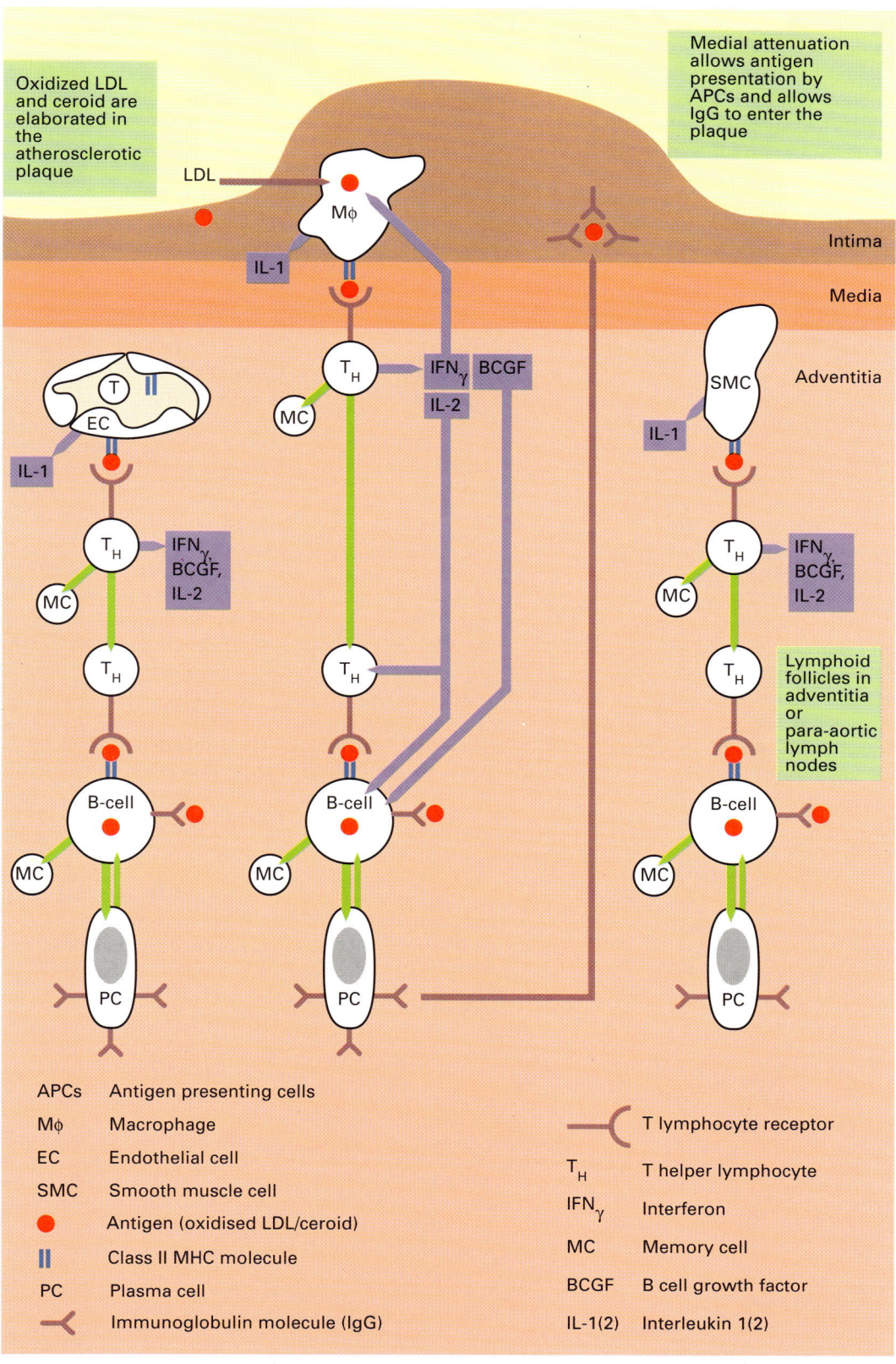

Oxidized LDL and ceroid are elaborated in the atherosclerotic plaque

Medial attenuation allows antigen presentation by APCs and allows IgG to enter the plaque

LDL

Mφ

IL-1

Intima

Media

T_H

IFN_γ BCGF

IL-2

MC

Adventitia

SMC

IL-1

T   EC

IL-1

T_H

IFN_γ, BCGF, IL-2

MC

T_H

IFN_γ, BCGF, IL-2

MC

T_H

T_H

T_H

Lymphoid follicles in adventitia or para-aortic lymph nodes

B-cell

MC

B-cell

MC

B-cell

MC

PC

PC

PC

APCs	Antigen presenting cells
Mφ	Macrophage
EC	Endothelial cell
SMC	Smooth muscle cell
●	Antigen (oxidised LDL/ceroid)
‖	Class II MHC molecule
PC	Plasma cell
Y	Immunoglobulin molecule (IgG)

⊥	T lymphocyte receptor
T_H	T helper lymphocyte
IFN_γ	Interferon
MC	Memory cell
BCGF	B cell growth factor
IL-1(2)	Interleukin 1(2)

Fig. 12.31 Schematic representation of the possible cellular interactions in chronic periaortitis that may generate increased numbers of lymphocytes and plasma cells in the adventitia.

peri-aortic mass. Isolated case reports have shown shrinkage of the peri-aortic mass in response to steroid therapy in IRF and in 'inflammatory aneurysm'. CT scans before and after biopsy diagnosis of IRF, have shown a decrease of peri-aortic size at follow-up, even though some patients had not been treated with steroids. This suggests that the mass in chronic periaortitis shrinks as part of its natural history. The variable proportions of cells and fibrous tissue in chronic periaortitis suggests that in its early stages the tissue is highly cellular and contains immature fibroblasts, and later evolves into predominantly fibrous tissue, contracting as it does so. This would account for the 'dragging' of mobile structures, like the ureters, medially towards the aorta. Ureteric obstruction in IRF may be relieved 'spontaneously' following surgery or even biopsy alone and this may be due to a rise in endogenous corticosteroids during surgery.

Terminology in clinical medicine may distort the facts to make them conform to the chosen words: 'When the dignity of time has conferred respectibility upon continued misuse, then everyone is quite happy.' The term 'idiopathic retroperitoneal fibrosis' is an example. It perpetuates the image of a disease of unknown cause, arising from somewhere in the retroperitoneum. The typical form of this condition always has a peri-aortic origin, and fibrosis is a variable component of the inflammation. It should be distinguished from the eccentric variants causing fibrosis of the retroperitoneum of different anatomical distribution, in all of which a causative agent can be found, such as endometriosis or neoplasia. The term 'inflammatory aneurysm' is another inaccuracy. It perpetuates the image of aneurysm secondary to an inflammatory process. While this may be the mechanism of mycotic aneurysm, which is very rare, both medial thinning, giving rise to aneurysmal dilatation, and adventitial inflammation are sequelae of atherosclerosis.

The term 'chronic periaortitis' is recommended to refer to the subclinical or clinically presenting adventitial inflammation associated with advanced atherosclerosis and medial thinning in dilated and undilated aortas, and has the advantage of pathological accuracy. In addition, 'textbook' chronic periaortitis, ('idiopathic retroperitoneal fibrosis' and 'inflammatory aneurysm') is surrounded by a substantial and mysterious fringe of clinical associations which are ill-defined and vary in severity and characteristics. Examples are pulmonary hyalinizing granuloma, lymphomatoid granulomatosis, Reidel thyroiditis, and sclerosing cholangitis. None of these associations were detected in recent large surveys of 'inflammatory aneurysm' and of 'idiopathic retroperitoneal fibrosis'. All could be pure coincidence.

In conclusion, the unifying concept of chronic periaortitis as a local complication of atherosclerosis brings together the conditions previously termed 'idiopathic retroperitoneal fibrosis', 'inflammatory aneurysm' and 'peri-aneurysmal retroperitoneal fibrosis' as part of a spectrum of the same disease. They all have in common advanced atherosclerosis, medial thinning, and adventitial chronic inflammation. In addition, our understanding of the cellular and non-cellular interactions in atherosclerosis, particularly the role of the macrophage and the role of lipids, is increasing. Light is being shed on the possible mechanisms of atherogenesis and also upon the mechanisms of the pathogenesis of atherosclerosis, the consequences of which we can still only visualize in terms of their 'clinical horizon' in our population.

12.3.5 Further reading

Baker, L. R. I., et al. (1988). Idiopathic retroperitoneal fibrosis; a retrospective analysis of sixty cases. Journal of Urology 60, 497–503.

Ball, R. Y., Carpenter, K. L. H., and Mitchinson, M. J. (1987). What is the significance of ceroid in human atherosclerosis? Archives of Pathology and Laboratory Medicine 111, 1134–42.

Bloor, K. and Humphreys, W. V. (1979). Aneurysms of the abdominal aorta. British Journal of Hospital Medicine 21, 568–83.

Brooks, A. P., Reznek, R. H., Webb, J. A. W., and Baker, L. R. I. (1983). CT in the follow up of retroperitoneal fibrosis. Clinical Radiology 38, 597–601.

Brown, M. S. and Goldstein, J. L. (1986). A receptor-mediated pathway for cholesterol homeostasis. Science 232, 34–47.

Crawford, J. L., Stowe, C. L., Safi, H. J., Hallman, C. H., and Crawford, E. S. (1985). Inflammatory aneurysms of the abdominal aorta. Journal of Vascular Surgery 2, 113–24.

Dixon, A. K., Mitchinson, M. J., and Sherwood, T. (1984). Computed tomographic observations in periaortitis: a hypothesis. Clinical Radiology 35, 39–42.

Dent, R. G., Godden, D. J., Stovin, P. G. I., and Stark, J. E. (1983). Pulmonary hyalinising granuloma in association with retroperitoneal fibrosis. Thorax 38, 955–6.

Goldstone, J., Malone, J. M., and Moore, W. S. (1978). Inflammatory aneurysms of the abdominal aorta. Surgery 83, 425–30.

Hansson, G. K., Jonasson, L., Lojsted, B., Stemme, S., Kocher, O., and Gabbiani, G. (1988). Localisation of T lymphocytes and macrophages in fibrous and complicated plaques. Atherosclerosis 72, 135.

Hansson, G. K., Holm, J., and Jonasson, L. (1989). Detection of activated T lymphocytes in the human atherosclerotic plaque. American Journal of Pathology 135, 169–75.

Megibow, A. J., Ambos, M. A., and Bosniak, M. A. (1980). Computed tomographic diagnosis of ureteral obstruction secondary to aneurysmal disease. Urologic Radiology 1, 211–15.

Mitchinson, M. J. (1984). Chronic periaortitis and periarteritis. Histopathology 8, 589–600.

Mitchinson M. J. (1986). Retroperitoneal fibrosis revisited. Archives of Pathology and Laboratory Medicine 110, 783–6.

Mitchinson, M. J. and Ball, R. Y. (1987). Macrophages and atherogenesis. Lancet, ii, 146–8.

Parums, D. V. (1990). The spectrum of chronic periaortitis. Histopathology 16, 423–31.

Parums, D. V., Chadwick, D. R., and Mitchinson, M. J. (1986). The localisation of immunoglobulin in chronic periaortitis. Atherosclerosis 61, 117–23.

Parums, D. V., Brown, D. L., and Mitchinson, M. J. (1990). Serum antibodies to oxidized LDL and ceroid in chronic periaortitis. Archives of Pathology and Laboratory Medicine 114, 383–7.

Pennell, R. C., et al. (1985). Inflammatory abdominal aortic aneurysms: a thirty year review. Journal of Vascular Surgery 2, 859–69.

Stratford, N., Britten, K., and Gallagher, P. J. (1986). Inflammatory infiltrates in human coronary arteries. Atherosclerosis 59, 271–6.

Van der Wal, A. C., Das, P. K., van de Berg, D. B., van der Loos, C. M., and Becker, A. E. (1989). Atherosclerotic lesions in humans. In-situ immunophenotypic analysis suggesting an immune mediated response. Laboratory Investigation 61, 166–70.

12.4 Ischaemic heart disease

N. Woolf

12.4.1 Clinical presentation

In clinical terms ischaemic heart disease expresses itself in a number of different forms:

1. stable angina;
2. unstable angina;
3. variant or Prinzmetal angina;
4. syndromes associated with acute myocardial necrosis;
5. sudden death;
6. chronic pump failure.

It is important to realize that these are not distinct entities but form a part of a spectrum of pathophysiological events of which the common pathological basis is stenosing atherosclerosis of the coronary arteries.

12.4.2 Some epidemiological considerations

Frequency

Ischaemic heart disease is, in quantitative terms, the single most important cause of death in relatively over-privileged Western communities. In the United Kingdom alone it accounts for some 140 000 deaths annually and is a major drain on the resources allocated for health care.

Risk factors

While no one would deny that certain inherited characteristics, such as genetically determined hyperlipidaemias and diabetes mellitus, play a part in the genesis of ischaemic heart disease (see Section 2.7), it is fair to say that many of the most significant contributions are not inherited and are encompassed by the 'life-style' both of the community and of individuals. The demonstration of geographical differences in the prevalence and incidence of ischaemic heart disease has been the first step in epidemiological research in this field and has provided the initial impetus for a large number of studies which have served to delineate 'risk factors' for ischaemic heart disease. Risk factors have been defined as 'habits, traits and abnormalities associated with a sizeable increase in susceptibility to disease associated with extensive and severe atherosclerosis'. This definition requires critical examination since it is clear that increasing age and male gender are both associated with an increase in risk for ischaemic heart disease and are hardly susceptible to modification. Nevertheless, the risk factor concept is a useful one which has yielded valuable data in a series of prospective incidence studies.

It would be impossible in this section to give a comprehensive account of the risk factors so far identified, but these are covered in detail in other publications listed below. The risk factors most extensively studied are as follows:

1. a raised plasma cholesterol concentration (most notably that fraction of cholesterol carried as part of the low-density lipoprotein molecule; see Section 2.7);
2. raised blood pressure;
3. cigarette smoking;
4. diabetes mellitus;
5. increased levels of certain clotting factors, most notably factors VII and VIII, and fibrinogen.

Data from the US 'Pooling Project' published in 1978 show the effects in males (in terms of incidence of myocardial infarction and sudden death) of being placed in different quintiles in respect of risk factors 1, 2, and 3; in terms of predictive value, these factors provide most information. This does not mean, however, that modification of other risk factors does not carry the potential for prevention of some cases of ischaemic heart disease.

So far as plasma cholesterol concentrations are concerned, major ischaemic episodes were 3.7 times as frequent in the top quintile as in the bottom one. Being in the top quintile of diastolic blood pressure conferred an increase in risk of 3.3 times, and being in the top quintile of smokers increased the risk by a factor of 5.2 as compared with the risk of the bottom quintile. Being in the top quintile for all three risk factors increased the risk by a factor of 8.6 times. The use of multiple logistic functions (taking multiple risk factors into account simultaneously) greatly increases the accuracy with which the relative risk of a clinical event can be predicted in all countries in which it has been applied. It is currently not possible to predict absolute risk for any individual on the basis of the risk factors so far identified. This may be because there are risk factors (e.g. susceptibility genes) which have still not been recognized or because of the difficulty in assessing the product of dose and time in relation to known factors. However, it is possible to identify individuals who have a relatively low or high risk in terms of variables which can be modified, and those in the second group can be offered advice and a regimen which offer the possibility of risk reduction.

Secular trends in the mortality from ischaemic heart disease, particularly in the United States since the late 1960s, show that a nihilistic attitude to such risk reduction is not justified. Since this time the death rates in the USA from ischaemic heart disease have fallen steadily and markedly. This decline has involved all sectors of the adult population. For individuals between the ages of 35 and 74 years the rate of mortality from ischaemic heart disease has fallen by more than 30 per cent, resulting in more than 800 000 lives saved between 1968 and 1984. In the 1960s the United States ranked second in the world (just behind Finland) so far as mortality from ischaemic heart disease was concerned. By the late 1980s the USA ranked eighth out of the 27 economically developed countries studied.

This decline in mortality has been accompanied by a marked increase in the number of people being treated for high blood pressure; by a fall in mean plasma total cholesterol levels of the order of 4.2 per cent; and by a steady decline in the proportion of the adult population who smoke cigarettes. There is evidence of a socio-economic connection in all these changes; the more 'educated' have changed their life-styles more than the less 'educated' (more and less 'educated' being correlated with whether one is a 'salaried' worker or whether one receives a weekly wage packet). The decline in the incidence of myocardial infarction and sudden death was twice as steep in the salaried individuals as in the 'wage' earners (38 and 18 per cent, respectively). Such data lend strong support to the view that improvements in life-style, and thus in life-style-related risk factors, can make a substantial contribution to reducing the mortality from ischaemic heart disease.

12.4.3   General physiological factors influencing the expression of ischaemia

Energy requirements

The requirements of heart muscle for energy generation are high since not only are large amounts of high-energy phosphates required for contraction, but there are considerable energy demands for the maintenance, firstly, of membrane integrity and, secondly, of the high concentration gradients in respect of sodium, potassium, and calcium ions that exist between the intracellular and the extracellular milieu.

Unlike 'white' muscle, cardiac muscle fibres are poorly supplied with endogenous fuel stores, have a highly developed blood supply, and are highly aerobic. These are the basic reasons why interruption to the blood supply of the myocardium, even for comparatively short periods produces catastrophic results, since there are such limited stores of endogenous fuels to be called upon. The mammalian heart, even at rest, removes some 80 per cent of the oxygen available in the coronary blood. Thus increased work loads, however they are brought about, necessitate a rapid increase in myocardial blood flow in order to satisfy the demand for fuel oxidation. The heart will use any fuel with which it is presented, and it is provided, normally, with a mixture of fuels. The relative proportions of these fuels in the blood varies with the physiological state of the animal; e.g. in the post-prandial state the concentrations of fatty acids will be low, while in states of starvation their levels rise. It is often stated that the heart has a predilection for fatty fuels. This is not a property specific in any way for heart muscle. Any tissue capable of oxidizing glucose and fatty acids will, when presented with a mixture of these, oxidize the fatty acids preferentially and there will be a decrease in glucose uptake and oxidation. This is simply inherent in the operation of the glucose–fatty acid cycle.

Patterns of myocardial blood flow

Perfusion of the myocardium via the coronary artery blood flow is of an unusual type in that, due to the compression of the intramyocardial vessels by contracting heart muscle during sys-

tole, flow ceases during this phase of the cardiac cycle. As diastole commences and the myocardium relaxes, blood is sucked into the intra-myocardial vessels from the epicardial arteries. This diastolic flow is driven by the difference between the pressure in the aortic root above the closed aortic valve (and transduced along the epicardial arteries) and that which obtains in the left ventricular cavity. While this flow is directly proportional to the pressure-dependent drive and the time for which this is allowed to operate, it is inversely related to the resistance in the myocardial vascular bed. Increases of intra-myocardial flow such as one experiences during exercise are mediated by relaxation of small arteries and arterioles within the myocardium, and changes in the calibre of the much larger epicardial arteries, in the disease-free state, do not contribute much to resistance.

In functional terms, the epicardial arteries are regional: each major branch supplies an identifiable segment of the myocardium. In the dead human heart it is possible to demonstrate anastomotic flow by injection of low-viscosity media. However, in man and in large animals, such as the pig or the dog, sudden blockage of a major coronary artery branch leads to necrosis of the segment of muscle supplied by that branch, indicating that these arteries are, functionally speaking, end arteries. In small animals, such as the rat, intramyocardial anastomotic flow is very great and it is correspondingly more difficult to produce regional ischaemic necrosis.

12.4.4   The general pathology of ischaemic myocardial injury

It is not easy in human ischaemic heart disease to obtain data relating to the time-related functional, biochemical, and ultra-structural changes which follow obstruction to a major branch of the coronary artery tree and the regional cessation of flow which is the consequence. Thus, most of our knowledge in this field is derived from studying the sequence of events set in motion by ligation of a major coronary artery branch in a relatively large animal, such as a pig or a dog. The most frequently used model is ligation of the left circumflex coronary artery in the dog. This artery is used rather than the anterior descending (interventricular) branch of the left coronary or the main right coronary since ligation of one of these invariably causes fatal ventricular fibrillation.

Within a few minutes of arterial ligation a portion of the lateral wall of the left ventricle ceases to contract and, in surviving animals, a signficant area of coagulative necrosis (myocardial infarct) develops over the next 12 h. The size of any such infarct is influenced by the coronary artery anatomy in the individual animal and on the degree of collateral flow. A considerable degree of variability exists and thus large numbers of animals must be used in any experiments designed to test therapeutic modalities for reduction in infarct size.

As already stated, the ischaemic muscle ceases to contract within a few minutes of coronary artery ligation. The development of necrosis may be inhibited if flow can be re-established within 20–40 min, but longer periods of ischaemia lead to irreversible myocyte necrosis.

Biochemical changes

Within seconds of coronary artery occlusion, oxygen tension within the affected area of myocardium falls, and mitochondrial respiration first declines and then ceases. Fatty fuels can only be utilized by processes that require oxygen, and thus anaerobic glycolysis of glycogen becomes the sole source of high-energy phosphates; this leads inevitably to a rise in lactate which, in the ischaemic state, cannot be removed readily. Endogenous glycogen stores within the heart are limited and anaerobic glycolysis is, in any event, an inefficient means for the production of ATP. Intracellular ATP concentrations fall steadily, reaching almost zero after 40–60 min, and the creatine phosphate content falls to zero after about 15 min of ischaemia. This, coupled with the inhibition of myosin ATPase by H^+ ions, leads to the cessation of contraction referred to above. During the period of ischaemia, oxidation of fatty acids in mitochondria is inhibited and this leads to an accumulation of fatty acyl-CoA (probably within mitochondria), fatty acyl-carnitine, and fatty acids themselves (mainly within the cytoplasm of the heart muscle cells). Both fatty acyl-CoA and fatty acyl-carnitine can act as powerful detergents and can both inhibit intracellular metabolic processes and disrupt cell membranes.

The key to whether ischaemic damage produces reversible or irreversible damage to heart muscle is the preservation of membrane integrity. This may be lost as a result of the action of a number of potentially cytotoxic mechanisms. These include lipid peroxidation of cell membranes, the target being unsaturated membrane lipids. The free radicals which initiate this could be generated in a number of ways. Superoxide anion can be generated in large amounts when electron carriers are highly reduced, such as is the case in ischaemia. Release of large amounts of endogenous catecholamine, which is also known to occur under these circumstances, may also be associated with free-radical generation; and other mechanisms, such as oxidation of hypoxanthine and xanthine by xanthine oxidase, may also produce superoxide and hydrogen peroxide. If such lipid peroxidation occurs in ischaemic myocardium, then a time of great potential danger is the phase of reperfusion, whether this is established by spontaneous or therapeutically induced (administration of streptokinase or plasminogen activator) thrombolysis. During reperfusion oxygen is readmitted to hypoxic tissues which contain high concentrations of NADH and hypoxanthine, and this combination of circumstances is likely to be associated with much free-radical generation and consequent lipid peroxidation of cell membranes. In experimental ischaemia, myocardial damage certainly occurs during the reperfusion phase and it might well be helpful in reducing such damage if methods for re-establishing flow through occluded coronary artery segments were to be accompanied by the administration of anti-oxidants such as superoxide dismutase and/or catalase (see Chapter 3.1 for further discussion of these mechanisms).

Ultrastructural changes occurring in ischaemic myocardium

Between 15 and 40 min after perfusion has ceased, rather characteristic ultrastructural changes appear. Not surprisingly, there is depletion of glycogen granules, and chromatin becomes increasingly dense at the nuclear margins. Mitochondria swell and cristae breaks can be noted. Amorphous, rather granular deposits appear within the mitochondria, a sign that is correlated with severe damage. Evidence of irreversible cell damage is expressed in the form of blebs in the sarcolemmal membrane, and small defects appear in the plasmalemma. Reperfusion causes the damage to become more severe; there is swelling of the muscle cells, the accumulation within mitochondria of hydrated calcium phosphate, and extensive sarcomere disturbance with smaller than normal distances between the Z bands. These 'contraction bands' are thought to be the result of the myocyte losing its ability to relax as a result of an abnormally high concentration of calcium within the cell.

Light microscopic changes

Changes cannot be seen on light microscopy until at least 4–8 h have elapsed after coronary artery occlusion. The first easily recognizable feature is the presence of neutrophils in the interstitial tissues. This may start as early as 4 h after occlusion and may last for some days. Macrophages begin to infiltrate the ischaemic zone after about 4 days. Individual muscle cells undergo coagulative necrosis and stain much more deeply with eosin, and this is followed by nuclear pyknosis and the loss of normal cross-striations. Within 4–5 days the dead cells disappear and the cell debris is phagocytosed by macrophages. Repair of the ischaemic tissue and its replacement by fibrous tissue depends on the ingrowth of granulation-tissue-type capillaries from the viable myocardium at the periphery of the ischaemic tissue. Collagen fibres begin to appear about the ninth day and repair is usually complete within 6 weeks.

12.4.5 The spectrum of ischaemic heart disease in man: 'variations on the theme of atherosclerosis'

Stable angina

Angina occurs when a need arises for the supply of oxygen to the myocardium which cannot be met. Circumstances under which this may occur include exercise, cold, eating, emotion, or a combination of some or all of these. Inability to meet the oxygen demands of the myocardium may occur when the oxygen demand is constant but the myocardial blood flow is diminished (for example by coronary artery spasm) or because of an increased demand for oxygen in the presence of a degree of coronary blood flow which cannot be increased. The term 'stable angina' is applied to the situation where it can be predicted that chest pain will occur once myocardial work and hence oxygen demand exceed a certain known level.

Coronary artery pathology in stable angina

Coronary artery angiography in patients with stable angina shows that these patients have segments of significant stenosis in one or more of the epicardial coronary arteries. The term 'significant' in this context means that the stenosed segment shows a reduction in diameter of the lumen of more than 50 per cent as compared with adjacent segments of 'normal' coronary artery. This degree of lumenal reduction equates with a reduction in cross-sectional area of 75 per cent. Studies of flow mechanics in tubes show that at a constant pressure, flow only begins to fall sharply when this degree of narrowing is present. The resistance to flow that an atherosclerotic plaque of such dimensions causes may be offset to a certain extent by a fall in resistance within intramyocardial vessels. However, there is a limit to this dilatation and eventually the plaque-mediated stenosis becomes flow-limiting, usually when there is an increase in myocardial oxygen demands. Post-mortem angiography of patients with clinical histories of stable angina often shows the presence of multiple segments of stenosis, but this may simply reflect the bias inherent in a study of patients who have died with their disease.

The morphology of stenoses: concentric and eccentric lesions

Two basic morphological patterns of plaque-mediated stenosis exist. In the first, 'concentric lesions', the intimal thickening involves the whole circumference of the affected vessel. As usual with atherosclerotic intimal thickening, there is atrophy of the medial smooth muscle beneath the plaque and, in the case of concentric lesion, this medial atrophy will also be circumferential. In addition, the concentric intimal lesion may exert a 'splinting' effect on the underlying media. An 'eccentric lesion' does not involve the whole circumference of the artery and there is a segment of normal, or near normal, artery wall opposite the plaque which may account for up to 50 per cent of the circumference. Often the internal elastic lamina below an eccentric plaque has been ruptured and, when the vessel has been perfusion-fixed at physiological pressures, the plaque may be seen to bulge outwards (Figs 12.32, 12.33, 12.34).

The preservation of an appreciable amount of normal medial muscle in relation to eccentric plaques, and the corresponding near complete loss of such muscle in concentric lesions, implies a marked difference in the vasomotor responses of such arterial segments. In eccentric lesions there is sufficient muscle remaining for significant contraction and dilatation to occur, while the reverse obtains in relation to concentric lesions. Angiographic studies in patients with stable angina have confirmed the validity of this view. The administration of vasoconstricting agents, such as ergonovine, causes eccentric stenoses to undergo a reduction in their diameter, while nitroglycerine or the calcium-blocking agent, Nifedipine, cause dilatation of such segments.

A post-mortem study of stenosed segments from patients with stable angina has shown concentric lesions to account for 76 per cent of the stenoses, the remaining 24 per cent being ec-

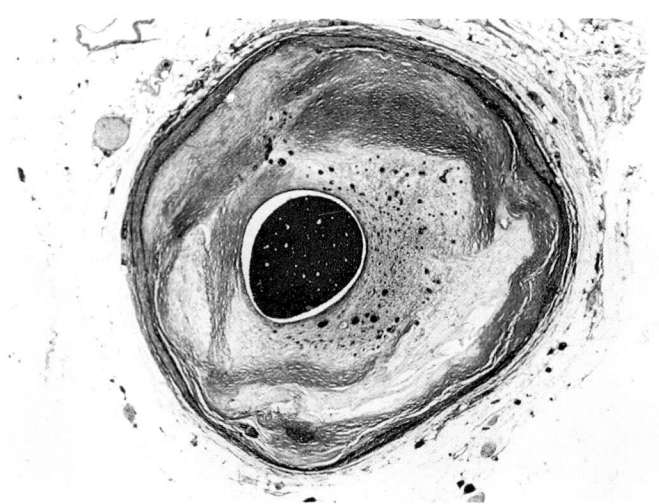

Fig. 12.32 Coronary artery which has been injected prior to fixation and which shows a centrally placed lumen with a more or less concentric thickening of the intima. (By courtesy of Professor M. J. Davies, St George's Hospital Medical School, London.)

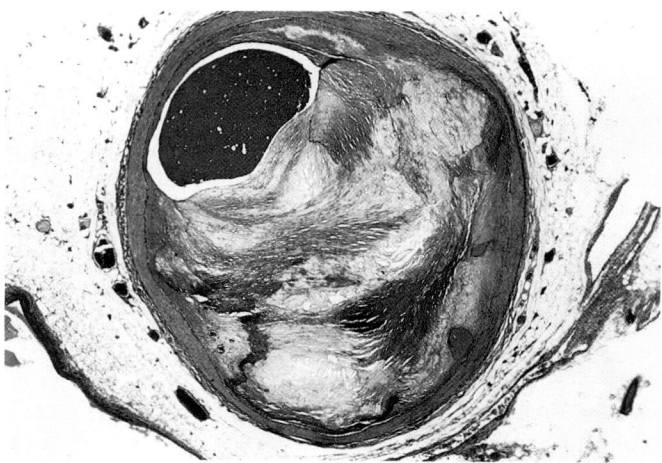

Fig. 12.33 A coronary artery showing an eccentrically placed lumen. A striking degree of connective tissue proliferation has taken place over approximately 75 per cent of the vessel circumference, the vessel wall in the remaining 25 per cent being virtually normal. (By courtesy of Professor M. J. Davies, St George's Hospital Medical School, London.)

centric. Over 60 per cent of the concentric lesions were fibrous plaques with insignificant lipid-rich atheromatous pools at their bases. In the case of the eccentric lesions, half had large lipid-rich pools and half were fibrous. In addition to the stenosed segments described above, a majority of patients with stable angina have segments in which the lumen is occupied by connective tissue in which there are multiple small vascular channels (Fig. 12.35). These have been interpreted as being segments in which occlusive thrombosis had occurred at some time in the past, the presence of the small vascular channels being the expression of recanalization of the thrombi.

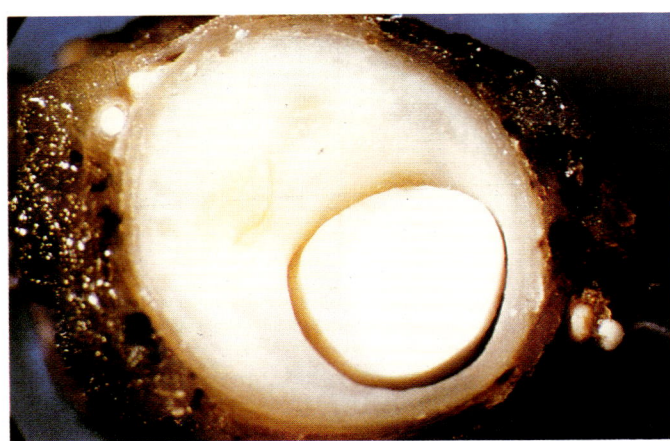

Fig. 12.34 A coronary artery following injection. This specimen shows the presence of a large eccentric plaque with a lipid-rich vessel pool. (By courtesy of Professor M. J. Davies, St George's Hospital Medical School, London.)

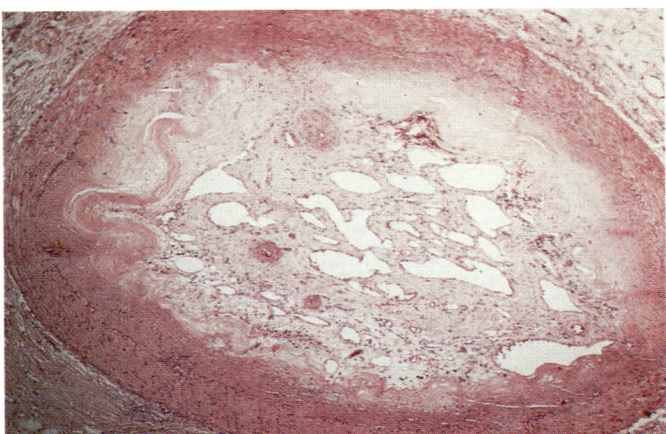

Fig. 12.35 Coronary artery showing complete replacement of the lumen by connective tissue in which many new vascular channels, formed as a result of recanalization, are present.

Unstable angina

The feature that differentiates between stable and unstable angina is the unpredictability of chest pain in the latter. This pain may occur at rest, and differs from time to time in frequency, intensity, and character. Over the first 3 months following the development of unstable angina, 4 per cent of the patients will die suddenly; 15 per cent will suffer a myocardial infarction; and many of the remainder will undergo spontaneous remission. Epidemiological studies have shown that treatment of unstable angina with aspirin reduces the frequency of sudden death and myocardial infarction, suggesting the involvement of a thrombotic element in the natural history. The existence of patients whose unstable angina persists for years raises the possibility that there is more than one underlying pathophysiological mechanism.

Stenosis morphology in unstable angina

Coronary artery angiography, both during life and in hearts obtained at post-mortem examination, show two distinct morphological variants. In the first of these (type I), the luminal outline of the stenosis is smooth and resembles what is seen in the vessels of patients with stable angina. The second form of stenosis (type II) shows a ragged luminal outline and/or overhanging edges, and the presence of contrast medium may be noted within the plaque substance (Fig. 12.36).

Detailed histopathological examination has shown that the type II lesion is a plaque in which acute changes are taking place. Most often they show splitting or fissuring of the plaque's connective tissue cap, and this is frequently associated with the presence of thrombotic material both within the soft material at the plaque base and within the lumen although the latter is not occluded at this stage. The myocardium of patients with unstable angina who have died and in whom such type II lesions are present not infrequently shows the presence of platelet microemboli in intramyocardial vessels downstream (Fig. 12.37).

Unstable angina associated with eccentric type I lesions is almost certainly due to localized spasm, and in a very few cases the clinical syndrome may occur on the basis of spasm of lesion-free coronary arteries (*variant angina*). Thus, unstable angina can be seen to be due to varying degrees of lumenal reduction; this may occur either as the result of the plaque complications which have been described above (see also Chapter 7) or because of vasomotor changes in relation to stable plaques.

Sudden death due to myocardial ischaemia

If the adjective 'sudden' is applied to deaths occurring within 6 h of the onset of symptoms in a previously symptom-free individual, then ischaemic heart disease (IHD) accounts for 60 per cent of such fatalities. Even if the time period is reduced to 15 min, the proportion of cases due to IHD does not change. Forty per cent of all deaths attributable to ischaemic heart disease fall into this category, a clinical problem of enormous magnitude when one considers the frequency of ischaemic heart disease as a cause of death. In addition, half the patients dying suddenly from IHD are said to have been unaware that they were suffering from cardiovascular disease. Quantitative data of this kind re-emphasize the importance of prevention as opposed to treatment of established disease, if signficant reductions in mortality—'the body count'—are to be obtained.

Pathophysiology of sudden death

Sudden death due to IHD is almost entirely due to the onset of fatal ventricular arrythmias, i.e. ventricular fibrillation usually preceded by the appearance of increasingly frequent ventricular ectopic beats. Of those patients who collapse in this way and are successfully resuscitated, only about 16 per cent develop a Q wave on electrocardiography and about 45 per cent show elevated concentrations of intracellular cardiac enzymes in their plasma. Thus, sudden ischaemic cardiac death is not merely a stage in the evolution of acute myocardial infarction, though in some cases it may be.

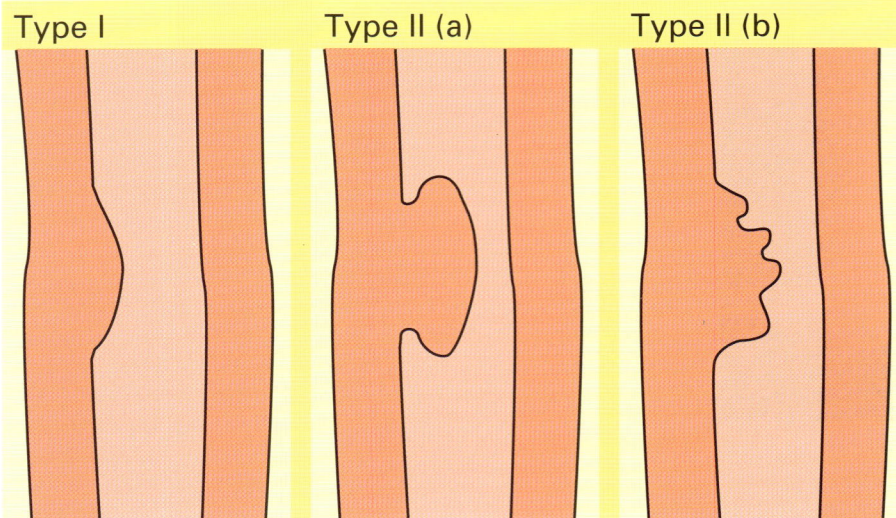

Fig. 12.36 A diagrammatic representation of type I and type II eccentric plaques, as seen on coronary artery angiography. Type I plaques have a smooth outline and slope upwards from the adjacent intima. Type II either show under-cutting of the plaque outline (a), or an irregular ragged lumenal edge (b).

Pathological changes in the coronary arteries in sudden death due to IHD

For many years the pathogenesis of sudden death with particular reference to thrombosis in the coronary artery bed has been a matter for controversy. Post-mortem coronary angiography followed by detailed histopathological studies of the stenosed or occluded segments have shown the presence of type II lesions with plaque fissuring and consequent thrombosis in more than 90 per cent of the cases examined. The frequency of occlusive thrombi is low (of the order of 30 per cent) but the remaining 70 per cent show mural thrombi of the type described in unstable angina. Intramyocardial platelet emboli and tiny foci of muscle necrosis have been found in up to 40 per cent of the cases. Such data show that there is a common pathological basis for a significant proportion of cases of unstable angina and for sudden cardiac death due to myocardial underperfusion—plaque fissuring—and emphasize the importance of gaining a better

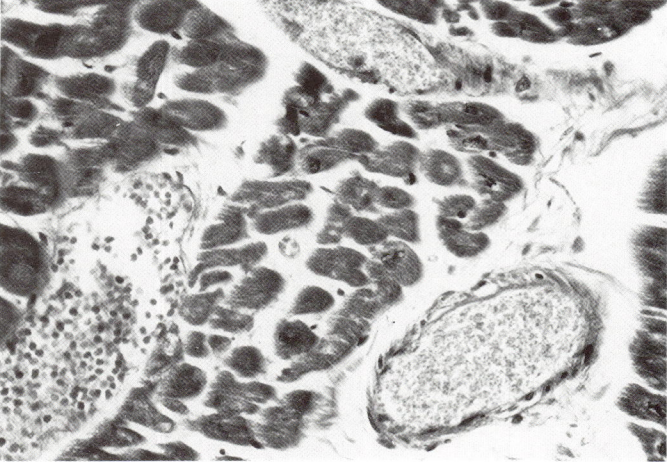

Fig. 12.37 A section of myocardium showing platelet microemboli in two of the small intramyocardial vessels. (By courtesy of Professor M. J. Davies, St George's Hospital Medical School, London.)

understanding of this key event in the natural history of atherosclerotic plaques.

Acute myocardial necrosis

The diagnosis of acute myocardial necrosis depends on the recognition of a set of morphological features, and no case of death due to IHD should be classified as a case of acute myocardial necrosis (infarction) in the absence of such morphological recognition. The importance of this, apparently banal, point is emphasized since failure to appreciate it has led to a long, pointless, and sterile controversy as to the pathogenesis of myocardial necrosis.

In animal models of myocardial necrosis, the characteristic morphological features cannot be recognized on light microscopic examination until 6–8 h have passed from the time of cessation of perfusion, and it is not likely that human heart muscle will behave differently. Thus, in any post-mortem series of rapidly occurring deaths due to IHD there will always be a number of cases in which a correct attribution cannot be made. In addition, there are different patterns of acute myocardial necrosis in which the underlying pathogenetic mechanisms are also different (see Chapter 7) and these patterns must be recognized.

Macroscopic delineation of acute myocardial necrosis This is most easily and effectively accomplished by the use of a simple histochemical technique in which differentiation between viable and non-viable myocardium depends on the presence or absence of intracellular respiratory enzymes, e.g. succinic dehydrogenase. Transverse slices of unfixed heart obtained at necropsy are immersed in a solution of nitro-blue tetrazolium, together with some sodium succinate (to provide excess substrate), and incubated at 37°C for 7–8 min. In those areas where the heart muscle has not undergone necrosis the intracellular dehydrogenases mediate the donation of hydrogen to the yellow, soluble nitro-blue tetrazolium. This leads to the precipitation of the dye as a purplish-blue insoluble 'formazan'.

The necrotic areas, lacking intracellular enzymes, appear colourless against the purplish-blue background.

Patterns of acute necrosis

Regional infarction

Regional infarcts are relatively large areas of coagulative necrosis in which the process has been confined to the territory of one major coronary artery branch. Thus, for example, occlusion of the anterior descending branch of the left coronary artery taking account of some variation in coronary artery anatomy will lead to necrosis of the anterior wall of the left ventricle and the anterior two-thirds of the interventricular septum (Fig. 12.38). Similarly, infarction of the posterior wall of the left ventricle and the posterior third of the septum is likely to be associated with occlusion of the right coronary artery.

Regional infarcts may be further subdivided on the basis of the amount (in terms of thickness) of ventricular wall which has undergone necrosis. Those which involve most of the thickness from endo- to epicardium are called *transmural*, although they usually show a very thin layer of non-necrotic myocardium just beneath the endocardium; the latter area is perfused directly from the ventricular cavity. Those which involve less than 50 per cent of the thickness of the ventricular wall, and in which the inner half of this wall is affected, are spoken of a *subendocardial* (Figs 12.39, 12.40). Subendocardial extension is often found at the margins of transmural infarcts.

Non-regional infarction

In non-regional infarcts the whole circumference of the left

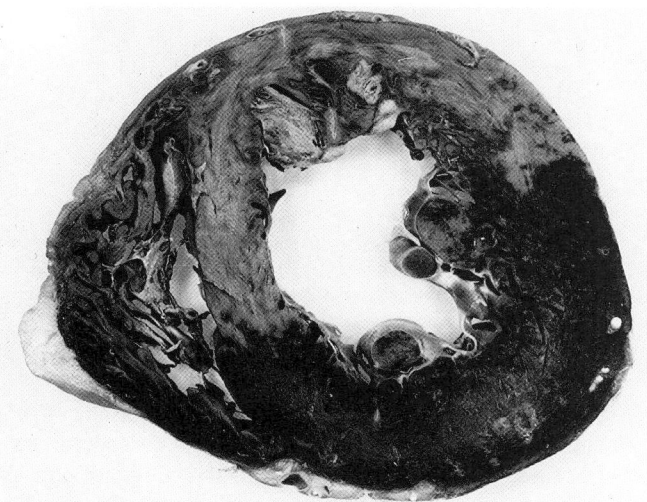

Fig. 12.38 This specimen from a patient dying with myocardial infarction is a section across the ventricles, which has been treated with nitro-blue tetrazolium which colours viable muscle a purplish-blue colour. The section shows loss of staining of the whole of the anterior wall of the left ventricle and the anterior two-thirds of the septum, indicating that this regional transmural infarct is almost certainly due to occlusion of the anterior descending branch of left coronary artery. (By courtesy of Professor M. J. Davies, St George's Hospital Medical School, London.)

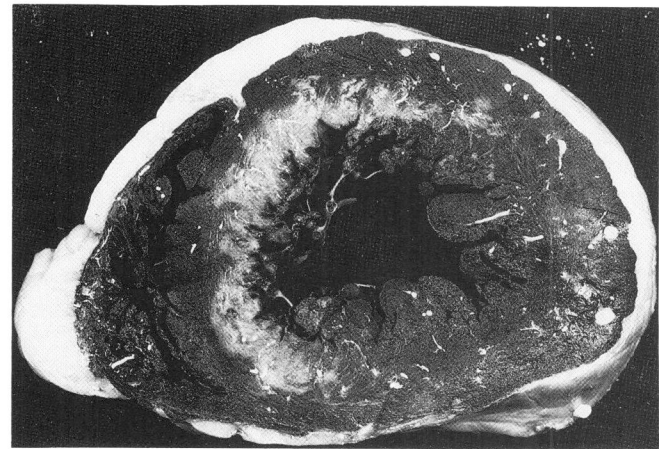

Fig. 12.39 A section through the ventricles which has been treated with nitro-blue tetrazolium. This shows an unstained non-viable area involving the inner one-third of the left ventricular wall in the distribution of the left anterior descending coronary artery. (By courtesy of Professor M. J. Davies, St George's Hospital Medical School, London.)

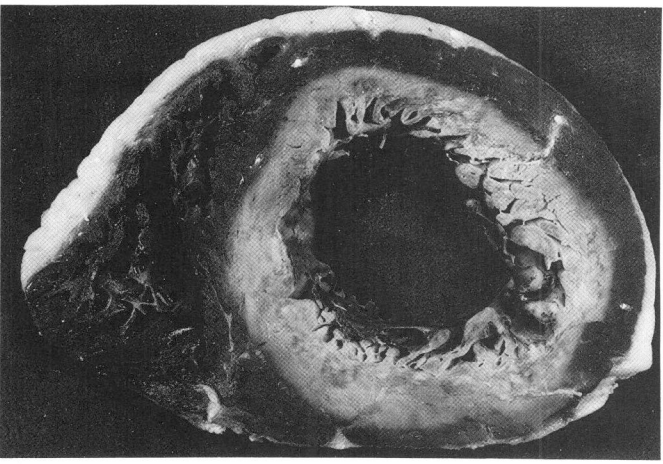

Fig. 12.40 A section through the ventricles which has been treated with nitro-blue tetrazolium, showing unstained non-viable myocardium in the inner half of the left ventricular wall, this time the damage being globally distributed and involving the whole of the left ventricular circumflex. (By courtesy of Professor M. J. Davies, St George's Hospital Medical School, London.)

ventricular wall is involved and these lesions are usually subendocardial (Fig. 12.40), although, in some instances, the necrosis may be more extensive and approach the epicardium in a curious 'saw-tooth' pattern. Satellite foci of necrosis may be seen in association with this diffuse subendocardial lesion, and in such cases the right ventricle may also be involved.

Coronary artery pathology in regional transmural infarction

The frequency with which coronary artery occlusion is causally associated with regional, transmural myocardial infarction has long been an area for debate. Not only have there been significant differences in the recorded prevalence of coronary artery occlusion but some workers have maintained that the thrombi found in arterial branches supplying infarcted areas have occurred as a consequence rather than as a cause of infarction. This long-running controversy should now be regarded as settled as a result of analysis of data obtained at clinical coronary angiography in patients developing regional infarcts. Within the first hour of the onset of pain and ECG changes, the artery subtending the area which later undergoes necrosis is totally occluded. In the hours that follow, some of the occluding thrombi undergo lysis, and within 12 h flow becomes restored in about 30 per cent of cases. At this point the previously occluded segment often shows the characteristics of a type II lesion. Thus, a post-mortem examination carried out on a patient who had survived for more than 24 h after the onset of symptoms need not accurately reflect the causal arterial pathology. Despite this reservation, more than 90 per cent of the cases of full-thickness regional infarction do show the presence of thrombotic occlusion of the subtending artery at post-mortem examination. It may well be that failure of thrombolysis and the resulting failure of any myocardial salvage may increase the risk of dying, and thus skew the post-mortem sample in the direction of those cases in which the thrombus persists.

Plaque fissuring and thrombus propagation The majority of these occlusive thrombi are associated with plaque fissuring (Figs 12.41, 12.42, 12.43). If the atherosclerotic plaque has a massive basal pool of liquid and tissue debris and a relatively thin connective tissue cap, the risks of fissuring are enhanced. The genesis of the basal necrosis is still poorly understood, though the presence of large numbers of activated macrophages within the plaque at a somewhat earlier stage of its natural history may provide a clue, since these cells may release lysosomal enzymes capable of lysing connective tissue, and initiate the generation of potentially damaging free radicals. The latter suggestion gains some support from the finding of conjugated dienes in the pool lipid.

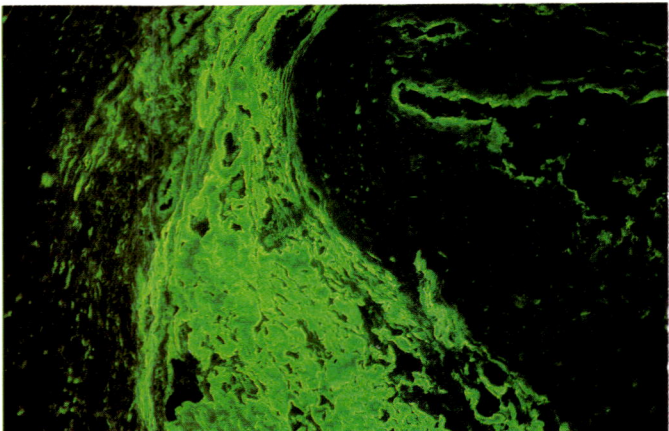

Fig. 12.42 Frozen section of a human coronary artery treated with fluoroscein-linked anti-human fibrin serum. The lumen is on the right of the photograph and the material beneath this is a non-fluoroscein area representing the tissue cap of the plaque. Deep to this is a large crescentic mass of fibrin representing intraplaque thrombus.

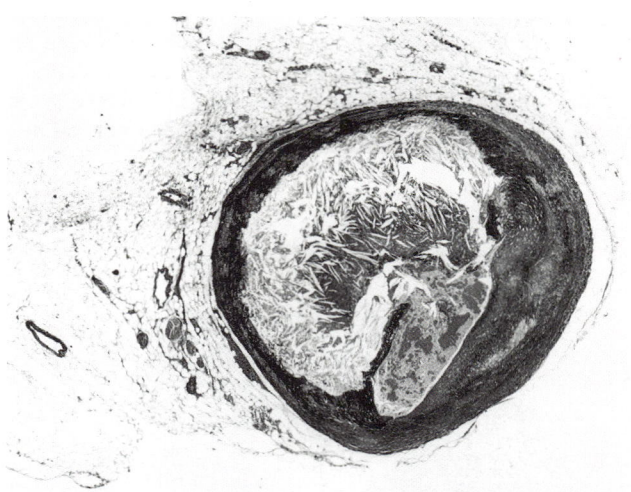

Fig. 12.43 Coronary artery showing loss of approximately 40 per cent of the very thin plaque cap. There is fresh platelet thrombus in the lumen and darkly staining thrombotic material admixed with the cholesterol-rich atheromatous debris. (By courtesy of Professor M. J. Davies, St George's Hospital Medical School, London.)

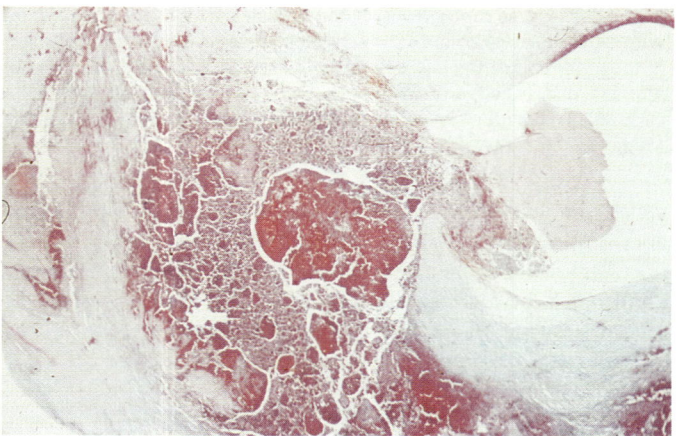

Fig. 12.41 This section shows rupture of the plaque cap, with a small platelet thrombus within the lumen on the right-hand side of the photograph. There is a larger thrombotic mass within the plaque substance.

In some cases the fissures are narrow while in others most of the plaque cap appears to have been lost. In either instance, the defect in the connective tissue cap is associated with a platelet-rich thrombus which has both intraplaque and intraluminal components. Downstream of the fissure and the platelet-rich plug, the thrombus consists predominantly of fibrin and incorporated red blood cells. These features suggest that thrombus propagation has occurred. This view gains support from the results of studies in which fibrinogen labelled with a radioactive compound is given intravenously to patients admitted to hospital within 4 h of the onset of symptoms of severe myocardial ischaemia leading to the development of infarction. In those patients who come to necropsy the radioactive label is found in the distal, fibrin-rich portion of the thrombus, while the platelet-rich portion shows no evidence of the laying down of the labelled fibrinogen. In a small number of cases, thrombosis develops in the absence of plaque fissures. Such thrombi form in areas of high-grade stenosis; and in a very small fraction regional transmural infarction has been documented as being due to spasm, usually in relation to a stenosed segment but very occasionally in the absence of stenosing atherosclerosis.

Regional subendocardial infarction

Aspects of the pathogenesis of this lesion still remain unclear, the position not being made easier by persisting uncertainties related to the electrocardiographic criteria on which this diagnosis is based during life.

There is a lower frequency of occlusive coronary artery thrombi at necropsy in these patients, and angiographic studies suggest that there is a greater degree of collateral flow than in hearts with regional transmural infarcts. Despite this, these patients run an increased risk of recurrent episodes of severe myocardial ischaemia.

A number of pathophysiological interpretations have been canvassed. These include the view that the pathogenesis is identical with that of transmural infarction but that better collateral flow protects the subepicardial regions; that lysis of occlusive thrombi has occurred at a time when full thickness damage has not occurred; and, lastly, that circumstances may arise (usually in patients with dilated ventricles and previous episodes of ischaemic damage) where the perfusion pressure is simply insufficient to fill both subepicardial and subendocardial vessels when both sets are maximally dilated.

Non-regional infarction (diffuse subendocardial necrosis)

Diffuse subendocardial necrosis occurs most frequently in patients with widespread coronary artery stenosis, but may be seen in the absence of coronary atherosclerosis. Occlusive thrombosis is found in no more than 15 per cent of patients with this pattern of necrosis who come to necropsy.

The pathophysiological basis of this lesion is a reduction in overall perfusion of the left ventricle. Any condition which tends to reduce perfusion pressure or significantly to reduce the diastolic interval will compromise flow to the myocardium and this always affects the subendocardial rather than the subepicardial muscle. The perfusion pressure will be reduced either through a fall in aortic root pressure (or a failure to transduce this pressure in severe coronary stenosis) on the one hand, or an increase in intraventricular diastolic pressure on the other. Such situations occur, for example, in severe aortic valve disease; in cardiogenic shock; in the end stages of dilated cardiomyopathy; or the presence of a very thick ventricular wall (Fig. 12.44).

In patients with a large transmural infarct there may be a fall in cardiac output (cardiogenic shock) and this can lead to a lowering in aortic root pressure and the development of diffuse subendocardial necrosis. Thus a vicious cycle may be estab-

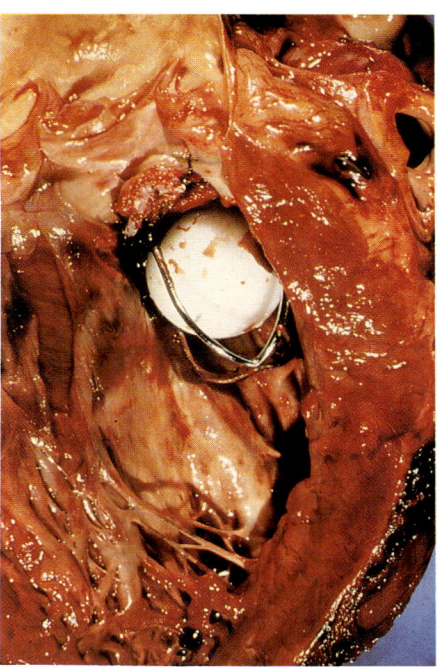

Fig. 12.44 A heart from a patient with a severely thrombosed left ventricle as a result of many years of mitral incompetence. The mitral valve was replaced with a Starr–Edwards prosthesis, but the heart was difficult to re-start at the end of the operation and the patient died within 24 h. Note the pale wash-leather appearance of the subendocardial necrotic muscle involving a large area below the prosthesis.

lished with ever falling cardiac output and ever increasing myocardial necrosis.

Histopathological evolution of myocardial infarcts

Attempting to determine the age of myocardial infarcts from the microscopic appearances is fraught with difficulties, since areas may be found in any individual lesion which are clearly at different stages of evolution both as regards necrosis and repair.

Most of the muscle cells in a regional, transmural infarct undergo the changes of coagulation necrosis, the most obvious early feature being a marked increase in the uptake of eosin. By the second day, loss of cross-striations is seen and the individual myofibrils begin to break down and appear as granular debris within the sarcolemma. These early signs of muscle damage are accompanied by an influx of acute inflammatory cells. These cells, chiefly neutrophils, may play a role in limiting the salvageability of the ischaemic myocardium. The initial ischaemia probably leads to stimulation of intramyocardial lysosomal proteases with cleavage of complement giving rise to chemotactic factors. The neutrophils become activated and release oxygen free-radicals which can cause lethal injury to cell membranes, a situation that is most likely to arise if reperfusion takes place. In experimental models of myocardial ischaemia, the extent of muscle damage can be reduced by pretreatment with non-steroidal anti-inflammatory drugs, or by rendering the animals neutropaenic before inducing ischaemia.

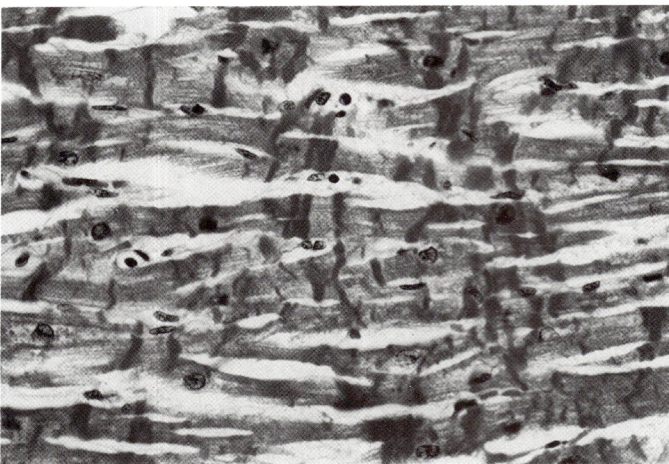

Fig. 12.45 Section through the left ventricular myocardium, showing many constriction bands running transversely across the muscle fibres. (By courtesy of Professor M. J. Davies, St George's Hospital Medical School, London.)

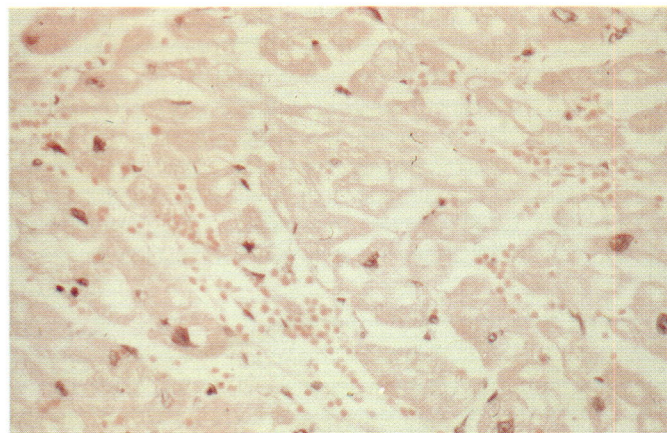

Fig. 12.46 Section of ischaemic myocardium showing a severe degree of vacuolation of the muscle fibres as seen in myocytolysis.

In some cases so-called 'contraction band' necrosis is evident. These localized, deeply eosinophilic areas within individual cells represent telescoping of sarcomeres, and tend to be seen most often where some degree of reperfusion has taken place (Fig. 12.45).

The speed with which demolition of the necrotic tissue and its replacement by fibrous tissue take place depends to a considerable extent on whether the ischaemia has rendered only the heart muscle cells necrotic or whether the underperfusion has been so severe as to involve the connective tissue stroma and the intramyocardial blood vessels. Where the latter have also undergone necrosis, the processes of demolition and repair through the medium of granulation tissue are retarded; dead muscle fibres may persist in the centre of the infarct for weeks or months and replacement of the whole area may be very slow indeed. In contrast, repair is much more rapid in those lesions where the stroma has not been rendered necrotic. Small, focal areas of necrosis are common, especially near the margins of large infarcts, and similar lesions may be seen, independent of the presence or absence of ischaemia in patients with very high catecholamine levels, low plasma potassium concentrations, and severe cardiac hypertrophy. Some cells show a curious appearance which has been termed 'myocytolysis'. They become enlarged and vacuolated and almost all the myofibrils disappear, although the nuclei stain normally and the cells still retain their intracellular enzymes (Fig. 12.46). These cells are thought to be teetering on the edge of survival but have lost their ability to maintain their normal volume, possibly through inhibition of the sodium–potassium ATPase pump.

Right ventricular infarction

The vast majority of cases of myocardial infarction affect the left ventricle alone and isolated right ventricular infarction is excessively rare and only occurs in patients who have a very marked degree of right ventricular hypertrophy. However, in patients who have large posterior infarcts due to proximal occlusion of the right coronary artery, some extension of myocardial damage to involve the right ventricle is not uncommon.

12.4.6 Complications of acute transmural infarction

Myocardial rupture

This catastrophic development may occur in three forms: external cardiac rupture associated with haemorrhage into the pericardial sac and resulting tamponade; rupture of the ventricular septum with the creation of a septal defect; and rupture of a papillary muscle.

External cardiac rupture

This is the third most common cause of death in patients with transmural infarcts, being responsible for 10–20 per cent of fatal cases. For reasons which are not clear, it tends to occur relatively more commonly in older women.

The diagnosis of cardiac tamponade at post-mortem is less easy than one might imagine. This is due to the fact that haemorrhage into the pericardial sac may, in some instances, be an agonal phenomenon associated with vigorous external cardiac massage in patients who have collapsed. However, the presence of a tense bulging pericardium due to an accumulation of blood of not less than 50 ml can be regarded as unequivocal evidence of true pericardial tamponade.

Early rupture (within the first two days) is associated with a slit like tear in the myocardium at the junction of the viable and non-viable muscle. More commonly, rupture occurs somewhere between 5 and 10 days after the onset of symptoms and, in these cases, the rupture can be seen to have taken place through the infarct itself, with the blood tracking through the wall between muscle bundles.

Rupture through the interventricular septum

Septal rupture occurs as a complication of antero- and postero-septal infarcts and may create a defect anywhere, of area from 1 to 3 cm^2. Such a defect imposes a sudden additional haemodynamic burden on a heart already compromised in function by the presence of a large transmural infarct, and it is thus not surprising that this complication carries a high mortality rate. Initially, the septal defect has a ragged outline but in those few patients who survive long enough to undergo surgical repair of the defect, the edges become smoothed out as the infarct heals and the fibrous tissue (which has by this time formed around the defect) provides an anchorage for the insertion of sutures.

Rupture of papillary muscle

Ischaemic damage to the papillary muscles is extremely common, being present in up to half the cases of posterior infarction and in a not insignificant proportion of cases of anterior infarction. In a very small minority of patients (less than 1 per cent of fatal cases) part or all of the papillary muscle becomes avulsed and is swept up towards the mitral orifice. This event is associated with the sudden onset of torrential mitral regurgitation.

Post-ischaemic atrophy of the papillary muscles is quite common and may be associated with the development of mitral incompetence.

Ventricular aneurysm formation

A true aneurysm of the left ventricle is a convex dilatation, the wall of which consists predominantly of collagen. Such lesions

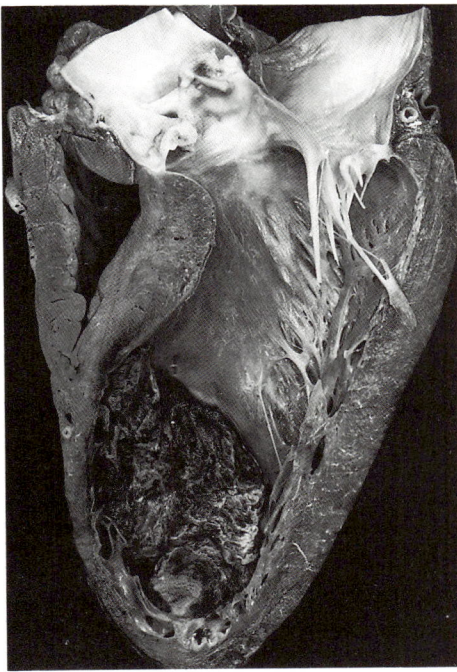

Fig. 12.47 A ventricular aneurysm; note the thinning of the ventricular wall which involves the apex of the left ventricle and the presence of a large mass of unorganized thrombus which now occupies the aneurysm cavity. (By courtesy of Professor M. J. Davies, St George's Hospital Medical School, London.)

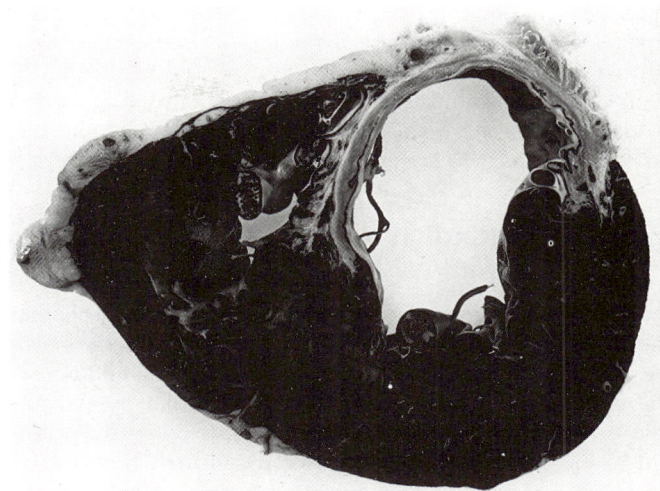

Fig. 12.48 A section across an area of old infarction stained with nitro-blue tetrazolium. Part of the ventricular wall has been reduced to a thin sheet of connective tissue with resulting formation of an aneurysm. (By courtesy of Professor M. J. Davies, St George's Hospital Medical School, London.)

are the result of full-thickness infarction and the stretching that can occur in the fibrous tissue which replaces the necrotic muscle. The term includes lesions with a wide base and which bulge diffusely from the ventricular wall, as well as saccular lesions which have a comparatively narrow neck. The patients may present with recurrent or persistent re-entry arrhythmias, cardiac failure, or with systemic embolization as a consequence of the mural thrombosis which often occurs within the aneurysm. The fibrous tissue wall occasionally undergoes extensive dystrophic calcification and this is particularly likely to occur when there is a thin layer of thrombotic material covering the luminal surface (Figs 12.47, 12.48).

12.4.7   Further reading

Davies, M. J. (1982). Ischaemic Heart Disease—the role of coronary thrombosis. *Hospital Update* **12**, 317–22.

Thomas, A. C., *et al.* (1988). Community studies of causes of 'natural' sudden death. *British Medical Journal* **297**, 1453–6.

Stehbens, W. E. (1985). Relationship of coronary artery thrombosis to myocardial infarction. *Lancet* **ii**, 639–42.

Bilia, L. M. and Willerson, J. T. (1987). The role of coronary artery lesions in ischaemic heart disease: insights from recent clinicopathologic, coronary arteriographic, and experimental studies. *Human Pathology* **18**, 451–61.

12.5   Hypertension

G. B. N. Lindop

Hypertension is raised pressure in a vascular bed. Used without qualification, hypertension means systemic arterial hypertension. However, there is also portal hypertension (see Chapter 17), and pulmonary hypertension (see Chapter 13). Hypertension affects about 15 per cent of the population in many developed countries and it is a major contributory factor to the high morbidity and mortality from cardiovascular diseases. Furthermore, it is easy to diagnose, monitor, and treat.

12.5.1 Distribution of blood pressure within a population

Epidemiological studies show that blood pressure in the population has a normal distribution curve which is slightly skewed to the right, hence any dividing line between normal and abnormal is arbitrary. However, mortality from cardiovascular disease is related to the level of blood pressure, even when it is within the range which is accepted as normal; this risk increases steeply in the hypertensive range of blood pressure where both the diastolic and the systolic blood pressure are predictors of cardiovascular complications.

12.5.2 Variability of blood pressure within individuals

Blood pressure has as diurnal variation; it also varies according to stimuli, such as exercise, assuming the upright posture, and exposure to cold and stress. Some subjects react to these stimuli with higher levels of blood pressure than others. The term 'labile hypertension' has been applied to this group, some of whom will develop sustained hypertension.

Blood pressure rises through childhood and reaches a plateau of normal adult levels in the third decade. In longitudinal studies of adults followed up over many years, those with lower initial blood pressures had the smallest rise in pressure with time. The higher the initial pressure, the steeper the rate of rise, whether in the hypertensive range or not. Therefore, those in the upper part of the normal range are more likely to become hypertensive later in life.

12.5.3 Definition

Working definitions of hypertension have been proposed by the WHO (Table 12.3).

Table 12.3 WHO working definitions of hypertension

Normotension	Systolic blood pressure ≤ 140 and Diastolic blood pressure ≤ 90
Hypertension	Systolic blood pressure ≥ 160 and/or Diastolic blood pressure ≥ 95
Borderline hypertension	Systolic blood pressure $>140 <160$ and/or Diastolic blood pressure $>90 <95$

Classification

Hypertension may be classified according to its clinical course and according to its cause. *Benign hypertension* is associated with few symptoms, and in most cases, a long clinical course. *Malignant hypertension*, if untreated, is usually fatal in under a year. Some forms of hypertension are the result of another disease, usually renal or endocrine disorders; this is known as *secondary hypertension*. In the great majority of cases of hypertension, no cause is found, so-called *essential hypertension*. Malignant hypertension may complicate either essential hypertension or secondary hypertension, but is much commoner in the latter group.

12.5.4 Benign hypertension

Clinical manifestations

Most patients with hypertension are asymptomatic; the diagnosis is usually made at a medical examination for another reason, or following one of the cardiovascular complications of hypertension. The commonest symptoms are non-specific; these are headaches, dizziness, and fatigue.

Pathology

Benign hypertension affects mainly the heart, the systemic arterial tree, and the kidney. The degree to which the heart and the arteries in the organs are affected varies greatly between individuals with similar levels of blood pressure. The clinical effects are mediated either by the pressure *per se* or by its accentuation of atheroma (see Section 12.2).

Heart

In response to the increased pressure load, the left ventricle undergoes hypertrophy which is usualy concentric (Fig. 12.49). The degree of hypertrophy is variable and correlates poorly with the degree of pressure. In some individuals the heart may double in weight, while others with similar levels of blood pressure may show only slight left ventricular hypertrophy after many years.

Cardiac hypertrophy *per se* has adverse functional effects: a hypertrophied ventricle is stiffer and therefore does not relax well enough for optimal filling in diastole; the centre of the hypertrophied myocyte is further from the capillary blood thereby increasing the diffusion distance for oxygen and nutrients, and, most importantly, hypertension is an important risk factor for ischaemic heart disease due to coronary artery atheroma. For these reasons, in the hypertensive population those with clinical evidence of severe left ventricular hypertrophy have a higher mortality than others; most dying of cardiac dysrhythmias.

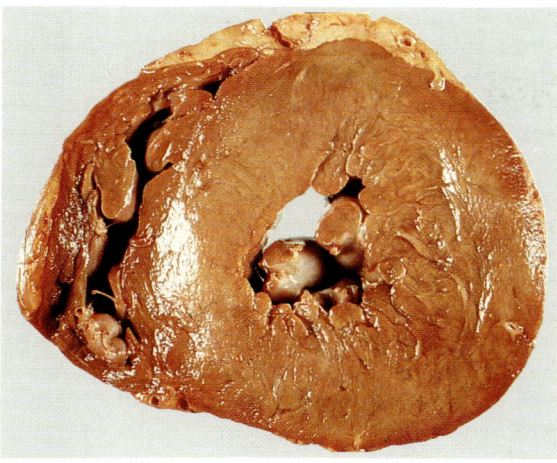

Fig. 12.49 A transverse section through a heart from a patient with long-standing benign hypertension. It shows concentric hypertrophy of the left ventricle.

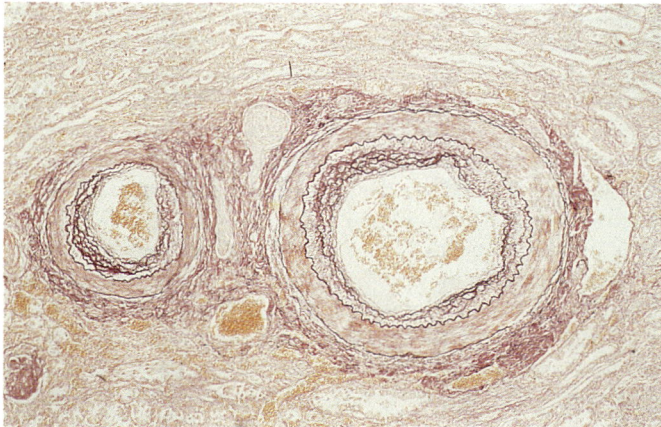

Fig. 12.50 Interlobar arteries in the kidney showing arteriosclerosis. There is intimal thickening with reduplication of the internal elastic lamina (seen as black wavy lines) but no significant narrowing of the lumen. (Elastic/van Gieson stain.)

Arteries

In all arteries and arterioles exposed to increased intraluminal pressure, the earliest change is thickening of the media due to both an increase in the size and in the number of medial smooth muscle cells. This has its greatest functional effect in the small resistance vessels where the increased smooth muscle mass causes the increased response to pressor agonists typical of some hypertensives. If the rise in pressure is long-standing, the hypertrophy of the media is replaced by the processes of arteriosclerosis in the large arteries and arteriolosclerosis in the arterioles. In large and medium-sized arteries arteriosclerosis is a normal feature of ageing, but it is accelerated in hypertension. The medial smooth muscle is replaced by collagen. This causes dilatation and lengthening of the aorta and its branches, accompanied by a loss of arterial compliance. This contributes to an increase in the systolic blood pressure. The dilatation is accompanied by thickening of the intima, and in medium-sized arteries there is reduplication of the internal elastic lamina (Fig. 12.50). Hypertension also causes an increase in glycosaminoglycans in the media of large arteries—'myxoid degeneration'. For this reason hypertension is the most important predisposing factor in dissecting aneurysm (see Section 12.6.9).

In the cerebral circulation, hypertension causes the formation of microaneurysms in the deep penetrating arteries of the cerebral cortex in the region of the basal ganglia, in the pons, and in the cerebellum. Rupture of these causes hypertensive cerebral haemorrhages. The increased presssure is also responsible for the rupture of berry aneurysms causing sub-arachnoid haemorrhage (Chapter 25).

Arterioles

Chronic hypertension causes arteriolosclerosis. Like the arteriosclerosis and myxoid degeneration of larger vessels, it is an accentuation of a process of ageing. It affects some vascular beds more than others; it is common in the arterioles of the abdominal viscera, retina, and adrenal capsule, and affects most severely the vessels of the kidney. It occurs rarely in the heart, skin, and skeletal muscle. In the kidney it affects mainly the afferent glomerular arterioles, which become thick-walled due to replacement of the smooth muscle cells by homogeneously staining hyaline material (Fig. 12.51) which, on light

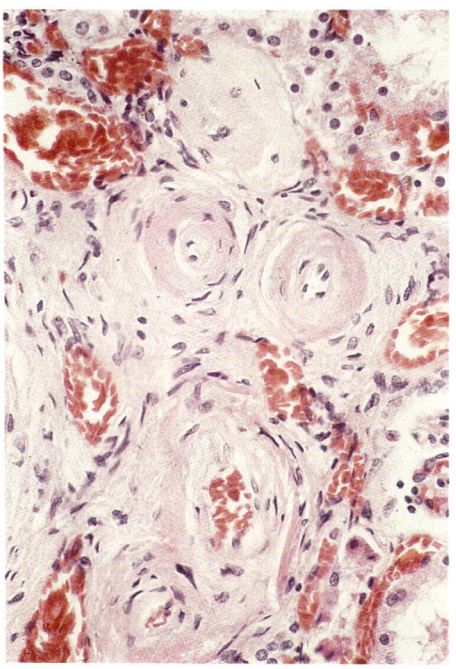

Fig. 12.51 An interlobular artery in the kidney shows arteriosclerosis. The media is thickened and medial smooth muscle cells are replaced by pink hyaline material. This has caused narrowing of the lumen. Two afferent glomerular arterioles also show arteriosclerosis.

microscopy, resembles the changes found in similar vessels in diabetes mellitus and amyloidosis. In all three diseases, proteins derived from the plasma are deposited in the walls of the blood-vessels by a process known as 'plasmatic vasculosis'. In this process there is accumulation of plasma protein in the blood vessel wall due either to increased permeability or to increased filtration pressure. Histochemical studies suggest that hyaline consists largely of glycoproteins; some of them are derived from the plasma but some may be due to excess basement membrane material. The outcome is loss of the medial smooth muscle cells, thickening of the wall, and narrowing of the lumen.

Arteriolosclerosis affects the kidney most severely. It is accompanied by sclerosis of glomeruli and atrophy of individual nephrons, which are then replaced by tiny scars. The loss of nephrons causes the kidneys to become smaller—the so-called 'granular contracted kidney' (see Chapter 19). In benign hypertension this gradual loss of nephrons causes only diminished functional reserve; unlike malignant hypertension (see below), it rarely causes renal failure and no effects have been defined in other affected organs.

In summary, in benign hypertension the first detectable change in the arterial tree is medial hypertrophy in the resistance vessels. This causes increased vascular resistance in response to the prevailing pressor stimuli. If the raised pressure is sustained, the hyperplasia is replaced by arteriosclerosis and arteriolosclerosis, which cause decreased compliance of the arterial tree, and a long-standing increase in resistance, respectively. Therefore, structural changes in the arterial tree will maintain raised arterial pressure regardless of its aetiology.

Complications and prognosis of benign hypertension

Many important complications of benign hypertension are due to the accentuation of atheroma; this causes ischaemic heart disease, cerebral infarction, aortic aneurysms, lower limb and mesenteric ischaemia. The other complications of hypertension are more directly related to the raised pressure. These are, cardiac failure, cerebral haemorrhage, subarachnoid haemorrhage, dissecting aneurysm, and the development of malignant hypertension. Some patients with benign hypertension may live a symptom-free life for several decades following diagnosis, but may die in middle age from one of the complications.

Treatment reduces the incidence of the common complications which are most directly related to the pressure, viz. cerebral haemorrhage, cardiac failure, and the transformation to malignant hypertension. Those caused by established atheroma are little affected by treatment. Thus myocardial infarction has replaced cardiac failure as the commonest cause of death in benign hypertension.

12.5.5   Malignant hypertension

Malignant hypertension is not a separate disease. To emphasize this, it is often called malignant-phase hypertension. Its clinical and pathological manifestations are different from benign hypertension simply because the blood pressure is so high

and/or its rise so steep that there is more severe damage to the arterial tree, sometimes with intravascular thrombosis and tissue damage. Malignant hypertension is defined on the cardinal clinical manifestations: high levels of blood pressure associated with retinal changes of papilloedema, exudates, and haemorrhages.

Malignant hypertension may complicate pre-existing benign hypertension, or it may appear to arise *ab initio*. The likelihood of developing malignant hypertension is increased in hypertensives who are young or Black; in patients whose hypertension is secondary to renal disease; and in those who smoke cigarettes. Malignant hypertension is unusual in the elderly, who can tolerate high blood pressures, possibly because the arteriosclerosis of old age protects the arterial tree from the effects of the high levels of blood pressure.

Clinical manifestations

Patients with malignant hypertension are usually symptomatic. They complain of headache and visual disturbances, and often have clinical manifestations of cardiac and renal failure. The blood pressure is usually greater than 220/140 and ophthalmoscopy shows retinal exudates, haemorrhages, and papilloedema. Rarely, altered consciousness or fits may occur due to cerebral oedema—*hypertensive encephalopathy*.

Pathology

There may be evidence of pre-existing benign hypertension in the form of left ventricular hypertrophy but often the heart is not enlarged. The histopathological hallmark of acute malignant hypertension is fibrinoid necrosis of small arteries and arterioles. Like the arteriolosclerosis of benign hypertension, this may affect many tissues, but the kidney is the principal target organ where the most commonly affected vessels are the afferent glomerular arterioles and the distal interlobular arteries.

Fibrinoid necrosis consists of a focal area of plasma insudation into an artery, leading to replacement of the normal structure of the media by homogeneous material which has the appearance and staining reactions of fibrin, so-called 'fibrinoid' (Fig. 12.52). Electron microscopy and immunocytochemistry confirm the presence of fibrin, but this is simply a marker for the accumulation of many other plasma proteins due to an increase in permeability. The insudation of plasma proteins is accompanied by cytological evidence of necrosis of the smooth muscle cells of the media. This is often accompanied by the extravasation of red blood corpuscles, which may be visible as tiny haemorrhages, and thrombosis of the lumen, which may result in small infarcts. When the afferent arteriole is affected, the fibrinoid necrosis may extend to the glomerulus and cause haematuria.

The other main arterial lesion in malignant hypertension is found mainly in the renal interlobular arteries, namely proliferative ('onion-skin') endarteritis; this has a variety of synonyms. The considerable thickening of the intima gives rise to a severe reduction in the lumen of the artery (Fig. 12.53).

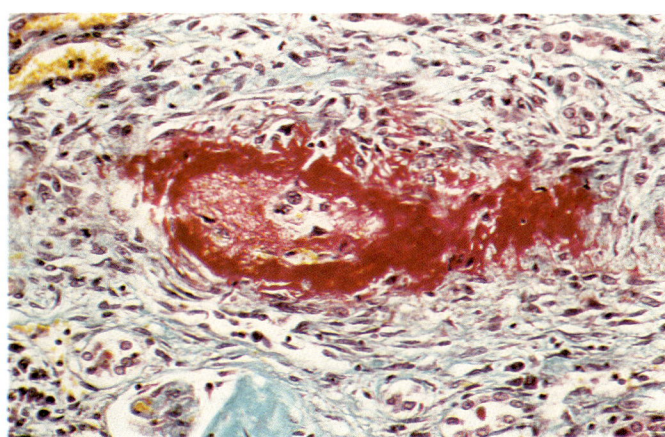

Fig. 12.52 An oblique section through a renal interlobular artery, showing fibrinoid necrosis. There is permeation of the full thickness of the vessel wall by fibrin (stained red) and a few red blood corpuscles (yellow) and the lumen is narrowed. There is an adventitial reaction but no significant inflammation. (Trichrome stain.)

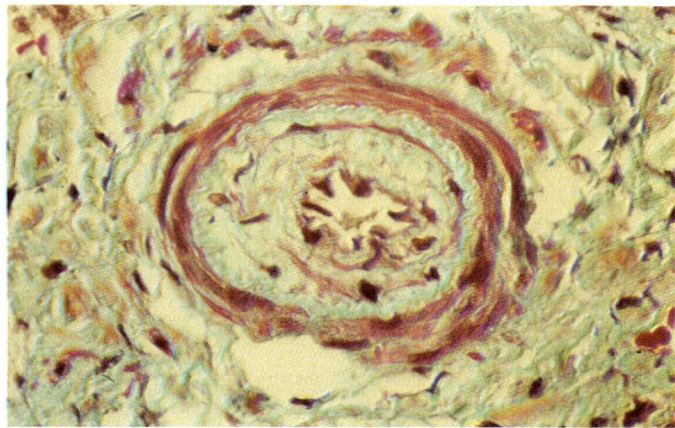

Fig. 12.53 A renal interlobular artery from a case of treated malignant hypertension showing severe 'onion-skin' endarteritis. The intima is thickened and contains concentrically orientated smooth muscle cells (red) and collagen (green). This has led to severe narrowing of the lumen and atrophy of the medial smooth muscle. (Masson stain.)

The diffuse damage to the vascular tree may be accompanied by intravascular coagulation which may accentuate the endothelial cell damage. Blood being forced at high pressure through a vascular bed with intravascular coagulation causes fragmentation of RBCs—microangiopathic haemolytic anaemia (MHA).

Pathogenesis of the arterial lesions

In response to a rising intraluminal pressure, the normal reflex vasoconstriction of an artery can be overcome. At first the failure to resist the pressure is focal; there is an area of increased permeability and dilatation associated with histological evidence of smooth muscle cell damage—fibrinoid necrosis. Then the dilatation and the increase in permeability extend along the length of the vessel. Flow increases as the upper limit of autoregulation is exceeded and tissue damage takes place. In the kidney, the pressure is transmitted to the glomeruli which undergo focal necrosis; the capillary loops also rupture, giving rise to haemorrhages into tubules, visible as 'flea-bite' haemorrhages on the surface of the kidney (see Chapter 19). This gives rise to proteinuria and haematuria, which are almost invariable in acute malignant hypertension.

The pathogenesis of the endarteritis in malignant hypertension is less well defined. It is best regarded as the healing stage of many types of arterial damage; these are intimal oedema, plasmatic vasculosis, and perhaps intravascular coagulation. All have in common endothelial cell injury. The cellular intimal thickening arises by the migration of smooth muscle cells through fenestra in the internal elastic lamina. The cells then orientate themselves circumferentially and secrete a connective tissue matrix; this is initially oedematous and rich in glycosaminoglycans but eventually becomes more collagenous. It is possible that the migration and proliferation of smooth muscle cells in this lesion could be augmented by the release of platelet-derived growth factor by platelets adhering to the damaged endothelium or released together with other growth factors and cytokines by the endothelial cells themselves (see Sections 12.2.7–8).

In malignant hypertension the arterial damage eventually causes renal ischaemia and stimulation of the renin-angiotensin system (see below). The high plasma levels of potent vasoconstrictors such as angiotensin II, noradrenaline, and vasopressin can, in some cases, lead to the development of a vicious circle. High levels of plasma aldosterone may also occur—'secondary hyperaldosteronism'.

In summary, in the earliest stages of acute malignant hypertension the arterial damage is caused by the failure of the vessel to resist the rise in pressure. The forced dilatation is associated with increased permeability and muscle cell necrosis. It remains to be determined which comes first, the increase in permeability or the necrosis of medial smooth muscle cells. Intravascular coagulation then occurs; this may augment the vascular damage and cause infarcts and MHA. The endarteritis is probably a healing response.

Clinical course and prognosis

In untreated malignant hypertension the average survival is less than a year. Renal failure is the usual cause of death. Now powerful antihypertensive drugs have revolutionized the prognosis. If patients can escape a cerebral haemorrhage or cardiac failure in the acute phase, most can be effectively treated. However, those who have sustained severe arterial damage often develop proliferative endarteritis which can cause renal failure due to ischaemia several years later.

12.5.6 Essential hypertension

Natural history

The onset of essential hypertension usually occurs between 35 and 45 years of age. The rate of rise in pressure varies according to the starting pressure; the higher the starting pressure the more rapidly it rises. Both systolic and diastolic blood pressure rise slowly over a number of years, then stabilize at about 55 years. In a few cases, the pressure may rise rapidly to high levels and give rise to malignant hypertension.

Aetiology

Genetic factors

The distribution of blood pressure in human populations is unimodal, suggesting a polygenic inheritance. In families with hypertensive and non-hypertensive parents the aggregation of high blood pressure in the offspring suggests a genetic component. This has been confirmed by twin studies and the comparison between the blood pressures of adopted and natural children with the same parents.

Racial factors

Hypertension is at least twice as prevalent in black Americans as in the white population; it also has a worse prognosis. Hypertensive black males have a death rate about six times that of white males with the same levels of blood pressure.

Age and sex

Essential hypertension usually begins between 35 and 45 years of age. It is commoner in females but has a better prognosis; the mortality rates for men are 1.5 to 2 times that of women.

Environmental factors

Stress Urban populations have higher blood pressures than rural populations and the adverse effects of urban living are confirmed by the rise in blood pressure of rural populations migrating to the cities. These and similar studies suggest an effect of stress. Experiments in which animals are subjected to a chronically stressful environment support this idea.

Diet The sodium intake of a population is culturally determined; it bears little relationship to physiological need. Epidemiological studies show that the prevalence of hypertension in a population is correlated with the salt intake. In some countries such as Japan there are large variations in the prevalence of hypertension and these are paralleled by the sodium intake, which may reach 400 mmol/day; in these regions the prevalence of hypertension reaches 40 per cent of the population. Animal experiments show that high salt intake will produce hypertension in most species. There is a wide variation in susceptibility, which is genetically determined and probably operates early in life. Transplant experiments indicate that the susceptibility to salt is conferred by the kidney. In spite of the compelling evidence from both epidemiological studies and animal experiments it remains controversial whether high salt diet causes hypertension in man.

Diets that are high in sodium are usually low in potassium and vice versa. Potassium supplements have been shown to ameliorate the effects of hypertension in animals. It is therefore possible that low potassium intake may be a significant factor in the tendency to hypertension in man. Other cations under

investigation are calcium and magnesium, as deficiency of both have been implicated in the development of hypertension.

There is also evidence that people with diets high in animal fats have higher blood pressures and that this can be lowered by substitution of unsaturated oils; also, the change from a Mediterranean diet to one rich in saturated fats caused an increase in blood pressure.

Smoking Cigarette smoking increases the risk of developing malignant hypertension in hypertensive patients, but this is far outweighed in importance by its effect as a major risk factor in ischaemic heart disease, and the other complications of atheroma.

In summary then, there is a genetic tendency to essential hypertension which is inherited as a polygenic characteristic. However, hypertension and its associated toll of cardiovascular diseases are rare in developing countries and common in 'Westernized' urban environments. Population migration studies show that the difference is environmental rather than genetic. Stress and diet are the main environmental factors that have been implicated; the former is difficult to define and the dietary factors remain controversial. This is a crucial area of research since it holds the hope of intervention through education and public health measures.

Blood pressure is controlled by many interlocking mechanisms; therefore, an alteration in one of them will produce secondary alterations in others. How the above aetiological factors operate is not known.

12.5.7 Pathophysiological abnormalities in hypertension

Cardiac output

Since arterial blood pressure is a product of cardiac output and peripheral resistance, theoretically, increases in either could cause hypertension. Some patients with labile and borderline hypertension have raised cardiac output, suggesting that some cases of essential hypertension begin with raised cardiac output, which subsequently falls to normal. However, most patients with established essential hypertension have a normal cardiac output and blood pressure is sustained by increased peripheral resistance.

The resistance vessel

The arteriolosclerosis of chronic hypertension is a consequence and not a cause of the raised pressure; it may contribute to the maintainance of the level of blood pressure in chronic hypertension. The earliest morphological change in the resistance vessels is hypertrophy. Hypertrophy has its greatest effect in the small resistance vessels where the thickening of the media has the greatest mechanical advantage. The increased 'sensitivity' of hypertensive patients to pressor agents is thus explained by this structural rather than a pharmacological mechanism.

Smooth muscle contractility and hypertrophy may also be linked at a molecular level. The binding of vasoconstrictors such as noradrenaline and angiotensin II to their receptors on the cell membrane activates the phosphoinositide system. This causes contraction of the smooth muscle cell by the release of free calcium within the cell. Activation of this second messenger system, which mediates contraction, also causes an increase in membrane diacylglycerol which participates in another signalling system. This acts via the enzyme protein kinase C which promotes cell growth. In this way activity of the system that causes contraction of the smooth muscle cell may also stimulate its growth. There is therefore current interest in the actions of hormones as growth factors for vascular smooth muscle cells, thereby causing hypertrophy.

Cell membrane abnormalities

Essential hypertension is associated with many abnormalities in membrane transport systems: these include channels for sodium, potassium, and calcium; exchangers for sodium/hydrogen and for sodium/calcium and pumps for calcium and for sodium/potassium.

The flux of ions through the cell membrane, the activity of the cationic pumps, the handling of calcium by the cell, and the fluidity of the membrane itself are all influenced by its lipid composition. Abnormalities of membrane lipids are now being described in hypertensive patients, and population studies show relationships between blood lipids, blood pressure, and membrane cation transport. A single abnormality of lipid metabolism may therefore underly the multiple abnormalities of cation transport by the cell membrane which are present in essential hypertension.

Central nervous system

In most models of experimental hypertension there is activation of the nervous system, and the hypertension in some models can be prevented by specific neurochemical and surgical manipulations of the brain. In man and in animals hypertension can be produced by stress via central mechanisms and, conversely, both man and animals can be trained to lower their blood pressure by awareness of their cardiovascular reflexes. Some vasoactive agents also have a central action, notably angiotensin II; this acts centrally to produce thirst and water retention.

Sympathetic nervous system

Much of the resting vascular tone is controlled by the sympathetic nervous system. While this is difficult to measure accurately, there is evidence of sympathetic overactivity in early essential hypertension and in some experimental models of hypertension. This could raise blood pressure by a variety of mechanisms: by a central action in the brain; by a direct vasomotor effect; or by acting in concert with the renin–angiotensin system, causing further constriction of resistance vessels or causing sodium retention by acting on the kidney. In hypertension the baroreceptor reflexes of the carotid sinus and the aorta are abnormal, being set too high. This is likely to be a secondary defect.

Sympathetic efferent nerves innervate the juxtaglomerular apparatus and their stimulation causes renin release mediated by a β-adrenergic receptor mechanism. Sympathetic nerves also contain a variety of neuropeptides, and some of them, such as neuropeptide-Y, are potent vasoconstrictors. Neuropeptides are likely to be important in regulating the cadiovascular system, and the mechanisms involved are under active investigation.

Circulating pressor agents

Catecholamines

High circulating levels of catecholamines cause hypertension in phaeochromocytoma; lower levels may be implicated in the stress reaction.

Renin–angiotensin system

In essential hypertension 60 per cent of patients have normal plasma renin; it is high in 15 per cent and low in 25 per cent. This may indicate that there is an imbalance between the renin–angiotensin system and the prevailing exchangeable sodium status. There is no clear evidence that the renin–angiotensin system is important in the pathogenesis of essential hypertension or in any of its complications other than in malignant hypertension.

Vasodilator systems

Renomedullary antihypertensive factors

The renal medulla contains a population of interstitial cells that contain osmiophilic secretory granules. These cells secrete at least two lipids that are potent vasodilators and reduce blood pressure. Bilateral nephrectomy causes hypertension, known as renoprival hypertension, which is cured by transplants of the renal medulla and medullary interstitial cells grown in culture. Difficulties in characterizing the medullary lipids have made it difficult to assess their contribution to the control of blood pressure in man.

Atrial natriuretic factor

Atrial peptides are secreted from the heart into the blood. They cause a potent diuresis and natriuresis and a drop in blood pressure, which is exaggerated in hypertensive subjects. They also directly antagonize the effects of the renin–angiotensin system, but there is no evidence as yet that they are involved in the pathogenesis of hypertension.

Natriuretic hormone

There is a low molecular weight natriuretic hormone circulating in human blood. It is not a peptide and its activity is increased by volume loading and high sodium intake. It is a sodium–potassium ATPase inhibitor and is probably secreted by the hypothalamus. It cannot account for all the abnormalities of membrane cation transport described in essential hypertension and its physiological significance remains uncertain.

Kalikrein–kinin and prostaglandin systems

Kinins and some of the prostaglandins are potent vasodilators.

Both systems can also interact with the renin–angiotensin–aldosterone system. They have a local function within the kidney and may contribute to the regulation of regional blood flow and electrolyte transport. However, there is no evidence that altered activity of these systems can cause or compensate for any type of experimental or human hypertension.

12.5.8   Secondary hypertension

Although hypertension has a high prevalence in the population, the proportion of cases in which an aetiology can be found is small, probably less than 5 per cent of an unselected hypertensive population and perhaps 15 per cent of patients referred to a hypertension clinic. Secondary hypertension is commoner in young patients, and the complete cure of some of these cases and the better control of others by surgery makes them worth identifying.

Renal hypertension

Renal disorders are about 10 times commoner than all other causes of secondary hypertension. There are two main groups of renal diseases that cause hypertension: renovascular disorders and renal parenchymal diseases.

Renovascular hypertension

The commonest cause is renal artery stenosis due to fibromuscular dysplasia (see Section 12.6.10) or atheroma of the renal artery, but similar mechanisms probably operate in other diseases that affect the intrarenal branches of the renal arterial tree (see below). The most common form of renovascular hypertension is due to a unilateral narrowing of one renal artery. Three phases can be discerned:

1. Immediately after constricting the renal artery there is a rise in the circulating levels of renin and angiotensin II associated with a rise in blood pressure; if the renal artery constriction or the ischaemic kidney are removed, there is a complete return to normal.

2. After some days or weeks blood pressure remains high in spite of somewhat lower renin and angiotensin levels; again, removal of the constriction or the affected kidney results in a fall of blood pressure to normal.

3. In the final stage, after many months or years, there is persistent hypertension but plasma renin and angiotensin levels are not above normal. The hypertension persists when the ischaemic kidney is removed, but can be cured by subsequent removal of the second kidney.

In the early phase of renal artery stenosis the blood pressure is directly influenced by the pressor action of plasma angiotensin II. In the intermediate phase the blood pressure is controlled by a slow action of angiotensin II. Therefore in both of these phases hypertension can be controlled by nephrectomy or by pharmacological blockade of the renin–angiotensin system. In the later stages the hypertension does not respond to removal of the ischaemic kidney because it is maintained by hypertensive

damage to the contralateral kidney. This view of the mechanism of renovascular hypertension is an oversimplification, since there is also increased activity of the sympathetic nervous system and evidence of an increased cardiac output in the early phase of the syndrome.

There is a group of diseases which cause narrowing and/or thrombosis of the renal arterial tree. These are the vasculitis syndromes, especially classical polyarteritis nodosa and progressive systemic sclerosis; chronic vascular rejection of renal allografts, radiation nephritis, and malignant hypertension. The mechanism of the hypertension in all of these conditions is probably analogous to renal artery stenosis.

Renal parenchymal disease

Glomerulonephritis This is the commonest renal parenchymal disease to cause hypertension. Even when acute glomerulonephritis resolves, the hypertension may occasionally persist. In chronic glomerulonephritis hypertension aggravates the glomerular damage caused by immune complex deposition by increasing the filtration pressure. It is therefore important to treat the hypertension of renal disease in order to slow the progression of renal failure. There is no association between acute pyelonephritis and hypertension.

Pyelonephritis In recurrent or chronic pyelonephritis hypertension is associated with renal scars. Many of these are caused by vesico–ureteric reflux and infection in childhood.

Diabetic and analgesic nephropathy Hypertension is present in about 60 per cent of patients with diabetic nephropathy. Blood pressure is raised in about half of the cases of analgesic nephropathy; it is possible that necrosis of the medullary interstitial cells raises blood pressure by a 'renoprival' effect (see above).

Polycystic disease In adult polycystic disease hypertension is almost invariable at some stage; about 50 per cent of sufferers die of its complications—myocardial infarction, cerebral haemorrhage, and congestive heart failure—rather than of renal failure. The hypertension in the late stages is due to renal failure with sodium and water retention. In the early stages the hypertension is probably caused by stretching of renal artery branches by the expanding cysts. Solitary cysts of the kidney can also cause high renin hypertension, which is cured by surgical excision or aspiration of the cyst.

Renal failure Hypertension is almost invariable in chronic renal failure from any cause, and it can be controlled by regulating the sodium balance by dialysis. It is likely that the hypertension of chronic renal failure is due to the failure of the sodium and water retention to suppress the renin–angiotensin system so that plasma levels of renin, angiotensin, and aldosterone are inappropriately high for the level of exchangeable sodium.

Adrenal causes of secondary hypertension

Phaeochromocytoma

Phaeochromocytoma causes hypertension mainly by creating

high levels of circulating catecholamines. The tumour may secrete noradrenaline, adrenaline, or dopamine, or a mixture of these, and in only 50 per cent of cases is the hypertension paroxysmal. Hypertension with similar symptoms can be due to catecholamine secretion by neuroblastoma or ganglioneuroblastoma.

Primary hyperaldosteronism (Conn syndrome)

This is due to an aldosterone-secreting adenoma of the adrenal cortex. The high plasma levels of mineralocorticoid cause sodium and water retention; in exchange for sodium the kidney excretes potassium and hydrogen ions. This causes hypokalaemia and a metabolic alkalosis. The expanded extravascular volume leads to hypertension and the increased potassium excretion leads to a fall in total body potassium, which causes muscular weakness. The raised sodium and extracellular fluid levels suppress renin synthesis and plasma levels of renin and angiotensin are low. These features allow this condition to be distinguished from 'secondary hyperaldosteronism'. This occurs in some cases of severe hypertension in which there are high levels of renin and angiotensin II, which stimulate the adrenal cortex. There is no oedema.

The hypertension almost always resolves with surgical excision of the adenoma.

Cushing syndrome

Hypertension occurs in about 80 per cent of cases of Cushing syndrome and about 90 per cent of Cushing disease; both the glucocorticoid and mineralocorticoid effects contribute to the hypertension.

Congenital adrenal hyperplasia

There are rare cases of hypertension in childhood due to congenital deficiencies of enzymes in the biosynthetic pathway of cortisol. Some of these result in the accumulation of salt-retaining precursors. Deficiency of cortisol causes the high plasma ACTH levels by failure of the negative feedback loop, and this is responsible for the hyperplasia of the adrenal cortex.

Other types of endocrine hypertension

One-third of patients with acromegaly have hypertension, and the level of blood pressure correlates with the plasma levels of growth hormone. A smaller proportion of patients with both hypo- and hyperthyroidism and with hyperparathyroidism are hypertensive, but the mechanisms remain obscure.

Hypertension in pregnancy

Most cases are due to pre-eclampsia, a disease characterized by oedema, proteinuria, and hypertension, which occurs after the 20th week of gestation and more usually nearer term. It is of uncertain aetiology and may progress to the more severe condition of eclampsia, characterized by higher blood pressure, coagulation disturbances, and fits, which may be fatal. Less often, essential hypertension or secondary hypertension are first manifest in pregnancy.

Hypertension in the elderly

If essential hypertension has not developed in middle age, mild to moderate elevation of blood pressure may occur, usually beginning after the sixth decade. The systolic blood pressure often rises disproportionately and sometimes solely. Arteriosclerosis and arteriolosclerosis probably play a part in its aetiology.

Iatrogenic hypertension

A slight rise in blood pressure occurs in most women taking the contraceptive pill; some of those with blood pressures in the upper part of the normal range therefore develop mild hypertension. Blood pressure returns to normal within 3–6 months on cessation. Hypertension may also complicate the therapeutic administration of glucocorticoids, as mentioned above. Acute hypertensive crises mimicking those of phaeochromocytoma may occur in patients taking monoamine oxidase inhibitors who consume foods that contain large amounts of tyramine.

Alcohol

There is a linear relationship between alcohol intake and blood pressure. Hypertension is commoner in habitual heavy drinkers, and blood pressure can sometimes be restored to normal following abstention. It returns to hypertensive levels on resumption of high alcohol intake; the mechanism of this effect remains unclear.

Renin-secreting tumours

The autonomous secretion of renin by tumours, so-called 'primary reninism', is a rare cause of hypertension. The classical renin-secreting tumour is the juxtaglomerular cell tumour. These are small benign tumours composed of renin-secreting juxtaglomerular cells. They cause severe hypertension due to the secretion of active renin which generates high levels of angiotensin II in the plasma. Hypertension is usually cured following removal of the tumour. Any mass in the kidney can cause hypertension by compression of the intrarenal arteries or by increasing the intrarenal pressure, however some cases of nephroblastoma and rare cases of renal cell carcinoma can also cause hypertension due to renin secretion by the tumour. Rarely, renin can be secreted 'inappropriately' by a variety of non-renal malignant tumours.

12.5.9 Further reading

Folkow, B. (1982). Physiological aspects of primary hypertension. *Physiological Reviews* 62, 347–504.

Kashgarian, M. (1987). Pathology of the kidney in hypertension. In *The kidney in hypertension* (ed. N. M. Kaplan, B. M. Brenner, and J. H. Laragh). Raven Press, New York.

Ledingham, J. (1971). The aetiology of hypertension. *Practitioner* 207, 5–19.

Lever, A. F. (1986). Slow pressor mechanisms in hypertension: a role for hypertrophy of resistance vessels? *Journal of Hypertension* 4, 515–24.

Lindop, G. B. M. and Lever, A. F. (1986). The anatomy of the renin–angiotensin system in the normal and pathological kidney. *Histopathology* **10**, 335–62.

Robertson, J. I. S., Morton, J. J., Tilman, D. M., and Lever, A. F. (1986). The pathophysiology of renovascular hypertension. *Journal of Hypertension* **4** (Suppl. 4), S95–S103.

Wiener, J. and Giacomelli, F. (1983). Hypertensive vascular disease. In *Hypertension* (2nd edn) (ed. J. Genest, O. Kuchel, P. Hamet and M. Cantin). McGraw-Hill, New York.

12.6   Arteritis

C. L. Berry

12.6.1   Polyarteritis, including polyarteritis nodosa

The systemic vasculitides are multisystem disorders characterized by arterial inflammation and often widespread vascular occlusion. The clinical manifestations are thus protean, but pyrexia of unknown origin and marked constitutional upset are common. Non-specific laboratory findings include an often marked leucocytosis and raised erythrocyte sedimentation rate (ESR).

Circulating immune complexes are demonstrated in many patients, including those with Wegener granulomatosis (see below), and a suggested pathogenesis is that these are deposited in the vessel wall, with subsequent inflammation and thrombosis. Whether deposition is found within the wall or not, endothelial cell damage following release of enzymes and oxygen radicals from leucocytes after phagocytosis of immune complexes is important, and damage to the subendothelial matrix appears to be a critical step in establishing a persistent lesion. Auto-antibodies against neutrophil cytoplasm are also present in Wegener granuloma and microscopic polyarteritis nodosa, apparently to an epitope associated with alkaline phosphatase. There are thus a number of possible modes of production of immune-mediated vascular damage.

Markers of infection by hepatitis B virus are found in 0–45 per cent of macroscopic polyarteritis nodosa (PAN). A role for the HBs antigen seems certain in some cases, and the liver disease accompanying PAN is probably due to infection rather than the vasculitis in many instances.

The progression of these diseases has often been monitored by the ESR but newer methods are now available. Factor VIII-related antigen is a large molecular weight glycoprotein produced by and stored in endothelial cells. Raised levels of the antigen may be found in vascular injury, notably in Wegener disease and polyarteritis, but not in the vasculitis which affects small vessels in the skin. Levels are raised in persisting disease but fall after therapy.

Polyarteritis nodosa (PAN)

This disease affects small and medium-sized muscular arteries in the heart in up to 80 per cent of fatal cases (Fig. 12.54), kidneys, gut, central nervous system, and muscle; lesions tend to occur at bifurcations. The pulmonary vessels are usually spared. There is a focal necrotizing arteritis of the wall and destruction of the structure occurs in a short segment, usually affecting the entire circumference. Fibrinoid necrosis is seen with a dense polymorphonuclear infiltrate in which eosinophils are prominent in the early phase (Figs 12.55, 12.56).

Later, fibrosis and resolution occurs and lymphocytes become

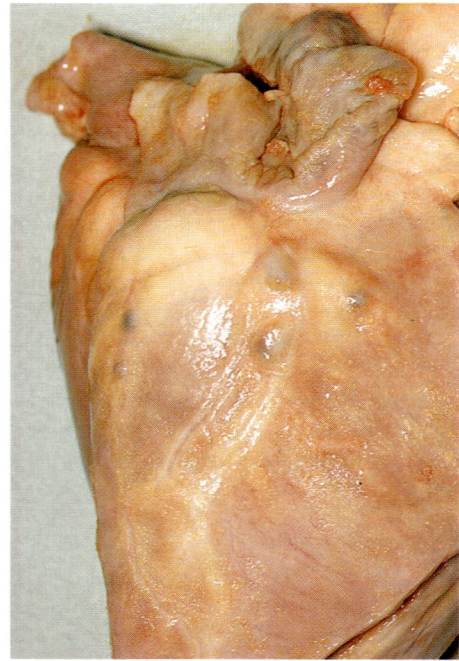

Fig. 12.54 Heart showing numerous aneurysms of the coronary arteries, appearing as dark blue dots.

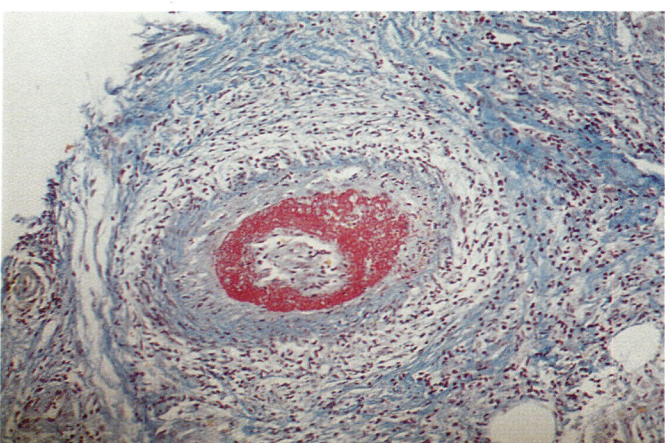

Fig. 12.55 Fibrinoid material in the wall of a vessel in the acute phase of polyarteritis. The fibrinoid material appears red. (MSB stain.)

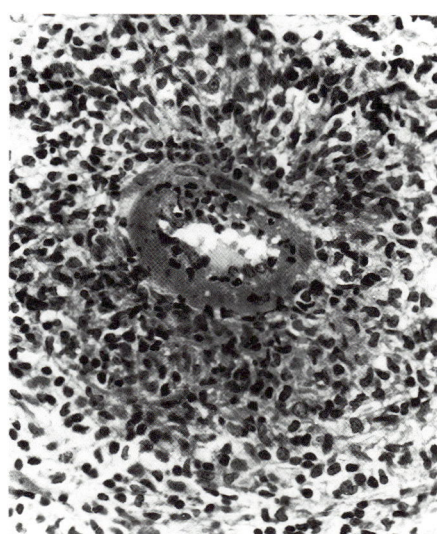

Fig. 12.56 Polymorphonuclear infiltrate most evident over an area of fibrinoid necrosis in PAN. There is inflammation and oedema of the vessel wall.

prominent. Lesions of different ages are found throughout the body.

Infarction is common in the acute phase of the disease, later fibrosis and scarring may cause further ischaemic damage to affected organs. Hypertension from renal lesions is an important cause of death in long-standing cases (Fig. 12.57).

Kawasaki disease

This particular form of polyarteritis occurs in infancy and childhood. Typically, in a child under 5 years of age, and usually about 1 year old, there is fever not responding to antibiotics, a variable rash on the trunk, and reddening and oedema of the palms and soles, with desquamation of the finger tips during convalescence. There are conjunctival congestion, changes in

the lips and oral cavity, and acute non-supparative swelling of the cervical lymph nodes. The disease is thus known as the 'muco-cutaneous lymph node syndrome'. It is clear now that more than 20 000 cases of the disease have been studied, that this is an infantile form of PAN, but that the prognosis is better than in the adult disease. Death occurs in less than 1 per cent of cases and is generally due to myocardial infarction from involvement of the coronary arteries (Fig. 12.58).

Wegener granulomatosis

This disease is probably related to PAN but more typically affects smaller vessels (including venules) with segmental glomerulonephritis and necrotizing granulomas of the lungs, nose, and para-nasal sinuses as major clinical presentations. There is necrosis with an extensive and florid inflammatory infiltrate in which giant cells may be seen (Fig. 12.59). The extent of tissue destruction may be severe (see also Chapter 13).

12.6.2 Arteritis in rheumatoid arthritis and other related conditions

In rheumatoid disease, arteritis may affect the aorta, pulmonary artery, or other major vessels. One of the first associations to be noticed was between aortitis and often severe aortic insufficiency in long-standing ankylosing spondylitis; similar changes may be seen in Reiter disease, relapsing polychondritis and, rarely, in Behcet syndrome. In classical rheumatoid arthritis, aortitis is generally associated with cardiac involvement but, unlike ankylosing spondylitis, the changes may occur early in the natural history of the disease and the degree of aortic insufficiency is generally moderate.

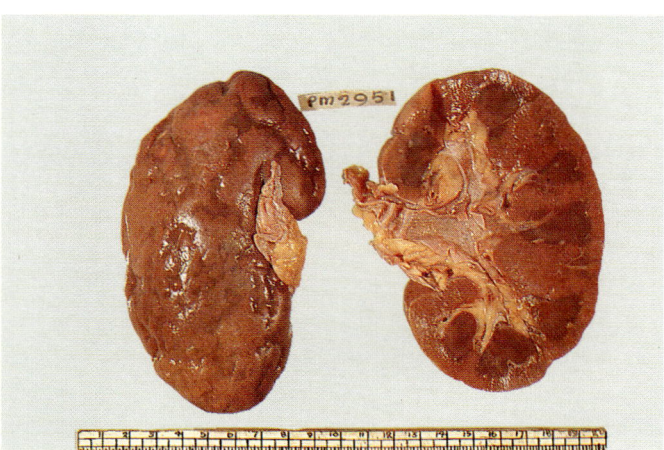

Fig. 12.57 Cut surface of a kidney in PAN showing extensive patchy and irregular infarction of the cortex.

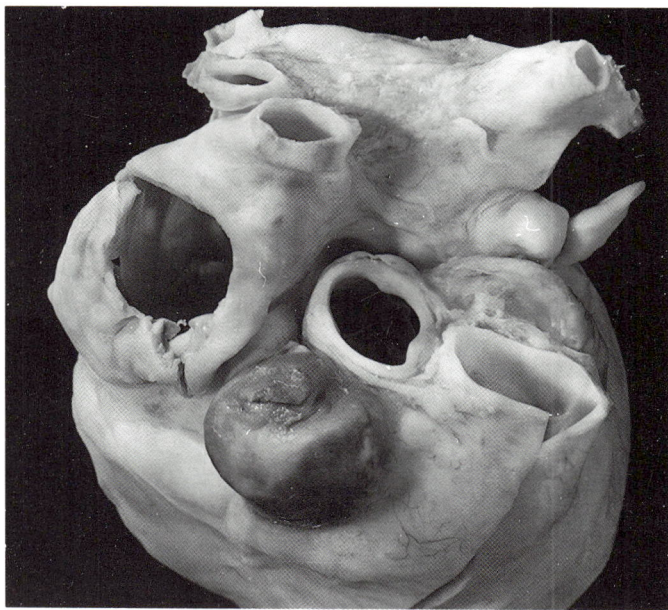

Fig. 12.58 Kawasaki disease. An infant heart with a large saccular aneurysm of the right coronary artery, which had ruptured causing cardiac tamponade. (Courtesy of Professor A. E. Becker.)

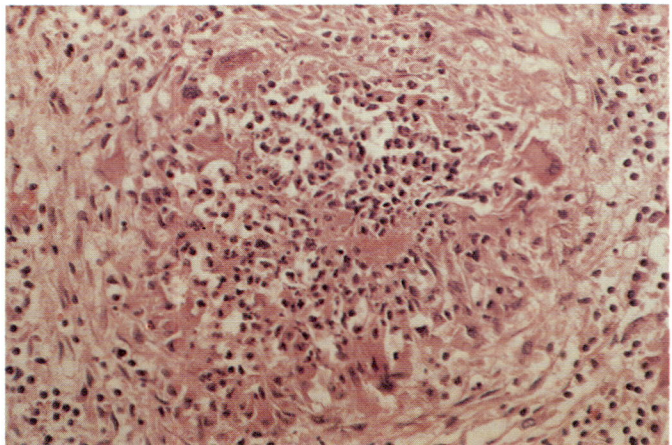

Fig. 12.59 Wegener granuloma of the lung. Acute arteritis with giant cell formation is evident.

In all these conditions the pathological findings are similar. Aortic involvement tends to be more marked proximally but patchy in distribution, affecting all vessel layers (fibrosis in the adventitia is common). The aortic valve may be affected directly by the inflammatory process. Histopathologically there is endarteritis obliterans of the vasa vasora but, unlike syphilis, with which the lesion may be confused, there are scattered areas of fibrinoid necrosis in the media and an acute inflammatory infiltrate in the intima with fibrosis in irregular bands, suggesting scarring of previously active areas.

12.6.3 Giant cell arteritis (temporal arteritis)

This term is used to describe a spectrum of inflammatory vascular diseases in which giant cells are found, but is probably better confined to the temporal arteritis/polymyalgia rheumatica complex. This is very rare under 50 years of age and shows a weak prediliction for women; the incidence is highest in North European populations. There are familial aggregates and an increased incidence of HLA-DR4 in affected individuals. The superficial temporal, occipital, facial, and ophthalmic arteries are most consistently involved.

The arteritis presents as a segmental inflammation of the media and internal elastic lamina (IEL); this pattern of involvement requires that biopsies of 10–20 mm should be taken for microscopic confirmation, as involved segments may be only 300–400 μm long. Macroscopically the vessels appear slightly thickened and may be nodular. On section, the IEL is disrupted with mononuclear and giant cell collections in affected areas. Thrombosis with occlusion of the lumen is common, associated with intimal thickening. In 40 per cent of cases biopsy fails to show giant cell change, but there may be intimal and medial fibrosis with defects in the IEL and some mononuclear cells, or non-specific intimal thickening with fragmentation of the IEL and microcalcification of the fragments (Fig. 12.60a, b).

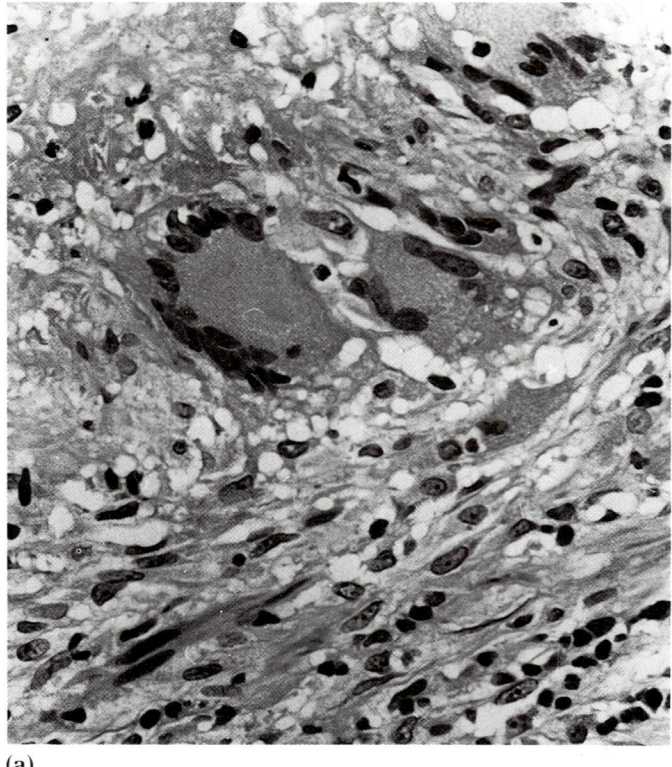

(a)

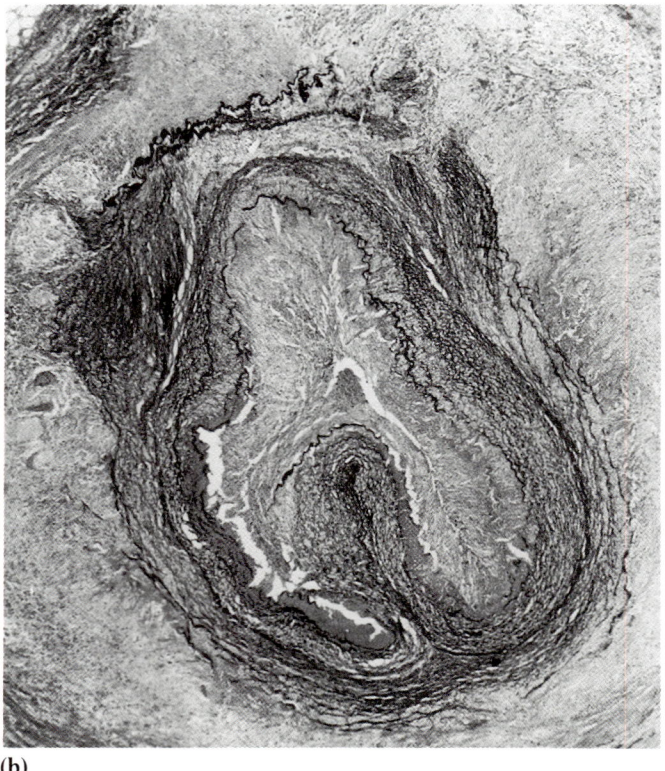

(b)

Fig. 12.60 (a) Giant cells and mononuclear inflammation in the wall of an artery with giant cell arteritis. (b) A more frequent finding is of a vessel showing intimal organization, disruption of the internal elastic lamina, and patchy calcification. (Elastic van Gieson (EVG) stain.)

The effects of arterial occlusion include necrosis of the scalp or tongue, but blindness is the most serious clinical complication. In general, the extent of the vascular changes are greater than the symptomatology would suggest. The great arteries may be affected and there may be an associated myocarditis.

Meticulous examination of biopsies is essential in this disease; overdiagnosis condemns an often elderly patient to some months of unnecessary steroid therapy, and non-diagnosis may result in blindness from involvement of the ophthalmic artery.

12.6.4 Takaysu disease

Sometimes referred to as 'pulseless disease', this condition is commoner in women (4:1) and typically presents before 40 years of age. It is a chronic inflammatory arteropathy which, in about half the cases, affects the arch of the aorta and its major branches, in particular, the post-vertebral subclavian artery. Splanchnic and renal artery involvement may occur and pulmonary involvement has been reported. The pathology has become better defined as the early stages of the disease can be examined in operative resections available as a result of advances in surgical therapy.

The hallmark of this condition is lumenal stenosis of the aorta without change in its external diameter. The affected vessel appears thick-walled and rigid with marked peri-vascular sclerosis and adherence to the surrounding tissues. Internally, the intimal surface is greyish white, thickened, and raised, obstructing the lumen. Non-involved vascular segments are clearly demarcated. Aneurysmal dilatation is rare and is not seen early in the course of the disease, although post-stenotic dilatation is common.

Histopathologically there is a chronic inflammatory process extending from the outer aspect of the artery and leading to occlusion, with most change seen in the adventitia and media (thrombosis is uncommon); the elastic structure of the media is destroyed and there is neovascularization (Fig. 12.61a,b). In the sheets of lymphocytes and macrophages that are seen, some giant cells are found and plasma cells may also be present. The intima is thickened by oedematous connective tissue with little cellular infiltration. Local lymph nodes show sinus histiocytosis and fibrosis.

The aortic valve may become thickened by the inflammatory process affecting the aorta, and this may affect its function. Coronary artery ostial stenosis may also develop.

In the later stages of the disease there will be a predominance of the fibrous component with scarring and shortening of affected vessels. Calcification occurs by this stage.

When the abdominal aorta or its major branches are involved, 'abdominal coarctation' or stenosing ostial lesions are common, and renal hypertension or intestinal ischaemia may occur. The disease is an important cause of renal hypertension in childhood.

Rupture of the vessel wall occurs infrequently in Takayasu disease; indeed, its occurrence should lead to the consideration of other diagnosis or raise the possibility of infection.

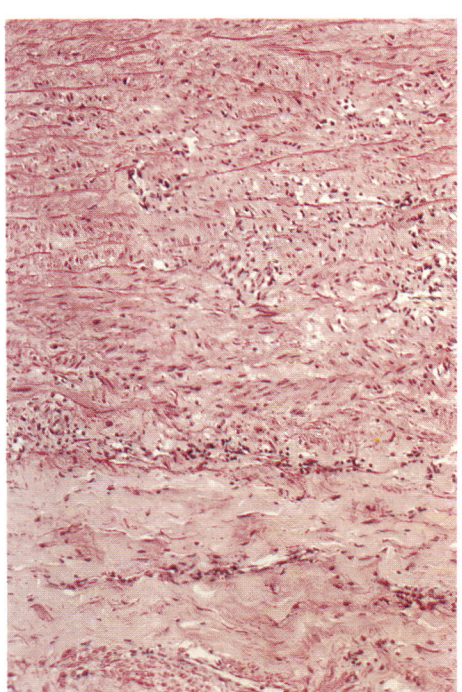
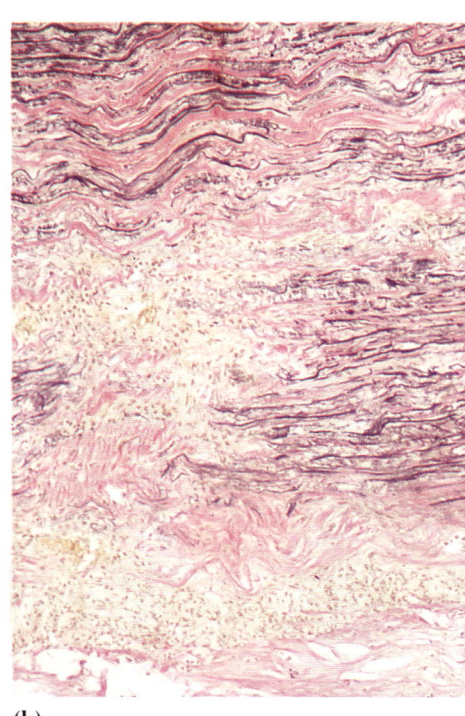

(a) **(b)**

Fig. 12.61 Takaysu disease. (a) Aortic media showing patchy infiltration by lymphocytes with early disruption of the media. (b) Loss of elastic tissue in another aorta with a more advanced lesion. Interruption of the lamellar structure is severe. (EVG stain.)

12.6.5 Systemic sclerosis

Systemic sclerosis is a systemic disease in which associated arterial damage is important in determining outcome, with progressive renal failure (with or without hypertension) a common cause of death. The interlobular and arcuate arteries and afferent arterioles are involved by a mucoid intimal proliferation, with concentric hyperplasia of intimal cells leading to narrowing of the vessels. Cortical infarction may occur. Morphometric studies separate these changes from those seen in hypertension alone; intimal thickening predominates rather than medial hypertrophy as the cause of arterial narrowing.

12.6.6 Syphilis

Historically, the chronic vascular complications of syphilis were major components of the symptomatology of many systems, in particular in the nervous system. The manifestations of syphilitic disease of large arteries are now rare, since they occur in the tertiary stage of the disease, which is now seldom untreated for the long periods necessary for the complications to occur, but they are still of interest. The way in which the disease affects arteries represents a paradigm of how selective destruction of the specialized structure of the vessel wall results in dilatation with aneurysm production or valvular incompetence.

Although the disease is now considered to be rare, it is important to note that it is not always easy to diagnose. Serological tests are negative in up to 28 per cent of cases.

There are four types of the disease affecting the aorta:

Syphilitic aortitis This is an active inflammatory process in which the medial structure of lamellar units is destroyed and replaced by fibrosis. The vasa vasora of the aorta are the primarily affected sites, and are surrounded by a lymphocytic infiltrate with some plasma cells present. There are occasional areas of necrosis and rare giant cells. The change is found primarily in the ascending aorta and the arch, but the descending thoracic aorta is often involved, although abdominal, and particularly infra-renal, involvement is uncommon, occurring in around 5 per cent of cases.

Typically, the intima shows a 'tree bark' appearance, with a thickened white surface with longitudinal and transverse fissures. However, this typical appearance is almost invariably obscured by concomitant atherosclerosis.

Syphilitic aortic aneurysm Aneurysms occur in around 40 per cent of cases of syphilitic aortitis, usually affect the thoracic aorta, and may be multiple. The proximal parts of major aortic branches may also be affected. The aneurysms are most frequently saccular and often contain laminated thrombi. Rupture may occur into the pleural cavity (usually the left) or into the oesophagus or mediastinum. Erosion of vertebral bodies may occur from vascular pressure.

Aortic insufficiency Insufficiency of the aortic valve occurs as a result of the destructive process of inflammation and fibrosis progressively removing the normal load-resisting structure of the aortic valve root. There is subsequent dilatation of the valve ring to more than the normal upper limit of 8.5 cm circumference. However, syphilis also affects the valve cusps directly. The thickening and fibrosis of the cusps, with rolling of their edges, commissural widening, and cusp contraction, are also important in causing incompetence.

Syphilitic coronary ostial stenosis The inflammatory process involves the coronary ostia with narrowing in 28 per cent of cases of aortic syphilis. Actual involvement of the coronary artery has been described very rarely. It is the intimal thickening and aortic wall fibrosis that are causal in producing functional stenosis. Myocardial infarction may occur.

12.6.7 Thromboangiitis obliterans (Buerger disease)

Thromboangiitis obliterans is an uncommon peripheral occlusive vasculitis, occurring almost exclusively in male smokers in the third and fourth decades. It affects both arteries and veins in a segmental manner. The legs below the knees are more often affected than the arms. Pain is a notable feature of the disease because of involvement of nerves in the inflammatory process that affects the neurovascular bundle. Pathologically, there is occlusion of the vessels by distinctive inflammatory thrombi with microabscesses and giant cells.

The causative role of smoking is emphasized by the occurrence of the disease in a saphenous vein graft used as a coronary artery in a man with the disease who continued to smoke. However, an idiosyncratic response may be critical. Familial cases occur and cell-mediated sensitivity to types I and III collagen may be found.

12.6.8 Degenerative arterial disease

Monkberg medial sclerosis

This is regarded by many as an ageing change rather than a disease entity. It is seen most extensively in the arteries of the limbs, head, and neck. The progressive replacement of medial smooth muscle by fibrous tissue, which accompanies age, is also associated with hyalinization and fine basophilic staining, suggesting early calcification. This may progress to sufficiently heavy calcification to show up on routine X-rays. There is no lumenal narrowing; the consequences of the change are those that attend the acquisition of a more rigid vascular system with age. Vascular calcification of this kind is not rare at other sites.

Marfan syndrome

This is a genetically determined generalized disorder of connective tissue transmitted as an autosomally dominant condition of variable expression. Patients are tall, have long thin fingers (arachnodactyly), chest deformities, and a high arched palate. Eye abnormalities are generally present with upward subluxation of the lens (found *in utero*), and myopia is frequent. Cardiovascular complications, mainly in the form of fusiform and dissecting thoracic aneurysms, are the major cause of death. However, valve disease, including prolapse of the mitral valve and aortic insufficiency, are also significant. Abnormal scleroproteins are produced in these individuals with poor performance under tension, possibly due to imperfect organization of collagen and or elastin. Urinary hydroxyproline is also increased, suggesting increased catabolism. However, the biochemical picture is variable, suggesting that this syndrome encompasses a group of related conditions. In 1991, the defective gene for some forms of Marfan syndrome was mapped to chromosome 15. The candidate gene encodes fibrillin, a protein involved in the supramolecular organization of elastin.

The lesion in the aortic wall is one where the normal pattern of medial lamellar units is destroyed; the wall is thinned; and pools of glycosaminoglycans are seen where the elastic structure of the wall is lost. The term 'cystic medial necrosis' was used by Erdheim to describe this lesion, but it should not now be used—there are no cysts and no necrosis. Similar changes, although less marked, may be seen in the pulmonary artery.

Raynaud disease and the Raynaud phenomenon

Typically, primary Raynaud phenomenon consists of spasm of the digital arteries with pallor and cyanosis, followed by a reactive hyperaemia occurring in episodes of 10–20 minutes' duration. It is cured by sympathectomy.

The phenomenon may occur secondarily in association with a large number of factors; this is the common form. These factors include the use of vibrating tools (when it is often unilateral): thromboangiitis obliterans; a late result of cold injury; sclerodema; and in association with neurological disorders and cervical ribs.

Raynaud disease is usually associated with proximal limb vessel disease or trauma, and should be diagnosed only when other potential causes of the syndrome have been eliminated. There are no typical pathological findings. When the phenomenon has been exhibited for years there may be intimal thickening and medial fibrosis with obstruction of the lumen.

12.6.9 Aneurysms and their pathogenesis

Aneurysms are permanent, irreversible localized dilatations of arteries. They are formed by vessel dilatation and their wall contains recognizable components of the vessel wall. False aneurysms result from rupture of the vessel and are organized perivascular haematomas in which no wall components are seen.

Many disease processes lead to the production of aneurysms; the fundamental lesion is destruction of the specialized load-bearing structure of the media. Arteries are not simple conduits for blood, but an important functioning unit. Certain aspects of endothelial and intimal functions and smooth muscle response in smaller vessels in hypertension are dealt with in Section 12.5. Here we concentrate on those load-bearing aspects of arteries that change with age and disease, which normally minimize cardiac work and ensure proper flow to the periphery.

The tangential tension in the aortic wall generated with each heart-beat is around 165 000 dynes/cm. This load is applied 100 000 times/day at average pulse rates. The structure of the media allows this load to be resisted and the work done by the heart in generating it to be utilized effectively. When pressure rises in the aorta after systole, the vessel distends, storing energy in its wall. This is then released, as pressure in the lumen falls and contributes to the maintenance of diastolic pressure. This elastic reservoir allows the heart to operate efficiently by varying stroke volume (cf. Starling's Law). If the heart were pumping into a rigid system of piping, the only way to increase cardiac output significantly would be an increase in pulse rate. For vigorous activity it would be necessary to raise this to rates which would not allow adequate time for the diastolic filling of the coronary vessels.

Changes in the medial structure produced by inflammation, necrosis, fibrosis, or erosion by the lesions of atherosclerosis result in replacement of a specialized load-bearing arrangement of fibrous tissue scleroproteins, which distends under tension. Dilatation follows and is progressive; as the radius of the vessel wall goes up the tension in the wall increases (at a given pressure). Aneurysms do not heal; they progress inexorably.

Atherosclerotic aneurysms

These are now much the commonest type of aneurysm and generally develop in those over 60 years of age. Males are 6–9 times more frequently affected. The lesions are commoner in smokers and predominantly affect the abdominal aorta (Fig. 12.62a,b). The descending thoracic aorta is more commonly affected than the arch or ascending part. Multiple aneurysms are common and ectasia of other large arteries is frequently seen. Expansion of the vessel is usually fusiform rather than saccular, and a ragged lining of thrombus and ulcerated atheromatous lesions is seen. Thrombotic or distal atheromatous embolization is common.

Aneurysms of this type increase in diameter at an average of around 0.4 cm/year (assessed by repeated tomography) but more rapid growth occurs. Rupture is common between aneurysmal diameters of 4–7 cm. Rupture is commonly retroperitoneal but this is clearly related to the site.

Syphilitic aneurysms

See Section 12.6.6.

Mycotic aneurysms

Mycotic aneurysms result from destruction of the load-bearing element of the arterial wall by infection. Historically, they were commonly due to septic emboli from subacute bacterial endocarditis but, as this has become less frequent, acute endocarditis in intravenous drug abusers or fungal infection in the immunocompromised have become more important. The term should

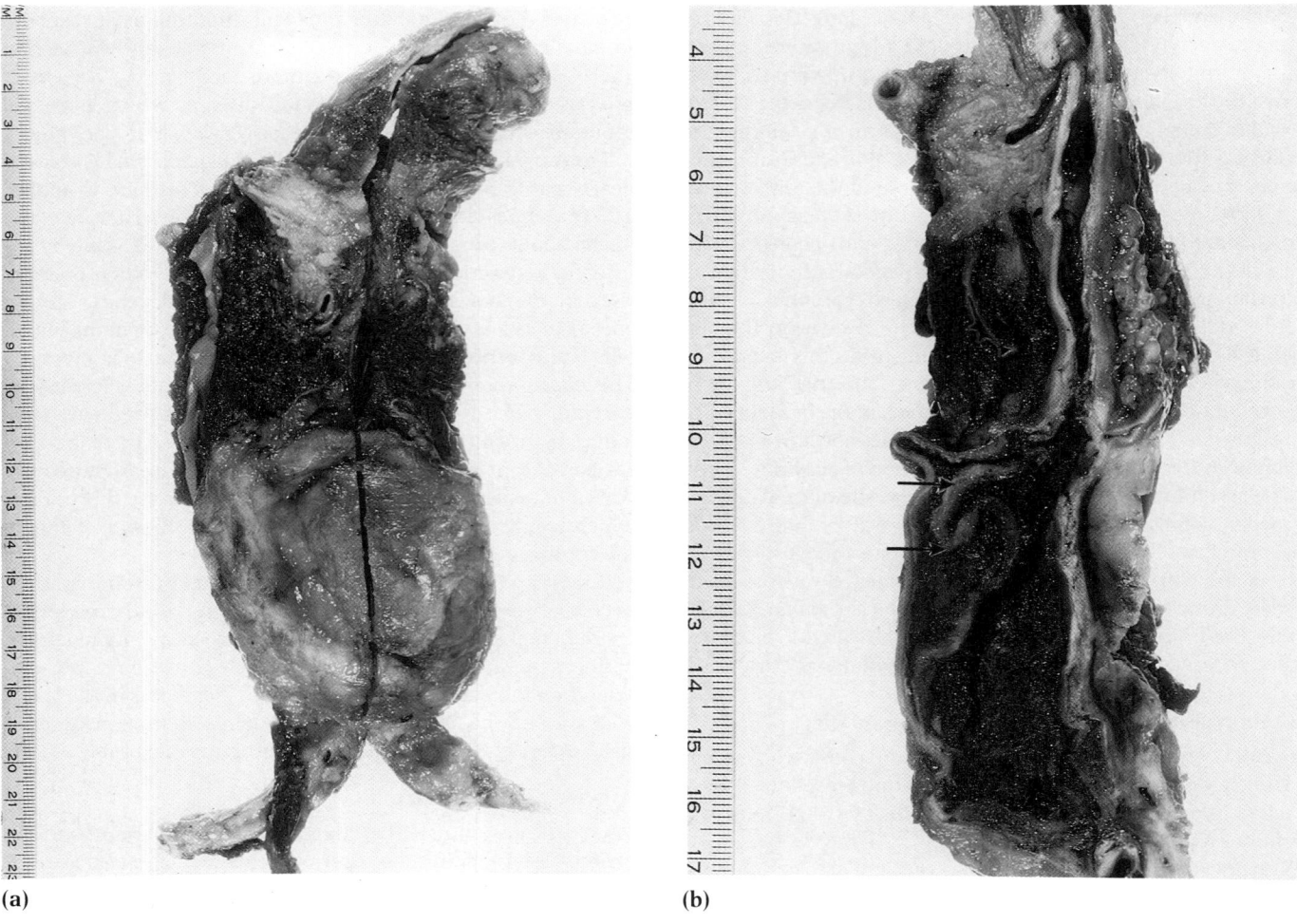

(a)   **(b)**

Fig. 12.62 (a) A large fusiform abdominal aneurysm showing the origin of the coeliac axis to the left of the incision. (b) Aortic aneurysm. The coeliac axis is at the top and the lumen of the aneurysm is filled with blood clot. Dissection into the wall has occurred (arrows).

only be used where infection has caused the damage leading to aneurysm formation. Infection of pre-existing aneurysms is not rare, with *Salmonella* and atherosclerotic abdominal aneurysms being the commonest combination. Bacterial and fungal infections are not uncommon at arteriotomy sites.

Vascular wall destruction (including the aortic wall) is not uncommon in military tuberculosis but mycotic aneurysms in this disease are more often due to spread from lymphadenitis to adjacent arteries.

Whatever the cause of a mycotic aneurysm, antibiotic therapy is ineffective and prophylactic excision avoids rupture.

Dissecting aneurysm

A dissecting aneurysm is the term used to describe the passage of blood into the wall through a generally transverse tear in the intima and inner media; subsequent tracking of blood longitudinally splits the layers of the outer media (Fig. 12.63). The new 'lumen' may then rupture externally or re-enter the aortic lumen, producing a tract which may endothelialize.

In more than half of the cases the transverse tear is in the first 2 cm of the aorta and dissection may progress around the arch (Fig. 12.64) or extend retrogradely with rupture into the pericardium, producing cardiac tamponade. Dissection may occlude the branch vessels, and when the coronary ostia are involved myocardial ischaemia with sudden death occurs.

Dissection is approximately twice as common in men as in women and is generally seen in those over 60 years. The majority of patients with dissection are hypertensive. Death occurs in more than 90 per cent of untreated patients, and is inevitable unless re-entry occurs.

Views of the pathogenesis of dissecting aneurysms have changed and the suggestion that the so-called 'cystic medial necrosis' (see above) is causative has been discarded. Longitudinal studies of the changes in medial structure and glycosaminoglycan (GAG) distribution with age have made it clear that the progressive breaking up of clearly defined elastic lamellae and accumulation of collagen and pools of GAG is an ageing phenomenon which may be exaggerated by stress, such as hypertension. The wall is weakened by these changes and

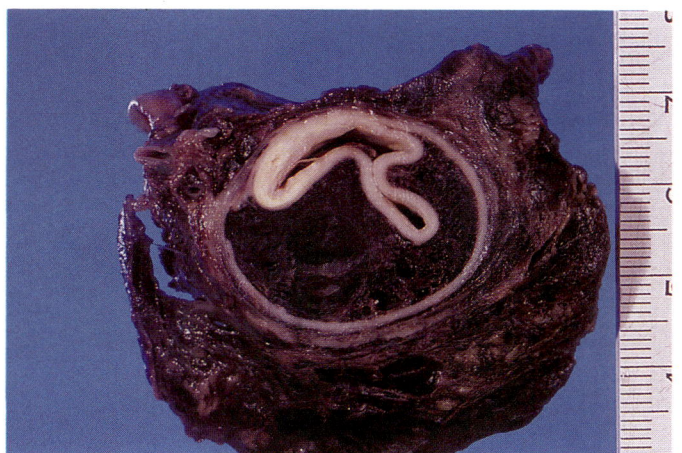

Fig. 12.63 Dissecting aneurysm of the aortic root showing blood clot separating the layers of the aortic media.

haemodynamic stress will result in intimal tearing, often facilitated by atherosclerotic lesions. Dissection is then the consequence of weakening of the network of scleroprotein which the normal media represents.

Dissection may occur as a result of closed chest injury as, for example, in road traffic accidents (Fig. 12.65)

'Congenital' aneurysms

Genuine congenital aneurysms (true aneurysms, present at birth) are extraordinarily rare. Most so-called aneurysms are examples of vascular malformations in which extensive arterio-venous communications occur with the formation of dilated venous sacs. These lesions are often referred to as cirscoid aneurysms and may be found in a number of conditions in which vascular malformations are part of a well-defined syndrome.

Aneurysm of the great vein of Galen develops in infants when there is communication between this vein and a posterior cerebral artery; pressure from the aneurysmal dilatation of the vein may obstruct the aqueduct, causing hydrocephalus, and shunting results in congestive heart failure.

However, there are a number of conditions where developmental defects in the vessel wall result in the formation of aneurysms in later life.

Berry aneurysms

The 'berry' aneurysms of the cerebral circulation are typically saccular, rarely found under the age of 40 years, and are slightly commoner in women. They are multiple in 20 per cent of cases and are usually a few millimetres in diameter and seldom larger than 1.5 cm (Fig. 12.66a, b). The apical angle of the bifurcation of the internal carotid artery or the origin of the posterior cerebral communicating artery are favoured sites. The fork formed by the anterior communicating artery with the anterior cerebral arteries, the branches of the middle cerebral

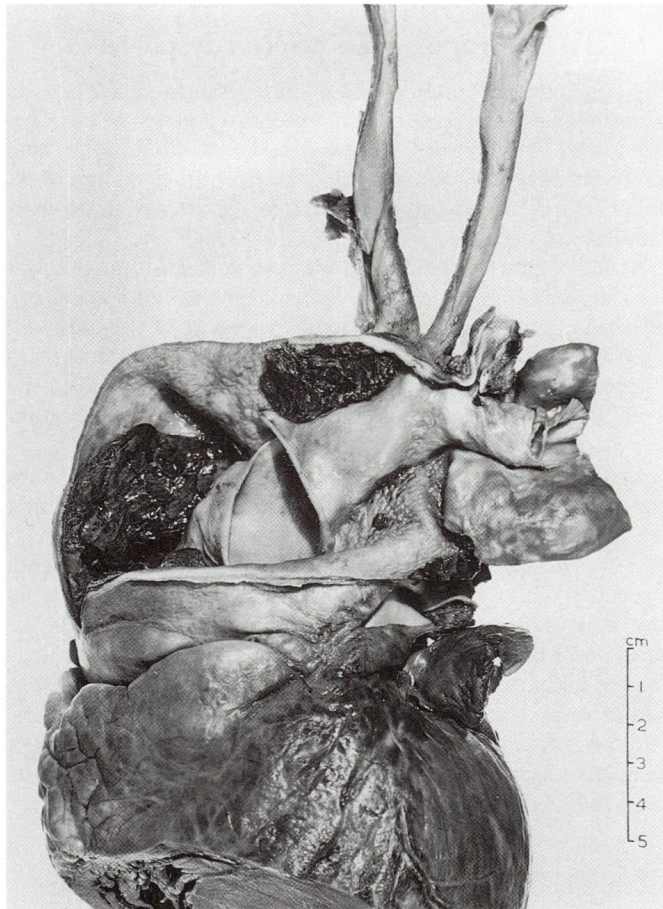

Fig. 12.64 Thoracic dissection around the arch of the aorta. Occlusion of the vessels to the head and neck was produced by this dissection.

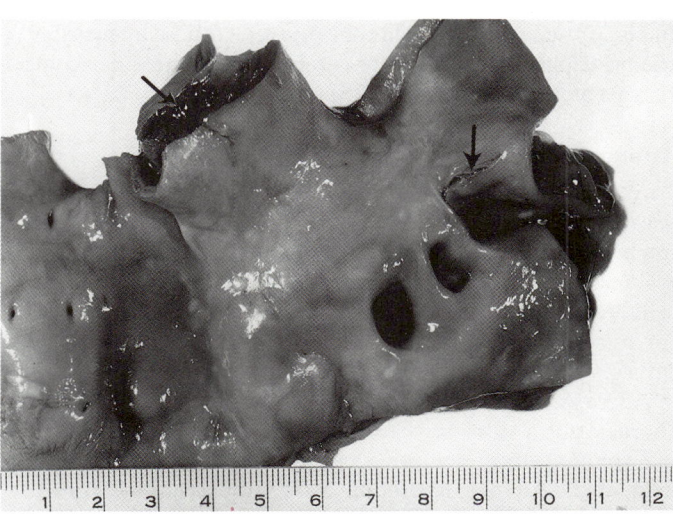

Fig. 12.65 Dissection produced by a traumatic tear in the arch of the aorta. The arrows show the tear and the blood clot in the vessel wall. The aorta is from a front-seat passenger in a head-on collision.

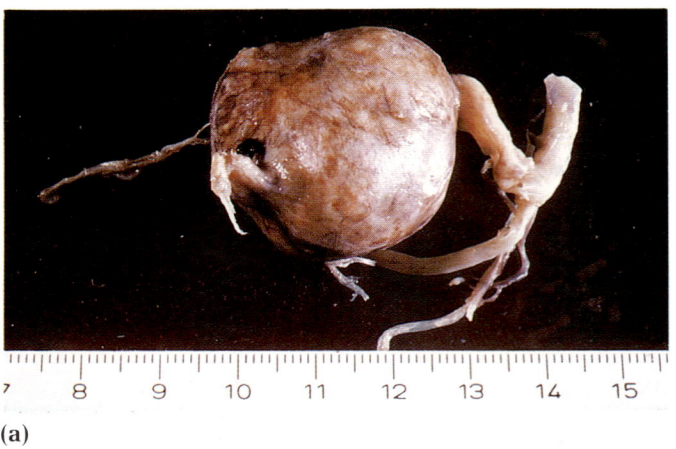
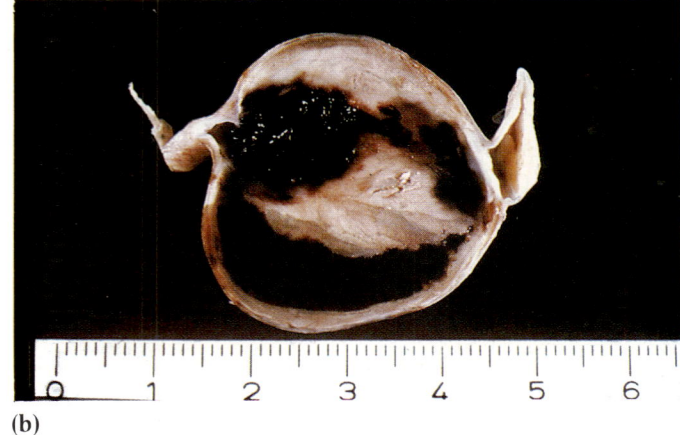

(a)   **(b)**

Fig. 12.66 (a) A large berry aneurysm of a basilar artery. (b) The aneurysm is filled by organized thrombus and blood clot.

arteries, and the bifurcation of the basilar artery are other common sites of occurrence.

Berry aneurysms are acquired lesions. In early life there is a defect in the muscle coat at the bifurcation of the vessel where the contiguous sides of the flow divider support each other in early development. Muscle is not laid down at this site as there is no haemodynamic stress; when the cerebral vasculature expands with the late developmental expansion of the cerebral hemispheres a defect is revealed. With the passage of time and elevation of blood pressure these defects develop into aneurysms.

Charcot–Bouchard aneurysms

These are small aneurysms of the cerebral microvasculature, mainly occurring in the basal ganglia, with diameters around 50–150 μm. Their pathogenesis is similar to that of berry aneurysms; it is possible to increase their frequency of occurrence and their size by raising the blood pressure of young animals. It is generally agreed that rupture of these aneurysms is the principle cause of massive cerebral haemorrhage in hypertensive patients (see Chapter 25).

Traumatic aneurysms

Any cause of vascular damage which results in loss of the specialized structure of the wall may result in true or false aneurysm formation; this includes surgery. Trauma from medical procedures has also produced aneurysms in the very young; a false abdominal aortic aneurysm has been produced in an infant following exchange transfusion via an umbilical artery.

Aneurysms may develop in the upper part of the descending thoracic aorta following closed chest injuries of the kind which are common in motor car accidents. If death does not occur from aortic rupture, laceration of the aortic wall will result in bleeding, with the immediate leakage limited by mediastinal and pleural connective tissue, forming a false aneurysm. Similar changes may occur in limb arteries.

Arteriovenous fistulae of any kind, including those formed deliberately, e.g. to facilitate dialysis, may dilate progressively and become aneurysmal.

12.6.10   Fibromuscular arterial dysplasia

This uncommon condition, first described in childhood, is important as a reversible cause of renal hypertension (see Section 12.5.8 and Chapter 19). It is found most often in the renal artery but may also occur in the arteries of the head and neck, the liver, spleen and gut, and rarely in the arteries of the legs. Familial cases occur.

At all sites the lesion is commoner in females. Although it has been described in a neonate, clinical presentation is usually between 25 and 50 years. The development of the effects of renal ischaemia with hypertension are the presenting signs in around 60 per cent of cases. The disease may be found in the renal arteries in non-hypertensive patients and clinical estimates of incidence are probably underestimated.

The disease may involve all layers of the arterial wall, with accumulation of cellular fibrous tissue in the intima obstructing the lumen, and splitting of the internal elastic lamina (Fig. 12.67). This form is common in younger patients but is often associated with the medial type. Here the normal medial structure is disrupted by fibroplasia and smooth muscle cells are plump and irregularly arranged, sometimes with the appearance of longitudinally arranged bands of muscle (Fig. 12.68). Aneurysmal dilatation may develop where deficiencies in the media occur and dissections are seen in the wall. Finally, a perimedial form may be seen where intensive fibroplasia in the outer half of the media may extend outside the vessel.

12.6.11   Pathophysiology of vascular disease

There are a number of obvious properties that must be possessed by vessels.

The endothelial surface must be non-stick and minimally

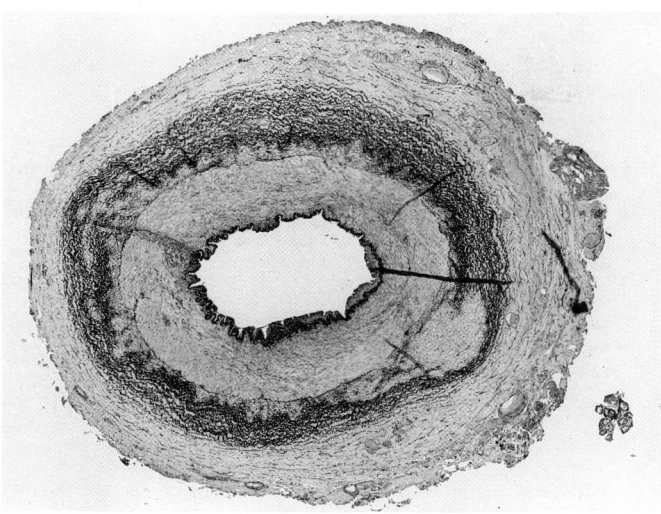

Fig. 12.67 A fibromuscular dysplasia involving all of the vessel coats. There is thickening of the intima and disruption of the elastic structure of the media. (EVG stain.) (Courtesy of Professor J.-P. Cammilleri.)

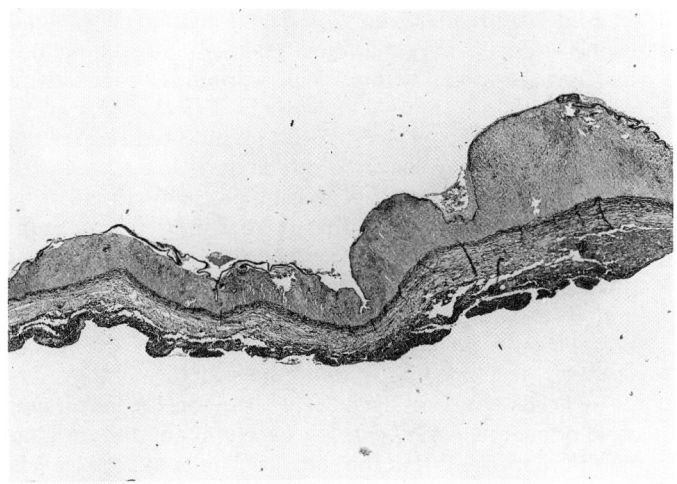

Fig. 12.68 Renal artery with bands of proliferating muscle in the media. (EVG stain.) (Courtesy of Professor J.-P. Cammilleri.)

thrombogenic, must not damage the cells circulating in the blood, and must be only selectively permeable, with a molecular sieve size that varies in different sites. These properties change in inflammation (see Chapter 5), may be altered by the introduction of prostheses into the circulation, or may be affected by degenerative disease.

The arterial media is a complex structure with a number of specialist properties which make a contribution to the efficient operation of the circulation. These depend critically on a nonuniformity of static mechanical properties; the proximal part of the circulation is much more distensible than the distal. The effects of this elastic nonuniformity are as follows:

1. The oscillatory component of the cardiac work is reduced. The presence of a proximal elastic reservoir which can store

energy allows the heart to work at a rate and stroke volume that is optimal for a given cardiac output (see Section 12.6.9).

2. The decrease in distensibility of more distal arteries greatly reduces a problem that exists with distensible systems; i.e. a tendency for oscillation to occur between various parts. This should not conjure up a vision of blood slopping to and fro in the arterial tree, but a tendency to this type of behaviour would exist and might damage arteries by the establishment of standing waves. These do occur in human arteries from the third decade, are established by reflection from bifurcations, and may damage the intima.

3. The pulse wave disturbance is continuously amplified as it moves distally and travels in less distensible vessel walls. The form of the pulse wave is critical in the function of some tissues and organs. For example, in the kidney, hypertension may develop if the organ is enveloped in a rigid wrapping; in experimental perfusion of isolated lungs gas exchange is more effective in the presence of pulsatile flow.

In smaller vessels, changes in pressure and flow tend to affect the viability of tissue in ways other than by affecting the adequacy of flow or the wave form. In limbs with an arteriovenous fistula there are changes in the circulation with temperature, and oxygenation problems and trophic changes in the skin. The effects on wound healing and blood flow of experimentally induced groin arteriovenous (A-V) fistulae are that wound healing occurs rapidly in proximal incisions on the treated side, but is less effective distally. These changes can be correlated with changes in flow, shown to be raised proximally and lowered distally (using radioactive ^{133}Xe). Distal venous stasis may be accompanied by ulceration, and venous diameter may increase by up to 80 per cent.

Some obvious examples of how medical intervention will compromise these essential arterial functions may be illustrated over a wide age-range. Figure 12.69 shows the aortic wall of an

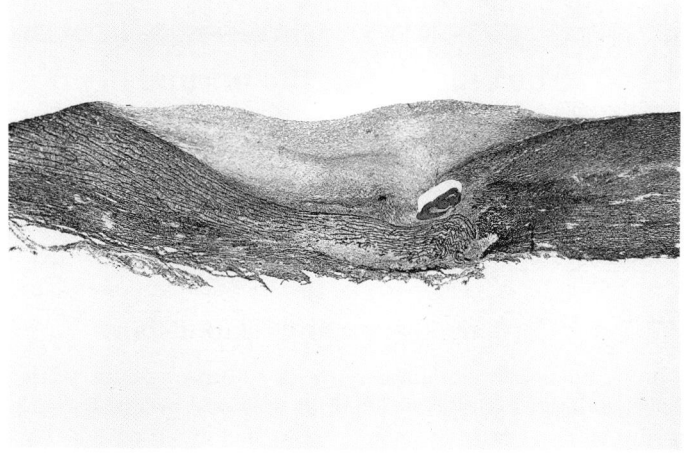

Fig. 12.69 Arterial wall following surgery for coarctation. Disruption of the normal media structure is evident, as is the presence of a collagen suture. (EVG stain.)

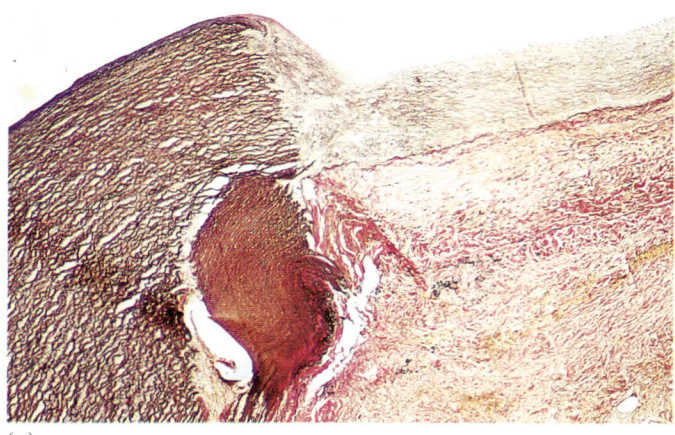

(a)

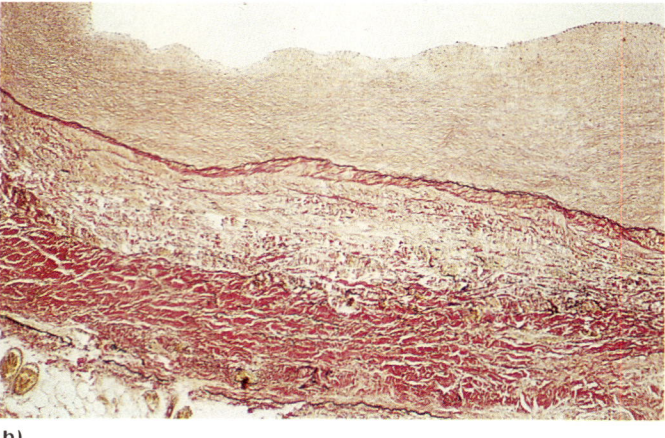

(b)

Fig. 12.70 (a) The anastomotic site between the wall of the aorta (left) and a coronary venous graft. The diference in the elastic contents of the two vessels is evident (note suture material is evident; EVG stain). (b) A vein graft after 10 days *in situ*. Gross thickening of the endothelium can be seen. (EVG stain.)

infant dying of a complex combination of congenital abnormalities after an aortic coarctation had been repaired. The wall has 'healed' but the new structure will not function as normal aortic media; changes of this kind may predispose to disease in later life. In Fig. 12.70 the changes that follow the grafting of a saphenous vein into the coronary circulation are illustrated. These venous segments do not perform as well, or remain patent as long, as arterial grafts where structure is more closely aligned to function.

12.6.12   Further reading

Cammilleri, J.-P., Berry, C. L., Feissinger, J. N., and Bariety, J. (1989). *Diseases of the arterial wall*. Springer Verlag, New York.
Silver, M. D. (ed.) (1983). *Cardiovascular pathology*. Churchill Livingstone, New York.

12.7   The anatomy of the normal heart

Robert H. Anderson

The normal anatomy of the heart is described as the necessary background for an understanding of congenital heart disease.

12.7.1   Cardiac position and relationships

Knowledge of cardiac anatomy starts with the position of the heart within the chest. The heart lies within its pericardial sack such that one-third of its bulk is to the right of the midline (Fig. 12.71). Its long axis is oblique, with the base in right-sided superior location and the apex extending well to the left. The right atrial appendage occupies the right border of the cardiac

silhouette, the pulmonary trunk forming the left superior border in anterior left-sided position relative to the aorta. The anterior interventricular groove marks the division of right and left ventricles, and is almost at the left border of the silhouette.

The heart is enclosed within the pericardium, a sack having an outer firm fibrous layer and an inner double serous layer. The inner layer of the serous sack fuses with the surface of the heart itself to form the epicardium. The outer layer fuses with the fibrous pericardium. The pericardial cavity therefore is between the epicardium and the tough fibrous pericardium. Within the overall cavity thus formed there are two distinct recesses named the oblique and transverse sinuses of the pericardium (Fig. 12.72).

Knowledge of the arrangement of the cardiac chambers themselves is facilitated by study of the structure of the short axis. The aortic root is wedged deeply between the mitral and tricuspid orifices (Fig. 12.73a). The expression of this wedging within the ventricles is that the subaortic outlet lifts the leaflets of the mitral valve away from the septum such that an extension of the outlet extends towards the diaphragmatic surface of the heart (Fig. 12.73b).

In contrast, the inlets and outlets of the right ventricle are widely separated by the muscular roof of the right ventricle (the supraventricular crest). When viewed anteriorly, therefore, the right ventricle occupies most of the cardiac surface, extending from the inferiorly located tricuspid to the superiorly positioned pulmonary valve (Fig. 12.74).

12.7.2   Morphology of the cardiac chambers

The right atrium possesses a venous component, an appendage, and an atrioventricular vestibule (Fig. 12.75). It is the appendage which most constantly retains its structure in congenitally malformed hearts, and which, therefore, is most reliable for identification. It is a triangular structure having a broad junction with the venous component marked externally by the ter-

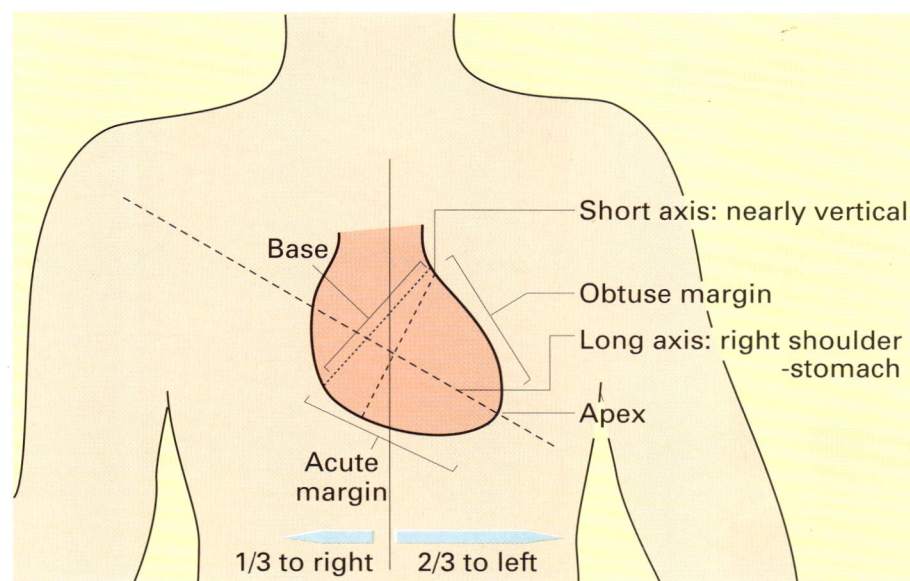

Fig. 12.71   Diagram showing the position of the heart within the chest and illustrating the landmarks of its silhouette. Note that the axes of the heart are at a considerable angle to those of the body.

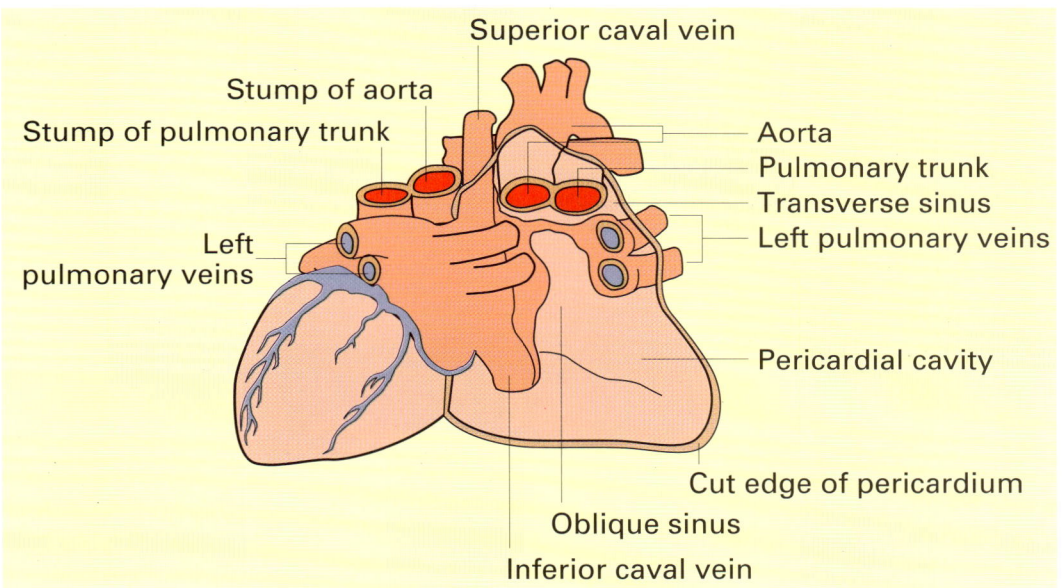

Superior caval vein

Stump of aorta

Stump of pulmonary trunk

Aorta
Pulmonary trunk
Transverse sinus
Left pulmonary veins

Left
pulmonary veins

Pericardial cavity

Cut edge of pericardium

Oblique sinus

Inferior caval vein

Fig. 12.72   Diagram illustrating how, following transection of the arterial pedicles and left pulmonary veins, the heart can be swung forward from its pericardial cradle, illustrating the oblique sinus of the pericardium behind the left atrium. The transverse sinus can also be seen, lying in the inner curve of the heart between the back of the great arteries and the front of the atrial chambers.

minal groove and internally by the terminal crest (Fig. 12.76a). The smooth-walled venous component receives the superior and inferior caval veins together with the coronary sinus. The venous orifices surround the septal surface of the right atrium, characterized by the broad rim and smooth floor of the oval fossa. The vestibule of the right atrium contains and supports the tricuspid valve with leaflets in septal, anterosuperior, and inferior (or mural) location.

The major distinguishing feature of the right ventricle is the coarse nature of its apical trabeculations, together with the fact that the septal leaflet of the tricuspid valve has extensive attachments distally to the ventricular septum, a feature lacking for the mitral valve. The outlet component is extensive, the leaflets of the pulmonary valve being exclusively attached to the ventricular musculature. This means that the larger part of the subpulmonary infundibulum can be completely removed from the heart without disturbing any left ventricular structures (Fig. 12.77).

The left atrium has an appendage, a venous component, and a vestibule (Fig. 12.78). The appendage is long and tubular,

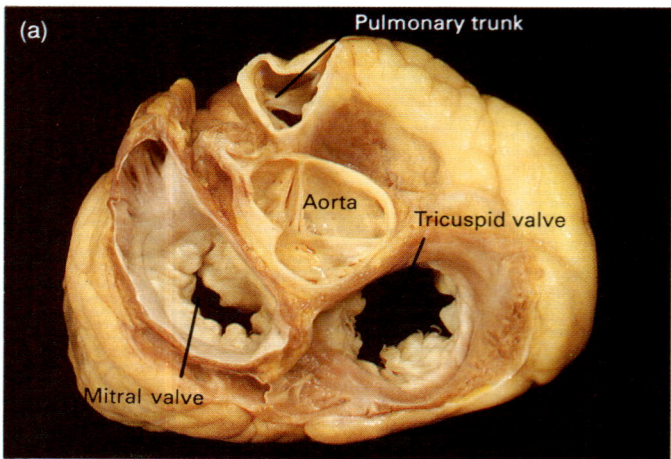

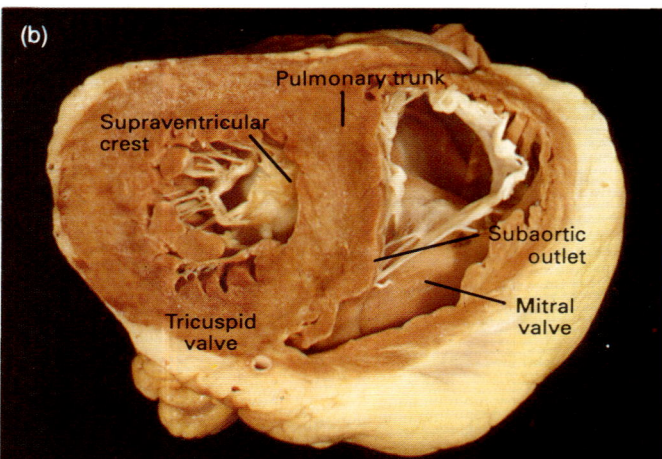

Fig. 12.73 The short axis of the heart at the level of the atrioventricular junction is seen (a) from the atrial and (b) from the ventricular aspects. (a) This has been prepared by removing the atrial chambers and arterial trunks. Note how the aortic valve is deeply wedged between the atrioventricular valves, producing a shamrock arrangement. (b) This represents a transection about 1 cm below the atrioventricular junction. Note that the tricuspid and pulmonary valves are separated by the supraventricular crest of the right ventricle and that the septal leaflet of the tricuspid valve hugs the inlet part of the septum. In contrast, the subaortic outflow tract lifts the mitral valve away from the septum and there is fibrous continuity between the aortic and mitral valves.

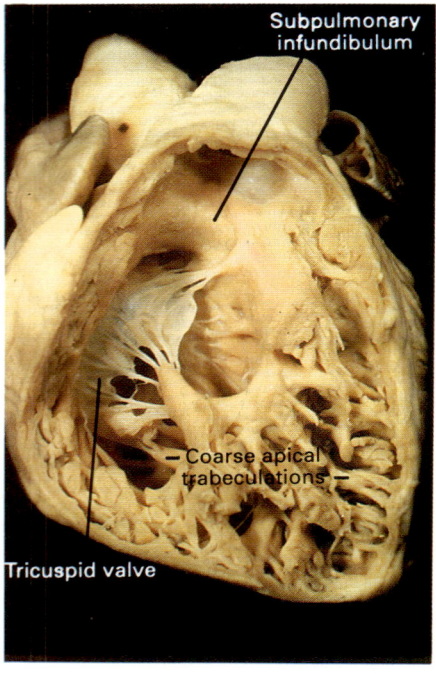

Fig. 12.74 This dissection of the anterior surface of the heart in its anatomical position shows how the right ventricle occupies the greater part of the cardiac silhouette, extending from the right-sided and inferior tricuspid to the left-sided and superior pulmonary valve. The two are separated by the muscular supraventricular crest which forms most of the subpulmonary infundibulum. Note also the characteristic coarse apical trabeculations.

usually crenelated, and has a narrow junction with the venous component of the atrium (Fig. 12.76b). The venous component receives the pulmonary veins at its corners. The vestibule supports the mitral valve with leaflets in mural and aortic position.

The left ventricle, like the right ventricle, is best described in terms of inlet, apical trabecular, and outlet components. The fine apical trabeculations (Fig. 12.79) are the most characteristic and constant feature of the left ventricle in congenitally malformed hearts. Both inlet and outlet components, however, have their own distinctive characteristics. The major distinguishing feature of the inlet is that the leading edges of the

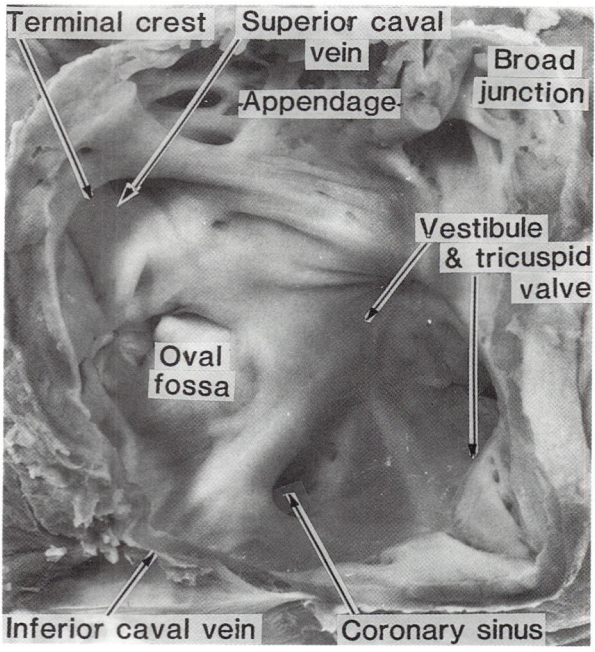

Fig. 12.75 This dissection shows the significant internal features of the morphologically right atrium.

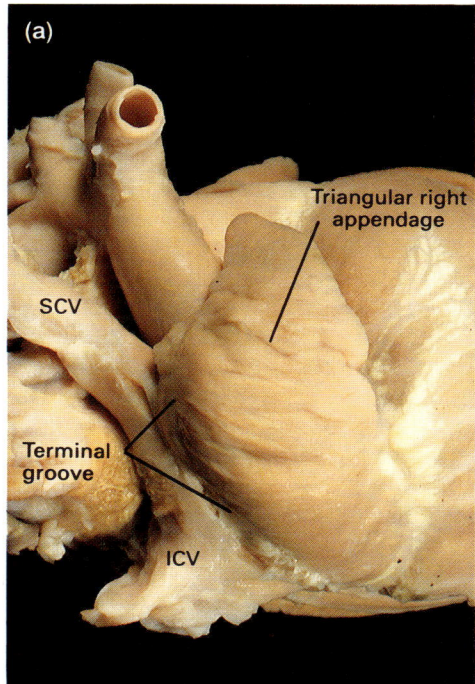
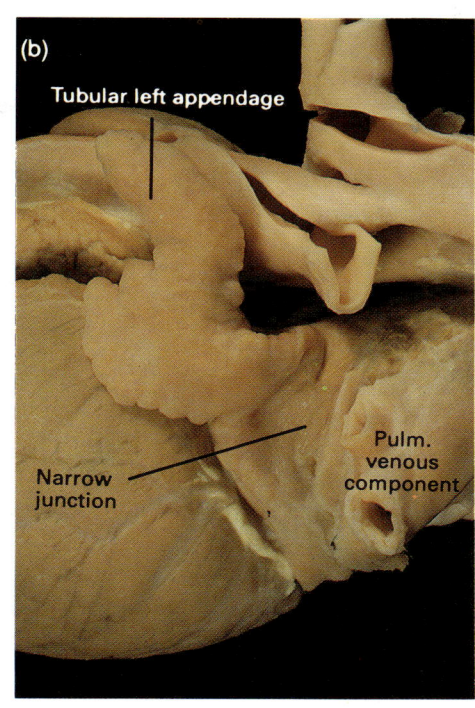

Fig. 12.76 These photographs of the right (a) and left (b) sides of the same heart show the significantly different shapes of the atrial appendages. SCV, ICV, superior and inferior caval veins.

leaflets of the mitral valve have no attachment to the septum. The tendinous cords from the leaflets are supported by paired papillary muscles (Fig. 12.79). The leaflets themselves are best described as aortic and mural. The aortic leaflet is so called because it is in direct fibrous continuity with the aortic valve. The mural leaflet, in contrast, is attached to the parietal part of the left atrioventricular junction. The leaflets have grossly dissimilar circumferential attachments, the aortic leaflet guarding

one-third and the mural leaflet two-thirds of the junction (Fig. 12.80). Usually the mural leaflet is divided into three components (called scallops), but this arrangement is variable. The feature of the outlet is its abbreviated nature. Unlike the pulmonary valve, the leaflets of the aortic valve are intimately related to the fibrous cardiac skeleton such that the circumference of the valvar orifice is partly fibrous. Despite this, the leaflets do not have an annulus in the sense of a complete ring.

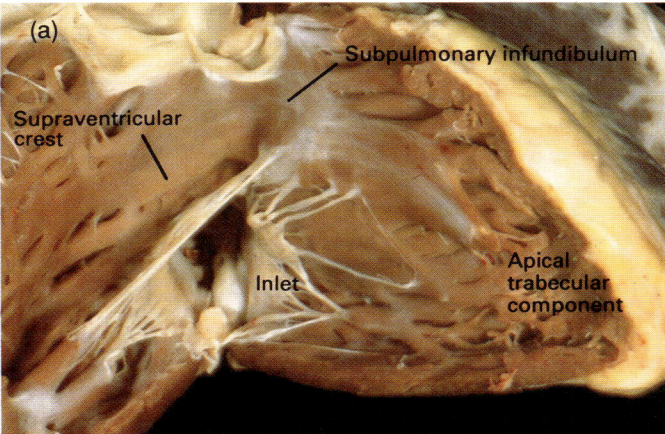
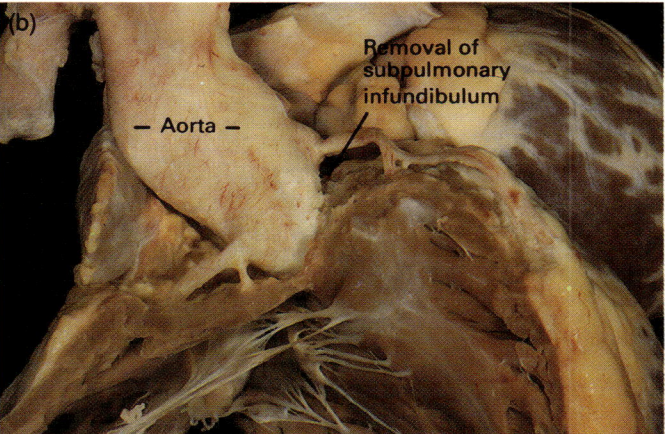

Fig. 12.77 The left panel (a) shows the opened morphologically right ventricle and illustrates its inlet, apical trabecular, and outlet components. Note the attachments of the tricuspid valve to the inlet septum. The dissection in the right panel (b) illustrates that most of the subpulmonary infundibulum is a free-standing muscular sleeve which can be removed without entering the left ventricle. It shows the central location of the aorta.

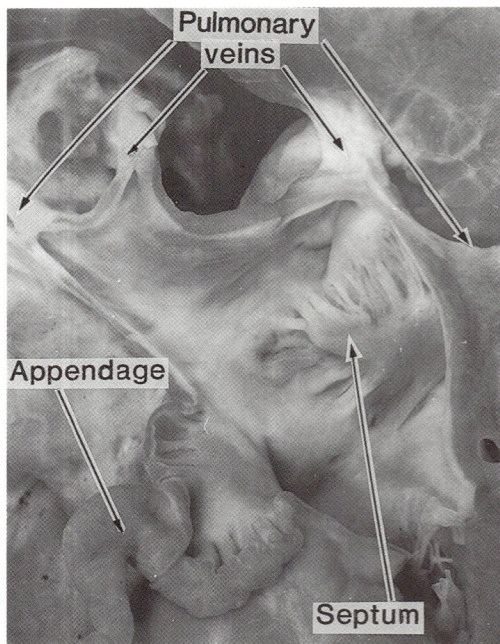

Fig. 12.78 This dissection demonstrates the distinguishing internal features of the morphologically left atrium.

support is conditioned by the semilunar attachments, the commissures being appreciably higher in the aorta than the troughs of the leaflets (Fig. 12.81).

12.7.3　The arterial trunks

The normal heart is characterized by a particular ascending of the trunks into the mediastinum called 'normal relations' (Fig. 12.78). The aorta springs from the middle of the cardiac base and is posterior and to the right relative to the pulmonary trunk. The trunks then spiral around one another to supply the systemic and pulmonary circulations, respectively. The arch of the aorta gives off brachiocephalic (innominate), left common carotid, and left subclavian arteries from its superior aspect, while the pulmonary trunk divides into right and left branches. An important channel connects the arterial trunks during fetal life, namely the arterial duct (ductus arteriosus). It runs from the left pulmonary artery to the aorta and marks the origin of the descending component of the aorta. The segment of the aortic arch between the left subclavian artery and the junction of the duct with the descending aorta is called the isthmus. The arterial duct stays patent only during fetal life and normally becomes constricted and closed in the first days after birth. Within the next six weeks it then becomes converted into the arterial ligament and, by adult life, is simply a fibrous cord.

12.7.4　The cardiac sub-systems

The conduction system (Fig. 12.82) generates and dissipates the cardiac impulse. The impulse is generated by the sinus node, a small cigar-shaped structure lying within the terminal groove. Preferential conduction from the node through the atrial musculature is governed by the geometric arrangement of the ordinary atrial muscle cells. There are no 'specialized' internodal tracts. The atrial impulse is distributed to the ventricular myocardium by the specialized atrioventricular conduction axis. The atrial component is the atrioventricular node, located within the triangle of Koch The axis penetrates through the central fibrous body at the apex of the triangle, being no more

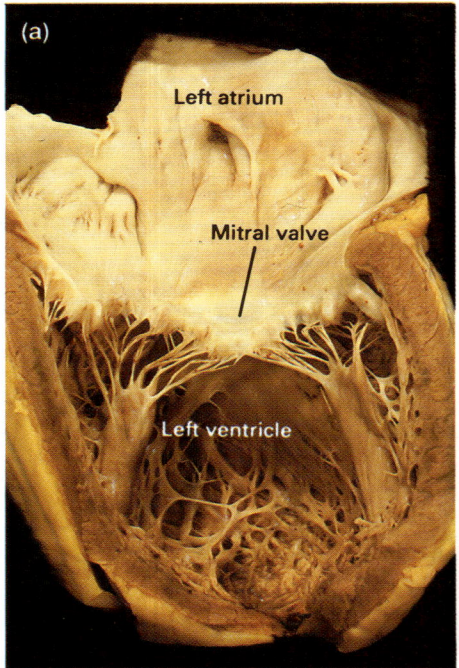

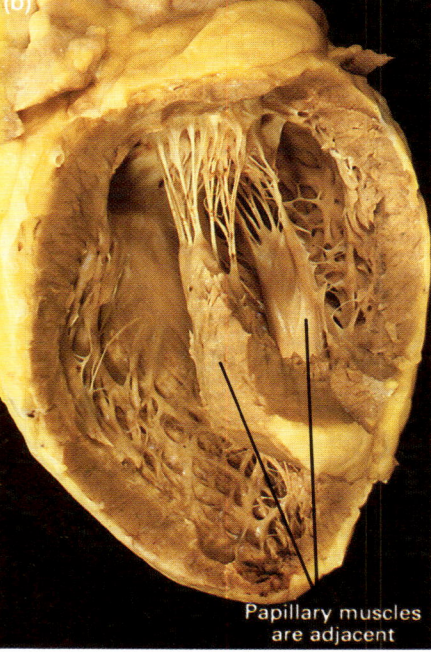

Fig. 12.79 The mitral valve has characteristically paired papillary muscles (a) and lacks any attachments to the inlet part of the ventricular septum. Note also the typical fine apical trabeculations of the morphologically left ventricle. When opened in the demonstrated fashion, however, the impression is gained that the papillary muscles are widely separated. When the same heart is dissected from the ventricular aspect without 'spreading' the atrioventricular junction, it can be appreciated that the papillary muscles are closely adjacent.

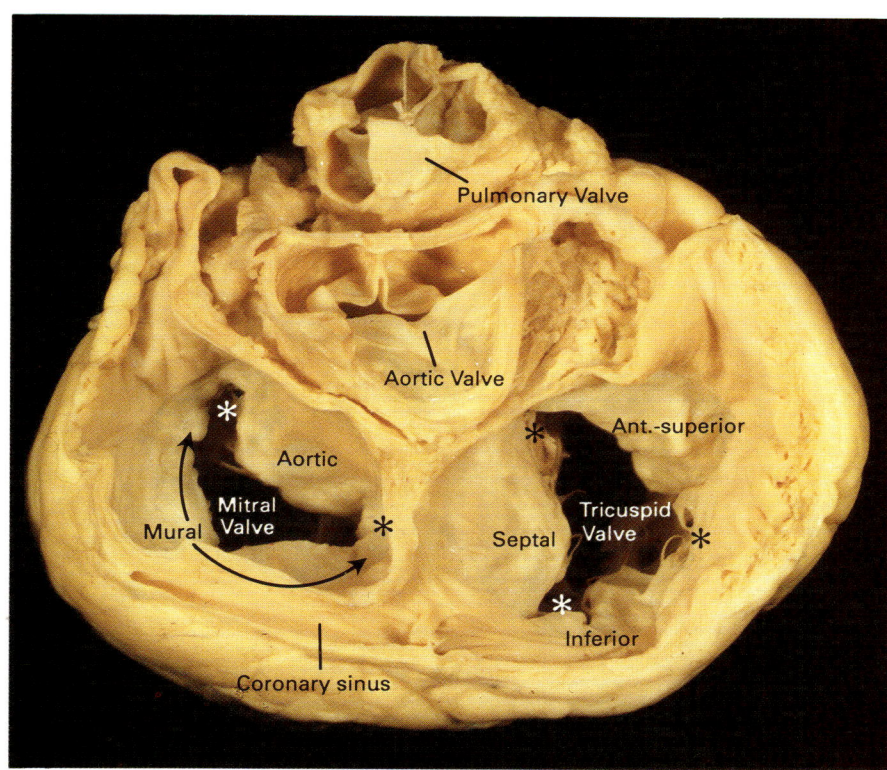

Fig. **12.80**   This dissection of the cardiac short axis illustrates the location of the leaflets of the atrioventricular valves. The two leaflets of the mitral valve are aortic and mural in their relationships; they guard grossly dissimilar proportions of the junction. The leaflets of the tricuspid valve are found in septal, antero-superior, and inferior locations. The asterisks mark the sites of the valvar commissures.

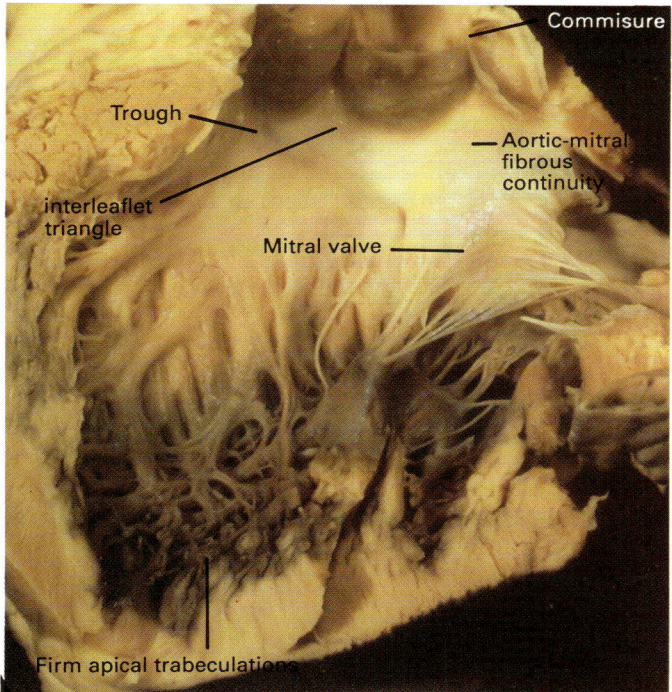

Fig. **12.81**   In this dissection the subaortic outflow tract is opened from its anterior aspect. Note the semilunar attachments of the leaflets of the aortic valve, which has no ring-like annulus. Note also the extensive area of fibrous continuity between the aortic and mitral valves and the fine apical trabeculations of the morphologically left ventricle.

than the size of a strand of cotton as it penetrates. Having penetrated, it reaches the subaortic outflow tract and branches into right and left bundle branches. The left branch spreads out in fan-like fashion while the right branch is a thin cord-like structure. Both branches pass out to the ventricular apices before arborizing into the myocardial masses as the so-called Purkinje networks.

The two major coronary arteries, right and left, arise from the sinuses of the aortic root which 'face' the pulmonary trunk (Fig. 12.83). The two main stem coronary arteries extend and branch from the sinuses so as to irrigate the atrioventricular and interventricular grooves. In most hearts, the right coronary artery encircles the right atrioventricular junction and descends within the posterior interventricular groove. In contrast, the left artery runs a very short course prior to branching into anterior interventricular and circumflex arteries. The interventricular branch occupies the anterior interventricular groove while the circumflex branch extends to varying points around the left atrioventricular junction. In a minority of individuals (perhaps one-tenth), it is the circumflex artery which reaches the crux and runs down into the posterior interventricular groove. The coronary veins also occupy the atrioventricular and interventricular grooves, returning blood into the coronary sinus, which itself runs along the left atrioventricular groove and opens into the right atrium.

In terms of nerves, the heart is supplied from both sympathetic and parasympathetic sources. The nerves monitor the function of the heart, being intimately related to the conduction

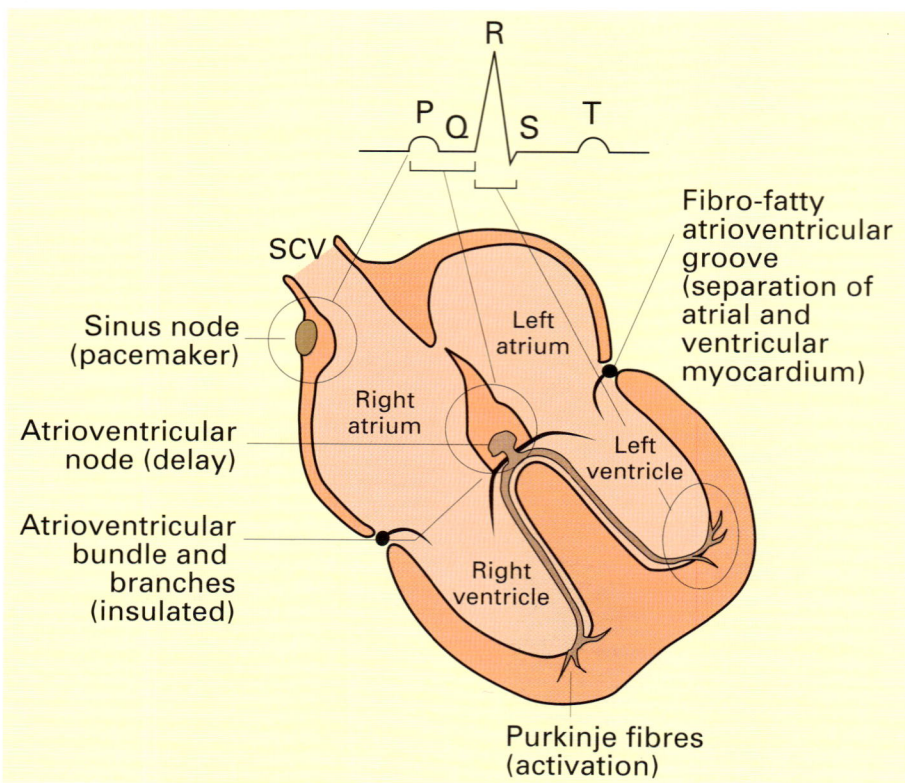

Fig. 12.82 This diagram shows the location of the components of the cardiac conduction system and some of their relations to the ECG.

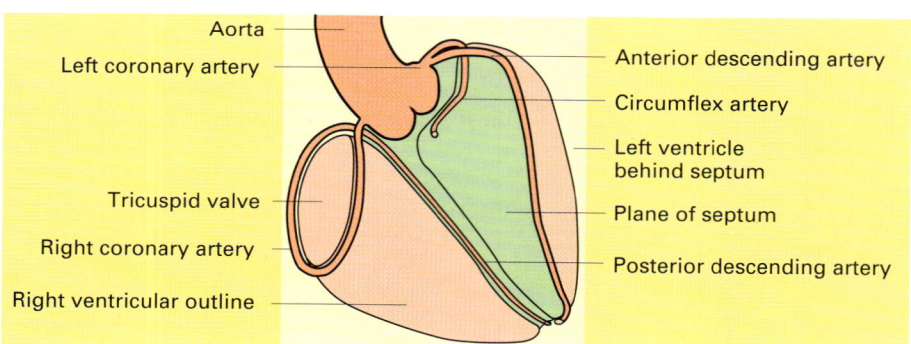

Fig. 12.83 This diagram represents the basic arrangement of the coronary arteries in the normal heart. The right and circumflex coronary arteries run within the atrioventricular grooves while the descending arteries occupy the interventricular grooves.

system, and are also widely distributed along the coronary arteries. The supply to the musculature of the heart itself is relatively limited compared with these richly supplied areas. The parasympathetic nerves come from the vagus and are relayed via ganglion cells confined to the atrial tissues. Indeed, there are few if any vagal fibres within the ventricles of the human heart. In contrast, the sympathetic fibres, derived from the cervical and upper thoracic ganglia of the sympathetic chains, are distributed more widely within the atria and ventricles, running primarily in concert with the branches of the coronary arteries.

12.8   The pathology of congenital heart disease

Robert H. Anderson

12.8.1   Introduction

In this section I give a brief overview of congenital cardiac malformations. The problems of space are made the more difficult since the potential combination of these lesions is almost limitless. Congenital heart disease has also tended to be considered as an arcane and difficult branch of cardiac pathology. This undeserved reputation was earned largely because of an unhealthy desire by early taxonomists to base their systems on embryological considerations. All of these are more or less speculative. Emphasis in this section will be placed upon the principles involved in examination and description of the congenitally malformed hearts—principles which ignore totally the role of cardiac development. Such an approach may not elucidate the aetiology of the malformations. It does greatly simplify their description.

12.8.2   Overall description of the congenitally malformed heart

Congenital lesions afflict the heart in various ways. There may be persistence of the fetal circulatory pathways, such as the oval foramen or arterial duct (ductus arteriosus). There may be anomalous defects of the septal structures or stenotic or regurgitant valves along the circulatory pathways. None of these are difficult to identify, although description of their variants may be more complicated. The most complex lesions, however, and those which give most problems in description and understanding, are those in which the cardiac chambers and arterial trunks are either abnormally positioned or abnormally connected one to the other. These lesions can then seem to be even more complicated should the abnormally constructed hearts themselves harbour the relatively simple anomalies outlined above. The first task of the pathologist, therefore, when searching for congenital cardiac malformations, is to establish the architectural make-up of the heart. If this is normal, then a catalogue is made of lesions within the established circulatory patterns of normality. If the cardiac connections are abnormal, this initial mapping of the chambers and arteries provides the necessary basis for determining the significance of the associated lesions. In addition, this systematic approach, called sequential segmental analysis, provides the rigour needed to identify each and every lesion. The approach demands that normality be proven rather than assumed.

12.8.3   The sequential segmental approach

In essence, the approach is to analyse cardiac construction in terms of three segments, namely, the atrial chambers, the ventricular mass, and the arterial trunks (Fig. 12.84). The make-up of each segment is determined in terms of the topological interrelationships of the contained chambers or great arteries but, perhaps more importantly, emphasis is placed on the way the structures in adjacent segments are, or are not, interconnected. Thereafter, note is taken of the morphology of the valves guarding the segmental junctions, the position of the heart is observed relative to the body, and full catalogue is made of the associated lesions. The pathologist should also note the arrangement of the thoracic and abdominal organs. This is

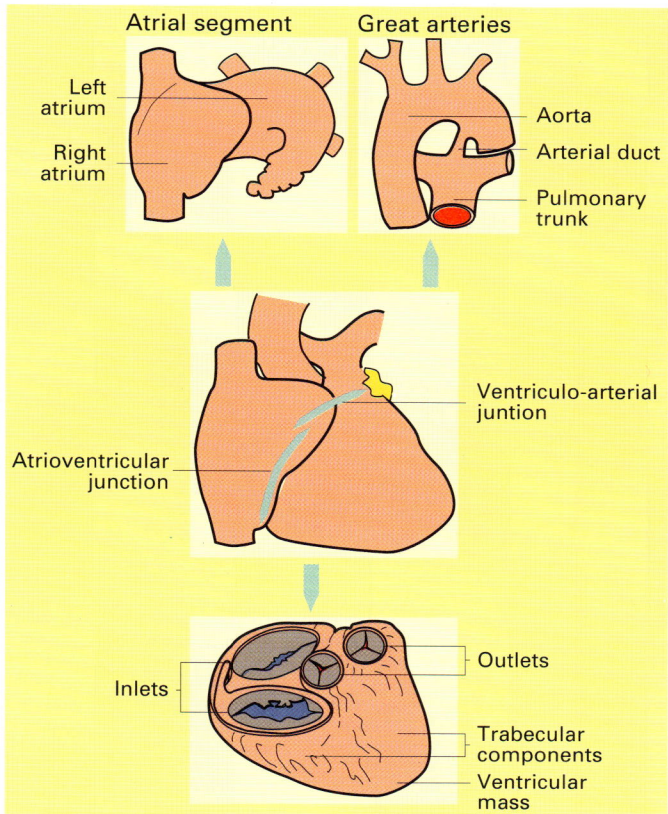

Fig. 12.84 The heart can be broken into three segments: atrial, ventricular, and arterial. Sequential analysis depends on recognition of the topological arrangements of each segment and description of the morphological connections at the atrioventricular and ventriculo-arterial junctions.

because there is usually, but not invariably, congruency between arrangement of the atrial chambers and the thoracoabdominal organs. In unusual situations, the location of each organ should be separately catalogued.

Sequential analysis always starts with the atrial chambers. According to the morphology of the appendage (see Section 12.7), atriums can only be of morphologically right or left type. The adjective 'morphologically' is often needed to describe these chambers since they are not always in the position anticipated for the normal heart. Because all hearts possess two appendages, there are four possible arrangements of the atriums (so-called 'situs'). These are the usual arrangement (solitus), its mirror-image variant (inversus), and two patterns in which both appendages are either of right or left morphology (Fig. 12.85). These latter variants are described as right or left atrial isomerism, respectively. As discussed above, almost always the thoracic-abdominal organs are in congruence with atrial arrangement. This is particularly important for the isomeric variants since the thoracic contents also show isomerism, while the abdominal contents are jumbled up (heterotaxic). Absence of the spleen accompanies right atrial isomerism in most cases

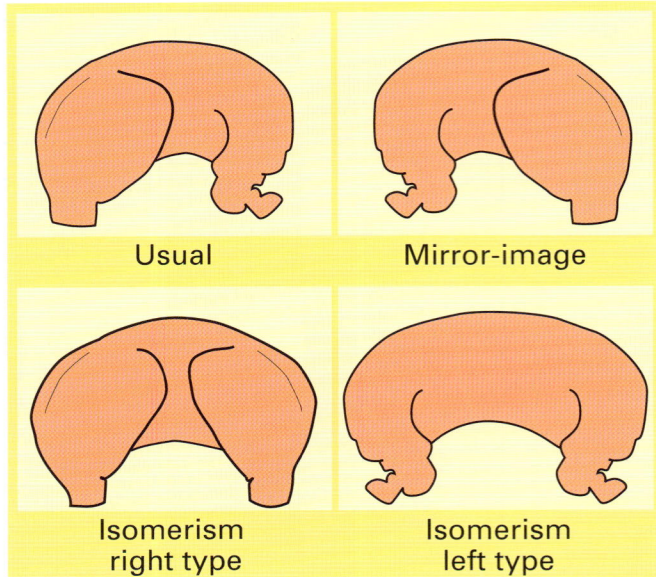

Fig. 12.85 All congenitally malformed hearts possess two atrial chambers, albeit that they may, on occasion, be a common structure because of lack of the atrial septum. Since each chamber can only be of right or left morphology, according to the pattern of its appendage, there are only four possible arangements, as shown.

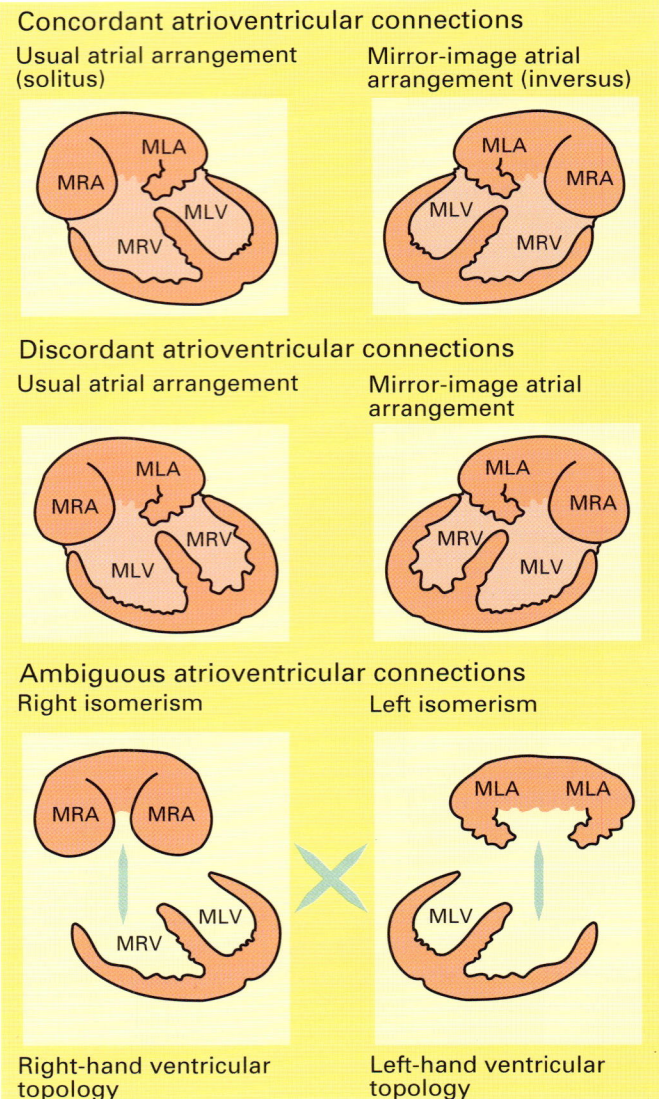

Fig. 12.86 When each atrium is connected to a separate ventricle (biventricular connections), there are three possibilities, as shown. Relationships of the ventricles can vary within each of these patterns. Abbreviations: M, morphologically; R, right; L, left; A, atrium; V, ventricle.

while multiple spleens are usually seen with left isomerism, but these latter associations are much less than perfect.

Having determined atrial arrangement, the next step in analysis is to ascertain how the atriums are connected to the ventricles and to note the effect this has on the morphology of the ventricular mass. In the majority of congenitally malformed hearts, each atrium connects to its own ventricle. There are three variants within this pattern (Fig. 12.86). The usual situation is called concordant atrioventricular connections. The reverse arrangement, with each atrium connected to a morphologically inappropriate ventricle, is termed discordant connection. These two variants can be found with usual or mirror-image atrial chambers, but not in the presence of atrial isomerism. Connection of each of isomeric atriums to separate ventricles results, of necessity, in ambiguous atrioventricular connections. There are then three further patterns of atrioventricular connection which are unified because the atrial chambers connect to only one ventricle. These are double inlet connection and absence of the right or left atrioventricular connection, respectively (Fig. 12.87). They can all exist with any atrial arrangement and with varying morphology of the ventricle connected to the atriums. When both atriums (or one atrium in the presence of an absent connection), are connected to a morphologically left ventricle, then the right ventricle is almost invariably present. But it is incomplete and hypoplastic because it lacks its inlet component. Similarly, if the atrial chambers are connected to a dominant morphologically right ventricle, the left ventricle is present within the ventricular mass but is incomplete and rudimentary. Rudimentary left ventricles are always postero-inferior to a dominant right ventricle

and usually left-sided, although they may be right-sided. Rudimentary right ventricles are antero-superiorly located relative to a dominant left ventricle but may be right- or left-sided with equal frequency (Fig. 12.88). Very rarely with double inlet or an absent connection, the atriums may be connected to a solitary ventricle. This can be because the right or left ventricle is so small as to be unrecognizable, but usually such a solitary ventricle has an apical trabecular pattern of neither right or left type. Instead it is very coarsely trabeculated and is described as having indeterminate morphology (Fig. 12.89).

Sequential analysis continues by determining how the arterial trunks are connected to the ventricular mass. When two

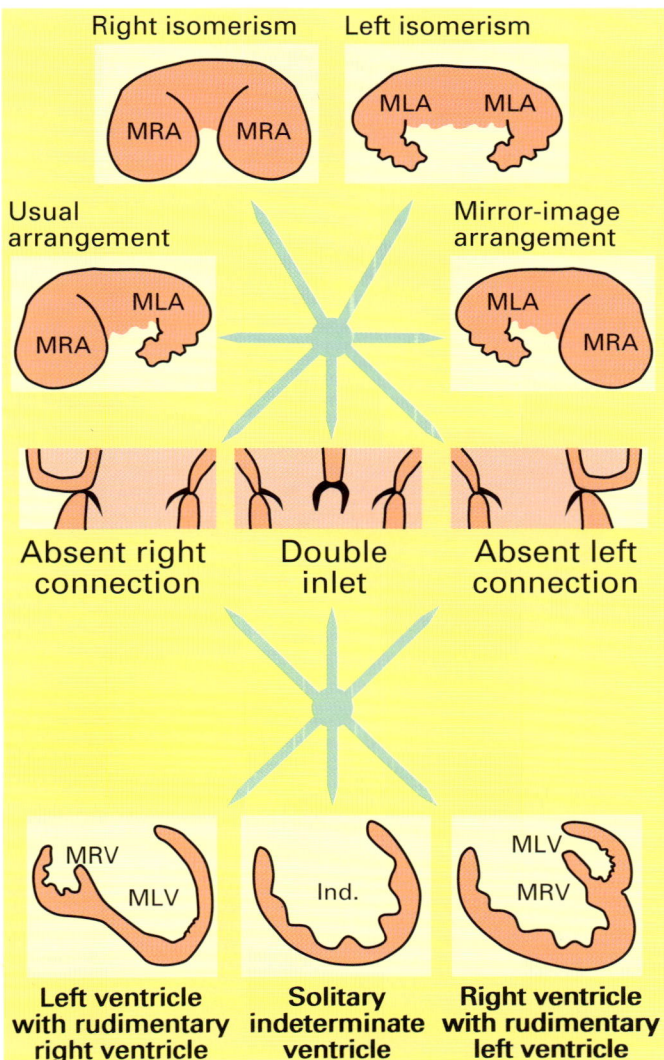

Fig. 12.87 This diagram depicts the possible combinations at atrioventricular level when there is a univentricular atrioventricular connection. It shows only the basic arrangement, taking no account of further variability possible in terms of ventricular relationships, ventriculo-arterial connections, and associated malformations. Abbreviations: M, morphologically; R, right; L, left; A, atrium; V, ventricle.

a single outlet of the heart. This can be simulated when there is atresia of one or other arterial trunk, but single outlet with arterial atresia is only described when the atretic trunk cannot be traced to its ventricular origin. This is very rare when the pathologist has the heart in his hands, although it may be a more common clinical diagnosis.

In terms of the morphology of the valves, similar patterns are found at atrioventricular and ventriculo-arterial junctions, the situation being more complicated at atrioventricular level because the atrioventricular valves have a tension apparatus. The possibilities are for there to be two valves or a common valve. One or two (or part of a common valve) can be imperforate, producing one variant of valvar atresia. This should be distinguished from absence of a connection. Either or both valves may override at arterial or atrioventricular levels. Atrioventricular valves can also straddle when their tension apparatus is attached to both sides of the septum. Overriding valves constitute a spectrum between different connections. So as to avoid intermediate categories when describing the connection, such valves are arbitrarily assigned to the ventricle supporting the greater part of their orificial circumference (the 50 per cent rule).

The above sequence will have determined the various arrangements of the heart, and will have permitted diagnosis of various lesions which exist by virtue of abnormal position or connections of their chambers (Table 12.4).

Abnormal position of the heart is described simply by noting whether the heart is predominantly in the left chest, the right chest, or midline, and by observing separately the orientation of the cardiac apex (to the left, right, or directly downward). Thereafter, it is necessary to catalogue associated lesions, proceeding again through the heart in sequential fashion so as to avoid missing any abnormality. Only the briefest review and illustrations can be given of the associated lesions.

ventricles are present, then the connection is almost always concordant but may be discordant (Fig. 12.90). Concordant or discordant ventriculo-arterial connections can exist with various arterial relationships which must be separately described. There are two further alternative ventriculo-arterial connections. A double outlet connection occurs when both arteries are connected to the same ventricle, which may be of right, left, or indeterminate morphology. The complimentary ventricle will then be incomplete since it will lack its outlet component. The other pattern is for a common trunk to exist, usually overriding the ventricular septum (Fig. 12.91) but occasionally connected exclusively to one or other ventricle. This latter setting produces

Table 12.4 Lesions characterized by anomalous position or connection of the segments

Lesion	Segmental morphology
Complete transposition	Concordant AV and discordant VA connections
Corrected transposition	Discordant AV and VA connections
Tricuspid atresia	Absent RAV connection with left atrium connected to dominant LV
Mitral atresia	Absent LAV connection with right atrium connected to dominant RV
Common arterial trunk	Concordant AV connection and common arterial trunk
'Single ventricle with outlet chamber'	Double inlet LV with incomplete and rudimentary RV
Atrial isomerism (splenic syndromes, visceral heterotaxy)	Isomeric atrial chambers with ambiguous or univentricular AV connection and varied VA connections

Abbreviations: AV, atrioventricular; VA, ventriculo-arterial; RV, right ventricle; LV, left ventricle.

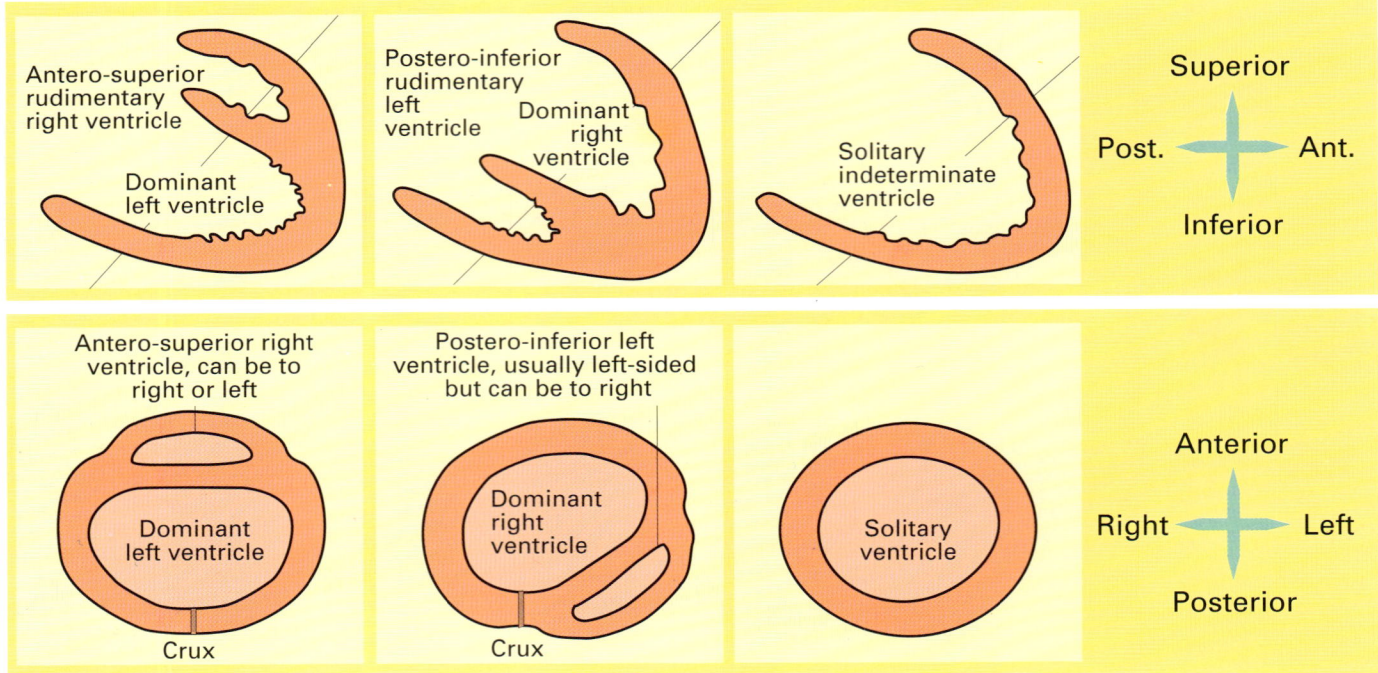

Fig. 12.88 The best guide to ventricular morphology in hearts having either double inlet or absence of one atrioventricular connection is usually the relationship between dominant and rudimentary ventricles. A rudimentary right ventricle is always positioned antero-superiorly, while a rudimentary left ventricle is found postero-inferiorly. Absence of a rudimentary ventrical is usually indicative of an indeterminate and solitary ventricle (the only true 'single' ventricle). Each anomaly is shown in two views (see direction indicator on right).

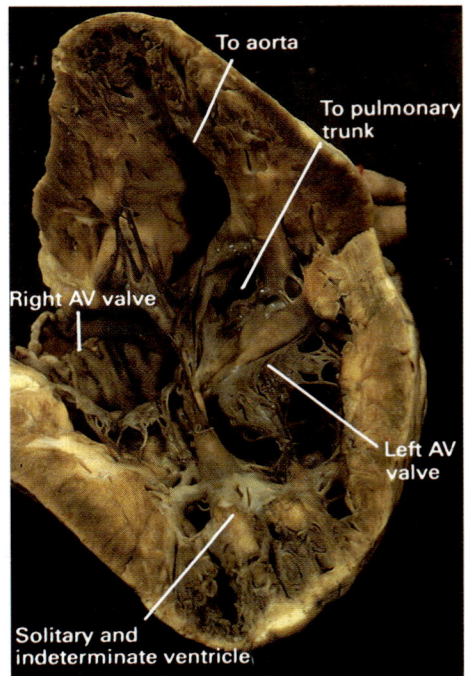

Fig. 12.89 This heart possesses a solitary ventricle of indeterminate morphology (very coarse apical trabeculations) which has a double inlet and a double outlet. It was not possible, even with most careful dissection, to find a second ventricle.

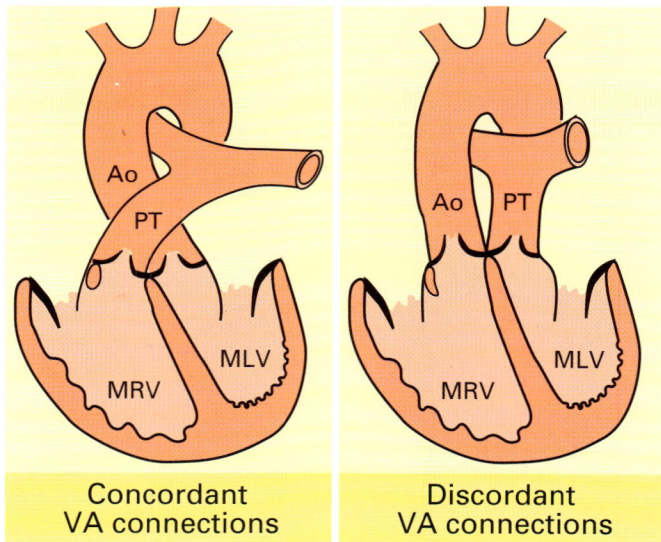

Fig. 12.90 The commonest ventriculo-arterial (VA) connection is a concordant one (left-hand panel). Usually this co-exists with normal arterial relationships [as shown with the aorta (AO) posterior and to the right] but can rarely be found with the aorta arising in anterior and left-sided position from the morphologically left ventricle (MLV). Discordant connections are shown in the right-hand panel. Arterial relationships are again variable, but most usually the aorta is anterior and right-side relative to the pulmonary trunk (PT), as illustrated. MRV, morphologically right ventricle.

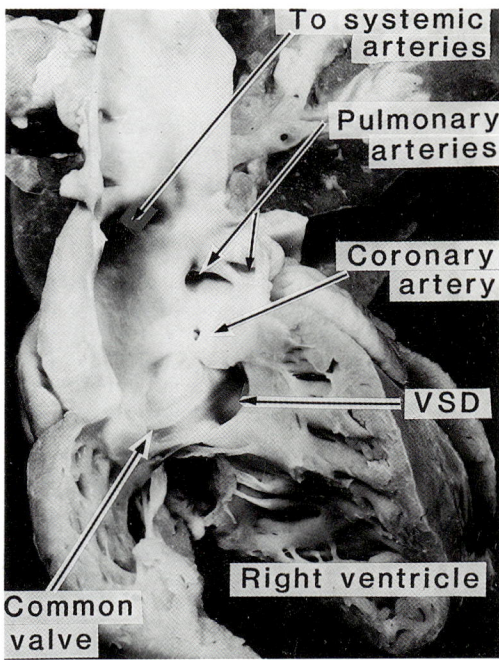

Fig. 12.91 This photograph of the opened right ventricle of a congenitally malformed heart shows a common arterial trunk overriding a subarterial ventricular septal defect (VSD) which is perimembranous (there is continuity between the tricuspid and truncal valves, arrowed). The arterial trunk is common because it supplies directly the systemic, pulmonary, and coronary arteries.

12.8.4 Anomalous venous connections

Either the systemic or pulmonary veins can be connected anomalously in whole or in part. Careful study should be made of the atrial appendages whenever anomalous venous connec-

tions are observed since such anomalous connections are an integral part of the syndrome of atrial isomerism. With usual or mirror-image arrangement, systemic venous anomalies are more usually isolated and may involve separately either the superior or inferior caval veins or the coronary sinus. Pulmonary veins may be anomalously connected in partial or complete fashion, the latter usually described as a totally anomalous connection. When found, it is important to note the site of anomalous drainage (Fig. 12.92) and check if it is obstructed. A divided atrial chamber ('cor triatriatum') can simulate, or coexist with, anomalous venous connections.

12.8.5 Septal defects

Holes between the chambers can be found at atrial level, at ventricular level, within the great arteries or at the site of the atrioventricular septum.

Atrial septum

Atrial defects (Fig. 12.93) are not all within the atrial septum. Only those within the oval fossa ('secundum' defects) are due to true septal deficiency. The sinus venosus defects exist because of biatrial connection of the caval and pulmonary veins. The coronary sinus defect is found when the party wall between sinus and left atrium is lacking.

Atrioventricular septum

The so-called 'primum' defect is, in reality, an atrioventricular septal defect. These fascinating lesions are found in the absence of both the muscular and membranous atrioventricular septal structures. Often called atrioventricular canal malformations (or endocardial cushion defects), their unifying feature is the presence of a common atrioventricular junction guarded by an

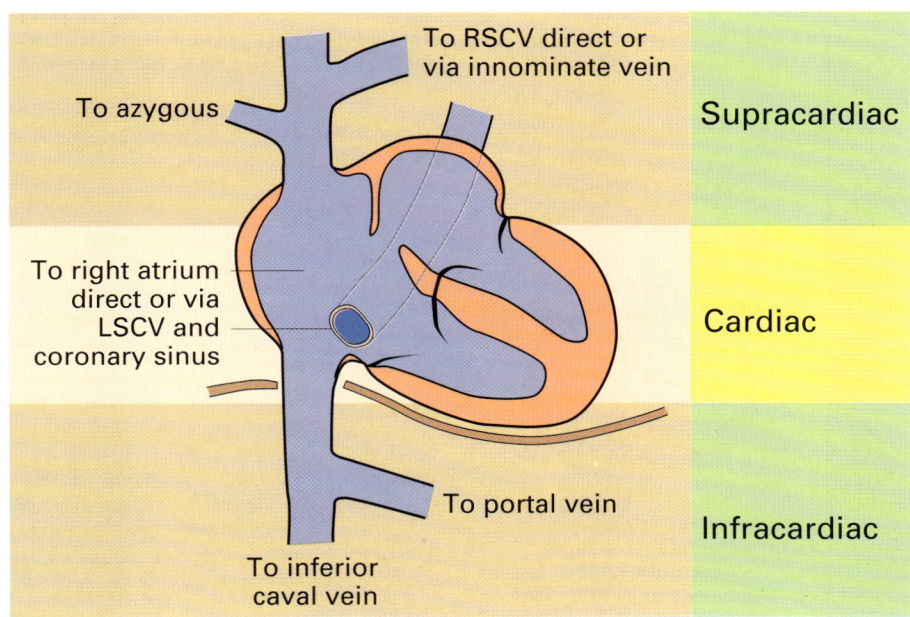

Fig. 12.92 This diagram illustrates the commonest categorization used to distinguish the different types of anomalous pulmonary venous connection. Abbreviations: R, right; L, left; SCV, superior caval vein.

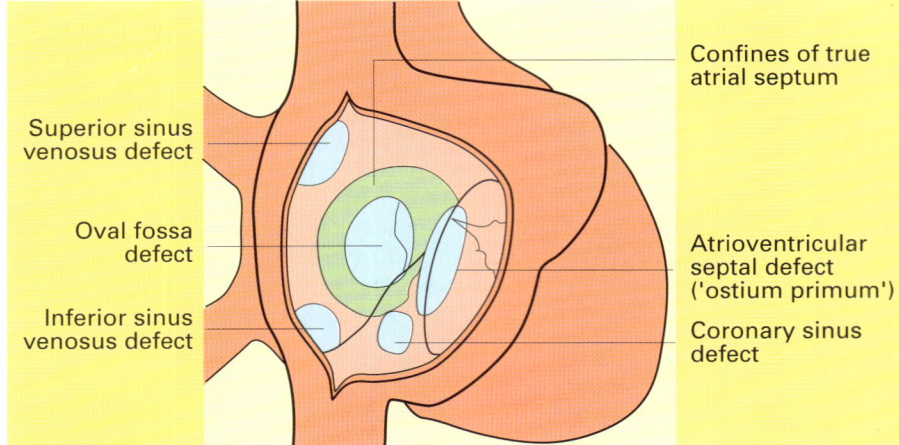

Fig. 12.93 There are four different types of hole which produce the potential for interatrial shunting of blood, but only those within the oval fossa are true septal defects. The so-called sinus venosus defects are found within the mouths of the caval veins which have a biatrial connection, usually in association with anomalous connection of the right pulmonary veins. The coronary sinus defect exists because of 'unroofing' of its course in the left atrioventricular groove. The ostium primum defect is an atrioventricular rather than an atrial septal defect (see Fig. 12.94).

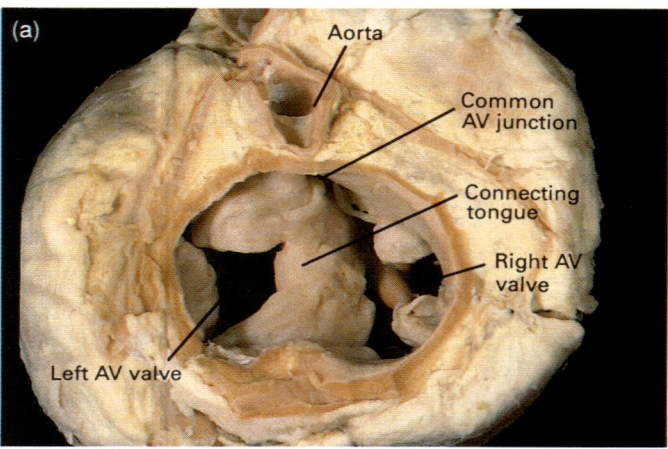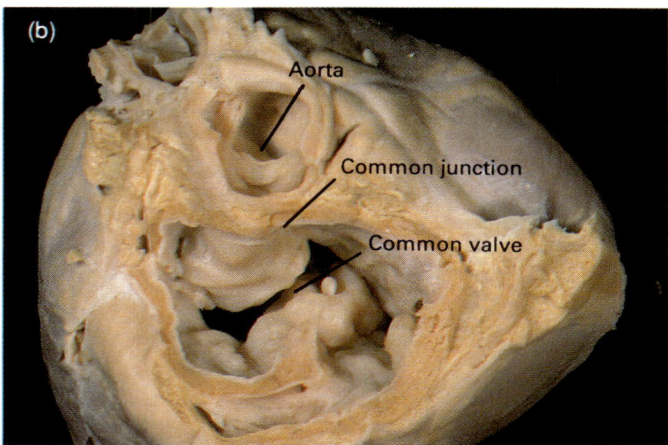

Fig. 12.94 These photographs are taken from the atrial aspects and show the short axis of (a) so-called 'ostium primum' defect and a 'complete atrioventricular canal'. Both exist because of absence of any atrioventricular septal structures. They are typified by a common atrioventricular junction and 'unwedging' of the subaortic outflow tract (compare with normal heart, Fig. 12.73). (b) In the 'complete' defect the common junction is guarded by a common valve. In contrast, the valve is separated into right and left components in the 'primum' defect (a) by a connecting tongue of valve tissue (arrowed). Note that the left valve in both lesions has three leaflets and bears no resemblance to a mitral valve (see Fig. 12.80). It is a mistake to interpret this left valve as a 'cleft mitral valve'.

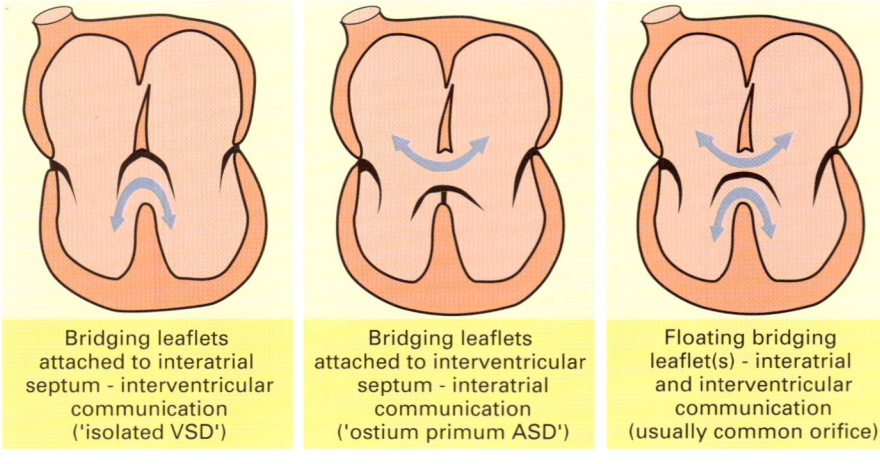

Bridging leaflets attached to interatrial septum - interventricular communication ('isolated VSD')

Bridging leaflets attached to interventricular septum - interatrial communication ('ostium primum ASD')

Floating bridging leaflet(s) - interatrial and interventricular communication (usually common orifice)

Fig. 12.95 This diagram shows how the relationship between the valve leaflets and the septal structures determines the anatomic potential for shunting in atrioventricular septal defects. Abbreviations: V, ventricular; A, atrial; SD, septal defect.

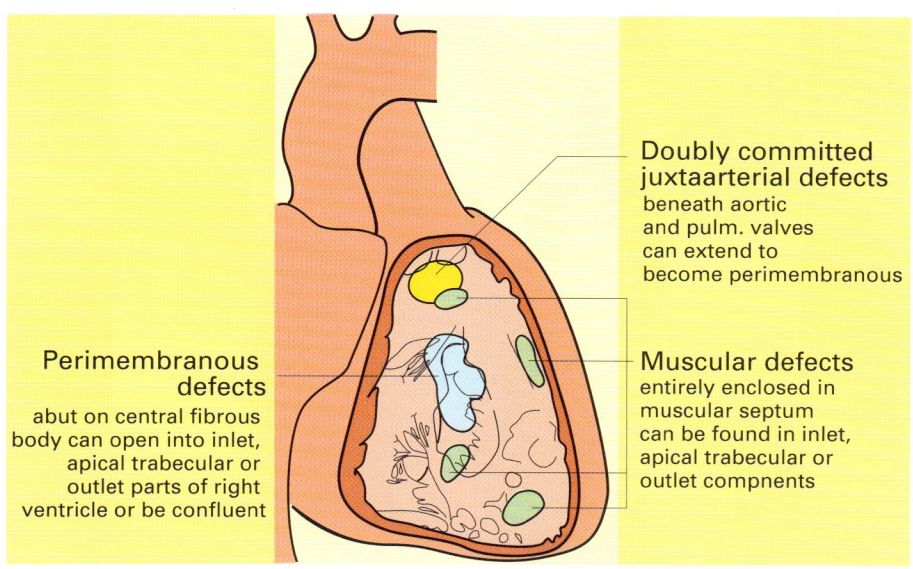

Doubly committed juxtaarterial defects beneath aortic and pulm. valves can extend to become perimembranous

Muscular defects entirely enclosed in muscular septum can be found in inlet, apical trabecular or outlet compnents

Perimembranous defects abut on central fibrous body can open into inlet, apical trabecular or outlet parts of right ventricle or be confluent

Fig. 12.96 This diagram shows how ventricular septal defects, according to their boundaries, can be placed into one of three groups: perimembranous, muscular, or doubly committed and juxta-arterial.

effectively common valve which may have either one orifice or separate right and left valve orifices (Fig. 12.94). Shunting through the defect depends on the relationship between the leaflets of the valve and the septal structures (Fig. 12.95).

Ventricular septum

Ventricular septal defects can exist in various parts of the septum. Three anatomic variants are recognized (Fig. 12.96). The majority are adjacent to the membranous component of the septum and are described as perimembranous. Others are within the muscular septum and are described simply as muscular defects. The third variant is between the outflow tracts and is characterized by fibrous continuity between the leaflets of the aortic and pulmonary valves. These are described as doubly committed and juxta-arterial.

Ventricular septal defects exist as part of many other lesions, such as complete transposition, double outlet ventricle, common arterial trunk, and so on. All can be described using the simple system outlined above.

Aortopulmonary septum

Defects at aorto-pulmonary level are readily recognized and usually described as windows.

12.8.6 Anomalies of the valves

The most obvious defects will have been detected when determining the segmental connections, and include straddling, overriding, and imperforate valves. Stenosis or regurgitation must be carefully assessed and their substrates determined. These include commissural fusion, leaflet prolapse, clefts, arcade lesions, Ebstein's malformation, and so on. Note should also be taken of the orificial arrangement. When assessing the atrioventricular valves, it is helpful to study separately the atrioventricular junction, the leaflets, and the tension appar-

atus, since different lesions afflict separate components of the valve. In terms of the arterial valves, attention will be focused on the leaflets but note should be taken of the supra- and subvalvar regions since these may be the sites of obstruction.

12.8.7 Ventricular malformations

The most obvious lesions within the ventricular mass produce imbalance in the size of the ventricles. This is seen with both double inlet ventricle and with atrioventricular valvar atresia, but these anomalies will have been noted during sequential

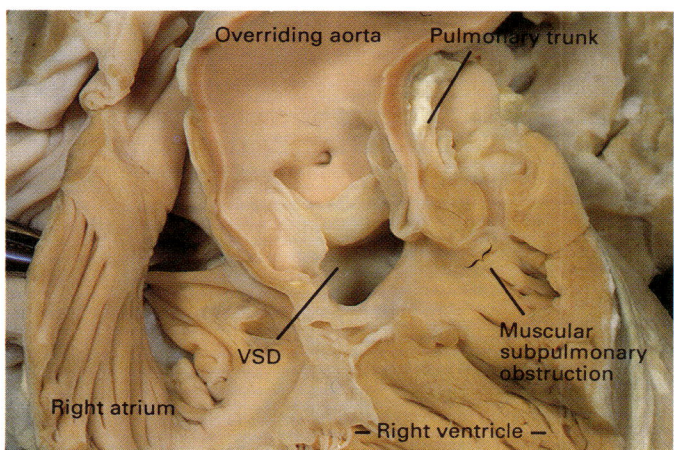

Fig. 12.97 This dissection of the right ventricle shows three of the cardinal features of tetralogy of Fallot—a subaortic ventricular septal defect (which, in this case, is perimembranous), overriding and biventricular connection of the aortic valve, and subpulmonary muscular obstruction. All of these relate to antero-cephalad deviation of the outlet septum relative to the rest of the ventricular septum ('malalignment'). The fourth feature of tetralogy (right ventricular hypertrophy) is a haemodynamic consequence of the anatomic derangement. VSD, ventricular septal defect.

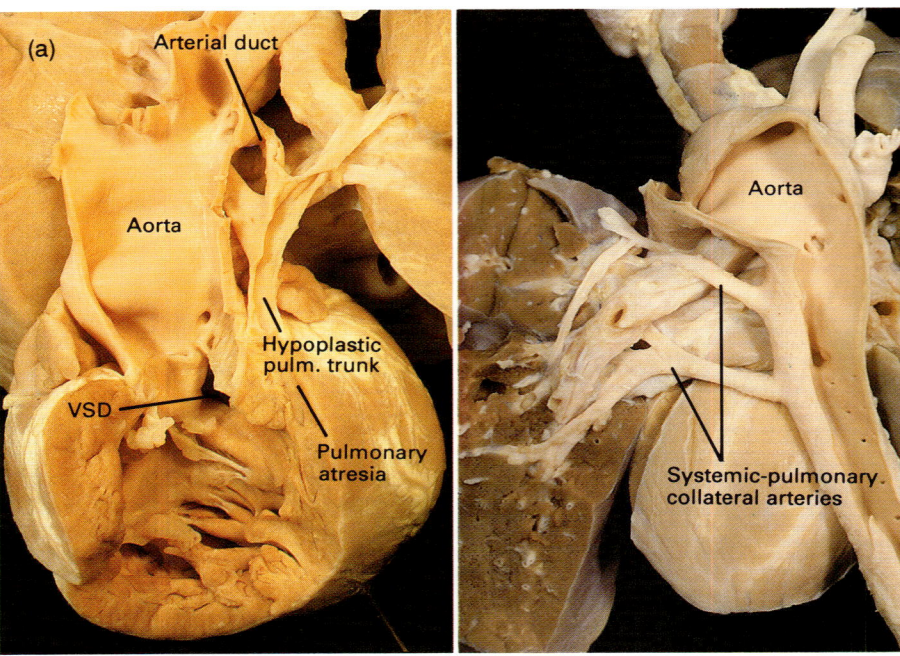

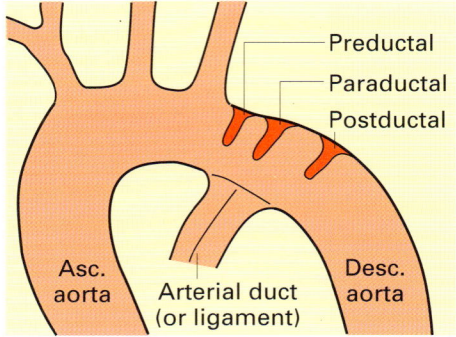

Fig. 12.98 The most important feature of hearts with pulmonary atresia co-existing with tetralogy of Fallot is the source of the pulmonary blood supply. These photographs show the commonest patterns, through either a patent arterial duct (a, arrowed) or via systemic-pulmonary collateral arteries (arrows in b).

analysis. The other primary lesions producing ventricular imbalance are atresia of either the aorta or pulmonary trunk in the setting of an intact ventricular septum. Careful note should be taken of ventricular pathology, the state of the atrial septum, and the organization of the arterial pathways in these malformations, irrespective of whether it is the aorta or pulmonary trunk which is atretic.

The typical morphology of tetralogy of Fallot is seen at ventricular level. It consists of antero-cephalad deviation of the outlet part of the muscular ventricular septum, producing a ventricular septal defect associated with overriding of the aortic valve and muscular subpulmonary stenosis (Fig. 12.97). The extent of deviation of the outlet septum determines the degree of pulmonary obstruction. If extreme, it results in pulmonary atresia. The vital feature is then the source of pulmonary arterial blood supply, which is usually achieved either through the arterial duct or by means of systemic to pulmonary collateral arteries (Fig. 12.98).

Fig. 12.99 Coarctation can be due to tubular hypoplasia of the aortic arch or, more usually, to a shelf-like obstruction within the aortic lumen. When the latter lesion is encountered, almost always it is in the environs of the arterial duct or, if this structure is closed, the arterial ligament. It can then be further described, as shown in this diagram, as being preductal, paraductal, or postductal.

12.8.8 Arterial malformations

Problems in the pulmonary circulation (such as stenoses, hypoplastic segments, or discontinuity of the pulmonary arteries) are seen as part of lesions, such as tetralogy, or can exist in isolation. Pulmonary arteries which are discontinuous can be fed by bilateral arterial ducts, or one may arise directly from the ascending aorta, the other being fed by a duct. Problems in the aortic pathways include coarctation (Fig. 12.99), interruption of the aortic arch and vascular rings. The various patterns of all these lesions are readily amenable to simple descriptive categorization.

12.8.9 Anomalies of the subsystems

Congenital anomalies can be found within the subsystems of the heart just as within the heart itself. Particularly important are congenital lesions of the coronary arteries. These can occur in isolation (as with anomalous origin of the left coronary artery from the pulmonary trunk) or as part of a congenital malformation (as with anomalous origin of the anterior descending from the right coronary artery in tetralogy of Fallot). Congenital lesions can afflict the myocardium, endocardium, or pericardium. Important congenital lesions afflicting the conduction system are ventricular pre-excitation and congenitally complete heart block. An anomalous course of the conduction system is also an integral part of several lesions, such as congenitally corrected transposition or double inlet left ventricle. Coverage of these, and many other lesions, is beyond the scope of this section. Interested readers are referred to more detailed texts (Anderson *et al.* 1987; Becker and Anderson 1981).

12.8.10   Further reading

Anderson, R. H., Macartney, F. J., Shinebourne, E. A., and Tynan, M. J. (1987). *Paediatric cardiology* (2 vols). Churchill Livingstone, Edinburgh.

Becker, A. E. and Anderson, R. H. (1981). *Pathology of congenital heart disease*. Butterworth, London.

12.9   The pathology of cardiac valves

M. J. Davies

12.9.1   Tissue responses of valves

The central core of dense collagen (fibrosa) within valve cusps has a high turnover rate but, being avascular, the morphological expressions of tissue damage are limited.

Excessive cusp fibrosis

Surface fibrosis

External to the core of the normal cusp is a layer of more loosely arranged collagen (spongiosa) rich in connective tissue mucins. This layer responds to mechanical trauma by the production of closely packed type III collagen fibrils, a process resulting in thickening of the apposition lines of the cusps with age; microscopic foci of platelet deposition occur at this point and organize to become fibrous filiform tags, particularly at the central point of each aortic cusp (Lambl's excrescences). The secondary surface fibrosis on cusps may be initiated by growth factors derived from platelets or endothelial cells. In regurgitant valves, surface fibrosis may alter the morphological appearance of the primary abnormality and further restrict cusp movement.

A specific form of fibrosis, affecting only the superficial layer of the pulmonary and tricuspid valve cusps occurs in carcinoid disease, restricting cusp movement and predominantly producing incompetence. The fibrosis is thought to result from the specific action of tumour products on the endothelial surface.

Rheumatic disease and cusp fibrosis

Acute rheumatic fever is the best example of an infectious disease which initiates an auto-immune process directed at normal tissues. Group A streptococcal infection of the pharynx is followed after a latent period of 2–3 weeks by a febrile illness with polyarthritis, pancarditis, and, on occasions, chorea. These manifestations are immune mediated and represent fortuitous sharing of human tissue antigens with components of the bacterial wall, a phenomenon known as molecular mimicry. Neither streptococci nor their antigens reach the heart, and circulating immune complexes are not involved in acute rheumatic fever, unlike post-streptococcal glomerulonephritis (see Chapter 19).

Most patients with acute rheumatic fever recover completely, but in a proportion the valvulitis initiates progressive fibrosis within the cusp, which becomes manifest as stenosis or regurgitation after a further latent period of years.

Clinical features of acute rheumatic fever   Acute rheumatic fever complicated approximately 3 per cent of attacks of group A streptococcal pharyngitis in the pre-antibiotic era. The systemic manifestations developing 2–3 weeks later have been classified as major, including pancarditis, polyarthritis, chorea, subcutaneous nodules, and erythema; or minor, including fever, a prolonged PR interval in the ECG, and an elevated ESR. Two major manifestations or one major and two minor manifestations are traditionally used (Jones' criteria) as confirming the diagnosis in a patient with evidence of preceding streptococcal throat infection. Fatality in the acute phase is rare and due to heart failure consequent upon myocardial involvement. The pancarditis, arthritis, and skin lesions resolve without long-term sequelae.

Acute rheumatic fever is most common between 5 and 8 years of age but well-documented first attacks up to young adult life are recorded. Patients who have had one attack are at very high risk in any subsequent episode of streptococcal pharyngitis. In the developed world the decline in frequency of acute rheumatic fever paralled the improvement of living conditions and began before the introduction of penicillin. In the Third World, in both tropical and temperate climates, acute rheumatic fever remains endemic and common. The disease had virtually vanished in countries with high socio-economic standards but there have been recent outbreaks in the USA, raising the possibility of the emergence of new, antibiotic-resistant strains of streptococci capable of inducing cardiac damage.

Pathology of acute rheumatic fever   The major target organ is the heart, which develops a pancarditis. The pericarditis is a non-specific acute inflammatory response; resolution is complete and there does not appear to be any risk of subsequent constricting fibrosis.

Myocarditis is responsible for conduction disturbances and heart failure, and thus death in the small proportion of fatal cases. The myocarditis has very specific histological features (Fig. 12.100). Throughout the interstitial connective tissue of the myocardium of all four chambers small microscopic granulomas (Aschoff bodies) develop. Each consists of a small focus of connective tissue which appears altered in its staining properties, and around which accumulate both small multinucleated giant cells (Aschoff cells) and cells with a single clear nucleus with a central bar of chromatin (Anitschkow myocyte). Whether these cells are of histiocytic or myocytic origin was controversial, but modern labelling techniques show that the

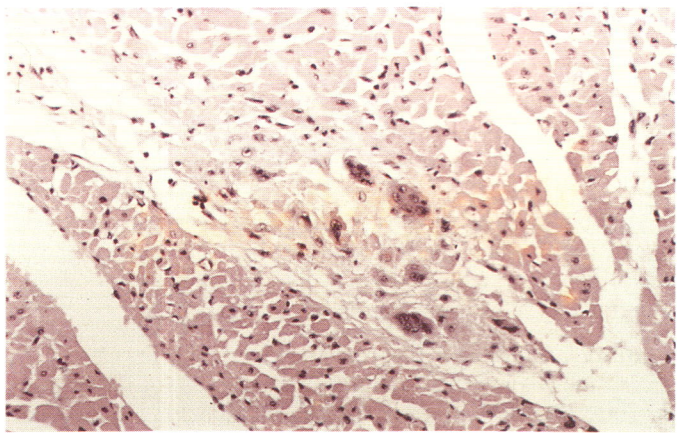

Fig. 12.100 Myocardial Aschoff body. There is a microscopic focus of altered connective tissue surrounded by a mixture of mononuclear and Aschoff giant cells.

cellular composition of Aschoff bodies is predominantly of macrophage origin with a population of T-lymphocytes, 90 per cent of which are T4 and 10 per cent T8. Most studies have not demonstrated bound globulins within the lesion. The tiny granulomas persist for years before ultimately becoming small fibrous scars; Aschoff bodies are thus a marker of previous acute rheumatic fever but give no indication of current activity.

In the acute stage the valve cusps become thickened by interstitial mucoid oedema and small sessile thrombi, never more than 1–2 mm in height and pale tan in colour, develop along the apposition lines of the aortic and mitral cusps. The thrombi consist predominantly of platelets and are the result of trauma at the apposition lines from the impact of slightly swollen cusps. The cusps contain a great excess of mononuclear chronic inflammatory cells and, rarely, Aschoff bodies form. Vascularization of the cusps is prominent. The small sessile vegetations of acute rheumatic fever do not act as a source of systemic emboli.

Heart failure in the acute stage of rheumatic fever is due to the myocardial involvement rather than valve damage; mitral regurgitation may occur but reflects a dilating left ventricle.

Immunology of acute rheumatic fever The fibrillary M protein of the streptococcal wall confers virulence by hindering phagocytosis and invokes antibodies that cross-react with human myocyte sarcolemma. Antibodies to the specific C carbohydrates, which confer the type A status, cross-react with a glycoprotrein present in human cardiac connective tissue. The 3 per cent of patients who develop acute rheumatic fever following group A streptococcal pharyngitis develop an exaggerated response to these antigens, as well as to the secretory products of streptococci, such as haemolysins. A high antistreptalysin O (ASO) titre is therefore a valuable diagnostic tool in acute rheumatic fever but has no direct pathogenetic role. The frequency of antibodies cross-reacting with cardiac tisue in acute rheumatic fever suggested initially that the disease might be humorally mediated but this simplistic view has not been sus-

tained. In experimental models of myocardial damage induced by injecting streptococcal antigens into mice, the tissue damage cannot be transferred by humoral antibodies but develops following injection of spleen cells from affected animals. The histology of the human Aschoff body is more akin to cell-mediated tissue damage. The current view is that patients who develop acute rheumatic fever have restriction elements on antigen-presenting cells, probably related to the class II major histocompatibility complex (MHC), with a high affinity for cross-reacting streptococcal wall components. The resulting cardiac damage is mediated by T-cells and the antibodies formed are an epiphenomenon.

Relation of chronic rheumatic valve disease to acute rheumatic fever Within days of an acute attack of rheumatic fever, blood vessels enter the base of the cusp and fibroblast activity is increased with deposition of collagen, particularly of type III. In the majority of cases this process is self-limiting, leaving a mildly distorted valve. In other cases fibrosis continues over years before causing sufficient disruption of cusp architecture to produce functional abnormality. The fibrosis thickens and retracts the cusp, reducing the overall area and hindering movement; this results in incompetence. A second major effect is fusion of the cusps at the commissures, leading to stenosis.

Fibrosis occurs throughout the cusp, effacing the normal architecture. Two mechanisms are postulated as responsible for the continuing production of excess collagen. Recurrent attacks of Group A streptococcal pharyngitis may invoke further immune-mediated damage. Many of these recurrences may be subclinical and are detected by elevation of ASO titres alone. In the Third World 'malignant' or juvenile mitral stenosis may develop before 20 years of age and represents this mechanism. The longer latent period between the acute attack and the development of chronic rheumatic disease seen in developed countries are more likely to reflect progressive secondary fibrosis in a distorted valve dependent on continuing deposition of platelets rather than direct immune damage.

In countries where acute rheumatic fever has virtually vanished, an increasing proportion of patients who present at 50 years of age with valves having the appearance of chronic rheumatic disease do not give a history of acute rheumatic fever. Thus there is no proof of a rheumatic aetiology, and other causes of an acute valvulitis, possibly viral, have been postulated to lead to the same end-stage morphology.

Valve calcification

Calcification occurs when the connective tissue of the valve is subject to excessive or long-standing stress, and develops in old age at the points of flexion in the aortic valve cusps, and in the mitral valve ring. Calcification with an identical distribution may occur at a younger age in subjects with abnormal calcium and phosphate metabolism, for example as a result of renal failure. A reduction in glycosoaminoglycan and increase in carboxyglutamic acid levels in valve tissue is associated with developing calcification.

Myxomatous change

Weakened connective tissue is a sequela of all the genetic defects of connective tissue synthesis, including Marfan disease and the Ehlers–Danlos syndrome. In the mitral and tricuspid valves, the cusps show a reduction in collagen and an increase in glycosoaminoglycan content, reflected histopathologically by fragmented collagen bundles between which lie pools of connective tissue mucin (Fig. 12.101). This appearance within the central fibrosa of the cusp is known as myxomatous degeneration or mucoid change. Cusps in which myxoid change is severe stretch, increasing cusp area, and chordae often rupture. Identical changes are found in the mitral valve of patients without obvious systemic connective tissue disease, and are known as 'floppy' valves. There is no evidence currently to suggest that the glycosoaminoglycans which accumulate are qualitively abnormal. Floppy valves are not vascularized and show no evidence of past or present valvulitis.

The isolated floppy mitral valve is often familial, and associated with minor skeletal abnormalities such as joint hypermobility. These patients may thus have minor abnormalities of connective tissue metabolism which is expressed predominantly in valve tissue that is subjected to high stress throughout life.

12.9.2 The pathology of functional abnormalities of individual valves

The incidence of different valve lesions varies with the geographic origin and age of the population being considered. Chronic rheumatic disease characterized by combinations of stenosis and regurgitation in the aortic, mitral, and tricuspid valves has virtually vanished in some populations, while remaining the biggest single cause of valve lesions in others. Lesions related specifically to old age will be under-represented in a study of surgical material and overrepresented in an autopsy series.

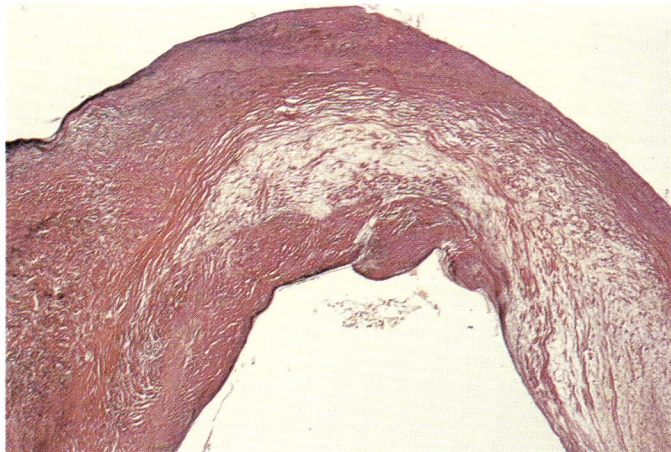

Fig. 12.101 The dense collagen of the fibrosa at the centre of the cusp is replaced toward the free edge by loosely arranged fragmented bundles of collagen interspersed by spaces which contain glycosoaminoglycans. Secondary surface fibrosis is superimposed on both aspects of the cusp. (Van Gieson stain.)

The aortic valve

The three cusps are contained within a short collagenous sleeve whose upper border is scalloped into three points, each marking a commissure where adjacent cusps meet. The upper border of the valve sleeve is inserted into the media of the root of the aorta and marked by the supra-aortic ridge on which the three commissures lie (Fig. 12.102). Behind the cusps the aortic sleeve bulges outwards as the sinuses of Valsalva. In the open position the cusps fold back into the sinuses; when closed the cusps abut on their ventricular faces, this being vital to prevent prolapse into the ventricle. The ventricular surface of each cusp has a central nodule from which radiates a ridge marking the apposition line with adjoining cusps. Above this line cusp tissue serves a strut-like function preventing cusp prolapse. Fenestration of this area of the cusp (lunula) is common but of no functional significance.

Between 1 and 2 per cent of normal subjects have two instead of three aortic valve cusps. The morphological appearances of these congenitally bicuspid valves is very variable. The cusps may be equal or unequal in size; in the latter case the larger cusp often has a central ridge indicating an abortive attempt to form a third commissure. One coronary artery may arise from each sinus or both from one sinus. In early life such bicuspid valves usually function normally but can be detected by echocardiography and, on auscultation, by a late systolic click.

Aortic valve stenosis

In congenital aortic valve stenosis there is a dome of fibrous tissue with a central fixed orifice. In the unicommissural form the orifice is placed peripherally and is elliptical in shape. In myxoid dysplasia the valve consists entirely of nodular masses

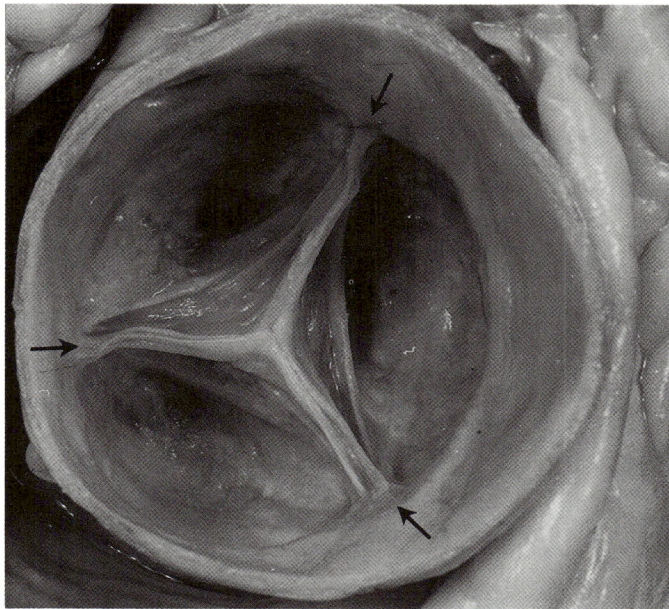

Fig. 12.102 Normal closed aortic valve viewed from the aorta. The commissures (arrows) lie on the supra-aortic ridge; behind each cusp is a sinus of Valsava.

of fibrous tissue containing connective tissue mucin without recognizable normal cusp tissue. In all these conditions stenosis is present at birth or developed in childhood.

The biggest single cause of isolated acquired aortic stenosis in adults is premature calcification of a bicuspid aortic valve (Fig. 12.103). Since up to 2 per cent of the normal population has a bicuspid valve, only a small proportion must develop enough calcification to cause stenosis. The typical patient with *bicuspid calcific aortic stenosis* develops a murmur by age 20–40 years and a significant stenosis between 40 and 60 years of age. Calcification develops as nodular masses within the cusp projecting into the sinuses, and is particularly severe in the raphe; the severity of stenosis is directly related to the degree of calcification. Nodular masses of calcium projecting into the sinuses may ulcerate and thrombosis occurs, simulating in appearance the vegetations of infective endocarditis. The calcific process is not due to previous cusp inflammation; there is no vascularization or commissural fusion. Patients with calcific bicuspid valves have neither more nor less coronary atheroma than equivalent normal subjects.

An identical form of calcification develops, given sufficient time, in tricuspid aortic valves. Significant obstruction is rare before 70 years of age, hence the term senile *tricuspid aortic valve stenosis* (Fig. 12.104). In familial hyperlipidaemia, similar cusp calcification appears much earlier in life; in addition, calcification in the supra-aortic ridge may produce supravalve stenosis.

In chronic rheumatic disease, fusion of all three commissures

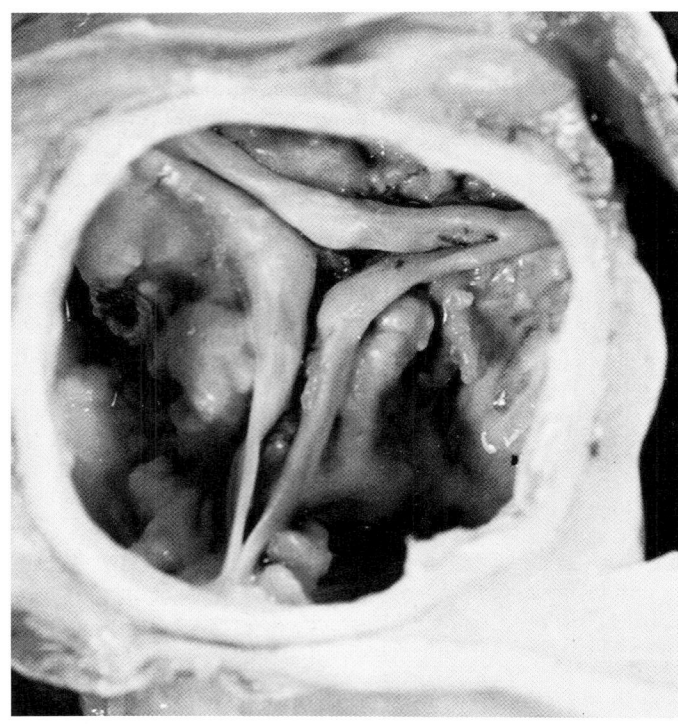

Fig. 12.104 Senile tricuspid aortic valve stenosis. All three cusps contain large nodules of calcium; commissural fusion is absent.

causes a fixed central orifice with stenosis and concomitant regurgitation (Fig. 12.105).

A minority of stenotic aortic valves in adults cannot be easily categorized. Bicuspid valves with commissural fusion are likely to represent coincidental rheumatic disease. Fusion of one commissure in a tricuspid valve only is usually regarded as rheumatic if the mitral valve is also abnormal; in isolation the pathogenesis remains uncertain.

Aortic regurgitation

Competence in the normal aortic valve depends on a critical relation between total cusp area and the cross-sectional area of the aortic root. The former must exceed the latter by at least 40 per cent to allow the cusps to abut and mutually support each other in the closed position. With slow enlargement of the aortic root, such as in old age, some compensatory increase in cusp area can occur, retaining normal function.

Aortic regurgitation due to cusp abnormality In chronic rheumatic disease the cusps are reduced in area by fibrosis which extends from base to free edge. The presence or absence of commissural fusion determines whether stenosis is also present. Perforations and tears in the cusp due to infective endocarditis destroy the integrity of one or more cusps, leading to regurgitation (Fig. 12.106). A small proportion of patients with a bicuspid aortic valve have a cusp structure that is inherently incompetent, with deeply notched or very unequal cusps.

Aortic regurgitation due to root disease Weakness of the aortic

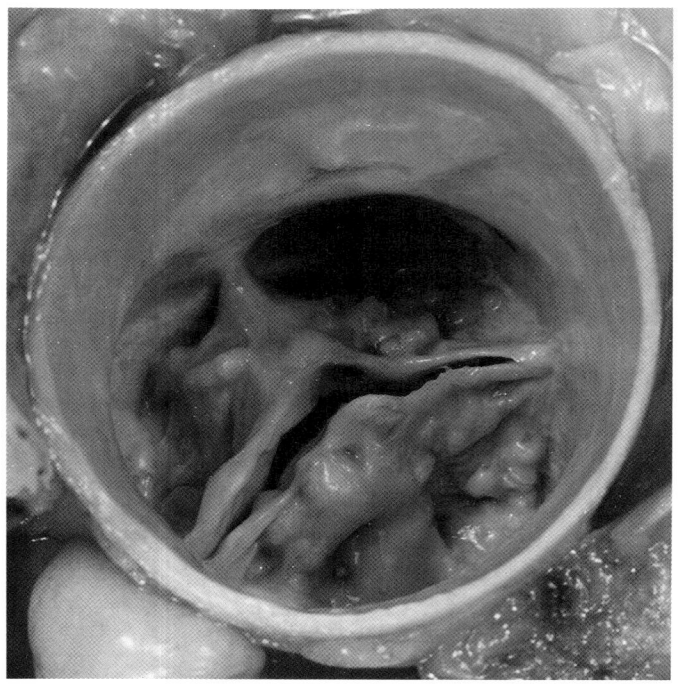

Fig. 12.103 Bicuspid calcific aortic valve stenosis. Both cusps contain nodules of calcium, the larger cusp has a raphe. The valve orifice is a transverse slit.

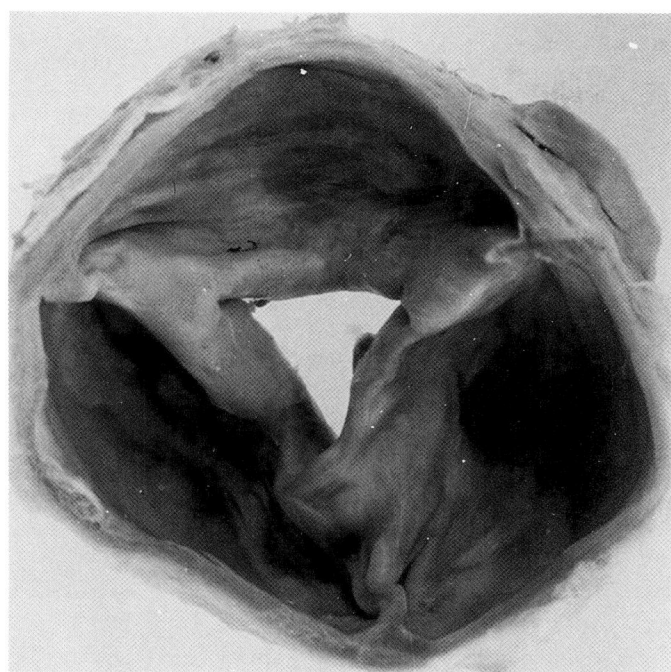

Fig. 12.105 Rheumatic aortic valve stenosis; there is fusion of the three commissures producing a fixed central triangular orifice.

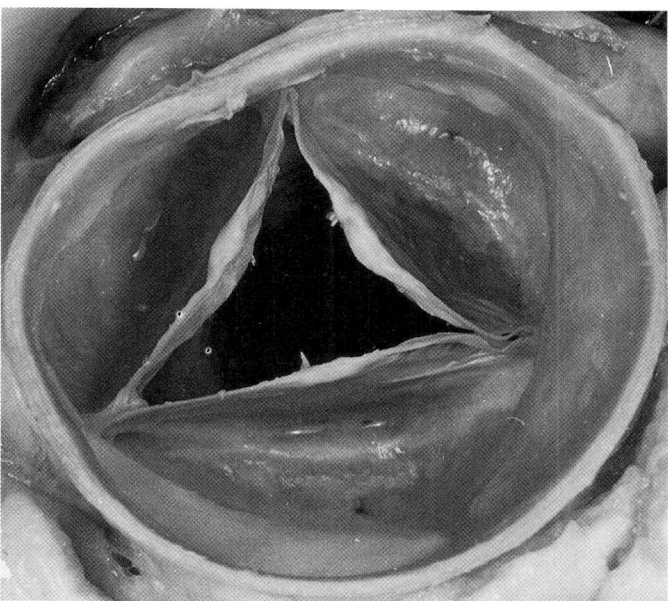

Fig. 12.107 Aortic regurgitation due to root dilatation; the cusps fail to meet, leaving a central orifice, when the valve is closed. Cusp morphology is normal apart from slight secondary thickening of the free edges.

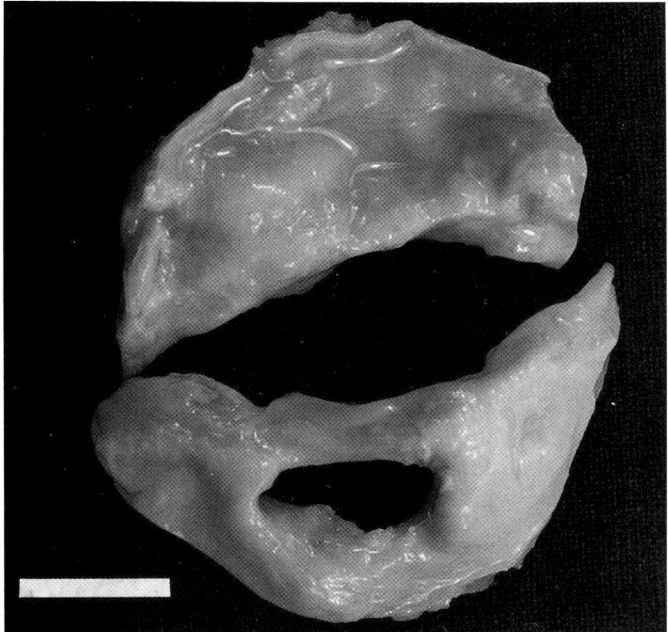

Fig. 12.106 Aortic regurgitation following bacterial endocarditis; one cusp of a bicuspid aortic valve has a large central hole.

root allows an increase in cross-sectional area above that which can be compensated for by an increase in cusp area. The cusps either fail to meet, leaving a central gap in the closed position (Fig. 12.107), or one cusp begins to prolapse downward due to lack of support.

The normal upper limit of the aortic root circumference at the supra-aortic ridge is 10.5 cm, and above this aortic regurgitation may occur; above 12 cm it is inevitable. The majority of patients with aortic root dilatation do not have any evidence of a general connective tissue weakness, but the condition may be familial. The condition is known either as idiopathic (primary) aortic root dilatation or annuloaortic ectasia, and has become the single most important cause of isolated aortic regurgitation in populations in which rheumatic disease has vanished. Histological examination of the aortic root reveals loss of both elastic and smooth muscle but no inflammatory element. In its mildest form smooth muscle is lost and the elastic laminae become straight and more closely packed; at the other extreme elastic tissue is fragmented and spaces containing connective tissue mucin appear. This extreme form, often known as 'cystic medial necrosis', is particularly common in Marfan disease.

Inflammatory aortic root disease is associated with syphilis (Fig. 12.108); the HLA-B27-related diseases such as ankylosing spondylitis or Reiter disease; and less commonly with rheumatoid disease. Destruction of the media is associated with an infiltration of lymphocytes and plasma cells, particularly around the vasa vasorum. Inflammatory root diseases, in general, causes more distortion of the cusps and their arrangement, with less root dilation, than non-inflammatory disease. In syphilis the commissures are widened and the cusps separate at the edges. Unless there is an actual gumma present, the cusps are only abnormal in having secondary fibrosis on the free edge.

In HLA-B27-related aortitis, fibrosis extends from the sinuses over the cusp bases themselves; a characteristic feature is that fibrosis also extends on to the base of the anterior cusp of the

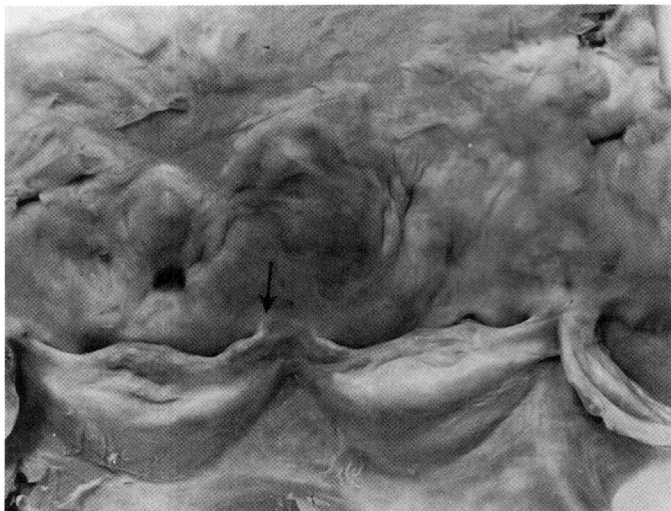

Fig. 12.108 Aortic regurgitation due to syphilis; the aortic root is dilated and the intima thickened; the valve cusps are separated at the commissures (arrow).

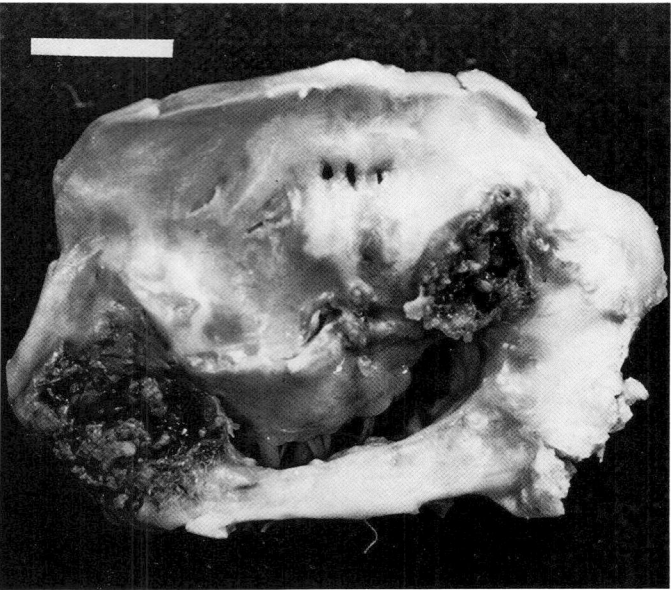

Fig. 12.109 Mitral stenosis; both commissures are fused and replaced by nodular masses of calcium which have undergone ulceration. The valve orifice is oval in shape.

mitral valve. Aortic incompetence may precede the appearance of joint disease. In rheumatoid disease a large granuloma may form at the base of a cusp.

The mitral valve

When fully open the mitral valve orifice is large enough to allow the left atrium and ventricle to form a single chamber; wide opening is dependent on freely mobile cusps. Below the mitral valve opening itself, the passage into the main body of the ventricle is around the papillary muscles and chordae.

Mitral valve stenosis

Mitral stenosis in adults is unique in that for all practical purposes there is one aetiology, chronic rheumatic valve disease. Stenosis, particularly in young subjects, may be due purely to fusion of the commissures, producing a restricted oval or 'fishmouth' opening. In such cases closed valvotomy with splitting of the commissures may produce a virtually normal valve. The degree of cusp fibrosis and rigidity, however, increases with age and significantly contributes to stenosis, particularly when dystrophic calcification develops within the cusp, making valve replacement necessary. The characteristic form of calcification is a nodular mass at one or both commissures (Fig. 12.109), but deposits within the cusp along the apposition lines also occur. In some cases of mitral stenosis commissural fusion is absent, but fibrosis and calcification so reduce cusp mobility that the valve orifice is fixed and crescentic in shape. The chordae in rheumatic disease thicken due to fibrosis and may become fused. The cusp and papillary muscles form fibrous pillars and the valve orifice leads into an inverted cone-shaped space, below the valve, from which access to the ventricular cavity is restricted by obliteration of the interchordal spaces.

Left atrial size and the presence or absence of thrombus in mitral stenosis is very variable. The myocardial muscle in large atria is replaced by fibrosis but whether this indicates an unusually severe acute rheumatic myocarditis or merely a late secondary change is uncertain. Other factors associated with large atria include concomitant regurgitation and atrial fibrillation. Atrial thrombus develops in mitral stenosis within the appendage or as a diffuse layer over the whole wall. Such layers of thrombi often develop an inner shell of calcification close to the endocardium. Atrial thrombus is more common in large atria and in association with atrial fibrillation.

Mitral regurgitation

Competence depends on the normal function of several components of the mitral valve. The cusps must be mobile enough to meet and abut. Prevention of cusp prolapse (due to the high pressure in the ventricle blowing the cusps into the atria) is dependent on support by the chordae (Fig. 12.110) but since the left ventricle is changing in shape during systole, the papillary muscles must constantly adjust the length of the papillary muscle–chordal–cusp axis to hold the cusps in exactly the correct position.

Restriction of cusp movement Chronic rheumatic disease both reduces total cusp area and fuses the chordae; both processes hindering normal cusp apposition. The mildest form is a reduction in the area of the posterior cusp, which becomes an immobile fibrous shelf. In more severe cases restriction of mobility of the anterior cusp is caused by fusion and shortening of the chordae (Fig. 12.111).

In the acute phase of systemic lupus erythematosus, fibrinoid necrosis occurs in the valve and vegetations form both on the apposition lines and in the angle between the posterior wall of

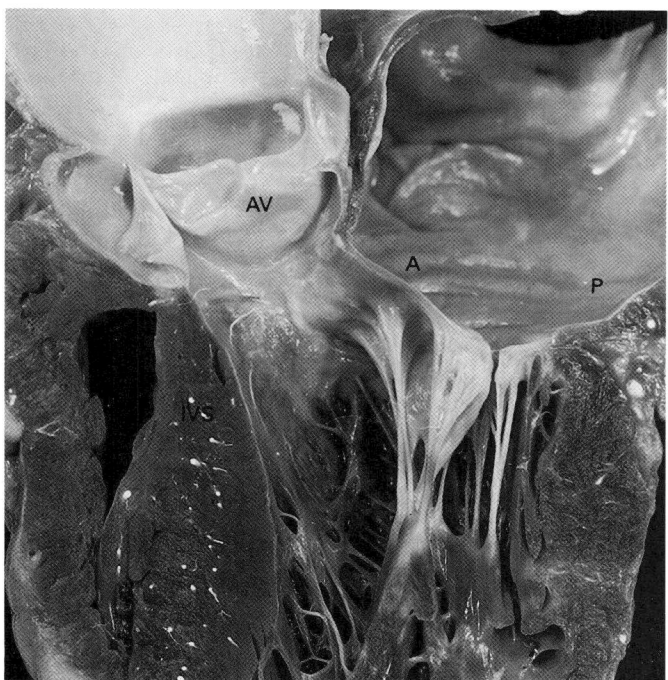

Fig. 12.110 Normal closed mitral valve; the valve has been transected in the long axis. The anterior (A) and posterior (P) cusps meet and are held at the same level by the chordae and papillary muscles. The anterior cusp is large, attached to the base of the aortic valve (AV) and forms one side of the left ventricular outflow tract, the other side being the interventricular septum (IVS).

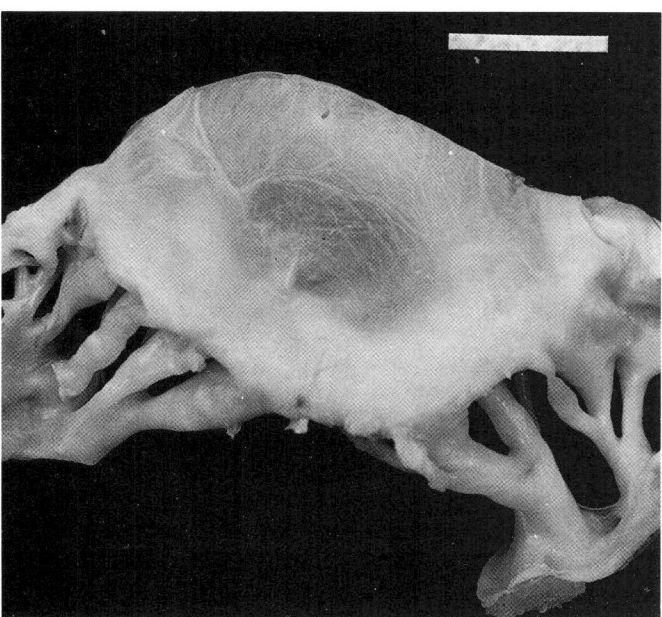

Fig. 12.111 Rheumatic mitral regurgitation; the chordae to the anterior cusp are very short and thick. Each represents fusion of several adjacent chordae.

the left ventricle and the cusp (Libman Sacks endocarditis). In the long term, vegetations organize by fibrosis to restrict movement of the posterior cusp. The final appearance simulates chronic rheumatic disease.

Systemic hypereosinophilia, particularly when the circulating eosinophils are degranulated, is associated with acute endocardial damage, which leads to deposition of thrombus over the inflow and apical portions of one or both ventricles. In the left ventricle thrombus is deposited particularly around the papillary muscles and chordae, to extend up, under the posterior cusp. Organization of the thrombus into fibrous tissue immobilizes the posterior cusp and incorporates the papillary muscles and chordae into a dense mass of fibrous tissue, obliterating the ventricular inflow and apex but sparing the outflow. Both mitral and tricuspid regurgitation are produced. This condition is often called Löeffler fibroplastic endocarditis, or non-tropical endomyocardial fibrosis, and is similar in its appearances to tropical endomyocardial fibrosis.

Loss of cusp integrity Bacterial endocarditis leads to the formation of vegetations which contain the organism on the valve. Following treatment by antibiotics, the vegetations diminish in size and vanish or become calcified sessile nodules. Cusp fibrosis develops, and organization of vegetations that have spread on to the ventricular face of the posterior cusp and into the angle between the cusp and ring, may lead to cusp immobilization. Infection with more virulent organisms is associated with destruction of the collagen beneath the vegetations, leading to perforations, aneurysms, or erosions of the cusp edges.

Aneurysms and clefts in the anterior cusp of the mitral valve also occur as congenital defects, particularly in association with atrioventricular canal defects.

Cusp prolapse Excessive cusp movement, with prolapse into the atria during ventricular systole, is a functional change identified by angiography or echocardiography, and is not caused by a single pathological process. It can be caused either by papillary muscle dysfunction, as in ischaemic disease, or by a structural abnormality of the cusp and chordae. When this structural abnormality results from excessive stretching due to myxoid change in the cusp collagen, it has become known as the '*floppy' mitral valve*. Echocardiography in living patients can only record cusp prolapse to be present, it does not define what component and how the valve is abnormal morphologically. It is, however, likely that the 5 per cent of the normal population that can be shown to have mitral valve prolapse by echocardiography do have minor degrees of a floppy mitral valve; what determines the minority of these subjects who will later progress to develop significant regurgitation is unknown, but chordal rupture is the most common factor precipitating significant mitral regurgitation.

When associated with significant regurgitation, floppy valves are easily recognized by the pathologist or surgeon. The cusp is enlarged, increased in area and dome shaped; it is thicker than normal but lacks the firm feel produced by rheumatic fibrosis, and the chordae are elongated rather than shortened. In the closed position a portion of cusp projects into the left atrium

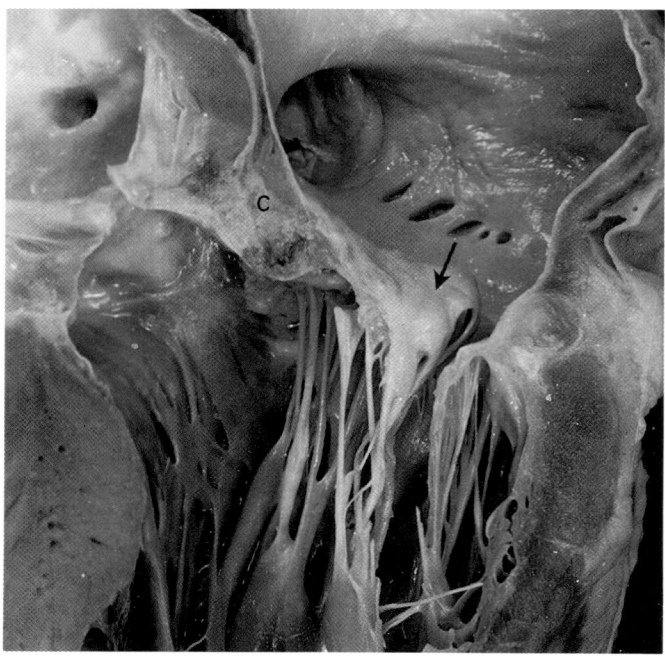

Fig. 12.112 Mitral regurgitation due to a floppy valve; the valve has been transected in the long axis. The anterior cusp (arrow) bulges into the left atrium above the posterior cusp. The base of the anterior cusp is calcified (C). Compare with Fig. 12.110.

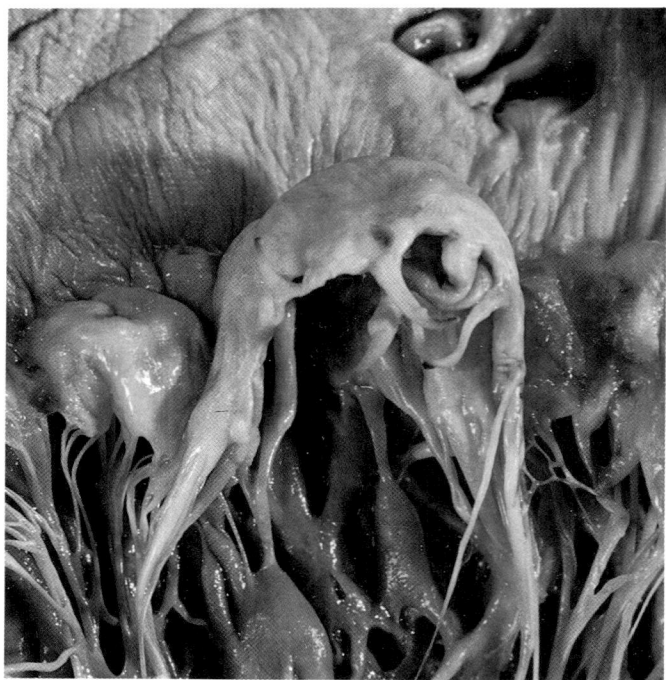

Fig. 12.113 Mitral regurgitation due to a floppy valve. The posterior cusp is ballooned or dome-shaped, with the stumps of ruptured chordae present.

(Figs 12.112, 12.113). The posterior cusp is more frequently involved; in such cases the anterior cusp may be macroscopically very close to normal. The excessive mobility of the cusps and chordae lead to constant friction and mechanical trauma; as a consequence surface fibrosis develops which, when extreme, can lead to considerable thickening of the cusp and of individual groups of chordae.

Two mechanisms have been postulated as responsible for chordal rupture. It may be that the chordae share, with the cusps, an inherent weakness of the connective tissue, based on a structural or biochemical abnormality. Alternatively, the chordae may be of normal length and merely elongate and rupture under increased stress in relation to the expanded and hypermobile cusps.

Microscopic thrombi develop on the apposition lines of floppy valve cusps due to excessive trauma in the hypermobile valve. Such tiny platelet thrombi are the source of transient embolic cerebral ischaemic attacks, and form a potential nidus for bacterial endocarditis. Large, macroscopically visible, thrombi on floppy valves are usually seen only with bacterial endocarditis. The risk of developing bacterial endocarditis in association with a floppy valve must, however, be very small, given that up to 5 per cent of a normal population have some degree of mitral prolapse.

Calcification may develop in the base of the cusp and ring in floppy mitral valves possibly due to excessive 'wear and tear' on the collagen.

Myxomatous degeneration and cusp expansion also occur in the tricuspid valve of most cases with a floppy mitral valve but are of very little functional significance. Aortic root dilation in association with floppy mitral valves is very rare outside known systemic disorders such as Marfan disease.

Chordal rupture in the floppy valve has been designated as spontaneous or primary type, in contrast to the secondary causes which include bacterial endocarditis, acute rheumatic fever, atrial myxomas, trauma, and numerous other rare causes recorded in the literature as individual cases.

Mitral ring disease In mitral ring calcification (Fig. 12.114) a mass of dystrophic calcification develops in the angle between the insertion of the cusp and the left ventricular myocardium. A bar of calcium extends across the posterior wall of the left ventricle, sometimes extending onto the ventricular septum at the medial commissure. The calcific mass pushes the base of the posterior cusp upward; minor regurgitation develops both as part of this upward shift and due to the calcification splinting the mitral valve ring. Clinically significant effects are rare unless the calcification is massive and causes an atrioventricular block by transecting the bundle of His. Mitral ring calcification is usually the result of old age, most cases being in women over 70 years of age. An identical lesion occurs in younger patients with hypercalcaemia and renal failure.

Papillary muscle disease Ischaemic papillary muscle damage has become a common cause of mitral regurgitation and ranges from a sudden catastrophic event to the insidious onset of trivial regurgitation. A degree of papillary muscle necrosis occurs in

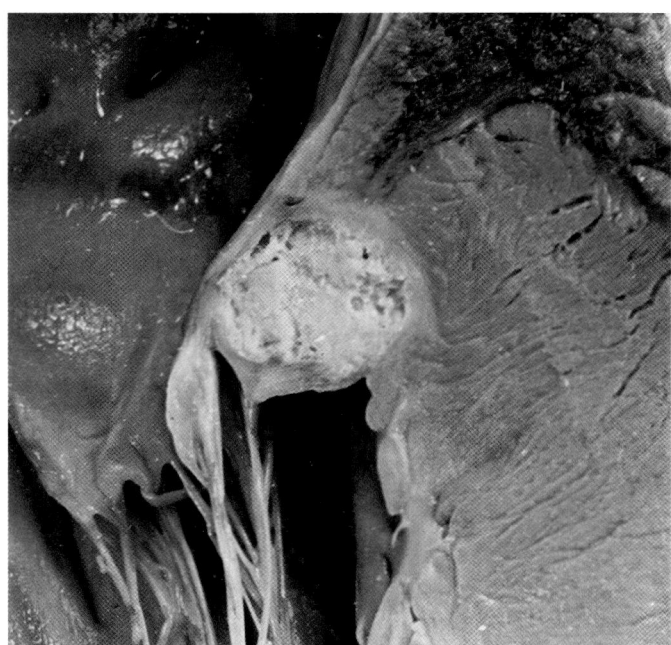

Fig. 12.114 Mitral ring calcification; a nodular mass is present in the angle between the base of the cusp and the left ventricular wall.

up to 50 per cent of acute regional myocardial infarcts; thus the potential for development of ischaemic mitral regurgitation is common. In the most severe form, the head of one papillary muscle avulses during an acute infarct to allow a flail-like movement of the stump, to and fro, across the valve orifice. The postero-medial papillary muscle ruptures 4–7 times more frequently than the antero-lateral. Fibrosis in an intact but infarcted papillary muscle leads to the formation of a thin elongated apical portion which allows upward movement of the cusp and is difficult to distinguish clinically from other causes of prolapse. Diffuse subendocardial fibrosis of any cause will also involve the papillary muscles and, particularly when the left ventricular cavity is dilated, leads to regurgitation. Mitral regurgitation is thus a feature of dilated cardiomyopathies.

Functional mitral regurgitation Mitral regurgitation which waxes and wanes with left ventricular function is often termed functional. It represents abnormalities which include a failure to reduce the mitral ring size with systolic contraction and alteration in the axis of the papillary muscle pull on the chordae as the ventricle dilates.

12.9.3 Infective endocarditis

Introduction

Infective endocarditis is the growth of micro-organisms on an endothelial surface, usually a valve, within the heart. The organism is present in masses of thrombus—vegetations—(Fig. 12.115) on the endocardium from which it can be recovered by culture. Infective endocarditis contrasts with acute rheumatic fever where bacteria are not present in the valve. Recognition that rickettsiae and fungi can also infect valves has led to the term 'infective' superseding bacterial endocarditis. In the past, stress was placed on distinguishing acute and subacute from chronic bacterial endocarditis. The former, caused typically by *Staphylococcus aureus*, developed on normal valves, progressed rapidly, and septic emboli led to pyaemic abscesses. The latter, characteristically caused by *Streptococcus viridans*, developed on previous abnormal valves, progressed slowly, and emboli led to bland infarction. It is the characteristics of the infecting organism that determine the clinical features in any particular patient, and it is now more usual to simply qualify the term 'infective endocarditis' by the name of the organism.

Pathogenesis

Animal models show that two factors are requisites of bacterial endocarditis; an episode of bacteraemia must coincide with small thrombi on the valve. Neither factor alone will initiate the disease. The virulence of the organism, the number injected intravenously, and the size of the thrombus on the valve also influence whether infection is established. Initially, organisms are deposited on the surface of the thrombus, followed by a lag period of 24 h before rapid bacterial growth occurs. This lag period is attributed to incorporation of the organism into a surface layer of fibrin, providing a protected site free from phagocytic neutrophils to which the term 'localized agranulocytosis' has been given.

Many aspects of the human disease suggest that such animal models do reflect the natural disease. Organisms such as *Streptococcus viridans* will only become established on previously damaged valves. The lesions at particular risk all involve high-pressure flow likely to lead to endocardial damage and the formation of platelet thrombi. Regurgitant valves are at a greater risk than stenotic valves. The site at which infection is initially established is often where the regurgitant jet hits the endocardium. High-pressure shunts, such as ventricular septal defects, are at greater risk than low-pressure shunts, such as the secundum atrial septal defect. All forms of prosthetic valve are at risk. Valves damaged by rheumatic disease were formerly responsible for the bulk of *Streptococcus viridans* endocarditis but bicuspid aortic and floppy mitral valves are now more commonly involved. Organisms such as *Staphylococcus aureus* can infect apparently normal valves but in this context it is pertinent that normal valves undergo age-related thickening in which tiny platelet thrombi occur. Thus even a valve which is clinically normal may be at risk either from very high levels of bacteraemia or from a virulent organism.

In man a known cause for bacteraemia precedes infection in approximately 50 per cent of cases. Dental work, known to produce a transient bacteraemia, still precedes about one-third of cases of *Streptococcus viridans* endocarditis, despite the recognition that antibiotic cover of such procedures is advisable. Skin sepsis, wound infections, and lung infection precede staphylococcal endocarditis; urogenital instrumentation, prostatectomy, and intestinal surgery precede enterococcal endocarditis.

Micro-organisms introduced in drug addicts by intravenous injection using contaminated needles leads to both pulmonary and tricuspid valve infective endocarditis, although aortic and mitral valve infection are also very common. It is estimated that two cases of infective endocarditis develop, per year, per 1000 intravenous drug addicts.

Incidence and prognosis

The mortality of 100 per cent in the pre-antibiotic era has been reduced, but it is still between 10 and 30 per cent. The decline in the number of patients at risk due to chronic rheumatic valve disease has been matched by the number at risk from prosthetic valves, intravenous injection, and immunosuppression, so that the overall incidence of infective endocarditis has not changed.

Causative organisms

The relative proportions of the different organisms causing infective endocarditis vary with patient selection (Table 12.5). When infection of natural (non-prosthetic) valves, in individuals who are not immunocompromised, is considered, up to 60 per cent of cases are due to streptococci and 15–25 per cent to staphylococci. Patients with prosthetic valves and drug addicts introduce a bias; the former have a far higher incidence of coagulase-negative *Staphylococcus albus*, the latter a high incidence of infection by Gram-negative bacteria and *Pseudomonas*. The commonest fungal cause of infective endocarditis is *Candida*; this occurs in drug addicts where the tricuspid valve is involved, in patients with prosthetic valves, and in immunocompromised individuals. Q fever endocarditis is caused by *Coxiella burnetii*; an acute influenzal-like illness is followed by

endocarditis after a long latent period and a preceding valve abnormality or prosthetic valve is almost always present.

Blood culture in infective endocarditis

The foundation for an assured clinical diagnosis is a positive blood culture, allowing bacteriocidal antibiotic therapy to be specifically tailored to the organism. Cases are encountered in which blood cultures are negative despite a high order of clinical suspicion. Some are due to rare organisms whose culture requirements have not been met. Surveys, however, suggest that the vast majority of 'culture negative' bacterial endocarditis is due to earlier inadequate antibiotic therapy.

The cardiac lesions in bacterial endocarditis

Gross appearances

The pathognomonic lesion is the vegetation, a large mass of thrombus adherent to the valve cusp or endocardium. Vegetations may be a single, sessile or polypoidal mass or a cauliflower-like mass covering the larger part of a cusp. Vegetations vary both in size and colour (Figs 12.115, 12.116); size is influenced both by the different haemodynamic properties of the valve and by the organism. Tricuspid and mitral vegetations tend to be larger and more polypoid than aortic lesions. Low-grade organisms, in particular *Coxiella*, form flat sessile vegetations. Vegetations may spread outside the cusp, either over the endocardium, particularly in the left atrium, or burrowing inward to form a paravalve abscess.

More virulent organisms destroy the underlying cusp, with perforations being particularly a feature of *Staphylococcus aureus* infection. The destruction of the cusp fibrosa may be due to proteases released by the polymorph response to the organism. In valves with infective endocarditis it may, or may not, be possible to recognize a previous abnormality; bicuspid aortic and floppy valves remain recognizable, the fibrosis that occurs in healing of bacterial endocarditis may, however, simulate rheumatic disease.

Table 12.5 Micro-organisms responsible for infective endocarditis

Organism	Proportion	
Streptococcus viridans		
Strep. sanguis	0–25%	
Strep. mitis	0–10%	
Strep. milleri		
Strep. mutans	0–15%	40–50%
Strep. salivarius		
Strain not specified	0–35%	
Group D streptococci		
Cocci, not specified	0–15%	
Strep. bovis	1–5%	
Strep. faecalis	5–10%	10–20%
Strep. faecium	<1%	
Staphylococcus		
Staph. aureus	10–15%	
Staph. epidermidis	5–10%	15–25%
Gram-negative bacilli	6–8%	
Coxiella	<1%	
Fungal	1–5%	
Others (*Pneumococcus, Meningococcus, Gonococcus,* etc.)	2–5%	
'Culture negative'-infective endocarditis	8–12%	

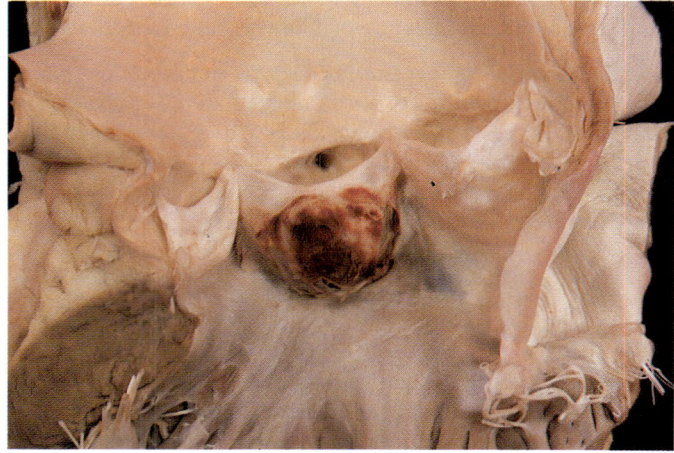

Fig. 12.115 Infective endocarditis; a red vegetation is present on one aortic cusp.

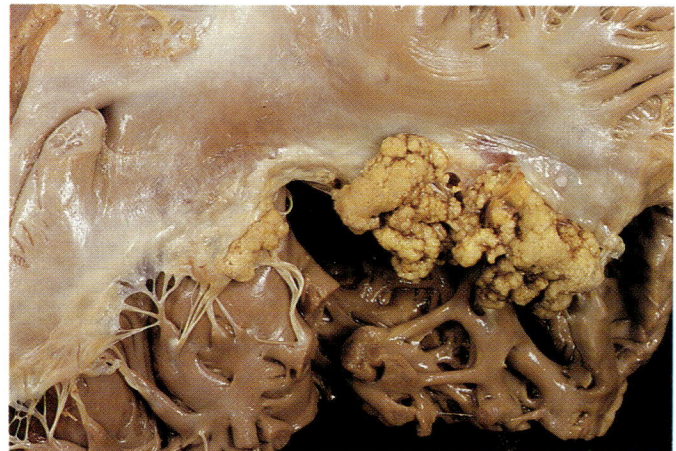

Fig. 12.116 Fungal endocarditis due to *Candida* in an immunosuppressed patient. The vegetations on the anterior cusp of the tricuspid valve are pale yellow.

Microscopic appearances

The most superficial layer in a vegetation is formed of agglutinated platelets; immediately beneath this there is a layer of densely packed fibrin, containing organisms (Fig. 12.117). Experimental models suggest that the most superficial bacterial colonies are dividing while deeper bacteria are inert but still viable. Very few polymorphs are present in the fibrin layer but beneath the vegetation itself the cusp tissue is heavily inflamed and vascularized. A wide range of cells is present, including macrophages and often small giant cells, but polymorphs predominate, particularly with pyogenic organisms such as *Staphylococcus aureus*.

Clinical course and complications

The mortality, the clinical signs, and symptoms of infective

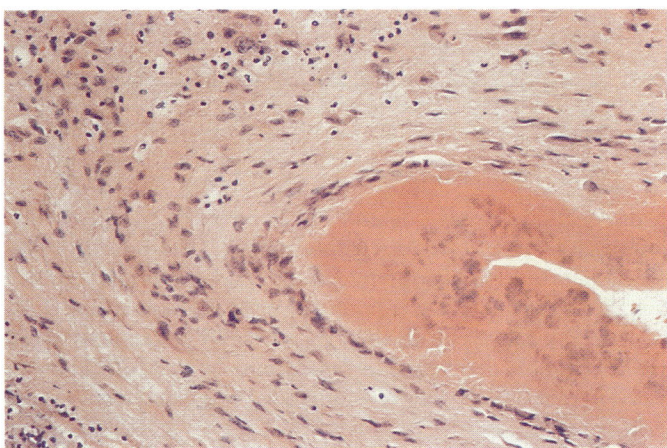

Fig. 12.117 Histopathology of staphylococcal endocarditis. The layer of fibrin, stained pink, contains numerous basophilic bacteria. The inflammatory response in the underlying cusp is florid but polymorphs have not penetrated the layer of fibrin.

endocarditis relate to cardiac failure, systemic emboli, and immunological manifestations.

Cardiac failure

The major factor responsible for cardiac failure is an acute volume overload on the left ventricle, imposed by increasing regurgitation as the valve cusps are destroyed. The rate at which cusp destruction develops is a direct consequence of the virulence and pyogenic potential of the organism. Rapid volume overloads are always poorly tolerated, but made worse by myocardial damage due both to embolic and immune mechanisms. Small intramyocardial emboli, consisting predominantly of platelets, are associated with multiple small foci of myocyte necrosis and are particularly common in aortic endocarditis. Emboli that contain viable pyogenic organisms form small intramyocardial abscesses. Even when small emboli cannot be recognized histologically, there is an increase in chronic inflammatory cells in the interstitial tissues of the myocardium, and often tiny foci of necrosis involving two or three myocytes. Such foci surrounded by chronic inflammatory cells were known as Braht–Wächter bodies and are associated with a low-grade vasculitis for which an immunological basis is likely (see below).

Major embolic complications

The friable nature of the vegetations, a constant exposure to high-pressure flow, and the cusp movement are responsible for the frequency with which emboli occur. When the organism is of high virulence, infected emboli give rise to metastatic abscesses; in contrast, lower-grade organisms are either not present, or cannot establish local growth after impaction of an embolus, and bland infarcts develop. While all the terminal branches of the systemic circulation, including spleen, mesentery, and kidney, are probably embolized, cerebral lesions account for most morbidity and mortality. Approximately 20 per cent of bacterial endocarditis will develop cerebal emboli. Renal emboli are thought to occur in up to 50 per cent of cases but are less significant in terms of mortality. Coronary emboli are rare due to the central flow through the aortic valve. Exceptions are infection of the aortic valve itself, particularly with ball and cage prostheses where flow is directed into the sinuses.

Imunological complications

The prolonged shedding of bacterial antigens into the circulation leads to immune complex formation which can be detected in the blood of close to 100 per cent of patients, along with low complement levels. High levels of circulating complexes are associated with arthritis, subungual splinter haemorrhages, purpura, and glomerulonephritis. The small red tender nodules (Osler nodes) in the skin are thought to be embolic rather than immunological in origin; in contrast, biopsy of purpuric skin lesions shows a vasculitis with deposition of immunoglobulin. Renal biopsy suggests that the majority of patients with infective endocarditis have immune complexes within the glomeruli; the most typical glomerular lesion is focal and proliferative glomerulonephritis but all gradations of severity up to a diffuse endocapillary form occur (see Chapter 19). Renal failure still accounts for up to 25 per cent of the mortality in acute endocarditis. 'Mycotic' aneurysms represent immune damage to larger arteries and range from being similar in size to the congenital cerebral berry aneurysm down to microscopic. The affected artery may, or may not, contain embolic material, but the characteristic feature is fibrinoid necrosis of the wall with a florid inflammatory response very similar to that seen in polyarteritis nodosa. Both rupture and thrombosis may occur, particularly in the cerebral circulation.

12.9.4   Further reading

General valve disease

Davies, M. J. (1980). *Pathology of cardiac valves*. Butterworth, London.

Fulkerson, P. K., Beaver, B. M., Auseon, J. C., and Grabler, H. L. (1979). Calcification of the mitral annulus. Aetiology clinical associations complications and therapy. *American Journal of Medicine* 66, 967–77.

Guiney, T. E., Davies, M. J., Parker, D. J., Leech, G. J., and Leatham, A. (1987). The aetiology and course of isolated severe aortic regurgitation: a clinical, pathological and echocardiograpic study. *British Heart Journal* 58, 358–68.

Nishimura, R. A., Schaff, H. V., Shub, C., Gersh, B. J., Edwards, W. D., and Takik, A. J. (1983). Papillary muscle rupture complicating acute myocardial infarction—analysis of 17 patients. *American Journal of Cardiology* 51, 373–8.

Olson, L. T., Subramanian, R., and Edwards, W. D. (1984). Surgical pathology of pure aortic insufficiency—a study of 225 cases. *Mayo Clinic Proceedings* 59, 835–41.

Perloff, J. K. (1982) Evolving concepts of mitral valve prolapse. *New England Journal of Medicine* 307, 369–70.

Perloff, J. K and Roberts, W. C (1972). The mitral apparatus. Functional anatomy of mitral regurgitation. *Circulation* 46, 227–39.

Roberts, W. C. (1973). Valvular, subvalvular and supravalvular aortic stenosis: morphological features. *Cardiovascular Clinic* 5/1, 97–126.

Savage, D. D., Garrison, R. J., and Devereux, R. B. (1983). Mitral valve prolapse in the general population 1. Epidemiological features: 2. Clinical features: 3. Dysrhythmias: the Framingham study. *American Heart Journal* 106, 571–86.

Rheumatic fever

Gotsman, M. S. (1984) Rheumatic fever in the eighties. In *The heart and rheumatic disease* (ed. B. M. Ansell and P. A. Simpkin), pp. 234–67. Butterworth's International Medical Reviews—Rheumatology 2.

Virmani, R. and Roberts, W. C. (1977). Aschoff bodies in operatively excised atrial appendages and in papillary muscle. Frequency and clinical significance. *Circulation* 55, 559–63.

Williams, R. C. (1985). Molecular mimicry and rheumatic fever. *Clinics in Rheumatic Diseases* 11, 573–91.

Infective endocarditis

Epidemiology

Bayliss, R., Clarke, C., Oakley, C. M., Somerville, W., Whitfield, A. G. W., and Young, S. E. J. (1983). The microbiology and pathogenesis of infective endocarditis. *British Heart Journal* 50, 513–19.

Ivert, T. S. A., Dismukes, W. E., Cobbs, C. G., Blackstone, E. H., Kirklin, J. W., and Bergdhal, L. A. L. (1984). Prosthetic valve endocarditis. *Circulation* 69, 223–32.

Reiseberg, B. E. (1979). Infective endocarditis in the narcotic addict. *Progress in Cardiovascular Diseases* 22, 137–44.

Skehan, J. D., Murray, M., and Mills, P. G. (1988). Infective endocarditis: incidence and mortality in the North East Thames Region. *British Heart Journal* 59, 62–8.

Pathogenesis

Freedman, L. R. and Valone, J. (1979). Experimental infective endocarditis. *Progress and Cardiovascular Disease* 22, 169–80.

Complications

Garnier, J. L., Touraine, J. L., and Colon, S. (1984). Immunology of infective endocarditis. *European Heart Journal* 5, 3–10.

Kauffman, R. H., Thompson, J., Valentijn, R. M., Daha, M. R., and Vants, L. (1981). The clinical implications and the pathogenetic significance of circulating immune complexes in infective endocarditis. *American Journal of Medicine* 71, 17–25.

Malquarti, V., Saradarian, W., Etienne, J., Milon, H., and Delahaye, J. P. (1984). Prognosis of native valve endocarditis—a review of 253 cases. *European Heart Journal* 5, 11–20.

Phair, J. P and Clarke, J. (1979). Immunology of infective endocarditis. *Progress in Cardiovascular Disease* 22, 137–44.

Fungal endocarditis

Walsh, J. T., Jutchins, G. M., Bulkley, B., and Mendelsohn, G. (1980). Fungal infections of the heart: analysis of 51 autopsy cases. *American Journal of Cardiology* 45, 357–66.

Q fever endocarditis

Geddes, A. M. (1983) Q fever. *British Medical Journal* 287, 927–8.

12.10   Non-ischaemic myocardial diseases

E. G. J. Olsen

12.10.1   Introduction

In this section cardiomyopathies and specific heart muscle diseases will be described. Much confusion has existed regarding the nomenclature of cardiomyopathies and several attempts to define and classify the conditions have been made in the past. Recognizing the problem, the World Health Organization and the International Society and Federation of Cardiology set up a task force in 1980. The recommended nomenclature will be used.

Definitions

Cardiomyopathies are defined as heart muscle diseases of unknown cause. They are classified into: dilated; hypertrophic;

restrictive types. One of the many difficulties that existed was the lack of uniformity as to what to include under the term 'secondary cardiomyopathies'. It was therefore recommended that the term should be replaced by 'specific heart muscle disease'. This is defined as: heart muscle disease of known cause or associated with disorders of other systems. It is classified as detailed in Section 12.10.5. Cardiomyopathies will be described first.

12.10.2 Dilated cardiomyopathy

When patients die in the end-stage of the disease the hearts are hypertrophied and often severely dilated, all cardiac chambers are affected. Despite the hypertrophy, measurements of ventricular wall thicknesses may be normal due to dilatation (Fig. 12.118a). The heart may be flabby and focal fibrosis may be noted. In over half the patients, endocardial thickening is usually found, together with thrombus superimposition. The coronary arteries are, with rare exceptions, normal.

Histopathology

Myocardial fibres are in normal alignment with nuclear changes of hypertrophy (pyknosis or vesicular change) but the fibre diameters may be normal or less than normal, due to stretching (Fig. 12.118b). Focal interstitial fibrosis of varying severity is frequently found together with foci of fibrous replacement of myocardial fibres. In some instances, evidence of myocarditis and myocyte degeneration may be evident (see below).

The extramyocardial coronary arteries rarely show significant arteriosclerosis and the small intramyocardial vessels are usually normal, although occasionally some intimal thickening may be identified.

Histochemically, an increase, normal, or decreased amounts of substances such as glycogen and succinic dehydrogenase may be present, depending to some extent on the length of history and the presence or absence of heart failure. Electron microscopy shows myocardial fibrils in regular, parallel arrangement, crenation of nuclear membranes, and an increase in mitochondria to more than one per two sarcomeres; degeneration of actin and myosin or more severe degenerative changes affecting groups of cells may be encountered. The morphological changes are therefore non-specific and diagnosis can only be achieved by excluding conditions that can result in a hypertrophied, dilated heart.

The features described above may not necessarily always be found as patients may die at any stage during the disease process and may therefore show only mild degrees of cardiomegaly.

Pathogenesis

By definition, the aetiology of dilated cardiomyopathy is unknown but several suggestions have been made, including the following: a decrease in succinic dehydrogenase; abnormalities of small vessels; a possible infective agent; and hypertension. Virus infection has also been implicated, as well as immunological disturbances. These aspects have been extens-

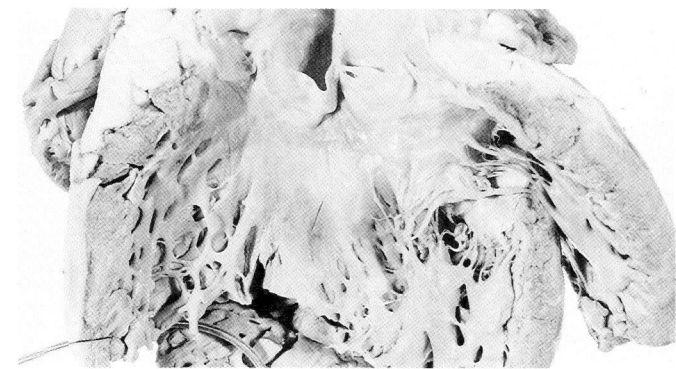

(a)

(b)

Fig. 12.118 (a) Dilated cardiomyopathy. The left ventricle has been opened, showing severe dilatation and thickening of the endocardium. Despite the heart weight of 750 g the walls of the ventricle are of normal thickness. (b) Photomicrograph showing myocardial fibres in regular alignment and nuclear changes of hypertrophy. The diameter of the myocytes is less than normal in many instances.

ively investigated in recent years by analysis of fresh endomyocardial tissue obtained by use of the bioptome. The apparatus consists essentially of a catheter and a cutting device (usually two opposing cups) which can be manipulated by an operating handle by means of a wire.

Analysis of the tissue samples thus obtained suggest possible pathogenic pathways. In patients with suspected dilated cardiomyopathy, myocarditis attributed to virus infection has been found in between 2 and 65 per cent. The author's own experience over 15 years is 28 per cent. Morphological, as well as clinical, diagnosis of myocarditis is exceedingly difficult (Olsen 1983). For this reason, a group of pathologists met in Dallas to define and classify myocarditis (Aretz et al. 1987).

Myocarditis

Definition Myocarditis is a process characterized by an inflammatory infiltrate of the myocardium, with necrosis and/or degeneration of adjacent myocytes not typical of the ischaemic damage associated with coronary artery disease. Based on sequential biopsies, these disorders have been classified as acute and resolving myocarditis.

Acute myocarditis This implies an inflammatory infiltrate and necrosis of adjacent myocytes. Some interstitial fibrosis may be present. Ongoing myocarditis is the term suggested if the degree of myocarditis is unchanged from the most recent previous biopsy.

Resolving (healing) myocarditis This implies reduction of the inflammatory cell infiltrate and fibrosis.

Resolved (healed) myocarditis This implies very little or no evidence of inflammation. Fibrosis may be extensive.

Although this classification is based on viral myocarditis, it applies to other forms of myocarditis as well (see below).

Evidence of virus infection causally related to myocarditis has, up to recent times, been based on neutralization tests, which have shown rising or high serum titres to coxsackie virus not only in cases with myocarditis, but also in biopsies showing the non-specific features of a hypertrophied, dilated myocardium (dilated cardiomyopathy). Despite many attempts, virus particles have only very rarely been isolated from endomyocardial biopsies. Recently, a virus-specific cDNA has been employed and coxsackie B virus RNA sequences have been demonstrated in biopsy tissue from 53 per cent of patients with myocarditis, and also in biopsies showing non-specific changes only (Bowles *et al.* 1986).

Extensive immunological studies, in recent years, have led to the following conclusions.

1. An immune disturbance exists in a significant number of patients.
2. Previous viral infection results in 'sensitization' of the myocardium or myocarditis.
3. Virus infection may trigger antibody production affecting suppressor cells.
4. Inactivity of T-cell receptors may interfere with normal B cell function resulting in production of antibodies.
5. T-cell suppressor cell dysfunction may also affect cell mediated immunity (Das *et al.* 1981).

Using right atrial strips between the venae cavae, a decrease in neuronal counts has also been found in patients with dilated cardiomyopathy (Amorim and Olsen 1982). It has been concluded that, in approximately half the patients with dilated cardiomyopathy, an infectious-immune mechanism is operative.

In some cases with dilated cardiomyopathy enlarged, ring-shaped mitochondria have been noted containing tubular cristae arranged in circular concentric lamellae, but the pathogenetic significance of this is unclear.

Peripartal heart disease

In the peripartal period extending to three months following childbirth, cardiomegaly and heart failure, identical to dilated cardiomyopathy, has been recognized, including some cases with myocarditis.

Infantile cardiomyopathy with histiocytoid change

In this rare condition, the hearts are hypertrophied and dilated and show yellowish nodules distributed haphazardly in the myocardium and cardiac valves. Histopathologically, those nodules contain cells resembling lipid-laden histiocytes but ultrastructurally these are myocytes.

Isolated endocardial fibro-elastosis

This disease is difficult to classify and is therefore conveniently described here. Two forms are recognized.

1. In the infantile form, heart failure becomes manifest within 6 months after birth. Usually the left or both ventricles are affected. The cardiac chambers are small and covered with thick, white endocardium.
2. In the adolescent form, cardiac hypertrophy and dilatation is typical. The pearly white, thick endocardium extends usually from the atria to the ventricles, involving valves, chordae, and papillary muscles. Trabeculation of the ventricular myocardium is strikingly prominent due to the thick endocardial covering. The outflow tract—unlike in endomyocardial fibrosis—is usually affected.

The histopathology in both forms is identical, consisting of regular bands of elastic tissue in the thick endocardium together with prominent smooth muscle if dilatation has been present. The aetiology is unknown but virus infection (intra-uterine), including mumps virus, has been implicated.

12.10.3   Hypertrophic cardiomyopathy

By contrast to dilated cardiomyopathy, characteristic features are discernible to the naked eye. Asymmetric hypertrophy of the interventricular septum is often severe and may exceed twice the thickness of the hypertrophied free left ventricular wall (Fig. 12.119a). Displacement of the anterior papillary muscle interferes with normal closure of the mitral valve and leads to mitral insufficiency, causing thickening of the valve leaflets. The anterior mitral valve leaflet may impinge on the thick septum, resulting in a mirror image of the valve leaflet forming on the thick endocardium.

The maximum bulge of the septum may be confined to the mid-region, the apex, or beneath the aortic valve. Varying degrees of fibrous tissue may be found. The coronary arteries are normal but despite this, infarct-like lesions, extending transmurally, have been described.

Controversy exists as to the diagnostic reliability of the asymmetric hypertrophy of the septum, as some asymmetric thickening may be found in the new-born and in congenital heart disease, and other cardiac conditions, particularly in right-sided involvement. In addition, concentric hypertrophy is also well recognized in cases with hypertrophic cardiomyopathy.

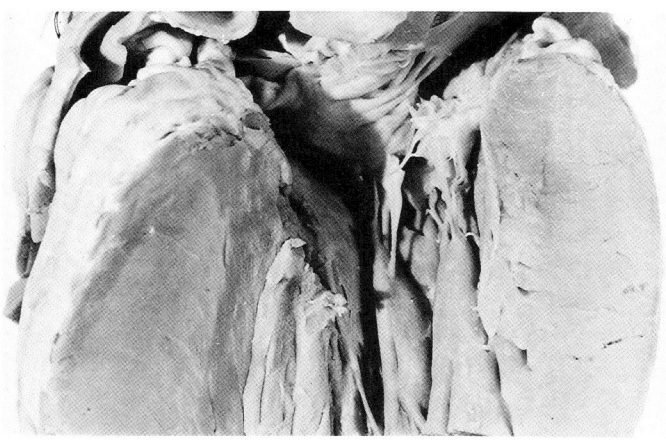

(a)

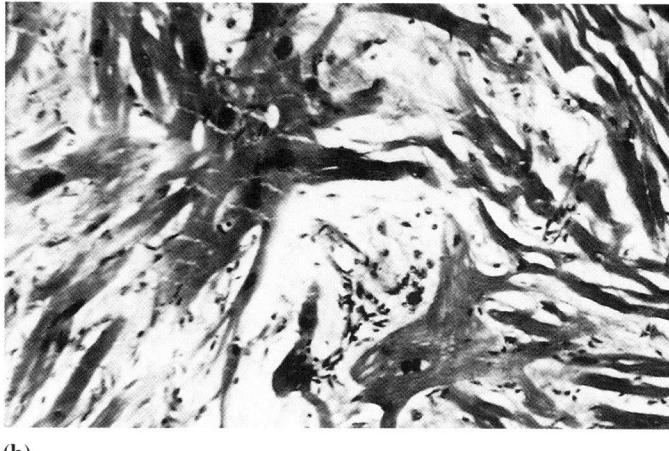

(b)

Fig. 12.119 (a) Hypertrophic cardiomyopathy. The left ventricle has been sectioned to show the asymmetrically hypertrophied interventricular septum (left side of the photograph). The free wall of the ventricle is also severely hypertrophied. (b) Photomicrograph of dissarray and severe hypertrophy of myocytes together with some bizarre-shaped nuclei. Note the cellularity of the interstitium, which also shows an increase in collagen tissue.

Histopathology

Disarray and short runs of myocardial fibres interrupted by connective tissue; large bizarre nuclei; fibrosis; degenerative muscle fibres with disappearing myofibrils (perinuclear halo); and disorganized myofibres (whorling) characterize the condition (Fig. 12.119b). By allocating a maximum of three points to each of these five features, and expressing the maximum 15 points as 100 per cent, the 'histological HOCM index' has been devised. Values of over 50 per cent permit diagnosis.

In addition, the disorganized myocytes are extremely hypertrophied and values of 100 μm diameter are not unusual. Disarray by itself, particularly if widespread, has been deemed characteristic by some workers, permitting diagnosis. This controversial topic has been extensively discussed in the literature (Olsen 1982; Maron 1983).

Intramyocardial vessels may show intimal thickening, particularly in the fibrous areas. These changes are likely to be secondary to fibrosis rather than primary in nature.

Histochemistry

Glycogen accumulation, particularly in the peri-nuclear regions, is often immense and is of diagnostic value. Succinic dehydrogenase, non-specific esterases, monamine oxidase, and phosphates are increased, probably due to the severe hypertrophy.

Electron microscopy

Disarray of myocardial fibrils coursing in all directions and an increase of inter- and intra-cellular connections is typical, forming a basket weave. This may explain the haemodynamic pathophysiology, namely failure of diastolic compliance. Nuclear changes of severe hypertrophy and focal accumulation of mitochondria (mitochondriosis), degeneration, and fibrosis complete the ultrastructural changes.

Hypertrophic cardiomyopathy with or without obstruction

At one time morphological differences were believed to exist in the distribution of the abnormal myocardial fibres, being confined to the thick septum if obstruction was present, and focally distributed throughout the myocardium if not. Complete overlap exists. Indeed, it has been questioned whether true obstruction is present.

Hypertrophic cardiomyopathy in association with other diseases

Hypertrophic cardiomyopathy has been found in association with other cardiac abnormalities, including hyperthyroidism, Friedreich ataxia, lentigenosis, and congenital heart disease. The aetiology is unknown. Genetic factors, hamartoma, increase in noradrenaline, abnormal muscle metabolism, hypertension, abnormal isometric contraction, and small vessel disease have been suggested.

12.10.4   Restrictive cardiomyopathy

At one time believed to be two separate entities, endomyocardial fibrosis was considered to be confined to the tropical and subtropical zones, whilst Loeffler endocarditis parietalis fibroplastica was believed to be restricted to the temperate zones and associated with eosinophilia. It is now known that both conditions are the same, irrespective of the geographical origin.

In the late phase of the disease the heart is hypertrophied and dilated with the brunt of the lesion appearing to have fallen on the endocardium, which is extremely thick. Left, right, or both ventricles may be involved. In left ventricular involvement, the inflow tract, the apex, and part of the outflow tract are affected. The posterior mitral valve leaflet, chordae, and papillary muscles may also be affected. The region below the aortic valve is usually spared. Thrombus is often superimposed. Fibrous septa extend into the myocardium. The coronary vessels are normal. In right ventricular involvement, the apex and an area beneath the tricuspid valve are affected. The apex becomes progressively obliterated (Olsen and Spry 1979).

Histopathology and pathogenesis

The thick endocardium is arranged in layers. Superficially, thrombus or fibrin is found, followed by a zone of dense collagen tissue. The deepest zone consists of loosely arranged connective tissue in which blood vessels and inflammatory cells, including some eosinophils, are seen. It is from this layer that the septa extend into the myocardium (Fig. 12.120a).

A retrospective study from cases in the temperate zone has shown progressive changes. With a short history of 5 weeks, on average, necrotic phase has been described, consisting of an often intense myocarditis rich in eosinophils and an arteriolitis. After an average duration of 10 months, the thrombotic stage is reached, consisting of frequently immense thrombus superimposition, some endocardial thickening (Fig. 12.120b) and a decrease in the severity of myocarditis. The intramyocardial vessels may contain thrombi. After 2.5 years (on average) the fibrous stage is found, which has been detailed above. Comparison of this stage with 75 hearts of cases obtained from the tropics showed no morphological differences. This permitted the suggestion to be made that both disease entities belong to the same disease spectrum, the origin of which could be traced back to the presence of eosinophils in the myocardium.

The cause of the eosinophilia was most frequently idiopathic, but in 25 per cent of cases the cause of eosinophilia could be attributed to asthma, Hodgkin disease, malignancy, and other acquired conditions. There are abnormal features in the eosinophils, consisting of vacuolation and degranulation. It has been demonstrated that if 15 per cent of eosinophils show degranulation, biopsy-proven cardiac involvement is invariably present.

Right ventricular arrhythmogenic dysplasia

This condition, characterized by severe fat infiltration, particularly of the right ventricle, is of unknown aetiology and can be classified under cardiomyopathies. The condition should be distinguished from Uhl's anomaly.

12.10.5   Specific heart muscle disease

Following the classification in Table 12.6, some of the conditions will be described. In many instances non-specific features are present in the heart. The various diseases are discussed under two headings: with or without diagnostic features.

Specific heart muscle disease with diagnostic features

Infective myocarditis

This may occur in association with endocarditis and pericarditis (see Section 12.9). Coxsackie viral myocarditis has been defined and classified in the section on dilated cardiomyopathy but the changes apply to any type of virus affecting the myocardium

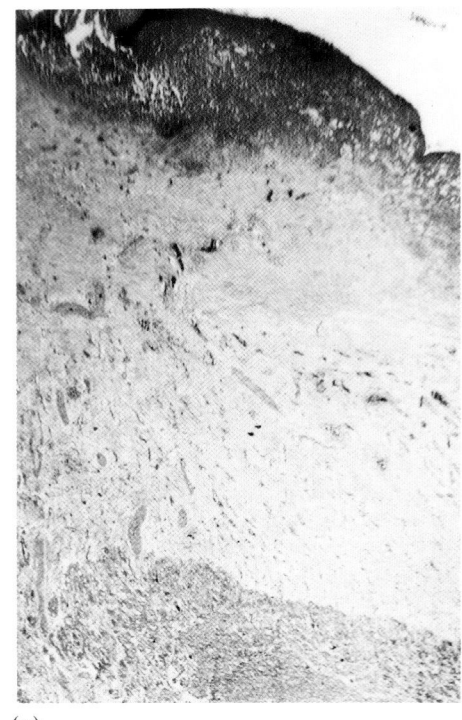

(a)

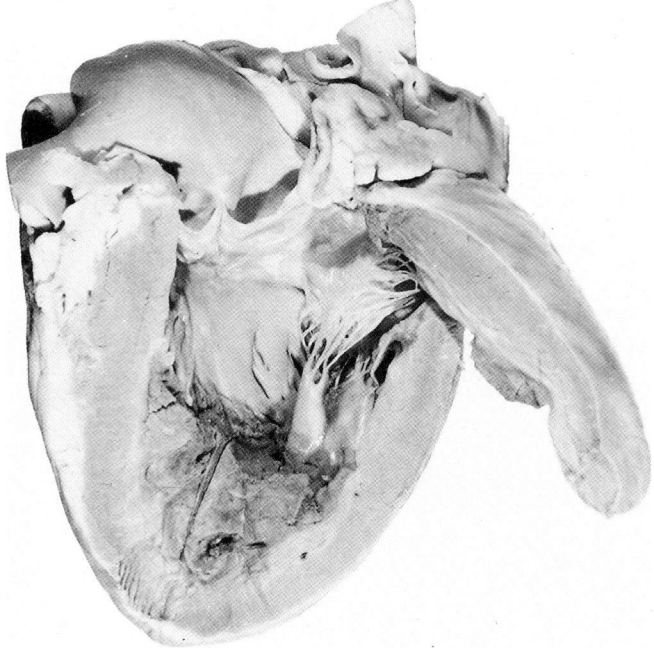

(b)

Fig. 12.120   (a) Endomyocardial fibrosis showing the histopathological features of the thick endocardium. Superficially, fibrin is superimposed followed by a layer of collagen tissue. The deepest layer abutting on to the myocardium is the granulation tissue layer. Note the septum extending into the myocardium. (b) A case of endomyocardial fibrosis in the thrombotic phase. The apex of the left ventricle is filled with thrombus; some endocardial thickening can already be noted.

Table 12.6 Specific heart muscle disease classification

Infective
  Viral myocarditis, e.g. coxsackie
  Rickettsial myocarditis, e.g. *Coxiella*
  Bacterial, e.g. staphylococcal
  Fungal, e.g. *Aspergillus*
  Protozoal, e.g. Chagas
  Metazoal, e.g. filaria
Metabolic
  Endocrine
    Thyrotoxicosis, hypothyroidism, adrenal cortical insufficiency, phaeochromocytoma, acromegaly
  Familial storage disease and infiltration
    Haemochromatosis, glycogen storage disease, Hurler syndrome, Refsum syndrome, Hand–Schüller–Christian disease, Fabry–Anderson disease, Morquio–Ullrich disease
  Deficiency
    Disturbances of potassium metabolism, magnesium deficiency, and nutritional disorders such as kwashiorkor, anaemia, and beri beri.
  Amyloid
    'Primary', 'secondary', 'familial': hereditary cardiac amyloidosis, familial Mediterranean fever, senile
General systemic diseases
  Connective tissue disorders
    Systemic lupus erythematosus, polyarteritis nodosa, rheumatoid arthritis, scleroderma, dermatomyositis
  Infiltrations and granulomas
    Sarcoidosis, leukaemia
Heredofamilial
  Muscular dystrophies
    Duchenne, dystrophia myotonica
  Neuromuscular disorders
    Friedreich ataxia
Sensitivity and toxic reactions
  Sulphonamides, penicillin, antimony, cobalt, emetine, alcohol, isoprenaline, anthracyclines, irradiation

and, indeed, to all other forms of myocarditis. Bacterial, fungal, protozoal, and metazoal forms of myocarditis will be described.

Bacterial myocarditis Any bacterial infection may affect the heart, particularly *Staphylococcus aureus*, haemolytic streptococcus, pneumococcus, meningococcus, *Haemophilus influenzae*, and spirochetes.

The hearts are usually hypertrophied and dilated. The myocardium is flabby and is often pale in colour. Streaky yellowish areas or microinfarcts may be discerned. Thrombus is often found; abscess formation can occur.

Initially a polymorphonuclear leucocyte infiltrate may dominate the interstitial infiltrate, later to be followed by lymphocytes, plasma cells, eosinophils, and mononuclear cells. Necrosis of myocytes is frequent in the acute phases and fibrosis is found in the later phases. Demonstration of the infective organism permits diagnosis. The morphological features are otherwise non-specific.

In tuberculosis, miliary, nodular, and diffuse morphological types are recognized. The condition is now rare.

Fungal myocarditis This type of myocarditis is rare but is found in association in patients on immunosuppresive agents, on chemotherapy, steroid therapy, or following irradiation or drug abuse. Any fungus may affect the heart, particularly *Candida*

and *Aspergillus*. Morphologically, nodules, white to yellow in appearance and up to 1.5 cm in diameter are typically randomly distributed in the myocardium. Microcolonies of radially arranged pseudohyphae, often in micro-abscesses, together with a chronic inflammatory infiltrate (which may be absent) are seen histologically.

In aspergillus myocarditis a fibrinopurulent infiltrate in the endocardium, extensive necrosis in the myocardium, and an acute inflammatory infiltrate are characteristic. Demonstration of the fungus permits diagnosis.

Protozoal myocarditis In toxoplasmosis, pseudocysts or macrophages crowded with the organism are found in areas of chronic inflammation within the myocardium.

'Chagas' disease is due to the transmission of *Trypanosoma cruzi* through the trimatid bug. The disease is confined to the South American continent. Three disease phases are recognized.

1. In the acute phase, pseudo-leishmanic cysts in myocardial fibres clinch the diagnosis. Myocarditis may be intense.
2. Little is known of the morphology in the latent phase, which may last 10–20 years.
3. The chronic phase is characterized externally by lymphoid hyperplasia and an apical aneurysm in up to 74 per cent of cases: fibrosis and chronic inflammation are usual but pseudo-leishmanic cysts are extremely rare; severe depletion of atrial neuronal cells is common.

Metazoal myocarditis Hydatid disease, usually due to *Echinococcus granulosus*, results in cysts located in any part of the heart inciting a strong fibrous reaction accompanied by some chronic inflammation. Calcification of cysts is frequent. Filariasis due to onchocerca incite an eosinophilic myocarditis. A causal link with endomyocardial fibrosis has been suggested.

Primary or isolated myocarditis

Three forms are recognized:

1. Diffuse myocarditis in which there is a mixed inflammatory infiltrate; the changes are non-specific.
2. Granulomatous myocarditis in which there are discrete giant cell granulomas scattered through the myocardium. Exclusion of granulomas of known causes is mandatory before the diagnosis can be made.
3. Giant cell myocarditis. In the mixed inflammatory cell infiltrate, giant cells of myogenic origin, of Langhans type, foreign body giant cells, and Touton giant cells abound. Association with thyroiditis has been reported.

Familial storage diseases

Haemochromatosis Macroscopically, brown discoloration giving a strong reaction to Perl's stain and fibrosis is found (Fig. 12.121a). Microscopically, iron deposition occurs at the nuclear poles extending longitudinally through the cardiac myocyte (Fig. 12.121b), resulting in necrosis of the fibre and

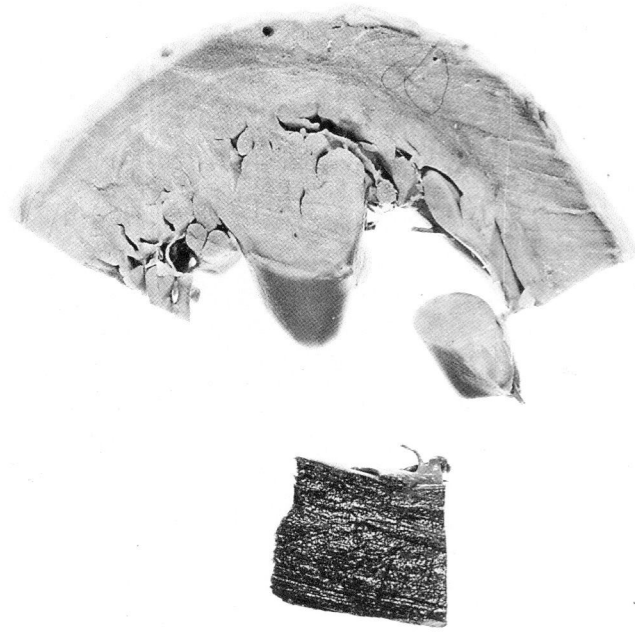

(a)

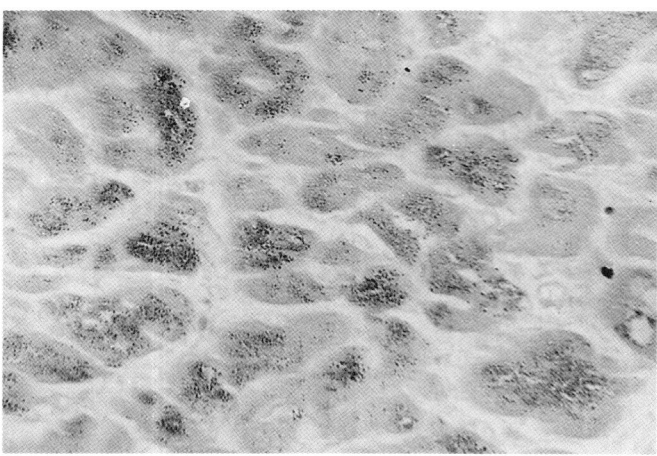

(b)

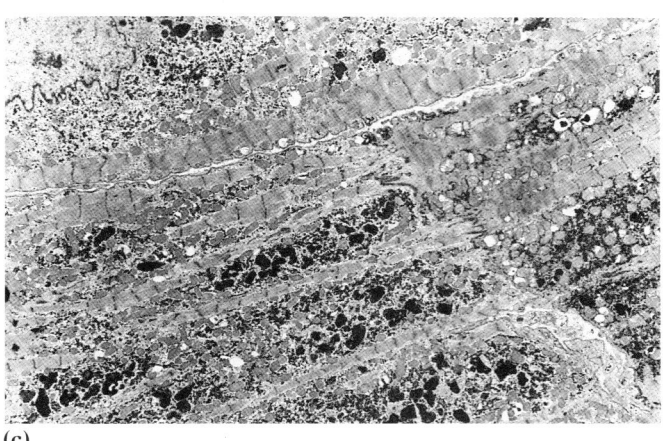

(c)

subsequent fibrosis. The conduction tissue may be involved. Valves and coronary arteries are spared. Electron microscopically, electron-dense particles of iron are located in lysosomes (Fig. 12.121c). The aetiology is unknown. Genetic factors and faulty iron handling have been suggested (see Chapter 17).

Haemosiderosis Transfusion siderosis is similar to haemochromatosis but necrosis and fibrosis is rare.

Glycogen-storage disease At least eight types of one or more deficiencies of enzymes involved in the synthesis and degradation of glycogen have been described. Heart involvement occurs in types II, III, or IV. In type II, Pompe disease, the heart is enlarged and microscopy shows a lace-like change in myocardial fibres. The 'empty' areas are filled with glycogen which is biochemically and ultrastructurally normal. Intralysosomal deposits of glycogen confirm the diagnosis electron microscopically. The defect is a deficiency of α1–4, glucosidase. In type III, glycogen is morphologically normal but biochemically abnormal; in type IV, abnormalities in both parameters are found.

Fabry–Anderson disease Deficiency of galactosidase A results in deposition of trihexosyl ceramide, especially in the mitral valve, left ventricle, and coronary arteries. Electron microscopically, osmophilic concentric laminar bodies in single-membrane-lined organelles are diagnostic.

Mucopolysaccharidoses Seven types of mucopolysaccharidoses have been described. Heart involvement occurs in Hunter, Hurler, and Scheie syndromes and in Morquio–Ullrich disease. Deposition of mucopolysaccharides (and glycolipids) occurs in vacuoles in myocardial fibres, in connective tissue, and in smooth muscle cells.

Amyloid

The heart is involved in the various types of amyloidosis (see Chapter 4). Macroscopically, the heart is overweight, firm, and has a glassy appearance. Myocardial, valvular, endocardial, epicardial, and vascular involvement occur. In the elderly it may be confined to the atria.

Microscopically, amyloid is deposited in a nodular form having a laminated appearance, or in a diffuse form distributed between fibres which often show necrosis. Areas of myocardium may eventually be replaced by sheets of amyloid. In the endocardium a stratified arrangement is typical. In valvular involvement extensive deposition beneath the covering endothelium may occur. The vascular walls are frequently affected (Fig. 12.122a). Microscopic recognition is by Congo red staining viewed with crossed polaroids (apple-green colour), methyl-violet stain (rose-violet), or thioflavine T under ultraviolet light

Fig. 12.121 (a) A slice of the left ventricle from a patient with haemochromatosis. The detached portion shows a positive Perl's reaction. (b) Photomicrograph showing iron deposition in the myocytes (black granules). (Perl's reaction.) (c) Electronmicrograph showing electron-dense iron deposition in lysosomes between myocardial fibrils.

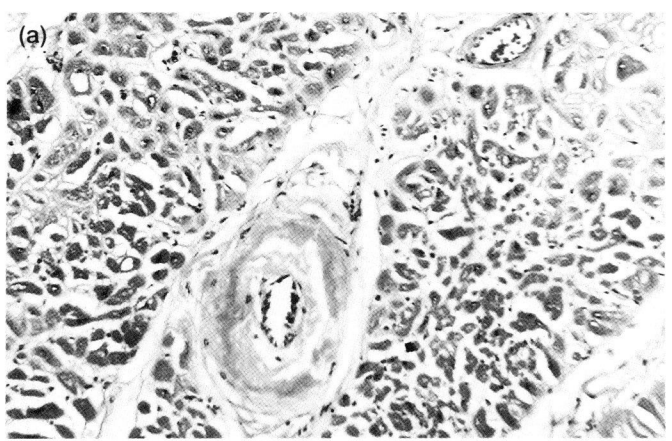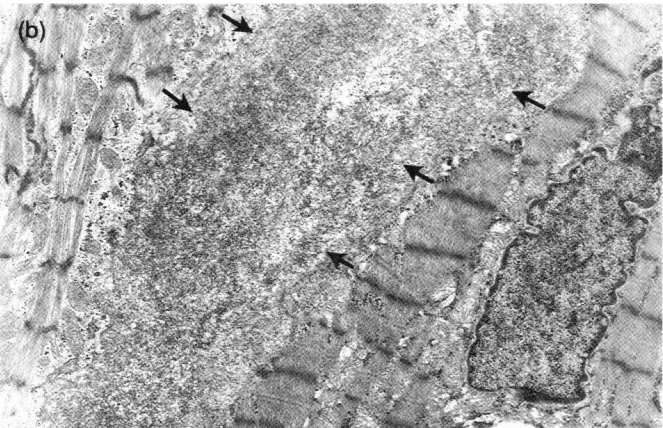

Fig. 12.122 (a) Amyloid heart disease having affected an arteriole (dark-staining material in the wall). The connective tissue (top right-hand corner of the illustration) also gave a positive reaction to Congo red. (b) Electronmicrograph of amyloid deposition clearly showing a fibrillar arrangement (arrows).

(yellow-green fluorescence). Good results have been reported with sodium sulphate–alcian blue (green staining).

Electron microscopic examination provides the definitive diagnosis, showing a fibrillary structure. Each fibril measures 5–30 nm and they are often laterally aggregated (Fig. 12.122b), with beading and a periodicity of 10 nm. They are located close to the basement membrane of muscle cells, blood-vessels, and connective tissue.

General systemic diseases

Heart involvement can occur in systemic lupus erythematosus, polyarteritis nodosa, rheumatoid arthritis, scleroderma, and dermatomyositis. These conditions are detailed elsewhere in this book.

Infiltrations and granulomas Leukaemic deposits and fatty infiltration are well-recognized conditions. In the latter condition, often in obese individuals, adipose tissue infiltrates the myocardium, particularly the right ventricle, leading to heart failure or even rupture. Microscopy shows fat cells insinuating between myocardial fibres, which may become atrophic.

Some granulomatous conditions have already been mentioned but sarcoidosis merits special mention. This systemic granulomatous disease of unknown aetiology affects many organs, including the heart (see also Chapter 13). This organ is usually overweight and dilated. Macroscopically, focal or massive involvement may be found, consisting of yellowish or white fibrous areas. Any part of the heart may be affected, especially the septum. Arteries and the conduction tissue may be involved. Microscopically, the lesions are discrete and resemble tubercles, though caseation is absent. Lymphocytes are fewer and giant cells larger. A histological classification into exudative, granulomatous, combined, and fibrotic forms has been proposed.

Specific heart muscle disease without diagnostic features

Endocrine diseases

In thyrotoxicosis, hypertrophy and heart failure may occur. In hypothyroidism basophilic degeneration of myocardial fibres is common, though non-specific. In phaeochromocytoma, myocytolysis, focal myocarditis, and glycogen accumulation may be found. In acromegaly, myocardial hypertrophy (not due to hypertension) and fibrosis is typical, often surrounding individual fibres which may become atrophic.

Deficiency diseases

Severe malnutrition, especially of protein, may cause kwashiorkor, resulting in small flabby hearts with dilation. Histology may show capillary dilation and interstitial oedema. In chronic anaemia, hypertrophy and dilation of the heart with 'thrust-breast' or 'tabby cat' appearances due to fatty change in myocytes may be found.

Beri beri This is due to deficiency of thiamine; it may also occur in chronic alcoholism, mimicking dilated cardiomyopathy. Endocardial thrombus, and extensive myocardial fibrosis may result.

Potassium deficiency This accompanies several diseases, including familial periodic paralysis, thyrotoxicosis, porphyrinuria, Faconi syndrome, and Conn syndrome. Diagnosis is achieved electrocardiographically. Extensive necrosis of myocardial fibres and focal inflammatory infiltrates have been described.

Keshan disease In certain regions of China, extending from the north-east to the south-west, selenium deficiency in the soil has been detected. The heart is frequently involved and morphologically resembles dilated cardiomyopathy. Haemorrhagic areas may be prominent.

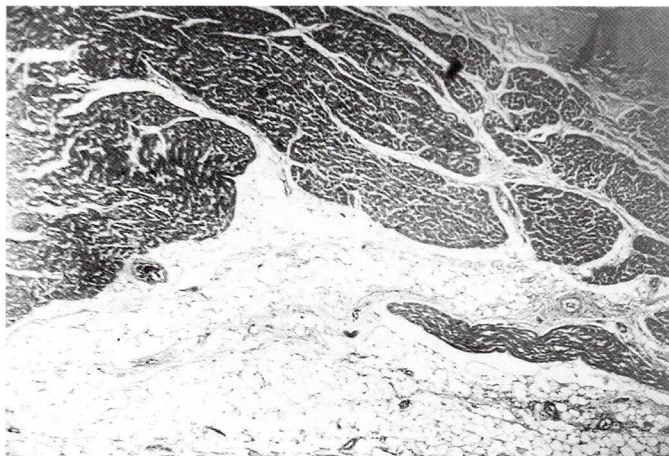

Fig. 12.123 A photomicrograph of the left ventricular myocardium from a patient with Friedreich ataxia. The left ventricular myocardium is extensely infiltrated with adipose tissue.

Carnitine deficiency also results in cardiac changes resembling dilated cardiomyopathy.

Heredofamilial diseases

Conditions such as muscular dystrophies, including Duchenne dystrophia myotonica, and neuromuscular disorders, such as Friedreich ataxia, show myocardial fibrosis, often band-like in the subepicardial region. Hypertrophy and extensive myocardial necrosis may be found. Fatty infiltration, in the form of adipose tissue, may be extensive, especially in Friedreich ataxia (Fig. 12.123). Small vessels may show intimal thickening, secondary to fibrosis.

Sensitivity and toxic reactions

Focal myocarditis, sometimes rich in eosinophils is typical; necrosis also occurs but these changes are not specific for any cause. In daunorubicin therapy nuclear changes of thick, intermediate, and thin filaments may be found, together with degenerative changes of the contractile apparatus.

After exposure to radiation, capillary damage resulting in ischaemic changes and fibrosis have been described.

Alcohol Alcohol abuse can lead to myocardial hypertrophy and dilatation morphologically indistinguishable from dilated cardiomyopathy. Many publications have described characteristic changes, including lipid accumulation in myocytes, all of which can be seen in dilated cardiomyopathy. However, distinction between the two conditions is possible on endomyocardial tissue obtained by bioptome using microenzyme analysis (Richardson and Atkinson 1980).

In beer-drinkers, hyaline necrosis and vacuolar degeneration in myocardial fibres has been noted as a result of excess cobalt. As cobalt content has now been reduced these changes are no longer seen.

For reviews of cardiomyopathies and specific heart muscle diseases see Olsen 1980 and Ferrans *et al.* 1987.

12.10.6 Bibliography

Amorim, D. S. and Olsen, E. G. J. (1982). Assessment of heart neurons in dilated (congestive) cardiomyopathy. *British Heart Journal* **47**, 11–18.

Aretz, H. T., *et al.* (1987). Myocarditis. A histopathologic definition and classification. *American Journal of Cardiovascular Pathology* **1**, 3–14.

Bowles, N. E., Richardson, P. J., Archard, L. C., and Olsen, E. G. J. (1986). Detection of Coxsackie-B-virus-specific RNA sequences in myocardial biopsy samples from patients with myocarditis and dilated cardiomyopathy. *Lancet* **i**, 1120–3.

Das, S. K., Stein, L. D., Reynolds, R. T., Thebert, P., and Cassidy, J. T. (1981). In *Congestive cardiomyopathy* (ed. J. F. Goodwin, A. Hjalmarson, and E. G. J. Olsen), pp. 87–93. Hassle, A. B., Molndal, Sweden.

Ferrans, V. J., Rodriguez, E. R., Tomita, Y., and Saito, K. (1987). *Pathophysiology of heart disease*, pp. 251–68. Martinus Nijhoff, Dordrecht.

Maron, B. J. (1983). Myocardial disorganisation in hypertrophic cardiomyopathy, another point of view. *British Heart Journal* **50**, 1–3.

Olsen, E. G. J. (1980). *The pathology of the heart* (2nd edn), pp. 178–99, 317–50. Macmillan Press, London.

Olsen, E. G. J. (1982). Myocardial disarray revisited. *British Medical Journal* **285**, 991–2.

Olsen, E. G. J. (1983). Myocarditis—a case of mistaken identity? *British Heart Journal* **50**, 303–11.

Olsen, E. G. J. (1985). *Hypertrophic cardiomyopathy*, pp. 1–18. Marcel Dekker, New York.

Olsen, E. G. J. and Spry, C. J. F. (1979). *Progress in cardiology*, Vol. 8, pp. 281–303. Lea & Febiger, Philadelphia.

Richardson, P. J. and Atkinson, L. (1980). *Myocardial biopsy, diagnostic significance*, pp. 97–101. Springer-Verlag, Berlin.

WHO/ISFC (1980). Report of the WHO/ISFC Task Force on the Definition and Classification of Cardiomyopathies. *British Heart Journal* **44**, 672–3.

WHO (1984) *Report of the WHO Expert Committee Technical Report Series E97*, pp. 47–50. World Health Organization, Geneva.

12.11   Pericardial disease

D. J. Evans

The pericardial sac is composed of connective tissue with a mesothelial lining. Its visceral layer is closely apposed to the heart, and in ordinary circumstances the cavity contains a small volume of fluid (about 30–50 ml).

The clinical manifestations of pericardial disease may take one of the following forms:

1. Precordial pain and a pericardial friction rub. These features are due to pericardial inflammation and may be accompanied by pyrexia.

2. Cardiac tamponade. The rapid accumulation of fluid within the cavity may interfere with venous return to the heart. This is particularly likely with haemorrhage into the pericardial sac, and in this case 200–300 ml of blood may be enough to cause death.

Tamponade may also occur with other types of effusion, especially those associated with malignancy or inflammation, but the quantity of fluid in the pericardial sac is usually much greater than in cases of pericardial haemorrhage. Even serous effusions sometimes present in this way.

3. Constrictive pericarditis. When pericardial fibrosis occurs, there may be interference with cardiac function which is usually due to impairment of diastolic filling. Although the features are somewhat similar to those of cardiac tamponade, the onset is insidious and signs of pericardial effusion are absent.

Effusion may occur in the absence of clinical symptoms and may be detected by imaging techniques, the most reliable of which appears to be echocardiography.

12.11.1 Pericardial effusion

Effusions may be of clear fluid, or may contain chyle, cholesterol, or blood.

Hydropericardium

Fluid accumulates in the pleural, peritoneal, and pericardial cavities in patients with congestive cardiac failure and in hypoproteinaemic states, such as the nephrotic syndrome. In these cases, the pericardial serosa is glistening and smooth and shows no evidence of inflammation. The effusion consists of a clear, translucent, straw-coloured fluid with a low protein content. The volume of effusion varies from case to case and is often several hundred millilitres.

An unexplained association of hydropericardium with myxodema has been observed.

Chylopericardium

This is a rare disorder in which the pericardial fluid appears milky due to the presence of chylomicrons. This is the consequence of leakage of lymph from the thoracic duct or its tributaries. It may be associated with congenital abnormalities, such as cystic hygroma or lymphangiectasis, but it may also be produced by traumatic rupture of the thoracic duct or injury to it during cardiac surgery. Tumour, tuberculosis, and thrombosis of the left subclavian vein are other documented associations.

Cholesterol-containing effusion

Although mentioned in most textbooks, this is extremely rare. About a quarter of the reported cases have been associated with hypothyroidism; tuberculosis and rheumatoid arthritis are other significant associations, but in half the cases the pathogenesis is obscure.

Haemopericardium

This is a fairly frequent post-mortem finding, most usually as a result of a ruptured myocardial infarct, or intrapericardial rupture of a dissecting aneurysm.

It may also follow trauma: this is most commonly a road traffic accident, but any direct wound to the heart may be responsible. In medical practice, intracardiac injections and attempted sternal marrow aspirations are occasional causes.

Rarely, haemorrhagic diatheses, malignancy, tuberculosis, or abscess may be responsible. Aneurysm of the coronary artery commonly presents by rupture into the pericardium, though it is, of course, uncommon.

12.11.2 Pericarditis

The classification of pericarditis is far from satisfactory. Because *in vivo* the material available for examination is an aspirate from the sac, there has been a tendency to categorize the lesions on that basis and to recognize serous, serofibrinous, fibrinous, purulent, haemorrhagic, or caseous pericarditis.

Serous effusions These are similar in appearance to transudates but they ordinarily have a higher protein content. They are associated with a pericardial inflammation, though this is usually only detectable by microscopy.

Fibrinous and serofibrinous pericarditis These differ from serous pericarditis in macroscopic appearances. Fibrinous exudates produce a characteristically shaggy appearance to the pericardial surfaces, sometimes described as 'bread and butter' pericarditis. Serofibrinous exudates are associated with a granular roughening of the serosal surfaces and strands of fibrin in the fluid. Microscopically, fibrinous and serofibrinous pericarditis appear similar. There is a surface deposit of fibrin (Fig. 12.124) and the underlying tissue shows dilated vessels. Scattered inflammatory cells may be present.

Purulent pericarditis This is associated with reddening and granularity of the pericardial serosa but the exudate varies

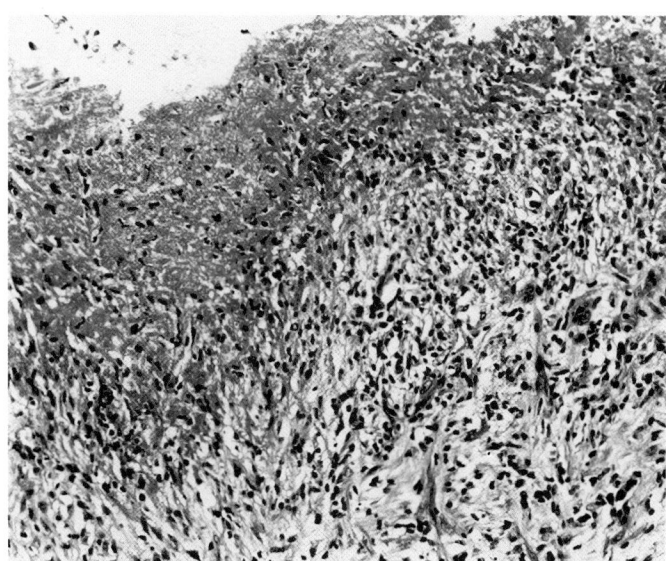

Fig. 12.124 Fibrinous pericarditis. There is a marked surface exudate of fibrin and deep to this the pericardium shows increased vascularity and a largely lymphoid infiltrate. In this instance the underlying condition was tuberculosis.

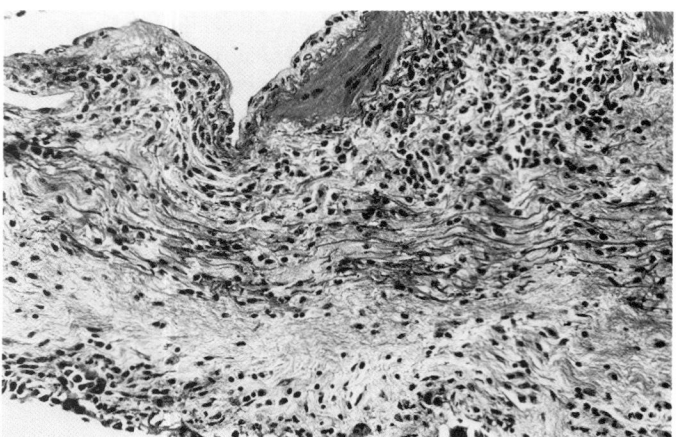

Fig. 12.125 Early purulent pericarditis. The epicardial layer is oedematous and contains many polymorphs. Some of these are penetrating between the mesothelial cells which show reactive changes. Macroscopically, the pericardial sac contained pus.

strikingly from case to case, both in volume and consistency, with the stage of the disease and the organism. Microscopically, the features are those of an acute inflammation (Fig. 12.125) with polymorphs in epicardial tissues. A surface exudate is usually present.

Caseous pericarditis This is sometimes seen in tuberculosis, but is not the most usual finding in that disease (see below).

Haemorrhagic pericarditis This differs from haemopericardium in that blood is mixed with an effusion. The pericardial appearances depend on the underlying causes: deposits of tumour or tubercles may be visible, though the latter finding is becoming increasingly rare.

The value of the above classification is limited by the fact that the same agent may produce different types of effusion. Thus bacterial infections may produce serous, serofibrinous, purulent, or haemorrhagic effusions. An alternative approach to classification on the basis of aetiology would be more satisfactory in theory. However, in some cases the nature of the disease process is not certain and in many cases the way in which the pericarditis is induced is obscure. Bearing in mind these limitations, we may recognize the following mechanisms.

Pathogenesis

Infections

Viral Sometimes chest pain and pyrexia lead to the discovery of a serous or serofibrinous effusion. Electrocardiographic changes, including arrhythmias, may be seen. Viral infections most commonly documented as associated are those of the coxsackie group, though others have sometimes been thought to be responsible, including adenovirus and echovirus 3. Proof of a causal association is difficult to obtain, expecially with common viruses such as infectious mononucleosis, mumps, and influenza. It seems likely that in most cases of viral pericarditis

there is associated myocardial inflammation (Proby *et al.* 1986).

A similar syndrome is sometimes seen in which no viral infection can be implicated—so-called primary pericarditis—though many such patients have clinical evidence (in the form of preceding URTIs) of a possible viral aetiology.

Bacterial This is frequently associated with clinically evident disease elsewhere and can be due to virtually any organism. The infection may reach the pericardium by surgical or traumatic means; as a part of a bacteraemic or septicaemic process; by lymphatic extension; or by spread from an adjacent organ, such as the lung.

On occasion the infection may appear primary: the organism usually involved is the meningococcus which may be presumed to have reached the pericardium during an initial bacteraemic phase. Initially, bacterial pericarditis may appear serous or serofibrinous, though it later becomes purulent.

Tuberculous pericarditis must inevitably be secondary to a focus of tuberculosis elsewhere in the body (usually the lung), but it is sometimes the dominant manifestation of disease (Strang *et al.* 1987) and, indeed, an active focus elsewhere may not be demonstrable. Like other forms of bacterial pericarditis, the features vary with the stage of the disease. Initially there is a fibrinous stage but this is followed by pericardial thickening and the development of tubercles (Fig. 12.126). At this stage there is an effusion which may contain lymphocytes as the predominant cell type. Later the pericardial thickening becomes more severe and caseation and tubercles more frequent, and eventually there may be fibrosis and calcification without residual tubercles. This sequence of events has been deduced from a study of many patients and should not, of course, be regarded as invariable in every individual; it should not be assumed that thickening fibrosis and calcification are pathognomonic of tuberculosis (see below).

Sarcoidosis has been observed to present with pericardial effusion. It may be argued that this is a disorder of unknown

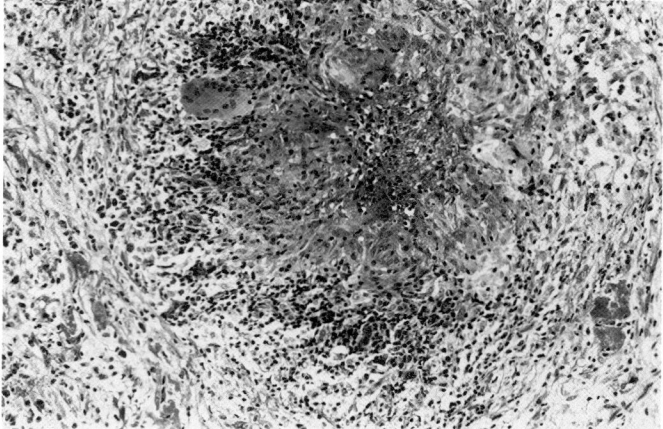

Fig. 12.126 Tuberculous pericarditis. A well developed tubercle in the deeper part of pericardium showing central necrosis and epithelioid and giant cells (from the same case as Fig. 12.124).

aetiology rather than an infection, and should not be included here: the subject is dealt with more fully elsewhere (Chapter 13).

Fungal These are uncommon. Coccidioidomycosis and candidiasis, and infection with *Aspergillus* have been described. Coccidioidomycosis leads to a granulomatous pericarditis. *Candida* and *Aspergillus* (Fig. 12.127a,b) are virtually restricted to immunocompromised subjects and pericardial involvement is rare as compared with pulmonary disease.

Others Hydatid involvement of the pericardium is a curiosity and toxoplasmosis is rare. Pericarditis due to percardial involvement from an amoebic liver abscess is a well-recognized complication present in up to 25 per cent of cases.

Pericarditis associated with 'immune-mediated' disease

A group of conditions exists in which the disease phenomena are accompanied by well-documented immunological abnormalities, although the exact mechanism of the disease is, in each instance, unclear.

Rheumatic fever This is dealt with elsewhere in more detail (Section 12.9). Pericarditis is present only in a minority of cases. Characteristically it is fibrinous or serofibrinous, and histopathologically the pericardium shows a mixed inflammatory infiltrate and Aschoff nodules. The disease has a clear-cut relationship to infection with β-haemolytic streptococci of Lancefield's group A, but the precise mechanisms involved are not determined.

Systemic lupus erythematosus (SLE) The classic description of these cases as 'collagen diseases' in the 1940s was of subserosal mucoid foci and fibrinoid necrosis. Subsequent studies of autopsy series also showed a high incidence of pericardial abnormality. There has, however, been a substantial change in the accepted view of the disease, which is now regarded as immune-complex-mediated, rather than as a primary disorder in collagen, and diagnostic criteria and management have changed substantially. In an echocardiographic study, only two out of 32 patients showed effusion, and clinical evidence of pericardial involvement is uncommon.

One of the problems with assessing the effect of SLE on the pericardium is that renal insufficiency is a common complication and pericarditis is a well-recognized consequence of uraemia.

Progressive systemic sclerosis and mixed connective tissue disease In progressive systemic sclerosis, evidence of pericardial involvement has been reported in more than 60 per cent of cases. Mixed connective tissue disease has been described as having associated pericardial effusion but the prevalence of this complication is not certain.

Rheumatoid arthritis In autopsy cases, pericardial fibrosis is frequent but fibrinous pericarditis and rheumatoid nodules are much less common.

Polyarteritis Pericardial lesions have been described in the Churg–Strauss syndrome but are otherwise uncommon in the arteritides.

Pericarditis associated with other conditions

Myocardial infarction After myocardial infarction, pericardial effusion may be demonstrated by echocardiography in between 40 and 60 per cent of cases. Symptoms of pericarditis are less often found (6–20 per cent). The effusion is often slow to resolve and is often demonstrable for up to a month.

In the 1950s Dressler described a syndrome in which pericarditis occurred as a late complication of myocardial infarction. There is controversy as to whether this syndrome is still seen clinically; it appears virtually to have vanished in Dressler's own hospital, and it has been suggested that it was related to the use of oral anticoagulants. It is of interest that it is still reported in centres using oral anticoagulants.

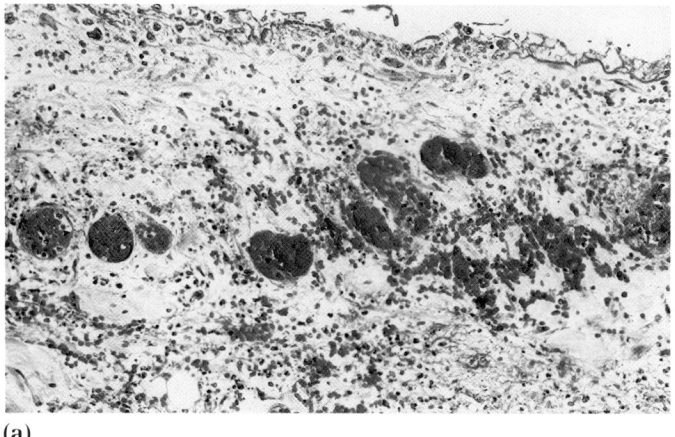

(a)

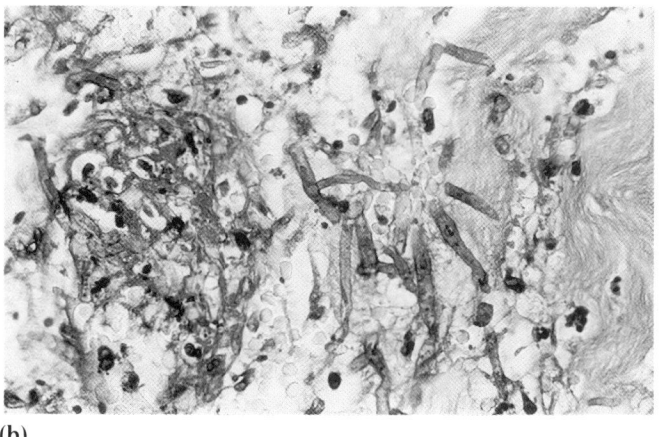

(b)

Fig. 12.127 Fungal pericarditis. (a) The pericardial surface shows reactive mesothelial cells and strands of fibrin. The deeper tissue is congested and shows nuclear debris. Hyphae of *Aspergillus* are difficult to see, but are easily visible on staining with periodic acid-Schiff (b) as branched septate hyphae.

Drug reactions Although pericardial reactions have been ascribed to several drugs—penicillin, phenylbutazone, and minoxidil—the evidence is less than convincing that the association is other than coincidental. With oral anticoagulants the evidence is anecdotal. Any effect observed might be due to the direct anticoagulant action of the drug, rather than a reaction to it.

Uraemia Pericarditis has been recognized as an accompaniment of terminal renal failure since the time of Bright, and although it is a less common finding now that renal replacement programmes are widespread, it is still seen in patients on dialysis. Although it is more commonly present in patients with poor control of uraemia, there is no direct relationship between its occurrence and the severity or duration of the uraemia.

The pericarditis is of the fibrinous type initially and, although it may resolve completely on therapy, cases have been reported which progressed to constrictive pericarditis.

Others A number of other conditions have been described as having associated pericardial effusion or pericarditis. In the case of inflammatory bowel disease, the finding is so infrequent as to cast doubt on the causal nature of the association. In the case of alcohol-induced pancreatitis, there is clear evidence on echocardiography that effusions are relatively frequent: however, in none of these cases was there clinical evidence of pericardial disease.

12.11.3   Chronic pericardial disease

Adhesions Although serous, serofibrinous, and fibrinous pericarditis may resolve completely, the latter may result in fibrous adhesions or even in complete obliteration of the pericardial sac.

Milk spots It is conventional to regard these focal patches of thickening as a consequence of local pericarditis, although they are so common as to throw suspicion on the view.

Constrictive pericarditis The clinical syndrome has been seen after a wide variety of insults to the pericardium. It has followed chylopericardium, coronary artery bypass surgery, rheumatoid arthritis, irradiation, sarcoidosis, and has been a late sequela of bacterial pericarditis. Although tuberculosis was formerly regarded as the major cause, this is no longer the case in Europe and the USA.

The histology is usually not of value in determining the cause. Fibrosis and calcification are the major findings and they are, of course, non-specific.

12.11.4   Pericardial tumours

Benign tumours

These are rare and of little clinical consequence. Pericardial cysts are unilocular cysts which contain clear fluid and are lined by mesothelium; they result from a developmental abnormality. Lymphangiomas and angiomas are occasionally

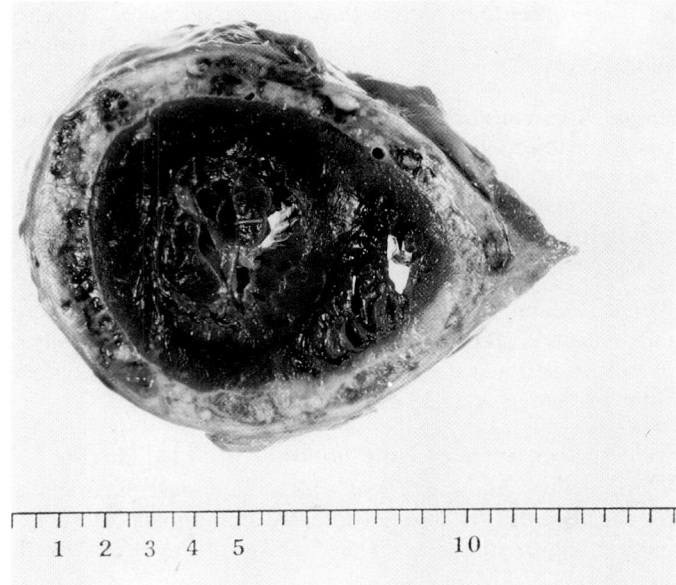

Fig. 12.128   Mesothelioma of the pericardium. Apex of the heart cut across to show tumour encasement of both ventricles by a primary mesothelioma.

recorded. Although lipomas also occur, it is hard to judge their frequency as they have excited little interest. Rarities and oddities reported include heterotopic tissue (thyroid, thymus, bronchial tissue), thymic neoplasms, and phaeochromocytoma.

Malignant pericardial tumours

Involvement of the pericardium by malignant tumours may result in a serofibrinous or haemorrhagic pericarditis. Most commonly, the tumour is metastatic with breast and lung the most frequent primary sites.

Mesothelioma may arise primarily in the pericardium but is rare. Although occasionally it forms a localized plaque, more characteristically it encases the heart (Fig. 12.128). Histopathologically it resembles the mesotheliomas of the pleura (see Chapter 13) and peritoneum.

12.11.5   Further reading

Lichstein, E., Arsura, E., Hollander, G., Greengart, A., and Sanders, M. (1982). Current incidence of post myocardial infarction syndrome. *American Journal of Cardiology* **50**, 1269–71.

Proby, C. M., Hackett, D., Gupta, S., and Cox, T. M. (1986). Acute myopericarditis in influenza A infection. *Quarterly Journal of Medicine* **60**, 887–92.

Rubin, R. H. and Moellering, R. C. (1975). Clinical, microbiologic and therapeutic aspects of purulent pericarditis. *American Journal of Medicine* **59**, 68–78.

Schiavone, W. A. (1986). The changing etiology of constrictive pericarditis in a large referral centre. *American Journal of Cardiology* **58**, 373–7.

Stanley, R. J., Subramanian, R., and Lie, J. T. (1980). Cholesterol pericarditis terminating as constrictive calcific pericarditis: follow-up study of patient with 40 year history of disease. *American Journal of Cardiology* **46**, 511–14.

Strang, J. I. G., Gibson, D. G., Nunn, A. J., Kakaza, H. H. S., Girling, D. J., and Fox, W. (1987). Controlled trial of prednisolone as adjuvant in treatment of tuberculosis constrictive pericarditis in Transkei. *Lancet*, 1418–22.

12.12   Tumours of the heart

Jeffrey M. Theaker

Primary tumours of the heart and pericardium are rare, whereas secondary tumours are common, being detected in approximately 10–20 per cent of patients dying with disseminated malignant disease.

12.12.1   Primary tumours of the heart

Approximately 75 per cent of primary tumours of the heart are benign, especially those arising within the left side. They are, however, of clinical importance since they can be difficult to diagnose clinically and, due to their position, can be life threatening. Almost any cardiac tumour can cause arrhythmias, sudden death, or cardiac failure.

Myxomata

These are the commonest type of primary heart tumour, accounting for about half of all benign tumours. They occur in all age-groups but most commonly present between the ages of 30 and 50 years. Although the majority occur sporadically, it has been noted recently that a small number of cases occur as part of a syndrome characterized by multiple lentigines, non-cardiac myxoid tumours, endocrine tumours, and a strong family history of cardiac myxomata (Vidaillet *et al.* 1987). Some of these patients have multiple cardiac myxomata.

The most common clinical presentation relates to obstruction to the flow of blood through the heart by these polypoid intra-cavity tumours, which often leads to the simulation of valvular disease, especially mitral dysfunction. Of note is that the murmurs produced are often variable and can be dependent upon the position of the patient. Myxomata are frequently friable and consequently embolic phenomena are the next most common mode of presentation. Since these tumours are most often located in the left atrium then embolism is generally systemic, and on occasion the diagnosis of cardiac myxoma is made following histopathological examination of surgically excised embolic material. Pulmonary emboli arising from right atrial myxomata are considerably more difficult to diagnose clinically.

Many patients with myxomata have general systemic constitutional effects, the cause of which remain unclear. These include fever, weight loss, anaemia, Raynaud phenomenon, raised erythrocyte sedimentation rate, and polyclonal hyper-gammaglobulinaemia.

In the past the detection of myxomata was difficult and often made either at autopsy or at operation for mitral valve disease. The introduction of echocardiography has enabled pre-operative diagnosis to be made in almost all cases, the most important factor being the consideration of this diagnosis.

Pathology

Myxomata can occur in any of the chambers of the heart but about 75 per cent originate within the left atrium and most of the remainder in the right atrium. In either instance, the majority are attached to the atrial septum in the region of the limbus of the fossa ovalis. Macroscopically, the tumours have a short, broad-based attachment to the endocardium and protrude into the cardiac chamber either as a mass of polypoid fronds or as a single, rounded, smooth-surfaced mass (Fig. 12.129). They generally have a soft, friable and gelatinous appearance, often associated with areas of haemorrhage and surface thrombus.

Microscopically, myxomata are characterized by abundant extracellular myxoid matrix, composed of acid mucopolysaccharides, enclosing collections of small polygonal, stellate, and spindled cells (Fig. 12.129). In addition, small blood-vessels and smooth muscle fibres can be seen and, commonly, there are degenerative features with areas of haemorrhage, thrombosis, calcification, and collections of haemosiderin-laden macrophages and other chronic inflammatory cells. Indeed, the latter

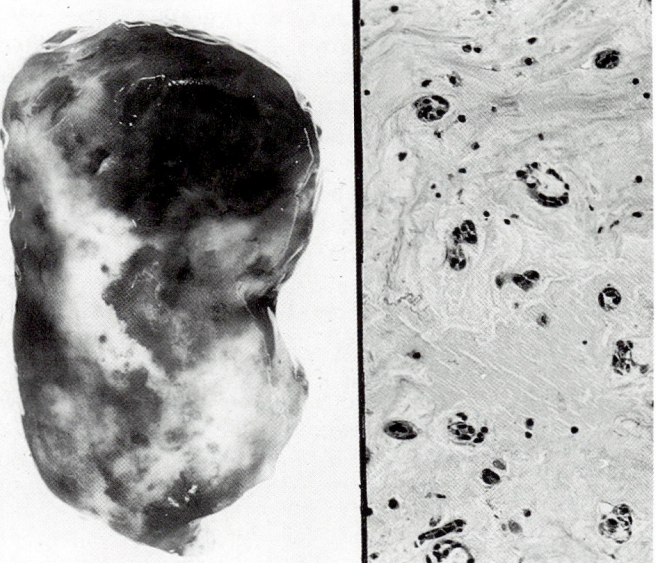

Fig. 12.129 This 115 g polypoid smooth-surfaced tumour was excised from the left atrium of a 78-year-old man who presented with pulmonary hypertension. The tumour was attached to the atrial septum by a short pedicle and herniated through a dilated mitral valve ring, causing blood flow obstruction and unusual heart murmurs. Histopathologically (right), the tumour had the typical appearance of a myxoma, with nests of small polygonal cells widely spaced by abundant myxoid matrix.

features have been used to support the theory that myxomata have a thrombotic origin, although the most commonly held view is that they are true benign neoplasms. Yet, the normal cell of origin of myxomata is still unknown despite careful study by light and electron microscopy and by immunohistochemistry. The multipotential mesenchymal cell of the subendocardium, endothelial cells, and neuro-endocrine cells are amongst those suggested as the cell from which these tumours originate.

Treatment of this benign tumour is by excision.

Rhabdomyoma

Cardiac tumours in childhood are even rarer than in adulthood, the commonest being the rhabdomyoma, which accounts for nearly half of all cardiac tumours in children less than 15 years of age. These tumours are commonly present at birth and are usually multiple. In approximately half of the cases the infant has other features of tuberous sclerosis. Three clinicopathological groups have been delineated. In some cases, large intracavity tumours are found in still births or in cases of neonatal death. In most of these cases other stigmata of tuberous sclerosis are not seen, although it is possible that they had not yet developed or were too subtle to be detected at autopsy. Such large rhabdomyomata can be detected antenatally by ultrasound examination of the fetus. In most of the cases clearly associated with tuberous sclerosis, the rhabdomyomata are small, multiple, and embedded within the myocardium, especially of the ventricles. In these cases there are usually few or no cardiac symptoms, the rhabdomyomata being found incidentally at autopsy and the clinical course being dominated by the other features of tuberous sclerosis. In the third group, the rhabdomyomata present symptomatically in older children without other stigmata of tuberous sclerosis, sometimes due to arrhythmias and sometimes due to obstruction to the flow of blood through the heart. These tumours can be successfully resected.

In all cases, the tumour consists of large, pale cells, some of which have a central cytoplasmic mass with thin extensions extending to the cell membrane, separated by glycogen-filled vacuoles (spider cells). Following careful examination, bundles of myofilaments showing cross-striations can be identified within the cytoplasmic masses, convincingly establishing the muscle origin of these lesions.

Since rhabdomyomata are commonly multiple, present at birth, and, in many cases, associated with tuberous sclerosis, it is thought that the lesions are not truly neoplastic but are hamartomatous in nature.

Other benign tumours

A number of common benign soft tissue tumours can also be found in the heart on rare occasions. These include fibromata, lipomata, haemangiomata, neurofibromata, and granular cell tumours.

Fibromata These are the second most common tumour type in children, are most frequently located within the ventricular myocardium, and can sometimes reach a large size and cause symptoms. Histologically, they are poorly cellular unencapsulated collagenous masses. The precise nature of these lesions is unclear. It has been suggested that they are hamartomata or alternatively, are part of the spectrum of fibromatosis.

Lipomatous hypertrophy of the atrial septum As well as simple lipomata, which occur very rarely in the myocardium, there is this unusual condition in which adipocytes, often of immature fetal type, accumulate diffusely within the atrial septum to form a large mass. Most examples are found in adults over 50 years of age, and although many cases are incidental autopsy findings, they do appear to be capable of causing arrhythmias or heart failure.

Papillary fibro-elastoma In addition to these common soft tissue tumours, there are several tumours more specific to the heart. The papillary fibro-elastoma (papillary tumour of cardiac valves) is an intracavity lesion derived from the endocardium, which appears macroscopically as an anemone-like structure with numerous long, thin papillary fronds. They may arise anywhere within the heart, although they are most commonly found on the valves, especially the aortic valve. Most cases are found incidentally at autopsy in adults. Histopathologically, the fronds recapitulate the normal structure of the endocardium, consisting of a fibrous core, containing elastic fibres, covered by plump endothelial cells. It is unclear whether these lesions are neoplastic, hamartomatous, or derived from thrombi. Similarly, the possible relationship to the very common valvular lesion known as Lambl's excrescence is controversial, although the distribution of these two lesions is somewhat different upon the valvular surface.

Mesothelioma of the atrioventricular node (congenital polycystic tumour). Rarely, a curious, small, poorly circumscribed nodule may be found in the atrial septum in the region of the atrioventricular node, in patients presenting with conduction defects or dying suddenly. Indeed, this is said to be the smallest human tumour capable of causing death. Microscopically, it consists of regular small cellular nests and tubular structures embedded within a fibrous stroma. The nature of these cells has also been controversial, with suggestions of an endothelial, endodermal, or mesothelial origin; the latter concept underlies one of the most commonly used names for this lesion—mesothelioma of the atrioventricular node. Ultrastructural and immunohistochemical study have provided clear evidence of an epithelial origin, although this does not distinguish between an endodermal or mesothelial origin. Morphological similarities to the mesothelial-derived adenomatoid tumours have been used to favour a mesothelial origin, although a recent immunohistochemical study (Fine and Raju 1987) supported an endodermal origin. Whatever their nature, it is believed that these lesions derive from 'epithelial-type' cells entrapped within the region of the atrioventricular node during fetal development.

Other 'tumours' On occasion, an intramyocardial cyst lined by respiratory-type epithelium, often with cartilage in its wall, may be detected, usually incidentally, at autopsy. Such endodermally derived bronchogenic cysts are also thought to represent a tissue heterotopia, following misplacement of tissue during embryogenesis. True benign teratomata, containing tissue representative of all three germ layers, have been described within the heart, and can reach a large size. Most have been described in young children.

Unilocular cysts lined by unremarkable mesothelial cells can be noted attached to the parietal pericardium. They are generally asymptomatic and are detected incidentally, either following chest radiography or at autopsy. Heterotopic thymic or thyroid tissue can also, on occasion, be detected within the pericardium.

Primary malignant tumours of the heart

Approximately 25 per cent of primary cardiac tumours are malignant, occurring predominantly in adults. The tumours tend to infiltrate freely through both myocardium and pericardium, and commonly produce large intracavity masses, such that blood flow is impeded. Since malignant tumours are more commonly right-sided than left-sided, one of the more common modes of presentation follows superior vena caval obstruction. Other modes of presentation include rapidly progressive heart failure, arrhythmias, and constitutional symptoms of malignancy. The prognosis, despite surgery, is very poor and at the time of death there is commonly direct spread outside the pericardium and distant metastases, especially pulmonary.

The most frequently diagnosed primary malignant tumours of the heart are angiosarcomata, rhabdomyosarcomata, and pericardial mesotheliomata. Other malignant tumours which have been documented as primary cardiac tumours, often in single case reports, include fibrosarcomata and malignant fibrous histiocytomata, malignant nerve sheath tumours, extraskeletal osteosarcomata, liposarcomata, synovial sarcomata, leiomyosarcomata, thymomata, and teratomata. Kaposi sarcoma occur in AIDS patients. The criteria used for the diagnosis of any of the sarcomata are identical to those used in general tumour pathology, such that the histological identification of an angiosarcoma depends upon the detection of vascular spaces formed from malignant tumour cells, and that of rhabdomyosarcoma upon the detection of cross-striations within the cytoplasm of malignant cells. Ultrastructural and immunohistochemical investigation may provide additional information regarding cellular differentiation. Even so, many tumours are so undifferentiated that they defy confident characterization.

Pericardial mesotheliomata are considerably rarer than their counterparts in the pleural and peritoneal cavities, and most commonly are of the spindle-cell rather than epithelial type. Since the tumour tends to encircle (see Section 12.11) and compress the heart or cause a pericardial effusion, the commonest mode of clinical presentation is with signs and symptoms of pericardial disease. Asbestos exposure is probably an important risk factor in their development.

Several examples of primary cardiac lymphoma have been described. By strict definition, the lymphoma should not involve any other organ other than the myocardium and pericardium since the heart is commonly secondarily involved in patients dying with disseminated lymphoma.

12.12.2 Secondary tumours of the heart

Metastatic tumours of the heart are common autopsy findings, and can be detected in up to 20 per cent of all patients dying of disseminated malignant disease. Essentially, almost any malignant tumour may metastasize to the heart. Numerically, the more common malignancies account for most cases, especially carcinomas derived from the bronchus, breast, and gastrointestinal tract. Furthermore, cardiac metastases have been reported in approximately 50 per cent of patients dying with disseminated lymphoma, leukaemia, and malignant melanoma. However, it is very much less common for the metastases to cause important clinical features during life, mainly because the clinical picture is dominated by other features of disseminated malignant disease. Tumour deposits, which may be only microscopic in size, may involve the myocardium or the pericardium, the latter being particularly associated with the development of a pericardial effusion. Cytological examination of a pericardial aspirate is commonly diagnostic in such instances. Myocardial involvement can lead to arrhythmias and cardiac failure, depending upon the size and location of the deposits.

The route by which a tumour reaches the heart is varied. Carcinoma of the bronchus and oesophagus, or pleural mesothelioma, may directly infiltrate into the pericardium and myocardium. Retrograde lymphatic permeation is a particularly important route of metastasis in carcinoma of the breast and bronchus, following replacement of the mediastinal lymph nodes by tumour, into which the lymphatic return of the heart also drains. In this instance, the patient commonly develops a pericardial effusion which may lead to life-threatening pericardial tamponade. Macroscopically, the pericardium may appear unremarkable or may show minor thickening only, yet histologically there is widespread permeation of pericardial lymphatics

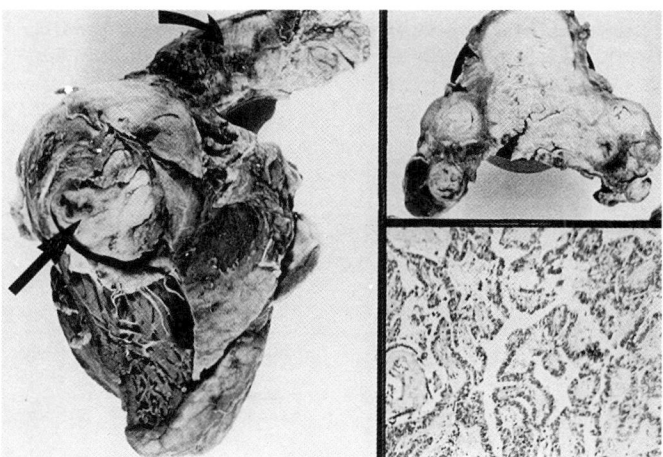

Fig. 12.130 A 40-year-old woman presented with superior vena caval obstruction. At autopsy, a tumour mass filled and distended the right atrium (straight arrow) and filled the superior vena cava (curved arrow). Tumour replaced much of her thyroid gland (top right). Histologically, this showed areas of papillary carcinoma (bottom right) admixed with areas of undifferentiated carcinoma.

by tumour, with focal pericardial invasion. At a later stage, there may be diffuse thickening of the pericardium which encases the heart, similar to a mesothelioma. Microscopically, tumours can also often be seen in lymphatics within the epicardium close to coronary arteries, and from here may then extend into the myocardium. Many intramyocardial metastases are haematogenous in origin; this applies particularly to malignant melanomata and lymphomata. In these cases the deposits are usually multiple. One of the less common, but more spectacular, routes of metastasis is by direct extension of a tumour via the vena cava into the right atrium. Most of these cases derive from a renal cell carcinoma, which commonly invades the main renal vein, but it is also occasionally seen in hepatocellular carcinoma, testicular tumours, and thyroid carcinomata (Fig. 12.130). Similarly, carcinoma of the bronchus may extend into the left atrium via the pulmonary vein.

12.12.3   Further reading

Davies, M. J. (1975). Tumors of the heart and pericardium. In *The pathology of the heart* (ed. A. Pomerance and M. J. Davies), pp. 413–39. Blackwell Scientific Publications, Oxford.

Fine, G. and Raju, U. (1987). Congenital polycystic tumor of the atrioventricular node (endodermal heterotopia, mesothelioma). A histogenetic appraisal with evidence for its endodermal origin. *Human Pathology* 18, 91–5.

Janigan, D. T., Husain, A., Robinson, N. A. (1986). Cardiac angiosarcoma. *Cancer* 57, 852–9.

McAllister, H. A. and Fenoglio, J. J. Jr (1978). Tumors of the cardiovascular system. In *Atlas of tumor pathology*, Fascicle 15, Second Series. Armed Forces Institute of Pathology, Washington, DC.

McCaughey, W. T. E., Kannerstein, M., and Churg, J. (1985). Tumors and pseudotumors of the serous membranes. In *Atlas of tumor pathology*, Fascicle 20, Second Series. Armed Forces Institute of Pathology, Washington, DC.

Vidaillet, H. J., Jr, Seward, J. E., Fyke, F. E., III, Su, W. P. D., and Tajik, A. J. (1987) 'Syndrome myxoma': a subset of patients with cardiac myxoma associated with pigmented skin lesion and peripheral endocrine neoplasms. *British Heart Journal* 57, 247–55.

12.13   Cardiac transplantation

Ariela Pomerance

12.13.1   Introduction

Although the first human heart transplant was carried out in 1967 (Barnard 1967) most centres (with the notable exception of Stanford) attempting this procedure rapidly abandoned it because of poor initial results. A decade later improved immunosuppressive drugs and the introduction of safe endomyocardial biopsy stimulated its revival, and heart transplantation is now an accepted treatment for end-stage heart disease.

12.13.2   The recipient heart

The overwhelming majority of heart transplants are for ischaemic heart disease and cardiomyopathy. Combining our experience from the two British transplant centres in 1975 (Pomerance and Stovin 1985) almost two-thirds of patients had ischaemic heart disease and almost one-third had dilated cardiomyopathy. Table 12.7 lists the recipient heart pathology in the first 500 heart transplants carried out at Harefield Hospital, UK. The less common pathology has included valvular and congenital heart disease, amyloid, adriamycin cardiotoxicity, and tumours. These conditions are fully described in this section.

The operative procedure for orthotopic transplantation involves joining donor and recipient hearts at the atria. Thus when received as surgical pathology specimens the upper atria and associated great veins and sino-atrial node are missing. Otherwise the recipient heart pathology does not really differ from post-mortem specimens.

Table 12.7 Original cardiac pathology in the first 500 heart transplant recipients at Harefield Transplant Unit (1980–8), UK

Ischaemic	Cardiomyopathies		Valve disease	Congenital	Other	
262	204		19	11	4	
	post-myocarditis	17			tumour	2
	adriamycin	7			trauma	1
	postpartum	6			arteritis	1
	restrictive	7				
	hypertrophic	6				
	amyloid	3				
	fibro-elastosis	4				
	familial	3				
	sarcoid	1				
	idiopathic	150				

12.13.3 Biopsy pathology

The introduction of safe and easy endomyocardial biopsies for monitoring rejection has been an important factor in the success of the present heart transplant programme. While microscopic examination of these tiny fragments is of undoubted value in identifying rejection, both pathologists and clinicians must be aware of the limitations. Rejection changes are patchy and focal. The heart is a large organ and biopsy samples are necessarily small. Even in deaths due to acute rejection, it is often easy to find biopsy-sized areas of subendocardial muscle without significant cellular infiltration in the post mortem sections. In practice though, if moderate rejection is present then even a single adequate biopsy fragment is likely to show diagnostic changes. The difficulties arise with minimal and mild cases where the chances of a positive biopsy clearly relate to the size and number of fragments of myocardium examined. Speigelhalter and Stovin (1983) calculated that with three negative fragments the chance of missing early rejection is about 50 per cent; four are needed to reduce the possibility of a false negative result to 2 per cent. Most centres now routinely take three or four fragments and cut multiple ribbons through them.

Acute rejection

The criteria for diagnosis and grading of rejection are still essentially those originally described by Billingham from the Stanford transplant unit (Billingham 1981, 1985).

Active acute rejection is characterized by a predominantly or entirely mononuclear interstitial and perivascular cellular infiltrate. The cells are large lymphocytes with cytoplasm which is lightly pyroninophic with methyl green pyronin (MGP) stains. Immunocytochemistry identifies the infiltrating cells as T-cells. In cyclosporin treated patients this population is a mixture of helper and suppressor cells. With conventional (i.e. azothiaprine and steroids) immunosuppression it consists mainly of suppressor cells (Weintraub *et al.* 1985; Rose and Yacoub 1987). Grades range from minimal, requiring observation rather than increased immunosuppression, through mild and moderate to severe, which (in our experience) is usually rapidly fatal.

Minimal and mild rejection

The earliest changes identifiable on routine haematoxylin and eosin sections are small, widely separated mononuclear cell infiltrates. Seen in cross-section they tend to form a 'necklace' of cells around individual myofibres (Fig. 12.131). The changes are often present in only one of several biopsy fragments and when sparse we grade the biopsies as minimal rejection.

Distinction between minimal and mild grades is entirely quantitative and therefore often rather subjective. In mild rejection the cellular foci are more numerous and larger than in minimal rejection, and oedema is often obvious. At the upper limit of mild rejection the cellular reaction cannot be distinguished quantitatively from moderate rejection and differentiation is based on the absence of obvious myofibre damage.

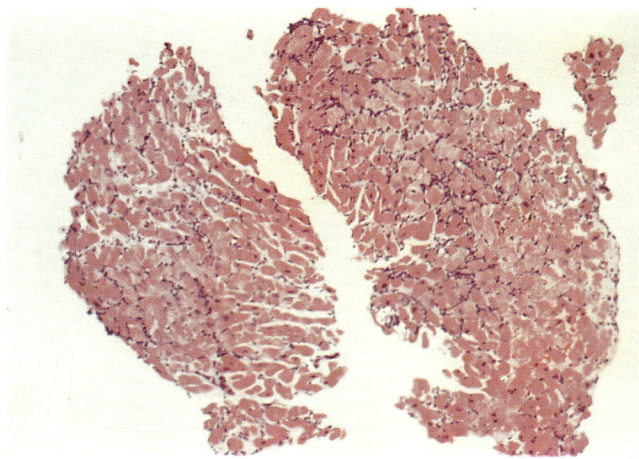

Fig. 12.131 Mild rejection. Focal mononuclear cell infiltration is present between myofibres. In cross-section the infiltrate appears as a 'necklace' around individual muscle fibres.

Moderate rejection

In moderate rejection (Fig. 12.132) cellular infiltrates are seen in all myocardial fragments. Although still focal, the foci are large, associated with oedema and often including polymorphonuclear leucocytes and occasionally eosinophils. The diagnostic feature is the presence of 'myocytolysis'. In the context of transplant biopsies this term refers to focal myofibre damage and disruption, not to the more traditional interpretation of myofibre vacuolation without cellular response. It is best demonstrated in PTAH-stained sections. Although the changes are striking, ultrastructural observations (Myles *et al.* 1987) suggest that they are not true necrosis, and normal structure is restored after treatment.

Severe rejection

In severe rejection (Fig. 12.133) frank myofibre necrosis and

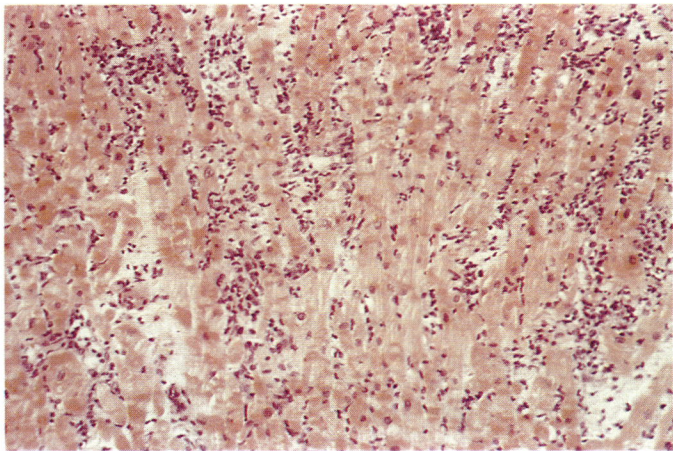

Fig. 12.132 Moderate rejection. Well-marked interstitial cellular infiltration and oedema involves the whole medium-power field and focal myofibre damage is present.

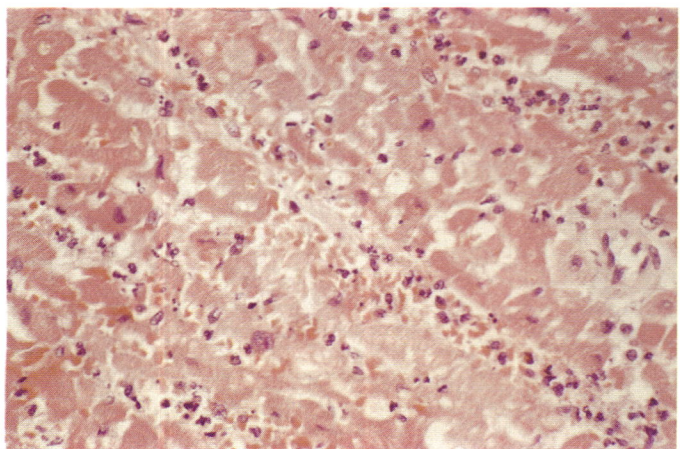

Fig. 12.133 Severe rejection. Well-marked myofibre necrosis with extravasated red blood cells and infiltration by both lymphocytes and polymorphs. This example is from a case of hyperacute rejection.

interstitial haemorrhage are added to the changes of moderate rejection.

Resolving rejection

With successful treatment, the infiltrating cells become fewer, smaller, and denser, pyroninophilia disappears and the interstitial oedema is replaced by loose connective tissue. Eventually the cellular infiltrate disappears completely and only fine focal interstitial fibrosis remains.

Persisting rejection

In cyclosporin-treated patients histological features of rejection are often seen for up to 3 weeks after treatment of the rejection episode. Beyond this period, if there is no evidence of resolution, biopsies are graded as persisting (ongoing) rejection.

Problems in interpretation of biopsy specimens

Because of the patchy distribution of diagnostic changes, at least three adequate sized 'bites' of assessable myocardium are needed for reliable assessment or exclusion of rejection. Often one or more of the pieces is not of suitable quality because of

1. fibrosis;
2. inclusion of previous biopsy site; or
3. presence of epicardial fat.

Large fragments of epicardial fat are not infrequent and may include pericardial surface mesothelial cells. Although evidence of perforation, this finding rarely has any clinical significance as the perforation is through the low-pressure ventricle and the pericardial cavity is usually obliterated by post-operative adhesions. Fibrosis merely reduces the amount of useful myocardium and is not a source of diagnostic confusion. However, biopsy sites and epicardial fat traumatized by surgery both include cellular reactions which may be confused with early rejection if the biopsy fragment includes just the edge of one of

these lesions. In most cases, examination of serial sections will reveal the underlying pathology and the MGP stain will show a high proportion of plasmacytic cells.

Effects of cyclosporin

The introduction of cyclosporin greatly reduced the incidence of acute rejection episodes and this drug is now the mainstay of treatment of almost all patients.

Although the established criteria for grading rejection still apply, we have not seen any biopsies which met all the criteria for severe rejection changes since cyclosporin was introduced. With the exception of hyperacute rejection, the rejection changes in patients on cyclosporin develop more slowly than in patients on conventional immunosuppression and minor episodes may resolve without any increase in immunosuppression. Indeed, about half the Stanford unit's patients with biopsy changes that had been graded as mild rejection had no evidence of rejection on the next biopsy even if untreated (Imakita *et al.* 1986). The microscopic changes of rejection also take longer to resolve than in conventionally immunosuppressed patients. Biopsies taken up to 3 weeks after an acute rejection episode may still show active rejection changes even though the patient's clinical response to treatment has been satisfactory.

A characteristic finding in many patients treated with cyclosporin is development of a dense endocardial mononuclear cell infiltrate (Fig. 12.134). This is predominantly lymphocytic, containing helper and suppressor T-cells in the same proportions as in the peripheral blood (Rose and Yacoub 1987). This finding seems unrelated to rejection, but the cells often infiltrate a short distance between the subendocardial myofibres and this may cause confusion if a biopsy fragment includes infiltrated subendocardial muscle without the diagnostic endocardium. The nature of this endocardial pathology is still not clear, although early cases tended to be associated with high blood cyclosporin levels. Once established, the condition does not seem to regress.

A specific type of fine interstitial fibrosis is associated with

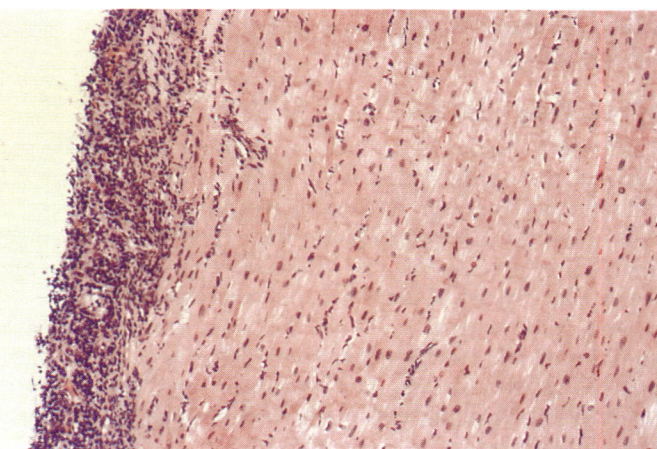

Fig. 12.134 Cyclosporin effect. A dense, band-like mononuclear cell infiltrate is present on the endocardial surface.

cyclosporin therapy. Electron microscopy showed this to consist of collagen (Billingham 1985). It was seen in a high proportion of the Stanford unit's patients but is dose-dependent and is now less evident with the lower cyclosporin levels currently used.

Other biopsy abnormalities

Previous biopsy sites

Heart transplant patients initially have several fragments of myocardium removed from their right ventricles at weekly intervals. It is therefore only to be expected that healing biopsy sites are frequently re-biopsied. Microscopically (Fig. 12.135) the appearances range from a patch of fresh thrombus over an endocardial defect, with early organization, to a small fibrous subendocardial scar with surrounding myofibres that have lost their normal parallel orientation. Inclusion of the edge of a recent lesion in a biopsy fragment may cause diagnostic problems, but the cells do not have the pyroninophilia of immunologically active lymphocytes and the serial sections usually disclose the previous biopsy site features.

Solitary granulomas

Small sub-endocardial giant cell lesions (Fig. 12.136) are occasionally seen in patients with no evidence of systemic disease. Some are clearly of foreign-body type and foreign material can often be identified, presumably introduced at a previous biopsy. Others are less specific and their nature undetermined.

Calcification

Focal calcification of isolated myofibres and small endocardial calcified foci have been seen in about 2 per cent of our patients, sometimes persisting over several months. The aetiology is obscure. We have found no correlation with recipient or donor age, cause of donor death, or ischaemic time. This finding does not appear to have any prognostic significance.

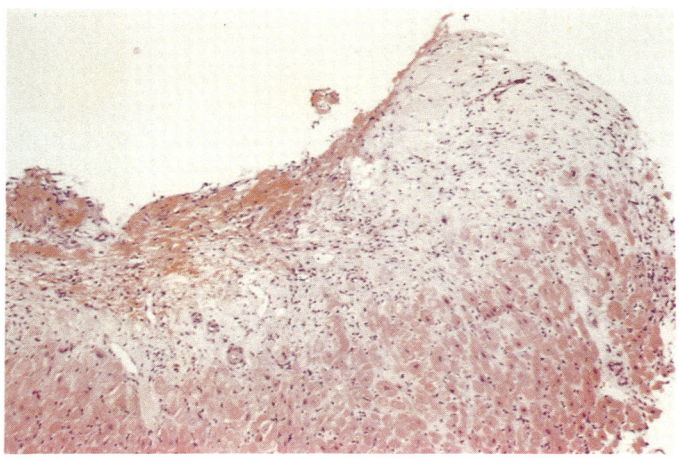

Fig. 12.135 Previous biopsy site. Subendocardial cellular infiltration, granulation tissue, and early fibrosis are present deep to a patch of adherent thrombus. Some cellular infiltration extends between the underlying myofibres.

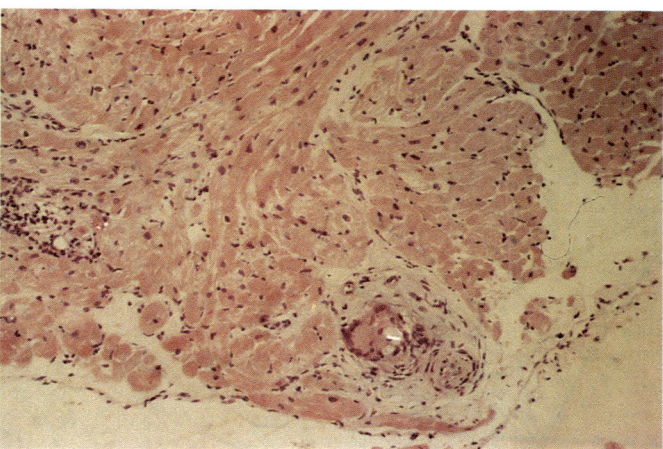

Fig. 12.136 Foreign-body granuloma in the subendocardium. Birefringent particles are present in the multinucleate giant cell.

Toxoplasma and other infective agents

Toxoplasma cysts and evidence of cytomegalovirus or fungus infection occasionally appear in a biopsy fragment. They may well only be seen in a few of the levels and the entire specimen should be examined very carefully if infection is suspected.

Chronic rejection

This term is generally applied to the coronary artery narrowing that develops in a high proportion of long-term cardiac transplant survivors. Some two-thirds of patients from the pre-cyclosporin era have developed angiographic evidence of coronary insufficiency or have died of coronary artery disease by the fourth post-operative year. The incidence is lower in patients treated with cyclosporin but is still about 25 per cent by the end of the fourth year (Reid 1988).

It is still not entirely clear why some patients develop the condition and not others. While most patients with chronic rejection were transplanted for ischaemic heart disease this is also the predominant pathology in heart transplant patients as a whole; there is no significant correlation between chronic rejection and the type of recipients' cardiac disease, triglyceride levels, or age. Donor age did, however, correlate with the development of chronic rejection, as did the number of rejection episodes (Reid 1988).

Chronic rejection is essentially post-mortem pathology, which is described below. Routine endomyocardial biopsies may show small foci of fibrosis and cellular infiltration but these are non-specific. Rarely an intramyocardial artery with intimal proliferation is included but the characteristic pathology occurs in the larger coronary artery branches; therefore endomyocardial biopsy is unhelpful in the diagnosis of chronic rejection.

12.13.4 Post-mortem transplant pathology

Apart from perioperative multisystem failure, almost all transplant recipient deaths have been due, predictably, to infection or rejection.

Infection

In our experience infection is mainly seen during the first few months after operation and has been uncommon after the first year. The pattern of infection is similar to that in other causes of immunodeficiency; infecting organisms are often multiple and commonly include *Candida* and other fungi and cytomegalovirus.

Rejection

Deaths from rejection have occurred at all stages from within 24 hours to over 7 years post-transplant. Rejection presents in hyperacute, acute, and chronic forms. Acute rejection deaths have mainly occurred during the first three postoperative months. The term hyperacute is used for the small number of patients who developed fulminating acute rejection shortly after operation. Most have had cytotoxic antibodies. Chronic rejection refers to the accelerated coronary atherosclerosis which has been responsible for most deaths after the first postoperative year.

In acute rejection the heart is overweight with a characteristic firm 'beefy' feel. On opening there is usually fine purple and yellow mottling under the ventricular endocardium and a sharp demarcation between normal recipient and intensely congested donor atrium at the anastomotic suture line. On section the myocardium is dark, often with fine yellow mottling. Microscopically the features are those of severe rejection, with numerous large foci of cellular infiltration, myofibre necrosis, and interstitial haemorrhage. In the hyperacute rejection cases haemorrhage has been more striking and the cellular infiltrate has included a high proportion of polymorphs (Fig. 12.133). Coronary arteries of all sizes may also show a well-marked mononuclear cell infiltrate in media, intima, and adventitia.

In chronic rejection the most striking macroscopic feature is thickening of the epicardial and large intramyocardial coronary artery branches (Fig. 12.137). The thickening is concentric, often strikingly yellow but without calcification or haemorrhagic occlusion. Microscopically (Fig. 12.138) there is marked concentric intimal fibroblastic proliferation. The thickened intima may contain lipid, and very rarely a little powdery calcification, but does not resemble the usual picture of spontaneous coronary atherosclerosis. In our experience the changes of chronic rejection are virtually confined to large coronary artery branches; involvement of small arteries by either cellular infiltration or intimal proliferation is unusual.

12.13.5 Non-cardiac cyclosporin-associated pathology

Lymphoproliferative disease

Lesions histologically indistinguishable from malignant lymphoma have been recognized in renal transplant patients since at least 1980 and similar pathology followed the introduction of cyclosporin into the routine treatment of heart transplant patients (Beveridge *et al.* 1984; Lancet 1984; Starzl *et al.*

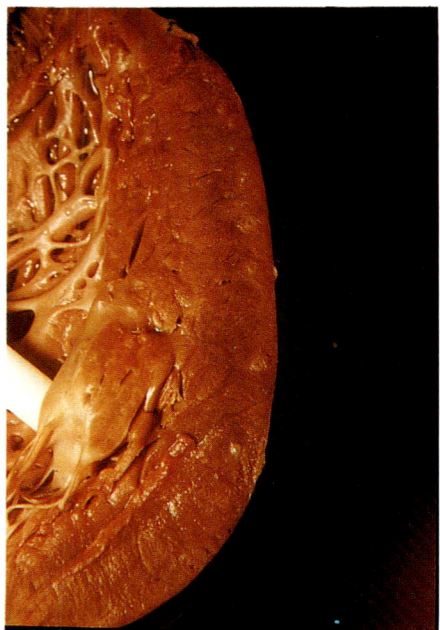

Fig. 12.137 Chronic rejection 3 years after transplantation. Thickened large intramyocardial arteries are seen on the cut surface of the left ventricle.

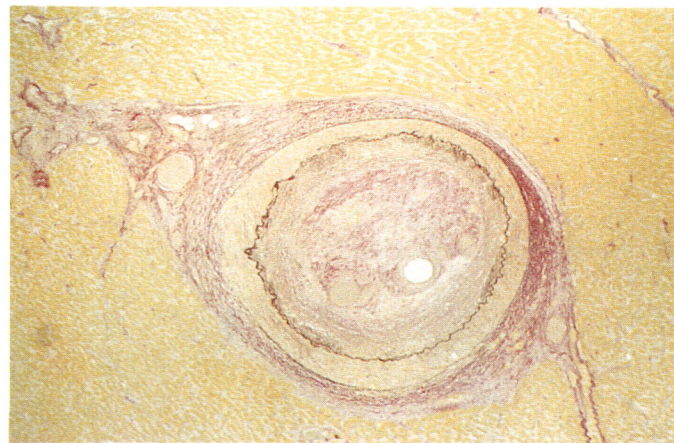

Fig. 12.138 Section of one of the thickened arteries shows almost complete occlusion of the lumen by fairly loose connective tissue. (van Gieson stain.)

1984). Unlike true malignant lymphomas, however, the lesions regress completely if cyclosporin is sufficiently reduced.

'Lymphomas' in cyclosporin-treated patients are associated with Epstein–Barr (EB) virus infection, either previously present in the recipient or, as in three of our cases, acquired from EB-positive organ donors. It is thought that cyclosporin's specific inhibitory action on suppressor T-cells affects the T-cells which restrain proliferation of the virus-infected B-lymphocytes (Nagington and Gray 1980). The condition develops in only a small proportion of cases. In our series it has appeared in three heart and two heart–lung transplant patients; an incidence of less than 1 per cent. All lesions regressed after cyclosporin was reduced. The incidence has been similar in the Papworth unit's patients, where two cases were found at post-mortem and the third is still alive almost 4 years after diagnosis (Stovin 1991, personal communication). The lesions are usually extranodal, becoming clinically apparent between 3 and 6 months after transplant. The microscopic appearances are those of non-Hodgkin B-cell lymphoma.

In spite of the histopathological features and the fact that most of these lesions are monoclonal, they are difficult to accept as true malignant lymphomas, if only because of the ease with which they can be made to regress. Although monoclonality is generally regarded as a hallmark of lymphoma, experimental studies have shown that monoclonal cell lines eventually result from polyclonal EB-virus-infected B-lymphocytes without developing neoplastic behaviour (Lancet 1984). For the present the term 'cyclosporin associated lymphoproliferative disease' seems preferable to lymphoma.

Gingival hyperplasia

This side-effect of cyclosporin treatment is common in transplant patients (Wysocki et al. 1983). It has affected about a quarter of our heart and heart–lung cases, developing between 3 weeks and 1 year after starting treatment (Seymour 1991, personal communication). The clinical picture and histological features are similar to those of phenytoin-associated hyperplasia (see Chapter 14), with elongated, attenuated rete ridges and marked submucosal fibroblastic proliferation and patchy, dense plasma-cell infiltration.

12.13.6   Bibliography

Barnard, C. N. (1967). A human cardiac transplant: and interim report of a successful operation performed at Groote Schuur Hospital, Cape Town. *South African Medical Journal* **41**, 1257–74.

Beveridge, T., Krupp, P., and McKibbin, C. (1984). Lymphomas and lymphoproliferative lesions developing under Cyclosporin therapy. *Lancet* **i**, 788.

Billingham, M. E. (1981). Diagnosis of cardiac rejection by endomyocardial biopsy. *Journal of Heart Transplantation* **1**, 25–30.

Billingham, M. E. (1985). Endomyocardial biopsy detection of acute rejection in cardiac allograft recipients. *Heart-Vessels* **1** (Suppl.), 86–90.

Imakita, M., Tazelaar, H., and Billingham, M. E. (1986). Heart allograft rejection under varying immunosuppressive protocols as evaluated by endomyocardial biopsy. *Journal of Heart Transplantation* **5**, 279–85.

Karch, S. and Billingham, M. E. (1985). Cyclosporin induced myocardial fibrosis: a unique controlled case report. *Journal of Heart Transplantation* **4**, 210–12.

Leading Article (1984). Lymphoma in organ transplant recipients. *Lancet* **i**, 601–3.

Myles, J. L., et al. (1987). Reversibility of myocyte injury in moderate and severe acute rejection in cyclosporin-treated cardiac transplant patients. *Archives of Pathology and Laboratory Medicine* **111**, 947–52.

Nagington, J. and Gray, J. (1980). Cyclosporin A immunosuppression, Epstein–Barr antibody, and lymphoma. *Lancet* **i**, 537.

Pomerance, A. and Stovin, P. G. I. (1985). Heart transplant pathology: the British experience. *Journal of Clinical Pathology* **38**, 146–59.

Reid, C. (1988). Chronic rejection in heart transplant patients, in preparation.

Rose, M. L. and Yacoub, M. H. (1987). The immunology of cardiac rejection in man. In *Immunology and molecular biology of cardiovascular diseases* (ed. C. J. F. Spry), pp. 177–97. MTP Press, Lancaster.

Speigelhalter, D. J. and Stovin, P. G. I. (1983). An analysis of repeated biopsies following cardiac transplantation. *Statistics in Medicine* **2**, 33–40.

Starzl T. E., et al. (1984). Reversibility of lymphomas and lymphoproliferative lesions developing under cyclosporin-steroid therapy. *Lancet* **i**, 583–7.

Weintraub, D., Masek, M., and Billingham, M. E. (1985). The lymphocyte subpopulations in cyclosporin-treated human heart rejection. *Journal of Heart Transplantation* **4**, 213–16.

Wysocki, G. P., Gretzinger, H. A., Laupacis, A., Ulan, R. A., and Stiller, C. R. (1983). Fibrous hyperplasia of the gingiva: a side effect of cyclosporin A therapy. *Oral Surgery* **55**, 275–8.

12.14   Aortocoronary bypass grafts

Sally P. Allwork

12.14.1   Introduction

Surgical operations to replace segments of arteries began about 100 years ago when the German surgeon, Gluck, used a vein graft in the carotid artery of a patient.

Operations to relieve angina by increasing the blood supply to the heart are among the commonest surgical procedures undertaken in the Western world at the present time. Unlike most surgical operations, they are palliative only, and do little or nothing to eliminate the underlying disease. Thus the hearts of patients coming to necropsy, either early or late after operation, may demonstrate both changes in the grafts themselves and, in the case of late death, there is almost always progression of the ischaemic myocardial disease (Fig. 12.139).

For a detailed account of the gross post-mortem appearances and early and late changes after operation, see Allwork (1991).

12.14.2   Bypass grafts

The long saphenous vein is commonly used to bypass an occluded or obstructed segment of coronary artery. However, the internal thoracic artery (usually called the 'internal mammary artery') is being used increasingly as the long-term patency is superior to that of veins. If neither of these is usable, arm veins, preserved umbilical veins, or man-made grafts must suffice. Saphenous veins are unsuitable as grafts if major varices are present, and the diameter of the internal mammary artery is usually too small in women to be usable. The internal thoracic artery is seldom used in old or obese people, as the dissection to

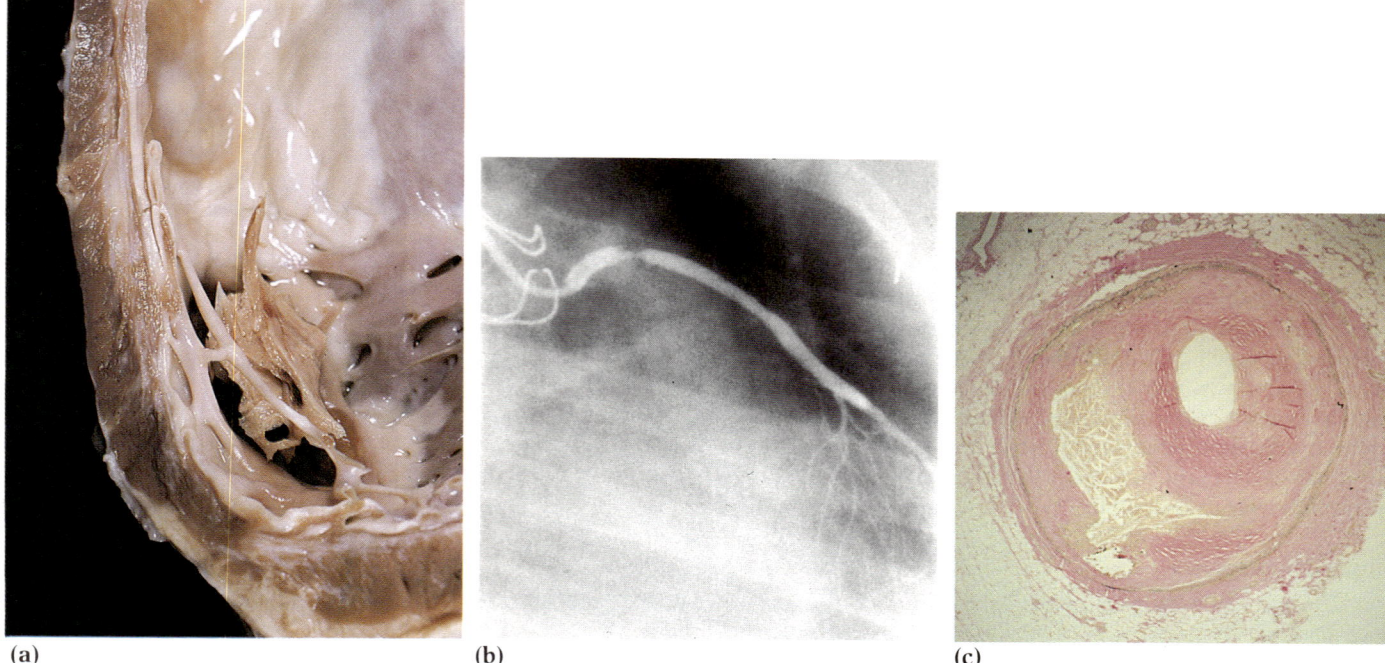

(a)   **(b)**   **(c)**

Fig. 12.139 (a) Apex of the left ventricle 3 years after triple bypass grafts. The grafts were widely patent, but there is marked fibrosis of the left ventricle as well as endocardial fibro-elastosis. (b) Cineangiocardiogram of a saphenous vein graft to the anterior descending branch of the left coronary artery, 7 years after grafting. There is an approximately 90 per cent stricture of the graft near its proximal insertion and other minor irregularities are seen along its length. The native artery at the distal anastomosis is patent, but there is a 'blush' of collateral vessels near the anastomosis. (c) Same patient as in (b). Section through a graft to the right coronary artery. There is both intimal hyperplasia and progression of the disease. The fibrous tissue cap is fissured, permitting the entry of phospholipids, giving the characteristic appearance of 'cholesterol clefts' between '7 o'clock and 11 o'clock'. (Elastic van Gieson stain.)

prepare it carries some morbidity, especially bleeding. Old age and obesity considerably enhance bleeding.

12.14.3   Graft failure

Early failure

In the early postoperative period the commonest cause of graft failure is poor 'run-off'. If the artery to be grafted is disproportionately small, or if there is downstream obstruction, myocardial infarction (sometimes very extensive), and/or thrombotic occlusion of the graft results at the distal anastomosis. Occlusion of the proximal (aortic) anastomosis by thrombus is rare. This is partly because the patients are anticoagulated in the early postoperative period. It is this, together with very early mobilization after such operations, which accounts for the very small incidence of pulmonary embolization in these patients.

When death occurs within a month of operation, areas of myocardial necrosis occur in the subendocardium of the left ventricle; necrosis is often proximate to haemorrhagic sites in up to a quarter of cases. Foci of contraction band necrosis and myocytolysis are scattered throughout the myocardium. Foci of both myocytolysis and necrosis occur in all hearts following cardiopulmonary bypass, so that this finding is not peculiar to graft operations.

Graft failure due to technical problems, such as kinking of a too long graft or dehiscence, are now very rare complications of this common operation. However, a small gap in the suture line, or a stitch cutting out may produce a relatively large false aneurysm. Localized dissecting aneurysms occur with relative frequency in both the artery and the vein at the distal anastomosis and may cause intraluminal obstruction.

Sepsis, although rare, may cause rupture and consequent haemorrhage at the site of the distal anastomosis. Aortocoronary bypass grafts do not predispose to infective endocarditis.

Late failure

Although the risk of occlusion of the graft due to acute thrombosis is permanent, as time from the operation advances the chances of graft failure due solely to thrombus recede, so that by the end of the first year it is uncommon. Instead, the graft may become narrowed or even occluded by diffuse fibrous thickening of the intimal layer (Fig. 12.140), and this may be exacerbated by thrombus. Fibrous hyperplasia (sometimes called 'fibro-intimal hyperplasia') occurs particularly in arteries from which a cast of atheromatous material was removed at operation ('endarterectomy') and in the adjacent vein graft.

The mechanism that causes fibrous hyperplasia is still incompletely understood. It apears to result from exaggerated proliferation of smooth muscle cells in the media due to injury

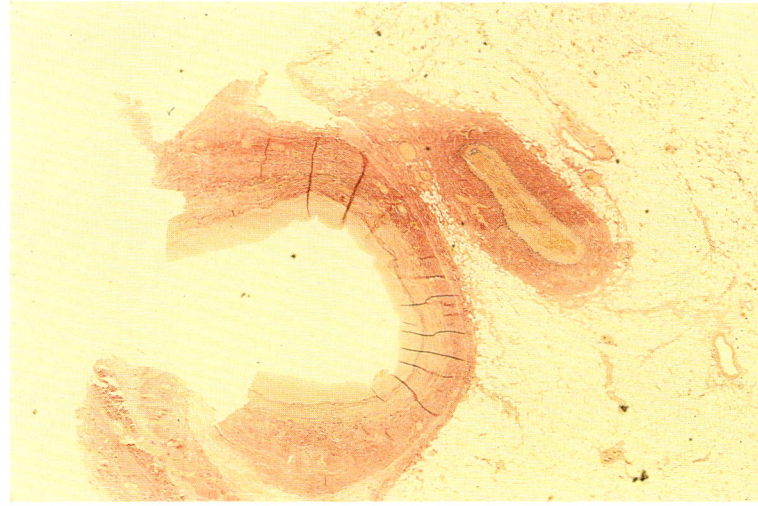

Fig. 12.140 Vein graft (opened longitudinally) at 3 months, and adjacent native coronary artery. There is intimal hyperplasia, and the media shows increased muscularity. The outer capsule of the graft consists mainly of fibrous tissue. The neighbouring native artery also has intimal hyperplasia as well as a recent thrombus. (EVG stain.)

(either acute or chronic) of the intimal endothelial cells. The process is mediated by the action of platelets.

Patients with underlying immunological vascular disease rapidly develop progressive atherosclerotic disease in vein grafts, which closely resembles atherosclerosis in native coronary arteries. In these patients the disease is concentric and diffuse, with a marked foreign-body reaction and transmural erosion by foam cells and atheromatous debris.

In the majority of patients with vein grafts the factors that favour the development of fibrous hyperplasia are:

1. surgical trauma (e.g. during dissection and preparation of the vein);
2. graft–artery mismatch;
3. haemodynamic changes, especially at the distal anastomosis;
4. local changes in arterial wall stress (e.g. due to the geometry of the distal anastomosis);
5. thrombosis of the vessel surfaces of both artery and vein;
6. imperfect endothelialization of the vein and adjacent artery.

In a proportion of graft failures the graft atrophies and may be represented as a fibrous cord on the epicardial surface of the heart. In this case the lumen of the aortic anastomosis is usually obliterated by fibrous tissue as well.

12.14.4 Healing of vascular grafts

The tissue that lies between the innermost layer of the graft and the lumen is called the inner capsule. It may consist of endothelial cells, smooth muscle cells, fibroblasts, fibrin, platelets, and collagen in variable combinations. A healed graft has an inner capsule of mature connective tissue, covered with endothelium. This type of intimal surface is a neointima. When the inner capsule is covered by other material (e.g. fibrin or collagen) a

pseudointima is present. Because smooth muscle cells adopt some of the characteristics of endothelial cells when they are exposed to flowing blood, it is necessary to demonstrate a product of endothelial cells, such as factor VIII (von Willebrand's factor) before naming the blood-contacting surface. The outer capsule of the graft is the coating of connective tissue on the outside.

The removal of a vein for grafting obligatorily results in stripping most of the adventitia. One consequence of this is that the intimal endothelium is lost as well, partly as the result of ischaemia due to the loss of the vasa vasorum and partly because of sudden exposure to arterial blood pressure. Reparative and adaptive changes take place to restore the intimal layer, thus initiating the process of healing. As the long saphenous veins of most mature adults have minor pathological changes, such as a degree of intimal thickening due to phlebosclerosis, the changes brought about by 'arterialization' are superimposed on the pre-existing state.

The luminal surface

The loss of the endothelium causes an acute but transient inflammatory cell reaction and oedema in the intima and immediately subjacent media. Specks of fibrin or thrombus are deposited on the intimal surface. Within one month to 6 weeks, proliferation of smooth muscle cells, fibroblasts, and endothelial cells produces a thickening of the intima, which attains maximal thickness after about 6 months. This new surface may be termed a neointima if it is composed of endothelial cells, but should be called a pseudointima if it consists of other elements, such as fibrin, collagen, smooth muscle cells, or platelets.

The medial layer

The media, like the intima, is adversely affected by the loss of its blood supply from the missing vasa vasorum, so that some of the smooth muscle cells die and are replaced by fibrous tissue.

The surviving smooth muscle cells hypertrophy so that by about 6 months the thickness of the media approximates to that of a native coronary artery.

The adventitial layer

Most of the native adventitia is lost when the vein is taken from the leg, and as time passes it is replaced by vascular scar tissue. Thus in the most successful operations, the graft has achieved its characteristic appearance; that is, a thickened wall with a widely patent lumen 9–12 months after grafting (Fig. 12.141).

12.14.5   Healing of other types of vascular graft

Internal thoracic artery

Grafted internal thoracic arteries demonstrate the same process of healing as vein grafts, but fibromuscular intimal hyperplasia occurs less frequently and is generally less severe in degree.

Umbilical vein

Umbilical vein grafts are enclosed in a fabric mesh and tanned in gluteraldehyde during preparation. The mesh is eventually incorporated into a sheath of connective tissue which is covered by a foreign-body reaction. The author has no experience of these grafts late after operation, but the late complications of biological valves (thinning, thickening, calcification, etc.) would seem to apply to these grafts as well.

Man-made grafts

The process of healing of man-made grafts is analogous to that of biografts but, unlike many other animals, man lacks the ability to endothelialize lengths much in excess of 10–15 mm. However, small areas such as intracardiac patches and the sewing rings of prosthetic heart valves heal so well as a rule that patches, in particular, are macroscopically indistinguishable from the surrounding tissue. Vascular grafts in man tend to

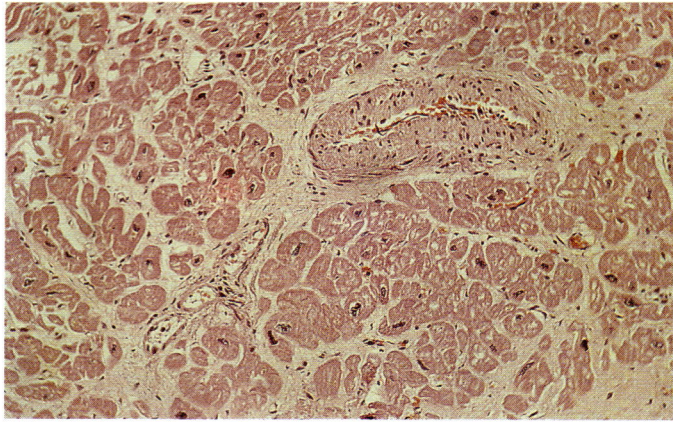

(a)

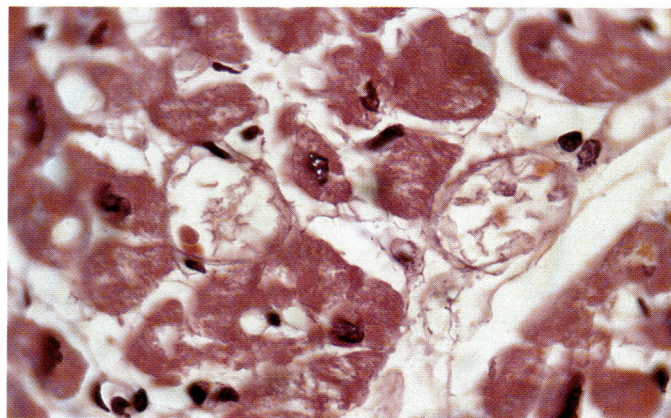

(b)

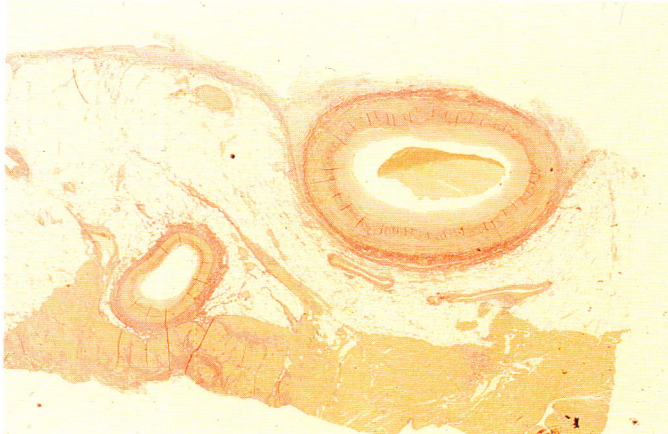

Fig. 12.141   Right coronary artery graft after 1 year. The adjacent native artery has some disease, but its proportions are similar to those of the graft. The graft has concentric hyperplasia which is absent in the native vessel. (EVG stain.)

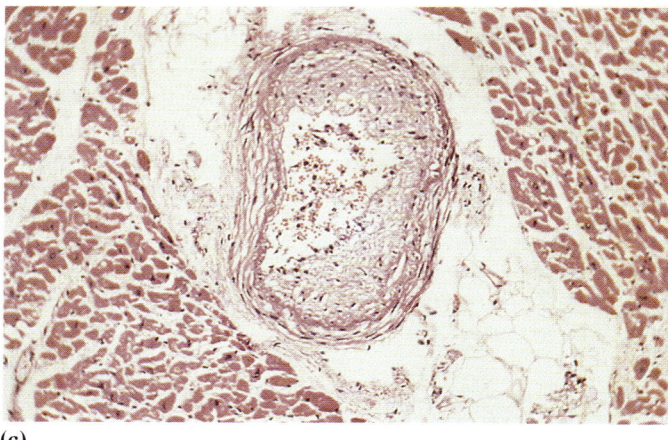

(c)

Fig. 12.142   (a) Intramuscular artery with developing fibrous tissue cap. There is also interstitial fibrosis, some oedema, and a few wavy eosinophilic bands, indicative of ischaemia. (b) Same patient. There is also dilatation of the lymphatics in this ischaemic myocardium. (c) Different patient at 4 years. A diseased collateral artery passes through fibrous myocardium which has myocytolysis and contraction band necrosis.

endothelialize completely only at, or close to, the anastomotic sites.

Low-porosity grafts heal by ingrowth of both endothelial and smooth muscle cells from the cut edges of the adjacent artery. Distal to the anastomosis, the 'intimal', blood-contacting layer is a pseudointima of platelet-fibrin aggregate.

Materials such as Dacron (polyester) and Gore-tex (polytetra-fluoroethylene, PTFE) permit the passage of fibrovascular constituents from the adventitial to the intimal surface, so that a potential exists for endothelial cells to migrate to the blood-contacting surface, creating a neointima. In some other animals endothelial cells pass rapidly to the inner layer by way of capillaries growing from the outer coat at considerable distances from the anastomotic site.

Like biografts, man-made grafts are prone to late failure due to intimal hyperplasia. In peripheral vascular grafts focal hyperplasia occurs at or near the anastomotic site without marked thickening of the inner capsule elsewhere; diffuse hyperplasia is commoner in coronary artery grafts. This results in concentric narrowing of the graft.

From the foregoing it is evident that most of the late pathology of vascular grafts is associated with exaggerated healing, expressed as fibrointimal hyperplasia. This may develop as early as 3 months after operation (see Fig. 12.140), or as late as 7 years, when it is associated with progression of the underlying disease (see Figs 12.139a–c and 12.141).

12.14.6   Collateral blood supply

The mechanism whereby the coronary collateral supply to the heart, present at birth, reopens or redevelops, is incompletely understood, but collateral channels are often to be found in association with both blocked and patent grafts. They are distinguishable from other intramyocardial arteries as they tend to pass parallel or obliquely to the muscle fibres, unaccompanied by either veins or nerves (Fig. 12.142a–c). At autopsy they are usually easy to see with the naked eye on the cut surface of the left ventricle.

Possession of a collateral circulation may contribute to improved immediate operative survival (Shimizu et al. 1986) but in the long term its efficacy in protecting against ischaemic changes demonstrated by electrocardiography is doubtful.

In addition to the coronary collateral supply, some individuals develop a non-coronary collateral circulation. It arises as tortuous vessels from the pericardial, mediastinal, and bronchial vessels and enters the pericardium by way of the vasa vasorum of the great arteries and veins, and the pericardial reflections. These small worm-like vessels are easier to indentify in the atrial than in the ventricular myocardium at autopsy, but in living patients the flow through them, although small, can adversely affect cardioplegia during bypass operations.

12.14.7   Further reading

Allwork, S. P. (1991). *Pathological correlation after cardiac surgery.* Butterworth–Heinemann, London.

Allwork, S. P. and Bentall, H. H. (1986). The usefulness of the phenomenon of histofluorescence in the identification of early myocardial necrosis. *Cardiovascular Research* **20**, 451–7.

Clowes, A. W., Kirkman, T. R., and Reidy, M. A. (1986). Mechanisms of arterial graft healing. Rapid transmural capillary ingrowth provides a source of intimal endothelium and smooth muscle in porous PTFE prostheses. *American Journal of Pathology* **123**, 220–30.

Echave, V., Koornick, A. R., Haimov, M., and Jacobson, J. H. (1979). Intimal hyperplasia as a complication of the use of the polytetrafluoroethylene graft for femoral-popliteal bypass. *Surgery* **86**, 791–8.

Shimizu, T., et al. (1986). A comparison of the results of aortocoronary bypass grafting in collateral and non-collateral groups. *Journal of Cardiovascular Surgery* **27**, 316–22.

Silver, M. D. and Wilson, G. J. (1983). Pathology of cardiovascular prostheses. In *Cardiovascular pathology* (ed. M. D. Silver), Vol. 2, p. 1280. Churchill Livingstone, New York.

12.15   Pathophysiology of heart disease

George Hart

This section contains a brief outline of the pathophysiology of heart disease in adults. Apart from a brief mention in connection with heart failure, ischaemic heart disease is not dealt with here because the pathophysiology of ischaemic heart disease is considered in conjunction with the pathology of this condition in Section 12.4.

12.15.1   Valvular heart disease

Valve disease in clinical practice tends to be classified first on the basis of the haemodynamic abnormality and then on the pathological process underlying the lesion, because the course and management of the patient often depend more on altered haemodynamics than on the means by which the lesion has been produced. The common disorders will be dealt with here (see also Section 12.9).

Valvar aortic stenosis

Although the aortic valve may be stenosed at birth, the commonest presentation of this condition is in the older age-group. Through a degenerative process the valve slowly becomes a fused, calcified structure enclosing a narrow orifice. Congenital abnormalities of the valve, such as a 'bicuspid' valve, may predispose to the development of stenosis in later life. Rheumatic disease of this valve usually results in a haemodynamically mixed lesion with a significant degree of incompetence as well as stenosis. Much rarer causes of aortic stenosis include hypercholesterolaemia (which is usually of the homozygous type II class with atheromatous deposits involving the aortic wall and the coronary ostia) and ochronosis.

The cross-sectional area of the aortic valve in the normal adult is approximately 3 cm². No systolic pressure gradient across the valve is normally detectable until the area of the valve orifice is reduced to about one-half of normal. With further narrowing, the left ventricular systolic pressure increases and hypertrophy develops, sarcomeres being added in series with those already present within the myocytes. A systolic gradient of approximately 50 mmHg, which is taken to indicate severe stenosis, is usually accompanied by a valve area of less than one-quarter of the normal sytolic value. Because of this non-linear relationship between valve area and pressure gradient and because resting cardiac output may be normal, symptoms usually appear late in the course of the disease and carry a poor prognosis unless the valve is replaced.

Left ventricular systolic function and cavity dimensions are normal at rest in aortic stenosis until the last stages of the disease; ventricular hypertrophy compensates for the raised systolic pressure and systolic wall tension remains normal. Hypertrophied ventricular myocardium is less compliant than normal, resulting in a raised left ventricular end-diastolic pressure and slower filling of the cavity in diastole. The contribution of atrial systole to ventricular filling becomes more important, and sudden clinical deterioration often follows the onset of atrial fibrillation.

The classical triad of symptoms experienced in aortic stenosis are angina, syncope, and effort intolerance. The epicardial coronary vessels are often large and free of atheroma. Coronary blood flow is increased but remains in proportion to ventricular mass. Angina may be attributable to subendocardial ischaemia but does not occur in hypertrophy from other causes without coexistent coronary disease. In aortic stenosis the higher ventricular systolic pressure increases oxygen requirement in addition to that imposed by the increased muscle mass, and the higher diastolic pressure and shorter diastole will reduce coronary filling.

Syncope and pre-syncope on effort probably result from the inability of systemic arterial pressure to rise normally on exercise because of the fixed outflow obstruction. In addition, arterial pressure may fall further because peripheral vasodilatation, which is normal on exercise, takes place through β_2-sympathetic activation and via vagal inhibition of the baroreceptor reflexes. These mechanisms are activated because of stimulation of ventricular stretch receptors by the elevated ventricular systolic pressure. It is possible that fatal arrhythmias may be triggered by myocardial ischaemia on exercise, but arrhythmias do not appear to be responsible for most of the documented attacks of syncope in this condition.

Ventricular systolic function may eventually decline in aortic stenosis, and this is usually associated with shortness of breath on effort. Congestive failure supervenes and, indeed, many patients first present in this way.

The clinical hallmark of valvar aortic stenosis is a slowly rising carotid upstroke; there is usually a diminished pulse pressure and a systolic murmur but the latter may be difficult to hear if the cardiac output is low. Left ventricular hypertrophy and strain may be evident on the resting electrocardiogram. Calcification of the valve and post-stenotic dilatation of the ascending aorta may be seen on the chest radiograph. Echocar-

diographic imaging (Fig. 12.143) demonstrates thickening and calcification of the valve and hypertrophy of the left ventricle. Aortic blood velocity measured by Doppler ultrasound is increased and a non-invasive estimate of the valvar gradient may be derived from the velocity envelope. Cardiac catheterization may be necessary in some cases when doubt remains from the non-invasive data about the degree of haemodynamic stenosis (and thus the pressure gradient needs to be measured directly) and in order to exclude coronary atheroma when angina is present.

Aortic regurgitation

Aortic regurgitation may arise through disorders of the valve itself, such as idiopathic or myxomatous degeneration, but in

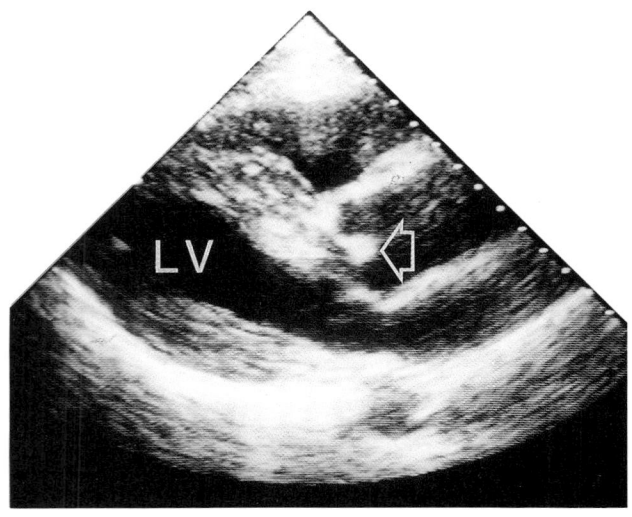

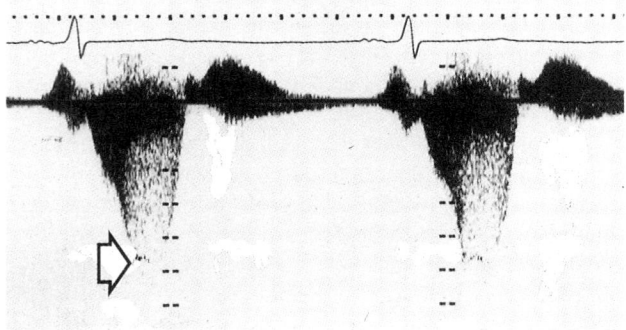

Fig. 12.143 Echocardiograms demonstrating features of valvar aortic stenosis. Upper panel: two-dimensional (2D) parasternal long-axis view. The arrow lies in the aortic root and points to the aortic valve which is thickened and calcified. See Fig. 12.145 for comparison. The wall of the left ventricle (LV) and the septum are hypertrophied. The marker dots on the right of the 2D echocardiograms in this section represent 1 cm. Lower panel: Doppler echocardiogram showing a high velocity jet in the aortic root. The double dash markers represent velocity increments of 1 m/s from the baseline downwards. The peak velocity (arrow) is nearly 5 m/s and represents a trans-valvar gradient of approximately 90 mmHg. The vertical markers in this and the remaining Doppler and M-mode figures of this section are spaced at 1 s intervals.

an increasing proportion of patients coming to aortic valve replacement, the regurgitation is secondary to dilatation of the aortic root (Table 12.8).

A primary adaptive response of the heart to chronic aortic regurgitation is an increase in end-diastolic volume; stroke volume increases to maintain ejection fraction and cardiac output. The heart dilates and hypertrophies with parallel replication of the contractile units. Left ventricular systolic wall tension and oxygen consumption increase. On exercise the increase in heart rate reduces the relative length of ventricular diastole and the regurgitant fraction diminishes. The fall in peripheral resistance with exercise (or following vasodilator therapy) acts to lower ventricular afterload. An increase in contractility may reduce end-systolic volume. By these mechanisms ejection fraction and cardiac output increase with exercise. Accordingly, moderate and even severe degrees of chronic aortic regurgitation may be well tolerated, without symptoms, for prolonged periods. Clinical features include a widened pulse pressure and associated signs, and Doppler ultrasound shows the reversed flow in diastole in the left ventricular cavity.

Eventually, as the ventricle progressively dilates, end-diastolic pressure rises, end-systolic volume increases, stroke volume is no longer maintained and congestive failure follows. In clinical practice valve replacement must be considered before the stage at which ventricular function becomes irreversibly damaged, although symptoms of effort intolerance may be slight and no reliable indicator currently exists of the degree of ventricular dilatation beyond which pump function is permanently impaired in the individual patient.

The physiology of acute aortic regurgitation (due, for example, to trauma or endocarditis) is rather different in that ventricular dilatation cannot take place acutely, so that end-diastolic pressure rises and stroke volume declines. Mitral valve closure takes place early (this is clearly demonstrated with ultrasound) and diastole is shortened. This clinical picture is that of a low-output state and an early diastolic murmur may be inapparent.

Mitral stenosis

Chronic rheumatic disease is usually held to be responsible for the process by which a normal mitral valve, which occupied an area of 4–6 cm^2, becomes progressively fibrosed and calcified and gives rise to a valve enclosing less than 1 cm^2 of orifice in severe stenosis. However, a history of acute rheumatic fever is obtainable in less than half of the affected patients, which are more frequently women. Obstruction to mitral diastolic flow raises left atrial pressure and gives rise to atrial hypertrophy and dilatation, pulmonary venous hypertension, and effort dyspnoea. Much more rarely, a similar clinical picture may result from other causes of left atrial hypertension, such as myxoma (see Section 12.12) or cor triatriatum.

Resting left ventricular end-diastolic pressure and volume are usually normal in mitral stenosis, although the ejection fraction may be reduced and regional abnormalities of wall motion are common, possibly indicating direct involvement of the left ventricular wall in the rheumatic process. Cardiac output rises less than normally during exercise because of the shorter diastole which accompanies a rise in heart rate. The mitral gradient increases approximately as the square of the flow rate and as the reciprocal of the square of the duration of diastole, so raising left atrial pressure as heart rate rises and reducing left ventricular filling.

Right ventricular and pulmonary artery systolic pressure rise on exercise, and later at rest as well. This takes place passively through back-pressure, through reflex pulmonary arteriolar vasoconstriction, and, in some cases, by obliterative changes in the resistance vessels of the lungs. Although pulmonary congestion is common in mitral stenosis, clinically severe pulmonary oedema is not (except perhaps when atrial fibrillation occurs for the first time), and it is possible that the rise in precapillary pulmonary vascular resistance may protect to some extent against the development of pulmonary oedema. Lung compliance is reduced. Right ventricular filling pressure rises and right ventricular hypertrophy develops, ultimately giving rise to right heart failure with peripheral congestion and organomegaly. The elevated right ventricular diastolic pressure frequently causes tricuspid regurgitation. Atrial fibrillation is common in haemodynamically moderate and severe mitral stenosis. With its onset there is often clinical deterioration because of the loss of atrial transport, which contributes more than normally to cardiac output in these patients, and also because ventricular rate rises. Atrial fibrillation and substantial left atrial enlargement constitute a considerable risk of peripheral embolization in rheumatic mitral stenosis (and incompetence), and anticoagulation is prescribed for rheumatic mitral valve disease which is other than mild.

Turbulent flow through the stenotic valve gives rise to the low-pitched apical diastolic murmur of mitral stenosis. Early ventricular filling is heralded by an opening snap as the (still mobile) valve leaflets are arrested by the chordae. An earlier

---

Table 12.8 Causes of aortic regurgitation

Disorders of the valve cusps
   congenital deformities (bicuspid valve; tetralogy of Fallot; VSD)
   rheumatic disease
   bacterial endocarditis
   ankylosing spondylitis
   rheumatoid arthritis
   calcific aortic valve disease
   trauma
Dilatation of the aortic root
   idiopathic
   aortic dissection
   systemic hypertension
   Marfan syndrome
   Ehlers–Danlos syndrome
   pseudoxanthoma elasticum
Inflammation of the aortic root
   non-specific aortitis
   ankylosing spondylitis
   rheumatoid arthritis
   syphilis
   Reiter syndrome

opening snap in diastole signifies higher atrial pressure. Echocardiography (Fig. 12.144) easily demonstrates the thickened leaflets which remain open for longer than normal in diastole. The posterior leaflet may move anteriorly at the onset of diastole. Doppler echocardiography reveals a slower rate of decline of mitral flow in diastole. The time taken for the velocity to fall to one-half of its initial peak value correlates with valve area and is an index of the severity of the stenosis.

Cardiac catheterization is not usually necessary other than to exclude coexistent valve or coronary disease. The progression of mitral stenosis, when not severe, is often very slow and operation is deferred until the patient's effort tolerance is substantially limited.

Mitral regurgitation

Partly because the mitral valve is a complex structure, connected to the ventricular myocardium via the chordae tendineae and papillary muscles, many different processes may produce regurgitation (Table 12.9). The fundamental haemo-

dynamic problem is ejection of part of the stroke volume into the left atrium in systole. A considerable proportion of this regurgitation takes place before aortic ejection, in the period at the beginning of systole when the heart normally contracts isovolumically. In order to maintain stroke volume and cardiac output, left ventricular end-diastolic volume and ejection fraction increase and the left ventricle hypertrophies. An incompetent mitral orifice reduces afterload and, as a result, wall tension and cardiac work diminish and indices of contractility may be enhanced. Factors which increase afterload, such as hypertension, aortic stenosis, or the development of congestion and further ventricular dilatation, may increase the degree of mitral regurgitation; treatment with diuretics and vasodilators reduces it.

The speed of development of mitral regurgitation affects the clinical picture by determining the response of the left atrium. In chronic cases the atrium dilates and its compliance increases. Atrial pressure does not rise substantially at rest until late and pulmonary vascular resistance is little changed. Atrial fibrilla-

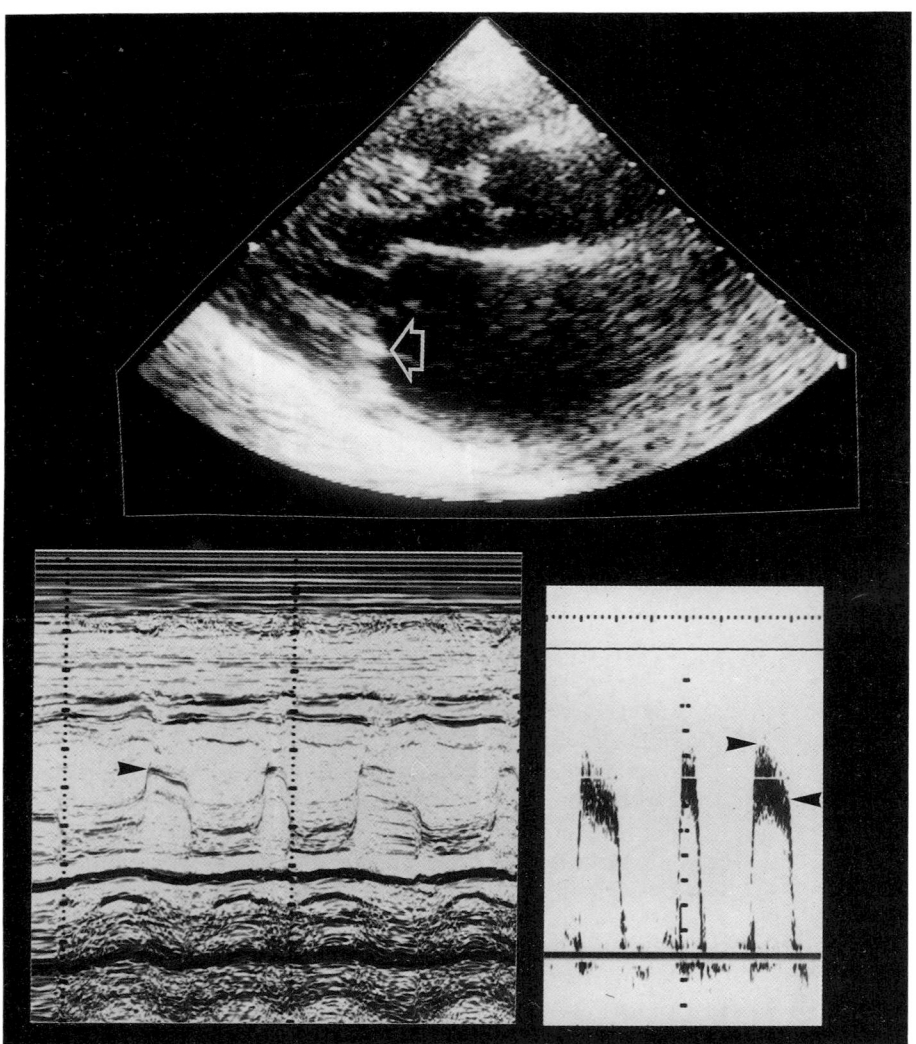

Fig. 12.144 Echocardiograms from a patient with mitral re-stenosis. Upper panel: two-dimensional parasternal long-axis view. The arrow, which lies in the left atrium, points to the posterior leaflet which is thickened and calcified. The left atrium is enlarged. Lower left panel: M-mode echocardiogram showing thickening and impaired mobility of the anterior mitral leaflet (arrowed) in diastole. Lower right panel: Doppler echocardiogram showing a slow decline of mitral flow in diastole. The arrows demonstrate how the pressure half-time is measured.

Table 12.9 Causes of mitral regurgitation

Disorders of the annulus
   ventricular dilatation causing enlargement of the valve ring
   calcification of the annulus
Disorders of the valve leaflets
   congenital (clefts, fenestrations, 'parachute' valve, atrial septal
     defects, transposition)
   myxomatous degeneration
   rheumatic disease
   infective endocarditis
   trauma
   Marfan syndrome
   Ehlers–Danlos syndrome
   pseudoxanthoma elasticum
Disorders of the chordae tendineae
   rheumatic disease
   myxomatous degeneration
   infective endocarditis
   chordal rupture (spontaneous, secondary to the above chordal
     pathologies and to trauma and myocardial infarction)
Disorders of the papillary muscles
   ischaemic heart disease
   cardiomyopathies
   rupture (ischaemia, trauma, infection)
Disorders of the left ventricular myocardium
   hypertrophic cardiomyopathy
   endocardial fibro-elastosis
   restrictive disorders (endomyocardial fibrosis; tumour infiltration of
     the myocardium)
Disorders of prosthetic valve
   paraprosthetic leak
   disease of biological valve leaflets
   infective endocarditis
   sticking in the open position of the ball or disc of a mechanical
     valve (due to pannus formation or vegetations)
   disc, ball, or poppet escape
   ring or strut fracture
   disc wear

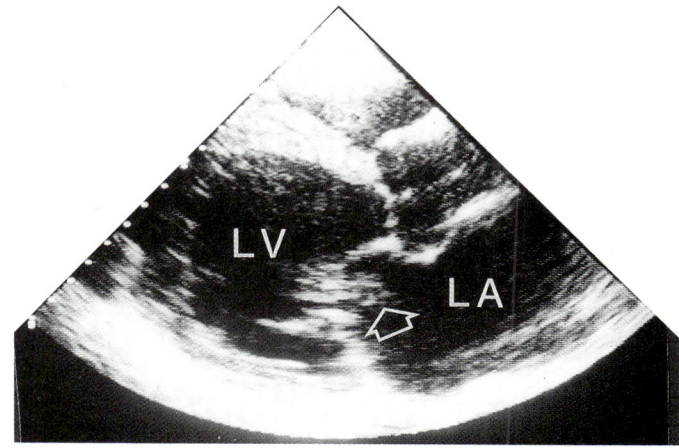

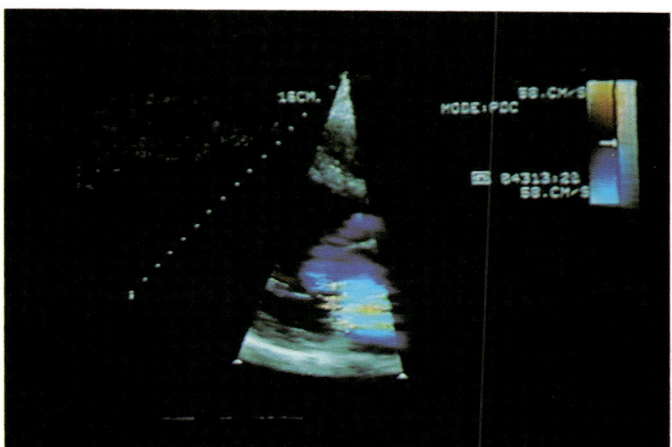

Fig. 12.145 Echocardiograms from a patient with mitral valve prolapse. Upper panel: two-dimensional parasternal long-axis view showing prolapse of part of the anterior leaflet of the mitral valve (arrowed) into the left atrium (LA) early in systole. Lower panel: colour Doppler study of the same view. A yellow jet indicating mitral regurgitation can be seen crossing the mitral valve from the left ventricle into the left atrium. LV, left ventricle.

tion is common. Severe chronic regurgitation may be well tolerated for several years until the left ventricle dilates further, the ejection fraction falls to normal or below, and end-systolic volume rises. Pulmonary artery pressure increases and right heart failure may follow. When a mitral valve is destroyed by endocarditis, or when acute regurgitation follows papillary muscle infarction, left atrial compliance is normal or reduced and, as a consequence, left atrial systolic pressure rises much more quickly. The rhythm is usually sinus. If the regurgitation is sudden and severe, pulmonary oedema and a low-output state may result. Less severe degrees of acute regurgitation may give rise to established pulmonary hypertension over the course of weeks or months.

   Clinically the diagnosis of mitral incompetence is made by hearing a systolic murmur, which may extend throughout systole or may be confined to mid or late systole, particularly if the degree of reflux is mild and due to mitral leaflet prolapse. Echocardiography may identify the structural change underlying the haemodynamic lesion (Fig. 12.145). Doppler and colour-flow imaging confirm the presence of a regurgitant jet, although quantitation of its severity with ultrasound may be difficult. At right heart catheterization, the pulmonary capillary wedge pressure shows an elevated systolic wave reflecting the mitral

regurgitation, which may be demonstrated directly by left ventriculography.

Tricuspid regurgitation

In most patients with tricuspid regurgitation the valve is structurally intact and the haemodynamic abnormality is secondary to a raised right ventricular filling pressure causing dilatation of the valve ring. Doppler echocardiography has shown that minor degrees of tricuspid regurgitation are very common. The most prevalent causes are the left-sided lesions producing pulmonary hypertension; tricuspid incompetence is a common accompaniment of congestive cardiac failure. Much more rarely, the lesion may be produced by intrinsic valve pathology such as infective endocarditis (e.g. in intravenous drug abusers), rheumatic fever, Ebstein's anomaly, trauma, carcinoid syndrome, myxomatous degeneration, and 'connective tissue' diseases. The degree to which these patients are functionally impaired is usually determined by the disorder giving rise to the tricuspid incompetence, for this lesion in isolation is often well tolerated. Characteristic findings are a raised jugular venous pressure having a pronounced systolic pulsation, and pulsatile hepatomegaly.

12.15.2 Congestive heart failure

Although the term 'heart failure' has eluded attempts at satisfactory definition, in clinical practice it is used when a patient develops oedema or congestion in association with cardiac disease or circulatory overload. The majority of cases of heart failure in developed countries arise from cardiac muscle damage secondary to coronary artery disease; other causes include (primary) cardiomyopathies, secondary disorders affecting the myocardium, valvular disease, hypertension (systemic and pulmonary), and congenital lesions. Conditions giving rise to 'high-output' heart failure include anaemia, arteriovenous fistulae, and Paget disease. We shall firstly consider those features which are common to most cases of cardiac failure, and then discuss the pathophysiology of the cardiomyopathies in more detail.

During the development of heart failure the body mounts a series of complex and interrelating pathophysiological responses which, rather teleologically, have been called 'compensatory mechanisms'. In the initial stages these may be viewed as acting to maintain cardiac output, but later in the course of the illness may give rise to the clinical manifestations of heart failure. The factors that determine the nature and extent of these reponses in heart failure remain poorly understood. For a full and up-to-date account of cellular and organ changes in heart failure, the reader is referred to the review volume edited by Swynghedauw (1990).

Systemic responses in heart failure

Raised ventricular filling pressure

An increase in filling pressure or preload is commonly found in heart failure and leads to a rise in cardiac output by the Frank–Starling mechanism, whereby stretch of the myocardium acts to increase the force of the heartbeat via an increase in Ca^{2+} released in the cardiac myocytes during systole. However, the rise in contractility with a given increment in diastolic pressure or volume is less in heart failure than in the normal heart, and this mechanism is likely to be less important still as failure worsens (Fig. 12.146). A raised filling pressure may be associated with a raised hydrostatic pressure in the capillaries of the pulmonary or systemic circulation and give rise to effort breathlessness and pulmonary oedema from left heart failure, and to oedema and organomegaly from right heart failure.

Ventricular hypertrophy

In response to chronic pressure or volume overload, the ventricular myocardium hypertrophies as new contractile units are added within the myocytes. The left side of the heart undergoes

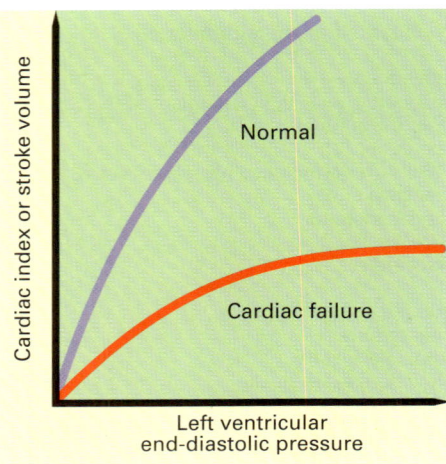

Fig. 12.146 Diagram illustrating the relationship between left ventricular performance (either cardiac index or stroke volume) and left ventricular filling pressure. For a given increase in left ventricular end-diastolic pressure (LVEDP) there is a greatly reduced increment in cardiac performance in heart failure compared with the normal heart.

a moderate degree of hypertrophy as a normal feature of ageing, and in dilated cardiomyopathies ventricular mass is usually raised, with a higher than normal proportion of fibrous tissue. The adaptive consequence of hypertrophy is to normalize systolic wall stress and to increase the capacity for ventricular work, so maintaining cardiac performance. At a cellular level, peak developed force is increased in moderate, early hypertrophy and reduced with severe hypertrophy and failure; relaxation is delayed and is slower than normal. Thus the pay-off for enhanced systolic work is increased stiffness of the ventricle in diastole, and this increases the resistance to ventricular filling and gives rise to an elevated filling pressure. The peak filling rate occurs later in the shorter diastole and the contribution of atrial systole to cardiac output is increased. Effort tolerance will deteriorate and pulmonary oedema may be precipitated in patients with left heart hypertrophy if atrial transport is lost with the onset of atrial fibrillation. Energy consumption is increased in hypertrophy and subendocardial ischaemia may contribute to the impairment of relaxation. The trigger for hypertrophy is not known, nor is its locus of action in the pathway from DNA to actin and myosin synthesis. Increased length of, or load on, the myocytes has been implicated; relative hypoxia, accumulation of metabolites, increased plasma catecholamines, and other circulating factors may be involved.

Adrenergic activation

Raised plasma levels of catecholamines are found initially on exercise and later at rest in patients with heart failure, and early in the progress of the disease may act to increase the force of cardiac contraction. The level of plasma noradenaline is correlated with the degree of ventricular dysfunction and with mortality. The sources of the raised levels include the adrenal medulla and the visceral innervation. Cardiac levels of catecholamines in patients with established heart failure are reduced, sometimes to less than 10 per cent of normal. In severe heart failure β_1-receptor density in the heart is reduced and the sensitivity of the myocardium to β-adrenergic stimulation (in terms of inotropic response and adenylate cyclase activity) is depressed, possibly as a result of the chronically raised plasma levels of catecholamines. The heart muscle responds normally to Ca^{2+} and to high concentrations of glycosides but cyclic AMP production is impaired (although adenylate cyclose remains normally sensitive to the direct activator forskolin). Thus although β-adrenergic activation may initially help to compensate for the ventricular dysfunction, these later changes may play an important part in the progression of contractile failure.

The role of the kidney

Sodium and water retention by the kidney may initially compensate by increasing circulating plasma volume, preload and, therefore, cardiac index. Indeed, an early observation was that sodium retention usually precedes the rise in venous pressure in heart failure. As the degree of failure progresses, however, renal mechanisms give rise to the oedema and congestion which characterize heart failure (see Chapter 7 for a discussion of the pathophysiology of oedema). Partly attributable to the raised catecholamines, vasoconstriction of the efferent arterioles in the kidney leads to an increase in filtration fraction through a greater decrease in renal plasma flow than in glomerular filtration rate. This in turn gives rise to increased Na^+ and water reabsorption in the proximal tubule because of an increase in colloid osmotic pressure and a fall in the hydrostatic pressure of the post-glomerular, peritubular blood. Furthermore, a fall in renal perfusion pressure leads to Na^+ retention via the renin–angiotensin system, as renin is released from the juxtaglomerular apparatus leading to angiotensin II production in the pulmonary circulation. In addition to promoting aldosterone secretion and thus increased Na^+ reabsorption in the distal tubule, angiotensin II increases afterload by increasing peripheral vasoconstriction. Diuretics are the cornerstone of symptomatic treatment in heart failure and these substances appear to increase plasma renin and aldosterone, so exacerbating the problems associated with renal Na^+ retention. Treatment with inhibitors of angiotension converting enzyme (ACE) has been shown to relieve symptoms in patients with treated heart failure and may also improve prognosis.

Other hormonal changes

Elevated plasma levels of arginine vasopressin in heart failure may increase water retention and lead to hyponatraemia (despite elevated total body Na^+), and also contribute to the vasoconstriction seen in these patients. Raised levels of atrial natriuretic peptide (ANP) have been found, in proportion to the rise in mean right atrial and pulmonary capillary wedge pressures. It appears unlikely, however, that this substance plays an important role in the pathophysiology of heart failure.

Changes in other organs in heart failure

Adrenergic overactivity gives rise to arteriolar vasoconstriction in the kidneys, liver, gut, skin, and skeletal muscles. Peripheral

resistance is raised and fails to fall as it normally does on exercise, partly, but not entirely, through the raised adrenergic tone. Skeletal muscle changes may contribute to the effort intolerance, breathlessness, and fatigue of heart failure patients, particularly in the later stages. There is a great increment in skeletal muscle aerobic and anaerobic metabolism as a function of work load in heart failure.

Venous tone is raised, particularly in the skin and mesenteric territories, reducing venous capacitance and raising right ventricular filling pressure.

Changes in the myocardial cell

It is established that impaired ventricular contractility in heart failure results from dysfunction of the ventricular myocytes and a number of abnormalities have been described. Diastolic calcium levels are increased and the Ca^{2+} transient is delayed, leading to impaired relaxation and the diastolic abnormalities described above. Calcium release by the sarcoplasmic reticulum (SR) is depressed and uptake by this organelle is slowed. The activity of isolated SR Ca^{2+}-ATPase is diminished, but the reason for this appears to be a fall in the number or volume of transport sites rather than a reduced specific activity of the enzyme. A change takes place in the myosin thick filaments with a switch to the synthesis of an isozyme having a lower ATPase activity. These changes combine to give rise to weaker and more long-lasting contractions. The stores of energy-rich compounds are preserved in the failing heart but accumulation of phosphate takes place and the myocytes begin to synthesize substantial quantities of peptides such as ANP. The significance of these findings is not known.

Arrhythmogenesis

The prognosis of patients who remain symptomatically limited after an episode of congestive heart failure is poor. The mode of death is sudden in nearly half of the cases and may be attributed to ventricular tachycardia or fibrillation, as Holter monitoring has shown a high incidence of malignant ventricular arrhythmias in these patients. Little is known of the detailed mechanisms of arrhythmogenesis associated with ventricular hypertrophy and dilatation. Reduced plasma K^+ and Mg^{2+} and raised catecholamine and angiotensin II levels have been implicated as contributory factors, together with the pro-arrhythmic effects of some cardioactive drugs. It is possible that membrane currents underlying the abnormal prolongation of the myocyte action potential may be important, and of particular interest in this regard is the oscillatory transient inward current which is activated by a rise in intracellular Ca^{2+}, and may be produced by sarcolemmal Na–Ca exchange.

It has been suggested that islands of fibrosis in chronic ventricular disease may alter the pattern of impulse conduction and myocyte repolarization, favouring the development of arrhythmogenic re-entry circuits. In contrast to patients with ischaemic ventricular damage, however, features such as late potentials, fractionated electrograms, and slow conduction appear to be infrequent in patients with failure due to other forms of chronic myocardial disease and suggest that re-entry may be less important in these patients.

Heart failure in ischaemic heart disease

In the acute phase of myocardial infarction the principal manifestations of heart failure are pulmonary oedema and cardiogenic shock; the presence and severity of such complications are directly related to the extent of the infarcted area of myocardium. Haemodynamic measurements show considerable variability in patients with myocardial infarction, but in a majority diastolic filling is impaired and left ventricular filling pressure increases, thus increasing pulmonary venous pressure and giving rise to breathlessness and pulmonary congestion. Abnormalities of systolic function include a fall in ejection fraction and in cardiac output. Patients whose cardiac index is less than 2.1 l/min/m² together with a pulmonary capillary pressure of greater than 18 mmHg have a worse prognosis. In patients suffering considerable loss of left ventricular myocardium (greater than aproximately 40 per cent), cardiogenic shock may supervene with systolic arterial pressure less than 80 mmHg and impaired organ perfusion giving rise to hypoxia, confusion, oliguria, and death in over 90 per cent of cases. Other complications associated with haemodynamic deterioration in acute infarction include rupture of the interventricular septum and the ventricular free wall (with the latter being usually fatal) and, less commonly, severe mitral regurgitation from infarction and rupture of a papillary muscle.

Chronic heart failure in the context of ischaemic heart disease is usually a reflection of the extent of myocardial loss. Heart failure is a common presenting symptom in patients who have developed a left ventricular aneurysm, which usually involves the antero-apical portion of the left ventricle and is associated with an occluded left anterior descending coronary artery.

12.15.3 The cardiomyopathies

In discussing the pathophysiology of the cardiomyopathies, it is helpful to group together conditions which behave in a similar haemodynamic way; three broad categories may be considered. For convenience we shall discuss these functional groups together as 'cardiomyopathies' whether or not a primary cause is apparent.

Dilated (congestive) cardiomyopathy

The clinical picture in this condition is of a patient who presents with the symptoms (effort dyspnoea, orthopnoea, noctural oedema, and lassitude) and signs (pulmonary and peripheral congestion, a raised venous pressure, organomegaly, a third heart sound, and possibly atrio-ventricular valve incompetence) of heart failure in association with a dilated left and right ventricle and evidence of global impairment of systolic ventricular function (Fig. 12.147).

Although ventricular function is often substantially depressed, at presentation there is considerable variation in the degree to which each ventricle may be involved. Investigation usually fails to reveal a primary cause, although it is important to exclude treatable disease; the known causes of this syndrome have been reviewed previously (Section 12.10). In addition to the features of heart failure described above, thrombus formation on the ventricular endocardial surface, with associated embolization, is a recognized complication of dilated cardiomyopathy.

Hypertrophic cardiomyopathy

In clinical practice this term embraces those patients with ventricular hypertrophy without discernible cause, usually involving the left ventricle and, in particular, the interventricular

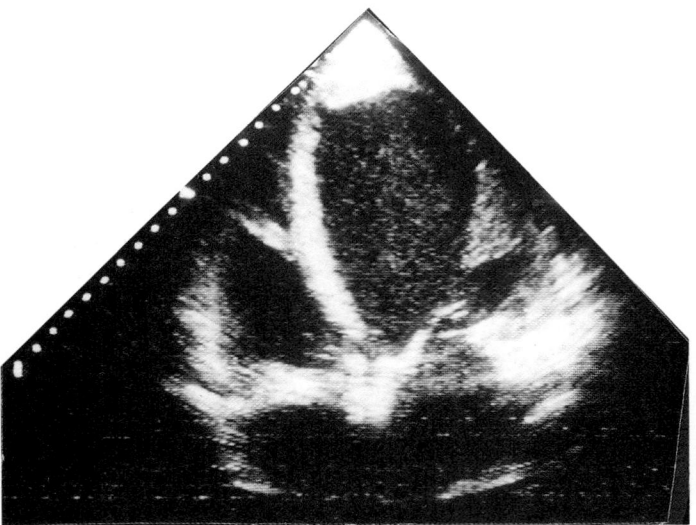
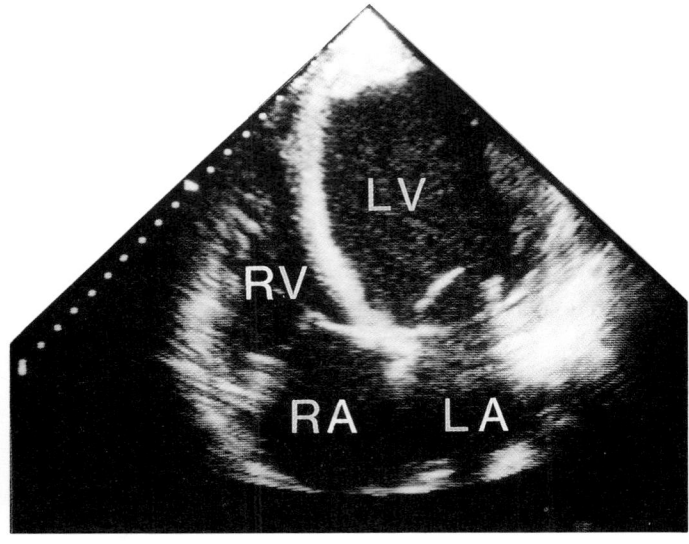

Fig. 12.147 Echocardiograms illustrating dilated cardiomyopathy. The patient was a man in his twenties whose left ventricular function deteriorated over several months following a viral myocarditis. The view is apical four-chamber and the panels are systole (left) and diastole (right). Symbols: LV, left ventricle; LA, left atrium; RV, right ventricle; RA, right atrium. The left ventricle is dilated. The papillary muscles move into view in systole but the left ventricular dimensions change only slightly, the overall ejection fraction being less than 10 per cent.

septum. A typical feature of hypertrophic cardiomyopathy is hyperdynamic ventricular contraction, with rapid emptying of the ventricle in the early part of systole and an ejection fraction at or above the upper end of the normal range. In about half of the cases there is a measurable gradient between the ventricular cavity and the aorta in systole. This appears to represent true obstruction to ventricular emptying when the mitral apparatus moves anteriorly in systole, towards a hypertrophied septum, at a time when ventricular emptying is not yet complete. These cases may also have a mild or moderate degree of mitral regurgitation. Another mechanism of gradient production appears to be rapid emptying with cavity obliteration, which may also be seen in association with systolic anterior motion of the mitral valve.

Hypertrophic cardiomyopathy shares some of the general features of cardiac hypertrophy detailed above. For example, ventricular relaxation is delayed and diastolic compliance is reduced, and some of the cellular features of this syndrome are also similar to those of secondary hypertrophy.

Symptoms in hypertrophic cardiomyopathy include chest pain, effort dyspnoea, and syncope. Between patients these may vary in severity from being absent to disabling. The majority of such patients have no atheroma in the epicardial coronary vessels to account for their chest pain. In those with typical angina and evidence of cardiac ischaemia, possible causes of pain include: inadequate capillary density relative to the degree of myocardial hypertrophy; external compression or intrinsic narrowing of small intramyocardial arteries; or a cellular metabolic reason associated with the raised metabolic requirements of hypertrophy. Breathlessness may be explained on the basis of the elevated ventricular diastolic and therefore pulmonary venous pressures, particulary on exercise, which result from the incompliant, hypertrophied ventricle.

Clinical findings include a brisk, jerky carotid upstroke, a sustained apex beat with a palpable atrial beat, and a harsh midsystolic murmur. Echocardiography (Fig. 12.148) is usually diagnostic in showing the ventricular hypertrophy, which is often asymmetrical, and the abnormalities of the mitral valve.

In the late stage, ventricular systolic function in hypertrophic cardiomyopathy may deteriorate, though the mode of death is commonly sudden. The degree of hypertrophy does not appear to correlate with prognosis, although in those patients showing non-sustained ventricular tachycardia on monitoring, treatment with the anti-arrhythmic drug, amiodarone, does appear to prolong survival.

Restrictive cardiomyopathy

This is a group of rare conditions which share clinical and pathophysiological features resulting from inability of the ventricles to fill normally in diastole, due to thickening and infiltration of the walls. In the West, amyloid deposition is perhaps the most common cause of the syndrome, which is also seen in haemochromatosis, sarcoidosis, hypereosinophilic syndrome, endomyocardial fibrosis, glycogen storage diseases, and other infiltrative disorders (see Sections 12.10.4–5). Peripheral and

pulmonary venous pressures are raised and the ventricular pressure trace shows a characteristic 'dip and plateau' appearance with a fall in pressure in early diastole, followed by a rapid rise to a plateau which is maintained for the remainder of diastole. Atrioventricular valve regurgitation is common. The most important differential diagnosis is constrictive pericarditis, which may be distinguished with the aid of echocardiography, CT, and magnetic resonance imaging.

12.15.4 Right heart failure and pulmonary hypertension

The pulmonary circulation provides for oxygenation and carbon dioxide excretion through a low pressure, high compliance circuit. Pulmonary artery systolic pressure is normally less than 30 mmHg but commonly rises as a secondary consequence of diseases affecting the left side of the heart, the lung vessels, and parenchyma. Causes of pulmonary hypertension are listed in Table 12.10.

A chronically elevated pulmonary venous pressure may give rise to reactive pulmonary hypertension in which pulmonary artery pressure rises so that pulmonary flow, at least in the early stages, remains normal. However, the extent to which such a rise in pressure occurs (in, for example, mitral stenosis) is extremely variable between patients, underlying our ignorance of some of the factors determining the behaviour of the pulmonary circulation. From work involving unilateral pulmonary occlusion in pulmonary hypertension, it appears that there is a neural component to the raised pulmonary vascular resistance. Other contributing factors include the consequent hyperplasia and hypertrophy of the vessel walls, so increasing luminal resistance, and interstitial oedema. Hypoxia produces a rise in pulmonary artery pressure through constriction of the smaller pulmonary arteries and arterioles. The mechanisms are thought to include a direct effect on the vascular smooth muscle, with a rise in intracellular calcium secondary to a reduction in energy-rich phosphate compounds, and indirect effects via the release of leukotrienes and histamine.

Pulmonary thromboembolism

The haemodynamic changes which result from an embolus, usually arising from the thigh or pelvic veins, lodging in the pulmonary arterial tree depend greatly on the size of the material, the rapidity with which it disperses into the smaller lung vessels, and the previous state of the heart and lungs. In massive embolization a tachycardia is invariably present and the right ventricle dilates. Pulmonary artery and right ventricular systolic pressures rise, but not usually in excess of 40–50 mmHg in the absence of pre-existing pulmonary hypertension. Right atrial pressure increases and the clinical picture may be that of hypoxia, shock, and oliguria, with associated metabolic acidosis. Left ventricular filling may be impaired secondary to right ventricular dilatation, and the ECG may show changes suggesting inferior ischamia.

Release of vasoconstrictive substances from platelets

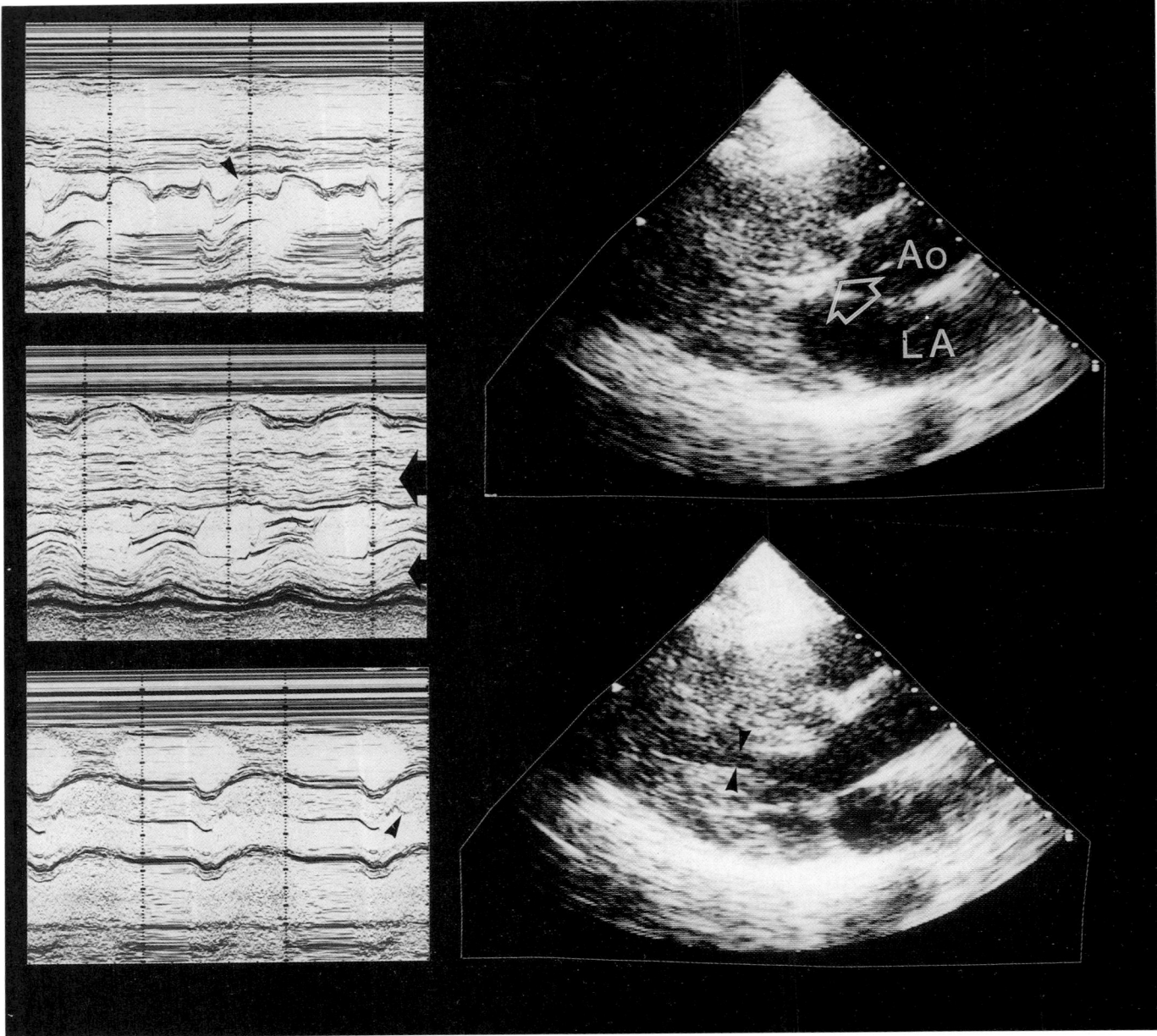

Fig. 12.148 Echocardiograms from a patient with hypertrophic cardiomyopathy. Left panel: M-mode echocardiograms showing, in the top record, systolic anterior motion of the mitral valve (the anterior leaflet is arrowed and moves forwards, i.e. towards the top of the record, in systole). The middle record shows asymmetrical septal hypertrophy; the septum (large arrow) is substantially thicker than the left ventricular free wall (small arrow). The bottom record shows mid-systolic closure of the aortic valve; the right coronary cusp is arrowed. Right panel: two-dimensional parasternal long-axis view of the same patient's heart. The upper record is taken very early in diastole when the aortic valve has just closed. The arrow shows the septum bulging into the left ventricular cavity which is almost obliterated at the end of systole. The lower record is at the end of diastole. The narrow ventricular cavity is outlined by the arrows.

increases pulmonary vascular resistance, which exacerbates the ventilation–perfusion mismatch existing as a consequence of the oxygenated but unperfused lung in the territory of the embolism. These substances, which include histamine, serotonin, and thromboxane A_2, also give rise to bronchoconstric-

tion, thus contributing to the dyspnoea which is often marked in the acute stages. Death may follow from a combination of hypoxia and right heart failure.

The clinical spectrum of pulmonary embolism embraces acute events of major or lesser severity and also repeated minor

Table 12.10 Causes of pulmonary hypertension

Disorders of the left heart and systemic circulation
    raised left ventricular end-diastolic pressure
        left ventricular failure
        reduced left ventricular compliance (e.g. from hypertrophy,
          ischaemia, tumour infiltration)
        systemic hypertension
    raised left atrial pressure
        mitral valve disease (stenosis, incompetence, prosthetic
          obstruction)
        constrictive pericarditis
        left atrial myxoma
        left atrial thrombosis
        cor triatriatum
    raised pulmonary venous pressure
        pulmonary veno-occlusive disease
        pulmonary venous obstruction (congenital; thrombotic)
        mediastinal fibrosis
Diseases of the lung tissue
    chronic bronchitis
    emphysema
    asthma
    bronchiectasis, including cystic fibrosis
    restrictive lung disease
    collagen vascular disease (scleroderma, systemic lupus
      erythematosus, rheumatoid arthritis)
    pulmonary fibrosis
    sarcoidosis
    bronchial tumours
    post lung resection
    cystic fibrosis
Disorders of the pulmonary circulation
    recurrent pulmonary emboli (thrombus, tumour)
    primary pulmonary hypertension
    increased pulmonary flow in left to right shunts; Eisenmenger
      syndrome
    schistosomiasis
    filariasis
    tropical eosinophilia
    sickle-cell disease
    pulmonary stenosis (congenital, or acquired from tumour)
    Takayasu disease
Disorders giving rise to alveolar hypoxia
    high altitude
    primary alveolar hypoventilation, sleep apnoea syndrome
    obesity and hypoventilation
Disorders of the thoracic cage
    kyphosis, scoliosis
    thoracoplasty
    pleural fibrosis
Diseases of the nervous and muscular systems
    poliomyelitis
    myasthenia gravis
    Guillain–Barré syndrome
    motor neurone disease (amyotrophic lateral sclerosis)
    myopathies, muscular dystrophies, spinal cord lesions

episodes which may go unnoticed by the patient, who may eventually present with the features of established pulmonary hypertension.

Primary pulmonary hypertension

Patients who present with established pulmonary hypertension and in whom there is no discernible cause for this disorder fall into the category of primary pulmonary hypertension. The dis-order is rare with a female preponderance and the prognosis is poor. Echocardiography is useful to exclude rare and clinically occult causes of secondarily raised pulmonary pressure, such as a left atrial myxoma and cor triatriatum, as well as the more common and clinically evident causes such a mitral stenosis and intracardiac shunts. Pathological lesions of intimal fibrosis, medial hypertrophy, plexiform lesions, and dilatations may be the result of long-standing and severe pulmonary vasoconstriction from unknown mechanisms. A response to vasodilating agents, and in particular to prostacyclin, has been described in some patients. The finding of *in situ* thrombosis in pulmonary vessels is common and, although there is little support for embolization in these patients, anticoagulation is associated with improved survival in some patients.

Cor pulmonale

This is a general term applied to the condition of patients in whom signs attributable to right heart failure, such as peripheral oedema, raised venous pressure, and hepatomegaly, occur in the setting of chronic hypoxic lung disease, chiefly chronic bronchitis and emphysema. The term itself suggests that the heart abnormalities are a crucial part of the picture and, indeed, the WHO definition of cor pulmonale (1961) was 'hypertrophy of the right ventricle resulting from diseases affecting the function and/or structure of the lung'. A traditional view of the pathophysiology of this condition has been that alveolar hypoxia, resulting from the lung disease, causes pulmonary arteriolar vasoconstriction and, together with destruction of lung parenchyma and associated vasculature, this results in secondary pulmonary hypertension. As a consequence, right ventricular hypertrophy and, ultimately, right heart failure and peripheral congestion develop. Recent work, however, suggests that such a straightforward scheme is difficult to reconcile with the clinical and pathological evidence in perhaps the majority of cases, and illustrates that much of the pathophysiology of this condition remains poorly understood.

In the clinical setting the diagnosis is usually readily made in a patient, usually a heavy smoker, who presents with breathlessness, central cyanosis, and severe airways obstruction. The majority of these patients have a raised arterial carbon dioxide tension and pulmonary function testing reveals a low forced expiratory volume, signifying airways obstruction, and a raised residual volume with respect to the total lung volume, indicating hyperinflation of the lungs. Often the illness features recurrent exacerbations characterized by increased breathlessness, lethargy, peripheral oedema, a raised jugular venous pressure, and hepatomegaly, sometimes associated with intercurrent lung infection. The prognosis is poor; three-quarters of the patients are dead 5 years after presenting with oedema. The cornerstone of therapy is domiciliary oxygen administration for prolonged periods, together with diuretics, bronchodilators, antibiotics, and physiotherapy as necessary.

Because systemic desaturation is invariable in established cor pulmonale, whether from alveolar underventilation or ventilation-perfusion imbalance, it has often been assigned a pivotal role in the development of the other features of the disease. Hypoxia acts as a pulmonary vasoconstrictor and chronic hypoxia in the experimental animal and in man (for example at high altitude) results in pulmonary hypertension and right ventricular hypertrophy, with some, but not all, of the structural changes in the pulmonary vasculature which may be found in cor pulmonale. Relief of hypoxia in cor pulmonale may cause some reduction of the elevated pulmonary vascular resistance, but the structural changes in the pulmonary arterioles remain, and do not show the slow reversal seen in simple hypoxic pulmonary hypertension. Thus the contribution of hypoxic pulmonary vasoconstriction in cor pulmonale remains uncertain. Furthermore, pulmonary artery pressure at rest in patients with cor pulmonale is only mildly elevated, except in acute exacerbations. However, the raised pulmonary vascular resistance (caused by arteriolar wall thickening and by destruction of the vascular bed in the lungs) means that stimuli such as exercise and hypoxia may transiently elevate the pulmonary artery pressure quite substantially. Cardiac output is usually normal at rest in cor pulmonale and right ventricular function remains good, although the end-diastolic pressure and volume may be elevated.

Right ventricular hypertrophy is not a constant finding in these patients either during life or at post-mortem. Thus it is difficult to find support for the hypothesis that the peripheral oedema in cor pulmonale is always necessarily attributable to back-pressure from a failing, hypertrophied right ventricle, although in acute exacerbations venous pressure is elevated and may lead to sodium retention through an increase in renal venous pressure. Impaired renal perfusion in cor pulmonale is associated with activation of the renin–angiotensin system, and in acute exacerbations of the disease with oedema, raised plasma levels of renin are usually found, leading to sodium and water retention by the kidney. There may be some redistribution of intracellular water to the extracellular space as intracellular cations are required to buffer the excess extracellular protons from the respiratory acidosis. These (and probably other) mechanisms may therefore contribute substantially to the signs found in cor pulmonale.

Other features of this condition include a loss of the normal drive to respiration on the basis of elevated carbon dioxide tension. These patients rely on arterial desaturation for their respiratory drive and may become apnoeic if this is corrected by too high a concentration of inspired oxygen. In addition, the carotid body becomes less sensitive to arterial hypoxaemia and proprioceptive afferents appear to play a substantial role in maintaining respiratory drive in cor pulmonale. In many patients an elevated red cell mass and packed cell volume are found, presumably secondary to the arterial hypoxaemia, and it is possible that a raised plasma viscosity may exacerbate the increased pulmonary vascular resistance.

12.15.5   Further reading

Ahumada, G. G. (ed.) (1987). *Cardiovascular pathophysiology*. Oxford University Press.

Braunwald, E. (ed.) (1988). *Heart disease* (3rd edn). W. B. Saunders, Philadelphia.

Bristow, M. R., *et al.* (1982) Decreased catecholamine sensitivity and β-adrenergic-receptor density in failing human hearts. *New England Journal of Medicine* **307**, 205–11.

Cooper, G. (1987). Cardiocyte adaptation to chronically altered load. *Annual Reviews of Physiology* **49**, 501–18.

Dalen, J. E. and Alpert, J. S. (eds) (1987). *Valvular heart disease* (2nd edn). Little, Brown and Company, Boston.

Harris, P. and Heath, D. (1986). *The human pulmonary circulation* (3rd edn). Churchill Livingstone, Edinburgh.

Ionescu, M.I. and Cohn, L. H. (eds) (1985). *Mitral valve disease: diagnosis and treatment*. Butterworth, London.

Parmley, W. W. (1985). Pathophysiology of congestive heart failure. *American Journal of Cardiology* **55**, 9A–14A.

Selzer, A. (1987) Changing aspects of the natural history of valvular aortic stenosis. *New England Journal of Medicine* **317**, 91–8.

Swynghedauw, B. (1990). *Cardiac hypertrophy and failure*. John Libbey & Co. Ltd, London.

Wigle, E. D., *et al.* (1985). Hypertrophic cardiomyopathy. The importance of the site and the extent of hypertrophy: a review. *Progress in Cardiovascular Diseases* **28**, 1.

Wilkinson, M., Langhorne, C. A., Heath, D., Barer, G. R., and Howard, P. (1988). A pathophysiological study of 10 cases of hypoxic cor pulmonale. *Quarterly Journal of Medicine* **66**, 65–85.

12.16   Veins

G. A. Gresham

12.16.1   Introduction

The structure, function, and pathology of the venous system have received comparatively little attention when compared to similar studies on the arterial system. This neglect is the result of a common tendency in medical thought: the presence of disease often dictates the need for fundamental studies of structure and function. Veins attract little attention except when they are involved in thrombosis or in abnormal dilatations such as varicosites in various parts of the venous tree. The object of this section is to illustrate the wide diversity of venous pathology that may be found in many disorders.

12.16.2   Structure and function

Venous structure is basically similar to that of arteries. There are intimal, media, and adventitial areas but they are often less clearly defined than those of arteries. Venous calibre is generally larger than that of arteries but the walls are thinner because of the presence of abundant collagen mingled with sparse amounts of muscle and elastic tissue. Unlike arteries, veins tend to collapse when not filled with blood. The internal elastic lamina is not well defined, being composed of irregularly arranged elastic fibres quite unlike the compact fenestrated internal elastic membrane of the arterial wall. Likewise, the medial smooth muscle bundles are loosely arranged and often separated by bands of collagenous tissue (Fig. 12.149).

The structure of veins is immensely variable and depends very much on mechanical conditions, such as the local intra-luminal pressure. Venous structure changes when mechanical conditions are altered as, for example, in varicose veins or in veins inserted into the arterial system as grafts to circumvent arterial obstruction. In normal circumstances veins that carry blood at higher pressure tend to have structures that approximate more closely to those of arteries. This is the case with the portal, pulmonary veins, and vena cava. In addition, flow in these veins is pulsatile rather than steady because of variation of intrathoracic and intra-abdominal pressure. In these large venous trunks the tunica media is thin but the adventitia is thick. Both contain smooth muscle fibres separated by collagen and a few elastic fibres. In the media the muscle tends to be arranged circularly and in the adventitia it is longitudinal. Such longitudinal adventitial muscle is also a feature of certain arteries, such as the common iliac vessels.

The structure of veins varies as one ascends the venous tree. The transition from capillary to venule is first indicated by the appearance of collagen fibres in the wall. Muscle fibres appear later in larger venules. Venules are essentially collagenous tubes lined by endothelium with occasional pericytes in the wall. Such small vessels are highly permeable and are sites of active fluid interchange between the tissue spaces and the circulation. Endothelial cells in this area have poorly developed junctions, thus accounting for their permeability. Post-capillary venules in the lymphatic system have an additional function. In the paracortical areas of lymph nodes they are lined by tall, rather than flattened, endothelial cells. This arrangement allows for the active intercellular passage of lymphocytes from the circulation into the tissues and vice versa.

As a general rule, muscle tends to be more apparent in larger veins. In those about 0.3 mm in diameter the muscle is a continuous layer of circularly disposed medial cells. Veins of the lower extremities have a thicker media than those of the upper parts of the body. This is particularly evident in the superficial veins of the lower limbs (Fig. 12.150). The development of the media and a thick collagenous adventitia depends largely on the intraluminal venous pressure. Pressure has a profound effect on the growth and development of any variety of blood vessel. Elastic fragmentation of the media of the pulmonary artery follows birth in normal infants. This is an expression of a fall of pressure which occurs when the postnatal circulation is established. In some ways the media of the pulmonary artery comes to resemble that of a vein. Also, the development of new vessels in canalized thrombi is an expression of the pressure in the thrombosed vessel. Canalizing vessels in thrombosed veins appear as venules and in arteries they appear as arterioles.

Veins that are especially rich in muscle include those of the gravid uterus and the umbilical vein, which has an inner longitudinal and outer circular layer, which also contains longitudinally oriented fibres. Veins of the gravid uterus also have intimal longitudinal muscle, which is also found in many limb veins and those of the mesentery of the intestine. Veins close to the heart, such as the vena cava and pulmonary veins, are peculiar in that circularly arranged cardiac muscle is found in the adventitia.

Some veins have no muscle and thus have no recognizable media. Examples are the cerebral and meningeal veins and the great dural venous sinuses. Retinal veins and those of bones also lack smooth muscle. The precise mechanical reasons for this are not clear. The distensible venous sinuses of the red pulp of the spleen are an extreme example of veins which consist only of permeable lining endothelium supported by reticulin fibres.

There is, then, a wide range of structure in veins, which may

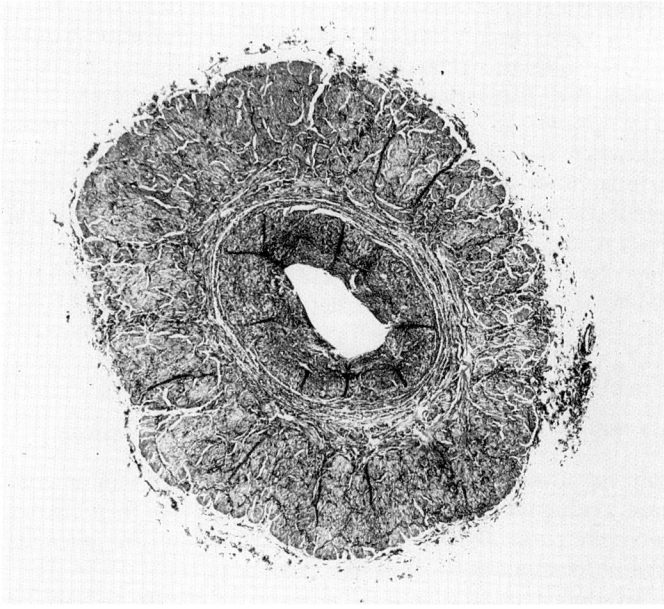

Fig. 12.150 Short saphenous vein showing well-defined muscle layers. (Weigert's resorcin fuchsin stain.)

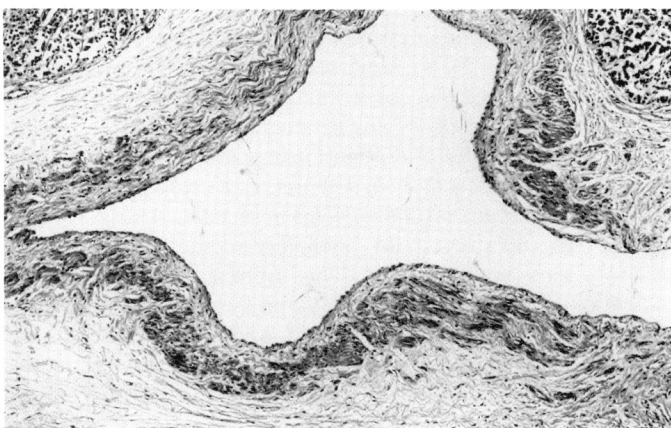

Fig. 12.149 Adrenal vein from a baby showing loosely arranged, dark-staining muscle separated by collagen. A clearly defined internal elastic lamina is not seen. (Weigert's resorcin fuchsin stain.)

change during life as haemodynamic conditions vary. Veins are essentially capacitance vessels that have little effect on peripheral resistance but do hold the greater part of the blood volume. However, they are not passive structures. They have a rich sympathetic innervation and, by constriction, can increase cardiac output and maintain circulating blood volume to essential organs. Venous pressure is an important consideration in the management of cardiac failure and other conditions. Collapsibility of peripheral veins makes pressure measurements unreliable and central venous pressure must therefore be determined. A lot of fundamental work remains to be done on veins. Comparative studies have shown great differences in the chemistry and metabolism of arterial and venous tissues. They differ in oxygen uptake, rates of glycolysis, proteoglycan metabolism, and prostacyclin production. Studies on arterial structure and function (which were impelled by widespread interest in arterial disease) have outstripped similar work on veins and provide an example of much needed research in this field.

Venous function depends a good deal on the presence of valves. Most veins over 2 mm in diameter have these structures; they are especially numerous in large veins of the lower limbs. They are not found in cerebral venous sinuses, meningeal veins, and visceral veins, with the exceptions of venae cavae and portal venous branches. Valves are paired intimal structures. They are essentially made of connective tissue, covered on both sides by endothelium. The connective tissue on the side away from the heart is rich in elastic fibres. Eddies occur at the sites of valves and it is not surprising that thrombi are found in valve pockets as a result of the turbulence. Recent use of veins as bypass grafts in coronary artery surgery and in microsurgery has led to studies on the distribution of valves in a variety of veins (Wyss *et al.* 1986).

Vasa vasorum are features of veins as well as arteries. They form capillary networks in the adventitia and, in the case of veins, extend deeply into the media. This is unlike the human arterial situation where vasa vasorum only supply the outer media. Part of the arterial wall is relatively hypoxic and this has been thought to be a factor in the development of arterial atherosclerosis. Atherosclerosis occurs rarely in veins but it is frequent in veins that have been inserted into the arterial circulation (Gresham 1983 and Section 12.14). This may be due, in part, to the increased pressure to which they are subjected. However, removal of the vein for grafting purposes may impair the blood supply of the vasa vasorum derived from neighbouring vessels. This may be another atherogenic factor in venous grafts.

12.16.3   Congenital and acquired anomalies

Congenital venous disorders are far more frequent than is commonly recognized. They become significant when they involve anomalous venous drainage and when abnormal arteriovenous communications are present in various organs.

Arteriovenous anastomoses are a normal feature and consist of direct connections between arteries and veins through which no interchange of blood and tissue fluids occurs. The ana-

stomoses consist of a layer of endothelium lying upon a tunica media composed of smooth muscle; this forms a sphincter. These muscle cells have an epithelioid appearance and have a rich autonomic innervation. Arteriovenous anastomoses occur in the exposed skin such as nose, lips, palms, and soles of the feet. They also occur in organs such as the thyroid and the alimentary system where intermittent function occurs and intermittent changes in blood supply are required. In some areas the anastomosis is surrounded by a sheath of connective tissue, forming a knot or glomus.

The nature, distribution, and possible roles of arteriovenous anastomoses in disease are summarized in a review by Sherman. The usual role of arteriovenous anastomoses is to regulate local circulation by rhythmic contraction and dilatation. If they remain persistently dilated, they may shunt blood away from parts of a tissue, and local ischaemia may result. The possible roles of arteriovenous anastomosis in gastroduodenal ulceration, diabetic gangrene, sclerodema, Raynaud disease, migraine, and shock have all been suggested.

Pathologically induced arteriovenous anastomoses are usually the result of trauma, developmental abnormality, vascular neoplasms, vasculitis, and degenerative disease. One of the more dramatic is rupture of an abdominal aortic aneurysm into the inferior vena cava. This is a rare event that leads to a precipitate rise of central venous pressure and rapid high-output cardiac failure.

Arteriovenous malformations are recorded in a variety of sites, including brain, lung, gut, and kidney. They are often symptomless and are only found when the excised organ is examined. Occasionally they produce clinical effects in life. In recent times, arteriovenous malformations of the colon have been recognized as a common cause of intestinal bleeding (see below).

Lung

Arteriovenous malformations in the lung occur most often in the lower lobes. They vary from tiny pin-point collections of vessels, often called telangiectases, to large cavernous spaces. Sometimes the lesion may replace the whole lobe of a lung which is supplied by an enlarged branch of the pulmonary artery. They consist of a collection of distended vessels fed by a dilated, thin-walled artery and drained by distended veins. The vessels that form the malformation resemble veins and often show intimal fibrosis and thrombosis. The presence of intimal thickening in abnormal dilated veins in sections of lung, kidney, or brain should suggest the possibility of the presence of an arteriovenous malformation. The intimal thickening is an indication of increased intravascular pressure. Large malformations cause cyanosis, polycythaemia, and finger clubbing, due to direct shunting of pulmonary arterial blood into the pulmonary veins, thus bypassing the capillary bed of the lung. Rupture of such malformations is not infrequent, leading to areas of surrounding haemorrhage and later deposits of haemosiderin.

Pulmonary arteriovenous malformations are sometimes associated with vascular lesions elsewhere in the skin, buccal mucosa, lips, respiratory, alimentary, and urinary tracts. Lesions may also occur in the liver, brain, or spleen. The lesions are often small telangiectatic structures but may coalesce to form larger lesions. This is Osler–Weber–Rendu disease, which is an autosomal dominant condition, though a family history is not present in about 20 per cent of cases. Histologically, the lesions consist of thin-walled venular and capillary spaces. Like the pulmonary lesions, they tend to bleed and this becomes more frequent with age, although it has little effect on life expectancy.

Colon

Unexplained bleeding from the lower intestinal tract is a not uncommon problem for the surgeon. Barium studies and endoscopy often reveal nothing abnormal and the assumption was that diverticula were the cause. However, the source of bleeding is often in the right side of the colon, whereas diverticula are much more common on the left side. Nothing may be found in the resected bowel by ordinary methods of examinations. However, vascular injection of the specimen will reveal the cause of bleeding. The lesions can also be seen in life by mesenteric angiography. Using this technique, lesions may be found without evidence of colonic haemorrhage. The incidence of colonic angiodysplasia is unknown and it is likely that lesions exist which do not produce any symptoms. It follows that the demonstration of angiodysplastic lesions in patients with melaena does not always imply that these lesions are the cause of colonic bleeding. Angiographic studies of the bowel in patients with intestinal bleeding reveal typical angiodysplastic lesions in some cases. Others have bled from vascular leiomyomas of the small bowel, or from inflammatory conditions such as Crohn disease and ischaemic colitis (see also Section 16.3.7).

Detection of angiodysplastic lesions in pathological specimens is difficult as the vessels collapse after bowel resection. Vascular injection with latex rubber often reveals surface lesions that can readily be seen by examining the surface of the colon with a dissecting microscope. The lesions vary from small focal early changes to multiple large lesions. The early lesions consist of dilated tortuous large submucosal veins with little dilatation of their mucosal tributaries. Later lesions show further dilatation of submucosal veins, with replacement of the overlying mucosa by various collections of dilated, thin-walled capillaries and venules which may rupture.

There is debate about the nature of angiodysplastic lesions. They have been variously thought to be congenital, neoplastic, or acquired. The lesions are small, multiple, and occur in elderly patients, suggesting that they are acquired abnormalities. The earliest change in the submucosal veins is likely to be due to chronic, partial, intermittent obstruction of submucosal veins where they penetrate the circular and longitudinal colonic muscle. Intermittent colonic contractions over the years lead to sporadic venous occlusions. Arteries are not affected and this leads to venous dilatation as the arterial input is maintained. Later, precapillary sphincters become incompetent and arteriovenous malformations result. Arterial dilatations are a late stage of the disease. It is thought that there is more tension in the wall of the more dilated parts of the large bowel. This may explain the occurrence of lesions in the right side of the colon. The finding of cholesterol emboli in arteries supplying the ectatic areas has led to a view that such emboli might be a cause. It is more likely that cholesterol emboli from the aorta are trapped in areas of low vascular resistance provided by angiodysplastic lesions.

Similar lesions occur in the stomach and duodenum, and a few cases have associated aortic valve disease. This is more likely to be an age associated phenomenon rather than implying some aetiological association.

Brain

Vascular anomalies of the brain, spinal cord, and their associated membranes are numerous. There is not space here to consider them in detail: a comprehensive review is given by Stehbens (1972). Vascular malformations of the brain and spinal cord are of three main types: capillary telangiectases; venous malformations, including cavernous and racemose angiomas; and arteriovenous malformations. They may exert clinical effects due to haemorrhage, thrombosis, or pressure on adjacent structures. Some have interesting effects, as with aneurysms of the great vein of Galen. These may present in neonatal life with intractable cardiac failure, hydrocephalus, and fits. An angiomatous network of adjacent arteries often feeds the aneurysm and this leads to arteriovenous shunting, causing the cardiac failure. In addition, the malformation 'steals' blood from parts of the brain causing cerebral infarction. The entire venous system within the skull, including the transverse and straight sinuses, are dilated and the onset of symptoms is determined by the size of the shunt and the size of the aneurysm, which may be up to several centimetres in diameter. Other arteriovenous shunts have been recorded between the anterior vessels of the circle of Willis and the straight sinus, and between a branch of the middle cerebral and the lateral sinus. Similar malformations occur over the cerebellum. The classical anomaly is Sturge–Weber syndrome (encephalofacial angiomatosis) where a vascular naevus in the territory of the fifth cranial nerve is associated with meningeal angiomatosis. Calcification of the adjacent brain is a feature, and deposits of iron and calcium encrust the affected meningeal vessels. A variety of clinical features may appear with increasing age: pareses, epilepsy, and neural retardation may occur. Isolated varices of cerebral veins are very rare, producing subarachnoid or intracranial haemorrhage.

Acquired arteriovenous communications may follow trauma to the head or rupture of an arterial aneurysm into an adjacent vein. Carotid-cavernous fistula can be produced in either way. The clinical features are dramatic with exophthalmos, pulsation of the eyeball, and the presence of a loud bruit.

Liver

Varicose lesions in and around the liver are numerous and their origins sometimes controversial. Peliosis hepatis consists of red foci scattered through the liver. Some foci consist of cysts, filled with blood, communicating with sinusoids. Others are phlebo-sclerotic with a fibrous wall and endothelial lining. They communicate with sinusoids and hepatic veins. Both types may occur together. The various associations suggested are pulmonary tuberculosis, androgenic steroid therapy, renal transplantation, and chronic haemodialysis.

Lesions of the portal vein may be congenital, such as obstructing valves and atresia and hypoplasia. Cavernomatous transformation of the vein is a major cause of portal hypertension in children. The vein is replaced by a sponge-like array of vessels. It may present with bleeding, splenomegaly, or pancytopenia. It may be an angiomatous malformation or may be secondary to intra-abdominal sepsis or umbilical sepsis. Catheterization of the umbilical veins has been noted as a cause. The association of congenital abnormalities, such as malformation of the biliary tract, a septal defect, and anomalies of the inferior vena cava, suggest a congenital origin.

Other lesions

Arteriovenous fistulas occur elsewhere in the body. They have been recorded in the neck, extremities, liver (haem-angioendothelioma), thorax, and lung. Other venous abnormalities consist of persistent remnants of embryonic structures. These occur in the venae cavae. Persistence of the right valve of the sinus venosus will produce a delicate network which may trap emboli or, rarely, prolapse into the orifice of the coronary sinus, giving rise to syncopal attacks (Fig. 12.151). Web-like structures in the inferior vena cava may lead to a Budd–Chiari syndrome. These webs may be congenital in origin or acquired by organization of pre-existent thrombi. This lesion is rare in Europe and North America but is common in Blacks and in some parts of India.

12.16.4   Varicose veins

Varicose veins are dilated, tortuous, thickened veins. They occur most commonly in the vessels of the lower extremities. They are not found in quadrupeds and their occurrence has often been cited as one of the many failures of man to adapt to the erect posture. About 17 per cent of the population has varicose veins: they vary from a small cluster of dilated vessels to extensive involvement of veins of the limb. The cause is probably an inherited defect in the venous valves or in the wall of the vein. This is supported by a familial incidence in about 43 per cent of cases, and in such families the same segment is sometimes affected in different members of the family. Elevation of venous pressure is a predisposing factor. Pressure of the gravid uterus or occupations involving prolonged standing are associated with varicose veins. Congestive cardiac failure with increased venous pressure is another factor, and thrombosis of pelvic veins will also predispose to venous varicosities in the lower limbs. Thrombosis of veins deep in the leg muscles can create varicosities in the superficial veins by causing blood to be deflected into them via the veins communicating between the deep and superficial vessels.

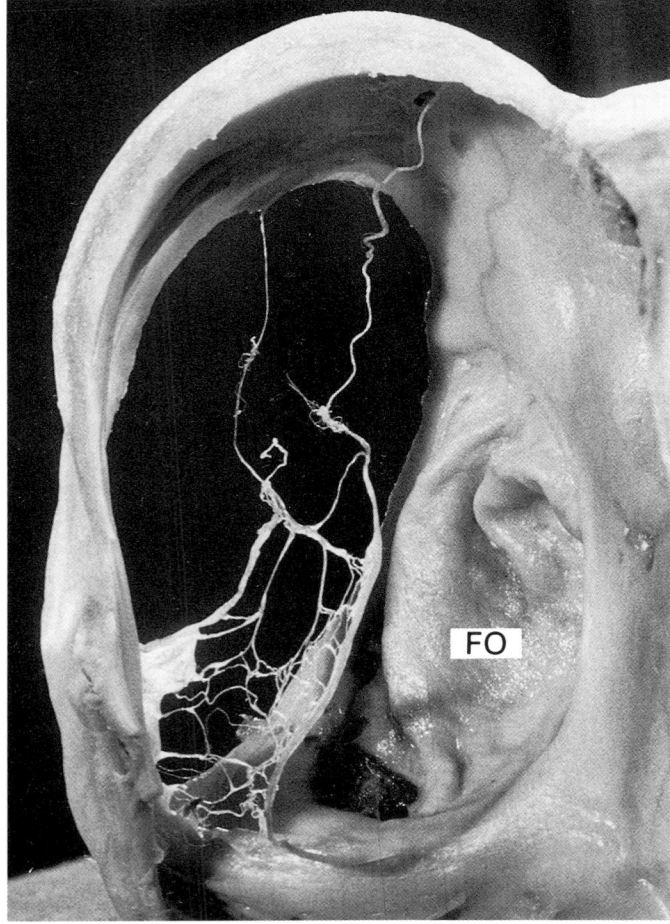

Fig. 12.151   Network of Chiari bridging the entrance of the inferior vena cava into the right atrium. Fossa ovalis (FO) to the right. The coronary fossa sinus is on the bottom edge of the picture.

The Klippel–Trenaunay–Weber syndrome provides an odd association of events that may indicate a primary defect as a cause of varicose veins. There is here an association between extensive cutaneous cavernous haemangioma, varicose veins, and hypertrophy of soft tissue and bones of a limb. The varicosities and limb hypertrophy develop later in life in children with such haemangiomas. The presence of arteriovenous shunts may be an explanation of the varicosities. Equally, a prime defect in the venous wall may be the cause.

Varicosities occur in ill-supported veins lying in loose connective tissue. The subcutaneous tissues of the leg are a favourite site and they also occur in other situations, such as the lower oesophagus, the anorectal junction, the pampiniform plexus of the spermatic cord, and in the parametrial veins.

Stagnation of blood in varicose veins leads to tissue oedema and hypoxia. In the legs the skin becomes atrophic and ulcerates. These lesions are difficult to heal because of the persistent hypoxia. This is aggravated by the leakage of fibrinogen, which polymerizes to fibrin, into the oedema fluid. This leads to an impermeable coat around cutaneous capillaries which impedes diffusion of nutrients to the skin and further aggravates tissue damage.

Varicose veins are subjected to factors that are known to promote arterial atherosclerosis. These are increased intraluminal pressure and hypoxia in the vessel wall. The veins respond, as do arteries, by thickening of the wall, a condition often called phlebosclerosis. In the early stages muscular hypertrophy occurs, and may develop in distinct longitudinal and circular layers (Fig. 12.152). Intimal fibro-elastic thickenings also appear, which may be the end-result of small organized thrombi. Later the thickened muscular wall becomes replaced by fibrous tissue, and foci of calcification and droplets of lipid appear in the thickened intima. Lipid is never as conspicuous as that seen in arterial atherosclerosis. Similar changes also appear, often in a few months, in veins used to bypass obstructions in the arterial circulation. Changes resembling arterial atherosclerosis have been described in veins used in aorto-coronary (Section 12.14) and popliteal artery bypass operations.

Venous thrombosis

The effects of venous thrombosis depend upon the vein involved. Adrenal vein thrombosis, which may occur in various bacterial septicaemias, can cause fatal adrenal infarction. Nowadays coliform bacilli are most often responsible. Cerebral venous sinus thrombosis is often associated with cerebral infarction. Thrombotic obstruction of the renal vein may produce overt infarction, although often this is not seen even though impairment of renal function occurs. In general, it is true that blockage of the entire venous network from an organ causes characteristic haemorrhagic infarcts. Blockage of deep and superficial veins in the legs causes swelling and pallor of the limbs (phlegmasia alba dolens). This occurs in the puerperium. The pallor is due to massive oedema associated with concomitant lymphatic obstruction. Deep venous thrombosis is

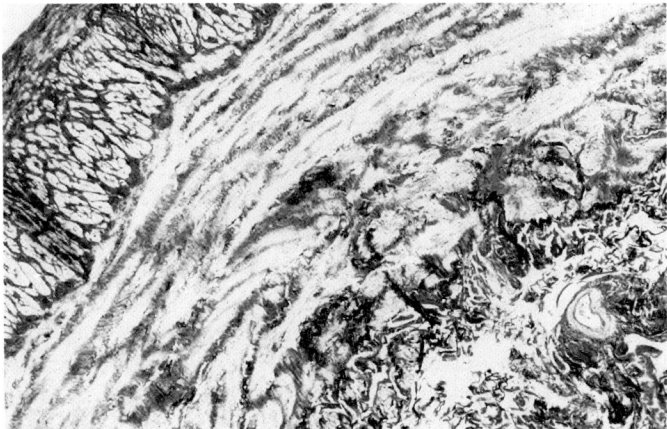

Fig. 12.152 Part of the wall of a varicose vein, showing a strip of intimal fibro-elastic thickening (top left) beneath it are vertical pillars of hypertrophied circular smooth muscle. Outer longitudinal muscle is loosely arranged. Adventitia bottom right. (Weigert's resorcin fuchsin stain.)

complicated by pulmonary embolism. These may be large and fatal, but repeated small emboli may occur, giving rise to progressive pulmonary hypertension. At autopsy the pulmonary artery contains adherent non-occlusive thrombi, some of which are organized to form fibrous tags and bands, on the intima of the vessel.

12.16.5 Thrombophlebitis and venous sclerosis

Infective

Any inflammatory process can extend into the adventitial coat of adjacent veins, giving rise to a thrombophlebitis. Ultimately, the process extends through the vein wall, causing endothelial damage and thrombosis. If the cause of the inflammation is bacterial, the thrombus becomes infected, liquefies, and fragments. Particles of thrombus laden with bacteria then embolize to the lungs and elsewhere; a process which is called pyaemia. This is illustrated by a chronic middle-ear infection extending into the adjacent lateral sinus, producing an infected thrombus, bits of which go to the lungs. Another example is portal pyaemia arising from an appendiceal abscess, extending into the portal tributaries, and ultimately producing hepatic abscesses. The commonest cause of hepatic abscess in the UK is due to *Streptococcus milleri* which derives from the vermiform appendix.

Inflammation arising directly in the vein wall is not frequent. It may be part of an allergic vasculitis or caused by external trauma or internal damage by plastic catheters.

A curious form of phlebitis affects the veins of the thoracoabdominal wall in the region of the breast. It is called Mondor disease. A chronic inflammatory reaction in the vein wall leads to progressive fibrosis which is concentric and leads to occlusion of the vessel. This produces tough fibrous cords which, with the passage of time, may disappear. The aetiology is obscure but local trauma has been suggested as a cause.

Buerger disease

Thromboangiitis obliterans (Buerger disease) is a well-known example of vasculitis affecting both arteries and veins. It is a disease mainly of males, arising in the third and fourth decades of life, involving segments of medium-sized arteries and veins of the lower limbs. Sometimes the upper limbs are involved. It is almost invariably associated with tobacco smoking and tends to improve when smoking is stopped. Resumption of smoking aggravates the disease. The disease is often associated with migrating thrombophlebitis (q.v.) and Raynaud phenomenon. The acute lesions affect arteries and veins and consist of diffuse inflammatory infiltrations of the vessel wall with microabscesses and giant cells in the thrombosed vessels.

The disease is more prevalent in the Middle and Far East than in the rest of Europe and is rare in women. Although the association with tobacco smoking is strong, the rarity of the disorder implies some additional aetiological factor. This is supported by occasional family incidence; association with certain HLA antigens; and immune reactions to human types I and III collagen. A report of the appearance of the disease in an arterial vein graft in a heavy smoker who had atherosclerotic disease of his coronary arteries is a provoking observation.

Idiopathic thrombophlebitis

Recurrent idiopathic thrombophlebitis (thrombophlebitis migrans) is a disorder characterized by recurrent episodes of thrombosis of superficial veins affecting different regions of the body surface. Occasional involvement of deep veins in the brain or viscera can produce infarction. It may continue to recur over many years. The aetiology is obscure though its association with malignant disease is well known. The histological appearances are similar to those of Buerger disease and the two diseases may be associated. However, occlusive arterial lesions are not a feature of thrombophlebitis migrans.

Systemic vasculitis

Various forms of systemic vasculitis involve veins. Hypersensitivity angiitis involving the skin begins as an acute necrotizing inflammatory process in small venules. Later, capillaries and arterioles are affected. In many cases an offending antigen can be identified and its removal leads to improvement of the condition.

Wegener granulomatosis

Wegener granulomatosis also affects small arteries and veins. Characteristic sites for the disease are upper respiratory tract, lungs, and kidneys. The lesion is an acute fibrinoid necrosis of vessel walls with associated giant-celled granulomas (see also Chapter 13).

Churg–Strauss syndrome

Allergic angiitis and granulomatosis (Churg–Strauss syndrome) is characterized by granulomatous vasculitis affecting many organs. The lesions resemble those of polyarteritis nodosa but are unique in that they involve blood-vessels of all sizes, including veins. Intravascular and extravascular granulomas and adjacent infiltrates of eosinophils are also characteristic. The disease is associated with severe asthma and an elevated blood eosinophil level.

Pulmonary veno-occlusive disease

Sclerosis or fibrous thickenings of veins occurs in several organs. Progressive reduction of the vascular lumen may give rise to clinical manifestations but venous sclerosis may also be totally asymptomatic.

Pulmonary veno-occlusive disease is a rare disorder of children and young adults. It causes pulmonary hypertension by obliteration of pulmonary venules and veins. This process is quite distinct from intimal venous fibrosis that occurs with increasing age or is associated with various forms of organic heart disease accompanied by reduced pulmonary blood flow, venous hypertension, and secondary polycythaemia. The lesions of pulmonary veno-occlusive disease are severe and there is no obvious predisposing cause. The veins and venules show profuse intimal proliferations of loose connective tissue; the thickening is sometimes nodular, suggesting an origin from organized thrombi. Venous involvement is extensive from the largest to the smallest branches and pulmonary hypertension with associated arterial hypertrophy is the result. Medial hypertrophy of the affected veins is also seen, and they come to resemble arteries in structure.

Most regard the disease to be due to widespread organizing thrombi. Viral and protozoal infections have been suggested as aetiological agents predisposing to venular thrombosis. The finding of IgG and complement suggests activation of coagulation processes by immune complexes generated by an infective agent. An association with chronic active hepatitis also suggests an immunological process. Other agents damaging the vein walls may be responsible and veno-occlusive disease has been described in patients receiving cytotoxic drugs such as bleomycin, Mitomycin C, and cisplatin. The finding of veno-occlusive changes in a 'cot death' indicates that other causes may exist.

Liver venous disease

Venular fibrosis occurs in branches of hepatic veins. It is an early indicator of the onset of cirrhosis in alcoholic patients. The lesion is perivenular with proliferation of myofibroblasts and collagen deposition around terminal hepatic venules. Intimal veno-occlusive disease may also be found in such cases, together with lymphocytic phlebitis of hepatic veins. Perivenular fibrosis seems to be the only venous lesion associated with progression to cirrhosis.

Veno-occlusive disease

Intimal hepatic veno-occlusive disease is seen in a variety of conditions. Most authors regard the initial lesion as endothelial damage followed by leakage of erythrocytes and plasma into the perivenular space. Some regard damage to the centrilobular hepatocytes as the initial event. Perivenular haemorrhage with hepatocyte necrosis is seen in right and left heart failure, which may lead to perivenular fibrosis: so-called cardiac cirrhosis.

Veno-occlusive disease of the liver was first described in Jamaica but sporadic cases and outbreaks occur in many parts of the world. The pyrrolizidine alkaloids contained in plants of the genera *Heliotropium*, *Senecio*, and *Crotalaria*, of which there are about 2000 species, cause the disease. Some 240 other genera contain varying amounts of the alkaloids. The seeds of such plants contaminate wheat and the alkaloids are ingested in the wheat flour. Early changes in the liver are periacinar congestion, haemorrhage, and hepatocyte necrosis. Quite early on, bands of collagen radiate from the central veins, which have undergone necrosis, and break up liver cell plates into small islets.

The initial event appears to be obstruction of central sinusoidal flow, caused by injured swollen hepatocytes associated with permeable, damaged vascular endothelium. A similar mechanism operates in veno-occlusive disease following bone marrow transplantation. An incidence of 21 per cent has been recorded in patients treated for myelogenous leukaemia.

Chemotherapy and irradiation are thought to be the causative factors. Thrombosis of hepatic veins and occlusive disease also occurs in polycythaemia and other high viscosity syndromes (Fig. 12.153) producing the Budd–Chiari syndrome.

Portal fibrosis with venous obliteration is a sequel of veno-occlusive disease. Similar portal lesions can occur without any other evidence of hepatic disease. In such cases portal tracts are expanded by fibrous tissue and veins are replaced by small capillary channels. Some have thought that mineral oil deposits in portal tracts cause fibrosis and venous obliteration; accumulation of oil may, however, be a secondary event to altered blood flow in sclerotic portal tracts. Isolated portal sclerosis often has no clinical effects, although it can be found in association with non-cirrhotic portal hypertension and with nodular regenerative hyperplasia of the liver (see Chapter 17).

'Auto-immune' venous sclerosis

Venous obliterations are a feature of the syndrome of multiple fibrosclerosis which includes Riedel thyroiditis, idiopathic retroperitoneal and mediastinal fibrosis, sclerosing cholangitis and pseudotumour of the orbit. The venous lesions are characterized by diffuse lymphocytic infiltration followed by sclerosis of the vein wall and fibrous obliteration of the vascular lumen. The changes occur in small and medium-sized veins. It has been proposed to be due to an auto-immune process but it is not clear if the phlebosclerosis is a primary or secondary event.

'Mucoid' degeneration

Degenerative changes in veins are rare, unless one includes intimal fibrosis which is a feature of many large veins with increasing age. Cystic and mucoid degenerations of leg arteries are well recognized. Similar changes have been reported only rarely in veins such as the femoral. In this condition cystic spaces in the vein wall protrude into the lumen and cause venous obstruction. The rarity of the condition in veins suggests that intraluminal pressure may be a factor in the genesis of mucoid degeneration of limb arteries.

12.16.6   Neoplasms in veins

Apart from venous metastases the vascular tumours discussed here are those found within, or arising from, large veins. These and other vascular tumours are discussed more fully in Section 12.18.

Venous metastases

Many malignant neoplasms permeate veins and metastasize by this route. Notable examples are renal cell carcinomas which spread along the renal vein and into the vena cava where a detached large mass of neoplasm may cause pulmonary embolism. Malignant tumours in adjacent lymph nodes may spread along small venous branches into the inferior vena cava, producing showers of tumour emboli and metastases in the lungs.

Carcinoma arising in the liver often penetrates portal and hepatic radicles to reach the main vessels (Fig. 12.154).

Classical patterns of metastasis are sometimes explicable by local venous arrangements. Malignant neoplasms arising close to the vertebral column often spread by way of the paravertebral venous plexus. For example, neuroblastomas of the adrenal often spread to the skull, and a similar venous pathway

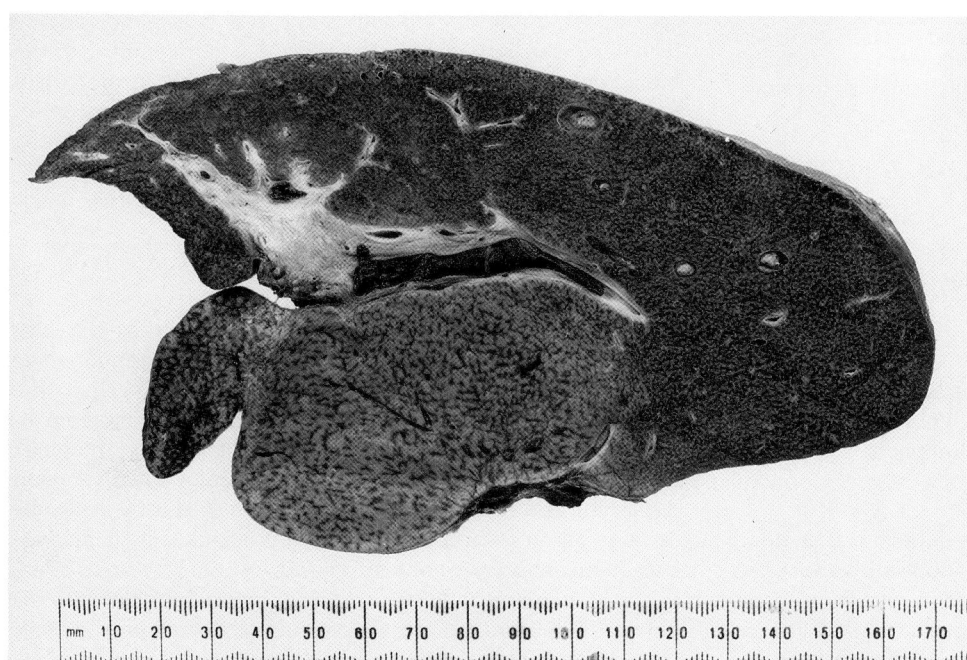

Fig. 12.153 Dark thrombus fills a main branch of a hepatic vein (centre); peripheral veins are also thrombosed. The adjacent liver and caudate lobe show severe congestion.

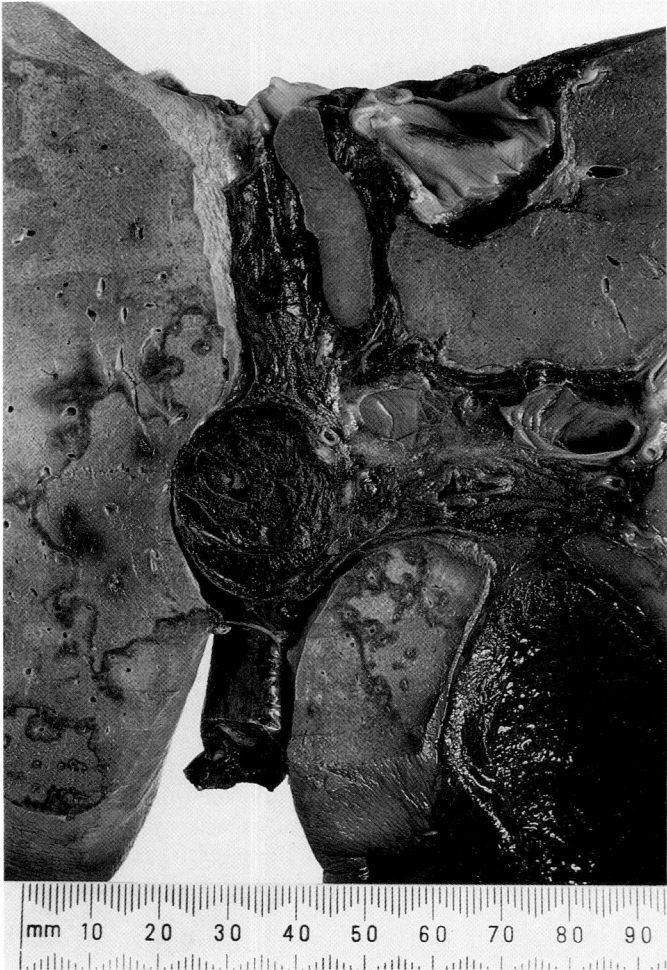

Fig. 12.154 Thrombosis of the main portal vein (centre); an unusual complication shown here is infarction of the adjacent liver. The thrombus in the vein contained fragments of metastatic pancreatic carcinoma.

may explain the distribution of metastases of carcinomas of the thyroid, prostate, and pancreas.

Benign neoplasms

Benign neoplasms of veins are rare.

Chemodectoma

Chemodectomas rarely arise from glomus bodies as in the jugular bulb. They develop slowly in the wall of the vein. Though prone to recur, they do not spread to distant parts.

Intravenous pyogenic granuloma

This is a benign lesion affecting the veins of the neck and upper extremities. The clinical course is short, about 2 months or so. The patient complains of a solid lump in the neck or upper extremity. At operation a 'tumour' is found in a vein and attached to the intima. Essentially it is an intravenous polyp composed of lobules of capillaries separated by a fibromyxoid stroma. The surface of the 'tumour' is clothed in endothelial cells and mitotic figures in endothelial cells in the lesion are frequent. A consistent finding is a small feeding muscular artery in the perivenous connective tissue opposite the stalk. In every respect the lesion resembles a cutaneous pyogenic granuloma.

Intravascular haemangioma Intravenous pyogenic granuloma is a distinct entity that needs to be distinguished from two other intravenous processes. Vegetant intravascular haemangioendothelioma is one of these, described by Masson in 1923. It appears to be an organizing thrombus composed of capillary vessels separated by cores of fibrin and erythrocytes which is later transformed to hyaline connective tissue.

Angiomatous nodule The other condition to be distinguished is the 'inflammatory' angiomatous nodule, more usually called angiolymphoid hyperplasia with eosinophilia. It is found on the ear and scalp. Blood-vessels, when involved, are more usually arteries than veins, though its occurrence in veins has been recorded. The lesion has an extensive inflammatory component of lymphoid cells and eosinophil leucocytes permeated by vascular channels lined by large endothelial cells which resemble epithelioid cells. The lesion infiltrates veins and may occlude the lumen but does not form a defined intraluminal polyp.

Malignant neoplasms

Angiosarcoma

See Section 12.18.15.

Systemic angioendotheliomatosis

This is a rare disorder which may be present in the skin. When systemic veins are involved the disease progresses rapidly. Biopsy of skin nodules reveals enlarged, rounded 'endothelial' cells in the lumina of capillaries and this is accompanied by thrombosis. In larger veins the process is not confined to the lumen but spread occurs through the vessel wall. In such cases tumour cells are pleomorphic and show mitoses. Angioendotheliomatosis may be purely intravascular, or may invade the vein wall.

This is almost certainly a lymphoproliferative disorder and is discussed more fully in Chapter 24.

Leiomyosarcoma

Leiomyosarcomas of veins are rare, although they are the commonest malignant tumour of these vessels. The commonest site is the inferior vena cava; they have been recorded in veins of the extremities and in the inferior mesenteric vein. Venous leiomyosarcomas of the limbs have been found most often in the lower extremity. The artery within the fibro-vascular sheath is often displaced and compressed, with luminal narrowing. The demonstration of this by angiography is often a clue to the presence of the adjacent venous neoplasm.

The lesions start in the vein wall but invariably grow into the lumen. Histologically they are typical leiomyosarcomas with a high grade of malignancy. The tumour cells are enclosed by reticulin; elastin is not present. Thin-walled angulate vessels are present, giving an appearance reminiscent of a pericytoma.

Electron microscopy reveals typical smooth muscle cells with actin myofilaments, focal elongate densities, and pinocytotic vesicles. Spread from the vascular sheath into adjacent fat and muscle occurs. Subsequent metastases to lungs and liver occur in the majority of cases.

12.16.7 Further reading

Cooper, P. H., *et al.* (1979). Intravenous pyogenic granuloma. A study of 18 cases. *American Journal of Surgical Pathology* 3, 221–8.

Dible, J. H. (1958). Organisation and canalisation in arterial thrombosis. *J. Path. Bac.* **75**, 1–8.

Gresham, G. A. (1983). The transplanted vessel. In *Biology and pathology of the vessel wall* (ed. N. Woolfe). Praeger, New York.

Heath, D., *et al.* (1959). The structure of the pulmonary trunk at different ages and in cases of pulmonary hypertension and pulmonary stenosis. *J. Path. Bac.* **77**, 443.

Mitsudd, S. M., *et al.* (1979). Vascular ectasis of the right colon in the elderly: a distinct pathological entity. *Human Pathology* **10**, 585–600.

Ogston, D. (1987). *Venous thrombosis. Causation and prediction.* A Wiley Medical Publication, Chichester.

Sherman, J. L. (1963). Normal arteriovenous anastomoses. *Medicine* **42**, 247–67.

Stehbens, W. E. (1972). *Pathology of the cerebral blood vessels.* The C. V. Mosby Co., St Louis.

Wyss, P., *et al.* (1986). Anatomy of the veins of the dorsum pedis with regard to their suitability as vascular grafts in reconstructive microsurgery. *Anatomy and Embryology* **175**, 199–204.

12.17 The lymphatics

Terence J. Ryan

12.17.1 Introduction

The lymphatics are the principal exit pathways from the interstitium. Lipid and protein, whether leaked from blood vessels or manufactured actively or passively by the disintegration of cells, are removed by a partnership between macrophages and lymphatics. In normal tissues almost all macromolecules and cells are cleared via the lymphatics. When this does not occur, pathology, such as is described below, is the consequence.

The primary role of this system is the control of the osmotic and hydrostatic pressure in the interstitium. Without such control the effluent that collects in the tissues causes oedema, hypoxia, fibrosis, and a loss of the normal responsiveness to changes in tissue tension.

12.17.2 The low-resistance pathways

It is not possible for cells and macromolecules to pass through all areas of the interstitium because of its complex fibrillar arrangement and compact 'ground substance'. But there are low-resistance pathways. These include septa, serous cavities such as the pleura or peritoneum, and, significantly, also within the tissues and nerves and the adventitia around blood-vessels. Elastin fibres are also a main preferential, or low-resistance pathway through the interstitium, along which cells migrate and protein or particulate matter tend to collect. This has been demonstrated in the mesentery and in the skin (Figs 12.155, 12.156).

Anionic domains that predominate in the wall of the lymphatic attract cationic proteins and serve, by their presence in the lymphatic wall, to act as a means of preferential selection, possibly unidirectionally into the lumen, and hence a low-

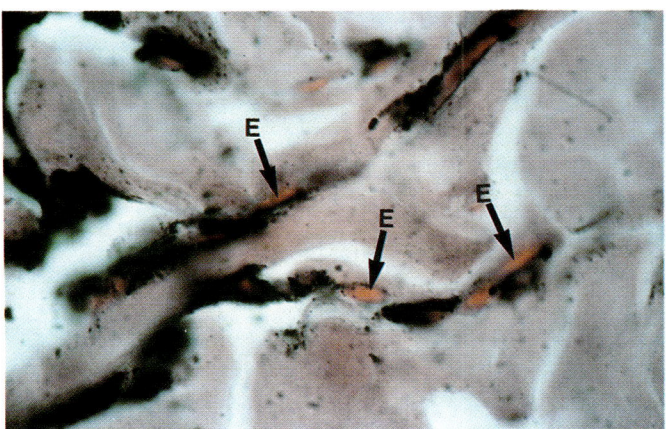

Fig. 12.155 The localization of carbon particles around elastic fibres. Following the inoculation of colloidal carbon into the dermis, it can be seen that the carbon (black colour) appears to preferentially localize along the elastic fibres (E). (Provided by R. L. Jones, P. S. Mortimer, and T. J. Ryan.)

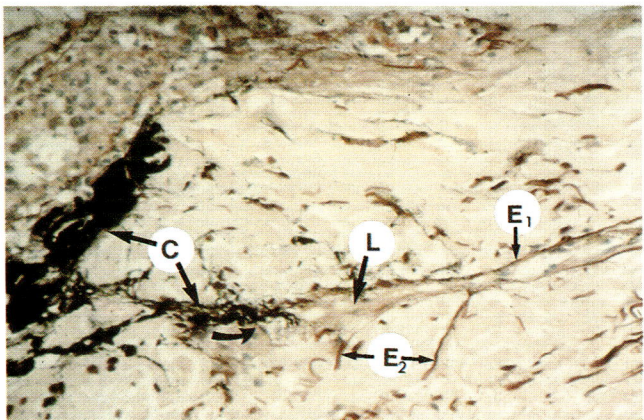

Fig. 12.156 The migration of colloidal carbon towards the initial lymphatic. Following the inoculation of colloidal carbon into the dermis, the carbon (C) appears to use the elastic fibres as a preferential pathway as it migrates towards the initial lymphatic. In this photomicrograph, the lymphatic (L) can be seen outlined by an envelope of elastic fibres (E_1). Elastic fibres (E_2) are also visible arising from the lymphatic wall and inserting into the surrounding connective tissues. (Orcein stain.) (From Jones 1985.)

resistance pathway. Low-resistance pathways for the migration of cells are important in wound healing and also for the spread of metastatic malignant cells.

12.17.3   Lymph flow

Lymph flow is determined by movement such as arterial pulsation, muscle contraction, massage, and any other factor tending to distort the tissue. Water and macromolecules are thus moved along low-resistance pathways into the lymphatics where the structures described below encourage flow away from the tissues. It remains uncertain whether tissue fluid leaked from blood-vessels acts by washing materials into the lymphatics or whether it is sucked by negative pressure into the initial lymphatics. Contractility of the lymphatic trunks is determined by intrinsic myogenic responses augmented by the autonomic nervous system and modified by local inflammatory mediators.

Anatomical distribution of lymphatics

The lymphatic system consists of lymphatic trunks which drain a network of initial lymphatics lying in the less compact areas of the peripheral tissues. The initial lymphatics have a much larger lumen than capillaries and, compared to the blood vascular network, the network is a loose mesh of low density.

Lymphatics are not present in the brain, bone, the eye, or in the centre of compact end organs, such as the fat lobule or some endocrine glands. To make up for this, there are special adaptations of blood vascular endothelium for the bulk transport of protein. This is best seen in the arachnoid villi or in the canal of Schlemm. In the brain, tissue plains, especially around major blood-vessels, allow lymph to exit from the enclosed environ-

ment of the skull. Organs such as the fat lobules normally have little need for a lymphatic system (except in the septa) because the metabolism of fat requires only that macromolecules are cleared by the rich vasculature that supplies the centre of the fat lobule, at which site macromolecules are only formed when fat is injured or when there is an excessive leakiness from the capillaries in inflammation, such as erythema nodosum or venous hypertension.

Lymph flows through a system of vessels which are normally only transiently filled and whose function determines that they are mostly empty. Indeed, if they are distended for prolonged periods, as in venous hypertension in the lower leg, then all sections of lymphatic vessels tend to leak and become incompetent. Flow through the lymph system is directed to

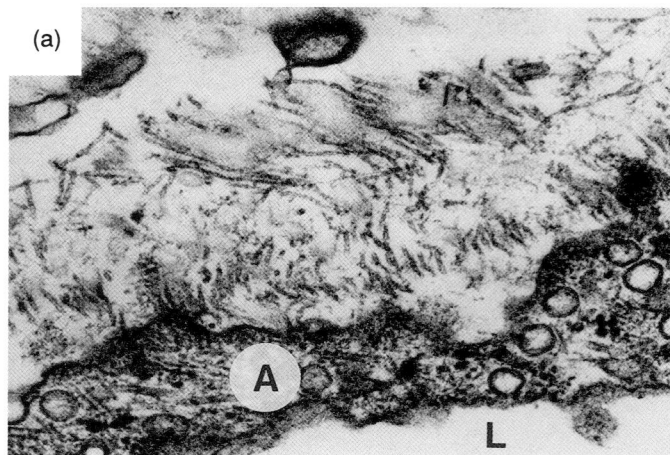

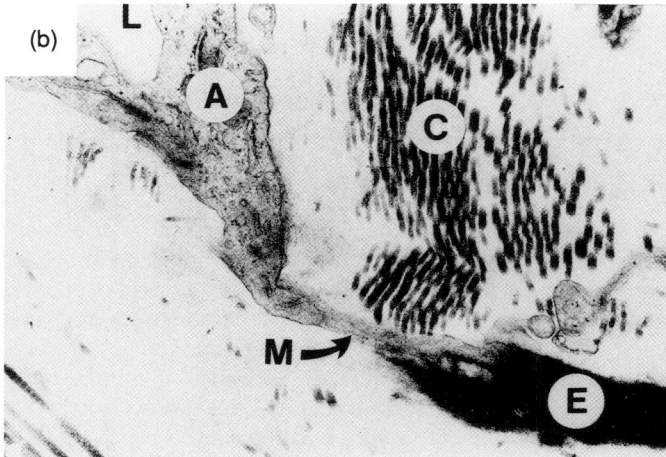

Fig. 12.158 The microfibrillar attachments to the lymphatic wall. (a) Anchoring filaments are visible running directly to the luminal surface of the dermal lymphatic endothelial cell (A). The filaments have a tubular substructure; they are 10–12 nm in diameter. L, lumen. (Provided by J. Daroczy, Bor-es Nemikortani Klinika, Budapest.) (b) The endothelium of the lymphatic (A) is attached by microfilaments (M) to an elastic fibre (E). This illustrates how the endothelium tends to be pulled away from the lumen (L) by the attachment to elastic fibres. C, collagen. (Phosphotungstic acid stain.) (From Jones 1985, Jones et al. 1986.)

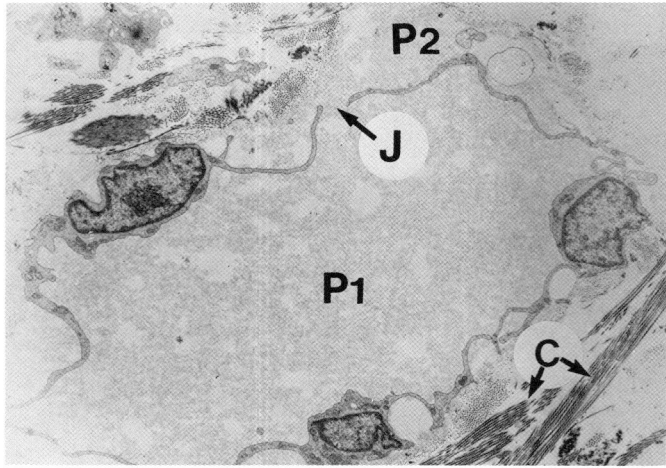

Fig. 12.157 The attentuated lymphatic endothelium. This electron micrograph of psoriatic human skin illustrates the extremely attenuated endothelium of a lymphatic capillary which lacks distinct supporting structures such as a basal lamina or pericytes. Electron dense granules of proteinaceous material are seen in the lumen (P1) and in the interstitium (P2) close to an open junction (J). C, collagen. (From Jones 1985.)

lymph nodes, in which or beyond which they may enter the bloodstream via lymphatic-venous anastomoses, of which the thoracic duct is the largest.

The initial lymphatic

The initial lymphatics are tissue spaces lined by an attenuated endothelium, the cells of which have relatively small nuclei compared to those of blood capillary cells. This lining function is an adaptation that encourages movement of fluid and cells into the lymphatics from the interstitium. There are wide gaps between the endothelial cells with overlapping lips of endothelium acting as valves (Fig. 12.157).

There is no barrier into the lymphatic lumen from the interstitium in the form of a basement lamina, but there are anchoring fibrillar materials attaching the endothelium to the connective tissues through which they are traversing. These microfilaments were at one time thought to be only composed of collagen but, at least in the skin, they are now thought to be more commonly related to elastin (Fig. 12.158a,b). Broad bands of elastin are attached to these anchoring fibrils and surround the lymphatic in the skin; they can be used to identify initial lymphatics from terminal blood capillaries (Fig. 12.159a–d).

The initial lymphatic contains valves which, in the blood vasculature system, is a feature of only larger venules and veins. These valves consist of endothelial cells flapping loosely into the lumen, with their nuclei projecting further into the lumen, often in clusters (Fig. 12.160).

Lymphatic network

The lymphatic network is a meshwork, lying superficially in the skin and on the surface of viscera, which allows collateral drainage through the lymphatic capillaries when deeper collecting vessels become obstructed. Compared to blood vasculature, the meshwork is wide and, in some sites, materials in the interstitium looking for an exit pathway have to travel as much as 1 mm in order to find a lymphatic.

The so-called collecting vessel is merely a slightly thicker-walled, more proximal vessel into which the network of initial lymphatics is drained. At a still more proximal level, thicker lymphatic trunks carry lymph to the lymph node. It is often insufficiently recognized that these lymphatic trunks are as numerous as veins and may be as thick walled (Fig. 12.161). For this reason, when their identity is complicated by inflammation, they become virtually indistinguishable from inflamed veins. Collecting vessels and lymphatic trunks follow arterio-venous routes and cross-sections of a neurovascular bundle will usually include a lymphatic (Fig. 12.162).

Phenotype of lymphatic endothelium and blood vascular endothelium

There has been considerable recent interest in the identification of lymphatics from blood vascular endothelium. It is not known whether endothelial cells retain an identity in all circumstances or whether they have a potential to change in response to an altered environment of inflammation and neoplasia. Blood-vessel endothelium has a great experience of both mechanical

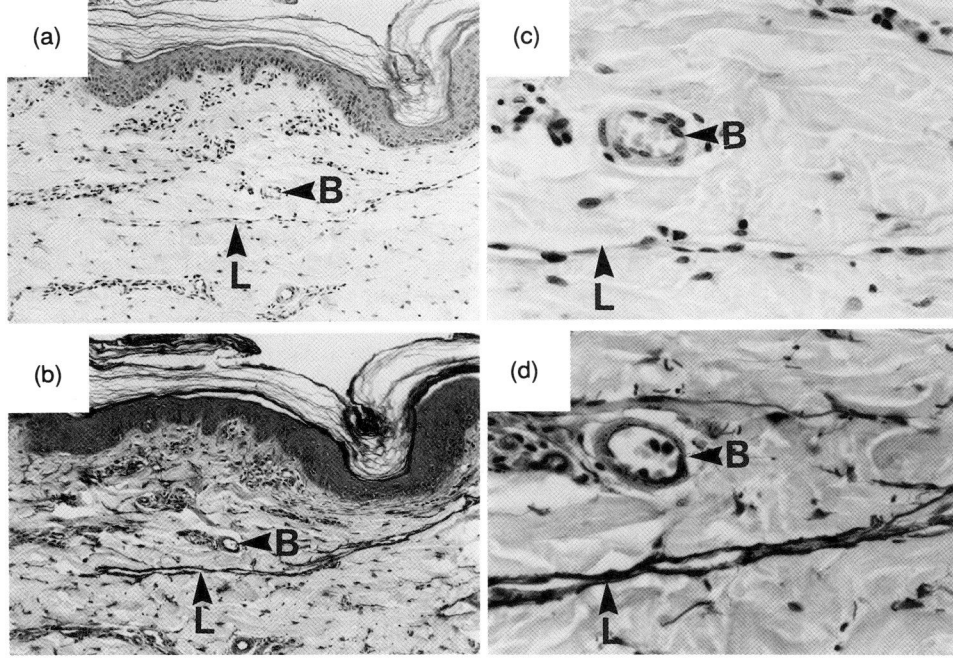

Fig. 12.159 A long, collapsed initial lymphatic. The lymphatics (L) are collapsed in normal skin and, compared to blood vessels (B), are extremely long. In routinely stained sections they may be difficult to identify, as shown in (a) and (c). However, an elastic fibre stain, (b) and (d), demonstrates the presence of an elastic fibre envelope or network surrounding the dermal lymphatics This technique can be used to help identify them. (Stains: (a) and (c), H & E; (b) and (d), orcein.) (Provided by R. L. Jones.)

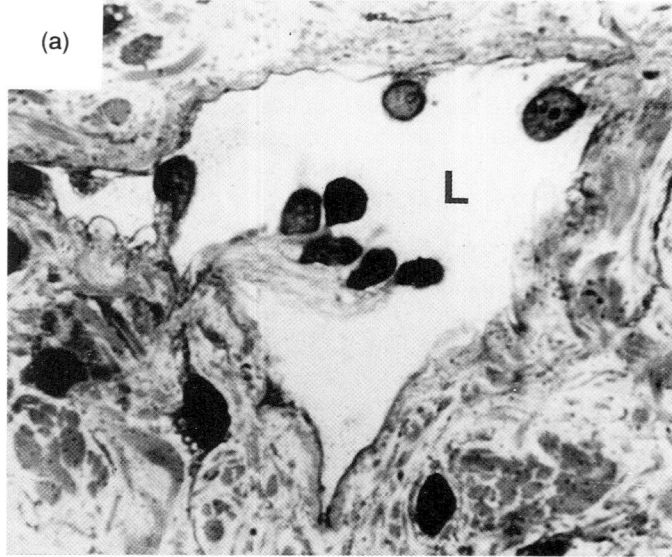

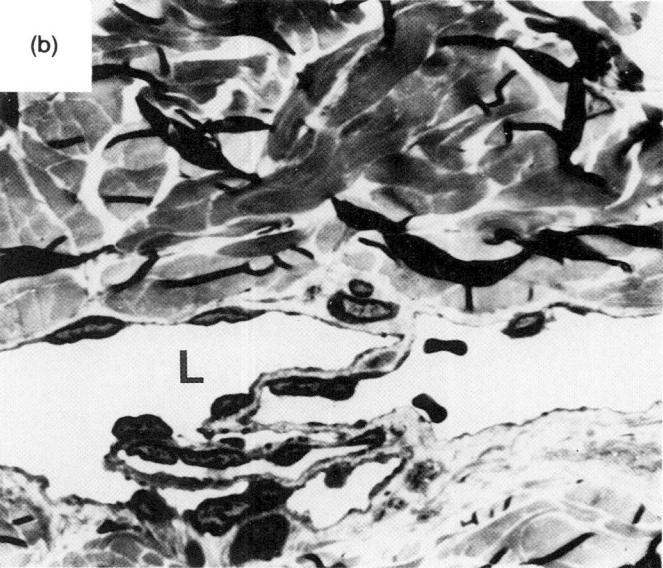

Fig. 12.160 Light microscopy of lymphatic valves (a) 'Tip cells' are visible along the edge of the valve protruding into the lymphatic lumen (L). (Semi-thin section; stain, toluidine blue; from Daroczy 1983.) (b) Tricuspid valve formation in the lumen (L) of a dermal lymphatic capillary. (Semi-thin section; stain, toluidine blue.) (From Daroczy 1984.)

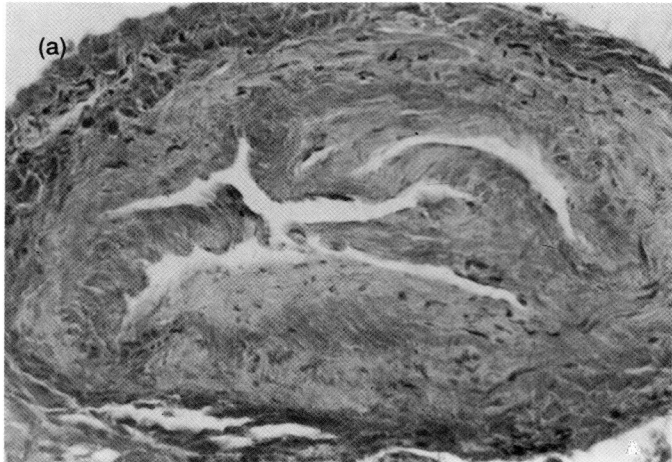

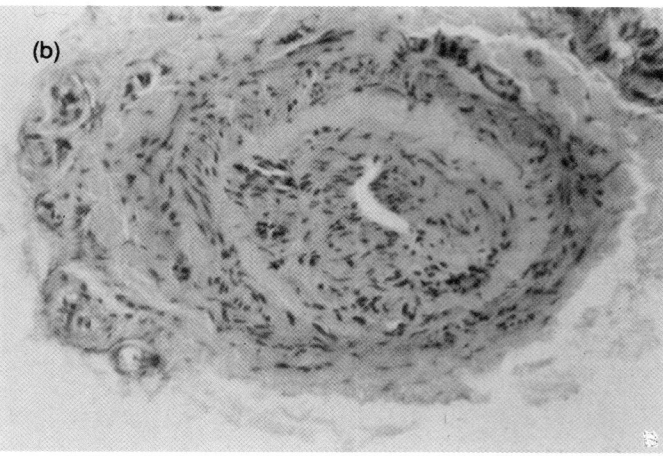

Fig. 12.161 (a, b) Two examples of great hypertrophy of the lymphatic trunk taken under direct vision from specimens on the dorsum of the foot by the late Professor Mannheimer (Vienna), showing a thick muscular wall. Especially when this becomes inflamed, as in lymphangitis, it becomes impossible to distinguish the vessel from bloodvessels of similar size.

and chemical properties of blood, to which it probably adapts with a greater number of possible activities, and hence identifiable characteristics. Only when lymphatic endothelium is exposed continuously to a similar environment may it adapt so that features like Weibel–Palade bodies, factor VIII positivity, or basement lamina formation are acquired. It is on the basis of such reasoning that some would argue that a lymphatic origin explains Kaposi's sarcoma, while others would look for a blood vascular origin, and yet others would argue that the endothe-

lium has features of both and no inevitable retention of any distinguishing mark.

The identification of lymphatic endothelium from blood vasculature endothelium in disease is impossible with any certainty. In health, the localization in, for example, the neurovascular bundle, or at certain sites known to be rich in lymphatics, may not be difficult to recognize. This is especially so when other features are taken into account, such as the attenuated walls; the elastin network and attachments; the presence of valves; and the absence of a basement lamina; together with lack of staining for factor VIII-related antigen and for collagen type IV or laminin in the basement lamina; Weibel–Palade bodies are also absent. However, in the larger normal collecting vessels such as the thoracic duct (as well as in embryo, wounds, and tumours) Weibel–Palade bodies and factor VIII-related antigen positivity are often present, although to a lesser degree

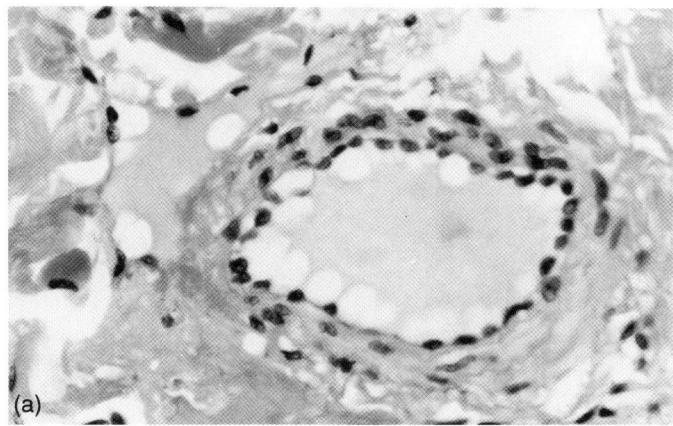

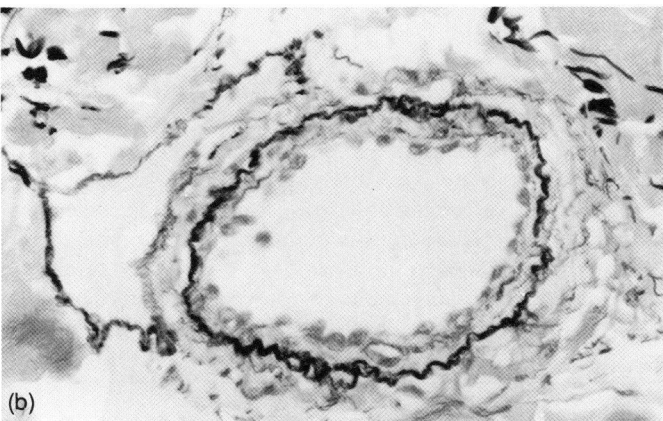

Fig. 12.162 A blood-vessel with an adjacent lymphatic. (a) Haematoxylin and eosin. The lymphatic on the left of the blood-vessel is not clearly defined. (b) Orcein stain, showing up very well the internal elastic lamina of the blood vessel, but it also delineates the lymphatic on the left.

than in blood vascular endothelium. Lymphatic endothelium also shares with blood vessel endothelium other markers, such as *Ulex europaeus* lectin binding and angiotensin converting enzyme.

12.17.4 Congenital disease

Lymphangiomas

Lymphangiomas are an extreme dilatation of lymphatics, usually due to a failure of emptying caused by proximal obstruction. Vesicular formation at the surface of the skin and of some internal organs is associated with sometimes quite deep cystic changes in dilated lymphatic trunks, most commonly found subcutaneously. The walls of such angiomas are often thickened and contain smooth muscle, in response to the development of high intravascular pressure within the closed and dilated lymphatic system. Spontaneous contractions can be observed in an attempt to overcome the obstruction.

Hygromata

These are especially large cystic and subcutaneous spaces, usually found in the flexures, especially around the neck. During development at the flexures, some degree of obstruction of developing lymphatic vessels may contribute to development of these abnormalities.

Status Bonnevie–Ullrich This is a condition of an aborted oedematous fetus with a cystic hygroma.

12.17.5 Lymphangiectasia

Lymphangiectasia is the appearance of dilated lymphatics, best recognized in the small intestine, where it is a cause of protein-losing enteropathy. Intestinal lymphangiectasia is a widespread dilatation of the lymphatic vessels of the submucosa, affecting mainly the small intestine. It may be asymmetrical. There is usually oedema, chyluria, chylothorax, chylous ascites, hypoproteinaemia, lymphocytopenia, and sometimes, hypocalcaemia. The oedema is often intercellular and interstitial, and intense. The cause is often unknown but it is assumed to be obstructive and can be shown to be made worse by any factors that could contribute to lymphatic block, including lipid from a fatty meal. Dilated abdominal lymph vessels have also been reported in restrictive pericarditis.

The yellow nail syndrome This is a condition of virtual cessation of nail growth in which occult or severe lymphatic hypoplasia and its consequences can be demonstrated.

12.17.6 Lymphatics and inflammation

The failure to clear macromolecules in the presence of any increase in vascular permeability predisposes towards the localization of inflammatory material, such as soluble immune complexes, bacterial endotoxin, or mediators of inflammation and coagulation products. The signs of inflammation are common at sites of impaired lymphatic function and become labelled with somewhat debated terms, such as erysipelas and cellulitis, which can be acute, subacute, or chronic. At the present time, these have become unsatisfactory labels for the less acute forms which are probably caused by bacteria, sometimes immune complexes, toxins, or sometimes merely by the accumulated proteins and cells. Studies of the unaffected limb in patients presenting with unilateral erysipelas or cellulitis have shown that a primary lymphatic ectasia or hypoplasia may exist (Stoberl and Partsch 1987).

Elastases produced by white cells may serve to destroy low-resistance pathways along elastin. Bacteria do not normally exit along lymphatics but are first detoxicated in the tissues by white cells and macrophages, which in the process tend to secrete elastase and destroy the exit pathway, thus containing inflammatory processes within the tissue. Only a few infections eventually involve lymphatic trunks and these include streptococcal lymphangitis and fungal sporotrichosis.

Granulomas, almost by definition, are problems of containment of inflammatory processes at local sites. In all granulomas there is a special problem of the development of aborted, low-resistance pathways for the clearance of macromolecules. Many granulomas have an enhanced vasculature which is excessively leaky and, at the same time, products of the breakdown of cells involved in inflammation produce a great deal of additional protein and lipid, some of which is antigenic.

Lymphatics and immunity

The immune system requires traffic and pathways for the lymphocyte and macrophage so that they can provide an effective immune system. It is assumed that exit pathways for cells, such as the Langerhans cell from the epidermis, always exist. In inflammation and neoplasia, more often than not, such pathways may be obliterated. Hence, antigen is not always carried to sites where it can be presented in an orderly way for cell recognition. Cellular immunity, delayed hypersensitivity, and graft rejection, for example, can be modified by section or ligature of the lymphatics.

12.17.7   Lymphatics and metastasis

Lymphatics are necessary for metastasis of cancer. Malignant cells have to find a pathway into the lymphatic and thence along the vessel and, ultimately, they need to survive in the lymph node. Studies of how many cells are transported and at what rate they enter or leave the lymphatic are relevant to the story of natural defences against cancer. Some cells, such as the melanocyte, seem to have a natural affinity for the low-resistance pathway of the elastin fibre into the lymphatic.

12.17.8   Lymphangitis

Lymphangitis results in thickening of the trunks, thrombosis, and recanalization. Often such trunks cannot be distinguished from a venulitis and this accounts for debates about the nature of the lymphatic or venous contribution to Mondor disease of the breast (see also Section 12.16.5) and certain fibrosclerotic conditions affecting the shaft of the penis. Inflammation of the collecting lymphatics seems to underlie these disorders. There is thrombotic occlusion and proliferation of all elements of the lymphatic wall, including endothelium, smooth muscle, and fibroblast, long thought to be a venous thrombosis. The fact that it was not recognized as lymphatic, probably depended on insufficient awareness of how thick-walled lymphatic trunks may become (see Fig. 12.161).

Fibrosis is an inevitable consequence of inflammation involving the lymphatics. It accounts for non-pitting oedema and some aspects of scarring around chronic inflammatory disease. It is described as sclerosing lymphangitis and also liposclerosis. Fibrosis of lymph nodes is often a precursor of lymphoedema, and atrophy of the high endothelium of the post-capillary venules may be a consequence of decreased traffic via the lymphatics. Atrophy is a consequence of disuse.

12.17.9   Lymphoedema

An older classification of lymphoedema was congenital and acquired but this has been overtaken by a more useful classification (Table 12.11), determined by the practical management of patients, which is based on the distinction between cancer, or non-cancer related lymphoedema. Worldwide, filariasis is the commonest cause of lymphoedema. The three causative parasites—*Wucheria bancrofti*, *Brugia malayi*, and *B. timori*—all produce disease in the lymphatic vessels in which they live. They are the most widespread and abundant of all human filarial worms.

One form of endemic elephantiasis found in Central Africa is believed to be due to lymph node fibrosis, consequent on the accumulation of silica absorbed through the skin of the legs.

Pathogenesis

Lymphoedema results when there is obstruction to the lymphatic pathway, either in the periphery or, even more commonly, within the lymph node, fibrosis of which may be a primary factor in the initiation of lymphoedema. Destruction of lymphatic valves by parasites or dilation of the lymphatics rendering the valves incompetent, also has to be taken into account when considering the pathogenesis of lymphoedema. Obstructive causes of lymphoedema are regarded as producing a low-output state. This can be compared to lymphoedema that

---

Table 12.11   Classification of lymphoedema

Cancer related
  I Acute
      post-operative
  II Chronic
      (a) direct infiltration of tumour in lymph nodes/compression of lymphatics
      (b) treatment associated
            block dissection of nodes
            post-radiotherapy
      (c) combination of (a) and (b) with recurrence of tumour after treatment

Non-cancer related
  I Acute
      post-operative
  II Chronic
      (a) congenital
            familial (Milroy disease)
            non-familial
      (b) primary lymphoedema
            (unexplained lymphoedema presenting after birth)
      (c) secondary lymphoedema
            associated with venous disease, e.g. leg ulcer
            others
              infection
                bacteria (erysipelas)
                parasite (filariasis)
              chronic inflammation
                dermatitis
                rosacea
              muscle disuse
              factitious

results from excessive permeability of the blood vessels with the flooding of the tissues by protein-containing fluid, as may occur in the lower leg due to venous disease and in many inflammatory states. This is known as a high-output lymphoedema. At one time, recurrent infection was thought to be an important cause of lymphoedema (but more emphasis is now made of the fact that an abnormality of the lymphatics may predispose to recurrent infection), perhaps due to exhaustion of macrophages; a failure to localize the bacteria causing the problem; and a loss of tissue immunity. Most particulate matter, such as bacteria, is first phagocytosed by macrophages before it finds its way into the lymphatics. There is doubt whether bacteria are frequently washed from the tissues to the lymph nodes. That inflammation is not the cause of fibrosis in the lymph nodes is supported by the observation that little fibrin is found at such sites.

The prevalence of lymphoedema following mastectomy varies from 7 to 63 per cent. Radiotherapy seems to be an important risk factor which may act either on the pre-lymphatics, the initial lymphatics, or the collecting vessels, and, of course, it can lead to fibrosis of the lymph node. In a large recent study in Norway (Petlund, personal communication) of 17 000 cases of carcinoma of the breast (of which 85 per cent were treated) 15 per cent developed lymphoedema. At the same time and in the same year (1991), 243 cases of carcinoma of the uterus were followed by a 10 per cent incidence of lymphoedema of the legs.

The consequences of lymphoedema

In lymphoedema there is stagnation of plasma proteins, lipid, fibrinogen, and many biochemical by-products of tissue metabolism. A large proportion of these are normally lysed by macrophages but macrophages can become exhausted or overloaded and there may be a failure of recruitment. The relationship between the lymphatics and the blood vessels becomes disorganized. Lymphatics become thick-walled and communications develop between the lymphatics and blood-vessels; physiologically, such communications are rarely found in healthy tissues except in the region of thoracic duct and, occasionally, in lymph nodes.

All tissues become oedematous, including nerves and vessel walls. Fibrinoid material and actual thrombosis block the lymphatic vessels and become deposited in the interstitium. There is proliferation of endothelium and fibroblasts in response to what is, in fact, a low-grade inflammatory state. At least a century ago, when elastin stains were first developed by pathologists

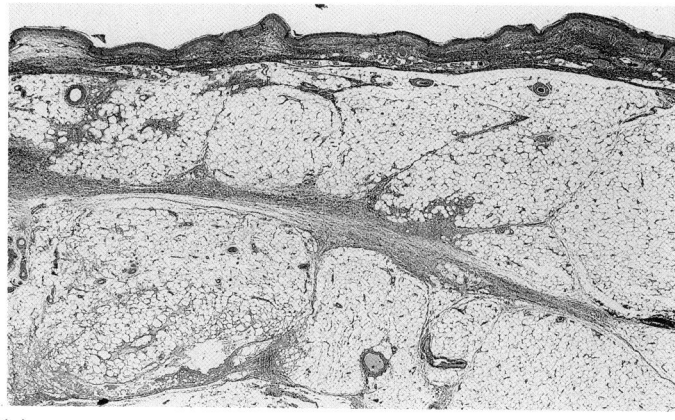

(a)

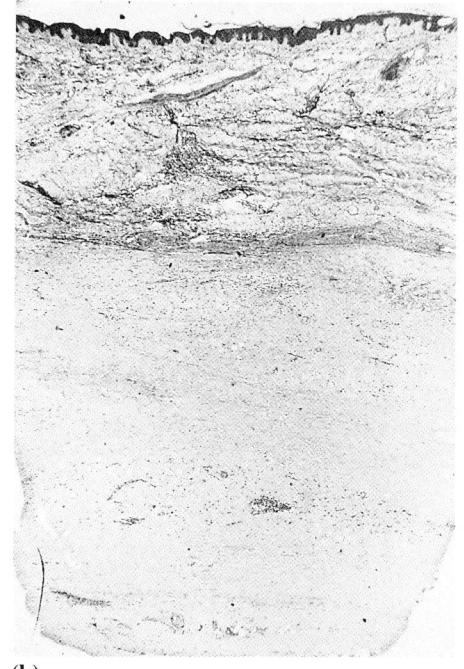

(b)

Fig. 12.163 Subcutaneous tissue is most affected by lymphoedema. Any chronic oedema is followed by fibrosis. (a) Septal fibrosis of fat; (b) complete fibrosis of fat; (c) chronic erythema nodosum or nodular vasculitis, in which a central vessel cannot, by current techniques, be confidently identified as either a vein or a hypertrophied collecting lymphatic. Only a minor degree of inflammation in the vessel wall would make it impossible to distinguish it from an artery. Elastin stains identifying internal and external elastic lamina are helpful in healthy tissue but veins can become arterialized in the lower leg and the elastic lamina of arteries can be destroyed by white cells. (From Ryan 1978.)

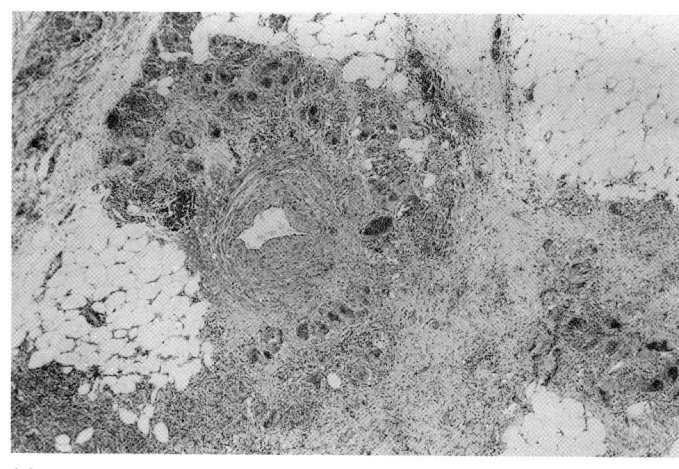

(c)

such as Unna, it was realized that elastin becomes disrupted quite soon after the development of oedema, leading to a loss of the anchorage dependence of the lymphatic endothelium, and perhaps facilitating its proliferation. It is the least compliant tissues that are protected from the effects of lymphoedema, while subcutaneous tissues and the deep dermis show the most marked changes, and it is at such sites in the skin that fibrosis becomes a final consequence (Fig. 12.163).

Ectatic lymph collectors develop an angioma-like configuration with increased smooth muscle and fibroblasts in their walls. A rise in pressure within these vessels gradually leads to opening up of lymphatic-lined free lymphatic pathways and the clinical appearance of vesiculation or lymphangioma. Other features of lymphoedema include an increased number of mast cells, deposits of fat, lymphaticovenous shunts, angiogenesis, and rarely, malignant endothelial transformation.

12.17.10   Lymphatic disease of special organs

While the lymphatics and their obstruction are discussed in each of the sections devoted to special organs, this section devoted to lymphatics would be incomplete without mentioning that there is an increasing literature devoted to the possibility that lymphatic disease can explain many previously unexplained disorders. This is based on experimental pathology induced by ligation of lymphatics producing changes in special organs. For example, removal of lipid by lymphatics is important in the arterial wall predisposed to atheroma. Ligation of thoracic lymphatics in rats fed high-fat diets enhances lipid deposition in the arterial wall. Protein oedema contributes to the fibrosis of cardiac fibro-elastosis and to interstitial pulmonary fibrosis.

There is considerable description in the older textbooks of lymphatic involvement in the lung as a consequence of tuberculosis or neoplasia. Lung lymphatics also feature in developmental defects of the new-born. High-protein oedema is a consequence of venous insufficiency, and hence lymphatic impairment is clearly important in portal hypertension.

Chronic inflammatory processes involving the lymphatics play some part in the development of chronic granulomatous diseases of the Whipple or Crohn type affecting the gut. Chronic fistulae, and recurrent infection give rise to, or are accompanied by, lymphoedema of the affected and adjacent tissues. Sporotrichosis, schistosoma, and filariasis also favour lymphatic vessels for their development.

Discussion of the compliance of the tissues causing stiffness that may result from a protein oedema and lymphatic fibrosis enters the descriptions of many forms of 'sclerosis'. This is relevant also to the 'fibrin cuff' theory of lipodermatosclerosis. Oedema that may be a consequence of lymphatic failure specifically contributing to disease, enters the literature devoted to a number of diseases, ranging from toothache to Menière disease. There is good evidence that hydrostatic pressure in these diseases builds up in a confined environment when drainage into lymphatics is impaired.

12.17.11   Further reading

Bollinger, A., Partsch, H., and Wolfe, J. H. N. (eds) (1985). *The initial lymphatics*. Georg Thieme Verlag, Stuttgart.

Daroczy, J. (1983). The structure and dynamic function of the dermal lymphatic capillaries. *British Journal of Dermatology* **109**, 99–102.

Daroczy, J. (1984). New structural details of dermal lymphatic valves and its functional interpretation. *Lymphology* **17**, 54–60.

DeLong, T. G. and Simmons, R. L. (1982). Role of lymphatic vessels in bacterial clearance from early soft-tissue infection. *Archives of Surgery* **117**, 123–8.

Foldi, M. and Casley-Smith, J. R. (eds) (1983). *Lymphangiology*. Schattaur Verlag, Stuttgart.

Hauck, G. (1982). The connective tissue space in view of lymphology. *Experientia* **38**, 1121–2.

Hendriks, H. R. and Eestermans, I. L. (1983). Disappearance and reappearance of high endothelial venules and immigrating lymphocytes in lymph nodes deprived of afferent lymphatic vessels: a possible regulatory role of macrophages in lymphocyte migration. *European Journal of Immunology* **13**, 663–9.

Jones, R. L. (1985). Elastic fibres and the lymphatics. A light microscopical study of their association in normal and leprous skin. Institute of Medical Laboratory Sciences.

Jones, W. R., O'Morchoe, C. C. C., Jarosz, H. M., and O'Morchoe, P. J. (1986). Distribution of charged sites on lymphatic endothelium. *Lymphology* **19**, 5.

Kinmouth, J. (1982). *The lymphatics* (2nd edn). Edward Arnold, London.

Kissin, M. W., Rovere, Q., Easton, D., and Westbury, G. (1986). Risks of lymphoedema following the treatment of breast disease. *British Journal of Surgery* **73**, 580–4.

Leak, L. V. (1986). Distribution of cell surface charges on mesothelium and lymphatic endothelium. *Microvascular Research* **31**, 18–30.

Marsch, W. C., Haas, N., and Stuttgen, G. (1986). 'Mondor's phlebitis'—a lymphovascular process. *Dermatologica* **172**, 133–5.

Mortimer, P. S. and Regnard, C. F. B. (1986). Lymphostatic disorders. *British Medical Journal* **293**, 347 (Leading article).

Mortimer, P. S., Cherry, G. W., Jones, R. L., Barnhill, R. L., and Ryan, T. J. (1983). The importance of elastic fibres in skin lymphatics. *British Journal of Dermatology* **108**, 561–6.

Mortimer, P. S., Jones, R. L., and Ryan, T. J. (1985). Human skin lymphatics: regional variation and relationship to elastin. In *Progress in Lymphology; Diagnostic, therapeutic and research approaches to lymphatic system structure and function* (ed. L. R. Sleim), pp. 59–64. Immunology Research Foundation, Newburgh, USA.

Mortimer, P. S., Simmonds, R., Rezvani, M., Robbins, M., Hopewell, J. W., and Ryan T. J. (1990). The measurement of skin lymph flow by isotope clearance—Reliability, reproducibility, injection dynamics and the effect of massage. *Journal of Investigative Dermatology* **95**, 677–82.

Olszewski, W. (1985). *Peripheral lymph: formation and immune function*. CRC Press, Boca Raton, Florida.

Parish, W. E. (1985). Cutaneous elastin degradation in ageing and inflammation. *Journal of Applied Cosmetology* **3**, 187.

Ryan, T. J. (1978a). Disorders affecting the lymphatic system. In *The physiology and pathophysiology of the skin*, Vol. 5 (ed. A. Jarrett), (2nd edn), pp. 1781–2008. Academic Press, London.

Ryan, T. J. (1978b). The lymphatics of the skin. In *The physiology and pathophysiology of the skin*, Vol. 5 (ed. A. Jarrett) (2nd edn), pp. 1755–1780. Academic Press, London.

Ryan, T. J. (1989). Structure and function of lymphatics. *Journal of Investigative Dermatology* **93**, 18S–24S.

Stoberl, C. and Partsch, H. (1987). Erysipelas and lymphoedema—egg or hen? *Zeitschrift für Haut Krankheiten* **62**, 56–62.

Wolfe, J. H. N. (1984). The prognosis and possible cause of severe primary lymphoedema. *Annals of the Royal College of Surgeons of England* **66**, 251–7.

12.18 Vascular tumours

C. D. M. Fletcher and P. H. McKee

12.18.1 Introduction

Vascular tumours represent one of the commonest groups of tumours to arise in skin or soft tissue. Readers are referred to the appropriate chapters for details of vascular neoplasms arising in other organs, such as the liver, spleen, and brain.

The overwhelming majority of these lesions are benign and it is frequently uncertain whether they represent true neoplasms, congenital malformations, or hamartomata. Traditionally, this group encompasses lesions derived from blood vascular endothelium, lymphatic endothelium, and specialized perivascular cells (glomus cells and pericytes); however, it should be noted that reliable distinction between the two types of endothelium is often impossible. Of the purportedly malignant tumours, Kaposi sarcoma has attained particular prominence in recent years, owing to its prevalence in patients with AIDS and its fascinating epidemiology.

12.18.2 Capillary haemangioma

Clinical features

Capillary haemangioma is the single commonest vascular tumour of infancy and, in this age-group, is known as a strawberry naevus. The strawberry naevus typically presents at birth as a small, fairly discrete red/purple patch in the skin, most often of the head and neck region although any cutaneous site may be affected. Females predominate over males. Following a period of growth, the majority of these lesions involve spontaneously by the age of 6 or 7 years.

Histopathology

These lesions are composed of multiple lobules in the dermis or subcutis. Each lobule comprises numerous small vascular channels which, in the early stages, are virtually uncanalized. They are lined by plump endothelial cells, often showing mitotic activity (Fig. 12.164). As the lesion matures, the vessels dilate to become thin-walled capillaries lined by flat endothelium. A small feeding artery or arteriole is often found at the base of the tumour.

Variants

Campbell de Morgan spots (cherry angiomas)

These present as tiny, discrete red macules, most often on the

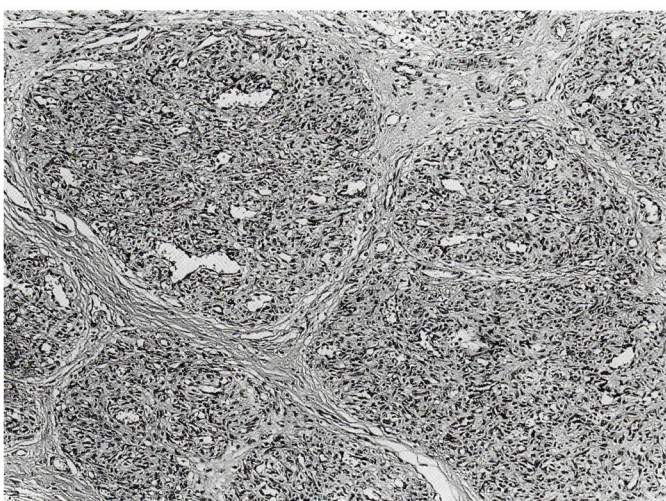

Fig. **12.164** Capillary haemangioma. Note the lobular architecture. Only a small number of vascular lumina are evident in this example, which was excised from a 4-month-old child.

skin of the trunk in middle to late adulthood. Histopathologically, they are composed of small dilated capillaries in the upper dermis.

Angiokeratomas

Typically present as a solitary raised nodule on the hands or feet of young adults. Microscopically, they resemble Campbell de Morgan spots with the addition of hyperkeratosis and acanthosis of the overlying epidermis. Multiple lesions, often located on the trunk, may be a feature of Fabry–Anderson disease.

Verrucous haemangioma

This affects the lower limbs of young children and is only distinguished from a strawberry naevus by the presence of overlying hyperkeratosis, papillomatosis, and acanthosis.

12.18.3 Cavernous haemangioma

Clinical features

The age, sex, and anatomical distribution of cavernous haemangiomas almost exactly parallel those of strawberry naevi. However, these lesions tend to be significantly larger, with ill-defined margins, and rarely, if ever, involve spontaneously. Furthermore, they may be associated with multiple enchondromas (Maffucci syndrome), a consumption coagulopathy due to platelet deposition within the tumour (Kasabach–Merritt syndrome) or vascular lesions in the alimentary tract (Blue rubber bleb naevus syndrome).

Histopathology

These tumours are composed of irregularly distributed, large, dilated vascular spaces, lined by flattened endothelium (Fig. 12.165). Intraluminal thrombosis is common and dystrophic calcification may be a feature.

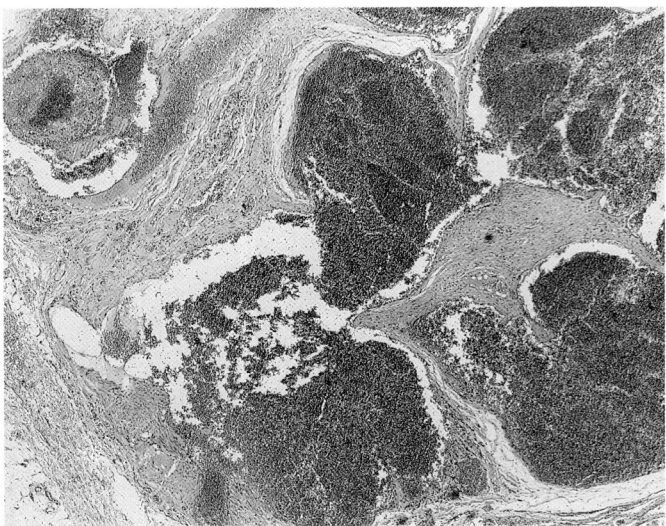

Fig. 12.165 Cavernous haemangioma. The vascular spaces are much larger than in a capillary haemangioma and are packed with red cells. One of the spaces (top left) contains partially organized thrombus.

12.18.4   Vascular ectasias

This group of lesions is characterized by the presence of dilated vessels of varying size, situated in the dermis. These vessels are normal in number, hence the designation ectasia rather than true haemangioma. Entities in this category include the salmon patch, port-wine stain, spider naevus, and angioma serpiginosum.

Naevus flammeus

This is the formal term applied to salmon patches and port-wine stains. The former are very common, congenital, pink/red macules in the head and neck region, which involute spontaneously. In contrast, the latter commence in a similar fashion but tend to extend steadily, right into adulthood, and only rarely involute. Port-wine stains may be associated with an ipsilateral intracranial vascular malformation (Sturge–Weber syndrome) or with hypertrophy and venous abnormalities of a limb (Klippel–Trenaunay syndrome).

Naevus araneus (spider naevus)

Spider naevi are extremely common lesions, which usually present as tiny, red puncta from which very small tortuous vessels radiate. They are most often seen in chronic liver disease, thyrotoxicosis, or pregnancy.

Angioma serpiginosum

This is a relatively uncommon lesion of childhood, characterized by innumerable, tiny red/purple puncta arranged in a gyrate or serpiginous pattern, most often on the lower limbs of female infants. There is usually unremitting progression into adult life.

12.18.5   Arteriovenous haemangioma

Clinical features

These tumours, also often known as cirsoid aneurysms or arteriovenous malformations, may be divided into two distinct groups. The deep type classically occurs in adolescence or early adulthood, is found most often in the limbs or head and neck region, is frequently large, and may be associated with significant arteriovenous shunting, pain, and soft tissue hypertrophy. The superficial type, in contrast, usually presents in the skin of the face or neck of middle-aged or elderly adults, is much smaller and is not associated with any appreciable circulatory disturbance.

Histopathology

The appearances are variable but, in general, comprise a poorly circumscribed mass of thick-walled vessels of varying calibre. An elastic stain is useful to demonstrate the admixture of arterial and venous channels, the latter usually being markedly predominant. Serial sections may reveal demonstrable arteriovenous anastomoses.

12.18.6   Deep haemangiomas

Haemangiomas may occasionally be found in a variety of deeply located sites, including skeletal muscle, joint cavities, lymph nodes, and peripheral nerves. Of these, the intramuscular tumours are much the commonest and most important.

Clinical features

Intramuscular haemangiomas (Allen and Enzinger 1972) may present at any age but are typically seen in adolescents and young adults. They are fairly evenly distributed between the trunk, limbs, and head and neck region. Most often there is a long history of a slowly growing mass, which is classically painful when the affected muscle is exercised. At least 20 per cent of cases recur locally, usually as a consequence of inadequate primary excision.

Histopathology

Microscopically, although traditionally divided into capillary, cavernous, or mixed types, these lesions often have a complex appearance of mixed vascular patterns, which may include venous, arteriovenous, or lymphangiomatous components (Beham and Fletcher 1991). Personal experience suggests that local recurrence is more closely related to adequacy of excision, rather than predominant histological subtype as was formerly suggested. Most cases have ill-defined, infiltrative margins (hence the risk of local recurrence) and they often lack a lobular pattern. There is frequently very marked fatty replacement of adjacent muscle, which has led some to describe these lesions as angiolipomata in the past.

Importantly, the capillary type, particularly if largely uncanalized and mitotically active, may be misdiagnosed as angiosarcoma. It can, however, be distinguished from the latter by the lack of pleomorphism or significant endothelial multi-layering and by the lack of irregular, ramifying, anastomosing thin-walled channels. In addition, it should be remembered that deeply located angiosarcoma is exceedingly rare.

12.18.7 Angiomatosis

Angiomatosis is a very uncommon condition, which typically presents in childhood. It is characterized by very extensive, diffuse proliferation of variably sized thin-walled vascular channels, often affecting very large areas of a limb and involving dermis, subcutis, muscle, and sometimes even bone. As with intramuscular haemangioma, there is frequently a prominent fatty component. Surgical management is often exceedingly difficult, owing to the extent of the lesion.

12.18.8 Pyogenic granuloma

This common lesion, which has recently been more appropriately redesignated lobular capillary haemangioma (Mills *et al.* 1980), has been a source of controversy for many years. It has long been uncertain whether this is a reactive phenomenon or a true neoplasm, although the latter appears more likely.

Clinical features

Pyogenic granuloma may arise at any age and shows a striking predilection for the oro-nasal mucous membranes and the skin of the head and neck region and finger. It classically presents as a polypoid, reddish nodule, which is often ulcerated and has almost always been present for less than 6 months. Often the tumour grows very rapidly and presents after only 6–8 weeks. Up to 10 per cent recur after local excision. A particularly rare subgroup, arising almost exclusively on the trunk of young boys, occasionally recurs with multiple tiny satellite nodules.

Histopathology

Characteristically, these lesions are exophytic and are surrounded on either side by a collarette of acanthotic epithelium (Fig. 12.166). They are composed of vessels almost identical to an ordinary capillary haemangioma, except that lobulation may be much more marked, with a prominent intervening myxoid stroma. Inflammatory cells are often very numerous in the stroma, especially in ulcerated lesions. This is a secondary phenomenon which heightens the resemblance to granulation tissue, but which is absent in the uncommon cases which arise in subcutaneous tissue or within a vessel (see below). Not surprisingly, in view of the rapid growth and effects of inflammation, normal mitotic figures are often plentiful.

Variants

Granuloma gravidarum is the term used to describe identical lesions, which arise on the gingivae of pregnant women and which involute spontaneously after delivery.

Intravenous pyogenic granuloma (Cooper *et al.* 1979) is a rare tumour, mainly affecting adults, which typically arises

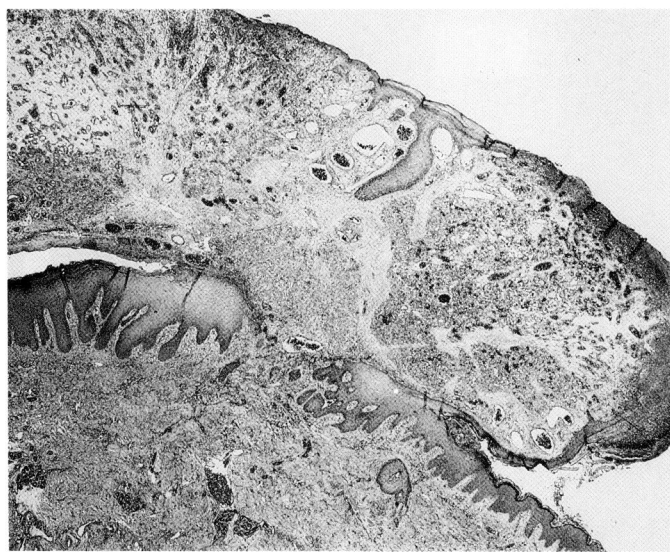

Fig. 12.166 Pyogenic granuloma. A characteristic exophytic lesion composed of lobules of capillaries showing surface ulceration and superficially resembling granulation tissue.

within veins of the upper limb or neck and behaves in an entirely benign fashion.

12.18.9 Intravascular papillary endothelial hyperplasia

Clinical features

This relatively common entity (Hashimoto *et al.* 1983), formerly known as Masson's vegetant intravascular haemangioendothelioma, is generally regarded as a reactive phenomenon which represents an infrequent form of organizing thrombus. When arising within a presumably damaged vessel, it typically presents as a reddish nodule in the finger or head and neck region of young to middle-aged adults, particularly females. However, a large proportion of cases are found in a pre-existent vascular lesion (such as a haemangioma or haemorrhoidal veins), in which circumstance the age, sex, and site are variable. Following excision, local recurrence is very unusual and is more often a result of regrowth of the preceding, causative lesion.

Histopathology

The appearances are both striking and characteristic (Fig. 12.167). Within the affected vascular channel are seen innumerable tiny papillae, having a central, rather hyalinized core covered by a single layer of bland, mitotically inactive endothelial cells. In more than 90 per cent of cases, this papillary proliferation is associated with adjacent thrombus and fibrin deposition, thought to be the initiating factor. Distinction from the papillary tufts of angiosarcoma is easily made by the purely intravascular location and the lack of endothelial pleomorphism, multilayering, or mitotic activity.

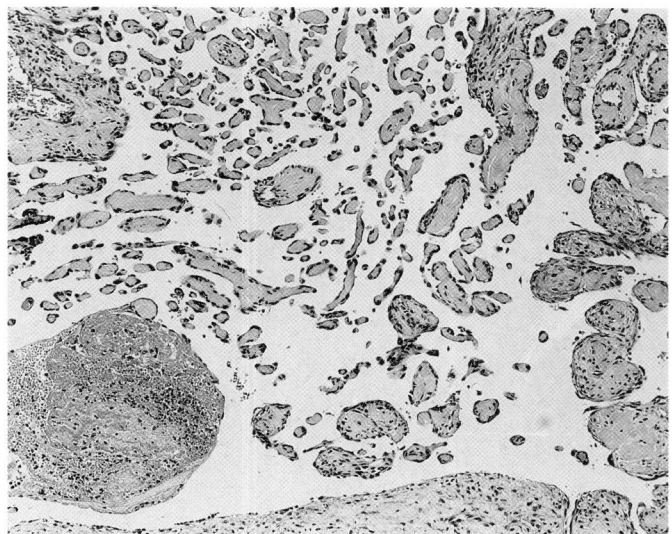

Fig. 12.167 Intravascular papillary endothelial hyperplasia. Note the multiple tiny papillae, each having a hyalinized core, situated within this blood-vessel. Associated thrombus is also present (bottom left), as is usually the case.

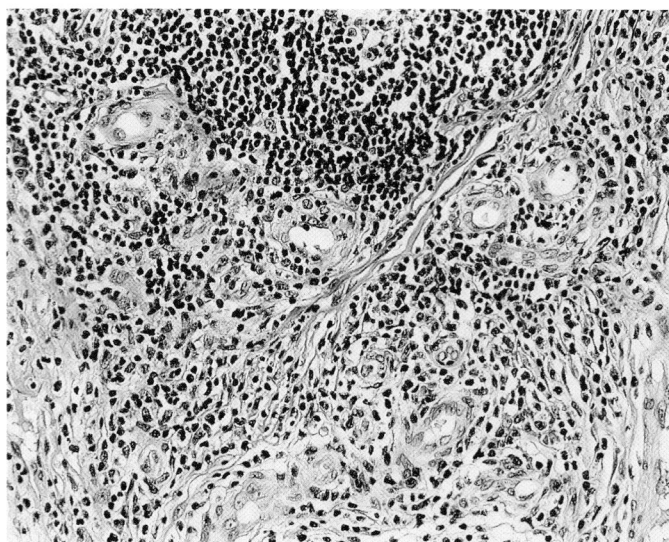

Fig. 12.168 Epithelioid haemangioma. Note the characteristically plump endothelial cells with large vesicular nuclei and the adjacent dense inflammatory infiltrate, which is composed mainly of lymphocytes and eosinophils.

12.18.10 Epithelioid haemangioma

This lesion (Urabe *et al.* 1987; Chan *et al.* 1989), also known as angiolymphoid hyperplasia with eosinophilia or histiocytoid haemangioma, is currently thought to be a true neoplasm (rather than a cutaneous reaction to varied stimuli), by virtue of the fact that it may arise at a wide variety of more deeply located sites and often recurs locally. Although this entity has been repeatedly confused with Kimura disease in the past, it is now clear that the latter is a quite different lesion, both clinically and pathologically, and probably represents an aberrant immunological reaction (Fletcher 1989).

Clinical features

This tumour typically presents as a reddish plaque or nodule in the head and neck region of middle-aged adults of either sex. Not infrequently there are multiple lesions, particularly in the periauricular area. Local lymphadenopathy and a circulating eosinophilia are uncommon. Up to 30 per cent of cases recur locally but metastasis is not a feature. In contrast, Kimura disease, which is more frequent in orientals, tends to affect rather younger patients, most often males, and is very often associated with lymphadenopathy and eosinophilia.

Histopathology

The majority of cases consist of a reasonably circumscribed intradermal or subcutaneous mass, composed of numerous, variably sized, proliferating vessels associated with a dense lymphocytic infiltrate (occasionally with germinal centres) and variable numbers of eosinophils. The cardinal feature is the plump epithelioid appearance of the endothelium lining the vascular channels (Fig. 12.168). These cells are cuboidal to round,

with copious eosinophilic cytoplasm and vesicular nuclei; they frequently protrude into the vessel lumen in a 'tombstone' or 'hobnail' fashion, and may show cytoplasmic vacuolation. Kimura disease, on the other hand, is usually more deeply located and tends to show much more fibrosis and far less in the way of vascular proliferation; epithelioid endothelium is not a feature.

12.18.11 Epithelioid haemangioendothelioma

This recently recognized tumour (Weiss *et al.* 1986) is confusingly named, since it is both clinically and histologically distinct from epithelioid haemangioma. As well as presenting in soft tissue, it may also arise in bone, liver, or lung, where it was formerly known as intravascular bronchioloalveolar tumour.

Clinical features

Cases in soft tissue most often present in the limbs of adults as a painful or tender mass. Up to 10 per cent recur locally after excision, but as many as one-third metastasize, particularly to lymph nodes. However, lymph node resection is often curative and only about 10 per cent of cases pursue a fatal course. As a consequence, this is often classified as a neoplasm of low-grade or borderline malignancy.

Histopathology

These tumours are composed of cords or nests of variably shaped, often rather epithelioid cells, which frequently radiate from a large central vessel. The cells only rarely form recognizable vascular channels, hence frequent misdiagnosis as a carcinoma, but intracellular microlumina are a striking feature (Fig. 12.169). There is typically a prominent myxoid or hyaline

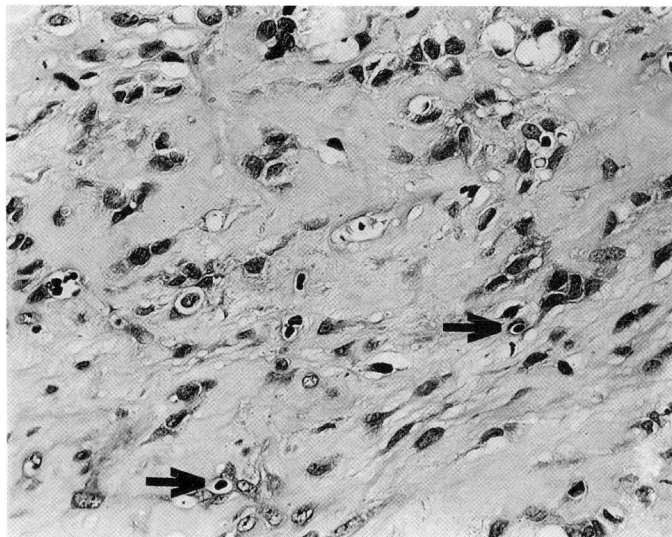

Fig. 12.169 Epithelioid haemangioendothelioma. The vascular nature of this tumour is not readily apparent. However, note the intracytoplasmic microlumina containing red blood cells (arrows).

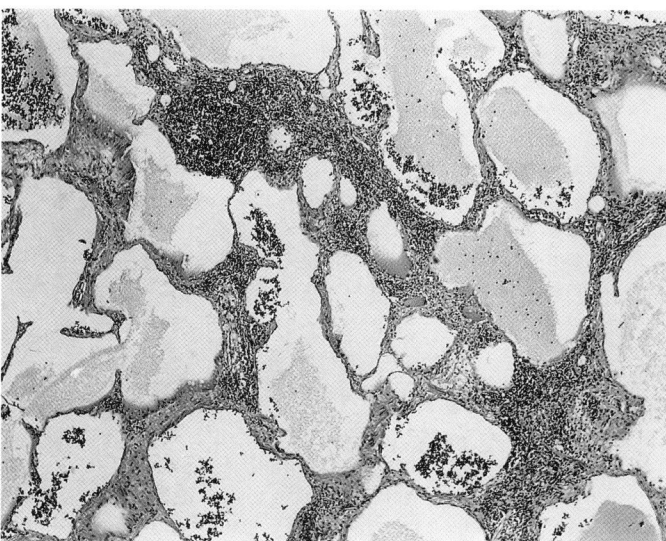

Fig. 12.170 Cavernous lymphangioma. The typical appearance of thin-walled, dilated lymphatic channels, associated with a prominent lymphoid infiltrate.

stroma. Unfortunately, there are no reliable means of distinguishing on histological grounds those cases that will behave aggressively.

12.18.12 Spindle cell haemangioendothelioma

This is another uncommon, recently described, vascular neoplasm (Weiss and Enzinger 1986) which typically arises in the distal extremities of adolescents or young adults. It is not infrequently multifocal and is very prone to local recurrence. However, metastasis is exceedingly uncommon and this is therefore also currently categorized as being of intermediate malignancy. Histologically, it consists of an admixture of thin-walled cavernous spaces and solid spindle-cell areas (the latter being possibly confused with Kaposi sarcoma). Within the spindle-cell areas, plump epithelioid endothelial cells, some of which show clear intracytoplasmic lumina, are often evident. Current evidence suggests that spindle cell haemangioendothelioma may be better regarded as a non-neoplastic lesion associated with abnormal local blood flow (Fletcher *et al.* 1991).

12.18.13 Lymphangioma

The majority of benign tumours derived from lymphatic endothelium are regarded as developmental malformations. They are classified into three principal types: cavernous lymphangioma, cystic hygroma, and lymphangioma circumscriptum.

Cavernous lymphangioma

As would be expected of a malformation, the majority of these lesions present at birth or in early infancy. The sex incidence is equal and the sites of predilection are the head and neck region, the axillae and groins. However, any site, including the abdominal cavity and retroperitoneum, may be affected. Most examples are manifest as an ill-defined, doughy mass. Local recurrence following excision is quite common.

Histologically, cavernous lymphangioma is composed of large numbers of fairly thin-walled, dilated lymphatic channels, situated in the subcutis, dermis, or skeletal muscle (Fig. 12.170). The endothelium is flat and monomorphic. Often the vascular spaces contain a layer of smooth muscle in their walls and there is frequently a prominent intraluminal and adventitial lymphoid infiltrate. Secondary haemorrhage into the lymphatic spaces is common and is not indicative of blood vascular origin.

Cystic hygroma

These lesions, for practical purposes, seem to represent variants of cavernous lymphangioma showing gross, cystic dilatation of their lymphatic channels. As a consequence, the clinical and other histological features are much the same as cavernous cases, although, for reasons which are unclear, cystic hygroma appears less prone to local recurrence.

Lymphangioma circumscriptum

This entity classically presents as a cutaneous, grouped collection of thin-walled, translucent vesicles. In its typical form, the vesicles appear at birth or in early infancy, are commonest around the limb girdles, and may cover an extensive area. In the less common, localized form, affecting only a small patch of skin, any site may be affected in any age group. Both forms are generally believed to represent a developmental defect, but occasional cases may be related to previous surgery or lymphatic obstruction.

Microscopically, the two types are indistinguishable and consist of markedly dilated lymphatic channels in the superficial (papillary) dermis, which often appear to extend into the epidermis. There is frequently adjacent acanthosis. Deeper involvement is occasionally seen and a fairly consistent finding is the presence of a thick-walled, muscular feeding vessel in the deep dermis. If the latter is not excised or ligated, the lesion may recur.

12.18.14   Lymphangiomyomatosis

This is a very rare condition (Basset *et al.* 1976), characterized by widespread proliferation of smooth muscle cells around lymphatic channels and lymph nodes, particularly in the mediastinum, lung parenchyma, and retroperitoneum. Females are exclusively affected, usually within the reproductive years, and they classically present with dyspnoea and pneumothorax. The disease pursues a relentless course with chylous effusions and is almost invariably fatal.

12.18.15   Angiosarcoma

The term angiosarcoma covers all lesions labelled haemangiosarcoma, lymphangiosarcoma, and malignant haemangioendothelioma, since it remains uncertain whether these lesions are derived from blood vascular or lymphatic endothelium, or perhaps from either. Other than visceral lesions (which are covered in the revelant sections), the vast majority of angiosarcomas arise in the skin. Deeply located angiosarcomas of skeletal muscle or of intra-abdominal origin are very rare.

Clinical features

Cutaneous angiosarcomas (Cooper 1987) are conveniently divided according to the absence or presence of pre-existent lymphoedema. Angiosarcoma without lymphoedema predominantly arises in the head and neck region (especially the scalp) of elderly patients of either sex. Angiosarcoma in a lymphoedematous limb classically arises in the arm of elderly females who have undergone mastectomy with axillary clearance 10 or more years previously (Stewart–Treves syndrome). In fact, it may arise in any long-standing lymphoedema, be it surgical, congenital, or filarial. Both types present as multifocal purplish plaques or papules, although head and neck lesions are also often nodular or ulcerated. Both pursue an aggressive course, the majority of patients dying with disseminated disease within 2 years.

Histopathology

Microscopically both types are very similar, although vascular differentiation is often more obvious in lymphoedema cases. Angiosarcoma is characterized by the development of innumerable, irregular anastomosing channels in the dermis or

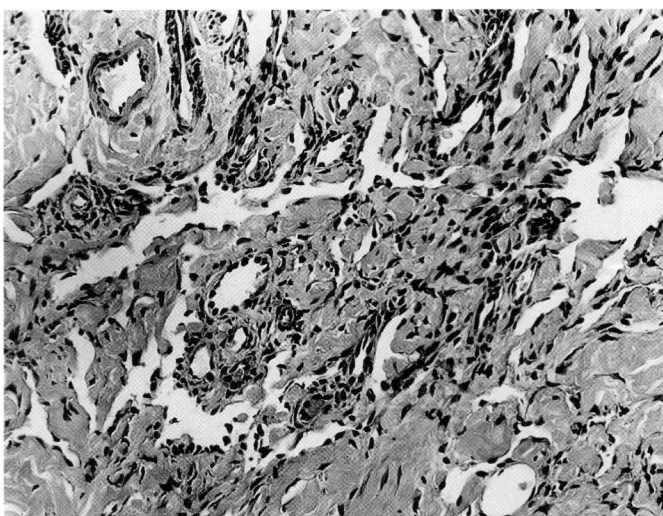

Fig. 12.171   Angiosarcoma. Irregular, anastomosing vascular channels lined by very hyperchromatic endothelial cells, are seen dissecting between dermal collagen bundles.

subcutis, which are lined by pleomorphic, hyperchromatic endothelial cells, often showing abnormal mitotic activity (Fig. 12.171). The endothelium frequently shows multilayering or a papillary growth pattern. A characteristic feature is the manner in which these channels dissect between the dermal collagen bundles. Some cases are poorly differentiated and consist mainly of spindle cells, in which circumstance electron microscopy (looking for Weibel–Palade bodies, pinocytosis, and basal laminae) or immunohistochemistry (for factor VIII-related antigen) or *Ulex europaeus* lectin binding may be of help. The rare cases arising in deep soft tissue often have an epithelioid appearance.

12.18.16   Malignant endovascular papillary angioendothelioma

This is a very rare neoplasm (Dabska 1969) which typically presents in the skin of young children and is histologically similar to well-differentiated angiosarcoma, except for the added presence of prominent glomeruloid papillary endothelial tufts. There may also be a prominent stromal lymphoid infiltrate. Although occasional cases metastasize to lymph nodes, no tumour-related deaths have been recorded to date and this is therefore best regarded as a very low-grade or borderline malignancy.

12.18.17   Systemic angioendotheliomatosis (angiotrophic lymphoma)

This exceedingly rare condition was, for some time, regarded as a multifocal, intravascular form of endothelial malignancy. There is now good evidence that it represents a malignant lymphoproliferative disorder, which is therefore not covered in this section (see Chapter 24).

12.18.18 Kaposi sarcoma

Attention has been centred on this fascinating lesion in recent years (Hutt 1984; Francis *et al.* 1986), owing to its recognition as a cardinal feature of the acquired immunodeficiency syndrome (AIDS). In fact, its unusual epidemiology had been apparent long before the recognition of AIDS. To this day the precise cell of origin is controversial, but most evidence currently supports derivation from lymphatic endothelium.

The distribution of Kaposi sarcoma is best appreciated by dividing cases into those of Western and those of African origin. Until about 1980, Western cases were uncommon and were virtually confined to elderly patients in whom the disease pursues an indolent, usually benign course. Recently, however, an increasing number of cases have been recognized in AIDS patients (mainly in the young male homosexual group) and in a small number of other immunocompromised individuals (e.g. transplant recipients). These cases tend to develop disseminated, often visceral disease which follows a rapidly progressive course. By way of contrast, in Sub-Saharan Africa, this tumour has been virtually endemic for many years and accounts for about 10 per cent of all malignancies. African patients fall into three categories: young children with rapidly fatal lymphadenopathic disease; adolescents and young adults, mainly males, with variably aggressive cutaneous disease; and middle-aged to elderly adults with usually indolent cutaneous disease. It is currently thought that the first two categories probably represent AIDS-related cases. Of particular importance, there is increasing evidence that Kaposi sarcoma is not, in fact, a neoplasm but is actually a multifocal, reactive, vascular proliferation (Bayley and Lucas 1990).

Clinical features

Elderly patients classically present with purplish plaques or nodules in the distal extremities. AIDS-related cases typically manifest multifocal cutaneous disease at almost any site, which ranges from tiny reddish blemishes to more obvious nodules. These individuals may also present with lymphadenopathy or symptoms referable to primary visceral involvement (particularly of the lung).

Histopathology

Three main forms exist, known as patch, plaque, and nodular types, of which the first two are virtually confined to AIDS patients and may overlap microscopically.

Patch-stage Kaposi sarcoma is easily mistaken for an inflammatory dermatosis. It is characterized by increased numbers of thin-walled vessels in the superficial dermis, often orientated parallel to the epidermis and lined by plump endothelial cells. Adjacent to these vessels there are scattered small spindle cells, plasma cells, lymphocytes, and extravasated red cells (Fig. 12.172).

Plaque-stage disease basically represents an exaggeration of patch-stage, in which the vascular and spindle-cell proliferation is much more extensive, often involving the deep dermis, and is

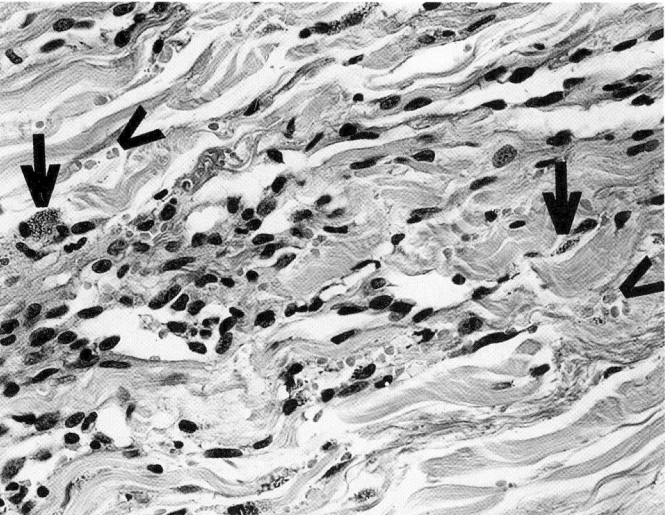

Fig. 12.172 Patch-stage Kaposi sarcoma. Small, thin-walled channels are lined by bizarre endothelial cells and there is an adjacent mild chronic inflammatory infiltrate. Note the haemosiderin deposition (arrows) and extravasated red cells (arrowheads).

typically associated with widespread haemosiderin deposition. The margins of the lesion are ill-defined.

Nodular Kaposi sarcoma is the most easily recognized and is typified by a relatively circumscribed intradermal mass, composed of fairly monomorphic, mitotically active spindle cells. Between these cells are irregular slit-like spaces containing numerous extravasated red cells (Fig. 12.173). Ectatic vascular channels are often apparent at the periphery of the nodule. In African and AIDS-related cases, intracytoplasmic eosinophilic hyaline inclusions may also be present in the spindle cells.

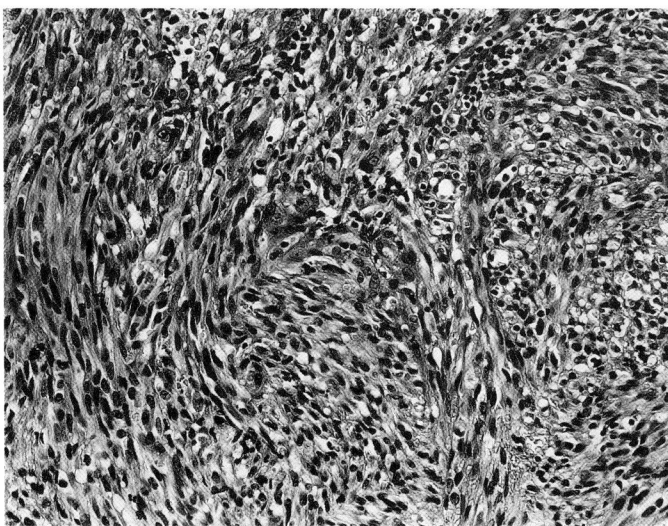

Fig. 12.173 Nodular Kaposi sarcoma. A mass of rather monomorphic spindle cells between which are many extravasated red cells. Note the sieve-like appearance on the right.

12.18.19   Epithelioid (bacillary) angiomatosis

This reactive lesion, which may clinically mimic Kaposi sarcoma, seems only to occur in immunocompromised individuals, particularly those with AIDS (LeBoit *et al.* 1989) and presents as multiple dermal, mucosal, or subcutaneous nodules. Histologically, the nodules consist of a lobular capillary proliferation, often lined by rather epithelioid endothelium, adjacent to which is a prominent stromal infiltrate of neutrophil polymorphs. Associated with the latter are clumps of granular material consisting of numerous bacteria (as revealed by the Warthin–Starry stain). These causative organisms are closely related to (if not identical with) the bacilli of cat-scratch disease.

12.18.20   Glomus tumour

This tumour (Tsuneyoshi and Enjoji 1982) is thought to originate from specialized contractile cells located in the wall of thermoregulatory arteriovenous anastomoses (glomus bodies).

Clinical features

These lesions typically arise in the hands (particularly the subungual region) of young adults, although they may occur at almost any mucocutaneous site. Classically, patients present with paroxysmal pain, often associated with cold or pressure. Occasional patients, usually children, have multiple lesions, which are less painful and are autosomal dominantly inherited. Local recurrence is uncommon.

Histopathology

Glomus tumours are characterized by a well-circumscribed mass of uniform, eosinophilic, rounded cells, arranged in nests or trabeculae around small, thin-walled vessels (Fig. 12.174). These cells often extend right up to the vascular endothelium. Cases containing prominent dilated vessels are known as glomangiomata, while uncommon examples containing large vessels and an intervening smooth muscle component are called glomangiomyomata.

12.18.21   Haemangiopericytoma

This tumour is derived from pericapillary modified smooth muscle cells and has both benign and malignant forms, differentiation between which may be very difficult.

Clinical features

Haemangiopericytomas (Enzinger and Smith 1976) most often present in middle to late adulthood as a deeply located mass, typically either in the lower limb or retroperitoneum. Occasional examples are associated with hypoglycaemia. Of these adult cases, between 20 and 30 per cent behave in a malignant fashion. Notable exceptions are infantile cases, which are

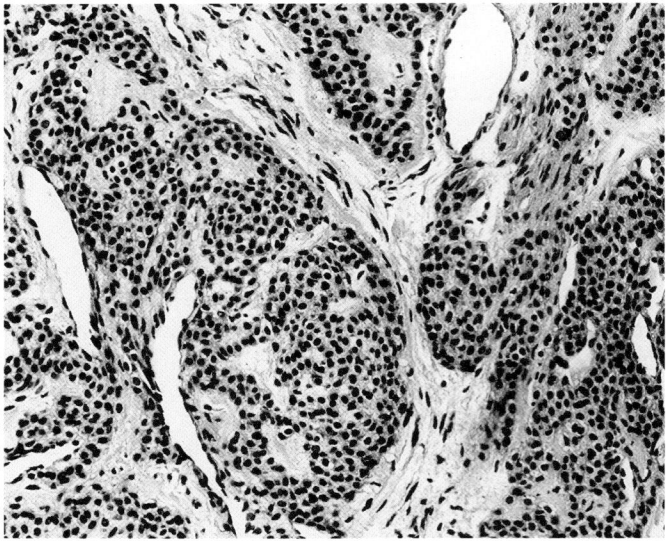

Fig. 12.174   Glomus tumour. A characteristic field showing clusters of uniform rounded cells, orientated around delicate vascular channels.

usually subcutaneous and only rarely metastasize, and tumours arising in the nose, which are invariably benign.

Histopathology

These neoplasms are usually well-circumscribed, multinodular masses, composed of relatively uniform, small basophilic cells, which are orientated around an extensive ramifying network of thin-walled capillaries (Fig. 12.175). The latter are often dilated and adopt a staghorn or antler-like configuration.

There is no endothelial atypia and a reticulin stain demonstrates the extravascular location of the tumour cells. The best criterion by which malignant examples are recognized is mitotic

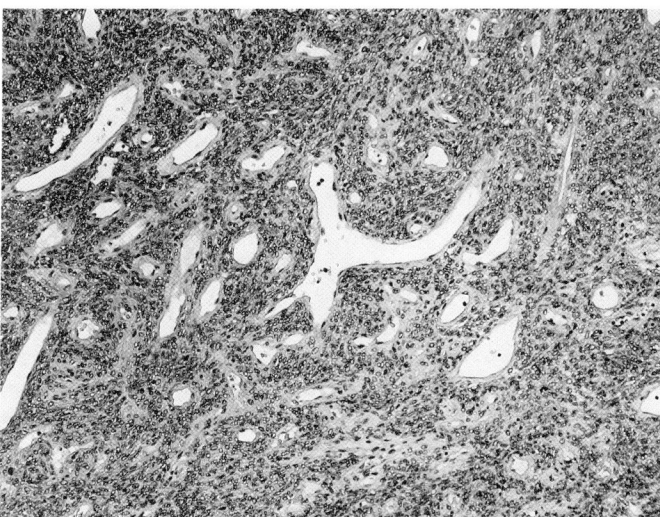

Fig. 12.175   Haemangiopericytoma. Non-cohesive sheets of small, round cells are arranged around numerous vascular channels, one of which shows a classical staghorn appearance.

activity of greater than 4 figures per 10 high power fields. It should be noted that many sarcomas, particularly synovial sarcoma and mesenchymal chondrosarcoma, may manifest a haemangiopericytoma-like appearance, underlining the need for extensive sampling of all soft tissue tumours (see Section 27.4).

12.18.22 Bibliography

Allen, P. W. and Enzinger, F. M. (1972). Haemangioma of skeletal muscle. An analysis of 89 cases. *Cancer* **29**, 8–22.

Bassett, F., Soler, R., Marsac, J., and Corrin, B. (1976). Pulmonary lymphangiomyomatosis. Three new cases studied with electron microscopy. *Cancer* **38**, 2357–66.

Bayley, A. C. and Lucas, S. B. (1990). Kaposi's sarcoma or Kaposi's disease? A personal reappraisal. In *The pathobiology of soft tissue tumours* (ed. C. D. M. Fletcher and P. H. McKee), ch. 7. Churchill Livingstone, Edinburgh.

Beham, A. and Fletcher, C. D. M. (1991). Intramuscular angioma: a clinicopathological analysis of 74 cases. *Histopathology* **18**, 53–9.

Chan, J. K. C., Hui, P. K., Ng, C. S., Yuen, N. W. F., Kung, I. T. M., and Gwi, E. (1989). Epithelioid haemangioma (angiolymphoid hyperplasia with eosinophilia) and Kimura's disease in Chinese. *Histopathology* **15**, 557–74.

Cooper, P. H. (1987). Angiosarcomas of the skin. *Seminars in Diagnostic Pathology* **4**, 2–17.

Cooper, P. H., McAllister, H. A., and Helwig, E. B. (1979). Intravenous pyogenic granuloma. A study of 18 cases. *American Journal of Surgical Pathology* **3**, 221–8.

Dabska, M. (1969). Malignant endovascular papillary angioendothelioma of the skin in childhood. Clinico-pathologic study of 6 cases. *Cancer* **24**, 503–10.

Enzinger, F. M. and Smith, B. H. (1976). Haemangiopericytoma. An analysis of 106 cases. *Human Pathology* **7**, 61–82.

Fletcher, C. D. M. (1989). Selected summaries: soft tissue tumours. *Journal of Pathology* **159**, 341–4.

Fletcher, C. D. M., Beham, A., and Schmid, C. (1991). Spindle cell haemangioendothelioma: a clinicopathological and immuno-histochemical study indicative of a non-neoplastic lesion. *Histopathology* **18**, 291–301.

Francis, N. D., Parkin, J. M., Weber, J., and Boylston, A. W. (1986). Kaposi's sarcoma in acquired immune deficiency syndrome (AIDS). *Journal of Clinical Pathology* **39**, 469–74.

Hashimoto, H., Daimaru, Y., and Enjoji, M. (1983). Intravascular papillary endothelial hyperplasia. A clinicopathologic study of 91 cases. *American Journal of Dermatopathology* **5**, 539–46.

Hutt, M. S. R. (1984). Kaposi's sarcoma. *British Medical Bulletin* **40**, 355–8.

LeBoit, P. E., Berger, T. G., Egbert, B. M., Beckstead, J. H., Yen, T. S. B., and Stoler, M. H. (1989). Bacillary angiomatosis. The histopathology and differential diagnosis of a pseudoneoplastic infection in patients with human immunodeficiency virus disease. *American Journal of Surgical Pathology* **13**, 909–20.

Mills, S. E., Cooper, P. H., and Fechner, R. E. (1980). Lobular capillary haemangioma: the underlying lesion of pyogenic granuloma. A study of 73 cases from the oral and nasal mucous membranes. *American Journal of Surgical Pathology* **4**, 471–9.

Tsuneyoshi, M. and Enjoji, M. (1982). Glomus tumor. A clinicopathologic and electron microscopic study. *Cancer* **50**, 1601–7.

Urabe, A., Tsuneyoshi, M., and Enjoji, M. (1987). Epithelioid hemangioma versus Kimura's disease: a comparative clinicopathologic study. *American Journal of Surgical Pathology* **11**, 758–66.

Weiss, S. W. and Enzinger, F. M. (1986). Spindle cell haemangioendothelioma. A low grade angiosarcoma resembling a cavernous haemangioma and Kaposi's sarcoma. *American Journal of Surgical Pathology* **10**, 521–30.

Weiss, S. W., Ishak, K. G., Dail, D. H., Sweet, D. E., and Enzinger, F. M. (1986). Epithelioid haemangioendothelioma and related lesions. *Seminars in Diagnostic Pathology* **3**, 259–87.

13

The respiratory system

13

The respiratory system

13.1 Normal structure and function

T. Creagh and T. Krausz

13.1.1 Development

Embryonic lung development begins at approximately 26 days after conception with evagination of the laryngotracheal groove to form a lung bud. A series of divisions occur until the bronchial tree is developed to the level of the segmental bronchi by 6 weeks after conception. The remainder of fetal lung development can be divided into separate stages as follows:

1. *Pseudoglandular phase, 7–17 weeks*: branching of the airways continues to the level of the terminal bronchiole. The airways have a glandular appearance and are lined by low columnar epithelium.

2. *Canalicular phase, 17–24 weeks*: the airways enlarge and the lining epithelium becomes cuboidal. An acinar framework is formed with development of saccules. The vascular system undergoes development, with formation of a capillary network.

3. *Terminal sac phase, 24 weeks–term*: the gas-exchanging surface of the lung greatly increases, together with the lung volume.

Alveoli become recognizable from about 32 weeks, with differentiation of the lining epithelium to *type 1 and type 2 pneumocytes*. A network of elastic fibres forms around the airways and within the alveolar septa. At birth, the number of alveoli is approximately 50×10^6, with up to 85 per cent being added in the first 2 years of life.

13.1.2 Structure

General considerations

The lungs are paired, asymmetric organs, with the right lung weighing 400–450 g and the left 350–400 g (Whimster and McFarlane 1974). They are covered by a serous membrane—*the visceral pleura*—which is reflected over the hilum to form the *parietal pleura* which covers the mediastinum, chest wall, and diaphragm. In normal individuals the parietal and visceral pleura are closely applied to each other.

Each lung is divided into *lobes* by *fissures* lined by the visceral pleura. The right lung is divided into three lobes, *upper, middle,* and *lower*, whereas the left lung is divided into an *upper lobe*, together with the *lingula* which extends anteriorly, and a *lower lobe* (Fig. 13.1).

The airways comprise the *trachea* which divides into the left and right main *bronchi* at the level of T4–5. The left main bronchus is narrower and is at a less acute angle than the right. The bronchi continue to branch dichotomously and asymmetrically within the lung for 8–25 generations until the *acini* are reached.

The lungs are traditionally divided into a number of structural units; these comprise:

1. *Bronchopulmonary segments*—that is, the unit of lung supplied by the first generation of bronchi (*segmental bronchi*) below the main bronchi (Figs 13.2, 13.3). This subdivision of the lobes is of value in thoracic surgery as the segments form limits of resection (Boyden 1955).

2. *Acinus*—the unit of lung supplied by a *terminal bronchiole* (Fig. 13.4). The acinus is the primary unit of lung function and all its components are involved in gas exchange. It comprises up to three generations of *respiratory bronchioles, alveolar ducts, alveolar sacs,* and *alveoli* (Pump 1969).

3. *Lobules*—these are polygonal structures outlined by connective tissue septa, which can be seen outlined on the pleural surfaces of the lung. They contain 3–5 acini each.

The airways

Bronchi

Bronchi are airways of greater than 1 mm diameter, which are reinforced by cartilage. The epithelial lining is pseudostratified, ciliated, and columnar, and lies on a basement membrane. The underlying lamina propria is composed of loose connective tissue and elastic fibres, arranged in bundles. The bronchi have a smooth muscle wall that is arranged in bundles which spiral down the airway in a loose coil. The bronchial glands lie in loose connective tissue between the muscular wall and the outer layer of the bronchi, which is composed of annular bundles of

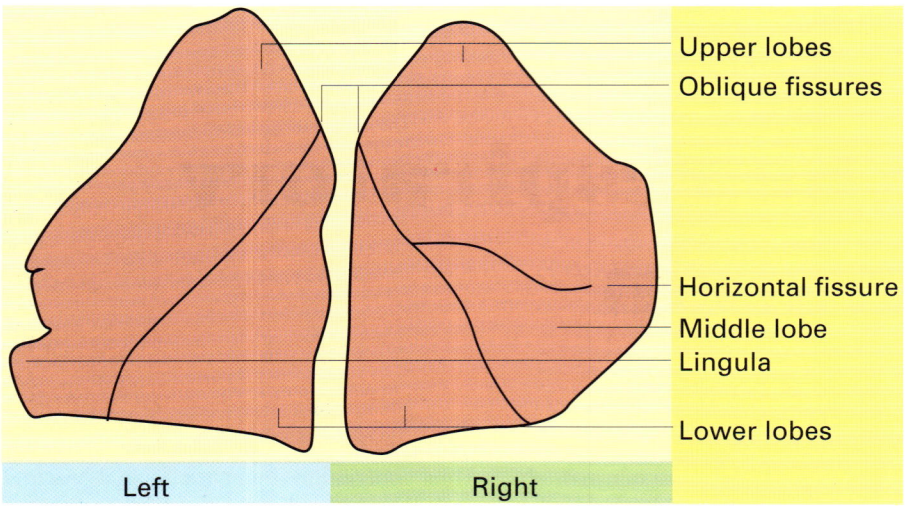

Fig. 13.1 Left and right lungs, lateral view.

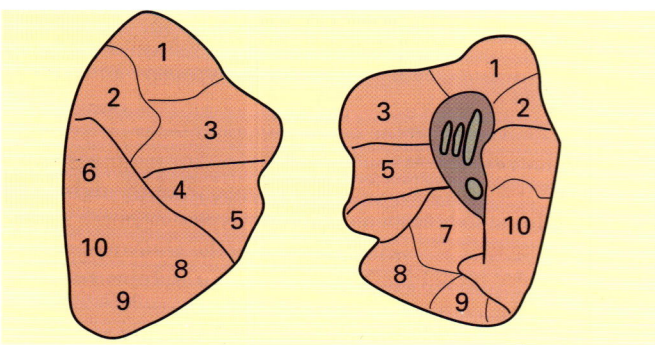

Fig. 13.2 Bronchopulmonary segments, right lung. Upper lobe: 1, apical; 2, posterior; 3, anterior. Middle lobe: 4, lateral; 5, medial. Lower lobe: 6, superior; 7, medial basal; 8, anterior; 9, lateral basal; 10, posterior basal.

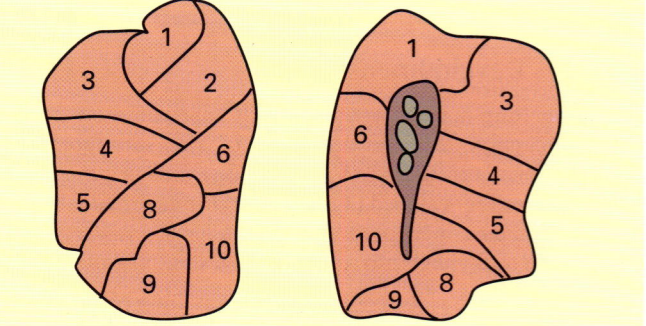

Fig. 13.3 Bronchopulmonary segments, left lung. Upper lobe; 1, 2, apico-posterior; 3, anterior. Lingula: 4, superior; 5, inferior. Lower lobe: 6, superior; 8, anterior basal; 9, lateral basal; 10, posterior basal.

collagen and cartilage. The cartilage is U-shaped in the trachea and extrapulmonary bronchi, forming rings which open dorsally, whereas in the intrapulmonary bronchi irregular islands of cartilage are present.

The bronchial epithelium is responsible for both the production and propulsion of mucus. It is covered by two layers of mucus: the *gel* layer, which forms a superficial visco-elastic barrier; and the *sol* layer, which lies beneath and is the layer in which cilia beat. The bronchial mucus contains antibacterial proteins, immunoglobulins, and proteinase inhibitors.

The epithelium is composed of three main cell types, comprising *basal, ciliated*, and *mucus-secreting cells*. Basal cells are the equivalent of reserve cells and are situated adjacent to the basement membrane. They are the stem cell of the bronchial

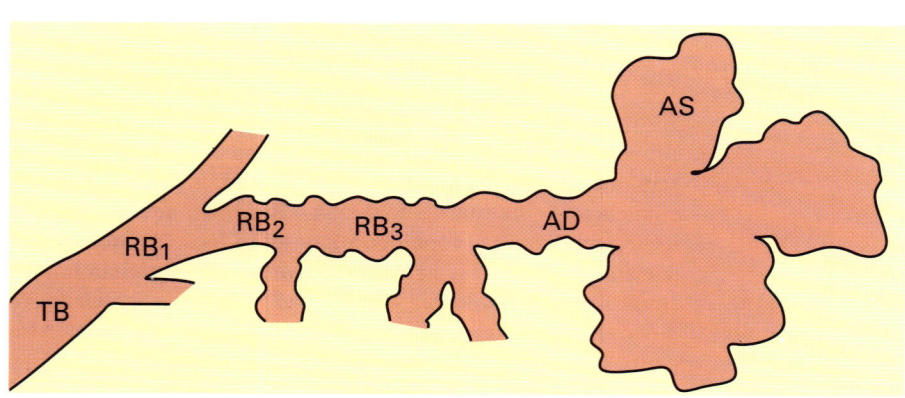

Fig. 13.4 The acinus. TB, Terminal bronchiole; RB, respiratory bronchiole; AD, alveolar duct; AS, alveolar sac. (Drawn after Thurlbeck 1968, with permission).

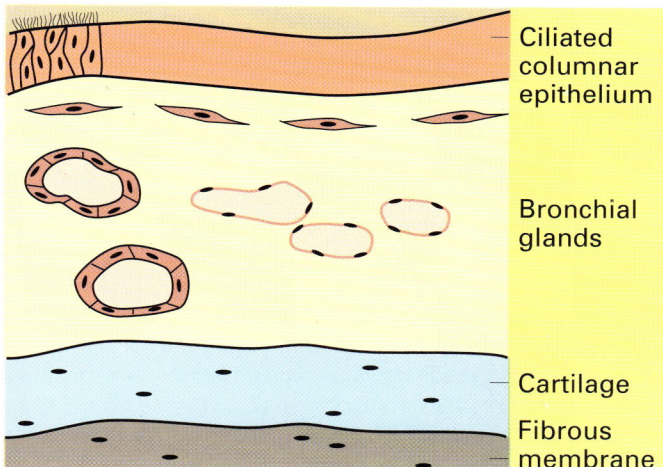

Fig. 13.5 Cross-section of bronchial wall.

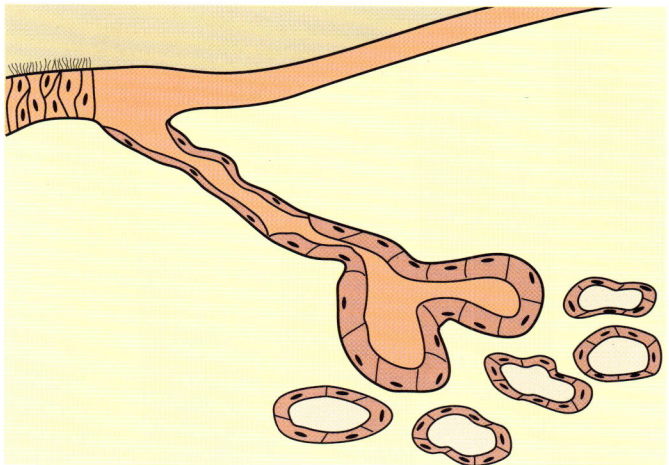

Fig. 13.7 Submucosal glands with collecting duct, lined by mucus cells in proximal portion and serous cells in terminal portion.

mucosa. After damage to the epithelium, initial regeneration takes the form of simple, stratified epithelium, with subsequent differentiation to columnar epithelium after approximately 3 weeks. Ciliated cells are columnar cells, the cilia being formed by membrane-covered extensions of the cell apex. The central axoneme (Fig. 13.6) arises from basal bodies in the apical cytoplasm and consists of nine pairs of microtubules arranged circumferentially around two single central tubules. Asymmetric arms, *dynein arms*, contain ATPase which provides energy for the beating of cilia. There are up to 200 cilia per cell (Gibbons 1981).

Mucus-secreting cells take the form of goblet cells and are partly responsible for the production of the gel layer of mucus. However, the submucosal glands produce the main part of bronchial mucus—these are tubules and acini formed by mucous, serous, and myoepithelial cells. The mucus discharges into the bronchial lumen via collecting ducts (Fig. 13.7) which are sited at a frequency of 1 per mm².

Neuroendocrine cells can also be identified in the bronchial

epithelium; these are sometimes termed Feyrter, Kulschitsky, or APUD (amine precursor uptake and decarboxylation) cells. They may be solitary or occur in clusters, where they are termed neuroepithelial bodies.

Bronchioles and alveoli

Bronchioles are airways (usually less than 1 mm diameter), which lack cartilage and submucosal glands, the wall being formed by smooth muscle surrounded by thin connective tissue. The epithelial lining is simple columnar and includes both ciliated and non-ciliated (*Clara*) columnar cells. They secrete the bronchiolar lining fluid, which is a hypophase covered by surfactant. Clara cells are the stem cells of the bronchiolar epithelium and proliferate in response to injury, with differentiation into ciliated cells. Respiratory bronchioles form a 'transitional' airway, being partly bronchiolar and partly alveolar in structure; they have smooth muscle, elastic fibres, and collagen coiled around their wall—uncoiling and subsequent elongation of the ducts occurs in inspiration.

The alveoli are formed by evaginations of the alveolar ducts and are arranged in an interlinked manner such that junctions of alveoli are formed by three alveolar walls. These walls consist of connective tissue, mesenchymal fibroblast-like cells, and networks of capillaries which are covered by a thin epithelial layer. Each alveolar wall (Fig. 13.8) is divided into 'thin' and 'thick' portions; in the thin portion the epithelial cells and the capillary endothelial cells are fused by basement membrane, whereas in the thick portion the epithelial and endothelial cells are separated by interstitium composed of elastic fibres, collagen, and mesenchymal cells.

The epithelial lining cells are divided into type 1 and type 2 pneumocytes. Type 1 (membranous) pneumocytes are simple, squamoid cells with an extensive, thin cytoplasm which covers most of the alveolar walls. Type 2 (granular) pneumocytes are cuboidal cells, with microvilli, which protrude into the alveolar space and only cover a small proportion of the alveolar wall. These cells contain secretory granules termed *lamellar bodies*,

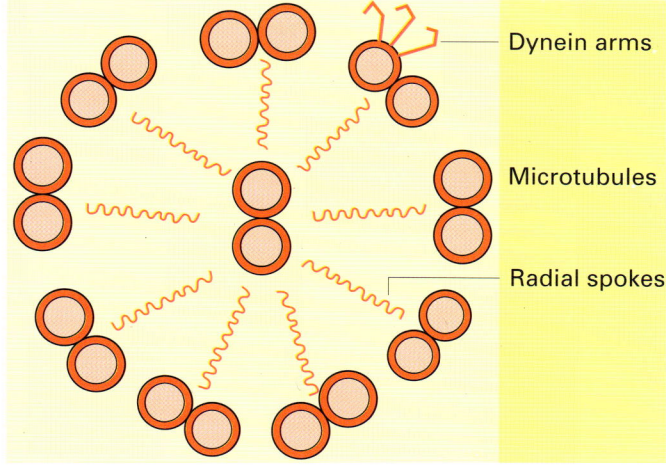

Fig. 13.6 Cross-section of central cilial axoneme.

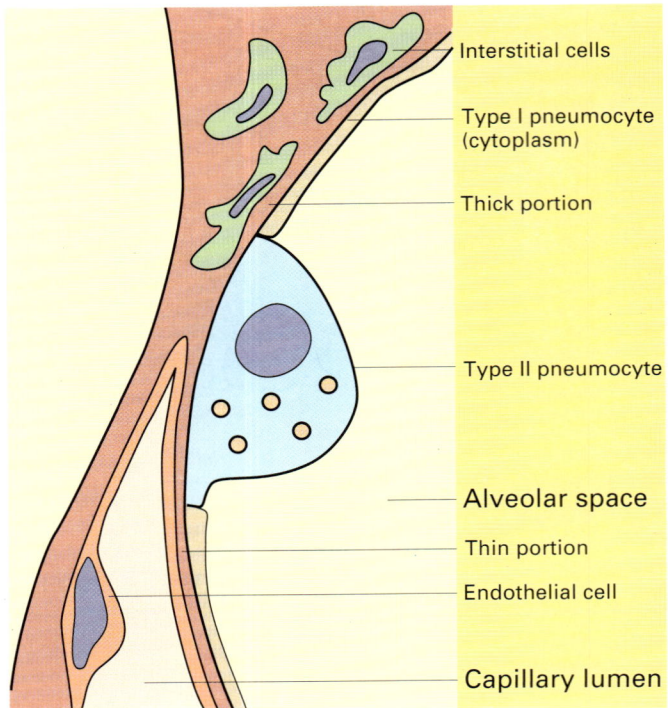

Fig. 13.8 The alveolar wall.

and are responsible for secretion of *surfactant*. This compound is composed of a mixture of protein and lipid. A layer of surfactant lines the alveolar spaces and lowers surface tension, preventing alveolar collapse (Askin and Kuhn 1971). Type 2 pneumocytes proliferate in response to injury, and subsequently differentiate into type 1 cells.

The alveolar walls are interrupted by round to oval 'pores' (*pores of Kohn*). The significance of these are unknown, and whether they are an anatomical or a pathological finding is also uncertain; in humans, however, they appear to increase with age, and are considered by some authors to be the earliest form of emphysema (Pump 1976).

Pulmonary circulation

The lung has a dual blood supply via the bronchial and pulmonary arteries. The bronchial arteries are at systemic pressure and supply the bronchial tree via the aorta, lying in the bronchial walls. The pulmonary arteries are at approximately one-sixth the systemic pressure and are divided into *elastic* and *muscular* arteries. Elastic pulmonary arteries include the pulmonary trunk, together with arteries with a diameter of 500 to 1000 μm or more. The media consists of multiple elastic laminae separated by smooth muscle. At birth, the pulmonary trunk and the aorta are of equal thickness; however, the laminae become increasingly fragmented, such that by 2 years of age an adult pattern is seen. The intrapulmonary elastic arteries, however, retain a concentric pattern. Muscular pulmonary arteries are 100–500 μm in diameter. The media is thin and lies between the internal and external elastic laminae.

The intima is not apparent in young adults, but with increasing age some proliferation and fibrosis occurs. Muscular pulmonary arteries branch with the bronchial tree and lie adjacent to the bronchioles, respiratory bronchioles, and alveolar ducts. At a diameter of approximately 70 μm they gradually lose their muscular coat, forming pulmonary arterioles. Serial cross-sections show muscularized segments alternating with segments containing no muscle—in the more distal portions the arteriole walls consists of a single elastic lamina lined by endothelium. The arterioles give rise to a complex capillary network which forms part of the interalveolar walls.

Pulmonary venules are indistinguishable from arterioles, initially having a single elastic lamina and eventually having a muscular media as they drain proximally. The pulmonary veins are muscular vessels which lie in the connective tissue septa separating lobules.

The pulmonary endothelium forms a characteristic pavement pattern and is responsible for gas exchange, fluid filtration, and metabolism of physiologically active compounds, such as nucleotides, vasoactive amines and peptides, prostaglandins, and lipoproteins. As the lung receives the entire cardiac output, the physiological effects may be considerable.

Lymphatic system

The pulmonary lymphatics are superficial and deep. The superficial lymphatics lie adjacent to the pleura, whereas the deep lymphatics lie in the interlobular septa and adjacent to the vessels and conducting airways. There are no lymphatics in the alveolar wall. Small collections of lymphoid cells may be found at the bifurcations of small bronchioles and respiratory bronchioles, and are also seen in proximity to lymphatics at the periphery of the acini. The lymph drainage is into hilar lymph nodes.

Innervation

The vagus nerve supplies the major motor and sensory innervation of the lung.

13.1.3   Functional anatomy

General

The lung can be divided into three functional zones, comprising the *conducting zone*, the *transitional zone*, and the *gas-exchanging zone*. The conducting zone includes the bronchi and bronchioles; the bronchial tree is arranged in a system of asymmetric dichotomous branching, such that the opposing needs of a low flow resistance and a minimal dead space can be met. The bronchial tree is widely thought of in 'generations', counting down from the trachea to the acini. The trachea is termed generation 0 and the main bronchi generation 1; there may be between 8 and 25 generations until the acini are reached (Horsfield and Cumming 1968). The transitional zone comprises the respiratory bronchioles. These usually branch symmetrically over three generations.

The respiratory, or gas-exchanging, zone includes the

alveolar ducts and alveoli (i.e. the distal acini). The number of alveoli varies between 200×10^6 and 600×10^6, and is thought to depend on height, giving an alveolar surface area of 70–80 m² (Angus and Thurlbeck 1972).

Pulmonary defence

Although ventilation and gas exchange are the two main functions of the lung, pulmonary defence mechanisms are also of importance.

1. *Clearance mechanisms.* Nasal clearance operates via trapping of inhaled particles and sneezing. Muco-ciliary clearance is important in the trachea and the bronchial tree and acts by the upward propulsion of mucus. This depends on both the consistency of the mucus and effective beating of cilia.

   Alveolar clearance is primarily by *alveolar macrophages*. These are derived from the bone marrow via circulating monocytes. They form an interstitial pool in the lung and accumulate and proliferate in the alveolar spaces. Besides phagocytosis, their function includes antigen presentation and production of secretory products, which include enzymes, complement, interferons, chemotactic factors, and mitogens (Brain *et al.* 1977).

2. Blood and lymph drainage.

3. Inflammatory response. *Immunoglobulins*: the bronchial mucus contains immunoglobulins, particularly IgA which is processed by mucinous and serous cells in the bronchial glands by forming dimers and adding the J-chain, the secretory component (McDermott *et al.* 1982). *Cell mediated response*: an immune reaction mediated by sensitized T-lymphocytes (Type IV response).

13.1.4 Bibliography

Angus, G. E. and Thurlbeck, W. (1972). Number of alveoli in the human lung. *Journal of Applied Physiology* **32**, 483–5.

Askin, F. B. and Kuhn, C. (1971). The cellular origin of pulmonary surfactant. *Laboratory Investigation* **25**, 260–8.

Boyden, E. A. (1955). *Segmental anatomy of the lungs. A study of the patterns of segmental bronchi and related pulmonary vessels.* McGraw-Hill, New York.

Brain, J. D., Goodleski, J. J., and Syroken, S. P. (1977). Quantification, origin and fate of pulmonary macrophages. In *Respiratory defense mechanisms II* (ed. C. Lenfent), pp. 839–89. Marcel Dekker, New York.

Dunnill, M. S. (1982). *Pulmonary pathology.* Churchill Livingstone, Edinburgh.

Gibbons, I. R. (1981). Cilia and flagella of eucaryotes. *Journal of Cell Biology* **91**, 1075–1245.

Horsfield, K. and Cumming, G. (1968). Morphology of the bronchial tree in man. *Journal of Applied Physiology* **24**, 373–83.

McDermott, M. R., Befus, A. D., and Bienanstock, J. (1982). The structural basis of immunity in the respiratory tract. *International Review of Experimental Pathology* **23**, 47–112.

Pump, K. K. (1969). Morphology of the acinus of the human lung. *Diseases of the Chest* **56**, 126–34.

Pump, K. K. (1976). Emphysema and its relation to age. *American Review of Respiratory Disease* **114**, 5–13.

Thurlbeck, W. (1968). Chronic obstructive lung disease. In *Pathology annual* (ed. S. C. Sommers), p. 377. Appleton-Century-Crofts, New York.

Thurlbeck, W. (1988). *Pathology of the lung.* Thieme, New York.

Whimster, W. F. and MacFarlane, A. J. (1974). Normal lung weights in a white population. *American Review of Respiratory Disease* **110**, 478–83.

Wigglesworth, J. S. (1984). *Perinatal pathology.* W. B. Saunders, Philadelphia.

13.2 Congenital malformations and perinatal respiratory disease

J. W. Keeling

13.2.1 Congenital malformations of the respiratory tract

The nose

The nares are absent in *cyclopia*, frequently associated with trisomy 13 and other chromosome anomalies. In some fetuses with cyclopia, a blind-ending proboscis is present above the orbits (Fig. 13.9) the brain is holoprosencephalic.

Choanal atresia, which may be unilateral or bilateral, results from failure of breakdown of the bucconasal septum. It may be familial.

Cleft lip and palate

Clefting of lip and palate, which may occur together or in isolation, is familial in one-third of cases. When lip clefting is bilateral and accompanied by total palatal cleft, then elevation of the midline nasal process ensues with consequent hypoplasia of midfacial bones and muscles. This anomaly is common in trisomies 13 and 18 (Fig. 13.10).

The Pierre Robin sequence, hypomandibulosis accompanied by glossoptosis and cleft palate, can effect airway obstruction in the neonate when the unduly floppy tongue is sucked back into the hypopharynx during inspiration.

Laryngeal stenosis and atresia

Obstruction of the larynx by muscle and cartilage or a membranous septum can occur in the subglottic region as a result of failure of canalization of the larynx. The laryngeal inlet is surprisingly normal. Pulmonary development is usually normal, but alveoli are distended by fluid. Rapid diagnosis at birth and tracheostomy are necessary for survival. Laryngeal atresia may accompany cardiac or renal defects.

Tracheal agenesis and stenosis

Absence of the trachea, with origin of main bronchi from the

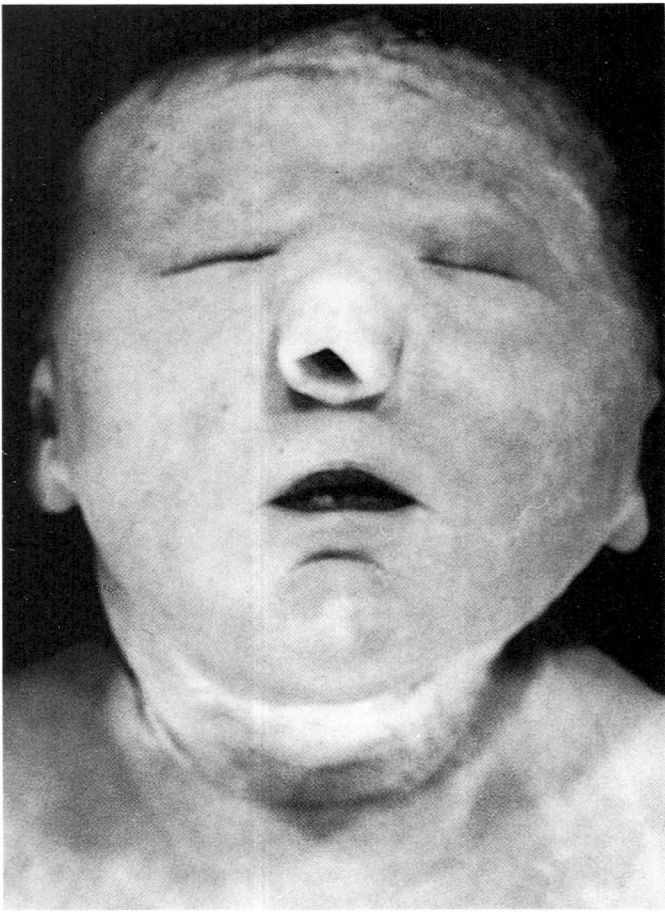

Fig. 13.9 Trisomy 13, there is a blind-ending proboscis replacing the nose. The brain was holoprosencephalic.

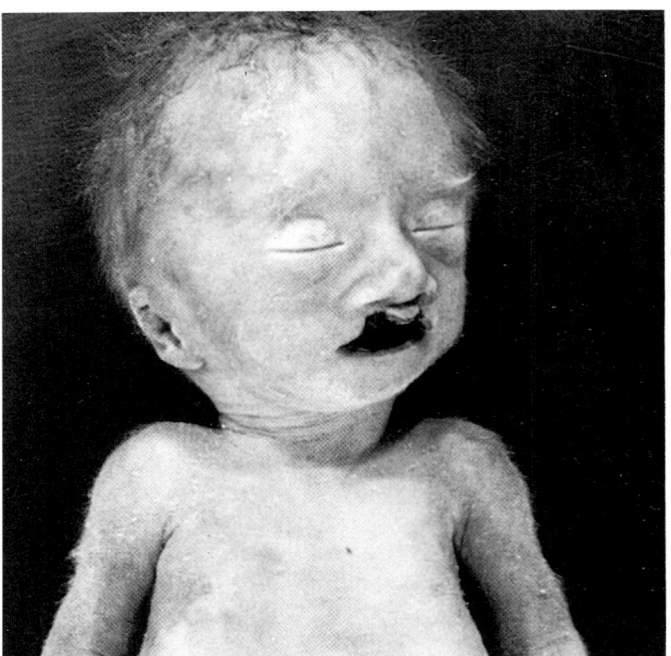

Fig. 13.10 Bilateral cleft lip and palate, permitting elevation of the mid-line nasal process, trisomy 18.

oesophagus, is a rare manifestation of the foregut anomaly which underlies tracheo-oesophageal fistula (see Chapter 15).

Localized stenosis of trachea or main bronchi may accompany anomalies of aortic or main pulmonary artery branching. An aberrant origin of a left pulmonary artery, which runs around trachea or right main bronchus (*pulmonary artery sling*), can compress the airway and is sometimes accompanied by a narrow trachea, having complete cartilagenous rings.

Anomalies of tracheal or bronchial cartilages

Focal absence of tracheal or bronchial cartilage is often seen in the vicinity of localized stenosis (see above). *Tracheomalacia* and *bronchomalacia*, floppiness of parts of the airway because of irregularity, narrowing, and excessive branching and interruption of cartilages, often accompanies oesophageal atresia and tracheo-oesophageal fistula. It can cause airway obstruction and pulmonary collapse, thus complicating postoperative management in these infants.

Deficiency of bronchial cartilage can give rise to *congenital lobar emphysema*.

Bronchial ciliary abnormalities

Cytoarchitectural anomalies of bronchial cilia result in *Kartagener syndrome* of sinusitis, bronchiectasis, and situs inversus, and the immobile cilia syndrome. Electron microscopic examination of cilia reveals absence or irregularity of dynein arms of microtubules. Ciliary abnormalities are inherited as autosomal recessive conditions.

Lungs

Agenesis

Bilateral pulmonary agenesis is very rare. Unilateral agenesis is more frequently seen; associated anomalies are radial aplasia and cardiac defects.

Sequestration

A sequestration is a circumscribed mass of lung without bronchial or pulmonary artery connection, receiving its blood supply from a systemic artery. It may be *intralobar* or *extralobar* in situation, extralobar sequestrations are seen with diaphragmatic hernia. Their increasing size may collapse adjacent lung, with ensuing respiratory embarrassment and predisposition to infection.

Adenomatoid malformation

This is a cystic hamartomatous anomaly which may involve all or part of a lobe or a whole lung. Three histological types are described which have different amounts of muscle, elastic tissue, and gland, and differing cyst size. The increasing size of the latter causes respiratory embarrassment postnatally and necessitates excision. Extensive lesions may present in fetal life, with polyhydramnios and fetal hydrops due to impaired venous return from the placenta consequent on raised intrathoracic pressure.

Pulmonary hypoplasia

Pulmonary hypoplasia is a common cause of perinatal death (Fig. 13.11). It is produced by a variety of congenital malformations and fetal disorders which reduce thoracic volume by their abnormal location (see Chapter 15), disordered skeletal growth (Fig. 13.12), or deformity, or which restrict respiratory movement *in utero* (Table 13.1). Pulmonary hypoplasia is defined in terms of its relationship to body weight: a ratio of $\leq 0.012:1$ indicates hypoplasia. Detailed studies show that bronchial branching is reduced and alveolar development normal. Histological examination of the hypoplastic lung shows crowding of airways. Hyaline membrane and massive pulmonary haemorrhage, disorders usually associated with fetal immaturity, are often present.

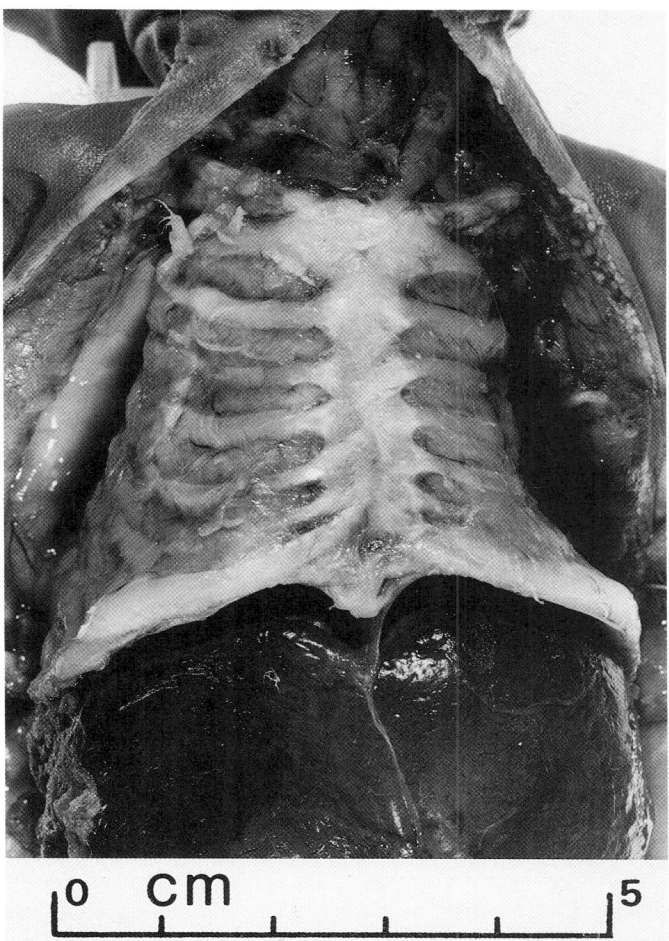

Fig. 13.12 Jeune's asphyxiating thoracic dystrophy, the chest is narrow and bell-shaped because of reduced rib growth.

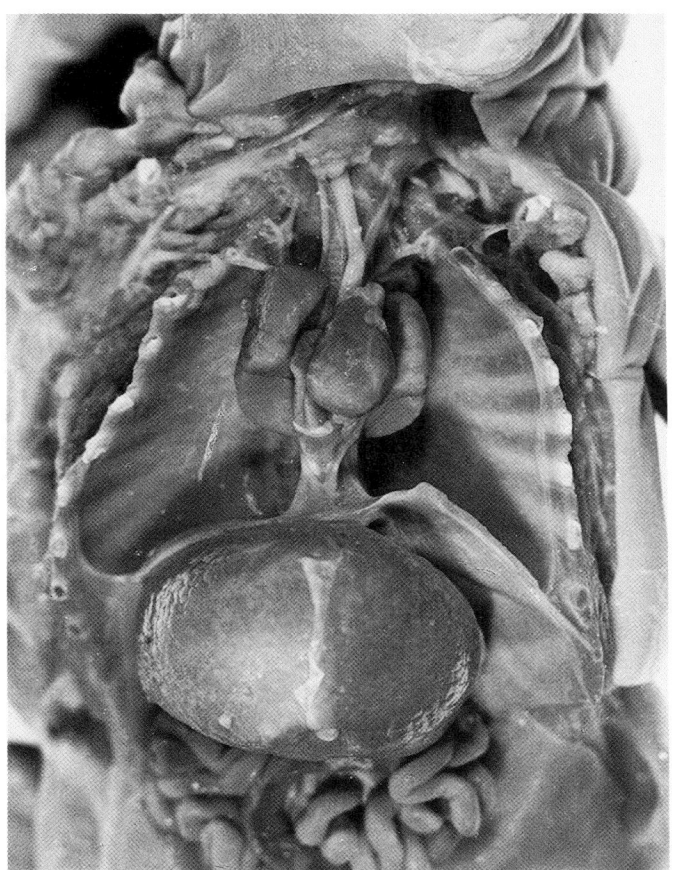

Fig. 13.11 Pulmonary hypoplasia, the lungs are very small when compared with the size of the chest. The cavities were filled with fluid (45XO karyotype).

Table 13.1 Causes of bilateral pulmonary hypoplasia

Condition	Effect
Diminished thoracic volume	
Diaphragmatic hernia	Abdominal viscera in chest
Mediastinal tumour	⎫ Increased thoracic visceral
Cystic lung malformation	⎭ volume
Large polycystic kidney	Elevation of diaphragm
Fetal hydrops	Pleural effusion
Skeletal dysplasias	Reduced rib length
Anencephaly/spina bifida	Reduced thoracic vertebrae
Large meningo-myelocoele	⎫
Amnion rupture sequence	⎬ Spinal and thoracic deformity
Thoracopagus conjoined twins	⎭
Reduced respiratory excursion	
Oligohydramnios	
Prolonged rupture of membranes	⎫ Increased external pressure on
Renal agenesis/dysplasia	⎭ chest wall
Congenital neuromuscular disorders	Hypotonia/diaphragmatic elevation

13.2.2   Perinatal and neonatal respiratory pathology

At necropsy in the perinatal or neonatal period, the lungs are often collapsed and dusky-pink or plum coloured. This appearance is common to a variety of conditions which can be distinguished by histological examination. These include *hyaline membrane disease, birth asphyxia, meconium aspiration, infection,* and *atelectasis*.

The lungs in stillbirth

Although the fetus makes breathing movements, these are not sufficient to expand alveoli, so that the terminal airways in antepartum stillbirths have a 'saw-toothed' or 'crumpled' outline. The histological appearance is uniform. This failure of expansion is often, inaccurately, termed *primary atelectasis* (atelectasis = collapse). If the fetus has been subjected to acute hypoxic stress, as, for example, in placental abruption, then it will respond by gasping and will take liquor amnii further down the respiratory tract, so that partial distension of some air spaces by squamous debris is seen (Fig. 13.13).

Birth asphyxia and meconium aspiration

The mature baby subject to hypoxic insult before birth will respond with bradycardia, passing urine and meconium, and making convulsive inspiratory efforts. A mixture of liquor amnii and meconium is both swallowed and drawn into the respiratory tract.

At necropsy, the skin is often meconium stained, the extremities cyanosed, and a fine petechial rash apparent over the face and neck. Meconium is often present in the oesophagus and stomach as well as in trachea and main bronchi. The lungs are collapsed and petechial haemorrhages are often visible through visceral and parietal pleura, and are present along the course of coronary arteries.

The histological appearance of the lung will depend on the extent of penetration of meconium into the respiratory tract and the length of survival. When meconium has not reached intra-pulmonary airways, then a pattern of irregular expansion of terminal bronchioles and alveolar collapse will be seen. When meconium has gained access to the lung, and particularly if the baby has survived or was resuscitated for some hours, then plugging of airways by meconium, desquamation of bronchiole and bronchiolar epithelium, and a diffuse inflammatory infiltrate within the parenchyma will be present (Fig. 13.14).

Pulmonary pathology in the preterm neonate

Respiratory distress syndrome, characterized by laboured respirations, ground-glass appearance of a chest radiograph, and surfactant abnormality, which requires respiratory support is a common problem in the neonatal period. It is strongly associated with prematurity, although other factors including hypoxia, acidosis, hypothermia, persistent fetal circulation, and prolonged patency of the ductus arteriosus contribute to its development or severity. Post-mortem examination of the lungs of babies dying from respiratory distress syndrome may exhibit the changes of hyaline membrane disease. It is important to remember that respiratory distress syndrome and hyaline membrane disease are not synonymous. The former is a clinical problem, which may be the manifestation of other types of pulmonary disease, such as *infection* or *meconium aspiration*. The latter is a pathological diagnosis. Although it is most often seen in preterm infants with respiratory distress syndrome, it may result from birth asphyxia in mature infants and accompany pulmonary hypoplasia. It is also seen as a complication of some viral infections and other disorders in older children and adults (see Section 13.3.1). Development of hyaline membranes within terminal airways takes time, so that very low birth weight babies with respiratory distress syndrome who die within 5 or 6 hours often do not contain characteristic membranes, although a similar pattern of overexpansion of terminal bronchioles with alveolar collapse is present.

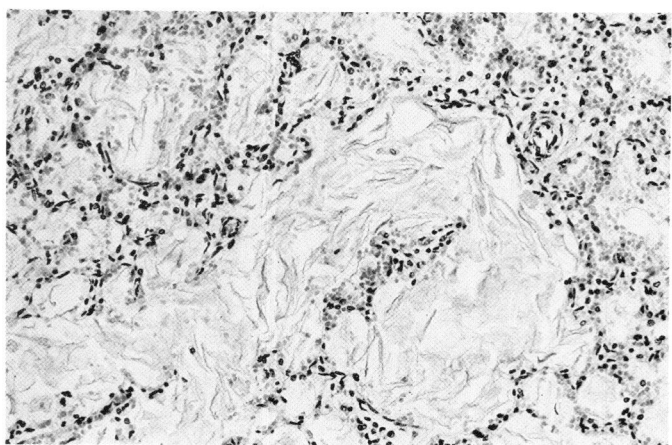

Fig. 13.13 Intra-uterine asphyxia, terminal airways are filled with squamous debris from inhaled amniotic fluid.

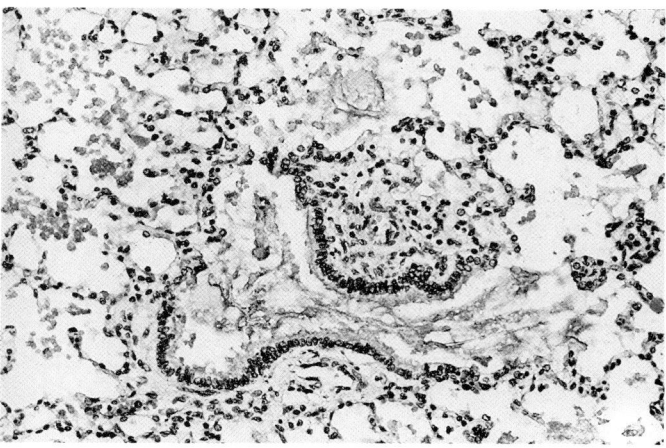

Fig. 13.14 Meconium aspiration; terminal bronchioles contain meconium. There is inflammatory cell infiltration in the adjacent parenchyma.

Hyaline membrane disease

The fully developed pathological picture of hyaline membrane disease is seen in babies surviving longer than 12 hours. The lungs are uniformly collapsed and congested, sometimes with discernible petechial haemorrhages in the pleural surface and a prominent pavement-like pattern of interlobular septa visible, expanded by oedema. The dense consistency of the lungs makes them easy to slice, and they sink when placed in fixative.

Histological examination reveals overexpansion of terminal bronchioles and alveolar ducts (Fig. 13.15). A dense acidophil exudate, often mixed with desquamated respiratory epithelium, lines terminal airways and some partly expanded alveoli (Fig. 13.16) while the majority of alveoli are collapsed.

Massive pulmonary haemorrhage

This condition is characterized clinically by outpouring of

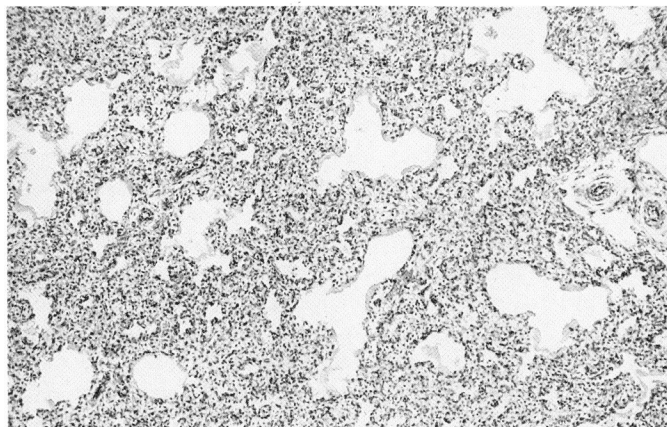

Fig. 13.15 Hyaline membrane disease. At low power the overdistension of terminal bronchioles and alveolar ducts is readily apparent. The intervening alveoli are collapsed.

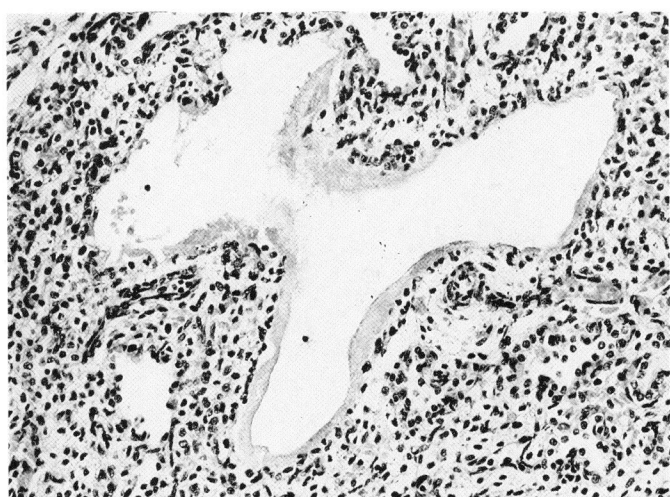

Fig. 13.16 Hyaline membrane disease. At high power the dense acidophil membrane is clearly seen on the surface of terminal air spaces. The lining epithelium has disappeared.

heavily bloodstained fluid from the lungs. Pathologically, the lungs are intensely congested and both alveoli and airways appear to be full of blood. The haematocrit of this fluid indicates that in most cases it is blood-contaminated oedema fluid, suggesting acute heart failure rather than haemorrhage as the underlying process. Precipitating factors are hypoxia and hypothermia, and this realization has led to a marked reduction in the frequency of this condition as a perinatal necropsy finding.

Iatrogenic pulmonary disease

The frequent need for respiratory support of some kind in the preterm infant means that related iatrogenic disease is a common finding in these babies.

The use of endotracheal tubes for ventilation can give rise to pressure necrosis of nasal cartilages, subglottic ulceration (Fig. 13.17), and erosion of tracheal epithelium, with consequent squamous metaplastic change to withstand the repeated trauma of contact with the endotracheal tube. In a few infants, laryngeal injury results in destruction of cartilages, or subglottic stenosis following healing of ulcers by fibrosis.

Mechanical ventilation at higher pressures of babies with

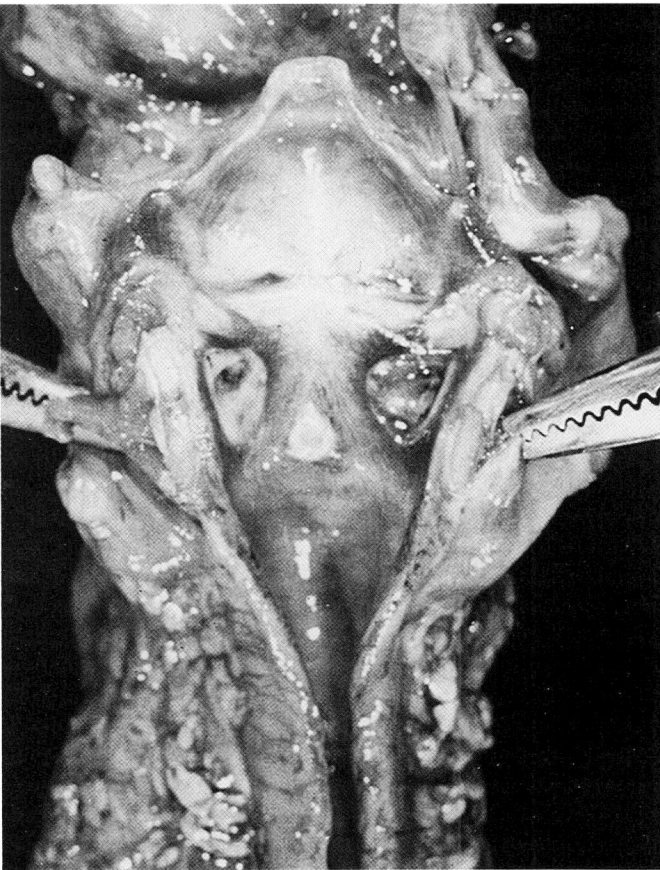

Fig. 13.17 Larynx opened posteriorly. There is ulceration in the subglottic region, in the mid-line, and laterally beneath the vocal fold because of movement of an endotracheal tube. (Keeling 1987.)

respiratory distress results in a high incidence of pulmonary interstitial emphysema, often followed by pneumothorax, causing further respiratory embarrassment (Fig. 13.18). The injudicious use of transthoracic cannulae to drain pneumothorax can perforate the lung (Fig. 13.19). This both renders them ineffective and can result in considerable haemorrhage from small vessel injury because of pulmonary congestion.

Bronchopulmonary dysplasia, a reaction to a combination of the use of oxygen and the barotrauma of ventilation, is a common sequel to respiratory distress syndrome in the very low birth weight baby. Pathological findings are related to length of

survival. In the first two weeks of life, these include squamous metaplasia of intrapulmonary bronchi, interstitial oedema with macrophage and fibroblast infiltration of alveolar walls, and persistence of hyaline membranes. Later, the alveolar lining regenerates and lining cells are cuboidal with eosinophilic cytoplasm; excess reticulin and collagen fibres are present in alveolar walls. The overall pattern is a mixture of lobular overdistension and collapse (Fig. 13.20).

Infection

Pulmonary infection in the new-born may be acquired before, during, or after birth. In the fetus, infection may be transplacental from maternal haematogenous infection (or rarely from a focus of infection within the uterus) or via the amniotic fluid. Transplacental infections that affect the lung include syphilis, *Listeria monocytogenes,* and some viral infections (Fig. 13.21). Infection acquired via the amniotic fluid is usually the result of ascending infection from the maternal genital tract, although iatrogenic introduction of organisms directly into the amniotic sac during amniocentesis or fetoscopy is occasionally responsible. Common vaginal contaminants are *Escherichia coli,* faecal streptococci, and the Group B β-haemolytic streptococcus; *Listeria monocytogenes* may also be acquired in this manner. Ascending infection is usually a complication of premature rupture of placental membranes, although infection can gain access to the amniotic fluid across intact membranes.

Bacterial contamination of the placental membranes provokes maternal polymorphonuclear response via the decidua. Organisms and maternal polymorphs pass into the amniotic fluid and thence gain access to the fetus via the respiratory and gastrointestinal tracts. The presence of polymorphs in the intrapulmonary airways of the fetus, often called *congenital pneumonia* (Fig. 13.22), is not sufficient for a diagnosis of pulmonary infection, it merely indicates opportunity of access. Pulmonary infection demands evidence of fetal response in the form of inter-

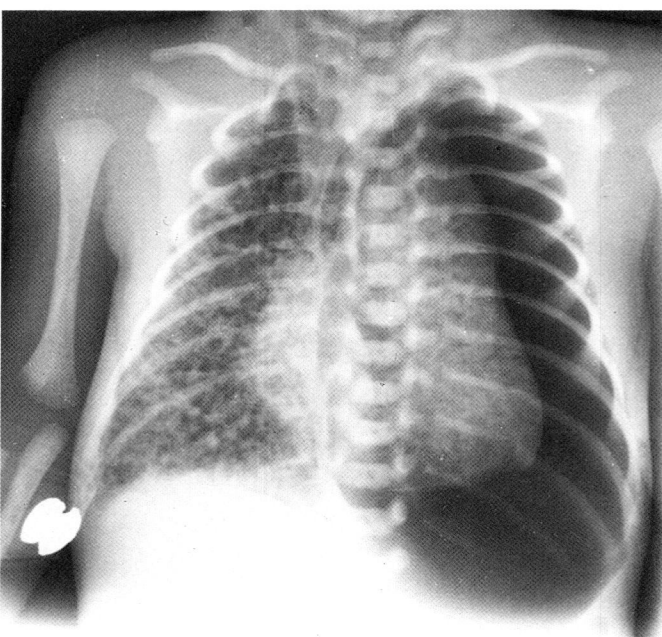

Fig. 13.18 Chest X-ray in hyaline membrane disease. Pulmonary opacity is apparent on the right, a large pneumothorax is present on the left.

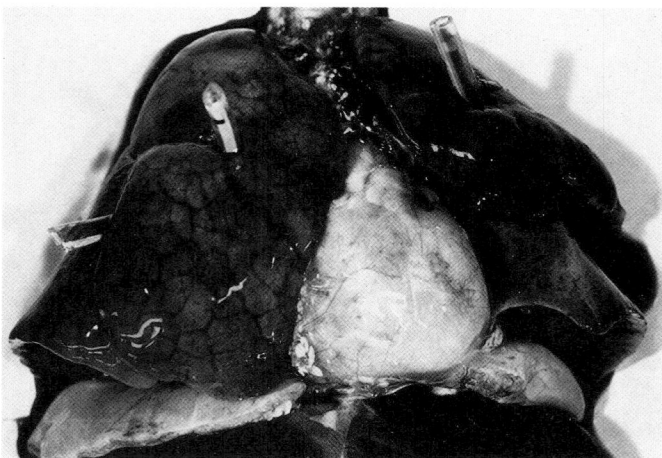

Fig. 13.19 The tips of three chest drain cannulae can be seen perforating the lungs.

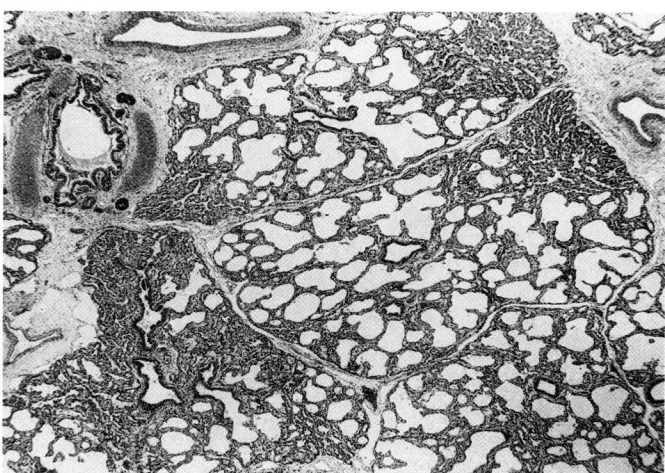

Fig. 13.20 Bronchopulmonary dysplasia. There is diffuse thickening of the alveolar walls and a lobular pattern of overdistension of air spaces and collapse.

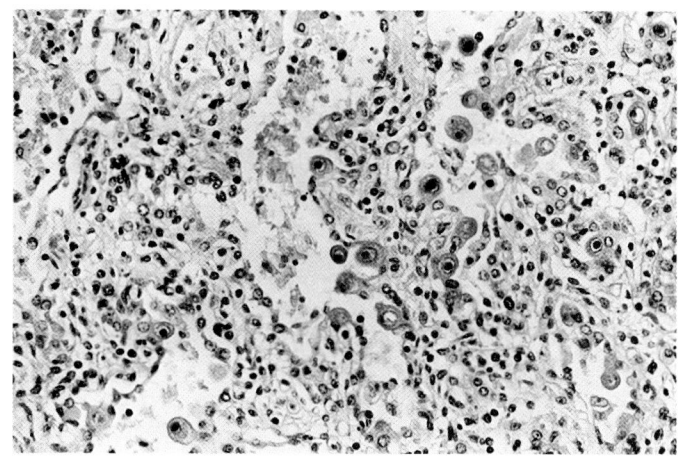

Fig. 13.21 Cytomegalovirus infection in a neonate. The alveolar walls are much thickened and there is a cellular infiltrate. Some alveolar lining cells are increased in size and dense inclusions are present within the nucleus.

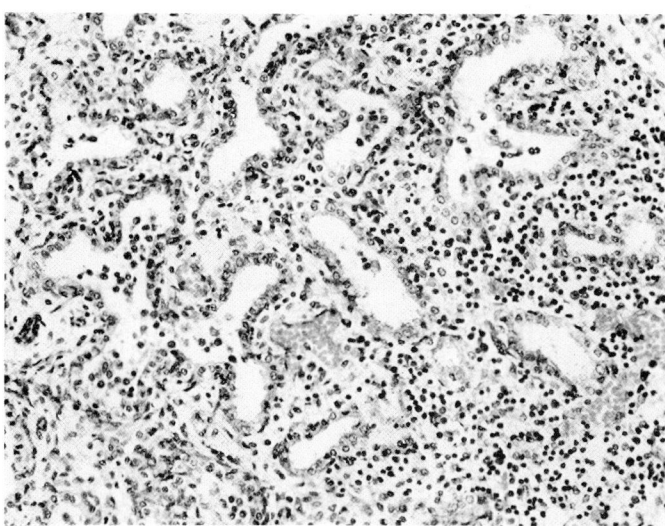

Fig. 13.23 Intra-uterine pneumonia. Maternal polymorphs are present within air spaces. There is a fetal response evidenced by inflammatory cell infiltration in airways parenchyma.

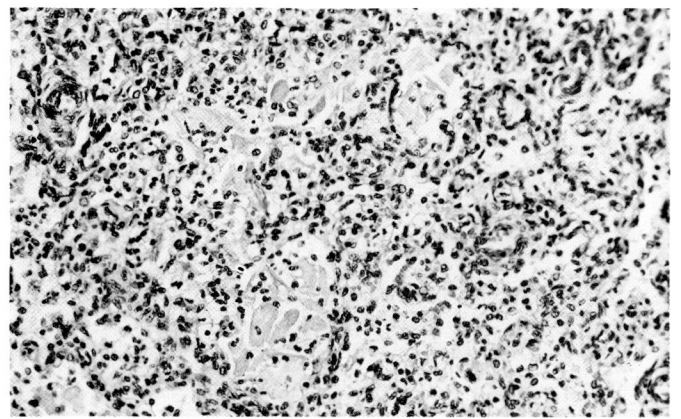

Fig. 13.22 'Congenital pneumonia'. Maternal polymorphs accompanied by polymorphs are present in the intrapulmonary airways.

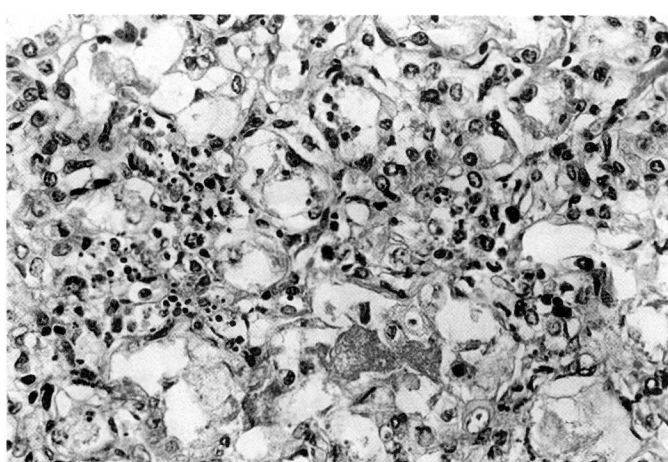

Fig. 13.24 Herpes virus infection. A focus of necrosis with much nuclear debris is present. There is little inflammatory cell infiltration. Such necrotic foci are scattered through the lungs and may be apparent on naked-eye examination.

stitial inflammatory cell infiltration, which may be predominantly mononuclear (Fig. 13.23).

The fetus can acquire pulmonary infection intrapartum when there is maternal genital tract disease such as herpes virus infection (Fig. 13.24), or from vaginal contaminants—Group B β-haemolytic streptococcus is an important fetal pathogen in this situation.

Neonatal pneumonia is a common problem in the preterm infant with poorly developed local defence mechanisms. Loss of integrity of the respiratory epithelium because of hyaline membrane disease, and contamination of ventilators and humidifiers by organisms such as *Pseudomonas aeruginosa* also play a part in the development of pulmonary infection in the neonate.

13.2.3 Further reading

Askin, F. (1991). Respiratory tract disorders in the fetus and neonate. In: *Textbook of Fetal and Perinatal Pathology* (ed. J. S. Wigglesworth and D. B. Singer), pp. 643–88. Blackwell Scientific Publications, Oxford.

Cox, J. (1989). The respiratory system. In *Paediatric pathology* (ed. C. L. Berry) (2nd edn), pp. 293–407. Springer-Verlag, London.

Godfrey, S. (1981). Growth and development of the respiratory system—functional. In: Davis, J., Dobbing, J., *Scientific foundation of paediatrics* (ed. J. Davis and J. Dobbing) (2nd edn), pp. 432–50. Heinemann, London.

Hislop, A. and Reid, L. (1981). Growth and development of the respiratory system—anatomical. In: Davis, J., Dobbing, J., *Scientific foundation of paediatrics* (ed. J. Davis and J. Dobbing) (2nd edn), pp. 390–432. Heinemann, London.

Keeling, J. W. (ed.) (1987). *Iatrogenic disease in fetal and neonatal pathology*, pp. 295–313. Springer, London.

Wigglesworth, J. S. (1984). *The respiratory system in perinatal pathology*, pp. 168–208. W. B. Saunders, Philadelphia.

13.3 Inflammation

13.3.1 Infection

J. B. Schofield and T. Krausz

Infections occur in the respiratory tract more frequently than at any other site. Most of these involve the upper respiratory tract and are caused by viruses, but lower respiratory tract infection, particularly pneumonia, remains an important cause of morbidity and mortality in all age-groups.

Acute bronchitis

Acute bronchitis is an inflammatory condition affecting the tracheobronchial tree, and is usually associated with a generalized respiratory tract infection. Most of these cases are due to viral infection and are more common in the winter. The viruses usually responsible for the common cold, e.g. rhinoviruses and coronaviruses, as well as influenza virus, parainfluenza virus, and adenovirus are the most often seen. *Mycoplasma pneumoniae, Bordetella pertussis,* and *Chlamydia psittaci* are also implicated, and bacterial superinfection may occur. Measles virus may cause a particularly severe acute bronchitis, and in the immunosuppressed, alcoholics, and patients with severe burns, herpes simplex virus may cause necrotic ulceration in the tracheobronchial tree. The role of *Streptococcus pneumoniae* and *Haemophilus influenzae* is unclear, as these are often commensal in the upper respiratory tract, but it is likely that they may cause bacterial superinfection. Diphtheria may involve the bronchi, either primarily or as a consequence of downwards extension of a pharyngeal or laryngeal infection, as discussed below. Acute viral laryngotracheobronchitis in infants is referred to as croup and is often caused by parainfluenza viruses.

Biopsy is rarely performed in acute bronchitis and uncomplicated fatal cases do not occur. Although influenza infection in the elderly may be fatal, the disease is not normally confined to the bronchi. Microscopically there is infiltration of the respiratory mucosa by inflammatory cells, particularly lymphocytes in viral infections but often mixed with polymorphs in the early phases. In influenza virus and parainfluenza virus infection there is often a *severe necrotizing bronchitis,* which is followed by organization and reparative changes, including *squamous metaplasia* of the respiratory epithelium. The infected epithelial cells may contain basophilic intracytoplasmic inclusions, but these are not specific. In adenovirus infection, specific intranuclear inclusions may be present in sloughed bronchial epithelium, but they are more often seen in alveolar cells in adenovirus pneumonia and are discussed below. Respiratory syncytial virus may cause ulcerative bronchitis, but more characteristically causes *bronchiolitis*. Measles virus causes bronchial epithelial hyperplasia and squamous metaplasia extending into submucosal glands, with scanty eosinophilic intracytoplasmic and intranuclear inclusions. *Mycoplasma pneumoniae* may cause a necrotizing bronchiolitis in severe cases, but is more commonly associated with a lymphoplasmacytic infiltrate in the bronchial and bronchiolar walls. In cases of bacterial superinfection, there is a neutrophil response, often associated with mucosal ulceration and exudation of purulent material on to the surface of the airways.

Diphtheria

Diphtheria is a localized infection of upper or lower respiratory tract, caused by a toxin-producing, club-shaped, non-motile, Gram-positive bacterium, *Corynebacterium diphtheriae*. The polypeptide exotoxin inhibits protein synthesis by blocking translation, and has both local and systemic effects, the latter including *myocarditis* and *peripheral neuropathy*. The disease is fortunately rare in the UK due to routine vaccination, but remains common in other parts of the world, where the peak age incidence is at 3 years, although children are at risk between the ages of 6 months and 15 years.

Spread is by inhalation of droplets from infected individuals who may be asymptomatic carriers. Once inhaled, the organism lodges on the epithelium of the respiratory tract (usually the posterior pharynx or fauces, and less commonly trachea or bronchus), multiplies and produces its toxin, which causes local necrosis. The necrotic material, together with inflammatory exudate containing neutrophils and fibrin, forms characteristic grey plaques known as *diphtheric pseudomembranes*. As the lesion progresses, the membranes become thicker and more yellow and adhere strongly to the underlying tissue; attempts at detachment lead to numerous small bleeding points, and haemorrhage causes darkening of the membranes. Membranes in the lower respiratory tree are thinner and separate more easily; these often slough and may lead to airway obstruction.

Absorption of the toxin leads to local effects, such as lymphadenopathy and oedema (*bull's neck*), and systemic effects, initially fever, tachycardia, and leucocytosis. In the second week of illness, myocarditis and, less commonly, peripheral neuropathy are seen; renal, hepatic, and adrenal involvement are rare. Myocarditis occurs in 50 per cent of patients and may lead to arrhythmias or heart failure. Peripheral neuropathy, usually manifested by weakness or paralysis of the soft palate or extra-ocular muscles, is seen in less than 25 per cent of cases and tends to resolve slowly, but occasionally may persist. The overall mortality is approximately 10 per cent in untreated cases, and death is most commonly due to a respiratory cause; early administration of antitoxin improves prognosis and mortality is rare in such cases.

Whooping cough

Whooping cough is caused by infection with *Bordetella pertussis*, a highly infectious bacillus which is responsible for endemic and epidemic upper respiratory tract infection. It usually presents in the under-6-year-old child, but is particularly dangerous in the under-1-year-old. The serious nature of the disease is related to the production of several toxins, the most important of which are *lipopolysaccharide endotoxin, heat-labile toxin,* and *pertussis toxin.* The toxins, as well as causing local damage, prevent phagocytosis of the organism, produce lymphocytosis by blocking lymphocyte recirculation into the lymphoid tissues, and may cause hypoglycaemia. A closely related organism, *Bordetella parapertussis* is responsible for up to 30 per cent of cases in some areas, particularly eastern Europe. *Bordetella bronchiseptica* causes disease in animals but rarely infects humans. Vaccination against *Bordetella pertussis* was introduced in the 1940s, causing a marked reduction in the disease incidence. In the 1970s, the rare but serious side-effects of vaccination were widely publicized, leading to a drop in the immunization rate and a consequently increased incidence of the disease in the late 1970s and early 1980s. The clinical illness is divided into three phases. In the *prodromal* (or catarrhal) phase there are mild non-specific features, including cough and rhinitis; during this phase the patient is highly infectious. The second *paroxysmal phase,* which lasts for up to 6 weeks, is marked by fits of coughing, often with the characteristic inspiratory whoop, and sometimes followed by retching. Rarely *encephalopathy,* probably due to hypoxia and small cerebral haemorrhages, supervenes at this stage and may lead to permanent brain damage or death. In the third or *convalescent phase* the symptoms gradually subside.

Microscopically there is *bronchitis* and *bronchiolitis,* and the organism, which is not invasive, remains attached to ciliated cells on the epithelial surface where it can be demonstrated by a Gram stain. The bronchial wall contains a lymphocytic infiltrate, and polymorphs are seen clustered around degenerate epithelial cells along the junction between the epithelium and underlying connective tissue. Sloughed degenerate epithelial cells and mucus may obstruct the airways but extension into the alveoli is uncommon. Pneumonia due to *Bordetella pertussis* is very rare and most cases of pneumonia are related to superinfection, usually by *Haemophilus influenzae.*

Bronchiolitis

Acute bronchiolitis is an infection of the lower respiratory tract occurring in the first 2 years of life (usually the first year). The commonest cause is viral infection, particularly respiratory syncytial virus (RSV) and, less commonly, parainfluenza virus; *Mycoplasma pneumoniae* has been implicated in some cases. As with viral bronchitis, there is a seasonal variation, with a higher incidence in the winter months. Microscopically there is lymphocytic inflammation of the bronchiolar epithelium, with subsequent necrosis and sloughing followed by epithelial regeneration with non-ciliated cells. Airways may become obstructed by necrotic debris, leading to adsorption collapse and, in severe cases, an *interstitial pneumonitis* may ensue. The disease causes

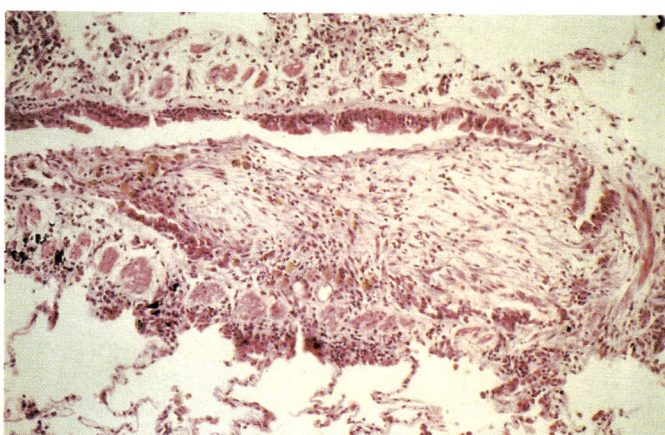

Fig. 13.25 Obliterative bronchiolitis; a polypoid mass of fibrous tissue protrudes into the bronchiolar lumen, causing obstruction.

marked respiratory distress and is rapidly progressive; hospitalization is often necessary but mortality is extremely low.

Bronchiolitis obliterans is a chronic inflammatory process involving the lower respiratory tract and is part of a continuum with organizing pneumonia. It results from repair of damaged small airways by the production of granulation tissue which forms polypoid masses obstructing the bronchiolar lumen (Fig. 13.25). It occurs in some children following *adenovirus infection* and in bone marrow transplant patients with *graft versus host disease,* but is not specific to these diseases and any agent causing damage in this area of the respiratory tract may give rise to a similar response, including inhalation of noxious fumes or gastric contents, organizing infections, allergic reactions, and connective tissue diseases. Microscopically there is plugging of bronchioles and alveolar ducts by oedematous polyps of granulation tissue. The bronchiolar wall is infiltrated by lymphocytes and there may be a polymorph exudate in the lumen. Lymphocytes and plasma cells may be seen within the alveoli. Many cases heal without long-term sequelae, but a few progress to chronic obstructive pulmonary disease.

Pneumonia

Until the introduction of antibacterial agents, pneumonia was often fatal, not only in the elderly and debilitated but also in many young people. Today the epidemiology of this disease has changed, partly because of advances in antimicrobial therapy but also because of changes in the groups most at risk. Increasingly important are immunosuppressed patients, either suffering from the results of cancer treatment or an immunosuppressive disease such as AIDS. This group is prey to a number of unusual infections, which have recently increased dramatically in importance. The classical lobar pneumonia of the pre-antibiotic era is now much less frequently encountered.

Development of pneumonia

The infecting organism is usually inhaled, but may rarely reach the lung by the bloodstream. Reactivation of latent infection in the lung is of particular importance in the immunosuppressed group.

The respiratory tract is normally sterile below the larynx. Various mechanisms are responsible for the clearance of infective particles; these are classically divided into mechanical and chemical mechanisms. Mechanical barriers include the *anterior nares* and *nasal turbinates*, which serve to remove large particles, and the *ciliary action* of the mucosa of the bronchopulmonary tree, which is responsible for removing the smaller particles. These smaller particles become embedded in respiratory mucus, produced by bronchial glands, and are wafted upwards by the beating of the cilia, until reaching the pharynx where they are swallowed. Humidification of the incoming air, which takes place principally in the nasal passages, is vital for the correct functioning of ciliary action. Chemical barriers include a variety of substances secreted by bronchial glands, including immunoglobulins (particularly IgA but also IgM and IgG), lactoferrin, and lysozyme. These agents possess antimicrobial activity and serve to maintain the sterility of the lower respiratory tract.

Infection occurs as a result of an imbalance between the virulence of an infecting organism and the ability of the host to resist infection. Resistance to infection relies on general factors, such as nutrition and normal immune function, and local factors such as bronchial obstruction, ischaemia, and trauma. Tissue damage by pulmonary pathogens occurs by two principal mechanisms. These are:

1. toxins, either derived from the cell walls of degenerate organisms (endotoxin) or by a specific chemical toxin elaborated by the organism (exotoxin); or more frequently by

2. a direct invasive cytolytic process.

Viral infection occurs exclusively by the latter mechanism, but is modified by host factors such as interferons. In both circumstances tissue damage with release of inflammatory mediators leads to an acute inflammatory response, and subsequent activation of the cell-mediated immune system.

Following an acute inflammatory reaction, there may be a range of possible outcomes depending on the extent of tissue damage, host factors, and organism virulence:

1. complete resolution;

2. destructive pneumonia—this may lead to lung abscess or empyema;

3. healing by fibrosis—there is subsequent loss of respiratory function;

4. chronic inflammation.

These processes will be considered in relation to specific infections.

Nomenclature and classification of pneumonia

The term *pneumonia* is used to denote an inflammatory condition affecting the lung parenchyma, usually caused by an infective agent. The term *pneumonitis* is often used synonymously with pneumonia, but tends to be reserved for interstitial inflammation, where the inflammatory cells are largely confined to the alveolar walls and septa. The distribution of inflammatory foci in pneumonia leads to two classical patterns: *lobar pneumonia*, which involves the whole of a lobe, and *bronchopneumonia*, in which there is patchy inflammation centred on lobules. The term 'consolidation' denotes replacement of airspaces by inflammatory exudate, giving the affected area a firm ('solid') airless consistency.

The classification of pneumonia has become increasingly complicated with advancing knowledge. The classical anatomical division into bronchopneumonia and lobar pneumonia is rather simplistic as both of these patterns may be caused by the same organism in hosts of differing ages and level of immune response; in the same way, classification by organism is not entirely satisfactory. We have chosen to discuss the pathological features of each disease under the causative factor.

It may be useful to distinguish between *primary pneumonia* when no predisposing factors are present, and *secondary pneumonia* when pre-existing structural or immunological abnormalities contribute, as a different range of pathogens is implicated in these two groups.

Primary pneumonias include the classical *pneumococcal lobar pneumonia*, other *primary bacterial pneumonias*, and *primary atypical pneumonias*. The concept of atypical pneumonia was proposed in the 1930s for a distinct syndrome of respiratory infection which did not respond to penicillin or sulphonamides, and was associated with patchy changes on chest X-ray. This group contains most of the non-bacterial causes of pneumonia, including *Mycoplasma pneumoniae*, *Rickettsia*, viruses, and *Legionella pneumophila*.

Secondary pneumonias include the pneumonia seen at the extremes of life, the frequently recurrent infections in patient with severe structural lung disease, such as cystic fibrosis, and pneumonia in the immunocompromised patient. Pneumonia in the surgical patient is also a topic of interest; these specific settings are discussed separately.

Acute pneumonia in the adult is most frequently due to bacteria (60–80 per cent), with *Mycoplasma pneumoniae* (10–20 per cent) and viruses (10–15 per cent) in the minority. Bacterial pneumonia in young healthy adults is infrequent but when it occurs it is usually caused by a *virulent pneumococcus*. Effective chemotherapy has made this disease much less common, and mortality is relatively rare (less than 5 per cent). Other bacterial causes of pneumonia in healthy adults are very uncommon, and as pneumococcal pneumonia has receded in importance, the group of primary atypical pneumonias has become more prominent.

The range of infective agents which may be responsible for acute pneumonia is extremely wide and these are listed in Table 13.2. Only the more common infections and those with specific pathological features will be discussed.

Bacterial pneumonias

Pneumococcal pneumonia is the most prominent example in this group and will be discussed in detail. Many other virulent bacteria can cause pneumonia if inhaled in sufficient quantity, although this is relatively uncommon. These may produce

Table 13.2   Infective agents causing pneumonia

Bacteria	Influenza virus types A, B
Common	Adenovirus types 4, 7
Streptococcus pneumoniae	Uncommon
Staphylococcus aureus	Adenovirus types 1, 2, 3, 5
Haemophilus influenzae	Cytomegalovirus
Pseudomonas aeruginosa	Varicella-zoster virus
Klebsiella pneumoniae	Herpes simplex virus
Escherichia coli	Measles virus
Enterobacter spp.	Epstein–Barr virus
Serratia spp.	Coxsackie virus
Legionella pneumophila	Echovirus
Anaerobes, e.g. *Bacteroides* spp.	Poliovirus
Fusobacterium spp.	Rhinovirus
Peptostreptococcus spp.	
Peptococcus spp.	Chlamydiae
Uncommon	*Chlamydia trachomatis*
Acinetobacter spp.	*Chlamydia psittaci*
Actinomyces spp.	*Chlamydia pneumoniae* (TWAR)
Aeromonas hydrophilia	
Branhamella catarrhalis	Mycoplasmas
Campylobacter fetus	*Mycoplasma pneumoniae*
Eikenella corrodens	
Francisella tularensis	Rickettsiae
Nocardia spp.	*Coxiella burnetii*
Pasteurella multocida	*Rickettsia rickettsii*
Proteus spp.	
Pseudomonas pseudomallei	Fungi
Pseudomonas mallei	*Aspergillus* spp.
Salmonella sp.	*Candida* spp.
Faecal streptococci	*Coccodioides immitis*
Streptococcus pyogenes	*Cryptococcus neoformans*
Yersinia pestis	*Histoplasma capsulatum*
	Mucor spp.
Mycobacteria	*Rhizopus* spp.
Mycobacterium tuberculosis	*Adsidia* spp.
Atypical mycobacteria	Parasites
	Pneumocystis carinii
Viruses	*Toxoplasma gondii*
Common	*Ascaris lumbricoides*
Respiratory syncytial virus	*Strongyloides stercoralis*
Parainfluenza virus types 1, 2, 3	*Paragonimus westermani*

either lobar or bronchopneumonia and are more frequently associated with metastatic spread than the pneumococcus.

Streptococcus pneumoniae *(pneumococcus)* This organism is classically cited as the cause of *lobar pneumonia*, although it is important to note that a number of these infections are less typical and may resemble *lobular pneumonia*.

Pneumococcal lobar pneumonia is an acute bacterial infection involving all of a lobe, caused by inhalation of a virulent type of *Streptococcus pneumoniae*. The organism is a Gram-positive encapsulated diplococcus, which grows as α-haemolytic 'draughtsman' colonies on blood agar and is noted for *optochin sensitivity*. Serotypes 1, 2, and 3 cause the majority of severe infections but 5, 7, and 14 are also implicated. The organism may be cultured from the nasopharynx for some days or weeks before causing pneumonia, which is often precipitated by a minor depression of host defences, such as a mild viral infection or an alcoholic binge.

An acute inflammatory reaction occurs which may be localized, or more frequently spreads rapidly to involve an entire lobe, with inflammatory oedema rich in pneumococci (Fig.

13.26). The rapid nature of the spread is due to bacteria passing through openings in the alveolar wall, the pores of Kohn (Fig. 13.27). An important factor is the inability of phagocytic cells to engulf the capsulated pneumococcus without prior opsonization; in the classical untreated case, the patients temperature

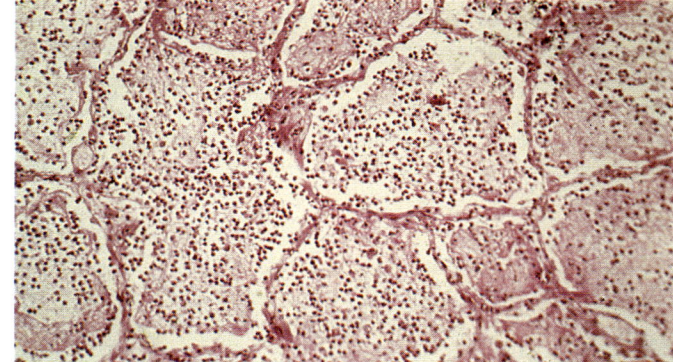

Fig. 13.26   Lobar pneumonia caused by *Streptococcus pneumoniae*; there is marked intra-alveolar oedema rich in neutrophils.

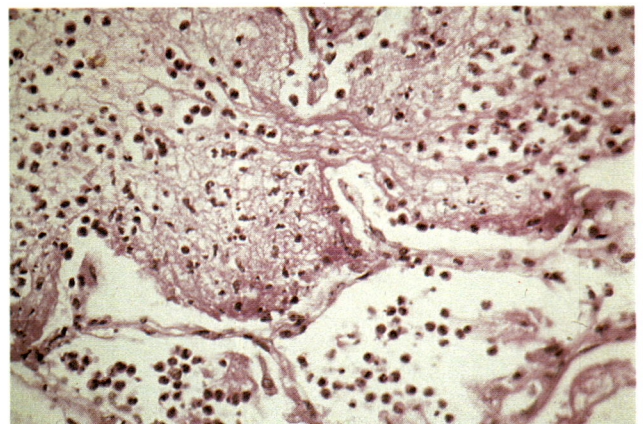

Fig. 13.27 *Streptococcus pneumoniae* pneumonia; inflammatory exudate spreading from one alveolus to another, probably through a pore of Kohn.

falls rapidly ('by crisis') at the stage when the opsonizing antibody concentration rises. A bacteraemia occurs early in the disease and may occasionally lead to metastatic deposits in the meninges, endocardium, or synovium.

The pathological features are classically described in four stages, although at any one time different areas of the same lung may show different stages in the evolution of the disease. This blurring of the classical pattern is accentuated by antibiotic therapy which may halt progression and accelerate resolution. The four stages are spreading *inflammatory oedema, red hepatization, grey hepatization,* and *resolution.* The term hepatization arose from a perceived macroscopic similarity between consolidated lung and liver tissue.

1. *Spreading inflammatory oedema.* This stage is not often seen microscopically and represents the early spreading of the organism. It normally lasts less than 24 hours and is characterized by accumulation of intra-alveolar oedema fluid containing numerous bacteria but only scanty macrophages and polymorphs. Vascular congestion is marked and the macroscopic appearance is that of a heavy, reddened lobe with a boggy texture.

2. *Red hepatization.* The lobe becomes firmer, airless, and brick red in colour, often with petechial subpleural haemorrhages and overlying *fibrinous pleurisy.* Microscopically, there is a precipitate of fibrin which fills the alveolar spaces, together with increasing numbers of polymorphs containing engulfed bacteria. Numerous extravasated red cells give the lobe the red colour and also account for the typical rusty colour of the sputum.

3. *Grey hepatization.* In this stage the lobe is firm and non-crepitant, covered by fibrinous exudate. Congestion has been reduced, partly due to compression of vessels by the distended airways which are now full of fibrin and degenerating polymorphs with only scanty red cells. Arterial and venous thrombosis also contribute.

4. *Resolution.* The onset of this stage (at 8–10 days in untreated cases) is marked macroscopically by a return of the normal pink colour of the lung as fibrin retracts from the alveolar walls and capillary circulation is restored. Enzymatic digestion of fibrin is accompanied by an influx of macrophages replacing and digesting the neutrophils and destroying the pneumococci. In most case complete resolution occurs and the lung parenchyma is restored to normal. The pleural reaction may also completely resolve but frequently a fibrous thickening or adhesion results. If resolution does not occur, there may be persistence of inflammatory activity, with subsequent organization of the intra-alveolar exudate (a process known as *organizing pneumonia* or *carnification*), with deposition of fibrous tissue (Figs 13.28, 13.29). Rare sequelae include local *suppuration* with *abscess formation.*

Diagnosis is usually confirmed by isolation of the organism from sputum or blood cultures. Pneumococcal vaccine is available, particularly for patients undergoing splenectomy who are susceptible to overwhelming pneumococcal septicaemia.

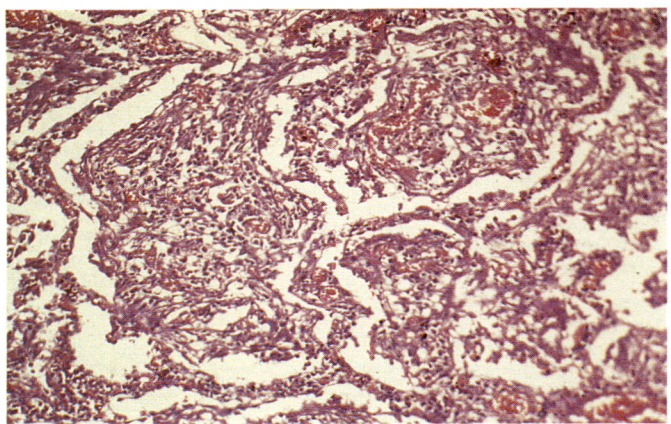

Fig. 13.28 In unresolved pneumonia, intra-alveolar inflammatory exudate is replaced by fibrous tissue.

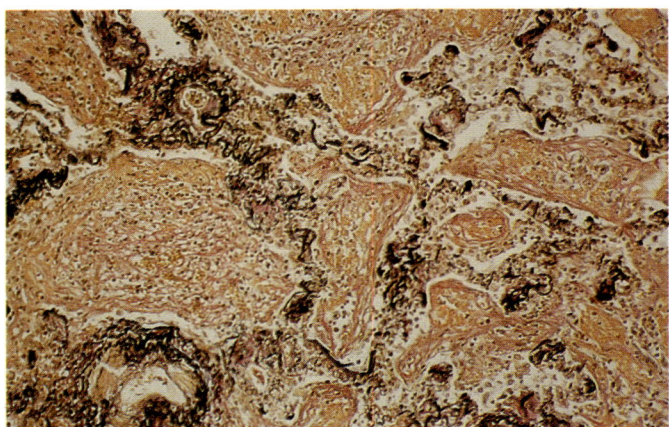

Fig. 13.29 Elastic van Gieson stain demonstrating collagenized intra-alveolar fibrous tissue (stained pink) in unresolved pneumonia.

Staphylococcus aureus This pathogen is most frequently encountered in babies and in elderly individuals debilitated by other diseases. *Staphylococcus aureus* causes a destructive pneumonia which usually follows a viral respiratory infection. The most severe and fulminating type complicates influenzal infection, particularly in young adults. It is also the predominant primary respiratory pathogen in children with cystic fibrosis. Intravenous drug abusers are prone to this infection as a result of injecting through infected skin lesions.

The organism, *Staphylococcus aureus* (previously known as *Staphylococcus pyogenes*) is a Gram-positive coccus which grows as golden-yellow colonies on blood agar, and produces *coagulase*, an enzyme which causes polymerization of fibrogen. This latter characteristic is used to differentiate the organism from the less virulent *Staphylococcus epidermis*.

Macroscopically, the areas of consolidation may be of lobar or lobular pattern. There is a high mortality, and at post-mortem the lungs are purple and heavy due to haemorrhagic pulmonary oedema. They may be covered by purulent exudate but there is no pleural reaction. There is an *ulcerative bronchitis* and *bronchiolitis*; the alveolar spaces are filled with oedema, fibrin, blood, scanty neutrophils, and many Gram-positive cocci (Fig. 13.30). If the patient survives the acute phase, focal suppurative lesions form and coalesce to produce multiple abscess cavities. *Empyema* and *pneumothorax* may occur after rupture of a peripheral abscess into the pleural cavity, or occasionally this may result in a *pneumatocele*.

Haemophilus influenzae. is most commonly associated with pneumonia in the older (over 50 years), alcoholic, or debilitated patient, but also may cause an acute pneumonia in young infants within 2 months of birth, and is often preceded by a viral infection. It is a small, Gram-negative, encapsulated rod which is a normal commensal in the upper respiratory tract, and six serotypes are recognized. It may be difficult to prove a causal relationship between isolation of the organism and infection unless it is found in pleural fluid or blood cultures. The pattern of pneumonic involvement may be either lobar or diffuse and there are no special pathological features. Cavitation, pleural effusion, and empyema may occur. In young children *Haemophilus influenzae* serotype b is especially important, causing otitis media and meningitis as well as pneumonia. Response to antibiotic therapy is usually good and mortality is low.

Legionella pneumophila Legionnaire's disease may present as an atypical pneumonia, but many cases mimic lobar pneumonia. The disease owes its name to an outbreak of severe pneumonia with a substantial mortality which occurred at an American Legion conference in Philadelphia in 1976. A previously unknown, slowly growing Gram-negative bacillus was identified as the cause. This group of organisms is called *Legionella pneumophila* and 10 serotypes are now recognized. There have been sporadic outbreaks world-wide, usually associated with institutions such as hotels and hospitals. The common factor is contamination of water storage tanks with legionellae and it is believed that aerosol production by showers and in air-conditioning units is the mechanism of spread. The disease is commonest in middle-aged men with a history of heavy drinking and smoking. As with other bacterial pneumonias, involvement of systems outside the respiratory tract is usual. Confusion and gastrointestinal symptoms are common modes of presentation, and the patient may progress to renal or hepatic failure. Macroscopically the appearances mimic the grey hepatization stage of pneumococcal lobar pneumonia. Lobes in both lungs may be affected and *fibrinous pleurisy* is usually seen.

Microscopically there is widespread haemorrhagic oedema limited by the alveolar septa, followed by fibrin deposition and an infiltrate of macrophages and neutrophils, the former frequently predominating. The organism can be directly visualized using an immunofluorescent technique or by Dieterle's silver staining method, but this is less reliable. Demonstration of the organisms in tissue section is important as culture is difficult. Although recovery may be complete, some cases progress to interstitial fibrosis with diminished pulmonary function. Other species of *Legionella* (originally called *atypical Legionella-like organisms, ALLO*) can cause an atypical pneumonia, or pneumonia in the immunocompromised.

Klebsiella pneumoniae Various members of the Enterobacteriacae may cause pneumonia; *Klebsiella* sp. causes a rare but serious form of lobar pneumonia, also known as *Freidlander's pneumonia*. Systemic upset is severe and there is a marked tendency to subsequent abscess formation. *Klebsiella* is a non-motile, capsulated, lactose-fermenting, Gram-negative rod, which produces characteristic mucoid, domed colonies when cultured on blood agar. Subclassification is by capsular (k) antigens into more than 70 types, 1, 2, and 3 being the most common. The disease usually occurs in males over the age of 50 with poor dental hygiene and often diabetes mellitus. Commonly involved sites are the posterior segment of the right upper lobe or the apical segment of the right lower lobe. This distribution suggests that the organism is seeded by inhalation.

The disease may progress to a chronic form, usually with

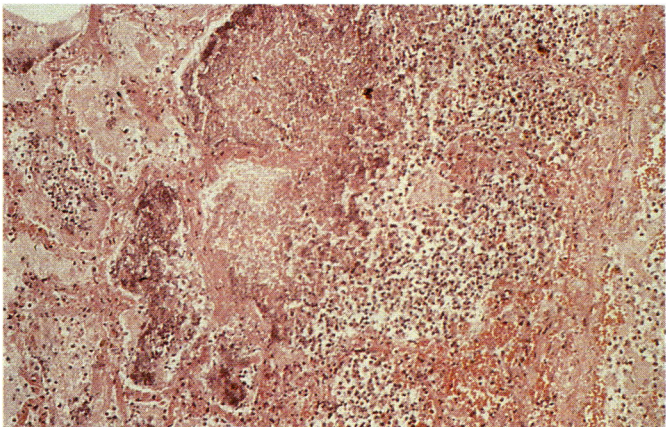

Fig. 13.30 Staphylococcal pneumonia; there is marked destruction of alveolar walls with abscess formation.

apical cavitation which may be difficult to distinguish from tuberculosis.

The consolidated areas are red to grey, with a sticky mucoid exudate in the bronchi which accounts for the redcurrant jelly sputum seen clinically. Initial microscopic features include copious oedema fluid and macrophages within the alveoli, but this rapidly gives way to a neutrophil exudate with destruction of the alveolar wall and replacement by granulation and fibrous tissue. There is also prominent interlobular oedema. As the disease progresses, multiple abscess cavities are formed, lined by granulation tissue and epithelial remnants. Secondary infection with other bacteria is common.

Pseudomonas aeruginosa and other Gram-negative organisms

Pneumonia due to *Pseudomonas aeruginosa* is almost exclusively seen in immunosuppressed and severely ill patients in the hospital setting, particularly in patients receiving artificial ventilation. The organism can often be isolated from the ventilator. Infection occurs in patients with severe burns, when the route of infection is via the bloodstream after cutaneous inoculation. It is an important pathogen in patients with severe structural lung disease such as *cystic fibrosis*. The pneumonia may be rapidly progressive and is often associated with bacteraemia.

Macroscopically, there are numerous haemorrhagic areas or scattered yellowish nodules with surrounding oedema. Microscopically, there is abscess formation with a predominantly mononuclear cell infiltrate and areas of necrosis with an associated *vasculitis*, often with *thrombosis* (Fig. 13.31). Bacteria can be demonstrated in the walls of arterioles and veins where they frequently cause haemorrhage. *Pseudomonas* is almost always associated with pulmonary haemorrhage for this reason. The abscesses are frequently multiple, may coalesce and, if large, are usually fatal. Prognosis in this disease is generally poor. Other Gram-negative organisms, such as *Proteus* sp., *Serratia* sp., and *Enterobacter* sp. may produce a similar pathological appearance.

Pneumonia caused by *Pseudomonas mallei* and *Pseudomonas pseudomallei* is considered with chronic pneumonias.

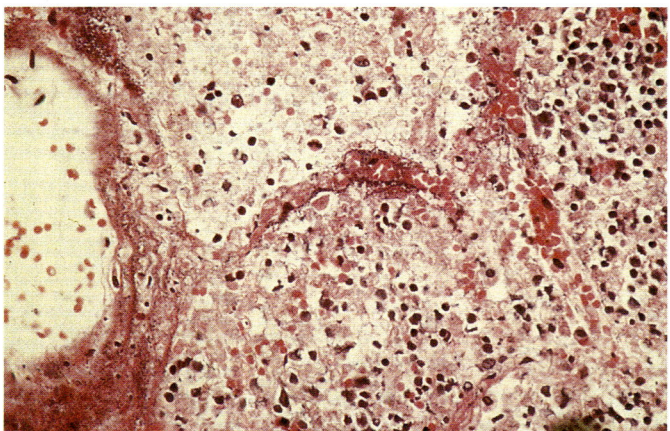

Fig. 13.31 *Pseudomonas aeruginosa* pneumonia; destruction and homogenization of the alveolar wall, which is colonized by the bacteria, with an associated haemorrhagic pneumonia.

Anaerobic organisms

These organisms are often found on mucosal surfaces, and particularly in the mouth. Although they may colonize bronchiectatic areas in the lung, they can cause *pneumonitis, necrotizing pneumonias,* and *lung abscesses*. Infection is usually seen in the context of aspiration of pharyngeal contents, e.g. following general anaesthesia or during unconsciousness, and multiple bacterial species are often involved. This is discussed further in the section on aspiration pneumonia. The common organisms encountered include *Bacteroides* sp., *Peptostreptococcus* sp., *Peptococcus* sp., and fusiform bacteria. The site of involvement reflects the importance of aspiration; posterior segments of upper and lower lobes are frequently involved, and the right lung more often than the left.

Necrotizing pneumonia is characterized by discrete areas of consolidation with microabscess formation, and often involves more than one lobe. Macroscopically the affected area is grey and airless, with fibrous thickening of the pleura, interlobular septa, and bronchi, often with *bronchiectasis*. There are numerous small cavities in the pulmonary parenchyma, Microscopically there are areas of fibrosis and organizing pneumonia with foci of necrosis and suppuration. Lung abscess and empyema frequently supervene.

Streptococcus pyogenes (Lancefield group A β-haemolytic streptococcus)

Fortunately, this disease is now rare and chiefly of historic interest. It usually follows a viral infection and was the predominant cause of death in the great influenza pandemic following the 1914–18 war. The disease has a rapid course, with a high mortality often within 72 hours. Macroscopically the lungs are oedematous and plum-coloured, with basal collapse secondary to bilateral pleural effusions. Extensive petechial haemorrhages are seen and bloodstained fluid fills the bronchi.

Microscopically there is shedding of the epithelium of bronchi and bronchioles and their walls contain a heavy polymorph infiltrate. The airways contain debris, pus cells, and oedema fluid rich in organisms. Many of the alveoli contain hyaline membranes. Abscess formation may occur if the patient survives the early disease.

Francisella tularensis

is a Gram-negative rod transmitted by rodents. The lungs are involved in a minority of cases of *tularaemia*. The pulmonary features are those of an ulcerative bronchiolitis with a fibrinous pneumonia.

Yersinia pestis

Plague is transmitted by the rat flea from an animal reservoir. The causative organism is *Yersinia pestis* and the pneumonic form of this disease produces a rapidly spreading haemorrhagic bronchopneumonia. Fortunately, the disease has disappeared from Europe and North Africa and is becoming rare in Asia and Africa. It is of historic interest as it was the cause of the Black Death in the fourteenth century. The last epidemic in England was over 300 years ago (the Great Plague of 1665) and the last reported case in the UK was over 70 years ago.

Bacillus anthracis

Anthrax is caused by *Bacillus anthracis*, which causes a severe infection in domestic animals. Man acquires the infection from an animal source, usually by inoculation of the skin which may be followed by septicaemia. The disease is usually cutaneous and the respiratory form of anthrax is rare but almost invariably rapidly fatal. Pulmonary anthrax was common in wool sorters following the inhalation of spores and was therefore known as *wool-sorter's disease*. In France it became known as '*la maladie de Bradford*'.

Few modern descriptions of the pathology exist. Macroscopically the hilar lymph nodes are enlarged with surrounding oedema and haemorrhage. There are bilateral haemorrhagic pleural effusions. The lungs are bulky and purple due to a haemorrhagic destructive pneumonia. No ulceration of the airways is seen and there is no neutrophil response. The oedema fluid contains huge numbers of the Gram-positive rods of *Bacillus anthracis*.

Acute non-bacterial pneumonias

Atypical pneumonia is defined as a syndrome of respiratory tract infection characterized by varied symptomatology, by radiological change of a patchy character, and by a lack of response to sulphonamides and penicillin. It is now known that most of these illnesses are due to non-bacterial agents. These include viruses (e.g. adenovirus), chlamydiae (e.g. *C. psittaci*), rickettsiae (e.g. *Coxiella burnetii*), and mycoplasmas (e.g. *Mycoplasma pneumoniae*). *Legionella pneumophila*, which is discussed in the previous section, is also a cause of atypical pneumonia. Rarely, fungi and protozoa may produce a similar clinical picture, particularly in the immunosuppressed.

Transmission is by inhalation of droplets or dust particles containing the organism. The term *atypical pneumonia* is now used to encompass those pneumonias that are not pyogenic and that can be defined as an acute febrile respiratory disease characterized by changes which are confined to alveolar septa and pulmonary interstitium. These changes are often referred to as interstitial pneumonitis. The causative agent remains obscure in up to a third of cases.

Mycoplasma pneumoniae is numerically the most important cause of *primary atypical pneumonia*. It appears that it was responsible for the outbreak of pneumonia in soldiers during the Second World War. Ultimately the organism was isolated from the sputum of such cases and called the 'The Eaton Agent', but it is now recognized as *Mycoplasma pneumoniae*. Outbreaks occur in families and institutions. The incubation period is approximately 2 weeks. Mycoplasmas are very small, pleomorphic organisms which will pass through antibacterial filters. Although they possess a limiting lipoprotein membrane, they lack a rigid cell wall. They can be grown in specific liquid or solid media enriched by serum and yeasts. In culture, *Mycoplasma pneumonia* is β-haemolytic for sheep red cells but grows very slowly. It can be stained by Giemsa but not by Gram's method, and can just be seen using the light microscope. Diagnosis is usually confirmed serologically; cold agglutinins to human group O red cells may be seen in up to 50 per cent of cases.

Infections with the organism are most frequently asympto-matic and as the disease is rarely fatal pathological descriptions are based on the unusual serious cases. Microscopically there is a predominantly interstitial infiltrate of lymphocytes, macrophages, and plasma cells with interstitial oedema. In very acute cases neutrophils may be present. Alveoli may be free of exudate but more commonly contain hyaline membranes similar to those seen in respiratory distress syndrome, reflecting diffuse alveolar damage. Superimposed bacterial infection may occur with typical features, but complete resolution is the rule.

Viruses Viral infection of the respiratory tract is often a precursor of bacterial pneumonias; however, true viral pneumonia may occur. Many groups of viruses have been implicated, including *influenza, parainfluenza, adenovirus, coxsackie, echovirus, varicella, vaccinia*, and *measles*. Any of these agents may cause mild upper respiratory tract infection, but more rarely produce an atypical pneumonia. It is uncertain why this extension occurs, but it is favoured by malnutrition and debilitating illness. Most viral pneumonias are relatively mild, having a mortality of less than 1 per cent, but in epidemics the infection may be more severe and may be complicated by secondary staphylococcal or streptococcal infection, with a consequent increase in mortality. The histological picture is analogous to that seen in mycoplasma pneumonia, but certain viruses produce specific appearances which are discussed below.

1. *Respiratory syncytial virus.* Respiratory syncytial virus (RSV) is a common cause of respiratory tract infection in the young child, in particular *bronchiolitis,* and is responsible for approximately 30 per cent of viral pneumonias in the under 3 years age-group. It is also recognized as a cause of outbreaks of respiratory infection in geriatric institutions. The disease is rarely fatal, except in immunosuppressed patients. Microscopically there is acute bronchiolitis which affects smaller airways, with desquamation of the epithelial cells followed by peribronchiolar lymphocytic infiltrate with oedema and plugging of the bronchioles with mucus and cell debris. This may lead to collapse or overinflation. *Interstitial pneumonitis* is seen, with an inflammatory cell infiltrate within the alveolar walls, with loss of alveolar lining cells and production of hyaline membranes. Regeneration occurs with non-ciliated epithelium.

2. *Adenovirus.* Adenovirus infection has a world-wide distribution and an increasing number of cases are reported. There are many reported fatalities in infants and young children. The virus causes a *severe bronchiolitis,* and types 4 and 7 are the most commonly encountered. In 50 per cent of cases of adenovirus pneumonia in children there are long-term clinical or radiographic abnormalities, with *bronchiectasis* or *bronchiolitis obliterans* in at least 25 per cent. It has been suggested that the pneumonia associated with whooping cough is due to concurrent adenovirus infection rather than a direct effect of *Bordetella pertussis.* Epidemics have also occurred in adults, particularly in military recruits.

Adenovirus is a DNA virus which produces a three-dimensional lattice in the nucleus of infected cells when viewed by the electron microscope. Growth of the virus leads to deformation of the nucleus. Microscopically there is ulceration of bronchiolar epithelium and production of PAS-positive hyaline membranes. There is a lymphocytic infiltrate which includes large hyperchromatic cells and spreads into the interstitium. The alveoli are filled by fibrinous material. Inclusion bodies of two different types (known as *Cowdray types A and B*) may be present in the epithelial cells, but are often scanty. The nucleus of an infected cell, may eventually disrupt, producing a characteristic 'smudge cell'.

Definitive diagnosis relies on virus isolation in tissue culture. Adenovirus infection may be associated with the production of cold agglutinins in 20 per cent of cases, compared with over 50 per cent of patients with mycoplasma pneumonia; other viral pneumonias do not show this phenomenon.

3. *Measles virus*. Asymptomatic chest X-ray changes are common in measles, but clinical infection is rare, except in immunosuppressed children. Measles infection normally involves the upper respiratory tract, but a severe and frequently fatal *giant cell pneumonia* may occur, particularly in the malnourished infant. The entities of measles and giant cell pneumonia are intimately related; giant cell pneumonia is seen in association with immunosuppression, and appears to be either reactivation or a primary infection with measles virus.

In this country measles virus pneumonia may be seen in association with leukaemia or chemotherapy, but world-wide it is commonest in Africa where severe malnutrition is widespread.

The disease causes formation of numerous small nodules which are scattered through the lung fields. Macroscopically the lungs are meaty with focal or lobar consolidation and haemorrhage. Microscopically there are changes in both airways and parenchyma, with degeneration and regenerative hyperplasia. There is a mononuclear infiltrate around bronchioles and extending into the alveolar septa. In the distal airways the epithelium becomes stratified, with multinucleate alveolar giant cells which may contain intranuclear and intracytoplasmic inclusions. These epithelial giant cells (Fig. 13.32) should be distinguished from the Warthin–Finkeldey lymphoid giant cells which are seen in the germinal centres of lymphoid tissue and are also characteristic of measles infection. The presence of measles virus in the giant cells can be demonstrated by immunofluorescence.

4. *Herpes viruses*. The herpes virus group, which includes *cytomegalovirus, varicella zoster virus*, and *herpes simplex virus,* is a common cause of pulmonary infection in the immunocompromised host.

Cytomegalovirus (CMV) is a complex DNA virus which produces cellular enlargement with characteristic inclusion bodies in both the nucleus and cytoplasm of infected cells. The severe form of this infection is also known as *cytomegalic inclusion disease*. The virus can infect any tissue, in particular salivary tissue, kidney, and lung. It is a cause of stillbirth and infant mortality. Severe cases of pneumonia occur almost exclusively in the immunosuppressed, and many of these are reactivations of infection acquired earlier in life. Fifty to sixty per cent of the population of London have been reported to be seropositive for CMV, the percentage rising with increasing age. In patients with AIDS, CMV may be associated with other infections, in particular *Pneumocystis carinii* pneumonia (PCP) and systemic fungal infections.

Macroscopically the lungs are heavy (up to 1000 g each), congested, and firm. Microscopically there may be a diffuse panlobular or a focal interstitial pneumonia. The former shows an extensive exudate of proteinaceous material into the alveoli (Fig. 13.33), with thickening of the alveolar walls and a lymphocytic infiltrate; hyaline membranes may be formed. Cytomegalic inclusions are infrequent, but are usually seen in endothelial cells and pneumocytes; however, the absence of inclusions does not exclude the diagnosis. The typical infected cells are very large with a central pinkish intranuclear inclusion surrounded by a pale halo, and resemble an *owl's eye* (Fig. 13.34). Cytoplasmic inclusions are particulate and much smaller, as confirmed by electron microscopy (Fig. 13.35).

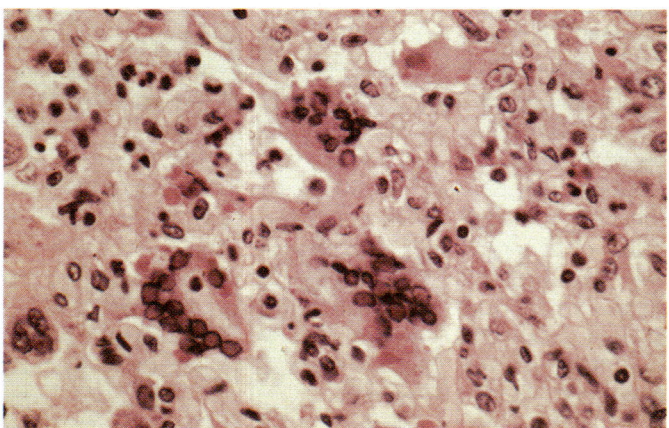

Fig. 13.32 Measles pneumonia; multinucleated epithelial giant cells with eosinophilic intranuclear viral inclusions.

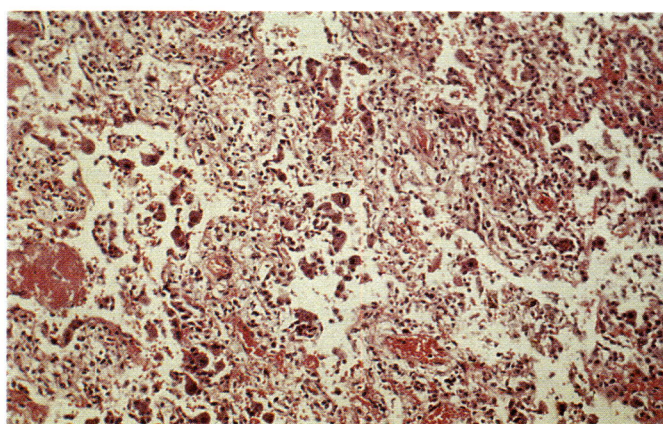

Fig. 13.33 Cytomegalovirus pneumonia (low-power view); the alveolar structure is disorganized with thickening of the alveolar wall. Some enlarged infected cells are seen in the alveolar spaces admixed with inflammatory cells and erythrocytes.

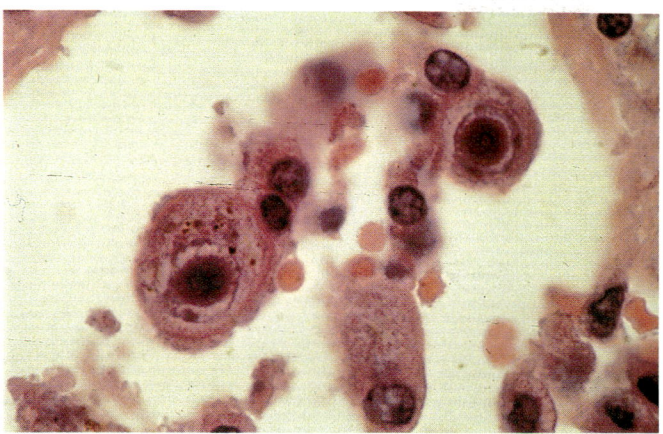

Fig. 13.34 Cytomegalovirus pneumonia (high-power view); typical owl's eye appearance of the enlarged nucleus. The intranuclear inclusion is separated from the nuclear membrane by a pale halo. Smaller intracytoplasmic inclusions are also seen in these massively enlarged cells.

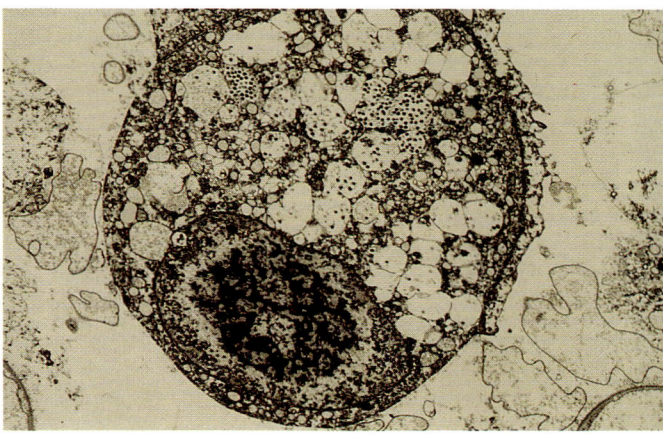

Fig. 13.35 Electron micrograph of a CMV-infected cell, highlighting the features seen in Fig. 13.34. Numerous viral particles are seen in the nucleus and the cytoplasm.

Rarely, pulmonary fibrosis has been described. Since latent infection is common, serology may be unhelpful and the diagnosis often relies on the identification of CMV in biopsy or aspirated material by the more sensitive immunocytochemical methods, or by virus isolation in tissue culture. Diagnosis is often easier when large amounts of tissue are available, for example open lung biopsy or at post-mortem.

Herpes simplex infection is less common but is also exclusive to the immunosuppressed, especially patients with severe burns. It produces an *ulcerative tracheobronchitis* and *focal pneumonia* with diffuse alveolar damage. The typical eosinophilic inclusions are often difficult to find, but may be seen in surviving alveolar epithelial cells.

Varicella zoster virus infections are usually self-limiting. However, chicken pox in the immunosuppressed, and occasionally in the normal adult, may be associated with *severe pneumonitis*

with a high mortality rate. Macroscopically, the lungs are heavy, plum-coloured, and oedematous, with focal pale areas of consolidation. The bronchi contain bloodstained mucus. Microscopically there is a interstitial mononuclear infiltrate with fibrinous oedema, haemorrhage, and hyaline membranes. Focal necrosis of alveolar walls and blood-vessels may be seen. Eosinophilic nuclear inclusions may be present in epithelial cells, but are usually very subtle. Bacterial superinfection may cause late mortality. Calcified nodules often appear after 1 year post-infection and persist for life.

5. *Influenza virus.* This is the commonest cause of lower respiratory tract infection in adults. It occurs in pandemic and epidemic forms, as well as in sporadic cases. Three serotypes (A, B, and C) are recognized; type A is the most common, and changes in the haemagglutinin and neuraminidase antigens (*antigenic drift and shift*) are responsible for epidemic and pandemic outbreaks of infection. Only influenza A and B cause pneumonia, influenza C causing sporadic upper respiratory tract infection.

Macroscopically, influenza A and B infection result in a *necrotizing bronchiolitis,* with *diffuse alveolar damage* and *hyaline membrane formation.* Basophilic inclusions may be seen in the epithelial cells. The picture is often complicated by concurrent or superadded bacterial infection.

6. *Parainfluenza virus* types 1, 2, and 3 are important causes of mild *upper respiratory tract* infections in adults. However, in children they cause 15 per cent of cases of pneumonia as well as approximately 35 per cent of cases of croup. Most children are infected at least once in the first 5 years of life with each of the four types of parainfluenza virus. The microscopic features of parainfluenza pneumonia are similar to those seen in influenza virus infection.

Chlamydiae Atypical pneumonia due to infection by group B chlamydiae causes the syndrome of ornithosis. *Chlamydia psittaci* can be carried and transmitted by many different species of birds. Psittacine birds (hence the term psittacosis) are the most dangerous, but in the UK infection is most frequently seen in poultry workers (over 60 per cent of workers in duck-processing plants show serological evidence of past infection). The route of infection is by inhalation of an aerosol of infected dried faeces from a sick or carrier bird. The other major group at risk is pigeon handlers. The illness ranges from a mild fever through a classical atypical pneumonia to a *fibrinous lobar pneumonia* with a severe typhoid-like clinical picture. The pathological features in the severe form of the disease (which has a mortality of 20 per cent) differ from other atypical pneumonias.

The lungs are bulky and show haemorrhagic consolidation, especially in the lower lobes, resembling that seen in β-haemolytic streptococcal pneumonia. Microscopically, in addition to the usual interstitial pneumonitis there is an intra-alveolar inflammatory response, predominantly of mononuclear cells, together with necrosis and sloughing of the alveolar epithelium. The alveolar walls become lined by rounded epithelial cells, many of which contain intracytoplasmic inclusion bodies.

Other chlamydiae have been implicated in severe pneumonias: *Chlamydia pneumoniae* (TWAR) has recently been recognized as a distinct species which causes outbreaks and sporadic cases of pneumonia in adults. *Chlamydia trachomatis* causes respiratory infection in neonates as a result of infection acquired from the female genital tract at the time of birth, and very rarely is seen in the immunosuppressed. *Chlamydia bedsoniae* is acquired from handling animal placentae (particularly cattle and sheep) during epidemic abortion in Africa.

Rickettsiae *Q fever* is an unusual type of pneumonic disease caused by the rickettsia *Coxiella burnetii*. The infection is endemic in cattle and sheep and the disease most common in animal handlers. Laboratory workers are at considerable risk, and for this reason routine isolation is not performed and the diagnosis is confirmed by demonstrating a rising specific antibody titre. The organism can cause infection by either inhalation or ingestion. Mortality is low, less than 1 per cent, but the organism may persist and can produce *endocarditis* years after the initial infection. Few records of the pathological features are available. The infection is systemic but pulmonary involvement is relatively uncommon and only seen in approximately 5 per cent of cases. The pathological changes appear to be similar to other cases of atypical pneumonia. Post-mortem material from a fatal case investigated by Whittacker showed greyish consolidation of the lower lobes with a *diffuse interstitial pneumonitis* and an intra-alveolar exudate containing pale, strap-like epithelial cells and lymphocytes. The causative agent may be identified in some cases.

Pneumonitis with interstitial pneumonia and alveolar infiltrates is seen in 15 per cent of cases of *Rocky Mountain spotted fever*, which is caused by *Rickettsia rickettsii*.

Protozoa

1. *Pneumocystis carinii pneumonia*. Parasitic pneumonia is uncommon except in the immunocompromised. Although it may be seen in any condition with reduced cellular immunity, recently it has been seen almost exclusively in patients with *AIDS*. It is estimated that 75 per cent of patients with AIDS will suffer from PCP at some stage and it is a major criterion for the diagnosis of this condition. The disease is caused by the protozoan, *Pneumocystis carinii*, which is world-wide in distribution and was associated with widespread disease in infants with severe malnutrition in Europe following the Second World War. The parasite is usually seen as a cyst, between 4 and 6 μm in diameter, which may be empty (in which case it may appear flattened or sickle-shaped, Fig. 13.36) or may contain up to eight intracystic bodies, known as *sporozoites*. There is some debate about the exact taxonomic position of the organism but most authors accept that it is a sporozoan rather than a fungus. Macroscopically there are two forms, *diffuse* and *focal*. The diffuse form is more common, and bilateral involvement is usually seen. There is widespread and extensive pink consolidation and the pale tissue may resemble pancreas. The pleura are usually normal. Microscopically the alveoli and airways are filled by frothy, eosinophilic, PAS-positive coagulum in which the

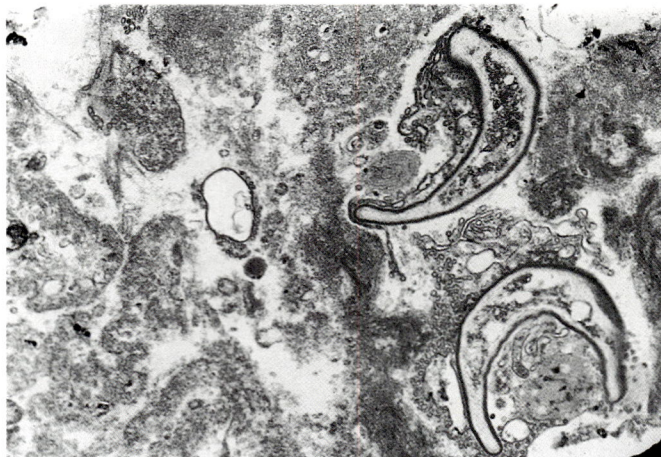

Fig. 13.36 Electron micrograph of *Pneumocystic carinii*; collapsed sickle-shaped cyst walls are seen.

'shadows' of the non-staining cysts may be seen (Fig. 13.37). A small basophilic dot may be seen within the cysts, which is the parasitic body. The cyst walls may be stained using Grocott's technique (Fig. 13.38). There is a diffuse, chronic, interstitial pneumonia but this may be minimal, particularly in AIDS, and the plasma cell infiltration initially described in the infantile form may be absent. Cysts may be scanty when treatment has been instituted before biopsy. *Cor pulmonale* has been reported as a sequela of interstitial fibrosis, although this is very uncommon. The diagnosis of PCP may be made on sputum or bronchoalveolar lavage fluid by demonstrating the cysts, and this may avoid the need for biopsy which is potentially hazardous.

2. *Toxoplasma gondii* may cause pulmonary infection in the immunosuppressed patient with systemic infection; pulmonary involvement is rare but has also been reported in infants with toxoplasmosis.

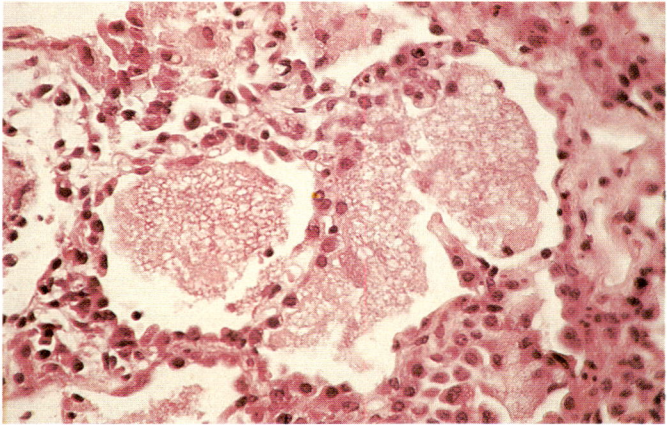

Fig. 13.37 *Pneumocystis carinii* pneumonia; foamy eosinophilic material representing the cystic organism (unlike fibrin which is fibrillary) fills the alveolar spaces. Occasional inflammatory cells are present in the interstitium.

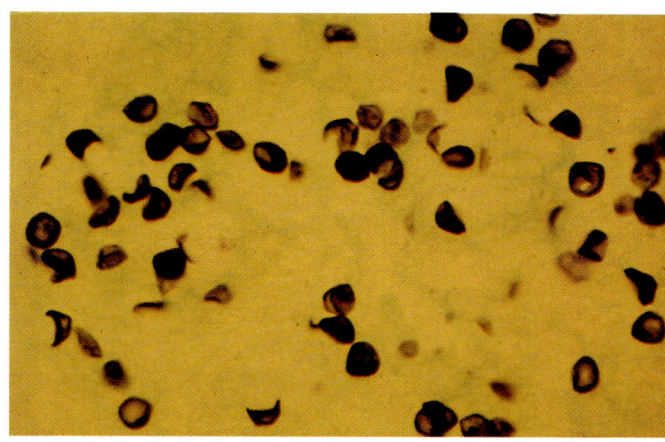

Fig. 13.38 *Pneumocystic carinii* appear as rounded black structures when stained with Grocott's methenamine silver technique.

Parasites

1. *Dirofilaria immitis*, the dog tapeworm, is a rare cause of focal caseating granulomatous disease in the lung, which is usually asymptomatic. Microscopically there are *necrotizing granulomas*, often with marked eosinophil infiltration, with large round worms usually seen in the damaged pulmonary arteries.

2. Other parasites. A number of other parasites have a pulmonary stage in their life cycle, including *Strongyloides stercoralis*, *Ascaris lumbricoides*, and *Paragonimus westermani*. These may be associated with an *eosinophilic pneumonia* (usually chronic) which results from a type I allergic reaction and may be part of *Loeffler's syndrome*.

Fungi A large variety of fungal organisms may, on occasion, produce *acute pneumonia*. Many of these infections occur predominantly in the immunocompromised or malnourished patients, in particular with *Aspergillus* sp., *Candida* sp., and *Mucor* sp. These fungi and many others may also produce chronic pulmonary changes which are considered later.

Pneumonia in specific clinical settings

Pneumonia in the debilitated patient

In the debilitated patient pneumonia is often caused by organisms normally commensal in the upper respiratory tract. The most important of these are pneumococci of low virulence and *Haemophilus influenzae*, but many organisms may be responsible. Predisposing factors are old age, infancy, terminal illness, and pre-existing respiratory disease, e.g. chronic bronchitis. *Pulmonary oedema*, whether due to heart failure, chest injury, or the inhalation of noxious gases, reduces host defences, and local airway obstruction by tumour or inhaled foreign body causes retention of secretions with subsequent infection. In these patients, the pattern of involvement tends to be patchy (*lobular pneumonia, bronchopneumonia*) and usually runs a prolonged relapsing course, depending on host factors and treatment. In

the absence of localizing factors, the disease tends to be patchy, basal, and bilateral.

Macroscopically the lesions are grey, firm, and initially 3–4 cm across, but may coalesce to form large areas of confluent pneumonia. Microscopically the bronchioles are filled with neutrophil-rich exudate, with some surrounding alveoli containing oedema with macrophages and polymorphs, while others contain fibrinous material with polymorphs. Some alveoli are collapsed due to bronchiolar obstruction and some show compensatory dilatation. It is often difficult to identify the bacteria.

Sequelae are similar to those seen in lobar pneumonia, and fibrosis, chronicity, or suppuration may occur. Complete resolution is seen less frequently in lobular pneumonia, and progressive fibrosis due to organization of the fibrinous exudate may be seen. There is frequent progression to a chronic stage with further pulmonary damage. Destruction of the bronchiolar wall leads to dilatation with retention of secretions and further infection. The end-stage of this process is *bronchiectasis*, which can be viewed as both cause and effect of pulmonary infection. Suppuration, abscess formation, and empyema complicating bronchopneumonia are most frequently encountered in the debilitated patient or in cases complicated by bronchial obstruction. Anaerobic bacteria, particularly *Bacteroides* sp., are implicated in many cases. Metastatic abscesses following bacteraemia can occur.

Pneumonia complicating structural disease

There are many situations where either there is a structural abnormality or a generalized diseases process which predisposes to pulmonary infection. Characteristically in these groups, organisms of low pathogenicity for normal individuals are responsible although, obviously, infections with more common pathogens also occur. In infection complicating pre-existing structural disease, patients with diffuse parenchymal disease are at greatest risk from lobular pneumonia, similar to that described in patients suffering from general debility. Patients with localized disease such as *bronchiectasis, cystic fibrosis*, and *chronic cavitating lung disease* (e.g. tuberculosis) are also at risk. In cystic fibrosis, *Pseudomonas aeruginosa*, which often becomes resistant to multiple antibiotics, and *Staphylococcus aureus* are particularly important.

Bacteria such as staphylococci, streptococci, pneumococci, and the Enterobacteriaceae, as well as anaerobes (e.g. *bacteroides*), are often isolated from the sputum of patients with bronchiectasis but it may be impossible to distinguish whether they are pathogenic or purely saprophytic.

Pneumonia in the immunosuppressed patient

It is important to note that although unusual agents cause infection in this group, common diseases also occur. Although infection with almost any agent may occur in this group, the pattern of infection varies according to the type of immune deficiency. If humoral immunity is predominantly impaired, there is a tendency to bacterial infection, whereas when cell-mediated immunity is reduced, viral, fungal, and protozoal infections predominate. This is rather a simplistic approach, as when T-cell function is deranged, B-cell activity is often depressed with consequent risk of bacterial infection. Neutropenia predisposes to bacterial and fungal infections.

There have been many medical advances in the treatment of malignant disease with the development of medical oncology and the increasing use of cytotoxic agents and radiotherapy. This, together with expanding organ transplantation programmes, has led to a marked increase in the number of immunocompromised patients. A number of unusual organisms cause disease in these circumstances, including *Pneumocystis carinii*, cytomegalovirus, herpes simplex virus, varicella zoster virus, *Nocardia* sp., *Mycobacterium* sp. (particularly the atypical varieties), *Aspergillus* sp., *Candida* sp., *Cryptococcus* sp., *Coccidioides* sp., *Toxoplasma gondii*, and phycomycete species.

The pattern of disease seen in the various groups differs. In particular, patients with AIDS are prone to develop relapsing *Pneumocystis carinii* pneumonia and are often treated with long-term prophylactic antibodies. Over 75 per cent of AIDS patients will develop PCP at some stage of their illness, and nearly half of this group initially present with PCP, which is a major criterion for the case definition of AIDS. Multiple infections are frequent and cytomegalovirus is often seen with PCP. This contrasts with the situation in neutropenic patients who are at particular risk from bacterial infection.

Pneumonia in the neonate

During birth there is a substantial risk of aspiration of amniotic fluid, particularly if labour is prolonged. Pneumonitis may result from a direct chemical irritant effect or from inspiration of potential respiratory pathogens. Bacteria usually implicated are *Haemophilus* sp., *Staphylococcus* sp., *Streptococcus* sp. (in particular Lancefield group B), and *Escherichia coli*. A blood-borne transplacental route is less common (less than 10 per cent) and usually results from maternal pyelonephritis. In view of the immaturity of both lung tissue and immune system, infection may be rapidly progressive and lead to death within 24 hours. Macroscopically there are few changes, but microscopically the alveoli are filled with polymorph exudate without fibrin. Inspissated amniotic contents may be seen. Pneumonia occurring after the immediate postpartum period parallels more closely that seen in older individuals.

Pneumonia caused by organisms of lesser virulence, such as *E. coli* or non-capsulated pneumococci, may occur, and spread is often more rapid and the disease more extensive than that seen in adults. The bacterial pneumonias tend to occur without prior viral infection and may be fulminating. A small number are due to aspiration of milk or gastric contents. If this occurs in hospital, it may precipitate a staphylococcal pneumonia which is usually fatal. Some very fulminant cases may show *haemorrhagic oedema* and *purulent bronchiolitis* but, if survival is prolonged, there is often abscess formation and empyema may result.

Haemophilus influenzae usually causes infection after 2 months of age when immunity conferred by the transplacental route has diminished. By the age of 5 years, children usually have high levels of antibody. Between these times *H. influenzae* is a common cause of *bronchiolitis* and *bronchopneumonia*, but the diagnosis may only be made with certainty by isolating the organism from blood cultures, as it is often found in sputum in the absence of disease.

Viral pneumonitis may occur in the neonate, for example in some babies congenitally infected with CMV, but is commoner after the first month. A variety of viruses, e.g. RSV, adenovirus and parainfluenza virus type 3, may be responsible and these produce very similar histological appearances. RSV is the commonest of these and can be identified in lung tissue by immunofluorescence. There are two principal pathological patterns which often overlap, *acute bronchiolitis* and *interstitial pneumonia*, and these are discussed in the section on viral pneumonias. Very small infants and children with *kwashiorkor* may develop parasitic infections such as PCP or viral infection, e.g. a herpes virus, as discussed above.

Sudden infant death syndrome is a mysterious and unresolved problem affecting children between the ages of 1 week and 4 months and is responsible for more than one-third of all postnatal deaths occurring in the first year of life in the United Kingdom. There is evidence in a minority of these patients of some viral infection, but the microscopic changes in the lungs vary between normality and well-established zones of interstitial pneumonitis. This may be associated with alveolar wall thickening; however, the changes rarely appear sufficiently severe to have caused death, and it has been postulated that viral infection may trigger apnoea or an anaphylactic reaction. It seems likely that this disease is multifactorial and that viral infection is just one of a group of disorders that may cause it.

Pneumonia in the hospitalized patient

Gram-negative bacteria are of foremost importance in serious pneumonia in the hospitalized patient. *Pseudomonas aeruginosa* is a common cause and is discussed in detail above. Less commonly, *Proteus* sp. and *Bacteroides* may produce a similar picture. Other Gram-negative organisms, such as *Serratia* sp. and *Enterobacter* sp., may be involved and usually reflect local hospital flora.

Patients with very severe illness who are hospitalized for protracted periods are subject to a number of pulmonary problems. In addition to the increased incidence of pneumonia, there is the additional risk of thrombo-embolic disease. Prolonged, broad-spectrum antibiotic therapy disturbs the normal flora, allowing overgrowth by organisms such as *Pseudomonas* sp. and *Candida* sp. Pathological features of the specific infections are discussed in the relevant sections.

Pneumonia in the surgical patient

Patients who undergo anaesthesia and surgery are at risk of various pulmonary complications. Aspiration may occur during or shortly after anaesthesia. In the immediate post-operative period there is a possibility of atelectasis with collapse of lobules or lobes, which can be complicated by infection, particularly with Gram-negative organisms. Pre-existing chest disease may be exacerbated and there is a higher incidence of thrombo-embolic phenomena.

Absorption collapse occurs following bronchial or bronchiolar obstruction by collections of mucus, usually following anaesthesia but also in the terminal stages of illness. Mucus viscosity may contribute, e.g. in cystic fibrosis. Inhaled anaesthetics tend to increase bronchial secretion. Other pulmonary problems in the surgical patient are exacerbation of chronic bronchitis and thromboembolism. Following severe trauma or surgery, shock lung may occur with or without secondary infection.

Aspiration pneumonia

Aspiration pneumonia is caused by inhalation of material from the pharynx (frequently regurgitated gastric contents) and may occur as a consequence of repeated vomiting from any cause. Depression of the cough reflex due to debilitation or unconsciousness increases the probability of aspiration; achalasia of the cardia and hiatus hernia are associated with an increased risk although silent aspiration may occur in sleep in normal individuals. Massive inhalation of stomach contents may lead to death by drowning, for example in alcoholics.

The consequences of aspiration are dependent on the nature of the aspirated material:

Vomitus rich in gastric acid produces a chemical pneumonitis which is manifest by immediate intra-alveolar oedema and haemorrhage. Later there is a polymorph infiltration and consolidation. Bacterial superinfection is common and lung abscess may ensue.

If infected material from the pharynx is aspirated, a mixed population of aerobic and anaerobic bacteria, e.g. *Bacteroides* sp., cause a destructive pneumonia.

If the gastric contents contain undigested food particles, the gastric acidity is often low and the bacterial content high. Obstruction of the airways by vegetable matter (which is radiolucent) leads to development of a *hypostatic pneumonia* with a foreign body and giant cell response. *Chronic foreign body granulomas* result, with the eosinophilic ghosts of the vegetable matter at their centre. This is a particular danger during anaesthesia for emergency surgery. Obstruction may cause abscess formation and anaerobes are usually responsible. Macroscopically a *putrefying pneumonia* ensues with *gangrene* of the lungs. There are ill-defined brown areas with central softening which becomes slimy and malodorous. Microscopically the central area contains spirochaetes and fusiform organisms and few polymorphs are seen. Material for microbiology can be obtained by bronchoscopy.

Aspiration of solid foreign bodies leads to a different response. The cough reflex may be counterproductive as the rapid inspiration preceding the cough may suck the material deeper into the respiratory tract. The response depends on the nature of the inhaled body and whether complete bronchial obstruction occurs. Vegetable matter, e.g. a peanut, is irritant due to hydrolysis of fat to form fatty acids. Metallic foreign bodies do not give rise to much initial reaction but may cause a chronic inflammatory disease locally. *Obstructive pneumonitis*

(absorption collapse) is a frequent sequela with subsequent risk of bacterial infection.

Chronic aspiration, as seen with achalasia, results in fibrosis of the lower lobes.

Obstructive pneumonitis

Obstructive pneumonitis may follow airway obstruction from any cause. There is reduction in lung volume as the alveoli become filled with oedema fluid and within 36 hours the alveolar capillaries are congested and there are many polymorphs. The obstruction predisposes to infection with a variety of organisms. These provoke an acute inflammatory response and pneumonia. If the obstruction is relieved, the resolution is rapid. If obstruction persists, then a more chronic type of inflammatory response supervenes with lymphocytes and macrophages with subsequent fibrosis replacing the exudate. Chronic suppurative foci often persist which are characterized by lipid-laden macrophages within the damaged alveoli (Fig. 13.39). This is referred to as *endogenous lipid pneumonia* and is seen most frequently following bronchial obstruction by carcinoma. It should be contrasted with exogenous lipid pneumonia, which follows inhalation of lipid material and is characterized by large lipid globules surrounded by inflammatory cells, mainly macrophages (Fig. 13.40).

Lung abscess and empyema

Lung abscess can be a consequence of *destructive pneumonia, bronchial obstruction, blood-borne infection*, a complication of *pre-existing lung disease*, or *direct local spread* from outside the lung. Causes of lung abscess are given in Table 13.3.

Inhalation abscess

This occurs after inhalation of infected material, usually during anaesthesia but also in other circumstances when the cough reflex is impaired. With improvements in anaesthetic techniques these are fortunately less frequent. Inhaled material

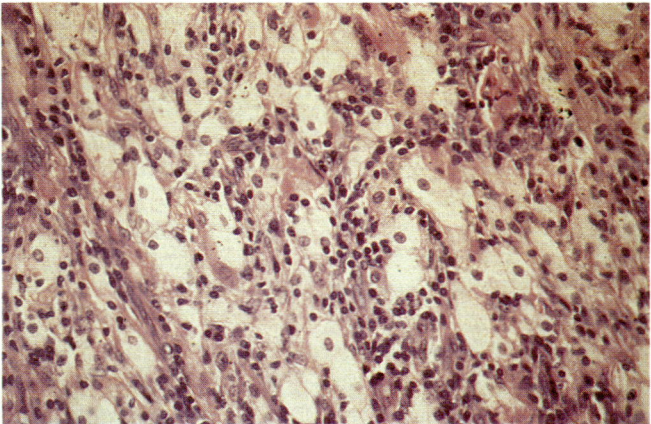

Fig. 13.39 Endogenous lipid pneumonia; macrophages contain finely divided lipid droplets, morphologically dissimilar from exogenous lipid pneumonia (see Fig. 13.40).

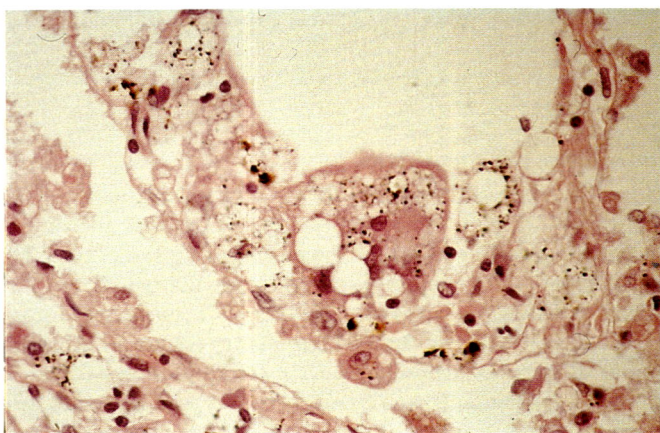

Fig. 13.40 Exogenous lipid pneumonia; varying sized vacuoles representing lipid dissolved during processing are seen in the alveolar macrophages.

Table 13.3 Causes of lung abscess

Inhalation of foreign bodies
Inhalation of pus, tooth, or tonsillar material
Complicating bronchial obstruction by neoplasm
Complicating bacterial pneumonia
Pyaemia and septic infarction
Trauma
Trans-diaphragmatic spread (including amoebic abscess)
Infected hydatid cyst
Cryptogenic (25%)

most frequently enters the axillary and posterior portions of the upper lobe or the apical part of the lower lobe, usually on the right side due to the relatively direct course of the right main bronchus. In most cases there is a mixture of aerobic and anaerobic bacteria, including *Klebsiella* sp., *E. coli, Pseudomonas* sp., *Bacteroides* sp., and *Streptococcus milleri*.

Lung abscess may occur at any site, but the upper parts of the right lung are favoured as discussed. Macroscopically there is an irregular ragged cavity filled with foul-smelling purulent material, which usually communicates with a bronchus. Rupture into the pleural space may occur, forming an *empyema* or *broncho-pleural fistula* and subsequent *pyopneumothorax*. Multiple abscesses are frequent. In chronic forms the wall becomes thick and fibrous. Microscopically the wall is formed of fibrous and granulation tissue surrounding necrotic tissue debris, organisms, and pus. Adjacent pulmonary arterioles show intimal fibrosis. In long-standing cases the cavity may become lined by columnar or squamous epithelium.

Abscess complicating a bronchial neoplasm

Over 10 per cent of all lung abscesses are associated with lung cancer, and this becomes even more significant in the older age-groups (up to 40 per cent). About a third of these are secondary to bronchial obstruction and two-thirds are due to necrosis and cavitation within the tumour. Squamous carcinoma is the most

likely to undergo cavitation and this should be distinguished from carcinoma arising within a pre-existing bronchiectatic cavity.

Abscess complicating bacterial pneumonia

Many bacteria may cause abscess formation as a complication of pneumonia. These abscesses are usually multiple but do not have the foul smell associated with some of the other varieties since anaerobes are rarely present. Certain bacteria are particularly likely to cause cavitation, including *Staphylococcus aureus*, *Klebsiella pneumophilia*, *Pseudomonas aeruginosa*, and, less commonly, the pneumococcus. *Escherichia coli* and *β*-haemolytic streptococci may be responsible in children.

Abscess complicating blood-borne infection

Blood-borne spread to the lungs can occur from remote areas of sepsis. Embolic abscesses may be produced by thrombophlebitis of a peripheral vein (usually pelvic) or associated with a central venous catheter. The abscesses are usually small, multiple, and subpleural. *Staphylococcus aureus* is the commonest causative organism and is important in intravenous drug users. Larger emboli may cause septic infarcts leading to formation of larger lung abscesses.

Traumatic lung abscess

This is very rare but may follow open or closed lung injury.

Trans-diaphragmatic spread

This may occur from subphrenic abscess or amoebic abscess of the liver. Fifteen per cent of amoebic liver abscesses spread to involve the adjacent lung. *Pulmonary hydatid cyst* may become secondarily infected, but this is rare.

Cryptogenic lung abscess

Up to 25 per cent of lung abscesses have no recognizable cause and these are referred to as *primary cryptogenic lung abscesses*. Complications of lung abscess include extension into the pleural cavity to form an *empyema, bronchopleural fistula*, and development of *brain abscess or meningitis* following *septic embolization*. Rarely, *secondary amyloidosis* is seen in association with chronic suppuration.

Chronic infections

Some organisms by their nature produce chronic infection rather than acute disease. Prominent amongst these is *Mycobacterium tuberculosis*, but many fungal infections also run a chronic course and these will be discussed in this section.

Mycobacterium tuberculosis

Tuberculosis may involve many different sites, but the most common is the lung. Tuberculosis in other sites is discussed under the relevant organ systems.

Pulmonary tuberculosis is the major cause of mortality and morbidity from tuberculous disease. The disease is prevalent in the Third World, particularly in overcrowded communities weakened by malnutrition. The disease has become much rarer in Western Europe and North America due to the eradication of the bovine strain of *Mycobacteria,* improved social conditions, and the development of effective treatment. The pathology of pulmonary tuberculosis is conventionally divided into *primary* and *secondary disease.*

Primary pulmonary tuberculosis The inhalation of *Mycobacterium tuberculosis* by a non-immune individual causes a focal non-specific inflammatory process at the lung periphery, usually in the lower lobe or the anterior segment of an upper lobe, known as the *Ghon focus.* There is rapid lymphatic spread of the bacteria to the regional lymph nodes, which become enlarged with marked *lymphadenitis.* The Ghon focus together with the involved hilar lymph nodes are known as the *primary complex.* The vast majority of cases heal at this stage to leave a *fibrotic scar.* Further development of the disease depends on the host response. In older people this stage of disease is often silent, although in some a pleural effusion may be present, and the condition resolves leaving a small area of calcification or fibrosis at the site of the primary complex. In the young (less than 2 years old) there is a tendency for the primary complex to be less well contained and it may rupture into a bronchus, causing *tuberculous bronchopneumonia,* or into a blood-vessel, causing *miliary tuberculosis.*

Microscopically the typical hallmark of tuberculosis is the tubercle (Fig. 13.41), a *caseating epithelioid granuloma* which contains multinucleated giant cells of *Langhans type, epithelioid histiocytes* (Fig. 13.42), and small lymphoid cells, surrounding an area of caseous necrosis. This is a manifestation of the *Type IV hypersensitivity reaction* and therefore is seen late in primary infection as well as in secondary (post-primary) infection. Mycobacteria can be identified by Ziehl–Neelsen staining as they resist decoloration by acid alcohol. The organisms can also be identified by the binding of auramine–rhodamine, a fluorescent dye, which is particularly helpful when the bacteria are scanty. It may be difficult to isolate the organism from a lesion in an individual with a good immune response. In patients with an impaired immune response, the organism is easier to see in

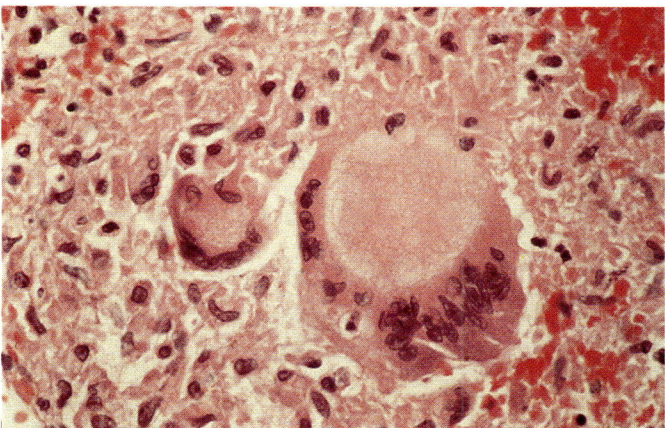

Fig. 13.42 Fibrocaseous tuberculosis; epithelial histiocytes and Langhans giant cells are seen in the inner layers of the fibrous well.

sputum and in tissue section after Ziehl–Neelsen staining, and to isolate on Lowenstein–Jensen medium.

Secondary pulmonary tuberculosis This is usually due to re-infection by *Mycobacterium tuberculosis.* It may also be due to reactivation of the primary lesion, but this is much less common, accounting for less than 10 per cent of cases. The lesion in the lung is almost always found in the subapical region of an upper lobe. The tissue damage is caused by a hypersensitivity reaction which leads to necrosis, around which lymphocytes, epithelioid histiocytes, and Langhans giant cells are seen. Outside this there is fibrotic reaction induced by a factor secreted by macrophages. Lymphatic spread is not a feature of secondary tuberculosis and the hilar nodes are not usually involved. The lesion described is referred to as a *tuberculoma,* which may become quiescent; in individuals with a normal immune response it may be difficult to isolate the organism. Alternatively, the lesion can enlarge and may erode through an adjacent bronchus; caseous infective material is discharged into the airways, resulting in open cavitating tuberculosis, with consequent risk of infection for contacts. The organism may be seen on Ziel–Neelsen or auramine–rhodamine staining of sputum, and cultured on Lowenstein–Jensen medium. As with primary tuberculosis, the contents of the tuberculous cavity may be inhaled to cause bronchopneumonia or may rupture into a vein (Fig. 13.43) producing miliary spread to another organ or organs. Erosion of blood vessels also leads to haemoptysis and may rarely result in fatal haemorrhage.

Miliary tuberculosis results from seeding of the organism via the bloodstream. Depending on the nature of the vessel involved, there may be diffuse pulmonary or systemic dissemination. The miliary foci are caseating granulomata (Fig. 13.44).

Epituberculosis is consolidation of a lobe, usually the right middle lobe, immediately following primary infection. This may be secondary to obstruction of the main bronchus by hilar node enlargement. Less commonly it may be due to a hypersensitivity

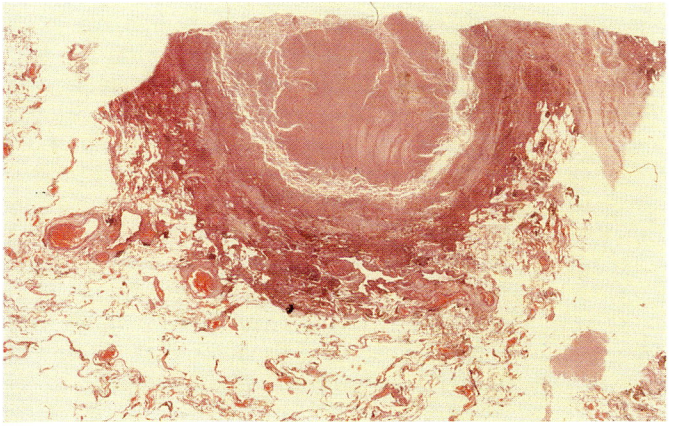

Fig. 13.41 Fibrocaseous tuberculosis; this pulmonary tubercle is surrounded by a thick fibrous wall and contains caseous material.

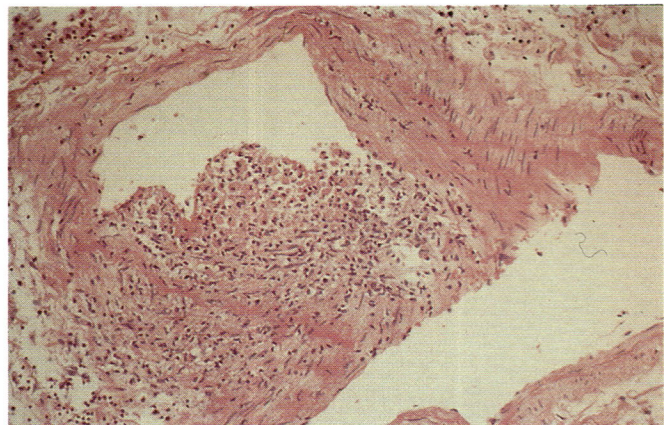

Fig. 13.43 Tuberculous vasculitis from a case of miliary tuberculosis.

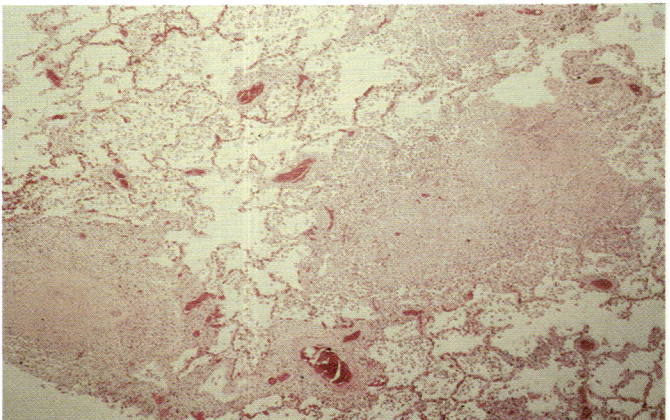

Fig. 13.44 Miliary tuberculosis; small nodules of granulomatous inflammation are scattered throughout the lung parenchyma.

reaction to the discharge of tuberculous products into the lobe or bronchus, exciting acute inflammatory changes in the affected lobe. This condition occurs predominantly in young children.

Tuberculous bronchopneumonia is usually seen in individuals with lowered immunity and is characterized by widespread caseous consolidation of the alveoli with little cellular response.

Atypical mycobacteria Non-tuberculous (atypical) mycobacteria have been recognized as a cause of pulmonary lesions for many years. The most important of these in human pulmonary disease are *M. kansasii* and *M. avium* complex (*M. avium intracellulare*). Although these organisms are of lower pathogenicity, they tend to be very resistant to treatment and therefore often cause severe disease and death. In the areas of the world where tuberculosis is rife the proportion of cases due to atypical mycobacteria is increasing. In the Western world these infections used to be associated with granulomatous lesions complicating chronic lung disease, particularly dust related; now they are

principally seen as an important infective agent in the immuno-compromised patient.

The range of histological appearances varies from those indistinguishable from classical caseating tuberculosis to a situation analogous to lepromatous leprosy when enormous numbers of organisms lie within macrophages with no apparent immune response. This latter appearance is seen particularly in association with AIDS where atypical mycobacterial infection tends to involve multiple sites.

Treponema pallidum

Pulmonary syphilis is usually seen in association with syphilitic disease affecting other organs. Congenital and acquired forms of the disease occur; both are virtually unknown in developed countries. *Congenital syphilis* is seen predominantly in tropical Africa where it usually causes stillbirth. The fetal lungs are firm and pale with diffuse fibrosis of alveolar septa, bronchial, and perivascular tissue. There is an interstitial infiltrate of lymphocytes and plasma cells, and abundant spirochaetes are present. The organism can be demonstrated by a silver impregnation technique.

In the *acquired form*, pulmonary manifestations include *tracheobronchitis*, *luetic pneumonia*, and *pulmonary gummas*. Luetic pneumonia is characterized by interstitial and intra-alveolar infiltration of plasma cells and histiocytes. Gummas vary in size, may be multiple or single, and are often associated with pulmonary fibrosis. They possess a fibrous capsule infiltrated by inflammatory cells (including numerous plasma cells) surrounding yellow to grey necrotic material. Only few epithelioid histiocytes are seen, and giant cells are exceptional. Another important feature is *vasculitis*, similar to that seen at other sites, which may affect the pulmonary artery or its branches.

Actinomyces israelii

Actinomyces israelii is associated with a *chronic granulomatous suppurative infection*. This may be a primary infection due to inhalation or, less commonly, secondary to direct spread from the liver or the cervical region. Primary infection occurs in the lower lobes and tends to be localized but may involve more than one lobe. The typical appearance is of a dense fibrotic lesion honeycombed with small abscess cavities containing yellow 'sulphur granules' which are masses of the organism.

Microscopically, these organisms appear as a basophilic mass of long filaments, with radiating eosinophilic club-shaped processes around the periphery. The cavities are lined by granulation and fibrous tissue with lymphocytes and plasma cells surrounding purulent abscesses containing the sulphur granules. Adjacent lung shows interstitial fibrosis and oedema. Diagnosis depends on identification of the organism, usually from the sputum, by Gram stain or by anaerobic culture on blood agar. Complications include *local invasive disease* with extension into pericardium or *fistulation* through the chest wall, *metastatic abscesses*, usually cerebral, and *amyloidosis*.

Nocardia

This is a similar organism to actinomyces but is aerobic. It is usually seen as an opportunistic pathogen in patients on steroids or otherwise immunosuppressed. Diagnosis is often difficult as the organism is not expectorated and may only be apparent at post-mortem. Acute or chronic infection may occur following inhalation of the organism. In the acute form there are multiple abscesses, grossly resembling the tubercules of miliary tuberculosis. Microscopically, the abscesses are lined by fibrous and granulation tissue containing polymorphs, lymphocytes, and plasma cells, with only few macrophages. Unlike actinomycosis, large colonies are not produced in the lungs and chronic infection leads to a lobar pneumonia resembling chronic interstitial pneumonitis with abscess formation. The organism is difficult to see in haematoxylin and eosin-stained sections but it is Gram-positive and usually acid-fast, in contrast to actinomyces.

Pseudomonas mallei and Pseudomonas pseudomallei

Pseudomonas mallei and *Pseudomonas pseudomallei* cause the diseases glanders and melioidosis. Both are extremely rare in humans. Glanders is primarily a disease of horses, mules, and donkeys, and human cases occur in animal handlers. It is a severe pyaemic infection in which the lungs may be involved.

Melioidosis may cause mild disease but can lead to *necrotizing bronchopneumonia* with *multiple lung abscesses*. The disease came to prominence in the Vietnam War where US servicemen were affected. Mortality is up to 50 per cent despite antibiotic treatment.

Fungi

Although there are many species of fungi, few cause disease in man. Some fungi are inherently pathogenic while others are usually saprophytic. The most pathogenic organisms, which include *Coccidioides, Blastomycetes, Paracoccidioides*, and *Histoplasma*, cause primary invasive pulmonary infections in healthy people. These diseases occur in well-defined geographical areas and are rare in the United Kingdom. Fungi which are usually saprophytic may be opportunist pulmonary pathogens especially in immunosuppressed individuals. These fungi include the genera *Aspergillus, Candida, Mucor*, and *Allescheria*.

The pathogenic fungi may produce a granulomatous response with tissue necrosis and destruction similar to tuberculosis or actinomycosis. In immunocompetent individuals, saprophytic fungi tend to cause hypersensitivity reactions to absorbed fungal products and frequently present as asthma. In the immunocompromised these normally non-invasive organisms may become invasive. The diagnosis of invasive fungal infection in life may prove difficult and may rely entirely on the identification of the fungus in biopsy specimens. The most valuable stains are the periodic acid-Schiff technique (PAS) and Grocott's methenamine silver impregnation technique. Sputum culture is unhelpful in distinguishing between invasive and saprophytic infection.

Coccidioides Coccidioidomycosis occurs in North America and is due to the inhalation of the spores of *Coccidioides immitis*. A subpleural lesion forms, closely resembling a small area of *acute bacterial pneumonia*. There is oedema and a polymorph infiltrate which is seen initially around the endospores in the alveoli. The endospores are double-contoured, spherical yeasts which stain with haematoxylin and eosin or periodic acid-Schiff. Within days macrophages replace the polymorphs, forming a granuloma, and subsequently fibrosis occurs, which may later calcify. This process closely resembles tuberculosis, and hilar lymph node involvement is common.

Although occasionally patients may develop widespread disease by a haematogenous route, most patients make an uneventful recovery. Immunosuppressed patients may develop a more extensive *coccidioidal pneumonia*. Approximately 1 per cent of patients develop chronic, cavitating disease. Macroscopically, satellite microabscesses are seen which may coalesce to form a large lobulated cavity surrounded by a thick fibrous capsule. Microscopically, the capsule is composed of hyalinized fibrous tissue infiltrated by lymphocytes and occasional multinucleate giant cells. The cavity is lined by granulation tissue surrounding necrotic material which contains the spores of *C. immitis*. Occasionally the filamentous forms, which are usually seen at lower temperature, may also be present. Frequently there is rupture into the bronchus and occasionally rupture into the pleural cavity, which may result in bronchopleural fistula. Secondary invasion of a tuberculosis cavity may occur and the two diseases may coexist. Diagnosis may be made by culture or sputum or lung tissue or by the histological appearance of resected lung. Precipitins are detectable within 10 days of the onset of symptoms and serological diagnosis by complement fixation test or agglutinins is available.

Blastomycetes and Paracoccidioides. Two types of blastomycosis are recognized:

1. 'North American' due to *Blastomyces dermatitidis*;
2. 'South American' due to *Paracoccidioides braziliensis*.

Both these diseases are caused by the inhalation of fungal spores which initially produce a small pulmonary lesion with lymph gland enlargement. They have the capacity to evolve into a chronic granulomatous process and may disseminate through the bronchial tree or by the invasion of blood-vessels. Both have a definite geographical distribution and do not occur in the UK. The histological appearances are similar to those seen in cryptococcosis, previously regarded as 'European' blastomycosis, which are discussed below.

Cryptococcus Cryptococcus neoformans is found world-wide in soil and bird droppings, especially from pigeons. Infection occurs by inhalation of the organism, and often presents as a meningitis following blood-borne dissemination. The infection is seen predominantly in immunosuppressed patients, in particular those with AIDS, malignancy (especially Hodgkin's disease), or receiving corticosteroid therapy.

There are three distinct pulmonary appearances caused by *Cryptococcus*:

1. A *primary complex* composed of a subpleural lesion with lymph node involvement. This may be associated with spread to involve the meninges. Usually the pulmonary lesion

becomes quiescent and heals with the production of a fibrous scar.

2. A *large solid granuloma* occupying most of a lobe, known as a *cryptococcoma*. This is most commonly see in the USA.

3. *Miliary dissemination* within the lung is usually fatal and is marked by massive oedema and haemorrhage resembling the red hepatization stage of pneumococcal lobar pneumonia. In this form cryptococci are exceedingly numerous.

Microscopically there is a granulomatous response with lymphocytes, macrophages, and multinucleate giant cells. The chronic granulomas are associated with extensive fibrosis. The organism is present in the granulomas as a capsulated, budding, small yeast, 25 μm in diameter. It is stained black with Grocott's stain and the capsule stains with periodic acid-Schiff or alcian blue. In wet preparations, e.g. cerebrospinal fluid (CSF), Indian ink is used for demonstration of the yeast bodies. Cryptococcal antigen may be detected in CSF or sputum. The organism can be cultured on specific media.

In the severely immunocompromised patient the infection tends to be disseminated with the organism scattered through the alveolar walls, often with minimal cellular reaction, or there may be non-caseating miliary granulomas. It is uncertain whether these cases represent primary infection or are a result of reactivation.

Histoplasmosis occurs in two forms:

1. North American (due to *Histoplasma capsulatum*);
2. African (due to *Histoplasma duboisii*).

The African form rarely causes pulmonary infection alone, though the lungs may be involved in the generalized disease. In contrast, *H. capsulatum* is predominantly a pulmonary disease and closely resembles tuberculosis with which it may be confused.

The infection is acquired by inhalation of the mycelial form of this dimorphic fungus which is present in the soil and in dust from animal droppings. In human histoplasmosis the organism exists in its yeast form, which is not infectious. The yeast is an oval body, 2–4 μm across, with clear central cytoplasm surrounded by a thick rigid cell wall. This structure is responsible for its apparent encapsulation when stained by Grocott's silver impregnation technique; in fact the organism does not possess a capsule, despite its name. Special stains are necessary to demonstrate the organism, which is usually invisible in haematoxylin and eosin-stained sections. Diagnosis may be helped by a positive histoplasmin skin test which denotes prior or current infection, but this may be of limited use in some areas (85 per cent of the population of Cincinnati are positive). Overwhelming infection may produce anergy with a false negative result, and the test may be falsely positive in other fungal infections.

As with tuberculosis, infection leads initially to the formation of a primary complex, which often settles with minimal symptoms. However, the disease may progress to a chronic form analogous to secondary tuberculosis, with cavitating or solid lesions, or to a diffuse apical infiltrate. Miliary disease may

occur, particularly in those with decreased immunity. Rarely, a solid 'coin' lesion (*a histoplasmoma*) may be removed as a bronchial neoplasm. *Sclerosing mediastinitis* also occurs rarely.

Histologically, the lesion may be difficult to differentiate from tuberculosis, sarcoidosis, or coccidioidomycosis. The only sure method is the recognition of the yeast forms by appropriate staining or cultural methods.

Aspergillus infection produces several different patterns of disease, depending on the degree of tissue invasion and the host response. These processes are allergic aspergillosis, invasive aspergillosis, and saprophytic aspergillosis.

The *allergic type* of bronchopulmonary aspergillosis is the commonest, and presents as asthma, usually in adults. Bronchospasm is caused by an allergic response to fungal proteins liberated from the inhaled organisms. Chest X-rays show patchy consolidation; peripheral blood eosinophilia is common and cutaneous testing for sensitivity to *Aspergillus* antigens is positive. Microscopically there is collapse and consolidation of the affected areas, with plugging of bronchi with eosinophil-rich mucus. Bronchi show goblet-cell hyperplasia and infiltration by eosinophils.

Invasive aspergillosis occurs almost exclusively in immunocompromised patients, although it has been reported rarely in apparently healthy individuals. It is particularly prevalent in patients with acute leukaemia or neutropenia and is usually fatal, although treatment with amphotericin B may achieve a cure if started early in the infection. The organism (*A. flavus, A. niger, A. fumigatus*, or a combination) is inhaled and invades the bronchial wall and lung parenchyma, producing a neutrophilic response, and frequently invades blood vessels, leading to thrombosis and infarction. The typical lesions are rounded with a haemorrhagic centre surrounding necrotic material (Fig. 13.45). The organisms are seen within the area of necrosis as slender branching septate hyphae (Fig. 13.46). The mode of branching (at 45°) is characteristic (Fig. 13.47). Identification is aided by PAS and methenamine silver techniques.

Aspergillus can colonize the cavities of tuberculosis or bron-

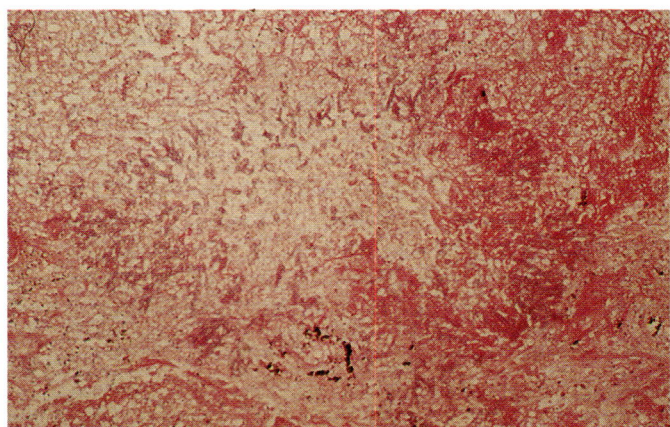

Fig. 13.45 Cavitating pneumonia due to *Aspergillus* sp.; a mass of fungal hyphae replaces the lung tissue with adjacent haemorrhage.

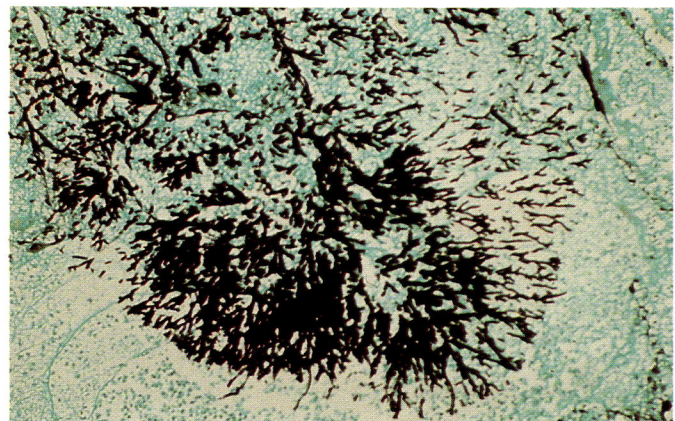

Fig. 13.46 *Aspergillus* hyphae stained with Grocott's methenamine silver technique.

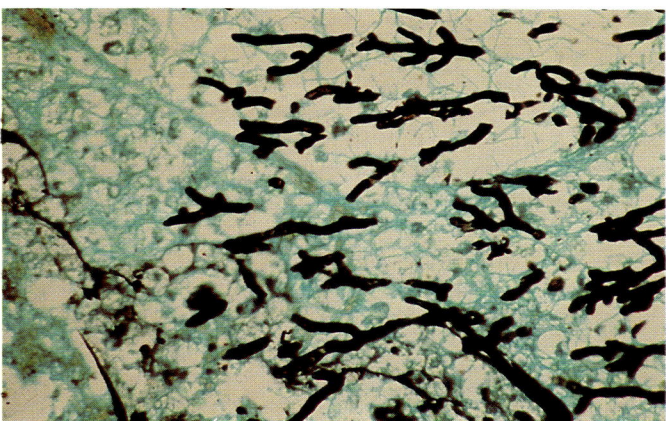

Fig. 13.47 *Aspergillus* hyphae (high power) demonstrating typical 45° branching pattern.

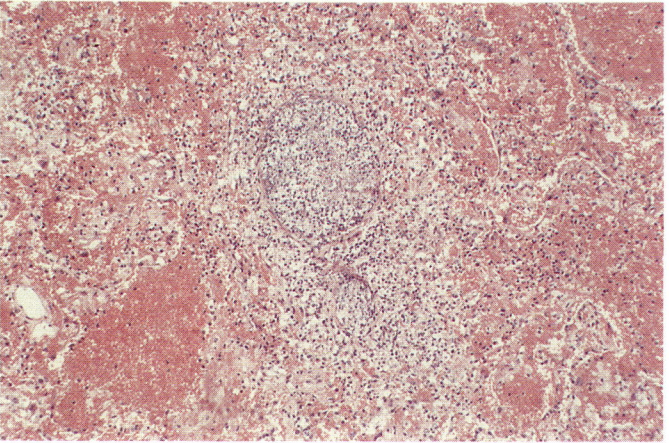

Fig. 13.48 *Candida albicans* pneumonia in a patient with disseminated candidiasis (low power); the alveolar architecture is completely destroyed by a haemorrhagic pneumonia with a pulmonary vessel (centre) containing numerous *Candida* spores.

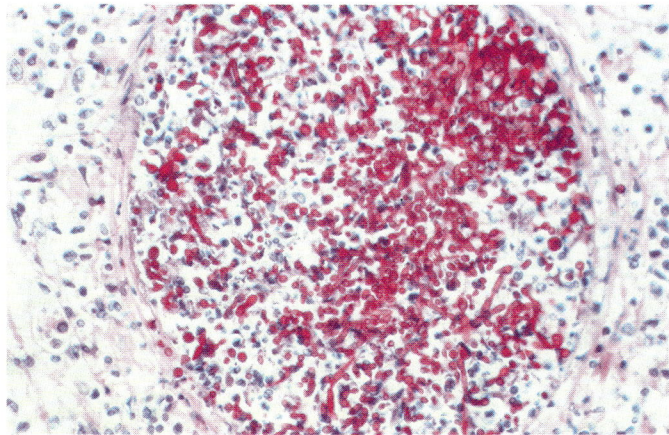

Fig. 13.49 *Candida albicans* (high power); periodic acid-Schiff stain showing pulmonary arteriole filled with budding spores.

chiectasis in a saprophytic role, causing an *aspergilloma*. This was first reported by Virchow in 1856. The lesion produces a characteristic radiological appearance of an opacity with a curved meniscus-like fluid level which moves on alteration of the patient's posture. Microscopically there is a thick fibrous-walled cavity containing necrotic debris, fibrin, and a mass of fungal elements, which may include fruiting bodies. Invasion of the wall rarely occurs, but occasional cases of 'semi-invasive aspergillosis' have been reported, with a cavitating pneumonia but without vascular invasion.

Candida albicans This is an uncommon cause of pneumonia which is seen in the severely immunocompromised and has a poor prognosis. The lung is usually involved as part of a disseminated candidosis, and the diagnosis can only be made definitely by identification of the organisms in tissue sections. In pulmonary candidosis following blood-borne spread, there are multiple miliary nodules with central necrosis and a variable inflammatory response, depending on the degree of immunosuppression.

The organism, a budding yeast with pseudohyphae, causes a *necrotizing pneumonitis* (Fig. 13.48) and can be seen in tissue sections. Identification is made easier by staining with PAS or methenamine silver (Fig. 13.49). An acute focal bronchopneumonia is seen following aspiration of *Candida* (which often colonizes the mouth in immunosuppressed patients), leading to abscess formation.

Mucor, Absidia, and Rhizopus The most important of this group is *Mucor*, which is most often seen in patients with diabetes or haematological malignancy. The pathological features are similar to those seen in invasive *Aspergillus* infection, but may be differentiated by the hyphal morphology; the hyphae of *Mucor* are thicker and show a characteristic 90° branching pattern (Fig. 13.50).

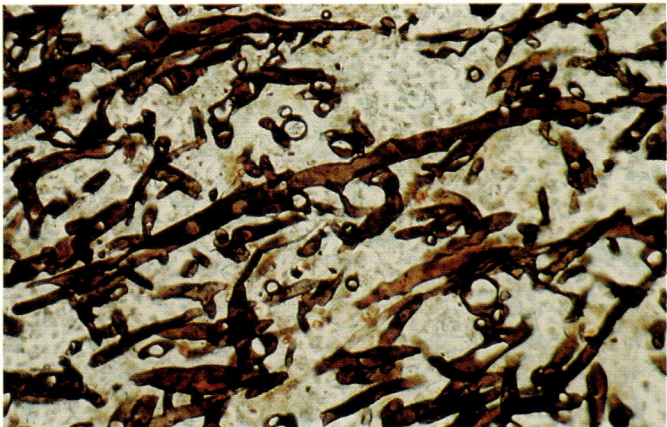

Fig. 13.50 Mucormycosis; broad fungal hyphae with 90° branching pattern. (Grocott's methenamine silver technique.)

Allescheria This is a rare fungal disease caused by one of the causative agents of maduromycetoma, *Allescheria boydii*. Only a few cases have been reported, and typically it causes fibrotic cavitating lesions.

13.3.2   Chronic obstructive airways disease

T. Creagh and T. Krausz

Chronic obstructive airways disease (COAD) is a term that encompasses a number of diseases which are characterized by an increase in resistance to airflow and which result in a reduced expiratory capacity. These include *chronic bronchitis, emphysema, bronchiolitis,* and *bronchiectasis.*

COAD is a major cause of morbidity and mortality throughout the Western world, causing nearly 62 000 deaths in 1983 and with an estimated 10 million affected in the United States. The most important factor implicated in the aetiology of COAD is *smoking*, causing approximately 90 per cent of cases.

Chronic bronchitis

Chronic bronchitis is defined as the production of sputum each day for greater than 3 months of the year, over two consecutive years. This is a clinical definition—the pathological equivalent is that of hypersection of mucus that results from enlargement of the mucus glands. There is an increase in the diameter of the acini and an increase in the proportion of mucous as compared to serous cells (CIBA Guest Symposium 1959).

A number of factors or conditions may be implicated in the pathogenesis of chronic bronchitis; these may be exogenous or endogenous (see Table 13.4) (Bake *et al.* 1982). *Irritant materials,* such as coal dust inhalation, results in hypersecretion of mucus and subsequent airway obstruction, although emphysema more commonly results. Other occupational hazards

Table 13.4   Aetiology of chronic bronchitis

Exogenous	Inhalation of irritant material
	Air pollution
	Occupational hazards, e.g. fumes
	Smoking
Endogenous	Asthma
	Cystic fibrosis
	Impaired defence mechanism
	Recurrent aspiration

include welding, inhalation of man-made fibres, coolants, and sulphur dioxide. *Smoking* is the commonest cause of chronic bronchitis and experimental evidence suggests that smoking induces mucous gland enlargement. The earliest and mildest abnormality found in smokers is a *respiratory bronchiolitis* (see below), which appears to be the precursor lesion in many cases of COAD. In *asthma*, mucus hypersecretion results from a combination of allergic response, recurrent infection, and bronchial hyper-reactivity. *Impaired defence mechanisms*, including immunodeficiency syndromes, such as hypogammaglobulinaemia and selective IgA deficiency, together with the immotile cilia (or Kartagener's) syndrome, predispose. Other ciliary abnormalities are commonly found in chronic bronchitis and may be implicated in the pathogenesis as mucociliary transport is severely impaired (Lungarella *et al.* 1983). Infection is thought to be secondary to mucus hypersecretion and probably plays a more causative role in communities where poor socio-economic conditions mean infection is common and less likely to be treated.

Mucous gland enlargement is one of the primary abnormalities in chronic bronchitis (Fig. 13.51). This can be measured quantitatively by two methods: the Reid Index and the volume proportion (Reid 1960). The Reid Index is the ratio of the thickness of the bronchial glands to the thickness of the bronchial wall (Fig. 13.52). In normal, non-bronchitic subjects the Reid Index is calculated as being between 0.36 and 0.41, whereas in bronchitics the Index is 0.44–0.79. The Reid Index has a number of disadvantages in that it is only of value if the mucosa

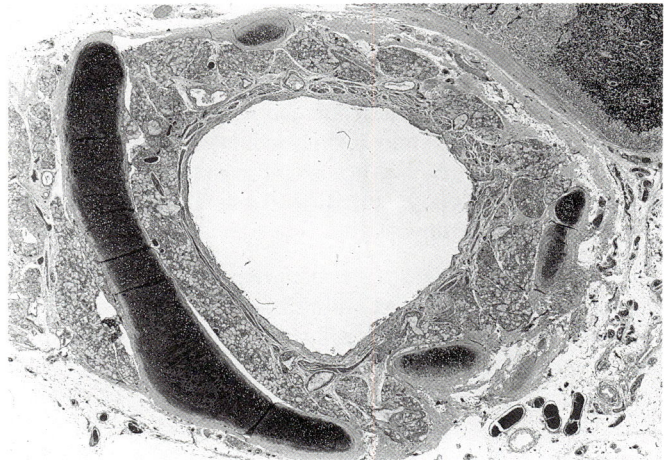

Fig. 13.51   Mucous gland hyperplasia in chronic bronchitis.

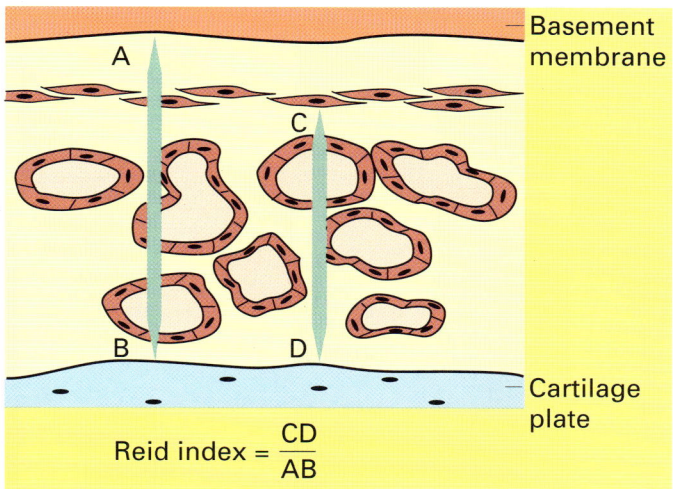

Fig. 13.52 Calculation of the Reid Index in chronic bronchitis.

$$\text{Reid index} = \frac{CD}{AB}$$

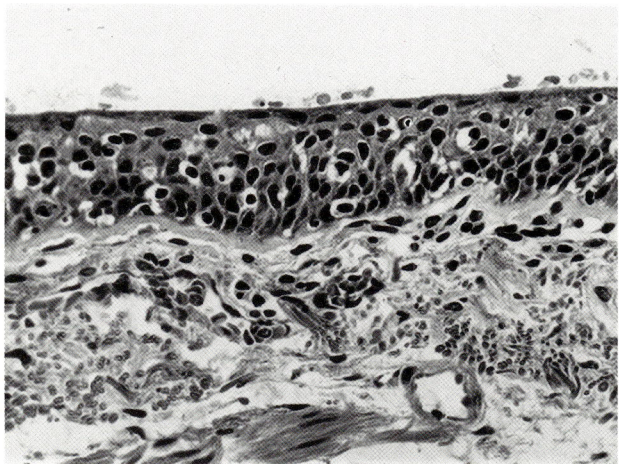

Fig. 13.54 Squamous metaplasia in chronic bronchitis.

is sectioned parallel to the cartilage, and this is infrequent. Also, glandular tissue often extends deep to the cartilage. In the volume proportion method, the mucous gland area is compared with the bronchial wall area by point counting (Dunnill *et al.* 1969).

Mucous gland enlargement is thought to cause bronchial obstruction by narrowing the lumen of the airways; however, mucus plugging of the bronchi is probably more important. *Goblet cell metaplasia* and a possible increase in the actual size of goblet cells add to the mucus hypersecretion and plugging (Fig. 13.53). Other changes include *squamous metaplasia* of the respiratory mucosa (Fig. 13.54).

The classical clinical picture of a chronic bronchitic is that of the 'blue bloater'. The patient is usually male, aged 40–45, with a long-standing history of productive cough and recurrent infections. The predominant airways obstruction causes failure of oxygenation in the alveoli and subsequent central cyanosis with a low P_{O_2}. The ventilation/perfusion inbalance leads to intrapulmonary shunting and development of right-sided heart failure (*cor pulmonale*). In reality, chronic bronchitis is often associated with emphysema and the differential diagnosis is not so clear-cut.

Emphysema

Emphysema is defined as the permanent, abnormal enlargement of any part, or all of the respiratory acinus, together with destruction of the lung tissue (Snider *et al.* 1985). Previously, airspace enlargement *without* destruction was also included; however, this is best termed *overinflation*, as the clinical syndrome of emphysema correlates best with accompanying lung destruction.

Emphysema is classified as to its anatomical distribution within the acinus:

1. *centrilobular (proximal acinar)*;
2. *panacinar*;
3. *distal acinar (paraseptal)*;
4. *irregular emphysema (paracicatricial)*.

Centrilobular emphysema

The hallmark of centrilobular emphysema is enlargement and destruction of the respiratory bronchioles (see Figs 13.55–13.58). Macroscopically, emphysematous spaces are seen midway between the centre and periphery of the lung lobules. The upper zones of the lungs are affected to a greater degree than the lower zone.

Centrilobular emphysema is the commonest form of emphysema and it is usually associated with smoking. There is often inflammation of the terminal and respiratory bronchioles, and the primary abnormality appears to be destruction of the lung parenchyma. A similar appearance is seen in *focal dust emphysema* (coal-worker's simple pneumoconiosis); however, here the primary abnormality is dilatation.

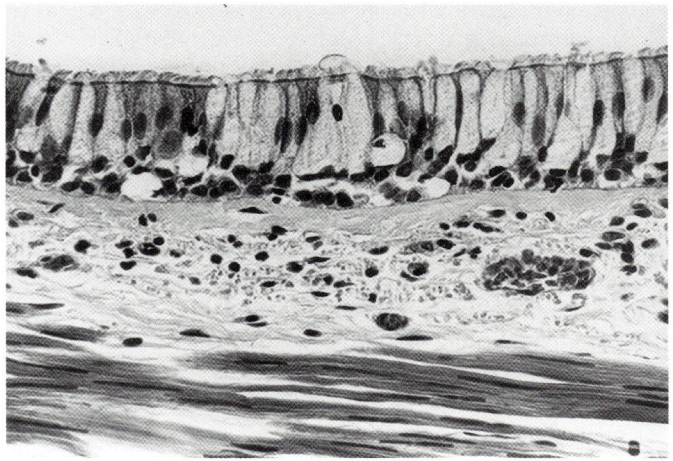

Fig. 13.53 Goblet cell metaplasia in chronic bronchitis.

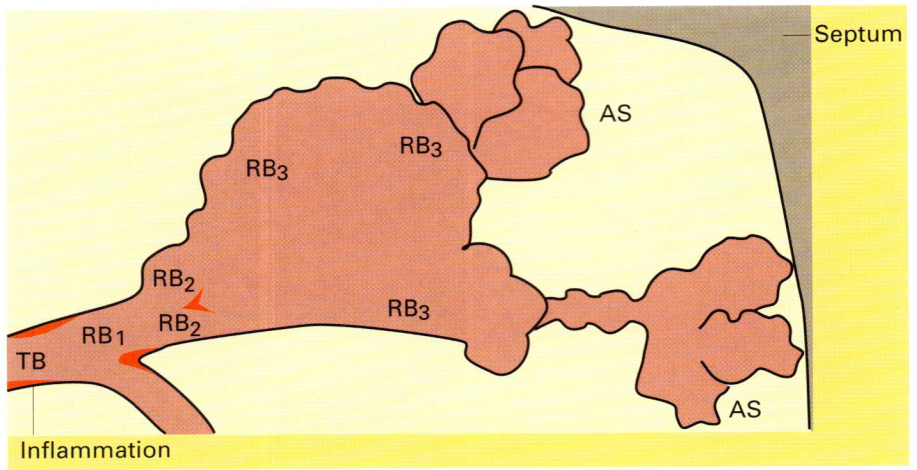

Fig. 13.55 Centrilobular emphysema; RB, respiratory bronchioles (order 1, 2, or 3); TB, terminal bronchiole; AS, alveolar sac.

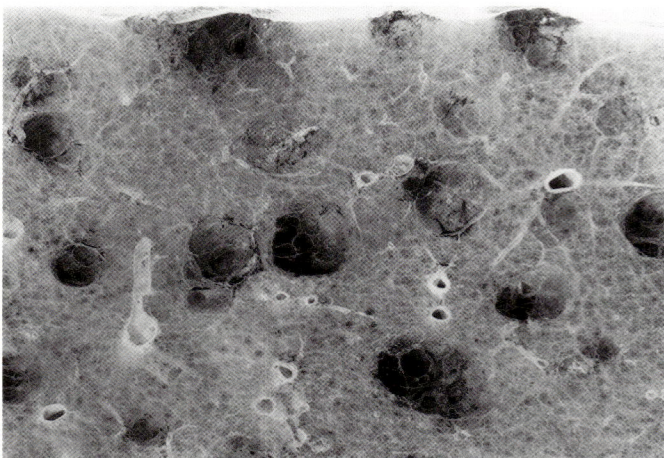

Fig. 13.56 Centrilobular emphysema. (Courtesy of Dr B. Heard.)

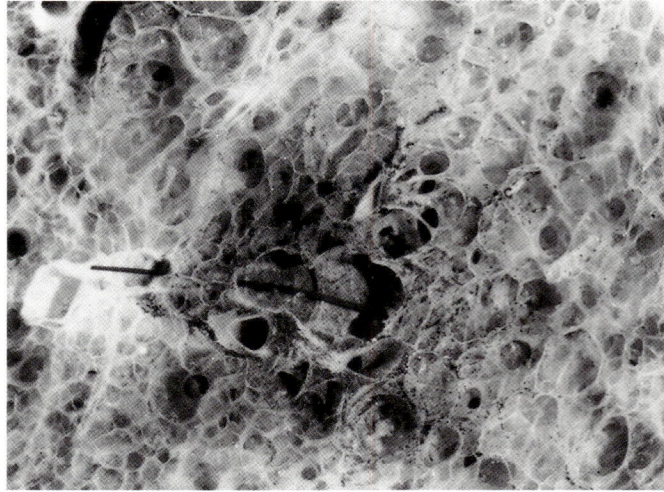

Fig. 13.58 Centrilobular emphysema. (Courtesy of Dr B. Heard.)

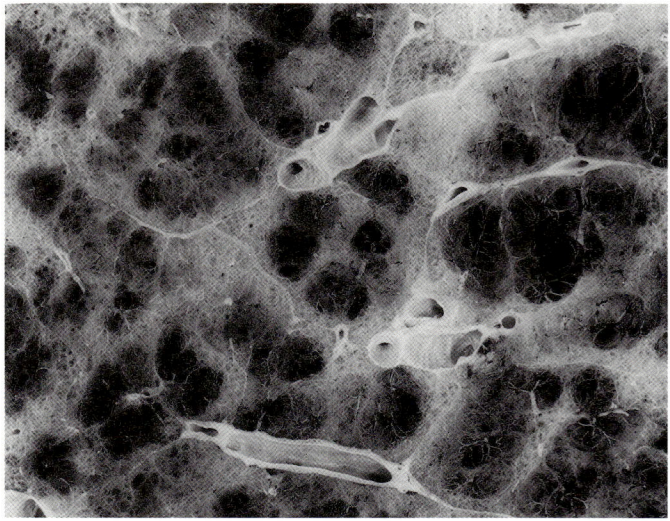

Fig. 13.57 Centrilobular emphysema, showing confluence of some lesions. (Courtesy of Dr B. Heard.)

Panacinar emphysema

Panacinar emphysema (see Figs 13.59–61) involves the entire acinus; although it is an uncommon form of emphysema, it includes most animal models and it is the type associated with *α-1-antitrypsin deficiency* (see below).

The early stages of panacinar emphysema involve the alveolar ducts and sacs and the morphological diagnosis may be difficult. This is facilitated by the examination of barium sulphate impregnated slices of lung. In the normal lung the alveoli are the smallest airspaces; they are multifaceted and are scattered amongst larger airspaces which represent a cross-section of the alveolar ducts and respiratory bronchioles. In early panacinar emphysema, the alveoli become enlarged and flattened, and distinction between them and the alveolar ducts is no longer possible. Later, the whole acinus becomes involved, including the respiratory bronchioles. The lower zones of the lung tend to be the most affected. Histologically, the severe loss of parenchyma is reflected (Figs 13.62, 13.63).

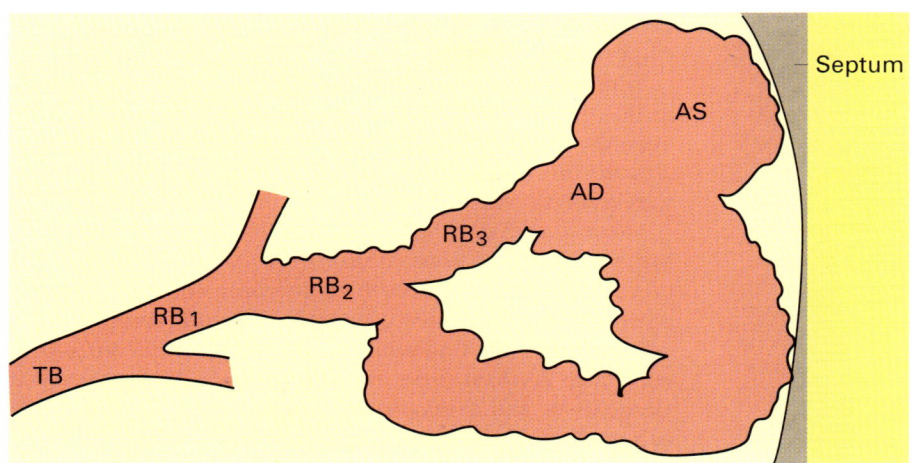

Fig. 13.59 Panacinar emphysema; RB, respiratory bronchioles (order 1, 2, 3); TB, terminal bronchiole; AD, alveolar duct; AS, alveolar sac.

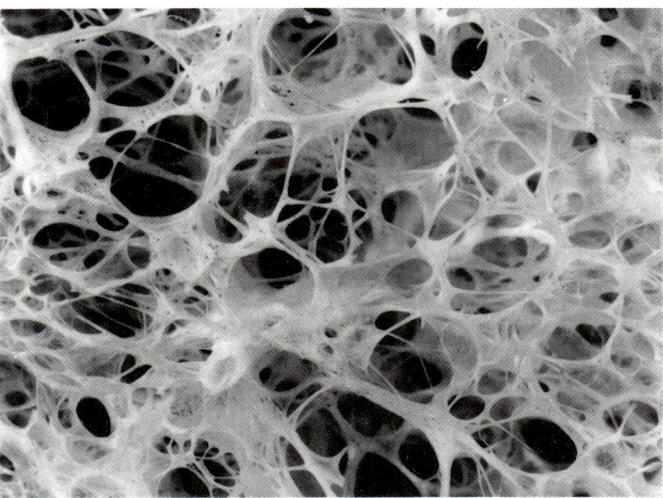

Fig. 13.60 Panacinar emphysema.

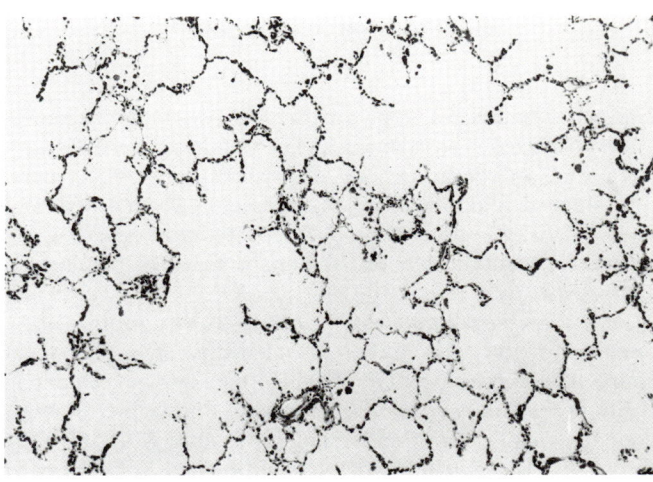

Fig. 13.62 Normal lung, ×90.

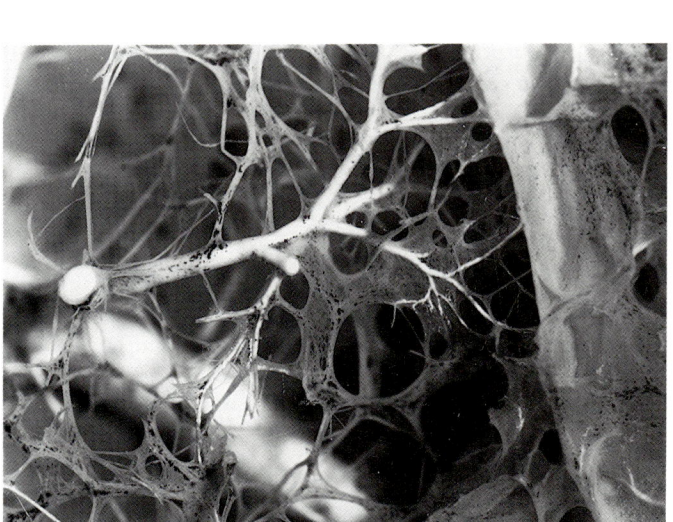

Fig. 13.61 Severe panacinal emphysema; arterioles injected with barium sulphate and gelatin mixture. (Courtesy of Dr B. Heard.)

Distal acinar emphysema (paraseptal)

This is the least common form of emphysema; it is subpleural and paraseptal in location and usually occurs at the posterior or anterior margins of the upper lung (see Figs 13.64, 13.65). These areas are exposed to the highest levels of intrapleural negative pressure and may be associated with the development of spontaneous pneumothorax in young adults. Distal acinar emphysema may also be seen in conjunction with panacinar or centrilobular emphysema (Fig. 13.65).

Irregular emphysema (paracicatricial)

Irregular emphysema is associated with scarring; the acinus is irregularly involved and it is thought that the airspace enlargement results from destruction of the alveolar walls (see Figs 13.66, 13.67).

Emphysema is a common condition and is thought to affect up to 50 per cent of the adult autopsy population—predominantly males. The aetiology of emphysema appears to involve several factors; however, a major advance in the understanding

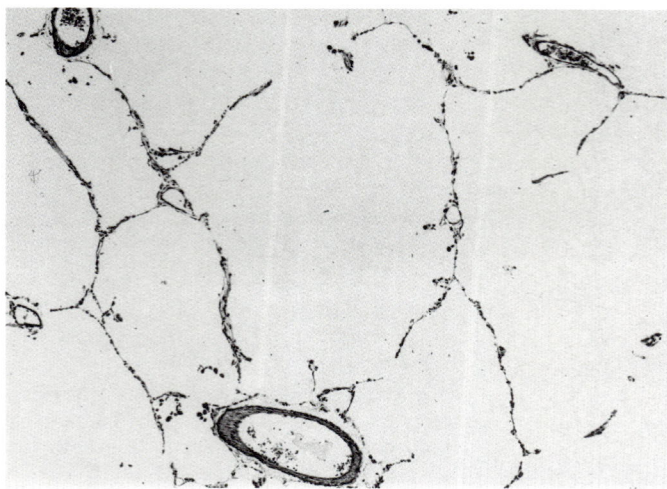

Fig. 13.63 Panacinar emphysema.

of its pathogenesis was made in the 1960s when two simultaneous discoveries were made: the first of these was the observation that on routine testing of patients with emphysema, some showed a diminished α-1-macroglobulin (Laurell and Eriksson 1963). Secondly, it was discovered that experimental intratracheal administration of papain in dogs resulted in emphysema (Gross *et al.* 1964).

The α-1-macroglobulin was identified as α-1-antitrypsin, a protease inhibitor. This protein is encoded for by a pair of co-dominant alleles (termed 'Pi') of which there are approximately 30 subtypes. The commonest of these is *PiM*, which is most frequently manifested in the homozygous state of *PiMM*. The subtype *PiZ* is associated with α-1-antitrypsin deficiency; in homozygotes the levels are approximately 10 per cent of normal, whereas in heterozygotes the levels are up to 60 per cent of normal. There is also a geographical variation in the frequency of the *PiZ* subtype, with 1 in 1000–5000 births in northern Europe being affected. The heterozygous state, *PiMZ*, affects 3 per cent of adults in the UK, as compared to 5–9 per cent of adults in the USA. α-1-Antitrypsin deficiency is associated with the development of *cirrhosis of the liver* in infancy, and *emphysema* in adults, which occurs at an early age; the risk of developing emphysema is increased by smoking and in these subjects

there is usually a mixture of both panacinar and centrilobular emphysema.

Administration of proteolytic enzymes by intratracheal installation was found to induce panacinar-type emphysema in animals; the enzyme had to have elastolytic activity (papain or elastase) and the severity of emphysema was dependent on both the elastolytic potency and the dose.

These two discoveries have been linked together to form the *protease–anti-protease imbalance hypothesis*. Protease activity in the lung is derived from neutrophils and macrophages, whereas anti-proteases include α-1-antitrypsin, serum α-1-macroglobulin and inhibitors in the bronchial mucus. An imbalance between these components leads to destruction of elastic tissue and development of emphysema; this may occur as a result of α-1-antitrypsin deficiency or smoking.

In smokers, increased numbers of neutrophils and macrophages accumulate in the walls and lumen of respiratory bronchioles, where they release proteolytic enzymes and chemotactic factors which attract further macrophages and neutrophils. The resulting respiratory bronchiolitis is the earliest lesion associated with chronic obstructive airways disease. Smoking also directly inhibits α-1-antitrypsin activity by oxidation of methionine. Continued protease–anti-protease imbalance eventually leads to the development of emphysema (Snider *et al.* 1986).

Pathological demonstration of emphysema

The pathological diagnosis of emphysema is best made from inflated and fixed lung tissue (Heard *et al.* 1979). A cannula is tied into the main bronchus and 10 per cent formalin is infused at a pressure of 25–30 cm of water over a period of 24–72 hours.

Examination of the fixed lung may be via barium sulphate impregnation of wet lung slices—the lung slice is first immersed in a barium nitrate saturated solution for 1 min, followed by immersion in saturated sodium sulphate—the normally translucent alveolar walls become opaque and easily visible; or by embedding in gelatin (*Gough–Wentworth sections*).

Emphysema can be measured quantitatively by various morphometric techniques.

Clinical features

As in chronic bronchitis, there is a classical clinical picture of

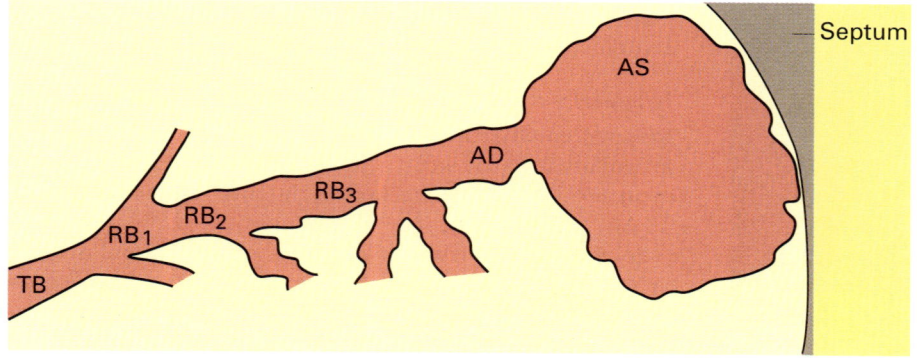

Fig. 13.64 Distal acinar (paraseptal) emphysema; RB, respiratory bronchioles (order 1, 2, 3); TB, terminal bronchiole; AD, alveolar duct; AS, alveolar sac.

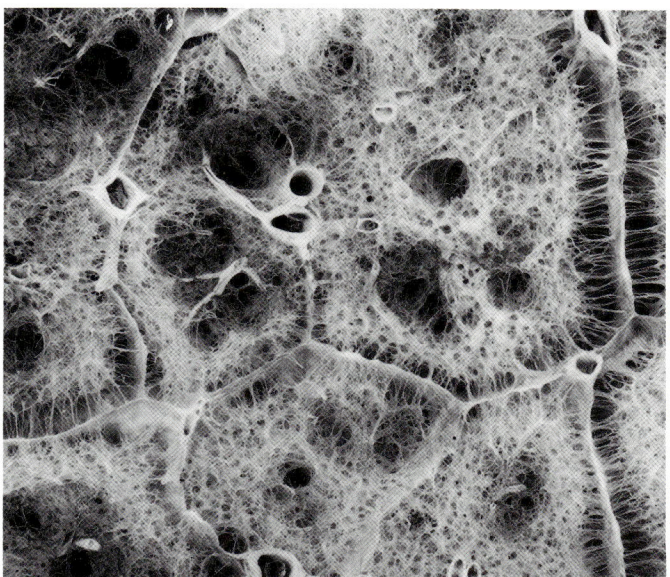

Fig. 13.65 Distal acinar (paraseptal) emphysema (with some centri-lobular emphysema). (Courtesy of Dr B. Heard.)

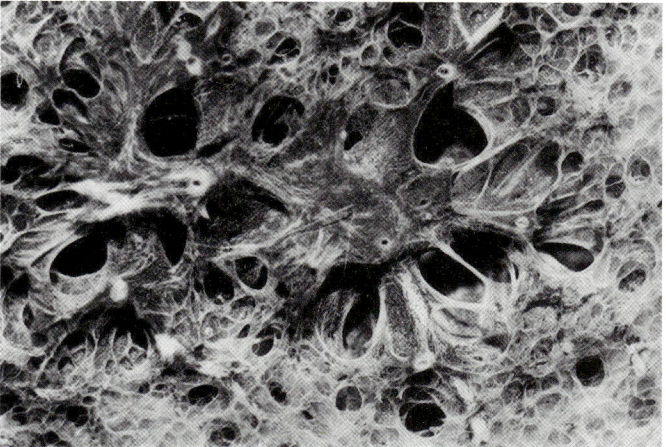

Fig. 13.66 Irregular emphysema; note the central scar.

emphysema—patients are termed 'pink puffers' and are usually male aged 50–75, with a history of early onset of severe dyspnoea. The predominant parenchymal destruction results in air being trapped in distal airways, with formation of a 'barrel chest'. Blood gases are usually well maintained; however, eventually the long-standing hypoxaemia and the decrease in the area of the pulmonary vascular bed may lead to pulmonary hypertension and cor pulmonale.

Emphysema is only detectable clinically when obstruction is severe, and at last one-third of the functioning pulmonary parenchyma has been destroyed.

Other conditions simulating emphysema

Overinflation Congenital—rapid overinflation of one lobe causes compression of the remaining lobes and acute respiratory distress.

Acquired Secondary to acute obstruction.

Ageing A number of changes occur in the lung, including 'rounding' of the lungs, with an increase in alveolar duct size and a loss of elastic and alveolar wall tissue. The overall alveolar surface area is diminished.

Bronchiolitis

As already mentioned, bronchiolitis or small airways disease is the earliest and mildest manifestation of chronic obstructive airways disease (Kerrebijn *et al.* 1982).

Bronchiolar inflammation, of which the commonest cause is smoking, has a number of consequences; these include bronchoconstriction (which may be reflexly mediated, or via release of mediators) and displacement of the bronchiolar lining material, which cause airways narrowing and airflow obstruction. Goblet cell metaplasia and hypersecretion of mucus cause further displacement of the surfactant layer.

The respiratory bronchiolitis caused by smoking may lead to protease–anti-protease imbalance (via neutrophil and macrophage accumulation) and progression to emphysema and/or goblet cell metaplasia and mucus hypersecretion with progression to chronic bronchitis. Often there is not a clear-cut distinction between emphysema and chronic bronchitis, and patients

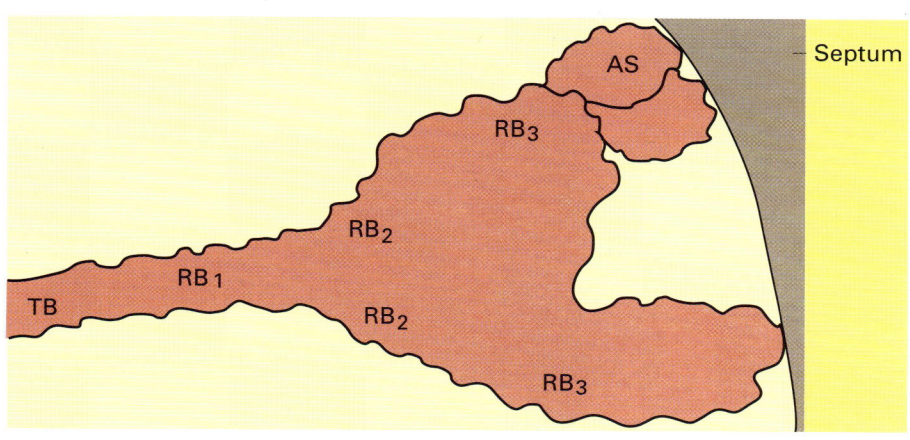

Fig. 13.67 Irregular emphysema; RB, respiratory bronchioles (order 1, 2, 3); TB, terminal bronchiole; AS, alveolar sac.

present with a combination of symptoms, signs, and pathological findings.

Other forms of bronchiolitis may be associated with rheumatoid disease, of unknown aetiology, a diffuse panbronchiolitis, or bronchiolitis obliterans. *Rheumatoid disease* causes inflammation of the small airways, together with occlusion of the lumen by loose fibrous tissue, which occurs patchily throughout the lung. The exact aetiology of this is unknown. *Cryptogenic bronchiolitis* shows chronic airway obstruction with a diminished FEV_1 of less than 60 per cent normal; however, no cause can be identified. This diagnosis is one of exclusion. *Diffuse panbronchiolitis* is a condition described in Japan, comprising severe, chronic inflammation of the proximal respiratory bronchioles with subsequent extension to more proximal bronchioles. The bronchiolar walls are thickened and fibrotic with an infiltrate of lymphocytes, plasma cells, and histiocytes. This leads to narrowing of the respiratory bronchioles and dilatation of more proximal airways such that the appearances resemble those of bronchiectasis. *Bronchiolitis obliterans* encompasses a spectrum of diseases, and is characterized by inflammation, plugging of the lumen by granulation tissue, and eventual obliteration. This may be idiopathic or associated with a number of conditions (Table 13.5).

Table 13.5   Types of bronchiolitis obliterans

Emphysema
Bronchiectasis
Toxic gases: nitrogen oxides, ammonia, sulphur dioxide
Infections: measles, adenovirus, mycoplasma
Allergic alveolitis
Eosinophilic pneumonia
Eosinophilic fasciitis
Sjögren's syndrome
Graft versus host disease
Heart–lung transplant
Connective tissue disease, especially rheumatoid arthritis
Penicillamine
Diffuse panbronchiolitis
Organizing pneumonia

Bronchiectasis

Bronchiectasis is an uncommon disorder today and can be defined as an abnormal and permanent dilatation of the bronchi. Clinically, bronchiectasis is often manifested in childhood with a history of recurrent chest infections, production of purulent sputum, and occasionally haemoptysis. Long-standing cases display finger 'clubbing'. The aetiology of bronchiectasis can be divided into focal and diffuse (see Table 13.6).

When associated with conditions such as cystic fibrosis, the lung findings are often not classified as bronchiectasis. In some post-infective cases the bronchial dilatation may revert to normal within several weeks and these should not be included under the heading of bronchiectasis.

Pathogenetically, a number of mechanisms are implicated. These include *atelectasis* and *traction* (Barker and Bardana 1988). In atelectasis, bronchiectasis evolves following collapse

Table 13.6   Aetiology of bronchiectasis

Focal
  Foreign body/tumour
  Lymphadenopathy
  Viscid secretions

Diffuse
  Aspiration/inhalation
  Post-infective
    TB
    Aspergillus and fungi
    Virulent bacterial/viral infection
  Abnormal host defence
    Immunodeficiency, e.g. panhypogammaglobulinaemia, ciliary dyskinesia
  Genetic disorders
    Cystic fibrosis
    Bronchial cartilage abnormalities
    Idiopathic

of a portion of the lung, which may be due to obstruction. If this is proximal, for example due to a tumour, there is compensatory expansion of the surrounding lung, mediastinal shift which results in an increase in the negative intrapleural pressure, and accumulation of secretions followed by secondary infection. In distal obstruction, for example in severe chronic obstructive airways disease, collapse of the affected lung occurs with dilatation of the proximal bronchi.

In established cases of bronchiectasis, parenchymal damage and fibrosis cause a traction effect which results in continued dilatation.

Pathologically, the lower lobes, especially the left lower lobe, are most often affected. The dilated bronchi may be described as *cylindrical* or *saccular*. *Cylindrical bronchiectasis* predominantly involves basal segments of the lung, the bronchi being filled with purulent material (Fig. 13.68). In *saccular bronchiectasis*, the dilated bronchi apear as rounded, blind-ending sacs, which may contain purulent mucus (Fig. 13.69). The normal longitudinal striations of the bronchial wall elastic fibres are lost and

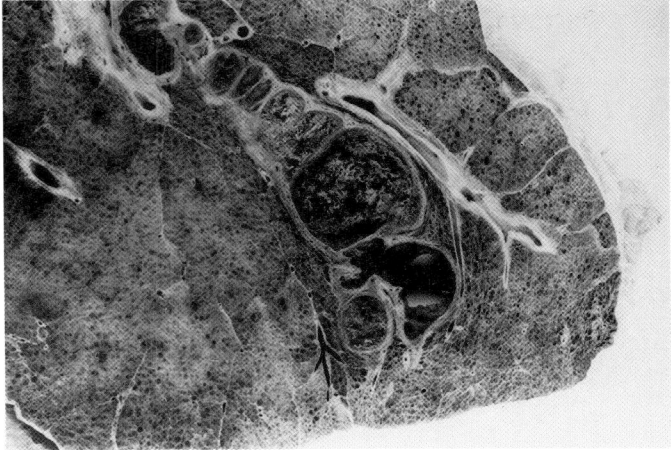

Fig. 13.68   Cylindrical bronchiectasis. (Courtesy of Dr B. Heard.)

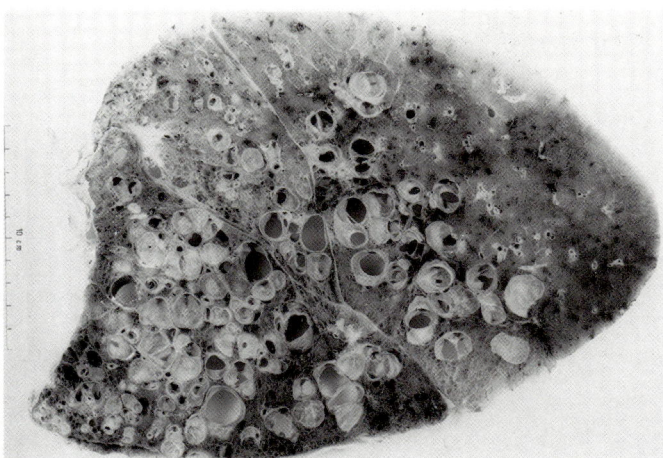

Fig. 13.69 Saccular bronchiectasis. (Courtesy of Dr B. Heard.)

transverse ridging is seen, together with obvious pitting of the walls due to dilatation of the mucous gland ducts.

Changes are also seen in the airways distal to the bronchiectactic areas—peribronchiolar fibrosis and lymphoid follicle formation are virtually pathognomonic of proximal bronchiectasis. 'Tumourlets' are seen adjacent to scarred bronchioles—these are small proliferations of the bronchial neuroendocrine (Kulschitsky) cells. The bronchial arteries are increased in size—they are responsible for supplying the inflammatory and fibrous tissue—and anastomoses develop between the pulmonary and bronchial arteries.

Microscopically, there is destruction of muscle, cartilage, and bronchial glands, the bronchial walls being formed by chronically inflamed fibrous tissue. Prominent lymphoid follicles are often present—this is sometimes termed *follicular bronchiectasis* (Fig. 13.70).

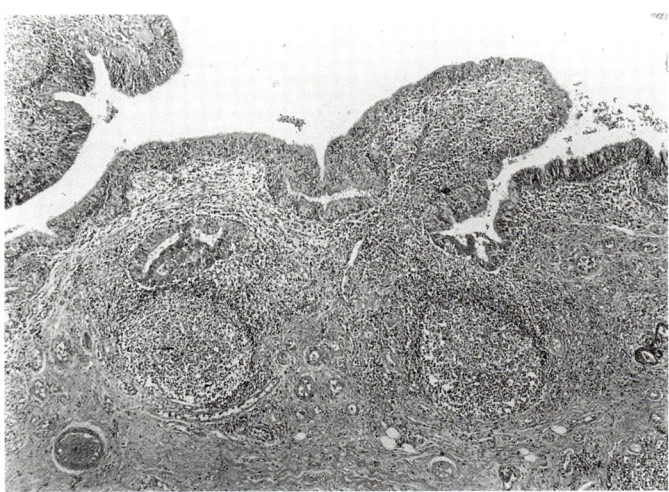

Fig. 13.70 Histology of follicular bronchiectasis. (Courtesy of Dr B. Heard.)

13.3.3 Asthma and allergic disease

M. H. Griffiths

Asthma

Asthma is an extremely common but potentially serious condition characterized by *paroxysmal wheezing* and *shortness of breath*. The wheezing is due to an acute, reversible increase in the resistance to airflow in the smaller airways so that increased respiratory effort is required for inspiration and expiration. Those prone to asthma can be shown to have airways which are hyper-reactive to inhaled irritants. This is demonstrated by challenging the patient with inhaled histamine or methacoline and observing an exaggerated reduction in the forced expiratory volume measured over a period of one second (FEV_1). Asthma may be precipitated by non-specific stimuli such as cold air, exercise, cigarette smoke, or viral infections, but in some, only exposure to a specific substance to which the patient has become allergic provokes an attack.

Asthma is responsible for much morbidity and, despite the many advances in its management, a certain mortality. There are approximately 2000 deaths in children and adults from asthma each year in England and Wales.

Clinical features

Patients tend to belong to one of three rather poorly defined groups. Patients with what is known as *extrinsic asthma* develop their symptoms in early childhood and the condition usually abates in adolescence or early adult life. Boys are affected more often than girls. There is, typically, a family history of atopy and these patients can often be shown to have hypersensitivity of the immediate type (type 1) to one or more specific allergens, such as certain pollens or the house dust mite *Dermatophagoides pteronyssinus*. It is thought that in these patients the bronchial response is triggered by the release of vasoactive amines from the resident mucosal mast cells which have been stimulated by a specific immunoglobulin of class E (IgE). *Intrinsic asthma*, on the other hand, tends to present in adult life and is more common in women. No history of allergy or atopy is obtained. Symptoms may be more chronic and less paroxymal than in extrinsic asthma. In a third clinical type, *extrinsic non-atopic asthma*, a hypersensitivity reaction of delayed type (type III) is important. Occupational asthma, e.g. hypersensitivity to flour and grain, is frequently of this type. The symptoms in these patients commence several hours after exposure to the allergen. The bronchial response is probably triggered by neutrophils in a reaction that involves complement fixation by immune complexes. Dual hypersensitivity reactions of types I and III occur in some instances.

Pathology

The airways obstruction in asthma is probably the result of a combination of the following factors:

1. *bronchial smooth muscle contraction;*

2. *an increase in bronchial mucosal thickness;* and

3. *exudate retention in the lumen.*

The relative importance of each of these factors is much debated.

Muscle The role of smooth muscle contraction in asthma is the most controversial of the three factors and widely divergent views have been expressed as to its importance in both acute and chronic asthma. Whatever its role, bronchial muscle hyperplasia is a constant finding in the airways of asthmatics and in this respect asthma differs from chronic bronchitis, the other major cause of obstructive airways disease. The increase in muscle bulk is not, however, necessarily evidence of chronic spasm, but may simply be a product of the trophic effects of locally released inflammatory mediators.

Mucosa Whether an asthma attack is initiated by inflammation or allergy, the result is a dilatation of mucosal blood vessels in response to released vasoactive amines. The mucosa becomes oedematous and thickened and the airways narrowed. Inflammatory cells such as neutrophils and eosinophils migrate from the capillaries into the mucosa, and goblet cells are stimulated to discharge mucus. Epithelial cells are shed into the lumen by a mechanism which is not completely understood but which may be caused by *eosinophil granule major basic protein*, a cytotoxic product of eosinophil granules, the presence of which has been demonstrated by immunofluorescence on damaged bronchial epithelium in asthma. Epithelial shedding leaves sections of the airways lined only by basal cells, which provide a poor barrier to the movement of tissue fluid and allow the leakage of proteinaceous inflammatory exudate into the lumen. Regeneration of the epithelium initially produces a lining of undifferentiated cells which lack cilia and do not participate in the clearance of mucus and exudate from the lumen.

Between asthma attacks histological examination of the mucosa reveals few changes. Goblet cells are increased in number in the bronchial epithelium at the expense of ciliated cells and may be found in bronchiolar epithelium where normally there is none. The basal lamina appears thickened (Fig. 13.71) due to deposition of collagen of types III and V beneath the basement membrane proper. This effect is also seen in chronic bronchitis. It has been attributed in asthmatics to fibroblast stimulation by mast cell and eosinophil products. The mucous portion of the submucous glands undergoes hypertrophy, increasing the bulk of the bronchial wall and increasing the volume of mucus in the lumen.

Exudate A study of the sputum reveals much about the contents of the airways in asthma and correlates with the findings in the bronchial mucus plugs which are found at post-mortem when death has occurred in *status asthmaticus*. The sputum contains thick mucus which may be organized into fibrillar spiral structures called *Curschmann's spirals* (Fig. 13.72) which are sometimes large enough to be visible with the naked eye. They probably represent casts of small airways. As well as

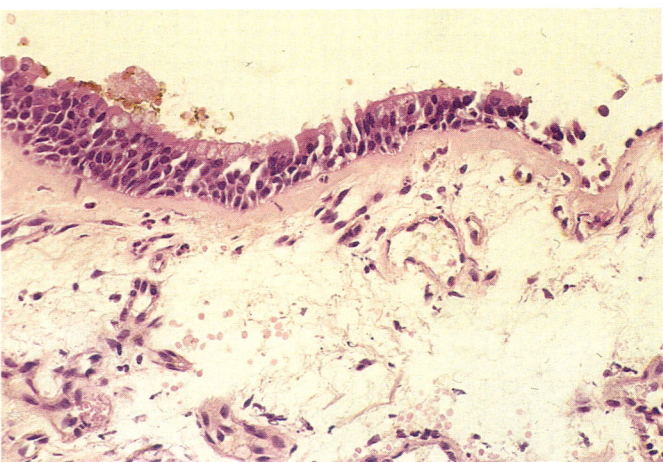

Fig. 13.71 Bronchial mucosa in asthma. There is epithelial shedding and an apparent thickening of the basement membrane due to the sublaminar deposition of collagen. Mucosal blood vessels are dilated.

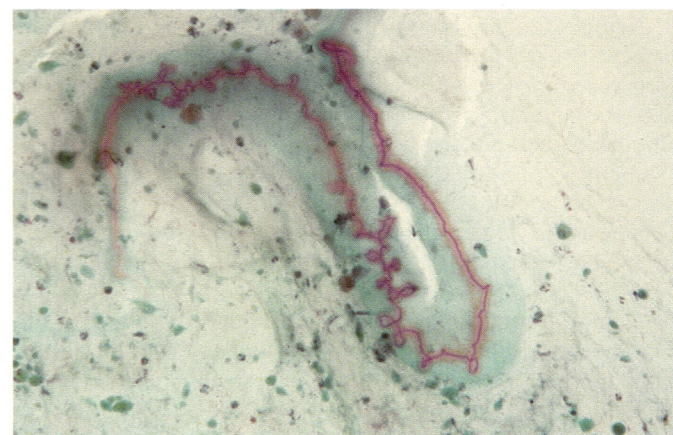

Fig. 13.72 A Curschmann's spiral in sputum from a patient with asthma. These intriguing structures are probably mucus casts of small airways. (Papanicolaou stain.) (Photograph courtesy of Dr G. Kocjan.)

mucus, the sputum consists of proteinaceous exudate in which shed epithelial cells are found, singly and in sheets and clusters (*Creola bodies*). Eosinophils in various stages of preservation may be numerous and may be accompanied by collections of *Charcot–Leyden crystals* (Fig. 13.73). These elongated hexagonal bipyramidal crystals are thought to be derived from the eosinophil granule membranes and, although characteristic of asthma, are also found in other conditions in which an infiltrate of eosinophils is present.

The main defect in the asthmatic bronchus is a failure to clear exudate, and factors which are important in the retention of exudate and mucus in the distal airways are:

1. an increase in production of mucus by mucous glands and goblet cells;

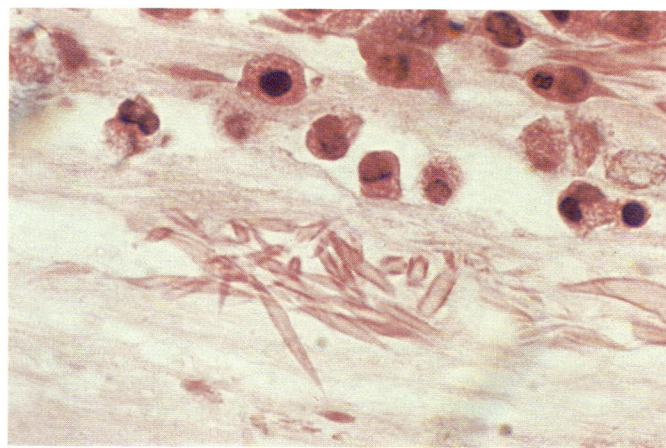

Fig. 13.73 Charcot–Leyden crystals. These bipyramidal hexagonal crystals, seen in the bottom half of the picture, are thought to be derived from eosinophil granule membranes.

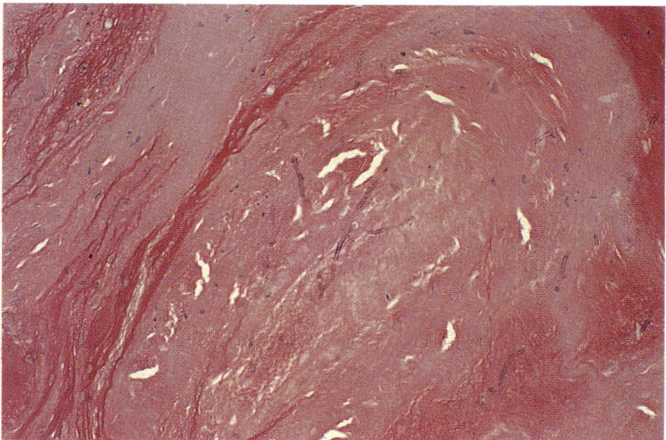

Fig. 13.74 *Aspergillus* hyphae in a mucus plug from an asthmatic patient with allergic bronchopulmonary aspergillosis.

2. less effective clearance of mucus due to a reduction in the population of ciliated cells through epithelial shedding and then their replacement, first by undifferentiated epithelium and then by an increased population of goblet cells;

3. the presence of a serous exudate which reduces the effectiveness of cilia in clearing mucus.

Status asthmaticus

This is the condition of extreme hypoxia and exhaustion caused by severe asthmatic bronchial obstruction and, although largely preventable, status asthmaticus is still responsible for a certain mortality. At post-mortem, the lungs, which normally collapse on opening the pleural cavities, fail to do so because of obstruction to the segmental and subsegmental bronchi and bronchioles by rubbery, grey plugs of mucus. The lung parenchyma is generally hyperinflated, although there may be scattered small areas of atelectasis, but it is structurally normal. There may be a degree of bronchiectasis.

Allergic bronchopulmonary aspergillosis

The airways of patients with chronic asthma are prone to colonization by fungi, usually of the *Aspergillus* species. Allergy may then develop to the fungus and the asthmatic response is compounded by a type III or immune-complex-mediated hypersensitivity reaction. Serum precipitins to *Aspergillus* species can be detected, and the blood eosinophil count is elevated. A distinctive type of proximal bronchiectasis may be present. As the fungal growth is entirely within the secretions in the airways (Fig. 13.74) and is therefore 'external', elimination of the fungus by systemic antifungal therapy is impossible but the symptoms do usually respond to systemic corticosteroids (see also Section 13.3.1).

Bronchocentric granulomatosis

Invasion of the bronchial wall by fungi such as *Aspergillus*

occurs rarely, but when it does it excites a granulomatous response in the wall of the bronchus or bronchiole and in the peribronchiolar tissues, hence the descriptive name of the condition. The majority of patients are chronic asthmatics and the airways affected are usually the distal airways. The fungal hyphae may be seen with the help of fungal stains within the necrotizing granulomas, but a careful search may be required and other causes of granuloma formation, such as tuberculosis and the necrobiotic nodules of rheumatoid lung disease, should be considered in the differential diagnosis.

Extrinsic allergic alveolitis

Extrinsic allergic alveolitis or hypersensitivity pneumonitis is the reaction of the lung parenchyma to inhaled organic dusts to which the individual has become hypersensitive. The condition is characterized histologically by a *diffuse granulomatous bronchiolo-alveolitis*. The hypersensitivity takes months or even years to develop, so it is usually in the context of occupational or domestic exposure to organic dust that the disease is acquired. The dusts which provoke this response usually contain particles of animal or vegetable protein, or vegetable matter which has been colonized by various micro-organisms. *Farmer's lung*, the disease associated with exposure to the dust of mouldy hay, was one of the first described and is the best known of the dozens of similar syndromes now recognized in association with an ever-growing number of occupations and interests, some of which are listed in Table 13.7. The clinical features and the pathology of all these conditions are similar.

Clinical features

The patient becomes acutely dyspnoeic 6–12 hours after exposure to the dust and may experience a dry cough, fever, and malaise. Because of the delay between exposure and the onset of the symptoms, the patient may not suspect the association, especially as the dust is invariably one to which he is habitually exposed. The cause may only be revealed by a carefully taken

Table 13.7 Some causes of extrinsic allergic alveolitis

Disease	Allergen	Source of allergen
Farmer's lung	Various thermophilic actinomycetes	Mouldy hay
Bird fancier's lung	Bird droppings or feathers	Pet birds
Bagassosis	*Thermoactinomyces sacchari*	Mouldy bagasse (sugar-cane fibre)
Air conditioner lung	Various thermophilic actinomycetes	Contaminated air-conditioning and heating systems
Mushroom worker's lung	*Thermoactinomyces vulgaris*	Mouldy compost
Furrier's lung	Animal fur dust	Animal pelts
Grain worker's lung	Unknown	Grain

clinical history. Continuous exposure to low levels of dust may sometimes produce more chronic, less episodic symptoms. The lung fields develop a variable degree of diffuse reticulate radiological shadowing.

Pathology

The histological triad of *bronchiolitis, diffuse interstitial pneumonitis,* and *scattered small non-necrotizing granulomas* is characteristic (Fig. 13.75). A cell-mediated or type IV hypersensitivity

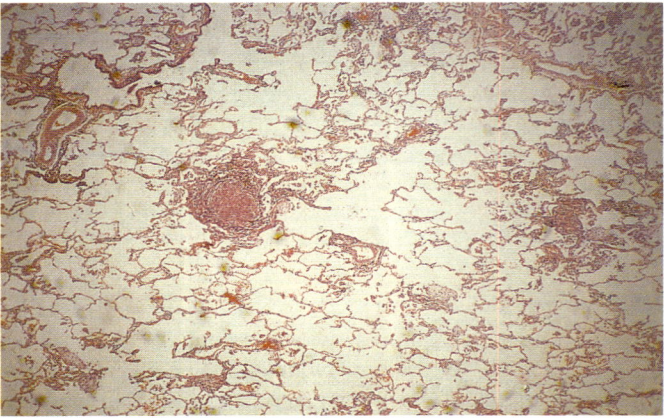

(a)

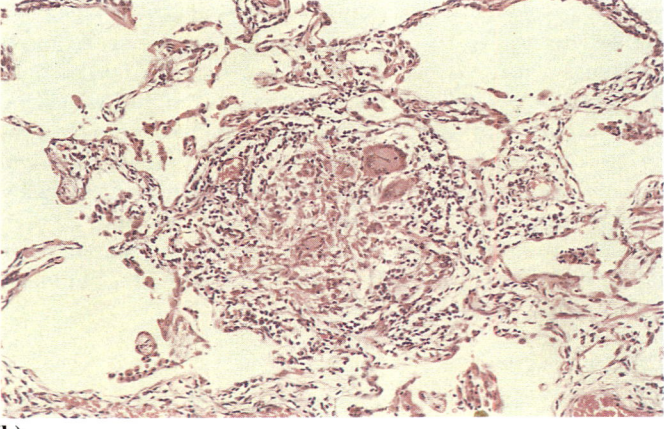

(b)

Fig. 13.75 Extrinsic allergic alveolitis. Low power (a) showing scattered non-caseating granulomas; and higher power (b) showing a granuloma and adjacent interstitial alveolitis. The patient kept budgerigars.

reaction is clearly involved in the development of the histopathological changes, i.e. granuloma formation, but a humoral reaction also occurs and precipitating antibodies to the provoking antigen can be demonstrated in the serum. The mere detection of these antibodies is of little diagnostic value as their presence simply correlates with exposure to the antigen, a fact already established from the clinical history, but a high titre of antibody, as measured by radioimmunoassay or enzyme-linked immunosorbent assay, does appear to correlate with the presence of disease. The humoral component of the reaction may be responsible for the asthma-like acute symptoms, possibly via a type III, immune-complex hypersensitivity reaction resulting from the local formation of immune complexes in the bronchial mucosa, complement fixation, and the release of factors chemotactic to neutrophils.

With continued exposure to the offending allergen, the changes in the lung parenchyma in some (but by no means all) patients may progress to irreversible diffuse interstitial fibrosis. Avoidance of the antigen, on the other hand, results in resolution of the inflammation and an excellent prognosis, hence the importance of recognizing the condition. The diagnosis must, of course, be based on firm evidence as it may lead to loss or change of occupation or to the abandoning of a favourite pastime, and a typical history plus a high serum antibody level are minimal requirements before recommending this course of action.

The diagnosis may be suggested for the first time by the findings in an open-lung biopsy taken to investigate interstitial lung disease of unknown aetiology. The histological differential diagnosis includes sarcoidosis, which in the early stages produces, as well as granulomas, an interstitial lymphocytic pneumonitis. Hypersensitivity to certain drugs, such as methotrexate, may also produce identical pathology.

Eosinophilic pneumonia

Acute eosinophilic pneumonia or Loeffler's syndrome

A transient and usually asymptomatic illness characterized by radiographic infiltrates and blood eosinophilia is known as *Loeffler's syndrome* after the Swiss clinician who described it in 1932. The illness resolves spontaneously within 4 weeks. Biopsy is rarely performed. In the tropics the condition is associated with intestinal infestation by worms such as *Ascaris lumbricoides*. The pulmonary infiltrates are a reaction to the migration of the *Ascaris* larvae through the pulmonary vasculature. A number of other causes of eosinophilic pneumonia, including certain drugs (see Section 13.3.5), are recognized but in most cases no cause is established.

Chronic eosinophilic pneumonia

Chronic eosinophilic pneumonia has, by definition, persisted for more than 4 weeks. It is characterized by peripheral pulmonary infiltrates, constitutional symptoms, and blood eosinophilia. The condition undoubtedly has an allergic basis but the underlying cause is rarely discovered. The natural history is very variable. It may persist for 6–8 weeks or for more than 3 months. Remission may occur spontaneously, or recurrence, or relentless progression to respiratory failure may follow. A response to corticosteroid therapy, should this become necessary, is the rule.

The histology of chronic eosinophilic pneumonia is of masses of eosinophils and macrophages filling the alveolar spaces, sometimes with small foci of necrosis in the exudate. Eosinophils, macrophages, lymphocytes, and plasma cells are present in the interstitium. The histology of the lung in Loeffler's syndrome, which is rarely biopsied, is probably similar.

13.3.4   Interstitial lung disease

M. H. Griffiths

Cryptogenic fibrosing alveolitis

Cryptogenic fibrosing alveolitis (diffuse interstitial pulmonary fibrosis, idiopathic pulmonary fibrosis) is an interstitial pneumonitis of unknown aetiology which usually progresses to diffuse lung fibrosis. The rate of progression is variable but may, to some extent, be predicted from the histological apearances in an open-lung biopsy. The course of the disease may sometimes be modified or even halted by steroids, especially when treatment is commenced in the early stages.

Clinical manifestations

The clinical features of the disease are those of progressive infiltrative lung disease, i.e. increasing exercise limitation by dyspnoea, a dry cough, malaise, and sometimes chest pain. The patients are usually middle-aged. Widespread crackles are audible on auscultation, and clubbing of the digits is usually present. Chest radiographs show bilateral reticular or reticulonodular shadowing, which is most pronounced at the lung bases. There is a rare, rapidly progressive form of the disease, which is sometimes known as the *Hamman–Rich syndrome* after the clinicians who first described it in 1935. The prognosis, even in cases with a more chronic presentation, is generally poor. The median survival of untreated patients is 4 years and the prognosis is improved in only a small proportion of patients by steroids and other immunosuppressant drugs.

Histology

There are two histological pictures associated with this condition, which are considered by many to represent the early and late phases of the same process. The early, or inflammatory, phase is characterized by widening of alveolar septa by an interstitial infiltrate of lymphocytes, plasma cells, and some eosinophils and neutrophils. The alveolar spaces are lined by prominent, cuboidal, type II alveolar epithelial cells, and may be filled with alveolar macrophages (Fig. 13.76). These macrophages were once thought to be desquamated alveolar epithelial cells, hence the term *desquamative interstitial pneumonia* (DIP), the name used for this histological appearance in America where it is often regarded as an entity separate from the less cellular, more fibrotic process known there as *usual interstitial pneumonia* (UIP). The diffuse pattern of DIP compared with the patchy involvement of UIP and the more favourable response of DIP to steroids are considered evidence that the two are different entities. In Britain, DIP and UIP are usually regarded as early and late phases of the same process. The late lesion (Fig. 13.77) is characterized by patchy interstitial fibrosis and a variable interstitial infiltrate of lymphocytes. Alveolar remodelling results in the formation of larger irregular alveolar spaces whose walls are thickened by the interstitial fibrosis and inflammation. The diffusing capacity of the lungs is therefore much impaired and their compliance reduced. The subpleural parenchyma is usually more severely affected than the central parts of the lung. Eventually, honeycombing (Fig. 13.78), an end-stage common to a number of interstitial pulmonary diseases, replaces much of the parenchyma, and the patient develops *pulmonary hypertension* and *cor pulmonale* or *respiratory failure*.

Pathogenesis

It seems likely that the process of interstitial fibrosis is promoted by alveolar macrophages activated by lymphokines and other factors to release the growth factors responsible for the proliferation in the interstitium of fibroblasts, myofibroblasts, and

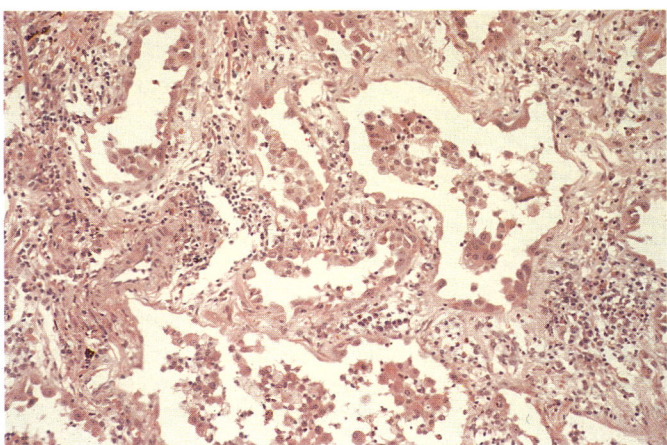

Fig. 13.76 Cryptogenic fibrosing alveolitis, early stage showing widening of alveolar septa by an inflammatory infiltrate and numerous macrophages in the alveolar spaces.

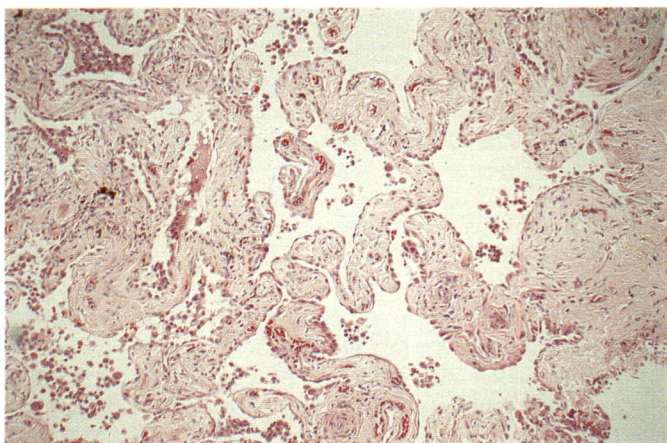

Fig. 13.77 Cryptogenic fibrosing alveolitis, late stage showing interstitial fibrosis.

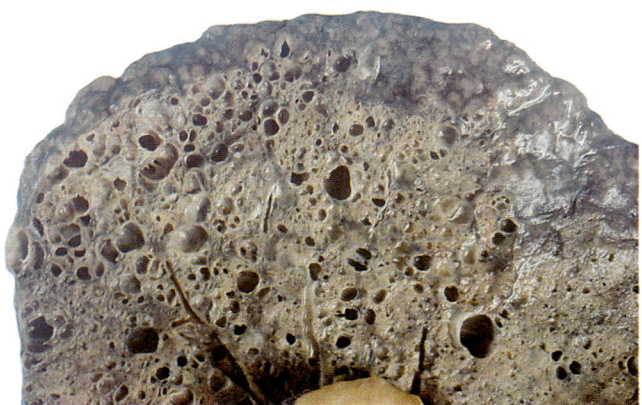

Fig. 13.78 Honeycomb lung, the end-stage of cryptogenic fibrosing alveolitis. Note the nodular pleural surface.

smooth muscle cells, and the subsequent laying down by these cells of reticulin fibres and collagen. The infiltration of inflammatory cells into the interstitium, the loss of type 1 pneumocytes and their replacement by type 2 pneumocytes, and the accumulation of macrophages in the alveolar spaces is probably a reaction to the initial insult. Viral infections, toxic damage, and immunological insults, all of which are known to cause pulmonary fibrosis, have been proposed as initiating agents. There are a number of immunologically mediated systemic illnesses, such as *rheumatoid arthritis, systemic lupus erythematosus*, and *ankylosing spondylitis*, that produce changes in the lung which are very similar to fibrosing alveolitis, but these similarities may merely reflect the limited repertoire of responses the lung tissue is capable of mounting to various forms of injury and do not necessarily imply common aetiology. A number of drugs are known to produce interstitial pneumonitis and fibrosis (see Section 13.3.5) but at the present time, in the majority of cases, the cause or causes of diffuse interstitial pulmonary fibrosis is unknown.

Lymphocytic interstitial pneumonia

Lymphocytic interstitial pneumonia is a chronic disorder characterized by a diffuse expansion of the pulmonary interstitium by mononuclear cells, chiefly mature lymphocytes, and probably represents a hyperplasia of the resident mucosa-associated lymphoid tissue (MALT) of the lung.

Clinical features

The condition is rare, usually affects women, and causes progressive dyspnoea or chronic cough. It may develop in the setting of *Sjögren's syndrome* or other auto-immune disease and is commonly associated with a dysproteinaemia. It is also a recognized feature of the acquired immunodeficiency syndrome (AIDS) in children. Radiologically, bilateral infiltrates of various decriptions are found, particularly in basal lung fields.

Pathology

Histologically, the entire interstitium is expanded by a mixed population of lymphocytes, plasma cells, and histiocytes. The lymphocytes may be arranged in nodules, sometimes forming germinal centres and there may be scattered granulomas. Bronchiolitis is not a feature. There are close similarities histologically with the primary malignant lymphoma of lung, low-grade B-cell lymphoma of mucosa-associated lymphoid tissue. The lymphoma may be distinguished by the immunohistochemical demonstration of light-chain restriction in the lymphocytic infiltrate or by gene rearrangement studies.

The course of lymphocytic interstitial pneumonitis is variable. It may remain static for many years or it may cause progressive destruction of alveolar tissue and scarring, resulting, ultimately, in *honeycomb lung* and *respiratory failure*. The response to steroid therapy and to immunosuppressive agents is also rather unpredictable.

Pulmonary alveolar proteinosis

Pulmonary alveolar proteinosis is a rare condition which causes progressive dyspnoea and bilateral radiological infiltrates due to the filling of the lung alveoli with dense proteinaceous fluid.

Clinical features

Those affected may be of any age but are usually middle-aged adults who notice dyspnoea developing insidiously over a period of months or years, associated with a cough productive of thick sputum. The radiological infiltrates are fine, diffuse, and perihilar, resembling pulmonary oedema.

Pathology

The histological appearances are very striking. The alveoli are filled with homogeneous eosinophilic proteinaceous fluid (Fig. 13.79) which stains with periodic acid-Schiff to give the characteristic magenta result. Degenerating cells and cholesterol crystals may be scattered here and there in the alveolar fluid. The protein-rich material contains a phospholipid which is similar in composition to surfactant, the substance produced by type 2 pneumocytes, which normally maintains low alveolar surface

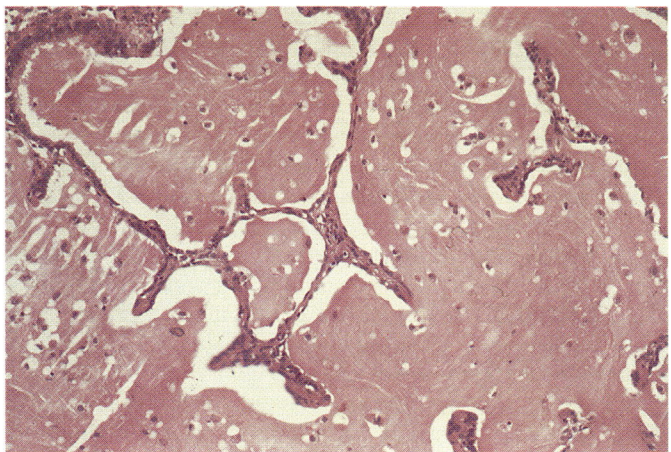

Fig. 13.79 Pulmonary alveolar proteinosis. The alveoli are filled with eosinophilic proteinaceous fluid.

tension. Indeed, with electron microscopy, lamellar bodies identical with those seen in the cytoplasm of type 2 pneumocytes may be found lying free in the fluid. The alveolar walls appear normal or show only very mild interstitial pneumonitis.

The disease is thought to be caused by an as yet unidentified defect of alveolar clearance mechanisms. In some patients the condition eventually clears spontaneously but the natural history is more often one of progressive filling of more and more alveolar tissue and the onset of respiratory failure. An effective treatment for this condition is *broncho-alveolar lavage*, a procedure in which saline is infused into the lung, one lobe at a time, via an endobronchial catheter and then drained away, removing the milky proteinaceous fluid. This procedure may produce prolonged clinical remission and can be repeated if the fluid reaccumulates, as is usually the case.

A reaction similar to pulmonary alveolar proteinosis is seen sometimes to opportunistic pulmonary infections in patients who are immunodeficient.

13.3.5 Lung disease caused by drugs and toxins

M. H. Griffiths

Introduction

A very large number of drugs and toxic substances have been reported to cause adverse reactions in the lung, but for only a proportion of these has the lung pathology been described in any detail. One of the problems of relating lung injury to a therapeutic substance is the usually non-specific nature of the reaction and it may be very difficult to decide whether a diffuse pulmonary abnormality has been caused by the drug in question, the disease being treated, a secondary condition such as infection, or by an unrelated event such as pulmonary embolism. Patients are often being treated with more than one drug,

and they may be receiving other potentially damaging therapy such as radiotherapy, the toxic effects of which may potentiate drug toxicity. Similar problems arise in the assessment of the effects of poisons of a non-therapeutic nature.

Some reactions are idiosyncratic, occurring only in certain susceptible individuals and involving the development of hypersensitivity, but other reactions are predictable, tending to occur with higher cumulative therapeutic doses or with deliberate intoxication. Those drugs for which a relationship between dose and toxicity has been established are indicated in the following tables with an asterisk.

Adverse reactions tend to fall into one of several histological patterns: *diffuse alveolar damage, interstitial pneumonitis, eosinophilic pneumonia, bronchiolitis obliterans, pulmonary haemorrhage, pulmonary oedema,* and *pleural inflammation and fibrosis,* all of which are described elsewhere in this chapter in association with other conditions. Several different adverse pulmonary reactions have been ascribed to some agents and these may involve several different pathogenetic mechanisms.

Diffuse alveolar damage

This is an acute reaction which involves alveolar capillary endothelial injury and, usually, alveolar epithelial necrosis and causes the clinical state known as the *adult respiratory distress syndrome*. The lungs are affected in a more or less generalized, if uneven, distribution. Drug toxicity is only one of many known causes of diffuse alveolar damage, and in most cases, no matter what the cause, the histological features of interstitial oedema, epithelial necrosis and regeneration, hyaline membrane formation, and interstitial fibrosis are similar (Table 13.8). Certain drugs produce additional changes which are more specific. *Busulphan, methotrexate,* and other cytotoxic drugs cause cytological atypia in the regenerating alveolar and bronchiolar epithelium. The cytomegally, nuclear pleomorphism, and nucleolar prominence may in fact be so dramatic as to simulate malignancy. Similar atypia is also seen in radiation injury.

Severe diffuse alveolar damage is rapidly fatal. Less severe damage may be reversible if the drug is discontinued and

Table 13.8 Drugs and toxins associated with diffuse alveolar damage

Cytotoxic drugs
  Bleomycin*
  Busulphan*
  Carmustine*(BCNU)
  Cyclophosphamide
  Methotrexate
  Mitomycin
Other agents
  Amiodarone*
  Amitriptyline overdose*
  Gold salts
  Hexamethonium
  Paraquat poisoning*
  Radiotherapy*

  * Dose related.

appropriate support therapy given, but there may be progression to diffuse interstitial fibrosis if the drug is continued.

Several different mechanisms of injury are recognized:

1. *Predictable injury* is usually dose-dependent. The toxic action may be direct or may involve the formation of intermediate products. There is experimental evidence that the toxicity of *bleomycin* is mediated through the generation of *superoxide radicals* (O_2^-). These reactive molecules are thought to participate in redox reactions, causing fatty acid oxidation and damage to cell membranes. Radiation can also generate reactive oxygen species, and it is of interest that the toxic effects of bleomycin on the lung can be potentiated by radiation or oxygen therapy. *Cyclophosphamide, nitrofurantoin*, and *paraquat* are also capable of generating oxidant molecules. These free radicals may also precipitate inflammatory reactions by oxidizing arachidonic acid, the initial step in the production of prostaglandins and leukotrienes. The activity of these oxidant molecules (which may be generated in many other ways, such as by cigarette smoke or by the activities of polymorphonuclear leucocytes and other phagocytes) is normally limited by antioxidant molecules. *Carmustine* and *cyclophosphamide* are thought to alter these antioxidase defences and to cause alveolar damage in this way. Fibrosis may be actively promoted by some drugs. *Bleomycin* has been shown experimentally to alter fibroblast growth and activity.

2. *Hypersensitivity reactions* are sporadic and unpredictable and are not dose related. *Methotrexate* toxicity, for example, is mediated via a hypersensitivity reaction, and *bleomycin* may sometimes act in this way. Corticosteroids may be effective in suppressing reactions of this type even when the drug is not discontinued.

Interstitial pneumonitis

Chronic interstitial pneumonitis is one of the more common adverse drug reactions (Table 13.9) and in many cases the pathological changes are those of the more chronic end of the spectrum of changes associated with acute diffuse alveolar damage, the mechanisms of injury being similar. It presents as breathlessness developing over weeks or months and associated with diffuse pulmonary radiological infiltrates. Histologically, lymphocytes, plasma cells, histiocytes, and sometimes eosinophils are seen in the alveolar interstitium. The alveolar septa are lined by cuboidal type 2 pneumocytes. Additional features characteristic of certain specific drugs or classes of drugs may be seen. *Methotrexate toxicity*, which is a hypersensitivity reaction, is associated with the formation of small non-necrotizing granulomas. Epithelial atypia is a feature typical of many cytotoxic drugs. *Amiodarone*, an anti-arrhythmic agent which is associated with pulmonary toxicity in a significant percentage of patients on higher maintenance doses, causes a pneumonitis characterized by the presence of foamy histiocytes in the interstitium and in the alveolar spaces (Fig. 13.80). The 'foamy' cytoplasm is seen by electron microscopy to be filled with membrane-bound lamellar inclusions, a change thought to represent an acquired lysosomal storage disease.

The interstitial pneumonitis in most cases resolves on discontinuation of the drug. In some cases a response to corticosteroid therapy has been recorded.

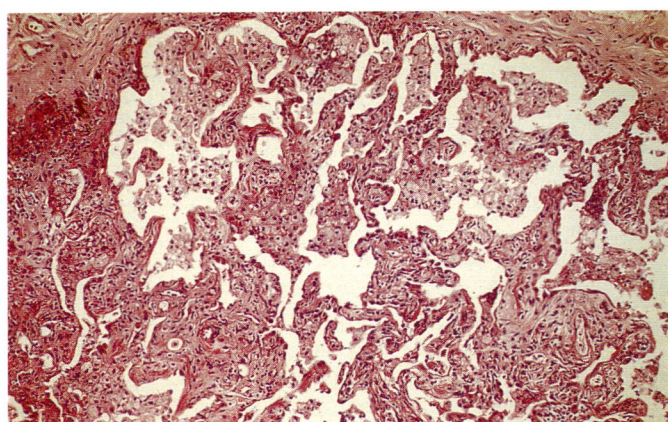
(a)

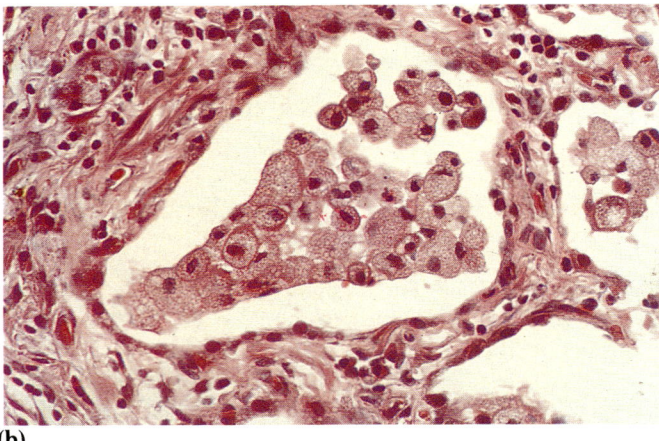
(b)

Fig. 13.80 Amiodarone lung. (a) Low power, showing interstitial pneumonitis. The alveoli are filled with foamy macrophages, seen in (b) at higher power, the result of a lysosomal storage disorder induced by the anti-arrhythmic drug, amiodarone.

Table 13.9 Drugs associated with interstitial pneumonitis

Cytotoxic drugs
  Busulphan*
  Carmustine (BCNU)*
  Chlorambucil
  Cyclophosphamide
  Methotrexate
  Procarbazine
Other drugs
  Amiodarone*
  Gold
  Nitrofurantoin

  * Dose related.

Eosinophilic pneumonia

The diagnosis of acute eosinophilic pneumonia usually rests on the discovery of radiological pulmonary infiltrates and an associated peripheral eosinophilia. Lung biopsy is rarely performed so the pathology is not well described. The infiltrates clear rapidly on discontinuation of the drug. Several drugs are associated with this condition (Table 13.10).

Table 13.10 Drugs associated with eosinophilic pneumonia

Bleomycin
Naproxen
Nitrofurantoin
Phenylbutazone
Pyrimethamine
Sulphasalazine

Bronchiolitis obliterans

Bronchiolitis obliterans, organizing pneumonia (BOOP) is a distinctive, if non-specific, reaction to a number of infective and toxic insults, including drugs (Table 13.11). It is recognized histologically by the proliferation within the lumens of the respiratory bronchioles and alveolar ducts of rounded masses of granulation tissue. There may be interstitial pneumonitis as well. Recovery on discontinuing the drug is the rule.

Table 13.11 Drugs associated with bronchiolitis obliterans

Amiodarone*
Gold
Methotrexate
Mitomycin

* Dose related.

Lung haemorrhage

Diffuse alveolar haemorrhage has been reported in a group of severely neutropenic patients who have been treated with a combination of *amphotericin B* and *leucocyte transfusion* (Table 13.12). It is also seen, rarely, as a complication of anticoagulation therapy and in drug-induced thrombocytopenia (*cyclophosphamide*) and thrombotic thrombocytopenia (*mitomycin*). Pulmonary haemorrhage is a serious side-effect of *penicillamine*

Table 13.12 Drugs associated with lung haemorrhage

Amphotericin B
Anticoagulants
Cyclophosphamide
Hydralazine
Mitomycin
Penicillamine*

* Dose related.

---

therapy used in the treatment of Wilson's disease, primary biliary cirrhosis, rheumatoid arthritis and other diseases. Haemoptysis and haematuria are the presenting symptoms of the 'pulmonary–renal' syndrome, which is fatal in up to 50 per cent of cases.

Pulmonary oedema

Various sedative drugs such as *chlordiazepoxide* (Librium), *paraldehyde*, and *ethchlorvinol* (Placidyl) have induced pulmonary oedema, usually after overdosage, and so, occasionally, have certain antipsychotic drugs. Intoxication with *salicylates* and opiates such as *heroin* and *codeine*, and with opiate antagonists, may cause pulmonary oedema (Table 13.13). It usually responds to supportive care. Pulmonary oedema is a relatively common side-effect of high-dose *cytosine arabinocide* therapy for acute leukaemia, a complication that is, again, usually reversible.

Table 13.13 Drugs associated with pulmonary oedema

Chlordiazepoxide*
Codeine*
Cytosine arabinoside*
Ethchlorvinol*
Heroin*
Hydrochlorothiazide
Methodone*
Mitomycine
Nalbuphine
Naloxone
Paraldehyde*
Propoxyphene*
Salicylates*
Tocolytic agents

* Dose related.

Pleural inflammation and fibrosis

Pleural inflammation may occur as part of a pulmonary toxic reaction (Table 13.14), e.g. *amiodarone, bleomycin, carmustine,* or as an independent manifestation of toxicity. The serotonin antagonist *methisergide* and the chemically related drugs *bromocriptine* and *mesulergine*, which are used in the management of Parkinson's disease, cause pleural fibrosis but are not toxic to the lung. *Hydralazine* is one of the drugs that causes pleurisy or pleuropericarditis as part of a *Lupus-like syndrome*.

Table 13.14 Drugs associated with pleural inflammation and fibrosis

Amiodarone*
Bleomycin*
Bromocriptine, mesulergine
Carmustine (BCNU)*
Hydralazine
Methysergide

* Dose related.

In all these conditions recovery is usual on discontinuing the drug responsible.

13.3.6 Sarcoidosis

A. R. Gibbs

Definition and clinical features

Sarcoidosis is a multisystem disorder of unknown aetiology characterized by *non-caseating granulomas* in various organs. The organs most commonly involved are intrathoracic (85 per cent), reticuloendothelial system (34 per cent), skin (34 per cent), ocular (27 per cent), nervous system (5 per cent), but almost any organ can be affected (James and Jones Williams 1985). In the majority of cases sarcoidosis is a benign and self-limiting disease, but about 3 per cent of patients die from its complications. The clinical presentation is dependent on which organs are involved, but cough, dyspnoea, erythema nodosum, and ocular symptoms are common. A considerable proportion of patients are asymptomatic but have an abnormal chest X-ray.

In Britain the incidence has been reported as between 0.21 and 0.54 per 10 000 population. Sixty per cent of cases occur in females. Any age may be affected, but 70 per cent of patients are less than 40 years old at presentation. In the USA, sarcoidiosis is many times more common in Blacks than in Whites.

There is an internationally agreed radiological classification system (Flint and Johnson 1986).

Type 0 normal chest X-ray (0–20 per cent) (extrathoracic sarcoidosis);

Type 1 bilateral hilar lymphadenopathy alone (40 per cent);

Type 2 bilateral hilar lymphadenopathy and diffuse pulmonary infiltration (25 per cent);

Type 3 diffuse pulmonary infiltration without hilar lymphadenopathy (10–15 per cent);

Type 4 pulmonary fibrosis (5–10 per cent).

Good prognosis factors include an abrupt onset, erythema nodusum, uveitis, arthralgia, and radiological types 1 and 2. The disease often remits spontaneously within 2 years of the onset. An insidious onset may be followed by progressive pulmonary fibrosis, the most frequent cause of death in this disease.

Diagnosis

Non-caseating granulomas, although characteristic, are not specific for sarcoidosis. Similar granulomas may be caused by a variety of agents (Table 13.15). It is mandatory to exclude a wide range of causative agents such as mycobacteria, fungi, and chemicals before sarcoidosis is diagnosed. All available clinical, radiological, microbiological, immunological, and histopathological information should be considered.

Table 13.15 Diseases characterized by granulomas

Bacteria, e.g. mycobacteria, *Yersinia, Brucella,* spirochaetes (*Chlamydia*)
Protozoa, e.g. *Toxoplasma*
Metazoa, e.g. *Schistosoma*
Viruses, e.g. cat-scratch disease
Fungi, e.g. *Aspergillus, Histoplasma*
Chemicals, e.g. beryllium, talc
Extrinsic allergic alveolitis, e.g. farmer's lung
Sarcoidosis
Crohn's disease
Vasculitides, e.g. Wegener's granulomatosis
Neoplasia, e.g. malignant lymphomas

The *Kveim–Siltzbach test* is frequently used in diagnosis. This consists of an intracutaneous inoculation of autoclaved or irradiated sarcoid material from spleen or lymph nodes. The area of inoculation is marked and biopsied 4–6 weeks later. The presence of sarcoid granulomas in the biopsy indicates a positive result. The overall rate of positivity is greater than 80 per cent; however, the rate may fall to 30 per cent in the chronic forms of sarcoidosis. Another useful investigation is the level of *serum angiotensin-converting enzyme,* which is raised in approximately 60 per cent of patients with sarcoidosis. *Broncho-alveolar lavage* with differential cell counts, although previously advocated by some investigators, does not appear to be reliable in diagnosing or monitoring the activity of sarcoidosis.

Pathology

The sarcoid granuloma is usually well demarcated and comprises a central collection of epithelioid cells interspersed with giant cells of both Langhans and foreign body type and a periphery of lymphocytes. Necrosis is absent or inconspicuous (Fig. 13.81). Reticulin is present within the centres of sarcoid granulomas, whereas it is absent in tuberculosis granulomas. Various

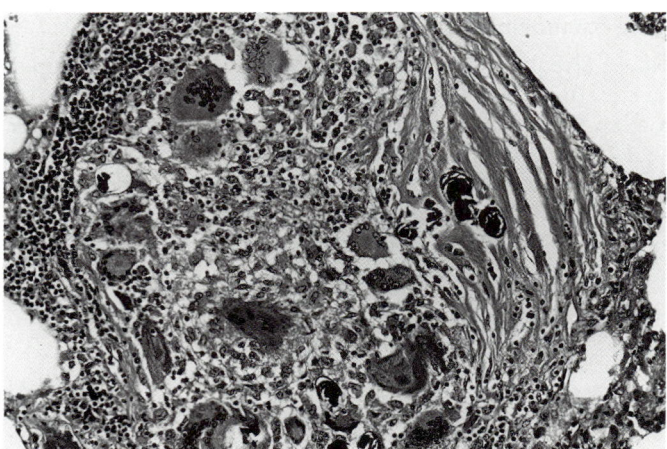

Fig. 13.81 A sarcoid granuloma containing epithelioid cells, giant cells of both Langhans and foreign body type and several Schaumann bodies. The periphery of the granuloma shows lymphocytes and fibrosis.

types of inclusion body may be present within the epithelioid and giant cells; these are more frequent in sarcoid than other granulomas, although not pathognomonic. These include

1. *Schaumann bodies*, which are large conchoidal basophilic bodies containing iron- and calcium-impregnated mucoprotein; and

2. *asteroid bodies*, which are bright eosinophilic star-shaped bodies composed of lipoprotein.

The sarcoid granuloma can either disappear or fibrose and become hyalinized.

Since the lungs are affected in more than 80 per cent of cases, transbronchial biopsy is highly effective in yielding sarcoid granulomas. It can be positive in those with apparently normal chest X-rays.

Macroscopically, in the acute form the lungs show multiple grey-white rounded lesions measuring 2–3 mm in diameter, but occasionally forming nodules up to 2 cm in diameter. In the chronic form the fibrosis is bilateral and maximal in the upper zones, often with honeycombing (see Section 13.4). Microscopically, the granulomas are well demarcated and located within the interstitium of the lung, around airways and vessels, interlobular septa, and subpleurally. They are frequently present in the submucosa of large bronchi and may cause *bronchostenosis*. Even in those lungs where fibrosis has become severe the granulomas persist in sarcoidosis, whereas in the chronic fibrotic stage of allergic alveolitis (hypersensitivity pneumonitis) the granulomas have frequently disappeared, a useful feature in differential diagnosis.

Pathogenesis

It is believed that the cause of the sarcoid granuloma is inhalation of an unknown antigen; putative agents include mycobacteria, viruses, mycoplasma, fungi, *Propionibacterium*, organic, and inorganic materials. The antigen, which is persistent or poorly degradable, is processed and presented by alveolar macrophage to T-lymphocytes, which then produce lymphokines, such as chemotactic factor for monocytes and interleukins 1 and 2. These

1. aid in *macrophage recruitment* from the blood;

2. prevent *macrophage migration* and;

3. *stimulate T4 helper cells.*

Thus the granuloma develops a centre of activated macrophages, which later form epithelioid cells and giant cells, and T-helper lymphocytes. The periphery of the granuloma comprises antigen-presenting interdigitating macrophages and T-suppressor lymphocytes. The T-helper cells cause the B-cells to produce immunoglobulins and antibodies. Interleukin-2 does not stimulate blood T-lymphocytes, which are reduced in number in the peripheral blood, and accounts for the relative T-cell anergy away from sites of disease activity (James and Jones Williams 1985; Schonfeld and Johns 1986).

13.3.7 Uraemic lung

A. R. Gibbs

Clinical manifestations

The patient who typically develops uraemic lung or pneumonitis is usually severely azotaemic and in acute rather than chronic renal failure (Rackow *et al.* 1978). The patient is dyspnoeic and rales are found at the lung bases. The chest X-ray shows a 'bat's wing' appearance.

Pathology

The changes in the lung are those of *diffuse alveolar damage* (see Section 13.4). The lungs are heavy and oedematous at autopsy. Microscopically, there is congestion of the alveolar septa and a fibrinous exudate within the alveoli, often with hyaline membrane formation (Fig. 13.82). In long-standing cases *bronchiolitis obliterans* may be observed. A quarter of the cases who come to autopsy with uraemic lung also show *fibrinous pleuritis* and *pericarditis*.

Pathogenesis

The factors involved in the production of these changes are complex, and include haemodynamic and permeability events. There is fluid retention in uraemia because there is impaired handling of ions and water by the kidneys and an element of left ventricular failure. This, combined with increased permeability of pulmonary capillaries, probably due to a toxic metabolite of the kidneys, results in leakage of protein-rich exudate from the capillaries into the lungs. Nowadays, with haemodialysis, this picture is rather uncommon and a more likely cause of pulmonary X-ray shadowing is infection.

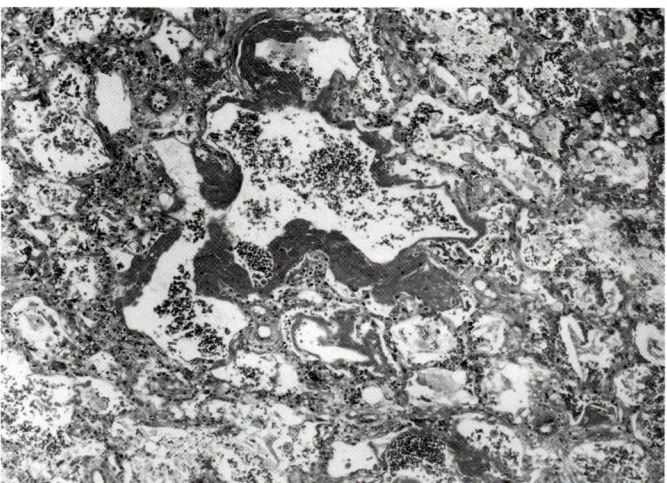

Fig. 13.82 Uraemic pneumonitis showing hyaline membranes, interstitial oedema and lymphoid infiltrate, and intra-alveolar collections of macrophages and red blood cells.

Calcinosis

Calcification of the lungs may occur in chronic renal failure when there is alteration of serum calcium and phosphorus levels. It is distributed along the alveolar walls and within vessels (Heath and Robertson 1977).

13.3.8   Rheumatoid lung disease

A. R. Gibbs

Rheumatoid disease is a systemic condition in which joint manifestations usually predominate but many other organs can be affected. The latex test demonstrates a rheumatoid factor titre greater than 1:160 in 80 per cent of patients. Rheumatoid disease is three times more common in women than in men. The association with pulmonary disease is well recognized and can take several forms (Table 13.16). The prevalence of lung disease is unknown, but it is greater in men than in women. The pulmonary manifestations can occasionally precede, but usually follow, the onset of rheumatoid joint disease. Signs and symptoms include dyspnoea, cough (which may be productive), fever, weight loss, weakness, wheeze, and cyanosis (Yousem *et al.* 1985).

Table 13.16   Forms of lung disease associated with rheumatoid arthritis

Pleural effusion and inflammation
Interstitial lung disease
Necrobiotic nodules
Rheumatoid pneumoconiosis (Caplan's syndrome)
Bronchiolitis
Vasculitis

Pleural effusion and inflammation

Pleurisy, which may be accompanied by effusion, occurs in up to 50 per cent of patients with rheumatoid arthritis (Walker and Wright 1968). The effusion is frequently unilateral, may be large, and persists over several months, although it eventually resolves spontaneously.

Pathology

The pleura shows an infiltrate of lymphocytes and plasma cells with a fibrinous exudate on the surface; in approximately half the cases pallisading of fibroblasts and histiocytes is seen, which is virtually pathognomonic of rheumatoid pleuritis (Fig. 13.83).

Interstitial lung disease

This occurs in approximately 1–2 per cent of patients with rheumatoid arthritis. Pulmonary manifestations usually appear within 4 years of the first joint symptoms. The severity of lung disease does not always parallel that of the joints. The most

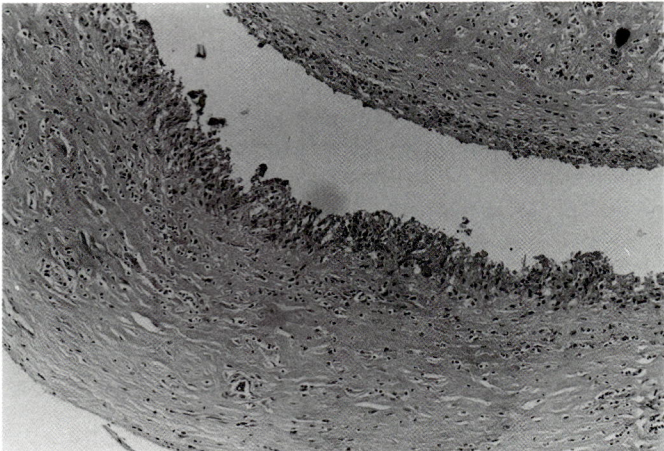

Fig. 13.83   Rheumatoid pleuritis, showing pallisading of fibroblasts, and macrophages at the surface.

important clinical symptoms and signs are cough, finger clubbing, and basal crepitations which may lead to respiratory failure and death. This form of rheumatoid lung disease carries the worst prognosis.

Pathology

The changes, which may include honeycombing, are most marked in the lower zones of the lungs and are identical to the *idiopathic form of diffuse interstitial fibrosis* (DIF). The fibrosis probably develops on the basis of diffuse alveolar damage (see Section 13.4). Immunoglobulins, but not complement, have been demonstrated in the lungs of some cases. The significance of these findings is unclear.

Necrobiotic nodules

Pulmonary necrobiotic nodules are uncommon. They are often multiple, discrete, located near to the pleura, and may spontaneously resolve, persist, or cavitate. They vary in size from a few millimetres to several centimetres. They are often asymptomatic and have a favourable prognosis.

Pathology

They are similar in appearance to rheumatoid nodules at other sites. They have a central zone of fibrinoid necrosis bordered by pallisaded histiocytes and fibroblasts.

Rheumatoid pneumoconiosis

The development, often rapidly, of multiple, rounded, and well-defined radiological opacities in coal-workers with rheumatoid arthritis was described by Caplan in 1953. Hence the eponymous term *Caplan's syndrome*. Caplan lesions do not usually cause any functional impairment.

Pathology

The opacities are due to nodules, measuring up to several centimeters in diameter, which show concentric laminations,

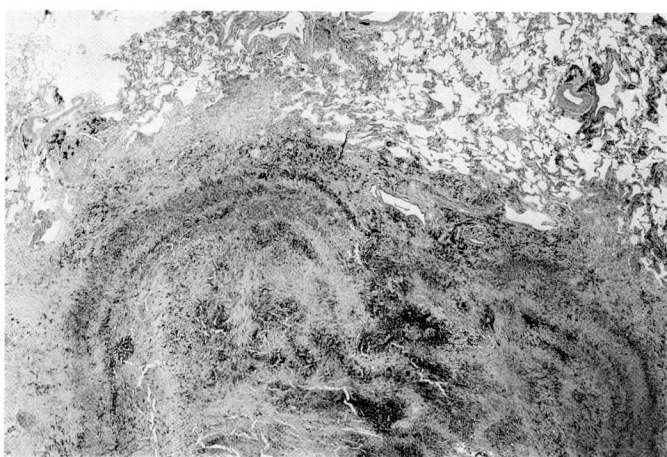

Fig. 13.84 A Caplan lesion in a coal-worker, showing laminated dust collections.

representing several dust layers formed by episodes of inflammatory activity. The central zone is necrotic and the peripheral zone contains lymphocytes and plasma cells (Fig. 13.84).

Bronchiolitis

Airway obstruction due to obliterative bronchiolitis is an uncommon but recognized complication of rheumatoid arthritis, which may cause death.

Pathology

The small airways less than 1 cm in diameter show a variety of changes, including mural fibrosis, hyperplasia of lymphoid tissue, and granulation tissue polyps within the lumen.

Vasculitis

Vasculitis affecting the lung is an extremely rare complication of rheumatoid disease.

13.3.9   Further reading

Chronic obstructive airways disease

Bake, B., Larson, S., and Mossberg, B. (1982). Chronic bronchitis in non-smokers. *European Journal of Respiratory Diseases* 63 (Suppl. 118).

Barker, A. F. and Bardana, E. J. (1988). Bronchiectasis. Update of an orphan disease. *American Review of Respiratory Disease* 137, 969–78.

CIBA Guest Symposium (1959). Terminology, definitions and classification of chronic pulmonary emphysema and related conditions. *Thorax* 14, 286–99.

Dunnill, M. S. (1982). *Pulmonary pathology*. Churchill Livingstone, Edinburgh.

Dunnill, M. S., Massarella, G. R., and Anderson, J. A. (1969). A comparison of the quantitative anatomy of the bronchi in normal subjects, in status asthmaticus, in chronic bronchitis and in emphysema. *Thorax* 24, 176–9.

Gross, P., Babjak, M. A., Tolkar, E., and Kaschak, M. (1964). Enzym-

atically produced pulmonary emphysema: a preliminary report. *Journal of Occupational Medicine* 6, 481–4.

Heard, B. E., Khatchatourov, V., Otto, H., Putov, N., and Sobin, L. (1979). The morphology of emphysema, chronic bronchitis and bronchiectasis. Definition, nomenclature and classification. *Journal of Clinical Pathology* 32, 882–92.

Kerrebijn, K. F., Sluiter, H. J., and Quarijer, Ph. H. (1982). Small airways and CARA. *European Journal of Respiratory Diseases* 63, (Suppl. 121).

Laurell, C. B. and Eriksson, S. (1963). The electrophoretic alpha 1-globulin pattern of serum in alpha 1-antitrypsin deficiency. *Scandinavian Journal of Clinical and Laboratory Investigation* 15, 132–40.

Lungarella, G., Fonzi, L., and Emini, G. (1983). Abnormalities of bronchial cilia in patients with chronic bronchitis. *Lung* 161, 167–57.

Reid, L. (1960). Measurement of bronchial mucus gland layer: A diagnostic yardstick in chronic bronchitis. *Thorax* 15, 132–41.

Snider, G. L., Kleineman, J., Thurlbeck, W. M., and Bengali, Z. (1985). The definition of emphysema. Report of a National Heart, Lung and Blood Institute, Division of Lung Diseases, Workshop. *American Review of Respiratory Disease* 132, 182–5.

Snider, L., Lucey, E., and Stone, P. (1986). Animal models of emphysema. *American Review of Respiratory Disease* 133, 149–69.

Thurlbeck, W. M. (1988). *Pathology of the lung*. Thieme, New York.

Whitwell, F. (1952). Study of pathology and pathogenesis of bronchiectasis. *Thorax* 7, 213–39.

Asthma and allergic disease

Dail, D. H. and Hamman, S. P. (1988). *Pulmonary pathology*. Springer-Verlag, New York.

Dunnill, M. S. (1987). *Pulmonary pathology* (2nd edn). Churchill Livingstone, Edinburgh.

Interstitial lung disease

Dail, D. H. and Hamman, S. P. (1988). *Pulmonary pathology*. Springer-Verlag, New York.

Drugs and toxins

Cooper, J. A. D., White, D. A., and Matthay, R. A. (1986). Drug-induced pulmonary disease. Part 1. *American Review of Respiratory Disease* 133, 321–40.

Cooper, J. A. D., White, D. A., and Matthay, R. A. (1986). Drug-induced pulmonary disease. Part 2. *American Review of Respiratory Disease* 133, 488–505.

Katzenstein, A.-L. A. and Askin, F. B. (1960). *Surgical pathology of non-neoplastic lung disease* (2nd edn). W. B. Saunders, Philadelphia.

Sarcoidosis

Flint, K. and Johnson, N. (1986). Intrathoracic sarcoidosis. *Seminars in Respiratory Medicine* 8, 41–51.

Gibbs, A. R. and Jones Williams, W. (1986). The pathology of sarcoidosis. *Seminars in Respiratory Medicine* 8, 10–16.

Gibbs, A. R. and Seal, R. M. E. (1982). *Atlas of pulmonary pathology*. MTP Press, Lancaster.

James, D. G. and Jones Williams, W. (1985). *Sarcoidosis and other granulomatous diseases*. W. B. Saunders, Philadelphia.

Schonfeld, S. A. and Johns, C. J. (1986). Sarcoidosis. In *Recent advances in respiratory medicine*, Vol. 4 (ed. D. C. Flenley and T. L. Petty), pp. 109–30. Churchill Livingstone, Edinburgh.

Williams, G. T. and Jones Williams, W. (1983). Granulamatous inflammation—a review. *Journal of Clinical Pathology* 36, 723–33.

Uraemic lung

Edelman, N. H. (1980). The lungs and ventilation in uremia. In *Pulmonary diseases and disorders*, (ed. A. P. Fishman), ch. 123. McGraw-Hill, New York.

Heath, D. and Robertson, A. J. (1977). Pulmonary calcinosis. *Thorax* **32**, 606–11.

Rackow, E. C., Fern, I. A., Sprung, C., and Grodman, R. S. (1978). Uremic pulmonary edema. *American Journal of Medicine* **64**, 1084–8.

Rheumatoid lung disease

Caplan, A. (1953). Certain unusual radiological appearances in the chest of coal miners suffering rheumatoid arthritis. *Thorax* **8**, 29–37.

Crofton, J. and Douglas, A. (1981). *Respiratory diseases* (3rd edn). Blackwell, Oxford.

Gibbs, A. R. and Seal, R. M. E. (1981). *Atlas of pulmonary pathology*. MTP Press, Lancaster.

Walker, W. C. and Wright, V. (1968). Pulmonary manifestations and rheumatoid arthritis. *Medicine* **47**, 501–20.

Yousem, S. A., Colby, T. V., and Carrington, C. B. (1985). Lung biopsy in rheumatoid arthritis. *American Review of Respiratory Disease* **131**, 770–7.

13.4   Lung fibrosis including dust diseases

Allen R. Gibbs and J. Christopher Wagner

Fibrosis of the lung can result from a wide variety of injuries and can range from *small focal scars*, such as those occurring after healing of a small pulmonary infarct, to *multifocal areas of fibrosis*, developing in relation to silica dust deposition, and to *diffuse interstitial fibrosis*. The latter may cause clinical disability and even death, while small focal scars have no clinical significance. In this chapter we shall concentrate on diffuse interstitial pulmonary fibrosis and certain dust diseases.

13.4.1   Diffuse interstitial fibrosis (DIF)

DIF may be the sequel to a wide range of insults to the lung (Fig. 13.85). It usually presents as extensive disease when the initial cause may be unrecognizable. When no clinical or pathological clues to the aetiology of DIF are present it is usually called *cryptogenic fibrosing alveolitis* or *fibrosing alveolitis* in this country. In North America it is called usual *interstitial pneumonia*. It is a diagnosis largely made by exclusion.

Pathology

The lungs from cases of DIF appear firm, heavy, and often shrunken. The external surfaces are frequently bosselated (Fig. 13.86). If the lungs are not inflated and honeycombing is absent, the fact that the lungs are abnormal can easily be missed since the cut surface may show only slight accentuation of the normal markings or induration. If honeycomb change is present, the abnormality is obvious. *Honeycomb lung* is both a radiological and pathological term for lungs which show fibrosis and enlarged air spaces which vary from a few millimetres to a centimetre or more in size (Fig. 13.86). Contrast this with emphysema where the walls of the enlarged spaces are thin and not fibrotic. Honeycombing is due to disorganization of the pulmonary architecture by fibrosis, with the formation of blind-

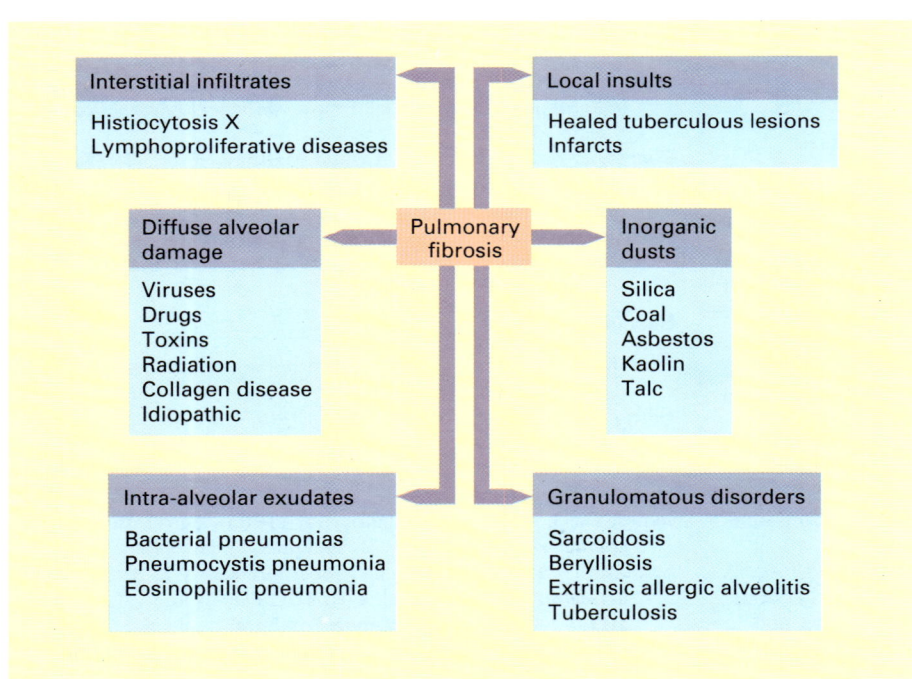

Fig. 13.85   Pathways to pulmonary fibrosis.

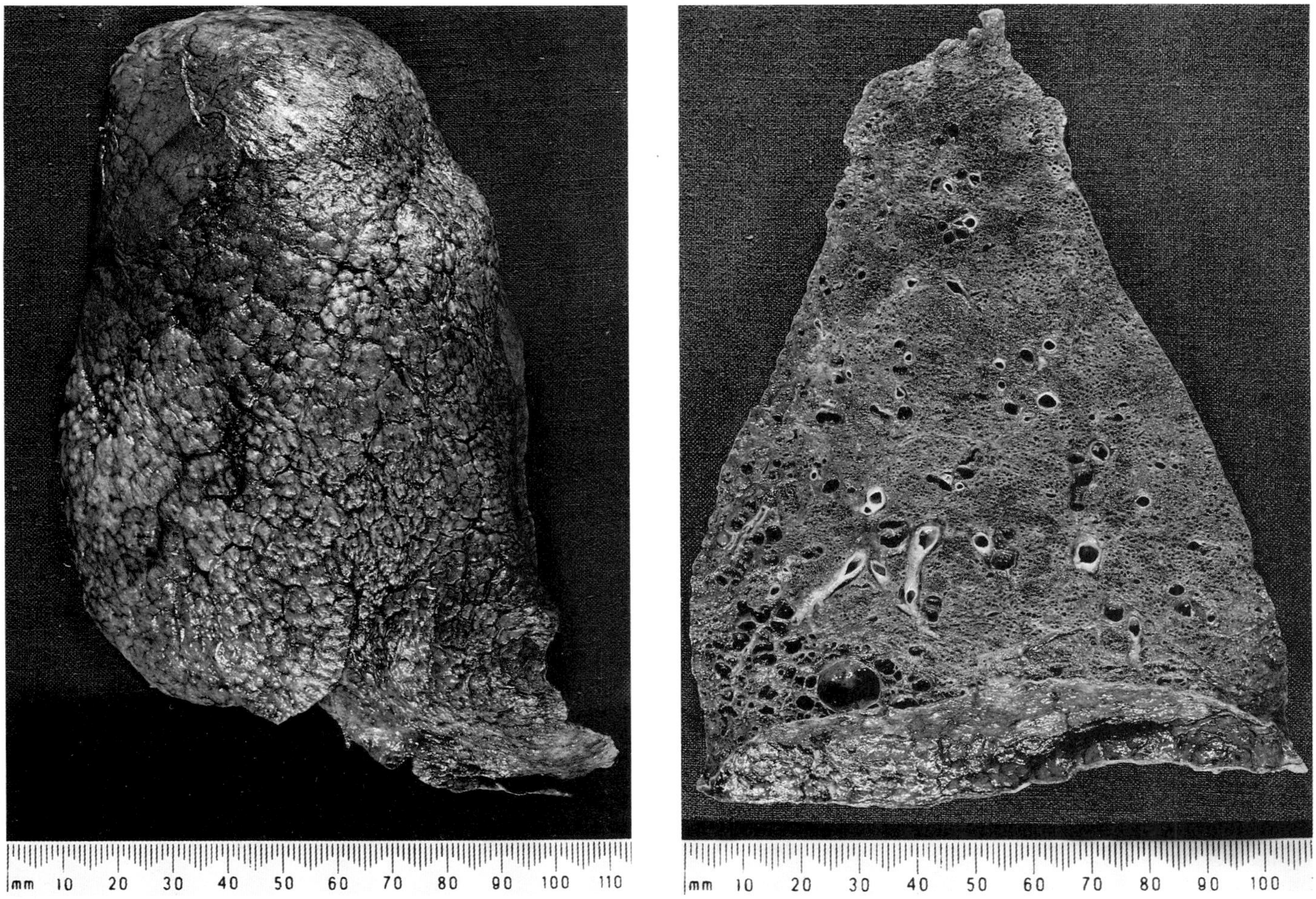

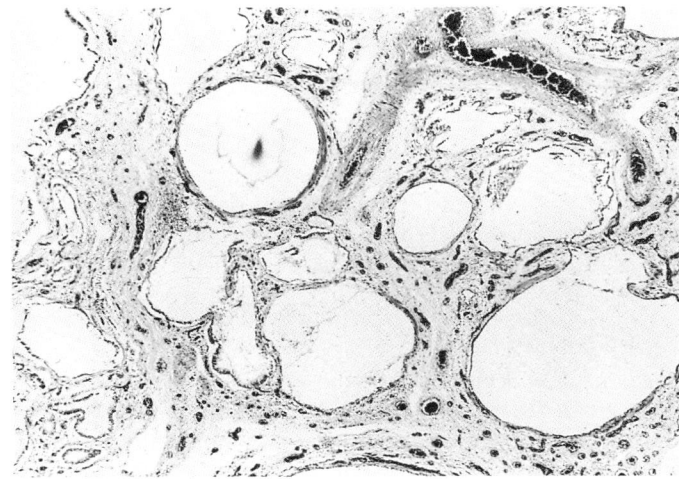

(a)   **(b)**

Fig. 13.86 (a) External surface of the lung from a case of cryptogenic fibrosing alveolitis, showing the typical bosselated appearance. (b) Cut surface of the lung, showing fibrotic lung with enlarged spaces (honeycomb lung) most severe in the lower zone.

ending, dilated bronchioles (Heppleston 1956). It can be seen in virtually any type of DIF, regardless of aetiology.

Microscopically, there are bands of fibrosis with reduction of alveoli and metaplasia of the epithelium of the dilated bronchioles to columnar or squamous types (Fig. 13.87). There are numerous lymphocytes and plasma cells present, sometimes with follicle formation within the interstitium. There is often muscle hyperplasia within the interstitium. There are varying numbers of mononuclear cells within the alveolar spaces, shown by electron microscopy to be macrophages and type 2 pneumocytes. If this intra-alveolar component is prominent in biopsies, the patient may show clinical improvement with corticosteroid treatment.

Clinical features

DIF is characterized by progressive and unremitting dyspnoea, dry cough, and fine crackles on auscultation. Finger clubbing is present in 60 per cent of patients. Any age can be affected, but

Fig. 13.87 Thickened fibrotic bands intermingled with dilated bronchiolar structures with loss of alveoli (from the same case as Fig. 13.86).

the majority of patients are between 40 and 60 years old. Sex incidence is equal. Radiological changes may be absent in the early stages, even when there is dyspnoea and when biopsy would reveal well-established interstitial fibrosis. Small irregular shadows with a basal distribution, sometimes with honeycombing, indicate advanced disease. Functional abnormalities include:

1. *a restrictive pattern* with decreased vital capacity and normal FEV/FVC ratio; and
2. *reduction in diffusing capacity.*

The prognosis is generally poor, with a mean survival from first symptoms to death of 6.0 years (Hay and Turner-Warwick 1986). In approximately 10 per cent of cases there is associated collagen disease, such as rheumatoid disease or systemic lupus erythematosus (SLE). A number of familial cases have now been reported.

Pathways to DIF

These can be considered under five headings.

Organization of intra-alveolar exudates

It is important to realize that interstitial fibrosis may originate from organization of an intra-alveolar exudate. If, for example, there is delayed resolution of a bacterial pneumonia, then fibroblasts may grow from the alveolar wall into the inflammatory exudate within the alveolar space so that the exudate becomes attached to the wall. Later there is retraction of the collagen, which causes the inflammatory exudate to become layered on the wall. The alveolar epithelium then grows over the exudate so that it now becomes incorporated into the interstitium. If the lung is examined at this stage, the intra-alveolar origin of the fibrosis will not be apparent.

Organization of interstitial infiltrates

Where there is an interstitial infiltrate with little intra-alveolar exudate, the collagen formation may develop within the interstitial space. A typical example is *histiocytosis X*.

Organization of granulomas

Granulomas are usually within the interstitium and organization of these can lead to interstitial fibrosis. Examples include *sarcoidosis* or *extrinsic allergic alveolitis*. However, a prominent interstitial inflammatory infiltrate is frequently present in addition to the granulomas, which also may undergo organization. This latter component is often more important than the granulomas in the development of fibrosis, particularly in extrinsic allergic alveolitis.

Incorporation of dusts

Dusts usually deposit within the alveolar spaces around the respiratory bronchioles. They are then phagocytosed by macrophages and some are taken by the macrophages to the interstitium between the alveolar walls and around the respiratory bronchioles. Depending on the fibrogenic properties of the dust, variable amounts of collagen are deposited. If the

fibrosis progresses, as it may well do in asbestosis, then the fibrosis extends out from the walls of the respiratory bronchioles to involve the walls of the adjacent alveolar ducts and alveoli. This may link up with fibrotic bands extending from the respiratory bronchioles of adjacent lobules. If this becomes widespread, the result is diffuse interstitial fibrosis, often with honeycombing.

Diffuse alveolar damage (DAD)

DAD is characterized by varying combinations of damage to the alveolar epithelium and endothelium of the alveolar walls. Many agents can cause this damage (Fig. 13.85), either directly or by the generation of toxic radicals or by the formation of immune complexes. The injurious agent may reach the lung via the airways or via the bloodstream. In individual cases the injurious agent is frequently not identified.

Ultrastructural studies have shown oedema of the type 1 pneumocytes and the endothelial cells, which often die within a few days. Since the type 1 pneumocytes have a much greater surface area than the type 2 pneumocytes, they are more liable to injury. The consequence of this is capillary congestion and intra-alveolar oedema, often with leakage of fibrin. After a day or two, hyaline membranes are formed by layering of a protein-rich exudate along the surface of the alveolar ducts and respiratory bronchioles (see Fig. 13.82). By about 3 days after injury, macrophages, type 2 pneumocytes, and red blood cells are conspicuous within the alveolar spaces, and lymphocytes and plasma cells within the interstitial space. At the end of about 1 week, the alveolar lining epithelial cells appear cuboidal in shape, whereas normally they cannot be visualized by the light microscope. This is due to proliferation and migration of the type 2 pneumocytes. After about 1 week, interstitial fibrosis becomes apparent, and after 2–3 weeks the changes may seem surprisingly chronic and merge with DIF.

Clinical features

DAD is characterized by severe dyspnoea, severe hypoxaemia, and diffuse pulmonary infiltrates on chest X-ray. A number of different names have been given to this syndrome occurring in various clinical situations, including *adult respiratory distress syndrome, acquired respiratory distress syndrome, shock lung,* and *respiratory insufficiency syndrome,* but they all have similar clinical, physiological, and pathological features. There are three possible sequelae to DAD:

1. resolution of the changes with recovery of the affected individual, which occurs if the damage is not too severe and if there are not repeated insults;
2. if the damage is severe, death may occur in the acute phase; or
3. if the damage smoulders on or there are repeated insults, then diffuse interstitial fibrosis may develop.

13.4.2   Asbestosis

Asbestosis is defined as diffuse pulmonary fibrosis caused by inhalation of asbestos dust. Its development requires heavy exposure and the *amphibole types* of asbestos are the most important in its causation (see Section 10.2).

Pathology

In the fully developed case the lungs will be reduced in size and show grey-white areas, most severe in the lower zones. Cystic spaces (honeycombing) may also be present in relation to the areas of fibrosis. Often pearly white parietal pleural plaques are also present, although they are not strictly part of the asbestosis picture. Microscopically, interstitial fibrosis will be seen which commences around respiratory bronchioles and extends to involve the alveolar ducts and alveoli and eventually results in gross distortion of the pulmonary architecture (Fig. 10.4, Section 10.2). The pathognomonic feature of asbestosis is the presence of yellow-brown beaded bodies (*asbestos bodies*) measuring greater than 30 μm in length, which are due to coating of the transparent asbestos fibres by protein and iron. Otherwise the changes are indistinguishable from cryptogenic fibrosing alveolitis.

Clinical features

There is dyspnoea, cough, weakness, cyanosis, weight loss, finger clubbing, and basal crackles. The disease is well advanced pathologically (usually more than a third of the lungs are involved) before clinical and radiological signs become apparent. The disease may present and progress long after the exposure has ceased.

13.4.3 Coal-workers' pneumoconiosis (CWP)

CWP requires prolonged exposure to coal dust, which usually contains less than 5 per cent of free silica. It shows distinct differences from silicosis, but the latter may develop in a minority of coal-workers who are exposed to coal dust with a high free silica content, for example hard-headers. CWP is commonly divided into two types: *simple* and *complicated*.

Pathology

Simple CWP is characterized by numerous black stellate macules situated most prevalently in the upper zones of the lungs (Fig. 13.88). They average a few millimetres in diameter and are usually surrounded by small spaces (*focal emphysema*) which are, in fact, *dilated respiratory bronchioles*. Since coal dust has a low fibrogenic potential, the macules are usually soft or impalpable and contain little collagen. The lesions consist of macrophages containing coal dust admixed with reticulin and a very small amount of collagen. By definition, no coal dust lesion exceeds 1 cm in diameter, although some authorities take 2 cm as the defining limit.

Complicated CWP, or progressive massive fibrosis (PMF), refers to conditions in which at least one coal dust lesion exceeds 1 or 2 cm in diameter. The PMF lesion is usually black, soft, and may reach 10 cm or more in diameter (Fig. 13.89). These lesions are usually located in the upper zones of the lungs and

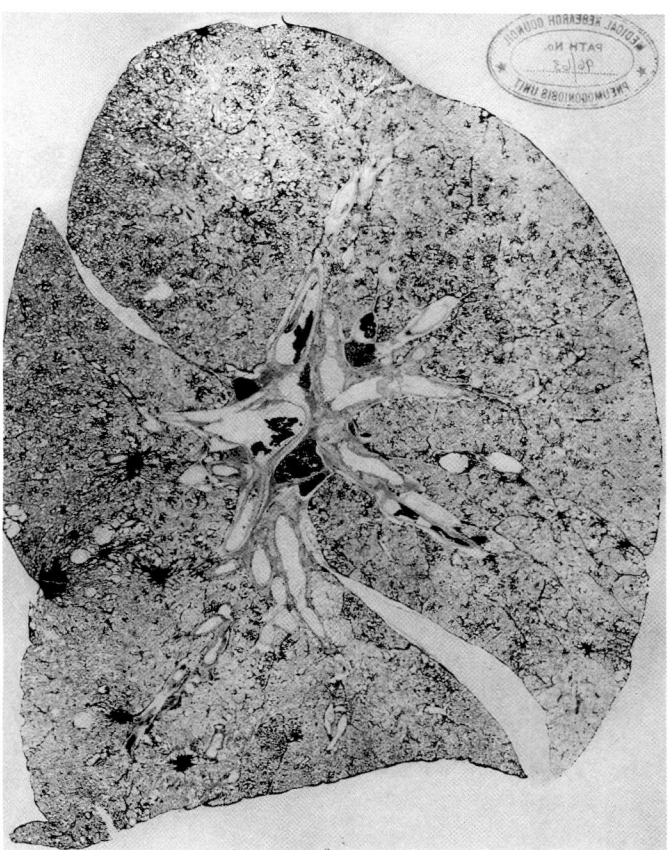

Fig. 13.88 Gough–Wentworth whole-lung section, showing simple CWP with numerous black macules and related emphysema. The macules average 2–3 mm in size, but there are five larger lesions in the lower lobe which measure up to 8 mm.

may extend across the oblique fissure into the other lobe. When large, they often cavitate. The background lung tissue usually shows numerous black macules, identical to those of simple CWP.

Clinical features

There is usually no clinical disability in coal-workers with simple pneumoconiosis, but disability may be present in complicated pneumoconiosis, particularly in those with large PMF lesions, which may lead eventually to cor pulmonale and death. In life, compensation is based on the radiological assessment of size and profusion of dust lesions; at death, compensation may be influenced by the pathological estimation of the extent and size of lesions in the lungs.

13.4.4 Silicosis

Silicosis is usually a slowly progressive disease characterized by the formation of rounded, whorled, hard nodules within the lungs (Fig. 13.90) and is caused by inhalation of dust containing a high percentage of free silica (usually quartz). As in CWP,

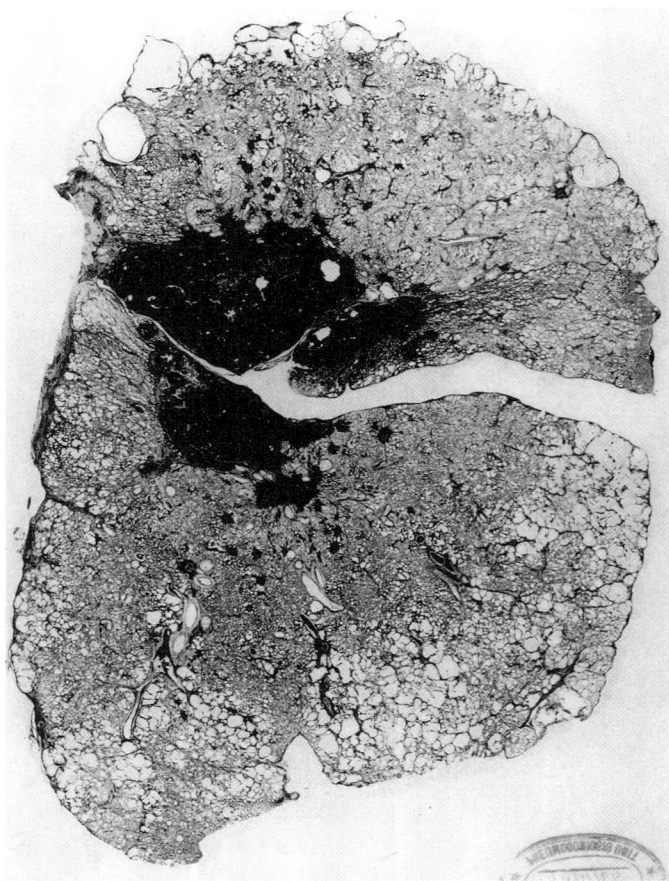

Fig. 13.89 Gough–Wentworth whole-lung section, showing complicated CWP (PMF) with a large, black lesion situated in the upper lobe and crossing the fissure into the lower lobe. There is also severe emphysema present.

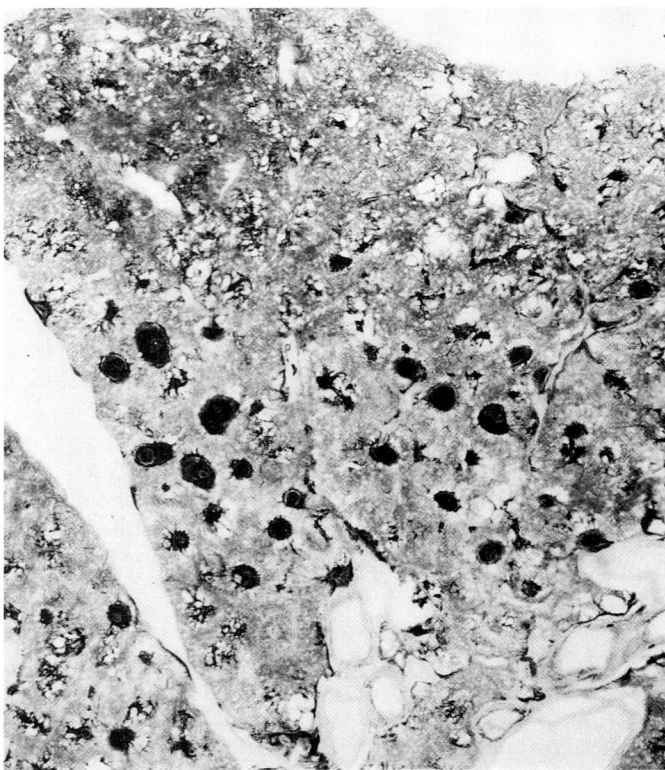

Fig. 13.90 Part of a Gough–Wentworth whole-lung section from a South African gold-miner, showing well-demarcated, whorled, rounded silicotic lesions.

it can be divided into simple and complicated types according to the size of lesions present within the lungs. Disability similarly relates to the complicated type. Simple silicosis may progress to the complicated form even after cessation of exposure. Silica is more fibrogenic than coal so silicotic lesions are more collagenous. The fully developed nodule consists of a central zone of concentrically arranged collagen with sparse macrophages, and a peripheral zone of more cellular dust containing macrophages (see Section 10.2). They are most prevalent in the upper zones of the lungs. Individuals with silicosis show an increased susceptibility to develop pulmonary mycobacterial infections.

13.4.5 Berylliosis

Sources of exposure include fluorescent lamp manufacture (prior to 1951), metalwork, ceramic manufacture, electronic industries, and the atomic energy industry. Inhalation of beryllium or its compounds can cause two types of disease, according to the intensity of exposure.

Acute berylliosis

This condition develops within a few weeks of exposure to a high dose and the manifestations are dyspnoea, tachycardia, and cyanosis, with diffuse miliary mottling on chest X-ray. Recovery may occur but in those who have succumbed the pathology has been that of DAD.

Chronic berylliosis

A chronic condition may develop after brief exposure and after a long latent interval. Diagnosis is therefore difficult. It shows clinical and pathological features which are very similar to those of sarcoidosis, but hilar lymphadenopathy is inconspicuous and the Kveim test negative. Local contact with the skin may cause dermatitis or chronic skin ulcers. It seems to have an immunological basis.

13.4.6 Further reading

Gibbs, A. R. and Seal, R. M. E. (1982). *Atlas of pulmonary pathology.* MTP Press, Lancaster.

Hay, J. G. and Turner-Warwick, M. (1986). Cryptogenic fibrosing alveolitis. In *Recent Advances in respiratory medicine*, Vol. 4 (ed. D. C. Flenley and T. L. Petty), pp. 131–52. Churchill Livingstone, Edinburgh.

Heppleston, A. G. (1956). The pathology of honeycomb lung. *Thorax* **11**, 77–93.

Jones Williams, W. (1977). Beryllium disease—pathology and diagnosis. *Journal of the Society of Occupational Medicine* **27**, 93–6.

Morgan, W. K. C. and Seaton, A. (1984). *Occupational lung diseases,* (2nd edn). W. B. Saunders, Philadelphia.

Parkes, W. R. (1982). *Occupational lung disorders* (2nd edn). Butterworths, London.

13.5   The pulmonary vasculature

C. A. Wagenvoort and W. J. Mooi

The vasculature of the pulmonary and systemic circulations differ essentially from each other in function, haemodynamics, and morphology. It is therefore not surprising that there are also considerable differences in pathological alterations in response to abnormal stimuli or circumstances.

The pulmonary vasculature receives the whole cardiac output, and therefore has an intimate relation with the heart. This implies that congenital as well as acquired cardiac conditions often result in some form of pulmonary vascular disease. Conversely, an effect on the right side of the heart is often apparent when there are advanced changes within the lung vessels. When these result from lung disease, this effect on the heart is often referred to as 'cor pulmonale', a somewhat unfortunate term since it is often ill-defined and does not distinguish between right ventricular hypertrophy and failure.

Pulmonary vascular pathology is particularly associated with pulmonary hypertension, which regularly induces lesions in the lung vessels, which in turn cause narrowing of lumina and, consequently, increased pulmonary vascular resistance and pressure. Some lesions in the lung vessels, however, are not related to an elevated pressure.

13.5.1   Normal pulmonary vasculature

Corresponding to the low resistance in the pulmonary circulation, the walls of pulmonary arteries are normally much thinner than their systemic counterparts. Also, the lumina of pulmonary arteries, capillaries, and veins are distinctly wider than comparable vessels in the systemic circulation. There is also a difference in wall structure between pulmonary and systemic arteries of similar size. This applies to the pulmonary trunk and main arteries, which are discussed elsewhere (p. 1024), but also to the intrapulmonary arteries down to their smallest precapillary branches (Harris and Heath 1986; Wagenvoort and Mooi 1989).

Lobar and segmental pulmonary arteries are of the elastic type, with regular parallel elastic laminae (Fig. 13.91) separated by occasional smooth muscle cells and a small amount of collagen. In contrast to the systemic circulation, where this type is found only in large arteries, pulmonary arteries maintain this type down to a calibre in the range of 1 mm or 0.5 mm, or even

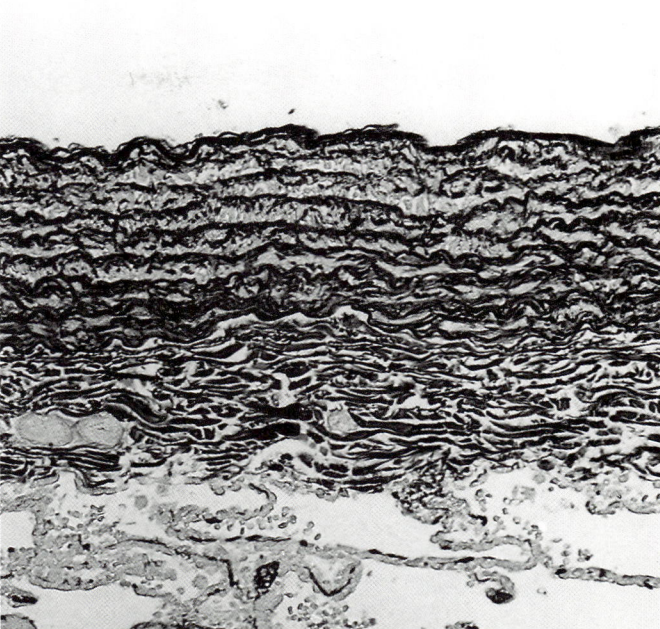

Fig. 13.91 Lobar pulmonary artery in a normal adult; there is a regular configuration of parallel intact elastic laminae. (Elastic van Gieson.)

much smaller in children. At this level, which corresponds roughly with the point at which the accompanying bronchus loses its cartilage to produce the terminal bronchioles, the arteries become muscular.

Normal muscular pulmonary arteries have a fairly thin adventitia, a media consisting of circularly arranged smooth muscle cells, and an intima consisting of a layer of endothelium resting on a basement membrane. The media is bounded on either side by an elastic membrane; the internal and external laminae separate the media from the intima and adventitia, respectively. The media is thin (Fig. 13.92), the average thickness being only 4 or 5 per cent of the external arterial diameter. Pulmonary arteries divide dichotomously with the bronchi they accompany, but there are also additional branches, which take an origin at right angles from their parent arteries: these vessels are designated supernumerary arteries.

When peripheral arterial branches have reached the level of the respiratory bronchioles, they branch further, to form networks of small intra-acinar arteries. These gradually lose their muscular coats, which peter out in radiating bundles of smooth muscle cells so that in cross-section only part of the walls are muscularized (Fig. 13.93).

From these alveolar networks, small pulmonary veins arise which merge to larger ones that enter the interlobular septa; in this way they keep the greatest possible distance from the bronchi and pulmonary arteries. The walls of normal pulmonary veins are thinner than those of the arteries, and consist of irregularly arranged elastic laminae, smooth muscle cells, and collagen fibres (Fig. 13.94). There may be an incomplete or even complete internal elastic lamina.

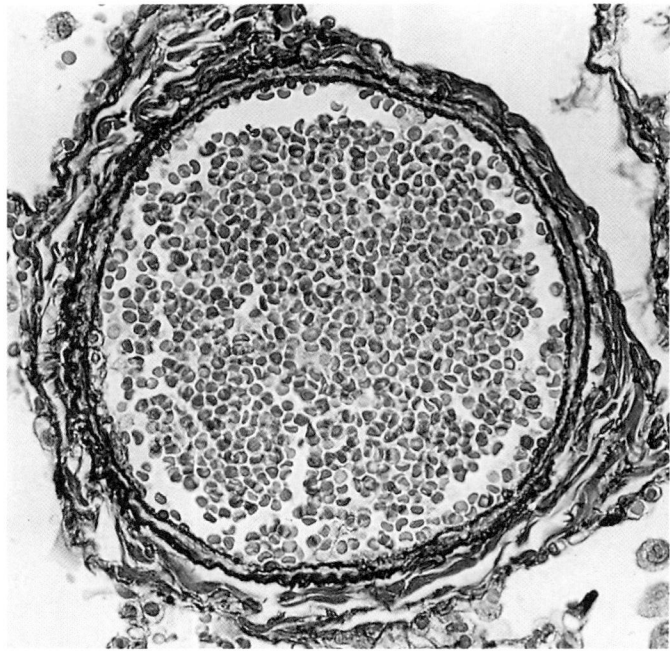

Fig. 13.92 Muscular pulmonary artery in a normal adult; the thin media is bounded by internal and external elastic laminae. (Elastic van Gieson.)

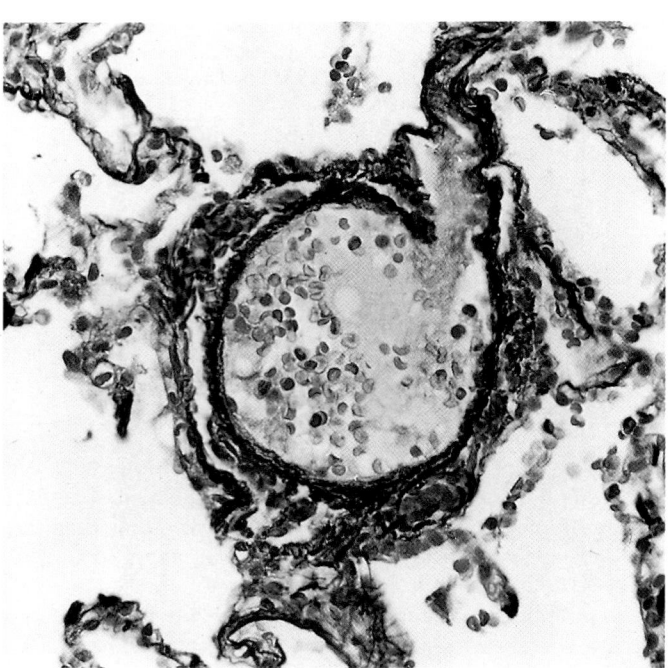

Fig. 13.94 Normal pulmonary vein with thin wall in which elastic fibres predominate. (Elastic van Gieson.)

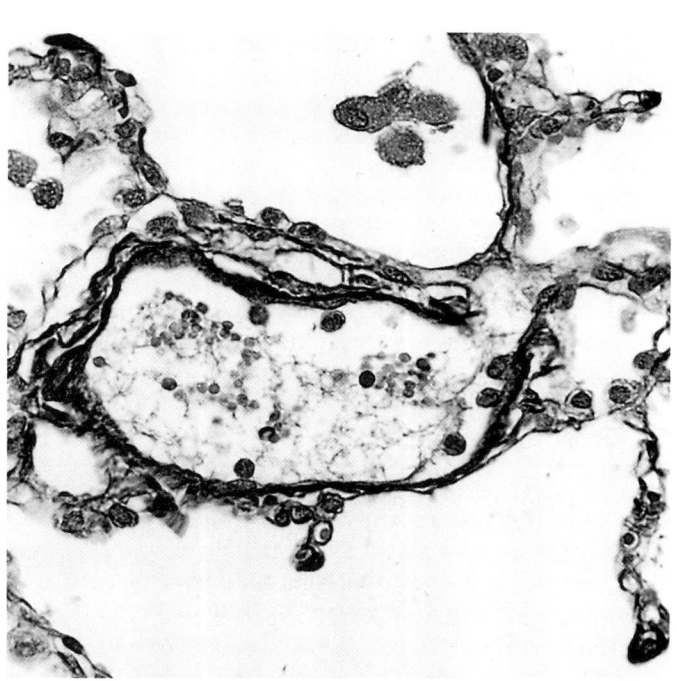

Fig. 13.93 Transition of an intra-acinar muscular pulmonary artery to a non-muscularized arteriole; a media bounded by elastic laminae is present on one side of the vessel only. (Elastic van Gieson.)

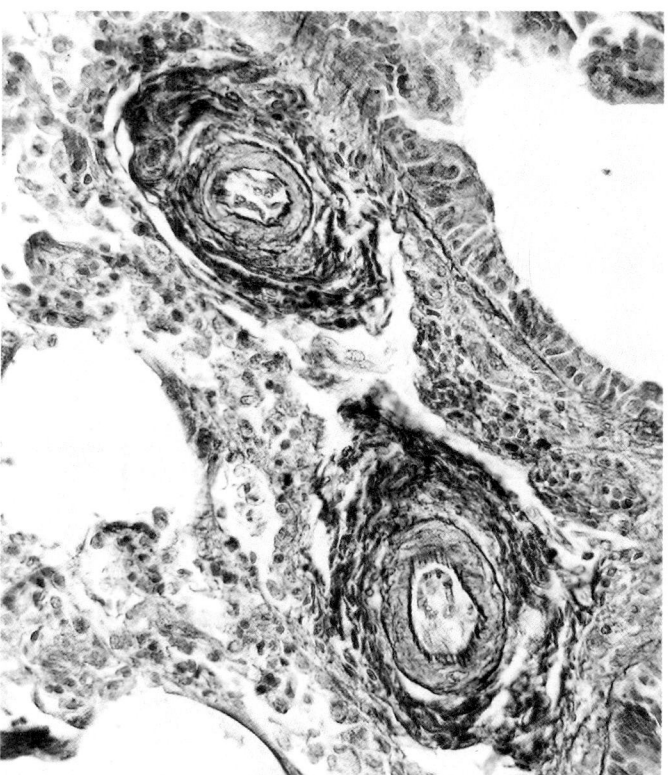

Fig. 13.95 Muscular pulmonary arteries in a stillborn infant; there is a thick media and a narrow lumen. (Elastic van Gieson.)

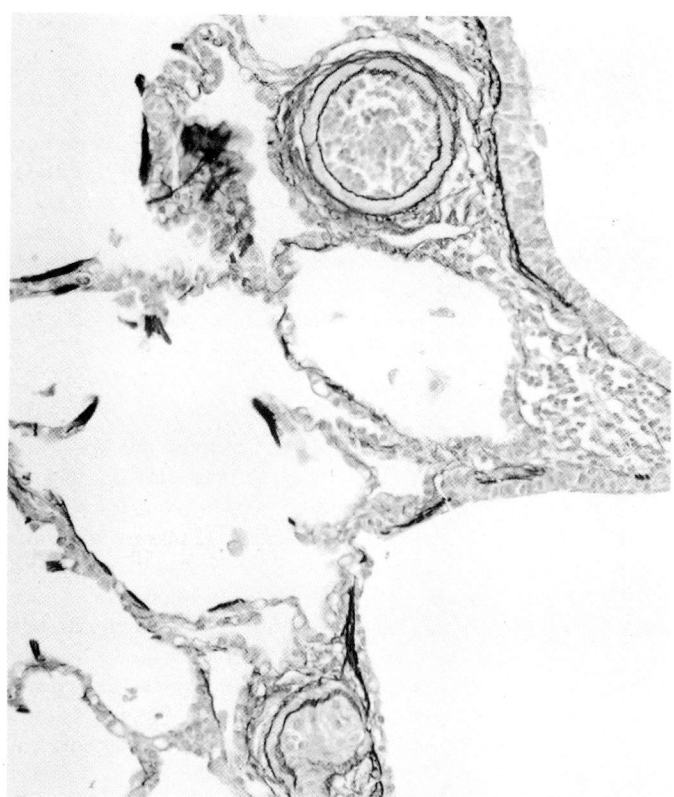

Fig. 13.96 Muscular pulmonary arteries in a new-born infant aged 3 weeks; the media has become thinner and the lumen considerably wider. (Elastic van Gieson.)

In late fetal life and in the new-born, muscular pulmonary arteries are very thick-walled, with narrow lumina (Fig. 13.95), reflecting the high resistance of the pulmonary vascular bed in the perinatal period. In the first 2–4 weeks of life, the medial thickness decreases rapidly (Fig. 13.96), followed by a further decrease during the subsequent year (Wagenvoort et al. 1961). In elderly individuals, mild intimal fibrosis of pulmonary arteries is regularly observed and can be considered an age change.

13.5.2 Pulmonary oedema and shock lung

In the normal lung, fluid constantly extravasates from the pulmonary arterioles, capillaries, and venules into the perivascular interstitial space. From there, it flows to the interlobular septa and the peribronchial interstitial space, and drains via the pulmonary lymphatics into the systemic venous circulation. *Pulmonary oedema*, i.e. accumulation of fluid within the pulmonary interstitium and alveolar airspaces, occurs when fluid leaves the pulmonary microvasculature more rapidly than it can be drained from the interstitium via the highly distensible lymphatics. Normal and abnormal fluid movements from the vessels into the interstitium depend on the hydrostatic and colloid osmotic pressures of the intravascular and extravascular

spaces, as well as on the permeability of the pulmonary vascular endothelium. The many causes of pulmonary oedema can often be understood in terms of changes in these parameters (Staub 1970, 1974).

Since the pathogenesis of pulmonary oedema depends on many factors, affecting the *microvascular blood pressure*, the integrity of the pulmonary endothelium and epithelium, the *colloid osmotic pressure*, the *interstitium*, and the *lymphatics*, there are many different causes of pulmonary oedema. The large majority of these causes can, however, be broadly subdivided into two main groups: those leading to *increased microvascular pressure* ('haemodynamic oedema') and those causing *microvascular damage* ('permeability oedema'); there is a small remaining group with poorly understood pathogenesis (e.g. neurogenic pulmonary oedema, high-altitude pulmonary oedema). It should be borne in mind that more than one factor may be involved at the same time in an individual patient: for instance, septic shock may cause pulmonary microvascular damage and permeability oedema, but may also lead to myocardial infarction causing increased pulmonary blood pressure and haemodynamic oedema; furthermore, the patient may require oxygen treatment because of respiratory failure, which in turn may contribute to pulmonary oedema formation. It is difficult to give exact figures for the immediate and long-term prognosis, because pulmonary oedema often occurs in the context of other life-threatening diseases. It is certainly often a direct cause of death when such patients succumb.

Pathology of pulmonary oedema and alveolar damage

Since several different factors may contribute to pulmonary oedema formation in a given case, the histopathology may be complex, various stages of the process being present at the same time. At the earliest phase, there is only an increase of fluid within the pulmonary interstitium, which may lead to some dyspnoea and radiographic signs of interstitial oedema, such as 'Kerley B lines' on the thorax radiograph, which represent oedematous interlobular septa. Histologically, interstitial oedema is evidenced by widening of alveolar septa, interlobular septa and peribronchial spaces, and dilated pulmonary lymphatics, which are normally inconspicuous.

When subsequently the alveolar airspaces become filled with fluid, *hypoxaemia* develops because of shunting of blood through these areas of oedematous lung tissue where gas exchange is no longer possible. Intra-alveolar oedema fluid may stain faintly eosinophilic (Fig. 13.97) because it often contains some protein; however, it may be difficult to visualize and, at autopsy, the lung weight may be a better parameter of early pulmonary oedema than histology. Often erythrocytes, together with sloughed endothelial and epithelial cells, are found in alveolar lumina. Alveoli that are partly filled with oedema fluid tend to collapse, because of increased surface tension caused by dilution and disappearance of the surfactant layer and by decrease of the circumference of the airspace.

After 1 or 2 days, *hyaline membranes* may develop in some cases: these consist of cellular debris within a fibrinous exudate, lining the alveolar septa. Subsequently, proliferation of type 2

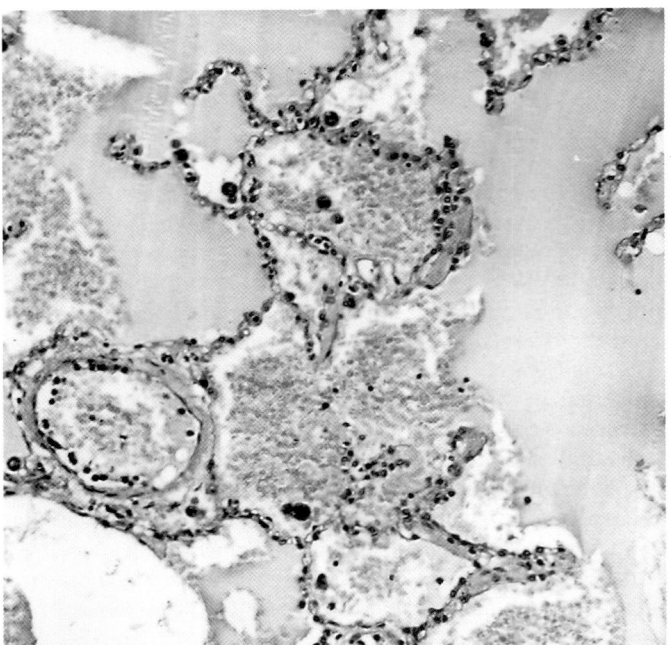

Fig. 13.97 Pulmonary oedema. Proteinaceous fluid has accumulated within alveolar airspaces, while there is intra-alveolar haemorrhage.

pneumocytes restores the continuity of the epithelial lining of the alveoli. These proliferating pneumocytes may overgrow the hyaline membranes, which thus contribute to the thickening of the alveolar walls. Intra-alveolar exudate may be resolved or may become organized to form loosely fibrotic masses within the alveolar lumina, sometimes extending through pores of Kohn into adjacent alveolar spaces. Within the alveolar septa, some chronic inflammatory infiltrate is usually present, and the interstitial exudate organizes, yielding thickened, fibrotic walls. Collapsed alveoli often become incorporated into the walls of larger, irregular air-filled spaces, so that the original delicate alveolar structure of the lung is lost. Obviously, the gaseous exchange is greatly impaired, because many capillaries have either obliterated or have become separated from the airspace by fibrotic tissue; also, ventilation of abnormally large distal airspaces is far less efficient than ventilation of intact lung parenchyma. Chronic respiratory insufficiency may therefore be the final outcome (Katzenstein and Askin 1982).

Increased microvascular pressure (haemodynamic oedema)

An abnormal increase in blood pressure in the pulmonary microvasculature can be caused by *left ventricular failure, mitral or aortic valve disease*, and, more rarely, by *cardiac myxomas, fibrosing mediastinitis, mediastinal tumours*, and other diseases narrowing the *large pulmonary veins*. Also, *overtransfusion*, especially in patients with hypoalbuminaemia (causing decreased osmotic pressure within the blood vessels, which

predisposes to fluid extravasation) is an important cause of pulmonary haemodynamic oedema.

Microvascular damage (permeability oedema)

Many different agents may cause damage to the pulmonary endothelium and epithelium: *infectious and toxic agents* (inhaled noxious gases and fumes), *ingested cytostatic agents* (the herbicide paraquat; heroin), *radiation*, and various causes such as *trauma, sepsis, shock, uraemia, heat, drowning*, etc. Many of these agents directly damage the pulmonary endothelium and epithelium, whereas others exert their effect mainly via activated polymorphonuclear leucocytes.

Shock lung

Traumatic and, more commonly, septic shock are important causes of pulmonary oedema. Severe trauma may produce air or fat embolism leading to pulmonary oedema, while trauma of the head leading to increased intracranial pressure may also cause pulmonary oedema. When there is also renal failure, overfilling with plasma expanders may lead to oedema. Therefore, in a patient suffering from pulmonary oedema after a severe trauma, there may be several factors beside the decreased blood volume and pressure, which may cause or contribute to the formation of pulmonary oedema. In septic shock, activation of polymorphonuclear leucocytes by bacterial endotoxins is probably the main pathogenetic factor. Released lysosomal enzymes or generated free radicals damage the endothelium, leading to permeability oedema.

13.5.3 Hypertensive pulmonary vascular disease

Pulmonary hypertension can result from a variety of causes, and may have different clinical manifestations. Similarly, hypertensive pulmonary vascular disease is not a histological entity but presents as a variety of distinct patterns of morphological lesions, each of these patterns being associated with a cause or with a group of causes for the pulmonary hypertension.

In some instances, the elevation of pressure in the pulmonary circulation results from an increased pulmonary blood flow, as observed in patients with congenital cardiac shunts, or from an increase in viscosity of the blood. In such cases, the lung vessels need not be significantly altered. More often, however, pulmonary hypertension is due to an increase in pulmonary vascular resistance, caused either by constriction of the vessels or by structural changes narrowing their lumina.

Causes of pulmonary hypertension include *congenital heart disease with a shunt, chronic hypoxia, recurrent pulmonary embolism, obstruction to the pulmonary venous flow* as a result of congenital or acquired heart disease, *pulmonary veno-occlusive disease*, and various forms of *vasculitis* and of *lung fibrosis* or *granulomatosis*. Sometimes the cause remains unknown despite extensive clinical and haemodynamic investigations, but such cases of unexplained or primary pulmonary hypertension, which may vary in morphology, are uncommon. Occurrence of lesions of two patterns simultaneously is not rare. Any of the histopathological forms of hypertensive pulmonary vascular disease may be complicated by lesions resulting from, e.g. thrombosis or pulmonary venous hypertension. The most important of these forms will be discussed.

13.5.4 Plexogenic arteriopathy

Terminology

Plexogenic pulmonary arteriopathy is a form of hypertensive pulmonary vascular disease with a characteristic pattern of vascular lesions, confined to the pulmonary arteries. A very striking and easily recognizable alteration, occurring in an advanced stage, is the *plexiform lesion* (p. 1004) It is important to realize that the term 'plexogenic arteriopathy' implies that the vascular disease may proceed to include these advanced lesions but not that plexiform lesions are necessarily present (Hatano and Strasser 1975). Indeed, plexogenic arteriopathy can often be diagnosed reliably in the absence of plexiform lesions (see below).

Aetiology

The aetiological factors involved in plexogenic arteriopathy are diverse. It is observed first of all in patients with *congenital heart disease* with a left-to-right shunt. This shunt may be *pre-tricuspid*, as in atrial septal defect, or *post-tricuspid*, as in ventricular septal defect or patent ductus arteriosus. In these conditions, the increased blood flow through the pulmonary circulation may lead to an increased pulmonary arterial pressure from birth. In the course of time, changes tend to develop, particularly in muscular pulmonary arteries, causing narrowing or obstruction of their lumina, so that increasingly severe pulmonary hypertension develops. If the pulmonary vascular lesions have advanced beyond a certain stage, the disease becomes irreversible and the patient inoperable. Eventually, right ventricular failure and death may ensue.

Severe hypertensive pulmonary vascular disease is uncommon in atrial septal defect and patent ductus arteriosus. It is more often found in ventricular septal defect, although advanced vascular lesions are uncommon before the age of 2 years. When more complicated congenital cardiac anomalies, such as atrio-ventricular septal defect or transposition of the great arteries with ventricular septal defect, are present, irreversible pulmonary vascular disease may develop in early infancy (Haworth *et al.* 1987).

A rare cause of plexogenic arteriopathy is *hepatic disease,* particularly when associated with portal hypertension (Edwards *et al.* 1987). It has been assumed that unknown substances, which are normally metabolized and inactivated in the liver, are bypassed in the presence of hepatic cirrhosis or other severe liver disease, and elicit the vascular disease in the lungs. Occasionally, portal vein thrombosis in the absence of liver parenchymal disease has a similar effect.

In *pulmonary schistosomiasis*, the ova of the parasites may embolize from the portal vein or inferior caval vein tributaries to the lungs, causing foreign-body granulomas and arteritis with obstruction of pulmonary arterial branches. However, in addition, the whole pattern of plexogenic arteriopathy may also be observed in such instances.

Finally, there is an unexplained or primary plexogenic arteriopathy, which is often referred to as primary pulmonary hypertension (p. 1020). This is an uncommon disease, affecting mainly young adults, with a female preponderance. With few exceptions, this disease runs a progressive course, eventually leading to death (Wagenvoort and Wagenvoort 1970).

Although the aetiology of primary plexogenic arteriopathy still remains to be elucidated, there is no lack of hypotheses. It has been maintained that thromboembolism is the initiating factor; however, the histological pattern of pulmonary vascular lesions caused by thromboembolism is totally unlike that of plexogenic arteriopathy (p. 1004). Therefore, it is highly unlikely that the changes of the latter pattern merely represent organized thrombi. It is conceivable that thromboemboli, upon their impact into the pulmonary arteries, trigger a reaction of these vessels which may lead to the patterns of plexogenic arteriopathy. However, if this happens at all, then only in a minority of patients with primary plexogenic arteriopathy.

Dietary factors have been suggested, because various herbaceous toxic products can cause pulmonary hypertension in animals. There is no evidence that this ever happens in man. However, plexogenic arteriopathy has been caused by the intake of certain appetite-suppressing drugs.

Immunological factors are probably also involved, at least in some patients with primary plexogenic arteriopathy. This disease is observed relatively often in association with various auto-immune diseases and Raynaud's phenomenon. Antinuclear antibodies have been found far more often in patients with primary plexogenic arteriopathy than in normal individuals or in patients suffering from various forms of secondary pulmonary hypertension. However, the search for immune deposits in lung tissue of these patients has rarely been successful.

The regular occurrence of familial cases points to the possibility of *genetic influences*. A dominant gene is supposed to be involved. Most probably, an increased reactivity of the pulmonary vascular smooth muscle to vasoconstrictive stimuli is genetically determined (Weir *et al.* 1974; Grover *et al.* 1975) and patients suffering from this form of pulmonary hypertension have hyper-reactive lung vessels. This would mean that a combination of endogenous and exogenous factors are responsible for the development of plexogenic arteriopathy.

Morphology and pathogenesis

Plexogenic arteriopathy develops as a sequence of morphological lesions, beginning with an increase in muscularity of the muscular pulmonary arteries (Edwards 1957), evidenced by medial hypertrophy of arteries possessing a muscular coat (Fig. 13.98), and peripheral extension of smooth muscle cells along small, previously non-muscularized branches. This latter process, known as *muscularization of arterioles* (Fig. 13.99), is based

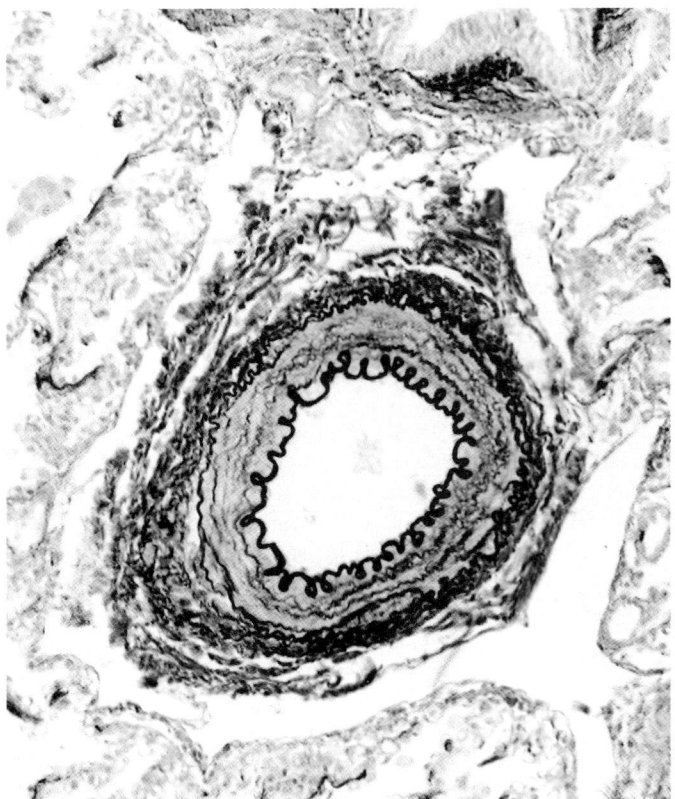

Fig. 13.98 Muscular pulmonary artery with prominent medial hypertrophy in plexogenic arteriopathy due to congenital heart disease. (Elastic van Gieson.)

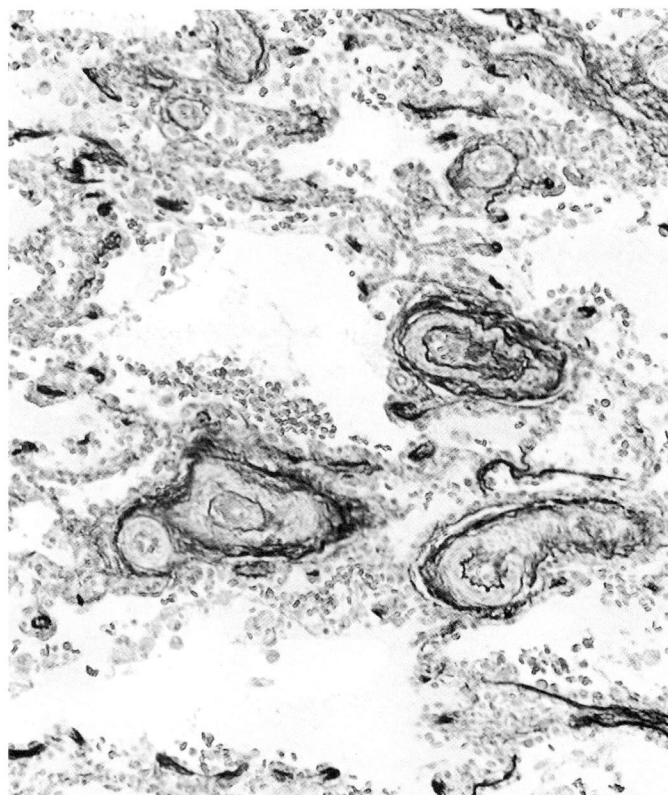

Fig. 13.99 Pulmonary arterioles with muscularizaton and narrow lumina in plexogenic arteriopathy due to congenital heart disease. (Elastic van Gieson.)

on an increase in number as well as in size of smooth muscle cells.

Such an increase in pulmonary arterial muscularity is usually the only vascular alteration in children under 2 years of age, and in patients with mild pulmonary hypertension. Also, experimental evidence indicates that it is the first change in this form of pulmonary hypertension. Since it is very likely that *vasoconstriction* plays a predominant role in the pathogenesis of plexogenic arteriopathy, the increased muscularity is probably related to a sustained increase in tone, and to arterial contraction, continuous or intermittent.

Intimal changes begin with *cellular proliferation* (Fig. 13.100). The cells constituting the intimal thickening are *myofibroblasts*; they have most of the characteristics of smooth muscle cells, but they are usually stellate or rounded rather than elongated. There is evidence that they are derived from the smooth muscle cells of the media, which may penetrate the internal elastic lamina.

Initially there are no or very few collagen fibres between the intimal cells, but they gradually increase in number, while elastic fibres may also be deposited. In this way there is a gradual transformation to intimal fibrosis, which has a peculiar *onion-skin appearance* (Fig. 13.101). This *concentric-laminar*

intimal fibrosis causes progressive narrowing and may eventually completely occlude the lumen (Wagenvoort 1985).

The more advanced lesions of plexogenic arteriopathy are always a sign of prominent pulmonary hypertension. With increasing pressure, the muscular coat of arterial branches may become incompetent, so that these vessels dilate and become exceedingly thin-walled, resulting in so-called dilatation lesions. These may be isolated 'vein-like branches' (Fig. 13.102) but often clusters of such wide, thin-walled arteries are formed (Fig. 13.103) (Heath and Edwards 1958). *Fibrinoid necrosis* of the arterial wall is particularly observed in a branch over a short stretch just distally to its origin from the parent artery (Fig. 13.104). It is usually accompanied by a clot of fibrin with an admixture of platelets in the lumen. Fibrinoid necrosis is probably caused by severe spastic constriction of the artery. *Arteritis* is sometimes seen in combination with this lesion, although it may occur independently (Fig. 13.105).

Plexiform lesions are found at the same locations as fibrinoid necrosis, and there is much evidence, also from experimental studies, that they develop in arterial segments thus affected. A plexiform lesion is a complicated structure, consisting of a plexus of capillary-like channels within a short, dilated portion of an arterial branch close to its origin from a larger parent

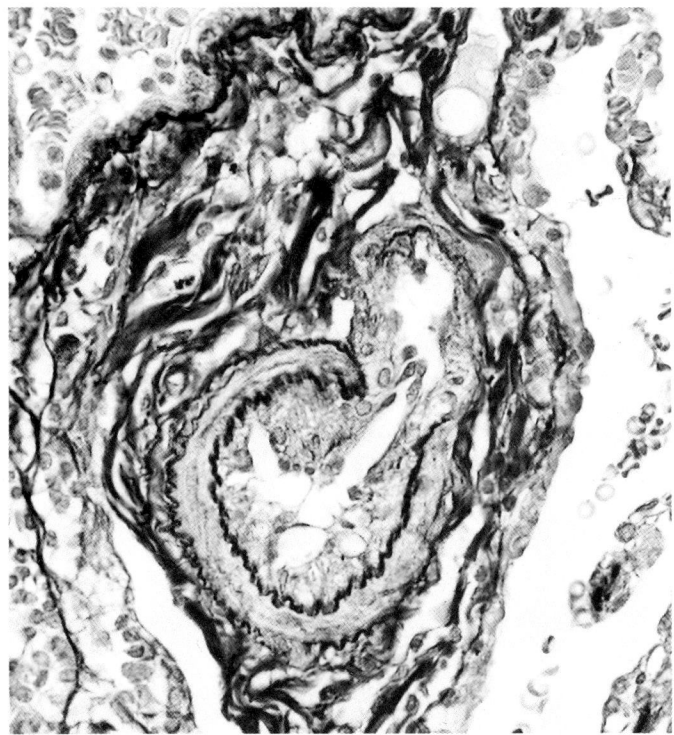

Fig. 13.100 Muscular pulmonary artery with cellular intimal proliferation causing severe narrowing of the lumen, in plexogenic arteriopathy. (Elastic van Gieson.)

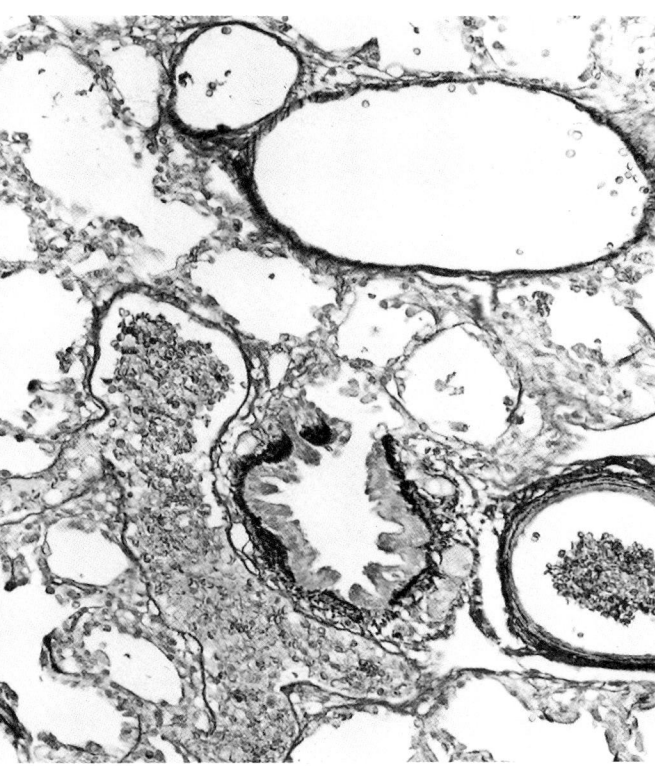

Fig. 13.102 Multiple pulmonary arteries arranged around a bronchus are severely dilated to form thin-walled 'vein-like branches'; in plexogenic arteriopathy. (Elastic van Gieson.)

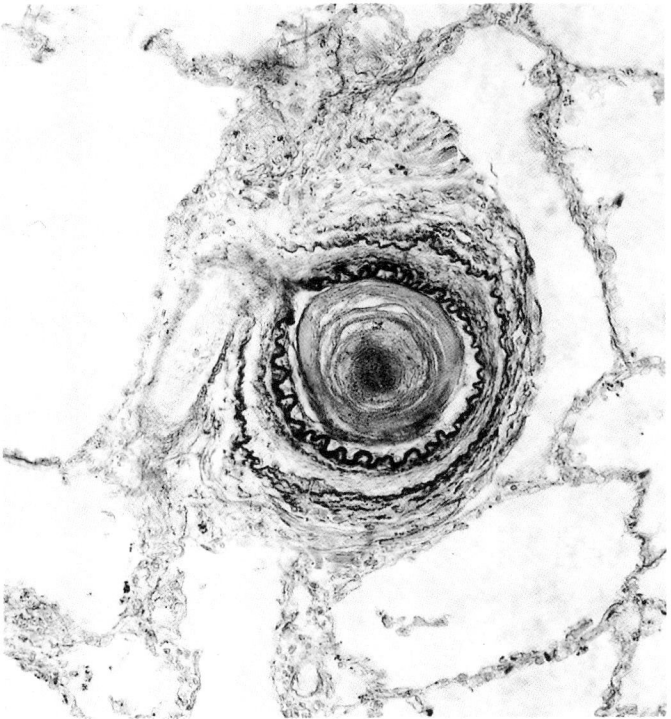

Fig. 13.101 Muscular pulmonary artery with concentric-laminar intimal fibrosis, obstructing the lumen in plexogenic arteriopathy. (Elastic van Gieson.)

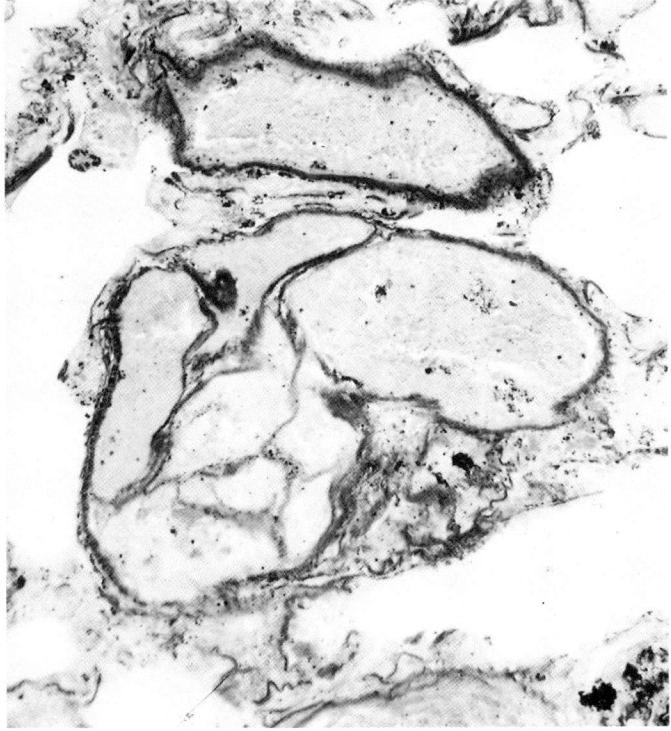

Fig. 13.103 Cluster of coiled branches of pulmonary artery forming a dilatation lesion; in plexogenic arteriopathy. (Elastic van Gieson.)

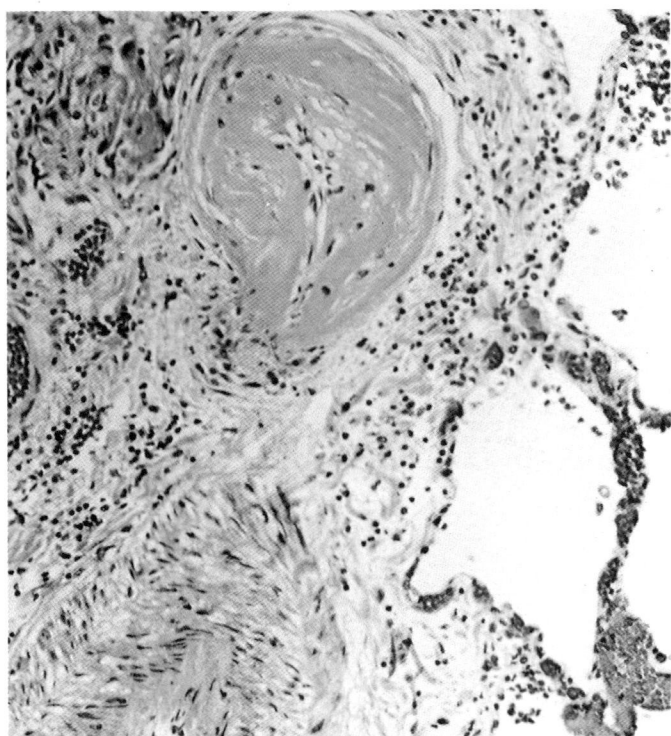

Fig. 13.104 Extensive fibrinoid necrosis in a branch of a large muscular pulmonary artery (bottom); in plexogenic arteriopathy.

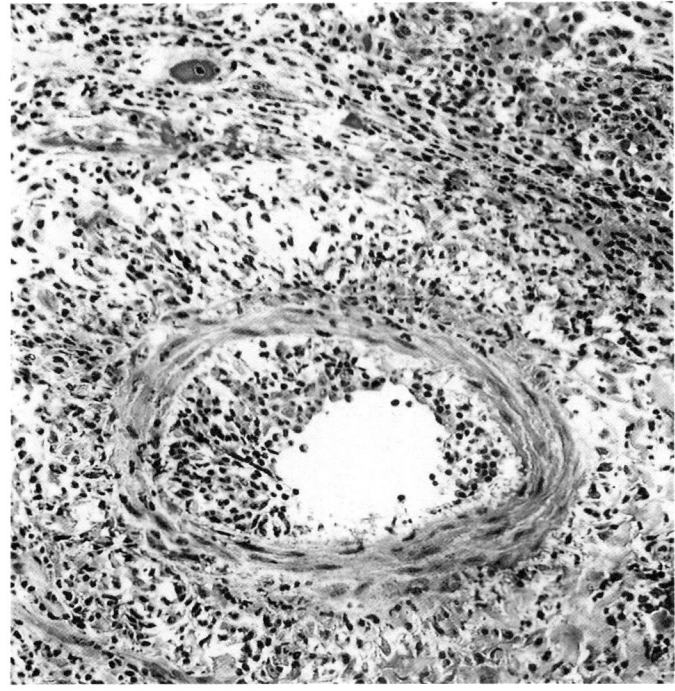

Fig. 13.105 Muscular pulmonary artery in plexogenic arteriopathy. There is severe arteritis extending well into the surrounding lung tissue.

artery (Fig. 13.106). The wall of the branch is thin and disorganized, with interrupted elastic laminae, as a result of previous necrosis. Distal to the plexus, the branch and its ramifications are usually also dilated and thin-walled (Fig. 13.107), but their walls are intact. The cells within the plexus have hyperchromatic nuclei; ultrastructurally, they show again the features of smooth muscle cells or myofibroblasts. Often remnants of fibrinoid material and platelet agglutinations can be recognized. Plexiform lesions are very striking alterations, especially when viewed in a haematoxylin stain (Fig. 13.108).

Although there is thus a sequence of changes in plexogenic arteriopathy, the rate at which these various lesions develop varies widely. In exceptional cases, the advanced alterations, including plexiform lesions, are observed at an age of 1 year or less. More often, there is a more protracted course and the advanced lesions may not develop at all.

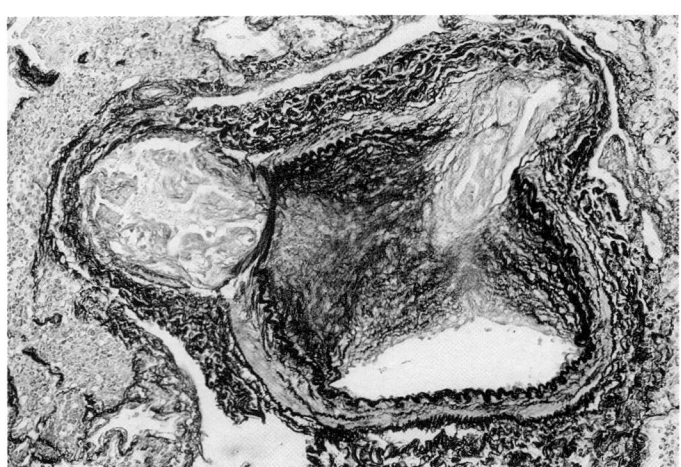

Fig. 13.106 Muscular pulmonary artery in plexogenic arteriopathy with plexiform lesions in two branches which have lost most of their normal wall structure. (Elastic van Gieson.)

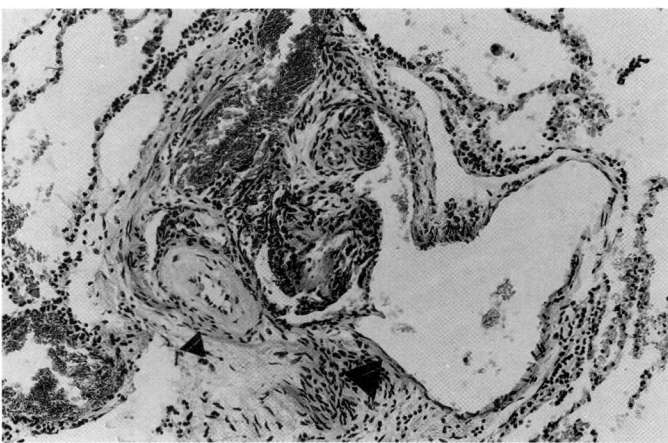

Fig. 13.107 Plexiform lesion in a branch of a pulmonary artery. This branch shows fibrinoid necrosis (small arrow) in its proximal part and marked dilatation (large arrow) in its peripheral part.

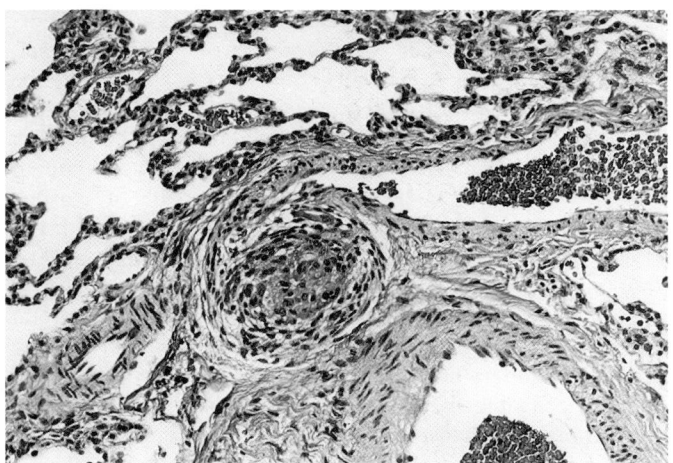

Fig. 13.108 Plexiform lesion in a branch shortly after its origin from a larger artery (bottom). The plexus is composed of cells with hyperchromatic nuclei.

Some of the vascular changes of plexogenic arteriopathy are reversible, as becomes evident in many cases of surgical repair of cardiac defects which had led to pulmonary hypertension. This applies to medial hypertrophy and cellular intimal proliferation, and also to mild concentric-laminar intimal fibrosis. Severe intimal fibrosis of this type, however, is irreversible, as are fibroid necrosis and plexiform lesions. Indeed, when these advanced lesions are present, there is progression of pulmonary vascular disease even when the cardiac defect is surgically closed (Wagenvoort *et al.* 1984).

The pulmonary veins are not affected in plexogenic arteriopathy, unless heart failure develops in a late stage of the disease and leads to pulmonary venous hypertension. Within the lung tissue there is often haemosiderosis, although usually not very pronounced.

13.5.5 Hypoxic arteriopathy

Mechanisms

Reduction of oxygen tension in the alveolar air causes pulmonary vasoconstriction, especially of small pulmonary arteries and muscularized or partly muscularized arterioles, and to a much lesser extent of small pulmonary veins. When there is alveolar hypoxia in only part of the lung, as in pulmonary atelactasis, such vasoconstriction is beneficial, since the blood flow is shunted away from these areas. This redistribution of flow minimizes a shunt of poorly oxygenated blood to the systemic side of the circulation. However, when most or all of the lung becomes hypoxic, the pulmonary vasoconstrictive response to hypoxia leads to pulmonary hypertension. Prominent pulmonary hypoxaemia may enhance hypoxic vasoconstriction, but probably has little effect on its own.

The mechanisms by which changes in oxygen tension alter the tone of the lung vessels have not yet been elucidated completely. A variety of cells has been implicated to produce vaso-constrictive mediators; however, no such mediator has been identified with certainty. Others presume that there is a direct effect of the alveolar oxygen tension on the smooth muscle cells of the pulmonary arterioles, which are in close contact with the alveolar spaces. It is supposed that a transmembrane calcium flux may be involved, since various calcium-channel-blocking agents can prevent the vascular response to hypoxia.

States of hypoxia

Various conditions of a completely different nature may cause alveolar hypoxia, e.g. by airway obstruction, impairment of respiratory movement, or low oxygen tension of ambient air.

Upper airway obstruction caused by enlarged adenoids occasionally leads to prominent pulmonary hypertension in children. In adults, the impediment to the air flow is usually localized in the bronchi and bronchioles, as in *chronic obstructive lung disease*. Pulmonary hypertension may develop, although this happens only in a small proportion of the patients.

Insufficiency of respiratory movements because of *muscular diseases* involving the thoracic musculature, or thoracic deformations such as *kyphoscoliosis*, may cause chronic hypoxia and pulmonary hypertension. Sometimes there is a central cause for impaired ventilatory drive, as in the *sleep-apnoea syndromes* and in the so-called *Pickwickian syndrome*, in which obesity of the patient is a contributory factor for hypoventilation. These patients may develop severe pulmonary hypertension and right cardiac failure.

A completely different cause of alveolar hypoxia is the low oxygen tension of the ambient air at *high altitude*. When lowlanders ascend to mountainous areas, particularly above 3000 m, they may develop acute mountain sickness and a rise in pulmonary arterial pressure, which usually subsides gradually within a few days but which sometimes requires oxygen treatment or return to sea-level. Normal high-altitude residents generally have a mild to moderate elevation of the pulmonary arterial pressure, which does not interfere with a healthy and active life, since they are acclimatized to the prevailing conditions. A special form of high-altitude disease is *high-altitude pulmonary oedema*: this is far more serious than acute mountain sickness and may be fatal if not treated by oxygen and rapid return to lower altitudes (Heath and Williams 1977).

Morphology and pathogenesis

The most striking morphological feature of hypoxic arteriopathy is an extensive muscularization of peripheral, originally non-muscular arterioles (Fig. 13.109). In contrast, the medium-sized and large muscular pulmonary arteries are usually normal (Fig. 13.110) or show only mild medial hypertrophy. This would suggest a direct action of the hypoxic alveolar air, because these small intra-acinar branches have a very thin adventitia, so that their medial smooth muscle cells are in close contact with the alveolar spaces and thus are most directly exposed to a possible direct vasoconstrictive effect of alveolar hypoxia. Larger arteries have a much thicker adventitia, and are located adjacent to bronchi and bronchioles.

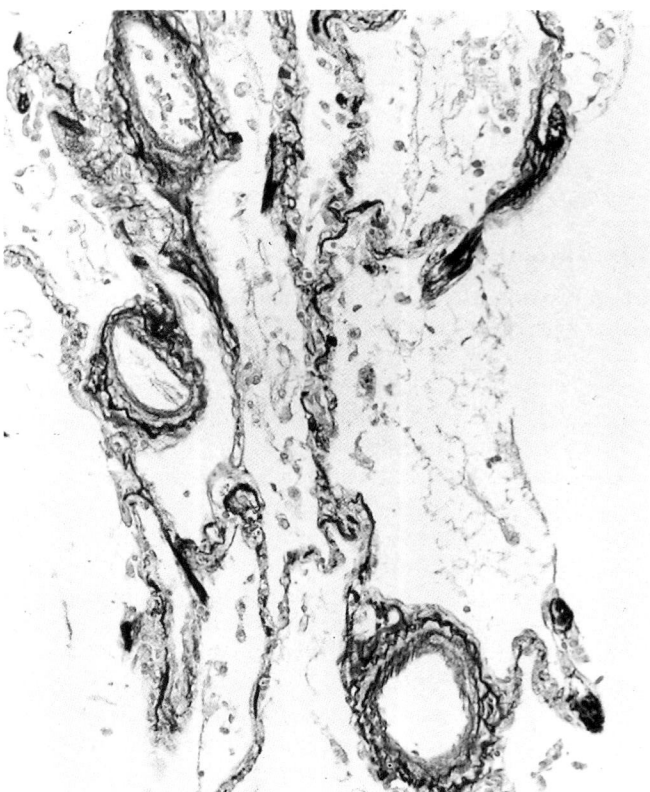

Fig. 13.109 Multiple pulmonary arterioles, normally devoid of smooth muscle, have become muscularized in hypoxic arteriopathy. (Elastic van Gieson.)

Not always do the muscular pulmonary arteries have a normal or near normal media: in some states of chronic hypoxia, such as chronic bronchitis or emphysema, there may be prominent *medial hypertrophy* and even *intimal fibrosis* of larger arteries. This, however, is related to concomitant inflammation or lung fibrosis, which is often present in such cases and known to induce these vascular changes independent of chronic hypoxia. Such complicating factors are usually absent in high-altitude residents or in patients with Pickwickian syndrome (Hasleton *et al.* 1968).

Development of longitudinal smooth muscle in the intima (Fig. 13.111), and to a lesser extent in the media, is regularly found in pulmonary arterioles. These cells, arranged in bundles or layers, probably enhance the vasoconstrictive effect of the circular medial smooth muscle.

The small pulmonary veins and venules also react to chronic hypoxia with an increase in thickness of their media, and occasionally with the development of intimal longitudinal smooth muscle cells. Constriction of small pulmonary veins may possibly play a role in high-altitude pulmonary oedema, although in these cases there is certainly also damage to the walls of the alveolar capillaries.

The pattern of histological vascular alterations in chronic hypoxia is not pathognomonic. Muscularization of arterioles occurs in most forms of hypertensive pulmonary vascular disease. The intimal longitudinal smooth muscle bundles in these arterioles are somewhat more characteristic, but they may

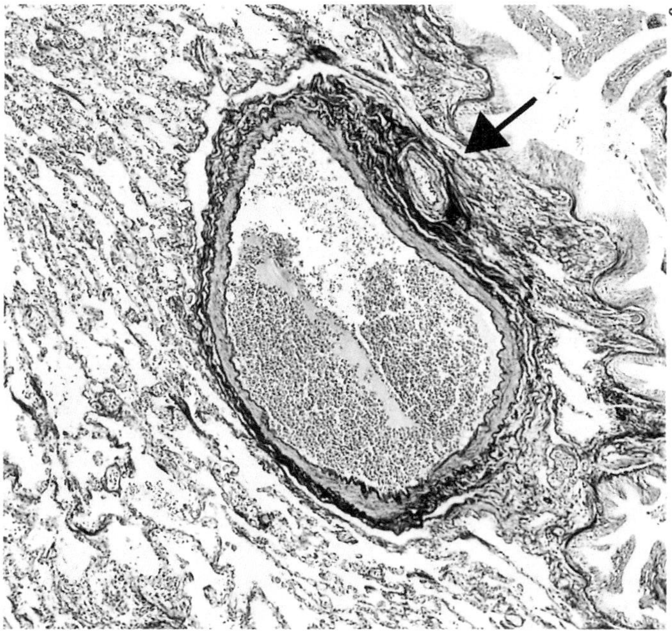

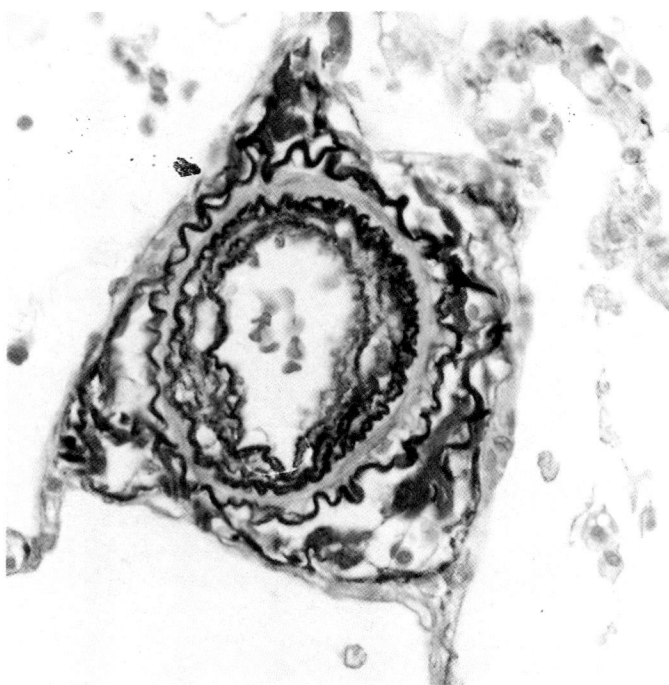

Fig. 13.111 Muscularized pulmonary arteriole in hypoxic arteriopathy. There is a distinct media between internal and external elastic laminae, while longitudinal smooth muscle cells in the intima are lying between elastic fibres. (Elastic van Gieson.)

Fig. 13.110 Muscular pulmonary artery with media of normal thickness in hypoxic arteriopathy. It gives rise to an arteriole (arrow) that shows distinct muscularization. (Elastic van Gieson.)

sometimes also be found in other forms, particularly in plexo-genic arteriopathy. It is especially the contrast between the distinct arteriolar changes and the absence of significant lesions in the larger muscular arteries, which suggests hypoxic arteriopathy.

13.5.6 Embolism, infarction, thrombotic arteriopathy

Pulmonary emboli usually consist of fragments of thrombi, detached from systemic veins or from the right side of the heart, swept into the pulmonary circulation and impacted in pulmonary arteries. Pulmonary thromboembolism is a rather common event which may have very serious consequences, particularly when the emboli are large enough to obstruct larger pulmonary arteries.

There are various other forms of pulmonary embolism in which pieces of tissue or other particles enter the pulmonary arteries, but none of these is as common as thromboembolism. Moreover, these forms usually remain asymptomatic, although in a few instances they can have serious consequences.

Tissue embolism

Pieces of bone marrow, sometimes with bone spicules (Fig. 13.112) or adipose tissue, or more rarely tissue of other organs, such as liver or brain, may lodge in pulmonary arteries following trauma or operation.

Tumour embolism

Fragments of tumour, which have invaded a systemic vein, may become detached and transported by the bloodstream. Within the lung most tumour cells will disintegrate and disappear, but some of these emboli may give rise to metastatic tumours. In some instances thrombosis of pulmonary arteries is elicited by the tumour tissue, causing obstruction of the pulmonary arterial bed and pulmonary hypertension (Fig. 13.113).

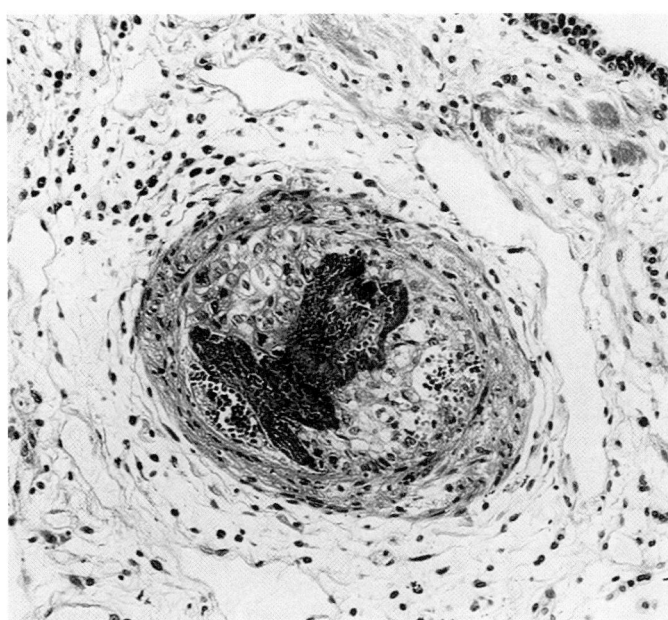

Fig. 13.113 Muscular pulmonary artery with tumour embolus from a gastric carcinoma, and a recent thrombus in the centre. (Periodic acid-Schiff.)

Foreign-body embolism

Not uncommonly, small particles of cotton wool or gauze fibres accidentally enter the circulation during intravenous injection or cardiac catheterization. They may cause *granulomatous arteritis* (Fig. 13.114) or *local intimal fibrosis* (Fig. 13.115), but have no further consequences. This is different when large numbers of foreign bodies are introduced: drugs intended for oral use and containing talc, starch, or fibres as filler material, are sometimes injected intravenously by drug addicts, and may cause widespread granulomatous pulmonary arteritis and pulmonary hypertension.

Fat embolism

During accidental or surgical trauma, fat from lacerated adipose tissue or from fractured bones may enter the circulation, and fat droplets may obstruct pulmonary capillaries and sometimes peripheral pulmonary arteries. Some of the droplets will pass through the pulmonary circulation to cause systemic fat embolism, as evidenced by the occurrence of petechial haemorrhages in the brain, skin, and kidneys. In some non-traumatic conditions, such as *diabetes* and *acute pancreatitis*, fat may be released from tissue to enter the bloodstream and cause fat embolism. The clinical symptoms of pulmonary fat embolism vary greatly, depending on the amount of fat released during the trauma, while assessment of the symptoms is often complicated by the general status of the patient. Undoubtedly, fat embolism is often asymptomatic, but in some patients it may cause dyspnoea, haemoptysis, coma, and death. At autopsy, the diagnosis can be made with fat stains on frozen sections.

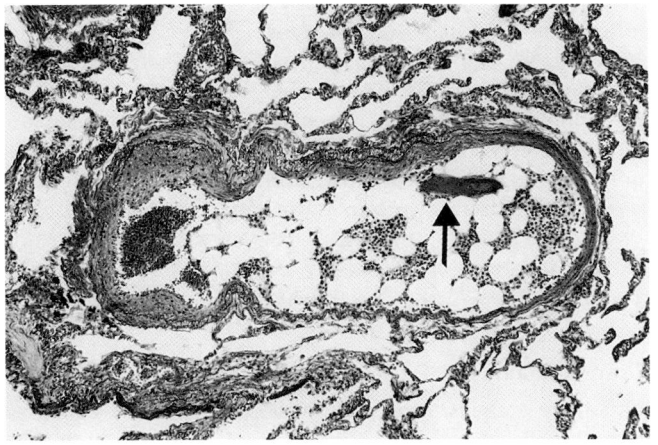

Fig. 13.112 Pulmonary artery with bone marrow embolus. Between the fat cells of the bone marrow lies a bone spicule (arrow).

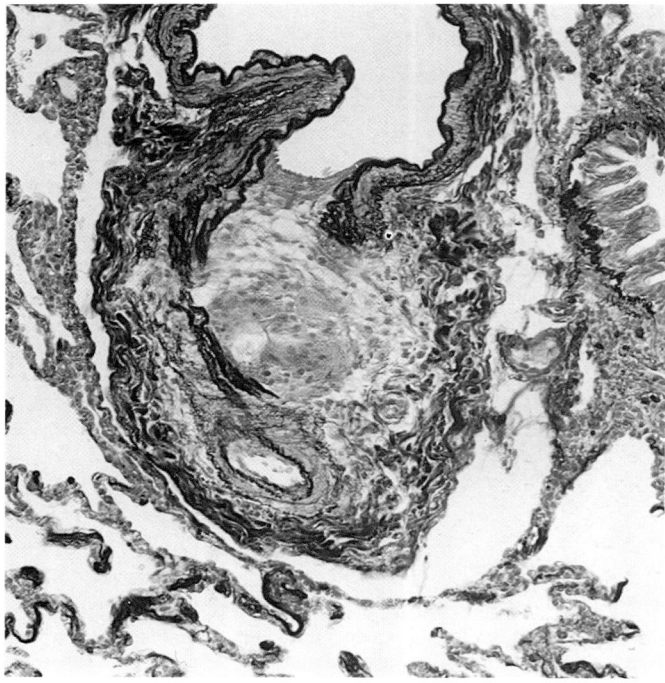

Fig. 13.114 Muscular pulmonary artery with foreign body (cotton wool fibre) granuloma which has interrupted the media. (Elastic van Gieson.)

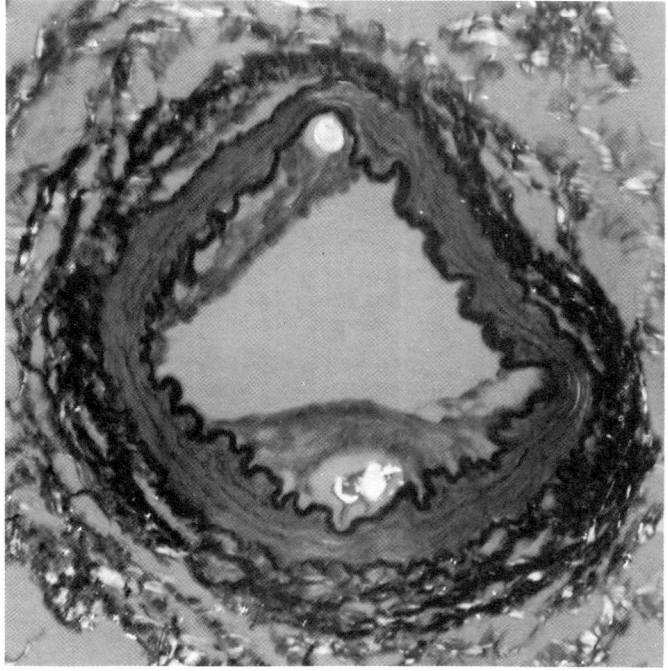

Fig. 13.115 Muscular pulmonary artery with two cross-sections of cotton wool fibre which has caused intimal fibrosis. (Elastic van Gieson, polarized light.)

Amniotic fluid embolism

During or following prolonged and difficult labour, pieces of tissue or cells from decidua or trophoblast may be forced into the maternal bloodstream and become lodged in the pulmonary arteries or capillaries. Sizeable emboli of this nature are uncommon, but isolated trophoblast cells trapped within alveolar capillaries are more often found. The significance of these forms of embolism is limited.

More important is *amniotic fluid embolism*. As a result of intense and prolonged uterine contractions, particularly after partial placental detachment, amniotic fluid may be forced into the maternal circulation. It causes obstruction of the lung vessels by different mechanisms, but only vascular blockage by its constituents such as fetal epithelial squames, lanugo hair, vernix, mucin, and meconium, conforms to the definition of embolism, since these can become impacted in the smallest arteries and in the capillaries of the maternal lungs. These particles can be identified histologically at autopsy.

Amniotic fluid embolism may lead to *severe respiratory distress, hypoxaemia, decrease in cardiac output* and in *systemic blood pressure,* and finally to *shock and death.* It is, however, questionable whether embolization of the contents of the fluid is most often and most prominently responsible for these symptoms. Other, non-embolic mechanisms are probably involved. It is likely that amniotic fluid contains substances that induce vasoconstriction of pulmonary arteries as well as thromboplastic substances; the latter cause widespread intravascular coagulation, particularly within the smallest lung vessels, sometimes leading to severe consumption afibrinogenaemia which may result in serious and sometimes fatal postpartum haemorrhage.

Air and gas embolism

Air or gas bubbles may enter the circulation in various ways, to be arrested eventually in pulmonary arteries or capillaries. Intravenous injections or infusions and accidental or surgical trauma involving the great systemic veins, particularly in the region of head and neck, are important causes. In *caisson disease,* gas bubbles, consisting mainly of nitrogen, are formed in the blood during rapid decompression.

Symptoms of air embolism depend on the amount of introduced air and especially on the rapidity by which it enters the circulation. In severe cases, acute pulmonary hypertension and decreased cardiac output may lead to death. In caisson disease the symptoms may appear either immediately or after an interval of up to 12 hours or more. At autopsy air bubbles present as empty round spaces in the blood-filled pulmonary arteries (Fig. 13.116); fat stains are necessary to distinguish them from fat emboli.

Thromboembolism

Pulmonary embolism generally involves thrombi, which are most often dislodged from systemic veins, particularly the deep veins of the leg and pelvic region, or from the right side of the heart, and are swept into the circulation, becoming lodged in

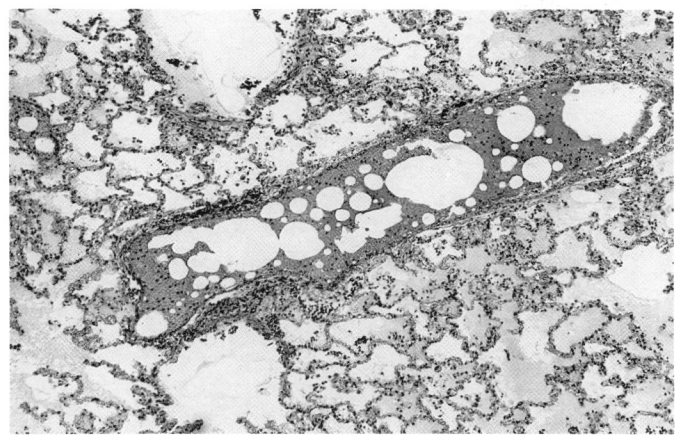

Fig. 13.116 Pulmonary artery in air embolism. There are multiple air bubbles of various size in the lumen.

the pulmonary arteries. Such thrombi may be up to 25 cm long and 1 cm thick.

Pulmonary thromboembolism is a very common phenomenon, but paradoxically, reliable estimates of its prevalence are lacking. Grossly recognizable thromboemboli are observed in 15–25 per cent of hospital autopsies of adult patients, and caused or contributed to the fatal outcome in most of these cases. When the lung vessels are screened histologically, post-thrombotic lesions are found in 60 per cent or more of cases. However, as we will see, it is difficult to exclude that some or even most of these thrombi have originated within the lung vessels (Moser 1979), since there are no differences between the sequelae of embolic and primary thrombi.

The effects of thromboemboli entering the pulmonary circulation depend largely on their size and number: small emboli generally remain clinically unnoticed, while very large ones are regularly fatal. An occasional thromboembolus of moderate size may have little effect, while numerous very small ones may cause pulmonary hypertension and death.

In acute as well as in chronic pulmonary thromboembolism, the clinical diagnosis usually poses great problems and is often not even suspected. The symptoms are generally non-specific. *Dyspnoea* is usually present; *cough, rales, tachycardia, haemoptysis, fever, and signs of pleuritis* may all occur in some patients but are absent in most. Invasive and non-invasive diagnostic methods are sometimes helpful but often inconclusive. This diagnostic inaccuracy is particularly unfortunate because adequate therapy is available and especially effective if applied promptly.

Massive pulmonary embolism

In normal lungs, occlusion of one pulmonary artery is well tolerated; the lungs have a great reserve capacity, so that 60 per cent or more of the pulmonary arterial bed can be occluded before pulmonary hypertension develops. In massive pulmonary embolism, the main pulmonary arteries (Fig. 13.117), the pulmonary trunk, and even the outflow tract of the right ventricle may be filled with masses of thrombi. In this situation the cardiac output is severely reduced and the right ventricular pressure increased. Death may occur instantaneously or after an interval of several hours or days, dependent on the suddenness and completeness of pulmonary arterial obstruction. Some patients survive and the clot is gradually resolved by thrombolysis. Unilateral massive occlusion of the pulmonary arteries may also be fatal in the presence of pre-existing cardiopulmonary disease or when there have been previous embolic events, which remained asymptomatic but which have blocked multiple arterial branches in both lungs. Large and long or V-shaped thrombi originating in the larger leg veins, may straddle the bifurcation of the pulmonary trunk or a main pulmonary

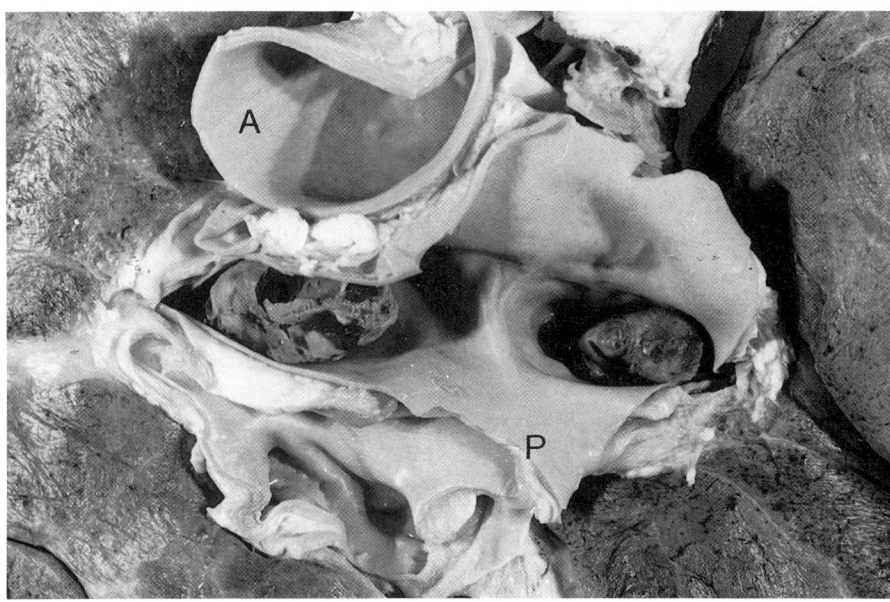

Fig. 13.117 Massive pulmonary thromboembolism with obstruction of both main pulmonary arteries by fresh thrombi. P, upper part of pulmonary trunk; A, aorta.

artery. Such saddle emboli are thereby prevented from becoming impacted in the arteries.

Recurrent pulmonary embolism

Medium-sized thromboemboli usually lodge in lobar, segmental, or more peripheral elastic pulmonary arteries. They may be symptomatic or not, but even if they produce symptoms, the diagnosis is often missed and the condition remains untreated. Small emboli obstructing muscular pulmonary arteries are generally asymptomatic in an initial stage. However, in all these instances of pulmonary embolism there is a strong tendency for recurrence over the years, and even if isolated events remain unnoticed, repeated episodes of thromboembolism may cause gradual obstruction of numerous elastic or muscular pulmonary arteries to such an extent that pulmonary hypertension develops. In cases of so-called *silent embolic pulmonary hypertension,* the symptoms of this serious complication are the first to draw attention to the underlying process (Messer 1984).

Sustained pulmonary hypertension as a result of recurrent thromboembolism is uncommon; silent embolic pulmonary hypertension is rare. The available evidence suggests that the cause of the elevation of pressure is mainly mechanical, due to extensive thrombotic obstruction of the pulmonary arterial tree. In some patients with pulmonary embolism, reactive arterial vasoconstriction may, however, contribute to pulmonary hypertension.

Since more than half of the pulmonary vascular bed must be obstructed before the pressure rises significantly, the number of emboli that occlude small arteries must indeed be very large. However, it must be realized that this process may extend over many years. Also, a single larger embolus may break down as a result of thrombolysis, resulting in many small ones.

Pulmonary infarction

Embolic occlusion of a major pulmonary artery causes ischaemia of lung tissue distal to it, with damage to the capillary endothelium. The dual blood supply of the lung ensures that this area still receives blood *via* the bronchial circulation, but this tends to leak out of the damaged capillaries so that the lung tissue becomes haemorrhagic. The term *pulmonary infarction* implies that there is necrosis of lung tissue, but this is far from common, certainly in view of the frequency of pulmonary embolism. Pulmonary infarcts are difficult to produce in experimental animals. In man, they are particularly observed in elderly patients and in those who have mitral valve disease or in whom the circulation is otherwise impaired. This suggests that an increased pulmonary venous pressure may be a contributing factor in the pathogenesis of an infarct.

Pulmonary infarcts are often multiple, and are more common in the lower lobes, as is to be expected since thromboemboli are somewhat more common and the pulmonary venous pressure is higher in the lower lobes. The infarcts are generally haemorrhagic, dark red-brown and sharply delimited (Fig. 13.118). In the necrotic area, the blood vessels lose their tone and, despite

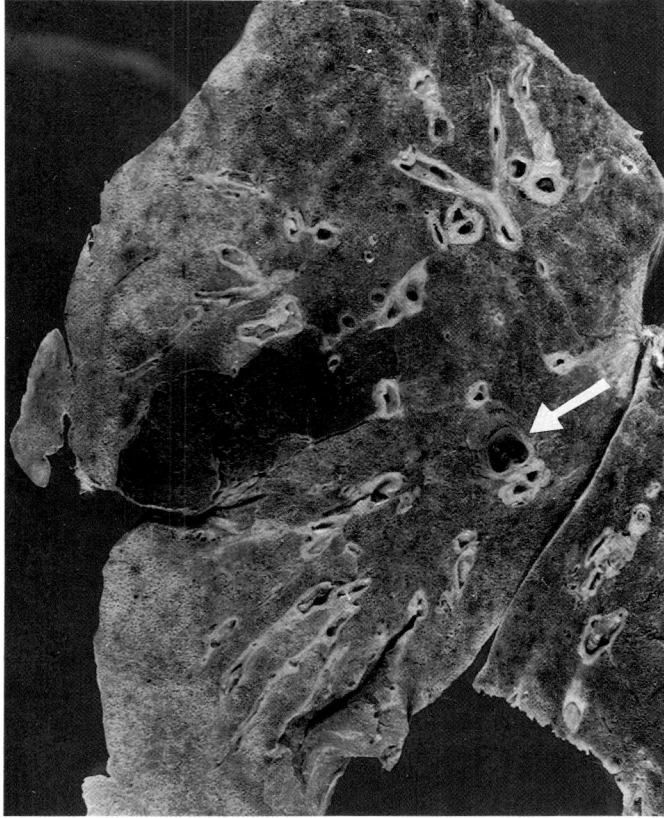

Fig. 13.118 Haemorrhagic pulmonary infarct, sharply delimited and bordering the pleura. A recent thromboembolus (arrow) occludes a pulmonary artery.

the interrupted arterial blood supply, they become dilated, engorged because of retrograde filling, and leaky. Since they correspond to the conical area supplied by the obstructed pulmonary artery, pulmonary infarcts are often wedge-shaped on cut section with the base bordering the pleura and the apex directed towards the hilum; their size varies widely. Within a few days, fibrinous pleuritis ensues, with its clinical signs of pleural pain and friction rub, which assist in establishing the diagnosis clinically. Occasionally a pulmonary infarct is pale with a red border; this appearance usually results from infection, as caused by an infected embolus. Such a septic infarction may turn into a lung abscess.

Histologically, the most impressive feature is the extensive haemorrhage; erythrocytes are distinct for the first 2 days until lysis sets in. A diagnostic feature is *necrosis of alveolar walls* and other structures, such as bronchioles and blood vessels (Fig. 13.119). The margins of an infarct usually show an inflammatory reaction, preceding organization of the necrotic tissue. Neutrophilic leucocytes are scarce except in septic infarcts, where they dominate the picture and are responsible for the pale colour. As long as there is no necrosis, pulmonary haemorrhages resulting from embolism are essentially reversible and may disappear completely. Infarcts, however, become organized and are gradually converted into collagen-rich scars which,

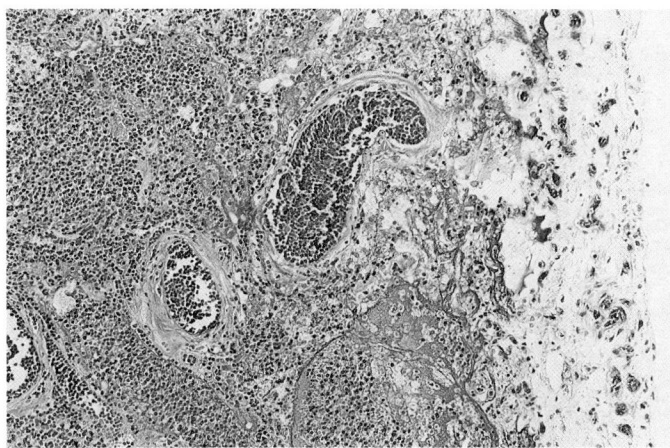

Fig. 13.119 Haemorrhagic pulmonary infarct, bordering the pleura. Alveolar walls and other structures are necrotic and alveolar spaces are filled with erythrocytes and fibrin.

as a result of retraction, are far smaller than the original infarct. They are therefore often missed at autopsy, unless the lungs are inflated through the bronchi, which makes the scar visible as a dimple at the pleural surface. A pleural adhesion may also mark its location.

Thrombotic arteriopathy

If the patient survives an episode of acute pulmonary thromboembolism, the fate of the thrombi within the pulmonary arteries varies greatly, regardless of whether the thrombi are large or small, or even whether they are embolic or primary in origin.

Thrombolysis may lead to disappearance, decrease in size, or fragmentation of thrombi. Thrombolysis is based upon proteolytic enzymes, particularly plasmin, which dissolve the fibrin in the thrombus. This process is an important factor in removing clots when these are still relatively fresh (Fig. 13.120). This can

happen within a few days; small thrombi are thereby probably much more rapidly dissolved than larger ones.

However, many thrombi do not dissolve, but become organized. Where the thrombus lies against the vascular wall, the endothelium becomes locally damaged and *myofibroblasts*, probably derived from the pulmonary arterial media, invade the thrombus. At the free ends of the thrombus, endothelial cells proliferate and cover its outer surface. The myofibroblasts form *collagen* and to a lesser extent *elastin*, thus replacing the thrombus by a fibrotic mass, which becomes incorporated into the arterial wall. Shrinkage of the fibrotic mass results in restoration of part of the lumen, leaving an eccentric patch of intimal fibrosis (Fig. 13.121). These intimal patches may occasionally show two or three layers, representing thrombi of different age, but there is no onion-skin configuration as in plexogenic arteriopathy. Total or subtotal obliteration of a pulmonary artery is frequent (Fig. 13.122), albeit usually over a short distance.

Next to shrinkage, recanalization of thrombi results in reduction of vascular obstruction (Fig. 13.123). Particularly in larger and occlusive thrombi, numerous capillaries invade the clots, together with myofibroblasts. These capillaries sprouted in part from the endothelial lining of the thrombus and in part from vasa vasorum of the arterial adventitia, form a network with each other and connect the arterial lumina on either side of the clot.

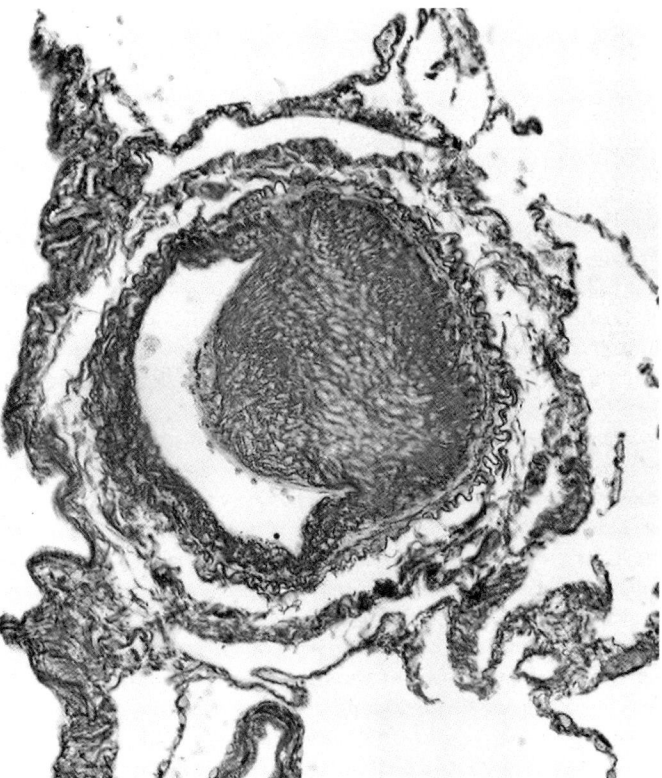

Fig. 13.121 Muscular pulmonary artery with eccentric intimal fibrosis in thrombotic arteriopathy. Although there had been severe pulmonary hypertension, the media is not increased in thickness. (Elastic van Gieson.)

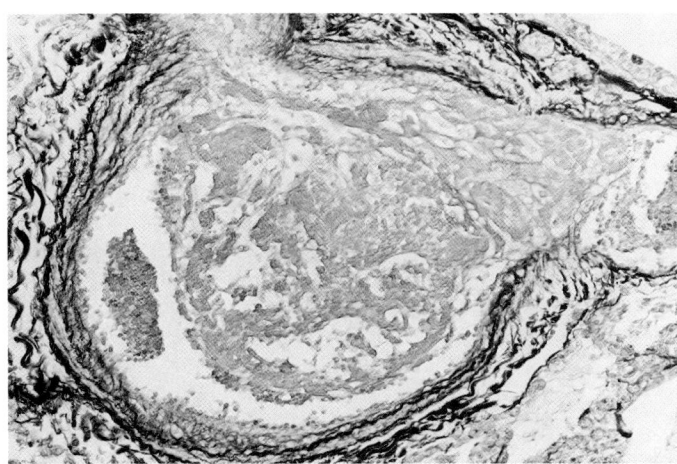

Fig. 13.120 Pulmonary artery with fairly fresh thrombus showing signs of disintegration, possible by fibrinolysis. (Elastic van Gieson.)

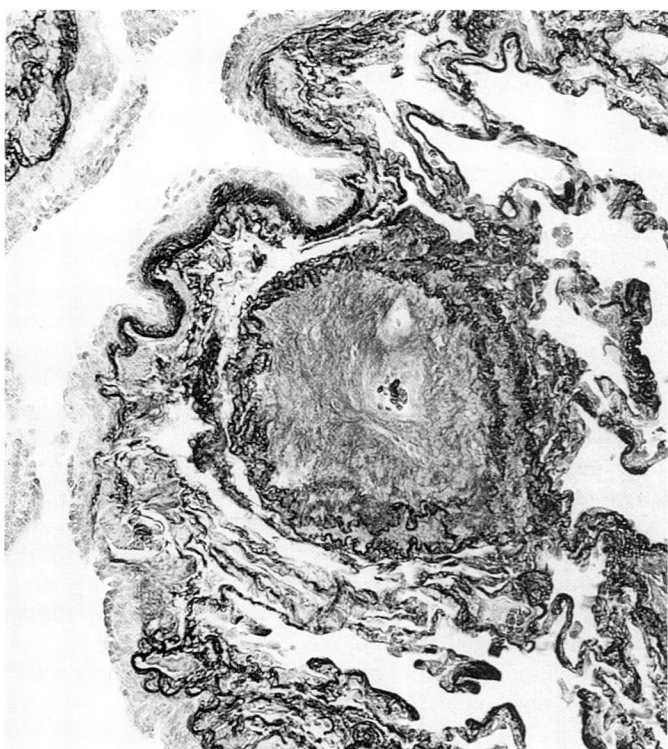

Fig. 13.122 Pulmonary artery almost completely occluded by intimal fibrosis in thrombotic arteriopathy; there is no concentric-laminar arrangement. (Elastic van Gieson.)

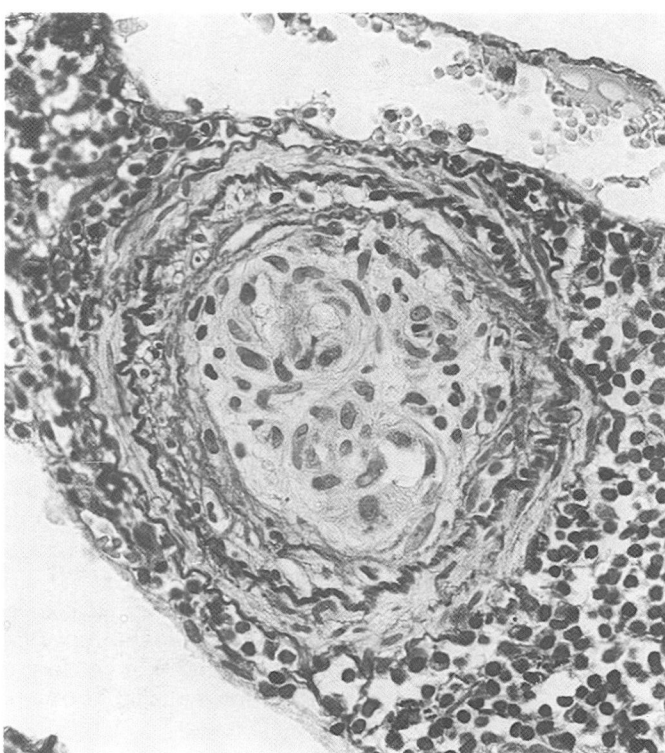

Fig. 13.123 Pulmonary artery obstructed by post-thrombotic intimal fibrosis with multiple small recanalization channels. There is some infiltrate of lymphocytes around the vessel. (Elastic van Gieson.)

These newly formed capillaries may dilate to form large channels, even to the extent that only fibrotic remnants of the thrombus remain as interconnected septa and lattices (Fig. 13.124). These intravascular septa are pathognomonic sequelae of thrombosis, whether embolic or primary. In the main pulmonary arteries and their largest branches they are grossly recognizable and known as *bands and webs* (Fig. 13.125). Sometimes subsequent emboli are trapped within these structures. They are far more common in smaller elastic arteries and particularly in muscular arteries.

Septic thromboemboli, containing pyogenic micro-organisms, may originate from an infected area and may be the cause of *pulmonary arteritis* and widespread *abscess formation.*

As we have seen, the occurrence of post-thrombotic lesions is exceedingly common, and may be found in the vast majority of autopsies on adult patients. Usually, however, their numbers are small in any given patient. An occasional patch of eccentric intimal fibrosis or intravascular septum has no clinical or haemodynamic significance, and the term thrombotic arteriopathy would not be justified. When they are more numerous, they may cause pulmonary hypertension, but this is difficult to predict from the histological picture. It may also be impossible to ascertain whether the lesions result from emboli or from primary thrombosis since, as discussed before, the resulting alterations are identical. Post-thrombotic lesions may also complicate other forms of vascular disease. They are common in

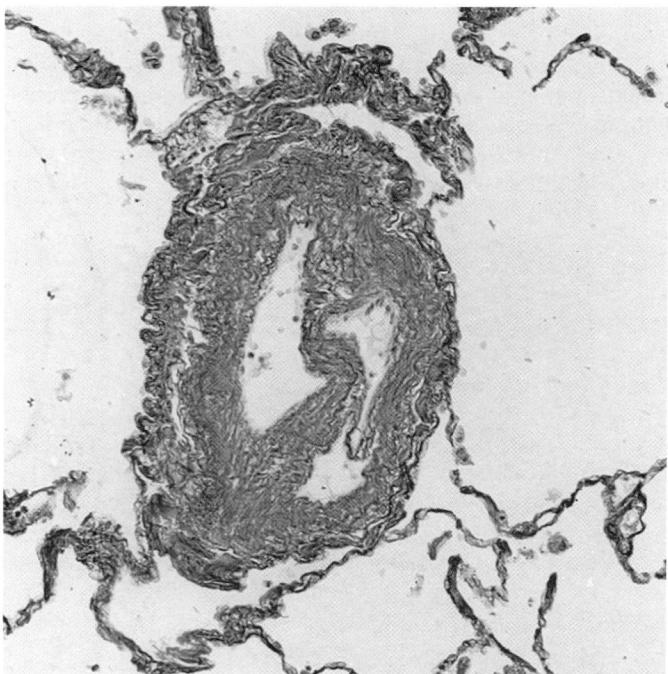

Fig. 13.124 Muscular pulmonary artery with intravascular fibrous septa due to organization and progressive recanalization of thrombus; in thrombotic arteriopathy. (Elastic van Gieson.)

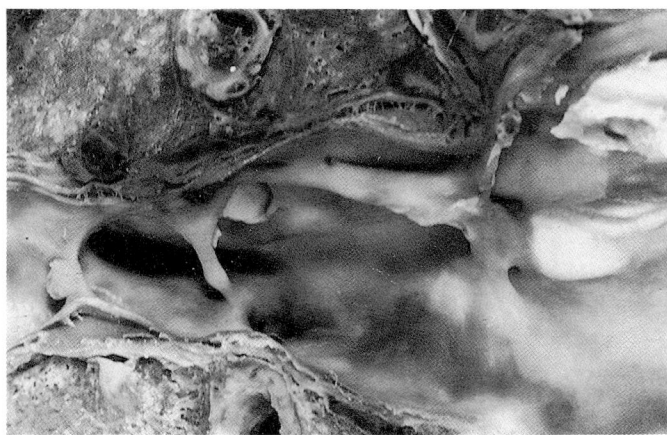

Fig. 13.125 Main pulmonary artery cut open close to the ramification of the pulmonary trunk. Remnants of organized and recanalized thrombi form band and web-like structures. A cross-section of a smaller branch (top) shows a more recent thrombus.

cases of diminished pulmonary flow, as in tetralogy of Fallot (p. 1020). They are also often seen in combination with plexogenic arteriopathy in patients with transposition of the great arteries who have an increased haematocrit, or in adult patients with primary plexogenic arteriopathy.

13.5.7 Congestive vasculopathy

Aetiology and mechanisms

Congestive vasculopathy is caused by an impediment to the pulmonary venous outflow. The obstruction may be localized in the large pulmonary venous trunks by a *congenital stenosis*, or caused by *pressure on the veins* from outside, as in mediastinal fibrosis. Far more often, the impediment is located in the heart: the most common causes for congestive vasculopathy are *rheumatic mitral stenosis and incompetence* and *left ventricular failure* resulting from coronary heart disease or systemic hypertension. Other acquired conditions that have a similar effect are *endocarditis, myocarditis, cardiomyopathies,* and *left atrial myxoma.* Congenital causes include *cor triatriatum* and *congenital aortic or mitral stenosis and atresia.*

In these cases of pulmonary venous hypertension, the pulmonary arterial pressure is raised disproportionally to that in the veins, and may even reach systemic levels. While this cannot result from transmission of pressure, it is not clear how the increased resistance in the pulmonary arteries is brought about; vasoconstriction and interstitial oedema of the arterial walls have both been implicated.

Interstitial oedema is a direct consequence of a rise in mean pressure, exceeding approximately 25 mmHg. Fluid accumulates in alveolar walls, in the peribronchial and perivascular connective tissue, and in the walls of lung vessels. Interlobular septa, which normally consist of loose connective tissue, are greatly distended by fluid and may show up on a chest radiogram as horizontal lines, so-called *Kerley B lines.* Throughout the lungs the pulmonary lymphatics are markedly dilated.

Morphology

In congestive vasculopathy the changes may vary considerably in severity but characteristically they are widespread, affecting pulmonary arteries and veins as well as the lung tissue. Often, the various lesions are striking. It is likely that long-standing interstitial oedema contributes to several of these alterations, since it induces deposition of collagen not only in lung tissue but also in vascular walls.

Muscular pulmonary arteries may show a marked thickening of the media (Fig. 13.126), which is often accompanied by muscularization of arterioles, although this may be much less conspicuous. The arterial media contains less smooth muscle and more collagen than a normal media, or a hypertrophied media in plexogenic arteriopathy. This medial fibrosis, which is an end-result of interstitial oedema, is probably responsible for the poor correlation between the severity of medial thickening and the degree of pulmonary arterial pressure and resistance seen in rheumatic heart disease. Often these histological changes are very pronounced while pressure and resistance are only mildly increased, or even within normal limits. The likely explanation is that in these instances, the muscularity of the arteries is not proportional to the medial thickness (Wagenvoort and Wagenvoort 1982).

Intimal fibrosis of pulmonary arteries is also often very pronounced and usually eccentric (Fig. 13.127). Even when it is circumferential, it does not exhibit an onion-skin configuration. In contrast to post-thrombotic intimal fibrosis (p. 1013), the intimal thickening in congestive vasculopathy generally extends over long distances. However, it virtually never

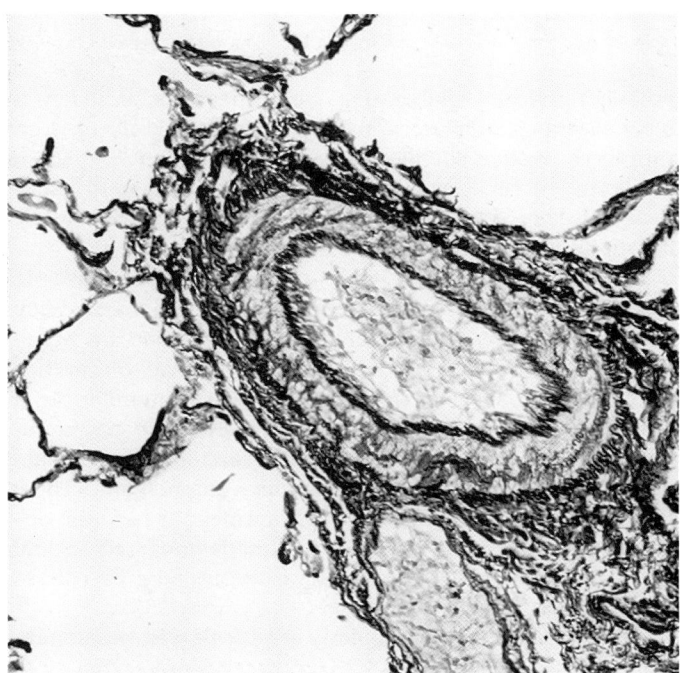

Fig. 13.126 Muscular pulmonary artery in congestive vasculopathy. There is severe medial hypertrophy. Dark areas within the media represent medial fibrosis. (Elastic van Gieson.)

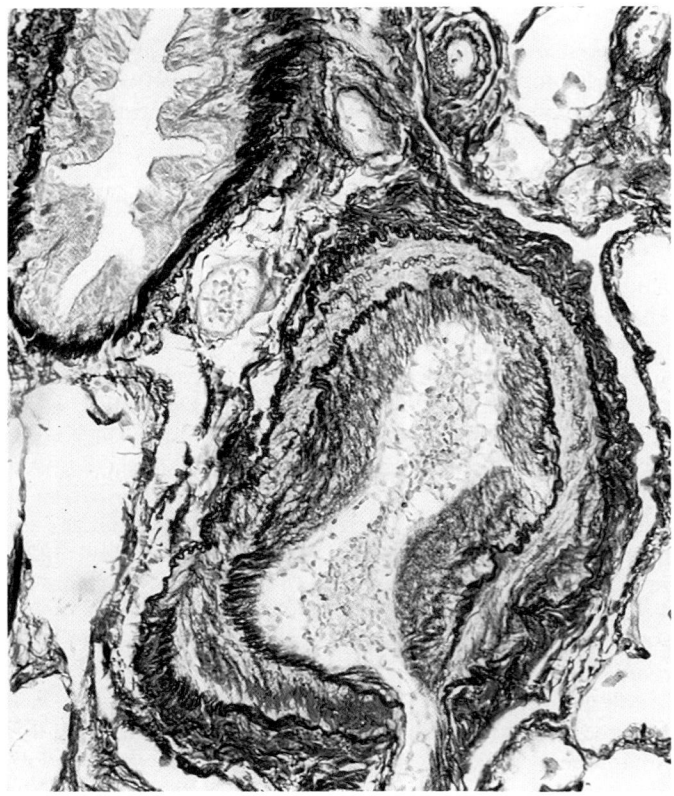

Fig. 13.127 Muscular pulmonary artery in congestive vasculopathy, showing medial hypertrophy and fibrosis and also prominent eccentric intimal fibrosis. At the top, a muscularized arteriole is seen. (Elastic van Gieson.)

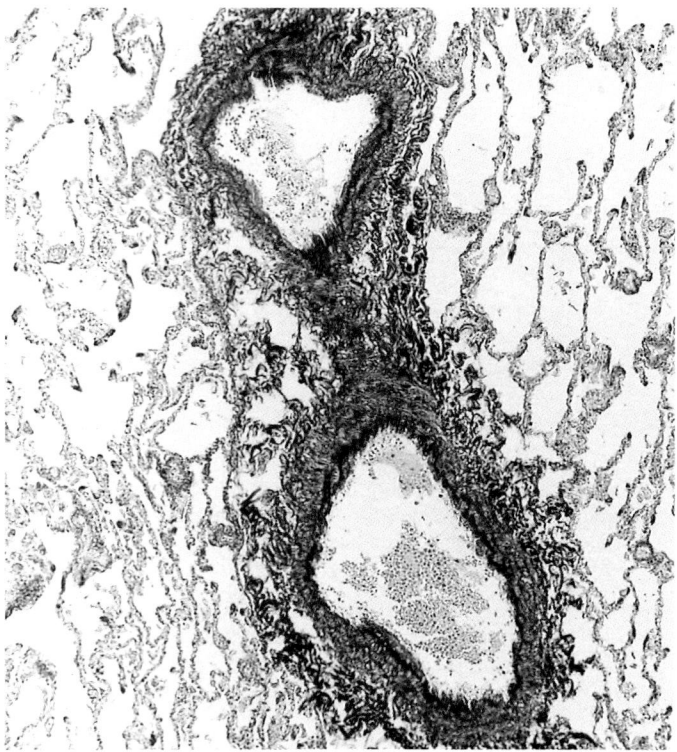

Fig. 13.128 Pulmonary veins with pronounced thickening of their walls, in congestive vasculopathy. (Elastic van Gieson.)

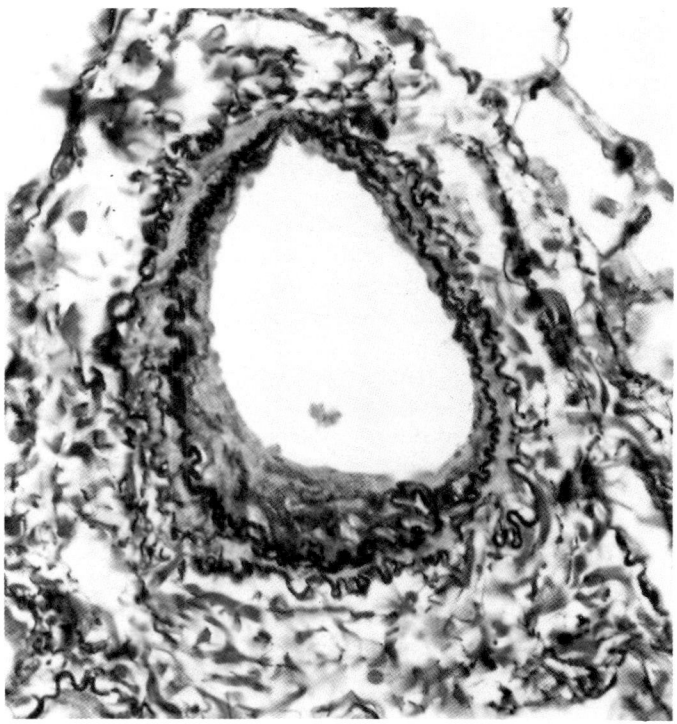

Fig. 13.129 Pulmonary vein in congestive vasculopathy with arterialization: distinct internal and external elastic laminae have developed; there is also mild intimal fibrosis. (Elastic van Gieson.)

produces complete obliteration and it has little tendency to recanalization. Pulmonary arteritis and fibrinoid necrosis are rare in congestive vasculopathy, while dilatation lesions and plexiform lesions do not occur, even when pulmonary hypertension is very severe. The adventitia of pulmonary arteries is fibrotic and greatly increased in thickness.

The walls of pulmonary veins are also regularly thickened (Fig. 13.128). In addition to medial hypertrophy, they develop arterialization, a striking change in configuration by which they acquire internal and external elastic laminae so that they resemble pulmonary arteries (Fig. 13.129). Intimal fibrosis of pulmonary veins is common but rarely severe. In approximately half of the patients with congestive vasculopathy there are additional alterations in the pulmonary parenchyma. These include interstitial oedema and fibrosis which, as has been discussed, affect almost all structures within the lungs. Interstitial fibrosis of alveolar walls may be very extensive (Fig. 13.130) so that the whole lung becomes firm.

Haemosiderosis is found regularly in patients with pulmonary venous hypertension (Fig. 13.131). Extravasated erythrocytes within the interstitium and alveolar spaces are ingested and broken down by macrophages, resulting in formation of haemosiderin. This is stored in the macrophages, which may show up in the sputum ('heart failure cells'). Some extracellular haemosiderin may be found in the interstitium. Haemosiderosis is easily recognized on gross inspection of the cut-surface of the lung. When combined with increased firmness due to interstitial fibrosis, the term 'brown induration' is used. These changes are generally associated with dilatation of lymphatics.

So-called *corpora amylacea* are commonly found in patients with pulmonary venous hypertension, although they are not specific for congestive vasculopathy. They are intra-alveolar, round or oval hyaline bodies, mostly varying in size from 50 to 100 μm, often with a structure of concentric rings (Fig. 13.132). They consist of glycoproteins, deposited around a central inclusion. Another concretion is the *osseous nodule*: a small nodular ossified body with a racemose form. Osseous nodules may be recognized on a chest radiogram, or a post-mortem pulmonary radiogram (Fig. 13.133).

Our knowledge about the reversibility of congestive vasculopathy is limited. Following mitral commissurotomy or valve replacement, pulmonary hypertension decreases in many patients with rheumatic heart disease. Sometimes this drop in pressure is sudden and large, even in patients whose preoperative lung biopsy specimen showed severe pulmonary vascular lesions. This almost certainly means that interstitial oedema of the vascular wall, notably of the intima, is involved in bringing about the increased pressure. Severe intimal thickening, causing pronounced obstruction to the pulmonary vascular bed, is unlikely to disappear or diminish instantly, if

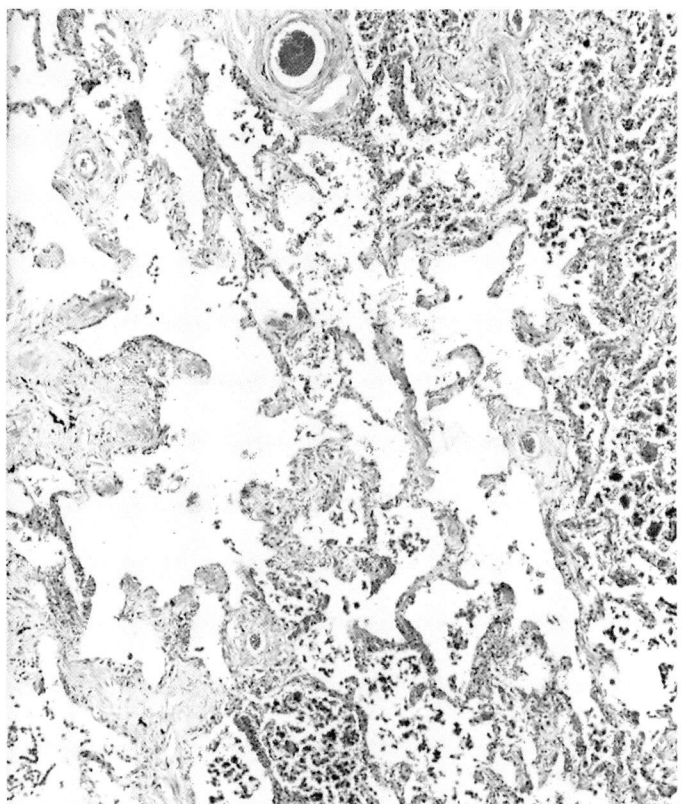

Fig. 13.130 Interstitial fibrosis of lung tissue, affecting the alveolar walls, in congestive vasculopathy.

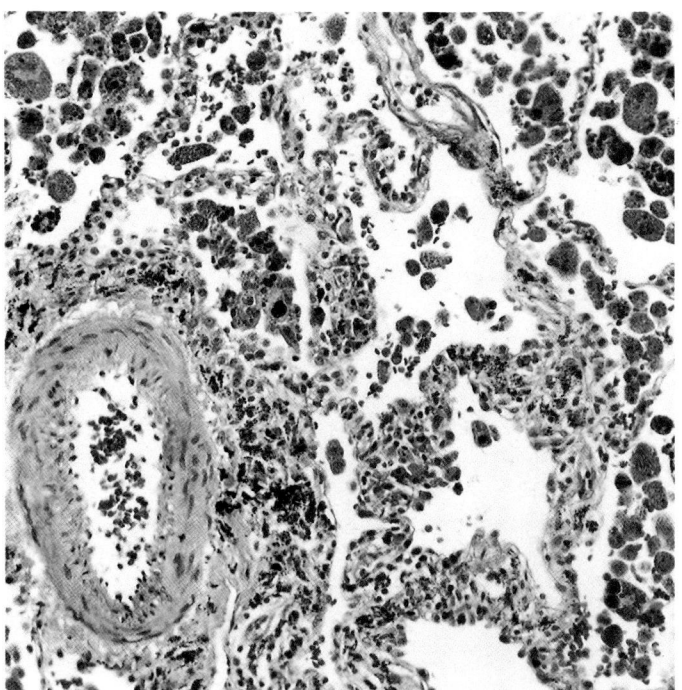

Fig. 13.131 Lung tissue with haemosiderosis; the iron pigment is deposited mainly in intra-alveolar macrophages.

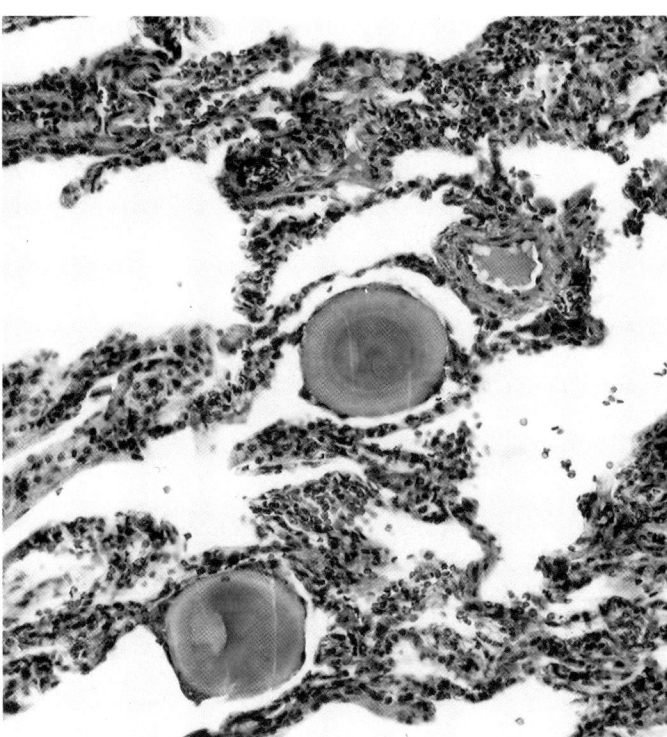

Fig. 13.132 Corpora amylacea with concentric laminar structure within the lung tissue; in congestive vasculopathy.

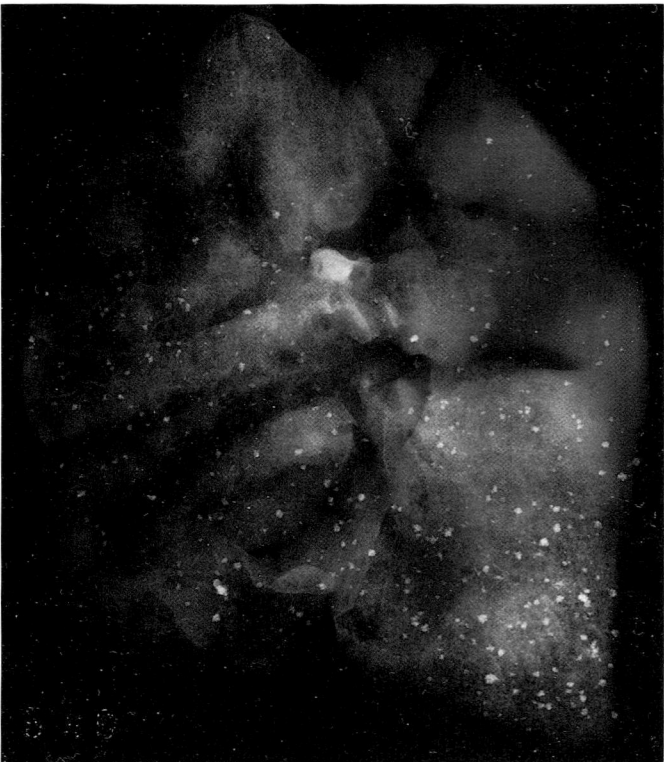

Fig. 13.133 Post-mortem radiogram of right lung with numerous osseous nodules from a patient with rheumatic mitral stenosis.

not by removal of interstitial fluid. In plexogenic arteriopathy due to a congenital cardiac shunt, the same degree of intimal thickening should be considered an irreversible lesion and, if present in multiple arteries, would constitute a contraindication for corrective surgery. There are indications that, in the long run, even severe medial hypertrophy and intimal fibrosis may regress completely or almost completely, when normal haemodynamics in these patients are restored.

13.5.8   Pulmonary veno-occlusive disease

Pulmonary veno-occlusive disease is a rare condition occurring at all ages from infancy to the seventh decade, with a highest incidence in children and young adults. In adults, males are approximately twice as often affected as females, but in children there is an equal sex ratio. The clinical diagnosis is difficult, since the signs and symptoms closely resemble those of primary plexogenic arteriopathy and silent recurrent thromboembolism. Together with these two conditions, it is usually listed as one of the three most important forms of 'primary pulmonary hypertension' (p. 1020). It has a progressive course, and is usually fatal within 1–3 years as a result of pulmonary hypertension and right cardiac failure.

Aetiology

The cause of pulmonary veno-occlusive disease is unknown, but there are strong indications that it is not an aetiological entity. It is likely that in some patients the disease may occur as a consequence of a viral respiratory infection. In other cases a toxic cause seems likely; several patients have developed veno-occlusive disease following chemotherapy for malignant conditions.

Morphology and pathogenesis

As the name suggests, the pulmonary veins, especially the smaller ones, become gradually narrowed and obliterated by *intimal fibrosis* (Fig. 13.134; Heath *et al.* 1966). The fibrosis initially has a loose texture, as a result of interstitial oedema, but gradually more and more collagen is deposited. Recanalization of the intimal fibrotic tissue is regularly observed (Fig. 13.135) and intravascular fibrous septa are common. In approximately half of the patients, the pulmonary arteries are involved, with similar histological changes (Fig. 13.136), although usually to a much lesser extent (Wagenvoort *et al.* 1985).

The intimal lesions are very probably the result of thrombosis. They are obliterative and subject to recanalization, while recent thrombi, although uncommon in the veins, are frequently found in the arteries, probably because these are affected in a later stage of the disease. In the lung tissue, haemosiderosis and, more characteristically, small areas of congestion and interstitial fibrosis are frequent (Fig. 13.137).

13.5.9   Arteriopathy in lung fibrosis

In the presence of lung fibrosis or granulomatosis, there are almost always prominent changes in the lung vessels, regard-

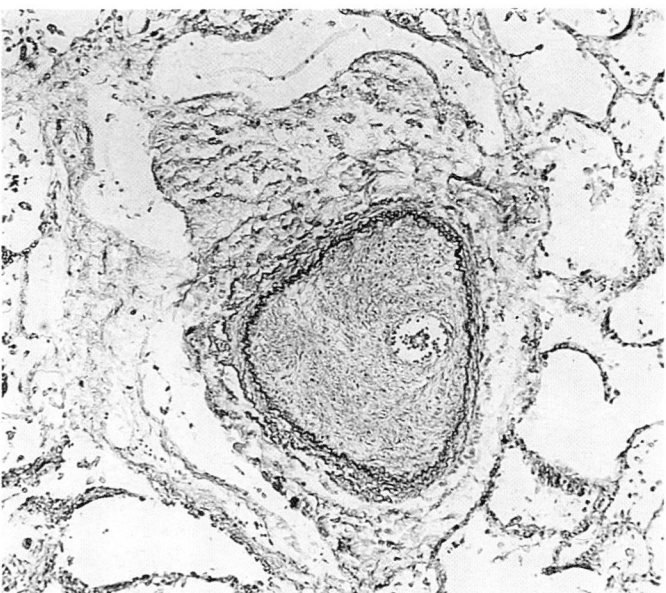

Fig. 13.134 Pulmonary veins in pulmonary veno-occlusive disease. The lumen is almost completely obstructed by loose intimal fibrosis. (Elastic van Gieson.)

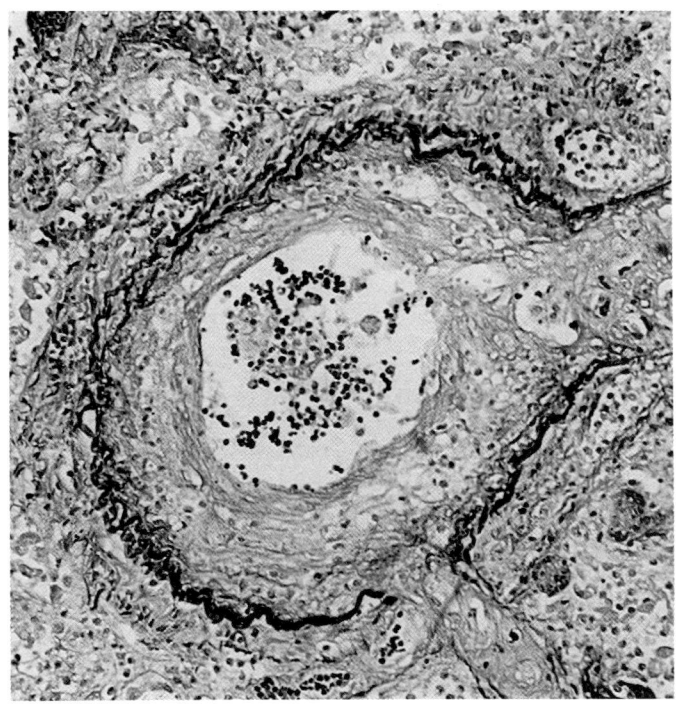

Fig. 13.135 Pulmonary vein in pulmonary veno-occlusive disease. Prominent intimal fibrosis with multiple small recanalization channels. (Elastic van Gieson.)

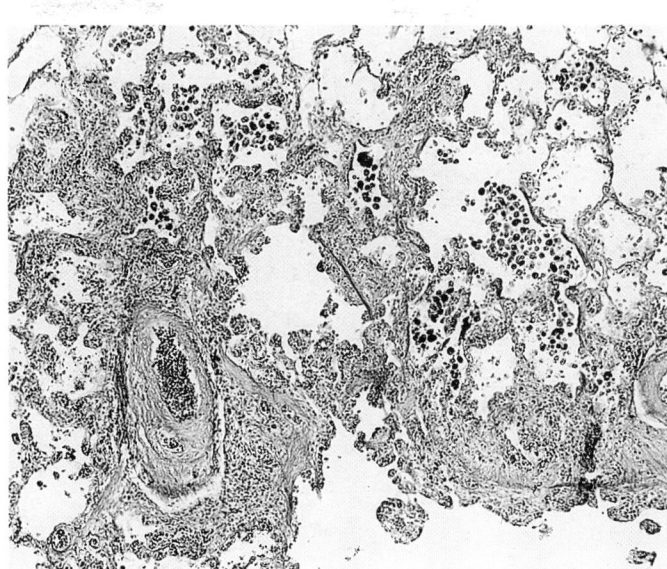

Fig. 13.137 Lung tissue in pulmonary veno-occlusive disease with a small area of interstitial fibrosis in combination with haemosiderosis. One vein is narrowed by intimal fibrosis. (Elastic van Gieson.)

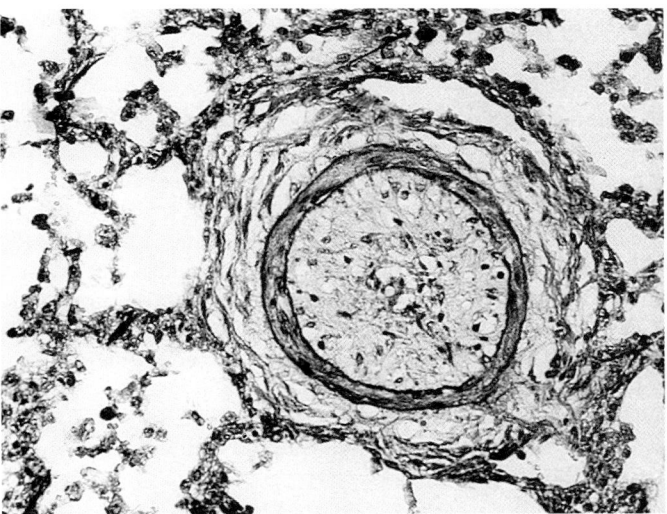

Fig. 13.136 Muscular pulmonary artery with subtotal occlusion of lumen by loose intimal fibrosis; in pulmonary veno-occlusive disease. (Elastic van Gieson.)

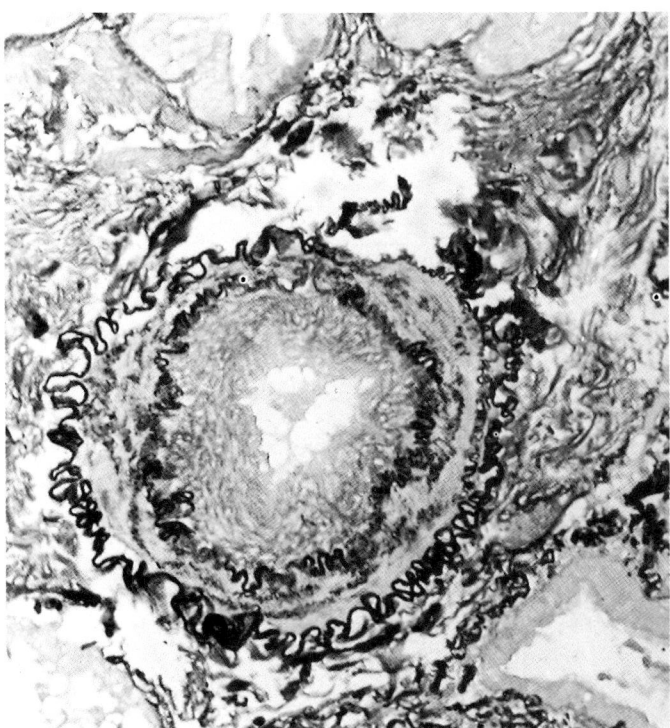

Fig. 13.138 Muscular pulmonary artery in a case of lung fibrosis. The artery, lying in a fibrotic area, shows severe medial hypertrophy and intimal fibrosis. (Elastic van Gieson.)

less of the type of the fibrosis or granulomatosis. The vascular lesions are limited to fibrotic areas or their immediate environment. In the muscular pulmonary arteries, medial hypertrophy and eccentric intimal fibrosis are usually severe, sometimes excessive (Fig. 13.138). The pulmonary veins also regularly show marked medial hypertrophy and intimal fibrosis (Fig. 13.139). Such vascular changes may be associated with pulmonary hypertension, but only when both lungs are extensively involved. The vessels in areas of lung tissue not affected by fibrosis are usually normal, and in most instances the pulmonary arterial pressure is within normal limits.

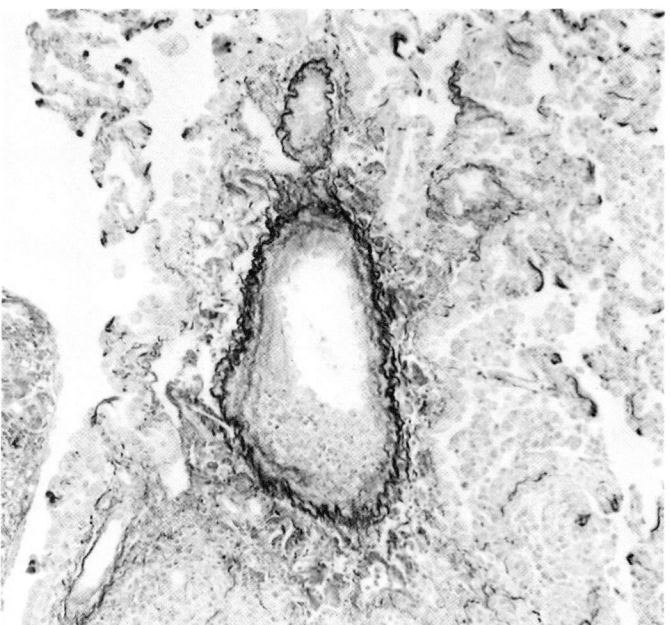

Fig. 13.139 Pulmonary vein in a case of lung fibrosis, with some medial thickening and prominent intimal fibrosis. (Elastic van Gieson.)

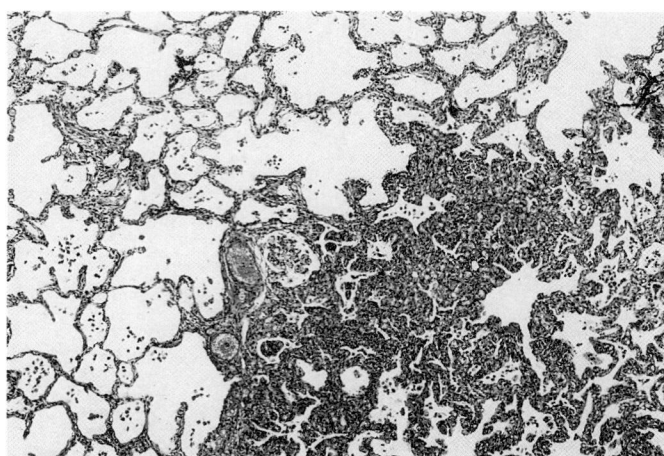

Fig. 13.140 Lung tissue with capillary haemangiomatosis; there is invasion of alveolar walls and spaces and of vessels by proliferating capillary-like channels.

13.5.10   Unexplained pulmonary hypertension

There are uncommon cases in which pulmonary hypertension can be demonstrated clinically, while the cause remains unsolved despite extensive clinical and physiological investigations. This occurs especially in three conditions: primary plexogenic arteriopathy (p. 1003), silent recurrent embolic pulmonary hypertension (p. 1012) and pulmonary veno-occlusive disease (p. 1018). The name 'primary pulmonary hypertension' has been proposed and is widely used for these cases, but this wrongly suggests that we are dealing with a single entity (Wagenvoort 1989). Moreover, the term is sometimes used for primary plexogenic arteriopathy alone. It is therefore more correct and less confusing to speak of unexplained pulmonary hypertension.

Very uncommonly, conditions other than the three just mentioned, provoke unexplained pulmonary hypertension. This may happen with an atypical case of a common disease in which the diagnosis is missed, or in very rare diseases such as *pulmonary capillary haemangiomatosis*. The latter condition is characterized by proliferation of capillary-like channels (Fig. 13.140) which may infiltrate not only interstitium, alveolar walls, and bronchi but also blood vessels, thus causing pulmonary hypertension (Wagenvoort *et al.* 1978).

13.5.11   Lung vessels in diminished pulse pressure and flow

In the presence of *pulmonary stenosis* there is a diminished pulse pressure in the pulmonary arteries, the systolic peaks being de-

creased, but the mean pressure is hardly influenced. As described below, a flattened pressure curve has a distinct effect on the media of pulmonary arteries.

Pulmonary stenosis is usually congenital; it may be infundibular or valvular. In *tetralogy of Fallot* there is also a diminished pulmonary flow, because blood is shunted from right to left through the ventricular septal defect. This, in combination with an increased haematocrit, causes a tendency to thrombosis and associated intimal changes.

Morphology

In diminished pulse pressure, the media of muscular pulmonary arteries may be thinner than normal (Fig. 13.141; Wagenvoort *et al.* 1967). Since the normal arterial media is already thin, the difference is not always obvious. However, in some cases there is complete *medial atrophy* so that internal and external elastic laminae make contact. Such extreme thinning is particularly observed in tetralogy of Fallot. The arteries are also regularly wider than normal, which becomes apparent when arterial diameter is compared to that of the adjacent bronchus or bronchiole. Especially in older children and adults with tetralogy of Fallot, recent thrombi are often present (Fig. 13.142). Organization of these thrombi may result in patches of eccentric intimal fibrosis (Fig. 13.143), often in combination with intravascular fibrous septa due to recanalization (Fig. 13.144). These septa are usually very thin and may be present throughout the arterial tree (Rich 1948). In pulmonary veins these post-thrombotic changes are uncommon. Usually there is an extensive development of collateral vessels (Rabinovitch *et al.* 1981).

13.5.12   Developmental anomalies of lung vessels

Congenital anomalies of the major lung vessels are uncommon and usually occur in the context of a more complicated

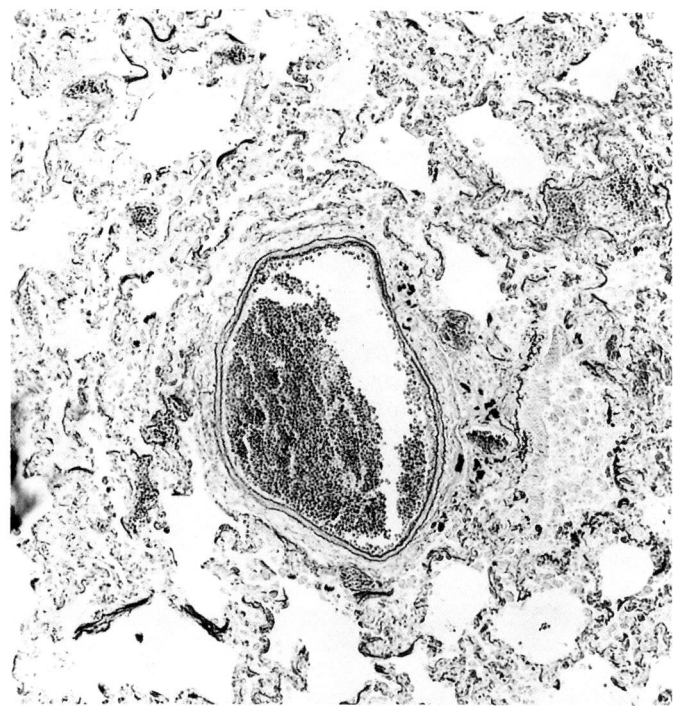

Fig. 13.141 Muscular pulmonary artery in tetralogy of Fallot; the artery is wide, as compared to the associated bronchiole, and extremely thin-walled. (Elastic van Gieson.)

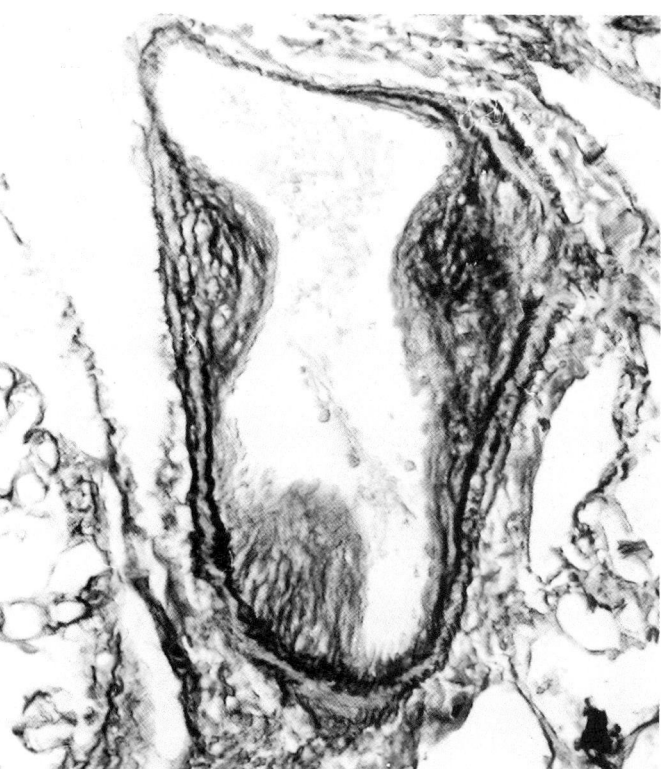

Fig. 13.143 Pulmonary artery in tetralogy of Fallot with eccentric patches of post-thrombotic intimal fibrosis. (Elastic van Gieson.)

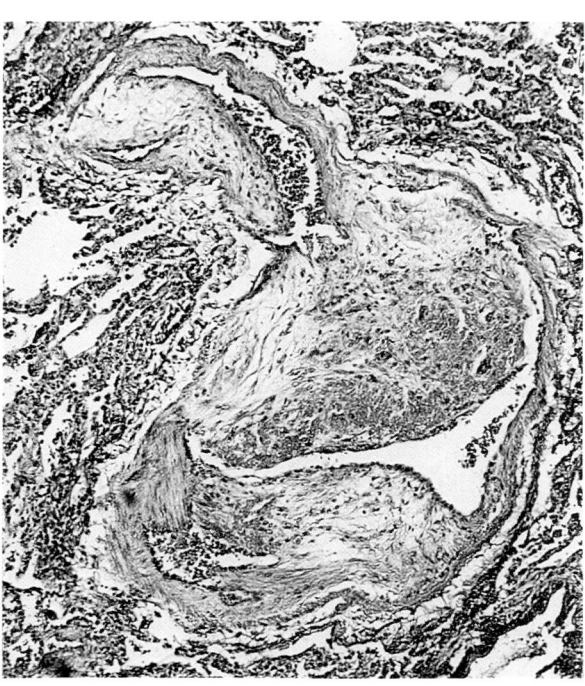

Fig. 13.142 Muscular pulmonary artery in tetralogy of Fallot with extensive thrombosis. The thrombus shows early organization.

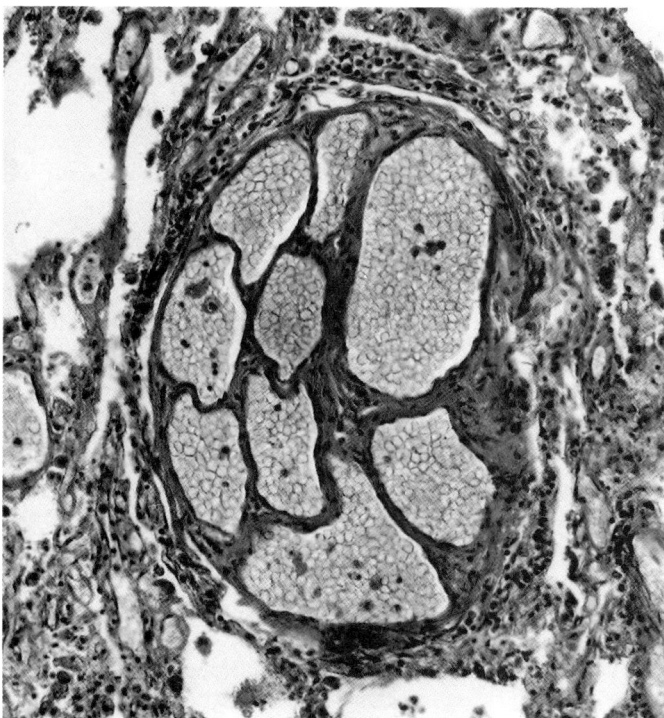

Fig. 13.144 Pulmonary artery in tetralogy of Fallot with multiple delicate interconnected fibrous septa resulting from recanalization of organized thrombus.

cardiovascular anomaly. Examples are *complete transposition of the great arteries, tetralogy of Fallot, truncus arteriosus,* and *total anomalous pulmonary venous connection.* In these situations any of the great pulmonary arteries or veins may be absent, abnormally connected, stenosed, or dilated. Some of these malformations are regularly associated with pulmonary hypertension (Edwards 1979).

Truncus arteriosus

In this malformation, a single artery arises from the heart, forming a common origin for aorta and pulmonary trunk, with a single semilunar valve. A ventricular septal defect is virtually always present so that this truncus arteriosus usually originates from a common ventricle. Truncus arteriosus is a very serious malformation, leading to *severe central cyanosis* and *pulmonary hypertension.* It is usually fatal within 1 or 2 months unless surgical correction is carried out. *Unilateral absence* or *stenosis of a pulmonary artery* is not unusual and may prevent the increase in pulmonary arterial pressure.

Aorto-pulmonary window

An aorto-pulmonary window or septal defect is a rare anomaly, providing a communication between aorta and pulmonary trunk just above the valves. This defect varies in size from some millimetres to a few centimetres. Clinically, it resembles a patent ductus arteriosus, which is also one of several possible associated malformations. If pulmonary hypertension develops in truncus arteriosus or aorto-pulmonary window, the hypertensive pulmonary vascular disease is of the plexogenic arteriopathy type.

Origin of coronary arteries from pulmonary trunk

In this rare condition it is usually the left coronary artery that takes its origin from the pulmonary trunk. In that case there is a blood flow from the aorta through the right coronary artery, which communicates with the left, and then retrogradely through the left coronary artery to the pulmonary trunk. This may cause myocardial infarction even in young infants, and surgical correction should be carried out as soon as possible. An origin of the right or of both coronary arteries from the pulmonary trunk is even more rare.

Absence of one pulmonary artery

This is a very unusual malformation, in which the pulmonary trunk has no bifurcation but continues as a single artery to the hilum of one lung. If the left pulmonary artery is absent, there is often an associated tetralogy of Fallot, while right-sided absence is commonly complicated by a patent ductus arteriosus. Unilateral absence often leads to pulmonary hypertension in the lung supplied by the pulmonary artery. The other lung derives its blood supply from a systemic branch of the aorta. Unilateral absence of a pulmonary artery also occurs when there is agenesis of one lung. In *pulmonary sequestration,* part of a lung, usually located in the left lower lobe, does not communicate with the rest of that lung: there is no connection of its bronchi with the normal bronchial tree nor is there a supply by the pulmonary artery. An anomalous arterial blood supply is derived from a branch of the aorta and the venous drainage is usually to the azygos system.

Pulmonary artery stenosis

A localized or segmental pulmonary arterial congenital stenosis, either as single or multiple lesions, may occur in the pulmonary trunk, in the main pulmonary arteries, and in intrapulmonary elastic arteries. Occasionally there is generalized hypoplasia of all or part of the pulmonary arterial tree.

Stenoses of the pulmonary artery are uncommon but not excessively rare, although there is little doubt that they are often not recognized clinically. Even at autopsy they may be easily missed when the vessels are opened lengthwise. A proximal stenosis or multiple stenoses lying more peripherally may be responsible for pulmonary hypertension as established by cardiac catheterization. Distal to the stenosis, however, the pulmonary arterial pressure is not increased and the arteries are normal or even thin-walled. The discrepancy between normal vessels and marked pulmonary hypertension may point to the correct diagnosis. There are often associated congenital malformations.

Pulmonary arteriovenous fistulae

A congenital arteriovenous fistula is an anomalous intrapulmonary direct communication between a pulmonary artery and a pulmonary vein without an interposed capillary bed (Fig. 13.145). These lesions, which consist of convoluted, dilated, thin-walled and blood-filled spaces, may be single or multiple and may vary considerably in size. Sometimes they occupy the greater part of a lobe, but they may also present as a number of small clusters. They are uncommonly bilateral. Small fistulae are referred to as *pulmonary telangiectases.* In *familial telangiectasia* or *Rendu–Osler–Weber disease,* such lesions occur in skin

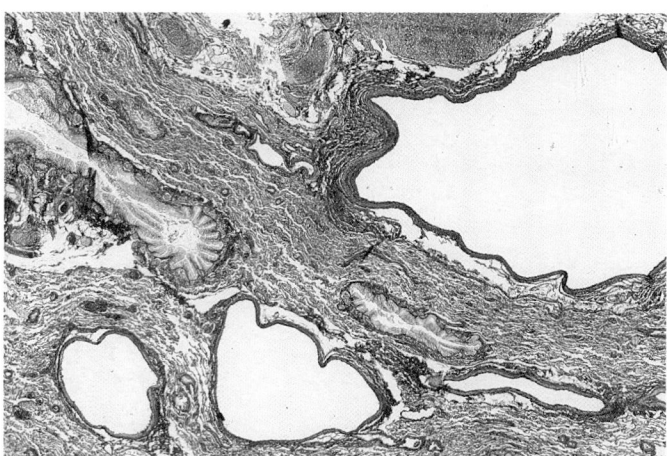

Fig. 13.145 Pulmonary arteriovenous fistula, consisting of a group of dilated vessels with a wall structure resembling in part that of arteries but mostly that of veins. (Elastic van Gieson.)

and mucous membranes, and may be particularly numerous in the lungs.

The clinical significance of arteriovenous fistulae and telangiectases depends partly on the size of the shunt of deoxygenated blood from pulmonary to systemic circulation. Thus, multiple small telangiectases may have just as much effect as a single large fistula. The symptoms, which often do not appear before young adulthood, include central cyanosis, if the shunt is large enough, haemoptyses, which are potentially life-threatening, and a continuous murmur over their site. Treatment consist of surgical removal, if possible.

Fistulae and telangiectases are more common in the lower than in the upper lobes, and often border the pleura. Demonstration of the smaller lesions by the pathologist may be difficult, particularly in collapsed lung tissue. Most of the tortuous, wide channels are thin-walled and resemble veins in structure. Usually a few cross-sections can be identified as pulmonary arteries. Without injection studies, proof of the presence of an arteriovenous anastomosis is not easily obtained.

Telangiectases may be acquired. This is rare except when associated with hepatic cirrhosis or fibrosis (Keren *et al.* 1983). The mechanisms involved are insufficiently explained but the clinical significance of these acquired telangiectases is probably very limited.

Cor triatriatum

In cor triatriatum, the left atrium is divided in two, as a result of failure of the common pulmonary vein to become incorporated in the atrium. The accessory chamber produced in this way is therefore actually part of the pulmonary venous system and receives the pulmonary veins. The membranous septum separating this chamber from the left atrium may contain several fenestrations or one wide opening. In most cases the pressure in the pulmonary veins is raised, leading to severe congestive vasculopathy in the lungs, even in young infants.

Anomalous pulmonary venous connection

In this anomaly all or part of the pulmonary venous drainage is directed to the right atrium or to the systemic veins connected with it. The variations are numerous. The pulmonary veins may drain into the left atrium, the left superior vena cava, the right superior vena cava, a coronary sinus, systemic tributaries of the inferior vena cava, or the portal veins.

In *total anomalous pulmonary venous connection* (Fig. 13.146), in which all the blood from the lungs enters the right atrium, there is always a *patent foramen ovale* or an *atrial septal defect,* so that both atria contain a mixture of oxygenated and deoxygenated blood. The abnormal venous return may be accompanied by some degree of obstruction, leading to pulmonary hypertension; *congestive vasculopathy* may then develop, even in infancy. If obstruction is absent or mild, and the communication between both atria adequate, symptoms may be absent or limited to mild cyanosis and dyspnoea. In *partial anomalous pulmonary venous connection,* usually the pulmonary veins of one lung drain normally on the left atrium, while those of the other

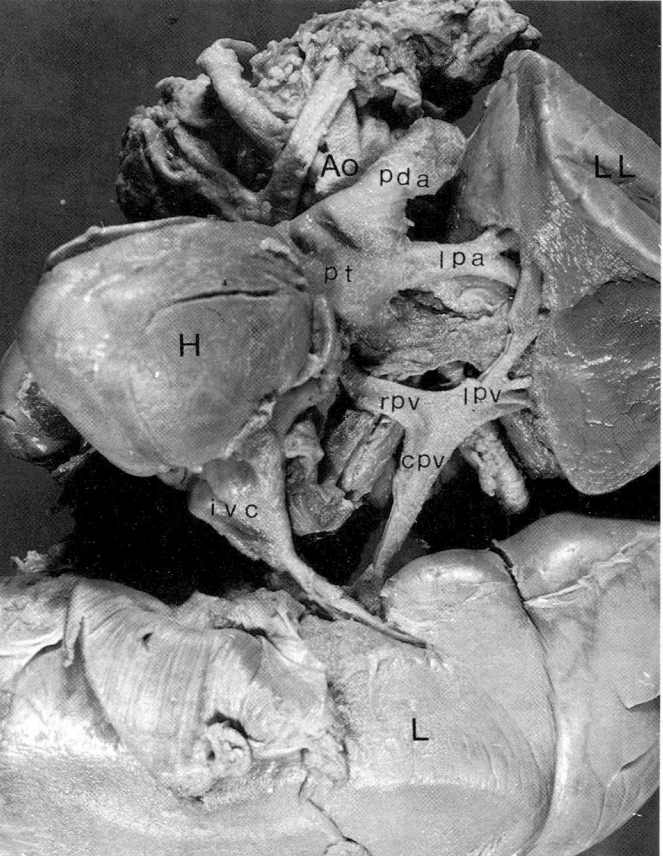

Fig. 13.146 Total anomalous pulmonary venous connection. The heart (H) is turned aside to show right and left pulmonary veins (rpv, lpv) joining to form a common pulmonary vein (cpv) which merges behind the liver (L) with the portal vein. LL, left lung; Ao, aorta; pt, pulmonary trunk; pda, patent ductus arteriosus; lpa, left pulmonary artery; ivc, inferior vena cava.

lung are abnormally connected; this happens far more often with the right than with the left lung. While the effect resembles somewhat that of an atrial septal defect, symptoms are usually minimal or absent, and corrective surgery, which is always indicated in the complete form, is often not necessary here.

A special form of partial anomalous connection is the '*scimitar syndrome*' in which the pulmonary veins of the right lung and more particularly of the right lower lobe, are connected with the abdominal caval vein by way of a venous trunk, penetrating the diaphragm. On a chest radiogram, this anomalous vessel impresses as a vertical, crescent- or scimitar-shaped shadow. There are, however, several other features in this complicated syndrome, including a bilobar right lung and a blood supply of the right lower lobe by one or more systemic arteries originating from the descending aorta, which may cause plexogenic arteriopathy in that lobe.

Congenital stenosis of pulmonary veins

Localized stenosis of one or more pulmonary veins is generally considered a congenital anomaly rather than an acquired lesion, since there are often associated cardiovascular malformations. Although the number of published cases is very limited, it may well be that these stenoses are not exceedingly rare, since they are often asymptomatic while the clinical diagnosis is very difficult and the pulmonary veins are rarely carefully inspected at autopsy. When multiple and large pulmonary veins are involved, pulmonary venous hypertension and congestive vasculopathy may result.

13.5.13   Lesions of major lung vessels

Acquired lesions of pulmonary trunk and main pulmonary arteries include alterations of media and intima related to changes in pressure, generalized dilatation and aneurysms, degenerative and metabolic lesions, and tumours. Pulmonary arteritis (Section 13.6) and thromboembolism (p. 1011) are discussed elsewhere. The pulmonary venous trunks are uncommonly affected by disease.

Pulmonary arterial medial thickness and structure

In prenatal life, the haemodynamic situation in systemic and pulmonary circulations is similar, and consequently the media of the neonatal pulmonary trunk closely resembles in thickness and structure that of the aorta. As in the aorta, the pulmonary trunk and main pulmonary arteries are of the elastic type with multiple parallel and regular elastic laminae.

In the postnatal period, the pulmonary arterial pressure decreases considerably relative to the systemic pressure, and the ratio in medial thickness between pulmonary trunk and aorta drops to approximately 3:5. Moreover, the elastic configuration of the extrapulmonary pulmonary arterial wall changes as the elastic laminae become interrupted and fragmented (Fig. 13.147), an alteration which does not occur in the intrapulmonary elastic arteries.

Medial changes of the pulmonary trunk are seen in pulmonary hypertension, particularly when present from birth, as in congenital heart disease. The medial thickness fails to decrease, so that it remains equal to that of the aorta. Also, the elastic configuration does not alter as it normally does, but even in adults the elastic laminae remain intact and regular (Fig. 13.148).

When pulmonary hypertension is acquired at a later age, the thickness of the media is also greater than normal but the elastic configuration is the same as in normal adults, with fragmentation of elastic laminae. In rheumatic heart disease a deposition of mucopolysaccharides and collagen contributes to the increase in thickness.

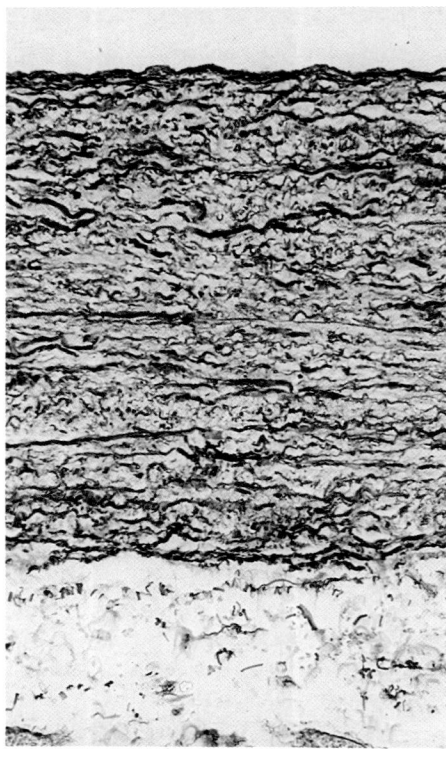

Fig. 13.147   Normal pulmonary trunk with irregular, interrupted elastic laminae. (Elastic van Gieson.)

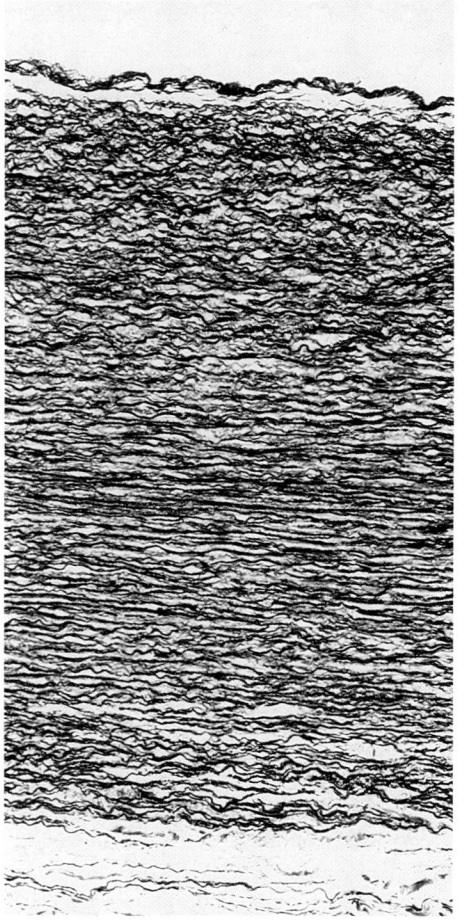

Fig. 13.148   Pulmonary trunk in pulmonary hypertension due to congenital heart disease. The wall is much thicker than normal, while there is an elastic configuration as in the aorta. (Elastic van Gieson.)

In patients with diminished pulmonary arterial pulse pressure and flow, as in tetralogy of Fallot, the pulmonary trunk may be very thin-walled, while fragmentation and disappearance of elastic fibres is even more pronounced (Fig. 13.149).

Intimal fibrosis, atherosclerosis

In normal adult individuals, particularly over the age of 40 or 50 years, intimal fibrosis and atherosclerosis are common in the pulmonary trunk and main arteries. However, such lesions are always mild: intimal fibrosis consists of a fairly thin layer, and atherosclerotic patches are small and mainly located at or near ramifications. In the presence of pulmonary hypertension, however, these lesions are much more severe (Fig. 13.150) and may even occur in young children. Ulceration and calcification may occur but are unusual. Atherosclerotic lesions may also be found in peripheral elastic pulmonary arteries. Equally severe atherosclerosis may result from hypercholesterolaemia.

Aneurysms

Some degree of generalized dilatation of pulmonary trunk and main arteries is seen regularly in various forms of pulmonary hypertension. Occasionally such a dilatation may be very striking.

Saccular or dissecting aneurysms of the major pulmonary arteries are uncommon. They sometimes develop in connection with bacterial endocarditis or after surgical closure of a patent ductus arteriosus. They are particularly associated with pulmonary hypertension (Fig. 13.151), which may be of any type. Aneurysms, either saccular or dissecting (Fig. 13.152), are also found occasionally in large intrapulmonary elastic arteries.

Tumours of major lung vessels

Tumours originating in major pulmonary vessels are rare. Most

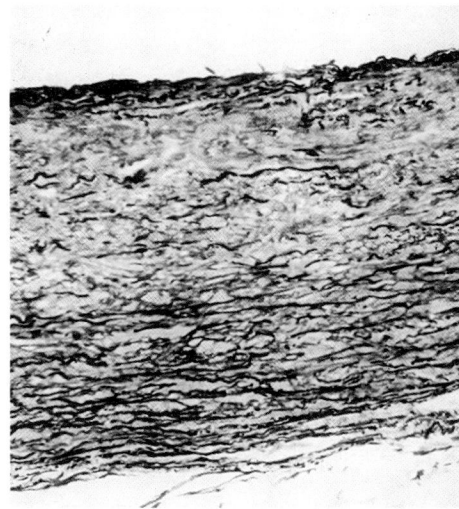

Fig. 13.149 Pulmonary trunk in tetralogy of Fallot. The wall is thinner than normal, while there is also more loss of elastic tissue. (Elastic van Gieson.)

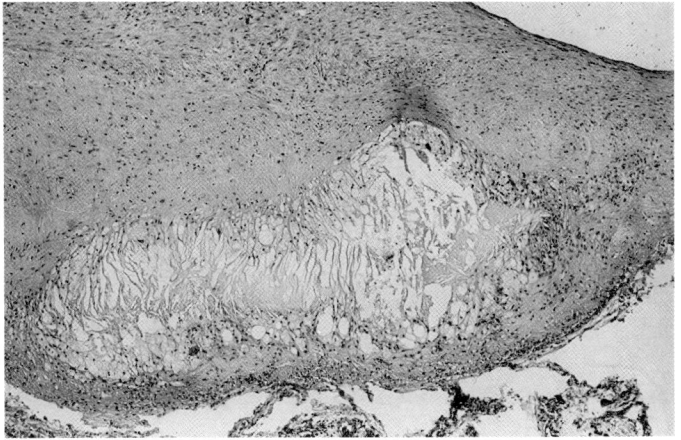

Fig. 13.150 Lobar pulmonary artery with a large patch of atherosclerosis; at this site the media has virtually disappeared.

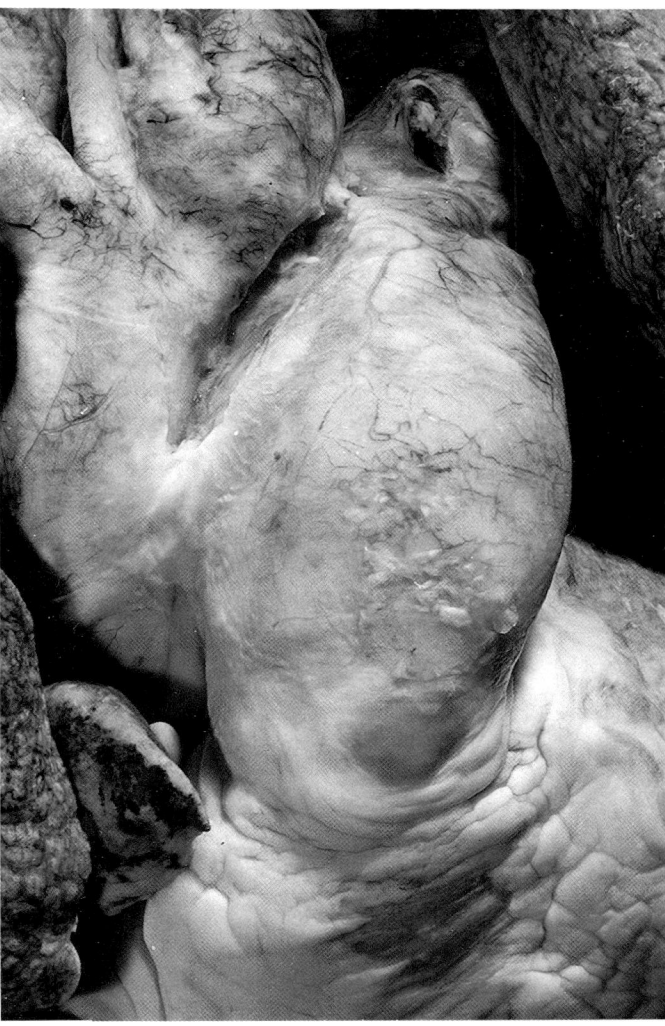

Fig. 13.151 Saccular aneurysm of pulmonary trunk in pulmonary hypertension due to congenital heart disease; to the left is the aortic arc.

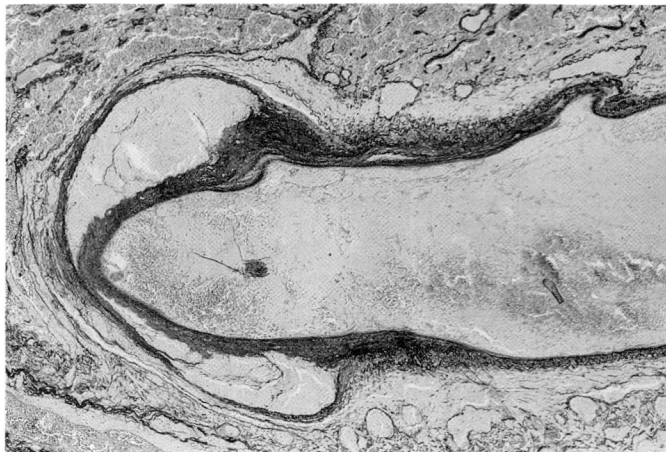

Fig. 13.152 Segmental pulmonary artery with dissecting aneurysm in chronic embolic pulmonary hypertension. (Elastic van Gieson.)

of them are sarcomas of various histological types, including *leiomyosarcomas, chondrosarcomas, or undifferentiated spindle-cell sarcomas,* involving the pulmonary trunk, although they may extend along the main pulmonary arteries or spread as tumour emboli to more peripheral vessels.

13.5.14   Bronchial vasculature

Bronchial arteries lie in the walls of bronchi, both outside the bronchial cartilage and in the bronchial mucosa; they usually run alongside a bronchial vein and a nerve bundle (Fig. 13.153). Their media is much thicker than that of a pulmonary artery; another difference is that there is no external but only an internal elastic lamina, as in all systemic arteries (Fig. 13.154). The very thin-walled bronchial veins contain valves.

A very common change in bronchial arteries is the development of longitudinal smooth muscle cells in bundles or layers within the intima. This often leads to severe narrowing or occlusion of the lumen (Fig. 13.155). They apparently develop in response to inflammatory, fibrotic, or other processes, and increase with age; they are not at all uncommon in otherwise normal individuals and their functional significance is probably limited.

Bronchial arteries become greatly enlarged and thick-walled in patients with *bronchiectasis* where the bronchial circulation is greatly increased. Wide bronchial arteries are also found in recurrent thromboembolism and particularly in tetralogy of Fallot, where they play a role in establishing a collateral circulation.

The bronchial veins, which communicate widely with pulmonary veins within the walls of bronchi, are dilated in chronic congestion.

13.5.15   Pulmonary lymphatics

Generalized dilatation of pulmonary lymphatics occurs whenever there is excess fluid within the interstitium of the lungs.

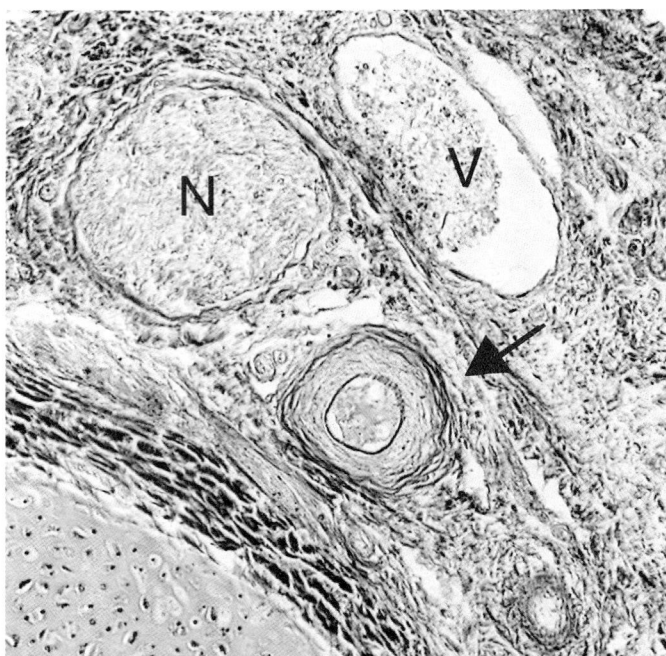

Fig. 13.153 Normal bronchial artery (arrow) associated with bronchial vein (V) and nerve bundle (N); cartilage of the bronchial wall is to the left. (Elastic van Gieson.)

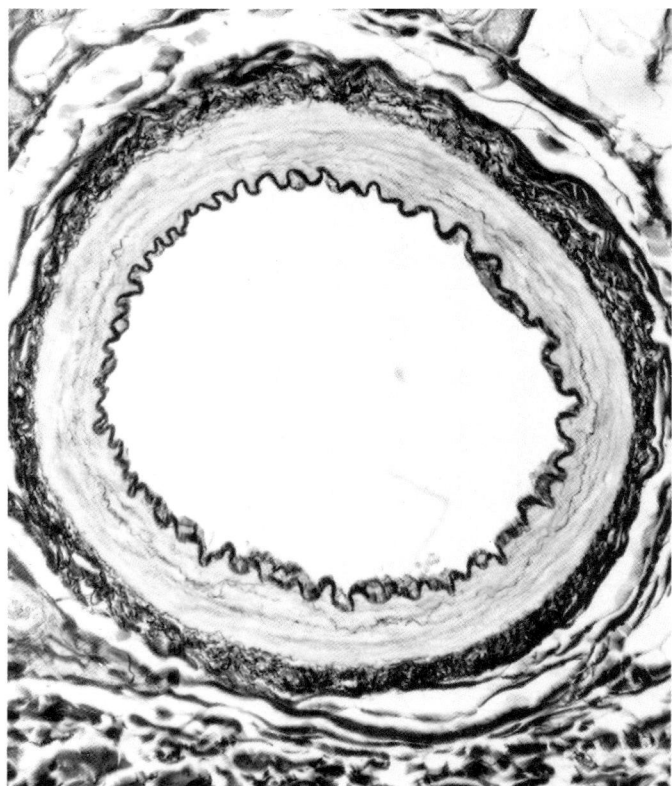

Fig. 13.154 Normal bronchial artery with rather thick media and intact internal elastic lamina, but without external elastic lamina. (Elastic van Gieson.)

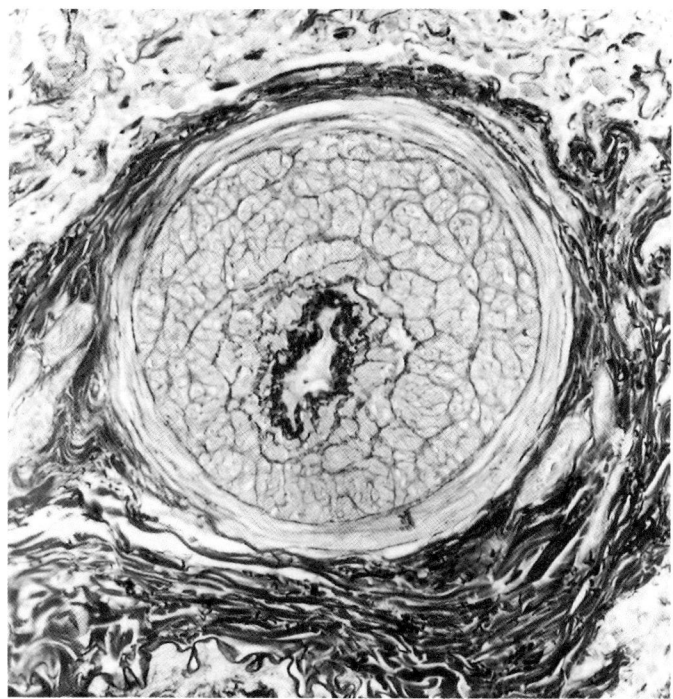

Fig. 13.155 Bronchial artery almost completely occluded by longitudinal smooth muscle cells, separated by elastic fibres. (Elastic van Gieson.)

Thus, in pulmonary venous hypertension and in any other situation in which pulmonary oedema occurs, the lymph vessels tend to be wide. Excessive dilatation, known as *lymphangiectasis*, occurs occasionally in infants with congenital heart disease, especially total anomalous pulmonary venous connection. Sometimes *focal lymphangiectasis* is observed in patients with chronic pulmonary venous hypertension.

13.5.16 Bibliography

Edwards, J. E. (1957). Functional pathology of the pulmonary vascular tree in congenital cardiac disease. *Circulation* **15**, 164–96.

Edwards, J. E. (1979). Congenital pulmonary vascular disorders. In *Pulmonary vascular pathology* (ed. K. M. Moser), pp. 527–71. Marcel Dekker, New York.

Edwards, B. S., Weir, E. K., Edwards, W. D., Ludwig, J., Dykoski, R. K., and Edwards, J. E. (1987). Coexistent pulmonary and portal hypertension: morphologic and clinical features. *Journal of the American College of Cardiology* **10**, 1233–8.

Grover, R. F., Will, D. H., Reeves, J. T., Weir, E. K., McMurphy, I. F., and Alexander, A. F. (1975). Genetic transmission of susceptibility to hypoxic pulmonary hypertension. *Progress in Respiration Research* **9**, 112–17.

Harris, P. and Heath, D. (1986). *The human pulmonary circulation* (3rd edn). Churchill Livingstone, Edinburgh.

Hasleton, P. S., Heath, D., and Brewer, D. B. (1968). Hypertensive pulmonary vascular disease in states of chronic hypoxia. *Journal of Pathology Bacteriology* **95**, 431–40.

Hatano, S. and Strasser, T. (eds) (1975). *Primary pulmonary hypertension*, Report of Committee. World Health Organization, Geneva.

Haworth, S. G., Radley-Smith, R., and Yacoub, M. (1987). Lung biopsy findings in transposition of the great arteries with ventricular septal defect: potentially reversible pulmonary vascular disease is not always synonymous with operability. *Journal of the American College of Cardiology* **9**, 327–33.

Heath, D. and Edwards, J. E. (1958). The pathology of hypertensive pulmonary vascular disease. A description of six grades of structural changes in the pulmonary arteries with special reference to congenital septal defects. *Circulation* **18**, 533–47.

Heath, D. and Williams, D. R. (1977). *Man at high altitude*. Churchill Livingstone, Edinburgh.

Heath, D., Segel, N., and Bishop, J. (1966). Pulmonary veno-occlusive disease. *Circulation* **34**, 242–8.

Katzenstein, A. L. A. and Askin, F. B. (1982). *Surgical pathology of non-neoplastic lung disease*, pp. 9–42. W. B. Saunders, Philadelphia.

Keren, G., Boichis, H., Zwas, T. S., and Frand, M. (1983). Pulmonary arterio-venous fistulae in hepatic cirrhosis. *Archives of Diseases in Childhood* **58**, 302–4.

Messer, J. V. (1984). Thromboembolic pulmonary hypertension. In *Pulmonary hypertension* (ed. E. K. Weir, and J. T. Reeves), pp. 169–249. Futura, Mount Kisco, New York.

Moser, K. M. (1979). Pulmonary vascular obstruction due to embolism and thrombosis. In *Pulmonary vascular diseases* (ed. K. M. Moser), pp. 341–86. Marcel Dekker, New York.

Rabinovitch, M., Herrera-de Leon, V., Castaneda, A. R., and Reid, L. (1981). Growth and development of the pulmonary vascular bed in patients with tetralogy of Fallot with or without pulmonary atresia. *Circulation* **64**, 1234–49.

Rich, A. R. (1948). A hitherto unrecognized tendency to the development of widespread pulmonary vascular obstruction in patients with congenital pulmonary stenosis (tetralogy of Fallot). *Bulletin of the Johns Hopkins Hospital* **82**, 389–401.

Staub, N. C. (1970). The pathophysiology of pulmonary edema. *Human Pathology* **1**, 419–32.

Staub, N. C. (1974). Pulmonary edema. *Physiological Reviews* **54**, 678–811.

Wagenvoort, C. A. (1985). Open lung biopsies in congenital heart disease for evaluation of pulmonary vascular disease. Predictive value with regard to corrective operability. *Histopathology* **9**, 417–36.

Wagenvoort, C. A. (1989). Terminology of primary pulmonary hypertension. In *Pulmonary circulation: advances and controversies* (ed. C. A. Wagenvoort and H. Denolin), pp. 191–7. Elsevier, Amsterdam.

Wagenvoort, C. A. and Mooi, W. J. (1989). *Biopsy pathology of the pulmonary vasculature*. Chapman & Hall, London.

Wagenvoort, C. A. and Wagenvoort, N. (1970). Primary pulmonary hypertension: a pathologic study of the lung vessels in 156 clinically diagnosed cases. *Circulation* **42**, 1163–84.

Wagenvoort, C. A. and Wagenvoort, N. (1977). *Pathology of pulmonary hypertension*. J. Wiley and Sons, New York.

Wagenvoort, C. A. and Wagenvoort, N. (1982). Smooth muscle content of pulmonary arterial media in pulmonary venous hypertension compared to other forms of pulmonary hypertension. *Chest* **81**, 581–5.

Wagenvoort, C. A., Neufeld, H. N., and Edwards, J. E. (1961). The structure of the pulmonary arterial tree in fetal and early postnatal life. *Laboratory Investigation* **10**, 751–62.

Wagenvoort, C. A., Nauta, J., Van der Schaar, P. J., Weeda, W. H. W., and Wagenvoort, N. (1967). Vascular changes in pulmonic stenosis and tetralogy of Fallot studied in lung biopsies. *Circulation* **36**, 924–32.

Wagenvoort, C. A., Beetstra, A., and Spijker, J. (1978). Capillary haemangiomatosis of the lungs. *Histopathology* **2**, 401–6.

Wagenvoort, C. A., Wagenvoort, N., and Draulans-Noe, Y. (1984).

Reversibility of plexogenic pulmonary arteriopathy following banding of the pulmonary artery. *Journal of Thoracic and Cardiovascular Surgery* **87**, 876–86.

Wagenvoort, C. A., Wagenvoort, N., and Takahashi, T. (1985). Pulmonary veno-occlusive disease. Involvement of pulmonary arteries and review of the literature. *Human Pathology* **16**, 1033–41.

Weir, E. K., Tucker, A., Reeves, J. T., Will, D. H., and Grover, R. F. (1974). The genetic factor influencing pulmonary hypertension in cattle at high altitude. *Cardiovascular Research* **8**, 745–9.

13.6   Pulmonary vasculitis

T. Creagh and T. Krausz

Pulmonary vasculitides comprise a group of inflammatory conditions affecting blood vessels; each condition forms a distinct clinico-pathological entity which may affect other organs. The lung is commonly involved due to its large blood supply and its accessibility to antigens via both the bloodstreams and inhalation. Pulmonary vasculitis may be classified as in Table 13.17.

Although the pulmonary manifestations are relatively heterogeneous, there is much diagnostic overlap between the granulomatous vasculitides, the related conditions bronchocentric and lymphomatoid granulomatosis, rheumatoid nodules, and fungal or tuberculous infection (Fig. 13.156).

13.6.1   Wegener's disease

Wegener's disease is classically characterized by a *necrotizing granulomatous vasculitis* affecting the upper and lower respir-

Table 13.17   Classification of pulmonary vasculitis

Granulomatous
  Wegener's
  Necrotizing sarcoid
  Allergic granulomatosis and angiitis (Churg–Strauss)
Hypersensitivity vasculitis
  Henoch–Schönlein purpura
  Connective tissue disease
  Infectious diseases
  Mixed cryoglobulinaemia
Takayasu's arteritis
Behcet's disease
Other related conditions
  Bronchocentric granulomatosis
  Lymphomatoid granulomatosis

atory tract, a *glomerulonephritis*, and *small-vessel vasculitis* (Godman and Churg 1954).

A limited form of Wegener's disease is also described when the lesions are confined to the lung and there is no glomerulonephritis; however, other organs, such as the skin, may be involved and it is probably best to describe this form by site.

The aetiology of Wegener's disease is unknown; however, the pathogenesis is thought to be immune-complex mediated. Clinically, adults tend to be affected, with 40 years being the mean age at presentation. Symptoms may be systemic, e.g. fever, malaise, arthralgia, and weight loss, or depend on the site of involvement (see Table 13.18).

Pathology

Macroscopically, discrete firm lesions are scattered across the lungs. There is usually central necrosis and cavitation and sometimes a necrotic blood vessel is seen.

The microscopic features are characterized by a *necrotizing*

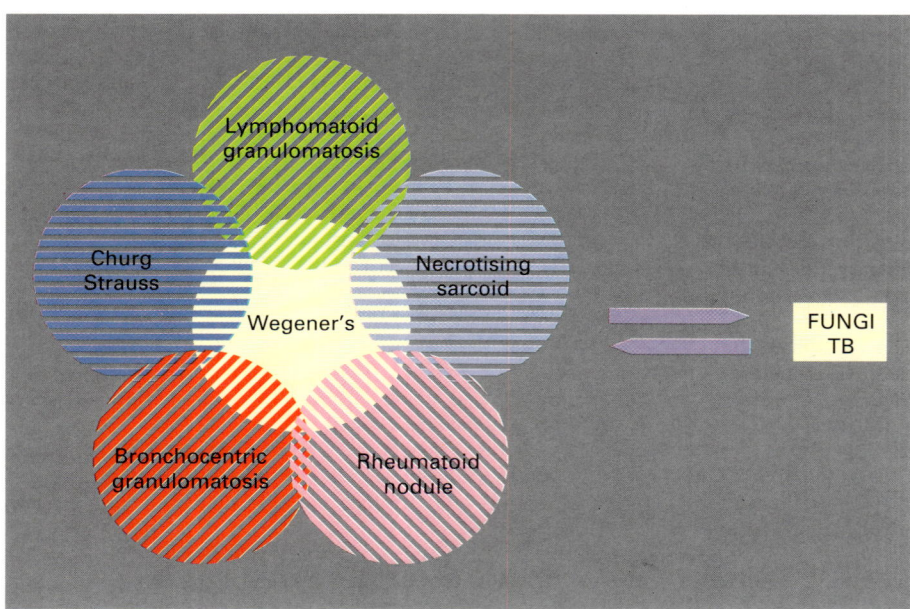

Fig. 13.156 Diagnosis overlap in pulmonary vasculitis and granulomatous disease.

Table 13.18 Organ involvement in Wegener's disease

Organ	System	Frequency
Lung	asymptomatic or cough and haemoptysis	94%
Paranasal sinuses	sinusitis	91%
Kidney	glomerulonephritis	85%
Joints	arthralgia	67%
Nose/nasopharynx	discharge, ulceration	64%
Ear	otitis media	61%
Eye	conjunctivitis, episcleritis, uveitis, retinal artery occlusion, nasolacrimal duct occlusion, proptosis secondary to retro-orbital inflammatory mass	58%
Skin	leukocytoclastic/granulomatous vasculitis	45%
Nervous system	mononeuritis multiplex, isolated cranial nerve abnormalities	22%
Heart	coronary vasculitis	12%

granulomatous inflammation which often appears geographic (Fig. 13.157). Both arteries and veins are affected (Fig. 13.158) by a *transmural infiltrate* with *necrosis of the vessel wall*. There is an adjacent infiltrate comprising polymorph neutrophils, lymphocytes, plasma cells, and histiocytes, which are often arranged in a palisaded manner around areas of necrosis, and *multinucleated giant cells* are present.

There is one histological feature that is considered to be pathognomonic of Wegener's disease; this is the presence of a vasculitis occurring in *uninflamed lung parenchyma*. However, this feature is rarely seen (Fig. 13.159).

13.6.2 Necrotizing sarcoid granulomatosis

At present it is uncertain whether this entity is related to sarcoidosis (see also Section 13.3.6): most of the evidence points to a separate condition with differing radiological and pathological features. However, the clinical features are more supportive of a

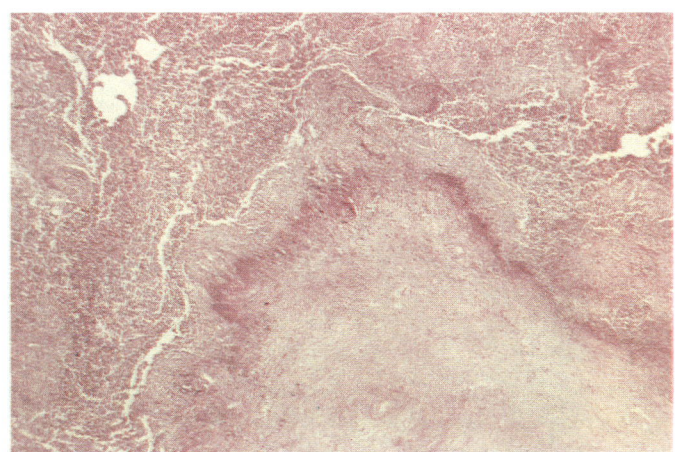

Fig. 13.157 Geographical nature of necrotizing lesions in Wegener's granulomatosis.

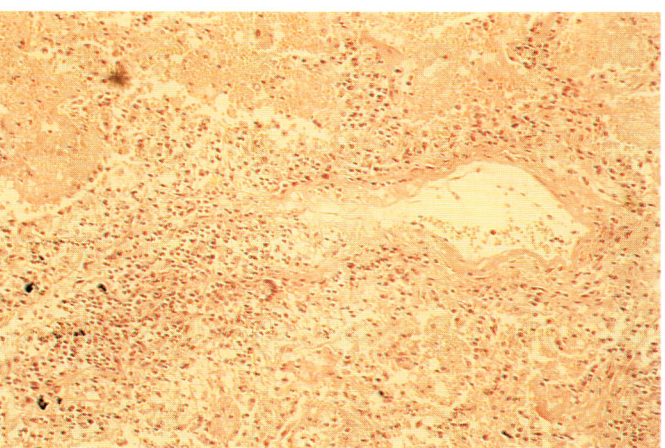

Fig. 13.158 Transmural inflammatory infiltrate destroying a medium-sized artery. The infiltrate includes neutrophils, polymorphs, lymphocytes, plasma cells, and occasional multinucleated giant cells.

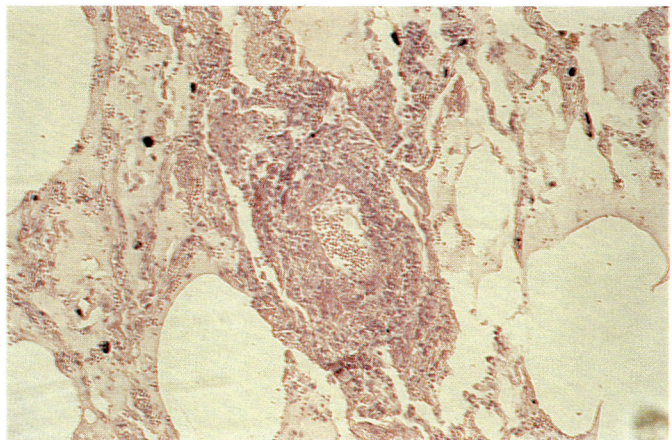

Fig. 13.159 Vasculitis occurring in an area of uninflamed lung parenchyma.

sarcoid-related entity. Young to middle-aged females are predominantly affected, presenting with systemic symptoms of fever, malaise, and weight loss, together with cough, chest pain, and dyspnoea. Up to 40 per cent of cases may be asymptomatic, with the diagnosis being made after a routine chest X-ray. Radiologically, bilateral rounded opacities are seen. Hilar lymphadenopathy is unusual. Extrapulmonary involvement is not generally described and necrotizing sarcoid granulomatosis is largely a self-limiting disease with a good prognosis—these findings are in contrast to sarcoidosis.

Histologically, there is an *extensive vasculitis* which involves arteries and veins; this is usually granulomatous (Figs 13.160, 13.161). However, in some cases the infiltrate does not include giant cells. Elsewhere in the lung there is formation of coalescent masses of sarcoid-like granulomas. Necrosis is usually seen in the centre of the aggregates (Fig. 13.162).

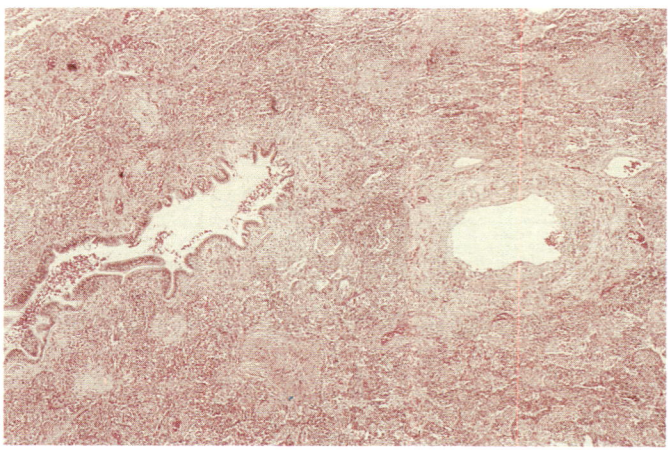

Fig. 13.160 Granulomatous vasculitis in necrotizing sarcoid granulomatosis—an adjacent bronchiole is unaffected.

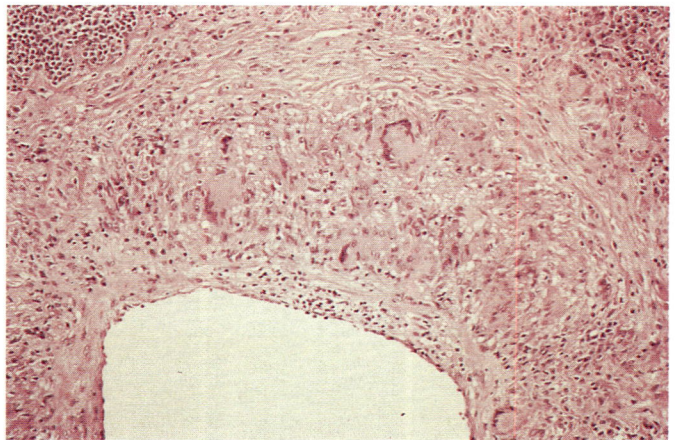

Fig. 13.161 'Sarcoid-like' granuloma seen in an artery wall.

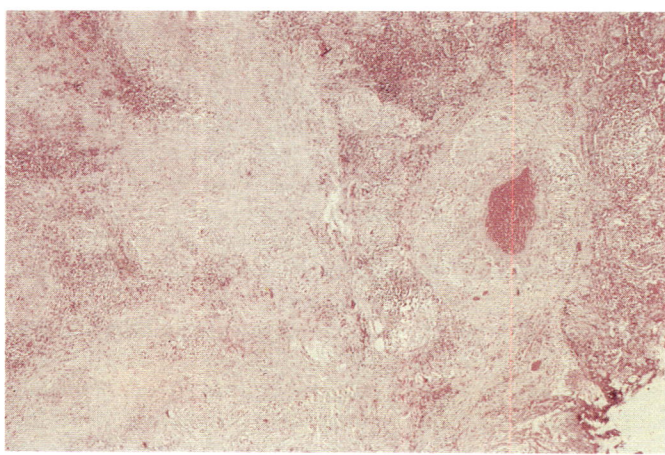

Fig. 13.162 Confluent granulomas surrounding an area of necrosis.

13.6.3 Allergic granulomatosis and angiitis (Churg–Strauss)

Churg–Strauss disease is a rare systemic disorder classically characterized by the following features:

1. *a vasculitis* involving capillaries, venules, and small and medium-sized arteries;

2. *granulomatous inflammation* which is both vascular and extra-vascular;

3. a peripheral and tissue eosinophilia; and

4. asthma (Churg and Strauss 1951).

Clinically, adults of any age are affected.

The lung is involved in virtually all cases by a vasculitis, which may or may not be granulomatous, together with necrotizing granulomatous destruction of the parenchyma. Eosinophils are present in large numbers (Fig. 13.163).

The major differential diagnosis is that of *polyarteritis nodosa* (PAN); however, although asthma and eosinophilia may occur in PAN, pulmonary involvement and extravascular granulomatous lesions are uncommon.

13.6.4 Rarer forms

Hypersensitivity vasculitides

These comprise a group of small-vessel vasculitides which are immune-complex mediated. They include vasculitides that occur in response to specific antigens (for example tumour antigens, certain drugs, and post-streptococcal upper respiratory tract infections), together with distinct syndromes such as Henoch–Schönlein purpura, connective tissue diseases, and mixed cryoglobulinaemia. The skin is predominantly affected by a *leukocytoclastic vasculitis*; however, any organ can be involved, with the most frequent being renal, joints, gastrointestinal, pulmonary, and neurological involvement.

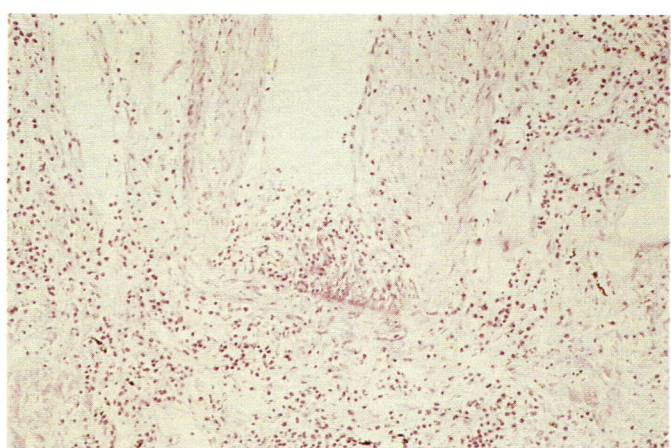

Fig. 13.163 Infiltration of a large-vessel wall by numerous eosinophils, with focal necrosis, in Churg–Strauss disease. The infiltrate extends into the lung parenchyma.

Takayasu's disease

This is a vasculitis of large vessels, most commonly affecting the aorta and its branches; however, the pulmonary arteries may be involved.

Behçet's disease

This syndrome is characterized by recurrent oral and genital ulceration, together with an associated uveitis, a synovitis, a meningoencephalitis, and/or recurrent venous and arterial thromboses.

Multisystem involvement may occur, with the skin being most frequently affected by a leukocytoclastic vasculitis. Rarely, a pulmonary vasculitis occurs, which may affect capillaries and small to large arteries in the form of thromboses, infarcts, and aneurysm formation.

In the related conditions, bronchocentric and lymphomatoid granulomatosis, the underlying pathology is *not* that of a vasculitis. Bronchocentric granulomatosis results from inflammation of the small bronchi and bronchioles, whereas lymphomatoid granulomatosis is thought to be a lymphoproliferative disorder in which the infiltrate is both angiocentric and angio-destructive.

Bronchocentric granulomatosis

Clinically, two groups of patients are affected: asthmatics, who tend to be young, and non-asthmatics, who are older. The disease is seen most frequently in asthmatics (see also Section 13.3.3), who usually present with symptoms of an acute chest complaint, and is associated with allergic bronchopulmonary aspergillosis (Koss *et al.* 1981).

There is a necrotizing granulomatous infiltrate centred around distal bronchioles, with subsequent destruction of the bronchiolar wall (Fig. 13.164). Polypoid masses of granulation tissue protrude into the bronchi (Fig. 13.165) and caseation may occur which can be seen macroscopically following the

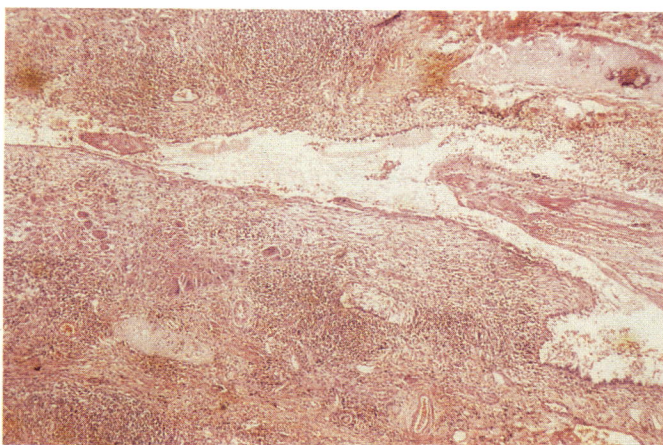

Fig. 13.165 Polypoid masses of granulation tissue protrude into the lumen of a large bronchus.

course of the bronchioles. Eosinophils are prominent and fungal hyphae may be present in the central necrotic areas (Fig. 13.166).

Although similar granulomas may be seen in other conditions (see Fig. 13.156), in bronchocentric granulomatosis *all* the granulomas are centred on bronchioles. In cases where the entire wall has been destroyed, this is determined by the site of the infiltrate adjacent to a pulmonary artery (Fig. 13.167).

Fungal infection and TB, particularly, must be excluded by special stains and culture.

Lymphomatoid granulomatosis

This condition usually affects middle-aged adults, being slightly more common in males. Presenting features may be chest-related only, but often include systemic symptoms. Extrapulmonary involvement is common, with the skin being affected in up to 40 per cent of patients, taking the form of subcutaneous nodules. The central and peripheral nervous systems, together with the kidneys, may also be involved (Liebow *et al.* 1972).

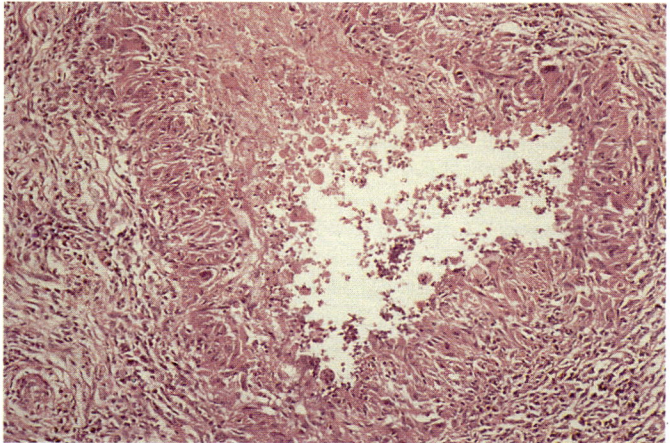

Fig. 13.164 Bronchocentric granulomatosis. A granulomatous infiltrate has completely destroyed a bronchial wall.

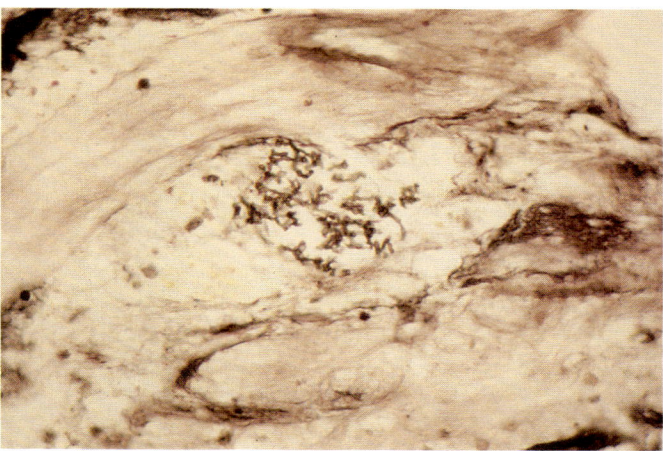

Fig. 13.166 Bronchocentric granulomatosis. Fungal hyphae. (Grocott.)

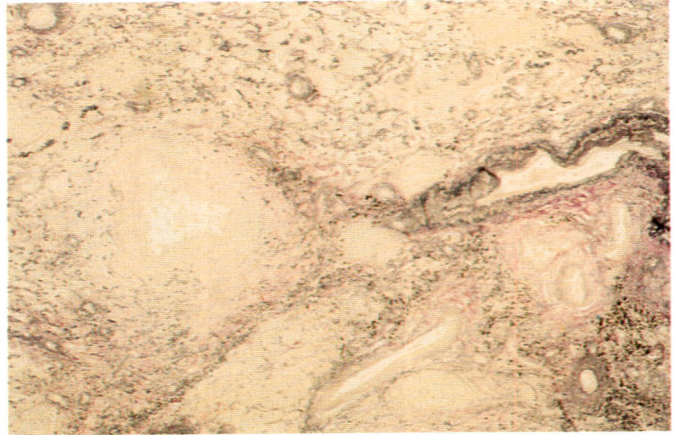

(a)

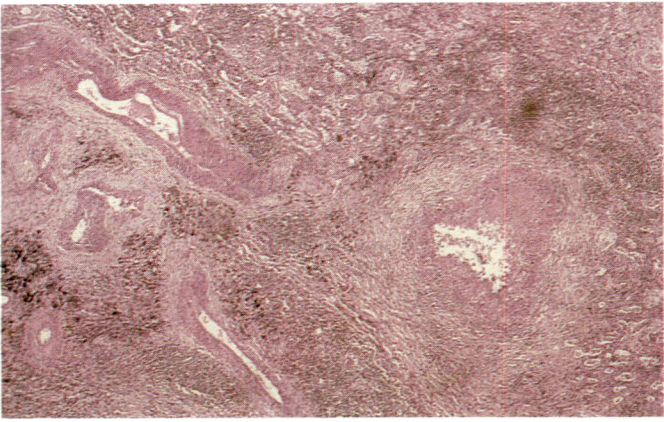

(b)

Fig. 13.167 A bronchus adjacent to a pulmonary artery which has been destroyed by the granulomatous process. [(a) H & E; (b) elastic van Gieson.]

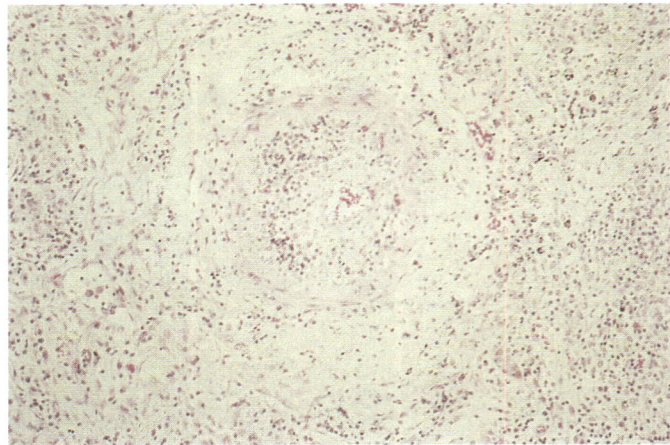

Fig. 13.168 Lymphoid infiltrate in lymphomatoid granulomatosis.

There is a *necrotizing, angiocentric, and angiodestructive infiltrative process* composed of small lymphocytes, plasma cells, histiocytes, and atypical lymphoid cells (Fig. 13.168). The necrotic component is prominent and results in extensive parenchymal destruction. True granulomatous inflammation, however, does *not* occur.

Lymphomatoid granulomatosis is now thought to be a form of *T-cell lymphoma*. Immunocytochemical staining demonstrates that the atypical cells stain with T-cell markers. There does appear to be a wide spectrum of appearances, ranging from mild atypia to frankly malignant cells, and it is possible that some cases represent a precursor form of T-cell lymphoma.

13.6.5   Further reading

Churg, J. and Strauss, L. (1951). Anergic granulomatosis, allergic angiitis and periarteritis nodosa. *American Journal of Pathology* **27**, 277–94.

Godman, G. and Churg, J. (1954). Wegener's granulomatosis: pathology and review of the literature. *Archives of Pathology* **58**, 533.

Katzenstein, A. (1980). Necrotizing granulomas of the lung. *Human Pathology* **11**, 596.

Katzenstein, A. L. and Askin, F. B. (1982). *Surgical pathology of non-neoplastic lung disease*. W. B. Saunders, Philadelphia.

Koss, M., Robinson, R., and Hochholzer, L. (1981). Bronchocentric granulomatosis. *Human Pathology* **12**, 632.

Leavitt, R. and Fauci, A. (1986). Pulmonary vasculitis. *American Review of Respiratory Disease* **134**, 149–66.

Liebow, A., Carrington, C., and Friedman, P. (1972). Lymphomatous granulomatosis. *Human Pathology* **3**, 457.

Thurlbeck, W. M. (1988). *Pathology of the lung*. Thieme, New York.

13.7   Tumours of the lung

K. C. Gatter and M. S. Dunnill

13.7.1   Malignant epithelial tumours

Carcinoma of the lung is now the leading cause of cancer mortality in the Western world (currently about 35 000 deaths annually in England and Wales). In the early years of this century carcinoma of the lung was a rare tumour and contemporary textbooks emphasized that the lung was usually the site for secondary deposits rather than for primary tumours. By the 1940s, however, lung cancer had increased in incidence and become one of the commonest malignancies encountered in clinical practice. This happened at a time of rapid advance in diagnostic methods, leading to questions whether this increased incidence was apparent rather than real. Careful epidemiological investigations by Doll and others in the 1950s showed this interpretation to be invalid. Incidence and mortality figures continued to rise in the 1960s and 1970s, leading to a concerted search for the cause or causes, of which cigarette smoking is the most notable and accepted.

Gross appearances and complications

Macroscopic features

The majority of lung cancers arise centrally from the major bronchi so that, for practical purposes, carcinoma of the lung is synonymous with carcinoma of the bronchus. A consistent finding of most studies is that the upper lobes are more commonly involved than lower lobes, and the right lung more than the left (Fig. 13.169). Due to their position, lung cancers give rise to a variety of local complications which may have important clinical effects.

Local complications

1. *Ulceration of bronchus.* Lung carcinomas frequently ulcerate the bronchus in which they arise, producing some degree of haemoptysis in up to 50 per cent of patients with the disease (Fig. 13.170).

2. *Bronchial obstruction.* The lumen of the bronchus is occluded in many patients with subsequent distal collapse and retention of secretions (Fig. 13.171). This may manifest itself clinically as dyspnoea, lead to secondary infection with an antibiotic-resistant pneumonia, or result in bronchiectasis and develop into a lung abscess.

3. *Central necrosis.* As a carcinoma enlarges and invades surrounding pulmonary tissue it frequently outgrows its blood supply, leading to central necrosis. In such patients fevers and night sweats may develop in the absence of overt infection, though the main danger is the production of *lung abscesses* when superinfection takes place. Lung abscess in an adult in the absence of known predisposing conditions is an ominous sign of an underlying carcinoma.

Clinico-pathological correlation

From a clinical standpoint the local complications such as those described above may give important clues towards an earlier diagnosis. *Haemoptysis,* *recurrent or antibiotic-resistant pneumonia,* and *unexplained pulmonary collapse* should all be investigated carefully to exclude an underlying carcinoma. However, it is unfortunately true that lung cancer frequently presents at an advanced stage, making therapeutic intervention difficult and rarely successful.

Spread of lung carcinoma Lung cancer commonly presents with symptoms of local invasion or distant spread which may well explain its poor prognosis and therapeutic resistance.

Local invasion of adjacent intrathoracic structures gives rise to a number of well-characterized clinical features. Involvement of the recurrent laryngeal nerve leads to *vocal chord paralysis* and hoarseness of the voice, whereas phrenic nerve infiltration leads to *unilateral diaphragmatic paralysis. Dysphagia* arises from extension around and compression of the oesophagus. Another common complication is *superior venal caval obstruction* due to direct invasion (or compression by hilar lymph nodes). This is manifested as venous engorgement of the head and neck (often best seen in the veins beneath the tongue), with oedema, breathlessness, and periodic loss of consciousness. Local involvement of the last cervical and first thoracic sympathetic nerves leads to *Horner's syndrome* (drooping eyelid, sunken eyeball, contracted pupil, and loss of sweating on the same side of the face). *Lymphatic spread* to hilar and peribronchial lymph nodes can compress the superior vena cava and adjacent bronchi, leading to complications as detailed above. Tumour cells spreading along the transbronchial lymphatics cause pleural seedlings which may give rise to pleural effusions with compression of the adjacent lung.

Distant spread is generally blood borne and may go to virtually any organ of the body. The commonest organs affected are the liver, bones (including bone marrow) and the adrenals. Brain, skin, kidney, and thyroid are also frequently involved in advanced cases. In fact, careful examination at autopsy will often demonstrate far wider dissemination of disease than was apparent during life.

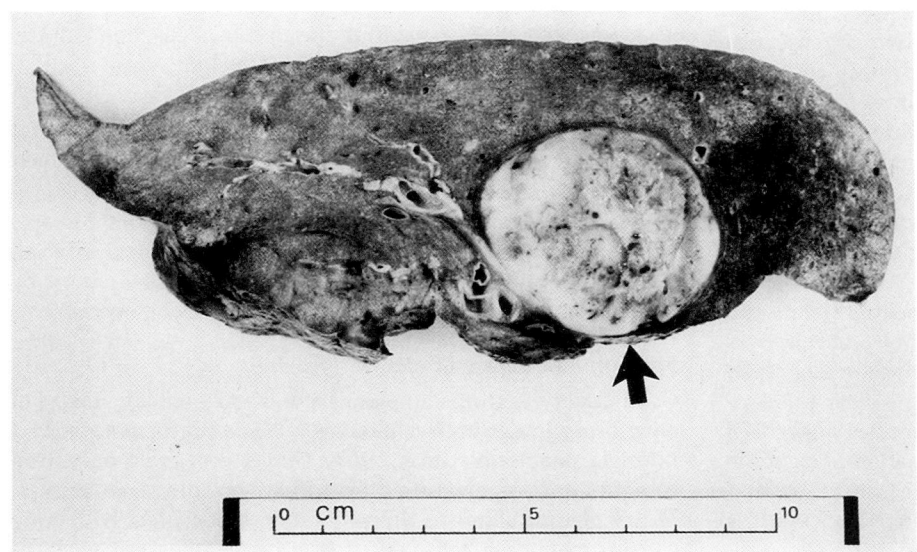

Fig. 13.169 This illustrates one of the most frequent macroscopic appearances of carcinoma of the lung. The tumour (arrowed) is relatively large, situated in the upper lobe and placed centrally.

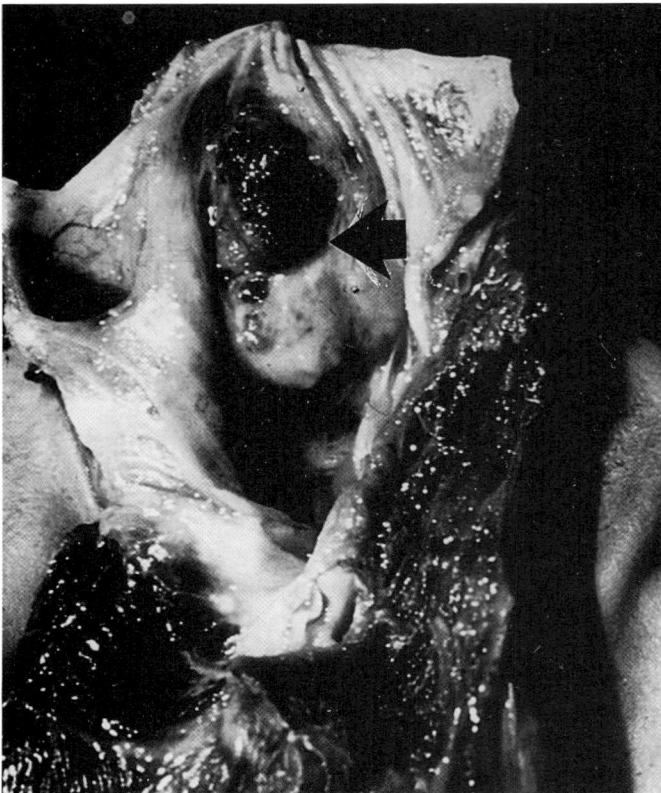

Fig. 13.170 A carcinoma of the lung arising in the bronchus (arrowed) has ulcerated the surface, causing bleeding which led to haemoptysis.

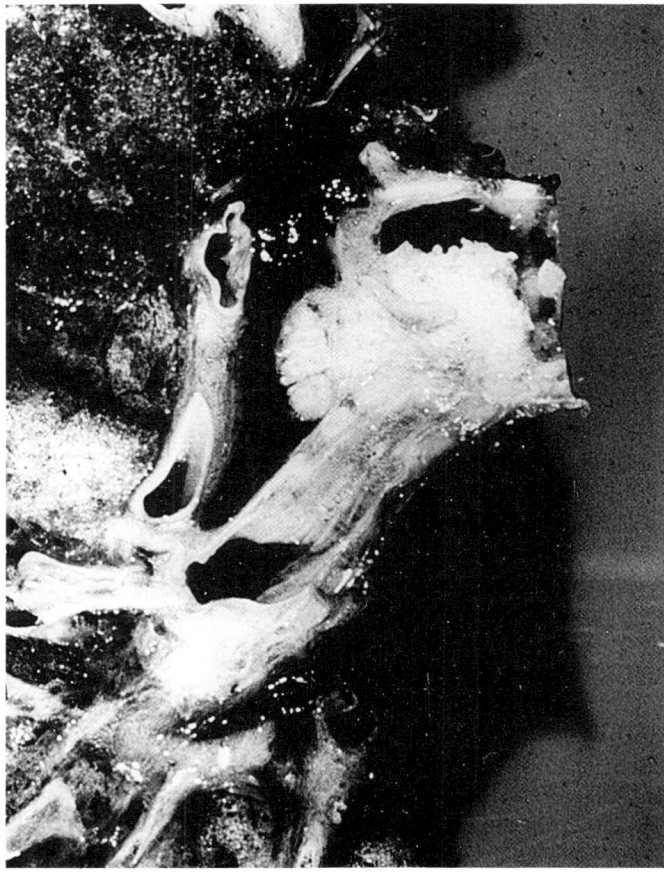

Fig. 13.171 Obstruction of the lower bronchus by a carcinoma of the lung has produced distal collapse with some consolidation of the lung.

Epidemiology

Cigarette smoking

During the 1930s and 1940s many studies implicated *tobacco smoking* as one of the causes of the rise in lung cancer, although there was considerable argument about its importance in relation to other factors, such as environmental pollution and occupational toxic hazards. The publication of two retrospective studies of the smoking habits of patients with lung cancer in 1950 by Wynder and Graham in the United States and Doll and Hill in the United Kingdom laid the foundation of the currently accepted thesis that cigarette smoking is the principal cause of lung cancer. Both studies showed that more than 95 per cent of their patients were regular smokers and that the proportion of heavy smokers (more than one pack per day) was particularly significant.

This led to the prospective study of the smoking habits and health of British doctors initiated in 1951 by Doll and Hill. Over more than 30 years this has confirmed the association between cigarette smoking and lung cancer, showing a clear relationship between the duration and amount of cigarettes smoked. Of particular importance is the finding that cessation of cigarette smoking leads to a continual decline in lung cancer, so that after 15 years an individual's risk of developing lung cancer is only slightly greater than that of a lifelong non-smoker.

Other aetiological factors

Beside cigarette smoking other factors pale into insignificance on a world-wide scale. However, there are well-recognized localized hazards, such as mining *radioactive ores*, exposure to *polycyclic aromatic hydrocarbons* amongst coal gas, and foundry workers, and mining or working with *asbestos*.

Diagnosis

It must be emphasized from the outset that no matter how suggestive the clinical or radiological picture may be, a firm diagnosis of lung cancer can only be made by microscopic examination. Material for diagnosis is generally obtained from sputum, pleural effusions, fine-needle aspiration biopsy, or by surgical biopsy using a bronchoscope or directly at operation.

Sputum cytology and pleural effusions

Good-quality sputum samples can be a most reliable means of diagnosing lung tumours. Studies indicate that, particularly if multiple samples are taken, up to 70 per cent of primary lung tumours can be diagnosed by careful sputum examination. When pleural effusions are present in association with lung cancer, malignant cells can usually be identified easily. Such effusions are easier to work with than sputum due to the much larger numbers of malignant cells present. However, the drawback is that only a small minority of lung tumours actually present with pleural effusions. In general, exfoliative cytology is better at making a distinction between benign and malignant pulmonary conditions than at subdividing various lung tumours.

Gray (1987) points out that the characteristics of malignant exfoliated cells are seen predominantly in their nuclei, and provides the following helpful list of their main features:

1. uneven distribution of chromatin;
2. hyperchromasia;
3. high nuclear-cytoplasmic ratio;
4. irregularity of nuclear membrane;
5. irregular nuclear contours;
6. abnormal nucleoli;
7. abnormal mitoses; and
8. nuclear pleomorphism.

Any combination of these features may be seen in a particular sample of malignant cells and no single one constitutes a diagnosis of malignancy by itself.

Fine-needle aspiration biopsy

This technique of withdrawing a sample of a tumour by needle aspiration is almost as old as histopathology itself. First developed in the 1880s, it was a popular technique in the early part of this century but fell into disuse with the rapid advances made in tissue processing as surgical pathology became a recognized speciality in the inter-war years. There were also reports of a high complication rate with the needles then in use, although this has virtually disappeared with the introduction of sterile disposable needles as used for taking blood samples. In the past decade or so there has been a considerable revival in the use of fine-needle biopsy, largely due to the perseverance of Scandinavian cytologists. Nowadays, with the vogue for early diagnosis augmented by sophisticated non-invasive investigations, fine-needle aspiration biopsy is taking an increasingly prominent role as a first-line investigation. It can certainly no longer be ignored by practising histopathologists. Fine-needle biopsy has the great advantage over exfoliative cytology that some architectural features of tumours are preserved and therefore are easier to compare with conventional histological sections. It still must be emphasized though that the technique is better suited to distinguish benign from malignant than to subdivide lung tumours. However, the combination of examination of exfoliative cytology with fine-needle biopsy under radiological or other control would probably allow the diagnosis of the majority of human lung tumours without recourse to other more invasive means.

Surgical biopsy

The gold standard of lung cancer diagnosis remains examination of the actual tumour, or at least a representative piece of it. The introduction of flexible fibre-optic bronchoscopes passed into the bronchial tree via the nasal passages has revolutionized this undertaking. Formerly it could be extremely difficult to obtain an adequate biopsy, particularly of distal lesions, without resort to open-chest surgery. Against this bright vista of technological progress, it seems almost churlish to bring up any problems. Nevertheless, accurate diagnosis of lung carcinoma from fibre-optic bronchiscopic biopsies can be difficult. The samples are small and may not contain tumour (thus only a positive result is definitive). Many small biopsies are fragile and easily crushed, either during the procedure or later handling, leading to undiagnosable specimens. Furthermore, examination of small specimens has similar sampling problems to those encountered with cytological preparations. Such preparations cannot take tumour heterogeneity into account, so there may be discrepancies between the classification of a tumour removed surgically and that diagnosed on bronchoscopic biopsy (which may or may not be relevant for the prognosis and therapy of individual patients).

Other techniques

There are a number of other techniques for obtaining material for diagnosis of lung tumours. Most are based on those detailed above, such as bronchial brushing or lavage via a bronchoscope. Others involve larger needles than those for fine-needle biopsy, such as the 'Trucut', or bronchial drill biopsy. All have their advocates, and their particular advantages and disadvantages depend as much on the situation and type of lesions being biopsied as on the individual experience and skills of those performing and reporting them.

Possible precursor lesions in the bronchi and lungs

Along with the increasing sophistication of non-invasive diagnostic techniques, such as fibre-optic bronchoscopy and computerized tomography, has come considerable interest in the possibility of an earlier diagnosis of cancer by recognition of premalignant changes. Pulmonary pathologists have sought to identify pre-invasive lesions similar to those recognized as intraepithelial malignancy in the cervix, breast, and gastrointestinal tract. Three types of cytological change have been investigated in the bronchi as possible precursors of later invasive malignancy. These are squamous metaplasia, basal cell hyperplasia, and bronchial dysplasia.

Squamous metaplasia

There is no squamous epithelium in the normal bronchial tree so that all squamous changes found are referred to as metaplastic. Such changes are frequently found in the epithelium adjoining bronchial squamous cell carcinomas and a careful examination of resection specimens often demonstrates a point where the tumour apparently arises from such epithelium. This naturally led to considerable excitement that squamous metaplasia was a consistent and required precursor for squamous cell carcinoma. Indeed many pathologists are of the opinion that a considerable number of such tumours do arise from metaplastic areas. Unfortunately, as a general principle this thesis is no longer tenable since many adenocarcinomas and small cell carcinomas also have a similarly close relationship to areas of squamous epithelium. This cannot be explained by the theory of a common origin of pulmonary tumours (see below) since a large number of other non-neoplastic conditions, such as asthma and severe influenza may also reveal extensive areas of squamous metaplasia. In fact there is now good experimental and clinical evidence that squamous metaplasia is part of the normal reparative process of the lung and that after damage or destruction of the bronchial mucosa, for whatever reason, regeneration occurs via the formation of stratified squamous epithelium. This differentiates into the usual columnar ciliated epithelium, provided that the initiating stimuli desist. Thus, in cigarette-smokers whose bronchial epithelium has shown evidence of squamous epithelium, repeat biopsy after a period of cessation of smoking frequently shows reversion to the normal mucosa.

Basal cell hyperplasia

This change in the bronchial mucosa is defined as stratified epithelium with retention of superficial ciliated cells (Fig. 13.172). Such changes have been reported to be much commoner in cigarette-smokers than in non-smokers, and often to be associated with significant dysplastic changes which may regress in those who cease to smoke. Unlike squamous cell metaplasia, there is no known pathophysiological role for basal cell hyperplasia in the lung, which partially accounts for its postulation as a malignant precursor. However, the lesion is not found in all, or even in the majority, of cases of carcinoma of the lungs, so that any pre-malignant role it may play must remain speculative for the moment.

Dysplasia

Dysplastic changes in the bronchial mucosa are not as well recognized and understood as those in the cervix uteri or bladder, which probably represents nothing more than the difficulty of obtaining sufficiently representative cytological or biopsy

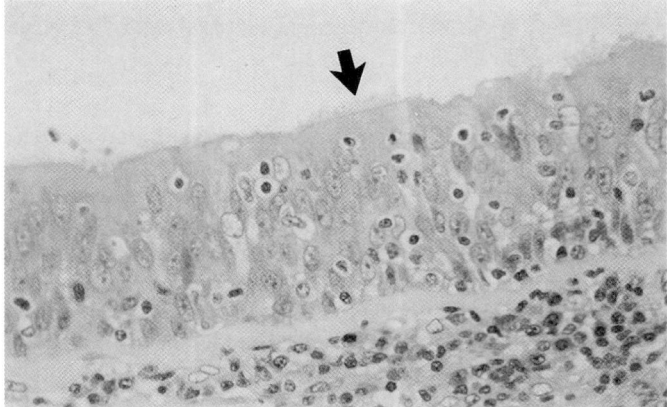

Fig. 13.172 An example of basal cell hyperplasia. Note the cilia present on the luminal surface (arrowed) which distinguishes this condition from squamous cell hyperplasia (see text for details).

material. Full thickness cellular disorganization with nuclear atypia and increased mitotic figures amounting to carcinoma *in situ* is seen from time to time and almost certainly represents a pre-invasive lesion. Whether there is a true hierachy of dysplastic change, as is well documented in cervical pathology, offering the possibility of early therapeutic intervention, is unknown (and is likely to remain so with currently available diagnostic techniques).

The classification of carcinoma of the lung

The task of classifying tumours is instantly appealing to those who like collecting butterflies or examining train timetables. Complexity provides interest. Butterflies and train drivers prefer direct recognition or simple schedules. Lung tumours are not exceptional amongst human malignancies in providing an example of these conflicting interests. There are those who believe that lung cancer is a single neoplasm manifesting a high degree of morphological diversity. Such people trace their view back to the eminent tumour pathologist, Willis, who concluded in 1948, based on a review of the clinical and pathological features of the disease, 'while these names all have descriptive value, and while many pulmonary cancers consist predominantly, sometimes exclusively of growth of a particular type, it must be emphasized that there is only one entity *carcinoma of the lung,* that individual tumours show various structural combinations, and that great pleomorphism is possible in one tumour'. It must be said in retaliation that there are those who believe Willis to have been a great champion of lost causes.

However, the post-war years have witnessed the recognition that lung cancer was endemic in the Western world and that it could be subdivided into several different entities of different cellular origin. This viewpoint has culminated in the WHO-sponsored classification scheme first published in 1967 and updated in 1982. This is a detailed system (Table 13.19) with more than 40 categories of neoplasm, 17 of these being malignant epithelial tumours.

The great advantage of this classification is that it has received broad acceptance from pulmonary pathologists as the baseline for typing lung tumours, whether or not they actually use it. This contrasts with lymphoma or testicular tumour classification where a standard scheme has been more difficult to attain. In practice, the WHO classification can yield a high degree of consistency amongst co-operating pathologists who accept and understand standard criteria for diagnosing individual lung tumour subtypes. Even amongst the experts, good inter-observer agreement is best on broad categories and worst on the fine print, particularly with regard to the poorly differentiated and anaplastic tumours. In view of the large numbers of lung tumours world-wide, and the fact that every pathologist has to deal with a certain number, practice has dictated a simpler approach to typing lung tumours, based on the WHO classification scheme. These are essentially similar and divide lung cancers into four groups, comprising *squamous cell carcinomas, adencarcinomas,* and *small and large cell carcinomas.*

Table 13.19 Revised WHO histological classification of lung tumours (1982)

I. Epithelial tumours
  A. Benign
    1. Papillomas
      a. Squamous cell papilloma
      b. 'Transitional' papilloma
    2. Adenomas
      a. Pleomorphic adenoma ('mixed' tumour)
      b. Monomorphic adenoma
      c. Others
  B. Dysplasia
    Carcinoma *in situ*
  C. Malignant
    1. Squamous cell carcinoma (epidermoid carcinoma)
      Variant:
      a. Spindle-cell (squamous) carcinoma
    2. Small cell carcinoma
      a. Oat-cell carcinoma
      b. Intermediate cell type
      c. Combined oat-cell carcinoma
    3. Adenocarcinoma
      a. Acinar adenocarcinoma
      b. Papillary adenocarcinoma
      c. Bronchiolo-alveolar carcinoma
      d. Solid carcinoma with mucus formation
    4. Large cell carcinoma
      Variants:
      a. Giant-cell carcinoma
      b. Clear-cell carcinoma
    5. Adenosquamous carcinoma
    6. Carcinoid tumour
    7. Bronchial gland carcinomas
      a. Adenoid cystic carcinoma
      b. Mucoepidermoid carcinoma
      c. Others
    8. Others

II. Soft-tissue tumours

III. Mesothelial tumours
  A. Benign mesothelioma
  B. Malignant mesothelioma
    1. Epithelial
    2. Fibrous (spindle-cell)
    3. Biphasic

IV. Miscellaneous tumours
  A. Benign
  B. Malignant
    1. Carcinosarcoma
    2. Pulmonary blastoma
    3. Malignant melanoma
    4. Malignant lymphomas
    5. Others

V. Secondary tumours

VI. Unclassified tumours

VII. Tumour-like lesions
  A. Hamartoma
  B. Lymphoproliferative lesions
  C. Tumourlet
  D. Eosinophilic granuloma
  E. 'Sclerosing haemangioma'
  F. Inflammatory pseudotumour
  G. Others

Criteria for the diagnosis and classification of lung cancers

Squamous cell carcinoma

These are defined on light microscopy as tumours exhibiting epithelial pearl formation, individual cell keratinization, or intercellular bridging ('prickles') (Fig. 13.173). The degree of differentiation should be determined by the extent of keratinization, which is recognized by a deep pink colour in the cytoplasm. In practice many pathologists prefer to base this diagnosis on a number of features such as overall morphology, degree of cellular pleomorphism, etc. so that there is considerable overlap between the categories. Also, and perhaps inevitably, the majority of tumours end up being called 'moderately differentiated' (Fig. 13.174).

On electron microscopy, well-differentiated squamous carcinomas are characterized by tonofilaments converging on well-developed desmosomes. Additional features are the deposition of keratin in keratohyaline granules and wide intercellular spaces bridged at desmosomal sites. These features are progressively lost as tumours become less differentiated.

Squamous cell carcinomas account for 50–70 per cent of surgical resections of lung tumours, but probably only 30–40 per cent overall. They are commonest growing centrally in or around major bronchi and many have a characteristic cheesy appearance on slicing. Microscopically, the cells grow in stratified or pseudoductal forms with small nests or 'pearls' in the centre of some of these. Giant pleomorphic nuclei and multinucleated cells are not uncommon. As the tumours enlarge, their centres develop a central necrotic mass of keratinous debris, accounting for the 'cheesy' appearance described above.

Adenocarcinoma

These are usually classified on light microscopical grounds as those tumours which demonstrate acinar or papillary differentiation (Fig. 13.175) in which at least some of the cells produce mucus, as demonstrated histochemically by Alcian blue/PAS staining. Ultrastructurally the main features are intracellular secretory vacuoles, well-developed endoplasmic reticula, prominent Golgi apparatus, and plentiful mitochrondria. Desmosomes are generally less developed than in squamous tumours.

Adenocarcinomas constitute 10–25 per cent of lung cancers and tend to be peripheral tumours in which it can be difficult to demonstrate a connection with an underlying bronchus. Primary pulmonary adenocarcinomas are sometimes indistinguishable from secondary tumours which must therefore be excluded by other means (consideration of the possibility is the first and most important). Adenocarcinomas may arise in preexisting pulmonary scars and tend to invade the overlying pleura. In the latter case a number of tumours, perhaps 10 per cent, will present with pleural effusions and may be difficult, both cytologically and histologically, to differentiate from malignant mesothelioma. If the WHO classification is strictly adhered to, adenocarcinomas should be split into four types: *acinar, papillary, solid, and bronchiolo-alveolar*. In practice, most pathologists only separate bronchiolo-alveolar tumours and

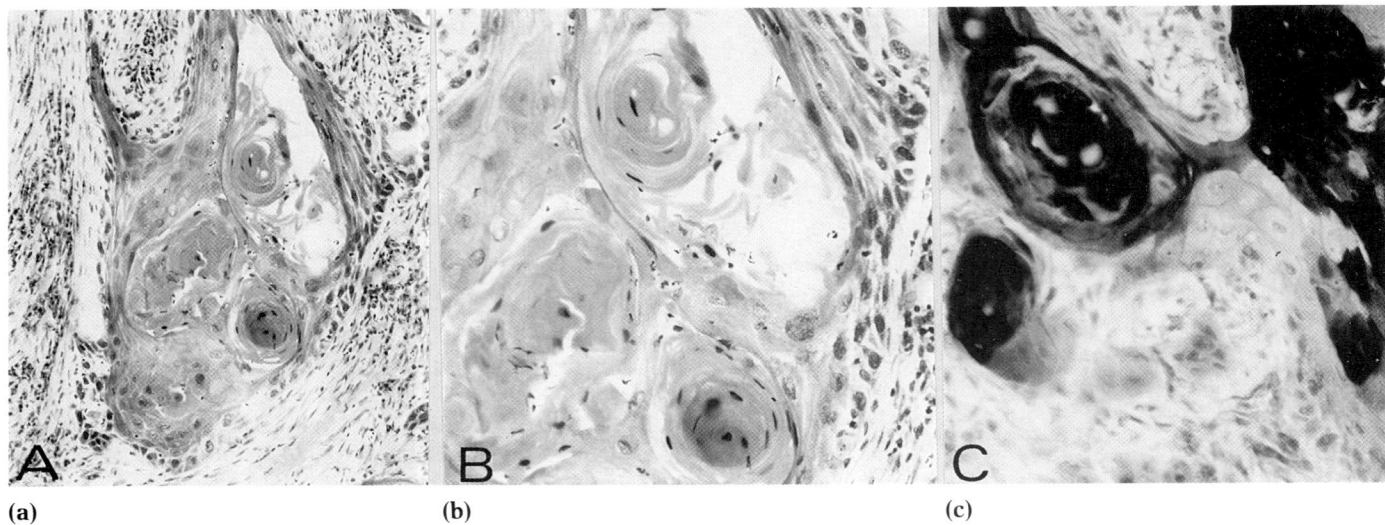

(a)   **(b)**   **(c)**

Fig. 13.173 Classical appearance of (a) well-differentiated squamous cell carcinoma with epithelial pearl formation. In (b) the pearls are illustrated at higher power, showing the central keratin formation which can be demonstrated to be high molecular weight keratin by immunostaining with appropriate monoclonal antibodies (as shown in c)).

treat the other three as one group. This is a perfectly reasonable thing to do since there is little or no evidence to suggest there is any difference in treatment, response, or survival amongst these different types.

Bronchiolo-alveolar carcinoma has a characteristic morpho-

logical appearance, with well-differentiated 'bland' cells growing along pre-existing alveolar airways (Fig. 13.176). It can at times be difficult to distinguish from hyperplastic regenerative alveoli, e.g. after a particularly severe viral pneumonia. Ultrastructural studies suggest that bronchiolo-alveolar tumours are themselves a heterogeneous group of neoplasms arising from mucus-secreting bronchial epithelial cells, type 2 pneumocytes, or Clara cells.

Small- or oat-cell carcinoma

On light microscopical grounds these tumours are recognized by their sheet-like composition of darkly staining cells with a

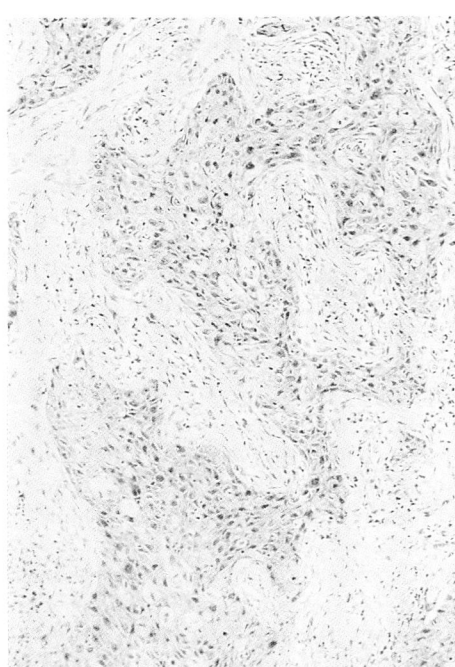

Fig. 13.174 Squamous cell carcinomas frequently lack such well-developed squamous features as illustrated in Fig. 13.173. Their more usual appearance is shown here, in which the overall architecture with rudimentary keratinization and tonofilament formation allows a diagnosis of moderately differentiated squamous cell carcinoma to be made.

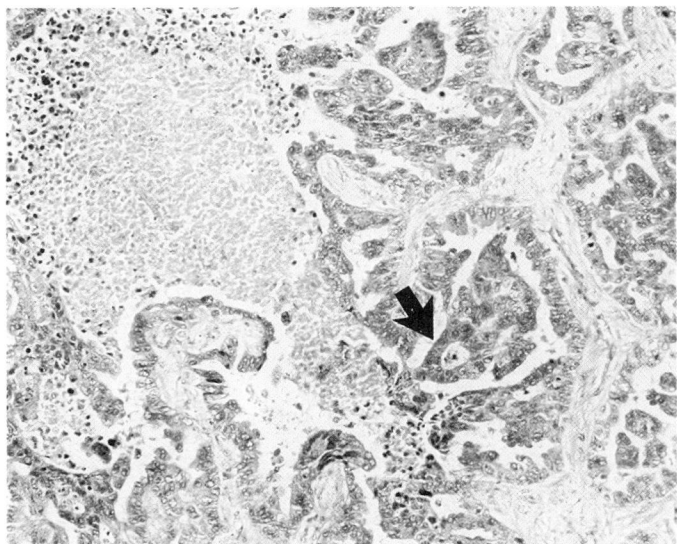

Fig. 13.175 Characteristic low-power features of an adenocarcinoma of the lung, showing the clear glandular formation (arrowed).

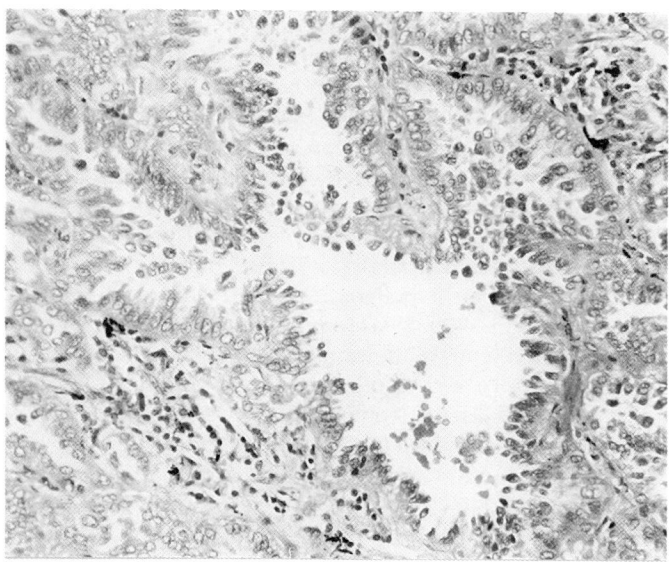

Fig. 13.176 A bronchiolo-alveolar cell carcinoma, illustrating the relatively bland tumour cells growing along pre-existing alveolar airways.

high nuclear to cytoplasmic ratio (Fig. 13.177). The term 'small cell carcinoma' is somewhat of a misnomer since careful morphometric studies have shown considerable variability in the size and shape of the tumour cells (leading to the subclassification of small cell carcinoma in the WHO classification illustrated in Table 13.19). In practice, many pathologists and oncologists do not distinguish the different subtypes and use the term 'oat-cell' carcinoma synonymously. There has been considerable argument whether oat-cell carcinoma is a distinct entity or just a form of poorly differentiated lung cancer. It is probably fair to say that Azzopardi established the entity morphologically with his detailed description of its characteristic features in 1959. These included the typical ribbon and stream growth pattern, the formation of rosettes and pseudorosettes, and the very characteristic deposition of DNA on blood vessel walls in necrotic areas. This latter feature is most commonly

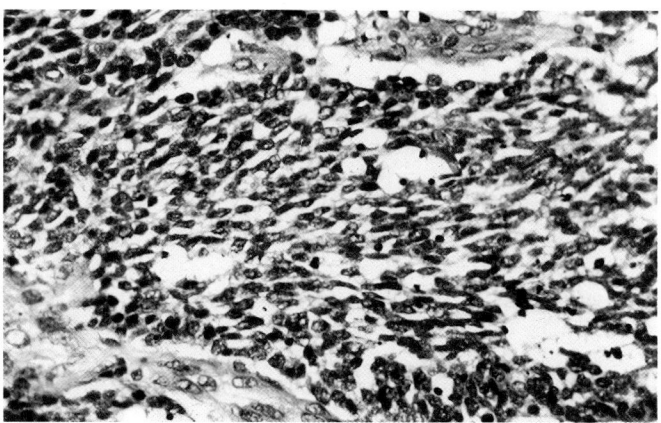

Fig. 13.177 Small cell carcinoma.

seen at post-mortem, when the tumours are more extensive than those seen at bronchoscopic biopsy.

Ultrastructurally, the only finding that has been claimed as distinctive is the presence of dense-core neurosecretory granules within the cells. However, these are by no means a consistent feature in all cases and a prolonged search has often to be undertaken to demonstrate any at all. In addition, such neurosecretory granules are not restricted to oat-cell carcinomas and its variants but may be seen in other lung tumours, a point that will be discussed in more detail later. Nevertheless, although it is difficult to give firm criteria for diagnosing oat-cell carcinoma, using the criteria of Azzopardi in a well-fixed and prepared biopsy it is a characteristic lesion, quite easily separable from the other classical types of lung cancer. Overlap between the different lung cancer types and the relevance this may have for treatment and prognosis will be discussed later in the section on lung tumour heterogeneity.

Large cell carcinoma

Although this comprises a separate entity in the WHO classification, it is in reality a term reserved for those malignant epithelial tumours which, on light microscopy, show none of the features described above as typical of squamous, adenocarcinoma, or small cell carcinoma. What remains are tumours composed of large cells, often arranged in sheets but with no other obvious forms of differentiation. If giant cells are plentiful, the tumour is often subclassified as *giant-cell carcinoma*. As is frequently the case with tumours diagnosed on grounds of exclusion, the more intensely they are studied the fewer they become. The introduction of electron microscopy into diagnosis has shown that most, if not all, large cell tumours have ultrastructural features of squamous cell or adenocarcinomas and can be classified as such.

Mixed tumours

There are a number of mixed tumour types in the WHO scheme, such as combined oat-cell or adenosquamous carcinoma. They are more commonly seen in resection specimens and at postmortem than in small biopsy specimens. For this reason many pathologists base their diagnosis on the predominant tumour type present, arguing that this is what determines the prognosis of the patient.

Heterogeneity of lung cancer and its relationship to histogenesis

It has been observed for many years, since the reports of Willis in the late 1940s and early 1950s, that more than one morphological pattern can be seen in any individual tumour (Fig. 13.178). Indeed, it has been argued that if a tumour is thoroughly studied in enough sections, heterogeneity will certainly be found. The advent of electron microscopy and immunocytochemistry with monoclonal antibodies has confirmed these histological observations, showing the presence of mucous, dense core granules and tonofilaments in tumours of all categories, with antigens of many different specificities being shared by all.

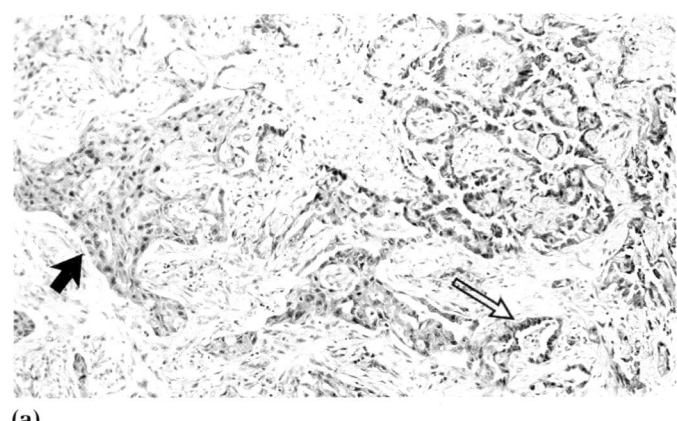

(a)

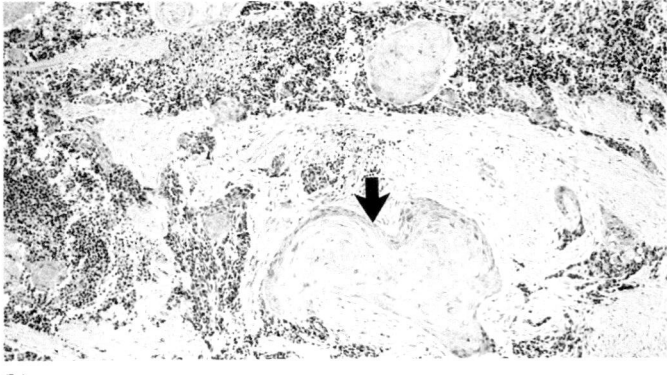

(b)

Fig. 13.178 Two examples of mixed tumours, illustrating the type of heterogeneity that may be seen in human lung tumours. (a) Shows on the left (solid arrow) typical squamous differentiation and on the right (open arrow) glandular (adeno) morphology. In (b) an area of typical keratinizing squamous cell carcinoma (arrowed) can be seen surrounded by characteristic small cell carcinoma.

Such studies have now led to the widespread acceptance of the following three conclusions:

1. *There is a close relationship between the different histological categories of lung tumour.*

2. *There is a heterogeneous differentiation pattern in many, if not most, lung tumours.*

3. *Lung tumours arise from a common stem cell and represent a single tumour with a tendency to differentiate along one or more pathways.*

What the nature of this pluripotent epithelial cell is remains unclear. It has been argued that only cells that can divide have the potential for undergoing hyperplasia, metaplasia, and neoplasia. In the bronchi there are only two obvious candidates which divide in the adult epithelium, the mucous cells and the basal cells. A further discussion of the experimental work, particularly of the response of animal tracheobronchial epithelium to injury, undertaken to elucidate the nature of bronchogenic carcinogenesis is beyond the scope of this chapter. Further details will be found in McDowell (1987).

Assessment of prognosis

It is widely held by pathologists that at best the lung tumour classification scheme distinguishes between carcinomas of bad and carcinomas of worse prognosis. Nevertheless, oncologists are of the view that small cell carcinoma is clinically different from other forms of lung cancer. Although there is little or no biological justification for such an abrupt division, the accumulation of therapeutic data over the years shows that operationally such a distinction has its uses. Typical small cell carcinoma is a highly proliferative malignancy with a tendency to present with metastatic disease. Such tumours are rarely cured by surgery and radiotherapy alone. Small cell lung cancers are generally more sensitive to chemotherapy than other lung tumours, which in limited disease (confined to one hemithorax) can increase median survival from 3 to 14 months.

There are, in our view, two problems with this simplistic clinical division. The first is that it only offers a positive therapeutic approach to at most 20 per cent of patients with lung cancer, i.e. those with small cell tumours. Apart from a small number of squamous and adenocarcinomas which are resectable, the clinical approach is palliative from the outset. A recent review of treatment for non-small cell carcinoma concluded that the use of chemotherapy was controversial (Anon 1988). Most trials were flawed by being uncontrolled or poorly randomized, and thus failed to give a definite conclusion. The other problem is that non-small cell carcinoma covers such a large spectrum of tumour types and differing proliferation rates that it is not surprising that clear answers are difficult to obtain. Recent studies of lung tumours using markers of proliferation and different aspects of differentiation are beginning to show patterns that might make a more rational approach to chemotherapy feasible. For instance, as a group, small cell lung cancer has a *high growth fraction*. So, too, does a significant percentage of squamous and adenocarcinomas. It would be valuable to ascertain whether these rapidly proliferating non-small cell tumours might behave similarly to small cell cancers, which would allow a radical approach to be taken to something approaching 50 per cent of human lung tumours. Nevertheless, at present the outlook for all human lung cancers is grim, with fewer than 30 per cent of patients in the most favourable categories surviving longer than 5 years.

Paramalignant disorders

Patients with lung cancer have a particularly high incidence of systemic symptoms, or paramalignant disorders, which are not obviously related to the physical presence of the tumour or its metastases. A knowledge of these is useful since it may lead to an earlier diagnosis, with the possibility of therapeutic intervention. Failure to recognize them certainly has a deleterious effect on prowess in medical examinations. The commonest of these are detailed in Table 13.20.

Endocrine manifestations, although not the commonest paramalignant disorder, have been more intensely studied than the others. Lung cancer cells are able to synthesize a variety of polypeptides that mimic virtually all the hormones produced by

Table 13.20 Paramalignant disorders associated with lung cancer

Unexplained weight loss of more than 6.4 kg	31%
Finger clubbing	29%
Fever	21%
Endocrine disorders	12%
Anaemia (microcytic or normocytic)	8%
Neuromyopathy	1.4%

the endocrine glands. Such ectopic secretions are responsible for many of the endocrine and metabolic manifestations experienced by some patients.

Ectopic adrenocorticotropin (ACTH) secretion, giving rise to a *metabolic Cushing's syndrome*, is probably the commonest endocrine disorder. Patients suffer from a *hypokalaemic alkalosis* which may be so acute that death can occur within a matter of weeks. Typical Cushing's syndrome is rare in lung cancer, probably due to the rapid production of the hormone giving little time for the development of the characteristic features. The syndrome is more commonly associated with small cell carcinomas, which probably reflects the amount of active ACTH produced rather than any fundamental difference from other tumour types. Elevated ACTH and pro('big')ACTH levels are a frequent finding in all types of lung tumour. There is evidence that plasma levels, particularly of proACTH, become elevated early in the course of a bronchial carcinoma and it has been suggested that this measurement would be useful in early diagnosis. This, of course, begs the question of who should be screened (or what therapy should be offered) even if it does have predictive value. Serum ACTH levels usually decline on surgical resection or successful therapy of the tumour. Reappearance usually means recurrence of the tumour.

Another common endocrine disorder is *inappropriate antidiuretic hormone (ADH) secretion* leading to intra- and extracellular overhydration, with the potential of cerebral oedema, fits, and coma if the serum sodium drops below 120 mmol/l. Most of these cases are associated with small cell carcinoma, which again may be related to rate of production, since the hormone has been demonstrated immunologically in other lung tumours. Other endocrine abnormalities include *hypercalcaemia from ectopic production of parathormone* (mainly squamous cell carcinomas), *hypercalcitoninaemia* (all tumour types), and the *ectopic production of human chorionic gonadotrophin (HCG)*, which occasionally leads to *gynaecomastia*. Many other peptides can be detected, such as serotonin, bombesin, gastrin-releasing peptide, and neurone-specific enolase, most of which are more important as potential diagnostic agents rather than for any clinical effect they have on patients.

13.7.2 Low-grade malignant and benign tumours

With the exception of the bronchial carcinoid tumour, all these neoplasms are extremely rare, so that the average diagnostician will only meet occasional examples (if at all) during a working lifetime. Provided that the malignant tumours described above are clearly recognized, there is little need for alarm with the remaining bronchial tumours, which can be diagnosed with specialist textbooks or sent for consultation.

Carcinoid tumours

These are the commonest tumours in this low-grade group and are classified as carcinomas in the WHO classification. Carcinoids frequently arise in young adults and appear to have no association with smoking behaviour. They were initially thought to be benign and were classified with a group of other uncommon tumours as *bronchial adenomas*. Carcinoids usually arise in the larger bronchi, possibly from the specialized *endocrine Feyrter or Kultschitsky-like cells* in the basal layer of the bronchial epithelium and mucous gland ducts. They usually present relatively non-specifically with cough or recurrent chest infections, or even on a routine chest X-ray. On resection many carcinoids have a characteristic gross appearance of a soft fleshy tumour extruding into the lumen of the bronchus in a 'dumbbell'-like fashion. Histologically, the tumour has a typical endocrine packeted appearance; often some attempt at rosette formation can be found in a diligent search. They resemble carcinoids in the gastrointestinal tract and have the same silver staining properties as foregut carcinoids, i.e. Grimelius (argyrophil) positive and Masson–Fontana (argentaffin) negative. Ultrastructurally, the tumour cells contain large numbers of dense-core neurosecretory granules. Carcinoids are characterized by a low number of mitotic figures and a small growth fraction. The tumours are locally invasive but only metastasize on rare occasions, when they may give rise to the carcinoid syndrome.

There is a somewhat controversial group of tumours of highly malignant phenotype which some authorities feel are *atypical carcinoid tumours*. These tumours arise in an older age-group, may well be associated with smoking, and have a light-microscopic appearance which does not resemble either carcinoid tumour or small cell carcinoma. These tumours, which are being increasingly recognized, do not as yet have a place of their own in the WHO classification. Whether they are truly a distinct group of tumours or represent a further example of the extreme heterogeneiety of lung tumours remains to be established.

Other low-grade malignant tumours

There are six other low-grade tumours previously recognized as part of the group of tumours called *bronchial adenomas*. These are *adenoid cystic tumour, mucoepidermoid tumour, pleomorphic adenomas, cystadenomas, oncocytomas,* and *acinic cell tumours*. These tumours are extremely rare and are not restricted to the lung, being much commoner in salivary and other minor secretory glands. Interested readers will find a detailed account of these in the sections on salivary tumours and tumours of the oropharynx, and in textbooks on these subjects.

13.7.3   Further reading

Anon. (1988). Lung cancer: when to give chemotherapy. *Drug and Therapeutics Bulletin* **26**, 29–30.

Dunnill, M. S. (1987). *Pulmonary pathology* (2nd edn). Churchill Livingstone, Edinburgh.

Gray, (1987). Pulmonary cytology. In *Pulmonary pathology* (ed. M. S. Dunnill), pp. 581–605. Churchill Livingstone, Edinburgh.

Horne, N. W. and Spiro, S. G. (1987). Tumours of the lung, mediastinum and pleura. In *Oxford textbook of medicine* (ed. D. J. Weatherall, J. G. G. Ledingham, and D. A. Warrell), pp. 15.145–15.158. Oxford University Press, Oxford.

McDowell, E. M. (ed.) (1987). *Lung carcinomas*. Churchill Livingstone, Edinburgh.

13.8   The pleura

F. Barker and T. Krausz

13.8.1   Inflammation

The pleura is the serous membrane that invests the surface of the lung and lines the pleural cavity. It is glistening and translucent when healthy but becomes opaque when inflamed, when it may be coated with a fibrinous or purulent exudate. The visceral and parietal layers meet at the hilum, and are lubricated by a watery fluid, the volume of which is normally less than 15 ml. The defining microscopical feature of the pleura is its lining of mesothelial cells; these may be cuboidal or flattened in shape and typically have microvilli on the free surface. The cytoplasm contains abundant glycogen. When exfoliated cells are examined in aspirates of pleural effusions, however, the individual cells are seen to have become rounded, and there is a tendency for the cells to form clusters. In the intact pleura, there is a submesothelial layer of connective tissue consisting of collagen and elastic fibres, with blood vessels, lymphatics, nerves, and submesothelial spindle cells. Elastic fibres are found in greatest density in those areas of the pleura associated with respiratory movements; the pleura contributes to the elastic recoil of the lungs.

Injury to or loss of the mesothelium is followed by *regeneration*. Evidence has accumulated that a population of *submesothelial reserve cells* exists, which proliferates in response to injury to the mesothelium and differentiates into replacement mesothelial cells (Bolen *et al.* 1986). The light-microscopical appearance of these cells is similar to that of fibroblasts, but in the reactive state the cells express keratins of low molecular weight as well as *vimentin* and *muscle-specific actin*. As these cells mature into mesothelial cells, vimentin is replaced by *keratin* of high molecular weight. The fibroblast-like cells have a tendency to align themselves parallel to the injured surface, unlike the malignant spindle cells in certain forms of mesothelioma (Battifora 1989).

Inflammation of the pleura may be *infectious* or *non-infectious*.

The majority of infections involving the pleura are secondary to an underlying infection of the lung, such as *pneumonia, tuberculosis, lung abscess,* and *bronchiectasis. A subphrenic abscess* may involve the pleura. *Primary infection*, reaching the pleura via the bloodstream, can also occur. Of the common pulmonary infections, *tuberculosis* is the one which is most likely to produce pleural inflammation. Secondary pleural inflammation of a non-infectious type may occur in *rheumatoid disease, systemic lupus erythematosus, vasculitides,* and *other auto-immune diseases*.

Inflammation of the pleura is associated with increased permeability of the capillaries, and therefore produces an *exudate*. If the volume of the exudate is sufficient to be clinically or radiologically detectable, it constitutes an effusion (see Section 13.8.4). Pleural inflammations may be classified according to the nature of the exudate, and for convenience are grouped into three; *serous, serofibrinous,* and *fibrinous exudates* make up one group, and *suppurative* and *haemorrhagic exudates* the second and third groups. Exudates which at the beginning are serous, tend to become fibrinous in time.

The serofibrinous type of inflammation may be found in a variety of clinical settings, which includes the infectious and non-infectious conditions mentioned above, as well as systemic infections, pulmonary infarction, renal failure, and neoplasms metastatic to the pleura or pulmonary lymphatics. By contrast, the other types of inflammation are less common and are associated with fewer clinical conditions.

When suppurative inflammation occurs, there is almost always bacterial or fungal infection of the pleura, usually because of direct extension from the lung. Occasionally, a subphrenic abscess may extend into the diaphragmatic pleura, and organisms from a distant focus of infection may reach the pleura by the lymphatic or haematogenous routes. The purulent fluid that accumulates will often yield an organism if cultured. *Empyema* (purulent fluid) usually proceeds to fibrous organization and sometimes calcification, which may restrict respiratory movement; the extent of this complication may be lessened if surgical drainage can be performed before organization takes place.

True haemorrhagic inflammation is rare; the red cells which are commonly present in aspirates of pleural fluid are usually introduced by the trauma of the aspiration and are responsible for the frequent but sometimes erroneous clinical suspicion of malignancy. Haemorrhagic inflammation occurs in malignant infiltration of the pleura, and in certain infections caused by rickettsia and viruses (Jones 1987).

13.8.2   Primary tumours and tumour-like conditions

A feature that distinguishes some of the primary pleural tumours and tumour-like conditions from most other tumours is that an aetiological agent, namely certain mineral dusts, is known. The most studied is *asbestos*, which is a group of inorganic silicates having infinite-chain silicate anions. The material tends to cleave into microscopical fibres, of which the longest and thinnest of those that reach the alveoli have the greatest carcinogenic potential. Fibres found in the alveoli have diameters of the order of 1 μm and lengths of tens of micrometres; larger fibres tend to be trapped by bronchial or nasal mucus and expelled. As fibre shape and size seems to be of greater significance than chemical composition, other inorganic fibres have become the subject of epidemiological study (Peterson *et al.* 1984; Wagner and Pooley 1986; Jones 1987). Asbestos bodies may be found in the lung, or less often in the pleura; the fibre is coated with iron-containing matter, producing a golden-brown, 'dumbell' shape (Fig. 13.179).

Pleural plaque

The pleural plaque is not a neoplastic condition. It is a sharply outlined, white or cream thickening of the pleura with a smooth or nodular surface. The area may be anything up to tens of square centimetres, while the thickness is usually not more than 0.5 cm. Patchy calcification may occur. The plaques are most commonly found on the central tendon of the diaphragm, and the posterolateral aspects of the parietal pleura. They do not produce symptoms. The X-ray appearance is of a veil-like soft tissue density, which is more noticeable if the plaque is calcified. The microscopical appearance is of almost acellular, dense connective tissue in which the collagen bundles lie parallel to the surface (Fig. 13.180). The presence of pleural plaques has a strong association with exposure to asbestos fibres, usually *amosite* and *crocidolite,* and certain other mineral dusts, which need not be severe. A number of pathogenetic mechanisms has been proposed to account for the formation of plaques, but there is no consensus (Jones 1987); there is a latent interval of roughly two decades between the exposure and the detection of plaques, which is usually incidental.

Solitary fibrous tumour of the pleura ('solitary fibrous mesothelioma')

These tumours are rare. While most cases are asymptomatic, large tumours may produce respiratory symptoms. A few

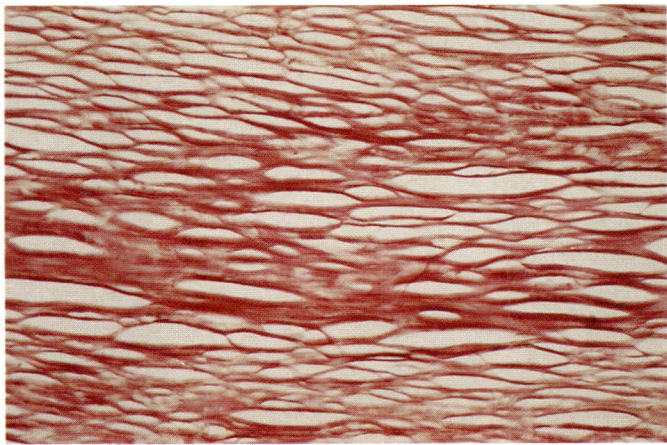

Fig. 13.180 A pleural plaque. The bundles of collagen fibres are arranged regularly in a basket-weave pattern.

tumours are associated with hypoglycaemia or an osteoarthropathy, which remit when the tumour is excised; the mechanism is unknown. Recurrence follows excision in about one-sixth of cases, but malignant behaviour, though well recognized, is not common.

Four-fifths of the tumours arise from the visceral pleura, while most of the remainder arise from the parietal pleura. A few develop in an interlobar fissure, or even wholly in the parenchyma of the lung. The tumours are sharply circumscribed, occasionally encapsulated, often pedunculated, and usually several centimetres across. The cut surface resembles that of a uterine 'fibroid' (Fig. 13.181). The microscopical appearance is of spindle cells intermingled with collagen bundles; a random arrangement is more common than a storiform pattern (Figs 13.182, 13.183). Mitoses are usually infrequent, but degenerative changes occur in the larger tumours. Frequent mitotic figures, large size, and necrosis are features that are associated with aggressive behaviour; pedunculated tumours, on the other hand, are usually benign, regardless of their microscopical features. The cellularity varies from case to case. Islands of

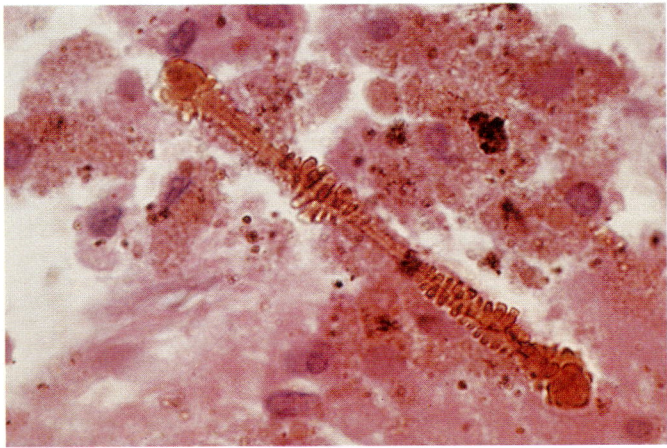

Fig. 13.179 An asbestos body. The mineral fibre is encrusted with brownish-yellow material which contains iron salts.

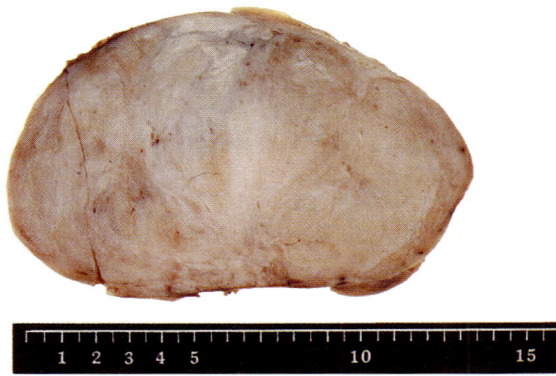

Fig. 13.181 A solitary fibrous tumour of the pleura. The cut surface shown here resembles that of a fibroid of the uterus.

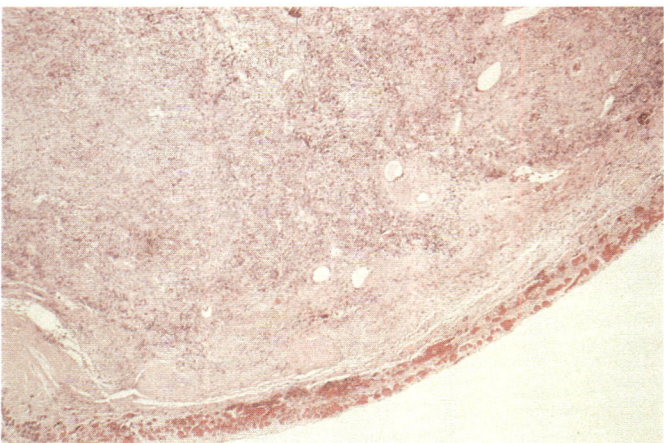

Fig. 13.182 A solitary fibrous tumour of the pleura. The tumour has a smooth margin.

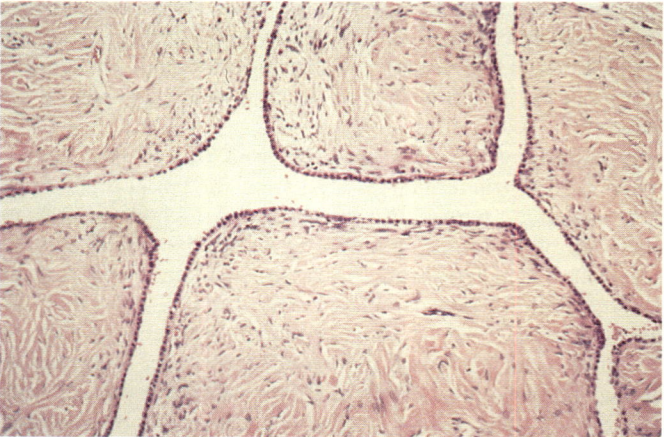

Fig. 13.183 A solitary fibrous tumour of the pleura. The cellularity of the collagenous stroma is low, the collagen bundles are arranged irregularly, and there is a single layer of entrapped respiratory epithelium.

epithelial cells can be found in a few of these tumours; it is suggested that they are derived from bronchial epithelium which has become incorporated into the tumour. Whether, as used to be thought, these tumours truly express mesothelial differentiation is disputed, as the modern histochemical and ultrastructural evidence suggests that the tumour cells are fibroblasts (Briselli *et al.* 1981; England *et al.* 1989).

Primary tumours—malignant

Malignant mesothelioma

The existence of this tumour as an entity was controversial until about 25 years ago, and although the tumour is now well documented, it remains one of the most difficult to diagnose in the living patient. Epidemiological evidence relating the development of the tumour to exposure to asbestos dust has accumulated, and has demonstrated a latent period, often of decades

(Wagner *et al.* 1960; Craighead 1987). *Crocidolite* appears to have the greatest carcinogenic potential, followed by *amosite,* and that in turn by *chrysotile* and *anthophyllite.* As exposure is usually occupational, most patients are male, but environmental exposure has produced the disease in women and children. A history of exposure to asbestos is not obtained in some cases of pleural malignant mesothelioma, even after detailed enquiry; this is often true of sporadic cases in children. It has been suggested that asbestos fibres from the mother may cross the placenta to reach the fetus, a theory for which there is some support in the form of animal experiments.

The clinical presentation of mesothelioma is usually that of persistent, dull, aching pain on one side of the chest. Often there is a pleural effusion, which may be bloodstained. Cytological examination of the fluid will generally demonstrate mesothelial cells, as well as red cells and inflammatory cells. The distinction between benign and malignant mesothelial cells is difficult and in many cases cannot be made with confidence; however, in malignant mesothelioma, the cells are more frequently bi- or multinucleated (Fig. 13.184), are arranged in clumps (Figs 13.185, 13.186), and the average nuclear and nucleolar sizes are larger, though morphometric assessment is necessary to demonstrate this last feature. The distinction from cells from a *metastatic carcinoma* is slightly easier. Only mesotheliomas with an epithelial component have a tendency to exfoliate cells into the pleural fluid. It is often necessary to resort to needle biopsy, and sometimes to open biopsy, to establish the diagnosis (Whitaker and Shilkin 1984).

The tumour grows preferentially over serosal surfaces, penetrating the interlobar fissures, and finally encasing the lung in a sheet of tumour which may be centimetres thick (Fig. 13.187). The tumour metastasizes via the lymphatics, producing distant foci in a quarter of cases. Deep extension into the parenchyma of the lung is uncommon.

Three principal histological types of mesothelioma are recognized, depending upon the relative amounts of epithelial and

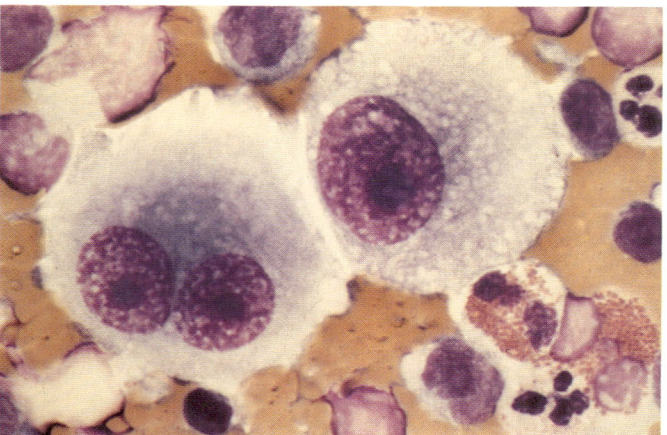

Fig. 13.184 A pleural effusion from a malignant epithelial mesothelioma. The two large tumour cells are adherent; one is binucleate, and the nucleoli are large. The chromatin is coarse; the cytoplasm is abundant. (Giemsa.)

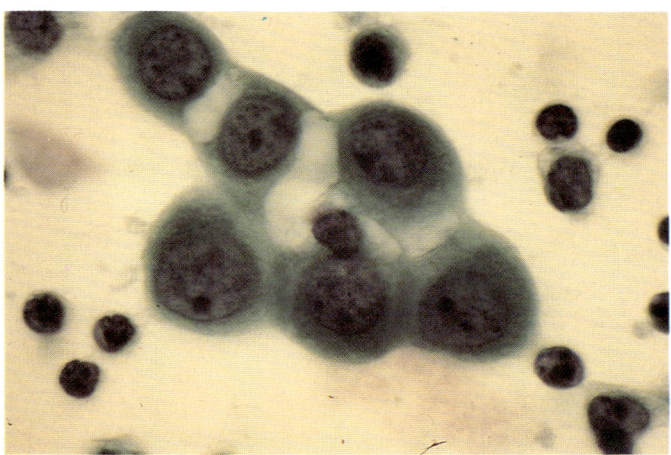

Fig. 13.185 The same effusion as Fig. 13.184. The 'windows' or pale spaces between the cells of this cluster are a frequent feature of mesothelial cells. These malignant cells have coarse chromatin and an increased nucleus/cytoplasm ratio. (Papanicolau.)

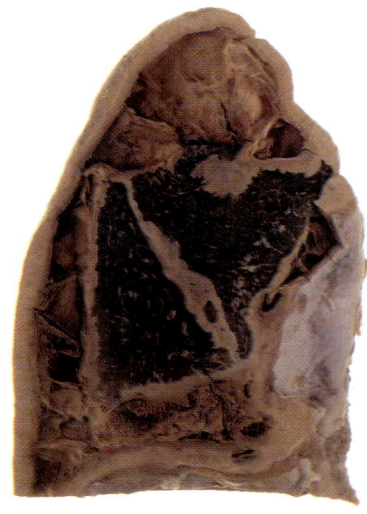

Fig. 13.187 A malignant epithelial mesothelioma. This parasagittal slice through the thoracic contents shows malignant growth over the parietal pleura, the encasement of the lung by tumour, and the growth of tumour along the interlobar fissure.

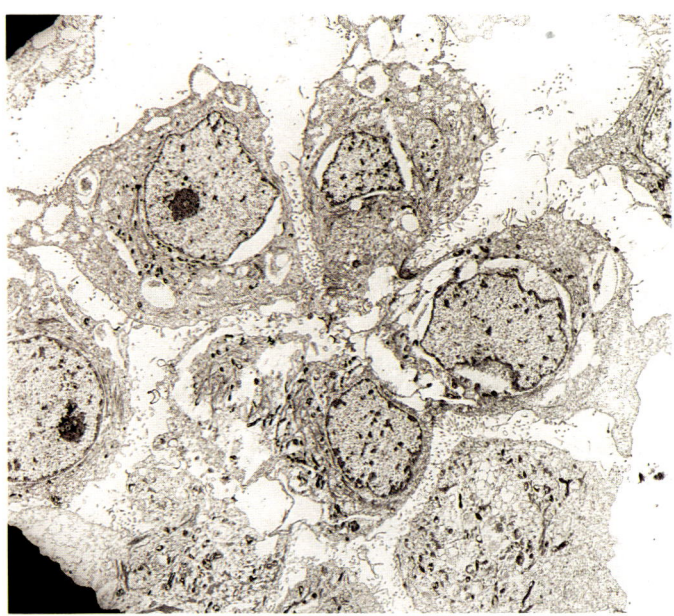

Fig. 13.186 A malignant epithelial mesothelioma. Intercellular spaces and abundant long, slender microvilli can be seen on the cell membranes in this clump of maglinant mesothelial cells. (E.M.)

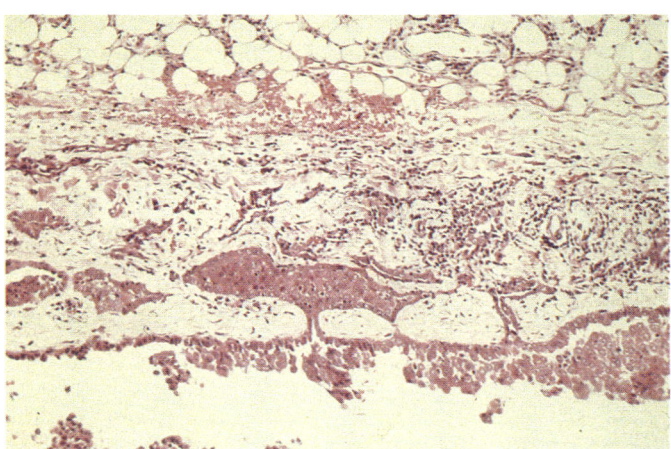

Fig. 13.188 A malignant epithelial mesothelioma. The tumour is present on the surface of the parietal pleura and has infiltrated the submesothelial tissue.

spindle cells, namely *epithelial*, *mixed*, and *spindle cell (sarcomatoid)*. On microscopical examination, the classical appearance is that of the mixed tumour, *a biphasic tumour* with epithelial and spindle-cell components. The former component has epithelial cells in tubules (Fig. 13.188), papillae (Fig. 13.189), or masses (Fig. 13.190), with acidophilic cytoplasm, and with round vesicular nuclei with a prominent nucleolus (Fig. 13.191). Cells in mitosis are infrequent. The spindle cells (Figs 13.192, 13.193) are set in a collagenous stroma which is often hyalinized; there may be clefts lined by spindle cells. If one or

other component predominates, a *monophasic tumour* of epithelial or spindle-cell type results. In large series, about two-thirds of tumours are epithelial, and one-quarter are mixed; fewer than one-tenth being spindle cell (Adams and Unni 1984).

Desmoplasia is a phenomenon which may be found in those mesotheliomas having a spindle-cell component (Fig. 13.194). The high proportion of collagen in desmoplastic mesotheliomas may cause confusion with solitary fibrous tumours, with reactive fibrosis, and with hyaline plaques, especially in small biopsy specimens (Cantin *et al.* 1982).

Electron microscopy may help to characterize a malignant pleural tumour. Mesothelial cells have long, slender microvilli (Figs 13.195, 13.196) which may be in contact with

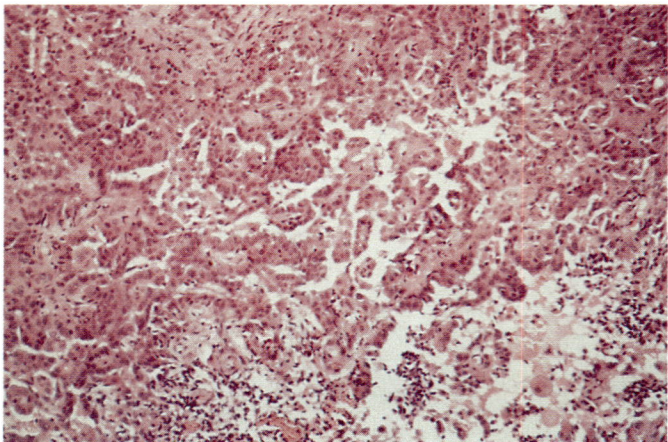

Fig. 13.189   A malignant epithelial mesothelioma. The tumour has a papillary growth pattern.

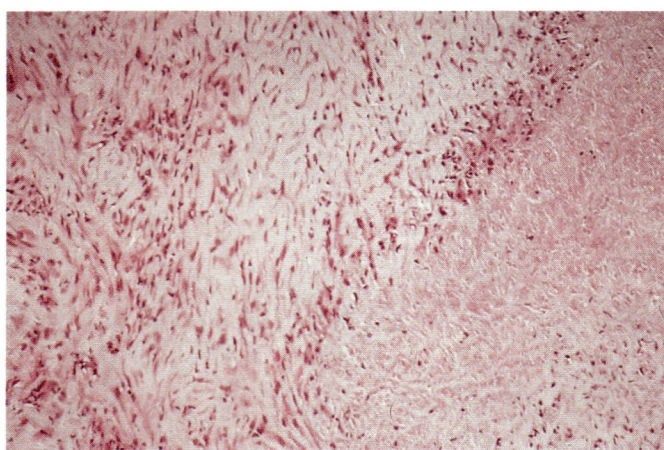

Fig. 13.192   A malignant sarcomatoid mesothelioma. The tumour has a spindle-cell growth pattern; there is an area of necrosis to the right.

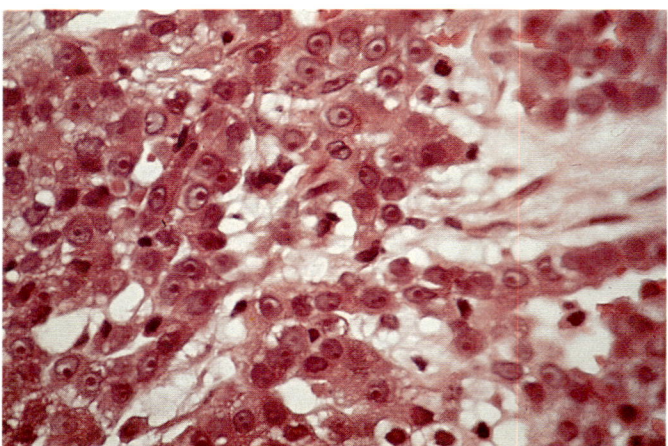

Fig. 13.190   A malignant epithelial mesothelioma. The tumour has a diffuse growth pattern.

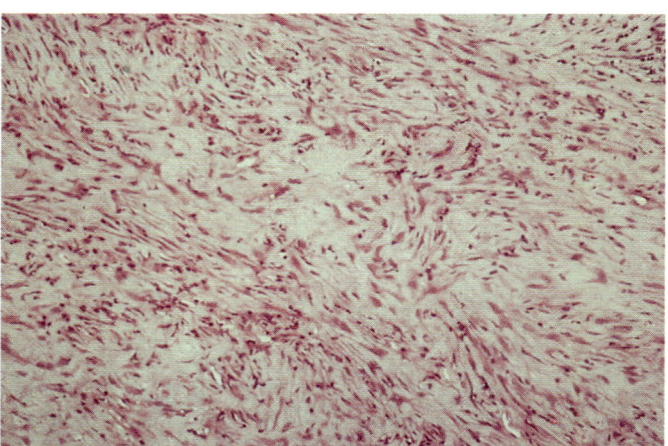

Fig. 13.193   A malignant sarcomatoid mesothelioma. The spindle cells are arranged at random.

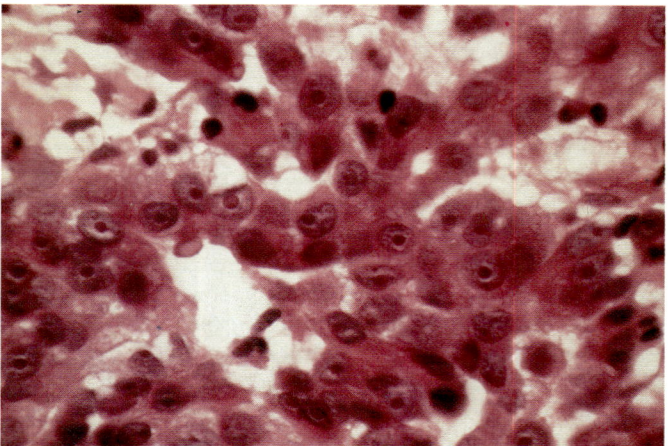

Fig. 13.191   A malignant epithelial mesothelioma. The nuclei are round, nucleoli are prominent, and the cytoplasm is abundant.

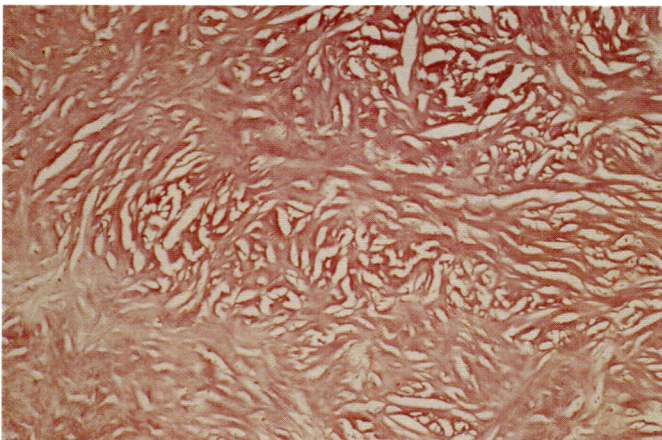

Fig. 13.194   A malignant sarcomatoid mesothelioma. The cells have undergone necrosis, leaving randomly arranged clefts in the collagenous stroma.

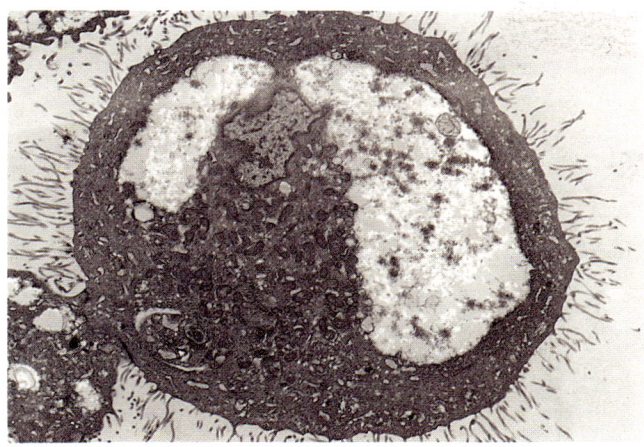

Fig. 13.195 A malignant epithelial mesothelioma. The long, thin microvilli on the cell membrane in this electron micrograph are characteristic of mesothelial cells.

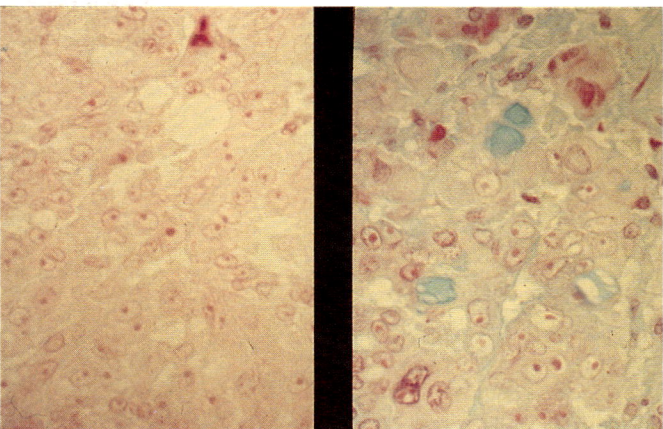

Fig. 13.197 A malignant mesothelioma. Both preparations were stained with alcian blue/PAS-diastase, but that on the right was pre-treated with hyaluronidase, which has prevented the blue staining by removing from the lumina the hyaluronic acid produced by mesothelial cells.

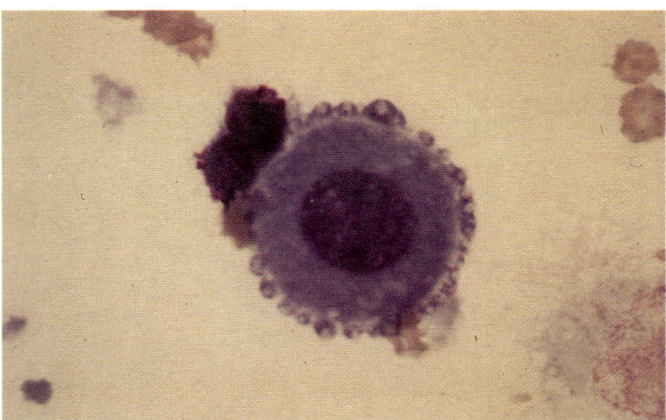

Fig. 13.196 A malignant epithelial mesothelioma. The ruffled border, corresponding to microvilli of the cell, is characteristic of mesothelial cells. (Giemsa.)

extracellular collagen as the basement membranes are incomplete, and often line intercellular spaces (Fig. 13.186). They often contain cytoplasmic glycogen, lipid, and bundles of intermediate filaments. Cells of an adenocarcinoma have short microvilli, and secretory vesicles in the cytoplasm. The basement membranes of carcinomas are more complete than those of mesotheliomas (Dewar *et al.* 1987).

Conventional histochemistry is used to identify epithelial and connective tissue mucins in cytoplasm or tubular lumina. The presence of *epithelial mucin*, which is best demonstrated by the PAS-diastase or mucicarmine techniques, confirms a diagnosis of adenocarcinoma. On the other hand, mesotheliomas produce varying amounts of *hyaluronic acid*, which is stained blue (as are other glycans) by the dye Alcian blue; the reaction is prevented by prior treatment with the enzyme hyaluronidase (Fig. 13.197). The presence of hyaluronic acid in the cytoplasm or in

tubular lumina is evidence of mesothelial differentiation. Unfortunately, the low reproducibility and sensitivity of the technique often lead to an inconclusive result. The hyaluronic acid concentration can be measured in the pleural fluid, which is an underused but helpful procedure (Battifora 1989).

Identification of *intermediate filaments* and *glycoproteins* by immunohistochemistry may help to distinguish malignant mesothelioma from other tumours, particularly adenocarcinomas of the lung. Most mesotheliomas express *cytokeratins*, many express *vimentin* and *epithelial membrane antigens*, while only rare cases express *carcino-embryonic antigen* (CEA), *Leu M1*, and *secretory component* (SC) (Figs 13.198–13.201). On the other hand, adenocarcinomas of the lung often express many or all of these antigens. It follows, therefore, that the combination of expression of cytokeratin with absence of expression of CEA, Leu M1, and SC supports a diagnosis of mesothelioma. The use of antibodies that can discriminate between high and low molecular weight cytokeratins has shown that low molecular weight cytokeratins are found in all histological types of mesothelioma, while high molecular weight cytokeratins are found only in mesotheliomas having epithelial differentiation (Bolen *et al.* 1986; Battifora 1989).

The prognosis for patients with mesothelioma is poor. No curative treatment is available, but palliation such as radiotherapy, chemotherapy, and pleurectomy may alleviate symptoms and prolong survival. Most patients die within 2 years after symptoms develop. The spindle cell type of tumour seems to have the worst outlook (Adams *et al.* 1986).

Sarcomas

Although rare, several types of sarcoma have been described arising in the chest wall. The difficulty of distinguishing a sarcoma from the spindle-cell component of a mesothelioma may be overcome by the techniques outlined above (Carter and Otis 1988; Andrion *et al.* 1989).

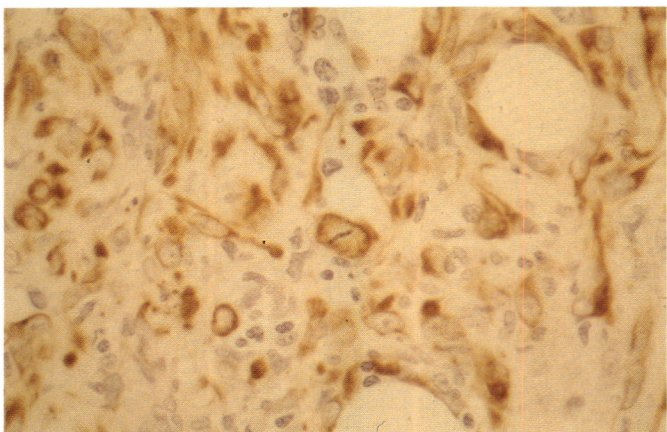

Fig. 13.198 A malignant sarcomatoid mesothelioma. The spindle cells in this sarcomatoid area contain cytokeratin (immunoperoxidase).

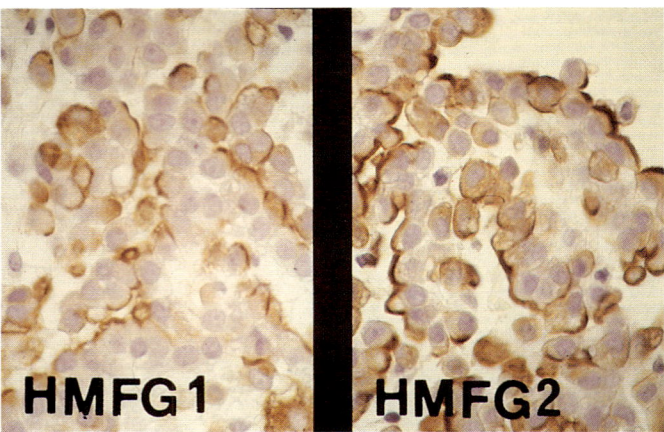

Fig. 13.200 A malignant epithelial mesothelioma. The cells express epithelial membrane antigens (HMFG1 and HMFG2) (immunoperoxidase).

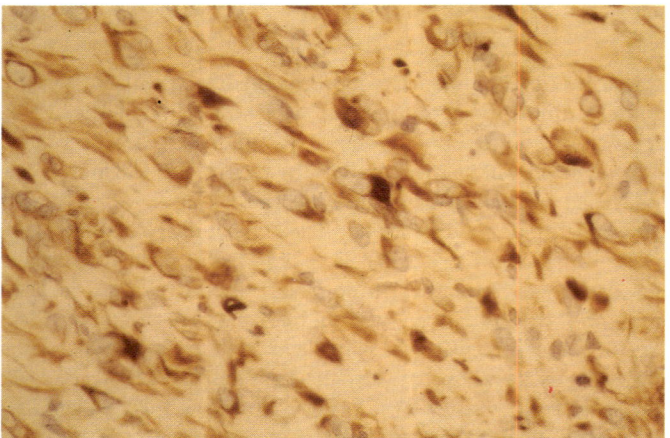

Fig. 13.199 The same lesion as in Fig. 13.198. The cells also contain vimentin (immunoperoxidase).

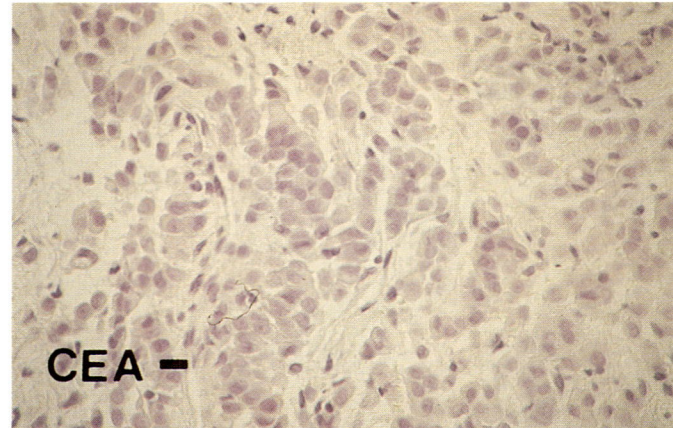

Fig. 13.201 The same lesion as in Fig. 13.200. The cells do not express carcino-embryonic antigen (immunoperoxidase).

Secondary tumours

Carcinomas commonly metastasize to the pleura and the incidence of metastatic tumour is much greater than that of the entities described above. Tumours of the lung and breast are particularly prone to do so, and they may closely resemble the epithelial component of a malignant mesothelioma. The accurate diagnosis of a pleural malignant neoplasm is of more than academic interest since a patient with a malignant mesothelioma may be entitled to compensation.

13.8.3   Pneumothorax

Air and other gases have a small but finite solubility in aqueous fluids and, in consequence, any trace of gas which might be present in the pleural cavity will be resorbed under normal conditions. During inspiration, the pressure within the thoracic cavity drops below that of the air outside, and this pressure difference forces air into the respiratory passages. The visceral and parietal pleurae are maintained in contact at all times by the absence of air from the pleural cavity. Physiologists loosely refer to a 'negative' intrathoracic pressure during inspiration; this pressure is negative only in that it is less than the atmospheric pressure outside; an *absolute* negative pressure, of course, is a physical impossibility.

Pneumothorax is the abnormal state in which air or another gas is present in the pleural cavity. This may occur *spontaneously*, as a *result of trauma*, or, formerly, as *a therapeutic procedure* in cases of tuberculosis. In all cases, the presence of the gas reduces the expansion of the lung, by an amount depending upon the volume of gas in the pleural cavity. In a chest X-ray, the lung can be seen to have retracted from the chest wall. At post-mortem, a pneumothorax may be demonstrated by piercing the intercostal muscle under water, when bubbles of gas will escape. The spontaneous type of pneumothorax most commonly occurs in association with diseases of the lungs, particularly those causing chronic airway obstruction, such as emphysema and asthma. Because of its destructive nature, *pulmonary tuberculosis* may also be complicated by pneumothorax. Pneumothorax develops when a communication is established between the respiratory passages and the pleural space, which may follow rupture of a subpleural bulla or abscess cavity; alternatively, air may track through the pulmonary interstitial tissue to reach the pleura, which may then be breached. Rarely, pneumothorax may develop in a subject who is apparently well, this situation being referred to as *spontaneous idiopathic pneumothorax*. This condition occurs in young adults and tends to recur.

If the defect in the pleura is a small one, it may heal and allow the gas to be reabsorbed naturally. However, if the volume of gas in the pleura is sufficient to cause respiratory embarrassment, it is usual to insert a chest drain, assisted, if necessary, by a small suction pump. A *tension pneumothorax* occurs when the pleural defect behaves like a clack valve and allows air to pass from lung to pleural cavity but not in reverse; respiratory embarrassment may be severe and require urgent treatment.

Trauma to the chest may produce a pneumothorax either through a penetrating injury of the chest wall, or through rupture of the visceral pleura, or both. Provided that the patient survives and the defect can be closed, spontaneous resorption of the air is usual (Thurlbeck 1988).

13.8.4 Pleural effusions

Pleural effusions may be formed by either of two mechanisms: *transudation* and *exudation*. The presence of an effusion can interfere with the expansion of the lung and, if of a significant amount, can cause a *compressive atelectasis*. Small effusions obscure the costophrenic angle in a chest X-ray, while larger effusions are easily seen because of their radiodensity.

Transudation

It has been estimated that the volume of fluid normally present in the pleural space is very small, amounting to only a few millilitres. This state is a dynamic equilibrium which is maintained by Starling's pressures in the parietal and visceral capillary blood vessels. A transudate accumulates if a pathological condition disturbs these pressures in such a way as to increase the rate at which fluid enters the space, or decrease the rate at which it is resorbed.

In the parietal pleura, the circulation is systemic and the mean capillary hydrostatic pressure is about 22 mmHg while, in the visceral pleura, the circulation is mainly pulmonary, with a mean capillary hydrostatic pressure of about 8 mmHg. As the oncotic pressures are similar in both circulations, and lie between the maximum systemic capillary hydrostatic pressure and the minimum pulmonary capillary hydrostatic pressure, there is a net movement of fluid across the space from the parietal to the visceral pleura. It follows that:

1. a rise in the systemic capillary pressure will increase the formation of fluid;

2. a rise in the pulmonary capillary pressure will hinder its resorption; and

3. a reduction in the oncotic pressure will increase formation and reduce resorption.

The subpleural lymphatics are a complicating factor; impaired movement of the chest wall or lung reduces the efficiency of lymphatic peristalsis, and will itself lead to the accumulation of an effusion.

Several conditions are associated with pleural transudates, of which the commonest is *biventricular cardiac failure*. This probably produces an effusion because of pulmonary vascular congestion, as it has been found that isolated right-sided cardiac failure does not ordinarily produce an effusion, presumably because parietal pleural lymphatics can resorb the transudate as it leaves the capillaries.

Less common causes of transudates include *cirrhosis*, *hydronephrosis*, and *peritoneal dialysis*. The mechanisms are uncertain, and may involve diaphragmatic or lymphatic communications between peritoneum and pleura.

Conditions that produce scarring with retraction of part of the lung are inevitably associated with a pleural transudate which fills the space created by the retraction. *Bronchiectasis* and *congenital malformations* with recurrent infections are examples.

Exudation

This form of effusion is quite different from transudation, and always involves an increase in capillary permeability, so that an exudate contains a relatively high concentration of protein, comparable to that of plasma (in the region of 30 g/l) and cells. When a pleural exudate develops, it is nearly always found in association with *pleural inflammation*, which may be acute (pleurisy), or chronic. *Tuberculosis, connective tissue diseases, pancreatitis,* and *subphrenic abscess* can cause chronic pleural inflammation with exudates.

Empyema is a particular form of exudate in which bacteria have reached the pleural space and elicited a purulent reaction. The decomposition of cellular material may produce an oncotic pressure greater than that of plasma, so that the fluid cannot be resorbed by the visceral capillaries. As the capacity of the lymphatics for reabsorption is often exceeded, the exudate accumulates, and the decrease in ventilation, occasioned by pain, aggravates the situation (Jones 1987).

13.8.5 Bibliography

Adams, V. I. and Unni, K. K. (1984). Diffuse malignant mesothelioma of the pleura: Diagnostic criteria based on an autopsy study. *American Journal of Clinical Pathology* 82, 15–23.

Adams, V. I., Unni, K. K., Muhm, J. R., Gett., J. R., Ilstrup, D. M., and Bernatz, P. E. (1986). Diffuse malignant mesothelioma of pleura; diagnosis and survival in 92 cases. *Cancer* 58, 1540–51.

Andrion, A., Massucco, G., Bernardi, P., and Mollo, F. (1989). Sarcomatous tumour of the chest wall, with osteochondroid differentiation. Evidence of mesothelial origin. *American Journal of Surgical Pathology* 13 (8), 707–12.

Battifora, H. (1989). *The pleura. Diagnostic surgical pathology* (ed. S. S. Sternberg), pp. 828–55. Raven Press, New York.

Bolen, J. W., Hammar, M. D., and McNutt, M. A. (1986). Reactive and neoplastic serosal tissue. *American Journal of Surgical Pathology* **10** (1), 34–47.

Briselli, M., Mark, E. J., and Dickersin, G. R. (1981). Solitary fibrous tumours of the pleura; 8 new cases and review of 360 cases in the literature. *Cancer* **47**, 2678–89.

Cantin, R., Al-Jabi, M., and McCaughey, W. T. E. (1982). Desmoplastic diffuse mesothelioma. *American Journal of Surgical Pathology* **6**, 215–22.

Carter, D. and Otis, C. N. (1988). Three types of spindle cell tumours of the pleura; fibroma, sarcoma and sarcomatoid mesothelioma. *American Journal of Surgical Pathology* **12**(10), 747–53.

Craighead, J. E. (1987). Current pathogenetic concepts of diffuse malignant mesothelioma. *Human Pathology* **18**, 544–57.

Dewar, A., Valente, M., Ring, N. P., and Corrin, B. (1987). Pleural mesothelioma of epithelial type and pulmonary adenocarcinoma: An untrastructural and cytochemical comparison. *Journal of Pathology* **152**, 309–16.

England, D. M., Hochholzer, L., and McCarthy, M. J. (1989). Localised benign and malignant fibrous tumours of the pleura; a clinicopathologic review of 223 cases. *American Journal of Surgical Pathology* **13**(8), 640–58.

Jones, J. S. P. (ed.) (1987). *Pathology of the mesothelium*. Springer-Verlag, Heidelberg.

Peterson, J. T., Greenberg, S. D., and Buffler, P. A. (1984). Nonasbestos-related malignant mesothelioma. *Cancer* **54**, 951–60.

Thurlbeck, W. M. (ed.) (1988). *Pneumothorax. Pathology of the lung*, pp. 775–80. Thieme Medical Publishers, New York.

Wagner, J. C. and Pooley, F. D. (1986). Mineral fibres and mesothelioma. *Thorax* **41**, 161–6.

Wagner, J. C., Sleggs, C. A., and Marchand, P. (1960). Diffuse pleural mesothelioma and asbestos exposure in the North Western Cape Province. *British Journal of Industrial Medicine* **17**, 260–71.

Whitaker, D. and Shilkin, K. B. (1984). Diagnosis of pleural malignant mesothelioma in life—a practical approach. *Journal of Pathology* **143**, 147–75.

14

The mouth, salivary glands, jaws, and teeth

14

The mouth, salivary glands, jaws, and teeth

14.1 Non-neoplastic disorders of the oral mucosa

W. J. Hume

14.1.1 Normal structure and function

The structure and function of oral mucosa resemble those of skin and other squamous epithelia. Structurally, it differs from skin in showing a range of cornification patterns, e.g. buccal mucosa, soft palate, and floor of mouth are non-cornified or weakly parakeritinized, whereas hard palate is orthokeratinized, dorsal tongue is parakeratinized and gingiva expresses both ortho- and parakeratin. Marked topographical differences exist in histological appearances, e.g. palate and gingiva have well-formed, slender epithelial rete ridges, whereas they are broader in the buccal mucosa. Floor of mouth, on the other hand, has a flat basement membrane and generally lacks rete ridges. These architectural differences are important for the proliferative organization of oral tissues. Evidence from rodent oral epithelia, both tongue and gingiva, suggest that rete ridges may represent functional units of proliferation, and there is evidence that basal cells can 'flow' along basement membranes and that basal cells overlying connective tissue papillae are more mature than those towards the tips of the epithelial rete ridges, e.g. in human palate and gingivae the former have a lower nuclear/cytoplasmic ratio, contain more cytoplasmic filaments, and have more desmosomes. These concepts are consistent with a hierarchy of keratinocytes within the basal layer consisting of long-lived stem cells, transient amplifying cells committed to maturation, and post-mitotic, maturing basal cells, as outlined on pages 1060–1061. In addition, bone marrow-derived Langerhans cells, which play a role in mucosal immunological responses, and melanocytes are present at all sites except junctional epithelium. Merkel cells are located towards the tips of epithelial rete ridges in epithelium of gingiva and hard palate. Whereas Langerhans cells and melanocytes are vimentin positive (i.e. they contain vimentin intermediate filaments in their cytoplasm), and Merkel cells contain simple keratins 7, 8, 18, and 19 (see Section 14.2.2), the keratin profile of oral mucosa is complex. Thus, areas showing cornification, e.g. hard palate, attached gingiva, and the filiform papillae of tongue, express keratins 1 and 10; whereas keratins 4 and 13 are found predominantly in non-cornified regions, such as buccal and interpapillary tongue epithelia. Keratin 16 is found in all sites: it is characteristic of rapidly turning-over epithelium. This is in keeping with higher cell desquamation and production rates for oral mucosa when compared with skin. Examples of the morphological differences between different sites are shown in Fig. 14.1.

14.1.2 Developmental abnormalities

Oral mucosa is subject to the same range of developmental abnormalities as skin and may also be involved in syndromes affecting the head and neck. In addition, there are abnormalities confined to the mucosa alone. Some of the more common developmental abnormalities will be described.

Fordyce's spots

The heterotopic development of sebaceous glands in oral mucosa produces yellowy-white nodules, usually on both buccal mucosae. They are of no significance but they may alarm the patient unduly.

Lymphoepithelial cyst

In addition to Waldeyer's ring of lymphoid tissue, the oral mucosa contains small lymphoid aggregates. These are superficially placed and may give rise to cyst formation, characterized by a lining of stratified squamous epithelium with lymphoid tissue in the cyst wall. They are usually found in the floor of the mouth.

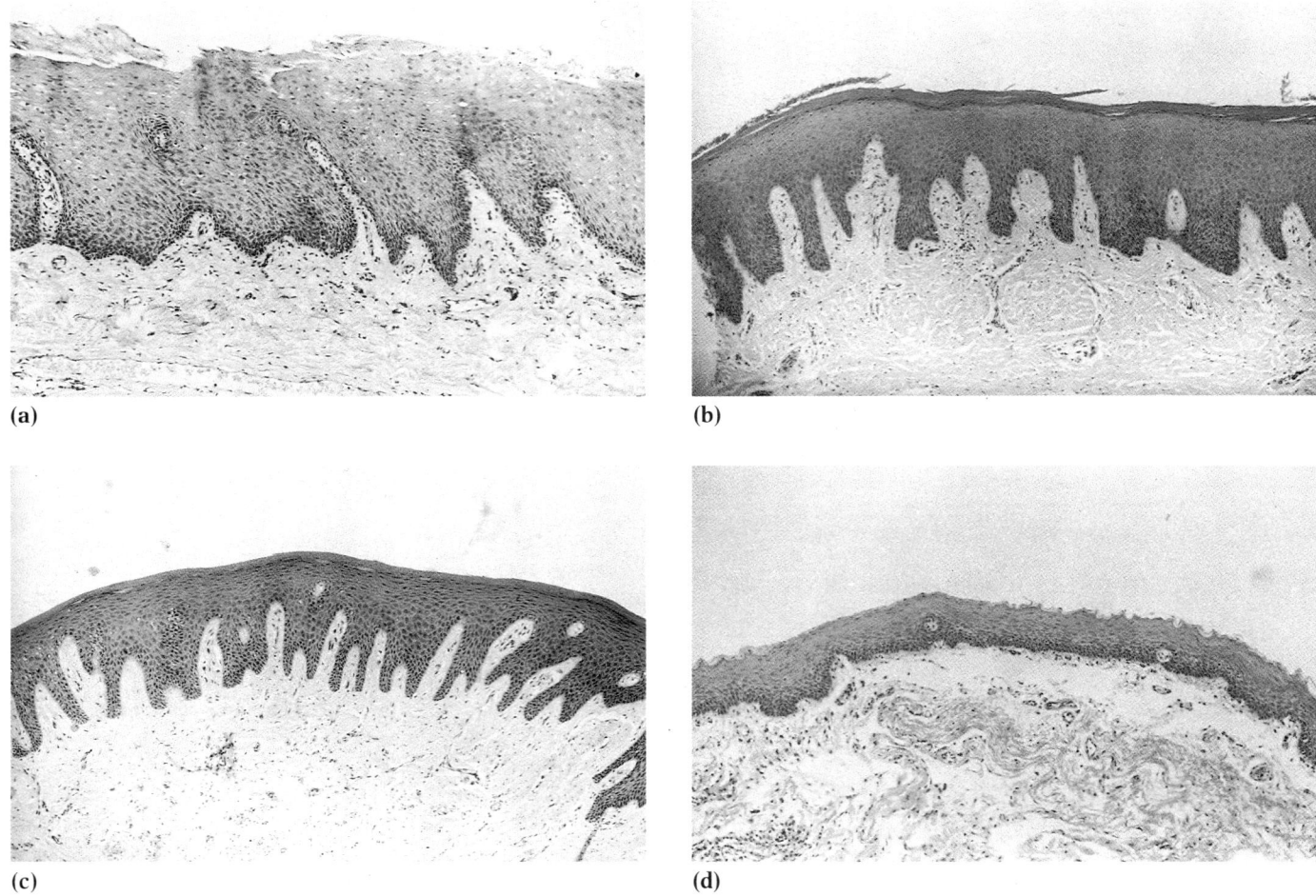

Fig. 14.1 Histological appearances of normal oral mucosa. (a) Buccal mucosa; (b) gingiva; (c) hard palate; (d) floor of mouth.

Hemifacial hypertrophy

This is a congenital condition in which the hard and soft tissues on one side of the face are larger than on the other. It may be noticeable at birth but becomes obvious as the child grows. The teeth on the affected side are larger and show an enhanced rate of development and eruption. The bony skeleton of the head may also be larger and the tongue may be similarly affected and show hypertrophy of papillae on the involved side. The skin may be rougher and the hair coarser.

Peutz–Jeghers syndrome

An autosomal dominant condition, it is one of several causes of melanotic macular pigmentation of the lips, skin, and oral mucosa. The main relevance of the syndrome is the small intestinal polyposis which rarely leads to malignancy.

Multiple endocrine neoplasia (MEN) syndrome

Several syndromes exist, characterized by neoplasms of endocrine glands. In MEN type 2B, phaeochromocytoma of the adrenal gland and medullary carcinoma of the thyroid gland are associated with multiple nodules of oral mucosa and eyelids. Histologically, these nodules resemble the haphazard collection of nerve fibres and perineurium seen in a traumatic neuroma. It is important that the significance of the oral lesions is recognized as they precede the development of endocrine gland neoplasia and can lead to early diagnosis of the syndrome.

Congenital epulis

This presents at birth as a mass attached to the gingiva and may be several centimetres in diameter. It mainly affects female babies. Histologically, there is a dense mass of large, granular cells covered by a uniform, stratified squamous epithelium lacking rete ridges. The origin of the granular cells is obscure, although pericytes have been suggested. The lesion resembles histologically, but is distinct from, the common granular cell tumour which is thought to be of Schwann cell origin.

Leukoedema

This term is used to describe a bilateral milky-white opalescence of the buccal mucosae which may also be thrown into folds

(Fig. 14.2). Stretching the cheeks causes the whiteness to disappear only to reappear when the tissues are relaxed. Histologically, the acanthosis and enlarged, vacuolated cells of the stratum spinosum are responsible for the whiteness. The condition is symptomless and of no prognostic significance.

White sponge naevus

An autosomal dominant inherited condition, white sponge naevus mainly affects the buccal mucosae, but may involve the lips and other oral tissues. The characteristic appearance is of a shaggy white patch which can be peeled off leaving an apparently normal mucosa (Fig. 14.3). Patients may be unaware of the condition but may seek advice because of the extensive desquamation of the superficial layers of the epithelium. The condition usually becomes apparent in childhood. Examination of siblings and parents may be helpful in establishing a diagnosis, in which case histological examination is unnecessary. However, this may not always be possible, and a family history is not detectable in all cases. Histologically, there is acanthosis, intra- and extracellular oedema of cells in the stratum spinosum, and parakeratinization (Fig. 14.4). The oedema within the superficial layers produces a weakening of intercellular adhesion so that a thick mass of squames can easily be rubbed off, leaving a thinner and, therefore, clinically less noticeable epithelium. However, the shaggy patch quickly becomes re-established. The epithelium is not dysplastic, the connective tissue shows no abnormality and is free of inflammation. Clinically, the condition can be distressing to the patient, but it does not give rise to neoplasia. The main lesions to be considered in the differential diagnosis are frictional keratosis, e.g. cheek biting, which also produces an irregular, shaggy white patch, but one that does not rub off, and acute pseudomembranous candidiasis, the white lesion of which can be wiped off. However, this produces bleeding from the connective tissue and diagnosis can be confirmed by finding hyphae in smears taken from the surface of the mucosa.

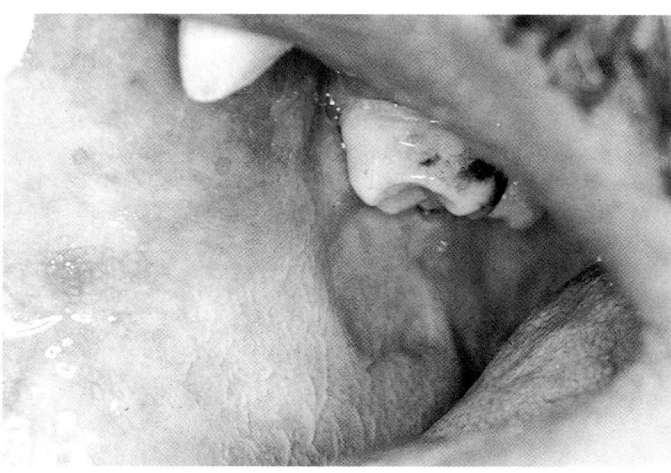

Fig. 14.2 Leukoedema, showing the characteristic faint white appearance of buccal mucosa.

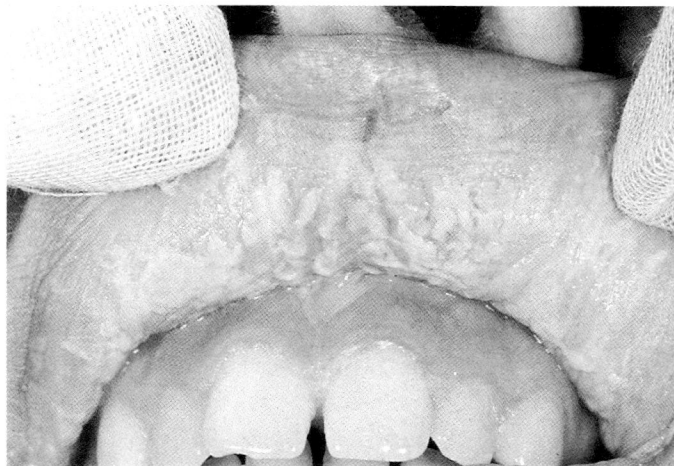

Fig. 14.3 White sponge naevus of oral mucosa. The white shaggy surface can be stripped off leaving a normal-appearing mucosa.

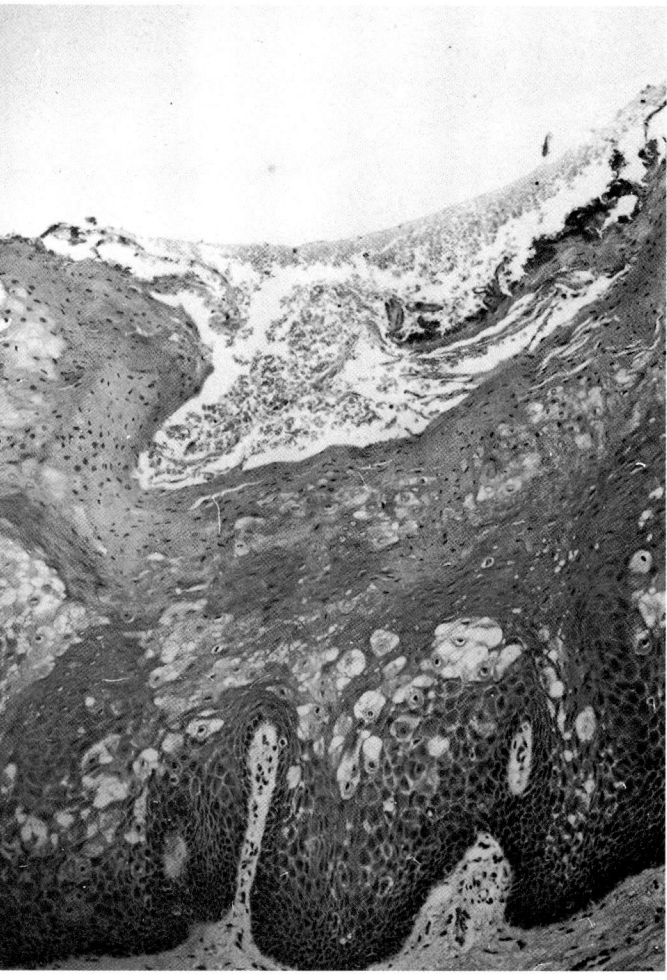

Fig. 14.4 Histology of white sponge naevus, showing marked oedematous changes in the stratum spinosum.

Other, less common examples of developmental oral white patches are *pachyonychia congenita*, in which finger nails, skin, and hair may be involved; *hereditary benign intraepithelial dyskeratosis* involving conjunctiva; and *dyskeratosis congenita*, which features skin pigmentation and nail dystrophy—in this condition there is a high incidence of oral cancer.

There are many causes of white patches in the mouth. It is important for the clinician to distinguish those that are premalignant from the majority that are not. This is not easy as the diagnosis of oral white patches can be difficult. Although histological diagnosis is often required, the patient should not need to be subjected to biopsy for lesions that can be easily diagnosed. It is worth remembering that it is no longer justifiable to use the term leukoplakia to indicate any white patch; instead, it should only be used for those white patches that cannot be rubbed off and cannot be diagnosed clinically or histologically as any specific condition. Even with this restricted definition, only a few per cent of oral leukoplakias become malignant and histologically the majority of lesions exhibit no dysplasia or only mild to moderate cellular atypia.

14.1.3   Infections

Infections of the oral mucosa are comparatively infrequent given the number and types of micro-organisms present and the tendency for injury.

Bacterial infections

Acute ulcerative gingivitis

In this painful condition there is ulceration of the interdental gingival papillae between the teeth, and sometimes this extends over the gingival surface. The ulcers have an irregular margin and are covered with a fibrinous exudate. There is characteristic halitosis and the teeth are painful to touch. The aetiology is unclear and is related in part to poor oral hygiene. A smear from the ulcers shows polymorphs, spirochaetes, and fusiform bacteria. Drug treatment, followed by oral hygiene, is effective but there tends to be an irreversible loss of gingival contour as a result of the destructive process. In conjunction with malnutrition, in tropical countries the disease presents as cancrum oris, an extensive necrosis of oral and perioral tissues.

Actinomycosis

Infection of oral tissues by *Actinomyces* presents as a brawny swelling of the mucosa which discharge the typical 'sulphur granules' on to the skin. The organisms are commensals in the mouth and frequently enter the tissues via an abrasion or a tooth extraction socket.

Tuberculosis

Infection of oral mucosa by tubercle bacilli is now uncommon but may still be seen in the elderly and in immigrants from parts of the world where the prevalence of the disease is high. Tuberculosis ulcers are usually secondary to pulmonary tuberculosis, they have an irregular outline and are frequently deep. The tongue is the most commonly involved site. Occasionally, infection with atypical mycobacteria occurs and even leprosy may have to be considered in the differential diagnosis.

Syphilis

Syphilitic infection of the oral mucosa is rare in this country. The chancre of the primary infection may occur on the lips or inside the mouth; mucous patches or snail-track ulcers can develop in the secondary stage of the disease, whereas in tertiary syphilis the gumma may affect the tongue or palate which may even perforate to give an oro-nasal fistula.

Viral infections

Herpes simplex

Primary infection with herpes simplex virus type 1 is generally subclinical. Only a few per cent of infected individuals present with primary herpetic gingivostomatitis and, although they are still likely to be children, the primary infection is seen more frequently in adults than was previously the case. The patient is unwell, has a raised temperature and develops vesicles on the oral mucosa on both sides of the midline, including lips and gingivae. The vesicles rupture, coalesce, and become secondarily infected. Healing occurs within two weeks. The haemorrhagic crusting of the lips is typical but may need to be distinguished from that in erythema multiforme, especially if the patient is adult. The secondary infection is usually a 'cold-sore' on the lip, although there may also be intra-oral vesicles and ulcers, and infrequently only the latter may be present. Recurrent infections may be associated with abnormalities of cell-mediated immunity.

Herpes zoster

The patient complains of pain affecting one or more branches of the trigeminal nerve. This is followed by vesiculation, erythema, and ulceration of skin and oral mucosa on one side of the midline. The protracted post-herpetic neuralgia is important in the differential diagnosis of facial pain in the elderly.

Herpangina

Infection by coxsackie virus A produces illness with fever, and vesiculation in the oro-pharynx.

Viral warts

Viral warts of the oral mucosa present as verruca vulgaris and condyloma accuminatum. Although features suggestive of a viral aetiology, such as koilocytosis, numerous mitoses, rete ridges inclined towards the centre of the lesion, and viral inclusions, may be present in some lesions, others can present few of these features. In such cases, diagnosis may be assisted by detecting human papilloma viral (HPV) DNA sequences within the tissues, by the technique of *in situ* hybridization on paraffin sections. Usually HPV types 6, 11, or 16 will be present.

Fungal infections

Candidiasis

Infection of the oral mucosa by *Candida albicans* is common and presents as one or more of the conditions listed below. As *Candida* is present as a commensal organism in the mouths of approximately one-half of the population, swabbing the mucosa in order to culture the organism is not helpful for diagnosis. Instead, a smear should be taken from the suspected area of mucosa and stained by the Periodic acid-Schiff method (PAS). The presence of hyphal forms, rather than spores, is usually indicative of candidal infection. In general, patients with recurrent oral infection should be given a thorough examination for anaemia, diabetes mellitus, abnormality of white cell number and function including immunodeficiency, and their drug history investigated, e.g. for recent antibiotic and immuno-suppressives.

Histological diagnosis of oral candidiasis is not necessary for most clinical presentations apart from chronic hyperplastic candidiasis. Candidal infection is strongly suggested by the accumulation of polymorphs as mico-abscesses in the superficial layers of the epithelium and is confirmed by demonstration of hyphal forms also within the superficial layers, although examination of several sections may be required to detect them. Penetration of hyphae deeper into the epithelium is most unusual even in patients with underlying systemic disease. Other conditions producing similar accumulation of polymorphs are much less common and include geographic stomatitis and recurrent trauma, e.g. from a denture.

Although the presence of hyphae in a mucosal biopsy indicates candidiasis, the organism may represent secondary pathology, e.g. candidal superinfection within the epithelium covering a connective tissue hyperplasia such as a fibrous epulis or denture-irritation hyperplasia.

Acute pseudomembranous candidiasis

This type of candidiasis, known as thrush, is seen in infancy and old age, but can occur at any age, especially if associated with systemic disease. Clinically, a white, thickened epithelial slough is present with a variable extent of erythematous mucosa. Rubbing off the slough leads to ulceration and bleeding.

Acute atrophic candidiasis

These patients often give a history of recurrent, painful mucosa following administration of antibiotics (antibiotic sore mouth). Clinically the mucosa is reddened and thinned.

Chronic atrophic candidiasis

This is the commonest form of the disease and is usually painless. It occurs in mucosa covered by a partial or complete denture, usually the palate, where the mucosa may be fiery red and oedematous. Although it is symptomless, treatment with antifungals is required to restore the mucosa to a healthy state to allow proper denture function and to prevent long-term damage that will make the fabrication of well-fitting dentures difficult.

Chronic hyperplastic candidiasis

Usually this presents on the buccal mucosa near the angle of the mouth as a thickened white area, often with a distinct nodular appearance. The mucosa around and within the lesion may show a variable degree of redness (Fig. 14.5). Although the initial diagnosis is often straightforward, a biopsy is necessary as this condition is pre-malignant. Histologically, in addition to the features mentioned earlier, there is parakeratinization, extensive acanthosis, an increase in mitotic figures within epithelium, and a chronic inflammatory cell infiltrate within the connective tissue. Fibrosis of superficial muscle may accompany long-standing candidiasis, especially in tongue. It is important to assess the degree of epithelial dysplasia, if present, and to exclude the presence of squamous cell carcinoma. Although there has been debate as to whether the *Candida* causes or is secondary to the white patch, the tendency for these lesions to resolve with long-term antifungal therapy supports the former theory. It is no longer acceptable to use the term candidal leukoplakia for this condition.

Median rhomboid glossitis

The presence of a lozenge-shaped area of depapillation in the midline, anterior to circumvallate papillae, was formerly thought to be developmental in origin. However, its absence in children, its frequent association with the wearing of a complete upper denture, the presence of candidal hyphae in biopsy and smears, and the tendency to resolve after antifungal treatment, suggest it to be a form of candidiasis.

Angular cheilitis

The fissuring and bleeding at the angles of the mouth is frequent in denture wearers, especially if the dentures are inadequate in their vertical dimensions and allow a bunching up of tissues with retention of moisture in tissue folds. The infective organism is often *Candida albicans*, although *Staphylococcus aureus* or

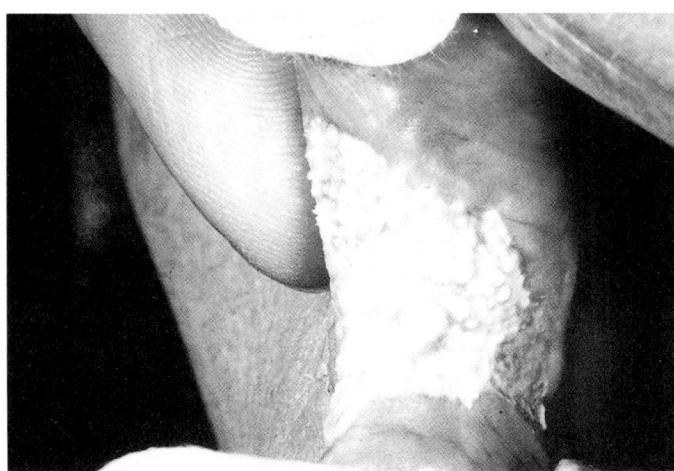

Fig. 14.5 Chronic hyperplastic candidiasis. The white thickened surface cannot be rubbed off.

streptococci may be the infecting agent. The condition is predisposed to by underlying disease such as haematinic and vitamin deficiency.

In addition to the above, the oral mucosa may be infected by *Candida* as part of a more widespread systemic candidiasis syndrome.

Acquired immuno deficiency syndrome (AIDS)

The presence of recurrent or uncommon infections in the mouth may occur in AIDS. These include candidiasis, perhaps in unusual sites such as the soft palate or oro-pharynx, herpes simplex virus (HSV) and human papilloma virus (HPV) infections. In 'hairy leukoplakia' there is hyperparakeratinization, acanthosis, and koilocytosis, on the lateral borders of the tongue. A reduction in Langerhans cell number, fungal infection, and Epstein–Barr virus may be present. This tongue lesion can be the first presenting feature of infection with human immunodeficiency virus (HIV).

14.1.4 Non-infective inflammatory conditions

Geographic stomatitis

This is a term to describe the yellowy-white and erythematous, serpiginous lesion of the oral mucosa. It usually affects tongue (geographic tongue) but can involve other oral sites. The lesion migrates with time across the mucosa and changes its shape and outline, hence its synonym of erythema migrans. Typically, in the tongue, the central zone is devoid of filiform papillae and is reddish in appearance, especially where it approaches the yellowy-white periphery (Fig. 14.6). The aetiology is obscure but many patients are nervous or anxious and cancerophobic. The condition may be painful and in such cases the burning sensation often develops *after* the patient first noted the unusual appearance. Following reassurance, the discomfort often sub-

sides and the condition may become less obvious or even disappear. Histologically, the filiform papillae are absent but the characteristic finding is the presence of large numbers of neutrophil polymorphs within the stratum spinosum (accounting for the yellow appearance), and dilated capillaries in the superficial connective tissue (Fig. 14.7). These appearances should be considered alongside candidiasis, in which the polymorphs are fewer and are located only within the most superficial layers of the epithelium, and psoriasis, which is extremely rare in the mouth. Clearly, the clinical appearances and site have to be considered in order to make the correct diagnosis.

Lichen planus

Although oral lichen planus is essentially the same as that affecting the skin, it frequently occurs in the absence of skin involvement and is usually symptomless. The characteristic clinical finding is the fine network of white lines, the Wickham's striae, which have small, white flame-like projections extending from them (Fig. 14.8). In these cases a biopsy is not necessary to establish the diagnosis. Sometimes the lesions are markedly erythematous and painful. Erosive lichen planus is particularly painful and produces extensive shallow ulceration of the mucosae. Long-standing lichen planus can develop into a solid, plaque-like area of keratosis, and squamous cell carcinoma may develop in a very few patients, especially with the erosive form of the disease. The histology is the same as for skin lesions, but the irregular keratinization patterns and the saw-tooth rete ridges are less common. In drug-induced lichen planus, e.g. following methyldopa, the presence of eosinophils in the inflammatory cell infiltrate is often suggestive of the aetiology. Graft versus host disease can produce the appearances of lichen planus, both clinically and histologically.

Inflammatory lesions of gingiva are common and include *hyperplastic gingivitis*; the identical *pyogenic granuloma* and *pregnancy epulis*; the *giant cell epulis* that histologically resembles the

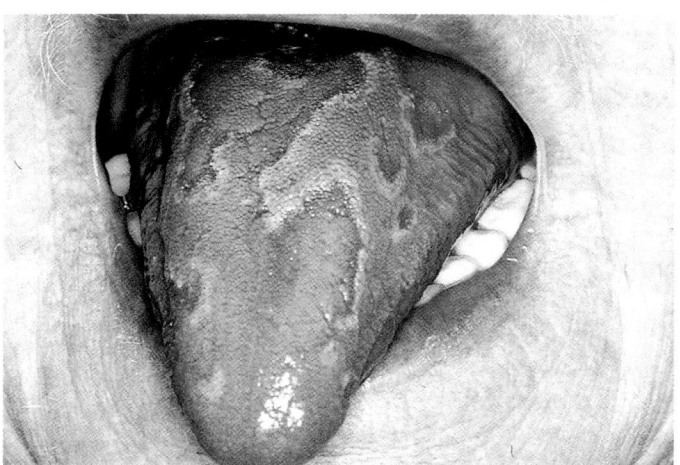

Fig. 14.6 Geographic tongue. The depapillated areas are surrounded by a yellowy-white margin. The appearance of the tongue changes with time.

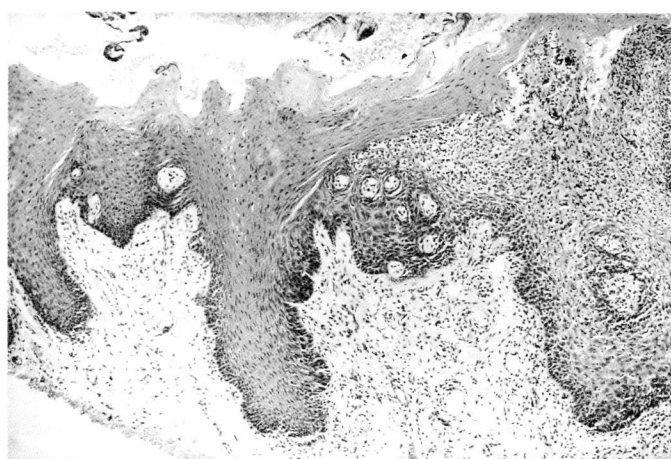

Fig. 14.7 Geographic tongue showing normal tongue epithelium on the left. On the right the epithelium is extensively infiltrated by polymorphs.

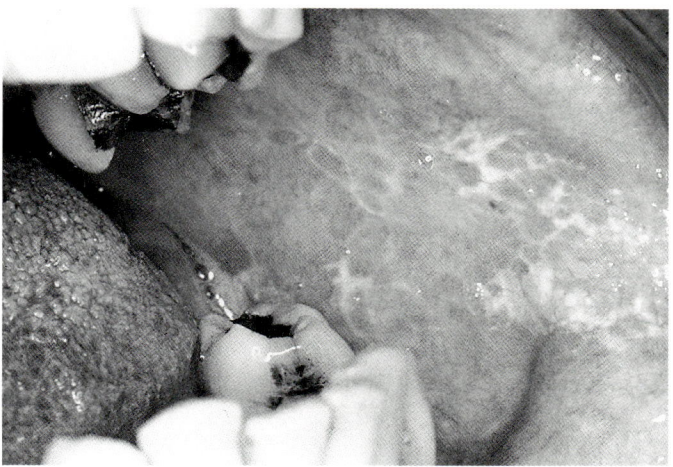

Fig. 14.8 Lichen planus of oral mucosa. The reticular appearance and small 'flame-like' projections comprise the characteristic Wickham's striae.

giant cell granuloma of bone, but arises from periodontium, and the *fibrous epulis* which is a chronically inflamed, cellular fibroblastic lesion that may exhibit metaplastic bone formation and dystrophic calcification.

14.1.5   Further reading

Shafer, W. G., Hine, M. K., and Levy, B. M. (1983). *A textbook of oral pathology* (4th edn). W. B. Saunders, Philadelphia.
Soames, J. V. and Southam, J. C. (1985). *Oral pathology*. Oxford University Press.

14.2   Neoplasms and precancerous conditions of the oral mucosa

P. R. Morgan

14.2.1   Introduction

Oral mucosa, in its structure and in its responses to certain disease processes, may be regarded as rather specialized skin, largely devoid of adnexal structures. However, the type and behaviour of oral neoplasms also reflect an affinity with other mucosal surfaces, especially of the oro-pharynx, oesophagus, and larynx. Overwhelmingly, the most important neoplasm of oral mucosa is squamous cell carcinoma, oral cancer. Currently, oral and oro-pharyngeal cancer combined rank sixth world-wide in terms of cancer incidence (fourth in males; eighth in females) but represent only about 2 per cent of cancer cases in the UK, a low-risk region. Despite the accessibility of the mouth to visual inspection, most oral cancers are detected late and their prognosis is comparable to that of carcinomas of the oesophagus or lung. Other primary malignancies of oral epi-

thelia are very rare. Benign neoplasms of oral epithelia are also rare, apart from papillomas (see below) and salivary neoplasms (see Section 14.3.7).

14.2.2   Oral squamous cell carcinoma

Clinical and macroscopic features

The most frequently affected sites for oral cancer in Western countries are the ventolateral aspect of the tongue and the floor of mouth, these accounting for over 50 per cent of cases. Other sites affected are buccal, retromolar, gingival, and soft palate mucosa, least commonly involved sites being the dorsum of the tongue (now that pre-malignant syphilitic leukoplakia has become so rare) and hard palate. The lip is the most commonly affected site in some communities, especially in white-skinned people exposed to prolonged sunlight, and shows a particularly high male predominance. In Eastern countries, and also in some Western communities indulging the 'snuff-dipping' habit, the buccal or commisural mucosa are the most frequent sites, at the point of contact with the topical tobacco mixture.

In any site, the earliest lesion is usually painless. Unfortunately, it is more usual for oral cancer to be detected when it has reached the stage of an ulcer with rolled margins and an indurated bed (Fig. 14.9), often with accompanying painless enlargement of one or more deep cervical lymph nodes. Infiltrated soft tissues are painfully immobilized but bone resorption and tooth mobility are more variable, occurring most consistently with carcinoma of the gingiva and alveolus. The gross appearance of the tumour cut surface is usually that of a white, striated mass showing an irregular border with adjacent tissues, often muscle.

Histological characteristics

The majority of oral cancers are well or moderately differentiated, according to generally agreed criteria. Keratin pearl formation is prominent (Fig. 14.10), especially in the more superficial parts of the tumour, prickle cell differentiation (a

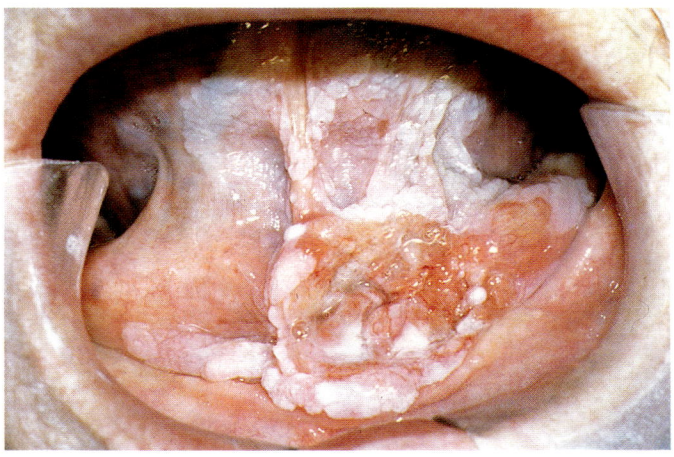

Fig. 14.9 Advanced oral squamous cell carcinoma of the floor of the mouth.

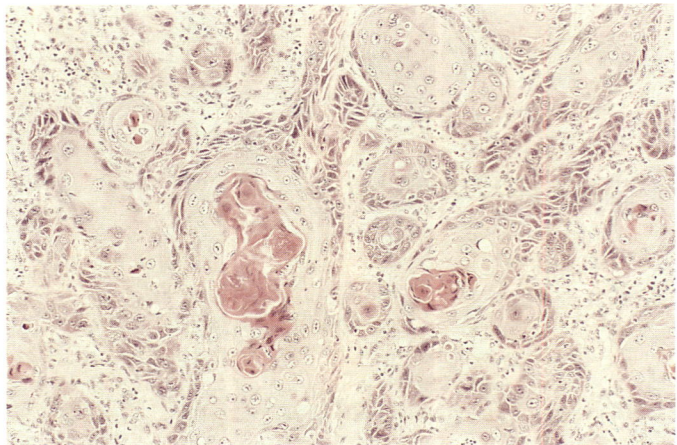

Fig. 14.10 Part of a large squamous cell carcinoma of this area showing prominent keratin formation in the infiltrating island.

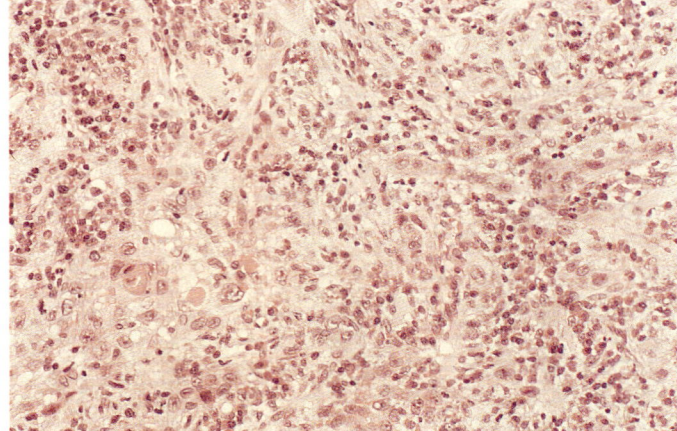

Fig. 14.12 Poorly differentiated squamous cell carcinoma of the tongue. There is an accompanying lymphocytic host response.

fundamental characteristic of keratinocytes) is usually conspicuous, and there is usually a strong host response of lymphocytes, plasma cells, and sometimes eosinophils in the connective tissue. The frequency of mitotic figures and the extent of cytological atypia such as nuclear hyperchromatism, anisonucleosis, and cellular pleomorphism vary in their extent but, paradoxially, bizarre forms are generally less in evidence in frank carcinomas than in dysplastic, non-invasive epithelium (see below). At the invasive front the carcinoma forms smaller islands and strands, some of which may lie at a distance from the main body of the tumour (Fig. 14.11).

Poorly differentiated squamous cell carcinomas, although the least common, are associated with a poorer prognosis than well- or moderately differentiated types, as is the general rule in other sites. Keratin formation is minimal and the malignant cells more uniform with loss of distinction between basal and supra-basal populations (Fig. 14.12). Mitoses are more fre-

quent and evenly distributed and the host response often less conspicuous than in better-differentiated carcinomas.

It must be stressed that these categories are not rigid nor objectively determined, so inconsistencies between behaviour and histological grade are common. Particularly with large oral carcinomas, there is often variation in the differentiation pattern from one part to another. It is arguable whether the grade of the malignancy should be defined by the majority of its composition or by the least well-differentiated areas which might be thought to govern its behaviour (compare Figs 14.10 and 14.13).

New markers of differentiation

It is now possible to define the differentiation patterns of squamous cell carcinomas by immunocytochemical means using antibodies (usually monoclonals) to molecules that are synthesized during the maturation of stratified epithelia.

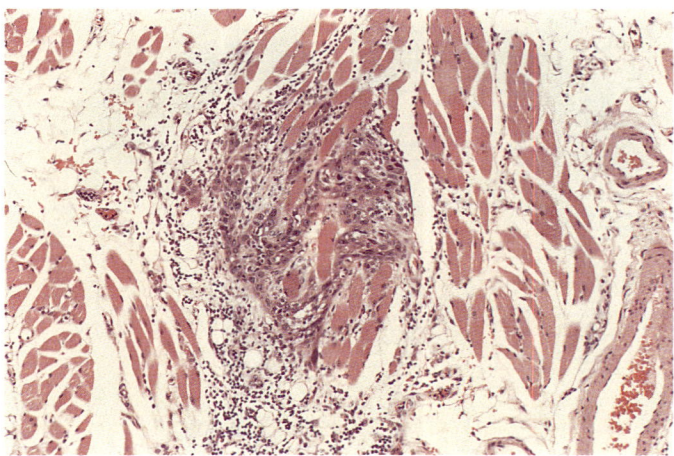

Fig. 14.11 A different case showing deep infiltration and disruption of lingual muscle fibres by squamous cell carcinoma.

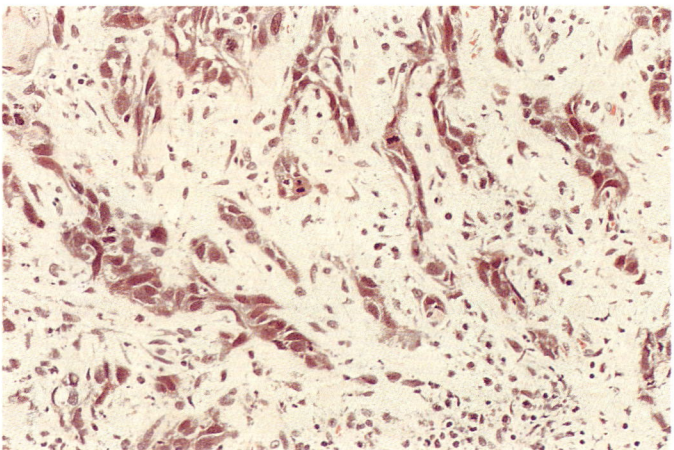

Fig. 14.13 Another part of the same tumour as shown in Fig. 14.10 but here showing loss of differentiation.

Examples are: involucrin, which forms a cytoplasmic envelope protein through cross-linking by a transglutaminase enzyme and constitutes a marker of terminal differentiation; cell surface carbohydrates, which can be visualized through the binding of specific sugar residues to different lectins (rather than antibodies); keratins, proteins of the intermediate filament system of epithelia. These last comprise a total of some 20 intermediate filaments of epithelium (excluding those of hair) expressed in various combinations in epithelial cells in a broadly, but not absolutely, tissue-specific manner and listed numerically by Moll *et al.* (1982). Stratified epithelia have the most complex pattern.

The distribution of keratins in normal oral epithelia has been mapped. Cornifying and non-cornifying sites are characterized by different pairs of keratins in the upper layers (1 and 10 and 4 and 13, respectively). These keratins are usually strongly expressed by well-differentiated oral squamous cell carcinomas (Fig. 14.14) but are detected as minor keratins in moderately and poorly differentiated tumours. Additionally, less well-differentiated carcinomas express some of the keratins that normally characterize simple epithelial cells, especially keratins 8 and 18 (Fig. 14.15), although not to the same extent as adenocarcinomas which arise from simple epithelia. In histologically equivocal anaplastic carcinomas, demonstration of the presence of keratins 5 and/or 14 indicates a squamous cell carcinoma rather than an adenocarcinoma.

Patterns of spread

Muscle and other connective tissues, including adipose tissue, tend to be invaded readily by oral squamous cell carcinoma, and submucosal spread poses problems for surgeons in establishing limits of excision, particularly in posterior regions of the mouth. Salivary tissue, for example in the floor of the mouth, is rarely invaded. Cancer in the floor of mouth tends to invade not in depth but *in breadth*, whereas in the tongue invasion is *in depth* and with submucosal spread. Bone may provide some resistance to invasion, especially the dense cortices of the

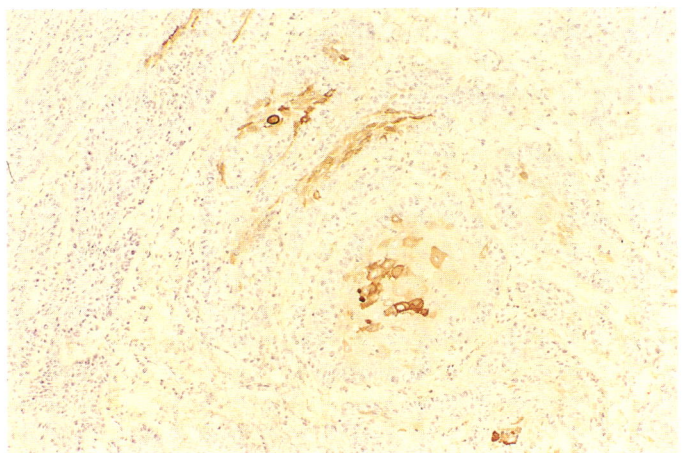

Fig. 14.14 Well-differentiated squamous cell carcinoma stained with a monoclonal antibody (immunoperoxidase technique) to keratin 10 to show cornifying cells in the neoplastic islands.

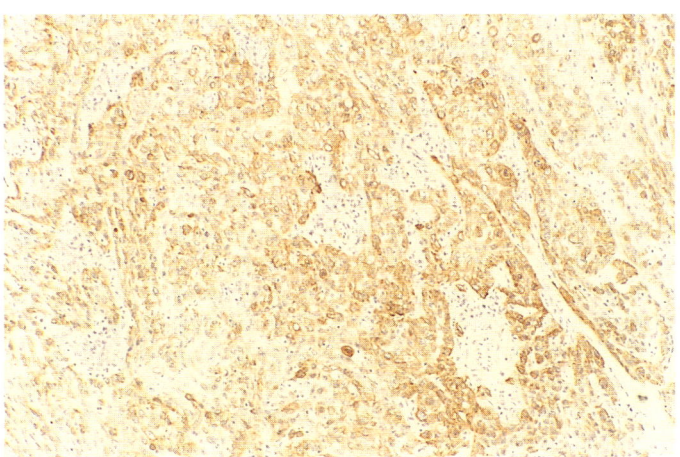

Fig. 14.15 Poorly differentiated squamous cell carcinoma stained with an antibody to keratin 18 (expressed normally by simple epithelia). Most tumour cells can be seen to express this keratin which is not extensively expressed in normal stratified epithelia or in well-differentiated squamous cell carcinomas.

mandible, but cortical defects in the edentulous alveolar ridges may provide a route of entry into the mandible, as may the inferior dental canal. Prior irradiation may also change the susceptibility of mandibular bone to invasion by tumour. There is less information on spread in the maxilla but the less dense and more vascular bone is likely to provide less resistance to invasion.

Lymph node spread is a relatively late feature of oral cancer. The pattern broadly follows the main anatomical drainage pathways from the site of the primary, the most commonly involved lymph nodes being one of the submandibular group, the jugulodigastric or the jugulo-omohyoid. Usually one large nodal metastasis is present rather than many small. However, positions of lymph node metastases are unpredictable and both clinically as well as in surgical resections all groups of nodes in the region should be examined.

Some oral carcinomas have a predominantly exophytic growth pattern, with minimal invasion and a negligible capacity for metastasis. First described as a separate form of oral cancer by Ackerman, *verrucous carcinoma* is characterized by its high degree of differentiation: an exophytic, keratotic surface beneath which are broad, aligned, acanthotic rete pegs, widest near the base and penetrating the underlying tissues by a 'pushing' process rather than by infiltration (Fig. 14.16). The basement membrane is intact, there are usually few cytological atypia, and the lesion is accompanied by a dense, lymphocytic or lymphoplasmacytic host response. Extensive areas of mucosa may be involved, buccal mucosa being the commonest site. Spread is slow and even local lymph node metastases are rare. Surgical resection is the treatment of choice and radiotherapy has been found to make the lesions more aggressive. In early reports, it was noted that many patients with verrucous carcinoma had used topically applied tobacco.

Mention has been made already of the variable capacity of

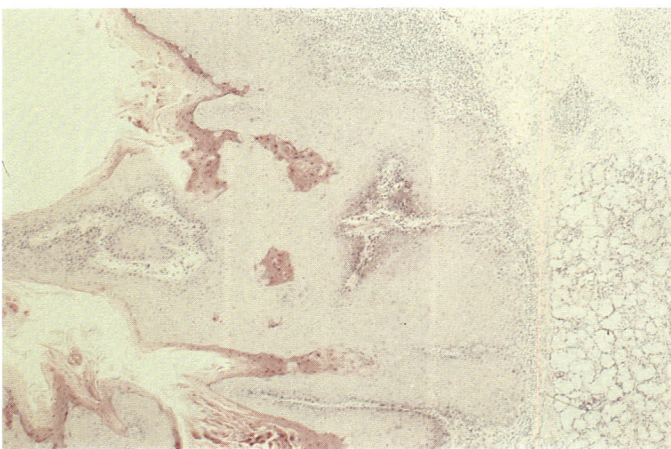

Fig. 14.16 Verrucous carcinoma of the floor of the mouth showing an exophytic growth pattern and broad-based, acanthotic rete processes.

oral squamous cell carcinomas to destroy bone. Some tumours are encountered which are characterized by a high degree of differentiation, usually with orthokeratin production, deeply penetrating and yet cohesive, acanthotic rete pegs, and well-ordered organization of the deeper epithelial layers such that it may be questioned whether the lesion is malignant at all (Fig. 14.17). Tumour stroma usually consists of cellular fibrous tissue and a dense, lymphoplasmacytic infiltrate, sometimes accompanied by polymorphs. The histological features of these lesions belie their aggressiveness, as cortical as well as cancellous bone is readily invaded, thus necessitating radical resection of what appears to be a low-grade tumour. Recurrence is frequent. Some of Ackerman's series evidently lay in this category. It is inappropriate for carcinomas of this sort to be classified as 'verrucous carcinomas' as this fosters the delusion of slow, superficial, non-infiltrative growth. In any large collection of oral carcinomas there will be some that have verrucoid features

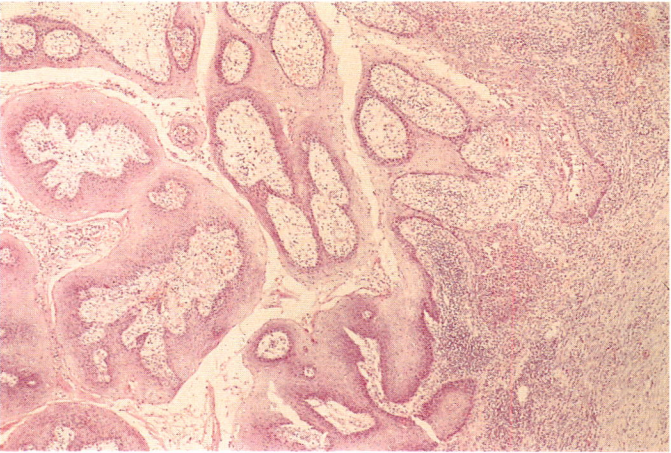

Fig. 14.17 A squamous cell carcinoma of the alveolar ridge infiltrating mandibular bone. This unusual type is well differentiated with a uniform papillomatous, cohesive but infiltrative growth pattern.

and yet show infiltrative growth. These, too, should not be termed 'verrucous carcinomas' as this diagnosis may lead to treatment that is insufficiently radical.

Epidemiological and aetiological factors

The incidence of oral cancer varies considerably between different parts of the world, with the highest levels on the Indian subcontinent and the lowest in Western Europe and North America. In these and other regions, however, the distribution is uneven. For example, the Bas-Rhin district of France has one of the highest incidences in the world, at about 16 cases per 100 000 population per annum. The mean incidence in Western countries is about 4 cases per 100 000 per annum, for both sexes combined.

Oral cancer is a disease mainly of the elderly, especially in Western countries, with an annual incidence in the over 70-year-olds of around 1 per 1000. In those countries of South-East Asia where the incidence is high it affects a somewhat younger population, but even in the West patients may present in their thirties or occasionally earlier. In all age groups and geographical locations there is a variable male preponderance (around 10 : 1 in parts of SE Asia) although the sex disparity has been reducing in England and Wales since the 1950s. Between 1950 and 1967 the male death rate due to oral cancer declined from 1200 p.a. to 550 p.a., while that for females remained constant at about 300 p.a. (these data refer mainly to *intra-oral* cancer as lip cancer is readily curable).

There is recent evidence that the incidence of oral cancer in many Western countries is rising after a steady post-war decline, at least in males. The increase seems to affect those born since about 1920 but the reason for this is not yet known.

The two major aetiological factors are tobacco and alcohol. Tobacco is the more important on a global basis, particularly in unsmoked forms such as snuff ('snuff-dipping' involves holding a moistened pad of tobacco in the buccal or labial sulcus often for long periods of time) or used as part of a mixture (pan) with areca nut and sometimes lime, a practice common in parts of South-East Asia. Ethanol itself seems not to be carcinogenic but other alcohols and impurities produced in the manufacture of beverages, especially home-brewed or illicit varieties, are probably implicated. It has been established that tobacco smoking and the consumption of alcoholic drinks have a potentiating action, increasing the risk of developing oral cancer many times over that from either factor alone.

Ultraviolet light is the dominant factor in the aetiology of lip cancer, which is thus of highest frequency on the lower lip of fair-skinned individuals living outdoors in regions with large amounts of sunlight. Chronic iron deficiency may render the epithelium atrophic and potentially more vulnerable to carcinogens and will be considered below. Other factors, some of which have been linked with malignant transformation in other sites, are more controversial as aetiological factors in oral cancer. They include chronic candidal infection, viruses (human papilloma virus, Epstein–Barr virus, possibly herpes simplex type I), and even chronic trauma.

Although only a minority of oral cancers occur in association with clinically detectable pre-malignant lesions and predisposing conditions, some of these have to be considered in their aetiology (see Tables 14.1 and 14.3).

Prognostic factors and staging

Compared with the favourable prognosis for lip cancer, whether treated by surgery, radiotherapy, or combined treatment (around 70 per cent five-year survival), that for intra-oral cancer is poor (around 40 per cent). According to a major retrospective study the other significant adverse factors determining survival are the size of the tumour at presentation (>4 cm in diameter), deep infiltration by tumour (>5 mm), fixed regional lymph nodes, evidence of distant metastases, old age (>70 years), and poor histological differentiation (anaplasia). Attempts have been made to incorporate site and histological grade of the primary tumour into staging systems for oral squamous cell carcinomas and may prove to have some prognostic value. The current TNM system revised in 1978 by Union Internationale Contre le Cancer is summarized in Table 14.2.

14.2.3   Oral pre-malignancy

Definitions

Few aspects of oral histopathology are more controversial than the attempts to assign degrees of malignant potential to the wide range of mucosal disorders in which squamous cell carcinoma has been shown to develop. The task is made easier by creating a division (Pindborg 1980) between pre-malignant *lesions*, which show clinically and histopathologically detectable mucosal changes in sites of oral cancer predilection, and pre-malignant *conditions*, more widespread or systemic disorders affecting oral mucosa where oral cancer is statistically more likely to develop although the site may be unpredictable. These categories are listed in Table 14.3.

Leukoplakia

This is a term best defined clinically to denote 'a white patch or plaque that cannot be characterized clinically or pathologically as any other disease' (WHO 1978). It is thus a diagnosis by exclusion and is a clinical rather than a pathological term, but the definition is more satisfactory than the ambiguity which otherwise attends the name. There is no doubt that under this definition leukoplakias are a heterogeneous group and therefore longitudinal surveys of their malignant potential have given widely varying results. It is generally accepted that the group as a whole gives an increased risk of malignant transformation of about 100 times over clinically normal oral mucosa, but the majority of oral squamous cell carcinomas are thought to develop in mucosa that is clinically normal.

Erythroplakia

Perhaps better termed 'erythroplasia', its earlier name, as it is not always a raised plaque, erythroplakia can be defined as 'a

Table 14.1   Summary of aetiological factors

Extrinsic agents
 Tobacco—unsmoked forms, some smoked
 Alcohol and associated impurities
 Areca nut/lime/betel mixtures (usually with tobacco), e.g. 'pan' or 'chewnam'

Infective and commensal agents
 Candida
 human papilloma virus $\left.\right\}$ speculative
 herpes simplex virus

Intrinsic conditions
 Chronic iron deficiency and other conditions listed in Table 14.3 under pre-malignant conditions
 Immune deficiency/suppression

Table 14.2   Summary of TNM staging

T Primary tumour
 T_0 no evidence of primary tumour
 T_1 2 cm or less in diameter
 T_2 between 2 cm and 4 cm in greatest diameter
 T_3 greater than 4 cm in diameter
 T_4 extension into bone and deeper tissues

N Regional lymph nodes
 N_0 no lymph nodes palpable
 N_1 clinically palpable nodes on same side as tumour; not fixed
 N_2 clinically palpable nodes contralateral or both sides; not fixed
 N_3 clinically palpable nodes which are fixed

M Distant metastases
 M_0 no evidence of distant metastases
 M_1 clinical and/or radiographic evidence of distant metastases

Grouping into stages

Stage	T	N	M
Stage I	T_1	N_0	M_0
Stage II	T_2	N_0	M_0
Stage III	T_3	N_0	M_0
	T_1, T_2, T_3	N_1	M_0
Stage IV	T_4	N_0, N_1	M_0
	Any T	N_2, N_3	M_0
	Any T	Any N	M_1

Table 14.3   Classification of oral pre-malignant lesions and conditions (modified from Pindborg 1980)

Pre-malignant lesions
 Leukoplakia: homogeneous or speckled
 Erythroplakia: homogeneous or speckled
 Sublingual keratosis
 Syphilitic leukoplakia
 Palatal changes associated with reverse smoking

Pre-malignant conditions
 Oral submucous fibrosis
 Sideropenic dysphagia and iron deficiency
 Lichen planus
 Discoid lupus erythematosus
 Dyskeratosis congenita
 Tylosis
 Xeroderma pigmentosum

persistent, predominently red mucosal patch or plaque which cannot be characterized clinically or pathologically as any other disease'. Erythoplakia is less common than leukoplakia but it has a much higher frequency of malignant transformation and hence is seen at those sites where oral cancer develops most frequently.

Epithelial dysplasia Sometimes still referred to as 'dyskeratosis' and not yet superseded by the name 'intra-epithelial neoplasia' now applied to several other mucosal sites, dysplasia is the term used to sum up various disturbances of epithelial proliferation and differentiation as seen by light microscopy. Individual features of dysplasia are often termed 'epithelial atypia'.

Certain specific features of a leukoplakic or erythroplakic lesion justify a high degree of suspicion. These include:

Site A lesion in an oral site which is prone to malignant transformation, e.g. lateral border of tongue, would give greater concern than one of similar appearance in a low-risk site, e.g. hard palate. An especially important site in this regard is the floor of mouth where reports have indicated that even clinically and histologically well-ordered keratotic epithelium may undergo malignant change within a period of months or a few years. This condition has now been termed 'sublingual keratosis' and should probably be separated from the other leukoplakias.

Colour and consistency A predominantly red or mixed red and white colour, usually indicating a degree of epithelial atrophy, should be regarded with suspicion and, particularly when there is induration, the lesion should be presumed malignant until the biopsy is examined.

Aetiological factors Notwithstanding the roles of the aetiological factors in oral cancer discussed above, it has been reported by several groups that leukoplakic lesions in non-smokers are more likely to undergo malignant transformation than those of smokers. Evidently, this suggests that tobacco induces lesions with variable malignant potential including 'smokers' keratosis' but also indicates that there are aetiological factors yet to be discovered.

Histological features of pre-malignant lesions

Apart from screening for actual malignancy, the role of histological examination lies in the assessment of the degree of dysplastic change in the epithelium. At risk of oversimplification, these changes can be considered to represent a variable combination of *disorderly maturation* and *disturbed cell proliferation*. Individually, they can be listed as:

- Disorderly maturation:
  hyperplasia or atrophy
  keratosis/parakeratosis
  drop-shaped rete processes
  irregular stratification/disordered cell polarity
  low level keratinization in single or small cell groups
  reduced epithelial cell cohesion
  cell pleomorphism

- Disturbed cell proliferation:
  loss of basal cell polarity
  basal cell hyperplasia
  increased nuclear:cytoplasmic ratio
  enlarged nucleoli
  nuclear hyperchromatism
  high-level mitoses
  anisonucleosis
  abnormal ('bizarre') mitoses

It is unlikely that all of these will be found on a single section. A readily identifiable and characteristic feature, whether the epithelium is atrophic or acanthotic, is a bulbous, or drop-shaped, rete pattern (Fig. 14.18) within which there is disturbed cell polarity. In normal and hyperplastic epithelium cells of the deep layers are orientated with their long axis at right angles to the plane of the basement membrane, whereas superficially they flatten, their long axis becoming parallel to the surface. This orderly transition is lost in dysplasia, the other features listed being exhibited to varying extents (Fig. 14.19). At the molecular level it is likely that these disturbances represent disruption of growth control and altered gene expression, probably including oncogenes. Reduced cellular cohesion sugests that intercellular contacts and communication are also disturbed. Indirect evidence of impaired epithelial function, or possibly the formation of new or altered molecules on the cell surface, is the almost invariable presence of a lymphoplasmacytic host response in the superficial connective tissue. Mitotic activity in dysplastic epithelium usually shows marked local variation; the further the dividing cells extend from the basal layer the more profound the disturbance in epithelial proliferation.

An assessment of the number of dysplastic features, their extent, and their severity constitutes the basis for attempts at grading the degree of epithelial dysplasia on a scale from mild, moderate, to severe, the latter merging with what may be described as carcinoma *in situ*. In oral epithelium it is rare to find

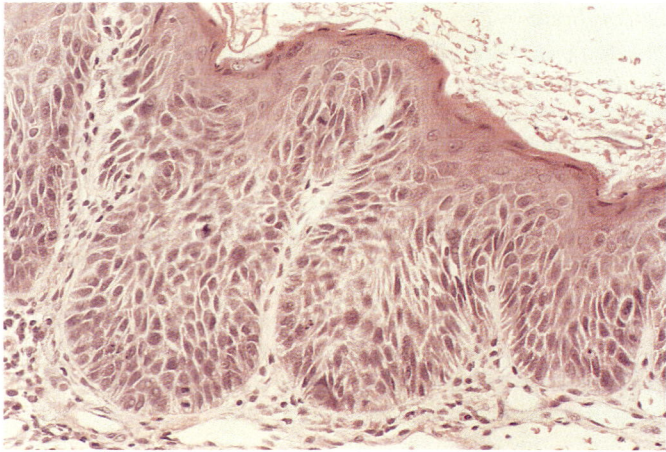

Fig. 14.18 Oral mucosa with atrophic and moderately dysplastic oral eithelium showing drop-shaped rete pegs, disordered cell polarity, and reduced cell cohesion.

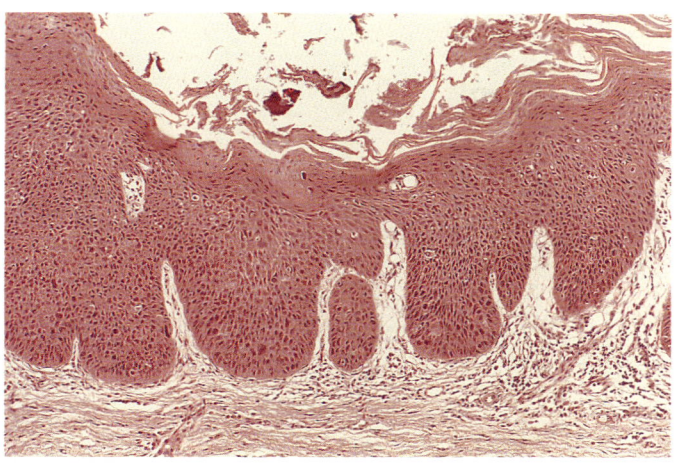

Fig. 14.19 Mucosa from the floor of mouth showing severely dysplastic, keratotic oral epithelium with markedly disordered cell polarity, low-level keratinization, nuclear hyperchromatism, and frequent and high-level mitoses.

the full-thickness dysplastic change seen, for example, in the uterine cervix (CIN 3), as the surface layers usually keratinize with little cytological evidence of pre-malignancy. Thus, exfoliative cytology has little value for routine oral screening in the diagnosis of pre-malignant change. Several attempts have been made to make the diagnosis of oral dysplasia more objective and reproducible, sometimes by 'weighting' certain features over others, but so far no reliable index exists. Some changes identical with those of mild dysplasia can be seen sometimes in epithelium unassociated with clinically suspicious lesions and may represent an age change in oral mucosa. Also some mild or even moderate dysplastic lesions undoubtedly regress, either spontaneously or following withdrawal of aetiological factors. Thus, epithelial dysplasia is not consistently a pre-malignant state. Nevertheless, malignant transformation amongst dysplastic lesions *as a group* is more common than in non-dysplastic epithelium and those lesions at the severe end of the range can be considered confidently as pre-malignant especially if they present at a high-risk site.

Pre-malignant conditions

The most important diseases of the oral mucosa in which there is a raised risk of malignant transformation are listed in Table 14.3. These will not be dealt with in depth here but a brief summary is appropriate.

Oral submucous fibrosis

This is a local disorder of collagen turnover and cross-linkage, causing progressive immobility of oral mucosa in response to a complex of factors. It is mainly confined to people of the Indian subcontinent, although cases also occur in other parts of South-East Asia. The epithelium overlying dense connective tissue of reduced vascularity is atrophic and may be dysplastic. There is now considerable evidence that it may undergo malignant transformation.

Chronic iron deficiency

This leads to sideropenic dysphagia (Paterson–Kelly or Plummer–Vinson syndrome) and has been linked with carcinoma of the upper alimentary tract, including the oral cavity, where leukoplakia may also be present. Many of the data have been obtained from Scandinavia and iron deficiency may help to account for the high female:male ratio for oral cancer in those countries.

Lichen planus

This is very common in oral mucosa and has been regarded only by some as a pre-malignant condition. With the benefit of careful follow-up studies it is now clear that there is an elevated risk of oral cancer in patients with long-standing lichen planus, particularly of the erosive (ulcerative) type. Lesions of discoid lupus erythematosus occur in the oral mucosa but the few cases of malignant transformation are confined mainly to the non-mucosal aspect of the lip.

Chronic epithelial atrophy

This is a common factor in the above conditions and may predispose to malignant transformation by carcinogens which might otherwise be without major effect. There are, in addition, several rare genetic conditions affecting the oral mucosa, in which the epithelium undergoes a relatively high rate of malignant transformation: these include dyskeratosis congenita, tylosis syndrome (intra-oral carcinoma), and xeroderma pigmentosum (lip cancer). It will be, perhaps, through the route of studying familial predispositions to oral cancer that some of the molecular mechanisms in its pathogenesis will be discovered.

14.2.4   Other oral neoplasms

Adenocarcinoma and adenosquamous carcinoma

When adenocarcinoma is found in oral mucosa it is likely to have arisen from minor salivary glands (see Section 14.3.7) and is, in any case, far less frequently encountered than squamous cell carcinoma. The adenosquamous carcinoma is even more unusual; it is a biphasic malignancy showing both squamous and glandular patterns of differentiation. It is possible that these too may originate from salivary tissue, but in the case illustrated (Fig. 14.20) the neoplasm arose on and invaded the edentulous lower alveolus. It metastasized to many cervical lymph nodes, showing both squamous and adenocarcinoma. This rare entity must be distinguished from the pseudoglandular (adenoid) vaiant of the squamous cell carcinoma, in which there is only an approximation to a gland-like morphology and a lack of mucin-positive epithelial cells.

Malignant melanoma

Melanotic lesions should be considered against a background knowledge of the range of pigmentation in normal oral mucosa. Only about 1 per cent of melanomas arise in the oral mucosa, but they may not be distinguishable clinically from other more

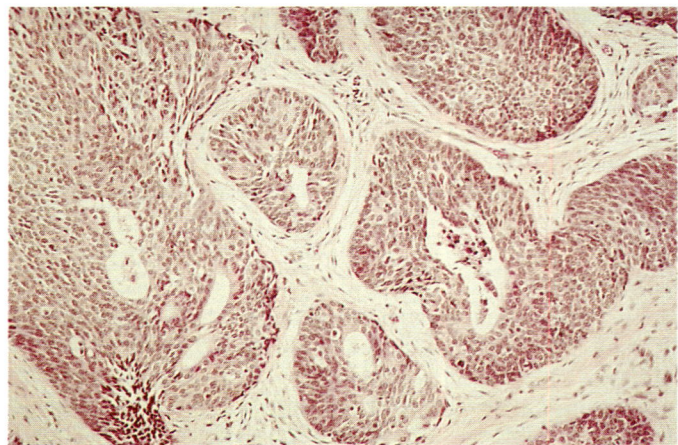

Fig. 14.20 Adenosquamous carcinoma from the alveolar mucosa. Keratin immunocytochemistry demonstrated two cell populations which were confirmed when separate adenocarcinoma and squamous cell carcinoma presented as lymph node metastases.

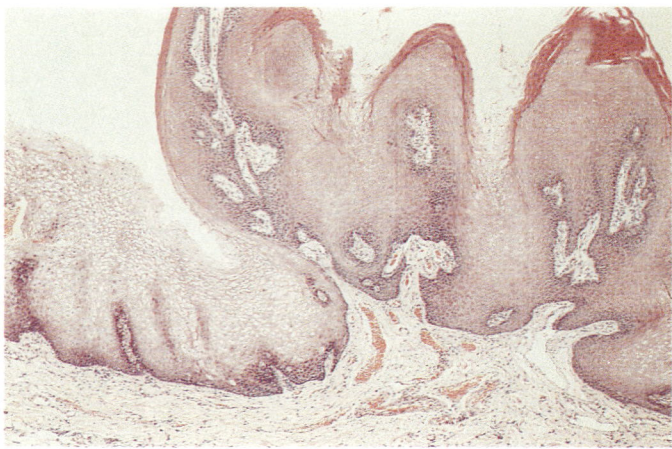

Fig. 14.21 Papilloma of the buccal mucosa, a pedunculated lesion showing typical acanthosis and hyperkeratosis.

common pigmented lesions (e.g. amalgam tattoos, haemosiderin deposits). Intra-oral melanomas are reportedly most frequent in the hard palate and in elderly males, but an enlarging or atypical pigmented lesion in any site should be excised for histological examination. The mucosal melanoma shows just as much histological variation as its cutaneous counterpart, including amelanotic variants, so they will not be described again here. Junctional activity is usually present in the adjoining epithelium, but in equivocal cases immunocytochemical tests to identify cells of neural crest origin are often of value. As the prognosis is poor, urgent definitive excision is essential. The possibility that the oral mucosal melanoma may be a metastasis rather than the primary neoplasm should also be borne in mind.

A similar range of naevi occur in oral mucosa as in the skin but they are much rarer and, although malignant transformation occurs, the majority of oral malignant melanomas seem to form in the absence of a pre-existing clinically detectable naevus.

Papilloma

The papilloma (squamous cell papilloma) is the commonest benign neoplasm of the oral mucosa. It can arise in any part of the oral mucosa but is most frequent in anterior parts of the mouth, often on the palate. It is pedunculated and has a white, folded surface. Histologically, it shows acanthotic, hyperortho- or parakeratotic epithelium, usually with many basal or parabasal mitoses of normal appearance. There are slender connective tissue papillae which generally do not contain inflammatory cells (Fig. 14.21). The presence of polymorphs superficially in the epithelium of large papillomas usually indicates an opportunist candidal infection of the irregular surface, and may contribute further to the high mitotic activity.

Neoplasms of connective tissue origin

Soft tissue tumours may occasionally present within or below the oral mucosa. Most are rare with no features unique to an intra-oral presentation, so the same principles of differential diagnosis apply as with those tumours presenting in other sites. Special mention should be made, however, of Kaposi's sarcoma in the oral mucosa, now a common manifestation of AIDS. It presents, often multifocally, as a purplish, macular or raised lesion, which may be ulcerated or covered by hyperplastic epithelium frequently containing numerous candidal hyphae (Fig. 14.22). As the oral mucosa is accessible to inspection, Kaposi's lesions excised from this site, at least in Western communities, tend to be in the early or angiomatous stages. A detailed description of Kaposi's sarcoma is given in Chapter 12.

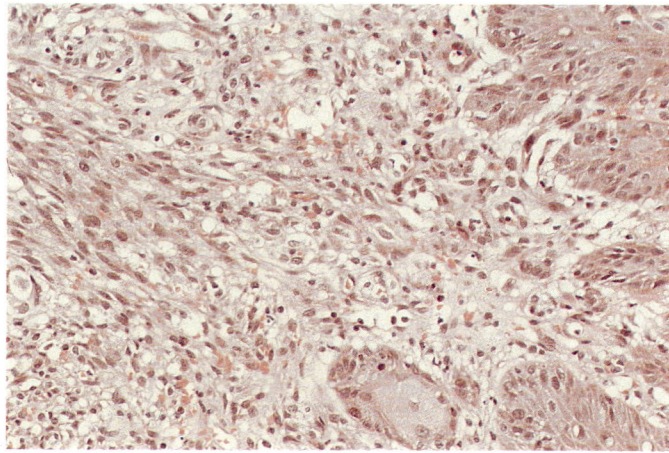

Fig. 14.22 Kaposi's sarcoma of the palatal mucosa: the superficial part of the lesion which is also associated with pseudo-epitheliomatous hyperplasia of the overlying epithelium.

14.2.5   Further reading

Ackerman, L. V. (1948). Verrucous carcinoma of the oral cavity. *Surgery* **23**, 670–8.

Anneroth, G., Batsakis, J., and Luna, M. (1987). Review of the literature and a recommended system of malignancy grading in oral squamous cell carcinomas. *Scandinavian Journal of Dental Research* **95**, 229–49.

Batsakis, J. G. (1979). *Tumours of the head and neck* (2nd edn). Williams and Wilkins, Baltimore.

Blot, W. J., *et al.* (1988). Smoking and drinking in relation to oral and pharyngeal cancer. *Cancer Research* **48**, 3282–7.

Boyle, P., Macfarlane, G. J., Maisonneuve, P., Zheng, T., Scully, C., and Tedesco, B. (1990). Epidemiology of mouth cancer in 1989: a review. *Journal of the Royal Society of Medicine* **83**, 724–30.

Brugere, J., Guenel, P., LeClerk, A., and Rodrigues, J. (1986). Differential effects of tobacco and alcohol in cancer of the larynx, pharynx and mouth. *Cancer* **57**, 391–5.

Eveson, J. W. (1983). Oral pre-malignancy. *Cancer Surveys* **2**, 403–24.

Moll, R., Franke, W. W., Schiller, D. L., Geiger, B., and Krepler, R. (1982). The catalog of human cytokeratins: patterns of expression in normal epithelial, tumours and cultured cells. *Cell* **31**, 11–24.

Moll, R., Krepler, R., and Franke, W. W. (1983). Complex cytokeratin polypeptide patterns observed in certain human carcinomas. *Differentiation* **23**, 256–69.

Pindborg, J. J. (1980). *Oral cancer and precancer.* John Wright and Son, Bristol.

Platz, H., Fries, R., and Hudec, M. (1986). *Prognoses of oral cavity carcinomas.* Carl Hanser Verlag, München, Wein.

World Health Organization Collaborating Centre for Oral Precancerous Lesions (1978). Definition of leukoplakia and related lesions: An aid to studies on oral precancer. *Oral Medicine, Oral Surgery, Oral Pathology* **46**, 518–39.

Oral cancer and pre-malignancy

Henk, J. M. and Langdon, J. D. (eds) (1985). *Malignant tumours of the oral cavity.* Edward Arnold, London.

Mackenzie, I. C., Dabelsteen, E., and Squier, C. A. (eds) (1980). *Oral premalignancy.* University of Iowa Press, Iowa City.

14.3   The salivary glands

P. M. Speight and S. Tinkler

14.3.1   Development, structure, and function

The salivary glands are usually considered in two groups—the paired bilateral major glands and the intra-oral minor glands. The major glands comprise the parotid, submandibular, and sublingual glands, while the minor glands are located beneath the epithelium in all parts of the mouth except for the attached gingivae and the anterior hard palate. Some knowledge of their development and structure is necessary in order to appreciate the pathological changes that may occur in disease.

Development

All salivary glands develop from proliferating downgrowths of embryonic oral epithelium which invades the underlying mesenchyme. The anlage of the parotid gland is the first to appear at about the fourth week of intra-uterine life, followed by the submandibular and sublingual glands at six and eight weeks. The distal portion of the downgrowths branch to form solid buds with bulbous terminals which will form the acini. The solid buds hollow out to form ducts by the sixth month but secretory activity does not commence until the early postnatal period. Later in development pluripotential epithelial cells appear and form two reserve cell populations which differentiate into mature cells of the secretory unit. The intercalated duct reserve cells give rise to acinar cells, intercalated and striated duct cells, and myoepithelial cells. The excretory duct reserve cells give rise to the columnar and squamous cells of the extralobular duct system. It has been proposed that all salivary gland neoplasms are ultimately derived from one or the other of the two reserve cell populations (Batsakis 1979).

Histology

The parenchyma of the salivary glands is divided into lobules by connective tissue septa which contain the blood vessels, nerves, and interlobular ducts. Within the lobules the gland tissue is arranged into secretory units composed of secretory endpieces and a series of ducts (Fig. 14.23).

Secretory endpieces

These produce most of the saliva and are composed of pyramidal cells arranged around a central lumen. In serous glands the endpieces are compact or 'grape-like' and are called acini, but in mucous glands they are elongated tubulo-acini. The parotid glands are serous while the glands of the palate and tongue are mucous. The submandibular gland is a mixed gland and is composed of serous acini with occasional mucous tubulo-acini, many of which are surrounded by serous cells arranged as caps or 'demilunes' (Fig. 14.24). The sublingual gland and the minor glands of the lips and cheeks are mainly composed of mucous cells with occasional serous demilunes.

The duct system

The endpieces open directly into short intercalated ducts composed of cuboidal or flattened epithelial cells surrounding a narrow lumen. These are continuous with the striated ducts which are predominantly intralobular and are composed of cuboidal or low columnar cells with prominent in-foldings of the basal membrane. These enclose many mitochondria and impart the striated appearance. The striated ducts blend imperceptibly with interlobular excretory ducts located within the connective tissue septae of the glands and which eventually unite to form the single extraglandular duct which drains into the mouth. The excretory ducts are similar in structure to striated ducts but also have occasional basal or reserve cells. Towards the orifice the main excretory duct becomes stratified prior to blending with the oral epithelium. As well as transporting the saliva, the duct system alters its composition by the selective reabsorption of electrolytes.

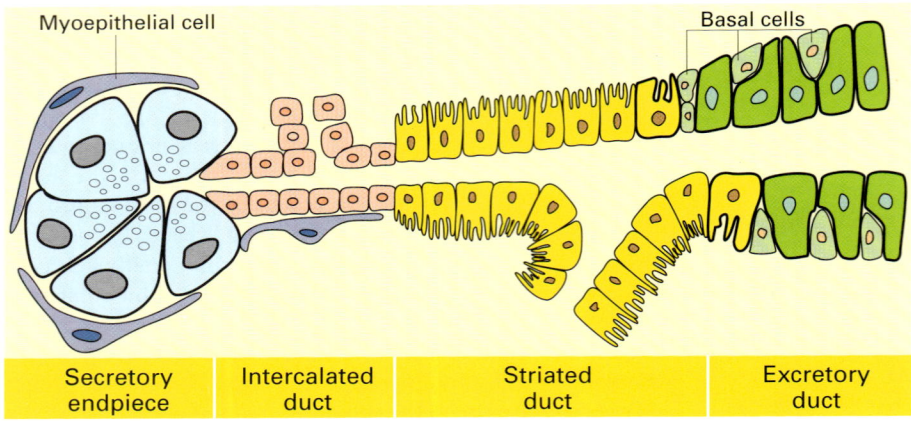

Fig. 14.23 Diagram of a secretory unit. Acinar cells, intercalated and striated duct cells, and myoepithelial cells are derived from a population of intercalated duct reserve cells. The columnar and squamous cells of the extralobular duct system arise from basally situated reserve cells in the excretory ducts.

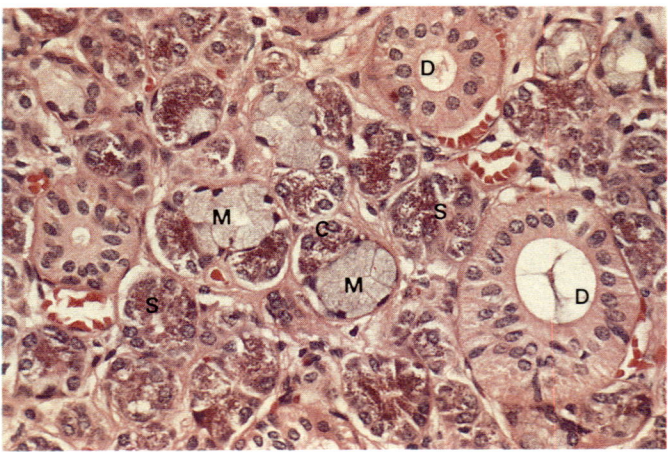

Fig. 14.24 Normal human submandibular gland. D, striated duct; S, serous acini; M, mucous tubulo-acini; C, serous cap or demilune.

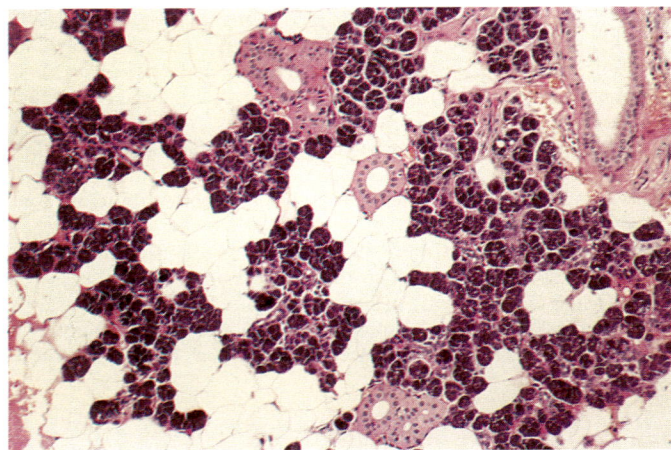

Fig. 14.25 Normal parotid gland from a patient aged 61. There is prominent replacement of the acinar cells by fat.

Myoepithelial cells

Myoepithelial cells lie within the basement membrane and have many branching processes which invest the secretory endpieces and intercalated ducts of most glands. Although these cells are epithelial in origin, they have many characteristics of smooth muscle, including parallel arrays of actin filaments. Contraction of myoepithelial cells may accelerate the onset of secretion by ejecting preformed saliva and rupturing cells packed with mucous secretory granules.

Age changes

The salivary glands undergo characteristic age changes which must be distinguished from pathological states. Gradual fatty replacement of the parenchyma is common and is most notable in the parotid gland, where the proportion of fat cells increases from less than 10 per cent at age ten to 20–30 per cent by the eighth decade (Fig. 14.25). Occasionally the fatty replacement is more marked and is referred to as interstitial lipomatosis. This may be localized or associated with general adiposity or diabetes mellitus. Lipomatosis must be distinguished from a lipoma which may rarely affect the parotid gland.

Oncocytic metaplasia is seen in about 80 per cent of glands by the age of 70 and is characterized by large eosinophilic cells with a granular cytoplasm which are found scattered among the acini and ducts. The granularity of the cells is due to an increase in the number of mitochondria, which are swollen and pleomorphic but still metabolically active. The cause of oncocytic metaplasia is unknown, but it is also seen in other glands including the pituitary gland, pancreas, and liver. When prominent it may cause gland enlargement and is referred to as oncocytosis. Oncocytes may also give rise to neoplasms, in particular the oncocytoma and adenolymphoma.

Other age changes include acinar atrophy, interstitial fibrosis, and infiltration of the gland by lymphocytes and plasma cells. These changes are usually mild but in diagnostic biopsies must be distinguished from sialadenitis. It is interesting that, despite the gradual replacement of salivary parenchyma, loss of secretory capacity or xerostomia is not associated with ageing in normal healthy individuals.

Function

The secretion of normal volumes of saliva is essential to the health of the oral cavity. The main functions of saliva are digestive and protective but it also plays a small role in excretion and is essential for the sense of taste. The lubricating properties of saliva, which are imparted by the high glycoprotein content, are essential for chewing, swallowing, and speech. Saliva also contains a number of non-specific antibacterial factors such as lysozyme, lactoperoxidase, and lactoferrin, which help to rid the mouth of pathogenic organisms. The integrity of the dental hard tissues is maintained by the buffering capacity of saliva which resists the action of acid-producing cariogenic bacteria. In addition, saliva has a high content of calcium and phosphate salts and acts as a supersaturated solution which prevents dissolution, and aids re-mineralization, of dental enamel.

The secretory immune system

Secretory IgA is produced by mucosa-associated lymphoid tissue (MALT) throughout the gastrointestinal and respiratory tracts and provides a significant barrier to micro-organisms and antigens. In the oral cavity the minor salivary glands produce about four times as much secretory IgA as the parotid glands. As part of the common immune system the salivary glands can produce a specific IgA response to gut antigens but, in addition, a local response can be initiated by instillation of antigen into the ducts of minor glands. There is thus increasing immunological and morphological evidence for a local duct-associated lymphoid tissue (DALT), analogous to that found in the gut and bronchi (GALT and BALT), which forms part of the common mucosal and secretory immune systems (see Section 24.13).

14.3.2   Congenital disorders

Congenital or developmental disorders including aplasia and hypoplasia are very rare but may be associated with developmental anomalies of the head and neck, such as hemifacial microsomia or mandibulo-facial dysostosis. Duct atresia, which refers to an absent or imperforate salivary duct, has occasionally been reported in the submandibular gland. In the floor of the mouth atresia of the ducts of the sublingual or minor glands may give rise to mucoceles (ranulae) which are sometimes seen in neonates.

A more common anomaly is the presence of aberrant salivary tissue. Although this may be located anywhere in the head and neck, common sites are within lymph nodes and in the lingual aspect of the mandible. In the latter case salivary tissue produces a lingual salivary gland depression which radiographically resembles a cyst and is called a Stafne's bone cavity. It can be differentiated from an odontogenic cyst because it is usually located towards the angle of the mandible and below the inferior dental canal. Tumours may develop in aberrant salivary tissue and reports of intra-osseous neoplasms suggest that salivary tissue may become entirely entrapped within bone during development.

14.3.3   Disorders of secretion

Xerostomia

Like sialorrhoea, xerostomia is a symptom and not a disease. It is important because of the devastating effects of reduced salivary flow on the health of the mouth. Xerostomia is accompanied by infection, ulceration, and rampant dental caries. In addition there is difficulty in eating, speaking, and swallowing. There are many conditions which may lead to a complaint of dry mouth. In some cases the flow rate is normal but there is a feeling of dryness due to local factors such as mouth breathing, smoking, or local infections. In other cases a real lack of flow is associated with stress, fear, or anxiety, and is a result of increased sympathetic activity. Xerostomia is also a common side-effect of many drugs, including tranquillizers, sedatives, antihypertensives, antihistamines, and anti-emetics. In these cases the functional capacity of the glands remains normal.

In some conditions the functional capacity of the salivary glands is reduced due to a loss of secreting cells. This occurs in irradiation sialadenitis when the salivary glands are damaged by therapeutic irradiation to the head and neck. As with other tissues the effects are dose dependent but the salivary glands, especially the parotid, appear to be particularly sensitive. Within a few days there is a reduction in salivary flow accompanied by gland swelling and tenderness. After a single dose the gland may recover but with a total dose of 20 Gy or over permanent damage will result. Thus severe and usually permanent xerostomia can be expected following all but palliative radiotherapy to the oral region. The resultant rampant dental caries and oral infections are often associated with osteomyelitis or osteoradionecrosis. These are important side-effects which may severely reduce the quality of life for some cancer patients. Careful planning, with a dental surgeon as part of the team, can ensure that oral and dental health are restored and maintained during treatment (Henk and Langdon 1985).

In Sjögren's syndrome the salivary glands are affected by an auto-immune sialadenitis which may lead to complete loss of acini and permanent and irreversible xerostomia. Other disorders that may lead to symptoms of dry mouth include those associated with a change in fluid balance, such as dehydration, diabetes, uraemia, or hypovolemic shock. It should be noted that sialadenitis and salivary calculi, which usually only affect single glands, are not usually associated with xerostomia. Tests of salivary gland function, useful in the diagnosis of xerostomia are discussed in the section on Sjögren's syndrome (p. 1073).

Sialorrhoea (ptyalism)

A true increase in salivary flow is rare but may be seen in mercury poisoning, rabies, and some neurological disturbances, including Parkinson's disease, myasthenia gravis, and epilepsy. It may also occur when the mouth is affected by an acute inflammatory disorder, such as herpetic gingivostomatitis or during tooth eruption. Apparent sialorrhoea, which manifests as persistent drooling, is due to loss of muscle control or of the swallowing reflex and may be seen in spastic children or following a stroke.

14.3.4   Salivary calculi

Salivary calculi, or sialoliths, are usually found in the large ducts of the major glands. They are more common in adults, and men are affected twice as often as women. Eighty per cent occur in the submandibular gland and, of the remainder, most are found in the parotid gland. The causes of salivary calculi are not known. They are not related to general disorders of calcium metabolism but appear to arise by local deposition of calcium and phosphate salts around a nidus of organic material composed of cell debris and precipitated glycoproteins. Organic and inorganic constituents may be deposited as alternating layers, producing a laminated structure which grows progressively to fill and eventually block the duct.

Submandibular calculi are probably more common because the saliva is viscous and the duct is long and tortuous. This may lead to stasis which favours deposition of both organic and inorganic constituents. Calculi may develop within the gland but about 70 per cent are found in the main excretory duct. Typically they are elongated, bullet-shaped stones which can be palpated in the floor of the mouth. They may grow to a large size before symptoms occur, and are therefore often discovered as a chance finding on a dental radiograph (Fig. 14.26). Occasionally they can be visualized as a pale yellow swelling in the floor of the mouth or may be seen protruding from the duct orifice. If the stone is not passed the duct eventually becomes obstructed, leading to the classical clinical sign of recurrent painful swelling associated with meals. Infection inevitably supervenes and leads to persistent chronic obstructive sialadenitis, the most common cause of submandibular swelling.

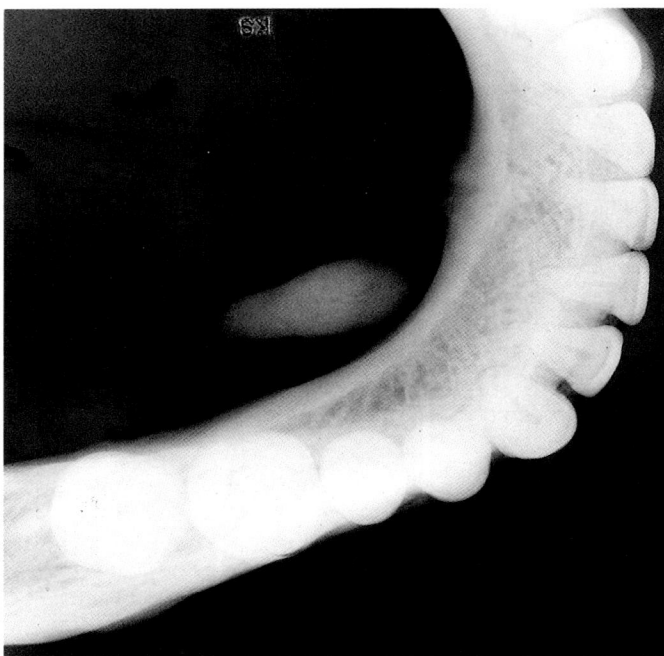

Fig. 14.26 A true occlusal radiograph of the mandible. There is a 'bullet-shaped' salivary calculus located in the anterior portion of the submandibular duct.

Parotid calculi appear to be much less common, but this is partly due to the fact that they are difficult to demonstrate since they may not be visible on a plain radiograph. Most are found within the parotid duct but, because of the watery nature of the secretion, do not give rise to swellings associated with meals.

14.3.5   Salivary cysts

Simple epithelial cysts of unknown cause may occasionally arise within the parotid or submandibular glands.

More commonly the minor glands are affected by mucus-filled cysts called mucoceles. About 80 per cent of these are mucus extravasation cysts and the remainder are mucus retention cysts.

Mucus extravasation cysts

These cysts are quite common in young adults and frequently present as soft blue swellings. Eighty per cent occur on the lower lip and most of the remainder are found in the cheeks or floor of the mouth. They arise due to trauma and rupture of the salivary duct with resultant leakage of mucus into the adjacent connective tissues. Histology of a well-formed cyst shows a mucus-filled cavity lined by connective tissue containing many inflammatory cells and macrophages (Fig. 14.27). The macrophages, which are filled with mucus and have a foamy cytoplasm, are often found within and lining the cystic lumen. Occasionally a more solid lesion, or mucus granuloma, may develop which contains mucus, inflammatory cells, macrophages, and multinucleated giant cells.

Mucus retention cysts

These are found in older age groups and are more evenly distributed among the intra-oral minor glands. Retention cysts may also have a traumatic origin, but in this case the duct becomes partially obstructed by stenosis or fibrosis. Microcalculi may also lead to mucus retention. As the pressure in the duct increases a cystic lesion develops which is filled with mucus and lined by a double-layered duct epithelium composed of cuboidal or columnar cells (Fig. 14.27). Occasionally there may be oncocytic change or squamous metaplasia of the epithelial lining.

Ranula

Ranula is the term used to describe a mucocele arising in the floor of the mouth. The name derives from the apparent resemblance of the lesion to the belly of a frog. Ranulae are often retention in type and are lined by a simple cuboidal epithelium. Usually they are about 2–3 cm in diameter but occasionally the mucus may extravasate below the mylohyoid muscle and extend through the fascial planes into the submandibular region and neck. Such a lesion may become quite large and is called a 'plunging ranula'.

14.3.6   Inflammatory disorders—sialadenitis

Inflammatory disorders are the most common diseases of the salivary glands and are usually bacterial or viral in origin.

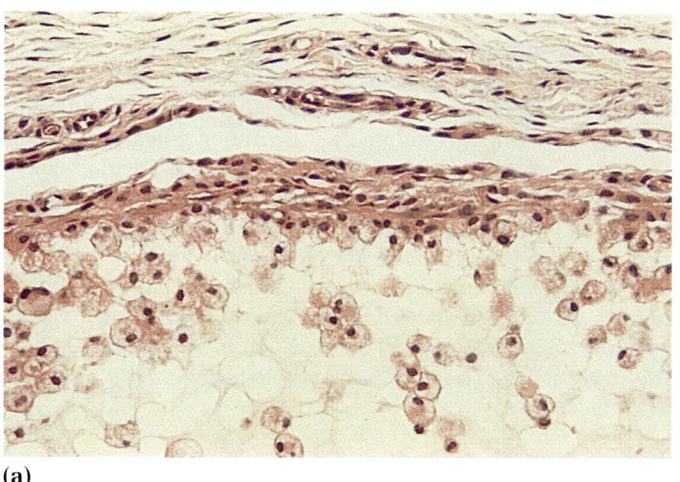

(a)

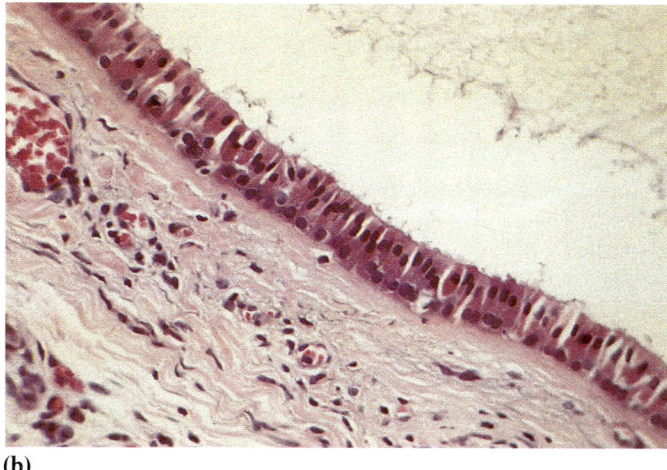

(b)

Fig. 14.27 (a) Mucus extravasation cyst. The cyst is lined by fibrous connective tissue containing inflammatory cells and macrophages. Macrophages containing mucus are seen within the lumen. (b) Mucus retention cyst. The cyst is lined by typical ductal epithelium composed of a basal layer of cuboidal cells and a luminal layer of columnar cells.

Acute sialadenitis

Acute sialadenitis is nearly always the result of an ascending infection from the oral cavity and is usually preceded by a diminished salivary flow. The parotid gland, which has a thin watery secretion, is more commonly affected than the submandibular gland. Acute parotitis used to be a common complication of the debilitation and dehydration that followed major surgery. Early mobilization, rehydration, and the use of antibiotics have rendered this unusual and acute parotitis is now more common in association with the severe xerostomia which results from therapeutic irradiation or from Sjögren's syndrome.

The causative organisms include those normally present in the mouth, such as *Streptococcus viridans* and occasionally *Staphylococcus aureus* or *Staph. pyogenes*. Typically, the disorder is of acute onset with tender, painful swelling of one or both parotid glands. The duct orifice may be red and swollen with pus discharging into the mouth. In some cases pus may localize to produce abscesses which discharge directly through the skin.

Chronic sialadenitis

Chronic parotitis may occur as a result of an unresolved acute parotitis. This usually follows a persistently reduced flow due to any of the previously mentioned causes. Occasionally there may be a calculus or stricture of the duct.

Chronic sialadenitis in the submandibular gland is relatively common and is usually the result of duct obstruction by a calculus. At first this is characterized by recurrent swellings due to retention of secretion, but as chronic infection supervenes the gland becomes inflamed and eventually fibrosed to produce a firm, tumour-like mass. Episodes of acute sialadenitis may occur and frequently the gland becomes functionless and requires removal.

Histologically the affected gland shows duct dilation and hyperplasia, acinar atrophy and fibrosis with a dense periductal and diffuse infiltrate of lymphocytes (Fig. 14.28). Noncaseating granulomata with multinucleate giant cells may occasionally be present, and are probably a reaction to extravasated mucus. Submandibular sialadenitis is presumed to be bacterial in origin but in many cases the aetiology is not clear. Chronic obstructive sialadenitis may sometimes produce such marked fibrosis that a hard swelling results which clinically is indistinguishable from a neoplasm. This has been termed chronic sclerosing sialadenitis or 'Küttner tumour'.

Chronic recurrent parotitis

This is a well-recognized entity which occurs either in young children between 5 and 10 years of age or in older, usually female, adults. In children there is a good prognosis but in some

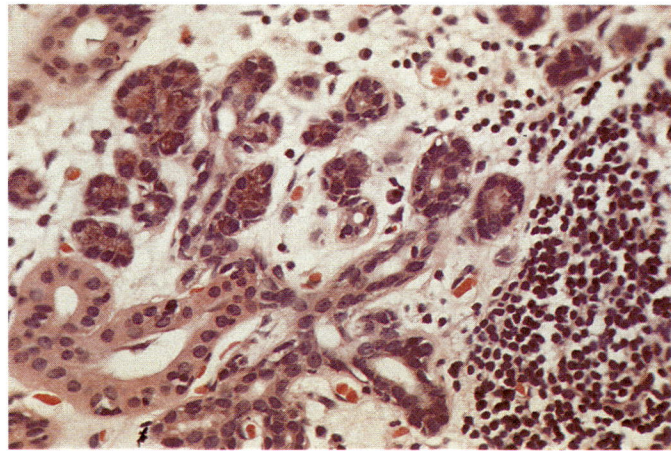

Fig. 14.28 Chronic sialadenitis of the submandibular gland. There is a dense infiltrate of chronic inflammatory cells associated with fibrosis, loss of acini, and proliferation of ducts. Compare with Fig. 14.24.

adults the disease persists and cannot be controlled by antibiotics. In these cases parotidectomy may be indicated. The disease is characterized by recurrent tender swelling of the parotid glands which lasts for 3–7 days and occurs at intervals of weeks or months. Each attack may be precipitated by an episode of illness and be accompanied by fever and malaise. In children the recurrent episodes become less frequent and usually cease at puberty. The cause of recurrent parotitis is uncertain. It is not associated with obvious obstruction, although congenital stenosis or stricture of the duct has been implicated. Other suggested aetiological factors include calculi, allergy, and infections by bacteria or viruses.

Histological examination shows proliferating and dilated ducts associated with acinar atrophy and fibrosis. The ductal changes are particularly prominent and are referred to as sialectasia. Sialography demonstrates this change particularly well since the dilated ducts become filled with radio-opaque contrast medium to give an appearance called globular or punctate sialectasis (Fig. 14.29). This is a useful diagnostic test which also has prognostic significance since those glands without prominent duct changes are more likely to resolve.

Specific bacterial and granulomatous lesions

Rarely the salivary glands may be involved in a specific inflammatory disorder, such as tuberculosis, syphilis, gonorrhoea, or actinomycosis. Of these, tuberculosis is the most common and often affects the parotid gland as a result of involvement of the intraparotid lymph nodes.

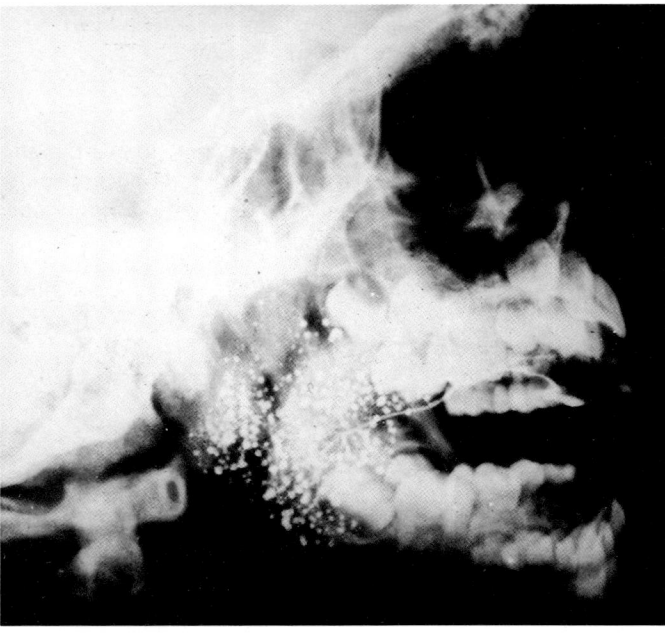

Fig. 14.29 A lateral sialogram in a young patient with chronic recurrent parotitis. The contrast medium fills the dilated ducts and extravasates into the adjacent tissues to give an appearance likened to a 'snowstorm' and called globular or punctate sialectasis. A similar appearance is seen in Sjögren's syndrome. (Courtesy of Professor G. R. Seward.)

As well as the specific infections, the parotid gland may be involved in up to 5 per cent of patients with sarcoidosis. In addition to the usual systemic manifestations there is painless, firm nodular swelling of the parotid glands which contain typical non-caseating granulomata. The minor salivary glands of the palate and lip may also be involved. A particular manifestation of sarcoidosis affects the uveal tract, the lacrimal and salivary glands, and sometimes the cranial nerves, and is called uveoparotid fever or Heerfordt's syndrome.

The term Mikulicz's syndrome is sometimes used in relation to bilateral salivary gland enlargement due to a known cause, such as tuberculosis, sarcoidosis, or lymphoid neoplasia. Since the term has no diagnostic or pathological connotations it is best avoided.

Mumps

Mumps is an acute infectious disease caused by a paramyxovirus which has a predilection for the parotid glands, although other organs may be affected, sometimes without parotid involvement. Mumps is the most common salivary gland disease and occurs most often in children of school age. The virus is transmitted by saliva droplets and, following infection, replicates in the oral cavity and upper respiratory tract. The salivary glands and other organs are infected by haematogenous spread following the primary viraemia. Typically, there is an incubation period of 2–3 weeks followed by sudden onset of painful parotid swelling, which in 75 per cent of cases becomes bilateral. This is usually accompanied by fever, malaise, and headaches. The swelling lasts for 7–10 days, but a patient's saliva may be infectious for a total of up to 6 weeks. The submandibular glands may be swollen in about 10 per cent of cases and other organs, most often the testes and pancreas, may also be involved. Widespread organ involvement is a particular feature of mumps in adults, and orchitis may be present in up to 30 per cent of cases. Central nervous system involvement in the form of a meningoencephalitis may also be a feature and may arise alone without evidence of salivary gland involvement.

Histologically the involved gland contains a dense infiltrate of lymphocytes and plasma cells throughout the interstitial connective tissues. This is associated with oedema and degeneration and vacuolation of acinar and duct cells. As the infection subsides the glands usually return to normal.

Cytomegalovirus infection

Cytomegalovirus is a ubiquitous herpes virus detectable in up to 80 per cent of adults. Infection is usually subclinical and, like other herpes viruses, the cytomegalovirus may remain latent until reactivated. Secondary infection may follow debilitating diseases, malignant neoplasms, immunosuppression, or acquired immunodeficiencies. Occasionally the primary infection is accompanied by fever, hepatosplenomegaly, and other symptoms resembling infectious mononucleosis.

A more common form of cytomegalovirus disease is prenatal infection due to transmission of the virus across the placenta following a primary infection in the mother. The parotid glands are involved as part of the generalized infection, which may also affect the brain, kidneys, liver, lungs, and pancreas. The histological appearances are diagnostic and include lymphocytic infiltration of the glands associated with multiple, giant epithelial cells within the ducts. These cells contain a large intranuclear inclusion body with a clear halo giving the characteristic 'owl's eye' appearance. Prenatal cytomegalovirus infection may lead to delayed fetal development and premature or still births. The parotid glands in up to 30 per cent of stillborn babies may contain cytomegalic inclusions.

Other viral infections

Occasionally sialadenitis of the parotid glands may be a feature of other infections, including influenza, infectious mononucleosis, and infections caused by coxsackie A and echoviruses. Usually the salivary gland features are similar to those seen in mumps. Bilateral parotid gland swelling, especially in children, has also been described as one of the features of HIV infection.

Irradiation sialadenitis

As mentioned previously, therapeutic irradiation for tumours of the head and neck may result in severe xerostomia, which is associated with a variable degree of sialadenitis. Histologically the irradiated gland contains an infiltrate of acute inflammatory cells associated with oedema and necrosis of acinar and ductal epithelial cells. After low doses these early changes are reversible but with higher doses there is epithelial atrophy with prominent fibrosis and permanent loss of secretory cells.

Sjögren's syndrome

Sjögren's syndrome is an auto-immune condition characterized by lymphocytic infiltration of exocrine glands, particularly the lacrimal and salivary glands, resulting in reduced secretion. The presence of dry eyes (keratoconjunctivitis sicca) and xerostomia is referred to as primary Sjögren's syndrome but in over half of cases one or both of these are accompanied by another auto-immune or connective tissue disorder leading to a diagnosis of secondary Sjögren's syndrome. In over 90 per cent of cases the associated disorder is rheumatoid arthritis, but others, including systemic lupus erythematosus, systemic sclerosis, polymyositis, and primary biliary cirrhosis are occasionally seen. About 15 per cent of patients with rheumatoid arthritis, 30 per cent with systemic lupus erythematosus, and over 70 per cent with primary biliary cirrhosis may suffer from Sjögren's syndrome.

Apart from the associated disorder, primary and secondary Sjögren's syndrome have other clinical, immunological, and genetic differences. Primary Sjögren's syndrome is associated with more severe eye and mouth symptoms, and has a higher incidence of salivary gland swelling and systemic manifestations, such as lymphadenopathy, Raynaud's phenomenon, myositis, and lung and renal involvement. Genetic factors also differ, since primary Sjögren's syndrome is strongly associated with HLA-DR3 while the secondary form is associated with HLA-DR4, which is also associated with rheumatoid arthritis

alone. Immunologically, both forms are characterized by B-cell hyperactivity and the production of many circulating auto-antibodies but the pattern of detectable auto-antibodies differs (Table 14.4). These genetic and immunological differences suggest that primary and secondary Sjögren's syndrome may be different disease entities.

Table 14.4 Auto-antibodies in Sjögren's syndrome

	Approximate frequency (%)	
	Primary SS	Secondary SS
Anti-SSA (Ro)	75	10
Anti-SSB (La)	40	5
Rheumatoid factors	95	100
Rheumatoid arthritis precipitin	5	85
Salivary duct antibody	25	70

Diagnosis

Most patients with Sjögren's syndrome are over 50 and 90 per cent are female. The diagnosis can only be made if two or three of the component parts are positively identified according to well-defined criteria as described by Manthorpe and Prause (1986). Keratoconjunctivitis sicca is diagnosed on the basis of reduced lacrimal secretion with associated inadequate tear film or filamentary keratitis visible on slit-lamp examination. Xerostomia is a result of reduced salivary secretion and the effects on oral health have been described previously. Diagnosis of the salivary component depends on being able to demonstrate a true loss of secretory capacity.

A number of tests of salivary gland function are currently in use. The simplest to perform is an estimation of salivary flow rate or sialometry. This can be a measurement of the stimulated parotid flow rate or of the whole saliva flow rate. Over 90 per cent of patients have a reduced salivary flow and, in general, it is more severely reduced in Sjögren's syndrome than in other causes of xerostomia. Sialography consistently shows punctate or globular sialectasis but is not specific since similar changes may be seen in sialadenitis (Fig. 14.29). Salivary scintiscanning is a technique whereby the salivary glands are examined with a gamma-camera after the intravenous injection of ^{99m}Tc pertechnetate, which is a radioisotope selectively concentrated and secreted by the salivary glands. Reduced uptake is an indication of reduced functional capaciy and is seen in over two-thirds of Sjögren's syndrome patients. Scintiscanning correlates well with the salivary flow rate and the degree of xerostomia, and also has the advantage of examining all the salivary glands at the same time.

Pathology

Histological examination of the salivary glands can provide direct evidence of gland damage. The parotid glands may be enlarged in about 75 per cent of primary and 15 per cent of secondary Sjögren's syndrome patients. The affected glands are diffusely infiltrated by lymphocytes and contain epimyoepithelial islands. The histopathology of the parotid lesions is identical to lymphoepithelial lesion and will be described later. Similar changes are seen in the minor salivary glands, which show focal lymphocytic sialadenitis in over 70 per cent of cases. The glands contain focal periductal infiltrates of lymphocytes but do not show features of non-specific sialadenitis such as acinar atrophy or fibrosis (Fig. 14.30). The foci of lymphocytes can be counted and a score of more than one focus per 4 mm² of salivary tissue, in the absence of non-specific changes, is considered consistent with the oral component of Sjögren's syndrome. However, similar changes are present in about 20 per cent of patients with rheumatoid arthritis and other connective tissue disorders, and in up to 5 per cent of normal glands. Thus, while biopsy of the minor glands of the lower lip is a useful indicator of salivary gland involvement, the results must be interpreted in conjunction with the other features of Sjögren's syndrome.

Aetiology and immunopathogenesis

The immunological features indicate that Sjögren's syndrome is auto-immune in nature but the initiating factors or mechanisms of tissue damage are unknown. The syndrome is characterized by B-cell hyperactivity and an abundance of non-organ specific auto-antibodies. The most prominent of these are rheumatoid factors and antinuclear antibodies, including anti-SS-A (Ro), anti-SS-B (La), and rheumatoid arthritis precipitin (RAP) (Table 14.4). Although salivary duct antibodies may be seen, these are not specific to Sjögren's syndrome and are only present in about 50 per cent of cases. Other features of hyperactivity include hypergammaglobulinaemia, and increased numbers of immune complexes and activated B-cells in the circulation. Many of the associated features of Sjögren's syndrome, including vasculitis, polyarthritis, and renal disease, are mediated by immune complex deposition, but the cause of the exocrine gland destruction is not clear.

In the salivary glands the lesions contain both T- and B-lymphocytes in varying proportions at different stages of the

disease. Overall, T-helper cells predominate and may be associated with a disturbance in immunoregulation, with inadequate T-suppressor activity and hyperstimulation of B-cells. There is little evidence for direct cell-mediated cytotoxic damage of salivary epithelial cells, and attempts to identify changes in the epithelium that may initiate an auto-immune response have largely failed.

There is evidence that viruses may initiate auto-immune disease by changing the cell surface and altering the antigenicity of host cells. In Sjögren's syndrome cytomegalovirus and Epstein–Barr virus have been subjected to rigorous study but, despite evidence that certain Epstein–Barr virus-related antigens may be found in the salivary glands, their role remains speculative.

It is likely that the aetiology of the disorder is multifactorial and that a disturbance in immunoregulation may be precipitated by an event such as a virus infection in genetically predisposed individuals.

14.3.7 Salivary gland neoplasms

Neoplasms of the salivary glands are uncommon, and in the United Kingdom comprise about 3 per cent of all tumours of the head and neck. A large survey of British salivary gland tumours (Eveson and Cawson 1985) has confirmed previous studies showing that about 85 per cent of neoplasms occur in the major glands and that of these 90 per cent are in the parotid, almost 10 per cent in the submandibular, and only very few in the sublingual. Of the 15 per cent that occur in the minor glands, over half (55 per cent) are in the palate, about 20 per cent in the lips, and the remainder distributed among the other sites. It should be noted, however, that although tumours in the minor glands are less common, 46 per cent were shown to be malignant compared to only 15 per cent in the parotid gland. In the most unusual sites almost all tumours were malignant—85 per cent in the sublingual glands, 92 per cent in the tongue, and 100 per cent in the alveolar ridge, tuberosity, and ethmoid regions. The submandibular gland is in an intermediate position with 37 per cent malignant tumours.

Salivary gland tumours are difficult to classify because of the wide variety of histological appearances and variability in behaviour. A new classification has recently been proposed by the World Health Organization and is summarized in Table 14.5. This is more detailed than the previous classification (Thackray and Sobin 1972) and attempts to distinguish tumours by their histopathological features, as well as by their prognosis and treatment.

At least 80 per cent of salivary gland tumours are benign and over 80 per cent of these are pleomorphic adenomas. Carcinomas comprise up to 20 per cent of total tumours and of these, the adenoid cystic carcinoma is the most common.

Pleomorphic adenoma

The pleomorphic adenoma is the commonest salivary neoplasm and is most often found in the superficial lobe of the parotid gland. Intra-orally the site of predilection is at the junction of

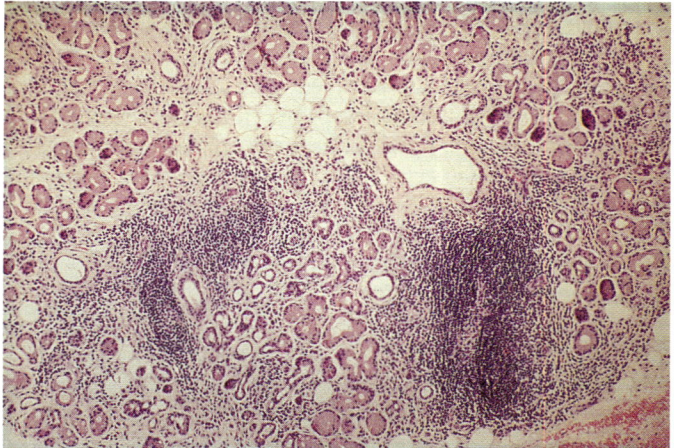

Fig. 14.30 A minor labial salivary gland from a patient with Sjögren's syndrome. This low-power view shows the focal, periductal nature of the inflammatory infiltrate.

Table 14.5 Histological classication of salivary gland tumours

1. Adenomas
   Pleomorphic adenoma
   Myoepithelioma
   Warthin tumour (adenolymphoma)
   Oncocytoma
   Basal cell adenoma
   Canalicular adenoma
   Sebaceous adenoma
   Duct papilloma
   Cystadenoma

2. Carcinomas
   Adenoid cystic carcinoma
   Mucoepidermoid carcinoma
   Acinic cell carcinoma
   Polymorphous low grade adenocarcinoma
   Epithelial-myoepithelial carcinoma
   Adenocarcinoma
   Squamous cell carcinoma
   Carcinoma in pleomorphic adenoma
   Other carcinomas

3. Non-epithelial tumours

4. Malignant lymphomas

5. Secondary tumours

6. Unclassified tumours

7. Tumour-like conditions
   Lymphoepithelial lesion
   Oncocytosis
   Sialosis
   Necrotizing sialometaplasia
   Salivary cysts
   Chronic sclerosing sialadenitis
   Cystic lymphoid hyperplasia in AIDS

Modified from Seifert *et al.* 1990.

hard and soft palate. The tumour can occur at any age but appears to be most frequent in the fifth and sixth decades, with an overall mean of about 48 years. Females are affected in 60 per cent of cases. Pleomorphic adenomas are typically slow growing, painless, smooth swellings, which are not fixed to surrounding tissue. They are usually about 2–3 cm in diameter but if left untreated may grow to enormous sizes. Occasionally a tumour may undergo a period of rapid growth and in some cases this may indicate malignant change.

Pathology

The excised specimen has a smooth, lobulated or nodular surface and is covered by a fibrous capsule which may be thin and incomplete. The cut surface shows a solid multinodular, grey-white tumour with bluish areas of chondroid or mucoid tissue. Although the lesion appears to be multifocal, studies of serial sections have shown that the apparently discrete nodules are joined to the main tumour mass by thin stalks. The tumour usually infiltrates the capsule and small foci may become walled off from the main mass. This is part of the normal growth pattern of the pleomorphic adenoma and does not indicate malignancy. However, small foci of cells may be left behind after simple enucleation and their continued growth is responsible for the high recurrence rate of this lesion.

Histologically the pleomorphic adenoma shows a variety of appearances, both in different areas of the same tumour and between tumours. A typical pattern is of epithelial cells arranged in sheets, strands, or duct-like structures embedded in a mucoid stroma (Fig. 14.31). The ducts contain mucus and are lined by cuboidal or flattened epithelial cells, often with an outer layer of smaller cells resembling myoepithelial cells. In some areas the epithelial cells form fine interlacing strands or exist as individual stellate cells which appear to blend into the background stroma. Such cells are considered to be myoepithelial in origin, and tumours in which this pattern predominates are sometimes referred to as myoepitheliomas. Squamous metaplasia, sometimes with prominent keratinization is quite often seen. Pleomorphic adenomas in the minor glands are often more cellular than those in the major glands and are composed of solid sheets and masses of polygonal epithelial cells.

The stromal changes in pleomorphic adenoma are characteristic. Although normal fibrous tissue may be present, more often this becomes hyalinized and apparently structureless. In most tumours there are areas of basophilic, mucoid, or myxochondroid material containing scattered epithelial islands (Fig. 14.32). Individual epithelial cells may become widely separated and embedded in the hyalinized stroma to produce a chondroid appearance resembling hyaline cartilage. Very occasionally the stroma may show areas of true cartilagenous or osseous metaplasia.

Histogenesis

The pleomorphic adenoma is often referred to as a mixed tumour but it is now believed that it is not a true mixed tumour but is of solely epithelial origin and that the connective tissue appearances are secondary. Thus, the term pleomorphic adenoma more aptly describes the lesion as an epithelial tumour of variable appearance.

The particular cell of origin remains uncertain. Immunohistochemical studies have shown that most of the cells are of ductal type but that myoepithelial cells may also be present and

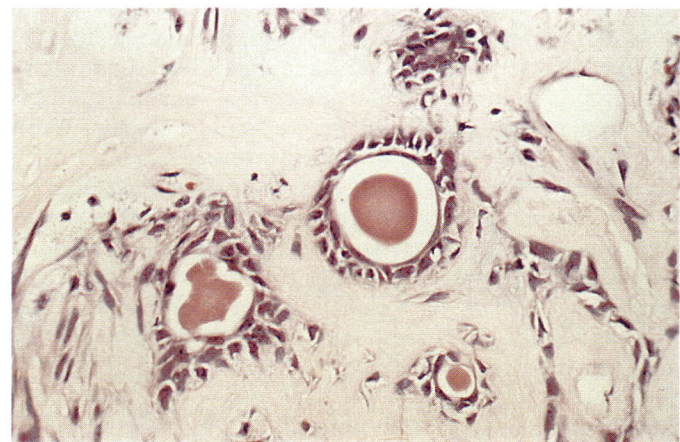

Fig. 14.31 Pleomorphic adenoma. The epithelial cells are arranged in strands and duct-like structures and are embedded in an amorphous mucoid stroma.

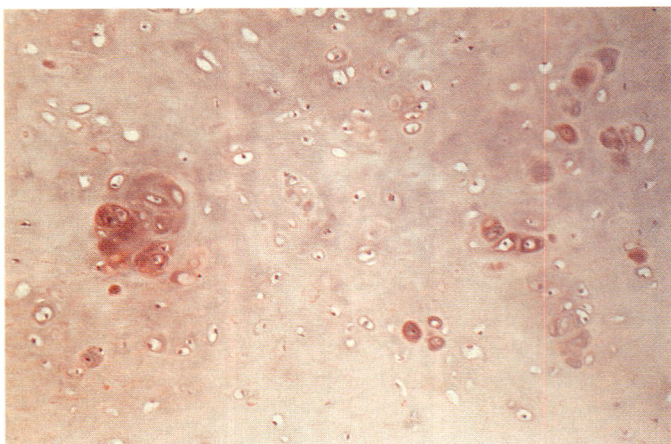

Fig. 14.32 Pleomorphic adenoma. The stroma may be mucoid or myxoid with few stellate cells. Centrally the cells are surrounded by a clear zone imparting a chondroid appearance.

in some tumours may predominate. Such findings would support an origin from intercalated duct cells, which are believed to act as reserve cells for ductal and myoepithelial cells. It is believed that the myoepithelial cells that are often found in mucoid areas may undergo a degree of mesenchymal differentiation and be responsible for the stromal appearances. Thus the presence of two cell types in varying proportions may explain the degree of histological diversity and results in a spectrum of appearances between monomorphic ductal tumours at one end and myoepitheliomas at the other. The modifying role of the myoepithelial cell is supported by the observation that the pancreas, which contains similar acinar and ductal cells but no myoepithelial cells, does not show such a diversity of neoplasms as the salivary glands.

Behaviour and prognosis

The pleomorphic adenoma is a benign tumour but has a reputation for recurrence. In early reports recurrence rates were of the order of 25–50 per cent and were probably due to continued growth of tumour nodules left behind after inadequate enucleation. Unlike primary tumours, recurrent tumours are often multifocal in their growth pattern and are notoriously difficult to remove, often resulting in repeated recurrences over many years with progressively more difficult and disfiguring surgery. For this reason the treatment of choice is adequate excision with a surround of normal tissue at the first operation. A small number of pleomorphic adenomas, between 1 and 5 per cent, may undergo malignant change and contain areas histologically identifiable as carcinoma. Carcinoma in pleomorphic adenoma will be discussed later.

Adenolymphoma (Warthin tumour)

This lesion comprises about 10 per cent of all salivary gland tumours. It is found almost exclusively in the parotid gland and arises most often in the sixth and seventh decades, with a mean

age of about 63. Early reports have suggested that over 90 per cent occur in males but more recent studies suggest a male:female ratio of about 2:1. The tumour presents as a slow-growing painless mass in the lower pole of the parotid. Unlike the pleomorphic adenoma the adenolymphoma is usually soft and cystic and in about 10 per cent of cases may be bilateral.

Pathology

Histologically the adenolymphoma is characterized by epithelial cells and normal lymphoid tissue (Fig. 14.33). Typically it is composed of numerous cystic spaces containing papillary ingrowths and lined by epithelium in a double layer of tall columnar cells and a basal layer of cuboidal cells. These have abundant eosinophilic granular cytoplasm and resemble oncocytes. The stroma of the tumour represents about 50 per cent of the total mass and is composed of well-organized lymphoid tissue with normal follicles and germinal centres. Long-standing tumours may lack a prominent lymphoid stroma due to progressive growth of the adenomatous component. Adenolymphomas are susceptible to infection and some tumours may show abscess formation. Fibrosis of the stroma and necrosis secondary to infarction may also be seen.

Histogenesis

The origin of the adenolymphoma is uncertain, but the juxtaposition of epithelial cells and lymphoid tissue suggests that it may arise within normal lymphoid tissue. Lymph nodes are often found within the parotid gland and they frequently contain salivary duct elements. The epithelium of the tumour resembles oncocytic change in striated ducts and it seems likely that most adenolymphomas arise from heterotopic ducts within the intraparotid lymph nodes.

Behaviour and prognosis

The adenolymphoma is benign, and adequate excision is curative. Recurrences have been noted occasionally but malignant change is exceedingly rare.

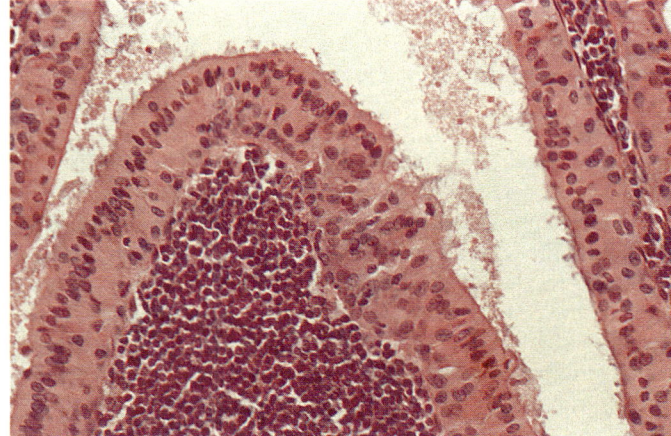

Fig. 14.33 Adenolymphoma (Warthin tumour). Cystic spaces are lined by a double layer of oncocytes supported by a dense lymphoid stroma.

Oncocytoma

The oncocytoma, or oxyphilic adenoma, comprises about 1 per cent of salivary tumours and usually presents as a painless swelling in the parotid gland. It is composed of columns and rows of large polygonal epithelial cells, which are identical to the oncocytes found in normal ageing salivary glands. It is a benign tumour which rarely recurs following adequate excision.

Other types of adenoma

These neoplasms share the features of benign behaviour and a uniform epithelial pattern (Fig. 14.34) and comprise 10–15 per cent of tumours. They are classified according to the cell type or by the predominant histological pattern and a number of tumours, including the basal cell adenoma, canalicular adenoma and sebaceous adenoma are recognized. The myoepithelioma is a tumour composed entirely of myoepithelial cells with a clear, spindle or plasmacytoid appearance. Similar cells are seen in pleomorphic adenoma and some regard the two tumours to be related. However, until the exact behaviour of myoepithelioma is established it is best regarded as a separate entity.

Mucoepidermoid carcinoma

Mucoepidermoid carcinomas comprise about 5 per cent of all salivary gland tumours and are the third most common type of minor gland tumour. Most lesions present in the parotid but the palate, alveolar ridges, and retromolar regions are frequent intra-oral sites. About 2 per cent of mucoepidermoid carcinomas have been reported to occur within the facial bones, most often in the molar region of the mandible. They can occur at any age but most arise in middle-age with a mean in the fifth decade. All mucoepidermoid carcinomas have a malignant potential but most present clinically like a benign lesion with a long history of a slow-growing painless mass. High grade lesions may be of rapid onset with pain, ulceration, and nerve paralysis, and may be accompanied by lymph node or distant metastases.

Pathology

The mucoepidermoid carcinoma is composed of two main cell types; mucus-secreting cells and epidermoid cells (Fig. 14.35). These are present in varying proportions but in most tumours, which are of low-grade malignancy, about half are mucus secreting. The mucous cells may be arranged in groups or clumps among the epidermoid cells but frequently they line cystic spaces. Epidermoid cells may also line the cysts but are more often found in solid sheets and masses. They are of squamous type with clearly visible intercellular bridges and may show keratinization. Occasional tumours contain many cells with abundant clear cytoplasm which does not contain mucus but appears to be distended with glycogen. These cells may predominate to produce the well-recognized clear cell variant.

In tumours of high-grade malignancy the cells are predominantly of the epidermoid type with few mucous cells and little cyst formation. There is often histological evidence of malignancy including nuclear and cellular pleomorphism, infiltrative growth, and invasion of lymphatics.

Histogenesis

Mucoepidermoid carcinomas are considered to arise from a reserve cell associated with the extralobular excretory ducts. Intra-osseous tumours may arise from salivary epithelium within a lingual salivary gland depression, but the origin of true intra-osseous lesions, surrounded by intact cortical plates, remains speculative. They may arise from salivary or oral epithelium entrapped during development, or it is possible that they arise from odontogenic epithelium.

Behaviour and prognosis

All mucoepidermoid carcinomas have a malignant potential

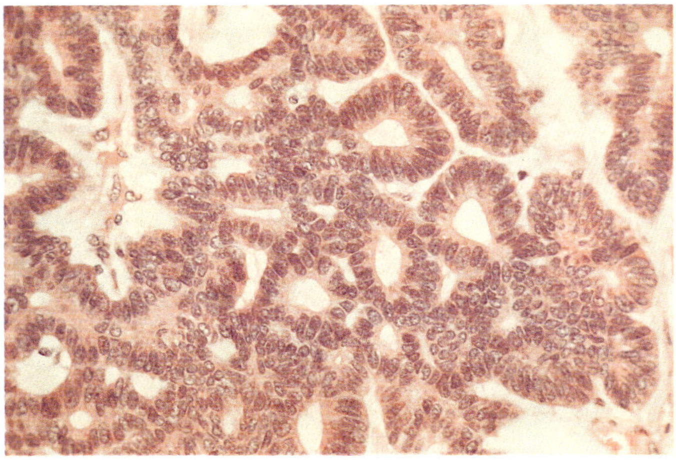

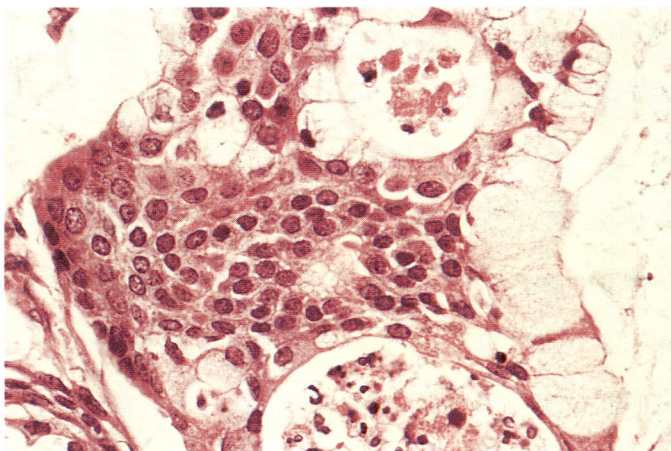

Fig. 14.34 Basal cell adenoma. The tumour is characterized by regular epithelial cells arranged in a uniform pattern throughout the lesion.

Fig. 14.35 Mucoepidermoid tumour. Epidermoid cells surround groups of mucous cells, which are also seen lining a cystic space.

and most authorities no longer use the term mucoepidermoid tumour. Overall, for all grades of tumour, about 10 per cent show lymph node or distant metastases and the five-year survival is 90 per cent or more. Well-differentiated tumours, which comprise about 65 per cent of the total, rarely metastasize and have a 100 per cent cure rate. For high-grade tumours regional lymph nodes may be involved in two-thirds of cases and distant metastases are seen in one-third. The five-year survival rate for these tumours is about 25 per cent.

Acinic cell carcinoma

This rare tumour arises almost exclusively in the parotid gland and is seen after middle age with a mean in the sixth decade. It may present in a similar fashion to pleomorphic adenoma as a slow-growing, painless swelling, but like the mucoepidermoid carcinoma some behave in a malignant fashion and occasional lesions present with pain and rapid growth.

Pathology

They are firm, solid tumours which are usually well encapsulated and rarely show cystic change. Histologically they are composed of polyhedral basophilic cells, similar in appearance to normal serous acinar cells. They may contain secretory granules but often these are not conspicuous and occasionally the cytoplasm may be completely clear. The cells are arranged in sheets or small clumps resembling acini. Ducts are not a feature, although primitive intercalated duct-like cells and spaces filled with secretion from the tumour cells may be seen. There is a fine, scanty fibrous stroma, and lymphoid tissue is sometimes present.

Histogenesis

The acinic cell carcinoma is presumed to arise from the intercalated duct reserve cell, since it is this cell which gives rise to normal acini.

Behaviour and prognosis

Overall about 10 per cent of lesions metastasize, resulting in a five-year survival of about 90 per cent. Local recurrence occurs in up to 20 per cent of cases and can be avoided by wide excision at the primary operation, which results in a significantly better prognosis.

Adenoid cystic carcinoma

This is one of the most common malignant tumours of the salivary glands and comprises 5 per cent of major gland lesions and up to 15 per cent of minor gland lesions. In the submandibular gland it is the second most frequent tumour after pleomorphic adenoma. Intra-orally the most frequent site is the palate, followed by the upper lip and buccal mucosa. Adenoid cystic carcinomas usually present after middle-age and often have a long history of a slowly growing, painless swelling. Eventually pain, ulceration, and infiltration of local tissues, including bone, supervene. Nerve infiltration, late metastases, and recurrence are also particular features of this tumour.

Pathology

The tumour is usually solid on section and infiltration of adjacent structures is often a prominent feature. It is composed of two cell types; duct cells, which are cuboidal or polyhedral with eosinophilic cytoplasm, and small, darkly staining myoepithelial cells. These are present in varying proportions and form three recognizable patterns. The most frequent and characteristic pattern is the cribriform or glandular type, consisting of cell masses containing cyst-like spaces filled with PAS-positive mucoid material (Fig. 14.36). The cells are mainly of the myoepithelial type and form a system of cystic spaces resembling a mass of intertwining cylinders, giving the tumour its alternative name of cylindroma. Occasional duct-like structures may be seen which are lined by duct cells with an outer layer of myoepithelial cells. The second pattern is the tubular type, which may also have cribriform areas but contains tubules lined by a multilayer of cuboidal duct cells surrounded by a hyaline stroma. Finally, some tumours may be solid or basaloid and are composed of solid sheets and cords of small, darkly staining epithelial cells containing small areas of necrosis. In all types mitoses and cellular atypia are not usually prominent and the stroma is usually scanty and fibrous, although hyalinization and mucoid changes may be seen.

Histogenesis

Immunocytochemical studies have confirmed the similarity of the cells in adenoid cystic carcinoma to normal intercalated ducts and myoepithelial cells. In this respect it is similar to the pleomorphic adenoma and would appear to arise from the intercalated duct reserve cells.

Behaviour and prognosis

The adenoid cystic carcinoma is a malignant tumour which infiltrates, invades, and metastasizes. Typically, in 50 per cent of cases the tumour exhibits late blood-borne metastases to

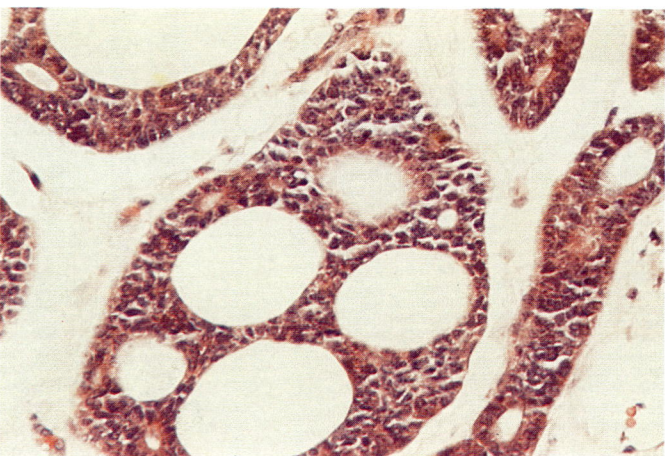

Fig. 14.36 Adenoid cystic carcinoma. Collections of small, darkly staining epithelial cells show the cribriform pattern characteristic of this tumour.

lungs, bones, liver, and brain. Regional lymph node involvement is less common but infiltration of adjacent structures, including bone and nerves (Fig. 14.37), is characteristic and results in frequent local recurrences. The histological appearances may be a good guide to the behaviour. The solid type has the highest incidence of metastases and a five-year survival of about 50 per cent, whereas in the glandular tubular types the five-year survival is of the order of 100 per cent. For all types the five-year survival is about 70 per cent but this lesion has a typically long course and survival drops to about 30 per cent after 15 years and 15 per cent after 20 years.

Carcinoma in pleomorphic adenoma

Carcinoma can arise in a pre-existing pleomorphic adenoma and is often referred to as a malignant mixed tumour. Usually the underlying pleomorphic adenoma has undergone one or more recurrences, but in a minority of cases they occur in a large, long-standing lesion not previously operated on. The incidence of malignant change in pleomorphic adenomas is estimated at about 5 per cent but this increases significantly in recurrent and older lesions. The concept of pleomorphic adenoma being a totally benign lesion should be held with caution and early and adequate surgery to the primary growth is always the treatment of choice. The average age of patients with a malignant lesion is about 65 years, which is 20 years later than pleomorphic adenoma. It typically presents as sudden and rapid growth in a previously slow-growing mass and may be accompanied by pain, ulceration, and nerve involvement.

Microscopically the tumour shows areas of typical pleomorphic adenoma which are partially, or almost totally, replaced by a histologically identifiable carcinoma. Usually this is an adenocarcinoma or undifferentiated carcinoma but mucoepidermoid carcinoma, adenoid cystic carcinoma, or squamous cell carcinoma may also be seen. The prognosis for patients with a carcinoma arising in a pleomorphic adenoma is poor, with an overall five-year survival of less than 25 per cent. At least 50 per cent of patients develop regional lymph node metastases and about 20 per cent have lung involvement. The metastases have the histological features of the carcinoma and do not show features of the underlying pleomorphic adenoma.

As well as carcinoma arising in pleomorphic adenoma, some lesions with the varied histological features of pleomorphic adenoma appear to be malignant from the outset. There is also a very rare tumour referred to as a true malignant mixed tumour, or carcinosarcoma, which has features of carcinoma and chondrosarcoma and appears also to arise from a pre-existing pleomorphic adenoma.

Other types of carcinoma

Many other types of carcinoma may arise in the salivary glands. The most frequently encountered are adenocarcinomas, squamous cell carcinomas, and undifferentiated carcinomas. Typically, they are of short duration, and pain, nerve involvement, and regional lymph node metastases may be present. The prognosis is poor, with an overall five-year survival between 25 per cent and 50 per cent. In addition to these well-recognized entities there are a number of rare carcinomas, including the epithelial-myoepithelial carcinoma (clear cell carcinoma), the polymorphous low-grade adenocarcinoma and malignant lymphoepithelial lesion. This latter is very rare but must be distinguished from lymphoepithelial lesion which is a distinct entity. The malignant lymphoepithelial lesion is found in the parotid gland and is composed of islands of anaplastic carcinoma embedded in a dense lymphoid stroma. Histologically it resembles nasopharyngeal carcinoma and has been termed undifferentiated carcinoma with lymphoid stroma in the new classification.

Non-epithelial tumours

Mesenchymal tumours arising in the salivary glands are rare, but when they occur the pathology is similar to that seen at other sites. In children haemangiomas are the most common salivary gland tumour and comprise up to 50 per cent of the total.

Lymphomas, both Hodgkin's and non-Hodgkin's, may arise within the lymph nodes associated with the parotid or submandibular glands or may be extranodal lymphomas within the gland itself. About 5 per cent of all extranodal lymphomas affect the salivary glands, and within the head and neck up to half of lymphomas arise within the salivary glands. Lymphomas may also be a complication of lymphoepithelial lesion, whether alone or in association with Sjögren's syndrome.

Metastatic lesions are rarely seen in the salivary glands, but when they do occur they are most often from a primary squamous cell carcinoma or malignant melanoma situated elsewhere in the head and neck. Rare cases of renal cell carcinoma have been described in the parotid gland.

Lymphoepithelial lesions

Lymphoepithelial lesions can be considered as a spectrum of clinicopathological entities characterized by persistant salivary

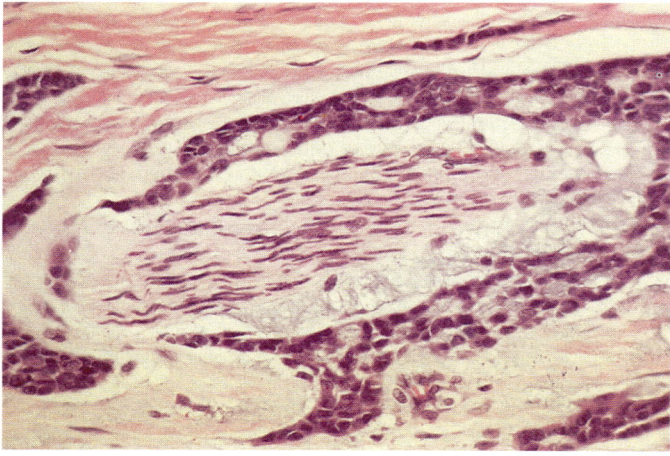

Fig. 14.37 Adenoid cystic carcinoma. A common feature of this tumour is perineural infiltration.

gland enlargement. The normal salivary gland structure is replaced by a dense lymphocytic infiltrate containing islands of proliferating epithelial cells. About 50 per cent of cases are associated with Sjögren's syndrome, but the remainder occur as isolated lesions without xerostomia or evidence of an auto-immune disease. Thus, although the lesions are histologically identical, lymphoepithelial lesion and Sjögren's syndrome can be considered as separate clinicopathological entities. Some authors, however, continue to use the terms synonymously and fail to differentiate between the two groups. Other terms used for this lesion include myoepithelial sialadenitis (MESA), benign lymphoepithelial lesion, auto-immune sialadenitis and Mikulicz's disease. This latter term should not be used since it may be confused with the syndrome of the same name.

Lymphoepithelial lesions, including those associated with Sjögren's syndrome, are usually seen in the parotid gland and comprise about 1.5 per cent of major gland tumours. Over 80 per cent of patients are female and most cases arise in the fifth or sixth decades. The parotid gland enlargement is typically soft and painless and may be bilateral. Histologically the affected glands show maintenance of the normal lobular architecture but are diffusely infiltrated by lymphoid tissue with total loss of acini. The ductal epithelium proliferates to form irregular masses of polyhedral cells embedded in a hyalinized stroma and infiltrated by lymphocytes (Fig. 14.38). These are usually referred to as epimyoepithelial islands but recent ultrastructural and immunohistochemical studies have shown them to be composed mainly of duct cells with few myoepithelial cells. The hyalinized areas are composed of basement membrane material.

The nature of the lesion remains uncertain but it is thought to represent a hyperproliferation or reactive hyperplasia of salivary lymphoid tissue. In the cases associated with Sjögren's syndrome the stimulus may be auto-immune but the pathogenesis of the localized lesions remains speculative. Immunohistochemical studies have shown that some lesions contain areas of monoclonal B-cell proliferation and it is thought that they may be low-grade localized lymphomas of mucosa-associated lymphoid tissue similar to those found in the gut. About 20 per cent of lymphoepithelial lesions progress to frank malignant lymphoma, and hence the designation of the lesions as benign is inappropriate (Falzon and Isaacson 1991). The lymphomas are almost exclusively non-Hodgkin's B-cell lymphomas (see Section 24.5). Risk factors and indicators of malignancy include unilateral gland involvement, rapid increase in swelling, and lymphadenopathy. Patients with evidence of an auto-immune disease are also at risk, and about 5–7 per cent of patients with Sjögren's syndrome develop lymphomas.

Sialosis

This is a benign, non-inflammatory, non-neoplastic bilateral swelling of the parotid glands. It presents as a slowly enlarging, soft, painless mass which is characterized histologically by hypertrophy of the serous acinar cells. Salivary scintiscanning shows an increased uptake of radioisotope and is useful in the differential diagnosis from lymphoepithelial lesion in which the uptake is reduced. The cause of sialosis is unknown but it is associated with a number of conditions including diabetes, alcoholic cirrhosis, protein deficiencies, and hormonal disturbances. It can also be induced by certain drugs, including phenylbutazone, iodine-containing compounds, some antibiotics, and adrenergic drugs. It is a completely benign condition and no treatment is necessary.

Oncocytosis

Oncocytosis refers to a unilateral enlargement of the parotid gland due to diffuse oncocytic metaplasia of both ducts and acini. It is very rare and appears to be due to hyperplasia of the oncocytes which are seen as a normal age change.

14.3.8 Bibliography

Batsakis, J. G. (1979). *Tumours of the head and neck* (2nd edn). Williams and Wilkins, Baltimore.

Eveson, J. W. and Cawson, R. A. (1985). Salivary gland tumours. A review of 2410 cases with particular reference to histological types, site, age and sex distribution. *Journal of Pathology* **146**, 51–8.

Falzon, M. and Isaacson, P. G. (1991). The natural history of benign lymphoepithelial lesion of the salivary gland in which there is a monoclonal population of B cells. *The American Journal of Surgical Pathology* **15**, 59–65.

Henk, J. M. and Langdon, J. D. (1985). *Malignant tumours of the oral cavity*. Edward Arnold, London.

Manthorpe, R. and Prause, J. U. (eds) (1986). Proceedings of the 1st International seminar on Sjögren's Syndrome 1986. *Scandinavian Journal of Rheumatology*, Suppl. 61.

Mason, D. K. and Chisholm, D. M. (1975). *Salivary glands in health and disease*. W. B. Saunders, London.

Nair, P. N. R. and Schroeder, H. E. (1986). Duct-associated lymphoid tissue (DALT) of minor salivary glands and mucosal immunity. *Immunology* **57**, 171–80.

Seifert, G., Meihlke, A., Haubrich, J., and Chilla, R. (1986). *Diseases of the salivary glands*. Georg Thieme Verlag, Stuttgart.

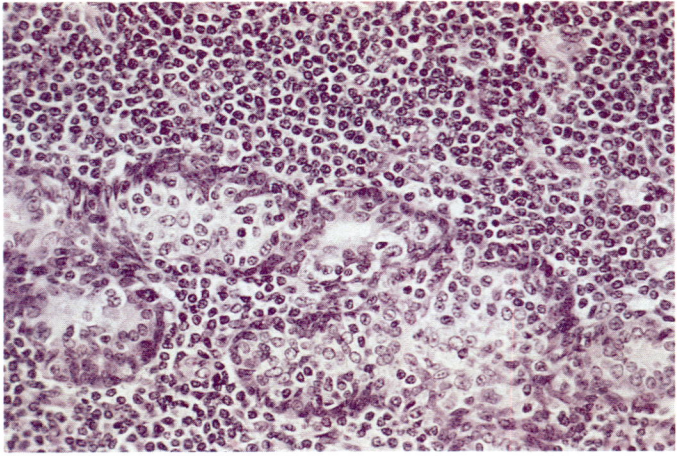

Fig. 14.38 Lymphoepithelial lesion. Proliferating islands of epithelial cells are surrounded and infiltrated by a dense lymphoid stroma.

Seifert, G., Brocheriou, C., Cardesa, A., and Eveson, J. W. (1990). WHO international histological classification of tumours: tentative histological classification of salivary gland tumours. *Pathological Research Practice* **186**, 555–81.

Thackray, A. C. and Lucas, R. B. (1974). *Tumours of the major salivary glands. Atlas of tumour pathology* (2nd series), Fascicle 10. Armed Forces Institute of Pathology, Washington, DC.

Thackray, A. C. and Sobin, L. H. (1972). *International histological typing of tumours. Histological typing of salivary gland tumours.* WHO, Geneva.

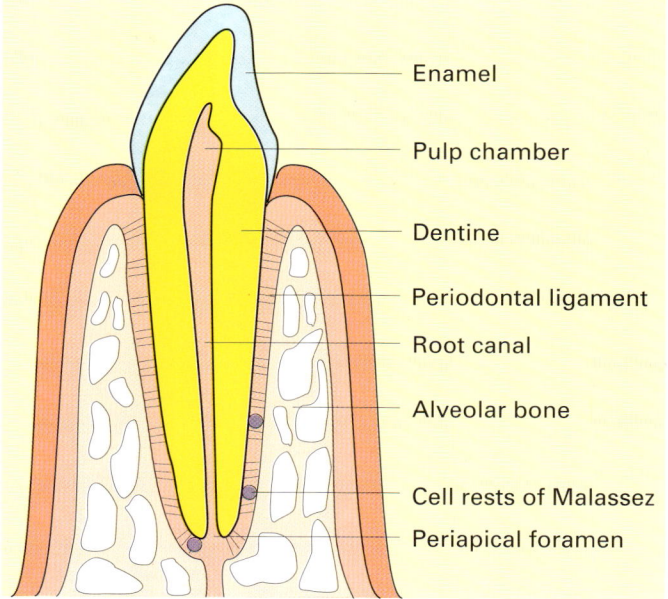

14.4   The jaws

S. Tinkler

14.4.1   Normal structure and function

The jaws are adapted anatomically for mastication. Movement of the horseshoe shaped mandible in relation to the maxilla is made via bilateral articulations at the tempero-mandibular joints and contact is made through the teeth which are borne in the alveolar processes. Dense compact bone covers the surface of the jaws and lines the tooth sockets, forming a radiodense layer or lamina dura which may be disrupted by inflammatory or neoplastic processes. The compact bone surrounds an inner supporting network of trabecular or spongy bone permeated by marrow spaces.

The teeth are maintained in their sockets by the periodontal ligament, a highly specialized collagenous connective tissue connecting the cementum covering the root surface to the alveolar bone (Fig. 14.39).

The nerve and blood supply for the teeth is carried via neuro-vascular bundles which run through the bone and pass into each tooth through a foramen usually located at the root apex, although supplementary foramina may occur at any point of the root surface. These foramina provide a ready pathway by which infection can spread from tooth to bone, and the peri-apical area is a common site for inflammatory phenomena.

Many of the cystic and neoplastic lesions involving the jaws result from aberrations of the dental tissues and are thus unique to the area. In addition, many of the processes occurring in tooth formation are reflected in the pathogenesis of these lesions. For this reason a basic knowledge of tooth development is essential in order to appreciate the pathology of this region.

Tooth development involves a complex series of tissue inter-actions that lead to production of the dental hard and soft tissues, and *in vivo* and *in vitro* studies involving recombination and manipulation of the various tissues have provided powerful models for studying epithelial–mesenchymal interactions. The sequential nature of morphodifferentiation and histodifferentiation ensures that aberration of a single step is likely to have a

Fig. 14.39 The tooth is held in its socket in the alveolar bone by a series of collagenous fibres known as the periodontal ligament. The blood and nerve supply of the tooth gain access by the periapical foramen. Sometimes subsidiary lateral foramina may also be present. Infection of the pulp, often resulting from dental caries, sometimes spreads through the root foramina to affect the deeper tissues of the jaws and periapical inflammation is a common occurrence. Epithelial remnants, known as the cell rests of Malassez present in the periodontal tissues may be stimulated into proliferation by inflammation and give rise to dental cysts.

profound effect on tooth development. An outline of normal tooth development is provided in Fig. 14.40.

The epithelium giving rise to cysts and neoplasms can arise from any point of development and the pathogenesis of some types of lesion is undisputed. For example, it is accepted that the dental follicle and reduced enamel epithelium give rise to the follicular cyst, and the cell rests of Malassez are particularly important in that they give rise to radicular cysts, which are very common. In contrast, the origin of other lesions is often more obscure. Some cysts and tumours may arise from dental lamina rests or reduced enamel epithelium and sometimes a congenitally missing tooth is replaced by a lesion, suggesting development from an aberrant tooth germ.

14.4.2   Inflammatory conditions of the jaws

Dental caries and periodontal disease are among the commonest diseases affecting man (see Sections 14.5 and 14.6) and spread of infection to the jaws is frequent and in the vast majority of cases the infections are mixed in nature. In addition, specific infections such as syphilis, tuberculosis, and cervicofacial actinomycosis may affect the jaws from time to time. The inflammatory conditions most frequently affecting the jaws, excluding periodontal disease, are outlined below.

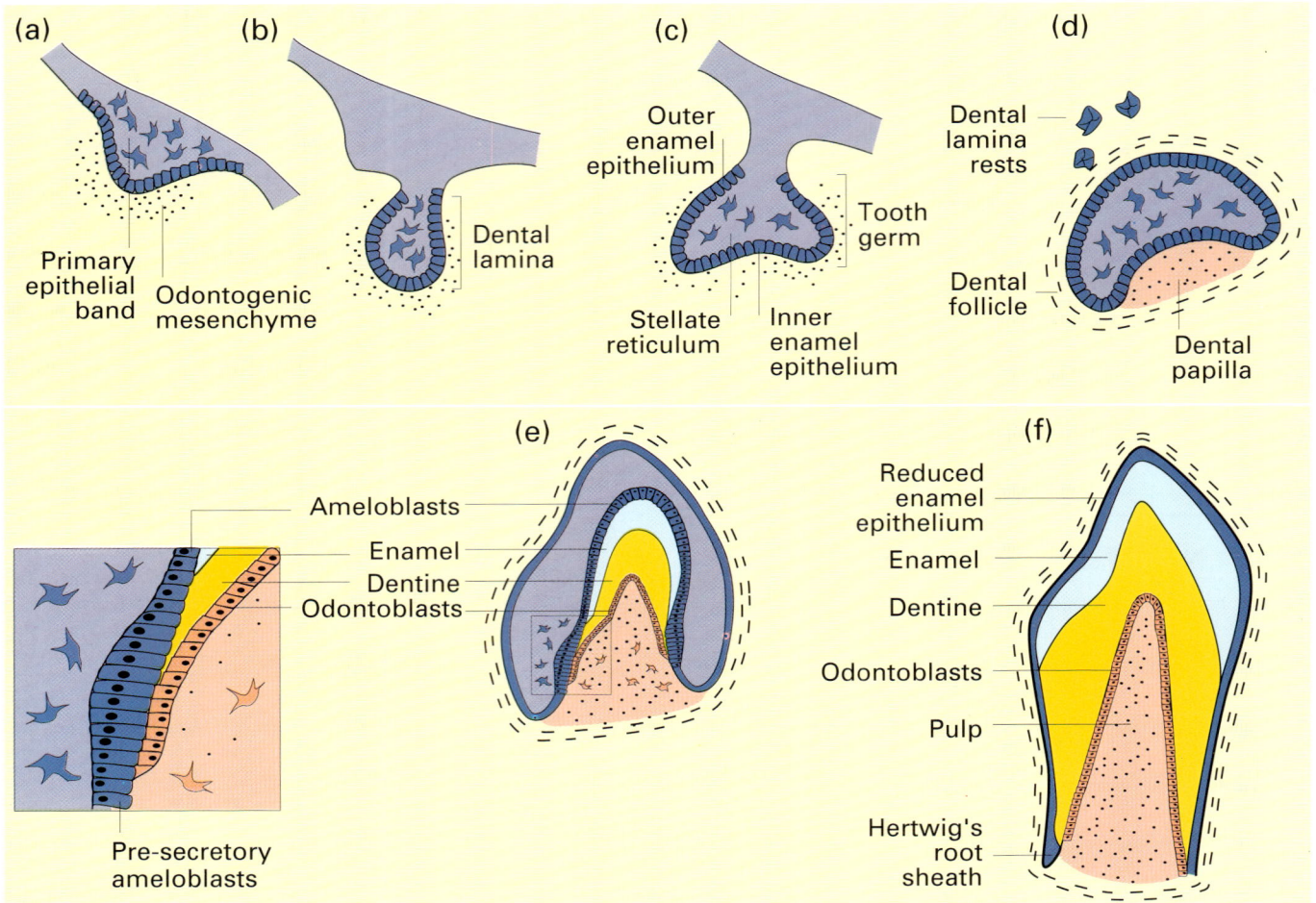

Fig. 14.40 (a) By six weeks *in utero* horseshoe-shaped thickenings within the ectoderm covering the maxillary and mandibular processes give rise to the primary epithelial bands. Development of these bands is dependent on the presence of underlying odontogenic mesenchyme which is of neural crest origin. (b) The primary epithelial bands grow inwards to produce the dental lamina which gives rise to the dentition. Localized proliferation within the dental lamina leads to the formation of a series of epithelial ingrowths, the tooth germs. (c) The tooth germ develops into a cap-shaped structure comprising an inner and outer layer of regular cuboidal epithelial cells, the inner and outer enamel epithelia. Sandwiched between the two layers is the stellate reticulum, which comprises loosely packed epithelial cells with prominent desmasomal junctions. (d) As the tooth germ develops, the odontogenic mesenchyme related to the concavity of the cap becomes densely cellular and forms the dental papilla, which will eventually give rise to the dental pulp. The ondotogenic mesenchyme immediately surrounding the tooth germ is known as the dental follicle and this eventually gives rise to the supporting tissues of the tooth, including cementum and periodontal ligament. (e) Regional differences in growth pressure cause folding of the inner enamel epithelium and the tooth germ becomes bell-shaped. The cuboidal cells of inner enamel epithelium elongate and their nuclei become aligned adjacent to the stellate reticulum (reversed polarity). Concomitantly, subjacent cells in the dental papilla line up below the inner enamel epithelium and differentiate into odontoblasts which start to elaborate dentine matrix. As the odontoblasts lay down matrix they move away from the inner enamel epithelium towards the centre of the papilla leaving behind them cytoplasmic extensions, the odontoblast processes. Dentine formation induces the cells of the inner enamel epithelium to mature into ameloblasts which start to move away from the dentine, secreting enamel matrix as they go. (f) As the ameloblasts move towards the outer enamel epithelium the stellate reticulum atrophies, and eventually the inner and outer enamel epithelia meet and combine to form the reduced enamel epithelium. Once enamel and dentine matrix have been laid down they quickly mineralize. Although enamel is confined to the crown, odontogenic epithelium is required to initiate dentine formation in the root. Cells derived from the reduced enamel epithelium proliferate downwards, forming Hertwig's root sheath which induces dentine formation and maps out the form of the root. Once the root sheath has initiated dentine formation it atrophies leaving behind it isolated epithelial islands, the cell rests of Malassez.

Periapical peridontitis

The commonest causes of inflammation in the supporting tissues are trauma, usually from biting on a newly inserted occlusal restoration that raises the bite, or passage of irritants from the pulp and root canal into the periapical tissues through the apical foramen. The latter is often a sequella to pulpitis and pulp necrosis resulting from dental caries, but another common cause is accidental extrusion of filling material or debris through the apex during endodontic procedures (conservative measures aimed at cleaning and sealing an infected root canal). Although the result of irritation depends on the type and severity of the stimuli and the tissue response, low-grade chronic inflammation is extremely common and usually produces a circumscribed lesion known as a periapical granuloma. These lesions are usually symptomless and often present as an incidental radiographic finding, where they produce a well-defined periapical radiolucency. Histologically they comprise a mass of granulation tissue often surrounded by a fibrous capsule. The granulation tissue is often vascular and haemosiderin deposits are common as are collections of cholesterol crystal clefts with associated foreign body type giant cells. Mixed inflammatory cells, often including large numbers of plasma cells and macrophages, reflect the level of inflammation. Periapical granulomas often contain arcades of hyperplastic squamous epithelium. These originate from the cell rests of Malassez (Fig. 14.39) which are stimulated to proliferate in response to inflammation. Most periapical granulomas will heal following adequate endodontic therapy or extraction; however, those which are neglected may progress to abscess formation or may develop into a radicular cyst.

Dental abscess

A paradontal abscess arises in the supporting tissues at the side of a tooth as a result of periodontal disease (see Section 14.5). The associated tooth is usually vital unless there is concomitant pulp disease. In contrast, periapical abscesses arise from irritants passing through the apical foramina and are thus related to a dead tooth and often arise in a pre-existing periapical granuloma or radicular cyst. In common with periapical granulomas, chronic periapical abscesses are often symptomless and usually present as a chance finding on a dental radiograph. In contrast, acute abscesses are usually painful and may not produce radiographic changes for several days. In both cases treatment involves drainage in conjunction with antibiotics as necessary. Drainage can often be achieved through the root canal so avoiding extraction, however, if pus has spread through bone and periosteum into the adjacent tissues then soft tissue incision may also be necessary. If neglected, most abscesses will drain naturally though a protracted course is likely until the cause (i.e. the offending tooth) is treated; sometimes, however, spreading soft tissue infections or osteomyelitis ensue.

Osteomyelitis

Fortunately osteomyelitis of the jaws is now relatively rare. As with osteomyelitis elsewhere in the skeleton, acute and chronic clinical forms are recognized, although these are often histologically indistinguishable. Osteomyelitis can arise in association with a dental infection or following trauma; however, it is most commonly encountered in the context of osteroradionecrosis following therapeutic radiation of the jaws for malignant disease. Radiation-induced endarteritis obliterans significantly reduces blood supply so impairing viability and lowering tissue resistance to infection. This is compounded by an increased risk of dental infection because radiation damage to the salivary glands reduces salivary flow, impairing natural cleansing and the caries rate is much increased. These patients are extremely prone to developing intractable chronic osteomyelitis with widespread bone necrosis, particularly following oral surgical procedures such as dental extraction. These problems are best anticipated before embarking on a course of radiotherapy and careful dental assessment with necessary treatment should be complete before radiotherapy is started. Once established, osteomyelitis in relation to osteoradionecrosis is extremely difficult to treat as response to antimicrobials is invariably disappointing.

Dry socket or alveolar osteitis occurs fairly commonly after tooth extraction, particularly if the extraction is difficult. It is usually confined to the lamina dura of the socket, parts of which may become necrotic and sequestrate, sometimes as a ring-shaped piece of dead bone. The condition is extremely painful and is usually accompanied by a foul discharge. Treatment is by saline irrigation and packing the socket with one of a variety of antiseptic preparations. Antibiotics do not appear to influence the course and healing is usually slow and uneventful.

Reactive bony change or condensing osteitis is sometimes seen in the jaws in response to low-grade irritation, particularly at the root apex. It produces a radio-opaque appearance on radiography which may persist following extraction. Histology of these lesions often reveals only a bony sclerosis with marrow fibrosis and scattered plasma cells and lymphocytes. A similar but more widespread process is designated 'diffuse sclerosing osteomyelitis'. This condition is more common in the mandibles of elderly patients where it produces a radiographic picture of diffuse sclerosis and patchy radiolucency. Symptoms are mild, and include vague pain and discomfort; however, acute episodes with suppuration and sinus formation may occur. Chronic periodontal disease may provide the source of infection in these patients.

Chronic osteomyelitis associated with proliferative periostitis is also known as Garré's disease. This condition, which usually involves the anterior surface of the tibia, also occurs in the jaws where it is commonest in the mandible of young people. It is a response to low-grade infection, often originating from the first permanent molar, but which spreads through the bone and produces a proliferative response in the adjacent periosteum. This results in a supracortical but subperiosteal mass, comprising trabeculae of woven bone rimmed by osteoblasts.

Neonatal maxillitis is a rare and serious form of acute osteomyelitis, resulting from infection possibly introduced during delivery or feeding. Treatment is urgent and the developing teeth are often destroyed.

Pericoronitis

Inflammation of the dental follicle and soft tissues surrounding a partially erupted tooth is known as periocoronitis. This extremely common condition is most often seen in relation to a partially erupted mandibular third molar. These teeth are the last to erupt and lack of space in the mandible often leads to their impaction and incomplete eruption.

Periocoronitis usually presents with pain and a bad taste. The overlying gum is frequently swollen and may become subject to trauma from the opposing maxillary tooth. Trismus and submandibular lymphadenopathy are often present in more severe cases. Treatment comprises extraction of the opposing maxillary third molar if it is causing trauma, control of infection, followed by extraction of the impacted tooth if normal eruption seems unlikely.

14.4.3   Cysts of the jaws

A cyst is a pathological cavity having fluid, semi-fluid, or gaseous contents and which is not produced by the accumulation of pus. Excluding the various types of soft tissue cysts, jaw cysts fall into two major categories: those possessing and those lacking an epithelial lining. Lesions in the latter group include the solitary bone cyst and the aneurysmal bone cyst. These lesions are rare in the jaws and do not differ significantly from when they occur at other sites. In contrast to the non-epithelial-lined jaw cysts the epithelial-lined variety is both extremely common and unique to the jaws.

Classification of epithelial-lined jaw cysts

Various methods of classifying epithelial-lined jaw cysts have been proposed, but one of the more widely accepted is that of the World Health Organization. However, since this classification was published several new entities have been described while the existence of others has been largely disproved. Main has recently suggested that the WHO classification be updated and it is his revision that is adopted here (see Table 14.6). The WHO classification of jaw cysts is based on the pathogenesis in so far as it designates the two major categories as developmental and inflammatory. The origin of the cystic epithelium is also taken into account and whereas all the inflammatory cysts and some of the developmental cysts are of odontogenic origin the latter category also includes cysts derived from non-odontogenic sources. It used to be thought that the non-odontogenic or so-called fissural cysts were derived from epithelium entrapped in mesenchyme during fusion of the embryonic processes. However, it is now accepted that the embryonic processes disappear as a result of expansile growth in the underlying mesenchyme rather than by their union, and the fissural cysts, including the globulomaxillary and median mandibular cysts, have been largely discredited. One exception to this is the mid-palatal cyst of infants which may arise from epithelium enclaved when the palatal processes combine. The developmental non-odontogenic cysts that are still recognized include the nasopalatine duct cyst which is thought to be derived from epithelium of the oro-nasal ducts, and the nasolabial cyst, which may originate from lacrimal duct epithelium.

Pathogenesis

Although there is a general consensus as to the derivation of cystic epithelium, the processes which initiate cyst formation are less well understood. In the case of the inflammatory jaw cysts initiation can be ascribed to inflammation stimulating epithelial proliferation within granulation tissue. However, inflammation is not a feature in developmental cysts and inception of these lesions remains uncertain. Nevertheless, it seems likely that for both inflammatory and developmental cysts epithelial proliferation gives rise to a mass in which hypoxia causes central necrosis and gives rise to a cavity lined by epithelium. The continued expansion of most cysts is thought to be brought about by a combination of osmosis, inadequate lymphatic drainage, and inflammatory exudation. The fluid in most cysts is hypertonic to tissue fluid and isotope-tracer studies have shown that the cyst wall acts as a semi-permeable membrane which allows fluid to diffuse into the cyst. Continued passage of fluid into the cyst produces increased pressure and leads to compression of the surrounding tissues, resulting in release of inflammatory mediators including bone resorptive factors. Elegant *in vitro* experiments have shown that most cyst walls produce prostaglandins, which are known to mediate bone resorption. Although the above theory goes some way to explaining the pathogenesis of many epithelial jaw cysts, it cannot explain expansion of the odontogenic keratocyst in which the fluid contains little soluble protein. However, autoradiographic studies following *in vitro* cell labelling with tritiated thymidine lesions suggests that in these lesions epithelial proliferation may be responsible for continued growth.

Histopathology

With the exception of the odontogenic keratocyst, the histology of the epithelial-lined jaw cysts is non-specific and conforms to a basic pattern consisting of a membranous connective tissue sac lined by epithelium (Fig. 14.41). However, the histological picture is extremely variable and is strongly influenced by inflammation. The cyst wall may vary from mature uninflamed fibrous tissue to a highly vascular granulation tissue containing large numbers of mixed inflammatory cells. Copious deposits of haemosiderin and collections of spindle-shaped cholesterol crystal clefts with associated foreign body giant cells are a common finding (Fig. 14.41d). The epithelial lining is usually stratified squamous in nature, although both mucous cells and respiratory epithelium are fairly common findings. In uninflamed specimens the epithelium is usually thin and lies on a flat basement membrane; however, when inflammation is a feature, epithelial hyperplasia is common and this may produce either generalized thickening or formation of complex arcades penetrating deeply into the cyst wall. In severely inflamed specimens the epithelium may be destroyed. Occasionally globular or hairpin-shaped eosinophilic lamellated bodies are seen in the epithelium or subepithelial connective tissue (Fig. 14.41e).

Table 14.6 Cysts of the jaws (Main's 1985 revision of the WHO classification)

Classification	Site	Suggested origin	Comments
1. Development			
(a) Odontogenic			
Odontogenic keratocyst	Usually mandibular angle or ramus	Dental lamina or tooth germ	Usually keratinizing. Prominent regular basal cell layer (see text). High recurrence rate
Follicular cyst	Around crown of unerupted tooth	Follicle and reduced enamel epithelium	Common
Eruption cyst	Around crown of unerupted tooth	Follicle and reduced enamel epithelium	Soft tissue analogue of follicular cyst
Lateral periodontal cyst	Periodontal ligament	Dental lamina rests or reduced enamel epithelium	Rare; associated tooth usually vital
Gingival cyst of adults	Gingiva	Dental lamina rests or reduced enamel epithelium	Rare; associated tooth usually vital
Alveolar cyst of infants	Gum pads	Dental lamina	Common, keratinizing and requires no treatment
(b) Non-odontogenic			
Nasopalatine duct cyst	Incisive canal and foramen	Oronasal duct epithelium	Neurovascular bundle often seen in wall; respiratory epithelium often present
Nasolabial cyst	Soft tissues of buccal sulcus adjacent to maxillary canines	Nasolacrimal duct epithelium	Respiratory epithelium often present
Mid-palatal cyst of infants	Midline palate	Epithelium of palatal processes	Common, keratinizing and requiring no treatment
2. Inflammatory			
Radicular cyst	Root apex	Cell rests of Malassez	Very common; associate tooth non-vital
Residual cyst	Edentulous alveolus	Cell rests of Malassez	A radicular cyst persisting after extraction of an associated tooth
Inflammatory lateral periodontal cyst	Periodontal ligament	Cell rests of Malassez	May arise in association with periodontal disease or a non-vital tooth with lateral root canals
Paradontal cyst	Adjacent to partially erupted tooth envolved with pericoronitis	Cell rests of Malassez or reduced enamel epithelium	
Inflammatory	Follicle of unerupted permanent tooth below infected deciduous predecessor	Follicle and reduced enamel epithelium	

These are known as Rushton or hyaline bodies and their origin is disputed. It has been suggested that they arise from breakdown products of extravasated erythrocytes, or alternatively they may be a secretory product of odontogenic epithelium. The fact that these bodies seem to be confined to odontogenic cysts would appear to support the latter contention.

In view of the non-specific histological findings in most cysts, diagnosis is usually impossible without adequate details of the clinical and radiographic findings. Factors such as relationship to, and vitality of, an associated tooth are of paramount importance if diagnostic errors are to be avoided.

Basic details of the different cysts are given in Table 14.7, while the more common and diagnostically important jaw cysts are considered in a little more detail below.

Follicular cyst

The follicular cyst is the commonest of the developmental cysts. As the name implies it forms within a dental follicle and is lined by epithelium derived from the reduced enamel epithelium. The cyst wall always envelops the crown of an unerupted tooth, usually a mandibular third molar, and attaches to the enamel–cement margin. Although these cysts are developmental they are often in continuity with the mouth and inflammation is

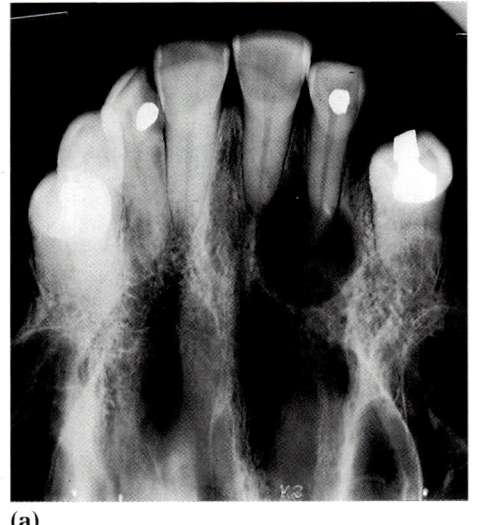

(a)

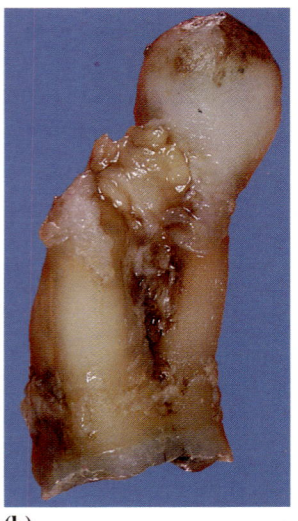

(b)

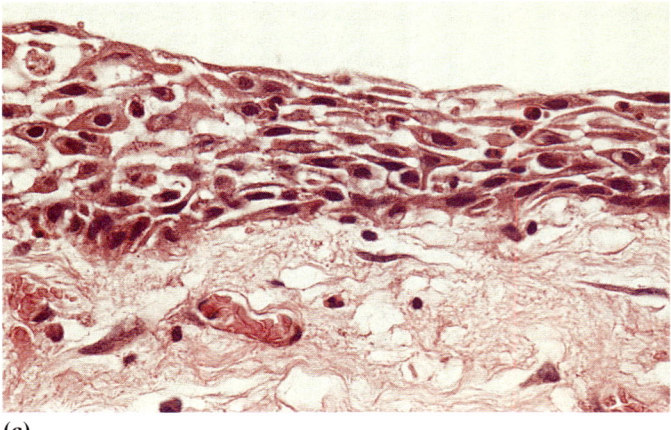

(c)

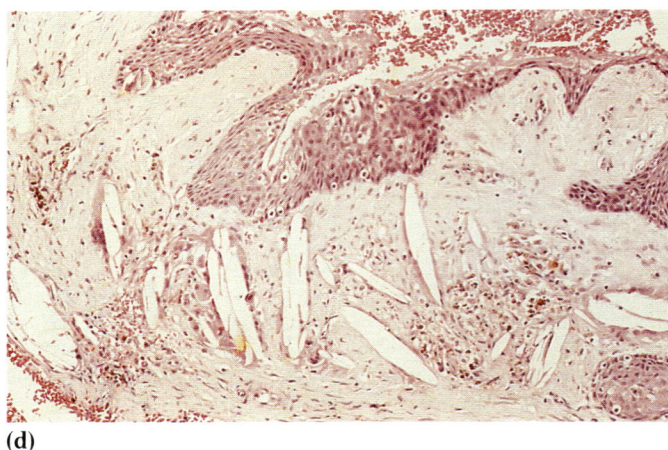

(d)

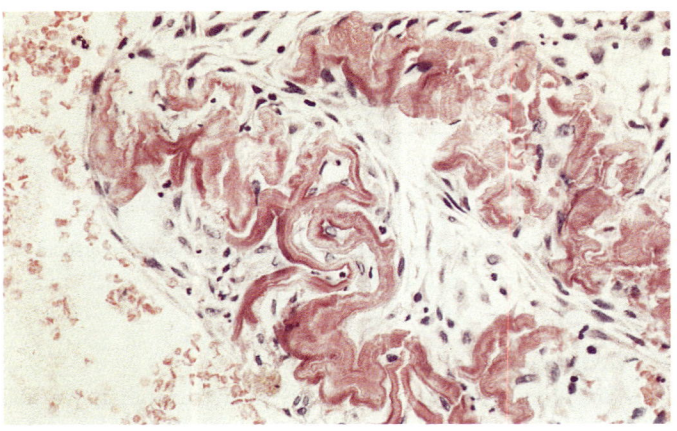

(e)

Fig. 14.41   (a) Radiographic appearance of a radicular cyst associated with the upper right lateral incisor tooth. The radiolucent area is periapical in position and its outline well defined. The tooth shows a filling. These features are not diagnostic but are compatable with a radicular cyst associated with a non-vital tooth. (b) Photograph of an extracted grossly decayed molar tooth with a radicular cyst attached to the periapical area of one root. (c) Photomicrograph of part of the wall of a radicular cyst showing fibrous tissue lined by non-keratinizing stratified squamous epithelium. (d) This radicular cyst wall shows a lining of non-keratinizing stratified squamous epithelium of variable thickness. The fibrous tissue cyst wall contains spindle-shaped cholesterol clefts and deposits of yellow-brown haemosiderin. (e) The epithelial lining of this radicular cyst contains lamellated eosinophilic bodies known as Rushton or hyaline bodies.

Table 14.7 Odontogenic tumours (after Lucas 1984)

Classification	Features
1. Lesions consisting of odontogenic epithelium	
Ameloblastoma	Benign neoplasm consisting of odontogenic epithelium arranged in a follicular or plexiform pattern within a fibrous stroma (see Section 14.4.4)
Adenomatoid odontogenic tumour	Strands or sheets of odontogenic epithelium in a fibrous stroma; tubule-like structures and amorphous calcifications may be present; may be cystic and often associated with an unerupted tooth; benign neoplasm or hamartoma
Calcifying epithelial odontogenic tumour	Sheets of eosinophilic polyhedral cells which often show marked atypia; deposits of amorphous hyaline material have some features of amyloid and show apple-green birefringence when stained with Congo red; this benign neoplasm is sometimes misdiagnosed as carcinoma
Calcifying odontogenic cyst	A benign cystic tumour lined by epithelial cells with indistinct outlines; the epithelial cells may lose their nuclei and undergo keratinization: these are known as ghost cells
Odontogenic carcinoma and malignant ameloblastoma	Rare malignant tumours of odontogenic epithelium
2. Lesions consisting of odontogenic epithelium and mesenchyme	
Ameloblastic fibroma	Cellular fibroblastic tissue containing strands and nests of epithelium resembling those seen in ameloblastoma but more scanty; behaves like an ameloblastoma
Ameloblastic sarcoma	Similar to the ameloblastic fibroma but the mesenchymal element is malignant
3. Lesions consisting of odontogenic epithelium and calcified dental tissues	
Ameloblastic fibro-odontoma	Similar to ameloblastic fibroma but containing enamel and dentine
Odontoameloblastoma	Similar to ameloblastoma but containing enamel and dentine
4. Lesions consisting of calcified dental tissues	
Complex and compound odontome	Mature dental tissues including enamel and dentine arranged haphazardly or as small denticles
Dens invaginatus	An abnormality in tooth morphology resulting from invagination of the inner enamel epithelium
Enalemloma	Isolated deposit of normal enamel on root surface
Dentinoma	Very rare benign tumour comprising deposits of dentine within a fibrous stroma
Cementoma	Subclassified into several types all comprising deposits of cementum within a fibrous stroma; some are benign neoplasms and some are developmental
5. Lesions consisting of odontogenic mesenchyme	
Odontogenic fibroma	Benign neoplasm comprising fibrous tissue resembling that seen in the dental follicle; sometimes contain scattered nests of odontogenic epithelium
Odontogenic myxoma	Similar to the odontogenic fibroma but the connective tissue is myxoid in nature and it behaves more aggressively and can show local invasion

common. Diagnosis depends on both histology and a knowledge of the relationship of the cyst to the tooth.

Odontogenic keratocyst

Although less common than the follicular cyst, the odontogenic keratocyst, also known as the primordial cyst, is of importance because of its high recurrence rate compared with other cysts. It occurs commonly in the mandibular ramus or at the angle of the jaw and, although growth is slow, it is progressive and can lead to extensive bony destruction with expansion (Fig. 14.42a). In contrast to the other types of jaw cyst, odontogenic keratocysts have a specific histological appearance (Fig. 14.42b). The cyst wall comprises loosely folded fibrous tissue while the epithelial–connective tissue junction is characteristically flat. The epithelial lining is thin, usually only 5–8 cell layers thick and, often though not invariably, shows keratinization. The most important diagnostic feature of the odontogenic keratocyst is not, however, related to keratin production, which can sometimes occur in other types of jaw cyst, but is the extremely regular appearance of the basal epithelial cells. These cells are cuboidal or columnar and often show a palisaded appearance. The nuclei are regularly aligned and are often orientated away from the basement membrane.

The presence of inflammation can significantly alter the appearance of odontogenic keratocysts and their distinguishing characteristics can be lost (Fig. 14.42c). In most cases, however, uninflamed areas persist and these retain the characteristic histology so that adequate sampling with careful scrutiny usually ensures correct diagnosis.

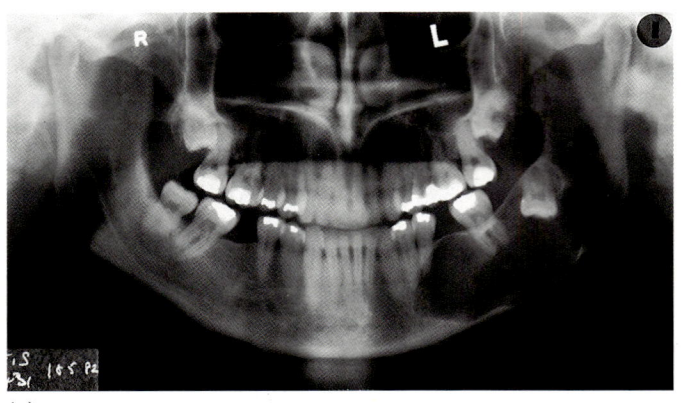

(a)

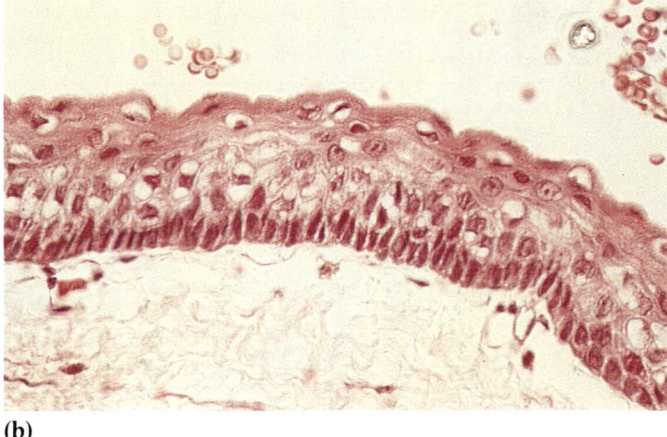

(b)

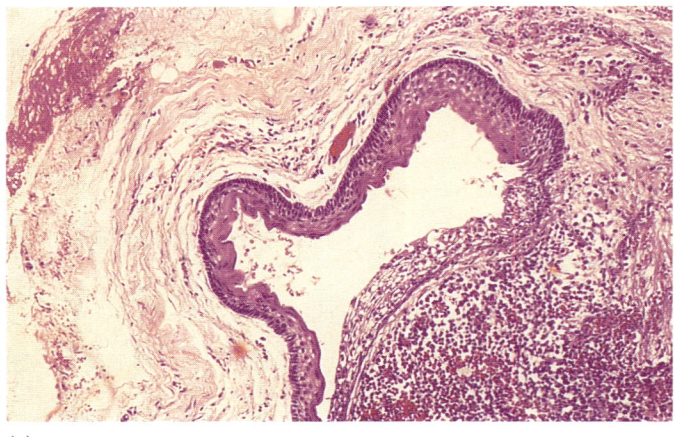

(c)

Fig. 14.42 (a) Radiograph of an odontogenic keratocyst occupying the body and angle of the left mandible and extending into the ramus. This cyst is associated with an unerupted molar tooth and on the radiographic evidence alone reliable diagnosis is impossible as this lesion could equally well be a follicular cyst. Histological examination would allow definitive diagnosis. (b) Photomicrograph of part of the wall of an odontogenic keratocyst showing thin parakeratinizing stratified squamous epithelium lining a fibrous tissue wall. Compare this picture with that of the radicular cyst (Fig. 14.41c) and note the regular palisaded basal cell layer in the odontogenic keratocyst. This is the most reliable feature when distinguishing keratocysts from other types of jaw cysts. (c) This photomicrograph illustrates how the presence of inflammation in the wall of an odontogenic keratocyst alters the lining epithelium so that the characteristic feature of a regular basal cell layer is lost. For this reason diagnosis of inflamed odontogenic keratocysts is often difficult and wide sampling is necessary.

Radicular cyst and other inflammatory cysts

The radicular cyst (Fig. 14.41) is by far the most common jaw cyst. It arises in relation to the apical foramen of a dead tooth and often forms in an apical granuloma (Figs 14.41a,b). Similar cysts may occur more coronally if lateral root canals exist; or inflammatory periodonal disease can be the precipitating factor, in which case the associated tooth is probably vital. The residual cyst is a radicular cyst which persists following removal of the tooth responsible for its formation, while the paradontal cyst is found in association with the crown of a partially erupted tooth involved with pericoronitis, usually a mandibular third molar. Another rare type of inflammatory odontogenic cyst is the inflammatory follicular cyst. This occurs when irritants from an infected deciduous tooth initiates cyst formation in the follicle of its permanent successor in the subjacent jaw.

14.4.4   Tumours of the jaws

The jaws are subject to the same range of tumours as occur elsewhere in the skeleton. In addition, the dental apparatus gives rise to the odontogenic tumours and, as is the case with the odontogenic cysts, an understanding of tooth development is necessary to appreciate the pathology of these lesions (Fig. 14.40). Furthermore, the jaws are also the site of a heterogeneous group of tumours which, while having no obvious odontogenic origin, appear to be confined to the maxilla and mandible.

Odontogenic tumours

These tumours (Table 14.10) comprise a spectrum ranging from developmental anomalies to benign neoplasms and include a minority which are frankly malignant. Their nomenclature and classification are both complex and confusing; however, the most satisfactory system in use at present is probably the scheme used by Lucas. This system (Table 14.10) divides these lesions according to their component tissues, both during their development and when mature, and takes into account the epithelial mesenchymal interactions which play a role in their pathogenesis. The first group of tumours comprise odontogenic epithelium within a fibrous stroma. The epithelium appears to have little effect on the surrounding connective tissue and neither odontoblast induction nor formation of dental hard tissue occurs. The second major category consists of odontogenic epithelium and fibroblastic mesenchyme that resembles dental papilla. The supposition is that the mesenchymal element is partially induced by the odontogenic epithelium, but that development is frozen before odontoblasts differentiate and therefore dental hard tissues do not form. In contrast to this, tumours in the third group show the full developmental sequence and consist of odontogenic epithelium, odontogenic mesenchyme, and dental hard tissues. The next group comprises mainly dental hard tissues, including dentine, enamel, and cementum; however, all that remains of the odontogenic epithelium responsible for their formation are small rests or a little reduced enamel epithelium. In the next group odontogenic epithelium is either absent or exists only as tiny rests, and the bulk of the tumour consists of connective tissue which resembles dental follicle or papilla. Most odontogenic tumours are extremely rare and only the ameloblastoma, which is the most common and diagnostically important, will be discussed in any detail.

Ameloblastoma

This benign neoplasm usually occurs in the mandibular molar region or ramus and presents as an incidental radiographic finding where it produces a uni- or multilocular radiolucency often associated with an unerupted tooth (Fig. 14.43a).

Histologically these tumours comprise islands and cords of odontogenic epithelium within a fibrous stroma (Fig.14.43b,c). Where islands of epithelium predominate the tumour is described as being follicular, whereas when the pattern is one of anastomosing cords the term plexiform is used. The epithelium in ameloblastomas resembles that seen in the tooth germ. The cells at the periphery are cuboidal or low columnar and have their nuclei orientated towards the centre of the follicle (reversed polarity) (Fig. 14.43c). These cells, which are generally regarded as being analogous to pre-secretory ameloblasts, surround more loosely packed epithelial cells with prominent spinous processes which resemble the cells of the stellate reticulum. Several variations within the basic follicular and plexiform pattern are recognized. For example, squamous metaplasia may occur within the epithelial islands and keratin formation is not unusual. Such ameloblastomas are described as acanthomatous. Granular and basal cell types are also described. These different patterns have no influence on behaviour or prognosis. Cystic degeneration is common in ameloblastoma and sometimes a large unilocular cyst forms. When this is associated with an impacted tooth these lesions are easily misdiagnosed as a follicular cyst. In these circumstances thorough sampling of the cyst wall frequently reveals islands of typical ameloblastoma or areas in which the basal epithelial cells are cuboidal or columnar and show reversed polarity.

The ameloblastoma is unencapsulated and is capable of local destruction and invasion. Although there are occasional reports of metastatic spread, these are usually lung deposits which represent seeding following tumour aspiration during surgery. Complete local excision is the treatment of choice.

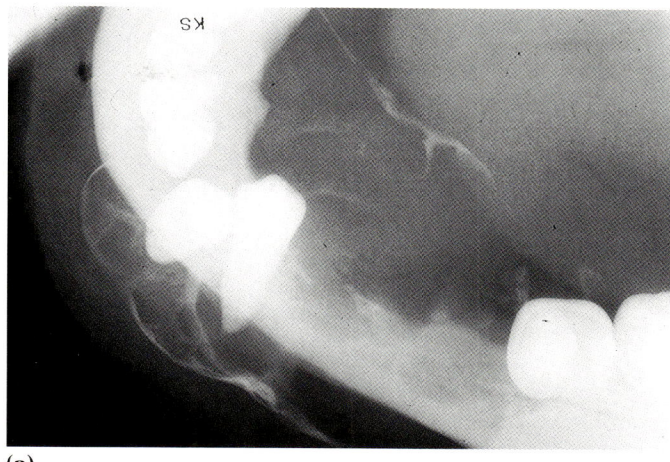

(a)

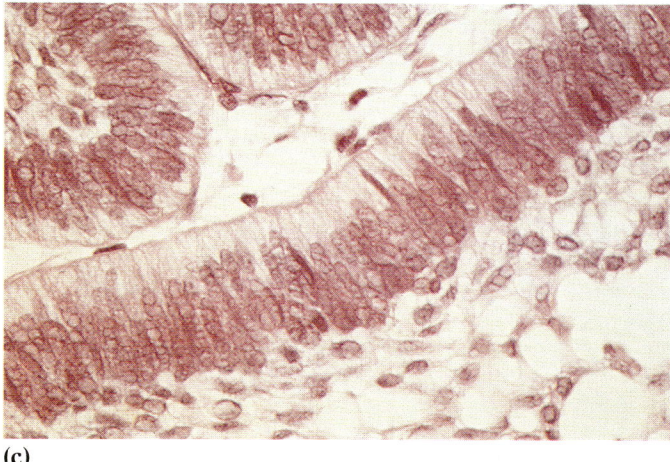

(b)

(c)

Fig. 14.43 (a) Radiograph of a mandibular ameloblastoma, showing the characteristic multilocular soap-bubble appearance of this lesion. (b) Low-power and (c) high-power photomicrographs of a follicular ameloblastoma, showing epithelial islands within a fibrous stroma. The peripheral epithelial cells are cuboidal/columnar with nuclei polarized towards the centre of the islands. These cells resemble the pre-ameloblasts of the tooth germ.

Miscellaneous jaw tumours

Fibro-osseous and giant-cell lesions in the jaws

This rather vague term is used to describe a number of jaw lesions, many of which are not obviously neoplastic or inflammatory in nature. It includes Paget's disease of bone and fibrous dysplasia as well as a number of lesions unique to the jaws. The basic histological pattern in fibrous dysplasia is of a replacement of normal bone by fibrous tissue containing irregular trabeculae of woven bone. The lesions are poorly demarcated and do not 'shell out' at surgery. Other rare jaw lesions are histologically similar to fibrous dysplasia but are circumscribed both radiographically and surgically. Those lesions in which the calcifications appear as trabeculae of woven bone are called ossifying fibroma, whereas those in which ovoid or spherical deposits of cementum-like material predominate are known as cementifying fibroma. Ossifying and cementifying show progressive growth and are regarded by some as benign neoplasms.

Some of the fibro-osseous lesions contain osteoclast-like giant cells and their differential diagnosis is important. The most common is the giant-cell granuloma. This lesion occurs in the tooth-bearing areas where it can present either as an exophytic gingival swelling (giant-cell epulis) (Fig. 14.44a) or as a radiolucent area within the bone (central giant-cell granuloma) (Fig. 14.44b). Microscopically the giant-cell granuloma is very similar to the giant-cell tumour that occurs elsewhere in the skeleton. Both tumours comprise collections of osteoclast-like giant cells within a highly vascular cellular stroma containing plump spindle cells and scanty collagen (Fig. 14.44c). Although it is often impossible to distinguish a giant-cell granuloma from a giant-cell tumour on an individual basis, the former generally contain fewer giant cells and these are less evenly distributed than in the giant-cell tumour. Important clinical differences also exist between these lesions. Although giant-cell granulomas are locally destructive, they follow a benign course and are usually cured by local excision or curettage, even when residual tumour is known to exist. In contrast, a significant number of apparently benign-appearing giant-cell tumours show persistent destructive local growth with frequent recurrences and distant metastases. Because of these differences in behaviour it is important to be aware that unequivocal giant-cell tumours of the jaws are extremely rare and that giant-cell lesions of the jaws are almost always benign.

Another lesion that is indistinguishable histologically from giant-cell granuloma is the brown tumour of hyperparathyroidism, and analysis of the serum biochemistry is obligatory in all giant-cell lesions of the jaws. Plasma calcium is raised significantly only in hyperparathyroidism.

In its early stages cherubism is very similar histologically to giant-cell granuloma. This condition is inherited as an autosomal dominant trait with variable expression. It usually first presents in early childhood as bilateral swellings in the molar and angle region of the mandible. The maxilla may also be affected. Lesions often enlarge rapidly in their initial stages but eventually become static and may regress during puberty and early adulthood. Although early lesions resemble giant-cell

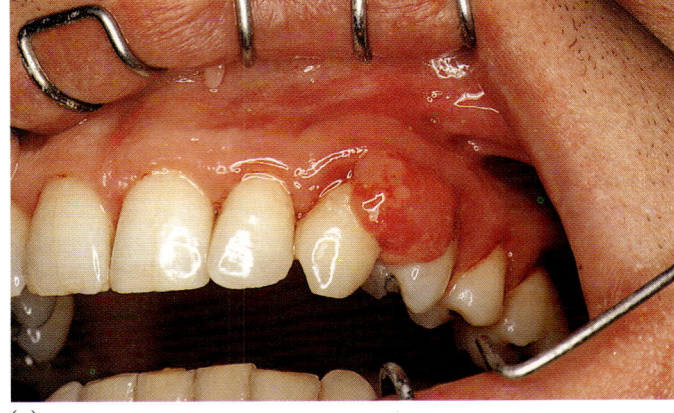

(a)

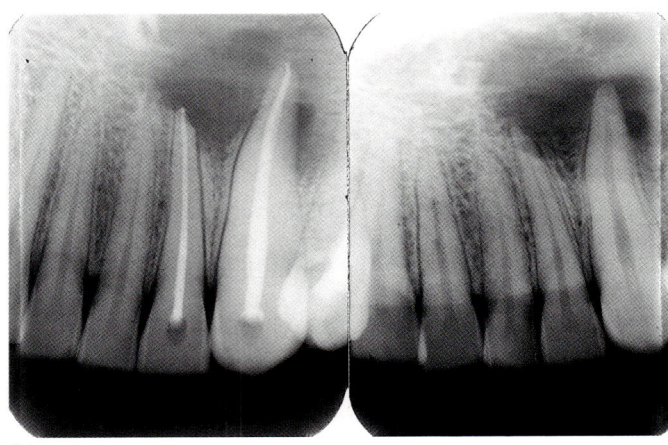

(b)

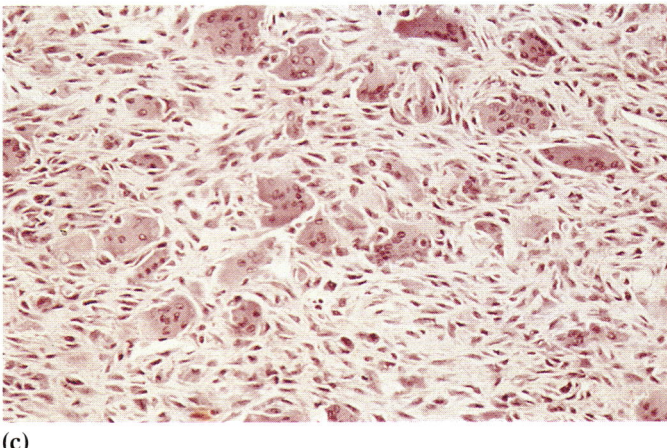

(c)

Fig. 14.44 (a) This haemorrhagic ulcerated gingival swelling between the canine and premolar teeth is a peripheral giant granuloma or giant-cell epulis. (b) Radiographs showing a mandibular radiolucency before (left) and after (right) root canal therapy of the lateral incisor and canine tooth. The lesion failed to resolve after root treatment and histological investigations revealed the lesion to be a central giant-cell granuloma. (c) Photomicrograph of a giant-cell granuloma, showing spindle cells and osteoclast-like giant cells within a vascular delicate connective tissue stroma.

granulomas, with maturation the vascular and giant-cell element diminish and the lesion becomes more fibrous and is eventually replaced by bone.

Tori and exostoses

Bony swellings comprising normal lamellar bone are common in the jaws. Those which are developmental in nature are called tori whereas those that arise in response to irritation are usually referred to as exostoses or enostoses depending on whether they are peripheral or central in location. The torus palatinus occurs in the midline of the hard palate, where it produces a lobulated or nodular ridge extending along the midline. The mandibular torus occurs on the lingual aspect of the mandible below the premolar teeth. These lesions require treatment only if they interfere with dentures.

Pigmented neuroectodermal tumour

This tumour, which is thought to be of neural crest origin, usually presents at birth or during the first year of life as a locally destructive mass in the maxilla, where it may displace developing teeth. The tumour consists of collections of small round cells similar to those seen in neuroblastoma. These cells are arranged in an alveolar pattern within a fibrous stroma. The alveoli are lined by cuboidal cells that elaborate melanin, which imparts a grey-blue colour to the tumour. Although these tumours often show rapid growth and are capable of local destruction, they can be adequately treated by local excision and show little tendency to recur.

Congenital epulis

These tumours are confined to neonates and present as a round or ovoid, sessile or pedunculated swelling, usually in the maxillary incisor region. Microscopically they consist of closely packed large granular cells which resemble those seen in the granular cell myoblastoma. However, ultrastructural and immunocytochemical studies do not support a common histogenesis for these tumours and suggest that granular cell myoblastoma is derived from Schwann cells while congenital epulis may be derived from smooth muscle.

14.4.5   Further reading

Harris, M., Jenkins, M. V., Bennet, A., and Willis, M. R. (1973). Prostaglandin production and bone resorption by dental cysts. *Nature* **245**, 213.

Lucas, R. B. (1984). *Pathology of tumours of the oral tissues* (4th edn). Churchill Livingstone, Edinburgh.

Main, D. M. G. (1985). Epithelial jaw cysts: 10 years of the WHO classification. *Journal of Oral Pathology* **14**, 1–7.

Pindborg, J. J., Kramer, I. R. H., and Torloni, H. (1971). *International histological classification of tumours No 5. Histological typing of odontogenic tumours, jaw cysts and allied lesions.* World Health Organization, Geneva.

Shear, M. (1985). Cysts of the jaws: recent advances. *Journal of Oral Pathology* **14**, 43–59.

14.5   Gingivitis and periodontal disease

D. M. Williams

14.5.1   Introduction

Gingivitis and periodontal disease constitute a group of destructive inflammatory conditions of the supporting structures of the teeth, triggered by the accumulation of dental plaque. Dental plaque comprises aggregations of bacteria embedded in a sticky matrix composed of bacterial products such as polysaccharides, and host products including salivary glycoproteins. It is now clear that plaque accumulation alone is insufficient to account for the disease and the subsequent pattern of destruction is believed to result from the interaction between microbial factors released from the plaque and the host response to them. Variation in the level of the host response between individuals and differences in microbial factors produced by plaque organisms lead to the development of recognizably different clinical patterns of disease.

14.5.2   Clinical manifestations

Inflammation may be longstanding and restricted to the gingival margin, producing a state known as chronic marginal gingivitis. This condition, which is widespread and painless, is characterized by swelling and redness of the marginal gingivae, associated with gingival bleeding, either spontaneously or in response to mild trauma (see Fig. 14.45). It is usually a stable condition that does not progress further in most individuals.

Destruction of the periodontal ligament and alveolar bone is less widespread than chronic marginal gingivitis; severe

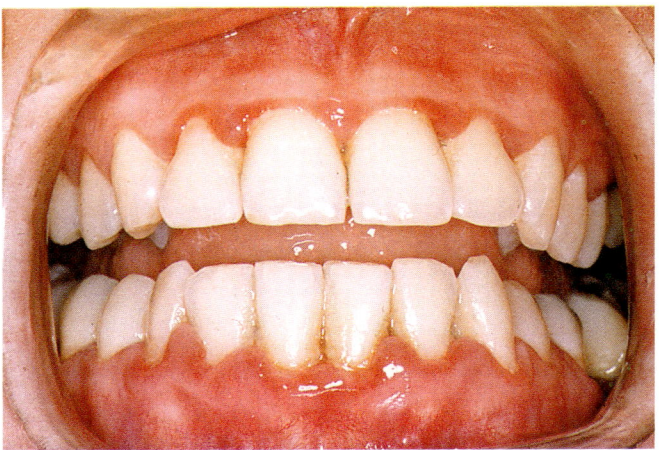

Fig. 14.45 Chronic marginal gingivitis. The interdental papillae in the upper incisor region are oedematous and reddened. The oedema extends around the entire gingival margin in some areas. More marked oedema is seen at the gingival margin in the incisor region of the lower jaw than is present in the upper jaw.

destruction and bone loss probably affects less than 10 per cent of the adult population. The most widespread form of the disease is chronic adult periodontitis (see Fig. 14.46), characterized by the presence of 'pockets' around the necks of a number of teeth, with associated loss of alveolar bone support. These pockets are usually 4–6 mm deep, although they may be much deeper in advanced disease. In most individuals bone loss is associated with gingival recession which exposes the roots of the teeth. As the disease becomes advanced the teeth loosen and may drift or become tilted. The disease, previously believed to be a slowly progressive condition, is now thought to advance in short bursts of rapid bone destruction separated by long periods of quiescence. Such destruction does not affect all teeth, but appears to involve only one or two sites in any burst of activity. The reasons for this selectivity are unclear.

In a much smaller proportion of adults destruction is more rapid, with widespread bone loss throughout the dentition. The teeth become loosened and are shed around the age of 40–50 years. This condition, known as rapidly progressive periodontitis, is generally painless and the degree of gingival inflammation is not marked. The factors which predispose certain individuals to this rapid destruction are not known, but are the subject of much active research.

A small number of children also develop a form of rapid periodontal destruction, which is highly characteristic and known as juvenile periodontitis. This condition, affecting between 0.1 per cent and 3.5 per cent of 10–19-year-olds, is limited to the permanent incisor teeth and the first permanent molars. It usually becomes apparent around 12–13 years of age and, if the disease is untreated, 50–75 per cent of the alveolar bone support is lost within 5 years, so that the teeth become loosened and are shed.

Although chronic inflammatory diseases of the gingiva and

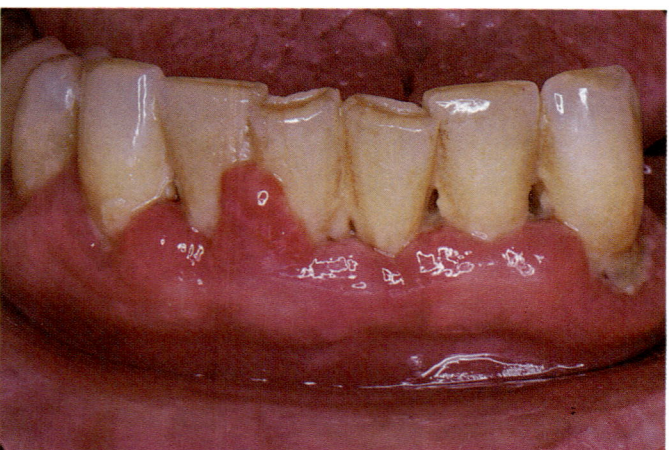

Fig. 14.46 Chronic adult periodontitis. To the left of the midline the interdental papillae are reddened, oedematous, and hyperplastic. On the right side fibrosis is evident, with superimposed oedema. There is extensive accumulation of dental plaque, especially beneath the contact areas between adjacent teeth. Associated with this there is pocket formation. The large spaces between adjacent teeth in this area are the consequence of resorption of alveolar bone accompanied by gingival recession.

periodontium predominate, acute diseases also occur. Patients with chronic adult or rapidly progressive periodontitis occasionally develop superimposed acute periodontal abscesses. These lesions result when the outlet of a periodontal pocket becomes obstructed; they are acutely painful and the accumulation of pus within the abscess is associated with rapid, dramatic bone loss.

The other principal acute condition is acute (necrotizing) ulcerative gingivitis (AUG). This is principally a disease affecting young adults which presents classically with acutely painful, necrotizing ulceration of the interdental papillae. The disease is accompanied by systemic symptoms of febrile illness and occasionally occurs in an epidemic-like fashion, its widespread occurrence among soldiers during the First World War leading to the condition being called 'Trench mouth'. However, there is no good evidence that AUG is a communicable disease, although a number of predisposing conditions that make the disease more likely to occur have been recognized. These include poor oral hygiene, smoking, and emotional stress. The latter may account for the apparent epidemics and is likely to be a significant factor in the increased frequency of the disease noted in students preparing for examinations. Recently a similar, though more chronic, form of ulcerative gingivitis has been reported in those infected with HIV.

14.5.3 The microbiology of gingivitis and periodontal disease

Within hours of cleaning the teeth dental plaque begins to accumulate at the gingival margin (see Fig. 14.47). The microbiology of this adherent supragingival plaque is discussed in the section on dental caries (see Section 14.6.3, Evidence for a microbial origin). Within 24 hours a complex plaque has become established, with significant numbers of Gram-negative anaerobic cocci (*Veillonella* spp.), facultative and obligate anaerobes (e.g. *Actinomyces* spp.). If the plaque is undisturbed, the flora continues to change with increased numbers of Gram-positive rods—especially *Actinomyces israeli*—and Gram-negative rods (e.g. *Bacteroides* spp.) appearing.

Of central importance to the establishment and progression of periodontal disease is the development of subgingival plaque (see Fig. 14.48) in the gingival sulcus and the developing periodontal pocket. This plaque develops by direct extension of the supragingival plaque and initially has a similar structure. However, the different conditions which prevail in the crevice lead to a marked change as it develops; crevicular fluid provides a ready source of nutrients, anaerobic conditions prevail, and salivary factors, particularly salivary IgA, have less influence on subgingival than on supragingival plaque.

In the plaque associated with chronic marginal gingivitis, steptococci account for about one-quarter of the microorganisms present, *Actinomyces* spp. for a quarter, and Gram-negative rods, such as *Bacteroides* spp. and *Fusobacterium*, for a further quarter. In the periodontal pockets of advanced periodontal disease the plaque microflora is composed overwhelmingly of anaerobes. By this stage Gram-negative rods have risen

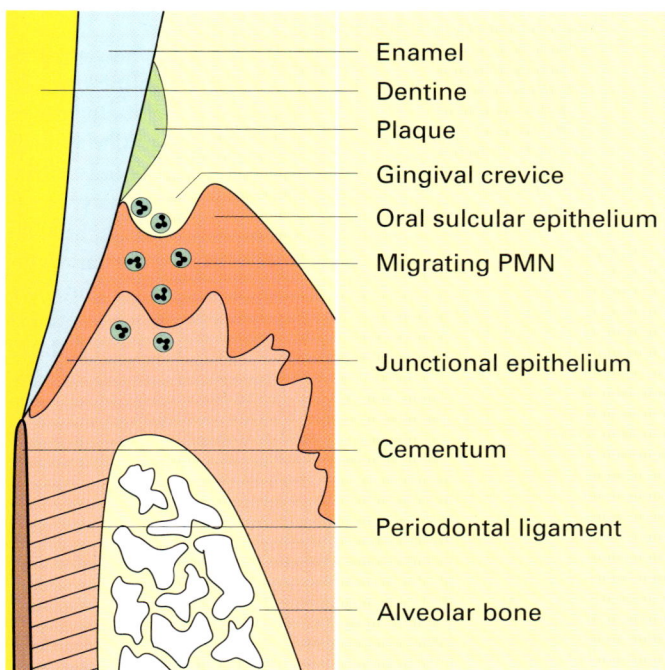

Fig. 14.47 Initial changes in the gingival crevice following accumulation of dental plaque. Within 2–4 days there is an increase in the flow of gingival crevicular fluid, accompanied by the emigration of PMN through the oral sulcular epithelium into the crevice.

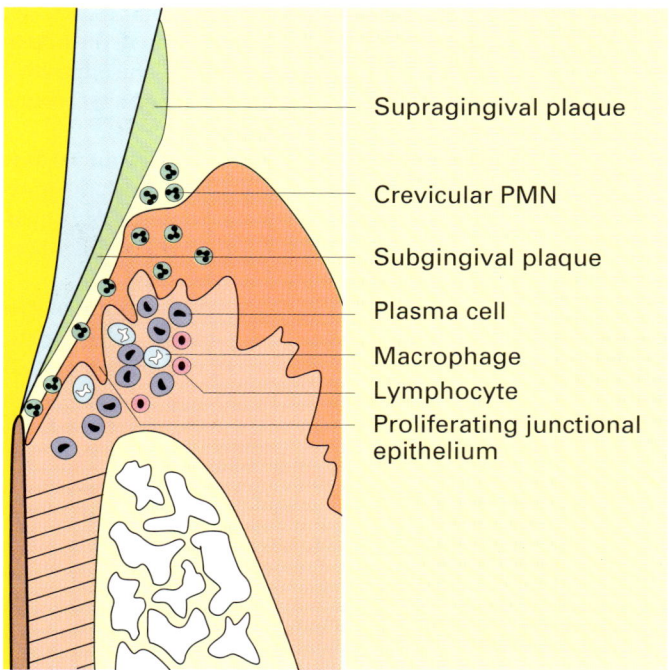

Fig. 14.48 Diagram of the gingival infiltrate in chronic marginal gingivitis. Rete peg proliferation is evident in the lateral part of the junctional epithelium. Emigration of PMN into the crevice continues, accompanied by a chronic inflammatory infiltrate in the underlying connective tissue. This infiltrate contains macrophages and T-lymphocytes, but plasma cells predominate.

from 25 per cent to 75 per cent and large numbers of spirochaetes (e.g. *Treponema* spp.) are also found, particularly at the advancing front of the plaque. These changes are associated with a compensatory reduction in the numbers of Gram-positive rods such as *Actinomyces*. In juvenile periodontitis the plaque contains the same basic types of micro-organisms as those described above but other species, including *Actinobacillus* (formerly *Actinomyces*) actinomycetemcomitans and *Capnocytophaga* spp., have also been identified. It is not clear, however, whether these organisms are of specific aetiological importance in this condition.

The subgingival plaque is less firmly adherent to the tooth surface than supragingival plaque, but the plaque micro-organisms are generally restricted to the gingival crevice and the periodontal pocket. Although plaque micro-organisms have been identified within the tissue abutting the periodontal pocket, this is thought to be neither a common nor an important occurrence.

Subgingival plaque, as with the supragingival plaque, may calcify, leading to the formation of subgingival calculus. This is generally more tenacious than supragingival calculus and an important aspect of current periodontal disease therapy is its thorough removal. Although not in itself pathogenic, it is thought that subgingival calculus acts as a site for the retention of plaque, thus preventing the resolution of inflammation in the pocket and contributing to chronicity.

It is unlikely from the available evidence that one organism alone is the specific cause of any of the clinically distinct forms of gingivitis and periodontal disease. The organisms most strongly implicated in destructive periodontitis include: *Actinomyces viscosus*; *Porphyromonas* (formerly *Bacteroides*) *gingivalis*; *Fusobacterium nucleatum*; *Bacteroides* spp.; Spirochaetes.

The organisms present in plaque produce a range of factors (see Section 14.5.5) and it is probable that variations between individuals in the response to these factors lead to the different clinical presentations which occur.

14.5.4 The histopathology of gingivitis and destructive periodontitis

The inflammatory and immunological responses to the accumulation of dental plaque are essentially similar to those occurring elsewhere in the body. There is a progressive transformation from an acute infiltrate, following the initial accumulation of plaque, to a chronic infiltrate with time. This transition is discussed in detail in the following sections.

Gingivitis

Within 2–4 days of the initial accumulation of plaque an acute inflammatory response occurs beneath the junctional epithelium. This results in the exudation of fluid from the gingival crevice—crevicular fluid—which has the typical constituents of an acute inflammatory exudate. This is accompanied by the migration of polymorphonuclear leucocytes (PMN) out of the vessels through the junctional epithelium and into the crevice (see Fig. 14.47). There is a degree of inflammation in the underlying connective tissue and, although the area of the infiltrate is small, there is significant loss of collagen, especially around blood-vessels.

If the accumulation of plaque persists, then by about 10 days a lymphocytic infiltrate begins to accumulate beneath the junctional epithelium. Associated with this infiltrate there is cytopathic alteration of resident fibroblasts, which has been attributed to direct lymphocyte-mediated cytotoxity.

In areas where plaque has been allowed to accumulate for 2–3 weeks the histological features associated with chronic marginal gingivitis are seen (see Fig. 14.48). Migration of PMN into the crevice persists and is more marked than in the earlier stages. Lymphocytes are present in the infiltrate beneath the junctional epithelium, with plasma cells predominating, and macrophages are also seen (see Fig. 14.49). The volume of this chronic inflammatory infiltrate increases with time, but it continues to abut the junctional epithelium. Immunoglobulin is present in the connective tissue and junctional epithelium. Loss of connective tissue seen in earlier stages of the disease continues, but alveolar bone loss is not apparent. A feature of long-standing chronic marginal gingivitis is lateral proliferation of the junctional epithelium.

Destructive periodontitis

This phase marks the transition from successful defence against the dental plaque and its products to marked immunologically mediated tissue destruction. The epithelial attachment moves apically on to the root surface, so that pocket formation is evident clinically (see Fig. 14.50). Ulceration of junctional epithelium may be present. Perivascular collagen loss persists, but is accompanied by fibrosis at a distance from the infiltrate. In addition to the histological features seen in chronic marginal gingivitis there is also evidence of alveolar bone destruction. The lesion is marked by periods of quiescence and exacerbation, but it appears that even during active bone resorption the inflammatory infiltrate does not abut directly on the alveolar bone. The histological features seen in chronic adult periodontitis, rapidly progressive periodontitis, and juvenile periodontitis are essentially similar.

14.5.5   Pathogenic mechanisms in gingivitis and destructive periodontitis

The histological features of gingivitis and destructive periodontitis are well established but the pathogenic mechanisms associated with each stage are less clear, although a number of

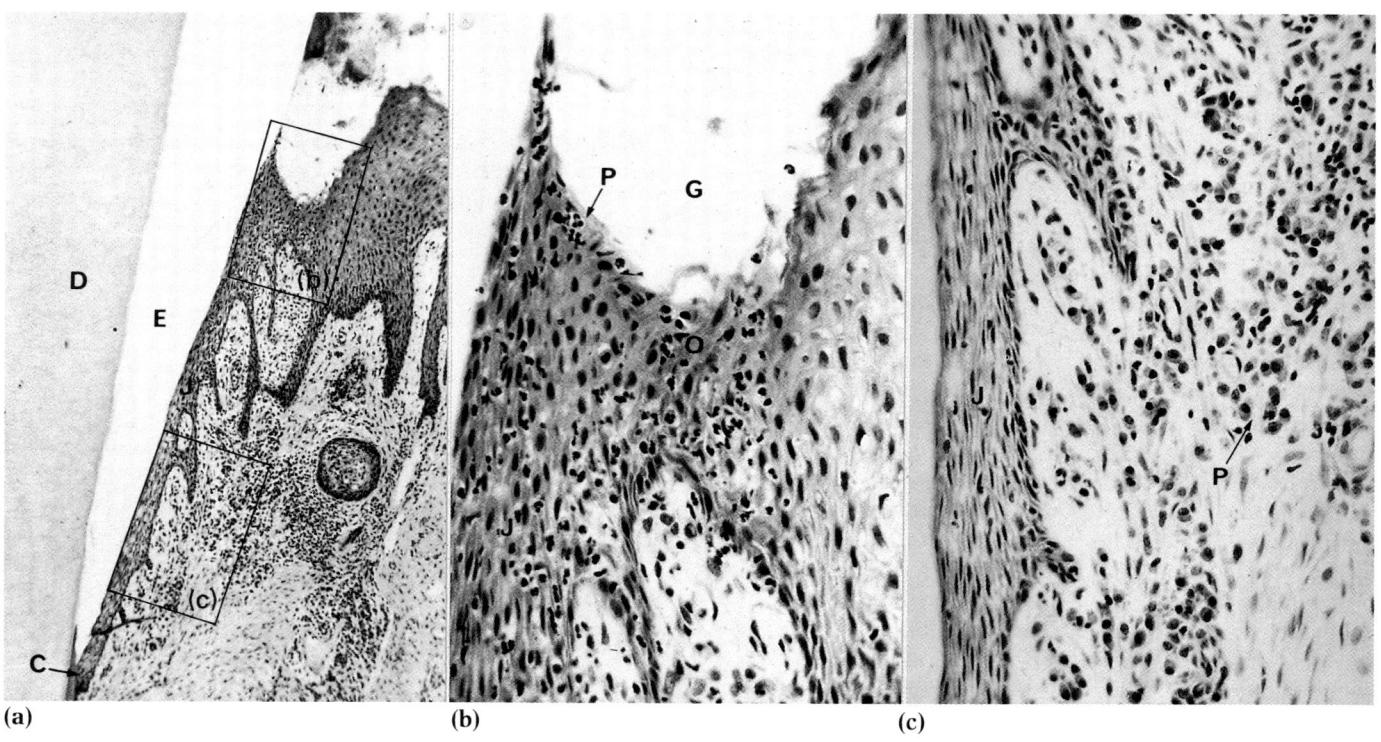

(a)   **(b)**   **(c)**

Fig. 14.49 Photomicrographs of the established lesion seen in chronic marginal gingivitis. (a) A medium-power view of the epithelial attachment area. The space (E) between dentine (D) and junctional epithelium (J) is the enamel space, produced by demineralization. The junctional epithelium extends on to cementum (C). (Original magnification × 25.) (b) Shows the area of the gingival crevice (G) at higher magnification. Numerous PMN (arrowed P) are seen migrating through the junctional epithelium and oral sulcular epithelium, which merge in the area of the crevice. (Original magnification × 40.) (c) Shows a representative area of the connective tissue infiltrate, bounded by proliferating junctional epithelium (J) on the left. Focal accumulations of plasma cells (arrowed P) predominate in this infiltrate. (Original magnification × 40.)

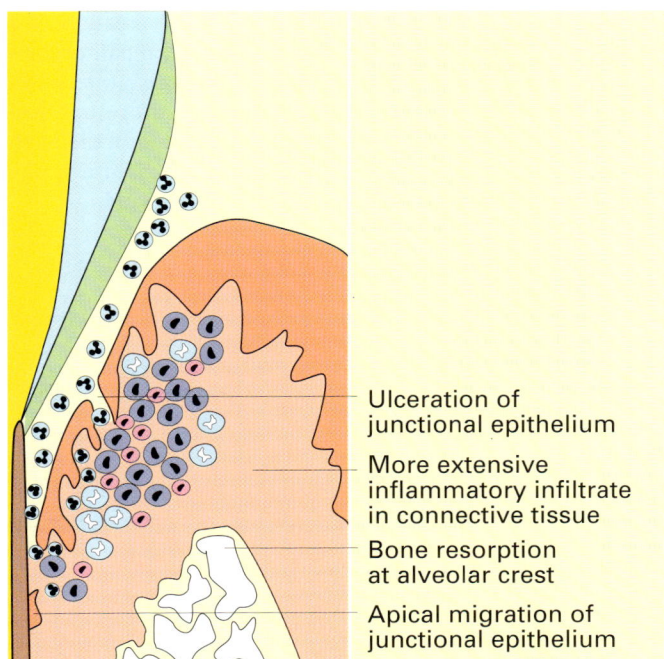

Ulceration of
junctional epithelium

More extensive
inflammatory infiltrate
in connective tissue

Bone resorption
at alveolar crest

Apical migration of
junctional epithelium

Fig. 14.50 Diagram of the changes seen in chronic adult periodontitis. The inflammatory infiltrate is more extensive than in chronic marginal gingivitis. Marked apical migration of junctional epithelium has been accompanied by loss of the connective tissue attachment leading to pocket formation. The most striking feature of the lesion, however, is resorption of alveolar bone, with loss of vertical bone height at the alveolar crest.

possibilities exist. The micro-organisms in dental plaque produce a range of factors which either damage the periodontal tissues directly or have an indirect effect, by initiating an inflammatory response. Amongst these are:

1. toxins, released from viable bacteria;

2. endotoxin, released on the death of bacteria and during their growth;

3. enzymes, including collagenase, hyaluronidase, and proteases;

4. lipoteichoic acid;

5. peptidoglycan.

The interaction between these factors and the inflammatory and immune response of the host are discussed in relation to gingivitis and destructive periodontitis.

Mechanisms in gingivitis

Events in the gingival crevice

The readily permeable junctional epithelium allows plaque products to diffuse freely into the tissues, activating complement and initiating a local inflammatory response. The classical pathway is activated by immune complexes containing IgG and IgM, and the alternate pathway is activated by endotoxins, pro-

duced by Gram-negative bacteria, and some polysaccharides. The results of this continued complement activation are histamine release, increased capillary permeability and leucocyte margination in the adjacent tissues, chemotaxis of neutrophil PMN and monocytes into the crevice, and enhanced phagocytosis of opsonized micro-organisms. Chemotactic factors in plaque also contribute to the accumulation of neutrophils in the crevice.

Neutrophil PMN are important in host defence within the crevice. They are involved not only in the phagocytosis and killing of bacteria, but also in extracellular release of enzymes. A further important function may be in causing detachment of bacteria from the tooth surface. The crucial importance of neutrophil PMN in an effective host response to plaque is indicated by the severe periodontal destruction seen in patients with neutrophil defects.

In the superficial part of the crevice, where salivary factors are able to gain access to the plaque, salivary IgA may be important in preventing plaque attachment to teeth and epithelial surfaces.

Events in the tissues

Because micro-organisms only rarely enter the tissues, the principal causes of the inflammatory cell accumulation in the tissues are diffusion of plaque antigens through the junctional epithelium and the damaging consequences of extracellular enzyme release from neutrophil PMN. The principal cell populations present in the connective tissue infiltrate are lymphocytes and macrophages.

In the early stages of disease T-lymphocytes predominate; these include cytotoxic T-cells, which interact with damaged fibroblasts, and immunoregulatory T-cells. Later, in the established lesion, B-cells are more numerous than T-cells and they secrete predominantly IgG specific for plaque antigens. The immune response to microbial antigens may be triggered directly as a result of their diffusion through junctional epithelium, or following antigen trapping by Langerhans cells (see Section 14.1.1) located in oral sulcular epithelium. Although immunoglobulin is present in the tissues, it diffuses into the crevice where it is important in opsonization and complement activation, as described in the preceding paragraph. Lymphokine-producing T-cells are also found within the tissues, their products including macrophage migration inhibition factor, γ-interferon, interleukin-1, and tumour necrosis factor, which may be important in the bone destruction which characterizes destructive periodontitis.

Macrophages in the tissues are engaged in phagocytosis and antigen presentation. A further function, which is probably of considerable importance, is the production of interleukin-1. The functions of this cytokine include immunoregulation, the enhancement of neutrophil function, and an indirect effect on bone resorption. The latter effect is probably important in the advanced lesion and the mechanisms of action may be via collagenase production, through the stimulation of plasminogen activator production, and by an indirect action on osteoclasts.

Mechanisms in destructive periodontitis

The transition from successful defence to immune-mediated destruction probably involves both host and microbial factors. However, because bone destruction is episodic it is difficult to obtain good evidence for the mechanisms that are involved at this stage. There are a number of microbial factors that have been shown to be capable of causing bone resorption *in vitro*. These include:

1. lipopolysaccharide;
2. peptidoglycan, the active component of which appears to be muramyl dipeptide;
3. capsular material, a water-soluble extract from Gram-negative micro-organisms which appears to consist largely of proteoglycan.

It is likely that host factors are more important in causing bone resorption than microbial factors though, and there is experimental evidence to support an active role for the following:

1. prostaglandins, especially PGE_2;
2. interleukin-1;
3. tumour necrosis factor.

It remains to be demonstrated whether these factors are implicated *in vivo* and their relative importance has still to be assessed. Following bone resorption, deposition of new bone occurs at periosteal and endosteal surfaces but it is unlikely that repair occurs at the alveolar crest. Thus loss of vertical bone height is irreversible, so that progressive bone loss may be inevitable with successive episodes of resorption, even when these are followed by repair.

14.5.6 Conclusion

Gingivitis and periodontal disease arise as the result of interaction between the micro-organisms and their products in dental plaque, particularly subgingival plaque, and host defence mechanisms. The processes occurring at this site are similar to those seen elsewhere in the body, but a number of aspects of the pathogenesis of these widespread diseases are poorly understood. In particular, it is not clear what causes the progression from established gingivitis to destruction of the periodontal ligament and the supporting alveolar bone. Current research is addressing this issue and attempting to elucidate why some individuals appear particularly predisposed to rapid periodontal breakdown.

The current emphasis of periodontal therapy is on the thorough removal of plaque by mechanical and chemotherapeutic means. The latter involves the introduction of antibiotics and anti-inflammatory agents directly into periodontal pockets, although this is still at an experimental stage, and the occasional use of systemic antibiotics. Deep pockets which progress in the presence of good oral hygiene, or which are too deep to allow the achievement of good oral hygiene, may require surgical elimination. The objective of such surgery is the restoration of an intact epithelial attachment and the creation of a cleansable area around the teeth. Whether bony repair accompanies this is contentious and there is considerable interest in the possibility of the implantation of materials to restore lost alveolar bone. In very advanced disease extraction of the teeth becomes inevitable and advanced periodontal disease is the principal cause of tooth loss in those over 30 years old.

14.5.7 Further reading

Lindhe, J. (1983). *Textbook of clinical periodontology*. Munksgaard, Copenhagen.

Page, R. C. and Schroeder, H. E. (1981). Pathogenesis of inflammatory periodontal disease: a summary of current work. *Laboratory Investigations* **33**, 235–49.

14.6 Dental caries

D. M. Williams

14.6.1 Introduction

Dental caries and periodontal disease—including gingivitis—(see Section 14.5) are universal dental diseases that dominate both the public perception and professional practice of dentistry. Dental caries is the decay of teeth due to destruction of the mineral phase by acid accompanied by breakdown of the organic matrix. Although painless in its early stages, advanced caries causes discomfort and toothache.

The disease predominantly affects the crowns of erupted teeth, causing destruction of dental enamel followed by dentine. The process begins typically in the pits and fissures of the occlusal surface or at the point of contact between adjacent teeth (approximal or smooth surface caries). However, it is increasingly being recognized that the process can also affect the roots of teeth which have been exposed as a consequence of advanced periodontal disease, with destruction beginning apical to the enamel–cemental junction and involving only cementum and dentine.

14.6.2 Epidemiology

Dental caries is a major public health problem in Britain. It has until recently been the major cause of tooth loss in Western societies and is also increasing in the developing world as a result of increased sugar consumption. Surveys of dental health in Britain in 1968 and 1973 showed the disease to be widespread in adults and children, with only three in 1000 adults free of dental caries. However, in the last decade there has been a fall of about 50 per cent in the incidence of dental caries in schoolchildren and the rate of tooth loss in adults due to caries has also begun to fall. The reasons for these trends are uncertain, but fluoridation of water supplies and toothpastes, together with changing dietary habits and improved oral hygiene, have been implicated.

14.6.3 Aetiology of dental caries

Evidence for a microbial origin

Both epidemiological studies and experiments using germ-free animals have demonstrated that dental caries is an infectious disease of microbial origin. Furthermore, *in vitro* studies have shown a number of micro-organisms to be capable of causing dissolution of enamel and dentine. Longitudinal epidemiological studies have demonstrated that the development of the disease in previously caries-free children and young adults is associated with the appearance of *Streptococcus mutans* in their mouths. Although a number of animal and *in vitro* studies have implicated other organisms, such as *Str. sanguis*, *Str. salivarius*, and *Actinomyces viscosus* in caries affecting smooth surfaces, pits, and fissures, epidemiological evidence for their importance is lacking.

Lactobacilli are found in large numbers in the mouths of those with active caries at a level proportional to the severity of the disease. However, evidence that the organism can actually initiate dental caries is poor and it is more likely that its association with active disease sites reflects an opportunistic colonization of a suitable ecological niche.

The aetiology of root caries is still poorly understood, but there is some evidence that *Str. salivarius* is more important than *Str. mutans* in the initiation of disease at this site. *Actinomyces* species have also been implicated in the process.

The role of dental plaque

When teeth erupt into the mouth their surface is rapidly covered by a layer called the pellicle, which is comprised predominantly of salivary glycoprotein. To the latter becomes attached dental plaque, which comprises aggregates of micro-organisms, embedded in an organic matrix, and food debris. The existence of plaque and products derived therefrom are central to the development of dental caries, gingivitis, and the periodontal diseases. Plaque varies between individuals in its thickness, composition, and the rates of formation. If left undisturbed, it becomes calcified, when it is known as *calculus*. Deposits of the latter are heaviest on the lingual aspects of the lower incisor teeth and on the buccal surfaces of the upper molar teeth opposite the opening of the parotid duct. Calculus *per se* is not implicated directly in disease, but it acts as a site for further plaque accumulation.

Coccal organisms predominate in the first-formed dental plaque and the extracellular matrix that they produce, together with salivary glycoproteins, forms a substrate permitting subsequent colonization by other species. In addition plaque acts as a diffusion-limiting membrane and probably leads to the characteristic appearance of the early enamel lesion. As plaque matures filamentous organisms begin to appear and anaerobic species predominate in the depths. Thus, established plaque has a complex ecology, and the interactions between the colonizing organisms are only poorly understood. Dental plaque is, however, highly variable in its composition, not only from individual to individual, but also from site to site within the same mouth. This variability has important implications for gingivitis and periodontal disease, as well as for dental caries.

The metabolism of dental plaque is complex, with many of the numerous micro-organisms having demanding growth requirements. The metabolic events which lead to certain micro-organisms being cariogenic involve the fermentation of carbohydrates, especially sucrose, to produce organic acids of which lactic acid appears to be produced in the largest quantities. Substantial amounts of extracellular polysaccharide are also produced and these serve as a reserve of carbohydrate and as a matrix permitting colonization by other species. The sharp fall in the pH which occurs within the dental plaque favours demineralization of the tooth surface. This is then followed by a slow rise in pH, permitting remineralization. It is the alternation between these two processes of demineralization and remineralization that gives rise to the characteristic appearance of the carious lesion in enamel. The frequent ingestion of significant quantities of sucrose is accompanied by episodes of demineralization with little opportunity for effective remineralization to occur. The clinical consequence of this is a high level of active dental caries.

To summarize, for dental caries to develop the appropriate micro-organisms need to be present on a susceptible tooth surface, with access to suitable substrates for a period of time. This complex interrelationship is shown diagrammatically in Fig. 14.51.

14.6.4 Enamel caries

The earliest macroscopic evidence of dental caries is the white spot lesion. This is most readily seen in the area of contact

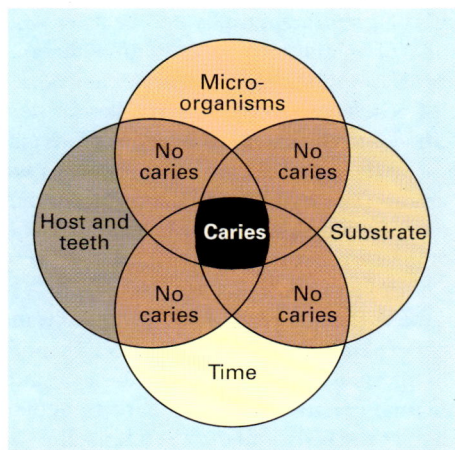

Fig. 14.51 Diagrammatic representation of the interaction of the aetiological factors involved in dental caries. Active disease only occurs when all of the factors interact together, depicted as the area where the four circles intersect.

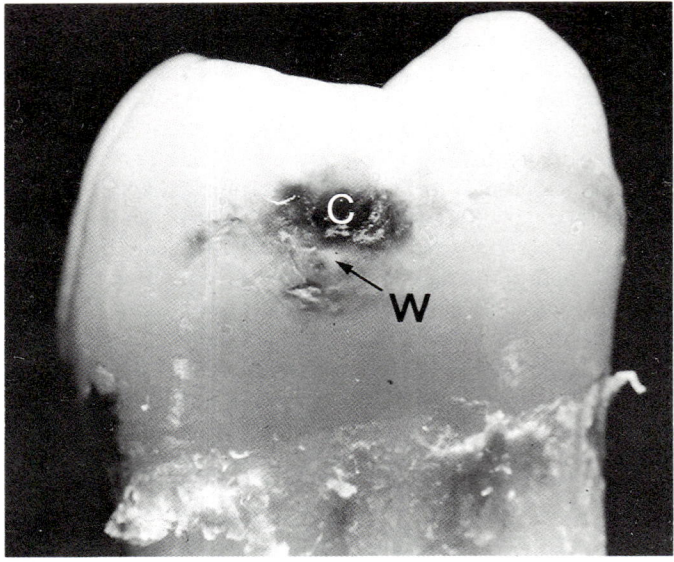

(a)

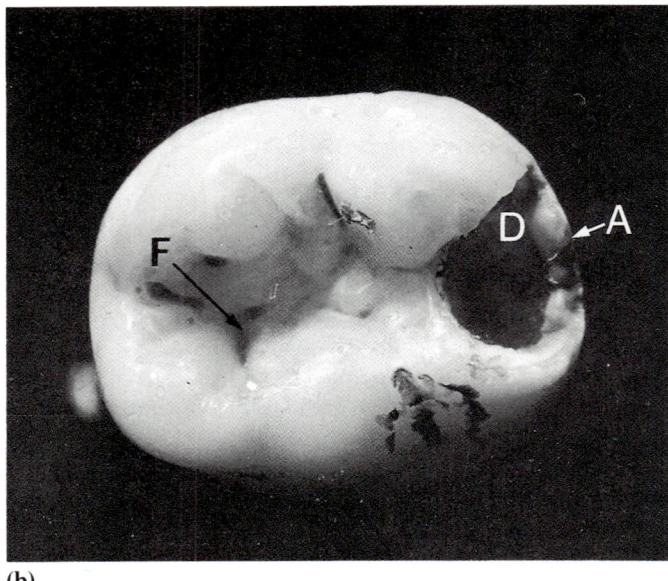

(b)

Fig. 14.52 (a) Side view of a premolar tooth, showing early dental caries at the approximal surface. The main lesion exhibits cavitation of enamel (C) below which a small white spot lesion (W) is also present. (b) Occlusal surface of a lower molar tooth. There is a cavitated lesion at the approximal surface (A) which has extended into dentine (D) causing extensive destruction. The overlying brittle enamel has collapsed causing a large cavity. At the opposite end of the tooth early dental caries is present within a fissure (F).

between adjacent teeth or near the gingival margin on a clean dry tooth surface (see Fig. 14.52a), but white spot lesions are also produced in pit and fissure caries. At this stage the tooth surface is smooth and intact, the opacity of the white spot lesion being due to subsurface demineralization, but as the lesion progresses to involve dentine, cavitation occurs (see Fig. 14.52b). The lesion in enamel is saucer-shaped or conical, with its base at the external surface of the tooth (Fig. 14.53), but as the amelo-dentinal junction is reached the lesion rapidly extends laterally along this interface. In this account a progressive lesion is described, but treatment may result in arrest and regression of the early lesion.

On the basis of microradiography and polarized-light studies, using a range of imbibition media with different refractive indices, a number of zones can be recognized in the white spot lesion (Fig. 14.53). These zones, which differ in their degree of demineralization and the extent to which remineralization also occurs, comprise the intact surface zone, beneath which is the body of the lesion. Deep to this is the dark zone and, in about 50 per cent of cases, a translucent zone is also seen at the advancing edge of the lesion.

The body of the enamel lesion accounts for the bulk of the early lesion and is the site of greatest demineralization, which reaches 25 per cent in the centre of the lesion. Demineralization in this region affects both interprismatic areas and the cores of individual enamel crystallites. In the dark zone demineralization is less than in the body and this represents the site at which demineralization of individual enamel crystallite cores has begun. In the translucent zone demineralization affects only the prism boundaries and there is little evidence of remineralization, in contrast to other zones of the enamel lesion.

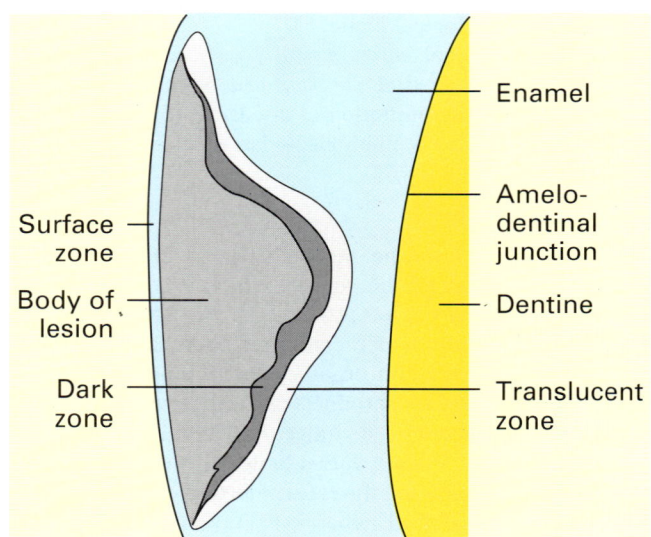

Fig. 14.53 White spot lesion in enamel. Early white spot lesion in enamel developing at the approximal surface. Beneath the intact surface zone is the body of the lesion, bounded on its inner aspect by the dark zone. The translucent zone is present deep to the dark zone and represents the farthest visible extent of the enamel lesion. Penetration to the amelo-dentinal junction is followed by rapid lateral spread along the amelo-dentinal junction.

The integrity of the surface zone, which is about 30 μm wide, has been attributed to special properties of surface enamel which confer upon it resistance to attack. However, *in vitro* studies have shown that if the outermost layer of enamel is removed prior to exposure to acid a surface zone still forms. This has led to the alternative explanation that this zone results from reprecipitation of calcium and phosphate ions released from demineralization deeper within the lesion. Remineralization occurs as the pH rises again within the plaque, and the diffusion-limiting membrane properties of the latter seem also to be important.

14.6.5 Dentine caries

Enamel is an extracellular secretion and does not contain any living cells, whereas the dentine is traversed by the cell processes of the odontoblasts that lie on its pulpal aspect. Thus, once caries begins to affect dentine the processes of acid dissolution of the mineral component and destruction of the organic matrix are accompanied by the defensive reaction of the pulp–dentine complex. The regions recognizable in the dentine lesion as it progresses are the result of the interaction between plaque micro-organisms and their products and the response of the pulp–dentine complex.

Even before cavitation of enamel has occurred, acid diffuses inwards from the surface to reach the dentine. The first response of the odontoblasts is the deposition of peritubular dentine on the wall of the dentinal tubules, resulting in their occlusion and the production of a translucent zone. Additionally, the odontoblasts form irregular secondary dentine—or reactionary dentine—on the roof or wall of the pulp chamber immediately beneath the carious lesion (see Fig. 14.54). The effect of these processes is to seal off the pulp chamber from the ingress of plaque micro-organisms and their products (see Fig. 14.55a,b). It is important to differentiate between the translucent zone seen in the early enamel lesion, which is the result of demineralization, and the translucent zone in dentine, which is due to increased mineralization.

In the absence of active or preventive treatment destruction will proceed with cavitation of the enamel, resulting in direct infection of the dentinal tubules by micro-organisms from the dental plaque. In areas of advanced destruction the dentine becomes softened and the micro-organisms are no longer contained within the dentinal tubules, but spread laterally into the intertubular dentine, forming liquefaction foci and transverse clefts (see Fig. 14.56). It is believed that proteolytic enzymes produced by plaque micro-organisms are involved in the destruction of the organic matrix of dentine which leads to this spread.

Little is known about the processes occurring in caries of exposed root surfaces, but the absence of a protective layer of enamel is likely to render the cementum and dentine more susceptible to destruction. It seems likely that the destruction of dentine which then occurs involves essentially similar stages to those just described.

As the defensive response of the odontoblasts is overwhelmed, an acute inflammatory reaction develops within the pulp (see Fig. 14.57). Initially this is localized beneath the lesion, but it gradually spreads to involve the pulp more extensively. With the further advance of destruction the translucent zone in the dentine is broken down and direct bacterial infection of the pulp occurs. In most instances this is followed by complete pulpal necrosis, with spread of infection and inflammation into the tissues around the root apex of the tooth and the formation of an apical abscess. These advanced stages of the disease are accompanied by severe pain, although the correlation between pathological events and clinical symptoms is poor. If infection spreads more widely, cellulitis and septicaemia may develop, with accompanying systemic symptoms. Alternatively, infection may track through overlying bone and soft tissues to form a sinus which usually discharges into the mouth, although in some instances the site of discharge may be the overlying facial skin. Once drainage is obtained, symptoms usually subside and

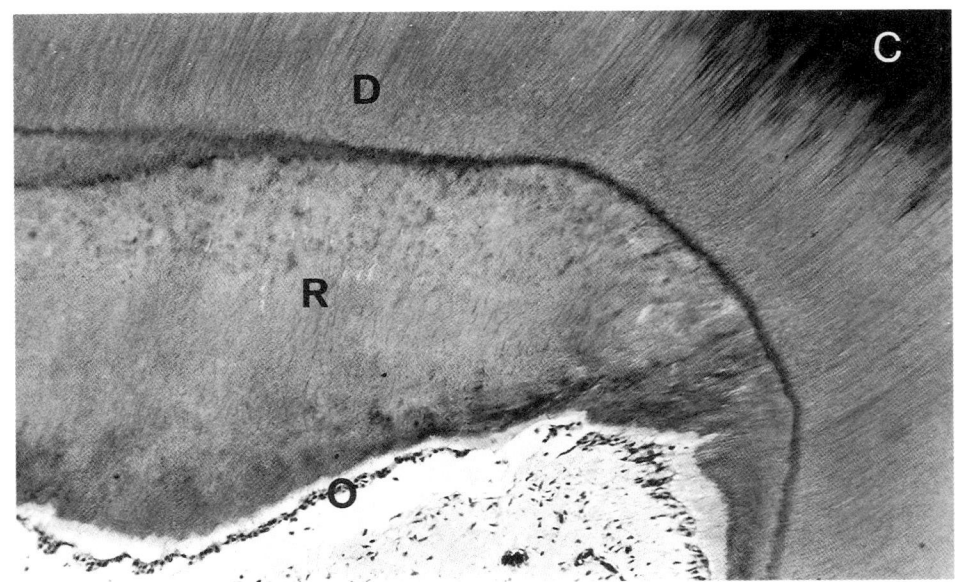

Fig. 14.54 Reactionary dentine (R) deposited on the roof of the pulp chamber in response to advancing dentine caries (C). The abrupt transition between normal dentine (D) and reactionary dentine is marked by a basophilic line. The regular odontoblast layer (O) is present on the deep surface of the reactionary dentine, separated from mineralized dentine by a narrow, pale-staining pre-dentine layer. (Haematoxylin and eosin stained decalcified section; original magnification ×50.)

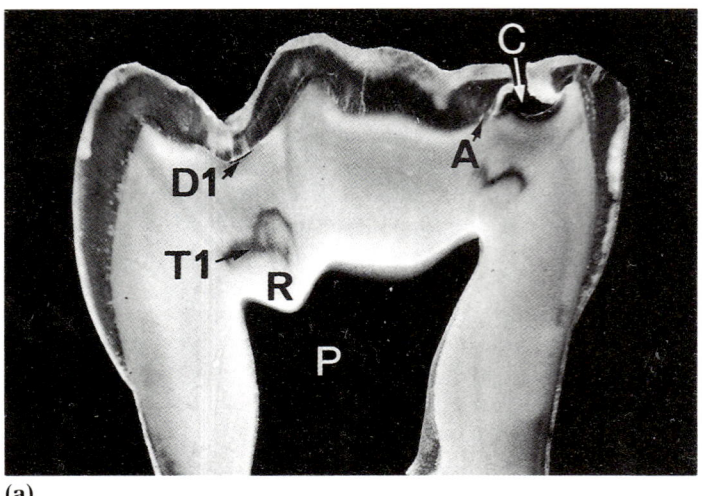

(a)

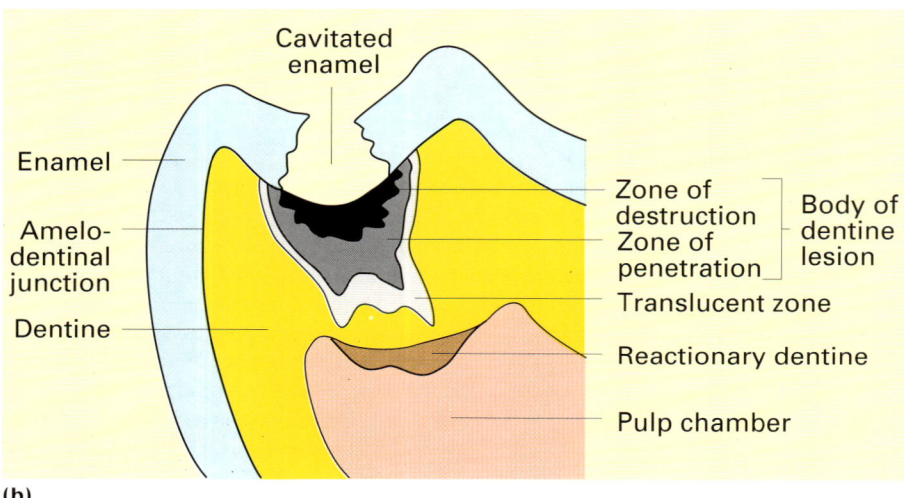

(b)

Fig. 14.55 (a) Ground section of a deciduous molar tooth with two carious lesions involving dentine (photographed by flashlight). The left-hand lesion shows a small area of destruction (D1), the translucent zone (T1) is particularly conspicuous on the deep surface of the lesion, and an area of reactionary dentine (R) is present on the roof of the pulp chamber (P). The lesion on the right-hand side of the tooth shows more marked destruction with cavitation of the enamel (C). Although the extent of cavitation on the outer aspect of the enamel is relatively slight, there has been extensive spread along the amelo-dentinal junction (A). (b) Advanced lesion in dentine, following development of dental caries in an occlusal pit. Prior to cavitation of enamel micro-organisms are unable to gain direct access to the dentinal tubules. However, once this has occurred micro-organisms infect the dentine as shown in the diagram. In the zone of destruction the dentine becomes grossly softened and micro-organisms spread laterally out of the tubules, forming liquefaction foci and transverse clefts. Their access to the pulp at this stage is prevented by the sclerosed dentinal tubules in the translucent zone. Deposition of reactionary dentine on the roof of the pulp chamber beneath the lesion constitutes a further defence response by the pulp–dentine complex.

a chronic lesion develops at the apex of the tooth. Usually this begins as an apical granuloma, but in a proportion of cases a dental cyst may form (see Section 14.4.3).

14.6.6   Conclusion

Dental caries results from the interaction between acids and enzymes produced in dental plaque and the dental hard tissues. Enamel caries involves the physiochemical processes of de-

mineralization followed by remineralization. Once the disease process enters the dentine, however, the defensive response of the pulp dentine complex is important in determining the pattern of destruction.

There is abundant evidence that reduction of dietary sugar intake, or replacing sugar with artificial sweeteners such as sorbitol and xylitol, reduces the incidence of dental caries. Supplementation of the water supply with fluoride to levels of 1 part per million also significantly reduces the incidence of dental

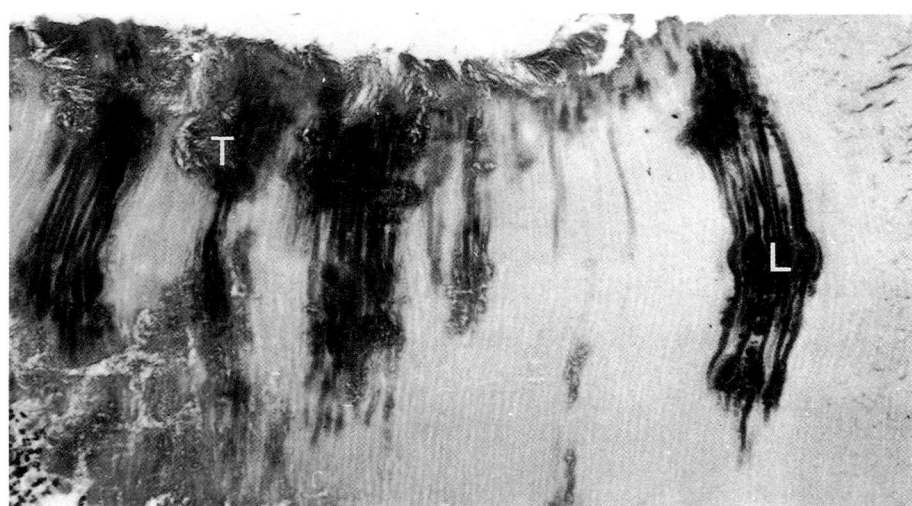

Fig. 14.56 Zone of destruction in the body of the carious lesion in dentine. The overlying enamel has been lost and micro-organisms, which stain darkly, have entered the dentinal tubules. Microbial demineralization of dentine has been accompanied by destruction of the organic matrix, leading to the formation of liquefaction foci (L) and transverse clefts (T). (Original magnification ×50.)

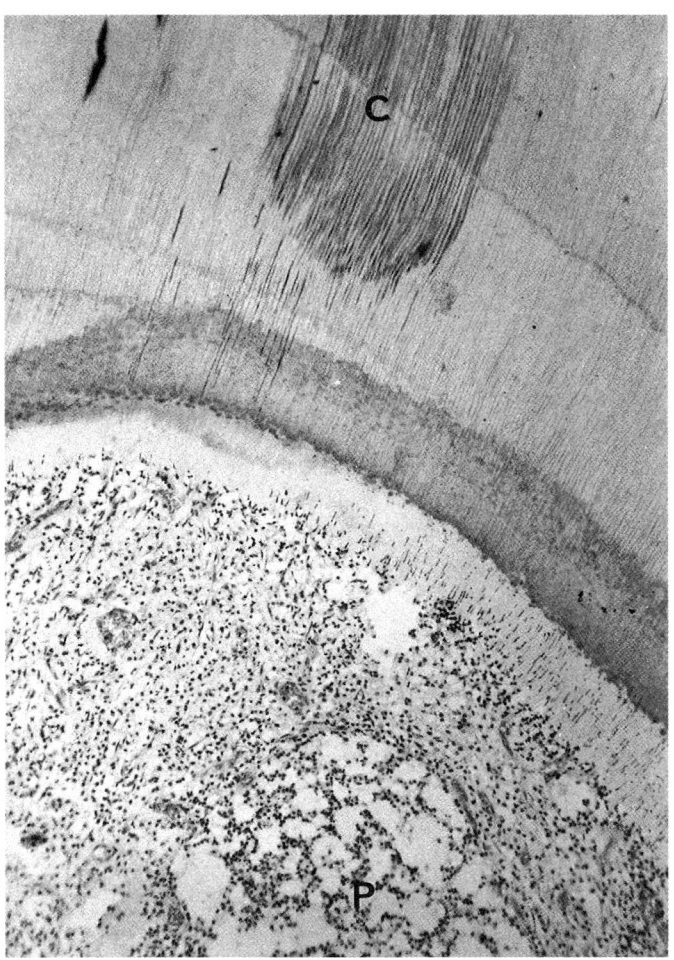

Fig. 14.57 Early pulp abscess formation (P) beneath advancing dentine caries (C). The central zone of necrosis is surrounded by an intense PMN infiltrate. A diffuse inflammatory infiltrate is present in the pulp adjacent to the abscess and the ondotoblast layer normally present at the pulp–dentine interface (see Fig. 14.54) has been lost. (Haematoxylin and eosin stained decalcified section; original magnification ×25.)

caries. In the absence of water fluoridation, fluoride tablets and topical application of fluoride gels are able to confer protection against dental caries. The mechanism of action of fluoride remains unclear, but its incorporation into hydroxyapatite crystals appears to increase their resistance to demineralization and favour remineralization. There is also increasing evidence that early carious lesions with an intact enamel surface zone can be 'healed' or arrested by the use of remineralizing solutions, modification of the diet, fluoride supplementation, and good oral hygiene. Even lesions which involve dentine may cease to progress.

Advanced progressive caries, with cavitation of enamel and infection of the dentine, usually requires excavation of the lesion and restoration of the tooth. Once necrosis of the dental pulp has occurred more advanced restorative treatment is required, involving root canal therapy, and gross destruction of the dental hard tissues may necessitate extraction. Dental abscesses may require incision and drainage, systemic symptoms being treated by antibiotic therapy using a broad-spectrum antibiotic such as penicillin. Apical granulomas and small cysts may respond to root canal therapy, but larger lesions usually require surgical enucleation.

14.6.7 Further reading

Kidd, E. A. M. and Joyston-Bechal, S. (1987). *Essentials of dental caries: the disease and its management*. Wright, IOP Publishing, Bristol.
Newbrun, E. (1978). *Cariology*. The Williams and Wilkins Company, Baltimore.
Silverstone, J. M., Johnson, N. W., Hardie, J. M., and Williams, R. A. D. (1981). *Dental caries: aetiology, pathology and prevention*. Macmillan, London.

15

Ear, nose, and throat

15

Ear, nose, and throat

15.1 Ear

L. Michaels

Disorders of hearing and balance are common in medical practice. In the following account consideration will be given to the main pathological changes in the middle and inner ears which produce these disorders.

15.1.1 Functional changes

Patients with ear disorders may complain of a wide variety of symptoms which include deafness, discharge, pain, itching, tinnitus, and vertigo. A careful examination of the tympanic membrane will elucidate many important pathological changes of external and middle ear diseases, but inner ear pathology is not reflected in this structure. A distinction between hearing loss derived from inner ear and that from middle ear disorders, can be made by hearing tests. In the clinic the tuning fork is utilized. A more refined approach is by the use of the audiometer which delivers electrically produced tones of variable frequency and intensity. Air conduction, i.e. reception of sounds transmitted through the ear canal and tympanic membrane, and bone conduction, i.e. reception of sounds transmitted through the skull bones are studied. In 'conductive' hearing loss, air conduction is reduced and a defect of the external or middle ear, including the ossicular chain can be expected. In 'sensorineural' hearing loss, bone conduction is reduced and a lesion of the cochlea itself or of the auditory system more central to the cochlea, may be assumed.

Investigation of the organ of balance (vestibular structures and semicircular canals) is carried out by observing nystagmus and also by eliciting and measuring it by means of temperature changes induced by injecting water into the ear canal (caloric test).

15.1.2 Anatomy

Middle ear

Since some knowledge of the anatomy of the middle and inner ear is required in understanding the pathological changes, a short review of this subject is presented.

The main features of the anatomy of the middle ear can be identified in Fig. 15.1 which is a photograph of a slice taken horizontally through the fixed but undecalcified left temporal bone. The photograph is of the upper surface of the slice. The ear canal (EC) passes medially and terminates at the tympanic membrane (TM) on the medial side of which is the middle ear. Outpouchings of the middle ear space are seen in the mastoid bone posterior to the ear canal and are known as mastoid air cells. The middle ear contains a chain of ossicles, the malleus, incus, and stapes, of which only the latter (St) is seen in the photograph. The Eustachian tube (E) passes anteriomedially from the middle ear and connects it with the nasopharynx. The stapes lies in the wall of the vestibule (a space unmarked in the photograph) and anteromedial to this are seen the coils of the cochlea, also unmarked in the photograph. The vestibule is innervated by the vestibular division of the eighth cranial nerve (V) and the cochlea by the cochlear division of the same nerve (C). The structures of the ear lie adjacent to the internal carotid artery (IC).

Inner ear

The bony cochlea consists of a bony tube coiled two-and-a-half times around a bony pillar called the modiolus. The cavity of the tube is incompletely divided into two chambers by a bony septum called the osseous spiral lamina, which is attached to the modiolus. The scala vestibuli opens into the vestibule and the scala tympani ends at the round window, an opening into the cochlea, which is separated from the middle ear by the secondary tympanic membrane.

The membranous labyrinth lies inside the bony labyrinth. It has three parts like the bony labyrinth:

1. three membranous semicircular canals inside the corresponding bony canals;

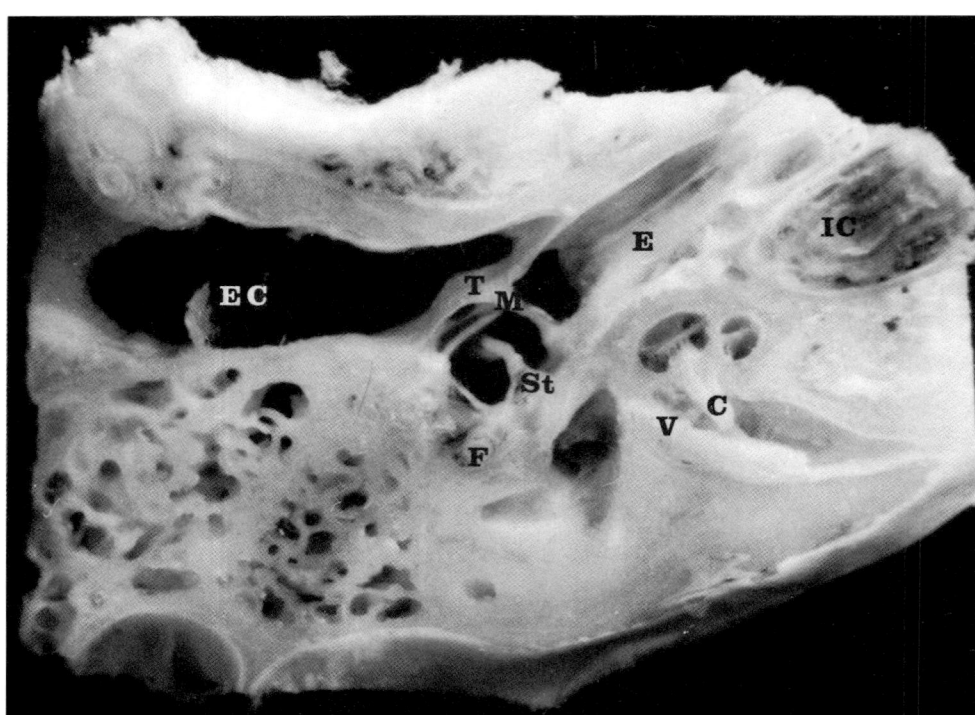

Fig. 15.1 Slice cut through undecalcified normal left temporal bone. For a description of the structures refer to the text.

2. two sacs, the utricle and saccule, within the bony vestibule. The saccule is joined to the cochlear duct by a narrow canal called the canalis reuniens. The utricle receives the five openings of the membranous semicircular canals. A small duct is given off from both utricle and saccule and these join to form the endolymphatic duct, which passes through the aqueduct of the vestibule, a bony canal, to the posterior surface of the petrous temporal bone when the duct dilates to form the endolymphatic sac;

3. the cochlear duct (scala media) within the canal of the bony cochlea. This duct contains the structures constituting the organ of hearing.

15.1.3 Important histological features

Tympanic membrane

The pars tensa consists of an external layer of skin, a central collagenous zone composed of two layers of collagen and fibroblasts, and an internal mucosal layer.

Cochlea

Modiolus

The modiolus is composed of spongy bone. It is penetrated by blood vessels and the nerve bundles of the cochlear branch of the eighth nerve. At the origin of the three cochlear coils and forming nests within the thin core of the modiolus lie the nerve cells of the spiral ganglion.

Spiral lamina

The spiral lamina (Fig. 15.2) separates the perilymph-containing space of the scala vestibuli (SV) from the similarly containing space, the scala tympani (ST). The inner zone of the spiral lamina is the osseous spiral lamina, which contains thin trabeculae of bone and nerve fibres. The outer zone of the spiral lamina is known as the basilar membrane. This bears the single row of inner hair cells (I), the three rows of outer hair cells (1, 2, and 3) and the tunnel cells enclosing the tunnel of Corti (TU) between them. The hair cells and their supporting cells are known as the organ of Copti. At the attachment of the basal lamina to the cochlear wall the periosteal connective tissue is thickened to form the spiral ligament (SL). An acellular, thick structure, the tectorial membrane (T), covers the hair cells of the organ of Corti.

Reissner's membrane

The cochlear canal is further subdivided by a thin membrane, Reissner's membrane (R), that extends from the spiral lamina to the outer wall of the bony cochlea, so producing an additional scala, the scala media or cochlear duct, which is inserted between the other two.

Stria vascularis

The outer vertical wall of the triangle of the cochlear duct formed on its other two sides by Reissner's membrane and the basilar membrane is the stria vascularis (S).

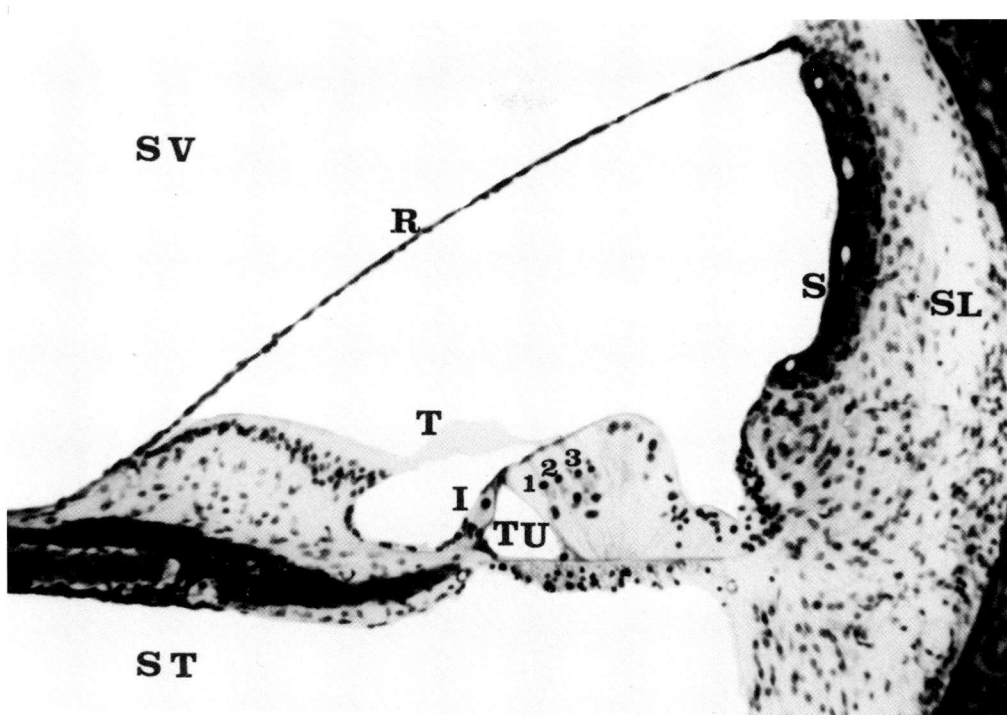

Fig. 15.2 Scala media and surrounding structures from the cochlea of a rhesus monkey. For a description of the structures refer to the text.

15.1.4   Infection

Otitis media

Otitis media is one of the most common of all diseases, particularly in young children.

Microbiology

In the acute phase *Streptococcus pneumoniae* and *Haemophilus influenzae* are the most common causative organisms. In the chronic phase, Gram-negative organisms, particularly *Proteus* and *Pseudomonas* are found. Although much less frequent than the above organisms, *Mycobacterium tuberculosis* may be the causative agent of chronic inflammation of the middle ear. In such cases the inflammatory reaction is quite distinct.

Acute otitis media

The incidence of severe acute otitis media as seen in hospital practice in developed countries has declined over the past 25 years because of the ready availability of antibiotics and improved socio-economic conditions. Children are more often affected than adults. The clinical features are general signs of infection, pain, particularly in the mastoid area, tenderness and swelling in the postauricular region, and oedema of the postero-superior wall of the external auditory meatus. The tympanic membrane is initially hyperaemic and then bulges as more pus collects in the middle ear, until eventually it may burst.

The mucosa of the mastoid air cells and main middle ear cavity is congested, oedematous, and infiltrated with neutrophils. Pus accumulates, fills the middle ear cavity and leads to the destruction of bone, the actual dissolution being carried out by osteoclasts. At the same time new bone formation takes place. The tympanic membrane shows marked congestion, the dilated vessels distending the connective tissue layer. The acute inflammation may spread deep into the temporal bone as osteomyelitis.

Chronic otitis media

This type of inflammation, while often indolent, may at times give rise to serious complications and even cause death by involvement of the brain. The hearing loss that is a constant concomitant also contributes to the immense socio-economic problem presented by chronic otitis media. It sometimes, but not always, follows an attack of the acute disease. The major feature is discharge from the middle ear. Sometimes polyps may occlude the external auditory meatus. The tympanic membrane is usually perforated in the pars tensa region.

The most characteristic feature of the pathology of chronic otitis media is the presence of inflammatory granulation tissue containing lymphocytes, plasma cells, and histiocytes. This tissue is particularly abundant in the medial wall of the middle ear and often protrudes through a perforation of the tympanic membrane to be seen in the ear canal as an aural polyp. Unlike other parts of the respiratory tract, where tubulo-alveolar glands containing mucous and serous elements are present, the middle ear is normally devoid of glands. Under conditions of chronic inflammation, however, the middle ear epithelium comes to resemble the rest of the respiratory tract by the formation of glands. The secretion derived from the glands is an important component of the aural discharge in chronic otitis media.

Yellow nodules are found in the tympanic cavity and mastoid in many cases of chronic otitis media. These are composed of cholesterol crystals (dissolved away to leave empty elongated clefts in paraffin-embedded histological sections) surrounded by foreign-body-type giant cells and other chronic inflammatory cells.

Tympanosclerosis is a special form of fibrosis which is often encountered in chronic otitis media. Deposits of dense white tissue are laid down following chronic suppurative otitis media on the crura of the stapes, within the tympanic cavity and sometimes in the mastoid. Microscopically the material is composed of hyaline collagen in the middle ear mucosa. Deposits of calcium salts, appearing as basophilic dust-like areas, are irregularly distributed through the collagen. Tympanosclerosis, although the result of otitis media, is not an ordinary form of fibrous tissue reaction, but resembles the type of collagen deposition seen in the silicotic nodules of the lung and leiomyomas of the uterus.

Cholesteatoma

Cholesteatoma is an important concomitant in from one-third to one-half of cases of chronic otitis media. It comprises the presence of keratinizing stratified squamous eipthelium within the middle ear cavity. It is possible to separate a congenital or primary form of cholesteatoma, in which epidermoid tissue is present behind an intact tympanic membrane, from an acquired form, in which there is a perforation of the tympanic membrane. There is evidence that the majority of congenital cholesteatomas arise from an epidermoid cell rest, which has been found to occur during development in the middle ear epithelium.

Typically in acquired cholesteatoma there is a foul smelling discharge and hearing loss with a perforation of the superior or posterosuperior margin of the tympanic membrane. The cholesteatoma appears as a pearly grey or yellow cyst-like structure in the middle ear cavity. Chronic inflammatory changes are always present. In most cases at least one ossicle is seriously damaged, so interrupting the continuity of the ossicular chain. Under the microscope the pearly material of the cholesteatoma consist of dead, fully differentiated anucleate keratin squames. This is the corneal layer of the squamous cell epithelium. The capsule of the epidermoid tissue is composed of fully differentiated squamous epithelium, similar to the epidermis of skin, and resting on connective tissue (Fig. 15.3).

The outer epithelium of the tympanic membrane and the epithelium of the adjacent ear canal have the property of migrating laterally, as a result of which a foreign body, such as an ink dot placed on the external epithelium, can be seen to move at a rate of about 0.07 mm each day from the ear drum laterally along the canal. The phenomenon of migration has been invoked to explain the origin of cholesteatoma from ear drum and external auditory epithelium.

Serous otitis media

In recent years a mild form of otitis media has become very widespread in young children. The symptoms are those of a

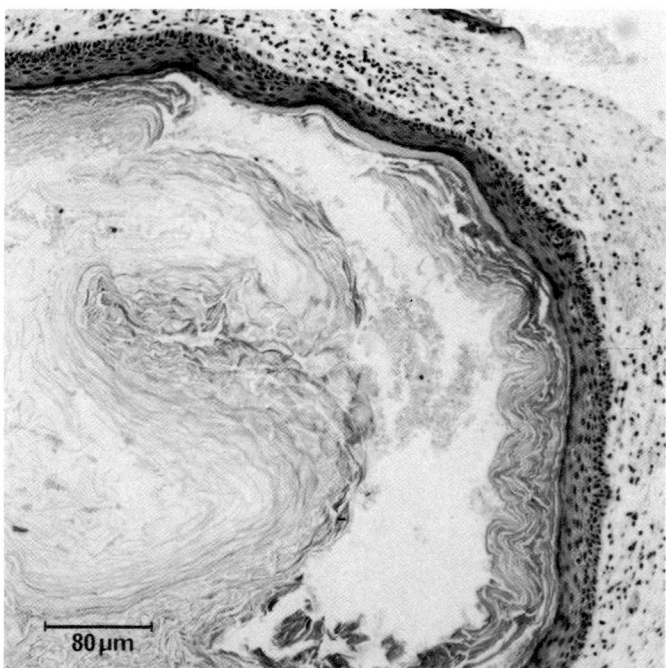

Fig. 15.3 Cholesteatoma sac, composed of squamous epithelium enclosing keratinous debris. (From Michaels 1987, with permission.)

mild chronic otitis media but the ear drum is usually not perforated. Pathological changes are similar to conventional otitis media in the few cases that have been studied at post-mortem. An exudate usually fills the middle ear, accounting for the designation 'serous' otitis media for the condition, but the exudate is usually thick and tenacious, which has given rise to the term 'glue ear' that is often applied to it.

15.1.5 Ototoxic damage to the inner ear

Ototoxic injury to the inner ear results from the damaging effect of chemical substances in the bloodstream. Such an effect has been observed with a variety of drugs. There are four classes of therapeutic substance of which the ototoxicity is clinically important because they are so frequently used in practice: (1) aminoglycoside antibiotics, (2) loop diuretics, (3) salicylates, and (4) quinine.

It would seem from numerous animal studies that the ototoxicity of aminoglycosides is the result of a direct effect of the drug on the sensory hair cells of the cochlea and vestibule. The ototoxicity of loop diuretics has been found to be due to damage to the stria vascularis. Little information is available as to the mechanism of salicylate and quinine ototoxicity.

15.1.6 Ménière's disease

Ménière's disease is an affection of both the hearing and balance organs of the inner ear, characterized by episodes of vertigo, hearing loss, and tinnitus. Its pathological basis is now firmly established as 'hydrops' i.e. distension of the endolymphatic spaces of the labyrinth by fluid. The cause of the hydrops in Ménière's disease is unknown. There are, however, other diseases of known aetiology in which hydrops may be present as a complication. The common feature of these conditions is the presence of inflammatory or neoplastic involvement of the perilymphatic spaces.

Pathology

The hydrops of Ménière's disease may affect one or both inner ears. In most cases the cochlear duct and saccule are involved, but the utricular and semicircular ducts are usually not. In the hydropic cochlear duct, Reissner's membrane, which is elastic, shows a variable degree of bulging. In the most severe cases, the membrane reaches the top of the scala vestibuli and may be in contact with a wide area of cochlear wall (Fig. 15.4). In the apical region it may bulge to such an extent that it fills the scala vestibuli and may even enter the scala tympani. The saccule swells up from its position on the medial wall of the vestibule and frequently touches the vestibular surface of the footplate of the stapes. The utricle may be compressed in the process. In some cases the swollen saccule may herniate from the vestibule into the semicircular canals.

Pathogenesis

Experimental ablation of the endolymphatic sac in guinea-pigs and cats results in endolymphatic hydrops within 3 months. In humans, operations for drainage of endolymph into the subarachnoid space are sometimes of value in the treatment of Ménière's disease. These facts suggest that obstruction of the endolymphatic duct may play a part in the pathogenesis of Ménière's disease. Endolymphatic duct obstruction is sometimes, but not consistently, present on histopathological examination of serial sections of temporal bones in cases of hydrops. More investigation on the pathology and pathophysiology of this common and disturbing ailment is required in order to attempt to control it in a rational way.

15.1.7 Presbyacusis

Presbyacusis is a term in current use to denote the hearing loss in aged people which cannot be ascribed to any known cause other than old age.

The deafness has the features of a sensorineural hearing loss particularly for high tones, which is found in all people above the age of 65 years. Two major pathological changes are present in the cochleas of old people, which account for the symptoms. The changes are: (1) atrophy of many of the outer hair cells and (2) giant stereociliary degeneration in some of those outer hair cells which have survived.

A severe degree of loss of outer hair cells is present in all coils of all cochleas from elderly patients. In addition, there is a complete loss of all hair cells of all rows, inner and outer, at the extreme lower end of the basal coil in every elderly cochlea.

The other change is the presence of enormously lengthened and thickened stereocilia emanating from some surviving hair cells. These giant structures are found to measure as much as 60 μm in length. They overlap many cells in the organ of Corti and sometimes cover the tunnel of Corti.

It is possible that giant stereociliary degeneration is a stage in the dissolution of the outer hair cells. Giant stereocilia have been seen in small numbers in human cochleas in people as young as 20 years of age. It has been shown that hair cells begin to disappear from an early age. Perhaps giant stereociliary

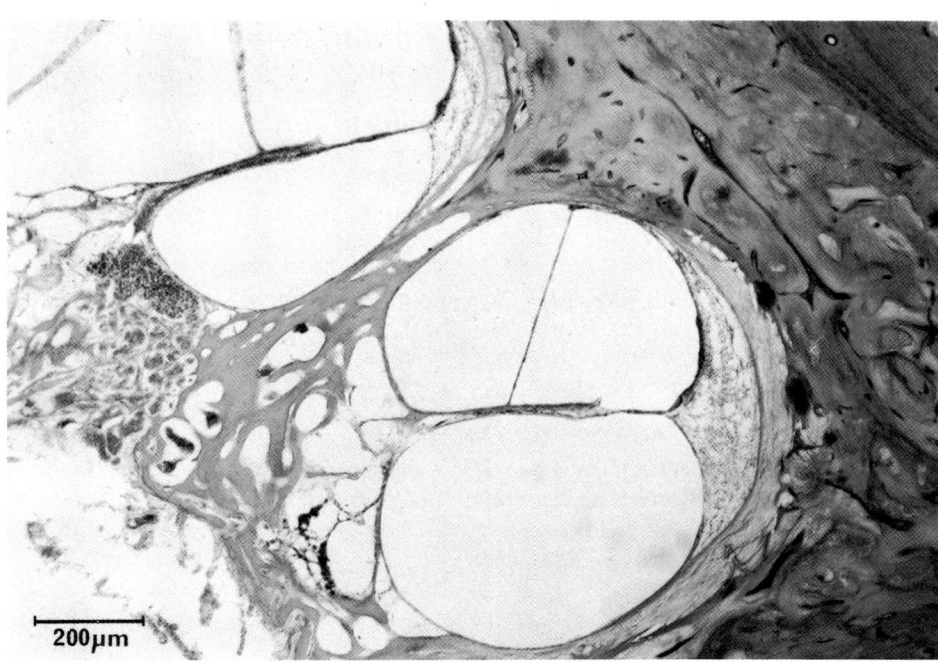

200μm

Fig. 15.4 Cochlear hydrops in Ménière's disease. The distended Reissner's membrane reaches the top of the scala vestibuli. (From Michaels 1987, with permission.)

degeneration is an alteration that is slowly taking place throughout life, resulting eventually in severe loss of stereocilia and presbyacusis, for it is not until the later years have been reached that hair cells will have been lost to a sufficient extent to produce significant deafness.

15.1.8   Otosclerosis

Otosclerosis is a common focal lesion of the otic capsule of unknown aetiology, which is found principally in relation to the cochlea and footplate of the stapes. Otosclerotic deposits, not associated with hearing loss, are detected in about 10 per cent of all adult temporal bones at autopsy of White people. Otosclerosis usually affects both ears symmetrically. The lesion attacks mainly Whites and is said to be unusual in Blacks and Mongolian people. The disease process is probably confined to the temporal bone. It is of clinical importance because of the conductive type of deafness that may occur in some patients with lesions of this disease.

Pathology

In cases with prominent otosclerotic involvement of the otic capsule the lesion may be seen as a smooth prominence of the promontory, the bony swelling over the basal coil which projects into the medial wall of the middle ear. The stapes is sometimes fixed. The pink swelling of the otosclerotic focus may sometimes even be detected clinically through a particularly transparent tympanic membrane.

In slices of temporal bones showing otosclerosis the focus appears well demarcated and pink. Blood vessels are prominent and evenly distributed. X-rays show the well-defined lesion as a patch of mottled translucency.

The histological characteristic of otosclerosis is the presence of trabeculae of new bone, mostly of the woven type. This contrasts with the normal temporal bone, the pathological bony tissue having a variable appearance, with areas of differing cellularity. In most places osteoblasts are very abundant within the woven bone. Marrow spaces contain prominent blood vessels and connective tissue. The commonest site for the formation of otosclerotic foci is the bone anterior to the oval window.

Otosclerotic involvement of the stapes footplate leading to functional fixation of the stapes, and so conductive deafness, may occur in two ways:

1. There may be actual participation by the stapes footplate in the formation of otosclerotic bone, so that the otic capsular focus of pathological bone is continuous with the former.

2. Frequently the footplate is not affected by the otosclerotic process, but the bone surrounding it proliferates to such an extent that the oval window is distorted and narrowed. The otosclerotic focus may also encroach on the round window, narrowing it in the same fashion.

Otosclerotic bone frequently reaches the endosteum of the cochlear capsule. In some cases it may lead to a fibrous reaction deep to the spiral ligament. Lesions of this type may give rise to a sensorineural hearing loss in addition to the more frequent conductive hearing loss of otosclerosis.

15.1.9   Neoplasms

Acoustic neuroma

Acoustic neuroma is the most frequent neoplasm in the temporal bone. It is a schwannoma of the eighth cranial nerve, but the term 'neuroma' is in most frequent usage.

Clinical features

Although the neoplasm usually grows from the vestibular division of the eighth nerve, most patients have hearing loss and tinnitus at presentation, while only a few complain of vertigo. Defective function of both the cochlea and the labyrinth are, however, elicited more often by the sophisticated procedures of audiometry and caloric testing.

Pathology

The neoplasm is of variable size and of round or oval shape. The larger tumours often have a mushroom shape with the two components, the stalk, an elongated intratemporal part and an expanded extratympanic part. The bone of the internal auditory meatus is often widened funnelwise by the slow growth of the neoplasm. The surface of the neoplasm is smooth and lobulated. The cut surface is yellowish, often with areas of haemorrhage. The nerve of origin is usually the vestibular division of the eighth nerve; it may be identified on the surface of the tumour and is often stretched by the latter. A fluid exudate may be observed in the cochlea and vestibule (Fig. 15.5).

Acoustic neuroma has the features of a neoplasm of Schwann cells with arrangement of the cells into a specific, almost organoid pattern. It is customary to define two areas of different appearance in the tumour as Antoni A and Antoni B types. The tumour cells in both areas are Schwann cells or their derivatives. Antoni A areas show the spindle cells of the neoplasm closely packed together. There is a tendency to palisading of nuclei, i.e. formation of nuclei of cells into rows which are aligned at right angles to the cells. Verocay bodies may be present in the Antoni A areas. These are whorled formations of palisaded tumour cells resembling tactile corpuscles. Antoni B areas show a loose reticular pattern, sometimes with histiocytic proliferation. Granular or homogeneous fluid exudate is usually present in the perilymphatic spaces of the cochlea and vestibule. This may arise as a result of pressure by the neoplasm on veins in the internal auditory meatus.

Middle ear neoplasms

The middle ear is only occasionally the site of a new growth. Because of its deep-seated position, primary malignant tumours of the middle ear do not usually manifest themselves until they are well advanced.

Adenoma

The epithelium of the middle ear has a propensity for gland

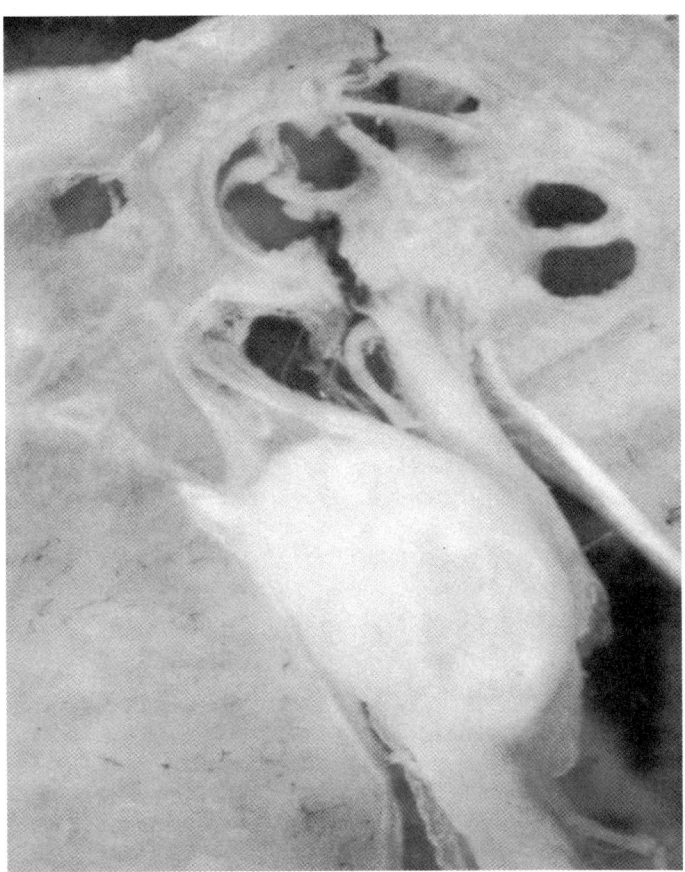

Fig. 15.5 Specimen of acoustic neuroma in the temporal bone at post-mortem. The neoplasm arises from the vestibular division of the eighth nerve and is compressing the cochlear division. Note the granular deposit lining the cochlea. (From Michaels 1987, with permission.)

formation in otitis media, and adenoma would seem to represent a benign neoplastic transformation of this epithelium along the same lines.

Adenoma is formed by closely apposed small glands with a 'back to back' appearance. The cells are regular, cuboidal, or columnar, and may enclose luminal secretion. Some middle ear adenomas give immunohistochemical reactions of neuro-endocrine type, so that the designation 'carcinoid of the middle ear' has been applied to them. Such neoplasms nevertheless behave in a benign fashion, like the non-neuro-endocrine ones.

Jugulotympanic paraganglioma

Synonyms of this neoplasm are glomus tumour and chemodectoma.

Most jugulotympanic paragangliomas arise from the paraganglion situated in the wall of the jugular bulb; a minority of the tumours arise from the paraganglion situated near the middle ear surface of the promontory. The distinction between jugular and tympanic paragangliomas can easily be made radiologically. The jugular neoplasm shows evidence of inva-

sion of the petrous bone. The tympanic neoplasm is confined to the middle ear. Jugulotympanic paragangliomas arise predominantly in females.

The neoplasm is a reddish sprouting mass at its external canal surface. In the jugular variety the petrous temporal bone is largely replaced by red, firm material and the middle ear space is occupied by soft neoplasm as far as the tympanic membrane. The bony labyrinth is rarely invaded by paraganglioma. The neoplasm in a typical section shows some resemblance to the carotid body tumour. Epithelioid, uniform cells are separated by numerous blood vessels. The tumour cells often form clusters or 'Zellballen'. Nuclei are usually uniform and small. Neurone-specific enolase and chromogranin, as demonstrated by the immunoperoxidase method, are present in the cells of this neoplasm.

Jugulotympanic paraganglioma is a neoplasm of slow growth. The jugular variety infiltrates the petrous bone, but distant metastasis is rare. Death usually results from spread of the tumour to the intracranial cavity.

Squamous carcinoma

Squamous carcinoma is very uncommon but, nevertheless, is the most frequent neoplasm of the middle ear.

In microscopic sections the tumour may be seen arising from the surface squamous epithelium, itself metaplastic from cuboidal epithelium. The neoplasm is an epidermoid carcinoma, similar in its range of keratinization and epithelial differentiation to neoplasms of the same histological type elsewhere in the upper respiratory tract.

The carcinoma tends to grow relentlessly and erode the thin bony plate surrounding the middle ear, eventually reaching the cranial cavity.

Metastatic tumours

The temporal bone is frequently the site of blood-borne metastasis from carcinomas originating in the following organs: breast, kidney, lung, stomach, larynx, prostate, and thyroid. The internal auditory meatus is a common location for such growth.

15.1.10   Further reading

Guild, S .R., Crowe, S .J., Bunch, C. C., and Polvogt, L. M. (1931). Correlations of differences in the density of innervation of the organ of Corti with differences in the acuity of hearing, including evidence as to the location in the human cochlea of the receptors for certain tones. *Acta Otolaryngologica* **15**, 269.

Michaels, L. (1986). An epidermoid formation in the developing middle ear; possible source of cholesteatoma. *Journal of Otolaryngology* **15**, 169.

Michaels, L. (1987). *Ear, nose and throat histopathology.* Springer-Verlag, London.

Michaels, L. and Soucek, S. (1990). Auditory epithelial migration: II. The existence of two discrete pathways and their embryologic correlates. *American Journal of Anatomy* **189**, 189.

Schuknecht, H. F. (1974). *Pathology of the ear.* Harvard University Press, Cambridge, Mass.

Soucek, S. and Michaels, L. (1990). *Hearing loss in the elderly. Audiometric, electrophysiological and histopathological consideration.* Bloomsbury Series in Clinical Science, Springer-Verlag, London.

15.2 Nose

A. D. Ramsay

15.2.1 Normal anatomy

The nose is a complex structure consisting of bony, cartilaginous, and soft tissue elements together with a system of air-filled spaces, the paranasal sinuses. The external nose has a bony framework composed of the nasal bone and frontal process of the maxilla and a cartilaginous framework comprising septal and alar cartilages. Internally the vomer bone and the perpendicular plate of the ethmoid join anteriorly with the septal cartilage to form the septum. The lateral wall consists of nasal bone, ethmoid bone, and sphenoid bone from front to rear, with inferior contributions from the maxilla and palatine bone. The occipital bone lies posteriorly, forming the roof of the nasopharynx. The three turbinates or nasal conchae are thin, curved bony laminae that arise from the lateral wall of the nose. The superior and middle turbinates originate from the ethmoid, and the inferior turbinate is an independent bone articulating with the nasal surface of the maxilla. At the roof of the nose the cribriform plates arise from the perpendicular ethmoid plate and run horizontally to connect with the lateral ethmoid masses. Olfactory nerve filaments pass from the olfactory epithelium to the olfactory bulb through small channels in the cribriform plates.

The paranasal sinuses comprise paired frontal, maxillary, and sphenoid sinuses and the ethmoid air cells. The frontal sinuses lie superior to the nose and drain through the frontonasal duct into the middle meatus, the channel between middle and inferior turbinates. The maxillary sinuses are lateral to the nose and the draining orifices lie in a curved gutter, the hiatus semilunaris, within the middle meatus. The sphenoid sinuses are posterior to the nose and superior to the nasopharynx and drain into the region behind the superior turbinate. The ethmoid 'sinuses' consist of a variable number of thin-walled cavities within the lateral ethmoid masses. They may be divided anatomically into posterior, middle, and anterior groups, and drain into the superior or middle meatus.

15.2.2 Normal histology

The anterior portion of the nasal cavity, the vestibule, is lined by keratinizing stratified squamous epithelium, with adnexal structures including sweat glands, sebaceous glands, and hair follicles. The nasal cavity proper commences at a depth of about 2 cm, and is lined by a ciliated pseudostratified columnar epithelium. Embryologically this lining has an ectodermal origin, and is distinct from the endodermally derived epithelium lining the larynx, trachea, and bronchi. The term 'Schneiderian' is sometimes applied to this nasal epithelium. The paranasal sinuses have a similar lining, although the cells are often more cuboidal than columnar, and goblet cells may be present.

Beneath the nasal epithelium there is a lamina propria composed of fibrous and elastic tissue, with underlying seromucinous glands and a deep vascular plexus. The vessels of this plexus show tremendous variation in luminal size, and hence the tissue is often labelled as 'erectile'. The sinuses lack this vascular network, and contain fewer seromucinous glands.

At the roof of the nose the specialized olfactory epithelium is a columnar epithelium containing olfactory neural cells, supporting (sustentacular) cells, basal cells, and small serous olfactory glands. The neural cells are bipolar primary sensory cells, the cell bodies lying at the base of the epithelium and the central processes running through the cribriform plate to synapse with the secondary sensory neurons in the olfactory bulb. The peripheral processes extend to the luminal surface where they form ciliated swellings, the olfactory vesicles, which serve as the sensory receptors.

15.2.3 Functional considerations

The rich vascularity of the nasal mucosa is reflected in the marked tendency for the nose to bleed. In addition, inflammation results in prominent oedema and swelling, leading to nasal blockage and polyp formation (see below). The thin bony trabeculae that make up the turbinates have a high potential for growth, and reactive new bone formation is a common finding in many nasal conditions. Similarly, the squamous epithelium of the anterior nose can show marked regeneration after damage (particularly adjacent to a septal perforation), sometimes mimicking dysplasia or carcinoma *in situ*. If the draining orifice of a sinus is blocked, the sinus cavity may become distended with mucin, forming a mucocoele, or sinusitis (see below) may result.

15.2.4 Infectious conditions

Acute rhinitis

Perhaps the commonest affliction of man, acute rhinitis may be produced by a wide variety of viruses, including rhinoviruses, adenoviruses, parainfluenza viruses, respiratory syncytial virus, influenza viruses, and others. The symptoms of the common cold are familiar to all, and the pathology consists of acute inflammation with oedema, glandular hypersecretion, and loss of surface epithelium.

Atopic rhinitis

This condition tends to afflict those individuals predisposed to atopy, and accompanies eczema or asthma. The nasal mucosa is hypersensitive to inhaled antigen (usually grass pollen, producing 'hay fever'), and contact with the antigen leads to IgE-mediated release of histamine from mast cells. This produces exudation and oedema, with concomitant nasal obstruction and watery rhinorrhoea. Histologically there is goblet cell hyperplasia in the epithelium; long-standing cases show a thickened basement membrane; and an inflammatory infiltrate, frequently with a high eosinophil content, is seen in the nasal connective tissue.

Sinusitis—acute and chronic

Following viral infection of the nasal mucosa, oedema of the sinus ostia often results in impaired drainage of secretions, and bacterial acute sinusitis can follow. Infection may also spread directly to the maxillary sinus from dental sepsis. *Haemophilus influenzae*, *Streptococcus pyogenes*, *Staphylococcus aureus*, and *Pneumococcus* are amongst the commonest causative organisms. Non-specific acute inflammation is the histological finding, with pus collecting in the sinus cavity.

Chronic sinusitis may arise following acute sinusitis. In the presence of compromised drainage and damaged sinus epithelium, the cavity is colonized by anaerobic bacteria, including corynebacteria, bacteroides, and anaerobic streptococci. Histologically there is usually mixed acute and chronic inflammation, with granulation tissue, fibrosis, and reactive new bone formation. Severe mucosal oedema may result in the development of inflammatory polyps.

Rhinoscleroma

Rhinoscleroma, or scleroma (the disease may involve sites other than the nose), is a chronic inflammatory condition occurring as a response to the organism *Klebsiella rhinoscleromatis*. It is most prevalent in Central and South America, Mexico, and parts of India, Africa, and the Middle East, affecting mainly young and middle-aged adults. The disease is found in rural rather than urban areas, and tends to accompany low socio-economic environmental conditions.

Clinically, rhinoscleroma presents with nasal blockage by firm, nodular intramucosal masses. The external nose is expanded, with airway obstruction, difficulty in speech, and loss of the sense of smell. Adjacent skin may be involved, and the disease can spread to nasopharynx, nasal sinuses, or larynx. Surrounding bone may be destroyed by compressive effects. There is slow and indolent progression but, despite the eventual development of severe deformities, the patients usually have no systemic symptoms, and feel quite well.

Histologically the pattern of rhinoscleroma is characteristic. The epithelium is usually intact, and the underlying tissues are expanded by a mixed inflammatory infiltrate. The latter consists of plasma cells, often showing cytoplasmic inclusions of immunoglobulin (Russell bodies), and cells known as Mikulicz cells (Fig. 15.6). Mikulicz cells are large (100–200 μm in diameter) vacuolated histiocytes with small hyperchromatic nuclei. In the advanced granulomatous (nodular) stage of the disease sheets of such cells are seen. Within the cytoplasm of the Mikulicz cells are numerous bacteria, which can be identified with Giemsa or silver deposition stains (e.g. the Warthin–Starry stain). Although there has been some dispute over the causative

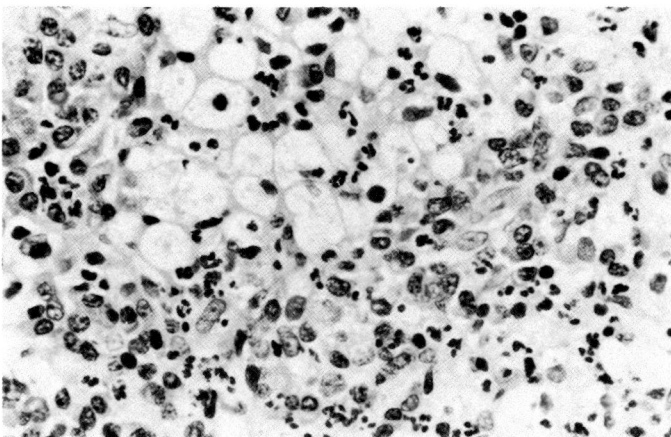

Fig. 15.6 Rhinoscleroma. High-power photomicrograph showing Mikulicz cells with abundant clear cytoplasm admixed with neutrophils and plasma cells.

organism, the bacteria are considered to be *Klebsiella rhinoscleromatis*. Other inflammatory cells, including neutrophils and eosinophils, may be seen, and there is a variable degree of accompanying fibrosis, which can be extensive in older lesions. Treatment is usually by antibiotic therapy, with surgical excision of obstructing or deforming masses.

The underlying pathogenesis of rhinoscleroma remains obscure. Large numbers of apparently intact bacteria inside macrophages suggests a parallel with mycobacterial infections and it may be that impoverished, undernourished patients are unable to mount an effective cell-mediated immune response to the organism.

Aspergillosis

Nasal disease in man can be produced by *Aspergillus fumigatus* and *A. flavus*. Aspergillosis may be seen as an acute necrotizing infection in immunosuppressed patients; as a non-invasive 'saprophytic' form in which the organism colonizes cavities, particularly the maxillary antrum; as a chronic granulomatous disease involving paranasal sinuses and orbit; and as an allergic form of paranasal aspergillosis.

In non-invasive aspergillosis (usually due to *A. fumigatus*) fungal hyphae form a brown or tan mass in the antral lumen. The mass is only loosely attached to the mucosa, and the patient presents with the features of chronic sinusitis, often with an opaque sinus X-ray. Histologically there is a mild inflammatory infiltrate around a tangle of interwoven fungal hyphae. The hyphae are typically septate, and branch dichotomously at an acute angle. Occasionally characteristic fruiting bodies or conidiophores are present at the ends of the hyphae. The usual treatment is sinus cleansing followed by re-establishment of normal drainage.

In chronic granulomatous aspergillosis the fungi invade the tissues around the sinuses, extending into cheek and orbit. There is a massive local reaction, with giant cells, granulomas, neutrophils, eosinophils, and widespread fibrosis. The firm, almost woody, texture of the inflammatory tissue, and the apparent invasion may lead to this variety of aspergillosis being mis-diagnosed as a malignant neoplasm. Histologically, fungal hyphae are difficult to see with routine stains, but special stains such as the Grocott–Gomori methenamine silver preparation reveal numerous short, irregular hyphal forms, often within giant cell cytoplasm (Fig. 15.7).

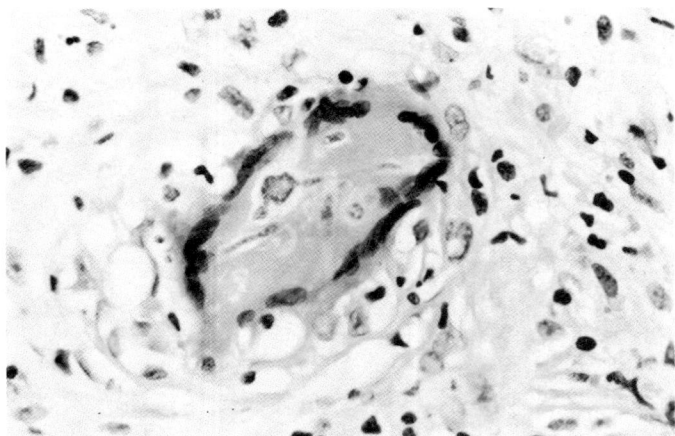

Fig. 15.7 High-power photomicrograph of chronic aspergillosis showing fragments of fungal hyphae within the cytoplasm of a giant cell.

Immunosuppressed patients with fulminant aspergillosis show extensive tissue necrosis, with fungi invading the blood vessels (angio-invasive aspergillosis) and leading to thrombosis. The infection may spread rapidly, and can extend into the cranial cavity with a fatal outcome.

Allergic paranasal aspergillosis shows dense, inspissated mucin rich in eosinophils. Charcot–Leyden crystals are present within this mucin, and special stains will show the characteristic fungal hyphae.

Zygomycosis

Nasal infection with fungi of the class Zygomycetes is seen in two forms. Rhinocerebral zygomycosis, or Mucormycosis, is a severe infection seen in acidotic diabetics and the immunosuppressed, and is caused by fungi of the *Rhizopus* and *Mucor* genera. Nasofacial zygomycosis is an infection of the nasal submucosa and adjacent tissues caused by the fungus *Conidibolus coronata*.

Mucormycosis is a rapidly progressing disease, presenting with severe headache, chills, and fever. It usually arises in the nasal turbinates and paranasal sinuses, and spreads to involve the meninges and brain, producing neurological changes and eventually death. Histologically there is extensive tissue necrosis with acute inflammation. The fungal hyphae are broad (10–15 μm diameter), irregular, and non-septate, and may be relatively few in number despite the extent of the damage. There is a marked tendency for the fungi to invade blood vessels,

and the resultant thrombosis is responsible for much of the necrosis.

Nasofacial zygomycosis is seen mainly in Africa and Asia in patients whose immune function appears normal. The infection causes a granulomatous inflammation of the nasal submucosa, spreading from the turbinates to the paranasal sinus, palate, pharynx, cheek, and nasofacial skin. The disease progresses in an indolent fashion, often with severe disfiguration, although dissemination is rare. Histologically there are giant cells, histiocytes, granulomas, neutrophils, and eosinophils. Necrosis is lacking, in contrast to Mucormycosis, but fibrosis is prominent. The few fungal hyphae seen are short, broad, and irregular, and are often surrounded by an eosinophilic deposit known as the Splendore–Hoeppli reaction. This consists of a precipitate of antigen, antibody, and plasma proteins, including fibrin. The fungal hyphae are seen as clear tubular structures in the centre of this eosinophilic deposit, and hyphal fragments can also be found within the giant cells.

15.2.5 Inflammatory disorders of the nose

Nasal polyps

Due to the highly reactive nature of the nasal mucosa, swelling and polyp formation is a prominent feature. Nasal polyposis is probably related to immediate (mast cell and IgE-mediated) hypersensitivity, and in some cases is associated with bronchial asthma. In young children the development of polyps can also be related to cystic fibrosis. In the majority of cases, however, the precise pathogenesis remains obscure, and no obvious allergen can be found. A specific form of polyp, the antrochoanal polyp arises from the mucosa of the maxillary sinus and bulges through the ostium into the rear of the nasal cavity and nasopharynx.

Nasal polyps are soft, pale grey-brown or pink translucent masses, usually between 0.5 and 2.5 cm in diameter. Their mode of removal frequently results in the presence of a stalk. Histologically they are composed of oedematous connective tissue with a myxoid stroma. Lymphatic channels are dilated, and the surface epithelium shows goblet cell hyperplasia and basement membrane thickening. In addition there is mucous gland hyperplasia, with distension of glandular lumina by excessive secretion. The stroma contains a variable inflammatory cell infiltrate, usually composed predominantly of eosinophils and plasma cells, with occasional collections of histiocytes. Longstanding polyps undergo fibrosis, and there may be squamous metaplasia of the surface epithelium. Pressure on the thin nasal bones may lead to new bone formation, and fragments of this new bone are frequently seen in polyps. Metaplastic bone or cartilage is seen rarely.

Wegener's granulomatosis

This systemic vasculitis classically involves upper respiratory tract (nose, nasopharynx, and paranasal sinuses), lung, and kidney, although the disease may not develop simultaneously at all three sites. Limited forms of Wegener's granulomatosis have been described in which only the lungs are affected, and severe disease can involve other sites including liver and skin. One should be wary of diagnosing Wegener's granulomatosis from a nasal biopsy in the absence of other evidence of disease, and a renal biopsy may be required to confirm the diagnosis prior to treatment with cytotoxics and/or high-dose steroids.

Wegener's granulomatosis produces mucosal thickening, with areas of ulceration in anterior nose or nasopharynx. The maxillary sinus may be blocked, with accumulation of pus in the antrum. Histologically there is a vasculitis affecting small arteries and veins, with acute inflammation and necrosis of the vessel walls, deposition of fibrinoid material, and occasional thrombosis. The distinctive feature of Wegener's granulomatosis is the presence of giant cells and granulomas. The latter show central necrosis (resembling caseation) surrounded by macrophages, giant cells, polymorphs, lymphocytes, and eosinophils (Fig. 15.8). These granulomas may be centred around the vessels, producing the distinctive granulomatous vasculitis. However, many nasal/nasopharyngeal biopsies in Wegener's granulomatosis are non-specific in appearance, showing only some of the features described, and in treated or 'burnt out' cases, the inflammation is replaced by dense fibrosis.

The renal lesion of Wegener's is a segmental glomerulitis, with focal necroses within the glomerular capillaries. There is no evidence of an immune complex aetiology for the disease, but recently autoantibodies directed against neutrophils have been identified in the serum, and these are being used as specific markers for Wegener's granulomatosis (Savage *et al.* 1987).

15.2.6 Epithelial neoplasms of the nose

Nasal papilloma

The squamous epithelium of nasal skin, nostril, and vestibule can give rise to benign stratified squamous papillomas that resemble those seen elsewhere in the body. However, the Schneiderian epithelium lining the nose gives rise to more specialized forms of nasal papilloma. These are usually divided into three types: the inverted papilloma, the everted papilloma, and the cylindric cell papilloma. There is some dispute as to whether these three lesions constitute distinct entities, and histologically there is some degree of overlap. However, most patients with papilloma can be grouped into one of these categories, and recurrent disease tends to have the same pattern as the original.

Inverted papilloma

The inverted papilloma typically arises from the lateral walls of the nose, or in the paranasal sinuses. Patients are usually adult males (the ratio is approximately 5 : 1 male : female), and this entity is the commonest benign epithelial neoplasm of nose and sinuses. Inverted papilloma is unrelated to nasal polyposis and allergy, and the aetiology remains obscure. The presenting symptom is usually nasal obstruction, which may be unilateral, and rare cases show facial deformity due to bone displacement. An affected sinus may be opaque to X-ray.

Macroscopically, inverted papillomas resemble nasal polyps, but are usually darker and less translucent. The surface is irregular, rather than smooth, and may show small pits where the epithelium is 'inverted'. Microscopically the lesion consists of squamous, respiratory or mixed epithelium with a loose connective tissue stroma. The lesion derives its name from the way in which the epithelium invaginates into the underlying tissue (Fig. 15.9). This 'inverted' growth pattern is quite marked, and may simulate invasion to the unwary pathologist. The invaginations are lined by a multilayered non-keratinizing squamous epithelium. Mitoses are present in the lower layers, and superficial layers show glycogen vacuolation. The epithelium bears a slight resemblance to urothelium, so that inverted papillomas were once referred to as 'transitional' papillomas. This term is now obsolete. The connective tissue element of these tumours may contain a chronic inflammatory infiltrate, and adjacent uninvolved nasal epithelium may show squamous metaplasia.

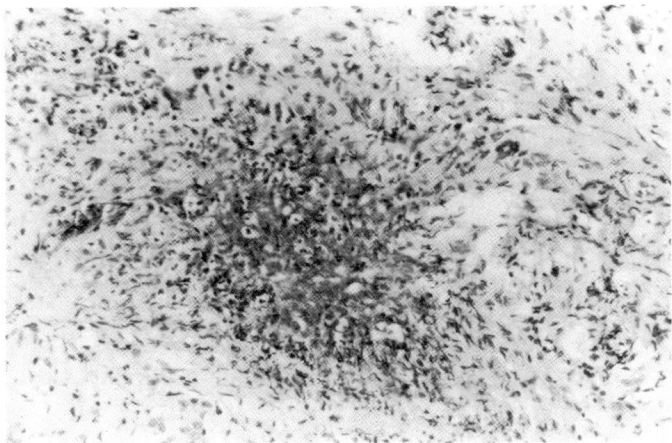

Fig. 15.8 Low-power photomicrograph of Wegener's granulomatosis involving the nasal mucosa. A granuloma is shown, with a central dark area of necrosis surrounded by macrophages and inflammatory cells.

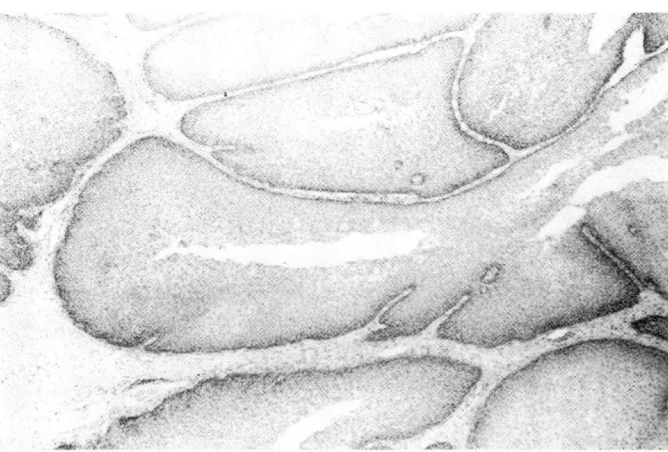

Fig. 15.9 Medium-power view of an inverted papilloma showing epithelial invaginations.

Treatment of inverted papillomas is by surgical excision, but there is a marked tendency to recur. This may be related to the inverting nature of the tumour, which makes complete excision difficult, but there is also a relationship between the mitotic rate of the tumour epithelium and recurrence rate. In tumours with more than two mitoses per high-power field, 88 per cent recur, whereas if mitoses are rare or absent the rate is only 37 per cent. There are reports of carcinomatous transformation in inverted papillomas, although in a series studied over 20 years at the Royal National Throat, Nose and Ear Hospital in London, none of 86 patients with inverted papilloma went on to develop carcinoma. However, most clinicians have seen cases in which squamous carcinoma has arisen in patients with recurrent inverted papilloma, and a small but definite risk of carcinomatous transformation must be assumed.

Everted papilloma

Usually arising from the nasal septum, the everted or fungiform squamous cell papilloma affects a younger age group than the inverted papilloma, but also shows a male predominance. Grossly the lesion has a warty, exophytic appearance, with a wide base. Microscopically it has finger-like papillae with a squamous epithelial surface and connective tissue core, and resembles squamous papillomas seen elsewhere in the upper respiratory tract. The epithelium may show keratinization and a granular layer, and the superficial cells tend to lack glycogen. Treatment is by surgical excision, and there is a 20 per cent recurrence rate. Malignant change has not been reported.

Cylindric cell papilloma

This entity has a variety of alternative names, including microcystic papillary adenoma, Schneiderian papilloma, and exophytic transitional papilloma. The usual sites are the lateral wall of nose and maxillary and ethmoid sinuses. It is the rarest of the nasal papillomas, affecting adults of either sex. Macroscopically the tumour is opaque, grey-yellow, and friable, with a granular surface. Microscopically it consists of a series of frond-like folds with a distinctive epithelial covering. The latter is a respiratory-type epithelium in which the cilia have been lost and the luminal cells have taken on an appearance resembling oncocytes, with homogeneous eosinophilic cytoplasm. Throughout the epithelium are scattered a variable number of rounded cystic spaces (microcysts) which contain mucin. As with other papillomas there is a tendency to recur after treatment, but malignant change does not occur in the cylindric cell papilloma.

Squamous cell carcinoma

Carcinoma of nasal squamous epithelium may affect the skin of the external nose and nasal vestibule or may originate from the nasal mucosa proper. Patients are predominantly male, and usually in the sixth or seventh decade. The tumour presents with symptoms of nasal or sinus obstruction. Disease that involves the nasal passages often presents at an earlier stage than that growing in the sinuses which spreads more extensively before causing symptoms. An occupational risk has been documented for those working in the nickel-refining industry, where workers have an increased incidence of nasal and bronchial carcinoma.

Macroscopically the tumour is seen as an irregular area of pale, thickened mucosa. Within the sinuses it forms solid white-yellow masses, often with patches of necrosis. Histologically the tumours usually show some keratinization, with keratin pearl formation. An origin from dysplastic surface squamous epithelium may be present, and 'prickles' can be identified between tumour cells. Less well-differentiated tumours are rare. The neoplasm tends to spread locally, eroding through bone to reach the orbit, oral cavity, or cranial cavity. Metastasis is usually confined to the cervical lymph nodes, and surgery is the normal mode of treatment, often in combination with radiotherapy.

Cylindric cell carcinoma

This relatively rare form of carcinoma is derived from the nasal respiratory (columnar or 'cylindric') epithelium, and is also termed transitional carcinoma and Schneiderian carcinoma. The clinical features resemble those of squamous cell carcinoma of the nose, but macroscopically the neoplasm shows an exophytic growth pattern. Microscopically the papillary surface is covered with a malignant epithelium composed of cylindric (columnar) cells, and strands and ribbons of tumour infiltrate the underlying connective tissue. In contrast to squamous cell carcinoma, the tumour may be seen to arise from respiratory epithelium. Areas within the cylindric cell carcinoma may show squamous metaplasia, and cause diagnostic confusion. Due to its rarity, the natural history of this tumour is uncertain.

Adenocarcinoma

Glandular carcinomas are reported to constitute approximately 6 per cent of all nasal carcinomas. Adenocarcinoma has a wide age-range, but predominantly affects men in the fifth decade. Such tumours arise high in the nasal cavity, frequently involving the ethmoid sinuses. An association between occupational exposure to the dusts of hardwoods and nasal adenocarcinoma has been reported, with furniture workers in the High Wycombe area of England showing a marked increase in incidence over the general population.

Nasal adenocarcinomas may be divided into low- and high-grade categories. Grossly they can be exophytic or infiltrative lesions, the lower-grade tumours tending to be more exophytic. Histologically these low-grade tumours are often papillary, and may resemble papillomas on examination at low power. At high power the tumour is seen to be composed of columnar cells forming regular glands, with occasional mitotic figures. The presence of the latter, together with the lack of connective tissue stroma usually enables the distinction from papilloma. High-grade tumours may also be papillary, but the cells show marked cytological atypia and numerous mitoses. Gland formation is irregular, and solid areas of tumour are often present. Both low- and high-grade tumours may be seen in woodworkers.

The prognosis of adenocarcinoma is related to the tumour

grade. Treatment is by surgical removal, and in both types local recurrence is more of a problem than metastatic spread. The five-year survival for low-grade adenocarcinoma is of the order of 50 per cent, whereas few patients with high-grade adeno-carcinoma survive beyond 3 years.

Neoplasms of nasal seromucinous glands

The nasal and sinus seromucinous glands can give rise to tumours more often associated with salivary glands. The pleo-morphic adenoma, adenoid cystic carcinoma, and mucoepi-dermoid carcinoma are the members of this group, and their histology and behaviour in this region resemble that of their salivary gland counterparts.

15.2.7 Non-epithelial neoplasms of the nose and nasal sinuses

Nasal glioma

The nasal 'glioma' is a developmental abnormality consisting of heterotopic deposits of cerebral tissue in the nose. In children such deposits may lie subcutaneously over the bridge of the nose, or may resemble nasal polyps high in the nasal cavity. In adults the heterotopic neural tissue is found in the middle tur-binate region. Brain tissues may also be seen in the nose as a result of herniation following nasal roof damage. Microscopic-ally such lesions contain astrocytic cells in a neurofibrillary background with occasional shrunken nerve cells.

Meninioma

Intranasal meningiomas are normally derived from intracranial meningiomas that extend directly from the cranial cavity. In rare instances where there is no intracranial tumour, the pri-mary nasal or sinus menigioma is presumed to arise from ec-topic arachnoid villi cells displaced during development. Grossly these tumours may resemble nasal polyps, but are opaque rather than translucent, and have a firmer texture. Histologic-ally the tumours adopt either a meningothelial or fibroblastic pattern, with concentric whorls of plump, epithelioid cells in the former, and similar whorls of spindle-shaped cells resembling fibroblasts in the latter. Calcified psammoma bodies may also be a feature. Nasal meningiomas are usually benign tumours, and are treated successfully by surgical removal.

Olfactory neuroblastoma

The olfactory neuroblastoma is a neoplasm unique to the nose, differing from neuroblastomas at other sites. It probably origin-ates from basal cells of the olfactory epithelium, and occurs in the upper nasal cavity. The ethmoid sinuses are usually involved, and the tumour may extend through the cribriform plate. There is an approximately equal sex incidence, and a wide age-range (9–66 in one study), with a median age of onset around 50. Presenting symptoms include nasal obstruction and epistaxis, and tumour spread may produce earache, visual dis-turbance, serous otitis media, cranial nerve palsies, or enlarged cervical lymph nodes.

Physical examination roveals a polypoid, granular red-pink mass high in the nasal cavity. Histologically the olfactory neuroblastoma has a characteristic appearance, containing dis-crete nests, trabeculae, and nodules of tumour cells, fibrillary (or neurofibrillary) material, and prominent collections of stromal blood vessels (Fig. 15.10). The uniform tumour cells have small, dark, round or oval nuclei, lack nucleoli, and show little cytoplasm. Mitotic activity is variable. The collections of tumour cells are well defined, and have an 'organoid' arrange-ment, usually lying around a knot of blood vessels. Some ex-amples contain pseudorosettes, tumour cells arranged in a cir-cular fashion around central areas of eosinophilic fibrillary material. The vascularity of the tumour may be so prominent as to suggest a blood vessel neoplasm. The eosinophilic fibrillary material consists of fine, pale-pink fibrils resembling neural tis-sue, and may show immunohistochemical staining with anti-body to S100 protein.

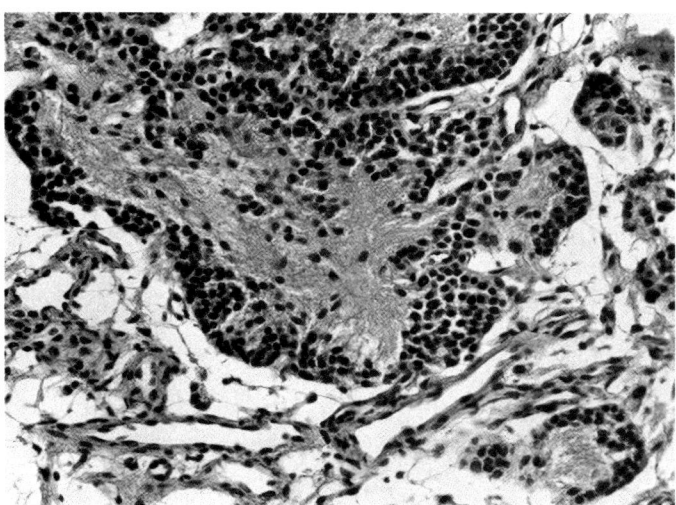

Fig. 15.10 Olfactory neuroblastoma. Medium-power H & E showing small, dark tumour cells surrounding fibrillary material.

The only histological feature of prognostic importance is the presence or absence of tumour necrosis, with cytological atypia and mitotic rate showing little relationship to long-term out-come. Treatment is primarily surgical, although radiotherapy is frequently added postoperatively. One study of 21 cases showed approximately a 50 per cent disease-free five-year survival. Local spread and recurrence are the main problems, but a per-centage do metastasize to cervical nodes.

Malignant melanoma

Although only a small fraction of all melanomas arise in the nasal passages, in elderly patients malignant melanoma ranks with lymphoma as one of the commonest non-epidermoid nasal malignancies. Nasal melanoma originates from the small number of normal melanocytes in nose and sinuses. Patients are usually over 60, although almost any age-group can be affected. Nasal bleeding and blockage are the commonest symptoms, and the tumour is usually found low in the nasal cavity, arising from septum or inferior turbinate.

Grossly the tumour forms a bulging polypoid mass which may have a brownish hue due to melanin pigmentation. Melanomas at all sites have a widely variable histological appearance, but most nasal melanomas are composed of large epithelioid cells with rounded nuclei and prominent eosinophilic nucleoli. Melanin pigment can often be identified within the cytoplasm of a proportion of cells, but special stains may be required to detect its presence. A proportion of nasal melanmas are amelanotic, and contain no identifiable pigment. In such cases electron microscopy can be used to search for the specific organelles of melanocytes, the melanosomes, and immunohistochemistry for S100 protein may help confirm the diagnosis.

The prognosis of nasal melanoma is poor, the disease spreading locally and distantly, with metastatic spread to lungs, skin, and brain. Surgical removal of tumour bulk is the primary method of treatment, and the overall five-year survival is given as between 11 per cent and 30 per cent.

Mesenchymal tumours

Benign soft tissue tumours of many types may be seen in the nose, including neurilemmoma and neurofibroma, pyogenic granuloma (frequently seen on the nasal septum) and haemangioma, leiomyoma, and benign fibrohistiocytic neoplasms. Such lesions do not differ from their counterparts elsewhere in the body.

Malignant soft tissue tumours of this region include rhabdomyosarcoma, and the rarer fibrosarcoma, leiomyosarcoma, and malignant fibrous histiocytoma. Rhabdomyosarcoma, a malignant mesenchymal tumour showing striated muscle differentiation, is the commonest sarcoma in the head and neck. The most frequent site of origin is the orbit, but the tumour also arises in the nasopharynx, nose, and nasal sinuses. It is essentially a tumour of childhood, with an average age of presentation of 7 years. Nasal bleeding and obstruction are the usual symptoms, and tumour growing into the nasal passages may produce the polypoid appearance termed sarcoma botryoides (resembling a bunch of grapes).

Histologically, rhabdomyosarcomas are divided into embryonal, alveolar, and pleomorphic subtypes. The embryonal rhabdomyosarcoma, the usual variety seen in the nose and nasopharynx, is composed of cells that resemble those found in developing muscle. Such rhabdomyoblasts may range from small, rounded cells with dark, hyperchromatic nuclei and a small amount of cytoplasm, to more differentiated, elongated, strap-like cells in which the cytoplasm shows cross-striations. The alveolar form consists of small cells with irregular hyperchromatic nuclei arranged in a loose alveolar pattern; and the pleomorphic form, which is more often seen in adults, contains large cells with marked nuclear irregularity and prominent eosinophilic cytoplasm. The diagnosis of rhabdomyosarcoma is based upon the detection of cytoplasmic cross-striations and

glycogen, the presence of thick (myosin) and thin (actin) cytoplasmic filaments by electron microscopy, or immunohistological demonstration of striated muscle components, including actin, myosin, and desmin.

Tumours of the hard tissues, bone, and cartilage, can also be seen in this region. Chondromas and chondrosarcomas are surprisingly rare despite the cartilaginous framework of the nose. Chondromas are circumscribed masses, with a grey-white glistening appearance, that are composed of histologically normal cartilage. Chondrosarcomas are lobulated tumours with varying degrees of cellularity and histological atypia. Osteomas are localized bony tumours that may represent focal overgrowth of bone rather than true neoplasms. They are relatively common in the paranasal sinuses, affecting persons in the third and fourth decades, and showing a slight male predominance. In Gardner's syndrome there is an association between osteomas of the skull and colonic polyps. Histologically such tumours are composed of mature bony trabeculae in fibrous tissue stroma. Osteosarcoma, a malignant neoplasm of bone-forming cells, usually arises in the long bones of adolescents, but may also arise from the maxilla and mandible, where they occur in an older age-group. These tumours present with jaw swelling, and X-ray shows bone destruction, soft tissue invasion, and calcified regions within the tumour mass. The histological hallmark of osteosarcoma is the presence of osteoid formed by the tumour cells. The cells themselves may be rounded or spindle-shaped, and show frequent mitoses. Cartilaginous and fibroblastic areas may also be present. The tumour shows rapid local invasion, but metastatic spread through the bloodstream occurs less commonly than with the long bone osteosarcomas. Treatment is by surgery with follow-up chemotherapy, and the overall five-year survival is in the order of 25 per cent.

Lymphoreticular neoplasms

Malignant neoplasms derived from lymphoid cells may be seen in the nasal region, usually of the non-Hodgkin's variety. (Hodgkin's disease rarely arises from or involves lymphoid tissue of nose or sinuses.) Clinically, nasal lymphomas are grouped into high-grade and low-grade varieties, the former usually receiving more aggressive chemotherapy. There are several pathological classifications of non-Hodgkin's lymphomas, with the Kiel classification being the most widely used in Europe (see Chapter 24). Most B-cell lymphomas are derived from cells normally found in the germinal centres of lymph nodes, and are termed follicle centre-cell lymphomas. Such lymphomas may show a follicular architecture. T-cell lymphomas are less well categorized, and there is evidence that many nasal lymphomas have a T-cell origin. Lymphomas are dealt with in detail in Chapter 24, but there are two entities in particular that are commonly found in the nasal region, namely plasmacytoma and the so-called malignant or 'lethal' midline granuloma.

Nasal plasmacytoma

This is a lymphoma composed of plasma cells and is categorized as malignant lymphoma, plasmacytic in the Kiel classification.

Plasma cell tumours are most often seen in bone marrow as part of multiple myeloma, but the nose is one of the recognized sites at which extramedullary plasmacytoma can arise. The tumours originate in the nasal septum or lateral wall, and patients present with an obstructing mass and localized mucosal thickening. Histologically the tumour consists of sheets of plasma cells, the nuclei showing a 'clock-face' or 'cart-wheel' pattern of nuclear chromatin (Fig. 15.11). The nucleus lies eccentrically in the basophilic cytoplasm, and there is often a perinuclear area of cytoplasmic clearing (the 'hof'). Binucleate forms and eosinophilic cytoplasmic inclusions of immunoglobulin (Russel bodies) are not uncommon, and there may be deposits of amyloid derived from light chains. Differentiation from reactive collections of plasma cells can be difficult, requiring immunocytochemical demonstration of light-chain restriction. The behaviour of these tumours varies, some being successfully treated by excision or local radiotherapy. Others metastasize to lymph nodes, skin, lungs, and liver. An overall ten-year survival in excess of 50 per cent has been described.

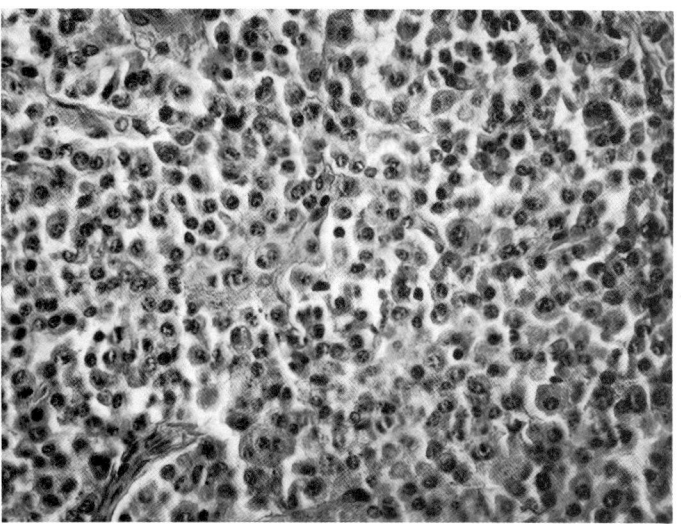

Fig. 15.11 High-power view of a nasal plasmacytoma showing a sheet of plasma cells.

Malignant (lethal) midline granuloma

In 1933 Stewart described 10 patients with severe nasal ulceration that progressed relentlessly until death, and the concept of 'lethal midline granuloma' was later devised to describe this condition. Although many entities, including tuberculosis, fungal infections, and Wegener's granulomatosis can cause this picture, an underlying disease could not be found in lethal midline granuloma. Also termed 'Stewart's granuloma', 'malignant midline granuloma', 'non-healing midfacial granuloma', and 'granuloma gangrenescens', patients present with ulceration and necrosis of nose and palate, and biopsies were interpreted as being inflammatory. In 1977 Michaels and Gregory re-assessed the biopsy findings and observed atypical cells in the inflammatory exudate. The term NACE (Necrosis with Atypical Cellular Exudate) was coined for this appearance. These atypical cells are now known to be lymphoid rather than histiocytic and 'idiopathic' lethal midline granuloma is considered to be a non-Hodgkin's lymphoma. Recent immunohistochemical studies indicate a T-cell origin for such neoplasms, and most cases of lethal midline granuloma are probably nasal T-cell lymphomas.

Miscellaneous nasal neoplasms

Although the commonest nasal tumours are discussed above, many other neoplasms can involve the nose and sinuses. Dental tumours can be seen in this region, in particular the ameloblastoma. Other bony tumours include the ossifying fibroma and its odontogenic equivalent, the cementifying fibroma, fibrous dysplasia of bone, histiocytosis X, and Ewing's sarcoma. Metastatic carcinoma can be also seen in the nose, in particular tumours originating from the kidney, lung, and breast.

15.2.8　Further reading

Binford, C. W. and Dooley, J. R. (1976). Diseases caused by fungi and actinomycetes—deep mycoses. In *Pathology of tropical and extraordinary diseases*, Vol. 2 (ed. C. H. Binford and D. H. Connor), pp. 551–99. Armed Forces Institute of Pathology, Washington, DC.

Calcaterra, T. A., Thompson, J. W., and Paglia, D. E. (1980). Inverting papillomas of nose and paranasal sinuses. *Laryngoscope* **90**, 53–60.

Chan, J. K. C., Ng, C. S., Lau, W. H., and Lo, S. T. H. (1987). Most nasal/nasopharyngeal lymphomas are peripherial T-cell neoplasms. *American Journal of Surgical Pathology* **11**, 418–29.

Harrison, D. F. N. (1984). Osseous and fibro-osseous conditions affecting the craniofacial bones. *Annals of Otology, Rhinology and Laryngology* **93**, 199–203.

Hyams, V. J. (1976). Rhinoscleroma. In *Pathology of tropical and extraordinary diseases*, Vol. 1 (ed. C. H. Binford and D. H. Connor), pp. 187–9. Armed Forces Institute of Pathology, Washington, DC.

Katz, A. and Lewis, J. S. (1971). Nasal gliomas. *Archives of Otolaryngology* **94**, 351–5.

Katzenstein, A.-L. A., Sale, S. R., and Greenberger, P. A. (1983). Pathologic findings in allergic aspergillus sinusitis. *American Journal of Surgical Pathology* **7**, 439–43.

Kjeldsberg, C. R. and Minckler, J. (1972). Meningiomas presenting as nasal polyps. *Cancer* **29**, 153–6.

McCluskey, R. T. and Fienberg, R. (1983). Vasculitis in primary vasculitides, granulomatoses and connective tissue diseases. *Human Pathology* **14**, 305–15.

Michaels, L. and Gregory, M. M. (1977). Pathology of 'non-healing (midline) granuloma'. *Journal of Clinical Pathology* **30**, 317–27.

Mills, S. E. and Frierson, H. F. (1985). Olfactory neuroblastoma. A clinicopathological study of 21 cases. *American Journal of Surgical Pathology* **9**, 317–27.

Mitchinson, J. M. (1984). The vasculitis syndromes. In *Recent advances in histopathology*, Vol. 12, pp. 223–40. Churchill Livingstone, Edinburgh.

Savage, C. O. S., Winearls, C. G., Jones, S., Marshall, P.D., and Lockwood, C. M. (1987). Prospective study of radioimmunoassay for antibodies against neutrophil cytoplasm in diagnosis of systemic vasculitis. *Lancet* **1**, 1389–93.

Stewart, J. P. (1933). Progressive lethal granulomatous ulceration of the nose. *Journal of Laryngology and Otology* **48**, 657–701.

15.3   Nasopharynx

A. D. Ramsay

15.3.1   Normal anatomy

The nasopharynx or nasal part of the pharynx lies behind the nose above the level of the soft palate. The superior and posterior walls are formed by the sphenoid and basilar occipital bone above and the first two cervical vertebrae below. The gap between the free edge of the soft palate and posterior wall of the nasopharynx is known as the pharyngeal isthmus, and is closed during swallowing by elevation of the soft palate and contraction of the pharyngeal sphincter muscles. The lateral walls of the nasopharynx contain the pharyngeal openings of the Eustachian tube, which lie approximately 1 cm behind and just below the posterior end of the inferior turbinate.

The pharyngeal tonsil consists of irregular collections of lymphoid tissue forming a bulge on the posterior wall of the nasopharynx. When enlarged in children this forms the mass known as 'adenoids'. During development the notochord occupies the region that gives rise to the basilar portion of the occipital bone, and so tumours originating from cranial notochord remnants can involve the nasopharynx.

15.3.2   Normal histology

The epithelial lining of the nasopharynx is partly columnar and partly squamous, the precise distribution being variable. Subepithelially there are seromucinous glands, particularly around the Eustachian tube orifices, and scattered lymphoid aggregates and follicles. Numerous plasma cells are present beneath the epithelium, and around nasopharyngeal crypts. In addition, there is a prominent population of dendritic reticulum cells. The nasopharynx has a role in mucosal immunity, processing foreign antigens encountered in the upper respiratory tract and producing IgA antibody for secretion on to the mucosal surface.

15.3.3   Functional considerations

Enlargement of the nasopharyngeal tonsil ('adenoids' in children) can block the posterior nose and prevent drainage of the paranasal sinuses, producing chronic sinusitis. Similarly, the orifices of one or both Eustachian tubes may be obstructed, producing a serous or secretory otitis media ('glue ear') and concomitant partial deafness. In adults Eustachian tube blockage is more likely to be due to a neoplastic process, and nasopharyngeal biopsy is therefore necessary in an adult with serous otitis media.

15.3.4   Neoplasms of the nasopharynx

Nasopharyngeal carcinoma (NPC)

Carcinoma of the nasopharynx usually arises from the region

behind the Eustachian tube outlet known as the fossa of Rosenmuller. Patients complain of hearing difficulties due to secretory otitis media, or epistaxis, headache, cervical lymph node enlargement, or cranial nerve palsies. NPC shows a male preponderance of approximately 2 : 1, and, although the disease may occur in the age-group of 10–20 years, it most commonly affects those in their sixth decade. There is a marked geographical variation, with the highest incidence being seen in the southern Chinese, an intermediate incidence level in North and East Africans, and a low incidence in Europeans and North Americans. There is evidence of an association with certain HLA haplotypes, and epidemiological studies of NPC have also indicated an association with the Epstein–Barr virus (EBV). Epstein–Barr nuclear antigen has been isolated from NPC cells, and high titres of IgA anti-EBV capsid antibody are seen in patients with NPC. In South-east Asia this antibody is used as a screening test for the presence of NPC.

There are three histological varieties of NPC; keratinizing squamous cell carcinoma, non-keratinizing squamous cell carcinoma, and undifferentiated carcinoma. In practice these entities form part of a spectrum of differentiation, and it may be difficult to distinguish non-keratinizing squamous cell carcinoma and undifferentiated carcinoma. The most common variety is the undifferentiated form, which consists of uniform cells with a poorly defined cytoplasmic border that gives the tumour a syncytial appearance. The nuclei are pale and rounded, with a distinct nuclear edge and one or two prominent eosinophilic nucleoli. Mitoses are common, and the tumour cells form trabeculae or solid sheets (Fig. 15.12). The reactive population of small lymphocytes that is usually seen between the tumour cells has led to the use of the term 'lymphoepithelioma' as a synonym for NPC in the past. Since the histological distinction between NPC and large cell (immunoblastic) lymphoma may be difficult, this confusing term should no longer be used. Electron microscopical examination of NPC reveals desmosomes, and immunohistochemistry detects cytokeratin production. Both

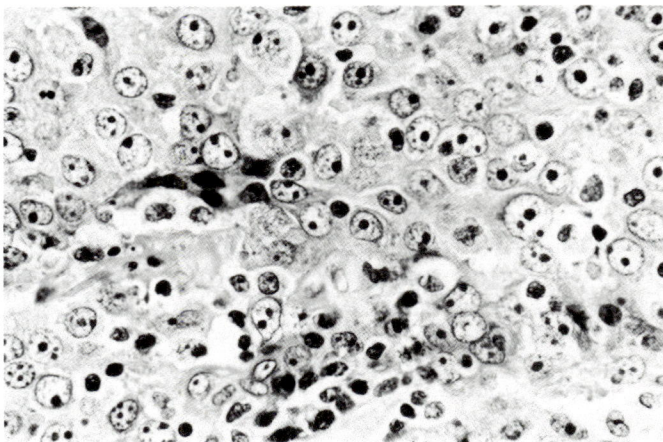

Fig. 15.12 Nasopharyngeal carcinoma; high-power H & E. The tumour cells have an indistinct cytoplasmic border and rounded nuclei with prominent nucleoli. Scattered small dark lymphocyte nuclei are present.

these features confirm the epithelial origin of the tumour, enabling its distinction from malignant lymphoma. It is of interest that the cells of NPC can be shown to express Class II MHC antigen (HLA-DR) on their surface. The keratinizing and non-keratinizing forms of NPC have a more conventional appearance, with intercellular bridges ('prickles'), a squamous epithelial pattern with flattened cells superficially, or keratin pearls.

NPC progresses by spreading both locally and distantly, invading the skull base and almost invariably metastasizing to cervical lymph nodes. The tumour is radiosensitive with local radiotherapy being the primary mode of treatment. The prognosis of NPC is related to the clinical stage; patients in which the disease is confined to the nasopharynx do well, but the outlook for those with cervical and more distant metastases is progressively worse.

Angiofibroma (juvenile angiofibroma)

This peculiar tumour of the nasopharynx, which may not be a true neoplasm, affects only males between 10 and 25 years of age. It has a vascular and fibrous component, and grows at the junction of posterior nasal cavity and nasopharynx, swelling to block the nasal airway. Although the tumour arises unilaterally, both sides of the nose are usually blocked at presentation. Epistaxis is common and in advanced cases orbital involvement may lead to proptosis. The development of angiofibroma frequently coincides with the pubertal growth spurt, and facial deformity may result from its effect on growing bones.

Grossly the tumour has a firm texture and a grey-pink cut surface which may be spongy due to dilated blood vessels. Histologically the lesion consists of thick- and thin-walled blood vessels in a fibroblastic stroma. The thick-walled vessels show an irregular muscular coat, and tend to be found in the centre of the tumour. The more peripheral vessels are thin and elongated, the endothelial cell nuclei protruding into the lumen in a 'hobnail' fashion. The stroma is collagenous, and the fibroblasts have large prominent nuclei that may look atypical, although mitotic activity is lacking (Fig. 15.13).

The histogenesis of angiofibroma is obscure, but the lesion resembles normal submucosal vascular tissue of the nose, and a disorder of growth of tissue in this region may produce the lesion. Treatment is by surgical excision, although the vascularity of the tumour can introduce technical difficulties. Preoperative embolization or oestrogen treatment can be used to decrease this vascularity, although the value of the latter is disputed. A number of angiofibromas recur after operation, and some need multiple resections. There is no evidence of malignancy, however, and metastatic spread does not occur.

Chordoma

This tumour is derived from notochordal remnants, and occurs at two main sites in the body, the sacro-coccygeal region and the base of skull. The latter tumours frequently extend forward from the spheno-occipital region to involve the nasopharynx, and so may present as nasopharyngeal masses. Patients can

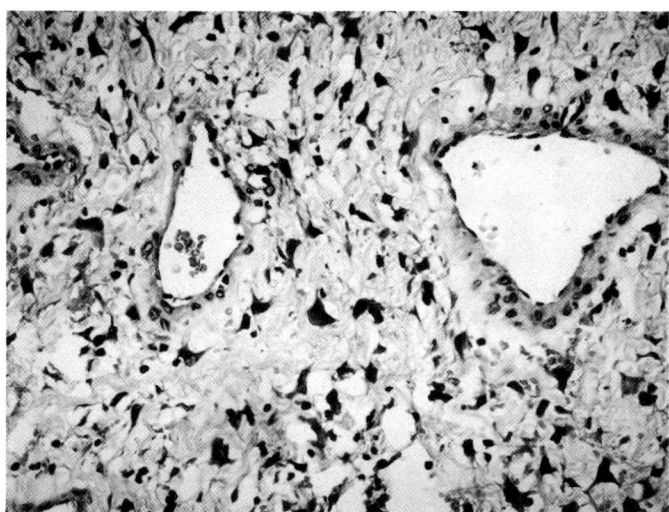

Fig. 15.13 Low-power H & E photomicrograph of nasopharyngeal angiofibroma. Thick-walled vascular spaces with prominent endothelial cells are present, and the stromal fibroblasts show large irregular hyperchromatic nuclei.

show cranial nerve palsies and X-rays will reveal the typical radiological appearance of the tumour, frequently with bony destruction at the skull base.

Macroscopically these tumours are grey-white with a mucoid texture, and under the microscope contain vacuolated cells and strands of epithelial-like cells in a myxoid stroma. Cytoplasmic vacuolation can impart a 'signet ring' or 'bubbly' (physaliferous) appearance to the tumour cells (Fig. 15.14). The nuclei are usually small and hyperchromatic, with few mitoses. The epithelial-like areas are formed by strands and alveoli of tumour cells. The neoplasm shows a lobular growth pattern, with a peripheral condensation of fibrous tissue forming a pseudo-capsule. The stroma is highly mucoid, and in some instances resembles that of cartilage. In contrast to cartilaginous tumours, chordoma cells express cytokeratin

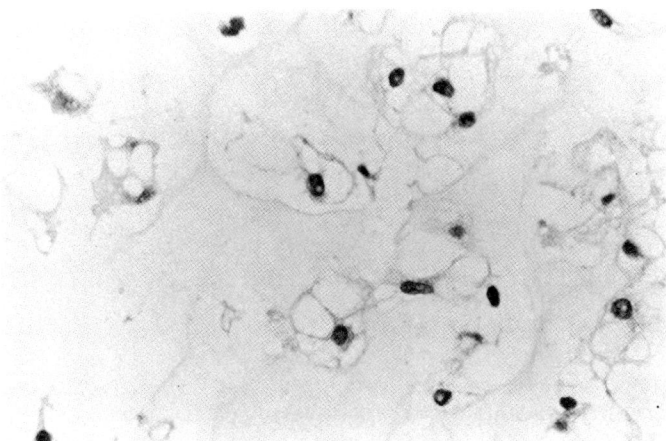

Fig. 15.14 Chordoma; high-power H & E. Physaliferous cells with 'bubbly' cytoplasm lying in a myxoid stroma.

immunohistochemically, and ultrastructural studies show the presence of desmosomal intercellular junctions.

Chordomas show wide local infiltration, but metastases are very rare. Surgical resection is the treatment of choice, but because of the site and extent of local spread of the lesion, complete removal is almost always impossible. However, patients may survive for many years with repeated incomplete excisions, and a mean survival of around 7 years has been documented for chordoma of the skull base.

Nasopharyngeal lymphoma

As with the nose, a variety of lymphoma may be seen in the nasopharynx, with a significant proportion being T-cell derived. Hodgkin's disease is rare in the nasopharynx but there are reports of the mixed cellularity subtype arising at this site.

Sarcoma of the nasopharynx

The nasopharynx is one of the commonest sites of origin for rhabdomyosarcoma, the clinical and histological features of which have been detailed in the section on the nose and paranasal sinuses. Other sarcomas are relatively rare, particularly liposarcoma which is almost unheard of in the head and neck region as a whole.

15.3.5   Further reading

Bosq, J., Gatter, K. C., Micheau, C., and Mason, D. Y. (1985). Role of immunohistochemistry in diagnosis of nasopharyngeal tumours. *Journal of Clinical Pathology* **38**, 845–8.

Chan, S. H., Day, N. E., Kunaratnam, N., and Chia, K. B. (1982). HLA and nasopharyngeal carcinoma in Chinese—a further study. *International Journal of Cancer* **15**, 171–6.

Chan, J. K. C., Ng, C. S., Lau, W. H., and Lo, S. T. H. (1987). Most nasal/nasopharyngeal lymphomas are peripheral T-cell neoplasms. *American Journal of Surgical Pathology* **11**, 418–29.

Zur Hansen, H., Schute-Holthausen, H., Klein, G., Henle, G., Clifford, P., and Santesson, L. (1970). Epstein–Barr virus DNA in biopsies of Burkitt tumours and anaplastic carcinoma of the nasopharynx. *Nature* **228**, 1056–8.

15.4   Palatine tonsil

A. D. Ramsay

15.4.1   Normal anatomy

The palatine tonsils are paired masses of lymphoid tissue lying in the lateral walls of the oral pharynx. Each tonsil occupies the sinus between the mucosa-covered arches of the palatoglossal and palatopharyngeal muscles (the anterior and posterior faucial pillars). Laterally the tonsils overlie the superior constrictor muscle, and extend inferiorly into the dorsum of the tongue and superiorly into the soft palate. The free medial surface contains the openings of 15–20 narrow channels, the tonsillar crypts, that penetrate deep into the underlying lymphoid tissue.

The palatine tonsil, together with the pharyngeal tonsil and lymphoid tissue at base of tongue (the lingual 'tonsil') form Waldeyer's ring. This constitutes a loose circle of lymphoid tissue around the upper end of the aerodigestive tract.

15.4.2   Normal histology

The mucosal surface of the tonsil, in common with the mouth and oropharynx, is covered by non-keratinizing stratified squamous epithelium. Intra-epithelial lymphocytes are present, and are particularly prominent in the crypt epithelium. The lymphoid tissue contains B-cell follicles, with germinal centres and mantle zones, and an interfollicular region of T-cells and plasma cells. The palatine tonsil functions similarly to the nasopharyngeal tonsil, foreign antigens stimulating B-lymphocytes within the crypts to produce antibody. The initial encounter with many antigens will take place in the upper respiratory tract, and Waldeyer's ring lymphoid tissue plays an important role in the body's immune defences.

15.4.3   Functional considerations

Reactive lymphoid hyperplasia can produce enlargement of the palatine tonsils. This is usually of little significance, but in some children can be so marked as to interfere with breathing, and result in attacks of sleep apnoea.

15.4.4   Infectious conditions

Tonsillitis

Despite the prevalence of tonsillitis, the microbiological processes involved have not been fully elucidated. Acute tonsillitis affects mainly children, but can occur in adults, and presents with sore throat, dysphagia, and fever. Some individuals have repeated multiple attacks of tonsillitis, and a retro-tonsillar abscess or quinsy can develop if pus does not drain from an inflamed tonsil. Complications of repeated tonsillitis include the post-streptococcal disease complex and the effects of tonsillar (and adenoidal) enlargement. The latter can produce attacks of apnoea during sleep and, in severe chronic cases, may result in pulmonary hypertension.

The organisms responsible for tonsillitis remain obscure, and viruses, bacteria, and fungi can be isolated from inflamed tonsils. Viral agents include adenoviruses, herpes simplex, and the Epstein–Barr virus. Bacterial organisms include *Streptococcus pyogenes* and *S. pneumoniae*, *Staphylococcus aureus*, *Haemophilus influenzae*, and anaerobic species. Some cases contain a mixture of these organisms. In addition *Candida albicans* has been found in inflamed tonsils, and colonies of *Actinomyces* are frequently seen in the crypts of both inflamed and uninflamed tonsils.

In acute attacks the tonsils and surrounding pharyngeal tissues are red and swollen, with pus exuding from the tonsillar crypts. Tonsils are removed after multiple acute attacks, and usually during a quiescent period. Macroscopically such resected tonsils may be larger than normal, and are often unequal in size. The tonsillar crypts are swollen, containing white-grey material that may be calcified in long-standing cases (tonsilloliths). Rarely there is some fibrosis, but most tonsils removed for repeated acute tonsillitis are essentially normal in appearance. Histologically the hallmark of acute tonsillitis is a neutrophil polymorph infiltrate beneath the crypt epithelium, often with extension of the exudate into the crypt lumen. The crypt epithelium may be ulcerated, and the lumina distended with pus, with occasional abscesses forming within the tonsillar substance. The lymphoid follicles are large and 'active', showing numerous mitoses, a high content of larger follicle centre cells (centroblasts), and prominent tingible body macrophages. Lymphoid hyperplasia can lead to obstruction of the crypts, which then fill with desquamated epithelial cell debris.

Infectious mononucleosis (glandular fever)

Infection of the tonsil by the Epstein–Barr DNA virus may be responsible for acute tonsillitis, and the histological changes this virus produces in lymphoid tissue can be mistaken for lymphoma. Patients show severe tonsillar enlargement with sore throat and fever, and can develop lymphadenopathy, hepatosplenomegaly, and skin rashes following ampicillin treatment. Heterophil antibodies against sheep red blood cells are present in the serum (detected by the Paul–Bunnell test), and a blood film shows abnormal circulating white cells. The virus infects B-cells and causes them to proliferate, and the response to these infected cells is a vigorous T-cell proliferation.

Histological examination of lymphoid tissue in infectious mononucleosis shows follicular hyperplasia in the early stages, but as the disease progresses the follicles are overrun by a paracortical proliferation of transformed lymphoid cells ('immunoblasts'). These cells show large nuclei, prominent nucleoli, and many mitoses. There may be areas of necrosis, and in the tonsil there is usually obstruction of crypt drainage. Seeing this active population of cells, some of which may resemble Reed–Sternberg cells, and an apparent loss of normal architecture, the examining pathologist may suspect malignant lymphoma. The clinical history, serological studies, and immunohistochemical examination of the cellular population within the tonsil (which does not show light-chain restriction) should enable the correct diagnosis to be achieved.

Other infections of the tonsil

Historically tuberculosis of the tonsil was seen following consumption of cow's milk infected with *Mycobacterium bovis*. A primary complex was produced which consisted of an inconspicuous tonsillar focus and enlarged cervical lymph nodes. Tonsillar tuberculosis is now rare due to the eradication of the bovine disease.

Corynebacterium diphtheriae pharyngitis involves the mucosa of the tonsil and surrounding soft palate, producing a 'membrane' of neutrophils, fibrin, bacteria, and squamous cells over the affected surfaces. The effect is due to a bacterial exotoxin, and immunization programmes generating effective antitoxin activity have virtually eliminated the disease in this country.

15.4.5   Neoplasms of the tonsil

Squamous cell carcinoma

Squamous cell carcinoma of the upper aerodigestive tract may affect the tonsil, although the larynx, tongue, and the floor of the mouth are more common sites. Tonsillar carcinoma is related to smoking and heavy alcohol consumption, shows a male predominance, and has a median age of onset of around sixty. Patients present with sore throat, swelling, and haemoptysis. Grossly one tonsil is usually swollen, and the lesion is exophytic or ulcerative. Histologically the features are those of typical squamous carcinoma, usually well or moderately differentiated, although occasional cases are so undifferentiated as to resemble nasopharyngeal carcinoma. Associated field changes of dysplasia or carcinoma *in situ* are frequently seen in the epithelium of the tonsil and surrounding structures. The tumour metastasizes early to lymph nodes in the cervical chain. Treatment is by means of local radiotherapy for disease confined to the tonsil, with surgical resection of the tonsil and adjacent involved tissue when tumour persists or recurs. Resection usually involves an accompanying radical neck dissection to remove tumour in lymph nodes, and the overall five-year survival is around 50 per cent.

Tonsillar lymphoma

The tonsil is a common site for malignant lymphoma, usually of the non-Hodgkin's variety, and most having a B-cell origin. In contrast, Hodgkin's disease is rare in the tonsil, and when it does occur is seen in association with disease in the upper cervical or pre-auricular lymph nodes. Any type of non-Hodgkin's lymphoma may arise in, or involve, the tonsil, including not only those commonly seen in peripheral lymph node, but also lymphomas of mucosa-associated lymphoid tissue (MALT) (see Chapter 24). The tonsil thus appears to participate in both peripheral and mucosal immunity.

15.4.6   Further reading

Barton, J. H., *et al.* (1984). Non-Hodgkin's lymphoma of the tonsil. A clinicopathologic study of 65 cases. *Cancer* **53**, 86–95.

Chan, J. K. C., Ng, C. S., and Lo, S. T. H. (1987). Immunohistochemical characterization of malignant lymphomas of the Waldeyer's ring other than the nasopharynx. *Histopathology* **11**, 885–99.

Saul, S. H. and Kapadica, S. B. (1985). Primary lymphoma of Waldeyer's ring. Clinicopathologic study of 68 cases. *Cancer* **56**, 157–66.

15.5   Larynx

L. Michaels

Diseases of the larynx are often of urgent concern to the patient because of involvement of the airway. Acute bacterial infection requires urgent diagnosis and treatment of the impending asphyxia. Carcinoma, on the other hand, may arise insidiously with only mild hoarseness at first, but prompt diagnosis is required for effective antitumour therapy to be instituted.

Clinical diagnosis of laryngeal disease is facilitated by the methods of laryngoscopy. There are two forms of this procedure. Indirect laryngoscopy is carried out by placing an illuminated mirror behind the tongue. Supraglottis, vocal cords, and even a small amount of subglottis may be inspected in this way. Direct laryngoscopy is carried out under general or local anaesthetic. The interior of the larynx is viewed under reflected light with a microscope, and instruments may be passed to obtain material for biopsy or to perform surgical procedures.

15.5.1   Anatomy

The larynx is basically a hollow tube with a flap at its upper end (the epiglottis), which serves to protect the airway from inspiration of food material, and highly mobile vocal cords lower down, which function in phonation.

Regions

Mainly for purposes of classification of neoplasms, the larynx has been divided into three regions: supraglottis, glottis, and subglottis. The supraglottis is that region above the true vocal cords, including the epiglottis, the false cords, the ventricles, and the saccules. The glottis comprises the vocal cords, the vocal processes of the arytenoids, and the anterior and posterior commissures. The subglottis is that region of the larynx below the true vocal cords down to the level of the lower border of the cricoid cartilage, below which the trachea commences.

Cartilages and elastic membranes

The complexity of laryngeal anatomy is the result of the curious relationships that exist among the five laryngeal cartilages. A useful approach to depicting these relationships has been made by Paff (1973), and is reproduced in Fig. 15.15. In this figure, the cartilages of the larynx are built up in their final relationship to each other. Diagram 1 shows the unembellished thyroid cartilage, the largest single cartilage in the laryngeal framework. In this diagram the thyroid cartilage is seen from behind. Below the anterior notch, a square area is depicted where the handle of the spoon-shaped epiglottis is attached (diagrams 2 and 3). The two false cords are inserted anteriorly at the pointed area and the true vocal cords are inserted into the two small oval areas below these. In diagram 4 the cricoid lamina (situated at the

back of the ring-shaped cricoid cartilage) is depicted from behind. The two lower facets are for articulation with the inferior cornua of the thyroid cartilage (as in diagram 5). The two upper facets are for articulation with the arytenoid cartilages. These are shown separately from behind in diagram 6, with the minute corniculate cartilage joined to the apex of each arytenoid. In diagram 7 the arytenoids are shown in position on top of the cricoid lamina, forming the cricoarytenoid joints. The arytenoids are thus in the posterior wall of the larynx. The hyoid bone is also related to the larynx by connection through ligaments and muscles. It is not shown in the diagram, but would be represented as a horseshoe-shaped structure, closed in front of the epiglottis and open behind.

Only the apical portion of the arytenoid and its lateral muscular process are shown in the posterior view. What is not shown is a short anterior projection from each arytenoid—the vocal process—which gives origin to the elastic tissue of the true vocal cord on each side. Beneath the mucosa of the larynx, superficial to the cartilage, an elastic membrane is present. (A similar structure is present in the trachea and bronchi.) The quadrangular membrane (the name given to the elastic membrane in the upper part of the larynx) is shown in diagram 8, stretching from the corniculate cartilage to the epiglottis above, and from the muscular process of the arytenoid to the lower part of the epiglottis below. The upper part represents the framework of the aryepiglottic fold. The recess between the lateral surface of the quadrangular membrane medially and the medial side of the thyroid cartilage lamina laterally on each side is occupied by the piriform fossa—a pouch of hypopharyngeal mucosa that serves for the passage of food and drink, on each side of the larynx. The quadrangular membrane ends inferiorly in the false cords. Beneath the false cords there is a gap in the elastic lamina of the larynx, which makes way for the ventricle of the larynx and its upward extension, the saccule. The core of the true vocal cord on each side is an elastic layer—the vocal ligament—which extends from the vocal process forwards to be inserted in the back of the thyroid cartilage (the oval area in diagrams 1, 3, and 5). From this elastic tissue of the true vocal cord the lower laryngeal elastic membrane—the conus elasticus, or cricothyroid membrane—extends downwards to be attached into the upper surface of the cricoid ring. Thus the upper part of the subglottic larynx, i.e. the part of the larynx below the true vocal cords but above the cricoid ring, is bounded anteriorly by the conus elasticus.

15.5.2   Some histological features

Epiglottis

The pear-shaped epiglottic cartilage contains elastic tissue and does not undergo ossification. The elastic cartilage is perforated in the lower two-thirds by numerous foramina, which are produced by seromucinous glands that open through the posterior epithelial surface. The mucosa lining the anterior epiglottic surface is stratified squamous epithelium in continuity with that of the posterior surface of the tongue (vallecula) and surrounding

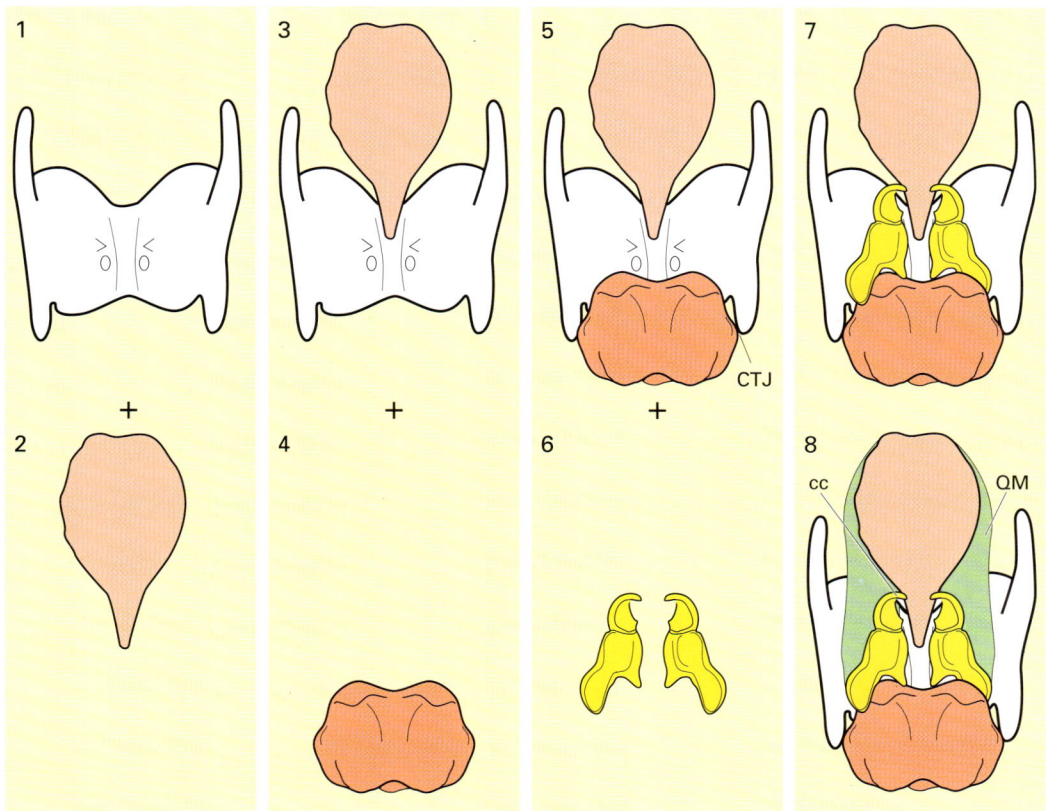

Fig. 15.15 The cartilaginous framework of the larynx. In this series of diagrams the cartilages of the larynx are built up into their actual relationships with each other. 1, the shape of the thyroid cartilage from behind. 2, the epiglottic cartilage, placed in position in 3. 4, the cricoid lamina from behind; the ring of the cricoid is not seen. 5, the position of the lamina in relation to the thyroid cartilage. The arytenoids are seen in 6 and are placed in position in 7. In 8, the elastic quadrangular membrane (QM) is in place. The vertically hatched part of this represents the aryepiglottic folds; cc, position of insertion of cuneiform cartilage at apex of arytenoid; CTJ, cricothyroid joint. (Drawn after Paff 1973, with permission.)

hypopharynx. The posterior (or laryngeal) epiglottis is covered by a similar stratified squamous epithelium in its upper half, but lower down this changes into the ciliated pseudostratified columnar type characteristic of most of the internal laryngeal lining. The submucosa of the lingual epiglottic surface is comparatively loose areolar tissue, compared with the dense compact connective tissue of the posterior epiglottic surface.

False cords

The epithelium of the false cords is of the respiratory type. However, squamous metaplasia is common. The submucosa is characterized by a large number of seromucinous glands embedded in a fibro-areolar stroma, which is admixed with strands of striated muscle fibres extending superiorly from the thyro-arytenoid (vocalis) muscle. These glands are also found within the loose fibres of the quandrangular membrane.

True vocal cords

The epithelium of the true vocal cord is of stratified squamous

variety. The lamina propria of the true vocal cord is bounded on its deep aspect by the vocal ligament, and at its upper and lower extents by respiratory mucosa. It contains no seromucinous glands. This vocal cord lamina propria is said to be deficient in lymphatic drainage and forms a space (Reinke's space). The vocal ligament (which is continuous below with the conus elasticus) is nodular thickening composed of elastic tissue to which the vocalis portion of the thyroarytenoid muscle is tethered.

15.5.3 Infections

The larynx is subject to infections caused by a wide variety of organisms, but only acute epiglottitis and acute laryngo-tracheobronchitis are seen in clinical practice with any frequency. The reason for this is partly that infection in general is now less common, with improved hygienic practices and much better methods of treatment. Other important reasons for the paucity of laryngeal infections are that few infecting organisms settle in the larynx, and those that do are efficiently eliminated.

The most important pathway for the exposure of organisms to the larynx is via the upper respiratory tract airway. The nose acts as a highly efficient filter of all large particles; only those smaller than 1 μm reach and settle in the lungs. Thus the great majority of dust particles or droplet nuclei containing bacteria, viruses, or fungi that enter the respiratory tract either remain in the nose or pass directly into the terminal part of the respiratory tree. Those organisms that do drop off at the level of the larynx are probably efficiently dealt with by the local mucous stream and by the standard immunological mechanisms. The slight tendency that the true vocal cords may have to act as a net for micro-organisms by virtue of their projection into the air flow is, no doubt, counteracted by the greater resistance to infection of the stratified squamous epithelium covering those structures.

The larynx is also subject to hypersensitivity reactions, which may mimic the effects of acute infection, so that these acute inflammatory conditions are best considered together.

Acute inflammation of the larynx

Acute inflammation may take a variety of forms in the larynx. There are four groups, each with a characteristic aetiological basis and pathological appearance, into which most cases would seem to fit:

1. Acute epiglottitis. This is usually caused by bacteria, in the majority of cases *Haemophilus influenzae* type B.
2. Acute laryngotracheobronchitis. This inflammatory lesion is probably caused by viruses, and the glottis and subglottic regions are particularly affected.
3. Allergic laryngitis.
4. Diphtheritic laryngitis.

The majority of cases are children in whom, because of the narrowness of the airway, the obstruction is serious and sometimes fatal.

Acute epiglottitis

Acute epiglottitis was not recognized as a pathological entity until the early 1940s, when the association with *Haemophilus influenzae* tybe B was noted in many cases.

Vague prodromata of upper respiratory infection are followed by sore throat and pain on swallowing. The voice is relatively unaffected and there is little cough. The condition progresses rapidly with shock, leading to severe respiratory obstruction within 1–24 h. The child's dyspnoea is exacerbated in the supine position. The clinical diagnosis is confirmed by observation of the fiery red, swollen epiglottis above the tongue.

Pathology At autopsy, not only does the epiglottis show signs of acute inflammation, but the adjacent tongue and pharyngeal structures are also swollen. Microscopic sections from fatal cases of acute epiglottitis show an acute inflammatory exudate with neutrophils, red cells, and fibrin infiltrating the anterior part of the epiglottis deep to the squamous epithelium. In all cases there is a lymphocytic exudate in the posterior epiglottic mucosa. Sections taken from the posterior part of the larynx,

hypopharynx, supraglottic larynx, including aryepiglottic folds, and vocal cord region show acute inflammatory exudate similar in intensity to the anterior epiglottic region affecting the vallecula, hypopharynx, and aryepiglottic fold region (Fig. 15.16). The exudate is also present in the deep tissues of the larynx, extending downwards deep to the thyrohyoid, thyroarytenoid, and interarytenoid muscles, but the false and true cord mucosae do not show this change.

Pathogenesis It is clear from the above description that acute epiglottitis does not originate as a laryngeal disorder, but as an acute inflammatory condition affecting the oropharynx and hypopharynx. The anterior mucosa of the epiglottis, the pre-epiglottic space, and the aryepiglottic folds are involved as part of this inflammatory process, and the inflammation tracks downwards through the deep muscular tissues of the larynx, but does not involve the mucosal surface of the larynx because the latter is on the airway side of the quadrangular membrane. Therefore, obstruction of the laryngeal airway takes place by pressure from outside. The clinical features of acute epiglottitis are in keeping with this distribution of the inflammatory pro-

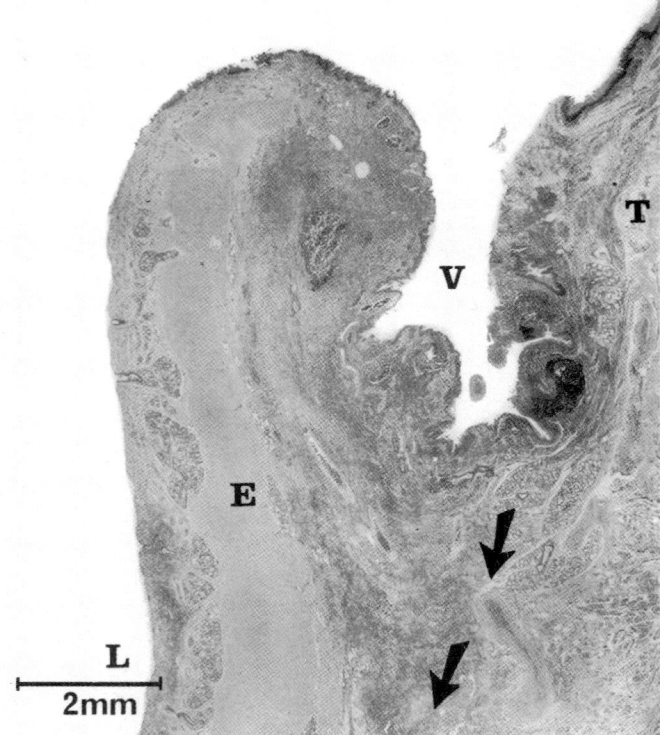

Fig. 15.16 Sagittal section through the epiglottis, vallecula, and posterior surface of tongue in a case of acute epiglottitis. Note severe accumulation of inflammatory exudate with a neutrophilic exudate in mucosa of anterior epiglottis, under vallecula, and in deeper tissue behind epiglottic cartilage. Posterior epiglottic mucosa is only mildly inflamed with a lymphocytic exudate. Arrows indicate the direction of spread of inflammation from vallecula into larynx. E, epiglottic cartilage; L, laryngeal cavity; T, back of tongue; V, vallecula. (From Michaels 1987, with permission.)

cess. Pain in the throat and difficulty in swallowing are important symptoms; hoarseness is not. Difficulty in breathing is a late symptom of acute epiglottitis, related to airway obstruction.

Haemophilus influenzae is a common organism in the normal upper respiratory tract flora. For reasons not understood the acquisition of the so-called B antigen conveys pathogenicity to this normally commensal organism. It is likely that this organism gains entry to the submucous tissues through the pharyngeal epithelium, perhaps through a crypt of the lingual tonsil, and, on finding a suitable soil in a particular case, induces a severe pharyngitis which eventually occludes the laryngeal inlet tissues in the way described. The reason why the condition has been given the designation acute epiglottitis, rather than pharyngitis, is that the epiglottic component is the most conspicuous one on observation of the tissues clinically and at autopsy. The actual airway obstruction is related to the deep extension of the acute inflammation in the larynx and not to the swelling of the epiglottis itself.

Acute laryngotracheobronchitis

The synonyms for acute laryngotracheobronchitis—subglottic laryngitis, non-diphtheritic croup, virus croup, and fibrinous laryngotracheobronchitis—indicate the likely aetiological and pathological bases as well as the characteristic anatomical location of this inflammatory disease.

The onset of the condition is more gradual than that of acute epiglottitis. When fully developed, there is a croupy cough with inspiratory and expiratory stridor, features which are not characteristic of the latter (see above).

A viral aetiology for this condition has been emphasized, but the evidence is not conclusive.

Pathology The mortality from acute laryngotracheobronchitis has been very low for many years. Thus, to obtain a description of the pathological appearances, it is necessary to refer to accounts given before the antibiotic era. According to the study of Brennemann *et al.* (1938), they are characterized by neutrophil exudate in the subglottis, accompanied by mucus and fibrin, with degeneration of epithelial cells. A gummy, rope-like exudate and crusting of necrotic epithelium are observed grossly. These changes take place mainly at the subglottic level in the larynx. There is a sparing of the seromucinous glands until late in the disease (unlike diphtheritic laryngitis, in which a specific necrosis of glands takes place with sparing of the surrounding tissue). The process extends downwards as tracheitis, bronchitis, and bronchiolitis associated with similar rope-like secretions and dried crusts. Interstitial pneumonia, atelectasis, and pulmonary oedema may also be present following the changes in the tracheobronchial tree.

In contrast to this earlier study, observations more recently have found 'round cell infiltration' of the inflamed tracheobronchial tree, more suggestive of a viral aetiology.

Allergic laryngitis

Although clinical features of laryngeal involvement are common in hypersensitivity reactions, there has been little opportunity for study of the pathological basis of allergic conditions.

A large number of possible inhaled allergens have been cited as relevant to allergic laryngitis, including house dust, moulds, feathers, animal dander, volatile oils, or emanations from plants. Food antigens have also been incriminated (Williams 1972).

The pathological feature of allergic laryngitis takes the form of varying degres of oedema involving the epiglottis, aryepiglottic fold, and vocal cords, the most severe being 'glottic oedema' related to anaphylactic reaction. In this condition the location of the oedema would seem to be similar to that of the acute inflammatory process of acute epiglottitis, i.e. the anterior surface of the epiglottis, aryepiglottic fold, base of tongue, and hypopharynx, and it seems possible that the respiratory obstruction is produced in a similar way by allergic oedema rather than by acute inflammatory exudate. Miller (1940) showed that the submucous areolar tissue extends from the base of the tongue continuously to the tip of the epiglottis, and the existence of a layer of such tissue could account for the spread of fluid in both allergic laryngitis and acute epiglottitis.

Angioneurotic oedema (angioedema)

In angioneurotic oedema, episodes of oedema take place in the larynx, principally in the epiglottis and supraglottis (for the anatomical reasons described above), and by prejudicing the airway, may endanger life. Two important forms may be recognized:

Angioneurotic oedema associated with urticaria This is the already mentioned acute form of allergic laryngitis. An external antigen such as pollen, food, or drugs, reacts with IgE to give rise to skin and laryngeal (and sometimes intestinal, particularly colicky) manifestations.

Hereditary angioneurotic oedema In this form there is no urticaria, but attacks of colic as well as laryngeal oedema are common. The condition is inherited as a autosomal dominant so that there is usually a strong family history. There is a deficiency of inhibitor of the serum complement factor C1. Complement factors C1, C4, and C2 are used up and their serum levels are very low. C1 inhibitor is also lacking in many of the relatives of the patients. The condition is treated by administration of an androgenic drug such as testosterone, which, surprisingly, raises the level of C1 inhibitor and prevents attacks of angioneurotic oedema.

Diphtheritic laryngitis

Diphtheria is an acute mucosal inflammation of the fauces, soft palate, and tonsils, produced by *Corynebacterium diphtheriae*. The mucosal inflammation of diphtheria may spread to, or may be confined to, the larynx. In these cases the epiglottis, false cords, and true cords are covered by a false membrane, a dull, greyish-yellow thickened layer which may extend down into the trachea.

Microscopically the false membrane is composed of fibrin and neutrophils with, in the early stages, large numbers of diphtheria bacilli. On the deeper aspects, the laryngeal epithelium is included with the membrane. Where this epithelium is respiratory columnar in type, the membrane peels easily off the basement membrane (it may indeed be coughed up), but in the squamous-epithelium-lined vocal cords the false membranes separates off with difficulty and airway obstruction may result.

The submucosal seromucinous glands underlying the diphtheritic membrane often show necrosis; in other forms of acute laryngitis this is said not to happen.

Tuberculosis

Tuberculosis of the larynx is a disease that is almost always associated with tuberculosis of the lungs. In common with pulmonary tuberculosis, laryngeal tuberculosis has become unusual in developed countries. The lesions are often nodular, sometimes ulcerated, and usually affect the vocal cords. Microscopic examination shows the fully developed appearance of tuberculosis with inflammatory tissue consisting of epithelioid cells, lymphocytes, and Langerhans giant cells. Caseous necrosis is present to a variable degree. Special stains may reveal acid-fast bacilli in some cases, but very often these are not seen due to their small numbers in the infected tissue.

15.5.4 Vocal cord polyp and Reinke's oedema

Reinke's space is a potential space of the true vocal cord situated immediately under the epithelium. In vocal cord polyp a localized grape-like swelling arises in the anterior part of the vocal cord from the exudation of blood products into Reinke's space. This condition is caused by excessive untrained use of the vocal cords which come together with undue force during phonation. Oedema of Reinke's space is caused by irritation of the vocal cords by cigarette smoking or industrial fumes. Hypothyroidism may cause a similar lesion. In oedema the full length of both Reinke's spaces are diffusely oedematous (Fig. 15.17).

15.5.5 Tumours of the larynx

Squamous cell papilloma

Squamous cell papillomas are polypoid protuberances of the epithelium, which are frequent in the larynx of adults. They are also present in children where, because of the much narrower diameter of the airway, the symptoms are more serious, and treatment is more urgent and difficult. By far the commonest site of occurrence of squamous papilloma of the larynx is the vocal cord. The anterior half of the cord is more frequently affected than the posterior.

Pathology

The papillary processes arise from the epithelium of the larynx as cylindrical projections, each with a vascular connective tissue core. In sections of some papillomas, smaller cylinders of squamous-cell-covered epithelium, each with its own fibrovascular core, are present in the vicinity of the larger papillae and are cut in various planes. These represent second- or even third-order branching of the papillary structures.

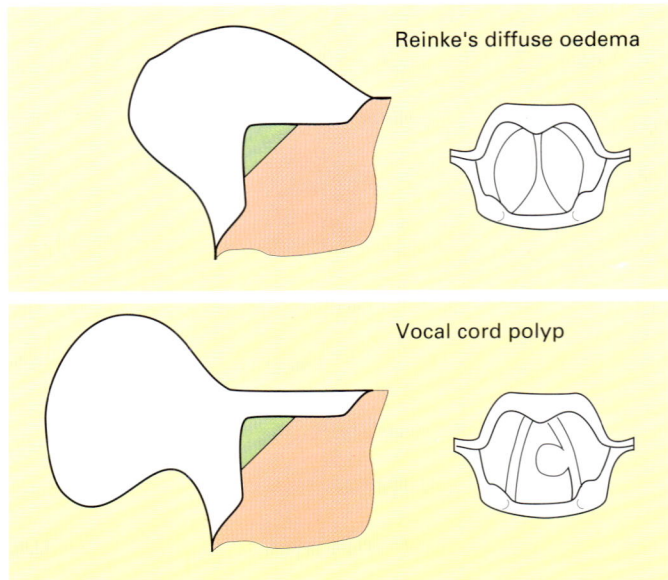

Fig. 15.17 Diagrams of coronal section (left) and direct laryngoscopic view to illustrate gross distinction between Reinke's diffuse oedema and vocal cord polyp. The coronal sections show (from left to right) Reinke's space, vocal ligament and thyroarytenoid muscle. In Reinke's oedema the full lenghts of both Reinke's spaces are diffusely oedematous. In the vocal cord polyp there is a localized swelling of Reinke's space on one side. (Drawn after Michaels 1987, with permission.)

A process of 'koilocytosis' is very frequently seen in squamous papillomas of the larynx. It consists of a spherical enlargement of the cells of the lesion, accompanied by perinuclear vacuolation, so that no stained cytoplasm is seen in the cell or, if it is, is present as a thin rim round the cell periphery. There may be moderate degrees of dysplasia. Koilocytosis is thought to be a feature of infection with human papillomavirus. Recently the technique of DNA hybridization has been used to detect the human papillomavirus genome (HPV) in laryngeal papillomas, and HPV types 6 and 11 have been found in the cells of most of these neoplasms.

Malignant change is an extremely rare development in the course of squamous papillomatosis.

Squamous cell carcinoma

Squamous cell carcinoma is by far the commonest neoplasm of the larynx, arising directly in many cases from the squamous epithelium covering the vocal cords; it also frequently arises from the covering epithelium of other parts of the larynx. It is well established that precancerous states (which can be recognized microscopically) frequently precede squamous carcinoma.

Epidemiological factors

As with carcinoma of the bronchus, there is strong evidence of a relationship between squamous carcinoma of the larynx and cigarette smoking. Evidence is growing also that alcohol excess may play a part in carcinoma of the larynx. Alcohol carcinogenesis is more difficult to explain than that due to cigarette smoking, in which known carcinogens are involved. The mechanism of carcinogenesis could involve alcohol-related nutritional deficiencies, such as zinc or vitamin A. Another possible mechanism could be a synergistic effect on a known carcinogen. There is a widespread clinical impression among laryngologists that the carcinogenic potential of cigarette smoking on the larynx is enhanced by excessive alcohol consumption. Another factor that may be found as a possible causative agent in carcinoma of the larynx is previous radiation to the area, either for an unrelated lesion of the neck or in the treatment of previous carcinoma of the larynx.

Carcinoma of the larynx occurs mainly in men, probably because of the higher incidence of heavy cigarette smokers among men.

It is likely that many cases of squamous carcinoma pass through a stage in which malignant changes are present for a time in the epithelium of the larynx without actual deep invasion. Such changes are termed precancerous, and it is important to consider them because it is possible that they represent the earliest treatable form of the malignant process. Squamous carcinomas in the larynx develop not only from the epithelium of the vocal cord, which is lined normally by squamous epithelium, but also from other areas, which are normally lined by respiratory epithelium.

Precancerous states

A severe degree of dysplasia and carcinoma *in situ* are the precancerous states, which can be recognized by microscopic examination of the laryngeal epithelium. Carcinoma *in situ* is a focal change in the squamous epithelium, in which whole thickness is replaced by dysplastic epithelium.

Dysplasia of squamous epithelium is the presence of cells that have features of malignancy but without the invasive properties of a carcinoma. The pathologist recognizes such cells by experience based on his repeated exposure to malignant tissues. A detailed analysis of such cells shows them to have many or all of the following characteristics:

1. nuclear hyperchromatism;
2. prominent nucleoli;
3. increase in nuclear–cytoplasmic ratio;
4. very large and very small nuclei;
5. irregularity in nuclear membranes;
6. increased numbers of mitoses;
7. the presence of mitoses in the upper epidermal layers (i.e. away from the basal layer); and
8. the presence of abnormal mitotic figures.

Taking the squamous epithelium as a whole, dysplastic epithelium shows the following overall structural changes:

1. hyperplasia of basal cells with disturbance of the normal maturational sequence; and (at a later stage)

2. the presence of 'drop-shaped rete processes'.

The rete processes normally taper progressively, or else form structures with almost parallel sides and blunt ends. Rete processes that are wider at their deeper part than superficially are described as 'drop-shaped' and occur frequently in dysplasic epithelia.

Observations have been made in the cervix uteri that have led to a classification of dysplasia by degrees of 'cervical intraepithelial neoplasia' (CIN) in which the highest, grade III, comprises lesions of both carcinoma *in situ* and severe dysplasia with surface maturation. Laryngeal dysplasia (LD) may be classified in a similar fashion. LD, grade I, shows a minor degree of atypical change confined to the basal third of the squamous epithelium. LD, grade III, embraces carcinoma *in situ* and is a better designation because not all cases go on to invasive carcinoma. It also embraces severe dysplasia, with and without surface keratosis, in which the atypical change involves at least two-thirds of the epithelium. LD, grade II, lies within the spectrum between LD grades I and III and shows involvement of one-third to two-thirds of the basal portion of the epithelium by the dysplastic change.

Invasive squamous cell carcinoma

Macroscopic appearances The commonest site for squamous carcinoma of the larynx is at the anterior part of the true cord. However, the lesion may be seen anywhere in the larynx. It is least frequent in a posterior situation. Whatever its size and situation, by far the most usual gross appearance is that of a flat plaque with a well-defined, somewhat raised, edge and a surface that ranges from occasional furrows to marked corrugation or even papillae. The cut surface reveals this structure to consist of a pale-grey well-defined band, of variable thickness (Fig. 15.18).

The anatomical routes of spread of squamous carcinoma arising from the epithelium of the laryngeal airway depend on the site of origin of the neoplasm within the larynx. The tumour usually invades outwards at right angles to the surface of origin. In advanced cancers the tumour is also markedly papillary and will tend to obstruct the airway of the larynx. Deep penetration of the cartilaginous framework of the larynx by tumour will eventually occur, allowing the neoplasm to escape into surrounding structures. Squamous cell carcinoma of the larynx has a high tendency to metastasize to cervical lymph nodes. This is particularly prominent in larger invasive tumours. In every post-mortem study on patients dying of carcinoma of the larynx, it has been found that the majority have bloodstream metastases, which are most common in the lungs. They are also frequently seen in the liver, bones, and mediastinal lymph nodes. In all cases showing bloodstream metastases, cervical lymph node metastases are present or have become manifest and have been treated.

Microscopic appearances The histological features of squamous carcinoma are extremely variable, and in a particular neoplasm result from the proportions of the different epidermoid components that are present. Like normal squamous cell

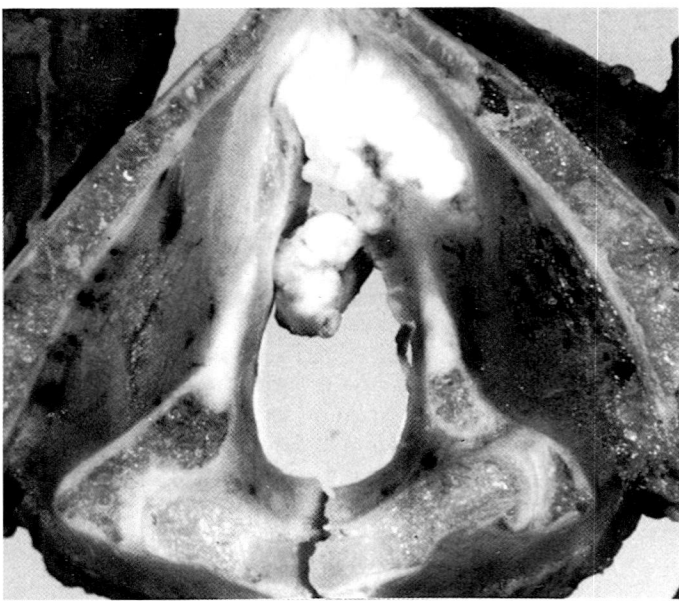

Fig. 15.18 Squamous carcinoma of the anterior glottic region. The neoplasm shows a papillary aspect as well as that of a flat plaque; (enlarged to 1.2 times actual size). (From Michaels 1987, with permission.)

epithelium, these include undifferentiated basal cells, intermediate 'prickle' cells, cells containing keratohyaline granules, and acellular keratinous material. Glycogen is also found frequently within the epithelial cells of a squamous carcinoma, which become large and appear empty. Unlike normal squamous epithelium invasive squamous carcinoma shows a confused assembly of component tissues and all of the individual cells show features of malignancy.

Special forms of squamous carcinoma

Spindle-cell carcinoma A form of squamous carcinoma of the larynx, which is often difficult to diagnose histologically because of its resemblance to sarcoma, is known as spindle-cell carcinoma (synonym: pseudosarcoma). The tumour usually arises from the vocal cord and is polypoid. Microscopically squamous carcinoma is present but gives way to a malignant cell mesenchymal neoplasm, which forms the bulk of the neoplasm. Diagnosis depends on the finding of malignant squamous epithelium in some parts of the tumour.

Spindle-cell carcinoma has a similar malignant potential to squamous carcinoma of similar size and position in the larynx.

Verrucous squamous carcinoma When invasive squamous cell carcinoma is very well differentiated it is difficult to distinguish it from a large squamous papilloma. This form of neoplasia is known as verrucous squamous cell carcinoma. The tumour has a prominent surface papillary component and deep invasion is by 'pushing' margins, composed of irregular rete ridges, not jagged narrow tongues of tumour as in conventional squamous carcinoma. A clue to the malignant neoplastic nature of the lesion lies in the especially large size of the cells of the malpighian layer. Verrucous squamous carcinoma grows slowly and invades and destroys the laryngeal wall, but neither lymphatic nor bloodstream metastases are to be expected.

Non-epidermoid epithelial tumours

These are rare in the larynx. Adenoid cystic carcinoma is seen rarely, as are other forms of adenocarcinoma. Mesenchymal tumours are even rarer.

15.5.6 Bibliography

Anderson, J. R. (ed.) (1980). *Muir's textbook of pathology* (11th edn). Edward Arnold, London.

Brennemann, J., Clifton, W. M., Frank, A., and Holinger, P. H. (1938). Acute laryngotracheobronchitis. *American Journal of Disease in Childhood* **55**, 667.

Michaels, L. (1984). *Pathology of the larynx*. Springer-Verlag, Berlin.

Michaels, L. (1987). *Ear, nose and throat histopathology*. Springer-Verlag, London.

Miller, V. M. (1940). Edema of the larynx. A study of the loose areolar tissues of the larynx. *Archives of Otolaryngology* **31**, 256.

Paff, A. G. E. (1973). *Anatomy of the head and neck*. Saunders, Philadelphia.

Williams, R. I. (1972). Allergic laryngitis. *Annals of Otology, Rhinology and Laryngology* **81**, 558.

16

The alimentary system

16

The alimentary system

16.1 Oesophagus

H. Thompson

16.1.1 Normal structure and function

The oesophagus is a muscular tube which is in a collapsed state most of the time although it distends to allow the passage of food, saliva, or gastric content during eating, swallowing, or regurgitation. The swallowing mechanism consists of relaxation of the sphincters accompanied by the passage of peristaltic waves of contraction through both striated and smooth muscle segments. The oesophagus extends from the pharynx at the level of the 6th cervical vertebra to the level of the diaphragm at the 11th or 12th thoracic vertebrae and it measures 24–30 cm in the adult, from 1.3 to 3 cm in its lateral diameter and approximately 1.9 cm in its anterior–posterior diameter. It is shorter, of course, in children and in women.

The entrance is encircled by the crico-pharyngeus muscle which acts as the upper oesophageal sphincter. On the other hand, the lower oesophageal sphincter at the gastro-oesophageal junction is a physiological entity rather than an anatomic stucture and it can be regarded as a 'closing segment'. The purpose of the sphincter is to prevent regurgitation of gastric contents into the oesophagus as well as to relax during swallowing to allow the passage of food. In the basal state in man the pressure is 12–30 mmHg above the intra-abdominal pressure level as determined by manometry. The sphincter can also be demonstrated radiologically.

The pharynx communicates with the oesophagus which then pursues a course down through the posterior mediastinum behind the trachea and left main bronchus through the left crus of the diaphragm into the stomach. In the empty state, the lumen contains numerous parallel longitudinal folds that smooth out on swallowing. There are four zones of relative narrowing in the oesophagus at the level of:

1. cricopharyngeus, 15 cm from the incisor teeth;
2. the aortic arch, 22 cm from the incisor teeth;
3. the left main bronchus, 27 cm from the incisor teeth; and
4. the diaphragm, 40 cm from the incisor teeth.

Foreign bodies larger than 2.5 cm in diameter can be arrested in those narrow zones.

The intra-abdominal segment of the oesophagus measures 1.2 cm in length. The endoscopic anatomy of the oesophagus is of considerable importance to the pathologist. The entrance to the oesophagus is located at a distance of 15–16 cm from the incisor teeth while the gastro-oesophageal junction is situated 36–42 cm from the incisor teeth. The oesophagus possesses the following layers, viz. mucosa, submucosa, muscularis propria, and a peri-oesophageal fibrous layer. The muscularis mucosa separates the lamina propria of the mucosa from the submucosa.

The oesophagus is lined by pale stratified non-keratinizing squamous epithelium. The basal germinative zone represents 10–15 per cent of the total mucosal thickness. Glycogen is present in the upper layers. The lower border with rete pegs interdigitates with the conical papillae of the lamina propria which may contain small numbers of chronic inflammatory cells and occasional lymphoid aggregates. Melanocytes, argyrophilic cells, and Langerhans cells can occur within the squamous mucosa. Ducts lead through the muscularis mucosa into submucous, racemose, mucin-secreting glands which resemble the minor salivary glands of the mouth and pharynx.

An important landmark is the crenated squamo-columnar junction (Z line or ora serratta) where the pale glistening oesophageal mucosa changes to a deeper red or orange colour with a more succulent appearance, representing the gastric columnar epithelium. It is situated 0–2 cm above the lower anatomical end of the oesophagus and it is usually within the lower oesophageal sphincter zone.

The upper oesophagus is encircled by striated muscle fibres over a distance of 6–8 cm merging with smooth muscle of the muscularis propria in the lower oesophagus. The vagus, glossopharyngeal nerve and sympathetic ganglia innervate the oesophagus. Neurones in the myenteric plexus are of two types, viz. arygrophil or arygrophobe. The arygrophil cells act as information-transmitting neurones and the arygrophobe cells are secretor neurones whose function is to produce acetylcholine to fire the muscle fibres when instructed by the arygrophil cell. The neural mechanisms interact with chemical messengers and the neuro-endocrine system.

The arterial supply of the oesophagus comes from the descending thoracic aorta, the inferior thyroid branch of the thyro-cervical trunk, the left gastric branch of the coeliac artery, and the left inferior phrenic branch of the abdominal aorta. The venous drainage involves the inferior thyroid veins, azygos, hemiazygos, accessory veins, short gastric, coronary, and vertebral veins. Communications between the lower oesophageal veins and the azygos veins can lead to the development of oesophageal varices in portal hypertension.

Lymphatic plexuses are distributed in the submucosa and in the muscle coat and drain at different levels into deep cervical, paratracheal, infrahyoid, posterior mediastinal (paratracheal), left gastric, and cardiac nodes, and also into the thoracic duct.

16.1.2 Developmental abnormalities

The oesophagus appears as a constriction separating the pharynx from the stomach around the 3rd week of gestation, when the embryo measures 2.5 cm in length. At 32 days (5 mm stage) it is a short tube and it rapidly elongates over the next 2 weeks. Lateral ridges of proliferating epithelium develop in the upper part, dividing the lumen into an anterior and posterior portion. Necrosis of epithelium in the septa and immigration of mesenchyme leads to separation of the trachea and oesophagus by the 36th day.

The original mucosal lining consists of simple pseudostratified columnar cells. The layers become thicker and at the 6 week stage (13 mm) extracellular vacuoles appear between the epithelial cells, leading to the formation of spaces. Ciliated cells appear among the columnar cells at 8 weeks (28 mm stage). Periodic acid–Schiff (PAS)-positive cells (non-ciliated cells) appear and occasional goblet cells are found and it is claimed that mucin-positive goblet cells become more numerous in the 4th-5th months. Further stratification occurs, associated with degeneration and sloughing of cells.

Squamous cells appear during the 5th-6th months (130–160 mm stage) spreading proximally and distally, replacing the ciliated mucin-secreting cells. Columnar cells may persist to birth in the upper oesophagus as well as small islands of mucin-secreting cells, viz. cardiac glands, which are superficial to the muscularis mucosa. Parietal and chief cells are occasionally represented. Deep submucosal glands develop about the 7th month.

The circular muscle coat can be identified at 6 weeks and the longitudinal muscle layer is evident at the 9th week (30–35 mm stage). The entire oesophagus is encircled by smooth muscle and scattered striated fibres appear in the upper oesophagus at about the 38 mm stage and encircle the upper oesophagus by the 5th month. Some smooth muscle fibres may persist.

Heterotopias
Gastric mucosa
Rector and Connerley found aberrant mucosa in 13.2 per cent of their autopsies in infants and children under 15 years of age. Approximately 50 per cent represented true mucinous cardiac glands which occur as oval pink patches in the mucosa of the upper oesophagus. Parietal cell glands were found in 2.6 per cent in the upper and mid-oesophagus. They probably represented metaplasia within cardiac glands.

Endoscopic assessment of the incidence of congenital ectopic gastric mucosa in the upper oesophagus varies from 0.1 to 4 per cent. Dysphagia due to cricopharyngeal spasm provoked by acid secretion from ectopic gastric mucosa has recently been documented.

Ciliated columnar cells
Rector and Connerley encountered patches of ciliated columnar cells in 4.3 per cent of their autopsies. They were absent in those dying after 3 days of life, although they were common in premature infants. They are evanescent and disappear rapidly after birth. Such patches are rarely encountered in adults.

Sebaceous glands
These may occur as solitary or multiple small yellowish papules in approximately 2 per cent of cases.

Congenital cysts and duplications
Congenital cysts
These may be bronchogenic, oesophageal, or enteric and are allegedly responsible for 6–10 per cent of mediastinal masses.

They are usually lined by ciliated columnar epithelium but squamous, cuboidal, or transitional epithelium may also be present. The cysts represent an abnormality of vacuolization during the septation process or alternatively originate from buds of embryonic epithelium.

Enteric cysts arise posteriorly and present as spherical cysts or as segmental cylindrical duplications which are often lined by gastric mucosa. Fibrous cords connect the lesion to the adjacent vertebrae and there may be associated vertebral anomalies. Two cases of carcinoma originating in duplication of the oesophagus have been reported in the literature.

Retention cysts
These represent dilatation of the ducts of submucosal glands due to blockage and they contain mucin. They are usually solitary and small in size, occasionally with inflammatory changes in their wall.

Oesophageal atresia and tracheo-oesophageal and broncho-oesophageal fistulas
The incidence of these abnormalities is from 1/2000 to 1/4000 births; other congenital anomalies are present in about 50 per cent. It represents a sporadic anomaly with a subsequent risk among siblings of 0.56 per cent. The most common abnormality is oesophageal atresia with a fistula connecting the distal

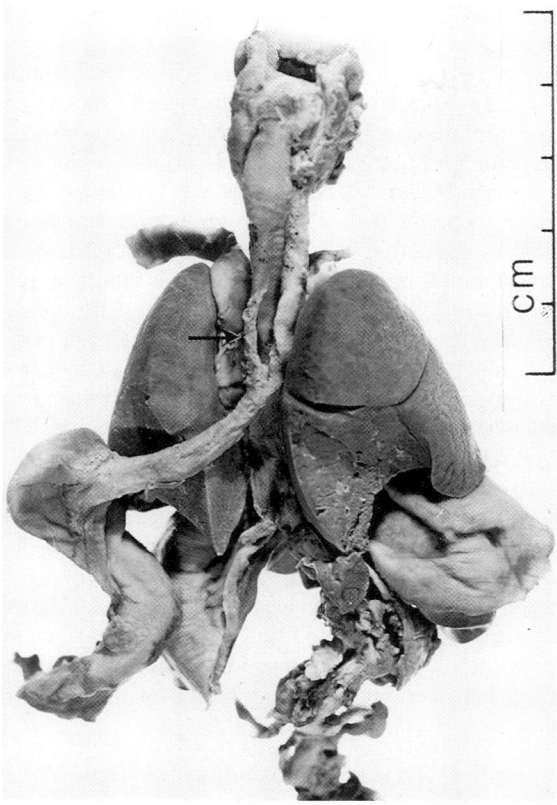

Fig. 16.1 Post-mortem dissection of a tracheo-oesophageal fistula (arrow) from a full-term infant.

oesophagus and trachea (Fig. 16.1). Septation of the oesophagus begins around the 21st day and is complete with separation of the oesophagus and trachea by the 36th day. A defect in the septation process can lead to the formation of a tracheo-oesophageal fistula. The associated atresia with a blind pouch is thought to be secondary to an oblique septation which extends more dorsally than normal, preventing normal development of the oesophagus.

Affected children develop symptoms within 24 h of birth. The inability to swallow saliva is responsible for excessive oral and nasal secretions. Air is forced through the distal fistula as a result of crying, causing abdominal and gastric distension with embarrassment of respiration. Regurgitation of air and gastric contents leads to chemical pneumonitis. Surgical correction of the anomaly is associated with survival figures of around 90 per cent.

Oesophago-bronchial fistulae can occur without atresia. They rarely persist into adolescent or adult life, presenting as a diagnostic problem suggesting that there may have been functional closure during childhood. Oesophageal fistulae may connect rarely with a pulmonary sequestration.

Congenital stenosis

This may represent a 'forme fruste' of atresia although it is usually more distal than the segment involved by atresia. It is

difficult to differentiate from acquired stenosis due to gastro-oesophageal reflux in early life.

Oesophageal webs and rings

Webs are described as thin membranes located on the anterior wall in the region of the crico-pharyngeus or as circumferential membranes that are thickest at this level. The membrane is thin, grey, and elastic, often with an eccentric lumen. They are most commonly encountered in the Plummer–Vinson syndrome, also known as the Patterson–Kelly syndrome, associated with sideropenic anaemia, dysphagia, koilonychia, glossitis, cheilitis, and splenomegaly, which occurs principally in middle-aged and elderly females. The dysphagia is intermittent in the early stages and restricted to solids. The syndrome is much less common now due to the improved health of the population. Histologically the membrane is lined by squamous epithelium.

Webs occur also in the absence of anaemia and, irrespective of associated anaemia, they may be asymptomatic. Webs and strictures have also been described in patients with benign pemphigus and in epidermolysis bullosa. Webs or membranes in the mid-oesophagus are rare but are frequently congenital in origin. Some webs or strictures, of course, in the mid-oesophagus are due to Barrett's syndrome.

Schatzki has described the radiological detection of a lower oesophageal ring which may be responsible for difficulty in swallowing when the diameter is reduced to 12 mm. It is seldom encountered before the age of 40 years and it is situated at the squamo-columnar junction as a thin, annular membrane associated frequently with a sliding hiatus hernia. The ring consists of loose connective tissue accompanied by overgrowth of the muscularis mucosa and covered by squamous or gastric mucosa. It is often grey and smooth above and pink below, as visualized during endoscopy. It probably represents an exaggeration of a normal ridge at the squamo-columnar junction. Most rings are asymptomatic but a food bolus, e.g. steak, may stick at the level of the ring, causing sudden dysphagia. This is sometimes referred to as the 'steakhouse syndrome'.

Pseudostrictures or rings can also cause diagnostic difficulty. The lower oesophageal sphincter may occasionally show up as a contractile ring on cinefluoroscopy. Muscle spasm and oedema due to reflux oesophagitis may cause a pseudostricture which will disappear following appropriate treatment. Other rare congenital rings which are completely covered by squamous epithelium have been described in the paediatric literature.

16.1.3   Functional disorders

Achalasia

This is a condition of debatable aetiology characterized by a large, dilated oesophagus (mega-oesophagus) (Fig. 16.2) which is due to failure of the lower oesophageal sphincter to relax in response to swallowing, as well as to the loss of peristaltic activity proximal to the sphincter. It is a neurogenic disorder and the majority of patients present between the ages of 35 and 45.

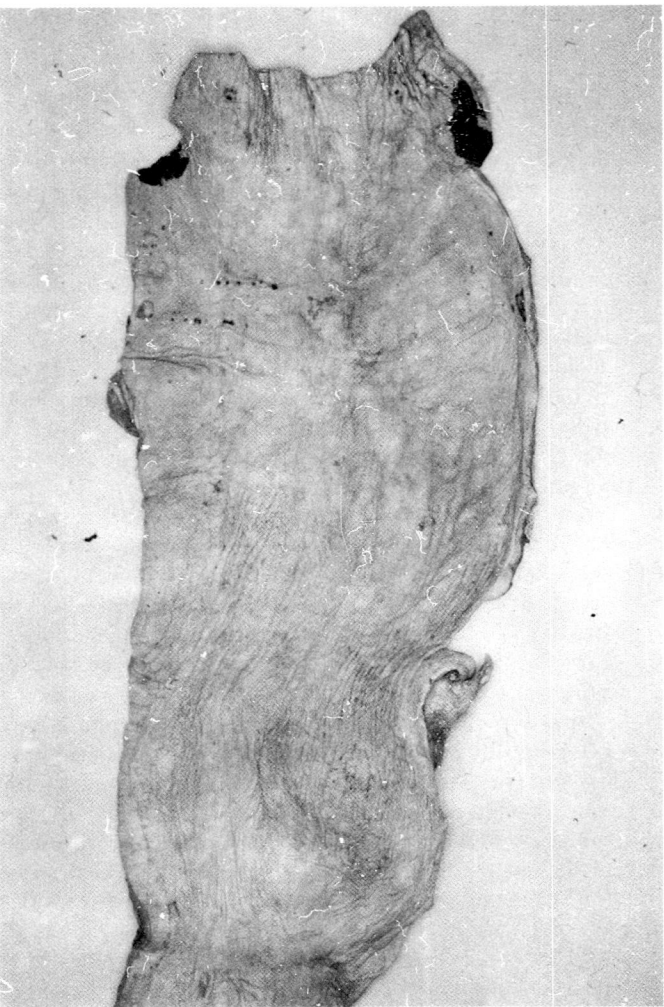

Fig. 16.2 A dilated mega-oesophagus from a case of achalasia.

Advanced cases at necropsy feature a short, distal narrow segment, 1.5–4.5 cm in length, with a normal thickness muscle coat or hypertrophied muscle, while the bulk of the oesophagus shows gross dilatation, elongation, and tortuosity. The oesophageal wall is thickened by muscular hypertrophy although thinning, atrophy, and non-specific sclerosis can also occur. Diverticula may be present. Retained food accumulates in the dilated oesophagus and the mucosa assumes the texture of crocodile leather. Retention and stagnation of food lead to oesophagitis with ulceration, leukoplakia, and papillomata in some cases. The patients complain of dysphagia, regurgitation of food, nocturnal coughing spells, substernal pain, and weight loss.

Achalasia is associated with the risk of aspiration pneumonitis, lipoid pneumonia, bronchiectasis, lung abscess, and pulmonary fibrosis. Non-tuberculous acid-fast bacilli may be found in the sputum of affected patients. Surgical treatment by Heller's operation of cardiomyotomy may be complicated by reflux oesophagitis. Squamous carcinoma is about seven times

more common in patients with achalasia than in the general population, and it may be of the verrucous type.

Ganglion cells are usually completely absent in the dilated segment and are present in reduced numbers distally. Occasionally a mononuclear infiltrate is present in and around Auerbach's plexus and there may be an associated proliferation of Schwann cells. Degenerative changes, viz. Wallerian degeneration and non-specific demyelination are present in vagal fibres and there is a reduction in, and abnormalities of, the neurones of the dorsal motor nucleus of the vagus. It is mainly arygrophil cells which are lost in the oesophagus and, if the arygrophil co-ordinating system has been destroyed, organized peristalsis cannot occur. Lewy bodies are present in a small proportion of cases. Pharmacological studies show hyperresponsiveness of the body of the oesophagus to cholinergic stimulation. There is also supersentitivity to gastrin. Vasoactive intestinal polypeptide (VIP)-containing nerve fibres, which cause relaxation of smooth muscle, are also reduced in achalasia. It has been suggested that a neurotropic virus may be responsible for the neurogenic lesion, and a recent serological study suggests an association between measles virus and achalasia. Ischaemia *in utero* or a toxic process have also been put forward as alternative hypotheses. Achalasia secondary to malignant disease interfering with oesophageal innervation has also been documented.

Diffuse spasm of the oesophagus: idiopathic muscular hypertrophy

This condition, which is characterized by marked thickening of the muscle coats of the oesophagus, is more common in males and it may be encountered as an unexpected, incidental, and asymptomatic finding at autopsy, although it may cause dysphagia and substernal pain in other patients during life. The oesophageal gastric junction is not involved and the hypertrophy involves predominantly the circular muscle coat. Fibrosis and lymphocytic infiltration may be present and ulceration has been described in occasional cases. The ganglion cells appear normal although the myenteric plexus may be infiltrated by chronic inflammatory cells. The term 'corkscrew oesophagus' is used by radiologists to describe the appearances on a barium-swallow examination. Occasional cases progress to true achalasia.

Crico-pharyngeal achalasia—oro-pharyngeal dysphagia

A group of disorders characterized by failure to relax, spasm, or other abnormality of swallowing or activity are included under this terminology. Crico-pharyngeal fibrosis can be demonstrated in some of these cases. Myotomy may be dramatically successful in the treatment of dysphagia.

Other motility disorders

Other neuromuscular disorders, if they present clinical problems, can be detected by manometry and other sophisticated tests. Patients with diabetes, muscular dystrophy, neurological disease, alcoholic neuropathy, peripheral neuropathy, amyloidosis, and disorders under treatment with ganglion-blocking drugs are prone to oesophageal motility disorder. Irradiation-induced motor disorder of the oesophagus has also been described.

Spontaneous rupture of the oesophagus

This is a serious complication of the act of vomiting, although cases have been reported following sudden increases in intra-abdominal pressure due to abdominal blows, parturition, epileptic seizures, straining at stool, asthma, prolonged hiccups, neurological disease, and accidental introduction of compressed air into the oesophagus. The tear usually occurs in the left posterior aspect of the oesophagus and it is usually linear in shape. Gastric contents escape into the mediastinum or pleural sac, leading to mediastinitis or empyema associated with interstitial emphysema and sometimes subcutaneous emphysema in the neck. There is a high mortality rate, even in cases treated by surgical repair. There is an association with alcoholism, although it can also occur in otherwise normal subjects.

Rarely, spontaneous mucosal tears are found in the mid- or distal oesophagus, associated with intramural dissection.

Mallory–Weiss syndrome

Another complication of the act of vomiting is the occurrence of fissure-like lacerations at the level of the cardia, which are further complicated by gastrointestinal haemorrhage. The tears range up to four in number and, although they involve the mucosa and submucosa, they do not penetrate into the muscularis propia. There may be an associated submucosal haematoma and the tears may extend into the oesophagus. There is a strong association with alcoholism and the tears are most common in middle-aged and elderly men, although they have been reported at all ages. Other precipitating factors include coughing, straining at stool, and prolonged severe hiccups. They may be responsible for up to 14.7 per cent of cases of massive gastrointestinal haematemesis.

Oesophageal apoplexy

Spontaneous bleeding into the wall of the lower oesophagus with submucosal haematoma formation produces severe retrosternal pain and it has a similar aetiology to spontaneous rupture. Intramucosal haematomas have also been described, complicating anticoagulant therapy.

Iastrogenic perforation of the oesophagus

Perforation can occur with the rigid oesophagoscope or with the flexible fibre-optic endoscope and it can also complicate other instrumental techniques, such as bougie or tube dilatation of a stricture or cancer. It may also complicate ingestion of a foreign body, e.g. fish bone etc. Large perforations have a high mortality rate and require surgical repair but small perforations can be treated successfully by conservative measures. Mediastinitis, pleurisy, cervical abscess, and emphysema may develop and prove difficult to treat. Small perforations of the oesophagus can be missed during barium-swallow examination and autopsy may expose unsuspected perforations.

Diverticula

Pharyngo-oesophageal diverticula represent acquired outpouchings in the crico-pharyngeal area and are the commonest variety of diverticula. They occur in late middle-aged or elderly patients and the symptoms are those of regurgitation of food that was swallowed earlier. A sweet taste is often noted and there is frequently a foul odour. Dysphagia, excessive salivation, intermittent hoarseness, and heartburn may also feature in the presentation and there is a risk of aspiration and pneumonitis. Hiatus hernia frequently coexists. The pathogenesis relates to premature relaxation of the crico-pharyngeus muscle during swallowing although this hypothesis is in dispute. The pharyngeal musculature propels food distally and forces out the posterior wall of the pharynx just above the horizontal fibres of the crico-pharyngeus. The diverticular sac is lined by mucosa and muscle, although this may be thinned out. Ulceration is rare but chronic inflammatory changes are common. Squamous carcinoma has been recorded as an additional complication in 0.31 per cent of cases.

Congenital diverticula of the crico-pharyngeal area are very rare. Acquired crico-pharyngeal diverticula have been described in infants following attempts to pass a nasogastric tube during spasm of the crico-pharyngeus or due to an obstetric problem during delivery. These diverticula appear to close spontaneously. Similar diverticula occur rarely in older children.

Diverticula of the mid-oesophagus close to the tracheal bifurcation were previously described as traction diverticula due to fibrosis in the vicinity resulting from tuberculosis or histoplasmosis of adjacent lymph nodes. Most cases nowadays are associated with motility disorder such as achalasia or diffuse spasm. Rare cases represent a 'forme fruste' of tracheo-oesophageal fistula complex. Isolated cases have followed foreign body penetration of the oesophageal wall.

Diverticula of the lower oesophagus are often described as epiphrenic and appear to be secondary to motility disorders, hiatus hernia, strictures, and webs. The acquired nature is endorsed by the presence of muscle in walls of the diverticula. A few have been associated with leiomyomas, possibly due to excavating ulceration. Isolated cases of squamous carcinoma originating within diverticula have been reported.

Intramural pseudodiverticulosis is characterized by the presence of multiple small collar-stud diverticula in the superficial layers of the oesophagus. There may be a history of mild dysphagia, suggesting that they are secondary to oesophagitis or strictures. The diverticula can be infected by candidiasis and abscesses are also described as a rare complication. These pseudodiverticula are formed by dilatation of the excretory portion of the ducts of the submucosal glands and they do not extend beyond the submucosa. There may be associated chronic inflammatory changes and fibrosis. The aetiology is debatable. Symptoms are usually due to an underlying oesophageal disorder and therefore the condition could be a secondary manifestation, but a congenital origin cannot be entirely excluded.

16.1.4 Inflammation

Reflux oesophagitis

Recurrent excessive regurgitation of acid gastric juice or alkaline secretions can lead to the histological consequences of gastro-oesophageal reflux and to erosive or ulcerative oesophagitis. Persistent regurgitation may then be complicated by the development of a peptic stricture or gastric-lined oesophagus (Barrett's oesophagus) is a small proportion of cases, with the additional small risk of adenocarcinoma.

Reflux oesophagitis (Fig. 16.3) is more common in middle-aged individuals, although it can occur in any age-group. Certain risk factors have been identified, which include hiatus hernia, obesity, duodenal ulcer, cigarette smoking, excessive vomiting, pregnancy, nasogastric intubation, systemic sclerosis, late fatty meals, diabetes, surgery at the gastro-oesophageal junction including vagotomy, pemphigus, epidermolysis bullosum, Zollinger–Ellison syndrome, delay in gastric emptying, duodenogastric reflux, recumbency, body-brace treatment for kyphoscoliosis, irritable bowel syndrome, alcohol abuse, radiation and drugs, e.g. oral contraceptives, aspirin and other non-steroidal anti-inflammatory drugs, theophyllin, anticholinergic drugs for Parkinson's syndrome, or anti-diarrhoeal drugs, tricylic antidepressants, and chemotherapeutic agents.

Gastro-oesophageal reflux is a normal physiological phenomenon associated with neutralizing and protective mechanisms that include the lower oesophageal sphincter, oesophageal clearing mechanisms, peristalsis, salivary and oesophageal gland secretions. The lower oesophageal sphincter may relax inappropriately in high-risk patients, allowing excessive reflux. There is also individual variation in the response of the oesophagus to recurrent and excessive reflux, and as the condition progresses it seems probable that the mucosa becomes more sensitive to the reflux of acid, pepsin, duodenal or intestinal contents, and bile.

Most patients suffer from heartburn, regurgitation or waterbrash, oesophageal pain or discomfort in response to alcohol, hot food, or beverage. Patients with more severe oesophagitis may develop dysphagia and pulmonary symptoms, viz. morning hoarseness, nocturnal cough, or asthma-like features. It is not uncommon to encounter patients with dysphagia who have little or no previous history yet investigations will reveal the presence of a peptic stricture or Barrett's oesophagus. Symptoms may have been tolerated by the patient or controlled by antacids.

The diagnosis of reflux oesophagitis is established by endoscopy and biopsy. Erosive and ulcerative oesophagitis can be clearly visualized during endoscopy. Additional tests may be necessary in some patients, such as Berstein's acid perfusion tests, manometry, scintography, oesophageal pH monitoring with capsule technique, etc.

Biopsies are helpful for confirmation of the diagnosis and, in the early stages, are probably more reliable than visual assessment. They are also essential for academic studies and for accurate comparisons on the response of the inflamed oesophageal mucosa to various therapeutic agents. At least two biopsies should be taken from levels more than 2.5 cm above the gastro-oesophageal junction; additional biopsies are, of course, valuable. It is desirable that the biopsies should include the lamina propria and for morphometric studies the biopsies should be flattened out on card or paper so that vertical sections can be prepared through the mucosa.

The best forceps biopsies are obtained through a rigid oesophagoscope but the Quinton suction biopsy instrument also provides excellent specimens. Small biopsies obtained by fibreoptic suction or punch technique have a more limited value. It is absolutely vital that the endoscopist should state the level of the biopsy site from the incisor teeth and additional information on the level of the ora serrata is of considerable value.

Oesophagitis can be classified as:

1. histological consequences of gastro-oesophageal reflux;
2. erosive or ulcerative oesophagitis;

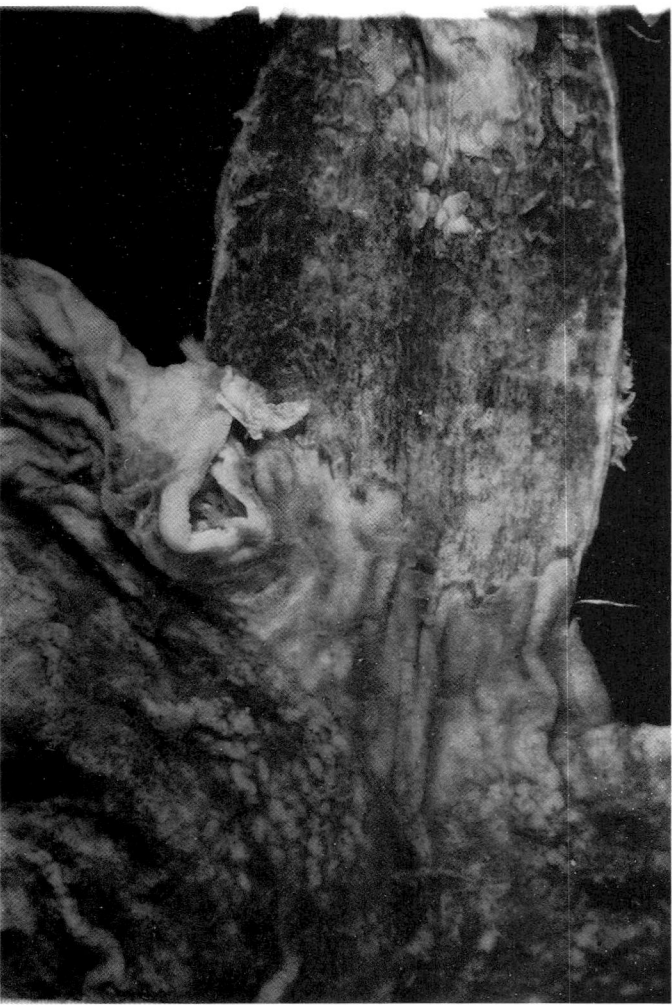

Fig. 16.3 The oesophago-gastric junction from a patient with severe reflux oesophagitis. There is intense congestion and superficial erosion of the distal oesophagus.

3. peptic stricture;
4. Barrett's oesophagus.

Histological consequences of gastro-oesophageal reflux

The histological changes characteristic of abnormal gastro-oesophageal reflux include basal cell hyperplasia, elongation of papillae, and the presence of neutrophils in subepithelial tissues. In recent years, these criteria have been subjected to close scrutiny and, although they are not specific, they are of considerable value in the context of gastro-oesophageal reflux.

Basal cell hyperplasia. The normal germinative zone of basal cells occupies 10–15 per cent of the epithelial layer thickness. Recurrent reflux and chemical irritation of the mucosa associated with desquamation of the superficial layers leads to regenerative changes and expansion in this zone (Figs 16.4, 16.5) so that it accounts for 20–60 per cent or more of the mucosal thickness. Glycogen staining by the PAS technique assists in

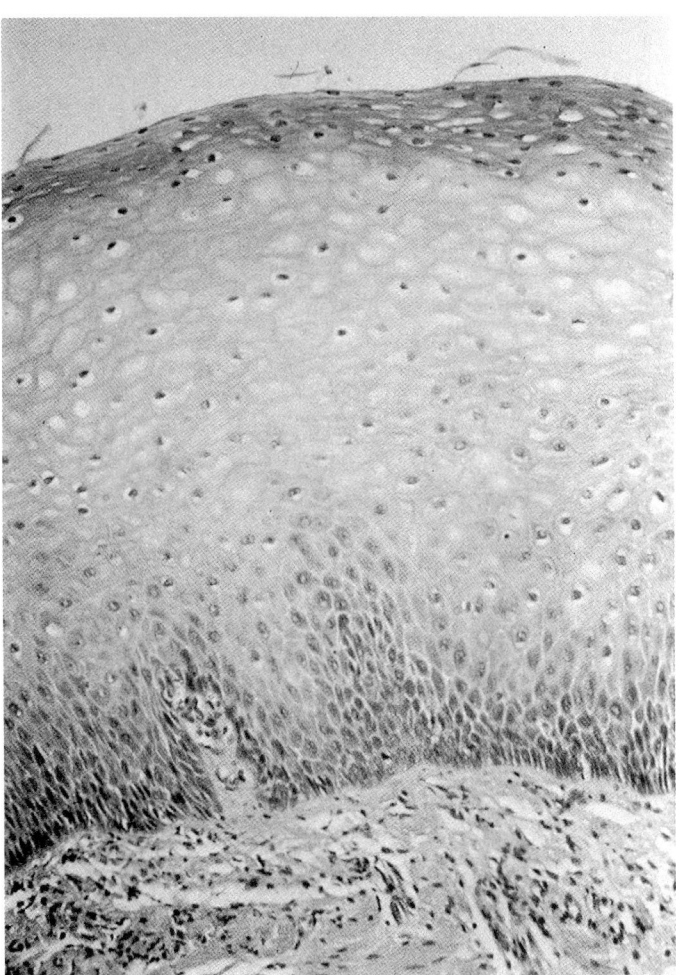

Fig. 16.4 Section of normal oesophagus showing that the basal cell layer accounts for less than 10 per cent of the thickness of the squamous epithelium.

interpretation of the percentage thickness, but this is disputed by some workers who consider it unnecessary. Measurements are taken by the micrometer eyepiece from the part of the biopsy where the zone is thickest, owing to the fact that the changes are often focal, provided that there is no evidence of tangential cutting. The claim that there is increased turnover of the basal cells is confirmed by labelling studies. The specificity of this feature has been questioned by some workers as probably representing a physiological response to reflux within the sphincter zone.

Elongation of papillae beyond the normal two-thirds is not such a constant feature but, none the less, when taken with basal cell hyperplasia it has diagnostic significance. Morphometry can also be applied, and thus it is also established that the diameter of the papillae is increased. It has been suggested that a papillary length greater than 50 per cent in at least two biopsies is significant.

Vascularization of papillae Markedly dilated capillaries and venules in the papillae are highly suggestive of reflux. Extravasated red cells may be present, as well as ingrowth of capillaries into the epithelium, margination, and diapedesis of granulocytes.

Neutrophils Polymorphonuclear leucocytes are encountered in subepithelial or intra-epithelial layers (Fig. 16.6) in 18–25 per cent of biopsies from patients with symptoms suggestive of gastro-oesophageal reflux. If the biopsy includes the lamina propria then they are found in more than half of the specimens showing basal cell hyperplasia. Polymorphs are a more reliable indicator of an inflammatory response but they have low sensitivity as a marker.

Eosinophils Intra-epithelial eosinophils are often found in reflux oesophagitis in children. Identification of eosinophils is assisted by the use of the stain Chromotrope 2R. In adult patients, this feature has low sensitivity.

Minor features Intra-epithelial lymphocytes appear to be increased in reflux oesophagitis. Langerhans cells and cytotoxic T-lymphocytes participate in this increased population of cells.

Erosive or ulcerative oesophagitis

More advanced established oesophagitis can be clearly visualized on endoscopy. Most patients have typical symptoms and dysphagia associated with muscle spasm may also be a feature. Biopsies show erosion of the mucosa, ulceration, acute and chronic inflammatory changes, as well as the usual histological changes of gastro-oesophageal reflux. Occasionally biopsies are disappointing and may show normal mucosa or slight abnormalities only. The severe degree of basal cell hyperplasia that is present in some patients rarely mimics severe dysplasia and cautious assessment is essential. Gastric metaplasia occurs in a proportion of patients. Slight fibrosis may be encountered in the lamina propria.

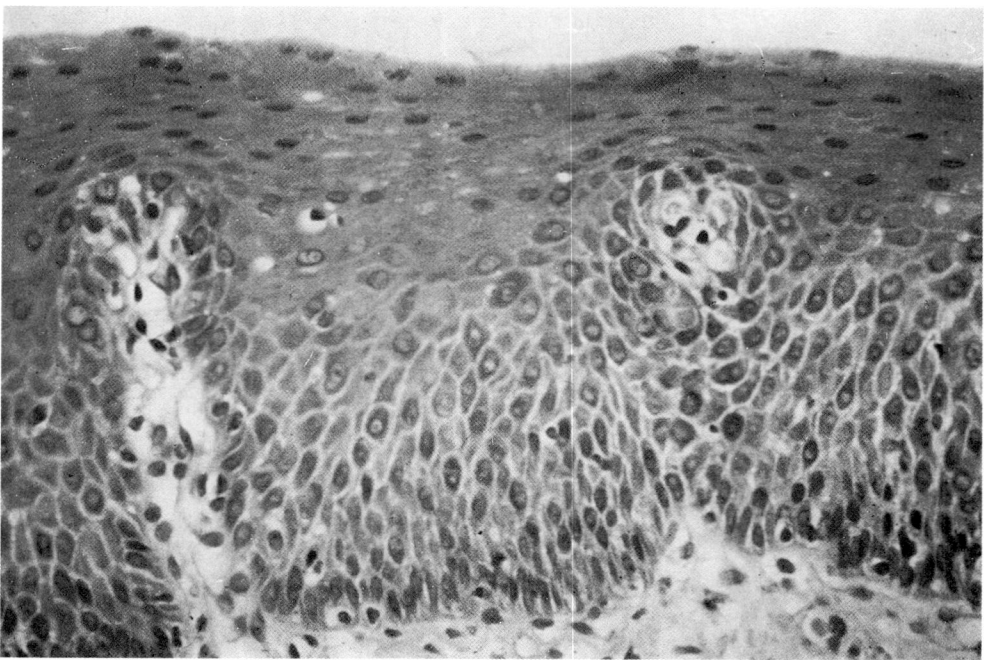

Fig. 16.5 Section of oesophageal mucosa from a case of reflux oesophagitis, showing a greatly expanded basal layer.

Peptic stricture

Severe oesophagitis with erosion formation or chronic ulceration is associated with fibrosis in the lamina propria, submucosa, muscle coat, and peri-oesophageal tissues. After a variable period of time, fibrous stenosis develops, leading to dysphagia. In the early stages of stricture formation, oedema and muscle spasm contribute to the dysphagia; this accounts for the fact that some strictures are reversible. Strictures are usually short, about 1 cm or so in length, but occasionally they measure up to 4 cm.

Strictures are more common in endentulous subjects and there is an association with non-steroidal anti-inflammatory drugs. There are two varieties of peptic stricture.

Chronic superficial oesophagitis This represents a more advanced stage of erosive or ulcerative oesophagitis. Resected specimens show circumferential fibrosis and frequently the gastric mucosa extends to a level of 2–4 cm above the cardia. The endoscopist may encounter pearly white plaques above the stricture, corresponding to foci of glycogenic acanthosis, which should not be mistaken for leukoplakia.

Chronic peptic ulcer Resected strictures may show one or two chronic peptic ulcer craters which penetrate the muscle coat as in gastric and duodenal ulcers. The muscularis mucosa and the muscularis propria merge at the edges of the ulcer crater and endarteritis obliterans occurs in the base of vessels. These chronic ulcers develop at the gastro-oesophageal junction or within gastric mucosa and may be referred to as Barrett's ulcers (Fig. 16.7). Gastric mucosa may reach levels up to 6 cm or more above the cardia, interdigitating with squamous mucosa.

Barrett's oesophagus

(Synonyms: columnar-lined oesophagus (CLO), columnar epithelial-lined oesophagus (CELO), gastric-lined lower oesophagus; Barrett's metaplasia, gastric metaplasia.)

Gastric mucosa with different histological patterns may extend in continuity from the stomach up into the lower oesophagus over a variable distance (Fig. 16.8). There is usually, but not always, clear evidence of reflux oesophagitis or a peptic stricture. Biopsies will reveal gastric mucosa proximal to the normal site of the gastro-oesophageal junction, which is located at a level of 36–42 cm from the incisor teeth There are two theories relating to the possible origin of gastric mucosa in the oesophagus, and it is probable that it represents an acquired lesion in the majority of cases.

Acquired origin

It has been suggested that recurrent ulceration due to reflux oesophagitis is followed by upward extension of gastric mucosa during the process of regeneration. Clear biopsy evidence has been obtained that glandular epithelium has appeared at levels previously occupied by squamous mucosa within a specified period of time, such as 32 months. Upward extension of gastric mucosa has been demonstrated in the animal model and as a complication of lye ingestion in the human subject. Gastric-lined lower oesophagus is usually an irreversible condition but anti-reflux operations stop the progressive ascent.

Congenital origin

The congenital theory cannot be excluded as a rare cause of the gastric-lined oesophagus but it is difficult to prove in individual

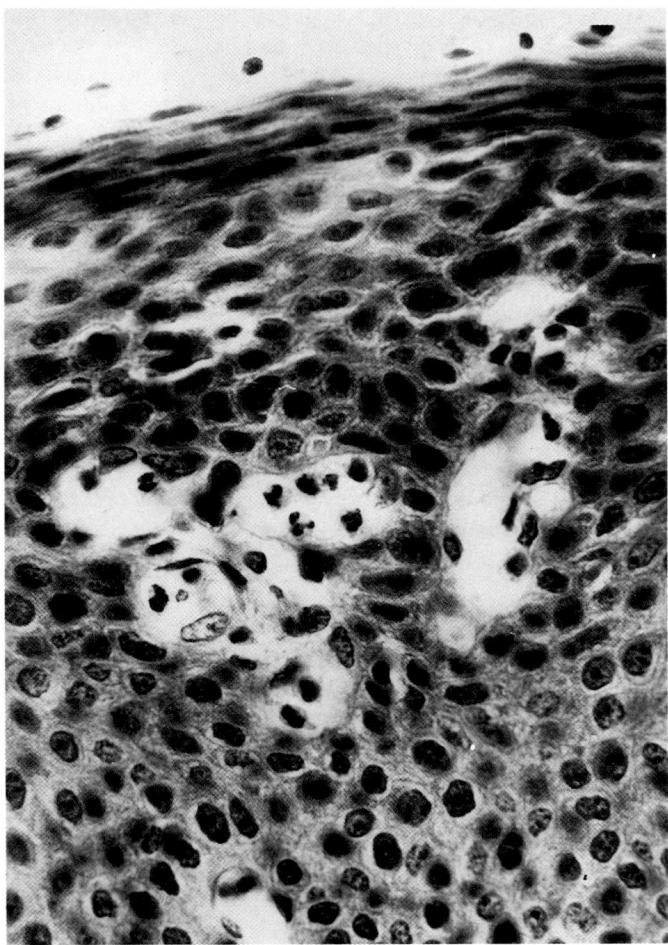

Fig. 16.6 Oesophageal epithelium from a case of reflux oesophagitis, showing intra-epithelial aggregations of neutrophils.

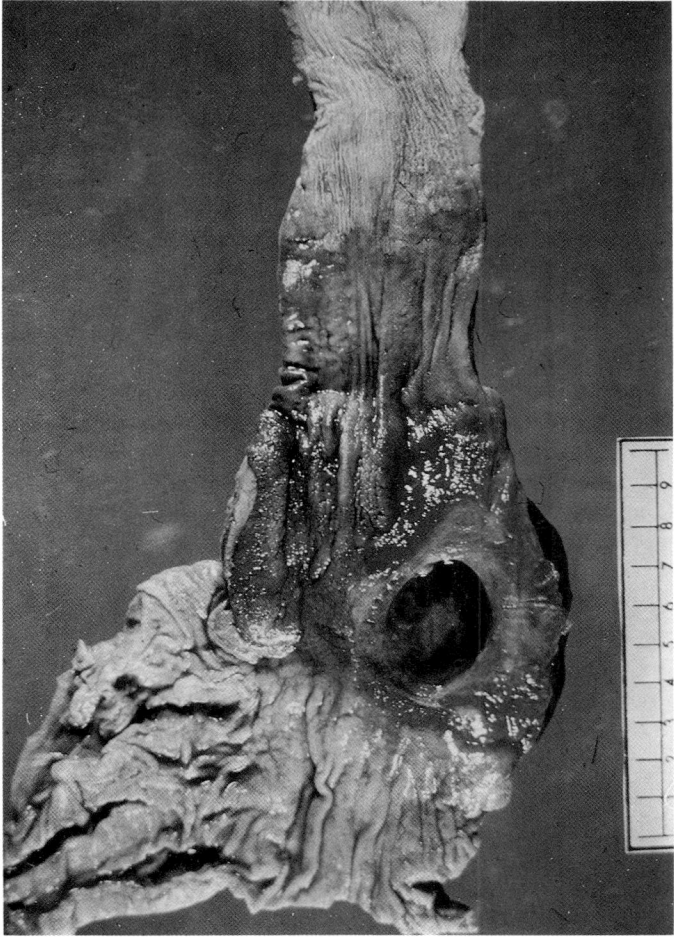

Fig. 16.7 Chronic peptic ulcer of the oesophagus.

cases. Since the oesophagus is lined by columnar epithelium at an early stage of development, it is possible that embryonic nests could persist into adult life. Persistent islets of columnar epithelium, most of which are located in the upper oesophagus, have been described in children. Rare cases of Barrett's oesophagus attributed to congenital origin are described in the literature.

Barrett's oesophagus has been reported in children with a history of excessive reflux during infancy. Occasional cases may be of congenital origin. It is surprising that there is an absence of Barrett's oesophagus in Black patients in the USA, and it is possible that genetic factors play a part. The incidence of Barrett's oesophagus in patients with endoscopic oesophagitis is recorded as 4–20 per cent, with an average of 10 per cent. It is possible that the lower figure is more accurate if one considers how common reflux oesophagitis is in the population; moreover there is often uncertainty regarding the location of the gastro-oesophageal junction and the distance of biopsies from the

incisor teeth. Higher incidences, up to 44 per cent, have been reported in association with peptic stricture.

The 'limited type' of Barrett's mucosa encircles the oesophagus in a circumferential manner up to mid-oesophageal level or to a distance of 30 cm from the incisor teeth. The 'extended type' reaches a higher level and rarely involves the whole oesophagus. Strictures can occur in the lower third or upper third of the oesophagus as well as at mid-oesophageal level, but in most cases there is a large component of muscular spasm rather than fibrous stenosis associated with ulceration, often at the squamo-columnar junction. An 'island' type has also been described which is associated with a significantly low incidence of ulcers, strictures, and motor abnormality.

Dissecting microscopy and electron microscopy are useful techniques in the demonstration of villi in resected specimens, biopsies, and necropsy material. Residual oesophageal submucosal glands can be identified histologically in the columnar-lined zone.

Three different types of mucosa have been described, viz.:

1. atrophic gastric fundic-type epithelium with parietal and chief cells usually in a distal location;

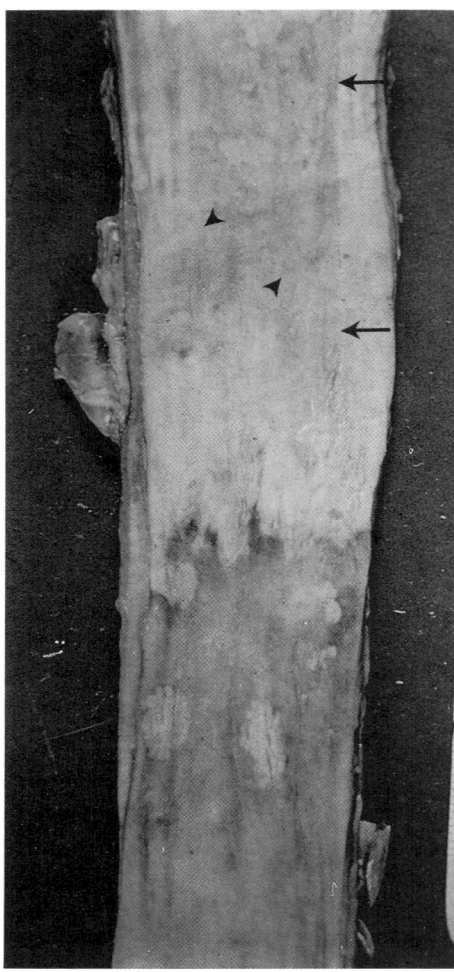

Fig. 16.8 A case of Barrett's oesophagus, showing columnar epithelium (arrow) extending up the oesophagus leaving isolated islands of squamous epithelium (arrowheads).

2. junctional-type epithelium with cardiac mucous glands; and

3. distinctive 'specialized' columnar epithelium, with villiform surface mucous glands and intestinal-type goblet cells, which is usually most proximal in location.

   Parietal cells (Fig. 16.9), Paneth cells, and chief cells occur in about 50 per cent of cases and acid pepsin mixture may be secreted by the mucosa. Intestinal metaplasia with villous formation (Fig. 16.10) is often a prominent feature. Cells intermediate between a mucous and an absorptive cell are present in the metaplastic mucosa and they can secrete either neutral mucins or sulphomucins. Type IIb, or type III, intestinal metaplasia has been cited as a cancer risk but it could also represent an associated phenomenon. Carcino-embryonic antigen (CEA) has been identified in columnar oesophageal epithelium but it is a poor marker of the cancer risk.

   Neuro-endocrine cells are numerous in Barrett's mucosa and they produce a wide variety of hormones, including gastrin, bombesin, substance P, somatostatin, and serotonin. Foci of

low-grade and high-grade dysplasia are encountered not uncommonly in resected specimens and biopsies from Barrett's mucosa. High-grade dysplasia (Fig. 16.11) is synonymous with carcinoma *in situ* but it is not necessarily an indication for resection because of the high mortality and morbidity rates associated with surgery. Oesophagectomy has been advocated for high-grade dysplasia if the patient is a good surgical risk. Dysplasia may undergo retrogression following anti-reflux surgery. There must be clear evidence of carcinoma in biopsy specimens, preferably with invasion, before surgical resection is undertaken. Dysplasia represents a recommendation for surveillance but there are opposing views on the cost-effectiveness and value of such programmes. Adenomatous polyps can also occur in Barrett's mucosa.

Specific types of oesophagitis

Bacterial oesophagitis due to pyogenic organisms or *Klebsiella* can develop in immunosuppressed or terminally ill patients, sometimes with pseudomembrane formation. Tuberculosis is a

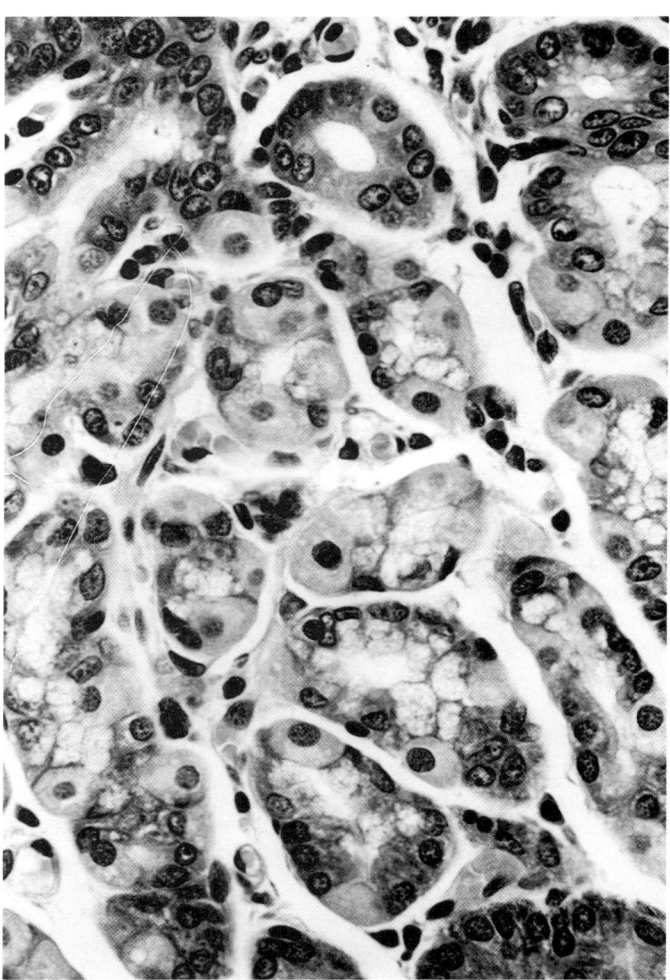

Fig. 16.9 Gastric-body-type mucosa from a case of Barrett's oesophagus.

rare cause of ulceration, and strictures in the oesophagus occur particularly in Asian subjects. Herpes virus infection can produce vesicles and small ulcers in the oesophageal mucosa; multinucleated cells and inclusion bodies are encountered in cytology smears. Herpes labialis or herpes zoster can be associated with or follow the oesophageal lesions. Cytomegalovirus and chickenpox can also induce oesophageal lesions. Post-irradiation oesophagitis is rare following high-dose radiation levels, usually of the order of 6000 rad. Arteritis with ulceration and stricture formation and Behcet's syndrome involving the oesophagus are very rare.

The incidence of gastro-oesophageal candidiasis (Fig. 16.12) in endoscopic series ranges from 4 to 8 per cent, with a high incidence in immunosuppressed, oesophageal cancer, and haemodialysis cases. Approximately 50 per cent of infected patients have white plaques on the oesophageal mucosa. Associated local pathology is present in nearly all patients, suggesting that candidiasis is secondary to underlying mucosal damage. Tissue invasion is uncommon. Other fungal infections which affect the oesophagus include aspergillosis, mucormycosis, etc.

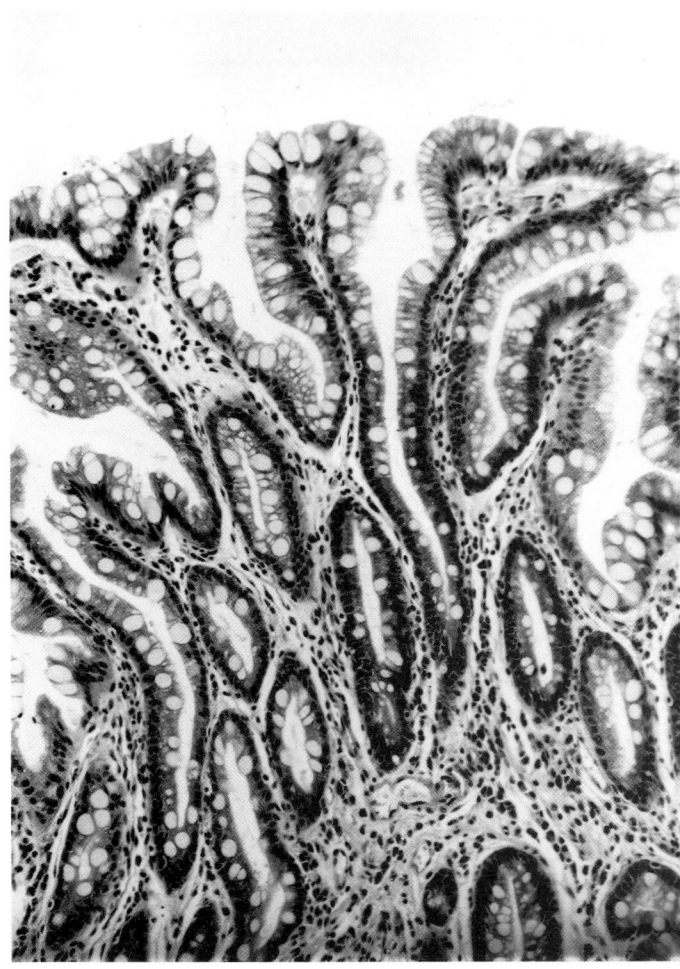

Fig. 16.10 Intestinalized epithelium from a case of Barrett's oesophagus.

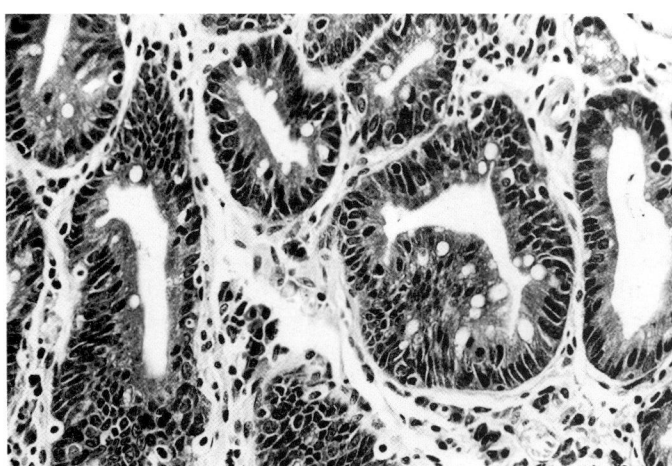

Fig. 16.11 A case of Barrett's oesophagus, showing high-grade dysplasia.

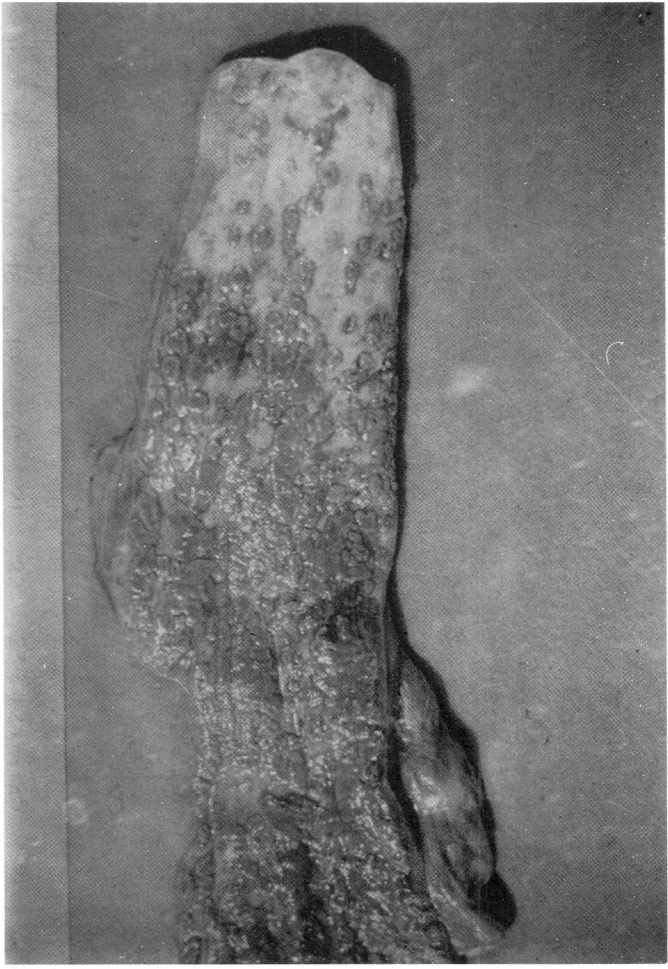

Fig. 16.12 Oesophagitis due to *Candida* infection.

A variety of skin disorders may be associated with oesophageal lesions. The most important of these include pemphigus, pemphigoid, and epidermolysis bullosum.

Apthous ulcers, extensive ulceration, stricture formation,
and granulomata have all been documented in rare cases of
Crohn's disease. Some of these patients have an associated
reflux oesophagitis.

Corrosive oesophagitis

Ingestion of strong caustic solutions, lysol, paraquat, acid or
alkaline solutions causes corrosive oesophagitis associated with
severe retrosternal pain and shock. Perforation and stricture
formation are well documented and carcinoma may complicate
lye strictures in later years.

Drug-induced oesophageal injury

A wide variety of therapeutic agents can cause erosions, ulceration, and pseudomembrane formation in the oesophagus. The
most commonly mentioned drugs are doxycycline, tetracycline,
clindamycin, potassium tablets, aspirin and other non-steroidal
anti-inflammatory drugs, emepronium bromide, clinitest tablets, and variceal sclerosants. Antibiotics have accounted for
more than 50 per cent of all cases reported in the literature.
Odynophagia and retrosternal pain occur in 75 per cent of
patients, while dysphagia is present in only 20 per cent. Remnants of the pill or capsule may be retained in the oesophagus,
providing a useful clue to the cause of injury. Enhancement of
radiation injury to the oesophagus has been observed with
chemotherapeutic agents, e.g. actinomycin D, adriamycin, etc.

16.1.5   Systemic disorders affecting the oesophagus

Systemic sclerosis

Reduced or absent peristalsis in the distal oesophagus and loss
or diminution of LES function can lead to obstruction or reflux
associated with dilatation of the oesophagus (Fig. 16.13). Oesophageal sclerosis is encountered in patients with Raynaud's
phenomenon who develop systemic sclerosis or scleroderma,
and may occur as a complication of the CREST syndrome, systemic lupus erythematosus, polymyositis, dermatomyositis,
other collagen disorders and, rarely, in the absence of any clinical disease or syndrome. Women are more frequently affected
than men.

Histological examination reveals atrophy of smooth muscle
and variable fibrosis accompanied by endarteritis of vessels.
Ganglion cells are normal in the early stages of scleroderma but
they are reduced in the late stages due to the ischaemia associated with the vascular changes. The striated muscle in the
upper part of the oesophagus is not usually affected unless there
is a severe generalized skeletal myopathy. The cause of atrophy
of smooth muscle is unknown but it has been suggested that
there is either an auto-immune basis or an ischaemic mechanism mediated by luminal narrowing or vasoconstriction, as
in Raynaud's phenomenon.

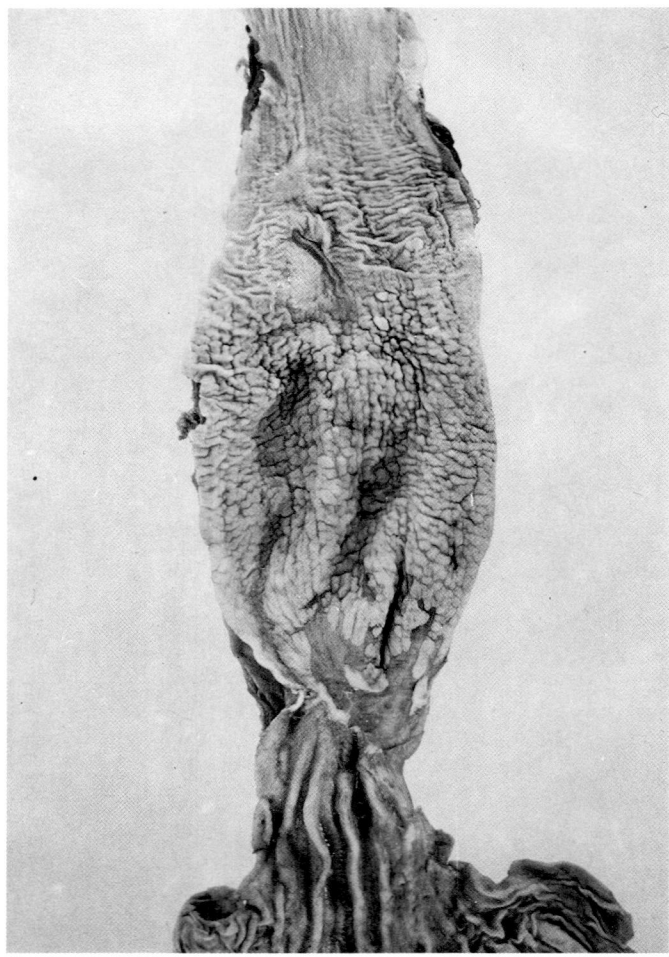

Fig. 16.13   The oesophagus from a case of systemic sclerosis showing
a dilated oesophagus with inflammation at the oesophago-gastric
junction due to reflux.

Patients present with dysphagia and heartburn and are
found to have dilatation of the oesophagus on radiological
examination. Reflux oesophagitis with erosions is usually present and it may progress to stricture formation.

Chagas' disease

Gross dilatation of the oesophagus or mega-oesophagus, occurring about 30 years after infection with *Trypanosoma cruzi* has
been reported in South America, Panama, Mexico, and the
southern United States. The disease is transmitted by the bite of
the *Triatoma megista* bug found in bedclothes and the thatched
roofs of village huts. Megacolon and dilatation of the ureters
and heart can also occur.

Smooth muscle fibres of the inner circular layer are hypertrophied at first but are thinned out as dilatation progresses.
There is a 90 per cent reduction in ganglion cells in mega-
oesophagus and 50 per cent reduction associated with
dilatation and functional disturbance. Pseudocysts release

neurotoxins which destroy the ganglion cells, leading to loss of peristalsis. Oesophagitis develops as a result of stasis and food decomposition.

Oesophageal varices

The oesophageal venous plexus communicates freely with the systemic venous system and the portal circulation, representing an anastomotic pathway. Submucosal veins enlarge into varices as a complication of portal hypertension accompanied by increased volume and flow in the splanchnic circulation. It has been suggested that a high LES pressure is protective and may account for the discrepancies in the incidence of varices in patients with portal hypertension.

Varices are most prominent below the aortic arch and appear as bluish, irregular, linear mucosal swellings or as obvious varicose veins running down towards the cardia. Spontaneous rupture of a varix leads to haematemesis or melaena and massive or persistent bleeding is often fatal. Injection sclerotherapy may cause thrombosis of varices, ulceration, fibrosis and, occasionally, stricture formation. Introduction of a Sengstaken tube or other device to arrest variceal haemorrhage may also be complicated by ulceration, ischaemic necrosis, etc.

Varices can occasionally develop in patients with the myeloproliferative syndrome, lymphoproliferative disorder, and Gaucher's disease. Obstruction of the superior vena cava can also create varices, which are often located in the upper oesophagus, as a complication of carcinoma of the lung, mediastinal fibrosis, substernal goitre, and carcinomas. Varices are sometimes encountered in patients with no background disease entity, and they can be termed idiopathic.

16.1.6 Tumours

Benign tumours

Polyps

These pedunuclated tumours, consisting of vascular fibroblastic tissue covered by mucosa which may show superficial erosion, project into the lumen. They occur at all levels in the oesophagus and rare cases have been described with an elongated pedicle which allowed the polyp to be regurgitated into the mouth and even hang outside it.

Leiomyoma

This is the commonest benign tumour, occurring in middle-aged and elderly males. It is encountered most frequently in the lower oesophagus as a polypoid mass or as a lobulated intramucosal tumour (Fig. 16.14). An ulcer crater may penetrate into the tumour. The cut surface of the tumour is greyish-white with a whorled fasciculated texture, often showing flecks of calcification. Occasionally two, three, or multiple tumours are present.

Histologically, smooth muscle tumours consist of interweaving bundles of spindle cells with myofibrils, in well-differentiated cases, which can be demonstrated by phosphotungstic acid haematoxylin stain or by electron microscopy. Distinction between benign and malignant smooth muscle tumours is extremely difficult and is based on the size of the tumour, number of mitoses, degree of nuclear pleomorphism, and evidence of local infiltration.

Leiomyomatosis
Confluent leiomyomatosis nodules involve the lower oesophagus and proximal stomach in this rare disorder associated with severe dysphagia. The nodules merge with

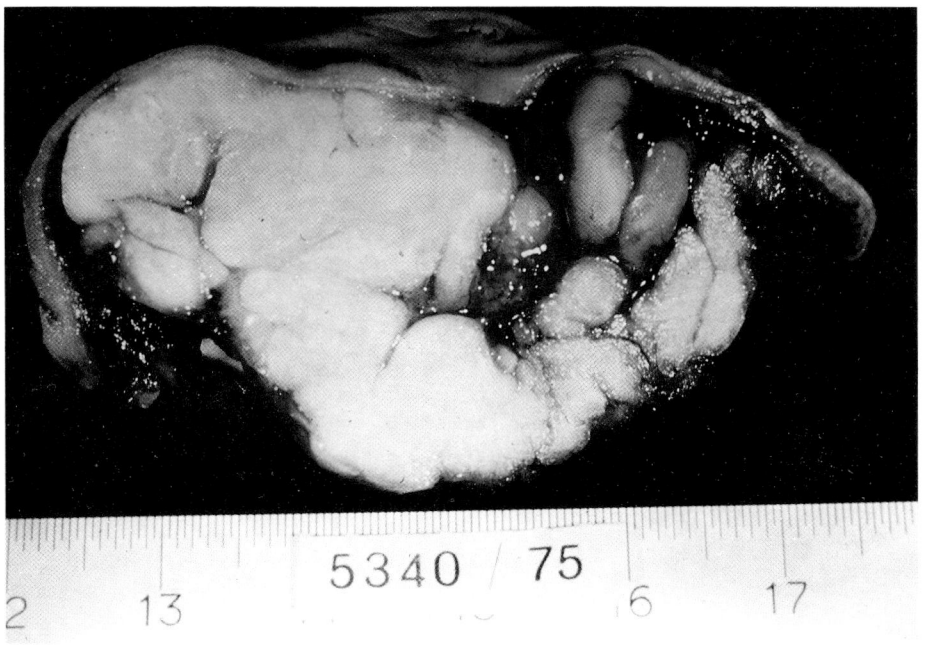

Fig. 16.14 An oesophageal leiomyoma.

hypertrophied circular muscle. There is an association with vulvar leiomyomatosis.

Neurofibroma

This is a rare submucosal tumour which can occur as a solitary lesion or as a feature of von Recklinghausen's disease.

Miscellaneous

Other benign epithelial and soft tissue tumours that occur rarely in the oesophagus include: papilloma, benign oesophageal papillomatosis, viral warts, lipoma, fibroma, haemangioma, lymphangioma, benign haemangio-endothelioma, chondroma, osteochondroma, granular cell myoblastoma, adenoma, fibromatosis, oncocytoma, etc.

Malignant tumours

Squamous carcinoma

The incidence in Britain and the USA varies from 5.2 to 10.4 cases per 100 000 of the population, representing between 2 and 5 per cent of all varieties of malignant disease. It is 1.5–3 times more common in men than in women, except in regions where there is an increased prevalence of the Plummer–Vinson syndrome. There is a high incidence in Northern China, the Caspian Sea littoral of Iran and Russia, and in South Africa among the native population. An increased incidence also occurs in Chile, Jamaica, Puerto Rica, Uraguay, Japan, India, France, Switzerland, West Kenya, and Zimbabwe.

Certain risk factors have been identified in different countries. Approximately 10 per cent of patients with the Plummer–Vinson syndrome will develop malignancy. The incidence of cancer in achalasia is seven times the expected incidence: oesophageal stasis due to lye stricture, peptic stricture, oesophageal webs, and diverticula also represents a hazard.

Alcohol abuse leads to an increased incidence among bartenders. Alcoholic beverages containing nitrosamines and zinc from utensils constitute a risk factor in West Kenya. The rare inherited disease, tylosis, is associated with a 95 per cent risk in the late-onset variety encountered in Liverpool. Tobacco smoking is widely recognized as a risk factor. There is an increased risk of carcinoma of the oesophagus in adult coeliac disease. Chewing seal skins in order to soften leather prior to stitching shoes is associated with an increased incidence in Alaskan Eskimo women, due to the fact that they swallow saliva mixed with ashes from the wood used to burn hairs from the skins. Betel nut chewing causes a high incidence of cancer in the middle third of the oesophagus in the young women of Ceylon. Diets high in nitrosamines or nitrates are a risk factor. Mouldy or pickled food contaminated by *Geotrichum candida* and *Fusarium* species are carcinogenic in China. Petrol contamination of water supplies and diterpine ester promoters have been incriminated as co-carcinogens in the Caribbean island of Curacao. Vulcanization workers have an increased risk of oesophageal cancer. Consumption of foods raised in soils deficient in trace elements, particularly molybdenum, is believed to be a factor. Diets deficient in vitamins C and A and riboflavin are also associated with an increased incidence. Environmental factors are clearly involved in high-incidence areas. Chronic oesophagitis involving the lower and middle third of the oesophagus occurs in Northern Iran and China, and it has been suggested that it could represent a precursor lesion of oesophageal cancer.

The majority of cases present at over 50 years of age and they

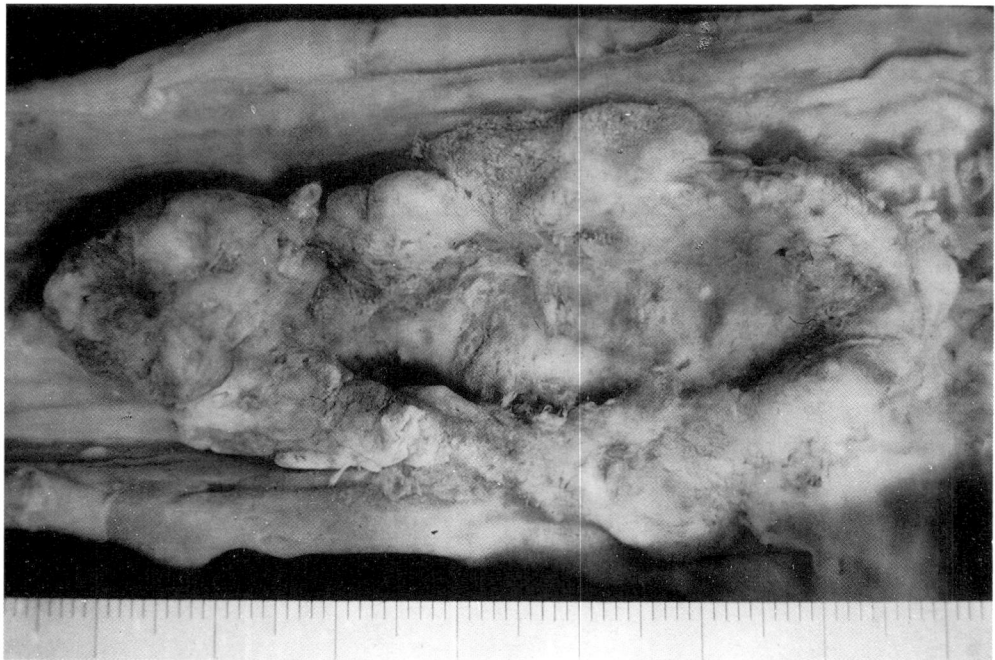

Fig. 16.15 Squamous cell carcinoma of the oesophagus presenting as a flat ulcerating growth.

are 1.5–3 times more common in men than women, except that postcricoid carcinoma occurs most commonly in a younger age-group, viz. 40–50 years as a complication of the Plummer–Vinson syndrome. The growth (Figs 16.15, 16.16) may present as a stricture or as a sessile, ulcerating or warty lesion. Microscopically the cancer spreads through the layers of the wall of the oesophagus to a variable depth then into the peri-oesophageal tissues, accompanied by lymphatic and vascular permeation. Most tumours are moderately well-differentiated squamous carcinomas with variable degrees of keratinization (Fig. 16.17), but well-differentiated carcinoma, poorly differentiated, spindle cell, and anaplastic variants are also encountered. Verrucous carcinomas are rare but they may appear in achalasia; multiple tumours are occasionally found. At presentation, lymph node metastases are present in 50–80 per cent of cases. In advanced cases, visceral metastases are found in 70 per cent of cases. The overall prognosis is poor and the five-year survival figures are rarely about 5 per cent although specialists in the field have obtained up to 20 per cent survivals. Superficial oesophageal carcinoma confined to the mucosa and submucosa

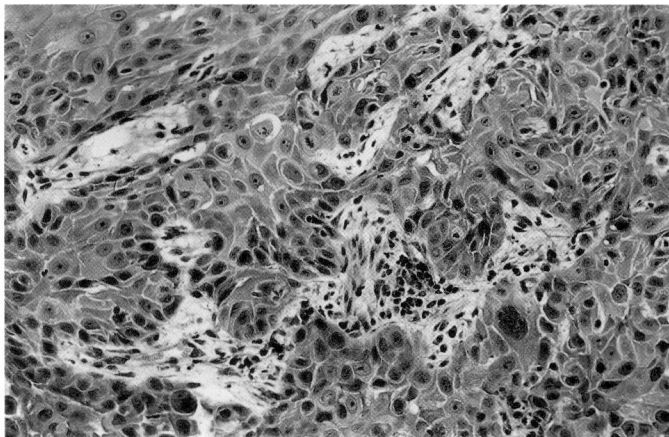

Fig. 16.17 Histological section from a case of moderately well-differentiated squamous cell carcinoma of the oesophagus.

is believed to have a prognosis comparable to that of early gastric cancer.

Mild, moderate, and severe dysplasia (synonymous with carcinoma *in situ*) may precede carcinoma or it may be associated with the growth at presentation. Low-grade dysplasia represents a recommendation for surveillance. High-grade or severe dysplasia constitutes a very difficult problem. Resection has been carried out for severe dysplasia in China where there is a high incidence of oesophageal cancer, but current programmes are therapeutic, with chemopreventive drugs, e.g. vitamins C, B2, anticancer B3, and tilorone, to prevent progression to cancer. In Britain, there is understandable reluctance to resort to surgery unless there is clear evidence of a growth or invasive cancer in the biopsy owing to the high mortality and morbidity rate of oesophageal surgery. Resection has, however, been carried out for high-grade dysplasia complicating tylosis.

Adenocarcinoma

The incidence is recorded as 10 per cent in most series, but if tumours of the cardia are included then the incidence is almost equal to that of squamous carcinoma in the lower oesophagus. Adenocarcinoma can originate in three different ways. First, as Barrett's adenocarcinoma; secondly, as gastric carcinoma spreading up into the oesophagus; and thirdly, as adenocarcinoma of oesophageal submucosal glands. Adenocarcinoma has also been documented as a rare complication of colonic interposition following oesophageal resections. The incidence of adenocarcinoma in the upper oesophagus is around 3 per cent.

Adenocarcinoma presents as a stricture or as a sessile or ulcerating lesion. The tumour spreads through the wall of the oesophagus in the same way as gastric cancer and there is an equally poor prognosis. The histological classification is comparable to carcinoma of the stomach, with intestinal and diffuse varieties. Tumours in the vicinity of the cardia may show an adenosquamous (mucoepidermoid, adenocanthoma, pseudoglandular) appearance. The clinical behaviour is just as aggressive as other adenocarcinomas.

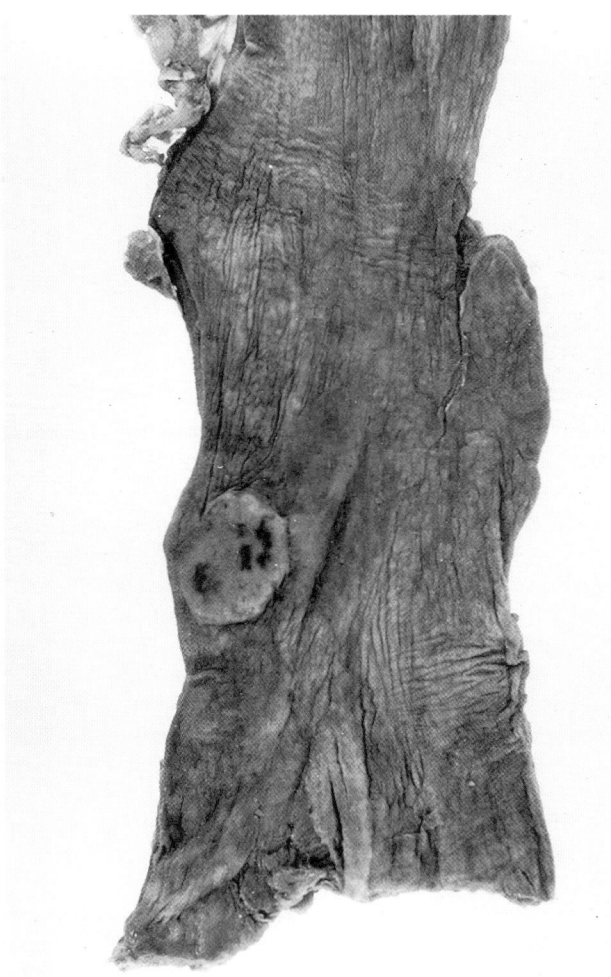

Fig. 16.16 A small, flat, wart-like oesophageal squamous cell carcinoma.

Adenocarcinoma in Barrett's oesophagus The incidence of Barrett's adenocarcinoma is believed to be around 5–10 per cent of oesophageal carcinomas. Intestinal (Fig. 16.18) and diffuse signet-ring cell carcinomas are encountered, with a predominance of the intestinal variety. Multiple cancers have been described and rare hormone-producing tumours have been documented.

The diagnosis in early cases is established by biopsy or brush cytology. More advanced cases will be evident on endoscopic or radiological examination. The increased life expectation in the general population has led to the diagnosis of increasing numbers of cases. Survival figures are poor, ranging from 0 to 7 per cent at 5 years. Occasional cases of squamous carcinoma complicating peptic oesophagitis, columnar-lined oesophagus, or gastric heterotopia have been recorded in the literature.

Diagnosis of squamous carcinoma and adenocarcinoma

Biopsy establishes the diagnosis with certainty, but a negative biopsy does not exclude carcinoma. Rare false positive reports have been described. Brush cytology (Figs 16.19, 16.20) is extremely valuable, and the combination of both techniques together raises the diagnostic accuracy rate to a high level. False positive cytology reports have also been documented, but in a properly organized department they are very rare and are therefore not a significant deterrent. Other cytology techniques have been used, such as balloon abrasion in China, etc.

Carcino-sarcoma

(Polypoid carcinoma with dominant spindle-cell elements, pseudosarcoma, polypoid carcinoma, pseudosarcomatous carcinoma).

This rare tumour is almost invariably polypoid, although a few have been ulcerative or constricting masses. They range in size up to 10 cm, or occasionally larger. The clinical presentation is usually with dysphagia and weight loss. The carcinomatous element may be clearly squamous, pseudoglandular, or undifferentiated. There has been considerable controversy over the spindle-celled component. Positive staining for keratin in the spindle cells by the immunoperoxidase technique

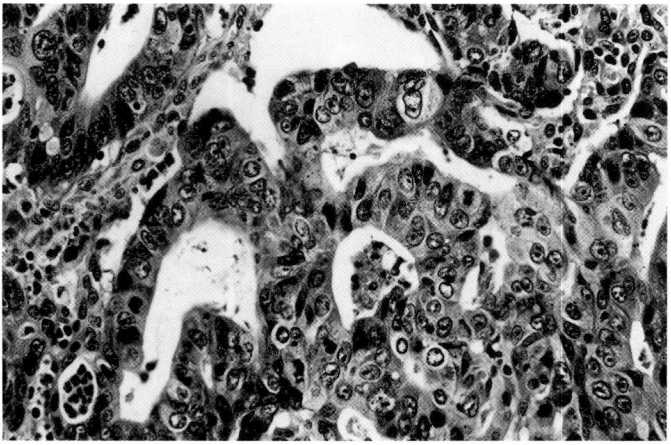

Fig. 16.18 Histology of a case of adenocarcinoma arising in a Barrett's oesophagus.

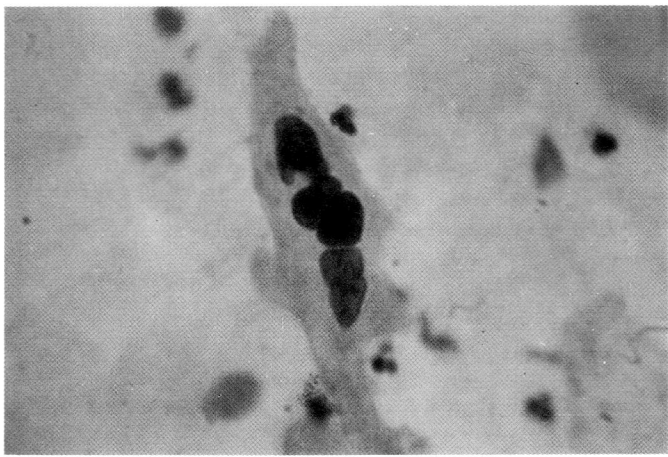

Fig. 16.19 Cytology smear made from brushings of a case of squamous cell carcinoma of the oesophagus.

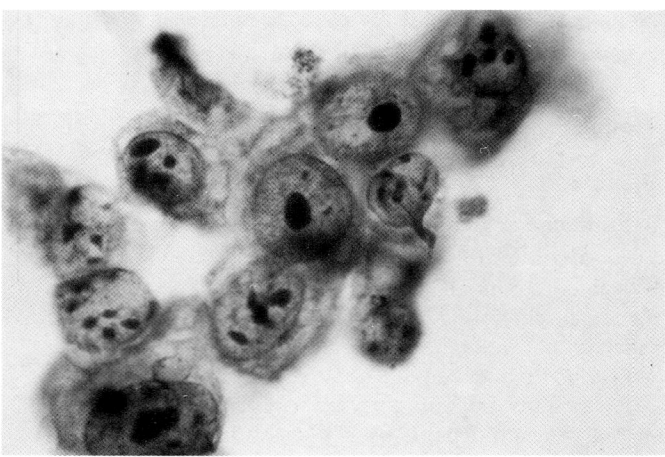

Fig. 16.20 Cytology smear made from brushings from a case of adenocarcinoma of the oesophagus.

strongly suggests that it represents spindle-cell squamous carcinoma, but some cases have been described as sarcoma. The literature indicates that these tumours are relatively benign, particularly if restricted to the mucosa and submucosa, but at least six have been recorded with metastases. The secondary deposits have been described as carcinomatous in most of the cases and as sarcoma in one case. There is, however, a significant postoperative mortality rate from surgical treatment.

Adenoid cystic carcinoma

Tumours comparable to those that occur in salivary glands and lung, with a cribriform or pseudoacinar pattern, basement membrane-like stroma, and occasional ducts, rarely involve the oesophagus. Mucin can be demonstrated using PAS and alcian blue techniques. Origin from the ducts of submucosal salivary glands has been postulated. Myoepithelial cells are a prominent feature. The majority have been located in the mid-oesophagus but they can arise at any level. They behave as aggressive invasive carcinomas with terminal metastases. The more aggressive tumours may represent basaloid squamous carcinoma rather than true adenoid cystic carcinoma.

Oat cell carcinoma

Carcinoma originating from embryonic nests of ciliated epithelium in the lower oesophagus is comparable to oat cell carcinoma of the bronchus in its clinical behaviour. Neurosecretory granules can be identified in the cells and, rarely, hormonal secretion has been responsible for clinical syndromes, e.g. ACTH production, etc. It is probable that a case of chorion epithelioma described in the literature, secreting urinary gonadotrophins, had a similar origin. A squamous component can occasionally be found in these tumours.

Malignant melanoma

This occurs as a sessile or pedunculated tumour in the lower or middle third of the oesophagus, originating from melanocytes in the squamous epithelium. Junctional change in the vicinity of the tumours endorses primary origin in the oesophagus. The lesions are encountered in elderly subjects.

Sarcoma

Leiomyosarcoma, fibrosarcoma, and rhabdomyosarcoma occur as rare tumours in the oesophagus.

Secondary malignant tumours

Local spread into the oesophagus can occur with gastric carcinoma and bronchial carcinoma. Metastatic lesions may complicate carcinoma of the breast, testis, prostate, pancreas, pharynx, etc. Malignant melanoma can give rise to multiple metastatic nodules; and other systemic forms of malignant disease, such as malignant lymphoma, leukaemia, myeloma, haemangioendothelioma, and Kaposi's sarcoma, can produce deposits in the oesophagus. Rarely, sarcomas can also metastasize to the oesophagus.

16.1.7 Further reading

Casella, R. R., *et al.* (1964). Achlasia of the oesophagus: pathology and etiologic considerations. *Annals of Surgery* **160**, 474–87.

Collins, B. J., Elliot, H., Sloan, J. M., McFarland, R. J., and Love, A. H. G. (1985). Oesophageal histology in reflux oesophagitis. *Journal of Clinical Pathology* **38**, 1265–72.

Hamilton, S. R. and Smith, R. R. L. (1987). The relationship between columnar epithelial dysplasia and invasive adenocarcinoma arising in Barrett's oesophagus. *American Journal of Clinical Pathology* **83**, 301–12.

Ismail-Beigi, F., Horton, P. F., and Pope, C. E. (1979). Histological consequences of gastroesophageal reflux in man. *Gastroenterology* **58**, 163–74.

Paull, A., Trier, J. S., Dalton, M. D., Camp, R. C., Loeb, P., and Goyal, R. K. (1976). The histological spectrum of Barrett's esophagus. *New England Journal of Medicine* **295**, 476–80.

Rector, L. E. and Connerley, M. L. (1941). Aberrant mucosa in the oesophagus in infants and children. *Archives of Pathology* **31**, 285.

Weinstein, W. M., Bogoch, E. R., and Bowes, K. L. (1975). The normal human esophageal mucosa: a histological reappraisal. *Gastroenterology* **68**, 40–4.

16.2 The stomach: developmental and inflammatory conditions

G. T. Williams

16.2.1 Normal structure and function

The human stomach is situated in the left upper quadrant of the abdominal cavity, inferior to the diaphragm and the liver. It has two major functions, the thorough mixing of ingested food, and the secretion of gastric juice rich in hydrochloric acid and proteolytic enzymes to facilitate the early stages of digestion.

It is conventional to divide the stomach into four anatomical regions (Fig. 16.21). The most proximal of these, immediately distal to the gastro-oesophageal junction, is the small and rather indistinct *cardia*. That part of the stomach which lies above a line drawn horizontally through the gastro-oesophageal junction is the *fundus*: it usually contains a bubble of ingested air. The proximal two-thirds of the remainder forms the *body*, while the *pyloric antrum* represents the distal one-third. The fundus and body act as a food reservoir and are primarily responsible for the secretion of gastric juice, while the pylorus is essentially a muscular funnel whose co-ordinated peristalsis is responsible for the mixing and grinding of gastric contents and their subsequent release into the duodenum. The stomach has anterior and posterior walls, which meet at the greater and lesser curvatures. The *incisura*, or angular notch, is the point on the lesser curve which roughly marks the junction of the body and pyloric antrum. The overall shape and capacity of the stomach vary considerably between individuals. They are also affected by posture, the activity of the abdominal wall muscles, and the tone of the gastric smooth muscle. When the stomach is empty the lining of the fundus and body is thrown into irregular muscosal folds, or rugae, which radiate from the lesser curvature; these disappear as the lumen fills.

Histological examination of the gastric wall reveals four layers. The luminal aspect is lined by a *mucosa* consisting of specialized epithelial glands in a loose connective tissue lamina

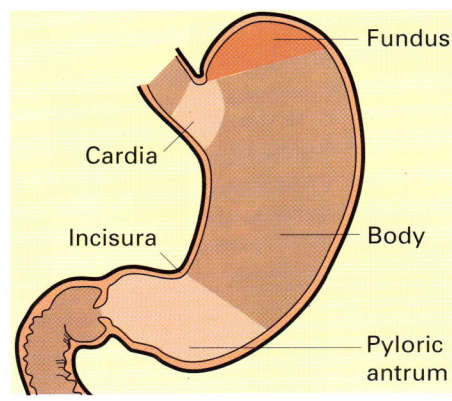

Fig. 16.21 The four anatomical regions of the stomach.

propria which contains scanty lymphocytes and plasma cells, fibroblasts, small lymphatics, capillaries, and nerve fibres (Figs 16.22–16.24). It is covered by a layer of mucus, measuring up to 300 μm in thickness, which has the two important roles of lubricating the gastric contents and protecting the underlying mucosa from their damaging effects. The surface columnar mucous cells of the mucosa produce most of this mucus and also secrete bircarbonate ions into it, so that a protective pH gradient is maintained through the mucus layer between the acidic gastric contents and the neutral mucosal cell surface. The mucous cells dip down into the underlying mucosa to form 2–3 million indentations called the *gastric pits or foveolae*. Opening into each of these are 1–4 specialized gastric glands which occupy the deeper parts of the mucosa and which vary in their histological appearances in the different regions of the stomach. In the cardia and pyloric antrum they are tubular or coiled racemose glands composed largely of mucus-producing cells (Fig. 16.23) whose secretions add to the surface mucous layer. Scattered endocrine cells are also present, most of those in the pyloric antrum producing either gastrin (predominantly) or somatostatin.

The straight, tightly packed tubular glands of the fundus and body contain a number of specialized epithelial cells (Fig. 16.24). These include large granular eosinophilic mitochondria-

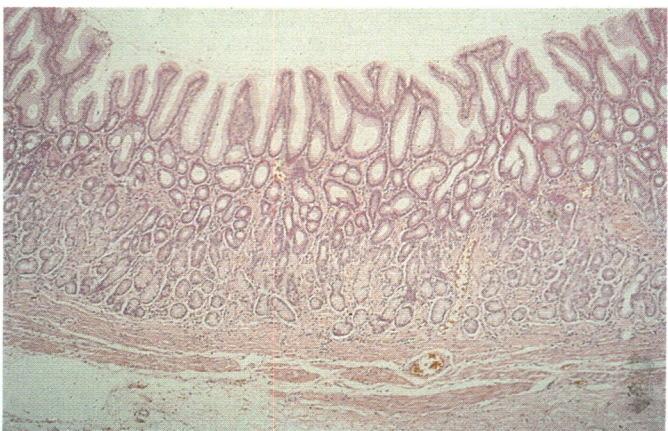

Fig. 16.23 Histological appearances of normal pyloric antral mucosa. The upper half is occupied by the foveolar zone while the lower half contains mucous glands. The smooth muscle fibres of the muscularis mucosae are seen at the bottom of the field.

rich *parietal or oxyntic cells* that produce hydrochloric acid and intrinsic factor; deeply basophilic cuboidal or triangular *chief cells*, containing abundant rough endoplasmic reticulum, prominent Golgi and secretory bodies that produce the pro-enzyme pepsinogens, which are converted to active proteolytic pepsins after secretion into the gastric lumen; columnar *mucous cells* identical to those of the mucosal surface and the foveolae; distinctive cuboidal *mucous neck cells* that contain neutral and (a little) sulphated mucin; and *endocrine cells* that contain a variety of dense-core peptide hormone granules, including gastrin (G-cells), somatostatin (D-cells), vaso-active intestinal polypeptide (D1-cells) and glucagon (A-cells). However, the hormone product of the majority of endocrine cells in the fundus and body, which resemble enterochromaffin cells morphologically (ECL-like cells), is unknown in the human, although they contain histamine in the rat.

The proportions of the various cell types vary at different levels of the gastric glands, so that although parietal cells are scattered throughout, the distribution of the other cell types allows three zones to be defined: an uppermost isthmus populated mainly by surface-type mucous cells, a neck zone containing the special mucous neck cells with their histochemically distinctive mucin, and a basal zone rich in chief cells and scattered endocrine cells (Fig. 16.22). There is evidence that all of the epithelial cells in the gastric mucosa arise from common precursor stem cells situated in the isthmic and neck zones of the glands, and undifferentiated cells can be recognized histologically in these sites. Most of their progeny migrate upwards towards the mucosal surface, differentiating into mucous cells, but some migrate more slowly downwards to differentiate into parietal cells, chief cells, or endocrine cells. A number of mechanisms may be involved in the control of cell renewal: humoral factors such as prostaglandins and epidermal growth factor are known to stimulate gastric mucosal proliferation and, by analogy with the intestine, the presence of food within the gastric lumen probably has a similar effect. Negative feedback control

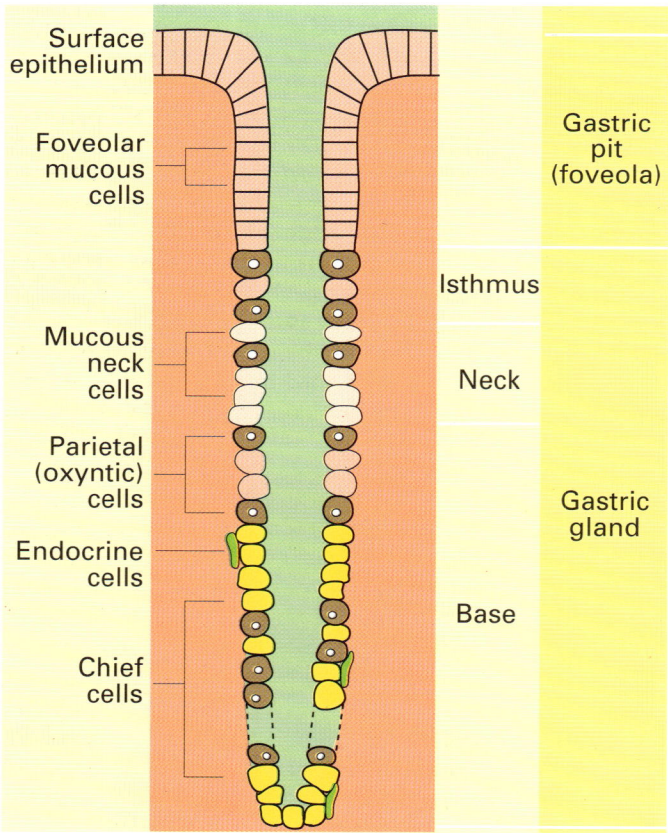

Fig. 16.22 Diagrammatic representation of the different zones of the gastric mucosal glands.

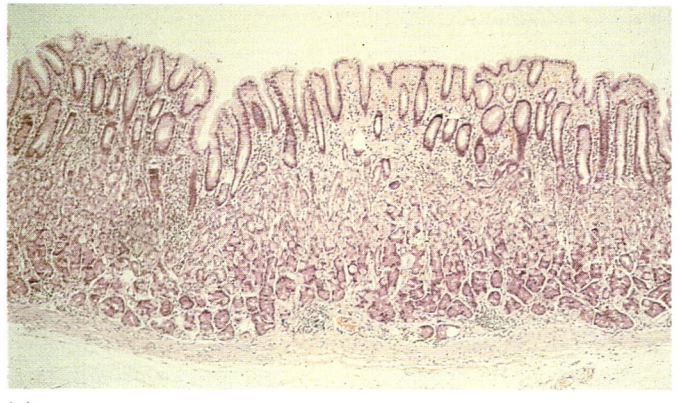

(a)

(b)

Fig. 16.24 Histological appearances of normal body mucosa. Lower magnification (a) shows a superficial foveolar zone and a much thicker deeper zone of specialized glands which on higher magnification (b) are composed of parietal cells with abundant pale cytoplasm (upper field) and more basophilic chief cells (lower field).

from the functional to the proliferative cells almost certainly also occurs.

At the deepest aspect of the mucosa there is a thin band of smooth muscle, the muscularis mucosae, which separates the mucosa from the *submucosa*, a zone of loose areolar connective tissue containing nerves, blood vessels, and lymphatics. Deep to this is the *muscularis propria*, the main smooth muscle coat of the stomach which is divided into an innermost oblique layer, an inner circular layer, and an outer longitudinal layer. The circular layer is thickened in the antrum to form the functional pyloric sphincter. On the outside is the *serosa* of the peritoneal

cavity, composed of loose connective tissue, blood vessels, lymphatics, and nerve fibres, covered by mesothelium.

The stomach receives a rich blood supply derived from branches of the coeliac, hepatic, and splenic arteries which anastomose freely within a submucosal plexus. This gives rise to the mucosal arteries, many of which are end arteries, especially along the lesser curvature. The venous drainage is mainly via the portal system, although there are portal–systemic anastomoses at the gastro-oesophageal junction which may distend to form gastric varices when there is portal hypertension (see Chapter 17). Small lymphatic channels in the mucosa form a plexus just above the muscularis mucosae which communicates with a more extensive submucosal plexus. From this, large lymphatic trunks follow the venous drainage of the stomach, first to lymph node groups along the greater and lesser curvatures, the porta hepatis and splenic hilum, and thence to the coeliac nodes around the coeliac axis. A detailed knowledge of this lymphatic drainage is essential for understanding the spread of gastric cancer and consequently for its rational surgical treatment. The nerve supply is from the terminal branches of the vagi and the sympathetic coeliac plexus; these contribute with peptidergic fibres to form two intramural plexuses, Meissner's plexus in the submucosa and Auerbach's plexus between the circular and longitudinal layers of the muscularis externa. Fine post-ganglionic nerve fibres from these plexuses innervate both the mucosa and the smooth muscle of the gastric wall.

The physiological control of gastric secretion is complex and involves nervous, endocrine, and paracrine mechanisms. Acetylcholine released by vagal stimulation, gastrin derived from antral endocrine cells, and histamine released from mucosal mast cells can all stimulate the parietal cells directly to secrete acid and, although the mechanisms are less well understood, almost certainly also stimulate the release of pepsinogens and intrinsic factor. Blocking of muscarinic cholinergic receptors by atropine, or of histamine receptors by H_2-antagonists, greatly reduces gastric acid secretion.

Secretion of gastric juice between meals is largely dependent upon tonic vagal activity: basal acid output is markedly diminished by vagotomy. Ingestion of food induces a dramatic increase in gastric secretion, up to 800 ml in volume This is achieved in three overlapping phases. In the cephalic phase the sight, smell, or taste of food results in vagal stimulation both of the parietal cells directly and of gastrin release by the antral endocrine cells, resulting in acid secretion even before food reaches the stomach. The gastric phase, during which secretion increases even more, results from the presence of food within the stomach: distension of the fundus and body stimulates gastric secretion via an intramural reflex, while the presence of intraluminal peptides and amino acids induces acid and enzyme production by direct chemical stimulation of the mucosa. In the intestinal phase the presence of peptides and amino acids within the duodenum stimulates the release of gastrin from the antral endocrine cells, and therefore maintains secretion for some time after feeding. The most potent physiological inhibitors of gastric secretion include a low pH in the antrum, which probably acts by releasing somatostatin locally, and the presence of hypertonic solutions or fat in the duodenum.

The factors controlling mucus and bicarbonate production by the surface epithelial cells are poorly understood. Vagal activity and release of endogenous prostaglandins are both known to increase their secretion but the most potent stimulant of mucus production is direct irritation of the luminal surface.

The motor functions of the stomach, whereby gastric contents are continually mixed and released in small quantities into the duodenum, result from the co-ordinated peristalsis of the smooth muscle coats of the distal body and pyloric antrum. Regular contraction waves, occurring at about 20 second intervals and lasting about 4 seconds, start from a pacemaker in the body near the mid greater curve and move distally, propelling a food bolus ahead of them. As each wave approaches the pylorus the leading portion of the bolus is forced into the duodenum. However, almost immediately afterwards the contraction wave reaches the pylorus itself and closes it, so that the majority of the gastric contents are trapped within the antrum and ground against the pylorus. Peristalsis is under neural control, being increased by vagal stimulation and suppressed by sympathetic activity. Gastric distension causes increased peristalsis, probably by vagal stimulation. The fundus and proximal body do not undergo peristalsis—they only act as the gastric food reservoir.

16.2.2 Developmental disorders

Infantile hypertrophic pyloric stenosis

This occurs in 3–4/1000 live births in the United Kingdom and affects boys five times more frequently than girls. Although the condition is not inherited in any classical Mendelian pattern, familial clustering of cases is well recognized. Racial variations in the incidence are also quite marked; commonest in Northern Europeans, the condition is rare in Africa and virtually unknown among the Chinese.

Infantile pyloric stenosis usually presents 2–6 weeks after birth, with severe and persistent projectile vomiting leading to dehydration and metabolic disturbances. It is remarkably rare in the new-born. The cause is a functional obstruction of the gastric outlet due to a pronounced concentric hypertrophy of the circular muscle coat of the pylorus. Often this localized thickening may be sufficiently marked to result in a 'tumour' being palpable on abdominal examination, and when palpated at laparotomy the pylorus has a hard, almost cartilagenous consistency. The pyloric obstruction leads to dilatation of the proximal stomach, whose wall is consequently thinned markedly. Infantile pyloric stenosis is simply and consistently relieved by surgical incision of the hypertrophied muscle coat (Ramstedt's pyloromyotomy). However, its aetiology is unknown. Studies of the autonomic innervation of the pylorus in this condition have been inconclusive. It is interesting to note than an identical condition may be induced in puppies by injecting pregnant bitches and their new-born offspring with the synthetic peptide hormone pentagastrin. Whether or not this is relevant to the development of the human condition remains to be seen.

Other developmental disorders

Other developmental disorders of the stomach are very uncommon. Anomalies in position result from malrotation of the developing gut, so that the stomach may come to lie within the thoracic cavity. Duplications, diverticula, and congenital cysts of the stomach are described rarely.

16.2.3 Gastritis

Although the term 'gastritis' is commonly used by the layman to encompass upper abdominal symptoms of epigastric discomfort or pain, distension, flatulence, and nausea, the correlation between such features of dyspepsia and histologically demonstrable inflammation within the gastric mucosa is extremely poor. A significant proportion of patients with dyspepsia have no obvious histological abnormality of the upper gastrointestinal tract, while many individuals with histologically proven gastritis are asymptomatic. In this section we will consider gastritis in the histological sense.

Inflammatory damage to the gastric mucosa may occur by a number of mechanisms. Most commonly it is caused by a luminal irritant, but endogenous factors, such as auto-immune destruction of the gastric epithelial cells and local ischaemia of the gastric mucosa, are also important sometimes. The luminal surface is vulnerable to damage by ingested irritants, both chemical and microbiological, and also by hydrochloric acid and proteolytic enzymes. Its integrity is dependent upon the existence of a number of protective mechanisms. The most important of these is thought to be the so-called mucus–bicarbonate barrier. This is a physical barrier of viscid mucus up to 300 μm thick which is produced by the gastric epithelial cells and separates the luminal contents from the epithelial surface. The arrangement of the mucus glycoprotein molecules is essential for this barrier function. Continued secretion of bicarbonate ions into the mucus layer by the surface epithelial cells ensures that it also forms a barrier to acid, with a pH gradient across it from pH 1 on the luminal side to pH 7 on the surface epithelial side (Fig. 16.25). Other protective measures include local immunological mechanisms and careful control of epithelial cell proliferation which allow a prompt regenerative response to cell damage. Locally released mediators, notably prostaglandins, are thought to be important in controlling this epithelial cell proliferation, and also the secretion of mucus and bicarbonate, and therefore appear to play a crucial role in maintaining mucosal integrity. However, since most of the protective mechanisms are ultimately dependent upon effective epithelial cell function, it follows that once these are overcome and epithelial cells are damaged a vicious cycle of perpetuating mucosal damage may ensue, leading to mucosal erosion and eventually to frank ulceration. It is not surprising, therefore, that factors involved in the causation of gastritis are also of importance in the aetiology of gastric ulceration (see below).

It is conventional to divide gastritis into acute and chronic forms, despite the fact that there is considerable overlap between the two conditions. Some forms of acute gastritis may progress to chronic gastritis, while in chronic gastritis there are

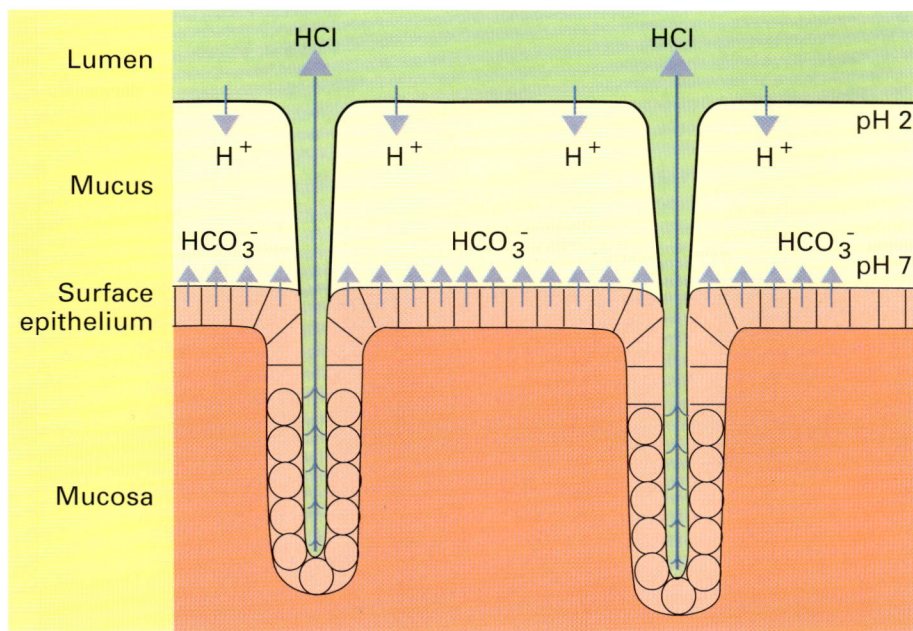

Fig. 16.25 The mucus–bicarbonate barrier. A pH gradient is maintained across the mucus layer by epithelial secretion of bicarbonate ions.

frequently episodes of superimposed acute inflammation, so-called active chronic gastritis. Nevertheless, there are enough distinctive aspects of each condition to warrant their separation here.

Acute gastritis

Acute gastritis is usually recognized clinically in three situations: in patients who have ingested irritant substances, in those who are extremely ill and debilitated for a variety of reasons (usually unconnected with the alimentary tract), and, rarely, in patients with a viral or bacteriological infection of the gastric mucosa. In some patients the inflammatory reaction produces symptoms of dyspepsia or vomiting, but others are remarkably free of symptoms and only present when haemorrhage from a severely damaged mucosa causes a massive haematemesis. In view of the fact that gastritis frequently fails to produce significant symptoms, it is possible that subclinical and self-limiting episodes of acute mucosal inflammation are common in the population.

Acute chemical gastritis

Chemical irritants causing acute gastritis include corrosives consumed accidentally or with suicidal intent, alcohol, drugs, and some spicy foods. Most irritants cause direct epithelial cell damage, the most toxic corrosives, such as phenol, lysol, and caustic soda, leading to severe coagulative necrosis or mucosal liquefaction. However, other mechanisms may be involved. The most important group of drugs causing gastritis, the non-steroidal anti-inflammatory drugs (including aspirin), not only cause direct epithelial damage but, by virtue of their action of inhibiting prostaglandin synthesis, reduce the mucosal concentrations of prostaglandins which have an important role in maintaining mucosal blood flow and are important mediators of

mucosal protective mechanisms. Aspirin also interacts with mucus glycoproteins, altering the physical properties of the surface mucus so that its viscosity, and consequently its effectiveness as a barrier, is greatly reduced. Mucosal damage therefore results from a combination of direct epithelial toxicity, back-diffusion of acid and pepsin from the gastric lumen, and relative mucosal ischaemia from local prostaglandin deficiency. Ingestion of many other drugs, including corticosteroids and some antibiotics, may be followed by acute dyspeptic symptoms, although in most cases it is not certain that they cause histological gastritis.

The gastric mucosa in acute chemical gastritis is oedematous, congested, and covered by large amounts of mucus. Intramucosal haemorrhage is the rule, varying in degree from petechial haemorrhages to the extensive mucosal bleeding of acute haemorrhagic gastritis (Figs 16.26, 16.27). Necrosis of the surface epithelium accompanied by exudation of fibrin and neutrophil polymorphs, the latter sometimes quite scanty, leads first to focal mucosal erosions (Fig. 16.28) (so-called acute erosive gastritis) and eventually to small acute ulcers, with sharp, well-defined edges and a grey base, that involve the full thickness of the mucosa. Massive haemorrhage may arise either from widespread oozing of blood from a diffusely haemorrhagic mucosa or when an acute ulcer penetrates the submucosa and erodes one of the plentiful small arteries and veins.

An acute gastritis with clinical and pathological features identical to chemical gastritis and resulting in massive gastrointestinal haemorrhage may occur as a life-threatening complication in severely ill patients following trauma, sepsis, major surgery, burns, or hypothermia. Progression from haemorrhagic gastritis to erosions and so-called acute 'stress' ulcers is common. A number of factors may be involved in its pathogenesis, including irritation by drugs, excess acid secretion

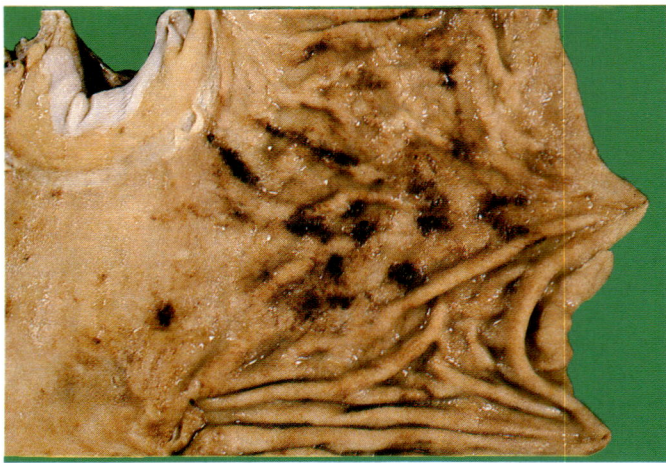

Fig. 16.26 Macroscopic appearances of acute gastritis, showing focal haemorrhages in the mucosa of the body of the stomach.

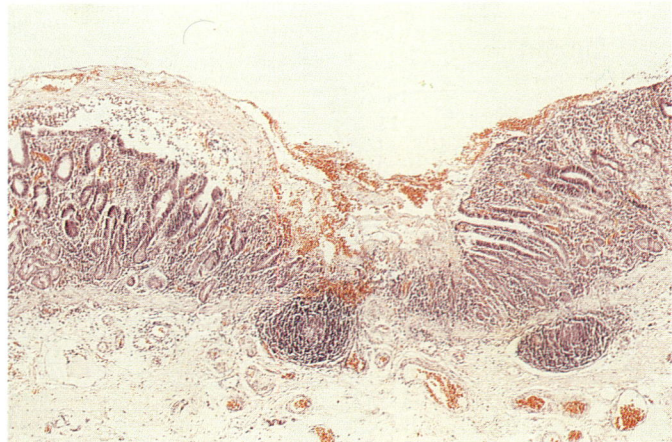

Fig. 16.28 Histological appearance of an acute mucosal erosion. There is necrosis of the superficial half of the gastric mucosa, covered by a haemorrhagic fibrinous exudate.

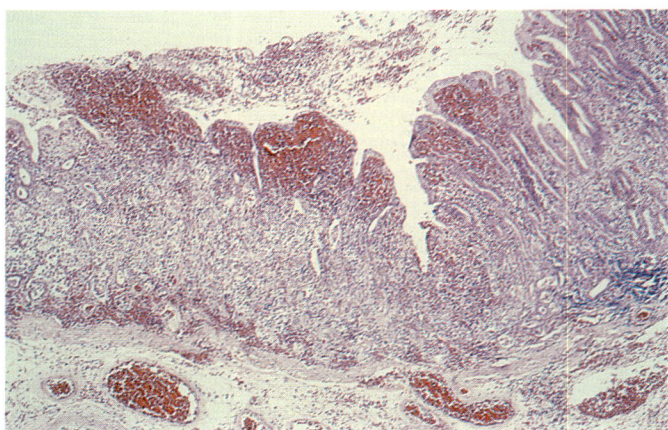

Fig. 16.27 Histological appearances of the mucosa from the specimen in Fig. 16.26, showing extensive haemorrhage in the foveolar zone, epithelial cell necrosis in the gastric glands, and early exudation of fibrin and polymorphs from the mucosal surface.

consequent upon hypergastrinaemia, reflux of bile and small intestinal contents into the stomach, and possibly infection (see below), but the most important is thought to be mucosal ischaemia, resulting from systemic shock and hypotension, which weakens the mucosal barrier and allows back-diffusion of acid through the damaged mucosal surface.

Acute infective gastritis

Infective causes of clinically significant acute gastritis are very uncommon. While it is possible that the epigastric discomfort and vomiting which occur in many viral illnesses are a consequence of gastritis, there are no histological studies to prove this. Apart from rare instances of proven gastric involvement in patients with *Salmonella* or *Yersinia* enteritis, infective gastritis in clinical practice is virtually confined to patients with immunodeficiency. Such patients may have cytomegalovirus or

herpes gastritis, which usually result in focal haemorrhagic erosions, but patients with chronic liver disease, especially alcoholics, may rarely develop a severe diffuse 'phlegmonous' gastritis from infection by bacteria, usually haemolytic streptococci. The intense inflammatory reaction in this condition often spares the mucosa and is centred on the deeper layers of the gastric wall which is intensely congested and covered by a fibrinopurulent serosal exudate.

In recent years interest in *Campylobacter pylori* (now known as *Helicobacter pylori*) as a cause of chronic gastritis (see below) has stimulated volunteers to ingest this organism experimentally, with subsequent examination of gastric biopsies. A relatively mild non-haemorrhagic acute gastritis associated with clinical features of dyspepsia may be induced, and can be either self-limiting or may progress to chronic gastritis. It now seems likely that *H. pylori* was responsible for episodes of transient acute gastritis with hypochlorhydria which were previously reported in healthy volunteers participating in studies of acid secretion, following contamination of intubation instruments by this organism.

Chronic gastritis

Chronic inflammation of the gastric mucosa is an extremely common finding in endoscopic biopsies from patients with upper gastrointestinal symptoms. However, the correlation between the severity of clinical features and the degree of gastritis is poor, and epidemiological studies have indicated that the condition is common among asymptomatic individuals, its frequency increasing with age. Geographic variations also occur: in one study it was recorded in 78 per cent of Japanese individuals aged over 50 years compared with 30 per cent of North Americans. When studied carefully in resection specimens, chronic gastritis is often found to be patchy and to show a poor correlation with the macroscopic appearance of the gastric mucosa. It may even be present in about 30 per cent of biopsies from endoscopically normal stomachs. The inconsistent relationship between chronic gastritis and both clinical and macroscopic features has led many to question its pathological significance, some regarding it merely as an ageing phenomenon. However, in recent years there have been advances in our understanding of the pathogenesis of chronic gastritis, and of its relationship to the two most important diseases of the stomach, namely peptic ulceration and carcinoma of the stomach. It is now possible to classify chronic gastritis into six quite well-defined varieties, although there is some overlap between them.

Auto-immune chronic gastritis

As the name suggests, this form of gastritis is associated with the presence of circulating auto-antibodies, nearly always to the parietal cells in the gastric glands, and often to intrinsic factor also. Auto-immune destruction of the gastric glands, predominantly in the body of the stomach, is accompanied by a mixed chronic inflammatory cell infiltrate of lymphocytes and plasma cells throughout the full thickness of the gastric mucosa, often with lymphoid follicles with active germinal centres. This histological picture has been called atrophic gastritis (Fig. 16.29) because of the loss ('atrophy') of the specialized glands in the deeper zone of the body mucosa. Auto-immune gastritis rarely produces clinical symptoms that can be related to the stomach. It is seen classically in pernicious anaemia, when defective secretion of intrinsic factor leads to vitamin B_{12} deficiency. Almost invariably there is also hypochlorhydria due to destruction of parietal cells, leading eventually to achlorhydria as the specialized glands of the body mucosa are completely destroyed. At this late stage the inflammatory infiltrate often diminishes to leave a paper-thin, transparent but non-inflamed, atrophic mucosa. The reduction in acid secretion stimulates hypergastrinaemia, another feature of auto-immune gastritis, and sometimes this has a trophic effect on the ECL

endocrine cells of the body mucosa, resulting in the formation of multiple, small, carcinoid tumours (see Section 16.17.5).

The chronic inflammatory destruction of the specialized glands of the gastric body mucosa is commonly accompanied by cystic change and metaplasia of the epithelium (Fig. 16.29). Often the change is from body type to one closely resembling pyloric antral mucosa (so-called pseudo-pyloric metaplasia), but more conspicuous is intestinal metaplasia, the appearance of enteric-type epithelium, including goblet cells, absorptive cells, Paneth cells, and intestinal-type endocrine cells, within the gastric glands. On rare occasions there may even be a villous architecture. The change can be demonstrated readily by mucin histochemistry, when the neutral mucin of normal gastric epithelial mucous cells contrasts with the acidic sialic acid-rich mucin of intestinal-type goblet cells (Fig. 16.30). Intestinal metaplasia may be divided into a complete type (type I), when the metaplastic glands consist exclusively of intestinal-type cells, and two less common incomplete types (types IIa and IIb), when intestinal cells are admixed with gastric-type cells within the same gland, sometimes with apparent hybrid forms. Type IIb intestinal metaplasia (now sometimes called type III) is characterized by the presence of sulphomucins within immature metaplastic cells (Fig. 16.31). Intestinal metaplasia is of particular interest to pathologists because of its association with gastric carcinoma. This link is particularly strong for the type IIb variant.

There is a considerable clinical overlap between auto-immune chronic gastritis and other organ-specific auto-immune diseases. Thus pernicious anaemia is associated with auto-immune thyroiditis (Hashimoto's disease), Addison's disease, and juvenile (type I) diabetes mellitus, or with a family history of these disorders.

Helicobacter-associated chronic gastritis

By far the commonest variety of chronic gastritis, this condition was known as chronic non-specific gastritis until 1983 when

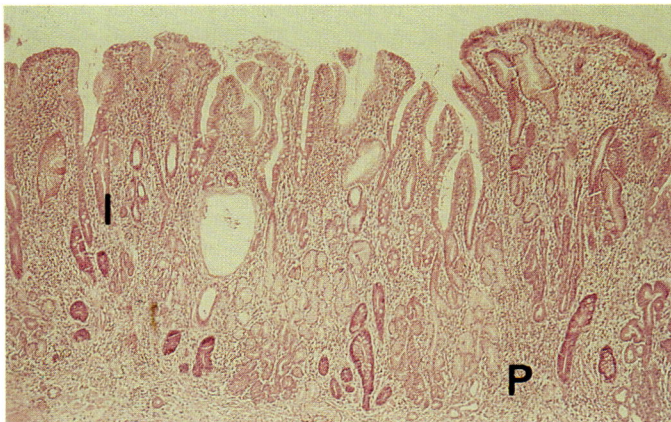

Fig. 16.29 Chronic atrophic gastritis in the body mucosa of a patient with circulating anti-parietal cell antibodies. A diffuse chronic inflammatory cell infiltrate is accompanied by destruction of the specialized glands and their replacement by small cysts, pyloric antral-type mucous glands (P) (pseudo-pyloric metaplasia), and intestinal-type glands (I) (intestinal metaplasia).

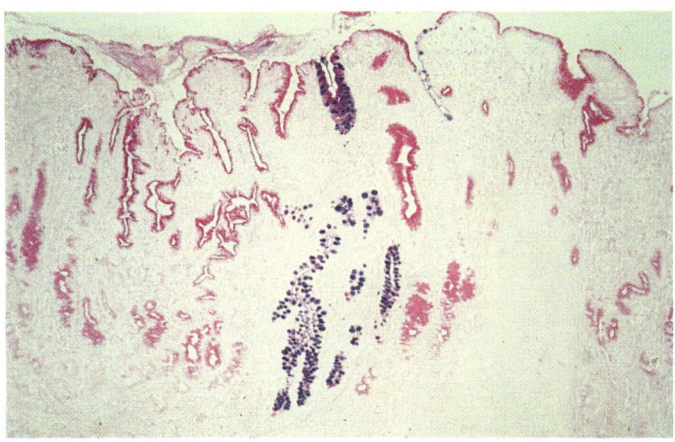

Fig. 16.30 Mucin histochemistry, using the alcian blue-periodic acid-Schiff technique, highlights the blue-staining sialic acid-rich mucin of intestinal metaplasia (centre) against the background of magenta-staining neutral mucin of the normal gastric epithelium.

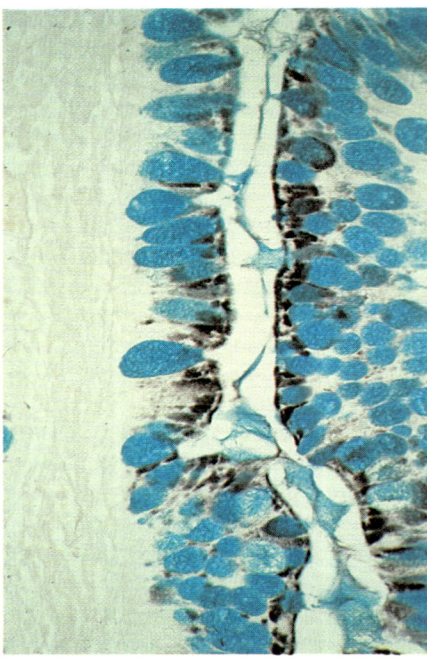

Fig. 16.31 Type IIb (more recently named type III) intestinal metaplasia stained by the high-iron diamine–alcian blue technique. Mature goblet cells containing blue-staining sialomucins are interspersed with immature cells containing black-staining sulphomucins.

Warren and Marshall pointed out its strong association with the presence of curved bacilli, later to be named *Campylobacter pylori* (and now renamed *Helicobacter pylori*) attached to the luminal surface of the gastric epithelial cells (Fig. 16.32). Its frequency increases with age and is largely responsible for variations in the overall incidence of chronic gastritis in different populations. The mucosa of the pyloric antrum is primarily affected, although extension into the body zone is not uncommon in long-standing cases. Histologically there is a chronic inflammatory cell infiltrate of lymphocytes and plasma cells

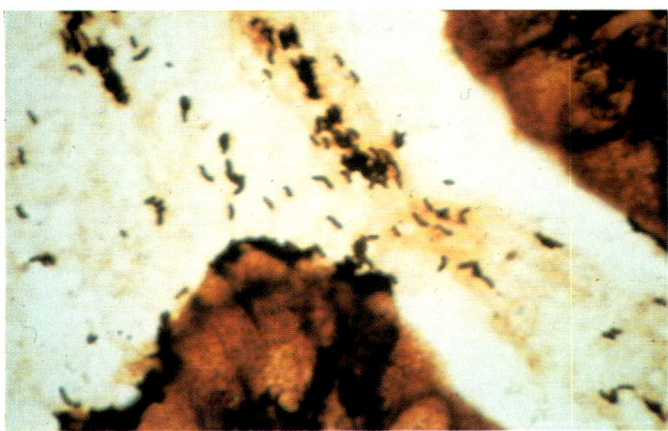

Fig. 16.32 *Helicobacter pylori* organisms, stained by the Warthin–Starry technique, are lying within the gastric mucus layer. Some (bottom left) are attached to the epithelial cell surface.

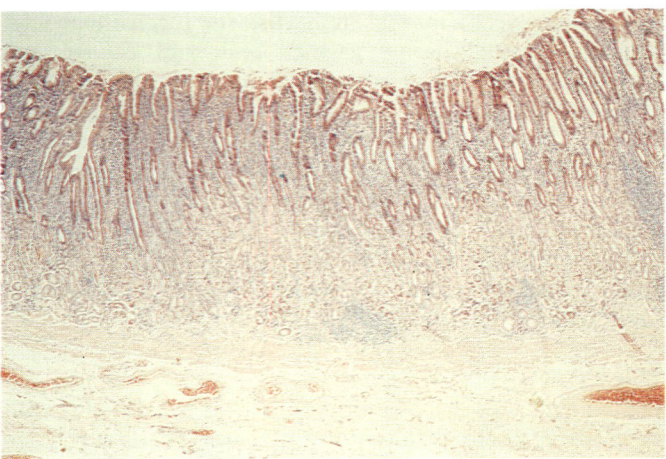

Fig. 16.33 *H. pylori*-associated chronic superficial gastritis of the antral mucosa. The inflammatory cell infiltrate is confined to the upper (foveolar) half of the mucosa.

which, in the early stages of the disease, are confined to the superficial (foveolar) part of the mucosa (Fig. 16.33), an appearance termed chronic superficial gastritis. However, with time the inflammatory process may extend more deeply to involve the whole mucosal thickness, resulting in a picture of chronic atrophic gastritis similar to that seen in the body of the stomach in auto-immune chronic gastritis. When this occurs, and when the process extends into the body mucosa, there is often some degree of hypochlorhydria, although this is only rarely accompanied by hypergastrinaemia. Intestinal metaplasia, of any of the types described above in auto-immune chronic gastritis, may also be found.

The chronic inflammation of *H. pylori*-associated chronic gastritis is often accompanied by a superimposed patchy acute inflammatory cell infiltrate of neutrophil and eosinophil polymorphs, largely confined to the superficial part of the mucosa and the surface epithelium (Fig. 16.34) and when this occurs the chronic gastritis is said to be 'active'. The acute inflammatory destruction of the superficial epithelial cells results in mucin depletion and stimulates regenerative hyperplasia in the isthmic and neck zones of the gastric pits. Sometimes the increased mitotic activity, accompanied by the appearance of conspicuous numbers of immature epithelial cells in the foveolae, can be sufficiently marked as to mimic a pre-invasive neoplastic epithelial cell proliferation or dysplasia (see Section 16.3.2).

H. pylori is a micro-aerophilic, curved, Gram-negative, urease-producing bacterium which is able to colonize the surface of the gastric mucosa, deep within the overlying mucus layer. Rather surprisingly, the organism is acid-intolerant, so that its survival is dependent upon the existence of the mucus–bicarbonate barrier. Infection is thought to occur during a meal, when there is relative hypochlorhydria, and once the organism is established in its ecological 'niche' it persists for months or years, resisting a local immune reaction that results in specific antibody secretion. The lymphoid cells that mediate

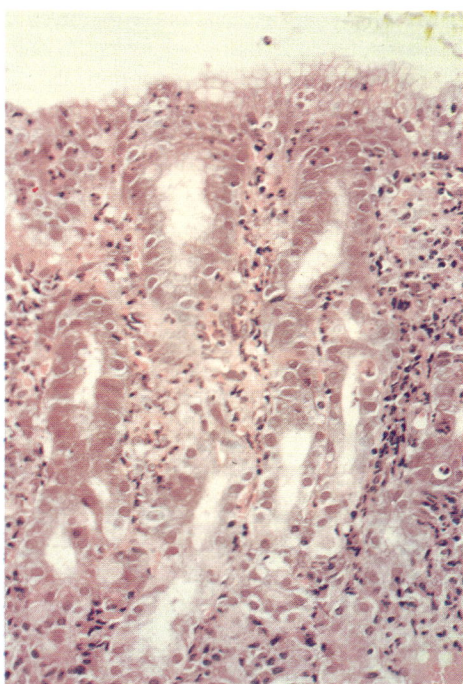

Fig. 16.34 Active chronic superficial gastritis associated with *H. pylori*. The field shows the luminal half of the mucosa, where there is a dense infiltrate of mononuclear cells and neutrophil polymorphs, the latter invading the surface epithelium. The foveolar epithelial cells show depletion of mucus and marked regenerative hyperplasia.

this immune response may well account for much of the chronic gastritis associated with the presence of the bacterium. Shifts in the balance between the organism and local mucosal defence mechanisms probably result in episodes of active gastritis, when abundant *H. pylori* can be consistently demonstrated, interspersed with periods of inactivity when the organisms are scanty or even absent. How epithelial damage occurs is not known, but suggestions include direct cellular toxicity by the bacterium or its products, damage from ammonia produced by virtue of the organism's urea-splitting capacity, and back-diffusion of acid from the gastric lumen resulting from disruption of the mucus–bicarbonate barrier by bacterial mucolytic enzymes. It is of interest that *H. pylori* does not attach to intestinal-type epithelium, and the intestinal metaplasia which frequently accompanies chronic gastritis is therefore spared.

Although it is clear that *H. pylori* is strongly associated with chronic gastritis, the evidence that it plays a causative role is not conclusive and it is conceivable that the organism is merely a commensal that colonizes inflamed mucosa. However, the fact that eradication of the organism is usually accompanied by a reduction or resolution of histological inflammation, and that human ingestion of the organism leads in some cases to chronic gastritis, strongly support a causative relationship. As with all chronic gastritis, the correlation between histological gastritis and gastric symptoms is poor, although some studies have

shown as association between active chronic gastritis and so-called non-ulcer dyspepsia.

Reflux (chemical) chronic gastritis

Persistent reflux of duodenal contents into the stomach produces a chronic gastritis which has a characteristic histological appearance manifested by foveolar hyperplasia, oedema, and vasodilatation in the lamina propria (Fig. 16.35). Inflammatory cells are remarkably scanty. This lesion is seen classically in gastric biopsies from post-gastrectomy patients, in whom duodeno-gastric reflux is common, but a similar lesion is seen in those with 'spontaneous' reflux and in patients receiving long-term non-steroidal anti-inflammatory drugs. This suggests that this form of gastritis represents a reaction to chronic chemical irritation of the gastric mucosa, and indeed the changes merge with those of acute chemical gastritis (see above). Bile acids and lysolecithin (produced by the action of pancreatic phospholipase on lecithin in bile) are both suspected of causing reflux gastritis, and the severity of histological abnormalities correlates with bile acid concentrations in fasting gastric juice. Clinical symptoms of dyspepsia in affected individuals are variable, but endoscopically the gastric mucosa is usually intensely hyperaemic and friable. Chronic occult blood loss is common, and the development of acute haemorrhagic erosions may result in massive haematemesis.

Chronic lymphocytic gastritis

This is a newly recognized variant of chronic gastritis, characterized by marked infiltration of the surface and foveolar

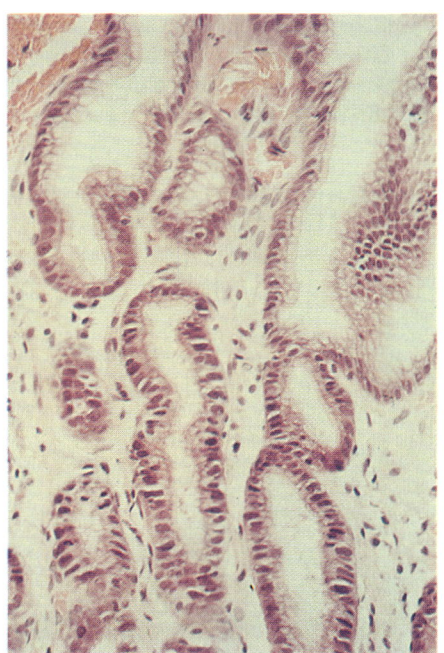

Fig. 16.35 Histological appearances of the superficial aspect of the antral mucosa in reflux gastritis. There is oedema of the lamina propria, capillary ectasia (upper field), and foveolar epithelial hyperplasia.

epithelium by mature T-lymphocytes. Its aetiology is unknown, but the lymphocytic infiltrate has been likened to that in the small bowel in coeliac disease. The body mucosa is mainly affected, and in many cases the endoscopic appearances are distinctive, with mucosal nodules bearing a central erosion, changes which have been termed chronic erosive gastritis or 'varioliform' gastritis. Not all cases with such chronic erosions have lymphocytic gastritis: however, similar lesions may occur in the antrum in Helicobacter-associated chronic gastritis (Fig. 16.36) and reflux gastritis.

Eosinophilic gastritis

This rare condition is characterized by a dense infiltrate of eosinophil leucocytes in the gastric mucosa, often extending into the deeper layers of the gastric wall where there is marked thickening by oedema. Within the stomach the pyloric antrum is chiefly affected, but in many patients the condition is part of a more widespread eosinophilic gastroenteritis. Peripheral blood eosinophilia and raised serum IgE levels are often present and affected patients frequently also suffer from asthma, suggesting that the condition is basically an allergic disorder. However, a definite allergen can only be identified in a minority of cases, and the precise mechanisms involved in this form of gastritis are unknown. Eosinophilic gastritis alone rarely causes impressive clinical symptoms but when the inflammatory infiltrate is particularly marked the eosinophils may invade and destroy the surface and foveolar epithelium, leading to focal necrosis and regenerative foveolar hyperplasia.

Granulomatous gastritis

Granulomatous inflammation of the gastric mucosa is uncommon, but is well recognized in sarcoidosis, tuberculosis, and histoplasmosis. Most examples are asymptomatic, although progression to ulceration or an inflammatory mass may occur. The stomach is affected in 1–2 per cent of patients with Crohn's disease, nearly always in association with intestinal involvement. The gross appearances are similar to those elsewhere in the gut, with patchy mucosal inflammation, fissuring ulceration, oedema, and thickening of the gastric wall. Histologically there is active chronic inflammation with transmural lymphoid aggregates, fibrosis, and non-caseating epithelioid granulomas. Ingested foreign materials and sutures may also incite localized granulomatous reactions. In some cases of granulomatous gastritis no cause is apparent. Although some of these may well represent cases of undiagnosed sarcoidosis or localized gastric Crohn's disease, only a minority subsequently develop typical lesions elsewhere.

16.2.4   Non-specific duodenitis

Although inflammatory diseases of the small intestine are discussed in full elsewhere in this book, it is appropriate to consider non-specific duodenitis here, because it is related both to chronic gastritis and peptic ulcer disease. The condition is termed 'non-specific' to distinguish it from 'specific' inflammatory lesions of the duodenum, notably coeliac disease and Crohn's disease. It is characterized by a diffuse chronic inflammatory cell infiltrate in the mucosa of the proximal duodenum (Fig. 16.37) and may be described as active or inactive, depending upon the presence or absence, respectively, of neutrophil polymorphs. The inflammation is accompanied by degeneration of the surface enterocytes, which may result in minor degrees of villous atrophy, and when it is severe there may be superficial mucosal erosions.

As with chronic gastritis, correlations between histological duodenitis and clinical symptoms or the endoscopic appearances of the duodenum are not good, although there is more than a tendency for patients with active duodenitis to give a history of dyspepsia and to show erythema, petechial haemorrhages, or erosions in the duodenum on endoscopy. There is a much stronger association between active duodenitis and peptic ulceration of the duodenum, and many authors consider the

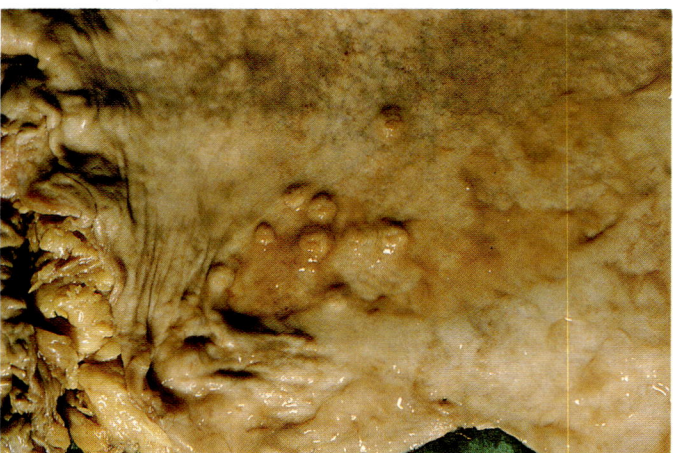

Fig. 16.36 Macroscopic appearance of so-called varioliform (chronic erosive) gastritis, in this case involving the antral mucosa, characterized by small nodules with a central dimple-like erosion. Helicobacter-associated gastritis was present in the background mucosa.

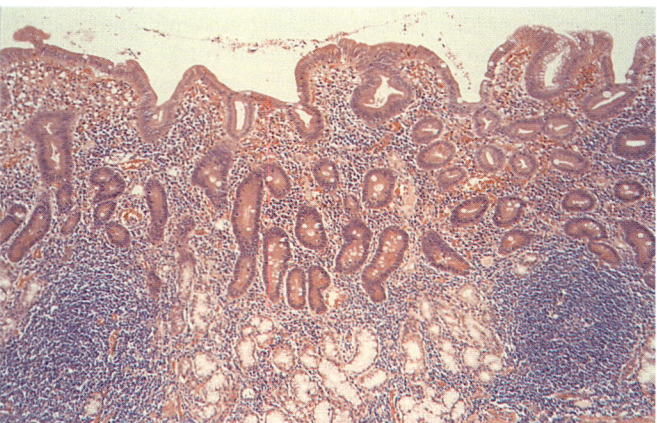

Fig. 16.37 Active chronic duodenitis. There is marked villous shortening, associated with a diffuse acute-on-chronic inflammatory cell infiltrate and lymphoid follicles.

two conditions to have a common aetiology. Many patients with duodenitis have excessive gastric acid output, and while this is certainly important it does not appear to be the only factor. Recently it has been suggested that *Helicobacter pylori* may be implicated in the pathogenesis of chronic duodenitis. It is well recognized that chronic duodenitis is frequently associated with metaplasia of the duodenal epithelium to one of gastric type and it is now apparent that this is often colonized by *H. pylori* organisms in active duodenitis: indeed, the condition is frequently accompanied by a *Helicobacter*-associated chronic gastritis. The overall evidence suggests, therefore, that while chronic hyperacidity is responsible for initiating chronic duodenitis and inducing gastric metaplasia, it is the colonization of the metaplastic epithelium by *H. pylori* that leads to active duodenitis by mechanisms analogous to those causing active chronic gastritis in the stomach. The consequent weakening of mucosal defence mechanisms may then allow progression to mucosal erosions, and possibly to frank peptic ulceration.

16.2.5   Peptic ulcer

This term is used to describe gastrointestinal ulceration in mucosal surfaces exposed to gastric acid and pepsin secretion. The great majority of peptic ulcers occur in the stomach and proximal duodenum, but other sites include the lower end of the oesophagus (see Section 16.1.4), the jejunum at gastroenterostomy stomas (stomal ulcers), and the ileum close to (or within) a Meckel's diverticulum containing heterotopic gastric mucosa (see Section 16.7.2). Patients with gastric hypersecretion due to the Zollinger–Ellison syndrome may develop multiple peptic ulcers throughout the duodenum and the jejunum.

Peptic ulcers are sometimes divided into acute and chronic types. By definition, the former involve the mucosa and submucosa only while the latter penetrate into, and often through, the main muscularis propria. Although obviously all chronic ulcers must have been superficial at one time, the two types present in sufficiently different clinical settings to warrant their continued separation.

Acute peptic ulcer

Acute peptic ulcers are usually seen as part of the spectrum of acute chemical gastritis either due to drugs (especially the non-steroidal anti-inflammatory agents) or in severely ill patients from extensive burns (Curling's ulcer), sepsis, trauma, surgery, or rapidly progressive intracranial disease (Cushing's ulcers). They are commonest in the stomach, especially the gastric body, but in severe cases the duodenum may also be affected. There appears to be a progression from acute haemorrhagic gastritis through gastric erosions to multiple small acute peptic ulcers, usually measuring less than 1 cm in diameter (Fig. 16.38), and haemorrhage from these, often considerable and even life-threatening, is frequently their first manifestation. However, a small minority progress rapidly to complete perforation and present with acute peritonitis. The pathogenesis of acute peptic ulcers is considered above with that of acute chemical gastritis.

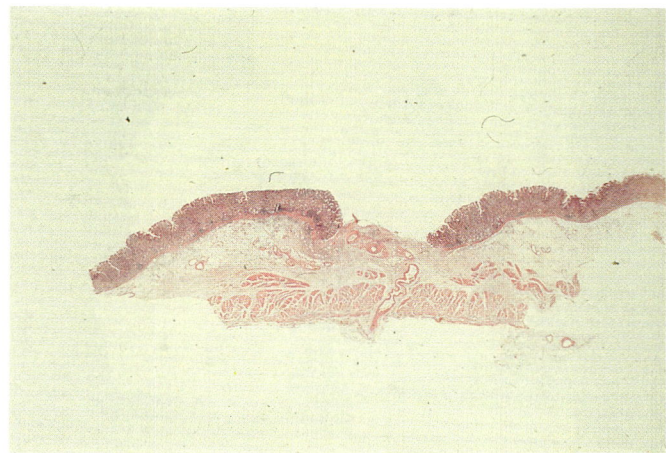

Fig. 16.38   Histological appearance of an acute gastric ulcer showing destruction of the full mucosal thickness. The ulcer base extends close to prominent submucosal vessels, and erosion of these may precipitate massive haemorrhage. The deeper layers of the gastric wall are normal, in contrast to a chronic peptic ulcer (cf. Fig. 16.41).

Chronic peptic ulcer

This is a very common condition which has been estimated to affect about 10 per cent of the population of the Western World at some time of their lives and leads to the loss of some 1.5 million working days every year in Great Britain. Nevertheless, the incidence in the UK appears to be falling, from a peak in the 1920s, and over the past 20 years significant advances in the development of drugs that influence gastric secretion and improve mucosal protection mechanisms, have resulted in a dramatic decline in hospital admissions. Mortality from peptic ulceration has also fallen markedly during this period, and nowadays is largely confined to the elderly or those who are debilitated from co-existing illness. Although mainly a disease of adults, it is well recognized in childhood. Most epidemiological data suggest that environmental factors are of greatest importance in the aetiology of peptic ulcers, but family studies have shown that first-degree relatives of peptic ulcer patients are affected with a frequency 2–3 times that of the general population, suggesting a genetic predisposition in some individuals. A positive association with blood group O and ABO(H) non-secretor status is also in keeping with this, although the nature of the genetic association is not known.

Chronic peptic ulcers can be separated into two major groups using clinical, epidemiological, and pathological criteria. The first group consists of ulcers in the first part of the duodenum and the most distal (prepyloric) part of the antrum. These occur much more commonly in males than females, in the younger age-groups (usually under 50 years) and in individuals in the higher socio-economic classes. Multiple ulcers are found in some 10–15 per cent of these cases (Fig. 16.39). The second group includes ulcers in the more proximal part of the stomach, classically situated on the lesser curve at the junction between the pyloric antrum and the body (Fig. 16.40), but occasionally on the anterior or posterior walls and rarely on the greater

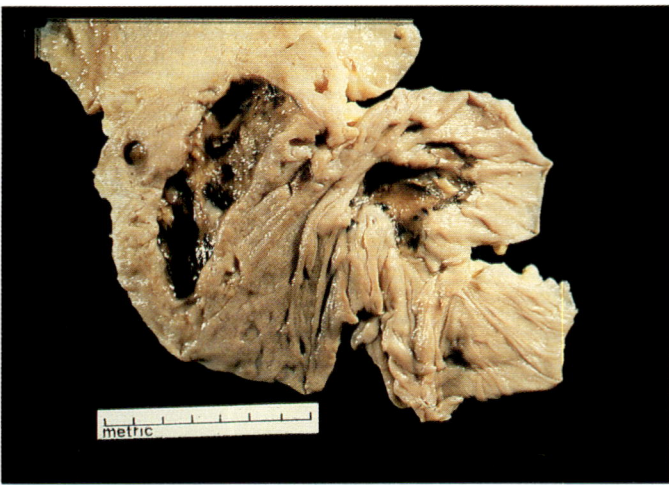

Fig. 16.39 Multiple chronic duodenal ulcers in the first part of the duodenum have a characteristic deep, punched-out appearance. There is a blood clot in the floor of the larger ulcer.

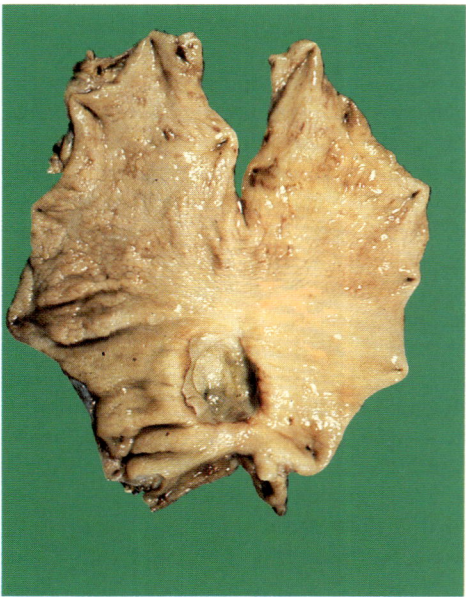

Fig. 16.40 Partial gastrectomy specimen opened along the greater curvature to demonstrate a 3 cm gastric ulcer in the antrum on the lesser curve. The floor of the ulcer is covered by pale slough and its margins are smooth and well demarcated.

curvature. These are usually solitary, occur with equal frequency in men and women, and are commonest in older individuals of lower socio-economic status. In a few patients the pattern of ulceration overlaps between the two main groups, with duodenal and proximal gastric ulceration either occurring synchronously or metachronously.

Morphological features

The macroscopic appearances of chronic peptic ulcers are similar irrespective of their anatomical sites. They are usually well

demarcated, round or oval, punched-out ulcers with distinct edges that are neither raised nor rolled, and have a firm grey-white floor that is covered by slough, or sometimes by blood clot (Figs 16.39, 16.40). The majority measure less than 2 cm in diameter, although some gastric ulcers, and a minority of duodenal ulcers, may be huge, reaching 10 cm or more. The ulcer base is indurated due to fibrosis that usually replaces the full thickness of the muscular coat and extends into the extramural fat causing an opaque puckering of the serosal surface which may be adherent to adjacent structures. The mucosa around the ulcer is often flat and atrophic, although sometimes fibrosis in the base of the ulcer results in prominent radiating mucosal folds which extend almost to the very edge of the ulcer. The regional lymph nodes often show moderate fleshy enlargement.

Histological examination of chronic peptic ulcers characteristically reveals four layers (Figs 16.41–16.43). The floor of the ulcer is covered by an *exudative zone* composed of fibrin, traces of tissue debris, and variable numbers of neutrophil polymorphs. Deep to this is the thin *necrotic zone* made up of amorphous eosinophilic necrotic tissue containing degenerate nuclei of inflammatory cells. Next is a thicker *granulation tissue zone* composed of neutrophil polymorphs, mononuclear cells, proliferating capillaries, and fibroblasts, and finally a *zone of cicatrization* composed of fibrous tissue which extends into or through the muscularis propria. Arteries within this fibrous tissue usually show a marked obliterative endarteritis (Fig. 16.43), and sometimes there is superimposed thrombosis. Another characteristic feature of benign peptic ulceration is fusion of the muscularis mucosae and the muscularis propria around the margin of the ulcer.

The mucosa around peptic ulcers regularly shows histological features of active chronic gastritis or duodenitis, and in the majority of such cases this is associated with the presence of *H. pylori*. Regenerative epithelial hyperplasia is usually marked at the very edge of the ulcer; it is often accompanied by apparent atypia of the immature epithelial cells and sometimes this can

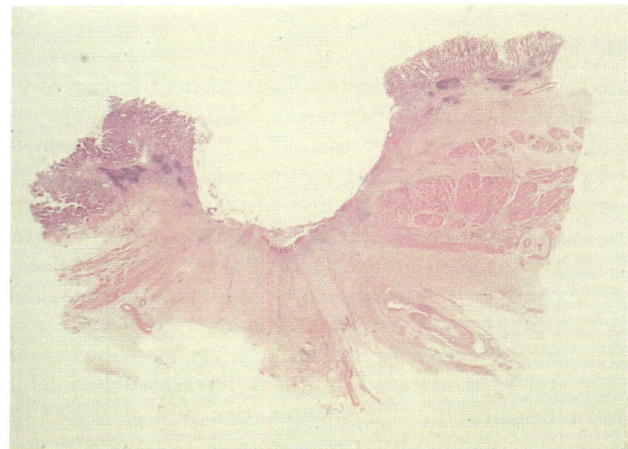

Fig. 16.41 Histological section through a peptic gastric ulcer showing complete destruction of the gastric wall and fibrous replacement of the muscular coat.

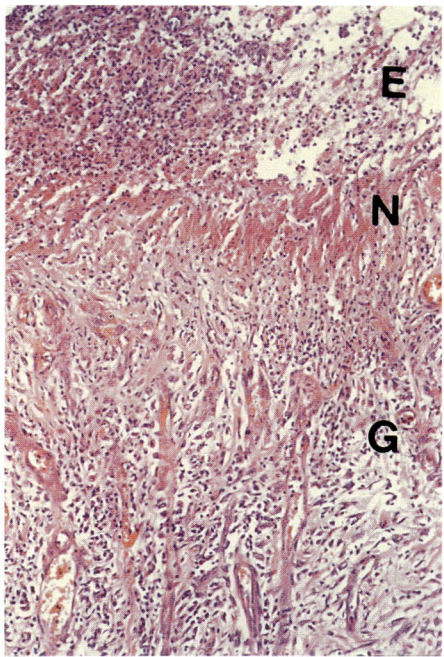

Fig. 16.42 The floor of a peptic ulcer is covered by a fibrinopurulent exudate (E), deep to which is a nectrotic zone (N) and a zone of inflammatory granulation tissue (G).

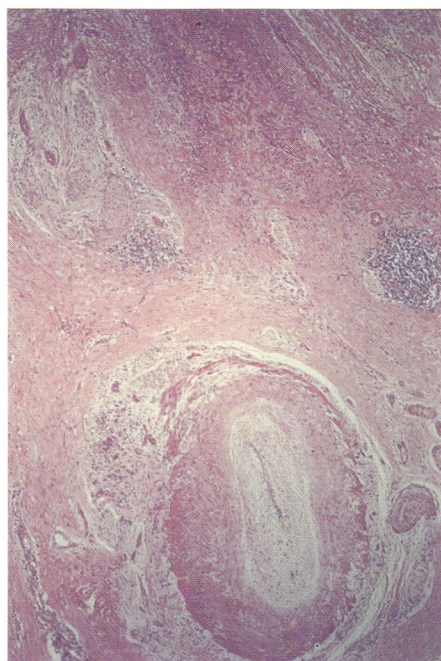

Fig. 16.43 An artery in the fibrotic zone at the base of a peptic ulcer shows marked luminal narrowing by endarteritis obliterans.

be sufficiently marked to mimic a neoplastic change. When healing of the ulcer begins, the regenerating epithelium migrates over the ulcer floor so that it is eventually covered by a single cell layer of rather undifferentiated columnar cells. With time these are replaced by more mature gastric-type mucous cells or intestinal-type goblet and absorptive cells and eventually there is differentiation to an incompletely developed, and rather thin atrophic glandular architecture. However, specialized epithelial cells such as parietal and chief cells virtually never return and the muscularis mucosae does not regenerate. Metaplasia is common, both intestinal metaplasia at the site of healed gastric ulcers and gastric metaplasia in healed duodenal ulcers. Epithelial regeneration is accompanied by organization and fibrous scarring in the deeper zones of the ulcer, but again the smooth muscle of the muscularis propria is irretrievably lost. It is possible, therefore, to recognize a healed ulcer by the submucosal and intramural fibrosis that replaces the muscle coats and the overlying atrophic mucosa. Grossly, this corresponds to a small mucosal depression covered by a thinned, translucent mucosa that overlies a pale, firm stellate scar (Fig. 16.44).

Complications

The natural history of chronic peptic ulcer disease is one of recurring cycles of relapse and remission. A number of studies have indicated that, even without specific medical therapy, over 40 per cent of peptic ulcers heal spontaneously over a period of 6 weeks, although nearly two-thirds of these will recur over the following 12 months. Although many peptic ulcers produce symptoms of dyspepsia, endoscopic studies have shown that a significant number are completely asymptomatic, so that the first clinical manifestation of an ulcer is with one of its potentially life-threatening complications.

The commonest complication of chronic peptic ulceration is *haemorrhage*. This can vary from relatively minor oozing from the floor of the ulcer, leading to chronic iron-deficiency

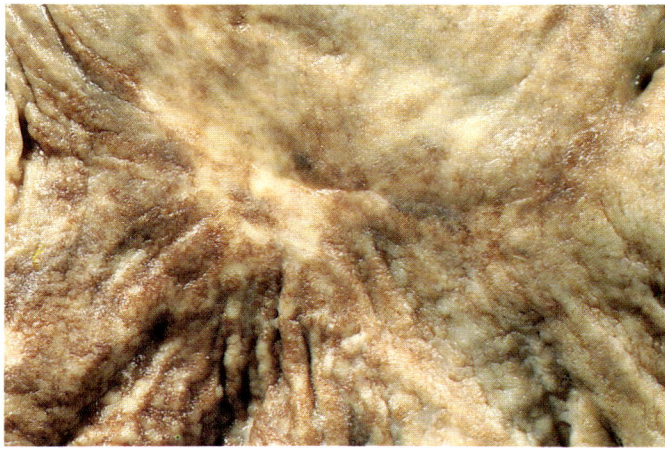

Fig. 16.44 Macroscopic appearances of a healed gastric ulcer, showing a pale stellate submucosal scar covered by thin, atrophic mucosa whose folds radiate from the central depressed area.

anaemia, to massive arterial bleeding from an eroded vessel presenting with haematemesis and melaena and leading rapidly to hypovolaemic shock. Such severe haemorrhage is particularly dangerous in the elderly, in whom bleeding peptic ulcers are an important cause of mortality. Although duodenal ulcers bleed more commonly than gastric ulcers, mortality from bleeding is greater in gastric ulcers because of their higher frequency in the elderly, whose circulation is less able to compensate effectively for a sudden fall in circulating blood volume. Endoscopy or macroscopic examination of resection or post-mortem specimens from such patients often reveals the affected artery in the floor of the ulcer, with a recent thrombus covering the eroded focus in its wall (Fig. 16.45).

The second acute life-threatening complication of chronic peptic ulcer is *perforation*, which leads to gastric or duodenal contents leaking into the peritoneal cavity, initiating an acute diffuse peritonitis. This complication is also commoner with duodenal and prepyloric ulcers, especially those on the anterior wall. Macroscopic examination usually reveals a small, neat round hole surrounded by a hyperaemic serosa that may be covered by a fibrinous exudate (Fig. 16.46). Although most perforated peptic ulcers produce dramatic acute abdominal symptoms and shock, this is not inevitable and 'silent' perforations are well recognized, especially in the elderly. Sometimes the perforation site is walled off by adherent omentum, so that the ensuing peritonitis is localized. Although the initial peritonitis following perforation of a peptic ulcer is a 'chemical' one caused by gastric acid, enzymes, bile, pancreatic juice, and partly digested food, there is usually concurrent bacterial contamination which can aggravate the inflammatory process, and progress to the development of intra-abdominal abscesses over the ensuing days or weeks.

A closely related complication to perforation is *penetration* of a peptic ulcer. Here there is also erosion of an ulcer through the wall of the stomach or duodenum but on this occasion it involves an adjacent viscus rather than the peritoneal serosa. The commonest example is posterior penetration of a chronic

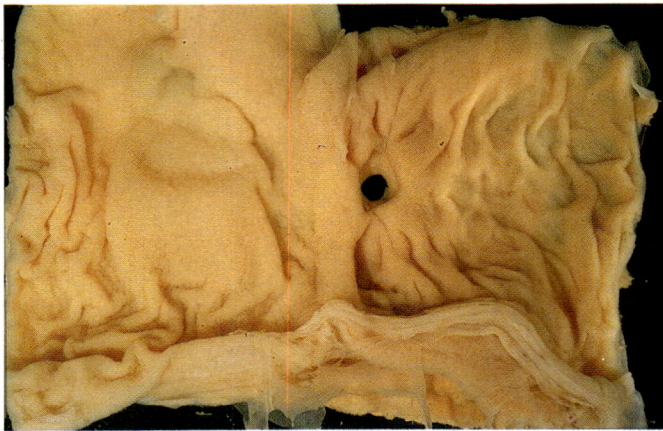

Fig. 16.46 A small perforated peptic ulcer situated on the anterior wall of the duodenum, immediately distal to the pyloric valve.

ulcer into the pancreas (Fig. 16.47) to produce a localized low-grade pancreatitis, but occasionally the splenic artery may be involved, resulting in acute haemorrhage. On other occasions a localized serositis over an active ulcer may cause the stomach or duodenum to adhere to the transverse colon; further extension of the ulcer may then lead to a gastrocolic or duodenocolic fistula.

Fibrosis, oedema, and muscular spasm occurring in association with chronic peptic ulceration is responsible for the fourth major complication, namely *stenosis* of the lumen of the stomach or duodenum. Although frequently occurring during the course of active ulceration, it may not present clinically until after the healing of an ulcer, when contraction of newly laid collagen bundles leads to cicatrization. It is not surprising that the commonest site to be affected is the distal stomach at the pylorus, when pyloric stenosis leads to intractable vomiting and electrolyte disturbances. Less common is duodenal stenosis or

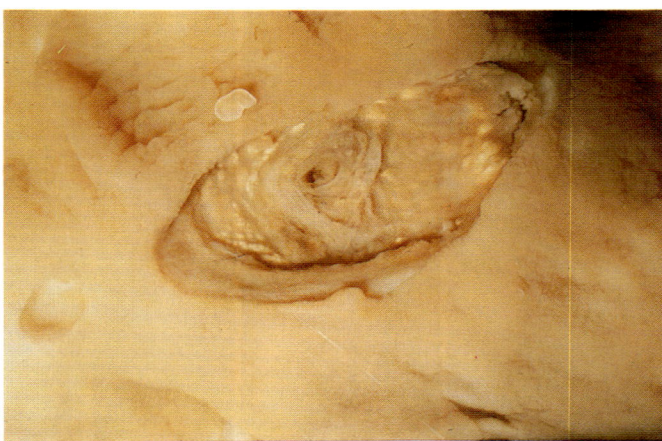

Fig. 16.45 An eroded artery, the defect in its wall covered with blood clot, is seen at the base of a chronic gastric ulcer. The specimen was obtained at autopsy from a patient who died of massive haemorrhage.

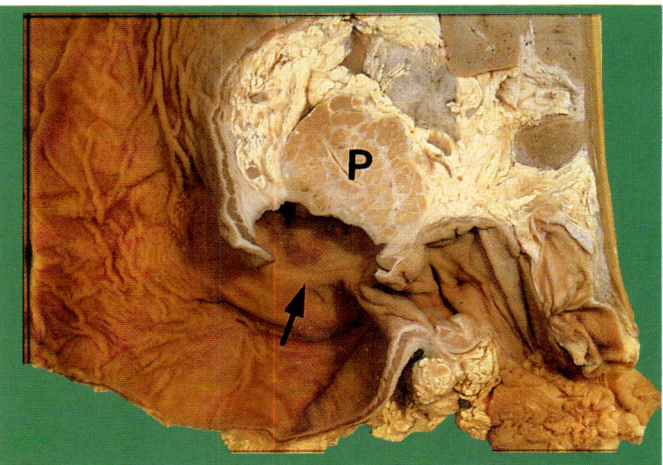

Fig. 16.47 A large posterior antral peptic ulcer has penetrated through the wall of the stomach to erode the anterior surface of the body of the pancreas (P).

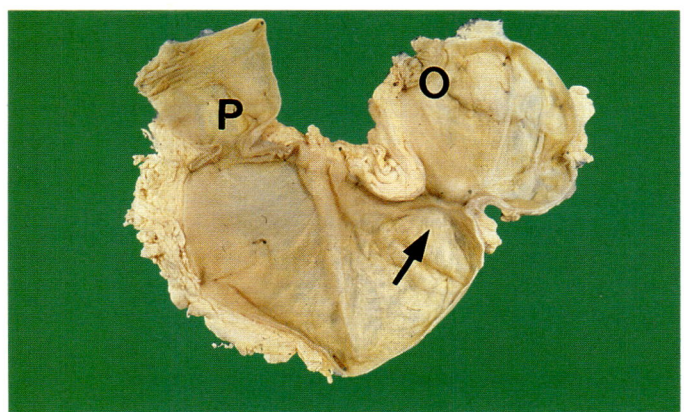

Fig. 16.48 An hour-glass stomach, caused by circumferential fibrosis of the wall of the body of the stomach at the site of a healed peptic ulcer (arrow). The gastro-oesophageal junction (O) and the pyloric valve (P) are marked.

concentric fibrosis in the stomach related to an ulcer in its middle portion, leading to a deformity known as the hour-glass stomach (Fig. 16.48).

The final complication of chronic peptic ulceration is the development of *carcinoma*, although this has been a rather controversial issue. While there is no evidence to suggest that malignancy may be a complication of chronic duodenal ulceration, there can now be little doubt that carcinoma may arise at the margin of a proportion of long-standing gastric ulcers. It is the frequency with which this complication occurs that is controversial. Earlier estimates suggesting that 30 per cent or more of gastric ulcers became malignant are now regarded as a gross over-exaggeration of the risk, because they failed to distinguish carcinomas which had undergone secondary ulceration from cancers arising in pre-existing ulcers (true ulcer-cancers). Furthermore it is likely that in some studies the florid regenerative epithelial hyperplasia that quite commonly occurs at the margin of a benign peptic ulcer was misdiagnosed as carcinoma. If careful histological criteria are used to define both invasive malignancy and the presence of a pre-existing peptic ulcer, the prevalence of carcinoma in ulcers is 1 per cent or less. In one study of 201 patients followed up for a mean of 5.7 years three gastric carcinomas were identified, only one of which was at the site of the original ulcer (Montgomery and Richardson 1975). Nevertheless, it is very important that the possibility of carcinoma is excluded in every patient with a gastric ulcer by multiple endoscopic biopsies and brush cytology, since the clinical management of gastric carcinoma is surgical while that of peptic ulcer is essentially medical. A considerable proportion of ulcer-cancers are tumours confined to the mucosa or submucosa and have an excellent chance of cure by surgery (see Section 16.3.2).

Aetiology

Despite extensive clinical and experimental research into peptic ulcer disease over many years, the aetiology and pathogenesis of the condition remain poorly understood. Disturbances in the balance between factors that damage the gastroduodenal mucosa, mainly acid and pepsin, and the integrity of local defence mechanisms, mainly the mucus–bicarbonate barrier and the surface epithelial cells, obviously underlie the ulceration process, but the relative importance of the different factors varies greatly both between and within the different types of peptic ulcer disease. Historically the factor that has received the greatest attention is excess gastric acid secretion, and the therapeutic success of acid-lowering drugs in all forms of peptic ulcer disease indicates that this factor is certainly of great importance. Nevertheless, the facts that gastric acid hypersecretion can be demonstrated in normal individuals without a history or endoscopic evidence of ulceration, and that some peptic ulcers occur in a background of hypochlorhydria, indicate that other mechanisms are also involved. Chronic ingestion of mucosal irritants is probably important in some individuals, but apart from the association between bleeding from peptic ulcers and the consumption of non-steroidal anti-inflammatory drugs, there is no proof of this and studies of dietary habits in peptic ulcer patients have been largely unrewarding. There is evidence that cigarette smoking has a detrimental effect on the healing of peptic ulcers, but a direct role in the primary disease process is unproven. Similarly, a possible link with stressful occupations has not been confirmed statistically. Peptic ulcers, especially duodenal ulcers, are commoner in patients with chronic lung disease, renal failure, and pancreatic insufficiency, but the reasons for these associations are unknown. Generally speaking, the available evidence suggests that gastric acid hypersecretion probably plays a major part in the type of peptic ulcer disease that is characterized by duodenal and prepyloric ulcers, while other factors leading to a failure in mucosal defence mechanisms are of greater significance in gastric ulcers. The recognition of a strong association between chronic peptic ulcer disease and *Helicobacter*-associated chronic gastritis has led to speculation of a central role for *H. pylori* in peptic ulceration, and this is discussed below.

Duodenal and prepyloric ulcers There is good evidence that gastric acid hypersecretion is important in chronic duodenal ulcer. Intubation studies have shown that up to 40 per cent of duodenal ulcer patients secrete excessive amounts of acid, not only in response to a meal but also in 'basal' conditions such as between meals and at night. Post-mortem studies have shown that there is an increase in the number of parietal cells within the stomach, while physiological studies have revealed these parietal cells to show an increased responsiveness to various secretagogues, including gastrin. In some duodenal ulcer patients there is also an exaggerated release of gastrin from the pyloric antrum following a protein meal, and a small minority, in whom there are multiple ulcers involving the whole of the duodenum and extending into the jejunum, have marked hyperacidity due to persistent hypergastrinaemia arising from either hyperplasia of antral G-cells or a gastrin-secreting tumour of the pancreas or duodenum (the Zollinger–Ellison syndrome, see Chapter 26). Recently, it has been demonstrated that about one-third of patients with duodenal ulcer disease have circulating auto-antibodies which stimulate the production of cyclic-AMP in parietal cells, in a manner similar to thyroid-stimulating antibodies in Graves' disease (see Chapter 26). It is possible that such receptor-stimulating antibodies play a role in inducing hyperacidity in some patients with duodenal ulcers.

The fact that more than 50 per cent of duodenal ulcer patients do not have demonstrable acid hypersecretion suggests that other mechanisms are also of importance in the aetiology. Some studies have suggested a role for other potentially damaging luminal agents, such as increased pepsin secretion by the stomach, others have postulated a causative role for the unusually rapid gastric emptying or the defective mixing of duodenal contents that can be demonstrated in some duodenal ulcer patients, and more recently attention has been drawn to an apparent failure of duodenal mucosal defence mechanisms, with defective secretion of bicarbonate by the duodenal mucosa. This latter finding may be related to the fact that chronic duodenal ulceration almost invariably occurs in a background of active non-specific chronic duodenitis associated with gastric metaplasia and colonization by *H. pylori* (see above). One current theory for the pathogenesis of duodenal ulcers suggests that duodenal hyperacidity first leads to chronic duodenitis and gastric metaplasia. Colonization of this gastric epithelium by *H. pylori* then sets up active inflammation with destruction of epithelial cells, and the ensuing failure of mucosal protection, allowing back-diffusion of acid and other luminal agents, leads first to duodenal erosions and then to overt duodenal ulceration. Very recently an even more crucial role of *H. pylori* has been suggested, which attributes the initial duodenal hyperacidity to gastric *Helicobacter* colonization—it is proposed that the powerful urease activity of this organism splits intragastric urea to produce ammonia at the cell surface, raising the pH of the gastric mucus layer and stimulating hypergastrinaemia, and thereby increased acid production. Preliminary reports of a dramatic reduction in duodenal ulcer relapses following eradication of *H. pylori* by antimicrobial therapy supports the view that the organism plays a very important role in the pathogenesis of the disease.

Gastric ulcers Most gastric ulcers occur on the lesser curve, in the vicinity of the junction between the antrum and the body of the stomach, and are accompanied by normal or low levels of gastric acid secretion, suggesting that factors decreasing mucosal protection are of primary importance in their pathogenesis. Nevertheless, hyperacidity is present in a few cases, and classically in gastric ulcers occurring in the Zollinger–Ellison syndrome. Gastric ulcers almost invariably arise in a background of active chronic gastritis, usually in association with *H. pylori*, and it is likely that this gastritis plays an important role in reducing mucosal resistance to the damaging actions of luminal acid and enzymes. On the other hand, the fact that *H. pylori*-associated gastritis is far commoner than gastric ulcer in the population indicates that additional factors are involved. Reflux of duodenal contents containing potentially irritant bile acids

and lysolecithin into the stomach has received the greatest attention, but its significance is controversial. Measurements of intragastric bile salt concentrations have shown higher levels in gastric ulcer patients than controls, but scintigraphic studies show that duodenogastric reflux also occurs in normal subjects, often to the same extent as in those with gastric ulcer. Even when reflux occurs in gastric ulcer it could be a consequence of motor dysfunction due to muscle damage by the ulceration process rather than a primary event. Nevertheless, even if duodenogastric reflux is not an underlying cause of gastric ulcer, it may well be of importance in aggravating the lesion and in preventing healing.

Chronic gastritis, either in association with *H. pylori* or duodenal reflux, involves the entire antrum, albeit patchily, while gastric ulcers are nearly always localized to the lesser curve. This suggests that factors specific to the lesser curve mucosa are also important in the pathogenesis of gastric ulcer. Two mechanisms have been postulated. Proponents of the importance of duodenogastric reflux in gastric ulcer have suggested that the jet of refluxing material is directed specifically at the mucosa of the proximal antrum on the lesser curve, at the precise site where gastric ulcer is commonest. Others have invoked regional mucosal ischaemia as an important predisposing factor, quoting anatomical studies showing that the blood supply to the lesser curve is by end arteries which arise directly from the left gastric artery, and is consequently more precarious than that of the remaining gastric mucosa which derives from a diffuse submucosal plexus.

16.2.6 Further reading

Dixon, M. F., O'Connor, H. J., Axon, A. T. R., King, R. F. J. G., and Johnston, D. (1986). Reflux gastritis: distinct histopathological entity? *Journal of Clinical Pathology* **39**, 524–30.

Goodwin, C. S., Armstrong, J. A., and Marshall, B. J. (1986). *Campylobacter pyloridis*, gastritis, and peptic ulceration. *Journal of Clinical Pathology* **39**, 353–65.

Haot, J., *et al.* (1986). Anatomo-clinical study of a series of chronic gastritis characterized by intraepithelial lymphocytic infiltration. *Acta Endoscopica* **16**, 69–74.

Imai, T., Kubo, T., and Watanabe, H. (1971). Chronic gastritis in Japanese with reference to high incidence of gastric carcinoma. *Journal of the National Cancer Institute* **47**, 179–95.

Kaye, M. D. (1987). Immunological aspects of gastritis and pernicious anaemia. *Clinics in Gastroenterology* **1**, 487–506.

Lam, S.-K. (1984). Pathogenesis and pathophysiology of duodenal ulcer. *Clinics in Gastroenterology* **13**, 447–72.

Montgomery, R. D. and Richardson, B. P. (1975). Gastric ulcer and cancer. *Quarterly Journal of Medicine, New Series* **45**, 591–9.

Peterson, W., Lee, E., and Skoglund, M. (1987). The role of *Campylobacter pyloridis* in epidemic gastritis with hypochlorhydria. *Gastroenterology* **92**, 1575.

Rees, W. D. and Turnberg, L. A. (1982). Mechanisms of gastric mucosal protection. A role for the mucus–bicarbonate barrier. *Clinical Science* **62**, 343–8.

Villako, K., Kekki, M., Tamm, A., and Savisaar, E. (1986). Development and progression of chronic gastritis in the antrum and body mucosa: results of long term follow-up examinations. *Annals of Clinical Research* **18**, 121–3.

Warren, J. R. and Marshall, B. (1983). Unidentified curved bacilli on gastric epithelium in active chronic gastritis. *Lancet* **i**, 1273–5.

Wyatt, J. I. and Dixon, M. F. (1988). Chronic gastritis—a pathogenetic approach. *Journal of Pathology* **154**, 113–24.

Wyatt, J. I., Rathbone, B. J., Dixon, M. F., and Heatley, R. V. (1987). *Campylobacter pyloridis* and acid-indiced metaplasia in the pathogenesis of duodenitis. *Journal of Clinical Pathology* **40**, 841–8.

16.3   Tumours of the stomach

J. R. Jass

16.3.1   Benign epithelial polyps

Any abnormal mass of tissue projecting into the lumen of the stomach may be described as a polyp; the term provides no insight into the underlying nature of the lesion. Cancers can be polypoid, but it is customary to consider polypoid carcinoma separately. Certain ill-understood forms of chronic gastritis (e.g. chronic lymphocytic gastritis) may present as multiple polyps or thickened gastric folds. Endocrine cell tumours (Section 16.17), lymphoid tumours (Chapter 24), neurogenic tumours (Section 16.16.3, smooth muscle tumours (Section 16.16.3), lipomas (Section 16.16.3), and inflammatory fibroid polyps (p. 1249) should also be considered in the differential diagnosis of polypoid lesions of the stomach. Gastric polyps are described in only 0.4 per cent of autopsies, but many are small and may be lost through autolysis. Higher figures of around 5 per cent are reported in endoscopic series. A classification of epithelial polyps is given in Table 16.1 and these are illustrated schematically in Fig. 16.49.

Hyperplastic polyps

Although traditionally regarded as the commonest type of gastric polyp, it is likely that the recently recognized fundic gland cyst polyps are very much more common, particularly in endoscopic practice. Hyperplastic polyps are rounded or lobulated and usually less than 1.5 cm in diameter. Smaller examples are sessile, but large polyps may become pedunculated. They can be single or multiple and may occur anywhere in the stomach. The

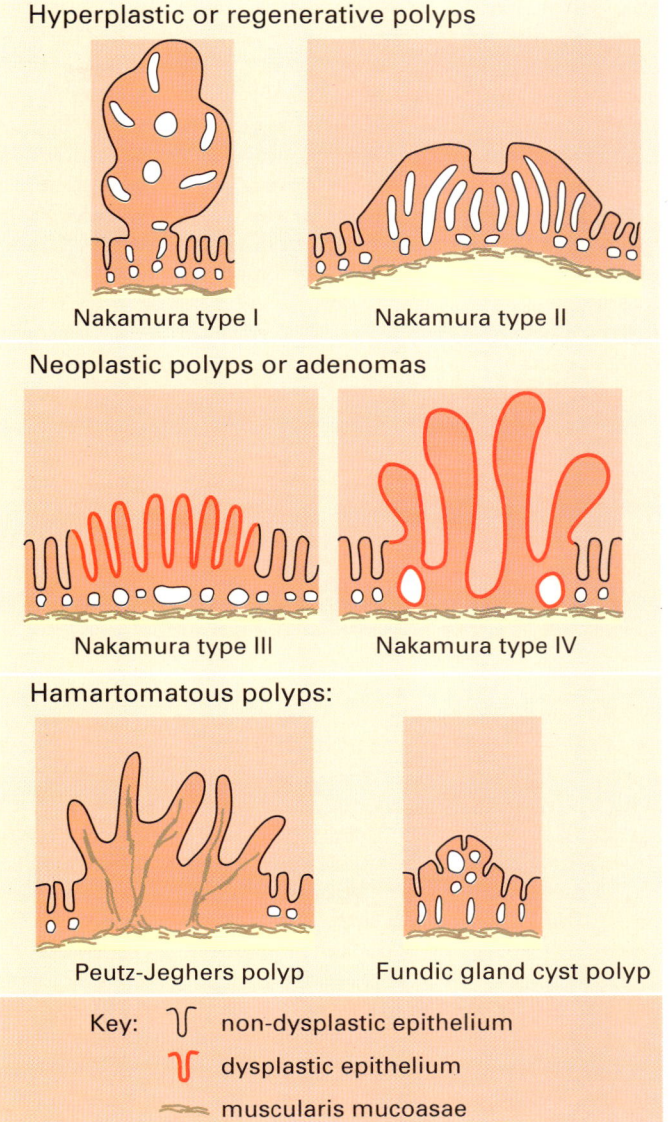

Hyperplastic or regenerative polyps

Nakamura type I   Nakamura type II

Neoplastic polyps or adenomas

Nakamura type III   Nakamura type IV

Hamartomatous polyps:

Peutz-Jeghers polyp   Fundic gland cyst polyp

Key: ⋔   non-dysplastic epithelium

⋔   dysplastic epithelium

〜   muscularis mucoasae

Fig. 16.49   The main types of gastric polyps.

majority occur in the antrum or intermediate zone—the sites of predilection for chronic gastritis. Multiple polyps may congregate in the intermediate zone between antrum and body.

The polyps are formed of elongated, branched, or cystic crypts, and groups of pyloric-type glands. Intestinal metaplasia is an infrequent and focal occurrence. The lamina propria is often oedematous and infiltrated by inflammatory cells. Plasma cells containing Russell bodies may be conspicuous. Bundles of smooth muscle may be prominent, especially in larger prolapsing polyps. The surface may show shallow erosions and it is important to distinguish inflammatory or regenerative epithelial changes (which are very common) from neoplasia (which is a rare complication).

The mucosa adjacent to hyperplastic polyps shows the

Table 16.1   Benign epithelial polyps of stomach

Underlying disorder	Type
Regeneration	Hyperplastic (Nakamura types I & II)
Neoplasia	Sessile tubular adenoma (syn: borderline lesion, type III polyp of Nakamura)
	Adenoma (syn: type IV polyp of Nakamura)
Hamartoma	Peutz–Jeghers polyp
	Juvenile polyp
	Fundic gland cyst polyp
Heterotopia	Ectopic pancreatic tissue

changes of chronic gastritis and in so doing mimics the histology of the polyp, though to a milder degree. This fact, together with the frequent occurrence of polyps at the site of gastric ulceration, erosions, or within gastroenterostomy stomas, suggests that the hyperplastic polyp arises through excessive regeneration following mucosal injury. Additional changes may be secondary to low-grade ischaemia, particularly in the larger prolapsing polyps. An unusual type of hyperplastic polyp (type II) has been reported from Japan. These polyps are often multiple and are characterized macroscopically by a central dimple and histologically by an onion skin arrangement of the hyperplastic crypts (Fig. 16.49). These probably represent an exaggerated form of epithelial regeneration following mucosal erosion.

Neoplastic polyps

Benign neoplastic polyps or adenomas are uncommon, particularly in low-risk areas for gastric cancer. Two types of adenoma are described which differ in their macroscopic and microscopic appearance as well as in their malignant potential.

Sessile tubular adenoma

This has been referred to as a borderline lesion in the Japanese literature and more recently as a type III polyp. It is the commonest variety of gastric adenoma but has no exact counterpart outside the stomach. The lesions are sessile, broad-based, and only slightly elevated. The surface is smooth or slightly papillary and may be lobular. They are either the same colour or darker than the surrounding mucosa. Most adenomas are single and the antrum is the site of predilection. Histologically they are composed of an upper compartment of dysplastic crypts and a lower compartment of normal or cystic pyloric glands. The dysplastic crypts are usually straight and unbranched and are lined by crowded, darkly staining cells with elongated, pseudostratified nuclei and small amounts of apical mucin (Fig. 16.50). The latter often stains brown with the high iron diamine/alcian blue technique, indicating the secretion of sulphated acid mucin. The surrounding mucosa usually shows extensive intestinal metaplasia of the incomplete variety (see p. 1155). The junction between adenoma and adjacent epithelium is sharply defined.

It is generally accepted that gastric adenomas have a significant potential for malignant change. However, recent evidence from Japan indicates that the malignant potential of sessile tubular adenomas, as described in this section, is very low.

Tubulovillous and villous adenomas

These rarely encountered neoplasms have been classified as type IV polyps. They are usually several centimetres in diameter with an irregular, shaggy surface. Unlike the sessile tubular adenoma described above, the entire polyp is composed of dysplastic epithelium (Fig. 16.49). The dysplasia is often severe and

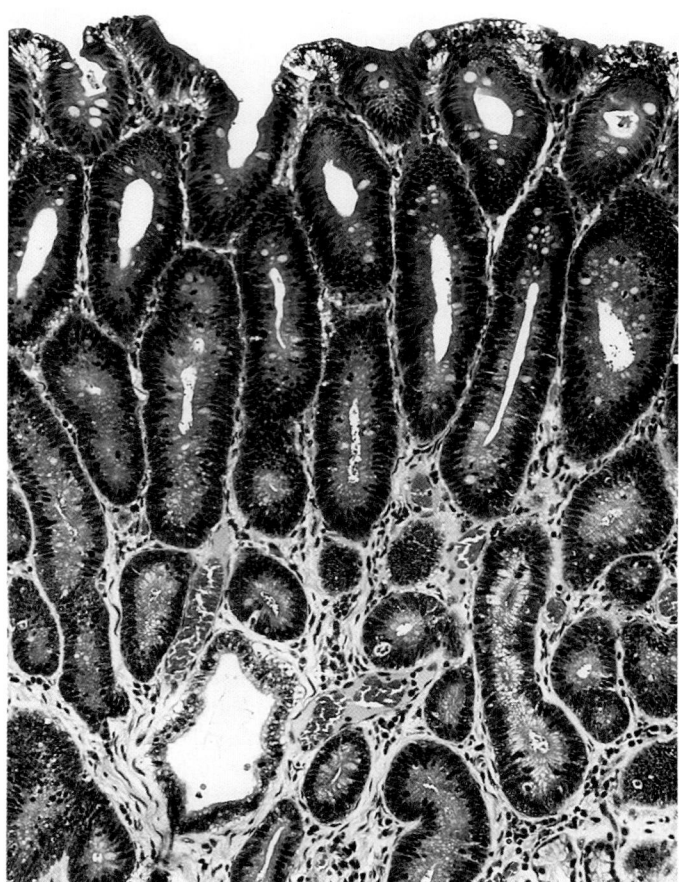

Fig. 16.50 Dysplastic crypts forming the upper part of a sessile adenoma.

the distinction from intramucosal carcinoma may not be straightforward. The potential for malignant change is high. These polyps may harbour an early carcinoma at the time of their discovery or adjoin an advanced gastric cancer. The surrounding mucosa may show complete or incomplete metaplasia but may also be gastric in type.

Hamartomatous polyps

Peutz–Jeghers polyp

Multiple hamartomas of the stomach and small bowel and circumoral pigmentation together constitute the Peutz–Jeghers syndrome, which is inherited as an autosomal dominant condition. The small intestinal polyps are of greater clinical significance because of their tendency to cause intussusception. There is an increased tendency to both gastric and small intestinal adenocarcinoma. Isolated gastric Peutz–Jeghers type polyps may occur in the absence of the syndrome. Peutz–Jeghers polyps are sessile and papillary. Histologically they reveal a characteristic tree-like branching of smooth muscle within the supporting stroma.

Juvenile polyps

These may occur in association with gastrointestinal juvenile polyposis, which may be either sporadic or inherited on an autosomal dominant basis. The polyps are rounded and may become pedunculated. Histologically they resemble their colorectal counterparts, showing cystic crypts and glands embedded in an oedematous lamina propria. The distinction from hyperplastic (regenerative) polyps may be difficult or impossible and the clinical background should be heeded when forming the final diagnosis.

Fundic gland cyst polyps

These have been described comparatively recently, but are probably the commonest type of epithelial gastric polyp. Their precise nature is not understood, but most authors group them with hamartomatous lesions. They appear on endoscopy as small, sessile, transparent polyps that are confined to the body of the stomach. They number from 10 to 30. Most patients have been middle-aged women, but they are probably found with increased frequency in patients with familial adenomatous polyposis. Histological examination reveals small cysts lined by mucus-secreting cells, parietal cells, and chief cells. The lesion appears to be without any clinical significance.

Heterotopic pancreas

Ectopic pancreas admixed with smooth muscle may present as a prepyloric polyp. Larger lesions may be associated with gastric outlet-obstruction ulceration or bleeding.

16.3.2 Gastric carcinoma

Although the incidence of gastric carcinoma is falling, it is still one of the major causes of cancer death world-wide. In England and Wales it is responsible for 11 000 deaths per year, making it the third commonest cause of death due to malignancy after cancer of the lung and colorectum. The five-year survival for patients with gastric cancer is around 5 per cent but screening programmes will hopefully lead to a reduction in mortality. In Japan screening is directed to the detection of early gastric cancer, which is usually curable. An alternative approach is to subject patients with precancerous conditions and lesions to careful follow-up surveillance.

Epidemiology

There are complex interrelationships between age, sex, site, geography, and pathological type of tumour, and it is therefore misleading to consider any of these variables in isolation. The incidence of gastric cancer increases progressively with age, most patients being between the ages of 50 and 70 years at the time of presentation. Gastric cancer can occur in young individuals when, regrettably, it is often a poorly differentiated and highly aggressive tumour. Gastric cancer is more common in males than females, but the male:female ratio increases with age, being 1:1 in young patients and at least 2:1 in the 60–70 age-group.

The incidence of gastric carcinoma shows considerable variation from country to country. High-incidence countries include Japan, China, Russia, Finland, Iceland, and Colombia. The lowest incidence is recorded in sub-Saharan Africa. There are also variations within countries, with populations inhabiting rural or mountainous regions being at greatest risk. Although the incidence of gastric cancer is falling progressively, the rate of this fall varies from one country to another. The decline has been most obvious in the USA, and is now beginning to be seen in Japan. It is unclear whether the improvement in Japan is due to the nationwide screening programme or the adoption of a Western-style diet by the more affluent Japanese.

The effect of the environment on the incidence of gastric cancer has been illustrated by studying migrant populations. The incidence of gastric cancer in Japanese who have moved to Hawaii has not shown an appreciable fall in the first generation but has done so in succeeding generations. This would suggest that populations are primed by exposure to environmental carcinogens in childhood or early adulthood.

There are interesting relationships between epidemiological variables and pathological types of gastric carcinoma. Laurén divided gastric carcinoma into 'intestinal' and 'diffuse' types (see p. 1170). Although the incidence of the intestinal type varies in high- and low-risk countries, the diffuse type is stable or less affected by environment. For example, the lowered incidence of gastric carcinoma found in the second-generation Japanese inhabiting Hawaii only implicates the intestinal type. Furthermore, the diffuse type affects the sexes equally and occurs in younger individuals. It is possible that genetic factors may play an important role in the aetiology of diffuse-type carcinomas.

Aetiology and pathogenesis

The epidemiological studies described above implicate environmental factors in the aetiology of gastric cancer, particularly the 'intestinal' type. Dietary practices are likely to be of crucial importance. The Japanese diet is characterized by a high intake of carbohydrate, pickled vegetables and dried, salted fish, and an absence of meat and fresh fruit and vegetables. In Finland high levels of polycyclic hydrocarbons have been found in smoked meat and fish. However, no single factor, common to all high-risk areas, has yet been identified. It is likely that a complex interplay of dietary factors is involved that would implicate not only the presence of promoting or initiating agents but also the absence of protective factors such as vitamins and trace elements.

Gastric cancer usually arises within a background of chronic gastritis, and the aetiology of the latter is clearly relevant to the present discussion. However, the precise aetiology of chronic gastritis remains as mysterious as that of gastric cancer itself. It is likely that the final mediators of gastric damage are hydrochloric acid and pepsin. Autodigestion is normally prevented by three mechanisms: the rapid regeneration of crypt and surface epithelium, the mucus–bicarbonate barrier, and the anti-inflammatory action of endogenous prostaglandins. In chronic gastritis these defences are presumably repeatedly compromised through the ingestion of cytotoxic dietary contaminants and possibly by superimposed infection with *Helicobacter pylori.* Cycles of injury and regeneration ensue, eventually producing the histological picture of chronic atrophic gastritis. Acid secretion is reduced in the atrophic stomach and the bacterial content of stomach is consequently increased. Bacteria are able to convert nitrates to nitrites, and nitrites may in turn be converted into carcinogenic N-nitrosamines. Epidemiological studies have correlated the incidence of gastric carcinoma with the level of nitrate in the water supply. The above hypotheses on the progression of chronic gastritis to cancer remain speculative, but it seems clear that the evolution of gastric cancer is a stepwise process that develops over many years, or even decades, and depends on the interplay of a variety of aetiological agents.

Genetic factors are also of some importance. Blood group A occurs with increased frequency in patients with gastric cancer. Pernicious anaemia is a precancerous condition and is known to be hereditary.

Precancerous conditions and lesions

A precancerous condition is a clinical state associated with an increased risk of cancer. A precancerous lesion is a histopathological abnormality in which cancer is more likely to occur than it its normal counterpart. In the stomach precancerous conditions include pernicious anaemia, chronic atrophic gastritis, previous gastric surgery, and possibly Ménétrier's disease. These conditions may or may not be accompanied by an identifiable precancerous lesion. The distinction between a condition and a lesion becomes somewhat blurred for chronic atrophic gastritis, which is an ill-understood clinicopathological entity. Within this entity, intestinal metaplasia (IM) is the lesion which appears to predispose to the development of gastric cancer. However, IM occurs too frequently to be clinically useful as a marker of precancer. On the other hand, epithelial dysplasia shows a very much more selective association with gastric cancer and is therefore regarded as a more important precancerous lesion.

Intestinal metaplasia (IM)

This may be defined as the replacement during adult life of gastric-type mucosa by a mucosa that is similar, if not identical, to that of normal small intestine (Fig. 16.51). The change develops in the context of advanced chronic atrophic gastritis and occurs with greater frequency in high-risk populations for gastric cancer. Extensive IM is seen in the mucosa adjacent to gastric carcinoma, notably the 'intestinal' type (p. 1170). IM is more frequent and more extensive in stomachs harbouring 'intestinal' type cancers than age-matched stomachs with 'diffuse' cancers or benign lesions. Incompletely differentiated forms of IM have been described. These lack Paneth cells and columnar mucus cells are seen in place of absorptive enterocytes. Variants of incomplete IM in which the columnar cells secrete sulphomucins show a selective association with intesti-

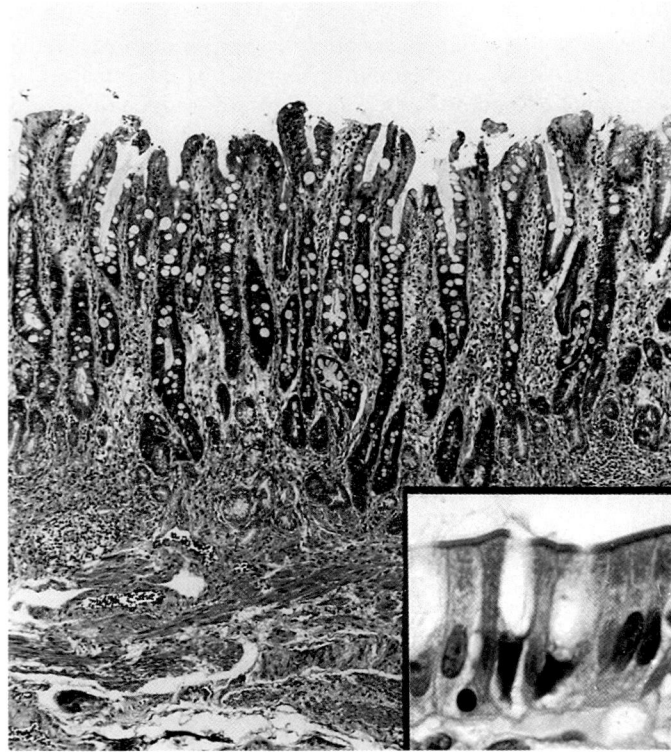

Fig. 16.51 Intestinal metaplasia of gastric mucosa. Inset shows intestinal-type goblet cells and enterocytes with a brush border.

nal-type gastric cancer. It is unclear whether such variants will assume clinical importance as precancerous lesions, but they may be of value in epidemiological studies.

Epithelial dysplasia

The term dysplasia identifies a lesion as being neoplastic but not having realized its increased potential to invade tissues in malignant fashion. It is therefore equivalent to 'intra-epithelial neoplasia'. Gastric dysplasia occurs in two forms. The first is as a circumscribed, raised lesion or adenoma. These are described on p. 1166. The second is as a diffuse, ill-defined, or patchy lesion that arises in flat mucosa, which usually shows the changes of chronic atrophic gastritis with or without intestinal metaplasia. The histological features of dysplasia include cytological atypia, failure of normal differentiation and maturation, and disordered architecture. Inflamed mucosa may show reactive changes that mimic dysplasia. Regenerating epithelium that is relining ulcers or erosions may also be mistaken for dysplasia (or even cancer). True dysplasia is a very uncommon lesion. It may be a cancer-associated lesion, and an accompanying malignancy must always be carefully excluded by repeated multiple biopsies and double-contrast barium studies. Patients must be carefully followed-up, because high-grade dysplasia can certainly progress to cancer. It may be difficult to distinguish severe dysplasia from intramucosal carcinoma, but gastrectomy should not be performed until a firm diagnosis of cancer has been made or there is a high level of suspicion that malignancy is present. Such a cautious approach will prevent unnecessary surgery.

Early gastric cancer

This does not represent a specific stage of the disease; rather the term 'early' is applied to cancers which are regarded on clinical grounds to be curable. The classification of early gastric cancer is based on the appearance of the tumour as visualized by either double-contrast barium meal or endoscopic examination (Fig. 16.52). Screening programmes in Japan have been directed towards the identification of early or curable gastric cancer rather than the prevention of cancer by diagnosing and treating precancerous lesions. A pathological classification of early gastric cancer is necessary if the results of treatment are to be compared and analysed. A cancer is designated as early if spread is limited to the mucosa or submucosa, but the lymph node status is irrelevant. Lymph node involvement is described in about 8 per cent of intramucosal carcinomas and 20 per cent of submucosal carcinomas. Five-year survival for early gastric cancer is shown in Table 16.2.

Early gastric cancers have been divided into two pathobiological types. The non-aggressive or superficial type spreads laterally and may remain confined to the mucosa for years, or may not invade at all. The aggressive or penetrating type may invade the submucosa when only a few millimetres in diameter. Paradoxically, the superficial type may be poorly differentiated and the penetrating type extremely well differentiated. Screening in Japan has resulted in the diagnosis of a relatively high ratio of early: advanced gastric cancers. However, some of this effort is negated by the fact that it is mainly the relatively non-aggressive early gastric cancers that are being detected whereas the aggressive early gastric cancers are slipping through the net and presenting as incurable advanced disease. The improving mortality figures for gastric cancer in Japan may reflect a declining incidence due to dietary modifications and are unlikely to be due to the screening programme alone.

Topography and macroscopic appearances of advanced gastric cancer

The antrum and lesser curve are the sites of predilection for gastric carcinoma. The cardia is the next most common site, but cardiac cancers share clinical and pathological features with adenocarcinomas of the lower oesophagus. Grossly, gastric cancers are either protuberant, ulcerated, or diffusely infiltrating. Ulcerating cancers typically have an irregular raised margin which contrasts with the 'punched-out' benign peptic ulcer (Fig. 16.53). They usually occur in the antrum or cardia. Protuberant cancers may be exceedingly bulky with a broad base and commonly arise in the body of the stomach. Diffusely infiltrating growths are poorly circumscribed and may extend widely, while producing little or no ulceration (Fig. 16.54). Rarely, the entire stomach is involved, giving rise to the shrunken leather-bottle stomach (linitis plastica). Widespread fibrosis results in the thickened, rigid gastric wall. Mucus production may be seen in any of the three morphological types; when mucus is abundant the cut surface of the tumour appears gelatinous.

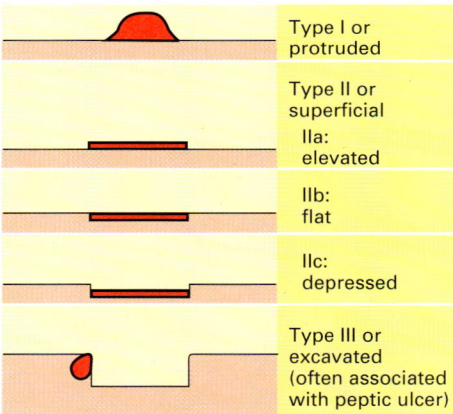

Fig. 16.52 Classification of early gastric cancer (EGC). Mixed varieties are common and early gastric cancer may be multifocal. Type I EGC is often a focus of malignancy in an adenoma. Peptic ulceration is the usual cause of an excavated EGC and is secondary to the tumour.

Table 16.2 Five-year survival for early gastric cancer

Intramucosal	
Lymph nodes negative	93%
Lymph nodes positive	91%
Submusocal	
Lymph nodes negative	89%
Lymph nodes positive	80%

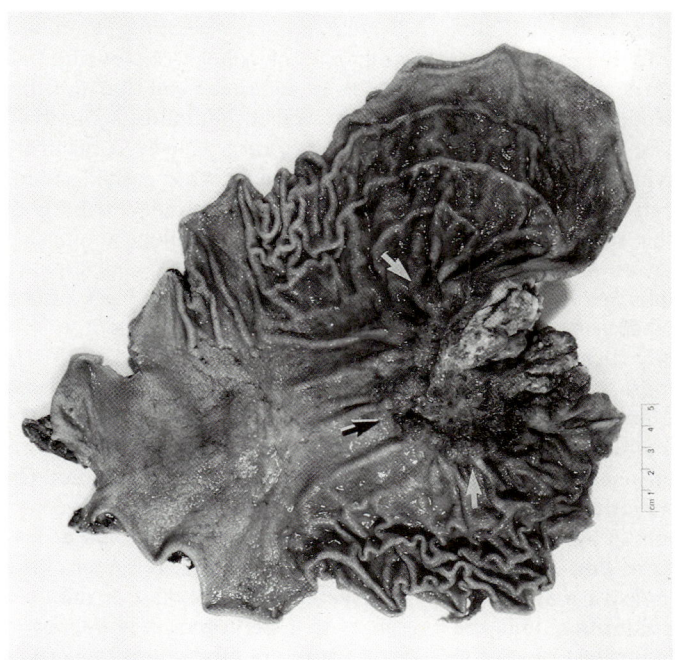

Fig. 16.53 Ulcerating carcinoma of the gastric cardia (arrows).

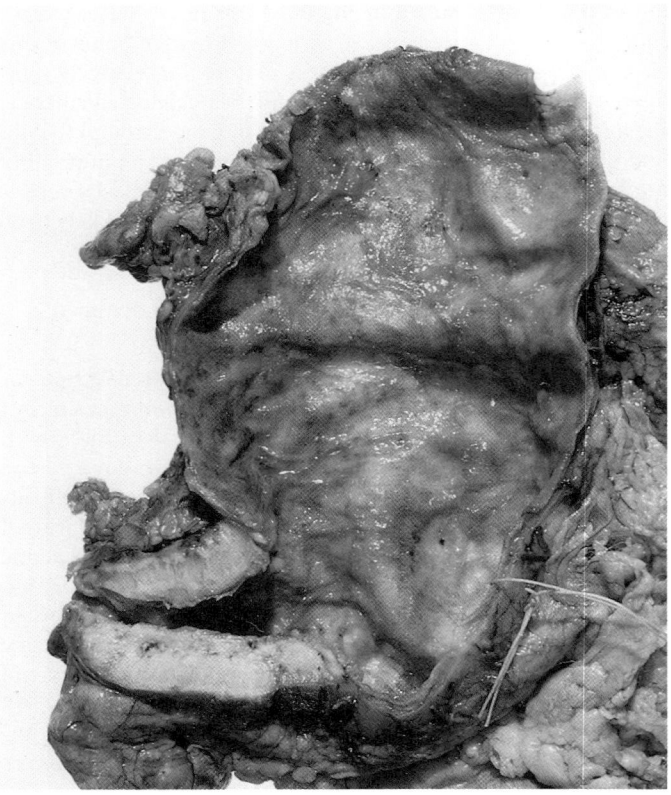

Fig. 16.54 Diffusely infiltrating carcinoma of the gastric antrum.

Table 16.3 Laurén's classification of gastric cancer; general characteristics of two main types of gastric cancer are listed

Intestinal type	Diffuse type
Glandular differentiation	Tumour cells single or in small clumps
Large cells with abundant cytoplasm and hyperchromatic nuclei	Small cells with inconspicuous cytoplasm and pyknotic nuclei
Intracellular mucus polarized to cell apex	Intracellular mucus not polarized (signet-ring cells)
Extracellular mucus within gland lumen	Extracellular mucus within stroma
Grows with expanding or pushing margin	Diffusely infiltrating growth pattern
Lymphocytes conspicuous	Lymphocytes inconspicuous
Frequent occurrence of intestinal metaplasia in adjacent mucosa	Intestinal metaplasia infrequent
M:F = 2:1	M:F = 1:1
Mean age 55 yr	Mean age 48 yr

of epidemiological importance. Laurén described two main types of gastric cancer, whose general characteristics are listed in Table 16.3, and whose histology is illustrated in Figs 16.55 and 16.56.

Laurén's classification has a number of drawbacks:

1. The terms 'intestinal' and 'diffuse' are not complementary and are potentially misleading.

2. The prognosis of the two types does not differ greatly,

Microscopic appearances

Adenocarcinoma is the most frequently encountered type of gastric malignancy and may be graded as well, moderately, or poorly differentiated. Adenocarcinomas secreting abundant mucus are described as mucinous or colloid. Signet-ring cell carcinoma is composed of poorly cohesive cells that are distended with accumulated mucin. Adenosquamous, squamous, and undifferentiated carcinomas are rare. However, accurate typing and grading is bedevilled by the fact that gastric adenocarcinoma is extremely heterogeneous, with different parts of the same tumour showing contrasting histological appearances. As a general rule, the exercise of tumour typing supplies information about the underlying histogenesis of a tumour, whereas grading of differentiation provides some insight into its biological aggressiveness. It is logical to type a tumour by its most well-differentiated areas, as these will have deviated least from the tissue of origin. For example, a tumour that includes glandular elements as well as sheets of undifferentiated cells is an adenocarcinoma and not an undifferentiated tumour. On the other hand, the grade of a tumour will probably be determined by its most poorly differentiated component. Other features that will influence prognosis include the character of the invasive margin, which may be either expanding or diffusely infiltrating, and the presence of a peritumoral lymphocytic infiltrate. The classification of Laurén not only has the merit of heeding the last two variables but provides information that is

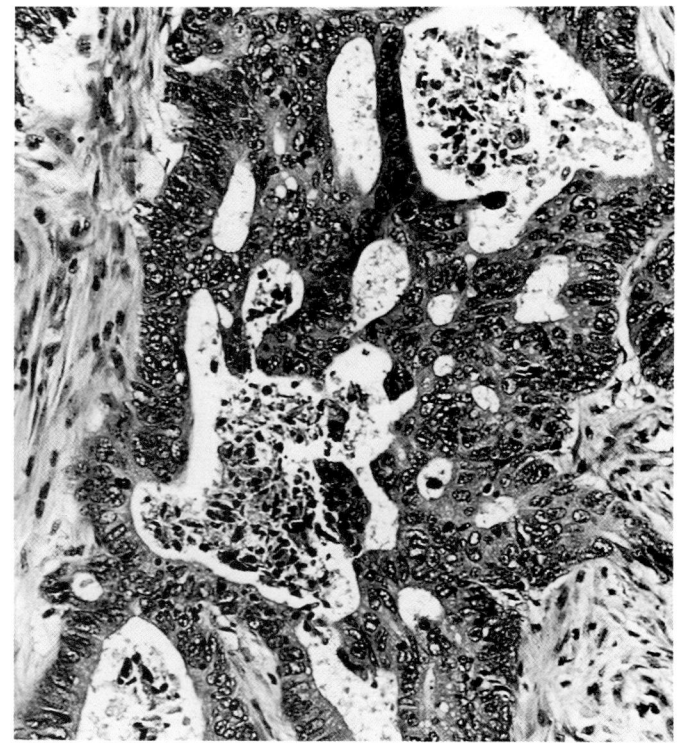

Fig. 16.55 Gland forming 'intestinal-type' carcinoma.

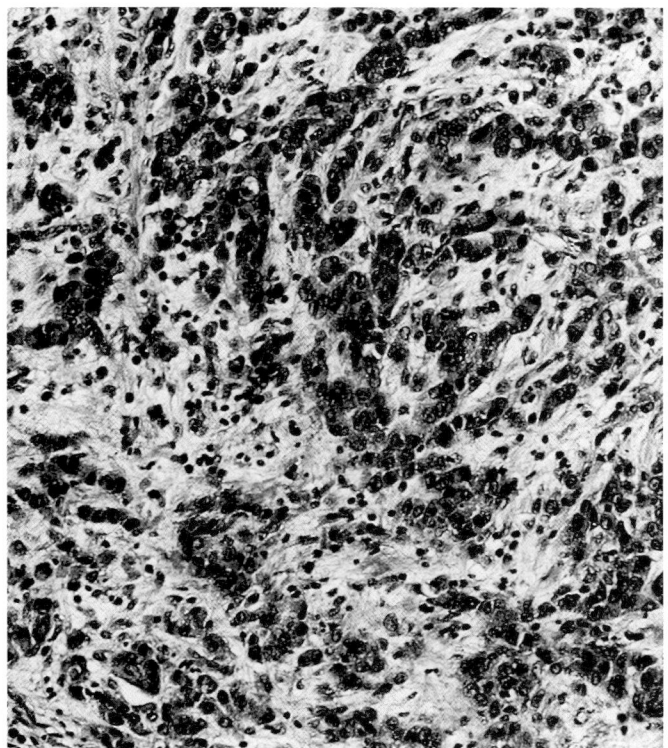

Fig. 16.56 Diffusely infiltrating carcinoma composed of irregular clumps of tumour cells.

although the intestinal type probably confers a small survival advantage.

3. Intestinal and diffuse features may be observed in the same tumour and a significant proportion of gastric cancers are therefore unclassifiable.

The term 'intestinal' implies a resemblance to cancers of the intestinal tract, notably the colorectum. It has no histogenetic implications. Thus intestinal-type cancers do not necessarily arise within intestinal metaplasia. Although mucin histochemical, enzyme histochemical, and ultrastructural studies commonly reveal the features of intestinal differentiation, this may reflect metaplasia within the tumour. Furthermore, 'diffuse' cancers may also show intestinal differentiation when subjected to detailed histochemical or ultrastructural study. It is in the field of epidemiological research that Laurén's classification has proved extremely useful.

The classification of Mulligan and Rember is similar to that of Laurén, except that they recognize a third type, the pylorocardiac carcinoma. These arise within the pylorus or cardia and the tumour cells may show a distinct resemblance to pyloric or cardiac gland cells. However, it is often difficult or impossible to distinguish pylorocardiac from intestinal-type carcinoma. Ming adopted a classification based on a single variable, namely the tumour growth pattern: expanding or infiltrating. Although similar to Laurén's classification, it is simpler and easier to use.

Spread

Direct

Gastric cancers typically show extensive spread. Most show spread in continuity beyond the external muscle coat into the serosal connective tissue. Penetration of the peritoneal membrane may result in invasion of adjacent organs, such as pancreas, spleen, liver, and transverse colon. Tumours at the cardia may extend upwards into the oesophagus, and pyloric cancers may show microscopic spread into the duodenum. It may be impossible to define the proximal and distal limits of spread by either observation or palpation. Diffuse intramural spread may extend beyond the macroscopically visible tumour to involve the resection margins; anastomotic recurrence is therefore frequent.

Lymphatic

Lymph node metastases are found in the majority of surgical specimens. The nodes of the lesser and greater curves are the first to be invaded and further spread may implicate para-aortic and coeliac axis nodes. Invasion of mediastinal lymph nodes may complicate cancers of the cardia, and splenic or pancreatic lymph node involvement may accompany tumours of the mid-stomach. The left supraclavicular node may be involved through spread along the thoracic duct. Enlargement of the left supraclavicular node is a well-known but rarely observed clinical sign. It is important to remove and examine all lymph nodes in a surgical specimen, as the number of involved nodes is an important prognostic variable.

Bloodstream

Tumour cells may invade tributaries of the portal veins and thereafter colonize the liver. Bloodstream spread may then continue to the lungs and on to other organs, such as skin and ovary. The liver and other organs may be involved in the absence of lymph-node metastasis.

Transperitoneal

A tumour which traverses the peritoneal membrane may give rise to multiple peritoneal seedlings throughout the abdominal cavity. Secondary ovarian tumours (Krukenberg) may result from transperitoneal spread, but may equally well be due to bloodstream spread.

Prognosis

The five-year survival following gastrectomy for advanced cancer is of the order of 20–30 per cent. The most important prognostic variables in patients having 'curative' surgery are the extent of direct spread in continuity, the number of involved lymph nodes, the character of the invasive margin (expanding versus diffusely infiltrating), and the presence or absence of a peritumoral lymphocytic infiltrate. Mucinous carcinomas have a poor prognosis but when well circumscribed they may be associated with prolonged survival.

16.3.3 Endocrine tumours

The reader is referred to Section 16.17 for an account of endocrine tumours of the gastrointestinal tract.

16.3.4 Non-epithelial tumours

The stomach is one of the commoner sites of gastrointestinal smooth muscle tumours. Most are small and innocent, occurring as incidental autopsy findings. Occasionally they may ulcerate and present with gastrointestinal haemorrhage. Small tumours present as mucosal nodules but larger examples may project into the gastric lumen or outwards into the serosa, or in both directions. On section, smaller tumours are well circumscribed and tan in colour. Large tumours are more likely to be malignant and may show cystic change, degeneration, and haemorrhage; solid areas may be white rather than tan.

A variety of patterns may be seen on histological examination, even within the same tumour. A common variety is characterized by bundles of spindle cells with eosinophilic cytoplasm and elongated, blunt-ended nuclei. The nuclei may become palisaded, mimicking a schwannoma. Individual nuclei may show bizarre changes, becoming enlarged, irregular in shape, and hyperchromatic. These changes are degenerative and not indicative of malignancy. The so-called epithelioid smooth muscle tumour consists of polygonal cells with a central round nucleus and pale cytoplasm that frequently shows artefactual vacuolation. Epithelioid and classical smooth muscle appearances may coexist in the same tumour.

It may be difficult, or indeed impossible, to predict whether a smooth muscle tumour will behave in a benign or a malignant fashion. In general, malignant tumours are larger, have a high nucleocytoplasmic ratio, contain areas of necrosis, may infiltrate surrounding tissues and, most importantly, show numerous mitotic figures (> 5 per 10 high-power fields). Malignant tumours invade adjacent organs and spread via the bloodstream to the liver. Lymphatic spread is uncommon.

Tumours of lymphoid tissue

The reader is referred to Chapter 24 for an account of lymphoid tumours of the gastrointestinal tract.

Tumours of nervous tissue

Schwannoma

These may occur as incidental findings, for example at autopsy, or may present with haemorrhage, pain, or an abdominal mass. They are usually single and can grow to a large size. They may project into the lumen, on to the serosa, or both. Microscopically they may be difficult to distinguish from smooth muscle tumours. Helpful features include encapsulation, nuclear palisading, and the presence of nerves. The rare granular cell tumour is derived from Schwann cells.

Neurofibroma

These may be solitary or a manifestation of generalized neurofibromatosis. Like smooth muscle tumours and schwannomas they may project into the lumen, towards the serosa, or both. The histological appearances are those of neurofibromas seen anywhere.

Tumours of connective tissue

Lipoma

Lipomas of the stomach are rare but they may be a source of haemorrhage or give rise to iron deficiency anaemia. They are single and may project into the gastric lumen as a lobulated mass. Histological examination reveals only normal-appearing adipose tissue.

Inflammatory fibroid polyp

This uncommon lesion is usually an incidental finding but larger examples may cause gastric outlet obstruction. They occur in adults of all ages and most are sited near the pylorus. They are solitary and may be sessile or pedunculated. Microscopically the tumour is composed of numerous small vessels set within connective tissue in which inflammatory cells, including eosinophils, are scattered. There may be a characteristic onion-skin arrangement of fibroblasts around the vessels.

Vascular tumours

Vascular malformations are rare, but may give rise to acute haemorrhage or iron deficiency anaemia. In hereditary haemorrhagic telangiectasia (Osler–Weber–Rendu syndrome) multiple lesions are seen at endoscopy.

Glomus tumours are uncommon. They usually arise in the antrum and bleeding is the typical presenting feature. Kaposi's sarcoma is being described more frequently than in the past as a complication of the acquired immune deficiency syndrome (AIDS). The endoscopic appearances range from purple-coloured macules to large nodular growths. Microscopic examination reveals bundles of spindle cells with interspersed thin-walled vessels and extravasated red blood cells.

Other tumours

Very rare malignant primary tumours of the stomach include choriocarcinoma, rhabdomyosarcoma, and haemangiopericytoma. Metastatic tumours are infrequent and usually asymptomatic, although they can be a cause of bleeding. The more usual primary sources include lung, breast, malignant melanoma, and thyroid. Leukaemic and lymphomatous spread to the stomach are also described.

16.3.5 Further reading

Day, D. W. (1987). The stomach. In *Systemic pathology*, Vol. 3: *Alimentary tract*, (3rd edn), (ed. B. C. Morson), pp. 149–228. Churchill Livingstone, Edinburgh.

Filipe, M. I. and Jass, J. R. (1986). *Gastric carcinoma*. Churchill Livingstone, Edinburgh.

Inokuchi, K., Kodama, Y., Sasaki, O., Kamegawa, T., and Okamura, T. (1983). Differentiation of growth patterns of early gastric carcinoma determined by cytophotometric DNA analysis. *Cancer* **51**, 1138–41.

Jass, J. R. (1980). Role of intestinal metaplasia in the histogenesis of gastric carcinoma. *Journal of Clinical Pathology* **33**, 801–10.

Laurén, P. (1965). The two histological main types of gastric carcinoma. Diffuse and so-called intestinal type carcinoma. An attempt at a histoclinical classification. *Acta Pathologica et Microbiologica Scandinavica* **64**, 31–49.

Ming, S.-C. (1977). Gastric carcinoma: a pathobiological classification. *Cancer* **39**, 2475–85.

Mulligan, R. M. and Rember, R. R. (1954). Histogenesis and biologic behaviour of gastric carcinoma. *Archives of Pathology* **58**, 1–25.

Nakamura, T. and Nakano, G.-E. (1985). Histopathological classification and malignant change in gastric polyps. *Journal of Clinical Pathology* **38**, 754–64.

16.4   Pathophysiology of the stomach

J. H. Baron

16.4.1   Normal physiology

The parietal cells of the body of the stomach secrete hydrochloric acid and intrinsic factor: zymogen chief cells secrete pepsinogens which are converted by gastric acid into proteolytic pepsins. The antral mucosa has different secretory functions; it does not secrete either acid or pepsins but has endocrine cells which synthesize and release polypeptide hormones, such as gastrin, in response to food. The surface epithelium and mucous neck cells of the body secrete alkaline mucus, as do the pyloric cells of the antrum.

The cephalic, gastric, and intestinal phases of gastric secretion overlap in time and are also related to each other in a complicated nervous and hormonal system.

There are many tests of gastric secretion, and they are used to answer three questions. First, how many parietal cells are there in this stomach? Maximal acid output is an expression of the number of parietal cells, the parietal cell mass. In man, 10^9 parietal cells produce about 23 mmol/h of acid. The number of chief cells is related to the number of parietal cells, so that acid is measured routinely, and pepsin only rarely. Secondly, are none, some, or all of these cells innervated by branches of the vagus nerves? Thirdly, are these parietal cells stimulated by excess gastrins?

In practice, gastric secretion is measured by continued aspiration through a naso-gastric tube in a fasting patient over a basal hour, followed by maximum stimulation with an agonist such as pentagastrin, possibly preceded by a vagal stimulus such as modified sham feeding (which has replaced, for safety and convenience, the older insulin test). The juice volume is measured, as well as pH and titratable acidity, so that acid output can be calculated. Corrections can be made for gastroduodenal loss, and for duodenogastric reflux. Alkaline secretion and mucus are not measured routinely.

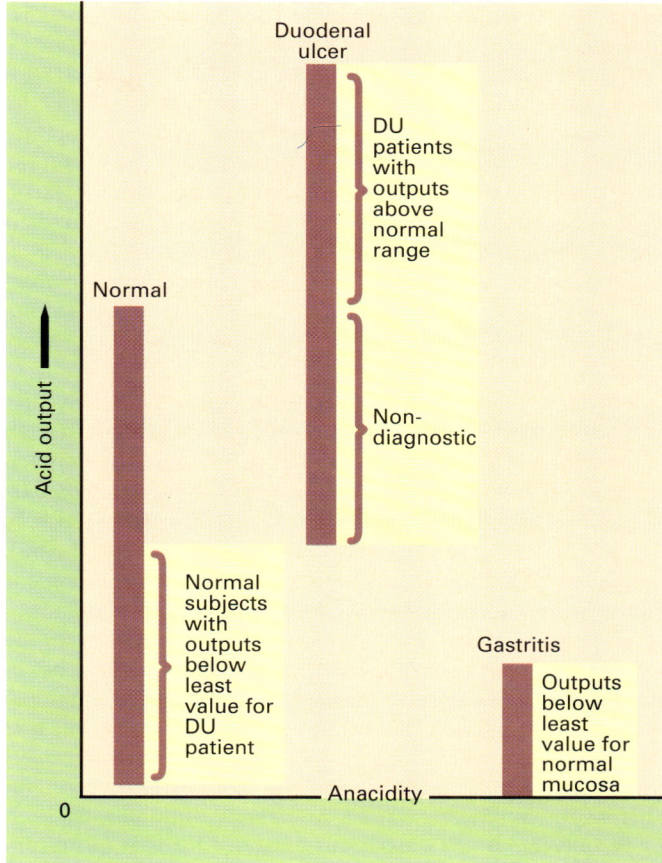

Fig. 16.57 Peak acid output in control subjects, patients with duodenal ulcer, and with gastritis. (Redrawn after Baron 1970, with permission of Universitatsvorlaget, Oslo.)

16.4.2   Abnormal physiology

Gastric secretion may be abnormal due to diseases. The abnormal secretions may be responsible for diseases. Hyposecretion of acid may impair absorption of organic iron. Decreased secretion of intrinsic factor causes B_{12} malabsorption and pernicious anaemia. Hypersecretion of acid and pepsin predisposes to duodenal ulcer disease.

Hyposecretion and gastritis

The histology of the mucosa of the body of the stomach is a determinant of basal and maximal acid output. There may be a hypersecretory phase in the early stages of superficial gastritis but later, and especially with atrophic gastritis and intestinal metaplasia, there is marked hyposecretion. In gastric atrophy, there is naturally anacidity. 'Anacidity' is defined as a pH not less than 7.0, even after maximal stimulation, and is preferable to the older terms 'no free acid' (which approximated to a pH more than 3.5) and 'achlorhydria', which was also imprecise.

In pernicious anaemia the gastritis of the body causes a reduction in secretion of acid and pepsin as well as of intrinsic factor. This auto-immune type A gastritis of pernicious anaemia may improve transiently after corticosteroids, with a temporary return of acid, intrinsic factor, and parietal cells. Similarly, with iron or folate deficiency from type B non-immune gastritis of the body, the mucosa and secretions may improve after appropriate haematinics. If the antrum and body both show gastritis (type B) than there will be few G-cells and thus a low serum gastrin. With a normal antrum but gastritis of the body (type A) and an intact feedback system, as in pernicious anaemia, anacidity leads to an alkaline antrum and therefore hypergastrinaemia.

16.4.3   Gastric ulcer

As a whole, patients with gastric ulcers have normal gastric secretion. However, ulcers in different sites are associated with different secretory patterns: the higher the ulcer up the stomach the lower the acid output. Almost without exception, peptic ulcers develop only in the presence of acid ('No acid, no ulcer'), and usually have parietal cells only above them (cephalad). Fundic mucosa rarely digests itself. Ulcers in the stomach occur almost always in pyloric-type mucosa just below (caudad) to the parietal cell mass. Thus, a stomach with a high ulcer, in the body, usually shows extensive gastritis, and therefore has hyposecretion. A stomach with an ulcer in the incisura (angulus) may have normal secretion, and a prepyloric gastric ulcer is often associated with hypersecretion, as in duodenal ulcer. Thus prepyloric ulcers could be caused by such hypersecretion, whereas the hyposecretion of a stomach with an ulcer high in the body is due to the gastritis associated with that ulcer, and not a cause of the ulcer.

16.4.4   Gastric cancer

Stomachs with cancer may have normal, low, or absent acid secretion. Absolute anacidity is found in only about one in five patients with gastric cancer, usually the large, infiltrating, or advanced forms.

16.4.5   Duodenal ulcer

The mean basal and maximal acid outputs of patient with duodenal ulcers are about double those of normal subjects, corresponding with a similar ratio between the number of parietal cells counted post-mortem in the stomachs of patients with and without duodenal ulcers.

In my model of the hypersecretory situation in duodenal ulcer disease, there is an overlap between patients and normal controls. Patients do not have duodenal ulcers in the absence of acid. There appears to be a threshold of acid secretion in patients with duodenal ulcers of about 15 mmol/h peak acid output, so that a proportion of normal subjects have acid outputs below this least value found in patients with duodenal ulcers.

On the other hand, about a quarter of patients with duodenal ulcers are hypersecretors, with outputs above the upper limit of normal range, which is about 40 mmol/h, but which depends on body build (especially height), age, and perhaps environmental factors such as smoking. If a patient has hypersecretion, he probably has, has had, or will have a duodenal ulcer (Fig. 16.58). Hyposecretors with a peak output of 0–15 mmol/h will probably never develop a duodenal ulcer. Most patients are normosecretors: other unknown factors determine whether they will develop a duodenal ulcer during their lifetime.

Basal interdigestive secretion   This is also abnormally high in about a quarter of patients with duodenal ulcer. Basal acid output is correlated with maximal secretion, so that basal hypersecretion can be due simply to an increased parietal cell mass. There are, however, data suggesting an increased 'drive' (vagal and/or hormonal) on the parietal cells of the stomach. Vagal drive, as estimated by the ratio of basal/maximal and of vagally/maximally stimulatable acid, has been suspected as being abnormally high in duodenal ulcer disease.

Meal-stimulated acid production is also a function of parietal cell mass, so that patients with duodenal ulcers secrete more acid after a meal than normal subjects and they also empty their meal buffer faster, so that titratable acid and hydrogen ions are over-rapidly emptied into the duodenum.

Hypersecretion of *pepsin* occurs with a similar overlap. However, pepsins are heterogeneous because pepsinogens are heterogeneous, and some pepsin fractions may be more ulcerogenic than others.

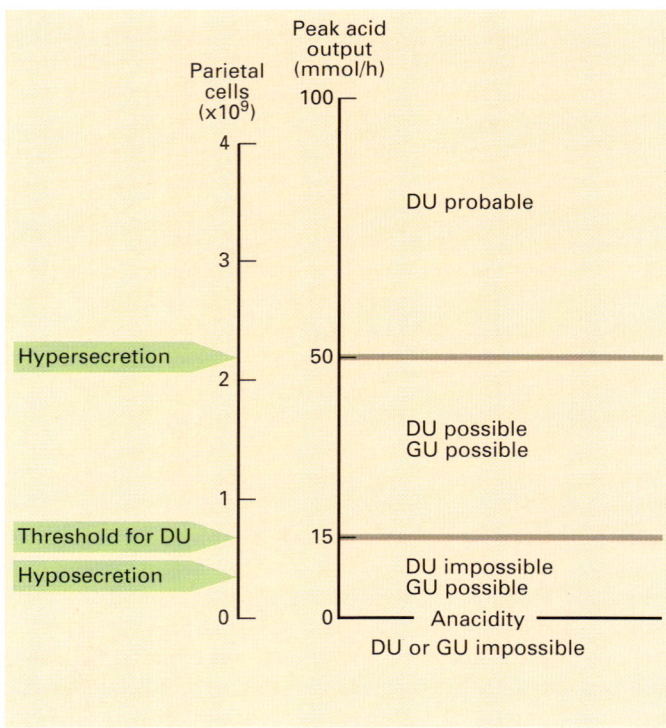

Fig. 16.58   Postulated parietal cell mass, peak acid output, and the secretory situation in peptic ulcers. (Redrawn after Baron 1972, with permission of Butterworths.)

Genetic and environmental factors each contribute about 50 per cent to the development of duodenal ulcers. Inherited tendency is probably transmitted by increased secretion of acid and pepsin, presumably from genetic control of parietal and chief cell mass.

Hormones Patients with duodenal ulcers tend to have higher than normal basal serum gastrin, and an abnormally high and more lasting post-prandial rise in serum gastrin. The absolute number of G-cells in the human antra (G-cell mass) is in some series twice normal, but with an overlap with the normal population as with acid secretion.

Patients with very high levels of fasting gastrin may have a gastrinoma, causing acid hypersecretion and usually associated with intractable peptic ulcer disease (Zollinger–Ellison syndrome). Some patients with hypergastrinaemia do not have a gastrinoma but have antral G-cell hyperplasia.

Other control factors The parietal cells with duodenal ulcers may be abnormally sensitive to endocrine and/or vagal stimuli. Gastrin released from the antrum after meals is inhibited by subsequent acidification. There are suggestions that there is a failure of this acid-inhibitory feedback in patients with duodenal ulcers.

Similarly, there are suggestions that there is a failure of duodenal inhibitory mechanisms in duodenal ulcer disease, leading to an over-rapid emptying of titratable acid and hydrogen ions into the duodenum in excessive and prolonged amounts after meals. Other deficiencies in duodenal control mechanisms that have been proposed include impaired bicarbonate secretion and impaired motility of the proximal duodenum, leading to decreased expulsion of acid down from the bulb.

Paracrine secretions There is little or no evidence of a deficiency of any measurable intestinal hormone after meals in patients with duodenal ulcers. However, there may be abnormalities of the paracrine secretions which diffuse from their cells of origin to the target cells. Thus the amount of stored histamine in the gastric mucosa of hypersecretors, such as patients with duodenal ulcers, is less than normal, which has been interpreted as due to an increased rate of formation and turnover of this stimulant of parietal cell H_2-receptors. Prostaglandin E_2 is found in the gastric mucosa, and may increase alkaline secretion in the mucus and inhibit gastric acid. There are some data suggesting that there may be deficiencies of mucosal-protective prostaglandins or excess of mucosal-damaging prostanoids, such as leukotrienes, in duodenal ulcer disease.

16.4.6 Further reading

Baron, J. H. (1970). The clinical use of gastric function tests. *Scandinavian Journal of Gastroenterology* **5** (Suppl. 6), 9–46.

Baron, J. H. (1972). Aetiology. In *Chronic duodenal ulcer* (ed. C. Wastell). Butterworths, London.

Baron, J. H. (1978). *Clinical tests of gastric secretion. History, methodology and interpretation.* Macmillan, London.

Baron, J. H. (1981). Pathophysiology of gastric acid and pepsin secre-

tion. In *Magen und Magenkrankheiten* (ed. W. Domschke and K. G. Wormsley). George Thieme Verlag, Stuttgart.

Baron, J. H. (1982). Current views on pathogenesis of peptic ulcer. *Scandinavian Journal of Gastroenterology* **17** (Suppl. 18), 1–10.

16.5 Normal structure and function of the small and large intestine

V. Sams

16.5.1 Small intestine

The small intestine stretches from the gastric pylorus to the ileo-caecal valve and occupies a central position in the abdominal cavity. It is one of the narrower parts of the gastrointestinal tract and has a length of approximately 5 m. The small intestine has two main functions—digestion and absorption.

Anatomy

The small intestine is composed of three main anatomical subdivisions, the duodenum, jejunum, and ileum. The duodenum is 20 cm long, largely retroperitoneal and roughly C-shaped. It is situated in the right upper quadrant of the abdominal cavity. It is conveniently subdivided into four parts. The first part corresponds to the duodenal 'cap', characteristically seen on upper gastrointestinal contrast studies. This part has the important posterior relations of the gastroduodenal artery, portal vein, and common bile duct. The second part of the duodenum is crossed by the transverse colon. The common bile duct and pancreatic duct enter this part of the duodenum posteromedially at the papilla of Vater. In 30 per cent of cases there is an accessory pancreatic duct which drains more proximally into the duodenal lumen. The superior mesenteric vessels cross the third part of the duodenum. The fourth part of the duodenum is variable in length and ascends to the duodenoljejunal flexure.

The rest of the small bowel is composed of the jejunum and ileum, the former occupies about 40 per cent of the remaining length of the small bowel. Both these parts are supported by a mesentery, the origin of which runs obliquely across the posterior abdominal wall from the duodeno-jejunal flexure to the right iliac fossa.

There is no recognized line of division between jejunum and ileum but there are some features that allow a degree of distinction to be made between the two macroscopically. The jejunal mesentery is less fat-laden than its ileal counterpart so that its long vasa recta are more readily apparent than the shorter vasa recta of the ileum. The jejunum feels much thicker than the ileum by virtue of the greater number of valvulae conniventes (plica circularis) present in the former compared to the latter (Figs 16.59, 16.60).

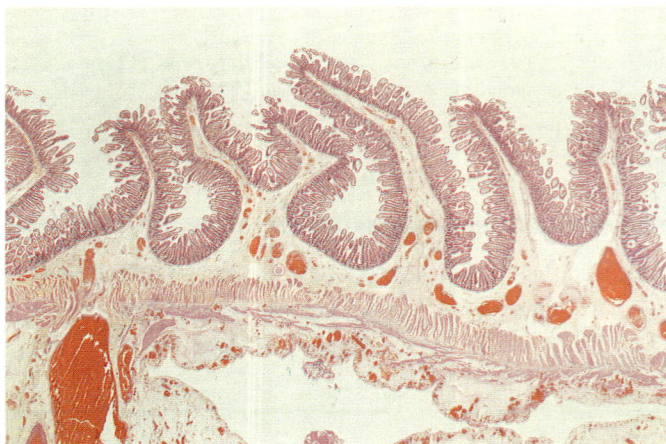

Fig. 16.59 A low-power view of the jejunum showing the greatly folded mucosa due to the many valvulae conniventes. Congested blood vessels highlight the submucosa and serosa, between which the inner circular and outer longitudinal layers of muscularis propria can be seen.

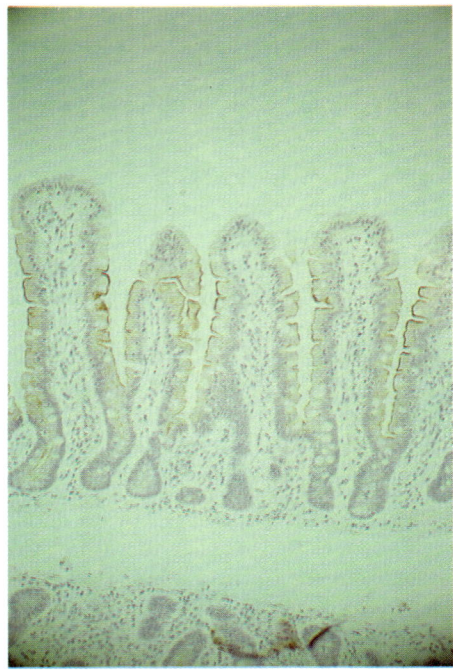

Fig. 16.61 This is a jejunal biopsy which has been immunohisto-chemically stained using an antibody to sucrase–isomaltase, shown here as a brown line in the region of the brush border on the villi.

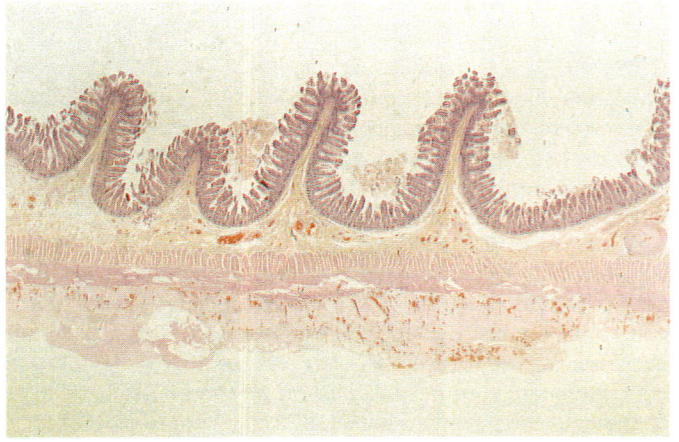

Fig. 16.60 A low-power view of the ileum showing a reduced number of mucosal folds compared to the jejunum (Fig. 16.59). Otherwise the architecture of mucosa, submucosa, muscularis propria, and serosa is similar to the jejunum.

Function

Small intestinal mucosal folds and villi provide an absorptive area of approximately 9 m². Interference with this absorptive function, whether due to obstruction or to mucosal disease, can cause severe changes in the fluid balance and nutritional status of an individual.

Small intestinal digestive processes have two phases: a luminal phase and a terminal (membrane) phase. The former is largely accomplished by pancreatic enzymes, the latter by enzymes which are integral proteins of the luminal membrane of the enterocyte (Fig. 16.61).

Histology

In keeping with the general structural organization of the gastrointestinal tract, the wall of the small bowel consists of mucosa, submucosa, muscularis propria, subserosal tissues, and serosa (Figs 16.59, 16.60).

The mucosa is composed of the surface epithelium and the underlying lamina propria. It has a complex architectural arrangement of villi and crypts (Fig. 16.62). Innumerable villi impart a velvety appearance to the mucosa. They are finger- or leaf-like mucosal evaginations which increase the absorptive surface by a factor of 10, and are unique to the small intestine. At their bases are epithelial invaginations called crypts which extend to the muscularis mucosae and are surrounded by a prominent fibroblastic sheath. Villi are normally 3–5 times longer than their crypts.

There is a heterogeneous epithelial cell population in the small intestine which varies between the villus and the crypt. On the villus there are absorptive cells, mature goblet cells, and a few endocrine cells. In the crypts there are goblet cells, endocrine cells, Paneth cells, and undifferentiated crypt cells.

Absorptive cells (enterocytes) are columnar cells and are the most abundant cells on the villus. These cells possess the enzymes necessary for the terminal digestion of carbohydrates (Fig. 16.61) and proteins and they are able to absorb various nutrients, including lipids, sugars, and amino acids. They have a conspicuous microvillus brush border (Fig. 16.63).

Goblet cells are present in the villi but are more abundant in the crypts. They derive their name from their supposed resemblance to a brandy goblet. They secrete ions and water in addition to mucus. Goblet cells increase in frequency along the

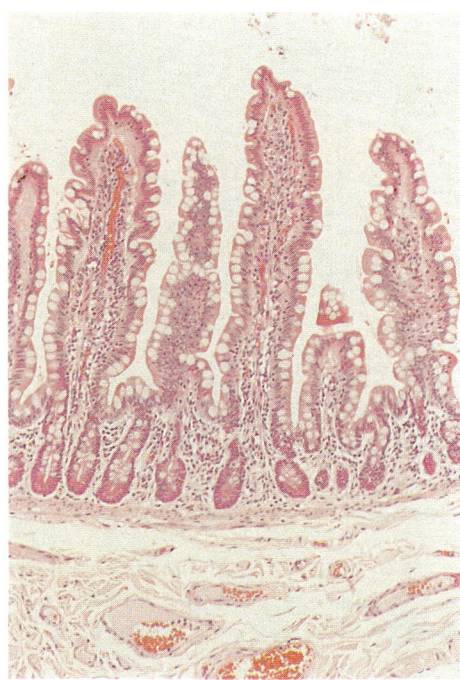

Fig. 16.62 A medium-power view of the jejunum showing the arrangement of villi and crypts. The length of the former can be seen to be at least 3–4 times that of the crypts, which is the normal crypt : villus ratio for jejunum. The bright pink Paneth cells are clearly visible at the base of the crypts.

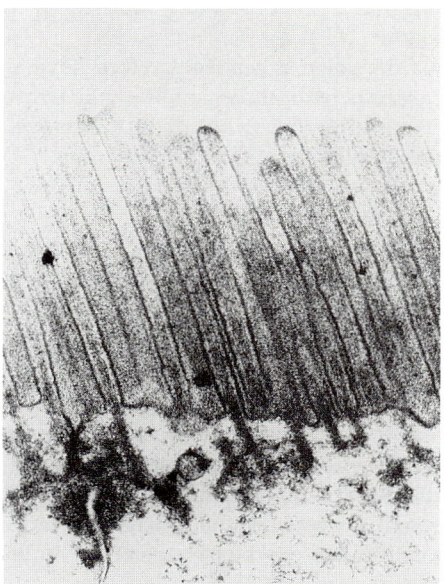

Fig. 16.63 This is an electron microscopic picture of the brush border of the jejunum showing the arrangement of the microvilli, the surface area of which is an important component in the total surface area of the small bowel available for absorption and digestion.

length of the small intestine, being most numerous in the lower ileum.

Endocrine cells are occasionally found on the villus but are more abundant in the crypts, particularly at the extreme ends of the small bowel. A more detailed analysis of these cells is found in Section 16.6.

Villus cells (goblet and absorptive) develop from undifferentiated cells found in the base of the crypts. Morphological and biochemical maturation occurs while cells migrate from the crypt on to the villus. The duration of proliferation and migration of these cells is approximately 5–6 days in most of the human small intestine.

In the base of the crypt is a further cell type, the rather conspicuous Paneth cell. Paneth cells are pyramidal in shape and are characterized by large membrane-bound acidophilic refractile granules in their apical cytoplasm. Lysozyme is believed to be secreted from these granules and is thought to play a role in bacterial protection since it can digest bacterial cell walls.

The pericrypt fibroblastic sheath is formed by cells that undergo a rapid turnover, similar to that of the epithelial cells. This co-migration of the epithelium and subjacent mesenchyme maintains an intimate relationship which enhances the structural integrity and functional efficiency of the intestinal mucosa.

The lamina propria penetrates the cores of the villi and takes along with it blood-vessels and delicate, loose connective tissue infiltrated by small numbers of various types of inflammatory cells. It also contains a central, blind-ending lacteal, and smooth muscle cells. The latter facilitate emptying of the former.

Lymphoid aggregates increase in number on passing distally in the small intestine and become confluent in the ileum, where they are known as Peyer's patches. Further details about the immune function of the small bowel are discussed in Chapter 24.

The submucosa of the small bowel is unremarkable except in the duodenum where it is largely filled by ramifying coiled tubular glands called Brunner's glands. Their excretory ducts penetrate the muscularis mucosae to open at the bases of the mucosal crypts. These glands secrete a thin, alkaline mucus which helps to neutralize the acid chyme as well as being protective against auto-digestion.

The muscularis propria is composed of two layers of muscle, an inner layer of circularly arranged fibres and an outer layer of longitudinally arranged fibres. Serosa and subserosal tissues encase the small bowel outside these muscle layers.

Blood supply

The duodenum is supplied by branches of both the coelic axis and the superior mesenteric artery. The jejunum is supplied by branches from the left side of the superior mesenteric artery, while the ileum is supplied both by similar branches of the superior mesenteric artery but, in addition, receives blood from branches of the ileo-colic artery, a branch from the right side of the superior mesentery artery. These branches ramify in the mesentery and reach the mesenteric border of the gut by vasa recta. These vessels then enter the intestinal serosa, divide, and pass round the bowel toward the anti-mesenteric border. Branches from these serosal vessels pierce the muscularis propria and form an extensive vascular plexus in the submucosa. Branches from the submucosal plexus form two groups: one which ramifies in a capillary network surrounding the crypt and the other group which continues to the villus. Venous pathways parallel the arterial ones.

Lymphatics

Lympatic drainage starts with the central lacteal and proceeds into the submucosal plexus from whence it drains, along with the veins, to extramural sites. Extramural lymph nodes of the duodenum consist of the pancreatico-duodenal group, the pyloric group, and the superior mesenteric group. This last group of nodes also receives lymph from the jejunum and ileum.

Innervation

The enteric nervous system is independent of the central nervous system. Sensory neurones detect fluidity, volume, chemical composition, and temperature of luminal contents. This information is processed and integrated within the interneural circuitry of the autonomic ganglia. Sympathetic ganglia are external to the gut wall lying in the coeliac, and superior and inferior mesenteric plexuses. Parasympathetic glanglia are located in both a submucosal plexus (Meissner's plexus) (Fig. 16.64) and in a myenteric plexus (Auerbach's plexus) (Fig. 16.65). The latter lies between the circular and longitudinal layers of muscularis propria. Stimulation of the parasympathetic gastrointestinal neurones usually increases circulation, secretion, and muscular activity. Stimulation of the sympathetic neurones has the reverse effect.

16.5.2   Large intestine

The large intestine begins at the ileo-caecal valve and ends at the anus. It is approximately 150 cm in length. Its two main

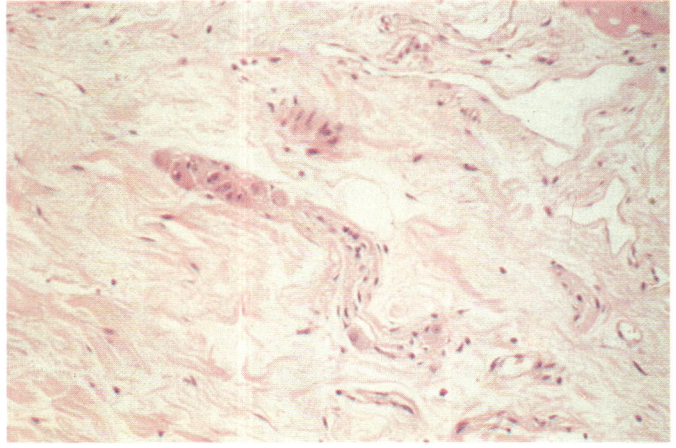

Fig. 16.64 Submucosa in which a group of ganglion cells are 'trailed' by some nerve fibres.

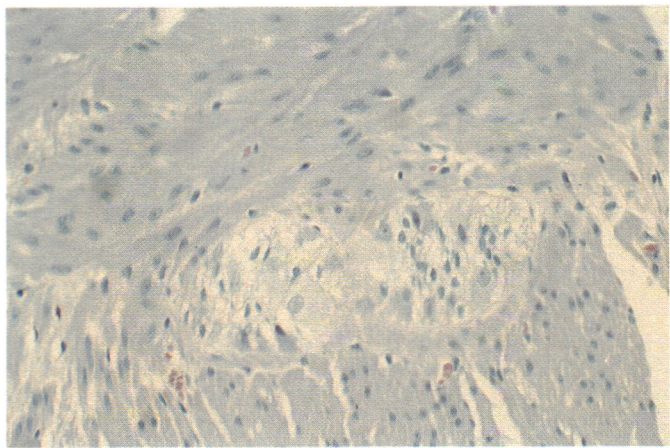

Fig. 16.65 Groups of ganglion cells between the inner and outer layers of the muscularis propria.

functions are the absorption of water and electrolytes, and the storage of faeces prior to their evacuation.

Anatomy

The large intestine is composed of six anatomical subdivisions. The first part of the large intestine is the caecum which lies below the ileo-caecal valve and from which the appendix arises. Next, the ascending colon passes from the ileo-caecal valve to the hepatic flexure. The transverse colon crosses from the hepatic to splenic flexure where the descending colon commences. The sigmoid colon arises in the left iliac fossa and has a mesentery which allows the bowel to assume a sigma-shaped configuration. The sigmoid becomes the rectum at the recto-sigmoid junction.

All parts of the colon except the rectum have a similar external appearance, with three longitudinal strips of muscle (taeniae coli) running their whole length, between which the bowel pouches into haustrations or sacculation.

Histology

As in the rest of the gastrointestinal tract, the wall of the large bowel consists of mucosa, submucosa, muscularis propria, subserosal tissues, and serosa.

The large intestinal mucosa is smooth and without villi. In contrast with the small intestine it has crescentic not circular folds (plicae semilunaris) (Fig. 16.66). The mucosal surface has a pitted appearance due to the openings of the glands or crypts of Lieberkuhn. These glands are straight and extend from the surface to the muscularis mucosae (Fig. 16.67). Mucin secretions flow from the crypt openings to cover the mucosa, providing a lubricated surface for the passage of the luminal contents which become increasingly solid as they pass from the right to the left colon.

Normal colonic epithelium consists of several different types of cells: mature absorptive cells, mature goblet cells, endocrine cells, and undifferentiated stem cells.

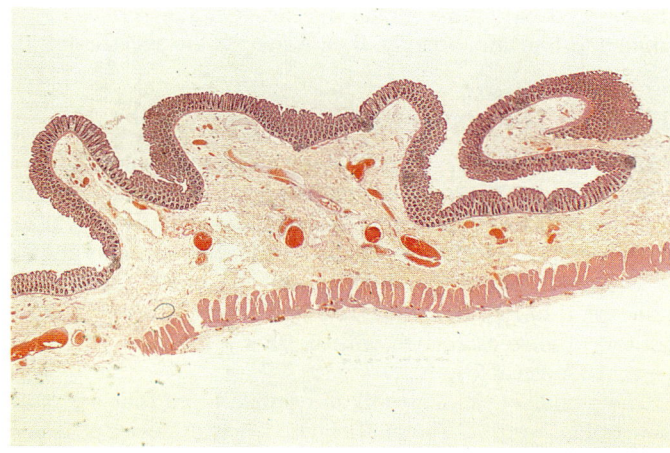

Fig. 16.66 Lower-power view of the colon showing the mucosal folding due to the semilunar folds in the large bowel. The submucosa contains congested blood vessels beneath which the muscularis propria is seen.

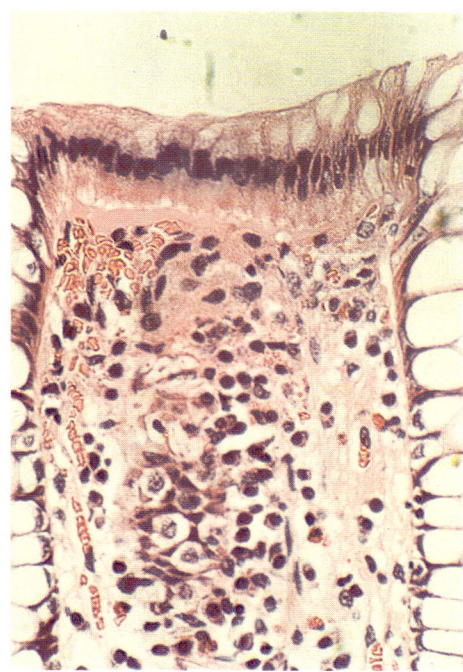

Fig. 16.68 A high-power view of the large bowel mucosa shows the presence of capillaries and scattered inflammatory cells in the lamina propria. Here absorptive cells are just seen between the goblet cells in the crypts but are more easily identified at the luminal surface.

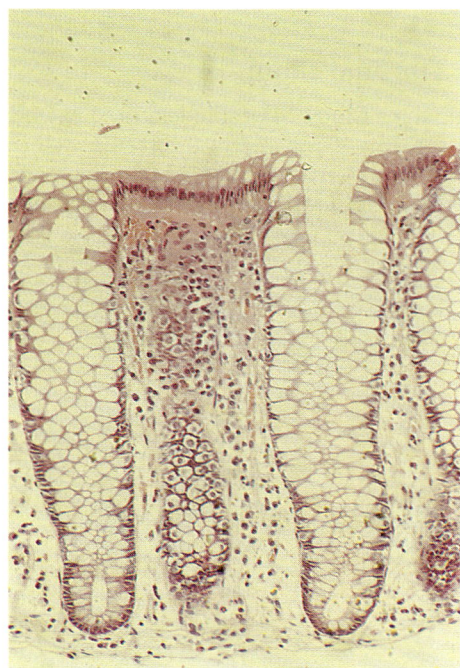

Fig. 16.67 The glands (crypts) of the large bowel are straight and appear to be lined solely by goblet cells.

Mature absorptive columnar cells absorb water and electrolytes. They have numerous short, regularly spaced microvilli, the density of which is significantly less than in the small bowel and the digestive capacity of which is minimal.

Goblet cells are numerous in the crypt epithelium but are, in fact, outnumbered by columnar (absorptive) cells by four to one. The goblet cells are responsible for the production of mucus (Fig. 16.68).

The colon has the least number of endocrine cells in the in-

testine. They are primarily located in the left side of the colon, particularly in the rectum. For further details see Section 16.6.

The undifferentiated stem cells give rise to columnar, goblet, and endocrine cells. They are located in the lowest two-thirds of the crypts. As in the small bowel, the large intestinal epithelial cells are a rapidly dividing cell population. Migration from this proliferative zone towards the gut lumen takes 3–8 days. The crypts are surrounded by a pericryptal fibroblast sheath which contributes to the integrity of the normal morphology and cellular dynamics of the colonic mucosa.

The lamina propria separates the colonic crypts and consists of loose reticular connective tissue containing fibroblasts, capillaries, and scattered mononuclear cells. These inflammatory cells present a barrier to entry by organisms and antigens to the interior of the body. Not surprisingly, therefore, their normal location is predominantly in the most luminal third of the lamina propria. The lamina propria also contains solitary lymphoid nodules that are often of sufficient size to displace the crypts, and extend into the submucosa. These lymphoid aggregates increase in number as the rectum is approached. The structure and function of these lymphoid cells is further discussed in Chapter 24.

The submucosa is similar to that described in the non-duodenal small intestine. The muscularis propria is composed of two layers of muscle, an inner layer of circularly arranged fibres and an outer layer of longitudinally arranged fibres. This latter layer is a continuous coat but it conspicuously thickened into three flat bands called taeniae coli, from the caecum to the rectum.

The serosal surface is incomplete since the ascending and descending portions of the colon are retroperitoneal. The serosa can contain lobules of fat that form pendulous projections, called appendices epiploicae.

Blood supply

The large bowel is derived embryologically from both the mid-gut and the hind-gut. The boundary between these portions being just to the left of the mid-point of the transverse colon. Correspondingly the caecum, the ascending colon, and the right part of the transverse colon are supplied by branches of the superior mesenteric artery. The remaining part of the transverse colon, the descending and sigmoid portions of the colon, and most of the rectum, however, are supplied by branches of the inferior mesenteric artery.

Vascularization of the colon is assured by a single marginal artery giving off vasa recta. However, there are critical areas of anastomotic supply where the colon is most vulnerable to ischaemia. These areas are in the region of the splenic flexure at the junctions between the superior and inferior mesenteric arteries, and in the rectum where the inferior mesenteric artery and the hypogastric vessels anastomose. Mucosal capillaries drain into venules at the luminal surface. Since one of the major functions of the colon is to absorb water it is not surprising that the vascular system is adapted to remove water absorbed by the epithelium and return it to the general circulation. Histologically one sees a well-defined capillary network between the functionally most mature absorptive cells at the luminal surface epithelium. This network functions as an intestinal glomerulus. In addition, the capillaries of the proximal colon have more fenestra as compared to those in the distal colon, which corresponds to the physiological emphasis on water reabsorption proximally.

Lymphatics

The lymphatics begin as a capillary plexus that wraps round the muscularis mucosae. From here they send small branches into the mucosa to reach no higher than the bases of the crypts of Lieberkuhn. These lymphatic vessels pass through the submucosa to form another plexus around the muscularis propria. Efferent collecting lymphatic trunks proceed from the paracolic lymph nodes to the intermediate lymph nodes in the mid portion of the mesentery. From the intermediate group large efferents reach the central or principal lymph node at the root of the mesentery.

Innervation

Like other areas of the bowel, the large bowel is innervated by the autonomic nervous system. Sympathetic innervation is mediated by fibres from the superior mesenteric ganglion and the hypogastric plexus. Parasympathetic fibres are derived from the vagus and pelvic nerves. All these fibres interconnect with the mural plexuses in a similar manner to that described in the small intestine and, broadly, their functions are also similar.

16.5.3   The appendix

The appendix develops as part of the midgut. In humans it is a vestigial organ. Its size is variable, being longest in infancy. The position of its tip in relation to the large and small bowel varies. Its only constant feature is that its base in the caecum is always at the point where the three taenia coli of the right colon coalesce. It has a small mesentery and often a number of other peritoneal folds associated with it, giving rise to a variety of para-appendiceal fossae.

The glands of the appendix are simple tubes that are often forked (Fig. 16.69). The epithelium is rich in goblet cells and endocrine cells. Lymphoid nodules are abundant and confluent (Fig. 16.70).

Its blood supply is derived from a branch of the superior mesenteric artery. Its nerve supply originates at the coeliac plexus and these fibres accompany the blood supply to the appendix.

16.5.4   The anal canal

The anal canal measures 2–3 cm in length. It extends from the perineal skin to the lower end of the rectum which is at the upper border of the internal sphincter at the anorectal ring. The junction between the anal canal and the perineal skin is known

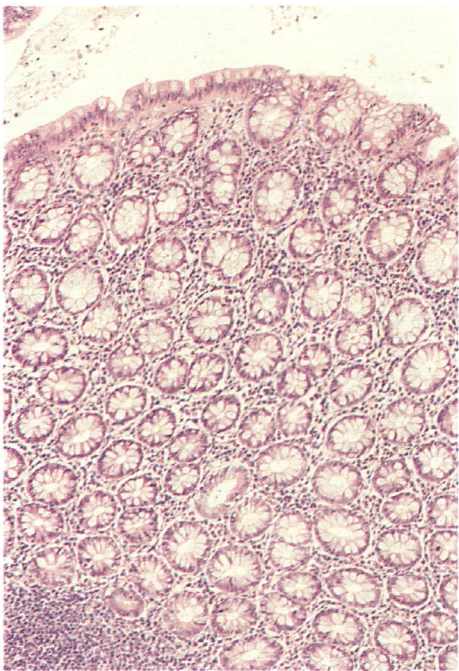

Fig. 16.69 A high-power view of the mucosa of the appendix showing many crypts cut in transverse section. Several of the crypts appear to be paired. This is the result of branching, which is common in the appendiceal mucosa.

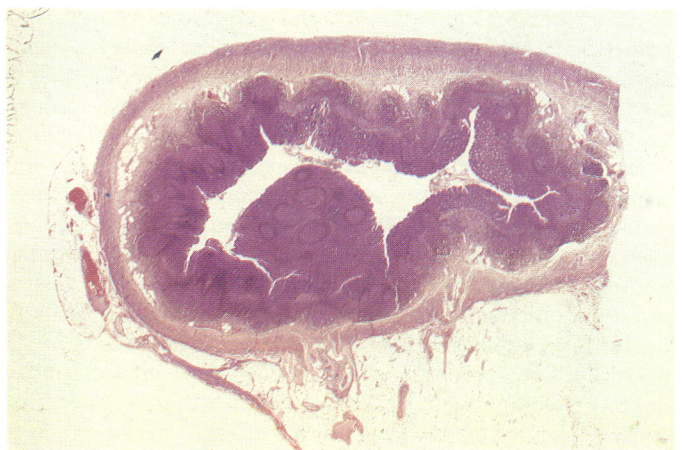

Fig. 16.70 A low-power view of a longitudinal section of the tip of the appendix, showing abundant lymphoid tissue.

as the anal verge. The dentate or pectinate line marks the junction between the anal canal and the rectum.

The lining of the anal canal varies throughout its length and is often described as a transitional mucosa or zone since its histology is variable (Fig. 16.71). In its upper part it is normal colorectal mucosa. There is then an area with scattered crypts between which the surface epithelium may be simple columnar, or a variety of non-keratinized squamous epithelium. Keratinized stratified squamous epithelium is found at the lower end of the anal canal. Melanin-containing cells are a regular finding in the squamous epithelium below the dentate line (Figs 16.72, 16.73).

The muscularis mucosae disappears at the pectinate line. The submucosa is highly vascular and contains the haemorrhoidal plexus. The veins in this plexus are particularly prone to develop varicosities.

The circular layer of the muscularis propria becomes thick-

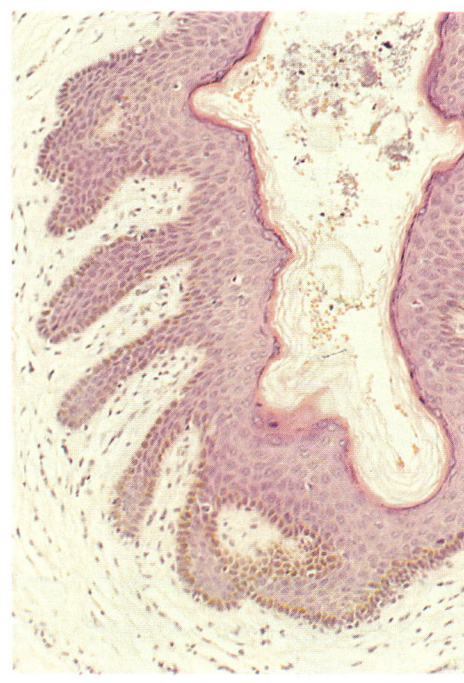

Fig. 16.72 The keratinized stratified squamous epithelium of the perianal skin.

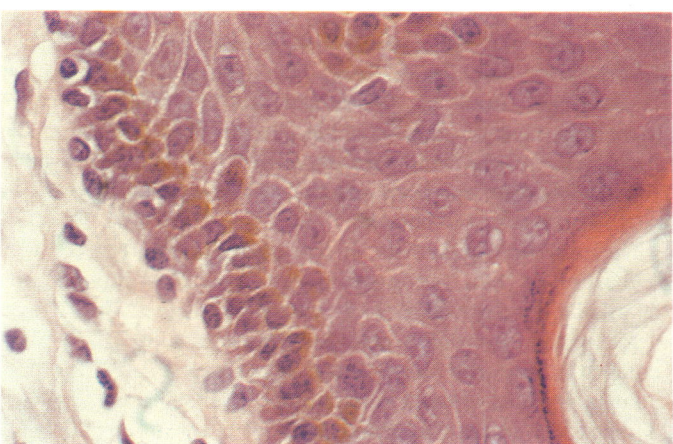

Fig. 16.73 A higher-power view of Fig. 16.72 showing the presence of melanin granules in the basal cells.

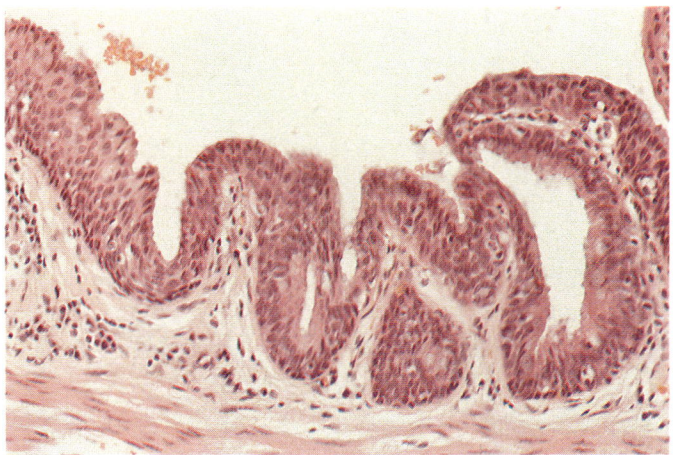

Fig. 16.71 Anal mucosa, the epithelium of which is transitional between the simple columnar epithelium of the rectum and the stratified squamous epithelium of the perineal skin.

ened to form the internal sphincter. The external sphincter is made of voluntary muscle arranged in three main groups: the subcutaneous, the superficial, and the deep or external sphincters. Between these groups strands of muscle derived from the longitudinal muscle layer of the rectum are found. The puborectalis muscle loops behind the bowel at the level of the anorectal ring.

The anal canal is the seat of faecal continence. Normally the anal canal is closed because of contraction of the internal sphincter. Rectal distension with faeces elicits a sensation signalling the urge to defaecation. Voluntary contraction of the external sphincter overcomes this reflex if social conditions are unfavourable but when a convenient time for defaecation is found it is accomplished by a series of voluntary and involuntary motions.

The blood supply to the anal canal is a watershed between the inferior mesenteric artery and the middle rectal vessels. The former drain via the portal venous system, the latter via the systemic venous system. The lymphatic drainage similarly exhibits a duality. The upper half of the canal drains to the lumbar nodes, while the lower half of the canal drains to the inguinal nodes.

Sympathetic nerve fibres to the anal canal arise from the inferior mesenteric ganglion. Parasympathetic fibres arise from the sacral cord. These fibres serve the emptying reflex and are antagonistic to the sympathetic fibres. The area below the dentate line has a rich plexus of sensory nerves which account for its extreme sensitivity.

16.6   Neuroendocrine system of the gut

J. M. Polak and S. R. Bloom

16.6.1   Introduction

The concept that the gastrointestinal tract carries out solely digestive functions was challenged at the turn of the century by the discovery, made by Bayliss and Starling, that extracts of duodenum elicit the release of bicarbonate from the pancreas. The concept of chemical substances acting at a distance from their site of origin was born and the name hormone (I arouse to activity) was then introduced.

The mucosal epithelium of the gastrointestinal tract was shown, more than 100 years ago, to contain scattered cells identifiable by their affinity for certain histological dyes. They were termed chromaffin cells by Heidenhain in 1870. Subsequently, these cells were found to correspond to those previously observed to react with ammoniacal solutions of silver. Modifications of silver-staining methods allowed the subclassification of enteroendocrine cells as either argentaffin or argyrophil, depending upon their ability to reduce silver ions alone or in the presence of a reducing agent, respectively. A considerable amount of research was dedicated to the discovery of the nature of the reducing substance (then termed enteramine) present in the argentaffin, so-called enterochromaffin (EC) cells. Eventually, pioneering work by Erspamer and associates led to the isolation from the cells of 5-hydroxytryptamine (5-HT), which was found to be identical to the previously described, vasoconstrictor substance, serotonin.

In addition, in the 1930s, Feyrter described gut endocrine cells as elements dispersed diffusely throughout the lining epithelium of the entire gastrointestinal tract. Feyrter observed the existence of similar cells in many other tissues of the body and thus introduced the concept of the 'diffuse endocrine system'.

The close anatomical and functional connections between this diffuse endocrine system and the autonomic/sensory nervous systems has led to the expansion of Feyrter's concept to that of a 'diffuse neuroendocrine system'. This system was also investigated extensively by Pearse, who described a number of common histochemical and functional properties for the components of the diffuse neuroendocrine system and grouped them under the heading of APUD (amine precursor uptake and decarboxylation) cells. Pearse also suggested a possible common neuroectodermal origin for the endocrine cells of the gastrointestinal tract and elsewhere. Although endocrine cells of tissues other than the gastrointestinal tract and pancreas (e.g. thyroid C cells, adrenomedullary cells) have an undisputed neuroectodermal origin, the general view is that the endocrine cells of the gut and pancreas originate from pluripotent endodermal cells.

Endocrine cells have a flask-shaped appearance, with the narrower end terminating in characteristic microvilli at the lumen of the gut and the secretory granules lying towards the basement membrane, where there are sometimes long basal processes. Numerous techniques are available nowadays for the identification of the endocrine cells of the gastrointestinal tract. These include the original methods of masked metachromasia, lead haematoxylin, and a variety of silver-impregnation methods (Fig. 16.74). Immunostaining using antibodies to 'general endocrine' markers are being used increasingly for the demonstration of gut endocrine cells. For example, antibodies to chromogranin (for details see Section 16.17) are particularly useful in demonstrating the entire endocrine apparatus of the gut. Ultrastructurally, the endocrine cells display a characteristic morphology, including the presence of specialized microvilli and electron-dense secretory granules, which are the storage site of peptide/amines as well as other substances. The secretory granules are morphologically heterogeneous and this permits differentiation between various endocrine cell types

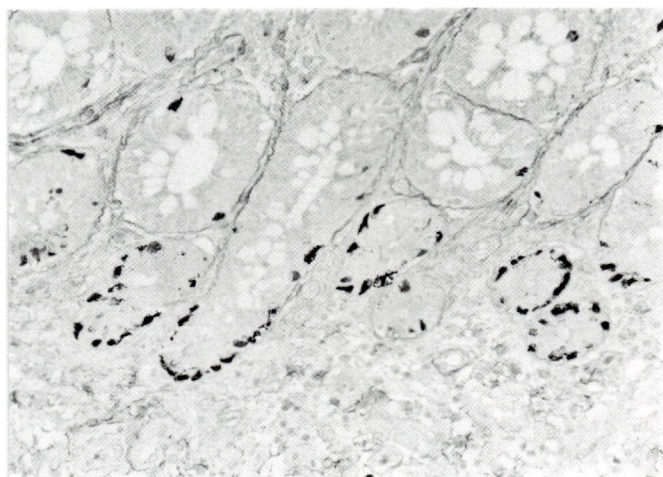

Fig. 16.74 Section of human small intestine with numerous argyrophil endocrine cells visualized by Grimelius' silver impregnation method. (Bouin's solution-fixed, 5 μm wax section.)

according to their granule size, electron density, and characteristics of the limiting membrane (Fig. 16.75).

Immunocytochemistry, applied both at light (Fig. 16.76) and electron microscopical levels (Figs 16.77, 16.78) and using specific peptide antibodies, permits a more 'functional' classifica-

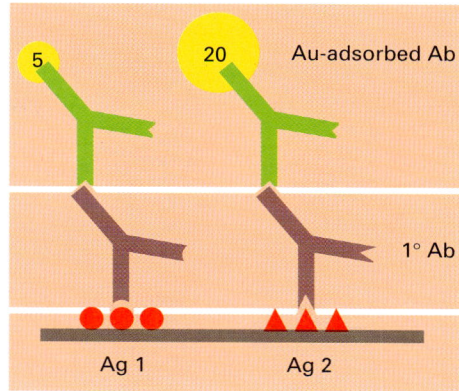

Fig. 16.77 Diagrammatic representation of the immunogold staining technique for electron microscopy. Visualization of the sites of attachment of primary (1°) antibodies (Ab) is achieved using second-layer antibodies labelled with colloidal gold adsorbed onto the Fc portion of the immunoglobulin molecule. Gold particles of different sizes can be used, e.g. 5 nm or 20 nm diameter, as shown.

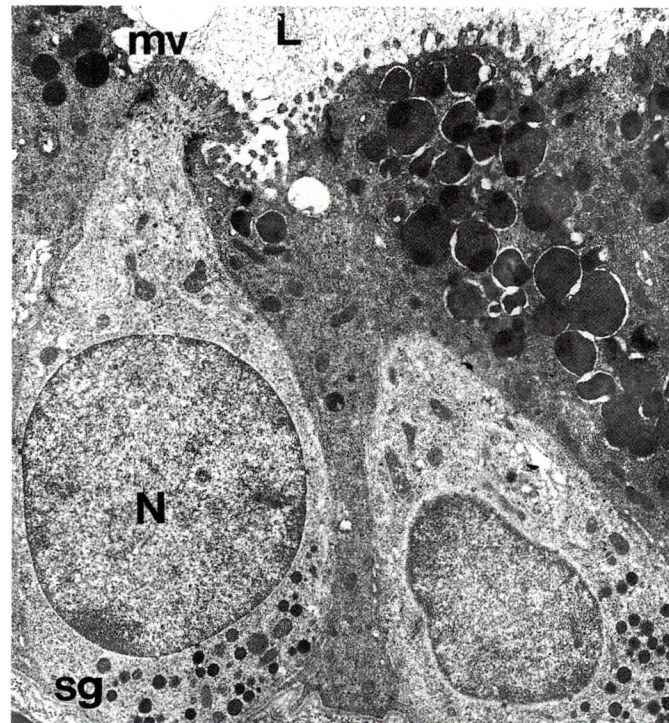

Fig. 16.75 Conventional electron micrograph of endocrine cells in human gastric mucosa. The cell on the left has been sectioned along its entire length. Microvilli (mv) can be seen projecting into the lumen (L). Secretory granules (sg) show a typical localization at the base of the cell. N = nucleus. (Glutaraldhyde-fixed, ultrathin Araldite section.)

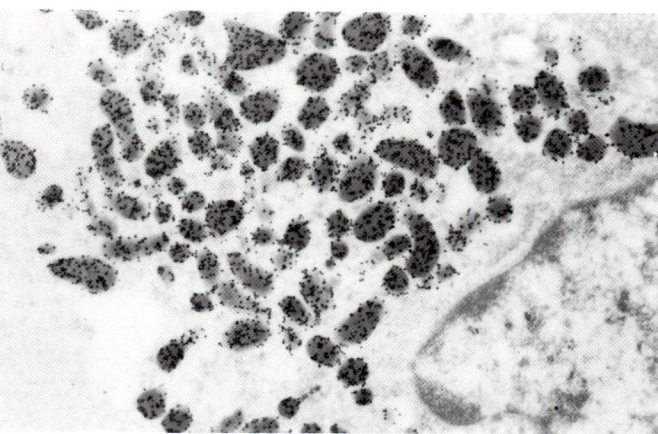

Fig. 16.78 An electron micrograph of a human enterochromaffin cell immunostained for chromogranin using the immunogold method described in Fig. 16.77. (Glutaraldehyde-fixed, ultrathin Araldite section.)

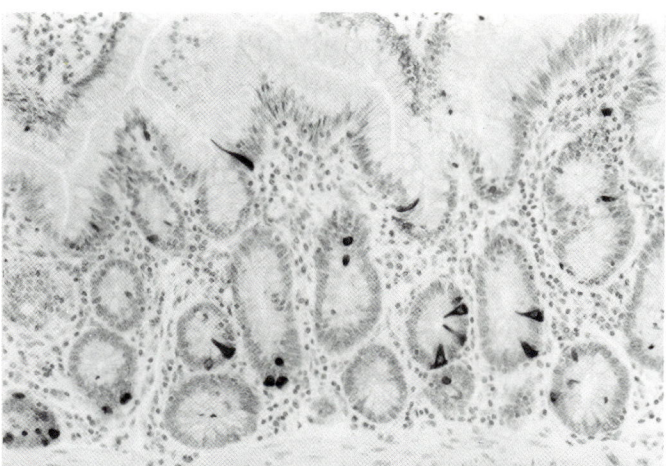

Fig. 16.76 Numerous endocrine cells scattered in the mucosal epithelium of human small intestine, demonstrated by immunostaining of the general endocrine cell marker chromogranin. (Bouin's solution-fixed, 5 μm wax section, peroxidase anti-peroxidase technique.)

tion of the endocrine cells of the gastrointestinal tract. Many types of endocrine cells of the gastrointestinal tract are now fully recognized, and correlative studies of light and electron microscopical immunocytochemistry permit their classification. The latest international classification of endocrine cells of the gastrointestinal tract was agreed in Cambridge in 1980. This correlates well with quantitative data provided by radioimmunoassay of tissue extracts. Using this technique it is possible to group the various extractable 'gut hormones' according to their anatomical distributions. For details of the most established gut peptides see Tables 16.4 and 16.5.

Gut functions are also regulated by enteric nerves of parasympathetic, sympathetic, and sensory nature. Until recently, it was only possible to visualize individual types of nerves at a given time, for example, by applying enzyme histochemistry

Table 16.4 Gut hormones, main distributions

Peptide	Cell type	No. of amino acids	Secretory granules mean diam. (nm)	Main actions	Fundus	Antrum	Duodenum	Jejunum	Ileum	Colon	Rectum
Gastrin	G	17	360	Gastric acid secretion		+	+				
	IG	34	175			+	+	+			
Somatostatin	D	28	310	Multiple inhibitory effects	+	+	+	+	+	+	+
Secretin	S	27	240	Pancreatic bicarbonate secretion			+	+			
Motilin	M	32	180	Motility			+	+			
CCK	I	34	250	Pancreatic enzyme secretion			+	+			
GIP	K	43	350	Insulinotropic			+	+			
Neurotensin	N	13	300	Hypotension					+		
Glucagon	EG	69	210	Gut metabolism and growth					+	+	+
PYY	EG	36	210	Inhibition of gastric acid and motility					+	+	+

CCK, cholecystokinin; GIP, gastric inhibitory polypeptide; pyy, peptide yy.

Table 16.5 Gut neuropeptides, distributed throughout the gastrointestinal tract

Peptide	No. of amino acids	Secretary granules mean diam. (nm)	Main actions	Main origin(s)
Bombesin (GRP)	27	NK	Multiple stimulatory effects, e.g. gastrin release	Local
CGRP	37	40	Gastric acid secretion, muscle constriction	Local and sensory
Galanin	29	NK	Muscle constriction	Local
Leu-enkephalin	5	83	Opiate effects	Local
Met-enkephalin	5	83	Opiate effects	Local
Neuromedin U	8 or 25	70	Muscle constriction, vasoconstriction	Local
NPY	36	85	Vasoconstriction	Local and sympathetic
PHM	27	90	Muscle relaxation, secretion	Local
Somatostatin	28	92	Inhibitory	Local
Substance P	11	82	Vasodilation, muscle constriction	Local and sensory
VIP	28	90	Vasodilation, muscle relaxation, secretion	Local

CGRP, calcitonin gene-related peptide; NPY, neuropeptide tyrosine; PHM, peptide histidine methionine; VIP, vasoactive intestinal polypeptide; NK, not known.

(cholinesterase staining) it was possible to demonstrate presumed cholinergic nerves or, by applying formaldehyde-induced fluorescence methods, it was possible to demonstrate sympathetic nerves. Nowadays, the use of antibodies to so-called neural markers, e.g. protein gene product (PGP) 9.5, neuron-specific enolase, or neurofilament triplet proteins permits the delineation of the entire enteric nervous system, the various subcomponents of which can then be demonstrated using either classical histochemical methods or specific antibodies to peptides. The latter are very useful since numerous peptides have been found to be present in enteric nerves. These include vasoactive intestinal polypeptide (VIP), the neurokinins, calcitonin gene-related peptide (CGRP), neuropeptide tyrosine (NPY), peptide histidine methionine (PHM), and bombesin. These peptides are found in parasympathetic, sympathetic, and sensory nerves (see Table 16.5, Figs 16.79, 16.80). Enteric nerves permeate all layers of the bowel and are characterized by an intermingled mesh of varicose nerve fibres, innervating vascular and non-vascular smooth muscle, mucosa, and

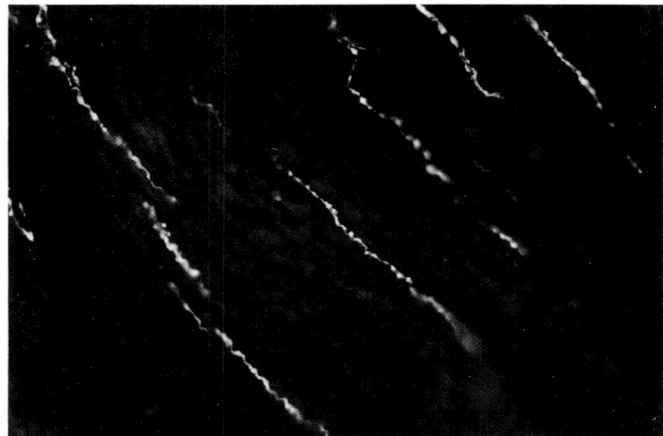

Fig. 16.79 VIP-containing nerves immunostained by the indirect immunofluorescence technique in a thick section of the smooth muscle coat of the rat colon. (Benzoquinone solution-fixed, 10 μm cryostat section.)

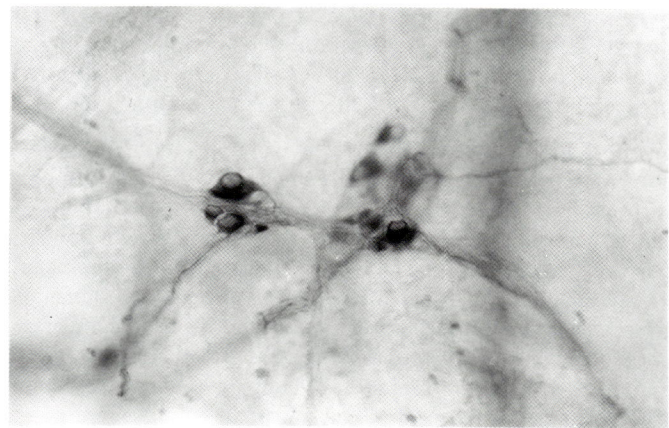

Fig. 16.80 A whole-mount preparation of the submucosa of the human colon immunostained for VIP. The submucous plexus can be seen, with numerous VIP-containing nerve fibres and ganglion cell bodies. (Benzoquinone solution-fixed tissue, peroxidase antiperoxidase technique.)

lamina propria. Peptide-containing perikarya are found in the two main ganglionated plexuses of the bowel.

16.6.2 Non-neoplastic conditions

(Neoplasms are discussed in Section 16.17.) Under this heading, a number of disease situations will be discussed in which an abnormal pattern of regulatory peptides has been detected.

Changes in circulating gut hormones (gut hormone profile)

Hormone levels have been investigated comprehensively in a wide variety of conditions using a standardized immunoassay technique. These levels reflect quite accurately the anatomical origin of a given diseased area of the gastrointestinal tract (Figs 16.81–16.84).

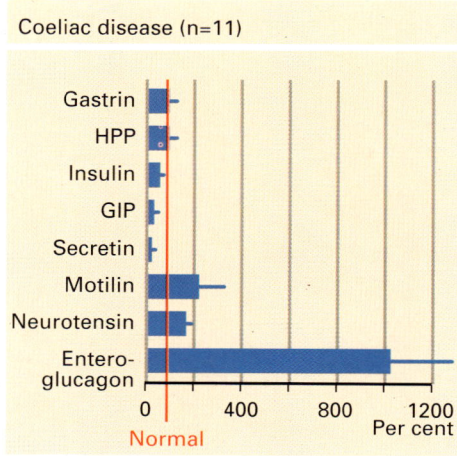

Fig. 16.81 The total three-hour integrated incremental hormone release after a 530 kcal breakfast in 11 subjects with active coeliac disease, expressed as the percentage of the mean normal response seen in healthy individuals.

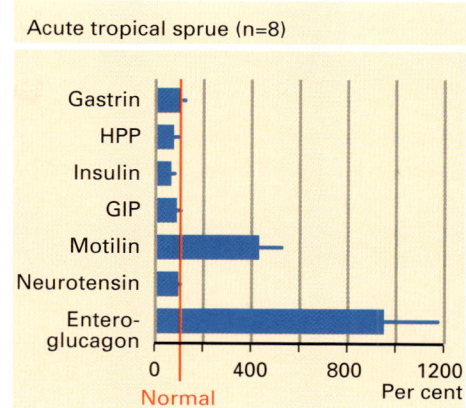

Fig. 16.82 The three-hour total integrated incremental hormone release following a 530 kcal mixed test breakfast in eight subjects suffering from acute tropical sprue (tropical malabsorption), expressed as the percentage of the mean normal response in healthy volunteers.

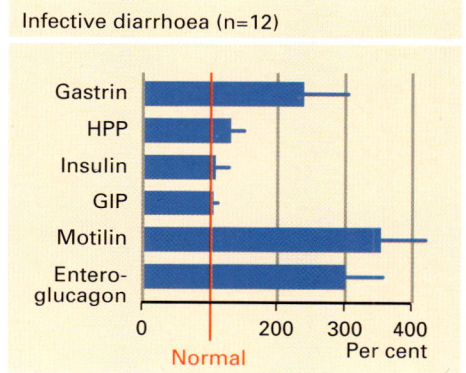

Fig. 16.83 The three-hour total integrated incremental plasma hormone release following a 530 kcal mixed test breakfast in 12 subjects suffering from acute infective diarrhoea, expressed as the percentage of the mean normal response in healthy individuals.

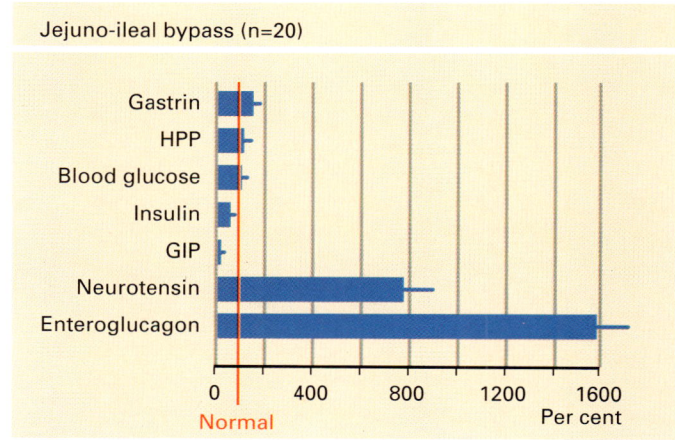

Fig. 16.84 The three-hour total integrated incremental hormone response following a 530 kcal mixed test breakfast in 20 subjects who had undergone 7" jejuno to 7" ileal gut bypass procedure as therapy for morbid obesity, expressed as the percentage of the mean normal response in healthy volunteers.

Endocrine cell abnormalities

Hyperplasia of endocrine cells has been found in a number of situations. These include the following:

Generalized endocrine cell hyperplasia

Hyperplastic endocrine cell changes, as delineated by immunostaining using the general endocrine cell marker chromogranin, have been noted in some diseases of the bowel, e.g. Crohn's disease (Fig. 16.85) and coeliac disease.

Hyperplasia of specific cell types

Gastrin (G) cells The entity of G-cell hyperplasia (Fig. 16.86) was first discovered using immunocytochemistry. Subsequently, functional studies were carried out and the condition has now been recognized to be a combined G-cell

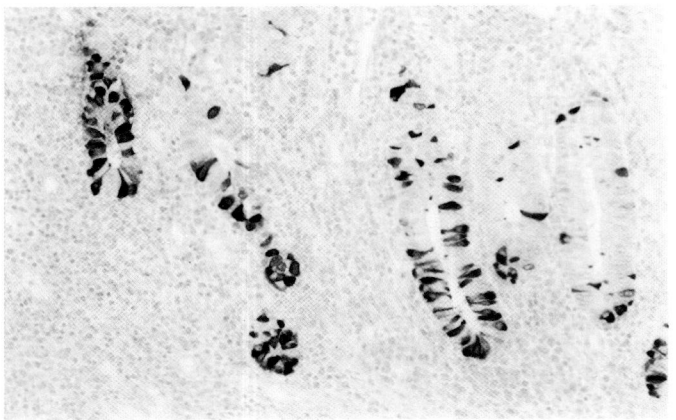

Fig. 16.85 Human ileal mucosal cells from a patient with Crohn's disease, immunostained for chromogranin. Chronic inflammatory changes can be seen in the lamina propria and, in the epithelium, abnormally high numbers of endocrine cells can be seen packed together. (Bouin's solution-fixed, 5 μm wax section, peroxidase antiperoxidase method.)

hyperplasia/hyperfunction. G-cell hyperplasia can be found in severe cases of duodenal ulceration, with symptoms closely resembling those of gastrinoma (although no tumour is found), or in atrophic gastritis with or without pernicious anaemia.

Secretin and CCK cells The presence of abnormally numerous immunoreactive endocrine cells in coeliac disease has been reported frequently. The findings of so-called secretin and CCK-cell hyperplasia are particularly relevant in this condition. It has been recognized for some time that anatomical abnormalities of the duodenal mucosa lead to an impairment of hormone release by intraluminal stimuli. Consequently, pancreatic bicarbonate and enzyme secretion is defective. By contrast, if secretin and CCK are administered intravenously the pancreatic response is normal. These findings suggest an impairment of gut hormone release in patients with coeliac disease, which explains the strongly immunostained endocrine cells previously interpreted as being hyperplastic. These findings fit in well with dynamic studies which indicate an impairment of hormone release after normal intraduodenal acid stimulus. Other endocrine cells have also been shown to be hyperplastic in this condition.

Enterochromaffin-like (ECL) cells A characteristic endocrine cell type has been reported to be present in the fundic mucosa. This cell, having a typically elongated shape with no luminal contact, was named the enterochromaffin-like (EC-like/ECL) cell. The peptide amine product of these cells, which contain characteristic secretory granules, is as yet unknown, but EC-like cells are stained by Sevier–Munger silver impregnation staining (Fig. 16.87). These cells have been shown to be sensitive to elevated gastrin levels, either due to hyperfunction of G-cells or the existence of a gastrinoma. In addition, exaggerated gastrin release from G-cells, resulting from the lack of gastric acid secretion (as is seen in pernicious anaemia), can lead to EC-like cell hyperplasia and subsequent micronodule and carcinoid tumour formation. These findings are becoming increasingly common as drugs capable of producing maximum gastric acid suppression (e.g. a new generation of H_2-receptor

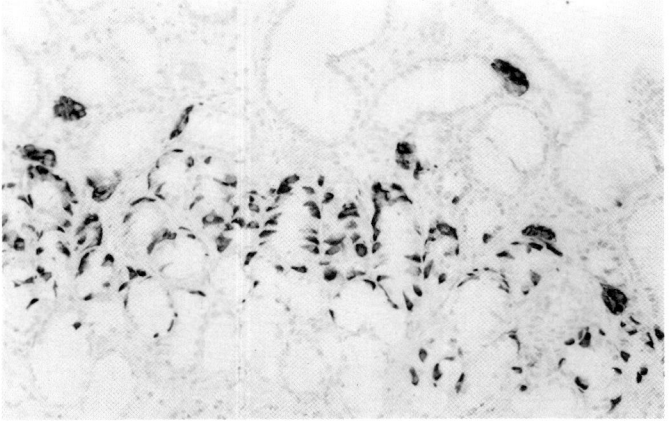

Fig. 16.86 A hyperplasia of gastrin cells in the antral mucosa of a patient with pernicious anaemia (achlorhydria). The cells can be seen to have formed abnormal clumps. (Bouin's solution-fixed, 5 μm wax section.)

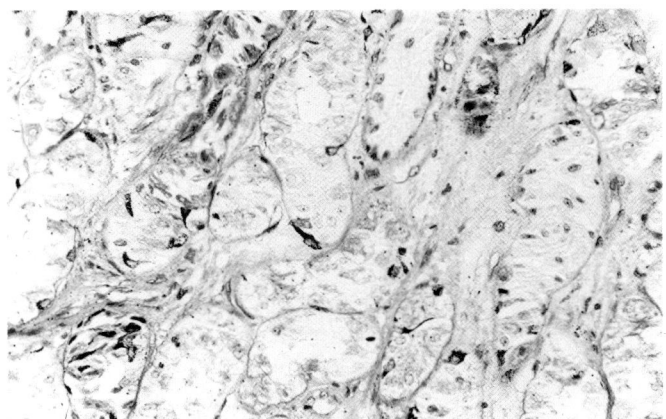

Fig. 16.87 Enterochromaffin-like cells demonstrated in the fundic mucosa of the human stomach, using the silver impregnation technique of Sevier and Munger. (Bouin's solution-fixed, 5 μm wax section.)

blockers, proton pump inhibitors, etc.) are now available for the treatment of duodenal ulceration and other hypersecretory conditions. These drugs, taken long-term, produce a complete blockade of gastric acid secretion and consequent oversecretion by G-cells, leading to chronically elevated circulating gastrin levels.

Glucagon-immunoreactive (EG) cells Hyperplasia and hyperactivity of EG cells has been found in situations of gut repair, e.g. intestinal resection.

Somatostatin cells A case of extreme somatostatin cell hyperplasia of the gastroduodenal mucosa, causing dwarfism, obesity, and goitre, has been described.

Hypoplasia of endocrine cells

Somatostatin cells, in particular, have been reported to undergo hypoplastic changes. They have been shown to be decreased in certain patients with excess gastric acid secretion and duodenal ulceration.

Neural abnormalities

Inflammatory bowel disease/Crohn's disease

Hyperplastic changes in nerves have been reported frequently to occur in the bowel of patients with Crohn's disease. These changes have now been shown to be due to abnormalities of the VIP/PHI-containing component of the enteric nervous system. VIP/PHI-containing nerves appear markedly hyperplastic, distorted, and brightly immunostained (Fig. 16.88). Since these changes are particularly evident in the mucosa and lamina propria, it has been suggested that VIP/PHI immunostaining could be a useful tool for diagnosing inflammatory bowel disease in endoscopic biopsies.

Chronic, intractable constipation

Peptidergic nerves of local origin (e.g. those containing VIP or substance P) have been shown to be present in abnormally low levels in diseases of the bowel associated with intractable chronic constipation and absence or degeneration of intrinsic neuronal cell bodies, e.g. Chagas' disease, Hirschsprung's disease, and grass sickness in the horse. By contrast, peptide-containing nerves of extrinsic origin (e.g. sympathetic nerves containing NPY), appear more numerous and densely immunostained. Normal levels of enteric peptide-containing nerves appear to be present in a generalized autonomic neuropathy, like that of the Shy–Drager syndrome, which shows no involvement of gut neuronal cell bodies.

16.6.3 Further reading

Bishop, A. E., Ferri, G. L., Probert, L., Bloom, S. R., and Polak, J. M. (1982). Peptidergic nerves. *Scandinavian Journal of Gastroenterology* **17**, 43–59.

Bloom, S. R. and Polak, J. M. (eds) (1981). Hormone profiles. In *Gut hormones* (2nd edn), pp. 555–60. Churchill Livingstone, Edinburgh.

Llewellyn-Smith, I. J. (1987). Neuropeptides and the microcircuitry of the enteric nervous system. *Experientia* **43**, 813–20.

Pearse, A. G. E. (1969). The cytochemistry and ultrastructure of polypeptide hormone-producing cells of the APUD series, and the embryologic, physiologic and pathologic implications of the concept. *Journal of Histochemistry and Cytochemistry* **17**, 303–13.

Polak, J. M. and Bloom, S. R. (1979). The diffuse neuroendocrine system. *Journal of Histochemistry and Cytochemistry* **27**, 1398–400.

Polak, J. M. and Bloom, S. R. (eds) (1985). *Endocrine tumours*. Churchill Livingstone, Edinburgh.

Solcia, E., Polak, J. M., Larsson, L.-I., Buchan, A. M. J., and Capella, C. (1981). Update on Lausanne classification of endocrine cells. In *Gut hormone* (2nd edn) (ed. S. R. Bloom and J. M. Polak), pp. 96–100. Churchill Livingstone, Edinburgh.

16.7 Congenital abnormalities of the small and large intestine

J. W. Keeling

16.7.1 Abnormalities of rotation

The normal process of intestinal rotation begins during the period of physiological intestinal herniation (15–48 mm stage) when most of the intestines lie in the extra-embryonic coelom, and is completed after the intestines return to the abdominal cavity. Failure of rotation may be complete (*non-rotation*) or, more usually, partial (*malrotation*).

Non-rotation

Non-rotation of the intestines accompanies exomphalos when part of the intestine fails to return to the abdominal cavity, and results in a diaphragmatic hernia. It is sometimes an incidental finding at surgery or necropsy. The normal 'C' configuration of

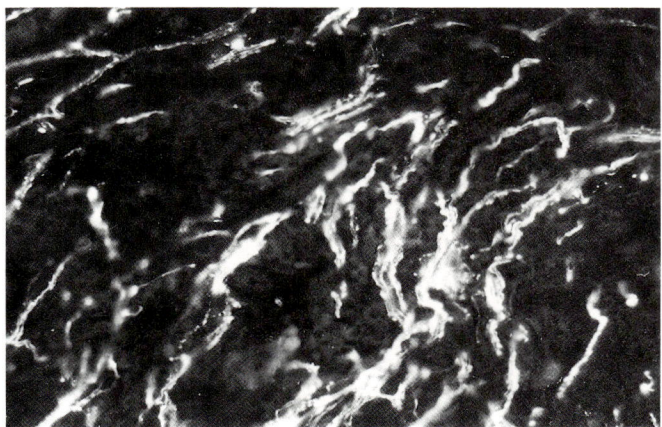

Fig. 16.88 Abnormally numerous, VIP-containing nerve fibres in the submucosa of the ileum taken from a patient with Crohn's disease. (Benzoquinone solution-fixed 10 μm cryostat section, indirect immunofluorescence.)

the duodenum is absent, the distal duodenum runs downwards, the small intestine lies in the right side of the abdominal cavity with caecum and colon to the left (Fig. 16.89).

Malrotation

Malrotation or incomplete intestinal rotation, occurs when coecal descent is arrested at any point along its normal route from the epigastrium anterior to the duodenum to the right iliac fossa. Failure of descent of the caecum reduces the length of the mesenteric root of the small intestine. This enhances the mobility of loops of small intestine and renders them liable to volvulus. Extrinsic duodenal obstruction can complicate malrotation. It can arise in two ways, either when the caecum lies directly in front of it, or as a result of peritoneal bands (Ladd's bands) running to the caecum when it lies just below the liver.

Malrotation occurs more frequently in individuals with autosomal trisomy (particularly of chromosomes 13, 18, and 21) and is part of some malformation syndromes.

16.7.2   Abnormalities due to persisting remnants

Vitello-intestinal remnants

A variety of anomalies result from persistence of all or part of the vitello-intestinal (omphalo-mesentertic) duct. This duct, the communication between mid-gut and yolk sac in the embryo, forms the apex of the herniated mid-gut loop. It normally becomes occluded and divides before the intestines return to the abdominal cavity. The defects are illustrated diagramatically (Fig. 16.90). Meckel's diverticulum accounts for 90 per cent of these anomalies, the rest are uncommon.

Meckel's diverticulum

Meckel's diverticulum is the commonest gastrointestinal congenital anomaly. It is present in 2–3 per cent of the population and represents persistence of the intestinal end of the duct.

This diverticulum is situated on the antimesenteric border of the terminal ileum. It is of similar construction and diameter to the ileum and their muscle coats are in continuity. Its mucosal lining is of small intestinal type, but focal heterotopic gastric mucosa is common. Gastric heterotopia are found in about half of surgically resected diverticula and 80 per cent of symptomatic cases. Gastric secretion by the heterotopic mucosa can produce peptic ulceration either within the diverticulum or in the ileum distal to it. These ulcers often bleed profusely. Perforation and its sequelae of adhesions or peritonitis is less common. Meckel's diverticulum may become the apex of an intussusception. It is occasionally the site of origin of tumour; carcinoid is the commonest tumour type. Complication of Meckel's diverticula are tabulated (Table 16.6).

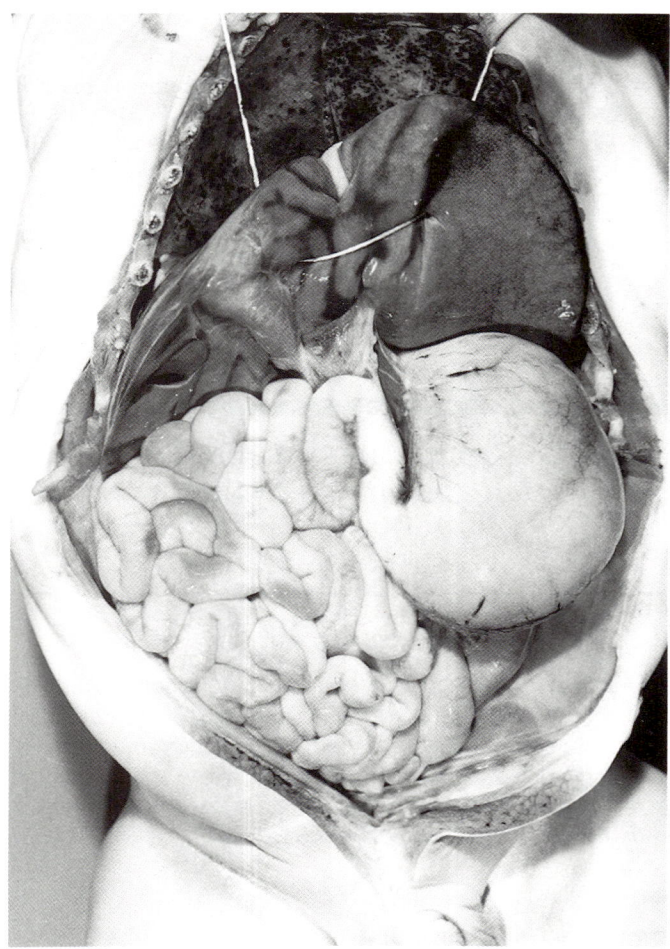

Fig. 16.89 Non-rotation of the intestines, small intestinal loops occupy the right side of the peritoneal cavity; incidental necropsy finding. (Reproduced from Keeling 1988, with permission.)

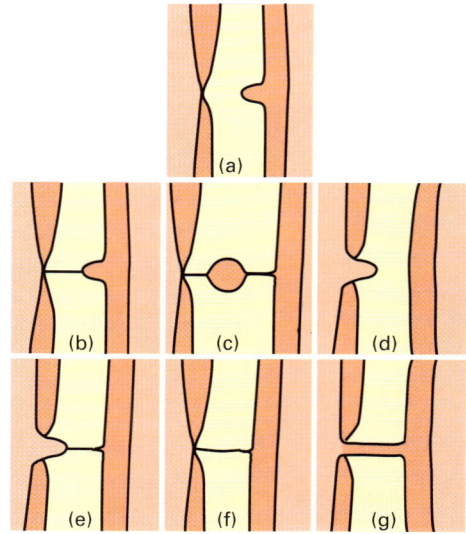

Fig. 16.90 Vitello-intestinal duct remnants: (a) Meckel's diverticulum; (b) diverticulum with fibrous cord; (c) enterocystoma; (d) umbilical sinus; (e) sinus with cord; (f) fibrous cord; (g) vitello-intestinal fistula.

Table 16.6 Complications of Meckel's diverticula

Presentation	Soderlund (1959)		Weinstein et al. (1962)
	Total	Children	
Peptic ulcer/haemorrhage	40	36	63
Bands/volvulus	40	28	28
Diverticulitis	24	13	29
Intussusception	19	19	15
Hernia	4	4	9
Umbilical fistula	15	15	8
Neoplasm	—		10
Total symptomatic	142	115	162
Incidental finding	271		560
Total	413		722

Intestinal duplication cysts (dorsal eneteric remnant)

Intestinal duplication are cystic structures lined by functional intestinal mucosa surrounded by smooth muscle. They may be spherical or cylindrical in shape and situated dorsal to the intestine at any point from the spinal cord to within the muscularis propria of the intestine, although most lie within the mesentery. Duplications can occur at any level of the gastrointestinal tract but about 50 per cent affect the small intestine, usually the terminal ileum. Cystic duplications vary in size from a few millimetres to 10–15 cm in diameter, tubular duplications can achieve a length of more than 30 cm. Increasing size is the result of mucus secretion into the lumen. They develop as a result of incomplete separation of the gut tube from the notocord leaving rests of endodermal cells along the line of normal gut migration.

Clinical presentation is often related to intestinal obstruction either because the intestine becomes stretched over the cyst (Fig. 16.91) or when a small, intramural cyst becomes the apex of an intussusception.

Cysts are usually lined by mucosa appropriate to the level of intestine at which they develop, but like Meckel's diverticula, they contain heterotopic gastric mucosa.

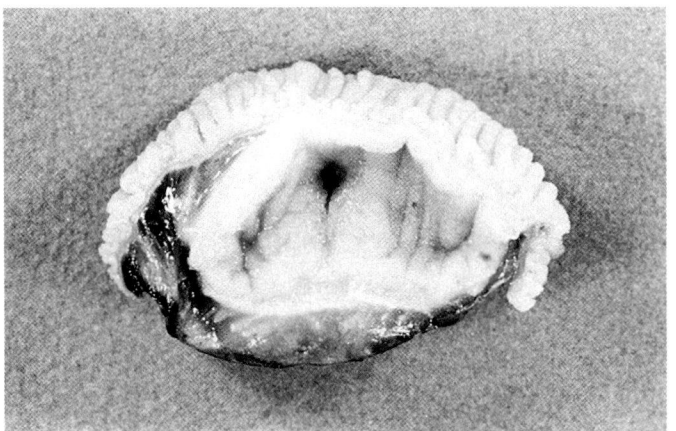

Fig. 16.91 Duplication cyst: small intestine is stretched over the cyst, there is a central communication with the intestinal lumen.

16.7.3 Intestinal atresia and stenosis

Intestinal atresia is a loss of continuity of the bowel lumen, either as a result of a diaphragm internal to the muscularis propria or because of loss of continuity between adjacent segments.

Atresia occurs most commonly in the duodenum (approximately 1/5000 live births), less commonly in the jejunum and ileum (together 1/6000 live births) and rarely in the colon. Stenosis is less common that atresia at any particular site and usually takes the form of a diaphragm with a small, central meatus.

Only in the duodenum is atresia the expression of disordered embryogenesis; at other sites it is the result of an intra-uterine catastrophe, usually of ischaemic origin, affecting a normally developed viscus. Supportive evidence for differing origins of atresia in different regions of the intestine is the co-existence of annular pancreas, the high incidence of other congenital anomalies, particularly tracheo-oesophageal fistula and congenital heart disease, and chromosomal abnormalities in babies with duodenal atresia. The abnormalities which predispose to intestinal volvulus, such as intestinal malrotation, gastroschisis, or meconium ileus, are common in babies with jejunal and ileal atresia. Furthermore, the presence of squamous debris and lanugo hairs in meconium distal to the obstruction indicates the patency of the mid-gut in the first half of the pregnancy. Jejunal and ileal defects have been produced in fetal animals by ligating branches of the superior mesenteric artery and allowing pregnancy to continue.

The usual presentation of duodenal atresia is vomiting when feeding is commenced. Radiographically, a double-bubble of gas is seen in the distended stomach and proximal duodenum separated by the pylorus (Fig. 16.92). Duodenal atresia may be diagnosed prenatally by ultrasound examination undertaken because of raised maternal serum α-fetal protein level. In the third trimester of pregnancy it may cause polyhydramnios because of defective fetal swallowing. Jejunal and ileal atresia present with abdominal distension and vomiting in the neonatal period. Peristalsis may be visible through the abdominal wall.

Types of intestinal atresia are illustrated diagramatically (Fig. 16.93). In the jejunum and ileum, type C is the most common (Fig. 16.94) and atresia is commonly multiple.

16.7.4 Volvulus

Torsion of loops of small intestine which disrupts local circulation leading to ischaemia and gangrene of the bowel can complicate a variety of abdominal malformations. It can occur prenatally and result in intestinal atresia or congenital short intestine, or in early life causing intestinal obstruction or abdominal pain. Predisposing conditions are malrotation, where a short mesenteric pedicle renders bowel loops unduly mobile, internal herniae, and intra-abdominal bands such as vitellointestinal remnants and various abdominal wall defects. Local intestinal abnormalities, such as duplications and abnormal

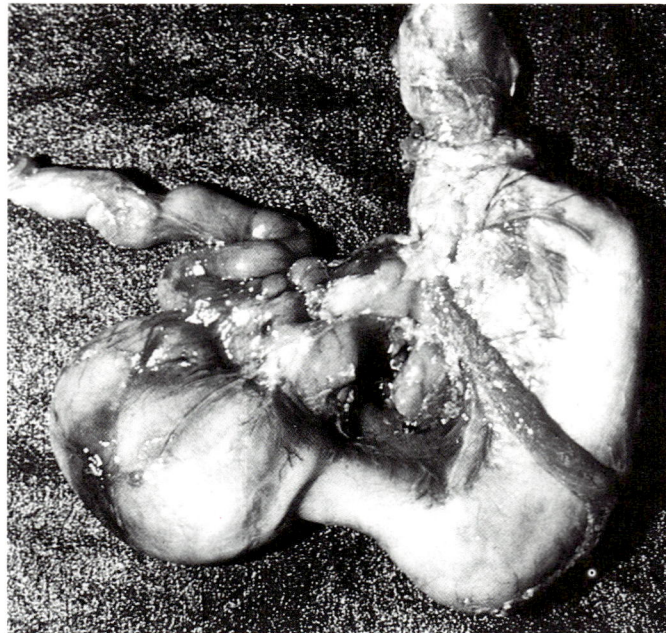

Fig. 16.92 Duodenal atresia: the proximal duodenum is very distended.

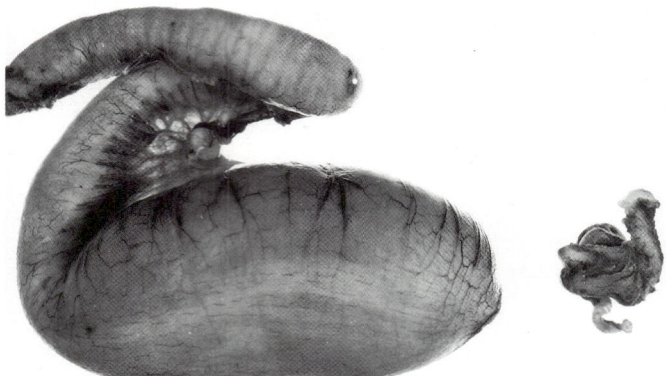

Fig. 16.94 Ileal atresia type C: proximal ileum is distended, distal loop is very narrow.

fective innervation of the distal intestine evidenced by absence of ganglion cells in both myenteric and submucosal plexuses, with hypertrophied nerve trunks within the plexus in rectum and sigmoid colon. The innervation defect interrupts intestinal peristalsis and effects a functional obstruction. The dilated, hypertrophied bowel is normally innervated, the aganglionic segment is of narrow calibre.

In 82 per cent of cases, aganglionosis is limited to the sigmoid colon and rectum (short segment disease). Four per cent of cases involve the ascending colon, in 13 per cent the whole colon is involved, and 1 per cent involves the whole of the small and large intestine (Fig. 16.95).

Diagnosis is made on rectal biopsy by absence of ganglion

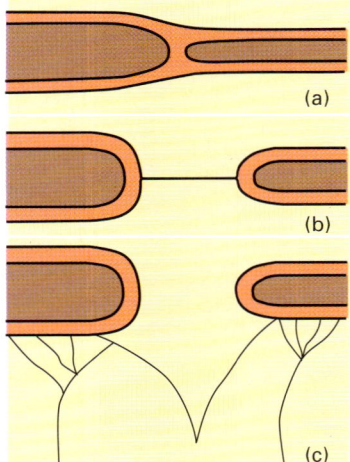

Fig. 16.93 Intestinal atresia: (a) lumen interrupted by musocal diaphragm; (b) loss of continuity of muscularis propria ends joined by fibrous cord; (c) gap between bowel loops and mesenteric defect.

intestinal contents as found in meconium ileus, also predispose to volvulus.

16.7.5 Neuronal abnormalities

Hirschsprung's disease

Hirschsprung described severe constipation from birth associated with megacolon sometimes progressing to fatal intestinal obstruction. Many years later, the defect was identified as de-

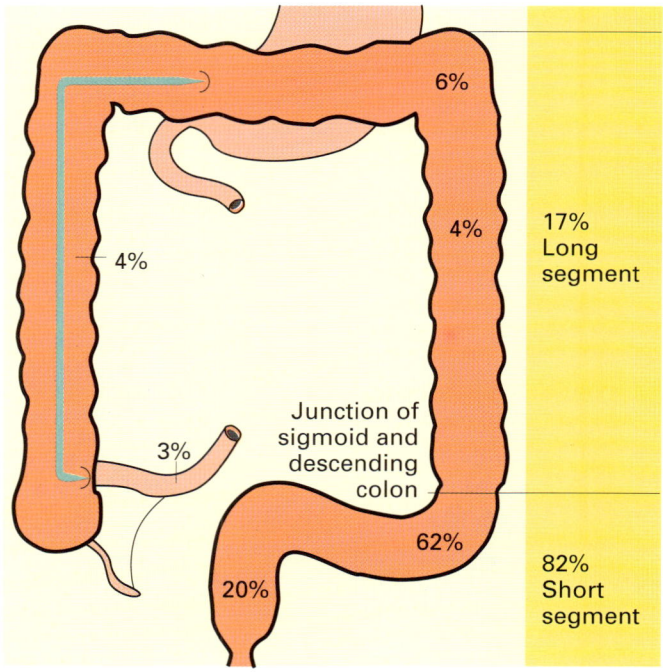

Fig. 16.95 Hirschsprung's disease: extent of aganglionic segment.

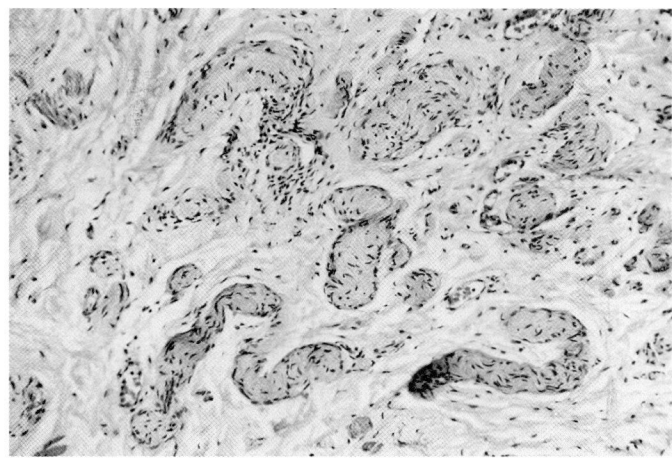

Fig. 16.96 Hirschsprung's disease: many hypertrophied nerve trunks are present in the submucosa of a rectal biopsy.

cells, presence of hypertrophied nerve trunks in the submucosa (Fig. 16.96), and an excess of cholinergic nerve fibres extending through the muscularis propria and into the lamina propria in most cases and demonstrable by acetylcholinesterase staining. In long segment disease, the plane of the mysenteric plexus is empty above the level of innervation by the sacral plexus.

Affected individuals usually present in early life with constipation from birth, although a few are seen in childhood and adolescence with a history of lifelong bowel disorder. The severity of symptoms is not related to the length of bowel involved, individuals with short segment disease may present with virtual intestinal obstruction in the neonatal period. Enterocolitis is a serious, sometimes fatal, complication both in untreated individuals and in the immediate postoperative period.

Ganglioneuromatosis

Individuals with multiple endocrine adenoma syndrome type IIB, inherited as an autosomal recessive disorder, have multiple ganglioneuromata of the gastrointestinal tract, producing nodular distortion of lips and palate margin and involving the submucosal plexus of the whole intestine. Neural plexi contain nodular expansions composed of nerve fibres and large numbers of ganglion cells. This altered innervation can produce constipation in early life.

Intestinal neuronal dysplasia

This is a recently recognized disorder of enteric parasympathetic innervation. There is hyperplasia of both submucosal and myenteric plexi and giant ganglion cells are found within the plexus. Isolated ganglion cells are found readily within the lamina propria and muscle coats away from the plexus. A localized form of this disorder is found within the ganglionated bowel of some children with Hirschsprung's disease. Diffuse involvement of the rectum and colon effects irregular bowel habit with abdominal distension and gross megacolon.

16.7.6 Heterotopias

Heterotopic gastric mucosa is commonly found in Meckel's diverticula and intestinal duplication. Heterotopic glandular tissue, resembling pancreatic acinar glands can be identified as creamish nodules beneath the serosa. They may be found in stomach and small intestine and are commonly found in autosomal trisomy, particularly trisomy 13.

16.7.7 Angioma

Intestinal angiomata present with rectal bleeding. They are usually cavernous angiomata, situated in the submucosa, thus liable to trauma. They are frequently multiple. An angioma may form the apex of an intussusception. Angiomata of the gastrointestinal tract often co-exist with similar lesions in other sites; cutaneous angiomata are common.

16.7.8 Muscle wall defects

Diaphragmatic hernia

The commonest diaphragmatic defect is that found in the posterolateral part of the diaphragm (Bochdalek hernia) resulting from failure of closure of the pleuroperitoneal canal. The defect is usually (80 per cent) left-sided, probably related to the earlier closure of the pleuroperitoneal cavity on the right side. Bilateral hernia are rare. Abdominal viscera pass through the defect into the hemithorax and the mediastinum is deflected to the opposite side (Fig. 16.97). The presence of abdominal viscera in the chest during fetal life restricts lung growth, particularly the ipsilateral lung which may weigh only 3–4 g (normal, 20 g). The liver is often excessively large because of increased abdominal volume available for growth, and may impede surgical return of the bowel to the abdominal cavity. Survival, despite earlier diagnosis and improved facilities for surgery, is poor and limited by the extent of lung development. Mortality is about 50 per cent amongst babies requiring surgery in the first day of life. Babies with large left-sided hernia often present at birth with respiratory problems. They are usually well grown with no dysmorphic features and, in the majority, this is the only defect. Some babies have co-existent cardiovascular anomalies. When the hernia is right-sided, small defects are often occluded by the liver and found only incidentally. Large right-sided defects which permit liver displacement into the thorax effect major distortion of great vessels which can obstruct venous return from the placenta and promote fetal hydrops.

Central, parasternal (Morgagni) hernias are much less common. Communication with the pericardial sac can be accompanied by large pericardial effusion and tamponade.

Abdominal wall defect

There are four types of abdominal wall defect which should be distinguished as their appropriate management requires awareness of concomitant disorders and risk of recurrence. Muscular

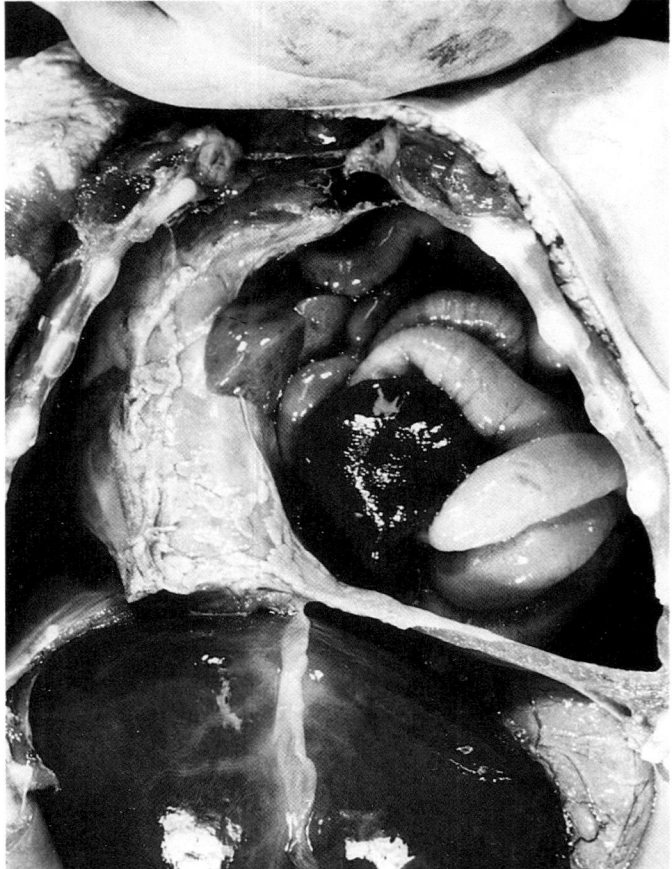

Fig. 16.97 Left-sided diaphragmatic hernia: the spleen and small intestine are in the left hemithorax, the mediastinum is displaced to the right. (Reproduced from Variend 1987, with permission.)

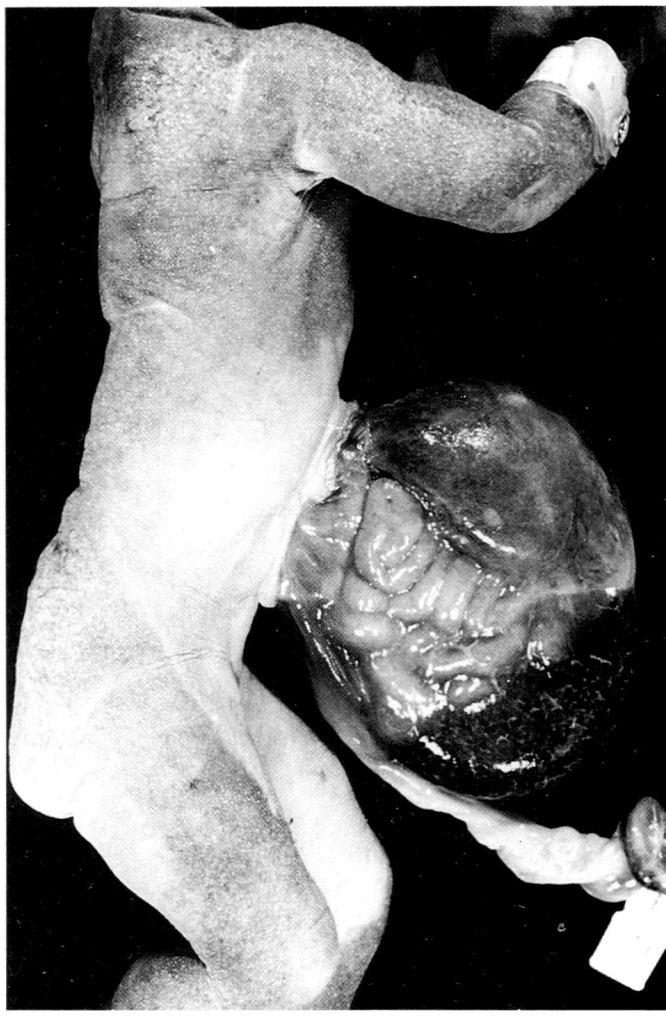

Fig. 16.98 Large exomphalos sac contains liver, loops of intestine, and free fluid, neonate with trisomy 18.

atrophy in fetal life can also produce abnormality of the abdominal wall.

Exomphalos (omphalocoele)

Exomphalos is a membrane-covered defect of the abdominal wall, of variable size and closely associated with the insertion of the umbilical cord. It is seen in 1:3500 live births. It represents failure of reduction of the physiological hernia. The sac consists of fusion of the peritoneum with the amniotic membrane continuous with that covering the umbilical cord. The neck of the sac is usually wide. Small defects contain bowel loops and are easily reducible. Large defects contain much of the liver in addition to intestines (Fig. 16.98) and may rupture during delivery. The intestine is always unrotated. Difficulty in returning viscera to the abdominal cavity is often experienced because the latter is poorly developed.

Babies with exomphalos often have malformations in other systems, particularly cardiac defects. Exomphalos is a frequent manifestation of autosomal trisomy, particularly of chromosome 13 but also chromosomes 18 and 21. It is present in the Beckwith–Wiedemann syndrome.

Gastroschisis

This is a small defect of the abdominal wall, almost always to the right of the cord insertion, separated from it by a few millimetres of normal skin, and without membranous cover. Its pathogenesis is unclear and most theories invoke premature vascular involution.

Loops of intestine pass through the defect and float freely in the amniotic cavity. During the last trimester they may become covered with a rind of fibrinous material which provokes adhesions when the gut is returned to the abdominal cavity. Associated defects are local; incomplete intestinal rotation, jejunal or ileal atresia, and short small intestine, may all be considered secondary to the gastroschisis. Recurrence is unlikely.

Body stalk anomaly

This is a large defect whose amniotic membrane covering is fused with that of the chorionic plate of the placenta. A very short umbilical cord runs within the sac wall. There is major fetal deformity with distortion of the spinal column and limb hypoplasia, abdominal, and sometimes thoracic, viscera lie within the sac.

This defect is thought to result from adherence of the embryo to the amnio-chorion in early fetal life (amnion rupture sequence). A predisposing factor is a collagen defect such as Ellers–Danlos syndrome or osteogenesis imperfecta. These disorders account for only a small proportion of cases, and for most families, recurrence is unlikely.

Vesico-intestinal fissure (lower midline defect)

This is a large, lower, central abdominal wall defect comprising a central portion of gut mucosa which communicates superiorly and inferiorly with the intestinal tract, flanked by bladder, each with one ureteric orifice. It is accompanied by imperforate anus and a variety of urogenital anomalies, sacral and lower limb defects.

Defective abdominal musculature (prune belly syndrome)

Atrophy of the abdominal wall muscles resulting in a lax, wrinkled abdominal wall is the result of gross, long-standing distension of the fetal abdomen. This is usually the result of bladder distension accompanying lower urinary tract obstruction usually due to urethral valves or stenosis, in the presence of functioning kidneys.

Examination of the abdominal wall in fetal life reveals necrosis of muscle fibres, focal calcification, and many macrophages. By term, all muscle may have disappeared.

16.7.9 Anorectal anomalies

Anorectal anomalies are seen in approximately 1/5000 live births; males are more commonly affected. Classification of this group of anomalies into high, intermediate, and low relative to the puborectalis sling of levator ani has practical significance. High defects are associated with spinal defects (50 per cent) and cardiovascular and tracheo-oesophageal abnormalities (VATER or VACTERL association). Fistulous communications between intestinal and genitourinary tract may occur with all levels of defect.

A defective dorsal cloacal membrane which fails to migrate appropriately towards the tail groove is thought to cause this spectrum of defects.

16.7.10 Mucoviscidosis (cystic fibrosis)

Mucoviscidosis is an important inherited disorder, producing major morbidity in childhood and adolescence which affects all exocrine glands. Its frequency is about 1/2000 live births in the UK. It is inherited as an autosomal recessive condition with a gene frequency of 4–5 per cent. The defective gene has been localized to the long arm of chromosome 7. There are abnormalities of both electrolyte transport in ductular epithelia and the composition of mucus. Functional and morphological ab-

normalities in this disorder are the result of abnormally viscid mucus.

About 15 per cent of affected individuals present in the neonatal period with intestinal obstruction due to meconium ileas. Many present in infancy and early childhood with signs or symptoms of malabsorption, others have recurrent chest infections. A small number of cases present as neonatal jaundice.

Meconium ileus

Small intestinal loops are distended by the accumulation of grey-green, putty-like, abnormally viscid meconium during the second half of pregnancy (Fig. 16.99). Volvulus, leading to intestinal atresia or stenosis, is a frequent complication, and intestinal perforation leads to meconium peritonitis. At birth the infant does not pass meconium, the abdomen is distended and doughy to palpation. An abdominal radiograph has a ground-glass appearance, with focal calcification of meconium in distended bowel loops. About 95 per cent of meconium ileus are manifestations of cystic fibrosis.

Histologically, small intestinal villi are flattened. Epithelial cells are distended by mucus and eosinophilic material is present within glands (Fig. 16.100). Peritonitis follows intestinal perforation; calcified flecks of meconium and a prominent eosinophil leucyte infiltrate are characteristic.

Pancreas

Inspissation of secretions within pancreatic glands and ducts leads to glandular atrophy with fibrosis and duct dilatation (Fig. 16.101). This results in malabsorption, particularly of fats, and poor weight gain.

At necropsy in the neonatal period, the pancreas may be palpably abnormal, firm with interlobular mobility, but this is not always the case and the pancreas from any neonatal death

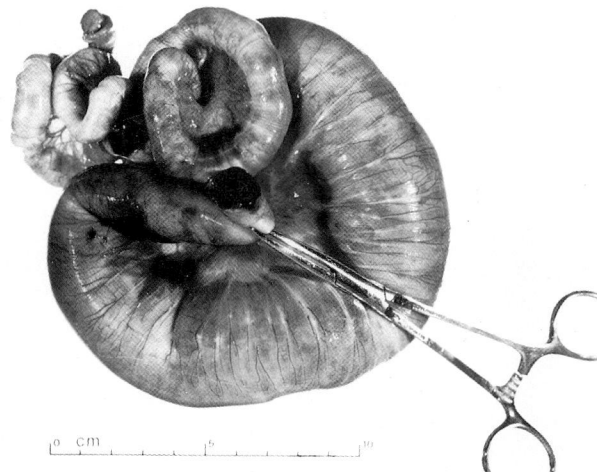

Fig. 16.99 Meconium ileus: the proximal ileus is distended by viscid meconium, the distal bowel is narrow. There is marked serosal congestion.

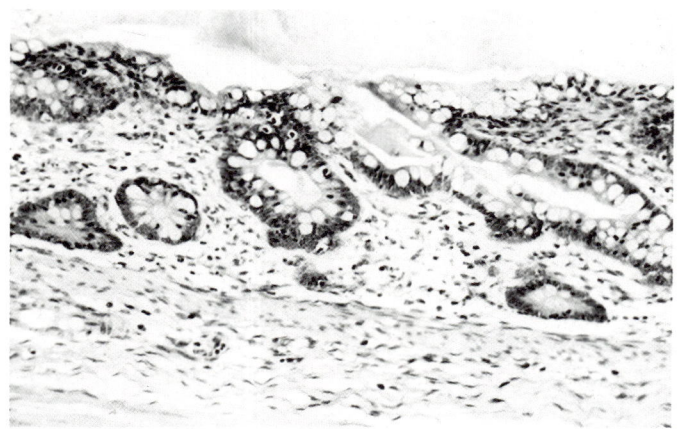

Fig. 16.100 Maconium ileus: intestinal villi are flattened, inspissated secretions are present in glands, and goblet cells are prominent.

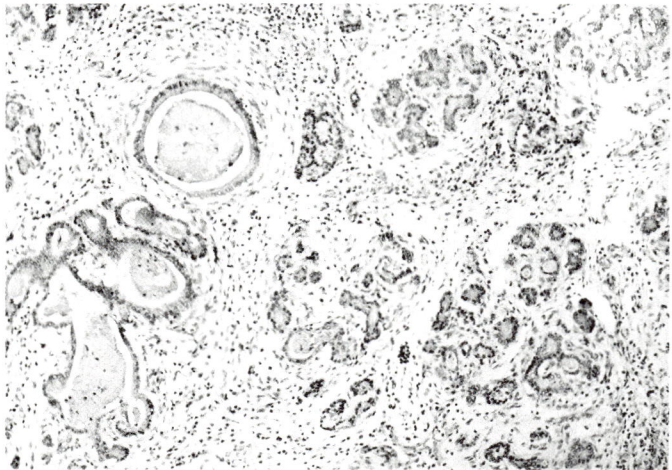

Fig. 16.101 Cystic fibrosis: within the pancreas in the neonatal period there is acinar atrophy, increased fibrosis, inflammatory cell infiltration, and duct dilatation.

should be examined histologically with cystic fibrosis in mind. As well as acinar atrophy and an increase in fibrous tissue, a patchy inflammatory infiltrate is usually present, duct dilatation is minor.

In the older child, the pancreas is very pale, acinar tissue being replaced by fat, within which islets of Langerhans and dilated, mucus-containing duct remnants are identified.

Neonatal jaundice

A small number of babies with cystic fibrosis present with conjugated hyperbilirubinaemia in the neonatal period. Liver biopsy shows portal expansion and duct proliferation, indicating large duct obstruction. Occasionally mucus plugs are seen in bile ducts within the biopsy, but this change is usually confined to the porta hepatis (see Chapter 17 for other hepatic manifestations of cystic fibrosis).

16.7.11   Bibliography

Dehner, L. (1987). *Pediatric surgical pathology* (2nd edn). Williams & Wilkins, Baltimore.

Keeling, J. W. (1988). Congenital abnormalities of the small intestine. In *Gastrointestinal pathology* (ed. R. Whitehead). Churchill Livingstone, Edinburgh.

Potter, E. L. and Craig, J. M. (1976). *Pathology of the fetus and the infant* (3rd edn), pp. 368–92. Year Book Medical Publishers Inc. Lloyd-Luke, London.

Soderlund, S. (1959). Meckels' diverticulum. A clinical and histologic study. *Acta Chir. Scand.* **118** (Suppl. 248).

Variend, S. (1987). Gastrointestinal tract and exocrine pancreas. In *Fetal and neonatal pathology* (ed. J. W. Keeling), pp. 318–24; 329–34. Springer, London.

Weinstein, E. C., Cain, J. C., and Remine, W. H. (1962). Meckels' diverticulum. *Journal of the American Medical Association* **182**, 251–3.

16.8   Malabsorption

F. D. Lee

16.8.1   Introduction

Malabsorption has been defined as any state in which there is a disturbance in the net absorption of any constituent across the intestinal mucosa. An important aspect of this definition is the recognition that although the absorption of most nutrients involves an active transport mechanism from the lumen of the intestine into the mucosa, with some substances, most notably water and electrolytes, there is a bidirectional flow across the epithelium. While most nutrients can be absorbed in any part of the small intestine, some, such as vitamin B_{12}, can only be absorbed in the ileum. The same is true of bile salts. An important consequence of this is that whereas the ileum may compensate for destruction or resection of the proximal small intestine the reverse is not the case. It must also be appreciated that in many intestinal diseases and, in particular, those in which there is an element of lymphatic obstruction, the effects of malabsorption may be compounded by the loss of protein into the intestinal lumen (protein-losing enteropathy).

Not all of the numerous causes of malabsorption are to be found in the small intestine. Digestive disturbances due to pancreatic or hepato-biliary disease, for example, are commonly implicated; indeed in some parts of tropical Africa chronic pancreatitis is a frequent, if not the most important, cause of malabsorption. In other parts of the tropics and in most of Europe and North America, however, the major causes do lie in the small intestine, tropical sprue and coeliac disease, respectively, being of outstanding importance. Nevertheless, practically any disease process primarily or secondarily affecting the small intestine is capable of causing malabsorption if the lesions are persistent and extensive. The mechanisms by which these disorders lead to impaired absorption are often far from being

Table 16.7 The causes of malabsorption

Mechanism	Disease
Inadequate digestion	Hepato-biliary disease; pancreatic insufficiency; gastric surgery
Intestinal mucosal damage	Dietary intolerance (expecially coeliac disease); tropical sprue; post-infective malabsorption; Crohn's disease, tuberculosis; parasitic disease; radiation enteritis; amyloidosis; drug treatment; intestinal lymphoma; Whipple's disease; immunodeficiency syndromes
Alteration in intestinal flora	Blind-loop syndrome; jejunal diverticulosis; chronic intestinal obstruction; progressive systemic sclerosis
Biochemical abnormality	Disaccharidase deficiency; abetalipoproteinaemia
Lymphatic obstruction	Intestinal lymphangiectasia (congenital or acquired)
Inadequate absorptive surface	Intestinal resection or bypass
Endocrine disturbance	Carcinoid syndrome; Zollinger–Ellison syndrome; Verner–Morrison syndrome; systemic mast-cell disease; chronic adrenal insufficiency
Circulatory disturbance	Mesenteric vascular insufficiency; congestive cardiac failure; constrictive pericarditis

completely understood. In Table 16.7 the more important malabsorptive diseases are grouped according to the putative mechanism thought to be predominantly involved in each instance. It has to be appreciated, however, that in some disease states more than one mechanism may be operating.

Many of the diseases mentioned are discussed in detail elsewhere; only those of particular relevance to the investigation of malabsorption, and particularly those which are likely to present abnormalities in intestinal biopsies, are considered in detail.

Intestinal biopsy

Intestinal biopsy is of central importance in the investigation of malabsorptive states. The biopsies can be taken in two different ways. First there is the biopsy capsule, which is introduced under radiographic control into the proximal jejunum and samples the mucosa in a random fashion. With the suction version, a single biopsy only can be taken but hydraulic versions capable of taking multiple biopsies at several levels of the small intestine are available. Secondly, multiple biopsies can be taken under direct vision with the fibre-optic endoscope, but these cannot at present be taken beyond the distal duodenum. Capsule biopsies provide more material but, through being random, suffer from the possibility of sampling errors. Endoscopic biopsies, to a large extent, overcome this problem but tend to be small and less amenable to morphometric analysis. That only the duodenal mucosa can be sampled is also a potential disadvantage, since normal morphology here may be affected by the presence of exuberant Brunner's glands or lymphoid aggregates

and high acid levels. Moreover, lesions tend to be atypical or poorly developed. In the distal duodenum, however, such disadvantages are minimal. It should be added that a capsule biopsy is preferred if enzymatic mucosal analysis or luminal bacterial sampling is contemplated (see later).

Two main groups of histological abnormalities can be detected by intestinal biopsy. The first of these is disturbance of the villous architecture (Figs 16.102–16.104). This usually takes the form of villous atrophy, in which there is a reduction of villous height, reflecting a fall in the enterocyte population. Under the dissecting microscope the normal, tall, finger-shaped villi are initially replaced by short ridges or convolutions (partial villous atrophy) but later the mucosa may become completely flat (sub-total villous atrophy). Villous atrophy is usually produced by accelerated enterocyte destruction (as in coeliac disease) in which case the crypts of Lieberkuhn are hyperplastic and ratio of crypt height to villous height is increased (crypt hyperplastic villous atrophy). Occasionally, however, villous atrophy is caused by disturbed enterocyte formation due, for example, to ionizing radiation, ischaemia, or vitamin deficiency. In such instances the crypts appear reduced in size (crypt hypoplastic villous atrophy).

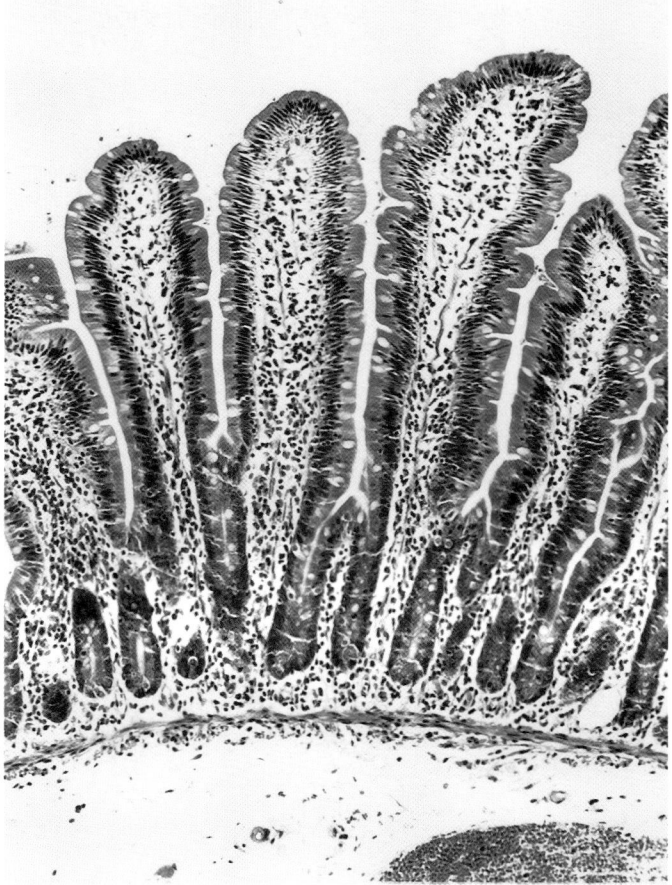

Fig. 16.102 The normal jejunal mucosa. Note the tall, finger-shaped villi, which are about three times longer than the crypts of Lieberkuhn.

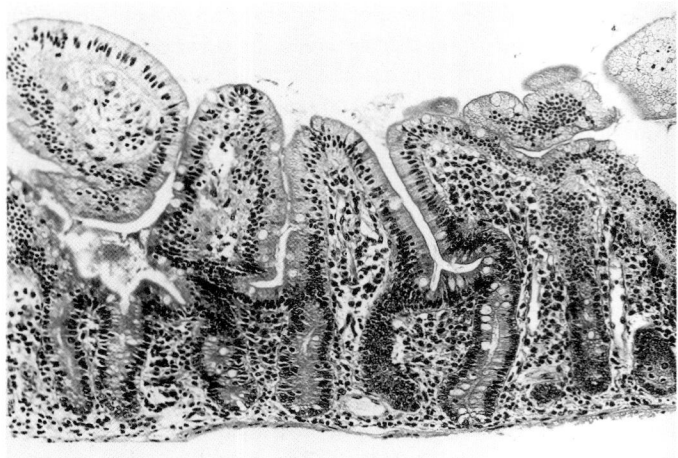

Fig. 16.103 Partial villous atrophy of crypt hyperplastic type, due to mefenamic acid toxicity. The villi are reduced in height and the ratio of crypt to villous height is abnormally increased.

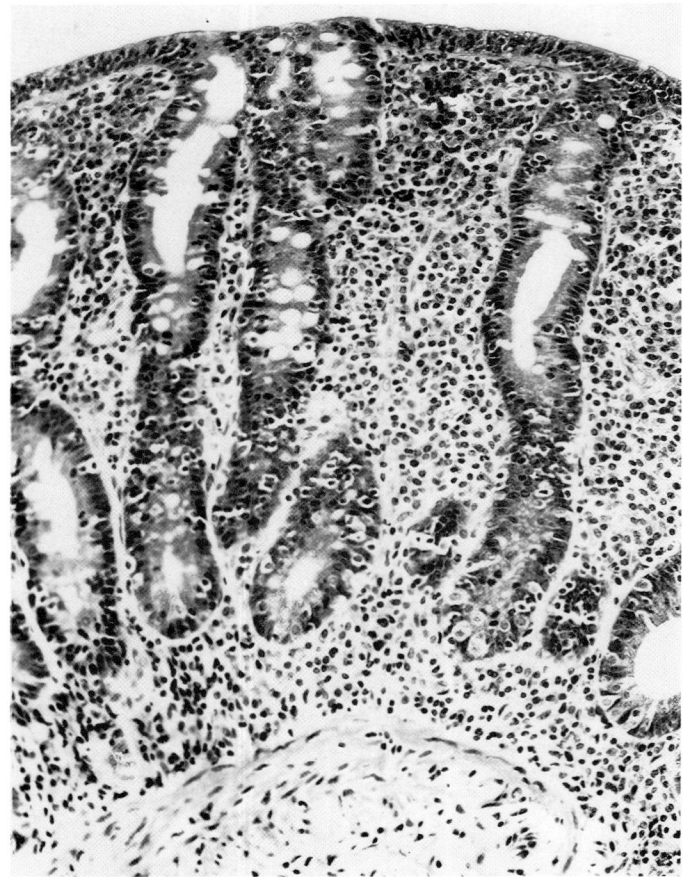

Fig. 16.104 Subtotal villous atrophy, crypt hyperplastic type, due to coeliac disease. The surface epithelium is abnormal and there is pronounced plasma cell infiltration in the lamina propria.

Secondly, intestinal biopsies may show distinctive changes not involving architectural disturbance. Included in this category are the presence of micro-organisms in the lumen, changes in the enterocytes, abnormal cellular infiltrates in the lamina propria, or alterations in the vasculature and lymphatics. Amyloidosis, although an uncommon cause of malabsorption, must always be kept in mind, especially in apparently normal biopsies.

Intestinal biopsy, of course, has its limitations. Focal or patchy disease (including Crohn's disease and most tumours) can seldom be detected: only diffuse diseases with distinctive mucosal lesions can be diagnosed regularly. More deeply situated lesions seldom come within the scope of biopsy pathology.

16.8.2   Coeliac disease

This disease may be defined as a malabsorptive state characterized by the presence in the upper small intestine of extensive and severe mucosal lesions, which show at least some histological improvement following removal of the wheat protein gluten from the diet, hence the alternative term, gluten-sensitive enteropathy. In global terms it is perhaps the most common cause of malabsorption, but it appears to be especially common in North-West Europe and it is likely that a genetic component is involved in its pathogenesis. In patients with coeliac disease presenting in adult life, there is an increased frequency of the histocompatibility antigens A1, B8, and the haplotypes D3/DQW2 and D7/DQW2. Despite these observations, there is evidence that the prevalence of the disease at all ages is falling, at least in the United Kingdom, suggesting that environmental factors also appear to be operating.

The mechanism whereby gluten, which is present not only in wheat but also in rye, barley, and possibly in oats, but seemingly not in maize, exerts its pathological effects in susceptible individuals is still uncertain. The initial hypothesis that it might be due to some kind of specific enzyme defect now seems unlikely, and although the idea that gluten might cause mucosal damage by acting as a lectin has its adherents, it has not been widely accepted. The more favoured view is that the mucosal damage is produced by a genetically determined cell-mediated abnormal immune response to gluten. It is notable that anti-gliadin antibodies (as well as anti-reticulin and endo-mysial antibodies) can often be detected in the serum of patients with coeliac disease. Serological tests, however, cannot as yet be regarded as specific for coeliac disease. Biopsy remains the primary diagnostic procedure.

The primary mucosal lesion in coeliac disease almost always takes the form of subtotal villous atrophy of crypt hyperplastic type (Fig. 16.104). The lesions are always most severe in the upper part of the small intestine and become progressively less marked distally. The villous atrophy is almost certainly due to premature enterocyte destruction, the crypt hyperplasia being a compensatory reaction. Evidence of enterocyte damage is thus invariably present in untreated cases and is always maximal at the villous extremity, being less pronounced, or even absent, in cells emerging from the crypts. Enterocyte damage is recognized by a reduction in cell height (below 30 μm), often associated with increased cytoplasmic basophilia or vacuolation and nuclear irregularity with loss of polarity. These changes may precede any alteration in villous architecture and may be found in the absence of villous changes. The elongated crypts show pronounced mitotic activity, and it can be shown that the mitotic index within the enterocyte population is substantially increased. While Paneth cells tend to become markedly decreased (or at least degranulated) during active phases of the disease, some endocrine cells [notably the enterochromaffin (EC) cells] show an increase in numbers.

Another important feature of coeliac disease is an increased prominence of the intra-epithelial lymphocytes (IEL). There is some controversy as to whether these cells are actually increased in number. There is no doubt that they are more numerous in relationship to the number of enterocytes, but in terms of mucosal area (as calculated by length of muscularis mucosae) their numbers are either normal or even slightly decreased. Some workers have shown that an increase in the mitotic index in the IEL population is much more characteristic of coeliac disease. This observation has not gone undisputed; none the less it is of considerable importance since the number of IEL in proportion to the enterocyte population may also be increased in other malabsorptive states, such as tropical sprue, post-infective malabsorption, cow's milk protein intolerance, hypogammaglobulinaemia, and the blind-loop syndrome. Only in tropical sprue, however, does the IEL/enterocyte ratio approach that in coeliac disease (see Fig. 16.105).

The lamina propria also shows a pronounced increase in leucocytic infiltration but this is almost exclusively due to an excess of plasma cells. While the pattern of immunoglobulin synthesis in this enhanced population is similar to that observed normally (IgA > IgM > IgG), only the IgM-producing cells are consistently increased both before and after treatment. It is by no means uncommon to find the occasional neutrophil in the lamina propria, especially during active phases of the disease. Eosinophils and histiocytes are invariably present, but are not usually increased in number. Histiocytes may, however, be conspicuous in the subepithelial location in the early phase of the disease.

A variety of other intestinal changes may also be encountered in coeliac disease. These include the deposition of lipofuscin (or, more accurately, ceroid) pigment in the smooth muscle of the muscularis propria, especially in the vicinity of the myenteric plexus, and of blood vessels. It may also be found in the lamina muscularis mucosae and is thus detectable in biopsies. There may also be excessive collagen deposition in the subepithelial location, and when this is severe it may render the lesions refractory to gluten withdrawal.

The most important diagnostic feature of coeliac disease is that a measurable improvement in villous architecture takes place when gluten is withdrawn from the diet. It is true that the signs of enterocyte damage respond much more rapidly to gluten withdrawal, but these are much less easy to quantitate. A measurable villous response may take some considerable time and is best assessed after a period of between 3 and 6 months.

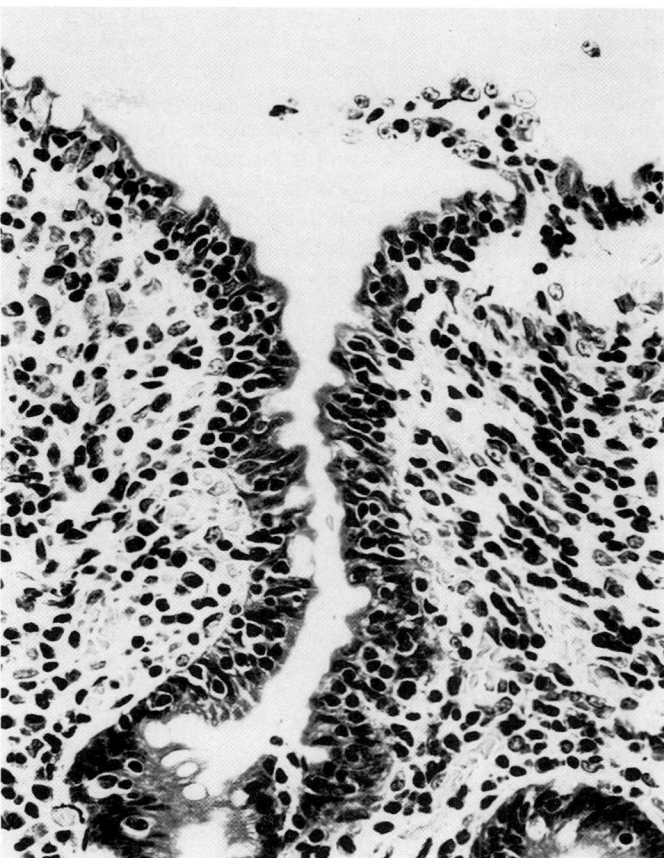

Fig. 16.105 Tropical sprue. There is partial villous atrophy and an apparently pronounced increase in lymphocytes within the villous epithelium.

While a return to complete normality is sometimes observed in childhood cases, this is much more unusual in cases diagnosed in adult life in which mild persistent villous atrophy with small foci of enterocyte damage at the villous extremity frequently persists. Some authorities insist that a diagnosis of coeliac disease can only be established unequivocally when mucosal damage can be demonstrated on gluten re-challenge. This, however, is only really necessary in cases where the diagnosis is in doubt.

The failure of a patient with putative coeliac disease to respond to gluten withdrawal even after a period of 6 months is an important clinical problem. Usually this is due to faulty dietary control, but if this can be excluded then the possibility of some complication needs to be seriously considered. The most important of these is the development of neoplasia. In the majority of cases this takes the form of a malignant lymphoma of T-cell derivation. This tumour usually arises in the proximal small intestine and it is important to note that many patients with this tumour do not give a history of pre-existing coeliac disease. In some instances the tumour is preceded, accompanied or even followed by ulceration of non-specific type (the so-called ulcerative jejunitis). It is not yet certain whether non-specific ulceration is always an expression of a neoplastic process or may occur in its absence. Even so, evidence of incipient ulceration, such as the presence of crypt abscesses, and of healed ulceration, e.g. gastric metaplasia, should be regarded with great suspicion, either in biopsies or in intestinal resections. Tumours other than lymphomas may arise in the small intestine as a complication of coeliac disease; there is, for example, an 80-fold increase in the incidence of small bowel carcinoma. There is also an association between certain types of extra-intestinal malignancy (e.g. oesophageal carcinoma) and coeliac disease. Another important cause of refractoriness to gluten withdrawal in a patient with subtotal villous atrophy is the presence of subepithelial collagen deposition (to which reference has already been made), a condition sometimes referred to as collagenous sprue, the implication being that in view of its unresponsiveness to gluten withdrawal it is in some way different from coeliac disease. Some patients with collagen deposition respond in the usual way to gluten withdrawal. Even when identifiable pathological complications have been eliminated, there are still cases with extensive and severe villous atrophy which prove completely unresponsive to all forms of treatment. The term 'refractory sprue' has been applied to such cases in view of the diagnostic uncertainty; it is at least probable, however, that these are incidences of coeliac disease in which, for reasons as yet unexplained, the intestinal lesions become irreversible.

It also has to borne in mind that dietary proteins other than gluten may induce crypt hyperplastic villous atrophy in early life. Most important in this regard are cow's milk protein and soya protein, although chicken, fish, and rice proteins have also been implicated. In most instances the lesions are transient and seldom persist beyond the age of 2 years. Sensitivity to both cow's milk protein and soya protein may be associated, however, with coeliac disease and might interfere with the response to gluten withdrawal even in later childhood or possibly in adult life.

Skin disease

There is little evidence that skin disease directly affects intestinal function. Should malabsorption complicate skin disease it is usually due to co-existent coeliac disease. This is certainly the case in dermatitis herpetiformis (DH) in which some degree of villous atrophy can be found in most cases. For reasons as yet not clear, the villous changes tend to be rather variable in expression, even within the same biopsy. None the less, the intestinal lesions respond to gluten withdrawal, as may some of the skin lesions if dietary restriction is sufficiently prolonged. However, whether the mechanism leading to intestinal damage is the same as that producing the skin lesions in DH is still uncertain.

16.8.3   Post-infective malabsorption

Even in temperate parts of the world some degree of mucosal damage may persist following intestinal infections, both of bac-

terial and viral type, especially in childhood. In some instances the mucosal changes, which usually take the form of crypt hyperplastic villous atrophy, are sufficiently severe to produce transient malabsorption, and there is a danger that such episodes may be mistaken for the onset of coeliac disease. Both the architectural and inflammatory changes tend, however, to be less pronounced than in coeliac disease. This is particularly true of the intra-epithelial lymphocyte population, which is rarely as conspicuous as it is in coeliac disease.

Tropical sprue

As its name implies, the essential feature of this disease is that a tropical environment appears to be an essential condition for its initiation. It is found especially in the Indian subcontinent, South-East Asia, Central America, and the northern part of South America. It is thought to be uncommon in Africa, but this may be due to a failure of recognition. The disease can affect those native to the tropics as well as visitors, and occasionally may become overt only after an individual has returned from the tropics. While the exact cause is uncertain, it has been shown that there is abnormal colonization of the lumen of the small intestine by aerobic enteric bacteria of variable type, seemingly this phenomenon being initiated by an acute intestinal infection. Tropical sprue differs from the more commonly encountered traveller's diarrhoea in that bacterial growth in the small bowel tends not only to be persistent but to be capable of producing significant pathological changes in the intestinal mucosa. Furthermore, the subsequent malabsorptive disorder is of sufficient severity as to produce nutritional disturbance, most notably folic acid and B_{12} deficiency. Indeed, haematinic deficiency may contribute to the perpetuation of the pathological lesions in the intestinal mucosa and the administration of folic acid, in addition to broad-spectrum antibiotics such as tetracycline, is recommended in the treatment of the disease.

Histological examination of intestinal biopsies reveals crypt hyperplastic villous atrophy which, in the majority of cases, is partial and only occasionally subtotal. There may, however be an increase in intra-epithelial lymphcytes, comparable in extent to that found in coeliac disease (Fig. 16.105). The mucosal changes are therefore similar in pattern, if not in degree, to those of coeliac disease and only minor differences have been described. Eosinophils, for example, may be conspicuous and a striking increase in argentaffin cells has been reported. It is also likely that although the lesions tend to be milder, they are also much more widely distributed throughout the small intestine than in coeliac disease.

16.8.4   Miscellaneous causes of malabsorption

Crohn's disease

Malabsorption is an important complication of this disease and may arise for a number of different reasons. The frequent involvement of the terminal ileum by transmural inflammation may impair absorption of such important substances as bile salts and vitamin B_{12}. This disturbance may be compounded by intestinal stasis induced by chronic ileal obstruction (see Section 16.13.3). In a small percentage of cases there is diffuse involvement of the ileum and jejunum in the disease process, with more severe malabsorption, often complicated by protein-losing enteropathy. In such cases there may be extensive chronic mucosal inflammation producing a structural change resembling subtotal villous atrophy, the presence of granulomas conferring upon it a distinctive, if not a diagnostic appearance. It should be mentioned that, apart from such severe disease, random jejunal biopsies in Crohn's disease may show focal inflammatory lesions which, in some instances, reveal a granuloma on repeated sectioning; such phenomena underline the point that in this disease mucosal involvement is more extensive than is generally realized.

Parasitic disease

While many protozoal and metazoal parasites are capable of colonizing the lumen of the intestine, only a few have been shown unequivocally to provoke malabsorption, and even then only in a minority of cases. There is no doubt, however, that deficiency of the immune system and, in particular, the cell-mediated component may greatly enhance the potential pathogenicity of these organisms. Indeed, the presence of heavy infestation with parasites such as *Giardia lamblia* should always lead the pathologist to consider the possibility of immunodeficiency.

Giardiasis

This disease is usually contracted by the ingestion of water contaminated with the protozoal parasite *Giardia lamblia* in its encysted form. The emerging vegetative form (trophozoite) proliferates mainly in the distal duodenum and upper jejunum, apparently because of the availability of bile salts which the organism requires for further development. Infestation has a variety of clinical consequences, ranging from an acute disease, which often masquerades as a form of traveller's diarrhoea, to a more chronic disturbance, which in a substantial proportion of cases is accompanied by malabsorption.

Although stool examination for the presence of cysts is the preferred method for detecting infestation, the diagnosis is often made in a biopsy using light microscopy. The trophozoites which reside in the intestinal lumen, often in close proximity to the epithelial surface, are readily recognized, even in H & E sections, as faintly basophilic, ovoid, or kite-shaped bodies, measuring 9–12 μm in length. The paired nuclei are usually visible, especially in Bouin-fixed biopsies (Fig. 16.106), but it may require oil immersion to detect the quadruple flagella. It is unlikely that the organism ever penetrates the epithelium, which in the great majority of cases appears undamaged (Fig. 16.106). Usually the villous pattern is normal and any inflammatory response minimal. There can be little doubt, however, that the parasite is capable of producing partial or even subtotal villous atrophy with an apparent increase in intra-epithelial lymphocytes in immunologically normal individuals. Such obvious villous changes appear to be more common in the

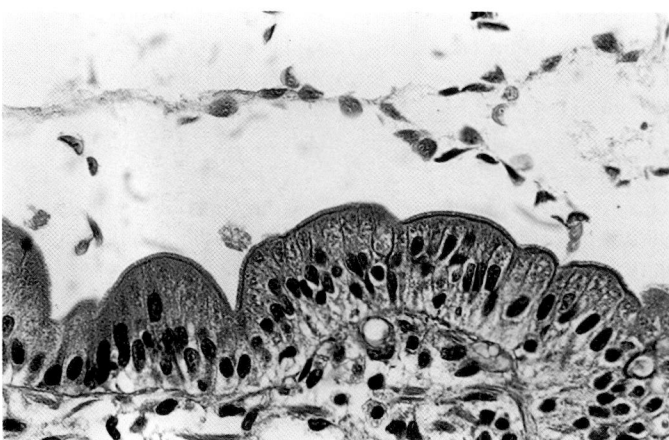

Fig. 16.106 Giardiasis. The characteristic trophozoites with paired nuclei are present in the intestinal lumen. Note that the epithelium appears normal.

tropics and tend also to be pronounced in immunodeficient individuals. Even so, the mechanism leading to malabsorption is far from clear. It is unlikely that mucosal damage is entirely responsible and the importance of other suggested factors, such as bile salt depletion, bacterial overgrowth, or physical occlusion of the enterocyte surface by parasites, has yet to be fully evaluated.

Other protozoal diseases

Coccidial protozoa, and in particular *Cryptosporidium* species, are known to be capable of producing mild self-limiting intestinal disturbance in normal individuals. In the presence of either congenital or acquired immunodeficient states the effects of infestation are much more severe and malabsorption is by no means unusual. Intestinal biopsies from immunodeficient patients with cryptosporidiosis may show partial villous atrophy associated with infiltration of the epithelium by neutrophils and an apparent increase in intra-epithelial lymphocytes. In H & E sections the organisms can be recognized as small, spherical, golden-brown bodies approximately 3 μm in diameter, attached to the enterocytes on the tips and sides of the villi but less often in the crypts. Giemsa staining shows the organisms in greatest detail.

Strongyloidiasis

Infestation with the nematode *Strongyloides stercoralis* is widespread in the tropics but is also endemic in parts of North America as far north as Canada. In most instances intestinal parasitization is symptomless but with heavy infestation there may be severe intestinal disturbance, including malabsorption, and the condition may be fatal. In such severe cases duodenal biopsies have shown marked mucosal inflammation with varying degrees of crypt hyperplastic villous atrophy, and the adult worms may be visible in the crypts. Extensive ulceration, both in the small intestine and colon, may be found in fatal cases.

It is now well recognized that overwhelming infestation with parasites is particularly likely to develop in immunosuppressed individuals, with correspondingly severe intestinal disturbance (hyperinfestation syndrome). These effects may be compounded by dissemination of larval forms beyond their usual habitat in the small intestine.

Radiation enteritis

The exposure of the small bowel to ionizing radiation, usually taking place during the treatment of intra-abdominal cancer, may have both immediate and long-term consequences. The immediate effects, usually taking the form of transient diarrhoea and malabsorption, are produced by damage to the rapidly dividing enterocyte precursors in the intestinal crypts. This leads to villous collapse of variable degree, although recovery usually takes place unless the effects are exceptionally severe.

It takes several months, and sometimes years, before the latter effects become clinically evident. Diarrhoea is the most common late manifestation and may be accompanied by malabsorption which is sometimes severe. The mechanism underlying these effects is progressive occlusion of the intestinal vasculature with the subsequent development of ischaemic damage. Should this affect the ileum, as is often the case, bile salt depletion and vitamin B_{12} malabsorption may ensue and may be compounded by the effects of intestinal stasis due to ischaemic stricture formation. Protein losing enteropathy, possibly due to lymphatic occlusion, may also be a feature.

Drugs

Although many therapeutic agents have been implicated in the causation of malabsorption, only in a few instances has this been accompanied and possibly mediated by clearly identifiable pathological changes in the intestinal mucosa. The antibiotic, neomycin, provided an early example of this association and, more recently, the anti-inflammatory agent mefenamic acid (Fig. 16.103) has been incriminated. The lesion produced in both instances is crypt hyperplastic villous atrophy (Fig. 16.103). It is now well recognized that malabsorption may arise during the administration of cytotoxic drugs, such as methotrexate, in patients with acute leukaemia, but there is seldom any significant villous disurbance. Focal enterocyte vacuolation and degeneration may, however, be detected by both light and electron microscopy in such instances.

Malignant lymphoma

It has been known for more than 50 years that malabsorption may develop in patients with malignant lymphomas (see Chapter 24) arising in, or involving, the intestinal tract. Several different mechanisms have been proposed to explain this association. At first it was thought that obstruction and compression of the mesenteric lymphatics by tumour was a major factor. There is no doubt that this does happen, albeit rarely, when a lymphoma (usually of the centroblast/centrocyte type, either follicular or diffuse) involves the retroperitoneal or mesenteric lymph nodes, either secondarily to a primary intestinal tumour or as part of a systematized disease process. Malabsorption may

also arise when the mesenteric lymphatics become obstructed by immunoglobulin (usually of IgM class) secreted by a lymphoplasmacytoid lymphoma when it infiltrates a mesenteric node.

In the condition now referred to as immunoproliferative small intestinal disease (IPSID), which includes the so-called Mediterranean lymphoma and its variant α-chain disease, there may be severe malabsorption, which has been attributed to mucosal involvement in the lymphoproliferative process. Intestinal biopsies carried out in this disease, which is mainly encountered in the Middle East and the Eastern Mediterranean littoral and is described more fully in Chapter 24, initially reveal intense infiltration of the lamina propria with plasma cells. In most cases these cells can be shown immunohistochemically to lack light chains and seem to be producing only the heavy chain of IgA immunoglobulin. This infiltrate is associated with varying degrees of villous blunting and fusion: there is, however, little evidence of enterocyte damage and the malabsorptive state responds at least initially to oral broad-spectrum antibiotics. This would suggest that abnormal bacterial colonization is of greater importance than lymphomatous infiltration in the pathogenesis of malabsorption.

In Europe and North America the most important cause of malabsorption in association with malignant lymphoma is the presence of diffuse abnormality of the intestinal mucosa, almost invariably due to pre-existing coeliac disease. This matter is discussed more fully in Chapter 24. It is important to note, however, that coeliac disease not only predisposes to the development of intestinal lymphoma but also to a number of extra-intestinal malignancies. This probably accounts for sporadic descriptions of malabsorption arising in association with a number of neoplasms apparently unrelated to the intestinal tract.

Whipple's disease

It has been apparent since its initial description in 1907 that this disease is an essentially systemic disorder in which the most impressive pathological changes take place in the small intestine. Malabsorption associated with diarrhoea and weight loss therefore tend to dominate the clinical picture, even though systemic symptoms such as fever, anaemia, skin pigmentation, peripheral lymphadenopathy, chronic cough, arthralgia, and signs of central nervous system involvement frequently accompany and may precede the intestinal disturbances. The disease responds to oral broad-spectrum antibiotics and it seems probable that it is caused by a specific micro-organism. Not having been cultured, however, its identity remains to be fully established. What also remains unexplained is the predilection of the disease for males approaching or passing middle age. The close similarity of the intestinal lesions to those observed in the acquired immunodeficiency syndrome (AIDS) complicated by atypical mycobacterial infection (Chapter 4) has revived interest in the possibility that there might be a disturbance of the microbiological defence mechanisms. Apart from reports of IgM deficiency or lymphopaenia in occasional cases, and an association with the histocompatibility antigen HLA-B27, there has never been evidence for more than a minor degree of immuno-deficiency. More recently, however, it has been suggested that macrophage dysfunction might be of greater pathogenic importance.

Histologically the pre-eminent intestinal lesion is a pronounced expansion of the lamina propria mucosae by an infiltrate of histiocytes with abundant finely granular and faintly basophilic cytoplasm, giving a diastase-resistant reaction with periodic acid-Schiff (PAS) which is much stronger than that usually observed in macrophages. Some histiocytes also contain haemosiderin. This infiltrate displaces the normal leucocytic population, which is still, however, detectable. In some cases neutrophils may be conspicuous, especially in the subepithelial location (Fig. 16.107). Another notable feature is the presence in the lamina propria of 'clear spaces' which sometimes appear to be lined by endothelium and may represent lacteals distended with fat lobules (Fig. 16.107). While the histiocytic infiltrate leads to marked villous distension and even, in places, villous fusion of such an extent as to produce an appearance resembling subtotal villous atrophy, there does not appear to be a significant alteration in enterocyte dynamics and the enterocytes, as a rule, show no evidence of damage.

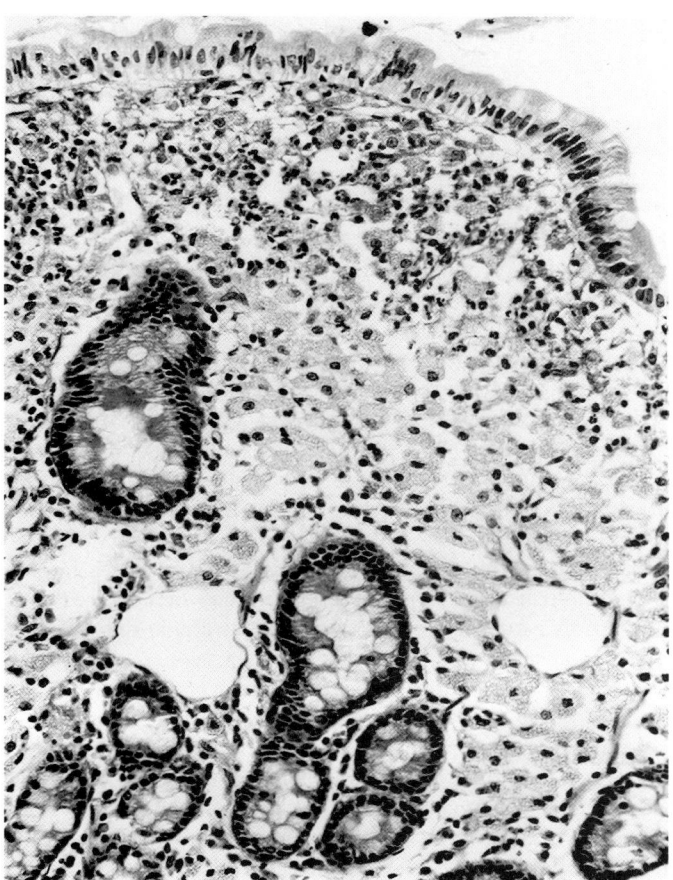

Fig. 16.107 Whipple's disease. The lamina propria mucosae is distended by an infiltrate of histiocytes with abundant granular cytoplasm. Neutrophils are present under the surface epithelium. Note also the 'clear spaces' with an apparent endothelial lining.

Electron microscopy reveals the presence of distinctive rod-shaped organisms measuring 1.5–2 μm in length throughout the lamina propria and even within the epithelium. The granules within the cytoplasm of the abnormal histiocytes represent phagosomes containing bacilliform bodies in varying states of disintegration. The organisms disappear on treatment but the histiocytes may persist for some considerable time.

In making a diagnosis of Whipple's disease other causes of mucosal histiocytosis have to be borne in mind. Of particular importance in this regard are mycobacterial infection in AIDS (Chapter 4) and histoplasmosis (Chapter 29). Foamy histiocytes may also be occasionally observed in association with immuno-deficiency or disorders of neutrophil function, as well as in association with rare metabolic defects. Conversely, Whipple's macrophages may be found without the small intestine, most notably in lymph nodes, heart valves, central nervous system, spleen, lungs, liver, kidneys, endocrine glands, and testis. They may also be found in the colonic mucosa, where they may be confused with the ubiquitous colonic histiocytes. The latter cells are also PAS-positive, but this is due more to the presence of ingested mucin than to bacterial debris.

Immunodeficiency syndromes

Malabsorption may be associated with defects either in the B- or T-cell components of the immunological system, especially if these are acquired rather than congenital. In either instance, however, intestinal biopsy may provide valuable diagnostic information.

In congenital sex-linked agammaglobulinaemia there is a complete absence of plasma cells from the lamina propria of the intestinal mucosa and the lymphoid aggregates are devoid of germinal centres. The villous pattern, however, is usually normal and intestinal disturbance is minimal. However, more serious forms of enteritis resulting from opportunistic infections such as cryptosporidiosis, may develop in patients with other types of congenital hypogammaglobulinaemia. Both plasma cells and intra-epithelial lymphocytes may be absent from the mucosa in *severe combined immunodeficiency*. In this condition large vacuolated macrophages showing some PAS-positivity have been found in the lamina propria. *Selective IgA deficiency*, which may be congenital or acquired, can only be identified in a biopsy by immunohistochemical means. There is, however, a substantially increased incidence of coeliac disease, characterized by subtotal villous atrophy which responds in the usual way to gluten withdrawal. Occasional cases of IgA deficiency have also been associated with nodular lymphoid hyperplasia (see below), giardiasis, or cryptosporidiosis.

Patients with primary acquired hypogammaglobulinaemia (variable immunodeficiency) show a variety of intestinal complications. Patients with severe depression of immunoglobulins of all classes are unusually prone to develop malabsorption. This may be accompanied by crypt hyperplastic villous atrophy of variable extent and severity. Characteristically, plasma cells are absent from the lamina propria. In some cases, the villous changes are undoubtedly due to co-existing coeliac disease which responds in the usual way to gluten withdrawal. In other instances, both the malabsorption and the mucosal lesions appear to be related to giardiasis and respond to appropriate drug therapy. There is, however, a residue of cases in which villous abnormality develops without an obvious cause being apparent. In another important group of patients in this category villous changes are less obvious, the most conspicuous mucosal abnormality being the lesion referred to as nodular lymphoid hyperplasia (NLH). In such patients there is severe depression of the serum IgA and IgM levels and a variable depression of IgG; and plasma cells are absent or can be found only with difficulty. Giardiasis is almost invariable and may lead to minor villous alterations and sometimes to malabsorption which responds to drug therapy. The lymphoid nodules do not, however, disappear on treatment. Why NLH should develop in some cases of hypogammaglobulinaemia and not others is far from clear; however, it has been postulated that NLH arises as a consequence of a maturation defect in the B-cell system and histologically the follicles often show deficient lymphocyte mantles. While the presence of NLH in the upper small bowel usually denotes an acquired defect in the B-cell system, it may on occasion represent a reactive change in immunologically normal individuals in association with conditions such as recurrent giardiasis.

Malabsorption associated with diarrhoea and weight loss may be an important feature of AIDS. In most instances the intestinal disturbance can be attributed to opportunistic infections, most notable those due to cytomegalovirus, coccidial protozoa or *Mycobacterium avium intracellulare*. In this last infection the lamina propria of the intestinal mucosa is infiltrated with foamy or vacuolated histiocytes containing numerous acid-fast bacilli. The overall appearance closely resembles that in Whipple's disease, although the histiocytes give only a weak PAS-positive reaction. Malabsorption may also be found in the absence of infection and, in such instances, the intestinal mucosa has been reported to show partial villous atrophy of crypt hyperplastic type, associated paradoxically with an increase in intra-epithelial lymphocytes.

Malnutrition

Apart from being an obvious consequence of malabsorption, impaired nutrition may itself have effects upon the intestinal mucosa. Quite severe forms of villous atrophy, closely resembling those seen in coeliac disease, may be found in association with severe protein calorie malnutrition (kwashiorkor), the intestinal mucosa returning to normal with improved nutrition. Both vitamin B_{12} deficiency and a folic acid deficiency may cause a mild crypt hypoplastic villous atrophy and it may be possible to detect cytomegalic change in the enterocyte population. Deficiencies of these two vitamins may also induce a hypoplastic phase in diseases such as coeliac disease and tropical sprue.

The stasis syndrome

The transit time of the small bowel contents plays a predominant role in maintaining the near sterility of the lumen, and any impairment of transit, if sufficiently prolonged, inevitably leads to bacterial overgrowth. Initially the normal sparse flora of Gram-positive organisms becomes replaced by coliform bacteria which, in turn, encourages the growth of anaerobes. These phenomena may have important functional consequences, especially if they take place in the upper small bowel. Malabsorption of fat and possibly other nutrients may be provoked by the degradation of bile salts by coliform bacteria, leading not only to bile salt depletion but also to the release of toxic bile acids capable of causing enterocyte damage or malfunction. In addition, anaerobic bacteria may take up vitamin B_{12} before it can reach its absorptive site in the distal ileum, thus leading to megaloblastic anaemia and the other effects of B_{12} deficiency.

These effects are sometimes collectively referred to as the stasis syndrome and are particularly likely to complicate structural alterations of long standing in the proximal small bowel, such as false jejunal diverticula, chronic intestinal obstruction, or surgical blind-loops. Damage to the intestinal musculature due, for example, to progressive systemic sclerosis or irradiation enteritis may have similar effects, and ganglion-blocking drugs have occasionally been incriminated.

The diagnosis of the syndrome is preferentially made by analysing the intestinal contents with a biopsy capsule but this is a difficult procedure and is not always feasible; confirmation is thus usually obtained by observing the respone of the malabsorptive state to the administration orally of broad-spectrum antibiotics. Mucosal biopsy is seldom helpful since at most only minor villous abnormalities are present and the sites involved are rarely accessible to biopsy.

Biochemical disorders

It is by no means uncommon for malabsorption to be caused by biochemical disturbances involving either the terminal phase of the digestive process at the enterocyte surface or the transport systems within the enterocyte itself.

Within the first category are the disaccharidase deficiencies. Most often these are congenital, the most important being lactase deficiency, which has a world-wide distribution and, especially in infancy, may produce quite severe diarrhoea due to the fact that unabsorbed lactose may retain excess fluid in the intestinal lumen. The intestinal mucosa, however, appears normal morphologically, the diagnosis being made by measurement of enzyme activity in homogenized mucosal biopsy material. Multiple disaccharidase deficiencies may be acquired as a result of the enterocyte damage found in conditions such as coeliac disease.

The second category includes the rare congenital disease usually known as *abetalipoproteinaemia*. Inherited as an autosomal recessive defect, it appears to be caused by the impaired formation of a protein required for the transport from the enterocyte to the villous lacteals of triglyceride resynthesized following the absorption of fatty acids and monoglycerides from the intestinal lumen. Tryglyceride thus accumulates within enterocytes and is discharged into the intestinal lumen when these cells come to the end of their life-span. The resulting steatorrhoea may be associated with malabsorption of fat-soluble vitamins. Other pathological effects of this disease

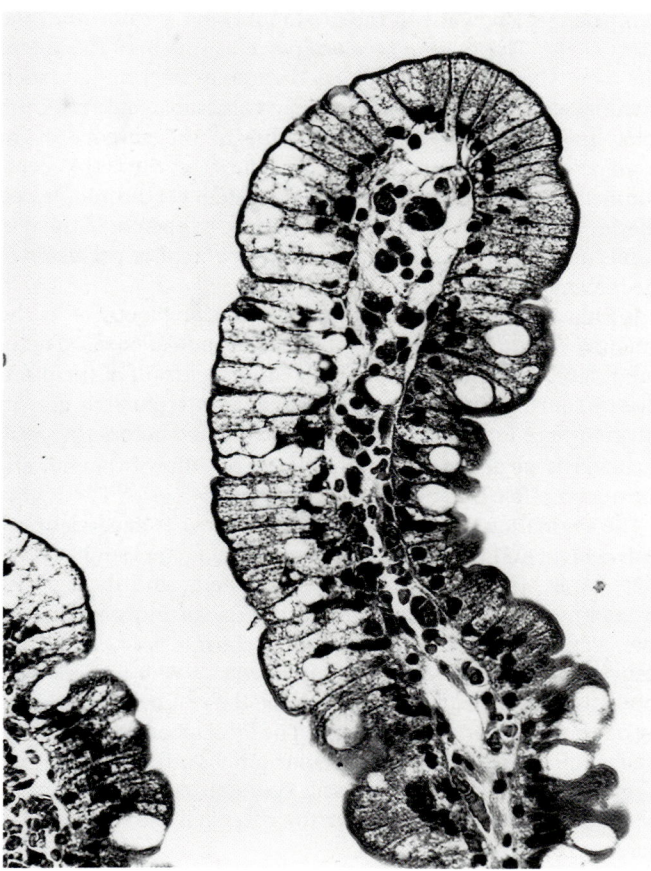

Fig. 16.108 Abetalipoproteinaemia. The villi are normal but the epithelial cells are vacuolated due to the accumulation of lipid.

include a curious, spiny, red cell defect (acanthocytosis), cerebellar dysfunction, and retinitis pigmentosa. The diagnosis is made readily in jejunal biopsies which reveal pronounced vacuolation of enterocytes at the villous extremity (Fig. 16.108). That this cellular change is due to lipid retention can be confirmed by the use of fat stains in frozen sections. The villous pattern is usually normal.

Intestinal lymphangiectasia

Interference with lymphatic flow from the intestinal mucosa is a not unimportant cause of malabsorption, especially if this is accompanied by enteric protein loss. Lymphatic obstruction may, for example, contribute to the impairment of absorption found in diseases affecting the mesentery and mesenteric lymph nodes, such as tuberculosis or malignant lymphoma, and may also be an important feature of Crohn's disease, in which there is often widespread lymphatic occlusion and obliteration by the granulomatous process. Lymphatic damage may also be a feature of a radiation enteritis, and some measure of lymphatic stasis may also be found in conditions such as congestive cardiac failure and constrictive pericarditis. In all of these conditions, dilatation of mucosal lymphatics may be conspicuous,

and lipid-containing histiocytes may be found not only in the dilated channels but throughout the lamina propria and in the submucosa. Under normal conditions, histiocytes of this kind are only found as a rule at the villous extremity.

The term *intestinal lymphangiectasia* usually refers, however, to a condition in which there is a congenital malformation of lymphatics in the small intestine and related mesentery. This is often accompanied by similar lymphatic disturbances elsewhere, especially in the limbs. The widespread dilatation of mucosal lymphatics, which is characteristic of the condition, leads to impaired fat absorption and to enteric loss of protein, which may be inferred from the presence of ceroid pigment in the intestinal musculature. There may also be enteric loss of lymphocytes of such a degree as to produce significant lymphopenia and predispose to opportunistic infection.

16.8.5 Further reading

Banwell, J. G., Kistler, L. A., Gianella, R. A., Weber, F. L., Lieber, A., and Powel, D. (1981). Small intestinal bacterial overgrowth syndrome. *Gastroenterology* **80**, 834–45.

Cook, G. C. (1984). Aetiology and pathogenesis of post-infective tropical malabsorption (tropical sprue). *Lancet* i, 721–3.

Cook, G. C. and Lee, F. D. (1966). The jejunum after kwashiorkor. *Lancet* ii, 1263–7.

Dobbins, W. O., III (1985). Whipples disease: a historical perspective. *Quarterly Journal of Medicine* **56**, 523–31.

Kotler, D. P., Gaetz, P. H., Lange, M., Klein, E. B., and Holt, P. R. (1984). Enteropathy associated with the acquired immunodeficiency syndrome. *Annals of Internal Medicine* **101**, 421–8.

Langman, M. J. S., McConnell, T. H., Spiegelhalter, D. J., and McCormack, R. B. (1985). Changing patterns of coeliac disease frequency: an analysis of Coeliac Society membership records. *Gut* **26**, 175–8.

Swinson, C. M., Slavin, G., Coles, E. G., and Booth, C. C. (1983). Coeliac disease and malignancy. *Lancet* **1**, 111–15.

Ward, H., Jalan, K. N., Maitra, T. K., Agarwal, S. K., and Mahalanabis, D. (1983). Small intestinal nodular lymphoid hyperplasia in patients with giardiasis and normal serum immunoglobulins. *Gut* **24**, 120–6.

Watt, J., Pincott, J. R., and Harries, J. T. (1983). Combined cows milk protein and gluten-induced enteropathy: common or rare? *Gut* **24**, 165–70.

16.9 Vascular disease of the small and large intestine

Helene C. Rees

16.9.1 Ischaemia

Introduction

Ischaemia occurs in the intestine when it receives less oxygenated blood than it requires to maintain proper structure and function. The intestine has a high metabolic rate and tolerates ischaemia poorly. Difficulties have arisen due to the many complex pathological entities that can be produced due to ischaemia and the various different names given to them. This range is the result of the variable effects produced by ischaemia depending on its severity, acuteness, and duration.

The main causes of ischaemia are vascular occlusion and hypotension, or a combination of both. The effect this will have on the bowel is very dependent on other factors, such as the degree and state of the collateral circulation, the bacterial flora of the gut, and the luminal pressure; for this reason a single event does not necessarily always give an identical outcome.

Many other diseases of the bowel can have similar histological appearances to ischaemia. Early, less severe ischaemic lesions with mucosal involvement alone can mimic non-specific colitis, infective colitis, or ulcerative colitis, and later stenotic ischaemic lesions can be very similar to Crohn's disease. It is therefore important to take into account the clinical findings and results of other investigations (see Table 16.8).

Pseudomembraneous colitis was initially thought to be ischaemic in nature but due to the isolation of *Clostridium difficule* a predominantly infective cause has been proven, but the macroscopic and microscopic ischaemic pseudomembranes can be very similar (Fig. 16.109).

Anatomy and physiology

The small and large intestine obtain their blood supply from the aorta via three main vessels: the coeliac axis, the superior mesenteric artery (SMA) and the inferior mesenteric artery (IMA). The circulation is very dependent on adequate pressure and flow. The upper and lower branches have good collateral supply from the extra coelomic vessels, so ischaemia in their distribution is rare, but the superior mesentertic artery is a functional end artery so acute occlusion of this vessel frequently results in ischaemic damage. Only the first part of the duodenum is supplied by the coeliac axis, the rest of the small and large bowel is supplied via the SMA and IMA (the SMA from the duodenum to a variable portion of the transverse colon and the IMA to the rest). The small bowel receives greater blood flow

than the large bowel and the proximal colon greater than the distal colon. The rectum receives twice as much as the colon. The watershed areas between each vascular distribution, such as the splenic flexure, are particularly vulnerable, but the entire colon has a greater susceptibility due to the absence of an arcuate system. The terminal branches of the IMA communicate freely with the internal iliac system via the middle and inferior haemorrhoidal arteries. Therefore ischaemia of the rectum is unusual unless there is stenosis or complete occlusion of the internal iliac arteries.

Within the bowel wall the main vascular plexus is in the submucosa and this has a good arteriolar anastomosis. Therefore infarction of the intestine following occlusion of the distal intestinal arteries is unusual. Due to a counter-current flow in the villi there is shunting of oxygenated blood across the base, particularly at decreased flow rates, so the tips of the villi are more susceptible to hypoxia.

The regulation of the intestinal blood flow is dependent on both central and peripheral factors. Central factors such as cardiac output, the autonomic nervous system, and the level of circulating catecholamines greatly influence intestinal blood flow. Peripheral factors are also important. These can cause both functional and reactive hyperaemia as well as pressure-flow autoregulation. This appears to be the result of factors acting on the pre-arteriole sphincters. The local blood flow pressure itself is thought to affect the vascular tone. Both metabolic and pressure effects cause decreased vascular resistance during reduction in arterial pressure or the reverse if the resistance is increased.

Pathogenesis

There are four major causes of intestinal ischaemia:

1. arterial occlusion;
2. non-occlusive states;
3. venous occlusion;
4. mural vascular pathology.

Table 16.8 Differential diagnosis of ischaemic colitis and inflammatory bowel disease*

	Ischaemic colitis	Ulcerative colitis	Crohn's disease
Age at onset	Elderly	Young	Young to middle-aged
Presentation	Always acute	Acute or chronic	Usually chronic
Segment involved	Splenic flexure (rectum rare, anus never)	Left-side or total (rectum always)	Anywhere (rectum usual, anus commonly)
Radiology	Thumbprints	Shortening	Spicules
	Stricture	Ulceration	Skip lesions
		Megacolon	Obstruction
Pathology	Fibrosis	Mucosal loss	Fissures
	Haemosiderosis	Crypt abscess	Granuloma
			Lymphadenopathy
Association conditions	Claudication	Iritis	Enteric fistula
	Angina	Arthritis	Anal involvement
	Stroke	Pyoderma	Failure of B_{12} absorption
		Malignant change	

*After Marston, A., (1985). *Clinics in Gastroenterology* **14**, 847–61; reproduced with permission.

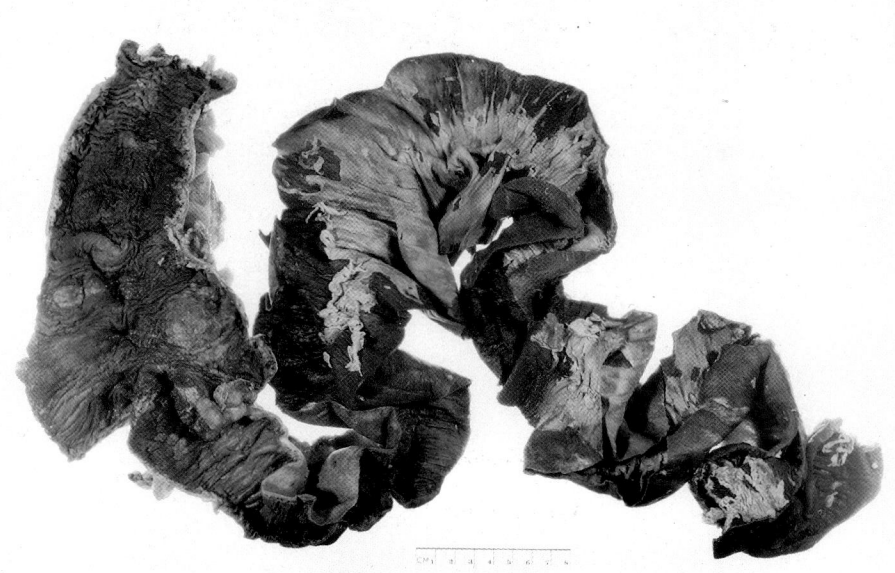

Fig. 16.109 Ileum and ascending colon. There is extensive haemorrhagic infarction of the small bowel with less severe changes in the caecum and ascending colon. The mucosal surface is covered with a pale pseudomembrane which easily separates from the deeply congested underlying tissue.

Arterial occlusion

Arterial occlusion due to atheroma is the commonest cause of ischaemia. It usually affects the main trunks at their ostia or in the proximal 2 cm of their course; superimposed thrombosis frequently precipitates the ischaemia. Most patients are in late middle age with vascular disease elsewhere, and males are more commonly affected than females. There is a correlation with ischaemic heart disease, diabetes, and hypertension. Blood flow studies show that there needs to be a very considerable reduction in diameter before the blood flow is reduced significantly, but once that point is reached only slight further diminution will produce a significant fall in blood flow. Stenosis of the SMA is commonly seen at post-mortem; in some it is just a coincidental finding, others will have a history of abdominal angina, and in some there will be intestinal infarction.

Thrombosis usually complicates atheroma. Other thrombotic disorders may predispose to vascular occlusion, including polycythaemia rubra vera, sickle-cell anaemia, and cryoglobulinaemia. In the neonate, thrombosis of the SMA can be associated with an indwelling umbilical arterial catheter.

Embolism is much less frequent and decreasing in incidence. It may be of cardiac origin due to atrial fibrillation, infective endocarditis, or from a mural thrombus in conjunction with a myocardial infarct. It may arise from the aorta overlying atheromatous plaques or in association with an aortic aneurysm. Less common causes of arterial occlusion are external pressure from tumours or the medial arcuate ligament, trauma, angiitis, or dissecting aneurysm of aorta.

Non-occlusive ischaemic infarction

This can be due to cardiac failure, hypovolaemic shock, splanchnic vasoconstriction, drugs, or trauma. Non-occlusive ischaemic infarction accounts for approximately 30 per cent of all cases of intestinal infarction. This is seen in older age-groups, usually with organic heart disease. The onset of intestinal ischaemia is often precipitated by a sudden drop in cardiac output due to myocardial infarction, the onset of cardiac arrythmias, or the additional stress of another illness, such as pneumonia or pulmonary embolus. Almost all are digitalized and this itself can cause splanchnic vasoconstriction. Cardiac surgery is a rarer cause. In patients with normal cardiac function intestinal ischaemia can develop as a result of hypovolaemic shock from blood loss or septicaemia.

Venous occlusion

Venous occlusion is less common but can result in infarction (Fig. 16.110). It is slower, with associated greater haemorrhage and oedema, but the final outcome is the same as it leads to arterial occlusion. It occurs most frequently from external pressure, such as compression from the edge of a hernial sac, volvulus, intersusception, or tumour. Thrombosis of the portal or mesenteric veins may, in younger females, be associated with the oral contraceptive pill or pregnancy. Hypovolaemia or malignancy may also predispose to venous thrombosis.

Pathology of mural vasculature

Any disease that affects small vessels can cause ischaemic

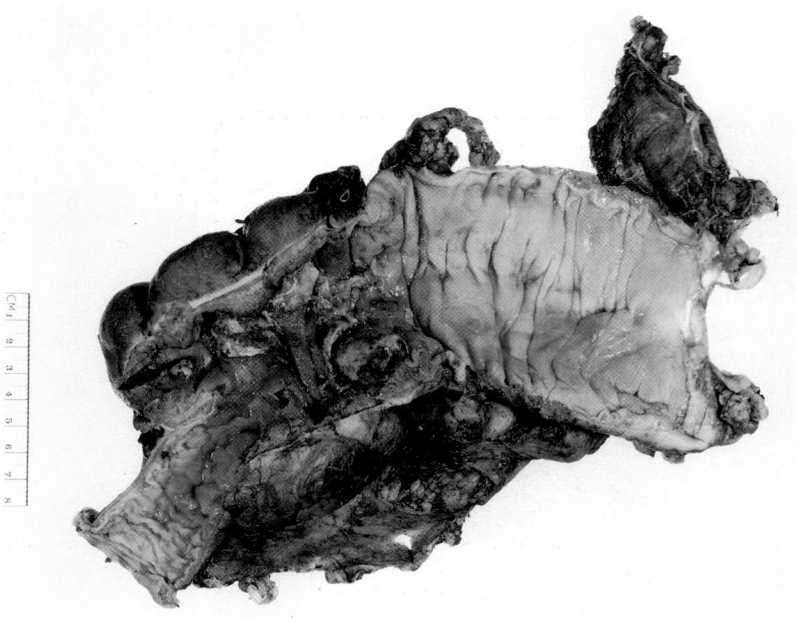

Fig. 16.110 Right hemicolectomy specimen shows marked thickening and haemorrhage of the caecal wall. The overlying mucosa is extensively ulcerated. These changes are the result of extensive mesenteric thrombosis.

lesions in the bowel. This is usually much less rapid in onset and there may be only very little evidence of ischaemic damage, if any.

Vasculitis is the predominant cause in this category; it can present with acute or chronic clinical features, and widespread or focal involvement.

Primary vasculitis due to immune complexes or collagen disease can affect the gut. Polyarteritis nodosa (PAN) involves the gastrointestinal tract in more than 50 per cent of patients at some time during the course of the disease. The small bowel is the most frequent site of involvement. A rare variant of PAN, Köhlmeier–Degos syndrome, is characterized by papular skin eruptions and intestinal perforations, associated with occlusive lesions of the small arteries. Vasculitis can be associated with rheumatoid arthritis and, when it is, it frequently involves the intestine. Systemic lupus erythematosus can affect the bowel and Henoch–Schönlein pupura most frequently involves the gastrointestinal tract in children. Less frequently, scleroderma, Wegener's granulomatosis, and dermatomyositis can affect the gut. Secondary vasculitis can occur due to infective causes such as tuberculosis, typhoid, or syphilis, or due to inflammatory conditions, like ulcerative colitis, Crohn's disease, or after irradiation.

Despite the numerous causes of ischaemia, the end result is similar. Experimentally it has been shown that there are two phases to ischaemic damage. The initial phase is due to hypoxia from lack of adequate blood supply. The second phase results from the secondary hyperaemia which occurs when blood seeps back into the ischaemic areas from the adjacent collateral circulation. This results in cytotoxicity from oxygen free radicals that have been formed as a result of various enzymes acting on intra-

cellular substrates. In the small bowel these radicals are produced by xanthine oxidase acting on hypoxanthine when oxygen becomes available during the reperfusion phase. In the colon other enzyme systems, such as aldehyde oxidase, are probably responsible, or polymorph neutrophils which are also a potent source of free oxygen radicals.

Pathology

Ischaemic infarction in the intestines is much less common than in the heart, brain, or limbs, but it has serious consequences particularly as mid-gut necrosis is almost always fatal.

Ischaemia is characterized by death of a variable thickness of intestinal wall, initially starting from the luminal aspect. The pathological features depend more on the severity and duration of the ischaemia than on its cause. Ischaemia may result either in haemorrhagic, gangrenous infarction usually associated with a major vessel occlusion, following which there is no chance of resolution, or ischaemic enterocolitis or colitis which is usually associated with a non-occlusive cause and which can be patchy or extensive. Ischaemic enterocolitis may lead to focal gangrene and perforation, transient ischaemic damage with complete resolution, or resolution but with the development of an ischaemic stricture.

Gangrenous infarction

The bowel is initially pale and contracted due to spasm. Later there is marked congestion and dilatation of vessels and the serosal surface becomes dull, dark plum red to black in colour with the development of a fibrinous exudate. The lumen contains thick, blood-stained fluid. The mucosal surface is dark red with a pseudopolypoid appearance and later develops irregular serpiginous ulceration which can extend to the submucosa. The muscle layer is thin and attenuated. There may be definite signs of perforation and associated peritonitis.

Microscopically the changes start at the mucosal surface and extend serosally. There is death of the surface enterocytes, damage to the basement membrane, and haemorrhage into the lamina propria with marked capillary dilatation. Finally, total necrosis of the mucosa supervenes with only a ghost outline remaining. Clusters of bacteria are seen in the dead tissue and polymorphoneutrophils gradually accumulate. The submucosa is oedematous with areas of haemorrhage. The deep muscle layer shows irregular staining with loss of nuclear detail and finally necrosis. Serositis is present. There is no possibility of resolution (Fig. 16.111).

Ischaemic enterocolitis

Although complete resolution is possible following ischaemic enterocolitis, up to 50 per cent will result in strictures. Complete resolution is only possible when the changes are confined predominantly to the mucosa. Microscopically there is oedema and congestion with areas of haemorrhage into the lamina propria and a gradual increase in polymorphonuclear cells. The tips of the villi and surface enterocytes show the first signs of necrosis. Often fibrin thrombi are seen in the small vessels. There can be areas of definite ulceration. Later, macrophages invade the area and, due to ingestion of red blood cells, will contain haemosiderin. Granulation tissue will form in areas of ulceration, and patchy fibrosis will supervene where the damage is too severe for complete resolution. Where the crypt bases still remain undamaged the crypt cells can proliferate to regenerate an intact mucosa.

Ischaemic strictures

Repair proceeds with the formation of granulation tissue and, if the muscularis mucosae is damaged, it is accompanied by splaying of the adjacent muscularis mucosae. Within the resulting fibrous tissue scattered clusters of haemosiderin-laden macrophages and foci of chronic inflammatory cells can be seen. The adjacent enterocytes attempt to cover the denuded surface (Fig. 16.112) but, if extensive, there will be a persisting ulcerated area. With time, a fibrous stricture develops with hypertrophy of the remaining muscle layer. These strictures are particularly frequent in the watershed areas such as the splenic flexure.

16.9.2 Other entities caused by an ischaemic basis

Necrotizing enterocolitis (NEC)

This condition is seen in very low-birth-weight babies but full-term infants may also be affected. There is patchy or widespread necrosis of small and large bowel mucosa and submucosa, most frequently seen in the terminal ileum or proximal colon. Gangrene and perforation can supervene. Factors involved in the pathogenesis appear to be mucosal ischaemia and damage, and

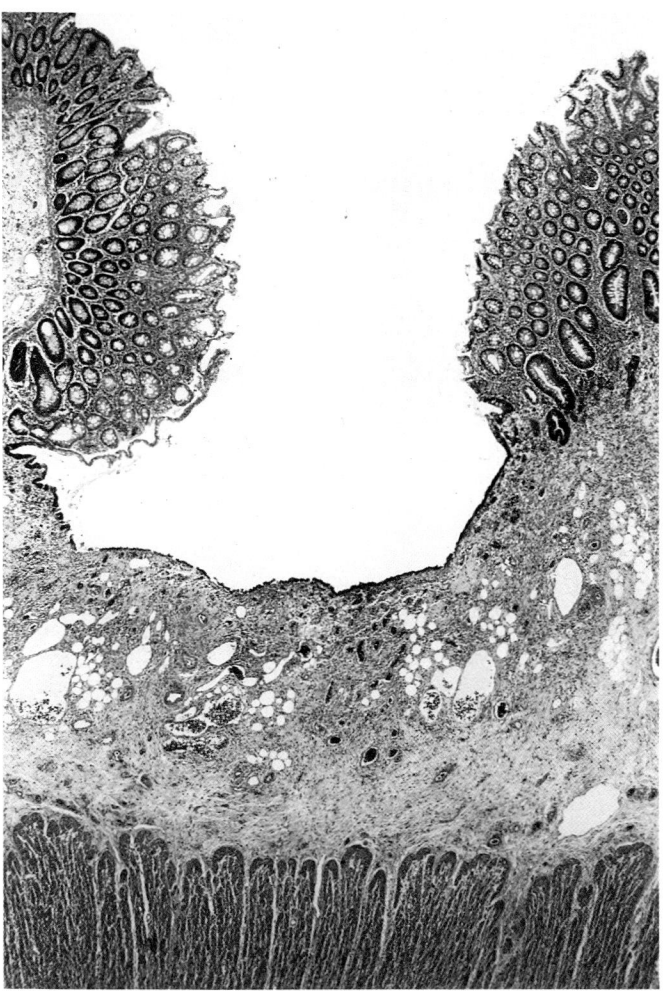

Fig. 16.112 Caecum. Repair processes taking place in an area of ischaemic ulceration.

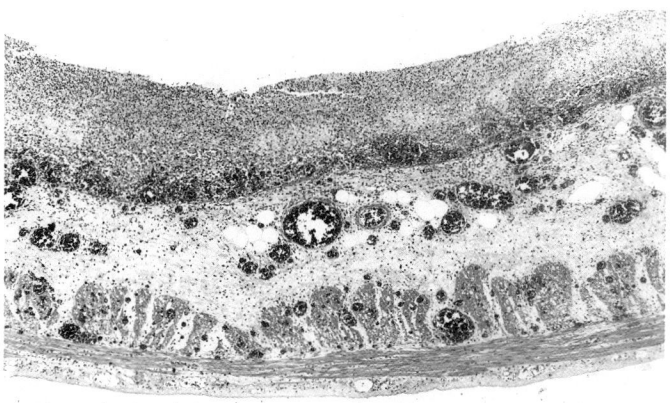

Fig. 16.111 Small bowel shows haemorrhagic infarction with complete necrosis of the mucosa, haemorrhage, congestion and eodema of the submucosa. The deep muscle layer shows patchy necrosis of the circular muscle.

bacterial colonization of the bowel lumen. It would seem that NEC is associated with overwhelming hypotensive ischaemic injury to the intestine, linked with enteric septicaemia, and that intestinal immaturity may aggrevate the situation. Other factors that help damage the mucosa, such as oral feeds, can play a part.

Macroscopically the bowel is dilated and markedly congested; this can be continuous or patchy, with or without associated serosal gas bubbles. Microscopically there is haemorrhagic infarction of the mucosa and a variable amount of submucosa with a range of inflammatory responses. Frequently there is pneumatosis intestinalis, especially involving the submucosa (Fig. 16.113). Often platelet fibrin thrombi can be seen in small capillaries. If the necrosis is limited to the mucosa and submucosa, healing with re-epithelization and variable amounts of fibrosis can take place. Often stricture formation follows.

Solitary ulcers in the small bowel

It is felt that ischaemia is an important factor in the aetiology of ulcers associated with ingestion of enteric coated potassium. In many cases the pathological features are entirely consistent with an ischaemic cause. Ischaemia can result from the relative hypotension as the blood pressure is reduced, or to arterial or venous spasms due to release of high concentrations of potassium locally.

Ulcers are also seen in association with the taking of non-steroidal anti-inflammatory drugs. This, again, is most likely ischaemic due to local vasoconstriction following the contact of a partially digested tablet with the small bowel mucosa.

16.9.3   Vascular anomalies

With more sophisticated diagnostic techniques, such as selective visceral angiography and good colonoscopy, the identification of these lesions has become easier, and their incidence has proved greater than previously thought. The lesions can be divided into five groups based on the type and size of the vessels involved and whether there are systemic or cutaneous associated lesions forming a syndrome. These groups are:

1. angioectasia (angiodysplasia);
2. multiple phlebectasia;
3. telangioectasia associated with various syndromes, such as hereditary haemorrhagic telangiectasia (Osler–Weber–Rendu syndrome);
4. haemangioma, divided further into type of vessel involved or associated syndrome;
5. disorders of connective tissue affecting blood vessels, such as Ehlers–Danlos syndrome.

All are exceedingly rare except for haemangiomas and angioectasia.

Angioectasia (Angiodysplasia)

In this condition there are small vascular ectasias involving the mucosa and submucosa of the bowel. Most frequently it is the caecum and ascending colon that are involved, but other areas of the colon and small intestine can be affected. The true incidence is not known but studies have revealed that they are a common cause of lower gastrointestinal bleeding in the elderly and post-mortem studies in asymptomatic patients have recorded an incidence of 1–2 per cent.

The aetiology is not known but the most acceptable explanation is that they are acquired degenerative lesions caused by chronic intermittent pressure obstructing veins as they penetrate the bowel wall. This is caused by contractions of the deep muscle layer and results in increased venous pressure causing dilatation of the submucosal and mucosal veins.

Macroscopically the lesions are difficult to see in resected specimens unless the vessels have been injected with a barium–gelatine mixture and examined under a dissecting microscope. They range from 0.5 to 1.5 cm, are often multiple, and are seen

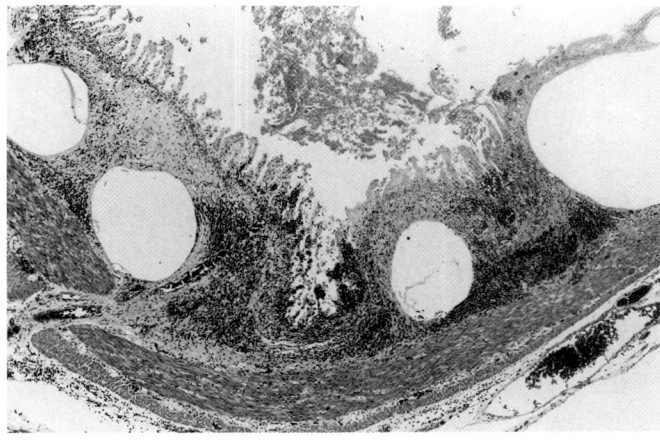

Fig. 16.113 Necrotizing enterocolitis of the small bowel. There is extensive mucosal and submucosal necrosis with haemorrhage and gas in the submucosa.

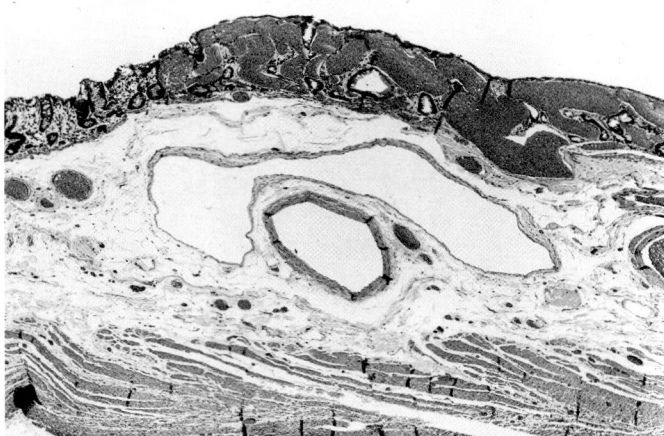

Fig. 16.114 Caecal angioectasia. The mucosa contains ectatic capillaries causing glandular atrophy and distortion. The underlying submucosa contains ectatic capillaries and venules. The vessels have been injected with a barium–gelatine mixture.

as a reef-like network of vessels in the mucosa. Microscopically the lesions consist of large, dilated capillaries in the mucosa causing atrophy of the adjacent glands. There are both ectatic capillaries and venules in the underlying submucosa. Only rarely are arterioles involved (Fig. 16.114).

Haemangiomas

These mainly involve the vessels of the submucosal plexus. They are rare apart from those associated with hereditary or congenital syndromes such as the autosomal dominant Blue rubber bleb naevus syndrome and the non-hereditary Klippel–Trenaunay–Weber syndrome.

Haemangiomas can be single or multiple: capillary, cavernous, or mixed. Sometimes cavernous haemangiomas of the rectum can be more diffuse and extend to involve the adjacent viscera or retroperitoneum.

16.9.4   Further reading

Boley, S., Sammartano, A., Adams, A., Diabiase, S., Kleihause, S., and Sprayregen, S. (1977). On the nature and etiology of vascular ectasias of the colon. *Gastroenterology* **72**, 650–60.

Camilleri, M., Chadwick, V. S., and Hodgson, H. J. F. (1984). Vascular anomalies of the gastrointestinal tract. *Hepato-Gastroenterology* **13**, 149–53.

Gentry, R., Dockerty, M. B., and Clagett, O. T. (1949). Vascular malformations and vascular tumours of the gastrointestinal tract. *International Abstracts of Surgery* **88**, 281–323.

Kliegman, R. M. and Fanaroff, A. A. (1984). Necrotizing enterocolitis. *New England Journal of Medicine* **310** (no. 17), 1093–103.

Kumar, P. and Dawson, A. M. (1972). Vasculitis of the alimentary tract. *Clinics in Gastroenterology* **1** (3), 719–43.

Kvietys, P. R. and Granger, D. N. (1986). Physiology and Pathophysiology of the colonic circulation. *Clinics in Gastroenterology* **15** (4), 967–85.

Marston, A. (1985). Ischaemia. *Clinics in Gastroenterology* **14** (4), 847–62.

Marston, A., Pheils, M. T., Thomas, M. L., and Morson, B. C. (1966). Ischaemic colitis. *Gut* **7**, 1–15.

Rees, H. C. and Wright, N. A. (1983). Angiodysplasia of the colon. In *Recent advances in histopathology* (ed. R. N. McSween).

Whitehead, R. (1972). The pathology of intestinal ischaemia. *Clinics in Gastroenterology* **1** (3), 613–39.

16.10   Small bowel infection

A. B. Price

16.10.1   Introduction

Inflammatory diseases of the small and large bowel can be divided into two basic patterns. First, specific inflammatory conditions due to proven infective agents in which there may be a recognizable pathological pattern and the organism identified, e.g. caseating granulomas in tuberculosis. Secondly, there is the non-specific inflammatory pattern. In this group the pathology is classified inflammatory by the nature of the cellular infiltrate but no recognizable infective agent is identified, e.g. ulcerative colitis, Crohn's disease. In time it seems likely that the non-specific group will diminish as specific causes are identified. For example, until 1973 pseudomembranous colitis was classified as a vascular disease but was then shown to be due to infection by *Clostridium difficile*. In a similar vein, *Campylobactor* spp. are now amongst the commonest causes of diarrhoea in Western Europe yet were grown for only the first time from stools in 1972.

The pathogenesis of intestinal infection, and consequently the pathological picture produced by any infective agent, depends on a variety of factors related to both host and organism. The route of entry is important, most are oral but infection can occur from sexual contact. Once within the intestinal tract there must be successful colonization before disease is evident and this depends on several mechanisms, amongst which are enterotoxins, enteroadhesion, and invasion aided by the production of cytotoxins. Some organisms are highly virulent and only a few are required to produce symptoms and damage, e.g. *Shigella* spp., while others have to be present in a large infecting dose, e.g. *Salmonella* spp. The pathogenicity of *Clostridium difficile* in the adult is due to production of certain toxins yet the organism and its toxins are non-pathogenic in the neonatal bowel. This is almost certainly because the neonatal gut epithelial cells lack the relevant receptors. In the acquired immunodeficiency syndrome (AIDS) alteration to the host's T-lymphocytes means that organisms, not normally pathogenic in the immunocompetent individuals, can cause disease, e.g. *Cytomegalovirus*, *Cryptosporidium*.

This balance of factors between host and organism is important to bear in mind when considering the pathology of intestinal inflammatory and infective conditions. Under normal circumstances the upper small bowel is populated by transient bacteria originating from the oral cavity. In the terminal ileum the flora approximates to that in the caecum. In tropical countries moderate numbers of organisms can be found in the jejunum. In the colon large numbers of bacteria are present, many of which have a role in human physiology. In particular, in the context of infection, many effectively compete to keep out pathogens. Moreover, antibiotics, although they may eliminate pathogens, also remove much of the normal protective flora thereby exposing the patient to a range of new pathogens, e.g. fungi, *Clostridium difficile*. The principal causes of specific intestinal inflammation are listed in Table 16.9.

In the clinical situation patients with enteric infections commonly present with acute watery diarrhoea, diarrhoea with blood, pus or mucus, systemic symptoms, or chronic diarrhoea and malabsorption. The first will often have non-invasive organisms and a short-lived attack. When blood is present it usually infers an invasive organism and colonic disease. Chronic diarrhoea, although it maybe due to *Giardiasis* or worms, is more likely to be one of the non-specific forms of inflammatory bowel disease, e.g. ulcerative colitis or Crohn's disease.

Table 16.9 Pathogens of the large and small bowel

Bacteria	Viruses
Aeromonas spp.	Adenovirus
Campylobacter spp.	Astrovirus
Chlamydia spp. [lymphogranuloma	Calicivirus
venereum (LGV) and non-LGV	Cytomegalovirus
immunotypes]	Herpes simplex virus
Coronavirus	
Clostridium spp. (*difficile, perfringens,*	*Norwalk virus*
septicum)	Rotavirus
Escherichia coli spp. (enterotoxigenic,	
enteroinvasive, enteropathogenic)	
Escherichia coli vero-toxigenic 0157	
Mycobacterium avium-intracellulare	
? Mycobacterium paratuberculosis	
Mycobacterium tuberculosis	
Neisseria gonorrhoea	
Pleisomonas spp.	
Salmonella spp.	
Shigella spp.	
Spirochaetosis	
Staphylococcus aureus	
Treponema pallidum	
Vibrio cholera	
Yersinia spp.	

Protozoans	Helminths	Fungi
Balantidium coli	*Anisakis*	*Actinomyces* spp.
Coccidia spp.	*Ankylostoma duodenale*	*Candida albicans*
Cryptospordium spp.	*Ascaris lumbricoides*	*Histoplasma* spp.
Isospora belli	*Capillaria philippinensis*	*Mucor*
Entamoeba histolytica	*Oxyuris vermicularis*	
Giardia lamblia	*Schistosoma* spp.	
Microsporidia	*Spirometra*	
	mansonoides	
Trypanosoma spp.	*(Diphyllobothrium)*	
	Strongyloides	
	stercoralis	
	Taenia spp.	
	Trichuris trichuria	

16.10.2   Bacterial infections

Cholera

Patients with cholera are described as having rice-water stools which are grey and opalescent due to the presence of mucus, inflammatory cells, and degenerate epithelial cells. The disease is caused by non-invasive toxigenic strains of *Vibrio cholera* and is endemic in parts of Africa and southern Asia. Pints of fluid are lost via the diarrhoea and severe dehydration results. It is a disease of the poor in conditions of inadequate sanitation, usually with seasonal outbreaks. Contaminated water from human carriers is the usual source of infection.

Pathology

Minor changes in the small intestine have been described. There may be desquamation of enterocytes over the tips of villi. The lamina propria is congested and there is a minor increase in inflammatory cells. However, the abnormalities are all mild and, indeed, may all be non-specific.

Pathophysiology

The excess intestinal secretion is due to cholera toxin. This is a protein, part of which is responsible for adherence of the organism to the enterocyte and part enters the cell to activate adenylate cyclase. This in turn affects the enzyme mechanisms that inhibit absorption and stimulate secretion of water and electrolytes.

Clostridial infections

There is a small group of ulcerating and necrotic conditions of the jejunum and ileum, commonly referred to by the term enteritis necroticans, that may be of clostridial origin.

Enteritis necroticans (Pig-bel)

This disease is a patchy necrotizing disease of the small bowel. The name Pig-bel derives from the hills of Papua New Guinea where the disease is a major cause of morbidity following ritual pig feasting. However, similar pathology has been described in outbreaks of disease in Germany and parts of Asia. Segments of small bowel show mucosal infarction (Fig. 16.115). There may be vascular thrombosis and gas cysts can be found in the bowel wall. This description is of the most severe form of disease and a less fulminant form can occur in which patients recover, with resolution leading to eventual strictures.

Clostridium perfringens type C is believed to be the pathogen in Papua. The pig is eaten along with sweet potato which contains a powerful trypsin inhibitor. Digestive proteases are inhibited, allowing the organisms to proliferate in the upper small bowel. In outbreaks of necrotizing jejunitis in Asian countries, *Shigella* spp., *Entamoeba histolytica*, and *Campylobactor* spp. have been identified. As these are mainly colonic pathogens it suggests that certain forms of necrotizing small bowel disease may simply be secondary to the metabolic effects of prolonged diarrhoea in these patients.

Escherichia coli infection

Three main groups of pathogenic *Escherichia coli* (*E. coli*) are capable of infecting the gut. These are enterotoxigenic *E. coli*,

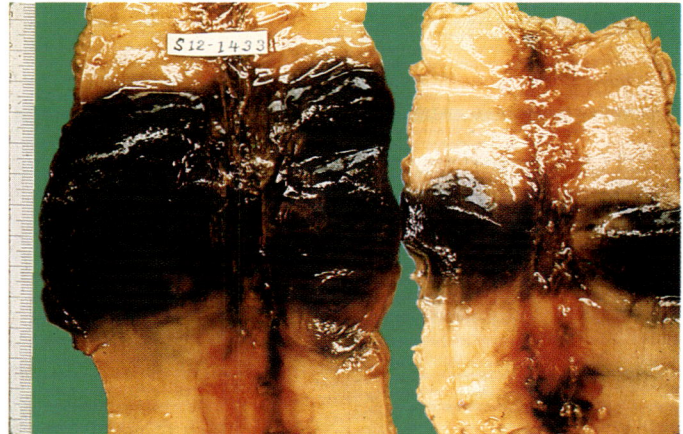

Fig. 16.115 Two lengths of ileum showing band-like zones of haemorrhagic necrosis. *Clostridium welchii* was implicated in this case.

enteropathogenic *E. coli*, and enteroinvasive *E. coli*. Recently an enterohaemorrhagic organism has been described (Section 16.12.2). Enterotoxogenic *E. coli* produce heat-stable and heat-labile toxins, the latter with an action similar to cholera toxin. This group is one of the commonest cause of travellers' diarrhoea but as yet no small bowel changes have been described. Enteropathogenic (enteroadherent) *E. coli* are a common cause of diarrhoea in infants and recent work has demonstrated adherence to enterocyte plasma membranes. Members of the enteroinvasive group resemble *Shigella* spp. and are colonic pathogens (Section 16.12.2).

Tuberculosis

Tuberculosis of the bowel can be divided into primary and secondary forms. In primary disease the organisms infect the mesenteric lymph nodes and bowel wall as the initial disease. In secondary tuberculosis the source of infection is swallowed sputum coughed up from an existing pulmonary lesion. This establishes re-infection in an already sensitized individual. Although it is an uncommon disease in the Western world, this is not the case in the United Kingdom immigrant Asian population. In this group gastrointestinal disease often presents in the years soon after arrival. Between 20 and 50 per cent of patients presenting with gastrointestinal tuberculosis will have pulmonary disease.

Macroscopic appearances

The distribution of disease tends to follow the localization of lymphoid tissue in the small intestine. Increasing in frequency from jejunum to ileum. In the pattern known as ulcerative tuberculosis, annular ulcers (Fig. 16.116), lying transversely and raised above the mucosa, are seen usually producing strictures. The cut surface may be white and friable. The local lymph nodes are invariably enlarged and may contain florid caseating granulomas when only small lesions are present in the gut. As fibrosis occurs there is a change to the hypertrophic or ulceroconstrictive form of disease. Here the bowel wall is thickened,

the mucosa is ulcerated, but fibrosis of the wall makes it firm (see Fig. 16.148). The strictures formed can be short, long, single, or multiple, and the appearances can be mistaken for Crohn's disease (Fig. 16.117) or malignancy. Tuberculosis is the commonest cause of an intestinal stricture in India.

Microscopy

The appearances at microscopy are no different to those seen in tuberculosis of any other organ. Granulomas, in which foci of caseation are nearly always found, occur in all layers of the bowel wall and regional nodes (Fig. 16.118). They are

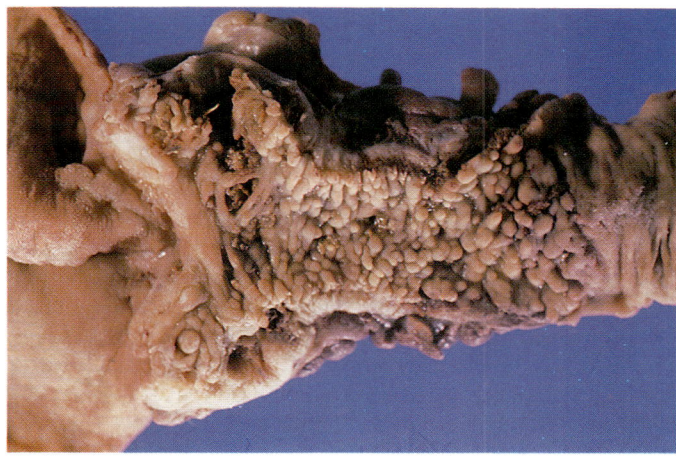

Fig. 16.117 Tuberculosis of the terminal ileum and caecum. There is ulceration around inflammatory mucosal projections and macroscopically this is difficult to distinguish from Crohn's disease.

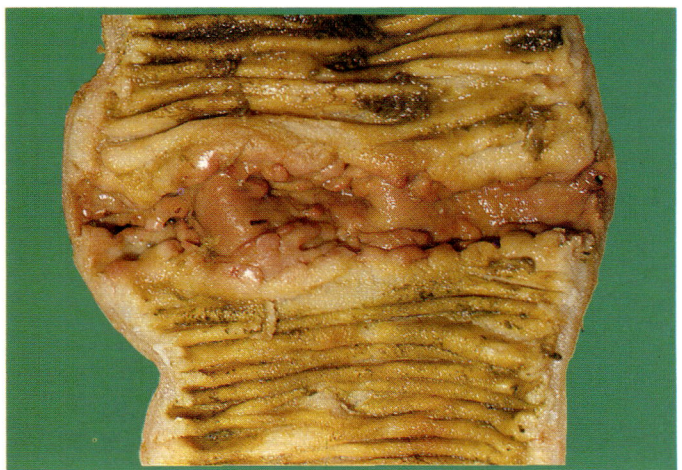

Fig. 16.116 Annular ulceration in a case of ileal tuberculosis.

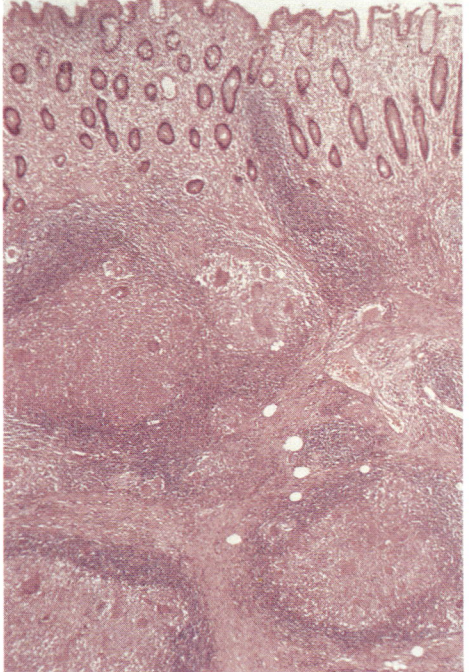

Fig. 16.118 Ileo-caecal tuberculosis showing confluent granulomas in the caecum.

especially common in Peyer's patches. In chronic tuberculosis caseation maybe absent and excess fibrosis present, which destroys the normal structure including the muscularis propria. Even granulomas can hyalinize and disappear in long-standing disease, leaving only small collections of lymphocytes. In such cases it is hard to distinguish the features from strictures due to ischaemia or Crohn's enteritis (Fig. 16.119). Furthermore, it may be difficult to demonstrate acid-fast bacilli in the bowel wall even after a prolonged search. Occasionally they may be more readily demonstrated in the local lymph nodes.

Typhoid fever

The incidence of typhoid fever has declined greatly in the West and the majority of cases documented by the Public Health Laboratories had contracted the infection while travelling outside Europe.

Pathogenesis

The typhoid bacillus, *Salmonella typhi*, reaches the small bowel in food or drink contaminated by infected excreta or from carriers of the organism. The organisms enter the bloodstream via Peyer's patches without producing damage and can be cultured from the blood during the first and second week of the illness. This septicaemia and toxaemia account for the clinical features and characteristic cutaneous rose spots. From the blood the bacilli are excreted by the liver into the bile, enter the gallbladder and then return back to the gut, where they can be cultured in increasing numbers from the stool from the third

week onwards. Urine culture may also be helpful. Specific agglutinating antibodies begin to appear in the blood at the end of the first week, reaching a peak towards the end of the third week. The serological test (Widal reaction) measures titres of serum agglutinins against the somatic (O) and flagellar (H) antigen. A rising titre has the most significance as false positives due to cross-reactivity with other Enterobacteriaceae are common. About 3 per cent of patients fail to clear the organism by 1 year and become chronic carriers.

Macroscopic appearances

Swelling and necrosis of lymphoid tissue produce scattered ulcers, most prominent in the terminal ileum and diminishing proximally in the upper part of the small bowel (Fig. 16.120). The ulcers are oval and arranged in the long axis of the bowel, in contrast to the transverse ulcers of tuberculosis. The ulcers are frequently raised above the mucosa and sharply demarcated with a black slough over the base. Healing occurs relatively swiftly after the acute illness subsides. There is no fibrosis and subsequent strictures or stenosis are rare. Local lymph nodes may be enlarged and show focal necrosis.

Microscopy

The typhoid ulcers are characterized by an infiltrate of large numbers of mononuclear cells, or modified histiocytes, rather than the neutrophil polymorph that is present in the base of most ulcers from other causes (Fig. 16.121). Plasma cells and lymphocytes are found alongside these mononuclear cells. The lesions contain large numbers of typhoid bacilli.

Complications

Perforation and haemorrhage are the two main complications. The former accounts for between 25 and 33 per cent of deaths due to typhoid. It is commonest between the second and third week, occurring usually in the terminal ileum. Bleeding is less common with modern therapy but occurs in the third week as the slough from the mucosal ulcers separate. Typhoid

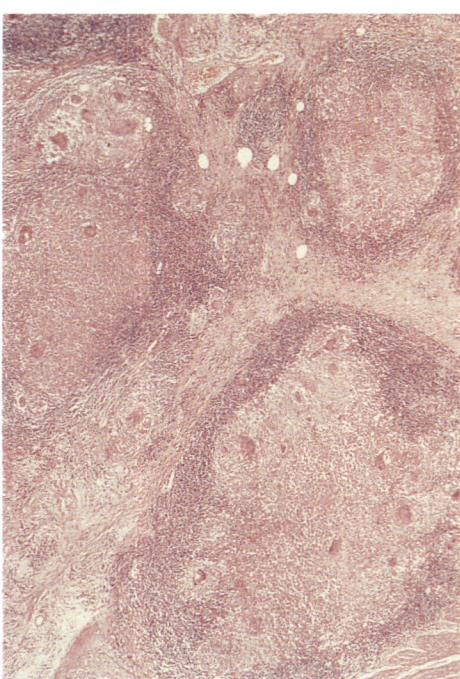

Fig. 16.119 This illustrates the large, closely packed granulomas typical of tuberculosis. In Crohn's disease the granulomas are smaller and more often single.

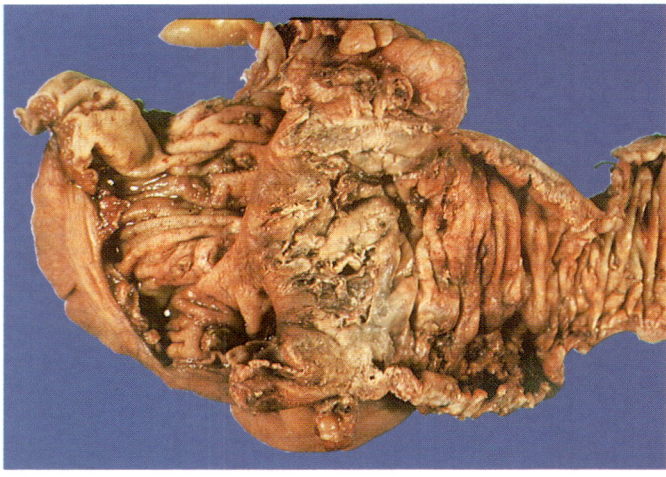

Fig. 16.120 Necrotic ulceration of the terminal ileum in a case of typhoid fever. (Courtesy Dr J. Newman.)

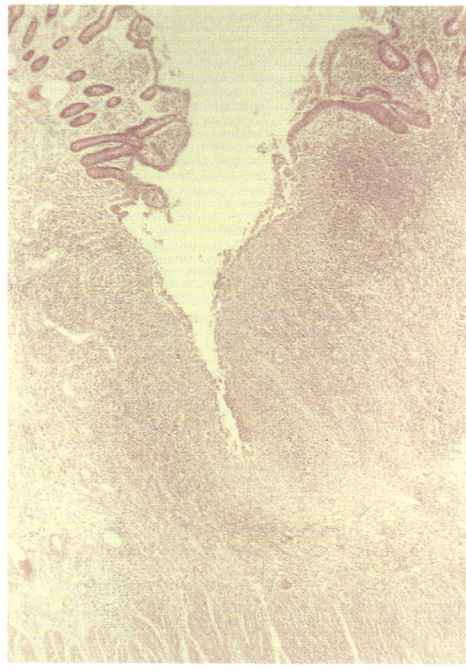

(a)

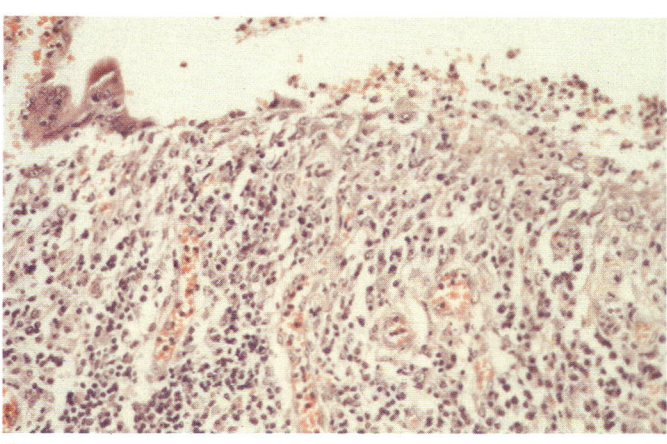

(b)

Fig. 16.121 (a) A penetrating typhoid ulcer with residual epithelium seen to either side towards the top of the picture. (b) The ulcer floor is made up by mononuclear cells in typhoid fever and there is a characteristic paucity of neutrophils.

cholecystitis is also a frequent complication. As well as gastro-intestinal complications, a range of systemic complications may occur, such as a myocarditis and focal necrosis in organs such as the kidney, liver, and testis.

Paratyphoid infection

Paratyphoid fever is a less severe illness caused by *Salmonella paratyphi*. In the West it occurs mainly as outbreaks of food-poisoning. The disease is milder with small ulcers usually restricted to the terminal ileum. It carries fewer complications than typhoid fever.

Other *Salmonella* infections

Salmonella outbreaks account for 10–15 per cent of all adult cases of infective diarrhoea. The organisms are widely distributed in the animal kingdom, including most domestic species and household pets. Infection is most often via the oral route following ingestion of food or drink contaminated by animal or human faeces. Eggs and egg products are commonly involved.

The changes produced in the gut by salmonellosis were believed to be predominantly in the small bowel but more recently it has become evident from biospy work that colitis is common. This correlates well with the observation of blood and pus in the stools of many patients with infection. Animal studies, however, suggest there is also small bowel dysfunction, possibly caused by an enterotoxin. Small bowel changes can be similar to typhoid though less severe. In the most severe cases other organs become involved, but this is rare.

Infection with *Yersinia*

The genus *Yersinia* includes four species. One is the historically famous plague bacillus and two, *Y. enterocolitica* and *Y. pseudo-tuberculosis* cause illness with major gastrointestinal manifestations in humans. The fourth is a pathogen of fish. They are Gram-negative coccobacilli.

Infection with *Y. enterocolitica* or *Y. pseudotuberculosis* is believed to be via the faecal–oral route with an incubation of 4–10 days. Contaminated water, milk, pork, and pet dogs have been shown to be the major sources. There is also considerable geographic variation in the incidence of infection, with the colder temperate climates, such as Scandinavia and Canada, having high infection rates.

Pathology

Both *Y. pseudotuberculosis* and *Y. enterocolitica* can cause a similar morphological picture of acute mesenteric adenitis with or without inflammation of the terminal ileum and appendix. In Sweden up to 5 per cent of children with appendicitis may have yersiniosis. The terminal ileum is thickened with ulceration of the mucosa over Peyer's patches, not unlike typhoid. Disease can extend into the caecum (Fig. 16.122). Local nodes are enlarged and often show small, yellow, necrotic micro-abscesses.

Characteristic microscopy is seen in the lymph nodes and in the follicles of the mucosa and submucosa of the terminal ileum. Granulomas are present which usually have a necrotic centre infiltrated by polymorphs with surrounding histocytes and epitheloid cells. This pattern of stellate microabscesses within granulomas and follicles (Fig. 16.123) is similar to that seen in cat-scratch disease. The muscle coat of the ileal wall is not involved.

Although *Y. enterocolitica* causes terminal ileal disease, it more commonly causes an acute self-limiting colitis resembling that seen with other invasive bacterial pathogens (Section 16.12.2).

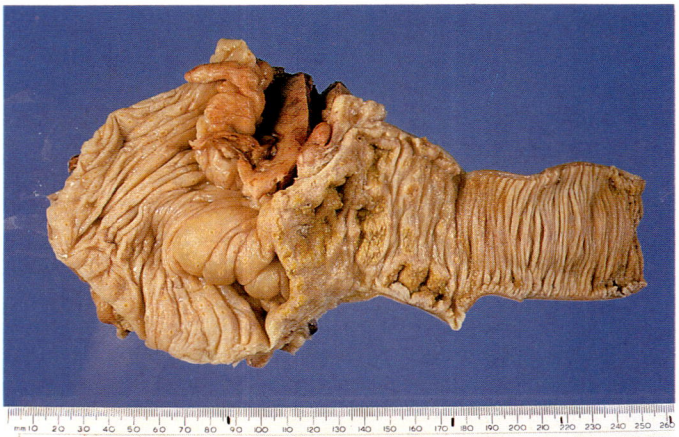

Fig. 16.122 Focal terminal ileal ulceration and caecal oedema in a case of yersiniosis. (Courtesy of Dr J. Newman.)

16.10.3 Viral infections

Viruses are important aetiological agents in acute gastroenteritis, which is one of the major causes of morbidity in the world. Indeed, pathogenic bacteria or parasites are only found in approximately 50 per cent of cases of acute gastroenteritis. The implication being that the majority of the remainder are likely to be of viral origin. In adults viral gastroenteritis is a major illness but amongst children it is a major cause of death. Diagnosis of viral enteritis is difficult, requiring electron microscopy of negatively stained stool specimens, latex agglutination, or polyacrylamide gel electrophoresis. The main viruses involved in gastroenteritis are listed in Table 16.10.

The pathology of viral infection is poorly documented, as most cases are self-limiting and the small bowel is relatively inaccessible. In general, there is minor villus blunting, lymphocytes may be increased in the lamina propria and, with appropriate methods, viral particles can be seen.

Cytomegalovirus

There is doubt whether Cytomegalovirus is a primary gut pathogen or simply a secondary invader in an already damaged bowel. Infection is mostly subclinical and overt disease rare. It is confined to patients with immunological impairment, particular patients with the acquired immunodeficiency syndrome

Table 16.10 The main viruses involved in gastroenteritis

Small round viruses and acute epidemic gastroenteritis (winter vomiting disease)
  (Norwalk and Hawaii viruses)
  Rota viruses (common in childhood)
  Fastidious adenovirus
Small round virus unassociated with acute epidemic gastroenteritis
  (Coxsackie A + B, Echovirus)
  Corono-virus
  Astro and Calici virus
  Cytomegalovirus

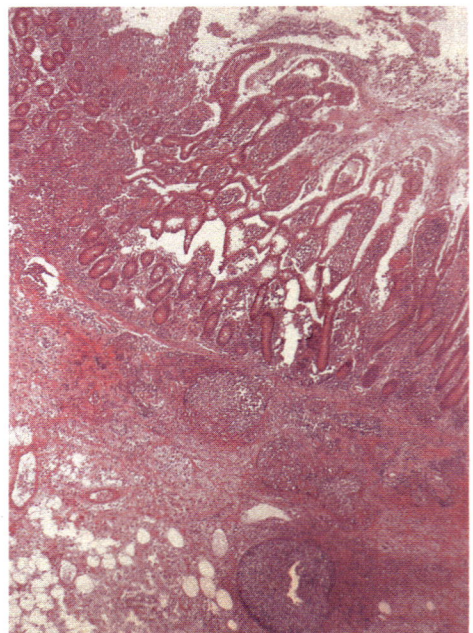

(a)

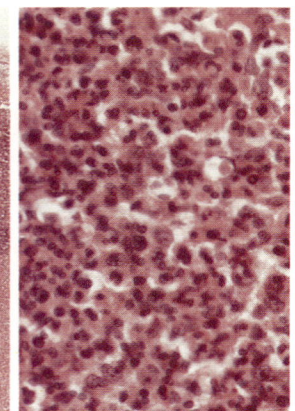

(b)

Fig. 16.123 (a) Ileal ulceration and mucosal inflammation in a case of yersiniosis. (b) The regional lymph nodes from (a) show necrotic lymphoid follicles, seen in the middle on the left, each with large numbers of central neutrophils (right).

(AIDS). The diagnosis depends on recognizing the characteristic intranuclear inclusions within macrophages or in endothelial cells of the vessel walls.

16.10.4 Fungal infections

Fungal disease of the small intestine is rare and invariably secondary to severe debilitating diseases, immunosuppression of any cause, and prolonged use of antibiotics or corticosteroids. *Mucorales*, *Candida*, and *Histoplasma* are the three likely to be encountered.

Secondary infection by *Candida* spp., whilst relatively common in the oesophagus or stomach, is exceptionally rare in the jejunum and ileum. Secondary infection by *Histoplasma* spp. has been documented in less than 80 cases and then usually at autopsy in patients with prolonged immunosuppression. Raised plaques are seen in the terminal ileum in association with the sites of lymphoid follicles. There can be obstruction and perforation by fungal balls. On microscopy, depending on the resistance of the host, the picture varies from severe necrosis to granulomas and fibrosis in the more immunocompetent individual. *H. capsulatum* appears as tiny basophilic objects of up to 3 μm in routine sections, whereas *H. duboisii* is 10–15 μm in diameter. The former is seen in the USA, the latter is more common in Africa.

Mucormycosis is a rarity in the small bowel, although the fungus is widely distributed in nature. It has non-septate, irregularly branching, broad hyphae. It is easily seen in ulcerated areas and can also produce a soft, mushroom-like fungal mass attached to the mucosa.

16.10.5 Parasitic infections

A large number of parasites, either protozoans or helminths can infest the jejunum and ileum. Diagnosis is made from the clinical evidence and examination of the stools for ova. Lassitude, abdominal pain, diarrhoea, and anaemia are common symptoms. Damage to the small bowel mucosa is often minor and, because infestations are common in Asiatic and African populations, it can be difficult to assess. This is because these populations show a wide range of variation in normal villus pattern.

Helminths

There are three main groups of parasitic helminths, the nematodes, castodes, and trematodes.

Ascariasis

This is the commonest and largest nematode infecting man. Its distribution is world-wide and it may reach a size of 20 cm. Most human cases are due to *Ascaris lumbricoides* but the larval stages of the dog and cat roundworm, *Toxicaris canis* and *T. cati*, respectively, can produce the syndrome of visceral larva migrans.

Infestation occurs through ingesting ova in food or drink. The hatched larvae penetrate the gut mucosa and via the portal system reach the lung. Here they mature and are coughed up to be swallowed and develop into adult worms in the small intestine.

Adult worms rarely produce symptoms of infection until there is a large load. They may then cause obstructive symptoms, especially in children, or precipitate nutritional deficiencies in malnourished groups (Fig. 16.124). The worms can migrate into the ducts of the pancreas or into the bile duct, in which case obstructive symptoms are likely.

In visceral larva migrans, humans ingest the eggs from the adult worms of a cat or dog. The larvae hatch in the small bowel and migrate around the body, producing symptoms and ab-

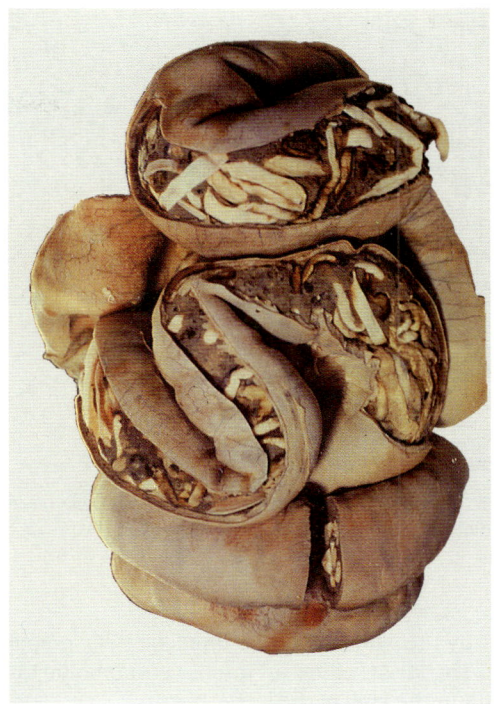

Fig. 16.124 A jejunum showing bolus obstruction due to ascariasis. (Courtesy Gower Medical Publishing and Dr D. R. Davies.)

normalities such as tender hepatomegaly, eosinophilia, and hypergammaglobulinaemia.

Ankylostomiasis (hookworm disease)

Ankylostoma duodenale and *Necater americanis* are the two species of hookworm that infect man. They are second to ascariasis as the commonest parasitic worm of man and have world-wide distribution, with possibly an increasing incidence in England. Cutaneous larva migrans is caused by larvae of animal species when man ingests the eggs. The larvae of *Ankylostoma* and *Necater* penetrate the skin and migrate via the lungs and pharynx to the small intestine. Here they develop into adults of about 1 cm length and attach themselves to the jejunal mucosa via their buccal capsule (Fig. 16.125). Large numbers of eggs are then passed in the stool.

From studies in the dog it has become clear that the adult changes its site of attachment every few hours. Although villus damage is produced, its recovery is swift and, although the worms can be seen in mucosal biopsies, villus abnormalities are usually minor.

Small worm loads are asymptomatic but, with large loads, iron deficiency anaemia from continual bleeding is common. Epigastric discomfort and tenderness can mimic peptic ulcer disease.

Anisakiasis

Infection is by larval forms of *Anisakis*, the host of the adult worm being the whale, seal, or dolphin. It is therefore a disease

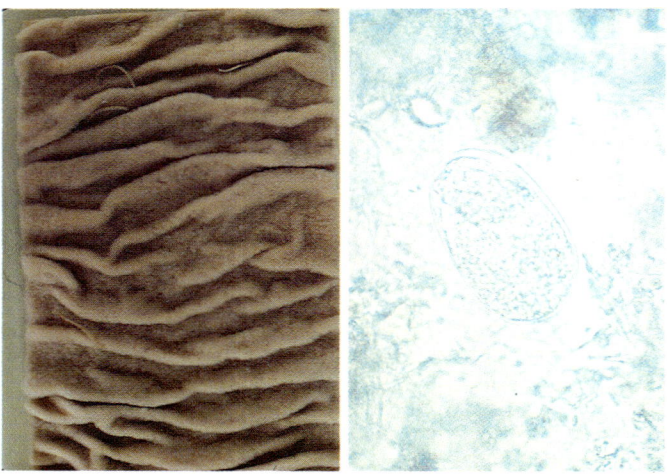

Fig. 16.125 Hookworm infestation of the small intestine. (Courtesy Gower Medical Publishing and Dr D. R. Davies.)

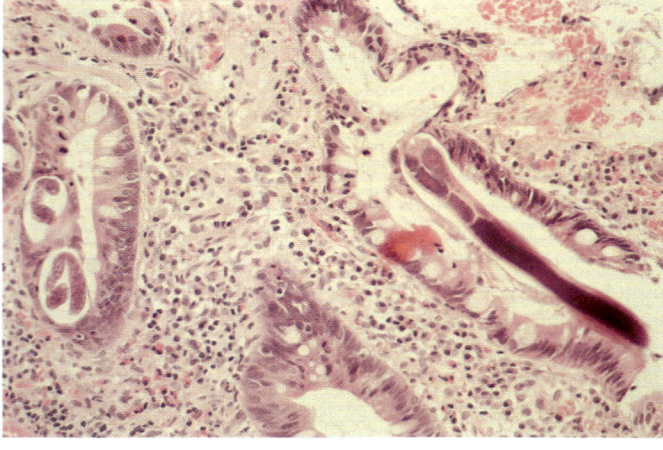

Fig. 16.126 Adult and larval forms of *Strongyloides stercoralis* in the jejunal mucosa.

of regions in the world that eat inadequately prepared salt-water fish. The larvae cause an intense eosinophilic infiltration and oedema in the wall of the lower ileum.

Capillariasis

Capillaria philippensis is a small nematode of length 3–4 mm restricted to coastal regions of the northern Philippines. It is acquired by eating raw fish infected with the larvae. The adult worm is found embedded in the jejunal mucosa and severe infection produces diarrhoea, malabsorption, wasting, and sometimes death.

Strongyloidiasis

This is caused by a small nematode that resides in the upper small intestine. It is 2–3 mm long and has a world-wide distribution very similar to that of hookworm. The adult female resides in the crypts of the duodenum and upper jejunum. The male is seldom seen. Eggs are produced and develop into rhabditiform larvae before being passed in the stools. Here they develop into infective filariform larvae which can then penetrate the skin. These migrate through the lungs maturing *en route* to be coughed up, swallowed, and the cycle completed by the worms colonizing the duodenum and jejunal mucosa. In immunocompromised patients, filariform larvae can develop within the gut. They can penetrate the mucosa of the colon or rectum and reinfection occurs. They may, however, disseminate widely to other organs, such as the liver and brain, producing a hyperinfection syndrome.

The worms are easily seen in small bowel biopsies (Fig. 16.126) and produce varying degrees of villus atrophy with an accompanying eosinophilic inflammatory cell infiltrate. It is interesting that auto-infection can occur in some asymptomatic individuals, for veterans of the Far Eastern campaigns of the

Second World War were shown to be infected some 30 years later.

Cestodes

The tapeworms are long, segmented, flat worms (Fig. 16.127) and the common ones that can become established in the small intestine of man are *Taenia saginata* (beef tapeworm), *Taenia solium* (pig tapeworm), and *Diphyllobothrium latum* (fish tapeworm). It is rare for the adult worms to cause symptoms. *Diphyllobothrium latum* can interfere with B_{12} absorption in the ileum and is a rare cause of megaloblastic anaemia. By contrast,

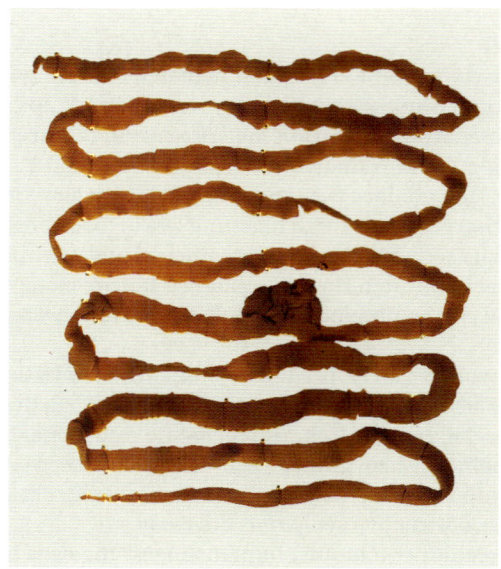

Fig. 16.127 A tapeworm. (Courtesy Gower Medical Publishing and Dr D. R. Davies.)

if man is infected by the larval stages of these worms from ingestion of the eggs, disseminated disease occurs and, for example, in cysticerosis (*Taenia solium*) central nervous system involvement is common.

Trematodes

These are the flukes, and the disease of main importance in the gut of man is schistosomiasis. It is considered in detail in Section 16.12.7, being mainly a colonic parasite.

Protozoal infections

The major pathogenic protozoa belong to four main classes: the Rhizopoda (*Entamoeba histolytica*), the Mastigophora (*Giardia lamblia*), the Ciliata (*Balantidium coli*), and the Sporozoa (*Coccidia-Cryptosporidium, Isospora,* and probably *Microsporidia*). *Entamoeba histolytica* and *Balantidium coli* are colonic pathogens and are considered in Section 16.12.6.

Giardiasis

Giardia lamblia is a motile flagellate protozoan with a world-wide distribution. It is commonest where sanitation is poor, and in 1–5-year-old children in Bangladesh prevalence rates of up to 51 per cent have been recorded. In the West incident rates are in the region of 5–7 per cent. It has an increased prevalence among homosexuals, is part of the gay bowel syndrome, and has a role in gastrointestinal infection in AIDS patients. There is a marked variation in the clinical response to *Giardia*. Although it can be entirely asymptomatic, *Giardia lamblia* is an established cause of acute diarrhoea amongst travellers, of malabsorption syndromes and vague non-specific upper gastrointestinal symptoms.

The organism exists in two forms, as a trophozoite or encysted. The trophozoite is pear-shaped with two nuclei and a ventral sucker, which is part of the mechanism by which it adheres to the enterocytes of the small intestinal villi. In the faecal stream trophozoites encyst and undergo division. Infection is by ingestion of contaminated water or food.

Similar to the clinical situation, the histological abnormalities produced by *Giardia* encompass a wide spectrum. Many biopsies are normal on light microscopy, the organisms seen lying between the villi and their shape varying with orientation (Fig. 16.128). All degrees of villus blunting can occur but seldom is there a completely flat biopsy as seen in a gluten-sensitive enteropathy (coeliac disease).

The variability in clinical response and morphological change to *Giardia* infections suggests that host immunity must play a major role. Hypogammaglobulinaemic subjects have a high incidence of infection, as do patients with low levels of secretory IgA. Experimental studies have shown that cellular immunity is involved via T-cells and, ultimately, organisms are engulfed by macrophages.

Coccidiosis

Within this group are the protozoans *Cryptosporidia* and *Isospora* (*I. belli* and *I. hominis*). Both are assuming increasing clinical

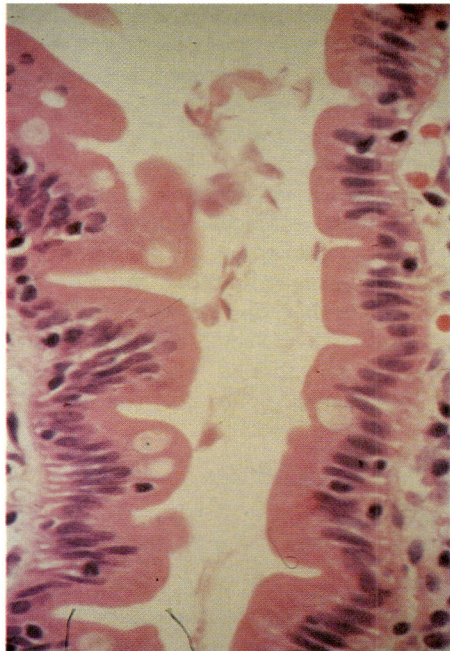

Fig. 16.128 *Giardia lamblia* in the crypts of the jejunal mucosa.

importance as opportunistic infections in AIDS cases. A third protozoan which is intracellular, *Microsporidia*, has also been observed in AIDS patients, but its precise taxonomy is not fully established.

Cryptosporidiosis and isosporiasis *Cryptosporidia* is a more common pathogen than *Isospora*, although it has a similar epidemiology and life cycle. The trophozoites reside on the surface of the enterocytes, either over the villi or deep in the crypts. They undergo repeated asexual divisions, or schizogony, before a sexual phase with gametes. Oocysts are passed in the faeces and infection is via faecal contamination of food or water. In

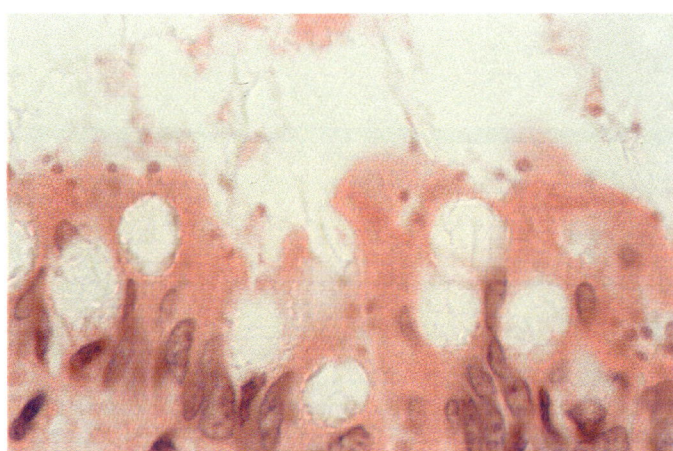

Fig. 16.129 Cryptosporidiosis on the surface of the jejunal mucosa.

most cases there is little damage to the villi of the small intestine, but partial villus atrophy can occur. Under the light microscope and routine haematoxylin and eosin staining the organisms appear as tiny bluish dots over the villus surface (Fig. 16.129), an appearance easily mistaken for stain deposit. *Isospora* can be intracellular.

Cryptosporidia produces a short attack of acute gastroenteritis in the immunocompetent individual, and is now a recognized cause of travellers' diarrhoea. In the immunosuppressed, chronic diarrhoea and malabsorption are more common. In parts of Africa and in Haiti up to 50 per cent of patients with AIDS are believed to be infected. *Isospora* produces similar infective symptoms and, though less common, is endemic in parts of South America and South-East Asia.

16.10.6　　Further reading

Binford, C. H. and Connor, D. H. (1976). *Pathology of tropical and extraordinary diseases*. Armed Forces Institute of Pathology, Washington.

Candy, D. C. A. and McNeish, A. S. (1984). Human *Escherichia coli* diarrhoea. *Archives of Diseases in Childhood* **59**, 395–6.

Casemore, D. P., Sands, R. L., and Curry, A. (1985). Cryptosporidium species: a 'new' human pathogen. *Journal of Clinical Pathology* **38**, 1321–36.

Day, D. W., Mandal, B. K., and Morson, B. C. (1978). The rectal biopsy appearances in *Salmonella colitis*. *Histopathology* **2**, 117–31.

El-Maraghi, N. R. H. and Mair, N. S. (1979). The histopathology of enteric infection with *Yersinia pseudotuberculosis*. *American Journal of Clinical Pathology* **71**, 631–9.

Gillon, J. (1984). Giardiases—review of epidemiology, pathogenetic mechanisms and host responses. *Quarterly Journal of Medicine* **53**, 29–39.

Igra-Siegman, Y., Kapila, R., Sen, P., Kaminski, Z. C., and Louri, D. P. (1981). Syndrome of hyperinfection with *Strongyloides stercoralis*. *Reviews of Infectious Diseases* **3**, 397–407.

Morson, B. C., Dawson, I. M. P., Day, D. W., Jass, J. R., Price, A. B., and Williams, G. T. (1990). *Gastrointestinal pathology* (3rd edn). Blackwell Scientific Publications, Oxford.

Tandon, H. D. and Prakash, A. (1972). Pathology of intestinal tuberculosis and its distinction from Crohn's disease. *Gut* **13**, 260–9.

Walker, P. D. (1985). Pig-Bel. In *Clostridia in gastrointestinal disease* (ed. S. P. Borriello), pp. 93–116. CRC Press, Boca Raton.

16.11　　Appendicitis

A. B. Price

16.11.1　　Acute appendicitis

Appendicitis is the commonest abdominal emergency in children and young adults. It is common in western Europe, North America and Australasia but rare in India and Africa. The peak incidence is in the second and third decade, it being uncommon before the age of 5 years. Death following appendicitis is rare,

although when it occurs it is usually in the elderly for the latter can have minimal symptoms despite severe disease.

Aetiology and pathogenesis

Apart from a small number of cases, acute appendicitis has not been regularly associated with any specific causative organisms. Bacteriological studies show a wide variety of organisms from amongst those normally to be found in the caecum. Antibody titres to mumps V antigen and *Yersinia* have been increased in some series.

Obstruction of the lumen is most likely to be the main precipitating cause. This may come about in several ways. The mucosa can become inflamed and oedematous; lymphoid tissue in the mucosa and submucosa can hypertrophy; foreign material and faecal debris can combine to form a laminated obstructing faecolith and finally the appendix itself may tort and be kinked. From experimental studies, infection of the appendix alone does not produce an acute appendicitis but if combined with obstruction then damage occurs.

It seems likely that the obstruction causes distension with accumulation of normal secretions; ischaemic damage to the mucosa ensues and then invasion by enteric pathogens.

Pathology

Initially the only sign is dilated vessels on the serosal aspect of the appendix. The distal segment then dilates and may contain purulent material. As inflammation spreads through the wall a patchy purulent exudate appears on the serosal surface (Fig. 16.130). The appendix then goes on to become soft, violaceous, and haemorrhagic with developing necrosis, culminating in gangrene and perforation.

On microscopy there is a transmural infiltrate of neutrophil polymorphs, ulceration of the mucosa with oedema, and congestion of the muscle (Figs 16.131, 16.132). Acute inflammatory cells spread across the serosa and out into the peri-

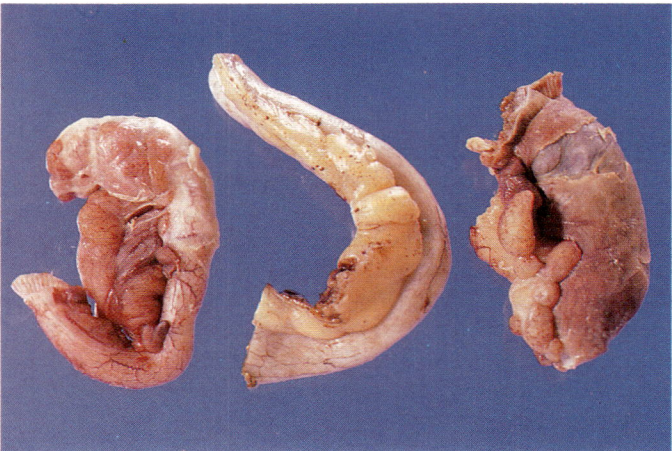

Fig. 16.130 At the centre is a normal appendix. On the left an appendix with pus covering the distal one-third. On the right the whole peritoneal aspect of the appendix is covered by a purulent exudate from a case of severe appendicitis.

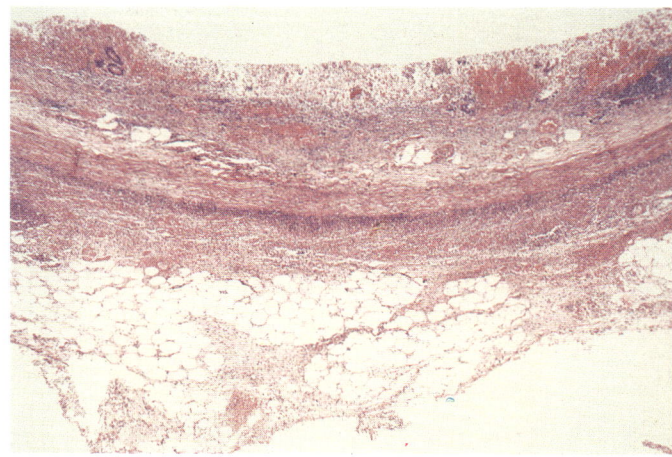

Fig. 16.131 Appendicitis showing haemorrhagic necrosis of the mucosa and full-thickness infiltration of the wall by inflammatory cells.

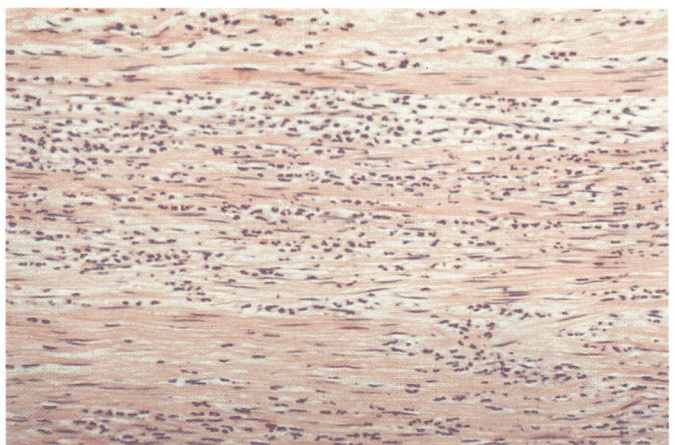

Fig. 16.132 Here the oedematous muscle coat of the appendix is seen infiltrated by neutrophil polymorphs.

appendicular fat. Vascular thrombi are present in severe cases, leading to ischaemia and gangrenous appendicitis. In a significant percentage of patients with clinical appendicitis the pathology shows inflammation limited to the mucosa without mural involvement. However, this limited degree of inflammatory change is also present in one-third of appendices at elective resections. The significance of inflammation limited to the mucosa is not clear, although in the animal model such mucosal lesions progress rapidly to peritonitis and gangrene.

Complications

The mortality from uncomplicated appendicitis is low, at around 0.1 per cent. However, in the elderly and very young once complications ensue it can rise to 6–12 per cent.

Perforation of the appendix is the most common and most serious, leading to generalized peritonitis (Fig. 16.133). Assum-

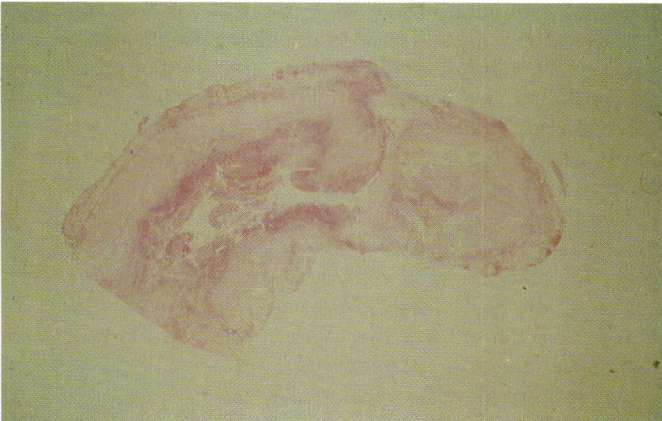

Fig. 16.133 A perforated appendix, the perforation is seen towards the tip on the upper wall.

ing the patient survives, pus can localize in the pelvis or under the diaphragm. If the appendix is retro-caecal or retro-colic, adhesions can occur, the perforation is walled off, and a local abscess forms. Abscesses may perforate into the rectum or vagina. Alternatively, a fistula may be produced between the appendix and the bladder, or elsewhere in the gastrointestinal tract. In women the end-result of perforation of the appendix can be tubal adhesions and infertility.

Occasionally, vessels in the mesoappendix can become infected and thrombosed. The thrombosis may propagate into larger vessels and, if infected clot reaches the liver, an hepatic abscess ensues.

Chronic appendicitis and obstructive appendicopathy

Chronic appendicitis is a controversial entity often referred to as a 'grumbling appendix'. It is not unusual at autopsy, or in right hemicolectomy specimens, to find a small shrunken appendix with fibrous obliteration of the lumen and atrophy of the lymphoid tissue (Fig. 16.134). This might suggest previous

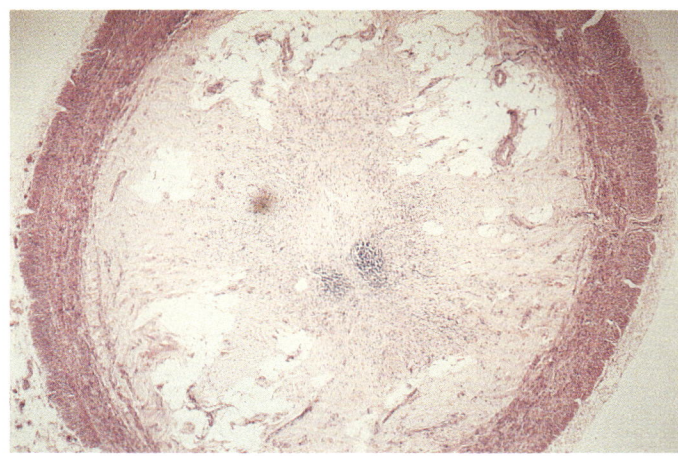

Fig. 16.134 Following an attack of appendicitis the lumen at the tip of the appendix may show fibrous obliteration.

attacks of inflammation but such findings are as common in patients with symptoms of a 'grumbling appendicitis' as in a symptomless population. The discovery of adhesions must indicate previous appendicitis, but not necessarily chronic appendicitis. This has to depend on demonstrating lymphocytes and plasma cells throughout the wall in the absence of neutrophil polymorphs. It is a rare finding.

Often there is a strong history of appendicular pain and a normal appendix. However, close inspection can reveal, in a proportion of cases, narrowing or obstruction of the lumen by a faecolith or foreign body. Alternatively, the lumen may be distended by packed faecal material. Either of these features may be the cause of symptoms and subsequent colicky pain known as obstructive appendicopathy.

16.11.2   Mucocele of the appendix

A mucocele refers to distension of the lumen due to the accumulation of mucin (Fig. 16.135). It is not a specific diagnosis but a gross appearance which may be the end-result of inflammation but may also be caused by a mucinous cystadenoma or carcinoma.

A simple mucocele is found in about 0.2 per cent of appendices examined at autopsy or operation. Post-inflammatory fibrosis and faecoliths are the commonest causes. On microscopy the mucosa may be flattened or show epithelial hyperplasia with features resembling a metaplastic polyp of the colon (Fig. 16.136). Any dysplasia indicates the presence of a cystadenoma.

Occasionally a mucocele can become infected and the appendix may rupture. This can result in the spread of mucin within the peritoneum or pseudomyxoma peritoneii. Excision of the appendix results in regression unless the mucocele was due to malignant change. In a small number of cases a mucocele of the appendix is associated with a cystadenoma in the ovary.

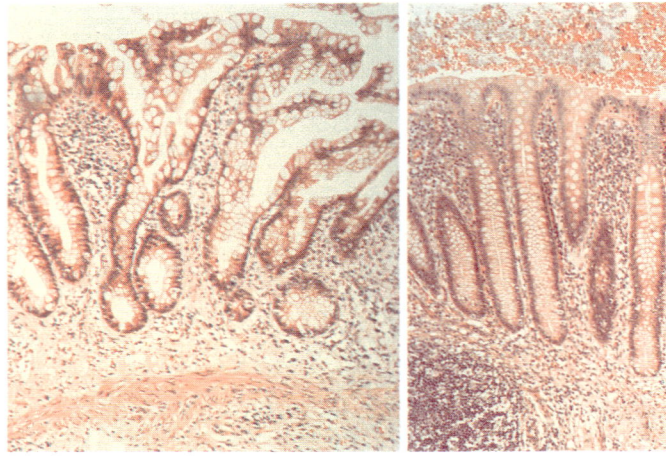

Fig. 16.136   The lining of a mucocele, before it becomes too distended and attenuated, often shows hyperplastic changes as seen on the left. A normal mucosa is seen on the right for comparison.

16.11.3   Other forms of appendicitis

Tuberculous appendicitis

This is seen as part of tuberculosis of the ileocaecal region. The pathology is similar to tuberculosis at any other site.

Crohn's disease of the appendix

Crohn's disease limited to the appendix is rare, although it can predate disease at distant sites. It is a common finding as part of

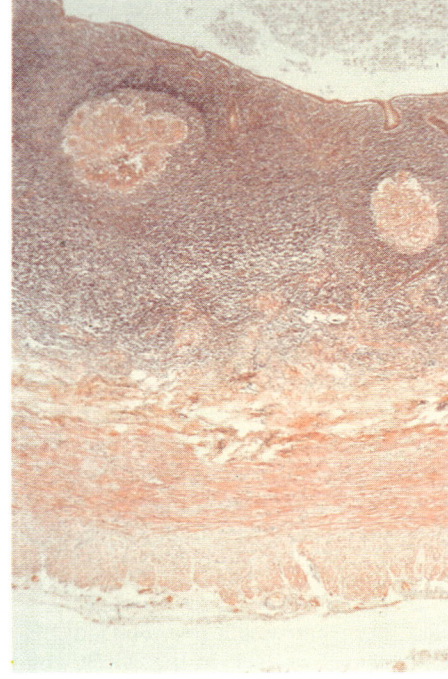

Fig. 16.137   Granulomas are seen in the mucosal lymphoid follicles. In this case no other pathology was present and the aetiology was unknown. Such examples have to be designated 'idiopathic'.

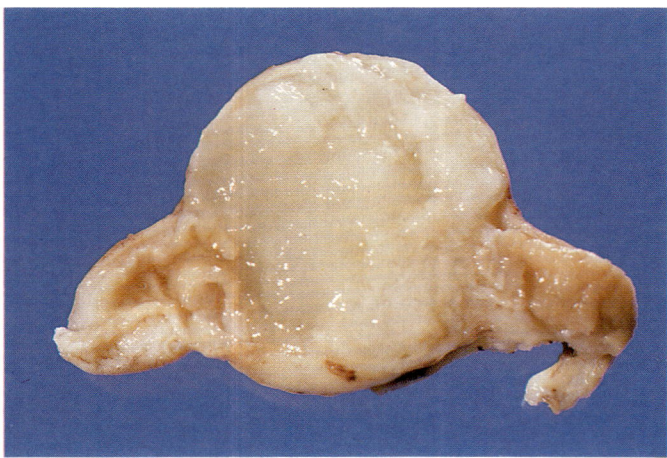

Fig. 16.135   A mucocele of the appendix.

terminal ileal Crohn's disease. In isolated appendicular Crohn's disease, less than 10 per cent develop more widespread disease. On microscopy the features are similar to Crohn's disease at any other site.

Ulcerative colitis in the appendix

The mucosa of the appendix is inflamed in about 50 per cent of patients with a total colitis. As the disease is confined to the mucosa it is asymptomatic and none of the normal complications of appendicitis arise.

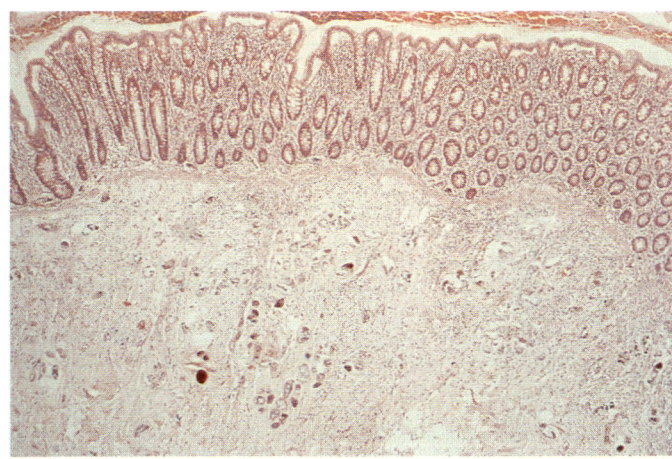

(a)

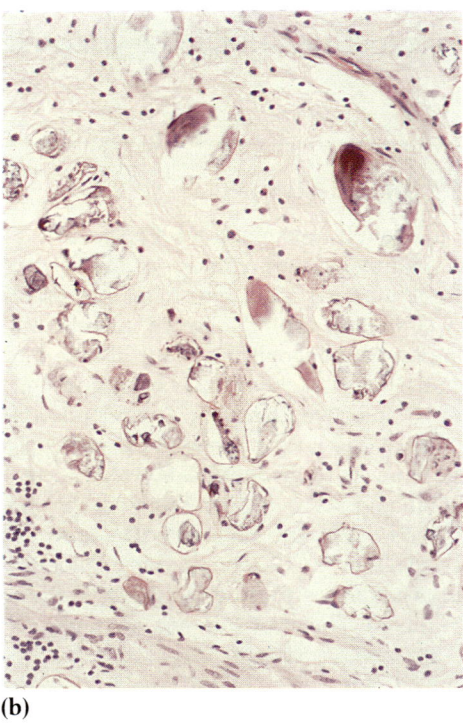

(b)

Fig. 16.138 (a) An appendix with a large number of schistosoma eggs in the submucosa and mucosa; (b) a higher magnification of (a).

Yersiniosis

Although infection with *Yersinia pseudotuberculosis* commonly affects the ileo-caecal region, the appendix is seldom involved. However, one investigation has shown that in patients with an acute abdomen in whom antibody titres for *Y. pseudotuberculosis* were positive, 31 per cent had appendicitis. The pathology is similar to that described in the terminal ileum (Section 16.10.2).

Granulomatous appendicitis

For the sake of completeness one must acknowledge that occasionally granulomas are found in a resected appendix. The accompanying pathology does not conform to any of the specific granulomatous diseases, no organisms are found, no foreign material, and no helpful serological findings or other clinical clues. The diagnosis must be of granulomatous appendicitis but of unknown aetiology (Fig. 16.137).

Actinomycosis

Actinomyces israeli is present in the mouth of about 5 per cent of normal people. It may survive passage through the gastric acid and reach the lumen of the appendix where it may remain without causing disease. It can only be considered a pathogen when it is in the midst of inflamed tissue. Acute appendicitis due to *A. israeli* is rare but when it occurs, unless diagnosed and adequately treated, chronic disease may follow. In this chronic disease, abscesses containing mycelia are found in the wall. There is often dense fibrosis and sinus tracts or fistulae develop between the appendix, adjacent bowel, other organs, or skin on the abdomen and perineum (see Section 16.12.4).

Schistosomiasis

Where schistosomiasis is endemic, 1–2 per cent of appendicectomy specimens contain schistosomes. Granulomatous appendicitis may develop during egg-laying. Alternatively, an obstructing appendicitis, the result of fibrosis around dead eggs,

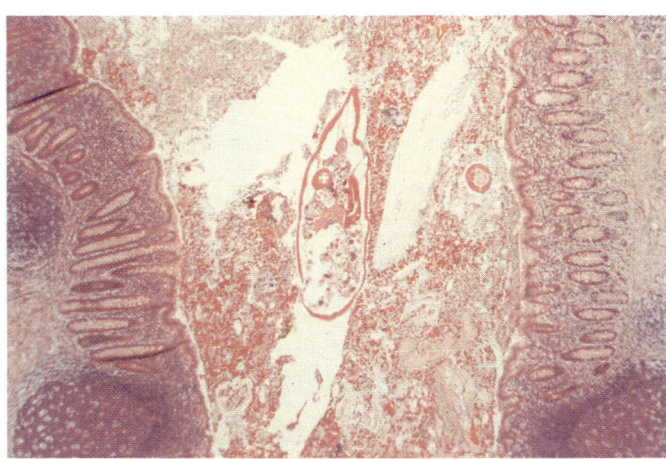

Fig. 16.139 *Enterobius vermicularis* in the lumen of an appendix.

occurs. The eggs then appear calcified in the appendicular wall (Fig. 16.138).

Miscellaneous forms of appendicitis

Appendicitis may be a complication of amoebic dysentry, strongyloidiasis, *Balantidium* infection, and pin-worm infestation (see below). Polyarteritis nodosa can present as acute appendicitis. Although not reported as a cause of appendicitis, spirochaetosis can be seen in the resected appendix. Interestingly, its incidence has been reported at a higher position in the non-inflamed appendix removed because of clinical suspicion

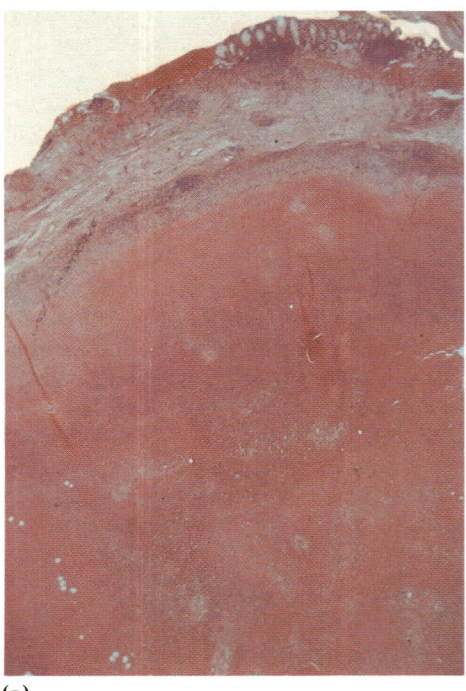

(a)

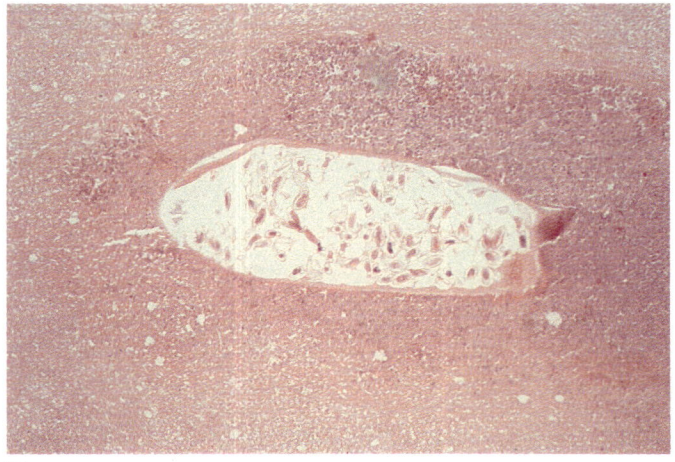

(b)

Fig. 16.140 (a) This illustrates an abscess in the rectal wall with overlying intact mucosa. (b) At higher power a gravid 'pin-worm' is seen at the centre of the inflammation.

than in those appendices removed incidently. In women, endometriosis may be found in conjunction with appendicitis.

Oxyuris/Enterobius vermicularis (pin-worms)

Pin-worms confined to the lumen of the appendix do not cause symptoms and are a common finding (Fig. 16.139). However, the gravid female worm migrates nocturnally to the anus in order to lay eggs in the perianal skin. This may cause intense pruritus ani and the consequent excoriation can result in implantation of the worm and eggs beneath the skin surface. This then results in inflammation and abscess formation (Fig. 16.140).

16.11.4   Further reading

Ariel, I., Vinograd, I., Hershlag, A., Olsha, O., Argov, S., Klausner, J., Rabau, M., Freund, V., and Rosenmann, E. (1986). Crohn's disease isolated to the appendix: Truths and fallacies. *Human Pathology* **17**, 1116–21.

Butler, C. (1981). Surgical pathology of acute appendicitis. *Human Pathology* **12**, 870–8.

Morson, B. C., Dawson, I. M. P., Day, D. W., Jass, J. R., Price, A. B., and Williams, G. T. (1990). *Gastrointestinal pathology* (3rd edn). Blackwell Scientific Publications, Oxford.

Williams, R. A. (1989). The appendix. In *Gastrointestinal and oesophageal pathology*, (ed. R. Whitehead), pp. 533–9. Churchill Livingstone, London.

16.12   Infections of the large intestine

A. B. Price

16.12.1   Introduction

The major problem in inflammatory diseases of the colon and rectum, for pathologist and clinician alike, is to distinguish infection from the two main causes of non-specific inflammatory bowel disease, Crohn's disease, and ulcerative colitis. Obviously a positive stool culture, or the detection of parasites, are paramount, but stool culture may be positive in only 50 per cent of cases of infective diarrhoea. Considerable reliance has therefore to be placed on the gross and microscopical appearances of the mucosa to distinguish between these two major divisions of inflammatory colonic pathology. Crohn's disease, ulcerative colitis, and other non-infective causes of colitis are considered in Section 16.13. The specific infections that mimic these latter conditions are those caused by bacteria that can invade the mucosa. The most common are *Campylobacter* spp., *Salmonella* spp., and *Shigella* spp. They produce a dysenteric illness with blood and mucus in the stools. In a proportion of patients, specific infections may precipitate the onset of Crohn's disease and ulcerative colitis and, conversely, patients with these conditions may suffer episodes of specific infection. It is impossible to distinguish between the individual infections on histology alone, microbiology being essential. As well as the effect on the colon, the majority of these bacteria produce toxins that interfere with small intestinal water and electrolyte metabolism, giving the diarrhoea a small intestinal component. In the United States the common bacterial diarrhoeas are referred to under the umbrella term of 'acute self-limiting colitis'. An additional term, transient colitis, has been used for patients with a clinical and microscopic picture of infective diarrhoea but in whom culture is negative. Table 16.9 lists the major intestinal pathogens.

16.12.2 Bacterial infections

Campylobacter infection

It was in 1972 that a medium was developed that allowed *Campylobacter fetus* sub-species *jejuni* and *coli*, to be identified in the stool. In the relatively short space of time since then, it has been appreciated that *C. jejuni* and *coli* are among the world's commonest causes of infective diarrhoea, particularly in the West. The bacterium is a Gram-negative spiral rod which, prior to 1964, was classified with the *vibrio* organisms. Infection with *C. jejuni/coli* is acquired from contaminated food, water, and also person-to-person spread. Frozen chickens are a commonly identified source. Abdominal pain, as well as diarrhoea, is a frequent clinical symptom, occasionally so severe that some patients may be subjected to a laparotomy. Indeed, appendicitis has been associated with *Campylobacter* infections. Overall, the disease itself is self-limiting. Rare instances of systemic symptoms such as arthritis have been reported. The aetiology of the diarrhoea is not fully established but is thought to have a small bowel secretory component, probably toxin-induced, as well as an invasive colonic phase. Macroscopically, changes may involve the whole colon or be limited to the sigmoid colon and rectum. Tiny ulcers may be seen scattered over the mucosa, with surrounding hyperaemia. The histological changes are considered alongside those of the other invasive colonic bacterial pathogens (see below).

Salmonella infection

Whereas *Salmonella typhi* and *S. paratyphi* cause a septicaemic illness, the large numbers of other species of *Salmonella* only produce a food poisoning pattern of illness confined to the gastrointestinal tract. Human salmonellosis is distributed worldwide and is amongst the commonest of the infective diarrhoeas. It is characterized by a 12–48 h incubation period and then colicky abdominal pain, copious watery diarrhoea, often bleeding, and general malaise. There is considerable variation in severity of the illness but in the old and very young the outcome can be fatal. Sigmoidoscopic examination rarely shows ulceration but the mucosa is oedematous, hyperaemic, and friable.

Transmission is invariably oral via food or drink contaminated with human or animal faeces. Chicken and turkey are incriminated most often and eggs or egg products are involved in many outbreaks. The increasing use of pre-cooked foods subsequently warmed-up has increased the danger of outbreaks, as

has the increase in fast-food restaurants. Unlike shigellosis, the infecting dose has to be large, but like most of the dysenteric organisms there is enterotoxin production that results in a defect in small bowel water and electrolyte transfer.

Autopsy studies on fatal cases have shown diffuse colonic inflammation and limited small bowel disease. Despite the fatalities, changes (both macroscopic and microscopic) appear minor. In routine clinical practice, rectal and colonic biopsies shows features similar to those of other bacterial diarrhoea, which are decribed below.

Shigella infection

There are four pathogenic species of *Shigella* (*S. dysenteriae*, *S. flexneri*, *S. boydii*, and *S. sonnei*) and for each only a small infecting dose of organisms is required. The small dose means that person-to-person contact is an effective route of transmission, though food and water can transmit the disease as well. Epidemics are common in Third World countries where there is a high population density coupled with poor sanitation and personal hygiene. Children are particularly susceptible to outbreaks. The virulence of the organisms depends on their ability to invade the colonic epithelial cells but a potent toxin is also produced. This toxin cross-reacts with the toxin produced by certain strains of *E. coli*, in particular strain O157 (see below), and *Vibrio cholera*. It, too, has a role in the pathogenesis of diarrhoea by its effect on the small bowel. The degree of colonic invasion partly determines whether the diarrhoea is bloody and how severe the dysenteric illness becomes. The incubation period is from 1 to 5 days and then intense abdominal cramps commence, accompanied by tenesmus and the frequent passage of small volumes of blood, pus, and mucus.

Pathology

Inflammation is most severe in the rectum and sigmoid colon but there is frequently a pancolitis. The mucosa is friable with small ulcers and adherent monopurulent exudate. The ulceration remains superficial, but in rare cases toxic megacolon with more penetrating ulceration may develop. Microscopy is similar to that of the other acute infective bacterial diarrhoeas (see below).

Escherichia coli infections and haemorrhagic colitis

Enteroinvasive *E. coli* spp. are closely related to *Shigella* spp. and produce a colitis similar to shigellosis. The enterotoxogenic and enteropathogenic species of *E. coli* are small bowel pathogens (Section 16.10.2). In recent years a predominantly right-sided haemorrhagic colitis has been associated with a serotype bearing antigens O157 and H7. This organism (enterohaemorrhagic *E. coli*) produces a Shiga-like toxin and is responsible for the haemolytic–uraemic syndrome.

The histopathology of infective colitis (acute self-limiting colitis)

Disease severe enough to warrant colectomy rarely occurs during the course of the common bacterial diarrhoeal illnesses (Fig. 16.141). The microscopic pathology has therefore been learnt

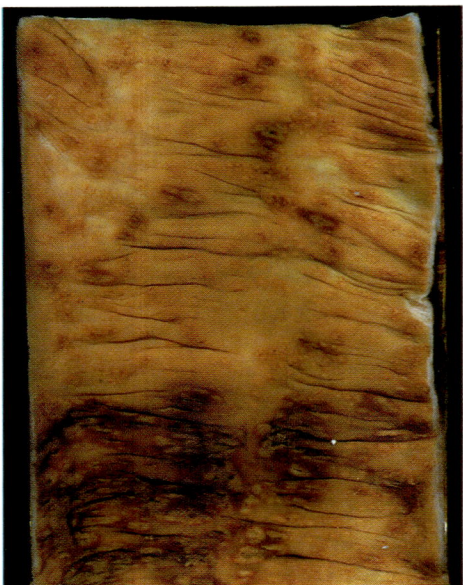

Fig. 16.141 Bacillary dysentry showing multiple small ulcers surrounded by haemorrhagic areas. (Courtesy of Gower Medical Publishing and The Royal College of Surgeons (England).)

from the study of colonoscopic and rectal biopsies. The mucosa shows focal clusters of neutrophil polymorphs in the lamina propria. It is characteristic to see many neutrophil polymorphs infiltrating and caught between the crypt epithelial cells and only a small number within the crypt lumen. Their presence in large numbers within the lumen is a feature more characteristic of ulcerative colitis (Fig. 16.142). The crypts remain aligned but the epithelium is flattened and degenerate, causing the crypt lumen to appear dilated. The mucosa is frequently oedematous.

Plasma cells and lymphocytes are increased but they are less striking than the number of polymorphs. The above features are sufficiently characteristic for a diagnosis of infective procto-colitis to be made from a biopsy, even in the face of a negative stool culture. The pattern of both crypt degeneration and neutrophil polymorph infiltration is unlike anything seen in Crohn's disease or ulcerative colitis (Figs 16.142, 16.143). In clinical terms the diagnosis is important for such cases should not be mislabelled ulcerative colitis or Crohn's disease. Both these are chronic lifelong disorders with important socio-economic implications for the patient. Infection, by contrast, is self-limiting and the bowel returns to normal.

Although a typical mucosal pattern of bacterial infection can be recognized, no histological distinction can be made between the common specific infections. Furthermore, the microscopy is only characteristic very early on in the attack, and even then the biopsy appearances can range from normal, through non-specific mild inflammatory changes, to the diagnostic pattern described. The reason for such a variable pattern is unknown but may relate to virulence factors present in the organism.

Infection due to clostridial organisms

Clostridial organisms are involved in several inflammatory and necrotizing diseases of the gut. *Clostridium perfringens* has been referred to in association with Pig-bel (Section 16.10.2) but this species can also cause a less severe food-poisoning illness in which there is a mild colitis. *Clostridium difficile* is the cause of pseudomembranous colitis and *Clostridium septicum* has been implicated in neutropenic colitis (Section 16.13.6).

Pseudomembranous colitis

In the old textbooks of pathology, pseudomembranous colitis appeared in the chapters on ischaemic bowel disease and was described as a necrotizing colitis. It is now known to be caused by the organism *Clostridium difficile* and its associated toxins. In

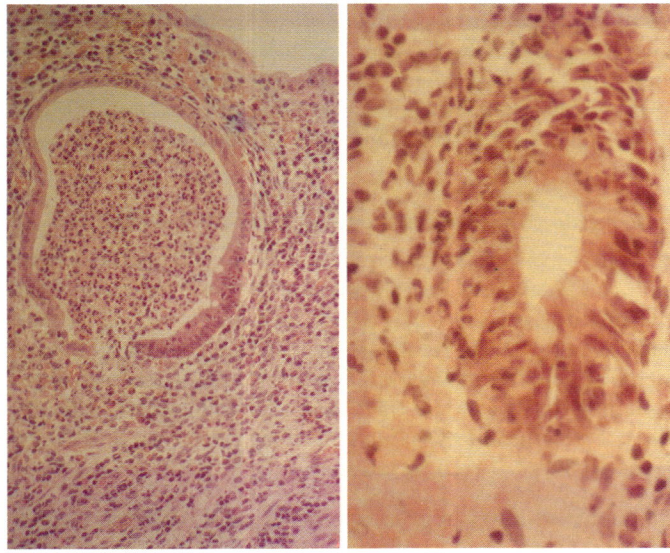

Fig. 16.142 On the right is an incipient crypt abscess, or cryptitis, with the neutrophil polymorphs entrapped between the epithelial cells of the crypt. On the left is a crypt abscess proper, with the majority of polymorphs within the crypt lumen.

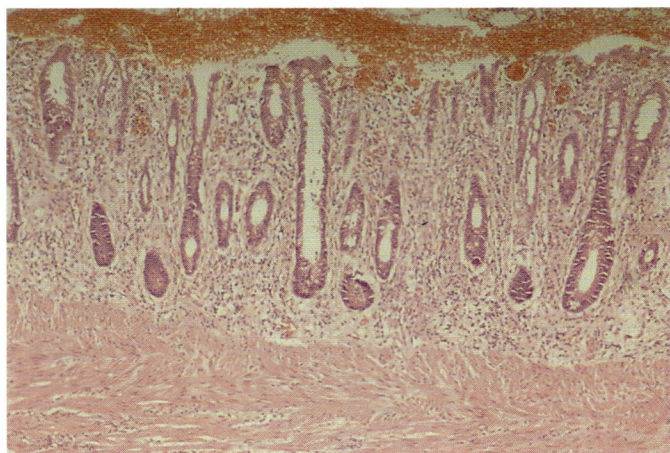

Fig. 16.143 The typical appearance of infective colitis. The crypts are aligned but many show degeneration of their epithelial cells, to a degree that some crypts seem to be dissolving away. Acute inflammatory cells are scattered across the lamina propria.

the early stages pseudomembranous colitis has very distinctive appearances, but these do eventually merge into a pattern of necrotizing colitis that is indistinguishable from those described in Section 16.9.1 in which ischaemia may also have a role. Some clostridial toxins can have vasoconstrictive properties thus combining an infective and ischaemic pathogenesis.

The large majority of cases of pseudomembranous colitis arise in patients who have had a recent course of antibiotics. However, it was described before the advent of these drugs, when it was seen mostly as a complication of intestinal surgery. In these early descriptions any site of the gut could be involved, but antibiotic-associated cases seem limited to the colon.

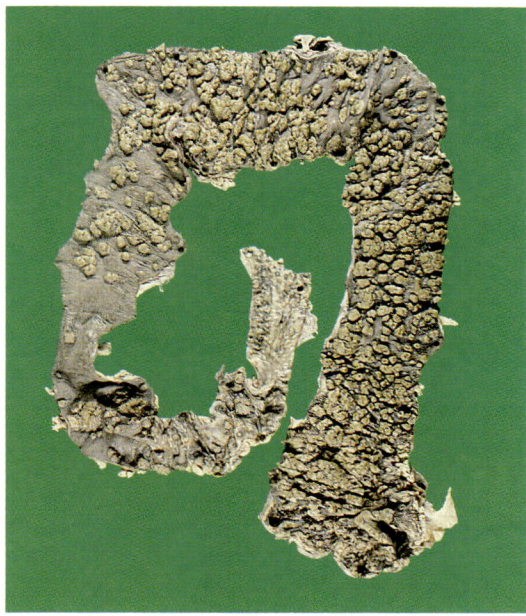

(a)

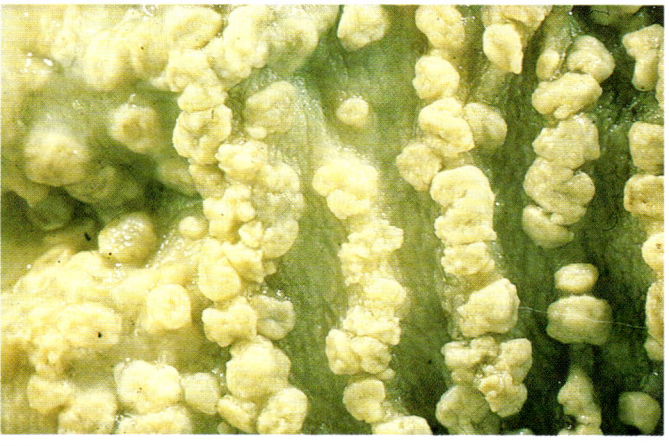

(b)

Fig. 16.144 (a) A colectomy showing the discrete yellow plaques on the mucosal surface that are diagnostic of pseudomembranous colitis. (b) This close-up of the colonic surface mucosa shows the yellow plaques separated by normal mucosa.

Pathology

Pseudomembranous colitis has a diagnostic morphological appearance and, while most cases are related to antibiotic therapy, the term is not synonymous with antibiotic-associated colitis nor antibiotic-associated diarrhoea (see below).

Macroscopic pathology The typical case shows discrete raised yellow/white plaques, from 1 to 5 mm in diameter, scattered over the mucosa (Fig. 16.144). The rectum is usually involved, but not invariably, and the colitis may be total or segmental. What controls the distribution of disease is not clear. With progressive damage the plaques coalesce and may form a continuous necrotic membrane over the mucosa (Fig. 16.145).

Microscopic pathology The microscopy corresponding to the discrete plaques is characterized by a focus of disrupted crypts. The luminal two-thirds of the crypts are distended, the epithelial cells are shed, and the group of damaged crypts is covered by fibrin, mucus, and inflammatory debris (Fig. 16.146)—the latter appearing as the surface yellow plaque. Although the crypts lose their cellular lining, their ghost outlines remain. Intervening mucosa between the plaques is either normal or shows a minor acute inflammatory cell infiltrate.

As the lesions enlarge damage becomes more complete, so that each focus joins an adjacent one and the mucosa is gradually replaced by an inflammatory membrane of necrotic epithelium, fibrin, and inflammatory cells. It is at this stage that there is confusion between pseudomembranous colitis and other conditions in which extensive mucosal necrosis occurs, e.g. ischaemia. The damage at all stages is confined to the mucosa and upper submucosa.

Prior to the development of the typical lesion, and prior to any recognizable macroscopic lesion, tiny intercryptal erosions may be present (Fig. 16.147). These are little more than a superficial collection of inflammatory cells, accompanied by a break in the surface epithelium and a wisp of fibrin at that site. A sequence can be traced from these early foci, through the distended and disrupted crypts, to complete mucosal necrosis.

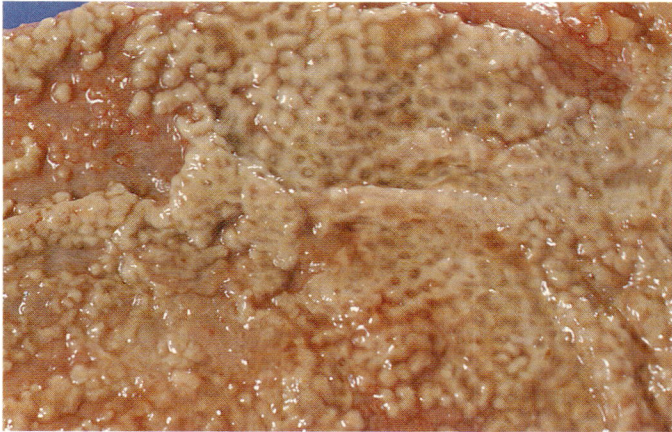

Fig. 16.145 At a more advanced stage of pseudomembranous colitis the plaques fuse to form a continuous necrotic membrane, as seen on the surface of this colectomy specimen.

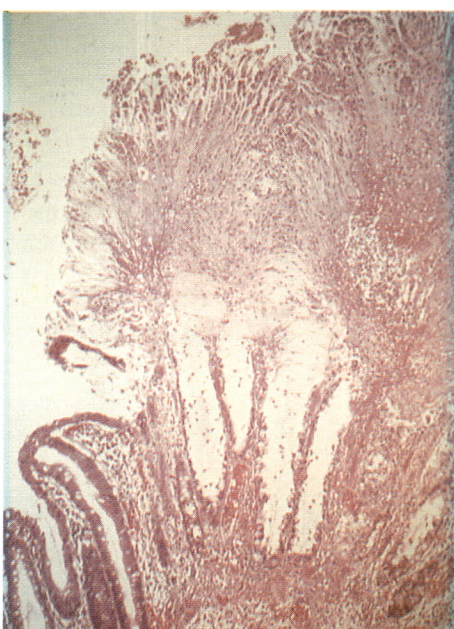

Fig. 16.146 Group of four crypts showing dilatation with loss of crypt cells and an overlying 'membrane' of inflammatory debris. This is the typical microscopy of pseudomembranous colitis.

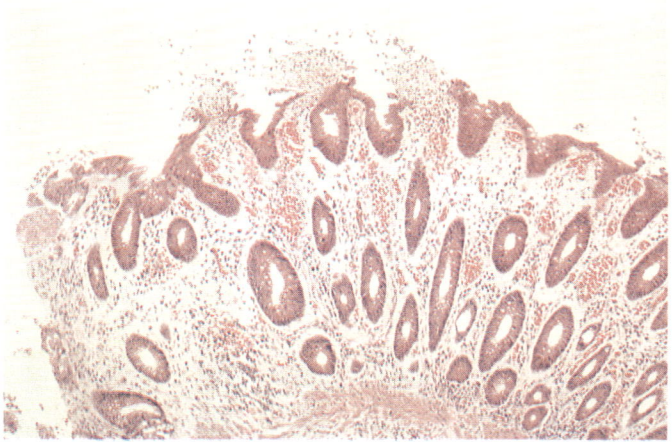

Fig. 16.147 The earliest lesion diagnostic of pseudomembranous colitis is seen here with two small intercryptal erosions, each with a cap of debris and inflammatory cells. The underlying mucosa shows a mild focal acute inflammatory cell infiltrate.

The role of *Clostridium difficile*

The organism is associated with pseudomembranous colitis in all but a few isolated case reports; and, again, in all but a few reports there is an antibiotic-related drug history. The disease can appear up to a month after the course of antibiotics has finished but onset is more usual during the course. Antibiotics alter the gut flora and micro-environment, making it susceptible to colonization by *Clostridium difficile*. Even so, the relationship between *C.. difficile* and the disease is complex. Thus, the

organism and its toxin are present in up to 64 per cent of healthy neonates and in a small proportion of healthy adults. It is known that, following a course of antibiotics, some patients will harbour the organism and its toxin without developing diarrhoea and, in others, who have diarrhoea, the organism is found but no toxin. Furthermore, not all patients develop the classical morphological picture of pseudomembranous colitis. Indeed it is more common, during a course of antibiotics, to experience only mild diarrhoea accompanied by minimal or no mucosal inflammatory changes. This wide spectrum of pathology is probably related to variations in the pathogenicity amongst strains of *Cl. difficile*. The organisms produce four toxins, the main ones being toxin A, a potent enterotoxin, and toxin B, a cytotoxin. Both are necessary for disease and variation in the ratio of these toxins would account for the variability in pathology.

There have been interesting observations in the experimental hamster model. These animals are normally very susceptible to antibiotic exposure, yet they will not succumb if maintained in sterile conditions, despite being colonized by *Cl. difficile*. Clearly, expression of the disease requires not only this organism but additional susceptibility factors to be present, either within the lumen or in the mucosa.

Antibiotic-associated colitis and diarrhoea

This term is restricted to patients with a colitis following exposure to antibiotics but in whom typical pseudomembranous colitis is not seen. On microscopy the picture resembles a mild form of infective colitis, described in Section 16.12.2. The correlation of this pattern of colitis with positive culture of *Cl. difficile* from the faeces is about 38 per cent, compared to 97–98 per cent in patients with morphological pseudomembranous colitis. In patients with antibiotic-related diarrhoea and a normal colonic or rectal mucosa the correlation is down to less than 10 per cent. Clearly, *Cl. difficile* must be only one of the causes of diarrhoea associated with antibiotics, even though it may be the sole cause of pseudomembranous colitis.

Tuberculosis

Tuberculosis of the gastrointestinal tract, whether primary or secondary, usually involves the terminal ileum and caecum (Section 16.10.2). The colon and rectum are rarely involved. When affected, a small number of large, well-defined ulcers are seen, with the adjacent bowel wall being thickened and indurated (Fig. 16.148). Miliary tubercles may be present on the serosal surface. Microscopy is the same as for tuberculosis more proximally (Section 16.10.2), it being important to make the distinction from Crohn's disease.

Other myobacteria are becoming important in immunosuppressed individuals and with the increase in AIDS. In this condition *Myobacterium avium-intracellulare* infection can be present (Section 16.12.3).

Yersinia enterocolitica infection

In addition to causing an acute ileitis (Section 16.10.2) *Yersinia*

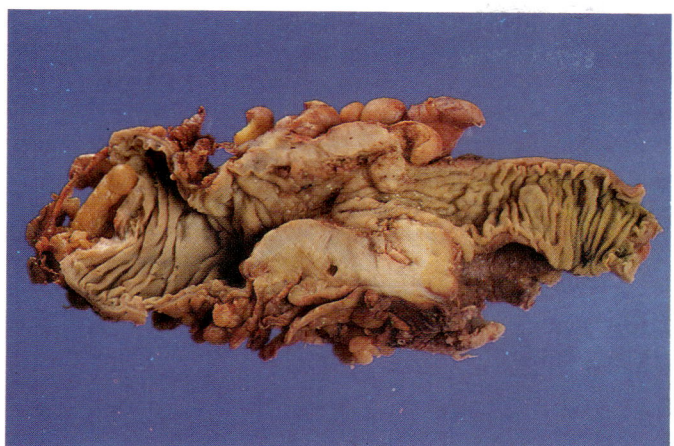

Fig. 16.148 In this case of tuberculosis the caecal wall is grossly thickened and fibrotic.

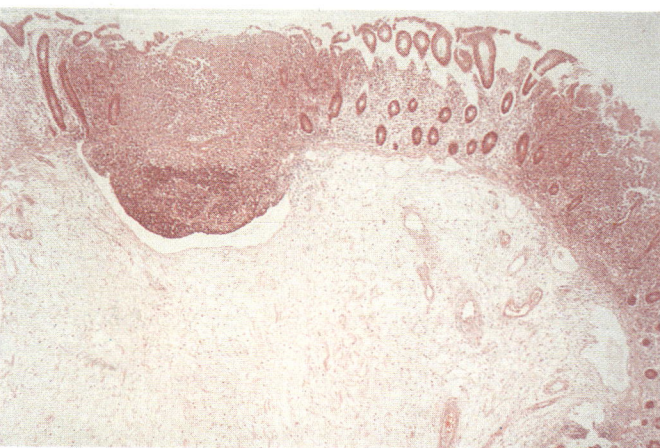

Fig. 16.150 In this case of yersiniosis focal ulceration is seen over lymphoid follicles in the caecal mucosa.

enterocolitica commonly produces a colitis which is usually self-limiting or one amenable to antibiotics. Children are most often affected. Occasionally there can be a range of systemic symptoms, such as myocarditis, arthritis, and erythema nodosum.

Affected individuals rarely come to surgery but in about half the cases colonoscopy demonstrates a patchy colitis with scattered, small, punched-out ulcers (Fig. 16.149). The rectum and sigmoid colon are often spared. Microscopy is that of non-specific inflammation and, unlike *Y. pseudotuberculosis*, granulomas are not a feature (Fig. 16.150).

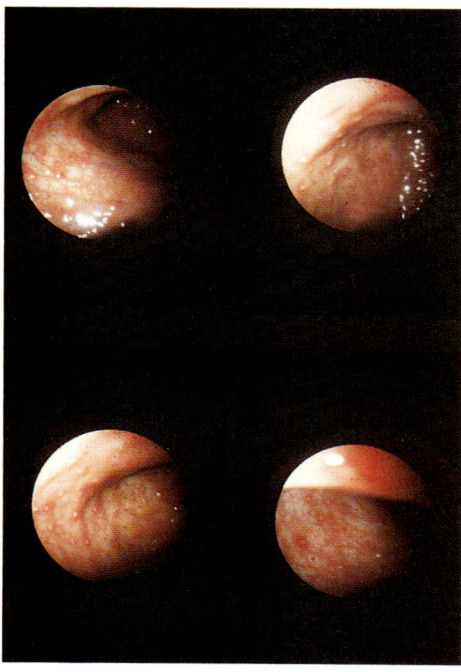

Fig. 16.149 Yersiniosis, showing multiple small mucosal ulcers in the colon. (Courtesy Professor Rutgeerts.)

16.12.3 Sexually transmitted intestinal disease

In addition to the well-known sexually transmitted diseases such as gonorrhoea and syphilis, it is now known that several other gastrointestinal pathogens can be sexually transmitted, e.g. *Salmonella* spp., *Campylobacter* spp. This group of infections and their symptoms have become known as the gay bowel syndrome because of their prevalence in the homosexual population. A small percentage of this group go on to develop AIDS. In this condition a variety of additional relatively new gastrointestinal pathogens can also be isolated (see below).

Gonorrhoea

In the male, rectal gonorrhoea is virtually always acquired through homosexual contact, although in the female spread can be from the urethra. In the majority of proven cases proctoscopic appearances and mucosal biopsy are normal. When abnormal, the abnormality is mild and generally limited to an increase in lymphocytes and plasma cells in the lamina propria. Very rarely is the picture of typical infective proctocolitis observed.

Detection of the gonococcus is best carried out by direct culture or via a mucosal smear. Proctoscopy and biopsy do not provide a diagnostic picture.

Syphilis

The primary lesion in syphilis occurs at the site of infection. The majority of cases occur in homosexuals as chancres of the anal canal. Lesions can occur in the rectum and mimic a carcinoma. If a lesion is biopsied, then organisms can be demonstrated by silver stains or by using an immunofluorescent antibody. Large numbers of plasma cells are characteristic surrounding proliferating capillaries lined by prominent epithelial cells.

In secondary syphilis there may be a proctitis, and occasionally the histological picture can resemble that of a typical bacterial infection. Sometimes small granulomas may be present.

Perhaps surprisingly, the mucosal inflammation in secondary syphilis is often more severe than that seen in rectal gonorrhoea.

Lymphogranuloma venereum (LGV) infection

This disease is due to the L1, L2, and L3 immunotypes of the obligate intracellular bacterium *Chlamydia trachomatis*. It should not be confused with granuloma venereum due to *Donovania granulomatis*, a Gram-negative cocco-bacillus. Although the disease was believed rare outside tropical countries, it is now appreciated as common in the homosexual populations of the West. Diagnosis is made by detecting changing serological antibody levels or by immunofluorescent staining of affected mucosa with monoclonal antibodies.

The proctitis caused by lymphogranuloma venereum in males is not normally preceded by the buboes seen in genital infections and is invariably related to homosexual practices. In females infection can spread from the vagina via lymphatics.

The initial stage of the infection presents as a mild proctitis or is asymptomatic. It seldom causes problems. A biopsy will show non-specific inflammatory changes and occasionally a granuloma. It is in the chronic phase that more severe pathology is seen. The rectal mucosa is granular and nodular with rigidity of the underlying tissue. This rigidity is due to extensive mural fibrosis which eventually gives rise to rectal stricturing. The mucosa is ulcerated and infiltrated by chronic inflammatory cells. Although the rectum is the main site of the disease, mild abnormalities can extend up to the transverse colon. Rarely a carcinoma may develop in long-standing strictures.

Chlamydia trachomatis proctitis

The non-LGV immunotypes of *Chlamydia trachomatis* are a very common cause of urethritis but may occasionally be responsible for a mild proctitis.

The gay bowel syndrome

This is a term to describe diarrhoea and symptoms of gastrointestinal disease caused by organisms that can colonize the gut of homosexual or bisexual individuals and spread as a result of sexual acts involving the ano-rectum. The most common pathogens are listed in Table 16.11 and many are also common to patients with AIDS who have gastrointestinal symptoms. The pathology of the gay bowel syndrome is simply that produced by the causative organism.

Acquired immunodeficiency syndrome (AIDS)

Infection of the small or large intestine is a common complication of infection with the human immunodeficiency virus (HIV). Diarrhoea and malabsorption are common symptoms, the precise clinical picture depending on the site and organism involved. At the time patients convert from sero-negative to sero-positive there is often an infectious mononucleosis-like illness with diarrhoea. Changes in the rectal mucosa have been described that resemble graft versus host disease (Section 16.14.3) with apoptosis of crypt cells and an infiltrate of lymphocytes. Viral particles have been demonstrated using *in situ* hybridization techniques.

Table 16.12 shows a list of possible pathogens that have been identified in patients with AIDS or with AIDS-related complex. *Cryptosporidia*, *Cytomegalovirus*, *Mycobacterium avium-intracellulare*, *Entamoeba*, *Giardia*, and *Campylobacter* are the commonest.

About 40 per cent of patients will show rectal and sigmoidoscopic abnormalities ranging from an ulcerative colitis-like picture (loss of vascular pattern, general inflammation, and friability) to discrete ulceration. Diagnosis depends on identifying the organism from stool culture or in a biopsy. In some cases it is difficult to assess if the presence of the organism is the cause of the symptoms as treatment may fail to produce a response.

Mycobacterium avium-intracellulare infection (*M. avium*)

M. avium is a ubiquitous micro-organism in the environment, being found in soil, carried by birds and by farm animals. Human infection is rare, although such infection can affect the skin. Systemic infection is only seen in patients with immune depression.

When infection of the gut is present, large numbers of phagocytic macrophages are seen in the lamina propria. These surround the crypts in the colon or distend the villi in the small intestine. These macrophages stain weakly with the periodic acid-Schiff reagent, and in this respect resemble the macrophages seen in Whipple's disease. However, unlike Whipple's disease, when stained by the Ziehl–Neelsen method or the Fite stain, the cells are seen to contain large numbers of acid-fast bacilli, *M. avium* (Fig. 16.151).

Spirochaetosis

Intestinal spirochaetes have been observed for many years by

Table 16.11 Common infections associated with the gay bowel syndrome

Campylobacter jejuni	Herpes simplex virus
Campylobacter-like organisms	HIV infection leading to AIDS
Chlamydia trachomatis (non-LGV)	*Neisseria gonorrhoea*
Clostridium difficile	*Salmonella* spp.
Entamoeba histolytica	*Shigella* sp.
Enterobius vermicularis	*Treponema pallidum*
Giardia lamblia	*Yersinia enterocolitica*

Table 16.12 Opportunistic infections associated with the acquired immunodeficiency syndrome

Small intestine	Large intestine
Crytosporidium spp.	
Cytometalovirus	
Isospora belli	
Mycobacterium avium-intracellulare	
Giardia lamblia	Gay bowel syndrome
Strongyloides stercoralis	Lymphogranuloma venereum
Sarcocystis hominis	Herpes simplex virus 1 and 2
Microsporidia	

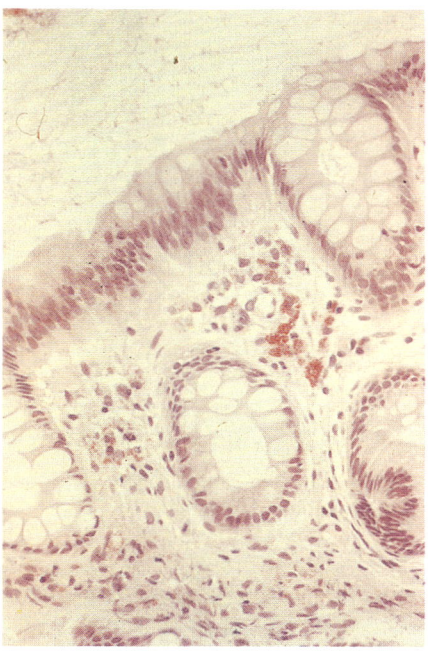

Fig. 16.151 Macrophages containing large numbers of acid-fast red-staining *Mycobacterium avium-intracellulare* are seen in the colonic mucosa. (Ziehl–Neelsen stain.)

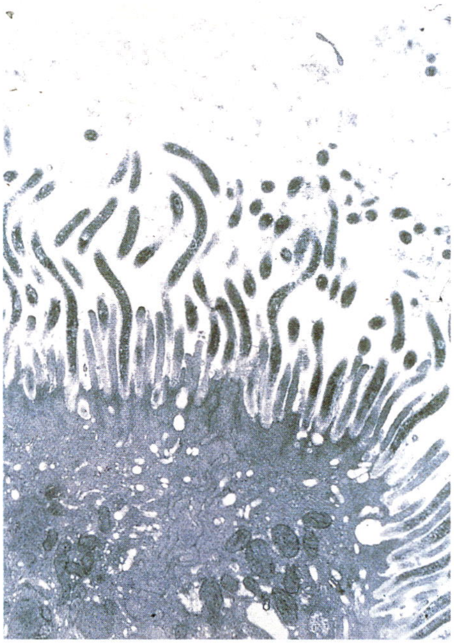

Fig. 16.153 On this electron micrograph, the spirochaetes are seen embedded on the colonic surface but not invading the colonocytes.

biologists studying the flora of the human gastrointestinal tract. In the stomach the old descriptions now match the recently discovered *Helicobacter pylori*, which is thought to be associated with gastritis. In the colonic and rectal mucosa spirochaetes can be demonstrated embedded along the surface epithelial cell borders in 3–7 per cent of populations attending gastroentero-logy clinics, and in up to 36 per cent of a homosexual popula-tion. The organisms appear as a blurred margin on the luminal aspect of the cell when using conventional histological stains. This is accentuated by silver staining (Figs 16.152, 16.153).

The organisms are unassociated with any inflammatory re-sponse but have been associated with depletion in the number of surface microvilli on colonocytes. It is still disputed whether these organisms are pathogens and responsible for symptoms. Indeed, there is still argument over their microbiological iden-tity. The natural category would be into the genus *Treponema* but details of their size and morphology suggest certain differ-ences and a new genus and species has been proposed, that of *Brachyspira aalborgi*. These organisms can also be found in the appendix.

16.12.4   Fungal infections

Actinomycosis

Actinomycosis is caused by the fungus *Actinomyces israeli*. It is most commonly found in the appendix (Section 16.11.3) and is rare in the large bowel. In the rectum it is often associated with anal fistulae (Fig. 16.154), and when present at this site is more commonly secondary to appendiceal disease than as a primary lesion. Macroscopically there may be a firm indurated stricture not unlike some carcinomas.

It is likely that actinomycosis is invasive only when the intest-inal wall has been breached by some other condition, such as a perforated diverticulum or trauma. Suture-line granulomas at the site of an anastamosis may contain actinomycetes. Abdom-inal intraperitoneal actinomycosis is occasionally associated with the use of the intra-uterine contraceptive device.

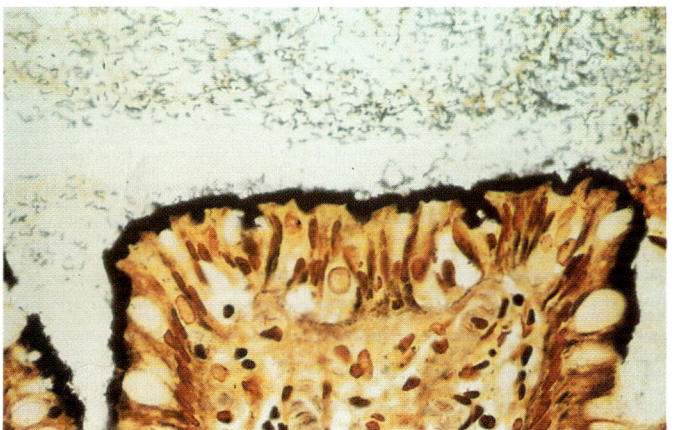

Fig. 16.152 A Warthin–Starry stain of colonic mucosa showing the thick luminal black line which is characteristic of spirochaetosis.

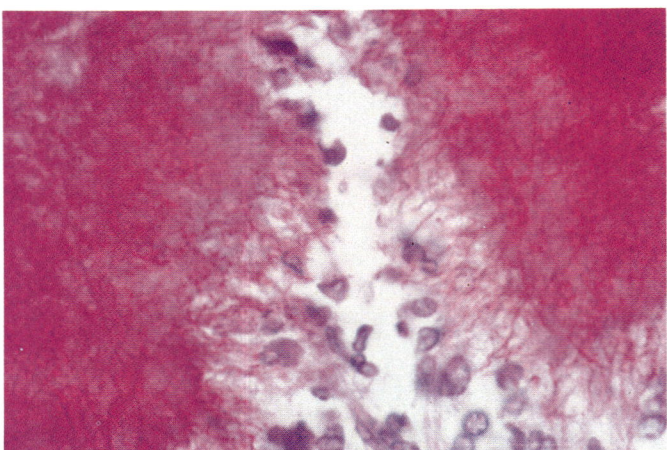

Fig. 16.154 Colonies of filamentous actinomycetes surrounded by inflammatory cells from a case of rectal actinomycosis. (PAS.)

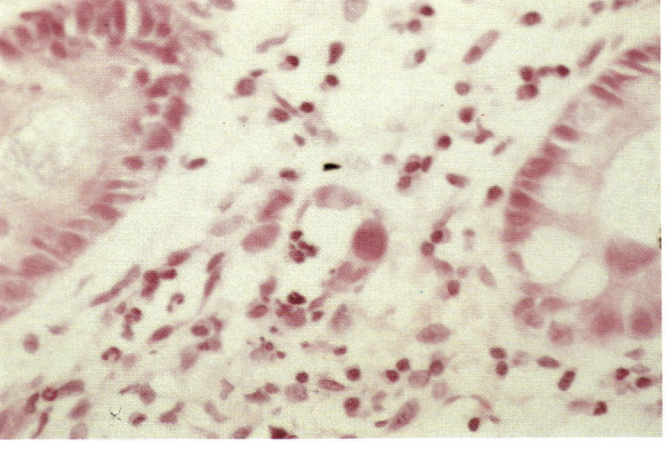

Fig. 16.155 Cytomegalovirus inclusions seen in an endothelial cell lining a capillary in rectal mucosa.

Other mycotic infections

There are a small number of case reports of mucormycosis, cryptococcosis, and histoplasmosis involving the large bowel. These are invariably in immunosuppressed patients. Candidiasis is a recognized rectal infection in patients with AIDS.

16.12.5   Viral infections

Cytomegalovirus

This is a herpes group of virus and an established colonic pathogen in immunosuppressed individuals, in particular those with AIDS. Its role as a primary pathogen of the colon in the immunocompetent is controversial. A self-limiting mild colitis has been described in a few such patients. In the immunodepleted, colonic infection is associated with ulceration. The ulcers can vary from minute to several centimetres in diameter, being discrete and punched out. Cytomegalovirus is seen in a small number of patients with ulcerative colitis and Crohn's disease almost certainly as a secondary invader, although it may interfere with healing. The presence of infection is recognized by characteristic 'owl-eye' intranuclear inclusions in macrophages or capillary epithelial cells (Fig. 16.155). Ill-defined cytoplasmic inclusions may also be present.

Herpes simplex virus

This virus may cause a limited distal proctitis in homosexuals, AIDS patients, and those immunosuppressed for other reasons. Characteristic multinucleate giant cells and intranuclear inclusions may be recognized on microscopy.

16.12.6   Protozoan infections

Entamoeba histolytica is the main protozoan parasite affecting the colon, although *Crytosporidia* spp. are now of growing importance with the increase in patients with AIDS (Section 16.10.5). *Balantidium coli* infection is rare and the enteromegaly of Chagas' disease (*Trypanosoma* spp.) is seldom seen in the West, in this the oesophagus is the major site of disease.

Amoebic dysentery

The normal habitat of *Ent. histolytica* is the crypts of the caecum and ascending colon. It has a world-wide distribution, and infection in Britian can be found in individuals who have not been abroad. Infection results from ingestion of cysts in food and water contaminated by faecal material. It is now appreciated that amoebiasis can also be a sexually transmitted disease, probably via the oral–anal route. The cysts develop into trophozoites in the small intestine and pass to their preferred ecological niche in the mucosa of the right colon. Trophozoites can be passed in the stools of affected individuals but survive for only short periods. It is the cysts that are the infecting agents.

Ent. histolytica, once in contact with intestinal epithelial cells, becomes adherent and causes cellular necrosis. The organisms ingest the lysed cells and invoke an infiltrate of neutrophil polymorphs. The amoebae are capable of invading all layers of the colonic wall and until comparatively recently it was a puzzle why some infected individuals failed to develop disease. Using starch-gel electrophoresis, virulence has now been shown to correlate with certain isoenzyme patterns. Twenty-two different zymodene types have been identified by this technique and only nine are associated with tissue invasiveness. However, it is still possible to be an asymptomatic carrier of a virulent zymodene type. Such individuals have positive serological findings, in contrast to carriers of non-pathogenic zymodene types.

Diagnosis is best made by identifying haematophagus trophozoites in fresh stools. The trophozoites quickly degenerate unless a fresh examination is performed. Serology is helpful, but it is difficult to distinguish between active disease, changes in the post-infection period, and asymptomatic carriers.

Pathology

The earliest lesions of amoebic colitis are yellow mucosal elevations produced by disintegrating surface epithelium. Ulcers then form which have an oval outline, overhanging edges, and lie in the transverse axis of the colon. They have a hyperaemic margin and yellow base. The right colon is the major site of disease (Fig. 16.156) but extension to the hepatic and splenic flexures is common. Diffuse colonic disease is the most dangerous form, from which major complications can arise. In such cases most of the mucosa may be shed (Fig. 16.157). In recovering mucosa entensive inflammatory polyps may form.

Microscopical examination shows that the mucosa is ulcerated and the ulcers are surrounded by a marked inflammatory response which frequently extends through the full thickness of the wall. There is oedema and vascular congestion, often with a prominent infiltrate of eosinophils. The organisms are to be found on or just beneath the surface of the ulcers in the overhanging margin. The ulcer is commonly covered by amorphous debris, the result of tissue necrosis (Fig. 16.158). In severe cases the organisms invade the bowel wall and may be observed in blood vessels. They are easily recognized on routine histological preparations, although recognition is enhanced by use of the periodic acid-Schiff reagent (Fig. 16.159). *Entamoeba* shows up as round organisms of 20–40 μm diameter and hence larger than other cells present. Ingested red blood cells are commonly seen within the cell cytoplasm. Erythrophagocytosis distinguishes *Ent. histolytica* from *Ent. coli* and other non-pathogenic intestinal amoebas. Often the organisms are only to be found in loose surface debris, and in biopsy work it is important to process and inspect all the material submitted.

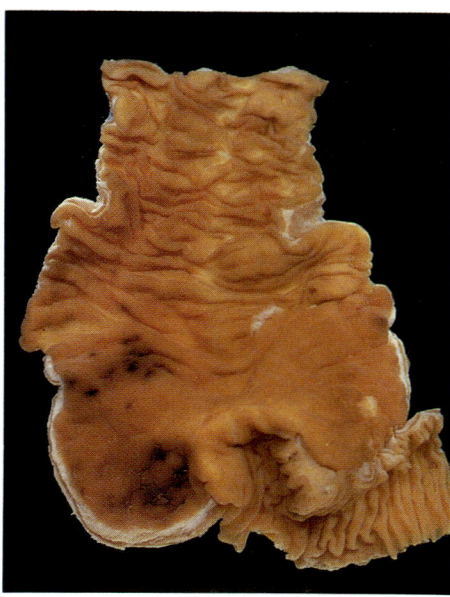

Fig. 16.156 Small raised yellow areas and tiny ulcers in the caecum of a case of amoebiasis. (Courtesy of Gower Medical Publishing and The Royal College of Surgeons (England).)

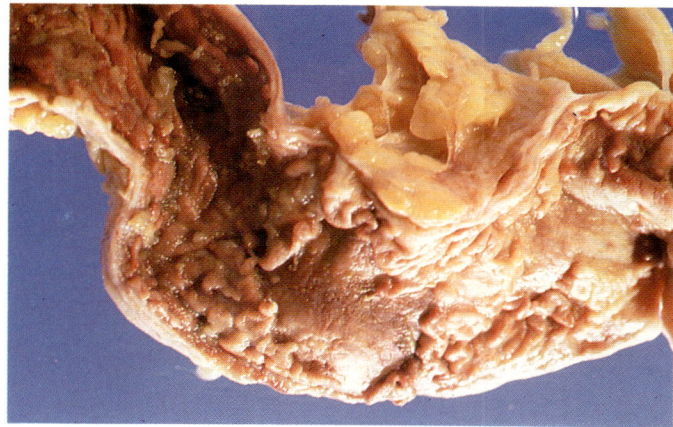

Fig. 16.157 In severe amoebiasis, as seen here, large areas of the mucosa are lost. The features are not that different from those seen in severe ulcerative colitis.

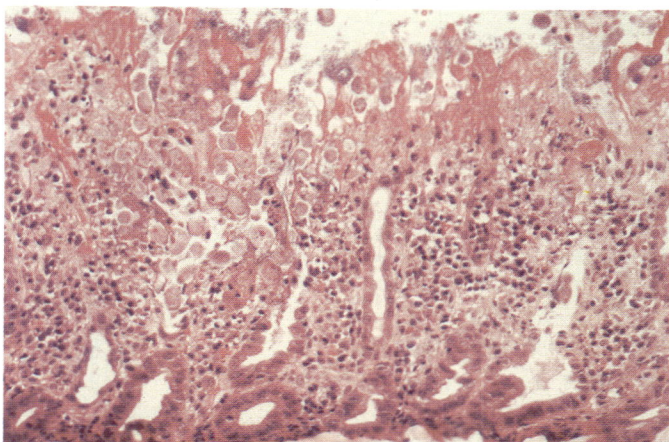

Fig. 16.158 An amoebic ulcer showing inflamed mucosa with debris and slough that contain numerous organisms (see Fig. 16.159).

Complications

These may be local or systemic. Local complications are the result of migration of amoebas through the colonic wall, and there is often superimposed bacterial infection. Progress from local ulceration to severe transmural disease and toxic dilatation can be subclinical. A common local complication is the formation of an amoeboma. This is a chronic form of disease in which localized secondary infection and fibrosis result in a circumscribed tumour. This may develop months or years after the initial infection. Amoebomas involve a short length of colon and are commonest in the caecum or rectum.

Invasion of veins leads to the most serious complication of amoebiasis, this is metastatic spread by the portal system to the liver with development of amoebic hepatitis or an amoebic liver abscess. In hepatitis there is marked portal-tract inflammation without necrosis or abscess formation. Organisms are not usually found. In a liver abscess small foci of necrosis coalesce to

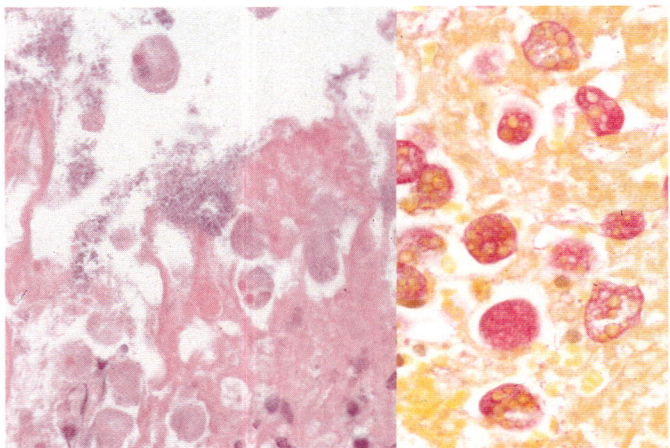

Fig. 16.159 *Entamoeba histolytica* organisms are clearly seen here with ill-defined nuclei and an occasional ingested red blood cell (left). On the right, these appearances are enhanced by using the periodic acid-Schiff reagent and added tartrazine.

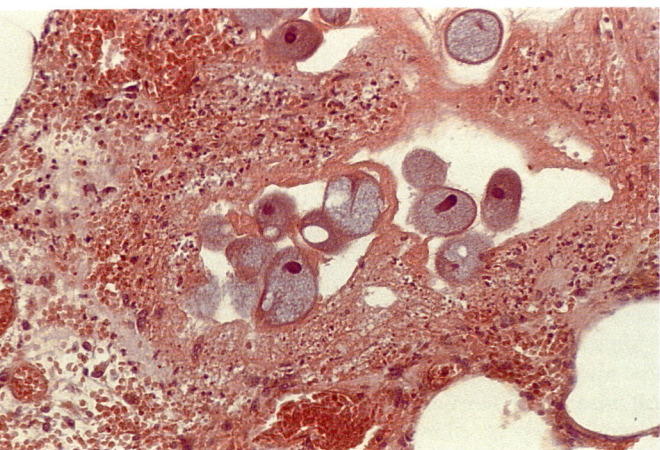

Fig. 16.160 The protozoan *Balantidium coli* in inflammatory debris overlying a colonic ulcer.

immune responses producing tissue damage. At this stage organisms are hard to find in tissue sections.

16.12.7 Inflammation due to helminths

Trichuriasis (whipworm)

This is believed to be the third most prevalent intestinal worm infestation after ascariasis and hookworm. The adult is between 2 and 5 cm in length and found predominantly in the caecum and right colon. Large numbers of eggs are passed each day and these develop into larvae over several weeks in moist warm soil. Infection is via ingested eggs from contaminated food and young children are most at risk. Larvae are set free in the small bowel, maturing to the adult in the right colon. The head of the worm buries itself in the mucosa and its body can be seen on colonoscopy, hanging from the mucosa. Infection is mostly asymptomatic, although in heavy infections a colitis can occur and, rarely, an appendicitis. An eosinophilia is a frequent accompaniment.

Oxyuriasis (*Oxyuris/Enterobius vermicularis*)

This is a common small nematode that inhabits the colon. It is seen most often by the pathologist in the lumen of the appendix and is considered further in Section 16.11.3.

Schistosomiasis

There are three main species of schistosomes that cause human infections, *Schistosoma haematobium*, *S. mansoni*, and *S. japonicum*. *S. haematobium* is mainly responsible for bladder disease, and *S. mansoni* and *S. japonicum* for colonic disease. *S. mansoni* is endemic in Africa and central South America, while *S. japonicum* is found in the Far East.

Infection occurs in man while wading or bathing in contaminated water in which the larval stage of the worm, the cercaria, are found. These can penetrate the skin and are carried by the bloodstream to the liver where they mature to adult

form a cavity filled with sterile pus. Bleeding often occurs into the cavity, to produce a reddish-brown colour likened to 'anchovy sauce'. Amoebas can be found in the abscess, except in very long-standing cases. If the abscess ruptures, dissemination (both local and distant) occurs, with brain and kidney lesions developing from bloodstream invasion.

Cryptosporidia and *Isospora*

These protozoans may be found in the colon as well as the jejunum and ileum (Section 16.10.5). The degree of colonic inflammation is usually mild.

Balantidium coli

This is a ciliated protozoan that produces changes similar to amoebas. Tissue diagnosis depends on recognition of the organism in histological sections (Fig. 16.160).

Chagas' disease—infection with *Trypanosoma cruzi*

Chagas' disease is endemic in certain parts of Latin America. The oesophagus is the major site of involvement in the gut, followed by the colon. Cardiac damage is the most frequent cause of death. *Trypanosoma cruzi* is a flagellate protozoan and disease is transmitted by the infective reduviid bug via a skin bite over which it subsequently defaecates. A parasitaemia follows.

Colonic damage is manifest in the chronic phase of the disease, occurring up to 15 or 20 years after the initial infection. There is chronic progressive constipation with the development of a megacolon. This is due to destruction of the myenteric plexus, in part by the organism and in part by the host's worms. It is thought that mature adults mate in the liver and then leave to lay their eggs at different sites, depending on the species. The eggs pass through the mucosa and out in the faeces. They hatch if deposited in warm fresh water, to release miracidial forms. These then infect freshwater snails. The cycle is completed by the snail releasing free-swimming cercaria that can re-infect man.

Pathology

The pathological changes in the gut in schistosomiasis are the result of the inflammatory reaction to the eggs in the intestinal wall. The severity depends on the balance between host immunity and the infecting dose. The eggs of *S. mansoni* are predominantly deposited in the left colon and rectum, those of *S. japonicum* are more common in the appendix and right colon.

Early on in the disease there can be acute proctitis and colitis, with haemorrhage and discharge of eggs into the lumen. In chronic infection a wide variety of appearances is possible, including ulceration, local and diffuse strictures, and inflammatory polyposis.

On microscopy the eggs are surrounded by histiocytes and giant cells forming granulomas (Figs 16.161, 16.162). In turn these granulomas are encompassed by an infiltrate of polymorphs, mainly eosinophils, and some fibroblasts. In time concentric fibrosis develops around the egg and the inflammation resolves. It is quite common to see the calcified remains of a schistosomal egg in the colonic mucosa or submucosa without any accompanying inflammation. The eggs of each of the species of *Schistosoma* are different and differentiation is possible on histological section. The eggs of *S. mansoni* are oval with a lateral spine. In *S. haematobium* infection (rare in the gut) spines are terminal, whereas in *S. japonicum* infection the eggs are spherical, but smaller than those of the other species, and have a small lateral spine. Eggs carried to the liver can promote portal fibrosis and eventual portal hypertension. In long-standing cases of schistosomiasis there is an increased incidence of colonic carcinoma.

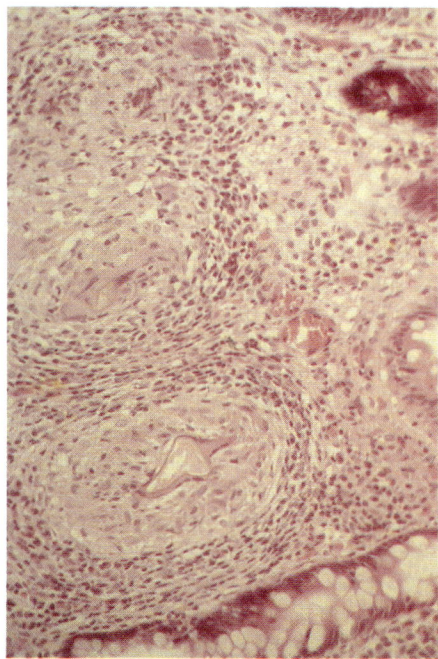

Fig. 16.162 A granuloma is visible containing a *Schistosoma* egg with a lateral spine, indicating that it is *S. mansoni*.

16.12.8   Further reading

Bartlett, J. G., Chang, T. W., Gurwith, M., Gorbach, S. L., and Onderdonk, A. B. (1978). Antibiotic-associated pseudomembranous colitis due to toxin-producing clostridia. *New England Journal of Medicine* **298**, 531–4.

Mathan, M. M. (1987). The large intestine: specific infections. In *Gastrointestinal and oesophageal pathology* (ed. R. Whitehead). Churchill Livingstone, London.

Morson, B. C., Dawson, I. M. P., Day, D. W., Jass, J. R., Price, A. B., and Williams, G. T. (1990). *Gastrointestinal pathology* (3rd edn). Blackwell Scientific Publications, Oxford.

Prathap, I. C. and Gilman, R. (1970). The histopathology of acute intestinal amoebiasis. *American Journal of Pathology* **60**, 229–45.

Price, A. B. (1980). Pseudomembranous colitis. In *Recent advances in gastrointestinal pathology* (ed. R. Wright). W. B. Saunders, London.

Price, A. B. and Davies, D. R. (1977). Pseudomembranous colitis. *Journal of Clinical Pathology* **30**, 1–12.

Schofield, J. B., Lindley, R. P., and Harcourt-Webster, J. N. (1989). Biopsy pathology of HIV infection: experience at St. Stephen's Hospital, London. *Histopathology* **14**, 277–88.

Surawicz, C. M. and Belic, L. (1984). Rectal biopsy helps to distinguish acute self limited-colitis from idiopathic inflammatory bowel disease. *Gastroenterology* **86**, 104–13.

Talbot, I. C. and Price, A. B. (1987). *Biopsy pathology in colorectal disease.* Chapman and Hall, London.

Weller, I. V. D. (1984). AIDS and the gut. *Scandinavian Journal of Gastroenterology* **20**, (Suppl. 114), 77–89.

Weller, I. V. D. (1985). The gay bowel. *Gut* **26**, 869–75.

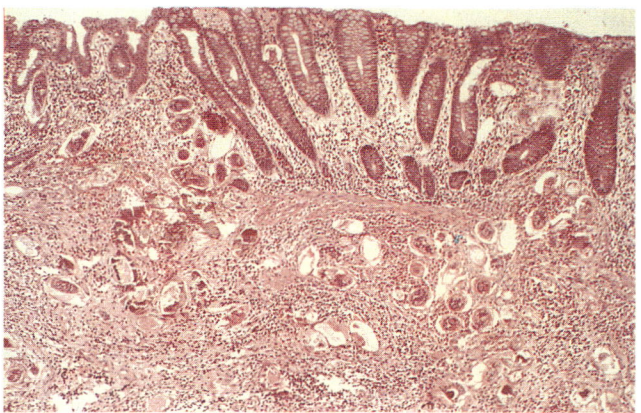

Fig. 16.161 *Schistosoma* eggs seen beneath the rectal mucosa.

16.13   Inflammatory bowel disease

A. B. Price

16.13.1   Introduction

In this section the non-infective patterns of inflammatory bowel disease are considered, including those in which infection is the suspected aetiology but not as yet the proven one. Ulcerative colitis and Crohn's disease are the two main entities but other rarer forms exist, e.g. collagenous colitis, neonatal necrotizing colitis. It seems likely that in time many of these will turn out to have an infective aetiology or be an atypical response to a particular commensal gut organism in susceptible individuals. Indeed, it is still a possibility that Crohn's disease and ulcerative colitis are one disease with different tissue reactions to a single aetiological agent. The different response being determined by the balance between the host's immunological profile, the putative pathogen, and the local environment. This concept is best understood by reference to leprosy. One patient group develops tuberculous leprosy with florid granulomas but in which few organisms are seen, others develop the lepromatous variety. In this pattern granulomas are not a feature but large numbers of organisms are present within the histiocytes that infiltrate the tissue.

Non-specific inflammatory bowel disease is the term generally used to cover these cases of chronic enteritis or colitis of obscure aetiology. Crohn's disease and ulcerative colitis have well-defined clinical and pathological patterns that emerge over a prolonged time-course. A diagnosis is reached from the amalgamation of the clinical, radiological, and pathological evidence collected over this period. There is no one parameter of either Crohn's disease or ulcerative colitis that is invariably present in one and invariably absent from the other.

16.13.2   Ulcerative colitis

Ulcerative colitis is a disease that commences in the rectum and, in a significant proportion of patients, spreads proximally to involve an increasing length of the colon. The disease spreads proximally but in continuity from the rectum and stops at the ileo-caecal valve. Inflammation does occur in the distal 10–20 cm of ileum but purely as a result of backwash through the ileo-caecal valve. It is a disease characterized by periods of exacerbation and remission, though a few patients may have more continuous low-grade activity. It is primarily an inflammatory condition of the mucosa and the deeper structures are spared, except in fulminating attacks when the whole wall is involved.

Epidemiology and incidence

The peak age incidence at presentation is the third decade, although very young children can be affected and it may pre-

sent in the elderly. Ulcerative colitis is common in most of the Anglo-Saxon communities of North-West Europe, New Zealand, and North America, and uncommon in eastern and southern Europe and the Third World. It has many epidemiological similarities with Crohn's disease. The incidence is higher in towns and urban communities than in rural society, and Jewish populations have a greater incidence than other groups. Overall, the incidence is reported as steady or rising slightly.

Aetiology and pathogenesis

The aetiology is unknown despite extensive research into likely causes, such as infection, diet, environmental factors, immunological defects, abnormalities of mucin, and genetic defects. It seems likely that, even if ulcerative colitis is found to have a single aetiology, the pathogenesis will be multifactorial.

A genetic factor is likely as siblings and first-degree relatives of patients with ulcerative colitis carry an increased risk of developing not only ulcerative colitis but also Crohn's disease. The risk has been calculated as approximately eightfold. Carriers of HLA-B27 and BW35 may also carry an increased risk.

The search for an infective agent has been pursued by trying to identify agents in stools and mucosa, by studying antibody titres to certain organisms in the serum, and by inoculating tissue filtrates into animals. No consistent abnormality has been found in the bacterial flora. *Escherichia coli* species in patients with ulcerative colitis have increased adhesive properties compared to control patients, and some workers have identified cell wall-deficient variants of several bacteria in colonic tissue. None of the common enteropathogens are consistently associated with ulcerative colitis, although in many patients the onset of disease is precipitated by an attack of infection. Bowel-wall filtrates from patients with ulcerative colitis have been shown to be cytopathic to cell-culture lines but positive proof that this effect is due to a virus has not been forthcoming. Inoculation of tissue filtrates into animals has produced several false positive trails, more so in the course of the investigation of Crohn's disease than ulcerative colitis.

Another line of investigation has been the study of goblet cell mucins. Mucus depletion of goblet cells is characteristic of ulcerative colitis. Although no primary abnormality has been demonstrated, one of the components of colonic mucin is reduced, even in cases in remission. In another approach non-smokers have been shown to be more susceptible to ulcerative colitis than smokers. The colonic mucosa of smokers exhibits enhanced glycoprotein synthesis, which may offer increased protection to the colonic-mucosal barrier.

Immunology

An immunological defect in ulcerative colitis is an attractive concept for either the aetiology or as part of the pathogenesis. Amongst early suggestions was one linking the disease with an allergy to cow's milk. This was based on demonstrating raised serum antibodies to milk protein. However, this was not confirmed subsequently and is now just one of a plethora of contentious findings in the immunology of inflammatory bowel disease. The field is littered with uncorroborated data because it is difficult to exclude technical artefact from much of the work. Immunological methodology is complex and, by necessity, carried out mostly *in vitro*. Furthermore, it is difficult to establish that an abnormality is primary and not secondary, for most correlate only with disease activity and are absent in remission.

Alll limbs of the immune system have been explored and no consistent abnormality demonstrated. Of particular interest is that circulating lymphocytes in ulcerative colitis are cytotoxic to colonic epithelial cells and this effect is blocked by a lipopolysaccharide extract of *Escherichia coli* OO19:B14. This extract will also activate normal lymphocytes. The mucosal as well as the circulating lymphocyte population also have this cytotoxic activity. Studies of plasma cells in the mucosa have produced inconsistent results but, in the main, demonstrate an increase in IgG-containing cells.

Abnormalities in B- and T-cell numbers in the serum and in the function of mucosal T-lymphocytes have been reported, but nearly all correlate with disease activity and are not prime defects. Animal models of colitis may be induced by immunological manipulations; for example, the injection of antibody–antigen complexes into a rabbit, preceded by rectal irritation with formalin. Many such models depend on the presence of the gut flora, and germ-free animals are unaffected.

Although some immunological abnormalities will no doubt play a role in the pathogenesis of ulcerative colitis, the range of abnormalities detected suggests that the disease will have a multifactorial basis.

Macroscopic appearances

Because ulcerative colitis is a mucosal disease, there is often little appreciation of involvement from inspection of the serosal surface. The length of the large bowel is commonly reduced, in particular the rectum (Fig. 16.163). When the bowel is opened in active disease the mucosa will be granular, congested, and friable, though surprisingly not necessarily ulcerated (Fig. 16.164). When ulceration is present it is patchy, but intervening mucosa is always microscopically abnormal, even though this may not be apparent macroscopically (Fig. 16.165). Ulceration can appear to be linear, aligned along the taeniae coli.

The mucosal changes in ulcerative colitis invariably involve the rectum. They may then spread proximally in continuity, involving greater lengths of bowel until there is a total colitis. However, not all regions of the colon may be equally active and this can give rise to patchy gross appearances which misleadingly suggest segmental disease (Fig. 16.166). Histology always confirms a continuous abnormality up to the proximal limit of disease (Fig. 16.167).

Fibrosis is not a feature of the pathology of ulcerative colitis and strictures are not seen. Quite commonly, polyps or mucosal tags are observed. They are inflammatory not neoplastic and are formed by irregular regeneration of the mucosa after severe

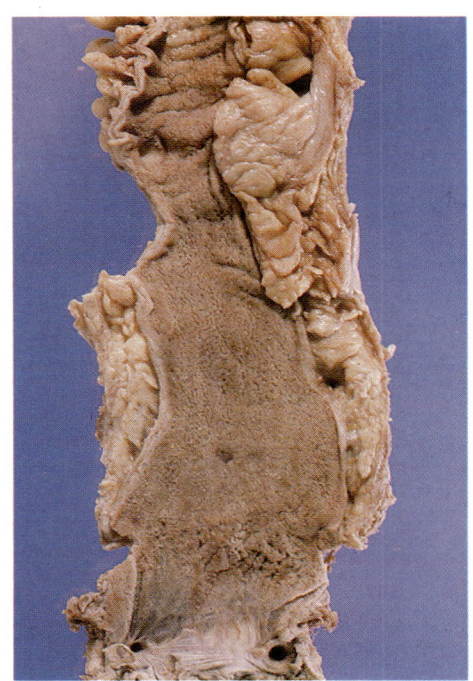

Fig. 16.163 The typical granular mucosa in the rectum in a case of ulcerative colitis.

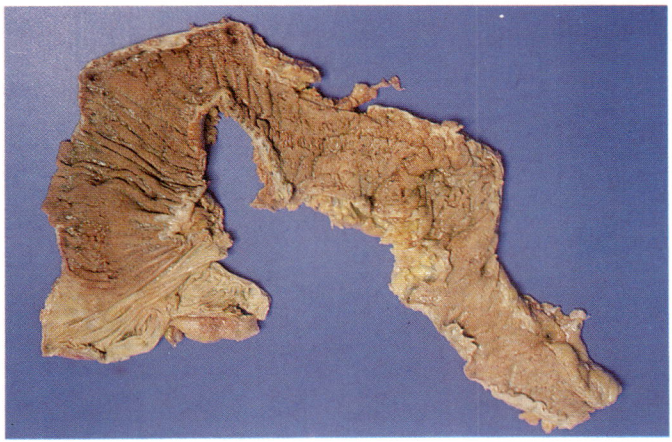

Fig. 16.164 Diffuse mucosal involvement in ulcerative colitis with sharp demarcation in the right colon.

ulceration. Obviously, a patient with ulcerative colitis may also have coincidental neoplastic polyps (adenomas). Occasionally large numbers of inflammatory polyps are seen, producing a pattern known as 'colitis polyposa' (Fig. 16.168). Approximately 10 per cent of colectomy specimens will show granularity and ulceration of the distal 10–20 cm of terminal ileum, the result of caecal backwash.

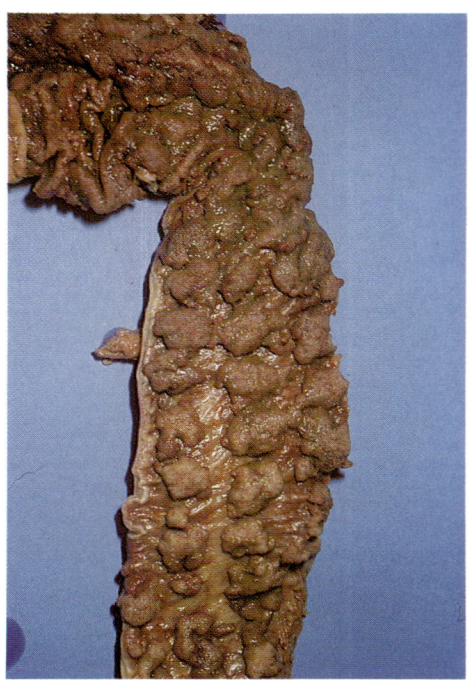

Fig. 16.165 Severe ulceration in ulcerative colitis. The ulcers surround surviving islands of granular mucosa.

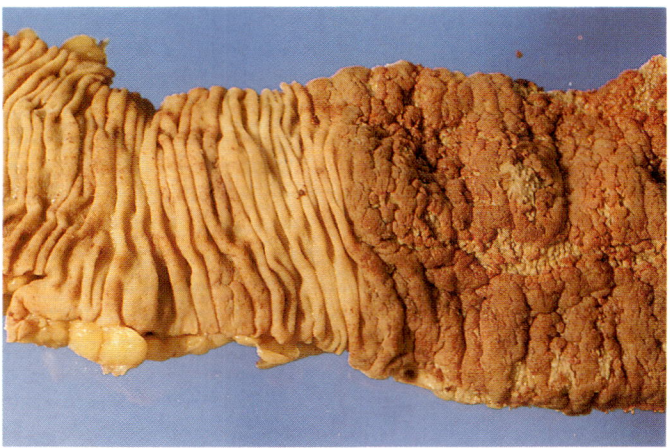

Fig. 16.167 The sharp demarcation between normal and abnormal mucosa in the transverse colon in a case of ulcerative colitis.

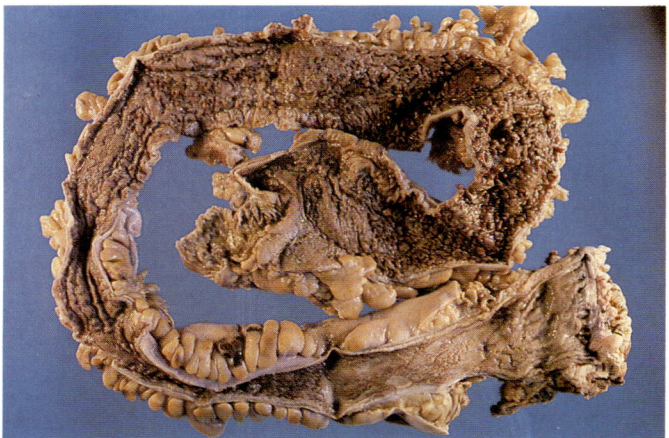

Fig. 16.166 A total colitis but the rectum is in a phase of remission partly induced by steroid enemas. This gives the impression of rectal sparing and segmental disease.

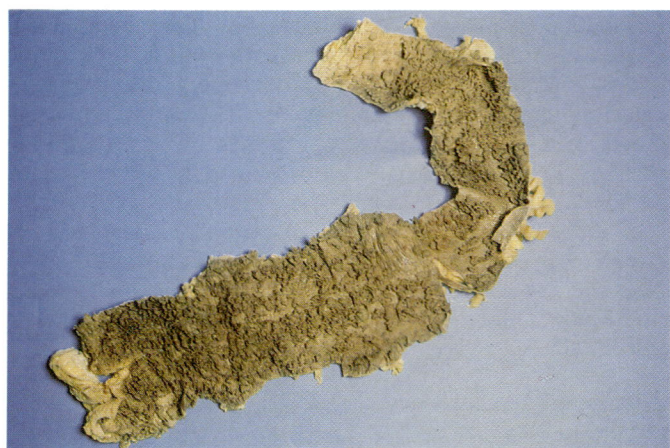

Fig. 16.168 Colitis polyposa in ulcerative colitis. There are extensive inflammatory polyps and mucosal tags throughout the colon.

Fulminant colitis

Approximately 5–13 per cent of patients with ulcerative colitis will have a fulminant episode, often resulting in an emergency colectomy. In such cases there is gross dilatation of the colon, mostly in the region of the transverse colon. The wall is thinned and there is extensive shedding of mucosa, with only scattered islands surviving (Figs 16.169, 16.170). Perforation is common in this phase of disease. Furthermore, in fulminant colitis not only is there mucosal disease but the whole thickness of the colonic wall, muscle included, is involved. Fulminant attacks of colitis with dilatation are a rare complication of many causes of inflammatory bowel disease, and macroscopically it is often impossible to distinguish between them at this time.

Ulcerative proctitis

Inflammation limited to the rectal mucosa can be caused by a large variety of inflammatory agents. Rectal disease is always the starting point for ulcerative colitis, or for what is more strictly termed ulcerative proctocolitis. Over a 10-year period in patients presenting with an initial proctitis the chance of spread to the sigmoid colon is about 30 per cent and to the whole colon between 5 and 10 per cent. There is some evidence that limited distal disease may predominate in the elderly population.

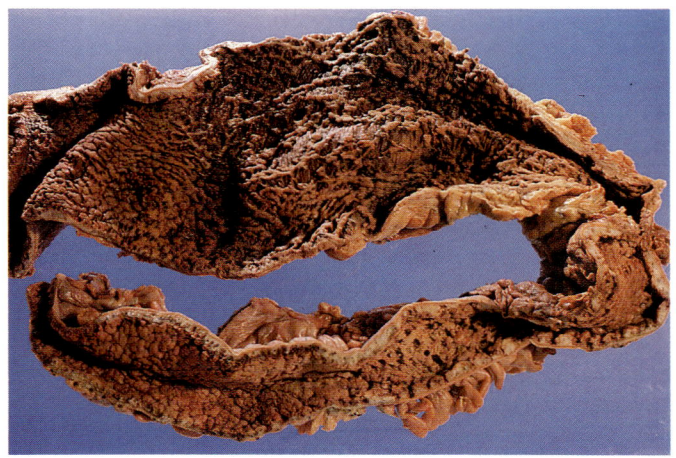

Fig. 16.169 Toxic megacolon with dilatation of the transverse colon.

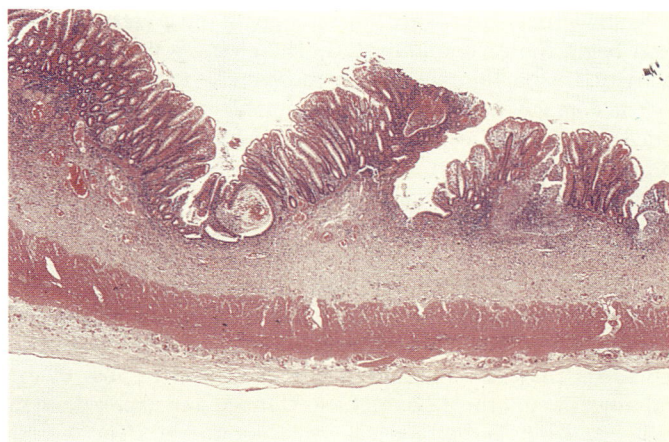

Fig. 16.171 Ulcerative colitis showing inflammation limited to the mucosa with associated distortion of the mucosal architecture.

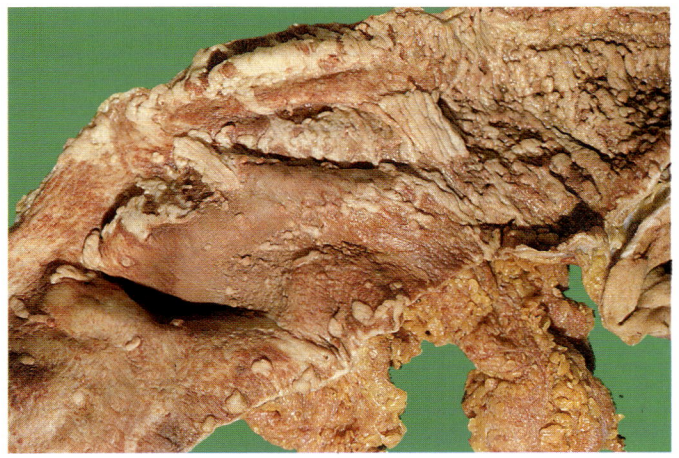

Fig. 16.170 Acute fulminant ulcerative colitis, showing dilatation of the transverse colon and extensive loss of the mucosa.

with congestion and dilatation of capillary blood vessels. A characteristic feature is the presence of crypt abscesses (Fig. 16.172). These are collections of polymorph neutrophils within the crypt lumen. They are not specific for ulcerative colitis and occur in a variety of inflammatory conditions. They are, however, particularly conspicuous in active ulcerative colitis, tending to identify the acute phase. It is likely that they are one of the many factors playing a role in ulceration of the mucosa, for bursting of the crypts disrupts the mucosa. Ulceration is a feature of active disease and can involve the full thickness of the mucosa, encroaching on the superficial submucosa. Accompanying the inlfiltrate of neutrophil polymorphs there is a heavy and diffuse infiltrate of plasma cells and lymphocytes throughout the lamina propria. Immunoglobulin studies of the plasma

Histopathology

The microscopic changes in ulcerative colitis are confined to the mucosa (Fig. 16.171) with the exception of fulminant disease (see below). It is also a continuous disease from its origin in the rectum to the proximal limit. Both these factors mean that mucosal biopsy is an accurate means of studying the pathology. Because it is a disease with periods of exacerbation and remission, it is convenient to divide the histological features into those of acute disease, resolving disease, and disease in remission.

Active colitis

The most striking feature is the diffuse inflammatory cell infiltrate of the mucosa, involving crypts and lamina propria, along

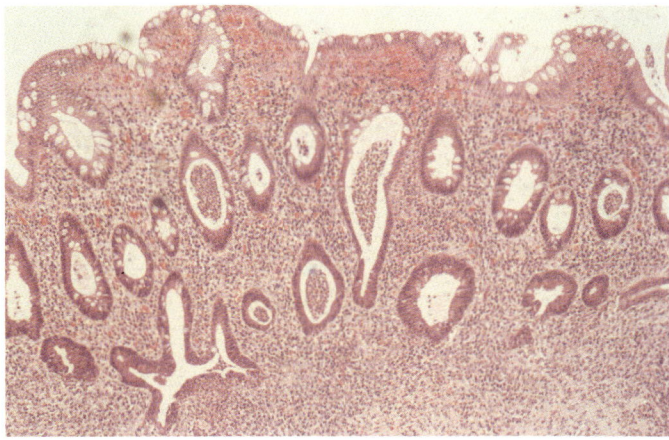

Fig. 16.172 The mucosa in active ulcerative colitis showing goblet cell depletion, diffuse inflammation of the lamina propria, and crypt abscesses.

cells show that all types are increased, with the greatest proportion being those containing IgG. The changes fluctuate with activity. Eosinophils may also be conspicuous in some cases.

The damage to the crypts with incomplete regeneration produces crypt architectural distortion, which results in crypt branching and shortening. The persistent architectural abnormality is particularly characteristic of ulcerative proctocolitis (Fig. 16.173).

Acute colitis—fulminant phase

This is the only stage in which inflammation extends beyond the mucosa to involve the submucosa and muscle wall (Fig. 16.174). There is extensive ulceration, involving loss of the submucosa, and the deep muscle is thinned and exposed, often only covered by a thin layer of granulation tissue. The muscle fibres appear vacuolated and are separated by oedema. There is

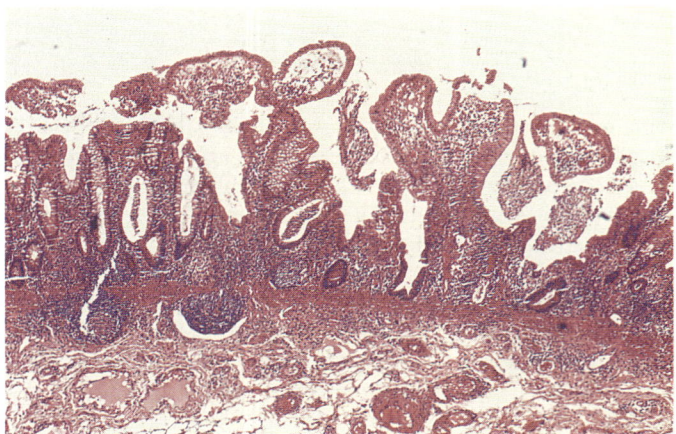

Fig. 16.173 Active ulcerative colitis, demonstrating the villiform mucosa with numerous crypt abscesses present. The inflammation is clearly limited to the mucosa.

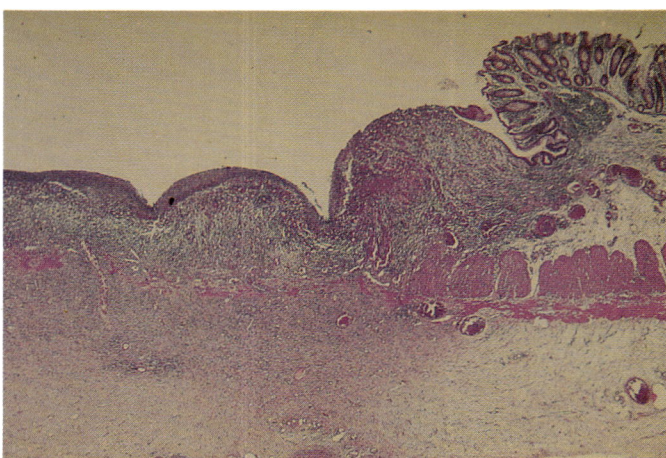

Fig. 16.174 Fulminant ulcerative colitis, illustrating the severe mucosal denudation along with transmural inflammation. Small clefts are apparent in the ulcerated regions.

intense capillary congestion. A regular pattern of splitting of the circular muscle coat is often seen, an appearance not to be mistaken for the fissuring that is characteristic of Crohn's disease (Figs 16.174, 16.175). Inflammatory cells of all types are seen scattered throughout the colonic wall.

Resolving and quiescent colitis

The waxing and waning nature of ulcerative colitis means that inflammatory changes may resolve without treatment. Because this can occur at different rates and different sites, there may be a false impression of segmental disease. With resolution the number of inflammatory cells diminish, and have a patchy distribution. Crypt abscesses are no longer seen but the crypt architectural damage remains (Figs 16.176, 16.177).

In quiescent disease, although the mucosa may no longer appear macroscopically abnormal, microscopic examination always reveals some hallmarks of previous inflammation. This usually takes the form of crypt atrophy. The crypts are shortened, few in number, and branched. There are few inflammatory cells remaining; indeed, the lamina propria may appear depleted of cells. In the quiescent phase Paneth cell metaplasia is often conspicuous, and increased numbers of argyrophil cells are noted. Lymphoid follicles may be prominent in the mucosa, an appearance termed 'follicular proctitis' (Fig. 16.178).

This whole spectrum of inflammatory change still occurs in the rectum after colectomy and ileo-rectal anastomosis.

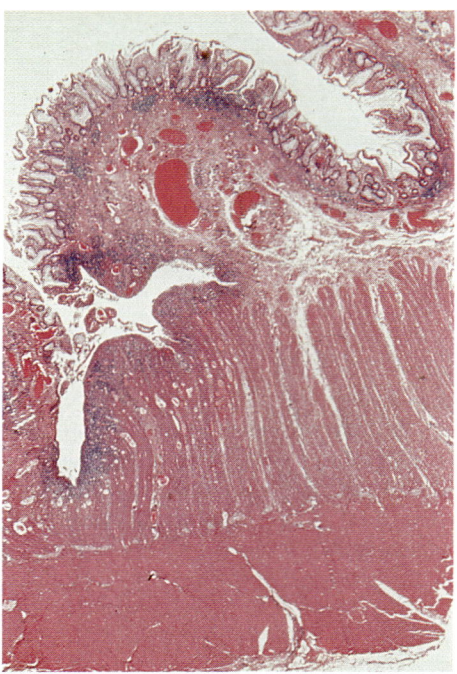

Fig. 16.175 Fulminant ulcerative colitis showing fissuring ulceration. In this phase of the disease these can no longer be considered reliable attributes for a diagnosis of Crohn's disease.

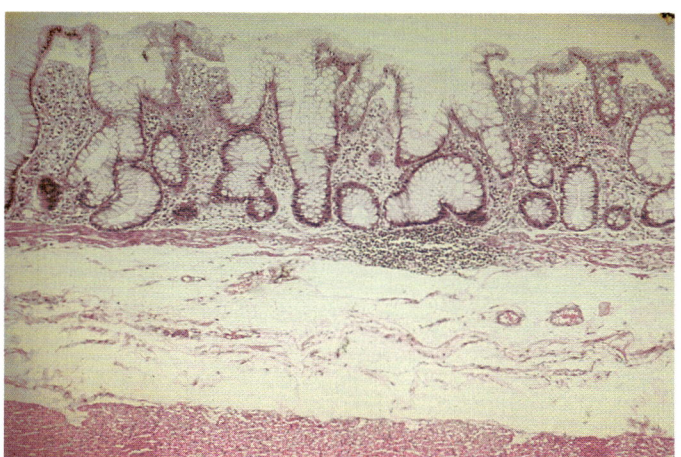

Fig. 16.176 Ulcerative colitis in remission with marked crypt distortion and a return of the goblet cell population.

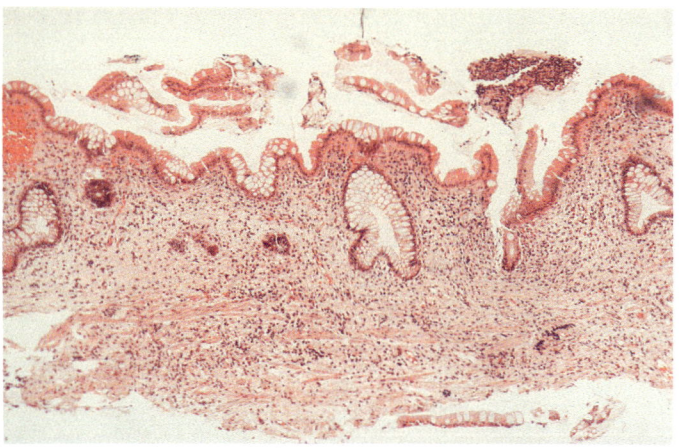

Fig. 16.177 Ulcerative colitis in remission, illustrating crypt atrophy and a paucity of inflammatory cells.

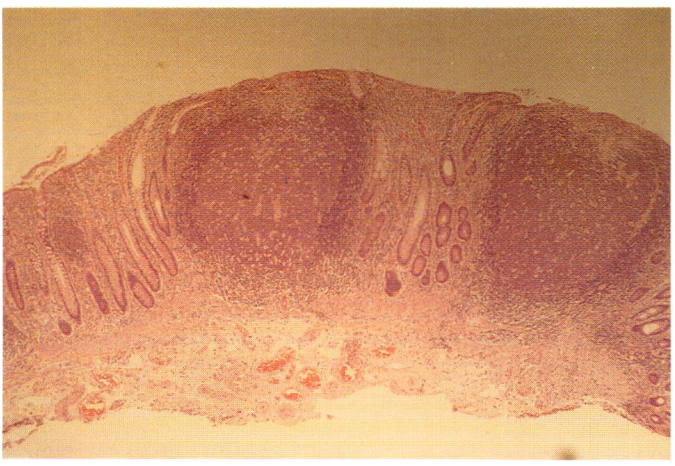

Fig. 16.178 Follicular proctitis in chronic ulcerative colitis with prominent lymphoid follicles.

Complications of ulcerative colitis

Cancer in colitis

Carcinoma of the colon and rectum is an accepted complication of ulcerative colitis. Two factors are of major importance, the duration of the disease and the extent of the disease. The risk is low when the history of colitis is less than 10 years' duration, but then increases, and patients with total colitis are at higher risk than those with limited, left-sided disease. The onset of disease in childhood is disputed as being an additional risk factor. Regardless of age of onset, the greatest risk of developing cancer occurs around the age of 50. The cumulative risk of cancer in ulcerative colitis varies depending on the cohort of patients under review, but is in the region of 7–9 per cent at 15 years and 13–17 per cent at 20–30 years. However, cancer in colitis accounts for less than 1 per cent of deaths from large bowel malignancies, and within the colitic population between 3 and 5 per cent may eventually develop a cancer.

In 1967 Morson and Pang drew attention to the detection of dysplasia in rectal mucosa as a precancerous phase in ulcerative colitis. The detection of dysplasitic mucosa at any site in the colon and rectum by colonoscopic and/or rectal biopsy is now a valuable method of surveillance for patients at risk of developing a carcinoma. Unfortunately, about 30 per cent of cancers in ulcerative colitis are not associated with dysplasia and, even when present, it is patchy. Colonoscopy is a necessary part of a surveillance programme, for the rectum is not invariably involved. The final problem is that dysplasia is not necessarily associated with a recognizable macroscopic lesion. Therefore a successful cancer screening programme for the 'at risk' population necessitates regular lifelong colonoscopic examination, with random biopsies at 10 cm intervals throughout the colon.

Macroscopic features of cancer and dysplasia in ulcerative colitis Cancer in colitis has the same distribution as cancer in the general population, although it is more frequently multiple and more frequently of a higher grade. It also differs by being more often flat with an ill-defined edge. Indeed, it resembles the macroscopic appearances of gastric carcinoma more than the common pattern of colonic carcinoma (Fig. 16.179).

Dysplasia in the colitic, as mentioned, may produce no visible lesions. More frequently it is marked by plaques, low nodules, or a velvety mucosal appearance (Fig. 16.180). There is therefore a marked contrast between the macroscopic appearances of dysplasia in the colitic and non-colitic population. Colonic dysplasia in the non-colitic population is polypoid, seen as a tubular adenoma or villous papilloma. It is therefore easily recognizable at endoscopy.

Microscopic feaures of dysplasia in ulcerative colitis Dysplasia is defined as 'an unequivocal neoplastic epithelial proliferation'. Its recognition is highly subjective and in the presence of active inflammation its distinction from reactive or regenerative change is extremely difficult.

The cytological and architectural criteria for a diagnosis of dysplaia in colitis are similar to those applied to other glandular epithelia. Within cells there is variation in nuclear position,

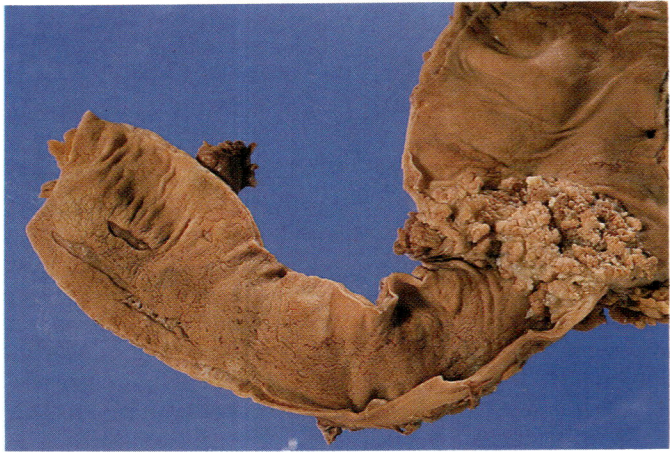

Fig. 16.179 This colectomy shows a cancer from a patient with long-standing ulcerative colitis.

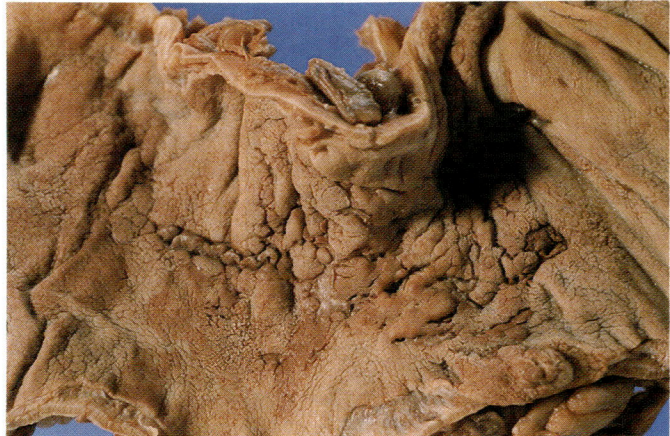

Fig. 16.180 The plaque-like appearance of dysplasia complicating ulcerative colitis.

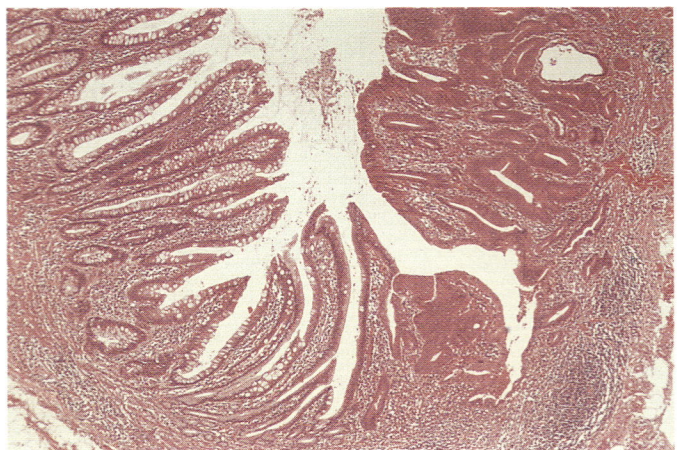

Fig. 16.181 In the left-hand half of this illustration there is villiform non-dysplastic mucosa, which contrasts with the right-hand field in which dysplasia is seen.

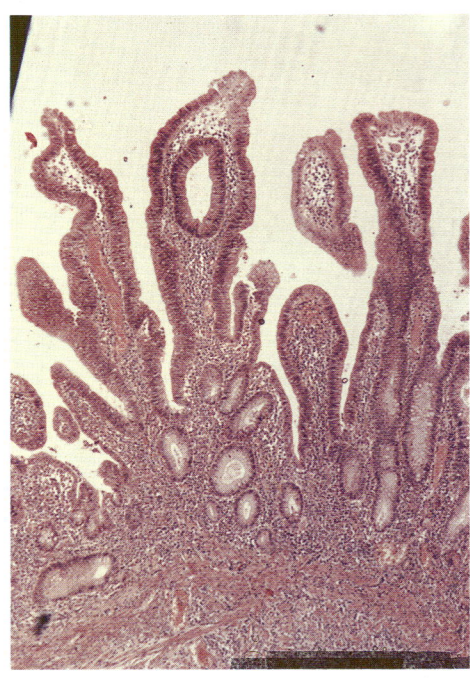

Fig. 16.182 Dyplastic mucosa covering the upper half of the mucosa with non-involved epithelium still lining the lower part of the crypts.

nuclear size, nuclear chromatin, and an increase in mitotic rate. Architectural abnormalities can produce thickening of the mucosa, which is often villiform due to elongation of the crypts. Cell maturation along the crypt is deranged.

The above changes can be graded according to their severity into high- and low-grade dysplasia (Figs 16.181–16.183). This is believed to relate to the risk of finding a concurrent carcinoma or to one developing subsequently. Because of the difficulties in the interpretation of inflammatory and dysplastic changes, an indefinite category also exists.

The clinical implications of dysplasia in colitis Data from various studies suggest that the maximum diagnostic yield of cancer based on finding severe dysplasia is 62 per cent. However, it must be appreciated that even if no cancer were found at colectomy, such a patient can be construed as a success for any cancer prevention programme. The major question then becomes the morbidity of colectomy versus the likelihood of developing cancer if no surgery was performed.

At the present time an unequivocal biopsy diagnosis of high-grade dysplasia calls for the immediate consideration of a proctocolectomy. Clinical management of low-grade dysplasia is less certain. In flat mucosa the patient can be kept under regular surveillance, but in the presence of a raised endoscopic lesion it has been shown that there is frequently a co-existing cancer and proctocolectomy must be considered. Patients falling within the indefinite group require careful follow-up. Most diagnostic problems centre on interpretation in the presence of

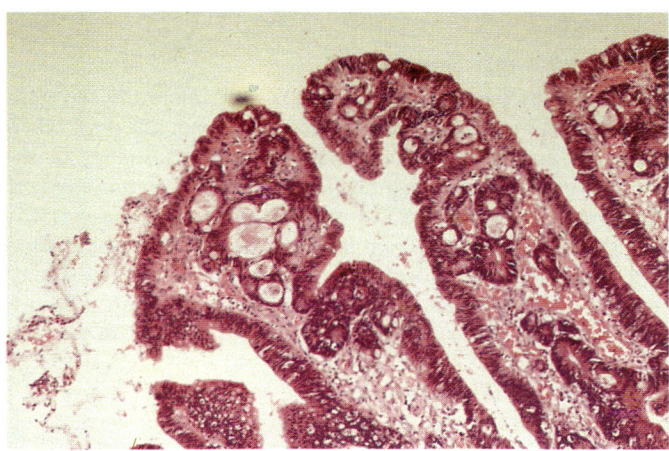

Fig. 16.183 Severe dysplasia verging on intramucosal carcinoma in villiform mucosa from a patient with long-standing ulcerative colitis.

inflammation, consequently repeat biopsies after a period of treatment often resolve the dilemma.

There is clearly a need for a specific objective marker that will recognize dysplasia. Quantitative and qualitative alterations in mucosal mucin histochemistry, the detection of aneuploidy by flow cytometry, and the study of the peanut lectin binding patterns have been the three main avenues investigated. Several oncogenes, such as c-*myc* and *ras*, have also been studied. At present none of these offer a viable alternative to subjective histological assessment.

Other complications of ulcerative colitis

The liver may be affected and liver function tests are frequently abnormal. Between 5 and 8 per cent of patients will have major problems, pericholangitis and sclerosing cholangitis being the two primary complications. Fatty change and viral hepatitis are also common, as most patients with ulcerative colitis will have been exposed to injections, infusions, and a hospital environment. Carcinoma of the bile ducts is a rare complication.

There are a large number of extra-intestinal manifestations of ulcerative colitis. These include arthritis, erythema nodosum, pyoderma gangrenosum, pericarditis, and uveitis.

The small bowel in ulcerative colitis

Although ulcerative colitis does not primarily involve the small bowel, it may become inflamed in certain situations.

Backwash ileitis

The occurrence of a backwash ileitis has already been referred to and is seen in up to 10 per cent of all colectomy specimens removed for ulcerative colitis. It is probably related to colonic contents entering the terminal ileum.

The ileum after colonic excision—'pouchitis'

Following removal of the colon and restorative surgery to fashion an ileo-rectal anastomosis, or some pattern of small bowel pouch, the small bowel mucosa commonly becomes the site of inflammation. In 'pouchitis' as it is termed, it may undergo 'colonization' to a degree that is indistinguishable from active ulcerative colitis. It is interesting that patients with familial adenomatous polyposis, who have similar operations, do not suffer this complication. Thus it is not simply a complication of therapy but is related to the underlying disease process.

16.13.3   Crohn's disease

It is likely that the first clearly recognizable account of this disease was by Dalziel in 1913, even though the paper in 1932 of Crohn *et al.* gave the name to the condition. In the early descriptions it was believed to be a disease limited to the small bowel, but in the 1960s disease of the colon, anus, and perianal skin was documented. It is now clear that all sites of the gastrointestinal tract can be involved, the mouth, oesophagus, stomach, and duodenum. In addition, there are many extra-intestinal manifestations, so that the concept of Crohn's disease must extend beyond the confines of the gut.

Aetiology and pathogenesis

The cause of Crohn's disease is unknown despite extensive research. Studies involving multivariant analyses on clinical and pathological parameters suggest that it may be a heterogeneous group of conditions rather than one, and the question of its relationship with ulcerative colitis has already been mentioned. The main pathways of investigation, as with ulcerative colitis, have been genetic, environmental, dietary, microbiological, and the use of experimental animal models.

A hereditary predisposition is likely as Crohn's disease can be up to 13 times more frequent in first-degree relatives than in unrelated groups. It has also been documented amongst twins. Because Crohn's disease is a relatively modern condition, it has triggered interest in environmental factors. The incidence is raised in both smokers and those with an increased sugar intake. Pathology indistinguishable from Crohn's disease is seen in a small number of patients taking the contraceptive pill. Dietary manipulation, such as the use of an elemental diet, will produce a remission in acute exacerbations of disease, and specific food substances, in particular wheat and dairy products, can precipitate symptoms in individuals in remission.

The presence of granulomas in approximately 60 per cent of Crohn's disease raises obvious comparisons with other granulomatous diseases and infections. Measurements of antibody titres to a wide range of bacteria have been undertaken, generally with conflicting results. Amongst those reported as raised are titres to *Eubacterium*, *Peptostreptocuccus*, and *Mycobacterium paratuberculosis*, the cause of Johne's disease (regional enteritis) in cattle.

Investigation of the gut flora and culture filtrates of intestinal tissue have drawn attention to cell-wall deficient bacteria, such as *Pseudomonas maltophilia*, and certain atypical *Mycobacteria*. One group claimed to have produced a lesion resembling Crohn's disease in a goat when injected with a mycobacterium isolated from a patient with Crohn's disease. Although considerable suspicion surrounds this group of organisms, the findings are far from reproducible.

At present, attempts to identify a viral agent have been unsuccessful and similar to the findings in ulcerative colitis. Considerable interest was generated by animal transmission experiments when granulomas were produced in the footpads of mice using Crohn's tissue. This effect was eventually shown to be due to the injection of foreign material.

Immunology

Much already written about ulcerative colitis (Section 16.13.2) applies also to Crohn's disease. The humoral and cellular limbs of the immune system have been investigated with no consistent defect found that could not be ascribed a secondary phenomenon. The granuloma, it can be argued, is a failure to clear the aetiological agent, and its absence in ulcerative colitis being evidence for two distinct disease entities. Such an argument is countered by those believing that ulcerative colitis and Crohn's disease are but one disease exhibiting an individual's capability for different immunological reactivity. Tuberculous and lepromatous leprosy are another example of this phenomenon.

Circulating immunoglobulins in Crohn's disease vary with activity, and numerous antibodies against host or foreign antigens have been documented. Those cross-reacting with *Escherichia coli* are best known. Circulating immune complexes can be found in Crohn's disease, with increased turnover of the complement system. However, although these abnormalities can be detected in ulcerative colitis, they may still have a role in the numerous extra-articular manifestations of Crohn's disease.

As with ulcerative colitis, circulating and tissue lymphocytes in Crohn's disease have been shown to be cytotoxic to colonic epithelium, this toxicity disappearing after colectomy. Study of T-cell subsets has yielded conflicting data, but there is a fundamental idea that a functional regulatory defect exists as a basis for the inflammatory changes. Mostly, however, the changes are secondary to activity of the disease.

It is most likely that the aetiology and pathogenesis of Crohn's disease are multifactorial. Genetic factors probably link with immunological ones to cause intestinal inflammation, operating via an environmental antigen, chemical or microbial. The granuloma, which is not invariably present, simply reflects the balance between these factors.

Epidemiology

Crohn's disease shares many epidemiological features with ulcerative colitis. The disease is becoming more common in Britain and Scandinavia, with the increase mainly in large bowel disease. There are two peak ages, one in the 20–40 age-group, the other in the 60–70 age-group. The disease is rare in southern Europe, Africa, and the Middle East. Like ulcerative colitis, there is a higher incidence in the Jewish population.

Pathology

Macroscopic appearances

The appearance of Crohn's disease is fundamentally the same whatever the level of the gastrointestinal tract affected. Differences are due to either local anatomy and physiology or the stage of the disease at the time of resection. The commonest site involved is the terminal ileum. As anorectal disease is frequently associated with both ileal and colonic disease, it ranks as the second most frequent site. Colonic disease is the next most common and becoming increasingly more frequent. Disease limited to the upper small bowel, stomach, or duodenum is less frequent.

There are three basic macroscopic patterns. First, ulceration may predominate; the ulcers are serpiginous, discontinuous, and in their earliest form present as small aphthoid lesions on the mucosa (Fig. 16.184). Colonoscopic studies suggest that these aphthoid ulcers progress to more typical linear ulceration over 2–3 years. Secondly, strictures may form. These can be short or long, multiple or single. A 'hosepipe' stricture of the terminal ileum is the classical appearance (Fig. 16.185) but such strictures can occur at any site. Thirdly is the pattern known as 'cobblestoning' (Fig. 16.186). This describes a mucosa divided into cobblestone-like areas by intercommunicating crevices or fissures surrounding islands of mucosa raised up by the underlying inflammation. Accompanying any of these patterns is the fissure, an important feature of both the macroscopic and microscopic pathology of Crohn's disease (Fig. 16.187). It is the pathological basis of fistulae, a frequent complication of the disease.

Whichever of the above patterns is present, and there is frequently a mixture, involvement of the bowel is discontinuous, there being areas of normal bowel (skip areas) separating diseased areas (Figs 16.188, 16.189). Because Crohn's disease is a transmural disease, the bowel wall is usually thickened, with involvement of the peri-intestinal fat and serosa. Approximately half of the cases of oesophageal Crohn's disease will have disease elsewhere in the gut.

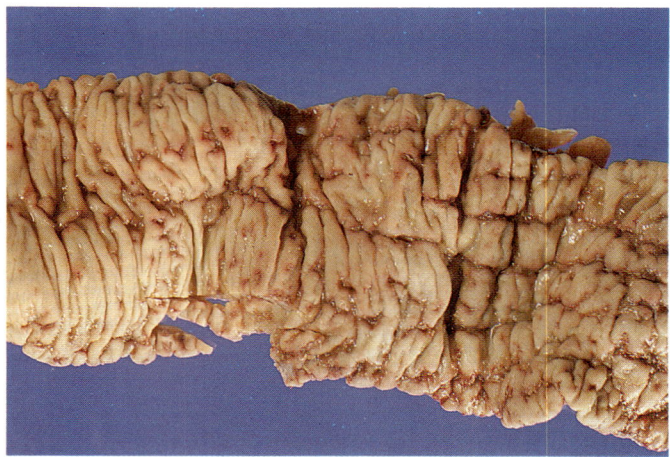

Fig. 16.184 This length of small intestine shows multiple aphthoid ulceration, seen as tiny, red, ulcerated foci.

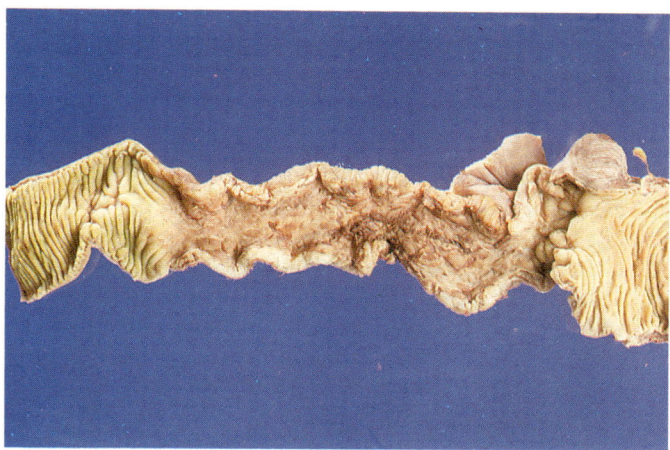

Fig. 16.185 Crohn's disease of the terminal ileum. The disease stops sharply at the ileo-caecal junction seen to the right of the picture.

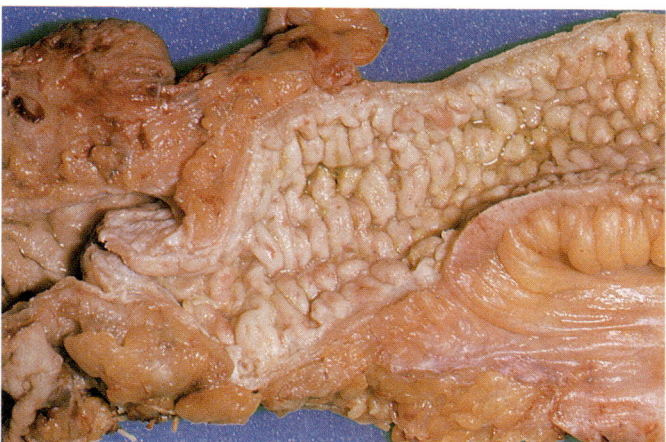

Fig. 16.186 Cobblestone ulceration in the terminal ileum in a case of Crohn's disease.

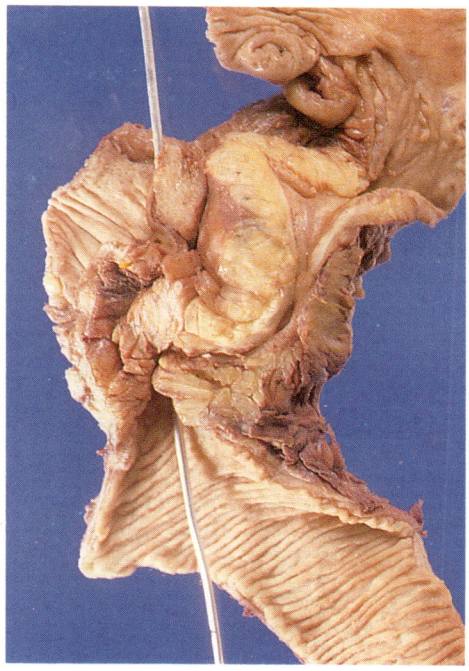

Fig. 16.187 The probe is inserted through an ileo-sigmoid fistula in Crohn's disease. A tight stricture is seen in the terminal ileum along the right-hand margin of the specimen, leading through the ileo-caecal valve into the caecum at the top right.

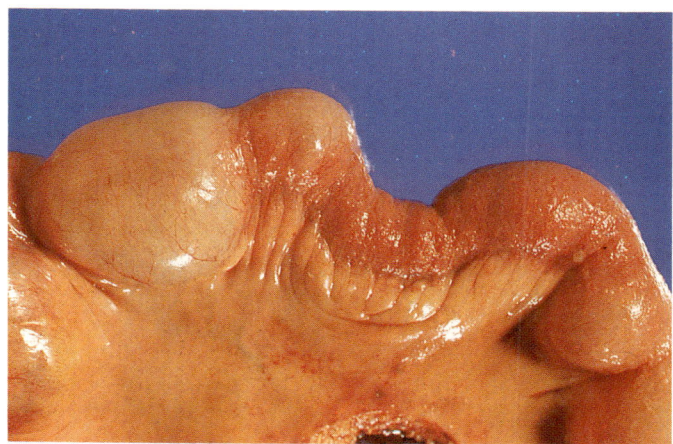

Fig. 16.188 A length of ileum inflated with formalin to accentuate the typical 'skip' lesions characteristic of Crohn's disease. Normal distended bowel is seen to either side of a stricture.

The oesophagus Oesophageal involvement is rare, the picture being one of ulceration and thickening, often indistinguishable from a malignant stricture.

Stomach and duodenum Between 0.5 and 4 per cent of patients with Crohn's disease have gastroduodenal involvement. Thickening and rigidity of the gastric wall is common, generally involving the antrum. The appearances are difficult to distinguish from linitis plastica. Rarely, the duodenum is the initial site, the wall appearing thickened with nodular mucosal folds and small irregular ulcers or erosions.

Small intestine The classical 'hosepipe' stricture of the terminal ileum is becoming less common as the diagnosis of Crohn's disease is now being made earlier in its natural history. Nevertheless, the terminal ileum is the primary site of the disease in about 50 per cent of cases. Several ileal strictures 5–10 cm long are the commonest pattern to observe. Between 25 and 30 per cent of cases involve the terminal ileum and right colon. About 5 per cent of patients may have extensive disease of the jejunum and ileum, and an equally small number have only jejunal disease.

Appendix The appendix may be involved in continuity with ileo-caecal disease, at a distance from other involved sites, or as the presenting site. The prognosis is good when it is the sole site involved at presentation.

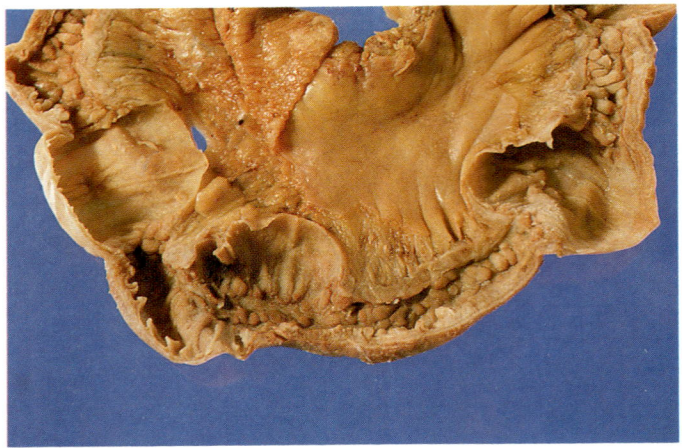

Fig. 16.189 The specimen seen in Fig. 16.188 opened to demonstrate the 'skip' lesions. Areas of diseased bowel are separated by normal areas.

Large intestine The pattern of inflammation in the large bowel can be divided into three: diffuse disease, segmental strictures, and distal rectal disease (Fig. 16.190). Any one of these varieties may be associated with small bowel involvement, although right-sided colonic disease is the commonest. These is accompanying small bowel disease in approximately 50 per cent of cases of colonic Crohn's disease.

The mucosal surface commonly shows discontinuous serpiginous ulceration or a longitudinal guttering-type of ulceration

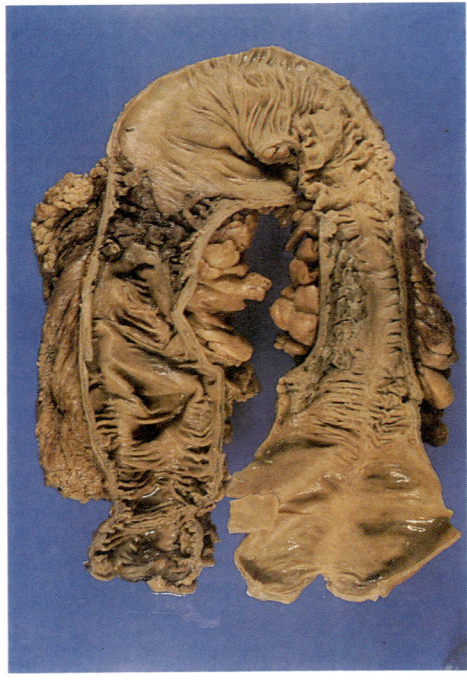

Fig. 16.190 Colonic Crohn's disease showing segmental disease in the descending colon and right colon, with an intervening length of normal bowel.

with intact oedematous mucosa alongside. Strictures are like those seen in the small intestine. In the rectum diffuse ulceration may be present with occasional foci of normal mucosa. The wall may be rigid or short strictures can be present.

Anus About 25 per cent of patients with small bowel disease and 75 per cent of those with Crohn's disease of the colon have anal disease at sometime in the natural history of the disease. It takes the form of a chronic fissure, an anal fistula, ulceration, or a characteristic perianal, dusky blue, oedematous appearance. Anal disease may be the presenting sign of latent disease elsewhere in the gut. It can be treated and cured prior to more proximal disease appearing. By contrast, resection of diseased segments does not necessarily improve the anorectal features.

Skin disease Ulceration of the perianal skin, spreading to involve the genitalia and groin, is common. Metastatic lesions can also occur at sites distant from the anal region. In these the typical granulomas of Crohn's disease are observed. Pyoderma gangrenosum, erythema nodosum, and eczema can also be complications of the disease.

Microscopic appearances

The most valuable diagnostic feature is the presence of an epitheloid cell granuloma, with or without giant cells (Figs 16.191, 16.192). This reaction, which is present in 50–70 per cent of all cases, is essentially the same as the tissue reaction in sarcoidosis, non-caseating tuberculosis, and beryllium poisoning. Large numbers of granulomas are present in some specimens, while in others only an occasional one is found after extensive searching. They can be found at any site in the bowel wall and at any level. It has been observed that more granulomas occur in the rectum than proximally and that the numbers diminish with the length of history of the disease.

Fissuring is a second important microscopic feature pointing to a diagnosis of Crohn's disease. Serpiginous clefts extend from the mucosal surface, which is invariably ulcerated, down into

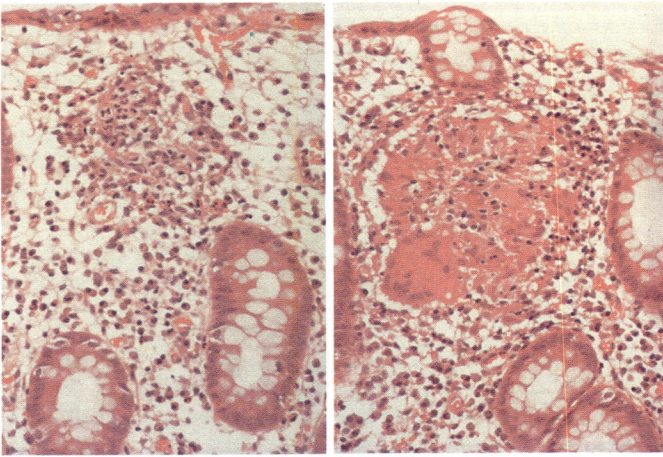

Fig. 16.191 A well-formed granuloma is seen in the mucosa of the colon on the right, with an ill-formed 'micro-granuloma' present on the left.

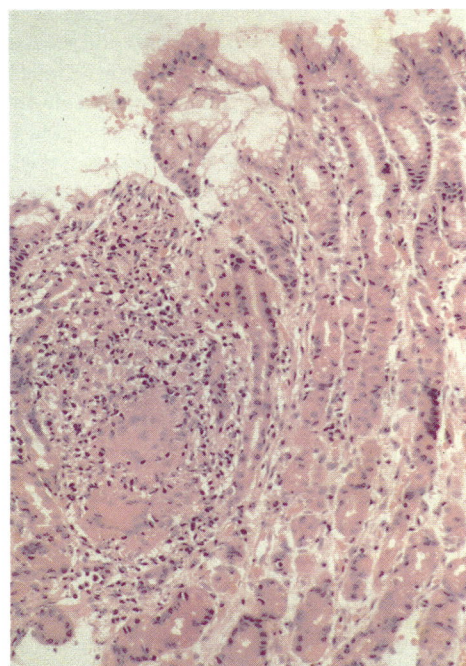

Fig. 16.192 Gastric Crohn's disease, showing a granuloma in the mucosa of the body of the stomach.

the submucosa and often beyond into the muscle and serosa. They are lined by inflammatory cells and are the histological basis for the formation of fistulae, characteristic of Crohn's disease (Fig. 16.193).

The diagnosis of Crohn's disease can still be made in the absence of both granulomas and fissures, as there is a distinctive pattern of transmural inflammation. The submucosa is frequently widened by oedema or is fibrotic. Focal aggregates of lymphocytes are scattered through all layers of the bowel wall and are often present as a bead-like line on the serosal surface

(Figs 16.194, 16.195). This pattern of inflammation is the most consistant of all the histological changes associated with Crohn's disease. These aggregates and granulomas may be intimately associated with small vessels. Other features such as ulceration, lymphangiectasia, neural hyperplasia, and pyloric gland metaplasia are non-specific, being seen in chronic inflammation of several causes.

Crypt abscesses in the mucosa are common but seen in fewer numbers than in ulcerative colitis. The goblet cell population is preserved to a greater degree than in ulcerative colitis, despite the presence of an inflamed mucosa. In addition, the crypt

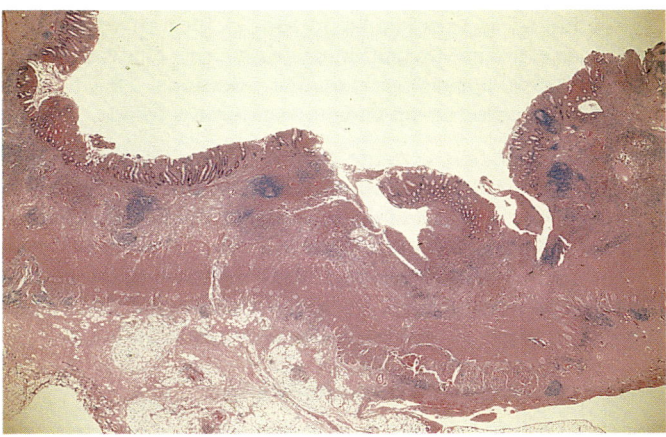

Fig. 16.194 Crohn's disease in the colon, showing transmural inflammation, lymphoid aggregates across the bowel wall, and early fissuring ulceration.

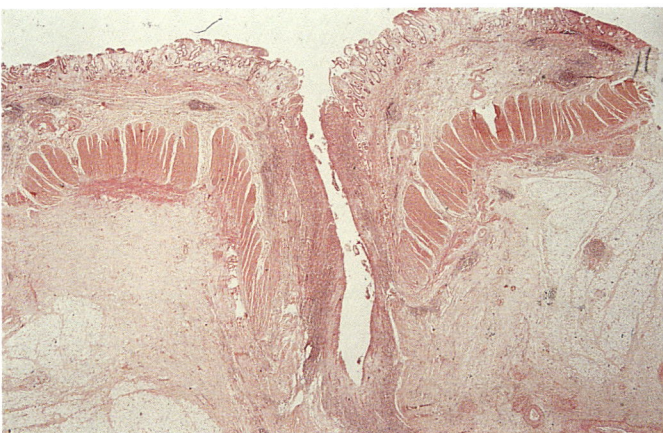

Fig. 16.193 A fissure passing through the full thickness of the bowel wall. This is typical of Crohn's disease and the histological basis for clinical fistulae.

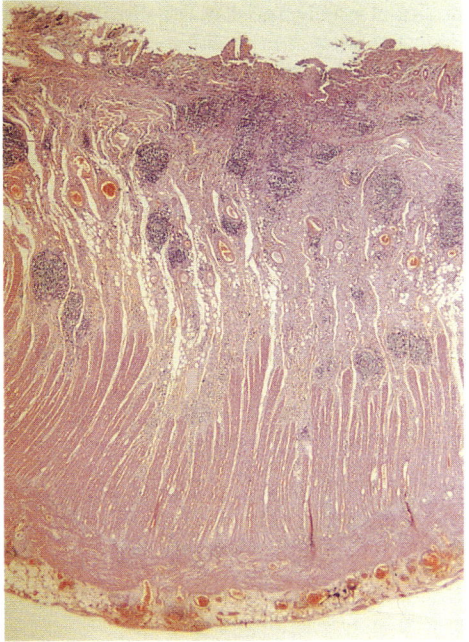

Fig. 16.195 In this section of ulcerated colon the lymphoid aggregates so characteristic of Crohn's disease are well seen distributed throughout the full thickness of the bowel wall.

alignment remains relatively intact. Aphthoid ulceration, already mentioned as one of the early macroscopic features of Crohn's disease, is seen on microscopy as small areas of ulceration over lymphoid follicles (Fig. 16.196).

Unlike ulcerative colitis, the histological patterns in Crohn's disease cannot be classified as active, remitting, and quiescent (Section 16.13.2). Indeed, in patients with Crohn's disease the clinicopathological correction is weak and some may be asymptomatic yet still have quite extensive ulcerating disease.

Acute Crohn's disease—toxic megacolon Acute dilatation of the bowel seems resricted to colonic Crohn's disease and may be seen at some point in the history of up to 11 per cent of cases. The pathology is very similar to that in ulcerative colitis. In this phase of disease the pathology of all forms of inflammatory bowel disease appear very similar (Sections 16.13.2 and 16.13.4). It represents an end-stage pattern of colitis.

Acute terminal ileitis Acute ileiti is a term used to describe patients with a brief acute illness and inflammation restricted to a short length of terminal ileum. About 11 per cent of cases of Crohn's disease present in this manner. Conversely, some 15 per cent of cases of terminal ileitis will eventually develop classical Crohn's disease. A large majority of these cases (60–80 per cent) are due to yersiniosis (Section 16.10.2).

Diagnosis of Crohn's disease by biopsy

Because Crohn's disease is a patchy disease and one that involves the full thickness of the wall of the bowel, superficial mucosal biopsies may be inadequate for diagnosis. The sampling error is overcome by multiple biopsies but, even so, many of the features are deep to the biopsy forceps. Furthermore, the commonest site of involvement is the distal ileum, which is a difficult region to biopsy. In the differential diagnosis of inflammatory bowel disease, finding a granuloma helps to eliminate the diagnosis of ulcerative colitis, but tuberculosis and schisto-

somiasis still require consideration. Care must also be taken when interpreting collections of histiocytes and even a giant cell when seen as a response to a damaged crypt. The clinical history and colonoscopic findings play a major role in decision-making and must always be considered alongside the biopsy data. In the correct clinical setting, a biopsy series showing predominantly right-sided disease, rectal sparing, patchy inflammation (both between sites and within a single biopsy sample), a regular crypt pattern, and only limited goblet cell depletion favours a diagnosis of Crohn's disease (Fig. 16.197). The transmural inflammation of Crohn's disease is often reflected in a biopsy by the presence of disproportionate inflammation. Here the submucosa appears as inflamed as, or more inflamed than, the overlying mucosa (Fig. 16.198).

Complications of Crohn's disease

These divide conveniently into those that are systemic reactions to the disease and those that are complications of the abdominal disorder.

Arthritis is a common manifestation, seen both as a 'colitic arthritis', which is a migratory asymmetrical arthritis, and as ankylosing spondylitis or sacro-ileitis. Colectomy does not necessarily cure the arthritis.

Skin lesions in Crohn's disease have already been mentioned. Uveitis and episcleritis can be found in up to 13 per cent of patients. Granulomas occur in the liver but serious liver disease is not a feature as it can be in ulcerative colitis. Amyloidosis, on the other hand, is a rare complication of Crohn's disease but not of ulcerative colitis.

Extensive Crohn's disease of the small intestine may lead to malabsorption, especially of vitamin B_{12} and bile salts. Malabsorption can also be a consequence of internal fistulae.

The following are focal rather than systemic complications. Subacute intestinal obstruction is a relatively common complication but acute obstruction is rare. Perforation of the gut

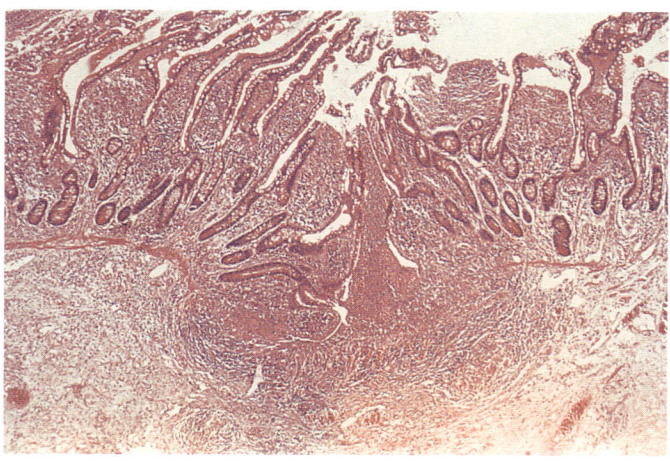

Fig. 16.196 Ulceration over a lymphoid follicle in Crohn's disease. This is the microscopy of an aphthoid ulcer (Fig. 16.163) and probably the earliest lesion in the development of the disease.

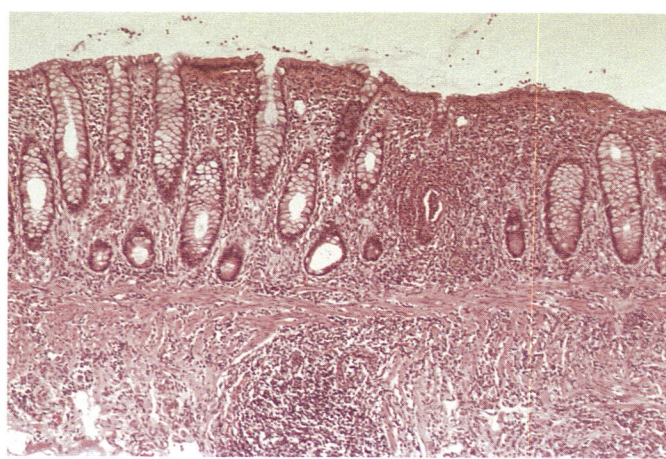

Fig. 16.197 The colonic mucosa in Crohn's disease, showing focal inflammation with an intact crypt pattern and good preservation of goblet cells.

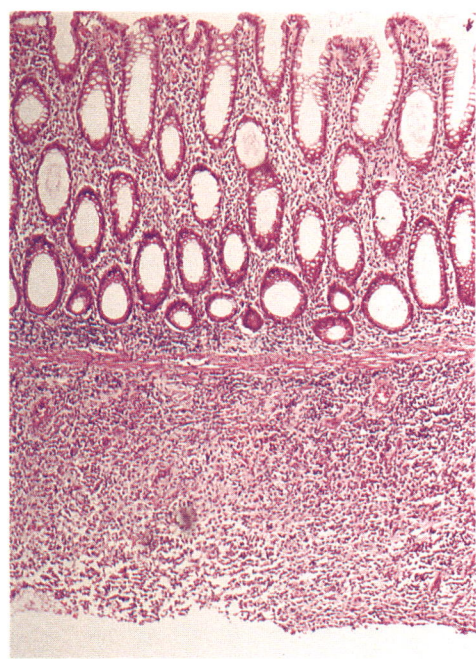

Fig. 16.198 In this biopsy disproportionate inflammation is well seen. The inflammation in the submucosa is greater than that present in the mucosa.

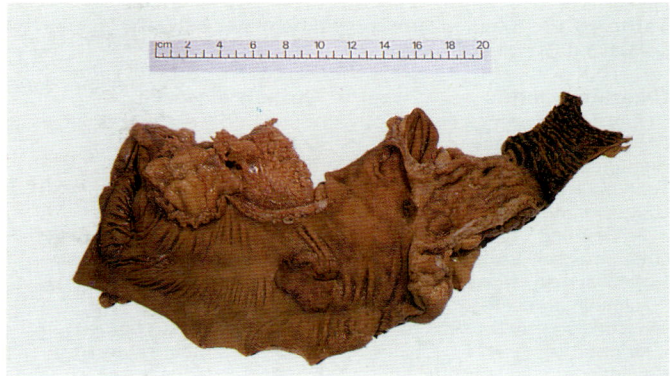

Fig. 16.199 A right hemicolectomy specimen in Crohn's disease, illustrating disease of the terminal ileum and a carcinoma in the right colon.

occurs in about 2 per cent of cases. Insidious penetration is more frequent and related to fissuring ulceration. This gives rise to peri-intestinal abscesses which can secondarily involve the bones of the pelvis to produce osteomyelitis. Loops of bowel may become adherent to each other, with subsequent fistulae involving a wide range of differing sites; for example, colo-vesical fistulae and fistulae onto the abdominal wall.

Cancer in Crohn's disease

There is a small but definite increase in the incidence of cancer throughout the gastrointestinal tract associated with Crohn's disease (Fig. 16.199). In the small bowel, cancer in Crohn's disease differs from that in the general population by occurring more distally and in a younger age-group. The history of Crohn's disease is usually a long one. In the colon the tumours are again in a younger age-group than colonic cancer in general, occur more proximally, and are more frequently multiple. The cancers in Crohn's disease tend to be at sites of macroscopic disease but may arise in bypassed segments.

The clinical recognition of intestinal cancer complicating Crohn's disease is difficult, and up to 60 per cent of such cancers are only recognized at the time of pathological examination of the resected bowel. If the data is restricted to small bowel cancers, then 44 per cent of these will be diagnosed for the first time by the histopathologist at the time of resection.

Dysplasia, so much a feature of cancer surveillance in ulcerative colitis, is extremely rare in cancer in Crohn's disease and there is no role for a similar cancer surveillance programme.

Prognosis

Although Crohn's disease may go into spontaneous remission in a small proportion of patients, the remission is seldom prolonged. Acturial analysis reveals that 20 years after the onset of symptoms 97 per cent of those at risk have had signs of recurrence. There are often long, disease-free intervals prior to recurrence which are commonly sited proximal to any anastomosis. Recurrence rates at 10 years range from 20 to 84 per cent for surgically treated ileo-colic Crohn's disease and 31–75 per cent for colonic disease.

There are no reliable histological features by which prognosis can be assessed, although many attempts to establish some have been made. The presence or absence of granulomas, for example, has no unequivocal prognostic significance, their role being disputed by several authors.

16.13.4 Colitis indeterminate

When all the distinguishing features between ulcerative colitis and Crohn's disease have been considered (Tables 16.13; 16.14), there will still be doubt about the diagnosis in approximately 10–15 per cent of resected cases, despite examination of the surgical specimen. These cases are generally those with extensive and severe mucosal ulceration in which surgery has been necessary because of incipient or actual colonic dilatation. In such cases there is invariably transmural inflammation, a regular pattern of fissuring or clefts from the ulcerated surface deep into muscle, and focal surviving mucosal islands. In the latter the inflammation may seem mild in comparison with the severity of adjacent disease and the goblet cell population is frequently well maintained. Although several of the above features are attributes suggesting Crohn's disease, in fulminant attacks of colitis they become unreliable and are present in ulcerative colitis and fulminant colitis of other causes (Figs 16.174, 16.175).

Thus the term 'colitis indeterminate' does not signify a specific entity, merely an admission that further pathological

Table 16.13 Main macroscopic differences between ulcerative colitis and Crohn's disease

Ulcerative colitis	Crohn's disease
Disease in continuity	Disease discontinuous
Rectum almost always involved	Rectum normal in 50%
Terminal ileum involved in 10%	Terminal ileum involved in 30%
Granullar and ulcerated mucosa; no fissuring	Discretely ulcerated; cobblestoning and fissures
Often intensely vascular	Vascularity less pronounced
Normal serosa (except in fulminating colitis)	Serositis common
Muscular shortening; fibrous stricture rare	Shortening due to fibrosis; fibrous stricture common
Never spontaneous fistula	Enterocutaneous fistula in 10%
Inflammatory polyposis common and extensive	Inflammatory polyposis less common
Malignant change and dysplasia well recognized	Malignant change rare
Anal lesions uncommon; acute fissures, excoriation	Anal lesions in 75%; fistulae and chronic fissures

Table 16.14 Main microscopic differences between ulcerative colitis and Crohn's disease

Ulcerative colitis	Crohn's disease
Mucosal and submucosal inflammation (except in fulminant colitis)	Transmural inflammation
Width of submucosa normal or reduced	Width of submucosa normal or increased
Intensely vascular; little oedema	Vascularity seldom marked; oedema marked
Focal lymphoid hyperplasia limited to mucosa	Focal lymphoid aggregates throughout wall
Crypt abscesses common	Crypt abscesses fewer
Mucus secretion reduced	Mucus secretion only slightly reduced
Paneth cell metaplasia common	Paneth cell metaplasia rare
No granulomas	Granulomas in 60–70%
Fissuring absent	Fissuring common
Dysplasia occurs	Dysplasia very rare
Anal lesions non-specific	Anal lesions often with granulomas

classification is not possible in this very acute stage of the disease process. Indeed, this fulminant pattern of colitis may occur during the course of most causes of inflammatory bowel disease. Often the clinical history or subsequent outcome of the case will permit a more confident diagnosis to be made. For example, biopsy of the rectal stump some time after a colectomy carried out for an attack of fulminant colitis may show the typical features of ulcerative colitis.

16.13.5 Miscellaneous inflammatory conditions predominantly involving the upper gastrointestinal tract

Eosinophilic infiltration of the gastrointestinal tract

Eosinophilic infiltration of the bowel occurs as a manifestation of many conditions which have an allergic basis and are accompanied by a defined clinical pattern. However, it can also accompany parasitic infestation and be part of a general tissue reaction in a range of conditions, such as ulcerative colitis, Crohn's disease, collagen diseases, and even lymphoma. It may also accompany certain systemic diseases, such as the vasculitides and Leoffler's syndrome.

The specific terms 'eosinophilic gastritis' and 'enterocolitis' are usually restricted to a recognizable clinical group in adults, whereas 'allergic gastroenterocolitis' is a pattern of disease often restricted to children. Inflammatory fibroid polyps were once thought to be a localized variant of eosinophilic infiltration but this is unlikely to be the case.

Eosinophilic gastroenteritis and colitis

This condition usually presents as recurrent bouts of pyloric or small bowel obstruction. It is commonest in patients between 30 and 60 years of age; 70 per cent will have a personal or family history of allergy and 90 per cent will have a blood eosinophilia.

Pathology

The bowel wall is thickened and oedematous, the mucosa is friable though seldom ulcerated. Short lengths of small bowel are the commonest sites to be involved, followed by the stomach and colon.

Histological examination shows that disease predominates in the submucosa with variable involvement of the mucosa and muscle coat (Fig. 16.200). The submucosa is oedematous and infiltrated by large numbers of eosinophils. A localized form of disease may exist in the rectum, termed allergic proctitis, in which the mucosa contains increased numbers of IgE-containing plasma cells. The presence of a vasculitis is not usually included in the strict definition of eosinophilic enteritis, such a change putting the features in the category of polyarteritis nodosa or other vasculitic entities.

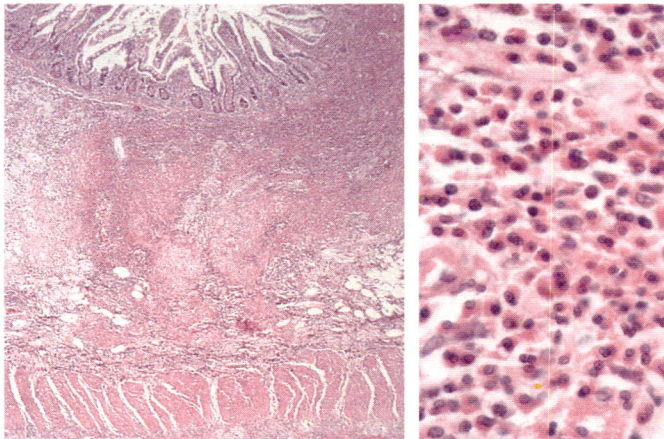

Fig. 16.200 Eosinophilic enteritis, showing the predominantly submucosal inflammatory infiltrate on the left which, in detail on the right, is almost entirely made up of eosinophils.

Aetiology

The aetiology of the condition is unknown. Unlike the infantile pattern (see below), a specific allergen has not been identified, although some cases are claimed to be due to ingestion of parasites, such as the worm *Eustoma rotundatum* caught from eating raw herrings. It is important to make the correct diagnosis for cases respond to sodium cromoglycate and steroids. They should not be incorrectly labelled ulcerative colitis or Crohn's disease.

Infantile allergic (eosinophilic) gastroenterocolitis

In children, in contrast to adults, it is common to identify dietary antigens. Cow's milk protein followed by soya and wheat protein are the commonest. Children present with a variety of clinical features: rectal bleeding and diarrhoea being frequent when there is a colonic disease; protein-losing enteropathy or a failure to thrive being associated with upper gastrointestinal tract involvement. Food-allergy colitis may well be the commonest cause of colitis in the first year of life.

The pathology is similar to that described in the adult, with widespread infiltration of the affected segment by eosinophils. In upper gastrointestinal involvement the antrum is more commonly affected than the jejunum.

Inflammatory fibroid polyp

The lesions have been described as eosinophilic granulomatous polyps. Although the aetiology is unknown, it is unlikely that they represent a localized pattern of eosinophilic gastroenteritis as originally believed. The polyps are usually single and found in all age-groups, but most commonly in adults. Obstruction or intussusception are common presentations, usually involving the small bowel and/or stomach.

Pathology

The polyps are sessile, ranging from 2 to 5 cm in diameter (Fig. 16.201). They originate in the submucosa and comprise

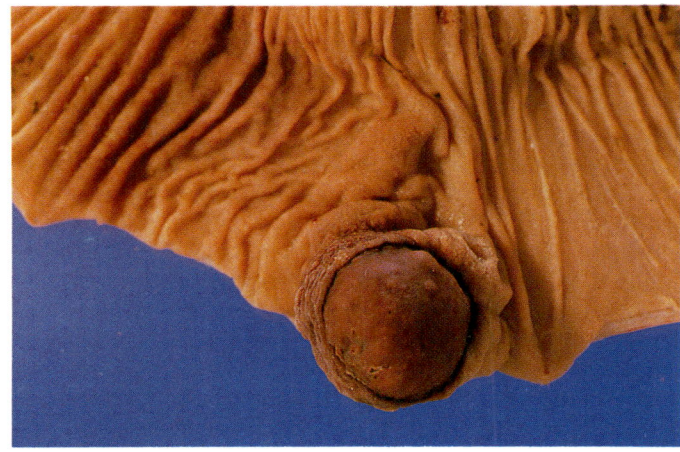

Fig. 16.201 A length of ileum showing an inflammatory fibroid polyp.

fascicles and whorls of loose fibroblastic connective tissue, throughout which is sprinkled an infiltrate of eosinophils and plasma cells (Fig. 16.202). The overlying mucosa is frequently ulcerated.

Solitary ulcers of the small intestine and drug-induced ulcers (potassium and non-steroidal, anti-inflammatory agents)

Isolated small intestinal ulceration is rare, but when it does occur it is both difficult to diagnose and to ascribe an aetiology. There is a long list of causes, broadly divided into congenital, vascular, inflammatory, neoplastic, and miscellaneous. Clinical presentation will depend on the precise cause, but in general the ulcers can occur at all ages and all sites. They are most common in the ileum. Patients present with haemorrhage and obstruction due to a stricture of perforation. Malabsorption as a presentation of small bowel ulceration is associated with the entity of chronic ulcerative jejuno-ileitis. More commonly, this clinical

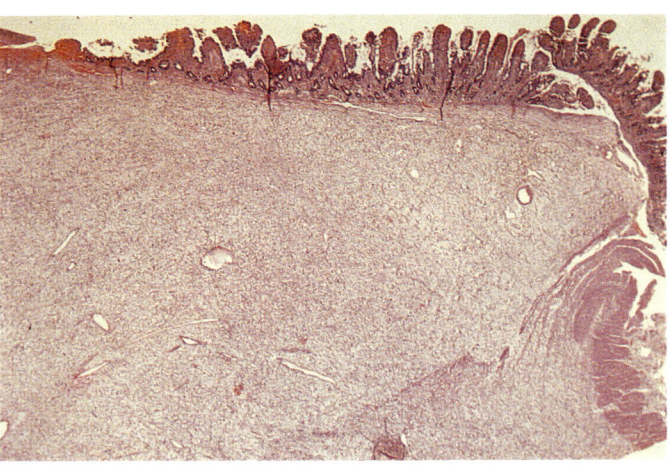

(a)

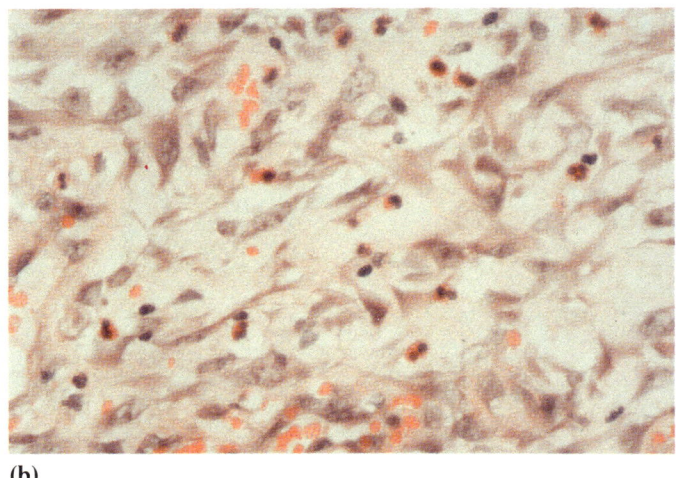

(b)

Fig. 16.202 (a) The microscopy of an inflammatory fibroid polyp, illustrating that the proliferating cells are in the submucosa with overlying mucosal ulceration. (b) At a greater magnification the mass of the polyp can be seen to comprise proliferating 'fibroblasts' and eosinophils.

presentation masks refractory coeliac disease or malignant lymphoma (Sections 16.8.2, 16.8.4).

Drug-induced ulceration has received particular attention, especially that due to potassium salts and non-steroidal anti-inflammatory preparations, both of which have widespread clinical use. Those ulcers associated with potassium ingestion are mostly single and have punched-out edges resembling a peptic ulcer (Fig. 16.203). The stricturing at the site usually produces an hour-glass deformity. Microscopy reveals changes confined to the mucosa and submucosa. There is ulceration with damage to adjacent villi. The mucosa is inflamed and the muscularis mucosae is frequently hypertrophic. A characteristic zone of submucosal fibrosis is present, restricted to the region of the ulcer (Fig. 16.204). Thrombi can sometimes be seen in nearby vessels. The muscle coat and serosa are not affected.

The aetiology of potassium-induced ulceration is believed to be ischaemic. High concentrations of potassium chloride can be liberated locally when a tablet impacts on the mucosa. This has a vasoconstrictive effect on local vessels. Slow-release potassium chloride tablets have reduced the incidence of this complication.

Non-steroidal, anti-inflammatory drugs, which are taken by large sections of the elderly population, also cause ulceration and perforation. The pathogenesis is likely to be via inhibition of pathways of prostaglandin metabolism and subsequent effects on mucosal cytoprotection. Occasionally this group of drugs has been associated with obstruction in which, rather than stenosing ulceration, the ileal lumen has become divided into a series

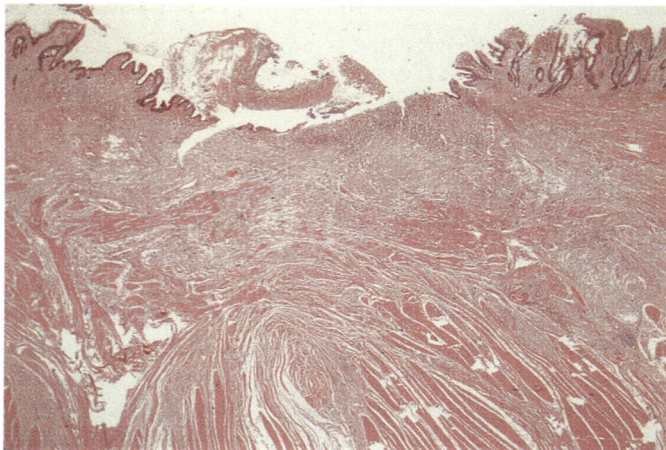

Fig. 16.204 The histology of a potassium-induced ulcer, showing the prominent submucosal fibrosis beneath the area of mucosal ulceration.

of short compartments by circular membranes of mucosa and submucosa, or by broader ridges. Often only a small pin-hole lumen will remain (Fig. 16.205). This pattern has been called 'diaphragm disease' because of the resemblance of the strictures to diaphragms placed across the bowel. On microscopy the 'diaphragms' resemble rigid *plicae circulares*, with a discrete zone of submucosal fibrosis at the apex of the fold. Overlying this is superficial mucosal ulceration. Similar pathology is seen in the less-dramatic ridges that can divide up the ileal lumen (Fig. 16.206a,b).

Gold therapy for rheumatoid arthritis is occasionally associated with either an enteritis or colitis. The picture is one of non-specific inflammation of the mucosa with none of the characteristic features of ulcerative colitis or Crohn's disease.

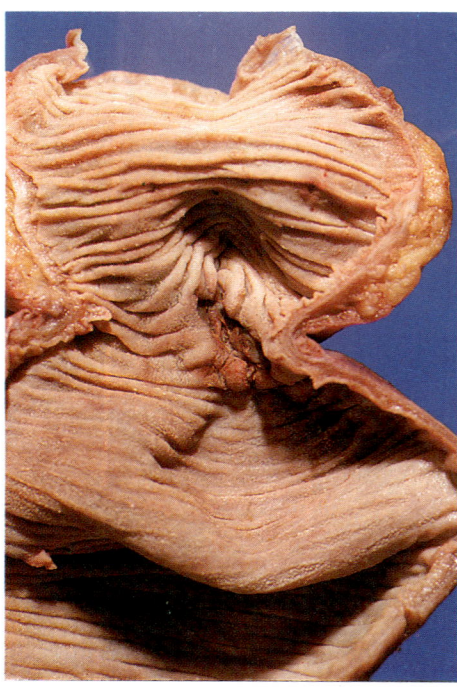

Fig. 16.203 A potassium-induced ileal ulcer, illustrating its punched-out appearance and the hour-glass deformity produced.

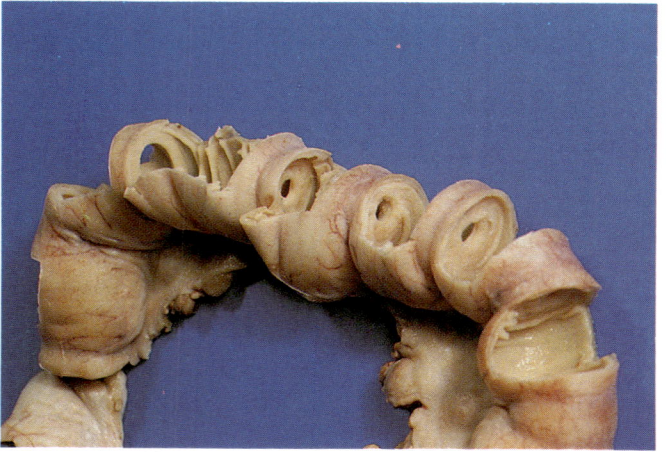

Fig. 16.205 Multiple 'diaphragms' in a length of resected ileum from a patient on long-term, non-steroidal, anti-inflammatory drugs.

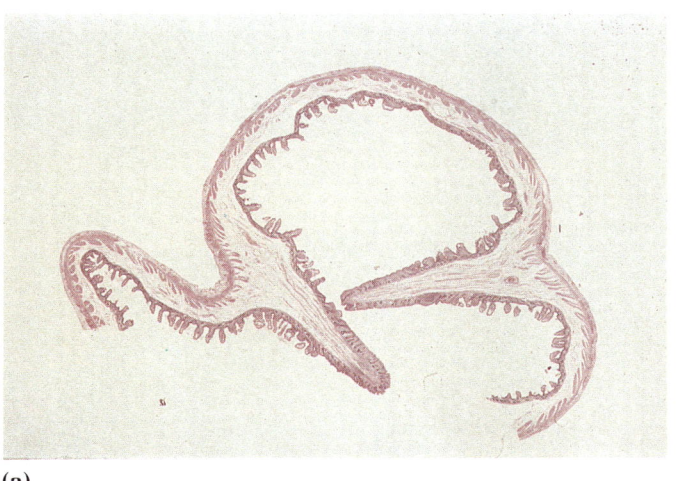

(a)

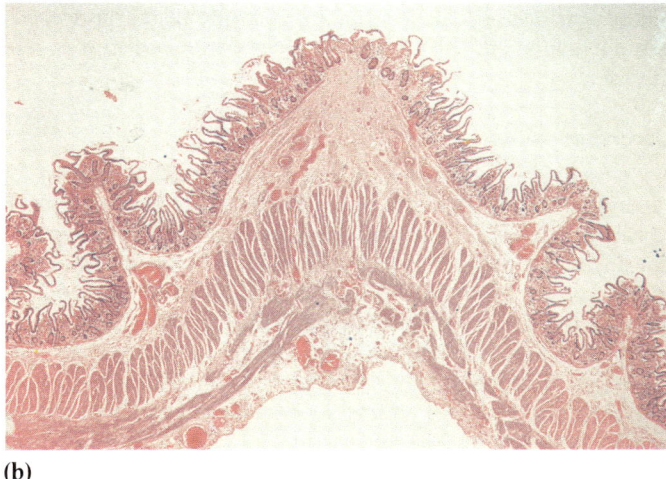

(b)

Fig. 16.206 (a) A cross-section through one of the 'diaphragms' showing their resemblance to *'plicae circulares'* with a small focus of fibrosis at the apex of each fold. (b) A focal area of submucosal fibrosis is seen in this illustration taken from an annular ridge across the ileum from a patient also on non-steroidal, anti-inflammatory drugs.

16.13.6 Miscellaneous inflammatory conditions predominantly involving the large intestine and rectum

Collagenous colitis

This condition is of unknown aetiology but is characterized by a prolonged history of intermittent diarrhoea over many years and an abnormal collagen band found beneath the surface epithelium of the colonic and rectal mucosa. The diagnosis relies on the identification of the band, for other investigations are usually unhelpful. The majority of the patients are women and, despite the long history of diarrhoea, no serious complications are known to occur.

Pathology

The abnormal collagen band can vary in thickness from just about the upper limits of normal, at 7–10 μm, to up to 70 μm. It is rarely continuous throughout the large bowel and several biopsies from the rectum and around the colon may be necessary to confirm the diagnosis. There is usually a non-specific inflammatory cell infiltrate in the mucosa that accompanies the abnormal collagen band (Fig. 16.207). A characteristic feature may be a large number of lymphocytes infiltrating the cryptal epithelium.

Like the aetiology, the pathogenesis of the diarrhoea is unknown, but the collagen plate may interfere with water absorption. Collagen is believed to be produced by the pericryptal fibroblasts and the basic disturbance is likely to be in these cells. Somewhat puzzling is the observation that a thick band of collagen can occasionally be seen during the course of other unrelated large intestinal diseases, e.g. carcinoma, diverticulitis. This has led to doubt whether collagenous colitis is a true entity rather than an epiphenomenon of several unrelated conditions.

Microscopic colitis

This term refers to a pattern of mild total colitis in which the history is very similar to that of collagenous colitis. Thus it is found in a predominantly female population who suffer chronic diarrhoea over a prolonged time-span but with no other complication. Minor inflammatory changes are seen in the mucosa, in the form of focal collections of lymphocytes, plasma cells, and crypt abscesses. Intra-epithelial lymphocytes are often a striking feature, and the term 'lymphocytic colitis' has been put forward as an alternative name.

In the small number of cases described, decreased colonic absorption of water and altered sodium, chloride, and bicarbonate exchange have been demonstrated. Some individuals eventually show evidence of an abnormal subepithelial collagen

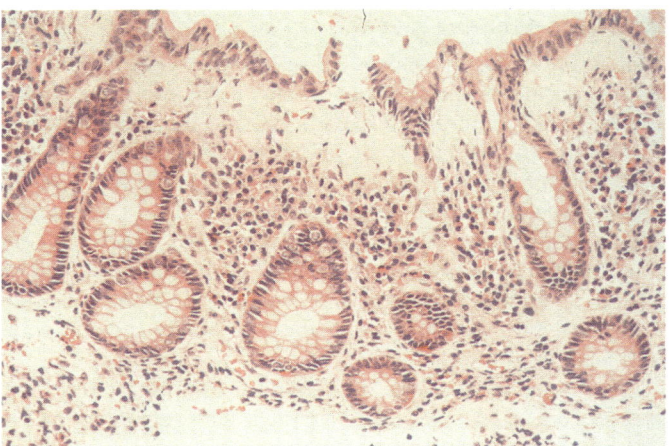

Fig. 16.207 A typical picture of collagenous colitis, illustrating the characteristic broad band of collagen beneath the surface epithelium.

band, and it seems likely that microscopic colitis and colla-genous colitis will turn out to be part of the spectrum of one disease.

Diversion colitis

As a temporary measure during the surgical treatment of inflammatory or neoplastic bowel diseases it is often necessary to carry out a defunctioning colostomy. A low-grade colitis can develop in the defunctioned segment. It is obviously important in the context of Crohn's disease and ulcerative colitis not to mistake this for an exacerbation of either of these two condi-tions. The mucosal inflammation resolves when bowel con-tinuity is restored. The aetiology of the inflammation is unknown, no bacterial pathogens have been identified, but an altered bowel flora, loss of essential nutrients, or prolonged mucosal contact with luminal toxins are possible mechanisms.

Necrotizing colitis

This term is used imprecisely to describe a severe but patchy gangrenous disease of the colon. Some cases are due to *Clost-ridium welchii* infection and in such instances the condition is clearly related to necrotizing small intestinal diseases such as Pig-bel (Section 16.10.2). However, it is difficult to distinguish primary clostridial infections from secondary involvement sub-sequent to ischaemic damage. This is made more difficult as some clostridial toxins are known to be vasoconstrictive.

There is a variable length of large bowel which is discoloured black or purple. The mucosa is either frankly gangrenous and covered by yellow-green slough or, in milder cases, can look congested and oedematous. On microscopy there are varying degrees of mucosal necrosis and haemorrhage. The muscle coat frequently shows signs of degeneration or myocytolysis. Clostridial organisms may be seen on Gram-staining, but as mentioned, their primary role evaluated against ischaemia is difficult to assess. This is made more difficult as most patients will be elderly, post-operative, and will have a chronic debilitating medical disease.

Neonatal necrotizing colitis

Neonatal necrotizing colitis is a disease of premature infants. It usually occurs in the first two weeks of life and after enteric feeding has commenced. Radiological demonstration of pneumatosis intestinalis is the hallmark of diagnosis.

Although the whole gut can be involved, the terminal ileum and the ascending colon are the commonest sites. The bowel is thickened due to the presence of gas-filled cysts which predom-inate in the submucosa (Figs 16.208, 16.209). There can be extensive mucosal necrosis and even perforation, although milder disease can exist, when there is simply inflammation with focal ulceration.

The precise aetiology is unknown. A role for bacteria has been the one most extensively pursued, with several species of *Clostridia* implicated, such as *Clostridium butyricum*, *Cl. difficile*, and *Cl. perfringens*. Overall, the condition resembles other similar forms of necrotizing intestinal disease, such as Pig-bel,

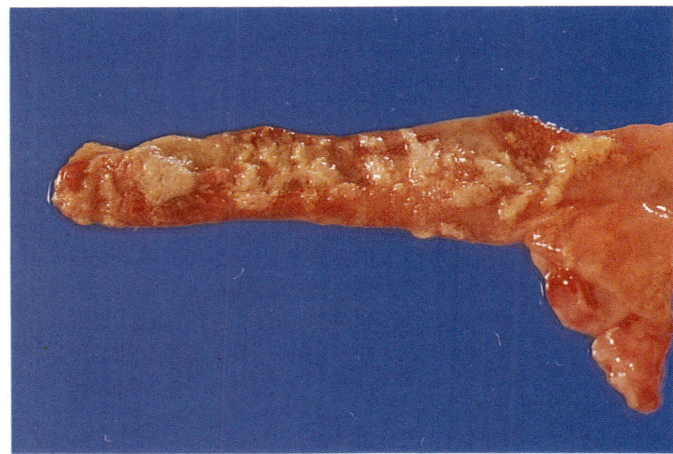

Fig. 16.208   Neonatal necrotizing enterocolitis in a premature infant, showing raised yellow areas corresponding to the submucosal cysts seen on microscopy.

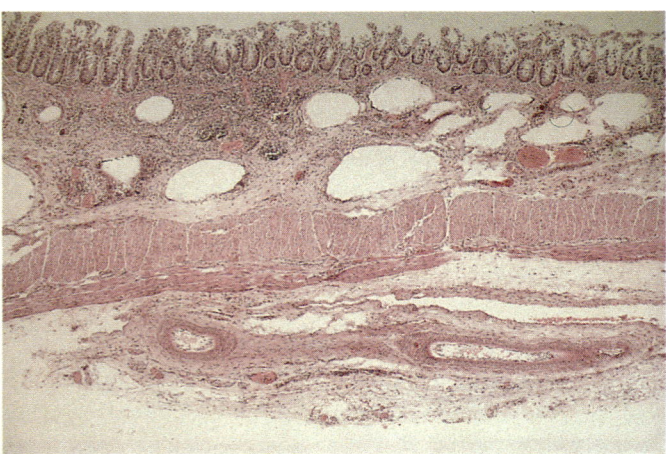

Fig. 16.209   In this illustration of a case of neonatal necrotizing enteritis the submucosal gas cysts are easily seen. The overlying mucosa is intact at this site.

neutropenic enterocolitis (see below), and pseudomembranous colitis (Section 16.12.2).

Neutropenic colitis

This is another segmental necrotizing disease, mostly affecting the right colon and terminal ileum, which is believed to be as-sociated with clostridial infection, namely *Cl. septicum*. It occurs in patients with neutropenia from a wide variety of causes, but mostly in those with leukaemia or receiving cytotoxic therapy. Clinically, the condition can mimic acute appendicitis.

The affected bowel is ulcerated with mucosal necrosis, haemorrhage, and considerable submucosal oedema. As with the other forms of necrotizing colitis described above, it can be difficult to separate the condition from primary ischaemic damage. Appreciation of the existence of neutropenic colitis is important, for in the correct clinical circumstances early administration of specific antibacterial therapy prevents a fatal outcome.

Cl. septicum is an inhabitant of the normal appendix, though not the colon. Mucosal damage, the result of leukaemic infiltration or haemorrhage in those with thrombocytopenia, may allow the organisms to breach the mucosa and initiate damage.

Phlegmonous enterocolitis

This rare pattern of inflammatory bowel disease is characterized by marked expansion of the submucosa. It is oedematous and infiltrated by large numbers of neutrophil polymorphs (Fig. 16.210). Gram-staining often reveals organisms, either Gram-positive cocci or rods. Group B β-haemolytic streptococci, *Escherichia coli*, and pneumococci have been grown from blood cultures in individual cases. The mucosa overlying the submucosa is usually intact, or shows just a small focus of ulceration. The disease seems to be a spreading cellulitis of the submucosa.

Variable lengths of colon or small intestine can be involved but the stomach is also affected. Although several bacteria have been implicated in this condition, what precipitates this unusual distribution of inflammatory change is not clear.

Mucosal prolapse syndrome (the solitary rectal ulcer)

The mucosal prolapse syndrome is a useful term that encompasses a recognizable spectrum of morphological change seen in the sigmoid colon and rectum and associated with several clinical conditions. The unifying event is mucosal prolapse of varying degree. The pathogenesis of the changes relates to recurrent ischaemic and mechanical damage caused by this prolapsing mucosa. At the severe end of the spectrum is complete rectal prolapse, the mucosa appearing through the anal sphincter. This is a condition of the very young or the very old. In a minor form, at the other end of the spectrum, the pathology is present in small areas of redundant mucosa around the opening of diverticula in sigmoid diverticular disease. However, in routine clinical practice the commonest presentation is the condition known as the solitary rectal ulcer.

Patients with the solitary rectal ulcer are usually young adults. They complain of pain, rectal bleeding, and the passage of mucus. A history of constipation with straining on defecation is common. The finding on rectal examination is an ulcer of diameter 0.5–5 cm, situated on the anterior rectal wall. It is flat, clearly delineated, and may be covered by white slough. However, ulceration is not invariable and the mucosa may simply appear reddened, friable, and even polypoid. When biopsied the mucosa is usually slightly villiform. The crypts are hyperplastic and there is goblet cell depletion. Superficial erosions are common on the surface. The lamina propria is partially obliterated by fibrosis and arborizing muscle fibres derived from the muscularis mucosae. Telangiectasia of the mucosal capillaries is common. On the deep aspect of the mucosa the base of the crypts may be caught up in the arborizing muscularis and even be seen extending into the submucosa (Figs 16.211, 16.212). This is known as focal colitis cystica profunda. Being hyperplastic, the unwary may misinterpret this appearance as invasive carcinoma.

Treatment is unsatisfactory and involves defecation measures to soften the stools and prevent straining on defecation. Genuine prolapse due to muscle problems of the perineal floor require surgical intervention.

There are several other situations in which mucosal prolapse is believed to be the basic defect. The pathological picture may be seen at the margins of a colostomy, at the apex of prolapsing

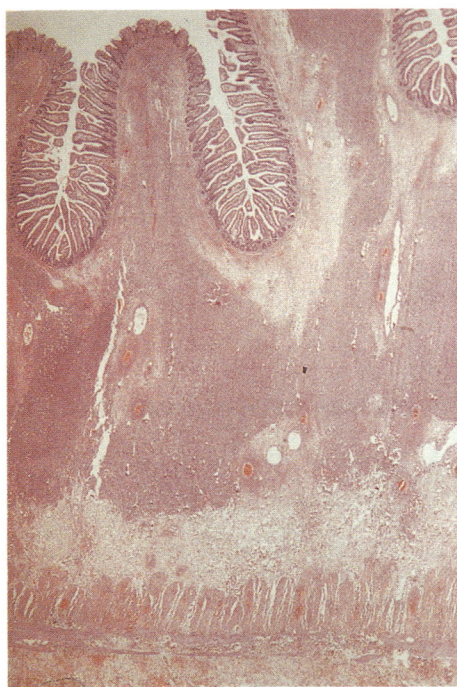

Fig. 16.210 Phlegmonous enteritis, showing marked expansion of the submucosa which is infiltrated by neutrophil polymorphs with an intact mucosa above.

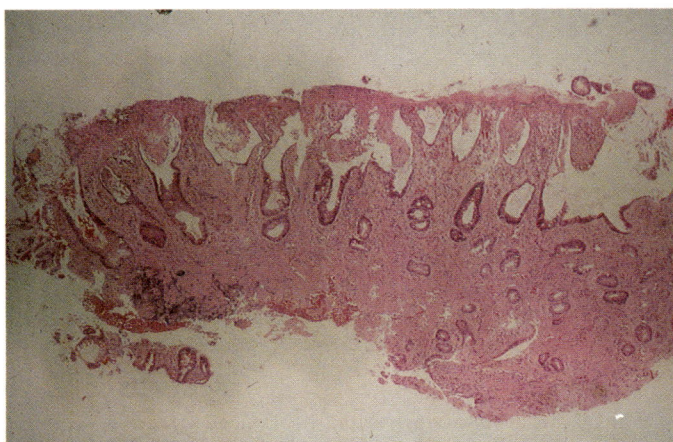

Fig. 16.211 A rectal biopsy from the mucosal prolapse syndrome showing prominent villiform mucosa with superficial ulceration of the villiform projections and fibrosis of the lamina propria.

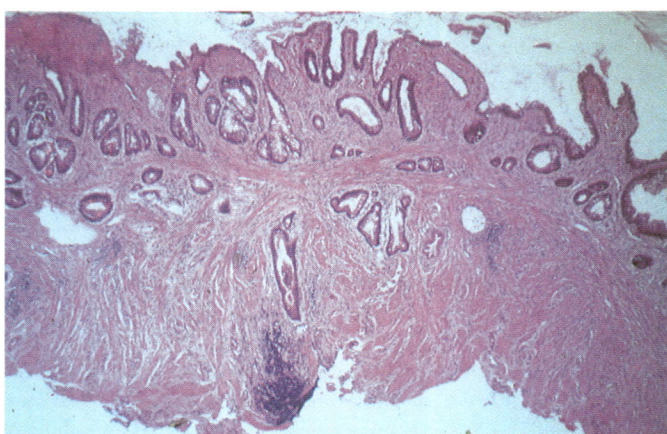

Fig. 16.212 In this example from a patient with a solitary rectal ulcer the fibrous obliteration of the lamina propria is well seen, along with telangiectasia. The crypts are irregular and hyperchromatic. In addition, the base of the crypts are seen caught up in the arborizing muscularis, giving an appearance that can be mistaken for carcinoma.

haemorrhoids, close to any polypoid lesions of the colon and, as mentioned earlier, in segments of diverticular disease at the margins of the diverticula.

The term 'inflammatory cloacogenic polyp' has been used to describe the mucosal prolapse syndrome presenting as a polyp at the anal margin, and the same pathology is probably the basis of the 'cap' polyps occasionally found in an otherwise normal sigmoid colon and, rarely, in association with ulcerative colitis.

The recognition of the pathological features of the mucosal prolapse syndrome is important to prevent patients being misclassified as having ulcerative colitis or Crohn's disease.

16.13.7   Further reading

Chambers, T. J. and Morson, B. C. (1979). The granuloma in Crohn's disease. *Gut* **20**, 269–74.

Crohn, B. B., Ginzburg, L., and Oppenheimer, G. D. (1932). Regional ileitis: a pathologic and clinical entity. *Journal of the American Medical Association* **99**, 1323–9.

Dalziel, T. K. (1913). Chronic interstitial enteritis. *British Medical Journal* **2**, 1068–70.

DuBoulay, C. E. H., Fairbrother, J., and Isaacson, P. G. (1983). Mucosal prolapse syndrome. A unifying concept for solitary ulcer syndrome and related disorders. *Journal of Clinical Pathology* **36**, 1264–8.

Farmer, R. G. (1987). Nonspecific ulcerative proctitis. *Gastroenterology Clinics of North America* **16**, 157–174.

Gilmour, H. M. (1989). Crohn's disease. In *Gastrointestinal and oesophageal pathology* (ed. R. Whitehead). Churchill Livingstone, London.

Hanauer, S. B. and Kraft, S. C. (1983). Immunology of Crohn's disease. In *Inflammatory bowel disease* (ed. R. N. Allen, M. R. B. Keighley, J. Alexander-Williams, and C. Hawkins), pp. 356–71. Churchill Livingstone, London.

Jessurum, J., Yardley, J. H., Giardello, F. M., Hamilton, S. R., and Bayless, T. M. (1987). Chronic colitis with thickening of the subepi-thelial collagen layer (collagenous colitis). *Human Pathology* **18**, 839–48.

Jewell, D. P. and Rhodes, J. M. (1983). Immunology of ulcerative colitis. In *Inflammatory bowel disease* (ed. R. N. Allen, M. R. B. Keighley, J. Alexander-Williams, and C. Hawkins), pp. 154–70. Churchill Livingstone, London.

Johnston, J. M. and Morson, B. C. (1978). Eosinophilic gastroenteritis. *Histopathology* **2**, 335–48.

King, A., Rampling, A., Wight, D. G. D., and Warren, R. E. (1984). Neutropaenic enterocolitis due to *Clostridium septicum* infection. *Journal of Clinical Pathology* **37**, 335–43.

Kirsner, J. B. and Shorter, R. G. (1982). Recent developments in non-specific inflammatory bowel disease. *New England Journal of Medicine* **306**, 837–48.

Lazenby, A. J., Yardley, J. H. Giardello, F. M., Jessurun, J., and Bayless, T. M. (1989). Lymphocytic (microscopic) colitis. *Human pathology* **20**, 18–28.

Lobert, P. F. and Appleman, H. D. (1981). Inflammatory cloacogenic polyp. A unique inflammatory lesion of the anal transitional zone. *American Journal of Surgical Pathology* **5**, 761–6.

Mayberry, J. F. (1985). Some aspects of the epidemiology of ulcerative colitis. *Gut* **26**, 968–72.

Mayberry, J. F. and Rhodes, J. (1984). Epidemiological aspects of Crohn's disease: a review of the literature. *Gut* **25**, 886–99.

Morson, B. C. and Pang, L. (1967). Rectal biopsy as an aid to cancer control in ulcerative colitis. *Gut* **8**, 423–34.

Morson, B. C., Dawson, I. M. P., Day, D. W., Jass, J. R., Price, A. B., and Williams, G. T. (1990). *Morson and Dawson's gastrointestinal pathology*. Blackwell Scientific Publications, Oxford.

Price, A. B. (1978). Overlap in the spectrum of non-specific inflammatory bowel disease—'colitis' indeterminate. *Journal of Clinical Pathology* **31**, 567–77.

Riddell, R. H., *et al.* (1983). Dysplasia in inflammatory bowel disease, standardised classification with provisional clinical applications. *Human Pathology* **4**, 931–68.

Rulter, K. R. P. and Riddell, R. H. (1975). The solitary ulcer syndrome of the rectum. *Clinical Gastroenterology* **4**, 505–30.

Talbot, I. C. and Price, A. B. (1987). *Biopsy pathology in colorectal disease*. Chapman and Hall, London.

Thomas, W. E. G. and Williamson, R. C. N. (1985). Non-specific small bowel ulceration. *Postgraduate Medical Journal* **61**, 587–91.

Tytgat, G. N. J. and van Deventer, S. J. H. (1988). Pouchitis—a review. *International Journal of Colorectal Disease* **3**, 226–8.

Whitehead, R. (1989). Ulcerative colitis. In *Gastrointestinal and oesophageal pathology* (ed. R. Whitehead), pp. 522–32. Churchill Livingstone, London.

16.14   Graft versus host disease

A. B. Price

16.14.1   Introduction

The gut, along with the skin and liver, is one of the main target organs for graft versus host disease (Chapter 4). For organ or bone marrow transplants to be successful patients are initially immunosuppressed by chemotherapeutic agents and irradiation. Damage to the gut can occur subsequently by one of three mechanisms. First, the pre-transplant conditioning itself is directly toxic; secondly, as a consequence of successful immunosuppression the gut is more susceptible to infection; and third, graft versus host disease can develop. In this condition donor lymphoid cells damage the host tissues. In clinical practice it is often difficult to be certain which of the above disease processes is present. Here the pathology of graft versus host disease is outlined only as it affects the gut, and a more detailed general account is given in Chapter 4.

16.14.2   Clinical features

Graft versus host disease can be divided into acute and chronic forms. Acute graft versus host disease commences 3–4 weeks after transplantation, whereas chronic graft versus host disease occurs between 80 and 400 days post-transplantation. Between 30 and 50 per cent of grafted patients develop some grade of acute graft versus host disease, and endoscopy will show changes in the terminal ileum and colon. Approximately 30 per cent of long-term survivors will develop chronic graft versus host disease which predominantly affects the oesophagus. Some 30 per cent develop chronic disease *de novo* but the majority have experienced an episode of acute graft versus host disease.

16.14.3   Pathology

Within the first 20 days of transplantation it is difficult to separate the toxic effects of pre-transplant conditioning from those of graft versus host disease. Chemoradiation therapy may produce diffuse mucosal abnormalities in small and large bowel. The stomach and oesophagus are more resistant. There are widespread abnormalities and atypicality of crypt cell nuclei, degeneration of crypt and surface epithelial cells in the colon, and villous architectural damage in the small intestine. These changes occur within 20 days of transplantation. Acute graft versus host disease rarely occurs before this time. Furthermore, whereas damage from chemoradiation tends to be a diffuse process, that due to graft versus host disease is more focal. In the colon the earliest visible event of graft versus host disease is focal crypt cell degeneration, also named an 'apoptotic body'. It is characterized by a single, or a small number of, necrotic crypt cells, often in a vacuole incorporating nuclear debris and a few inflammatory cells. There may be adjacent crypt abscesses and some epithelial nuclear atypicality. As the disease progresses whole crypt can be involved, degenerate, and be lost (Figs 16.213, 16.214). For the degree of crypt damage there is a very limited inflammatory cell infiltrate in the lamina propria, a point in contrast to the inflammation seen in inflammatory bowel disease. In severe cases the whole of the mucosal epithelium may be lost. Despite the cryptal damage, the argentophyl cells at the base of the crypts survive in small isolated nests. As well as the colon, the jejunum and ileum are commonly involved, but these are much harder sites to study outside autopsy series.

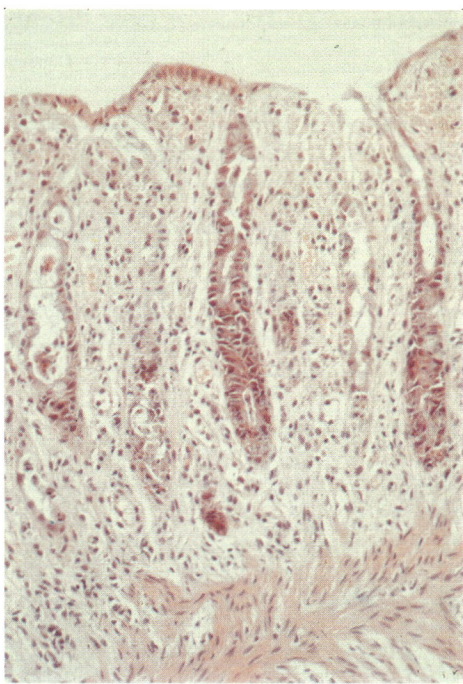

Fig. 16.213   This shows the degeneration and loss of whole crypts in graft versus host disease. There is very little inflammation present and a characteristic cluster of surviving argentaffin cells are seen centrally, just above the muscularis mucosae.

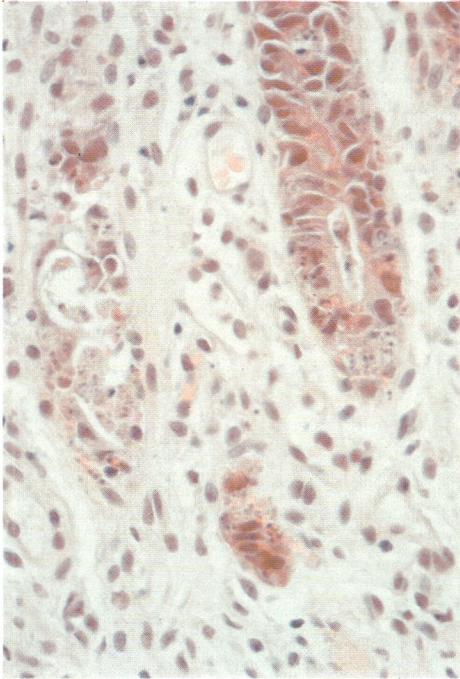

Fig. 16.214   In this illustration an apoptotic body is seen at the base of the crypt to the right. The crypt to the left is severely damaged by a similar process and persisting argentaffin cells are present in the central lower half of the field.

16.14.4   Chronic graft versus host disease

Upper gastrointestinal damage, in particular in the oesophagus, is common in chronic graft versus host disease, in contrast to the lower gastrointestinal involvement in the acute condition. The clinical presentation can include dysphagia, painful swallowing, retrosternal pain, aspiration, and insidious weight loss.

Pathology

The oesophageal lesions of chronic graft versus host disease may include desquamation of the squamous epithelium, oesophageal webs, ring-like narrowing, and strictures. Most of the changes involve the proximal rather than the distal oesophagus.

On microscopy the oesophageal mucosa is infiltrated by lymphocytes, neutrophils, and eosinophils in amongst the degenerate and desquamating squamous epithelium. Most characteristic, and accounting for the strictures, is the submucosa fibrosis. This does not involve the muscle or neuronal elements as occurs in scleroderma, the other condition in which there is extensive submucosa oesophageal fibrosis.

Infection in graft versus host disease

Because of immunosuppression and persistent immunological dysfunction, infection is common in chronic graft versus host disease. The infecting agents are of a similar spectrum to those seen in AIDS (Section 16.12.3). For example *Candida*, Cytomegalovirus and Herpes simplex virus are the common infections in the oesophagus. In the stomach, as well as these, fungi such as *Aspergillus* and *Histoplasma* can occasionally be found. Infections of the large and small intestine include Cytomegalovirus, *Clostridium difficile* (pseudomembranous colitis), *Cl. septicum* (a cause of neutropenic colitis), giardiasis, and cryptosporidia.

16.14.5   Pathogenesis

This is dealt with in greater detail in Chapter 4. Several hypotheses exist for the explanation of mucosal necrosis in graft versus host disease. It might be that allogeneic reactions against host lymphoid cells in the mucosa cause the release of toxic lymphokines; that an immunodeficiency state exists from a donor–host lymphoid cell interaction; but most likely that donor T-lymphocytes react with antigens on the surface of host crypt cells. The primary event appears to be direct T-lymphocyte-mediated crypt cellulitis, as removal of mature T-lymphocytes reduces the incidence of graft versus host disease.

16.14.6   Further reading

Epstein, R. J., McDonald, G. B., Sale, G. E., Shulman, H. M., and Thomas, E. D. (1980). The diagnostic accuracy of the rectal biopsy in acute graft-versus-host disease: a prospective study of thirteen patients. *Gastroenterology* **78**, 764–71.

McDonald, G. B., Shulman, H. M., Sullivan, K. M., and Spencer, G. D. (1986a). Intestinal and hepatic complications of human bone marrow transplantation. Part I. *Gastroenterology* **90**, 460–77.
McDonald, G. B., Shulman, H. M., Sullivan, K. M., and Spencer, G. D. (1986b). Intestinal and hepatic complications of human bone marrow transplantation. Part II. *Gastroenterology* **90**, 770–84.

16.15   Diverticular disease

N. A. Shepherd

16.15.1   Introduction

The term 'diverticular disease' includes both diverticulosis, the presence of numerous outpouchings of mucosa through the bowel wall, and diverticulitis, in which the diverticula are the source of inflammation. Although solitary and multiple diverticula occur elsewhere in the colon, and indeed in the small intestine, diverticular disease is most common in the sigmoid colon. In approximately 60 per cent of cases the sigmoid is the only site of the diverticula. Diverticular disease never occurs in the rectum. The disease is prevalent in the aged population of Western societies: it has been estimated that 66 per cent of the population over the age of 80 suffer from the disease. It is very rare in rural Africa and Asia.

16.15.2   Diverticular disease of the sigmoid colon

Pathogenesis

Epidemiological evidence shows that there is an inverse relationship between fibre content of the diet and the prevalence of diverticular disease. Thus, in rural Africa, where diverticular disease is most unusual, the diet is high in fibre. Burkitt has shown that the traditional African village diet contains about four times more fibre than the average British diet. The lack of a large residue within the lumen of the bowel leads to prolonged contraction of the circular layer of muscle and this in turn raises the intraluminal pressure. The effect of the raised intraluminal pressure is to force pockets of mucosa through the weaker areas in the colonic wall where the arteriovenous bundles traverse the muscularis propria.

The primary pathogenic mechanism in diverticular disease is not the formation of the mucosal outpouchings themselves but an abnormality of the muscularis propria. There are three main theories which have been put forward to explain the characteristic muscular thickening. It has been suggested that an increase in muscle bulk, either by hyperplasia or hypertrophy, may occur. Although this mechanism would certainly cause muscular thickening, there is no good evidence that this occurs. Certainly, individual muscle cells appear morphologically normal with no evidence of hypertrophy. Prolonged muscular spasm is the second theory but in basal conditions the intraluminal pressure of the sigmoid colon in patients with diverticular disease is normal and thus prolonged spasm is unlikely. A recent finding of elastosis in the longitudinal muscle, the *taeniae coli*, supports the third theory that the bowel wall is shortened in diverticular disease. The taeniae coli act as a scaffold upon which the circular muscle contracts. If the longitudinal muscle is shortened due to elastosis then the effect is to cause gross thickening of the circular muscle. This third theory of muscular shortening or contracture holds sway currently but, whatever the precise mechanism, there is little doubt that a low residue diet and a consequent muscular abnormality are the predeterminants for the development of diverticular disease.

Pathology

Macroscopically the consistent abnormality is a thickening of both the circular and longitudinal layers of the muscularis propria. This may be so marked that the muscle layers, especially the taeniae, become almost cartilaginous in appearance. The thickened interdigitating bands of the circular layer restrict the lumen and cause the characteristic concertina-like appearance (Fig. 16.215). There is a striking redundancy of the mucosa and this may further narrow the lumen of the colon. The diverticula penetrate the muscularis at the point where the blood vessels pass into the bowel wall, and are arranged in two longitudinal rows between the mesenteric taenia coli and the two antimesenteric taeniae. These outpouchings protude through the circular muscle into the pericolic tissues, although they are often lined by an attenuated layer of the longitudinal muscle. It should be emphasized that, although the diverticula do not represent the primary pathology, the complications of diverticular disease are usually associated with the presence of diverticula.

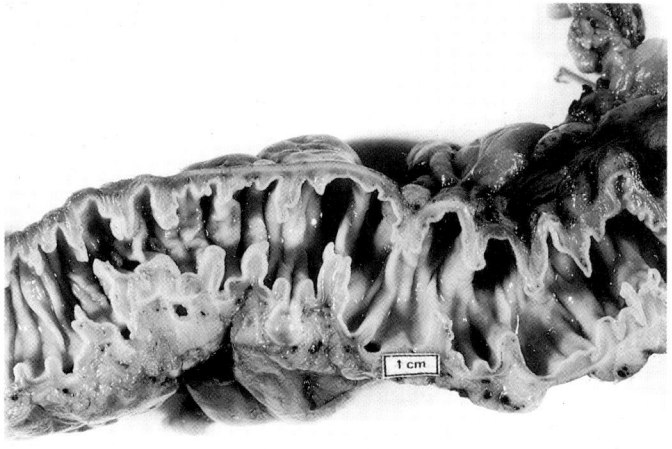

Fig. 16.215 Diverticular disease of the sigmoid colon. The bowel shows the typical concertina-like configuration, the muscularis is thickened, and there are several diverticula penetrating into the serosal tissues.

Complications

Diverticulitis and abscess

The great majority of patients with diverticular disease are symptomless, and the occurrence of acute inflammation in the diverticula is surprisingly rare. Only about 0.5 per cent of patients with diverticular disease require operative intervention because of diverticulitis. The inflammatory process is nearly always restricted to one diverticulum. The inflammation is the result of mucosal ulceration of the pouch secondary to erosion by inspissated faecal debris. The inflammatory focus may remain localized to the wall of the diverticulum or may enlarge to form a pericolic abscess (Fig. 16.216). The involvement of the peritoneal surface causes a localized peritonitis. Chronic diverticulitis leads to extensive fibrosis in the serosal tissues. The pericolic tissues then become hard and distorted: often the surgeon is unable to differentiate between complicated diverticular disease and carcinoma.

The histological features of diverticulitis are usually non-

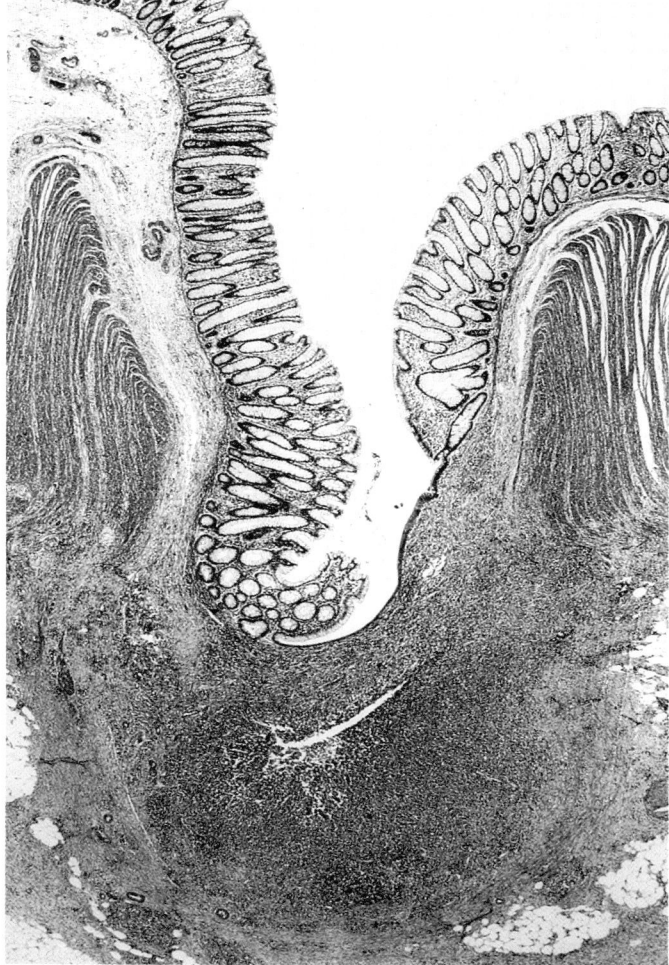

Fig. 16.216 Section of active diverticulitis with abscess formation. The inflammation is centred on the apex of the diverticulum. The muscularis propria is markedly thickened.

specific. There is active inflammation in and around the diverticulum and often a foreign body giant cell reaction to faecal debris within the serosal tissues is seen. The inflammatory focus starts at the apex of the diverticulum and spreads into the surrounding serosal tissues (Fig. 16.216). Suppuration and microabscess formation may occur and a localized peritonitis is characterized by a fibrinous exudate with mesothelial cell degeneration and active inflammation.

Perforation and haemorrhage

Perforation leading to localized or generalized peritonitis is rare: it is occasionally due to penetration of the bowel wall by a sharp object, such as a chicken bone. Haemorrhage is due to ulceration of the mucosa within the diverticulum. Occasionally, hard inspissated faeces within the diverticula may erode into one of the larger blood vessels adjacent to the diverticulum and this may lead to life-threatening haemorrhage.

Fistula

Fistulae may complicate an acute diverticulitis; the inflamed colon, usually with a pericolic abscess, becomes stuck to an adjacent organ and an inflammatory track communicates between the two viscera. Colovesical fistulae are the most common, although fistulae to the skin, small intestine, uterus, and vagina can all occur. Fistula to the bladder causes the characteristic symptom of pneumaturia and cystitis inevitably results.

Intestinal obstruction

Although obstruction of the colon does occur in diverticular disease, small intestine obstruction is more common. The inflammatory mass in the sigmoid leads to numerous fibrous adhesions which tether and stenose loops of small bowel. Large intestinal obstruction is the result of gross muscular thickening and the mucosa redundancy that accompanies it.

Right-sided diverticulosis

The presence of numerous diverticula in the ascending colon is generally known as right-sided diverticulosis. This disease is more common in Japan and Hawaii than in Western races and occurs in a younger age-group than sigmoid diverticular disease. Dietary factors are probably responsible for these differences. The pathological features of right-sided diverticular disease are broadly similar to those of sigmoid diverticular disease. Complications include abscess, fistula, haemorrhage, and obstruction.

Solitary diverticulum of caecum and ascending colon

This term is something of a misnomer, for diverticula are seldom solitary. It is not unusual to find a few diverticula in the caecum or ascending colon. They are usually asymptomatic but may, on occasion, give rise to diverticulitis which clinically simulates the presentation of acute appendicitis. The diverticulitis may be complicated by haemorrhage, peritonitis, and abscess formation. As with acute diverticulitis of the sigmoid colon, it may

be difficult to differentiate the condition from carcinoma on macroscopic examination.

Small intestinal diverticula

These are most commonly seen in the duodenum and are rarely symptomatic. Multiple diverticula may be seen in the jejunum in elderly patients. As in sigmoid diverticular disease, the diverticula occur at the point where blood vessels penetrate the muscularis propria and are therefore always present in an orderly row at the mesenteric aspect of the intestine. Jejunal diverticula are usually symptomless, most often being an unexpected finding at autopsy. Rarely, they may be a cause of the blind-loop syndrome due to alterations in the bacterial flora of the bowel.

16.15.3 Further reading

Heaton, K. W. (1985). Diet and diverticulosis—new leads. *Gut* **26**, 541–3.

Painter, N. S. (1975). *Diverticular disease of the colon*. William Heinemann, London.

Painter, N. S. and Burkitt, D. P. (1971). Diverticular disease of the colon: a deficiency disease of Western civilisation. *British Medical Journal* **2**, 450–4.

Parks, T. G. (1975). Natural history of diverticular disease of the colon. *Clinics in Gastroenterology* **4**, 53–70.

Whiteway, J. and Morson, B. C. (1985). Elastosis in diverticular disease of the sigmoid colon. *Gut* **26**, 258–66.

16.16 Epithelial and mesenchymal tumours of the small and large bowel

J. R. Jass

16.16.1 Benign epithelial polyps and polyposis syndromes

The term polyp describes a circumscribed lesion that projects into the bowel lumen. It is a descriptive term and not a final diagnosis. Epithelial polyps are classified according to the process that is thought to underlie their development (Table 16.15). Non-epithelial polyps and polypoid carcinoma will be considered separately.

Hyperplastic or metaplastic polyp

Little is known of the aetiology, nature, or epidemiological significance of this lesion. It is the only epithelial polyp of the gastrointestinal tract that is peculiar to the large bowel and appendix, being especially prevalent in the distal colon and rectum. They are rarely seen in low-risk populations for large bowel cancer (such as Japanese), but become more prevalent in Japanese who have migrated to high-risk Hawaii. This would

Table 16.15 Histological classification of epithelial polyps of the small and large bowel

Underlying disorder	Usual name of polyp	Polyposis syndrome
Defective maturation	Hyperplastic (metaplastic)	Hyperplastic polyposis
Neoplasia	Adenoma Tubular Tubulovillous Villous	Familial adenomatous polyposis
Hamartomatous malformation	Juvenile Peutz–Jeghers	Juvenile polyposis Peutz–Jeghers Cronkhite–Canada
Inflammation	Inflammatory	Inflammatory polyposis

suggest that environmental factors, perhaps dietary, are important in their aetiology.

Some insight into the underlying disorder is provided by ultrastructural and cell kinetic studies. As in normal large bowel mucosa, immature proliferating cells occupy the crypt base. While migrating upwards the cells mature, cease to divide, and are ultimately shed from the surface of the polyp. However, morphological features which accompany the normal process of differentiation are expressed prematurely and in an exaggerated form in hyperplastic polyps. At the same time cellular migration occurs more slowly and cells are retained longer than their normal counterparts.

Hyperplastic polyps present as sessile, pale mucosal nodules, rarely exceeding 5 mm in diameter. Small adenomas may be indistinguishable from hyperplastic polyps and the final diagnosis must therefore be a histological one. Occasionally the polyps are large and pedunculated, but the head remains pale (unlike the adenoma). Hyperplastic polyps are often clustered in large numbers around carcinomas of the sigmoid colon and rectum. Histological examination reveals a slightly thickened mucosa. The lower third of the crypt, respresenting the proliferative zone, may be lengthened and dilated. Above this zone the crypts assume a characteristic serrated or saw-tooth contour and are lined by mucus-secreting columnar cells but relatively few goblet cells (Fig. 16.217).

It is generally accepted that the hyperplastic polyp is not an important precancerous lesion.

Hyperplastic polyposis

This describes a condition in which numerous hyperplastic polyps occur throughout the colorectum and may be more than the usual 5 mm in diameter. Patients are mostly aged between 20 and 50 years. Unlike familial adenomatous polyposis (FAP) (see below), the condition is not thought to be precancerous, though there are a few reports of associated malignancy. Hyperplastic polyposis is of some clinical importance. First, it may be mistaken for FAP, both radiologically and endoscopically. Secondly, there may be co-existing adenomas that would be difficult to identify and remove. On the other hand, the chance removal of an adenoma might lead to an erroneous diagnosis of

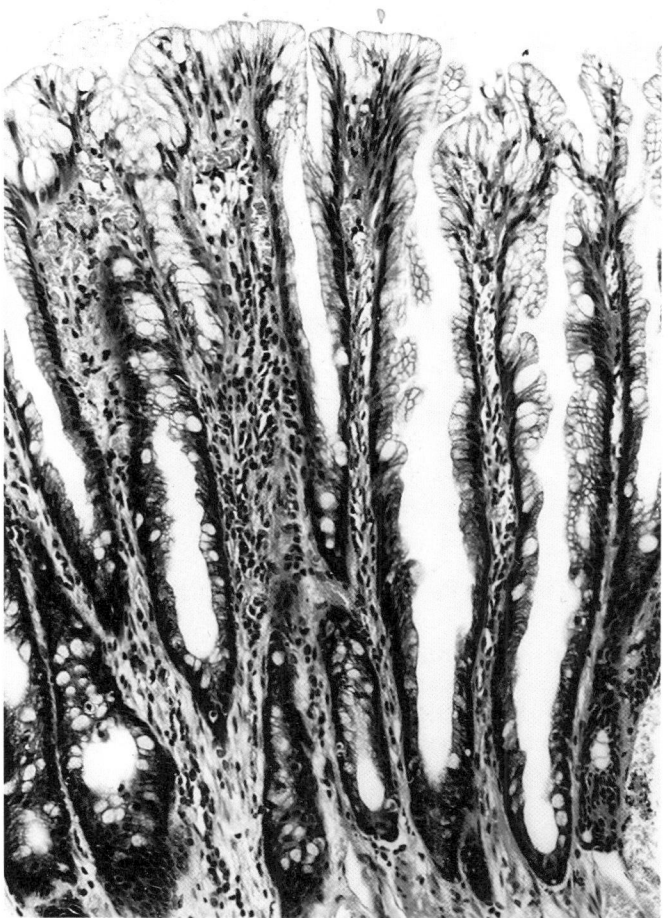

Fig. 16.217 Hyperplastic (metaplastic) polyp.

FAP and precipitate an unnecessary colectomy. It is therefore essential to examine several polyps, especially in 'new' cases of polyposis. Finally, the few descriptions of adenomatous change within hyperplastic polyps (mixed polyps) have often been in patients with hyperplastic polyposis.

Adenoma

Definition and neoplastic nature of adenoma

The adenoma is essentially a circumscribed focus of epithelial dysplasia (intra-epithelial neoplasia). The majority present as polyps, either sessile or pedunculated, but they are occasionally only slightly raised or even flat (Fig. 16.218). They may occur in the small intestine, particularly in the vicinity of the ampulla of Vater, the appendix, but are very much more common in the large intestine. Their importance lies in their increased potential for malignant change, although only about 5 per cent of large bowel adenomas will become malignant. They rarely produce symptoms, but larger adenomas may bleed.

Genetics

It is likely that the progression from normal to adenoma to

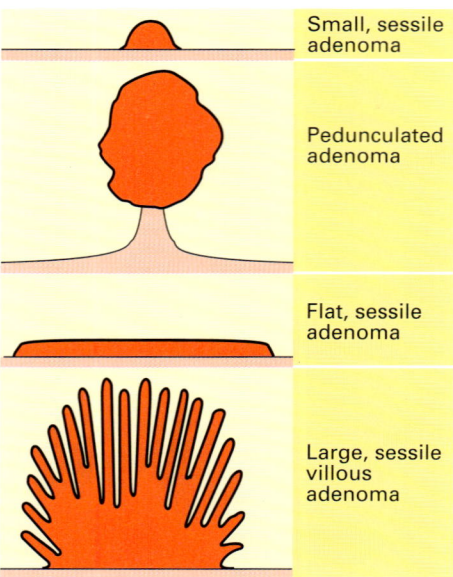

Small, sessile adenoma

Pedunculated adenoma

Flat, sessile adenoma

Large, sessile villous adenoma

Fig. 16.218 Gross appearances of adenomas.

carcinoma results from a stepwise accumulation of genetic lesions. Cytogenetic and DNA flow cytometric studies have shown that the genetic constitution of a series of adenomas is extremely heterogeneous. Most adenomas are small, show minimal histological deviation from the normal, and have a normal karyotype. An abnormal DNA content, indicating gross aneuploidy, characterizes larger, severely dysplastic adenomas. The steps that initiate the evolution of the adenoma are probably small deletions or point mutations that are not associated with changes of karyotype. A deletion in the long arm of chromosome 5 gives rise to the dominantly inherited condition familial adenomatous polyposis. Loss of the homologous gene appears to be required for the progression from .adenoma to carcinoma. Sporadic adenomas may arise and progress to cancer through somatic mutations at the same locus. A point mutation has been demonstrated at codon 12 of the dominant oncogene c-Ki-*ras,* though only in a proportion of colorectal cancers and adenomas. The progression from normal to adenoma to carcinoma implicates other mutations also, notably in the short arm of chromosome 17 (p53 gene) and the long arm of chromosome 18. Not only are we beginning to identify the genetic lesions that underlie the development of colorectal neoplasms, but it may in future become possible to define and classify these lesions accordingly.

Epidemiology

Adenomas of the large intestine are found with greater frequency, are larger, and show more severe dysplasia in populations at high risk of large bowel carcinoma. In North America they may be found in as many as 50 per cent of autopsy examinations of the large bowel, whereas an equivalent series of autopsy examinations in Africa may disclose not a single example. There is a very close association between the prevalence of adenomas and the incidence of colorectal cancer in different populations. They occur with greater frequency in males, but are described as being relatively larger and more dysplastic in females.

Topography

Most small bowel adenomas occur in the vicinity of the ampulla of Vater. Adenomas of the appendix are typically diffuse, occupying a comparatively large part of the mucosal lining. Although large bowel cancer occurs with greatest frequency in the sigmoid colon and rectum, it is of interest that adenomas show no such predilection, being distributed uniformly within the large bowel. However, the largest and most dysplastic adenomas are located in the distal colon and rectum. This may simply be because adenomas of the distal colon and rectum develop at an earlier age and therefore have more time to grow.

Histogenesis

Normal intestinal crypts are populated by stem cells, differentiating cells that are capable of division, and mature cells. The most immature cells are located at the crypt base, whereas mature cells are found in the upper crypt and surface epithelium. The adenoma probably results from a stem cell defect which leads to a monoclonal proliferation of immature cells. These eventually populate the entire length of the crypt. The unicrypt adenoma so-formed may divide and ultimately give rise to a visible mass.

Macroscopic appearances

The smallest adenomas present as sessile nodules and are the same colour as the surrounding mucosa. As they increase in size, the head darkens and the polyp usually become pedunculated. When the head becomes larger than 1 cm in diameter it is often furrowed and assumes the appearance of a miniature cauliflower. Occasionally adenomas remain as sessile growths, though they may reach a considerable size. Such tumours often have a shaggy or velvety surface (villous adenomas) (Fig. 16.219).

Microscopic appearances

Most adenomas are formed of branched tubules lined by an epithelium which can be distinguished from the normal by a number of cytological features. The nuclei are enlarged, elongated, crowded, and pseudostratified. Mitoses are seen at all levels of the crypt. Mucus production is reduced and this, together with the increased nuclear:cytoplasmic ratio, makes the epithelium appear dark in H&E sections (Fig. 16.220). The architectural and cytological changes together with the impairment of differentiation are collectively described as epithelial dysplasia. Dysplasia may be graded subjectively as mild, moderate, and severe. The majority of adenomas are composed of mildly dysplastic epithelium, which differs little from the normal. A minority show severe dysplasia, which approximates to carcinoma *in situ.* The grading of dysplasia probably represents the morphological counterpart of the stepwise accumulation of genetic errors described above.

Adenomas may differ architecturally from the above descrip-

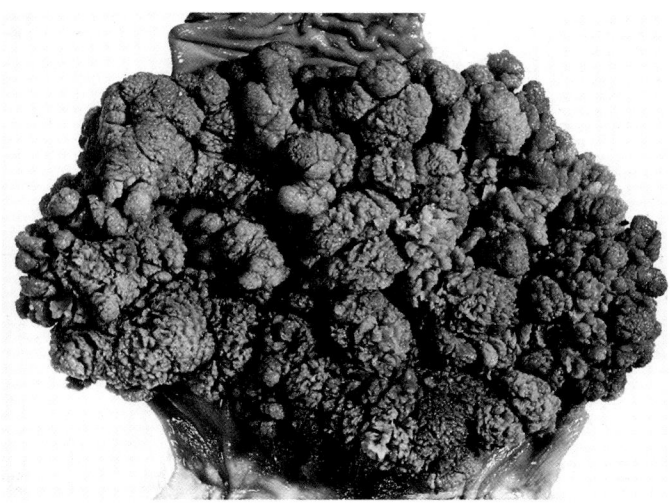

Fig. 16.219 Villous adenoma of rectum.

tion in having a surface epithelium that is thrown into complex folds. Such villous adenomas are uncommon. The villi are often lined by a well-differentiated mucus-secreting epithelium. This may be associated with such an abundant passage of mucus per rectum that the patient becomes depleted of water and electrolytes. Adenomas may also show an intermediate architecture when they are described as tubulovillous.

As well as showing a loss of normal functional activities such as the secretion of mucin and secretory component, adenomas may express certain antigens inappropriately or in excess of

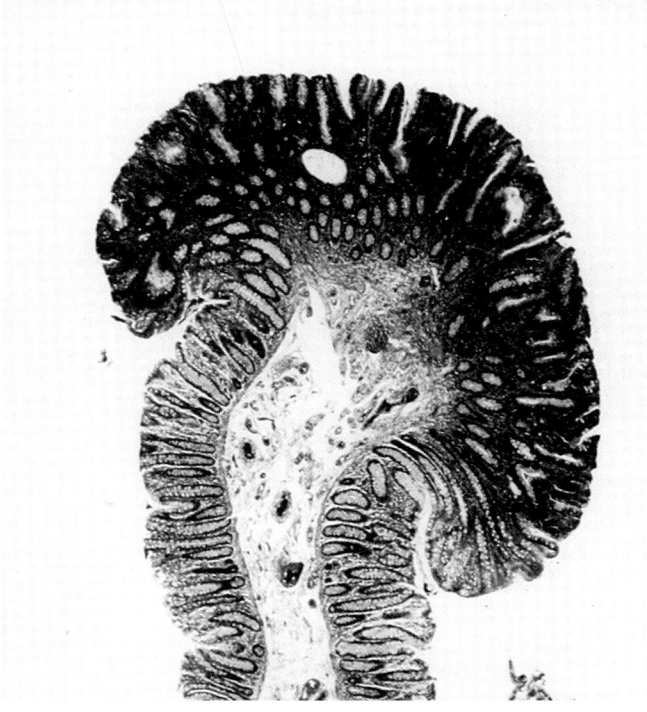

Fig. 16.220 Tubular adenoma of rectum.

normal. Notable examples include carcino-embryonic antigen and blood group antigens. These changes may result from the defective synthesis of normal cell products or the activation of genes that are normally repressed. Most of the antigenic changes occur late in the evolution of the adenoma when the epithelium has become severely dysplastic. These epiphenomena have not yet been shown to be of diagnostic or clinical value.

Malignant potential of adenomas

The majority of adenomas will not become malignant, perhaps only 5 per cent. This is an average figure and the risk is probably considerably higher for rectal adenomas. If a series of large bowel adenomas is examined, those which are most likely to contain a focus of cancer will be large, severely dysplastic, and have a villous architecture. It is likely that the majority of carcinomas arise in a pre-existing adenoma. Certainly, the systematic removal of adenomas appears to remove or greatly diminish any further risk of cancer. The rare adenomas that avoid detection through being small and flat may account for reports of so-called *de novo* carcinoma.

Multiple adenomas

Some patients present with multiple adenomas, say between 3 and 30. Such patients are at increased risk of developing additional adenomas and carcinoma. There are reports which suggest that a proneness to adenomas may be dominantly inherited, and it is possible that a proportion of patients with multiple adenomas have an incomplete form of familial adenomatous polyposis. These may account for some reports of familial colorectal cancer.

Adenomas of the appendix

In this organ adenomas are usually diffuse lesions with a villous configuration. The appendix may become distended by the secreted mucus, forming a cystadenoma. The lining adenomatous epithelium is often flattened, making distinction from a simple mucocele (p. 1220) extremely difficult. Most appendiceal adenomas are symptomless, but some present as acute appendicitis. Rupture of a distended cystadenoma may result in pseudomyxoma peritonei.

Familial adenomatous polyposis

In this rare condition the tendency to produce hundreds or thousands of colorectal adenomas is inherited on an autosomal dominant basis. Colorectal cancer is an inevitable complication which is prevented by prophylactic colectomy. Index or propositus cases present in the third or fourth decade with altered bowel habit and the passage of mucus and blood per rectum, and at least one large bowel cancer is usually found. A careful family history must be taken and the patient's siblings and children should be screened for the disease. Screening usually begins in the teens and the great majority of patients develop adenomas by the age of 20 if they are carrying the abnormal gene. It is essential to obtain histological proof of the disease,

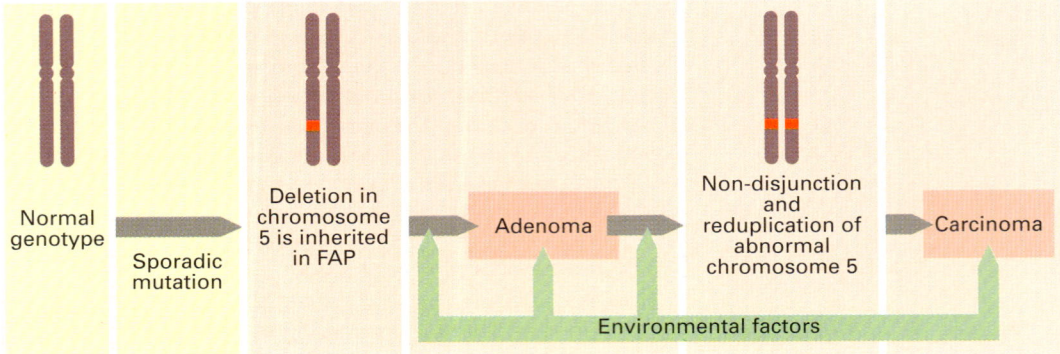

Fig. 16.221   Model for the genetic evolution of colorectal neoplasia.

this rule applying to call-up cases as well as the propositus. Now that the polyposis gene has been located on the long arm of chromosome 5, it should soon become possible to achieve early diagnosis through the technique of gene tracking within families. If the disease has arisen as a new mutation, there will be no history of polyposis or cancer in the patient's parents, grandparents, or siblings, but any children will have a 50 per cent of inheriting the defective gene.

It is likely that the discovery of the polyposis gene will provide important insight into the genetic defects which underlie the evolution of colorectal neoplasia (Fig. 16.221). It now seems probable that familial adenomatous polyposis is due to the deletion of a gene which controls growth and differentiation. Furthermore, loss of the normal homologous gene may be an important step in the progression from adenoma to carcinoma. The same genetic lesions may be implicated in at least some sporadic colorectal cancers, but as somatic rather than inherited mutations.

Macroscopic examination of a colectomy specimen for polyposis reveals numerous adenomas, whose size and number will be influenced by the age of the patient (Fig. 16.222). Microscopic study discloses not only typical adenomas with varying degrees of epithelial dysplasia but also microadenomas and even unicrypt adenomas that are invisible on gross inspection. The intervening mucosa is morphologically normal but there are reports of alterations in cell function implicating the composition of goblet cell mucus and epithelial turnover. Not all of these claims have been substantiated, and it is more likely that the primary expression of the defective gene is an all-or-none focal abnormality, namely the unicrypt adenoma.

The defective gene is, of course, present in all somatic cells of an affected individual, yet its expression is limited to particular organs. This is presumably because the gene is linked specifically to the control of intestinal differentiation. Extracolonic manifestations do occur, however, and some are of major clinical significance, notably abdominal fibromatosis and duodenal adenoma and carcinoma. The latter arise mainly in the periampullary region. The association between familial adenomatous polyposis and certain minor lesions, including osteomas of the skull and mandible and cutaneous cysts, has been described

as Gardner's syndrome. It is preferable to consider familial adenomatous polyposis as a single entity in which a variety of extracolonic manifestations occur with a frequency yet to be determined.

Juvenile polyps and polyposis

This polyp is usually limited to the large bowel except in patients with juvenile polyposis (see below). It is considered to be a hamartoma since it is formed of tissue indigenous to the site of origin but arranged in a haphazard manner. Most occur in childhood and are either solitary or present in small numbers. A

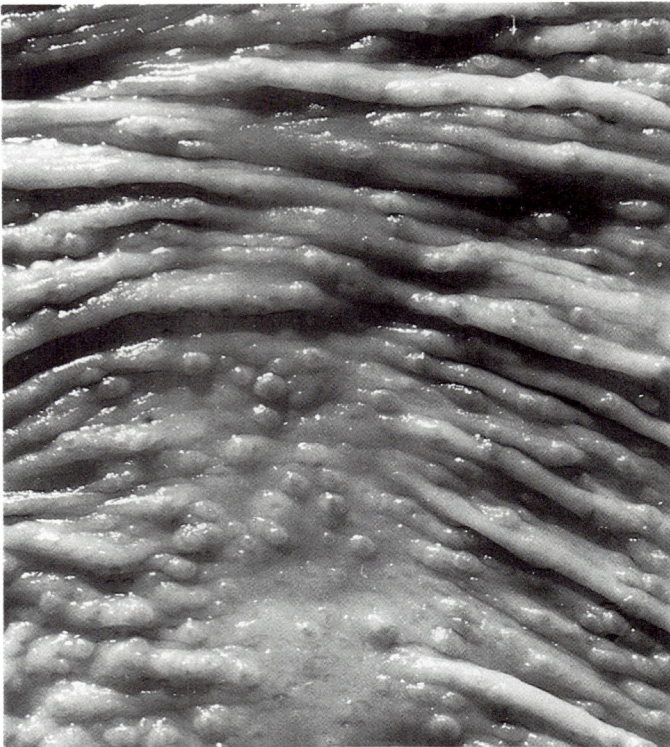

Fig. 16.222   Numerous small colorectal adenomas in a specimen of familial adenomatous polyposis.

child of either sex will typically present with rectal bleeding. Occasionally the head may autoamputate and be recovered by the parent. The polyp has a smooth, red head and a narrow stalk. Microscopically the polyp is formed of epithelial tubules which may be cystic and are lined by essentially normal epithelium. The tubules are embedded in an abundant and oedematous lamina propria that is devoid of smooth muscle (Fig. 16.223). The surface often shows superficial ulceration.

Juvenile polyposis is a very rare condition which may present in a number of ways. One is as a severe and life-threatening disease of infancy characterized by diarrhoea, haemorrhage, malnutrition, and intussusception. Juvenile polyps are found throughout the gastrointestinal tract but are most numerous within the colon and rectum. The disease may be likened to an infantile form of the Cronkhite–Canada syndrome (see below). A more usual presentation is that of an older child or young adult with brisk bleeding per rectum. The condition may be sporadic or dominantly inherited. Sporadic cases are frequently associated with congenital defects, including abnormalities of the cranium and heart. There is a greatly increased risk of colorectal cancer, and this complication is recorded mainly in young patients aged 20–40 years. The polyps of juvenile polyposis can be unusually large, multilobated, and papillary. Histological examination reveals less lamina propria than in the typical variety, and foci of epithelial dysplasia are seen not uncommonly.

Peutz–Jeghers polyps and syndrome

This syndrome is inherited as an autosomal dominant trait and is characterized by circumoral pigmentation and multiple hamartomatous polyps in the stomach, small bowel, and colon. The polyps are largest in the stomach and small bowel. Those within the latter organ are responsible for the main presenting feature, which is intussusception. The diagnosis is usually made in the first or second decade. There are reports of associated tumours, both gastrointestinal and in other organs such as the breast and cervix. Sex cord tumours of the ovary occur sufficiently commonly to be considered part of the syndrome. There is without doubt a significant excess of small bowel adenocarcinoma. Although this complication will affect only a small proportion of Peutz–Jeghers patients, it should be recalled that small bowel adenocarcinoma is otherwise extremely uncommon. It should be stressed, however, that innocent epithelial misplacement is a frequent and often florid finding in Peutz–Jeghers polyps of the small bowel. Epithelium may even extend through the bowel wall into the serosa. This must be carefully distinguished from genuine malignancy.

The polyps range in appearance from small nodules to large pedunculated tumours indistinguishable from large bowel adenomas. Histologically the core of the polyp is formed by a tree-like branching of the muscularis mucosae. This is covered by essentially normal intestinal epithelium. Isolated Peutz–Jeghers-type polyps may occur in either the small or large bowel in patients who do not have the syndrome.

Cronkhite–Canada syndrome

In this condition polypoid changes occur in the mucosa of the stomach, small intestine, and colon and are associated with a protein-losing enteropathy. Accompanying ectodermal lesions include alopecia, atrophy of the nails, and hyperpigmentation. The polyposis is diffuse as opposed to a multiplicity of discrete polyps. Histologically the mucosal changes resemble those of the juvenile polyp.

Inflammatory polyps and polyposis

Chronic inflammatory bowel disease is characterized by alternating phases of ulceration and healing. Inflammatory polyps may arise when mucosa becomes undermined and later transformed into a mucosal tag, or when granulation tissue becomes organized and re-epithelialized. Surviving islands of mucosa in a severely ulcerated bowel may appear polypoid but should be distinguished from true inflammatory polyps. Inflammatory polyps are often finger-like and may become fused to form bridges. Florid examples are described as bizarre or giant inflammatory polyposis and may mimic a villous adenoma.

Mixed polyps

Occasionally it may not be possible to classify a polyp as one of the entities discussed above. For example, the head of a polyp may be partly adenomatous and partly hyperplastic (metaplastic). It is not known whether such hybrids occur by chance or whether they indicate relationships between lesions that have previously been regarded as disparate.

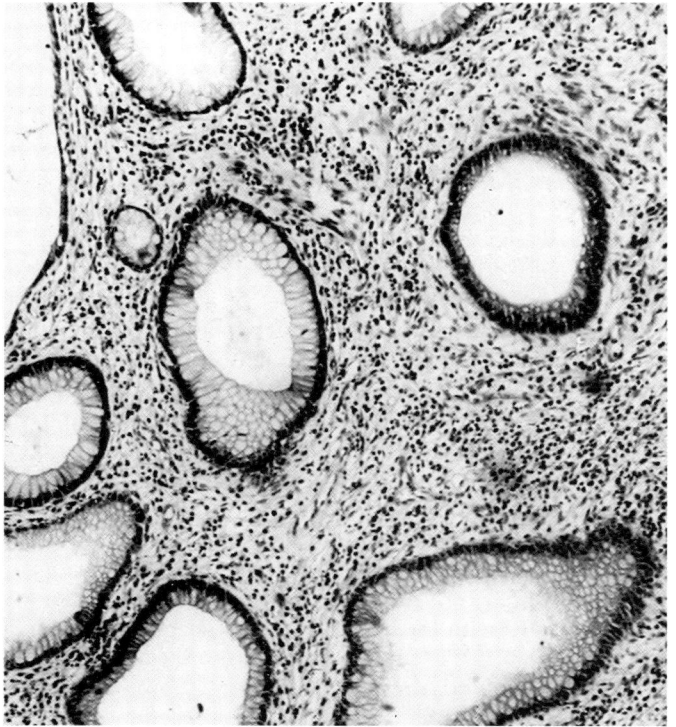

Fig. 16.223 Juvenile polyp.

Other forms of polyposis

The preceding sections will include many but by no means all the conditions that present with multiple intestinal polyps. Benign lymphoid polyposis (p. 1282) is a cause of small and large intestinal polyposis. Malignant lymphomatous polyposis (Chapter 24) is another, although it is extremely rare. Secondary deposits of tumour, notably malignant melanoma, may present with multiple polyps, particularly of the small intestine. Finally, there are other rare and poorly characterized epithelial polyposis syndromes.

16.16.2   Carcinoma

Carcinoma of the large bowel is one of the leading causes of cancer death in the West and accounts for about 19 000 deaths in the United Kingdom each year. The actual incidence of the disease is higher because patients with relatively early disease may be cured by surgery. Although at least 50 per cent of patients undergoing potentially curative surgery are in fact cured of the disease, many patients die of the presenting complications, have inoperable disease, receive palliative surgery only, or are not even referred for surgical treatment. In effect, only about 25 per cent of patients who develop the disease are cured by surgery. Colorectal cancer cannot therefore be regarded as a form of malignancy with a favourable outcome. Small bowel carcinoma is, by contrast, an uncommon malignancy. This presumably reflects differences in the composition and transit time of luminal contents of each organ. The following account will concentrate on cancer of the large bowel.

Epidemiology

There are marked geographical variations in the incidence of colorectal cancer. The disease is common in Western Europe, North America, and Australasia but is uncommon in South America and Asia, and extremely rare in Africa. Incidence rates show a good correlation with meat consumption. Migration studies reinforce the importance of environmental factors, Japanese Hawaiians and Black Americans having the same high risk as their fellow countrymen. Time-trend studies help to show how changes in the life-style of different populations may influence the incidence of the disease. The most rapid increases with time are seen in those populations who formerly had a low incidence, but are rapidly converting to a Western life-style. Japan is a good example of this phenomenon. There may be differences in the epidemiology of right- and left-sided large bowel cancer. It is often stated that the incidence of cancer of the right colon is increasing in high-risk populations. This appears to be particularly noticeable in elderly females and could be an age-related effect only.

Age and sex incidence

Colorectal cancer becomes more frequent with increasing age, but is by no means a disease of extreme old age. The mean age at diagnosis is around 60 years. The disease is more common in men than women, but this difference depends upon both age and the site of the disease. Rectal cancer is more frequent in males and this difference increases with age. Cancer of the right colon appears to show a slight predilection for females.

Aetiology

Both environmental and inherited factors play a role in the aetiology of colorectal cancer. Although epidemiological studies provide clear evidence of the importance of the environment, a number of important inconsistencies need to be addressed. It should be appreciated that most inhabitants of high-risk areas will not develop the disease, despite indulging in dietary indiscretions, and that some individuals in low-risk areas will be affected. Maori and non-Maori New Zealanders take equivalent diets, but the incidence of colorectal cancer is much higher in non-Maoris. Although population studies may clearly implicate specific agents, such as faecal bile acids, in the aetiology of the disease, no differences are found when individual cases are matched with controls. These observations point to the existence of inherited factors which could operate in a number of ways. Cancer is a genetic disease arising on the basis of a stepwise accumulation of genetic errors. One of these steps may be inherited and this has been shown to be the case in familial adenomatous polyposis (Chapter 2). Inherited factors may also act in less direct ways, such as through DNA repair defects or by influencing the metabolism of potential mutagens or promoting agents. Evidence for the latter mechanism is provided by the association of the fast acetylator phenotype and colorectal cancer.

The interplay of inherited and environmental factors has been related to the morphological development of cancer through the normal–adenoma–carcinoma sequence. It has been suggested that the tendency to form adenomas is inherited (a parallel with familial adenomatous polyposis) whereas the development of the adenoma and its progress to cancer will be influenced by environmental mutagens and promoting agents. This concept receives some support from the study of a colorectal cancer family kindred in which the production of adenomas was inherited as an autosomal dominant trait.

Dietary fat is regarded as an important factor in tumour promotion. It may have a direct influence by increasing epithelial turnover. Alternatively, fat may act indirectly through its metabolism to bile acids in the liver. Bile acids are then excreted and converted into tumour promoters by bacteria in the bowel lumen. The role of dietary fibre may be to bind with fats and bile acids or simply to inhibit their promotional activity by a dilutional effect. Acidification of the stool also seems to be protective, perhaps by reducing the bacterial hydroxylation of bile acids. The bacterial fermentation of fibre to short chain fatty acids within the right colon will contribute to the acidification of the stool. A high consumption of unrefined carbohydrate has been associated with the presence of both adenoma and carcinoma. Calcium has been implicated as a protective factor by virtue of its ability to convert fats into inert soaps. Cruciferous vegetables and the anti-oxidant trace metal selenium may also be protective.

Precancerous lesions and conditions

It is generally believed that the majority of adenocarcinomas of the intestinal tract arise within pre-existing adenomas. Adenoma and carcinoma may be regarded as stages in a disease continuum caused by a stepwise accumulation of genetic errors. It is clear, therefore, than an understanding of the cause and evolution of adenocarcinoma must begin with the study of adenomas.

Patients with precancerous lesions or conditions are at an increased risk of developing cancer and may therefore require close surveillance. The screening of high-risk groups may lead either to the prevention of cancer or to its detection at an early, and therefore curative stage. There is little evidence that patients who produce a single adenoma are at increased risk in developing carcinoma in the future. However, patients who have multiple adenomas, with or without a synchronous carcinoma, are more likely to produce additional neoplasms. Familial adenomatous polyposis is an important, though rare, precancerous condition and juvenile polyposis is now regarded in a similar light. The risk of cancer in ulcerative colitis is currently thought to be around 5 per cent for patients who have had extensive colitis (radiological or endoscopic involvement at least as far as the hepatic flexure) for 20 years. This is lower than earlier estimates, but patients may develop cancer at an unusually young age. Thus colitics aged 30–40 years will be at least 60 times as likely to develop colorectal cancer as an age-matched cohort without colitis. Cancer in colitis can often be shown to develop within a pre-existing epithelial change, known usually as dysplasia. Crohn's disease is a precancerous condition also, but it is small intestinal malignancy, normally extremely rare, that shows the greatest relative increase in incidence. This is true also for the Peutz–Jeghers syndrome.

Patients with a first-degree relative with large bowel cancer have about three times the normal risk of developing the disease themselves. This is an average figure, however, and will vary according to the age of the first-degree relative. When relatives are in their sixties, the risk is probably not increased at all. When they are less than 45, the risk may be considerably more than three times the expected figure. This is because cancer often occurs at an unusually early age in members of so-called colorectal cancer families. Clinical and pathological features of the colorectal cancer family syndrome have been extrapolated from observations based upon a number of well-studied kindreds. Cancers are stated to show a predilection for the right colon, to be multiple, and, at least in some families, to be associated with extracolonic malignancy, notably of breast and uterus. The alleged absence of adenomas in these patients is probably incorrect. In fact, adenomas appear to occur with increased frequency in members of colorectal cancer families. It has been suggested that mucinous carcinoma occurs with increased frequency in colorectal cancer family kindreds.

Topography

About 50 per cent of large bowel cancers arise in the sigmoid colon and rectum. The caecum and lower part of the ascending colon are the next sites of predilection. The rest are distributed evenly throughout the remainder of the colon. In ulcerative colitis these regional differences are less obvious and cancers are often multiple. As noted above, the right colon may be implicated more frequently in affected members of colorectal cancer families. The ampullary region of the duodenum is the preferred site of small bowel cancer. Cancer in Crohn's disease may occur in any region of the small or large bowel that is affected by the disease.

Early colorectal cancer

The term 'early' is essentially a clinical judgement indicating that a tumour is likely to be at a curative stage. An early cancer cannot be defined in precise clinicopathological terms. In the colorectum the term has come to imply that the tumour is not only curable, but may be cured by local means as opposed to radical forms of surgery. Early colorectal cancers may adopt four macroscopic forms. Two of these, the malignant adenoma and the small polypoid carcinoma, may be removed endoscopically. On the other hand, the large, sessile adenoma with a focus of malignancy and the small ulcerating carcinoma will usually require surgical excision. Local removal is regarded as adequate treatment provided that excision is complete, the tumour is not poorly differentiated, and there is no obvious invasion of vessels by tumour.

Macroscopic appearances

Cancer of the intestinal tract may appear as a protuberant mass, as an ulcer with a rolled, everted edge (Fig. 16.224), or as a diffusely infiltrating tumour. The latter may be a relatively small, annular growth which produces a tight stricture or a larger plaque-like lesion. The prognosis is influenced by the appearance of the tumour, being most favourable for well-circumscribed, protuberant tumours and least good for diffusely infiltrating growths. There are relationships between site, presenting features, and appearance. Large, protuberant tumours often occur in the caecal area and patients typically present with iron deficiency anaemia (due to chronic blood loss) and a mass in the right iliac fossa. The splenic flexure is the site of predilection for stricturing tumours and patients present with the signs of intestinal obstruction. The majority of rectal cancers are ulcerating, and patients may present with bright red bleeding per rectum, tenesmus, or altered bowel habit.

Microscopic appearances

Most intestinal cancers are adenocarcinomas (Fig. 16.225). About 10 per cent of large bowel cancers are distinguished by an abundant secretion of mucin. These are of two main types. One is relatively well differentiated and often arises within a villous adenoma. The other is poorly differentiated, has a poor prognosis and affects relatively young patients. The signet-ring cell carcinoma is an example of a poorly differentiated mucinous carcinoma. The signet appearance is due to the nucleus being pushed to the periphery of the cell by accumulated intracytoplasmic mucin. It is important to distinguish

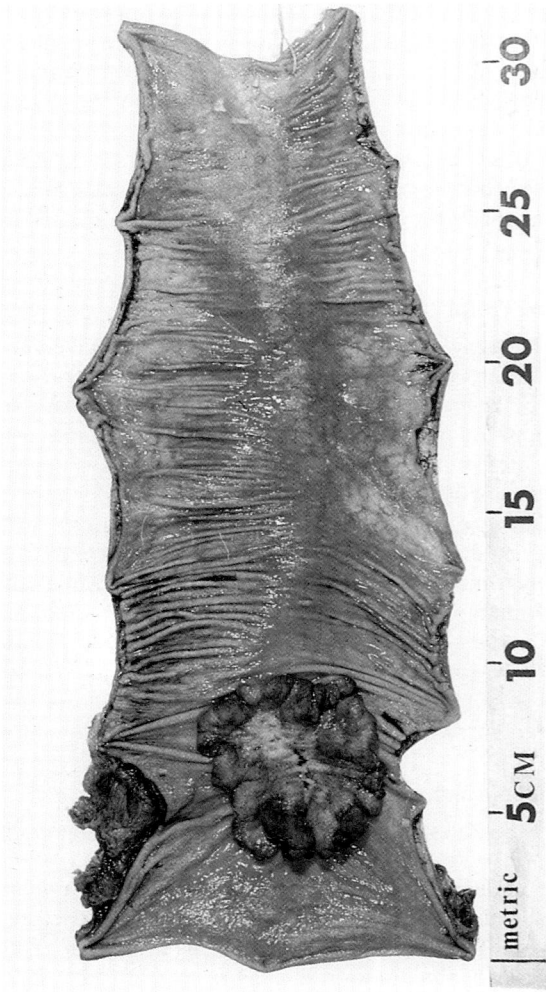

Fig. 16.224 Ulcerating carcinoma of the rectum.

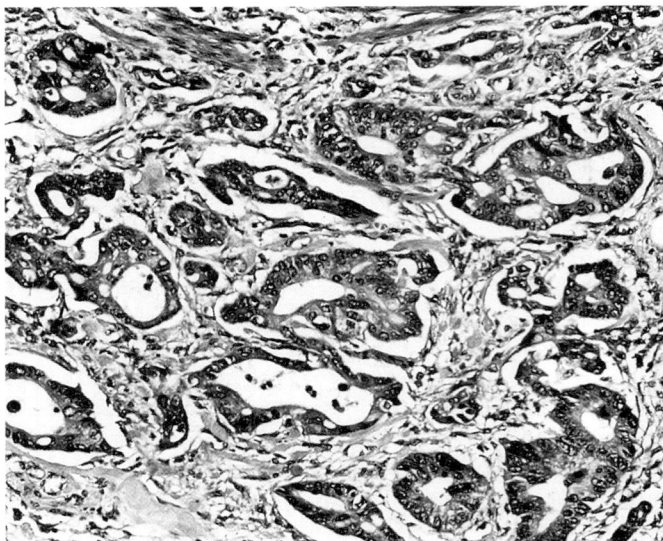

Fig. 16.225 Typical moderately differentiated adenocarcinoma of the large bowel.

Special techniques for studying tumour cells

The techniques of histochemistry and immunocytochemistry have uncovered numerous functional differences between normal and cancerous cells. These changes implicate mucins, blood-group antigens, class II histocompatibility antigens (HLA-DR), and enzymes (brush border and cytoplasmic). Normal differentiation antigens, such as secretory component, are lost, whereas oncodevelopmental antigens [e.g. carcinoembryonic antigen (CEA), stage-specific embryonic antigen 1] show increased expression. These changes are of some interest, but none seems to provide important insight into the pathogenesis of the disease or to be clinically useful as a diagnostic or prognostic marker. The measurement of serum CEA may help to monitor recurrence of cancer, and monoclonal antibodies to CEA and other tumour-associated antigens may be of value in clinical staging through the technique of radioimmunolocalization.

The DNA content of tumour cells can be measured by techniques such as flow cytometry. Colorectal cancers are classified as near diploid when the DNA content deviates little from normal, and aneuploid when there is a marked excess of DNA and therefore chromosomes. About 65 per cent of colorectal cancers are aneuploid and these have a somewhat poorer prognosis than diploid tumours. Tumour heterogeneity exists at the molecular level. Up to 40 per cent of colorectal cancers are homo- or hemizygous for chromosome 5. This means that through a mitotic defect, such as non-disjunction, the tumour cells have come to lack one member of the chromosome 5 pair (Fig. 16.221). Another equally interesting heterogeneity is provided by the demonstration of a mutation at codon 12 of the c-Ki-*ras* oncogene in a proportion of colorectal cancers. These observations point to the existence of different molecular path-

between primary signet-ring cell carcinoma and secondary spread from a site such as the stomach. Colorectal cancers may occasionally be formed of aggregates of large undifferentiated cells, but careful sampling will usually reveal areas of glandular differentiation. Squamous and adenosquamous carcinomas are excessively rare. Endocrine tumours are described in Section 16.17. The rare small cell, undifferentiated carcinoma resembles the oat cell carcinoma of the lung both histologically and in terms of its behaviour. It disseminates early and is therefore treated by chemotherapy rather than by surgery.

About 80 per cent of large bowel adenocarcinomas are well or moderately differentiated, whereas 20 per cent are poorly differentiated. The latter term signifies little or no glandular formation by the tumour and confers a poor prognosis. Diffusely infiltrating cancers also have a poor prognosis, whereas the presence of a lymphocyte-rich stroma at the invading edge of the tumour confers a favourable outlook.

ways in the pathogenesis of large bowel cancer, but these differences have not yet been shown to be of prognostic significance.

Spread

Spread of intestinal cancer occurs by direct growth through the bowel wall, through invasion of lymphatic and venous channels, and transperitoneally when cancer traverses the serosa. Direct spread occurs via the routes of least resistance. The submucosa offers little resistance, but the external muscle coat is a dense structure and tumour passes through the gaps in this layer which provide a pathway for the blood supply to the mucosa. The peritoneum also provides a tough barrier to direct spread.

Tumours which have spread as far as the submucosa are associated with a 4 per cent risk of lymph node spread only. This risk rises to about 12 per cent for tumours which invade the external muscle coat. However, once cancers traverse the muscle coat and penetrate the serosal or mesenteric fat, the risk of lymph node involvement rises to 60 per cent. Neoplasms confined to the mucosa are not associated with lymph node metastases and it is therefore the practice of many pathologists to withold a diagnosis of cancer unless there is evidence of invasion across the line of the muscularis mucosae into the submucosa. Failure to adhere to this policy may result in patients receiving needlessly radical surgery.

Prognosis is influenced by the number of lymph node metastases. Positive nodes are obviously not dangerous if no distant or local tumour is left after surgical treatment. However, the more positive lymph nodes there are, the greater is the risk of incurable, occult metastasis in distant sites such as the liver. Veins must provide an important, direct route of spread to the liver. However, the demonstration of tumour within veins does not appear to exert an independent influence on survival in the presence of other prognostic variables.

Staging and prognosis

The Dukes classification, proposed in 1932, is a simple pathological staging system which provides a guide to prognosis in patients undergoing surgical treatment for large bowel cancer (Fig. 16.226). The figures published by Dukes were based on a series of operable rectal cancers which included palliative as well as radical ('curative') cases. It is now appreciated that curative and non-curative operations should be grouped separately. Non-curative operations are those in which there is distant spread, or there has been incomplete local removal, or the bowel has been perforated (spontaneously or operatively), carrying the theoretical risk of extramural dissemination by tumour cells. The distinction between curative and non-curative cases requires information from the surgeon and histological confirmation by the pathologist whenever this is feasible. The prognosis for 'curative' cases will depend on whether there is occult residual disease, usually in the form of occult liver metastases. The latter have been demonstrated by a sensitive scanning technique, but this lacked the specificity that would be required of a diagnostic procedure. Since distant spread cannot be demonstrated accurately at the present time, the ability to offer a prognosis depends on being able to predict whether there is occult disease. There is no internationally agreed system of prognostic classification, but it is clear that it should be based on a small number of objective and independent variables. Until there is such agreement, the ABC system of Dukes should continue to be used as a guide to prognosis.

Carcinoma of the appendix

These are rare tumours which presents either as an acute appendicitis or as a mass in the right iliac fossa in a middle-aged patient. They may arise in a pre-existing cystadenoma. The tumour is then described as a mucinous cystadenocarcinoma and presents as a mucocele. This may rupture and give rise to

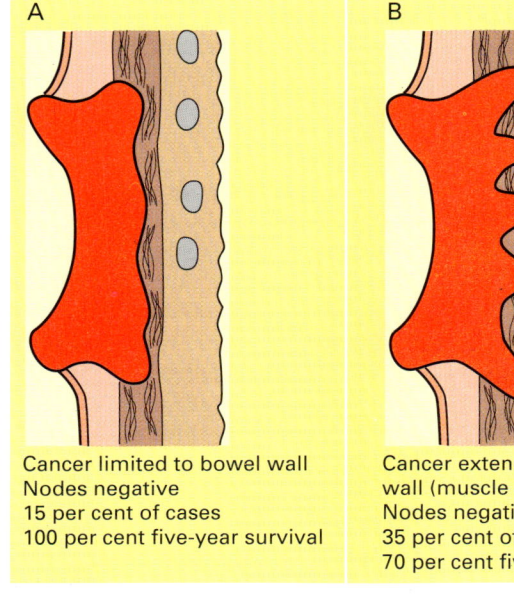
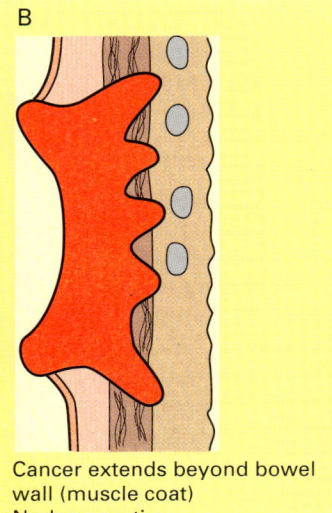
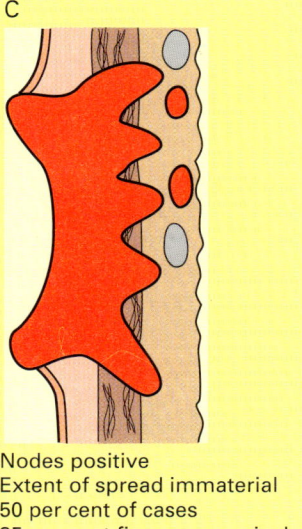

A

Cancer limited to bowel wall
Nodes negative
15 per cent of cases
100 per cent five-year survival

B

Cancer extends beyond bowel wall (muscle coat)
Nodes negative
35 per cent of cases
70 per cent five-year survival

C

Nodes positive
Extent of spread immaterial
50 per cent of cases
35 per cent five-year survival

Fig. 16.226. Dukes classification of large bowel cancer.

pseudomyxoma peritonei. More rarely, the tumour arises in a conventional adenoma and forms a papillary or tubular adenocarcinoma without abundant mucus production. The tumour spreads like a colorectal adenocarcinoma and may be staged by the Dukes classification.

Secondary carcinoma

The stomach is one of the commonest sources of secondary deposits in the intestines. Other tumours giving rise to intestinal secondaries include carcinoma of the breast, ovary, cervix, kidney, lung, bladder, and malignant melanoma.

Endocrine tumours

The reader is referred to Section 16.17 for an account of endocrine neoplasia in the gastrointestinal tract.

16.16.3   Non-epithelial tumours

Smooth muscle tumours

These may present as small mucosal polyps or as larger masses which may be intraluminal, intramural, or both intramural and extramural (dumb-bell) in position. The small mucosal tumours arise from the muscularis mucosae and are benign. The larger tumours arise from the external muscle coat and a proportion behave in a malignant fashion.

Neurogenic tumours

It is often difficult to determine whether a neurogenic tumour is a genuine neoplasm or a hamartomatous malformation. Of the following, schwannoma, paraganglioma, and ganglioneuroma are considered to be neoplasms, but the latter two are excessively rare.

Schwannoma

These are similar to their gastric counterparts.

Neurofibromatosis

Involvement of the intestinal tract should be considered when patients with neurofibromatosis (von Recklinghausen's disease) present with gastrointestinal bleeding or obstruction. Histologically, neurofibromas are made up of loose fibrous tissue with a wavy appearance interspersed with occasional nerve fibres. Solitary intestinal neurofibroma is excessively rare.

Ganglioneuromatosis

A diffuse form of intestinal ganglioneuromatosis occurs in association with medullary carcinoma of the thyroid, phaeochromocytoma, multiple mucosal neuromas, and a characteristic facial appearance, which together constitute the dominantly inherited syndrome of multiple endocrine adenomatosis type IIB. The affected segment of intestine is often ulcerated and may resemble Crohn's disease macroscopically.

Histological examination reveals an abnormal proliferation of nerves and ganglion cells in the myenteric and submucosal plexuses.

Polypoid ganglioneuromatosis differs from the above in that the neural proliferation lies within the lamina propria and gives rise to mucosal polyps. This condition has been described in the large intestine in association with juvenile polyposis.

Solitary ganglioneuromas and paragangliomas are extremely rare and some may be misdiagnosed examples of gangliocytic paraganglioma (see below). Solitary ganglioneuroma occurs more frequently in the large bowel than elsewhre in the gastrointestinal tract. Segments of the intestinal tract, usually small intestine, may show a diffuse ganglioneuromatosis in the absence of any of the syndromes described above. However, a proportion of these may be examples of burnt-out Crohn's disease.

Gangliocytic paraganglioma

These rare tumours occur in the duodenum and patients are usually middle-aged and present with gastrointestinal bleeding or abdominal pain. The lesion appears as a polyp a few centimetres in diameter, which may be ulcerated. Histological examination reveals endocrine cells, spindle-shaped Schwann cells, and ganglion cells in varying proportions. The lesion has been described in patients with neurofibromatosis.

Tumours of connective tissue

Inflammatory fibroid polyps

These may occur in the small bowel and result in intussusception. They are indistinguishable from their counterparts in the stomach (p. 1249).

Lipoma

Lipomas of the intestinal tract may present with intestinal bleeding but are uncommon. Hyperplasia of fat may affect the ileo-caecal valve and this is a fairly common, incidental finding in operation specimens.

Vascular tumours

Most vascular tumours of the intestinal tract are malformations or hamartomas rather than true neoplasms. Cavernous haemangiomas may occur in the small intestine, colon, or rectum, and present with haemorrhage or anaemia. Angiodysplasia is now understood to be one of the commonest causes of gastrointestinal bleeding. Multiple vascular ectasias may occur in a variety of syndromes, notably Osler–Weber–Rendu or hereditary haemorrhagic telangiectasia.

Lymphangiomas are extremely rare. In lymphangiectasia the lymphatics within a variable length of small bowel are dilated and the condition may give rise to malabsorption. Solitary or multiple lymphatic cysts may occur in the bowel wall or mesentery. These are usually harmless.

Kaposi's sarcoma may affect the intestinal tract in patients with the acquired immuno-deficiency syndrome.

Lymphoid tumours

The reader is referred to Chapter 24 for an account of gastro-intestinal tumours of lymphoid tissue.

16.16.4   Further reading

Bodmer, W. F., *et al.* (1987). Localization of the gene for familial aden-omatous polyposis on chromosome 5. *Nature* **328**, 614–16.

Bos., J. L., *et al.* (1987). Prevalence of *ras* gene mutations in human colorectal cancers. *Nature* **327**, 293–7.

Burt, R. W., Bishop, T., Cannon, L. A., Dowdle, M. A., Lee, R. G., and Skolnick, M. H. (1985). Dominant inheritance of adenomatous colonic polyps and colorectal carcinoma. *New England Journal of Medicine* **312**, 1540–4.

Dukes, C. E. (1932). The classification of cancer of the rectum. *Journal of Pathology and Bacteriology* **35**, 323–32.

Goh, H. S. and Jass, J. R. (1986). DNA content and the adenoma-carcinoma sequence in the colorectum. *Journal of Clinical Pathology* **39**, 387–97.

Haggitt, R. C. and Reid, B. J. (1986). Hereditary gastrointestinal polyposis syndrome. *American Journal of Surgical Pathology* **10**, 871–87.

Hill, M. J. (1982). Genetic and environmental factors in human colo-rectal cancer. In *Colon carcinogenesis* (ed. R. Malt and R. William-son), pp. 73–82. MTP, Lancaster.

Jass, J. R. (1987). The large intestine. In *Alimentary tract, systemic pathology* (3rd edn), (ed. B. C. Morson), pp. 313–95. Churchill Livingstone, Edinburgh.

Jass, J. R., *et al.* (1986). The grading of rectal cancer: historical perspectives and a multivariate analysis of 447 cases. *Histopatho-logy* **10**, 437–59.

Jass, J. R., Love, S. B., and Northover, J. M. A. (1987). A new prog-nostic classification of rectal cancer. *Lancet* **i**, 1303–6.

Muto, T., Bussey, H. J. R., and Morson, B. C. (1975). The evolution of cancer of the colon and rectum. *Cancer* **36**, 2251–76.

Solomon, E., *et al.* (1987). Chromosome 5 allele loss in human colo-rectal carcinomas. *Nature* **328**, 616–19.

Solomon, E. (1990). Colorectal cancer genes. *Nature* **343**, 412–14.

Vogelstein, B., *et al.* (1988). Genetic alterations during colorectal-tumor development. *New England Journal of Medicine* **319**, 525–32.

Williams, G. T. (1987). The vermiform appendix. In *Alimentary tract systemic pathology* (3rd edn), (ed. B. C. Morson), pp. 292–312. Churchill Livingstone, Edinburgh.

Williams, G. T., Arthur, J. F., Bussey, H. J. R., and Morson, B. C. (1980). Metaplastic polyps and polyposis of the colorectum. *Histo-pathology* **4**, 155–70.

16.17   Endrocrine tumours of the gut

J. M. Polak and S. R. Bloom

16.17.1   Introduction

Various terms have been used to describe tumours arising from the diffuse neuro-endocrine system and there is as yet no con-sensus on their terminology. Oberndorfer in 1909 proposed the term 'carcinoid' to describe tumours with a 'carcinoma-like' structure. However, this term became associated with tumours producing defined clinical features which were later attributed to the production and release of serotonin. It is now known that this class of tumour may or may not produce serotonin and thus, in certain circumstances the word carcinoid may be mis-leading. Since these tumours originate from the so-called 'diffuse neuro-endocrine system' the name neuro-endocrine tumours has been suggested. APUDomas is an alternative term not much favoured. These tumours are defined as being derived from cells of the APUD (amine precursor uptake and decarboxy-lation) system. The term APUD was coined by Pearse to describe certain cytochemical and functional characteristics of cells belonging to the diffuse neuro-endocrine system. Although these tumours often produce more than one regulatory peptide (mixed endocrine tumours), usually one circulating peptide is responsible for the associated clinical syndrome. In such cases, the name of this active secretory product is used to describe the tumour, e.g. gastrinoma, insulinoma. The most commonly used terminology, however, is that of peptide-producing endo-crine tumours, or just simply endocrine or neuro-endocrine tumours.

16.17.2   Clinical and biochemical features

It is difficult to assess the true incidence of endocrine tumours, but well-recognized functioning tumours are clearly uncom-mon. Schein and co-workers calculated an incidence of less than 1 in 100 000 per year. Clinically silent, non-secreting tumours, however, are found in approximately 1 per cent un-selected autopsies. Endocrine tumours are often characterized by the hypersecretion of active regulatory peptides which are responsible for their clinical manifestation. However, clinical features induced by some functional tumours may be obscured by the presence in the circulation of more than one regulatory peptide with counter-active effects. In addition to hormonal effects, non-specific manifestations, depending on site, size, and invasion, may be present. Clinical suspicion is usually aroused when more common diseases have been excluded. This some-times delays diagnosis with adverse effects on the prognosis. Many pre-operative, non-invasive techniques are also widely used, including a series of stimulation and suppression tests for the particular hormone. Further, a series of localization tech-niques, in particular angiography, ultrasound, or isotope scan-ning and high-resolution computerized tomography, are used. Percutaneous, trans-hepatic portal and pancreatic venous sam-pling, with parallel measurement in systemic blood, may also be useful. Other localization techniques include radioisotope-tagged, specific antibodies and nuclear magnetic resonance. Highly sensitive and specific radioimmunoassays for the measurement of regulatory peptides in blood and tissue are readily available, allowing early diagnosis of functioning tumours. Thus, very small tumours may be diagnosed clinically and biochemically, presenting a challenge to specialists in 'localization techniques' and to surgeons. However, it must be remembered that circulating levels of active peptides can be elevated in diseases other than tumours, for example, gastrin in atrophic gastritis. Such cases must be excluded before making the diagnosis of endocrine tumour.

16.17.3 Histology

The growth pattern of endocrine tumours is quite characteristic. The tumours are composed of uniform cells with little atypia and few mitoses, arranged in irregular masses, ribbons, or glandular structures (Fig. 16.227). It has been claimed, in the past, that a specific growth pattern may have some diagnostic significance in the typing of tumours. However, this view is not uniformly accepted and, in our experience and that of others, the criterion of growth pattern has proved unreliable for precise diagnosis. The use of antibodies to neurone-specific enolase and to chromogranin (Fig. 16.228), as well as silver

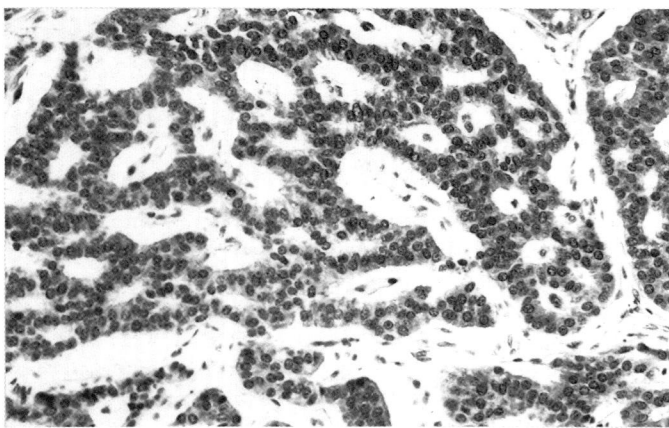

Fig. 16.227 Haematoxylin and eosin stain of a pancreatic β-cell (insulin-producing) tumour. Regular cells with round to ovoid nuclei are arranged mainly in ribbons, separated by fine tissue stroma.

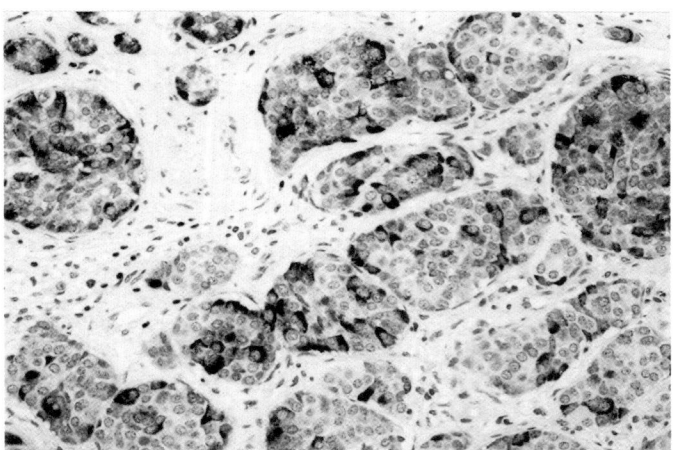

Fig. 16.228 A mid-gut carcinoid tumour immunostained for chromogranin A using the peroxidase anti-peroxidase technique. Tumour cells are arranged in nests within which scattered immunoreactive cells can be distinguished. (Haematoxylin counterstain.)

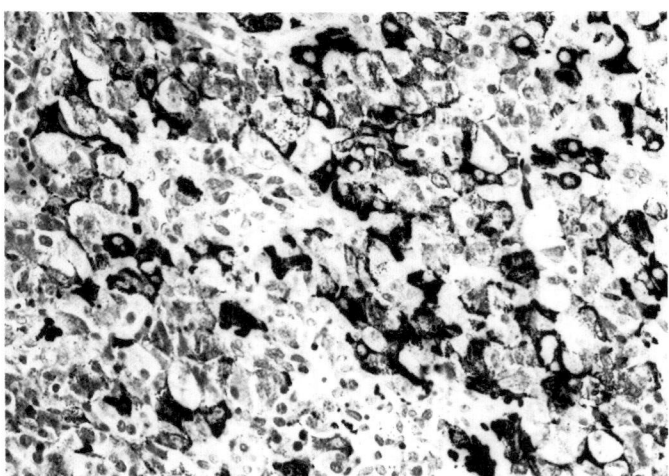

Fig. 16.229 A pancreatic A-cell (glucagon-producing) tumour stained using the silver impregnation technique of Grimelius. Argyrophil cells are full of black deposit. (Haematoxylin counterstain.)

impregnation methods, in particular Grimelius's silver impregnation technique (Fig. 16.229), are of good diagnostic value. Hyalinization of the tumour stroma is common and sometimes extensive. It is seen particularly in some classes of tumours, such as insulinomas, medullary carcinomas of the thyroid, VIPomas, etc. It was first noted that parts of the hyalinized areas were positive for amyloid stains and ultrastructurally possessed the characteristic fibrillary processes. It has been claimed that this substance is related to the hormone produced by the tumours. Classical histochemical stains for amyloid (e.g. tryptophan and tyrosine) are negative and therefore it is possible that this amyloid is chemically different from classical amyloid. Specific names have been proposed, such as APUD amyloid or endocrine- or tissue-associated amyloid. Chemical characterization of this amyloid has revealed that in certain tumours (e.g. medullary carcinoma of the thyroid) part of the pro-hormone sequence is found. In others, however, e.g. insulinomas, a characteristic protein has been isolated which shows partial sequence homology with a novel neuropeptide, termed calcitonin gene-related peptide. Assessment of malignancy may be difficult histologically. This class of tumours is slow growing and, unless there is clear-cut evidence of massive infiltration into neighbouring tissue or the presence of metastases, it may be impossible to predict behaviour. A more functional criterion of malignancy has been proposed recently. This is the production and release of alpha human choriogonadotrophic hormone (HCG) by many malignant endocrine tumours, in particular pancreatic endocrine tumours, although 30 per cent of those which behave malignantly show no reactivity for HCG. In other sites, for instance the lung, this criterion is even less reliable, for benign carcinoid tumours of the lung frequently react on immunocytochemistry to antibodies to α-HCG. Tumours with mixed endocrine cell types seem to respond better to chemotherapy (e.g. streptozotocin).

16.17.4 Techniques for demonstrating neuro-endocrine differentiation

Accurate determination of neuro-endocrine differentiation is achieved routinely by the application of specialized methods, including silver impregnation procedures and conventional electron microscopy. Immunocytochemistry may be applied, at both light and electron-microscopical levels, and can be directed at specific markers (e.g. peptide/amine) and more general ones (e.g. neurone-specific enolase, chromogranins). Peptide-producing endocrine cells are frequently unevenly distributed within a tumour. It is therefore very important to sample a large number of specimens taken randomly throughout the tumour mass.

Silver impregnation methods

The procedures most frequently used can be subdivided broadly into argyrophil and argentaffin reactions. Cells displaying argyrophilia take up silver ions from the impregnation solution, but visible metallic silver only appears after a subsequent reducing process brought about by an external agent or agents. Cells showing argentaffinity contain one or more chemical substances which retain silver ions from ammoniacal silver solution and reduce them to metallic silver. In contrast to the argyrophil reaction, the chemistry of argentaffin staining is better understood. It would appear that serotonin (5-hydroxytryptamine, 5-HT) reacts with paraformaldehyde to cause a silver reaction. Some variants of the original Masson argentaffin reaction are frequently used. Numerous argyrophil stains have been proposed. Of these the most reliable and commonly used is that introduced by Lars Grimelius which stains most endocrine cell types and tumours. The staining is characteristically granular and is positive in most granule-containing endocrine cells or tumours. Poorly granulated tumours are rarely argyrophilic.

Electron microscopy

By electron microscopy, endocrine tumours can be seen to contain variable numbers of secretory granules (Fig. 16.230) but often peptide-producing tumour cells store less peptide than their normal counterparts. Neurosecretory granules of APUD-omas are, in general, spherical or polymorphic (average size ranging from 100 to 350 nm) and are surrounded by a limiting membrane that is either closely apposed or loosely attached, leaving a clear halo between the electron-dense core and the membrane. It is generally accepted that a poorly granulated tumour reflects high secretory activity and poor storage capacity. The former frequently correlates with the presence of abundant ribosomes, rough endoplasmic reticulum, and prominent Golgi apparatus. Moreover, early studies have shown that poorly granulated tumours are characterized biochemically by significantly elevated levels of circulating hormones. This suggests that one of the metabolic defects in the endocrine tumour cell resides in the control of synthesis and secretion. Partial or complete loss of control of secretion by the tumour cells results in inappropriate production and secretion of peptides. At

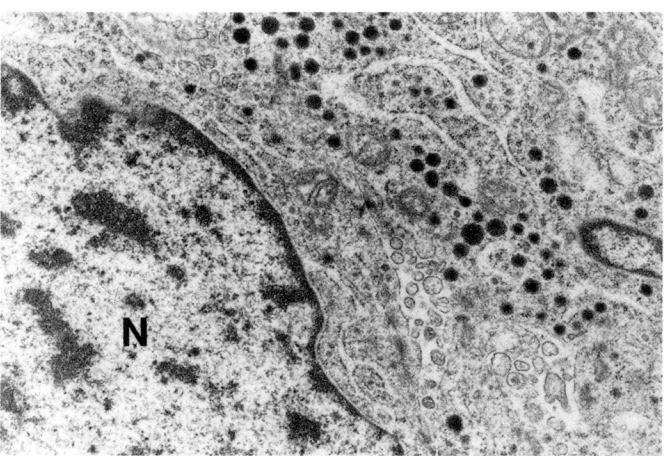

Fig. 16.230 Electron micrograph of a gastric microcarcinoid, showing typical electron-dense secretory granules lying in the cell cytoplasm (N = nucleus).

present, the process behind the defective conversion remains unknown.

Immunocytochemistry

Immunocytochemistry has revolutionized the study of neuro-endocrine tumours. Polyclonal sera and monoclonal antibodies are now widely available and staining can be performed, mostly using conventional fixation and embedding procedures, for both light and electron microscopy. Antibodies are now available to a number of intracellular antigens, grouped under the term of 'general neuro-endocrine markers'. Furthermore, region-specific antibodies to regulatory peptides are now widely and commercially available.

Antibodies to 'general neuro-endocrine markers'

Neurone-specific enolase (NSE) Neurone-specific enolase is an isoenzyme of the glycolytic enzyme enolase, originally extracted from the rat brain and subsequently found by immunocytochemistry to be localized to neurones. Antibodies to NSE were later found to immunostain all components of the diffuse neuro-endocrine system. NSE is an enzyme unrelated to the presence of secretory granules. In view of its putative involvement in metabolism and its non-granular cytoplasmic localization, its presence may indicate the functional state of an endocrine cell or tumour. The staining is often rather diffuse in the cytoplasm, with poorly defined areas. It is important to be selective when choosing antibodies to NSE as it is a large protein, of molecular weight 78 000, and therefore populations of antibodies are likely to react to many separate epitopes of the molecule. The protein, which has not yet been produced synthetically, is currently extracted from animal or human brain. Therefore, it is likely that the antigen will be contaminated with material other than pure NSE and thus spurious staining of non-neuronal elements could be expected. Monoclonal antibodies to NSE are now becoming available and it is predicted that a good mixture of high-quality monoclonal antibodies which would recognize several epitopes of the molecule will be of excellent value for morphologists.

Chromogranins, pancreastatin, GAWK, and CCB The acidic soluble proteins of chromaffin granules have been collectively named chromogranins. During the last few years these chromogranins have been analysed and characterized in great detail, their physico-chemical properties and biosynthetic pathways established, and, in 1986, the primary DNA sequence of pre-pro-chromogranin was obtained. The physiological functions of these characteristic proteins is, however, still unknown. Originally, it was thought that these proteins are involved in a storage complex with catecholamines. More recent studies, demonstrating a widespread distribution of chromogranins not only in catecholamine-containing but also in endocrine cells and nerves of the 'diffuse neuro-endocrine system' have, however, called this finding into question.

Chromogranin is the generic term, which includes a number of separate proteins. These have been variously named but an agreed classification for the chromogranins has been proposed at a meeting of the New York Academy of Sciences. Chromogranins are now divided into three main classes: chromogranin A (= parathyroid secretory protein I), chromogranin B (= secretogranin 1), and chromogranin C (= secretogranin 2). Chromogranin A is abundant in chromaffin tissue and corresponds to at least 50 per cent of the protein of the bovine chromaffin granule matrix. It has been shown recently, by both biochemical and cDNA analysis, to show close similarity to parathyroid secretory protein I. Chromagranin A is present in the central and peripheral nervous systems, in the anterior pituitary, the parathyroid gland, and in peptide-producing endocrine cells of the 'diffuse neuro-endocrine system'. The other chromogranins are less abundantly present and show a more limited distribution either in chromaffin or non-chromaffin (e.g. pituitary) tissue. Chromogranin immunoreactivity is found in the storage granules of cells of the diffuse neuro-endocrine system, and the presence of chromogranin in peptide-producing endocrine tumours has been reported by many workers. Secretion of chromogranin-immunoreactive material into plasma can be found in a variety of neuro-endocrine neoplasms. Deduction of the cDNA sequence of bovine chromogranins revealed within the structure of chromogranin A the presence of pancreastatin, a 49 amino-acid peptide originally extracted from the porcine pancreas and shown to inhibit glucose-induced insulin release; and from the structure of chromogranin B, two further peptides: GAWK, a peptide originally extracted from the anterior pituitary, and a peptide termed CCB (C-terminal carboxyl peptide of chromogranin B).

Protein gene product 9.5 (PGP 9.5) is a recently extracted soluble brain protein of molecular weight 27 000. It would appear to be a reasonably good marker for the immunocytochemical identification of neuro-endocrine tumours, although it is possibly less reliable than chromogranins or NSE, due to its broader immunoreactivity and presence in non-neuro-endocrine tissue.

7B2 (APPG) is a large protein originally discovered by Chretien's group in the anterior pituitary of the pig, hence its alternative name APPG. Its name derives from the initial chromatographic peak obtained during analysis of extractable pituitary material. Antibodies to a segment of this protein have now been raised and used in radioimmunoassay and immunohistochemical procedures. 7B2 immunoreactivity is present in most neuro-endocrine cells and derivative tumours, in particular β-cells and insulinomas.

Synaptophysin or P38 is a Ca^{2+}-binding, glycosylated polypeptide of molecular weight 38 000 that is an integral component of pre-synaptic vesicles of a variety of mammalian species. This protein also exists in a range of normal neuro-endocrine cells and their derivative tumours.

Region-specific peptide antibodies

The structures of a number of regulatory peptides and prohormones have been disclosed by molecular biological techniques in recent years, frequently by the use of extracts of neuro-endocrine tumours. This is not surprising since the production of regulatory peptides by tumours is a well-recognized phenomenon. The ability to develop peptide antibodies, recognizing various portions of the pro-molecule is advantageous for the study of neuro-endocrine tumours, both from biochemical and morphological viewpoints, since some tumours are known to produce, store, and release abnormal molecular forms of peptides. Furthermore, these antibodies have been used successfully at the ultrastructural level, in particular by gold-immunolabelling procedures.

16.17.5 Main features of gastrointestinal neuro-endocrine tumours

The marked heterogeneity observed in endocrine tumours of the gastrointestinal tract reflects the variety of endocrine cell types producing peptides/amines present in the mucosal epithelium. It was thus with foresight that Williams and Sandler in 1963 re-evaluated the variety of endocrine tumours of the gastrointestinal tract and proposed a classification according to their morphological features, functional capacity, and embryological origin. These authors divided the neoplasms into three main groups: foregut, endocrine tumours arising from the tracheo-bronchial tree, stomach, duodenum, and pancreas; midgut tumours, originating from the duodenum, ileum, appendix, ascending colon, and sometimes Meckel diverticulum; and hindgut tumours arising from transverse, descending, or sigmoid colon and rectum. The authors also pointed out that midgut carcinoid tumours were in general argentaffin (as well as argyrophil), whereas foregut carcinoid tumours were argyrophilic but not argentaffin and hindgut carcinoids were mostly negative for silver stains. Although the advent of novel technology and better knowledge of the nature of these tumours suggested that this classification represents an oversimplification, it still provides a useful frame of reference in dealing with most carcinoid tumours. Ultrastructurally, midgut carcinoid tumours have cells with large, dense, polymorphic, argentaffin secretory granules; foregut carcinoid tumour cells have small, round granules, frequently with a prominent halo between the electron-dense core and the membrane; and hindgut carcinoids have larger, round granules with a tightly apposed membrane. Endocrine tumours of the gut, although of slow growth and spread, can metastasize to many parts of the body.

The histological and cytological appearance of endocrine tumours is not a reliable criterion to determine their malignant potential, since many malignant carcinoid tumours, primary and metastatic, lack cellular atypia and have very low mitotic rates. The only reliable indication for malignancy is the presence of distant metastases, extensive invasion of adjacent tissues, or permeation of vascular tissue. It is nowadays accepted that most, if not all, endocrine tumours carry the potential for long-range malignant behaviour. Their behaviour is not identical in all endocrine tumours of the gastrointestinal tract, thus only 1–10 per cent of appendiceal carcinoid tumours metastasize and 8 per cent of rectal, 28 per cent of gastric, 50 per cent of colonic, and 47–75 per cent of ileal carcinoid tumours. Tumours of less than 1 cm in diameter only rarely mestatasize, whereas a large proportion of tumours measuring more than 2 cm in diameter frequently show distant spread to lymph nodes and liver.

Foregut endocrine tumours

Endocrine tumours of the foregut are rare. They constitute only about 4 per cent of the total number of gastrointestinal tumours. However, the frequency of carcinoid tumours of the duodenum related to that of other tumours is quite high (about 30 per cent) since, for unknown reasons, the duodenal mucosa is quite resistant to the development of non-endocrine adenocarcinomas. There have been a few reports on the occurrence of the carcinoid syndrome, Zollinger–Ellison syndrome, and Cushing's syndrome due to hormone secretion from gastric and duodenal carcinoid tumours but, on the whole, endocrine syndromes from these tumours seem to be infrequent and unpredictable. Foregut carcinoid tumours may arise in the oesophagus, stomach, duodenum (including ampulla of Vater), pancreas, biliary tree, bronchial tree and lung, and, rarely, thymus. A number of foregut carcinoid tumours from stomach, pancreas, and bronchial tree have been associated with a peculiar atypical carcinoid syndrome, characterized by a red rather than cyanotic flushing, probably caused by the release of 5-hydroxytryptophan and, in some cases, histamine. Tumours of the foregut are, in general, argyrophil by both Grimelius' and Sevier–Munger's silver impregnation method, and nearly always negative with methods for agentaffinity. The incidence of foregut tumours is now increasing or, at least, this entity is more readily recognizable. This may be due partly to the development of therapeutic regimes for the treatment of gastric hypersecretion associated in particular with duodenal ulceration. A number of drugs are used nowadays (e.g. H$_2$ receptor blockers) and, in particular, a new generation of drugs aimed at

total blockade of gastric acid secretion (e.g. proton-pump inhibitors), which produce marked hypochlorhydria and subsequent reactive hypergastrinaemia. This drug-induced hypochlorhydria is analogous to that seen in atrophic gastritis, with or without association with pernicious anaemia, which also shows secondary hypergastrinaemia. Gastrin is trophic to the gastric mucosa and in particular to a specific endocrine cell-type, prevalent in the fundic mucosa, termed the enterochromaffin-like (ECL or EC-like) cell. This cell has a characteristically elongated shape with no lumenal contact. The peptide product of ECL cells, which contain characteristic secretory granules, is as yet unknown, but ECL cells in rodents have been shown to produce histamine. ECL cells are stained specifically by argyrophil silver impregnation methods or by immunocytochemistry with antibodies to general neuro-endocrine markers, e.g. chromogranins. These cells have shown various degrees of proliferation from micronodular formation up to the clear development of carcinoid endocrine tumours of the body of the stomach (Fig. 16.231). These tumours may extrude towards the lumen of the stomach (polypoid type) or grow towards the gastric wall (scirrhous or infiltrating type). The peptide or amine product of this gastric carcinoid tumour remains to be elucidated. These tumours tend to be multiple and their development is sometimes preceded by diffuse and nodular hyperplasia of ECL cells.

Antral and duodenal carcinoid tumours are less frequent than those of the non-antral stomach; these tumours are usually argyrophil and non-argentaffin, do not display formalin-induced fluorescence, and are devoid of serotonin. They tend to produce multiple peptide hormones, among which gastrin and somatostatin are found most frequently. The histogenesis of duodenal carcinoid tumours may be difficult to establish. If the tumour is growing in the surrounding tissues, it cannot be determined with certainty whether it has arisen from endocrine cells of the duodenal mucosa, pancreatic ducts, or from pancreatic islets. Since the initial observation of a somatostatinoma in the pancreas and the duodenum, 18 cases of somatostatinomas have so far been reported in the duodenum. Gangliocytic

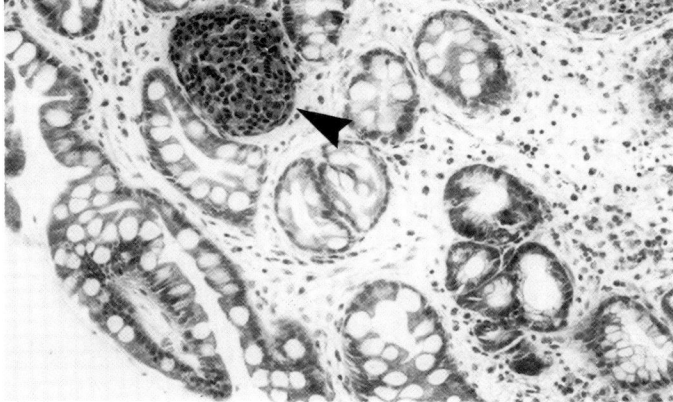

Fig. 16.231 Lower-power micrograph of gastric epithelium showing extensive intestinal metaplasia. A carcinoid tumour nodule can be seen in the lamina propria (arrow) immunostained for chromogranin A. (Peroxidase anti-peroxidase method with haematoxylin counterstain.)

paragangliomas of the duodenum with psammomatous bodies have also been reported. Neurogenic tumours of the gastro-intestinal tract, including duodenal paragangliomas (Fig. 16.232) are uncommon. The tumours are usually found in a second part of the duodenum and often cause abdominal pain, discomfort, or gastrointestinal bleeding. Sometimes these may be incidental findings at surgery or autopsy. The histologic features vary, with characteristics resembling paraganglioma, ganglioneuroma, and carcinoid tumours.

The reported average age for presentation with a benign duodenal lesion is 56 years. Usually, the tumours have a polypoid appearance and can thus be identified on endoscopy. The frequent finding of pancreatic polypeptide immunoreactivity in these duodenal paragangliomas supports the hypothesis that duodenal paragangliomas are hyperplastic or neoplastic proliferations of endodermally derived epithelial cells originating from the ventral primordium of the pancreas. Furthermore, somatostatin immunoreactivity was found in both epithelial and ganglion cells, a finding that further supports the postulated pancreatic origin of this tumour. Most of the foregut tumours tend to grow slowly and allow lengthy survival.

Midgut carcinoid tumours

Midgut carcinoid tumours form a remarkably homogeneous group, both from the morphological and functional viewpoints, in spite of the fact that numerous hormones are produced by separate endocrine cell types in this anatomical area of the gut. This variability is also remarkable considering that their biological behaviour differs considerably. Whereas appendiceal carcinoid tumours seldom show malignant features and are frequently incidental discoveries, up to one-half of ileal carcinoid tumours show malignant behaviour at one point or other. Grossly, midgut carcinoid tumours appear as yellow-greyish masses which are often located in the submucosa and protrude into the lumen of the gut. Appendiceal carcinoid tumours are usually discovered during surgery and most are located at the tip of the appendix and may or may not be visible on gross examination of the outer surface. Histologically, midgut carcinoid tumours show nests and sheets of uniform, polygonal cells with abundant cytoplasm and round central nuclei, separated by slender strands of fibrovascular stroma. Mitoses and atypias are rare. After silver impregnations, midgut carcinoid tumours, as a rule, are both argentaffin and argyrophil (Fig. 16.233). Ultrastructurally, the electron-dense secretory granules are polymorphic, very dense and large if the cells are argentaffin, and round with closely apposed membrane and of various sizes and lesser electron density if the cells are argyrophilic. Tumours of the midgut may produce a variety of regulatory peptides but they are mostly associated with the production of serotonin and neurokinins. Primary midgut carcinoid tumours are clinically 'silent' as a rule, except when massive metastases occur in the liver or in the lung, in which case they may be associated with a syndrome. The carcinoid syndrome encompasses a spectrum of clinical and biochemical manifestations associated with the presence of some functional carcinoid tumours, and includes skin flushing, episodic watery diarrhoea, and fibrotic changes in the heart. The physiopathology of the syndrome has been discussed extensively but not fully elucidated.

Hindgut carcinoid tumours

Hindgut carcinoid tumours are rare in the colon but relatively more frequent in the rectum, where they are often discovered incidentally during routine rectal examination. Grossly, rectal carcinoid tumours appear as rounded, somewhat elastic masses, located in the submucosa and covered by a reddened, sometimes friable or bleeding mucosa. Histologically, hindgut carcinoid tumour cells display a typical arrangement in nests and cords, often showing extensive areas with a trabecular pattern, which characterize these tumours elsewhere. Application

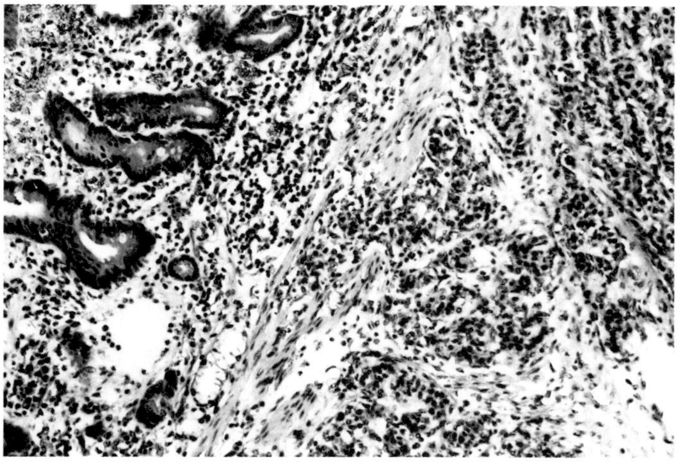

Fig. 16.232 Haematoxylin and eosin stain of a submucosal duodenal gangliocytic paraganglioma. This benign tumour is not encapsulated and consists of a mixture of spindle and paraganglion-like cells with scattered ganglia.

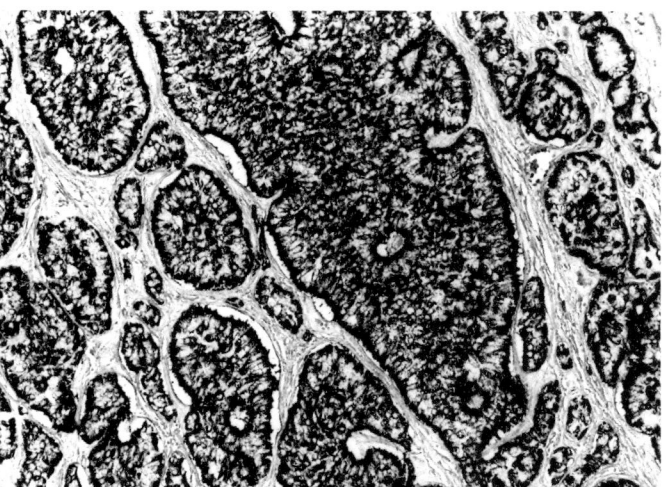

Fig. 16.233 A low-power micrograph of a midgut carcinoid tumour with cells arranged in typical sheets and nests. Dense argyrophilia is shown by Grimelius' silver impregnation technique.

of silver stains is, in general, unrewarding and a variety of regulatory peptides, in particular those of the glucagon and pancreatic polypeptide families, have been reported to be associated with these tumours. Functionally, the great majority of hindgut carcinoid tumours are clinically 'silent'. The symptoms sometimes associated with the presence of these tumours include pain, bleeding, and occasional bouts of diarrhoea. These can be attributed readily to the mechanical trauma inflicted by the passage of solid faeces.

Mixed exo/endocrine tumours

The association of non-endocrine and endocrine proliferations in tumours has been reported frequently in the gastrointestinal tract and a number of terms have been used, including amphicrine tumour, mucocarcinoid tumour, etc.

16.17.6 Further reading

Ch'ng, J. L. C., Polak, J. M., and Bloom, S. R. (1985). Endocrine syndromes. In *Endocrine tumours. The pathobiology of regulatory peptide-producing tumours* (ed. J. M. Polak and S. R. Bloom), pp. 264–80. Churchill Livingstone, Edinburgh.

Doran, J. F., Jackson, P., Kynoch, F. A. M., and Thompson, R. J. (1983). Isolation of PGP 9.5, a new human neurone-specific protein detected by high resolution two-dimensional electrophoresis. *Journal of Neurochemistry* 40, 1542–7.

Fischer-Colbrie, R., Hagn, C., and Schober, M. (1987). Chromogranins A, B and C: Widespread constituents of secretory vesicles. *Annals of the New York Academy of Sciences* 493, 120–34.

Grimelius, L. and Wilander, E. (1985). Silver impregnation and other non-immunocytochemical staining methods. In *Endocrine tumours. The pathobiology of regulatory peptide-producing tumours* (ed. J. M. Polak and S. R. Bloom), pp. 95–115. Churchill Livingstone, Edinburgh.

Hakanson, R. and Sundler, F. (ed) (1986). Mechanisms for the development of gastric carcinoids. *Digestion* 35, S1.

Hamid, Q. A., *et al.* (1986). Duodenal gangliocytic paragangliomas: A study of 10 cases with immunocytochemical neuroendocrine markers. *Human Pathology* 17, 1151–7.

Heitz, P. U., Kasper, M., Kloppel, G., Polak, J. M., and Vaitukaitis, J. L. (1983). Glycoprotein-hormone alpha-chain production by pancreatic endocrine tumours: a specific marker for malignancy. *Cancer* 51, 277–82.

Lasson, A., Alwmark, A., Nobin, A., and Sundler, F. (1983). Endocrine tumours of the duodenum. *Annals of Surgery* 197, 393–8.

Pearse, A. G. E. (1969). The cytochemistry and ultrastructure of polypeptide hormone-producing cells of the APUD series, and the embryologic, physiologic and pathologic implications of the concept. *Journal of Histochemistry and Cytochemistry* 17, 303–13.

Pearse, A. G. E., Ewen, S. W. B., and Polak, J. M. (1972). The genesis of apudamyloid in endocrine polypeptide tumours: Histochemical distinction from immunamyloid. *Virchows Archiv B Cell Pathology* 10, 93–107.

Polak, J. M. and Bloom, S. R. (1979). The diffuse neuroendocrine system. *Journal of Histochemistry and Cytochemistry* 27, 1398–1400.

Polak, J. M. and Marangos, P. J. (1984). Neurone-specific enolase, a marker for neuroendocrine cells. In *Evolution and tumour pathology of the neuroendocrine system* (ed. S. Falkmer, R. Hakanson, and F. Sundler), pp. 433–80. Elsevier, Amsterdam.

Polak, J. M. and Van Noorden, S. (eds) (1986). *Immunocytochemistry: modern methods and applications* (2nd edn) John Wright and Sons, Bristol.

Polak, J. M. and Varndell, I. M. (eds) (1984). *Immunolabelling for electron microscopy*. Elsevier, Amsterdam.

Williams, E. D. and Sandler, M. (1963). The classification of carcinoid tumours. *Lancet* i, 238–9.

16.18 The anus

N. A. Shepherd

16.18.1 Haemorrhoids

Haemorrhoids (piles) are the commonest cause of anorectal bleeding. They result from dilatation of the vascular spaces of the internal haemorrhoidal plexus. Whether these vessels represent dilated and varicose veins or arterio-venous communications is controversial. It is probable that haemorrhoids are enlarged anal cushions, normal structures containing blood vessels, connective tissue, and smooth muscle, which contribute to anal canal closure by close apposition to each other. The histological appearance of the anal cushion is like that of erectile tissue, which normally contains numerous arterio-venous communications. There is further evidence against the theory that haemorrhoids are merely ectatic veins of the haemorrhoidal plexus: haemorrhoids are not a significant feature of portal hypertension and the vascular spaces within haemorrhoids have abundant smooth muscle which is far in excess of that normally seen in veins of the equivalent size.

Macroscopic appearances

Haemorrhoids are plum-coloured soft swellings which are consistently positioned in the right anterior, right posterior, and left lateral quadrants of the anus. They may have both an internal component in the anal canal and an external component at the anal verge. These two components have vascular connections. Chronic haemorrhoids may cause skin tags at the anal verge, and fibrous anal polyp, a pedunculated polyp lined by squamous epithelium which arises from the dentate line, probably represents an atrophied haemorrhoid.

Microscopic appearances

Histological examination of haemorrhoids reveals thick-walled vascular spaces in the submucosa of the anal canal. The vessels have abundant smooth muscle in their walls. They frequently contain thrombi at various stages of organization and there is often extensive stromal haemorrhage (Fig. 16.234). The overlying mucosa may include both rectal- and anal-type epithelium and there may be ulceration, squamous metaplasia of rectal-type mucosa, and the histological changes of mucosal prolapse.

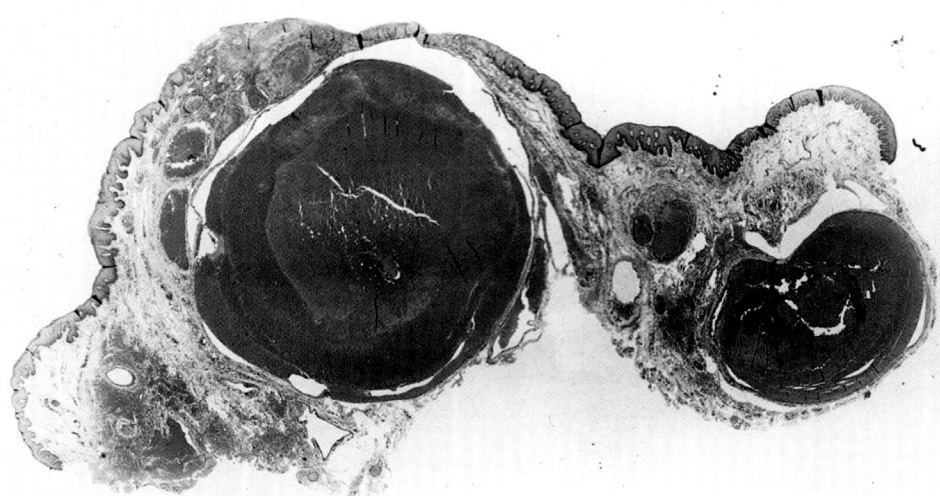

Fig. 16.234 A photomicrograph of a thrombosed haemorrhoid. There is extensive stromal haemorrhage.

Complications

Complications of haemorrhoids include haemorrhage, thrombosis, strangulation with ischaemic necrosis, prolapse, and infection. Haemorrhoids may cause significant anaemia due to chronic blood loss and very occasionally the haemorrhage may be life-threatening.

16.18.2   Inflammation

Fissures

A fissure is the commonest form of anal ulceration. It is usually seen in young adults but may occur in children. Although they can occur at any point on the circumference of the anal canal, fissures are most often common in the midline posteriorly. Anterior fissures are more often seen in females. The cause is uncertain but the passage of hard faeces with subsequent trauma is a factor. Patients are not, however, always constipated and fissure *in ano* may be associated with diarrhoea. Fissures are accompanied by spasm of the internal sphincter and treatment is aimed at relaxation of this sphincter.

A fissure appears as a longitudinal elliptical ulcer in the squamous mucosa of the lower anal canal. Frequently there is an oedematous polyp at the lower edge of the fissure, the sentinel pile. The edges of the ulcer may be undermined. Histologically the ulcer bed is lined by granulation tissue and there is non-specific chronic inflammation and oedema in the adjacent stroma. It is mandatory to examine all tissues excised or curetted from anal fissures for epithelioid cell granulomas: fissures are the commonest anal manifestation of Crohn's disease. Other conditions, such as tuberculosis, syphilis, anal Paget's disease, and anorectal sepsis, may also be associated with fissure *in ano*.

Anorectal sepsis—abscesses and fistulae

These conditions are best considered together as they often co-exist and the pathogenesis is similar. Anorectal sepsis is prob-

ably most commonly caused by infection of the anal glands. Microbiological evidence indicates two major groups of patients. One group comprises the anal equivalent of cutaneous abscesses, are caused predominantly by staphylococci, never develop into fistulae, and are adequately treated by simple drainage. The second group, which causes more morbidity, is often associated with fistula formation and the causative organisms are usually enteric Gram-negative bacilli. The study of both conditions requires an understanding of the anatomy of the anal canal and the interested reader is referred to Goligher's *Surgery of the anus, rectum and colon* (1984) for an excellent clinical anatomic account. There are five main types of anorectal fistula and five major sites of anorectal abscess. These are demonstrated in Fig. 16.235. The distinction between these five types of fistula is not always exact. It should be emphasized that low fistulae, the subcutaneous and intersphincteric types, are much commoner than the extensive, and often complicated, high-level fistulae.

Pathogenesis

True anorectal abscesses and fistulae are the consequence of infection of the anal glands, which in turn may be caused by obstruction due to faecal material, foreign bodies, and trauma. The glands are predominantly submucosal and infection of these glands results in the low-level submucosal fistulae. A few glands, however, penetate the internal sphincter and inflammation of these glands may cause the extensive high-level type of fistula. Most fistulous tracts have their internal opening at the site of an anal gland orifice. The anal gland ducts are lined by prominent lymphoid tissue which may act as a focus of inflammation. Hyperplasia of this lymphoid tissue has led to comparisons with the lymphoid tissue of the tonsil and nasopharynx and the epithet of anal tonsil.

Microscopic features

The fistula tracts are lined by granulation tissue although re-

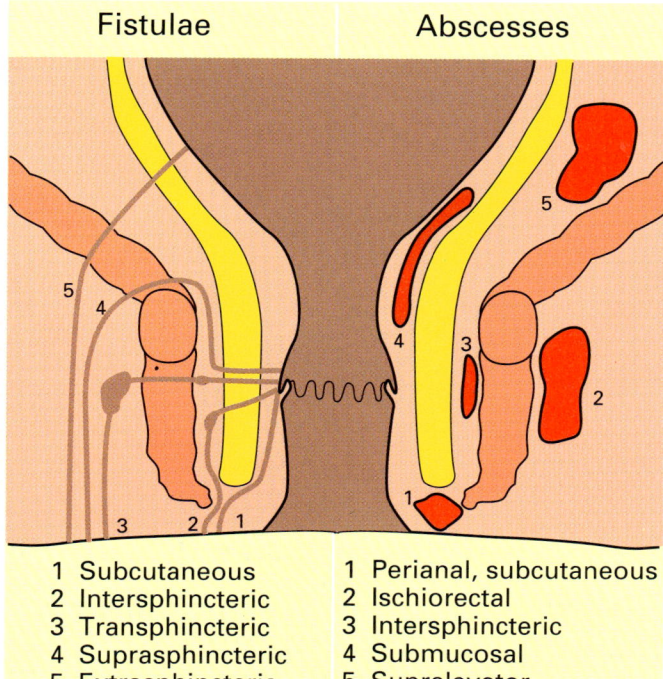

Fistulae

1 Subcutaneous
2 Intersphincteric
3 Transphincteric
4 Suprasphincteric
5 Extrasphincteric

Abscesses

1 Perianal, subcutaneous
2 Ischiorectal
3 Intersphincteric
4 Submucosal
5 Supralevator

Fig. 16.235 The five main types of anorectal fistula and five major sites of anorectal abscess.

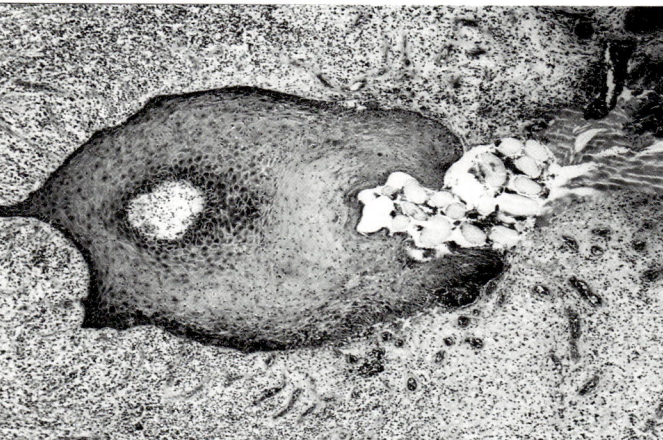

Fig. 16.236 Histological appearance of a pilonidal sinus. The sinus is lined by stratified squamous epithelium and numerous hair shafts are present. There is granulation tissue around the sinus.

epithelialization by both squamous and rectal-type mucosa may occur. A foreign body giant cell reaction to faecal debris and undigested food particles is not an unusual feature. Oleogranulomas, foci of foamy macrophages containing lipid vacuoles, are the result of packing of the tracts with oily liniments. Fistulae may be a manifestation of anal Crohn's disease and epithelioid cell granulomas may be seen in the inflamed tissues. Mucinous adenocarcinoma is a rare complication of anorectal fistulae.

Pilonidal sinus and abscess

Pilonidal sinus is most common in young adults, particularly men. Hirsutism and chronic irritation are aetiological factors and the lesions are thought to be the result of penetration of the skin of the natal cleft by hair shafts. Single or multiple pits are seen in the skin in this region. Secondary infection leads to abscess formation. Histologically a sinus lined by stratified squamous epithelium and granulation tissue is seen and hair shafts, with an associated foreign body giant cell reaction, are usually, though not invariably, present (Fig. 16.236).

Crohn's disease

One-quarter of all patients subsequently diagnosed as Crohn's disease present with anal disease. At least half of all patients with colorectal Crohn's disease have accompanying anal pathology. Anal Crohn's disease is less common in patients with small bowel involvement alone. In a series of 127 patients with anal Crohn's disease studied at St Mark's Hospital, 59 had a fissure,

34 had a fistula or abscess, and 22 had skin tags. A characteristic macroscopic appearance of anal involvement is a blue-crimson discoloration of the skin. High-level fistulation is most commonly caused by Crohn's disease.

Histological examination of anal Crohn's disease reveals focal but extensive surface ulceration. Transmural inflammation, which is so characteristic of small and large intestinal Crohn's disease, may be seen, but is often less marked in the anal canal. Fissuring ulceration is common and granulomas are more often present in anal Crohn's disease than in intestinal Crohn's disease. The granulomas may contain a central focus of necrosis and this should not be taken as evidence of tuberculosis.

Hidradenitis suppurativa

This chronic suppurating and scarring skin condition predominantly affects those areas where apocrine sweat glands are concentrated. Axillae, breast, genitalia, and perianal skin are the common sites. The disease has been considered as a primary inflammation of apocrine sweat glands, although more recently a primary folliculitis has been postulated. Certainly the inflammation is centred on hair follicles but the disease is rare in regions where apocrine sweat glands are absent. Hidradenitis suppurativa is more common in males, and hormonal factors have been implicated in the pathogenesis. The persistent active inflammation that characterizes the conditon may lead to extensive scarring. The histological appearances are not specific but include an active inflammation in and around skin adnexae, including hair follicles and sweat glands, focal chronic inflammation of the dermis, and extensive fibrosis.

16.18.3 Specific infections

Syphilis

Primary chancres are relatively common in the anus and perianal skin of homosexuals and may mimic fissures, fistulae, or malignant tumours. Histological examination is not usually undertaken and the diagnosis is established by examination of a smear under dark-ground illumination, where the motile spirochaetes will be seen.

Tuberculosis

Anal tuberculosis is now very rare in Britain, although it is on occasion seen in immigrants from those countries where pulmonary and intestinal tuberculosis are still relatively common. Patients may present with anal ulceration, nearly always secondary to tuberculosis elsewhere, usually in the lungs. Tuberculosis may cause chronic abscesses and complex fistulae. Again, this type is usually secondary to pulmonary tuberculosis. Histological examination reveals the classical features of tuberculosis. There are epithelioid cell granulomas, Langhans-type giant cells and extensive caseous necrosis. In the acute, ulcerating form of anal tuberculosis, acid-fast bacilli are easy to demonstrate on Ziehl–Neelsen staining, whereas in the most chronic form with fistulae, they may be sparse or absent and it may be difficult to differentiate tuberculosis from Crohn's disease.

Lymphogranuloma inguinale

Lymphogranuloma inguinale, a tropical and subtropical chronic scarring disease, more commonly affects the rectum, particularly in females, but may result in fissures, fistulae, and extensive fibrosis of the anal canal, with obstruction of lymphatics leading to perianal elephantiasis. The aetiological agent is *Chlamydia* sp. The histological features of lymphogranuloma inguinale are not specific, but include chronic inflammation, wth numerous lymphocytes and plasma cells, and extensive fibrosis.

Herpes simplex infection

Anal and perianal herpes simplex infection may accompany herpetic infection of the genital region and has similar appearances. It is particularly common in homosexuals. Herpes simplex infection is also the commonest anal manifestation of the acquired immunodeficiency syndrome (AIDS). Herpetic infection in AIDS causes extensive but rather superficial ulceration of the anal canal and perianal skin (Fig. 16.237) and the ulcer beds are lined by fibrinous debris. The condition responds relatively well to topical antiviral chemotherapy.

16.18.4 Tumours

Benign tumours and precancerous conditions

Leukoplakia

Leukoplakia is a clinical diagnosis describing white plaque-like lesions, and the term should not be used as a pathological diagnosis. The clinical condition of leukoplakia produces a wide spectrum of histological appearances, which vary from entirely benign squamous metaplasia overlaying prolapsing haemorrhoids to gross hyperplasia of the perianal skin which may be

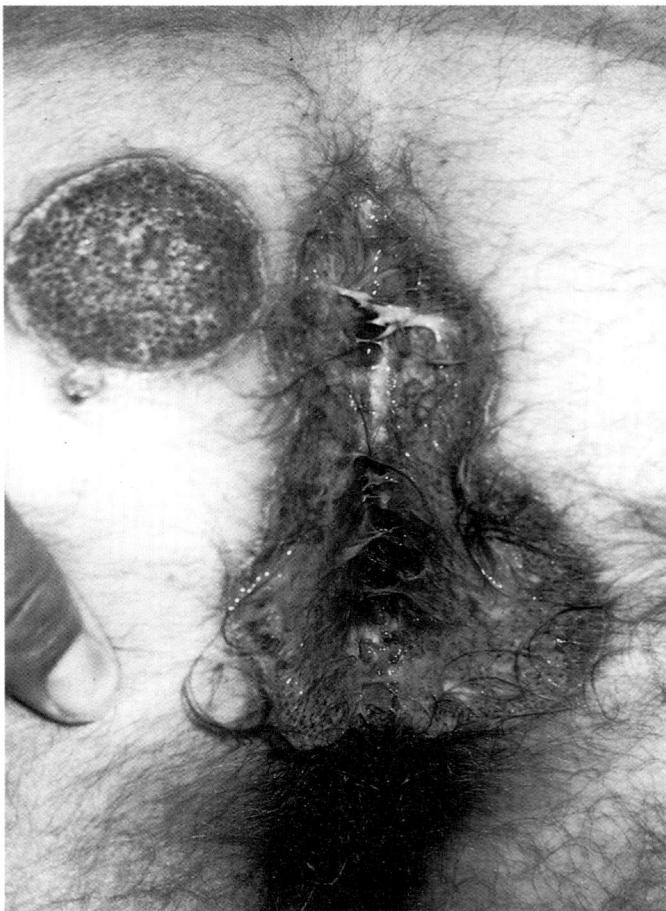

Fig. 16.237 Herpes simplex infection of the perianal region in an AIDS patient.

associated with dysplasia and carcinoma of the squamous epithelium. In the latter condition there is hyperkeratosis, a thickening of the prickle-cell layer of the epidermis (acanthosis), often with an irregular 'saw-tooth' outline, and a band-like chronic inflammatory cell infiltrate in the upper dermis. The appearances are similar to those of lichen planus of the skin and mucous membranes.

Viral warts (condylomata acuminata)

Condylomata acuminata are raised, red, warty growths which are found in the perianal skin and rarely extend into the anal canal. They are caused by human papilloma virus types 6 and 11 and are sexually transmitted. More than half of the male patients with anal condylomata acuminata are homosexuals. The histological features include papillomatous outgrowths of the acanthotic and parakeratotic squamous mucosa. The granular layer of the epidermis is prominent and there is an associated chronic inflammation of the dermis. Vacuolation of cells (koilocytosis) in the upper layers of the epidermis is characteristic. When viral warts are treated with topical podophyllin, the resulting cytological abnormalities may mimic dysplasia of the squamous mucosa.

It is probable that condylomata acuminata represent the benign end of a spectrum of squamous neoplasia of the anal region which includes a clinically progressive but cytologically benign lesion, giant condyloma of Buschke and Lowenstein, and a low-grade squamous cell carcinoma, known as verrucous carcinoma. Human papilloma viruses have been implicated in the aetiology of all these conditions.

Dysplasia, squamous carcinoma in situ, and Bowen's disease

Intra-epithelial neoplasia, including dysplasia, squamous carcinoma *in situ*, and Bowen's disease, is rare in the anal canal. Bowen's disease of the perianal skin is identical, both clinically and histologically, to that seen elsewhere in the skin (Chapter 28). Dysplastic changes are most commonly seen in the transitional zone of the anal canal, the area of the anus associated with the highest incidence of malignancy. Histologically the changes are identical to those seen in the cervix, vulva, and penis, and a classification, based on that in use for the cervix (Chapter 21), has been proposed for the anal canal. Thus grades of ACIN (anal canal intra-epithelial neoplasia) 1, 2, and 3 represent mild, moderate, and severe dysplasia, respectively, squamous cell carcinoma *in situ* being included in ACIN 3.

Malignant tumours

Squamous cell carcinoma

Squamous cell carcinoma encompasses the majority of primary malignant tumours of the anal canal and perianal skin. It includes the commonest tumour of the upper anal canal, the so-called basaloid or cloacogenic carcinoma, and also those of the lower anal canal and perianal region. Anal carcinoma is a rare malignant tumour in Britain and accounts for less than 5 per cent of all malignant tumours of the anorectum removed by synchronous combined excision of the rectum. It is more common in northern coastal Brazil and areas in India, where it is associated with conditions of extreme poverty and poor hygiene. There is increasing evidence linking anal carcinoma with anal papilloma virus (HPV) infection. The DNA of HPV type 16 has been detected in a high percentage of these tumours. Anal carcinoma is associated with homosexual activity and it is of interest that cases of anal cancer occurring at an unusually young age have been observed in patients with AIDS. The common link between these findings and the association of anal carcinoma with multicentric dysplasia and carcinoma of the lower female genital tract is sexual transmission of HPV.

It is important to differentiate between squamous cell carcinoma of the anal canal and of the anal margin and perianal skin. These tumours have quite different clinical, pathological, and prognostic characteristics. Anal canal carcinoma is approximately three times as common as perianal squamous cell carcinoma and is more commonly seen in women, whereas perianal carcinoma is four times commoner in men.

Macroscopic appearances Most carcinomas within the anal canal arise at or above the dentate line and commonly present as lower rectal rather than as anal tumours. This is because downwards spread of tumour is limited by the fibrous ligaments that connect the mucosa at the dentate line to the underlying internal sphincter. Only about one-quarter of anal canal carcinomas arise from the true squamous epithelium of the anal canal. Carcinomas of the anal verge arise at the junction of the squamous mucous membrane of the anal canal and the hair-bearing perianal skin. Anal carcinomas present as ulcerating, protruding, or verrucous tumours.

Microscopic appearances Carcinomas of the anal verge and perianal skin are predominantly well-differentiated squamous cell carcinomas with keratinization. Carcinomas of the lower anal canal are also of squamous cell type but usually lack keratinization. Tumours of the upper anal canal, the most common site, are most often of basaloid or cloacogenic type. These tumours arise from the transitional epithelium, which lies between the rectal-type mucosa and the stratified squamous mucosa of the anal canal and morphologically resembles the transitional epithelium of the urinary tract. The tumour cells are small and darkly staining, there is minimal keratinization and the tumour grows in clumps which show a striking peripheral palisading and central necrosis (Fig. 16.238). The histological appearances resemble those of a basal cell carcinoma of the skin. The division of squamous cell carcinoma of the anal region into basaloid and classical squamous carcinoma is somewhat artificial, as it is the site, grade, and stage of the carcinoma that relates to prognosis. There is an increasing body of opinion for adoption of a similar classification for anal carcinoma as that applied to carcinoma of the cervix uteri. In this classification there are three histological types of carcinoma: small cell non-keratinizing, large cell keratinizing, and large cell non-keratinizing.

Spread, prognosis, and treatment Anal canal carcinomas may spread locally into the lower rectum due to anatomical factors

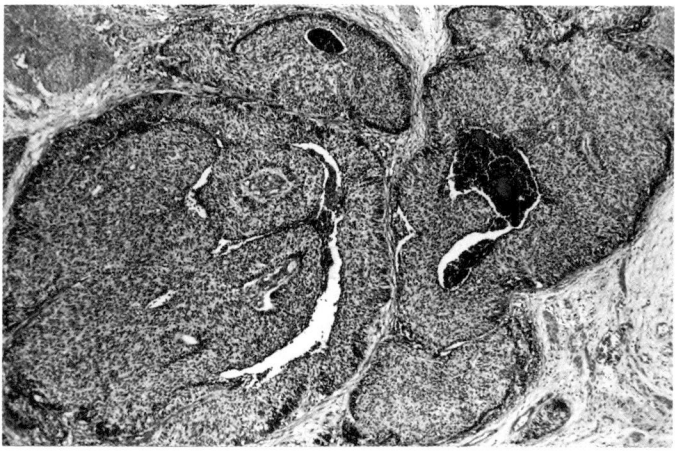

Fig. 16.238 A basaloid (cloacogenic) carcinoma of the anal canal. There are islands of tumour cells with peripheral palisading and focal central necrosis.

(see above). Lymphatic spread is preferentially to the haemorrhoidal lymph nodes in the lower rectum and later to superficial inguinal lymph nodes. Carcinomas of the anal verge and perianal skin metastasize to inguinal lymph nodes and spread to haemorrhoidal nodes is distinctly unusual. The prognosis of anal carcinoma is primarily dependent upon staging parameters, particularly lymph node involvement. Whereas formerly most carcinomas of the anal region were treated by synchronous combined excision of the rectum, management of these tumours is now directed toward preservation of anal function. Thus, therapy for most tumours is radiotherapy, often combined with chemotherapy, particularly 5-fluorouracil and mitomycin. Local excision is reserved for small perianal tumours.

Malignant melanoma

Malignant melanoma accounts for approximately 10 per cent of all malignant tumours of the anus. It is usually of the nodular type and, due to late presentation and advanced stage, is associated with a particularly gloomy prognosis. The tumour may present as a rectal mass, for anal melanomas are usually centred above the dentate line. The microscopic features are variable but are broadly similar to those of cutaneous melanomas (Chapter 28). Anal melanomas are often lacking in melanin pigment and therefore the diagnosis is often unsuspected clinically.

Adenocarcinoma

Adenocarcinoma of the anal canal is usually the result of local spread from a primary tumour of the rectum. Adenocarcinoma of anal glands is very rare, but can be associated with extramammary Paget's disease. Mucinous adenocarcinoma may arise in anorectal fistulae.

Perianal Paget's disease

This rare condition presents with a perianal scaly eczematous eruption in elderly patients, both male and female. Histologically the epidermis of the perianal skin is infiltrated by groups of large vacuolated cells which contain abundant mucin. The mucin can be demonstrated by periodic acid-Schiff (PAS) and alcian blue stains. The infiltrate also involves the pilosebaceous units and the ducts of apocrine sweat glands. The disease is thought to be due to epidermal invasion from an underlying low-grade carcinoma of sweat glands, although infiltration of the dermal tissues is rare in the early stages of the disease. Intraepidermal spread from an adenocarcinoma of the lower rectum or anal canal may closely mimic genuine Paget's disease. The natural history of perianal Paget's disease is one of repeated local recurrences before late metastasis.

Rare tumours of the anal region

Keratoacanthomas, although more frequent on sun-exposed skin (Chapter 28), may occasionally be seen in the perianal skin. Its pathological import is that it may be misinterpreted as a squamous cell carcinoma, with which it shares many histological features. The perianal skin is a rare site of basal cell carcinoma (rodent ulcer). The pathological features are the same as those elsewhere in the skin (Chapter 28) and local excision is adequate treatment. Benign lymphoid polyps may be found in the upper anal canal, although these are more frequent in rectal mucosa. Bowenoid papulosis is an unusual condition of the anogenital region. It affects young adults and presents as a papular eruption. Although there are worrying histological features, similar to those seen in Bowen's disease, there appears to be no malignant potential. Bowenoid papulosis is a further example of HPV-associated pathology in the anal region. Other unusual benign tumours of the anal region include sweat gland tumours, smooth muscle tumours of the anal sphincters, and lipomas.

Primary malignant lymphoma of the anal canal is excessively rare, but it is occasionally seen as a complication of AIDS. Leukaemic deposits may occur in the anus, while ulceration of the perianal skin is a relatively common accompaniment of acute leukaemia. Tumours of the retrorectal or presacral space may occasionally manifest as anal tumours. These include cystic teratomas, ependymomas (of both myxopapillary and papillary types), and a rare multicystic lesion, the retrorectal cystic hamartoma (anal gland cyst hamartoma). It is uncertain whether the latter represents a hamartomatous condition or is secondary to infection of anal glands and fistulae. The condition may recur if inadequately excised but there is no malignant potential.

16.18.5   Further reading

Haemorrhoids and inflammation

Eykyn, S. J. and Grace, R. H. (1986). The relevance of microbiology in the management of anorectal sepsis. *Annals of the Royal College of Surgeons of England* **68**, 237–9.

Goligher, J. (1984). *Surgery of the anus, rectum and colon* (5th edn). Baillière Tindall, London.

Nicholls, R. J. and Glass, R. E. (1985). *Coloproctology*. Springer-Verlag, Berlin.

Parks, A. G., Gordon, P. H., and Hardcastle, J. D. (1976). A classification of fistula-in-ano. *British Journal of Surgery* **63**, 1–12.

Tumours

Adam, Y. G. and Efron, G. (1987). Current concepts and controversies concerning the etiology, pathogenesis, diagnosis and treatment of malignant tumours of the anus. *Surgery* **101**, 253–66.

Fenger, C. and Nielsen, V. T. (1986). Intraepithelial neoplasia in the anal canal. The appearance and relation to genital neoplasia. *Acta Pathologica Microbiologica et Immunologica Scandinavica* **94**, 343–9.

Morson, B. C., Dawson, I. M. P., Day, D. W., Jass, J. R., Price, A. B., and Williams, G. T. (1990). Section VII/Anal Region. In *Gastrointestinal pathology* (3rd edn), pp. 651–86. Blackwell Scientific Publications, Oxford.

Palmer, J. G., Scholefield, J. H., Coates, P. J., Shepherd, N. A., Jass, J. R., Crawford, L. V., *et al.* (1989). Anal cancer and human papillomaviruses. *Diseases of Colon and Rectum* **32**, 1016–22.

Shepherd, N. A., Scholefield, J.H., Love, S. B., England, J., and North-over, J. M. A. (1990). Prognostic factors in anal squamous carcinoma: a multivariate analysis of clinical, pathological and flow cytometric parameters in 235 cases. *Histopathology* **16**, 545–55.

16.19 The peritoneum

N. A. Shepherd

16.19.1 Inflammatory conditions

Acute peritonitis

Acute infection of the peritoneum may be localized or diffuse. This depends upon the load and virulence of the microorganisms involved and the site of the primary infective focus. Although the peritoneal sac is continuous, there is potential compartmentalization of the peritoneal cavity due to serosal folds around the viscera, and this may influence localization of the infective focus. Acute diffuse peritonitis is a common condition and still causes much morbidity and mortality. It is most usually the result of perforation of a hollow viscus, and acute appendicitis and perforated peptic ulcers are the most common causes. Peritonitis may also be caused by trauma and surgical procedures, including laparotomy and peritoneal dialysis. Infection derived from the female genital tract is a rare cause of peritonitis, and haematogenous spread of infection to the peritoneum is distinctly rare. Although most cases of acute peritonitis are caused by bacterial infection, occasionally the condition may result from escape of gastric secretion, bile, and pancreatic enzymes. In all of these conditions, however, secondary bacterial infection by enteric organisms is likely.

Bacteriology

Acute peritonitis due to a ruptured viscus is usually caused by Gram-negative organisms, in particular *Escherichia coli*. However, the infection is often mixed, and other organisms implicated include streptococci, anaerobic organisms (especially *Bacteroides*), *Proteus*, and *Pseudomonas*. Infection by a single organism is unusual. It does occur in so-called primary peritonitis, but this disease is seen less often than in former years. It usually occurs in children and is caused by *Streptococcus pneumoniae*. In adults, primary peritonitis is nearly always a complication of ascites due to cirrhosis.

Pathology

In early acute peritonitis there is congestion of the blood vessels in the connective tissue beneath the peritoneum, which loses its normal sheen. Soon a fibrinous exudate lines the peritoneum, matting together loops of bowel and omentum (Fig. 16.239). At this stage histological examination reveals a fibrinous exudate with degeneration of the mesothelial cells that line the peritoneal cavity. Soon an intense polymorph infiltrate supervenes and

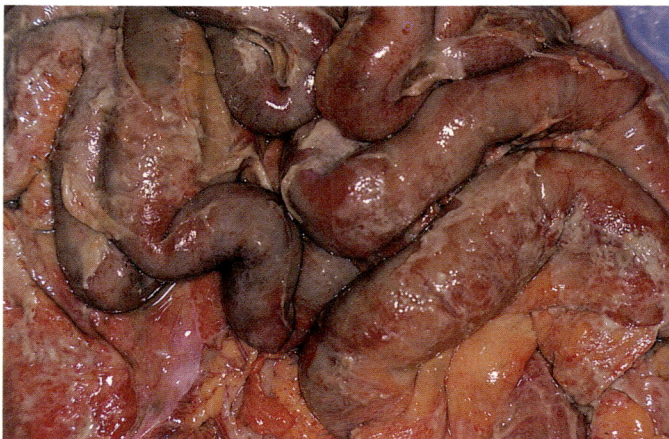

Fig. 16.239 Acute peritonitis secondary to ruptured colonic carcinoma. Loops of small intestine are congested and the peritoneal surface is lined by a fibrinous exudate.

granulation tissue containing numerous small blood vessels forms. If the patient survives the acute insult, there is organization with fibrosis, and a variable number of fibrous adhesions may be formed between the viscera.

Complications

Acute diffuse peritonitis is a grave condition, if not adequately treated, and is associated with a high mortality. The most serious complications of acute peritonitis are paralytic ileus and toxaemia. These conditions are usually interrelated. Paralytic ileus is due to the toxic effects of the bacteria within the abdominal cavity which cause the bowel to lose its peristaltic activity, leading to complete functional intestinal obstruction. The bowel dilates and appears dark and dusky as a result of venous stasis. Gross fluid and electrolyte disturbances then supervene. Absorption of bacterial endotoxins through the inflamed peritoneum causes endotoxaemia, which may also result from septicaemia. This combination of endotoxic shock and gross fluid and electrolyte imbalance is the cause of the high fatality rates of untreated acute bacterial peritonitis.

Localized abscess formation may result from peritonitis. These occur most often in the subphrenic space, after perforation of the stomach or upper small intestine, or in the pelvis after perforation of the appendix or a diverticulum in the sigmoid colon. Fibrous adhesions are a chronic complication of peritonitis. Adhesions may cause bowel obstruction and strangulation.

Chronic peritonitis

Chronic inflammation, in the absence of bacteria, within the peritoneal cavity results in hyperplasia of the mesothelial lining and fibrosis. This may be particularly marked on the capsules of the liver and spleen, which become thickened and white. The term 'sugar icing' is used to describe this change. Patients with asbestosis of the lung may develop fibrous plaques in the peritoneum as well as the pleura. Talcum powder, formerly used on surgical gloves, causes a chronic granulomatous fibrosing peritonitis. Concato's disease is a chronic serositis in which hyaline thickening is seen throughout the peritoneal cavity. In Pick's disease there is fibrosis of the peritoneum, especially around the liver, associated with pericarditis. Chronic infective peritonitis may be caused by tuberculosis (see below), actinomycosis (secondary to appendiceal or uterine infection), fungi, or worms. Drugs, such as practolol, are an occasional cause of fibrosing obliterative peritonitis.

Tuberculous peritonitis

Tuberculous peritonitis is less common than in former years, although it may be seen in immigrants from parts of the world where tuberculosis is endemic and in immunodeficient patients. The disease usually results from a tuberculous focus in a caseous mesenteric lymph node or in the fallopian tube. Occasionally it is due to haematogenous spread. It is very rarely caused by direct spread from a tuberculous enteritis. The appearances of tuberculous peritonitis vary from multiple small tubercles disseminated throughout the peritoneal cavity to large caseous masses within the abdominal cavity, particularly involving the omentum. The appearance of disseminated tuberculous peritonitis may closely mimic peritoneal metastases. Occasionally there are few tubercles and the disease is then characterized by multiple fibrous adhesions and a peritoneal effusion. The histological appearances vary from florid granulomatous inflammation with extensive caseation to chronic inflammatory changes with fibrosis and relatively few granulomas.

Ascites

The accumulation of fluid within the peritoneal cavity is known as ascites. Traditionally the fluid is described as a transudate, with a low protein content, or an exudate with a protein content exceeding 25 g/l. Transudates are most often the result of vascular disturbances, especially portal hypertension and congestive cardiac failure, due to a rise in portal venous pressure which exceeds the osmotic pressure of the blood. Exudates are the result of infection and of involvement of the peritoneum by malignant tumours. In both cases there is an inflammatory focus and plasma proteins leak from small blood vessels. Chylous ascites, a milky fluid due to the presence of lymph, may follow obstruction of the lymphatics of the thoracic chain and is usually caused by tumours.

16.19.2   Tumours and tumour-like proliferations

Cysts and benign tumours

Cysts are quite common within the peritoneal cavity and are of mesothelial, lymphatic, and developmental types. Benign soft tissues tumours seen in the peritoneal, mesenteric, and retroperitoneal tissues include lipomas, smooth muscle tumours, and fibromatoses. Lipomas of the peritoneum usually arise from the fat of the appendices epiploicae, but rarely produce symptoms. Fibromatoses are benign but locally aggressive fibrous proliferations which may occur in the mesentery and retroperitoneum. Sporadic cases are unusual and the disease is most commonly seen in familial adenomatous polyposis (see Section 16.16.1). Also known as desmoids, these lesions are associated with much morbidity, in particular small bowel obstruction, and a significant mortality, usually related to extensive bleeding, especially after surgical intervention. Deposits of endometriosis are often found in the peritoneal cavity and, in particular, in the pouch of Douglas and uterovesical angle. Although these are not strictly tumours, they may mimic intraperitoneal tumours and are associated with extensive haemorrhage. The histopathological features are similar to those seen in the gynaecological tract (Chapter 21).

Retroperitoneal fibrosis

This idiopathic condition usually affects middle-aged adults. There is extensive fibrosis in the retroperitoneal space and this leads to ureteric obstruction. The condition may be diagnosed on intravenous urogram as the ureters are displaced medially; most other space-ocupying lesions in the retroperitoneum push the ureters laterally. There is a spectrum of histopathological appearances, ranging from dense fibrosis to a chronic inflammatory cell infiltrate with numerous lymphoid follicles and germinal centres. Although the cause of the condition is largely unknown, it has occurred after use of the drugs, methysergide and practolol. Retroperitoneal fibrosis is associated with chronic fibrosing conditions in other organs: pseudotumour of the orbit, sclerosing cholangitis, Riedel's thyroiditis, and mediastinal fibrosis.

Papillary mesothelial hyperplasia

Mesothelial hyperplasia is a common result of a localized focus of peritoneal irritation, including abscess, tumour, and ascites. This hyperplasia may be either solid or papillary. In both cases it may be difficult histologically to differentiate mesothelial hyperplasia from malignant mesothelioma. Papillary mesothelial hyperplasia shows finger-like processes lined by a single layer of mesothelial cells (Fig. 16.240).

Pseudomyxoma peritonei

The spread of mucous material within the peritoneal cavity secondary to rupture of a mucinous cyst is known as pseudomyxoma peritonei. This may occur spontaneously or during surgical removal. Rupture of non-neoplastic mucocoeles and benign mucinous cystadenomas, especially of the appendix and ovary, usually causes a localized and self-limiting tissue reaction. However, rupture or intraperitoneal spread of a mucinous cystadenocarcinoma of ovarian, appendiceal, or gall-bladder origin, results in a progressive obliteration of the peritoneal cavity with intestinal obstruction, and is often fatal.

Malignant mesothelioma

Peritoneal malignant mesothelioma is a tumour of middle to late adulthood and, like mesothelioma of the pleural cavity, is

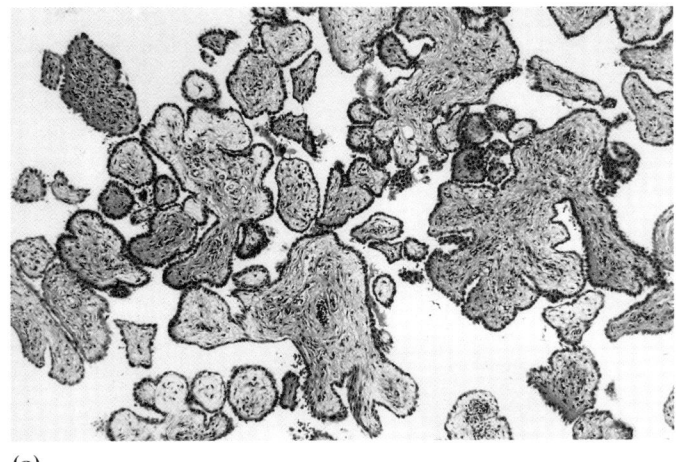

(a)

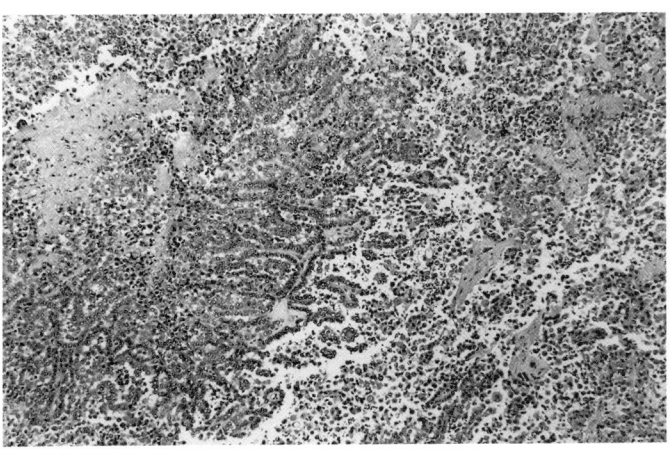

(b)

Fig. 16.240 (a) Papillary mesothelial hyperplasia; finger-like stromal processes are lined by a simple mesothelial layer. (b) Malignant peritoneal mesothelioma; although papillary, the tumour is very cellular and there are more solid areas.

associated with asbestosis. The tumour is much rarer in the peritoneum than in the pleural cavity. At presentation the tumour is often extensive, involving loops of intestine and often filling and obliterating the peritoneal cavity. There are three main histopathological patterns of malignant mesothelioma: epithelial, sarcomatous, and mixed. The epithelial pattern usually predominates in peritoneal mesothelioma, often with a papillary configuration (Fig. 16.240). The prognosis, like that of its pleural counterpart, is appalling.

Secondary carcinoma

Secondary carcinoma is the commonest malignancy of the peritoneum. Carcinomatous involvement of the peritoneal cavity occurs by direct spread, by transcoelomic spread, or by spread in the lymphatics of the subperitoneal connective tissue. Direct spread is most often seen in carcinomas of the gastrointestinal tract and ovary, and transcoelomic spread is characteristic of carcinomas of the stomach and ovary. Haematogenous spread to the peritoneal cavity is unusual, although malignant melanoma has a particular affinity for spread in the abdominal cavity.

Three patterns of intraperitoneal spread of carcinoma are seen. In the first type, numerous small tubercle-like nodules are present throughout the cavity and these may mimic tuberculous peritonitis. Massive spread filling and ablating the peritoneal cavity occurs in metastatic adenocarcinoma, usually of mucoid type, from the ovary or colon. Finally, diffuse carcinoma of the stomach produces a thickening of serous membranes and numerous thick fibrous plaques. Histopathological examination reveals signet-ring cell carcinoma embedded in an abundant fibrous stroma.

16.19.3   Further reading

McCaughey, W. T. E., Kannerstein, M., and Churg, J. (1985). *Tumors and pseudotumors of the serous membranes*. Fascicle 20, Second series, Armed Forces Institute of Pathology, Washington.

Morson, B. C., Dawson, I. M. P., Day, D. W., Jass, J. R., Price, A. B., and Williams, G. T. (1990). Section VIII/Peritoneum. In *Gastrointestinal pathology* (3rd edn), pp. 687–732. Blackwell Scientific Publications, Oxford.

17

The liver and biliary system

17

The liver and biliary system

17.1 Normal liver: structure and function

James O'D. McGee

17.1.1 Gross structure

The liver is the largest organ in man (approximately 1.5 kg), and constitutes about 2.5 per cent of body weight. It lies in the right upper quadrant of the abdomen under the ribs and is generally not palpable except under the right costal margin and xiphisternum, particularly on inspiration. Anatomically, it consists of four lobes; right, left, quadrate, and caudate. On the basis of vascular supply and biliary drainage, a more useful functional definition of structure is the right and left hemiliver. A line visualized between the inferior vena cava superiorly and the gall bladder inferiorly separate the right and left functional domains. This is important when surgical decisions about partial hepatic resections are considered, e.g. in patients with primary or secondary tumours.

Blood supply

This is summarized in Figs 17.1–17.3.

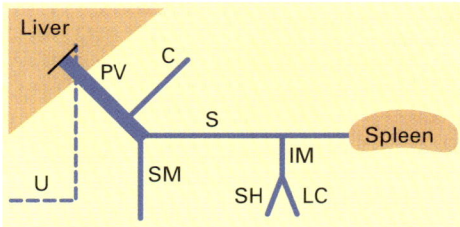

Fig. 17.1 Prehepatic portal venous system. The portal vein (PV) is formed by the union of the superior mesenteric (SM) and the splenic veins (S). The splenic also usually drains the inferior mesenteric vein (IM). SH = superior haemorrhoidal vein. LC = left colic vein. U = umbilical vein; this is not patent in normal adult life. C = coronary vein.

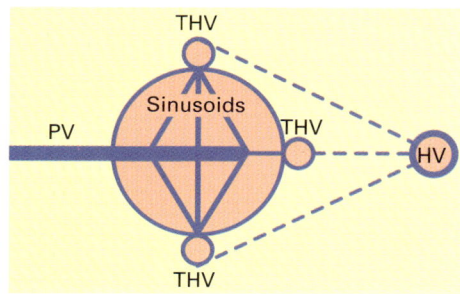

Fig. 17.2 Intrahepatic venous distribution. The portal venous radicles (PV) feed into the sinusoidal system and thence into the terminal hepatic venules (THV), and finally into the main hepatic veins (HV). In this diagram, the portal venous supply is present at the centre of the acinus and the terminal hepatic veins (central veins) are at its periphery.

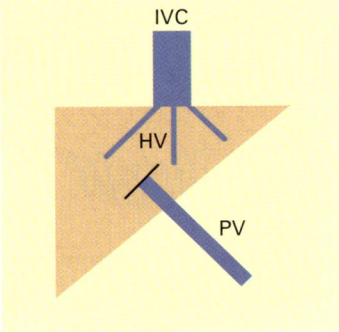

Fig. 17.3 Posthepatic venous exit. The right, middle, and left hepatic veins (HV) drain the corresponding segments of the liver into the inferior vene cava (IVC).

The portal vein

This is formed by the union of the superior mesenteric and splenic veins, and delivers blood through the hilum. This vein then progressively divides into smaller terminal branches which supply about 70 per cent of oxygen to the liver parenchyma.

The hepatic artery

The hepatic artery is a branch of the coeliac axis, and variations in its anatomy are common. This artery arborizes in portal tracts, alongside the portal vein, and delivers about 30 per cent of the oxygen to the liver. The terminal branches of the hepatic artery form two plexuses before delivering their blood into sinusoids; one plexus is around small portal vein radicles and the other around small bile ducts. The plexus around the bile ducts may modify the constituents of bile by reabsorption of bile contents (e.g. in obstructive jaundice), and influence secretion of bile duct epithelium.

From the terminal portal veins and hepatic arterioles sprout small side branches which feed directly (or sometimes indirectly from the hepatic artery plexuses) into the hepatic sinusoids where blood from both sources mixes in the intercommunicating complex of sinusoids.

Hepatic sinusoids

These are unique vessels in man (Figs 17.4–17.6). They are lined by endothelial cells and Kupffer cells which are predominantly phagocytic or potentially so. Unlike other vascular linings, there are no tight junctions between endothelial cells and/or Kupffer cells. Holes (fenestra) are frequent in endothelial cells and these tend to occur in groups known as sieve plates; the fenestra do not have an occluding diaphragm present in many other endothelia. Unlike other endothelia, there is no anatomically identifiable basement membrane under the sinusoidal lining cells. These three structural attributes—no tight interendothelial junctions, fenestra, and no basal lamina—allow direct access of plasma from the sinusoidal lumen to the surface of hepatocytes. This arrangement is probably important

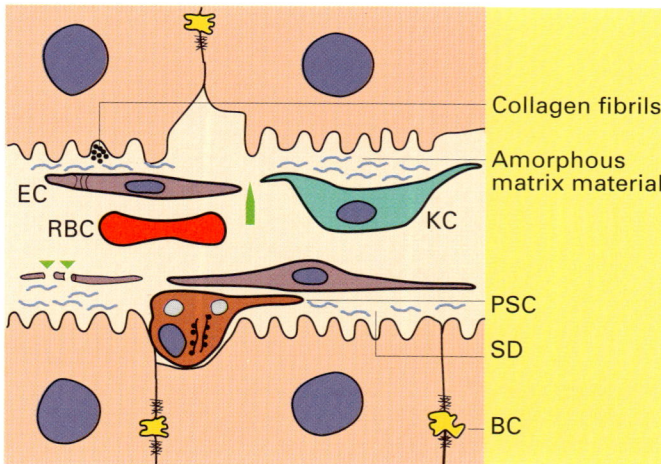

Fig. 17.4 Diagrammatic representation of the ultrastructure of hepatic sinusoid and adjacent hepatocytes. Hepatic sinusoids are unique in that there are no tight junctions between endothelial cells (EC), and/or endothelial cells and Kupffer cells (KC). There is, therefore, free access of plasma (arrow) to the space of Disse (SD). There is also relatively free access through fenestra and sieve plates in endothelial cells (arrowheads). A perisinusoidal cell (PSC) is shown in a hepatic recess; this cell contains fat vacuoles in which there is vitamin A. This cell also contains a lot of rough endoplasmic reticulum and probably functions as a matrix-producing cell. BC = bile canaliculus.

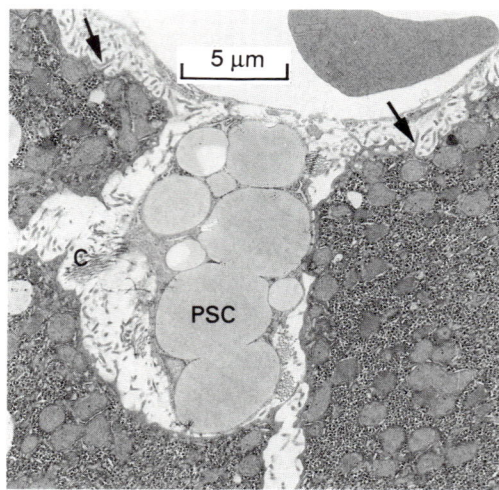

Fig. 17.5 Electron micrograph of hepatic sinusoid and adjacent hepatocytes. There are gaps in the sinusoidal lining and a perisinusoidal cell (PSC) filled with fat vacuoles in a hepatic recess. The microvillous surface of the hepatocytes (arrows) aids in absorptive function of these cells. There are scattered bundles of collagen fibrils and amorphous material probably composed of matrix components (such as laminin, proteoglycan, etc.) in the space of Disse which lies between the sinusoidal lining and the microvillous surface of the hepatocyte. (See also Fig. 17.61a.)

in the free bilateral uptake and exchange of materials between hepatocytes and plasma (Figs 17.5, 17.6).

Although normal human sinusoids do not have an anatomical basal lamina, small bundles of collagen fibrils and other extracellular matrix components do exist in the space (of Disse) between the sinusoidal lining and the hepatocyte surface. These matrix components may be produced by perisinusoidal cells (Ito cells) which are rich in vitamin A and lie in the space of Disse (Fig. 17.5). Hepatocytes may also be involved in the physiological manufacture of extracellular matrix in the space of Disse. In liver disease associated with fibrosis it may be that increased matrix deposition in this space modifies hepatocyte and perhaps also sinusoidal function (see Section 17.11).

Hepatic veins

Sinusoidal blood drains slowly, and perhaps intermittently, because of postulated pre- and post-sinusoidal sphincters, into terminal hepatic veins. These microscopic veins join up to form the main hepatic veins which empty into the inferior vena cava just below its junction with the right atrium (see Fig. 17.3).

Biliary system

Unlike the hepatic vascular supply, the biliary system conducts secretion out of the liver in the reverse direction to afferent blood supply. This conduit arises from bile canaliculi formed between apposing lateral surfaces of two hepatocytes. The canaliculi are 'sealed' from the sinusoidal border of the hepatocytes by tight junctions; normally, bile does not pass through these junctions but other molecules may do so (Fig. 17.6c). The

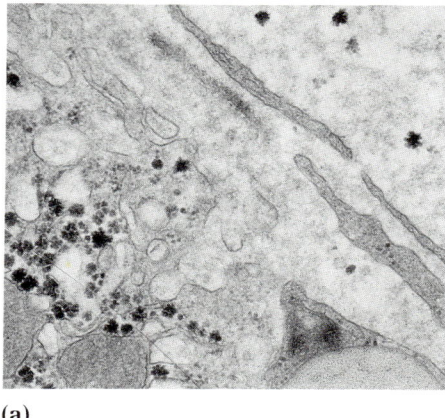

(a)

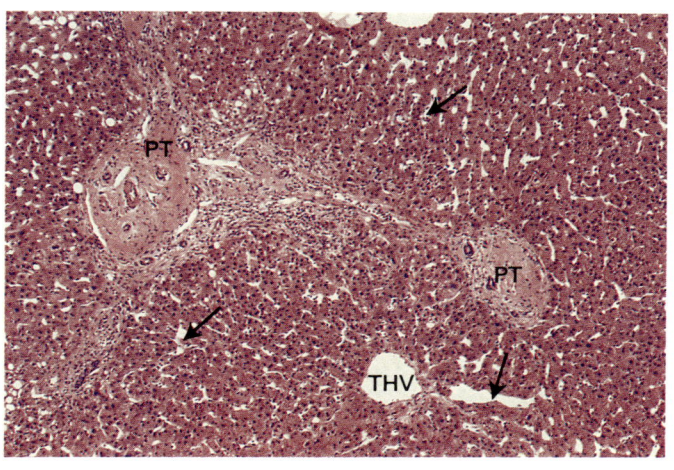

(b)

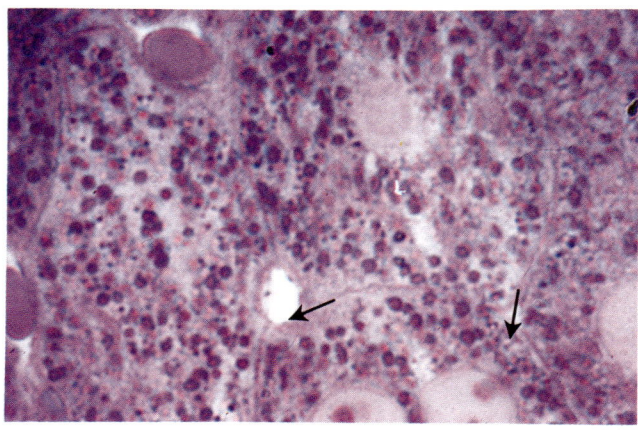

(c)

canaliculi course between adjacent hepatocytes to the portal tracts, where they exit through the limiting plate of hepatocytes into bile ductules (ducts of Hering), and thence into small bile ducts and onward into the right and left hepatic ducts which join to form the common bile duct at the liver hilum. The common bile duct empties its contents into the second part of the duodenum at the level of the head of the pancreas; the pancreatic duct frequently drains into the common bile duct before it exits into the duodenum at the ampulla of Vater. The gall bladder, which stores bile between meals, drains into the common bile duct via the cystic duct just below the hilum of the liver (see also Section 17.15.1).

17.1.2 Microanatomy

The liver is composed of three structures; portal tracts, hepatic parenchyma, and hepatic outflow veins (Figs 17.6, 17.7). Each portal tract contains a branch of the portal vein and hepatic artery, a bile duct, lymphatics, and, occasionally, recognizable nerves. All of these are enclosed in a sheath of connective tissue. Hepatocytes arranged in intercommunicating one-cell thick plates, radiate from portal tracts towards terminal hepatic venous radicles. The sinusoids lie between, and on each side, of these plates of hepatocytes.

The description of these microscopic structures is agreed but there is debate about how they are organized into functional units. In the first half of the twentieth century, the functional unit was construed as the liver lobule with a hepatic (central)

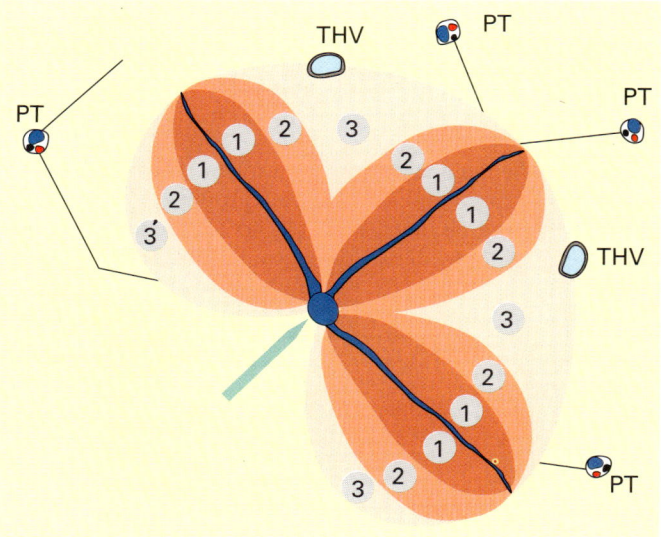

Fig. 17.6 (a) Electron micrograph of a hepatic sinusoid. Endothelial cells lining this sinusoid have intercellular gaps. This allows free exchange between plasma and hepatocytes. Glycogen rosettes are prominent in hepatocytes. (b) Low-power view of a normal liver, showing portal tracts and hepatocytes with intervening sinusoids (portal tracts, PT; terminal hepatic venules, THV; sinusoids are indicated by arrows). (c) Plastic section (1 μm) of normal liver. Bile canaliculi are easily seen between hepatocytes (arrow).

Fig. 17.7 Diagram of three acini (red) and their relation to liver lobules. Two lobules are partially outlined (black lines) with portal tracts (PT) and terminal hepatic ('central') veins at their periphery and centre respectively. Simple acini occupy sectors in both lobules. The centre of the acinus is the terminal portal vein (large arrow); blood from these and hepatic arterioles supply the parenchyma. Zone 1 is best oxygenated and zone 3 least. Zone 3 abuts on THVs and small sectors around portal veins. THVs drain adjacent acini.

vein at its centre and several portal tracts at the lobule periphery (Fig. 17.7). In the 1950s, the concept of the liver acinus was introduced by Rappaport as the basic/primary functional unit. This conceives that the portal tract (with its feeding vein and artery etc.) is the backbone of the acinus. From here, blood is dispersed outwards towards the terminal hepatic (central) venules.

The zone of hepatic tissue immediately adjacent to the portal tract (zone 1) is rich in oxygenated blood, while the peripheral zone 3 around the hepatic venule is relatively oxygen poor. Zone 2 is an arbitrary zone between zones 1 and 3, and corresponds to the midzone of the lobular model.

The acinar model is now generally accepted, since it is based on functional studies of hepatic blood distribution and also because it more readily explains the microscopic distribution of hepatic disease. In carbon tetrachloride poisoning, for example, there is necrosis of hepatocytes in zone 3. These tracts of damage are present not only in the most anoxic area around the terminal hepatic venule but in equally anoxic zone 3 areas which abut on portal tracts (Fig. 17.8). The microscopic distribution of this single lesion cannot be explained easily using the lobule as the functional unit of liver structure. The acinar model will be used throughout this chapter to describe hepatic pathology.

For comparison, the lobular and acinar terminologies, as they relate to microanatomy and pathology, are summarized in Table 17.1.

17.1.3   Liver function

Tests of liver function will be summarized briefly here since they are alluded to throughout this chapter.

Protein synthesis

The liver is the main site of plasma protein synthesis (with the exception of Igs). Albumin, fibrinogen, prothrombin, other clotting factors, and ceruloplasmin (Table 17.2) are synthesized almost exclusively by hepatocytes. Routine tests of hepatic syn-

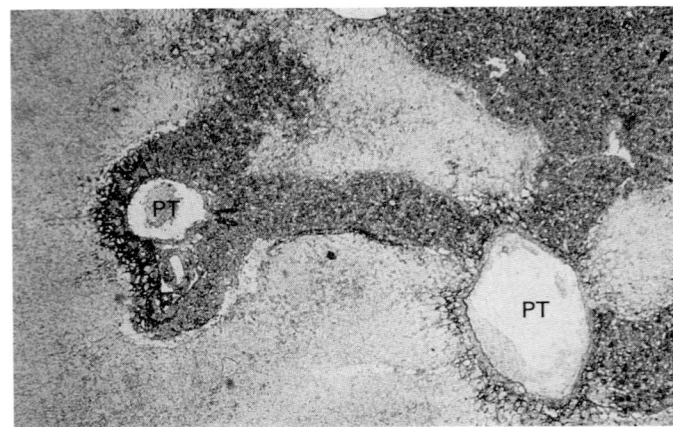

Fig. 17.8 Carbon tetrachloride poisoning. This photomicrograph illustrates in practice one of the reasons for preferring the acinar to the lobular concept. There is an area of necrosis linking terminal hepatic veins. These areas of necrosis surround and abut on a portal tract (PT). This distribution of necrosis, which was traditionally regarded as centrilobular, cannot be explained on the basis of the lobular concept; it is more readily explained using the acinar concept. This is an autoradiograph showing [^{3}H]amino-acid uptake (black) by surviving hepatocytes.

thetic function rely on measuring albumin and prothrombin (normally measured as the prothrombin index). The normal liver makes about 10 g albumin/day but in end-stage liver disease production is reduced to 4 g/day. Since the half-life of albumin is about 22 days, the level of this protein drops slowly in serum in acute liver disease but is usually permanently low in chronic end-stage liver disease (cirrhosis). The prothrombin index is a much more sensitive test of hepatocyte synthetic function because prothrombin has a much shorter half-life.

Ceruloplasmin and α-1-antitrypsin (AAT), also produced by hepatocytes, are measured particularly in disorders in which they are specifically deficient, viz. Wilson disease and AAT deficiency. Although the plasma levels of these proteins are decreased in these disorders, both proteins are acute-phase reactants. In hepatocellular disease, the levels of both proteins may

---

Table 17.1   Acinar and lobular terminologies compared

Acinar	Lobular
Simple acinus	Parts of two lobules
Terminal portal vein	Small portal vein
Terminal hepatic vein	Central vein
Acinar zone 1; periportal	Peripheral zone; periportal
Acinar zone 2	Midzone
Acinar zone 3; perivenular	Centrilobular; central zone; central
Panacinar	Panlobular
Mutliacinar necrosis	Multilobular; massive, submassive necrosis
Periacinar bridging necrosis/fibrosis around periphery of two acini	Central–central bridging necrosis/fibrosis
Portal–portal bridging necrosis/fibrosis	Portal–portal bridging necrosis/fibrosis
Periacinar bridging necrosis/fibrosis within one acinus	Central–portal bridging necrosis/fibrosis

Table 17.2 Serum liver function tests*

Protein synthesis	Microsomal function/ biliary secretion	Enzymes
Albumin	Bilirubin	
Prothrombin	Bile salts	ALT
Fibrinogen	Cholesterol	AST
α-1-Antitrypsin	γ-GT	LDH
Ceruloplasmin	Alkaline phosphatase	
Transferrin	5'-Nucleotidase	
α-Fetoprotein		
α2-Macroglobulin		
Complement components (C3, C6, C1)		

* See also Section 17.16.
Abbreviations: γ-GT, γ-glutamyltransferase; ALT, alanine aminotransferase;
AST, aspartate aminotransferase; LDH, lactate dehydrogenase.

be normal in spite of an inherited deficiency state. Some complement components produced in the liver are also acute-phase reacents and behave similarly.

Other hepatocyte proteins helpful in diagnosis are transferrin and α-fetoprotein (AFP). The former, which transports iron, is normally not fully saturated but is 90 per cent saturated in idiopathic haemochromatosis. AFP is the fetal counterpart of albumin and is present at very low levels in adult plasma but is characteristically grossly elevated in primary hepatocyte malignancy.

Carbohydrates, amino acids, and fat metabolism

The liver is the interface between absorbed glucose, amino acids, lipids, and the systemic circulation. The liver stores glucose as glycogen (see Fig. 17.6). Lipids, on the other hand, are oxidized in the liver and/or linked with triglyceride for transportation in plasma. These functions, which are dependent on many other factors (e.g. insulin and glucagon, in the case of blood glucose levels), are not measured routinely as parameters of hepatocyte function.

Bile secretory function

Bilirubin, alkaline phosphatase which outlines bile canaliculi, bile salts, copper, and cholesterol (among many other compounds) are secreted by hepatocytes into bile. Bilirubin is conjugated mainly with glucuronide within hepatocytes before secretion. It would be predicted, therefore, that unconjugated bilirubin would appear in the plasma in increased amounts when the functional capacity of the hepatocyte for handling it is overloaded, as in haemolysis, or where there is severe hepatocyte death with consequent disappearance of a corresponding proportion of the bilirubin conjugation mechanism. Similarly, the level of conjugated bilirubin rises in bile duct obstruction, presumably by reabsorption from bile ducts via the capillary plexus around these structures. In like manner, the serum levels of bile salts which give rise to itching, cholesterol which may produce skin xanthomas, and alkaline phosphatase become

elevated when there is significant obstruction to the outflow of bile from the liver.

Copper, coupled with copper-binding protein, accumulates in hepatocytes in biliary obstructive lesions and in cirrhosis of non-biliary types.

Other enzyme tests

The liver, like heart, kidney, and muscle, is rich in aspartate aminotransferase (AST)—a mitochondrial enzyme—and the cytosolic enzyme, alanine aminotransferase (ALT). In hepatocyte damage both enzymes are elevated. In acute liver disease and in ongoing hepatocyte destructive disorders, elevations of ALT and AST roughly reflect the extent of hepatocyte damage or death.

γ-Glutamyltransferase (γ-GT) is probably derived from hepatocyte microsomes. It is elevated in patients with biliary obstruction and usually parallels alkaline phosphatase levels in the serum. Parenthetically, it can be used to confirm that an elevated alkaline phosphatase level is liver derived; the latter is also elevated in bone and gut disease. γ-GT had a vogue as a 'specific' indicator of alcoholic liver disease; it may be induced in microsomes by alcohol abuse. However, many other factors influence the level, so it cannot be considered specific for alcohol abuse; about one-third of alcohol abusers have a normal level.

Singly, not one of these tests is a satisfactory measure of 'liver' function, for reasons which are given above. Together, they give a more accurate assessment of what may actually be happening in a diseased liver. At this time, there are no satisfactory serum tests for liver mononuclear phagocyte system (MPS) function, or extracellular matrix production, both of which are important aspects of many liver disorders.

17.1.4   Further reading

Arias, I. M. (1990). The biology of hepatic endothelial cell fenestra. In *Progress in liver disease* (ed. H. Popper and F. Schaffener), pp. 11–26. Saunders and Co., London.

Boyer, J. L. (1990). Physiology of bile secretion and cholestasis. In *Progress in liver disease* (ed. H. Popper and F. Schaffener), pp. 237–60. Saunders and Co., London.

MacSween, R. N. M. and Scothorne, R. J. (1987). Developmental anatomy and normal structure. In *Pathology of liver* (ed. R. N. M. MacSween, P. P. Anthony, and P. J. Scheuer), pp. 1–45. Churchill Livingstone, Edinburgh.

17.2   Congenital liver disorders

Bernard Portmann

This section covers a variety of structural abnormalities affecting the liver, its vasculature and the extra- and intrahepatic segments of the biliary tree. It embraces the fibro-cystic liver changes associated with polycystic disease, for which the reader will find additional information on the renal changes in Chapter 19. Biliary atresia, neonatal hepatitis, and paucity of the intrahepatic bile ducts are discussed in proximity to one another as part of the differential diagnosis of cholestatic syndrome in infancy.

17.2.1 Anatomical anomalies

These have been reviewed recently by Ishak and Sharp (1987). In situs inversus totalis or abdominalis, the liver lies in the left upper quadrant. It is symmetrical and has a transverse position in the asplenia syndrome.

Atrophy of the left lobe commonly follows excessive regression after closure of the umbilical vein and ductus venosus at birth.

Supernumerary lobes are relatively frequent on the inferior surface of the liver. They are usually of no clinical significance, except for Riedel's lobe, a tongue-like projection of the right lobe which may be palpated in the right hypochondrium.

In an autopsy series, Michels (1951) found variations of the conventional pattern of the hepatic artery in 45 per cent of cases. The main anomalies were replacement of, or accessory, left or right branches; and the common hepatic artery originating from the superior mesenteric artery.

Congenital anomalies of the portal vein include a preduodenal location and a variable degree of hypoplasia and atresia. In cavernous transformation, the portal vein is replaced by a spongy mass of anastomosing channels. This cause of portal hypertension in children may represent a sequel of portal vein thrombosis following umbilical sepsis and catheterization; or an angiomatous malformation, as suggested by a third of the cases having other congenital abnormalities.

Hepatic vein thrombosis (Budd–Chiari syndrome) has been associated with partial membranous obstruction or a web in the adjacent portion of the inferior vena cava. The latter represents a possible congenital anomaly or a residuum of thrombosis.

Anomalies of the bile ducts, such as duplication, accessory ducts, and anomalous junction with the pancreatic duct, are mainly asymptomatic findings detected by cholangiography. There are case reports of congenital bronchobiliary fistula.

17.2.2 Congenital dilatation of the bile ducts

This infrequent anomaly is classified into five types, according to the shape and location of the cysts (Crittenden and McKinley 1985). The main anatomo-clinical forms are choledochal cyst proper, and Caroli disease.

Choledochal cysts may vary considerably in size, and may contain as much as 10 litres of bile. The wall consists of dense connective tissue with little, if any, smooth muscle. When present, the epithelial lining is cuboidal or columnar. Chronic inflammation is often seen near the distal end of the common bile duct, which may be narrowed, particularly in the infantile form. Complications include recurrent ascending cholangitis, rupture, gallstone formation, secondary liver changes with bili-

ary fibrosis or cirrhosis, and carcinoma development. The clinical presentation may mimic that of biliary atresia or include the classic triad of abdominal pain, right upper quadrant mass, and jaundice. More than half the patients will not be diagnosed before adulthood (see also Section 17.15.2).

Caroli disease is characterized by the presence of multiple intrahepatic cysts (1.0–4.5 cm in diameter) communicating freely with the bile ducts. They are lined by normal, ulcerated, or focally hyperplastic biliary epithelium. Severe chronic inflammation and abundant mucous glands are often observed in the fibrotic wall, and the lumen may contain bilirubin calculi. The disease most often presents in adults as recurrent cholangitis. Liver abcesses, sepsis, and the development of carcinoma are other major complications. A number of cases are associated with congenital hepatic fibrosis and/or medullary sponge kidney, and therefore merge with the spectrum of disease seen in childhood polycystic disease.

Childhood polycystic disease and congenital hepatic fibrosis

Although these two conditions may differ sharply in terms of symptoms and age at clinical presentation, there are frequent intermediate forms and the hepatic changes are qualitatively the same.

Macroscopically, the liver may be normal or show a variable degree of enhanced portal tract markings and anastomosing fibrous bands. Histopathologically, there is an increased number of excessively branching bile ductules set in a variable amount of porto-septal fibrosis. The ductules may be dilated and contain bile-stained concretions (Figs 17.9, 17.10). A unique feature is that the ductal structures are often cut in such a way as to draw elongated profiles with cleft-like lumens, a pattern closely resembling the earliest form of bile duct or ductal plate in the embryo. This suggests that not only an excessive proliferation but also a lack of involution of the embryonal plate may have contributed to the lesion, for which the term 'ductal plate malformation' has been proposed.

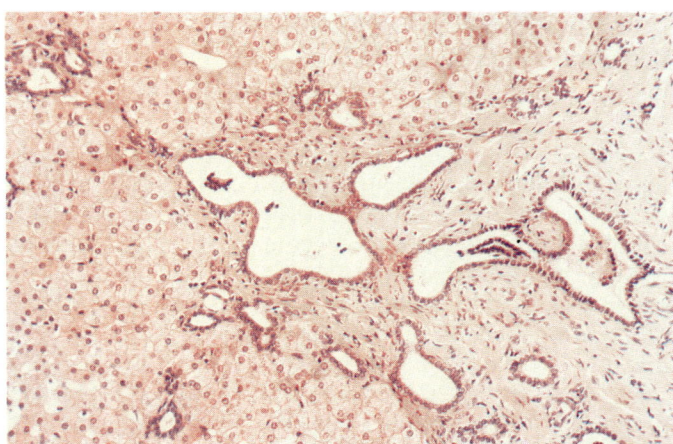

Fig. 17.9 Infantile polycystic disease. Irregularly branching ducts are lined by cuboidal cells and set in a fibrous matrix.

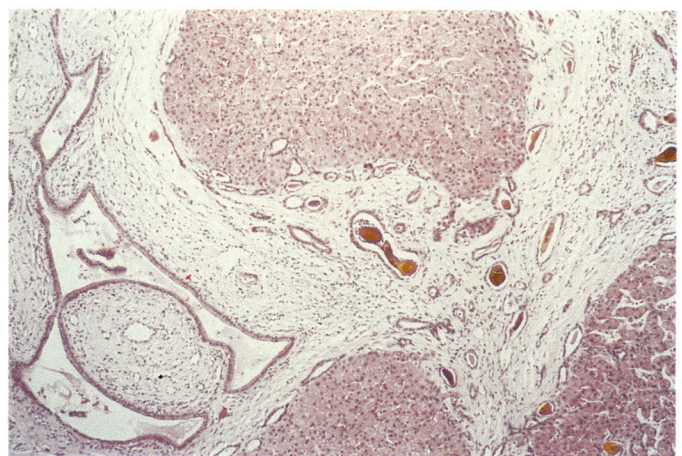

Fig. 17.10 Congenital hepatic fibrosis. Bridging fibrous septa contain numerous dilated ducts, some filled with bile. Note the circular shape of a larger duct in the lower left-hand corner.

Childhood polycystic disease refers to those patients presenting with renal failure due to replacement of both kidneys by radially arranged fusiform cysts. The condition, which is inherited in an autosomal recessive manner, has been divided into four types—perinatal, neonatal, infantile, and juvenile—according to age at presentation and degree of renal involvement. There is a trend to a smaller number of renal cysts and a greater degree of hepatic fibrosis as patients grow older. Late infantile and juvenile cases may develop portal hypertension, and are indistinguishable from congenital hepatic fibrosis.

Congenital hepatic fibrosis affects predominantly children and adolescents, who present with hepatosplenomegaly or bleeding oesophageal varices due to portal hypertension. Periportal fibrosis may be prominent, with broad fibrous septa delineating irregularly shaped islands of intact liver parenchyma. There may be superimposed cholangitis, particularly in the variant associated with Caroli disease. The kidney may show the changes of childhood polycystic disease; more often there is medullary tubular ectasia detected radiologically. Others have nephronophthisis. In nearly half of the patients there is no detectable renal abnormality.

Adult polycystic disease

This condition is inherited as an autosomal dominant character. Adult-type polycystic kidneys are associated with few or numerous hepatic cysts in 16–21 per cent of autopsy cases; whereas about half of the patients presenting with polycystic liver also have polycystic kidneys.

The liver is diffusely (less often focally) cystic. The cysts vary in size from the barely visible to more than 10 cm in diameter. They do not communicate with the biliary system. They contain a clear, colourless or light yellow fluid. Microscopically, the cysts are lined by columnar or cuboidal, often flattened, epithelium, supported by thin bands of connective tissue. Biliary microhamartoma (von Meyenburg complexes) are frequently associated; these consist of periportal collections of small bile

ducts set in a round or irregularly shaped area of collagen (Fig. 17.11).

Clinically, the symptoms are those of a benign hepatic mass presenting in adulthood, the moribidity and mortality being essentially related to the renal involvement.

17.2.3   Cholestatic syndrome in infancy

The syndrome of conjugated hyperbilirubinaemia with darkening of the urine and reduction in stool pigmentation may present at, or shortly after, birth and is always pathological.

Except for an association with α-1-antitrypsin deficiency in up to 20 per cent of the patients, very few cases have a recognized infectious or metabolic cause. In most instances the aetiology and pathogenesis remain unknown, and the disorders are broadly classified into three categories:

1. those having structural defects of the biliary tree (extrahepatic biliary atresia);

2. those due primarily to parenchymal damage (neonatal hepatitis); and

3. those associated with a reduced number of intrahepatic bile ducts (paucity of the intrahepatic bile ducts).

Extrahepatic biliary atresia

Approximately a third of infants presenting with prolonged cholestatic jaundice have biliary atresia, the overall incidence being estimated at 1 in 14 000 live births. The condition is characterized by obstruction, destruction, or absence of segments of the extrahepatic biliary tree, due to a sclerosing inflammatory process.

Transverse sections of the biliary stump removed at surgery reveal variably inflamed connective tissue with single or multiple duct lumens lined by altered biliary epithelium; peripheral glands with or without duct remnants; or concentrically arranged lamellae of collagen without epithelial components.

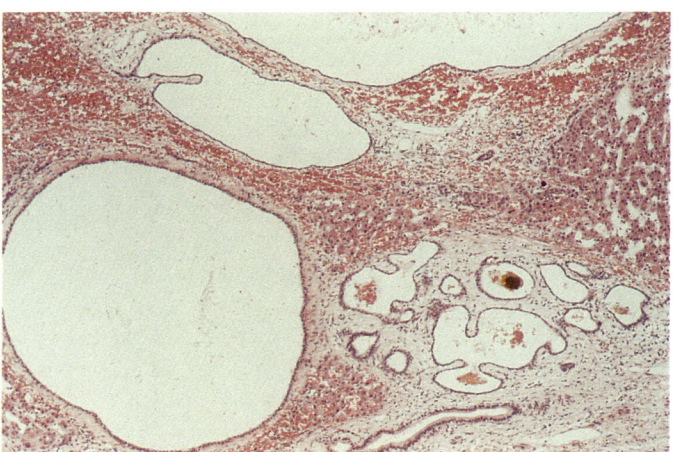

Fig. 17.11 Adult polycystic disease. Hepatic cysts, lined by flattened epithelium, are separated by little parenchyma; a biliary microhamartoma is also present in the lower right-hand corner.

Within the liver there is widening of the portal areas due to oedematous fibrous tissue deposition and a characteristic proliferation of tortuous ducts and ductules (Fig. 17.12). Cholestasis is invariably severe and often includes ductular bile casts. Giant cells are present in about half of the cases. Fibrosis is progressive, with periportal septum formation, linkage of portal areas, and eventual development of a secondary biliary cirrhosis.

Without surgical correction, death from complications of cirrhosis and portal hypertension usually occurs by 1 or 2 years of age. Following hepatic porto-enterostomy (Kasai procedure), 70–80 per cent of infants clear their jaundice and there is a 90 per cent chance of survival through to 10 years of age, providing surgery is performed before eight weeks of age. This emphasizes the need for an early diagnosis, which is achieved by combining clinical features, biopsy appearances, and imaging techniques using hepatobiliary radiolabelled compounds.

The aetiology of biliary atresia is unknown. There is no support for a genetic basis. Abnormalities in other organs found in 25 per cent of cases may have resulted from concomitant, yet undetermined, insults to the embryo. Ischaemia, biliary reflux of pancreatic enzymes, and immune-mediated damage have been proposed as initiating mechanisms. More recently viral infection has been suggested as a cause, particularly reovirus 3; this virus damages murine bile duct epithelium and produces a biliary atresia-like lesion in weanling mice.

Neonatal hepatitis

The term 'neonatal hepatitis' embraces a heterogeneous group of conditions associated with hepatic parenchymal damage and inflammation. An infective cause, such as cytomegalovirus, rubella, herpes simplex, varicella, hepatitis B, coxsackie or echo virus, toxoplasma, and treponema, is rarely identified. In very few instances galactosaemia, fructosaemia, and tyrosinaemia may present as neonatal hepatitis; in these cases fatty change is superimposed on the basic histopathological changes. In the vast majority of patients no cause is found.

The gross pathology comprises an enlarged cholestatic liver with splenomegaly and a frequently thin, but patent extrahepatic biliary system. Microscopically, multinucleated giant hepatocytes are prominent, associated with cholestasis and a variable degree of ballooning degeneration, cell necrosis, and loss of hepatocytes. There are foci of haemopoiesis, some haemosiderosis, and usually mild portal inflammation (Fig. 17.13).

The overall prognosis is favourable, although the infants appear more severely ill than those with biliary atresia. Progression to cirrhosis occasionally occurs, particularly in the rarer familial cases.

Paucity of the intrahepatic bile ducts

This pathological category encompasses patients in whom liver biopsy reveals an absence or reduced number of interlobular bile ducts. Biliary hypoplasia may occur in association with genetic disorders, in particular α-1-antitrypsin deficiency and impaired cholic acid synthesis, and in trisomy 17, 18, and 21. Exceptionally, it occurs after intra-uterine viral infection.

Excluding these associations, patients with this disorder can be divided into two groups:

1. the rare syndrome of arterio-hepatic dysplasia (Alagille syndrome) which is associated with a characteristic facies and a range of cardiovascular, skeletal, and ocular anomalies;

2. the extremely rare form not associated with these extrahepatic abnormalities.

Morphologically, the ratio of interlobular bile ducts to portal tracts is markedly reduced, cholestasis is prominent, and there may be focal giant cell transformation and a mild portal fibrosis (Fig. 17.14). Progression to cirrhosis is rare in Alagille syndrome.

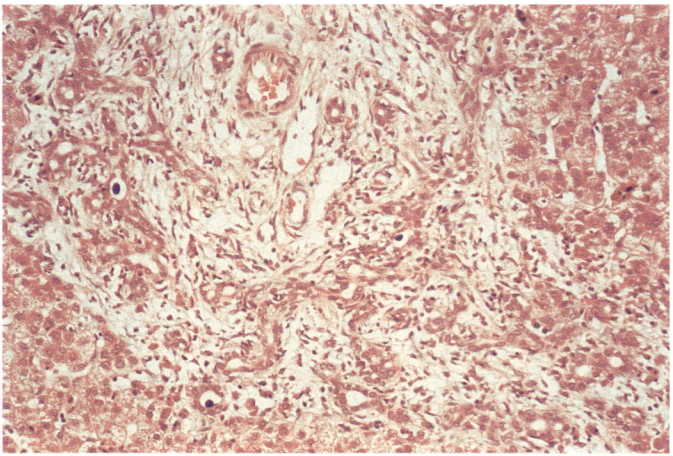

Fig. 17.12 Extrahepatic biliary atresia. The fibrotic and oedematous portal tracts contain proliferated ducts, some with luminal bile plugs.

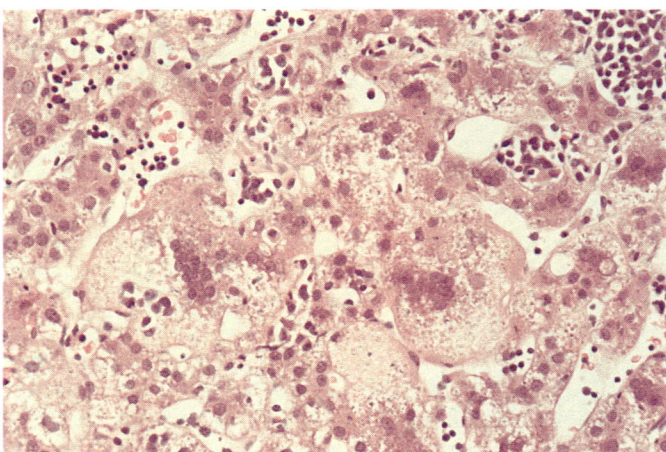

Fig. 17.13 Neonatal hepatitis. There is a marked disarray of the liver cell plates due to focal cell loss and multinucleated giant cell transformation. The liver is also infiltrated with haemopoietic and inflammatory cells.

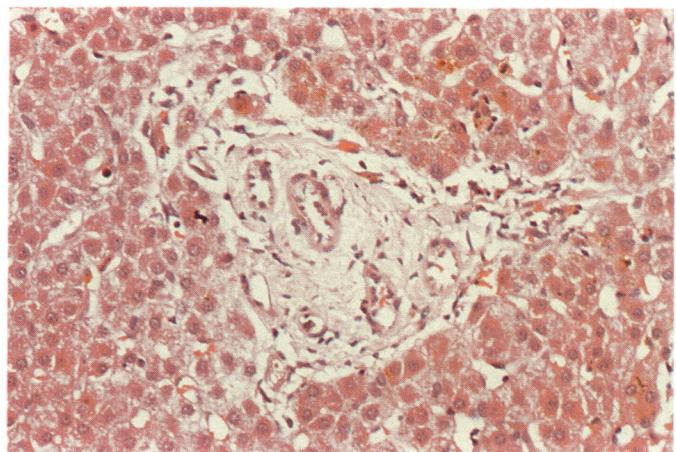

Fig. 17.14 Paucity of the intrahepatic bile ducts. A mildly oedematous and inflamed portal tract is devoid of a bile duct.

α-1-Antitrypsin and cholestasis in infancy

α-1-Antitrypsin deficiency is mentioned here as being the most common single association, found in up to 20 per cent of the infants presenting with prolonged cholestasis. Histopathologically, there may be paucity of the intrahepatic bile ducts, neonatal hepatitis with usually fewer giant hepatocytes, and/or portal changes. These changes mimic those of biliary atresia but occur in the absence of an extrahepatic bile duct lesion, and usually there is less cholestasis. α-1-Antitrypsin granules may be difficult to detect on biopsy obtained before 3 months of age, and the diagnosis has to be confirmed by determination of the α-1-antitrypsin serum phenotype (see Section 17.9.8).

As a group, infants with α-1-antitrypsin deficiency have a worse prognosis, cirrhosis developing in approximately 50 per cent of the patients.

17.2.4 Further reading

Alagille, D., Estrada, A., Hadchouel, M., Gautier, M., Odièvre, M., and Dommergues, J. P. (1987). Syndromic paucity of interlobular bile ducts (Alagille syndrome or arteriohepatic dysplasia): review of 80 cases. *Journal of Pediatrics* **110**, 195–200.

Balistreri, W. F. (1985). Neonatal cholestasis—medical progress. *Journal of Pediatrics* **106**, 171–84.

Blyth, H. and Ockenden, B. G. (1971). Polycystic disease of kidneys and liver presenting in childhood. *Journal of Medical Genetics* **8**, 257–84.

Chung, E. B. (1970). Multiple bile duct hamartomas. *Cancer* **26**, 287–96.

Crittenden, S. L. and McKinley, M. J. (1985). Choledochal cyst—clinical features and classification. *American Journal of Gastroenterology* **80**, 643–7.

Dalgaard, O. Z. (1957). Bilateral polycystic disease of the kidneys. A follow-up of 284 patients and their families. *Acta Medica Scandinavica* **328**, 13–225.

Fauvert, R. and Benhamou, J. P. (1974). Congenital hepatic fibrosis. In *The liver and its diseases* (ed. F. Schaffner, S. Sherlock, and C. M. Leevy), pp. 283–8. Intercontinental Medical Book Corporation, New York.

Gautier, M. and Eliot, N. (1981). Extrahepatic biliary atresia. Morphological study of 98 biliary remnants. *Archives of Pathology and Laboratory Medicine* **105**, 397–402.

Glaser, J. H. and Morecki, R. (1987). Reovirus Type 3 and neonatal cholestasis. *Seminars in Liver Disease* **7**, 100–7.

Ishak, K. G. and Sharp, H. L. (1987). Developmental abnormality and liver disease in childhood. In *Pathology of the liver* (2nd edn) (ed. R. N. M. MacSween, P. P. Anthony, and P. J. Scheuer), pp. 66–98. Churchill Livingstone, Edinburgh.

Jørgensen, M. J. (1977). The ductal plate malformation. *Acta Pathologica Microbiologica Scandinavica* **257**, 1–88.

Mercadier, M., Chigot, J. P., Clot, J. P., Langlois, P., and Lansieux, P. (1984). Caroli's disease. *World Journal of Surgery* **8**, 22–9.

Michels, N. (1951). The hepatic, cystic and retroduodenal arteries and their relation to the biliary ducts. *Annals of Surgery* **133**, 503–24.

Mowat, A. P. (1984). Alpha-1-antitrypsin deficiency in liver disease. In *Gastroenterology*, Vol. 4, 1, Butterworth's International Medical Reviews (ed. R. Williams and W. C. Maddrey). Butterworth, London.

Mowat, A. P. (ed.) (1987). *Liver disorders in childhood* (2nd edn). Butterworth, London.

Ohio, R., Hanamatsu, M., Mochizuki, I., Chiba, T., and Kasai, M. (1985). Progress in the treatment of biliary atresia. *World Journal of Surgery* **9**, 285–92.

Puente, S. G. and Bannura, G. C. (1983). Radiological anatomy of the biliary tract: variations and congenital abnormalities. *World Journal of Surgery* **7**, 271–6.

Voyles, C. R., Smadja, C., Shands, C., and Blumgart, L. H. (1983). Carcinoma in choledochal cysts. *Archives of Surgery* **118**, 986–8.

Wagget, J., Stoll, S., Bishop, H. C., and Kurtz, M. B. (1970. Congenital bronchobiliary fistula. *Journal of Pediatric Surgery* **81**, 1–13.

17.3 Viral hepatitis

17.3.1 Pathology of viral hepatitis

Peter J. Scheuer

Introduction

Viral infections of the liver may be due to one or more of a number of hepatotropic agents (the hepatitis viruses) or to other viruses which affect many organs including the liver. The hepatitis viruses are considered first. These are listed in Table 17.3. The hepatitis A virus (HAV) is an RNA enterovirus which can be demonstrated in faeces and liver of infected patients. The corresponding antigen, HAAg, is demonstrable in the liver by specific immunocytochemistry.

The best-studied hepatitis virus is the agent of type B hepatitis, HBV, discovered in the 1960s following the demonstration of the surface antigen (HBsAg) by Blumberg. The virus is a member of the hepadna family. It consists of a central core containing DNA, surrounded by an envelope or coat of surface material. The complete virus is known as the Dane particle. In addition to HBsAg, two further antigens can be demonstrated;

Table 17.3 The hepatitis viruses

Virus	Characteristics	Predominant mode of spread
Hepatitis A (HAV)	RNA enterovirus	Faecal–oral; sporadic or epidemic
Hepatitis B (HBV)	DNA hepadna virus	Parenteral; blood, venereal, perinatal transmission
Hepatitis C (HCV)	RNA, flavivirus-like	Parenteral: blood and blood products; may also be sporadic
Hepatitis D (HDV; the delta agent)	Defective RNA virus	Parenteral: only in the presence of HBV
Hepatitis E	RNA calicivirus	Faecal–oral; epidemic or sporadic
? Other non-A, non-B viruses	Unknown	Blood and blood products; also sporadic

core antigen (HBcAg), and the associated 'e' antigen (HBeAg). The significance of these antigens and their corresponding antibodies is further discussed in the next section of this chapter.

An apparently unique virus, the delta agent (hepatitis D virus; HDV), is found in some patients infected with HBV. The delta virus is an incomplete or defective RNA virus which is unable to replicate in the absence of the surface material of HBV. It is therefore only found in patients who are also infected with HBV. It can infect patients simultaneously with HBV (co-infection), or complicate existing chronic type B hepatitis (superinfection). Superinfection with HDV is an important cause of acute fulminant hepatitis, a very serious and often fatal condition.

Lastly, there is a group of viruses collectively known as the non-A, non-B (NANB) viruses. Two of these have been identified. The agent of hepatitis C, a major cause of transfusion-related hepatitis, was identified in the late 1980s by the techniques of molecular biology applied to RNA from infected plasma. Infection is diagnosed by detection of serum antibodies to viral proteins and PCR tests. The other virus, usually designated as hepatitis E virus, is responsible for outbreaks of epidemic hepatitis spread by sewage-contaminated water. It also causes sporadic hepatitis.

All these viruses can cause acute hepatitis, the pathological features of which are broadly similar whichever virus is responsible. In addition, HBV, HDV, and the parenterally transmitted NANB viruses are important causes of chronic liver disease, sometimes culminating in cirrhosis. The relationship between HBV and primary liver cancer is discussed separately.

The pathology of viral hepatitis

The pathological features of acute viral hepatitis differ from those of classical acute inflammation for two principal reasons: first, the cellular reaction is predominantly lymphocytic and monocytic because it is driven by viral antigens rather than by the chemical mediators of classical inflammation; and secondly, because the liver is a solid parenchymal organ, the cells of which are themselves the targets of immunological or viral onslaught, so that hepatocellular damage is an essential feature of hepatitis. It is the variable mixture of these two components that determines the exact pathology of the acute hepatitis in each individual patient.

Macroscopic features of acute hepatitis

The changes found in the milder, non-fatal forms of acute hepatitis are not well documented, because the organ is rarely seen with the naked eye. Clinical examination and imaging techniques indicate swelling of the organ. Observation by laparoscopy confirms the swelling and shows a reddened, oedematous capsular surface exuding serous fluid. In patients with much cholestasis, the surface becomes yellow or green, while focal areas of liver cell destruction are seen as irregular subcapsular depressions. When necrosis is widespread, as in fatal fulminant hepatitis, the liver shrinks and the capsule becomes wrinkled. Sectioning at autopsy then reveals either uniform destruction of the hepatic parenchyma, or irregular dark areas of necrosis alternating with paler areas of surviving parenchyma (Fig. 17.15). These surviving areas are often rounded as a result of regenerative hyperplasia, especially in patients who die some weeks or months after onset, from complications of the hepatitis rather than from liver failure. The appearances in such livers somewhat resemble those of cirrhosis. Recovery from acute hepatitis leaves the liver looking macroscopically normal or, if there has been much necrosis and collapse, irregularly scarred.

Microscopic features of acute hepatitis

Infiltration with lymphocytes, plasma cells, and macrophages is seen diffusely throughout the hepatic parenchyma, but is usually most severe in perivenular areas, in acinar zones 3 (Fig. 17.16). It is accompanied by evidence of hepatocellular injury

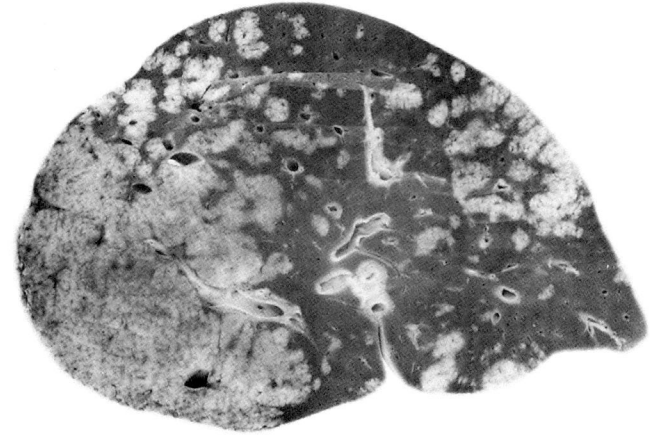

Fig. 17.15 Viral hepatitis with severe hepatic necrosis. Cross-section of a liver showing dark areas of collapse and paler, nodular zones of surviving and regenerating liver parenchyma.

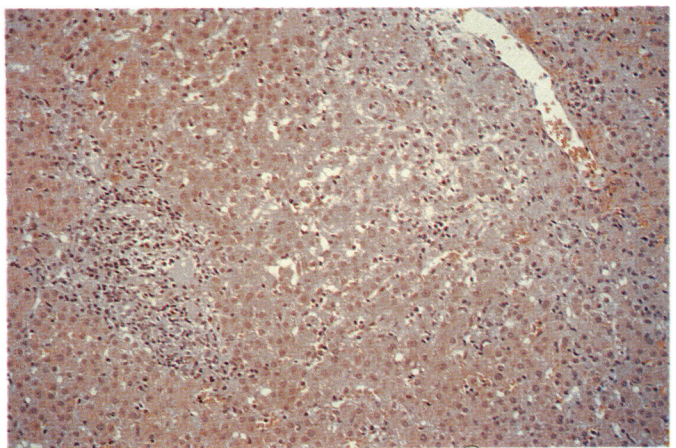

Fig. 17.16 Acute viral hepatitis. The parenchyma and portal tract (left) are infiltrated with inflammatory cells. Liver cell swelling is most severe near the terminal hepatic venule (top right).

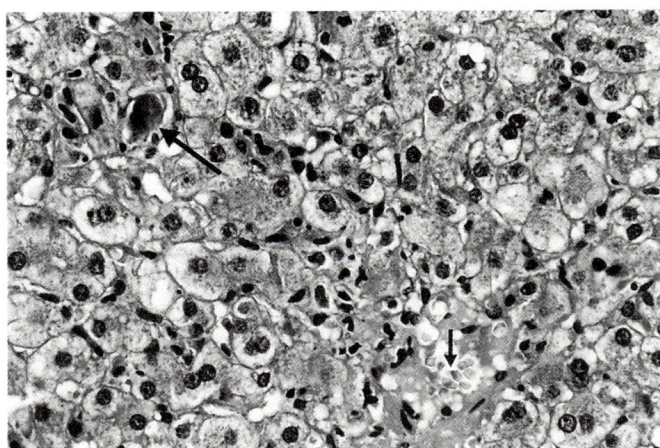

Fig. 17.17 Acute viral hepatitis. This high-power view shows swollen liver cells near a terminal hepatic venule (short arrow). Liver cell plates are irregular because of cell swelling and loss. An acidophil body is seen top left (long arrow). There are scattered inflammatory cells.

and death. Cell injury takes various forms. The commonest is cell swelling, corresponding ultrastructurally to intracellular oedema with dilatation of the cisternae of the endoplasmic reticulum. This type of injury is probably the precursor of cell lysis. Other hepatocytes show acidophilic change, with increased density and eosinophilia of their cytoplasm. Acidophil bodies, dense round or ovoid bodies with or without a nuclear remnant, are found lying free in the sinusoids, space of Disse, or liver cell plates (Fig. 17.17). These, the Councilman bodies first described in yellow fever, probably represent examples of the process of apoptosis (Section 3.1). Further evidence of liver cell damage is provided by the presence of bile in liver cell cytoplasm and canaliculi, suggesting interference with normal bile secretory mechanisms. Loss of hepatocytes, whether by lysis or apoptosis, leads to disruption of the liver cell plates and a phagocytic reaction. Dead cells are quickly removed, so that little or no dead tissue is seen under the microscope, in contrast to the process of infarction; thus hepatic necrosis in hepatitis is recognized less by cell death than by its precursor—cell injury—and its sequel—phagocytic scavenging. The presence of activated phagocytic Kupffer cells is readily shown in tissue sections by the periodic acid-Schiff method after digestion with diastase to remove liver cell glycogen.

Histological changes in acute hepatitis are also found in the portal tracts, which are infiltrated with a variety of inflammatory cells, mainly of the lymphocyte series, and are thus enlarged. Small bile ducts sometimes show irregularity of their epithelium, or inflammatory infiltration.

The distribution of the above changes, and their severity, varies. Most often, the hepatocellular necrosis is focal or spotty, with isolated foci of cell loss within damaged but surviving parenchyma. This is sometimes referred to as the classical form of acute hepatitis. The integrity of the liver cell plates is maintained by the surviving cells, and there is little or no collapse of the connective tissue framework of the acinus. In more severe cases, confluent necrosis results from the death of groups of

adjacent hepatocytes, usually next to or near a terminal hepatic venule. If this confluent necrosis is sufficiently severe to affect the whole of zone 3 of an acinus, a necrotic bridge develops between the terminal hepatic venule and a portal tract, since acinar zone 3 touches both these structures (Fig. 17.18). Bridging necrosis of this kind is important for several reasons. First, it denotes a hepatitis of more than usual severity. Secondly, it usually undergoes collapse, thus distorting the normal acinar structure and blood-vessels. In patients who subsequently develop chronic liver disease, this structural distortion is one of the factors that hasten the onset of cirrhosis. Thirdly, portal blood may find its way through the initially collapsed vascular channels of a necrotic bridge, to reach the terminal hepatic venule without filtering through intact hepatic parenchyma. Thus the anatomical basis is provided for portal–systemic venous shunting within the liver, one of the factors

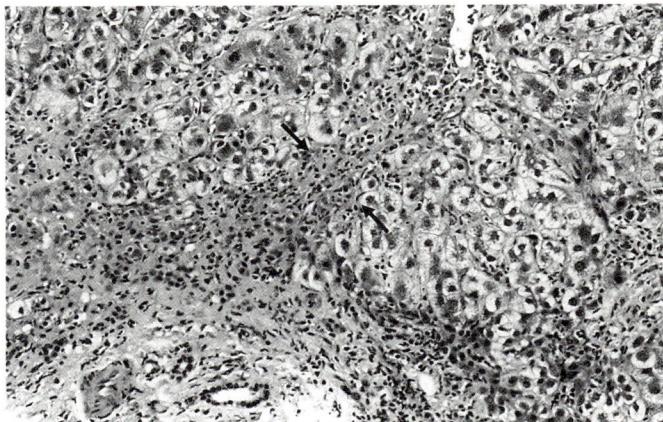

Fig. 17.18 Acute viral hepatitis with bridging necrosis. The arrows outline a necrotic bridge linking the portal tract (below left) to a terminal hepatic venule (above right).

that determine the onset of hepatic encephalopathy. In a minority of patients, confluent necrosis affects not only acinar zone 3, but also zones 2 and 1, so that whole acini are destroyed. This process of panacinar necrosis is seen most commonly in patients with life-threatening, fulminant hepatitis, in whom it affects much of the liver. The term 'submassive necrosis' is sometimes applied to this lesion. For reasons which are poorly understood, the panacinar necrosis may spare substantial portions of the hepatic parenchyma; these then form the basis for regenerative hyperplasia. Lastly, in addition to classical hepatitis, hepatitis with bridging necrosis, and hepatitis with panacinar necrosis, there is a form in which the necrosis develops mainly around enlarged, inflamed portal tracts, in acinar zones 1—hepatitis with periportal necrosis.

As already noted, all the hepatitis viruses cause fundamentally similar changes, and a firm aetiological diagnosis cannot be made on purely histological grounds. There are, however, certain patterns or trends associated with the individual viruses. In type A hepatitis, a periportal pattern is common and is sometimes associated with much perivenular cholestasis but little perivenular inflammation or necrosis. There is evidence to suggest that the cholestasis is partly the result of the amputation of small bile ducts and ductules involved in the portal and periportal inflammation and necrosis. The histological cholestasis is sometimes associated with a clinically and biochemically cholestatic course. In type B hepatitis, infiltration of the parenchyma by lymphoid cells is prominent, and these may be seen closely attached to or even apparently within hepatocytes, processes respectively called peripolesis and emperipolesis. In chronic carriers of the hepatitis B virus who are superinfected with the delta virus, hepatitis is usually severe and may be fulminant. In hepatitis C, infiltrating lymphocytes in the portal tracts often form follicles with or without germinal centres, resembling the follicles normally found in the cortex of a lymph node. Bile-duct damage is sometimes a prominent feature. Many lymphocytes are also found in the acinar sinusoids, and acidophil bodies are plentiful. Hepatitis E has been reported to resemble hepatitis A in its pathological features. It must be emphasized that the above patterns are not consistently present, and that all the hepatitis viruses may give rise to a wide variety of histological changes. Furthermore, viral hepatitis is closely mimicked by the idiosyncratic form of drug-induced liver injury (see Section 17.7).

Course and sequelae

In most patients, acute hepatitis runs its course over a period of several weeks, and then gradually regresses. As inflammation subsides and surviving hepatocytes divide to replace lost parenchyma, the histological appearances become less specific and eventually normal. Recent hepatocellular loss may sometimes be deduced from small areas of collapse or foci of activated, hypertrophied macrophages in acini and portal tracts. In patients with severe necrosis of bridging or panacinar type, corresponding areas of collapse are large, and may eventually turn into fibrous scars; however, considerable removal and remodelling of scars is possible.

In a minority of patients with type B and a substantial proportion of those with parentally transmitted NANB hepatitis, the disease becomes chronic. Chronicity is defined as continuing inflammation without improvement, of at least 6 months' duration. The various types of chronic hepatitis and their relation to cirrhosis and hepatocellular carcinoma are discussed in Section 17.5. It is sufficient here to note that chronicity is associated with very varied severity, some patients having virtually normal livers by light microscopy. In others there is severe inflammation and necrosis. Two causes of hepatitis appear to be associated with a high frequency of chronic disease: transfusion-related NANB hepatitis including hepatitis C, and the combination of HBV and HDV infection. The HBsAg-rich, ground-glass hepatocytes, which are characteristic of chronic HBV infection, are not found in acute type B hepatitis, although small amounts of HBsAg can sometimes be demonstrated by immunocytochemical methods early in an acute attack.

Other viral infections

In some viral infections the liver is merely one of several organs affected. However, in some of these other infections hepatic necrosis plays a substantial part. An example is yellow fever, the disease in which Councilman first described the shrunken, rounded liver cells which bear his name. Councilman bodies are apoptotic hepatocytes.

Cytomegalovirus infects the liver in the neonatal period or in adult life. In the latter, immunocompromised patients are most at risk of infection, which may be subclinical. Histological examination reveals varying degrees of infiltration with inflammatory cells, together with the characteristic inclusions in bile duct epithelium, liver cells, and endothelial cells.

The viruses of herpes simplex and of herpes zoster/varicella (chickenpox) are also more likely to involve the liver in patients with inadequate immune responses, in whom they cause focal areas of hepatic necrosis. In infectious mononucleosis the liver is infiltrated by atypical lymphocytes, even in patients without symptoms or signs of hepatic involvement. Granulomas are occasionally found. Serious liver disease due to the Epstein–Barr virus is rare. Adenoviruses and echoviruses occasionally involve the liver.

Infection of the neonatal liver by cytomegalovirus has already been mentioned. Other causes of neonatal infection include the rubella virus and reovirus. All three have been postulated as causes of bile duct damage with consequent loss of intrahepatic bile ducts (vanishing bile duct syndrome, paucity of intra-hepatic bile ducts) or hepatic bile ducts (extrahepatic biliary atresia).

A large variety of infective agents may be found in the livers of patients with the acquired immunodeficiency syndrome (AIDS), as well as in other patients with an inadequate immune response. Among the common bacterial agents are *Mycobacterium tuberculosis* and another mycobacterium, *M. aviumintracellulare*. Other organisms responsible for liver lesions in AIDS are cytomegalovirus, the fungus *Histoplasma*, and the protozoan *Cryptosporidium*.

17.3.2 The hepatitis viruses: virology and immunobiology

H. C. Thomas and J. Monjardino

Hepatitis A virus (HAV)

Although hepatitis A (infectious hepatitis) has been known as a clinical entity for many years, it was only in 1973 that the virus was first identified. Recently, both the use of genetic engineering technology and the identification of *in vitro* systems for virus propagation have provided a new impetus for active research in this field, leading to the structural characterization of the virus and further elucidation of its biology.

Structure

Hepatitis A virus is a small, non-enveloped RNA virus of the Picornaviridae family, genus Enterovirus. Poliovirus is the prototype of this family but the genomic and growth characteristics of HAV appear to be quite unique. The mature virions are approximately spherical, about 27 nm in diameter, and of icosahedral symmetry, with a sedimentation coefficient of 156S and a density of 1.325 g/cm³. The particles are remarkably heat resistant when compared to other picornaviruses, and will remain stable at 60 °C.

The genome is a molecule of single-stranded RNA about 7500 nucleotides long, with a polyA tail at the 3′ terminus. The genome comprises a long 5′ untranslated region, an open reading frame, and a short 3′ untranslated region. The virus particle contains three major structural polypeptides (VP1, VP2, VP3), ranging in size from 24 000 to 34 000 Da, and a minor one (VP4) of less than 8000 Da (Fig. 17.19). Recent molecular cloning of HAV cDNA from different virus isolates has shown more than 95 per cent identity in nucleotide sequence and over 98 per cent homology in predicted amino-acid sequence for the genomic regions analysed, but no homology with the genomes of other members of the picornavirus family. The amino-acid changes observed between different strains so far analysed appear to occur in the capsid, and particularly within VP1. Recent studies have implicated this polypeptide as having a major role in the immune response against HAV, but cross-neutralization studies have failed to show any antigenic differences between isolates of different geographic origins, implying that the amino-acid changes lie in non-antigenic regions of VP1. Although different in nucleotide sequence when compared to other picornaviruses, HAV RNA shows clear similarities in genomic organization with other members of this family. These include a central open reading frame flanked by untranslated regions at both the 5′ and 3′ ends and a 3′ polyA tail. The same applies to the viral proteins which, in spite of very limited homology with those of other picornaviruses, retain an analogous ordering of their respective genes in the open reading frame. Other gene products are thought to include proteins involved in replication, and include an RNA polymerase and a protease thought to carry out the processing of the polyprotein made from the polycistronic mRNA in a manner similar to that documented for poliovirus.

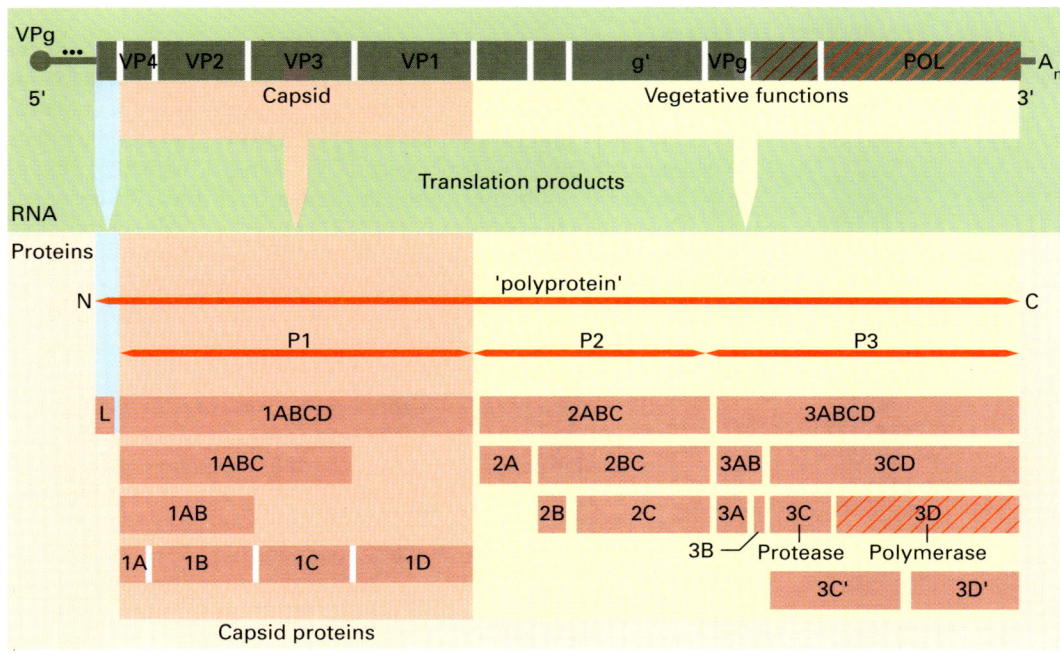

Fig. 17.19 The HAV genome.

Replication and expression of viral genes

Little is known at the molecular level about the replication of HAV RNA and the assembly of new virions. Most *in vitro* systems used so far produce poor virus yields and do not undergo cell lysis (cytopathic effect). The infection appears to spread to adjacent cells by an unknown mechanism and cell lines remain persistently infected, in contrast to the *in vivo* infected hepatocytes which undergo lysis during the self-limiting course of acute infection.

Immunobiology

The virus replicates within the liver, is excreted in the stool, and evokes a strong antibody response. A rapid rise in IgM antibody titre occurs at onset and is of diagnostic use (Fig. 17.20). This antibody lasts for 3–6 months. IgG antibodies are present in high titre from the clinical onset and remain for life, conferring protective immunity. The virus-neutralizing antibody is directed to a conformational determinant, including sequences from the VP1 structural capsid peptide. The majority of the antibodies are directed to a limited number of epitopes. In North America and Western Europe, by middle age, approximately 40 per cent of people have immunity. The prevalence of infection increases by 10 per cent per decade of life. The infection rate is greater in developing countries. In most tropical areas more than 90 per cent of the population will have immunity by 10 years of age.

It is suspected that hepatitis A virus (HAV) replicates initially in the intestinal mucosa and then subsequently in the liver. This is supported by the observation that in marmosets immunosuppressed with prednisolone, HAV antigens can be detected in the enterocytes of the upper jejunum. There is an IgA-class antibody response within the intestinal mucosa, and it is likely that this is important in conferring protective immunity against enteric challenge.

Cell-mediated immunity to the virus capsid antigens has been demonstrated. Whether the liver damage is caused by a cyto-

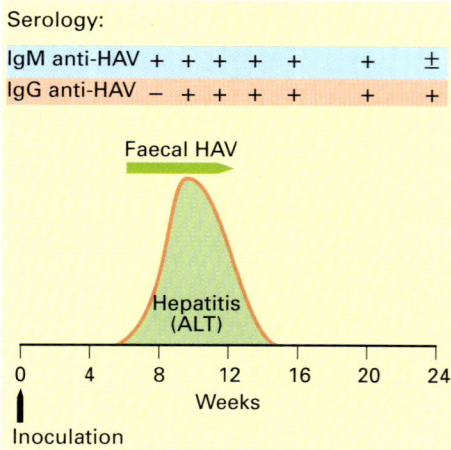

Fig. 17.20 The immune response to HAV. HAV virus is shed into the faeces before the development of humoral immunity (IgM anti-HAV) and before the hepatitis.

pathic effect of the virus or by cell-mediated immune responses directed to viral determinants on the infected hepatocytes has not been established.

During the acute phase of the infection, serum IgM concentrations increase and large amounts of circulating immune complexes are present. Low-titre smooth muscle antibody is often present. Low-titre IgM-class liver membrane antibodies (LMA) are found in most sera and may be causatively related to the piecemeal necrosis that is seen in most of these patients. It should be emphasized, however, that chronic infection and chronic hepatitis are not seen.

Hepatitis B virus (HBV)

The discovery in 1965 by Blumberg and co-workers of the Australian antigen and of its significance as a serum marker of human hepatitis B virus infection was followed by the identification of the virion by Dane in 1970 and by major contributions during the early 1970s to our understanding of the structure and antigenic make-up of the virus particle. Although sensitive and reliable diagnostic tests were developed at this time, which led to the characterization of the natural history and epidemiology of the disease, the molecular events underlying viral replication, pathogenesis, and persistence were still largely unknown, due to the lack of suitable *in vitro* cultured cells that would support viral replication. Progress in this area eventually came in the 1980s from the application of the new technologies of genetic engineering and from the identification and subsequent study of related viruses, which together with hepatitis B make up the new group of hepadna viruses. This group presently includes the human heptatitis B virus (HBV), woodchuck hepatitis virus (WHV), ground squirrel hepatitis viris (GSHV), and duck hepatitis B virus (DHBV).

Structure

Hepadna viruses are small DNA viruses with a marked hepatotropism. They contain a partially double-stranded, circular genome about 3.2 kilobases long and made up of a complete minus strand (discontinuous at one point) and an incomplete plus strand (50–70 per cent of full length), which are maintained in a circular configuration through the 200 base pair overlap of the 5′ termini (Fig. 17.21). At both sides of the cohesive region there is an 11 base pair repeat, conserved in all HBV genome sequences, and termed DR1 and DR2. The viral envelope is made of a major surface antigen polypeptide in both glycosylated and non-glycosylated form, and of small amounts of two larger polypeptides (also present in glycosylated form) which are co-terminal with the major surface polypeptide at the carboxyl end but differ at the amino end (Fig. 17.22). The nucleocapsid of the virion contains both a core polypeptide, closely bound to the viral genome, and DNA polymerase activity, which can extend the incomplete strand of viral DNA.

Of the two strands of the genome, the longer strand has been shown to contain all the coding potential of the virus, and four open reading frames have been identified from the DNA sequences published for the different subtypes. Of these, two have been positively assigned as the surface and core genes; one

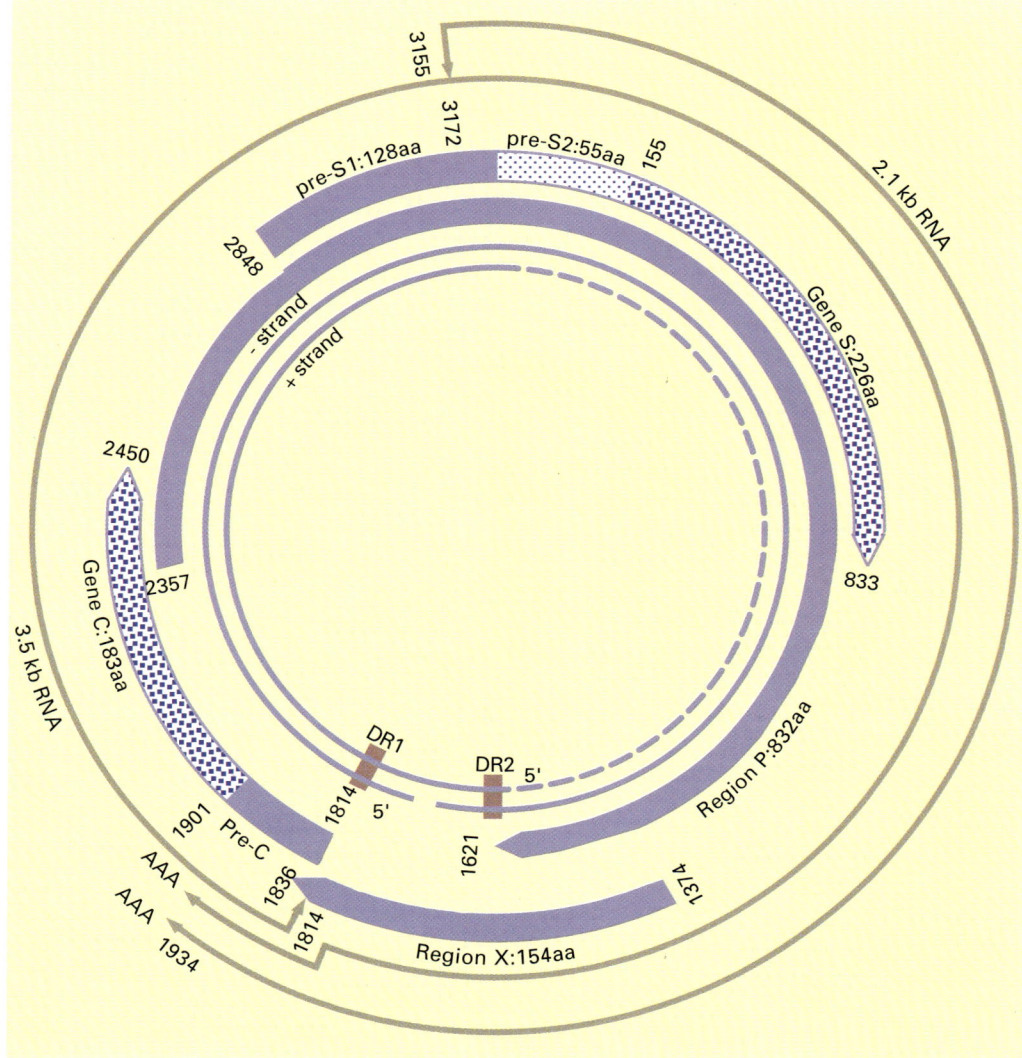

Fig. 17.21 The HBV genome. See text for abbreviations.

is presumed to code for the DNA polymerase; and the fourth, or X, gene corresponds to a gene product of unknown function (Fig. 17.21). The open reading frame of the surface antigen gene extends upstream in the same reading register by 489 nucleotides (ayw3 subtype) and provides coding potential for 163 additional amino acids. In HBV, this pre-S region contains two AUG codons. These two initiation codons subdivide the pre-S region into pre-S1 and pre-S2, and polypeptides initiating from them constitute the minor envelope components described above (Fig. 17.22). The core gene is similarly extended by a pre-core region with the potential for coding for 29 additional amino acids.

Viral particles present in blood comprise both the fully infectious 42 nm Dane particle and excess viral coat material in the form of 20 nm spheres and 20 nm diameter tubules, which do not contain DNA and are, therefore, not infectious (Fig. 17.23). Large amounts of a core-related peptide (e antigen) are also found in serum in association with viral replication. This soluble antigen is generated from the pre-core containing core polypeptide by proteolytic cleavage at the amino and carboxyl ends.

Replication and expression of virus genes

Recently, it was reported that the virus receptor involved in attachment to the hepatocyte is contained predominantly within the pre-S1 region. Both the nature of the hepatocyte viral receptor and the mechanism by which the virus enters the hepatocyte are largely unknown. Progress in this area is likely to have significant clinical implications, both in prevention and control of the infection.

The strategy of replication of HBV was partially elucidated by the elegant studies carried out by Summers and Mason on the duck hepatitis virus, subsequently confirmed by investigations of the human and other hepadna viruses, and is schematically

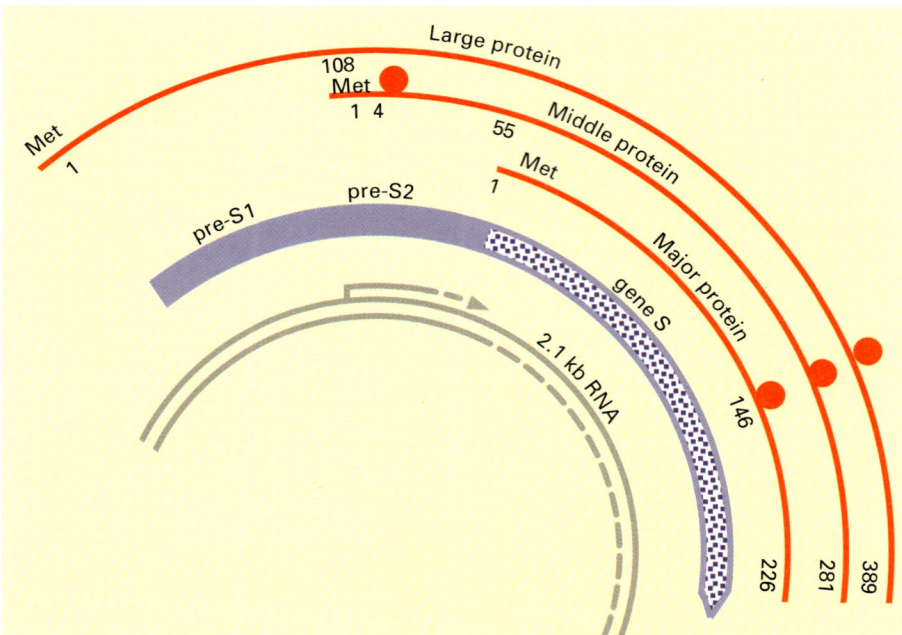

Fig. 17.22 HBV envelope proteins (large, middle, and small). ●, glycosylation sites.

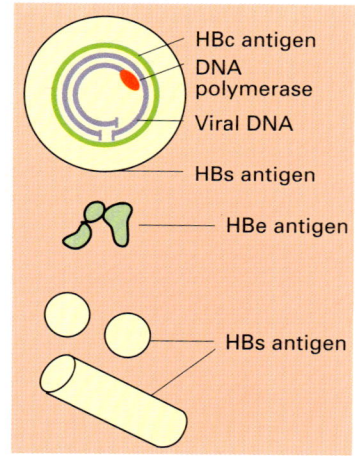

Fig. 17.23 Diagrammatic appearance of HBV (particles, non-infectious spheres and tubules of HBsAg, and HBeAg).

depicted in Fig. 17.24. The replication of viral DNA is initiated by the uncoating and filling in of the infecting viral genome to generate a circular, double-stranded template for the synthesis of a pre-genomic RNA, presumably by the host RNA polymerase II. This pre-genomic RNA, which is terminally redundant by about 120 nucleotides (i.e. present at both ends of the molecule), becomes associated with immature core particles and serves as a template for the reverse transcription of the minus viral DNA strand, which initiates from a protein primer within the DR1 direct repeat. The completed minus strand, which is terminally redundant by about 8 nucleotides, serves in turn as the template for the synthesis of the plus strand, which

initiates from a transposed RNA primer derived from the 5′ end of the pre-genomic RNA. This RNA primer base pairs, via its DR1 direct repeat, to the direct repeat sequence DR2. The enzyme copies the region adjacent to the DR2 sequence first and proceeds to the 5′ end of the template minus strand where it stops before switching via the terminal redundancy to the 3′ end of the minus strand, which it then proceeds to copy. In the case of HBV, the growing plus strand is never completed and, upon reaching a critical length, a conformational change must take place in the closely associated core which will trigger the ordered intracytoplasmic transit of the core particles and their ultimate coating and release.

Analysis of viral messenger RNA during HBV replication shows a similar pattern in all hepadna viruses. In HBV-infected cells two major transcripts have been identified, one 2.1 kb long associated with the synthesis of the major HBsAg polypeptide, and a larger, terminally redundant transcript of about 3.4 kb, which appears to serve as the messenger RNA for the synthesis of both core and polymerase, as well as to constitute the pre-genomic RNA template required for replication. Both these major transcripts terminate at the same point on the circular DNA under the control of a polyA termination sequence mapping at about 1900, although the longer transcript is only processed at this point when the polymerase passes through it a second time (Fig. 17.21). Both the 3′ and 5′ ends have been mapped for the two major mRNA species and starting codons have been identified for the synthesis of the major surface and core peptides, as well as the other minor peptides which share with surface and core the carbonyl end but differ at the amino end (pre-S and pre-core). Recent studies have shown that pre-core sequences contain as a signal peptide, directing the core peptide towards the endoplasmic reticulum (ER) membrane

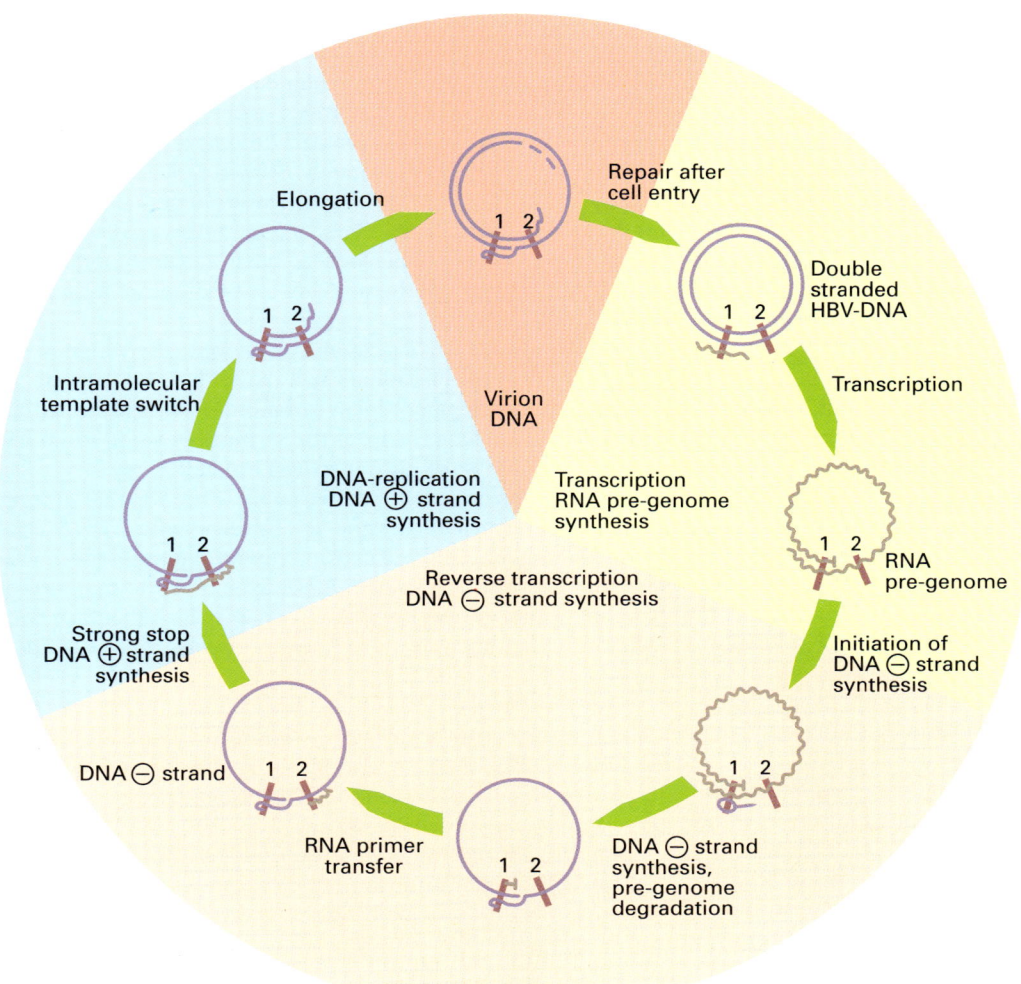

Fig. 17.24 Proposed model for replication of HBV. Replication is divided into three stages: transcription, reverse transcription, and DNA replication. After entry into the hepatocyte and uncoating the partially double-stranded virion, DNA is made fully double-stranded and serves as a template for transcription of a long terminally redundant RNA pregenome as well as other viral transcripts. The minus strand of HBV DNA is synthesized by reverse transcription of pregenomic RNA, and is primed by a virus-coded protein positioned within the repeat sequence DR1. The RNA template is progressively degraded as DNA synthesis proceeds (by RNAse H activity associated with the enzyme) but a short oligoribonucleotide from the 5′ end of the RNA, comprising DR1, is retained. The latter is transposed by a poorly understood mechanism to base-pair with the DR2 region of the minus DNA strand close to its 5′ end. Synthesis then proceeds to the end of the 5′ end of the template (strong stop of DNA plus strand synthesis) before an intramolecular strand switch which allows the molecule to become circular, and positive strand synthesis to proceed. Before completion of the second strand the core particles become coated with surface antigen and exit the cell.

where it interacts with the surface antigen complex in the process of virion assembly and where HBeAg is secreted into the lumen of the ER following proteolytic cleavage of core peptide during rapid viral replication.

The enzyme DNA polymerase has not yet been solubilized from purified Dane particles and its amino-acid sequence is inferred from the DNA sequence of the open reading frame which has been tentatively ascribed to it. The enzymatic activity can, however, be assayed in permeabilized cores and has been used extensively as a marker of serum infectivity and viral replication. The product of gene X is unknown. The gene codes for 154 amino acids, corresponding to a polypeptide of molecular weight 16 560, and recent evidence has shown that it is more related to genes of eukaryotic cells than to the other genes of HBV (or viral genes in general), and suggests that it may be a 'late' acquisition from the cell genome, with a regulatory function.

Immunobiology

HBV is parenterally transmitted, usually during therapeutic use of blood or blood products, sexual contact, or sharing of needles during drug abuse. The incubation period is 3–6 months.

When infection occurs in adult life it may result in acute hepatitis, varying in severity from asymptomatic to fulminant hepatitis, or, in 10 per cent of cases, in chronic infection with development of chronic hepatitis. More rarely, extrahepatic syndromes, including polyarteritis nodosa, membranoproliferative glomerulonephritis, polyneuropathy, papullar acrodermatitis, and mixed-cryoglobulinaemia, may occur (Fig. 17.25).

In Japan and China, infection usually occurs at birth. The child born to a chronic carrier mother who has viraemia (HBe antigenaemia) at the time of birth will almost certainly be infected, and more than 95 per cent of these patients develop chronic infection (Fig. 17.25). In these communities between 10 and 20 per cent of the population is chronically infected.

The acute infection is diagnosed by the presence of HBs antigen and IgM anti-HBc in high titre. The patients are often asymptomatic but may develop jaundice and even liver failure (Fig. 17.25). Acute hepatitis is common after exposure in adult life but rare during neonatal infection.

Patients developing chronic infection initially exhibit high levels of viral replication, marked by HBe antigenaemia, and this indicates a state of relatively high infectivity. Patients in this phase often have only mild liver disease, but as the infection continues, over the years, the patient will develop chronic active and lobular hepatitis (Fig. 17.26). This inflammatory activity represents immune clearance of infected liver cells and is accompanied by a falling level of viraemia. Eventually, the virus will be cleared from the peripheral blood but hepatitis B surface antigenaemia will continue because of the presence of hepatitis B virus sequences integrated in the DNA of the liver cells. These two phases of active viral replication and integration of the virus can be differentiated by the presence of HBe antigen and antibody in the serum (Fig. 17.26).

After 20–30 years of chronic infection these patients, who have developed severe chronic liver disease with cirrhosis, run the risk of developing hepatocellular carcinoma.

Recently, randomized controlled trials have shown that lymphoblastoid and recombinant α-interferon will terminate HBV replication in approximately 50 per cent of patients acquiring the infection in adulthood. These patients then show a marked improvement in their inflammatory liver disease. Patients acquiring the infection at birth are more difficult to treat, but prednisolone therapy followed by interferon appears to be promising.

Once hepatocellular carcinoma is present, the prognosis is poor. The majority of patients will die within 3–6 months of diagnosis. Early hepatocellular carcinoma can be detected by monitoring for α-fetoprotein in the serum. For small tumours, hepatic resection is the only effective form of therapy.

The envelope proteins of the virus have been prepared from plasma of viraemic patients and also by recombinant DNA techniques. These proteins will evoke a humoral immune response and this is effective in preventing infection in the majority of patients. A small minority, particularly of older patients or subjects with other diseases, have failed to respond to the vaccine.

Delta hepatitis virus (HDV)

Delta hepatitis virus is a defective, naturally occurring human virus first described by Rizzetto in 1977, which requires hepatitis B virus for its transmission. This dependence on HBV has meant that experimental studies have been limited to the chimpanzee. Successful co-infection with delta hepatitis virus and the HBV-related virus from the woodchuck (WHV) recently reported, has now provided a more accessible animal model for the study of HDV.

Structure

Delta hepatitis virus is a small RNA virus consisting of spherical 36 nm diameter particles. The outer coat consists of surface antigen material provided by HBV and surrounds a circular single-stranded RNA genome of about 1700 nucleotides and the delta antigen. Three complete cDNA sequences have been reported, showing significant genetic heterogeneity between

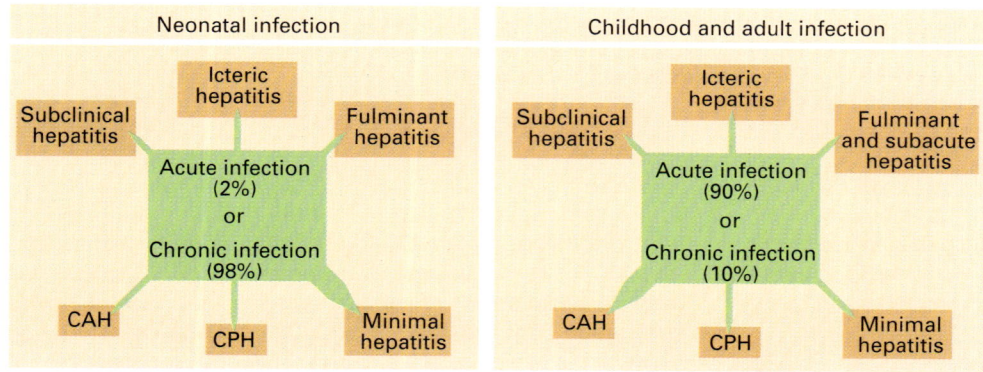

Fig. 17.25 Clinical syndromes following HBV infection. CAH, chronic active hepatitis; CPH, chronic persistent hepatitis.

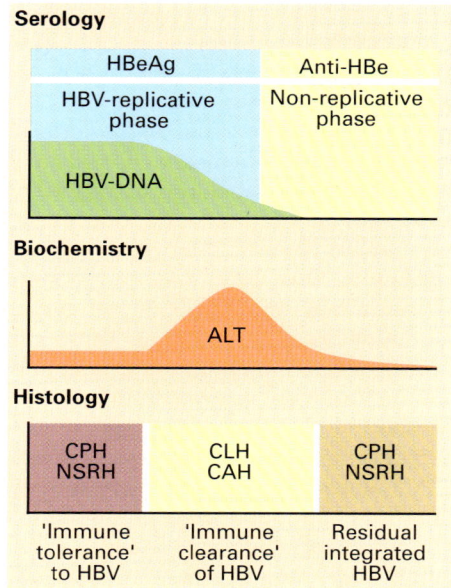

Fig. 17.26 Natural history of chronic HBV infection. During the period of viral replication, HBeAg is present in the patient's serum. Continued production of HBs antigen after cessation of HBV replication indicates the presence of hepatocytes that contain integrated HBV sequences. CPH, chronic persistent hepatitis; CLH, chronic lobular hepatitis; CAH, chronic active hepatitis; NSRH, non-specific reactive hepatitis.

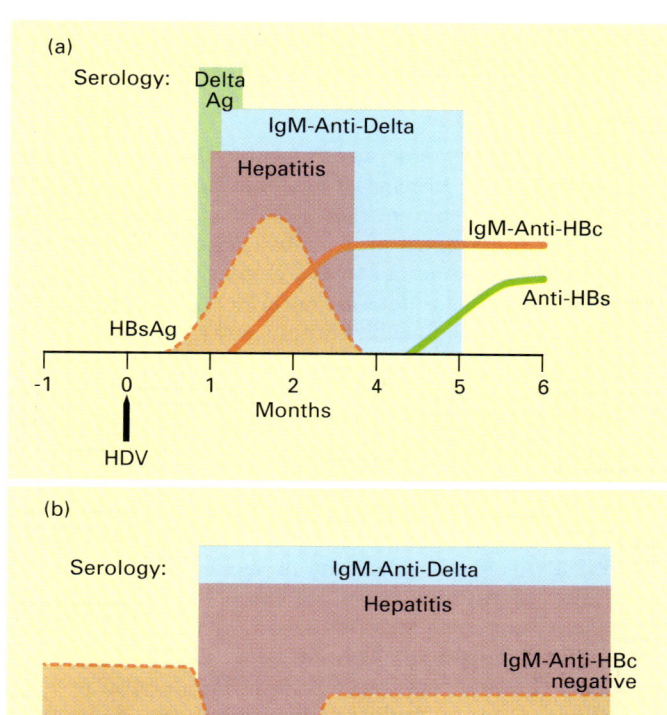

Fig. 17.27 Co-infection and superinfection with HDV. (a) Co-infection results in the development of IgM anti-HBc and IgM anti-HDV. (b) Superinfection of an HBV carrier with HDV results in IgM anti-HDV in the absence of IgM anti-HBc.

isolates, particularly between the directly derived human sequences and that from virus sequentially passaged in the chimpanzee. The viral RNA shows a high degree of self-complementarity and its unusual properties resemble those of viroids and virusoids that infect plants. Analysis of the sequence predicts several open reading frames, and one on the antigenomic strand has been assigned to the gene coding for the delta antigen.

Replication and expression of viral genes

Based in the evidence referred to above and on the observation that eukaryotic ribosomes do not translate circular RNA, it has been suggested that delta virus is a minus-strand RNA virus, requiring the synthesis of functional linear mRNA from the circular genomic template. Antigenomic RNA has also been postulated to be required as a replicative intermediate template for the synthesis of the new viral genomes. The enzyme(s) involved in these reactions have not been identified and the mechanism of replication has not been established.

Immunobiology

Both HDV and HBV may be introduced in the same inoculum (co-infection) (Fig. 17.27) and give rise to acute hepatitis with a 5–10 per cent chance of chronicity. In other cases, delta virus superinfects an established chronic HBV carrier and causes an acceleration of the course of the chronic hepatitis, so that the patient rapidly progresses to cirrhosis. Both co-infection and superinfection can, in the acute phase, be diagnosed by the demonstration of delta antigen or IgM anti-delta in the serum. In co-infection, but not in superinfection, high-titre IgM anti-HBc is also present. In chronic delta virus infection, higher-titre IgG antibody is found, and continuing IgM antibody responses are observed.

Non-A, non-B hepatitis virus infection

The non-A, non-B viruses are an important cause of epidemic (enterally transmitted) and post-transfusion (parenterally transmitted) hepatitis. The diagnosis depended upon the exclusion of HAV and HBV infection by demonstrating the absence of IgM anti-HAV and IgM anti-HBc, respectively. Epstein–Barr virus and cytomegalovirus infection were also excluded by IgM antibody tests.

In 1989–91 one parenterally and one enterally transmitted

non A, non B virus have been isolated, the genomes cloned and sequenced, and diagnostic tests developed.

Hepatitis C virus

In 1989 one of the parenterally transmitted viruses was cloned and sequenced from infected chimpanzee blood. The virus was pelleted from the serum, nucleic acid extracted and amplified, and sequences expressed in a lambda bacteriophage library. Clones expressing immunoreactive proteins of the hepatitis C virus were identified by immunological techniques using globulin pooled from patients with chronic post-transfusion non-A, non-B hepatitis. It was assumed that these patients had in their serum an antibody to at least one of the components of the non-A, non-B virus. This assumption turned out to be correct in that the group identified one clone which expressed a fragment of a non-structural protein of hepatitis C virus. Subsequently further clones were identified, and the complete genome was sequenced. The genome consists of a molecule of single-stranded RNA of positive polarity of about 9400 nucleotides, and contains a single open reading frame encoding a polyprotein of approximately 3010 amino acids. From this polyprotein, nucleocapsid, matrix, envelope, and non-structural (presumed enzyme) proteins of HCV are produced. The long, open reading frame is flanked by two sequences, one of about 320–340 nucleotides at the 5′ end and one of about 40–60 nucleotides at the 3′ end. Comparison of published sequences from several isolates shows overall homology ranging from 70 to 90 per cent at nucleotide level, and higher homology at amino acid level. Computer genome homology searches have shown this agent to be distantly related to the Flaviviridae and Pestiviridae. Both the hydrophylicity/hydrophobicity analysis and the identification of 'signature' sequences for signalases and RNA replicases suggest that, as with members of those genera, structural proteins are encoded from the 5′ end, and follow the order capsid-matrix-envelope downstream before a series of 5 non-structural polypeptides (Fig. 17.28). The latter include both proteases for processing the polyprotein and the polymerase at the 3′ end of the coding region.

Currently, acute and chronic HCV are diagnosed by the appearance of an antibody to one of the non-structural proteins (NS4). Following acute non-A, non-B hepatitis, about half the patients make a complete recovery, and the remainder progress to chronic liver disease. Antibody to the NS4 protein is found in 90 per cent of the chronic group and half the acute resolving group after about 24 weeks. The seroprevalence of this antibody in chronic post-transfusion non-A, non-B hepatitis varies from 71–88 per cent and in chronic sporadic non-A, non-B hepatitis from 58–75 per cent. Between 60 and 90 per cent of haemophiliacs and intravenous drug abusers, and 20 per cent of dialysis patients have been found to be anti-HCV positive. However, only 8 per cent of homosexuals and 6 per cent of the sexual contacts of intravenous drug users were seropositive. This suggests that HCV is not as readily transmissible as HBV or HIV following sexual contact. Most seroprevalence studies in healthy populations have been undertaken in collaboration with blood transfusion services. A British survey examined 1100 blood donations and found 6 to be anti-HCV positive (0.55 per cent). Similar seroprevalence rates have been described elsewhere in Europe and North America.

The late occurrence of the antibody to the non-structural (NS4) protein in acute hepatitis limits the diagnostic usefulness of this test. PCR amplification systems have been used to detect viral genomes in serum, and this test demonstrates that the patient with acute hepatitis C virus infection has viraemia for several weeks before the appearance of this antibody. Antibodies to the nucleocapsid region of HCV occur a little earlier but there is still a period of viraemia preceding the appearance of this antibody.

Patients with chronic hepatitis C virus infection are capable of transmitting the virus by blood donation or by close personal contact resulting in transfer of body fluids. There are problems with false positivity with existing tests, and not all patients with serological evidence of HCV infection necessarily have viraemia as detected by the polymerase chain reaction.

From a clinical point of view the hepatitis C virus is an important infective agent. Although the acute illness is mild, 20–80 per cent of patients develop chronic infection, and in some cases this ultimately leads to cirrhosis and hepatocellular carcinoma. The parenterally transmitted viruses are probably cytopathic. Low-titre smooth muscle antibody occurs, but hyperglobulinaemia is not evident until cirrhosis is present.

Patients with hepatitis C virus-induced chronic hepatitis may be treated with intramuscular α-interferon. Protracted periods of treatment from 3–12 months control viraemia and result in normalization of liver function tests. However there is a high relapse rate even after one year of therapy with α-interferon and the long term response rate is of the order of 30 per cent.

A second parenterally transmitted non-A, non-B virus may exist—HCV appears to account for only 90 per cent of cases of post-transfusion hepatitis.

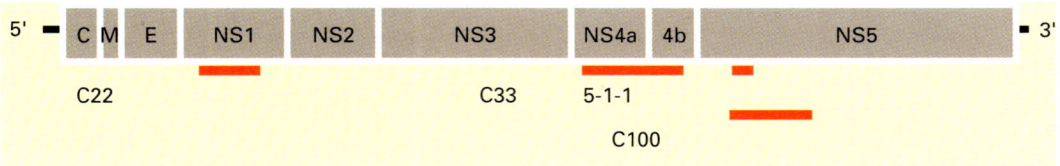

Fig. 17.28 Genome of HCV putative viral proteins encoded within the single open reading frame are: C–nucleocapsid; M–matrix; E–envelope; NS1, NS2, NS3, NS4, NS5–non-structural proteins. Current diagnostic tests detect anti-NS4 (C100); future tests will detect anti-C22 and anti-C33.

Epidemic non-A, non-B hepatitis (hepatitis E) virus

This form of hepatitis was first described in Kashmir and North Africa. The disease is similar to acute HAV infection. The hepatitis is usually self-limiting but in 20 per cent of cases follows a cholestatic course. Chronic infection and chronic hepatitis do not occur. The epidemic form is particularly severe in pregnant women. The disease is transmitted by the faecal-oral route. A virus particle has been identified in the faeces of infected patients, and a serum antibody response is seen. Most recently the virus has been isolated, cloned, and sequenced. The sequence of the virus suggests homology to the Caliciviruses which are positive stranded RNA agents. Viral nucleic acid has been detected in infected liver cells, and virus particles in bile and faeces. Diagnostic tests have been developed, and an IgM antibody is present in acute phase sera. No treatment is necessary.

17.3.3 Further reading

Pathology of viral hepatitis

Dienes, H. P., Popper, H., Arnold, W., and Lobeck, H. (1982). Histologic observations in human hepatitis non-A, non-B. *Hepatology* 2, 562–71.

Dienes, H. P., Hütteroth, T., Bianchi, L., Grün, M., and Thoenes, W. (1986). Hepatitis A-like non-A, non-B hepatitis: light and electron microscopic observations of three cases. *Virchows Archiv A* 409, 657–67.

Rizzetto, M., Bonino, F., and Verme, G. (1988). Hepatitis delta virus infection of the liver: progress in virology, pathology and diagnosis. *Seminars in Liver Disease* 8, 350–6.

Scheuer, P. J. (1987). Viral hepatitis. In *Pathology of the liver* (2nd edn), (ed. R. N. M. MacSween, P. P. Anthony, and P. J. Scheuer). Churchill Livingstone, Edinburgh.

Wilkins, M. J., Lindley, R., Dourakis, R. P., and Goldin, R. D. (1991). Surgical pathology of the liver in HIV infection. *Histopathology* 18, 459–64.

Zuckerman, A. J., (1989). The elusive hepatitis C virus: a cause of parenteral non-A, non-B hepatitis. *British Medical Journal* 299, 871–3.

Zuckerman, A. J. (1990). Hepatitis E virus. The main cause of enterically transmitted non-A, non-B hepatitis. *British Medical Journal* 300, 1475–6.

Hepatitis A

Baroudy, B. M., Miele, T. A., Ticehurst, J. R., Maizel, J. V., Purcell, R. W., and Feinstone, S. M. (1985). Sequence analysis of HAV cDNA coding capsid proteins and RNA polymerase. *Proceedings of the National Academy of Sciences USA* 82, 2143.

Emini, E. A., Schlief, W. A., Colonno, R. G., and Wiemer, E. (1985). Antigenic conservation and divergence between the viral specific proteins of poliovirus type 1 and various picornaviruses. *Virology* 140, 182–4.

Fasel-Felley, J. (1986). A specific immune response to purified HA antigen demonstrated by leucocyte migration inhibition in patients recovering from viral hepatitis A. *Journal of Hepatology* 2, 237–44.

Feinstone, S. M., Kapikain, A. Z., and Purcell, R. H. (1973). Hepatitis A: detection by immune electron microscopy of a virus like antigen associated with acute illness. *Science* 182, 1026–8.

Karayiannis, P., *et al.* (1986). Hepatitis A virus replication in tamarins

and host immune response in relation to pathogenesis of liver cell damage. *Journal of Medical Virology* 18, 261–76.

Thomas, H. C. (1981). T cell subsets in patients with acute and chronic HBV infection, primary biliary cirrhosis and alcohol-induced liver disease. *International Journal of Immunopharmacology* 3, 301–8.

Thomas, H. C., *et al.* (1978). Immune complexes in acute and chronic liver disease. *Clinical and Experimental Immunology* 31, 150–9.

Ticehurst, J. R. (1986). Hepatitis A virus: clones, cultures and vaccines. *Seminars in Liver Disease* 6 (1), 46–55.

Wiedmann, K. H., Bartholomew, T. C., Brown, D. J. C., and Thomas, H. C. (1984). Liver membrane antibodies detected by immunoradiometric assay in acute and chronic virus induced and autoimmune liver disease. *Hepatology* 4, 199–204.

Hepatitis B

Almeida, J. D., Rubenstein, D., and Stott, E. J. (1971). New antigen/antibody system in Australia antigen associated hepatitis. *Lancet* ii, 1225.

Blumberg, B. S., Harvey, J. A., and Visnich, S. (1965). A new antigen in leukaemic serum. *Journal of the American Medical Association* 191, 101–10.

Dane, D. S., Cameron, C. H., and Briggs, M. (1970). Virus-like particles in serum of patients with Australia antigen-associated hepatitis. *Lancet* i, 695–702.

Fowler, M. F., Thomas, H. C., and Monjardino, J. P. (1986). Cloning and analysis of integrated HBV-DNA of the adr subtype derived from HCC. *Journal of General Virology* 67, 771–5.

Macdonald, J., *et al.* (1987). Diminished responsiveness of male homosexual chronic HBV carriers with HTLV-III antibodies to recombinant alpha interferon. *Hepatology* 7, 719–23.

Neurath, A. R., Kent, S. B., Strick, N., and Parker, K. (1986). Identification and chemical synthesis of a host receptor binding site on HBV. *Cell* 46, 429–39.

Seeger, C., Ganem, D., and Varmus, H. (1986). Biochemical and genetic evidence for the hepatitis B virus replication strategy. *Science* 232, 477–84.

Summers, J. and Mason, W. S. (1982). Replication of the genome of a hepatitis B like virus by reverse transcription of an RNA intermediate. *Cell* 29, 403–15.

Tiollais, P., Pourcel, C., and Dejean, A. (1985). The hepatitis B virus. *Nature* 317, 489–94.

Will, H., *et al.* (1987). Replication strategy of human hepatitis B virus. *Journal of Virology* 61, 904–11.

Hepatitis C

Bamber, M., *et al.* (1981). Short incubation non A, non B hepatitis transmitted by Factor VIII concentrates in patients with congenital coagulation disorders. *Gut* 22, 854–61.

Bradley, D., McCaustland, K., Cook, E., Scable, C., Ebert, J., and Maynard, J. (1985). Post-transfusion non-A, non-B hepatitis in chimpanzees. Physicochemical evidence that the tubule-forming agent is a small enveloped virus. *Gastroenterology* 88, 773–9.

Choo, Q.-L., Kuo, G., Weiner, A., Overby, L., Bradley, D., and Houghton, M. (1989). Isolation of a cDNA clone derived from a blood-borne viral hepatitis genome. *Science* 244, 359–62.

Dienstag, J. L. (1983). Non A, Non B hepatitis: i) recognition, epidemiology and clinical features. *Gastroenterology* 85, 439–62.

Dienstag, J. L. (1983). Non-A, Non-B hepatitis: ii) experimental transmission, putative virus agents and markers, and prevention. *Gastroenterology* 85, 743–68.

Hoofnagle, B. J., Mullen, K. D., and Jones, B. (1986). Treatment of chronic NANB hepatitis with recombinant human alpha interferon. *New England Journal of Medicine* 315, 1575–8.

Jacyna, M. R., Brook, G., Loke, R. H., Main, J., Murray-Lyon, I. M., and Thomas, H. C. (1989). A controlled trial of lymphoblastoid interferon in chronic NANB hepatitis: short term results. *British Medical Journal* **298**, 80–2.

Takamizawa, A., *et al.* (1991). Structure and organization of the hepatitis C virus genome isolated from human carriers. *Journal of Virology* **65**, 1105–13.

Hepatitis D

Chen, P. J., *et al.* (1986). Structure and replication of the genome of the hepatitis delta virus. *Proceedings of the National Academy of Sciences USA* **83**, 8774–8.

Makino, S., *et al.* (1987). Molecular cloning and sequencing of a human hepatitis delta virus RNA. *Nature* **329**, 343–6.

Rizzetto, M., *et al.* (1977). Immunofluorescence detection of a new antigen/antibody system (anti delta) associated to the hepatitis B virus in the liver and the serum of HBsAg carriers. *Gut* **19**, 997–1003.

Saldanha, J. A., Thomas, H. C., and Monjardino, J. P. (1990). Cloning and sequencing of RNA of hepatitis delta virus isolated from human serum. *Journal of General Virology* **71**, 1603–6.

Wang, K.-S., *et al.* (1986). Structure sequence and expression of the hepatitis delta virus genome. *Nature* **323**, 508–13.

Hepatitis E

Kane, M. A., *et al.* (1984). Epidemic non A, non B hepatitis in Nepal. *Journal of the American Medical Association* **252**, 3140.

Khuroo, M. S. (1980). Study of an epidemic of non-A, non-B hepatitis. *American Journal of Medicine* **68**, 818.

17.4 Non-viral causes of inflammation

Peter J. Scheuer

Inflammation of the liver may result from infection with bacteria, fungi, viruses, or parasites, or it may, like inflammation in other organs, be non-infective. Viral hepatitis was considered in Section 17.3. One of the most important causes of non-infective inflammation is bile duct obstruction.

17.4.1 Bile duct obstruction

When a large bile duct is obstructed at any point in its course within or outside the liver, several gross and microscopic changes follow. The ducts themselves dilate and are filled with abundant bile, which may become infected. The liver enlarges and becomes bile-stained. Under the microscope, this bile-staining is seen to correspond to the accumulation of bile in canaliculi as well as in hepatocytes and macrophages (Fig. 17.29). The major site of this cholestasis is zone 3 of each acinus, the area least well supplied with blood and nearest to the efferent (terminal) hepatic venules. The zonal distribution of the cholestasis is partly an artefact of paraffin embedding, and partly attributable to mechanical factors and differences in

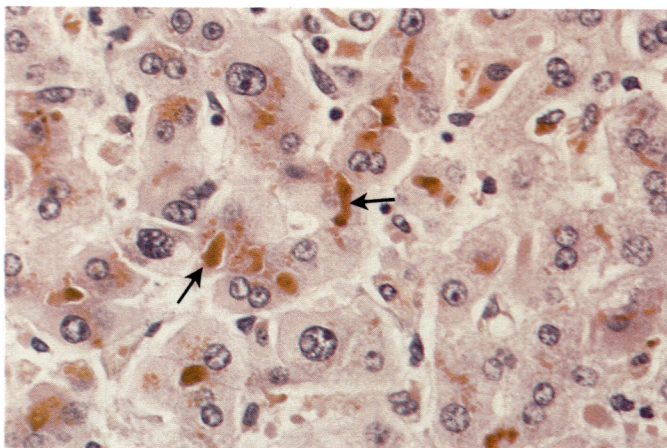

Fig. 17.29 Cholestasis. Bile plugs (arrows) are seen in dilated bile canaliculi between hepatocytes, in the liver of a patient with bile duct obstruction.

function between hepatocytes in the various acinar zones. Within a few days of the onset of biliary obstruction, alterations are found in the portal tracts; these, together with the cholestasis, produce a characteristic histological picture of acute obstruction. The portal tracts become swollen as a result of oedema of the connective tissue and infiltration by polymorphonuclear leucocytes, a classical acute inflammatory reaction attributed to the action of toxic bile salts reabsorbed from the bile by small bile ducts. The latter elongate, becoming tortuous. They are thus seen in two-dimensional sections as multiple cross-sectional profiles, mainly at the periphery of the tracts (Fig. 17.30). This is loosely referred to as bile duct proliferation. Leucocytes are seen not only around but even within the bile duct wall. This histological cholangitis does not necessarily denote bacterial infection of the bile, with a true ascending cho-

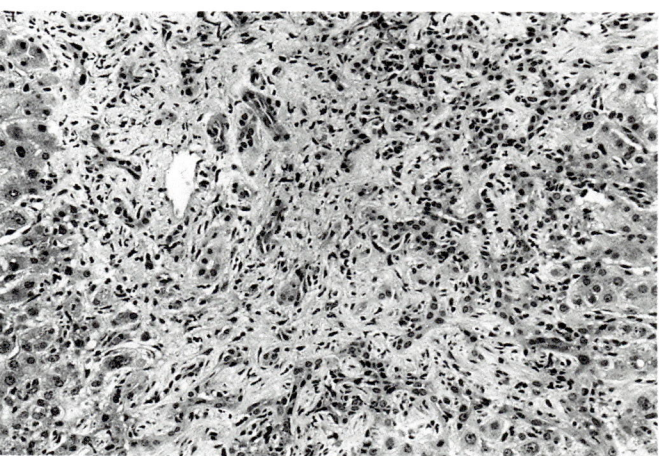

Fig. 17.30 Liver in bile duct obstruction. Most of the field is occupied by an inflamed, enlarged portal tract in which there are many proliferated bile ducts and inflammatory cells. Liver parenchyma is seen on either side.

langitis. In the latter, which may complicate biliary obstruction, far greater numbers of inflammatory cells are found, many of them within the lumens of the small ducts (Fig. 17.31). Bacterial cholangitis can lead to the formation of localized abscesses.

Relief of the duct obstruction is followed by rapid resolution of these changes. If the obstruction is not relieved, or if the patient suffers repeated attacks of obstruction or cholangitis, the portal inflammation persists and becomes chronic. There is increasing fibrosis around ducts and extending between adjacent portal tracts. Focal hepatocytic hyperplasia is shown by thickening of liver cell plates. Eventually biliary cirrhosis may develop. This is discussed in Section 17.11.3.

17.4.2   Bacterial infection of the liver

Cholangitis complicating biliary obstruction has been described in the preceding section. A particular form of cholangitis prevalent in the Far East, primary recurrent pyogenic (oriental) cholangitis, is of uncertain cause, although parasitic infestation of the biliary tract may be responsible. Abscesses may form in the liver in the absence of an obvious predisposing cause, such as bile duct obstruction. The infecting organisms may be aerobic or anaerobic. Upper abdominal peritonitis with perihepatitis is found in some patients with chlamydial or gonococcal infections of the genital tract, the Fitz-Hugh–Curtis syndrome.

The liver is involved in many systemic bacterial infections. When tuberculosis spreads by the bloodstream, granulomas commonly form in the liver (Fig. 17.32). They resemble tuberculous lesions elsewhere in the body, but do not always undergo necrosis. Mycobacteria may be very scanty. In tuberculoid leprosy there are also granulomas in the liver, whereas in the lepromatous form, in which cell-mediated immunity is low, focal accumulations of foamy macrophages within the acini contain large numbers of organisms. A variety of lesions, including gummas, have been described in the liver in patients with syphilis.

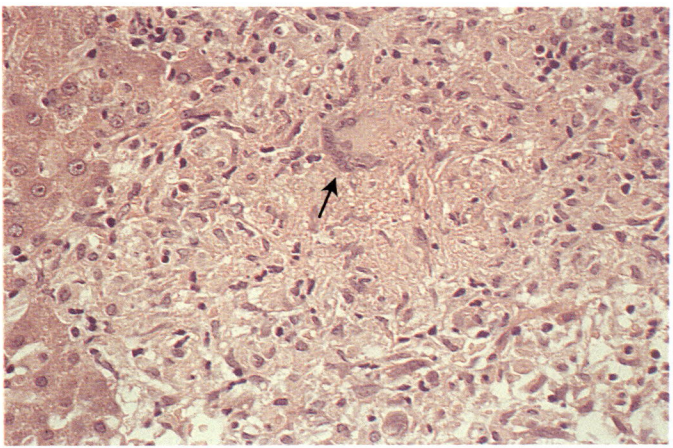

Fig. 17.32 Hepatic tuberculosis. An epithelioid-cell granuloma is seen within the hepatic parenchyma. It contains a multinucleated giant cell of Langhans type (arrow).

In Weil disease, caused by infection with *Leptospira*, conventional stains show only non-specific changes, such as focal necrosis, cholestasis, and increased liver cell mitoses, but a specific bacterial antigen can be demonstrated by immunohistochemical methods. In typhoid fever, the liver contains localized accumulations of mononuclear macrophages, the typhoid nodules. Hepatic granulomas are seen in brucellosis and in Q fever; in the latter, caused by *Coxiella burnetii*, the lesions sometimes have a distinctive and diagnostic 'fibrin-ring' or 'doughnut' appearance, with fibrin and inflammatory cells arranged around a central fat vacuole (Fig. 17.33).

17.4.3   The liver in sepsis

Patients with systemic infections, particularly when caused by Gram-negative organisms such as *E. coli*, are often jaundiced,

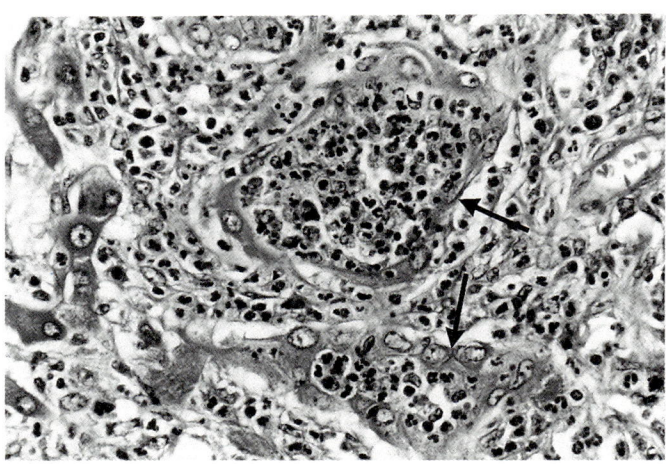

Fig. 17.31 Acute cholangitis. Two small bile ducts (arrows) are filled with pus cells, which also infiltrate their walls.

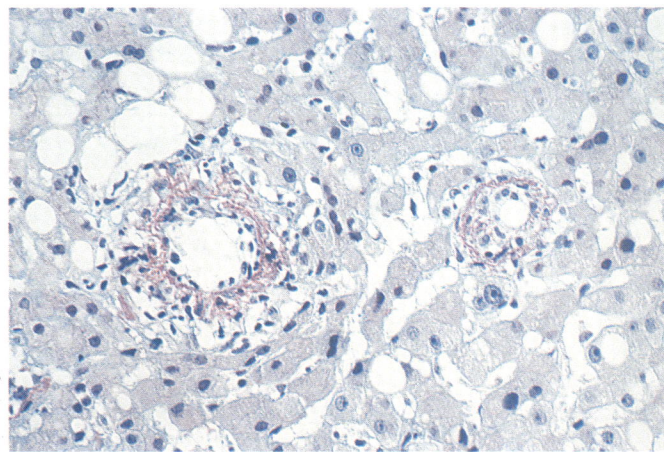

Fig. 17.33 Liver in Q fever. Two granulomas are seen within fatty liver parenchyma. The lesions consist of centrally located fat around which there are deeply stained rings of fibrin, epithelioid cells, and neutrophil leucocytes.

possibly because of circulating bacterial endotoxins. There is morphological cholestasis in the form of bile plugs or thrombi in dilated bile canaliculi. In some patients inspissated bile accumulates in inflamed and dilated small bile ducts at the margins of portal tracts. In the toxic shock syndrome, caused by a circulating staphylococcal exotoxin, polymorphonuclear leucocytes are found in and around bile ducts within portal tracts, mimicking ascending bacterial cholangitis.

17.4.4   Parasitic diseases

Protozoal diseases

Malaria

The pathological changes in the liver in malaria depend not only on the parasite species but also on the patient's immune status. When a non-immune patient is infected with *Plasmodium falciparum*, the most widespread and dangerous of the different species, the organisms parasitize the patient's erythrocytes, which are then engulfed by macrophages, including the Kupffer cells of the liver. Haemozoin, derived from haemoglobin in the erythrocytes, accumulates in the Kupffer cells in the form of fine, dark, pigment granules. Because Kupffer cells migrate towards the portal tracts, the pigment is gradually cleared from the acini and is eventually found only in portal macrophages. In endemic areas, some infected patients develop the tropical splenomegaly syndrome, characterized by high serum levels of malarial antibodies and infiltration of the hepatic sinusoids and portal tracts by lymphocytes.

Leishmaniasis

Systemic leishmaniasis, or kala-azar, is caused by the protozoan, *Leishmania donovani*. The organisms, about 3 μm long, are found in large numbers in the cytoplasm of macrophages in liver, spleen, lymph nodes, and bone marrow (Fig. 17.34). In some patients epithelioid-cell granulomas are seen in the liver.

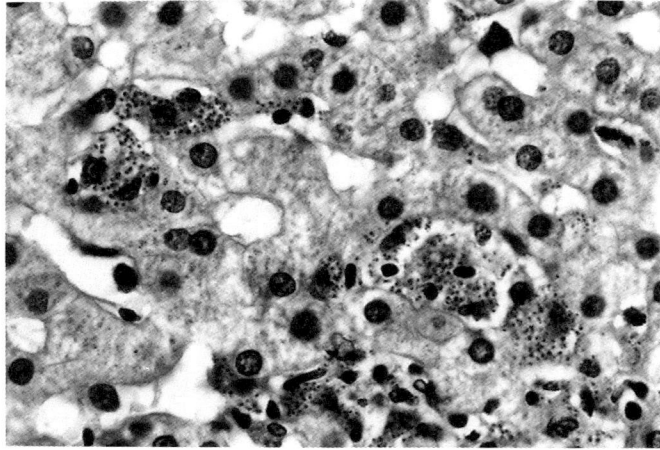

Fig. 17.34   Systemic leishmaniasis (kala-azar). Kupffer cells contain numerous Leishman–Donovan bodies.

Amoebiasis

Entamoeba histolytica reaches the liver by the portal bloodstream. Some patients, but by no means all, have overt amoebic colitis which provides a source of the parasites. If these are able to proliferate within the liver, focal abscess-like lesions develop, usually in the right lobe. The hepatic parenchyma is destroyed, and ragged cavities form, surrounded by a wall of granulation and fibrous tissue (Fig. 17.35). The cellular response to the parasite is predominantly histiocytic and lymphocytic. Trophozoites can be identified in the wall. They are rounded structures up to 60 μm in diameter, with a single nucleus and multiple cytoplasmic vacuoles, which reflect the amoeba's phagocytic activity. Amoebae may spread beyond the liver by the bloodstream into the peritoneal cavity, or via the diaphragm into pleura, lung, or pericardium.

Helminthic diseases

Schistosomiasis

Schistosomiasis is a disease of great importance in Africa, South America, and eastern Asia. Serious hepatic involvement is most often ascribed to *Schistosoma mansoni*, which lives in the portal venous system. Ova laid by the mature female worm are deposited in the liver, where they excite an inflammatory reaction. In patients with chronic schistosomiasis this usually takes the form of granulomas in the portal tracts (Fig. 17.36). These often have an orderly structure, with a central ovum surrounded by palisaded histiocytes and giant cells, and an outer mantle of fibrous tissue. The whole lesion is infiltrated by inflammatory cells, among which eosinophils are prominent.

Some patients chronically infested with *S. mansoni* develop portal hypertension. This is associated pathologically with extensive portal fibrosis and fibrous obliteration of intrahepatic portal vein branches. Portal tracts become linked by fibrous septa, which surround islands of hepatic parenchyma (Fig. 17.37). The hepatocytes themselves are not usually affected, and liver function remains normal, in contrast to many examples of cirrhosis. Because of the macroscopic resemblance of the thickened portal veins and tracts to the stems of clay pipes, the lesion is often described as pipestem fibrosis.

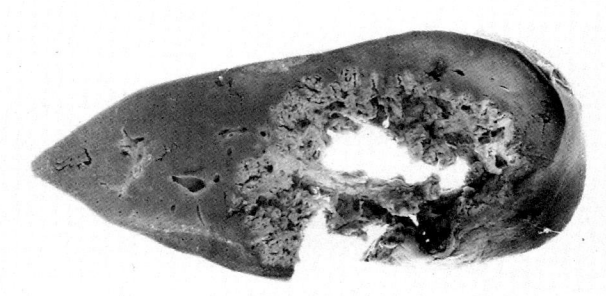

Fig. 17.35   Hepatic amoebiasis. Ragged cavities are seen within the liver parenchyma. They are the result of invasion by amoebae, and hepatocellular necrosis.

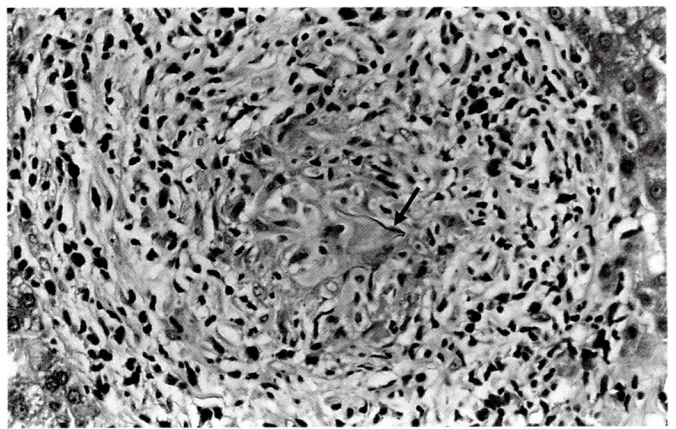

Fig. 17.36 Schistosomiasis. A granuloma has formed in a portal tract around an ovum, the remnants of which are marked by the arrow.

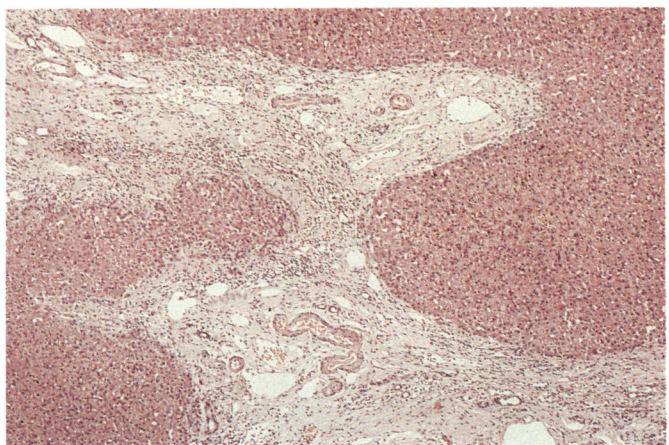

Fig. 17.37 Schistosomiasis: pipestem fibrosis. Broad fibrous septa link portal tracts and surround irregular islands of relatively normal liver parenchyma. The septa contain abundant vascular channels.

Opisthorchiasis

This infestation, formerly known as clonorchiasis, is important because the flukes, which inhabit the larger bile ducts, stimulate hyperplasia of biliary epithelium. The hyperplasia may then develop into adenocarcinoma. *Opisthorchis sinensis*, the Chinese liver fluke, is acquired by eating raw or undercooked fish.

Fascioliasis

The common liver fluke *Fasciola hepatica* is a parasite of sheep and cattle which occasionally infests man. Outbreaks of fascioliasis can sometimes be traced to the eating of wild watercress, contaminated by animals. The route of entry of *Fasciola* into the liver is unexpected for a parasite which, like *Opisthorchis*, inhabits the large bile ducts; ingested parasites migrate from the gut through the peritoneal cavity and penetrate the liver capsule. Here they give rise to focal subcapsular areas of necrosis and granuloma formation which may be mistaken for meta-

static tumour. The larvae then migrate deep into the liver and finally settle in the bile ducts, causing obstruction and inflammation. Unlike *Opisthorchis* they do not appear to cause carcinoma of the biliary tree.

Hydatid disease

The common type of hydatid disease in man is caused by the larval form of a tapeworm, *Echinococcus granulosus*, whose primary host is the dog. Secondary hosts, including man, are infected as a result of ingesting ova. The embryos pass from the intestine to various organs, including liver, where they develop into cysts (Fig. 17.38). These have an inner germinative layer which eventually proliferates to form daughter cysts with scolices. Outside this layer is a laminated membrane of parasite origin, surrounded in turn by a host capsule of inflammatory and fibrous tissue. Rupture of a cyst results in further spread of the parasite. Other complications include secondary bacterial infection of the cyst. Old cysts containing dead parasites often calcify. The much less common form of hydatid disease, alveolar echinococcosis, is caused by *E. multilocularis*.

Ascariasis

The roundworm *Ascaris lumbricoides* may involve the liver during its initial migratory larval phase, giving rise to granulomas, necrosis, and infiltration by neutrophil and eosinophil leucocytes. The adult worms inhabit the intestines and, when abundant, may find their way from the duodenum into the biliary tree where they cause obstruction and cholangitis.

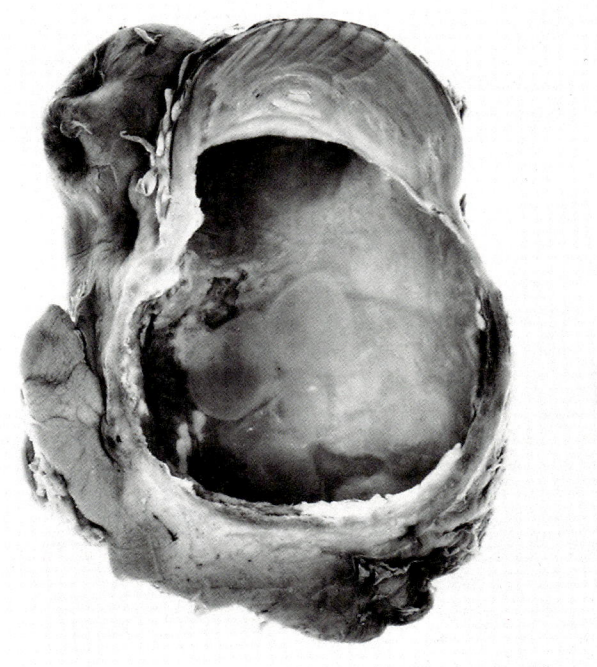

Fig. 17.38 Hydatid disease of the liver. Within this surgically excised hydatid cyst, several pale, translucent, thin-walled daughter cysts are visible.

17.4.5 Other types of hepatitis

James O'D. McGee

Granulomatous hepatitis

Many disorders can produce a granulomatous hepatitis. This is characterized by the focal accumulation of epithelioid cells and multinucleate giant cells in the hepatic parenchyma and/or portal tracts (see Figs 17.32 and 17.33). The commonest causes in Europe and the USA are tuberculosis, sarcoidosis, drug reactions, and primary biliary cirrhosis. The causes of granulomatous hepatitis are listed in Table 17.4 (see also Section 17.4.2). In about 30 per cent of cases it is impossible to discern the aetiological agent. In a case where granulomatous hepatitis is suspected, or in one which is rebiopsied, it is useful to send a piece of the tissue for microbiological analysis.

In sarcoidosis, hepatic granulomas are found in as many as 66 per cent of cases but liver dysfunction is rare. The granulomas may be found in any location within the liver but are commonest in portal tracts and around terminal veins. Schaumann

bodies and asteroids are rare findings in sarcoidosis of the liver. Typically the granulomas do not undergo necrosis but small foci of fibrinoid at their centres are not uncommon. On morphological grounds only, it is frequently impossible to differentiate the granulomas found in tuberculosis, primary biliary cirrhosis, and other disorders which cause granulomatous hepatitis.

Non-specific reactive hepatitis

The liver reacts to a number of disparate stimuli by producing the picture of non-specific reactive hepatitis, the most common cause being a febrile illness. It is a frequent finding on biopsy, and may be provoked by any systemic or severe local infection and by a variety of drugs. It is characterized by prominent sinusoidal cells and a mild infiltrate of lymphocytes and mononuclear cells in portal tracts, although not all portal tracts are equally involved. There might also be small foci of necrosis and mild fatty change in hepatocytes. The portal tract infiltrate is not associated with piecemeal necrosis, and this should not be confused with CAH (chronic active hepatitis) but may be difficult to distinguish from CPH (chronic persistent hepatitis) (see Section 17.5).

It is important to emphasize to the clinician that this is not a primary liver disease but a reaction of the liver to extrahepatic stimuli.

17.4.6 Further reading

Desmet, V. J. (1987). Cholestasis: extrahepatic obstruction and secondary biliary cirrhosis. In *Pathology of the liver* (2nd edn) (ed. R. N. M. MacSween, P. P. Anthony, and P. J. Scheuer). Churchill Livingstone, Edinburgh.

Patrick, R. S. and McGee, J. O'D. (1988). Hepatitis associated with non-viral infections. In *Biopsy pathology of the liver* (2nd edn). Chapman and Hall, London.

Simson, I. W. and Gear, J. H. S. (1987). Other viral and infectious diseases. In *Pathology of the liver* (2nd edn) (ed. R. N. M. MacSween, P. P. Anthony and P. J. Scheuer). Churchill Livingstone, Edinburgh.

Table 17.4 Causes of granulomatous hepatitis

Infections	Drugs
Actinomycosis	Allopurinol, aspirin, cephalexin,
Amoebiasis	diazepam, halothane, isoniazid,
Ascaris	methyldopa, nitrofurantoin,
Aspergillosis	oxyphenylbutazone, penicillin,
Blastomycosis	phenytoin, quinidine,
Candidiasis	sulphonamides
Coccidioidomycosis	
Cryptococcosis	**Immunological disorders**
Cytomegalovirus	Aids (atypical mycobacteria, TB, etc.)
Fascioliasis	Granulomatous disease of childhood
Granuloma inguinale	Polyarteritis nodosa
Giardiasis	Temporal arteritis
Histoplasmosis	Wegener granulomatosis
Hydatid disease (granulosa)	
Infectious mononucleosis	**Neoplasms**
Kala-azar	Hodgkin disease
Leprosy	Liver reaction to extrahepatic
Listeriosis	neoplasms
Meliodosis	Non-Hodgkin lymphoma
Mucormycosis	
Nocardiosis	**Foreign material**
Opisthorchiasis	Barium, beryllium, intravenous drug
Paracoccidioidomycosis	abuse, mineral oil, silica, starch,
Psittacosis	suture material, talc, thorotrast
Pyogenic infections	
Q fever	**Miscellaneous**
Schistosomiasis	Biliary obstruction
Strongyloidiasis	Crohn disease
Syphilis (secondary and	Jejuno–ileal bypass
tertiary)	Lipogranulomas (alcohol-induced)
Toxoplasmosis	Primary biliary cirrhosis
Toxocariasis	Sarcoidosis
Tuberculosis (and atypical	Whipple disease
mycobacteria)	
Tularaemia	
Typhoid	

17.5 Chronic hepatitis

V. J. Desmet

17.5.1 Introduction

In the broad sense, the term chronic hepatitis can be applied to a number of hepatic disorders of diverse aetiologies. These may be characterized by partly distinctive histopathological features in liver biopsy material and may show highly variable clinical courses and outcome. However, they all share the feature of chronic or recurrent inflammation in the liver, based on presumed immunologically mediated mechanisms. The most important groups of liver disorders in this broad category comprise: chronic hepatitis *sensu stricto*, primary biliary cirrhosis, primary sclerosing cholangitis, and alcoholic liver injury. These subgroups should be considered rather as syndromes, subject to further division into several subcategories and/or stages, rather than specific disease entities. They will be further analysed in the following sections, except for alcoholic liver disease. Because of its clear relation to alcohol intake, the latter is discussed in Section 17.6.

17.5.2 Chronic hepatitis

Definition

Chronic hepatitis is defined as chronic inflammatory disease of the liver, continuing for at least 6 months. The arbitrary time period of 6 months is included in order to avoid overdiagnosis on interpretation of liver biopsies taken near an acute attack of viral hepatitis. Chronic hepatitis can be diagnosed sooner if the clinical situation warrants, for instance in the 'auto-immune' type, or in Wilson disease (see below).

Clinical features

Since the term 'chronic hepatitis' refers to a spectrum of different disease variants, it is not surprising that there are no specific clinical features.

Some patients have no symptoms at all. The most frequent symptom is fatigue. Biochemical tests show variable increases in serum bilirubin, transaminases, and gammaglobulin values, which often bear little relation to liver biopsy features.

The lack of specific clinical and biochemical features emphasizes the importance of needle liver biopsy in establishing the diagnosis of chronic hepatitis.

Aetiology

Since the original description of chronic forms of hepatitis by Kalk in 1947 it has become clear that chronic hepatitis may be caused by various agents and mechanisms.

Hepatitis viruses

Hepatitis B virus (HBV) infection is an important cause of chronic hepatitis; generally, about 5–10 per cent of HBV-infected persons develop chronic forms of hepatitis. In several European countries, about two-thirds of cases of chronic hepatitis are HBV-related; the incidence of HBV-positive chronic hepatitis varies in different geographical areas.

Hepatitis delta virus (HDV) is an RNA virus which needs HBV as a helper virus for replication. HDV infection thus only occurs in HBV-positive patients. Superinfection by HDV may lead to chronic HDV-positive hepatitis and aggravation of the underlying HBV-positive chronic hepatitis. HDV is more widespread than originally thought from its first discovery in Italy in 1977.

Hepatitis non-A, non-B (NANB) viruses; hepatitis C virus The term non-A, non-B (NANB) hepatitis was adopted around 1975 to designate those cases of viral hepatitis that were serologically unrelated to any known hepatotropic virus. Two NANB viruses were identified in recent years. The 'parenterally transmitted form' of NANB hepatitis is caused by a newly identified RNA virus: hepatitis C virus (HCV). Infection with HCV may lead to chronic hepatitis in up to 50 per cent of cases, although the disease often has an indolent course; cirrhosis develops in about 25 per cent of patients with chronic hepatitis C over 5–10 years. HCV appears to be a major cause of chronic liver disease in the Western world. The 'enterically transmitted form' of NANB hepatitis is caused by a newly identified RNA virus: hepatitis E virus (HEV). Infection with HEV does not lead to chronic liver disease, and is therefore similar to infection with hepatitis A virus (HAV).

Drugs

Several therapeutic drugs may cause chronic hepatitis; examples include oxyphenisatin, α-methyldopa, isoniazid, nitrofurantoin, dantrolene, sulphonamides, propylthiouracil. A drug history should always be taken in any patient with suspected chronic hepatitis (see Section 17.7).

Metabolic disease

Some metabolic disorders may present the clinical and histopathological features of chronic hepatitis. These include Wilson's disease and α-1-antitrypsin deficiency.

Auto-immunity

In a number of patients, chronic hepatitis appears to be an auto-immune disorder. To this category belongs the type of chronic hepatitis described by Waldenström in 1950, occurring in young women with severe liver disease, endocrine dysfunction, and hyperglobulinaemia. In recent years, the incidence of auto-immune chronic hepatitis appears to be declining.

Classification and histopathology

Introductory note

As chronic hepatitis represents a broad spectrum of clinical disease variants and histopathological lesions, there is a need for classification in order to allow a reasonable comparison between clinical studies and treatment results from different centres.

Although end-stage liver disease (cirrhosis) may develop from chronic hepatitis, attempts are made to distinguish as far as possible between chronic hepatitis and cirrhosis, since cirrhosis by itself carries its own symptoms and complications. It is recognized that the disease processes constituting chronic hepatitis may continue to operate and to further damage a liver which is already in the cirrhotic stage; this situation is indicated by the terms 'chronic active hepatitis with cirrhosis' or 'active cirrhosis' (see Section 17.12).

In 1968, a group of liver pathologists proposed a simple classification of chronic hepatitis. Distinction was made between chronic persistent hepatitis (CPH), a mild category, and chronic aggressive hepatitis (CAH), a more severe variant with higher propensity for cirrhogenic evolution. In subsequent years, additional variants have been described, but the main grouping still distinguishes mild from severe inflammatory liver disease.

In recent years, the validity of the histopathological classification of chronic hepatitis has been questioned in view of the progress of serological diagnosis of viral hepatitis (chronic viral hepatitis B, C, and D) and its treatment with antiviral agents (e.g. interferon). The actual usefulness of histopathological variants of chronic hepatitis is considered later.

Classification

The subgroup of milder variants of chronic hepatitis comprises chronic persistent hepatitis, chronic lobular hepatitis, non-specific reactive hepatitis, and chronic septal hepatitis.

Chronic persistent hepatitis This variant corresponds to the originally defined type of mild chronic hepatitis, and morphologically represents 'portal' hepatitis. Portal tracts are infiltrated by mononuclear cells, mainly lymphocytes, which remain restricted within the confines of the portal connective tissue (Fig. 17.39). The parenchyma shows no, or only minor, inflammatory lesions, in the form of occasional focal necrosis.

The histopathological picture of 'portal hepatitis' is not specific; it may also be observed as a late residue of resolving acute hepatitis, and in less representative biopsies from chronic active hepatitis (CAH), primary biliary cirrhosis, and primary sclerosing cholangitis. Therefore, a histopathological picture of 'portal hepatitis' should only be interpreted as chronic persistent hepatitis after consideration of the clinical and biochemical features.

Chronic lobular hepatitis This term was introduced in 1971 to describe lobular lesions of necrosis and inflammation as observed in classical acute hepatitis, but on a chronic time scale (Fig. 17.40). The diagnosis of chronic lobular hepatitis can only

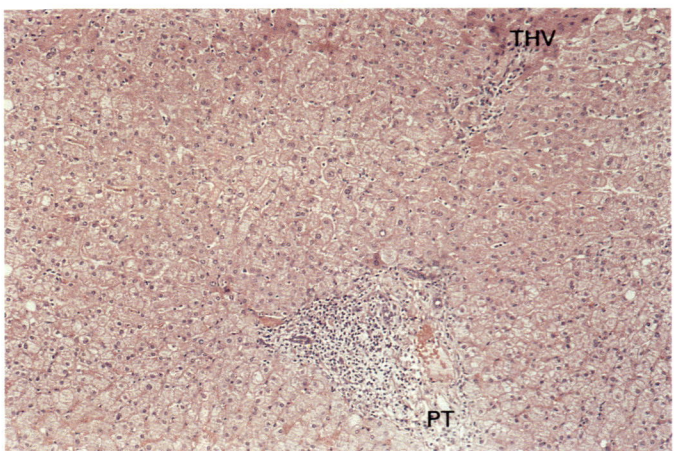

Fig. 17.39 Chronic persistent hepatitis. Overview of portal tract and parenchyma. The portal tract (PT) shows moderately dense mononuclear cell infiltration, which remains confined within the limits of the portal tract. Apart from some mild inflammatory infiltration near the terminal hepatic venule (THV), the parenchyma reveals no appreciable changes.

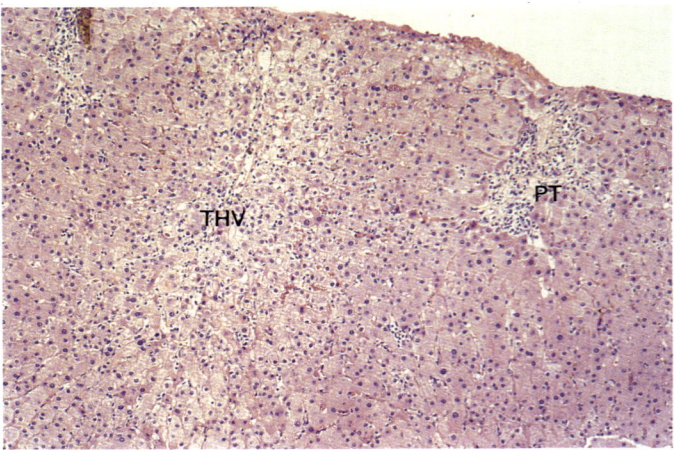

Fig. 17.40 Chronic lobular hepatitis. Liver biopsy from a patient with a mild rise in transaminases for over 6 months. The liver biopsy shows features of mild acute hepatitis: mild mononuclear cell infiltration in the portal tract (PT); slight liver cell pleomorphism and mononuclear cell infiltration around the terminal hepatic venule (THV); and occasional foci of lymphocytic infiltration in the remaining parenchyma.

be made after consideration of the clinical history of the patient. Chronic lobular hepatitis may be caused by hepatitis viruses B and C and carries a variable prognosis.

Non-specific reactive hepatitis (NSRH) A subgroup of patients with chronic hepatitis has been described with a more fluctuating course than in classical chronic persistent hepatitis.

Such biopsies are characterized by low-grade, or minimal, changes (like occasional foci of necrosis, mobilization, and increase of Kupffer cells) and mild portal inflammation, usually in only some portal tracts. In short, the lobular lesions are milder than in chronic lobular hepatitis and the portal infiltration less than in chronic persistent hepatitis; it may correspond to a remission phase of chronic lobular hepatitis. NSRH is also frequently found in systemic (particularly febrile) illness. In these cases, NSRH represents a reaction of the liver to systemic disease (or drugs) and the prognosis is that of the initiating illness (see Section 17.4.5).

Chronic septal hepatitis can be considered as a remission phase of chronic active hepatitis, during which the disease activity has regressed to the lower level of chronic persistent hepatitis. The previously more vigourous disease activity is reflected in the presence of periportal connective tissue septa which are burned-out scars of previously more active inflammation (Fig. 17.41). The prognosis of chronic septal hepatitis is not as good as that of simple chronic persistent hepatitis.

Chronic active hepatitis The more severe forms of chronic hepatitis are designated chronic active (aggressive) hepatitis.

The *elementary lesions* in chronic active hepatitis comprise piecemeal necrosis, focal necrosis, confluent necrosis, parenchymal regeneration, bile duct lesions, and fibrosis.

Variants of chronic hepatitis with higher disease activity are

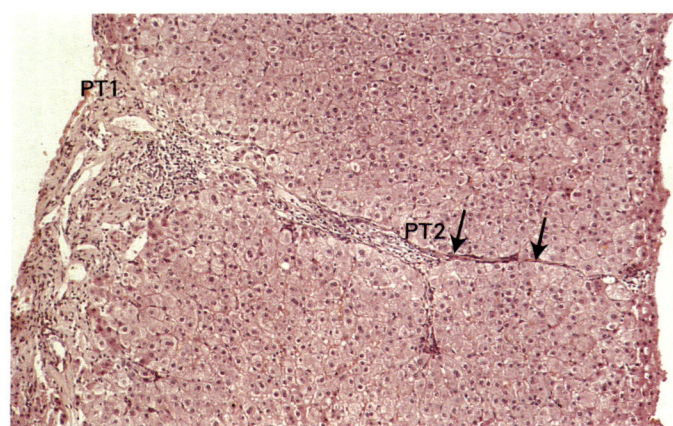

Fig. 17.41 Chronic septal hepatitis. Besides mild lymphocytic infiltration in larger (PT1) and smaller (PT2) portal tracts, the latter are also characterized by fibrous extensions ending into the parenchyma (arrows). Liver parenchymal cells reveal no striking alterations.

termed chronic active or aggressive hepatitis. The histopathological hallmark of this group is piecemeal necrosis, which itself may be present in mild or extensive degree.

The term *piecemeal necrosis* refers to liver cell necrosis in close association with mononuclear inflammatory cell infiltration at the junction between interstitium (portal tracts or connective tissue septa) and parenchyma (Fig. 17.42). Chronic active hepatitis thus morphologically corresponds to periportal (and periseptal) hepatitis. The predominant lymphocyte subset in piecemeal necrosis in viral chronic hepatitis is suppressor/cytotoxic lymphocytes. Liver cell necrosis in areas of piecemeal necrosis occurs by apoptosis, an immunologically mediated mode of cell death (see Section 3.1).

In parenchymal territories 'invaded' by piecemeal necrosis, hepatocytes become surrounded by lymphocytes and are sequestrated from the remaining part of liver cell plates (trapping of hepatocytes). Such sequestrated liver cell groups often acquire a swollen, pale appearance, and group themselves around a central lumen: liver cell rosettes (Fig. 17.43). They become surrounded by pericellular fibrosis, and are interpreted as attempts at regeneration in an unfavourable environment. Piecemeal necrosis thus leads to erosion of the limiting plate, progressive extension of wedge-shaped areas of inflammation into the parenchyma, and subsequent fibrosis.

Lesions of the parenchyma also occur to a variable extent in chronic active hepatitis. The most important are focal necrosis and confluent necrosis.

Focal (spotty) necrosis is recognized as a small accumulation of lymphocytes in a focal area where one or more parenchymal cells have disappeared or are still visible as small, eosinophilic cytoplasmic fragments (Fig. 17.44). The mode of cell death in focal necrosis appears to correspond to apoptosis.

Confluent necrosis refers to necrosis of groups of liver cells; the necrosis is of the lytic type, with disappearance ('drop-out') of the affected parts of the parenchyma. This leads to denudation of the reticulin framework, which may collapse when the necrosis affects larger areas.

Confluent necrosis occurs preferentially in the microcirculatory periphery of the functional liver units, leading to portal-central bridging necrosis when it is located in the microcirculatory periphery (zone 3) of simple acini (Fig. 17.45). Multiacinar necrosis is a more severe degree of necrosis which affects several adjacent liver acini (Fig. 17.46). The term 'bridging hepatic necrosis' has been proposed to indicate confluent necrosis which links portal tracts and terminal veins, or terminal veins with each other. Recent experimental evidence suggests that confluent lytic necrosis of larger parenchymal territories may be caused by humoral immune mechanisms involving circulating antibodies and/or immune complexes.

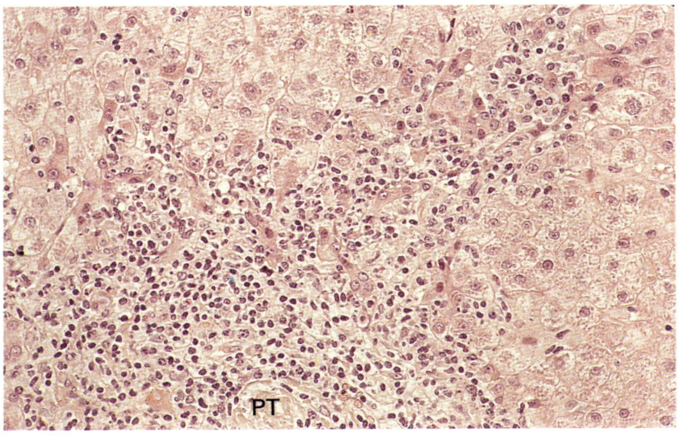

Fig. 17.42 Piecemeal necrosis. Detail from liver biopsy with chronic active (aggressive) hepatitis. The portal tract (PT) is densely infiltrated by mononuclear cells, mainly lymphocytes. The latter infiltrate beyond the connective tissue–parenchymal interface, and create irregular, wedge-shaped extensions into the periportal parenchyma. Hepatocytes disappear in the inflammatory areas.

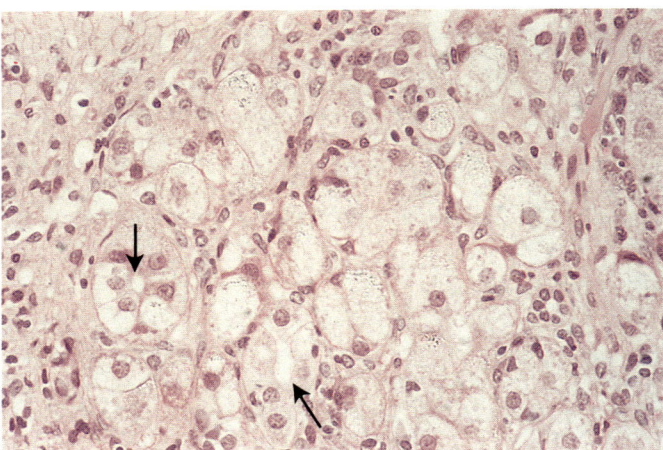

Fig. 17.43 Liver cell rosettes in periportal area from liver biopsy with chronic active hepatitis. Small groups of mostly pale and swollen hepatocytes are separated by pericellular fibrosis and some infiltrating lymphocytes. Some of the groups are arranged around a recognizable lumen (arrows).

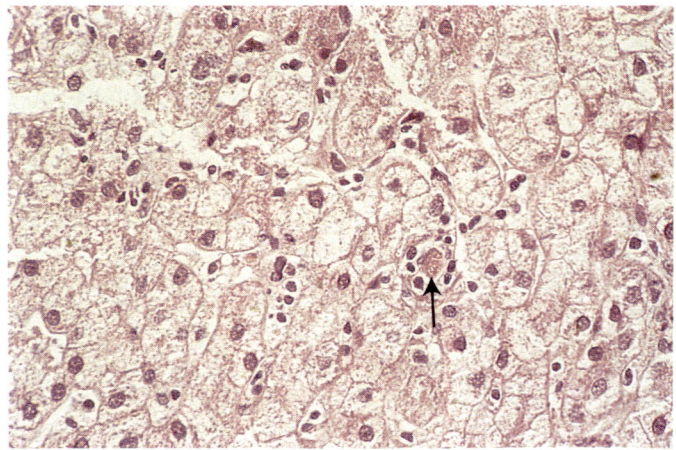

Fig. 17.44 Focal necrosis. Detail of the acinar parenchyma from liver biopsy with mild chronic active hepatitis. Small groups of mononuclear cells and lymphocytes are scattered throughout the parenchyma. In one, an acidophil (apoptotic) body, representing a necrotic hepatocyte, can be identified (arrow).

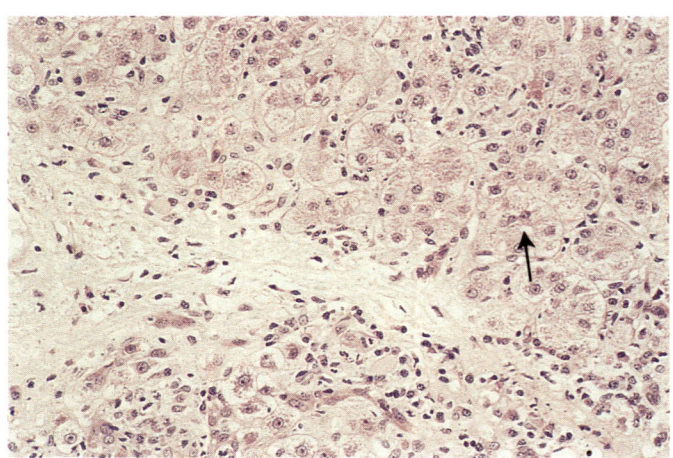

Fig. 17.45 Portal-central bridging hepatic necrosis. A streak of necrosis extends from a portal tract (outside picture) to a terminal hepatic venule (outside picture). Note inflammatory infiltration towards the portal side of the 'bridge'. The adjacent parenchyma shows signs of regeneration in the form of tubular arrangements of hepatocytes (arrows). The reticulin framework in the necrotic bridge has already largely collapsed.

Loss of liver cells is compensated for to a variable degree by *liver cell regeneration*. The latter may be recognized as actual liver cell mitoses, the appearance of small basophilic hepatocytes near the edge of confluent necrosis, the appearance of double cell-thick plates and nodular parenchymal masses, and in some instances (e.g. drug-induced chronic hepatitis), the appearance of multinucleated parenchymal giant cells.

A peculiar lesion of *interlobular bile ducts* has been described in chronic hepatitis, especially in more severe variants and in chronic hepatitis due to HCV. This lesion is observed in portal

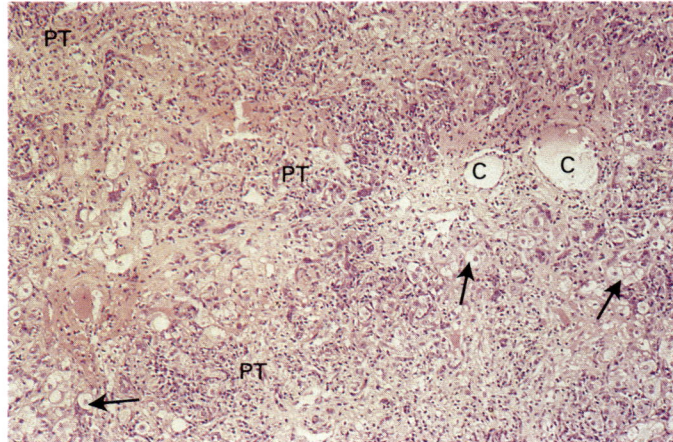

Fig. 17.46 Multiacinar necrosis in liver biopsy with severe chronic active hepatitis. There is lymphocyte infiltration in and around portal tracts (PT); most of the parenchyma has disappeared; some scattered swollen hepatocytes (examples: see arrows) remain. C, draining veins.

tracts with dense lymphocytic infiltration, often with lymphoid follicle formation. The affected duct shows swelling and stratification of its lining cells, permeated by lymphocytes and mononuclear cells (Fig. 17.47). The basement membrane remains intact, and real duct destruction does not seem to occur. On ocassion, this lesion may be difficult to differentiate from bile duct lesions in primary biliary cirrhosis (see below).

Fibrosis in chronic active hepatitis is mostly of the septal type. Septal fibrosis may occur as 'active' and 'passive' septa. Active septa correspond to connective tissue sheets rich in inflammatory cell infiltration and accompanied by irregular piecemeal necrosis at their interface with the parenchyma. They are

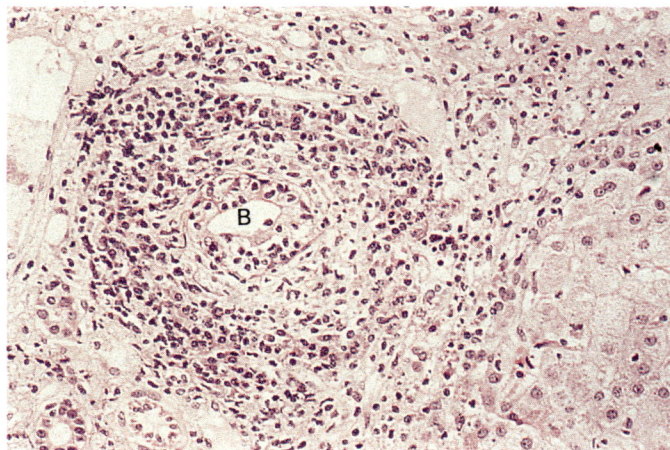

Fig. 17.47 Hepatitic type of bile duct lesion in severe chronic active hepatitis. The portal tract is densely infiltrated by mononuclear cells, including lymphocytes and plasma cells. Piecemeal necrosis is seen in the right part of the picture. The bile duct (B) shows vacuolization and some multilayering of its lining cells, with numerous infiltrating lymphocytes.

thought to originate from extensive piecemeal necrosis, invading in a wedge-shaped fashion into the parenchyma and eventually linking adjacent portal tracts, or by extension of piecemeal necrosis along areas of confluent necrosis, carrying the inflammatory infiltrate deep into the acini.

'Passive' septa correspond to connective tissue sheets carrying few or no inflammatory cells, being sharply delineated from the adjacent parenchyma. They are mainly derived from passive collapse of the reticulin framework and subsequent scarring in areas of confluent necrosis. Multiacinar confluent necrosis results in extensive areas of postnecrotic scarring, in which the approximated pre-existing portal tracts may still remain identifiable.

The relentless occurrence of piecemeal necrosis and confluent necrosis with associated fibrosis, counteracted by more or less successful attempts at parenchymal regeneration, lead to progressive distortion of the normal acinar architecture. In this way, chronic active hepatitis is associated with increasing degrees of nodular transformation of the parenchyma with intersecting septal fibrosis, imperceptibly merging with the stage described as cirrhosis. In the cirrhotic stage, the disease activity (in terms of inflammation and necrosis) may continue, speeding up a fatal outcome by liver failure (active cirrhosis), or may burn out, establishing a quiescent state in a structurally and haemodynamically altered liver (inactive cirrhosis).

Liver biopsy evaluation in chronic hepatitis should try to specify not only the degree of disease activity, but also the stage of structural derangement of acinar architecture. The latter may be difficult to recognize in needle biopsies from macronodular cirrhosis, emphasizing the usefulness of laparoscopy.

Classification of chronic active hepatitis Even chronic active hepatitis is not a single disease but a spectrum of conditions, often with a fluctuating course.

Chronic active hepatitis with minimal activity is borderline to chronic persistent hepatitis. It is characterized by mild piecemeal necrosis, moderate spotty necrosis, and normal liver architecture. Chronic active hepatitis of moderate activity is typified by moderate piecemeal necrosis, marked focal necrosis, and essentially preserved lobular architecture. Chronic active hepatitis of severe activity displays the most marked necroinflammatory lesions, with marked piecemeal necrosis, liver cell rosettes and active septa, bridging and/or multiacinar confluent necrosis, possibly passive septa, and in some instances bile duct lesions of the hepatitic type. According to the stage of advancement of the disease, liver architecture may be more or less severely disturbed.

Histopathological assessment of disease activity

It is difficult to assess degrees of disease activity from long morphological descriptions. Attempts have been made to quantitate the elementary lesions in numerical scores, and to express this evaluation by a 'histopathological activity index'. This may prove useful in comparative studies of therapeutic results. One should bear in mind, however, that the scores of such an 'index' result from arbitrary values attributed to histological

changes, the biological impact of which cannot be measured quantitatively.

Histopathological markers of aetiology

Histopathological and immunohistochemical markers are helpful in defining the aetiology of chronic hepatitis. In recent years, *in situ* hybridization techniques (see Section 30.4) for hepatitis B viral DNA have further extended the possibility of aetiological diagnosis on tissue sections.

Hepatitis B virus can be recognized as the aetiological agent by the finding of ground-glass hepatocytes and sanded nuclei. Ground-glass hepatocytes are parenchymal cells with a pale, homogeneous appearance on hematoxylin–eosin stained sections (Fig. 17.48). This appearance is due to hypertrophy of the endoplasmic reticulum. One should realize, however, that a ground-glass appearance of hepatocytes may also be produced by several other causes.

Sanded nuclei correspond to liver cell nuclei with peripheral margination of their chromatin around a central, finely granular, eosinophilic mass. This nuclear change is brought about by massive accumulation in the nucleoplasm of hepatitis B core particles.

Immunohistochemical techniques (fluorescence, peroxidase) are more sensitive for detecting hepatitis B surface and core antigens in biopsy specimens. They may reveal these antigens in various cellular locations: cytoplasmic and membranous (for hepatitis B surface antigen) and nuclear, cytoplasmic, or membranous (for hepatitis B core antigen) (Figs 17.49, 17.50, 17.51).

Non-A, non-B viral hepatitis, now identified as HCV, has been reported to be characterized by mild fatty change, abundance of acidophil bodies, dense intra-acinar lymphocytic infiltration, parenchymal giant cells, dense aggregates of lymphoid cells and even lymph follicles in portal tracts, and the hepatitic type of bile

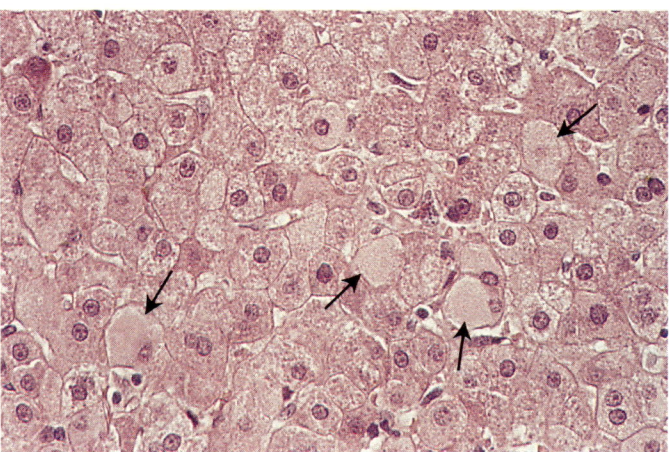

Fig. 17.48 Detail of liver parenchyma in a liver biopsy with hepatitis B virus-positive chronic persistent hepatitis. Several ground-glass hepatocytes are scattered between normal-appearing parenchymal cells (arrows).

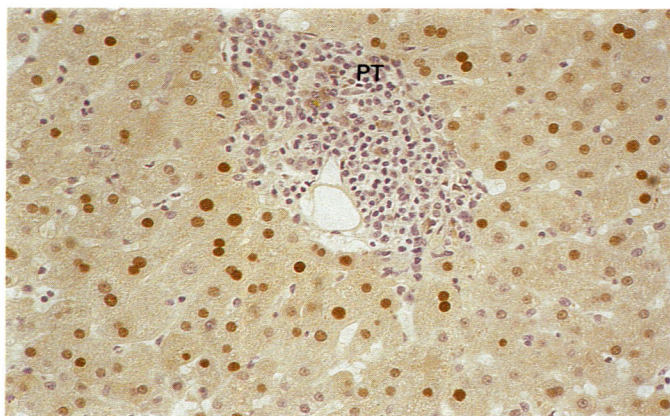

Fig. 17.49 Hepatitis B virus-positive chronic persistent hepatitis, replicative phase. Section stained for HBcAg. The portal tract (PT) is infiltrated by mononuclear cells. The darker-appearing nuclei in numerous hepatocytes contain HBcAg. (Immunoperoxidase stain for HBcAg; counterstain with haematoxylin.)

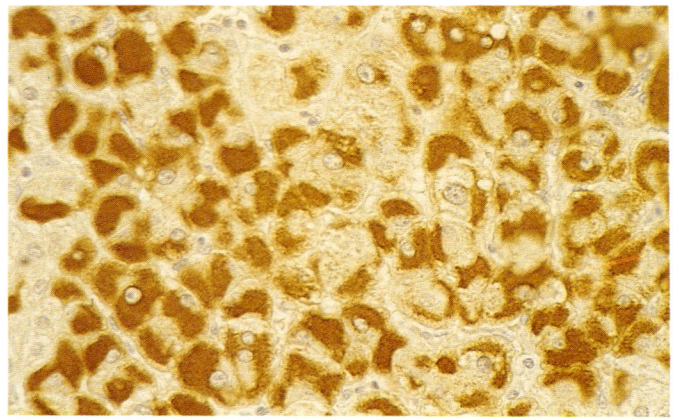

Fig. 17.51 Hepatitis B virus-positive chronic hepatitis, non-replicative phase. Detail from liver biopsy with minimal inflammatory changes. This section, stained for HBsAg, reveals large numbers of hepatocytes with massive cytoplasmic staining for this viral antigen. (Immunoperoxidase stain for HBsAg.)

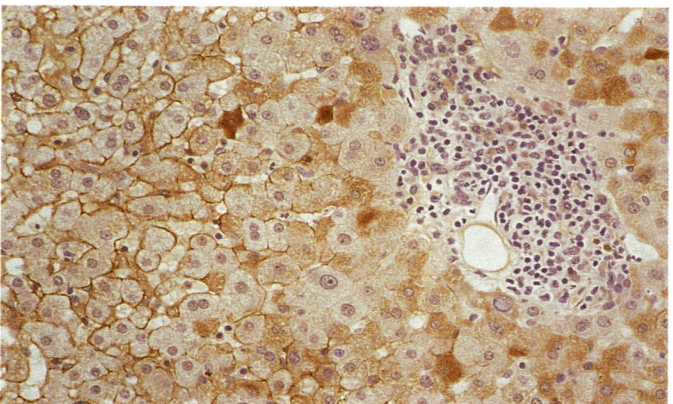

Fig. 17.50 Hepatitis B-positive chronic persistent hepatitis, replicative phase. There are small numbers of cells with cytoplasmic HBsAg, and larger numbers with membrane localization of antigen. (Immunoperoxidase for HBsAg.)

duct lesion. However, no single pathognomonic lesion exists to allow for a reliable distinction of this type of viral hepatitis. Also, ultrastructural changes described in nuclei and cytoplasm of hepatocytes in hepatitis C lack confirmation of specificity and rather represent cellular changes associated with active replication of several RNA viruses as seen in other cell types. Reagents (antibodies) allowing reliable immunohistochemical demonstration of HCV antigens in liver tissue are to be expected soon.

Delta virus hepatitis can be recognized on liver tissue sections by immunohistochemical demonstration of hepatitis delta antigen. Delta infection in chronic viral hepatitis type B is usually characterized by more severe parenchymal and portal inflammatory activity.

Drug-induced chronic hepatitis may be suspected on the findings of eosinophils in the inflammatory infiltrate, cholestasis, possibly parenchymal giant cells and granulomas.

Wilson disease should be suspected in a biopsy which, besides features of chronic hepatitis, also shows steatosis, vacuolated nuclei, Mallory bodies, and possibly copper accumulation, especially in younger patients.

α-1-Antitrypsin deficiency is recognizable by the occurrence in periportal hepatocytes of coarse eosinophilic cytoplasmic inclusions of variable size; these inclusions are PAS positive and diastase resistant, and show immunoreactivity for α-1-antitrypsin on immunohistochemical stains (see Section 17.9).

Natural history of chronic viral hepatitis type B and its modulation

In the 1970s, classification of chronic hepatitis was an important base for therapeutic decisions; treatment with steroids and immunosuppressive drugs was used for active forms of chronic hepatitis. Around 1980, however, several studies indicated that steroid therapy was not advantageous, and was even harmful, in chronic viral hepatitis type B. New forms of treatment (immunomodulation, antiviral agents) are under investigation. The distinction between mild and severe variants of chronic hepatitis remains important, as appears from new insights into the natural course of chronic hepatitis B viral infection, which can be divided into three phases.

The first phase is a period of 'immune tolerance' to the hepatitis B virus, associated with a high viral replication rate (high replicative phase of chronic viral hepatitis type B). Clinically and biochemically, the disease is mild. Liver biopsy shows only low inflammatory activity, corresponding to chronic persistent hepatitis or non-specific reactive hepatitis. Immunohistochemical staining for viral antigens reveals HBcAg in numerous liver cell nuclei and HBsAg in liver cell membranes (see Figs 17.49, 17.50).

After a variable time period of months or years, the patient's immune system succeeds in eliminating substantial numbers of virus-infected cells ('immune-clearance phase'). This phase is preceded or associated with a rise in serum transaminases. Histopathologically, one observes more impressive necro-inflammatory lesions, recognizable as chronic active hepatitis of variable severity.

The ensuing third phase is a 'non-replicative phase' with hepatitis B viral DNA integrated into hepatocyte DNA. The disease becomes mild, transaminases are only slightly elevated, and the liver reveals only mild inflammatory lesions of chronic persistent hepatitis. In this phase, immunohistochemistry for viral antigens reveals only a few or no liver cell nuclei positive for HBcAg, but numerous hepatocytes show massive staining for HBsAg (ground-glass hepatocytes) (see Fig. 17.51).

The course of chronic viral hepatitis type B may be modulated with variations in degree of disease activity by superinfection with hepatitis A, D, and C viruses and by therapeutic interventions (immunosuppression, immunostimulation, antiviral agents). Superinfection with other non-B viruses occurs, especially in high-risk groups such as drug-abusers and multiply transfused patients. It thus appears that the prognosis of chronic hepatitis depends not only on the degree of disease activity and structural changes (chronic persistent or active hepatitis), but also on serology (type of serological viral markers), therapy, and risk factors.

One may conclude that the 'old' classification of chronic hepatitis, reflecting the degree of necro-inflammatory activity in terms like CPH and CAH, is still valid. Indeed, the degree of disease activity on initial biopsy appears to be one of the factors determining the response to interferon treatment in hepatitis B, and also determining the risk of progression to cirrhosis in hepatitis C. One must bear in mind, however, that the denominations CPH and CAH do not indicate distinct disease entities, but only levels of disease activity. Throughout the course of the disease, a patient may fluctuate from CPH to CAH, and back again to CPH.

In conclusion, the full evaluation of a patient with chronic hepatitis requires consideration of the histopathological lesion, supplemented with immuno-localization of viral antigens, identification of the aetiological agent(s), study of the serological profile, and consideration of the life style of the patient. An example of a full diagnosis would be: chronic persistent hepatitis, viral type B, replicative phase, in homosexual patient with HIV superinfection.

17.5.3 Primary biliary chirrhosis

Definition

Primary biliary cirrhosis (PBC) is a relatively uncommon disease, occurring most frequently in middle-aged women. The aetiology is unknown, but many features indicate that it may be an auto-immune disease.

Only the later stages of the disease correspond to a true cirrhosis; a presymptomatic and precirrhotic stage may exist over several years. The initial lesions are more accurately described by the term 'chronic non-suppurative destructive cholangitis'; indeed, the basic disease process consists in a progressive disappearance of intrahepatic bile ducts caused by a destructive inflammatory process distinct from purulent cholangitis. The disease runs a progressive course, usually over many years, leading to cirrhosis and death in liver failure.

Clinical features

The initial symptoms are usually intense pruritus with increasing skin pigmentation and eventually cholestatic jaundice. Portal hypertension and xanthomas may become apparent before the patient has cirrhosis. The most striking serum abnormalities include elevation of alkaline phosphatase and gamma-globulins, especially IgM. The most helpful diagnostic test is the demonstration of antimitochondrial antibodies.

Primary biliary cirrhosis is not uncommonly associated with other 'auto-immune' disorders, such as the 'sicca complex', CREST syndrome (calcinosis, Raynaud's phenomenon, oesophageal dysfunction, sclerodactyly, and telangiectasis), rheumatoid arthritis, renal tubular acidosis, and interstitial pulmonary fibrosis.

In recent years, increasing numbers of asymptomatic patients are recognized as suffering from PBC by the incidental discovery of hepatomegaly, raised serum alkaline phosphatase, and a positive antimitochondrial antibody test.

Pathological features

Early lesions

The initial injury affects medium-sized interlobular bile ducts 45–75 μm in diameter. The early lesions are focal, involving only segments of the bile ducts. The portal tracts are infiltrated by mononuclear, mainly lymphocytic cells in close proximity to the bile ducts. The latter show distinctive abnormalities. Their lining epithelium is swollen and may become stratified. The basement membrane is focally disrupted and lymphocytes and plasma cells infiltrate the epithelium (Fig. 17.52). In serial sections, rupture of the bile ducts may be recognized, which causes a phagocytic reaction with the appearance of ceroid-loaded macrophages and multinucleate giant cells.

The smaller portal tracts usually show a mononuclear inflammatory infiltrate of variable density, even within the same biopsy. Some portal tracts carry well-formed secondary lymphoid follicles; others show mixtures of lymphocytes, plasma cells, and also eosinophils. In others, focal aggregates of epithelioid cells or epithelioid granulomas are found; the latter may lie close to the bile duct or surround it (Fig. 17.53). The bile duct epithelium shows degenerative changes as described above.

In the smallest portal tracts, there is also a lymphoplasmocytic infiltrate; bile ducts of 20–30 μm in diameter are affected early on in the disease, with degenerative epithelial changes and inflammatory infiltration.

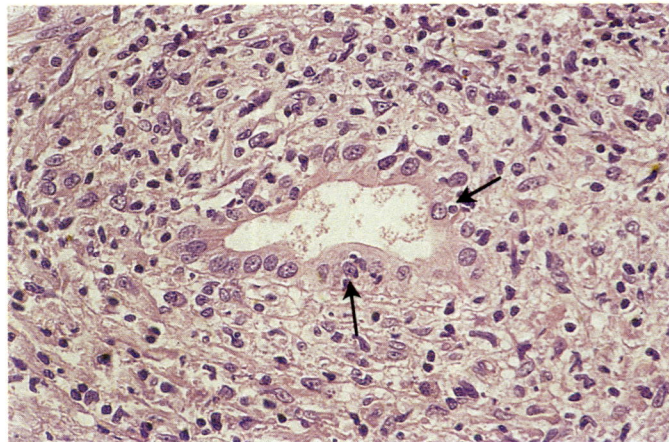

Fig. 17.52 Primary biliary cirrhosis; detail of portal tract. The figure shows a bile-duct of about 100 μm (longer outer diameter); some of the lining cells are vacuolated and lifted from the basement membrane by infiltrating inflammatory cells (arrows). The duct is surrounded by a moderately dense infiltration of lymphocytes, histiocytes, and plasma cells.

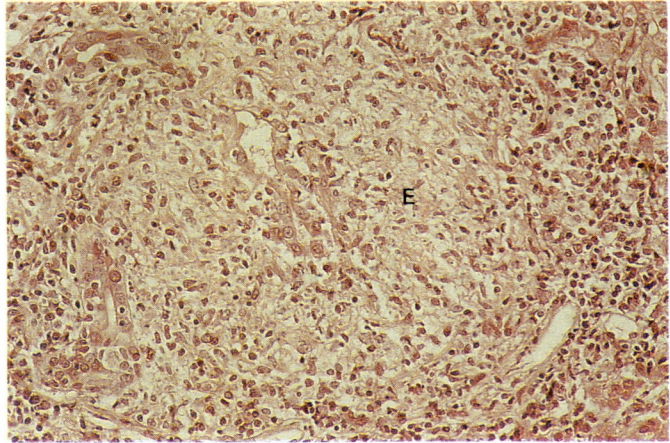

Fig. 17.53 Primary biliary cirrhosis; detail of portal tract. The bile duct (centre of picture) shows degeneration and necrosis of its lining epithelial cells; it is encased by a mass of epithelioid cells (E) surrounded by a dense mononuclear infiltrate.

The damage of the bile duct radicles leads to destruction and eventually disappearance of bile duct segments, usually without leaving a recognizable scar. Sections through affected portal tracts in this stage reveal hepatic artery branches which are not accompanied by a bile duct of comparable size (Fig. 17.54), constituting a useful marker for loss of ducts (ductopenia).

The parenchymal changes are mild; focal epithelioid granulomas may be found in some 25 per cent of biopsies. The usual conspicuous feature is focal Kupffer cell hyperplasia and sinusoidal lymphocytic infiltration. Cholestasis is not observed in the early stages of the disease.

The bile duct lesions in the early phase are those that are

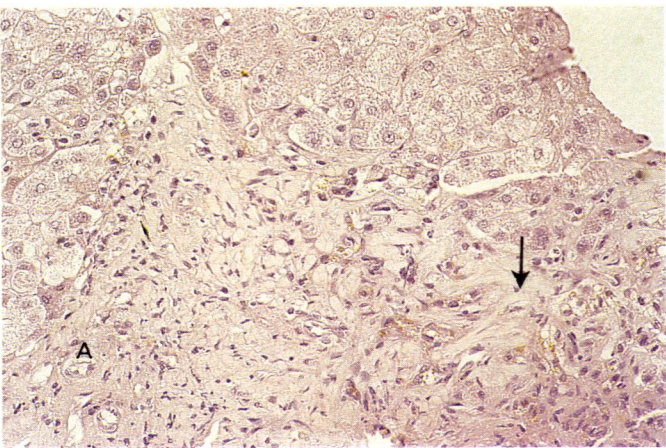

Fig. 17.54 Primary biliary cirrhosis. Sclerosing portal tract with peri-portal fibrosis (arrow). No bile-duct can be recognized. A, hepatic artery branch.

characteristic for PBC and on which a definitive histopathological diagnosis can be based. The differential diagnosis includes chronic active hepatitis, primary sclerosing cholangitis, and—in the presence of epithelioid granulomas—sarcoidosis. The similarity of the bile duct lesions in PBC to those observed in graft versus host disease and liver allograft rejection has been emphasized (see Section 17.4).

Progress of liver injury and histological staging

The subsequent progression of the disease is the result of the continuous involvement of further bile duct segments and of the increasing extent to which the necro-inflammatory process also involves the parenchymal cells, possibly as part of the same immunological assault that destroys the bile duct radicles. The consequences of progressive bile duct loss are ductular increase, chronic cholestasis, and progressive fibrosis; whereas parenchymal destruction paves the way for nodular regeneration and additional fibrosis.

Evidence of progressive liver injury is observed at the margins of the portal tracts: the limiting plates are interrupted by extending inflammatory infiltrate and increasing numbers of ductular structures. The latter originate not only from ductular proliferation, but to a large extent also from ductular metaplasia of acinar zone 1 hepatocytes. The 'ductular reaction' is accompanied by fibroblastic proliferation, increased deposition of collagen and other matrix components, oedema, and polymorphonuclear infiltration. These complex changes occurring at the interface between portal tract and acinar zone 1 parenchyma create an irregular borderline and have been termed 'biliary piecemeal necrosis' (Fig. 17.55).

The latter can be differentiated from classical (or lymphocytic) piecemeal necrosis of CAH by its higher content of ductules and polymorphonuclear leucocytes. Furthermore, it is associated with signs of chronic cholestasis in the acinar zone 1 hepatocytes. These parenchymal cells show swelling with perinuclear condensation of their cytoplasm and pale appear-

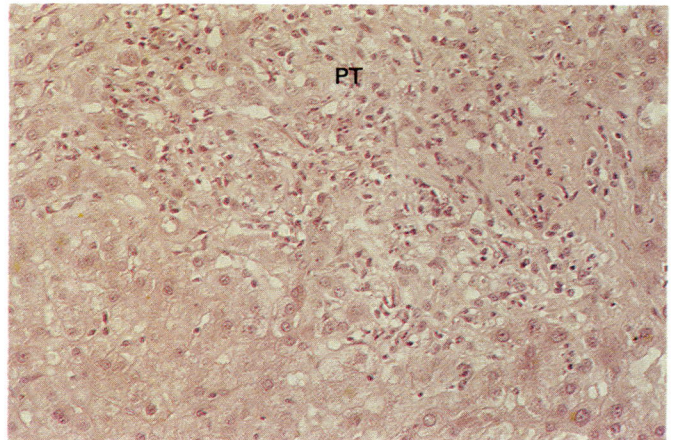

Fig. 17.55 Primary biliary cirrhosis. Irregular borderline between sclerosing portal tract (PT) and adjacent parenchyma. The irregularity is due to oedema, increase in ductules, and inflammatory infiltration, including neutrophils (so-called biliary piecemeal necrosis).

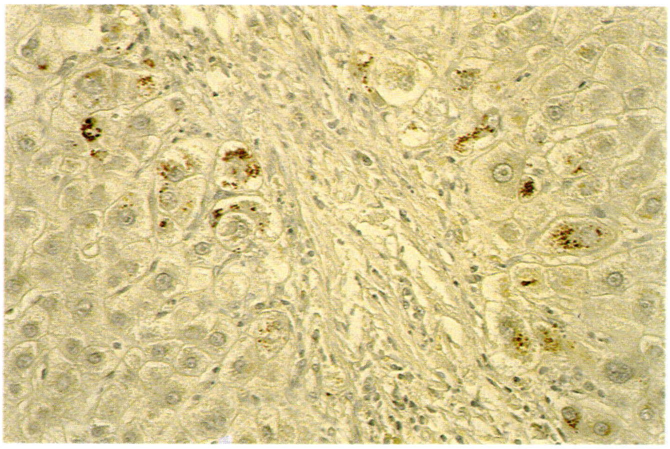

Fig. 17.56 Primary biliary cirrhosis. Sclerosing portal tract without identifiable bile duct. The periportal hepatocytes are swollen and contain dark-staining copper granules (so-called cholate-stasis). (Rhodamine stain (for copper).)

ance of the peripheral parts of the cell. This change is associated with progressive accumulation of coarse granules, which correspond to lysosomes loaded with copper, complexed with copper-binding protein or metallotheonein. These granules stain positive with Shikata's orcein stain (metallotheonein) and rhodanine (copper) (Fig. 17.56). Mallory bodies may develop in these cells, reflecting a severe disturbance in the composition and organization of intermediate filaments of the cytoskeleton. In later stages, bilirubin inclusions may also be observed. These hepatocellular changes are characteristic for chronic cholestasis, and are presumably caused by the detergent effect of retained bile salts, which explains the term 'cholate-stasis'. Biliary piecemeal necrosis and cholate stasis lead to progressive destruction of parenchyma in acinar zone 1, accompanied by extending periportal inflammation and fibrosis. A progressive disturbance of the liver architecture ensues, associated with nodular parenchymal regeneration, eventually resulting in established cirrhosis.

Several authors have proposed slightly different systems to divide the histological evolution of PBC into successive stages (Table 17.5). Histopathological staging is useful for prognostic purposes, since it helps to evaluate the stage of progression of primary biliary cirrhosis in a particular patient. However, one must realize that the prognostic usefulness of staging is only relative, and is hampered for several reasons. Since the progression of the disease is often variable within the liver, there may be considerable overlap between the stages described. Furthermore, there is variation in the speed of progression of the disease from one patient to the next; some patients progress for some time, but may then stabilize in the same stage for a long time, even years.

Clinically, the development of jaundice is a bad prognostic sign. Histopathologically, the presence of portal–portal bridging fibrosis is inversely correlated with survival. Whether the presence of epithelioid granulomas indicates a more favourable outlook remains an unsettled question.

In spite of its limitations, histopathological staging in PBC has proved to be useful in selecting patients with terminal PBC as candidates for liver transplantation. Furthermore, semi-quantitative scoring of histopathological changes is used for the evaluation of treatment efficacy in controlled clinical trials of new treatment modalities (e.g. urso-deoxycholic acid).

Table 17.5 Histopathological staging systems in PBC

Author	Stage 1	Stage 2	Stage 3	Stage 4
Rubin *et al.* (1965)	Damage to intrahepatic bile ducts	Ductular proliferation	Ductular proliferation	Cirrhosis
Scheuer (1967)	Florid bile duct lesion	Ductular proliferation	Scarring	Cirrhosis
Popper and Schaffner (1970)	Cholangitis	Ductular proliferation and destruction	Precirrhotic stage	Cirrhosis
Ludwig *et al.* (1978)	Portal hepatitis	Periportal hepatitis	Bridging necrosis or fibrous septa or both	Cirrhosis

Mixed forms of chronic active hepatitis and primary biliary cirrhosis

The histopathological differentiation between chronic active hepatitis and PBC may be difficult, since lymphocytic piecemeal necrosis may also be seen in PBC, and the diagnostic features of bile duct lesions and epithelioid granulomas may be missed in a needle biopsy. Additional helpful features in favour of PBC are biliary piecemeal necrosis, marked ductular proliferation, cholate-stasis, and marked variability in the appearance of portal tracts.

However, some patients seem to suffer from a disease that corresponds to a mixed form of CAH and PBC. In this mixed type, there is more severe liver injury with distinctive features of both PBC and CAH. In contrast to 'pure' PBC, more bridging necrosis and earlier progression into cirrhosis has been described, whereas intense ductular proliferation marks a difference with 'pure' CAH.

The subtype pattern of antimitochondrial antibodies has also been used to classify PBC into different subgroups. The presence of anti-M8 or anti-M4 may indicate a more progressive and rapid course of the disease.

17.5.4   Primary sclerosing cholangitis

Definition, aetiology, pathogenesis

Primary sclerosing cholangitis (PSC) is a disorder characterized by non-specific inflammation and progressive fibrosis in the wall of the biliary tract, leading to irregular narrowing of both the intra- and extrahepatic bile ducts. In some instances, intrahepatic bile duct involvement can occur in the absence of extrahepatic bile duct disease. The disease has to be distinguished from secondary sclerosing cholangitis; hence, sclerosing lesions following biliary surgery, treatment of echinococcal cyst, cholelithiasis, congenital bile duct abnormalities, and bile duct carcinoma have to be excluded.

There is a male:female preponderance of 2:1; the disease is most frequent between 20 and 50 years of age. PSC may occur alone, but in 50–70 per cent of patients it is associated with chronic ulcerative colitis. In recent Norwegian and Swedish studies, the association is even up to 100 per cent. Conversely, 4–5 per cent of patients with ulcerative colitis suffer from PSC. Occasional cases may be associated with Crohn colitis, chronic pancreatitis, retroperitoneal and mediastinal fibrosis, and other conditions of obscure aetiology.

The aetiology of PSC is not known. Because of its frequent association with ulcerative colitis, portal toxaemia and bacteraemia have been considered, but lack supporting proof. Chronic inflammatory bowel disease does not seem to cause PSC: the two diseases can occur independently; PSC may become symptomatic before the chronic inflammatory bowel disease; and colectomy does not improve PSC. Some familial cases have been reported, and a close association with HLA antigens B8 and DR3 has been observed, suggesting a possible auto-immune origin of the disease. Viral infections and toxic bile acids have also been proposed as possible aetiologic factors.

Clinical features

A patient with PSC usually presents with fatigue, vague upper abdominal pain and progressive jaundice; less commonly, recurrent attacks of cholangitis herald the beginning of the disease. Most patients develop secondary biliary cirrhosis with progressive liver failure, deepening jaundice, and death within 5–7 years after diagnosis. A more benign course and long survival has been observed in some cases.

The liver function tests show abnormalities similar to those seen in PBC, except for a higher increase in serum transaminases, no marked increase in serum IgM, and absence of antimitochondrial antibodies.

The disease is diagnosed with increasing frequency since the introduction of endoscopic retrograde cholangiopancreatography (ERCP) and percutaneous transhepatic cholangiography (PTC) in the mid-1970s. Cholangiography reveals irregular areas of stricture and dilatation (beaded appearance) of the bile ducts; in 80 per cent of the patients, both the intra- and extrahepatic bile ducts show these abnormalities. In later stages, the biliary tree shows an attenuated pattern ('pruned tree' appearance).

Asymptomatic cases are discovered with increasing frequency (up to 10 per cent in some series) because of an isolated rise of alkaline phosphatase and changes on cholangiography. It is of interest that several recent studies have demonstrated the occurrence of PSC in the paediatric age group.

Pathological features

Macroscopically, the extrahepatic bile ducts appear as thickened cords with a thick wall and narrow lumen. The histopathological changes in PSC are not pathognomonic, since similar lesions can be observed in chronic secondary cholangitis and in PBC.

The distinctive lesion is concentric periduct fibrosis ('onion-skin' type) around medium-sized or larger bile ducts, with degeneration and atrophy of their epithelial lining (Fig. 17.57). Eventually, bile ducts are replaced by fibrous cords. A disease variant exists in which only the small, intrahepatic bile ducts are affected and become replaced by remarkably prominent fibrous scars. This picture of fibrous-obliterative cholangitis, accompanied by reduced numbers of interlobular bile ducts, is the feature most suggestive of PSC. However, it is found in only 40 per cent of biopsies at most.

In other cases, the portal tracts show a diffuse mixed inflammatory infiltrate of lymphocytes, plasma cells, and neutrophils, often tending to be more dense around the bile ducts. Lymphoid aggregates and even lymphoid follicles may be found, but no epithelioid granulomas. The smaller bile ducts may show degenerative epithelial changes, such as anisocytosis, nuclear pyknosis, cytoplasmic shrinkage or vacuolation, and shedding from the basement membrane, and often are surrounded by a ring of oedema, thickening of the basement membrane, or hyaline fibrosis. In many portal tracts bile ducts disappear without any residual trace.

As the disease advances the inflammation has a tendency to

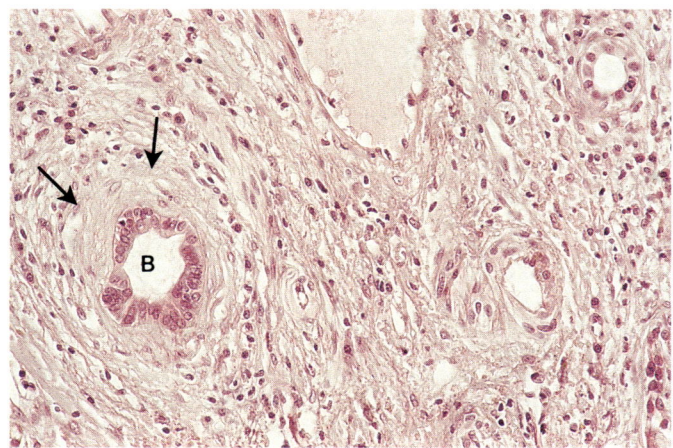

Fig. 17.57 Primary sclerosing cholangitis. Detail of portal tract with sclerosing connective tissue and sprinkling of mononuclear cells. The bile duct (B) shows irregularity of its lining epithelium, and concentric periductal fibrosis (arrows).

subside, leaving portal tracts carrying hepatic artery branches unaccompanied by bile ducts (paucity of intrahepatic bile ducts). One may find variable degrees of portal and periportal fibrosis and ductular proliferation (Fig. 17.58). Variability in this picture presumably determines the degree of obstruction caused by narrowing and obliteration of bile duct radicles.

Parenchymal bilirubinostasis is an early and more frequent finding in PSC than in primary biliary cirrhosis. Changes of cholate-stasis gradually develop as in primary biliary cirrhosis, with parenchymal zone 1 accumulation of copper and copper-binding protein. Further progression is characterized by increasing periportal fibrosis with formation of portal–portal septa and eventual development of cirrhosis of the biliary type.

The distinction between PSC and primary biliary cirrhosis on histopathological appearances alone may be impossible:

Wiesner *et al.* (1985) reported that histopathology allowed a reliable distinction in only 28 per cent of a series of 318 patients who had one of these two syndromes. Especially in smaller, less representative biopsies, differentiation from chronic hepatitis (CPH, CAH) may be difficult or impossible. Such less distinctive portal inflammation has been described under the term 'pericholangitis' but this term should be abandoned.

A new entity described in 1988 as 'Idiopathic Adulthood Ductopenia' resembles PSC clinically and histologically, but is not associated with inflammatory bowel disease.

In a few patients with undoubted PSC on cholangiography, the lesions may be unexpectedly mild on liver biopsy; conversely, histopathological lesions of PSC may be observed in patients with chronic inflammatory bowel disease but with a still normal ERCP. This indicates the necessity for performing both cholangiography and liver biopsy to reach a reliable diagnosis: each of these techniques provides information on different segments of the biliary tree. Histopathological staging of PSC (basically according to the scheme of Ludwig *et al.* in Table 17.5) has been introduced since the increased use of liver transplantation in the treatment of terminal PSC.

Adenocarcinoma of the bile ducts may develop in patients with long-standing PSC and ulcerative colitis.

17.5.5   Further reading

Chronic hepatitis

Bianchi, L., *et al.* (1971). Morphological criteria in viral hepatitis. *Lancet* i, 333–7.

Bianchi, L., *et al.* (1974). Guidelines for diagnosis of therapeutic drug-induced liver injury in liver biopsies. *Lancet* ii, 854–7.

Bianchi, L., *et al.* (1977). Acute and chronic hepatitis revisited. *Lancet* ii, 914–19.

Bianchi, L., Spichtin, H. P., and Gudat, F. (1987). Chronic hepatitis. In *Pathology of the liver* (2nd edn) (ed. R. N. M. MacSween, P. P. Anthony, and P. J. Scheuer), pp. 310–41. Churchill Livingstone, Edinburgh.

Bradley, D. W., Krawczynski, K., Beach, M. J., and Purdy, M. A. (1991). Non-A non-B hepatitis: toward the discovery of hepatitis C and E viruses. *Seminars in Liver Disease* 11, 128–46.

Callea, F., De Vos, R., Togni, R., Tardanico, R., Vanstapel, M. J., and Desmet, V. J. (1986). Fibrinogen inclusions in liver cells: a new type of ground-glass hepatocyte. Immune light and electron microscopic characterization. *Histopathology* 10, 65–73.

Conn, H. O. (1976). Chronic hepatitis: reducing an iatrogenic enigma to a workable puzzle. *Gastroenterology* 70, 1182–4.

De Groote, J., *et al.* (1968). A classification of chronic hepatitis. *Lancet* ii, 626–8.

Desmet, V. J. (1986). Histopathology of chronic viral hepatitis. In *Viral hepatitis* (ed. F. Callea, M. Zorzi, and V. J. Desmet), pp. 32–40. Springer-Verlag, Berlin.

Desmet, V. J. (1990). Liver reaction patterns in infections. In *Infectious diseases of the liver* (ed. L. Bianchi, K.-P. Maier, W. Gerok, and F. Deinhardt), pp. 31–47. Kluwer Academic Publishers, Dordrecht.

Desmet, V. J. (1991). Immunopathology of chronic viral hepatitis. *Hepatogastroenterology* 38, 14–21.

Desmet, V. J. and De Vos, R. (1985). Ultrastructural findings in non-A, non-B viral hepatitis. In *Hepatology, a Festschrift for Hans Popper* (ed. H. Brunner and H. Thaler), pp. 159–75. Raven Press, New York.

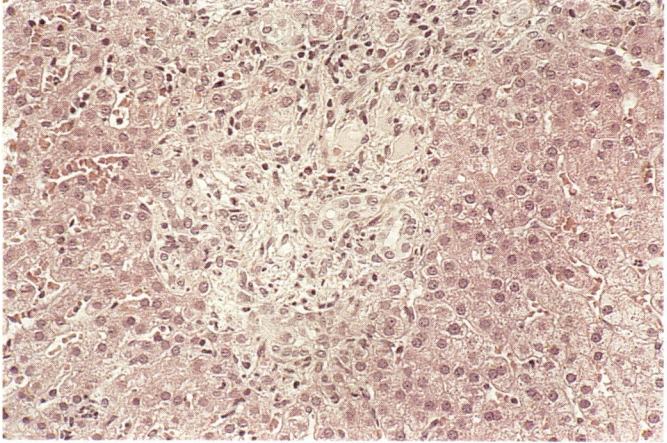

Fig. 17.58 Primary sclerosing cholangitis. A smaller portal tract shows oedema and ductular proliferation accompanied by inflammatory cells, including neutrophils (so-called cholangiolitis).

Genesca, J., Esteban, J. I., and Alter, H. J. (1991). Blood-borne non-A, non-B hepatitis: hepatitis C. *Seminars in Liver Disease* 11, 147–64.

Gerber, M. A. and Vernace, S. (1974). Chronic septal hepatitis. *Virchows Archiv (A)* 353, 303–9.

Ishak, K. G. and Sharp, H. L. (1987). Metabolic errors and liver disease. In *Pathology of the liver* (2nd edn) (ed. R. N. M. MacSween, P. P. Anthony, and P. J. Scheuer). Churchill Livingstone, Edinburgh.

Kalk, H. (1947). Die chronischem Verlaufsformen der Hepatitis Epidemica im Hinblick auf ihre klinische Symptomatologie. *Deutsche Medizinische Wochenschrift* 72, 471–6.

Knodell, R. G., *et al.* (1981). Formulation and application of a numerical scoring system for assessing histological activity in asymptomatic chronic active hepatitis. *Hepatology* 1, 431–5.

Liaw, Y. F., Chu, C. M., Chen, T. J., Lin, D. Y., Chang-Chien, C. S., and Wu, C. S. (1982). Chronic lobular hepatitis: a clinicopathological and prognostic study. *Hepatology* 2, 258–62.

Liaw, Y. F., Chu, C. M., Su, I. J., Huang, M. J., Lin, D. Y., and Chang-Chien, C. S. (1983). Clinical and histological events preceding hepatitis B e antigen seroconversion in chronic type B hepatitis. *Gastroenterology* 84, 216–19.

Liaw, Y. F., Sheen, I. S., Chu, C. M., and Chen, T. J. (1984). Chronic hepatitis with nonspecific histological changes. Is it a distinct variant of chronic hepatitis? *Liver* 4, 55–60.

Popper, H. and Schaffner, F. (1971). The vocabulary of chronic hepatitis. *New England Journal of Medicine* 284, 1154–6.

Poulsen, H. and Christoffersen, P. (1972). Abnormal bile duct epithelium in chronic aggressive hepatitis and cirrhosis. A review of morphology and clinical, biochemical and immunologic features. *Human Pathology* 3, 217–25.

Rizetto, M., Bonino, F., and Verme, G. (1988). Hepatitis delta virus infection of the liver: progress in virology, pathobiology and diagnosis. *Seminars in Liver Disease* 8, 350–6.

Scheuer, P. J. (1986). Changing views on chronic hepatitis. *Histopathology* 10, 1–4.

Zimmerman, H. J. and Ishak, K. G. (1987). Hepatic injury due to drugs and toxins. In *Pathology of the liver* (2nd edn) (ed. R. N. M. MacSween, P. P. Anthony, and P. J. Scheuer), pp. 503–73. Churchill Livingstone, Edinburgh.

Primary biliary cirrhosis

Berg, P. A. and Klein, R. (1987). Immunology of primary biliary cirrhosis. *Clinical Gastroenterology* 1, 675–706.

Berg, P. A. and Klein, R. (1991). Autoantibody patterns in primary biliary cirrhosis. In *Autoimmune liver diseases* (ed. E. L. Krawitt and R. H. Wiesner), pp. 123–42. Raven Press, New York.

Desmet, V. J. (1986). Current problems in diagnosis of biliary disease and cholestasis. *Seminars in Liver Disease* 6, 233–45.

Desmet, V. J. (1987). Cholangiopathies: past, present, and future. *Seminars in Liver Disease* 7, 67–76.

Klöppel, G., Seifert, G., Lindner, H., Dammermann, R., Sack, H. J. and Berg, P. A. (1977). Histopathological features in mixed types of chronic aggressive hepatitis and primary biliary cirrhosis. *Virchows Archiv A* 373, 143–60.

Ludwig, J., Dickson, E. R., and McDonald, G. S. (1978). Staging of chronic nonsuppurative destructive cholangitis (syndrome of primary biliary cirrhosis). *Virchows Archiv für Pathologische Anatomie* 379, 103–12.

Popper, H. and Schaffner, F. (1970). Non-suppurative destructive chronic cholangitis and chronic hepatitis. In *Progress in liver diseases*, Vol. III (ed. H. Popper and F. Schaffner), pp. 336–54. Grune and Stratton, New York.

Portmann, B. and MacSween, R. N. M. (1987). Diseases of the intrahepatic bile ducts. In *Pathology of the liver* (2nd edn) (ed. R. N. M. MacSween, P. P. Anthony, and P. J. Scheuer), pp. 424–53. Churchill Livingstone, Edinburgh.

Poupon, R. E., Balkau, B., Eschwège, E., Poupon, R., and UDCA-PBC Study Group (1991). A multicenter, controlled trial of ursodiol for the treatment of primary biliary cirrhosis. *New England Journal of Medicine* 324, 1548–54.

Rubin, E., Schaffner, F., and Popper, H. (1965). Primary biliary cirrhosis. Chronic non-suppurative destruction cholangitis. *American Journal of Pathology* 46, 387–407.

Rudzki, C., Ishak, K. G., and Zimmerman, H. J. (1975). Chronic intrahepatic cholestasis of sarcoidosis. *American Journal of Medicine* 59, 373–87.

Scheuer, P. J. (1967). Primary biliary cirrhosis. *Proceedings of the Royal Society of Medicine* 60, 1257–60.

Vierling, J. M. (1990). Primary biliary cirrhosis. In *Hepatology. A textbook of liver disease*, Vol. II (2nd edn) (ed. D. Zakim and T. B. Boyer), pp. 1158–205. W. B. Saunders, Philadelphia.

Primary sclerosing cholangitis

Baptista, A., *et al.* (1983). Histopathology of the intrahepatic biliary tree. *Liver* 3, 161–75.

El-Shabrawi, M., *et al.* (1987). Primary sclerosing cholangitis in childhood. *Gastroenterology* 92, 1226–35.

Fausa, O., Schrumpf, E., and Elgjo, K. (1991). Relationship of inflammatory bowel disease and primary sclerosing cholangitis. *Seminars in Liver Disease* 11, 31–9.

Ludwig, J., Wiesner, R. H., and La Russo, N. F. (1988). Idiopathic adulthood ductopenia. A cause of chronic cholestatic liver disease and biliary cirrhosis. *Journal of Hepatology* 7, 193–9.

Ludwig, J., La Russo, N. F., and Wiesner, R. H. (1990). The syndrome of primary schlerosing cholangitis. In *Progress in liver disease*, Vol. IX (ed. H. Popper and F. Schaffner). W. B. Saunders, Philadelphia, pp. 555–66.

MacSween, R. M. N., Burt, A. D., and Haboubi, N. Y. (1987). Unusual variant of primary sclerosing cholangitis. *Journal of Clinical Pathology* 40, 541–5.

Wiesner, R. H., Larusso, N. F., Ludwig, J., and Dickson, E. R. (1985). Comparison of the clinicopathologic features of primary sclerosing cholangitis and primary biliary cirrhosis. *Gastroenterology* 88, 108–14.

17.6   Alcoholic liver disease

James O'D. McGee

Alcohol toxicity has been known for at least 5000 years. This is due almost entirely to ethanol and its metabolites, particularly acetaldehyde. Other constituents of alcoholic drinks such as colourants and other congeners are probably irrelevant to disease production; a possible exception is the presence of high iron levels in some wines and beers.

In the past half century, and particularly in the past two decades, the incidence of alcohol-induced disease has increased alarmingly. There is a direct link between the alcohol consumption per capita and end-stage alcoholic liver disease, viz. cirrhosis. Alcoholic cirrhosis is the fourth commonest cause of death in men and the fifth commonest in women in the USA in the age-group 35–54. Alchoholism and its related diseases are now a major health problem; together they constitute the third largest health problem in the USA, causing about 200 000 deaths per year.

17.6.1 Ethanol metabolism

Ethanol is rapidly absorbed from the stomach and small intestine; the absorption rate is reduced by food. About 95 per cent is metabolized in the liver to acetaldehyde and acetate and the remainder is excreted as ethanol in urine and breath (Fig. 17.59). The urine concentration is usually $1.3 \times$ that of blood, while the breath:blood ratio is 1:2300.

Other consequences of ethanol oxidation in the liver relate mainly to the increased NADH:NAD$^+$ ratio (see Fig. 17.59).

1. There is lactic acidosis due to increased lactate production and decreased utilization. The acidosis, besides causing clinical problems *per se*, is also associated with reduced renal uric acid secretion and secondary hyperuricaemia.

2. Hypoglycaemia may result from reduced gluconeogenesis from amino acids. Hypoglycaemia may be fatal in adults but particularly in children, who may be particularly susceptible to relatively small quantities of alcohol.

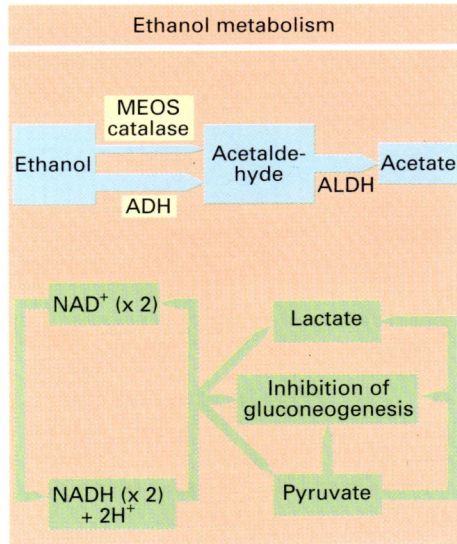

Fig. 17.59 Approximately 95 per cent of ethanol is oxidized to acetaldehyde and acetate and the remainder is excreted unchanged in the urine and, to a lesser extent, in breath and through the skin. Ethanol is metabolized to acetaldehyde by a NAD$^+$-dependent hepatic alcohol dehydrogenase (ADH); a small proportion is oxidized by the microsomal ethanol-oxidizing system (MEOS) and the catalase pathway. MEOS activity may be increased by chronic alcohol abuse and by enzyme-inducing drugs, and this may explain the increased ethanol tolerance observed in heavy drinkers. Acetaldehyde is oxidized via the NAD$^+$-dependent enzyme, aldehyde dehydrogenase (ALDH), to yield acetate. Ethanol metabolism results in accumulation of free NADH, increase in the NADH:NAD$^+$ ratio and inhibition of hepatic gluconeogenesis; the lactate:pyruvate ratio increases and hyperlactataemia occurs.

3. H$^+$ ion increase depresses fatty acid oxidation by competing with fatty acids as the energy source for liver mitochondria. In long-standing alcohol abuse, protein synthesis, which is necessary for triglyceride transport from hepatocytes, is inhibited. These two mechanisms together cause fat retention in hepatocytes.

4. Steroid (including oestrogen) metabolism in liver is also disturbed. This may account for some of the hormonal problems in chronic alcoholism.

Alcohol also induces microsomal hypertrophy and 'drug'-inducing enzymes. This has important clinical consequences (see Section 17.16).

17.6.2 Alcoholic liver disease

Alcohol induces a spectrum of liver disorders, with fatty change at the benign end of the spectrum, alcoholic hepatitis in the middle, and cirrhosis, with or without hepatic cancer, at the other end of the spectrum. The risk of developing chronic liver disease correlates only broadly with the level of alcohol consumption and its duration; heavy drinking always worsens the prognosis whatever the pathology. Fatty change, however, is an exception (see below).

Fatty change

Clinical presentation

Fatty change is present in about 90 per cent of patients presenting for treatment of alcoholism. There may be no signs or symptoms referrable to the liver. Asymptomatic hepatomegaly or a mild abnormality in LFTs may be discovered at a routine medical check. Non-specific digestive symptoms may be a problem, but this is probably due to the effects of ethanol on the alimentary tract. Sudden death may occur rarely in patients who only have severe fatty change at autopsy. Blood alcohol levels in these patients may be relatively low (< 50 mg/100 ml) and it has been postulated that death is due to alcohol withdrawal.

Fatty change is the only form of alcohol-induced liver disease that is predictable and probably dose-related. From studies on acute alcohol consumption in healthy (non-alcohol-dependent) volunteer medical students, it has been concluded that most individuals who consume large amounts of alcohol (more than 180 g spread over one day) develop fatty change. This condition, however, is reversible and the liver returns to normal if alcohol intake is stopped. There may be one exception to this rule; patients with perivenous fibrosis (see below) may progress to chronic liver disease.

Pathology

Fat, in the form of triglyceride accumulates in hepatocytes throughout the acinus but may be accentuated in zone 3 (Fig. 17.60). The lipid accumulates in a single vacuole, displacing the nucleus—so-called large droplet fatty change. Occasionally, lipid accumulates as 'small droplet fatty change'; this mimics the appearances seen in tetracycline toxicity and fatty liver of pregnancy.

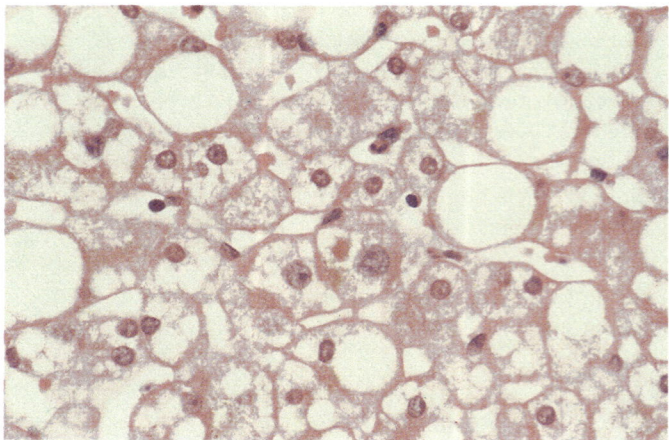

Fig. 17.60 Fatty change in an alcoholic liver. Many of the hepatocytes contain single, large, fat vacuoles. A megamitochondrion is present in one hepatocyte (centre of field).

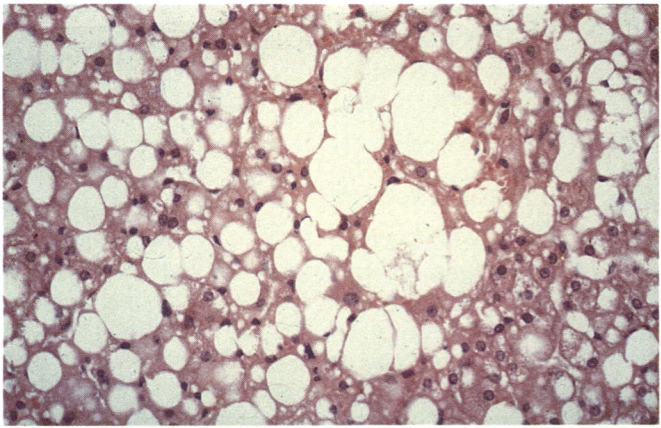

Fig. 17.61 Fatty change of large and small droplet type in acute alcoholic liver disease. Large fat droplets are evident in many cells, together with fat cysts due to coalescence of fat in adjacent hepatocytes.

Fatty change *per se* is not diagnostic of alcohol abuse. None the less, fatty change appears almost invariably in hepatocytes within 3–7 days of heavy alcohol consumption. The fat probably disappears within 3–4 days, but may take weeks in severe cases. In alcoholics, therefore, some fatty change would be expected unless there is proven, prolonged alcohol abstinence. Fatty change, without other hepatic pathology, in Western adults should raise the possibility of alcoholism and this should be positively excluded before other aetiologies are investigated robustly.

Fatty change also occurs in obesity, diabetes mellitus, Crohn disease, ulcerative colitis, methotrexate and steroid therapy, congestive cardiac failure, abetalipoproteinaemia, and malnutrition states such as intestinal bypass and kwashiorkor.

Fatty cysts and lipogranulomas result from the coalescence of fat vacuoles in adjacent hepatocytes and rupture of fat vacuoles/cysts, respectively. The formation of fat cysts (Fig. 17.61) correlates broadly with the degree of fatty change. Lipogranulomas (Fig. 17.62) consist of a central fat-filled space surrounded by mononuclear cells, with or without multinucleate giant cells and eosinophils. These lesions occur anywhere in the acinus, including portal tracts. Both of these lesions probably have little functional significance, although focal fibrosis has been ascribed to healing of lipogranulomas. Fat accumulation in portal tract macrophages, presumably due to lipid release from hepatocytes, is also common.

Perivenular fibrosis This lesion can accompany simple fatty change. Attention was first drawn to it in baboons chronically fed alcohol. Perivenular fibrosis was present in these animals with fatty change only. Some of these baboons apparently progress to alcoholic cirrhosis without going through an acute alcoholic hepatitis phase and it has been suggested that perivenular fibrosis is a 'marker' for progression to cirrhosis.

Perivenular fibrosis is defined as the presence of fibrosis

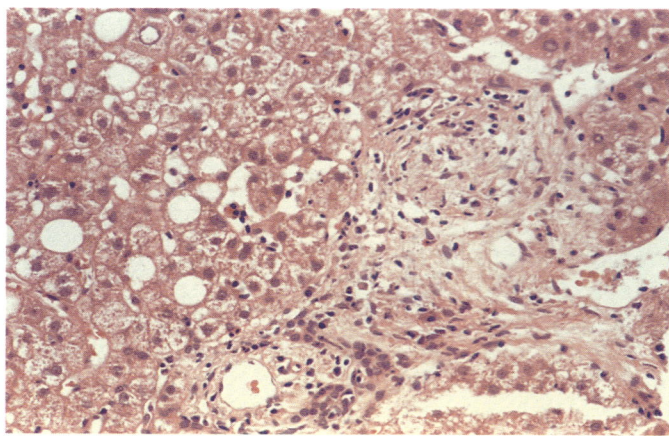

Fig. 17.62 Lipogranuloma in alcoholic liver disease. There is a lipogranuloma in a portal tract. There is also fatty change of large droplet type in hepatocytes.

around two-thirds of the circumference of terminal hepatic venules; the fibrous layer being at least 4 μm thick. It is usually associated with pericellular fibrosis in zone 3 (Fig. 17.63). Follow-up of patients with fatty liver and perivenular fibrosis by serial liver biopsy has shown that about 75 per cent develop more severe liver fibrosis and a few develop cirrhosis within 4 years when the patients continue to abuse alcohol. At this time, it is presumed that patients with this lesion at the fatty liver stage are at higher risk of subsequently developing more severe liver disease and they should be counselled accordingly.

Zieve syndrome (triad) of hyperlipidaemia, haemolytic jaundice, and pancreatitis occurs rarely in alcoholic liver disease. It may be associated with fatty change only or cirrhosis, but the diagnosis is based not on hepatic pathology but the triad of features listed.

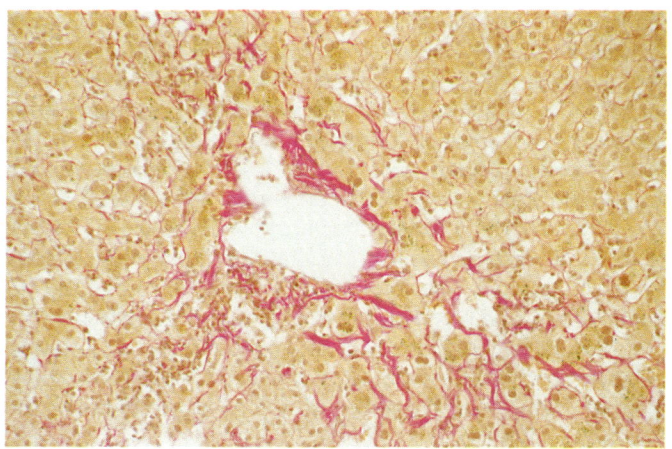

Fig. 17.63 There is quite prominent perivenular fibrosis in this acute alcoholic liver disease. There is also pericellular fibrosis radiating out from this terminal vein around individual hepatic sinusoids and hepatocytes themselves. This is a van Gieson preparation to demonstrate collagen fibres, in red.

Pathogenesis and prognosis

Lipid accumulates in hepatocytes for the reasons mentioned earlier: decreased lipoprotein synthesis, increased fatty acid accumulation, and increased mobilization of triglyceride from peripheral fat stores to the liver. Fatty change only is entirely reversible. If associated with perivenous fibrosis, the latter feature may indicate that the individual is at higher risk of developing cirrhosis if alcohol abuse continues.

Alcoholic hepatitis

Clinical presentation

This term was introduced about 30 years ago to define a clinico-pathological syndrome. However, the liver pathology of acute alcoholic hepatitis may be associated with a variety of clinical signs and symptoms. This pathology may be asymptomatic but it is usually associated with hepatomegaly, raised transaminases, and vague digestive symptoms. The distinctive clinical picture of the syndrome as first described is uncommon and is present only occasionally in patients whose liver shows the characteristic feature of hepatitis; jaundice, fever, abdominal pain, neutrophil leucocytosis, coagulation defects, renal impairment, tender hepatomegaly, and occasionally encephalopathy characterize this clinical syndrome. It has a high morbidity and mortality.

Alcoholic hepatitis can only be diagnosed reliably by biopsy. On the other hand, the clinical presentation and severity cannot be reliably predicted by the severity of the pathology.

Pathology

This is characterized by: liver cell damage in the form of ballooned hepatocytes which frequently contain Mallory bodies (MBs, alcoholic hyaline); focal neutrophil polymorph and mononuclear cell infiltration usually associated with ballooned

hepatocytes which may or may not contain MBs; and fatty change. Fatty change in hepatocytes is a relatively constant feature but is variable in degree; it is identical in morphology to fatty change only, described above.

Ballooned hepatocytes may be four times the diameter of a normal hepatocyte. Ballooning is usually maximal around terminal hepatic veins. The cytoplasm is 'empty' and contains fine eosinophilic strands of cytoplasm, which are probably precursors of fully formed Mallory bodies. MBs are often present in the same cells. Ballooning of hepatocytes is characteristic of alcoholic liver disease and its presence alone is highly suggestive of an alcohol aetiology (Fig. 17.64).

MBs are discrete eosinophilic structures in hepatocytes which usually also show balloon degeneration to a greater or lesser degree (see Fig. 17.64b). The MB-containing cells occur throughout the acinus, and are characteristically located around terminal veins in acute alcoholic hepatitis, but in cirrhosis they are present in highest numbers in cells immediately adjacent to fibrous septa. MB-containing cells may be surrounded by polymorphs, mononuclear cells, and lymphocytes,

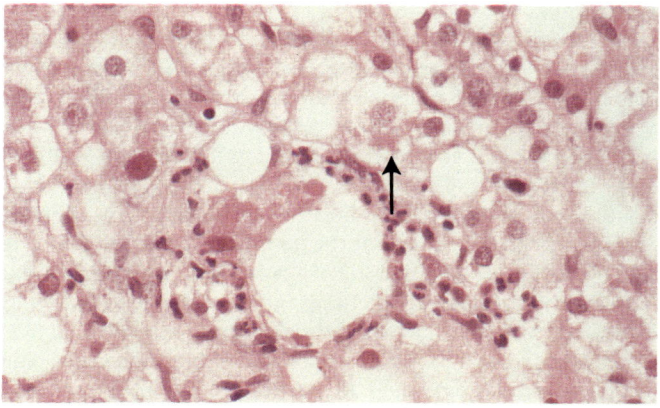

(a)

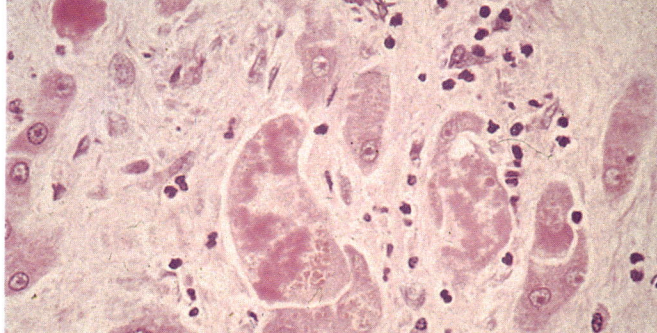

(b)

Fig. 17.64 (a) Acute alcoholic hepatitis. A fat-filled hepatocyte is surrounded by polymorphs. There is also a Mallory body present in a ballooned hepatocyte (arrow). (b) Mallory bodies in ballooned hepatocytes.

from which the designation 'hepatitis' derives. However, these inflammatory cells may be associated with focal areas of hepatocyte drop-out and MBs are frequently not evident within the foci of inflammation.

MBs in the context of fatty change, ballooning of hepatocytes, and inflammatory cell infiltration are strong pointers to an alcohol aetiology of the liver disease. However, MBs are also found in primary biliary cirrhosis, diabetes mellitus, Wilson disease, Indian childhood cirrhosis, intestinal bypass, rarely in long-standing bile duct obstruction, abetalipoproteinaemia, and perhexiline therapy. They have also been reported in obesity, but these patients may also be covert alcohol abusers.

Another feature of hepatocytes is megamitochondria. These giant mitochondria may be as large as hepatocyte nuclei (Fig. 17.65). They probably indicate recent heavy drinking and do not disappear from the liver until sobriety has been restored for about 1 month. Giant mitochondria are sometimes found in small numbers in normal liver so their presence *per se* is not pathognomonic of alcohol abuse; however, in large numbers they are highly suspicious. Systemic sclerosis is also associated with large numbers of megamitochondria in hepatocytes but their pathogenesis is unknown.

Perivenular and pericellular fibrosis are almost always present, together with a variable degree of portal tract fibrosis. Since alcoholic hepatitis is commonly most prominent in zone 3, pericellular fibrosis usually affects perivenular hepatocytes. Individual hepatocytes gradually disappear and larger foci of fibrosis are formed, eventually resulting in solid, often stellate, septa of fibrous tissue radiating from the terminal hepatic veins. There is usually pericellular fibrosis at the periphery of these septa. This form of fibrosis is characteristic of alcohol, and has considerable diagnostic importance. Sometimes these scars extend to link up with portal tract fibrous tissue, thus dissecting the normal liver architecture. The fibrosis does not inevitably indicate a poor prognosis with progression to cirrhosis, as it may regress if alcohol is discontinued.

Central sclerosing hyaline necrosis This condition was described in the early 1960s and represents a severe degree of alcoholic hepatitis in which perivenular fibrosis ('central sclerosis'), MBs ('hyaline'), and hepatocyte damage/death ('necrosis') are more pronounced than in the condition described above. In the most severe cases, the perivenular/pericellular fibrosis links with portal tract fibrosis and in the process destroys and isolates hepatocytes (Fig. 17.66). At this stage, the liver may be almost completely replaced by fibrous tissue. At autopsy, the liver is brick-hard and white due to fibrous tissue, and regenerating nodules are not apparent. This full-blown picture is, fortunately, not common and is associated with marked portal hypertension and ascites due to the perivenular lesion. When jaundice is evident at presentation the mortality is about 50 per cent within 2 years.

Prognosis

The outcome is probably most dependent on whether the patient can be persuaded to stop consuming alcohol. In those patients who continue to abuse alcohol, about one-third will develop cirrhosis within 2 years. Those who stop drinking may show complete resolution of their liver pathology within 2 years.

Full-blown central sclerosing hyaline necrosis has a bad prognosis (see above) but it has not been established whether this lesion can resolve when alcohol is discontinued.

Alcoholic cirrhosis

This is the commonest form of cirrhosis in Europe and the USA. It is the fourth commonest cause of death in American men, and fifth in women, in the age-group 35–54 years. Now it is not uncommon to make this diagnosis in late 20- or early 30-year-olds.

Twenty to thirty years ago, alcoholic cirrhosis was described as a fine 'nutritional cirrhosis', the normal liver architecture being replaced by small regenerating nodules (1–3 mm) which

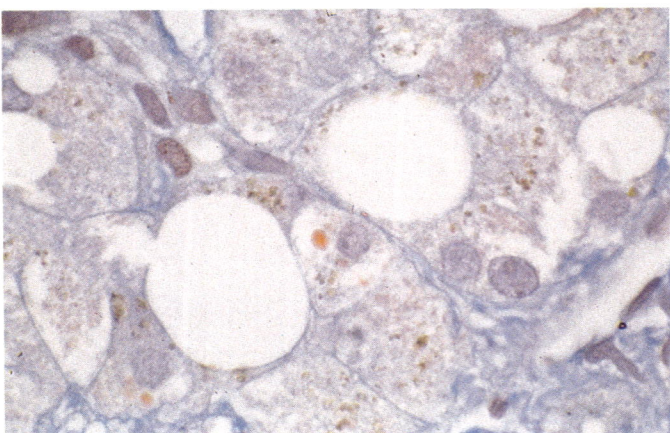

Fig. 17.65 Megamitochondria in acute alcoholic liver disease. A megamitochondrion is stained red with this trichrome preparation (arrow). There is also large droplet fatty change in adjacent hepatocytes.

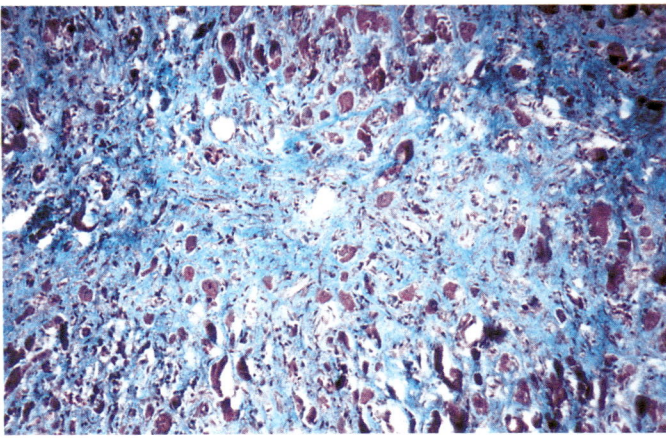

Fig. 17.66 Central sclerosing hyaline necrosis. There is marked fibrosis around a terminal hepatic venule. Fibrous tissue is blue in this trichrome preparation.

were yellow due to their lipid content (Fig. 17.67). Now, alcoholic cirrhosis often presents as a mixed type or as macronodular cirrhosis. In the latter form of cirrhosis, the regenerating nodules are approximately 1 cm in size, and may not be yellow because they lack fatty change.

Microscopically, the liver architecture is destroyed by the formation of large amounts of connective tissue, and hepatocytes show regenerative changes (Fig. 17.68). The special features that distinguish alcoholic cirrhosis from cirrhosis of other aetiologies (see Section 17.11) are Mallory bodies, giant mitochondria, and increased iron storage in hepatocytes (see below). Acute alcoholic hepatitis may be superimposed on an established cirrhosis. Fatty change is usually not as florid as in acute alcoholic liver disease, and fat may be absent.

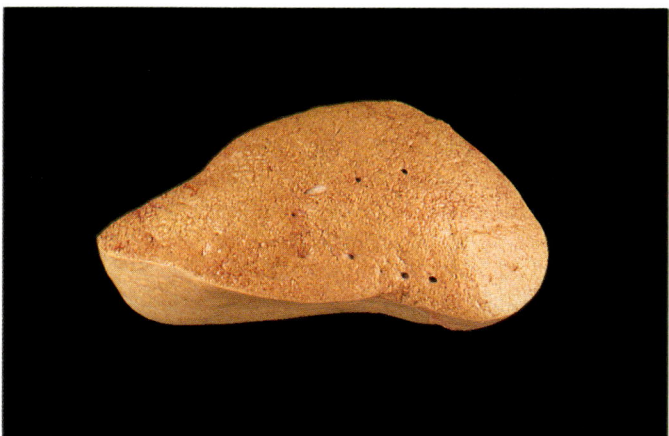

Fig. 17.67 Gross appearance of a micronodular cirrhosis in an alcoholic. The liver is extremely yellow due to the presence of fat in hepatocytes. The liver is broken up into small nodules by the formation of connective tissue and regenerated hepatocytes.

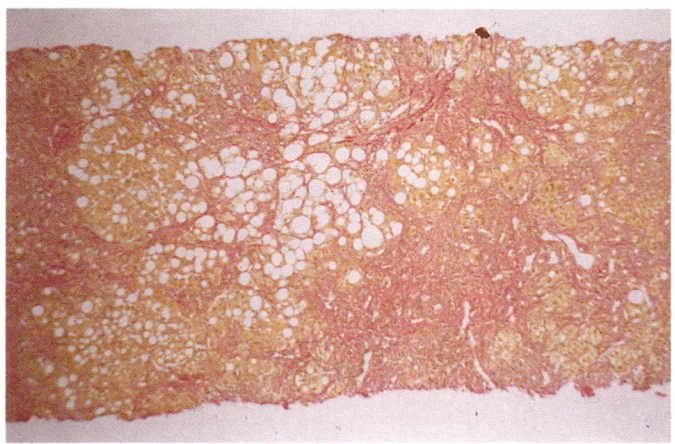

Fig. 17.68 Micronodular cirrhosis in an alcoholic. The liver is dissected by red connective tissue which is isolating small regenerated nodules of hepatocytes. Some of these hepatocytes contain large vacuoles of fat. This is a van Gieson stain to demonstrate connective tissue; hepatocytes are yellow.

In established alcoholic cirrhosis, a chronic active hepatitis picture, with piecemeal necrosis, inflammatory cell infiltration, and bile ductular proliferation, is sometimes present at the junction of regenerating nodules and fibrous septa.

Prognosis

Cirrhosis is an irreversible condition and most patients will ultimately die from a direct complication of cirrhosis, e.g. portal hypertension and bleeding, infection, etc. (see Section 17.11). Alcohol abstinence is probably the only factor that affects prognosis. Five-year survival in patients who continue to drink is about 40 per cent, while about 70 per cent survive for 5 years (and much longer) when they curtail or stop drinking. Until specific therapy for collagen productive disorders are introduced, abstinence is the only treatment, apart from the usual supportive measures.

Other alcohol-induced liver disorders

Cholestasis

Alcoholic liver disease may present with clinical and biochemical features of a large duct obstruction, including right upper quadrant pain, jaundice, fever, elevated serum bilirubin, and alkaline phosphatase. Large duct obstruction and alcoholic pancreatitis can be excluded by ultrasound and endoscopic retrograde cholangiopancreatography (ERCP) and serum amylase.

For unknown reasons, severe cholestasis sometimes occurs with 'large droplet' fatty change, in association with 'small droplet' fatty change, alcoholic hepatitis, decompensated cirrhosis, and Zieve syndrome (see above).

Hepatic iron overload (siderosis)

Usually only mild iron overload occurs, if at all, in alcoholic liver disease. The iron is present in hepatocytes in the form of haemosiderin, an insoluble iron protein complex which stains blue with Perl's stain. Haemosiderin may occur in hepatocytes in any part of the acinus but it rarely occurs throughout all cells (grade 4 iron overload).

Iron overload in alcoholics has been ascribed to increased iron absorption from the gut in the presence of a normal iron intake. Increased absorption from alcoholic drinks rich in iron, such as wine and the beer drunk by Bantus, may possibly also be a factor; with these possible exceptions, it does not seem to correlate with the type of alcoholic beverage consumed. When siderosis is severe (i.e. is present in all hepatocytes, bile duct epithelium, and portal tract collagen) idiopathic haemochromatosis should be excluded. The latter is associated with HLA A3, B7, and B14 and is a genetic disorder of iron metabolism. It is important to exclude this disorder because it is treatable; siblings (and parents) should be investigated (see Section 17.10) and treated to prevent chronic liver disease.

Porphyria cutanea tarda

This is a disorder of haem metabolism (Section 17.9) which presents with photosensitivity. The condition is often brought to light by alcohol consumption and the patient develops cutaneous and hepatic abnormalities. The liver abnormalities include fatty change, usually some degree of siderosis, and red autofluorescence of hepatocytes due to the contained porphyrin. There is dramatic clinical and biochemical amelioration of the condition when alcohol is withdrawn.

Hepatocellular cancer

Primary liver cancer occurs in 15–30 per cent of alcoholic cirrhotics. The cirrhosis is usually of macronodular type. It may rarely occur in alcoholics without cirrhosis. There is no evidence that alcohol is a direct carcinogen but it could conceivably act as a promoter because it is a potent inducer of hepatic microsomal p450s. In HBV-positive patients, alcohol consumption may reduce by about 10 years the average age at which hepatic cancer occurs in these cases; i.e. at age 50 rather than at 60 years of age.

Pathogenesis of alcoholic liver disease

As pointed out earlier, alcohol produces a spectrum of liver disease, ranging from fatty change to alcoholic hepatitis and cirrhosis. These categories are helpful in patient categorization and in predicting prognosis, but it should be realized that fatty change can blend with alcoholic hepatitis which, in turn, can be present in established cirrhosis. Similarly, the individual morphological correlates of alcohol, e.g. MBs and megamitochondria, may occur throughout the spectrum.

Hepatocyte damage

Ethanol, in sufficient dosage, is a direct hepatotoxin. In nonalcoholic volunteers, liver damage in the form of fatty change, proliferation of smooth endoplasm reticulum (SER), and mitochondrial abnormalities are evident within 2–4 days. The mechanisms for lipid accumulation have been discussed. The proliferation of SER is an adaptive response which is responsible for increased alcohol tolerance in alcoholics. It also increases acetaldehyde production. Drug metabolism is enhanced and the hepatotoxic effects of drugs may be potentiated; this can be a serious clinical problem.

Mitochondrial abnormalities may be due to acetaldehyde accumulation and the shift in redox potential due to the altered $NAD^+/NADH$ ratio consequent on ethanol oxidation. The extent to which mitochondrial abnormalities and megamitochondria contribute to perpetuation of liver damage is not clear.

There is hepatic glutathione depletion and evidence of lipid peroxidation in association with chronic alcohol abuse. Lipid peroxidation and generation of free radicals are a conceivable mechanism for balloon degeneration of hepatocytes and cell death. The evidence for this, however, is not strong.

Mallory bodies are composed of clumps of intermediate filaments and other unidentified subcellular organelles. In spite of intense activity in this area of research, it is still not clear what function intermediate filaments serve. It is probable that they are involved in maintaining 'architectural cytoplasmic integrity'. Since Mallory bodies occur in a large number of other

conditions, it seems unlikely that ethanol is directly responsible for intermediate filament disorganization and accumulation in alcoholic liver disease. The intermediary between ethanol and filament disorganization is unknown. The notions that Mallory bodies result from microtubular failure and vitamin A deficiency are not credible.

There is circumstantial evidence that immune mechanisms may play some part in alcoholic liver disease. In acute alcoholic hepatitis, lymphocytes (mainly T-cells) accumulate at sites of hepatocyte drop-out; HLA class I antigens, which are not normally detectable on hepatocytes, can be detected on hepatocytes in alcoholic hepatitis; hypergammaglobulinaemia (particularly IgA) is found in some patients with alcoholic liver disease. These observations have provoked speculation, but no firm testable hypothesis for the role of immune mechanisms in the genesis of chronic alcoholic liver disease has emerged.

The mechanisms underlying hepatic fibrosis and liver cell regeneration—the cardinal features of cirrhosis—are considered later, in Sections 17.11 and 17.12, respectively.

Alcohol consumption and cirrhosis

It has been shown that there is a relationship between the risk of alcoholic cirrhosis and dose and duration of consumption. However, the relationship is not linear. In some studies, only 25 per cent of patients drinking more than 220 g/day developed cirrhosis after 10 years! On the other hand, it is claimed that some women and certain ethnic groups develop cirrhosis with doses as low as 20–40 g/day. These observations point clearly to other important factors, such as a susceptibility gene(s) or other unknown superimposed agent(s), which determine whether any individual will progress beyond fatty liver. At this time, we are ignorant of what these other factors might be.

17.6.3   Further reading

Fleming, K. A. and McGee, J. O'D. (1984). Alcohol induced liver disease. *Journal of Clinical Pathology* 37, 721–33.

Hall, P. de la M. (1987). Alcoholic liver disease. In *Pathology of the liver* (ed. R. N. M. McSween, P. P. Anthony, and P. J. Scheuer), pp. 281–309. Churchill Livingstone, Edinburgh.

17.7   Drug- and toxin-induced disease

K. Weinbren

17.7.1   Introduction

A variety of changes may develop in the liver as a result of toxic effects of chemicals, and there have been various attempts to organize the accumulated data. One is to categorize the effects according to whether the changes are considered to represent hepatocellular damage (hepatitic) or to interfere with the excretion of bile pigment (cholestatic). Another approach attempts to distinguish the liver cell type primarily affected. Most commonly the hepatotoxic reactions are assessed according to whether an intrinsic or direct-acting toxicity is inferred or whether the reaction is regarded as idiosyncratic.

Hepatotoxic reactions

Hepatotoxic reactions have, for many years, been separated into two main groups. Type I includes those that are predictable and dose-related, in which a high proportion of subjects exposed to high enough doses are affected, and the offending agent is often found to be hepatotoxic in experimental animals. Type II refers to those reactions that are unpredictable, not dose-related, in which a very small number of patients at risk are affected, and where the effects are not readily reproducible in experimental animals.

In general, idiosyncratic hepatotoxicity (type II) refers to reactions in which only a small number of specially sensitive subjects are affected, some of whom may possess a special metabolic activity that permits accumulation of toxic compounds or increased synthesis of hepatotoxic metabolites.

Evidence has now accumulated which suggests that the distinction between these two types of reactions is not always clear-cut. It is known, for example, that although it is usual for hepatotoxicity from paracetamol (acetaminophen) to develop after doses in excess of 15 g, unpredicted instances of toxic liver injury are reported after therapeutic doses in some patients. These subjects are considered to be more susceptible, either because of enzyme induction or depleted glutathione. In addition, some compounds may cause two entirely different reactions, as cholestasis and tumours are both associated with anabolic steroids.

Minor abnormalities in serum hepatic-derived enzyme levels may be found in up to even 20 per cent of patients taking chlorpromazine, a drug usually associated with the low-incidence unpredictable reactions (type II).

This overlap makes it difficult to place drug reactions in watertight compartments and, although the general guidelines suggested in the past are useful, it is not reasonable to rely entirely on the approach.

The possibility of immune-mediated idiosyncratic hepatotoxicity was raised by the discovery of antibodies in the blood of patients suffering from halothane hepatoxicity and, in lesser amounts, in the case of several other inhalation anaesthetics. Neoantigens have been detected in halothane treated humans, rats, and rabbits, all of which appear to have the same hapten derived from a reactive metabolite, trifluoroacetyl chloride (TFA). The combination of the TFA hapten and cellular protein form the neoantigen. Similar changes occur with other compounds, including ethanol and methyldopa, but the mechanisms underlying the production of the neoantigen are not yet defined.

Hepatotoxic chemicals

Hepatotoxic chemicals have also been divided into those compounds that require metabolism by the liver for their toxic effects and those that do not. Some of the former depend on mixed function oxidase activity or cytochrome p450s.

While it is reasonable to classify hepatotoxic chemicals using information that relates to these metabolic pathways, the relevant data are not always available when assessing a clinical or pathological problem of suspected drug toxicity. None the less, in attempting to analyse the mechanisms involved, this separation of hepatotoxins on the basis of how they are metabolized is sometimes helpful.

Most drugs presented to liver are lipophilic and the first reaction is usually an oxidation forming a hydroxyl group (phase I reaction) and the second is a conjugation (phase II reaction) generally with sulphate or glucuronic acid and usually at the site of the hydroxyl group. The compound becomes water-soluble as a result. The phase I enzymes, known as p450s, because of their absorption at 450 nm, have been found in most species and include several, sometimes heterogenous, forms; some phenotypes are good metabolizers and some are poor. The amino acid sequence of the p450s vary, but some have significant homology in some regions, which has led to p450s being grouped in gene families, the suffixes 'I', 'II', or 'III' being added to p450. The differences in catalytic activity of the different p450s are probably associated with most instances of idiosyncratic hepatotoxicity. In some circumstances, a compound may be converted into a toxic metabolite by the p450 system, the activity of which often varies between different individuals.

It is sometimes possible to check the gene families involved, by testing with certain compounds known to distinguish between poor and active metabolizer phenotypes and an approach to the toxicity developed. For example, debrisoquine has been used to indicate poor metabolizers and perhexiline toxicity is noted more commonly in this group. On the other hand, there is suggestive evidence that some patients who are less liable to be affected by paracetamol toxicity, become susceptible when members of the gene family p450II are induced by some other compound, in particular, alcohol.

Specific structural lesions associated with drug toxicity

Changes that are found in relation to drug- or toxin-induced liver injury are, in many respects, similar to those associated with other pathogens, in that a primary lesion affecting one cell type may provoke reactive changes in the remaining tissue and a complex lesion may result (Table 17.6). It is usually possible to identify the main cell type involved. Therefore, lesions that are interpreted, for example, as affecting primarily hepatocytes, will be associated with a greater or lesser degree of accompanying alterations in other components, including macrophages, canaliculi, bile duct epithelium, and even other surviving hepatocytes.

Many different therapeutic agents have been suspected of causing liver toxicity. The development of symptoms attributable to liver dysfunction in the absence of other causes, and the development in high incidence of raised levels of liver-derived enzymes in the serum of symptom-free subjects in clinical trials or in those treated with therapeutic doses of the drug, are regarded as evidence of a probable causal relationship. There

Table 17.6 Structural changes in hepatotoxicity

Structure	Process	Lesion	Agent example*
Hepatocyte	Necrosis (coagulative)	Confluent	Paracetamol, *Amanita phalloides*
	Necrosis (cytolytic)	Hepatitis-like	Isoniazid, methyldopa
		Mononucleosis-like	Hydantoin, para-aminosalicylic acid
	Hypersensitivity	Hepatitis-like	Halothane
		CAH-type	Oxyphenisatin, methyldopa
	Chronic steatosis	Macrovesicular	Alcohol, methotrexate
		Microvesicular	Tetracycline, valproic acid
	Phospholipidosis	Storage	Perhexiline maleate, amiodarone
	Pigment	Lipofuscin	Phenothiazines, phenacetin
Biliary passages	Canalicular cholestasis (pure)	Bile inspissation	Anabolic steroids
	Canalicular and hepatocellular damage	Inspissation and inflammation	Phenothiazines, sulphonylureas, erythromycin estolate
	Bile duct necrosis	Necrosis and cholestasis	Paraquat, ajmoline, benoxyprofen
Vascular	Sinusoidal change	Dilatation	Contraceptive steroids
		Peliosis	Anabolic steroids
		Fibrosis	Vinyl chloride monomer, thorotrast
Hepatic veins	Radicles and sublobular: occlusion	Veno-occlusive	Azathioprine, 6-thioguanine
	Main veins: occlusion	Thrombosis	Contraceptive steroids
	Perisinusoidal cells: activation	Fibrosis	Vitamin A, alcohol
Mononuclear phagocyte system	Kupffer cells and histiocytes: phagocytosis	Storage	Polyvinol pyrrolidone
		Lipogranuloma	Mineral oil
		Granuloma	Carbamazepine, butazolidin
Tumours	Hepatocyte neoplasia	Adenoma	Contraceptive and androgenic steroids (carcinoma with Fanconi anaemia)
	Biliary neoplasia	Cholangiocarcinoma	Thorotrast
	Vascular neoplasia	Angiosarcoma	Vinyl chloride monomer

* Several hundred agents have been suspected; only a sample are listed. See Zimmerman (1990) for longer list.

are circumstances when the evidence supports only the possibility rather than the probability of hepatotoxicity in man, but it is usually difficult to deny the relationship in case reports without knowledge of the circumstances. Animal hepatotoxicity does not prove a causal relationship between a drug and hepatic injury in man, although properly conducted experimental studies support the probability when suspicions are raised in man. Hundreds of agents have been incriminated but only a few of the more acceptable examples are mentioned. Almost every class of therapeutic agent includes compounds that are considered possible or probable hepatotoxins and, in most instances, the lesions simulate those caused by other pathogens. The type of lesion does not always correlate with the class of toxic compound, but there are examples where a pattern emerges. Thus, anaesthetic agents and narcotic analgesics are usually associated with hepatocellular damage; phenothiazines with cholestasis; anabolic agents with hepatocellular adenoma. It is necessary, however, to exclude other causes in cases of suspected drug toxicity, even when the toxic effect is of a type associated with a particular class of drugs. In each class of drugs there are some agents that produce cholestasis and others that lead to hepatocellular damage.

17.7.2 Hepatocyte lesions

Hepatocyte necrosis

This is evidenced, on the one hand, by eosinophilic change with the features of coagulative necrosis, probably representing denaturation of cytoplasmic protein, or, on the other hand, by loss of cells that have undergone cytolytic necrosis. The exact determinants of the coagulative or the cytolytic variants of necrosis are not defined and it is not clear whether this difference is related to dosage. The distribution of the damage varies with different toxic agents, but in most instances the severest changes can be recognized in perivenous regions. Confluent coagulative necrosis may involve the liver to different degrees in different parts and the lesions show changes with time. The lesion may extend so that more than a perivenous band of cells is involved, but portal tracts are not included in the necrotic change. The associated inflammatory reaction consists, in most instances, of mononuclear cells, including lymphocytes and macrophages. The accumulation of such inflammatory cells may be separately identified in juxtaposition to recognizably necrotic hepatocytes, or may replace necrotic tissue that has been phagocytosed and the tissue organized. Confluent tracts of coagulative necrosis are not a frequent finding in drug toxicity, but this is reported in instances of paracetamol overdosage or poisoning by *Amanita phalloides*. Carbon tetrachloride is sometimes associated with groups of coagulative necrotic cells, usually accompanied by steatosis.

The pathogenetic mechanisms involved in this form of hepatotoxicity have not yet been explained in spite of intensive investigations. Metabolism by the cytochrome enzyme system results in the generation of a variety of possible products which may cause lethal cell injury, but the particular cellular site that is primarily damaged is not certain. Carbon tetrachloride (CCl_4) and paracetamol (acetaminophen) have attracted particular attention. Hepatotoxicity of CCl_4 may result from metabolism by the p450 phase I reaction which is essentially reductive and is inhibited by oxygen. Several isoforms of p450 produce a variety of toxic species including primary and secondary free radical metabolites, which may cause lipid peroxidation and the destruction of membranes, lesions which are located mainly perivenously, where among other factors, the oxygen tension is low. Therefore, it is usual to attempt to treat CCl_4 poisoning with oxygen in some form.

The mechanisms underlying paracetamol toxicity are also not fully understood, but the extent of damage is generally related to dosage (intrinsic hepatotoxicity), the amount of p450 oxidation to the toxic metabolite *N*-acetyl-*p*-benzoquinone imine (NAPQI) which involve a major clearance metabolic pathway and the cellular content of glutathione (see also Sections 3.1, 3.3). In this regard, glutathione conjugates electrophilic metabolites, with excretion mainly as mercapturic acid. The balance between glutathione synthesis (from L-cysteine, L-glutamate, and glycine) and its destruction or transport from the liver determines its availability for the hepatocyte and depends on many factors including fasting and hormonal levels. This significantly affects the detoxication of paracetamol.

The other form of necrosis encountered is a cytolytic necrosis in which confluent coagulative change is not observed. Mononuclear phagocytes often mark a focus from which hepatocytes have disappeared, having undergone cytolytic necrosis. These usually affect perivenous regions predominantly but other parts of the hepatocyte plates are also the site of mononuclear accumulation, often referred to as 'spotty necrosis' even though actual necrotic hepatocytes are no longer present. At the same time, the loss of damaged cells may stimulate a proliferative response of other less affected hepatocytes and the compensatory hyperplasia (sometimes evidenced by plate thickening usually, at first, more striking in periportal regions) may increase the mass of hepatocytes with an apparent reduction of the necrotic regions.

The combination of necrosis, inflammation, and compensatory hyperplasia occurs with drug hepatotoxicity as well as with other forms of hepatocyte damage, and it is sometimes difficult to distinguish lesions associated with the administration of toxins from those caused by hepatitis viruses. This is particularly relevant in instances of cytolytic necrosis and is less confusing when toxin-induced coagulative necrosis is observed.

So far as the extent of necrosis is concerned, the lesions may vary from involvement of a relatively small number of cells, with a greater or lesser degree of macrophage activity, to survival of only biliary and vascular structures and an occasional hepatocyte in a sea of lymphocytes and macrophages. In other than the most affected regions, hepatocytes may show features of compensatory hyperplasia and provide an appearance either of restoration or of less severe involvement of liver parenchymal cells. Cytolytic necrosis without coagulative change may thus involve the perivenous region, a substantial part of the acinus, or appear to affect the parenchyma irregularly.

'Submassive' and 'massive' necrosis are terms sometimes used to indicate a very severe form of perivenous toxic injury. Caution ought to be exercised in the use of these terms. If a patient dies after taking a toxin, the hepatic lesion is usually exaggerated by post-mortem autolysis so that perivenous lesions may, in such circumstances, be reported as 'diffuse', 'submassive', or 'massive' as a result of this combination of effects.

The question of whether a compound is associated with a zonal perivenous lesion or a diffuse lesion may relate to severity, but several authors tend to distinguish categories of drug toxicity on this basis. Thus, it is indicated that hepatocyte necrosis is usually zonal in instances of direct intrinsic toxicity varying from involving nearly whole acini or lobules to small foci, depending on dosage. In most instances, if there is to be any survival, periportal hepatocytes will remain (as seen in paracetamol, chloroform, or halothane toxicity) and the predominant perivenous damage has generally been ascribed to the greater concentration of the drug-metabolizing enzymes that mediate the production of toxic metabolites from these compounds or to reduced oxygen tension. This is not always so, as evidenced from the case of allyl alcohol, which affects periportal regions primarily and is metabolized in both periportal and perivenous regions. In most instances in which loss of hepatocytes is observed after exposure to a toxin, isolated eosinophilic necrotic cells are also encountered, but these are not necessarily confined to the perivenous zones. Drugs and toxins that have been reported as causing perivenous necrosis include paracetamol, paraquat, halothane, chloroform, aflatoxins, phalloidin, and many others, sometimes with associated steatosis.

The finding of shrunken, eosinophilic cells with the characteristics of apoptotic cells, including the chromatic condensation, macrophage recognition, and evidence of protein synthesis (see Chapter 3.1), is also reported in instances of toxic injury, but apoptosis seems to occur with lower concentrations of toxins. It is not known why some cells undergo apoptosis in toxic injury. Scattered dark cells are also seen in the livers of patients subjected to toxic injury. These are eosinophilic but may not necessarily show the features regarded as essential for categorization as apoptotic. It is not clear how these relate to apoptosis.

Viral hepatitis-like lesion

In some instances, hepatocytes are lost by cytolytic necrosis, with collections of lymphocytes and macrophages probably representing the residual inflammatory reaction to this cellular damage or 'spotty necrosis'. In addition, some hepatocytes show changes that are regarded as stages towards cell death and take the form of hepatocyte swelling. There are also scattered eosinophilic necrotic cells. Together with the variable accumulation of lymphocytes in portal tracts and reactive macrophages, the microscopical features may resemble viral hepatitis and there may be difficulty in distinguishing between the two conditions (Figs 17.69, 17.70).

The pathogenetic basis for this particular lesion is not known; it is clear that hepatocytes undergo cytolytic necrosis and that phagocytosis of cellular debris and lymphoid accumulation develop. The precise pathway to lethal cellular injury has not been defined, but these hepatitis-like changes are not described in mushroom poisoning, carbon tetrachloride damage, or para-cetamol toxicity, and the part played by lymphocytes is not known. Drugs that have been reported as leading to this lesion include phenylbutazone, sulphonamides, para-aminosalicylic acid, isoniazid, often enhanced by rifampicin. In some instances, an immunological mechanism is supported by the presence of skin rashes and eosinophilia, but it is difficult to separate a primary immunological event from that which is secondary to necrosis of the liver. There is evidence from the presence of IgG antibodies in patients with halothane jaundice, but not in halothane-treated patients with minor abnormalities of serum enzyme levels, that an immunological component may play a part in severe halothane liver damage.

Acute mononucleosis-like lesions

In some instances, evidence of cellular necrosis is slighter although eosinophilic necrotic cells are seen, but there are also heavier accumulations of portal lymphocytes and striking intra-sinusoidal lymphocytosis. A clinical syndrome with lymph-adenopathy, fever, and sore throat may be reported. Drugs that have been associated with this lesion include diphenyl-hydantoin and dapsone.

Chronic active hepatitis

The morphological features of chronic active hepatitis (CAH), with conspicuous portal and periportal inflammatory change and necrosis of hepatocytes, have been described with administration of a variety of therapeutic agents since the recognition of the development of these changes in patients receiving oxyphenisatin, a compound that was used in laxative preparations.

The lesions usually resemble those of CAH (Figs 17.71, 17.72, 17.73). Hyperglobulinaemia is frequently present and antinuclear antibodies are sometimes found. There is extensive fibrosis, within and outside portal tracts, and cirrhosis may develop. The lesions are found after the offending drug has been

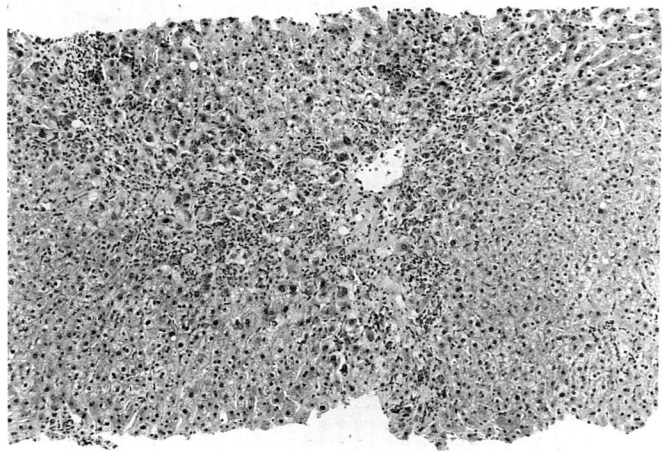

Fig. 17.69 Viral hepatitis-like hepatotoxicity. Loss of perivenous cells, hepatocyte swelling, and accumulation of lymphocytes with foci of 'spotty necrosis' in a patient who had taken the non-steroidal anti-inflammatory agent Sudoxicam.

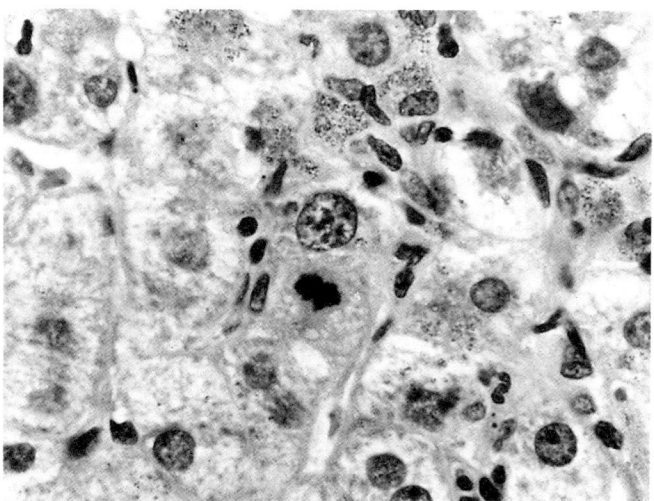

Fig. 17.70 Accumulation of pigment granules in Kupffer cells, and hepatocyte mitoses in the same patient as illustrated in Fig. 17.69.

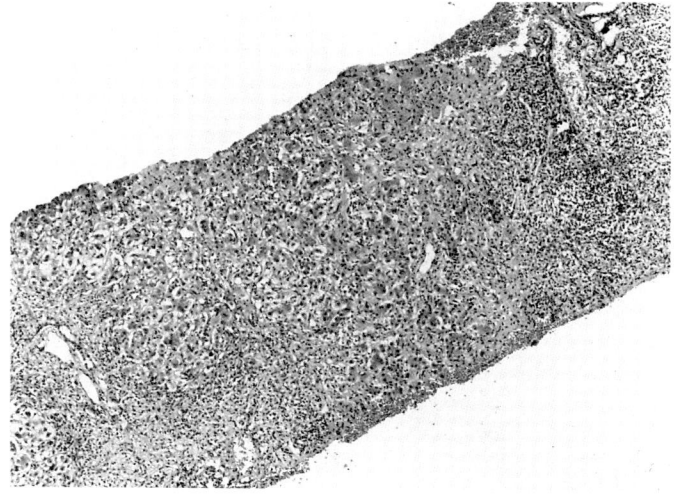

Fig. 17.71 Drug-induced chronic active hepatitis in a patient treated with α-methyldopa. There are extensive accumulations of lymphocytes in portal tracts and between hepatocyte plates.

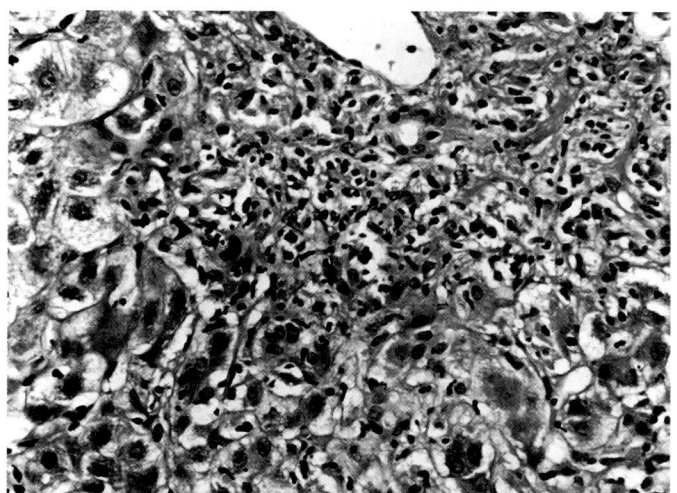

Fig. 17.72 Extension of inflammatory cells beyond the limiting plate with swelling of hepatocytes arranged in two-cell-thick plates and pseudo-acini. Taken from the same patient as illustrated in Fig. 17.71.

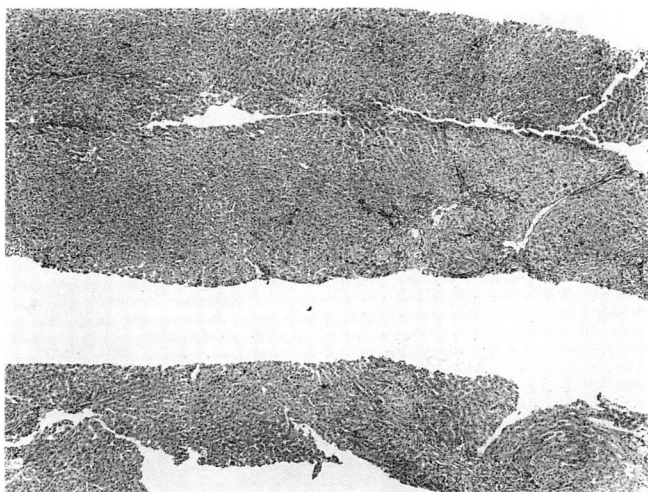

Fig. 17.74 Less severe inflammation 6 months after cessation of treatment with α-methyldopa. Taken from the same patient as illustrated in Figs 17.71–17.73.

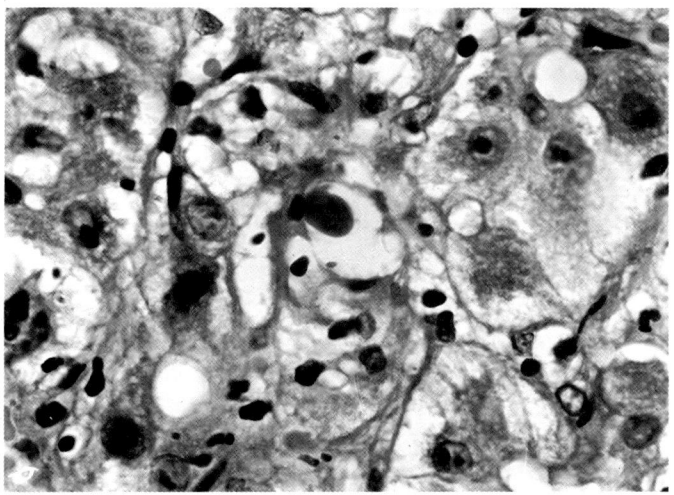

Fig. 17.73 Eosinophilic necrotic cell between hyperplastic plates of swollen hepatocytes. Taken from the same patient as illustrated in Fig. 17.71.

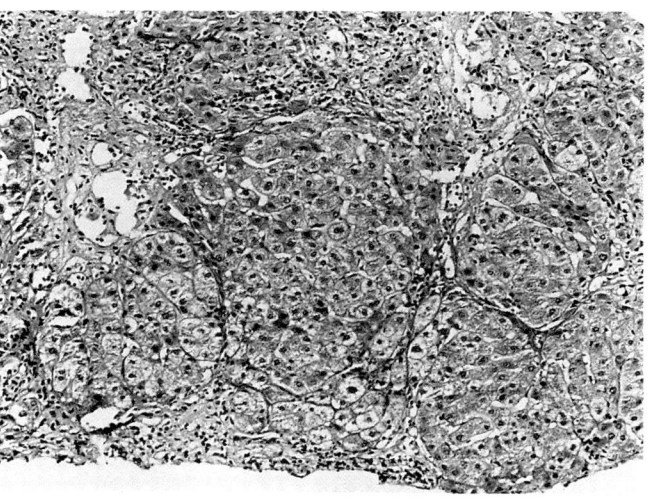

Fig. 17.75 Less inflammation, but some residual activity, some fibrous bands, and two-cell-thick hepatocyte plates in late needle biopsy specimen. Same section as illustrated in Fig. 17.74.

administered for a long time, but several of the suspected agents may also be associated with a pattern closer to acute viral hepatitis.

Withdrawal of the relevant compound is followed by recovery of biochemical, serological, and structural changes, although this is not invariable (Figs 17.74, 17.75). Unfortunately, the drug may be continued even after hepatic injury has been sustained, largely because of lack of recognition of the cause, and it may be that the chronic lesion is related to this phenomenon. The pathogenesis of drug-induced CAH is not known. Besides the features of CAH, sometimes features of acute hepatitis are present. Although this combination is helpful for diagnosis, no

indications of a mechanism are suggested. The incidence of the entity is not known but reports on female patients outnumber those on males. Although the reports are not always well based, it seems that at least 2 months of therapy precede the development of CAH and therapy had been maintained after evidence of liver damage was noted. An allergic or hypersensitivity mechanism is not strongly supported, but this is not excluded.

The incriminated therapeutic agents include oxyphenisatin and α-methyldopa, the evidence for which is convincing, but there are also several other suspected compounds, including isoniazid, nitrofurantoin, dantrolene, and, rarely, sulphonamides.

Subacute hepatic necrosis

This condition consists of hyperplastic liver tissue with fibrosis and evidence of repair, loss of hepatocytes, portal tract survival, and proliferation of small bile ducts (Figs 17.76, 17.77). This condition was associated with exposure to toxic chemicals used in the munitions industry during wartime (e.g. dinitrobenzene, trinitrotoluene, tetrachloroethane) but has also been ascribed to the effects of viral hepatitis. While it is clear that liver cells are destroyed in this condition, it is not understood why patients do not survive with these large islands of hyperplastic hepatocytes. Impaired regeneration has been postulated in cases associated with viral infection, but this does not appear to be well based so far as toxicity is concerned. Drugs that have been reported as causing this condition include a variety of different compounds, usually in a very low incidence and probably by virtue of some idiosyncratic pathway. α-Methyldopa, benoxyprofen, and

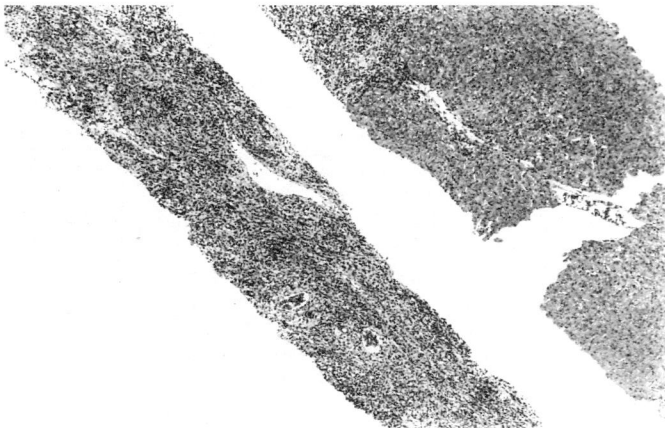

Fig. 17.76 Subacute hepatic necrosis in a patient taking α-methyldopa. Jaundice 3 months previously. One part of this needle biopsy specimen shows only bile ducts and inflammatory cells, the other shows evidence of hyperplasia.

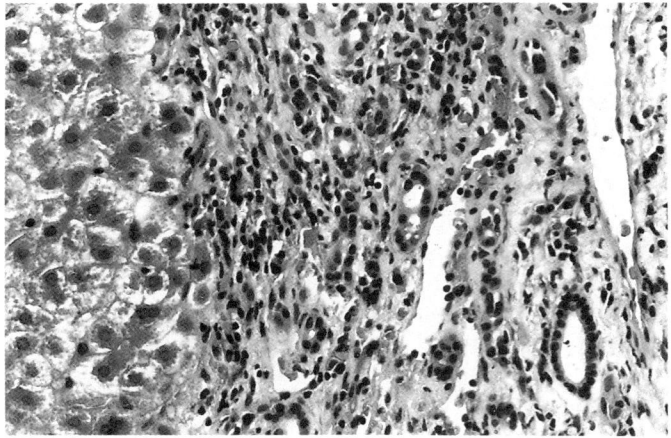

Fig. 17.77 Juxtaposed necrotic region from which hepatocytes have disappeared (right) and hyperplastic plates of compensatory hyperplasia on left. Same section as illustrated in Fig. 17.76.

cinchophen have been incriminated, but it is often not clear whether other factors (such as viruses and alcohol) played a part.

Cirrhosis

The development of cirrhosis in patients suffering from active chronic hepatitis is well established and it appears that the type of CAH caused by drug toxicity may sometimes also be associated with cirrhosis, probably if therapy is continued in the presence of liver damage.

There are also other instances of drug-induced cirrhosis that do not involve the CAH pathway. Changes found with several therapeutic agents resemble those associated with chronic alcoholic liver disease and, although not always validated, cirrhosis is reported.

The pathogenesis of the condition is not understood and may parallel that postulated for the development of alcoholic cirrhosis. The drugs that are associated with this type of cirrhosis are perhexiline maleate and amiodarone, both associated with phospholipidosis cellular inclusions and both possessing amphophilic chemical properties. The cirrhosis associated with methotrexate toxicity is considered in the section concerned with steatosis.

The question of whether cirrhosis is a sequel to the effect of a single episode of substantial liver necrosis is confusing but, in general, the probability of the development of the structural changes of cirrhosis, together with portal hypertension and possible liver failure, is very low. Patients who survive after paracetamol overdosage do not appear to develop cirrhosis, and microscopical findings, even shortly after recovery, indicate an acinar pattern of survival which, with hyperplasia, is likely to retain vascular relations, as opposed to the nodules of cirrhosis in which vascular relations are lost.

Other forms of toxic injury involving hepatocytes include steatosis and accumulation of pigments and other intracellular material.

Macrovesicular steatosis

Many toxins have been associated with the development of hepatocyte steatosis, of which two varieties are usually recognized. Macrovesicular steatosis usually involves the production of a single, large, fat-containing globule, compressing the nucleus and cytoplasmic organelles, while the hepatocytes in microvesicular steatosis contain many fine, fat-containing globules which surround the nucleus. Of the compounds associated with macrovesicular steatosis, most notable is ethanol (Fig. 17.78), which is an exceedingly common cause in many parts of the world. Macrovesicular steatosis is encountered in many forms of malnutrition, or even in prolonged fasting, and it is sometimes difficult to ascribe the changes to drug toxicity. Apart from ethanol, with which other characteristics of alcoholic liver disease are found, high doses of corticosteroids, perhexiline maleate, and L-asparaginase are associated with macrovesicular steatosis. Methotrexate is associated with foci of hepatic steatosis as well as portal and extraportal fibrosis, the former considered to be reversible, but the latter sometimes

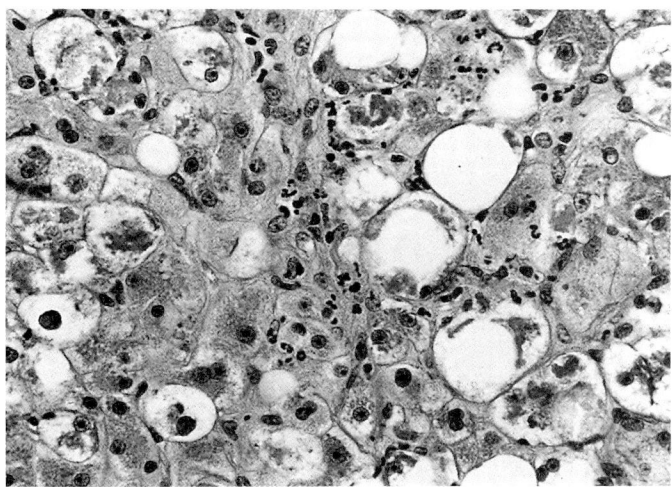

Fig. 17.78 Macrovesicular steatosis in a patient with alcoholic hepatitis. Note the abundant alcoholic hyalin.

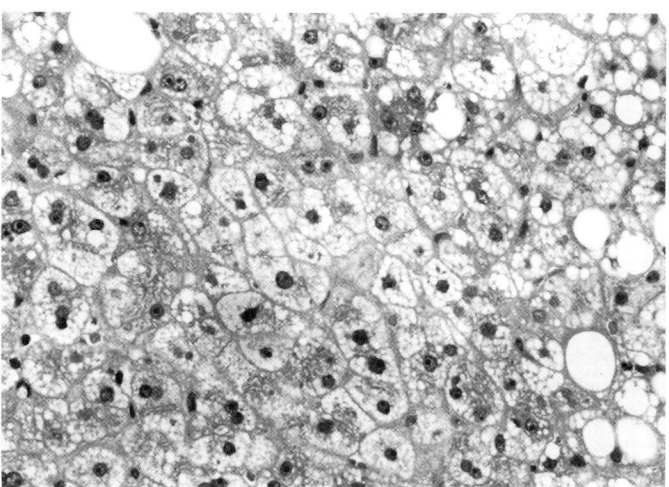

Fig. 17.80 Diffusely distributed, fine, fatty droplets without displacement of nuclei. Same section as illustrated in Fig. 17.79.

extending into cirrhosis. Withdrawal of treatment after a total of 1.5–2 g may be indicated by the hepatic structural changes, but the efficacy of the compound may not be reproducible with other therapy, particularly in patients suffering from psoriasis. Other toxins are frequently associated with this form of steatosis.

Microvesicular steatosis

This form of steatosis is generally distinguished from macrovesicular steatosis although, in some forms of alcohol abuse, a form of microvesicular steatosis is seen. The cytoplasm in microvesicular steatosis is filled with small, fat-containing globules (Figs 17.79, 17.80) that surround the nucleus, which thus retains its central position.

This curious lesion is also noted in acute fatty liver of preg-

nancy, with no known associations with a drug or toxin (Fig. 17.81), and also in patients who have taken valproic acid or tetracycline (usually intravenously). The lesion has also been ascribed to other toxins in particular circumstances, and there may be a link between this form of steatosis and aspirin toxicity in Reye syndrome (but this is not certain).

The pathogenesis of hepatic steatosis is defined in instances of alcohol-induced macrovesicular change. The accumulation of fat is essentially a consequence of the depression of lipoprotein synthesis and decreased fatty oxidation. Fatty acids are consequently trapped in the liver, and it is likely that similar mechanisms operate in the case of other forms of macrovesicular steatosis.

Microvesicular fatty change is not as well understood and, although mitochondrial abnormalities are observed in some

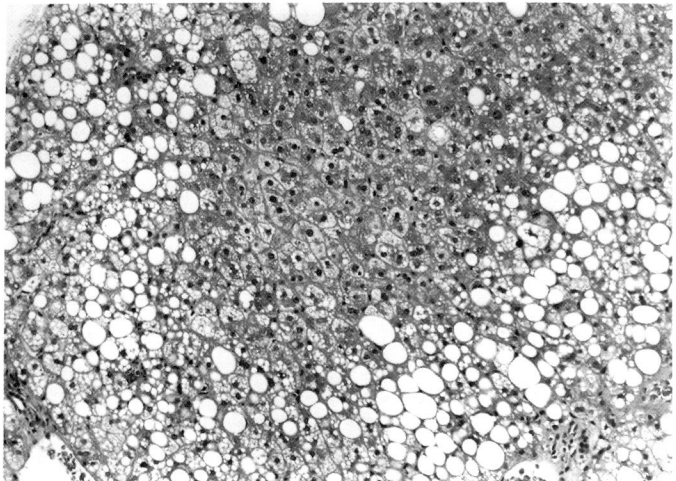

Fig. 17.79 Microvesicular steatosis and macrovesicular steatosis in a patient who had taken oral tetracycline.

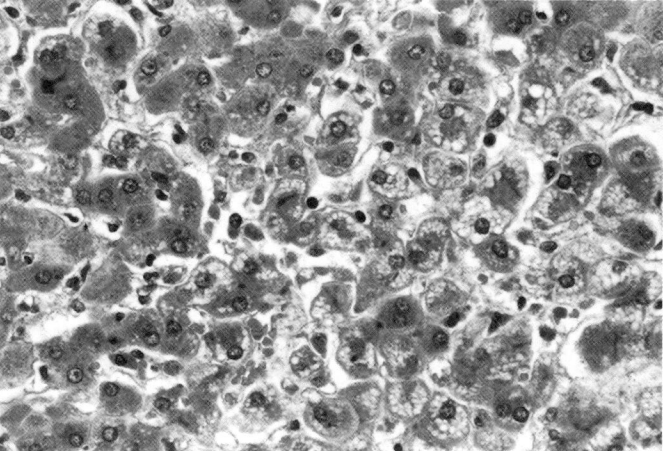

Fig. 17.81 Microvesicular steatosis in a patient with acute fatty liver of pregnancy, showing steatotic cells confined to perivenous regions, survival of periportal cells, and bile pigment inspissates.

instances, this is not invariable. It is also not clear why this reaction is similar to that seen in acute fatty liver of pregnancy. It is possible that tRNA is affected and the formation of a protein carrier for lipoprotein is inhibited by the antibiotic toxins.

Other hepatocyte changes

These include a variety of changes within cells so that the hepatocytes are still identifiable. They fall mainly into two groups of lesions, some of which may occur acutely and may accompany other acute, apparently more lethal, cellular lesions; and others that occur after more chronic exposure to the toxin. The more acute lesions usually involve swelling of hepatocytes, similar to that noted in viral hepatitis. The exact nature of the swelling is not clear. The more chronic lesions include phospholipidosis, often associated with the administration of amphophilic compounds, such as amiodarone or clofibrate; and the development of Mallory hyalin, a cytological change, usually associated with alcoholism, but now described with other compounds causing toxicity in man, particularly perhexiline maleate. Other chronic changes affecting the hepatocyte may involve a ground-glass transformation of the cytoplasm (Figs 17.82, 17.83), generally based on a diffuse hypertrophy of the smooth endoplasmic reticulum and associated with increased microsomal enzyme activity; this change, although resembling that associated with HBsAg carriers, does not stain with orcein and the cells are referred to as orcein-negative ground-glass cells. In general, this change is regarded as a form of adaptation and is similar to that known to occur in small experimental animals given high doses of drugs that are metabolized by p450s. There appears to be a similar form, which may be attributable to the effects of cyanamide or disulfuram treatment used for aversion therapy in alcoholics. These pale inclusions are also orcein-negative.

Lipofuscin is increased in pericanalicular perivenous hepatocyte lysosomes in some instances of drug toxicity, usually after

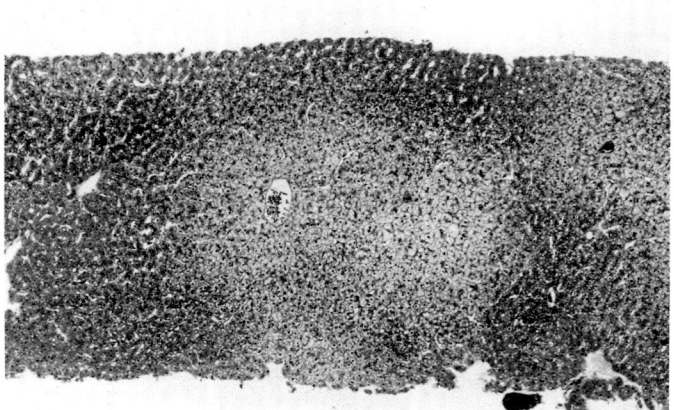

Fig. 17.82 Perivenous hepatocyte hypertrophy; ground-glass appearance in a patient with evidence of hepatic enzyme induction after long-term medication with a variety of compounds.

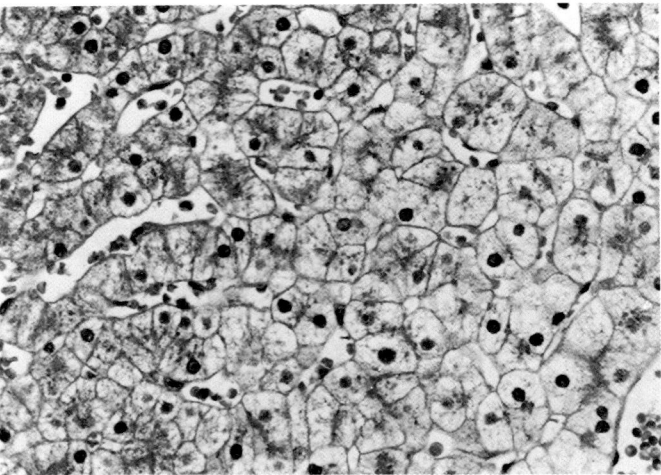

Fig. 17.83 Pallor and enlargement of perivenous hepatocytes, arranged in two-cell-thick plates. Same section as illustrated in Fig. 17.82.

long-term administration of phenacetin, chlorpromazine, or cascara sagrada. The exact mechanism underlying this change is speculative. Copper accumulation is found in chronic cholestasis and thus may mark the effects of chronic cholestatic drug toxicity. So far, mitochondrial and peroxisome proliferation, described as indicators of chronic drug toxicity by clofibrate and related substances experimentally, have not been reported in this context in patients.

17.7.3   Changes involving biliary pathways

Intracanalicular inspissates of bile-containing material are frequently observed in many different liver diseases, including acute viral hepatitis, duct obstruction, and vascular abnormalities, and in these circumstances other pathological changes are usually present. In some forms of drug toxicity the outstanding feature consists of such 'bilirubin casts' and the clinical features suggest an arrest of the normal flow of bile, or 'cholestasis'. In some instances, the inspissates are accompanied by a mild portal inflammatory response and evidence of focal damage to hepatocytes in the form of overt cellular change or ceroid pigment accumulation within macrophages; in other instances there is little evidence of hepatocyte damage, the lesion is accompanied by very few lymphocytes and mononuclear phagocytes, and is apparently confined to the canaliculi. This form of canalicular change is associated in the main with administration of anabolic, androgenic, or contraceptive steroids, and is sometimes referred to as 'bland' or 'steroid' cholestasis, while the lesions associated with chlorpromazine, other phenothiazines, and other drugs, including sulphonylureas, are conveniently referred to as 'hepatocanalicular' cholestasis, because of evidence of accompanying hepatocyte damage (Fig. 17.84). There have been reports of occasional instances of drug cholestasis that continue for a prolonged period and simulate primary biliary cirrhosis (PBC).

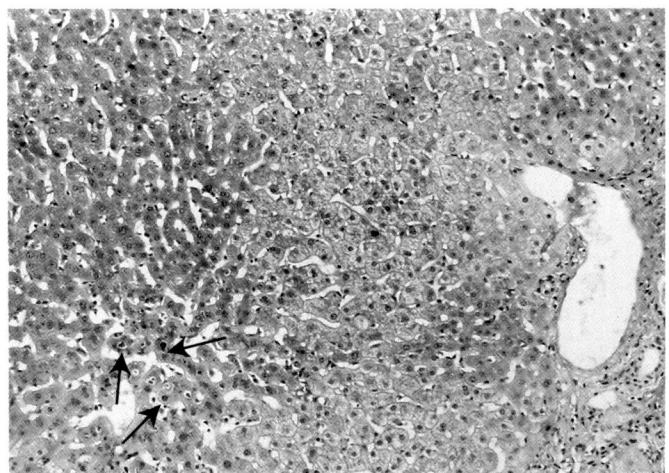

Fig. 17.84 Drug cholestasis with perivenous canalicular inspissates of bile (arrows).

The basis for the development of drug-induced cholestasis relates to current understanding of the cellular mechanisms involved in the formation and excretion of bile by the liver cell. The extraction of water and solutes from sinusoids occurs across the basolateral cell membrane where the energy for the extraction is derived from Na^+, K^+-ATPase activity. Bile acids form the main component transported across the cell membrane and their movement across the cell to canalicular excretion correlates well with bile-flow. Several factors modulate the flow-rate including competitive inhibition by other anions, the osmotic effect of the bile acid micelles, and the availability of unsaturated transport carrier. The carrier proteins have not been identified *in vivo*, but glutathione S-transferase and 3 alpha hydroxysteroid dehydrogenase bind to bile acids *in vitro*. Another carrier has been identified at the apical or canalicular membrane where the bile is excreted, and pericanalicular actin filaments may also play a part at this site. It is not clear what contribution is made to the process by other intracellular organelles. There are thus several sites of potential defect in the process of bile formation by the hepatocyte. Of the many compounds which have been reported as causing cholestasis, several groups have been investigated in attempts to localize the cellular defect. One group includes the androgenic and oestrogenic steroids, particularly those with alkyl substitution at the 17 alpha position. In their case, the liver lesion is usually limited to acinar zone 3 canalicular stasis without extensive hepatocyte necrosis, although individual hepatocytes may show feathery change. *In vivo* transport studies indicate the main effect on basolateral membrane fluidity with decrease Na^+, K^+, -ATPase activity, with less evidence to support an effect on transcellular passage. It is not clear why alkyl substitution at the 17 alpha position increases the likelihood of cholestasis with the sex steroids.

Another group of compounds is typified by chlorpromazine which is associated with cholestasis in 1–2 per cent of re-cipients. Characteristically, it produces microscopical changes which include the accumulation of eosinophils and mild hepatocellular damage. It appears to affect both basolateral membrane transport and also pericanalicular actin filaments. p450 catalytic activity is suggested as a basis for this cytotoxicity, one phenotype tending to promote rapid formation of toxic metabolites and slow generation of nontoxic intermediates. Cytotoxicity is expressed at the site of cellular uptake and also at the site of canalicular excretion.

Erythromycins, especially the estolate and some tricyclic antidepressants, including amitriptyline, also cause cholestasis, but, so far, damage has not been localized at the uptake basolateral membrane, or in the transcellular transport system, or at the excretory cytoskeletal canalicular region. In both groups, the possibility of the binding of a toxic metabolite to liver cell membranes or other hepatocyte components leading to an immune mediated cholestasis has been raised.

Different mechanisms therefore form the basis of drug-induced cholestasis for steroid hormones (hepatocyte uptake), phenothiazines (intrinsic toxicity at several sites), and erythromycin estolate and some tricyclic antidepressants (immune mediated).

There is also a curious, ill-understood lesion characterized by bile pigment inspissation and showing evidence of destruction of cells lining small ducts at the margins of portal tracts. Bile inspissation without necrosis is associated with sepsis but the toxic lesion involves necrosis (Fig. 17.85). The reasons for the necrosis are not clear and, in general, the pathogenesis of ductular cholestasis has not been elucidated. These lesions have been associated with the drugs or toxins paraquat, ajmaline, 4'4-diamino-diphenylmethane (a flour contaminant) and cooking oil. The subsequent development of the damaged ducts in this form of 'cholangio destructive toxicity' proceeds to a form of sclerosing cholangitis.

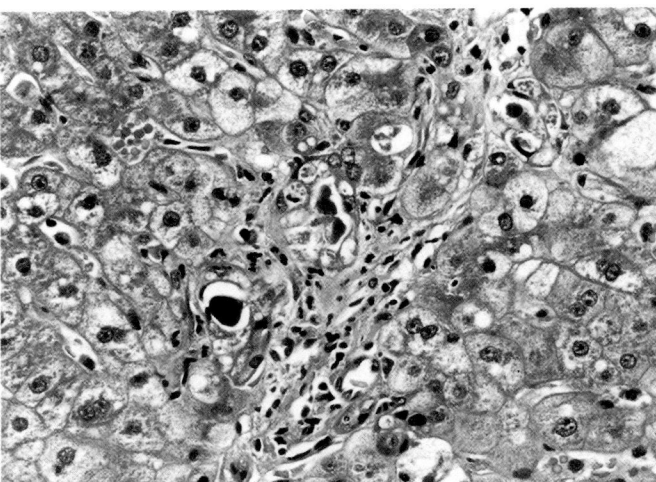

Fig. 17.85 Necrosis of small bile ducts with inspissation of bile ('cholangio destructive toxicity') in a patient given a high dose of intravenous contrast medium.

17.7.4   Lesions involving vascular pathways

Major arterial or portal venous lesions are not usually ascribed to drug toxicity, apart from drug-associated polyarteritis. Thrombosis of portal vein branches is not a common drug-induced lesion, even though hepatic venous thrombosis is a well-known side-effect of chemical contraception in women.

Sinusoids

Sinusoids are sensitive to the effects of drugs and toxins, and the development of marked sinusoidal dilatation, especially in a non-perivenular location, has been correlated with the administration of contraceptive steroids; this contrasts strikingly with the effects of thrombotic or other physical occlusion of a large branch of the portal vein, when perivenous sinusoids dilate with associated atrophic hepatocytes. A more striking and more irregular distortion of sinusoids, in which these structures take on the appearance of irregular blood-filled cavities which are sometimes devoid of recognizable endothelium, is referred to as 'peliosis', which is also found in some patients receiving steroid therapy of one form or another. The association of this condition with anabolic steroids is well recognized, but it occurs also with tamoxifen and even stilboestrol. A considerable fibrosis of the endothelial lining is described in toxicity from vinyl chloride monomer, and is known to occur after exposure to arsenicals in Italian vineyard workers and also many years after injections of thorotrast as a contrast medium. The mechanism underlying sinusoidal changes is not understood.

Ito cells

These fat-storing perisinusoidal cells also have the capacity to form collagen. Perisinusoidal collagenosis may be seen in patients suffering from hypervitaminosis A and may be associated with fat-filled Ito cells.

Hepatic veins

Obstruction to hepatic venous outflow pathways may develop as a result of a drug- or toxin-associated lesions at different sites in the hepatic venous tree. Thrombotic occlusion of large tributaries, particularly in relation to the ostia of the main hepatic veins, may be associated with the use of contraceptive steroids. In such circumstances, the microscopical changes of sinusoidal and perisinusoidal accumulations of erythrocytes are accompanied by atrophy or loss of perivenous hepatocytes and evidence, usually, of hyperplasia of periportal hepatocytes. More long-standing changes include perivenous or linear fibrosis, sometimes with obliteration of the lumen of the hepatic venous radicle. Sometimes there are striking conformational changes in the liver, with regions (the drainage of which is uncompromised) undergoing conspicuous compensatory hyperplasia. This is particularly noted in caudate lobes that drain separately from the three main hepatic veins into the inferior vena cava.

Lesions affecting mainly the smaller sublobular veins or venous radicles consist of proliferation of connective tissue together with intramural entrapment of erythrocytes charac-

teristic of the condition known as veno-occlusive disease (VOD), the parenchyma undergoing changes that resemble those associated with hepatic venous occlusion. In this condition, the sinusoids are distended in the acute phase, with erythrocytes and atrophic or absent perivenous hepatic plates contrasted with surviving periportal cells, which are often arranged in two-cell-thick plates. This condition was first associated with pyrrolizidine alkaloids but is known also to reflect the toxic effects of certain drugs, including azathioprine, 6-thioguanine, and cytosine arabinoside (Fig. 17.86). Similar lesions are reported after supervoltage irradiation and a series of small vein lesions have been noted with high frequency in chronic alcoholic liver disease (see Section 17.6).

17.7.5   The mononuclear phagocytic system

An inflammatory reaction, usually in the form of accumulations of lymphocytes and proliferation of macrophages, sometimes containing pigment granules, occurs frequently in drug toxicity. This is expected and reflects the consequences of hepatocyte necrosis, irrespective of its cause. In some circumstances the inflammatory reaction may contain a high proportion of neutrophils, notably the lesions caused by ethanol intake. The reasons for this difference in response are not clear.

In general, the inflammatory reaction subsides when the affected cells are phagocytosed or have disappeared and only residual pigmented macrophages remain, but, in some instances, persistence leads to features of chronic active hepatitis. The pathogenesis is not clear, apart from the appreciation that repeated administration is necessary.

A second form of drug-induced injury in which the inflammatory reaction is associated with a chronic lesion, mainly involving portal tracts in this instance, is the development of periportal fibrosis and features suggestive of primary biliary cirrhosis. This has been reported in cases of long-standing treatment with phenothiazines, such as chlorpromazine. This is an

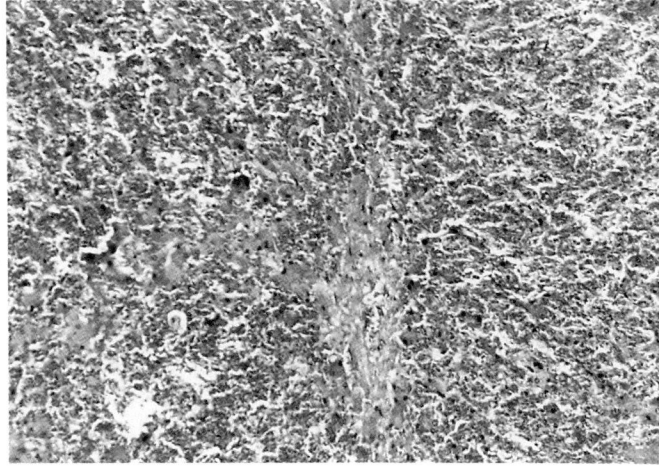

Fig. 17.86 Veno-occlusive disease. Thickened wall of hepatic vein with occluded lumen and surrounded by accumulations of erythrocytes in a patient treated with 6-thioguanine.

unusual complication, but so far no microscopical details have been identified as differentiating this condition from non-drug-induced primary biliary cirrhosis. A far more frequent reaction of the mononuclear phagocytic system is the formation of histiocytic granulomas, drug toxicity now being regarded as responsible for 29 per cent of hepatic granulomas (Fig. 17.87). Structural differences may sometimes be identified between drug-induced and infective or other granulomas, and these relate mainly to the site (usually portal in drug-induced), to the fibrous content (usually devoid of fibrous bands in drug-induced), and the content of eosinophils (usually increased in drug-induced). Many different drugs have been implicated, including sulphonamides, phenylbutazone, phenytoin, and carbamazapine.

Factors governing the formation of granulomas associated with drug toxicity are not defined. Some form of hypersensitivity is suspected in view of the small number of patients who are affected, and because of the increased incidence of eosinophils; but the reasons for the portal localization and deficient fibrous structure are not clear. The granulomas do not appear to represent a response to hepatocyte necrosis, as residuals in the form of necrotic cell fragments or phagocytosed pigment are not usually reported.

Lipogranulomas are noted, both in portal and perivenous locations, and are ascribed to animal oil in food or as medication. Kupffer cell storage of circulating substances is sometimes reflected in foamy change of the cytoplasm of enlarged Kupffer cells. Compounds associated with this change include the vehicle 1-vinyl-2-pyrrolidone (povidone) which is poorly absorbed from the gastrointestinal tract but is stored in histiocytes of the liver and spleen.

17.7.6 Tumours

The development of hepatic tumours as a result of exposure to drugs or toxins is well established in experimental animals, but there appears to be a limited number of acceptably documented carcinogens in man.

Hepatocellular tumours are recognized as a complication of cirrhosis, irrespective of the cause of the cirrhosis. Cirrhosis that is ascribed to the repeated administration of certain chemical agents may also be associated with the development of hepatocellular carcinoma and, as a result of this, the tumour is sometimes regarded as drug induced. The most common relationship is between tumour, cirrhosis, and the intake of ethanol.

Hepatocellular tumours in humans are associated with the administration of steroid hormonal agents. Hepatocellular adenomas are described in a higher than control incidence in women taking contraceptive steroids. This soft, unencapsulated, rather vascular tumour (Fig. 17.88), consists of thick plates of uniform, large, pale hepatocytes, usually with regular nuclei but without portal tracts, bile ducts, or firmly identifiable Kupffer cells (Fig. 17.89). The plates are separated by vascular spaces like sinusoids which, in general, are associated with normal-looking reticulin fibres. Intracytoplasmic globules of α-1-antitrypsin have been reported in some tumours, and necrosis or haemorrhage are noted frequently. Malignant tumours are rarely ascribed to contraceptive steroids and neither necrosis nor haemorrhage within the tumour are pointers in this direction.

Hepatocellular tumours are also reported after administration of anabolic/androgenic steroids, a striking example of which is represented by the development of hepatocellular tumours in young patients suffering from Fanconi anaemia who are treated for long periods with anabolic compounds. In such circumstances, the tumour may show characteristics of malignant change. The use of anabolic or androgenic steroids is also associated with the development of hepatocellular tumours in adults, notably in patients undergoing surgery for sex change

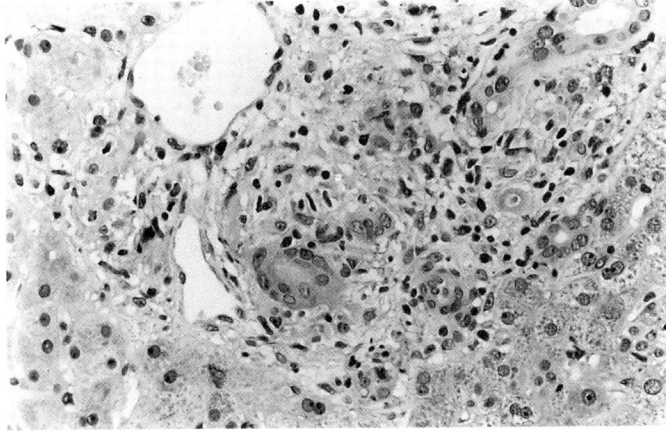

Fig. 17.87 Histiocytic portal granuloma with giant cells, no fibrosis, and accompanying eosinophils in a patient treated with carbamazapine.

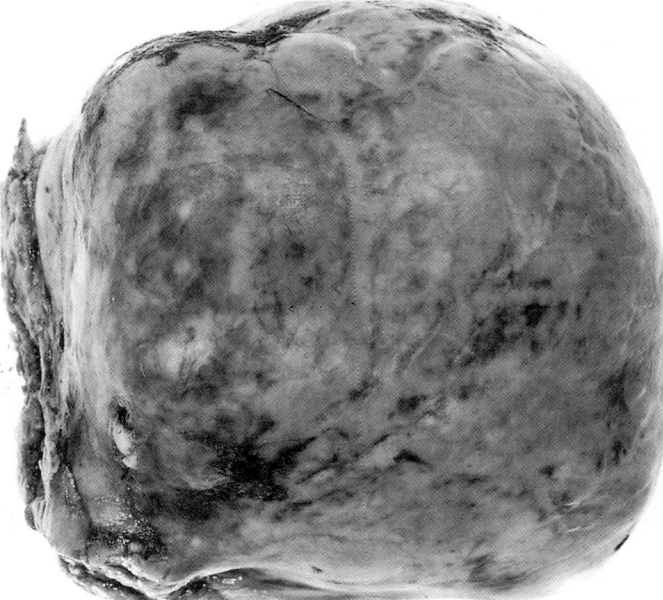

Fig. 17.88 Hepatic adenoma in a patient using oral contraceptive agents for 5 years. No evidence of recurrence 5 years after surgical resection.

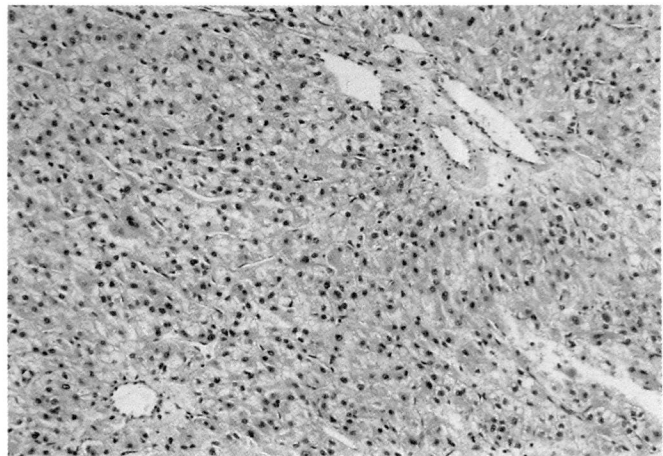

Fig. 17.89 Hepatic adenoma. Pale cells without portal tracts or identifiable Kupffer cells, and with large vessels, in a patient using oral contraceptive agents for 10 years.

or those in whom body building or muscle hypertrophy is considered advantageous for athletic or other competitions. The tumours are similar in many respects to the liver cell adenomas associated with contraceptive pills and no instances of malignant change with invasion or metastases are reported. Cytologically however, there may be striking abnormalities, with variations in nuclear size, sometimes bizarre nuclei, and even mitoses, but these have not so far been associated with biologically malignant activity. In addition, there are several instances reported of regression of the tumours on cessation of the steroid therapy.

The development of hepatocellular carcinoma and of adenocarcinomas of bile duct origin has been ascribed to exposure to thorotrast and thorotrast particles are sometimes found in relevant tissue bearing such tumours.

Although other chemicals are demonstrably carcinogenic in experimental animals, and epidemiological evidence indicates that occupational and other exposure may be suspected with such tumours, the suggestions that these compounds are carcinogenic in man are not strongly supported in individual case studies. Thus drugs that are mutagenic *in vivo*, or carcinogenic in experimental animals, may be withheld from patients so that they remain only suspect hepatic human carcinogens.

Angiosarcoma, now clearly associated with exposure to vinyl chloride monomer, is reported as occurring with increased frequency in patients who have been treated with arsenical solutions and also in patients who have been injected with thorotrast. Other compounds that have been suspected as causing haemangiosarcoma include androgenic-anabolic steroids, but this may be a chance association.

17.7.7   Further reading

Bagheri, S. A. and Boyer, J. L. (1974). Peliosis hepatis associated with androgenic-anabolic steroid therapy. *Annals of Internal Medicine* **81**, 610–18.

Beermann, B., *et al.* (1971). Transient cholestasis during treatment with ajmaline and chronic xanthomatous cholestasis after administration of ajmaline, methyl testosterone and ethinylestradiol. *Acta Medica Scandinavica* **190**, 241–50.

Black, M. (1984). Acetaminophen hepatotoxicity. *Annual Review of Medicine* **35**, 577–93.

Black, M. and Raucy, J. (1986). Acetaminophen, alcohol and cytochrome P450. *Annals of Internal Medicine* **104**, 427–92.

Boyer, T. D. (1989). The glutathione S-transferases: an update. *Hepatology* **9**, 486–96.

Burk, R. F., Reiter, R., and Lane, J. M. (1986). Hyperbaric oxygen protection against carbon tetrachloride toxicity in the rat: association with altered metabolism. *Gastroenterology* **90**, 812–18.

Devalia, H. and McLean, A. E. M. (1983). Covalent binding and the mechanism of paracetamol toxicity. *Biochemical Pharmacology* **32**, 2602–3.

Dincsoy, H. P., Weesner, R. E., and MacGee, J. (1982). Lipogranulomas in non-fatty human liver: A mineral oil induced environmental disease. *American Journal of Clinical Pathology* **78**, 35–41.

Falk, H., Thomas, L. B., Popper, H., and Ishak, K. G. (1981). Arsenic-related hepatic angiosarcoma. *American Journal of Industrial Medicine* **2**, 43–50.

Farber, J. L. and Gerson, R. J. (1984). Mechanisms of cell injury with hepatotoxic chemicals. *Pharmacological Reviews* **36**, 715–55.

Gan, T. E. and van der Weyden, M. B. (1982). Dapsone-induced infectious mononucleosis-like syndrome. *Medical Journal of Australia* **1**, 350–1.

Guengerich, F. P. (1989). Characterization of human microsomal cytochrome p450 enzymes. *Annual Review of Pharmacology and Toxicology* **29**, 241–64.

Hoyumpa, A. M. and Connell, A. M. (1976). Methyldopa (Aldomet) hepatitis: report of a case and review of the literature. *Drug Intelligence and Clinical Pharmacology* **10**, 144.

Ishak, K. G. and Rabin, L. (1975). Benign tumors of the liver. *Medical Clinics of North America* **59**, 995–1013.

Jacqz, E., Hall, S. D., and Branch, R. A. (1986). Genetically determined polymorphism in drug oxidation. *Hepatology* **6**, 1020–32.

Lee, F. I. (1982). Vinyl chloride-induced liver disease. *Journal of the Royal College of Physicians of London* **16**, 226–30.

Lewis, J. H., Tice, H., and Zimmerman, H. J. (1983). Budd–Chiari syndrome associated with oral contraceptive steroids. Review of treatment of 47 cases. *Digestive Diseases and Sciences* **28**, 673–83.

Loomus, G. N., Aneja, P., and Bota, R. A. (1983). A case of peliosis hepatis in association with tamoxifen therapy. *American Journal of Clinical Pathology* **80**, 881–3.

Lullman, H., Lullman-Rauch, R., and Wasserman, O. (1975). Drug-induced phospholipidosis. II Tissue distribution of the amphiphilic drug chlorphenteres. *CRC Critical Reviews in Toxicology* **4**, 185–218.

McMaster, K. R. and Hennigar, G. R. (1981). Drug-induced granulomatous hepatitis. *Laboratory Investigation* **44**, 61–73.

Mays, E. T. and Christopherson, W. (1984). Hepatic tumors induced by sex steroids. *Seminars in Liver Disease* **4**, 147–57.

Mullick, F. G. and Ishak, K. G. (1980). Hepatic injury associated with diphenylhydantoin therapy: a clinicopathologic study of 20 cases. *American Journal of Clinical Pathology* **74**, 442–52.

Nebert, D. W. (1979). Multiple forms of inducible drug-metabolizing enzymes; a reasonable mechanism by which any organism can cope with adversity. *Molecular Cell Biochemistry* **27**, 27–46.

Neuberger, J. and Davis, M. (1983). In *Recent advances in hepatology*, (ed. H. C. Thomas and R. N. M. MacSween), p. 59. Churchill Livingstone, London.

Pessayre, D., *et al.* (1979). Perhexilene maleate-induced cirrhosis. *Gastroenterology* **76**, 170–7.

Pessayre, D. and Larrey, D. (1988). Acute and chronic drug-induced hepatitis. *Bailliere's Clinical Gastroenterology* **3**, 385–422.

Peters, R. L. (1986). In *Liver pathology* (ed. R. L. Peters and J. R. Craig), p. 340. Churchill Livingstone, New York.

Phillips, M. J. and Satir, P. (1988). The cytoskeleton of the hepatocyte: organization, relationships, and pathology. In *The liver. Biology and pathobiology* (2nd edn) (ed. I. M. Arias, W. B. Jakoby, H. Popper, D. Schacter, and D. A. Shafritz), pp. 16–22. Raven Press, New York.

Popper, H., *et al.* (1978). Development of hepatic angiosarcoma in man induced by vinyl chloride, thorotrast and arsenic. Comparison with cases of unknown etiology. *American Journal of Pathology* **92**, 349–69.

Portmann, B., *et al.* (1975). Histopathological changes in the liver following a paracetamol overdose: correlation with clinical and biochemical parameters. *Journal of Pathology* **117**, 169–81.

Puppala, A. R. and Ro, J. A. (1979). Possible association between peliosis hepatis and diethylstilbestrol: Report of two cases. *Postgraduate Medicine* **65**, 277–8, 280–1.

Reed, G. B. and Cox, A. J. (1966). The human liver after radiation injury. A form of veno-occlusive disease. *American Journal of Pathology* **48**, 597–612.

Reichen, J. and Simon, F. R. (1988). Cholestasis. In *The liver. Biology and pathology* (2nd edn) (ed. I. M. Arias, W. B. Jakoby, H. Popper, D. Schacter, and D. A. Shafritz), pp. 1105–24. Raven Press, New York.

Reynolds, T. B., Peters, R. L., and Yamada, S. (1971). Chronic active and lupoid hepatitis caused by a laxative, oxyphenisatin. *New England Journal of Medicine* **285**, 813–20.

Rubel, L. R. and Ishak, K. G. (1982). Thorotrast-associated cholangiocarcinoma: an epidemiologic and clinicopathologic study. *Cancer* **50**, 1408–15.

Russell, R. M., Boyer, J. L., Bagheri, S. A., and Hruban, Z. (1974). Hepatic injury from chronic hypervitaminosis A resulting in portal hypertension and ascites. *New England Journal of Medicine* **291**, 435–40.

Satti, M. B., Weinbren, K., and Gordon-Smith, E. C. (1982). 6-Thioguanine as a cause of toxic veno-occlusive disease of the liver. *Journal of Clinical Pathology* **35**, 1086–91.

Smith, D. J. and Gordon, E. R. (1988). Role of liver plasma membrane fluidity in the pathogenesis of estrogen-induced cholestasis. *Journal of Laboratory and Clinical Medicine* **112**, 679–85.

Solis-Herruzo, J. A., *et al.* (1984). Hepatic injury in the toxic epidemic syndrome caused by ingestion of adulterated cooking oil (Spain, 1981). *Hepatology* **4**, 131.

Starko, K. M. and Mullick, F. G. (1983). Hepatic and cerebral pathology findings in children with fatal salicylate intoxication: Further evidence for a causal relation between salicylate and Reye's syndrome. *Lancet* i, 326–9.

Vasquez, J. J., Guillen, F. J., and Zozaya, L. M. (1983). Cyanamide-induced liver injury. A predictable lesion. *Liver* **3**, 225–31.

Vergani, D., *et al.* (1980). Antibodies on the surface of halothane-altered rabbit hepatocytes in patients with severe halothane-associated hepatitis. *New England Journal of Medicine* **303**, 66–71.

Watkins, P. B. (1990). Role of cytochromes p450 in drug metabolism and hepatotoxicity. *Seminars in Liver Disease* **10**, 235–50.

Weitz, H., *et al.* (1982). Veno-occlusive disease of the liver in patients receiving azathioprine. *Virchows Archives of Pathology and Anatomy* **395**, 245.

Williams, A. T. and Burk, R. F. (1990). Carbon tetrachloride hepatotoxicity: an example of free radical-mediated injury. *Seminars in Liver Disease* **10**, 279–84.

Zimmerman, H. J. (1990). Update of hepatotoxicity due to classes of drugs in common use: non-steroidal drugs, anti-inflammatory drugs, antibiotics, antihypertensives, and cardiac and psychotropic agents. *Seminars in Liver Disease* **10**, 322–38.

Zimmerman, H. J. and Ishak, K. G. (1987). Hepatic injury due to drugs and toxins. In *Pathology of the liver* (ed. R. N. M. MacSween, P. P. Anthony, and P. J. Scheuer), p. 503. Churchill Livingstone, London.

17.8 Vascular disorders of the liver

R. S. Patrick

17.8.1 The liver in circulatory failure

Right-sided heart failure

Hepatic congestion occurs in right-sided heart failure from any cause, acquired or congenital. The cut surface of the enlarged, firm liver presents a characteristic mottling, like that of a cut nutmeg, because of dark zone 3 congestion and pallor of periportal liver tissue, which may be accentuated by fatty change. Congestion is readily confirmed microscopically, with wide sinusoidal openings into dilated terminal veins. Adjacent hepatocytes undergo atrophy and contain lipochrome pigment or they may disappear. Macrophages containing haemosiderin or ceroid pigment may appear in these zones. A minority show bile capillary cholestasis; jaundice is a clinical feature of these cases but can be due also to excess bilirubin production from haemorrhagic infarcts in the lungs and elsewhere.

In cardiac failure of acute onset, usually following massive myocardial infarction (cardiogenic shock), haemorrhagic necrosis may be found around terminal veins. This may be accompanied by neutrophil polymorph infiltration.

Left-sided heart failure

Reduced arterial blood flow causes atrophy or necrosis of the oxygen-sensitive hepatocytes, especially in the relatively hypoxic zone 3, where there is also sinusoidal dilatation but no congestion. (Similar sinusoidal dilatation of uncertain cause is seen occasionally in association with various infections and Hodgkin disease.)

Shock

Hepatic changes similar to those found in acute cardiac failure may be found in shock from other causes—trauma, haemorrhage, pulmonary embolism, etc., especially in cases lasting longer than 24 hours. It is probably a factor in the development of jaundice following surgery for non-hepato-biliary diseases and cardiac bypass surgery ('post-pump' jaundice) but in some of these cases the pathogenesis is not known.

Factors other than circulatory failure can contribute to liver damage in certain types of shock; excessive production of endotoxin in Gram-negative bacterial infections or failure by Kupffer cells, damaged in various ways, to detoxify endotoxins may cause severe hepatocyte damage. In some cases, including endotoxic shock and heat stroke, there is cholangitis and intra-hepatic cholestasis. The latter is sometimes prominent in dilated ductules adjacent to portal tracts; these channels seem to end blindly, as interlobular and septal bile ducts are not involved (Fig. 17.90).

17.8.2 Cardiac 'cirrhosis'

In some cases of prolonged cardiac insufficiency, especially mitral stenosis and constrictive pericarditis, fibrosis develops in congested zone 3 and spreads throughout the liver. The liver retains its congested appearance but becomes shrunken and there is fibrous thickening of Glisson's capsule.

Microscopic examination confirms zone 3 congestion and fibrosis, the latter forming bridges with adjacent fibrotic zones. Here, the hepatocytes have disappeared or have undergone atrophy to resemble biliary epithelium lining small channels. Surviving parenchyma surrounds portal tracts and has, in turn, a margin of developing fibrous tissue. This gives a pattern of 'reversed lobulation' (Fig. 17.91). Very rarely, there is nodular hyperplasia of surviving parenchyma which produces a fine micronodular cirrhosis (true cardiac cirrhosis). By contrast, some cases of nodular regenerative hyperplasia of liver without fibrosis occur in cardiac failure (see Section 17.12.5).

17.8.3 Other types of impaired hepatic venous outflow

Budd–Chiari syndrome

This unusual form of hepatic congestion arises from obstruction of hepatic veins at their ostia or of the inferior vena cava. The disease is always associated with severe ascites and hepato-megaly, but jaundice is often slight or absent. Many are mis-

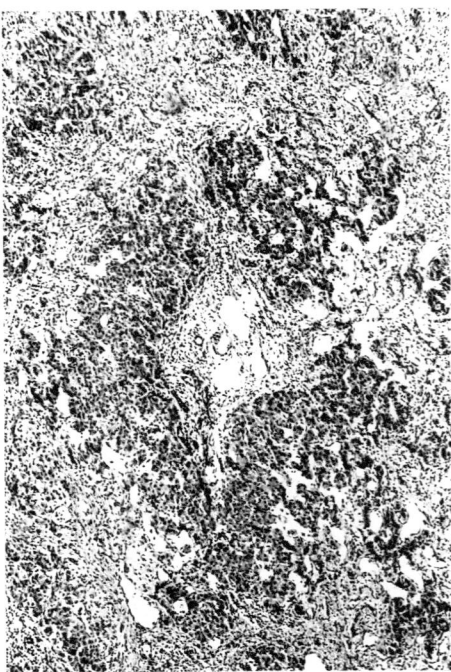

Fig. 17.91 Reversed lobulation in cardiac 'cirrhosis'. The portal tract is surrounded by dark-stained parenchyma with sinusoidal dilatation. At the periphery there is bridging of zones by pale connective tissue containing atrophic liver cells, some of which form tiny tubular structures. (Periodic acid, Schiff stain.)

diagnosed as cirrhosis or tumour but hepatic and inferior vena caval venography will reveal the obstruction. The majority of cases are due to thrombosis, which may be of sudden onset and cause severe illness but many develop insidiously with organiz-ation of the lesion. Recanalization and relief of the obstruction is possible but occurs rarely. Thrombosis may be idiopathic or may have some recognized cause, such as trauma or a clotting tendency, especially polycythaemia and paroxysmal nocturnal haemoglobinuria, and some are attributed to oral contraceptive intake. The obstruction can be a fibrous web, usually fenestrated, which stretches across the venous ostia or vena cava. Rarely, there is invasion by tumour, or pressure on vessel walls by tumour or abscess.

The changes in the liver are similar to those found in congest-ive cardiac failure, and fibrosis may supervene. A striking but unusual feature is compensatory hypertrophy of the caudate lobe, which has its own hepatic venous outflow and could therefore escape obstruction (Section 17.12.3, Fig. 17.133).

Veno-occlusive disease

This disease is well known in the Caribbean, especially among children, but persons of all ages can be affected and outbreaks or sporadic cases have been reported from all parts of the world. There is usually gross abdominal swelling from ascites and hepato-splenomegaly, and death may supervene from liver failure or haemorrhage. Some cases undergo spontaneous remission and others may develop hepatic fibrosis.

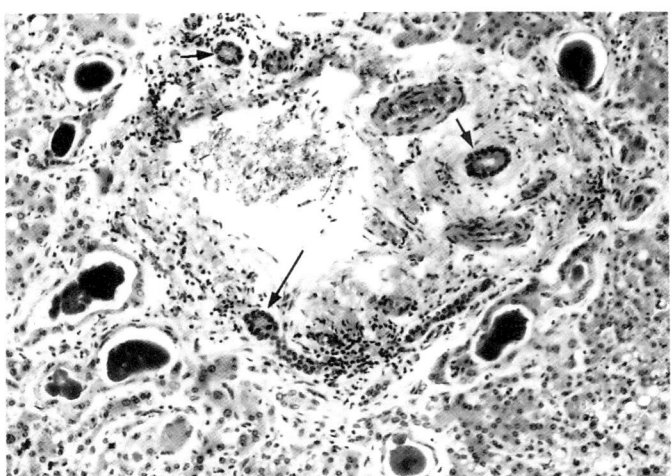

Fig. 17.90 Liver in endotoxic shock. Bile ductules adjacent to the portal tract are grossly distended with bile pigment. Interlobular bile ducts (arrows) are not involved.

Unlike Budd–Chiari syndrome, hepatic venous obstruction in this disease is localized to intrahepatic vessels. It seems to begin with deposition of fibrin in centrilobular sinusoids, but thrombosis is not apparent, vascular constriction being due to subendothelial growth of loose connective tissue (Fig. 17.92). This causes severe sinusoidal congestion and dilatation with hepatocyte atrophy or necrosis around terminal venules.

There are various causes, the most important being ingestion of pyrrolizidine alkaloids present in senecio and crotalaria plants used in the manufacture of bush teas and herbal medicines. Cattle grazing on pastures containing these plants may suffer from similar liver damage. Other causes include urethane, immunosuppressive agents such as azathioprine, certain cancer chemotherapeutic drugs, and irradiation therapy applied to the region of the liver. It occurs in some cases of graft versus host disease following bone marrow transplantation. Recognition of the cause and its removal may lead to regression but in many the prognosis is poor.

Central hyaline sclerosis

This is present in some cases of severe alcoholic hepatitis; there is fibrous narrowing or obliteration of many terminal venules extending into adjacent sinusoids (Section 17.6.2, Fig. 17.66). Subendothelial connective tissue proliferation in larger veins, similar to veno-occlusive disease, is seen occasionally in these alcoholic cases.

Sinusoidal obstruction

It is possible that hepatocytes swollen by hydropic degeneration or fatty change may obstruct sinusoidal blood flow and aggravate liver cell damage. It is suggested that this is an important factor in alcoholic hepatitis, but it is not generally accepted. The significance of obstruction by tumour or inflammatory cells is likewise controversial. In sickle-cell anaemia, severe liver dysfunction with focal necrosis, often mistaken clinically for viral hepatitis, can follow a sickle-cell crisis when liver sinusoids are blocked by clumps of abnormal erythrocytes, fibrin, and platelets, which become ingested by swollen Kupffer cells (Fig. 17.93).

17.8.4   Lesions of the portal venous system

Causes of portal hypertension (see also Section 17.16.3)

Portal venous obstruction

Thrombosis from various causes, such as splenectomy, may spread from splenic or mesenteric veins or originate in portal vessels outwith or within the liver. It may take the form of suppurative pyelophlebitis, which rarely complicates intra-abdominal inflammation such as acute appendicitis or cholecystitis. There may be extensive infiltration by tumour, especially hepatocellular carcinoma or angiosarcoma. In advanced schistosomiasis, many portal vessels are blocked by numerous parasite eggs which induce a chronic inflammatory reaction and eventually extensive obliterative fibrosis ('pipe-stem fibrosis') of affected veins.

Other liver diseases

Cirrhosis of any type or cause is associated with portal hypertension. Vascular injection studies of cirrhotic liver reveal distortion of portal vein branches by expanding nodules, and kinking of vessels where they pass under the edges of fibrous membranes. Arteriovenous shunts develop and augment the hypertension. However, hypertension may be modified by the development of anastomoses between portal and hepatic veins, whereby some blood entering the liver bypasses sinusoids; this, incidentally, contributes to hypoxic hepatocyte damage in cirrhosis. (This is discussed more fully in Section 17.11.4.) Diffuse nodular hyperplasia of liver and portal hypertension coexist,

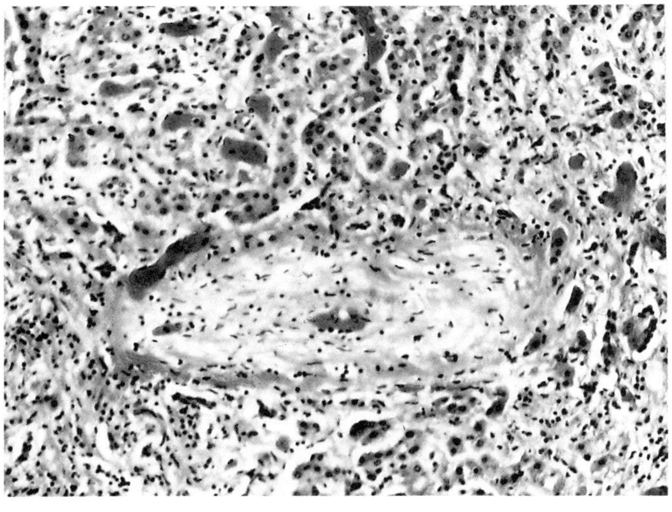

Fig. 17.92 Veno-occlusive disease induced by urethane. The lumen of this terminal vein is grossly narrowed by proliferation of subendothelial connective tissue.

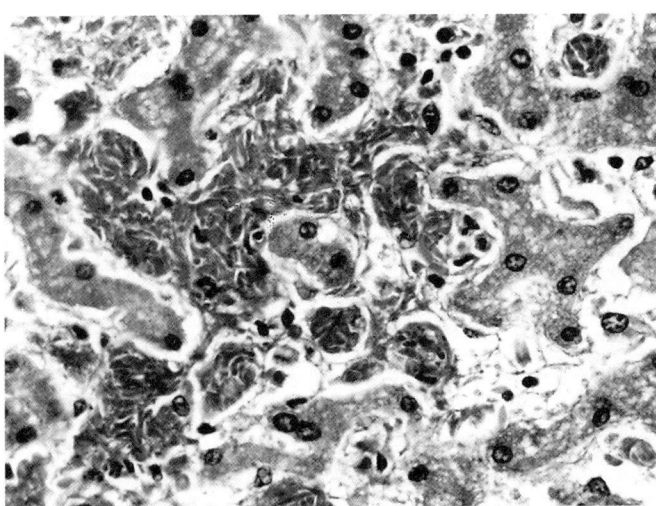

Fig. 17.93 Sickle-cell anaemia. Liver sinusoids are occluded by clumps of abnormal erythrocytes. (Provided by Dr F. D. Lee.)

but whether by cause or effect is uncertain. Partial nodular transformation of liver in the porta hepatis region presumably acts by compression of portal vessels.

Impaired hepatic venous outflow, as discussed above, causes severe portal hypertension. It is particularly significant in alcoholic hepatitis with central hyaline sclerosis.

Other liver diseases with portal hypertension are unusual. They include non-cirrhotic but fibrotic conditions such as congenital hepatic fibrosis, mucoviscidosis, some cases of sarcoidosis and fibrosis attributable to arsenical compounds, excess vitamin A intake, etc.

Developmental anomalies of the portal vein

These include fibrous strictures and aplasia (which is not always fatal). Two special anomalies are recognized.

Cavernomatous transformation of the portal vein In the porta hepatis, the vein is replaced by a spongy mass of small anastomosing blood-vessels. This may be a congenital malformation or acquired following portal vein thrombosis, especially in neonates subjected to umbilical vein catheterization.

Cruveilhier–Baumgarten syndrome This is persistence of the umbilical vein in the falciform ligament, which links the portal vein with dilated vessels in the anterior abdominal wall. A similar condition may develop in established portal hypertension from cirrhosis and other causes.

Increased portal venous blood flow

This may occur in splenomegaly unrelated to primary liver disease, such as polycythaemia, myelofibrosis, leukaemia, etc. Arteriovenous fistula within or outwith the liver, due to trauma, ruptured aneurysm, etc., is a rare cause.

Idiopathic

Portal hypertension may occur in patients with normal liver structure and with no recognizable extrahepatic cause. Others may show varying degrees of portal vein fibrous thickening, chronic portal hepatitis, or septal fibrosis, but it is impossible to state whether these changes are the cause or result of elevated portal pressure. Many cases in whom portal venous thrombosis or fibrous obliteration may be prominent have been reported from India, and this has been referred to as non-cirrhotic portal fibrosis or hepato-portal sclerosis. The same condition is probably fairly common in all parts of the world (Fig. 17.94) and there may be various causes. It seems possible that some are the end result of chronic hepatitis, perhaps related to steroid therapy.

Infarction from portal venous occlusion

Zahn's infarcts are usually dull-red in colour and triangular in shape, with the base at the capsular surface. Portal vein occlusion by thrombus, etc. may be seen near the apex. The red colour is due to severe sinusoidal congestion and there is

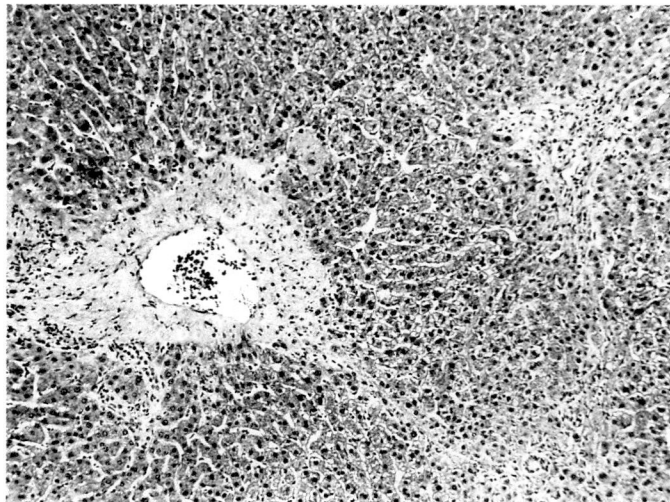

Fig. 17.94 Non-cirrhotic portal fibrosis. There is gross fibrous thickening of the portal vein wall, and thin fibrous septa bridge adjacent portal areas.

atrophy of intervening liver cell plates (Fig. 17.95). Similar lesions are sometimes caused by hepatic venous obstruction.

Porto-caval shunts

Extrahepatic shunting between portal vein and a large systemic vein is sometimes undertaken with success in the treatment of portal hypertension. The procedure is not without risk, as susceptibility to hepatic encephalopathy is increased. There may also be some deterioration of liver function but severe parenchymal damage or infarction are rare. The absorption of iron is enhanced, causing haemosiderin deposition in liver cells and at other sites.

Intrahepatic portal hepatic venous shunts develop in cirrhotic livers.

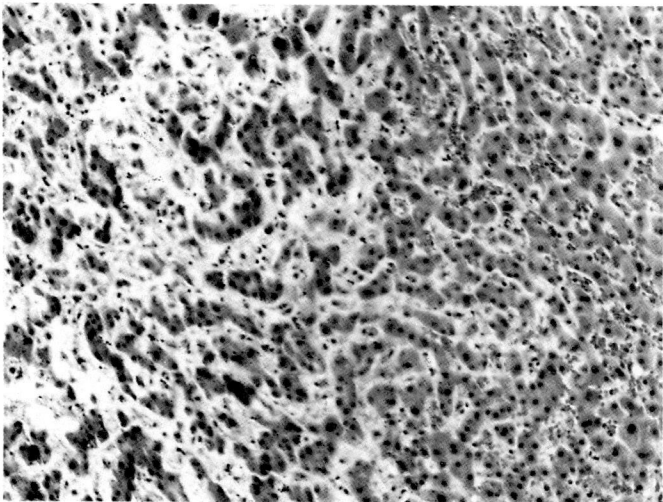

Fig. 17.95 Zahn's infarct (left) from portal venous obstruction.

17.8.5 Hepatic arterial lesions

Systemic arterial diseases

Conditions such as diabetic arteriolosclerosis and amyloidosis can involve the hepatic arteries. The liver is affected fairly frequently in polyarteritis nodosa, and some of these cases may be related to HBV infection. Dissecting aneurysm of the aorta can spread to the hepatic artery but this is very rare.

Arterial occlusion

The vessel or its branches may be occluded rarely by tumour or embolus. Surgical occlusion may be accidental or used in the treatment of aneurysm or primary liver cancer.

Liver infarction occurs in only a minority of cases, and is variable in extent and distribution. This may be explained by the additional portal venous blood supply and by variations in the hepatic arterial system; accessory arteries may be present that arise from the superior mesenteric artery or the left gastric artery. Hepatic infarcts are pale and irregular in shape. Histologically, there is coagulation necrosis and a margin of attempted organization in those who survive for several days.

17.8.6 Miscellaneous

Vascular lesions in transplanted liver

These include arterial thrombosis and venular endotheliitis in acute rejection, and infiltration of arterial walls by foamy macrophages in chronic rejection. They are described in Section 17.14.

The liver in toxaemia of pregnancy

Severe liver damage is rare in pre-eclampsia but present in about 50 per cent of cases of fully developed eclampsia. It consists of patchy sinusoidal obstruction by fibrin thrombi and related haemorrhagic necrosis, usually having a periportal distribution (Fig. 17.96). The lesion may arise from sinusoidal-lining cell damage and has the character of disseminated intravascular coagulation. Subcapsular haemorrhage and rupture of liver may follow minor trauma.

Peliosis hepatitis

This very rare condition occurs in patients with advanced wasting disease, such as tuberculosis, or in those receiving steroid therapy. The liver is filled with blood-containing spherical cysts measuring up to 1 cm in diameter, and has a remarkable mottled appearance. Most cysts are in direct communication with sinusoids. Some may undergo thrombosis or fibrosis. The pathogenesis is unknown (Fig. 17.97).

More irregular focal sinusoidal dilatation may be seen within some primary liver cancers or in the vicinity of tumours. It may be a feature of hairy-cell leukaemia in which the normal sinusoidal lining is replaced by tumour cells. Focal periportal sinusoidal dilatation is associated with oral contraceptive intake.

Inherited telangiectasia (Rendu–Osler–Weber syndrome)

This is a rare autosomal dominant disease affecting various organs, the liver being involved in only a minority of cases. There are multiple cavernous haemangiomas and bundles of tortuous arteries and veins, often encased in fibrous tissue. Over

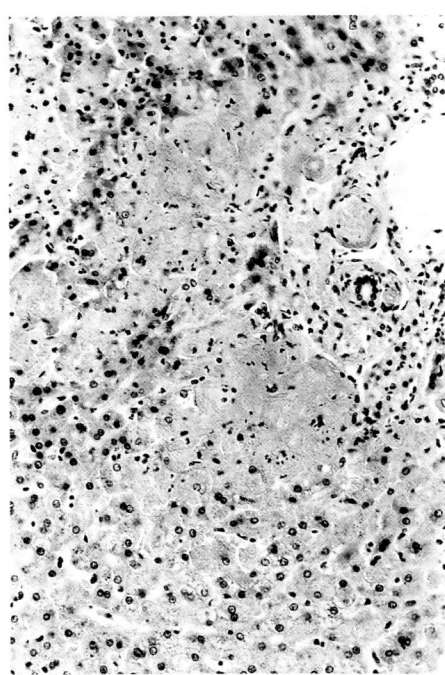

Fig. **17.96** Liver in eclampsia. There is an area of haemorrhagic necrosis adjacent to the portal tract.

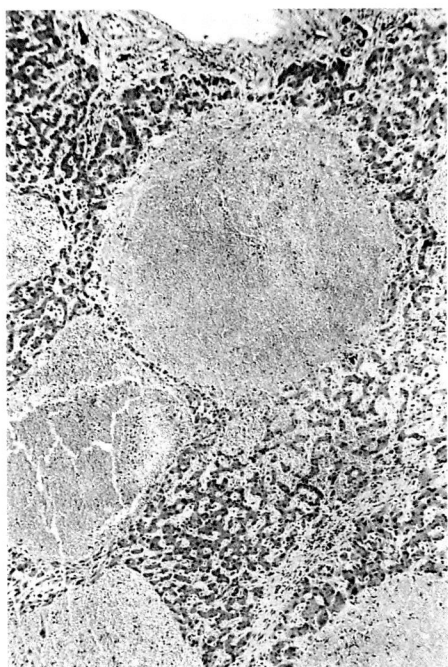

Fig. **17.97** Peliosis hepatis. There are several blood-filled cystic spaces in direct communication with sinusoids.

the years, it can spread within the liver and terminate in a cirrhotic condition. There are usually multiple arteriovenous fistulas within these lesions.

17.8.7   Further reading

Bras, G., Jelliffe, D. B., and Stuart, K. L. (1954). Veno-occlusive disease of liver with non portal type of cirrhosis, occurring in Jamaica. *Archives of Pathology* **57**, 285–300.

Nolan, J. P. (1981). Endotoxin, reticulo-endothelial function and liver injury. *Hepatology* **1**, 458–65.

Okuda, K., *et al.* (1984). Clinical study of eighty-six cases of idiopathic portal hypertension and comparison with cirrhosis with spleno-megaly. *Gastroenterology* **86**, 600–10.

Vidins, E. I., Britton, R. S., Medline, A., Blendis, I. M., Israel, Y., and Orrego, H. (1985). Sinusoidal caliber in alcoholic and non-alcoholic liver disease; diagnostic and pathogenic implications. *Hepatology* **5**, 408–14.

Ware, A. J. (1978). The liver when the heart fails. *Gastroenterology* **74**, 627–8.

17.9   Metabolic disorders

P. P. Anthony

17.9.1   Introduction

The scientific study of inherited metabolic disorders may be stated to have begun with the brilliant work of Sir Archibald Garrod on alkaptonuria and like disorders, which he summarized in his classic monograph, *Inborn errors of metabolism*, in 1923. He observed that most of these conditions showed a tendency to cluster in families amongst whom there was a high incidence of consanguinity. Garrod suggested that the cause in most instances was an inherited one and it could be explained in terms of the recently rediscovered laws of Mendel. The 'one gene—one enzyme' concept was established by Beadle and Tatum and by Ephrussi in the 1940s on the basis of experiments on the *Drosophila* fly and the bread mould, *Neurospora crassa*. The molecular basis of an inherited disorder was first established by Pauling and Ingram during their studies of sickle-cell disease in the 1950s. The pace of progress soon accelerated and it has, in recent years, become a veritable flood of new knowledge, as testified by subsequent volumes of the compendium, *The metabolic basis of inherited disease* by Stanbury and others which first appeared in 1960.

17.9.2   General considerations

The clinical expression, course, and severity of this group of disorders are extremely variable, but symptoms and signs referable to the liver and the central nervous system are common. This is hardly surprising as the liver plays a part in most meta-bolic processes and the central nervous system is uniquely susceptible to the effects of any disturbance of the internal milieu. Thus, many patients present in early life with failure to thrive, organomegaly particularly enlargement of the liver and spleen, hypotonia, convulsions, and, as the child grows older, gross mental retardation. Survival to adulthood is possible in some cases or subtypes of a disease but almost never without symptoms. Early death is a common outcome.

The diagnosis in some cases is strongly suggested by the clinical symptoms or some physical sign unique to the disease, such as a characteristic facial appearance, changes in the eye, a skin lesion, and so forth, but confirmation requires laboratory investigation. This includes enzyme assays on red or white blood cells, identification of accumulated or missing metabolites in blood or urine, and chemical analysis of tissue samples. Cell culture, most commonly of skin fibroblasts, has proved to be almost invariably useful in demonstrating enzyme defects, while recombinant DNA technology has enabled the identification of the gene responsible in a growing number of cases. These techniques are extensively reviewed by Stanbury *et al.* (1983) and Antonarakis (1989). As many inherited metabolic disorders produce readily identifiable changes in tissues, histopathological examination of a biopsy is often the quickest method for arriving at the diagnosis or at least for suggesting the most likely group of disorders. A sample of liver obtained by percutaneous needle biopsy can be most informative. It must be delivered fresh to the laboratory so that it may be examined by special methods if required. These are histochemical and immunological techniques, polarized or ultraviolet light microscopy, and electron microscopy. These methods demonstrate lipids, carbohydrates, pigments, crystals, and metals. The general morphological appearances that may be seen in a liver biopsy are described in detail by Ishak and Sharp (1987) and the ultrastructural changes by Phillips *et al.* (1987).

Prevention of inherited metabolic disorders is now possible by genetic counselling, screening for heterozygotes, and prenatal diagnosis by amniocentesis and chorionic villus biopsy. Treatment is possible in a few instances, if the condition is recognized at or near birth, by dietary restriction, replacement of the deficient end-product, depletion of a stored abnormal metabolite, or use of a metabolic inhibitor, amplification of enzyme activity, and organ transplantation. Ultimately, direct replacement of an abnormal gene may correct the disorder. This is still a theoretical possibility only but it may be realized by the end of the century.

Table 17.7 lists the main features, mode of inheritance, and enzyme defect of some inherited metabolic diseases, many of which involve the liver (see below).

17.9.3   The porphyrias

Classification

The porphyrias constitute a group of disorders with varying clinical features that result from specific enzyme defects in the biosynthesis of haem. It is customary to divide them into two

Table 17.7 Summary of metabolic disorders

Disease	Inheritance	Defect	Metabolite stored (mishandled or deficient)	Organ involved	Manifestations
Porphyrias					
Acute intermittent porphyria	AD	Porphobilinogen deaminase	(Porphobilinogen, δ-aminolaevulinic acid)	Nervous system, liver, intestine	Neurovisceral manifestations, often precipitated by drugs; cirrhosis, liver cell carcinoma
Porphyria cutanea tarda	AD	(Uroporphyrinogen decarboxylase)	(Uroporphyrin)	Skin, nervous system, liver	Photosensitivity, skin rash, peripheral neuropathy, cirrhosis, liver cell carcinoma
Erythropoietic protoporphyria	AD	Ferrochelatase	(Protoporphyrin)	Skin, liver	Photosensitivity, skin rash, cirrhosis
Disorders of carbohydrate metabolism					
Glycogen storage diseases					
Type I (von Gierke)	AR	Glucose-6-phosphatase deficient or ineffective	Glycogen	Liver, kidney, intestine	Hepatomegaly, hypoglycaemic convulsions, gout, liver cell tumours
Type II (Pompe)	AR	Lysosomal α-1,4-glucosidase (acid maltase)	Glycogen	Generalized	Cardiomegaly, hypotonia, respiratory failure
Type III (Forbes Cori)	AR	Amylo-1-6-glucosidase (debrancher enzyme)	Dextrin-like	Liver, muscle, leucocytes	Variable, hepatomegaly, hypoglycaemia, muscle weakness, infections
Type IV (Andersen)	AR	α-1,4,-Glucan: α-1,4-glucan-6-glycosyl transferase (brancher enzyme)	Amylopectin-like	Generalized	Hepatosplenomegaly and ascites due to cirrhosis, hypotonia, anaemia
Type V (McArdle)	AR	Muscle phosphorylase	Glycogen	Muscle	Painful muscle cramps on exercise, myoglobinuria
Type VI (Hers)	AR	Liver phosphorylase	Glycogen	Liver	Hepatomegaly
Type VII (Tarui)	AR	Phosphofructokinase	Glycogen	Muscle	Painful muscle cramps on exercise, myoglobinuria
Type VIII	XR	Phosphorylase kinase	Glycogen	Liver, brain	Hepatomegaly, progressive brain damage, early death
Galactosaemia	AR	Galactose-1-phosphate uridyl transferase, galactokinase, epimerase	Galactonate, galactitol, galactose-1-phosphate	Liver, kidney, lens	Diarrhoea, vomiting, liver failure, mental retardation, cataracts
Hereditary fructose intolerance	AR	Fructose-1-phosphate aldolase or 1,6-diphosphatase	(Fructose, uric acid, lactate)	Liver, kidney, intestine	Vomiting, hypoglycaemia, hepatomegaly, liver failure, convulsions
Glycoprotein and glycolipid storage disorders					
Mucopolysaccharidoses					
Type I (Hurler)	AR	Specific lysosomal enzymes responsible for metabolism of dermatan sulphate, heparan sulphate, and keratan sulphate, singly or in combination	Dermatan sulphate, heparan sulphate, keratan sulphate	Generalized	Mental retardation; involvement of bone, joint, eye, ear, skin common; cardiovascular malfunction and respiratory insufficiency frequent; liver, spleen may be enlarged; most forms display characteristic clinical features, e.g. dwarfism, gargoyle-like facies; they are all progressive but severity of effects vary
Type II (Hunter)	XR				
Type III (Sanfilippo)	AR				
Type IV (Morquio)	AR				
Type V (Scheie)	AR				
Type VI (Maroteaux-Lamy)	AR				
Type VII (Sly)	AR				

Abbreviations: A, autosomal; X, X-linked; D, dominant; R, recessive; ACD, acquired.

Table 17.7 (*cont.*)

Disease	Inheritance	Defect	Metabolite stored (mishandled or deficient)	Organ involved	Manifestations
Mucolipidoses: Types I–IV	AR	Multiple defects in lysosomal acid hydrolases	Mucopoly-saccharides and lipids	Generalized	Clinical manifestation and tissue changes similar to those seen in the mucopolysaccharidoses
α-Antitrypsin deficiency	AR or ACD	Inability of liver cells to release enzyme	α-1-Antitrypsin	Liver, lung	Neonatal 'hepatitis', cholestatic jaundice, cirrhosis, liver cell carcinoma, panacinar emphysema
Disorders of amino acids					
Phenylketonuria	AR	Phenylalanine hydroxylase	(Phenylalanine)	Brain	Mental retardation, convulsions, eczema
Alkaptonuria (ochronosis)	AR	Homogentisic acid oxidase	(Phenylalanine, tyrosine)	Connective tissue, joints	Arthritis
Tyrosinaemia	AR	Fumaryl acetoacetate hydrolase or tyrosine amino transferase	(Tryosine)	Liver, kidney	Type I: liver failure, liver cell carcinoma, renal tubular dysfunction Type II: mental retardation, corneal changes, hyperkeratoses
Cystinosis	AR	? Lysosomal transport defect	L-Cystine	Kidney, eye, lymph nodes, bone marrow, viscera	Renal failure, corneal opacities
Homocystinuria	AR	Cystathione synthetase and others metabolizing methionine	Homocysteine, methionine	Brain, eye, bones, blood-vessels	Mental retardation, ectopia lentis, bony abnormalities, thromboembolic phenomena
Hereditary oxalosis	AR	Excessive synthesis of oxalic acid	(Oxalic acid)	Kidney, liver, spleen many viscera, bone	Progressive renal failure
Lipid storage disorders Gangliosidoses					
GM1: infantile, juvenile, and adult forms	AR	Lysosomal acid β-galactosidase	GM1 ganglioside	Liver, spleen, kidney, heart, brain, and eye	Infantile: hepatosplenomegaly, rapid neurological decline to early death, multiple bony abnormalities. Juvenile: mainly neurological manifestations, spasticity, ataxia, convulsions, death in first decade of life. Adult: progressive cerebellar symptoms, not fatal
GM2: infantile (Tay–Sachs and Sandhoff), juvenile, and adult forms	AR	Lysosomal hexosaminidase A or B or both	GM2 ganglioside	Liver, spleen, kidney, heart, brain, and eye	Infantile (Tay–Sachs): psychomotor retardation, blindness, megalocephaly; (Sandhoff): similar Juvenile: ataxia, rigidity, convulsions Adult: similar but less rapidly progressive
Fabry disease	XR	Lysosomal α-galactosidase A	Glycosphingolipids, mainly ceramide trihexoside	Body fluids and most viscera, predilection for vascular endothelium	Angiokeratomas in skin and mucous membranes, cerebral vascular disease, myocardial infarction, renal failure
Metachromatic leucodystrophy (infantile, juvenile, and adult forms)	AR	Lysosomal arylsulphatase A	Galactosyl sulphatide	Brain, kidney, gall bladder	Dementia, paralysis, incontinence

Abbreviations: A, autosomal; X, X-linked; D, dominant; R, recessive; ACD, acquired.

Disease	Inheritance	Defect	Metabolite stored (mishandled or deficient)	Organ involved	Manifestations
Gaucher disease	AR	Lysosomal glucocerebrosidase	Different forms of glucocerebroside (glucosyl ceramide)	Reticuloendothelial cells in liver, spleen, bone marrow, nerves in children	Adult type is chronic with hepatosplenomegaly and bone lesions; infantile and juvenile types are acute or subacute, and neurological symptoms predominate
Globoid cell leucodystrophy (Krabbe disease)	AR	Lysosomal galactosylceramidase	Galactosylceramide	Brain, peripheral nerves	Demyelination with characteristic 'globoid' cells in white matter leads to psychomotor distrubances, blindness, deafness, paralysis, and early death
Niemann–Pick disease (types A–E)	AR	Lysosomal sphingomyelinase	Sphingomyelin	Liver, spleen, bone marrow, lung, brain	Hepatosplenomegaly, mental retardation, convulsions, anaemia, blindness
Wolman disease, cholesterol ester storage disease (CESD), and cerebrotendinous xanthomatosis (CTX)	AR	Lysosomal acid lipase (Wolman, CESD), mitochondrial C27 steroid 26-hydroxylase (CTX)	Cholesterol esters and triglycerides (Wolman, CESD), cholesterol and cholestanol (CTX)	Liver, spleen, bone marrow, lymph nodes, intestine (Wolman, CESD), brain, and nerves (CTX)	Wolman disease: hepatosplenomegaly, adrenal calcification, death in infancy CESD: hepatomegaly, premature atherosclerosis in adult life CTX: dementia, cataracts, xanthomas
Refsum syndrome	AR	Phytanic acid α-hydrolase	Phytanic acid	Brain, nerves, eye, liver, kidney	Manifestations are variable and mainly neurological with visual and hearing defects
Diseases of metal storage					
Idiopathic haemochromatosis	AR	Unknown	Iron	Liver, pancreas, myocardium, endocrine organs	Cirrhosis, liver cell carcinoma, diabetes, cardiac failure, hypogonadism
Wilson disease	AR	Unknown	Copper	Brain, eye, liver, kidney	Liver disease, progressive brain damage, corneal rings, renal failure, heamolytic anaemia
Disorders of bilirubin metabolism					
Unconjugated hyper-bilirubinaemia syndromes					
Crigler–Najjar disease Types I and II	AR	Bilirubin UDP-glucuronyl-transferase is absent or reduced	(Bilirubin conjugation defective or fails completely)	Blood, brain	Type I: severe jaundice due to unconjugated hyperbilirubinaemia, death in infancy or childhood from kernicterus. Type 2: mild jaundice and/or neurological symptoms in adult life
Gilbert syndrome	AD	Bilirubin UDP-glucuronyltransfer-ase is reduced	(Bilirubin conjugation impaired)	Blood	Mild, episodic jaundice
Conjugated hyper-bilirubinaemia syndromes					
Dubin–Johnson syndrome	AR	Impaired hepatocellular secretion of conjugated bilirubin	(Conjugated bilirubin, porphyrin)	Blood, liver	Chronic or intermittent jaundice; pigmented liver
Rotor syndrome	AR	Impaired hepatocellular secretion of conjugated bilirubin	(Conjugated bilirubin, porphyrin)	Blood	Chronic or intermittent jaundice, normal liver

Table 17.7 (*cont.*)

Disease	Inheritance	Defect	Metabolite stored (mishandled or deficient)	Organ involved	Manifestations
Benign recurrent intrahepatic cholestasis	?	?	(Bilirubin and bile acids)	Blood, liver	Recurrent attacks of cholestatic jaundice and pruritus
Byler disease	AR	? Defective canalicular bile acid transport	(? Lithocholic acid)	Liver	Progressive liver failure
Miscellaneous					
Cystic fibrosis (mucoviscidosis)	AR	Cell membrane transductance protein	(Systemic secretory defect)	Pancreas, lung, intestine, liver, gall bladder, genital tract	Steatorrhoea, chronic obstructive lung disease, meconium ileus, biliary cirrhosis, gallstones, infertility
Myoclonus epilepsy (Lafora disease)	AR	Unknown	Abnormal poly glucosan inclusions	Brain	Grand mal convulsions, myoclonus, dementia
Cerebro-hepato-renal syndrome of Zellweger	AR	Defects of phospholipid biosynthesis	(Peroxisomal and mitochondrial function)	Brain, bone, soft tissues, liver, heart, kidney, pancreas	Characteristic facies, mental retardation, convulsions, hypotonia, hepatomegaly, cardiovascular anomalies, renal cysts

Abbreviations: A, autosomal; X, X-linked; D, dominant; R, recessive; ACD, acquired.

subgroups according to the site of origin of the abnormal metabolite, which may be the liver or the bone marrow. The hepatic porphyrias include acute intermittent porphyria and porphyria cutanea tarda, both of which are uncommon; variegate porphyria (virtually confined to South Africa) and hereditary coproporphyria, are also rare. The erythropoietic porphyrias are erythropoietic protoporphyria, which is uncommon, and congenital erythropoietic porphyria, which is rare. Inheritance is thought to be autosomal dominant in all but the last named, which is autosomal recessive. All the porphyrias, except acute intermittent porphyria, are associated with photosensitivity. All the hepatic porphyrias manifest neurological symptoms: colicky abdominal pain, intestinal pseudo-obstruction, peripheral neuropathy, as well as psychiatric disturbances; these are often precipitated by barbiturates, oral contraceptives, or alcohol, which induce hepatic haem synthesis. Anaemia occurs only in congenital erythropoietic porphyria and is due to haemolysis of damaged red cells.

Liver pathology

Liver involvement occurs in three of the porphyrias, as listed in Table 17.7. The changes in acute intermittent porphyria and porphyria cutanea tarda are similar and include deposition of fat and iron, abnormalities of mitochondria, fibrosis, and cirrhosis. Hepatocellular carcinoma may be a late complication. Needle-shaped crystals, which are birefringent under polarized light, are seen in liver cells in porphyria cutanea tarda. The most severe liver damage, however, is seen in erythropoietic protoporphyria. The liver is macroscopically black, due to the accumulation of a dense, dark-brown pigment in Kupffer cells, canaliculi, and portal tracts (Fig. 17.98) which is birefringent

with a characteristic Maltese-cross pattern and shows intense red autofluorescence. This pigment is most likely protoporphyrin. Electron microscopy shows a radiating 'star burst' pattern of numerous slender crystals. Gallstones may also develop. Cirrhosis is a common but late complication.

Hepatic porphyria-like syndromes are sometimes seen in patients suffering from alcoholic liver disease, cirrhosis, and hepatocellular carcinoma.

17.9.4   Glycogen storage diseases

Inherited defects of the many enzymes involved in the synthesis and degradation of glycogen give rise to a wide range of clinical manifestations, but chiefly involve the liver and muscle. Their prevalence varies from 1 in 100 000 to 1 in 500 000 live births. All those listed in Table 17.8 are autosomal recessive conditions, except Type VIII which is X-linked. Further types, i.e. IXa, b, c, X, 0, and multiple enzyme defects in the same individual, have also been described. They are all characterized by the accumulation of normal or abnormal glycogen in cells of affected organs, chiefly the liver (Fig. 17.99).

Type I glycogenosis (von Gierke disease)

This is the commonest form of glycogenosis. It can be further subdivided into type Ia, in which glucose-6-phosphatase is grossly deficient, and type Ib, in which there is a defect in transport, probably through the cell membrane, of the same enzyme. The two subtypes are, however, clinically indistinguishable. Hepatomegaly is detectable at birth and hypoglycaemic convulsions occur in the neonatal period. Stunted growth is noticeable

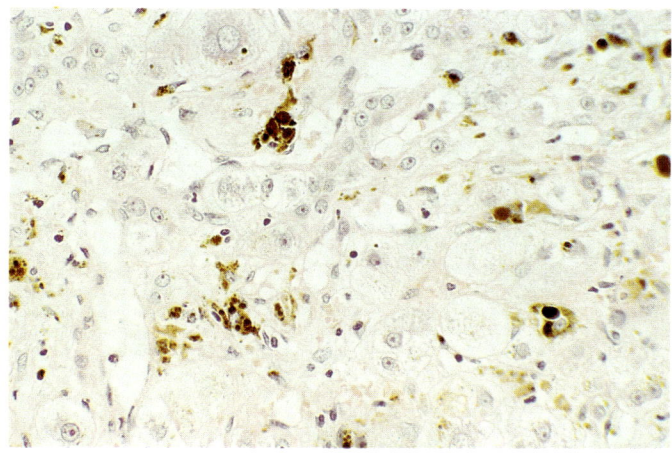

Fig. 17.98 Erythropoietic protoporphyria. Grossly disorganized liver cell plates contain swollen hepatocytes separated by sinusoids. Dark-brown deposits of pigment are shown in canaliculi and Kupffer cells. The patient died at the age of 46 from hepatic failure due to cirrhosis.

by one year of age. Obesity, skin xanthomas, a bleeding tendency, proneness to infection, and gout develop in time as affected children progress towards adulthood. Some patients ultimately develop multiple hepatocellular adenomas or, rarely, carcinoma. Frequent glucose feeds have some effect on symptoms and successful liver transplantation has been reported.

Laboratory investigations show periodic hypoglycaemia, chronic lactic acidosis and elevated levels of transaminases, cholesterol, fatty acids, triglycerides, and uric acid.

Large quantities of glycogen accumulate in the liver and kidneys, which become greatly enlarged, and in intestinal mucosa. Hepatocytes are uniformly swollen and show a 'regular mosaic' pattern with a clear cytoplasm in routine sections (Fig. 17.100). This swelling is due to large amounts of glycogen, which can be confirmed by periodic acid-Schiff stain or Best's carmine (preferably on material fixed in alcohol) and by electron microscopy. Cytoplasmic lipid vacuoles are usually also present. Histochemistry demonstrates the absence of glucose-6-phosphatase in the classical type Ia but near normal activity in type Ib. Renal tubular and intestinal mucosal epithelium show similar appearances.

Type II glycogenosis (Pompe disease)

This disease may first develop in infancy, childhood, or adult life. The infantile form corresponds to the classical entity described by Pompe and is characterized by massive cardiomegaly and hypotonia. Cardiorespiratory failure usually results in death during the first year of life. Children present with a muscular dystrophy-like disease and adults with weakness of limbs. Liver disease is not a feature in any of these forms. Lymphocytes and muscle fibres (skeletal, cardiac, and smooth muscle) show glycogen-filled vacuoles in lysosomes. The cause is deficiency of 1,4-glucosidase (acid maltase) in all organs, but the variability in the severity of manifestations is unexplained.

Type III glycogenosis (Forbes disease, Cori disease)

There are six subtypes of this disease identified by various combinations of enzyme deficiency in liver and muscle. The result is an abnormal glycogen molecule which has excessive numbers of branching points. This accumulates in liver, muscle, and leucocytes. The manifestations are somewhat similar to those of

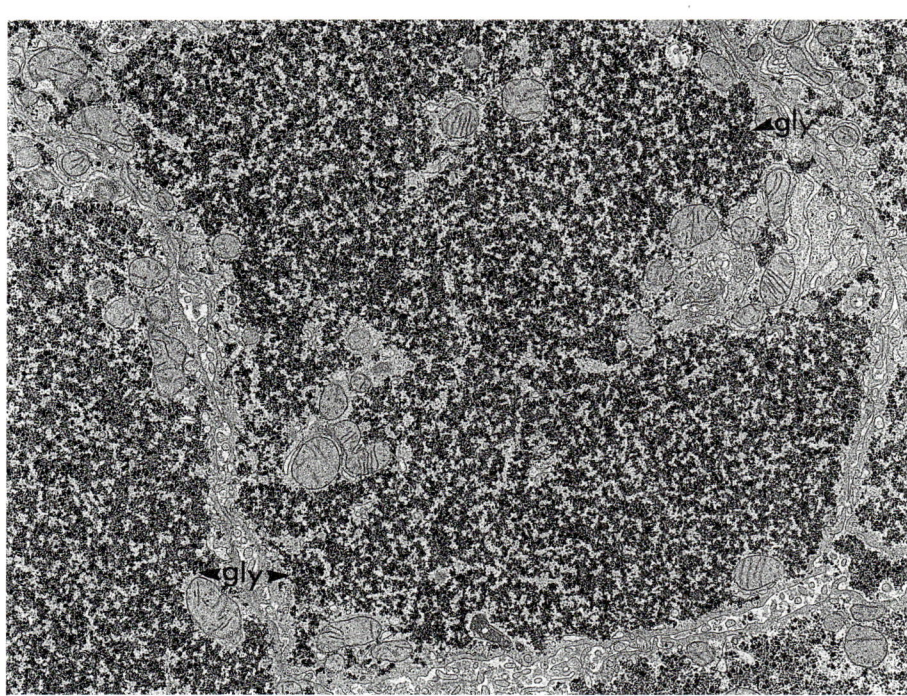

Fig. 17.99 Glycogen storage disease. The patient was a 3-year-old girl with massive hepatomegaly. Note the vast amounts of glycogen deposits (gly) which displace organelles to the margins of liver cells. (Courtesy of Professor M. J. Phillips, University of Toronto.)

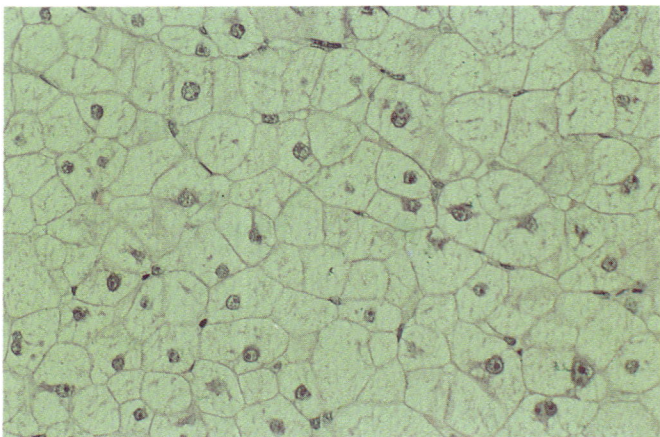

Fig. 17.100 Type I glycogenosis (von Gierke disease). Hepatocytes are uniformly swollen with centrally placed nuclei and a clear cytoplasm from which glycogen has leached out during fixation in aqueous form-alin. Note the regular mosaic pattern characteristic of this disease.

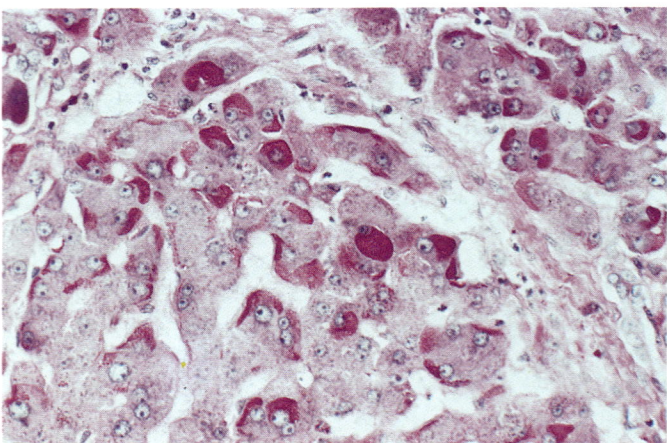

Fig. 17.101 Type IV glycogenosis (Andersen disease). Liver cells contain large cytoplasmic inclusions of bright purple colour.

type I but the onset is later in childhood, hypoglycaemia is rarely severe, and lactic acidosis does not occur. The histological appearance of the liver is also similar to type I but fibrosis is more likely and cirrhosis may develop. Many patients survive into adulthood.

Type IV glycogenosis (Andersen disease)

This disease is characterized by the generalized deposition of large abnormal glycogen molecules with decreased branching points, reminiscent of the amylopectin found in starch. Patients present early in infancy with failure to thrive, hepatospleno-megaly, hypotonia, anaemia, and osteoporosis. Death usually results from cirrhosis. Liver cells contain large cytoplasmic inclusions which stain with periodic acid-Schiff reagent, Best's carmine, and Lugol's iodine (Fig. 17.101). Similar inclusions, however, may also be seen in myoclonus epilepsy (Lafora disease) and following cyanamide administration. The three types of inclusion can be distinguished by electron microscopy.

Type V glycogenosis (McArdle disease)

Skeletal muscle only is affected in this condition. Symptoms do not usually develop until the late teens or early twenties. Physical activity is reduced by painful muscle cramps. Myo-globinuria, severe enough to cause renal failure, may follow strenuous exercise. The normal rise in venous lactate after muscle exercise fails to occur and muscle cells contain an in-creased amount of glycogen. Liver disease is not a feature of this disorder.

Type VI glycogenosis (Hers disease)

In this condition only the liver is affected. Hepatomegaly and growth retardation are the presenting features but serious dis-turbance of liver function does not develop and patients survive into adulthood. The microscopic appearances of the liver are

similar to those in type I disease but the outline of hepatocytes produces an 'irregular mosaic' pattern.

Type VII glycogenosis (Tarui disease)

The manifestations of this disease are identical to those of Type V.

Type VIII glycogenosis

This is the only X-linked recessive form of glycogenosis and is therefore only seen in males. The clinical picture is one of hypo-tonia, hepatomegaly and progressive brain damage which results in death during childhood. Deactivation of the phosphorylase system is responsible for the accumulation of glycogen in liver and brain.

17.9.5 Galactosaemia

'Classical' galactosaemia is due to deficiency of galactose-1-phosphate uridyl transferase. This results in the accumulation of galactonate, galactitol, and galactose-1-phosphate in the liver, kidneys, lens, and other organs. The prevalence is 1 in 62 000 live births. All the clinical manifestations are directly related to the ingestion of galactose which leads to failure to thrive, diarrhoea, vomiting, liver failure, a bleeding tendency, albuminuria, cataracts at an early age, and mental retardation. A diet low in galactose alleviates most symptoms. The diagnosis is suggested by the finding of galactose in blood or urine and is confirmed by the demonstration of the enzyme deficiency in peripheral blood cells.

Liver biopsy shows fatty change, cholestasis, and bile-duct proliferation in the early stages, followed by pseudoglandular transformation of liver cell plates, fibrosis, and cirrhosis as time goes on (Fig. 17.102). The identity of the metabolite that is responsible for liver and brain toxicity is not known, but galacti-tol is thought to be the cause of cataracts.

Absence of galactokinase leads to a mild disease characterized by juvenile cataracts. Its prevalence is 1 in 100 000 live births.

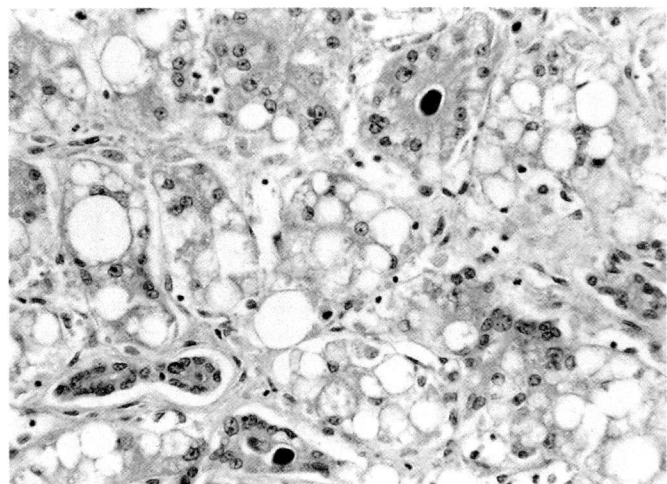

Fig. 17.102 Galactosaemia. Advanced changes of fatty vacuolation, bile-duct proliferation, pseudoglandular transformation of liver cell plates, bile plugs in canaliculi, and diffuse fibrosis with loss of sinusoids.

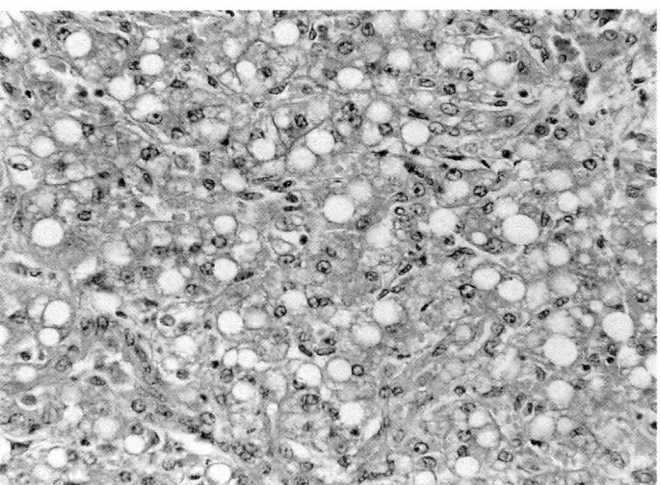

Fig. 17.103 Hereditary fructose intolerance. This shows a fairly non-specific picture seen in many inborn metabolic disorders. There is fatty change, some disorganization of liver cell plates, and diffuse fibrosis.

The third form of galactosaemia is due to epimerase deficiency. Seven variants have been described, and all are rare. The clinical course is generally benign.

17.9.6 Hereditary fructose intolerance

The usual cause of this disease is deficiency of fructose-1-phosphate aldolase, of which three types are known. Absence of A leads to muscle involvement, B to liver disease, and C to brain damage. It is commonest in Switzerland, where it occurs in 1 in 32 000 live births, and is uncommon elsewhere. Deficiency of fructose-1,6-diphosphatase is rare but the effects are serious. Essential fructosuria, due to deficiency of fructokinase is a benign condition.

Symptoms are precipitated by ingestion of fructose and depend on the age at which fructose is first introduced into the diet. In infants below six months of age there is vomiting, jaundice, convulsions, and they soon develop hepatomegaly and liver failure. Laboratory investigations reveal fructosaemia, fructosuria, hypoglycaemia, lactic acidosis, hyperuricaemia, and aminoaciduria. After six months of age, the symptoms and biochemical abnormalities are less severe. An intravenous fructose tolerance test and demonstration of the enzyme defect establish the diagnosis. Patients remain healthy on a fructose-free diet.

Structural changes in the liver include a neonatal hepatitis-like syndrome with giant cell transformation, fatty change, and fibrosis, the latter appearances being rather similar to those seen in galactosaemia or tyrosinaemia (Fig. 17.103). True cirrhosis is rare, but acute hepatic necrosis may occur. Ultrastructural changes include characteristic concentric membraneous arrays of the smooth endoplasmic reticulum, irregular lucent areas ('fructose holes'), and increased numbers of cytolysosomes.

17.9.7 Glycoprotein and glycolipid storage diseases

The mucopolysaccharidoses and mucolipidoses are uncommon or rare generalized disorders with variable clinical manifestations.

Mucopolysaccharidoses

The group comprises seven different disorders, each with its own set of distinctive clinical features. Their prevalence varies from 1 in 24 000 to 1 in 150 000 live births, but only a handful of examples are known of type VII. All are autosomal recessive conditions except type II, which is X-linked. They represent generalized, single or combined, deficiencies of lysosomal enzymes responsible for the metabolism of glycosaminoglycans (mucopolysaccharides), namely dermatan sulphate, heparan sulphate, and keratan sulphate. The result is the accumulation of incompletely degraded forms of these in various organs, usually in macrophages. They are also excreted in the urine. The enzyme deficiency in each type of mucopolysaccharidosis can be demonstrated in white blood cells and in skin fibroblasts in culture. All but type IV show characteristic bony changes known as dysostosis multiplex. Joint stiffness, corneal opacity, deafness, hirsutism, cardiovascular and respiratory problems, and hepatosplenomegaly are common. Death commonly occurs in childhood but some survive to adulthood.

Type I (Hurler, Scheie, and Hurler–Scheie syndromes)

This is the prototype disorder in this group. It is characterized by early development of a coarse, gargoyle-like facies (Fig. 17.104), dwarfism, hepatosplenomegaly, cardiovascular disease, corneal opacity, and severe mental retardation. Death usually occurs by 10 years of age.

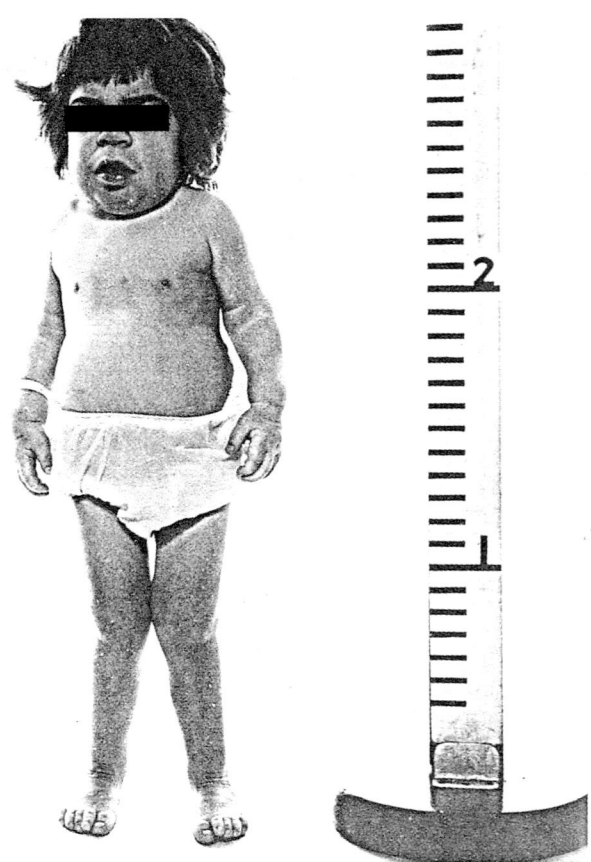

Fig. 17.104 Mucopolysaccharidosis, type I (Hurler syndrome). The patient was a 3-year-old girl. Note the coarse, 'gargoyle'-like facies, swollen abdomen, and grossly stunted growth. (Courtesy of Dr A. H. Fensom, Guy's Hospital, London.)

Type II (Hunter syndrome)

This, too, is a serious disorder. It only affects boys. Failure to thrive, mental deficiency, a coarse facies, joint contractures, hepatosplenomegaly, and deafness are the usual manifestations by 2–4 years of age.

Type III (Sanfilippo disease)

Four different enzyme defects are known but the clinical manifestations are the same. Mental retardation, coarse features, and hepatosplenomegaly develop in childhood and few patients survive to adult life.

Type IV (Morquio syndrome)

The predominant feature is a multiplicity of skeletal abnormalities. Damage to the spinal cord is common and atlanto-axial subluxation may cause paralysis and death. Mental impairment is absent or minimal.

Type V (Scheie syndrome)

This is now classified under Type I, alone or in combination.

Type VI (Maroteaux–Lamy syndrome)

The clinical picture is similar to type I but is less severe.

Type VII (Sly syndrome)

This is exceedingly rare. It is, again, rather similar to type I. Pulmonary infections are singularly common.

The light microscopic and ultrastructural changes in the mucopolysaccharidoses are similar and they cannot be distinguished by morphology alone. The stored material is leached out by aqueous fixatives such as formalin and special care is required in handling biopsies. All tissues and organs in the body are affected in the form of lysosomal inclusions, which can be demonstrated by the colloidal iron method and digested away by hyaluronidase. On electron microscopy, aggregates of electron-lucent material are seen in lysosomes. Neuronal degeneration, 'pseudoatherosclerosis', and liver cirrhosis are frequently found at autopsy.

Mucolipidoses

This is a group of closely related disorders of lysosomal acid hydrolases (glycosidases, sulphatases, cathepsins). They are all rare. Four types are known at present: a Hurler syndrome-like condition; I-cell disease (so-called after the inclusions seen in fibroblasts); one resembling Maroteaux–Lamy syndrome; and an extremely rare form confined to Ashkenazi Jews. The basic defect in these disorders is in the enzyme pathway that phosphorylates mannose residues in newly synthesized acid hydrolyses, and this leads to their functional failure. Connective tissues are primarily affected and cultured skin fibroblasts have proved to be very useful for elucidating the biochemical defects. All four types of mucolipidosis are inherited in an autosomal recessive manner.

Clinical manifestations include mental retardation, gargoyle-like facies, dysostosis multiplex, corneal opacity, and hepatosplenomegaly. Death occurs in childhood or early adult life.

The main histopathological findings are vacuolation of fibroblasts, liver and Kupffer cells, renal tubular epithelium, and peripheral nerves. Electron microscopy shows both fibrillogranular material and lipid droplets or membranous lamellae. Thus, some similarity is seen both to the mucopolysaccharidoses and the gangliosidoses.

17.9.8   α-1-Antitrypsin (AAT) deficiency

AAT deficiency is one of the commonest forms of inherited metabolic disease amongst Caucasians, with an estimated prevalence of 1 in 3500 live births. The enzyme is the major component (approximately 90 per cent) of α-1-globulin in the serum. It is a single polypeptide which is produced by the parenchymal cells of the liver. It is secreted by them into the bloodstream at a rate sufficient to maintain a concentration of 1.5–2.0 g/l. AAT is an acute-phase reactive protein that inhibits a variety of proteases, including trypsin, chymotrypsin, plasmin, and thrombin. Its most specific function, however, is directed against neutrophil polymorph elastase, a broad-spectrum protease capable of degrading most structural proteins in the extracellular matrix of the body. Thus, AAT protects tissues against injury. Affected individuals produce AAT normally and the profound deficiency in serum (10–15 per cent of normal) results from the inability of the liver cells to release it. In some populations the fault lies in a single amino-acid substitution, namely lysine for glutamic acid, in the AAT molecule, but mutations elsewhere in AAT have similar clinical consequences. The clinical effects are pulmonary emphysema in adults and liver disease in both children and adults. The reasons for the localization of damage to just these two organs are unknown.

Phenotypes

The pattern of inheritance of AAT deficiency is complex and some 33 genotypic variants are known. These form the basis of the Pi (protease inhibitor) system which was initially worked out by starch gel electrophoresis of serum and, more recently, by isoelectric focusing and the use of monoclonal antibodies. Variants are designated according to their relative mobility on electrophoresis as F (fast), M (intermediate), S (slow), or Z (very slow), or as subtypes of these and as abbreviations of the city where the discovery was made. A single autosomal allele is inherited from each parent. Most combinations express a normal phenotype, i.e. a normal level of AAT in the serum. The commonest is PiMM which is present in 80–90 per cent of the population. An abnormal phenotype is usually associated with PiZ and may be inherited in a recessive (PiZZ) or a codominant (PiMZ, PISZ, etc.) pattern. The former is much more likely to be associated with disease. Severe deficiency of AAT and organ involvement are also seen in Pi null individuals (Pi − −) and in those who are hemizygotes for PiZ and Pi − (PiZ −). Treatment is now possible by replacement therapy using purified AAT from pooled normal plasma and by liver transplantation which corrects the phenotype to that of the normal donor.

Liver disease in infancy and childhood

Large-scale population studies carried out in Sweden suggest that the majority (approximately two-thirds) of infants who have a genotype that includes PiZ develop some form of liver impairment. The manifestations vary from asymptomatic abnormalities of liver function tests to clinically evident disease. Neonatal cholestatic jaundice is the commonest presentation and, if it persists beyond 6 months of age, it is likely to lead to cirrhosis, liver failure, and death during childhood (see also Section 17.2). The rate of progress is variable but only 25 per cent are thought to recover. Chronic liver disease may also present during childhood or adolescence in the absence of a history of prolonged jaundice in infancy but this is much less common.

The differential diagnosis includes various forms of neonatal hepatitis as well as biliary 'atresia'. Liver biopsy shows gross histological cholestasis, portal fibrosis, and bile duct proliferation. AAT globules in the cytoplasm of liver cells may be difficult to demonstrate up to 6 months of age by the periodic acid-Schiff technique, but they are detectable by immunological methods and by electron microscopy. Older children present

with hepatosplenomegaly, ascites, or bleeding from oesophageal varices, and may be labelled as having chronic active hepatitis or 'cryptogenic' cirrhosis. AAT globules are usually demonstrable by all special methods and the true diagnosis should not be missed. Recovery at this stage has not been documented.

The genotype should always be identified, not only for the confirmation of the diagnosis but also for the purposes of genetic counselling.

Liver disease in adults

Estimates of the risk of liver disease in adults with an abnormal phenotype, i.e. a low serum level of AAT, vary with the sensitivity of the methods used, but the most recent studies, particularly from Sweden, indicate that it is significant. Liver disease in adults is not associated with emphysema. Patients are older than those with lung involvement and usually present in the sixth decade of life, or even later, with hepatosplenomegaly, ascites, and varices. A history of persistent neonatal jaundice is rarely obtained. The level of alcohol consumption, infection with hepatitis viruses, or exposure to hepatotoxic agents such as halothane do not seem relevant. Liver biopsy shows cirrhosis with large amounts of AAT in a conspicuous globular form in the cytoplasm of hepatocytes near fibrous septa. These are visible even in routinely stained sections as pale pink bodies and stain intensely with the periodic acid-Schiff reagent and by enzyme-labelled antibodies against AAT (Figs 17.105, 17.106). Electron microscopy also readily demonstrates dilated sacs of endoplasmic reticulum filled by moderately electron-dense, finely granular, or homogeneous material (Fig. 17.107) that can be identified as AAT by immunoperoxidase or immunogold labelling. Hepatocellular or cholangiocellular carcinoma may develop, usually in males and not in females. The magnitude of this risk is in dispute but it may be as high as 30 per cent in those with established cirrhosis. Curiously, neoplastic liver cells do not contain AAT globules.

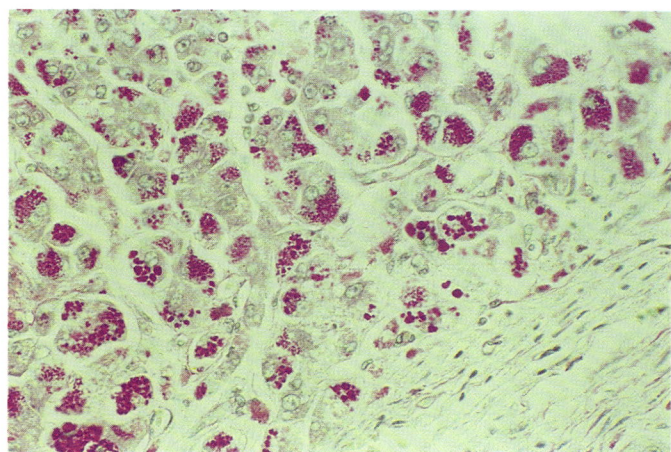

Fig. 17.105 α-1-Antitrypsin deficiency in an adult of PiZZ phenotype. The liver is cirrhotic and large, purple, PAS-positive globules are seen in the cytoplasm of hepatocytes, particularly near fibrous septa.

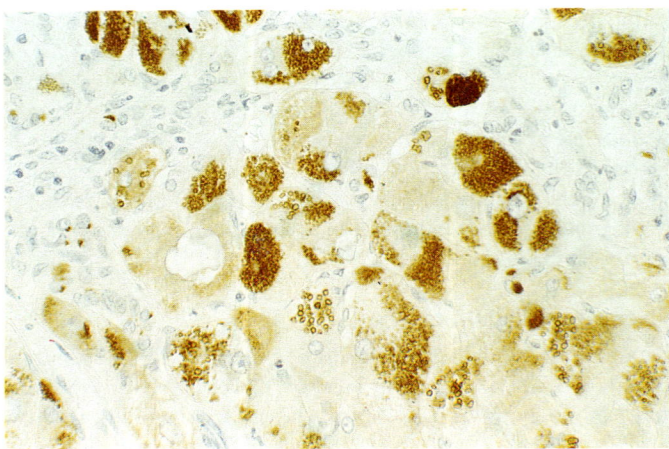

Fig. 17.106 The nature of the globules as α-1-antitrypsin is confirmed by an enzyme-labelled antibody technique which produces a brown-coloured reaction product.

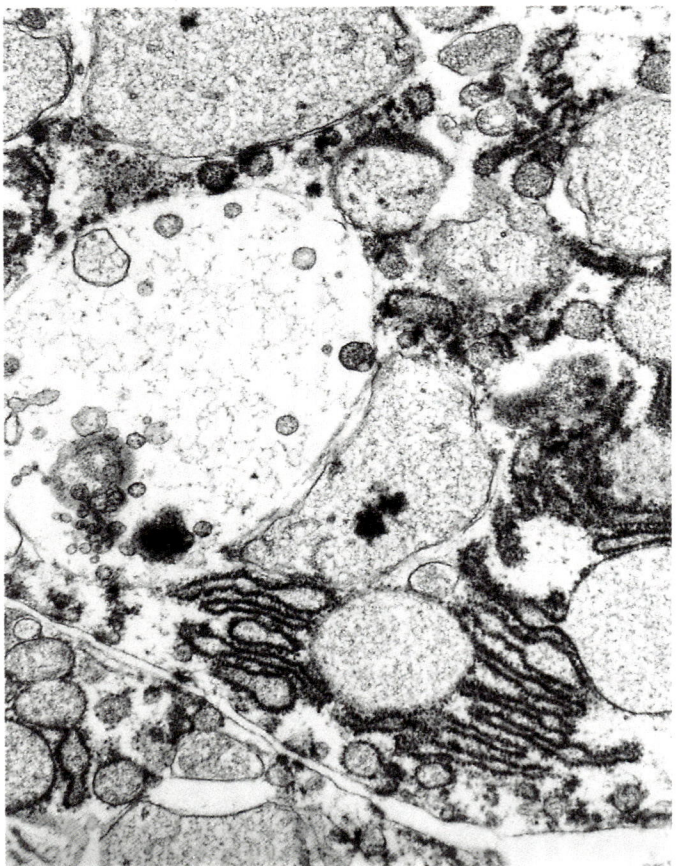

Fig. 17.107 α-1-Antitrypsin deficiency. The endoplasmic reticulum of liver cells is distended by large, finely granular material which corresponds to the globules seen on light microscopy. Specimen obtained at autopsy.

In summary, disease of the lung and liver is a significant risk in PiZ individuals but the variability in age at presentation, the dissociation of emphysema from cirrhosis, and the absence of both in many cases constitute an unresolved mystery.

17.9.9 Disorders of amino acids

A large number of conditions have been described under this heading, comprising 24 major groups, most of which have multiple subtypes. Table 17.8 lists six of the commoner disorders and those that are associated with liver disease are discussed below.

Tyrosinaemia

There are two main forms.

Type I

This has a prevalence of 1 in 100 000 live births. The main deficiency is that of fumaryl acetoacetate hydrolase, which leads to accumulation of tyrosine precursors in the liver and kidneys. Acute and chronic manifestations are known. The former are mainly due to liver disease. There is failure to thrive with vomiting, diarrhoea, hepatosplenomegaly, a tendency to haemorrhage, and infections. Death occurs from liver failure by 1 year of age. The chronic manifestations are growth retardation, multiple renal tubular defects, rickets, episodes of acute intermittent porphyria, and liver disease. Death usually occurs during the first decade of life.

Laboratory investigations show elevated levels of tyrosine, hypoglycaemia, aminoaciduria, phosphaturia, and albuminuria.

The microscopic changes in the liver are similar to those seen in galactosaemia and hereditary fructose intolerance, namely fatty change, cholestasis, pseudoglandular transformation of hepatic cell plates, fibrosis, and cirrhosis. Approximately one-third of patients who survive beyond 2 years of age develop hepatocellular carcinoma.

Type II (Richner–Hanhart syndrome)

This is due to deficiency of tyrosine aminotransferase. It is rare. The liver and kidneys are not affected. The most constant features are corneal changes, erosions of the palms and soles, and hyperkeratoses. Mental retardation occurs sometimes.

Cystinosis

This disorder occurs in 1 in 100 000 live births. It is characterized by the accumulation of cystine crystals in many sites, including the eye, kidneys and cells of the reticuloendothelial system, including Kupffer cells. Three clinical forms are recognized.

Nephropathic (infantile) cystinosis

This has been the one most thoroughly studied. Renal involvement predominates. The characteristic features are the tubular defects of Fanconi syndrome, vitamin-D-resistant rickets, chronic acidosis, crystal deposits in the conjunctiva and cornea, depigmentation of the retina, severe growth retardation, and, ultimately, death from renal failure in the first decade of life. Renal transplantation has been successful in prolonging survival.

Late onset (intermediate or adolescent) cystinosis

This is a milder form of the disease with survival into the second decade of life.

Benign cystinosis

Accumulation of cystine is minimal and patients have a normal life expectancy. Cystine deposits are readily recognizable by microscopic examination of biopsies from conjunctiva, liver, kidney, lymph nodes, or bone marrow. They are best visualized by polarized light or phase contrast in unstained frozen sections or in sections fixed in alcohol, where they appear as rectangular or hexagonal crystals, usually in macrophages such as the Kupffer cells of the liver (Fig. 17.108). Electron microscopy is a useful adjunct in cases where no crystals can be seen by light microscopy.

Cystinosis must be distinguished from *cystinuria*, a relatively common autosomal recessive disorder (prevalence 1 in 7000 live births) whose only clinical manifestation is urinary tract calculi, and from the serious condition of *homocystinuria*.

Hereditary oxalosis (primary hyperoxaluria)

This comprises two rare disorders, types I and II, with different enzyme defects but similar clinical manifestations. There is overproduction of oxalic acid in both, with hyperoxaluria and recurrent calcium oxalate stones in the urinary tract, which lead to renal failure in early adult life. Oxalosis is unsuitable for treatment by renal transplantation as recurrences develop rapidly. Oxalate crystals accumulate in many tissues (including liver) but the kidneys are the only organs that suffer damage. They appear as round or rhomboid crystals arranged in rosette-like formations and are brilliantly birefringent when viewed by polarized light.

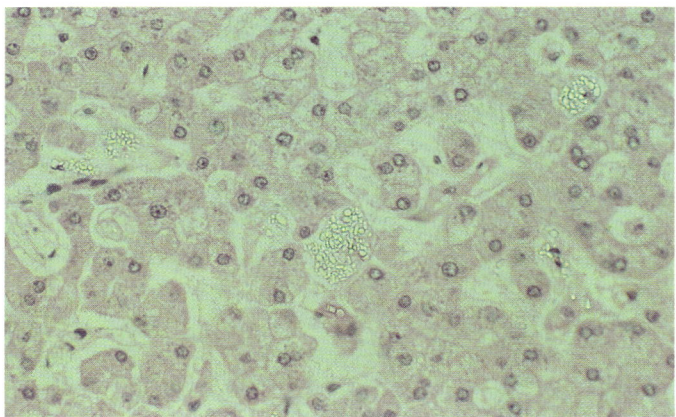

Fig. 17.108 Cystinosis. Brightly refractile crystals of cystine are shown in the Kupffer cells of the liver.

17.9.10 Lipid storage disorders

These disorders generally result from deficiencies of lysosomal enzymes that are responsible for the metabolism of complex lipids. Inheritance is autosomal recessive in all of them except in Fabry disease, which is a sex-linked condition. They are generally rare except in communities such as Ashkenazi Jews amongst whom there is a high rate of consanguinous marriages.

The gangliosidoses

Gangliosides are sialidated glycosphingolipids that are mainly found in neurones. Brain involvement therefore predominates in this group of disorders.

GM1 gangliosidoses

This group includes patients with acute onset of symptoms in infancy and rapid decline to death at one end of the spectrum, and normal intelligence and survival to adulthood at the other. Acid β-galactosidase exists in several forms, and the differing manifestation of its deficiency may be explained by better or worse residual activity for one substrate than another. All GM1 gangliosidoses are rare.

The infantile form, type I manifests itself during the first 6 months of life, with progressive neurological deterioration leading to blindness, deafness, and decerebrate rigidity, hepatosplenomegaly, multiple bony abnormalities, and 'cherry-red spots' on the retina. Death supervenes by 2 years of age. Foamy histiocytes are seen throughout the reticuloendothelial system. Neurones are ballooned with lipid deposits. Liver cells, renal glomerular and tubular epithelial cells, and myocardial muscle fibres are finely vacuolated. Electron microscopy shows large lysosomes containing finely granular or fibrillary material and, occasionally, concentrically arranged lamellae (Fig. 17.109).

The juvenile form, type II presents at about 1 year of age with ataxia, rigidity, and convulsions. Visceral involvement and bony abnormalities are minimal. Death usually occurs between 3 and 8 years of age.

The chronic adult form, type III is not fatal. Mental development is normal and cerebellar ataxia may be the only symptom.

GM2 gangliosidoses

These, too, are heterogeneous and manifestations vary according to defects in the activity of lysosomal hexosaminidases A, B, or both. They all lead, however, to neuronal damage.

The infantile form exists in two phenotypic variants.

Type I (Tay–Sachs disease) is the most common. The heterozygote frequency is 1 in 30 in Ashkenazi Jews and 1 in 300 amongst Gentiles, producing a 1 in 3000 prevalence rate amongst the former. Both heterozygote identification and prenatal diagnosis are now possible. The common presenting features are psychomotor retardation, megalocephaly, spasticity, paralysis, and convulsions. A typical 'cherry-red spot' is seen in

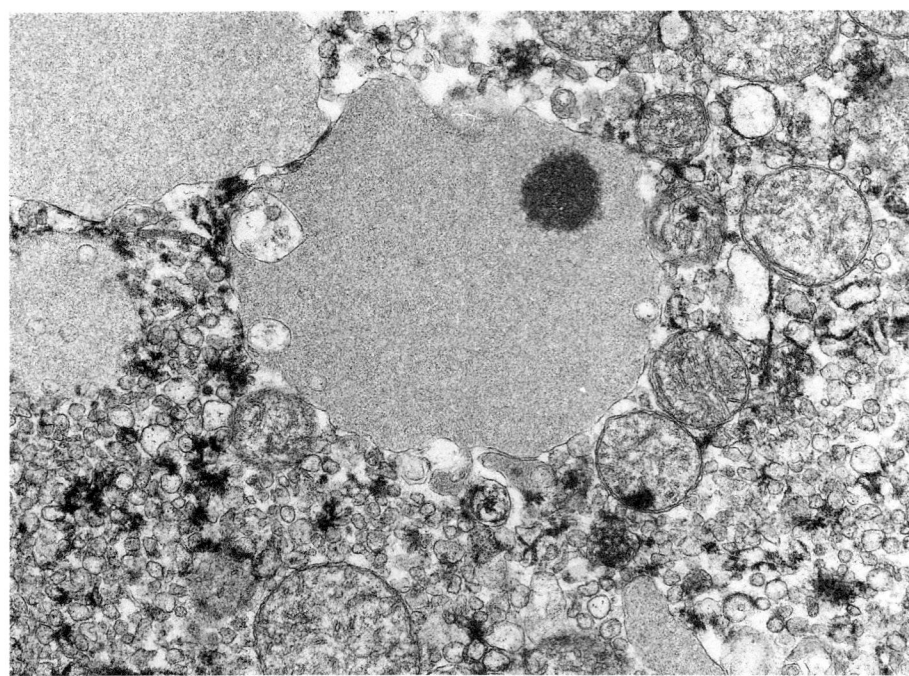

Fig. **17.109** GM1 gangliosidosis. Enlarged lysosomes in a liver cell contain finely granular material with a 'two-tone' appearance. (Courtesy of Professor M. J. Phillips, University of Toronto.)

the macular region of the retina. Blindness soon develops and death occurs by the third year of life.

Type II (Sandhoff disease) also presents in infancy. It shows no ethnic predilection. The clinical features and course are similar to those of Tay–Sachs disease. Lysosomal lipid accumulation is seen in both diseases in neurones, the retina, reticuloendothelial cells, myocardium, and the kidneys. Electron microscopy shows large lysosomal inclusions which contain parallel arrays of densely stained membranes ('zebra' bodies).

Type III The juvenile form follows a more protracted course but severe neurological manifestations develop by the end of the first decade of life. 'Cherry-red spots' are absent and blindness may not develop. The adult form, *type IV*, is less progressive still. These latter two variants are rare.

Fabry disease

This is an X-linked recessive disorder that affects hemizygous males. The prevalence is 1 in 40 000 live births. Heterozygous females are usually asymptomatic but some show an attenuated form of the disease or, rarely, severe symptoms. Affected males present in childhood or adolescence with paraesthesiae and pain in the extremities, cutaneous and mucosal vascular lesions (angiokeratoma corporis diffusum), and corneal opacities. Renal failure, hypertension, myocardial infarction, strokes, and lymphoedema develop later in life and death results from renal or cardiovascular complications. Confirmation of the clinical diagnosis requires the demonstration of deficient α-galactosidase A activity in serum, urine, or leucocytes.

The substance that accumulates in myocardium, liver,

spleen, and other organs is mainly ceramide trihexoside. There is a marked predilection for blood-vessels in all organs. Electron microscopy shows concentrically laminated inclusions in lysosomes.

Metachromatic leucodystrophy

The main manifestations of this disorder are due to demyelination and are mainly neurological in character (see Chapter 25). There are three forms, determined by age of onset. Their total prevalence is 1 in 100 000 live births.

The infantile form is the most common and presents with mental deficiency, paralysis, blindness, and urinary incontinence. Death usually results from infection in early childhood. Those affected by the juvenile form may survive to early adult life and show psychotic behaviour in addition. In the adult form dementia is the predominant feature.

The enzyme deficiency is demonstrable in leucocytes and skin fibroblasts, and large amounts of sulphatides are found in the brain, peripheral nerves, liver, gall bladder, kidneys, and other organs, as well as in the urine. Microscopic examination of tissues shows metachromatic granules in macrophages and parenchymal cells. These are contained in lysosomes and the 'prismatic' ultrastructural appearances are quite characteristic.

Gaucher disease

This was one of the earliest reported inborn metabolic disorders, described clinically in the late nineteenth century. The prevalence is quite high in Ashkenazi Jews, approximately 1 in 2000 live births. Three types are recognized, all of which are due to deficiency of the enzyme, glucocerebrosidase.

Type I (adult or chronic non-neuronopathic) Gaucher disease

This is the classical form. It presents during late adolescence or early adult life with hepatosplenomegaly and, in a minority, with skeletal symptoms such as bone pain, spontaneous fractures, and arthritis. A characteristic expansion of the distal femora (Erlenmeyer flask) is seen on X-ray in about two-thirds of patients. Brownish pigmentation of skin over the lower extremities is a common finding. Neurological signs are rare.

Type II (infantile or acute neuronopathic) Gaucher disease

This is first manifested by neurological signs and later by hepatosplenomegaly.

Type III (juvenile or subacute neuronopathic) Gaucher disease

This presents with gradual mental deterioration.

Types II and III affect Gentiles and are usually fatal but those with the classical type I may survive to old age.

The diagnosis of Gaucher disease may be made by finding typical Gaucher cells in the bone marrow, liver, or spleen, and confirmation is readily obtained by measuring the amount of glucocerebroside in these tissues or by demonstrating deficient enzyme activity in leucocytes or skin fibroblasts. Tartrate-resistant acid phosphatase is elevated in the serum. Detection of heterozygotes and prenatal diagnosis are now possible and bone marrow transplantation has been tried for treatment.

The Gaucher cell is a macrophage loaded with glucocerebroside. It is large, up to 100 μm, with a pyknotic nucleus and abundant, faintly striated or crinkled cytoplasm, best demonstrated with a trichrome or periodic acid-Schiff stain (Fig. 17.110). Intense acid phosphatase activity is usually present. In the liver they may block sinusoidal spaces and compress liver cells, causing their atrophy. Portal hypertension is the result. Electron microscopy shows rod-shaped lysosomal inclusions which, in cross-sections, consist of numerous small tubules. Cells with the same appearance are found in the bone marrow and spleen. The exact mechanism of tissue injury, particularly in the nervous system in Types II and III, is not fully understood.

Globoid cell leucodystrophy (Krabbe disease)

This is a rapidly progressive, invariably fatal disease of infants. The prevalence is 1 in 50 000 live births in Sweden but is much lower elsewhere. The cause is deficient activity of lysosomal galactosylceramidase, the result of which is accumulation of the substrate in the brain, peripheral nerves, and many organs (including liver), but the chief clinical manifestations are due to severe loss of myelin. Affected infants of 3–6 months of age develop irritability, spasticity, peripheral neuropathy progressing rapidly to paralysis, blindness, and deafness. Death usually occurs by 2 years. Diagnosis is possible during life by demonstrating the enzyme deficiency in serum, leucocytes, or cultured skin fibroblasts.

Numerous multinucleated 'globoid' cells are found in the cerebral white matter at autopsy. These are macrophages that

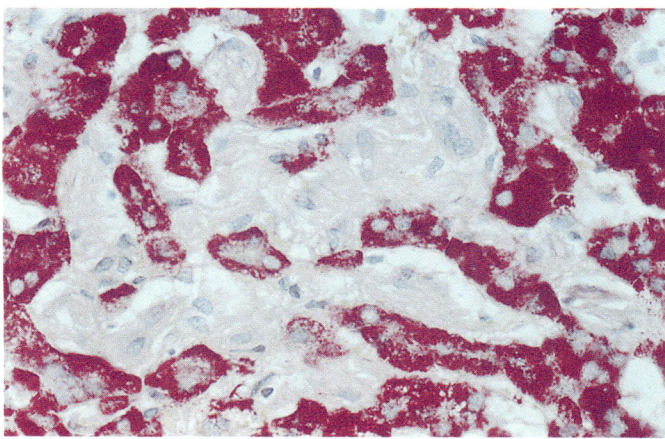

Fig. 17.110 Gaucher disease. Hepatocytes are stained purple due to their glycogen content and Kupffer cells are large and pale (Gaucher cells). The faintly crinkled appearance of the cytoplasm is characteristic. Compare with Fig. 17.111.

contain large amounts of galactosylceramide in lysosomal vacuoles. The cells are periodic acid-Schiff positive. Electron microscopy shows irregularly crystalloid tubular profiles which often have longitudinal striations. Severe myelin loss and gliosis complete the picture.

Niemann–Pick disease

Five types of this disorder are presently recognized, the first three of which occur almost exclusively in Ashkenazi Jews with a prevalence of 1 in 25 000 live births.

Type A

Type A represents the majority of patients. It presents in infancy with severe central nervous system manifestations and hepatosplenomegaly. A 'cherry-red spot' on the retina is seen in about one-third of cases. Anaemia, thrombocytopenia, lung infiltrates, osteoporosis, and a sallow olive discoloration of skin are frequent. Death generally occurs by 4 years of age.

Type B

Type B differs from A by the absence of neurological manifestations, but visceral involvement is extensive. Patients may attain adulthood in reasonably good health.

Type C

Type C shows a more prolonged course than A, but manifests both central nervous system involvement and hepatosplenomegaly. It is usually fatal by the age of 20 years.

Types A, B, and C are all autosomal recessive disorders due to different mutations that impair the activity of lysosomal sphingomyelinase. Affected siblings in the same family always manifest the same type of disease. The diagnosis is made by measuring enzyme levels in leucocytes, skin fibroblasts, or other tissues. Heterozygotes can be recognized and prenatal diagnosis is possible.

Type D

A sphingomyelin lipidosis that occurs in Nova Scotia and in a few Spanish American families has been called type D. It is similar to type C but sphingomyelinase is not deficient.

Type E

Type E refers to occasional adult patients who have been found incidentally with moderate sphingomyelin excess in the liver and spleen but no neurological abnormalities.

The hallmark of Niemann–Pick disease is the presence of large foam cells in the liver, spleen, and bone marrow (Niemann–Pick cells). In the liver, these are Kupffer cells (Fig. 17.111) which progressively increase in number and, at the same time, liver cells also become vacuolated. In time, the two types of cell may become indistinguishable. Electron microscopy shows large, pleomorphic inclusions of lipids, which include sphingomyelin as well as cholesterol and lipofuscin, all enclosed in concentric or parallel lamellae (Fig. 17.112).

Wolman disease, cholesterol ester storage disease, and cerebrotendinous xanthomatosis

These disorders are discussed together as the enzyme deficiencies are not well defined and they may well represent phenotypic variants of the same basic defect of lysosomal acid lipase function. They are, however, clinically different. They are all rare.

Wolman disease

This presents in infancy with failure to thrive, hepatospleno-

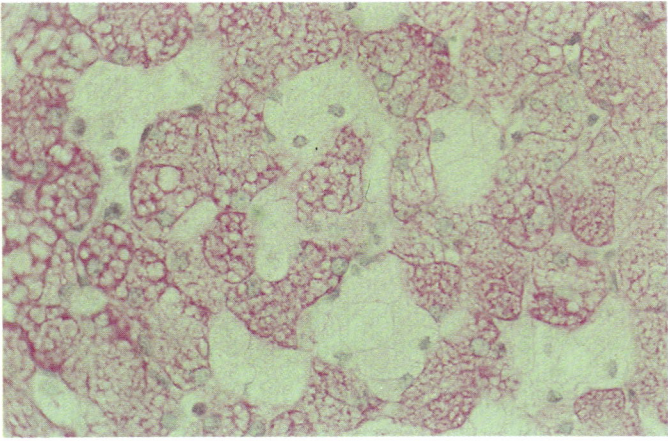

Fig. 17.111 Niemann–Pick disease. Liver cells are vacuolated. Kupffer cells are pale and their cytoplasm appears finely granular (Niemann–Pick cells). Compare with Fig. 17.110.

megaly, and calcified adrenals on X-ray. Death usually occurs by 6 months of age. Cells of the reticuloendothelial system contain large amounts of cholesterol and triglycerides and their acid lipase content is greatly reduced. Fatty change in hepatocytes and cholesterol crystals are evident in Kupffer cells.

Cholesterol ester storage disease

This shows a more benign course. Affected individuals develop early atherosclerosis. Cholesterol in both conditions is best visualized in frozen sections under polarized light, when they appear as birefringent, needle-shaped crystals, or by electron microscopy which also demonstrates lipid droplets of varying density and lipofuscin granules.

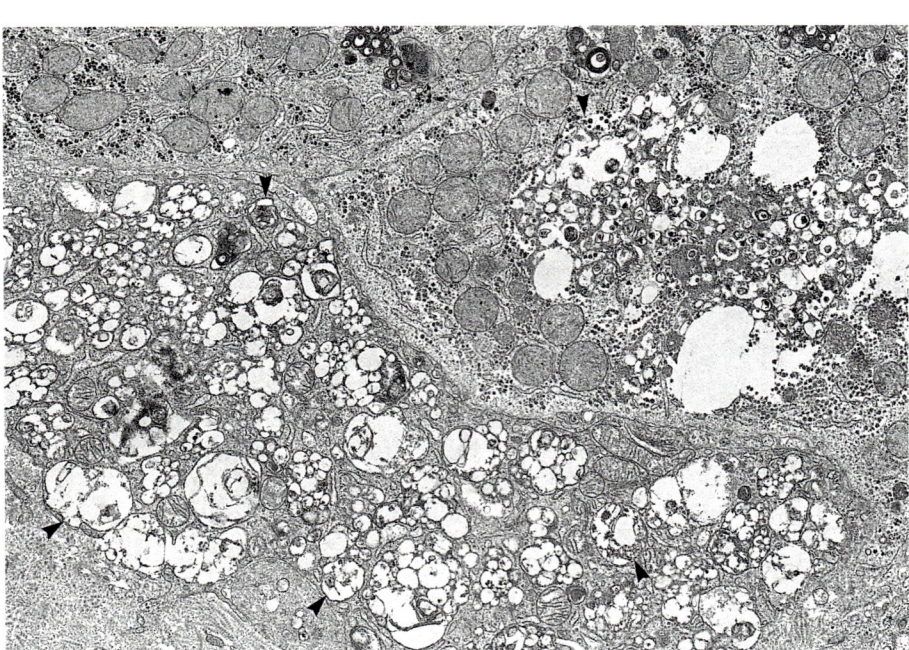

Fig. 17.112 Niemann–Pick disease. Sphingomyelin deposits are indicated by arrowheads. They are composed of concentric lamellae alternating with electron-lucent areas in lysosomes. (Courtesy of Professor M. J. Phillips, University of Toronto.)

Cerebrotendinous xanthomatosis

This condition is manifested by excessive deposition of cholesterol and cholestanol in almost all tissues of the body. Patients develop dementia, cataracts, and skin xanthomas.

These patients have liver biopsies to establish the presumptive diagnosis.

Refsum syndrome

The manifestations of this rare syndrome result from the deposition of exogenous phytanic acid in the central and peripheral nervous systems, including the eye. They include cerebellar ataxia, peripheral neuropathy, and retinitis pigmentosa, as well as deafness and anosmia. Hepatomegaly and skin and bone changes develop in time. The most characteristic pathological finding is hypertrophic neuropathy, as seen in a peripheral nerve biopsy. Treatment with diets low in phytanic acid (the main sources are milk, butter, and bovine fat) brings about a significant improvement in symptoms.

17.9.11   Diseases of metal storage

Idiopathic haemochromatosis and secondary haemosiderosis are dealt with in Section 17.10.

Wilson disease (hepatolenticular degeneration)

Pathogenesis

Wilson disease, first described in 1912, is due to an inborn error of copper metabolism that is transmitted in an autosomal recessive manner. The prevalence is 1 in 100 000 live births. Heterozygotes can now be identified with a reasonable degree of certainty. Copper homeostasis normally depends on a balance between intestinal absorption and biliary excretion. Caeruloplasmin, a protein present in the blood, binds free ionic copper, and one of its probable roles is copper transport from the intestine to the tissues. Copper is an integral component of a number of important enzymes, such as cytochrome oxidase, tyrosinase, and dopamine hydroxylase, and it is essential for health. Free ionic copper, on the other hand, is highly toxic. The exact metabolic defect in Wilson disease is still not known but the effects are. These are a low level of caeruloplasmin in the blood, decreased biliary and increased urinary excretion of copper, and the gradual accumulation of toxic ionic copper in the liver, brain, cornea, and other tissues.

Presentation

The clinical manifestations of Wilson disease vary according to the age of the patient and the stage of the disease. The accumulation of copper begins at birth but symptoms and signs do not appear until the end of the first decade of life. Liver involvement may be manifested in several ways. Acute hepatitis develops in about a quarter of cases and may mimic a viral infection. At its most severe, it may be fulminant, causing death. Chronic hepatitis, usually seen in adolescents, may masquerade as auto-immune chronic hepatitis. Cirrhosis in adult life, however, remains the commonest initial presentation in about half of all cases. Sudden release of ionic copper tends to precipitate haemolytic crises with renal failure, which may complicate any of the above. An important, but late, clinical sign is the appearance of characteristic Kayser–Fleischer rings (which consist of copper) in the cornea. Involvement of the lenticular nuclei of the brain is manifested by involuntary movements, loss of co-ordination, mental deterioration, pseudobulbar palsy, and other neurological signs, which are progressive and ultimately fatal in middle or early old age. Renal tubular dysfunction, osteoporosis, and arthropathy may also develop.

The diagnosis depends on an awareness of the condition. Wilson disease should be considered a possibility in all children and adolescents with liver disease and in adults with symptoms referable to the basal ganglia. Once the condition is recognized, treatment with D-penicillamine is effective but takes time. No single test is pathognomonic, and investigation should include slit-lamp examination of the cornea, measurements of serum copper, caeruloplasmin, urine copper, and a liver biopsy. It is also mandatory to examine all siblings since, if they are affected, they are at risk of an acute and possibly fatal attack of liver disease or haemolytic crisis.

Liver pathology

Liver biopsy in the precirrhotic stage shows fatty change. The nuclei of liver cells appear 'empty' (Fig. 17.113). This is due to the presence of large amounts of glycogen which tends to dissolve in the course of tissue processing.

Kupffer cells often contain haemosiderin which is probably due to subclinical haemolytic anaemia. Increasing amounts of copper accumulate in time (Fig. 17.114).

Changes that are indistinguishable from chronic hepatitis of viral, auto-immune, or other aetiologies may be seen. Fibrosis and, ultimately, cirrhosis develop. The latter is characteristically macronodular (Fig. 17.115). Liver cell carcinoma has been recorded in a few cases. Ultrastructural findings are, in themselves, not diagnostic. Abnormalities of mitochondria

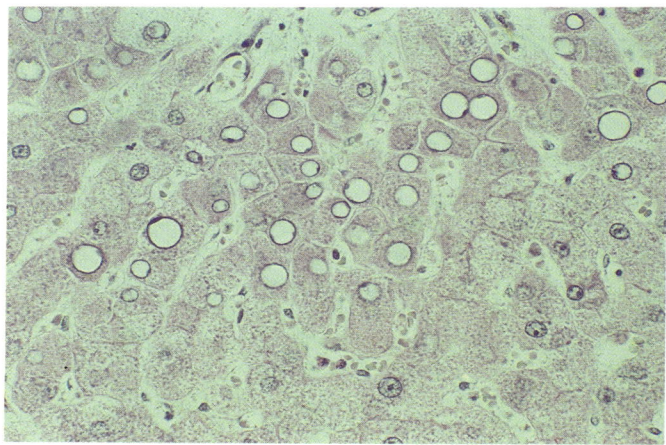

Fig. 17.113 Wilson disease. Empty-looking 'glycogenated' nuclei in hepatocytes.

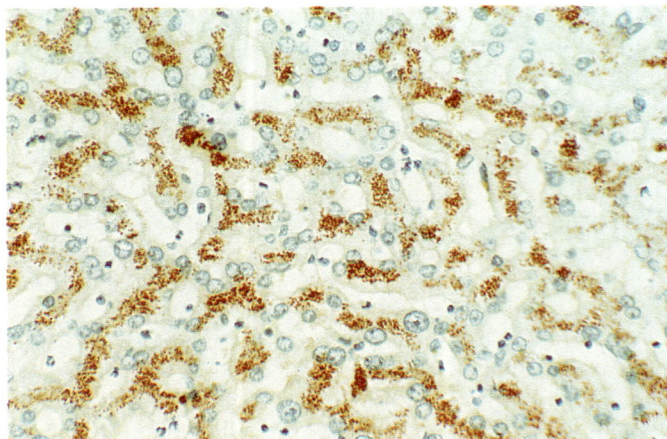

Fig. 17.114 Wilson disease. Orange-brown staining lysosomal copper granules are seen in liver cells.

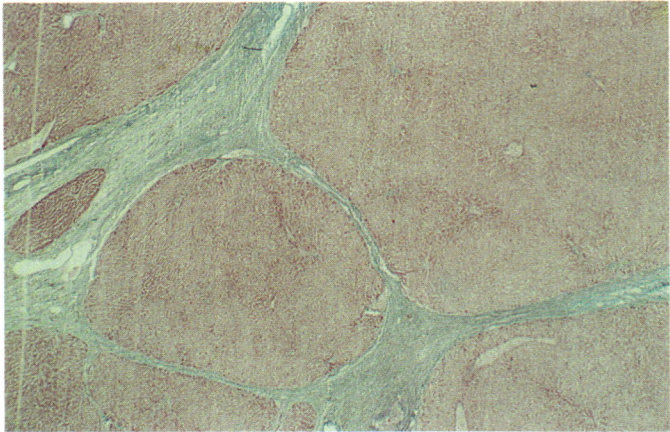

Fig. 17.115 Wilson disease. Macronodular cirrhosis.

predominate and are the most distinctive. They include variability in size and shape, separation of membranes, and the presence of various inclusions. Other alterations include an increased number of peroxisomes, copper, lipofuscin, lipids in lysosomes, and Mallory bodies, which may also be seen by light microscopy.

Menkes disease

This is a rare, sex-linked recessive disorder of copper metabolism that is different from Wilson disease. It probably results from defective absorption of copper from the intestines and is, in effect, a copper deficiency state. Menkes disease presents in infancy with a characteristic facies; kinky, 'steely' hair; hypothermia; jaundice; arterial degeneration; and progressive brain damage that leads to early death.

Indian childhood cirrhosis

This is a progressive, fatal, and sometimes familial, disorder that is largely restricted to Asia. Affected children have normal levels of caeruloplasmin but liver biopsy shows an extremely high concentration of copper in the liver. Fatty change is common and Mallory bodies are numerous. Cirrhosis eventually develops and death results from liver failure in early life.

Finally, quite large amounts of copper may be found in liver biopsies of cirrhosis from any cause but particularly in primary biliary cirrhosis and primary sclerosing cholangitis. These conditions are characterized by progressive destruction of the intrahepatic bile ducts, which results in an inability to excrete a normal dietary intake of copper by the usual biliary route.

17.9.12   Disorders of bilirubin metabolism

Bilirubin is an orange-coloured pigment that is derived mainly from the breakdown of erythrocyte haemoglobin. It is a waste product that is eliminated from the body by the liver through excretion into bile. The essential step is conjugation of water-insoluble bilirubin with mono- and diglucuronic acid, which renders the molecule water soluble. This is effected largely by the enzyme bilirubin UDP-glucuronyltransferase. High levels of free, unconjugated bilirubin are toxic to the brain, particularly in infancy, but conjugated bilirubin is relatively harmless.

Unconjugated hyperbilirubinaemia syndromes

The effects of these vary from the rapidly fatal to the chronic and benign.

Crigler–Najjar disease

This rare disorder exists in two forms.

Type I is due to absence of bilirubin UDP-glucuronyltransferase. It is inherited in an autosomal recessive manner. Affected infants are deeply jaundiced from birth, and severe unconjugated hyperbilirubinaemia leads to toxic damage of immature neurones in the basal ganglia of the brain (kernicterus). Death occurs in infancy.

Type II is a benign disorder in which mild jaundice and/or neurological symptoms may develop in adolescence or adult life. Bilirubin UDP-glucuronyltransferase activity is reduced but the enzyme may be induced by phenobarbitone, and the condition ameliorated.

Liver biopsy in Crigler–Najjar syndrome shows cholestasis only.

Gilbert syndrome

This is a heterogeneous group of benign conditions that are probably inherited in an autosomal dominant manner. The prevalence is 1–2% live births. Impaired hepatic uptake of bilirubin and reduced activity of bilirubin UDP-glucuronyltransferase lead to mild unconjugated hyperbilirubinaemia that is manifested as episodic jaundice. This may be provoked by fasting, which has been claimed to be a diagnostic test for the condition. Liver biopsy shows an increased amount of lipofuscin pigment and/or haemosiderin.

Conjugated hyperbilirubinaemia syndromes

These rare conditions are all benign except Byler disease and its variants, which are fatal.

Dubin–Johnson syndrome ('black liver jaundice')

This autosomal recessive condition is characterized by chronic or intermittent jaundice due to a failure to excrete conjugated bilirubin into bile. There is also an unexplained abnormality of coproporphyrin metabolism. The most important laboratory test for diagnosis is impaired excretion of bromsulphtalein (BSP). The liver is black, due to the accumulation of coarse, dark-brown pigment in the pericanalicular region of hepatocytes where it is contained in lysosomes. The nature and origin of this pigment are unknown. It shares some staining reactions with both melanin and lipofuscin but it is, in fact, neither (Fig. 17.116). The pigment is the result, rather than the cause, of the hepatic excretory defect but it is highly characteristic of the condition.

Rotor syndrome

This benign autosomal recessive condition is clinically similar to Dubin–Johnson syndrome but the liver looks normal and BSP kinetics and coproporphyrin excretion are different.

Benign recurrent intrahepatic cholestasis

This comprises a number of conditions which may be related and do have similar clinical manifestations.

Benign recurrent intrahepatic cholestasis (Summerskill–Tygstrup disease) occurs sporadically or, occasionally, in isolated communities or in families. Episodic jaundice may be quite severe but resolves without any liver damage.

Intrahepatic cholestasis of pregnancy The high prevalence of this condition in certain parts of the world, such as Scandinavia, Poland, and Chile, suggests a hereditary predisposition. Jaundice develops during the last trimester of each pregnancy and may be preceded by pruritus gravidarum, which also

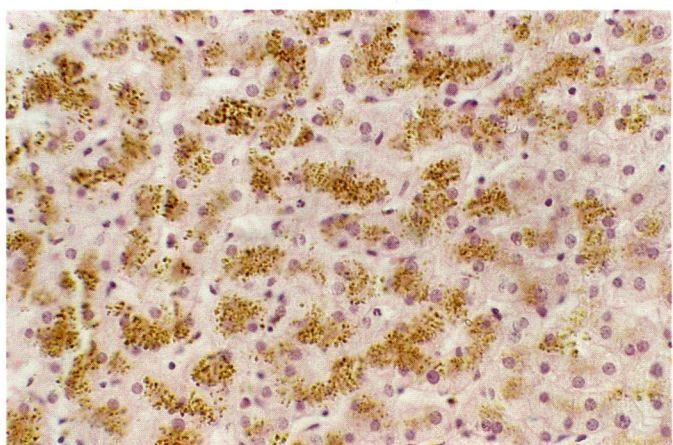

Fig. 17.116 Dubin–Johnson syndrome. Coarse brown granular pigment is present in the pericanalicular region of hepatocytes.

occurs by itself as a variant without jaundice. Vomiting may be severe and prolonged. There is an increased incidence of premature delivery, still birth, and postpartum haemorrhage. The condition promptly resolves after delivery, leaving no ill-effect. Such individuals are also unusually liable to cholestatic jaundice from oral steroid contraceptives.

Familial benign chronic intrahepatic cholestasis This rare form appears to be inherited in an autosomal recessive manner and is associated with abnormalities of skin, hair, nails, and cornea, which suggests a defect in cytokeratin intermediate filament metabolism. It has only been described in Sweden so far.

In all forms of benign cholestasis the liver shows canalicular plugs of bile during an attack of jaundice but is normal otherwise.

Byler disease

This rare, autosomal recessive disorder progresses to cirrhosis during infancy or early childhood. It was first described in a close Amish community in the United States but it occurs elsewhere. A defect in canalicular bile acid transport has been suggested as the cause. The liver shows cholestasis, ductular proliferation, and fibrosis. Excess amounts of copper and Mallory bodies may be seen. Somewhat similar conditions have also been described in Norwegian and North American Indian families.

17.9.13   Miscellaneous

A number of hereditary syndromes exist which do not fit easily into a classification. The most important of these by far is mucoviscidosis.

Mucoviscidosis (cystic fibrosis of the pancreas)

The term mucoviscidosis is perhaps more appropriate than cystic fibrosis of the pancreas since other organs are also involved and because it expresses the essence of the disease which is the secretion of abnormally viscid mucus by all glandular epithelia. Mucoviscidosis is the commonest inherited disease in Caucasians. The prevalence is 1 in 2000 live births and it is inherited in an autosomal recessive manner. The defective gene, on chromosome 7, encodes a cell membrane transductance protein.

Presentation and diagnosis

Mucoviscidosis is characterized by a clinical triad of chronic obstructive lung disease, pancreatic exocrine deficiency, and abnormally high sweat electrolytes, which is present in most patients by adolescence. The earliest presentation is 'meconium ileus' in the neonatal period but this is relatively uncommon. The intestinal tract is filled with a thick, jelly-like material that is adherent to the mucosal surface and causes obstruction. Removal by irrigation may only be partially effective. Perforation and peritonitis may occur and strictures can develop. Exocrine pancreatic insufficiency with steatorrhoea, wasting, and stunting of growth develops in childhood or adolescence.

Chronic obstructive lung disease is manifested at about the same time, with persistent or recurrent infections, caused especially by *Staphylococcus pyogenes* and *Pseudomonas* species. The lung parenchyma is progressively destroyed by infection, bronchiectasis, and fibrosis. As a result, respiratory failure, pulmonary hypertension, and cor pulmonale with congestive cardiac failure are common causes of death. Clinical liver disease develops in only 5–15 per cent of patients but microscopic abnormalities are present in the majority. Gallstones are increasingly frequent in those surviving beyond the first two decades of life. Infertility is common, particularly in males, and is due to atresia of the vasa deferentia.

Laboratory diagnosis depends on the demonstration of an elevated concentration of chloride in sweat. The generally accepted upper limit of normal (up to adolescence) is 60 mmol/l. Values above 50 mmol/l in children and between 60 and 80 mmol/l in adults are suspicious and the test should be repeated. Pancreatic enzymes may be normal in 10–20 per cent of patients but stimulation tests reveal markedly diminished water and bicarbonate secretion. The earliest liver function abnormality is an elevated level of alkaline phosphatase.

Liver pathology

The progression of the disease has been well studied in liver biopsies. Fatty change is frequent and iron may be deposited in liver cells. 'Focal biliary fibrosis', however, is the most characteristic finding and is pathognomonic of mucoviscidosis. Portal tracts are expanded by fibrosis in which cholangioles proliferate. These are dilated and contain plugs of inspissated mucus stained variably with bile (Fig. 17.117). Some of these mucus plugs ultimately develop into concretions. Areas of focal biliary fibrosis join up with the passage of time and a coarse macronodular cirrhosis develops, which may result in death from liver failure and/or the effects of portal hypertension.

Changes in other organs, such as the lung and pancreas, mirror those seen in the liver. Bronchioles and ducts are obstructed by inspissated mucus plugs. The results are infection, rupture of small airways, and destruction of the parenchyma by fibrosis. Treatment of all the manifestations of mucoviscidosis is purely supportive.

Myoclonus epilepsy (Lafora disease)

This rare autosomal disorder starts in adolescence with epileptic fits, followed by myoclonus and mental deterioration. The histopathological hallmark is the presence of distinctive cytoplasmic inclusions (Lafora bodies) in neurones, liver cells, and muscle fibres. They consist of an unusually branched polyglucosan and their appearance and staining reactions are similar to those seen in type IV glycogenosis (Fig. 17.101).

Cerebro-hepato-renal syndrome of Zellweger

Zellweger syndrome is a rare autosomal recessive condition in which the main defects are those of peroxisomal and mitochondrial function, resulting in abnormalities of phospholipid synthesis. A whole variety of congenital abnormalities are present,

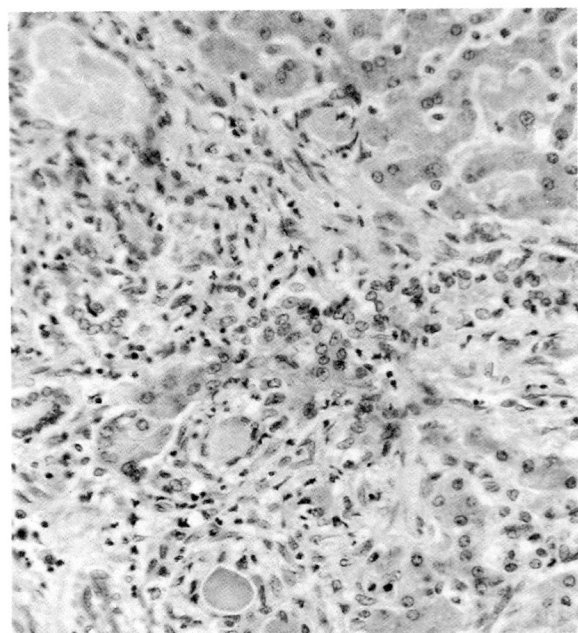

Fig. 17.117 Mucoviscidosis. 'Focal biliary fibrosis' consists of portal tracts expanded by fibrosis in which many bile ducts are present. Some are dilated and contain plugs of thick mucus.

which include a characteristic facies, cerebral dysgenesis, and cardiac, ocular, and genital malformations. Hepatomegaly, renal cysts, and hypotonia are common. Death usually occurs by 6 months of age. Absence of peroxisomes in liver cells and abnormal mitochondria are the characteristic ultrastructural findings.

17.9.14 Acquired metabolic disorders

These are numerous and only some, namely those affecting the liver, are described briefly below.

Reye syndrome

The syndrome of 'encephalopathy and fatty degeneration of the viscera' was described 25 years ago in Australia and many cases have been reported since then from all parts of the world. The disease occurs almost exclusively in children and is usually preceded by a viral infection, particularly influenza B or varicella. Initial symptoms are lethargy, confusion, and vomiting. The liver is not enlarged and jaundice does not develop. Laboratory tests show hypoglycaemia, hyperammonaemia, and hypoprothrombinaemia. Neurological symptoms predominate, coma develops, and death ensues unless steps are taken to correct the metabolic abnormalities and to reduce cerebral oedema. Early diagnosis is essential and the liver biopsy changes are pathognomonic in the appropriate clinical setting. Hepatocytes are swollen and are packed with tiny lipid vacuoles that are so small that they may only be demonstrated by special stains, such as Oil Red O, or by osmication. Necrosis and inflammation are rarely seen. Electron microscopy shows gross abnormalities of mitochondria. Microvesicular fatty change, similar to that seen in the liver, is present in many organs at autopsy.

Reye syndrome resembles other diseases, such as inheritable urea cycle defects and acute fatty liver of pregnancy, as well as drug reactions and toxicity syndromes associated with tetracycline, aflatoxin, margosa oil, valproic acid, and, indeed, aspirin. Many of these children have been given various drugs, including salicylates, for the preceding viral illness and for vomiting. There is increasing circumstantial evidence for a role of aspirin which is now considered inappropriate and dangerous for the symptomatic treatment of viral infection in childhood. It is unlikely, however, that aspirin is directly responsible for the condition.

Kwashiorkor

The term in the Ga language of the Gold Coast of Africa means 'red boy' but the name varies in different parts of the world. It is widely prevalent in tropical countries. Children are most commonly affected 6–18 months after weaning when they are fed a carbohydrate diet that is adequate in calories but is deficient in protein. This is catastrophic at a time when the growing body of the child requires a high intake. The hair is depigmented, thin, and soft; the skin shows a dusky red, flaky appearance (hence the name); and the liver is often enlarged. This is due to the accumulation of vast amounts of neutral lipid in hepatocytes, which take on the appearance of fat cells. Necrosis, inflammation, or fibrosis do not develop. The pancreas, thymus, lymph nodes, muscle, and salivary glands atrophy. Normal immune responses are depressed and children commonly die of intercurrent viral infections, malaria, or tuberculosis. All features of kwashiorkor rapidly regress on adding protein to the diet, most often skimmed milk, and there are no sequelae.

Diabetes mellitus and obesity

The main structural alterations are seen in the microvasculature of the retina, kidney, and the peripheral nervous system, but the disease affects many organs, including the liver. Fatty change is seen and is common, particularly in type II diabetes of adults, and its extent seems related to the degree of accompanying obesity. Liver cell nuclei appear empty, due to a large amount of glycogen in them. Liver cell necrosis and inflammation may develop and mimic alcoholic hepatitis. Cirrhosis is 2–3 times more frequent in diabetics than in the rest of the population. Fatty change, hepatitis, and fibrosis may also be seen in obese people, mainly middle-aged or elderly and female, in the absence of overt diabetes.

Intestinal bypass operations

Rapid weight loss observed after major intestinal resections led to the practice of jejuno-ileal or jejuno-colic shunt operations in the treatment of gross obesity. Enthusiasm has waned for these procedures as it soon became evident that serious liver disease was a frequent complication. Fatty change is universal after surgery; hepatitis, which again resembles that due to alcohol, develops in 10–15 per cent, and cirrhosis, hepatic failure, and

death may follow. The metabolic base of liver disease after intestinal shunt operations is complex. Many nutrients, including amino acids, are poorly absorbed, bile salts pass to the colon instead of being reabsorbed by the small intestine, and bacteria grow in the excluded segment.

Parenteral nutrition

Liver disease is increasingly being recognized in critically ill patients on prolonged intravenous feeding regimens of any kind. Cholestatic jaundice is the most frequent manifestation in infants and may proceed to fibrosis and cirrhosis in a few months. Factors that are likely to play a part are duration of therapy, prematurity, and sepsis. Adults are less likely to suffer serious liver damage. Fatty change is common, cholestasis is rare, and fibrosis is mild. Complete recovery is the rule in most cases.

17.9.15 Further reading

General

Antonarakis, S. E. (1989). Diagnosis of genetic disorders at the DNA level. *New England Journal of Medicine* **320**, 153–63.

Bianchi, L., Gerok, W., Landmann, L., Sickinger, K., and Stalder, G. A. (1983). *Liver in metabolic diseases*. MTP Press, Lancaster.

Holton, I. (ed.) (1987). *The inherited metabolic diseases*. Churchill Livingstone, Edinburgh.

Ishak, K. G. (1986). Hepatic morphology in the inherited metabolic diseases. *Seminars in Hepatology* **6**, 246–58.

Ishak, K. G. (1990). Pathology of inherited metabolic disorders. In *Pediatric hepatology* (ed. W. F. Balistreri and J. T. Stocker), pp. 77–158. Hemisphere, New York.

Ishak, K. G. and Sharp, H. L. (1987). Metabolic errors and liver disease. In *Pathology of the liver* (2nd edn) (ed. R. N. M. MacSween, P. P. Anthony, and P. J. Scheuer), pp. 99–180. Churchill Livingstone, Edinburgh.

Phillips, M. J., Poucell, S., Patterson, J., and Valencia, P. (1987). *The liver: an atlas and text of ultrastructural pathology*, Chapter 5, pp. 239–391. Raven Press, New York.

Stanbury, J. B., Wyngaarden, J. B., Fredrickson, D. S., Goldstein, J. L., and Brown, M. S. (1983). *The metabolic basis of inherited disease* (5th edn). McGraw-Hill, New York.

Porphyrias

Bengtsson, N. O. and Hardell, L. (1986). Porphyrias, prophyrins and hepatocellular cancer. *British Journal of Cancer* **54**, 115–17.

Elder, G. H. (1986). Metabolic abnormalities in the porphyrias. *Seminars in Dermatology* **5**, 88–98.

Lefkowitch, J. H. and Grossman, M. E. (1983). Hepatic pathology in porphyria cutanea tarda. *Liver* **3**, 19–29.

MacDonald, D. M., Germain, D., and Perrot, H. (1981). The histopathology and ultrastructure of liver disease in erythropoietic protoporphyria. *British Journal of Dermatology* **104**, 7–17.

Glycogen storage disorders

Greene, H. L. (1982). Glycogen storage disease. *Seminars in Liver Disease* **2**, 291–301.

McAdams, A. J., Hug, C., and Bove, K. E. (1974). Glycogen storage disease, types I to X. Criteria for morphologic diagnosis. *Human Pathology* **5**, 463–87.

Fructose intolerance

Odievre, M., Gertil, C., Gautier, M., and Alagille, D. (1978). Hereditary fructose intolerance in childhood. *American Journal of Diseases of Children* **132**, 605–8.

Glycoprotein and glycolipid disorders

Callahan, J. W. and Lowden, J. A. (eds) (1981). *Lysosomes and lysosomal storage disease*. Raven Press, New York.

van Hoof, F. (1974). Mucopolysaccharidoses and mucolipidoses. *Journal of Clinical Pathology* **27** (Suppl. 8), 64–93.

α-1-Antitrypsin deficiency

Eriksson, S., Carlson, J., and Velez, R. (1986). Risk of cirrhosis and primary liver cancer in alpha-1-antitrypsin deficiency. *The New England Journal of Medicine* **314**, 736–9.

Fagerhol, M. K. and Cox, D. W. (1981). The Pi polymorphism: genetic, biochemical and clinical aspects of human alpha-1-antitrypsin. *Advances in Human Genetics* **11**, 1–62.

Garver, R. L., *et al.* (1986). Alpha-1-antitrypsin deficiency and emphysema caused by homozygous inheritance of non-expressing alpha-1-antitrypsin genes. *The New England Journal of Medicine* **314**, 762–6.

Sharp, H. L. (1984). Alpha-1-antitrypsin: an ignored protein in understanding liver disease. *Seminars in Liver Disease* **2**, 314–27.

Sveger, T. (1978). Alpha-1-antitrypsin deficiency in early childhood. *Pediatrics* **62**, 22–5.

Amino-acid disorders

Carson, J. A. J., Biggart, J. D., and Bittles, A. H. (1976). Hereditary tyrosinaemia. *Archives of Disease in Childhood* **51**, 106–13.

Hardwick, D. F. and Dimmick, J. E. (1976). Metabolic cirrhosis of infancy and early childhood. In *Perspectives in paediatric pathology*, Vol. 3 (ed. H. S. Rosenberg and R. P. Bolande). Year Book Medical Publishers, Chicago.

Morris, M. C., Chambers, T. L., Evans, P. W. G., Malleson, P. N., Pincott, J. R., and Rose, G. A. (1982). Oxalosis in infancy. *Archives of Disease in Childhood* **57**, 224–8.

Seegmiller, J. E. (1973). Cystinosis. In *Lysosomes and storage diseases*, (ed. H. G. Hers and F. van Hoof), pp. 485–518. Academic Press, New York.

Lipid storage disorders

Brady, R. O. and King, F. M. (1973). Gaucher's disease. In *Lysosomes and storage diseases* (ed. H. G. Hers and F. Van Hoof), pp. 381–93. Academic Press, New York.

Brady, R. O. and King, F. M. (1973). Niemann–Pick disease. In *Lysosomes and storage diseases* (ed. H. G. Hers and F. van Hoof), pp. 439–52. Academic Press, New York.

Brady, R. O. and King, F. M. (1975). Fabry's disease. In *Peripheral neuropathy*, Vol. 11 (ed. P. J. Dyck, P. K. Thomas, and E. H. Lambert), pp. 914–27. Saunders, New York.

MacFaul, R., Cavanagh, N., Lake, B. D., Stephens, R., and Whitfield, A. E. (1982). Metachromatic leukodystrophy: review of 38 cases. *Archives of Disease in Childhood* **57**, 168–75.

O'Brien, J. F. (1983). The lysosomal storage diseases. *Mayo Clinic Proceedings* **57**, 192–7.

Petrelli, M. and Blair, J. D. (1971). The liver in gangliosidosis types 1 and 2. *Archives of Pathology* **99**, 111–16.

Copper disorders

Scheinberg, I. H. and Sternlieb, I. (1984). *Wilson's disease*. Saunders, Philadelphia.

Stromeyer, F. W. and Ishak, K. G. (1980). Histology of the liver in Wilson's disease: a study of 34 cases. *American Journal of Clinical Pathology* **73**, 12–24.

Bilirubin disorders

Blanckaert, N. and Schmid, R. (1982). Physiology and pathophysiology of bilirubin metabolism. In *Hepatology, a textbook of Liver Disease*, (ed. D. Zakim and T. D. Boyer), pp. 246–72, Saunders, Philadelphia.

Crigler, J. F. and Najjar, V. A. (1952). Congenital familial nonhemolytic jaundice with kernicterus. *Pediatrics* **10**, 169–79.

De Vos, R., De Woolf-Peeters, C., Desmet, V. J., Egermont, E., and Van Acker, K. (1975). Progressive intrahepatic cholestasis (Byler's disease). *Gut* **16**, 943–50.

Dubin, I. N. and Johnson, F. B. (1954). Chronic idiopathic jaundice with unidentified pigment in liver cells. *Medicine* **33**, 155–97.

Eriksson, S. and Larsson, C. (1983). Familial benign chronic intrahepatic cholestasis. *Hepatology* **3**, 391–8.

Golan, J. L. (ed.). (1988). Pathobiology of bilirubin and jaundice. *Seminars in Liver Disease* **8**, 105–99.

Reyes, H. (1982). The enigma of intrahepatic cholestasis of pregnancy: lessons from Chile. *Hepatology* **2**, 87–96.

Tygstrup, N. (1960). Intermittent possibly familial intrahepatic cholestatic jaundice. *Lancet* **1**, 1171–2.

Cystic fibrosis

Isenberg, J. N. (1982). Cystic fibrosis. *Seminars in Liver Disease* **2**, 302–13.

Oppenheimer, E. H. and Esterly, J. R. (1975). Pathology of cystic fibrosis: review of the literature and comparison with 146 autopsied cases. *Perspectives in Pediatric Pathology* **2**, 241–78.

Park, R. W. and Grand, R. I. (1981). Gastro-intestinal manifestations of cystic fibrosis: a review. *Gastroenterology* **81**, 1143–61.

Reye syndrome

Bove, K. E., McAdams, A. J., Partin, J. C., Partin, J. S., Hug, G., and Schubert, W. K. (1975). The hepatic lesion in Reye's syndrome. *Gastroenterology* **69**, 605–97.

Crocker, J. F. S. (1982). Reye's syndrome. *Seminars in Liver Disease* **2**, 340–52.

Partin, J. S., Daugherty, C. C., McAdams, A. J., Partin, J. C., and Schubert, W. K. (1984). A comparison of liver ultrastructure in salicylate intoxication and Reye's syndrome. *Hepatology* **4**, 687–90.

Diabetes mellitus

Stone, G. B. and van Thiel, D. H. (1985). Diabetes mellitus and the liver. *Seminars in Liver Disease* **5**, 8–28.

Intestinal bypass

O'Leary, J. P. (1983). Hepatic complication of jejuno-ileal bypass. *Seminars in Liver Disease* **3**, 203–15.

Parenteral nutrition

Bower, R. H. (1983). Hepatic complications of parenteral nutrition. *Seminars in Liver Diseases* **3**, 216–24.

17.10 Iron overload of the liver

R. W. Chapman

17.10.1 Introduction

The syndrome of diabetes mellitis, hyperpigmentation, and cirrhosis with iron overload was first discribed by Troisier in 1871. Eighteen years later, the term 'haemochromatosis' was proposed by von Recklinghausen because he believed that the excess pigment was derived from the breakdown of the blood. Haemochromatosis has been used ever since to describe the syndromes of iron overload associated with tissue damage. It refers to a group of disorders of different aetiologies, in which there is a progressive increase in total body iron stores. Excess iron is deposited in the parenchymal cells of the liver, heart, pancreas, and other organs, eventually resulting in cellular damage and functional insufficiency of the organs involved. In the liver, progressive parenchymal iron deposition leads to fibrosis and eventually cirrhosis. The group of disorders that give rise to the clinico-pathological syndrome of haemochromatosis are listed in Table 17.8.

17.10.2 Normal iron metabolism

Iron balance

Iron plays an essential role in a wide variety of metabolic processes in the body. The largest amount is required for haemoglobin synthesis, but all cells have an active iron metabolism and iron forms an integral part of many enzymes and is a cofactor for others. An equilibrium normally exists between the demands of erythropoiesis and those of other tissues, and iron balance is regulated so that there are adequate but not excessive amounts within the body.

The normal adult has a total body iron content of about 4–5 g, of which some 75 per cent is present in haemoglobin and 3 per cent in myoglobin. Apart from small amounts contained within various enzyme systems (10 mg), circulating in plasma and the extracellular fluid attached to transferrin (4 mg), the remainder of the body's iron is stored either as intracellular deposits of soluble ferritin or an insoluble haemosiderin.

Iron balance is unusual in that there is no major excretory pathway for iron. In a balanced state, iron requirements are largely determined by the amount lost from the body. Normally the small obligatory loss due to desquamation from epithelial surfaces, biliary and urinary excretion, and gastrointestinal blood loss amounts to less than 1 mg daily. Menstrual blood loss in women normally averages about 15–20 mg monthly.

Homeostasis is maintained by physiological adjustments of the absorption mechanism so that the amount of iron crossing the small intestinal epithelial barrier is related to internal iron status. Approximately 12 mg of iron daily will compensate for all physiological losses.

Absorption of iron

Iron is absorbed both as haem and non-haem iron. There are three main phases in the absorption of iron from the gut:

1. the intraluminal phase, where food is digested by the gastric and pancreatic enzymes and iron is released in a soluble form;

2. the mucosal phase, in which iron is taken up by the mucosal cell and transported across the cell or retained as ferritin;

3. the corporeal phase, in which iron is taken up by transferrin in plasma on the serosal side of the mucosal cell and carried to the liver and haemopoietic tissues.

Despite intensive investigation, the mechanism by which the body regulates iron absorption by the intestine remains a mystery. Current evidence suggests that the primary control of iron uptake and transport lies within the enterocyte, which is then influenced by other factors such as the amount of ongoing erythropiesis and the total body iron content.

Iron transport and delivery to tissues

The exchange of iron between tissues is mediated by the protein, transferrin. Each molecule can bind two atoms of iron at specific sites on the protein. Transferrin synthesis in man occurs mainly in the liver and the protein is then released into the plasma where it is distributed throughout most of the extracellular fluid. The primary function of transferrin is to transport iron from cells throughout the body where iron is utilized. The most important site of iron delivery is to erythroid cells in the bone marrow. The interaction between transferrin and the erythroid cell involves three main steps: first, binding of the iron-transferrin complex to specific receptors on the erythroid cell; secondly, internalization of the iron–transferrin–receptor complex through the cell membrane; and, thirdly, the iron is released within the cell. Following delivery of the iron, transferrin is released by the recipient cell to recirculate. Specific transferrin receptors have been identified in reticulocyte membranes and in liver cell membranes.

Iron storage

In addition to being the main site of transferrin synthesis, the liver is the major iron storage depot in the body, containing

---

Table 17.8 Classification of hepatic parenchymal iron overload syndromes

Idiopathic haemochromatosis (primary, genetic)
Secondary haemochromatosis
  Anaemia/ineffective erythropoiesis/haemolysis, (e.g. thalassaemia, sideroblastic anaemia)
  Liver disease with secondary iron overload, (e.g. alcohol, porphyria cutanea tarda, porto-caval shunt)
  Excessive iron ingestion/increased absorption, (e.g. Bantu, medicinal iron ingestion)

about one-third of the total body iron content. Within the liver, iron is stored in both the parenchymal cells and the Kupffer cells. Iron is stored as the large soluble protein, ferritin, and also as haemosiderin, a relatively insoluble molecule made up of ferritin aggregates. All cells appear to have the capacity to synthesize ferritin, which has a protective and a storage function. A protective role is required because intracellular free iron is toxic. Small amounts of ferritin circulate in the serum and, in general, the serum ferritin concentration is proportional to body iron stores. The origin and function of serum ferritin is unknown, however.

17.10.3   Pathogenesis of iron overload

Iron overload can arise through two main mechanisms.

1. An increase in body iron stores can occur through an increase in iron absorption. This may arise either through an increase in the amount of dietary iron or through increased absorptive activity by the gut epithelium. It is unclear whether significant iron overload can result in normal individuals from a prolonged increase in dietary iron intake. Although there have been reports of excess oral iron intakes leading to parenchymal liver damage, it is uncertain whether the affected subjects were carrying the idiopathic haemochromatosis gene. In the condition known as 'Bantu siderosis', South African blacks develop iron overload, caused by drinking large amounts of native or 'kaffir' beer. This concoction, brewed in iron pots, contains massive amounts of iron in combination with alcohol, which in itself has effects on iron metabolism.

In primary or idiopathic haemochromatosis (IHC) the absorption of iron by the enterocyte is inappropriately high and over many years iron stores insiduously increase. The mherited defect in iron regulation in IHC is unknown but probably lies within the enterocyte. Excess iron absorption also occurs in disorders of erythropoiesis, particularly conditions with ineffective erythropoiesis such as thalassaemia major and sideroblastic anaemia. The iron overload is made worse in these conditions by the need for frequent blood transfusions in order to maintain haemoglobin concentrations. An additional factor, which may worsen liver damage in these patients, is the high prevalence of viral hepatitis, both hepatitis B and C.

2. Parenteral iron administration also results in iron overload. This can be produced either by repeated blood transfusions or by multiple injections of iron preparations. The excess iron is first processed by the reticuloendothelial (RE) system before being made available to other tissues. The iron is initially stored in the RE system as haemosiderin, which is less harmful than parenchymal iron loading where tissue damage occurs at an earlier stage.

Various degrees of iron overload occur in different types of chronic liver disease, such as in cirrhotic patients after a portocaval shunt operation, and in alcoholic liver disease. The mechanism of iron overload is often unclear in these patients and may be multifactorial. The amounts of excess iron are seldom high enough, however, to merit treatment.

Iron toxicity

The direct role of excess iron in producing the pathological changes of acute iron toxicity is not disputed. However, the pathogenesis of the tissue damage observed in chronic iron overload has remained a controversial topic for many years.

The hepatic lesion of acute iron toxicity seen in humans, viz. periportal fat deposition leading to frank necrosis of liver cells, can be reproduced in experimental animals. The body of evidence suggests that in such cases the iron acts as a metabolic poison. In constrast, the difficulty in chronic iron overload was that until recently there was a lack of direct experimental evidence to support the widely held concept that chronic iron overload produces tissue damage. However, there is strong circumstantial clinical evidence based on several observations. First, in chronic iron overload there is an association between both the localization and degree of iron deposition and the development of fibrosis. Secondly, the removal of excess iron produces a clinical and histopathological improvement in both primary and secondary haemochromatosis.

Intracellular mechanisms of tissue damage in iron overload

Despite intensive investigation, the intracellular mechanisms by which iron causes tissue damage is unknown. Research has been hindered by the lack of animal experimental models for haemochromatosis. A number of studies over the past decade, however, have suggested possible mechanisms by which iron may produce cellular damage and fibrosis. Ultrastructural and biochemical studies suggest a role for the lysosome in the pathogenesis of tissue damage. Reduced stability of lysosomal membranes, associated with increased haemosiderin deposition, has been demonstrated in liver biopsies from patients with both primary and secondary iron overload. Lysosomal integrity was restored after iron removal by phlebotomy. It was proposed that the progressive accumulation of haemosiderin that occurs in haemochromatosis (up to values one-hundredfold above normal) is responsible for disrupting the lysosome and releasing cell-damaging enzymes into the cytosol.

An alternative hypothesis for iron toxicity is that intracellular membrane damage is initiated by peroxidative degradation of membrane lipids. Recently, levels of hepatic iron overload approaching those found in human haemochromatosis were achieved in the rat by the oral administration of carbonyl iron. Evidence of peroxidation *in vivo* was found in microsomal and mitochondrial lipids by detection of conjugated dienes, products of peroxidative damage of polyenoic fatty acid consittuents of membrane phospholipids. Although the biochemical mechanisms responsible for lipid peroxidation in iron overload are unknown, it is possible that the organelle damage may be caused by the generation of free radicals by unbound ferrous iron. Normally, the hepatocyte maintains iron in a non-toxic protein-bound ferric (Fe^{3+}) form. Neither hypothesis, however, accounts for the fact that in iron overload, hepatic fibrosis occurs in the absence of marked hepatic necrosis and inflammatory infiltrate. Increased liver cell fibrosis was found on biopsy in thalassaemic children in the first few years of life, before body stores of iron are greatly increased. Iron is required as a cofactor in collagen synthesis at the stage of proline and lysine hydroxylation. It has been suggested, therefore, that the increased fibrosis that occurs in haemochromatosis may be due to a direct effect of iron on collagen deposition as well as a secondary reaction to liver cell necrosis.

None of the three theories of chronic iron toxicity that have been discussed are mutually exclusive, and it is possible that all these factors may be operating in the development of tissue damage.

Patients with IHC who also abuse alcohol tend to develop fibrosis and cirrhosis at lower levels of storage iron than patients who do not take excess alcohol. This observation suggests that there may be synergism between the hepatotoxic effects of excessive iron and alcohol, although it remains to be proved experimentally.

17.10.4   Idiopathic haemochromatosis

The first comprehensive description of the classical clinical triad of idiopathic haemochromatosis, viz. skin pigmentation, hepatomegaly, and diabetes, was provided in a seminal review of 345 cases by Sheldon in 1935. Sheldon also proposed the concept that haemochromatosis results from an inborn error of iron metabolism which, over many years, leads to a progressive increase in body iron stores. This hypothesis was not universally accepted for some decades but recent genetic studies have confirmed that Sheldon's theory, based solely on sound clinical deduction, is correct.

The iron accumulation in IHC is caused by an inappropriately high absorption of iron by the duodenal mucosa, at physiological levels of intraluminal iron. This leads to an increase in serum iron, a decrease in serum transferrin concentration, and consequent increase in transferrin saturation, with preferential donation of transferrin-bound iron to parenchymal cells. Tissue iron accumulation is slow as iron absorption is only increased from the normal 1 mg/day to 2–4 mg/day, leading to a net accumulation of 500–1000 mg/year. The disease does not normally present until after the age of 40 years when iron stores are usually greater than 20 g, compared with the normal

1 g of storage iron. Physiological iron losses through menstruation and pregnancy explain the tendency for the clinical manifestations to present at a later age (often greater than 50) in women.

The term idiopathic, hereditary, or genetic haemochromatosis should be employed in those patients in whom there is parenchymal iron loading and evidence of a positive family history of haemochromatosis. In clinical practice, when a definite family history is often lacking, the diagnosis is based on the exclusion of other conditions predisposing to iron overload. With the advent of improved diagnostic techniques, patients are increasingly being diagnosed at much earlier stages before organ damage occurs. Such patients are referred to as having 'latent' or 'precirrhotic' haemochromatosis.

It is still unclear whether this increase in absorption is due to a primary defect in the enterocyte or a generalized defect of iron metabolism. It is also possible that there may be an abnormality in reticuloendothelial cell function which secondarily affects iron absorpotion.

Inheritance of idiopathic haemochromatosis

HLA typing studies of patients with clinical haemochromatosis have confirmed that IHC is inherited as a single gene autosomal recessive disorder (Fig. 17.118). The gene frequency may be as high as 1 in 10 to 1 in 20 in some Anglo-Saxon populations; the calculated homozygote frequency is about 1 in 400. This makes IHC one of the three most prevalent human genetic disorders commoner, for example, than cystic fibrosis, which has a gene frequency of 1 in 50.

In 1976, the close association was discovered between IHC and the histocompatibility antigen HLA-A3, which is present in about 75 per cent of IHC, compared with 28 per cent in control populations. Weaker associations, probably due to linkage disequilibrium, have been described with HLA-B7 (44 per cent v. 26 per cent) and -B14 (26 per cent v. 7 per cent) but these show geographic variations (Fig. 17.119). These studies, which have been confirmed in Anglo-Saxon and Celtic communities throughout the world, have placed the IHC susceptibility gene on chromosome 6 in close proximity to the A locus. IHC is much rarer in other population groups such as Asians and Arabs.

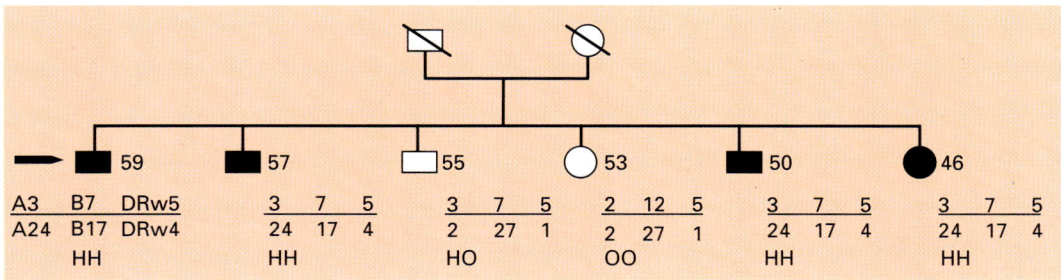

Fig. 17.118 Haemochromatosis family tree showing affected siblings with HLA haplotypes identical to those of the proband (arrowed). HH, homozygote for the haemochromatosis allele; HO, heterozygote for the haemochromatosis allele; OO, homozygote. (Modified from Basset *et al.* 1979.)

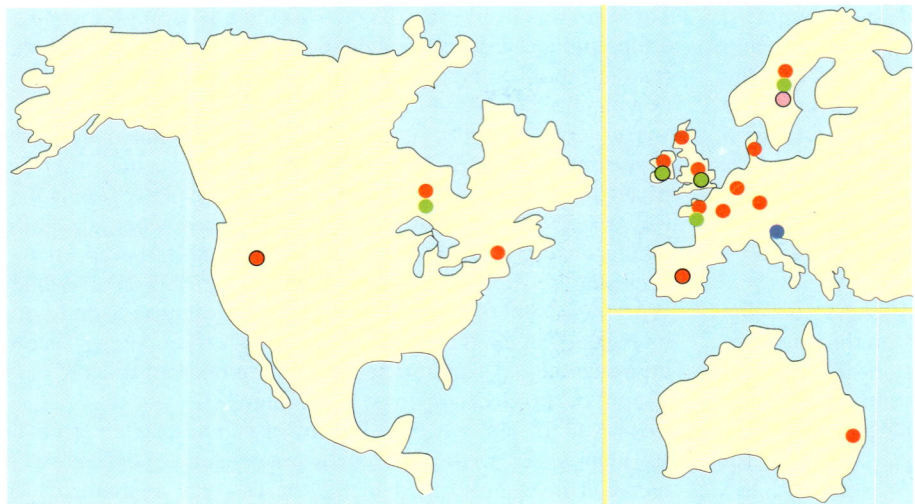

Fig. 17.119 HLA marking of IHC throughout the world by A3, B7 (red dots), A3, B14 (green dots), A3, B35 (blue dots), A1, B8 (pink dots). (From Simon *et al.* 1987, with permission.)

Since homozygotes require two such alleles for expression of IHC, it has become possible to identify heterozygotes. These subjects may develop biochemical expression of this disease (increased transferrin saturation) but do not develop progressive iron overload or clinical evidence of IHC.

Pathogenesis of iron overload in IHC

It is unfortunate that the putative protein that controls iron metabolism, and which is coded for (or probably modified) by the IHC gene, has not been identified. It is clear, however, that the transferrin gene, which is found on chromosome 3, is not implicated. Transferrin structure, function, and turnover in IHC patients is identical to controls. Also, there is no increase in transferrin receptors in the intestinal mucosa in IHC patients, and transferrin receptors are decreased on the hepatocyte membranes of IHC patients. This decrease is appropriate in the presence of hepatocyte iron loading.

DNA sequences coding for the ferritin subunit H have been localized on several chromosomes. Interestingly, one of these genes is located on the short arm of chromosome 6. Initial studies of polymorphism patterns suggested a significant difference between IHC patients and controls. However, further studies have failed to confirm any alteration in the H ferritin genes between idiopathic haemochromatosis patients and controls. Moreover, other structures of ferritin metabolism have not shown any differences between IHC and control subjects. The significance of the specific polymorphism for the ferritin H subunit on chromosome 6 remains to be determined.

Current evidence for the cause of IHC favours an abnormality in intestinal mucosal control of iron uptake, so that iron absorption increases inappropriately at an early stage as a result of increased iron transfer across the enterocyte. This process causes a slight increase in iron absorption from the diet which leads to a gradual accumulation of iron over many years. Confirmation of this hypothesis has come from the inappropriate up-regulation of transferrin receptors on the enterocyte in the presence of increased body iron stores in primary haemochromatosis, whereas in secondary iron overload appropriate down-regulation occurs. In contrast, hepatocyte transferrin receptors are appropriately down-regulated in both primary and secondary haemochromatosis in the presence of excess hepatic iron.

Pathological effects of iron overload

As discussed previously, in fully established IHC the total body iron content may exceed 20 g. The heaviest iron deposition occurs in the liver and pancreas; in these organs the iron concentration may be increased fifty or one-hundredfold. In other organs, such as the skin, cardiac muscle, and pituitary gland, the degree of iron overload is less marked, being increased from 5 to 25 times the normal tissue iron concentration. The pathological effects of the excess iron content on the various organs involved in IHC will be discussed below.

Liver

The liver becomes enlarged and firm in consistency. On biopsy, the liver in patients with IHC characteristically shows iron deposition, together with dense fibrous septa surrounding groups of lobules. Eventually, a fully established cirrhosis develops. In IHC, unlike secondary haemochromatosis, the iron deposits characteristically first appear in the periportal hepatocytes (Fig. 17.120). Later on, excess iron is found in the biliary epithelium and collagen of portal tracts and Kupffer cells (Fig. 17.121). There is usually little evidence of inflammation or cell death. Some IHC patients who also abuse alcohol will also show evidence of alcoholic liver damage (see Section 17.6). Iron overload due to haemolysis is characteristically present in Kupffer cells (Fig. 17.122), although when massive it is also evident in hepatocytes.

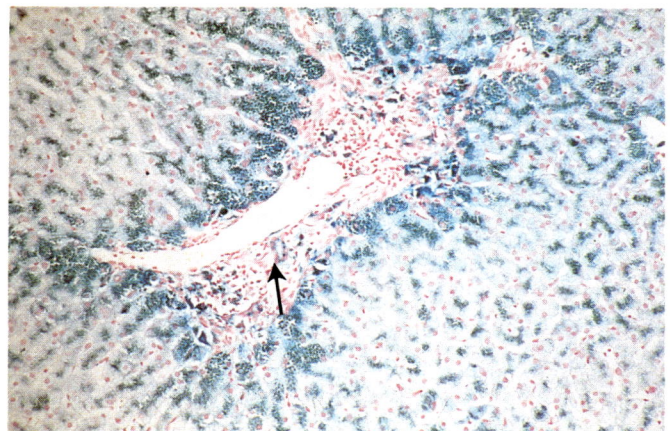

Fig. 17.120 Iron deposition in the form of haemosiderin in idiopathic haemochromatosis. The iron, which has been stained with Perl's reagent to make it blue, is most prominent in the hepatocytes, immediately around the portal tract. There is a little haemosiderin present in the portal tract itself, on collagen fibres, and also in a bile duct (arrow). This is an early stage of idiopathic haemochromatosis.

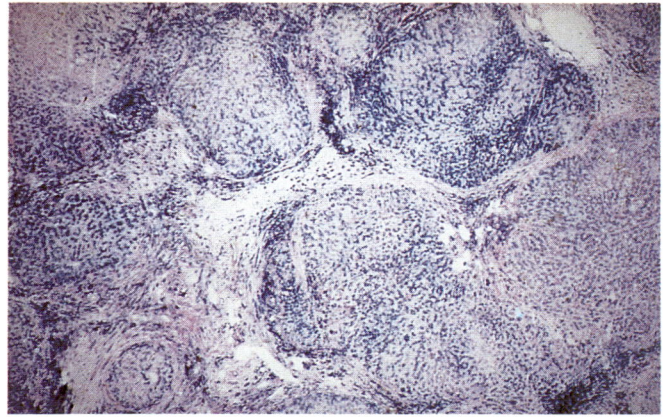

Fig. 17.121 Established cirrhosis in idiopathic haemochromatosis. There is iron present (blue) in virtually every hepatocyte and also in the connective tissue septa which surround regenerated nodules.

Despite gross iron excess, leading to the development of cirrhosis, liver function is usually well maintained until the disease reaches a very advanced stage. Similarly, portal hypertension usually occurs late in the clinical course of IHC. In patients with secondary haemochromatosis, the pathological changes are similar except that iron deposits are more prominent in the Kupffer cells.

Pancreas

Histological examination of the pancreas usually reveals the presence of heavy deposits of iron in the acinar cells and in the islets of Langerhans. In addition, the numbers of islets are decreased. Marked fibrosis is often observed, together with an increased in acinar cells, which may show degenerative changes. Although the islet damage contributes to the develop-

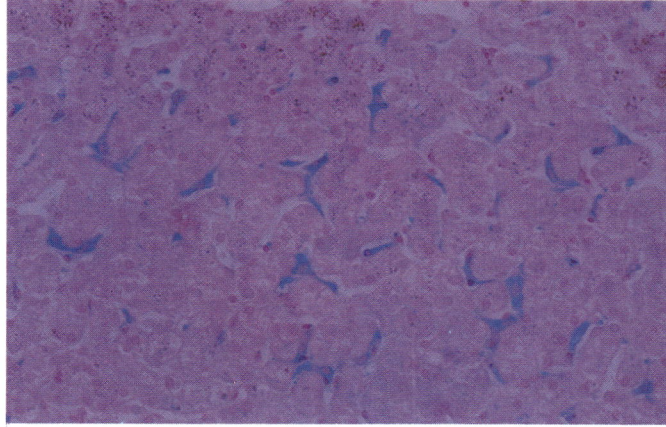

Fig. 17.122 Haemosiderin deposition in Kupffer cells. This is a form of secondary iron overload in a patient with haemolytic anaemia. The iron is present exclusively (in this case) in sinusoidal lining cells.

ment of diabetes mellitis, which is found in about two-thirds of patients with IHC, it is not the sole determinant of the impaired glucose tolerance. Other factors, such as familial disposition to diabetes mellitus and the presence of cirrhosis, also play a role in the glucose intolerance.

Skin

It is not commonly recognized that the characteristic slate-grey hue of the skin which is seen in patients with IHC is primarily due to increased melanin deposition in the dermis. Iron deposition in the skin is, by contrast, rather patchy in distribution, tending to occur around sweat glands. Atrophic changes may be seen in the basal layer. Pigmentation due to melanin may also be seen in the lips, tongue and gums, and in the cornea and retina.

Heart

Iron in the form of haemosiderin is found in the muscle fibres of the heart in established IHC; the haemosiderin is arranged around the poles of the nuclei. Surprisingly, fibrosis is relatively uncommon. Haemosiderin is also deposited in the conducting system of the heart, being preferentially laid down in the atrioventricular node rather than the sinoatrial node. This may explain why patients with established IHC develop cardiac arrhythmias.

Joints

An arthropathy occurs in about 20–50 per cent of patients with IHC. The arthropathy is unrelated to either the extent or duration of iron overload, and occasionally may be the presenting feature. It is characterized by the deposition of iron and calcium pyrophosphate in the synovium. Although a number of small and large joints may be involved, the most common sites are the first and second metacarpophalangeal joints and the knee joints. Chondrocalcinosis occurs in about 50 per cent of patients with arthropathy; the knee is most commonly involved, with calcification present in the menisci and hyaline cartilage. The histological changes consist of scanty deposits of calcium pyrophosphate with deposition of haemosiderin in the synovial lining cells and phagocytic cells. The relationship between iron overload and the pathogensis of the arthopathy is unclear (see also Chapter 27).

Other organs

Iron is also deposited in other organs, such as the pituitary, thyroid, parathyroids, and the adrenal gland. Of these endocrine organs only the function of the pituitary is impaired to any degree. Although impaired testicular function is a common feature of IHC, the iron content of the testes is relatively low and the depressed gonadal function results from pituitary rather than testicular dysfunction.

Clinical features and their pathogenesis

The clinical features of IHC (bronze diabetes) are characteristic in advanced stages of the disease. Patients may present with one or more of a variety of symptoms and signs, shown in Table 17.9. Weight loss, tiredness, and malaise are almost invariable at presentation, and, on direct questioning, impotence and arthritic symptoms may antedate the diagnosis of IHC by many years. Abdominal pain is common, and in about 10 per cent this is the presenting symptom. Cardiac or hepatic failure are rare at the outset. Liver function tests are well preserved with serum aminotransferase values elevated to no more than twice normal in the majority of patients, in spite of fibrosis and cirrhosis usually being present at the time of diagnosis. Liver function tests are often normal in precirrhotic patients.

Table 17.9 Clinical manifestations of IHC

Malaise, weight loss, abdominal pain (100%)
Hepatomegaly (95%)
Pigmentation (90%)
Hypogonadism (70%)
Diabetes mellitus (65%)
Arthropathy (50%)
Congestive heart failure (15%)

Diagnosis of IHC

Early diagnosis and therapy of IHC can prevent or delay fatal complications and, therefore, there is increasing interest in this important aspect of IHC. The minimum criteria for diagnosis are increased iron stores with predominantly parenchymal cell distribution, in the absence of a cause for secondary iron overload. A family history of iron overload is also useful in diagnosis.

Routine non-invasive tests The most useful non-invasive screening tests for iron overload are the serum iron, transferrin saturation, and serum ferritin concentration, measured by radioimmunoassay (Fig. 17.123). The characteristic pattern in IHC is an elevated serum iron concentration together with a decreased serum transferrin concentration leading to an

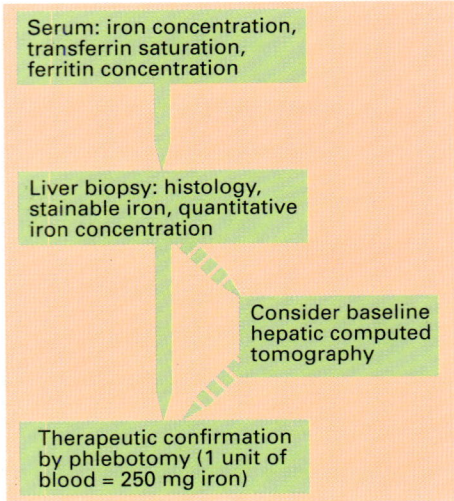

Fig. 17.123 The evaluation of iron stores in idiopathic haemochromatosis.

increased transferrin saturation. The serum ferritin concentration is also markedly elevated. All have the advantage of being highly sensitive but the inherent disadvantage of low specificity. Elevated serum ferritin concentrations in the absence of iron overload may be found in other conditions such as hepatocellular necrosis, malignant neoplasms, and lymphomas.

In practice, a combination of serum iron, transferrin saturation, and serum ferritin concentration should be used for the screening of all first degree relatives. If any one of these tests are abnormal, then a liver biopsy should be performed to accurately quantitate the liver iron concentration. In contrast, if serum ferritin and transferrin saturation are both normal, then significant iron overload can be excluded. HLA typing is useful for identifying relatives who are at increased risk of developing IHC but the procedure is costly, time consuming, and cannot be recommended for routine screening.

Quantification of iron stores by liver biopsy The diagnosis of IHC should always be established by a liver biopsy. Although the degree of stainable iron present is helpful, measurement of chemical liver iron concentration is the most accurate means for determining liver iron stores. Most symptomatic patients with IHC have values in excess of 1000 μg/100 mg (normal 20–140 μg/100 mg). Liver biopsy has the added advantage of allowing histological assessment of the degree of liver damage and the presence of cirrhosis.

Alternative non-invasive methods In view of the problems with specificity of the established non-invasive tests discussed previously, two alternative methods for assessment of iron stores have recently been under investigation:

1. Hepatic computed tomography. The relative electron density of iron is high compared with other hepatic cellular constituents. Liver iron may be quantitated by determining the linear attenuation coefficient of the liver (CT number), as there is a direct linear relationship between the liver iron concentration, as determined chemically, and the CT number in patients iron overload.

Recent studies have compared CT with the serum ferritin concentration in the detection of iron overload. Serum ferritin proved to be more sensitive, but a high CT density was highly specific for iron overload. The relative lack of sensitivity of CT may be due to coexisting hepatic fat deposition in patients with excess alcohol intake, obesity, or diabetes mellitus (which lowers hepatic CT density).

CT scanning may be useful in the following situations:

(a) patients with liver disease and suspected IHC in whom a diagnostic liver biopsy is contraindicated;
(b) children with iron overloaded (e.g. thalassaemia major) in whom liver bipsy may be undesirable;
(c) monitoring iron removal therapy; and
(d) detecting unsuspected iron overload on abdominal CT scans.

2. Nuclear magnetic resonance: the paramagnetic properties of ferritin and haemosiderin have been used recently for the measurement of hepatic iron stores in a few patients with iron overload. Further studies are needed to confirm the usefulness of this new technique.

The problem of iron overload in alcoholic liver disease The differentiation of IHC in the alcoholic from alcoholic liver disease with iron overload can be a difficult problem for the clinician. The confusion has arisen as a result of several factors:

1. 25–40 per cent of patients with IHC have excessive alcohol intakes;

2. the misinterpretation of the significance of stainable liver iron as a measure of tissue iron concentration; and

3. the low sensitivity and specificity of indirect tests for iron overload in alcoholics.

It is now recognized that slight to moderate stainable iron (grades 1–2) is common in normal livers and may not reflect increased iron stores. In addition, alcoholic patients with cirrhosis and increased stainable liver iron can be divided into two groups. First, those patients who have a mild to moderate increase in stainable iron with normal (66 per cent) or mild increase in body iron stores (33 per cent). These patients do not have IHC and are not heterozygotes for the disease. Secondly, alcoholic patients with gross iron deposition and increased total body iron stores of the magnitude seen in IHC (liver iron concentration > 1000 $\mu g/100$ mg dry weight; $15–50$ g total iron stores). HLA and other family studies have shown that these patients probably have IHC. Diagnostic difficulties can still arise in young homozygotes, who may still have hepatic iron levels less than 1000 $\mu g/100$ mg. Recent studies have shown, however, that when the chemical liver iron concentration is corrected it still distinguishes early homozygous haemochromatosis from alcoholic siderösis and IHC heterozygotes. In young asymptomatic homozygotes, there will be an excess of hepatic iron present but exactly how much will have accumulated depends on age, sex, and dietary factors. It has been found that the hepatic iron index, defined as hepatic iron in micromoles per gram dry weight divided by age in years, clearly differentiates between homozygotes and alcoholic liver disease patients with increased hepatic iron. All homozygous patients with idiopathic haemochromatosis have values greater than 2.0, whereas the highest value for alcoholic liver disease subjects is 1.4. In the majority of alcoholics with IHC the hepatic histology is indistinguishable from that of non-alcoholic IHC.

The detection of IHC in the alcoholic population is important as phlebotomy benefits patients with IHC but does not improve clinical, biochemical, or pathological markers in patients with alcoholic liver disease and iron overload.

Treatment of idiopathic haemochromatosis

Excess iron in IHC is removed by phlebotomy. Regular weekly venesection, removing 1 unit of blood, is performed until complete mobilization of excess body stores is achieved. Each unit of blood removed contains about 250 mg of iron and it may take up to 2 years to deplete the iron stores. Chelation therapy with desferrioxamine only removes 10–20 mg/day. Iron removal may be monitored by progressive measurements of the serum ferritin, as plasma iron and haemocrit do not fall until the serum ferritin is reduced below 50 mg/ml. Weekly phlebotomy is stopped when the serum ferritin reaches 10 mg/ml or the haemoglobin drops to 10 g/dl. Iron removal can be confirmed by serial CT scan measurements. Following iron depletion, 1 unit of blood is removed by venesection at approximately three-monthly intervals to maintain iron stores at normal levels.

No controlled prospective trials of phlebotomy have been performed in IHC, and for ethical reasons it is unlikely that such a trial will ever be carried out. Two large studies, using a retrospective control group, found that venesection, in cirrhotic patients with IHC, improved five-year survival from 18 per cent to 66 per cent and 85 per cent, respectively. Coexistent alcohol abuse appears to worsen survival, predisposing to early death from congestive cardiac failure secondary to cardiomyopathy.

Symptomatically, phlebotomy usually produces a rapid improvement in lethargy and malaise. Hepatomegaly and skin pigmentation decrease; liver function tests and cardiac function improve. Congestive cardiac failure is the one indication for adjuvant chelation therapy with desferrioxamine in addition to phlebotomy in IHC.

Phlebotomy does not produce any clear-cut effect on the diabetes mellitus associated with IHC; only 30 per cent of patients show any improvement in carbohydrate tolerance.

Unfortunately, hypogonadism and arthropathy do not improve with iron removal.

Cause of death in IHC

The causes of death in treated and untreated patients are shown in Table 17.10. Treatment has reduced mortality from hepatic failure and variceal bleeding. However, as the patients are

Table 17.10 Causes of death in treated/untreated idiopathic haemochromatosis

Cause of death	Treated (%)	Untreated (%)
Primary liver cell cancer	33	19
Other cancers	20	—
Hepatic failure	8	27
Variceal bleeding	3	15
Heart failure	15	12
Myocardial infarct	7	8
Bacterial infection	5	11
Diabetic coma	1	8
Others	8	—

living longer, the proportion of patients developing liver cell cancer and other adenocarcinomas is increasing.

Precirrhotic IHC patients have a normal life expectancy. Moreover, in general, development of primary liver cancer in IHC is confined to patients with cirrhosis. Only two cases of liver cancer have been reported in precirrhotic patients. These facts provide an important rationale for detecting and treating precirrhotic IHC patients with phlebotomy. Unfortuanately, iron removal does not prevent the development of primary liver cancer in cirrhotic patients, which may occur up to 15 years after complete iron depletion by venesection.

17.10.5   Secondary (acquired) haemochromatosis

The causes of secondary (acquired) haemochromatosis are shown in Table 17.9. The pathogenesis of the iron overload has been discussed earlier.

Haemolytic anaemias

The increased iron absorption and iron overload which results from the haemolytic anaemias associated with ineffective erythropoiesis, such as thalassaemia major, can produce the full clinico-pathological syndrome of haemochromatosis, which has been described earlier. Regular chelation therapy with subcutaneous desferrioxamine can significantly reduce the excess body iron stores and slow the onset of tissue damage. The treatment procedure is inconvenient and expensive.

Liver disease with secondary iron overload

The relationship between alcohol abuse and iron metabolism has been discussed earlier. Increased body or hepatic iron stores occur in patients with cirrhosis from causes other than alcohol, e.g. after porto-caval shunt. However, the levels of excess iron rarely, if ever, reach levels that cause tissue damage.

Porphyria cutanea tarda

Porphyria cutanea tarda is the most common form of porphyria. It is characterized by chronic skin blistering, hirsutism, and hyperpigmentation in the areas exposed to sunlight. The disease is caused by diminished activity of hepatic uroporphyrinogen decarboxylase, which in turn causes excessive hepatic production of uroporphyrin-1. Porphyria cutanea tarda is almost invariably associated with liver disease, usually alcoholic, and the presence of increased hepatic iron stores. However, only a small percentage of patients with this form of liver disease develop symptomatic porphyria. This suggests that the decreased activity of uroporphyrinogen decarboxylase has a separate aetiological basis, perhaps genetic in nature, and that in these susceptible patients iron facilitates the biochemical expression of the underlying enzyme deficiency.

The removal of excess iron stores by phlebotomy decreases the hepatic overproduction of porphyrins and has a beneficial effect on both the skin and hepatic abnormalities. Interestingly, phlebotomy is effective in relieving the skin disorder even in patients with normal iron stores.

17.10.6   Further reading

Bassett, M. L., Halliday, J. W., and Powell, L. W. (1979). Early detection of idiopathic haemochromatosis: relative value of serum ferritin and HLA typing. *Lancet* **ii**, 4–7.

Sheldon, J. H. (1935). In *Haemochromatosis*. Oxford University Press, London.

Simon, M. and Brissot, P. (1988). The genetics of haemochromatosis. *Journal of Hepatology* **6**, 116–24.

Simon, M., *et al.* (1987). *American Journal of Human Genetics* **41**, 89–106.

Tavill, A. S. and Bacon, B. R. (1986). Haemochromatosis: how much iron is too much? *Hepatology* **6**, 142–4.

17.11   Cirrhosis

James O'D. McGee

17.11.1   Definition

Cirrhosis is the generic term for chronic end-stage liver disease. It is the end result of many liver disorders and is irreversible. In a significant, but decreasing proportion of patients, the aetiology (or preceding disease process) cannot be deduced from the pathology or other clinical data. Many of the diseases described so far in this chapter, on their own or in combination with a concomitant process, can produce end-stage liver disease.

Cirrhosis is best defined as a chronic irreversible disease of the liver in which the normal architecture of the entire liver is destroyed by the deposition of connective tissue and the formation of regenerated nodules. The important points in the definition are:

1. The entire liver is involved.

2. The architectural destruction is due to regenerated nodules

of hepatic parenchyma which are surrounded by connective tissue.

3. Within regenerated nodules the normal vascular relationship of portal tracts and terminal hepatic veins no longer exist. If the vascular architecture is not entirely destroyed, the diagnosis of cirrhosis should be avoided, in spite of pronounced fibrosis. While the vascular architecture is preserved, the liver has the capacity to resorb large amounts of connective tissue and return to microscopic normality.

17.11.2   Clinical presentation

In a patient known to be suffering from a disease likely to proceed to cirrhosis, the clinical presentation is characterized by the nature of the preceding disease itself, e.g. alcohol abuse. Irrespective of the disorder that leads to end-stage liver disease, cirrhosis carries with it features that are 'grafted' onto the primary liver disease. These are palmar erythema, spider naevi (most obvious over the upper trunk), gonodal atrophy, and gynaecomastia, particularly in alcoholics. All of these are attributed to hyperoestrogenism secondary to impaired oestrogen metabolism. Dupuytren's contracture occurs in alcoholism. Finger clubbing is common, but the mechanism is unknown. These and other features of hepatocyte dysfunction are listed in Table 17.11. In some cases, cirrhosis is asymptomatic throughout its development until a major complication comes to light.

The ultimate cause of death in cirrhotics is related to other complications of the condition, viz. portal hypertension and ascites; progressive failure of hepatocyte and sinusoidal functions; and hepatocellular cancer.

17.11.3   Pathology

In the past, classifications of cirrhosis were numerous because there were few objective tests available from which to deduce the aetiology of the condition. The simplest classification currently in vogue is still useful if only to alert the clinician to the correct aetiological diagnosis. This classification is based mainly on the size of regenerated nodules.

Micronodular cirrhosis Here the nodules are uniformly small (<3 mm) and the surrounding fibrous bands are thin and relatively uniform in thickness (Fig. 17.124).

Macronodular cirrhosis The nodules are larger than 3 mm and may be 1 cm or larger. The fibrous bands are of variable thickness (Fig. 17.125a). Frequently, these large nodules are broken up by microscopic (or just macroscopically visible) fibrous septa.

Mixed cirrhosis Since neither the micro- nor macronodular form can be accurately defined, this category includes those forms of cirrhosis in which the nodules are of variable size (Fig. 17.125b).

The usefulness of this classification lies only in that some types of liver disease produce a characteristic type of cirrhosis. Alcohol formerly produced a micronodular cirrhosis, and ethanol should be the first agent considered in this type of cirrhosis. However, alcoholics, who now survive much longer frequently have a mixed or macronodular cirrhosis. This presumably simply reflects the ability of hepatocyte nodules to grow in size with time.

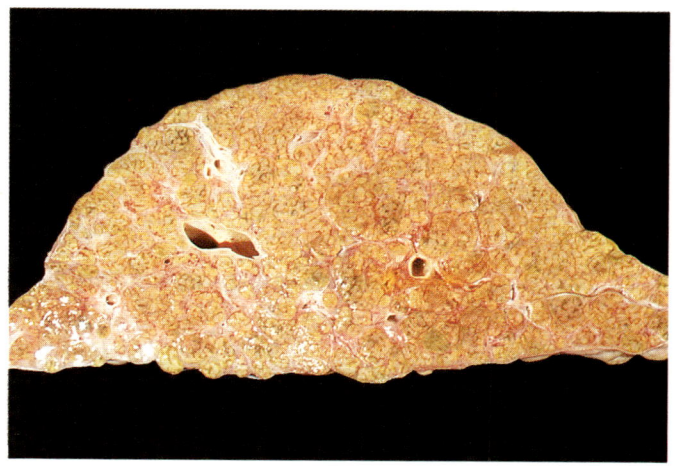

Fig. 17.124   Cross-section of a micronodular cirrhosis. Very small nodules (pale yellow) are surrounded by thin connective tissue septa.

Table 17.11   Complications of end-stage liver disease

Hepatocyte failure	Portal hypertension	Sinusoidal failure
Hypoalbuminaemia	Portal systemic shunts	Hepatic dysfunction (due to sinusoidal
Decreased synthesis of prothrombin, fibrinogen,   oesophageal varices   collagenization)
factors V, VII, IX, X	other shunts	MPS dysfunction and infection (due to
Hyperbilirubinaemia	Encephalopathy	intrahepatic shunting)
Increased ALT, AST (due to hepatocyte damage)	Coma	
Hyperoestrogenism (gonodal atrophy etc.)	Ascites	
Inability to conjugate other hormones (e.g. aldosterone) and drugs	Splenomegaly (hypersplenism)	
Urea defects; hepatorenal syndrome		

* Abbreviations: MPS, mononuclear phagocyte system; ALT, alanine aminotransferase; AST, aspartate aminotransferase.

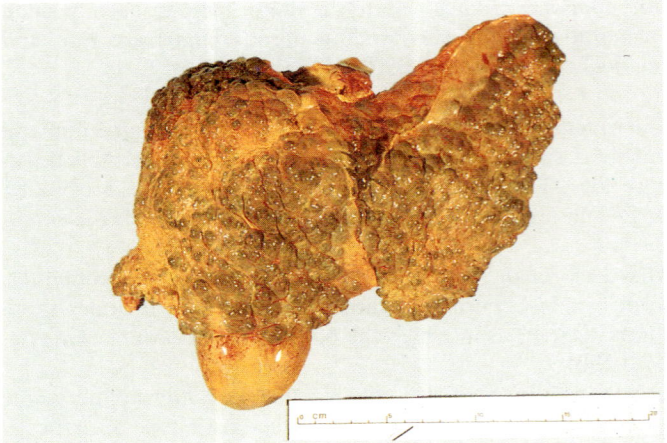

(a)

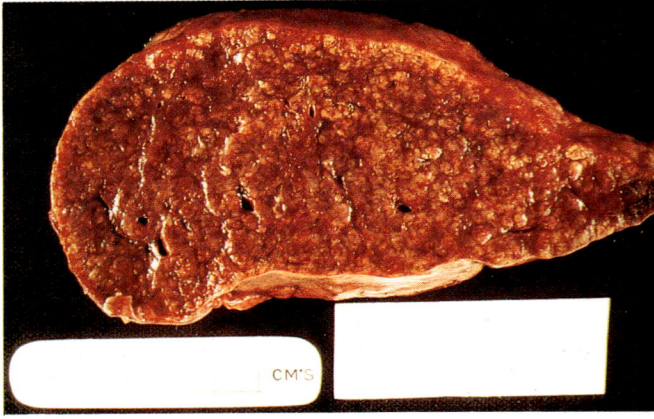

(b)

Fig. 17.125 (a) Macronodular cirrhosis. The surface of the liver is replaced by large regenerating nodules, many of which are 1 cm or more in diameter. The gall bladder is evident at the bottom left of the liver. (b) Predominantly macronodular cirrhotic liver with micronodular components. Many of the nodules are 1 cm in diameter but the nodule size varies from a few millimetres to more than 1 cm.

Classification is relatively easy at laparotomy, laparoscopy, or autopsy but is more difficult on a needle biopsy. This is due to the nature of the needle biopsy sample, which is 1 mm thick and can therefore not enclose a complete 'macronodule'. A much more satisfactory classification of end-stage liver disease is a pathogenetic one and this is presented in Table 17.12. Here the aetiological agent or mechanism (e.g. duct obstruction) is correlated with the usual macroscopic type of cirrhosis and also the microscopic features which enable the aetiological diagnosis to be made on biopsy. The approximate frequency of the various pathogenetic types of cirrhosis are given in Table 17.13.

Most of the diseases that result in cirrhosis have been described in detail earlier; only the morphological pointers to aetiology are summarized in Table 17.12.

Table 17.12   Morphological correlates of pathogenesis in cirrhosis

Pathogenesis	Predominant type	Characteristic morphological features
Alcohol	Micronodular, (macronodular in advanced stages)	Fatty change; Mallory bodies; hydropic swelling; siderosis
Viral hepatitis (HBV, HCV)	Macronodular, mixed	Acidophilic cells; ground-glass changes; HBV antigens in hepatocytes
Large bile duct obstruction	Micronodular	Jigsaw pattern; cholestasis; bile ductular proliferation
Primary biliary cirrhosis	Micronodular†	Absence or reduction of medium-sized bile ducts; lymphoid aggregates; granulomas; peripheral cholestasis; Mallory bodies sometimes present; excess copper and copper binding protein
Haemo-chromatosis	Micronodular	Haemosiderin in hepatocytes, ductular epithelium, macrophages in septa. Kupffer cells contain haemoderm particularly in secondary iron overload
α-1-Antitrypsin deficiency	Micro-macronodular or mixed	PAS-positive diastase-resistant granules and globules in hepatocytes
Wilson disease	Macronodular	Excess copper in hepatocytes; glycogenic vacuolation of nuclei; fatty change; Mallory bodies sometimes present
Toxins and drugs	Macronodular or mixed	Variable
Intestinal bypass	Micronodular	Fatty change; Mallory bodies may be present
Venous outflow impairment	Micronodular	Reversed lobulation; passive congestion
Other inborn errors of metabolism*	Micronodular	Accumulation of carbohydrates and lipids; pseudoglandular appearance of liver cell cords; ductular proliferation; giant cell transformation; intrahepatic inclusions
Cystic fibrosis	Micronodular	PAS-positive secretion in proliferating ductules: biliary pattern may be only focal
Hereditary haemorrhagic telangiectasia	Macronodular	Dilated vessels in septa
Indian childhood cirrhosis	Micronodular	Severe hepatocellular degeneration; Mallory bodies: creeping fibrosis

* Enzymatic deficiencies in infants and children. Glycogenosis (types III and IV), galactosaemia, hereditary fructose intolerance, hereditary tyrosinaemia.
† In early cases there is no true cirrhosis but a fibrotic change with preservation of hepatic parenchymal architecture.

Table 17.13 Pathogenetic types of cirrhosis and incidence

Pathogenesis	Incidence*
Alcohol	60–70%
Postviral (postnecrotic): HBV, HCV	10–15%
Biliary (primary biliary, primary sclerosing cholangitis, other duct obstructions)	5–10%
Pigment anomalies (iron overload)	5%
Metabolic disorders (Wilson disease, α-1-antitrypsin deficiency, etc.)	<1%
Idiopathic (unknown aetiology)	10–20%

* These figures give an approximate range for Europe and the USA.

General microscopic features of cirrhosis

The generic diagnosis is made on three features: fibrosis, regenerated nodules, complete vascular/microanatomical distortion of the liver acinus.

Excessive fibrous tissue is readily identified on routine histopathological stains. There are three chemically non-specific tinctorial properties of connective tissue which are helpful in cases where the diagnosis is not easy—reticulin, van Gieson, and trichrome staining (Figs 17.126, 17.127). Fibrous septa

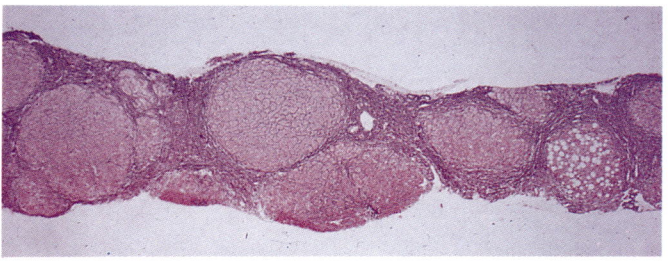

Fig. 17.126 A micronodular cirrhosis in an alcoholic. These small nodules (on a needle biopsy) are surrounded by black connective tissue stained with reticulin. Note that only one nodule (right) contains fat.

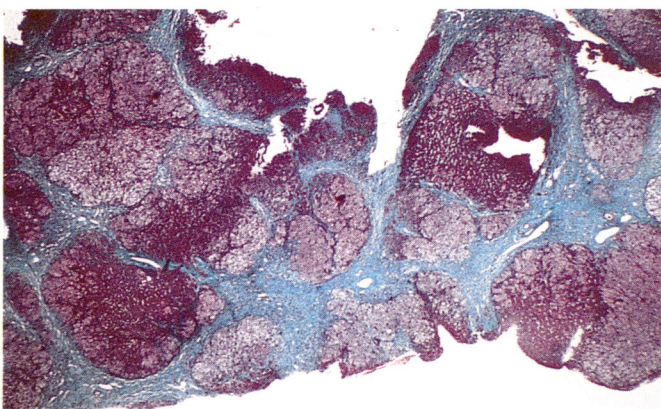

Fig. 17.127 A mixed cirrhosis in a patient with hepatitis B virus infection. The regenerated nodules are outlined in blue connective tissue stained with a trichrome method. The nodules vary in size from less than 1 mm to 5 mm. This micrograph was taken at the same magnification as that in Fig. 17.126.

may be thick or thin, and contain large venous radicles, bile ducts, and arteries, but anatomical portal tracts are not present. In needle biopsies, which are frequently fragmented, fibrous tissue may only be evident around the periphery of regenerated nodules; this is particularly so in macronodular types of disease.

Regenerated nodules are usually easy to pick out because they are delineated by connective tissue. The constituent hepatocytes are two cells thick in most places (Fig. 17.128). In fully established cirrhosis, many plates may be one cell thick so the diagnosis is not precluded by this; twin plates will always be found to predominate, however. In children, two-cell-thick hepatocyte plates persist from birth to about 6 years. The adult, one-cell-thick plate, is found thereafter. It is important to bear this in mind in diagnosis of cirrhosis in this age-group.

Within regenerated nodules, normal hepatic veins and portal tracts are not present. In macronodular cirrhosis, an excessive number of venous channels are commonly found but their origin (either from the portal or hepatic venous system) is unknown. Occasionally, portal tracts, albeit hypoplastic, are present in macronodules. This is presumably because the nodule was formed by encirclement of several acini by fibrous tissue, or perhaps (and less likely) these tracts were formed as a micronodule grew larger.

In developing cirrhosis, there is a stage when the vascular/microanatomy is not completely deranged and in these cases the designation 'developing' cirrhosis is used; the author's preference, however, is to use the term 'extensive fibrosis with regeneration which will probably lead to cirrhosis'. This is perhaps conservative but it concedes that if the pathogenetic mechanisms responsible for complete liver architectural destruction were blocked, the disease could be reversed. This may well be more than academic in the future when specific therapies become available for fibrotic liver disorders.

The two exceptions to the statement that 'architectural distortion' should be complete are biliary cirrhosis and cardiac cirrhosis (see Sections 17.15 and 17.8, respectively). In biliary cirrhosis, fibrosis starts and spreads from portal tracts to

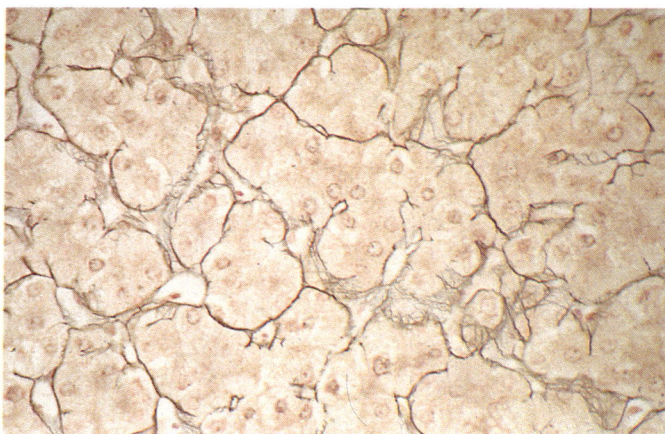

Fig. 17.128 Evidence of regenerative activity in a cirrhotic nodule. All of the hepatocyte plates are more than one cell thick. Each plate is outlined in black by a reticulin stain.

surround simple and complex acini, and terminal veins may still be evident in the regenerating nodules. In cardiac cirrhosis, the reverse is so.

Activity in cirrhosis and non-specific features

In any cirrhosis, there is a variable number of inflammatory cells in fibrous septa, some of which may be relevant to the disorder which eventuated in end-stage liver disease. On the other hand, an intense infiltrate of lymphocytes, polymorphs, and plasma cells at the junction of nodules and septae is taken as continuing activity of the cirrhotic process. This may be associated with piecemeal necrosis and pericellular fibrosis (Fig. 17.129). There is debate as to whether to call this lesion 'activity' or chronic active hepatitis in a cirrhotic liver; which is correct cannot be answered by science at this time. None the less, patients with an 'active cirrhosis' do sometimes have an amelioration of symptoms on steroids whether or not their cirrhosis had its origin in a preceding chronic active hepatitis.

Non-specific changes in cirrhotic livers are mainly bile ductular proliferation, copper-binding protein in hepatocytes, occasionally cholestasis; and, in autopsy liver, central necrosis in nodules. Dysplasia (Fig. 17.130) and adenomatous hyperplasia in nodules have a presumed preneoplastic significance and are discussed later (Section 17.13).

Differential diagnosis

The main disorders that may masquerade as cirrhosis clinically and on biopsy are listed in Table 17.14.

17.11.4   Pathogenesis of cirrhosis

The three phenomena to be considered are architectural distortion with resultant portal hypertension; connective tissue formation; and the formation of regenerated nodules.

It is easy to conceive how hepatic architecture becomes destroyed. In almost all diseases that lead to cirrhosis, there is con-

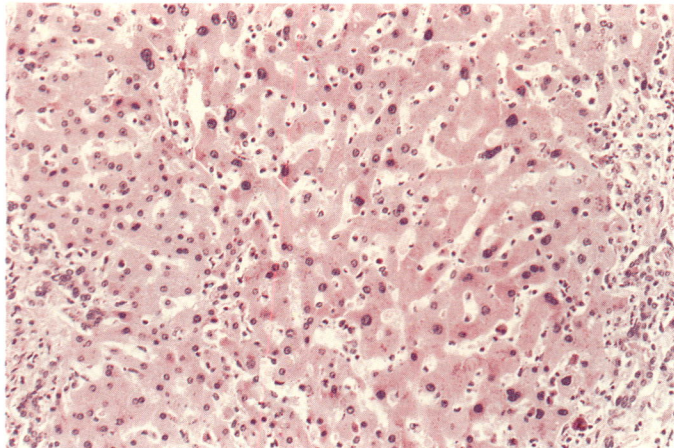

Fig. 17.130   Dysplasia in a cirrhotic liver. The nodule occupying most of the right side of the field shows very large pleomorphic nuclei.

Table 17.14   Differential diagnosis of cirrhosis*

Clinical	Biopsy
Chronic active hepatitis	'Central' hyaline schlerosis in alcoholics
Congenital hepatic fibrosis	Focal nodular hyperplasia
Granulomatous hepatitis	
Budd–Chiari syndrome	Veno-occlusive disease
Blood dyscrasias	Radiation damage
Schistosomiasis	Schistosomiasis
Tropical splenomegaly	
Partial nodular transformation of liver	Diffuse nodular hyperplasia
Non-cirrhotic portal hypertension in India and Japan	
Portal vein thrombosis (with Cruveilhier–Baumgarten syndrome); splanchnic A-V fistula	Congenital hepatic fibrosis
	Non-cirrhotic portal hypertension

* All of these conditions, except focal nodular hyperplasia, produce portal hypertension.

nective tissue deposition around perivenous areas and in portal tracts. The fibrosis extends out from these structures and, by extending around zone 3 of the acinus, hepatic veins and portal tracts link up. Alternatively, or at the same time, connective tissue radiates directly from either perivascular or portal tracts into the acinus and subsequently join up. The result of all of these mechanisms is that portal blood flows directly into the hepatic venous system without traversing the acinus. This occurs via the large vessels characteristic of fibrous septa.

Another consequence of this shunting is that the vascular supply of the residual nodules is relatively compromised. It has been proven also that hepatic arterioles and portal venous structures anastomose in fibrous septa. A very apt demonstration of this is that the blind end of the portal vein at the liver hilum, after surgical portal systemic shunt operations, has an arterial pulse. This shunting contributes to portal hypertension. Of more significance there is increased peripheral resistance

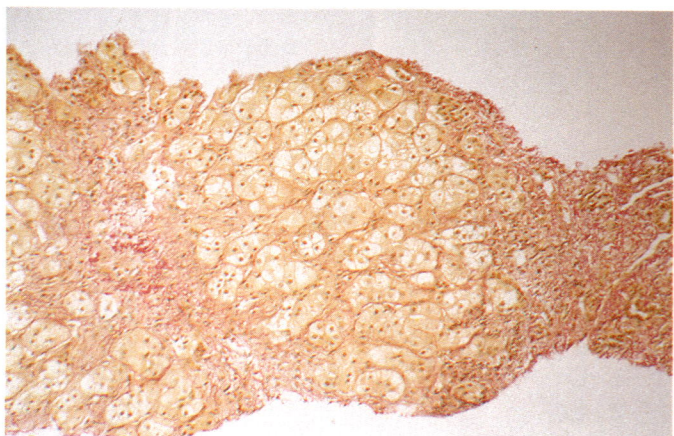

Fig. 17.129   An active cirrhosis. There is inflammatory cell infiltration at the edge of a micronodule. This is associated with extension of pink fibrous tissue (van Gieson's stain) around and between hepatocytes, which are yellow.

within the liver due to kinking and distortion of portal and hepatic veins as they course under or over fibrous septa; this has been shown in reconstruction studies. The collagenization of sinusoids in the cirrhotic liver convert an open sinusoidal system to a closed system and this is probably also of importance in the genesis of portal hypertension. The major points in the vascular system at which resistance is increased in portal hypertension in cirrhosis are shown in Fig. 17.131. Portal hypertension results in the formation of shunts between the portal and systemic veins outwith the liver. The most important site is at the oesophagogastric junction (Fig. 17.132). Ascites, another consequence of cirrhosis, is discussed in Section 17.16.

Fibrous tissue deposition in end-stage liver disease is due to a net increase in the amount of collagen and other matrix components in the liver. This discussion will be restricted to collagen since it has been best studied, but it is probable that glycosaminoglycan, laminin, etc. synthesis is also increased in developing and established cirrhosis. It might seem self-evident, when there is such a massive increase in collagen in liver, that this would be due to increase of collagen production in end-stage liver disease. However, this was not generally acknowledged until the late 1960s. Before that, it had been conceived (and still is by some) that collagen septae in the liver are generated by collapse of preformed hepatic matrix, presumably following hepatocyte death. Since massive hepatocyte death is infrequent in the 'run up' to cirrhosis, this seems unlikely. In fact, there is no scientific evidence that collapse generates collagen septa in a cirrhotic or fibrotic liver. Collagen septa are generated by increased collagen synthesis, either by an increase in the amount of collagen produced per synthetic cell, or by an increase in the number of collagen-productive cells, or by both mechanisms. It is also theoretically possible that decreased degradation of collagen might also result in a net increase in collagen, but the evidence is against this; rather, it would appear that collagen degradation is increased in the precirrhotic and cirrhotic liver.

The increase in synthesis of collagen may be induced by collagen-stimulating factors which have not been properly characterized. The factors that are responsible for the increase in the number of collagen-productive cells have been ascribed to macrophage-derived factors and other cytokines. Transforming growth factor B might also be involved. The evidence for the relevance of these *in vivo* is weak.

Finally, the nature of the cells responsible for collagen production in the normal and cirrhotic liver is also debated. The consensus view is that portal tract fibroblasts and perisinusoidal cells (Ito cells) are responsible for the physiological production of collagen and perhaps other matrix components. It is probable also that both cell types increase in number in diseases that lead to cirrhosis. Of more conjecture is whether hepatocytes generate collagen and matrix physiologically and in disease. There is good evidence that hepatocytes *in vitro* synthesize collagen under isolated conditions. It is also true, however, that isolated

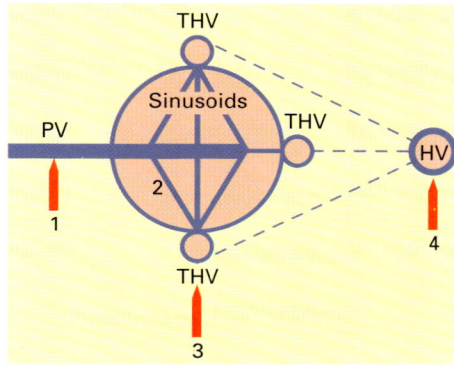

Fig. 17.131 Intrahepatic obstruction of the portal venous system in cirrhosis. Blocks (arrows) may occur in portal venous radicles (1), sinusoids (2), terminal hepatic veins (3), or in hepatic veins (4). See the text for mechanisms of obstruction. PV, portal venous radicles; THV, terminal hepatic venules; HV, hepatic veins.

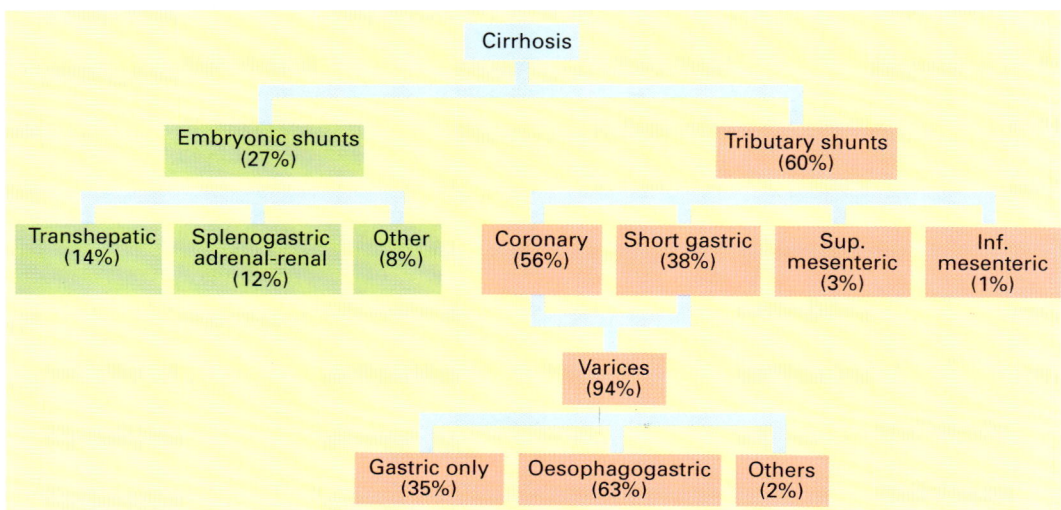

Fig. 17.132 Distribution of sites of portosystemic shunts in cirrhosis.

hepatocytes very rapidly (within 2 h) change their intermediate filament type from cytokeratin ('epithelial' type) to vimentin ('mesenchymal' type). Given the latter, one has to wonder seriously whether the production of collagen by hepatocytes *in vitro* is an artefact of the cell being removed from its normal environment. Having criticized the interpretation of these types of experiment, I would not be surprised to find that *in vivo* hepatocytes may well produce, and also modulate, the matrix in which they function, but the proof of this is not yet available.

The major collagen types in normal liver are I, III, IV, V, and VI; types I and III comprise about 66 per cent of the total, and the other third is comprised by the minor types. All are increased in end-stage liver disease but the minor types may be increased about tenfold. The problems to be addressed, therefore, in understanding the regulation of collagen production are not only those mechanisms that increase collagen production but also those regulating the molecular type produced.

Regeneration, and its regulation, are even more problematic than collagen regulation in the genesis of cirrhosis. This is the subject of Section 17.12.

17.11.5   Further reading

Montgomery-Bissell, D. (1990). Cell-matrix interaction and hepatic fibrosis. In *Progress in liver disease* (eds H. Popper and F. Schaffner). Saunders Inc., Philadelphia.

17.12   Hepatocyte hyperplasia

K. Weinbren

17.12.1   Introduction

When part of the liver is affected by disease, resected, or damaged by vascular compromise or toxins, surviving liver cells undergo a remarkable proliferative response, sometimes referred to as regeneration. This growth occurs in all species so far tested and substantial data have now accumulated about the structural and biochemical changes that develop. The underlying mechanisms are not understood; it is not clear what enzymatic and humoral factors are relevant; and recent observations on growth factors and oncogenes require further analysis.

17.12.2   Proliferation of hepatocytes

After partial hepatectomy there is a measurable increase in DNA; the rate of incorporation of precursors into DNA and the incidence of hepatocyte mitoses also increase. There are sometimes microscopic rearrangements of hepatocytes in a liver that

has undergone hyperplastic changes, and these may provide a means of recognizing the process in tissue sections. While it is possible to detect cellular proliferation after evident damage to liver tissue, proliferation of liver cells may also be observed in other conditions and it is necessary to distinguish compensatory hyperplasia from somatic growth, chemically induced adaptive growth associated with enzyme induction, and neoplasia. The term 'compensatory hyperplasia' encompasses two components, the meanings of which are generally agreed. 'Hyperplasia' refers to the process by which a stimulus-dependent increase in the rate of DNA synthesis is effected *in vivo*. 'Compensatory' indicates that the stimulus for this activity involves a loss of, or damage to, functioning liver tissue, with a predominant involvement of hepatocytes in most cases. The widely used synonym 'regeneration' clearly derives from this latter consideration, but there is no blastema or undifferentiated cell formation at the site of the defect, as there would be in reptilian limb regeneration. There are forms of liver cell proliferation also, which might not be associated with loss of, or damage to, functioning liver tissue. In these conditions, the terms 'compensatory hyperplasia' and 'regeneration' are not appropriate, and the stimulus for proliferation should be sought in some other change.

The term 'hypertrophy' is sometimes applied to liver enlargement observed on a macroscopical level, and sometimes to cellular enlargement noted on microscopical examination. The *Shorter Oxford Dictionary* lists hyperplasia as a form of hypertrophy accompanied by cell division. This clearly indicates organ enlargement by the term 'hypertrophy', and the microscopical component by the reference to cell division. When 'hypertrophy' is applied to microscopical changes, it implies increased cellular mass (apart from storage) without substantial DNA synthesis, and represents a process strikingly different from hyperplasia, and one which is regulated by different mechanisms.

One of the main characteristics of compensatory hyperplasia is that, after part has been removed, the surviving hepatocytes throughout the remaining liver appear to take part in the response, so that growth is never confined to the resection surface, and there is no single focus of hepatocyte proliferation. The presence of a single mass of compensatory hyperplastic tissue without evidence of a proliferative reaction in healthy hepatocytes in other parts of the organ has not been validated in the human liver, and the focal nodules observed in carcinogenicity studies in rodents are probably related to a phase in the neoplastic process.

The superimposition of compensatory hyperplasia on another proliferative process is an obvious possibility since it is conceivable that an acute injury or disease may affect a young growing individual or acute toxic damage may develop in an organism in which adaptive proliferation of liver cells is already in progress in association with enzyme induction. It has become customary to consider the development of hepatocyte plates which are more than one cell thick in a human adult as representing the effects of hyperplasia, and in most instances a reflection of compensatory hyperplasia.

Observations on hepatic and other changes in subjects in whom compensatory hyperplasia was known to be taking place

The involvement of the whole remnant, the timing and magnitude of the DNA synthetic response, the spatial distribution of the hepatocytes exhibiting mitoses, the proportion of cells taking part in the acute proliferative response after two-thirds partial hepatectomy at different ages in the rat, and a wide variety of biochemical changes are generally not disputed. Biochemical changes include, among others, increases in water, fat content, and cyclic AMP, and ornithine decarboxylase activity. Certain physical changes are reported and there are changes in endocrine organs and in the serum. These include increases in somatomedin C and α-fetoprotein and a decrease in VLDL, as well as serum factors which are not characterized. The serum of humans, dogs, and rats which have undergone partial hepatectomy, and the serum of patients suffering from fulminant hepatitis stimulate hepatocyte proliferation. In addition, the expression of c-myc and c-fos is increased tenfold for a short time after partial hepatectomy, a more prolonged rise being noted in rats. Studies on p53 suggest a role for this gene in the regulation of hepatocyte growth, but this is not yet certain. In general, most studies on gene transcription and translation in the liver remnant after partial hepatectomy have not yielded qualitative changes when compared with controls, but quantitative increases in the expression of genes which are normally expressed at low levels in resting hepatocytes are reported.

Attempts made to modify the proliferative response by *in vivo* manipulation

Duct and vascular occlusion, deviation of portal blood flow, endocrine ablation, and administration of hormones and chemical substances, are among the many procedures which have been attempted. The considerable experimental activity in this field has not yet yielded a consensus view about the main *in vivo* growth mechanism. What seems to have emerged is that several hormones are capable of modulating the proliferative response to partial hepatectomy in the experimental animal, but so far no individual compound, including those that may show conspicuous biological activity in other respects (such as insulin, glucagon, heparin, epidermal growth factor, and nerve growth factor), appears to be the certain initiator of compensatory hyperplasia as tested *in vivo*.

In vitro studies to identify growth factors for the hepatocyte

The conditions governing the growth of hepatocytes *in vitro* usually require precise control, and changes are effected by chemical and physical variations, even without addition of putative stimulating or inhibitory factors. There are several attributes of monolayer cultures, apparently closely related to cellular proliferation, which are incompletely understood and which complicate the interpretation of changes that may be observed on addition of compounds under test. One such phenomenon, known as contact inhibition, is reflected in the progressive decrease in synthesis of macromolecules as cellular monolayers fill an area, and is reversed by experimentally creating a separation between the cells. Suggested mechanisms include changes in the rate of diffusion of molecules between cells that depend on confluency, or reduced pinocytosis and uptake of mitogenic serum molecules in contacting neighbour cells, but contact inhibition has so far not provided an understanding of the initiation of the compensatory hyperplastic response.

A second phenomenon is related to the dependency of the culture on the addition of fresh medium. A change of medium is often associated with a wave of division in cultures and has been considered to be due to a serum factor that reduces contact inhibition, or by a change in pH or by an alteration in the availability of surface receptors, possibly due to proteolytic activity of fresh medium. This, so far, has not provided the key to hyperplasia, but has led to the important suggestion that tumour cells probably release 'autocrine' or self-growth-promoting factors. It is possible that cells undergoing hyperplasia may also release autocrine growth factors.

Several factors have been found to be effective in stimulating DNA synthesis in density-inhibited hepatocyte cultures; these include some of the known hormones, and other substances that are not conventional hormones. The established hormones with mitogenic effects on cultured cells include insulin, glucagon, growth hormone, thyroxine, and cortisol, all of which stimulate adult or neonatal rat hepatocyte DNA synthesis or [³H]dT incorporation into DNA.

A second class of proliferogenic compounds, which are not conventional hormones, have been grouped together on the basis of their property of stimulating DNA synthesis in cultured hepatocytes. These are generally peptides: epidermal growth factor (EGF), insulin-like growth factor (IGF I and II), and somatomedin C. These factors possess a number of common properties, besides the capacity to stimulate rat hepatocyte DNA synthesis *in vitro*, which include a single-chain polypeptide structure of molecular weight about 7500 Da, insulin-like activity on adipocytes, and the ability to stimulate cartilage growth *in vitro*; all react strongly with IGF receptors and weakly with insulin receptors. They generally cross-react extensively, apart from IGF-II.

Epidermal growth factor, first extracted from salivary glands, is a proliferogenic factor whose effect is reproducibly demonstrable in culture systems. Many studies of this peptide have now been made, and it appears to be active early in the cell cycle, and shows conspicuous biological synergism with glucagon, IGF-I, and IGF-II. EGF is grouped with the transforming growth factors, TGF-α and TGF-β, which are derived from transformed cells. They appear able to transform or stimulate growth in other cells. Both EGF and TGF-α are effective as growth stimulators in culture, but TGF-β appears to be more potent in regulating differentiation than in stimulating proliferation.

A third, rather less compact, group of proliferogenic factors has been described as showing effects on some cell culture systems, but not all appear to have been tested or are found to be active in hepatocyte systems. These include platelet-derived growth factor (PDGF) contained in the α-granules of platelets, and able to induce proliferation in a variety of cells, and fibro-blast growth factor (FGF), derived either from pituitary or brain, which is similar in some respects to PDGF.

A compound derived from rat platelets is also a potent mito-gen for cultured hepatocytes, and has been reported in the serum of patients with fulminant hepatic failure. It is referred to as 'hepatocyte growth factor', its amino-acid sequence has been determined and shows considerable homology with plasmino-gen. While it appears to be possible that this mitogen is involved in the proliferative response, it is not clear what other factors may modulate this response. It seems that some effects have been ascribed to 'receptor masking factors'; it is thought that noradrenaline might be a masking factor for TGF-β, but the others are not yet defined. It is not even known if they represent an effect of the cell dispersion procedure, as they are not reported in collagenase-free EDTA preparations. There are thus a number of positive and negative growth factors which are detectable using hepatocyte monolayer cultures. An assess-ment of their significance *in vivo* is difficult, because of the characteristics of density-inhibited monolayer cultures. In addi-tion to this the effects of extracellular factors or the extracellular matrix ought to be considered, including the proteoglycans, collagen, and glycoprotein, because differences have been observed between the activities of cells on plastic or glass, and those of cells on collagen.

The mechanism for the response in cell cultures has not been elucidated, but ther is agreement that the binding of the growth factor as ligand and the relevant membrane receptor leads to the receptor/ligand undergoing endocytosis and possible de-gradation by lysosomes. It is not clear how the proliferogenic complex is further processed, but tubules, actin filaments, orni-thine decarboxylase activity, and protein kinases associated with receptors play a part. Complicating factors include possible 'down-regulation' or blocking of receptor-sites by related mo-lecules, changes in the passage of nutrients into cells with increased membrane activity, and, of course, familiar technical problems like temperature variation and proteolytic activity in the serum which may expose receptors or make membranes more permeable. The culture system is difficult to interpret, but it has underlined the importance of ligand-receptor complexing as the primary event. None the less, although it is possible to identify a cellular response to specific proliferogenic stimuli in hepatocyte cultures, it is disturbing that the response generally involves a single cycle of mitoses after exposure to the putative growth factor, whereas after partial hepatectomy several waves of mitoses are observed. This constant difference between *in vivo* and *in vitro* reactions has cast doubt on the usefulness of the monolayer culture, but recently the addition of nicotinamide together with EGF was found to convert the response to multiple waves. By supplying factors which may be deficient in culture systems, therefore, it may be possible for *in vivo* conditions to be more closely simulated. But interpretation of culture systems remains complicated although ligand-receptor complexing, and some hormonal effects are likely to operate also *in vivo*. At pres-ent, however, not all *in vitro* activity is detected in the living organism.

Attempted correlations between *in vitro* and *in vivo* observations

Alterations in the liver tissue undergoing hepatocyte hyper-plasia are similar in several respects to those noted in culture systems. Notable are increased activity in the ornithine de-carboxylase (ODC)–putrescine system and increased lipid, α-fetoprotein (AFP), actin filaments, and electrical charge. Of these changes, it seems reasonable to regard most as reflecting the proliferating process in which the cells are involved, either in the organ *in situ*, or in a monolayer system, and it is not likely that any of these changes represents the factor that initiates the replicating process with such reproducibility and precision.

Irreversible inhibition of ODC by the administration of difluoromethylornithine was found to block DNA synthesis *in vivo*. This was restored in regenerating liver by the addition of putrescine. A comparable decrease in the rate of DNA synthesis *in vitro* has been observed by inhibition of the polyamine synthetic pathway by diaminopropane and DL-hydrazine-amino-valeric acid, but this cannot be regarded as evidence in favour of the regulating molecule being a substance involved in the ODC–polyamine pathway, as polyamines, spermine, and putrescine do not appear to initiate cellular proliferation when administered *in vivo*.

In a comparable way, insulin has been administered to intact animals without the desired effect of initiating a wave of hepato-cyte proliferation, but an interesting anomaly has been observed in relation to the administration of insulin to rats pre-viously rendered diabetic by the administration of alloxan. In such circumstances, after 30 days of diabetes, administration of insulin was associated with the initiation of DNA synthesis in the hepatocytes, by a mechanism that is so far not clear. It may be that there is a form of insulin receptor upregulation *in vivo* after 30 days of diabetes, and that hepatocytes may be more responsive to the ligand in these circumstances. But there is insufficient evidence that insulin is the initiator of the compen-satory proliferative response even though it is also mitogenic in cultures.

The administration of various amines, either in combination with other factors or in the form of isoproterenol, has also been attended by a proliferative response in hepatocytes. The sub-stance is strikingly associated with an increase in cell size and also in DNA synthesis in the salivary gland as well as in the liver. Mediation by the autonomic nervous system has been excluded and the phenomenon suggests a parallel to that noted after exposure to phenobarbital or other enzyme inducers. In such circumstances proliferation of endoplasmic reticulum, sometimes in the perivenous regions and sometimes in other regions, accompanies DNA synthesis and mitoses in the same regions of the acinus. None of these findings, however, sheds light on the mechanism underlying the initiation of DNA syn-thesis after liver cells have been damaged or destroyed. They do indicate that the process of cellular proliferation, once initiated, may be influenced by a variety of factors and that several differ-ent circumstances may lead to hepatocyte DNA synthesis even when liver tissue has not been destroyed or damaged.

To date, hypotheses derived from *in vivo* and *in vitro* data include the possible combined activity of several factors. EGF, TGF-α, insulin, and glucagon have been suggested as the main stimuli of hepatocyte proliferation, with indirect effects from parathyroid hormone and calcitonin, which do not affect cultured hepatocytes, and VLDL which might be inhibitory. It is not known what initiates the process *in vivo* or what inhibits growth after a certain mass is achieved. The mechanism involved in the translation of *in vivo* damage to liver cells into a stimulus for DNA synthesis has also eluded identification. The replicative response develops after partial resection, hepatocyte necrosis, or atrophy, three very different effects on the liver cell. The response is similar after each of these different forms of injury, although the possibility has been raised that toxic necrosis may elicit an effect different from that following resection.

17.12.3 Thick hepatic plates in the human

The question of the morphological expression of cells which have proliferated in the human liver has already been raised, and since the general acceptance of the view that plates consisting of two layers of hepatocytes might represent the effects of cellular division in the adult, this feature has been increasingly referred to in disease states and usually interpreted as the result of hepatocyte hyperplasia. Unusually, however, such changes may reflect the outcome of processes other than hyperplasia.

Liver plates which are two cells thick are observed in the human in a wide variety of pathological conditions, and very often impart characteristic macroscopic appearances which may be encountered during surgical procedures or in biopsy. The characteristic first noticed about hyperplastic liver was the

pallor as compared with normal liver tissue, and next was the proliferative phenomenon, which imparts a convexity to the part of the lobe or the surviving liver that is thus affected. These two attributes are found in many liver diseases and an appreciation of their significance may sometimes help to assess the underlying condition.

The conditions with which hyperplasia is associated include changes in the liver in which cellular damage or loss plays some part, but this feature is sometimes difficult to identify amidst the other processes, such as inflammation and repair, macrophage activity, necrosis, or atrophy. However, the presence of thick hepatocyte plates may represent compensatory hyperplasia which may be consequential to a variety of lesions, including cellular necrosis of coagulative or cytolytic types, caused by vascular insufficiency, toxins, viral infection, or tumour replacement. In all these circumstances hyperplastic tissue may be found as diffuse or zonal changes, usually depending on the degree of severity and survival of hepatocytes in different regions of the liver.

Obstruction to tributaries or ostia of hepatic veins results in severe changes in cells and sinusoids surrounding hepatic venous radicles with periportal hepatocyte survival and hyperplasia, as well as hyperplasia of liver cells in regions with intact hepatic venous drainage systems. These last regions may undergo striking cellular hyperplasia, sometimes seriously distorting liver contour and substance. Caudate lobes are frequently reported as undergoing much enlargement, in some cases of ostial occlusion, because of the separate venous drainage of the caudate lobe directly into the inferior vena cava (Fig. 17.133).

It is generally agreed that occlusion of portal venous branches, if involving large-enough regions, is associated with

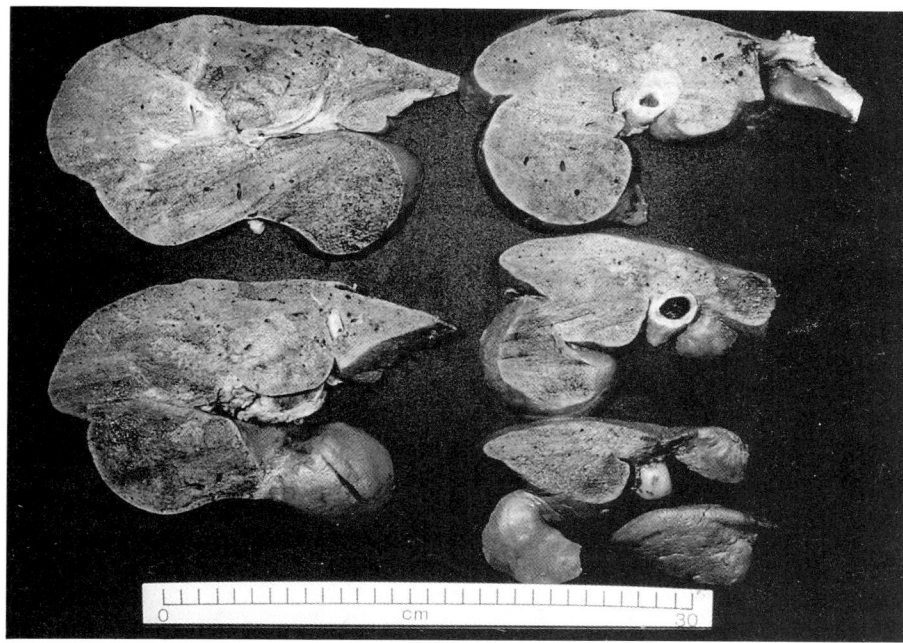

Fig. 17.133 Marked compensatory hyperplasia of caudate and quadrate lobes of liver with occlusion of main hepatic veins.

hyperplasia of liver tissue in which portal blood flow is maintained, in both experimental animals and man. There is some disagreement about the nature of the exact changes that develop after deprival of portal blood flow to part or all of the liver. Some reports stress the atrophy of the parenchyma without particular development of cellular necrosis, but others that the main change is a form of 'shrinkage necrosis', by means of which separate hepatocytes become necrotic without a general reaction and with only a minor component of atrophy. Deprivation of portal blood may exert its effect by decreased protein synthesis or by increased lysosomal–autophagosomal activity, since both probably occur with reproducible regularity, and analytical procedures have been devised for quantifying the autophagosomes.

The incidence of hyperplastic changes is therefore moderately frequent, being noted in many chronic liver diseases and clearly anticipated after major injury or surgical resection, or other forms of hepatocyte trauma. The recognition of these hyperplastic changes in terms of structural alteration is made only when the hyperplastic process has been of sufficient intensity to result in the formation of thick hepatocyte plates, many minor hepatocyte losses being repaired and cells being replenished without diffuse conformational changes. In some cases it is possible to distinguish between forms of hyperplasia on the basis of the position of the plates affected, such as 'diffuse hepatocyte hyperplasia' or 'periportal hepatocyte hyperplasia'. The prognostic importance of the integrity of vascular supply and drainage in chronic liver disease is generally agreed, and a further categorization of the hyperplastic changes therefore depends on the identification of a normal spatial relationship between portal tracts and efferent veins. Thus, diffuse thickening of 'hyperplastic' plates associated with normal vascular relations is referred to as 'lobular or acinar hyperplasia' and that in which a normal vascular relationship is lost, as 'nodular hyperplasia', the latter term including a range from large nodules, as seen in some forms of cirrhosis, to very small nodules, usually noted in diffuse nodular hyperplasia. The types of chronic hepatic disease associated with thickening of liver plates, usually considered to represent compensatory hyperplasia, include almost any condition in which substantial cellular damage or destruction is known to have taken place, such as direct toxic action of chemicals like paracetamol (acetaminophen), accidental trauma or surgical resection (Fig. 17.134), replacement of tissue by tumour, inflammatory destruction of liver cells in duct obstruction (Fig. 17.135), and also conditions in which loss of liver cells is presumed to have taken place, such as cirrhosis. Thick plates are also noted occasionally in circumstances in which evidence of previous cellular necrosis is not persuasive or is completely lacking, such as focal nodular hyperplasia. It is probable that plates will remodel to one cell thickness if the stimulus abates, but this is not proven in man; it seems unlikely, however, that recovery and restitution to single-cell-thick hepatocyte plates will occur if cirrhosis is present. It may be that the vascular distortion found in cirrhosis maintains a stimulus to hyperplasia because of the constant hypoperfusion or necrosis. The question of progression of hyperplastic plates

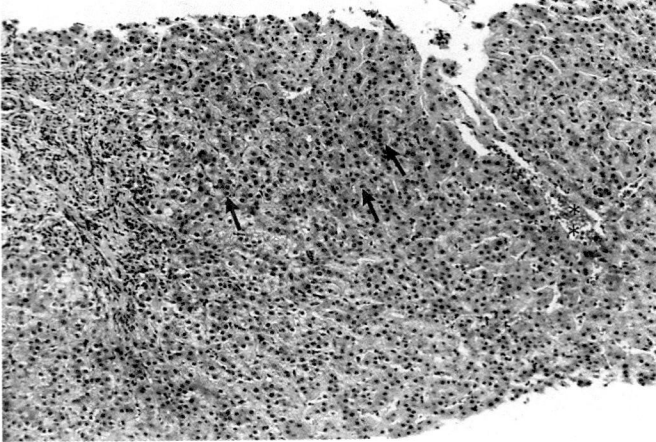

Fig. 17.134 Diffuse acinar hyperplasia in a needle biopsy specimen of the left lobe of the liver after resection of the right lobe following trauma. Note the thick hepatocyte plates (arrows) and the hepatic venous radicle (asterisk).

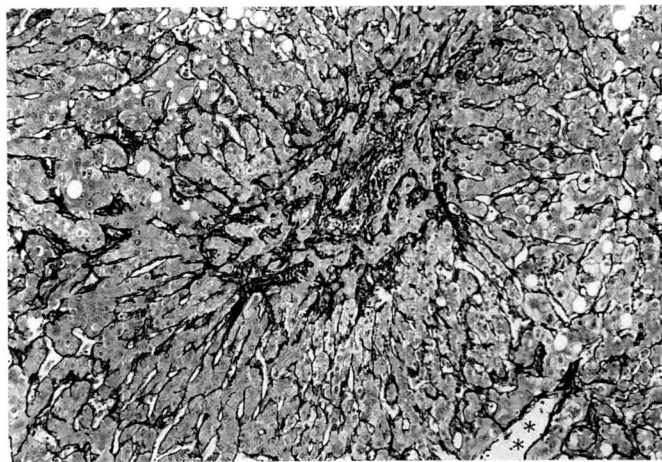

Fig. 17.135 Diffuse acinar hyperplasia in chronic obstructive biliary disease. Note the hepatic venous radicle (asterisks).

was raised nearly 80 years ago, but there is as yet no acceptable evidence that the hyperplastic process may be converted into a neoplastic lesion *sui generis*. In general, in instances of apparent conversion of hyperplastic nodules into neoplasms, another factor such as a virus or a toxin operates, or at least such intervention is not excluded.

A severe distortion may also be a reflection of compensatory hyperplasia of part of the liver, and anatomical landmarks and visceral relations may be difficult to assess during imaging or other investigative or therapeutic procedures. This is not a new observation and, for well over a century, compression atrophy of part of the liver has been known to result in a compensatory elongation of the right lobe of the liver, a phenomenon not known to be associated with clinical symptoms.

The recognition of hyperplastic plates does not indicate the basis of the process or even the diagnosis. It usually implies that hepatocytes have been stimulated to proliferate. The thick plates are probably a more accurate indication of hyperplasia even than the presence of mitoses within liver cells. The main reason for this preference is that it is often impossible to exclude the phenomenon of 'mitotic arrest' as a result of toxins or metabolites and the incidence of mitoses may reflect accumulation of incomplete divisions. The preferred site of the hyperplastic plate-change is generally the periportal region, and in more severe instances this phenomenon may be diffuse, involving also perivenous hepatocytes, irrespective of the cause. Only occasionally are perivenous regions preferentially involved and the diagnosis of enzyme induction is possible, although the selective effect on cellular populations in different acinar sites has been challenged.

17.12.4 Focal nodular hyperplasia

Focal well-demarcated hepatic masses, distinguished from surrounding liver tissue, have been referred to by several different names, these mainly reflecting the notions of pathogenesis of different authors. The term introduced by Edmondson in 1956, 'focal nodular hyperplasia' (FNH) seems to have attracted most support but the other synonyms include 'benign hepatoma', 'adenoma', 'cholangiohepatoma', 'solitary hyperplastic nodule', and 'focal cirrhosis'. There was a good deal of confusion between this lesion and hepatic adenoma at first, a confusion that extended into the attempted definition of the relationship between this change and the use of oral contraceptive agents, but the entity is now reasonably well recognized and is diagnosed in clinical practice, with particular emphasis on imaging and angiographic characteristics.

The structural changes that are usually found in this lesion include the presence of a well-demarcated, usually subcapsular, tan mass, which is firmer and paler than the adjacent parenchymal tissue but is not completely surrounded by a fibrous capsule (Fig. 17.136). The dimensions of the lesions range from a few millimetres to greater than 15 cm and the edge of the lesion is bosselated with several smaller convexities protruding and ir-

regularly distorting the junction between the lesion and the surrounding liver parenchyma; irregular convexities may distort the capsule. There is usually no rim of atrophic parenchyma surrounding the lesion of FNH, a contrast to the darker atrophic liver tissue so frequently found adjacent to metastatic neoplastic lesions. The cut surface of FNH is made up of small subunits of pale parenchyma, varying in diameter from 0.1 to 0.5 cm, usually separated from each other by thin strands of fibrous tissue, which arborize from a central, rather thicker band of fibrosis. While the fibrosis is striking in most of the lesions encountered, it may not be evident in smaller lesions, those approximately 1–2 cm. The site of the lesion is not constant. Of the larger examples recorded, there are different experiences reported as to the lobe of liver most frequently involved, but authors agree that most lesions are subcapsular. In 20 per cent of instances, lesions are multiple.

On microscopy, hepatocyte plates which are thicker than those usually found in the adult liver are separated by recognizable sinusoids, but normal vascular relations are not identifiable. Fibrous foci containing irregular duct-like structures, sometimes with vascular components, resemble portal tracts, usually without organized triads (Fig. 17.137). Frequent thick-walled fibromuscular vessels are encountered, some with internal elastic laminae and some without. Enlarged nerve fibres are sometimes noted enmeshed between connective tissue fibres and close to dilated lymphatics. The fibrous tissue that courses between these parenchymal nodules is otherwise unremarkable, sometimes loose and oedematous and in some parts moderately dense. The hepatocytes that comprise FNH are not reported as differing from those in the remaining liver parenchyma, apart from the observation that the hepatocytes of the lesion did not store iron-containing particles while such storage was found in surrounding tissue. Normal complements of fat and glycogen are usually reported, although sometimes there is striking steatosis. Ploidy changes have not been noted and nuclei resemble those of diploid normal hepatocytes. Mitochondria are present and not enlarged or strikingly abundant. Both endothelial and Kupffer cells are present within sinusoids, but so far

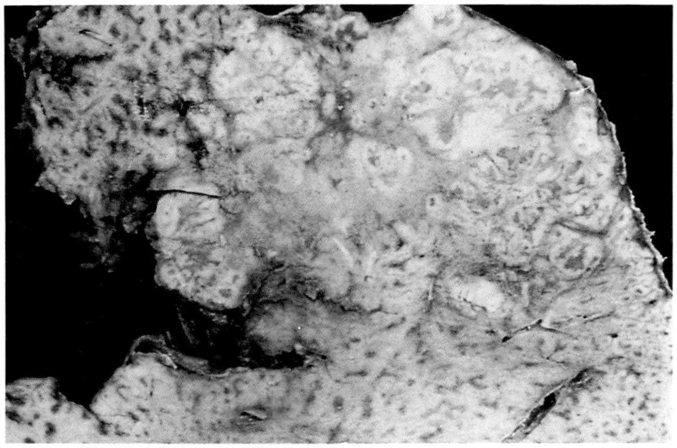

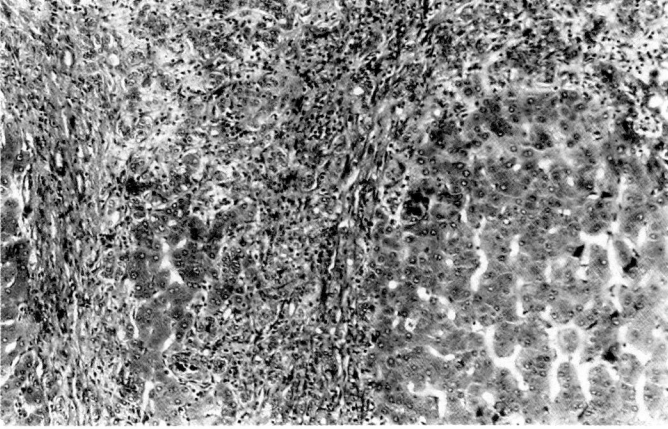

Fig. 17.136 Focal nodular hyperplasia. A resection specimen showing an irregular pattern and fibrous bands.

Fig. 17.137 Mature fibrosis incorporating abundant duct-like structures between thick hepatocyte plates in focal nodular hyperplasia.

perisinuoidal fat-storing (Ito) cells have not been reported. Intracanalicular cholestasis is sometimes noted. The biliary structures within the fibrous tissue are sometimes recognizable as normal-appearing ducts and sometimes as irregular collections of bile duct cells not organized into well-established ductal tubes. Sometimes they resemble the proliferating marginal bile ducts associated with large duct obstruction, consisting of cuboidal to columnar duct cells forming about narrow lumens.

Accumulations of lymphocytes are often found in these fibrous regions. Hepatic venous radicles are not found regularly between fibrous portal regions, and therefore normal acini are not definable, thus justifying the use of the appellation, 'nodular'. Thickening of the plates, which resembles the effects of hyperplasia in other conditions, is another characteristic of this local lesion, but not all descriptions have included the observation that most hepatocyte plates are thick, although in many reports and illustrations this seems to be the case. One other structural aspect noted by several authors is the presence of prominent vessels in adjacent parenchyma, sometimes coursing over the lesion and sometimes present within the larger fibrous septa. The lesion is not accompanied by cirrhosis and there is a reported incidence of 20 per cent with cavernous angioma.

The cause of this lesion is not known. It has been found in patients of all ages, about 8 per cent of those reported occurring in children. In children there seems to be a striking female preponderance (probably fourfold) but not in reports on adults. It is usually detected in life by accident at surgery or by an imaging procedure. No relationship has so far been reported with exposure to chemicals or viruses and, in particular, it is generally agreed that this lesion is not caused by administration of oral contraceptive agents. The pathogenesis of this lesion is also not clear. It is postulated by some that the presence of large arteries may lead to the changes noted by means of 'hyperarterialization' of parts of the liver tissue, and by others that these changes may be the result of focal damage and focal regenerative healing. A third possibility is that these are hamartomatous lesions, and the vascular anomalies may represent another aspect of the hamartomatous change. The persistence of thick liver plates may reflect some failure in development, as these should, of course, convert to single-cell-thick plates as children pass the age of 5 or 6.

The lesions are benign, none ever having been reported to develop characteristics associated with malignant change. It is not known if they heal with fibrosis and whether they present a risk if the patient uses oral contraception. This last point has been raised because of the associated vascularity in lesions found in young women, in which cases it is suggested that FNH may be more sensitive to the effects of such compounds.

A distinction is made between FNH and hepatic adenoma and it is unusual now for these lesions to be confused. The structure of the adenoma is strikingly different, containing no ducts or tracts; its prognosis is that of a neoplasm; it is associated with administration of the oral contraceptive and is accordingly found predominantly in women of child-bearing age. It also differs from vascular anomalies such as haemangioma, which shows no hepatocyte change; from congenital hepatic fibrosis, a diffuse lesion with retained vascular relations and single-cell-thick plates; from haemorrhagic telangiectasia, which consists of vascular lesions without focal parenchymal masses; and from diffuse nodular hyperplasia, which is diffuse and without severe fibrosis or ductal anomalies.

Reference has occasionally been made to the possibility of confusion with hepatocellular carcinoma. This resemblance is usually difficult to recognize as the hepatocellular carcinoma is made up of tumour cells and not normal-appearing hepatocytes, does not contain ductal structures in its substance, and although there may be fibrous bands coursing through the tumour, these do not contain abundant ductal structures or duct cells, abnormal thick-walled vessels, or an abundance of nerves.

Among the childhood lesions that are sometimes reported as resembling FNH, it is distinguishable from hepatoblastoma by its normal-appearing hepatocytes, presence of biliary structures and other cell types, and absence of mesodermal tumour elements; from haemangioendothelioma by consisting predominantly of hepatocytes rather than crowded endothelial cells with islands of ducts and hepatocytes; from embryonal (undifferentiated) sarcoma because of the difference in cell type; and from mesenchymal hamartoma by the predominantly cellular mesenchyme and paucity of hepatocytes in this last condition.

17.12.5 Diffuse nodular hyperplasia

This condition, sometimes referred to as nodular regenerative hyperplasia, is characterized also by a striking thickening of hepatocyte plates which is not confined to a single or focal mass. The main clinical features are related to an increased level of portal venous pressure, which are similar to those observed in other conditions associated with portal hypertension (Fig. 17.138).

The structural changes observed in this condition consist of a diffuse replacement of single-cell-thick plates by plates that are two cells thick. For the most part, a normal relationship

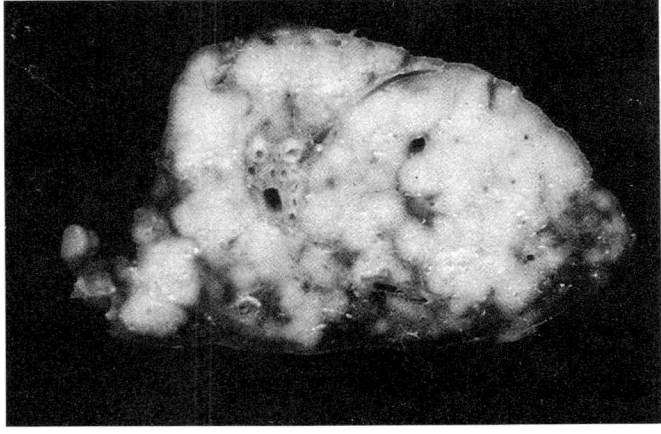

Fig. 17.138 Diffuse nodular hyperplasia. Wedge resection specimen showing multiple pale irregular foci.

between portal tracts and hepatic venous radicles is noted, but many rounded foci are observed. These subacinar nodules are smaller than recognizable hepatic acini and do not include hepatic venous radicles. They appear to compress surrounding hepatocyte plates and these form the basis of the structural changes which extend throughout the liver tissue. This mixture of thick hepatic plates associated with retention of vascular relations, together with interspersed small nodules without hepatic venous radicles, is characteristic of diffuse nodular hyperplasia (DNH) (Figs 17.139, 17.140). The nature of these subacinar or small nodules is not clear. They may represent a single or simple acinus. They do not appear to surround extensions of portal vein branches, but these may not be recognizable. The constancy of their small size suggests that these may, indeed, indicate a particular structural component, but the reason for their prominence is not clear. Increased fibrosis and thickened

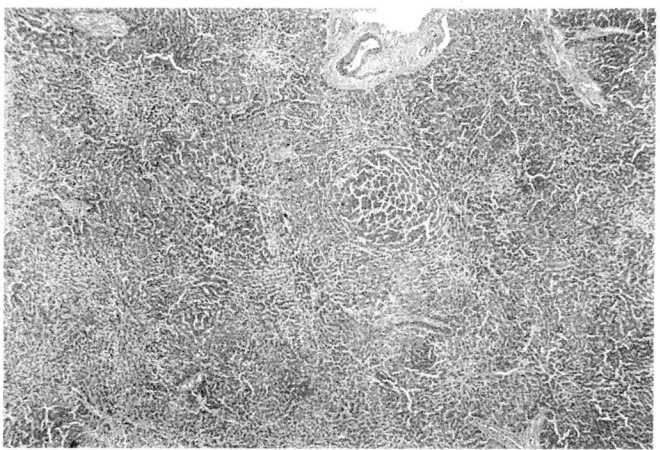

Fig. 17.139 'Sublobular' nodules in an autopsy liver from a patient with diffuse nodular hyperplasia.

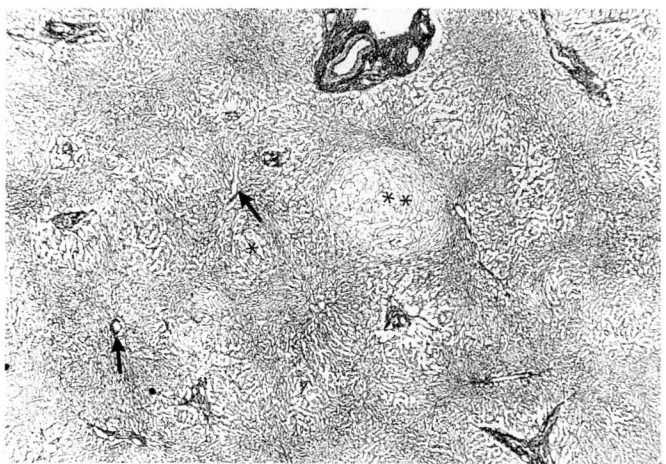

Fig. 17.140 Diffuse nodular hyperplasia. Reticulin impregnation to show small nodules (asterisks) and recognizable hepatic venous radicles (arrows). This is the same specimen as that illustrated in Fig. 17.139.

sinusoidal reticulin are not usually found, except in foci where hepatic plates are apparently compressed between adjacent small nodules. In these regions hepatocytes are smaller than elsewhere, but the atrophied cells are generally arranged in plates that are two cells thick.

DNH is distinguishable from other conditions in which thick hepatocyte plates are observed: in particular, congestive cardiac failure and hepatic venous occlusion, in both of which the hyperplasia is generally periportal; compensatory hyperplasia after damage or chronic obstructive biliary disease, in which vascular relations are normal; and cirrhosis, in which the vascular relations are lost and there is generally much irregular fibrosis.

Quantitative changes in small portal veins are described, but these are not always observed and quantitatively similar changes are sometimes noted in patients in whom there is no evidence of DNH.

The cause of DNH is not known. Other diseases sometimes associated with this condition include congestive cardiac failure, myeloproliferative conditions, Felty syndrome, and rheumatoid arthritis. Occlusion of small portal vein branches has been suggested as a possible cause, but this suggestion is not supported in all cases at present. This possibility is not excluded and lesions involving occlusion to very small portal veins may become more evident with the use of quantitative procedures.

17.12.6 Further reading

Bucher, N. L. R., Patel, V., and Cohen, S. (1978). Hormonal factors concerned with liver regeneration. In *Ciba Foundation Symposium* 55, pp. 95–110. Elsevier, Amsterdam.

Bucher, N. L., Robinson, G. S., and Farmer, S. R. (1990). Effects of extracellular matrix on hepatocyte growth and gene expression: implications for hepatic regeneration and the repair of liver injury. *Seminars in Liver Disease* 10, 11–19.

Demetriou, A. A., Seifter, E., and Levenson, S. M. (1983). Ornithine decarboxylase as an early indicator of *in vitro* hepatocyte DNA synthesis. *Journal of Surgical Research* 35, 163–7.

Du Bois, R. D. (1990). Early changes in gene expression during liver regeneration: what do they mean? *Hepatology* 11, 1079–82.

Fausto, N. and Mead, J. E. (1989). Regulation of liver growth: proto-oncogenes and transforming growth factors. *Laboratory Investigation* 60, 4–13.

Gospodarowicz, D. and Mescher A. L. 1980). Fibroblast growth factor and the control of vertebrate regeneration and repair. *Annals of the New York Academy of Sciences* 399, 151–74.

Ham, R. G. (1981). Survival and growth requirements of nontransformed cells. *Handbook of Experimental Pharmacology* 57, 13–88.

Harkness, R. D. (1957). Regeneration of liver. *British Medical Bulletin* 13, 87–93.

Huber, B. E., Heilman, C. A., Wirth, P. J., Miller, M. J., and Thorgeirsson, S. S. (1986). Studies of gene transcription and translation in regenerating rat liver. *Hepatology* 6, 209–19.

James, R. and Bradshaw, R. A. (1984). Polypeptide growth factors. *Annual Review of Biochemistry* 53, 259–92.

Kleinman, H. K., Klebe, R. J., and Martin, G. R. (1981). Role of collagenous matrices in the adhesion and growth of cells. *Journal of Cell Biology* 88, 473–85.

Knowles, D. M. and Wolff, M. (1976). Focal nodular hyperplasia of the liver. *Human Pathology* 7, 535–45.

LaBreque, D. R. (1982) *In vitro* stimulation of cell growth by hepatic stimulator substance. *American Journal of Physiology* **242**, 289–95.

Leffert, H. L., *et al.* (1982). Hepatocyte regeneration, replication, and differentiation. In *The liver: biology and pathobiology* (ed. I. Arias, H. Popper, D. Schachter, and D. A. Shafritz), pp. 601–14. Raven Press, New York.

Leffert, H. L., *et al.* (1990). Cellular and molecular biology of hepatocyte growth, regeneration and gene expression. *Advances in Second Messenger Phosphoprotein Research* **24**, 352–8.

McGowan, J. A., Strain, A. J., and Bucher, N. L. R. (1981). DNA synthesis in primary cultures of adult rat hepatocytes in a defined medium: effects of epidermal growth factor, insulin, glucagon and cyclic AMP. *Journal of Cellular Physiology* **108**, 353–63.

Makino, R., Hayashi, K., and Sugimura, T. (1984). c-*myc* transcript is induced in rat liver at a very early stage of regeneration or by cycloheximide treatment. *Nature* **310**, 697–8.

Michalopoulos, G., Houck, K. A., Dolan, M. L., and Luetteke, N. C. (1984). Control of hepatocyte replication by two serum factors. *Cancer Research* **44**, 4414–19.

Milland, J., Tsykin, A., Thomas, T., Aldred, A. R., and Schreiber, G. (1990). Gene expression in regenerating and acute-phase rat liver. *American Journal of Physiology* **259**, 310–17.

Mitaka, T., Sattler, C. A., Sattler, G. L., Sargent, L. M., and Pitot, H. C. (1991). Multiple cell cycles occur in rat hepatocytes cultures in the presence of nicotinamide and EGF. *Hepatology* **13**, 21–30.

Moesner, J., Baunsgaard, P., Starklint, H., and Thommesen, N. (1977). Focal nodular hyperplasia of the liver. Possible influence of female reproductive steroids on the histological picture. *Acta Pathologica et Microbiologica Scandinavica Section A* **85**, 113–21.

Morley, C. G. D. and Royse, V. L. (1981). Adrenergic agents as possible regulators of liver regeneration. *International Journal of Biochemistry* **13**, 969–73.

Popper, H. (1987). Cell necrosis in cirrhosis. In *Liver cirrhosis*, Falk Symposium 44 (ed. J. L. Boyer and L. Bianchi), pp. 9–18. MTP Press, Lancaster.

Poso, H. and Pegg, A. E. (1982). Effect of alpha-difluoromethylornithine on polyamine and DNA synthesis in regenerating rat liver: reversal of inhibition of DNA synthesis by putrescine. *Biochimica et Biophysica Acta* **696**, 179–86.

St Hilaire, R. J. and Jones, A. L. (1982). Epidermal growth factor: its biologic and metabolic effects with emphasis on the hepatocyte. *Hepatology* **2**, 601–13.

Schlessinger, J. and Geiger, B. (1981). Epidermal growth factor induces redistribution of actin and alpha-actinin in human epidermal carcinoma cells. *Experimental Cell Research* **134**, 273–9.

Sporn, M. B. and Roberts, A. B. (1985). Autocrine growth factors and cancer. *Nature* **313**, 745–7.

Steiner, P. E. (1959). Nodular regenerative hyperplasia of the liver. *American Journal of Pathology* **35**, 943–53.

Thompson, L., *et al.* (1986). Sequential protooncogene expression during rat liver regeneration. *Cancer Research* **46**, 3111–17.

Vecchio, F. M., *et al.* (1984), Fibrolamellar carcinoma of the liver: the malignant counterpart of focal nodular hyperplasia with oncocyte change. *American Journal of Clinical Pathology* **81**, 521–6.

Wanless, I. R. (1986). Nodular regenerative hyperplasia of the liver. A morphometric study of 23 cases. *Laboratory Investigation* **54**, 67A.

Wanless, I. R. (1987). The use of morphometry in the study of nodular and vascular lesions of the liver. *Analytical and Quantitative Cytology and Histology* **9**, 39–41.

Wanless, I. R. (1990). Micronodular transformation (nodular regenerative hyperplasia) of the liver: a report of 64 cases among 2500 autopsies and a new classification of benign hepatocellular nodules. *Hepatology* **11**, 787–97.

Weinbren, K. and Mutum, S. S. (1984). Pathological aspects of diffuse nodular hyperplasia of the liver. *Journal of Pathology* **143**, 81–92.

Weinbren, K., Hadjis, N. S., and Blumgart, L. H. (1985). Structural aspects of the liver in patients with biliary disease and portal hypertension. *Journal of Clinical Pathology* **38**, 1013–20.

Yamada, K. M. (1983). Cell surface interactions with extracellular materials. *Annual Review of Biochemistry* **52**, 761–99.

Yanker, B. A. and Shooter, E. M. (1982). The biology and mechanism of action of nerve growth factor. *Annual Review of Biochemistry* **51**, 845–68.

17.13   Hepatic tumours

R. S. Patrick

Because of the association of liver cell adenoma with focal nodular hyperplasia, the two conditions are described together (see Section 17.12).

17.13.1   Hepatocellular carcinoma

Incidence

There is a remarkable variation in the incidence of this tumour throughout the world. The areas of high frequency, where it is undoubtedly the commonest type of malignant disease, include sub-Saharan Africa and the Orient, especially South-East Asia and much of China. This is in sharp contrast to most of Europe and the American and Australasian continents, where the incidence can be less than 5 cases per 100 000 persons per annum. The incidence is also low among many generations of white settlers in South Africa, but this tumour is probably not genetically determined as its incidence falls among Negroes living in low-incidence countries; when familial clustering of cases occurs there is probably some local environmental factor, such as hepatitis B virus (HBV) infection.

Where the incidence is low, the tumour often affects middle-aged or elderly males, many of whom suffer also from cirrhosis, usually of mixed or macronodular type. In some cases of cirrhosis, hepatocyte dysplasia has been regarded as a premalignant condition. It affects groups of cells which are enlarged with prominent cytoplasm and hyperchromatic nuclei, sometimes multiple, pleomorphic, or folded (Fig. 17.141). Dysplasia is common in experimental animals during the induction of liver tumours by chemical carcinogens. However, it is not present in all human liver cell cancer cases and is often found in the absence of tumour.

In high-incidence areas, the tumour tends to develop more rapidly and in younger patients, usually males. Cirrhosis is less frequent but nevertheless the association with dysplasia is more convincing.

Over the past 30–40 years, there has been a small but significant rise in incidence in many Western countries, possibly related to the rising incidence of chronic alcoholism.

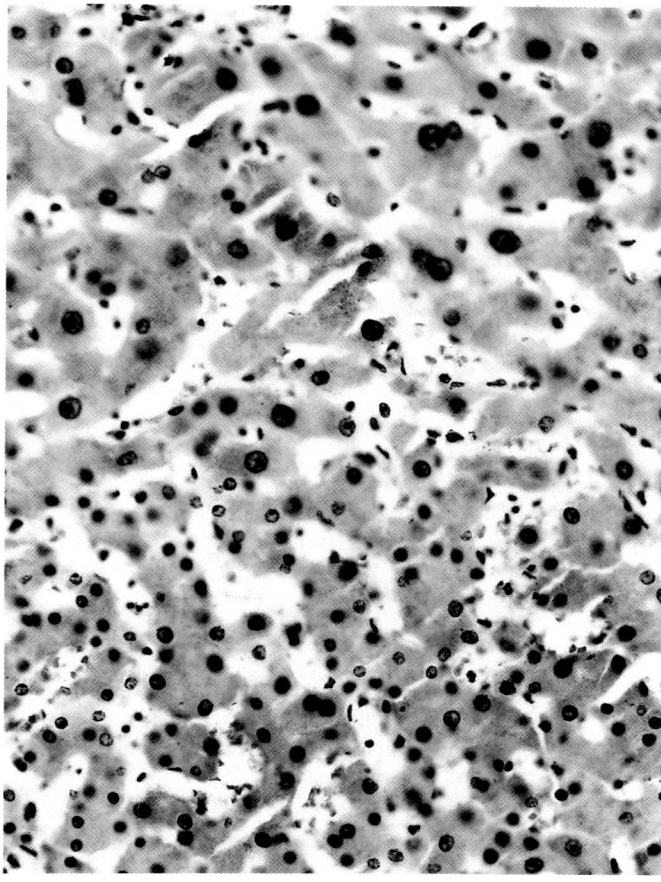

Fig. 17.141 Hepatocyte dysplasia (above) for comparison with normal liver cells (below).

Aetiology

Many cases are idiopathic, but the following factors have been implicated.

HBV infection

There is now much circumstantial evidence linking the two conditions. The high-incidence localities throughout the world of the infection and of the tumour correspond very closely. The tumour is relatively common in HBV carriers and in those with HBV-induced chronic hepatitis and cirrhosis. There is a close association between the infection and hepatocyte dysplasia. Viral antigens are detected in the blood of many hepatocellular cancer cases, and both surface and core antigens may be demonstrated in hepatocytes of tumour-bearing livers, even in low-incidence countries. Fragments of HBV genome have been detected in hepatocyte nuclei during tumour development and in liver cancer cells. A hepadna virus similar to HBV can infect woodchucks, causing hepatitis, and some of these animals later develop primary liver cancer, but without cirrhosis.

Of course, none of these observations provide absolute proof of a primary oncogenic function for HBV, and it has been argued that cancer is merely a consequence of macronodular cirrhosis which develops from the infection. However, this would not explain the occurrence of tumours in non-cirrhotic liver in localities where the incidence of both tumour and infection is high. Possibly the viral DNA incorporated into hepatocyte nuclei initiates neoplastic change which remains latent until promoted by other factors at a later date.

Other viral infections

Antibodies to hepatitis C virus (HCV) have been found in the sera of many cases of hepatocellular cancer in localities where the infection is common, and only a minority of these cancer patients have evidence of additional HBV infection. A similar association between HCV and other chronic liver diseases unrelated to tumours would suggest that the infection may be acquired only by chance. However recent studies of sera stored for many years have shown that HCV infection invariably precedes the development of liver cancer, and that the viral antibody level is maintained throughout the long period of chronic hepatitis and cirrhosis until the appearance of the tumour.

There is at present no convincing evidence to link hepatocellular cancer with hepatitis virus A, D (delta), E, or other known liver viral infections.

Aflatoxins

These toxins are derived from the mould *Aspergillus flavus*, which can contaminate ground-nut meal and cereals stored under hot, humid conditions in the tropics. Aflatoxins can induce acute liver injury and tumours in various experimental animals. There is a possibility, therefore, that aflatoxins are related to the development of human liver cell cancer, but this is still unproven.

Other toxins and drugs

A wide range of chemicals may induce primary liver cancer when fed to experimental animals, especially rats. These include paradimethylaminoazobenzene (butter yellow), 2-acetyl-aminofluorine, and other aromatic amines, nitrosamines, and nitrosamides, such as dimethyl nitrosamide, ethionine, thioacetamide, and many others. These are valuable in studies on carcinogenesis, but, with the possible exception of nitrosamines, their relevance to human liver tumours is doubtful. A few chemicals, such as vinyl chloride are more commonly associated with angiosarcoma. Oral contraceptives, especially mestranol and ethinyl oestradiol, and androgenic/anabolic steroids used to treat sexual disorders and refractory anaemias, have very rarely been associated with benign and possibly malignant liver tumours. The fact that some 'cancers' regress when the androgenic/anabolic steroid therapy is terminated throws some doubt on their malignant nature. (See also Section 17.7.6.)

Alcohol

It could be assumed that cirrhosis from this cause might be complicated by malignancy, especially those macronodular cases that may develop following periods of abstention.

However, not all alcoholics with hepatocellular carcinoma have cirrhosis. The importance of malnutrition, which occurs in some alcoholics and from other causes, is unknown.

Metabolic disorders

The incidence of primary liver cancer is raised in patients with certain inherited metabolic disorders, such as tyrosinosis, type I glycogen storage disease, and, probably, α-1-antitrypsin deficiency in adults. The incidence is also relatively high in advanced idiopathic haemochromatosis (but this may relate to the long-standing cirrhosis and frequency in males) and in Bantu siderosis, probably associated with HBV infection.

Inferior vena caval obstruction

In South Africa and Japan an association has been noted between the tumour and chronic Budd–Chiari syndrome, due to obstruction of the upper inferior vena cava by membranous bands or fibrosis. The reasons for this association are unknown.

Clinical features and diagnosis

In high-incidence countries, the illness can begin suddenly with severe abdominal pain related to a large tender liver, followed by rapid deterioration and death within a few weeks. Most cases in Western countries have a more insidious onset and may be suspected by physical deterioration in patients with cirrhosis. Nodularity of an enlarged liver is not invariably present. Isotope scanning, ultrasonography, and angiography are of value in detecting intrahepatic lesions and in localizing the optimum position for aspiration needle biopsy. Jaundice is often mild or absent, and the presence of relatively low serum bilirubin with high serum alkaline phosphatase is characteristic.

The detection in the circulation of unusual products of cancer cell origin, especially α-fetoprotein, is of greater diagnostic value. α-Fetoprotein is a glubulin produced during the early stages of fetal development but is barely detectable in normal children or adults. Levels above 500 μg/l serum are found in 80–90 per cent of hepatocellular cancer patients, but much smaller amounts can be detected in some cases of hepatitis or liver regeneration. Acidic isoferritin is another oncofetal protein of similar diagnostic value, but not carcino-embryonic antigen. Prolyl hydroxylase, the enzyme essential for collagen 'maturation', may be produced in large amounts, even by tumours with little fibrous stroma. Rarely, there is production of substances with humoral effects, such as an erythropoietin-like material causing erythrocytosis; chorionic gonadotrophin and placental lactogen, sometimes with sexual effects; and parathormone causing hypercalcaemia; etc. Metabolic disorders may be complex; thus hypoglycaemia is not usually due to the production of an insulin-like substance, but may be a consequence of impaired gluconeogenesis or glycogenolysis.

Pathology

Macroscopic appearances

The liver is nearly always enlarged, sometimes to a remarkable degree, especially in high-incidence countries. In low-incidence regions, a multinodular distribution throughout a cirrhotic liver is the usual pattern. The tumour nodules are mostly well demarcated, one or more centimetres in diameter, and of fairly uniform size and paler than the surrounding liver. Necrosis and haemorrhage can be extensive and bile-staining, when present, is pathognomonic. Nodules are generally of soft consistency and tend to bulge from the cut surface and under Glisson's capsule which they may invade; but, unlike secondary cancer, umbilication is unusual.

Less commonly, the liver is non-cirrhotic and contains a large tumour mass usually occupying much of the right lobe. It can be well defined or infiltrate the surrounding tissue, commonly with numbers of small pale and discrete satellite nodules.

A diffuse type infiltrating the entire organ is also described but is quite rare. Nodularity is absent or barely detectable and the condition may be mistaken for diffuse fibrosis or fine micro-nodular cirrhosis.

Tumour invasion of portal or hepatic veins may be seen, which can extend into the inferior vena cava. Invasion of a large bile duct occurs rarely in patients who give a history of obstructive jaundice. Oesophageal varices and ascites are often prominent, even in non-cirrhotic cases. Rupture of tumour with peritoneal bleeding and deposits on the peritoneal surface, or direct invasion of surrounding tissue, may be evident. In about 50 per cent of cases, metastatic deposits are found, especially in abdominal lymph nodes, lungs, and bone marrow.

Routine examination of a cirrhotic liver at autopsy may reveal one or more small, firm, pale areas which are small foci of malignancy, but the rate of development of these is not known. In Japan, minute tumours, each surrounded by a thick avascular capsule, are not uncommon, sometimes within livers shrunken by advanced cirrhosis. Very rarely, a pedunculated and readily resectable liver cell cancer occurs, attached by a narrow band of tissue to a cirrhotic liver not otherwise affected by tumour.

Microscopic appearances

In many cases, tumour cells have eosinophilic cytoplasm and round, vesicular nuclei with distinct nucleoli; apart from a slightly larger size, they bear a close resemblance to normal hepatocytes. Mitotic activity is variable. They are arranged typically in plates or trabeculae, usually several cells thick, and separated by sinusoidal channels which have an endothelial and very scanty reticulin lining, but Kupffer cells are not seen (Fig. 17.142).

In some tumours or parts of tumour there is an acinar pattern of cells around small channels, which represent bile canaliculi and may contain bile pigment. Occasionally these channels are distended with bile-stained fibrin or hyaline material and resemble thyroid acini. Glycogen is common in tumour cell cytoplasm and granules of bile pigment are found much less frequently. In cases associated with idiopathic haemochromatosis, haemosiderin is absent from tumour cells. In about 15 per cent of cases there are prominent, rounded hyaline bodies within tumour cells or lying extracellularly (Fig. 17.143); immunohistochemistry reveals that these consist of various

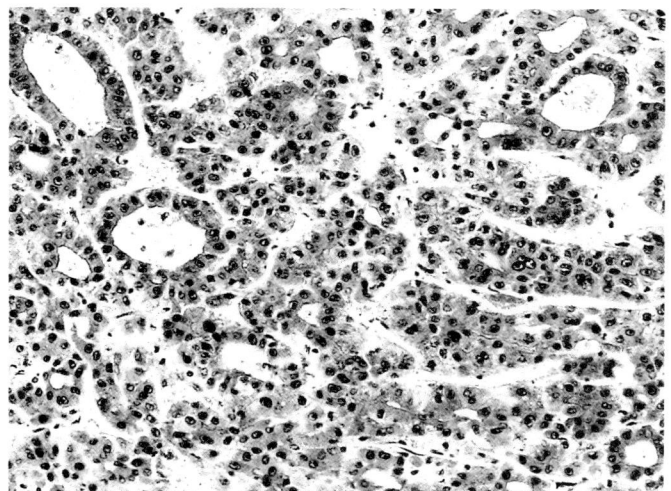

Fig. 17.142 Hepatocellular carcinoma. There is a typical arrangement of well-differentiated tumour cells into trabeculae and acini.

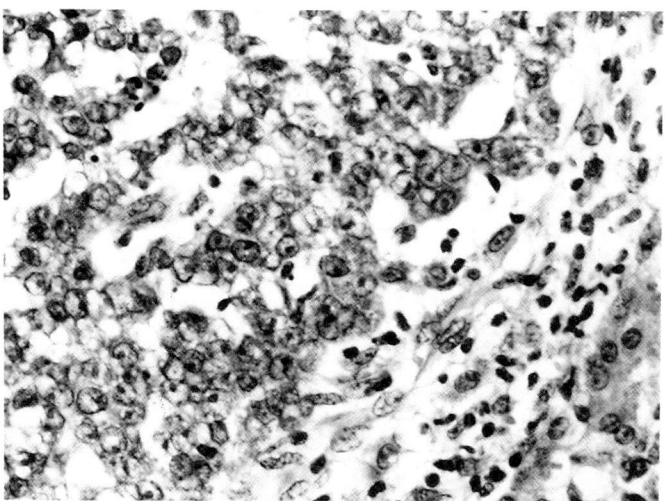

Fig. 17.144 Hepatocellular carcinoma. Small cell type with vacuolated cytoplasm.

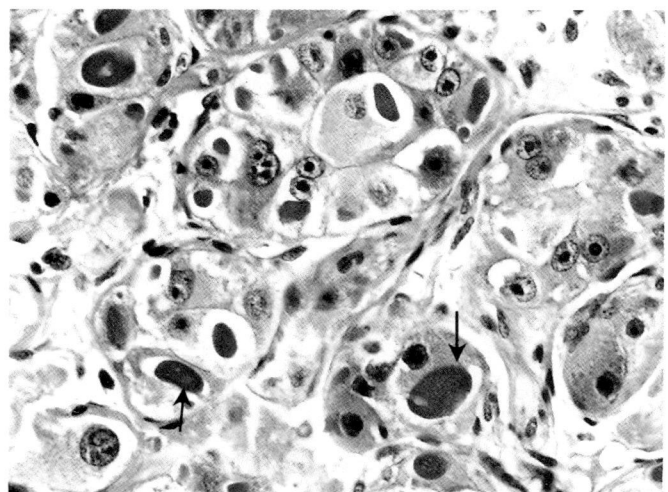

Fig. 17.143 Hepatocellular carcinoma. Many tumour cells contain large, well-demarcated inclusion bodies (arrows).

proteins, such as α-fetoprotein, α-1-antitrypsin, albumin, etc. Less frequently, there are Mallory bodies in cell cytoplasm, sometimes in alcoholic patients. An irregular distribution of fatty change affects some tumours.

Less well-differentiated tumours may contain solid masses of cells, sometimes pleomorphic or with giant multinucleated forms. Some consist of small, round cells with scanty cytoplasm, which may be vacuolated because of excess glycogen (Fig. 17.144).

A connective tissue stroma is usually inconspicuous but a minority are sclerotic and sometimes associated with hypercalcaemia. There can be a distinct pattern of collagen bands separating columns of prominent polygonal tumour cells with eosinophilic and granular cytoplasm; these cells can be

regarded as oncocytes, being rich in mitochondria. This is the *fibrolamellar* type of *hepatocellular carcinoma* (Fig. 17.145); it is worthy of distinct recognition not only for its structural character but for its tendency to occur in a younger age-group and always in a non-cirrhotic liver. Successful resection is sometimes possible, and it has a better prognosis than other types of hepatocellular cancer.

Prognosis

This is very poor as only a small number of non-cirrhotic cases, especially fibrolamellar cancers, are suitable for resection. Death usually occurs well within a year of establishing the diagnosis. Causes of death include liver destruction by tumour, oesophageal bleeding from portal hypertension caused by cirrhosis or by vascular invasion with tumour, rupture of tumour

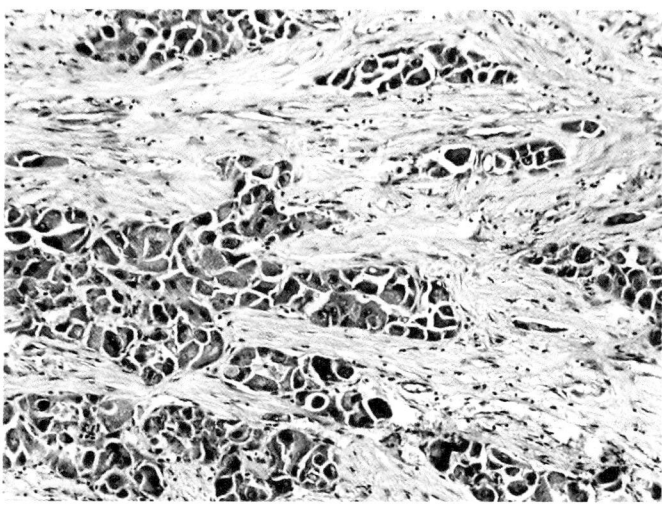

Fig. 17.145 Hepatocellular carcinoma. Fibrolamellar type.

with massive haemorrhage, tumour metastases, hypogly-caemia, and other humoral effects.

17.13.2   Tumours derived from bile duct epithelium

Tumours with similar pathological features can arise in extra-hepatic bile ducts (see Section 17.15.10).

Benign biliary tumours

Bile duct adenoma, papilloma, cystadenoma

Adenoma forms a small pale nodule, usually subcapsular, and consists of small ducts lined by cuboidal epithelium. It is with-out clinical significance. Papillomas within bile ducts tend to be multiple and may cause obstruction; they may recur after re-section, and malignancy can supervene. Biliary cystadenoma resembles similar ovarian tumours as it can grow to a large size, contain multilocular cysts with mucinous fluid, possess a cystic lining of cuboidal or columnar epithelium and a compact cellu-lar stroma, and has a tendency to malignant change. All these biliary tumours are rare.

Cholangiocarcinoma

Aetiology

This is a rare tumour in all parts of the world except the Orient where there is a clear association with two liver fluke infesta-tions, *Opisthorchis sinensis*, found in South and East China, and *Opisthorchis viverrini*, found in Thailand and Malaysia. Their presence within bile ducts induces striking adenomatous epithe-lial proliferation followed, in some cases, by neoplasia.

In other countries there is an association with sclerosing cholangitis, usually complicating ulcerative colitis, but such cases are rare.

Clinical features

Depending on tumour location, two distinct types are recog-nized. Both carry a poor prognosis.

Hilar carcinoma   This grows slowly, causing progressive obstructive jaundice. There is a risk of cholangitis which may be fatal.

Peripheral intrahepatic carcinoma   The features are similar to hepatocellular carcinoma, although hepatomegaly and portal hypertension are often less prominent. There is no association with HBV infection and no elevation of α-fetoprotein. A few tumours produce parathormone, causing hypercalcaemia in the absence of bone metastases.

Pathology

Hilar tumours   These may form hard strictures of bile ducts in the porta hepatis and can be difficult to distinguish from scler-osing cholangitis which can coexist. Others are more friable intraluminal growths. Both cause biliary obstruction and tend to invade surrounding hepatic tissue. The liver, but not the tumour, is bile-stained and peripheral ducts may be dilated or show evidence of suppurative cholangitis. Secondary biliary cir-rhosis can occur in slowly growing tumours.

Microscopically, these are scirrhous adenocarcinomas. The friable cases are usually papillary and pre-invasive malignant change may be seen in adjacent bile duct epithelium. Some may originate in extrahepatic ducts and spread along these into the liver.

Peripheral tumours   Usually, there is a solitary pale tumour, several centimetres in diameter, sometimes ill-defined, and lying within a non-cirrhotic liver. Compared with hepatocellu-lar cancer, they are usually quite scirrhous and avascular and never bile-stained. Tumour necrosis and vascular invasion are less common.

Again, these are adenocarcinomas, usually fairly well differ-entiated with infrequent mitotic figures (Fig. 17.146). The cells are cuboidal or columnar with small round nuclei and clear cytoplasm. Mucus secretion is common but may be scanty. The fibrous stroma may be extensive and contain acidic mucopoly-saccharide or calcium deposits. There is a tendency to grow

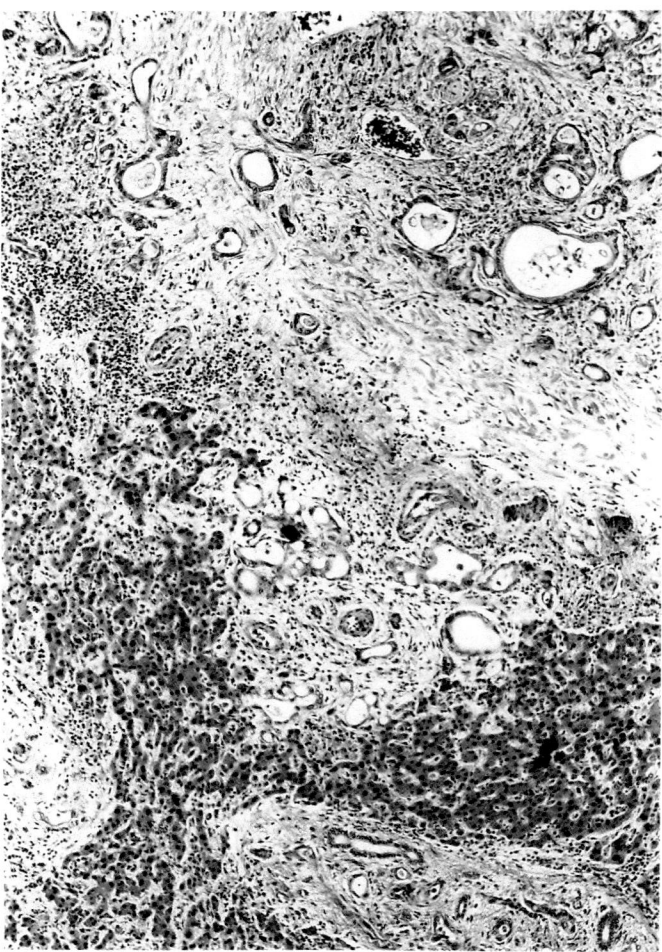

Fig. 17.146   Cholangiocarcinoma arising in the periphery of liver. It is a scirrhous adenocarcinoma invading liver parenchyma and spreading within a portal tract (below).

along adjacent liver sinusoids and to spread peripherally in portal lymphatics; these may be lined by tumour cells which also project into dilated lumens as small, blunt papillae. It will be appreciated that the differential diagnosis from secondary adenocarcinoma may be impossible, especially in biopsies.

Metastases are often found in abdominal lymph nodes and may be blood-borne to the lungs and elsewhere.

17.13.3 Other malignant biliary tumours

Cholangiolocellular carcinoma

This consists of trabeculae of small cuboidal cells in a scirrhous stroma and may originate in canals of Hering. They behave as for cholangiocarcinoma.

Squamous cell cancer

This may arise from biliary-type epithelium lining hepatic cysts.

Carcinoid tumour

Carcinoid tumour may originate in argentaffin cells within bile duct walls. All are very rare.

Mixed bile duct and liver cell cancer

This is also rare. Possibly these are 'collision' tumours arising by chance in the same organ. A transitional cell type is also described. Both behave as hepatocellular carcinoma.

17.13.4 Vascular tumours

Haemangioma

These common tumours, cavernous in type, form small, dark-red or purple areas under the liver capsule. Rarely, they measure several centimetres in diameter and form tender palpable masses, sometimes associated with thrombocytopenia or hypofibrinogenaemia. Multiple lesions should not be confused with hereditary telangiectasia or peliosis hepatis.

Infantile haemangioendothelioma

These are rare single or multiple tumours occupying much of the liver in young infants. They have a spongy brown appearance with central fibrosis. Microscopically, they consist of vascular channels lined by plump endothelial cells which can also form solid masses. There is variable fibrous stroma containing biliary channels and foci of haemopoiesis. Similar lesions at other sites, such as lungs, bone, or skin, are of multicentric origin and not metastases, as the tumours are essentially benign. Nevertheless, death is usual because of liver destruction or high-output cardiac failure, often mistaken clinically for congenital heart disease with systemic congestion. Coagulative disorders may also coexist. Cases who survive undergo extensive fibrosis, often with calcification.

Angiosarcoma

Incidence

This is a very rare tumour in all parts of the world, with its highest incidence in elderly males.

Aetiology

Most are idiopathic, but an association is recognized with the following, which are related also to hepatocellular carcinoma and cholangiocarcinoma.

Thorotrast This is 20 per cent thorium dioxide, used as a contrast medium in radiology until discontinued over 30 years ago, but liver tumours from this cause still appear occasionally. Thorotrast may also induce hepatic fibrosis and portal hypertension. It appears in liver sections as dull grey granules which emit α-radiation tracks detectable by autoradiography.

Arsenical compounds These may be absorbed by persons who work with certain insecticides, or by patients with skin disease treated with Fowler's solution.

Vinyl chloride The incidence of hepatic angiosarcoma is relatively high in workers with this material in the manufacture of synthetic rubber, spray paints, insecticide aerosols, etc. The finished polymer, polyvinyl chloride, is harmless. There may be a prolonged incubation period before the tumour is manifest when there is liver dysfunction and portal hypertension. Liver biopsy may then reveal dysplastic changes in hepatocytes and sinusoidal cells, together with perisinusoidal, portal, and subcapsular fibrosis.

Clinical features

There is abdominal pain and a large tender liver with progressive liver failure, including jaundice and malaise. Death is usual within 6 months, often from severe internal haemorrhage following tumour rupture. As in other vascular tumours, there may be coagulation defects.

Pathology

The liver is grossly enlarged with numerous dark tumours or blood-filled cystic spaces. These can be minute or measure many centimetres in diameter. They may be well defined but are not encapsulated. They may bulge out from the capsular surface of the liver, and rupture may be evident. A minority of cases are cirrhotic. Blood-borne metastases may be found, especially in bone marrow.

Microscopically the tumour cells are spindle-shaped and hyperchromatic (Fig. 17.147). They line blood-filled spaces or form solid masses, with poorly defined margins. They appear to grow along sinusoids, replacing the normal lining cells, and these channels dilate as the intervening hepatocyte plates atrophy or disappear; however, small groups of liver cells, each with a lining of tumour cells, may survive within blood-filled spaces. Tumour invasion of hepatic and portal veins may be evident and there may be islands of haemopoietic cells.

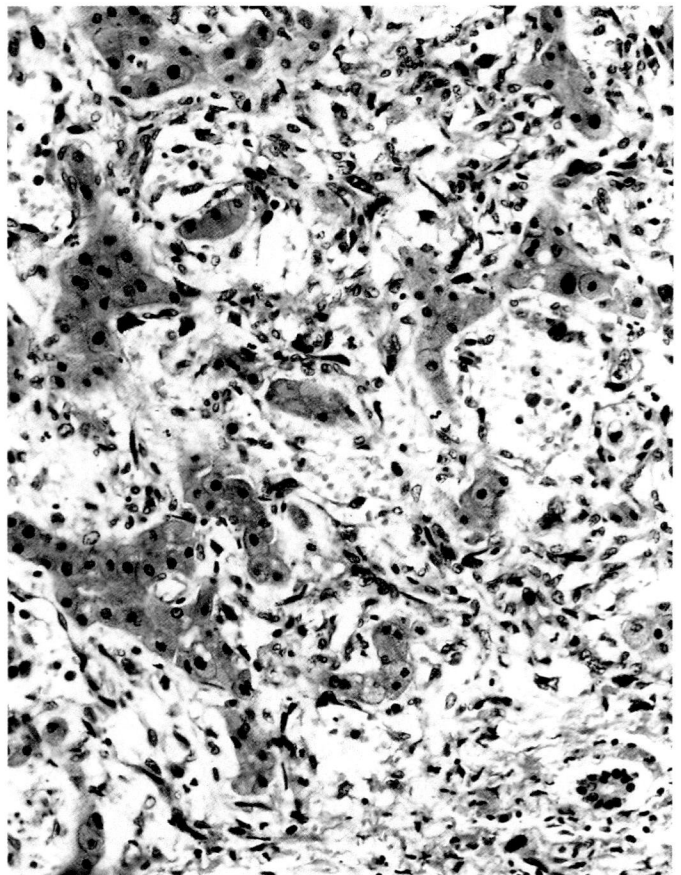

Fig. 17.147 Angiosarcoma of the liver. Surviving hepatocyte plates are separated by pleomorphic or spindle-shaped tumour cells set in a loose connective tissue stroma.

Epithelioid haemangioendothelioma

This uncommon tumour can occur in adult liver as multiple, firm, pale nodules. Microscopically, it is often mistaken for cholangiocarcinoma because of its scirrhous nature and epithelioid cells. These cells tend to form clumps or grow along sinusoids or within veins. Cytoplasmic vacuolation of groups of cells may give a pseudoacinar pattern and erythrocytes may be seen in some of these. Other tumour cells are elongated (dendritic) and lie within a dense fibrous stroma which may be calcified. The tumour is invasive and may form metastases but growth is slow compared with other malignant hepatic tumours. Its vascular nature may be demonstrated by its content of factor VIII-related antigen (Fig. 17.148).

17.13.5   Malignant tumours of childhood

Hepatoblastoma

Incidence

With few exceptions, this rare tumour occurs within the first 3 years of life and may be found in the fetus. It is commoner in males.

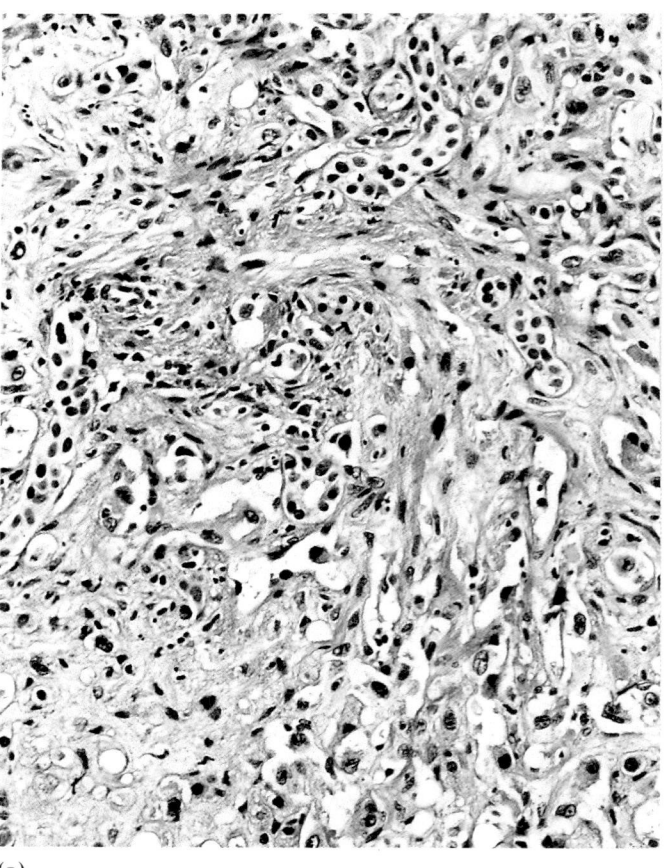

(a)

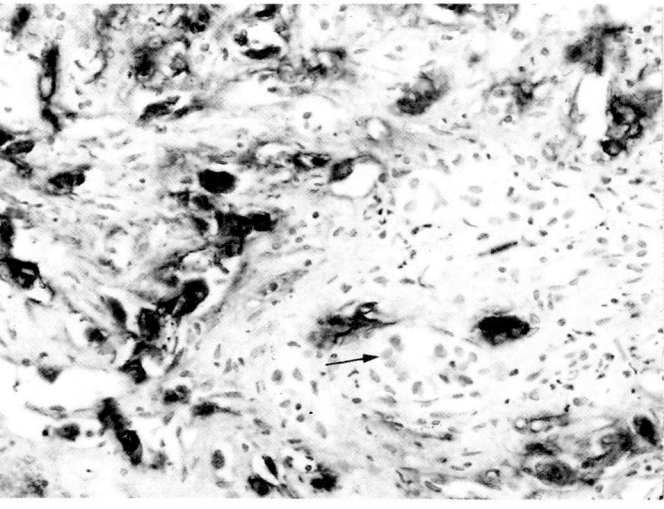

(b)

Fig. 17.148 Epithelioid haemangioendothelioma of the liver. (a) There is sinusoidal invasion by columns of epithelioid tumour cells and a few spindle-shaped dendritic cells. (b) Tumour cells contain factor VIII-related antigen shown by the immunoperoxidase method. Note that bile duct epithelium (arrow) does not stain.

Clinical features

There is a grossly enlarged liver which is firm and tender, smooth or nodular. The child fails to thrive and jaundice is unusual. Serum α-fetoprotein levels are usually high. Cardiac defects and other developmental anomalies may coexist and, rarely, there is sexual precocity from secretion of chorionic gonadotrophin by the tumour. Prognosis is very poor as few are resectable.

Pathology

Two types are described, viz. epithelial and mixed epithelial and mesenchymal. Both form a single large mass, usually in the right liver lobe. It is well circumscribed and sometimes encapsulated with prominent vessels on the capsular surface. The cut surface is pale grey and may be lobulated and partly calcified, especially the mixed type. Necrosis and haemorrhage can be extensive.

Microscopically (Fig. 17.149) much of the epithelium consists of fetal-type hepatocytes, slightly larger than normal liver cells. They are arranged in plates, usually two cells thick, separated by thin-walled sinusoids. Mitotic figures are rare but foci of haemopoiesis are quite common. More primitive embryonic

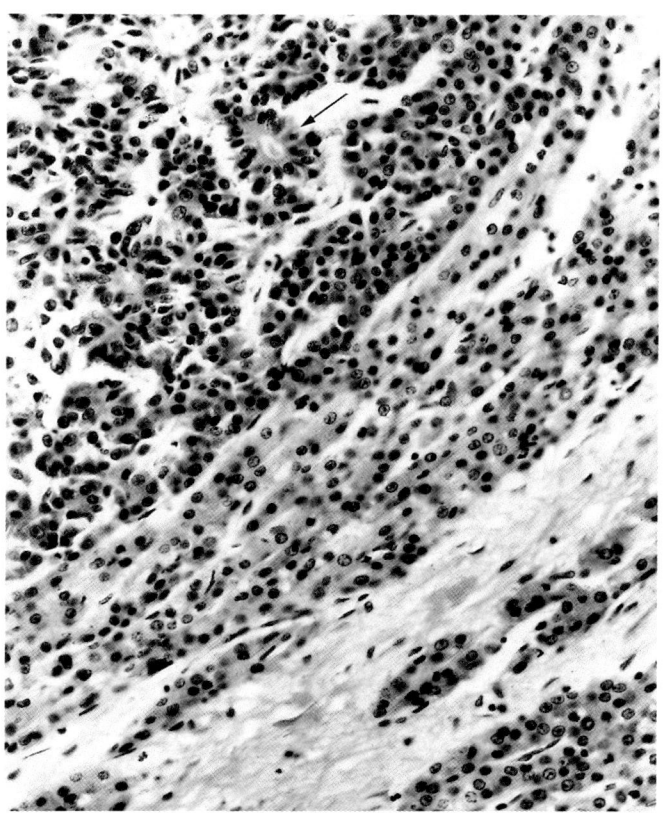

Fig. 17.149 Hepatoblastoma. A band of fetal-type hepatocytes runs diagonally from top right to bottom left and is separated from similar cells, bottom right by a mesenchymal component of the tumour. Embryonic-type cells including a rosette (arrow), are present above, top left. (Provided by Dr F. D. Lee.)

hepatocytes occur in groups and may blend with fetal cells. These are poorly differentiated with poor cohesion and may form acini, rosettes, or papillae. Their nuclei are rich in chromatin and mitotic figures are numerous.

The mesenchymal component of mixed tumours is variable in amount. It consists of primitive elongated connective tissue cells set in a myxomatous stroma. More mature young fibroblasts with a parallel orientation may be present adjacent to collagen fibres. Islands of osteoid tissue and foci of calcification may be present, but cartilage and muscle cells are rarely recognized. It should be noted from recent immunohistochemical studies that cells embedded in osteoid matrix are not typical osteoblasts as they possess certain features of epithelium.

Undifferentiated (embryonal) sarcoma

This is also rare with a poor prognosis, but affects patients in the 6–15-year age-group. The tumour forms a large solitary mass with a pseudo-capsule. The cut surface is gelatinous or cystic, with extensive necrosis and haemorrhage. It is a myxomatous tumour with hyperchromatic cells, atypical mitoses, and cytoplasmic vacuoles, which may contain PAS-positive inclusions. The tumour cells may be arranged in whorls and part of the lesion may be very vascular. Small groups of hepatocytes and bile ducts may be included at the periphery of the tumour.

Embryonal rhabdomyosarcoma has many similar features but arises from the walls of bile ducts and presents with obstructive jaundice.

17.13.6 Miscellaneous primary tumours

These include fibroma, lipoma, leiomyoma, neurilemmoma and their malignant counterparts, together with mesothelioma and fibrous histiocytoma. Mixed and mesenchymal hamartoma and teratoma are recorded. Adrenal cortical tumour may arise from nests of adrenal cells situated within the liver close to the right gland. All are very rare.

17.13.7 Secondary tumours

The liver is a very common site for secondary carcinoma from any source, especially alimentary canal, breast, and bronchus. These are discrete tumour nodules of variable size; rarely, there is diffuse infiltration with tiny nodules and much fibrosis ('carcinomatous cirrhosis'). In many cases it is impossible to state the primary tumour site from the gross or microscopic appearances, but some do have characteristic features, such as follicular carcinoma of thyroid containing thyroglobulin, clear-cell carcinoma of kidney, malignant melanoma, etc.

Hodgkin and non-Hodgkin lymphoma and leukaemia also involve the liver frequently. In some of these there are also chronic non-specific inflammatory changes and granulomas, which should not be overinterpreted as tumours. Cholestasis is not infrequent and is also of uncertain pathogenesis, as not all cases can be explained by excessive blood destruction and bilirubin production, or by biliary obstruction by tumour.

17.13.8   Further reading

Anthony, P. P., Vogel, C. L., and Barker, L. P. (1973). Liver cell dysplasia; a premalignant condition. *Journal of Clinical Pathology* **26**, 217–23.

Bassendine, M. F. (1984). Hepatitis B virus and liver cell cancer. In *Recent advances in histopathology* no. 12 (ed. P. P. Anthony and R. N. M. MacSween), pp. 137–46. Churchill Livingstone, Edinburgh.

Baxter, P. J., Anthony, P. P., MacSween, R. N. M., and Scheuer, P. J. (1980). Angiosarcoma of the liver; annual occurrence and aetiology in Great Britain. *British Journal of Industrial Medicine* **37**, 213–21.

Farber, E. (1982). Neoplastic transformation. In *The liver; biology and pathology* (ed. I. Arias, H. Popper, D. Schachter, and D. A. Shafritz). Raven Press, New York.

Hodgson, H. J. F. (1987). Fibrolamellar carcinoma. *Journal of Hepatology* **5**, 241–7.

Ishak, K. G., Sesterhenn, I. A., Goodman, Z. D., Rabin, L., and Stromeyer, F. W. (1984). Epithelioid haemangioendothelioma of the liver; a clinicopathologic and follow-up study of 32 cases. *Human Pathology* **15**, 839–52.

Johnson, P. J. and Williams, R. (1987). Cirrhosis and the aetiology of hepatocellular carcinoma. *Journal of Hepatology* **4**, 140–7.

Keating, S. and Taylor, G. P. (1985). Undifferentiated (embryonal) sarcoma of the liver. *Human Pathology* **16**, 693–9.

Kiyosawa, K., *et al.* (1990). Hepatitis C virus and hepatocellular carcinoma: additional evidence of a causal link. *Hepatology* **12**, 671–5.

Van Eyken, P., Sciot, R., Callea, F., Ramaekers, F., Schaart, G., and Desmet, V. J. (1990). A cytokeratine–immunohistochemical study of hepatoblastoma. *Human Pathology* **21**, 302–8.

Weinberg, A. G. and Finegold, M. J. (1983). Primary hepatic tumours of childhood. *Human Pathology* **14**, 512–37.

Weinbren, K. and Mutum, S. S. (1983). Pathological aspects of cholangiocarcinoma. *Journal of Pathology* **139**, 217–38.

General

Okuda, K. and MacKay, I. (eds) (1982). *Hepatocellular carcinoma*, UICC Technical Report Series, Vol. 74. International Union against Cancer, Geneva.

17.14   Pathology of liver transplantation

Bernard Portmann

Liver transplantation is now widely accepted as a modality of treatment of various forms of liver disease. Following the first successful liver transplantation in man by Starzl in 1963, there were approximately 1000 grafts inserted world-wide over the next 20 years; a number which is now attained yearly. Increased interest in this procedure has coincided with the 50 per cent one year survival rate achieved by steady improvement in surgical techniques, organ preservation, patient selection, and immunosuppression.

Pioneer work in the pathology of the liver graft was mainly based on animal experiments and human autopsy material. More recently, liver biopsy has become an important component of patient assessment and the ever increasing number of biopsies forwarded to the pathologist has allowed a better discrimination of the changes due to graft rejection from those due to other complications.

17.14.1   Acute rejection

Acute allograft rejection is characterized by a dense portal tract accumulation of small and large lymphocytes, eosinophils, and smaller numbers of plasma cells and neutrophils. The interlobular bile ducts may be obscured by the cell infiltrate or exhibit a variable degree of epithelial swelling and eosinophilic shrinkage with nuclear pleomorphism, multilayering, or loss. Both portal and hepatic venules may show endotheliitis with attachment of lymphocytes to their endothelial lining (Figs 17.150, 17.152). Perivenular hepatocyte necrosis and loss are usually minimal; when severe it may reflect ischaemic damage inflicted on the graft prior to revascularization in the host, or secondary to thrombotic occlusion of, or rejection changes in, medium-sized arteries.

Acute rejection occurs commonly at 7–15 days, less often later after surgery. The changes usually subside following steroid therapy. Hyperacute rejection, as observed within minutes or hours of a kidney transplant, has not been documented in liver allografts. However, antibody-mediated haemorrhagic necrosis may occur within a week or so of a liver having been transplanted across major ABO blood group barriers.

17.14.2   Chronic rejection

Chronic rejection classically comprises arterial lesions in the form of intimal accumulation of foamy, lipid-laden macro-

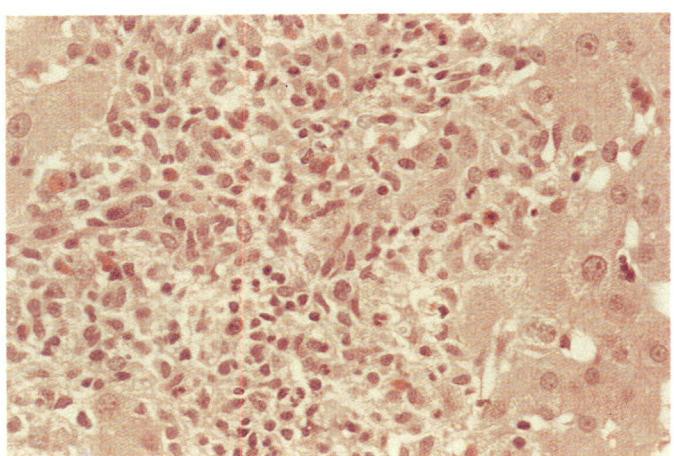

Fig. 17.150 Acute rejection in liver allograft. A dense mixed-cell infiltration obscures the portal tract structures.

phages (Fig. 17.151) and an on-going degeneration with progressive disappearance of the interlobular bile ducts, named the vanishing bile duct syndrome.

Canalicular cholestasis is consistently present. Some perivenular cell loss seems to parallel the degree of arterial changes and may progress to perivenular fibrosis and periacinar septum formation. An accelerated form of the vanishing bile duct syndrome may develop fully within a few weeks of surgery, in which case the changes of both acute and chronic rejection coexist (Fig. 17.152). More commonly the course is subacute, evolving over months, and the cellular infiltrate grows less as the bile ducts disappear. In advanced stages, mildly fibrotic portal tracts are devoid of bile ducts and contain only occasional mixed inflammatory cells or groups of foamy macrophages filling terminal vascular branches (Fig. 17.153). Unlike the changes of acute rejection, the disappearance of the bile ducts

cannot be arrested by medical treatment and in most instances the lesion will progress to graft failure requiring retransplantation.

An additional form of chronic rejection seems to remain static or to progress very slowly over years. The histopathology resembles chronic persistent hepatitis and/or non-suppurative destructive cholangitis (Fig. 17.154). In these instances, one considers the differential diagnosis of chronic non-A, non-B hepatitis, or recurrence of the primary disease for which transplantation was performed, e.g. primary biliary cirrhosis.

17.14.3   Mechanisms of rejection

The pattern of liver graft rejection is in keeping with T-cell mediated damage to the tissue components which normally

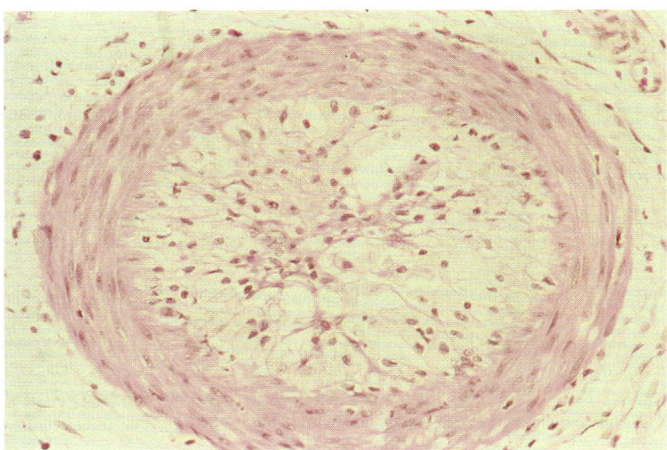

Fig. 17.151   Chronic rejection in liver allograft. A medium-sized artery is occluded by subintimal accumulation of foamy-looking macrophages.

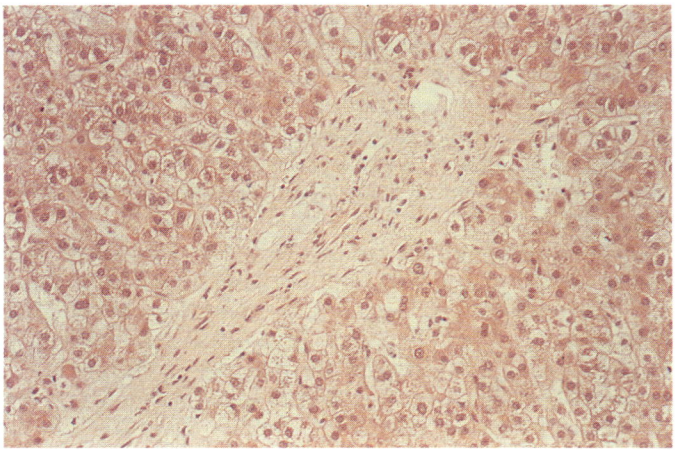

Fig. 17.153   Chronic rejection (vanishing bile duct syndrome). A mildly fibrotic portal tract contains very few inflammatory cells and small vascular spaces, one occluded by foamy macrophages. There is no identifiable bile duct.

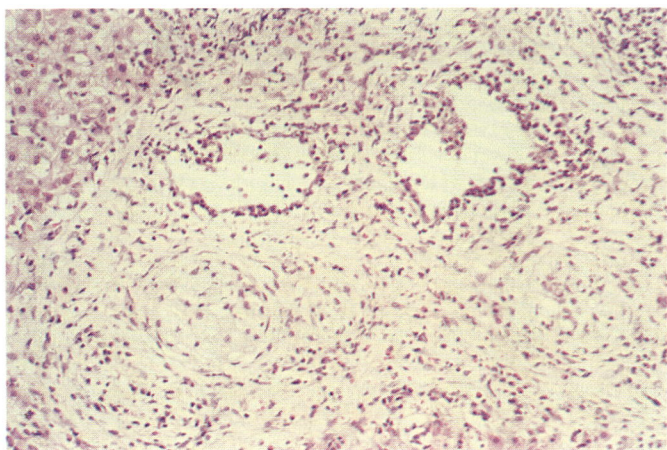

Fig. 17.152   Accelerated chronic rejection. There is coexistence of portal venular endotheliitis, arteriolar occlusion by foam cells, and a mixed-cell infiltrate most prominent at the site of a vanished bile duct (top right-hand corner).

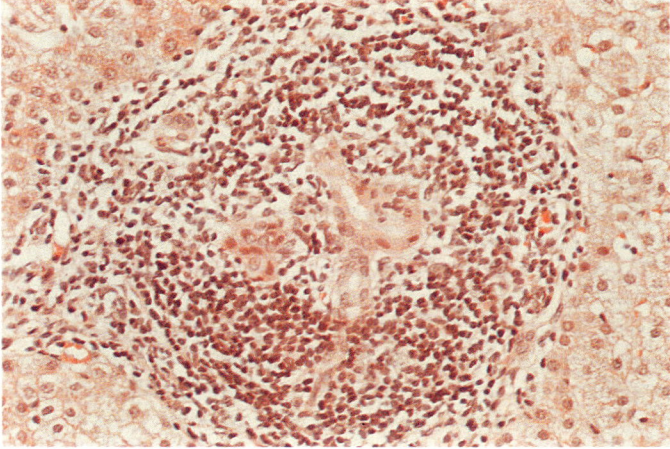

Fig. 17.154   Late lesion in an allograft 2 years after transplantation. There is a destructive cholangitis with a dense, predominantly lymphocytic infiltrate.

express the major histocompatibility class II antigens, namely the bile duct epithelium and the vascular endothelium. Normal hepatocytes, the essential functional units of the liver, do not have detectable DR antigens, which may explain why the liver appears less aggressively rejected than other organs.

The lack of cellular infiltration late in the course of chronic rejection may represent a fading response after complete disappearance of the bile ducts, the triggering antigens; or the additional involvement of a humoral mechanism. That an immunological process is responsible for the duct damage is further supported by the similarity of the bile duct changes observed during both liver graft rejection and graft versus host reaction after bone marrow transplantation.

17.14.4   Differential diagnosis

As with other grafted organs there is a number of potential complications to be considered in the differential diagnosis of rejection. Severe graft infarction in the early postoperative course may follow arterial thrombosis or uncontrollable haemorrhage. In the rare cases with apparently patent vessels, kinking of arterial branches, accelerated rejection, or a Shwartzman-type reaction have been proposed as alternative explanations.

Cholangitic changes are commonly seen secondary to biliary sludging, stricture, or leak, with or without ascending infection. There is portal oedema with marginal ductular proliferation and predominantly polymorphonuclear cell infiltration. These may be superimposed on the changes of acute rejection.

Opportunistic infections do not differ from those encountered in vigorously immunosuppressed patients in general. The liver graft is at risk of being infected by viruses, a situation which, in turn, may trigger a rejection episode via new display of HLA antigens induced by interferon. The risk is particularly high with cytomegalovirus (of which a large proportion of the population are carriers), and with the non-A, non-B agent(s) because of the large amount of blood transfused during transplantation. From the third week after surgery viral infection is suspected where lobular hepatitis with an attenuated inflammatory cell response is present.

In addition to the conditions described above, severe and prolonged cholestasis may occur without a satisfactory explanation, so-called 'functional' cholestasis. Cholestasis may also be associated with sepsis, in which case cholangiolar bile casts with surrounding neutrophils may be added to the picture.

Recurrence of the original liver disease has been extremely frequent, particularly when the primary disease was malignancy, suggesting that minute extrahepatic growths were present, but undetected at the time of surgery. Furthermore, thrombosis has been documented in a patient with the Budd–Chiari syndrome. Recurrence of hepatitis B serum markers with variable hepatitic changes in the graft has been almost the rule; in approximately a fifth of the patients, hepatitis recurrence is associated with a severe cholestatic and fibrosing hepatitis which rapidly progresses to liver failure. Recurrence of primary biliary cirrhosis is still not proven because of the difficulty of histopathological interpretation, whereas auto-immune chronic active hepatitis appears to be controlled by the immunosuppressive regime. There is, as yet, no definite evidence of graft reinfection in patients transplanted for fulminant viral hepatitis.

17.14.5   Further reading

Davies, S. E., et al. (1991). Hepatic histological findings after transplantation for chronic hepatitis B virus infection, including a unique pattern of fibrosing cholestatic hepatitis. Hepatology 13, 150–7.

Demetris, A. J., Lasky, S., Van Thiel, D. H., Starzl, T. E., and Dekker, A. (1985). Pathology of hepatic transplantation. A review of 62 adult allograft recipients immunosuppressed with a cyclosporin/steroid regimen. American Journal of Pathology 118, 151–61.

Fennell, R. H. and Roddy, H. J. (1979). Liver transplantation: The pathologist's perspective. In Pathology Annual, Vol. 14 (Part 2), (ed. S. C. Sommers and P. P. Rosen), pp. 155–82. Appleton-Century-Crofts, New York.

Ludwig, J., Russel, H. W., Batts, K. P., Perkins, J. D., and Krom, R. A. F. (1987). The acute vanishing bile duct syndrome (acute irreversible rejection) after orthotopic transplantation. Hepatology 7, 476–83.

McDonald, G. B., Shulman, H. M., Wolford, J. L., and Spencer, G. D. (1987). Liver disease after human bone marrow transplantation. Seminars in Liver Disease 7, 210–29.

Polson, R. E., Portmann, B., Neuberger, J., Calne, R. Y., and Williams, R. (1989). Evidence for disease recurrence after liver transplantation for primary biliary cirrhosis. Clinical and histological follow-up studies. Gastroenterology 97, 715–25.

Porter, K. A. (1969). Pathology of the orthotopic homograft and heterograft. In Experience in hepatic transplantation (ed. T. E. Starzl), pp. 422–71. W. B. Saunders, Philadelphia.

Portmann, B. and Wight, D. G. D. (1987). Pathology of liver transplantation (excluding rejection). In Liver transplantation (2nd edn) (ed. Sir Roy Calne), pp. 437–70. Grune and Stratton, London.

Portmann, B., Neuberger, J. M., and Williams, R. (1983). Intrahepatic bile duct lesions. In Liver transplantation (1st edn) (ed. R. Y. Calne), pp. 279–87. Grune and Stratton, London.

Portmann, B., O'Grady, J., and Williams, R. (1986). Disease recurrence following orthotopic liver transplantation. Transplantation Proceedings XVIII, 5 (Suppl. 4), 136–41.

Snover, D. C., et al. (1984). Orthotopic liver transplantation: a pathological study of 63 serial liver biopsies from 17 patients with special reference to the diagnostic features and natural history of rejection. Hepatology 4, 1212–22.

Snover, D. C., Freeze, D. K., Sharp, H. L., Bloomer, J. R., Najarian, J. S., and Ascher, N. L. (1987). Liver allograft rejection. An analysis of the use of biopsy in determining outcome of rejection. American Journal of Surgical Pathology 11, 1–10.

Starzl, T. E., Marchioro, T. L., Von Kaulla, K. N., Hermann, G., Brittain, R. S., and Waddell, W. R. (1963). Homotransplantation of the liver in humans. Surgery Gynecology & Obstetrics 117, 659–76.

Starzl, T. E., Iwatsuki, S., Shaw, B. W., and Gordon, R. D. (1985). Orthotopic liver transplantation in 1984. Transplantation Proceedings 17, 250–8.

Wight, D. G. D. and Portmann, B. (1987). Pathology of liver transplantation. In Liver transplantation (2nd edn) (ed. Sir Roy Calne), pp. 385–435. Grune and Stratton, London.

17.15 The gall bladder and biliary tract

Peter Kelly

17.15.1 Normal anatomy, development, and function

The biliary tract carries the bile from the liver to the duodenum. The major intrahepatic bile ducts unite to form two main hepatic ducts, left and right, each of which carries the bile from the corresponding lobe of the liver. The two hepatic ducts emerge from the porta hepatis and join together about 2 cm distal to the porta to form the common hepatic duct. The common hepatic duct is about 4 cm long and joins the cystic duct to form the bile duct (usually called the common bile duct). The bile duct is about 8 cm long and 0.8 cm in diameter. It descends in the free edge of the lesser omentum to pass behind the duodenum to enter the posteromedial wall of the descending or second part of the duodenum at the hepatopancreatic ampulla or ampulla of Vater where it is joined, in about 70 per cent of people, by the main pancreatic duct (of Wirsung). In the remainder, the pancreatic duct enters separately. In the distal part of its course the bile duct may be embedded in the pancreatic parenchyma.

The cystic duct (4 cm) is an extension of the neck of the gall bladder. The gall bladder is a pear shaped sac, 7–10 cm long, with a capacity of about 50 ml. It consists of three parts—neck, body, and fundus—and lies on the inferior surface of the liver in a depression between the quadrate and right hepatic lobes known as the gall bladder bed or fossa. The surface of the gall bladder that is not apposed to the liver is covered by peritoneum, which is reflected off the surface of the liver. The mucosa of the neck of the gall bladder is thrown into corkscrew-like folds to form the spiral valves of Heister. Frequently in surgical specimens, a small diverticulum of the neck of the gall bladder, directed towards the fundus, is found. This is known as Hartmann's pouch. Although a common finding, it is not seen in normal gall bladders but only in those showing other abnormalities, especially gallstones.

The arterial blood supply to the gall bladder is discussed below. The veins of the gall bladder, along with those of the hepatic ducts, proximal bile duct, and cystic duct usually enter the liver directly. There is thus no cystic vein to correspond to the cystic artery.

The gall bladder and biliary tract are lined by tall columnar epithelium. Associated with this, in the neck of the gall bladder and in the bile ducts, are simple tubulo-alveolar mucus glands. These are not found in the fundus or body of the gall bladder. The mucosa of the gall bladder is thrown into numerous delicate folds which give a fine honeycomb appearance to the luminal surface. The mucosa is supported by a delicate fibrovascular lamina propria, beneath which is the muscularis propria which is composed mainly of longitudinally arranged fibres but with a few circular fibres as well. There is no submucosa in

the gall-bladder. The rest of the extrahepatic biliary tree contains few muscle fibres, except at the distal end where circular muscle fibres in the bile duct itself, the distal pancreatic duct, and the ampulla proper combine to form a sphincter—the sphincter of Oddi. The mucosa of the bile duct at the ampulla shows a complex pattern of folding. Outside the muscle layer of the gall bladder is a loose connective tissue adventitia containing elastic fibres which, on the free surface, is covered by serosa.

Luschka's ducts are small aberrant ducts lined by columnar epithelium, which are found in the adventitia of the gall bladder. They are sometimes in continuity with bile ductules in the contiguous liver and may thus be the source of seepage of bile from the gall bladder bed following cholecystectomy. They do not communicate with the lumen of the gall bladder. On the other hand, Rokitansky–Aschoff sinuses are small diverticula of gall bladder mucosa between the muscle fibres of its wall. They are sometimes found in normal gall bladders but much more frequently in disease states—especially chronic cholecystitis.

Embryologically, the epithelium of the liver and biliary tree is derived from the endoderm. In the third week, the hepatic diverticulum forms at the junction of fore- and midgut. Later this divides into two branches, the cranial, which gives rise to the hepatocytes, intrahepatic ducts, and the bile duct, and the caudal, which forms the gall bladder and cystic duct. The mesenchymal supporting tissues of all these structures are derived from mesoderm.

The hepatic bile contains water, the inorganic anions Cl^- and HCO_3^-, bile acids and their salts, bilirubin, cholesterol, lecithin and other phospholipids, unesterified cholesterol, excreted hormones, and drugs and their metabolites. Mucus is secreted into the bile by the biliary epithelium. The gall bladder stores bile between meals and concentrates it to as little as 10 per cent of its original volume by absorption of Na^+, Cl^-, HCO_3^-, and water by active transport of the ions. The ordinary epithelial cells of the gall bladder have a microvillous luminal surface consistent with their absorptive function. It is probable that the bile ducts can secrete a clear alkaline fluid and that they can also, in their distal portion, concentrate bile. In addition to its storage and concentration functions, the gall bladder, in co-ordination with the distal bile duct and sphincter of Oddi, delivers bile into the duodenum in response to the entry of fatty food into the duodenum. At rest, the sphincter of Oddi is contracted, thus preventing exit of bile through the ampulla and reflux of duodenal contents into the biliary and pancreatic ducts. Gall bladder contraction and relaxation of the sphincter of Oddi occur in response to a rise in plasma levels of the hormone cholecystokinin (CCK) which follows entry of fat into the duodenum. CCK is the major hormone involved in control of the gall bladder and sphincter of Oddi, but other local hormones such as motilin, secretin, vasoactive intestinal polypeptide, and pancreatic polypeptide also have specific roles. Neural control is of little importance.

Bile acids and their salts are an important constituent of the bile. They contribute, with phospholipids, to the formation of micelles containing cholesterol which is not soluble in water, and thus prevent its precipitation into crystals, especially when the bile is concentrated in the gall bladder. In the lumen of the small intestine, the bile salts form micelles with dietary fat and fat-soluble vitamins, which are then actively transported across the mucosa of the distal ileum into the portal bloodstream. This enterohepatic circulation of bile salts is of particular importance as the liver cannot synthesize sufficient bile salts *de novo* to re-plete the pool if there is marked impairment of ileal absorption of bile salts. This will lead to progressive malabsorption of fats and fat-soluble vitamins. On the other hand, obstruction of the normal flow of bile into the duodenum will lead to retention of bile salts, as well as bilirubin and cholesterol, again with, among many other consequences, failure to absorb fats from the intestine.

17.15.2   Congenital anomalies of the biliary tract

A large number of different congenital anomalies of the biliary tract have been described. Major anomalies are rare but as many as half of all patients presenting with gallstones show a significant variation from 'normal' biliary anatomy. The anom-alies may lead to stasis with consequent inflammation or stone formation but their major importance is to radiologists and sur-geons, as failure to recognize anatomical variants may lead to injury to the bile duct or cystic artery in the course of surgery for biliary tract disease. The anomalies are generally grouped into those of the gall bladder, those of the bile ducts, and those of the cystic artery. In general terms, anomalies of the biliary tract are due to abnormalities in the growth of the hepatic diverticulum, which includes reduplication, or in failure of a lumen to form in the solid bud of proliferating epithelium.

Gall bladder

Among anomalies of the gall bladder, agenesis is very rare. It may dispose to development of stones in the bile duct. It is often associated with major congenital anomalies in other systems, including tracheo-oesophageal fistula, polycystic kidneys, and cardiac defects. Reduplication of the gall bladder may occur and, rarely, triple gall bladders have been described. The extent of duplication varies from the presence of a longitudinal septum in an externally normal gall bladder to bilobed gall bladder, the two lobes sharing a single cystic duct, to two complete gall bladders each with a short cystic duct which join to enter the bile duct in a common cystic duct. These variants constitute the split cystic primordia group. In the multiple cystic primordia group two completely separate gall bladders are found, each of which has its own cystic duct which enters the bile duct separately at a variety of different sites.

The gall bladder may rarely be found in an abnormal posi-tion, so-called ectopia of the gall bladder. It may be completely intrahepatic either in the right or the left lobe. It may be left-sided, in which case insertion of the cystic duct may be anom-alous. Left-sided displacement is sometimes associated with situs inversus. It may lie transversely, and in some cases of transverse gall bladder the hepatic ducts open directly into it.

The retrodisplaced gall bladder is found behind the right lobe of the liver. When a gall bladder has a long mesenteric attachment to the liver or is completely covered in peritoneum it is said to be floating, a condition that renders it susceptible to torsion.

The Phrygian cap deformity of the gall bladder is relatively common and consists of partial folding over of the fundus. The gall bladder may be multiseptate, being divided into a number of intercommunicating locules by thin septa. The hour-glass deformity is usually acquired as a result of localized post-inflammatory fibrosis.

Bile ducts

The cystic duct may be abnormally long, in which case it enters the common hepatic duct distally and is sometimes twisted around it. On the other hand, it may have a high insertion at the level of the right hepatic duct or the junction of the right and left hepatic ducts. Absence of the cystic duct is usually associ-ated with agenesis of the gall bladder, although rarely the gall-bladder opens directly into the common hepatic duct. Failure to recognize any of these variants may lead to inadvertent ligation of the right hepatic duct or bile duct during surgery.

Accessory hepatic ducts form separate supplementary chan-nels between the right lobe of the liver, or, rarely, the left, and the extrahepatic biliary tract. They may open into the common hepatic duct or the gall bladder itself. Inappropriate surgical handling of accessory ducts may lead to segmental biliary obstruction following ligation, on the one hand, or bile leakage, on the other, if a small accessory duct is not recognized during dissection of the gall bladder.

Abnormalities of the common hepatic and bile ducts include low fusion of the hepatic ducts, which in the extreme case leads to double common duct. The cystic duct may fuse with the right hepatic duct. The right hepatic duct may, rarely, drain directly into the gall bladder.

Anatomical variations at the lower end of the bile duct have been touched on earlier. Some are so common as to be con-sidered normal variants rather congenital anomalies. The com-monest variation is separate insertions of the bile duct and main or ventral pancreatic duct (of Wirsung) into the duodenum. Less commonly, the dorsal pancreatic duct of Santorini becomes the dominant pancreatic duct. Variations in the relationship of the bile duct and pancreatic ducts are of interest in the study of the pathogenesis of acute pancreatitis and the role of gallstones in that process.

Cystic artery Normally, the blood supply to the gall bladder is provided by the cystic artery which branches off the right hep-atic artery in a plane posterior to the hepatic ducts. Variations of this arrangement are very common and, interestingly, com-moner in those with gallstones. An accessory cystic artery may be indavertently divided during cholecystectomy, leading to haemorrhage. The cystic artery or right hepatic artery may be located anterior to the hepatic ducts. Another common vari-ation is the recurrent right hepatic artery in which the vessel follows the cystic duct before giving off the cystic branch and turning upwards to the porta. If not recognized, it can be mistaken for the cystic artery and divided.

Ectopic tissues

Ectopic tissues are an unusual finding in the gall bladder. Liver tissue may be found within the wall, as may pancreatic tissue, which may include both endocrine and exocrine elements. Gastric-body mucosa may also be seen; sometimes in continuity with the mucosa, sometimes deep within the wall. This should not be confused with gastric antral metaplasia (see below) when examining surgical specimens of diseased gall bladders.

Congenital dilatation and cystic diseases of the bile ducts

Pathological dilatation may occur anywhere in the biliary tree, intrahepatic or extrahepatic. Cystic dilatations of the bile ducts are usually discussed as a separate disease entity, although it should be recognized that there is some overlap of this group with biliary atresia, on one hand, and, on the other, with the complex group of dysplastic liver diseases, which includes congenital hepatic fibrosis (see Secton 17.2). Classification of dilatation and cystic diseases of the bile ducts depends on

1. the site of the dilatation(s), whether intra- or extrahepatic;
2. the type of dilatation—saccular, fusiform, or diverticular; and
3. whether it is solitary, multiple, or diffuse.

On this basis five types are recognized:

I. dilatation of the (common) bile duct; there are three subtypes, (a) large saccular, (b) small localized, and (c) diffuse fusiform;
II. diverticulum of the common bile duct or gall bladder;
III. choledochocele—a dilatation which involves only the intraduodenal portion of the bile duct;
IV. multiple intra- and extrahepatic dilatations; and
V. fusiform intra- and extrahepatic dilatations.

Type I is the commonest and is usually referred to as choledochal cyst, although types II and III may be included under this heading. The condition of cystic dilatation of the intrahepatic biliary tree is more commonly known as Caroli disease.

The aetiology of this group of diseases is obscure. Among the possible mechanisms are congenital weakness or deficiency in the wall of the bile duct with obstruction of the duct distally. The obstruction may be due to incomplete canalization of the duct, to congenital inflammation, a congenital valve in the distal duct, or angulation of the insertion of the bile duct into the duodenum. The disease is much commoner in females and occurs more frequently in the Japanese. The typical clinical presentation of choledochal cyst is with a triad of jaundice, pain, and a mass in the right upper quadrant. Although congenital, the disease rarely presents in neonates and is often not apparent until early adulthood.

The cysts vary enormously in size, with a volume ranging from a few millilitres to 10 litres. The wall is composed mainly of fibrous tissue. It is often inflamed. Some residual islands of a columnar epithelial lining may be found but it is usually absent.

Complications include: cyst perforation leading to bile peritonitis, ascending cholangitis, hepatic abscess, and, in cases of prolonged obstruction, secondary biliary cirrhosis. Adenocarcinoma or, more rarely, squamous carcinoma may arise in the cyst wall.

Extrahepatic biliary atresia

In extrahepatic biliary atresia, bile excretion is prevented by the destruction or obstruction of the bile ducts in their extrahepatic course or in their major intrahepatic branches. The site of involvement and its extent are very variable. The rarer 'surgically correctable' cases are defined as those in which there is residual patent extrahepatic bile duct in continuity with the intrahepatic system. This term is misleading, however, as even in cases where the common hepatic or right and left hepatic ducts are atretic, there are often hypoplastic bile ducts draining to the porta hepatis which offer a route of excretion in the surgical procedure of hepatic porto-enterostomy. The disease is rare, affecting about 1 in 10 000. It is much commoner in females.

Pathologically, the process is characterized by the presence of intense inflammation, fibrosis, and necrosis of the epithelium. In the early stages, the inflammation is acute while, later, chronic inflammatory cells predominate. In some instances, there is no inflammation, only fibrosis, and bile duct epithelium is absent with no residual lumen. The intrahepatic bile ducts are rarely involved early on and remain patent to the porta hepatis until about 2 or 3 months after birth, but as the disease progresses they are obliterated. The liver shows changes of giant cell transformation, cholestasis, and inflammation of the portal tracts. These are also found in in neonatal hepatitis. However, in extrahepatic biliary atresia there is marked proliferation of interlobular bile ducts. As the disease progresses, there is increasing fibrosis of the portal tracts, culminating in secondary biliary cirrhosis, even in the first year of life.

Clinically, the disease presents with jaundice, and the differential diagnosis is with other causes of conjugated hyperbilirubinaemia in infancy, including neonatal hepatitis, which may closely resemble it. The distinction between the two will depend on a combination of clinical, biochemical, radiological, histopathological (liver biopsy), and, ultimately, surgical findings. Early diagnosis is essential because the progresssion to cirrhosis is often rapid, with death before 2 years of age in the majority of untreated cases. Paucity of the intrahepatic bile ducts (formerly known as intrahepatic biliary atresia) may also present with conjugated hyperbilirubinaemia in the neonatal period. This condition differs sharply from extrahepatic biliary atresia in its pathology, associated conditions, aetiological factors, and prognosis. It is discussed in greater detail elsewhere (Section 17.2).

The aetiology of extrahepatic biliary atresia is unknown. The weight of evidence favours the conclusion that, in the great majority of cases, the condition results from a destructive inflammatory process acquired, generally, *in utero* rather than from a primary maldevelopment. Indeed, in a few cases there is good evidence that the biliary tree was intact in the immediate postnatal period and that there was subsequent destruction of the bile ducts. That there are many similarities, clinical, biochemical, and pathological, between extrahepatic biliary atresia and neonatal hepatitis has been mentioned earlier (Section 17.2). This has led some to suggest that they, and possibly choledochal cyst as well, are different manifestations of the same basic disease process, called 'infantile obstructive cholangiopathy', which is possibly a viral infection with hepatitis viruses, cytomegalovirus, reovirus type 3, or rubella among the proposed agents. The evidence implicating reovirus type 3 is particularly strong. The condition has been found to be associated with a variety of chromosomal abnormalities (trisomy 17, 18, or 21; Turner syndrome) intra-abdominal vascular anomalies, and, most frequently, polysplenia syndrome. It is rarely familial.

In spite of advances in diagnosis and surgical treatment, the prognosis is still guarded, with death, usually from the effects of cirrhosis, occuring early in life. However, some long-term survivals following surgical treatment have been reported.

Spontaneous perforation of the bile duct

This is a rare cause of biliary peritonitis in neonates or infants. The aetiology is unknown. It may be related to congential weakness of the wall.

17.15.3   Gallstones

Gallstones are concretions formed from normal or abnormal constituents of the bile. The term used to denote the presence of gallstones in the biliary tract is cholelithiasis. Cholelithiasis is very common in Western societies and it has been shown in autopsy studies that about 20 per cent of the population have gallstones. The incidence is increasing and, in some Western countries, cholecystectomy is the third commonest general surgical operation, following appendicectomy and herniorrhaphy. Gallstones are common in women and rare in children.

The major constituents of gallstones are cholesterol, pigment as calcium bilirubinate, and calcium carbonate. If stones are composed of one constituent only they are said to be pure, although this should not be taken to imply strict chemical purity. About 10 per cent of all gallstones are pure and of these, in Western societies, cholesterol stones are the commonest. They are composed of crystalline cholesterol monohydrate. They are usually solitary and vary greatly in size, measuring up to 5 cm in diameter. They are spherical or ovoid and are translucent white or pale yellow in colour. The surface of larger stones is often bosselated. On the cut surface, they have a radiate crystalline structure (Fig. 17.155). Pure cholesterol stones can float in bile. Pigment stones are usually multiple. They occur in two forms: black pigment stones, which are small and featureless and form in the gall bladder. They are commoner in those suffering from cirrhosis and chronic haemolysis, although most patients found to have this type of stone suffer from neither. They are not associated with infection. Brown pigment stones, by contrast, are larger and are lamellated on the cut surface.

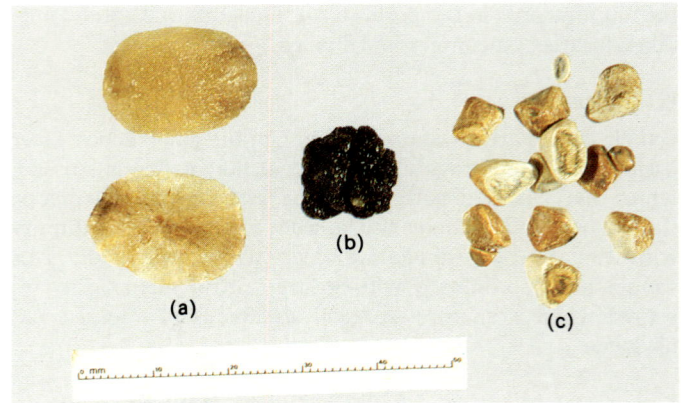

Fig. 17.155   Gallstones: (a) cholesterol, (b) pigment, (c) mixed.

They can form in the biliary tree outside the gall bladder and occur in association with stasis and infection. Black pigment stones are the commoner type in Western societies. Both types are composed essentially of calcium bilirubinate. Calcium carbonate stones are rare. They are smooth surfaced and, if they are multiple, the surface may be faceted. They are opaque and grey-white.

About 90 per cent of gallstones contain significant amounts of two or more constituents. Combined or compound stones account for about 10 per cent of all gallstones and consist either of a relatively pure core with a mixed outer shell or vice versa. The remaining 80 per cent of gallstones are mixed. In these, the individual components are much more intimately admixed although they are by no means homogeneous. They are almost invariably multiple and are often found in very large numbers in a gall bladder. They vary greatly in size from tiny, gritty particles to stones several centimetres in diameter. In any individual case, stones of the full range of sizes may be found. While some mixed stones have a lobulated 'mulberry' appearance, they are usually faceted. Their colour varies from yellow to brown-green. On the cut surface or on surfaces which have been worn down by rubbing against other stones, they have a lamellated appearance—the different lamellae corresponding to different compositions of the precipitate from the bile with time (Figs 17.155, 17.156). Many mixed stones have a soft homogenous brown core. In some, this is replaced by a central cavity filled with gas which gives rise to a characteristic appearance on radiographs. Mixed stones generally contain 50–70 per cent cholesterol and are therefore considered to be a variant of cholesterol stones.

Apart from the three major constituents, most gallstones contain varying amounts of other substances such as proteins, mucopolysaccharides, and bile acids. While these minor constituents may not be quantitatively important, they may be of great importance in providing a nucleus around which the stone may form (see below).

Only about 10–15 per cent of all gallstones are radio-opaque, this property being largely dependent on the calcium content. Cholesterol stones are generally radiolucent, 10–15 per cent

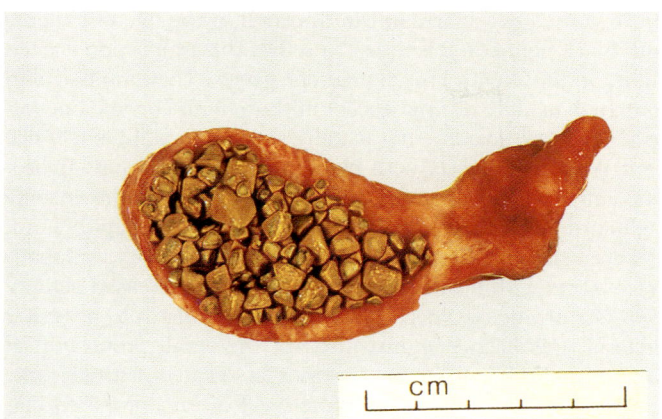

Fig. 17.156 Cholelithiasis. The gall bladder is packed with faceted mixed gallstones. The wall is fibrotic.

of mixed stones and 50 per cent of pigment stones are radio-opaque.

Aetiology and pathogenesis of gallstones

While some general observations can be made about the pathogenesis of all gallstones, it should be remembered that cholesterol and pigment gallstones differ markedly in their specific aetiological and pathogenetic factors, including their disease associations.

In general, three factors contribute to the formation of gallstones regardless of type. They are:

1. abnormal composition of the bile;
2. stasis; and
3. infection.

The importance of the individual factors and their interplay is usually impossible to establish in individual cases. Much more is understood of the pathogenesis of cholesterol (and mixed) gallstones than of pigment stones.

Gallstones develop in three stages. These are the formation of saturated bile; nucleation, i.e. the formation of a core on which the stone can continue to grow; and, finally, growth—the increased in size of the stone by continuing aggregation or precipitation to clinically significant size. The aetiological factors of abnormality of bile composition, stasis and infection, will come into play at different stages of, and make a variable contribution to, this sequence of events in lithogenesis. So, for example, cholesterol, mixed, and black pigment stones very rarely form outside the gall bladder, and abnormalities of bile composition play a relatively important part in their formation, whereas brown pigment stones often form in the bile ducts and infection plays a large part in their development. Stasis may be important both in allowing tiny early stones to persist in the biliary tree and grow, and in predisposing to infection.

Cholesterol gallstones

Cholesterol is insoluble in water and if the cholesterol excreted by the liver were not held in solution by the formation of micelles, it would precipitate out. Micelles are formed by the combination of bile salts, which have detergent properties, and phospholipids, especially lecithin and cholesterol. The relative concentration of each of these components is important, for cholesterol will only remain in micellar solution within a certain narrow range of relative concentrations. If these are related to each other as in the ternary phase diagram in Fig. 17.157, it can be seen that cholesterol may precipitate out where the bile is abnormal because there is relative excess of cholesterol or a relative lack of bile salts or phospholipids. The line separating the one-phase or 'stable' zone (micellar solution) from the two-phase supersaturated or 'labile' zone (micellar solution and cholesterol crystals) is designated the equilibrium limit of solubility. There is not, however, a sharp transition from stable to labile, and a so-called 'metastable' zone (cross-hatched area in diagram) immediately below the equilibrium line is recognized. In solutions that fall into this zone, very slow precipitation of cholesterol crystals may occur. In addition, a protein with nucleation inhibitory properties may be present in gall bladder bile which increases the degree and duration of metastable supersaturation.

Factors that may result in the production of a bile of abnormal composition include the rate of bile acid secretion by the liver, as it has been shown that when this rate is low the ratio of bile acid to cholesterol decreases, as does that of phospholipid to cholesterol.

The absolute concentration of cholesterol in the bile is related to the rate of its synthesis. The rate-limiting enzyme is 3-hydroxy-3-methyl-glutaryl coenzyme A reductase (HMG CoA reductase). This enzyme appears to have higher activity

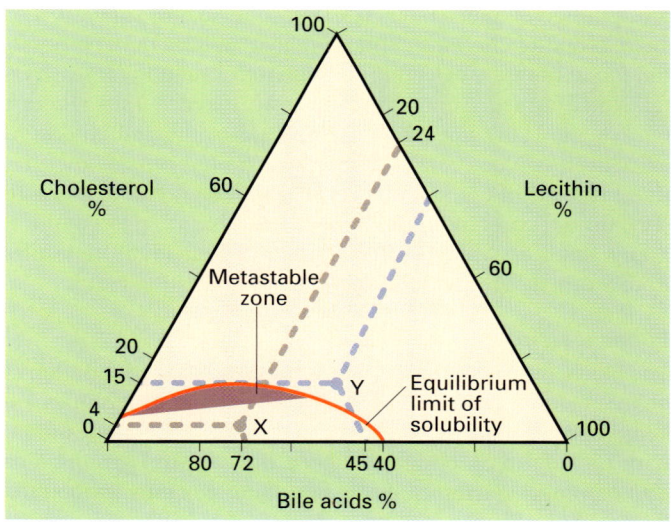

Fig. 17.157 Ternary phase diagram of bile composition and solubility. Concentrations of the three major constituents are expressed as mole percentages (totalling 100 per cent). Concentrations plotted below the equilibrium limit of solubility outside the metastable zone, such as X, are in micellar solution. In the metastable zone cholesterol precipitates slowly from supersaturated bile. Concentrations plotting above the equilibrium limit of solubility, such as Y, fall into the labile zone in which cholesterol crystals can form. (After Carey and Small 1978.)

in those with gallstones than in controls. Other factors that may contribute to higher biliary levels of cholesterol are increased ingestion and absorption; mobilization of cholesterol from tissue pools, such as may occur in catabolic states; or reduced conversion of cholesterol to bile acids.

Relative bile acid concentration may be reduced due to increased loss from the body, such that hepatic synthesis can no longer replace the loss—this only seems to occur in cases of severe malabsorption. Bile acid synthesis may be reduced either in the inborn error of metabolism, cerebrotendinous xanthomatosis, or if there is reduced responsiveness of the normal feedback increase in bile salt synthesis to reduction in the pool. Conditions in which reduced phospholipid synthesis or secretion could contribute to gallstone formation have not been identified.

Supersaturation of bile with cholesterol is probably insufficient *per se* for formation of gallstones. Such bile is often found in normal subjects. Random coalescence of cholesterol molecules to form a nucleus for further growth is called homogeneous nucleation and occurs only in highly supersaturated bile and is probably of limited clinical importance. Precipitation of cholesterol around some particle other than a cholesterol crystal is called heterogeneous nucleation and can occur at a lower relative concentration of cholesterol. Heterogeneous nucleation requires particles of 10–100 nm diameter. It has been noted earlier that nearly all cholesterol stones have a pigmented centre. Recent animal studies have shown that increased secretion of mucus occurs as an early response to the presence of supersaturated bile in the gall bladder. There is evidence that gall bladder mucin may act as a 'pronucleation' factor. Nucleation may be of particular importance in causing precipitation of 'metastable' bile. Recent evidence suggests that aggregation of cholesterol-phospholipid vesicles may be essential for initiating nucleation of cholesterol monohydrate crystals. Once formed, a microlith must grow to reach a size where it may be clinically apparent. If emptying of the gall bladder is efficient, it will be expelled before this can happen. If however, there is stasis of the gall bladder, the microlith can increase in size. Growth may occur by two mechanisms: aggregation of many small crystals, or precipitation of individual molecules from a supersaturated solution on to a pre-existing nidus.

Pigment stones

The biochemical alterations in bile that lead to the formation of pigment stones are not fully known. Black pigment stones are composed of a highly cross-linked polymer of bilirubinate anion, with Ca^{2+} forming bridges between the carboxyl groups. The also contain calcium bilirubinate and calcium carbonate. Brown pigment stones consist mainly of calcium bilirubinate and calcium soaps of fatty acids. Both types contain up to 60 per cent by weight of a glycoprotein matrix.

The bilirubin in pigment gallstones consists almost entirely of the calcium salts of unconjugated bilirubin. Unconjugated bilirubin is largely insoluble in water. Calcium forms highly insoluble salts with unconjugated bilirubin anions. It has been shown that there is a higher proportion of unconjugated bilirubin to conjugated bilirubin than normal in the bile of patients with black pigment gallstones, and that this proportion is even higher in those with brown pigment stones. The total bilirubin content is usually normal except in those with chronic haemolysis. The calcium content is usually normal. In gall-bladder bile from Western subjects with black pigment gallstones, hydrolytic activity for conjugated bilirubin, probably by the enzyme β-glucuronidase derived from hepatocytes or biliary epithelium, had been shown. Normal bile shows no such activity. In Japanese subjects with brown pigment gallstones, increased activity of β-glucuronidase, derived from *Escherichia coli* or other bacteria, has been demonstrated. In the small proportion of patients with black pigment stones associated with chronic haemolysis, an increased absolute level of unconjugated bilirubin can arise as a proportion of the increased total bilirubin level without any increase in the rate of enzymatic hydrolysis of conjugated bilirubin. Regardless of how it comes about, the presence of large amounts of unconjugated bilirubin in the bile can be considered to be analogous to saturation with cholesterol.

The mechanism of polymerization of bilirubin in black pigment stones is not known. Nor is it known whether polymerization occurs as a separate event to nucleation. It has been shown, however, that bilirubin binds to the mucin glycoprotein of gall bladder bile. Parasites or their ova are often found to form the nidus of brown pigment stones.

Pigment and cholesterol gallstones do not form simultaneously in the same individual. It has been shown that in model solutions cholesterol solubility is reduced by addition of bilirubin and, conversely, that bilirubin solubility is reduced in the presence of solubilized cholesterol.

Specific risk factors for the development of gallstones

Cholesterol stones

Obesity Obese individuals have a higher bile cholesterol saturation than matched non-obese controls. This has been shown to be due to high biliary cholesterol secretion, reflecting an increase in synthesis. These findings accord with the epidemiological observation of increased frequency of cholesterol gallstones in obese persons.

Diet There is a higher incidence of gallstones in those with a high calorie intake. This is associated with higher biliary cholesterol secretion. Paradoxically, some individuals on low calorie diets have been shown to have an increased bile cholesterol saturation. This may be due to excretion of cholesterol mobilized during adipose tissue breakdown. A modest increase in bile cholesterol saturation has been noted in those with high dietary cholesterol intake. Dietary fibre has not been shown to have much effect on cholesterol metabolism in man, although high bran diets have been shown to be associated with a reduction in cholesterol saturation in those with gallstones.

Demography Some American Indian tribes have a very high prevalence of cholesterol gallstones. There is also a relatively high prevalence in northern Europe, North and South America compared with the Orient. These differences may be due to differences in biliary cholesterol content.

Intestinal disease Bile acids are actively absorbed from the distal ileum. There is increased prevalence of cholesterol gallstones in patients who have ileal disease, such as Crohn disease, or who have had ileal resection or bypass. Failure to absorb bile acids leads to faecal losses which exceed the synthetic capacity of the liver, with consequent reduction in the bile acid pool. As a result of this, bile saturation increases.

Female sex hormones There is an increased prevalence of gallstones among women of reproductive age. Biliary cholesterol secretion is increased and this may be related to a decrease in the chenodeoxycholic acid content of bile. This substance is known to decrease biliary cholesterol secretion. This effect occurs both with endogenous oestrogens and with exogenous oestrogen, usually taken as oral contraceptives.

Drugs There is an increased incidence of gallstones among patients taking clofibrate. This is associated with increased biliary cholesterol secretion.

Pigment stones

It has already been noted that the pathogenesis of pigment gallstones is different to that of cholesterol stones. The conditions that predispose to the development of pigment stones are also different.

Demography Bilirubin stones are rare in American Indians, in contrast to cholesterol stones. Pigment gallstones, especially brown pigment stones, are commoner in rural Japan, although the prevalence is declining while that of cholesterol stones is increasing. This may be due to reduction in the prevalence of parasitic infestation together with the adoption of a Western diet.

Haemolysis The high prevalence of pigment gallstones in patients suffering from haemolytic anaemia has already been discussed.

Cirrhosis There is a higher incidence of pigment lithiasis in cirrhotics. The mechanism is not known.

Infection and infestation In Japanese patients with brown pigment gallstones, the bile is frequently infected, usually with *E. coli*. While it may be argued that infection is secondary to the presence of stones, in Western patients with pigment gallstones, the bile is much less frequently infected. It is also known that β-glucuronidase, produced by *E. coli*, increases the level of unconjugated bilirubin, which is a predisposing factor to development of pigment stones.

Age The prevalence of both cholesterol and bilirubin gallstones increases with age.

The pathological and clinical consequences of cholelithiasis

In uncomplicated cholelithiasis, the gall bladder may be normal, especially if the stones are pure cholesterol or pigment. In

many cases of cholesterol gallstones, the gall bladder shows changes of cholesterolosis (see below). A gall bladder containing stones may show hypertrophy of the muscularis. Especially if mixed stones are present, there may be varying degrees of chronic inflammation of the wall of the gall bladder, ranging from a scattering of chronic cells to fully developed chronic cholecystitis with fibrosis. Clinically, cholelithiasis may be completely asymptomatic, so-called 'silent gallstones'. Patients found to have silent gallstones incidentally in the course of screening or other investigations have a relatively low chance of becoming symptomatic or developing complications (18 per cent after 15 years). There is, nevertheless, controversy about what advice to give to such patients. Emergency surgery in older patients who have developed complications carries a significant mortality and there is also a small risk of developing carcinoma.

Traditionally, flatulent dyspepsia has been regarded as a symptom of cholelithiasis but it has been shown that dyspepsia is as common in subjects without gallstones as it is in those with, and it is therefore not a specific feature of cholelithiasis. The association of hiatus hernia, diverticulosis of the colon, and cholelithiasis is known as Saint's triad. There may be a underlying disorder of gastrointestinal motility in such patients.

The complications of cholelithiasis include acute and chronic cholecystitis. These are discussed below. Smaller stones, 0.5–1 cm in diameter, may migrate into the cystic duct or bile duct, giving rise to the symptom of biliary colic. Sometimes the stone may pass on into the duodenum. However, if a stone impacts in Hartmann's pouch or in the cystic duct, it may give rise to acute cholecystitis or, if there is complete obstruction to the passage of bile, the condition of hydrops of the gall bladder may develop. The gall bladder becomes distended by a clear secretion from the wall, the bile having been resorbed. If the fluid is mucoid, the term mucocele is used (Fig. 17.158). The gall bladder is enlarged and tense. The wall is thinned and the mucosa may be atrophic. Stones may be present. Rarely, hydrops of the gall bladder develops in children in the absence of

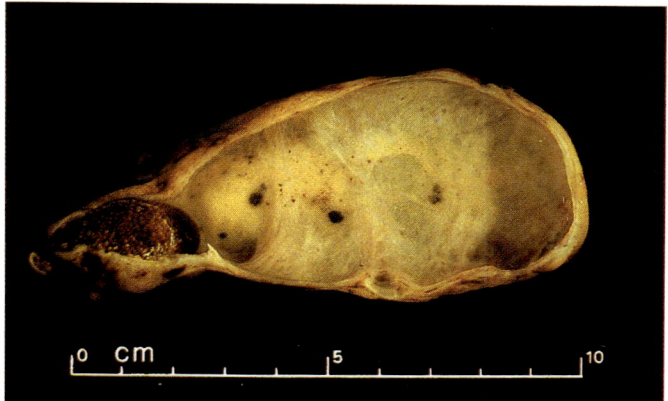

Fig. 17.158 Mucocele of the gall bladder. A stone is impacted in the neck of the gall bladder, obstructing outflow. The gall bladder is distended, the mucosa is atrophic, and the wall fibrotic. The gall bladder was filled with mucus.

stones or obstruction of the cystic duct. In most of such cases there is associated systemic infection. The condition is self-limiting. Rarely, a mucocele of the obstructive variety may rupture and lead to pseudomyxoma peritonei. If acute inflammation complicates obstruction of the cystic ducts, the gall bladder becomes distended by pus, giving rise to empyema. The wall is usually intensely inflamed. In many cases, the content is not, in fact, pus but appears turbid owing to the presence of calcium carbonate and cholesterol crystals. A stone lodged in the bile duct may impact in it, especially at the ampulla of Vater, and give rise to obstructive jaundice. In this condition of stasis, infection is a frequent complication, causing cholangitis which may spread to the intrahepatic ducts as ascending cholangitis. This may lead to the development of multiple abscesses in the liver. Prolonged obstruction of the bile duct, from whatever cause, may culminate in the development of secondary biliary cirrhosis. Fibrous stricture of the bile duct may develop at the site of damage by a stone.

In the Mirizzi syndrome a stone impacted in the neck of the gall bladder or cystic duct leads to stricture of the common bile duct or common hepatic duct by direct mechanical compression or by the associated inflammation. The condition can be further complicated by the formation of a fistula between the gall bladder or cystic duct and the common bile duct, common hepatic duct, or even the contiguous intestine. The condition may mimic carcinoma clinically and radiologically.

Because cholelithiasis is so frequently associated with chronic cholecystitis, in which the wall of the gall bladder is rendered indistensible by fibrosis, the association of obstructive jaundice with a palpable, distended gall bladder is taken to indicate that the cause of the obstruction is neoplastic rather than calculous. There are, however, so many exceptions to this principle, which is usually known as Courvoisier's law, that full investigation should always be carried out to determine the cause of the obstruction. Occasionally a stone impacted in Hartmann's pouch may cause sufficient local inflammation and oedema to lead to transient obstruction of the bile duct with jaundice.

Gallstones have been implicated in the pathogenesis of some cases of acute pancreatitis. It is probable that a gallstone, passing along the biliary tree, causes temporary obstruction of the ampulla of Vater, allowing reflux of bile in the pancreatic duct in those with the usual anatomical arrangement of the ampulla. The refluxing bile activates pancreatic enzymes such as trypsin, phospholipase, and lipase, which usually remain in their inactive form while still in the pancreas. The activated enzymes then proceed to digest the pancreas itself, in turn liberating more enzymes and activating other systems, such as the clotting and complement cascades.

If an inflamed gall bladder containing stones adheres to an adjacent hollow viscus, an internal biliary fistula may form between the two viscera by a combination of continuing inflammation and the pressure effects of the gallstones. The small intestine, especially the duodenum, is usually involved, although a fistula may form between the gall bladder and colon, stomach, or, rarely, the bile duct. Other processes may also give rise to biliary fistulae. These include especially Crohn disease,

carcinoma of either organ, peptic ulcer, or, rarely, trauma. Gallstones may, of course, enter the intestine through such a fistula and, in perhaps 10 per cent of cases, if the stone is large enough (2.5–4 cm), it may impact in the intestine, usually the distal ileum, to give rise to mechanical obstruction of the intestine, gallstone ileus. Less commonly, the stomach or colon may be involved. Sometimes an adhesion forms between the gall bladder and the abdominal wall and may give rise to an external biliary fistula. This can also arise as a complication of biliary surgery. Gallstones are found in about 70 per cent of cases of carcinoma of the gall bladder.

17.15.4 Cholesterolosis of the gall bladder

Cholesterolosis is a condition of abnormal accumulation of cholesterol in the mucosa of the gall bladder. It is quite common, being found in about 12 per cent of autopsies and up to 25 per cent of surgically removed gall bladders. It is commonest in women and has a peak incidence in middle age.

On inspection, the mucosal ridges of the gall bladder are flecked with yellow deposits of cholesterol to give a honeycomb or granular appearance (Fig. 17.159). It may be diffuse or localized. If diffuse, it is often called 'strawberry gall bladder', although, in fact, the mucosa between the deposits is usually green, unless it is hyperaemic. Microscopically, the mucosal ridges are found to be distended by accumulations in the lamina propria of foamy macrophages containing the cholesterol ester (Fig. 17.160). The pathogenesis of cholesterolosis is uncertain. It is probably caused by increased uptake of cholesterol from the bile. Supersaturated bile is present in cholesterolosis and cholesterol gallstones are found in about 50 per cent of cases.

The clinical significance of cholesterolosis is uncertain. Some patients have symptoms of abdominal pain, nausea, vomiting, and food intolerance. In some patients in whom no other abnormality could be found, the symptoms disappeared after cholecystectomy. Cholesterolosis should not be confused with cholesterol polyps (q.v.).

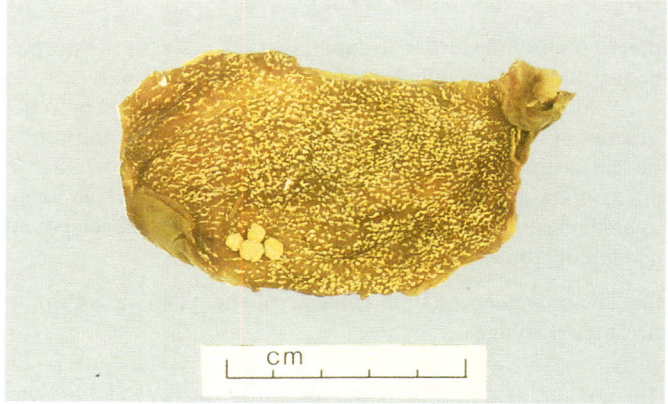

Fig. 17.159 Cholesterolosis of the gall bladder. Several small cholesterol stones are also present.

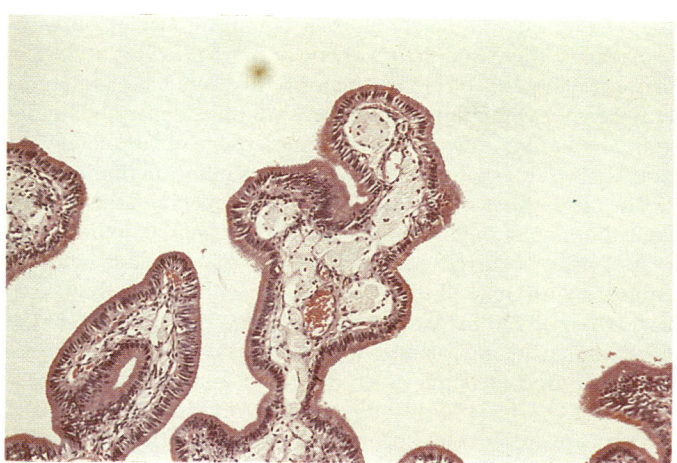

Fig. 17.160 Cholesterolosis of the gall bladder. The lamina propria of the mucosal ridges contains collections of foamy macrophages containing cholesterol ester.

17.15.5 Inflammation of the gall bladder— cholecystitis

Acute cholecystitis

The great majority of cases of acute cholecystitis are associated with gallstones. However, in a minority, 5–10 per cent, of patients with acute cholecystitis no stone is found. This so-called acalculous cholecystitis may arise in a variety of circumstances, in some of which the mechanism is not understood. It is commoner in men. In about half of the cases, no cause is found. In some, the cause is a specific infection, most commonly *Salmonella typhi*. *Salmonella typhi* may remain in the gall bladder for a long time after an acute episode of typhoid fever, without giving rise to symptoms. Live organisms may be excreted in the faeces by such chronic asymptomatic carriers. Other organisms that have been implicated include *Leptospira*, *Brucella*, *Vibrio cholerae*, *Streptococcus*, *Mycobacterium tuberculosis*, and *Actinomyces*. There is a higher incidence of acalculous cholecystitis following severe burns or trauma, prolonged labour, or major surgery even when it is non-abdominal. Prolonged parenteral feeding increases the risk of developing acalculous cholecystitis in these circumstances. In a third group of cases, the underlying insult appears to be ischaemia due to embolism, polyarteritis nodosa or other vasculitides, or systemic lupus erythematosus. Finally, the cystic duct may be obstructed by tumour, fibrosis, or kinking.

In the majority of cases of acute cholecystitis, at least one gallstone is found in the gall bladder. Most suffers are female and the peak incidence is at 50–70 years. There is often a history of previous attacks of biliary colic. Presenting symptoms include right upper quadrant pain often referred to the interscapular area or right shoulder. There is anorexia, nausea, and vomiting. On examination, there is fever with tenderness in the right upper quadrant. A gall bladder mass may be palpable. There may be mild jaundice. The neutrophil count is raised.

The gall bladder is usually enlarged with oedema and congestion, even haemorrhage of the wall, which is markedly thickened. There is often an exudate on the serosa which is fibrinous or even purulent (Fig. 17.161). The lumen contains cloudy bile containing pus or blood. A stone is often found impacted in Hartmann's pouch. The mucosa shows congestion and focal or widespread necrosis. In gangrenous cholecystitis necrosis is widespread and may extend through the wall. If the lumen is filled with pus, the condition is described as empyema of the gall bladder. Histologically, a prominent feature of early acute cholecystitis is congestion and haemorrhage of the mucosa and the wall (Fig. 17.162). There is a variable neutrophil infiltration, ranging from scanty to very marked. Necrosis may be seen. Intramural microabscesses may be found.

In specimens obtained at interval cholecystectomy, the acute inflammation will have started to resolve and granulation tissue may be present in the wall. Eosinophils become prominent and lymphocytes, plasma cells, and macrophages are also found.

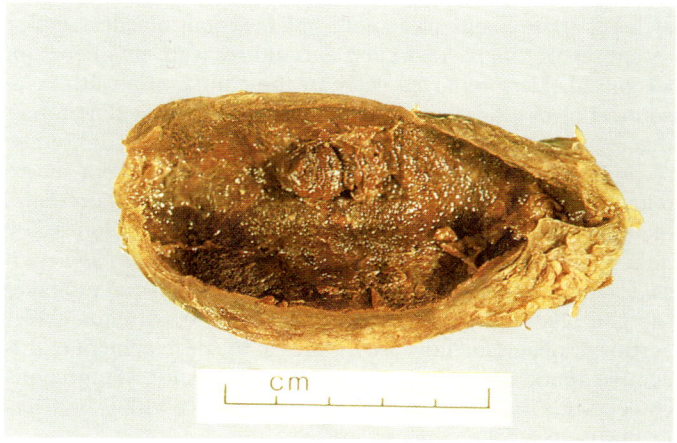

Fig. 17.161 Acute cholecystitis. The wall of the gall bladder is thickened and haemorrhagic. The mucosa is necrotic and sloughing off.

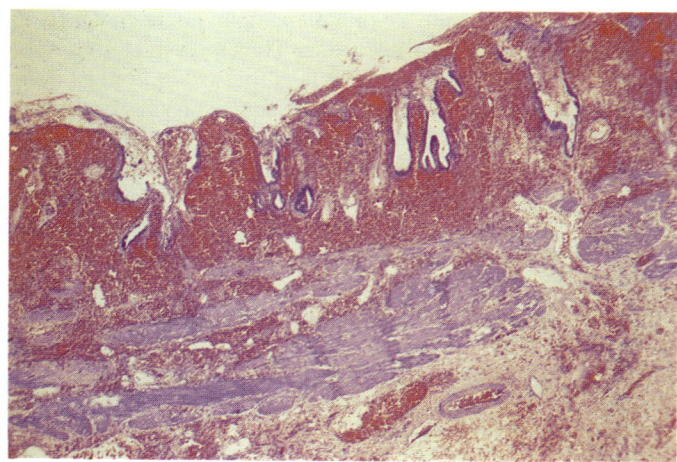

Fig. 17.162 Acute cholecystitis. There is extensive haemorrhage into the mucosa of the gall bladder.

Collections of foamy macrophages, some of which contain bile pigment, are frequently found in the wall. This appearance is described as resolving acute or subacute cholecystitis.

The pathogenesis of acute cholecystitis has not been fully elucidated. The single most important factor is impaction of a stone in the neck of the gall bladder which probably results in damage to the mucosa. Patients who are taking thiazide diuretics have a higher risk of developing acute cholecystitis. It is likely that the subsequent inflammation is primarily chemical in nature—due to the irritant effect of bile, especially bile salts, which has breached the mucosal barrier. One postulated mechanism is that phospholipase from the lysosomes of gall bladder epithelial cells is released by trauma to the mucosa caused by a stone. Lecithin in the bile is then converted to lysolecithin by the phospholipase. Lysolecithin is an active detergent which is known to be toxic to mucosa. Bacterial infection may then occur secondarily. The histological appearance of the gall bladder in very early acute cholecystitis lends support to this hypothesis as there is little polymorph infiltration but very marked vascular reaction. However bacteria are cultured from at least 50 per cent of acutely inflamed gall bladders and a recent report that positive bacterial cultures were obtained from all gall bladders removed early in the course of an attack of acute cholecystitis casts some doubt on the chemical irritation theory. In gangrenous cholecystitis, infarction is thought to be secondary to thrombosis of vessels, which results from severe inflammation and distension of the gall bladder. Occasionally, in gangrenous cholecystitis the necrotic tissues are colonized by anaerobic gas-forming organisms, especially *Clostridium welchii*, which results in formation of gas in the wall and lumen of the gall bladder, so called emphysematous or gaseous cholecystitis. Diabetes mellitus predisposes to the development of this complication, which has a significant mortality. Gangrenous cholecystitis may, of course, also complicate vasculitis or arterial obstruction following torsion.

Clinical course and complications of acute cholecystitis

In many instances, acute cholecystitis resolves spontaneously with fibrosis of the wall. The relationship of acute cholecystitis to chronic cholecystitis is uncertain. They have in common the the strong aetiological factor of cholelithiasis but in most cases of chronic cholecystitis a history of acute attacks is not given. Empyema and hydrops have been discussed already. Acute inflammation is not necessarily a precursor to hydrops. Perforation of the gall bladder occurs in about 5 per cent of cases, especially in the setting of gangrenous cholecystitis. Usually, the perforation is contained by omentum and remains localized but free perforation into the peritoneal cavity will lead to the life-threatening complication of biliary peritonitis.

Chronic cholecystitis

Chronic cholecystitis is much commoner than its acute counterpart. It, too, is much more common in females and has the same peak age of incidence. Gallstones are present in an even higher proportion of cases. Bacteria can be cultured from the bile of only a minority of cases of chronic cholecystitis. In some cases, there is a history of one or more previous attacks of acute cholecystitis but in the majority this is not so. Symptoms may be very vague, the commonest are right upper abdominal pain and flatulent dyspepsia with intolerance of fatty foods. On oral cholecystography, the gall bladder is non-functioning.

The appearance of the gall bladder will depend on the relative contributions of inflammation and fibrosis. When acute cholecystitis has occurred in the past the gall bladder may be enlarged with marked thickening of the wall, which may be so florid that, on initial inspection, carcinoma is suspected. On the other hand, the gall bladder may be shrunken with a thin fibrotic wall and atrophic mucosa, which may appear trabeculated (Fig. 17.156). Gallstones, usually multiple, of the mixed variety, are present in 95 per cent of specimens. The histological appearance is equally variable. There may be heavy chronic inflammation with a so-called cholegranulomatous reaction, consisting of foamy macrophages, some containing pigment, and including multinucleate giant cells surrounding clefts which contained cholesterol crystals. Rokitansky–Aschoff sinuses may be prominent and some may contain concretions of bile (Fig. 17.163). At the other end of the spectrum, there may be little inflammation, just fibrosis of the wall and atrophy of the mucosa (Fig. 17.164). Small arteries in the wall may show endarteritis obliterans. Follicular cholecystitis is a variant of chronic cholecystitis in which there is a prominent infiltrate of lymphocytes in the mucosa, with associated germinal centres. The wall of the gall bladder may show focal or diffuse dystrophic calcification. If it is diffuse, the condition is described as 'porcelain gall bladder'. The wall is usually smooth, thin, and brittle. There is an increased incidence of carcinoma in gall bladders which show this change, much in excess of that observed in chronic cholecystitis generally. In addition to the cholegranulomatous reaction described above, a number of other characteristic inflammatory variants are recognized. These generally consist of collections of macrophages containing various components of bile or its breakdown products, and other inflam-

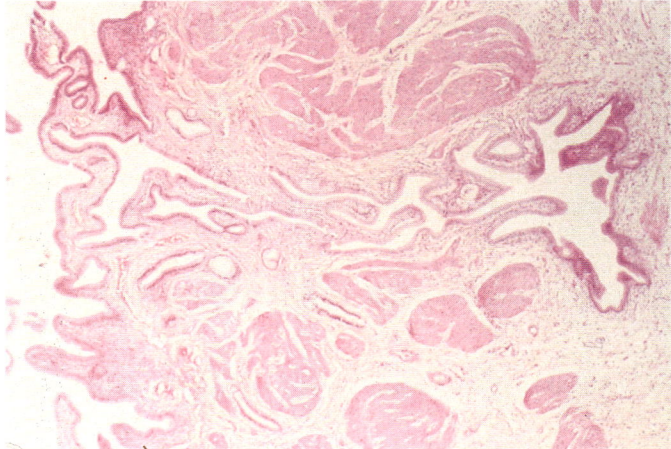

Fig. 17.163 Chronic cholecystitis. A Rokitansky–Aschoff sinus extends through the muscularis into the subserosal connective tissue.

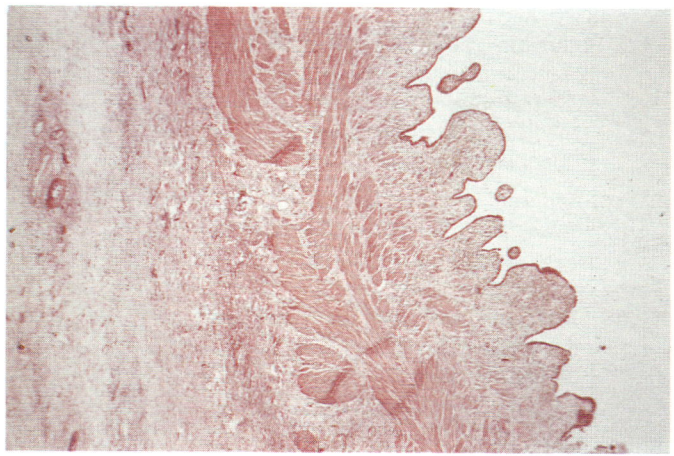

Fig. 17.164 Chronic cholecystitis. The mucosa is atrophic. There is fibrosis of the wall.

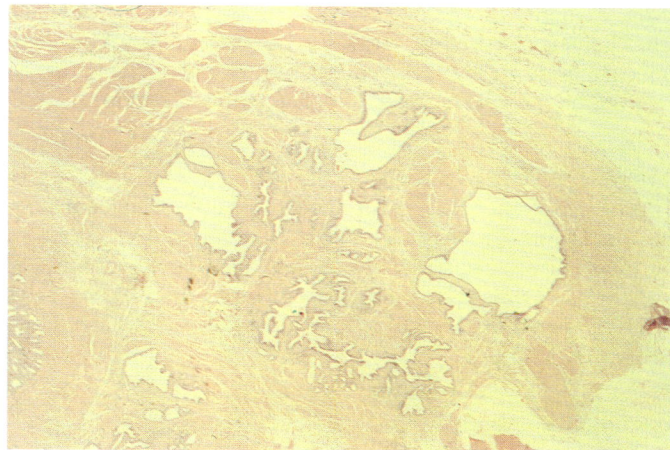

Fig. 17.165 Adenomyosis of the gall bladder. Mucosal diverticula interdigitate between bundles of hypertrophic smooth muscle.

matory cells. In xanthogranulomatous cholecystitis, abundant foamy macrophages are present. In ceroid granuloma, ceroid pigment, related to the 'wear and tear' pigment lipofuscin, is found in abundance in macrophages which are collected in the lamina propria. Macroscopically, they are seen as brown masses in the wall. Malakoplakia (q.v.) of the gall-bladder is unusual but well recognized. These lesions differ from cholesterolosis in that they appear to be a response to previous inflammation which has resulted in extravasation of bile into the wall of the gall bladder.

17.15.6 Diverticular disease of the gall bladder

These conditions are characterized by the presence of multiple diverticula of gall bladder epithelium between the smooth muscle bundles of the wall. The smooth muscle is usually hypertrophied, often markedly so. The condition may be diffuse or localized. The diffuse type is known as adenomyomatosis or cholecystitis glandularis proliferans. The localized variety is called adenomyoma and is most commonly located at the fundus. Both types are usually recognized macroscopically. The diverticula, which often contain bile concretions, may extend to beneath the serosa. The wall of the gall bladder is often markedly thickened by the hypertrophic smooth muscle. Gallstones are frequently present. Histologically, the mucosal outpouchings may show a complex pattern of ramification between muscle bundles (Fig. 17.165). There is frequently associated inflammation, acute or chronic, including cholegranuloma. The relationship of this entity to the isolated Rokitansky–Aschoff sinuses of chronic cholecystitis is debatable. They are, however, often found in a similar setting. The pathogenesis of these lesions is uncertain. They are not neoplastic and probably arise as pulsion diverticula with secondary hypertrophy of smooth muscle, analogous to diverticular disease of the colon (q.v.). In some cases there is evidence of obstruction to gall bladder outflow. The collective term, diverticular disease of the gall bladder, for these lesions is preferable to the alternative

hyperplastic disease or even the portentous hyperplastic cholecystosis, neither of which sheds much light on the pathogenesis.

17.15.7 Infestation of the biliary tree

A variety of metazoan parasites have been found in the biliary tree and, in some parts of the world, especially China and South-East Asia, they are an important cause of morbidity and mortality. The bile ducts are much more frequently involved than the gall bladder. The commonest parasites are the liver flukes *Fasciola hepatica* and *Opisthorchis sinensis*. Their presence leads to chronic cholangitis which may, in turn, give rise to intrahepatic abscesses and hepatic fibrosis. They are an important factor in the pathogenesis of brown pigment gallstones in the bile ducts. Carcinoma of the biliary tree is often associated with *Opisthorchis* infestation and has also been reported with opisthorchiasis. *Ascaris lumbricoides* is occasionally found in the bile ducts. The usual tissue response to these parasites is eosinophil polymorph infiltration and fibrosis. Granulomatous inflammation is seen in response to ova of *Ascaris lumbricoides*, schistosomes, and *Fasciola hepatica*. Hydatid cysts may rupture from the liver into the bile ducts.

17.15.8 Infections

Specific bacterial infections have been discussed in the section on acalculous cholecystitis. A variety of other infections of the gall bladder, viral, protozoal, and fungal, may also occur. These include cytomegalovirus in patients who have had liver transplants, giardiasis, candidiasis, and aspergillosis.

17.15.9 Miscellaneous lesions

Torsion or volvulus of the gall bladder

A floating gall bladder (see above), especially one that contains stones, may twist on its pedicle. If the torsion is severe, the arterial supply is occluded. Elderly patients are most susceptible. The clinical presentation is that of acute cholecystitis. The histological appearance ranges from congestion and haemorrhage to infarction with varying degrees of acute inflammation.

Vascular lesions

These have already been mentioned in the discussion of acalculous and gangrenous cholecystitis. The gall bladder may also be involved by a vascular lesion, so-called 'localized visceral angiitis', which is histologically identical to small vessel polyarteritis nodosa but which, as its name implies, is confined to a single organ.

Haemobilia

Haemobilia denotes the presence of blood in the biliary tree following haemorrhage resulting from the presence of a pathological communication between the vascular system and the biliary tract. The condition may result from trauma or diseases such as cholelithiasis, inflammation, or tumours. In most cases, the source of bleeding is the liver but it may also originate from the gall bladder. Percutaneous needle biopsy of the liver is an increasingly common cause of haemobilia.

The presentation will depend on the rate of bleeding. Very minor haemobilia may go completely unnoticed. More severe bleeding will lead to melaena or haematemesis. If blood clots form in the biliary tract, biliary colic may ensue. Very heavy bleeding will results in shock and death from exsanguination.

Cholesterol polyps

Occasionally polyps which have a multilobular yellow appearance are found in the gall bladder. One or more such polyps may be present. They are attached to the mucosa by a narrow stalk, although they may become detached and be found floating in the bile. They measure up to 1 cm in diameter. Histologically, they consist of aggregates of macrophages with foamy cytoplasm beneath the biliary epithelium. The foamy appearance is due to the presence of cholesterol. Such cholesterol polyps are not usually associated with the cholesterolosis. They may give rise to right upper quadrant pain and dyspepsia.

Benign strictures of the biliary tract

Fibrosis of the wall of the bile duct may follow injury to, or inflammation of, the duct and can lead to narrowing of the lumen with consequent obstruction to the passage of bile from the liver.

Typically, a benign stricture is localized and confined to a short length of the bile duct not more than 1–2 cm in extent. Although the mucosa in the area of narrowing may be ulcerated, the typical cholangiographic appearance is one of a smooth, tapered narrowing of the duct lumen. The ducts proximal to the stricture are dilated and, if the obstruction continues, the liver will show an increasing degree of portal fibrosis, eventually culminating in secondary biliary cirrhosis.

The causes of such benign bile duct strictures are listed below.

1. Injury to bile ducts:
   (a) following operations on or in the vicinity of the gall bladder and biliary tree;
   (b) Post-traumatic:
      (i) blunt abdominal trauma;
      (ii) penetrating wounds.
2. Post-inflammatory strictures associated with:
   (a) gallstones (see also Mirizzi syndrome);
   (b) penetrating duodenal ulcer;
   (c) chronic pancreatitis;
   (d) subhepatic inflammation or abscess;
   (e) infestation with parasites;
   (f) post radiotherapy;
   (g) pyogenic cholangitis.
3. Papillary stenosis:
   (a) primary;
   (b) associated with cholelithiasis;
   (c) iatrogenic.
4. Localized primary sclerosing cholangitis.
5. Congenital biliary atresia.

By far the commonest cause of benign biliary stricture is injury sustained during cholecystectomy. The incidence of damage to the biliary tree during cholecystectomy is about 1 in 500 operations. Factors that increase the possibility of such injury occuring include anatomical variations in the biliary tree, inflammation and oedema in the region of the cystic duct, and porta hepatis, especially if the gall bladder is small and fibrotic.

Papillary stenosis is an obstructive lesion of the papilla of Vater which is due to inflammation and fibrosis in that area or, rarely, to adenomyosis. The vast majority of cases are ascribable to gallstones, pancreatitis, duodenal ulceration, or surgical handling. In a small number of cases of so-called primary papillary stenosis no cause can be identified.

Primary sclerosing cholangitis

This is discussed in detail elsewhere (Section 17.5.4).

Limy bile

If the concentration of calcium salts in the bile is sufficiently high, they may precipitate to cause opacification and sludging of the bile, 'limy bile'. The radio-opaque calcium salts will produce a cholecystogram on plain abdominal radiographs. Limy bile is more likely to be found in the setting of hydrops of the gall bladder.

Hyperplasias and metaplasias of gall bladder epithelium

A variety of metaplastic changes have been described in the gall bladder mucosa in association with inflammatory disease. The finding of mucous glands in the body or fundus of the gall bladder is known as mucous gland hyperplasia or metaplasia (Fig. 17.166) which is often considered to be a form of gastric antral metaplasia. Goblet cells are sometimes found in the surface epithelium or the mucous glands, and this goblet cell metaplasia becomes commoner with increasing age. Paneth cells

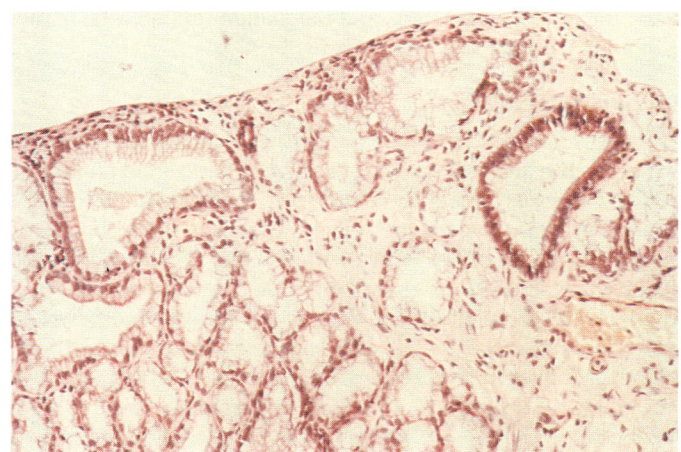

Fig. 17.166 Mucous metaplasia of the gall bladder epithelium. Mucous glands, resembling those found in the gastric antrum, in the gall bladder mucosa.

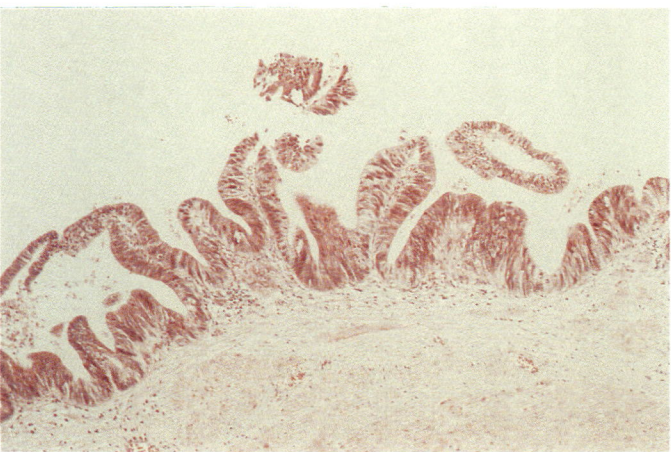

Fig. 17.167 Dysplasia of the gall bladder. The epithelium shows papillary hyperplasia with moderate nuclear atypia.

and enterochromaffin cells are also found in gall bladder surface epithelium or mucous glands with increasing frequency with age. The various combinations of goblet cell, enterochromaffin cell, and Paneth cell metaplasias, often in association with gastric antral epithelium, are grouped together as intestinal metaplasia of the gall bladder, although true intestinal metaplasia, as defined by the presence of columnar cells with a high brush border, is a rarity. The incomplete form of intestinal metaplasia, including mucous gland metaplasia, is a common incidental finding in inflamed gall bladders. The frequent coexistence of goblet cells, enterochromaffin cells, Paneth cells, and mucous glands in the same mucosa suggests that their appearance is part of the same process. Much less common than mucous gland hyperplasia, but often associated with it, is focal mucosal hyperplasia. This may occur primarily, in which case no other abnormality is found in the gall bladder, or secondarily, when it is associated with other disorders of the gall-bladder including cholesterolosis. Focal mucosal hyperplasia is also classified according to the architecture of the hyperplastic epithelium. Thus, in villous hyperplasia mucosal folds are long, irregular, and ramifying, whereas in adenomatous or spongioid hyperplasia a reticulate appearance is found. Villous hyperplasia may be a precursor of cholesterolosis of the gall bladder.

Regardless of the histological subtype, mucosal hyperplasia may be difficult to identify on gross examination but, typically, the mucosa appears thickened, often with an irregular surface. In older patients adenomatous hyperplasia is sometimes found in association with mucous gland hyperplasia. Primary focal mucosal hyperplasia may, however, be seen in patients of all ages.

Epithelial hyperplasia of the gall bladder occurs in which the epithelium shows pseudostratification with nuclear crowding and taller than normal columnar epithelium. A proportion of such cases show areas of atypical hyperplasia or dysplasia, in which there is loss of normal architecture, sometimes with micropapillae and nuclear atypia (Fig. 17.167). Some cases of

atypical hyperplasia may progress to carcinoma *in situ* and a proportion of these to invasive carcinoma (see below).

17.15.10 Tumours of the gall bladder and biliary tree

Benign tumours

Benign tumours of the gall bladder are rare. Two entities sometimes considered under this heading are not true neoplasms at all. They are: cholesterol polyps (see above) and inflammatory polyps or pseudotumours.

Benign true neoplasms of gall bladder epithelium are classified according to their pattern of growth. They are usually polypoid and may be sessile or have stalks. They may be multiple. Like intestinal polyps, a spectrum of growth patterns is seen, ranging from a solid adenomatous polyp or tubular adenoma to a predominantly papillary lesion which may resemble a villous adenoma of the large intestine. The tubular adenoma consists of tubules or acini proliferating within the substance of the polyp, where they are surrounded by a loose fibrous stroma (Fig. 17.168). The papilloma consists of branching fronds covered by columnar epithelium with a connective tissue core (Fig. 17.169). A mixed growth pattern is not unusual in these tumours. Like adenomas of the intestine, varying degrees of dysplasia of the epithelium are seen, although their potential for malignant transformation is uncertain. Remnants of adenoma are sometimes found, however, in gall bladders containing invasive cancer.

A large variety of non-epithelial tumours of the gall bladder have been reported. These include granular cell tumour, amputation neuroma, paraganglioma, leiomyoma, and lipoma.

Benign tumours of the extrahepatic bile ducts are especially rare. Among lesions, which may present like tumours, are rare hamartomas around the ampulla and heterotopic pancreatic tissue. Benign epithelial neoplasms are similar to those of the gall bladder.

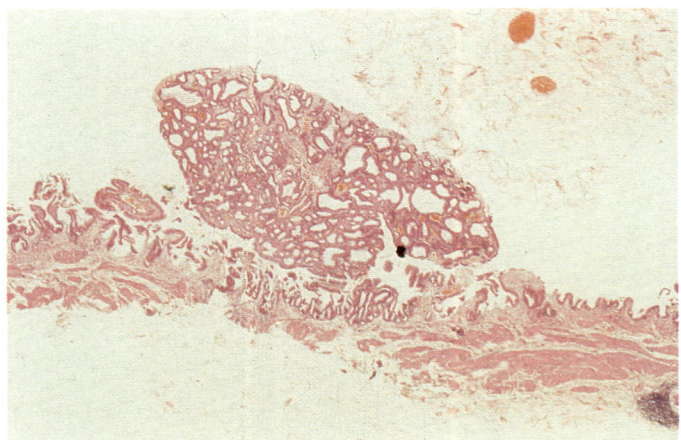

Fig. 17.168 Tubular adenoma of the gall bladder.

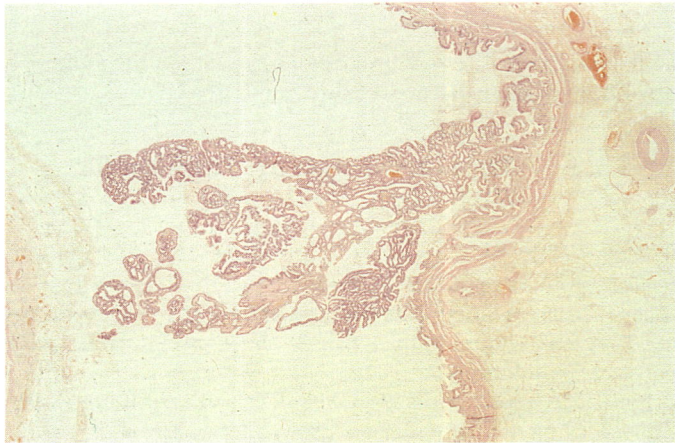

Fig. 17.169 Papilloma of the gall bladder.

Biliary cystadenoma is a rare benign tumour of the bile ducts, which occurs more commonly in the liver but which may also be found in the extrahepatic ducts. Multiple tumours, both intra- and extrahepatic, occurring in the same patient have also been reported. Most present as an abdominal mass or with large bile duct obstruction. The tumours are multiloculated, thin-walled cysts, measuring up to several centimetres in diameter and containing fluid, which may be serous or mucoid. Microscopically, the cysts are lined by a single layer of columnar or cuboidal epithelium.

Papillomatosis

Very rarely, multiple papillary tumours are found in the biliary tract. The usual presentation of this condition, papillomatosis, is with obstructive jaundice. The tumours may be distributed extensively throughout the biliary tree, including intrahepatic ducts and the gall bladder. Histologically, the tumours show a complex branching pattern and may be cytologically benign or show degrees of atypia up to and including carcinoma. Treatment is difficult because of the extensive involvement of the tract, the tendency to recur, and the malignant potential of the tumours.

Malignant tumours

Primary malignant epithelial neoplasms of the biliary tree are not at all unusual and account for up to 3 per cent of all malignancies. They are the fifth commonest gastrointestinal malignancy. Their peak age of incidence is in the eighth decade. The incidence related to sex varies with the site. Those of the gall bladder are about three times commoner in women whereas, among those of the bile ducts, there is a slight preponderance of men. Carcinomas of the bile ducts are less common than those of the gall bladder. There is a relatively higher incidence of carcinoma of the biliary tree among American Indians and Japanese.

The aetiology of carcinoma of the biliary tree is unknown. Gallstones are found in about 75 per cent of patients with gall bladder cancer but the association is much weaker, at about 32 per cent, in those with bile duct cancer. There is a higher incidence of gall bladder cancer in chronic typhoid carriers. There is a particularly high risk of gall bladder cancer in those with chronic inflammatory bowel disease. In the case of bile duct cancer, other aetiological associations include parasitic infestation (*Opisthorchis sinensis*, *O. viverrini* or *O. felineus*), primary sclerosing cholangitis, and long-standing choledochal cyst.

Gall-bladder

Carcinomas of the gall bladder will usually have grown to considerable size by the time they produce symptoms. As a result they are often inoperable at the time of surgery. Most cases are not diagnosed before surgery. The usual presentation is with upper abdominal pain, weight loss, and jaundice.

Grossly, the usual appearance of carcinoma of the gall bladder is of a diffusely infiltrating tumour which occupies a variable proportion of the gall bladder (Fig. 17.170). The infiltrating tumour is usually scirrhous and is therefore firm in consistency and gritty on sectioning. Less commonly, the tumour is polypoid or fungating, growing into the lumen. At the time of presentation, most tumours involve the entire gall bladder, and in only 10 per cent of cases at presentation is the tumour completely confined to the gall bladder. In another 15 per cent of cases, the local spread is limited to regional lymph nodes and the gall bladder fossa. The polypoid type carries the best prognosis, as invasion is often minimal at the time of diagnosis.

Histologically, 80 per cent of the tumours are adenocarcinomas. They are usually moderately differentiated and have a desmoplastic stroma (Fig. 17.171). They may show mucinous foci and some tumours, especially those that have a polypoid appearance macroscopically, have a well-marked papillary growth pattern. Less than 5 per cent of tumours are squamous, and mixed adeno- and squamous carcinomas are also rarely found. Another 5 per cent of tumours are anaplastic and among these are found a small number of small-cell or oat-cell carcinomas. Other rarities include intestinal-type adenocarcinoma

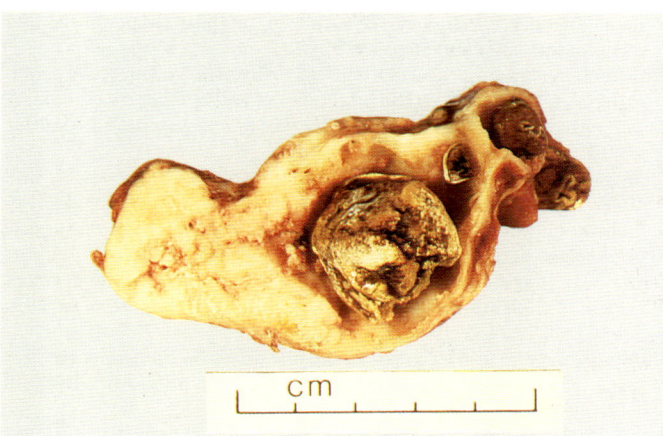

Fig. 17.170 Carcinoma of the gall bladder. There is marked thickening of the wall by a diffusely infiltrating tumour which has destroyed the mucosa. Note the presence of gallstones.

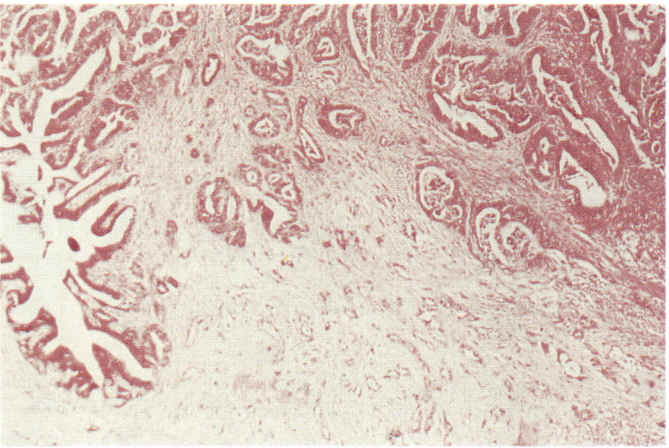

Fig. 17.171 Carcinoma of the gall bladder. The tumour has destroyed the muscularis.

(with goblet cells), giant cell adenocarcinoma, and adeno-carcinoma with choriocarcinoma-like areas, which are, nevertheless, negative on immunohistochemical staining for human chorionic gonadotrophin. If the mucosa of the gall bladder close to an invasive carcinoma is examined, areas of mucosal dysplasia and carcinoma *in situ* are sometimes found. These lesions are also found with increased frequency in populations which are at high risk of developing gall bladder carcinoma. In these, invasive carcinoma has not yet developed or is only identifiable microscopically. This has led to the suggestion that at least some carcinomas arise through a progression from epithelial hyperplasia through atypical hyperplasia or dysplasia then carcinoma *in situ* of which some cases become invasive carcinoma.

Extensive direct invasion of the tumour into adjacent liver is a common finding at surgery. Other neighbouring viscera may also be directly invaded which may result in the formation of a

malignant fistula. The tumour also spreads by lymphatic or vascular metastasis, growth along the ducts, perineural infiltration or intraperitoneal seeding. Distant metastatis usually occurs late in the disease, typically to lung and bone.

Other rare primary tumours of the gall bladder include carcinosarcoma, sarcoma—including haemangiosarcoma and leiomyosarcoma—malignant melanoma, and, very rarely, primary lymphoma. Carcinoid tumours may also occur.

Secondary tumours are found in the gall bladders of about 6 per cent of patients dying with carcinoma.

Malignant tumours of the bile ducts

These tumours are usually smaller at presentation than gall bladder carcinoma because even relatively small lesions in the bile ducts may give rise to symptoms resulting from obstruction, partial or complete, of bile outflow. These are usually slow-growing. In spite of this, the prognosis for carcinoma of the bile ducts is very poor, with most patients dying within a year of diagnosis.

The clinical presentation, gross appearance, histology, treatment, and prognosis of these tumours varies with the position at which they arise in the biliary tract. Conventionally, three zones of origin are considered: the proximal ducts, including the hilum; the mid-ductal region, including the common bile duct, cystic duct, and supra- and intrapancreatic segments of the common bile duct, and finally the ampullary region. About 50 per cent of tumours of the extrahepatic bile ducts arise in the proximal third.

The majority of tumours present with cholestasis. If obstruction is incomplete or intermittent, the patient may not be jaundiced and the only biochemical abnormality may be a marked rise in serum alkaline phosphatase. At operation, the findings depend on the site of the tumour. Those in the distal part of the bile duct usually produce marked dilatation of the proximal biliary tree, including the gall bladder, whereas those promixal to the cystic duct are associated with an enlarged, turgid liver and empty, collapsed bile duct and gall bladder.

On gross examination, three macroscopic subtypes can be identified. These are sclerosing or diffuse, nodular, and papillary. The sclerosing or diffuse type consists of firm thickening of the duct. It is usually found in the proximal zone and may extend diffusely along the biliary tree into the substance of the liver. Tumours of this sort, arising at the confluence of the bile ducts, are often designated 'Klatskin tumours'. They are notoriously difficult to diagnose as, even at laparotomy, they may be mistaken for sclerosing cholangitis, benign stricture, or, in some instances, carcinoma of the gall bladder. If the hilum of the liver is not dissected at laparotomy, a small sclerosing carcinoma of the proximal ducts may be missed completely. In this group, the more localized sclerosing subtype often shows local invasion of surrounding tissues, whereas the diffuse type typically spreads linearly along the ducts.

The nodular type is found most commonly in the middle third. The tumour forms a nodule which projects into the lumen of the bile duct. The papillary or polypoid type shows mainly intraluminal growth. It is found most commonly in the distal third and, in that region, most frequently at the ampulla of Vater where it is included among the group of ampullary and periampullary tumours. Because of special considerations in the diagnosis and treatment of these tumours, they are discussed separately.

Microscopically, these tumours resemble those of the gall bladder. The range of special types and variants is similar to that of the gall bladder although the proportion of well-differentiated tumours is higher.

The most important mode of spread of carcinoma of the bile ducts is by direct invasion of adjacent tissues. Perineural invasion is often prominent. They may also grow along the bile ducts into the liver. Extension into the pancreas or duodenum occurs with tumours arising in the distal third. Metastasis is most commonly to regional lymph nodes or liver.

Ampullary and periampullary tumours

Tumours in this region can originate from:

1. the distal common bile duct;
2. the ampulla of Vater proper;
3. the periampullary duodenum; and
4. the head of the pancreas.

They are grouped together because of similarities in their clinical presentation and in the approach to their diagnosis and treatment. Although it is often difficult to do so, an effort should be made to establish the site of origin of a tumour in this region as the survival following surgery is much longer for the first three types than for carcinoma of the head of the pancreas. The latter tumour is often inoperable at the time of diagnosis. On the other hand, true ampullary tumours and tumours of the distal common bile duct, because of their anatomical location and also because of their frequently papillary, intraluminal growth pattern, give rise to symptoms early on, before extensive local invasion has occurred. Typically, pancreatic adenocarcinoma is moderately to well differentiated and shows a tubular growth pattern with mucus production. Many cases of ampullary and lower bile duct cancer show a polypoid, papillary structure but scirrhous types can occur. Ampullary carcinoma can develop in a villous adenoma of the ampullary region. On the other hand, well-differentiated adenocarcinoma of the pancreas can show a papillary growth pattern on the luminal surface. Duodenal carcinoma typically resembles adenocarcinoma elsewhere in the intestine. Reliance cannot be placed, therefore, on the histological appearance of biopsy material to establish a pre-operative diagnosis of the tumour site of origin, and clinical, radiological, endoscopic, and histological findings should be considered together.

17.15.11   Further reading

Alagille, D. (1984). Extrahepatic biliary atresia. *Hepatology* **4** (1), 75–105.

Albores Saavedra, J., Alcantra-Vazquez, A., Cruz-Ortiz, H., and Herrera-Goepfert, R. (1980). The precursor lesions of invasive gall bladder carcinoma. Hyperplasia, atypical hyperplasia and carcinoma-*in-situ*. *Cancer* **45**, 919–27.

Albores-Saavedra, J., Cruz-Ortiz, H., Alcantra-Vazquez, A., and Henson, D. E. (1981). Unusual types of gall bladder carcinoma. A report of 16 cases. *Archives of Pathology and Laboratory Medicine* **105**, 287–93.

Albores-Saavedra, J., Manrique, J. de J., Angeles-Angeles, A., and Henson, D. E. (1984). Carcinoma *in situ* of the gall bladder. A clinicopathologic study of 18 cases. *American Journal of Surgical Pathology* **8**, 323–33.

Bennion, L. J. and Grundy, S. M. (1978). Risk factors for the development of cholelithiasis in man. *New England Journal of Medicine* **299**, 1161–7, 1221–7.

Blumgart, L. H. (1988). Cancer of the bile ducts. In *Surgery of the liver and biliary tract* (ed. L. H. Blumgart), pp. 829–53. Churchill Livingstone, Edinburgh.

Carey, M. C. and Small, D. M. (1978). The physical chemistry of cholesterol solubility in bile: relationship to gallstone formation and dissolution in man. *Journal of Clinical Investigation* **61**, 998–1026.

Christensen, A. H. and Ishak, K. C. (1970). Benign tumours and pseudotumours of the gall bladder. *Archives of Pathology* **90**, 423–32.

Claesson, B., Holmlund, D., and Maetzsch, T. (1984). Biliary microflora in acute cholecystitis and the clinical implications. *Acta Chirurgica Scandinavica* **150**, 229–37.

Elfving, G., Lehtonen, T., and Teir, H. (1967). Clinical significance of primary hyperplasia of gall bladder mucosa. *Annals of Surgery* **165**, 61–9.

Elfving, G., Palmu, A., and Teir, H. (1968). Cholesterolosis and mucosal hyperplasia of gall bladder. *Annales Chirurgiae et Gynaecologiae Fenniae* **57**, 28–30.

Gracie, W. A. and Ransohoff, D. F. (1982). The natural history of silent gallstones. The innocent gallstone is not a myth. *New England Journal of Medicine* **307**, 798–817.

Ishak, K. G., Willis, G. W., Cummins, S. D., and Bullock, A. A. (1977). Biliary cystadenoma and cystadenocarcinoma. Report of 14 cases and review of the literature. *Cancer* **38**, 322–38.

Jacyna, M. R. and Bouchier, I. A. D. (1987). Cholesterolosis: a physical cause of 'functional' disorder. *British Medical Journal* **295**, 619.

Knight, M. (1981). Anomalies of the gall bladder, bile ducts and arteries. In *Surgery of the gall bladder and bile ducts* (2nd ed) (ed. R. Smith and S. Sherlock), pp. 97–117. Butterworth, London.

Kozuka, S., Tsubone, M., Yasui, A., and Hachisuka, K. (1982). Relation of adenoma to carcinoma in the gall bladder. *Cancer* **50**, 2226–34.

Laito, M. (1983). Histogenesis of epithelial neoplasms of human gall bladder I and II. *Pathology Research and Practice* **178**, 51–6, 57–66.

Landing, B. (1974). Considerations on the pathogenesis of neonatal hepatitis, biliary atresia and choledochal cysts—the concept of infantile obstructive cholangiopathy. In *Progress in paediatric surgery*, Vol. 6 (ed. A. M. Bill and M. Kasai), pp. 113–39. University Park Press, Baltimore.

Longmire, W. P., Mandiola, S. A., and Gordon, H. E. (1971). Congenital cystic disease of the liver and biliary system. *Annals of Surgery* **174**, 711–24.

MacPherson, B. R., Pemsingh, R. S., and Scott, G. W. (1987). Experimental cholelithiasis in the ground squirrel. *Laboratory Investigation* **56**, 138–45.

Ostrow, J. D. (1984). The etiology of pigment gallstones. *Hepatology* **4**, (5), 2155–225.

Schriever, C. E. and Jungst, D. (1989). Association between cholesterolphospholipid vesicles and cholesterol crystals in human gallbladder bile. *Hepatology* **9**, 541–6.

Sjodahl, R., Tagesson, C., and Wetterfors, J. (1978). On the pathogenesis of acute cholecystitis. *Surgery, Gynaecology and Obstetrics* **146**, 199–202.

Soloway, R. D., Balistreri, W. F., and Trotman, B. W. (1980). The gall bladder and biliary tract. In *Recent advances in gastroenterology*, Vol. 4 (ed. I. A. D. Bouchier), pp. 251–90. Churchill Livingstone, Edinburgh.

Weedon, D. (1984). *Pathology of the gall bladder*. Masson, New York.

Weinbren, K. and Mutum, S. S. (1983). Pathological aspects of cholangiocarcinoma. *Journal of Pathology* **139**, 217–38.

Welton, J. C., Marr, J. S., and Friedman, S. M. (1979). Association between hepatobiliary cancer and typhoid carrier state. *Lancet* **i**, 791–4.

17.16   Pathobiology of liver disease

Joan Trowell

17.16.1   Hepatic failure

Acute

Acute hepatic failure occurs when there is massive necrosis of hepatocytes. It may be caused by many agents, which may be either chemical hepatotoxins, such as carbon tetrachloride or an overdose of drugs, such as paracetamol (acetaminophen), or an infection, commonly viral, which attacks the hepatocytes; hepatic necrosis also occurs with anoxia and with physical damage, such as that caused by irradiation.

It is a rapidly progressive illness in patients whose liver function was previously normal, and, if fulminating, it may cause death in coma in a few days or weeks from the first symptoms.

The mortality from fulminating liver failure is 80 per cent, with about one-third of the patients under 25 years old recovering. The prognosis deteriorates with increasing age and few patients over the age of 60 years survive.

The abnormal biochemical investigations characteristic of acute hepatic failure are very high levels of those serum enzymes that indicate cell necrosis, such as lactate dehydrogenase (LDH), aspartate aminotransferase (AST), and alanine aminotransferase (ALT). These may rise to over 1000 international units and may be as high as 5000 IU. These levels are found in the serum early in the illness when the serum bilirubin has risen little above the normal range. Within a few days the serum bilirubin level rises steeply, but in acute hepatic failure this is more an indication of the duration of the illness than of the severity of the hepatic necrosis or even of the outcome of the illness. At a later stage, when the acute necrosis has ceased, the serum enzymes fall to much lower levels, below 500 IU. This fall in the serum enzyme level does not provide any guide to the prognosis, as this depends on the extent of the hepatic necrosis and on the number of functioning hepatocytes that remain. If the patient survives the initial period of hepatic necrosis but dies days or weeks later of a complication (Fig. 17.172)—coma, secondary infection, haemorrhage—the liver may show evidence of regeneration at autopsy.

The best guide to prognosis in acute hepatic failure is the level of coagulation factors in the circulation (see below). Measurement of the prothrombin index will aid a diagnosis of acute hepatic necrosis as it will be severely impaired and may be the first evidence of hepatic failure found on investigating a confused or comatosed patient. Prothrombin levels below 5 per cent of a control value indicate a very poor prognosis and a patient who will not survive without radical treatment. In contrast, a lesser impairment of the prothrombin index in a patient with signs of hepatic encephalopathy suggest that the patient has cirrhosis with an acute complication rather than acute liver

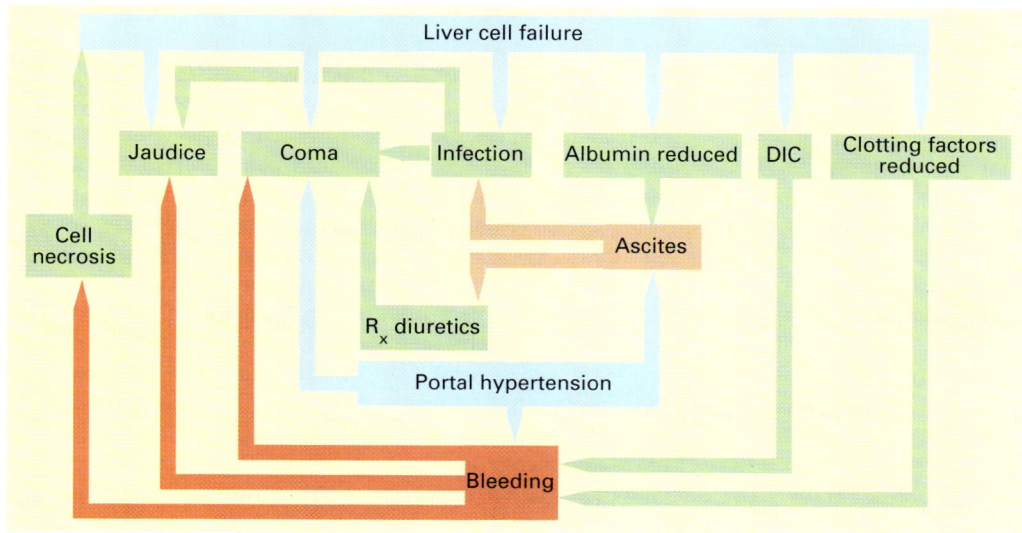

Fig. 17.172 Complications of hepatic failure.

failure. Normal or minimally impaired coagulation in a patient with AST or LDH levels over 2000 IU suggests that the site of cell necrosis is outside the liver.

Chronic

Patients with chronic liver disease and cirrhosis may be well for months or years with few, if any, symptoms and, if their liver function is well compensated, they may have no abnormalities of the standard liver function tests until there is an acute deterioration and hepatic failure occurs. This deterioration may be precipitated by progression of the underlying disease process, or by one of a number of different factors, e.g. infection, gastrointestinal haemorrhage, or alteration of the normal serum electrolyte concentrations, especially hypokalaemia. This most often occurs as a result of diuretic therapy. Hypokalaemia may also occur in cirrhotics in the absence of diuretic treatment; in these patients it is associated with inappropriately high serum levels of aldosterone.

The deterioration in the patient's clinical state may occur very rapidly, with symptoms of confusion, stupor, and even coma occurring in a few hours. This rapid change in the conscious level occurs especially in cirrhotics with infection or gastrointestinal haemorrhage, or fluid or electrolyte imbalance following a rapid diuresis. But, if the precipitating cause is treated, clinical recovery may be equally rapid. This dramatic change in clinical state may be secondary to anoxia following the hypovolaemia due to haemorrhage or diuresis. It may not be due to any change in the number of functioning hepatocytes but may be due to alterations in cellular metabolism. These changes are complex but lead to a metabolic acidosis, which is often associated with a high level of serum lactate; the latter is normally metabolized by liver cells. The mechanism that triggers this acute deterioration in hepatic function is not fully explained but it is associated with the shunting of portal venous blood away from the liver. In portal hypertension there is also an irregular pattern of perfusion within the nodular cirrhotic liver. This leads to regions of relative anoxia within the nodules of the cirrhotic liver and these same cells are also deprived of substances such as glucagon, which are carried in the portal blood and which normally play a part in regulating hepatocyte metabolism.

This shunting of portal venous blood also allows into the systemic circulation compounds that are normally removed from the portal venous blood by the liver cells, either completely on a first pass, or progressively on recirculation. These substances have distant effects on other organs, such as the brain, causing alteration in the conscious level in hepatic encephalopathy, and the kidney, causing the alterations in cortical and medullary blood flow that may contribute to the accumulation of ascites and lead to the impaired renal function of end-stage liver disease and to hepato-renal failure.

On administration of a drug to a patient with hepatic failure, the pharmacokinetics of the drug will be altered if the liver is the site of either activation or elimination of that drug. Many drugs are metabolized or excreted by the liver, and in hepatic failure

the plasma half-life of such drugs will be prolonged. If normal doses of the drug are given at standard intervals, blood levels will rise progressively. This leads to an increase in the side-effects of the drug and increasing toxicity. Patients with cirrhosis also have an increased sensitivity to opiates and benzodiazepines (see below).

If no acute complications occur in a patient with cirrhosis, the deterioration may be insiduous over weeks or months, with an increase in lassitude and fatigue the only symptoms noted. In these patients the diagnosis is overlooked until either there is some dramatic complication, such as haemorrhage or infection, or some incidental event brings the deterioration to medical attention. Such patients may be diagnosed as cirrhotic at an elective or emergency laparotomy for a related or an unrelated condition.

Whichever is the case, such patients have a stormy course after operations, with the development of jaundice, deficiencies of clotting factors and bleeding, ascites, and encephalopathy. They also have poor wound-healing, a high incidence of wound and chest infections, and of wound dehiscence. The postoperative problems are reduced if fluid overload is prevented by limiting fluid intake to 1 litre/day, avoiding infusions of saline, reducing the dose and frequency of any sedation to the minimum required, and ensuring an adequate intake of protein and calories in the postoperative period to maintain protein balance and avoid hypoalbuminaemia. This is usually achieved with infusions of 20 per cent or 50 per cent glucose and salt-reduced human albumin 20 per cent. This regime reduces the problems with ascites but, even so, ascites may still accumulate and require diuretic therapy.

17.16.2   Bleeding in liver failure

Acute hepatic failure and the acute decompensation of patients with chronic liver disease have different aetiologies and a different time-course, but they have common features with a common pathogenesis. Bleeding is one such feature. This may be a generalized tendency due to inadequate production of the clotting factors that are produced in the liver: fibrinogen, factors II, V, VII, IX, X, XI, XII, and XIII can all be affected. Synthesis of factors II, V, IX, and X is dependent on vitamin K, and the prolonged steatorrhoea that can be associated with bile duct obstruction or chronic liver disease leads to vitamin K malabsorption (Fig. 17.173). This may contribute to the bleeding problems and is improved by giving vitamin K intravenously.

In acute liver failure the illness is too short for the body stores of vitamin K to be depleted and the clotting factors with the shortest half-life in the plasma disappear most rapidly from the circulation. In severe fulminating liver failure factor VII falls rapidly as it has a half-life of about 6 hours. Initially fibrinogen levels are well preserved but these fall if the liver cell damage is more prolonged and severe. Fibrinogen levels are also reduced when disseminated intravascular coagulation (DIC) occurs; this may complicate fulminating hepatic failure and occurs in patients with cirrhosis, especially when they develop septicaemia or another infection. In addition to low fibrinogen

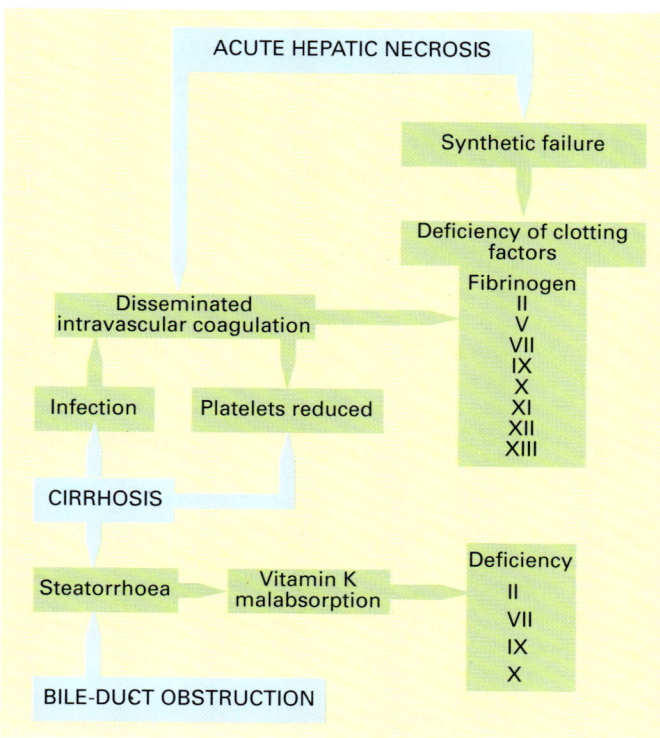

Fig. 17.173 Coagulation abnormalities in hepato-biliary disease.

levels, DIC is associated with a low platelet count, below 100×10^9, and with the finding of fibrin degradation products (FDP) in the blood and urine. DIC is not helped by treatment with heparin, and little helped by giving transfusions of clotting factors and blood, although transfusion may be necessary if there has been significant blood loss. DIC is halted by treating any precipitating factor, such as infection. As this infection can be occult in patients with cirrhosis, the finding of evidence of DIC should lead to bacteriological culture of blood, urine, ascites, and any other appropriate sites; after this, broad-spectrum antibiotic therapy should be given until the results of the cultures become available, when the appropriate antibiotic is substituted.

Haemorrhage into the upper gastrointestinal tract is associated with portal hypertension. This classically occurs as haematemesis or melaena due to bleeding from varices in the lower oesophagus or fundus of the stomach. But in patients with portal hypertension varices may occur in any part of the gastrointestinal tract, and any of these may be the site of clinically significant haemorrhage. Haemorrhage from the oesophagus, stomach, or duodenum can also be due to acute erosions or a chronic peptic ulcer; both of which have an increased prevalence in patients with cirrhosis. As the management of these conditions differs, it is important to investigate the patient to determine the site of haemorrhage. This is most usefully done endoscopically, and if oesophageal varices are found to be bleeding, they can be treated at the same time by injecting sclerosant

into or around the vein to reduce the risks of continued and recurrent bleeding.

17.16.3   Portal hypertension

Portal hypertension may be the result of obstruction to the flow of blood in the portal vein, either within or outside the liver.

Intrahepatic

Portal hypertension occurs most commonly in association with cirrhosis when only 13 per cent of the portal blood flow can be recovered from the hepatic veins after passing through the liver. The most important mechanisms in the production of portal hypertension is the shunting of blood from portal vein into hepatic veins, and the development of shunts between portal veins and hepatic arterioles.

In those parts of the world where it is endemic, schistosomiasis is a frequent cause of intrahepatic portal hypertension (Section 17.4). Other causes are congenital hepatic fibrosis (Section 17.2) and idiopathic non-cirrhotic portal hypertension (Section 17.8). These causes of non-cirrhotic intrahepatic portal hypertension still permit excellent liver function, and for this reason patients with these conditions are often misdiagnosed as having extrahepatic portal hypertension.

Transient

Portal hypertension can occur without hepatic fibrosis in the presence of severe acute liver disease due to viral hepatitis, alcoholic hepatitis, or fatty liver. In these patients the raised portal venous pressure may be too transient for collaterals to form but varices may be seen in acute liver failure. In those patients who survive, these resolve spontaneously as the portal pressure falls to normal when the liver heals.

Prehepatic

Portal hypertension from extrahepatic causes is much less common. It is frequently associated with a leash of veins in place of the portal vein (see Section 17.8.3). This has led to speculation that this caverous transformation is a congenital malformation. However, many of these small vessels may be collaterals formed from the venae comitantes of the portal vein which dilate to carry the portal venous blood to the liver. Portal vein thrombosis can occur following intra-abdominal or umbilical sepsis, and also after splenectomy. The majority of patients with extrahepatic portal hypertension present in childhood.

Obstruction by malignant tumour either of the portal vein itself or of the splenic vein near the pancreas, with or without a secondary portal vein thrombosis, may cause a prehepatic portal hypertension.

Posthepatic

Portal hypertension occurs with obstruction to the flow of blood in the hepatic veins and inferior vena cava. This occurs most often in patients whose primary disease is outside the liver, such as disseminated malignant disease and renal carcinoma; or haematological diseases that cause a generalized thrombotic tendency, such as polycythaemia. It has been seen as a thrombotic complication of the oral contraceptive pill. Patients with cardiac failure may have splenomegaly secondary to portal hypertension; constrictive pericarditis presents with ascites as the result of posthepatic portal hypertension. In patients who have liver disease the hepatic veins may be obstructed within the liver. The portal pressure is raised in patients with hyaline sclerosis, which occurs around the central veins in alcoholic liver disease (see Section 17.6) and in hepatic veno-occlusive disease (see Section 17.8), which occurs as a toxic effect of pyrrolizidine alkaloids from bush teas or herbal medicines.

Complications of portal hypertension

Porto-systemic shunts

The collateral blood vessels that distend to form varices in patients with portal hypertension are at the sites of anastomoses between the portal and systemic venous systems. The most important of these are at the gastro-oesophageal junction between the left gastric and short gastric veins (portal) and the intercostal, diaphragmatic, and azygos veins (systemic), and at the anus, between the superior haemorrhoidal veins (portal) and the middle and inferior haemorrhoidal veins (systemic). Collateral vessels also ocur in the falciform ligament between the porta hepatis and the umbilicus (the umbilical vein of the fetal circulation), and in the retroperitoneal space, around the spleen, the kidneys, the ascending and descending colons, and the duodenum.

Haemorrhage

Bleeding into the gastrointestinal tract is the most acute and life-threatening. This is most often from oesphageal varices or other sites of portal and systemic anastomoses.

Patients who have had previous abdominal surgery and who have developed adhesions have additional collateral vessels therein. These may give rise to troublesome bleeding at any further laparotomy as the portal venous pressure may rise to 20 mmHg.

Ascites

Fluid retention with ascites occurs in the presence of portal hypertension and is discussed in detail later.

Portal-systemic encephalopathy

This occurs in the presence of shunting of portal blood into the systemic circulation and may occur in patients with cirrhosis or extrahepatic portal hypertension. It may be the result of spontaneously occurring shunts but occurs in varying degree in all patients who have had surgical porto-systemic shunts as treatment for variceal bleeding.

Shunting of the portal blood also affects drug metabolism and contributes to the increased incidence of infection in patients with portal hypertension.

All these features are discussed in more detail in Sections 17.16.2 and 17.16.4–7.

17.16.4   Ascites

This is a frequent presenting symptom in patients with decompensated cirrhosis. They become aware of increasing abdominal distension and discomfort if the accumulation of the ascites is rapid (Fig. 17.174). If the fluid accumulates more slowly, abdominal pain may draw attention to the ascites only when it becomes infected. This spontaneous bacterial infection occurs in cirrhotics with ascites and, if untreated, it progresses to septicaemia and the patient may be confused or comatosed when first seen.

A small quantity (about 50 ml) of the ascitic fluid should be aspirated and examined. In cirrhosis, the ascites is a clear fluid with a yellow tinge that depends on the degree of jaundice. In the presence of infection, it becomes turbid with an increased number of polymorphs in the ascitic fluid (more than 250 cells/mm^3). The fluid may be bloodstained; this may follow a traumatic tap, other local trauma (such as liver biopsy), or may, very rarely, occur spontaneously in cirrhotics with poor clotting. More often, bloodstained ascitic fluid occurs in a patient with a tumour: a benign hepatic adenoma in a woman taking the contraceptive pill, a malignant hepatoma complicating cirrhosis, or another malignant tumour whether or not in a patient with cirrhosis.

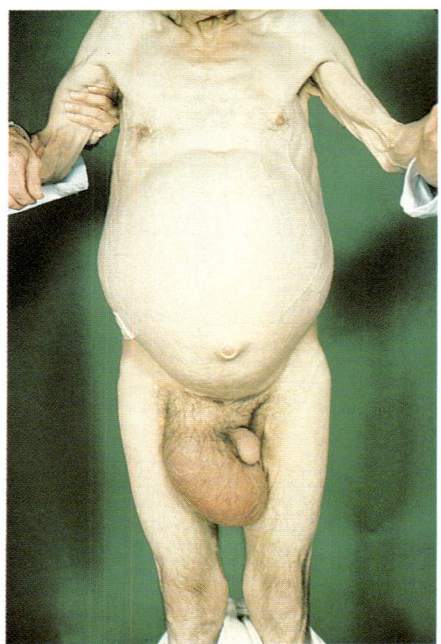

Fig. 17.174 Patient with massive ascites and a communicating hydrocele.

The protein content of the ascitic fluid should also be measured. In uncomplicated cirrhosis both the albumin and total protein content is low, not exceeding the plasma concentration, as it is a transudate, and rarely more than 20 g/l. A raised ascitic protein indicates an exudate due to an inflammatory process in the peritoneum, or a tumour (Fig. 17.175). The low-protein ascitic fluid can also differentiate hepatic ascites from those due to hepatic vein occlusion (Budd–Chiari syndrome) and constrictive pericarditis, both of which may present with high-protein ascites. Pancreatic ascites also has a raised protein level and it is diagnosed by finding a high amylase level in the ascitic fluid. Ascitic fluid should also be stained and examined for cells and micro-organisms; a raised polymorph count suggests an acute bacterial infection and bacteria, frequently Gram-negative rods, may be seen on a Gram stain; a raised mononuclear count in ascitic fluid suggests tuberculosis of the peritoneum, which has an increased incidence in cirrhotics, especially alcoholics, and tubercle bacilli may be seen on Ziehl–Neelsen staining. Cytological stains may show malignant cells in the ascitic fluid when the ascites is due to disseminated malignant disease, but malignant cells are not always found and the failure to find malignant cells does not exclude malignancy as the cause of the ascites.

Pathogenesis

Hepatic ascites is caused by several different factors, which each contribute to the accumulation of fluid in the peritoneal cavity (Fig. 17.175). In cirrhotic patients the single most important factor contributing to the formation of ascites is portal hypertension. Cirrhotics also have a tendency to sodium and water retention because of their functional renal impairment (see below): they have impaired albumin synthesis in the liver, leading to a low serum albumin level; and they have an increased production of hepatic lymph secondary to portal hypertension, some of which passes from the surface of the liver into the peritoneal cavity. In a cirrhotic patient who does not have portal hypertension, such as a patient who has had a porto-caval shunt operation, ascites tends to be absent and the excess fluid retained becomes gravitational, with oedema of the feet and legs, or the sacrum and abdominal wall in those patients who are confined to bed.

Salt and water retention

The retention of sodium in cirrhosis is associated with high levels of aldosterone in both urine and blood in some of the patients who have ascites, although not in all of these patients. These high levels of aldosterone are not found in cirrhotics without ascites. Altered rates of both the secretion and clearance of aldosterone occur in cirrhotics with ascites. Although aldosterone is metabolized only in the liver, and although the rate of clearance is reduced in cirrhotics, the level of the plasma aldosterone is much more dependent on the rate of secretion. This correlates closely with the plasma renin activity and the plasma concentration of angiotensin II. The increased aldosterone level is mainly secondary to increased activity of the renin–angiotensin system.

The glomerular filtration rate can be normal in patients with sodium retention, and this is therefore considered to be due to increased tubular reabsorption of sodium. Aldosterone acts on the distal convoluted tubules and the collecting tubules. However, increased sodium reabsorption from the proximal tubule may be the more important mechanism, as little sodium would reach the distal tubule. Variation in the circulation influences proximal tubular reabsorption of sodium; increased circulating blood volume decreases sodium reabsorption, and decreased circulating blood volume increases sodium reabsorption. This

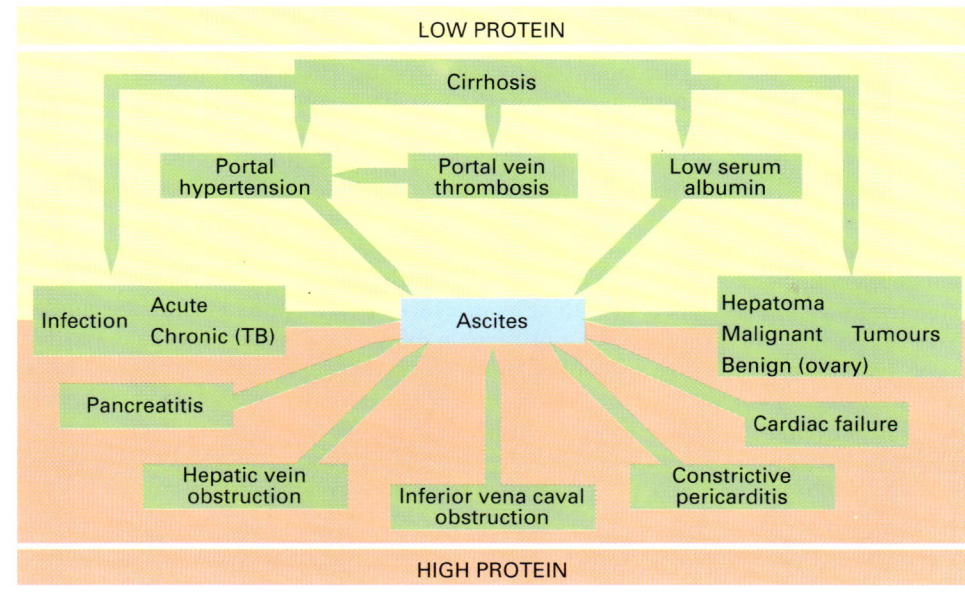

Fig. 17.175 Pathogenesis of ascites.

may be a direct effect or mediated by humoral natriuretic factors. Renal sympathetic nervous activity also increases proximal tubular sodium reabsorption, and plasma norepinephrine levels are increased in cirrhotic patients. This may explain the increased sodium retention that occurs in cirrhotic patients after they have bled from varicies.

Cirrhotics are frequently unable to excrete a water load. This is proportional to a reduction in the glomerular filtration rate and to the proximal sodium reabsorption. They also have an increase in the plasma antidiuretic hormone (ADH) in spite of a reduced plasma osmolality, and this increased level of ADH is not suppressed in cirrhotics by a water load. This is probably because of failure of inhibition of vasopressin by prostaglandin E_2, which is synthesized in the epithelium of the collecting tubules, with a correspondingly low urinary excretion of prostaglandin E_2 in cirrhotics with ascites, as the high plasma ADH level probably inhibits the synthesis of prostaglandin E_2. Non-steroidal, anti-inflammatory drugs inhibit prostaglandin synthesis and enhance the antidiuretic effect of antidiuretic hormone, thus reducing the ability of a cirrhotic patient with ascites to excrete a water load.

The mechanism stimulating the rise in aldosterone and ADH is complex. The sodium retention precedes ascites formation and these patients have an increased circulating blood volume. However, they have a decreased peripheral resistance and a low arterial pressure, which indicates an 'effective' hypovolaemia related to splanchnic vasodilatation thought to be due to portal hypertension.

17.16.5   Hepato-renal failure

Patients with liver disease often have a low blood urea. This is secondary both to a low intake of protein due to anorexia and dietary restriction; and, in advanced liver disease, to the failure of hepatocyte metabolism and the resulting deficiency of urea synthesis. In many cirrhotics (65 per cent), the blood urea rises in the terminal phase of the illness. This may be precipitated by diuretic therapy, by infection, or by haemorrhage, especially massive bleeding into the gastrointestinal tract. It also rises in fulminating hepatic failure (55 per cent). In both groups the renal blood flow is severely reduced, and functional renal failure and acute tubular necrosis occur with equal frequency, and carry a high mortality.

The functional renal failure of cirrhotics and patients with acute liver failure is characterized by sodium retention and the inability to excrete a water load. Thus, although the total body sodium is high, the serum sodium level is often reduced and the serum osmolarity is low. Urinary sodium excretion is very low in cirrhotic patients with ascites (often between 3 and 10 mEq/l urine). These patients tend to be oliguric, with an elevated blood urea. This may rise steeply with a rapidly fatal outcome in patients with severe hepatic impairment, or may plateau and remain elevated but constant for months. There are no structural abnormalities in these patients' kidneys, which have been shown to function normally when transplanted into a patient with renal failure but normal liver function. The functional

renal failure also improved following a successful liver transplant. It is improved by expanding the circulating blood volume, by albumin infusions, or following the insertion of a peritoneo-venous shunt. This indicates that it is brought about by changes in the renal circulation secondary to liver failure. It can be induced by non-steroidal, anti-inflammatory drugs that act by inhibiting renal prostaglandin synthesis. This renal impairment normally reverts rapidly on stopping the drug.

Renal failure in cirrhotics may be due to other causes, of which the most common is acute tubular necrosis following massive variceal haemorrhage. This also gives a low urinary sodium, but can be distinguished by the very high urinary β_2 microglobulin in the presence of severe renal tubular damage; this protein is normally almost completely reabsorbed by the proximal tubules.

17.16.6   Encephalopathy

Diagnosis

The most dramatic presentation of hepatic encephalopathy is a comatose patient. In grade 4 coma a patient is unrousable by any stimulus. The conscious level may have deteriorated rapidly over hours or even minutes and may improve equally rapidly if appropriate therapeutic measures are taken. Less extreme degrees of encephalopathy result in a confused, drowsy, or stuporose patient with poor co-ordination and a flapping tremor of the outstretched hand (asterixis). The speech of these patients is slurred, and they may perseverate. They have a characteristic, rather sweet, fetor. Such patients are often thought to be sleeping rather more than normal during the day and have an inverted sleep pattern with wakefulness at night. There may be intellectual impairment often in patients who appear superficially to be fully conscious. This may show on simple arithmetic testing. Disturbances of spatial perception and an associated constructional apraxia result in changes in handwriting and an inability to perform simple tasks, such as copying spirals and five-pointed stars. In chronic liver disease personality changes may occur. This often results in immature patterns of behaviour, with a previously pleasant patient becoming truculent and noncompliant. These patients may also have a facile and rather euphoric attitude to their illness and their other responsibilities. Extreme examples of chronic neurological and psychiatric syndromes have been reported.

The diagnosis of hepatic encephalopathy is made by finding mental changes involving impairment of consciousness in a patient with other evidence of liver failure. Finding the characteristic fetor or flapping tremor may suggest the diagnosis, but the former is not always present, and the latter also occurs in patients with chronic carbon dioxide retention and in uraemia. The electroencephalogram (EEG) is useful in confirming the diagnosis, and shows a slowing from the normal alpha rhythm to a delta rhythm of below four cycles/s. However, it also is not specific as this pattern is found in other metabolic conditions, such as uraemia.

Other investigations are unhelpful. The cerebrospinal fluid

(CSF) is under normal pressure and has a normal cell count (unless there is a secondary infection and meningitis has occurred). The CSF protein level may be raised. Blood ammonia levels are raised in many patients with hepatic encephalopathy, but the raised levels correlate poorly with the clinical state and the EEG changes. They do not give any guide to prognosis and add little to the clinical assessment of the patient. They are therefore of limited value and rarely performed.

Pathogenesis

The development of encephalopathy is related to cerebral oedema, to structural abnormalities in the brain, and to changes in the composition of the cerebrospinal fluid. Substances that can cross the blood–brain barrier from the plasma increase as the result of the elevated plasma levels of normal and abnormal metabolites, secondary both to hepatocyte failure and to shunting of the portal venous blood away from the liver to the systemic circulation.

The commonest finding in the brain of a patient dying with hepatic encephalopathy is of cerebral oedema. This may be part of the generalized tendency to retain salt and water, but it has also been linked with positive-pressure ventilation, as it occurs in most of the patients who die with fulminating liver failure having been treated in an intensive care unit. The other structural changes involve the astrocytes, which become enlarged. These changes occur within a few days and are reversible in the early stages, but in patients with long-standing chronic encephalopathy they become irreversible and the patients' clinical condition does not respond to treatment. However, the clinical state in most patients is so variable that structural changes are less important than metabolic ones.

Many metabolic changes have been demonstrated in patients with hepatic encephalopathy, although the mechanism for these may not be understood. The alteration of the concentration in the blood of many compounds can alter the conscious level of a patient in liver failure. The simplest of these, and one of clinical importance, is the infusion of potassium into a hypokalaemic encephalopathic patient. An equally rapid clinical improvement occurs when bicarbonate solution is infused into a comatosed patient with acute liver failure.

Ammonia has been investigated in patients with hepatic failure. Ammonia toxicity alters cerebral metabolism, increasing glutamine synthesis and interfering with the reductive amination of ketoglutarate. Ammonia also depresses cerebral blood flow. Both these are compatible with the findings in hepatic coma, but there is no clear correlation between blood and brain ammonia levels and the conscious level in hepatic encephalopathy. This may be because the blood–brain barrier is more permeable to ammonia if an alkalosis is present. This may explain the observation that encephalopathy worsens after a brisk diuresis which precipitates a hypokalaemic alkalosis.

If ammonia toxicity is implicated in hepatic coma, it is only one of several factors. For example, methionine precipitates hepatic coma without changes in blood ammonia levels. The fetor of hepatic coma is related to mercaptans which are derived from methionine.

Serum levels of aromatic amino acids (tyrosine, phenylalanine, and tryptophan) are increased in liver disease, due to reduced hepatic deamination. The ratio between the level of these and of the branched-chain amino acids (valine, leucine, and isoleucine), which are decreased, has been related to the development of hepatic coma. The relative concentration in the brain of these precursor amino acids controls neurotransmitter synthesis, but this ratio appears to be reduced in cirrhosis whether or not encephalopathy is present. However, attempts have been made to treat hepatic encephalopathy with infusions and oral feeding of branched-chain amino acids.

Changes in neuroreceptors in the brain have been shown in experimentally induced hepatic failure. The inhibitory neurotransmitter, γ-aminobutyric acid (GABA), has been shown to be raised in the serum of patients with hepatic encephalopathy. It is a product of the action of gut bacteria on protein in the bowel. The increased serum levels of GABA are the result of impaired hepatic metabolism and shunting of portal venous blood. GABA only crosses the blood–brain barrier if it is defective. In experimental hepatic coma increased numbers of GABA-binding sites have been demonstrated on post-synaptic neuromembranes. There are also increased numbers of binding sites for drugs such as barbiturates and benzodiazepines. This may explain the observation that patients with liver disease are sensitive to the sedative effect of these drugs.

17.16.7 Other complications of liver failure

Infection

Secondary bacterial infections are extremely common in both fulminating liver failure and patients with chronic liver disease. These may be respiratory, urinary, or related to intravenous infusion sites. Cirrhotics also develop infection of their ascites without any precipitating factor (so-called 'spontaneous bacterial peritonitis').

The infection may present with fever or other classical symptoms related to the site, such as cough or dysuria. However, it is often merely a general deterioration in the patient's condition, especially an increase in jaundice or encephalopathy, which brings the problem to attention. For this reason bacterial cultures of blood, urine, ascites, and, where possible, sputum should be taken from any patient with either acute or chronic liver failure in whom there is any unexplained clinical deterioration. Infections may be with Gram-negative or Gram-positive organisms, and they may be opportunistic infections with organisms not normally the cause of pathogenic infections. In addition to the clinical deterioration and fever, the presence of infection may also be suggested by the finding of a raised neutrophil leucocyte count.

Tuberculosis has a increased incidence in patients with chronic liver failure, both in the peritoneum and other sites.

The increased incidence of infections is due to impairment of phagocytic activity of the reticuloendothelial system and to alteration in neutrophil activity. The former may be due to shunting of the portal venous blood which bypasses the Kupffer cells lining the hepatic sinusoids and prevents them from filtering out any bacteria present in the portal blood. There is a decrease in Kupffer cell function but not cell number. Neutrophil function is also altered with reduced adherence. Deficiencies of complement, of serum opsonization, and of chemotaxis have also been demonstrated and may contribute to the increased susceptibility to infection in patients with liver failure.

Hypoglycaemia

Clinically significant hypoglycaemia occurs in acute fulminating liver failure and in cirrhotics whose liver function is deteriorating rapidly. If untreated, it may be the cause of death, especially in children with Reye syndrome. In alcoholics after a bout of very heavy drinking hypogycaemia can cause death with massive fatty infiltration of the hepatocytes. The low blood glucose, if suspected, can be confirmed rapidly by dextrostix, and corrected by an intravenous injection of 50 per cent dextrose, and the blood glucose maintained by an infusion of 10 per cent or 20 per cent dextrose until liver function improves.

The low blood glucose is the result of failure of hepatic gluconeogenesis and of high insulin levels. These are both the result of hepatic necrosis and of shunting of portal venous blood. This prevents insulin from being metabolized by liver cells and it prevents glucagon from exerting its normal regulatory effect on hepatic metabolism.

17.16.8   Jaundice

Jaundice is due to the accumulation of bilirubin in tissues as the result of either an increase in its production or an abnormality in its excretion.

Bilirubin is produced in reticuloendothelial cells as the end-product of haemoglobin and myoglobin catabolism. Unconjugated bilirubin is transported in the plasma bound to albumin. It is conjugated in the hepatocyte microsomes to bilirubin monoglucuronide and then to the diglucuronide before excretion into the bile canaliculus. This is an active process against a concentration gradient and the conjugated bilirubin then passes into the bile and thus to the duodenum. The bilirubin diglucuronide is water-soluble and, if the level in the plasma rises, it is filtered by the renal glomerulus and is present in the urine. Bilirubin diglucuronide is not absorbed from the small intestine and passes into the colon where it is hydrolysed by bacterial β-glucuronidase and reduced to urobilinogens. This is minimally absorbed from the colon and it is then re-excreted by the liver forming an enterohepatic circulation. In liver disease, if the level of urobilinógen rises in the blood, it passes in increased amounts into the urine.

Pathogenesis

The simple mechanistic classification of jaundice is into prehepatic, hepatic, and posthepatic causes (Fig. 17.176), but the

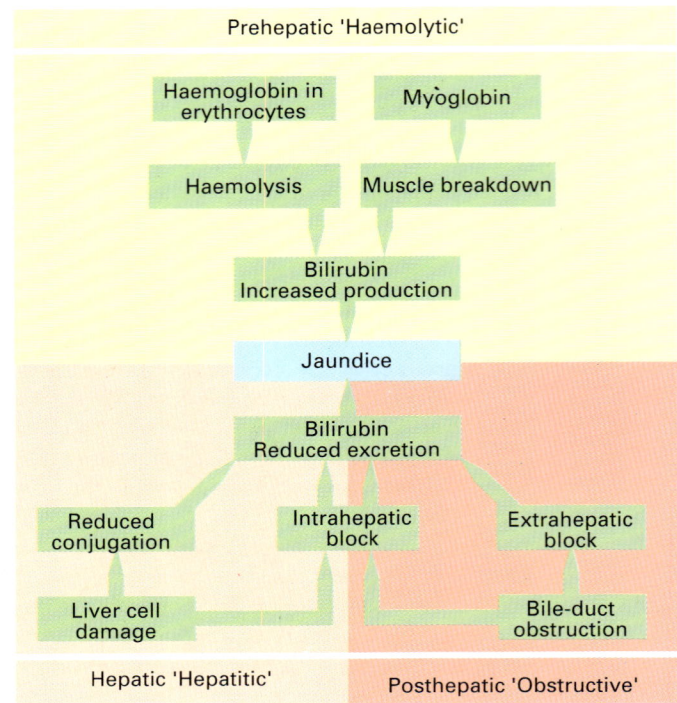

Fig. 17.176   Mechanisms of jaundice.

situation is usually more complex, as the elevation of the serum bilirubin and the resulting jaundice may be due to a problem at one of more than six different stages: an increased rate of production of bilirubin from increased red cell destruction; a failure of uptake or conjugation of bilirubin in hepatic microsomes; a failure of excretion of bilirubin by the liver cells; or from an obstruction to the flow of bile in the bile canaliculus or in the intrahepatic or extrahepatic bile ducts. These mechanisms may be grouped into the classification given above but in an individual patient there is often more than one cause and the distinction then becomes difficult.

Prehepatic jaundice

This occurs with haemolysis which may be due to a haematological disorder (Chapter 23) or to destruction of erythrocytes in the tissues as occurs after a pulmonary embolus. It is associated with a high unconjugated bilirubin, and the absence of bilirubin in the urine (acholuric jaundice), although, predictably levels of urobilinogen in urine may be increased; the liver has a large reserve for conjugation of bilirubin, with a consequent increase in gut urobilinogen. Other tests of liver function are little disturbed, although the AST may be a little above the normal range and the LDH shows a greater increase. A similar biochemical picture is found in defects of bilirubin conjugation, such as Gilbert syndrome; this is a common benign condition which is often discovered as a chance finding of an elevated bilirubin at routine screening or during the investigation of unrelated pathology. It is due to a defect in membrane uptake and/or conjugation of bilirubin. It is not associated with any liver disease and does not have any mortality or morbidity. Crigler–Najjar syndrome, a rare congenital defect of bilirubin conjugation (Section 17.9) also produces unconjugated hyperbilirubinaemia. The latter and, more commonly, haemolytic disease in the new-born, lead to kernicterus (Chapter 25).

Hepatic jaundice

In hepatic failure, this is due to the failure of liver cells to metabolize and excrete bilirubin. In the early stages of acute liver failure the bilirubin is little raised but as the days pass it increases by an increment each day which reflects the severity of the liver damage. Both the unconjugated and the conjugated bilirubin are raised in the serum. In these patients the serum AST is very high and the prothrombin time is prolonged if the liver damage is severe. Bilirubin and increased urobilinogen are present in the urine.

In chronic liver disease the bilirubin is often little raised, and clinical jaundice may be slight or absent. However, if the rate of destruction of hepatocytes increases, for example in alcoholics who increase their alcohol consumption, or patients with chronic active hepatitis who reduce their steroid therapy, the serum bilirubin level increases with a parallel increase in the jaundice. In any one of these patients there are often prehepatic, hepatic, and posthepatic causes of the jaundice. The serum unconjugated and conjugated bilirubin rise, and the AST and alkaline phosphatase may both be raised, but the low serum albumin is the clue to the chronicity of the liver damage.

Sometimes in both acute and chronic liver disease there is marked distortion of the normal hepatic architecture and this adds intrahepatic obstruction to the excretion of bile. This causes an obstructive jaundice with an increase in the serum alkaline phosphatase, and the clinical features of an obstructive jaundice: pale stools due to an absence of bile pigments in the stool, and itching of the skin which is associated with an increase in bile acid levels. The urine may be dark due to bile pigments, and urobilinogen is normally found in the urine as the obstruction is rarely complete in chronic liver disease and some bile does reach the colon.

This intrahepatic cholestasis also occurs in patients with viral hepatitis after the initial phase of hepatic necrosis. In these patients, the rise in the serum alkaline phosphatase together with a rising bilirubin occurs when the AST has fallen from the initial very high level. If the serum enzyme levels are measured for the first time at this point, the obstructive pattern of liver function tests may lead to confusion in the diagnosis and the jaundice may be erroneously attributed to an extrahepatic pathology. At times the absence of urobilinogen in the urine may add to this confusion, but the absence is rarely complete for long, and the return of urobilinogen is a predictor of early recovery.

Sometimes in liver disease, erythrocyte survival is reduced and the increased rate of haemolysis contributes to the bilirubin load and the level of jaundice. This also happens when a patient receives a blood transfusion, as the transfused erythrocytes have a shortened survival time in the circulation. In these patients the raised serum bilirubin is present together with a slight elevation of the AST, but the LDH will also be raised and examination of the blood film may show evidence of haemolysis. As the raised bilirubin is predominantly unconjugated and is transported in the blood bound to albumin, it is not filtered by the glomerulus and is not found in the urine. However, when haemolysis complicates liver failure, the jaundice is multifactorial, and some bilirubin can be detected in the urine.

Dubin–Johnson syndrome, Rotor syndrome, and other disorders (see Section 17.9) are rare causes of (predominantly) conjugated hyperbilirubinaemia.

Extrahepatic jaundice

This form of jaundice is due to obstruction of the bile ducts outside the liver. It is important to differentiate this from other types of jaundice as its management requires the removal or bypass of the mechanical obstruction. Common causes of extrahepatic jaundice include gallstones, strictures of the bile duct, which are frequently malignant, and pathology (especially carcinoma) of the head of the pancreas. Extrahepatic jaundice has the clinical features of obstructive jaundice: pale stools, dark urine, and itching (see above). The bilirubin elevation is predominantly conjugated (probably due to reabsorption from biliary channels in the liver), the alkaline phosphatase level is usually raised, but may not be if the obstruction is intermittent and due to gallstones.

Other abnormalities of liver function are present only if the obstruction has been present for a long time and secondary liver damage has occurred. When this happens the AST may rise; the prothrombin time becomes prolonged but corrects with intravenous vitamin K, at least until severe chronic damage with secondary biliary cirrhosis has occurred. If the problem continues untreated, the serum albumin falls. This is associated with dilated bile ducts proximal to the level of the obstruction. The urine contains bilirubin, but urobilinogen may be absent from the urine if the obstruction is complete and no bilirubin is reaching the colon.

As the treatment requires either endoscopic intervention or laparotomy, the precise localization of the site of the obstruction is necessary and can be obtained by scanning with ultrasound or CAT, or by visualizing the bile ducts using percutaneous or endoscopic retrograde cholangiographic techniques. The endoscopic techniques can also be used to remove a gallstone or pass a stent through a stricture in the bile duct.

Investigation of the jaundiced patient

The assessment of a jaundiced patient must start with a careful history. Although much will be learnt by further investigation, clues to the aetiology will be missed if attention is not paid to the points listed in Table 17.15.

The history is particularly important in hepatic jaundice, which may be due to toxic agents such as drugs in which case further prescription and damage will only be prevented by discovering the cause. Not every patient with liver disease presents with a symptom such as jaundice which directs attention to the

Table 17.15 Hepatic and biliary disease, historical data

Jaundice	Occupation, current and past
Itching	Alcohol, consumption (pattern and
	duration)
Pain	social consequences
Fever, rigors	financial problems
Nausea, anorexia	legal problems
Pale stools, dark urine	Drugs (prescribed and illicit)
Abdominal swelling, ascites	Travel overseas
Oedema	Transfusion (blood and blood
	products)
Haematemesis, melena	Contact history
Drowiness, confusion, coma	Family history

Table 17.16 Signs suggestive of liver disease

Jaundice	Abdominal tenderness
Fever	Ascites
Spider naevi	Oedema
Palmar erythema	Bruises
Dupuytren's contractures	Tremor ('flap'/asterixis)
Xanthomata	Fetor
Hepatomegaly/splenomegaly	Confusion (drowsiness/coma)

liver. In these patients the examination may discover physical signs suggestive of liver disease (Table 17.16).

The history and physical examination influence further investigations. These may be performed on a blood sample or may be more invasive with increased risks to the patient (Table 17.17). Which investigations are performed on any patient will be decided in the knowledge of the history, examination, and the investigations already available. The aim is to discover enough to diagnose and treat the patient with a minimum of risk to the patient.

Table 17.17 Investigation of hepatic and biliary disease

Primary	Secondary
Essential blood tests	Scans
liver function tests	ultrasound
prothrombin time/clotting	CAT
factors	Isotope
full blood count	NMR
Other blood tests	Liver biopsy
virology (HBsAg, HAAb,	blind
HCAg, etc.)	guided
immunology	Endoscopy
(immunoglobulins, auto-	upper gastrointestinal tract
antibodies)	Cholangiography
alcohol	ECRP
serum iron/iron-binding	percutaneous
capacity/ferritin	Angiography
ceruloplasmin/copper	mesenteric
α-1-antitrypsin	portal venography
α-fetoprotein	
Urine	
bilirubin	
urobilinogen	
Stools	
bile pigments	
blood	

17.16.9 Further reading

Arroyo, V., Rimola, A., and Rodes, J. (1986). Pathogenesis and treatment of ascites. In *Recent advances in hepatology*, 2 (ed. H. C. Thomas and A. E. Jones). Churchill Livingstone, Edinburgh.

Berk, P. D., *et al.* (1986). Update on bilirubin metabolism. In *Recent advances in hepatotogy*, 2 (ed. H. C. Thomas and A. E. Jones). Churchill Livingstone, Edinburgh.

Gimson, A. E. S. and Williams, R. (1983). Acute hepatic failure: aetiological factors, pathogenic mechanisms and treatment. In *Recent advances in hepatology*, 1 (ed. H. C. Thomas and R. N. M. MacSween). Churchill Livingstone, Edinburgh.

Sherlock, S. (1989). *Diseases of the liver and biliary system* (8th edn). Blackwell Scientific Publications, Oxford.

18

The exocrine pancreas

J. Rode

18

The exocrine pancreas

J. Rode

18.1 Introduction

The pancreas is a relatively inaccessible retroperitoneal organ and as such impossible to palpate clinically. Both its exocrine and endocrine components possess a large reserve capacity. Disease processes involving the gland may therefore go unnoticed for a long period until in an advanced stage, or become obvious only when involving adjacent structures as the stomach, duodenum, or common bile duct.

The organ was already known to the ancient Greek anatomists of the Alexandrian School of medicine as long ago as the third century BC, *pan* meaning 'all' and *creas* 'flesh', which pertains to its solid parenchymatous nature. Its gross anatomy, however, was not studied until the late Renaissance and knowledge about its physiology started to emerge only at the beginning of modern times. The lack of an English term for the human organ may reflect its long obscure function and symptomatology when diseased.

Surgery was rarely performed on the pancreas until the introduction of Whipple's two-stage operation in 1935. Previously, the investigator of pancreatic histology and pathology had to rely on animal models or cadaverous material. Examination of pancreatic autopsy tissue is highly unsatisfactory because of autolysis commencing soon after demise. It follows that the study of human pancreatic diseases is just beginning to gain impetus with the introduction of safer interventive procedures and sophistication of non-invasive imaging techniques.

It is the custom to regard the pancreas as two entirely separate organs, an exocrine and an endocrine gland fortuitously put together in one anatomical site. Its disease processes are taught and dealt with by different groups of specialists. However, both components develop from the same embryological structures and an intimate functional relationship between the two compartments becomes increasingly apparent.

18.2 Normal structure and function

18.2.1 Embryology

The human pancreas develops from a ventral and a dorsal embryological bud of the primitive duodenum. The bilobed ventral bud rotates clockwise around the gut until it comes to lie next to the larger part derived from the dorsal bud (Fig. 18.1). The two elements normally fuse during the 7th week of fetal life, forming a single organ. In the mature pancreas the larger part of the head, uncinate process, the neck, body, and tail are derived from the embryological dorsal element while a smaller

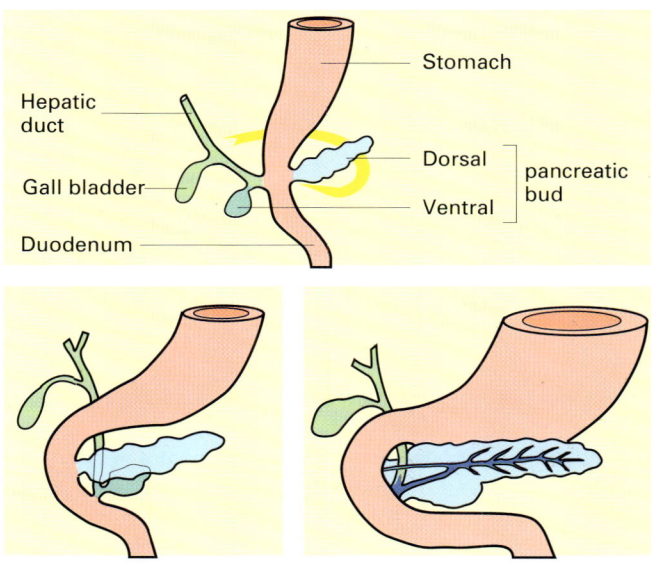

Fig. 18.1 Development of the human pancreas. (Drawn after Cubilla and Fitzgerald 1984 and Klöppel and Heitz 1984, with permission.)

portion of the posterior head derives from the ventral bud. In most instances, the two main ducts of these primordia fuse forming a duct system which drains the organ via the major ampulla (ampulla of Vater) alone or via both the major and minor ampullae.

After fusion of the ventral and dorsal *anlagen* during the 7th week, the pancreas is formed by an increasing number of endo-dermally derived branching epithelial tubules which terminate in solid cords and cell clumps. Intervening mesodermal cells differentiate into fibroblasts and form the primitive pancreatic stroma. The solid side-branches give rise to islet cells and then acini. Between weeks 8 and 16 the pancreas organizes into lobes and lobules and the vascular network increases around the acini. By the end of the 5th month the acinar cells resemble those of the adult pancreas.

18.2.2   Gross anatomy

Gross appearance and dimensions

The gland is divided into a head, neck, body, and tail part, although there is no anatomical division between these regions. A groove on the posterior surface accommodates the terminal part of the superior mesenteric vein and the beginning of the portal vein. This part of the pancreas is regarded as its neck, joining the head and body. A hook-shaped process (uncinate process) projects from the lower part of the head upwards behind the superior mesenteric vessels and the gland neck.

In the new-born the pancreas weighs 2–3 g. Its weight increases to 7 g by the end of the first year and reaches approximately 40 g by the age of 15. In the adult the weight ranges from 70 to 150 g and its length from 15 to 25 cm.

The pancreas has a firm rubbery consistency and is distinctly lobulated. Depending on its functional state, it is slightly pink or yellowish-white. It is surrounded by a thin condensation of retroperitoneal connective tissue forming a pseudocapsule. The anterior surface of the head and body possess a serous periton-eal covering whereas the posterior surface is in direct contact with adjacent anatomical structures, allowing direct spread of pathological processes involving the gland.

Position

The pancreas lies transverse within the posterior deep abdom-inal cavity across the upper lumbar vertebrae. The head is tucked into the loop of the duodenum and together with the body lies behind the lesser sac of the peritoneum. The tail turns forwards into the lienorenal ligament and reaches the hilus of the spleen.

The pancreas is in intimate contact with important organs and vital blood vessels. Stomach, duodenum, transverse colon, spleen, kidneys, and suprarenal glands are viscera in close rela-tionship to the gland. It lies close to blood vessels such as the aorta, vena cava, hepatic artery, portal vein, and splenic ves-sels. The head embraces the coeliac trunk and superior mesen-teric artery and vein. The lower 3–5 cm of the common bile duct runs in a groove in the posterior surface of the head.

The topographical relationships of the pancreas have impor-tant clinical implications. Inflammatory processes and sequelae of trauma are liable to involve the lesser sac. Any of these struc-tures may be invaded by cancers of the pancreas and the prominence of the lumbar spine renders the organ vulnerable to abdominal contusion injuries. Furthermore, the deep location and close relation to blood vessels impede surgical access.

Duct system

The main pancreatic duct in the mature gland (Wirsung's duct) is formed by the duct of the original ventral pancreas and the distal portion of the embryological dorsal duct. It is made up in the tail by the convergence of a number of small duct radicles. In the body region the main duct receives tributaries from the lobules that join it in more-or-less right angles, giving it the typical herring-bone pattern seen on pancreatograms, whereas in the head the arrangement of the tributaries is more irregular.

Wirsung's duct and the common bile duct form the ampulla of Vater prior to their drainage into the duodenum. The angle of their confluence and the length of the common channel is vari-able. The relationship of the two ducts in the ampulla has been found to be of considerable clinical significance, especially in regards to bile reflux into the pancreatic duct system when blockage occurs in this region. In a number of cases the two ducts remain separate and open independently but adjacent to each other on the tip of the major papilla.

The accessory duct (Santorini's duct) derives from the prox-imal remnant of the embryological dorsal duct and drains the anterior portion of the head and the uncinate process. It is pres-ent in 99 per cent of subjects and opens into the duodenum at the minor papilla, which is situated 1–3.5 cm rostral and slightly anterior to the major papilla. Rarely, the duct ends blindly in the minor papilla. In 5–10 per cent of cases the ac-cessory duct replaces Wirsung's duct as the main route of drain-age. There are a number of variations from the main ductal patterns (Fig. 18.2). It is conceivable that disturbances during embryogenesis and, especially, anomalies of the draining duct system may lead to pathological processes later in life, affecting only parenchymal sectors derived from either primordium.

Both major and accessory ampullae are invested with true sphincter muscles. Although the sphincter of the major ampulla (sphincter of Oddi) has been described in detail, little is found in the literature pertaining to the muscle surrounding the access-ory ampulla.

Blood supply and lymphatics

Commensurate with its role as an endocrine and exocrine se-cretory gland, the pancreas is endowed with a rich blood sup-ply. This is basically derived from branches of the coeliac trunk above the neck of the pancreas and the superior mesenteric artery below the neck. Arterial arcades are formed between the major supply arteries, and there are numerous anastomoses within the substance of the pancreas. The location of the prin-cipal arteries in relation to the pancreas is remarkably constant

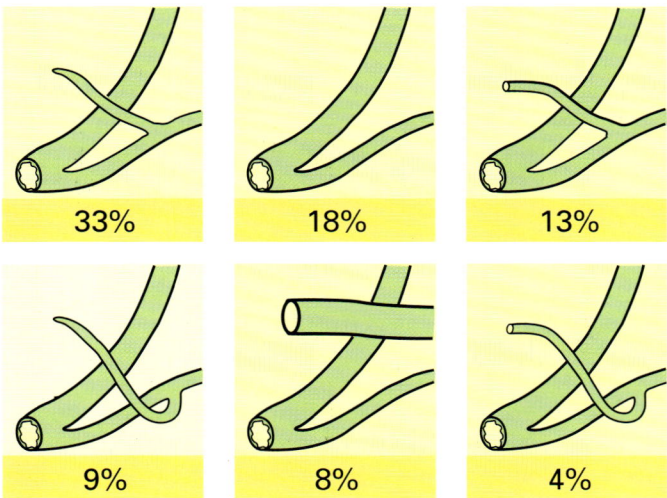

Fig. 18.2 Pancreatic and common bile duct drainage patterns in the human pancreas. (Drawn after Stolte, M. (1984). *Chronischepankreatitis*. Erlangen: Perimed-fachbuch-Verlagsgesellschaft, with permission.)

but there is a great variability in the origin and course of their branches.

Within the pancreas the arterial branches form an interlobular plexus in the connective tissue of the interlobular septa. From these plexus single intralobular arteries pass into each lobule where they form glomerula-like tufts supplying individual islets of Langerhans and then continue to adjacent acini. Thus a portal type of system is formed where the exocrine pancreas receives blood rich in islet-cell hormones.

The veins of the pancreas correspond in general to the arterial pattern. The blood drainage is collected into the portal venous system behind the neck of the gland where the portal vein is formed.

The pancreas possesses an extensive lymphatic drainage. The deep lymphatic plexus originate from a periacinar and perilobular capillary network and pass to the surface accompanying the blood vessels in the connective tissue septa. Lymph nodes usually lie adjacent to the gland in association with major supply arteries. A primary chain of nodes stretches along the splenic artery serving to drain the bulk of the head and tail. Other primary nodes are grouped anterior and posterior in the sulcus between the head of the organ and the duodenum.

Nerves

Both exocrine and endocrine pancreatic function is regulated by complex humoral and nervous influences. The rich innervation of the organ is via autonomous sympathetic and parasympathetic fibres, forming three different plexus around acini, blood vessels, and islets. Intrapancreatic ganglia within the interlobar connective tissue appear to play a central role in integrating cholinergic, adrenergic, and peptidergic nerve impulses.

Parasympathetic innervation is by the vagus nerves, which reach the pancreas via the coeliac plexus. The vagus fibres provide part of the secretory stimulus both for the endocrine and exocrine compartments, and regulate the capillary blood flow. Only a small proportion of the vagal nerve fibres are efferent. At least 90 per cent of fibres are afferent and are involved in the duodenal pancreatic reflex.

The sympathetic innervation of the organ reaches it via the greater splanchnic nerves and coeliac ganglia. The majority of fibres pass along the major arteries to the pancreas and supply the pancreatic vasculature. Stimulation of the splanchnic nerves results in vasoconstriction and in ischaemia of the exocrine and endocrine parenchyma. Pain-mediating fibres in the pancreas appear to accompany sympathetic fibres. Little is known about the stimuli for pancreatic pain, and alleviation of these debilitating symptoms associated with some pancreatic diseases poses a major challenge in modern medicine.

18.2.3 Histology

The secretory units of the exocrine pancreas are numerous small glands, the acini, which are aggregated into lobules, which in turn form lobes. The lobules are separated by delicate connective tissue septa and are macroscopically recognizable. The well-developed interlobar connective tissue contains ducts, nerve fibres, ganglion cells, lymphatics, and blood vessels.

The pancreatic enzymes are synthesized in the acinar cells. These are truncated, pyramidal cells grouped around a small central lumen. The enzymes are stored in the form of acidophilic zymogen granules within the luminal basophil cytoplasm. The granules are released into ductules, solubilized and diluted by pancreatic juice, and discharged as pancreatic secretion into the duodenum.

Conventionally, the pancreatic architecture is conceived to resemble a bunch of grapes in which the acini (Latin, 'grapes') form terminal spheroidal buds on intercalated ductules derived from the progressive division of the main duct (Fig. 18.3). However, recent reconstruction studies of serial sections and scanning electron microscopy after silicon rubber injection into the duct system have altered this view. Acini may be spheroidal, tubular, or irregular in outline. They may not necessarily terminate the glandular system but intercalated ductules can be

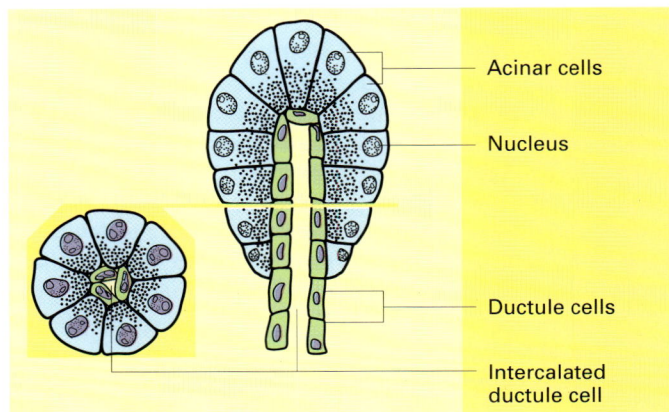

Fig. 18.3 Conventional concept of the exocrine pancreatic acinus as a terminal structure. (Drawn after Cubilla and Fitzgerald 1984, with permission.)

formed on the other side of acini and these may thus form swellings in an anastomosing and looping ductal system (Fig. 18.4).

Morphological changes that take place during a wide range of pancreatic diseases, such as in cystic fibrosis, chronic pancreatitis, and adenocarcinoma, are now understandable through these findings.

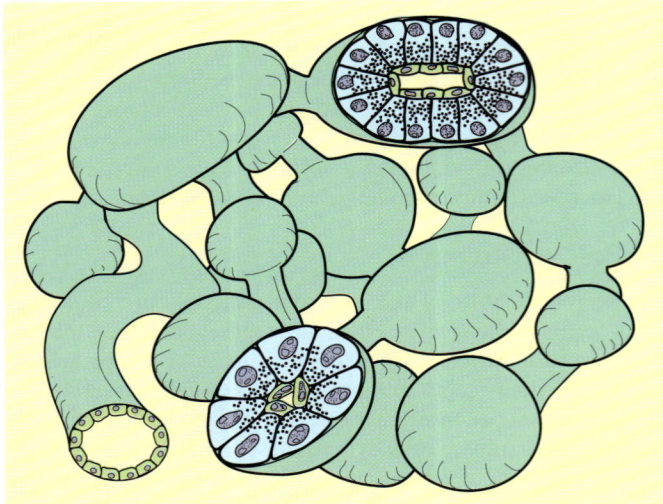

Fig. 18.4 Three-dimensional conceptualization of exocrine pancreatic architecture. There is continuity of the lumina through ductules and acini by the formation of loops and anastomoses. (Drawn after Akao *et al.* 1986, with permission.)

18.2.4 Physiology

The secretion of the exocrine pancreas, the pancreatic juice, consists of enzymes and water together with electrolytes. There are at least 22 digestive enzymes: proteolytic enzymes, including elastase; several amylases; lipolytic enzymes, including phospholipase; and nucleolytic enzymes. The function of the secretion ranges from breakdown of food and decrease of the duodenal content acidity to maintenance of cellular growth of the small intestinal mucosa. The two components are secreted independently. The water and electrolytes originate from the cells of the duct system. The enzymes are contributed by the acinar cells. All enzymes are produced as inactive precursors and are activated in the duodenum on contact with its content.

The secretory activity is well adjusted to the volume and constituents of the intestinal content. Its regulation is complex and involves an intricate interplay between humoral mediators and neurogenic reflexes. The process, initiated by a cephalic phase, such as smell, sight, or chewing of food, is continued by a gastric phase and an intestinal phase, the entrance of acid gastric content and foodstuff into the duodenum where two duodenal hormones, secretin and cholecystokinin, are released into the bloodstream. These are the most potent mediators of pancreatic secretion and increase the flow of pancreatic juice and its enzyme content. Fat and alcohol, particularly, stimulate secretion and may play a role in the aetiology of some pancreatic

disorders by initiating secretion exceeding the capacity of the draining duct system.

Hormal influences probably play the most important role in exocrine pancreatic regulation. However, there is evidence that vagal stimulation leads to secretion of enzyme-rich pancreatic juice and local cholinergic enteropancreatic reflexes mediate pancreatic enzyme secretion. Structural evidence for neural control mechanisms is provided by the occurrence of cholinergic axon terminals in close association with many of the acinar cells.

Besides excitatory regulation of the external pancreatic secretion, evidence of the existence of neurohormonal inhibitory factors is emerging. These may play a significant role in the balance exerted on the gland through hormones and the autonomous nervous system. At present, knowledge of physiological inhibitor substances is still fragmentary, but somatostatin and pancreatic polypeptide (PP) are possible candidates.

There is a close functional relationship between the exocrine and endocrine pancreas. The exocrine compartment receives its blood supply after it has passed through the islets. Insulin and glucagon influence enzyme synthesis and release by the acinar cells. Insulin potentiates amylase secretion whereas glucagon exerts an inhibitory effect on the secretory response of the exocrine gland. Insulin has been shown to have a trophic effect on the gland, and glucagon has been shown to induce atrophy.

18.2.5 Further reading

Adda, G., Hannoun, L., and Loygue, J. (1983). Development of the human pancreas: variations and pathology. A tentative classification. *Anatomica Clinica* **5**, 275–83.

Akao, S., Bockman, D. E., de la Porte, P. L., and Sarles, H. (1986). Three-dimensional pattern of ductuloacinar associations in normal and pathological human pancreas. *Gastroenterology* **90**, 661–8.

Baldwin, W. M. (1911). The pancreatic ducts in man, together with a study of the microscopical structure of the minor duodenal papilla. *Anatomical Record* **5**, 197–227.

Cubilla, A. and Fitzgerald, P. J. (1984). Tumors of the exocrine pancreas. In *Atlas of tumour pathology*, Armed Forces Institute of Pathology, Second Series, Fascicle 19. Washington, DC.

Go, V. L. W., Gardner, J. D., Brooks, F. P., Lebenthal, E., DiMagno, E. P., and Scheele, G. A. (eds) (1986). *The exocrine pancreas: biology, pathobiology and disease*. Raven Press, New York.

Henderson, J. R., Daniel, P. M., and Fraser, P. A. (1981). The pancreas as a single organ: the influence of the endocrine upon the exocrine part of the gland. *Gut* **22**, 158–67.

Klöppel, G. and Heitz, P. U. (eds) (1984). *Pancreatic pathology*. Churchill Livingstone, Edinburgh.

18.3 Congenital anomalies

18.3.1 Aplasia and hypoplasia

Total congenital absence of the pancreas (aplasia or agenesis) is very rare and frequently associated with other severe malformations. If compatible with life, the leading clinical symptoms are steatorrhoea and diabetes mellitus. More often aplasia of the ventral or dorsal pancreas has been described, with hypoplasia of the gland as consequence. Aplasia of the dorsal anlage is the more common anomaly.

18.3.2 Annular pancreas

In annular pancreas a ring of pancreatic tissue encircles the descending duodenum (Fig. 18.5) or, rarely, the junction of the first and second parts of the duodenum. The annulus derives from the ventral primordium of the gland, as demonstrated by its islets rich in pancreatic polypeptide. Its prevalence is not clear but it has been calculated to occur in 1 in 20 000 individuals. Males are affected predominantly. Annual pancreas may be associated with other congenital abnormalities, especially with trisomy 21. Its presentation tends to be bimodal, with approximately equal peaks in neonatal life and in the fourth and fifth decade. Neonatal presentation is usually with congenital duodenal obstruction. The most common adult symptom is upper abdominal pain due to chronic inflammation affecting the annulus.

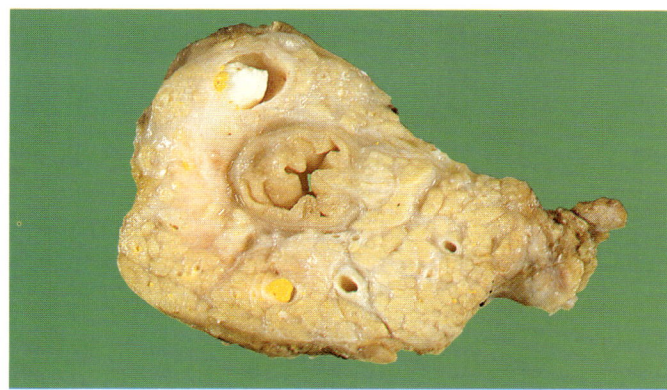

Fig. 18.5 Annular pancreas. This is a horizontal section through a Whipple's operation specimen from a 28-year-old male patient who suffered periodic epigastric pain for 10 years. The annulus is fibrosed as a result of chronic pancreatitis, a stone is seen impacted in the markedly dilated duct of the ring. (The yellow material filling some of the ducts is post-operatively injected radio-opaque resin.)

18.3.3 Anomalies of the duct system

At times congenital abnormalities of the pancreatic duct system can become of clinical importance. Isolated atresia or congenital obstructions of the main pancreatic duct at the duodenum are rare lesions and are generally associated with other malformations of the pancreatico-biliary system. The major pancreatic duct may drain into the common bile duct, producing a long common channel that predisposes to reflux into the biliary or pancreatic system. An abnormally high orifice of the major pancreatic duct in the duodenum may be accidentally ligated during surgery in this region, resulting in serious complications.

Fusion of the two embryological duct systems may not occur. In this condition the ducts of Wirsung and Santorini persist as totally separate structures (pancreas divisum) and the major part of the gland is drained via the accessory papilla. The incidence of pancreas divisum is between 5 and 10 per cent in Western society. Recently, it has been reported that chronic pancreatitis and pain is more prevalent in individuals bearing this anomaly. Pancreas divisum pancreatitis has been shown to be a segmental disease involving almost exclusively the dorsal derived gland (Fig. 18.6). This suggests inadequate drainage of Santorini's duct at its outlet at the accessory papilla in patients suffering from this form of pancreatitis.

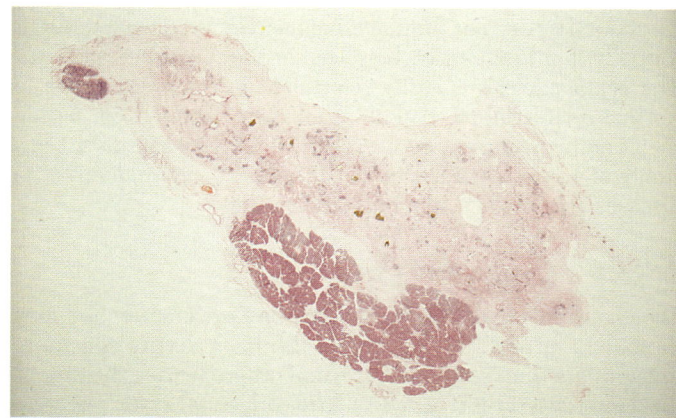

Fig. 18.6 Pancreas divisum pancreatitis. This whole-mounted H & E stained section through the pancreatic head of a Whipple's operation specimen from a young woman with pancreas divisum shows severe segmental pancreatitis with fibrosis and complete loss of exocrine parenchyma involving the dorsally derived pancreas. The part derived from the ventral gland is completely unaffected.

18.3.4 Heterotopia of pancreatic tissue

An aberrant or ectopic pancreas consists of pancreatic tissue outside its usual location and without contact with the normal pancreas. Its composition can vary in the amount of its exocrine, endocrine, ductular, and smooth muscle constituents. It possesses its own duct system and a separate blood supply. Ectopic pancreas results from heteroplastic differentiation of parts of the embryonic endoderm that normally do not produce pancreas, or from aberrant extension of otherwise normal pancreas into adjacent structures. Heterotopic pancreas is found in about 2 per cent of all autopsies. Infants with trisomy 18 are often affected. The most frequent sites are the stomach, duodenum, jejunum, ileum, Meckel's diverticulum, and other intestinal diverticula. Rarer reported localizations are the gall-bladder, liver, mesentery, spleen, and omentum. Pancreatic tissue has also been documented in benign mediastinal teratomas.

The heterotopic pancreas is usually a firm, yellow-white nodule with a granular or ulcerated surface. It can measure from a few millimetres to several centimetres in diameter. The most common site within the intestinal tract is the submucosa, followed by the muscle layer, and less frequently the subserosa.

At times it has been confused at surgery with tumours of a more sinister nature.

Ectopic pancreatic tissue is rarely symptomatic. It can cause pyloric obstruction, ulceration, haemorrhage, and intestinal invagination or pain when inflamed. Within the ampulla of Vater it may give rise to obstructive pancreatitis, obstructive jaundice, cyst formation, or suspicion of cancer when seen by modern imaging techniques. Carcinoma and islet-cell tumours are said to be more common in the aberrant pancreas.

18.3.5 Heterotopia of spleen within the pancreas

In about 10 per cent of individuals accessory splenic tissue is found within the hilus of the spleen or the tail of the pancreas. The ectopic spleen is easily recognized by its resemblance to normal splenic tissue. Usually it measures about 1 cm in diameter and possesses its own capsule. Accessory spleens are virtually of no clinical importance, although they are involved in disease processes affecting the main organ.

18.3.6 Congenital cysts

True congenital cysts of the pancreas are uncommon and may be solitary or multiple. Solitary congenital cysts are difficult to differentiate from retention cysts and originate from dysgenetic focal duct strictures (Fig. 18.7). The congenital cystic pancreas is most commonly associated with polycystic disease of the kidneys and liver, or with malformations of the central nervous system (von Hippel–Lindau disease).

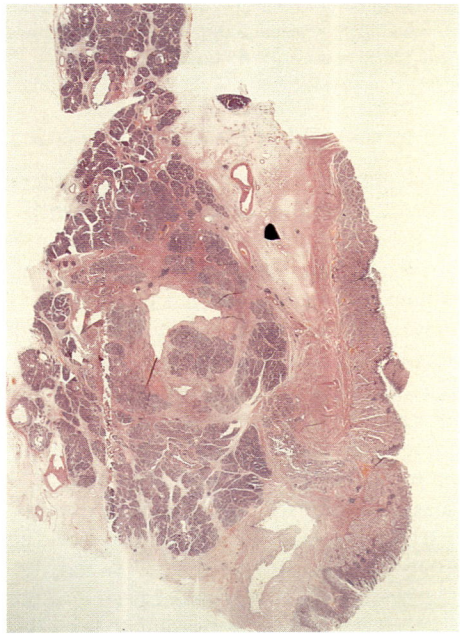

Fig. 18.7 A true congenital cyst within the head of the pancreas in a whole-mounted, H & E stained section of a Whipple's specimen removed from a 25-year-old male for pancreatic pain. Also seen is a duodenal wall cyst below the major papilla.

18.4 Regressive changes and atrophy

18.4.1 Lipomatosis

Lipomatosis of the pancreas is a condition in which the parenchyma is dispersed by adipocytes (Fig. 18.8). In its severest form the gland is greatly increased in size by fat tissue and there is a deceptive impression of an actual parenchymal loss. The cause of lipomatosis of the pancreas is not known. It is associated with age and obesity. Interstitial pancreatic adipocytes normally increase in number in adult life, when they are found confined to the embryologically dorsal gland element. This may point to an endocrine component in the pathogenesis of lipomatosis, since this part of the gland is the main site within the pancreas of insulin production. Lipomatosis is a common finding in adult-type diabetes mellitus which is often associated with obesity.

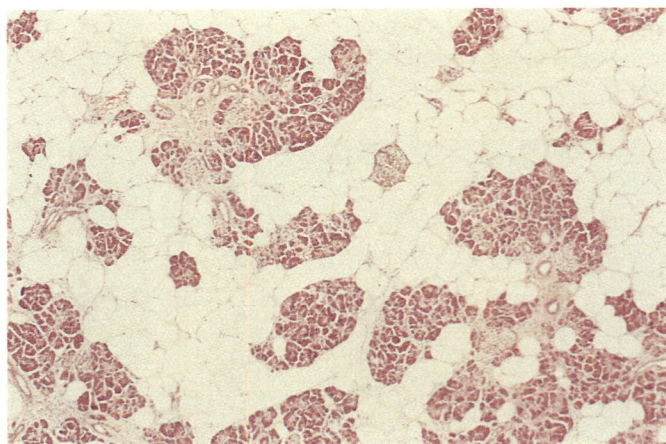

Fig. 18.8 Lipomatosis of the pancreas. This section is from the enlarged pancreas of a diabetic patient. The parenchyma is widely separated by adipose tissue.

18.4.2 Lipomatous atrophy

True loss of pancreatic parenchyma is seen in 'lipomatous atrophy', which is also termed 'lipomatous pseudohypertrophy' of the pancreas because of the massive fatty infiltration of the gland. It is a rare condition, occurring in infants, and is characterized by pancreatic insufficiency, bone marrow dysfunction, and skeletal abnormalities (Shwachman syndrome).

18.5 The pancreas in systemic diseases

18.5.1 Cystic fibrosis

Cystic fibrosis is the most common inherited disease of Caucasian people in North America and Central Europe. Early descriptions of the condition in the first three decades of this century only focused attention on clinicopathological disturbances involving the pancreas until its systemic nature was recognized.

The pathological findings in the pancreas depend on the age of the patient and the severity of the disease. At birth there is usually no gross abnormality of the gland, except for a firmer consistency. Progressive fibrosis accentuates this firmness thereafter. In patients with long-standing disease the pancreas is small, hard, and nodular, or at times lipomatous, which needs differentiation from lipomatous atrophy. Only occasionally is there stenosis or obstruction of a large duct. In general, the obstruction involves smaller ductules leading to the formation of small, turbid, white, fluid-filled cysts.

The microscopic features are most marked in patients who have survived longest. In premature babies and infants who have died of meconium ileus no recognizable abnormalities may be detected. The histological changes result from the accumulation and inspissation of a concentrated, viscous secretion within acini and ductules, leading to their progressive cystic distension. The cysts are lined by flattened, cuboidal epithelium and contain eosinophilic calcium-rich mucus. Other acini atrophy severely and, as compensation, the intra- and interlobular fibrous connective tissue increases, and this may be associated with replacement by fatty tissue. There is often a mild chronic inflammatory cell infiltrate. The islets are usually normal in number but are irregularly scattered throughout the altered parenchyma, similar to the pattern seen in chronic pancreatitis. Islet tissue may also proliferate in a way akin to nesidioblastosis.

The pathogenesis of the morphological changes in the pancreas show similarities to chronic obstructive pancreatitis as, for instance, seen in carcinoma of the head of the pancreas or in the model of pancreatic duct ligation. In these conditions pancreatic enzymes are not involved in the destruction of acinar parenchyma and inflammation is, in general, only mild.

18.5.2   Haemochromatosis

In primary haemochromatosis the pancreas may be slightly larger than normal and is of a deep brown colour with a rusty tint. The colour is due to the non-iron pigment haematoidin, and haemosiderin. The cell overload with haemosiderin causes cell damage followed by progressive atrophy of the exocrine parenchyma and increasing fibrosis of the organ. The degree of atrophy and fibrosis may be extensive but exocrine pancreatic insufficiency is rarely observed.

Histologically the iron is mainly deposited within the cytoplasm of the acinar and duct cells, but also to a lesser degree within endocrine cells and cells of the interstitial tissue. Within the endocrine cells haemosiderin accumulates exclusively within β-cells but usually the islets appear structurally preserved. This points against β-cell loss as the mechanism primarily responsible for the diabetes, the so-called bronze diabetes, affecting over half of the cases.

18.5.3   Malnutrition

The pancreatic changes associated with protein-caloric malnutrition tend to be found in tropical regions (kwashiorkor) but are occasionally also encountered in affluent countries. The basic pathology affects the exocrine pancreas, which progressively atrophies and is eventually replaced by fibrous tissue without signs of inflammation. In severe cases the pancreatic lesions may be irreversible.

18.6   Inflammations

18.6.1   Introduction

Although the effects of inflammations of the pancreas have been known for more than 100 years, there was little information as to the pathological changes involving the gland itself. The pathologist distinguished between acute and chronic pancreatitis and recognized an overlap of the two. However, histopathological material from cases of acute pancreatitis is rarely available and the morphological descriptions of the condition are largely based on tissue derived at autopsy or unsatisfactory surgical material. Tissue diagnosis of chronic pancreatitis was also rare in the past and comprehensive post-mortem descriptions of the disease were not published until the mid-1940s. It is not surprising that pancreatitis was pathologically ill-defined. Clinical definitions and diagnosis of these disorders were a matter of confusion and controversy for a long time. Recent attempts have therefore been made to come to a consensus in order to avoid misunderstandings, and to create a common basis on which to accumulate data.

18.6.2   Classification

The first attempt at an internationally uniform classification dates to 1963. It is referred to as the Marseille classification after the venue of the meeting of pancreatologists when it was proposed. The classification was based purely on clinical findings. Twenty years' experience with this classification showed some of its deficiencies and led to the revised Marseille classification of 1984.

In the new Marseille classification the need to include histological morphological criteria is recognized. Pancreatitis in its acute and chronic form is defined. Acute pancreatitis may take a mild or severe clinical course. Chronic pancreatitis is subdivided on a morphological basis into:

1. chronic pancreatitis with focal necrosis;

2. with segmental or diffuse fibrosis; and

3. pancreatitis with or without calculi.

A special form is separated from these three on a patho-aetiological basis,

4. obstructive pancreatitis.

This last condition differs from the previous in that the changes seen within the pancreas are potentially reversible or improve when the cause of the obstruction is removed, whereas the changes in the first group are progressive and irreversible.

Aetiological factors are not considered in the Marseille classification and verification and determination of the inflammatory process by histological means, though desirable, constitute a potentially hazardous procedure for the patient. A classification similar to the Marseille classification but stipulating the inclusion of aetiological factors whenever this is possible was proposed during a workshop held in Cambridge in 1983. Pancreatitis is defined by clinical, biochemical, and imaging criteria, and reference to histological verification is omitted. In this classification recognition of a separate entity is proposed. This special form of chronic pancreatitis is thought to be more prevalent in patients bearing the congenital abnormality of an unfused duct system, so-called, pancreas divisum pancreatitis.

Ideally, a classification of pancreatitis with the aim to promote our knowledge of the disease should include aetiology, histology, clinical data as to severity and number of attacks, outcome of treatment, results of exocrine and endocrine function tests, and morphological data obtained by radiological and other imaging techniques.

18.6.3   Acute pancreatitis

Definition

Acute pancreatitis is characterized clinically by acute onset of abdominal pain accompanied by increased pancreatic enzymes in blood or urine or both. It may present as a single episode or recur. In its mild form there is peripancreatic fat necrosis and interstitial oedema, but pancreatic necrosis is absent. In its severe form there is extensive necrosis within and around the pancreas and haemorrhage, often leading to shock and death. Only rarely does acute pancreatitis lead to chronic pancreatitis.

Epidemiology and aetiology

The incidence of acute pancreatitis amongst hospital admissions has been estimated at about 1 per cent. In the general population its incidence is 5–11 per 100 000. Acute pancreatitis may be encountered at any age, but is rare in children. It usually affects adults between the ages of 30 and 70 years, with a mean age of about 55 years. Men and women appear to be equally affected but there is a wide range reported between the male to female ratios, which most likely reflects local variations in the involved causative factors.

Because the pathogenesis of acute pancreatitis is still poorly understood, evidence of a causal relationship between assumed aetiological factors and acute pancreatitis is mainly epidemiological. It is therefore preferable to refer to these as associations rather than causes. The factors most commonly associated with acute pancreatitis are biliary tract diseases, such as gallstones or inflammation of the gall-bladder or bile ducts, and alcoholism. Together these are found in 80–90 per cent of cases. The remaining patients have the disease either in the absence of any other known associated process (idiopathic) or in association with various known or suspected single factors or combinations of factors, such as infections (e.g. mumps, coxsackie virus, and viral hepatitis), trauma, toxic substances including drugs (e.g. diuretics, methyldopa), acquired and inherited metabolic abnormalities (e.g. uraemia and hyperlipidaemia types I and V), endocrine (e.g. hyperparathyroidism) and nutritional factors, vascular disorders (e.g. ischaemia, shock), and congenital or acquired ductal abnormalities. Unexplained hereditary influences and abnormal immune responses may also play some part.

There are considerable geographical variations in the distribution of the associated factors. In countries with a high prevalence of alcoholism, biliary tract disease becomes a less important denominator. Alcoholism continues to be listed as one of the main causes of acute pancreatitis, although it must be assumed that an acute attack in chronic alcoholics is often only the first manifestation of chronic pancreatitis. In many instances an alcoholic patient who experiences his first episode of pancreatitis may have acute pancreatitis clinically, but presumably already has chronic pancreatitis histologically. Idiopathic acute pancreatitis constitutes the third largest group affected. With more thorough investigations and identification of apparent associated factors the number in this group is on the decline.

Pathogenesis and pathophysiology

The pathogenesis of acute pancreatitis remains a confused subject despite extensive investigations and numerous proposed theories. The pancreas synthesizes a variety of digestive enzymes, such as proteases and phospholipases, that are capable of tissue damage. There is evidence that in some forms of acute pancreatitis the underlying process is autodigestion affecting the adipose and interstitial tissues as well as the pancreatic parenchyma.

Normally, the enzymes are present in the pancreas only in the form of inactive proenzymes, or zymogens. Activation occurs in the duodenum, where the brush-border enterokinase catalyses the conversion of trypsinogen to trypsin, while trypsin, in turn, activates other zymogens. If acute pancreatitis is indeed an autodigestive disease, the question is unsolved at what level activation of the enzymes occurs, and the mechanisms preceding these events are largely unsolved.

Current thinking favours an intracytoplasmic activation within acinar cells, resulting from a variety of aetiological factors producing cell injury. However, if the disease is the result of intraparenchymal zymogen activation, it might be expected that in the majority of patients acute pancreatitis would progress to the more severe form, since it is unclear by what mechanisms this process might be turned off once initiated. This is clearly not the case, and these unsolved questions are of extreme importance and have obvious therapeutic implications.

Recent experimental studies have shown that bile, alcohol, or drugs may reduce the ductal barrier and allow diffusion of ductal content without zymogen activation. Similarly, ductal rupture as a result of duct hypertension following duct obstruction may lead to extravasation of pancreatic juice into the parenchyma of the gland. Leakage and diffusion of the fluid give rise to interstitial oedema with an inflammatory response and scattered focal areas of fat necrosis but without parenchymal necrosis.

It is therefore reasonable to suspect that there may be two separate forms of acute pancreatitis, although in clinical practice it is almost impossible to distinguish these conditions. Morphologically the distinction is usually clear. Occasionally, however, the features may be mixed. The majority of patients suffer from a mild form affecting mainly the interstitial tissue and soon get well. The induced pancreatic changes invariably regress. A small minority of patients are affected by a severe form, with tissue necrosis and haemorrhage, and die or develop inflammatory masses. Only occasionally will the interstitial form of pancreatitis progress to the haemorrhagic form.

Morphology

In the acute interstitial (oedematous) form of pancreatitis the gland is firm, swollen, and scattered foci of fat necrosis may be seen. On histology, there is patchy oedema of the interstitium. Some acini are dilated, the acinar cells are flattened and their zymogen granule content is reduced. Small amounts of inspissated secretions are evident in the acinar and small ductal lumina. If fat necrosis is present, it usually involves the interstitial adipose tissue.

In the severe, haemorrhagic form of acute pancreatitis the gland shows areas of grey-white necrotic softening, areas of blue-black haemorrhage, and yellow-white foci of chalky fat necrosis. The extent of haemorrhage is variable. In the severest cases the pancreas is converted into a mass of blood clot. The peripancreatic fatty tissue, as well as any of the fat deposits within the abdominal cavity, may also be involved by fat necrosis. In rare cases areas of fat necrosis are found within the subcutaneous adipose tissue and the bone marrow. In the process of fat necrosis neutral fats stored within adipocytes are broken down, glycerol is reabsorbed, and the fatty acids combine with calcium salts of the extracellular fluids to form calcium soaps (saponification).

A zone of acute inflammatory cells is present around the foci of pancreatic necrosis but this is, in general, less marked than the amount of tissue damage would suggest. After a few days secondary infection may supervene and areas of suppuration and abscess formation now dominate the picture. If the patient survives, reparative fibrosis occurs. Liquefied areas are walled off and pseudocysts of varying size result.

18.6.4   Chronic pancreatitis

Definition

Chronic pancreatitis is a persistent, usually progressive, inflammatory condition characterized by irregular sclerosis of the gland with destruction and loss of exocrine parenchyma. Clinically, it is associated with recurrent or persistent abdominal pain but may also be present without pain. The exocrine and endocrine pancreatic functions may be impaired. The morphological changes in the pancreas can be focal, segmental, or diffuse, and are irreversible.

Epidemiology and aetiology

Chronic pancreatitis is less frequent than acute pancreatitis. Its incidence in different countries varies considerably. It is reported to be on the increase in industrialized nations, possibly in parallel with the increasing consumption of alcohol. In England its incidence accounts for approximately 3 cases per year per population of 100 000. Males are, in general, more prone to develop chronic pancreatitis. The average age of onset in Western society is 40 years. Chronic pancreatitis is more prevalent in tropical countries where protein malnutrition in infancy is endemic. In these countries the disease is usually encountered in individuals of less than 20 years of age and the male to female ratio is equal.

In one distinct form of chronic pancreatitis characteristic calcifications develop in the duct system (chronic calcifying pancreatitis). This is the main form of pancreatitis encountered in tropical countries, whereas in temperate areas of the world alcohol consumption is considered its main cause. Chronic alcoholism accounts for 60–85 per cent of the Euro-American type of chronic pancreatitis, its incidence varying from country to country. A large variety of other aetiologies have been implicated for the remainder. These are either metabolic or manifestations of systemic diseases.

There is a large proportion of patients with chronic pancreatitis where no aetiological factor is apparent. Consequently, this 'idiopathic' form constitutes the second largest group, with an incidence reported between 9 and 41 per cent.

The Marseille classification drew attention to chronic obstructive pancreatitis. The importance of this condition is twofold. It is the only form of chronic pancreatitis that may improve following definitive surgery to relieve the obstruction. A wide range of lesions can lead to major duct obstruction, including congenital and acquired duct abnormalities, duodenal or periampullary cysts, and ectopic pancreas, intraductal papillomata, and pancreatic or Vaterian carcinomas, and neuroendocrine tumours. Especially in the latter cases cure may be achieved if resection is performed at an early stage.

Pathogenesis and pathophysiology

Only a few people indulging in excessive alcohol intake develop chronic pancreatitis. This variable susceptibility in chronic alcoholics suggests additional individual host factors so far unknown. The primary event appears to be alcohol-induced hypersecretion rich in enzymes and calcium. The juice precipitates as protein plugs within the duct system, leading to obstruction and calculus formation. It has been suggested recently that reduced secretion of 'stone protein' that normally holds calcium in solution is the primary cause of the calcification.

The resulting ductal obstruction is thought to induce secondary changes in those acini where drainage is impeded. The acinar cells lose their zymogen granules and height. Eventually they assume a ductal epithelial appearance and form 'tubular complexes', followed by an intense fibrotic reaction. Some corresponding morphological features encountered in the non-alcoholic forms of pancreatitis suggest that similar pathogenetical mechanisms play a role. The histological hallmark in alcohol-related chronic pancreatitis is a patchy and focal distribution of the lesions, in contrast to an even distribution seen in obstructive pancreatitis upstream from the obstructive cause in the ampullary or major duct regions. There is some evidence of participation of auto-immune mechanisms in at least some patients suffering from idiopathic chronic pancreatitis.

Continuous or intermittent severe and often debilitating abdominal pain is one of the cardinal symptoms in patients suffering from chronic pancreatitis. Effective medical measures for pain relief may involve potentially addictive drugs. The mechanisms playing a role in the production of this pain are entirely unclear.

Malabsorption with steatorrhoea and development of diabetes mellitus are regular features in the late stage of chronic pancreatitis. Steatorrhoea is usually a sign of severe pancreatic deficiency and occurs when pancreatic lipase output has been reduced in excess of 90 per cent. Endocrine pancreatic insufficiency develops in up to 70 per cent of patients with chronic pancreatitis, despite preservation of the endocrine gland component in this process. Satisfying explanations of the processes involved in pancreatic diabetes are still lacking. Insulin, but also glucagon, secretion may be impaired.

Extrahepatic biliary tract obstruction with jaundice develops in 5–10 per cent of patients with chronic pancreatitis. The distal common bile duct traverses the head of the pancreas before joining the main pancreatic duct. Fibrosis of the head of the gland, or compression of the choledochus by a pseudocyst or abscess following an acute exacerbation of pancreatitis, may be the cause of the obstructive jaundice seen in some of the patients.

Morphology

In the early stage of the disease the pancreas may appear grossly normal but later the organ can become enlarged and hard due to ensuing fibrosis and ductal dilatation. Unless the disease is far advanced the increase in size is diffuse or segmental. With progressive severity the gland eventually shrinks. The surface becomes smooth and grey-white. When exocrine parenchyma is still preserved the gland will show a variegated tan and white cut surface, which later becomes uniformly white as a consequence of complete fibrous replacement.

The main duct and its side branches are frequently irregularly dilated and contain clear juice or proteinaceous floccular material. In cases of the calcifying form of pancreatitis, the inspissated calculi may vary in size from millimetres to several centimetres. Often the diseased pancreas contains cysts. These are either retention cysts or pseudocysts. Retention cysts develop from obstructed ducts into which secretion continues to drain. These cysts are initially lined by ductal-type epithelium but when they increase in size they may lose their lining and become surrounded by chronically inflamed connective tissue. In this case they are difficult to distinguish from necrotic pseudocysts which result from attacks of necrotizing pancreatitis.

Microscopically, there is irregular loss of acini and an apparent increase of ductules, which are separated by fibrous tissue. The ductules are at times lined by atypical epithelium which is difficult to distinguish from carcinoma. With progressive fibrosis the ductules disappear. In some cases fibrosis involves predominantly the perilobular space widely separating the lobules (Fig. 18.9).

Embedded within the fibrous tissue are the preserved endocrine cell islets, which may even increase in size and number. Occasionally neoformation of islet cells can be observed when islet cells appear to sprout out of preserved ductules, events reminiscent of those taking place during embryogenesis (Fig. 18.10). The pancreatic nerves have been shown to increase in size and are focally surrounded by aggregates of chronic inflammatory cells (Fig. 18.11).

Focally, the irregularly ectatic ducts are inspissated by hyaline proteinaceous material. The ductal epithelia often flatten or become metaplastic and hyperplastic with mucinous and squamous differentiation. Hyperplastic, neutral mucus-producing glands are seen to surround the major ducts in many cases. In obstructive pancreatitis the ductal wall may be formed by loose, concentrically arranged laminated fibrous connective tissue.

Pancreas divisum pancreatitis is a special form of segmental pancreatitis. It occurs in some but not all individuals who possess a congenital unfused duct system. The disease involves diffusely and exclusively the embryological dorsal derived portion of the gland (see Fig. 18.6). A likely cause of this condition is a relative obstruction of Santorini's duct in the region of the accessory papilla.

Recently, a further variant of segmental pancreatitis has been identified. In this form the part of the head of pancreas that lies

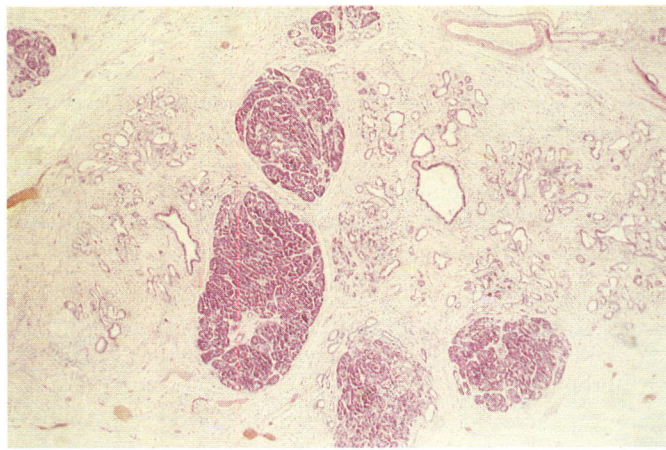

Fig. 18.9 Chronic pancreatitis. Some unaffected parenchymal lobules are widely separated by marked fibrosis. The lobular ducts are dilated.

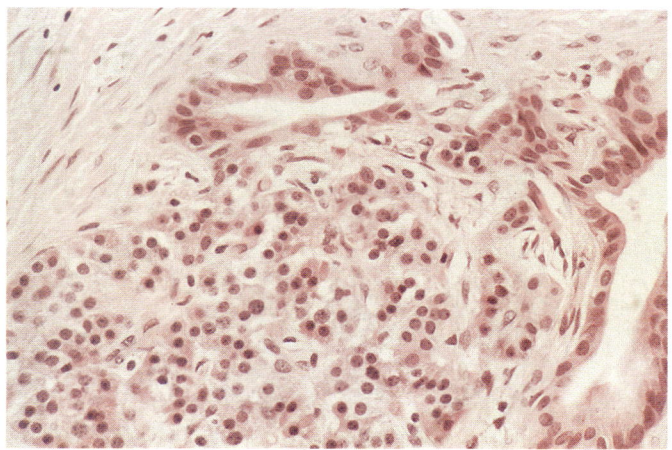

Fig. 18.10 Chronic pancreatitis. In this field there is apparent neo-formation of islet-cell tissue from surviving ductules.

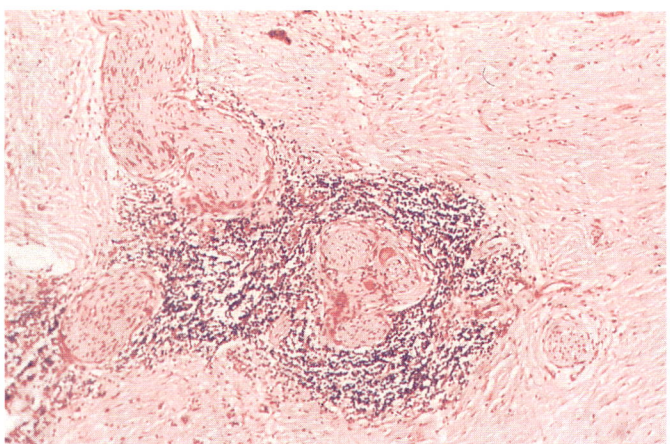

Fig. 18.11 Chronic pancreatitis. Nerves within the fibrous tissue are prominent and surrounded by chronic inflammatory cells.

in the 'groove' between the duodenum and common bile duct is affected. 'Groove pancreatitis' is said to occur in approximately one-quarter of all surgically duodenopancreatectomy specimens resected for chronic pancreatitis. Very commonly duodenal wall cysts or cysts within the pancreatic head are found in this condition, suggesting a possible aetiological association. Preceding diseases of the biliary system, peptic ulcers, or gastric resections are other, often associated factors. This form of pancreatitis may present with duodenal stenosis, and a 'tumour' within the proximal pancreatic head is detected radiologically. This may lead potentially to an erroneous diagnosis of cancer.

18.6.5 Further reading

Cotton, P. B. (1985). Pancreas divisum—curiosity or culprit? *Gastro-enterology* **89**, 1431–5.

Foulis, A. K. (1984). Acute pancreatitis. In *Recent advances in histo-pathology,* No. 12 (ed. P. P. Anthony and R. N. M. MacSween), pp. 188–96. Churchill Livingstone, Edinburgh.

Frey, C. F. (1986). Classification of pancreatitis. *Pancreas* **1**, 62–8.

Sarles, H. (1985). Chronic calcifying pancreatitis. *Scandinavian Journal of Gastroenterology* **20**, 651–9.

Yatto, R. P. and Siegel, J. H. (1984). the role of pancreatobiliary duct anatomy in the etiology of alcoholic pancreatitis. *Journal of Clinical Gastroenterology* **6**, 419–23.

18.7 Non-endocrine tumours

18.7.1 Introduction

In its strictest application the Latin term 'tumour' simply refers to a swelling of tissue, which may be reactive, inflammatory, or neoplastic in nature. The following section deals with tumours in the sense of 'neoplasms' or 'new-growths', and the two terms will be used interchangeably. The non-neoplastic tumours of the pancreas are dealt with elsewhere in this chapter. In this connection, non-neoplastic tumours are important in so far as they have to be included in the differential diagnosis of neoplasms and require different treatment.

Classically, we distinguish between benign and malignant neoplasms. The majority of benign neoplasms of the pancreas are islet-cell tumours. Epithelial adenomas of the pancreas are rare. Even rarer are benign connective tissue neoplasms. Metastatic carcinomas involve the gland more frequently than primary neoplasms. Malignant epithelial tumours, in particular adenocarcinomas, account for more than 90 per cent of the primary pancreatic non-endocrine tumours. There have been only sporadic reports of sarcomas and lymphomas arising in the pancreas as the primary site. Adenocarcinomas of the pancreas possess an abysmal prognosis. This may be the prime reason why several classifications of pancreatic neoplasms have received little attention so far, because there is widespread doubt as to the clinical and biological significance of distinguishing different subgroups. However, with progress in diagnostic techniques and treatment of these neoplasms several entities with a more optimistic outlook have emerged.

18.7.2 Classification

Histological typing and subtyping of primary exocrine pancreatic tumours represent an attempt, in addition to staging and grading, to form a basis for therapy selection and prognostic assessment. Use of these methods also aims to further our knowledge of the natural history of these diseases. The majority of tumour classifications are based on microscopic appearances. Correlation of morphology to structures and cells normally occurring at the same site should not imply a relationship through histogenesis. Most current classifications emphasize the histogenetical approach and there is much argument as to the cell of origin. Many studies assume that epithelial tumours of the pancreas derive differentially from ductal or ductular cells and acinar cells. Unequivocal transition of such cells to *in situ* or invasive carcinoma has so far not been demonstrated. Furthermore, there is a group of neoplasms where the appearances of the composite cells defeat such speculations. It should be borne in mind that all epithelial elements of the pancreas, including its endocrine component, are derived from endodermal stem cells. It is therefore not surprising that epithelial tumours of the gland can show differentiation of varying grades and directions, and neoplasms of mixed composition occur.

A simplified classification of benign and malignant tumours of the exocrine pancreas is given in Table 18.1.

Table 18.1   Classification of primary neoplasms of the exocrine pancreas

Benign neoplasms	Malignant neoplasms

Adenoma
   Papillary adenoma
	Adenocarcinoma
	   Histological variants
	      Ductal type adenocarcinoma
	      Acinar cell type carcinoma
	      Adeno-squamous carcinoma
	      Giant cell type carcinoma
	      Mixed cell type carcinoma

	Squamous cell carcinoma Small cell anaplastic carcinoma

Cystadenoma
   Serous (microcystic)
      cystadenoma
	Cystadenocarcinoma
	   Mucinous cystadenocarcinoma

	Solid and cystic tumour
	Pancreatoblastoma Osteoclast-type tumour
Benign connective tissue tumours	Sarcoma Lymphoma

18.7.3   Hypertrophy, hyperplasia, metaplasia, dysplasia, and pancreatic neoplasia

Since most neoplasms of the exocrine pancreas are adenocarcinomas, changes that may be associated or precede these tumours are of great interest. Most frequent epithelial alterations involve the ducts, ductules, and acini. Commonly seen are mucous-cell hypertrophy, goblet-cell metaplasia, proliferations of glands, and epithelial papillary and pseudopapillary hyperplasias. Under mucous-cell hypertrophy an enlargement of ductal epithelial cells with accumulations of considerable amounts of supranuclear mucus is understood which usually occurs within wider-calibre ducts. Glandular proliferations are commonly seen surrounding larger ducts and are reminiscent of the neutral mucin-producing glands within the gastric pyloric region. Metaplastic conversion of epithelial cells to goblet cells is mainly encountered in ductules (Fig. 18.12) and acini, whereas papillary and pseudopapillary hyperplasias are found in large and medium-sized ducts. The latter changes are usually accompanied by mucous-cell meta- and hyperplasia.

The alterations described above occur more commonly in the pancreatic head than in the distal pancreas. They are more

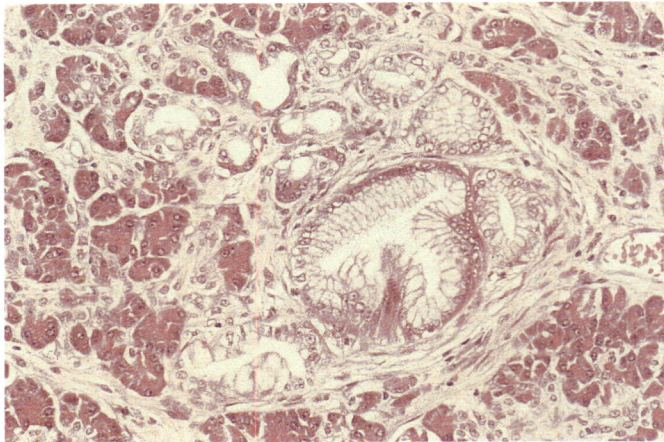

Fig. 18.12   Mucinous metaplasia of small-duct epithelium. The cause for this change was not evident in this case.

prevalent in chronic pancreatitis, especially of the obstructive type, and in age. Carcinoma of the pancreas often leads to ductal obstruction. This may account for the frequent finding of these changes in cancerous glands. Carcinoma, in addition, is more prevalent in the older age-group in which these changes are also more commonly found. This would explain the seeming association of ductal meta- and hyperplasias with adenocarcinoma. On the other hand, a high proportion of pancreatic cancer cases show atypical ductal hyperplastic changes of varying severity, including carcinoma *in situ* in other parts of the gland (Fig. 18.13) away from the frank invasive tumour, in addition to benign-appearing hyperplasias. This has been argued as evidence in support of the concept of a sequential or multistep evolution of pancreatic carcinoma from hyperplasia via metaplasia to dysplasia. However, the point of transformation from benign hyperplasia to neoplasia has not been established and distinction between the two can be difficult. Features in support

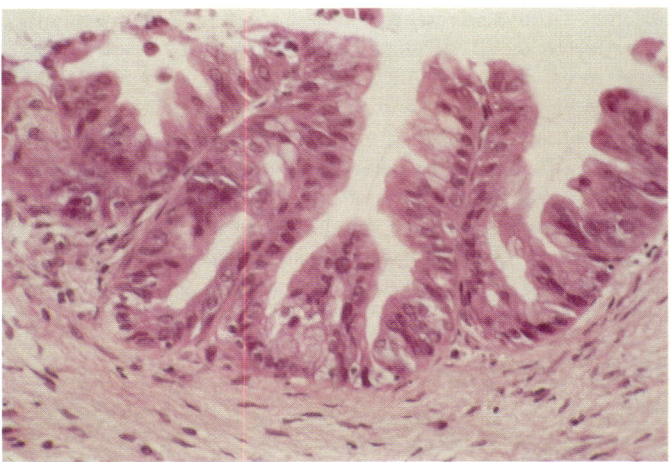

Fig. 18.13   Ductal epithelial hyperplasia with severe dysplasia. In other parts of the gland there was poorly differentiated adenocarcinoma.

of a diagnosis of neoplasia include papillary projections with fibrous cores, cell stratification, and nuclear pleomorphism, as well as a switch in the cellular mucin composition from production of neutral mucins by the reactive lesions to mixed acid as well as neutral mucins in the neoplastic epithelium.

Ductal epithelial squamous metaplasia is not uncommon and is found mainly in medium-sized ducts. It is more frequent in older individuals and has been associated with chronic pancreatitis where, in the calcifying form, it is often found in the region of the calcerous ductal impactions. Atypia has not been observed in squamous metaplasia. There appears to be no association between squamous metaplasia and pancreatic carcinoma, and in particular not with its squamous or adenosquamous variants.

Focal aggregates of dilated ductules of varying calibre, lined by cells ranging from columnar to cuboidal or goblet-cell types, are frequently found in chronic pancreatitis (Fig. 18.14). These 'ductular complexes' do not represent a benign or premalignant neoplastic process but are areas of parenchyma where acinar cells have lost their zymogen granule complement and have transformed to cells with epithelial features. Recognition of this entity if important in order to avoid a misdiagnosis of carcinoma. This is particularly likely in glands with florid chronic inflammation, where the cells lining the ductules may assume rather worrisome features.

Acinar cells may undergo various changes. Most common are focal, well-demarcated nodules composed of acinar cells possessing a pale eosinophilic cytoplasm devoid of zymogen granules and with pleomorphic or small dense nuclei. The relevance of these lesions is unclear. They have been observed in association with a variety of conditions and are sometimes referred to as 'acinar-cell dysplasia'. However, considering their relevant frequency and the rarity of carcinomas with acinar-cell features, an association between the two would be unlikely.

In surgical pancreatic specimens removed for chronic pain

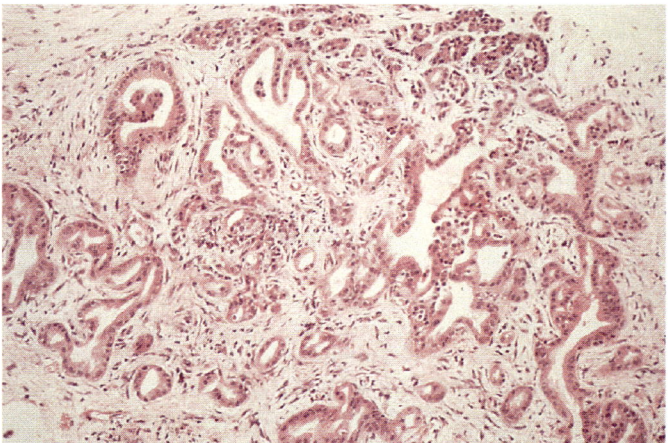

Fig. 18.14 Focal aggregate of ductules in chronic pancreatitis. It is important to recognize this reactive change and not to misdiagnose carcinoma.

but showing little evidence attributable to fibrosis and inflammation, a focal or diffuse conversion of acinar cells with characteristics of centroacinar cells is not uncommon (Fig. 18.15). The significance of this type of metaplasia is unclear. A reported association with pancreatic adenoma and, in particular, serous cystadenoma is purely speculative.

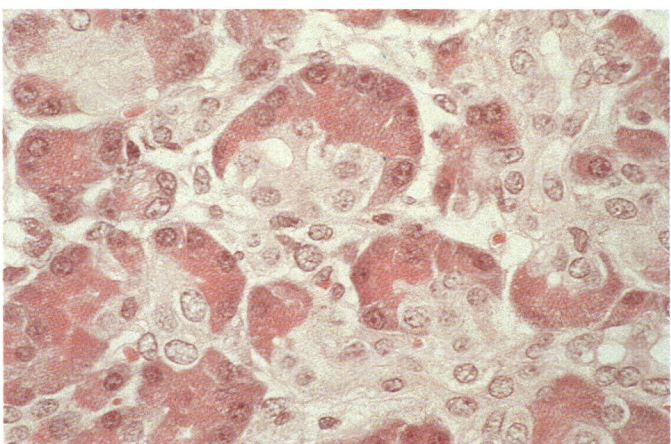

Fig. 18.15 Centroacinar cell metaplasia in a pancreas removed for pain. The significance of this change is unclear.

18.7.4 Benign neoplasms

Adenoma

In the literature two types of lesions are sometimes erroneously referred to as pancreatic adenomata, namely duct adenoma and acinar-cell adenoma. The first lesion is not a true neoplasm. It is composed of small focal aggregates of dilated ductules which are frequently found in chronic pancreatitis specimens. The second type of lesion is also not uncommon. It is a focal, demarcated area where the acinar cells are converted to cells with a diminished complement of cytoplasmic zymogen granules and therefore appear paler. The cell nuclei in these aggregates may be pleomorphic or appear pyknotic. A capsule surrounding these areas is not seen. The cause and significance of this type of lesion is not clear but features of a neoplastic process are lacking. Research workers have been able to produce similar changes in laboratory animals.

Papillary adenoma

Pancreatic intraductal papilloma (papillary adenoma) is an uncommon neoplasm. Patients with this type of tumour are usually in their fifth to seventh decade of life. Men and women are equally affected. The most frequent presenting symptoms are upper abdominal pain, diarrhoea, and weight loss. In the majority of cases reported in the literature the tumours arose in the main pancreatic duct in the head region of the gland. Some tumours were multiple and involved the duct of Wirsung from the ampulla of Vater to the body portion of the pancreas. Papillary adenomas are soft and friable, and distend and obstruct the ductal lumen. There is marked dilatation of the duct system distal to the tumour and, as a result, chronic obstructive pancreatitis with marked fibrosis ensues. Histologically, the tumours resemble the tubulo-villous adenomas of the large bowel (Fig. 18.16). Like these, the lining mucus-secreting epithelium of the papillary projections and tubules show a spectrum of cellular atypia up to a degree indistinguishable from carcinoma *in situ*. Atypical epithelial proliferations extending into smaller side-branches may be extremely difficult to distinguish from invasive carcinoma. The malignant potential of this type of neoplasm appears to be low. Metastatic spread has not been observed in any of the reported cases. Long-term follow-up studies have shown total pancreatectomy to be curative.

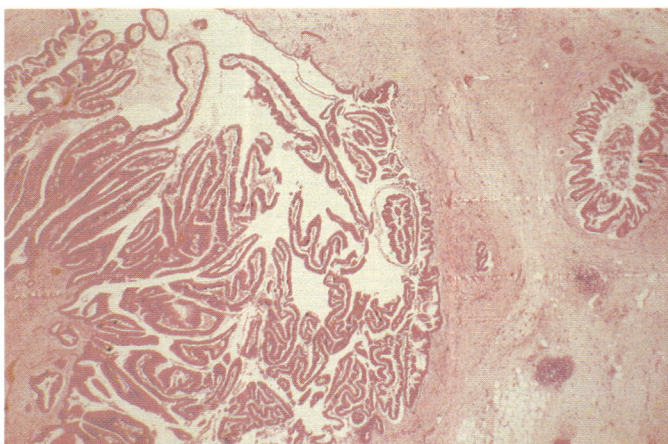

Fig. 18.16 Papillary adenoma of the main pancreatic duct. The tumour resembles villous adenoma of the large bowel. Epithelial proliferations are seen to extend into a smaller side-branch. There was severe chronic pancreatitis distal to the tumour.

Cystadenoma

The majority of pancreatic cysts are non-neoplastic. Distinction of these cysts is important because of their different management. Most clinically evident cysts of the pancreas are 'pseudocysts' which are acquired and inflammatory in nature. The next most common cysts are retention cysts which may be single or multiple. In most instances retention cysts are secondary to inflammation and duct obstruction. True congenital cysts are rare and can be single or multiple. Congenital cysts may be associated with cysts involving other organs, as is the case in von Hippel–Lindau disease.

Serous cystadenoma

Serous cystadenoma of the pancreas is an uncommon, benign tumour, which derives its name from the water content of its cysts. It is also referred to as 'microcystic adenoma' or 'glycogen-rich adenoma'. It comprises 4–10 per cent of all cystic lesions of the pancreas. The tumour shows a predilection for elderly women in the seventh decade of life. Identical lesions of the pancreas have been observed in association with von Hippel–Lindau disease. About a third of the tumours involve the head of the pancreas, although they may occur anywhere in the gland. In rare cases the entire pancreas may be diffusely involved. Most of the serous cystadenomas are incidental findings at autopsy without having given symptoms during life. However, when localized in the pancreatic head they may cause biliary and gastrointestinal obstruction or bleeding. The majority of tumours can be treated conservatively because of their benign nature. This will avoid unnecessary complications following surgical intervention.

Macroscopically, the tumours are roundish with an average size of 6–10 cm. Cut surfaces are honeycomb-like with numerous small cysts. Many tumours fibrose or occasionally calcify centrally, aiding the radiological diagnosis (Fig. 18.17). Histologically, the cysts vary in size and configuration. They are lined by flattened cuboidal epithelium which may form papillary projections (Fig. 18.18). The cytoplasm of the epithelial cells is clear and contains abundant glycogen. Stains for intracellular mucins are negative.

Mucinous cystic neoplasms

Traditionally, mucinous cystic neoplasms of the pancreas have been differentiated into a benign and a malignant variant, i.e. mucinous cystadenoma and cystadenocarcinoma. However, even benign-appearing mucinous cystic tumours have been shown to possess a high malignant potential and should be treated as carcinomas. Virtually all such tumours will reveal areas of atypia or carcinomatous transformation when extensively sampled. Consequently, the designation mucinous cystadenoma should be abandoned.

Solid and cystic tumour

Solid and cystic tumour of the pancreas is a distinctive neoplasm recognized with increasing frequency. In the past, neoplasms of this type were often misinterpreted. There are various designations under which it is found in the literature. These include 'childhood adenocarcinoma of pancreas', 'papillary-cystic tumour', and 'papillary and solid neoplasm'. Although most of these terms are purely descriptive, others express speculations as to the tumour's histogenesis, such as 'non-functioning islet cell tumour'. The tumour was originally described by Frantz in 1959, under whose eponym reports on the neoplasm are increasingly found in the literature.

Solid and cystic tumour of the pancreas shows a striking female preponderance and has been described in adolescent girls and young women with an age range from 10 to 35 years. Its almost exclusive involvement of young women in a particular age-group and recent reports of significant levels of oestrogen and progesterone receptors on the tumour cells suggest an involvement of hormonal factors in the pathogenesis of this type of tumour of the pancreas.

The patients are often asymptomatic but may show gradual abdominal enlargement. Some women experience vague

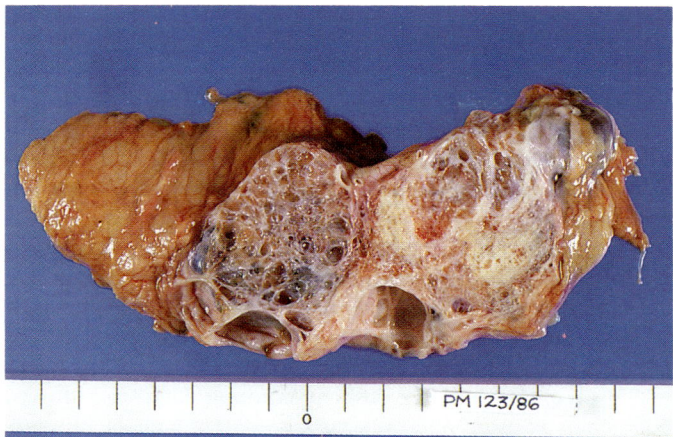

Fig. 18.17 Large serous cystadenoma of the body and tail of the pancreas. This tumour was symptomless and found incidentally at autopsy.

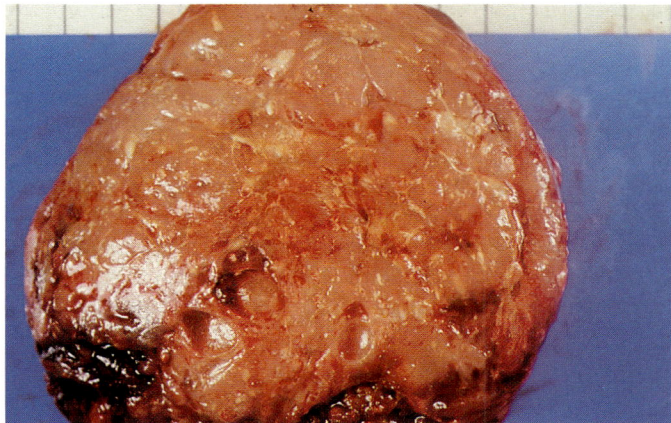

Fig. 18.19 Solid and cystic tumour of the pancreas. This was a large, encapsulated and pedunculated tumour arising in the pancreatic body region in a 23-year-old woman. The cut surface shows solid, degenerative cystic, and haemorrhagic areas.

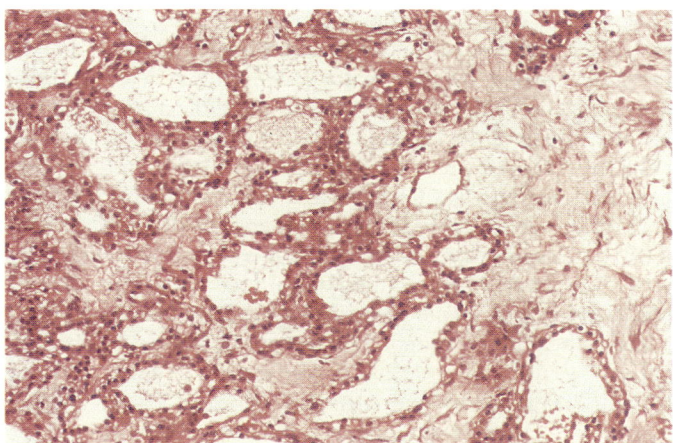

Fig. 18.18 Serous cystadenoma of pancreas. The tumour is composeo of cysts of varying size lined by cuboidal epithelial cells. The cytoplasm of some cells appears clear in this H & E stained section after their glycogen has leached out.

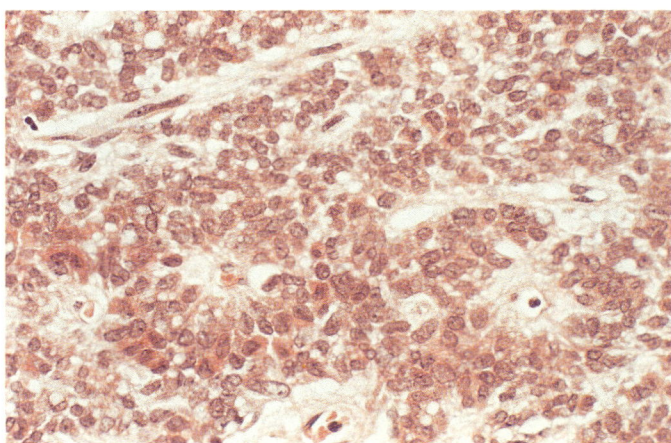

Fig. 18.20 Solid and cystic tumour of the pancreas. The cells are uniform and arranged around fibrovascular connective tissue cores.

abdominal pain or discomfort. No functional symptoms are known to occur in association with these tumours. It is important that most patients were cured by adequate tumour resection. Few cases with local recurrences are reported but metastases are exceptional. In the vast majority of cases these tumours can therefore be regarded as benign.

Solid and cystic tumour occurs anywhere in the pancreas and tends to grow towards its outside. They are large, round tumours with an average diameter of 9–10 cm. The cut surface may be predominantly solid or show areas of cystic degeneration with haemorrhage into the tumour centre (Fig. 18.19). Histologically, the tumour is composed of solid sheets of uniform, polygonal cells, suggesting an islet-cell tumour. The cells are arranged around delicate or hyalinized fibrovascular stalks, forming pseudorosettes in places (Fig. 18.20). The microscopic hallmarks of this neoplasm are pseudopapillae and microcysts resulting from tumour degeneration.

18.7.5 Malignant neoplasms

Carcinoma

Incidence

The incidence of pancreatic cancer is steadily increasing in developed countries. In England and Wales the number of patients suffering from the disease has approximately doubled in the past four decades. In most Western countries there is now an annual incidence of between 9 and 10 cases per 100 000 of the population. Males show a slight preponderance over females. The steady increase in the incidence of pancreatic cancer is only partly explained by increased longevity. The cancer is unusual before the age of 45, while 80 per cent of patients are older than 50 years and about 50–60 per cent are over 65 years. The incidence and mortality rates are almost identical since survival rates for pancreatic cancer are still abysmally low. Currently, pancreatic carcinoma ranks as the fourth most common cause of cancer-related deaths in the United States with roughly equal predilection for men and women. It is exceeded only by cancer of the lung, colorectum, and breast. About 25 000 people die of pancreatic cancer in the USA each year. Consequently, this type of cancer poses a major community health problem and a challenge to identify associated specific aetiological factors and means of prevention.

Aetiology

Despite extensive epidemiological, demographic, and experimental studies there are many open questions as to the aetiology of pancreatic carcinoma. The increased incidence in the older age group suggests a slow process in pancreatic carcinogenesis. A higher incidence in American Blacks and the occurrence of the disease in siblings may point to a genetic predisposition. Families at high risk for pancreatic cancer have been reported, but available data do not suggest an association with a specific blood group or HLA type. Although in most countries the incidence in males is almost double that in females, higher ratios for females are recorded in Latin American women in Texas. No consistent differences by geographical location have been found in the USA. Environmental influences may play a role in addition to genetic factors. Immigrants to the USA of all major ethnic groups adjust their incidence rate to that of the host country and share a uniform risk of developing pancreatic cancer.

In cigarette-smokers the risk of developing cancer of the pancreas is higher than in non-smokers but the strength of this association is much less than for lung cancer or other smoking-related cancers. Both alcohol and coffee were initially incriminated to play an aetiological role. In more recent studies this association could not be confirmed. Also implicated have been chronic pancreatitis, diabetes, and biliary disease, but the case against these conditions has now been abandoned. A number of chemicals are known to induce pancreatic cancer in laboratory animals. Such a process may also be operating in man but no particular carcinogen has been identified so far. Preliminary evidence suggests that dietary constituents may be of importance. Especially, dietary fats have been implicated while vitamins and dietary fibre are reported to protect against cancer of the pancreas.

Clinical symptoms and course

The outcome of treatment is dismal for pancreatic cancer. Its five-year survival rate is 1–2 per cent and is the lowest of all cancers. The symptoms of carcinoma of the pancreas are vague in the early stages of the disease. The mean time lapse between onset of symptoms and admission to hospital is 15 weeks. By the time diagnosis is made most cancers are already in an advanced stage. As a result the average interval from the appearance of symptoms and death is only 7.5 months. A high degree of sus-

picion is an essential prerequisite if pancreatic cancer is to be discovered at an early stage.

The presenting symptoms of pancreatic carcinoma vary with the location of the growth. The first symptoms produced by tumours of the pancreatic head are pain, jaundice, and weight loss. Jaundice is the earliest symptom in ampullary cancers and abdominal pain is predominant in tumours of the body and tail. Pain elicited by carcinomas of the body and tail of the pancreas is related to invasion of adjacent organs, in particular the peritoneum and stomach. By the time these carcinomas are detected almost all of them have therefore widely metastasized.

Other symptoms associated with carcinoma of the pancreas are rare or non-specific. Some patients may complain about back pain or flatulent dyspepsia and nausea. Migratory thrombophlebitis is more often an associated symptom of tumours involving the body and tail rather than head carcinomas. Anaemia is not an early feature in cancer of the pancreas.

When diagnosis is established about 80 per cent of pancreatic carcinomas are already inoperable. In the remaining patients, radical resection prolongs life and is followed by an overall survival time of 10–32 months. Factors influencing prognosis are site, stage, and size of the carcinoma. Cancer of the head of the pancreas treated by pancreatoduodenectomy bears a better prognosis than that of the body and tail after distal pancreatectomy. Stage of the carcinoma and regional lymph node involvement are related to the size of the primary tumour. Spread to lymph nodes is less frequent and survival time is longer in stage I tumours of less than 3 cm diameter. Poorly differentiated adenocarcinomas are reported to have a poorer prognosis than well-differentiated carcinomas, but in most cases the ultimate prognosis is not significantly influenced by the histological grade of the primary tumour. Furthermore, with adequate sampling differentiation of various grades may be found in the same tumour. However, certain subtypes show a definitely better prognosis. Cystadenocarcinomas behave in an excellent fashion after resection, provided that the tumour has not already spread.

In inoperable cases biliary bypass procedures or choledochal stenting together with chemotherapy or radiotherapy or both influence survival. Relief of jaundice offers significant palliation during the survival period.

Morphology

The most common site of adenocarcinoma of the pancreas is the head region where 60–70 per cent of these tumours are found (Fig. 18.21). About 15 per cent are located in the body and approximately 10 per cent in the tail. The remainder may arise in a combination of sites, or precise localization is impossible to assess. Some carcinomas of the head may have arisen from the epithelium of the intrahepatic portion of the common bile duct. Their morphological features, presenting symptoms, and clinical behaviour are identical to most adenocarcinomas of pancreatic origin. The incidence of carcinoma arising in aberrant pancreas is difficult to determine since its true origin in the stomach, duodenum, or small intestine is easily missed.

Carcinomas of the pancreatic head tend to be smaller than

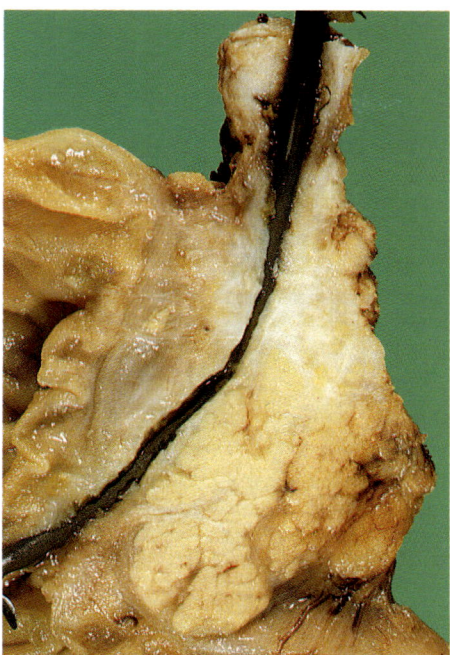

Fig. 18.21 Adenocarcinoma of the head of the pancreas. The hard, fibrotic, grey tumour has infiltrated the intrapancreatic portion of the bile duct. The marked biliary obstruction is relieved by a stent which had been inserted endoscopically through the major ampulla.

those of the body and tail but the difference is not marked. In autopsy material the size of carcinomas of the pancreatic head averages 5.5 cm and that of the body or tail about 7 cm. Carcinomas of the pancreatic head are often obstructive thus attracting earlier surgical intervention than distal tumours. In Whipple's specimens resected for head carcinomas the median diameter of these tumours is in the order of 2.5–3.5 cm. Macroscopical identification of small tumours may be difficult and only possible due to focal induration of the parenchyma, dilatation of ducts in the vicinity, or circumscribed narrowing of the common bile duct.

Some abnormality of the outer surface of the pancreas is often seen, usually in the form of a circumscribed enlargement of the gland which feels hard to palpation. When incised the tumours are poorly demarcated and are grey-white or yellowish. Small cystic spaces containing turbid or brown fluid are quite common.

Direct spread beyond the pancreas involves primarily retroperitoneal spaces and peritoneum, with subsequent spread throughout the peritoneal cavity. The mesenteric and splenic vessels may become infiltrated, resulting in their fixation and splenic infarction. Adjacent organs such as spleen, the left adrenal and kidney, and the gall-bladder can be invaded in advanced disease, and extension into the duodenum, stomach, and transverse colon may lead to gut obstruction.

Lymphatic spread occurs early in the course of the disease and usually precedes haematogenous spread. In nearly all carcinomas microscopic examination reveals infiltration of peri-

neural spaces and lymph channels. Lymph-node groups involved at an early stage by secondary carcinoma are found posterior to the duodenum and along the upper and lower margin of the pancreatic head. Carcinomas of the body and tail preferentially metastasize to the superior body and pancreatic head groups and often show pleural and lung carcinomatosis. Common sites of haematogenous spread are the liver, lungs, adrenals, kidneys, and bone, whereas skin and brain are rarely affected.

Microscopically the majority of adenocarcinomas of the pancreas strongly resemble pancreatic duct structures. Typically these carcinomas elicit a marked desmoplastic reaction which accounts for their firm consistency (Fig. 18.22). Embedded within the dense fibrous stroma are well-differentiated duct-like structures; less mature, irregular, solid and tubular arrangements; or poorly differentiated carcinoma, comprising single or groups of mucin-producing signet ring cells, clear cells, and anaplastic bizarre or giant-cell forms. An uncommon pattern is seen in mucinous or 'colloid' adenocarcinomas. In these tumours clusters of neoplastic cells are seen floating in pools of mucin. Some poorly differentiated carcinomas are compact and made up of sheets of large pleomorphic mononuclear and multinucleated cells (giant-cell carcinoma) (Fig. 18.23). However, it is not uncommon to identify neoplastic gland- or duct-like structures, even in this type. Carcinomas with an extensive pleomorphic spindle or sarcomatoid cell pattern may simulate a soft-tissue neoplasm such as malignant fibrous histiocytoma. These poorly differentiated carcinomas tend to be larger than

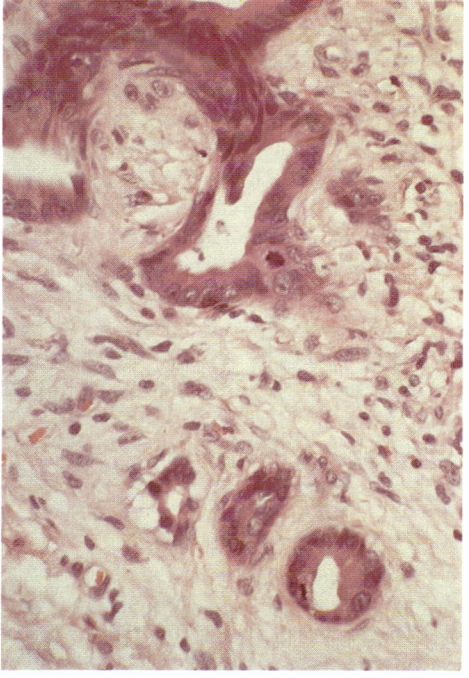

Fig. 18.22 Adenocarcinoma of the pancreas. This fairly well-differentiated carcinoma resembles pancreatic duct structures. It has elicited a marked desmoplastic reaction.

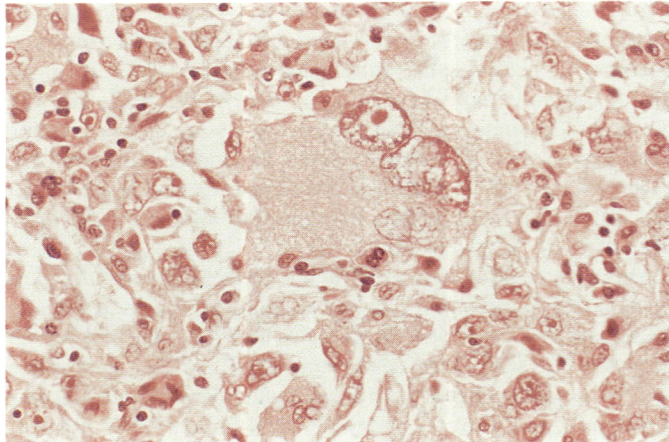

Fig. 18.23 Pleomorphic or giant-cell carcinoma of pancreas. This poorly differentiated carcinoma consisted of sheets of mononuclear and multinucleated giant cells. In some areas of the tumour neoplastic gland-like structures could be identified.

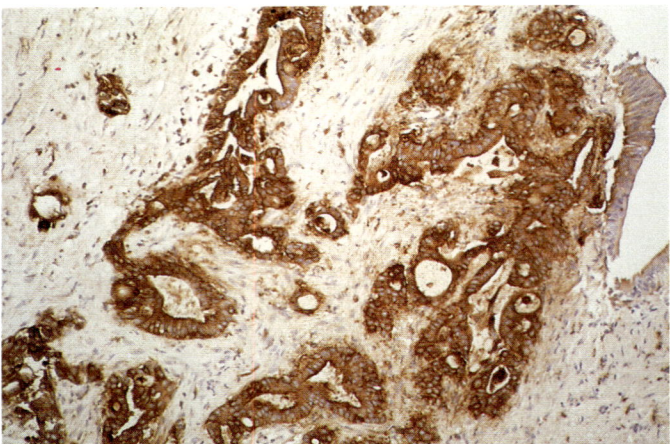

Fig. 18.24 Adenocarcinoma of the pancreas. The carcinoma shows positive immunocytochemical staining for carcino-embryonic antigen (CEA) as demonstrated here by the brown reaction product. Non-neoplastic ductal epithelium (upper left) does not stain for CEA.

the usual variants. Necroses are common and a fibrous reaction is only slight. Anaplastic small-cell carcinomas are rare. Metastases from oat cell carcinoma of the lung, which they resemble, and from similar cancers of other sites are more common. With adequate sampling, many tumours defeat categorization into one specific tumour type and grade with well-differentiated patterns accompanying poorly differentiated components.

At times well-differentiated carcinoma may be difficult to distinguish from reactive ductules found in chronic pancreatitis. Helpful diagnostic criteria in this case are variations in nuclear size, nuclear hyperchromasia, prominent nucleoli, and perineural invasion. Histochemical stains with the PAS method and alcian blue technique at low pH for neutral and acid mucins often differentiate neoplastic epithelium from the normal by revealing acid, probably sialomucin, production by carcinoma cells. Immunocytochemistry employing monoclonal antibodies directed against carcino-embryonic antigen (CEA) may also prove to be of value. In the majority of cases CEA is expressed in carcinoma but not in reactive ductal epithelium (Fig. 18.24).

The use of a number of cancer-associated monoclonal antibodies has been disappointing at the tissue level. Adenosquamous or pure squamous differentiation is not uncommon in carcinoma of the pancreas. Applying markers for high molecular weight keratins will reveal this type of keratin in a high proportion of carcinomas, even in those without an obvious squamous phenotype.

Mucinous cystadenocarcinoma

Mucinous cystic neoplasms account for about 1–2 per cent of all pancreatic exocrine tumours. Although some mucinous cystic tumours of the pancreas appear to be histologically benign, even after extensive sampling, it is advisable to treat them as carcinomas because of their high malignant potential. The neoplasm affects women six times more often than men. Its peak presentation is in the fifth decade of life. Most patients present

with epigastric pain or discomfort. In cases where the tumour has been completely excised the prognosis seems to be favourable in more than 50 per cent of patients.

Mucinous cystadenocarcinomas may develop in any part of the pancreas, but the region of the tail seems to be most likely involved. The uni- or multilocular cysts are usually large, measuring on average 10 cm in diameter, and are filled with sticky mucin (Fig. 18.25). The dense, fibrous capsule of the tumours may contain dystrophic calcifications and residual atrophic exocrine and endocrine pancreatic tissue.

Histologically, the cysts are lined by intestinal-type columnar epithelium that may contain goblet cells, Paneth cells, and a variety of endocrine cells. Amongst the latter, serotonin-producing cells are the most common. Focally the columnar epithelium forms intracystic papillary projections, and atypical epithelium or frank invasive adenocarcinoma may be observed. If metastasis occurs, the histological pattern may vary from

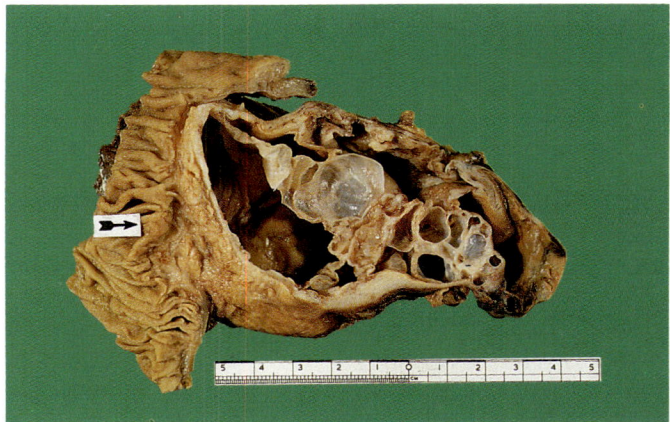

Fig. 18.25 Mucinous cystadenocarcinoma of the pancreas. The multiloculated tumour arose in the head of the gland. The arrow points to the major papilla in the opened duodenum of this Whipple's specimen.

well-differentiated cystic structures to poorly differentiated adenocarcinoma.

Rare cancers

Pancreatoblastoma

Pancreatoblastoma is a rare pancreatic neoplasm initially believed to occur exclusively in young children, but rare adult cases have now been reported. The tumour has distinctive histological features, being composed predominantly of small primitive cells with the formation of organoid 'squamoid corpuscles' in places. The histological pattern varies somewhat from case to case, and mesenchymal components such as foci of chondroid, osteoid, and bone have been observed. The tumour involves both sexes equally and may be found in the head, body, or tail of the pancreas, either encapsulated or non-encapsulated, with extension into adjacent organs. There are suggestions that some forms of this cancer behave in an indolent fashion and have a favourable prognosis.

Carcinomas with mixed acinar, duct, and islet-cell features

Taking into consideration the common embryological origin of acinar, ductal, and islet cells from foregut endoderm it is not surprising that carcinomas of the pancreas may variously express features of any of these cell types, and mixed carcinomas occur. In practice, these tumours are rare. Relatively well-differentiated examples may be easily recognized but others often require elaborate electron-microscopical and immunohistochemical testing before allocation to a particular category. The value of such classification for treatment and prognosis has to be awaited. Carcinomas with pure, well-differentiated acinar cell features are uncommon. They are usually large and the stroma is scanty, rendering them soft to palpation. Poorly differentiated forms of this type and carcinomas with mixed acinar–ductal, acinar–islet, and ductal–endocrine differentiation have been described.

Osteoclast-type giant-cell tumour

Giant-cell tumours of the pancreas composed of benign-appearing giant cells resembling osteoclasts in a background of a pleomorphic sarcomatous stroma should be distinguished from pleomorphic carcinomas containing bizarre multinucleated giant cells. The two types of tumours have been occasionally confused in the literature. Only a few cases have been recognized so far. The tumour resembles giant-cell tumour of bone and seems to bear a somewhat better prognosis than the usual bizarre giant-cell carcinoma.

Techniques of investigation for carcinoma

Failure to detect early, potentially curable cancer by conventional non-interventive methods has compounded the abysmally low survival figures. In order to achieve better survival rates identification of individuals at risk and those patients bearing early resectable pancreatic cancer would be desirable. Immunological tumour markers for pancreatic cancer-associated antigens released into the bloodstream are currently under investigation. Determination of serum CEA has attracted wide interest, especially in combination with other gastrointestinal cancer-associated antigens such as CA19-9, a monosialosyl Lea blood-group antigen. High serum levels usually indicate advanced disease, while about half of the patients with small resectable carcinomas have elevated levels. Patients with benign pancreatic and biliary disease also show raised values. At present the sensitivity and specificity of these tests are too low for screening of an asymptomatic population.

In the symptomatic patient the clinical diagnosis of pancreatic cancer will be supported by the results of imaging techniques. Accuracy in the diagnosis of pancreatic cancer by retrograde pancreatography, ultrasonography, computerized tomography (CT), and angiography has been reported to be as high as 70–90 per cent. However, in spite of the recent advances in these techniques the differential diagnosis of carcinoma versus pancreatitis remains a difficult area. Confirmation of carcinoma and identification of potentially treatable rarer benign or less-aggressive lesions is therefore desirable.

A number of cytological methods have been developed to obtain pancreatic cells by duodenal aspiration, endoscopic cannulation of the pancreatic duct after secretin simulation or abrasive brushing, and by a direct percutaneous approach using fine-needle aspiration under ultrasound or CT guidance. The disadvantages of these methods are the requirement of a highly specialized cytology service, the low sensitivity and accuracy rate, and often the failure of the cytology to provide precise information as to cell type and tumour origin.

Biopsy provides an objective diagnosis of pancreatic cancer and identifies resectable tumours and those conditions suitable for conservative or palliative treatment only. Several methods of obtaining tissue of the pancreas evolved in the past but did not gain popularity because of the potential hazard for the patient, especially fistula formation. Recently a new, safe, image-guided percutaneous pancreatic core biopsy technique has been introduced. This method takes advantage of a spring-loaded biopsy device. The size of the needle chosen and the high speed under which the device operates prevents haemorrhage and fistula formation but guarantees adequate tissue sampling. This method promises to overcome previous reservations about the performance of diagnostic pancreatic biopsies and allows hitherto unavailable insights and special histological investigations of this organ.

Sarcoma and lymphoma

Although malignant soft tissue tumours of all types can be expected to involve the pancreas as the primary site, reports of such sarcomas are exceedingly rare in the literature. Most of these reports are of single cases. Fibrosarcoma, leiomyosarcoma, rhabdomyosarcoma, malignant haemangiopericytoma, malignant fibrous histiocytoma, and sarcoma of unknown histogenesis are described.

Lymphomas arise only rarely in the pancreas but secondary involvement of the pancreas by advanced lymphoma is not uncommon. In advanced Hodgkin's disease the pancreas has been found to be involved in 20 per cent of cases at autopsy but no patient has been recorded in which the pancreas was the primary site of origin.

Tumours of the ampulla of Vater

Tumours arising in the region of the ampulla of Vater are not pancreatic tumours in the strictest sense. However, they are commonly discussed along with pancreatic tumours because of their similarity in effect and appearance and have to be included in the differential diagnosis of pancreatic head neoplasms. In some instances it is impossible to ascertain whether a tumour arose in the head of the pancreas, distal bile duct, ampulla of Vater, or peripapillary duodenum.

The vast majority of ampullary and peripapillary tumours are adenocarcinomas. There are a small number of carcinoid and other neuroendocrine tumours, including gangliocytic para-gangliomas. Adenomyomas and cysts in this region are probably not true neoplasms but hyperplastic or reactive sequelae to aberrant and inflamed pancreas or to duodenal wall cysts and diverticula.

Ampullary adenocarcinomas resemble their pancreatic counterparts. When they arise within the ampulla or terminal bile duct the tumour may be extremely small when detected. In these cases their size varies from 0.5 to 2 cm. Obstructive symptoms are produced at an early stage by scirrhous infiltration and thickening of the ampullary and common bile duct wall (Fig. 18.26). Larger tumours are found protruding as polypoid

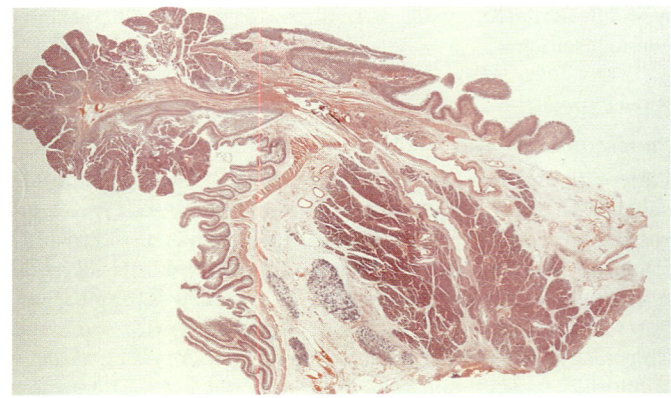

Fig. 18.27 Tubulovillous adenoma of the major papilla. Whole-mounted section of a drawn-out pedunculated adenoma arising from the ampullary and duodenal mucosa. Preceeding adenoma can be recognized in about one-third of ampullary carcinomas.

masses into the duodenal lumen, or arising from the major papilla. In about 20–30 per cent of cases a sessile polyp of the duodeno-ampullary mucosa precedes the infiltrating carcinoma. Morphologically these adenomas resemble tubular or tubulovillous adenomas of the large bowel (Fig. 18.27). A high prevalence of adenomatous polyps of the duodenal papilla has been reported in familial adenomatous polyposis.

Histologically these carcinomas show a spectrum of differentiation. Well-differentiated carcinomas may produce an exophytic papillary growth which has to be distinguished from a preceding villous adenoma. Infiltrating carcinomas spread into the sphincter muscle of Oddi, the duodenal mucosa, and submucosa. Metastases to regional lymph nodes primarily involve the retroduodenal group of nodes and are found in approximately 40 per cent of resected specimens.

Prognosis of adenocarcinoma of the ampullary region is better than that for carcinoma of the pancreas. Five-year survival figures of 18–40 per cent have been reported. The reasons for this more optimistic outlook are most likely anatomical. Tumour size is of importance. The critical size of the primary carcinoma with regard to survival appears to be 2 cm.

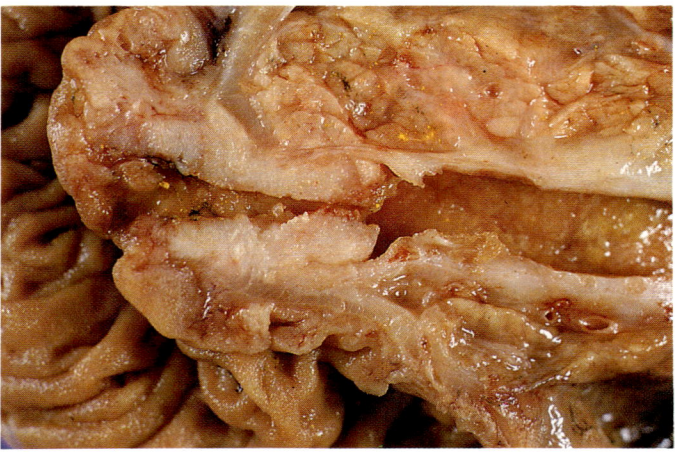

Fig. 18.26 Adenocarcinoma of the ampulla of Vater. The carcinoma has infiltrated the wall of the ampulla. The obstructed bile duct (towards right) is dilated and its wall is inflamed and thickened. The major papilla is lacerated after endoscopic attempts to relieve the obstruction.

18.7.6 Further reading

Lack, E. E. (1989). Primary tumors of the exocrine pancreas. Classification, overview, and recent contributions by immunohistochemistry and electron microscopy. *American Journal of Surgical Pathology* **13** (Suppl. 1), 66–88.

19

The kidney

19

The kidney

19.1 Normal structure

Nicholas A. Wright

The kidney is a complex organ, which subsumes several important functions; of course the formation of urine is its most obvious role, but also implicit in this is its vital co-ordination of water and salt metabolism and acid–base balance. In addition, renal hormones regulate blood pressure and stimulate erythropoiesis. This functional richness is reflected in a complex structure.

The gross anatomy of the kidney is, however, straightforward. On section, the kidney is divided into a cortex which varies somewhat in thickness, but is generally about 15 mm thick. The medulla is divided into renal pyramids, at the tips of which are the renal papillae. The urine passes into one of 12 minor calyces, which in turn form two or three major calyces. These then communicate with the ureter, and hence with the urinary bladder.

In man the pronephros and mesonephros regress, although the excretory duct of the pronephros, the Wolffian duct, goes to form the collecting system. The metanephros provides nephrons for the adult kidney. These developmental divisions are reflected in the several congenital anomalies affecting the kidney (see below).

The nephron is usually divided into the glomerulus and the tubules. It is perhaps best to appreciate the glomerulus as an invagination of an original epithelial vesicle or sac (Bowman's capsule) by a ball-shaped collection of capillaries and mesenchyme. Thus, the invaginated epithelium becomes closely associated with the capillaries, and is called the visceral epithelium, while the epithelium that remains on the outside (the parietal epithelium) confines the space (Bowman's space) into which the glomerular filtrate passes. This schema allows a listing of the structures through which filtration occurs; first, of course, the filtrate passes through the endothelium, a specialized form that contains fenestrations, each about 90 nm in diameter, followed by the glomerular basement membrane, some 300 nm in thickness, which on electron microscopy consists of three layers, a central electron-dense layer, the *lamina densa*, on both sides of which are the electron-lucent *lamina rara interna* and *externa*. Distal to the basement membrane are the *visceral epithelial cells*, commonly called *podocytes*, which possess complex interdigitating processes closely associated with the lamina rara externa. These *foot processes* are separated from one another by *filtration slits*; the *slit diaphragm* bridges across each filtration slit. These structures are shown in Fig. 19.1.

The *mesangium* forms a supportive branching framework for the glomerular tuft, and consists of mesangial cells, which are stellate, embedded in a matrix (Fig. 19.1).

The primary function of the glomerulus is production of the glomerular filtrate, being remarkably selective in this filtration process; almost completely excluding most plasma proteins while allowing small solutes and water free passage. The glomerular basement membrane is the main structure responsible for this differential molecular size segregation. Glomerular damage leads to passage of macromolecules into the glomerular filtrate. The mesangial cells appear phagocytic and may clear away any macromolecules which may pass the filter, and, by actively contracting, may also regulate glomerular blood flow.

The glomerular filtrate passes into the *proximal tubule*, whose cells are possessed of long apical microvilli, adapted for their main function of reabsorption of solutes such as sodium, potassium, phosphate, glucose, and, of course, water. The tubule loops backwards towards the glomerulus, becoming the distal tubule, eventually carrying the urine towards the collecting tubules and the calyces.

The main renal arteries carry about 25 per cent of the cardiac output to the kidneys. The *interlobular arteries* carry most of this blood to the cortex, which is richly vascularized. *Arcuate arteries* run between cortex and medulla, giving off the *interlobular arteries* running perpendicular to the cortical surface. These, in turn, furnish the *afferent arterioles*, which enter the glomerulus, and from which the capillaries are derived. The *efferent arteriole* emerges from the glomerulus, and peripheral arterioles give rise to a rich peritubular vascular network of capillaries; deep glomeruli provide the straight *vasa recta*, which supply the medulla.

At the point where the afferent arteriole enters the glomerulus, is the juxtaglomerular (JG) apparatus, consisting of modified granular smooth muscle cells occupying the media of the afferent arteriole: the *juxta-glomerular cells*, which secrete the hormone *renin*. The *macula densa* are specialized distal tubular cells adjacent to the parent glomerulus, where cells are crowded and interdigitated. In the region between the glomerulus, the macula densa, and the afferent arteriole are the mesangial-like

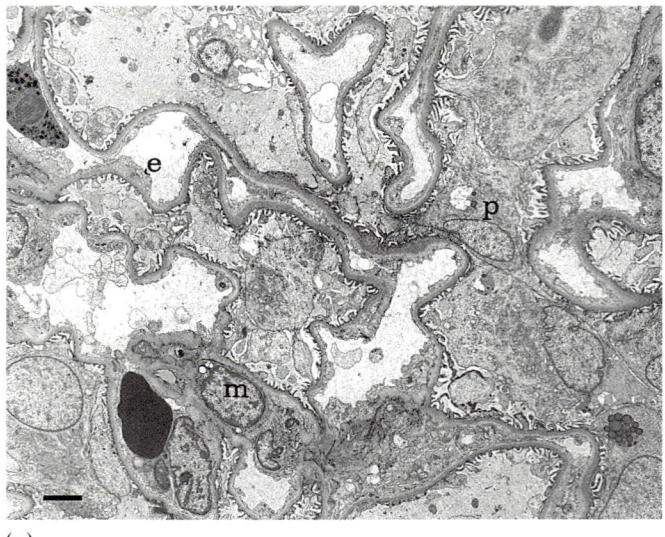

(a)

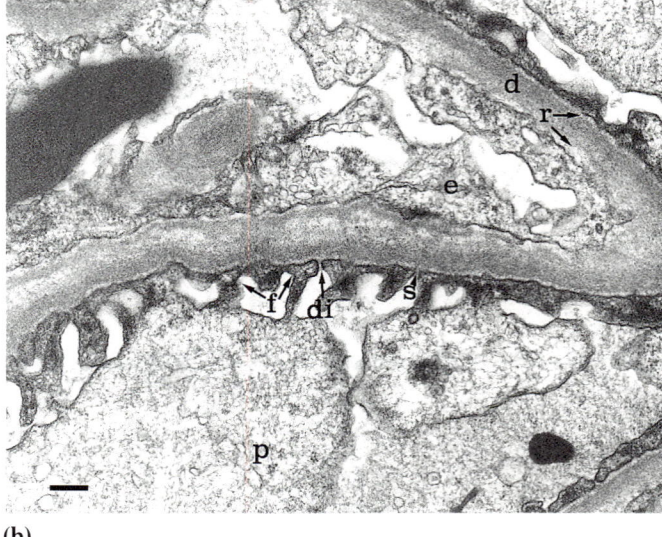

(b)

Fig. 19.1 (a) A low-power electron micrograph of the human renal glomerulus: e, endothelial cell; p, podocyte; m, mesangial cell. (b) The fenestrated endothelium. d, basement membrane, lamina densa; r, basement membrane, lamina rara, externa and interna; e, endothelial cell; f, foot processes; di, slit diaphragm; s, filtration slit; p, podocyte; magnification bar = 0.3 μm. (Courtesy Dr C. Sarraf.)

non-granulated or *lacis cells*. The JG apparatus is ultimately concerned with blood pressure regulation.

The *interstitial space* of the kidney is occupied by capillaries, fibroblasts, and mucopolysaccharides, and is often involved in renal diseases.

19.2　Congenital diseases of the kidney

A. R. Morley

The *ureteric bud* grows from the *mesonephric duct* headwards to become attached to the *metanephros*. The tip divides to form generations of *ampullae* which give rise to the *pelvis, calyces*, and *collecting tubules*. In the adjacent area (the *renal blastema*) the ampullae induce *nephron* formation, with the production of *glomeruli* in the outer zone. Abnormalities of these processes result in a wide range of malformations, displacements, and incomplete development of the bladder, kidney, and the collecting system. Many present *in utero* or in childhood and congenital malformations in other systems are commonly seen. The diseases considered are listed in Table 19.1 and in greater detail by Risdon (1981).

19.2.1　Atresia

Bilateral absence of the kidneys is rare and is usually found in stillbirths although survival until delivery may occur. The 'Potter' face, comprising large, low-set ears, 'parrot beak' nose, and

Table 19.1　Congenital diseases of the kidney

Atresias
Displacements and fusion ('horseshoe kidney')
Dysplasia
Infantile polycystic kidney
Adult polycystic kidney
Multicystic disease in renal transplants
Solitary cortical cysts
Medullary sponge kidney
Uraemic medullary sponge kidney
Congenital nephrotic syndrome

receding chin are found in this group, as well as in those with bilateral dysplasia and infantile polycystic kidney.

Unilateral atresia is found in 1:1000 of the population and is compatible with normal existence. This makes demonstration of a second kidney essential before nephrectomy or renal biopsy. The single kidney shows compensatory hypertrophy and is more liable to trauma.

19.2.2　Displacements and fusion (horseshoe kidney)

The kidney may be displaced in its cephalic journey. In *simple ectopia* the kidney remains on the correct side but its final position is at the level of the pelvic brim, and rarely entering the abdominal cavity. In *crossed ectopia* the kidney crosses the midline, remaining at the pelvic brim or rising to fuse with the orthotopic kidney. Failure of rotation may result in the pelvis facing anteriorly rather than medially.

The '*horseshoe' kidney* is a combination of fusion of the lower poles of the kidneys in front of the great vessels and with some degree of caudal displacement, sometimes forming a single pelvic mass of renal tissue (Fig. 19.2).

All forms of displacement and fusion are associated with abnormalities of the ureters, either in their course, or with abnormal openings into the bladder or urethra. Infections and stone formation are common in patients with ectopia and fusion.

19.2.3 Dysplasia

Disturbed differentiation of nephrogenic tissue results in the persistence in the child or adult of tissues that are normally only found in the embryo. Dysplasias may be bilateral or unilateral and, in extreme forms, are incompatible with life. Such dysplastic kidneys are often cystic, with distorted structure and poor or absent function. Tissues common to a wide range of dysplastic kidneys are:

1. *undifferentiated mesenchyme*, which is prone to produce cartilage;

2. *embryonic tubules* surrounded by a concentric sheath of primitive mesenchyme; and

3. *primitive glomerular structures.*

In some cases, islands of undifferentiated small spindle cells, forming tubular structures, may be found beneath the capsule, occasionally sheathing the entire kidney. This tissue closely resembles that of the *Wilms tumour (nephroblastoma)* and is termed *nephroblastomatosis*. Despite this similarity, malignant change is rare.

Dysplastic kidneys may have multiple cysts of varying size. It cannot be emphasized too strongly that the term 'polycystic' is reserved for inherited disorders with bilateral cystic kidneys which do not contain dysplastic tissues, and that unilateral cystic kidneys are almost invariably dysplastic.

Cystic dysplasia is often associated with abnormalities of the urinary tract, particularly the ureters. Obstruction is common, and when this occurs early in fetal life it may be associated with dysplastic tissue. For example, *posterior urethral valves* may be associated with cystic dilation of the tubules confined to the outer cortex.

19.2.4 Infantile polycystic kidney

Infantile polycystic kidney is inherited as an *autosomal recessive*. There is therefore no family history, but siblings may also have the disease. It is only found in children and results in renal failure within 1–2 years after birth. It is being increasingly recognized that some patients have lesser degrees of damage, compatible with prolonged survival; consequently a number of genetically distinct disorders may be present.

The disease is always bilateral, with marked enlargement of the kidneys which may impede delivery. The normal renal outline is maintained, but on section the cortex and medulla are replaced by radially orientated fusiform clefts of uniform size and rarely more than a few millimetres wide (Fig. 19.3). The cysts are thought to be derived from dilated collecting ducts.

Cysts of the liver and focal proliferation of bile-ducts are always present in such patients.

19.2.5 Adult polycystic kidney

Adult polycystic kidney is the commonest inherited renal disorder leading to renal failure, and accounts for some 10 per cent of the patients on maintenance dialysis. It is inherited as an *autosomal dominant* and there is usually a family history of renal failure or death from hypertension in several generations. The gene causing this disorder has recently been located on chromosome 16, and genetic probes are being developed which allow intra-uterine prediction of the disorder.

Both kidneys are greatly enlarged, weighing several kilograms and up to 30 cm in length. The cysts are largely spherical and vary from microscopic dimensions to several centimetres in diameter (Fig. 19.4). Haemorrhage into cysts is common. Dilatation involves all sections of the nephron, including Bowman's capsule.

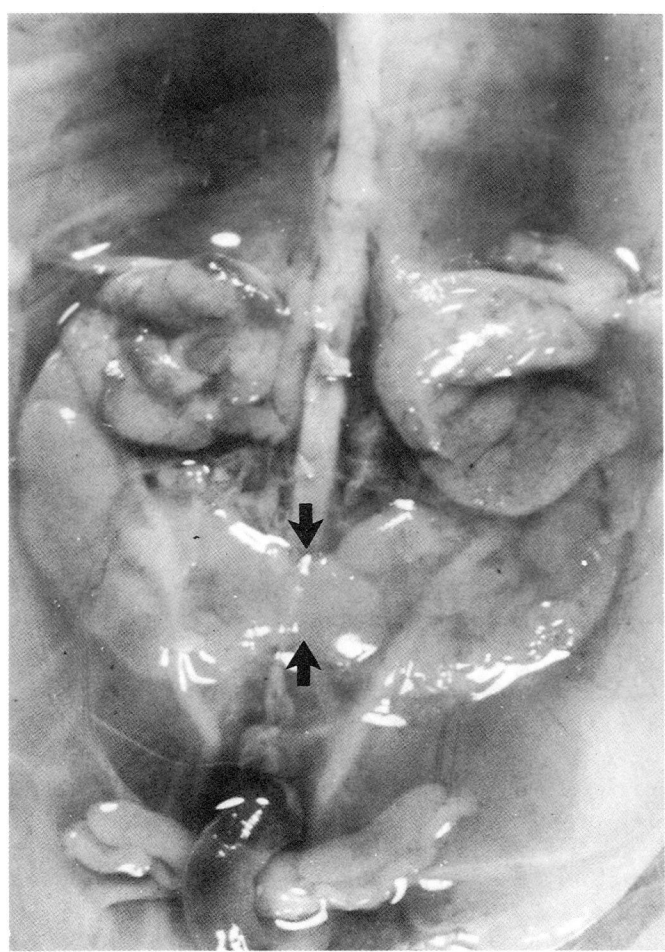

Fig. 19.2 Horseshoe kidney. Posterior abdominal contents of a stillborn fetus, showing the interconnecting bar between the lower poles (between arrows) of the kidneys. Note anterior displacement of ureters.

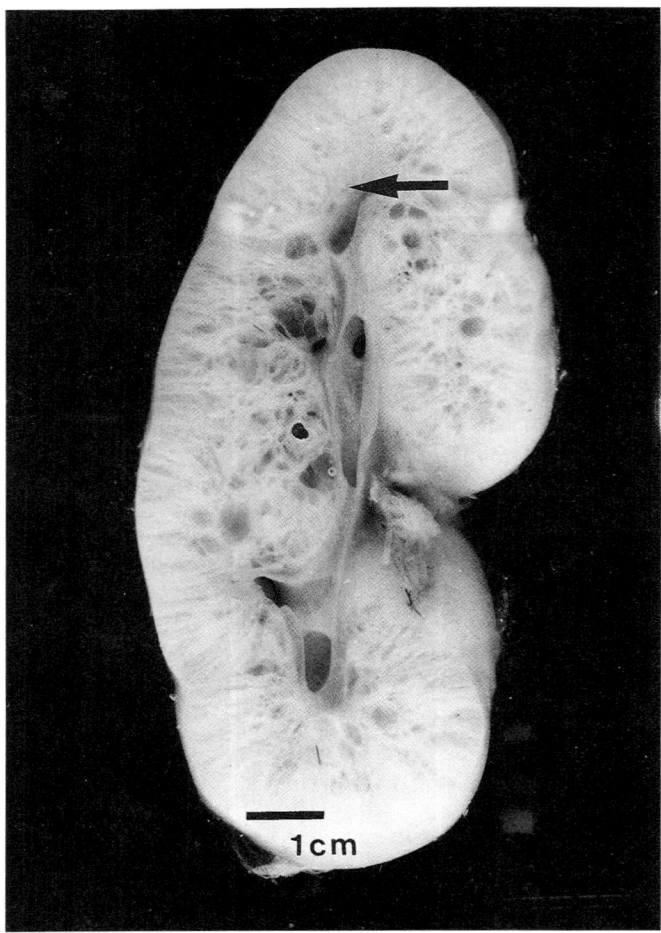

Fig. 19.3 Infantile polycystic kidney. Right kidney with radial honeycomb pattern of uniform-sized cysts formed from the collecting tubules.

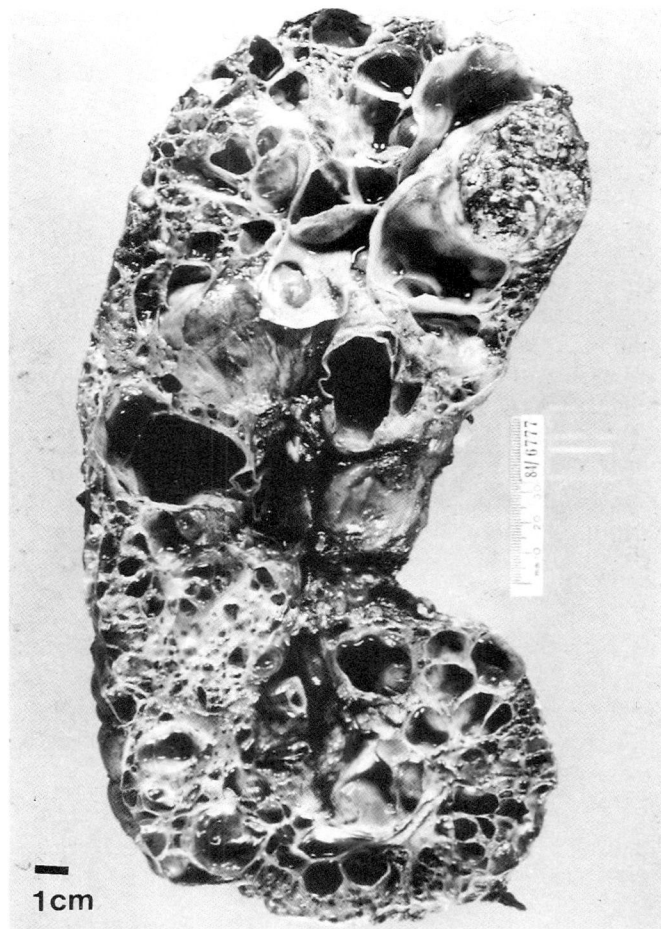

Fig. 19.4 Adult polycystic kidney. A greatly enlarged kidney with spherical cysts up to 6 cm in diameter, and dark areas of haemorrhage.

The cysts may be detected by ultrasound in asymptomatic patients, but the usual presentation is in the fourth decade with hypertension or haematuria, which proceed to renal failure within a decade. Some patients present with subarachnoid haemorrhage, since about 1 in 6 of the patients have a berry aneurysm. As in infantile polycystic kidney, cysts of the liver and biliary duct hamartomata may be found.

Multicystic kidney disease in transplant patients

With increasing numbers of renal transplant patients, it has been found that residual kidneys in patients whose primary disease was not adult polycystic kidney undergo fibrosis and cyst formation. Multiple small tubular adenomas develop and some of these may become malignant, leading to an increased incidence of renal cell carcinoma.

Solitary renal cysts

Cysts lined with a simple cuboidal epithelium are common in the cortex. They are filled with clear watery fluid and may reach

a diameter of 5–10 cm. They are occasionally mistaken for malignant tumours but are readily detected with ultrasound.

19.2.6 Medullary cystic diseases

There are two diseases in which cysts are found in the medulla.

Medullary sponge kidney

This is a common disorder with a male predominance. The lesions are usually bilateral. Diagnosis is generally made by radiology, which shows the presence of clumps of contrast medium in the medulla.

Most patients are in the 40–60 age-group, and present with renal colic, dysuria, or haematuria as a result of the passage of small stones. Renal failure is rare.

Multiple small cysts are found in the medullary collecting tubules. These are lined by columnar or cuboidal epithelium (Fig. 19.5). The cysts contain laminated concretions composed of calcium phosphate.

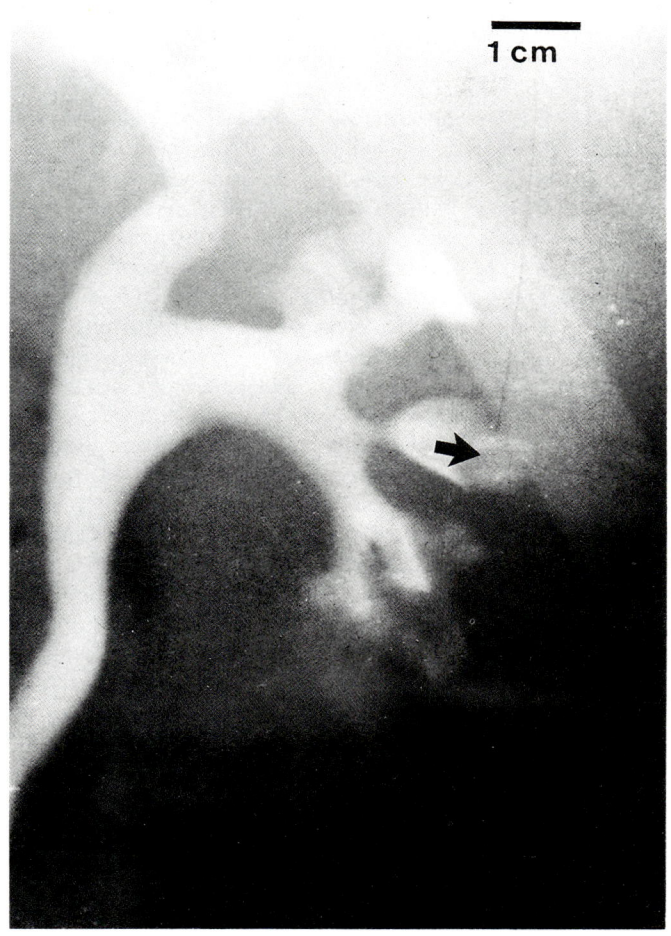

Fig. 19.5 Medullary sponge kidney. Retrograde pyelogram showing extension of contrast medium into the dilated collecting ducts.

Uraemic medullary sponge kidney

This condition is found up to the age of 20–30 years. Renal failure develops and this may be associated with a salt-losing nephropathy. A family history may be present, but the mode of inheritance is not clear.

The kidneys are small, and the medulla contains numerous cysts, similar to those found in medullary sponge kidney.

19.2.7 The congenital nephrotic syndrome

In the first year of life the chief cause of the nephrotic syndrome is inherited as an *autosomal recessive*. It follows that although there is no family history, siblings may develop the disease. This disorder can be identified in the prenatal period by a high level of α-fetoprotein in the amniotic fluid, which is not associated with spinal abnormalities. The condition is most common in Finland and is usually fatal within 1–2 years.

On examination, the kidneys show dilatation of the proximal tubules and vacuolation. Glomeruli may be enlarged and show extensive loss of the podocyte foot processes. Tubular lipid accumulation and interstitial foam cells may be found, indicative of heavy proteinuria.

19.2.8 Further reading

Risdon, R. A. (1981). Diseases of the kidney and lower urinary tract. In *Paediatric pathology* (ed. C. L. Berry), pp. 395–450. Springer-Verlag, Berlin.

19.3 Glomerulonephritis

D. R. Turner

19.3.1 General considerations

Glomerulonephritis is a major cause of chronic renal failure, requiring treatment by renal dialysis and renal transplantation. These therapies are better than the alternative (death) but may have considerable consequences for the quality of life of the individual as well as major economic consequences in health care terms.

A variety of reactions are described in the glomerulus which are included under the general term of glomerulonephritis, although the evidence of inflammation in some forms is relatively obscure. This is largely due to the specialized structure of the glomerular tuft which determines the range of possible reactions that can be elicited. In most organ systems, inflammation is a reaction that occurs predominantly in the perivascular connective tissue. There is, however, no loose areolar tissue within the normal glomerular tuft. There are two zones that need to be considered as the nearest equivalents of perivascular connective tissue; that are the region of the *glomerular capillary basement membrane*, through which the main filtration function occurs, and the central branching core of *mesangial matrix and mesangial cells* which support the capillary loops.

The normal glomerular capillary wall is modified to provide a major blood filtration function, which occurs through the *fenestrated endothelium*, the *semi-permeable basement membrane*, and the *split-pore membranes* between adjacent epithelial cell foot processes, thereby gaining access to the urinary space. Consequently, there is a very limited distance in which an inflammatory reaction could take place, but, on the other hand, the capillary walls are subject to continuous, very high blood flow rates and are therefore maximally exposed to any noxious substances that may be present in the circulation. It has also been suggested that the tortuous nature of the glomerular capillary loops may enhance the possibility of blood-borne material becoming entrapped there.

The second zone to be considered as a possible site where inflammation may occur is the mesangium. This is the

Table 19.2 Definitions of clinical presentation in glomerulonephritis

Proteinuria
  The identification of more than 0.3 g of protein in a 24 h urine specimen

Nephrotic syndrome
  Heavy proteinuria, usually in excess of 3.5 g/24 h, together with a low serum albumin and generalized oedema; hypercholesterolaemia is usually also present

Haematuria
  Any blood in the urine is abnormal; it may be microscopic or macroscopic and of either glomerular or non-glomerular origin; phase-contrast microscopy by skilled observers may assist with this distinction

Nephritic syndrome
  Haematuria together with some proteinuria; a reduction of glomerular filtration rate and a tendency to hypertension and generalized oedema

Acute renal failure
  Classically described as the sudden onset of uraemia with oliguria (less than 400 ml/24 h) but a significant proportion of cases are non-oliguria

Chronic renal failure
  A slowly developing uraemia (which, however, may present acutely in a patient with, say, dehydration from another cause)

branched supporting structure of the glomerular capillary loops and consists of a semi-permeable basement membrane-type material, or mesangial matrix, secreted by the mesangial cells which are embedded within it. The mesangial cells are modified smooth muscle cells and are thought to control the flow of blood through the glomerular capillaries.

A third potential site for inflammation is the glomerular capsule, which is directly related to the surrounding connective tissue.

Before considering the detailed aspects of how individual types of glomerulonephritis affect either the capillary walls or the mesangium, or even the glomerular capsule, the major clinical consequences of glomerular disease need to be considered. From a knowledge of glomerular structure and function, it is evident that several different effects could be induced by disease.

If the glomerular filters are damaged such that they become more permeable, they will allow protein to be lost into the urine (*proteinuria*). More severe damage will increase the proteinuria, which may be sufficient to induce a full nephrotic syndrome (Table 19.2) involving a net reduction of serum albumin and generalized oedema. If the capillary walls are disrupted by disease, red blood cells will pass into the urine, causing haematuria. When there is both an increase in general permeability of the glomerular basement membrane (proteinuria) together with leakage of red blood cells into the urine, the combination is referred to as the nephritic syndrome (Table 19.2) and may be accompanied by generalized oedema and mild hypertension.

Renal failure means a failure of the normal excretion of substances such as urea, creatinine, and potassium which then accumulate in the blood. This may be a sudden event, due to obstruction of the glomerular filters in an acute glomerulonephritis, or may develop slowly over many years as a consequence of progressive scarring of glomeruli (*chronic renal failure*).

It would be most convenient if one could deduce from the clinical presentation what form of glomerulonephritis was present. Sometimes this is possible, but frequently there are several possibilities (Table 19.3) and a renal biopsy is required to analyse the morphological features and investigate whether there are immune deposits present in the glomerular tufts. These findings can then be used to assess the prognosis for the patient and the most appropriate treatment.

Although it had originally been thought possible to classify glomerulonephritis according to the aetiological factors responsible, this has not proved to be at all satisfactory since, first, the aetiological agent can be very difficult or impossible to identify and, secondly, one agent may be capable of inducing widely different forms of glomerulonephritis. Therefore, the current classification of glomerulonephritis is based on the morphological changes seen and then subclassified according to the presence or absence of immunoglobulins and other immune reactants. This has so far proved to be the most reliable method for assessing prognosis and treatment, although it has to be appreciated that the renal biopsy only identifies what is happening at a given moment in time and may fail to predict future changes.

Table 19.3 Common modes of presentation of glomerulonephritis

	MIN. C.H.	AC. DIFF. PROLIF.	MEMBRAN.	M.C.G.N. I and II	MESANG. PROLIF.	FOCAL PROLIF.	FOCAL SEG. SCLER.	CRESC.	END-STAGE
Proteinuria	+		+		+	+	+		
Nephrotic syndrome	+		+	+	+	+	+	+	
Haematuria					+	+	+		
Nephritic syndrome		+		+		+	+		
Acute renal failure								+	
Chronic renal failure			+	+		+	+		+

MIN. C.H., Minimal change nephropathy; AC. DIFF. PROLIF., acute diffuse proliferative glomerulonephritis; MEMBRAN, membranous glomerulonephritis; M.C.G.N., mesangiocapillary glomerulonephritis; MESANG. PROLIF., mesangial proliferative glomerulonephritis; FOCAL PROLIF., focal segmental proliferative glomerulonephritis; FOCAL SEG. SCLER., focal segmental glomerulosclerosis; CRESC., diffuse crescentic glomerulonephritis.

19.3.2 The basic morphological patterns of glomerulonephritis

These are listed below:

1. minimal change nephropathy (lipoid nephrosis);
2. acute diffuse proliferative glomerulonephritis (post-infectious glomerulonephritis);
3. membranous glomerulonephritis;
4. mesangial proliferative glomerulonephritis;
5. focal segmental proliferative glomerulonephritis;
6. mesangiocapillary glomerulonephritis (membrano-proliferative glomerulonephritis);
7. diffuse crescentic glomerulonephritis;
8. focal segmental glomerulosclerosis (and hyalinosis);
9. diffuse global sclerosis (end-stage disease).

It has proved useful to define some of the terms used in the above list. Thus:

1. *Focal* is taken to mean less than 70 per cent of glomeruli affected (in a given histological section).
2. *Diffuse* is taken to mean 70 per cent or more of glomeruli affected.
3. *Segmental* is taken to mean a portion or lobule of the glomerular tuft showing obliteration of capillary lumens by disease.
4. *Global* is taken to mean that all portions of a given glomerular tuft show capillary obliteration.

19.3.3 Minimal change disease

Also known as minimal change nephropathy or lipoid nephrosis.

Typically, a young child presents with generalized oedema and is found to have heavy proteinuria (> 3.5 g/l) together with a low serum albumin (the nephrotic syndrome, Table 19.2). Despite the fact that there has been a major change in permeability of the glomerular capillary walls, the appearance of all glomeruli by light microscopy is surprisingly normal (Fig. 19.6). Detailed morphometric studies have indicated minor changes in the mesangial areas, which is why the condition is termed 'minimal change disease'. No significant deposition of immunoglobulins or complement components can be demonstrated, although in mesangial areas a minority of cases show a few flecks of IgM and C3, which are regarded as non-specific. Electron microscopy shows a change in the epithelial cells that normally make contact with the outer aspect of the glomerular capillary wall by a series of cytoplasmic projections called *foot processes* or *podocytes*. In minimal change disease the epithelial cells have reduced their surface area by withdrawing their foot processes, with the result that the cell bodies are applied directly to the external aspect of the capillary basement membrane (Fig. 19.7). This appears to represent the basic withdrawal response of a cell that has been damaged: therefore, it is not surprising to

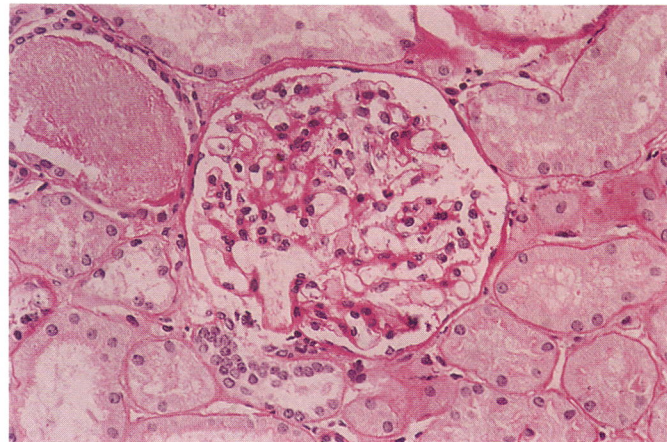

Fig. 19.6 Minimal change disease with a glomerulus showing no abnormal features by light microscopy. (PAS.)

find that it is a non-specific effect which occurs in other forms of glomerular disease.

Experimental studies in rats, using an aminonucleoside called *puromycin*, which is a glomerular poison, have shown that a nephrotic syndrome can readily be induced with minimal morphological changes. The same loss of epithelial cell foot processes is seen by electron microscopy. In the human disease the 'toxic' material responsible has not so far been identified, although there is evidence of T-lymphocyte dysfunction and lymphokines could be responsible for the altered permeability of the glomerular capillary wall (Silva and Hogg 1989). A variety of aetiological factors have been proposed, suggesting that a circulating inflammatory substance is responsible for the change in permeability of the glomerular capillary basement membrane. A small proportion of cases does show an association between minimal change disease and allergies to bee stings and pollen.

The normal glomerular capillary wall bears a heavy negative charge due to the presence of molecules such as *heparan sulphate* and *sialic acid*. There is evidence of a reduction of this charge in puromycin nephropathy, which would presumably allow negatively charged proteins such as albumin to pass through more readily than normal.

Corticosteroid drugs are used to control minimal change disease in the human and are usually effective within 8 weeks. This is due, in part at least, to their known effect of reducing capillary permeability. The prognosis for minimal change disease is excellent in that although recurrent episodes are common, progression to renal failure is unknown. In severe attacks patients may be vulnerable to episodes of shock as a consequence of hypovolaemia due to massive protein loss. Heavy protein loss also leads to an increased susceptibility to infection. Although the typical patient affected is a young child, minimal change disease can occur at any age.

The alternative name of 'lipoid nephrosis' describes the considerable accumulation of lipids that may occur in the proximal convoluted tubule and in the urine. This corresponds to the

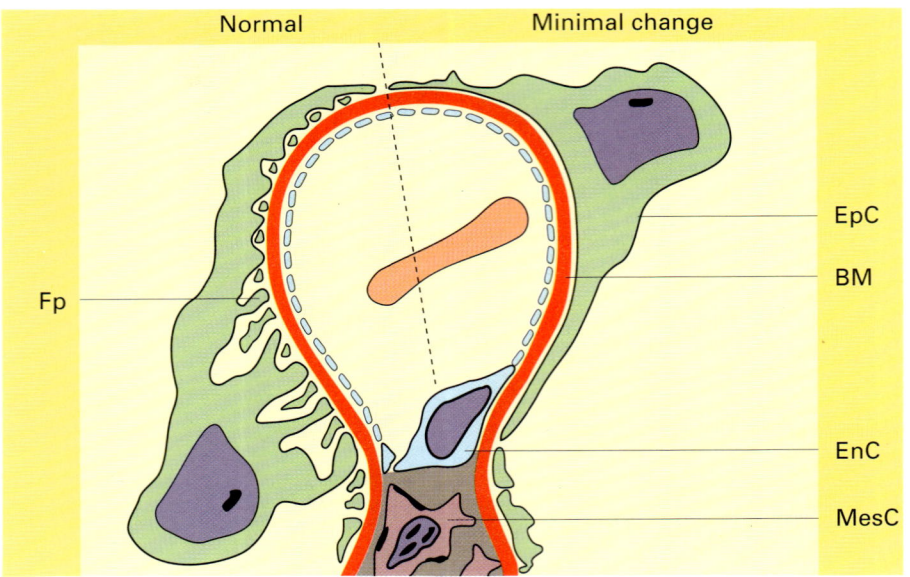

Normal   Minimal change

Fp

EpC

BM

EnC

MesC

Fig. 19.7 Diagrammatic representation of a glomerular capillary loop to contrast normal foot processes on the left with so-called 'fusion' of foot processes in minimal change disease. EpC, Epithelial cell; BM, basement membrane; EnC, endothelial cell; MesC, mesangial cell; Fp, foot process.

hyperlipidaemia, which is due to an increased secretion of lipoproteins by the liver, due in turn to the low oncotic pressure caused by heavy albuminuria.

19.3.4 Acute diffuse proliferative glomerulonephritis

Also known as acute post-infectious glomerulonephritis or acute diffuse endocapillary glomerulonephritis.

This is an important condition in terms of understanding glomerular disease but is now relatively uncommon in Europe. Classically, the patient has a history of a sore throat followed some 10 days or so later by feeling generally unwell with haematuria, proteinuria, hypertension, and some generalized oedema ('nephritic syndrome'). *Group A streptococcal infection* was thought to be the main cause of this phenomenon but a variety of other organisms, including *Streptococcus pneumoniae*, staphylococci, and viruses, may occasionally induce the same response. All glomeruli show dramatic changes by light microscopy (Fig. 19.8), with marked hypercellularity due to a combination of infiltration by neutrophils and monocytes and proliferation of cells intrinsic to the glomerular tuft (mesangial cells particularly). Immune complexes accumulate in the glomerular capillary walls (subepithelial site particularly) and are thought to be responsible for recruiting the neutrophils and monocytes (Fig. 19.9). Since the inflammatory cells remain for the most part within the capillary lumens and there is swelling of the endothelial cell cytoplasm, the blood flow through the tuft may be sufficiently impeded to cause acute renal failure in severe cases. However, despite the apparent ferocity of the process, complete resolution is the usual outcome, although it may take many months before the glomeruli are morphologically normal. Occasionally a *diffuse crescentic glomerulonephritis* may develop in the acute phase on top of the basic process of endo-

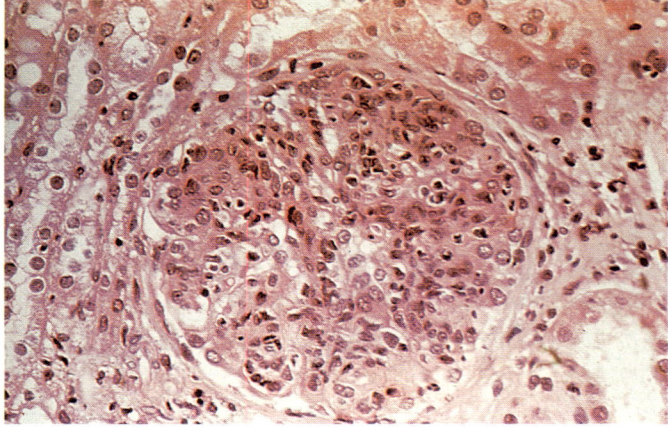

Fig. 19.8 Hypercellular glomerular tuft in acute diffuse proliferative glomerulonephritis. (Silver impregnation, H & E counterstain.)

capillary proliferation. This proliferation of epithelial cells may also occur in association with several different forms of glomerulonephritis and is described in more detail under the heading 'Diffuse crescentic glomerulonephritis' (see Section 19.3.9).

The best experimental model of acute proliferative glomerulonephritis is *acute serum sickness* which can be induced in rabbits by a single large dose of bovine serum albumin injected intravenously (Wilson and Dixon 1986). As the rabbit's antibody levels rise (around 7–10 days) so antigen in the circulation is bound to form immune complexes of various sizes. Large complexes tend to be taken up by the macrophage/monocyte phagocytic system and are removed from the circulation, but intermediate-sized complexes are deposited in the mesangial and subendothelial areas of glomeruli, where activated complement components attract neutrophil pholymorphs and macrophages. Small complexes seem to pass through the glo-

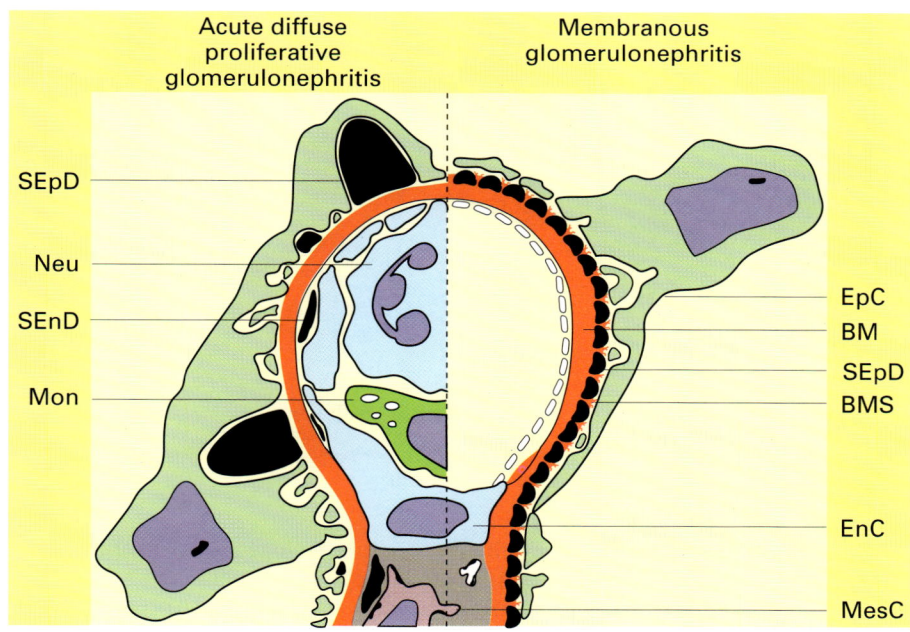

Fig. 19.9 Diagrammatic representation of a glomerular capillary loop to contrast changes seen in acute diffuse proliferative glomerulonephritis with membranous glomerulonephritis. SEpD, subepithelial deposit; Neu, neutrophil; SEnD, subendothelial deposit; mon, monocyte; BMS, basement membrane 'spike'; BM, basement membrane; EnC, endothelial cell; MesC, mesangial cell.

merular capillary basement membranes and accumulate in the subepithelial position. In fact, many of these small immune complexes dissociate and reaggregate in order to reach the subepithelial position, though whether they all do is not established. Other factors that may encourage the formation of subepithelial deposits are the markedly anionic nature (negative charge) of the outer layer of the glomerular capillary basement membrane and the cationic nature (positive charge) of some immune reactants. In addition, it has been demonstrated that low-affinity antibody is more likely to be associated with the formation of subepithelial deposits, probably because the immune complexes will more readily dissociate and this then facilitates their passage through the glomerular capillary basement membrane.

In the human disease the presumption is that a bacterial antigen takes the place of the foreign antigen. Immune deposits of IgG, C3, and C1q can be localized by both immunocytochemical studies and by electron microscopy to the external aspect of the glomerular capillary basement membrane in particular, but are also to be found in the subendothelial space and mesangial matrix (Fig. 19.9). Electron microscopy shows large electron-dense masses at these sites, consisting of a complex lattice of IgG, C1q, and C3, together with the relevant antigen. However, elution studies to isolate and identify the antigen have proved to be very difficult, which may mean that the relative proportion of antigen present is very small (perhaps less than 1 per cent). In view of the large size of the 'deposits', one must assume that they develop by accretion *in situ*, with the constituent components passing through the glomerular capillary basement membrane which has been rendered more permeable by the inflammatory process. Total haemolytic complement and C3 are low in the serum during the first 2 weeks of the illness, indicating their involvement in the acute process before return-

ing to normal levels. Indeed, the acute episode relates to a critical event in the immune process where antibody levels are rising at the same time as antigen is progressively being eliminated, so the tendency to deposit immune complex components in the glomeruli is short-lived and the patient soon begins to recover. In morphological terms there may be significant mesangial cell proliferation with some increase in mesangial matrix material, and this may persist for many months, along with mesangial deposits of C3 and some minor proteinuria. Although the long-term prognosis is considered to be excellent, some examples of residual focal glomerular scarring have been seen in cases biopsied many years later.

19.3.5 Membranous glomerulonephritis

The usual presentation of this relatively common form of glomerulonephritis is either with the nephrotic syndrome or isolated proteinuria. The incidence of membranous glomerulonephritis is much higher in adults than in children and the cause is usually not identified. However, about 20 per cent of cases are associated with a specific antigen in the circulation, as in persistent hepatitis B, Epstein–Barr virus infections, and tumour antigens in malignant disease (Table 19.4).

Table 19.4 Antigens that have been shown to induce membranous nephropathy

Antigens from neoplasms
Penicillamine
Gold
Hepatitis B
Epstein–Barr virus infection
Mercury
Syphilis

Early glomerular changes can be difficult to identify using conventional light microscopy, since increased thickness of the glomerular capillary walls which develops in all glomeruli can be quite subtle at first. However, modern techniques of immunocytochemistry readily demonstrate the presence of immune reactants such as IgG and C3, and other immunoglobulins may also be present. The immune deposits are identified on the external aspect of the glomerular capillary wall, forming a pattern of fine granules outlining the glomerular capillary loops (Fig. 19.10). By electron microscopy the immune deposits appear as large, electron-dense masses on the external aspect of the glomerular capillary basement membrane beneath the epithelial cells, which often show some loss of the normal foot processes (see Fig. 19.9).

A surprising feature of membranous glomerulonephritis is the lack of an inflammatory cellular reaction despite the presence of immune complexes, which is, of course, in marked contrast to what occurs in acute diffuse proliferative glomerulonephritis. Thus, there is no infiltration of the glomerular tuft by neutrophils or monocytes, no endothelial cell swelling, and no mesangial cell proliferation, despite the activation of complement which has been shown to be responsible for the proteinuria that occurs (Fig. 19.11). Perhaps the subepithelial location of the deposits is sufficiently separate from the circulating blood that neutrophils are not attracted. The only glomerular reaction of note is the increased production of glomerular capillary basement-membrane material, which results in a series of projections or 'spikes' extending outwards between adjacent subepithelial immune deposits (see Fig. 19.9). These 'spikes' can be impregnated with silver for identification by light microscopy and contribute to the main morphological feature of the disease, namely, a *diffuse thickening of glomerular capillary walls*. In more advanced cases, the basement membrane thickening may completely envelope the immune deposits.

Membranous glomerulonephritis is generally regarded as a chronic immune-complex disease. Evidence from several different experiments strongly suggests that the immune complexes are formed *in situ* on the external aspect of the glomerular capillary basement membrane, as a consequence of circulating

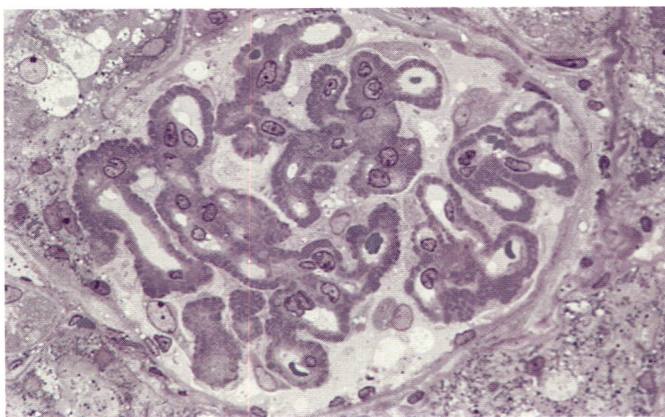

Fig. 19.11 Membranous glomerulonephritis. Resin-embedded section stained with toluidine blue.

antibodies reacting with either endogenous glomerular antigens or antigens implanted from the circulation.

Heymann nephritis is a well-established model of membranous glomerulonephritis which has been investigated in considerable detail by many workers (Eddy and Michael 1989). It can be induced in rats by immunizing them with a homogenate of kidney cortex from homologous rats. Antibodies are formed to an antigen which is normally located in the brush border of renal proximal convoluted tubular cells. It is referred to as the *Heymann antigen* and is a glycoprotein of molecular weight 330 kDa, which has also been identified on the cell membrane of the glomerular epithelial cell foot processes. Thus, if circulating antibodies to the Heymann antigen can penetrate the glomerular capillary basement membrane, they will encounter the Heymann antigen in the subepithelial position, which is precisely where the immune deposits develop. It has been suggested that the Heymann antigen on the glomerular epithelial cells represents an *endocytosis receptor*, which could explain the granular localization of the subepithelial deposits.

In idiopathic membranous glomerulonephritis, approximately 75 per cent of cases process slowly to chronic renal failure over several years, with the development of *glomerular sclerosis*, *focal tubular atrophy*, and *interstitial fibrosis*. The other 25 per cent appear to remit spontaneously, with loss of proteinuria, dissolution of the electron-dense deposits, and gradual restoration of the thickened basement membrane to normal. The failure to fully appreciate this variable outcome has confused the interpretation of some major therapeutic trials. Where a known antigen or hapten can be eliminated, the membranous glomerulonephritis can be expected to resolve, with gradual reduction of the proteinuria and return to normal glomerular morphology over a period of several months.

19.3.6 Mesangial proliferative glomerulonephritis

This form of glomerular damage represents the simplest proliferative change, which can be induced by a wide range of disease

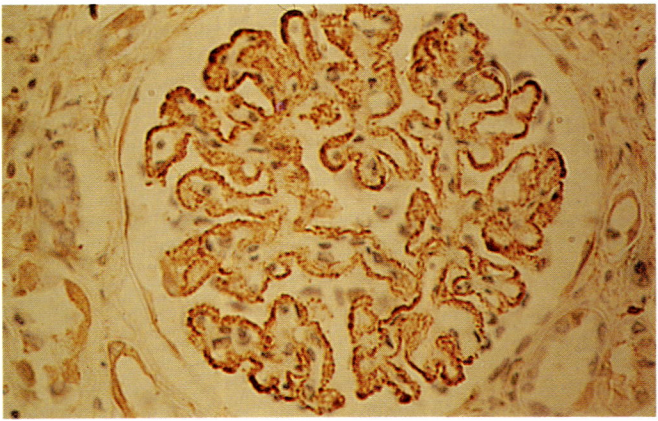

Fig. 19.10 Membranous glomerulonephritis, stained with anti-IgG and revealed with peroxidase.

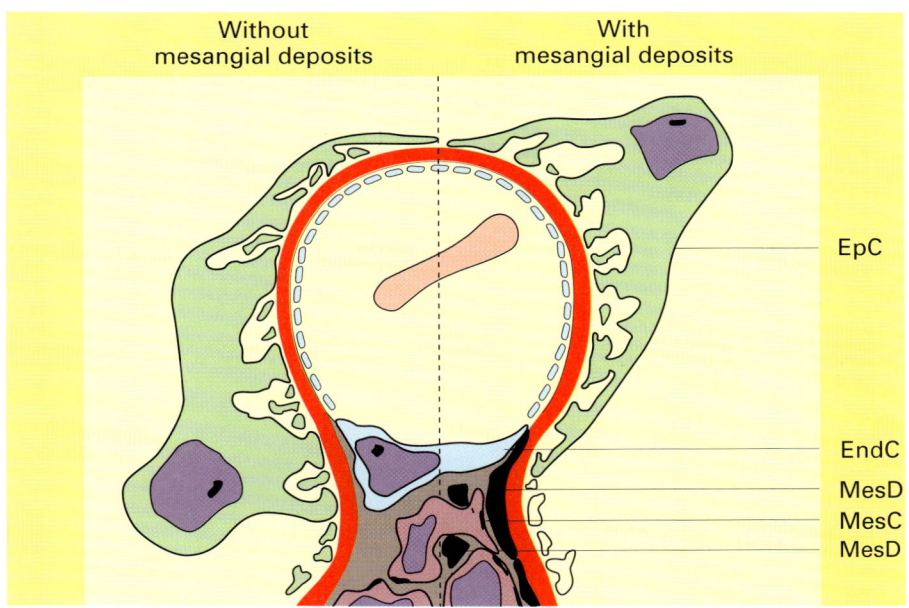

Without mesangial deposits

With mesangial deposits

EpC

EndC
MesD
MesC
MesD

Fig. 19.12 Diagrammatic representation of a glomerular capillary loop in mesangial proliferative glomerulonephritis with and without mesangial immune deposits. EpC, Epithelial cell; EndC, endothelial cell; MesC, mesangial cell; MesD, mesangial deposit.

processes, including *IgA disease, Henoch–Schönlein syndrome, systemic lupus erythematosus, bacterial endocarditis, shunt nephritis,* and *Alport's syndrome.* Most, if not all, glomeruli show a widening of the mesangial stalk, which may be due to an increase in matrix, mesangial cells, immune deposits, or a combination of these (Fig. 19.12). In practice, it may be difficult to separate mild mesangial proliferation from normal glomeruli by conventional light microscopical techniques, particularly in badly prepared renal biopsy material. The insistence on well-stained thin sections is essential for accurate assessment (Fig. 19.13). In reality, the finding of immunoglobulins and complement in the mesangial areas using immune studies will often confirm the impression of mesangial proliferation and thereby solve the dilemma. Furthermore, the nature of the immunoglobulins will give a strong indication of the precise nature of

the disease process that has induced the mesangial reaction (Fig. 19.14).

The mesangial region is peculiarly available to access by molecules within the circulation, since there is no basement membrane between the lumen of the glomerular capillary and the mesangial matrix. Experimental studies have shown that macromolecules readily accumulate within the mesangial matrix after injection into the circulation. It is no great surprise to find that immune complexes, particularly those formed with high-affinity antibody, can also enter and be deposited in the mesangial matrix. Experimentally, it has been shown that immunizing mice by the oral route with ovalbumin causes a rise in serum IgA levels, and IgA deposits develop in the mesangium in the majority of cases (Emancipator *et al.* 1983). This phenomenon was enhanced by reticuloendothelial blockade. If a monoclonal antibody prepared against Thy-1 antigen (which is also present on normal rat mesangial cells) is injected into rats, a florid mesangial reaction develops with heavy proteinuria (Wilson *et al.* 1988). The mesangial matrix is disrupted and subsequently cell proliferation occurs. Thus, either or both of these mechanisms involving preformed immune complexes or antibody directed against mesangial antigens could induce a mesangial proliferative glomerulonephritis.

Mesangial proliferative glomerulonephritis may be associated with *proteinuria,* a *nephritic syndrome,* or even a *full nephrotic syndrome,* which perhaps indicates the depth of current ignorance of the basic causes of these phenomena.

IgA nephropathy

The most well-recognized form of mesangial proliferative disease is characterized by the presence of IgA in the mesangium of all glomeruli, without clinical evidence of involvement of other organs. Biopsies in which there is also segmental involvement of capillary loops would be classified as a *focal proliferative*

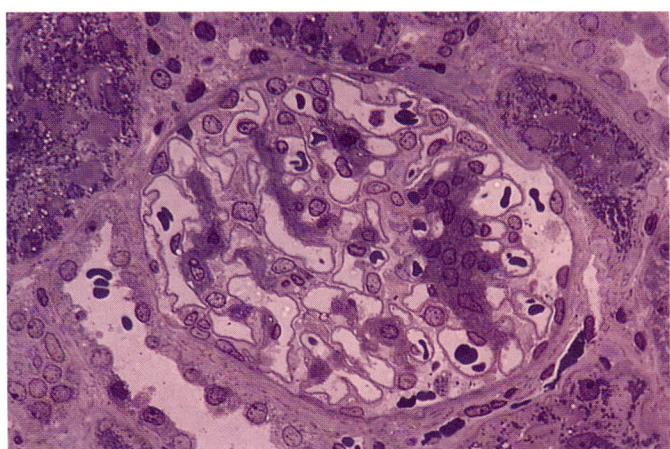

Fig. 19.13 Mesangial proliferative glomerulonephritis. Resin-embedded section stained with toluidine blue.

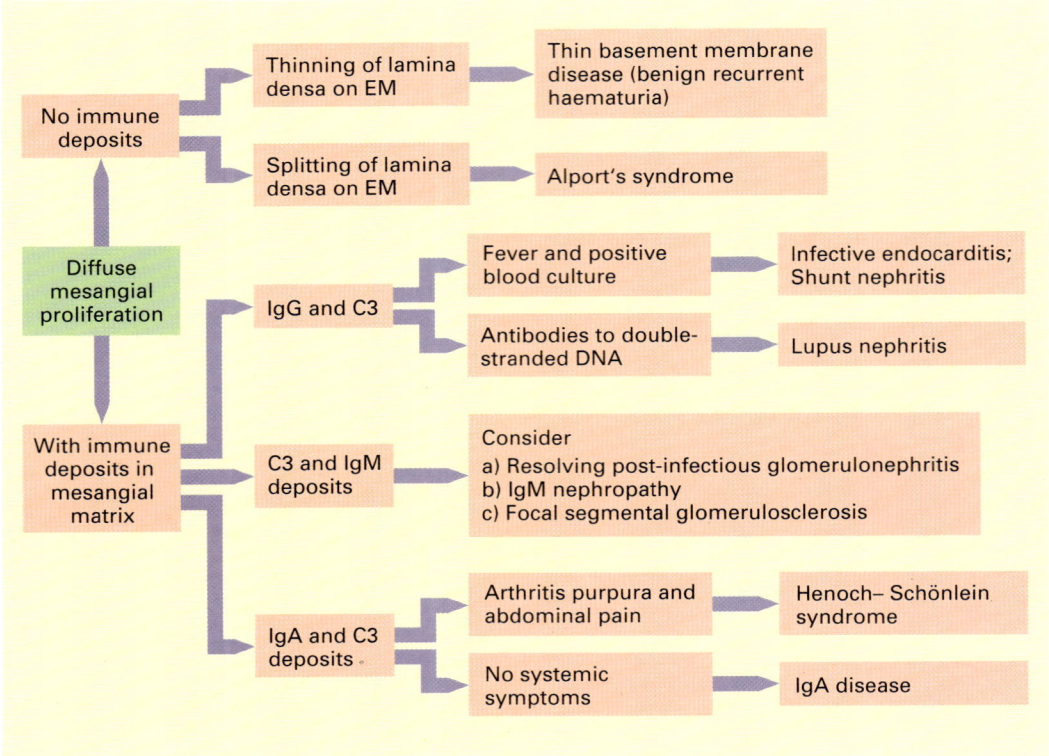

Fig. 19.14   Analysis of mesangial proliferative glomerulonephritis.

glomerulonephritis (see Section 19.3.7). In either case, the patients (particularly children) commonly present with a clinical syndrome of recurrent attacks of macroscopic haematuria triggered by a sore throat or other infective illness. In adults, IgA nephropathy may occur without macroscopic haematuria and, instead, may present either because hypertension or proteinuria are detected on routine testing, or a full nephrotic syndrome may develop.

The association of gastrointestinal diseases such as cirrhosis, coeliac disease, and tonsillitis with IgA disease could explain the raised serum levels of IgA which are frequently recorded. The presence of IgG, IgA, and C3 in the mesangial deposits suggests that immune complexes are being formed, and recent evidence suggests that, in some cases at least, the IgG is specifically directed against mesangial antigens, which could explain the mesangial proliferation.

The general view of IgA nephropathy is that it has a good prognosis, particularly when the disease is limited to mesangial areas. Overall, this is true, although a significant proportion (10–20 per cent) of patients develop more severe glomerular disease, together with proteinuria and hypertension, leading finally to chronic renal failure; consequently a guarded prognosis is necessary in the presence of proteinuria and hypertension. IgA disease is a common form of glomerulonephritis, but many children with recurrent haematuria alone are not sub-jected to renal biopsy and such cases will not therefore appear in pathological analyses.

19.3.7   Focal segmental proliferative (and necrotizing) glomerulonephritis

This term includes two different basic patterns of glomerular reaction which superficially resemble each other. One represents an exaggeration of diffuse mesangial proliferative glomerulonephritis described above, in which the same range of mesangial reactions with immune deposits has extended segmentally in the subendothelial spaces into one or more lobules of some glomeruli, so that the capillary loops of some segments of a proportion of glomeruli are occluded (Fig. 19.15). This mesangial proliferative type is therefore associated with a similar range of clinical conditions, *Henoch–Schönlein disease, systemic lupus, bacterial endocarditis, shunt nephritis*, as well as IgA disease (Fig. 19.16). Since the mesangial proliferation is diffuse, the term 'focal' is perhaps misleading but is well established.

The other variety of focal proliferative glomerulonephritis lacks demonstrable immune deposits in the glomerular tuft and lacks generalized mesangial cell proliferation. The segmental lesions are often *necrotizing*, showing leakage of fibrin into the urinary space and *crescent formation* due to epithelial cell proliferation. The remainder of the glomerular tuft appears starkly

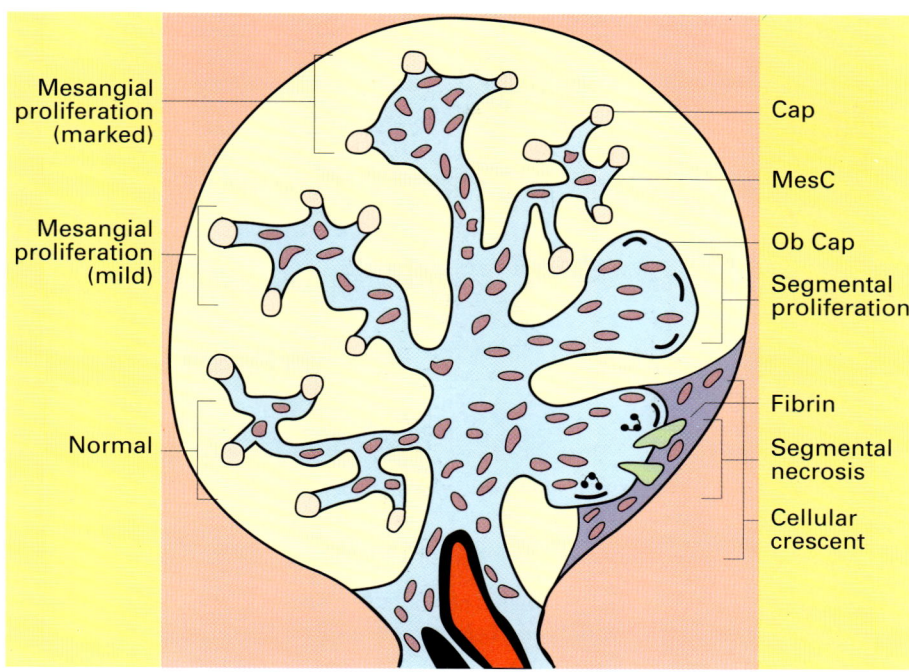

Mesangial proliferation (marked)

Mesangial proliferation (mild)

Normal

Cap

MesC

Ob Cap

Segmental proliferation

Fibrin

Segmental necrosis

Cellular crescent

Fig. 19.15 Diagrammatic representation of a glomerulus, showing varying degrees of mesangial proliferation, the formation of segmental lesions, and segmental necrosis with crescent formation. Cap, Capillary; MesC, mesangial cell; ObCap, obliterated capillary loop.

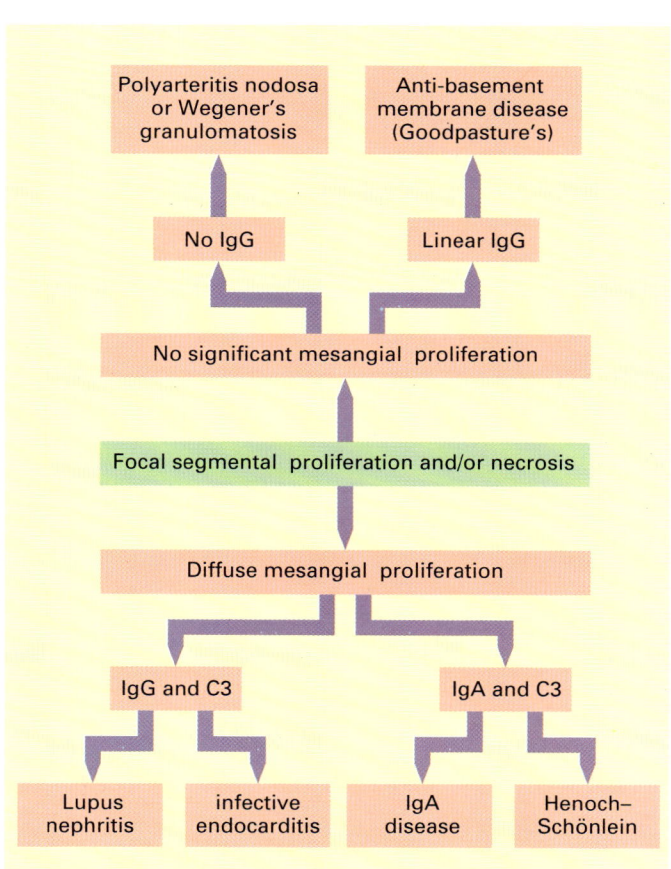

Polyarteritis nodosa or Wegener's granulomatosis

Anti-basement membrane disease (Goodpasture's)

No IgG

Linear IgG

No significant mesangial proliferation

Focal segmental proliferation and/or necrosis

Diffuse mesangial proliferation

IgG and C3

IgA and C3

Lupus nephritis

infective endocarditis

IgA disease

Henoch–Schönlein

Fig. 19.16 Analysis of focal segmental proliferative glomerulonephritis.

normal by comparison (Fig. 19.17). This form of focal segmental glomerulonephritis is usually associated with *polyarteritis nodosa*, *Wegener's granulomatosis*, and *Goodpasture's syndrome* (or anti-basement membrane disease), and is more truly 'focal'.

19.3.8 Mesangiocapillary glomerulonephritis (membrano-proliferative glomerulonephritis)

This section deals with a diffuse pattern of severe glomerular alteration which may be associated with a variety of systemic disorders, such as *systemic lupus, haemolytic-uraemic syndrome, shunt nephritis, IgA disease,* and *cryoglobulinaemia,* or may occur in an idiopathic form with only renal involvement (Table 19.5). The majority of idiopathic cases (about 80 per cent) are included under the term *type I,* or *subendothelial deposit type of mesangiocapillary glomerulonephritis.* The minority group is termed *type II mesangiocapillary glomerulonephritis,* or *linear dense deposit disease.* Although the presentation, course, and outcome of these two conditions are similar, there are some significant differences in morphology and associated aspects.

Type I: mesangiocapillary glomerulonephritis (subendothelial deposit type)

Typically an adolescent or young adult presents with a nephrotic syndrome (haematuria and proteinuria) and low serum C3 levels, perhaps following a sore throat, and is presumed to have an acute diffuse proliferative glomerulonephritis (postinfectious glomerulonephritis). However, instead of resolving over the next few weeks as anticipated, the proteinuria

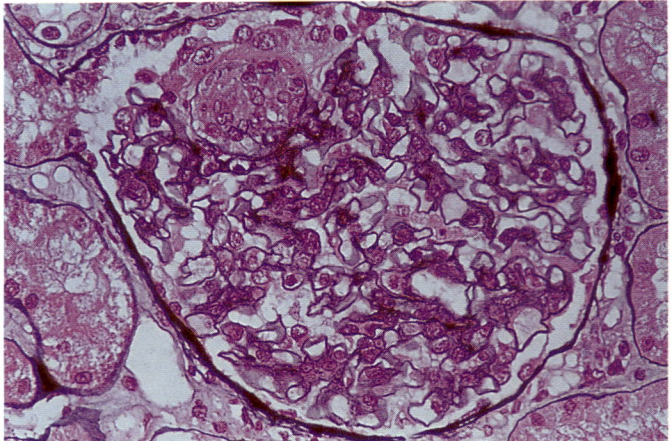

Fig. 19.17 A segmental proliferative and necrotizing lesion with relative normality of the remainder of the glomerular tuft. (Silver impregnation, H & E counterstain.)

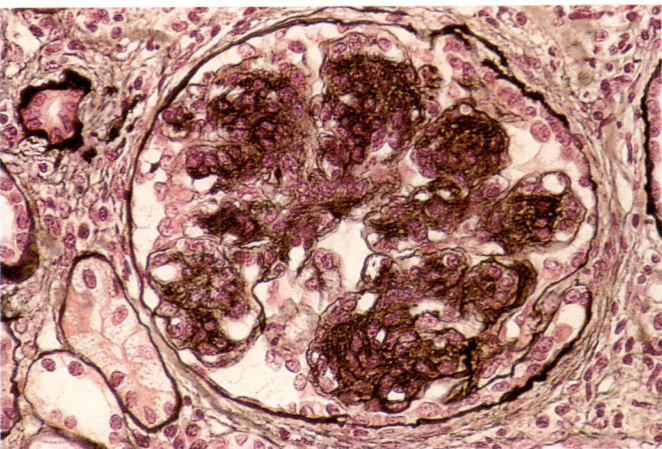

Fig. 19.18 Mesangiocapillary glomerulonephritis type I with marked lobular pattern. (Silver impregnation, H & E counterstain.)

increases and a full nephrotic syndrome is likely to develop. A renal biopsy is necessary to establish whether a mesangiocapillary pattern of glomerulonephritis is present. This shows a profound modification of glomerular structure, with marked mesangial cell proliferation and a corresponding increase in the surrounding mesangial matrix, which considerably enhances the lobular arrangement of the normal glomerular tuft (Fig. 19.18). In addition, the capillary walls are thickened to several times their original width by a complicated process of complement deposition and extension around the capillary loops of mesangial cell processes, which have subsequently secreted an additional layer of matrix material in the subendothelial zone (Fig. 19.19). The cellularity of the glomerular tufts may be further increased by infiltrating neutrophils and monocytes, and sometimes by epithelial cell proliferation forming crescents. Silver impregnation methods demonstrate a double-layer or 'tram-track' appearance of the glomerular capillary wall by light microscopy, which is characteristic (but only *diagnostic* of mesangiocapillary disease when it is widespread).

The complement deposits appear electron dense by electron microscopy, and are most obvious in the subendothelial position, where they can be of considerable size. Smaller dense deposits may also be identified in the mesangium and occasionally

in the subepithelial position. In all of these sites lesser quantities of IgG, IgM, and IgA may also be identified.

The aetiology and pathogenesis of type I mesangiocapillary glomerulonephritis are unclear but a few clues have been identified. Thus patients often have low levels of C3 in the serum, and the blood often contains an auto-antibody (called *C3 nephritic factor*) which can break down C3, resulting in persistent complement activation. As mentioned above, C3 is a major constituent of the subendothelial deposits and there is circumstantial evidence that the alternative pathway of complement activation is involved, since *properdin* can often be identified in the complement deposits. In many cases there is also circumstantial evidence of immune complex formation and involvement of the classical pathway of complement activation. The precise relationship, however, between these observations remains unclear.

Type II: mesangiocapillary glomerulonephritis (linear dense deposit type)

This variety of mesangiocapillary glomerulonephritis has a similar clinical presentation to type I but, in addition, some patients also have a *partial lipodystrophy* (absence of subcutaneous fat in the upper half of the body), which, along with the

Table 19.5 Analysis of mesangiocapillary glomerular alteration

Type I		Type II	(Type III)
Idiopathic	Secondary to		
Large subendothelial deposits containing C3 predominantly but also some IgG in most cases	(1) Infective endocarditis and shunt nephritis (2) Lupus nephritis (3) Henoch–Schönlein syndrome (4) Haemolytic-uraemic (5) Toxaemia of pregnancy (6) Scleroderma	Linear dense deposit recurs in transplants, may be associated with partial lipodystrophy	Similar to Type I but with the addition of subepithelial (membranous) deposits. Probably should be included in with the Type I

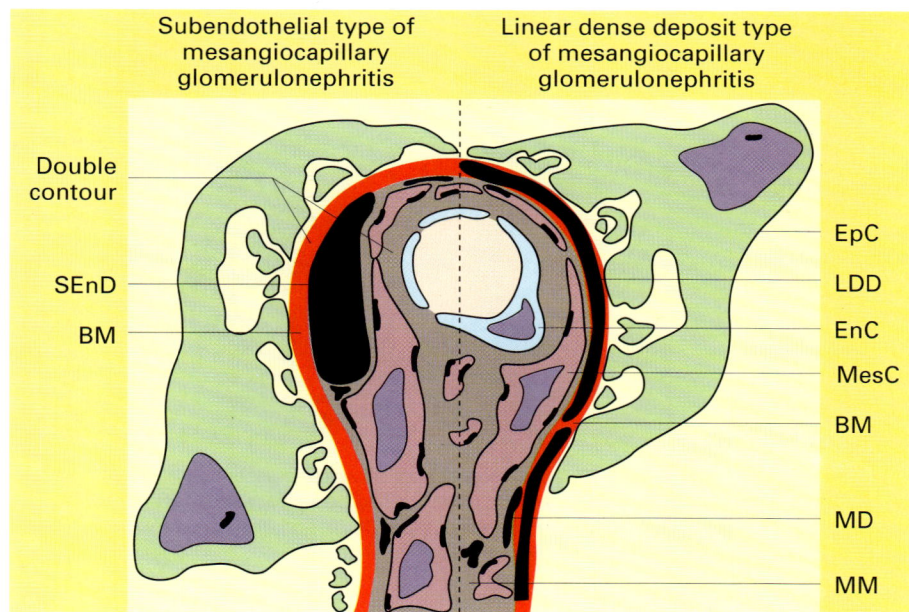

Fig. **19.19** Diagrammatic representation of a glomerular capillary loop, contrasting the changes seen in mesangiocapillary glomerulonephritis of the subendothelial deposit type with the linear dense deposit type. SEnD, Subendothelial deposit; MesC, mesangial cell; EpC, epithelial cell; LDD, linear dense deposit; EnC, endothelial cell; MD, mesangial deposit; MM, mesangial matrix; BM, basement membrane.

low serum C3, may precede the onset of renal symptoms by several months or even years. The morphological features show a superficial similarity to the type I pattern, with mesangial cell proliferation and marked capillary wall thickening due largely to mesangial cell interposition; however, the electron-dense deposited material, instead of being in the subendothelial zone is located within the substance of the glomerular capillary basement membrane (Fig. 19.19). Silver impregnation largely fails to demonstrate the original basement membrane so that only the irregular new layer of matrix material secreted by the mesangial cell process is clearly shown. Indeed, the appearance of the glomerular capillary walls may be confused with a late-stage membranous pattern, particularly when the mesangial proliferation is relatively mild (Fig. 19.20).

The linear dense deposit can also be demonstrated within the basement membrane of Bowman's capsule and the first part of the proximal convoluted tubule. Immune studies show posivity for complement only and, even then, there are suggestions that it is only the surface of the dense deposit which reacts. Some further electron-dense deposits may also be found within the mesangial matrix and occasionally in the subepithelial position.

The association of low levels of C3 in the serum, the presence of C3 nephritic factor, and the identification of complement in the linear dense deposits suggests that continued complement activation by C3 nephritic factor is an important pathogenetic mechanism (Donadio 1988).

The clinical course for both types of mesangiocapillary glomerulonephritis is much the same, with about a 50 per cent survival at 10 years, despite the use of a range of therapeutic regimes, involving anti-inflammatory agents, anti-platelet drugs, and alternate-day steriods, which all have their protagonists. Both types may recur following renal transplantation, and it is the linear deposit type which is particularly prone to do this. Surprisingly, the linear deposit is often not accompanied by the rest of the glomerular changes, and if renal function deteriorates, it is mainly due to rejection rather than recurrent disease.

As was mentioned at the beginning of this section, a mesangiocapillary pattern of glomerulonephritis may develop in association with a range of other disorders in which deposited material accumulates in the subendothelial zone of the glomerulus. In the majority of these cases there is strong evidence of a chronic antigenaemia and immune-complex deposition (systemic lupus, chronic liver disease with IgA deposition, cryoglobulinaemia, and shunt nephritis). In other cases, such as the *haemolytic-uraemic syndrome* and *pre-eclampsia*, there is evidence of fibrin deposition in the subendothelial zone. Thus, with the

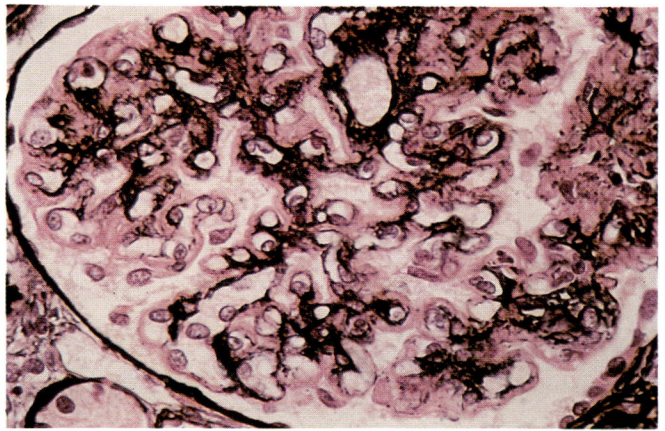

Fig. **19.20** Mesangiocapillary glomerulonephritis type II. (Silver impregnation, H & E counterstain.)

exception of linear dense deposit disease, the mesangiocapillary pattern seems to develop under conditions where either complement, immune complexes, fibrin, or a combination of these are continually deposited in the subendothelial zone of glomeruli.

19.3.9   Diffuse crescentic glomerulonephritis

At one time this pattern of glomerular disease was called rapidly progressive glomerulonephritis and that is certainly how it tends to behave clinically. From the morphological aspect, the striking feature is the massive proliferation of cells in Bowman's space, affecting a high percentage of glomeruli (Fig. 19.21). There has been controversy about the precise cellular constitution of these crescentic masses of cells, which seem to develop as a consequence of leakage of fibrin into the urinary space. Certainly, they comprise both epithelial cells and macrophages, the proportion of the latter increasing with the severity of the disease process.

Diffuse crescentic glomerulonephritis represents a particularly severe form of the several basic types of glomerulonephritis described, but the dramatic appearance of cellular crescents may mean that the associated glomerular tuft changes are overlooked. In fact, diffuse crescentic change may complicate acute diffuse proliferative glomerulonephritis, mesangiocapillary nephritis (both type I and type II), and any of the varieties of

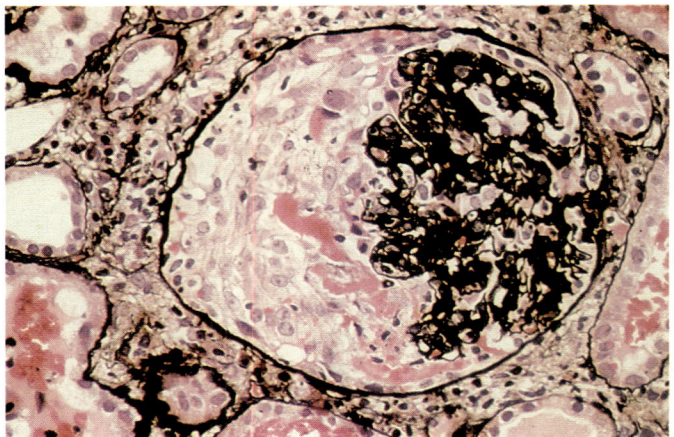

Fig. 19.21   Glomerulus from a case of crescentic glomerulonephritis, with half Bowman's capsule filled by a crescentic mass of proliferating epithelial cells admixed with fibrin and inflammatory cells. (Silver impregnation, H & E counterstain.)

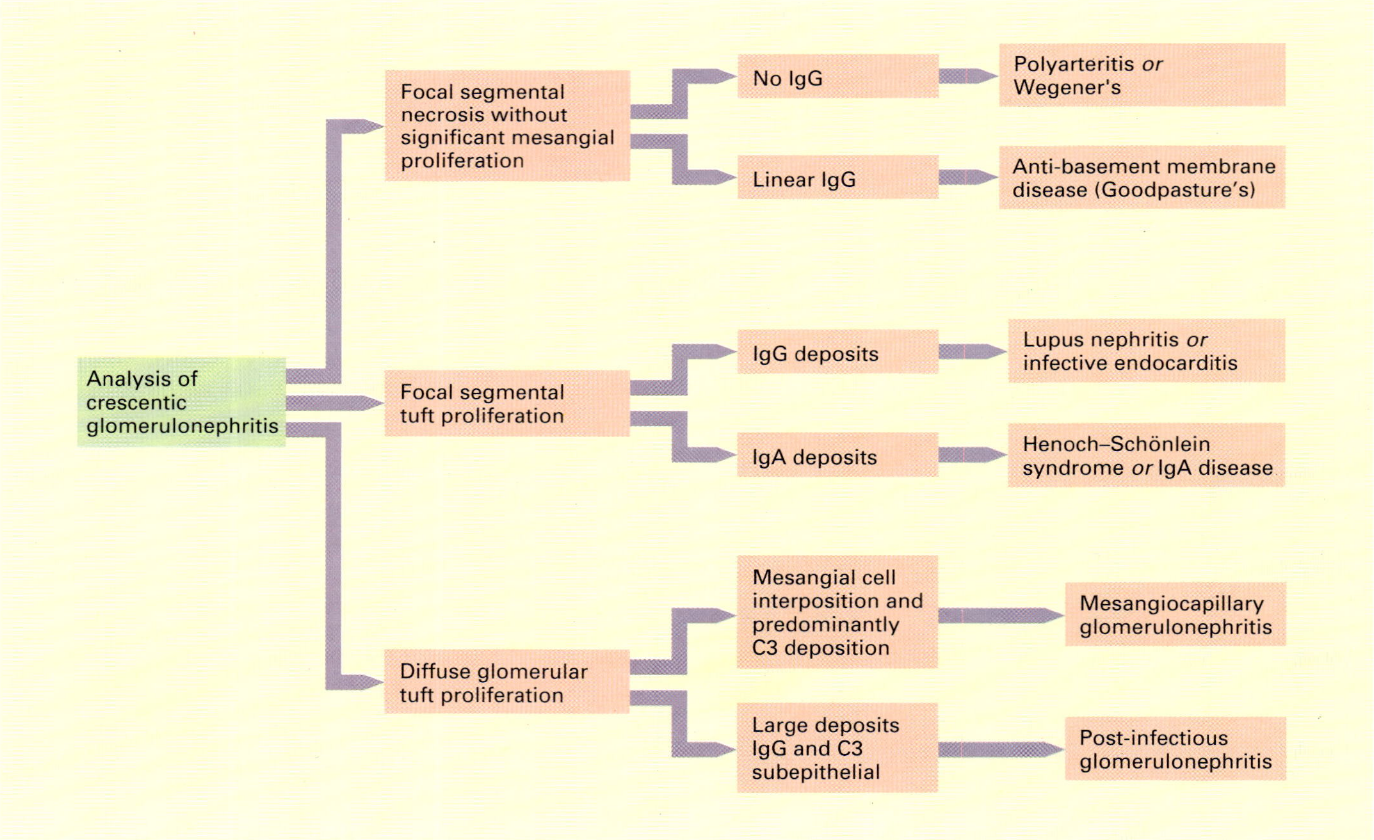

focal segmental proliferative glomerulonephritis (with or without mesangial proliferation and deposits). Thus, careful examination of the glomerular tuft should enable the renal biopsy to be more accurately classified (Fig. 19.22). In view of the rapidly progressive nature of crescentic nephritis, these patients are

Analysis of crescentic glomerulonephritis			
Focal segmental necrosis without significant mesangial proliferation	No IgG	Polyarteritis *or* Wegener's
	Linear IgG	Anti-basement membrane disease (Goodpasture's)
Focal segmental tuft proliferation	IgG deposits	Lupus nephritis *or* infective endocarditis
	IgA deposits	Henoch–Schönlein syndrome *or* IgA disease
Diffuse glomerular tuft proliferation	Mesangial cell interposition and predominantly C3 deposition	Mesangiocapillary glomerulonephritis
	Large deposits IgG and C3 subepithelial	Post-infectious glomerulonephritis

Fig. 19.22   Analysis of crescentic glomerulonephritis.

usually subjected to intensive therapeutic regimes including steroids, cytotoxic drugs, and anticoagulants, and, if started at a sufficiently early stage, may produce dramatic improvement. Alternatively, without treatment the glomeruli become rapidly destroyed, developing sclerosis over a period of a few weeks or so. The only subcategory with a relatively better prognosis is post-infectious glomerulonephritis with diffuse crescents.

19.3.10 Focal segmental glomerulosclerosis (and hyalinosis)

This is a controversial category, with opinions varying considerably as to whether it should be regarded as a disease entity, represents the bad end of the spectrum of minimal change disease, or is simply scarring due to a variety of causes. However, it does have a readily recognizable morphological pattern and a fairly predictable prognosis when identified, early in the course of a disease in which the patient presents with the nephrotic syndrome. The proteinuria is usually non-selective, and microscopic haematuria and hypertension frequently occur. The typical biopsy appearance is that an occasional glomerulus in the renal biopsy contains an abnormal segment with excessive matrix material (sclerosis) and large protein masses within capillary loops (hyalinosis) (Figs 19.23, 19.24). These lesions may be situated at any part of the circumference of the glomerulus but are most common adjacent to the proximal tubule. Early segmental lesions may show little more than some intracapillary foam cells and a small adhesion to Bowman's capsule. Although direct proof is lacking, it may be that these early lesions are potentially reversible. Once the fully developed lesions are present, however, it would seem that progression to chronic renal failure is inevitable, although the rate of progres-

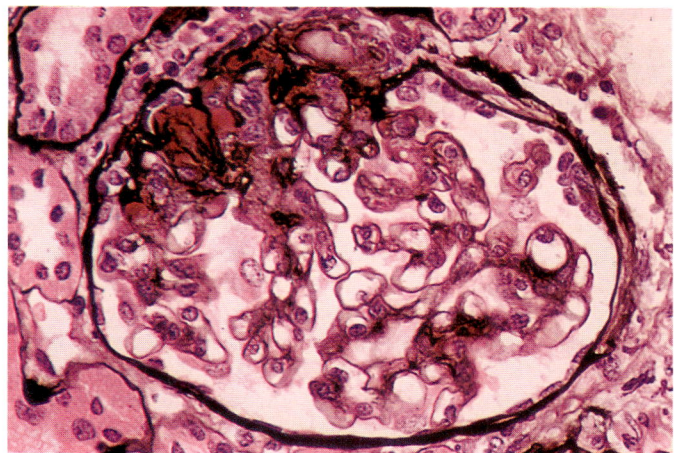

Fig. 19.23 Glomerulus showing a segmental sclerosing lesion with hyalinosis adjacent to the hilum. Silver impregnation.

sion varies considerably from case to case, being anything from 2 to 20 years. The identification of focal tubular atrophy in addition to the glomerular lesions is a useful indication of progressive disease.

Immune studies show non-specific staining for IgM and C3 limited to the segmental lesions. Part of the argument for the specificity of focal segmental glomerulosclerosis comes from the evidence of rapid recurrence of the disease in some patients who have received renal transplants. On the other hand, there is no doubting the fact that identical lesions are seen complicating other forms of glomerular disease, such as *diabetic glomerulosclerosis* and *membranous glomerulonephritis*. Furthermore, they may also be found in other forms of progressive renal damage,

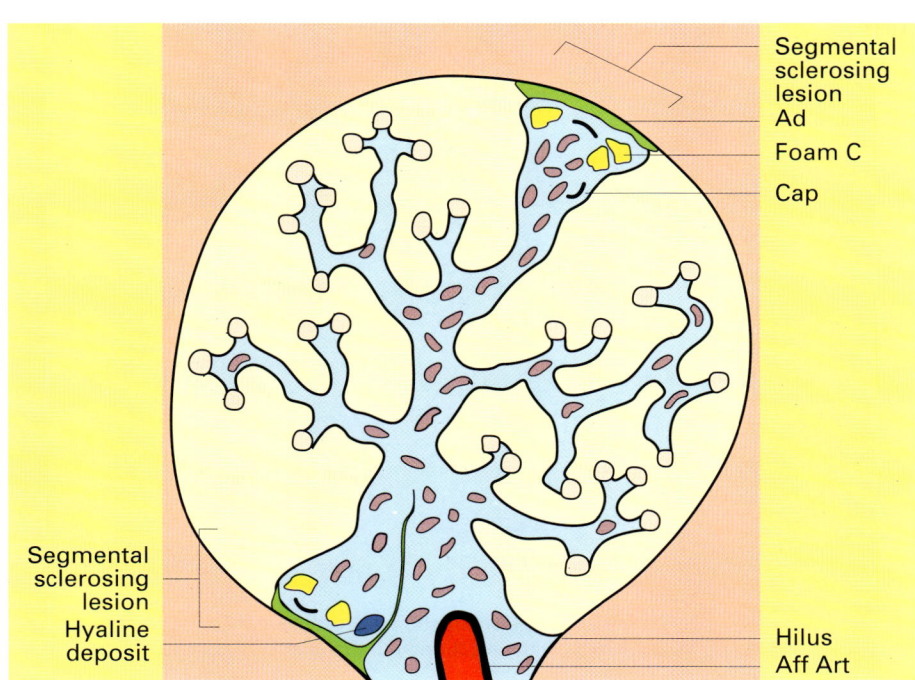

Fig. 19.24 Diagrammatic representation of glomerulus, showing segmental sclerosing lesions, both peripheral and parahilar. Ad, Adhesion; Foam C, foam cell; Cap, capillary (occluded); Aff Art, afferent arteriole.

such as *chronic atrophic pyelonephritis, analgesic nephropathy*, and *essential hypertension*, which fits with the idea that they are related in some way to progressive loss of nephrons. Whether they are cause or effect is uncertain. It has been proposed by Brenner (1983) that they can be induced by hyperfiltration, which occurs when renal reserve is significantly reduced; in turn the formation of these segmental sclerosing lesions causes further glomerular loss, reducing the renal reserve still further and establishing a vicious circle. It is not easy to understand how this relates to the situation in which focal segmental glomerulosclerosis and hyalinosis occurs as the only finding at an early stage in a patient with the nephrotic syndrome. Possibly there is a functional abnormality producing the effect of hyperfiltration in a proportion of glomeruli, which then develop the segmental lesions. As was noted many years ago, the affected glomeruli tend to be those situated in the juxta-medullary zone of the renal cortex, which are known to differ haemodynamically from the glomeruli which lie further out in the cortex. Despite the various criticisms and the introduction more recently of the term 'glomerular tip lesion' for early lesions at the periphery of the tuft, it still seems appropriate to use the category of focal segmental glomerulosclerosis to describe those cases in which patients present with heavy proteinuria, show segmental sclerosing lesions in renal biopsy, and progress relentlessly to chronic renal failure.

19.3.11   End-stage glomerulonephritis

This occurs when there has been extensive global sclerosis of glomeruli (Fig. 19.25). Much of the scarring is due to increase in basement membrane and mesangial matrix material, rather than fibrillar collagen, although fulminating crescentic glomerulonephritis may be associated with destruction of Bowman's capsule and ingrowth of collagen to replace the cellular crescent. Sclerosis of glomeruli may occur for many reasons, but when it is secondary to glomerular disease the residual cells

within the mass of sclerotic material tend to be larger with more prominent nuclei than in, say, ischaemic glomeruli. As the glomeruli become progressively sclerosed, so the accompanying nephrons undergo the same fate, with cellular atrophy, basement membrane thickening, and interstitial fibrosis. Vascular changes of arteriosclerosis and intimal thickening of arteries also occur, resulting finally in granular contracted kidneys.

19.3.12   Systemic disorders with glomerular involvement

Systemic lupus erythematosus

In this auto-immune disorder, antibodies to DNA and a variety of other 'self' antigens are formed and many different organs may be affected, including the kidney. However, the degree to which the kidney is attacked varies considerably, not only from one case to another and from one time to another but also between different glomeruli in the same biopsy. The diagnosis has usually already been established clinically, including testing the serum for antibodies to double-stranded DNA. The value of a renal biopsy is to assess the degree of renal involvement so that prognosis can be gauged and treatment planned if appropriate. A variety of proliferative patterns may be seen in glomeruli, ranging from diffuse mesangial proliferation through focal segmental proliferative glomerulonephritis (Fig. 19.26) to diffuse proliferative glomerulonephritis with crescentic formation (see above). The complexity of the disease is emphasized by the fact that a membranous pattern of glomerulonephritis can be superimposed on any or all of the proliferative patterns. Immune deposits of all types (immunoglobulins, complement components, properdin, etc.) can be identified in the mesangium, subendothelial space, and also in a typical membranous distribution, indicating that a variety of immune mechanisms are involved. In addition, there is frequently a degree of interstitial nephritis, which may contribute significantly to nephron loss.

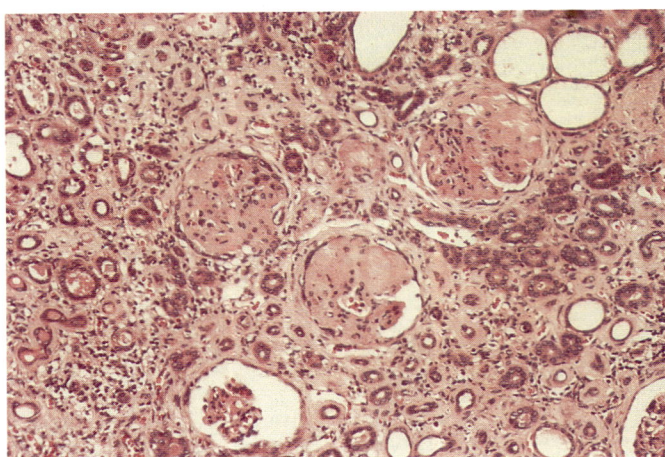

Fig. 19.25   Renal tissue, showing end-stage sclerosing glomerulonephritis with surrounding tubular atrophy and interstitial fibrosis.

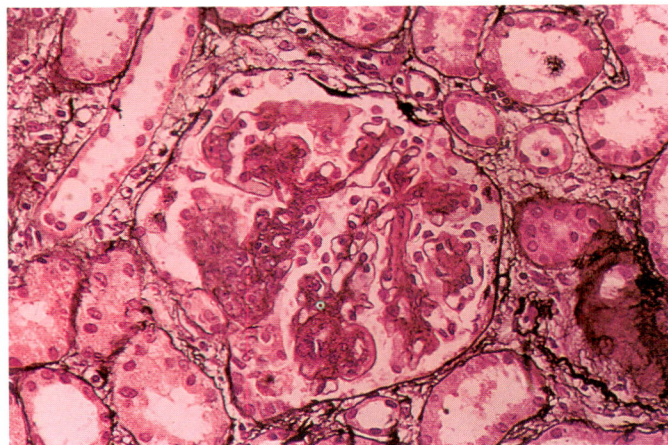

Fig. 19.26   Glomerulus showing focal segmental proliferative glomerulonephritis with an adhesion to Bowman's capsule. (Silver impregnation.)

A *spontaneous lupus-like disease with glomerulonephritis* has been well documented in both rats and mice and, indeed, an auto-immune response to DNA with anti-DNA antibodies has been confirmed. However, it is less than clear that the glomerular reactions in these animals are entirely due to the deposition of immune complexes of this type. A variety of studies suggest that some additional immune-complex systems play a role in the pathogenesis of lupus nephritis. In particular, there is now good evidence of a general disturbance of immune regulation with polyclonal B-cell activation. This type of reaction can also be induced by the injection of lipopolysaccharides (bacterial products), and may also occur in trypanosomiasis and after viral infections. Furthermore, it can also be induced by drugs and graft versus host disease.

The Henloch–Schönlein syndrome

This condition consists of episodic attacks of a characteristic purpuric rash, abdominal pain, arthritis, and haematuria of glomerular origin, occurring particularly in children. The glomeruli show patterns of proliferation with IgA deposits which are virtually identical with those described in IgA disease (see above). The reason for renal biopsy is usually to assess the severity or stage of the renal disease rather than to establish the diagnosis. Mild cases demonstrate IgA deposits in the mesangium with an associated mesangial cell proliferation. More severe cases show focal segmental proliferation superimposed on mesangial proliferation, often with associated small cellular crescents and fibrin deposition. The proliferation of cells within the glomerular tufts may become diffuse and be associated with numerous large cellular crescents, when the prognosis must be guarded. When focal segmental proliferation involves a greater percentage of the glomerular tuft, the changes may approach those seen in mesangiocapillary glomerulonephritis (type I).

Anti-basement membrane disease (Goodpasture's syndrome)

This is a rare condition in which an IgG auto-antibody to glomerular basement membrane is present in the circulation and capable of binding to the Goodpasture antigen, which is a constituent of normal glomerular basement membrane (Fig. 19.27). The effect of this is to cause either a focal segmental proliferative glomerulonephritis with crescents, or a diffuse crescentic glomerulonephritis. The dominant feature in the histology is the development of cellular crescents. In more severe cases the glomerular basement membrane may be extensively disrupted such that it may be difficult in immune studies to identify clearly the linear deposition of IgG along the membrane, which is characteristic of anti-basement membrane disease. In addition, cross-reaction of the antibody with pulmonary basement membranes can induce intrapulmonary haemorrhage, which may be life threatening. Exposure to hydrocarbons and virus infections have been implicated as factors in the development of anti-basement membrane disease, presumably by altering the pulmonary basement membrane

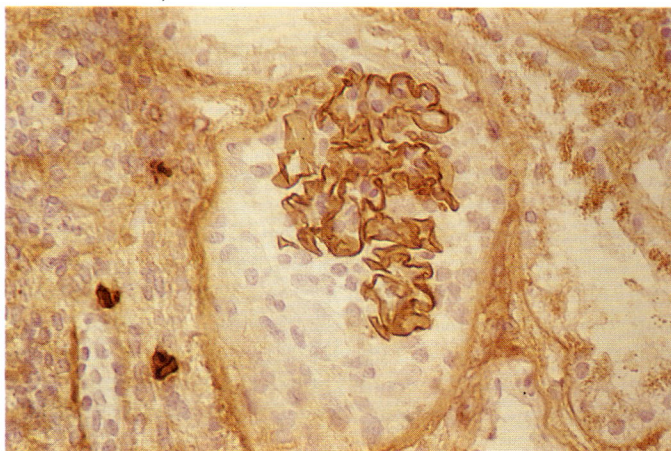

Fig. 19.27 Goodpasture's syndrome, with linear staining for IgG along the glomerular basement membrane revealed by peroxidase.

sufficiently to induce the formation of an auto-antibody which cross-reacts with the glomerular basement membranes.

Animal experiments have resulted in the development of several models of anti-basement membrane disease based on injecting heterologous antibody directed against antigens in the glomerular basement membrane (nephrotoxic nephritis) (Wilson and Dixon 1986). The antibody binds to the glomerular basement membrane in a linear distribution and induces proteinuria and a proliferative glomerulonephritis with recruitment of polymorphs, platelets, macrophages, and cellular crescent formation. Recent evidence suggests that eicosanoids produced by inflammatory cells may play an important role in the production of the glomerular lesions. The severity of the glomerulonephritis is enhanced by the development of a secondary reaction caused by the animal forming antibodies against the injected heterologous antibody, and binding to it on the glomerular basement membrane. This is referred to as *the autologous phase*. If the animal has been pre-immunized with IgG from the species that has been used to prepare the anti-glomerular basement membrane antibody, then an accelerated nephrotoxic nephritis occurs, with increased influx of inflammatory cells. Although these models are clearly artificial, they are closely related to an auto-immune or experimental allergic glomerulonephritis (*Steblay nephritis*) in which the animals have been immunized with either heterologous or homologous glomerular basement membrane antibodies which induce glomerulonephritis. If combined with a noxious stimulus to the lung, intrapulmonary haemorrhage may also occur as in Goodpasture's syndrome, forming a closely analogous situation with the human disease.

Much of the experimental work on glomerulonephritis has demonstrated the involvement of humoral immunity. By contrast, cellular immunity is much less apparent. However, in nephrotoxic nephritis, and particularly in the accelerated form, macrophages play a significant role in the reaction, and experimentally this can be shown to be T-cell mediated. It is also worth noting that in several forms of glomerulonephritis the macrophages that are normally resident in the glomerulus are increased in number and could play a part in the afferent limb of the immune response.

Polyarteritis nodosa

A systemic disorder affecting blood vessels of various sizes. A destructive arteritis develops in short segments of blood vessels and the symptoms and signs produced will depend on the precise location of the vascular lesions. This condition tends to affect older people, although it is occasionally seen in children and young adults. Haematuria is evidence of renal involvement and the patient may also develop hypertension, eosinophilia, and raised erythrocyte sedimentation rate. The glomeruli often show segmental necrotizing lesions, with associated cellular crescent formation (so-called *microscopic polyarteritis*) (Fig. 19.28). Despite strong circumstantial evidence suggesting an immune-complex aetiology for this condition, in the vast majority of cases no immune deposit or complement components are identifiable in the glomeruli. A strongly positive result for fibrin is seen in the necrotic segments and associated cellular crescents. Thus, the glomerular disease is classifiable either as a *focal segmental necrotizing glomerulonephritis with crescents* or a *diffuse crescentic glomerulonephritis*, according to its extent and severity.

Wegener's granulomatosis

This is a more chronic form of systemic vasculitis which involves the lungs, nasal passages, and kidneys particularly. The glomerular changes seen in renal biopsy in this condition are virtually identical with those seen in polyarteritis nodosa and therefore need no further description. Recently, an interesting finding has been the presence of a circulating auto-antibody to neutrophils in cases of active Wegener's granulomatosis, though whether this is important in the aetiology of the condition, or simply an indicator of disease activity, is not yet clear.

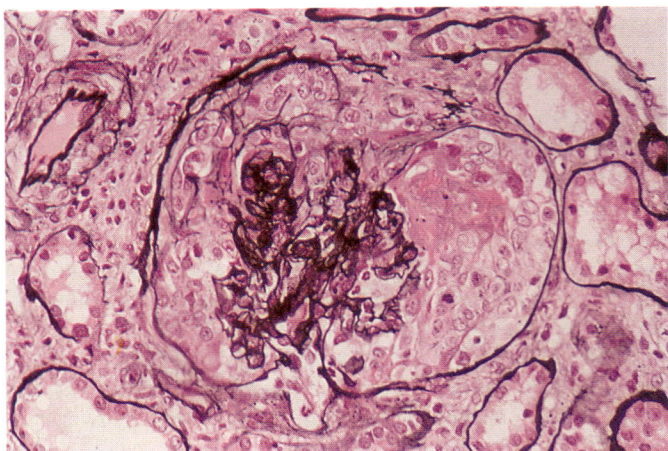

Fig. 19.28 A 'collapsed' glomerulus, with segmental necrosis on the left side and large cellular crescent, in polyarteritis nodosa. (Silver impregnation.)

Infective endocarditis and shunt nephritis

These conditions may be associated with glomerulonephritis. In both conditions the scene is set for a chronic immune-complex disease with infection of a heart valve or prosthetic shunt by an organism of relatively low virulence shedding antigen into the circulation and stimulating antibody formation. Haematuria, with or without significant proteinuria, is a strong indication of renal involvement. The glomeruli classically show a generalized mesangial cell proliferation with mesangial deposits containing IgG and C3. In addition, there are focal segmental proliferative and necrotizing lesions, which may have associated cellular crescents. Where the organism is of low virulence the pattern of glomerular disease is more likely to resemble the type I mesangiocapillary glomerulonephritis. Clearly the progression or resolution of the glomerular disease depends upon the speed of diagnosis and treatment of the primary infecion, but in any event there is likely to be some residual scarring in the kidney.

19.3.13 Bibliography

Brenner, B. M. (1983). Haemodynamically mediated glomerular injury and the progressive nature of kidney diseases. *Kidney International* **23**, 647–55.

Donadio, J. V. (1988). Membrano-proliferative glomerulonephritis. In *Diseases of the kidney* (ed. R. W. Schrier and C. W. Gottschalk), pp. 2035–60. Little Brown, Boston.

Eddy, A. A. and Michael, A. F. (1989). Immunopathogenetic mechanisms of glomerular injury. In *Renal pathology* (ed. C. C. Tisher and B. M. Brenner), pp. 111–55. Lippincott, Philadelphia.

Emancipator, S., Gallo, G., and Lamm, M. (1983). Experimental IgA nephropathy induced by oral immunisation. *Journal of Experimental Medicine* **157**, 572–82.

Silva, F. G. and Hogg, R. J. (1989). Minimal change nephrotic syndrome. In *Renal pathology* (ed. C. C. Tisher and B. M. Brenner), pp. 265–339. Lippincott, Philadelphia.

Wilson, C. B. and Dixon, F. J. (1986). The renal response to immunological injury. In *The kidney* (ed. B. M. Brenner and F. C. Rector), pp. 800–90. Saunders, Philadelphia.

Wilson, C. B., Yamamoto, T., Moullier, P., and Blanty, R. C. (1988). Selective glomerular cell immune injury—anti mesangial cell antibodies. In *Nephrology* (ed. A. M. Davison), pp. 509–22. Baillière Tindall, London.

19.4   Renovascular diseases

G. B. N. Lindop

19.4.1   Renal artery stenosis

Renal artery stenosis causes ischaemia of the kidney and, since ichaemia is one of the commonest histological changes seen in renal pathology, renal artery stenosis provides a useful model for its study. The condition is produced experimentally by placing a constricting clip on one renal artery; this is one of the best-studied causes of stimulation of the renin–angiotensin system and of hypertension. Renal artery stenosis is one of the most important causes of secondary hypertension in man.

Causes

In almost two-thirds of cases, atheroma is the cause of renal artery stenosis, especially in diabetics. Occasionally, the ostium of the artery is narrowed by a plaque of aortic atheroma. The remaining cases are almost all due to *fibromuscular dysplasia* (p. 1472). This mainly occurs in women during the reproductive years, while atheroma usually affects patients more than 45 years old. Rarely, renal artery stenosis is caused by dissecting aneurysm (Section 12.6.9) or aortitis (Section 12.3.4).

Clinical manifestations

Renal artery stenosis is usually diagnosed during the investigation of hypertension associated with high plasma levels of *renin* and *angiotensin—renovascular hypertension*. It often causes malignant hypertension and hypertension that is difficult to control pharmacologically. Renal artery stenosis may be suspected by the presence of an abdominal bruit on auscultation, or delayed excretion of the contrast medium of an excretory urogram, but the definitive investigation is angiography (Fig. 19.29). If bilateral, it can cause renal failure.

Gross appearances

Since the glomerular filtration rate is the main determinant of renal workload, renal artery stenosis causes *atrophy of the kid-*

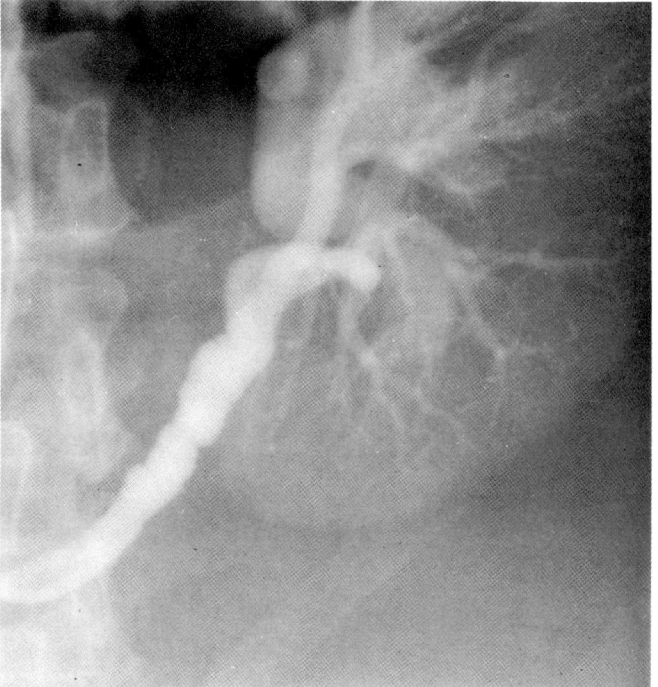

Fig. 19.29 An angiogram from a case of renal artery stenosis due to fibromuscular dysplasia. It shows a 'string of beads' appearance with alternating constrictions and dilatations; see Fig. 19.31.

ney. It becomes uniformly smaller, often by as much as 50 per cent. If a segmental artery or a branch of the renal artery is affected, then the area supplied will shrink and form a smooth, depressed area below the surface of the surrounding kidney (Fig. 19.30a); in a previously normal kidney the surface is smooth. On section, the cortex is narrowed with loss of the normal demarcation between cortex and medulla.

Microscopic appearances

Renal atrophy predominantly affects the tubules, which collapse and lose their lumen. The cells become smaller and lose their specialized features and the atrophied tubules are surrounded by a thickened basement membrane. The tubular atrophy causes the glomeruli to appear crowded together. Each glomerular tuft shrinks due to the falling filtration pressure. The collapsed capillaries at first have a small lumen and a wrinkled basement membrane. Later, the tuft becomes completely solidified and Bowman's space becomes filled with basement membrane material and mesangial matrix; the whole glomerulus is then replaced by a fibrous ball which shrinks and eventually disappears. Only the contralateral kidney is subjected to hypertensive damage; the arteries in the ischaemic kidney are protected from the pressure by the stenosis.

The ischaemic kidney responds to the fall in perfusion by hyperplasia of the *juxtaglomerular apparatus* (JGA) giving rise to an increase in plasma and renal renin (Fig. 19.30b). The increased generation of *angiotensin II* causes raised plasma aldosterone levels and suppression of renin synthesis in the contralateral (non-ischaemic) kidney. Some cases with *malignant hypertension* develop *hyponatraemia* due to *pressure natriuresis* from the contralateral kidney. The low sodium then stimulates further renin release, causing a vicious circle of further elevations of plasma renin and angiotensin II levels and blood pressure. Eventually, the contralateral kidney may become damaged by the hypertension and may itself become ischaemic. This stimulus overrides the suppressive effect of raised plasma angiotensin II levels, and it, too, may secrete renin which perpetuates the hypertension.

These considerations are important in deciding which patients with renal artery stenosis will benefit from surgery. Renal vein blood samples will show higher levels of renin in kidneys with high secretion rates. However, since the renal vein renin concentration is also dependent on the renal plasma flow, there will be a tendency to have artificially high levels in ischaemic kidneys, and these measurements are now interpreted with caution. Revascularization of an ischaemic kidney can produce reversal of the atrophy and, in some cases, achieve a useful degree of function; hence the operations of *angioplasty* and *renal artery bypass* are undertaken with greater frequency than nephrectomy. The proportion of patients cured by surgery depends mainly on the care with which they are selected. Those patients whose blood pressure does not fall to normal following surgery can often be treated more effectively by drugs.

Fibromuscular dysplasia

This is a group of arterial diseases of confusing nomenclature

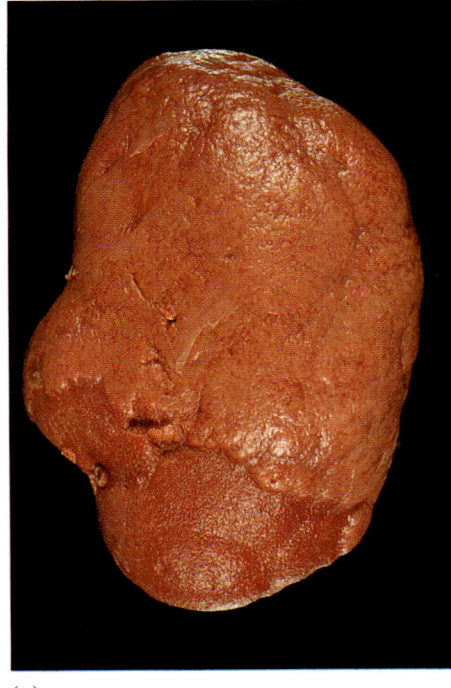

(a)

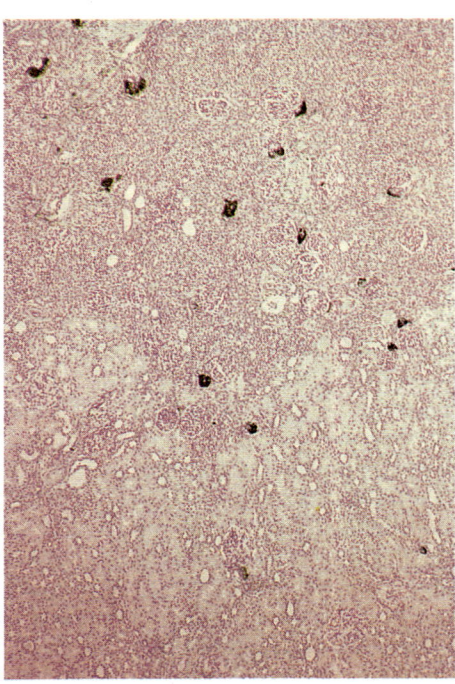

(b)

Fig. 19.30 (a) A kidney with stenosis of the renal artery branch supplying the upper pole; the ischaemic area is dark, smooth, and is sunken below the surface of the normal kidney. (b) The junction between the ischaemic and the normal kidney stained with an immunoperoxidase technique and a renin antiserum, which stains the renin-secreting cells brown. Almost all of the immunostainable renin is present in the ischaemic area, which also shows severe atrophy of the tubules.

and uncertain aetiology. The diseases are characterized by focal abnormalities in the structure of the arterial wall.

Clinical features

Fibromuscular dysplasia may be found in children, but is commonest in young and middle-aged adults. Women are affected twice as often as men. Fibromuscular dysplasia affects medium-sized arteries in many organs, but almost always presents clinically as hypertension due to renal artery stenosis.

Pathology

Fibromuscular dysplasia may be unilateral or bilateral. Any layer of the vessel wall can be affected, and the abnormality can be localized or extend along the length of the artery into its branches. Excess smooth muscle and/or fibrous tissue with thickening of the wall causes stenosis; alternatively, deficiencies of elastic or fibromuscular tissue cause aneurysms (Fig. 19.31) or dissection. Although the aetiology is unknown, a congenital malformation of the artery seems a likely explanation.

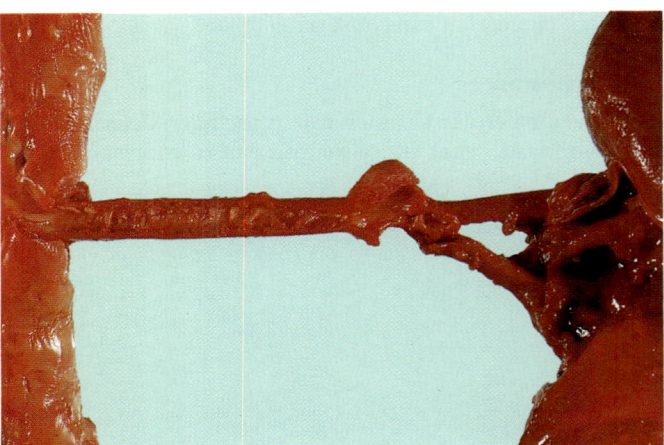

Fig. 19.31 The left renal artery is opened longitudinally to show fibromuscular dysplasia, with circumferential bands of thickened fibro-muscular tissue alternating with thinned. One of the latter has given rise to an aneurysm at the bifurcation of the artery.

19.4.2   Renal artery thrombosis and embolism

Thrombosis of the renal artery is a complication of renal artery stenosis and its treatment; it also occurs in dissecting aneurysm and following renal transplantation. It causes acute renal failure if bilateral. Emboli are usually derived from the heart and are caused by diseases such as *myocardial infarction* (mural thrombus), *chronic rheumatic heart disease*, or *infective endocarditis*. The remaining cases are due to complicated atheroma in the aorta. Microscopic evidence of atheromatous embolism from ruptured atheromatous plaques can be found in the kidneys of 15 per cent of elderly patients (Fig. 19.32).

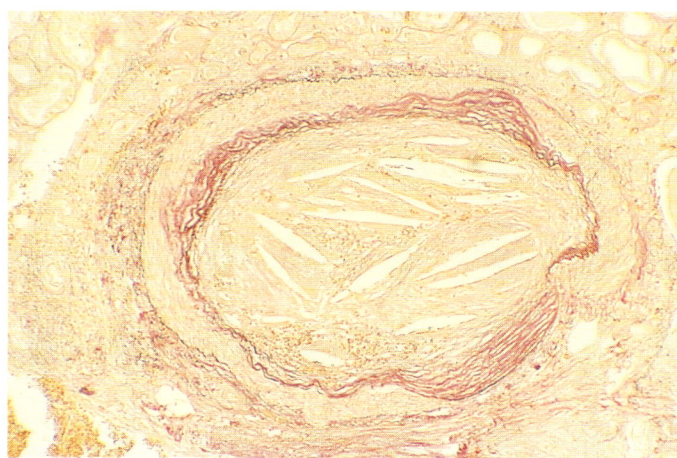

Fig. 19.32 Atheromatous embolism of a renal artery branch which is occluded by organized thrombus-containing clefts. These were occupied by cholesterol crystals which have been dissolved out by the solvents during tissue embedding. (Elastic van Gieson stain.)

19.4.3 Renal vein thrombosis

Thrombosis of the renal veins has predisposing factors similar to those that operate in other vascular beds (p. 509). An *acute form* occurs most commonly in infants with *severe dehydration*, usually due to *vomiting and diarrhoea*. The thrombosis probably begins in the renal vein radicles. Propagation proximally and distally can lead to venous infarction of the whole kidney, and death if bilateral. A more gradual onset is commoner in adults. The renal vein is often occluded by tumour thrombus due to invasion by *renal cell carcinoma*. Other cases of renal vein thrombosis are associated with the *nephrotic syndrome*. Careful study of well-documented cases, especially those in which the thrombosis is unilateral, indicates that venous thrombosis is usually a complication of the nephrotic syndrome rather than vice versa. Renal amyloid (Section 19.9.1) is also a recognized association of renal vein thrombosis.

Clinical features

Acute renal vein thrombosis can present as renal infarction, with loin pain and haematuria. In adults, renal vein thrombosis is more often asymptomatic, and is usually diagnosed in the investigation of proteinuria or the nephrotic syndrome. The outlook is then governed by the prognosis of the underlying renal disease.

Pathology

The acute form with venous infarction gives rise to a large, swollen, deeply congested kidney, while in the chronic form the kidney is enlarged, oedematous, and pale. The microscopic features of venous infarction are seen in the acute form, while in chronic cases there is interstitial fibrosis with dilated and atrophied tubules. The glomeruli show no significant abnormality.

19.4.4 Infarction

The kidney is usually infarcted by occlusion of an artery; venous infarction (Section 19.4.3) is rare. Although there are anastomoses with the vessels supplying the capsule and the renal pelvis, the arteries of the kidney are best considered as end arteries. Large infarcts affect all regions of the kidney, but small infarcts usually spare the renal medulla, since this area has a lower oxygen requirement and has a richly anastomosing blood supply.

Clinical feautures

The clinical symptoms of acute infarction are pain and haematuria; small infarcts are usually asymptomatic.

Pathology

Small infarcts are roughly conical and have a base on the renal capsule. When recent, they are reddish in colour. The necrotic area changes to greyish-yellow over a few days, leaving a residual red edge of vascular congestion (Fig. 19.33). Within a few days all of the structures in the infarcted zone are necrotic. At the edge of the infarct there is vascular congestion and a slight acute inflammatory response, then organization proceeds as in coagulative necrosis in other sites (p. 147). At the edge of the infarct there is transient hyperplasia of the renin-secreting cells in the JGA of the surviving but ischaemic glomeruli. This may cause high plasma renin levels and transient hypertension.

19.4.5 Vasculitis

Polyarteritis

The kidney is affected in 70 per cent of cases of polyarteritis. The classical form, *polyarteritis nodosa*, affects large branches of the renal artery—interlobar and arcuate arteries; smaller arteries and glomeruli are only rarely affected. In the acute phase, the acute inflammation and/or aneurysms can lead to arterial

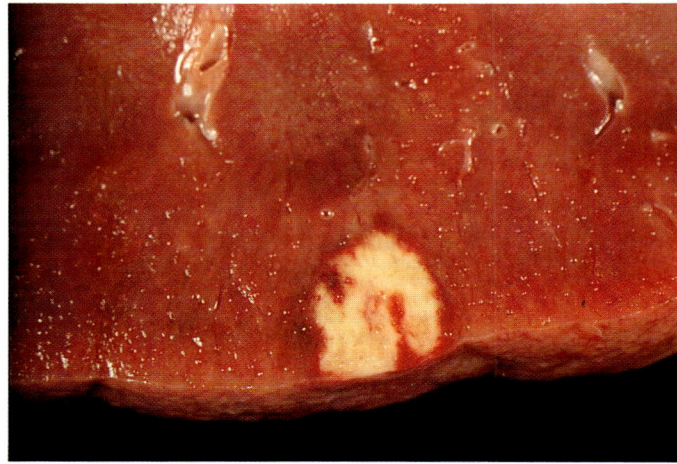

Fig. 19.33 A small recent renal infarct, which is slightly swollen. The yellow, necrotic renal cortex has a congested border.

thrombosis with infarction of the kidney or haemorrhage. Alternatively, in the quiescent phase the endarteritis caused by healing of the arterial inflammation gives rise to multifocal ischaemia of the kidney. In the areas of ischaemic renal cortex subtended by an affected artery there is focal hyperplasia of the JGA and histological changes identical to those of renal artery stenosis. Therefore, classical polyarteritis nodosa is usually accompanied by hypertension at presentation. At post-mortem the kidney may show multiple infarcts or be coarsely scarred, and small aneurysms may be visible in the renal arterial tree.

By contrast, *microscopic polyarteritis* affects mainly glomerular capillaries and arterioles and, occasionally, distal interlobular arteries. The predominant presentation is therefore acute renal failure without hypertension. This is due to a focal or diffuse crescentic glomerulonephritis (see Section 19.3.12). The kidney is similarly affected by *Wegener's granulomatosis*, which also causes a small vessel vasculitis and a necrotizing crescentic glomerulonephritis, often accompanied by granulomas in the interstitium. Unlike polyarteritis, Wegener's granulomatosis responds well to immunosuppressive therapy. Granulomatous vasculitis and glomerulonephritis also occur in *allergic granulomatosis* (Churg–Strauss syndrome), where they are associated with large numbers of eosinophils, and as part of a drug reaction.

Vasculitis resembling the spectrum of polyarteritis occurs in patients with sero-positive *rheumatoid disease* who have high titres of rheumatoid factor, in *systemic lupus erythematosus*, and in other connective tissue diseases. *Henoch–Schönlein purpura* is the commonest of the group of hypersensitivity vasculitides that affect the kidney. It usually causes a focal glomerulonephritis, which has a very good prognosis in childhood, but is less benign in adults in whom the change to rapidly progressive glomerulonephritis is commoner (see Section 19.3.12).

The renal arteries are rarely affected by Takayasu's disease (p. 845), giant cell arteritis (p. 844), and the arteritis of rheumatic fever (p. 843).

19.4.6   Hypertension

The nature of the arterial changes in hypertension and their pathogenesis are described on p. 833. The arterial lesions may be widespread but always affect the kidney most severely.

Chronic benign hypertension

Gross appearances

In most cases the kidney appears macroscopically normal, but in some cases the kidneys are reduced in size and have a finely granular surface.

Microscopic appearances

Arteriosclerosis (p. 798) affects the renal artery branches down to the interlobular arteries, but usually has no significant effect on flow. The most important lesion is *hypertensive arteriolosclerosis* (p. 803). This causes thickening of the wall and narrowing of the lumen of afferent glomerular arterioles (Fig. 19.34); less

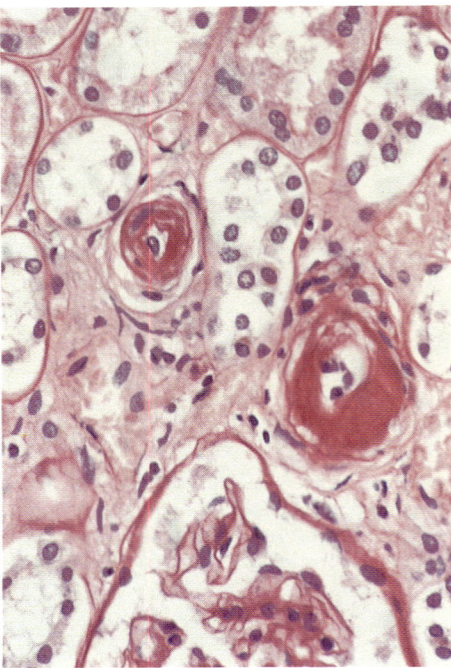

Fig. 19.34   Two renal arterioles from a case of benign hypertension. One shows early and the other more advanced hyaline arteriosclerosis. This has caused thickening of the wall and narrowing of the lumen. The PAS stain shows replacement of the smooth muscle cells by accumulation of proteins, derived mainly from the plasma.

severe changes are found in the efferent vessels. Arteriolosclerosis is associated with *obsolescence of the glomerulus*. When the glomerulus ceases to filter, its tubule atrophies leaving a small scar. The many scars caused by nephron-loss, combined with intervening nodules created by the hypertrophied tubules of each surviving nephron, are responsible for the granular surface of the kidney, *granular contracted kidney* (Fig. 19.35a,b).

The loss of individual nephrons, 'nephron fallout', is a normal age change (a loss of up to 25 per cent of nephrons may occur in normal adults). It is accelerated and more severe in hypertension. If severe, the nephron loss can cause the kidney to shrink to two-thirds of its normal size. The increased glomerular filtration rate in the surviving nephrons stimulates hypertrophy of the tubules, but, paradoxically, increased perfusion of glomeruli also causes glomerulosclerosis. Hyperperfusion of glomeruli may therefore accelerate the nephron loss in the population of residual nephrons.

Histologically identifiable atheromatous embolism from ruptured plaques in the aorta is common in autopsy kidneys (p. 521). This has led some to believe that complicated atheroma in the aorta may also be important in causing nephron loss by microembolism.

In conclusion, the nephron loss in chronic hypertension may be caused in some cases by hypertensive arteriolosclerosis and in others by microembolism. In all cases, when the population of functioning nephrons becomes small enough the glomerulo-

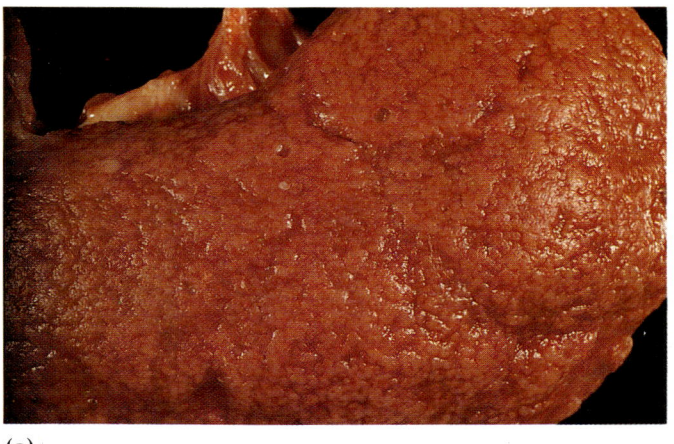

(a)

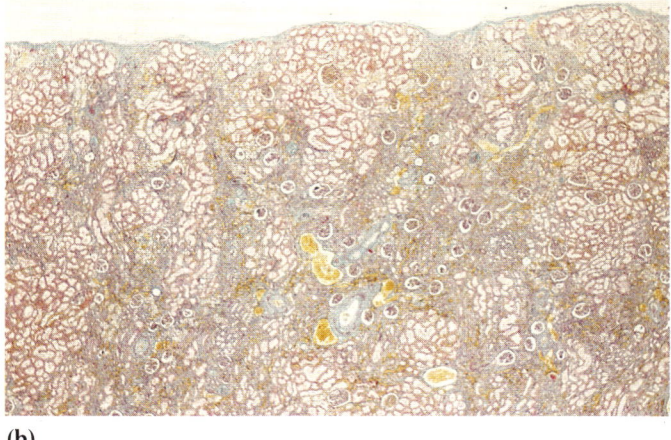

(b)

Fig. 19.35 (a) The surface of the kidney from an elderly person with long-standing benign hypertension. It has a finely granular surface. (b) A histological section showing that this appearance is due to small scars caused by nephron loss alternating with raised nodules of hypertrophied tubules of the surviving nephrons. (Masson's trichrome.)

sclerosis and associated nephron loss are accelerated by hyperperfusion of the surviving glomeruli.

In contrast to *malignant hypertension* (see below), in chronic benign hypertension the arterial lesions develop over a period of many years and renal failure is rare. The main clinical importance of chronic hypertensive damage to the kidney is the loss of functional reserve; if severe, this may cause renal failure if renal perfusion falls, most often following the onset of cardiac failure.

Malignant hypertension

Gross appearances

This depends on the stage of the disease and whether there has been pre-existing chronic benign hypertension (p. 834). In acute malignant hypertension, apparently arising *ab initio*, the kidney is slightly swollen and oedematous. The surface is spotted with 'flea-bite' haemorrhages (Fig. 19.36) and on section

there may be small infarcts. If malignant hypertension supervenes on long-standing benign hypertension, the kidney may be slightly smaller and have a finely granular surface. In treated cases who survive for several years, the kidney is also small but the surface is coarsely granular.

Microscopic changes

In acute malignant hypertension, the most characteristic lesion is *fibrinoid necrosis* of small arteries and arterioles. This affects predominantly the afferent arterioles and the distal interlobular arteries. The commonest sites are at the branching point of an afferent arteriole from the interlobular artery and the point at which the afferent arteriole enters the glomerulus. In the latter case the fibrinoid necrosis may extend into the glomerular tuft (Fig. 19.37). This can cause rupture of the tuft and haemorrhage into the tubule. When interlobular arteries are affected, small infarcts may occur; for these reasons haematuria is common in acute malignant hypertension. Fibrinoid necrosis is also

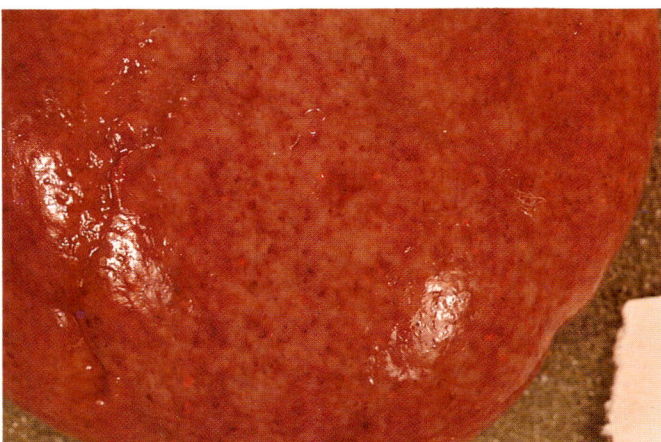

Fig. 19.36 The surface of a kidney from a case of acute malignant hypertension. The kidney is swollen, oedematous, and is covered with tiny haemorrhages—a 'flea-bitten' kidney.

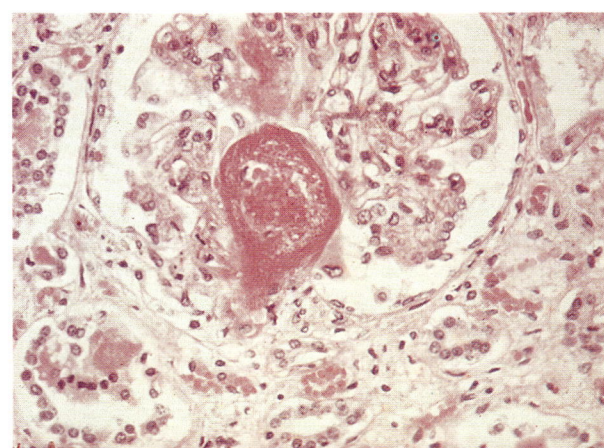

Fig. 19.37 A case of malignant hypertension, showing a renal glomerulus with fibrinoid necrosis and thrombosis of its afferent arteriole.

associated with *intravascular coagulation* and fragmentation of circulating red blood corpuscles—*microangiopathic haemolytic anaemia.*

The lesions of fibrinoid necrosis are often seen in combination with *endarteritis*, and in some cases endarteritis may predominate and fibrinoid necrosis may be scanty or absent. The effect of both arterial fibrinoid necrosis and endarteritis is to cause renal ischaemia. This leads to stimulation of renin release from the juxtaglomerular apparatus and the high levels of plasma renin and angiotensin II, which are common in malignant hypertension.

Fibrinoid necrosis and endarteritis are also found in a variety of other diseases in which arterial damage is associated with intravascular coagulation. The histological appearances may be indistinguishable from the arterial lesions caused by irradiation, progressive systemic sclerosis, haemolytic-uraemic syndrome, thrombotic-thrombocytopenic purpura, postpartum renal failure, or renal transplant rejection (see below).

19.4.7   Intravascular coagulation

More than 20 per cent of the cardiac output passes through the kidney; consequently, in diseases associated with disseminated intravascular coagulation, renal manifestations often predominate. Capillary thrombi are usually seen in the glomerular capillaries (Fig. 19.38) and the breakdown products of fibrin formed in the circulation are easily detected in the urine. In addition, intravascular coagulation occurs in several renal diseases and certainly plays a secondary role in the pathogenesis of some of them; for example, in malignant hypertension the primary event is vascular damage due to the pressure-rise, and in haemolytic-uraemic syndrome it is likely that the primary vascular damage is induced by a virus infection or by the immune response which it elicits. However, the intravascular coagulation that occurs in these conditions contributes to the renal failure and causes microangiopathic haemolytic anaemia. Also, experimentally produced intravascular coagulation causes renal vasoconstriction and histological lesions indistinguishable from those seen in many renal diseases. It is likely that the coagulation cascade and the endothelial cell interact in a complex way to produce the clinical and histological manifestations of diseases in which intravascular coagulation occurs (p. 519).

Thrombotic microangiopathies

The renal vasculature is susceptible to a number of diseases that can produce lesions indistinguishable from those described in malignant hypertension. In *haemolytic-uraemic syndrome*, *thrombotic-thrombocytopenic purpura*, and *postpartum acute renal failure*, *fibrinoid necrosis* of small arteries and arterioles with *intravascular coagulation* and haemolytic anaemia dominate the clinical picture; these have been called *thrombotic microangiopathies*. In other diseases (such as *renal allograft rejection*, *scleroderma*, and *irradiation*) *endarteritis* and *hypertension* are more prominent.

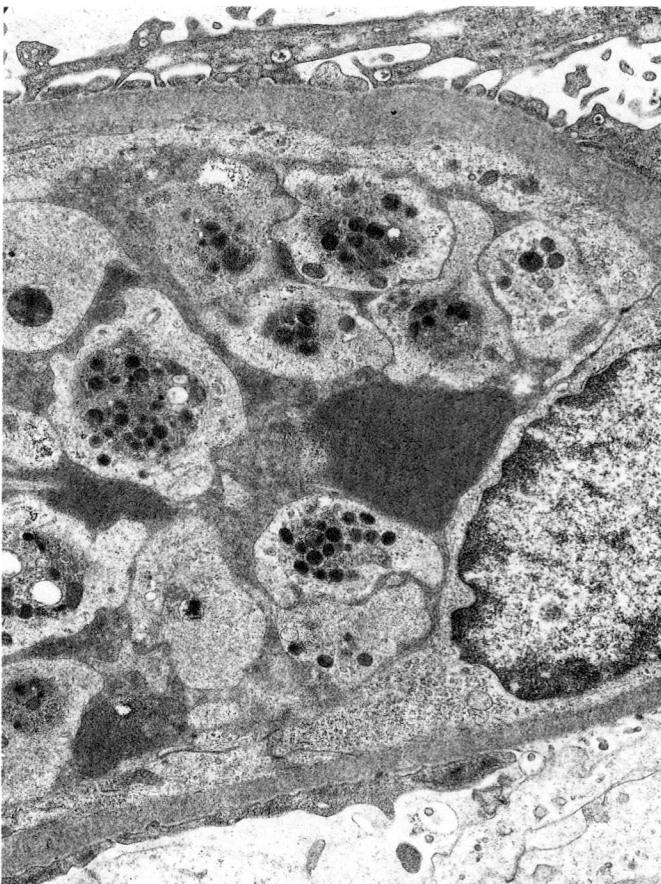

Fig. 19.38   A glomerular capillary from a case of intravascular coagulation. The capillary lumen is plugged with platelets, some of which have discharged their granules.

Haemolytic-uraemic syndrome

This syndrome can affect adults but is most common in children under 4 years of age. It occurs up to 2 weeks after gastrointestinal or upper respiratory infection when there is an illness characterized by vomiting, purpura, melaena, and haematuria. There is evidence of intravascular coagulation and renal failure. Fatal cases may show patchy cortical necrosis of the kidneys, often with petechial haemorrhages. The arterioles have plasma protein in their walls (*plasmatic vasculosis*) and *luminal thrombosis* (Fig. 19.39), which also often, and sometimes predominantly, affects the glomeruli. This is associated with microangiopathic haemolytic anaemia. The interlobular arteries sometimes show oedematous intimal swelling. Subsequent *endarteritis* may give rise to severe narrowing and cause malignant hypertension in cases that recover; those who do not, die of renal failure.

Thrombotic-thrombocytopenic purpura

There are histological changes of intravascular coagulation in the kidney in patients with thrombotic-thrombocytopenic pur-

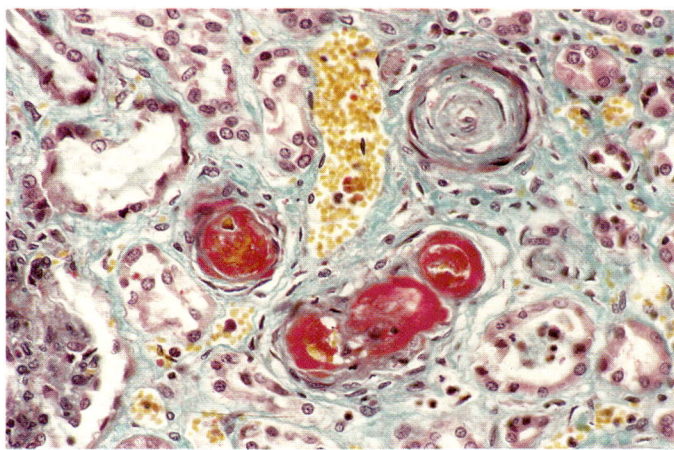

Fig. 19.39 A case of haemolytic-uraemic syndrome showing fibrinoid necrosis and intravascular coagulation in arterioles. In addition, there is 'onion-skin' endarteritis of an interlobular artery, appearances indistinguishable from malignant hypertension.

pura, but the haematological complications are more prominent than in the haemolytic-uraemic syndrome. While renal failure may occur, involvement of the coronary and cerebral circulations are usually more important clinically.

Similar changes in the renal vascular tree occur in *renal allograft rejection*, *acute postpartum renal failure*, and in some patients treated with the cytotoxic drugs *cisplatin* and *bleomycin*. It is likely that the histological similarity of these conditions is due to a common pathogenetic mechanism. A likely candidate is *endothelial damage*. This could be caused by pressure, by infectious agents, by immunological mechanisms, by intravascular coagulation, or by a combination of these factors.

Scleroderma (progressive systemic sclerosis)

Patients with scleroderma often have hypertension; in 5 per cent of cases this is malignant hypertension. The range of vascular changes in the kidney may be indistinguishable from malignant hypertension. The mechanism of the arterial damage in scleroderma is not clear but is presumed to be immunological in nature.

In conclusion, it is likely that intravascular coagulation is both a cause and an effect of renal damage in a range of disorders in which there is endothelial cell damage; increased vascular permeability and fibrinoid necrosis occur in the acute stage, while endarteritis predominates in the healing phase. The histological appearances are similar in these diseases because the vascular tree has a limited range of responses to injury, regardless of aetiology.

19.4.8   Further reading

Tischer, C. C. and Bremner, B. M. (1989). *Pathology of the kidney.* J. B. Lippincott Co., Philadelphia.

19.5   Pyelonephritis

M. J. Wilkins and D. J. Evans

Pyelonephritis is an infection of the kidney which affects the parenchyma, the pelvis, and the calyces. Both acute and chronic forms may occur and may be found with or without obstruction to the urinary tract. There is a twentyfold increased incidence of pyelonephritis associated with *obstruction*.

19.5.1   Urinary-tract infection (UTI)

Infection may reach the kidney via the *bloodstream* or by *ascent from the lower urinary tract*. Ascending infection is usually deemed the more important mechanism, though bloodstream spread to the kidney has probably been underemphasized in the past, since a transient bacteraemia occurs with lower tract infections.

At first presentation, the most common pathogenic organisms responsible for a urinary-tract infection are bacteria of the coliform group, mainly *Escherichia coli* and *Enterobacter*, more rarely *Klebsiella*, *Pseudomonas*, and *Proteus*. *Staphylococcus albus* may occur in girls between the ages of 10 and 16 years, and *Klebsiella* and *Enterobacter* are more common in neonates. Other bacteria occur more commonly in recurrences; in cases in which sulphonamide or antibiotic therapy has been used, especially in cases with obstruction, and particularly those in which instrumentation has been used. These include various species of *Proteus* (especially *Proteus mirabilis*), *Enterococcus*, *Pseudomonas*, *Staphylococcus*, and *Candida*. Serotyping using O antigens shows that for *E. coli* infection, the urinary pathogens are usually present in the patient's own faecal flora. It also appears that certain serotypes of *E. coli* are more likely to produce infection. This probably reflects both their relative prevalence in faeces and their pathogenicity. Serotype O_6 appears more pathogenic than other types and this may be related to its ability to adhere to the urothelium.

Recurrent UTIs due to *E. coli* usually show different O serotypes in each recurrence. The controversial role of *protoplasts* in recurrent UTI should also be mentioned here. Protoplasts develop when the cell wall of an organism is disturbed so that the organism loses its usual form and becomes spherical. These forms can survive well in the hypertonic renal papillae and may persist at this site, especially in the presence of pre-existing renal damage. Since they are devoid of cell walls, they are also resistant to many antibiotics used to treat UTIs. It is important to realize that even the apparently healthy urethra frequently harbours organisms that may initiate an infection if carried to the bladder during, for example, catheterization, and these organisms are probably also important in the pathogenesis of recurrent UTIs.

Several normal defence mechanisms are important in preventing UTIs. These include:

1. The urethral length itself (greater and more effective in the male).
2. The presence of a competent valvular mechanism at the insertion of the ureter into the bladder.
3. The voiding mechanism (which allows clearance of organisms).
4. The low pH of urine (which renders it a poor culture medium).
5. The intrinsic antibacterial properties of the urethral and bladder mucosa.
6. The batericidal action of prostatic fluid.
7. The presence of cervico-vaginal antibodies which coat faecal enterobacteriacae and protect against periurethral colonization.

The role of serum antibodies is yet to be established. They may be produced only in response to infection.

Diagnosis of UTI and pyelonephritis

In testing urine samples for evidence of infection, counts of $>10^5$ bacteria/ml almost certainly indicate infection, while probably one-third of those $<10^5$/ml are also associated with true bladder infection. Contamination of urine samples may occur due to the normal distal urethral flora in both catheter and early stream samples. Asymptomatic bacteriuria, i.e. bacterial infection of the urinary tract with no clear clinical symptoms, occurs in 1 per cent of female children and <1 per cent of male children, but is of significance because those children with persistent bacteraemia have a higher incidence of renal scarring. Asymptomatic bacteriuria is also found in 3.4–6.9 per cent of pregnant women and some patients develop overt attacks of acute pyelonephritis later in pregnancy. However, it appears that bacteriuria in the adult rarely leads to progressive kidney damage.

Finally, *sterile pyuria*, in which pus cells are present in the urine in the absence of a positive bacteriological culture, while classically seen in renal TB and calculous disease, may also be seen in bacterial infection of the kidney.

When urine is infected it may be difficult to determine whether the kidney is infected. The following criteria have been proposed for determining whether this is the case:

1. elevated C-reactive protein in the serum;
2. raised levels of serum antibodies;
3. pus casts in the urine;
4. antibodies to Tamm–Horsfall protein;
5. coating of bacteria in the urine by antibodies.

Aetiology and pathogenesis of pyelonephritis

Infection of the kidney occurs more frequently when urinary stasis is present. Causes of stasis include:

1. benign senile hyperplasia of the prostate;
2. congenital valves of the posterior urethra;
3. renal calculi;
4. urinary tract primary neoplasm;
5. carcinoma of the cervix with involvement of the lower end of the ureter;
6. pregnancy, or after damage to, or disease of, the spinal cord, when there is atonia and dilatation of the ureters;
7. obstruction distal to the bladder (especially likely to result in infection because of increased catheter use and residual urine in the bladder).

Renal infection may occur by *haematogenous spread* or by *ascending infection* from the bladder via the ureters.

The normal kidney is very resistant to blood-borne organisms, especially *E. coli* and other common urinary pathogens. However, some organisms will produce infection in normal unobstructed kidneys. *Staphylococcus aureus* is the most common of these, e.g. in staphylococcal endocarditis or as part of a bacteraemia from a boil or carbuncle.

Actinomyces species, fungi, yeasts, *Mycobacterium tuberculosis*, and *Brucella* species will also produce infection in a normal kidney via the bloodstream. However, if the kidney is injured, especially by obstruction, blood-borne organisms will localize much more readily, and haematogenous transmission of Gram-negative organisms is recognized as an occasional complication of urethral instrumentation.

The most common pathway for renal infection is by ascent from the bladder. Though the normal human bladder and bladder urine are sterile, organisms do colonize the urethra and vaginal vestibule in the female. The extent of colonization may be influenced by host and bacterial factors.

Distal organisms may gain entry to the bladder with *urethral instrumentation* and *catheterization*, but in the absence of instrumentation urinary tract infections are much more common in females, ascent favoured by the shorter urethra. Once in the bladder, infection may occur and is favoured by the presence of a residual volume of urine following micturition as may occur with lower urinary tract obstruction or the presence of stagnant urine in bladder diverticula.

Once within the bladder, organisms remain localized in the majority of individuals but in some individuals they may pass up the ureters during micturition due to *incompetent vesico-ureteral valves*, either due to deformity or due to delayed maturation, i.e. *vesicoureteral reflux (VUR)*. In normal individuals, VUR is prevented by the oblique insertion of the ureters into the bladder, so that the ureter is compressed and closed during voiding. VUR is present in at least 0.5 per cent of neonates and is probably more common in males. In most children further maturation of the vesicoureteral junction leads to disappearance of VUR by adolescence.

Primary VUR appears to be due to a congenital defect in which the intravesical portion of the ureter is shortened and situated more laterally than normal. There are numerous reports of reflux occurring in families and in different generations of the family, but the mode of inheritance of this abnormality remains uncertain. Reflux is seen in 30–50 per cent of children with recurrent UTIs. Secondary VUR may occur as a result of trauma or surgery, and is present in up to 25 per cent of paraplegics with neurogenic bladder. Bladder infection itself can cause or accentuate VUR especially in children.

In the more severe cases of VUR, the infected urine can gain access to the renal parenchyma by intrarenal reflux in certain individuals. It has been demonstrated than an abnormality of the renal papillae is the basis upon which this occurs. Two populations of papillae are present.

1. *Simple (or convex) papillae,* in which the collecting-duct orifices are slit-like and close in response to a rise in intrapelvic pressure, as occurs in VUR, hence preventing reflux of urine into the renal parenchyma.

2. *Compound papillae,* with a concave surface and round or oval orifices which cannot be closed off, are found in 75 per cent of normal human kidneys. It is significant that in man these potentially refluxing papillae are located mainly in the upper and lower poles; the most common sites for pyelonephritic scarring.

Thus VUR followed by intrarenal reflux is a major mechanism whereby bacteria can be delivered from the infected bladder into renal parenchyma.

19.5.2 Acute pyelonephritis

Clinically, patients present with sudden onset of lumbar pain and tenderness, fever, and malaise. Dysuria and frequency occur if a lower UTI is also present. Predisposing factors are often present: *urinary obstruction, instrumentation, VUR, pregnancy, developmental anomalies of the kidney,* and *diabetes mellitus.* Thirty per cent of *pregnant women* with bacteriuria will subsequently develop acute pyelonephritis.

Gross appearance

The kidney is enlarged with a bulging cut surface and an adherent capsule. Small, raised, yellow-white abscesses with a haemorrhagic rim which vary in size, are seen on the surface, situated mainly in the cortex (Fig. 19.40). Other parts of the cortex show large areas of confluent inflammation and the papillae draining these areas show straight yellow streaks corresponding to large collecting ducts filled with polymorphs. Where obstruction has occurred, or in cases where there has been severe reflux, the parenchyma may be generally thinned and the papillae blunted. In such cases the most pronounced changes are seen in the upper and lower poles. When abscesses are widespread throughout the parenchyma, blood-borne infection is more likely. The pelvic and calyceal mucosal surfaces are frequently congested, and where obstruction or reflux has occurred the pelvic wall is thickened and the calyces dilated.

When the obstruction is total or almost complete, the suppurative exudate can fill and greatly distend the pelvis—*pyonephrosis.*

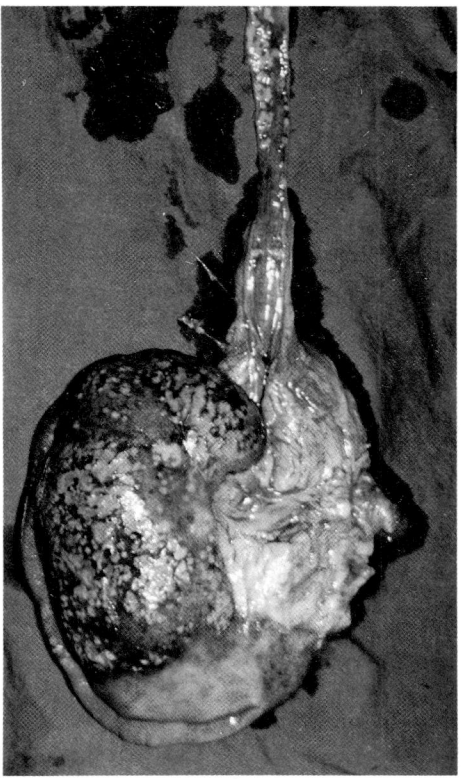

Fig. 19.40 Acute pyelonephritis, showing multiple cortical abscesses.

Microscopic appearance

There is extensive destruction of the parenchyma in infected areas by an acute inflammatory process, particularly in the cortex. The interstitium is infiltrated by polymorphs which sometimes burst into the tubules, and there is loss of varying numbers of proximal convoluted tubules (Fig. 19.41). Chronic inflammatory cells may also be present. Usually arteries, arterioles, and glomeruli show considerable resistance to infection. In adjacent areas there is a less pronounced acute reaction.

Abscesses are found in the outer part of the medulla, and polymorphs accumulate in collecting ducts in the inner part. The pelvic and calyceal epithelium also show acute inflammatory changes. However, extensive tracts of parenchyma show no inflammation whatsoever, so that there are discrete wedge-shaped areas of involvement with no spread of inflammation outside them. Occasionally, but especially in diabetics and those with obstruction, *papillary necrosis* may occur and one or all of the pyramids of an affected kidney may be involved.

In uncomplicated acute pyelonephritis, resolution occurs after the acute phase with a rapid return to the asymptomatic state, though bacteria may persist in the urine. In others, *interstitial fibrosis* and *tubular atrophy* ensues. The cortical surface becomes depressed, while the underlying calyx becomes distorted, expanded, and club-shaped. Acute pyelonephritis progresses to chronic pyelonephritis in only a small number of cases.

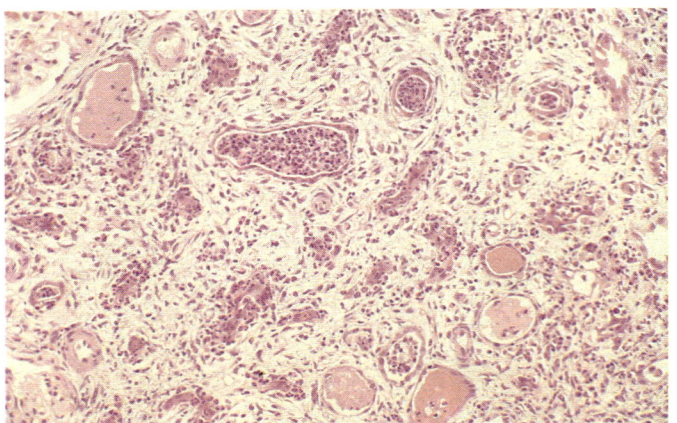

Fig. 19.41 Acute pyelonephritis, showing tubules filled with polymorphs and much interstitial oedema.

19.5.3   Chronic pyelonephritis

Chronic pyelonephritis accounts for 10–20 per cent of end-stage renal disease. It is a *chronic tubulointerstitial disorder* in which renal scarring is associated with pathological involvement of the calyces and renal pelvis. The diagnostic criteria are:

1. irregular scarring (asymmetric if bilateral);
2. inflammation, fibrosis, and deformity of calyces underlying the parenchymal scars;
3. predominantly tubulo-interstitial histological damage.

Bacterial infection associated with VUR or obstruction plays a role in most cases of chronic pyelonephritis. There are two broad forms:

Chronic obstructive pyelonephritis

Recurrent infections superimposed on obstructive lesions lead to recurrent bouts of renal inflammation and scarring, resulting in a picture of chronic pyelonephritis. However, the effects of obstruction lead to parenchymal atrophy and it may be difficult to differentiate the effects of the infection from obstruction alone.

Chronic reflux-associated pyelonephritis

This is the much more common form of chronic pyelonephritis, and is also sometimes termed *reflux nephropathy*. Renal involvement occurs very early in childhood due to VUR and intrarenal reflux, of urine which is infected. Whether VUR causes damage in the absence of infection (*sterile reflux*) is uncertain. The result is dilatation of one or more calyces accompanied by an overlying scar.

In cases in which VUR has been very severe there may be generalized pelvicalyceal dilatation with generalized thinning of the parenchyma (*back-pressure type*) in addition to focal scarring, and the latter may appear less prominent.

Clinically, chronic pyelonephritis has an insidious onset and may present as chronic renal failure or hypertension.

Gross appearance

The kidney is irregularly scarred and, if there is bilateral disease, the involvement is asymmetrical. Coarse, discrete cortico-medullary scars are seen overlying a blunted or deformed calyx, and these scars mostly involve the upper and lower poles.

The scars are large because the compound refluxing papillae drain large areas of parenchyma. The intervening unscarred areas are smooth or granular (related to hypertensive changes of small arteries). Varying degrees of pelvic or calyceal dilatation, with an overlying thinned parenchyma, are present when obstruction or severe reflux has been present. The pelvic epithelium is thickened and finely granular.

It is of the utmost importance to examine the calyceal system and its relationship to scars and to correlate with the clinical aspects of the case in making a diagnosis of infection as the main aetiological agent, since the microscopic picture is essentially one of chronic interstitial nephritis and the histology may be impossible to distinguish from an ischaemic or obstructive cause.

Microscopic appearance

Scarred areas are often composed entirely of dilated atrophic tubules, with normal renal parenchyma abutting on to the scarred area. The affected areas are often very extensive and, in some cases, no normal tissue may remain.

The glomeruli show very variable changes, including thickening of Bowman's capsule, fibrosis outside the capsule, collapse or solidification of the tuft, eccentric sclerosis or hyalinosis of the tuft, proliferative changes, and necrosis. In late stages the changes are indistinguishable from advanced ischaemic obsolescence.

There is destruction of tubules, especially the proximal convoluted tubules, which may disappear completely or show atrophy and shrinkage of epithelial cells with thickening of the basement membrane. The most characteristic picture is that of tubules lined by atrophic epithelium and containing homogeneous eosinophilic casts, some being much dilated with an appearance likened to thyroid tissue. Chronic inflammatory cells are scanty in these areas and the atrophic tubules may occupy much of what was cortex and extend out to the capsule of the kidney. These *thyroid-like areas* were once claimed to be specific for pyelonephritis, but may also be seen, on a similar scale, in ischaemic kidneys (Fig. 19.42).

In some cases there is considerable infiltration of the interstitium by chronic inflammatory cells (lymphocytes, plasma cells, and eosinophils), especially in cases with relatively little loss of parenchyma, but inflammatory cells are inconspicuous or absent in cases with heavy scarring. Lymphoid follicles are useful indicators of previous infection and can be very useful in differentiating scars following infection from those of other causation. There is a variable degree of interstitial fibrosis. The arteries and arterioles may show medial and intimal thickening in many cases, especially in those associated with hypertension, but this is a late change. Sections through the renal pelvis show an infiltrate of chronic inflammatory cells in which plasma cells

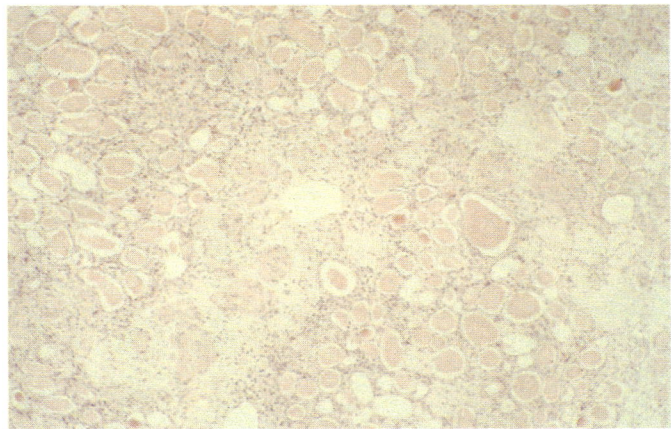

Fig. 19.42 Chronic pyelonephritis, showing interstitial fibrosis and dilated tubules filled with casts—so-called 'thyroidization'. (Courtesy of Dr M. Thompson.)

are prominent. In non-scarred tissue the glomeruli, arteries, and arterioles may show hypertensive and ischaemic changes. Otherwise, the tubules and interstitial tissue is unremarkable.

Formation of new radiological scars in adults is very uncommon, even if reflux persists, yet in some patients a progressive decline in renal function occurs, independently of ongoing reflux or obstruction, and is accompanied by hypertension and proteinuria. This is due to the development of a glomerular lesion—*focal and segmental hyalinosis and sclerosis* (FSHS). One popular theory for the development of FSHS is that the glomerular lesion is related to prolonged 'hyperfiltration' in the residual glomeruli (see Section 19.3.11).

19.5.4 Other infective renal disease

Renal tuberculosis

Once a common disease, renal TB is no longer common in the Western world due to prompt and effective treatment of cases of tuberculosis. Almost all renal TB is haematogenous in origin, usually originating in the lung. Initial lesions are usually cortical, bilateral, and mostly within glomeruli. These then either completely heal, leaving small fibrous scars, or progress focally, explaining why renal TB is usually unilateral. The progressing lesion spreads into pyramids and into calyces. The lesions vary from minute to large cavitating masses. Therapy induces healing and fibrosis and this can cause obstruction, usually at one of three places: the neck of the calyx, ureteropelvic junction, or ureterovesical junction.

Xanthogranulomatous pyelonephritis

This is a chronic infective condition of the kidney which is never bilateral. It is important because it may be mistaken for cancer of the kidney. It occurs more commonly in females than males and may occur at any age. Symptoms include fever, weight loss, lassitude and nausea, and vomiting. A palpable mass may be present. Urine culture shows *Proteus* (implicated in over 60 per

cent), *E. coli*, *Klebsiella*, *Pseudomonas*, and *Enterobacter*, in decreasing order.

Gross appearance

The kidney is enlarged with adhesions to adjacent retroperitoneal tissue and perirenal fibrosis. The pelvis is dilated and often contains a *staghorn calculus*. The calyces are also dilated and lined by a yellowish zone which is friable on the inner aspect. Often abscesses with a surrounding yellowish zone can be seen in the parenchyma. The cortex is reduced in thickness and firm in consistency.

Microscopic appearance

The yellow areas noted macroscopically are composed of an admixture of large, finely granular foam cells which contain lipid, smaller cells with an eosinophilic granularity, plasma cells, fibroblasts, and polymorphs with or without foreign body giant cells. Near the calyx there is much necrotic debris, and polymorphs are prominent in the areas abutting on the non-infected parenchyma. There is a proliferation of fibroblasts and fibrous tissue. Focal calcification is a frequent finding.

19.5.5 Further reading

Becker, G. (1986). Urinary tract infection and reflux nephropathy in adults. *Medicine International* 2 (33), 1337–43.

Hodson, J. and Kincaid-Smith, P. (eds) (1979). *Reflux nephropathy*. Masson Publishing, New York.

Kincaid-Smith, P. and Becker, G. (1978). Reflux nephropathy and chronic atrophic pyelonephritis: a review. *Journal of Infectious Diseases* 138, 774–80.

Malek, R. S. and Elder, J. S. (1978). Xanthogranulomatous pyelonephritis: A critical analysis of 26 cases of the literature. *Journal of Urology* 119, 589–93.

Smellie, J. and Normand, C. (1986). Urinary tract infection and reflux nephropathy in children. *Medicine International* 2 (33), 1344–50.

19.6 Interstitial nephritis

M. J. Wilkins and D. J. Evans

Inflammatory cells may migrate into the interstitium and this may be accompanied by the development of oedema and/or fibrosis. There is a variable degree of tubular damage, hence the term *tubulo-interstitial nephritis* is sometimes used. There is little evidence that the interstitium itself is a primary target.

Both acute and chronic forms occur. In both there is an infiltrate of lymphocytes, plasma cells, and other mononuclear cells, generally with few neutrophil polymorphs. The interstitium is oedematous in the acute form and fibrotic in the chronic form. Interstitial nephritis can be divided into *primary* where there is no glomerular lesion and *secondary* where there is a coexisting glomerular lesion. It is as well to note, however, that glomerular solidification may occur as a secondary phenomenon in chronic cases.

19.6.1 Acute interstitial nephritis

Situations in which acute interstitial nephritis occurs are:

1. reactions to drugs;
2. infections;
3. accompanying glomerulonephritis;
4. as a complication of transplantation.

The histological picture is generally non-specific, though occasionally a clue to the underlying aetiology may be present. Immunological mechanisms, either through anti-tubular basement membrane (anti-TBM) antibodies or by deposition of immune complexes in TBMs or peritubular capillaries, can contribute to a tubulo-interstitial nephritis.

Drug-induced acute interstitial nephritis

An acute interstitial nephritis may occur between 2 and 40 days (average 15 days) after exposure to certain drugs, and is a hypersensitivity reaction. Drugs that have been implicated include:

1. *antibiotics*: sulphonamides, synthetic penicillins, rifampicin;
2. *diuretics*: thiazides, frusemide;
3. *non-steroidal anti-inflammatory drugs*: phenylbutazone;
4. *cimetidine*.

Patients present with fever, eosinophilia (which may be transient), haematuria, mild proteinuria, sterile pyuria, and a skin rash in 25 per cent of cases. About 50 per cent show rising creatinine or acute renal failure with oliguria; this typically resolves on withdrawal of the drug, though it may take several months for the renal function to return to normal.

Grossly the kidneys are usually enlarged. The major histological changes are in the interstitium which is oedematous, causing separation of tubules, and most commonly contains an infiltrate of lymphocytes, plasma cells, and macrophages. Some cases show eosinophils and neutrophils in large numbers. Interstitial giant cells and granulomas may be seen, especially in cases related to methicillin and thiazides. Tubular changes include atrophy, dilatation, and focal epithelial cell loss with regeneration. Tubular casts may be seen. The glomeruli and blood vessels are usually normal. Electron microscopy and immunofluorescent studies are usually normal, although occasionally linear IgG and C3 are seen along the tubular basement membrane without glomerular changes.

It seems likely that the primary damage is to tubules and that a secondary reaction in the interstitium follows.

Infections

The reaction in acute pyelonephritis is a form of interstitial nephritis, with neutrophils predominating in this setting. Interstitial nephritis is also seen with *Mycoplasma pneumonia*, toxoplasmosis, leptospirosis, and brucellosis. The mechanism of production of the inflammatory infiltrate is not always clear; however, direct invasion of the kidney is likely.

19.6.2 Chronic interstitial nephritis (chronic interstitial fibrosis)

This non-specific parenchymal reaction results from a large number of stimuli. Some examples of chronic interstitial nephritis have passed through an acute stage—bacterial infections being the best example of this. Most take on a chronic pattern from the beginning. In some cases interstitial changes follow tubular atrophy and loss.

Chronic interstitial nephritis occurs in:

1. bacterial infection;
2. obstruction of the outflow of urine, either outside or within the renal parenchyma, e.g. gout;
3. analgesic nephropathy (secondary to papillary damage);
4. radiation injury;
5. Sjögren's syndrome;
6. sarcoidosis (with non-caseating granulomas containing giant cells);
7. nephronophthisis and medullary cystic disease;
8. Balkan nephritis.

The overall picture is one of diffuse interstitial fibrosis with tubular atrophy and a residual chronic non-specific inflammatory cell infiltrate.

19.6.3 Further reading

Heptinstall, R. H. (1976). Interstitial nephritis: a brief review. *American Journal of Pathology* **83**, 213–36.

19.7 Papillary necrosis

M. J. Wilkins and D. J. Evans

Papillary necrosis is not a disease entity *per se* but is a distinct clinico-pathological syndrome that develops in the course of other diseases, which directly or indirectly affect the kidney in general, and the renal medullary vasculature in particular, leading to focal or diffuse ischaemic necrosis of various segments of the renal medulla. The necrosis is always limited to the inner zone of the medulla and is usually restricted to the papillae.

The clinical course of papillary necrosis that develops is variable. It may present as an acute devastating illness, e.g. in *diabetes mellitus* or *obstruction*, that results in the rapid demise of the patient, or it may pursue a more protracted course of months or years, such as in *analgesic nephropathy*. The exact mechanism by which papillary necrosis develops remains uncertain, the basic pathophysiological process appears to be ischaemic necrosis.

Development of papillary necrosis

The main conditions associated with papillary necrosis are:

1. analgesic abuse;

2. diabetes mellitus;

3. pyelonephritis, which often presents in association with other diseases, although it may be the only cause;

4. urinary tract obstruction—obstruction leads to increased tubular dilatation, leading to compression of the interstitium containing the pyramidal blood vessels; the compromised blood flow then results in ischaemic necrosis of the papillae; the significance of infection in this connection, while important, remains undefined;

5. sickle-cell haemoglobinopathies.

19.7.1 Analgesic nephropathy

This is a chronic renal disease caused by excessive intake of analgesic mixtures, characterized morphologically by *papillary necrosis* and chronic *tubulo-interstitial nephritis*. First reported in Switzerland in 1953 and now recognized world-wide, there is a high incidence in Australia and Western Europe. Damage was first ascribed to *phenacetin* but the mixtures consumed often contained, in addition, *aspirin, caffeine, codeine,* and *acetaminophen,* a metabolite of *phenacetin*. It appears that the minimum requirement is 2–3 kg of phenacetin over 3 years, with an average of 10 kg consumed over 13 years. The disease accounts for approximately 15 per cent of end-stage renal disease in Australia.

Pathogenesis

There is much debate on this subject and it is thought that the main problem lies with the analgesic mixture, the weight of evidence favouring phenacetin, aided by another drug in the mixture. A recent multicentre case control study found an increased risk of chronic renal disease in association with the use of analgesic mixtures that contained phenacetin. The long-term daily use of acetaminophen, the major metabolite of phenacetin, was associated independently with an increased risk of chronic renal disease. There was no increase in risk associated with regular aspirin use.

In experimental animals, phenacetin (or its derivatives) and aspirin alone can cause papillary necrosis but only when given in very large doses. It is, however, readily induced by mixtures of aspirin and phenacetin, usually combined with water depletion, resulting in an increased concentration in the medulla. It is now clear that the papillary damage occurs first and that the cortical tubulo-interstitial nephritis is a secondary phenomenon. The initial injury is to the vasa recta and peritubular capillaries.

The phenacetin metabolite acetaminophen binds covalently to cellular proteins and depletes *renal glutathione*, and thus may injure cells by covalent bonding and damage to oxidative systems. The ability of aspirin to inhibit prostaglandin synthesis suggests that it may induce its potentiating effect by inhibiting the vasodilatory effects of prostaglandin, thus inducing an ischaemic component. Thus the papillary damage may be due to a combination of the direct toxic effect on tubular and endothelial cells and ischaemic injury. This postulate is consistent with the synergistic effects of these drug combinations.

Gross appearance

In the late stage of the disease there is total papillary necrosis and the kidney is often reduced in size. The subcapsular surface shows alternating depressed areas and raised nodules, the latter often assuming a characteristic ridged form. Depressed areas correspond to cortex in continuity with necrotic papillae that have undergone secondary atrophic changes. Nodules or ridges correspond to areas of cortex in direct line with the columns of Bertin, hypertrophy having taken place in these areas. Many of the papillae are totally necrotic, shrunken and withered with a yellow–brown colour. Calcification of necrotic papillae is sometimes apparent on cutting the kidney, and bone formation may occur. Some papillae may have separated, leaving a raw surface and radiologically dilated calyx. Sloughed papillae may be located in the pelvis or passed down the ureter.

Microscopic appearance

Confluent papillary necrosis is seen with dystrophic calcification, with or without bone formation. Less severe changes are present in the proximal medulla. There is only a minimal polymorphonuclear reaction to the necrosis, and the dead and healthy tissue merge almost imperceptibly one with the other. Overlying cortical changes include loss and atrophy of the convoluted tubules with interstitial fibrosis and variable numbers of chronic inflammatory cells. Lipofuscin often accumulates in atrophic tubular cells. These changes in the cortex are non-specific, also appearing in chronic infection, ischaemia, and urinary tract obstruction.

The cortical atrophy is probably due to obstruction of the loops of Henle, i.e. interference with continuity of the tubular system. The relative sparing of the columns of Bertin is due to the fact that they drain into forniceal regions of the calyx, thus avoiding the necrotic papillae.

Early and intermediate stages also exist. In the early stage the kidneys have a normal weight, the papillae are firmer than normal and show a series of yellowish lines radiating from the tips of the papillae, separated by darker areas. There are patchy changes concentrated around groups of collecting ducts, consisting of necrosis of interstitial cells, loops of Henle, and peritubular capillaries. The necrotic areas alternate with healthy areas.

In the intermediate stage the kidneys may still be of normal weight, the papillae are now shrunken and show an almost uniform yellow–brown discoloration which extends to the junction of the inner and outer medulla. Micro-confluent areas of necrosis occur in the inner medulla, which involve all the elements but the collecting ducts. The patchy necrosis seen in the early stage extends to the outer medulla. The cortex may show patchy tubular atrophy, interstitial fibrosis, and patchy chronic inflammation.

Clinical aspects

The disease is more common in females than males (usually in a 3:2 ratio), and has been found to occur most often in those suffering from chronic headaches and psychoneuroses. Clinical symptoms are often slight before the onset of renal insufficiency. If renal function tests are done, the earliest change is inability to produce a concentrated urine, as would be expected in a papillary lesion.

Headache, gastrointestinal symptoms, and hypertension are common accompaniments of analgesic nephropathy. Pyuria is very common, although the urine is often sterile.

Sloughing of the tips of the papillae leads to haematuria, renal colic, and ureteric obstruction. Progressive lesions will lead to chronic renal failure; however, if drugs are withdrawn and infections treated promptly, the renal failure may stabilize and improve slightly.

Urothelial transitional cell carcinoma

There is a definite association between analgesic abuse and transitional cell carcinoma of urothelial surfaces, especially the renal pelvis. Most of these patients have analgesic nephropathy, but this is not invariable. Risk does not appear to reduce with cessation of analgesics after the nephropathy is established. Cases of cancer, reported several years after the peak incidence of papillary necrosis, suggest that a prolonged period is necessary for malignancy to develop. There is often widespread urothelial atypia. Bilateral nephroureterectomy should be carried out with transplantation for end-stage analgesic nephropathy.

19.7.2 Papillary necrosis and diabetes

Papillary necrosis is particularly prevalent amongst diabetic patients. It is usually a terminal event in diabetes, with rapid onset of acute renal failure, although recovery does occasionally occur. Reasons for this are the impaired circulation to the papillae and propensity for infection. Papillary necrosis occurs in 25 per cent of patients with diabetes and acute pyelonephritis.

Gross appearance

The disease is bilateral, the kidney is enlarged, normal, or (more rarely) reduced in size, and the subcapsular surface is granular in cases with arterial narrowing. There are small, white abscesses on the subcapsular surface, as in acute pyelonephritis.

Small cortical abscesses are present on the cut surface, with thin yellow lines coursing to the papillae if there is infection of any magnitude. Varying numbers of papillae show yellow or grey–red, sharply defined lanceolate or box-shaped areas, involving as a rule the distal two-thirds. There is a congested border to the necrosis.

Microscopic appearance

Necrotic tissue is separated from the living tissue by a dense zone of polymorphs. In the necrotic area, tubular epithelium has usually disappeared. Powdered nuclear material and bacteria are often present in the necrotic tubules. Dead interstitial tissue is usually free from inflammatory cells. The surface epithelium over the papilla is lost, particularly at the tip. In the non-necrotic medulla adjacent to the polymorph zone there may be evidence of acute pyelonephritis. The remaining kidney parenchyma may show stigmata of acute or chronic pyelonephritis, or diabetes. The cortex may also exhibit tubular loss and atrophy, with increased fibrosis and increased numbers of chronic inflammatory cells.

19.7.3 Further reading

Abel, J. A. (1971). Analgesic nephropathy: a review of the literature, 1967–1970. *Clinical Pharmacology and Therapeutics* **12**, 583–98.

Eknoyan, G., Quinibi, W. Y., Grissom, R. T., Tuma, S. N., and Ayus, J. C. (1982). Renal papillary necrosis: an update. *Medicine* **61**, 55–73.

Sandler, D. P., *et al.* (1989). Analgesic use and chronic renal disease. *New England Journal of Medicine* **320**, 1238–43.

19.8 Renal transplantation

M. J. Wilkins and D. J. Evans

Renal transplants are classified into four groups according to the genetic relationship between the donor and recipient:

1. *autograft*, the donor and recipient are the same individual;

2. *isograft*, the donor is of the same genotype as the recipient (an identical twin);

3. *allograft*, the donor is of the same species as the recipient but of a different genotype;

4. *xenograft*, the donor is of a different species from the recipient.

Autografts and isografts are accepted by the recipient. Allografts and xenografts induce an immune response which, if not circumvented or suppressed, will lead to destruction of the transplanted kidney.

Only renal allografts have been used extensively. The patient's tendency to reject the graft is counteracted by immunosuppressive treatment. The sole or main agent generally used now is cyclosporin A, though prednisolone and antilymphocyte antibodies may also be required. Azothioprine is less used than formerly. The recipient is usually tissue-typed and the best-matched kidney available for transplantation is chosen.

19.8.1 Renal allografts

Without intervention, allografts rarely function for more than several days. In contrast to the minimal transient cellular invasion that occurs in autografts, in allografts and isografts there is a progressive infiltration with cells and oedema fluid, followed by widespread tubular necrosis. The transplant acts as multiple foreign antigens, provoking an actively acquired immunity in the host. The rejection of allografts is determined by genetic factors; the survival varies directly with the antigenic similarity between the donor and the recipient, defined in terms of the extent of human leucocyte antigens matching.

The most important genetic region controlling the rejection of kidney grafts is called the major histocompatibility complex. In man this complex is known as the HLA system because transplantation antigens were first identified in peripheral blood leucocytes and were thus designated as human leucocyte antigens (abbreviated HLA). The closely linked genes of the HLA system are grouped on a very small segment of the short arm of chromosome 6. Four loci, designated A, B, C, and D, control transplantation antigens. The antigens at locus D originally were defined by mixed lymphocyte culture. When typing for these antigens is carried out serologically with natural isoantibodies, the antigens are termed D-related, or HLA-DR. The association of HLA-D and HLA-DR is very close, and they may be separate sites on the same HLA antigen molecule that are recognized serologically (DR) and by cellular responses (D).

There is an enormous degree of genetic polymorphism in the HLA system and with well over 60 antigens coded for by the HLA system, the number of possible phenotypes is huge.

The A, B, and C antigens of HLA are found on the surface of most nucleated cells, as well as on platelets, including the renal vascular endothelium, particularly large vessel endothelium, and within renal tubular, interstitial, and mesangial cells (proven by immunofluorescence studies using monoclonal antibodies). The HLA-D antigens exist on the surfaces of the B-lymphocytes, some T-lymphocytes, and on monocytes and macrophages. HLA-DR is found in renal endothelial cells, particularly the endothelium of the intertubular capillaries, and is induced on renal tubular, interstitial, mesangial, and possibly glomerular epithelial cells. Proteins other than those of the HLA system are involved in transplant rejection, though to what extent is not yet established.

Much experimental work in dogs has been undertaken in the past to study the sequence of events and mechanisms resulting in the rejection of a renal transplant without immunosuppression, when it is rare for a kidney to survive longer than 20 days.

However, with the use of powerful immunosuppressive drugs and selection of a graft which by HLA typing is most compatible with the recipients antigens, graft survival is considerably prolonged in the transplantation programmes undertaken today. Tissue matching is certainly worthwhile in choosing the best

donor for an intrafamilial renal graft, since there is a 25 per cent change of a sibling inheriting the same chromosome from each parent, but HLA compatibility has a less dramatic effect on the outcome of cadaveric renal grafts.

Until recently, patients received blood transfusions prior to transplantation since this induced a state of immune unresponsiveness and hence improved graft survival. However, with the improved drug regimens used today, the benefits of immunosuppression resultant on prior blood transfusion are outweighed by the problems of sensitization.

Rejection is commonly classified clinically as *hyperacute*, *acute*, or *chronic*.

19.8.2 Hyperacute rejection

This occurs in red cell ABO group incompatibility or when, as a result of *pregnancy*, *blood transfusion*, or a *previous transplant*, the recipient has developed cytotoxic HLA antibodies reactive with the donor's cells, i.e. circulating antibodies are already present at the time of transplantation. The speed with which the graft is rejected depends largely on the degree of sensitization and the magnitude of the mismatch between the donor and recipient.

Hyperacute rejection can be avoided by ensuring that the donor and recipient are ABO compatible, screening the recipient for antidonor antibodies, looking for cold agglutinins, cross-matching donor cells in pooled plasma that is to be used to perfuse the donor kidney, and undertaking a final cross-match before transplantation. These procedures ensure that hyperacute rejection is a rare event today. In the rare circumstance when this does occur on re-establishing the blood flow to the transplanted kidney, it becomes pink but does not develop normal tone. After 10–20 min the organ progressively softens and mottled blue areas appear on its surface. Blood flow quickly falls and diuresis does not occur. Within a few hours urine flow ceases. Over the next day or so *progressive cortical necrosis* occurs.

Early biopsies of hyperacutely rejecting allogenic kidneys show a linear localization of IgG and C3 on the glomerular and intertubular capillary walls. Soon afterwards, neutrophils line the capillary walls, the platelets degranulate, and fibrin appears in the capillary lumens. Soon most of the intrarenal capillaries and arterioles are blocked by microthrombi (Fig. 19.43). After a few days there is complete cortical necrosis.

It appears that hyperacute rejection is mediated solely by a humoral mechanism. In recently reported cases the antibodies have been mainly anti-endothelial and not picked up by the screening procedures mentioned above. Treatment is rarely helpful and most surgeons remove a hyperacutely rejected kidney as soon as the diagnosis is established.

19.8.3 Acute rejection

Despite continuous immunosuppressive therapy, many patients with renal allografts undergo one or more clinical episodes of acute rejection. These episodes are common during the first few weeks after transplantation and, although they may occur at

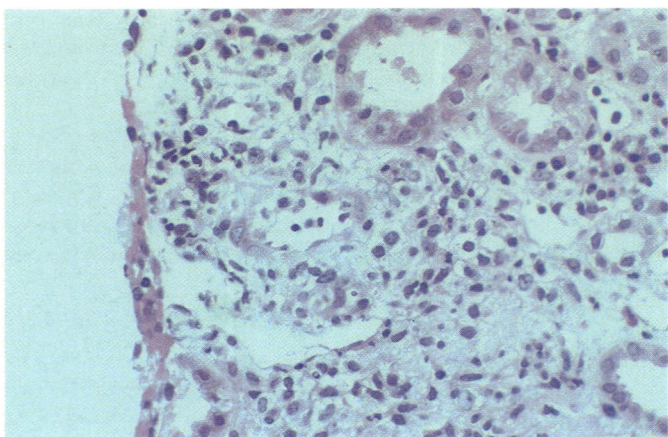

Fig. 19.43 Hyperacute rejection. Microthrombi are present in capillary lumina. (Courtesy of Dr M. Thompson.)

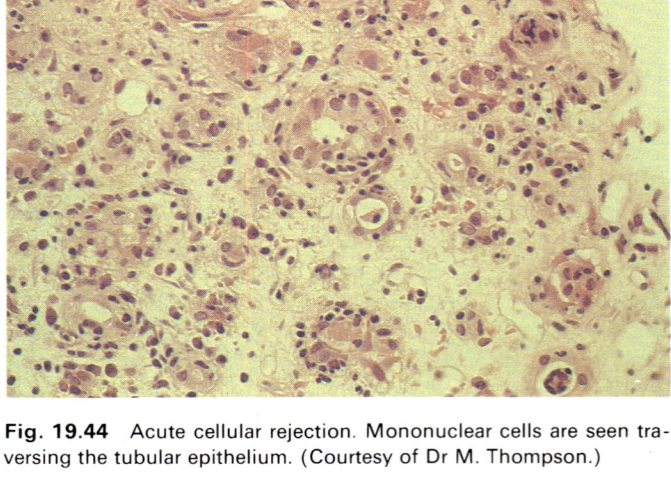

Fig. 19.44 Acute cellular rejection. Mononuclear cells are seen traversing the tubular epithelium. (Courtesy of Dr M. Thompson.)

any time during the life of a graft, they are uncommon after one year.

In severe cases the patients develop fever, swelling and tenderness of the kidney, anorexia and oliguria, increased blood pressure, and proteinuria. There is decreased creatinine clearance and increased blood urea. Generally, however, acute rejection presents as failure of the kidney graft to function adequately or as a deterioration in renal function.

Gross appearance

The graft is swollen and heavy with a pale cortex, bulging cut-surface, and tiny haemorrhagic foci scattered throughout the cortex, often with medullary congestion and haemorrhage.

Microscopic appearance

A wide spectrum of changes is seen with varying degrees and

combinations of cellular- and antibody-mediated damage. The exact pattern produced depends on many factors.

In predominantly *cellular rejection*, which occurs early after transplantation, the main site of damage is to the epithelium, and mononuclear cells are seen traversing the tubular epithelium (Fig. 19.44). There is accompanying oedema and a chronic inflammatory cell infiltrate of the interstitium. This type of rejection responds well to treatment with immunosuppressive drugs and the prognosis is good.

In predominantly *vascular rejection*, which tends to occur some time later after transplantation, the prognosis is poor unless diagnosed early, since the process is difficult to reverse with steroids. The walls of small arteries and arterioles are infiltrated by mononuclear cells (Fig. 19.45), the endothelial cells become swollen and necrotic and there is focal fibrinoid necrosis of the vessel walls. Microthrombi then adhere to the damaged areas, with eventual obliteration of the lumina. There is accom-

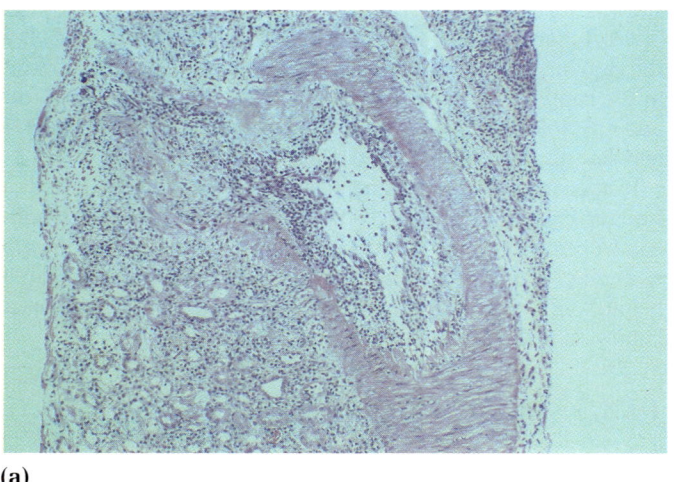

(a)

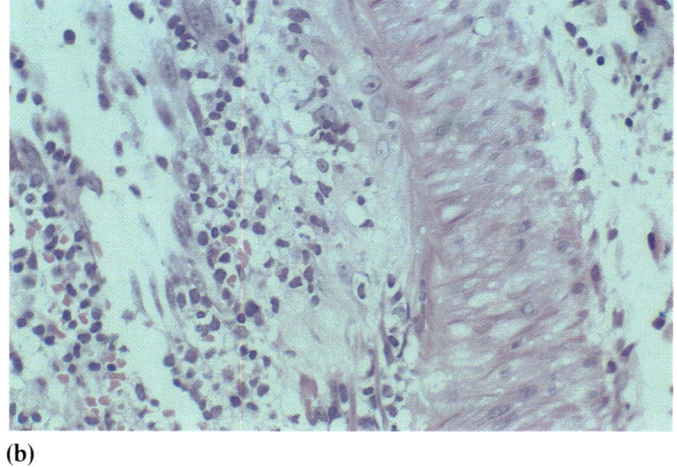

(b)

Fig. 19.45 Acute vascular rejection. Note vessels are infiltrated with mononuclear cells: (a) low power; (b) high power. (Courtesy of Dr M. Thompson.)

panying interstitial oedema and focal haemorrhage. Uncontrolled progression of these changes leads to cortical necrosis.

19.8.4 Chronic rejection

The changes of chronic rejection may occur as a sequel to one or more episodes of acute rejection, only partially responsive to high-dose steroid therapy. Under these circumstances chronic rejection is sometimes seen relatively early after transplantation. Usually the first indication of chronic rejection is a gradual deterioration in renal function some months or years after transplantation, without any obvious clinical episode of rejection.

Gross appearance

The kidney is of normal size or small. It is pale and usually smooth but there may be depressed scars of old infarction.

Microscopic appearance

There is arterial narrowing and glomerulopathy, separately or in combination. Both are usually associated with tubular atrophy and interstitial fibrosis with a patchy mononuclear cell infiltrate (Fig. 19.46). The juxtaglomerular apparatus is frequently hyperplastic. Arteriolar walls are thickened by large subendothelial hyaline deposits containing immunoglobulins and complement, and the lumina are narrowed and sometimes occluded as a result of continual or intermittent formation of platelet and fibrin aggregates on the vessel wall. Ischaemic changes are most marked in the superficial cortex, and sometimes infarcts are produced.

Glomerular changes seen include thickening of glomerular capillary walls and expansion of the mesangial matrix in a focal and segmental pattern. Segmental sclerosis, with or without hyalinosis, is common. There may be epithelial crescents. These changes are called *transplant glomerulopathy*.

These changes of chronic rejection pursue a relentless but variable downhill course which is resistant to treatment.

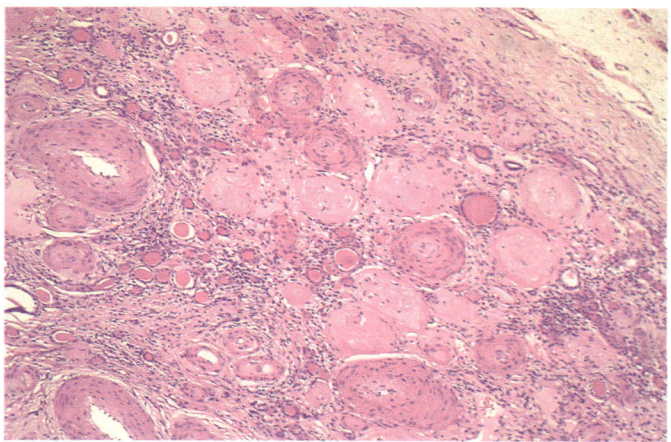

Fig. 19.46 Chronic rejection, showing tubular atrophy and interstitial fibrosis. (Courtesy of Dr M. Thompson.)

19.8.5 Other complications of renal transplantation

1. *Acute renal failure* in the period immediately after transplantation.

2. *Infections.* Immunosuppression leads to opportunistic infections, e.g. by cytomegalovirus, fungi, and various bacteria.

3. *Hypertension.* There is a high incidence in the first or second month following transplantation, especially in those recipients whose blood pressure is raised before transplantation. Causes include rejection, stenosis of the renal artery of the graft, the presence of the patient's own diseased kidneys, recurrent glomerulonephritis, and steroid excess.

4. *Lipid abnormalities,* a consequence of chronic renal failure, continue to affect many patients after transplantation.

5. *Gastrointestinal complications,* peptic ulcer, multiple superficial gastric erosions, etc., probably steroid-related.

6. *Malignant neoplasia.* There is an excess of squamous-cell carcinoma of the skin and fatal lymphoproliferative disorders, many of which are Epstein–Barr virus related, show a considerably increased incidence.

7. *Recurrence of glomerulonephritis.* Glomerulonephritis can be transmitted from host to graft. Sometimes it may be difficult to differentiate between transmission of glomerulonephritis, glomerulonephritis occurring as part of the rejection process, and glomerulonephritis arising as a new disease involving antigens unrelated to the recipient's original glomerulonephritis and unrelated to graft antigens. Examples of glomerulonephritis that recur in the transplanted kidney include:
   (a) anti-glomerular basement membrane mediated glomerulonephritis;
   (b) Berger's disease (IgA nephropathy);
   (c) type II mesangiocapillary glomerulonephritis;
   (d) focal segmental glomerulosclerosis;
   (e) membranous glomerulonephritis (rare).

8. *Recurrence of other diseases*: primary oxalosis, cystinosis, amyloidosis.

9. *Transmission of disease to the recipient by the graft.* Occasionally infection, e.g. viral hepatitis, is transmitted from the donor to the recipient. Rarely, cancer, unsuspected in the donor at the time of transplantation, has grown and spread in the recipient.

19.8.6 Further reading

Balch, C. M. and Diethelm, A. G. (1972). The pathophysiology of renal allograft rejection: a collective review. *Journal of Surgical Research* **12**, 350–77.

Cameron, J. S. and Turner, D. R. (1977). Recurrent glomerulonephritis in allografted kidneys. *Clinical Nephrology* **7**, 47–54.

Herbertson, B. M., Evans, D. B., Calne, R. Y., and Banerjee, A. K. (1977). Percutaneous needle biopsies of renal allografts: The relationship between morphological changes present in biopsies and subsequent allograft function. *Histopathology* **1**, 161–78.

19.9   Acute tubular necrosis

A. R. Morley

Acute renal failure may be caused by a wide range of factors which can be divided two main groups.

Ischaemic, which may occur in association with *hypotension, hypovolaemia, intravascular coagulation*, and *bacteraemia shock*. This is much the larger group and is of considerable clinical importance. When these abnormalities persist, cortical necrosis may occur. In this group tubular epithelial cell damage may be found, but tubular epithelial cell necrosis is not common. However, the term 'acute tubular necrosis' is commonly used by clinicians to indicate renal failure due to hypovolaemia. It must be clear from the outset that this term perpetuates a theory for the causation of acute renal failure and has little experimental support. It must, however, be admitted that the term 'ischaemic' is also open to criticism.

Nephrotoxic, caused by agents having a direct effect on the tubular epithelial cells. The considerable metabolic activity of tubular cells and their ability to absorb agents by pinocytosis from the lumen makes them vulnerable to many toxic agents excreted via the kidney. Furthermore, crystalline products within the lumen can lead to obstruction and to further tubular damage. In this group of diseases acute renal failure can indeed be related to 'acute tubular necrosis'.

19.9.1   The pathological changes in acute renal failure

Renal failure associated with shock ('ischaemic')

This condition is popularly termed *acute tubular necrosis* (ATN). As a widely used label it is unlikely that the use of this term will disappear, even though it is becoming clear that this process is not the main cause, or pathological finding.

Macroscopic examination reveals little beyond pallor of the cortex and some swelling of the cut surface. Microscopy shows normal glomeruli, some of which may contain eosinophilic material. In the latter stages, ingrowth of tubular epithelium (*tubular metaplasia*) is common. Tubules show a wide range of changes, which have been accorded variable importance. These include flattening of the epithelium, fewer nuclei per unit length of tubule, and occasional mitotic figures. Pyknotic nuclei and the eosinophilic cytoplasm of necrotic cells are rarely seen. Occasionally, rupture of tubular basement membranes may be seen. Sometimes these changes are most marked in the distal convoluted tubules, which may contain cellular debris. Pigmented iron-containing casts may be found, and are common in the collecting ducts. The role of casts as a cause of obstruction is not generally accepted, although there is evidence that Tamm–Horsfall protein, found in hyaline casts, can cause an inflammatory reaction if released by tubular damage into the interstitium.

In the medullary sinusoids in all forms of acute renal failure, primitive marrow cells may be found, chiefly nucleated red blood cells and myelocytes. Interstitial oedema is present in variable amounts. Scattered lymphocytes, plasma cells, and histiocytes are found in small numbers.

Electron microscopy has revealed widespread loss of the brush-borders in the proximal tubules, and considerable emphasis has been placed on the finding of spaces, indicating the loss of epithelial cells. Such changes may support the postulated back-flow of glomerular filtrate in renal failure.

Nephrotoxic acute renal failure

The changes are exemplified by *acute mercurial poisoning*, in which necrosis of proximal tubular epithelium predominates. Microdissection studies have shown that necrosis may be sharply localized to a particular segment of the nephron. Basement membranes of the tubules remain intact and may serve as a scaffolding for regeneration. Necrotic epithelial cells desquamate into the lumen, and there may be extreme pleomorphism and mitotic activity (Fig. 19.47).

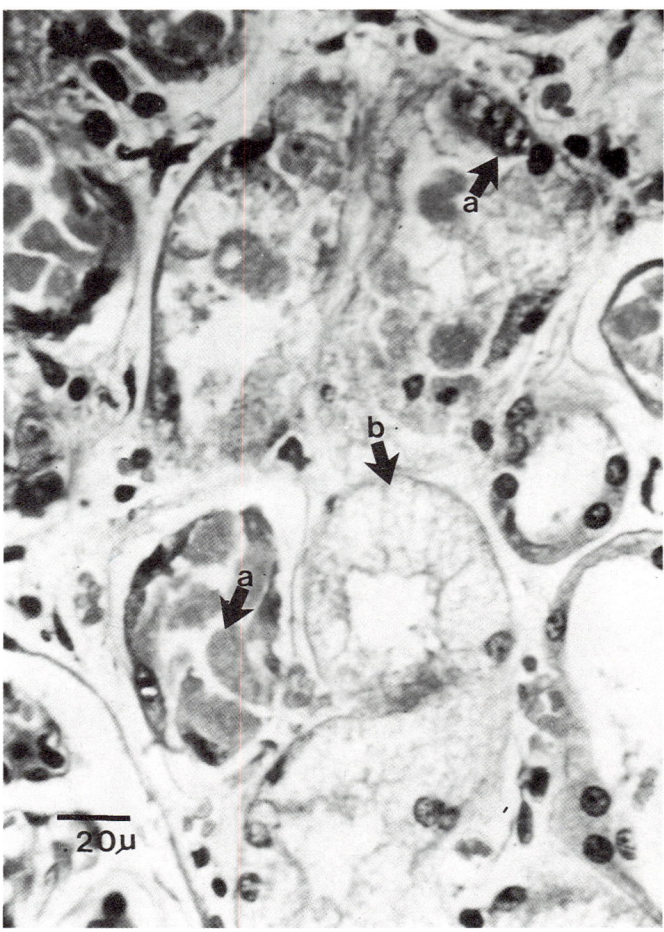

Fig. 19.47 Renal cortex in a patient with acute tubular necrosis following mercury chloride ingestion. Necrotic cells and pleomorphic tubular nuclei are present (a). Other tubular cells show foamy cytoplasm characteristic of dextrans and osmotic diuretics (b).

Tubular cytoplasmic vacuolation may be prominent. Unilocular vacuoles are found in association with hypokalaemia. In many patients therapeutic measures, such as the administration of *dextrans* or mannitol as volume expanders, can lead to widespread isometric vacuolation.

In *ethylene glycol (antifreeze) poisoning*, the presence of large numbers of oxalate crystals between tubular cells and in the lumen are a characteristic feature.

Cyclosporin A is now widely used as an immunosuppressant in transplantation of the kidney, heart, and liver. In high dosage it is nephrotoxic, producing widespread tubular vacuolation, vascular hyalinization, and, ultimately, interstitial fibrosis and tubular atrophy.

19.9.2   Renal cortical necrosis

The kidney, with its large circulation, nearly all of which passes through the cortex and glomeruli, is particularly susceptible to ischaemia. This may involve arteries and/or arteriolar obstruction, which can be caused by the wide range of vascular

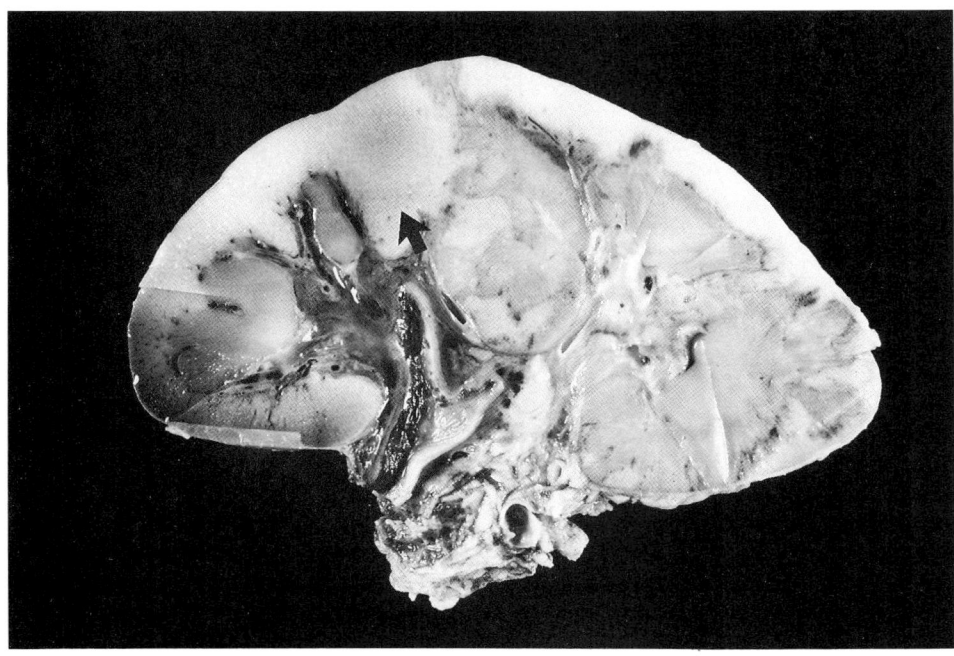

Fig. 19.48 Partial cortical necrosis as a result of severe vascular rejection. Note the triangular shape of cortical infarcts and involvement of the column of Bertin (arrow).

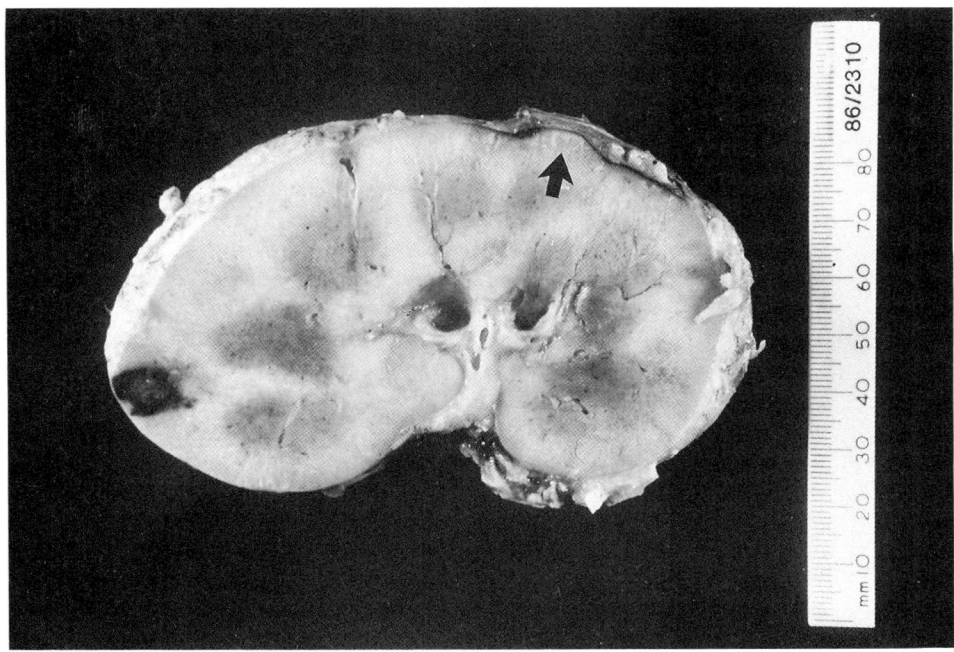

Fig. 19.49 Cortical calcification (arrow) in renal transplant 6 weeks after severe vascular rejection.

mechanisms described in Section 19.4. In the past, postobstetric and postoperative shock were the major causes; today renal transplantation and rejection must be added. In addition, cortical necrosis may be associated with intravascular coagulation related to *snake venom*, and the *haemolytic-uraemic syndrome*. In the tropics, dehydration and fluid loss in gastrointestinal disease may result in cortical necrosis.

Renal appearances in cortical necrosis

Cortical necrosis can be divided into *minor*, *focal*, *patchy*, *confluent*, and *complete forms*. These will depend on the severity and prolongation of the precipitating factors. In general, it can be expected that where more than half of the renal cortex is destroyed, the patient will develop renal failure. Conversely, the minor forms are usually a chance observation with less evidence of renal damage.

In the localized forms of cortical necrosis, the areas of necrosis are seen as white patches in the cortex. On section, areas of cortical pallor are seen of triangular outline (Fig. 19.48). It should be remembered that the columns of Bertin extend into the inner renal zone and may also show cortical necrosis. The pale areas are surrounded by rims of congestion and haemorrhage. At the viable margins of necrotic areas, infiltration of neutrophils is seen. Within necrotic areas, glomeruli and tubules are seen but lack nuclear staining or show pyknotic nuclei. Detachment of tubular epithelium from the basement membranes is similar to that seen on post-mortem degeneration.

In the more severe forms of cortical necrosis, recovery of function is rare. Within 2–3 weeks of onset, the development calcification appears as a cortical rim which may be seen on X-ray (Figs 19.49, 19.50). In a few patients some recovery occurs after an interval of weeks or months, this is rarely maintained and hypertension may develop.

19.9.3   Further reading

Dische, F. (1984). *Concise renal pathology. Acute renal failure*, pp. 92–105. Castle House, Tunbridge Wells.

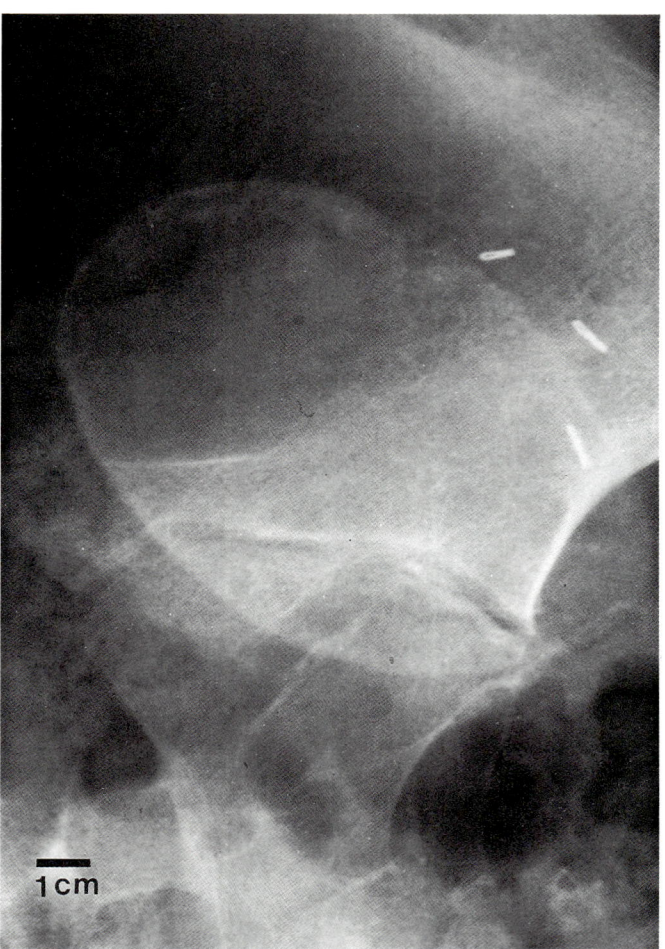

Fig. 19.50 Radiograph of calcified renal transplant following cortical necrosis.

19.10   Metabolic diseases

D. J. Evans

19.10.1   Amyloid

Amyloid is the name that was given to a family of proteins which are deposited in interstitial tissues and may cause disease because of consequent cellular atrophy or because of interference with basement membrane functions (see Section 5.5). The name was selected by Virchow because of their 'starch-like' affinity for iodine, which is due to the carbohydrate groups they contain.

All amyloids appear histologically as eosinophilic intercellular deposits which usually have an indefinite margin. They stain with Congo red, and after staining show green and yellow dichroism when viewed with crossed polaroids. Other staining reactions, such as metachromasia with methyl violet and applegreen fluorescence with thioflavine T, are either less sensitive (as with the former), or less specific (as with the latter).

Ultrastructurally, amyloids consist of a matrix in which there is a *major fibrillar component*, with fibrils of varied length but 8–10 nm diameter (Fig. 19.51), and a minor component (*P component*) which resembles a pentagonal doughnut, 8 nm in diameter, with a hollow core. The fibrils differ chemically and in their origin in different types of amyloid (Cohen and Connors 1987). Thus, in the systemic amyloids related to chronic infection, some tumours, and familial Mediterranean fever (secondary amyloids), the fibril is related to *a serum apoliprotein* (SSA) and the fibril protein is known as *fibril protein AA*.

A variety of other amyloids exists, but the only one commonly to affect the kidney is derived from immunoglobulin light chain (*amyloid fibril protein, AL*). This may occur in patients

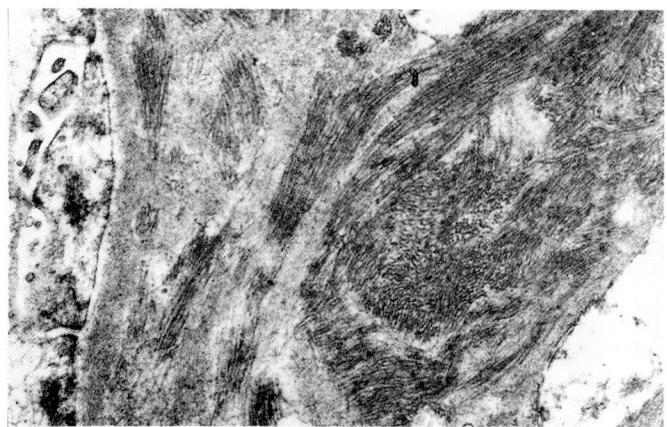

Fig. 19.51 High-power electron micrograph showing the fibrillar structure of amyloid. In this example, the parallel orientation is an unusual feature.

with myeloma, or more frequently in patients with *monoclonal gammopathy (primary amyloid)*. The various types of amyloid may be distinguished from each other by immunohistology as well as by clinical features.

The clinical manifestation of renal amyloid is usually due to glomerular involvement and consequent proteinuria. The proteinuria may initially be slight and highly selective, or severe and associated with nephrotic syndrome (Watanabe and Saniter 1975). Progression to glomerular destruction usually results in renal failure within a few years (Kyle and Bayrd 1975). *Renal vein thrombosis* is a relatively common complication and may be associated with deterioration of renal function or with acute renal failure.

It is common for renal failure to occur with kidneys that are enlarged, although, occasionally, shrunken kidneys are seen in patients dying with renal failure.

Histologically, the extent and distribution of amyloid vary from case to case and during the course of the disease. Glomerular deposits may be small and inconspicuous initially, and confined to mesangium, but eventually obliterate individual capillaries or complete tufts (Fig. 19.52). The deposits may then be found in any site in the glomerulus and often cross the basement membrane (Fig. 19.53).

Arterioles, interlobular arteries, tubular basement membranes, and interstitial tissues may also show involvement. With amyloid AL, vascular involvement is particularly common and often occurs in the absence of glomerular deposits.

Immunofluorescence findings in glomerular amyloidosis are variable. Small amounts of immunoglobulin are present in the deposits as a result of absorption, and these are sometimes detectable by fluorescence. AL amyloid is usually derived from λ light chains but, because it is from the variable portion, antisera against λ light chains may fail to stain it. In some cases, irregular granular deposits of immunoglobulin are present in the glomeruli, unrelated to the amyloid deposits: their significance is uncertain.

Localized amyloid

Isolated deposits of amyloid may be found in the renal pelvis or ureters without evidence of involvement of the renal parenchyma. Such deposits may produce haematuria, pain, infection, or even renal failure (Mariani *et al.* 1978). The amyloid is often of the AL type and is presumably analogous to amyloid tumours elsewhere, such as in the lung.

19.10.2 Myeloma

The commonest form of renal involvement in myeloma is by the formation of tubular casts derived from the abnormal immunoglobulin light chain, which passes from the serum into

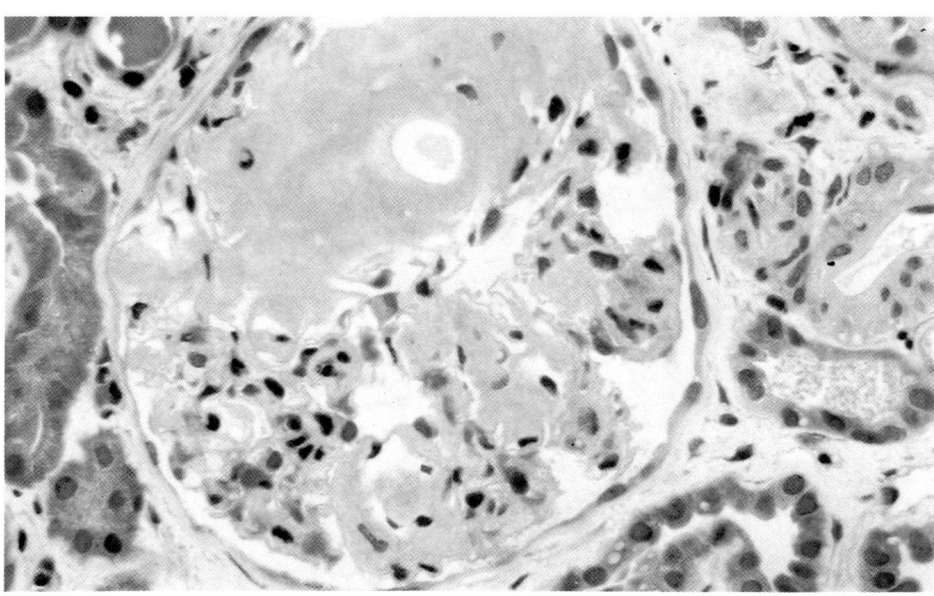

Fig. 19.52 Glomerulus showing a large segmental deposit of amyloid and other smaller deposits. Some trapped nuclei are visible in the large deposit but many cells have been lost. The amyloid is also encroaching on capillary lumina.

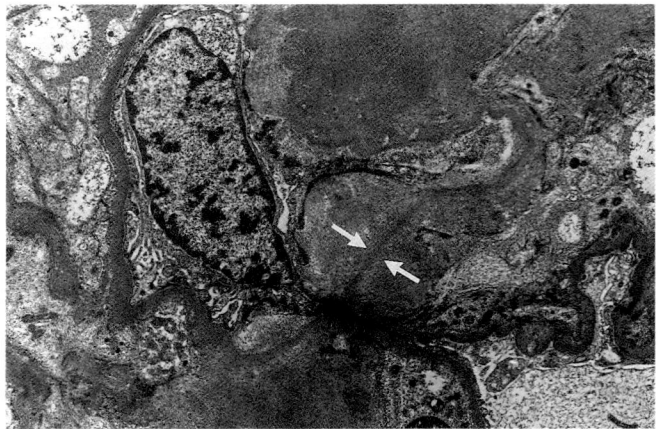

Fig. 19.53 Electron micrograph showing amyloid on both sides of a glomerular basement membrane (arrows).

the glomerular filtrate, and may be detected in the urine as Bence–Jones protein.

On histological section, the casts are usually present in the distal convoluted tubules (Fig. 19.54). and collecting tubules. Less commonly, they are seen in proximal convoluted tubules or in Bowman's space. They appear as eosinophilic and sharply outlined: sometimes they are cracked, laminated, or calcified, and sometimes they contain polymorphs. A surrounding giant-cell response is often present. Occasionally protein crystals may be formed (Fig. 19.55).

Dilatation or atrophy of the tubules is common, as is accompanying interstitial fibrosis with focal lymphocytic infiltration: this may be a consequence of tubular obstruction by the protein casts. Glomeruli are usually normal.

The usual clinical presentation is with insidious onset of renal failure. *Acute renal failure* may occur (De Fronzo *et al.* 1975),

especially following dehydration, and there is a particular hazard to *intravenous pyelography* in these patients.

Other changes

Amyloidosis (q.v.), *nephrocalcinosis* (consequent upon hypercalcaemia), and *pyelonephritis* (due to impaired immunity) are other possible consequences. Rarely, there may be seen a glomerular change rather similar on light microscopy to that of diabetes (Fig. 19.56): this is a consequence of deposition of a paraprotein fragment in the tissues. Most usually this is a κ light chain. The deposits may be seen in the glomerular capillary basement membrane or in the mesangium. Tubular basement membranes and vessels are also affected. Deposits are strongly PAS-positive. Ultrastructurally, they are granular and electron dense, and quite different from amyloid.

Another occasional occurrence is tubular loss of phosphate, glucose, and amino acids, similar to that of the De Toni–Fanconi syndrome.

19.10.3   Diabetes

Renal failure is an important cause of mortality and morbidity in diabetes. Almost 50 per cent of type I diabetics develop renal failure and this is usually due to glomerular involvement. Several different glomerular lesions may be seen microscopically.

The nodular lesion (Kimmelstiel and Wilson 1936): this is pathognomonic of diabetes. It varies in size and appears as a homogeneous eosinophilic mesangial nodule, typically with a rounded outline and usually acellular (Fig. 19.56). The number of lesions is quite variable, as is the proportion of glomeruli affected: individual glomeruli may have no nodules, a single nodule, or multiple nodules. They are relatively well

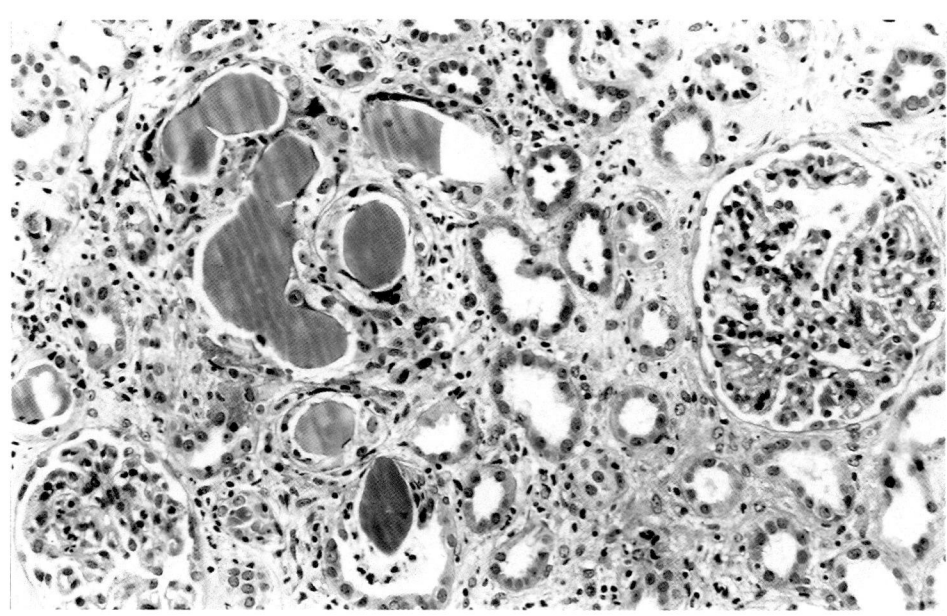

Fig. 19.54 Myeloma kidney. The glomeruli are normal but the tubules show atrophy and there is some interstitial fibrosis and inflammation. Prominent, deeply eosinophilic casts are present and are exciting a giant-cell reaction.

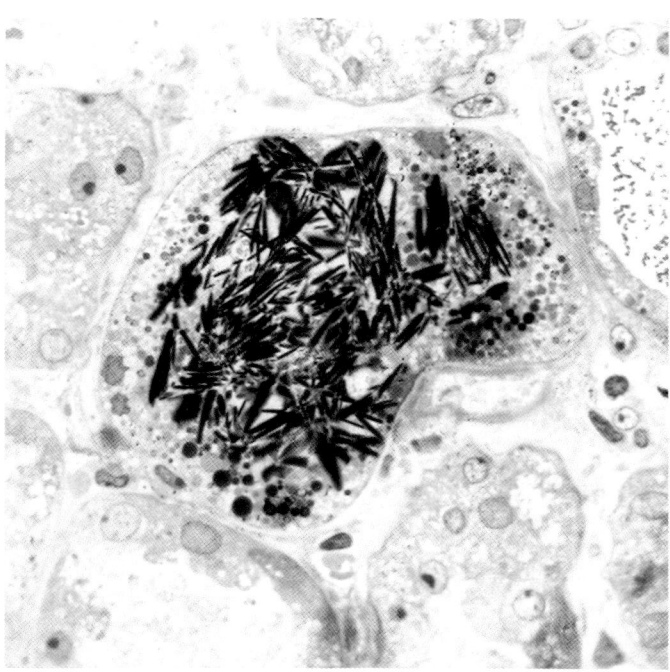

Fig. 19.55 Biopsy from a myeloma kidney, showing needle-shaped paraprotein crystals within the lumen of a tubule.

demarcated. Although they stain with PAS, the strength of the reaction varies. The lesion correlates poorly with proteinuria or renal impairment.

The diffuse lesion (Spühler and Zollinger 1943): this term is used in different ways by different authors, and covers cases of diabetes where there is a diffuse increase of mesangial matrix in the absence of any obvious thickening of the peripheral capillary wall, and others where thickening of both capillary wall and mesangium occur together (Fig. 19.57). The lesion correlates better with proteinuria than the nodular lesion. It is not uncommon for the diffuse and nodular lesions to occur together.

The exudative lesion (Barrie *et al.* 1952): this is not confined to diabetes. It consists of brightly eosinophilic, strongly PAS-positive (periodic acid–Schiff), and PTAH-positive (phosphotungstic acid–haematoxylin) material, apparently lying in capillary lumina on light microscopy (though in fact subendothelial), and often at the margin of the lobule. Sometimes it can be seen to contain lipid. The deposits are *not* rounded, as their configuration depends on that of the capillary lumen. The lesion is readily distinguished from the nodular lesion by its shape and staining properties (Fig. 19.58).

The capsular drop lesion: this is pathognomonic of diabetes. It is a highly eosinophilic small nodule on Bowman's capsule, with similar staining properties to the exudative lesion (Fig. 19.57).

Blood vessel changes

Severe hyaline arteriolosclerosis is common in diabetes, and both afferent and efferent arterioles may be involved.

Tubular changes

Tubular changes in diabetes are usually non-specific with atrophy and basement membrane thickening, or accumulation of lipid.

Immunohistology

In the diffuse glomerular lesion, linear IgG and sometimes IgM are seen. This is thought to represent non-specific trapping since eluted antibody will not bind to basement membrane (Gallo 1970) and albumin is also present. In the exudative lesion, IgM, C3, lipid, and fibrinogen may be found.

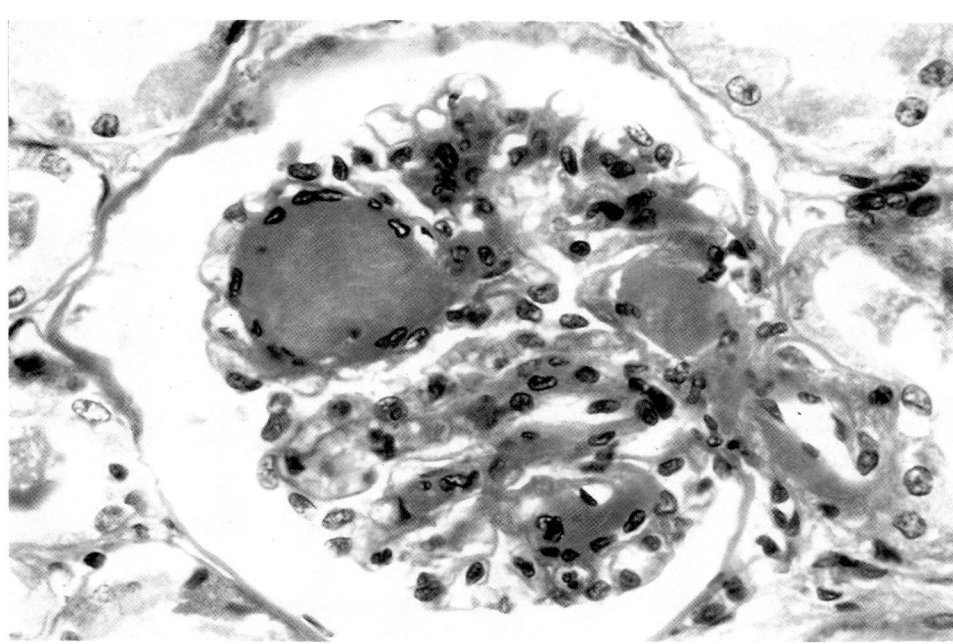

Fig. 19.56 Nodular diabetic glomerulosclerosis. This glomerulus also shows hyaline change in an afferent arteriole.

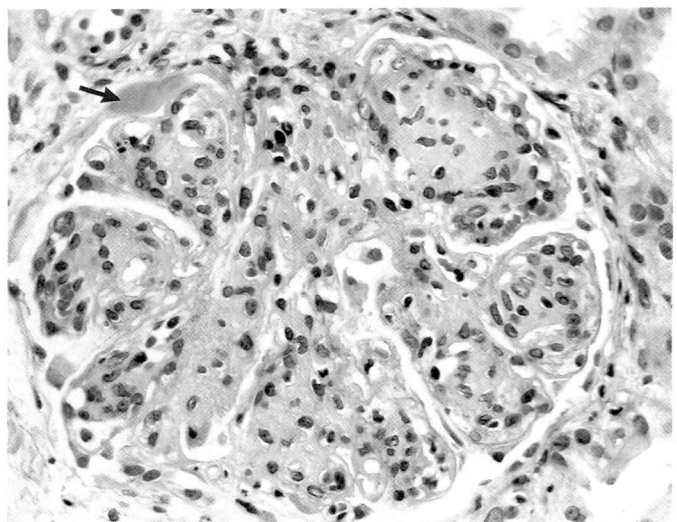

Fig. 19.57 Diffuse diabetic change mainly affecting the mesangium. A capsular drop is also present (arrow).

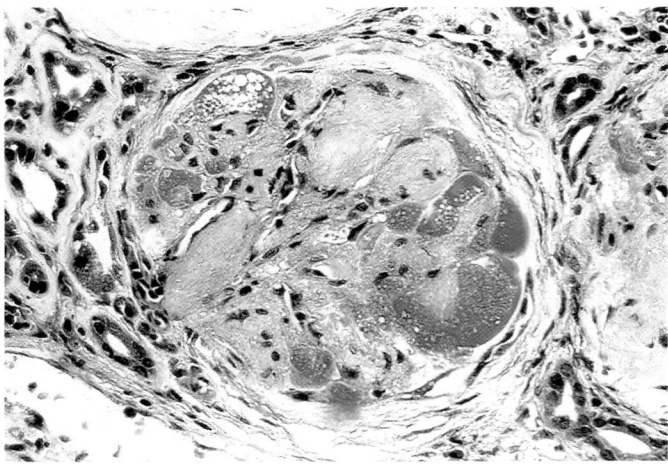

Fig. 19.58 Exudative diabetic change. The glomerular destruction is advanced: there are large eosinophilic and lipid-containing deposits, apparently in the capillary lumina, but these are superimposed on sclerotic changes.

Pathogenesis

This is still quite obscure. The immunohistology gives little support to the view that the glomerular lesions are immune-complex- or antibody-mediated.

Many diabetics have elevated glomerular filtration rates on presentation and attempts have been made to relate the lesions to glomerular hyperfiltration (Hostetter *et al.* 1982). However, the distinctive histology is against this.

Another proposed mechanism involves the non-enzymic glycosylation of proteins with impairment of turnover (Kanwar *et al.* 1983), possibly involving 'browning reactions' which cross-link proteins (Monnier *et al.* 1986). More recently there has been a revived interest in the possibility of disturbed polyol

metabolism, with high plasma glucose leading to a deficiency in myoinositol, which is an important component of cell membranes (see *Metabolism* 1986).

The long-held view that diabetics are particularly prone to urinary infections may not be true for ambulatory patients, though urinary infections are fairly frequent in autopsy cases. *Papillary necrosis* is prevalent among diabetics and often has a fatal outcome (Lawler *et al.* 1960).

19.10.4   Renal stones

The commonest renal stones consists of *calcium phosphate, calcium oxalate*, or *a mixture of the two*. 'Infection stones' (triple phosphate stones) are no longer as common as they were. *Uric acid stones* are less frequent than the two former types, and *cystine stones* are a rarity.

Calcium-containing stones

Several factors have been identified which predispose to the formation of calcium-containing stones.

Hypercalciuria

Idiopathic hypercalciuria is most frequent in males and appears to be due to increased intestinal absorption of calcium (Ritz and Massry 1977). About one-third of patients with calcium oxalate stones have idiopathic hypercalciuria.

Secondary hypercalciuria occurs when bone calcium is mobilized as a result of *primary hyperparathyroidism, sarcoidosis, Cushing's syndrome, hypertension, renal tubular acidosis*, or *prolonged bed rest*, and may result in stone formation. Different workers give strikingly different figures for the importance of hyperparathyroidism as a cause of renal stones, ranging from under 1 per cent to nearly 10 per cent of cases.

Hyperuricosuria

This is present as an isolated finding in nearly 15 per cent of cases with calcium oxalate stones, although its role in stone formation is unproven (Coe 1978).

Hyperoxaluria

Primary hyperoxaluria results from recessive inheritance of a metabolic abnormality (Williams 1978), and is associated with widespread deposits of oxalate in the kidney and oxalate deposits in other tissues. *Secondary hyperoxaluria* is due to increased absorption of dietary oxalate and may be seen in patients with *jejuno-ileal bypass* or *inflammatory bowel disease*. Both groups have an increased incidence of oxalate stones, but in primary oxalosis progressive destruction of renal tissue and renal failure develop inexorably.

'Infection stones'

These stones are also called *struvite stones* or *triple phosphate stones* and contain magnesium ammonium phospate and carbonate apatite. They are found in infected urines in which alkaline urine is produced by urea-splitting organisms, though other factors may also be involved (Howard 1954).

Uric acid stones

These stones form in an acid urine: about a quarter of affected patients have *gout*, but in most other cases hyperuricosuria is not present.

Cystine stones

These are almost always associated with cystinuria and are found in childhood or early adult life.

General comments

The initiation of stone formation is incompletely understood: the suggestion that they begin as plaques on the medulla has received little support. There is little evidence to support the view that stasis is of importance, and infection appears relevant only to struvite stones.

The consequence of stone formation depends on the size and positions of the stone. Ureteric or pelvic obstruction may produce *hydronephrosis* and *atrophy*. *Associated infections* may contribute to renal damage, but even in their absence there may be loss of useful renal function.

19.10.5   Gout

The subject is a confusing one, both with regard to the nomenclature and with regard to the effects on the kidney.

Secondary gout is the name given to the syndrome in which there is overproduction of uric acid associated with breakdown of purines derived from the cells of associated lymphomas, leuk-

aemias, or myeloproliferative disorders. Affected patients do not show gouty tophi or arthritis: acute impairment of renal function, which is probably due to precipitation of uric acid crystals in renal tubules, is the main clinical feature.

Primary gout is a metabolic disorder in which there are increased levels of uric acid in the blood, accompanied by clinical manifestations of gout, i.e. attacks of *gouty arthritis* or the presence of *gouty tophi* (tissue deposits of monosodium urate monohydrate).

Renal handling of uric acid/urate is complex. After being filtered by the glomerulus, there is resorption in the proximal part of the proximal convoluted tubules, followed by excretion more distally. A reduction in glomerular filtration rate may therefore contribute to an elevation in serum uric acid, and specific interference with tubular excretion (such as may be produced by lead poisoning and by diuretics) has a similar effect.

Renal failure is a fairly common finding in the gouty patients described in the literature (Barlow and Beilin 1968), and is present in up to 40 per cent of cases, but in many of these the appearances in the kidney closely resemble those of *ischaemia* and lack specific features, so it is difficult to be certain that the gout is responsible for the renal damage. Indeed, many cases of gout show no evidence of progressive renal impairment when followed over many years.

Could the impairment of renal function precipitate the gout rather than vice versa? Against this it is often argued that gout is rare in chronic renal failure, but in that case there is impairment of polymorph function, which may be partly responsible for the absence of gouty arthritis.

The specific changes described in the gouty kidney consist of *microtophi*, occurring mainly in the interstitium near the collecting tubules (Fig. 19.59a, b). These are often said to have

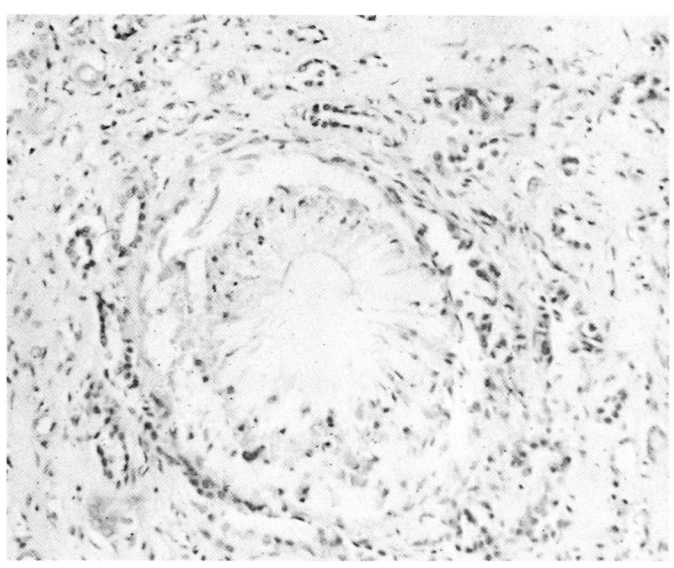

(a)

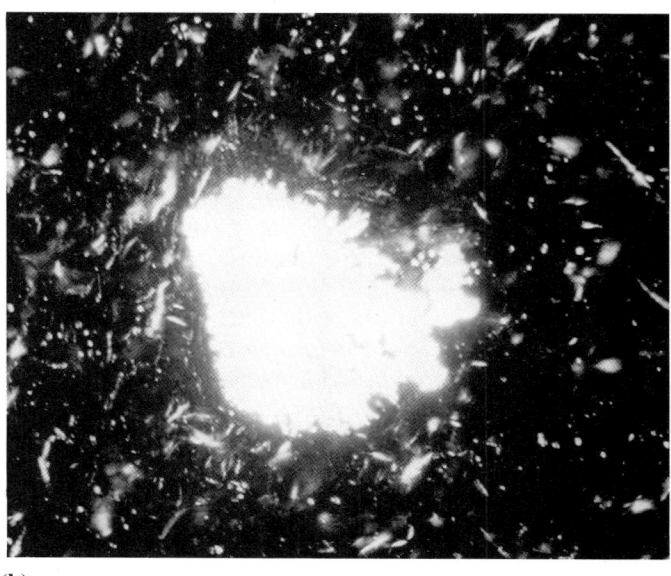

(b)

Fig. 19.59   Gouty kidney. (a) The urate deposit has been virtually dissolved during processing and only the ghost of a microtophus can be seen. (b) Frozen section showing birefringent sodium urate crystals in a microtophus. Some of the other crystalline material may be an artefact of section production.

originated from tubular precipitates, but this view may not be correct. Histological evidence of residual tubules is usually absent: moreover, microtophi consist of acicular crystals of sodium urate which tend to form at round pH 7.4, whereas tubular deposits are of amorphous uric acid which form below pH 5.7, and there is no good evidence of transformation from the one to the other.

Proof that the kidney can be damaged specifically in abnormalities of urate metabolism is provided by study of patients with deficiency of *hypoxanthine guanine phosphoribosyl transferase (HGPRT)*. In these cases, elevated output can be compensated for by elevated urinary excretion, with blood levels remaining normal. Formation of uric acid stones may be seen, but the level of uric acid excretion is not the only factor concerned: a possible additional factor is the habitual fluid consumption and urine output.

Episodes of acute impairment of renal function may be noted, especially in the neonate and following dehydration: because this is reversible by induction of diuresis and administration of alkali, it appears likely to be due to tubular blockage with uric acid. Recurrent tubular blockage might well be responsible for the tubular atrophy and interstitial fibrosis seen in cases with chronic renal damage: indeed uric acid casts as well as microtophi are usually demonstrable in such cases (Emmerson and Row 1975).

19.10.6   The kidney in pregnancy

Eclampsia and pre-eclampsia

During normal pregnancy there are substantial changes in renal blood flow and glomerular filtration rate, and the kidney increases in size. The glomerular filtration rate (GFR) increases by as much as 50 per cent; renal plasma flow is most increased in the first two trimesters (by up to 80 per cent) and remains elevated until delivery (Davison and Dunlop 1980); the kidney increases in weight by about 50 per cent.

Despite these large physiological changes, most pregnancies are not accompanied by the development of proteinuria. However, in a minority of individuals *eclampsia* (fits) occur and these are associated with *proteinuria, oedema,* and *hypertension*. Those patients who have the last three features are said to be *pre-eclamptic*, since they are at risk of developing fits.

Where the patient is known to have normal blood pressure and urine at the beginning of pregnancy, the diagnosis presents little difficulty; but pre-existing hypertension or glomerulonephritis may cause diagnostic problems in patients presenting late in pregnancy. Hypertension itself may redispose to eclampsia.

On a world-wide basis there are substantial differences in the prevalence of pre-eclampsia (Dieckmann 1952). In some nations about a quarter of women have been affected; in others only a fraction of 1 per cent.

Pre-eclampsia is about seven times as common in first as in other pregnancies: a proportion of affected women have recurrences in subsequent pregnancies, but this is only so in a minority of cases, and some workers believe that in multiparous women the disorder has a different natural history.

In most cases, onset of pre-eclampsia is after the 30th week (although it may be earlier in patients with hydatidiform mole). Proteinuria is ordinarily quite moderate in degree, and rarely reaches nephrotic levels. Occasionally acute renal failure is seen, but, usually, falls in GFR and renal plasma flow rate are of moderate degree, and levels may not reach pre-pregnant levels.

Following delivery, evidence of renal damage resolves. There is less agreement on the long-term effect on blood pressure, but the balance of the evidence indicates that pre-eclampsia has no adverse long-term effects (Chesley 1978).

Microscopy

The changes are virtually confined to the glomeruli. These appear somewhat enlarged and bloodless and the capillary lumina show partial occlusion by the cytoplasm of swollen endothelial cells. There is some expansion of the mesangium, but cellular proliferation is not a feature. Several authors describe the occurrence of mesangial interposition, with double-contours in peripheral capillary loops seen on silver staining (Tribe *et al.* 1979), but this is by no means a universal finding.

Immunohistology

Variable results have been reported. The most constant finding has been the presence of fibrin. IgM has been found quite commonly but IgA, IgG, and C3 are less frequently reported.

On electron microscopy the most striking finding is the swelling of the endothelial cells and, to a lesser extent, the mesangial cells. The subendothelial zone is usually widened and translucent, though it may also contain denser deposits. Mesangial interposition is also reported as occurring.

The pathogenesis of the disorder is not understood. It has been suggested that the lesions are the consequence of *intravascular coagulation*, or alternatively of an *immune complex disease*, but the evidence for both suggestions is unconvincing.

Postpartum haemolytic-uraemic syndrome

This is an uncommon entity occurring after delivery. It is not related to previous pre-eclampsia. Patients develop progressive renal failure, often, though not invariably, with severe hypertension. *Microangiopathic haemolytic anaemia* is usually demonstrable at least transiently. Recovery of renal function is rare and restricted to those cases that do not have changes in the interlobular arteries.

Microscopically, the changes are usually similar to those seen progressive systemic sclerosis or malignant hypertension. There is subintimal thickening of interlobular arteries which is widespread. Fibrinoid necrosis of arterioles and interlobulars are less frequently seen. Glomeruli show shrinkage of their tufts and convolution of the basement membrane, probably as a result of the ischaemia, and tubules become atrophic (Fig. 19.60).

Occasional cases have been reported in which the vessels are normal and the glomeruli show changes similar to those seen in milder varieties of the haemolytic-uraemic syndrome (Section 19.4.7).

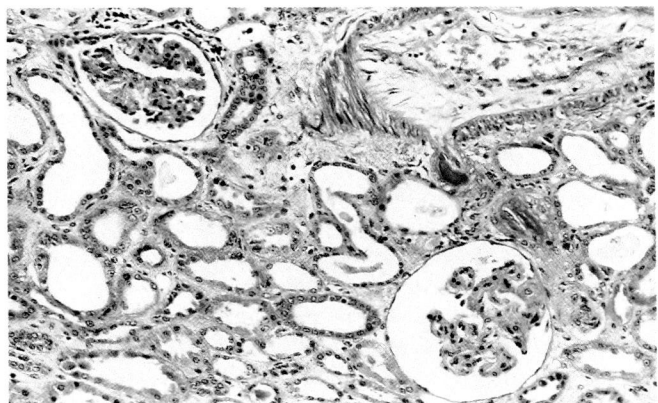

Fig. 19.60 Haemolytic-uraemic syndrome post-pregnancy. There is some tubular atrophy, and the Bowman's spaces appear unduly wide: an interlobular artery shows marked subintimal mucoid change and there is fibrinoid necrosis of an afferent arteriole.

Ultrastructurally the glomeruli show expansion of the subendothelial space with an absence of dense deposits in it. Immunohistochemistry shows staining for fibrin in the subendothelial space: otherwise the findings are often negative in the glomeruli, although immunoglobulins and C3 have been reported.

The pathogenesis of this condition is quite unknown.

19.10.7 Cryoglobulinaemia

Cryoglobulinaemia can be recognized by collecting and separating blood at 37 °C and then keeping the serum at 4 °C for 72 h. Any precipitate that forms is then separated and can be redissolved and analysed for its immunoglobulin content.

Cryoglobulins are usually classified as suggested by Brouet *et al.* (1974):

1. type I, isolated monoclonal immunoglobulin;

2. type II, mixed monoclonal and polyclonal immunoglobulins;

3. type III, mixed polyclonal.

Isolated monoclonal cryoglobulins are found in a variety of B-cell disorders—*lymphomas, chronic lymphatic leukaemia, Waldenstrom's macroglobulinaemia,* and *multiple myeloma.* They have occasionally been found to be associated with a *mesangiocapillary glomerulonephritis* (the cryoglobulin and complement being present in subendothelial deposits) but nephritis is much less frequent than with type II cryoglobulinaemia.

In type II cryoglobulinaemia, the monoclonal component is a *rheumatoid factor* (usually of the IgM κ variety) and the polyclonal IgG is the antigen of the immune complex, though occasionally monoclonal components of other classes are found. The monoclone may be associated with an overt B-cell disorder.

Disease in these patients can be attributed to the large amounts of circulating immune complexes and is commonly manifest as arthropathy, vasculitis (particularly skin purpura), and nephritis. Kidney involvement may be a presenting feature but more commonly follows several years of purpura or arthropathy.

Histologically, the renal disease usually takes the form of a mesangioproliferative or mesangiocapillary nephritis, although focal segmental nephritis is also described. Sometimes intracapillary 'thrombi' are a prominent feature.

Vasculitic changes are quite commonly present and are most usually seen in the interlobular arteries or afferent arterioles. The appearances vary with the stage of evolution, from a necrotizing arteritis through to a scarred vessel with disrupted elastica.

Immunohistology may be negative in mesangioproliferative disease but where there is a mesangiocapillary picture the components of the mixed cryoglobulin (usually IgM and IgG) and C3 may be demonstrable in a granular pattern around the capillary loops and in the mesangium, often outlining lobules. In the acute phase of involvement vessels may contain IgM, IgG, and C3.

Ultrastructurally the findings are similar to those of mesangiocapillary glomerulonephritis type I (Section 19.3.8), but the subendothelial deposits may have a structured appearance. With IgM and IgG cryoglobulinaemia, this consists of curved cylinders and rings with spokes. Other types of cryoglobulin may show different appearances (Feiner and Gallo 1977).

It is not clear whether the subendothelial deposits of cryoglobulins form *in situ* or are derived from microprecipitates formed in the blood. Microprecipitates formed experimentally are rapidly phagocytosed, so it appears more likely that there is subendothelial precipitation, perhaps as a result of the plasma concentration occurring during glomerular filtration.

Type III cryoglobulins contain polyclonal IgG and polyclonal rheumatoid factor. They commonly occur in *systemic lupus erythematosus, systemic infections, sarcoidosis,* and certain types of *glomerulonephritis.* They are present in low concentrations and are thought not to have a pathogenetic role in the nephritis in most cases.

Waldenstrom's macroglobulinaemia

Proteinuria is quite a frequent finding in this condition, but except where there is associated amyloidosis, renal symptomatology is rarely prominent. Because the monoclonal protein is an IgM and of high molecular weight, it is rarely present in the urine. However, light chains may be excreted: they may be demonstrable as a Bence–Jones protein and may cause a 'myeloma' type of lesion in the tubules.

Glomerular histology may show striking capillary 'thrombi'. These are, in fact, large subendothelial deposits of macroglobulin and may be prominent even when there has been little clinical evidence of renal involvement. Glomerular proliferative changes are rare.

19.10.8 Fabry's disease (angiokeratoma corporis diffusum)

This rare X-linked metabolic disorder is due to a deficiency of a *specific α-galactosidase*, which is involved in glycosphingolipid metabolism, and as a result there is accumulation of *ceramide trihexoside* in various cells (Desnick *et al.* 1973).

The patients affected are usually males, although heterozygous females sometimes show symptoms (Farge *et al.* 1985). Presentation is usually in childhood, with attacks of fever, paraesthesiae in the hands and feet, and a skin rash consisting of purple or reddish macules or papules. At this stage proteinuria and haematuria may not be demonstrable, but subsequently renal symptomatology may dominate the picture and death from renal failure or hypertension is the usual outcome unless there is intervention.

Histologically, the earliest change to be seen is that of foamy vacuolation of the podocytes. Tubular cells, small arteries, and arterioles are also involved, though less dramatically. Layer in the course of the disease the glomeruli show changes resembling those of focal segmental sclerosis and hyalinosis (Fig. 19.61).

Ultrastructural studies and histochemistry show a more widespread involvement of cells than is seen on conventional microscopy, including mesangial and endothelial cells.

19.10.9 Lecithin cholesterol acyltransferase deficiency

This rare metabolic abnormality produces disease only in homozygotes. Characteristic corneal opacities develop, a target cell haemolytic anaemia is present, and renal failure may occur in the fourth and fifth decades of life. The renal failure is due to glomerular destruction but the mechanism of this is not well understood. It may be due to lipid infiltration, but extensive lipid infiltration can be present without proteinuria or renal failure (Fig. 19.62). The development of renal symptoms does not relate well to overall levels of lipids or to specific lipid fractions (Borysiewicz *et al.* 1979).

19.10.10 Aminoaciduria

A. R. Morley

The appearance of amino acids in the urine is an indication of a *disorder of tubular reabsorptive function*. The proximal tubule is an important site for reabsorption, and abnormalities of this function may be the result of an inborn error of metabolism, with high plasma levels resulting in an excess in the glomerular filtrate leading to overflow or as result of toxic damage to the epithelial cells (Table 19.6). Aminoaciduria may also result from a failure of tubular transport. Many of these conditions appear in childhood associated with renal impairment or failure to thrive.

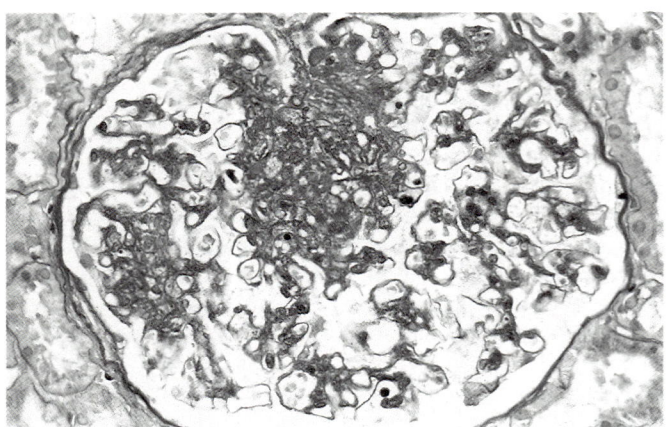

Fig. 19.61 Segmental sclerosis in a glomerulus from a case of Fabry's disease. The podocytes show vacuolation.

Table 19.6 Causes of aminoaciduria

Inborn errors	Toxins
Cystinuria	Cadmium
Phenylketonuria	Lead
Fanconi's syndrome; cystinosis	Solvents
Hartnup's disease	Galactosaemia
Maple syrup urine	Wilson's disease
Glycogen storage disorders	
Tubular glycosuria	

Cystinuria

This disease, which affects some $50/10^6$ of the population, is characterized by the formation of cystine stones. Affected patients secrete 600–1200 mg/24 h. There is defective transport of cystine, arginine, and ornithine in both the small intestinal mucosa and in the proximal tubule. Inheritance is recessive but the presence of stones may not be manifest until the age of 30–40 years. Stones may be bilateral and are poorly radioopaque. Cystine is particularly precipitated by nocturnal urinary acidity. Treatment includes alkalinization of the urine,

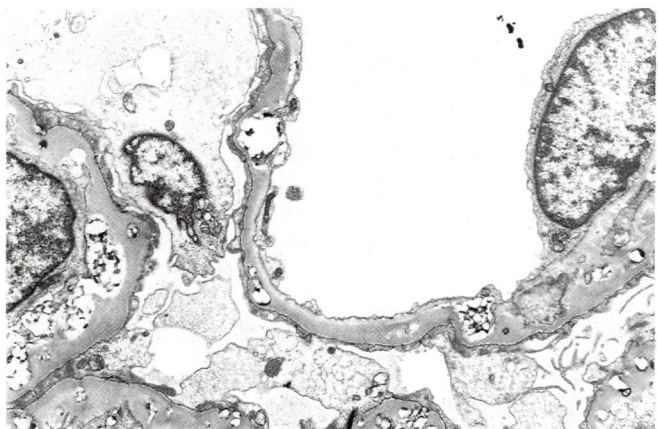

Fig. 19.62 Electron micrograph of part of a glomerulus from a patient with lecithin cholesterol acyltransferase disease. Lipid-containing deposits are present subepithelially, subendothelially, and within the glomerular basement membrane.

increasing urinary volume, as well as treatment with penicillamine and captopril leading to the production of soluble mixed disulphides. Apart from the dangers of obstruction, there are no systemic effects of this disorder.

De Toni–Fanconi syndrome: cystinosis

Generalized aminoaciduria is an indication of tubular damage and may be found in many of the conditions listed above. The term 'Fanconi's syndrome' is now used to embrace this wide range of disorders, some acquired, others genetically determined. The commonest disorder associated with Fanconi's syndrome is *cystinosis*. In contrast to cystinuria there is a poor prognosis due to renal failure. The disease presents in the first year with polyuria, vitamin-D-resistant rickets, excretion of a wide range of amino acids, and glycosuria. Cystinosis results from a generalized lysosomal disorder of cystine metabolism. Extensive deposition of cystine crystals in the tissues results. Formation of stones is rare. Renal failure, metabolic disturbances, or infection result in death in the first decade.

Examination reveals that the deposits of cystine are widespread in the reticuloendothelial system, retina, cornea, and in the interstitium of the kidneys (Fig. 19.63). A 'swan neck' deformity of the proximal tubule at the exit from the glomerulus has been described, but the specificity of this lesion is doubtful. There is extensive tubular atrophy in those reaching renal failure, and the disease has been treated by renal transplantation. Survival for up to 10 years without disease recurrence has been recorded.

Other inborn errors of metabolism

Inherited abnormalities of enzymes involved in amino-acid metabolism result in a number of syndromes characterized by excretion of a specific amino acid. The commonest of these is *phenylketonuria* which affects some $100/10^6$ of the population and is inherited as a recessive. In this disease the deficiency of *phenylalanine hyroxylase* leads to accumulation of phenylalanine, and its overflow into the urine. In *maple syrup urine disease* there is overflow excretion of *leucine, isoleucine,* and *valine* in the urine. Both these conditions are associated with mental deficiency. *Hartnup's disease* has an incidence of $40/10^6$, with autosomal recessive inheritance. There is a tubular defect with excretion of a very wide range of amino acids, including *alanine, glutamine, histidine, and serine.* There is also a defect of intestinal absorption of tryptophan. *Cerebellar ataxia* and a *pellagra-like skin disorder* are found. Of the glycogen storage disorders, only *glycogenosis type I* (von Gierke's disease) involves the kidney, with glycogen in the proximal tubule and aminoaciduria, but no disorder of renal function.

Tubular glycosuria is important because it is common and may be confused with diabetes mellitus. It is due to an isolated failure of tubular glucose reabsorption without hyperglycaemia. Renal function and tests of glucose tolerance are normal.

Toxins and aminoaciduria

Lead poisoning may occur from industrial exposure or ingestion

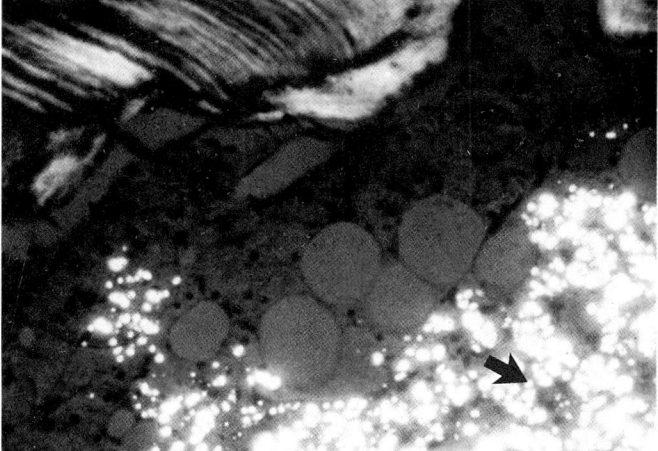
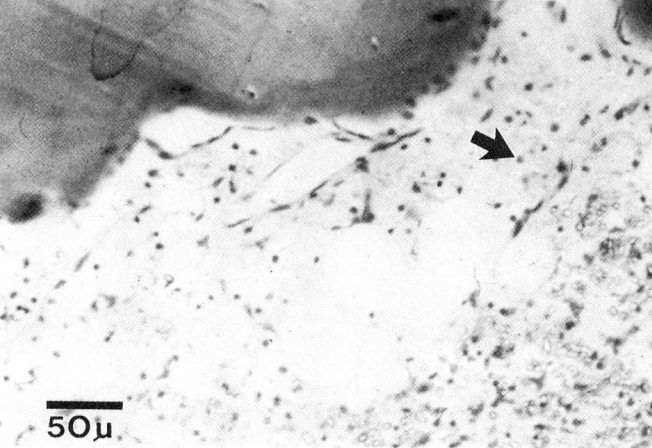

Fig. 19.63 Marrow from a 7-year-old female with cystinosis. Note the refractile crystals demonstrated by polarized light (arrow).

of lead-containing paint in children, with resulting glycosuria and aminoaciduria. Industrial exposure to *cadmium* may cause similar problems.

Solvents, such as carbon tetrachloride and toluene, cause liver and renal damage. Toluene is a component of many of the glues used by 'glue sniffers', and tubular damage with defects of amino-acid excretion have been described in such patients.

Galactosaemia is caused by an inherited deficiency of the enzyme required for the conversion of galactose-1-phosphate to glucose-1-phosphate. The disease appears in the homozygote. Liver disease, jaundice, cataracts, and mental retardation occur unless lactose and galactose are excluded from the diet. Both aminoaciduria and proteinuria occur. The nature of the tubular lesion is uncertain.

Wilson's disease (hepato-lenticular degeneration), an autosomal recessive condition, results from an inability to secrete copper in the bile. Copper is then deposited within renal tubules. Deposition of copper within the basal ganglia causes neurological disorders and liver accumulation is associated with cirrhosis.

Focal renal tubular damage occurs in association with copper deposition. Treatment with the chelating agent, penicillamine, may result in membranous nephropathy.

19.10.11 Bibliography

Barlow, K. A. and Beilin, L. J. (1968). Renal disease in primary gout. *Quarterly Journal of Medicine* **37**, 79–96.

Barrie, H. J., Azkanazy, C. L., and Smith, G. W. (1952). More glomerular changes in diabetes. *Canadian Medical Association Journal* **66**, 428–31.

Borysiewicz, L. K., Soutar, A. K., Evans, D. J., Thompson, G. R., and Rees, A. J. (1979). Renal failure in familial lecithin: cholesterol acyltransferase deficiency. *Quarterly Journal of Medicine* **204**, 411–26.

Brouet, J. C., Clauvel, J. P., Danon, F., Klein, M., and Seligmann, M. (1974). Biologic and clinical significance of cryoglobulins. *American Journal of Medicine* **57**, 775–88.

Browne, J. C. M. (1958). The significance of hypertension in the pregnant woman. In *Symposium on non-toxaemic hypertension in pregnancy* (ed. N. F. Morris and J. C. M. Browne), p. 75. Little, Brown and Co., Boston.

Chesley, L. C. (1978). Hypertension disorders in pregnancy. Appleton Century Crofts, New York.

Churg, J., Bernstein, J., Risdon, R. A., and Sobin, L. H. (1987). Renal disease: Classification and Atlas. In *WHO developmental and hereditary disorders*, Part II, ch. 16, pp. 204–37. World Health Organization, Tokyo.

Coe, F. L. (1978). Hyperuricosuric calcium oxalate nephrolithiasis. *Kidney International* **13**, 418–26.

Cohen, A. S. A. and Connors, L. H. (1987). The pathogenesis and biochemistry of amyloidosis. *Journal of Pathology* **151**, 1–10.

Davison, J. M. and Dunlop, W. (1980). Renal haemodynamics and tubular function in normal pregnancy. *Kidney International* **18**, 152–61.

De Fronzo, R. A., Humphrey, R. L., Wright, J. R., and Cooke, C. R. (1975). Acute renal failure in multiple myeloma. *Medicine* **54**, 209–23.

Desnick, R. J., Allen, K. Y., Desnick, S. J., Raman, M. K., Bernlohr, R. W., and Krivit, W. (1973). Fabry's disease: enzymatic diagnosis in hemizygotes and heterozygotes. *Journal of Laboratory and Clinical Medicine* **81**, 157–71.

Dieckmann, W. J. (1952). *The toxaemias of pregnancy* (2nd edn). Mosby, St. Louis.

Emmerson, B. T. and Row, P. G. (1975). An evaluation of the pathogenesis of gouty kidney. *Kidney International* **8**, 65–71.

Farge, D., Nadler, S., Olfe, L. S., Barre, P., and Jothy, S. (1985). Diagnostic value of kidney biopsy in heterozygous Fabry's disease. *Archives of Pathology and Laboratory Medicine* **109**, 85–8.

Feiner, H. and Gallo, G. (1977). Ultrastructure in glomerulonephritis associated with cryglobulinaemia. *American Journal of Pathology* **88**, 145–62.

Gallo, G. R. (1970). Elution studies in kidneys with linear deposition of immunoglobulin in glomeruli. *American Journal of Pathology* **61**, 377–85.

Hayslett, J. P. (1985). Post-partum renal failure. *New England Journal of Medicine* **312**, 1556–9.

Hostetter, T. H., Rennke, H. G., and Brenner, B. M. (1982). The case for intrarenal hypertension in the initiation and progression of diabetic and other glomerulopathies. *American Journal of Medicine* **72**, 375–80.

Howard, J. E. (1954). Clinical and laboratory research concerning mechanisms of formation and control of calculous disease by the kidney. *Journal of Urology* **72**, 999–1008.

Kanwar, Y. S., Rosenzweig, L. J., Linker, A., and Jabubowski, M. L. (1983). Decreased *de novo* synthesis of glomerular proteoglycans in diabetes. Biochemical and autoradiographic evidence. *Proceedings of the National Academy of Sciences USA* **80**, 2272–7.

Kimmelstiel, P. and Wilson, C. (1936). Intercapillary lesions in glomeruli of kidney. *American Journal of Pathology* **12**, 83–98.

Kyle, R. A. and Bayrd, E. D. (1975). Amyloidosis. Review of 236 cases. *Medicine* **54**, 271–99.

Lawler, D. P., Schreiner, G. E., and David, A. (1960). Renal medullary necrosis. *American Journal of Medicine* **29**, 132–56.

Mariani, A. J., Barrett, D. M., Kurtz, S. B., and Kyle, R. A. (1978). Bilateral localised amyloidosis of the ureter presenting with anuria. *Journal of Urology* **120**, 757–9.

Metabolism **35** (Supplement) (1986).

Monnier, V. M., Vishwanath, V., Frank, K. E., Elmets, C. A., Dauchot, P., and Kohn, R. R. (1986). Relation between complications of Type I diabetes mellitus and collagen linked fluorescence. *New England Journal of Medicine* **314**, 405–8.

Ritz, E. and Massry, S. G. (1977). The kidney in disorders of calcium metabolism. *Contributions to Nephrology* **7**, 114–27.

Spühler, O. and Zollinger, H. U. (1943). Die diabetische glomerulosklerose. *Deutsche Archiv für Klinische Medizin* **190**, 321–79.

Tribe, C. R., Smart, G. E., Davies, D. R., and MacKenzie, J. C. (1979). A renal biopsy study in toxaemia of pregnancy: using routine light and electron microscopy linked with immunofluorescence and immune electron microscopy. *Journal of Clinical Pathology* **32**, 681–92.

Watanabe, T. and Saniter, T. (1975). Morphological and clinical features of renal amyloidosis. *Virchows Archiv A. Pathological Anatomy* **366**, 125–35.

Williams, H. E. (1978). Oxalic acid and the hyperoxaluric syndromes. *Kidney International* **13**, 410–17.

19.11 Renal tumours

A. J. D'Ardenne

19.11.1 Renal adenoma

The existence of renal adenomas is controversial. Small renal epithelial tumours are quite common incidental findings at post-mortem examinations and in nephrectomy specimens, but distinguishing those that are benign from those that are malignant presents a problem. The capacity of such tumours to manifest malignant behaviour, namely to metastasize, is partly related to their size. It was once suggested that all renal epithelial tumours less than 3 cm in diameter should be regarded as 'adenomas' and all tumours greater than 3 cm in diameter are 'carcinomas'. As with most such arbitrary rules, there are exceptions, metastatic behaviour having been reported in tumours which would have been classified as 'adenomas' on the basis of size alone. Since renal 'adenomas' and 'carcinomas' probably represent different stages in the life history of the same tumour, many believe that all such neoplasms should be regarded as at last potentially malignant and termed 'carcinoma'. It is worth noting, however, that in the majority of cases, the incidental discovery of small tubular neoplasms in nephrectomy specimens should give little cause for further concern for the patient. An alternative view, therefore, is that many can be classified as 'adenomas' provided additional criteria to size are taken into account. These include absence of cytological or architectural atypia, absence of necrosis or haemorrhage, and absence of invasion (Mostofi and Davis 1986).

19.11.2 Renal carcinoma

Renal carcinomas are malignant tumours derived from renal tubular epithelium. Alternative terms are renal adenocarcinoma and renal cell carcinoma. In the past this tumour has also been called Grawitz tumour (after the description of a case by Grawitz in 1893) and 'hypernephroma', a name attributable to its previous putative origin from adrenal cortical rests.

Incidence

Renal carcinomas account for less than 2 per cent of all cancer deaths. They occur 2–3 times more frequently in males than in females, and have an increasing incidence with age. There is some geographical variation in the incidence of renal carcinoma, with a higher incidence in Jews.

Renal carcinomas also occur in other mammals and frogs. In some species of frog the incidence may be as high as 25 per cent. These tumours are caused by a herpes virus (Lucké tumour virus). There is no evidence of a viral aetiology in man.

Clinical features

The classic symptoms of renal carcinoma are haematuria (60 per cent of cases), loin pain (56 per cent), and a mass (20 per cent). Other modes of presentation include non-specific symptoms such as fever, malaise, weight loss, nausea, and vomiting. Patients may also present with symptoms related to metastases. Up to one-third of patients have metastatic deposits at presentation.

On investigation, the most common finding is gross or microscopic haematuria. Many patients are anaemic, but a small proportion have *polycythaemia*, believed to be due to production of erythropoietin by the tumour. Approximately one-third of patients with renal carcinoma have an elevated plasma renin concentration. This tends to be associated with high-grade, high-stage tumours. Elevated plasma calcium is also often present. This may be related to bony metastases, to production of a vitamin-D-like substance, or to production of a parathormone-like substance. Other hormones reported to have been produced by renal carcinoma include glucagon (Gleeson *et al.* 1970) and gonadotrophins (Goble *et al.* 1974). Production of these substances is probably rare.

Diagnosis is primarily radiological.

Gross appearances

Renal carcinomas are usually roughly spherical or lobulated (Fig. 19.64). The majority have an expansile pattern of growth,

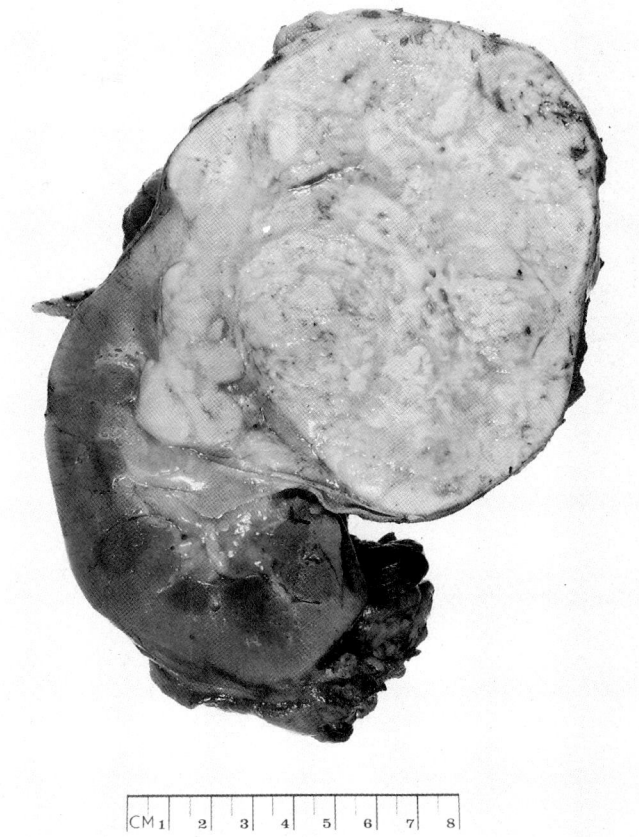

Fig. 19.64 Renal carcinoma with pale variegated cut surface and a little subcapsular haemorrhage.

compressing adjacent renal parenchyma into a pseudocapsule. The more malignant varieties may display infiltrative growth. The tumour may arise in upper, middle, or lower poles of the kidney. The cut surface is often haemorrhagic and may be bright yellow due to a high lipid content. Other areas may appear greyish-white or cystic. There is a wide variation in size, as noted above, but tumours that have become clinically apparent tend to be at least 5 cm in diameter. Carcinoma may be seen invading through the renal capsule, into the renal pelvis, or along the renal vein. It may also be found in regional lymph nodes.

Histological appearances

The variegated gross appearance of renal carcinomas is reflected in their histology. There are three main cell types, which may be arranged in varying patterns. The commonest cell types are the *clear cell* and the *granular cell* varieties (Fig. 19.65). Clear cells have an apparently empty cytoplasm due to their high content of lipid, which is removed during processing for embedding in paraffin wax. They also contain glycogen. Granular cells have an eosinophilic cytoplasm with a particulate appearance. This is due to a high content of mitochondria, which may be identified on electron microscopy. Clear cells and granular cells

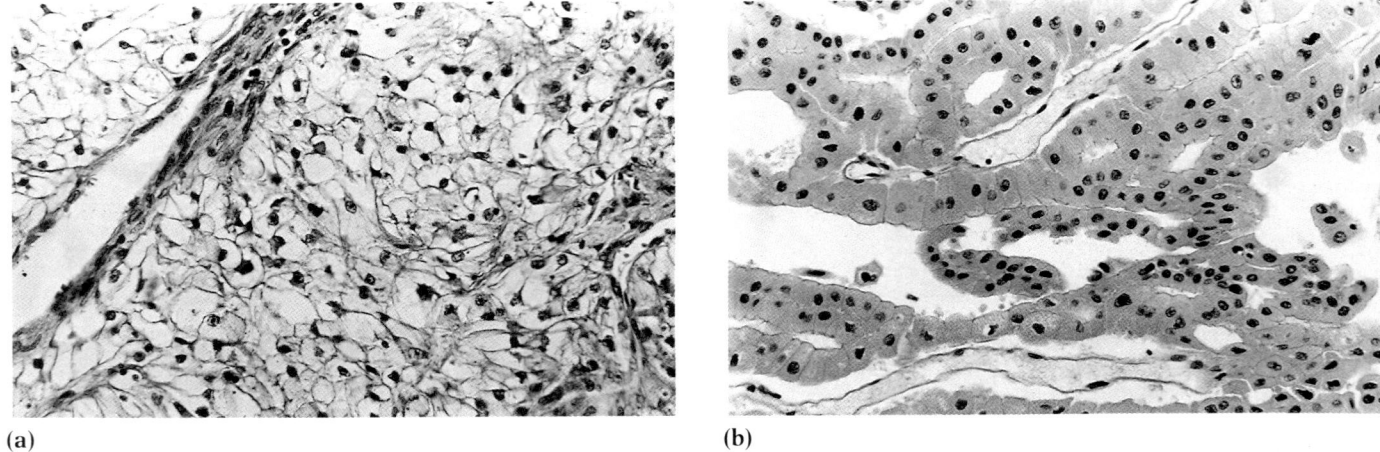

(a)   (b)

Fig. 19.65   Renal carcinoma histology: (a) 'clear cells' with apparently empty cytoplasm; (b) 'granular cells' arranged in tubular structures around thin-walled blood vessels.

tend to be arranged in a tubular or acinar pattern, but some-times display papillary features, especially within cysts. The tumours are usually highly vascular. The rarer, third cell type is the *spindle cell* tumour. These are often hard to distinguish from spindle cells seen in mesenchymal tumours and tend to be arranged in a sarcomatoid pattern. Sarcomatoid tumours account for 1–1.5 per cent of renal carcinomas and are highly aggressive.

Histological features carrying prognostic significance are cellular and nuclear pleomorphism, nuclear hyperchromatism and mitotic activity, and the presence of necrosis. Most clear and granular cell tumours have regular nuclei with infrequent mitoses, in contrast to spindle-cell tumours which are often highly pleomorphic and exhibit many mitoses. The proportion of clear and granular cells in a tumour is not prognostically significant, nor is their architectural arrangement. Different histological grading systems classify renal carcinomas into two, three, or four categories, distinguished mainly by nuclear characteristics.

Renal oncocytomas

Tumours composed entirely of uniform packets of eosinophilic granular cells with small condensed nuclei, very few mitoses, and no necrosis have been termed oncocytomas by analogy with similar tumours elsewhere (salivary gland, thyroid, para-thyroid, and adrenal). They have been associated with a very good prognosis and thus separate classification has been con-sidered justifiable. However, exceptions have been reported and their ability to metastasize noted. These tumours are probably best regarded as well-differentiated renal carcinomas.

Metastatic spread

Renal carcinoma has three main routes of spread: *direct exten-sion* through renal capsule, via *lymphatics* to regional nodes, and along *the renal vein*. Blood-borne metastases are most com-monly encountered in the lungs, but may also be found in other

sites. In approximate order of frequency these include bones, brain, liver, adrenals, skin, and thyroid.

There are several staging systems for renal carcinoma, each carrying prognostic significance. A convenient system is that of Robson *et al.* (1969): *in stage I*, the tumour is confined within the renal capsule; *in stage II* there is extension through the renal capsule (and possibly into the adrenal gland); *in stage III* there is involvement of the renal vein and/or regional lymph nodes; and in *stage IV* there is involvement of adjacent organs (other than the adrenal) or distant metastases. There is a marked difference in survival between stage I and stage IV disease. In stage I up to 70 per cent survive 10 years, but in the presence of widespread metastases survival is very poor (mean 12 months). It is improved if metastases are confined to the lungs, and by re-moval of the primary tumour (Maldazys and deKernion 1986). There are several case reports of spontaneous regression of indi-vidual metastases after nephrectomy. Solitary metastases are not unusual and resection of these may also improve survival.

Histogenesis

Renal carcinoma is derived from renal tubules. Ultrastructural studies have favoured origin from proximal tubular epithelium, since tumour cells may have a readily demonstrable brush border. Immunohistological studies have mostly supported this view, although the findings have not been conclusive. A wide variety of monoclonal antibodies have been produced with specificity for different regions of the nephron. Although the majority of renal carcinomas express antigens normally con-fined to proximal tubular epithelium, many express antigens normally confined to distal tubules. The pattern of antigenic expression is variable, but both distal and proximal tubular antigens may be found within the same tumour. Possible ex-planations include aberrant differentiation by malignant cells as well as the origin of renal carcinomas from varying parts of the nephron. No correlation has been demonstrated between the pattern of antigenic expression and histological type.

Aetiology

Little is known about the aetiology of renal carcinoma, but cigarette smoking, tobacco smoking, and obesity have all been incriminated as significant risk factors for the development of this neoplasm (Bennington 1973; Yu *et al.* 1986). Abuse of analgesics containing phenacetin has also been associated with renal carcinoma, although much less commonly than with transitional cell carcinomas of the urinary tract (Lornoy *et al.* 1986). The majority of renal carcinomas develop in normal kidneys but there is a significantly increased risk of their occurrence in acquired cystic disease. This is found in about 35 per cent of patients on long-term dialysis, and approximately 6 per cent of cases develop renal epithelial neoplasms (Dunnill *et al.* 1977; Hughson *et al.* 1986). The majority of these tumours are found incidentally at post-mortem or in nephrectomy specimens but some are clinically aggressive and metastasize. There is no evidence to suggest that renal tumours develop in end-stage kidneys *per se*.

Heredity

Renal carcinomas have been associated with the autosomal dominant form of *inherited polycystic disease* as well as with *acquired cystic disease*. A more direct familial association is with the rare *von Hippel–Lindau syndrome*. This condition is inherited as an autosomal dominant gene with variable penetrance, and one-third of patients develop renal carcinoma. Its other manifestations include retinal angioma, haemangioblastoma of cerebellum and spinal cord, angiomatous or cystic lesions of kidneys, liver, pancreas, lung, skin and epididymis, and adrenal phaeochromocytoma. Renal carcinomas occurring in this syndrome are frequently bilateral and develop at a relatively young age.

19.11.3   Wilms' tumour

Wilms' tumour is an embryonic tumour derived from metanephric mesenchyme.

Incidence

Wilms' tumour is mainly a tumour of childhood, although it can occur in adults. It has a peak incidence at 3–4 years of age. It accounts for approximately 6 per cent of malignancies in children under 15. There is an equal sex incidence and a stable and equal geographical incidence throughout the world. Roughly a third are heritable, including all those that are bilateral or multifocal. Associated abnormalities may include *sporadic aniridia* (1 per cent), *hemihypertrophy* (3 per cent), and *genitourinary abnormalities* (5 per cent).

Clinical features

The majority of cases present with an abdominal mass. They are often otherwise asymptomatic. Others may suffer from abdominal pain, anorexia, nausea, vomiting, or constipation. In 10 per cent, symptoms are attributable to metastases. Clinical signs may include microscopic haematuria, fever, and hypertension.

Diagnosis is dependent on radiology.

Gross appearances

A proportion of tumours are bilateral, but the majority are unilateral. The left kidney is affected more often than the right. Grossly the tumour appears demarcated but not encapsulated. It is often lobular with a greyish-white cut surface (Fig. 19.66). As with renal carcinoma, there may be invasion of hilar lymph nodes and of the renal vein.

Histological appearance

Microscopically, Wilms' tumour has elements resembling those in developing fetal kidney. These are present in varying proportions and include *undifferentiated blastema*, *primitive tubular* and *glomeruloid structures*, and *stromal elements* (Fig. 19.67). These three elements are not invariably all present in each tumour, and it is not uncommon to find tumours possessing only blastemal and stromal components. In addition to structures normally seen in developing kidney, there may be differentiation towards ectopic epithelia, such as squamous, basal, and mucus-secreting, or differentiation of stroma to striated muscle, cartilage, fat, or bone. Striated muscle fibres in particular are seen quite frequently, and may produce an appearance similar to *rhabdomyosarcoma*. Wilms' tumours with heterotopic elements are distinguishable from teratomas in that there is no attempt at organoid differentiation.

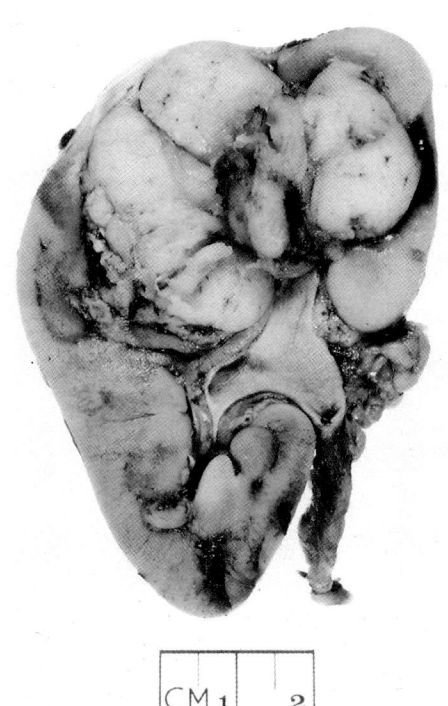

Fig. 19.66   Wilms' tumour with pale, lobated, cut surface.

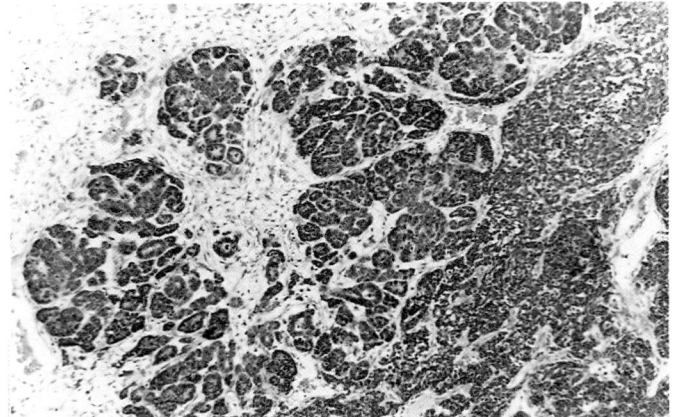

(a)

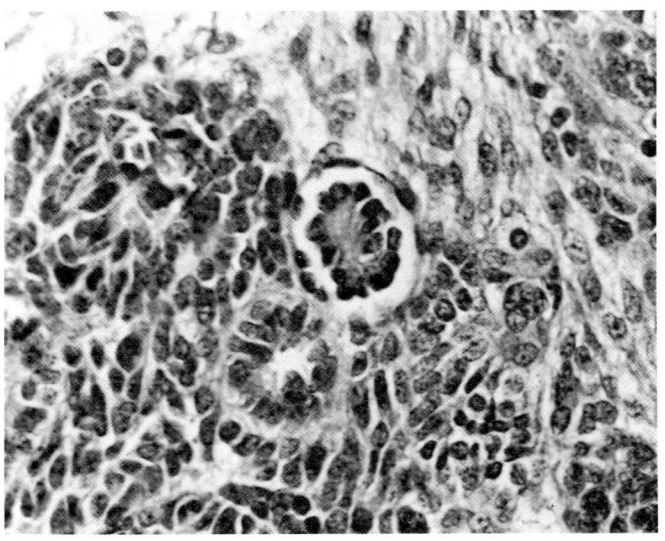

(b)

(c)

Fig. 19.67 Wilms' tumour histology: (a) low magnification, demonstrating stromal, tubular, and blastemal components; (b) higher magnification, demonstrating well-formed tubules in undifferentiated blastema; (c) primitive glomeruloid body.

Prognostic features

In the third American National Wilms' tumour study, the only histological feature associated with a poor outcome was that of *extreme cellular anaplasia* (Beckwith 1983). Anaplastic Wilms' tumours are defined as having easily identified, large and hyperchromatic nuclei and abnormal mitoses. They constitute less then 5 per cent of Wilms' tumours. The remainder are described as having 'favourable histology'. *Tubular differentiation* was associated with improved prognosis in one series (Marsden *et al.* 1984), but not in the American study.

Spread and staging

As with most tumours, the extent of spread at operation is of prognostic significance. More than one staging system has been devised, based on presence and extent of intra-abdominal spread at the time of operation and the presence of metastatic deposits in lymph nodes or elsewhere. The lung is the commonest site for blood-borne metastases, but there may also be spread to brain and bone. The liver may be involved, either by direct spread or via the bloodstream.

Outcome

The outlook for children with Wilms' tumour has improved dramatically in recent years. In the group with favourable histology, i.e. the majority, a 90 per cent cure rate can be achieved using two-agent chemotherapy alone. Unfortunately, at present, there is no evidence to suggest that more intensive therapy improves the outlook for patients with anaplastic tumours (Beckwith 1986).

Aetiology

The aetiology of Wilms' tumours has generated considerable interest and genetic factors have been demonstrated to be of paramount importance.

Nephroblastomatosis

Nephroblastomatosis is defined as the *persistence of metanephric blastema beyond 36 weeks of gestation*, or *its presence in the wrong place or amount before that time*. It is not in itself malignant but is seen in more than 20 per cent of patients with Wilms' tumours, as opposed to an overall incidence of less than 1 per cent in infant autopsies. It is therefore believed to be a precursor of Wilms' tumour, although only a small percentage of patients with nephroblastomatosis will develop the neoplasm. Nephroblastomatosis can be classified according to its site in the kidney; *the commonest site is superficial and subcapsular*, where most nephronogenesis occurs during renal development. The risk of developing Wilms' tumour with each type of nephroblastomatosis is not known. If nephroblastomatosis is discovered incidentally in a kidney removed for a non-neoplastic condition, there is probably no cause for concern and follow-up is unnecessary. However, if it is found in a kidney which is also the seat of a Wilms' tumour, there is a significantly increased risk of developing another Wilms' tumour in the contralateral kidney, and careful follow-up with ultrasound has been recommended (Beckwith 1986).

Heredity

Wilms' tumour occurs in childhood in both inherited and sporadic forms. In a percentage of both, including most cases associated with sporadic aniridia, a specific deletion of band p13 of chromosome 11 has been observed. The tumours are homozygous for abnormality at this site. In inherited disease, the chromosome from one parent already carries the deletion or an invisible mutation. It thus only requires a single second mutation or 'hit' (Knudson and Strong 1972) to acquire homozygosity. The tumour is the result of deletion or inactivation of both copies of the wild-type genetic locus. The precise molecular mechanisms are still unknown. However, the 11p- deletion is close to the site of an oncogene and may result in loss of regulatory sequences or 'anti-oncogenes' (Knudson 1985) (see Chapter 2).

In sporadic nephroblastoma, it is assumed that two 'hits' (mutations or deletions) at the genetic locus must occur. The chance of two such events occurring in the same cell is considerably less than the chance of a single mutation occurring in any cell. This is all that is required for tumour production in inherited disease, since one chromosome already carries the abnormality. It has been suggested that the increased incidence of nephroblastomatosis in Wilms' tumour is morphological evidence that one mutation has already occurred.

Trisomy and teratological syndromes

Wilms' tumour has also been associated with other chromosomal abnormalities, including *trisomy 18*, and with *Beckwith's syndrome* in which a trisomy of part of chromosome 11 is sometimes found. In these conditions there are many other somatic abnormalities and the mechanisms are not understood.

Other renal tumours of childhood

In the past, nearly all renal tumours of childhood were classified as Wilms' tumours. Recently, important new entities have been defined. These are probably of different histogenesis to Wilms' and, importantly, have a different behaviour pattern and therapeutic requirements.

Congenital mesoblastic nephroma

Congenital mesoblastic nephroma is a tumour of the neonatal period, unlike Wilms' tumour which is uncommon in the first year of life. It presents as a large abdominal mass without pain or haematuria. *In utero,* it may give rise to polyhydramnios. There is an equal incidence in both kidneys. Grossly, it has a cut surface resembling that of a uterine fibroid, greyish-white and whorled. Sometimes it may appear yellowish-brown or cystic. Histologically, it consists of spindle or smooth muscle cells interdigitating with normal nephrons. These tumours are nearly always benign, although a rare sarcomatous variety may exist. The margins are locally infiltrative and radical resection of the kidney is advocated to prevent local recurrence.

Bone-metastasizing renal tumour of childhood (clear-cell sarcoma)

Bone-metastasizing renal tumour of childhood accounts for about 5 per cent of primary renal childhood tumours. It has about the same age distribution as Wilms' tumour, but is commoner in males. It has a distinctive and deceptively innocent histological appearance, being composed of ovoid or polygonal cells with inconspicuous cytoplasm, pale nuclei with a prominent nuclear membrane, and inconspicuous nucleoli. There are few mitoses. The tumour cells are usually separated by a vascular stroma. Variants of this classical pattern have been described.

The importance of bone-metastasizing tumour lies in its worse prognosis than Wilms' tumour. Early studies indicated an incidence of bone metastases of 40–60 per cent and a death rate of 50 per cent. There is now evidence that the outcome may be improved by more intensive chemotherapy (unlike anaplastic Wilms' tumour).

The histogenesis of the tumour is unknown.

Malignant rhabdoid tumour

Malignant rhabdoid tumour accounts for 2 per cent of childhood renal tumours and tends to affect a younger age-group than Wilms', with a mean age at diagnosis of 13 months. Microscopically, it is composed of cells with abundant eosinophilic cytoplasm and nuclei with single prominent nucleoli. They were originally thought to resemble rhabdomyoblasts and hence the name. However, ultrastructural and immunohistological studies have failed to show any relation to rhabdoid cells and the histogenesis of this tumour is unknown.

Its significance lies in its extremely aggressive behaviour, with an associated 90 per cent mortality.

Multilocular cystic nephroma

Multilocular cystic nephroma has an equal frequency in children and adults. It is an encapsulated tumour, which, as the name suggests, is composed of multiple cysts. Microscopically, these are lined by columnar to flattened epithelium and there is a fibroblastic stroma. In infants the stroma may contain *foci of nephroblastoma*. These tumours have a good prognosis even if nephroblastomatous foci are present, and they are adequately treated by nephrectomy alone.

19.11.4   Other renal tumours

Medullary fibroma

Medullary fibromas are extremely common incidental findings at post-mortem. They are small, white, well-circumscribed nodules, 0.1–0.3 cm diameter and are usually found in the mid-portion of the renal medulla. Microscopically, they are composed of unencapsulated bundles of stromal cells in a collagenous matrix. Ultrastructural studies have indicated that the constituent cells are derived from medullary interstitial cells rather than fibroblasts. The significance and aetiology of these common tumours is uncertain, and they may represent nodules of hyperplasia rather than true neoplasms.

Angiomyolipoma

Angiomyolipomas are uncommon tumours. They are hamartomatous malformations rather than neoplasms and they are benign. They are of interest because of their association with *tuberous sclerosis*, although 50 per cent of cases occur in patients who do not have this condition. Between 40 and 80 per cent of patients with tuberous sclerosis have angiomyolipoma. The tuberous sclerosis syndrome was described by Bournville in 1880 as a triad of *mental retardation, epilepsy*, and *adenoma sebaceum*. It is inherited as an autosomal dominant gene with variable penetrance and is associated with a number of anatomical abnormalities. These include *hamartomatous malformations of glial cels and neurones in the brain, known as 'tubers', astrocytomas* (less often), *visceral angiomas, cardiac rhabdomyoma*, and *cutaneous lesions (adenoma sebaceum)*.

Angiomyolipomas show considerable variation in size and number, ranging from small unilateral lesions to massive bilateral renal involvement. Clinically they may present with a renal mass, haematuria, or flank or abdominal pain related to haemorrhage or extrarenal extension. Microscopically, they consist of a varying mixture of adipose tissue and thick-walled blood vessels surrounded by irregularly disposed sheets of smooth muscle. The smooth muscle component may show hyperchromatic and pleomorphic nuclei with frequent mitoses. These features have sometimes led to an erroneous diagnosis of malignancy.

Juxtaglomerular tumour

Juxtaglomerular tumours are rare, but important, since they can give rise to *severe hypertension* and *hypokalaemia*. This is associated with *high levels of plasma renin and secondary aldosteronism*. They occur in a younger age-group then renal carcinoma (mean 19 years). Macroscopically, they are small, well-circumscribed tumours arising in the renal cortex. Histologically, they are composed of fairly uniform cells with regular nuclei. These cells are arranged in packets or sheets separated by a rich vascular bed. They are characterized by prominent cytoplasmic granules which may be visualized by electron microscopy. Immunostaining indicates that the granules contain renin, and renin has been extracted from these tumours. They probably arise from juxtaglomerular cells, which in turn are derived from modified smooth muscle of arteriolar media. *As such they are analagous to haemangiopericytomas*. However, they have a less aggressive behaviour and none has been reported to invade or metastasize. This may be because they present early due to their production of renin.

Mesenchymal tumours

Benign

The most common mesenchymal tumours of the kidney are benign tumours of fat and smooth muscle, i.e. lipomas and leiomyomas. These are usually of no clinical importance and are identified incidentally at post-mortem.

Malignant

Sarcomas of the kidney are rare, accounting for only 2–3 per cent of malignant renal tumours. Over half of the sarcomas arising in kidney are leiomyosarcomas. Microscopically, renal sarcomas have features found in sarcomas in other sites. They may appear very similar to the sarcomatoid variants of renal carcinoma. Immunohistochemistry and electron microscopy may be of assistance in distinguishing between these neoplasms.

Haemopoietic and lymphoid neoplasms

The kidney is commonly infiltrated in lymphoma and leukaemia, although the incidence of renal involvement varies with the type. Leukaemic infiltrates tend to be diffuse, affecting mainly outer cortex, whereas lymphomatous infiltrates, including those of Hodgkin's disease, are more often nodular. Both may cause renal enlargement and, on occasion, renal impairment. Symptoms may be produced by urinary outflow obstruction. In most cases, however, lymphomatous infiltration of the kidney is clinically silent and found only on radiological investigation or at post-mortem. Rarely, renal involvement by lymphoma presents as a solitary mass, resembling the presentation of renal carcinoma.

Occurrence of primary renal lymphoma is controversial, but cases in which lymphoma appears to have been confined to the kidney at the time of presentation have been described (Osborne *et al.* 1987).

Deposits of multiple myeloma may also occur in the kidney, but this tends to be of minor clinical importance compared with other renal complications of the disease.

Metastatic carcinomas

The kidney is a common site for metastases and it has been estimated that these are approximately twice as frequent as primary renal carcinoma. The most common source of metastases are breast and lung, but they may also come from many other primary sites. Metastatic carcinoma is usually clinically silent, although it may present as a renal mass or with haematuria.

19.11.5   Bibliography

Beckwith, J. B. (1983). Wilm's tumour and other renal tumours of childhood: a selective review from the National Wilm's Tumour Study Pathology Centre. *Human Pathology* **14**, 481–92.

Beckwith, J. B. (1986). The John Lattimer Lecture. Wilm's tumour and other renal tumours of childhood: an update. *Journal of Urology* **136**, 320–4.

Bennington, J. L. (1973). Cancer of the kidney—aetiology, epidemiology and pathology. *Cancer* **32**, 1017–29.

Bennington, J. L and Beckwith, J. B. (1975). *Tumours of the kidney, renal pelvis and ureter*. Fascicle 12, Armed Forces Institute of Pathology, Washington.

Berry, P. J. (1987). Paediatric solid tumours. In *Recent advances in histo-*

pathology, Vol. 13 (ed. P. P. Anthony and R. N. M. MacSween), pp. 203–32. Churchill Livingstone, Edinburgh.

Dunnill, M. S., Millard, P. R., and Oliver, D. (1977). Acquired cystic disease of the kidneys: a hazard of long term intermittent maintenance haemodialysis. *Journal of Clinical Pathology* **30**, 868–77.

Gleeson, M. H., Bloom, S. R., Polak, J. M., Henry, K., and Dowling, R. H. (1970). An endocrine tumour in kidney affecting small bowel structure, motility and function. *Gut* **11**, 1060.

Goble, D. W., Schambelan, M., Weintraub, B. D., and Rosen, S. W. (1974). Gonadotrophin secreting renal carcinoma. *Cancer* **33**, 1048–53.

Hughson, M. D, Buchwald, D., and Fox, M. (1986). Renal neoplasia and acquired cystic disease in patients receiving long-term dialysis. *Archives of Pathology and Laboratory Medicine* **110**, 592–601.

Knudson, A. G. (1985). Hereditary cancer, oncogenes and anti-oncogenes. *Cancer Research* **45**, 1437–43.

Knudson, A. G. and Strong, L. C. (1972). Mutation and cancer. A model for Wilm's tumour of kidney. *Journal of the National Cancer Institute* **48**, 313–24.

Lewi, H. J. E., Alexander, C. A., and Fleming, S. (1986). Renal onco-cytoma. *British Journal of Urology* **58**, 12–15.

Lornoy, W., *et al.* (1986). Renal cell carcinoma, a new complication of analgesic nephropathy. *Lancet* i, 1271–2.

Maldazys, J. D. and deKernion, J. B. (1986). Prognostic factors in metastatic renal carcinoma. *Journal of Urology* **136**, 376–9.

Malek, R. S, Omess, P. J., Benson, R. C., and Zincke, H. (1987). Renal carcinoma in von Hippel–Lindau syndrome. *American Journal of Medicine* **82**, 236–8.

Marsden, H. B. and Lawler, W. (1980). Bone-metastasizing renal tumour of childhood. Histopathological and clinical review of 38 cases. *Virchow's Archiv A* **387**, 341–51.

Marsden, H. B., Lawler, W., Carr, T. F., and Kumar, S. (1984). A scoring system for Wilm's tumour: pathological study of the second Medical Research Council (MRC) trial. *International Journal of Cancer* **33**, 365–8.

Mostofi, F. K. and Davis, C. J. (1986). Tumours and tumour-like lesions of the kidney. *Current Problems in Cancer* **10**, 53–114.

Osborne, B. M., Brenner, M., Weitzner, S., and Butler, J. J. (1987). Malignant lymphoma presenting as a renal mass: four cases. *American Journal of Surgical Pathology* **11**, 375–82.

Robson, C. J., Churchill, B. M., and Anderson, W. (1969). The results of radical nephrectomy for renal cell carcinoma. *Journal of Urology* **101**, 297–301.

Yu, M. C., Mack, T. M., Hanisch, R., Cicioni, C., and Henderson, B. E. (1986). Cigarette smoking, obesity, diuretic use and coffee consumption as risk factors for renal cell carcinoma. *Journal of the National Cancer Institute* **77**, 351–6.

19.12 Pathophysiology of renal failure

P. J. Ratcliffe and J. G. G. Ledingham

The division of renal failure into *acute and chronic* may be difficult, especially when there is an acute deterioration in a chronic condition, but the majority of cases of acute renal failure evolve over a period of hours or days, whereas most cases of chronic renal failure are presumed to have evolved over a period of years. Only a minority of cases are observed to progress over a matter of weeks and these are generally termed 'rapidly progressive'. In considering the pathophysiology of excretory loss, the distinction between 'acute' and 'chronic' is of paramount importance, since in chronic renal failure the principal reason for organ failure is a severely reduced number of nephrons, whereas in acute renal failure we have to consider the reason why a substantially normal number of nephrons may fail to function. Furthermore, in most cases of acute renal failure, the nephron is not irreversibly damaged, so that if the aetiological process is self-limited or can be reversed, potential for recovery is present, whereas in chronic renal failure this is not the case.

19.12.1 Aetiology of acute renal failure

A list of causes of acute renal failure is given in Table 19.7. For a detailed account of the individual disease the reader is referred to other sections of this chapter. Two syndromes, 'pre-renal failure' and 'acute tubular necrosis', which account for the majority of cases, require special explanation.

Table 19.7 Some causes of acute renal failure

Pre-renal failure	Cardiogenic shock, e.g. severe myocardial infarction Blood loss Plasma loss, e.g. burns Salt and water loss, e.g. G-I losses, diabetic ketoacidosis Septicaemic shock
Acute tubular necrosis	*Haemodynamic* (as for pre-renal failure) *Toxic*: heavy metals (e.g. mercuric salts), organic solvents (e.g. carbon tetrachloride), polyene antibiotics, aminoglycoside antibiotics, haem proteins, immunoglobulin light chain, dextrans, radiographic contrast, animal venoms, *Amanita phalloides*
Renovascular and thrombotic diseases	Persisting renal vasoconstriction, e.g. hepatorenal syndrome Cyclosporin A Renal artery stenoses, bilateral, single kidney Renal artery occlusion, e.g. dissecting aneurysm Microangiopathic conditions, e.g. haemolytic uraemic syndrome, thrombotic-thrombocytopenic purpura Malignant hypertension Cortical necrosis, e.g. in abruptio placentae
Glomerulonephritis	
Interstitial nephritis	Infective, e.g. leptospirosis Drug induced, e.g. penicillins, non-steroidal anti-inflammatory drugs Papillary necrosis
Crystalluria	Urate Oxalate Sulphonamides
Urinary obstruction	Ureteral obstruction with a single kidney or bilateral ureteral obstruction, e.g. stones, retroperitoneal fibrosis, tumour Urethral obstruction, e.g. prostatic disease, urethral disease

Table 19.8 Classical urinary biochemistry in different types of acute renal failure

	Pre-renal failure	Acute tubular necrosis	Acute glomerulonephritis
Urine volume	Anuria or oliguria	Oliguria to polyuria (any volume except anuria)	Anuria or oliguria
Urinary [Na$^+$]	<20 mmol/l	>40 mmol/l	<20 mmol/l
Fractional excretion of sodium	<1%	1–10%	<1%
Urine osmolarity	>500 mOsm/kg	<400 mOsm/kg	<400 mOsm/kg
Urine to plasma creatinine ratio	>40	<20	<20

Pre-renal failure

Pre-renal failure is present when poor renal perfusion accounts for the failure of renal function, and the diagnostic hallmark is the rapid return of renal function when perfusion is restored. It is implied that the nephrons themselves are undamaged and, classically, the urinary biochemistry reflects the response of normal tubules to impaired renal perfusion. There is avid retention of sodium and water, producing a low urinary sodium concentration and high urinary urea, creatinine, and osmolarity (Table 19.8). However, these features are not invariably present, possibly because of a minor degree of pre-existing or coexisting tubular disease, exposure to diuretic drugs, or interference with the generation of medullary osmotic gradients at very low solute filtration rates.

Reduced renal perfusion from any cause may give rise to pre-renal failure (Table 19.7). It may occur when cardiac output is insufficient for systemic perfusion, when there is depletion of circulatory volume due to loss of blood, plasma, or salt and water, or when there is a generalized failure of peripheral circulatory control such as may be induced by septicaemia. In addition to the systemic perfusion pressure, the renal circulation is influenced by a number of vasoconstrictor and vasodilatory influences, which act to differing degrees on afferent and efferent arteriolar tone to influence renal blood flow and glomerular

Table 19.9 Some renal vasoactive substances. A physiological role in the renal circulation has been not proven beyond doubt for all of these substances

Vasoconstrictors
  angiotensin II
  catecholamines
  renal nerve activity
  vasopressin
  thromboxanes
  leukotrienes
  adenosine

Vasodilators
  prostaglandins (E$_2$ and I$_2$)
  bradykinin
  atrial natriuretic peptide
  glucagon
  vasoactive intestinal peptide

filtration (Table 19.9). Predictably, there is no simple relationship of pre-renal failure to systemic blood pressure. Pre-renal failure will almost invariably be present when the mean systemic blood pressure is less that 50–60 mmHg, but, presumably reflecting changes in the renal haemodynamics, it frequently occurs at much higher systemic blood pressures. The importance of particular renal vasoactive substances is demonstrated by the occurrence of reversible renal failure in response to certain pharmacological inhibitors. For instance, prostaglandin synthetase inhibitors will often produce a striking reduction in renal function when the renal circulation is already compromised. When the threat to renal perfusion is local, such as with stenosis of the major renal arteries, angiotensin converting enzyme inhibition will often cause severe but reversible renal failure, probably because maintenance of glomerular capillary filtration pressure is dependent on maintenance of efferent arteriolar tone by angiotensin II. Why this reaction should occur more commonly when the threat to renal perfusion is local rather than systemic as, for instance, in severe cardiac failure, is unclear.

Certain poorly understood conditions involving persistent renal vasoconstriction may be considered as specific types of pre-renal failure, since they are not reversed even when systemic perfusion pressure is restored. In hepato-renal syndrome, advanced liver failure is complicated by an unusual form of acute renal failure in which the urinary biochemistry is similar to that in classical pre-renal failure, yet improvement of systemic perfusion does not result in return of renal function. The kidney itself is undamaged and will function if transplanted into a normal recipient. The syndrome is believed to arise from persisting renal vasoconstriction, the aetiology of which remains undefined: treatment with vasodilators such as dopamine, phentolamine, and converting enzyme inhibitors, has been ineffective.

A more recently defined cause of persistent renal vasoconstriction is the immunosuppressive drug cyclosporin A, where, likewise, the mechanism of persisting vasoconstriction is unclear.

Acute tubular necrosis (ATN)

Acute tubular necrosis is a form of acute renal failure that occurs in seriously ill patients, usually when there has been a severe haemodynamic disturbance or exposure of the kidney to toxic substances. Unlike pre-renal failure, it is not immediately reversible by correction of the haemodynamic disturbance. Since the aetiology is not always clear, the justification for regarding acute tubular necrosis as a single entity is clinical; the syndrome has recognizable clinical features, essentially a loss of excretory function combined with urinary abnormalities suggestive of tubular dysfunction (Table 19.8), it complicates specific clinical settings, and has a definable prognosis: recovery within days or weeks of removal of the initiating cause. Confusion has been generated by the variety of alternative names, which includes lower nephron syndrome, vasomotor nephropathy, traumatic anuria, ischaemic nephropathy, post-ischaemic acute renal failure, and acute intrinsic renal failure. We shall use the term 'acute tubular necrosis', since it is entrenched in medical parlance and not because it accurately reflects the pathology. Frank necrosis of tubular cells is not usually extensive and may not be present at all. Although injury to the tubules is a consistent feature, this may not be discernible morphologically.

A conventional list of aetiological factors for acute tubular necrosis is included in Table 19.7. Although most of these associations are well established, for many the mechanism by which the kidney is damaged is not clearly proven. What is established beyond doubt is that the clinical syndrome of acute tubular necrosis, and an experimental form of acute renal failure resembling it, can be produced reliably by complete renal ischaemia of a certain duration, or by exposure to direct-acting nephrotoxins, such as heavy metal salts. It is usually presumed that the factors listed in Table 19.7 cause renal damage by similar mechanisms.

Thus, haemodynamic risk factors are presumed to cause renal damage by ischaemia. The causes of pre-renal failure may all give rise to acute tubular necrosis and it is probable, but unproven, that this reflects more severely impaired renal perfusion causing ischaemic damage to the renal tubules in established ATN. As with pre-renal failure, there is no simple relationship to systemic blood pressure. Furthermore, the risk of progression from pre-renal failure to ATN is much greater in certain situations, such as traumatic or septic shock or in pregnancy, than it is in cardiogenic shock or gastrointestinal haemorrhage, possibly reflecting differences in the renal circulatory response to shock of different aetiologies.

It is not clear why the kidney in particular should be susceptible to ischaemic damage in these situations. Susceptibility to ischaemic damage during hypoperfusion would not be predicted from the high renal blood flow and low arteriovenous oxygen extraction of the kidney under normal physiological conditions. To account for the peculiar susceptibility to ischaemic damage, inefficient regional intrarenal oxygen delivery and sensitivity to disproportionately severe rises in renal vascular resistance have been proposed. Evidence for both mechanisms exists and they are not mutually exclusive. Unfortunately, at present, there is no simple means of detecting the time of precise onset of renal ischaemia. Thus, although it seems likely that renal ischaemia is responsible for the occurrence of ATN in many situations, this, along with the exact reasons for its occurrence cannot be proven.

Direct nephrotoxicity is often presumed when no hemodynamic disturbance seems likely. For some factors, such as heavy metal salts, organic solvents, and polyene antibiotics, a consistent association with acute tubular necrosis is observed in man and can be reproduced in experimental animals, so that the status of the nephrotoxin is beyond question. For many more commonly implicated risk factors, the clinical association is less consistent and more difficult to reproduce experimentally. Radiographic contrast media, haem proteinuria, Bence–Jones proteinuria, and aminoglycoside antibiotics fall into this category. For example, aminoglycoside antibiotics will, if given for a sufficient period at sufficient dosage, reliably produce acute renal failure in experimental animals. They are never used at these doses in man, where at therapeutic doses they consistently alter urinary enzyme excretion but do not consistently cause renal failure. Renal failure does occur sporadically and may be dependent on a coincidence of risk factors, such as a coexisting impairment of perfusion leading to coincident ischaemia. Experimental evidence supports the possibility that the ischaemically damaged renal tubule is more susceptible to aminoglycoside injury, but this is unproven in man. In another situation, haem proteinuria, the association with acute tubular necrosis, although well established, also occurs inconsistently and it is difficult to produce renal damage in experimental animals, even using high doses of haem proteins. Possible explanations in this case are that the haem proteins are only a marker for the presence of more toxic substances released during cellular breakdown, or that, again, an interaction of factors is required for renal damage, either at the cellular level or within the lumen, such as might be produced by precipitation of the protein at low urinary pH.

In fact, most cases of acute tubular necrosis arise against a complex clinical background in which multiple risk factors coincide and interactions are likely. The complexity of the situation usually makes it difficult to draw firm aetiological conclusions about individual risk factors from clinical surveys.

19.12.2 Mechanisms of excretory failure in acute renal disease

Each nephron functions as a unit, requiring tubular integrity as an anatomical conduit and transporting epithelium, as well as a blood supply to a filtering glomerulus. The mechanism of failure in such a system will depend on the aetiology of the renal disease.

For many conditions, such as obstruction of the major renal vessels or the ureter, the mechanism of excretory failure is clear. Pre-renal failure is, by definition, consequent on failure of renal perfusion and presumably arises simply from glomerular capillary hypotension. In acute glomerulonephritis, filtration failure due to glomerular damage is the principal abnormality.

In contrast, great controversy surrounds the mechanism by which the major manifestation of diseases principally affecting the renal tubules is an apparent failure of glomerular filtration.

Most attention has been given to acute tubular necrosis, where a massive literature has arisen on the experimental pathophysiology—though similar considerations and arguments could be applied to other conditions, such as acute interstitial nephritis, and certain forms of transplant rejection where the primary pathology is tubulo-interstitial.

The principal mechanisms proposed to explain excretory failure in acute tubular necrosis are a persistent alteration of renal blood flow, an alteration of kidney capillary ultrafiltration, obstruction of the renal tubules, and backleakage of filtrate from damaged tubules. We shall discuss each mechanism separately and then consider how they may interact, since, as was first suggested in the original description by Bywaters, it is likely that several factors contribute to the excretory failure.

Renal perfusion

Persisting alterations in renal blood flow have been proposed to account for loss of filtration in acute tubular necrosis. However, the persisting reduction in total renal blood flow, both in man and in experimental models of acute tubular necrosis, is slight in comparison to the apparent reduction of glomerular filtration rate. Theoretically, abnormal renal perfusion could still account for loss of filtration if a subtly balanced reduction in efferent arteriolar tone and increase in afferent arteriolar tone occurred, or if blood was shunted through an aglomerular circulation. In practice, no such shunt pathway or redistribution of arteriolar tone has been demonstrated.

Glomerular ultrafiltration coefficient

In most, but not all, models of ATN, the glomerulus is structurally normal but reduction in the glomerular ultrafiltration coefficient (Kf), which may be due to a change in the capillary hydraulic conductivity (Lp) or a change in the filtering surface area, may be present without morphological abnormality. Reduction in Kf cannot be assessed in man but has been demonstrated in a variety of animal models of ATN.

Alterations in renal perfusion or in the glomerular-capillary ultrafiltration coefficient could arise from direct injury, for instance from endothelial cell swelling in ischaemia or from circulating or locally generated vasoactive substances, such as angiotensin II. Much interest has, however, surrounded the possibility that they could also arise as a secondary consequence of tubular injury and be mediated via tubuloglomerular feedback mechanisms arising from the macula densa, comprised of specialized tubular cells in the distal nephron which are in close juxtaposition with the glomerulus and afferent arteriole. A clear demonstration of the existence of such a feedback system operating at a single nephron level has emerged from micropuncture experiments, but its role in acute renal failure remains unproven and it is doubtful whether the reduction in filtration achieved by maximal activation of the tubular glomerular feedback mechanism could account for the near total failure of filtration which is often apparent.

Backleakage of filtrate

In experimental models of acute tubular necrosis, backleakage of filtrate can be demonstrated directly by the loss of filtration markers following microinjection into the renal tubules, where it correlates with the presence of structural damage to the renal tubules. In man, the persisting dense nephrogram sometimes seen in acute tubular necrosis after intravenous urography is thought to reflect persisting filtration, with accumulation of contrast in the kidney arising from backleakage of filtrate from damaged tubules.

Tubular obstruction

Obstruction to the renal tubules was originally suggested by the occurrence of intratubular casts of cellular debris and precipitated proteins. It is now realized that obstruction may occur simply as a consequence of tubular cell swelling. Direct demonstration of tubular obstruction in some models of ATN is provided by micropuncture measurements of rises in proximal intratubular pressures to stop flow pressures.

It is clear, first, that all these mechanisms may have some role in the pathogenesis of acute tubular necrosis and, secondly, that none can completely account for the syndrome. Different mechanisms operate at different times during the course of acute tubular necrosis. For instance, obstructing intratubular debris, raised proximal intratubular pressures, and leakage of microinjected inulin can explain the severe oliguric renal failure in the first 1–2 weeks following 60 min of occlusion of the renal artery in the rat, on the basis of tubular obstruction and backleakage of filtrate. These abnormalities then resolve, but renal function nevertheless remains quite severely impaired, presumably for other reasons, for at least 4–6 weeks. Factors may also operate concurrently and this may be difficult to detect. For instance, in the presence of tubular obstruction, proximal intratubular pressures will not rise if there is a coincident tubular backleakage or lowering of the glomerular filtration pressure.

It is important to realize that the mechanisms described do not necessarily imply the existence of frank cell necrosis. Nevertheless, the notoriously poor correlation, particularly in human 'acute tubular necrosis', between the severity of renal failure and morphological tubular damage requires some explanation. Two possibilities have been put forward. First, the function of a nephron may be critically impaired by a single, and perhaps very small, area of damage, not necessarily in the field of view. Secondly, in the kidney, large transtubular fluid movement may continue immediately prior to histological fixation, so that with conventional means of fixation, examination of the fixed tissue may not accurately reflect the tubular hydrodynamic situation pertaining *in vivo*; and subtle renal tubular damage is difficult to detect.

The consensus view is thus that tubular injury, but not necessarily tubular necrosis, is central to the development of this form of acute renal failure. It is likely that, in most cases, several of the mechanisms described combine to produce a profound loss of renal function.

19.12.3 Aetiology and mechanisms of excretory failure in chronic renal disease

A list of causes of chronic renal failure is given in Table 19.10. Specific renal diseases are described in other sections, but in the majority of patients presenting with established severe chronic renal failure no specific cause can be identified. Even when there is a history of preceding renal disease, such as glomerulonephritis or childhood pyelonephritis, it is often uncertain how much of the progressive loss of renal function is due to continued disease activity, and how much is due to self-generating mechanisms of progressive nephron loss. Most patients with a creatinine clearance less than 25 ml/min will run an inexorably progressive course to end-stage renal failure, even when there is good evidence that the initiating disease is inactive. In all chronic renal diseases, failure is largely explained by a reduction in the number of functioning nephrons. As far as can be judged from animal studies, surviving nephrons appear to behave in a regulated way, although a larger spread of single nephron glomerular filtration rate (SNGFR) is found than in normal kidneys. In glomerular diseases a reduced ultrafiltration coefficient lowers SNGFR in affected glomeruli, but adaptive changes tend to restore it in these and SNGFR may be elevated in less affected or unaffected nephrons.

The progression of chronic renal failure

Possible reasons for progression of chronic renal failure include hyperfiltration injury from glomerular or systemic hypertension or the intrarenal deposition of retained substances, such as phosphate and calcium, urinary phosphate excretion, hyperuricaemia, hyperlipidaemia, hyperoxalaemia, and production of local growth promoting factors in glomerali. Of these the leading contenders are probably still glomerular hypertension and the deposition of calcium and phosphate.

In response to a reduction in the functioning renal mass, an adaptive change occurs in the remaining nephrons which has been characterized in experimental models of ablative nephropathy (although not in other animal models of renal failure) using micropuncture techniques (Brenner et al. 1982). Afferent arteriolar vasodilation leads, in non-diseased glomeruli, to an increase in single nephron perfusion, glomerular transcapillary hydraulic pressure, and SNGFR. A similar adaptive mechanism may occur in diffuse glomerular disease to limit the expected reduction in single nephron glomerular filtration rate. It is postulated that this adaptive increase is responsible for self-generating renal damage manifest as glomerulosclerosis, proteinuria, and progressive renal failure, since both the haemodynamic adaption and these effects can be ameliorated by protein restriction, both in experimental models and perhaps also in man. Inhibitors of angiotensin converting enzyme will also reduce proteinuria, glomerulosclerosis, and progression of disease in some experimental models of chronic renal failure. In some examples the effects coincide with a reduction in efferent arteriolar tone and thus a reduction of trans-capillary pressure and glomerular blood flow; in others the beneficial effects of ACE inhibitors may be mediated by a reduction in the traffic of small molecules across glomerular capillaries independent of pressure and flow. Proof of benefit in man by use of ACE inhibitors even in diabetic nephropathy (for which evidence is best) is still incomplete.

Systemic hypertension is a frequent complication of renal disease and may itself damage the kidney. In considering hypertensive renal damage, an important distinction must be made between so-called 'benign' and 'malignant' hypertension. In malignant hypertension, the severely raised pressure disrupts the vascular endothelium, leading to permeation, swelling, and necrosis of the arteriolar wall. In the kidney this causes rapidly progressive renal failure. Lowering the blood pressure allows healing of the fibrinoid necrosis and may result in a considerable recovery of renal function. The relationship of benign hypertension to renal damage is less clear, but it is widely believed that benign hypertension also contributes to the progression of renal disease. This is true in many experimental models of glomerular disease, but convincing evidence in man is only present in diabetic renal disease, where hypertension is associated with the development and progression of diabetic glomerulosclerosis, and treatment of hypertension limits progression. It is likely that systemic hypertension short of the malignant phase and the haemodynamic adaptations to reduced renal mass in surviving nephrons summate to produce physical damage to glomerular capillaries and associated mesangial tissue.

It has also been suggested that the phosphate retention which accompanies chronic renal failure may contribute to progressive loss of renal function by facilitating calcium phosphate deposition in renal tissue. Calcification is often observed in end-stage kidneys, and renal calcium deposition may exacerbate

Table 19.10 Some causes of chronic renal failure

Glomerular disease	Primary glomerulonephritis, e.g. proliferative membranous, membrano-proliferative, mesangial IgA
	Focal glomerulosclerosis
	Glomerulonephritis in systemic disease, e.g. systemic lupus erythematosus, polyarteritis, endocarditis
	Diabetic glomerulosclerosis
	Hypertensive glomerulosclerosis
	Amyloidosis
	Hereditary glomerular disease, e.g. Alport's syndrome
Renovascular and thrombotic diseases	As in acute renal failure, unresolved
Interstitial diseases	Interstitial nephritis, unresolved
	Papillary necrosis, e.g. diabetes, sickle-cell anaemia, analgesic nephropathy
	Pyelonephritis (scarring in childhood)
	Deposition, urate, oxalosis, cystinosis
	Myeloma kidney
	Hypercalcaemic syndromes
Cystic diseases	Adult polycystic kidney disease
	Medullary cystic disease
Urinary obstruction	As in acute renal failure, unresolved

injury by generating damaging inflammation and scarring. The probability that the critical factor influencing microscopic calcification is the plasma calcium : phosphate product has led to attempts to retard the progression of renal disease with dietary phosphorus restriction and agents that decrease gastrointestinal absorption of phosphate. In experimental models of chronic renal failure, dietary restriction of phosphate can limit both development of renal calcification and progression of renal failure (Ibels *et al.* 1978) but clear evidence of preservation of renal function by phosphate restriction in man is lacking.

19.12.4 Pathophysiological consequences of renal failure

The complex manifestations of renal failure stem from three important disturbances: failure of water and electrolyte homeostasis, retention of toxic substances, and failure of renal endocrine function. Additionally, certain homeostatic adaptations to renal failure may themselves have adverse effects, a concept known as the 'trade-off' hypothesis.

Electrolyte homeostasis in renal failure

To maintain homeostasis for water and electrolytes when glomerular filtration is diminished, tubular reabsorption is altered so that the kidney excretes a much larger fraction of the filtrate. Additionally, to correct a given electrolyte imbalance, a very much larger change in fractional excretion is required—an adaptation known as the magnification phenomenon. These adaptations are much more complete in chronic renal failure than in acute renal failure. Thus in chronic renal failure most patients are able to avoid a *severe* disturbance of sodium, potassium, water, and acid : base homeostasis until glomerular filtration falls to a very low rate, often less than 10 ml/min, whereas in acute renal failure severe abnormalities develop rapidly.

The mechanisms of the adaptations are poorly understood. Animal studies of single nephron physiology have demonstrated that similar changes in tubular reabsorption are present in nephrons with widely differing filtration rates—a phenomenon known as glomerular tubular balance. Homogeneity of tubular function is often retained across both kidneys, even in unilateral models of renal disease, implying the existence of some co-ordinating systemic stimulus. However, no adequate explanation for this phenomenon exists and it appears that different mechanisms are involved in the adaptive increases in fractional excretion of different electrolytes.

Sodium and water

The fractional excretion of sodium rises from approximately 1 per cent in health to values approaching 50 per cent in severe chronic renal failure. These changes cannot arise from alterations in single nephron GFR, which may be low, normal, or high. Possible explanations include osmotic diuresis from retained solutes, altered Starling forces in peritubular capillaries, such as loss of the normal rise in post-glomerular plasma oncotic pressure at low filtration fractions, or the retention of natriuretic substances. A damaged kidney can retain sodium normally, provided a healthy contralateral organ prevents a uraemic environment and maintains normal body fluid volumes. Levels of atrial natriuretic peptide are high in chronic renal failure. Studies of cation fluxes in blood cells have suggested the presence of an inhibitor of sodium–potassium ATPase in uraemic patients; such an inhibitor might also act on the renal tubular cells to promote sodium excretion.

Sodium homeostasis is usually well preserved until the GFR falls below 10–20 ml/min, provided changes in dietary intake are not extreme. At lesser levels of renal function, most patients retain sodium and water with a consequent increase in plasma volume, extracellular fluid, and total body water, resulting most commonly in 'volume-dependent' hypertension. Oedema is unusual unless there is coincident impairment of cardiac function or hypoalbuminaemia. A few patients, usually those with interstitial or tubular, rather than glomerular disease (e.g. obstructive uropathy, pyelonephritis, analgesic nephropathy, nephronophthisis, or polycystic disease) are incapable of conserving sodium even when dietary intake is normal. The resulting volume depletion results in a reversible exacerbation of renal failure because of impaired renal perfusion.

Changes in fractional excretion of sodium are usually matched by parallel changes in water-handling by the kidney. Indeed, the capacity to dilute the urine is well preserved until renal function is grossly depressed; but maximal urinary concentration is lost with GFRs as high as 60 ml/min. This concentration defect is probably largely due to the increased load of solute presented to surviving nephrons and may be substantially, but not completely, restored when dialysis has reduced solute load per nephron. Scarring of medullary tissues must contribute in those rare patients in whom chronic renal disease is associated with obligatory water loss, amounting to a secondary nephrogenic diabetes insipidus. This syndrome has been observed, particularly in nephronophthisis, but also in obstructive nephropathy, pyelonephritis, nephrocalcinosis, polycystic disease, and renal amyloidosis.

Potassium

Plasma potassium concentrations are usually maintained within normal limits until late in chronic renal failure unless there is acidosis or hyperkalaemia is precipitated by a high dietary intake, by the use of potassium-retaining diuretics, or the presence of adrenal insufficiency or inactivity of the renin–angiotensin–aldosterone system. Fractional potassium excretion increases *pari passu* with the fall in GFR in chronic renal diseases, and may, on occasion, exceed 100 per cent. The compensatory mechanisms that allow this to take place include increased delivery of sodium to the distal tubular exchange sites, increased capacity to secrete potassium by the distal nephron, perhaps mediated by a rise in cortical and outer medullary Na-K ATPase in basolateral tubular membranes, and adaptations by the large bowel such that its mucosal secretory capacity for potassium is enhanced. The importance or otherwise of aldosterone in potassium adaptation is uncertain. Although plasma potassium concentrations may rise at end-stage chronic renal failure, total body potassium is not necessarily increased. Oliguria much increases the risk of hyperkalaemia sufficient to provoke cardiac arrest.

Acid : base

Metabolic acidosis in chronic renal failure may be the result of a failure to excrete ammonium and titratable acid, or because of renal tubular dysfunction leading to urinary bicarbonate losses. The traditional view is that acidosis is more often due to decreased urinary buffer (principally phosphate) and capacity to secrete ammonium, rather than to bicarbonate leakage; but Muldowney has produced persuasive evidence that impaired proximal tubular reabsorption of bicarbonate (and sodium) are more commonly the cause (Muldowney et al. 1972). There is some evidence that parathyroid hormone contributes to such bicarbonate wastage.

Studies of proton balance in renal failure have indicated that patients with renal disease are persistently in positive proton balance long before systemic acidaemia is detected, and it has been suggested that the buffering occurs in the bone minerals; an effect that might contribute to renal osteodystrophy.

Overt metabolic acidosis leads to respiratory compensation by hyperventilation. Acidosis also contributes to the development of hyperkalaemia by causing a shift of cellular potassium into the extracellular space. Terminally, uncompensated acidosis leads to myocardial depression and coma.

Uraemic toxins

The response of many manifestations of renal failure to dialysis has implicated toxic dialysable substances in the pathogenesis of 'uraemia'.

Many features of the uraemic syndrome can be ameliorated by protein restriction and exacerbated by catabolic states, implying that some aspects of nitrogen metabolism are important. Urea retention itself is relatively unimportant, since raising the plasma urea artificially mimics the uraemic syndrome poorly. Other retained low molecular weight substances include, in addition to creatinine, guanidines, products of nucleic acid metabolism such as urate, aliphatic and aromatic amines, indoles, phenols, amino acids, small peptides, and isocyanate. Many substances of higher molecular weight are also retained, including peptides, polyamines, carbohydrate derivatives, and low molecular weight proteins.

It is likely that different substances are responsible for the many different manifestations of the uraemic syndrome (Table 19.11). For instance, many aspects of the uraemic syndrome are improved rapidly by haemodialysis using membranes with a high clearance of substances of molecular weight up to approximately 300, implicating a low molecular weight toxin; but others, such as neuropathy, appear to respond only to prolonged haemodialysis, to correlate poorly with concentration in plasma of low molecular weight markers such as urea and creatinine, and to respond better to treatment by peritoneal dialysis. These observations gave rise to the *middle molecule hypothesis*, that substances of molecular weight 300–2000, which are not cleared well by conventional haemodialysis

Table 19.11 Some manifestations of 'uraemia'

Nausea, vomiting
Diarrhoea

Itch
Skin pigmentation

Serositis (including pericarditis)

Impaired erythropoiesis
Platelet dysfunction
Impaired immunity

Accelerated atheroma
Cardiomyopathy

Osteodystrophy
Myopathy
Arthropathy

Hiccup
Myoclonus
Convulsions
Coma

Neuropathy

membranes, were responsible at least for some of the manifestations of uraemia; but a single or even predominant 'uraemic toxin' has yet to be identified (Bergstrom and Furst 1983).

More recently, retention of a substance of even higher molecular weight, a β_2-microglobulin (molecular weight 11 500), has been implicated in the pathogenesis of an arthropathy in dialysis patients, involving deposition of β_2-microglobulin amyloid.

19.12.5 Erythropoiesis in renal failure

A normochronic normocytic anaemia occurs in the vast majority of patients with severe chronic renal failure, developing in most cases when creatinine clearance declines below approximately 25 ml/min. Anaemia is often milder in patients with large polycystic kidneys and is more severe after bilateral nephrectomy. Recently, the renal hormone erythropoietin has been synthesized by recombinant DNA techniques and full correction of anaemia by doses of exogenous erythropoietin, not vastly greater than expected physiological rates of production, has demonstrated the central importance of erythropoietin deficiency in the anaemia of chronic renal failure. The precise mechanisms whereby damaged kidneys fail to secrete erythropoietin are not yet known. The hormone stimulates erythropoiesis and is principally active on the colony-forming units (CFU-E) in the erythrocyte progenitors.

A number of other factors exacerbate the anaemia of chronic renal failure. Depression of erythropoiesis and shortening of red cell survival by uraemic toxins have been demonstrated. Blood loss may be increased, particularly in patients receiving haemodialysis treatment. Deficiencies of iron and of folate may occur. Aluminium intoxication from contaminated dialysate or aluminium-containing phosphate-binding drugs causes a severe microcytic anaemia, and retention of aluminium or other trace elements, even at low levels, may impair erythropoiesis.

In acute renal failure, anaemia also develops rapidly, but the precise role of erythropoietin deficiency has not yet been clarified. Coincident systemic disease such as bleeding and infection are common and also contribute to anaemia.

19.12.6   Renal osteodystrophy

Chronic renal failure is often, but not always, complicated by a bone disease termed renal osteodystrophy. The prevalence of this complication depends on the method of diagnosis. It is very common if bone biopsy is performed, less common radiologically, and least common of all (perhaps some 5 per cent) if symptoms are the criterion. Osteodystrophy is most likely to occur at or around puberty. Within a very complex disturbance of bone metabolism, two disorders, parathyroid stimulation and deficiency of $1,25(OH)_2$ cholecalciferol, have a well-established role. In addition, derangements of acid–base status, magnesium metabolism, aluminium retention, the serum calcium:phosphate product, calcitonin, and steroid hormones may all contribute to renal osteodystrophy. Similar metabolic abnormalities are also present in acute renal failure, but it is in chronic renal failure, particularly when it has been slowly progressive over many years or when life has been prolonged by dialysis, that the clinical importance of renal osteodystrophy is fully realized.

Parathyroid stimulation

The stimulus for excess parathyroid hormone secretion in chronic renal failure is controversial. As glomerular filtration declines, fractional excretion of phosphate increases, but, in contrast with the position for sodium and potassium, this adaptation is relatively incomplete, so that phosphate retention occurs rather earlier and is commonly observed when creatinine clearance declines below about 25–30 ml/min. It has been proposed that phosphate retention leads to depression of the serum calcium and thus stimulates parathyroid hormone secretion. Raised levels of parathyroid hormone promote phosphate excretion and thus phosphate balance is preserved at the expense of a raised level of parathormone—a commonly quoted example of the 'trade-off' hypothesis. Recently, doubts have arisen about this explanation, since parathyroid hormone levels are commonly raised before any disturbance of serum calcium and phosphate is detected, and can be suppressed by $1,25(OH)_2$ cholecalciferol therapy without increasing ionized calcium. In this context, the presence of receptors of $1,25(OH)_2D_3$ in parathyroids and the demonstration that this D metabolite can suppress parathyroid hormone secretion is pertinent.

In chronic renal failure, continuous parathyroid stimulation leads to parathyroid hyperplasia, and in some cases normal control of parathyroid hormone secretion is lost, leading to persistent secretion in the face of hypercalcaemia, a poorly understood phenomenon (perhaps dependent in part on the mass of parathyroid cells) known as tertiary hyperparathyroidism.

Secondary hyperparathyroidism plays a major role in the pathogenesis of renal osteodystrophy, giving rise to osteitis fibrosa, with increased bone reabsorption and excess collagen synthesis. Additionally, parathyroid hormone has been implicated as a uraemic toxin, contributing to such diverse complications as neuropathy, cardiomyopathy, and impaired erythropoiesis.

Vitamin D metabolism

Production of the most active form of vitamin D_3, $1,25(OH)_2$ cholecalciferol requires 1-hydroxylation of 25-OH cholecalciferol. The 1-hydroxylase enzyme is present almost exclusively in kidney, where it has been isolated from the mitochondria of the proximal tubule. For reasons that remain unclear, levels of $1,25(OH)_2$ cholecalciferol are reduced early in chronic renal failure. In addition to its role in the pathogenesis of parathyroid stimulation, $1,25(OH)_2$ cholecalciferol deficiency might itself be expected to impair bone mineralization, leading to osteomalacia. Bone histology confirms the frequent concurrence of osteomalacia and osteitis fibrosa, and both may respond well to treatment with $1,25(OH)_2D_3$. In some cases osteomalacia is not present even when levels of $1,25(OH)_2$ cholecalciferol are very low, and in others there may be a failure to respond to $1,25(OH)_2$ cholecalciferol therapy. Other factors, such as hypophosphataemia or aluminium retention, are probably important in these cases.

19.12.7   Hypertension in renal disease

Hypertension is only common in specific types of acute renal failure. For instance, it is common in acute glomerulonephritis, where sodium retention is of paramount importance, but rare in acute tubular necrosis. In chronic renal failure the incidence of hypertension is high, particularly with glomerular disease, and both the incidence and severity increase as renal disease advances.

Sodium retention, abnormalities of the renin–angiotensin system, and increased sympathetic activity, are all important in the pathophysiology.

A degree of sodium retention is generally present in patients with mild renal failure and hypertension, and both may progress as renal function declines. Nevertheless, the correlation of sodium balance with blood pressure is not tight and sodium depletion by diuretics, diet, or dialysis fails to achieve adequate control of hypertension in a significant minority of patients. In these patients an important role for the renin–angiotensin system is postulated, which does not appear to be appropriately controlled in relation to sodium balance, so that hypertension may arise from an abnormal renin/sodium relationship. Support for this hypothesis is provided by evidence that the pressor response to angiotensin II is positively correlated with sodium balance, and that the hypotensive response to pharmacological interruption of the renin–angiotensin system is negatively correlated with sodium balance. In addition to interacting with sodium balance, the renin–angiotensin system interacts in a complex way with the autonomic nervous sytem, and increased sympathetic activity may also contribute to pathogenesis of hypertension in renal disease.

Hypertension due to renovascular disease requires separate consideration. It accounts for a small minority of patients with renal disease and hypertension but has attracted a great deal of interest because of its relationship to the classical experiments of Goldblatt and colleagues, and because it may, in certain cases, be amenable to surgical cure by renal revascularization. It is clear that activation of the renin–angiotensin system is of central importance in the acute development of hypertension after experimental renal artery constriction, and presumably this is also the case in man. However, hypertension usually persists into a chronic phase despite reduction in plasma renin. Sodium retention, an abnormal sodium/renin relationship, and interactions between the renin–angiotensin and autonomic nervous systems have again been postulated, but as with hypertension in chronic renal parenchymal disease, the precise importance of these factors is unclear.

19.12.8 Further reading

Anon. (1991). Dialysis amyloidosis. *Lancet* **338**, 349–56.

Badr, K. F. and Ichikawa, I. (1988). Prerenal failure: a deleterious shift from renal compensation to decompensation. *New England Journal of Medicine* **319**, 623.

Bergstrom, J. and Furst, P. (1983). Uraemic toxins. In *Replacement of renal function by dialysis* (ed. W. Drukker, F. M. Parsons, and J. F. Maher), pp. 354–90. Martinus Nijhoff, The Hague.

Beutler, B. and Cerami, A. (1987). Cachectin: more than a tumor necrosis factor. *New England Journal of Medicine* **316**, 379–85.

Blythe, W. B. (1983). Captopril and renal autoregulations. *New England Journal of Medicine* **308**, 390–1.

Brezis, M., Rosen, S., Silva, P., and Epstein, F. M. (1984). Renal ischaemia: A new perspective. *Kidney International* **26**, 375–83.

Bricker, N. S. (1972). On the pathogenesis of the uremic state. An exposition of the 'trade-off hypothesis'. *New England Journal of Medicine* **286**, 1093–9.

Clive, D. M. and Stoff, J. S. (1984). Renal syndromes associated with non-steroidal anti-inflammatory drugs. *New England Journal of Medicine* **310**, 563–72.

Coburn, J. W. and Slatopolsky, E. (1986). Vitamin D, parathyroid hormone and renal osteodystrophy. In *The kidney* (3rd edn) (ed. B. M. Brenner and F. C. Rector), pp. 1657–729. W. B. Saunders, Philadelphia.

D'Amico, G. and Sanna, G. (1991). Lipid abnormalities in renal disease. *Kidney International* **Suppl. 32**, S1–S72.

El Nahas, A. M. (1989). Glomerulosclerosis: insights into pathogenesis and treatment. *Nephrology, Dialysis and Transplantation* **4**, 843–53.

Eschbach, J. W. (1989). The anemia of chronic renal failure: pathophysiology and the effects of recombinant erthropoietin. *Kidney International* **35**, 134–48.

Fine, L. G. (1988). Preventing the progression of human renal disease: have rational therapeutic principles emerged? *Kidney International* **33**, 116–28.

Harris, R. C., Meyer, T. W., and Brenner, B. M. (1986). Nephron adaptation to renal injury. In *The kidney* (3rd edn), (ed. B. M. Brenner and F. C. Rector), pp. 1553–85. W. B. Saunders, Philadelphia.

Hostetter, T. H. and Brenner, B. M. (1983). Renal circulatory and nephron function in experimental acute renal failure. In *Acute renal failure* (ed. B. M. Brenner and J. M. Lazarus), pp. 67–90. W. B. Saunders, Philadelphia.

Miller, T. J., *et al.* (1978). Urinary diagnostic indices in acute renal failure: A prospective study. *Annals of Internal Medicine* **89**, 47–50.

Muldowney, F. P., Donohoe, J. F., Carroll, D. V., Powell, D., and Freaney, R. (1972). *Quarterly Journal of Medicine* **41**, 321–42.

Powell, J. S. and Adamson, J. W. (1985). Hematopoiesis and the kidney. In *The kidney, physiology and pathophysiology* (ed. D. W. Seldin and G. Giebisch), pp. 847–66. Raven Press, New York.

Slatopolsky, E. (1990). Update on vitamin D. *Kidney International* **Suppl. 29**, S1–S68.

Smith, M. C. and Dunn, M. J. (1986). Renovascular and renal parenchymal hypertension. In *The kidney* (3rd edn) (ed. B. M. Brenner and F. C. Rector), pp. 1221–51. W. B. Saunders, Philadelphia.

Solez, K. (1983). Acute renal failure (acute tubular necrosis, infarction and cortical necrosis). In *Pathology of the kidney* (3rd edn) (ed. R. H. Heptinstall), pp. 1069–148. Little Brown and Co., Boston.

Takabatake, T. and Thuram, K. (1991). Tubulo-glomerular feedback system. *Kidney International* **Suppl. 32**, S1–S152.

Trueta, J., Barclay, A. E., Daniel, P. M., Franklin, K. J., and Prichard, M. M. L. (1947). *Studies of the renal circulation*. Blackwell Scientific, Oxford.

19.13 Urinary outflow tract

D. Griffiths

19.13.1 Normal structure and function

The *urinary outflow tract* extends from the renal pelvis to the external meatus of the urethra and is adapted for the transport, storage, and excretion of urine. The tract is lined by *transitional epithelium* that extends continuously from the renal pelvis to the proximal urethra. A layer of connective tissue—*the lamina propria*—separates the epithelium from the muscularis, the outermost layer of the tract.

Renal pelvis, ureter, and bladder

The muscularis of the renal pelvis consists of bundles of smooth muscle arranged in a spiral continuous with the muscularis of the ureter. In the upper ureter the muscularis is organized as interlacing bundles without layers but in the lower ureter, two layers, an *inner longitudinal* and an *outer circular*, are present. Contraction of the muscle produces the stellate lumen that is seen when the ureter is viewed in histological cross-section. Urine is propelled down the ureter by *peristalsis*, at its termination the ureter enters the bladder at an angle, forming a valve-like structure at the orifice that prevents reflux of urine into the ureter during micturition. Disorders of peristalsis can lead to urinary obstruction even without luminal occlusion.

The muscularis in the bladder forms the *detrusor muscle* and is thicker than that of the ureter, being made up of a meshwork of interlacing smooth muscle bundles separated by loose, vascular connective tissue. The muscle bundles in the inner layer are thicker than the bundles in the outer layers. In men, muscle is concentrated at the bladder neck where it forms the *internal or preprostatic sphincter*. Organized reflex contraction of the detrusor, in association with relaxation of the outlet sphincters, result in *micturition*. Only the start of this process is under voluntary control. Neurological disease, at any level from the cerebral cortex to the sacral plexuses, may result in loss of coordinated micturition, resulting in a 'neurogenic bladder' causing retention of urine or irregular detrusor activity. This may result in *bladder hypertrophy*, *vesicoureteric reflux*, and *ascending infection*.

The muscularis is separated from the epithelium by a layer of loose connective tissue; this is thin in the renal pelvis and thicker in the ureter and bladder. By anatomical convention— because of the absence of a well-formed muscularis mucosae— this is designated the lamina propria, although some authors have used the term submucosa. Recent studies of normal bladders have shown that some bladders do have a *muscularis mucosae* (Ro *et al.* 1987). The presence of muscle in the subepithelial connective tissue has implications for the staging of bladder cancer.

The urinary-tract epithelium, termed the *urothelium* or *transitional epithelium*, lies on a basement membrane and is 3–6 cells thick. In the bladder the thickness depends on the degree of distension at fixation. Small basal cells with scanty cytoplasm are attached to the basement membrane, cells with rather more cytoplasm lie in the mid-zone beneath specialized surface cells. These specialized cells at the luminal surface, the 'umbrella cells', provide a barrier between the lumen and the underlying tissue: they have abundant cytoplasm, tight epithelial junctions to adjacent cells, and have a specialized surface membrane containing glycoproteins. These features are thought to confer properties of both waterproofing and resistance to bacterial adherence to the urothelium.

The important anatomical relationship of the bladder are the *uterus, cervix, and vagina in females*, and the *prostate and rectum in males*. There is a small peritoneal surface at the dome that offers contact with the small and large bowel. Tumours or inflammatory lesions at these sites may involve the bladder and/or produce vesical fistulae.

Urethra

The male urethra is divided into four anatomical sections: the *prostatic* and *membranous urethra* make up the proximal or posterior urethra, while the *bulbous and penile urethra* form the distal or posterior urethra. The prostatic urethra is lined with transitional epithelium and contains the ostia of *prostatic* and *ejaculatory ducts*. In the membranous urethra the epithelium changes to a *stratified columnar epithelium*. The main secretory duct of the *bulbo-urethral (Cowper's) glands* enter the bulbous urethra. Squamous epithelium continuous with that of the glans penis lines the distal penile urethra.

In the female urethra there is a similar transition from urothelial to stratified columnar epithelium and then to squamous epithelium near the external meatus. Mucous glands are present in the urethral wall.

Normal epithelial variants

Epithelial variants in the bladder are common but are important to the pathologist because they can resemble some disease processes and may sometimes be incorrectly attributed to disease. Weiner *et al.* (1979) studied 100 grossly normal bladders obtained at autopsy. *Brunn's nests* were found in 90, *cystitis cystica* in 60, and *squamous metaplasia* in 22.

Brunn's nests are nests of small urothelial cells lying in the lamina propria adjacent to or in continuity with the overlying epithelium. Occasionally they may show squamous metaplasia and appear as squamous islands in the lamina propria. They probably originate from buds of urothelium growing down into the lamina propria.

Cystisis cystica refers to cystic structures of varying sizes in the lamina propria, often in continuity with the urothelium or adjacent to a Brunn's nest. The cysts are lined by simple or stratified epithelium, the stratified type resembles a Brunn's nest with a central lumen (Fig. 19.68). The single layered type, which is a form of glandular metaplasia, may contain mucoussecreting cells (*cystitis cystica glandularis*). Large cysts or large areas of glandular metaplasia were not seen in the normals and these should be considered abnormal.

Squamous metaplasia consists of partial or complete replacement of the epithelium by mature squamous epithelium. This exists in two forms: the *non-keratinizing form* resembles vaginal epithelium and is commonly found in the trigonal region of mature and post-menopausal women (Fig. 19.69). The other form, *keratinizing squamous metaplasia*, is not seen in bladders without disease and is associated with chronic inflammation, lithiasis, diverticuli, or schistosomiasis.

19.13.2   Congenital lesions

The embryonic development of the urinary tract involves the co-ordinated growth of several different embryonic structures, including the *mesonephron*, the *cloacal membrane*, the *urorectal septum*, and *adjacent mesoderm*. Disorders of this growth produce a wide range of congenital abnormalities. Very few are genetic-

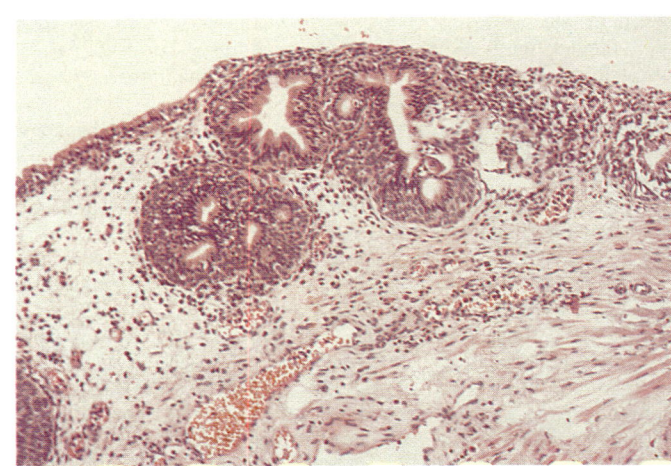

Fig. 19.68 Cystitis cystica in a bladder with no other abnormality.

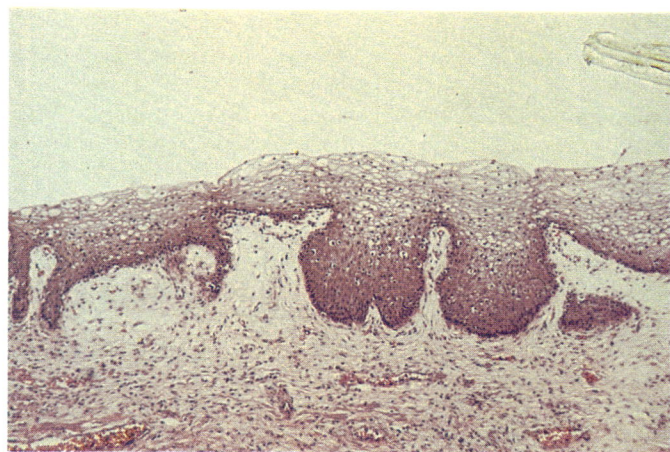

Fig. 19.69 Squamous metaplasia, non-keratinizing, from the trigone of a woman aged 24 years.

ally determined, although severe urinary-tract abnormalities are sometimes associated with major chromosomal abnormalities. Any congenital urinary-tract obstruction may be responsible for *coexistent renal dyplasia*. Many abnormalities are minor and may be asymptomatic for many years, only coming to light as an incidental finding on radiology, at autopsy, or when a predisposition to urinary tract infection is noted.

Renal pelvis and ureters

Idiopathic pelviureteric junction obstruction

This is a relatively uncommon disorder where there is obstruction to the flow of urine at the pelviureteric junction (PUJ) but no intrinsic lesion can be identified. It is more common in males and often presents in childhood, up to 30 per cent of cases are bilateral. Familial cases have been reported. The condition results in *hydronephrosis* of the affected side. Some cases may have an anatomical explanation: they may be due to an *aberrant renal vessel* compressing the renal pelvis, or *a high insertion of the ureter into the pelvis* may cause kinking of the ureter at this site. In the majority of cases no such physical obstruction can be identified and obstruction has been assumed to be due to a failure of peristalsis. Abnormalities of the pelviureteric muscle have been seen in some cases, although it is not known if this is the cause of the obstruction or the result of it.

Ureteral duplication

Ureteral duplication is often found as an incidental radiological or autopsy finding. A wide variety of variations on the theme of duplication are described and the American Pediatric Association has made a recent attempt to standardize the confusing terminology of these abnormalities (Glassberg *et al.* 1984). The defects seen range from a *bifid renal pelvis* to *complete duplex systems*. Duplex systems have either a normal and a supernumerary kidney or a single kidney with two pelvises (*duplex kidney*) draining into the bladder via completely separate ureters; the ureter draining the upper part of the renal mass usually enters the bladder below the normal ureteric orifices on the trigone. Incomplete duplications lead to *Y-shaped ureters* or *ureteric diverticula*. Ureters draining into the bladder via a ureteric orifice at an abnormal site are susceptible to reflux. When this occurs only the part of the kidney drained by the abnormal system would be affected by reflux nephropathy. Ureters, duplicated or solitary, may rarely drain into other organs, for example urethra, vagina, or seminal vesicles. *Renal dysplasia* and *infection* are common complications of these ectopic ureters.

Bladder

Extrophy

Although rare, with an incidence of 1 per 20 000 live births, *extrophy of the urinary bladder* is a serious condition responsible for considerable morbidity and mortality in affected individuals. Extrophy results from the failure of growth of the mesoderm into the cloacal membrane and the consequent persistence of this membrane on the anterior abdominal wall. With increasing fetal growth the membrane ruptures and the bladder beneath everts and lies on the anterior abdominal wall with the urothelium exposed. In *large superior defects* the bladder mucosa is exposed through a defect in the anterior abdominal wall and, in addition, the urethra is usually open and runs, in the male, along the top of the penis, in the female the clitoris is usually bifid and the open urethra runs between the two halves. With severe defects there is usually failure of fusion of the symphysis pubis and associated pelvic abnormalities. Small inferior defects in the male may lead to degrees of *epispadias* alone.

After birth the exposed extrophic bladder epithelium becomes inflamed as a result of trauma, infection, and of cellular damage caused by an inappropriate environment. Inflammation is often so severe that the mucosa comes to resemble granulation tissue. Histologically there is ulceration, inflammation, and both squamous and glandular metaplasia. *Glandular metaplasia* that is histologically similar to *colonic epithelium* can cover a large part of the exposed bladder muscosa.

The most severe early consequence of extrophy is ascending urinary tract infection, and early closure or urinary diversion prevents the inevitable renal damage that occurs with this complication. The major serious late complication of untreated bladder extrophy is *adenocarcinoma* that originates from the metaplastic glandular epithelium. This occurs in 5–15 per cent of untreated cases and is unusual before 20 years of age.

Persistent urachus

The urachus is an embryonic structure connecting the urogenital sinus to the allantois via the umbilicus. Embryonic remnants of the urachus lie in a line along the anterior abdominal wall from the umbilicus to the dome of the bladder. Careful dissection and microscopic examination reveals some persistent tubular structures in about a half of all adults at autopsy. These are themselves of little significance. The two main disorders are the *persistence of the lumen* and the development of *neoplasia in urachial remnants*.

Persistence of the complete urachus leads to drainage of urine from the bladder to the umbilicus. Urinary-tract infection commonly complicates this abnormality. Persistence with closure at one end or the other results in a *urachal pouch* at the umbilicus or a *urachal diverticulum* at the dome of the bladder. Closure at each end but persistence of a large part of the lumen results in a potential space which may come to clinical attention as a *urachal cyst* if secretions accumulate.

Neoplasia in urachal remnants is rare (less than 1 per cent of bladder carcinomas are thought to be of urachal origin) and usually develops in remnants that have been clinically silent. This suggests that the remnants present in most individuals present a very low risk of becoming malignant. Carcinomas may occur at any site along the urachal tract, but tumours at the umbilicus and the dome of the bladder are more common than tumours at intermediate sites. About 90 per cent are adenocarcinomas and these are assumed to originate from the columnar metaplasia present in many urachal remnants (Fig. 19.70).

When the tumour develops in the anterior abdominal wall or umbilicus, the diagnosis of urachal origin is rarely in doubt, but when the tumours arise in the dome of the bladder the distinction from a primary vesical neoplasm may not be so straightforward, as urachal tumours are histologically indistinguishable from other adenocarcinomas of the bladder. The distinction is important as urachal carcinomas tend to spread along the urachal tract, so the surgical approach is to remove the tract along with the dome of the bladder. Criteria proposed to determine whether a tumour is of urachal origin include:

1. the tumour site at the dome or on the anterior wall of the bladder;

2. the presence of an associated urachal remnant; and

3. the absence of any abnormality of the urothelial mucosa from which an adenocarcinoma could have developed.

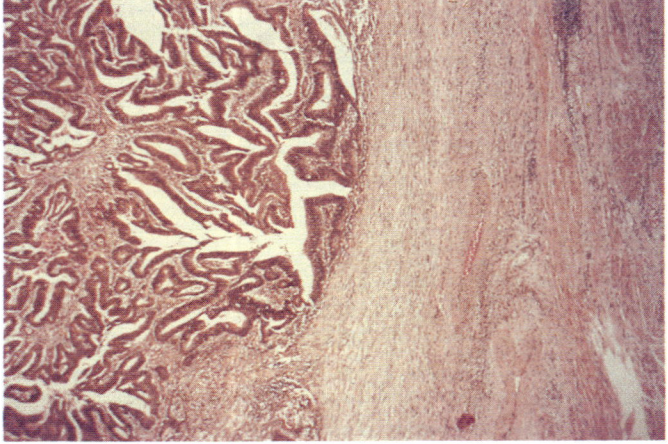

Fig. 19.70 Adenocarcinoma of the urachus, from a man aged 40 years; the tumour is present deep in the bladder wall at the dome. Muscle bundles (right) separate the tumour (left) from the urothelium.

Others

Ureteral and urethral valves are structures that obstruct the normal flow of urine but not retrograde flow. Most are due to redundant mucosa forming a flap within the lumen. They usually present early in life with urinary tract obstruction and its complications.

Congenital bladder diverticula are rare lesions due to a defect in the detrusor muscle alongside the ureteric orifice. Bladder mucosa forced through the defect by the intravesical pressure forms a para-ureteric diverticulum. This is usually associated with severe vesicoureteric reflux.

Ureterocoeles are cystic dilations of the intravesical ureteral segment; they form cystic ballooning structures bulging into the bladder and are most commonly associated with ureteric duplication and ectopic ureteric orifices.

19.13.3   Inflammatory disorders

Infective cystitis

Urinary-tract infection is common; about 20–30 per cent of all women will suffer at some time during their lives. The organisms are usually coliforms that inhabit the bowel or the perineal area; *Escherichia coli*, *Proteus*, and *Klebsiella* are the most common. The main predisposing factors and the more serious renal consequences are discussed with pyelonephritis (Section 19.5.1). A symptomatic urinary-tract infection with dysuria, frequency, and urgency is usually associated with a *bacterial colony count of more than* 10^5 *per ml of urine*. In an attack of acute cystitis the bladder mucosa is oedematous, shows vascular congestion, and incorporates an infiltrate of neutrophil polymorphs. In more severe infection there may be mucosal ulceration with inflammation extending into the muscularis. On recovery the histological changes usually resolve but a mild chronic inflammatory infiltrate, consisting mainly of lymphocytes, may persist for some time. Persistent or repeated infections may lead to *follicular cystitis* while severe infections in some predisposed individuals may cause *emphysematous or gangrenous cystitis*. Continued chronic inflammation may also lead to *metaplasias of the bladder epithelium*.

Follicular cystitis

The term 'follicular cystitis' describes the presence of *lymphoid follicles with germinal centres* in the lamina propria; this is usually associated with chronic inflammation of the lamina propria. Similar changes can also occur elsewhere in the urinary tract. Grossly, the mucosa is granular and thickened and there may be some associated fibrosis of the muscularis, leading to a reduction in the bladder volume. The condition usually results from chronic or repeated infection, although occasionally lymphoid follicles can be found without other evidence of inflammation.

Emphysematous cystitis

Emphysematous cystitis is characterized by the presence of *gas bubbles* in the lamina propria. The gas is produced by bacteria, usually *E. coli* or *Enterobacter aerogenes*. Microscopically the gas bubbles are identified as spaces in the lamina propria surrounded by foreign body giant cells. There is commonly acute inflammation in the adjacent tissues. The condition is most frequently seen in the elderly and debilitated and in diabetics, when the gas-forming bacteria invade the bladder wall.

Gangrenous cystitis

Infarction of the mucosa and part of the muscle of the bladder wall may occur in a severe infection when the organisms invade the bladder wall and when the associated inflammatory oedema compromises blood flow. Other prejudicial factors are almost always present and include *extrinsic pressure* (gravid uterus, obstructed labour, impacted faeces), *intrinsic pressure* (bladder outflow obstruction), and a generally *compromised circulation* (severe altherosclerosis of the abdominal aorta, shock). The mucosa slough off and this, together with the fibrinous exudate, may give it a *membranous or diptheroid appearance*. The necrosis may allow the spread of infection to perivesical tissues. This severe cystitis was probably more common before antibiotic therapy was available and is now mostly seen in elderly patients. There is a high mortality, but it is unclear whether this is primarily due to the cystitis or the predisposing condition.

Tuberculosis and granulomatous cystitis

Urinary-tract TB is now rare in the developed world. The ureter and bladder are infected by seeding from a *post-primary focus in the kidney*. The initial lesion in the ureter is usually at the pelviureteric junction. In the bladder the ureteric orifice and trigone are usually involved.

Histologically, *classical caseous granulomas* are present in the lamina propria, these discharge into the lumen to produce sharply demarcated ulcers. As the disease advances there is often considerable scarring, which is responsible for ureteric stenosis with *obstructive uropathy* or *bladder contraction*, leading to disabling frequency of micturition. Occasionally fibrosis of the bladder may hold the ureteric orifice open leading to vesicoureteric reflux.

Other forms of granulomatous cystitis are rare: granulomas can sometimes be seen after urinary-tract instrumentation, and iatrogenic granulomas are present in the lamina propria following treatment of carcinoma *in situ* of the bladder with *intravesical BCG*.

Schistosomal cystitis

Schistosoma haematobium causes urinary bilharzia. The live adults in veins do not provoke an inflammatory response, but the eggs do. The eggs tend to be deposited and accumulate in discrete sites; they are usually most numerous in the bladder, the resulting inflammation producing red, fleshy masses. Histologically, there is a diffuse inflammatory reaction with numerous eosinophils and neutrophils associated with discrete granulomas of epithelioid and giant cells around the eggs. *The only pathognomonic feature is the presence of eggs.* The lesions heal by fibrosis, the eggs may become mineralized and, when they are numerous, this produces a characteristic radiological appearance. *Obstructive uropathy* due to fibrosis of the bladder can occur; however, mid-ureteric obstruction is usually due to an acute lesion and this is reversible with treatment. In long-standing infection the transitional epithelium can undergo metaplasia to intestinal-type epithelium or to keratinizing squamous epithelium. The development of carcinoma is a recognized late complication, although the relative risk is unknown. About half the tumours are squamous carcinomas, usually well differentiated and keratinizing, about 10 per cent are adenocarcinomas, and the remainder are transitional or mixed type.

Non-infective inflammation and miscellaneous conditions
Non-infective painful bladder disease

The majority of individuals who have frequency and dysuria have a bacterial cystitis. If bacterial infection cannot be identified, and if symptoms persist, cystoscopy is usually carried out to determine the cause. In most cases no cause is found and the condition is self limiting. A few patients will have a specific cause, such as urinary stone or tumour, while the remainder will have an idiopathic inflammatory disease of the bladder, such as interstitial cystitis or eosinophilic cystitis.

Interstitial cystitis This rare condition occurs typically in middle-aged and elderly women who present with suprapubic pain, frequency, nocturia, and urgency, usually of many months', if not years', duration and who have repeatedly had negative urine cultures. Cystoscopic appearances are said to be characteristic with small scars or ulcers, usually multiple, scattered over the bladder mucosa. When the bladder is distended these rupture and bleed. In severe or late disease there may be a large ulcer (*Hunner's ulcer*) with associated fibrosis of the bladder wall, leading to a decrease in the bladder volume. Histologically, all cases show focal ulceration with local acute inflammation, together with diffuse chronic inflammation affecting the whole of the bladder and the full thickness of the bladder wall. The infiltrate consists predominantly of lymphocytes with variable numbers of plasma cells, neutrophils, and eosinophils. Mast cells are usually prominent, particularly within the muscle. The inflammation in the muscle is sometimes associated with focal necrosis of muscle cells and partial or complete fibrosis of muscle bundles. It is this replacement of the muscle by fibrosis that leads to the contraction of the bladder seen in advanced disease. The aetiology of the condition is unknown (Fall *et al.* 1987).

Eosinophilic cystitis The term 'eosinophilic cystitis' describes an idiopathic inflammation of the bladder in which the eosinophil polymorph is a prominent cell in the inflammatory exudate. The condition occurs in two clinical settings: in the one there is evidence *of allergy*; in the other there is previous *bladder injury or urinary obstruction*. In the allergic type the patient is usually young or middle-aged, has a history of allergic phenomenon, and often has a blood eosinophilia (Hellstrom *et al.* 1979). In the bladder injury type, the patient is usually an elderly male with a history of prostatic disease, transurethral resection, or other bladder trauma. In both types the cystitis presents as sudden onset of severe dysuria, frequency, and sometimes haematuria; remission may be followed by episodic recurrence. At cysto-scopy during an episode the whole bladder is involved with gross mucosal oedema, producing masses of oedematous folds and polyps. Characteristic microscopic features may only be present during an episode and consist of mucosal oedema and a mixed inflammatory infiltrate in which eosinophils are promi-nent. The inflammation extends into muscle, and focal muscle necrosis and fibrosis may be seen. In prolonged disease, fibrosis of the detrusor may be prominent and the bladder volume con-sequently reduced. The more severe and advanced disease resembles interstitial cystitis, which may also show an inflitrate of eosinophils.

Metaplasias and related phenomenon

Endometriosis The bladder is one of the commoner extragenital sites for endometriosis. The deposits are commonly found on the serosa, but are more rarely found in the muscle or mucosa of the ureters or bladder. Urinary obstruction has been recorded due to endometriosis of the ureter; however, the most common symptom of urinary endometriosis is haematuria. Histologic-ally, the appearances are usually typical, with glands within the endometrial stroma, but diagnostic problems can occur if there is extensive haemorrhage into the endometriotic cyst. About 50 per cent of cases of urinary endometriosis have a history of pelvic surgery or injury and are probably due to implantation.

Squamous metaplasia Although small areas of non-keratinizing squamous metaplasia on the trigone of women is a normal finding, extensive squamous metaplasia, particularly of the keratinizing type, usually occurs as a response to chronic inflammation. It occurs most commonly in association with cal-culi, especially in the renal pelvis and in bladder diverticula; it is also seen in extrophy of the bladder and in chronic schistosome infestation. Keratinous debris produced by squamous meta-plasia may obstruct the ureter or be passed as masses in the urine. This form of squamous metaplasia is associated with an increased risk of subsequent squamous cell carcinoma (Hertle and Androulakakis 1982).

Glandular metaplasia Small foci of cystitis cystica are found in many normal bladders. In the presence of chronic inflammation such glandular metaplasia becomes more common and more extensive. It is particularly extensive in bladder extrophy. The metaplasia arises from downgrowths of the urothelium (Brunn's nests) which undergo columnar change (*cystitis cystica*) and then may become populated with goblet cells (cyst-itis cystica glandularis) (Fig. 19.71). In advanced cases this can resemble colonic epithelium. Glandular metaplasia causes problems in two ways: first some glands may fill with secretions and distend to produce a space-occupying lesion which can ob-struct the ureter (*ureteritis cystica*) (Fig. 19.72). Secondly, any large area of the colonic type of metaplasia appears to confer a high risk of development of adenocarcinoma (Bullock *et al.* 1987).

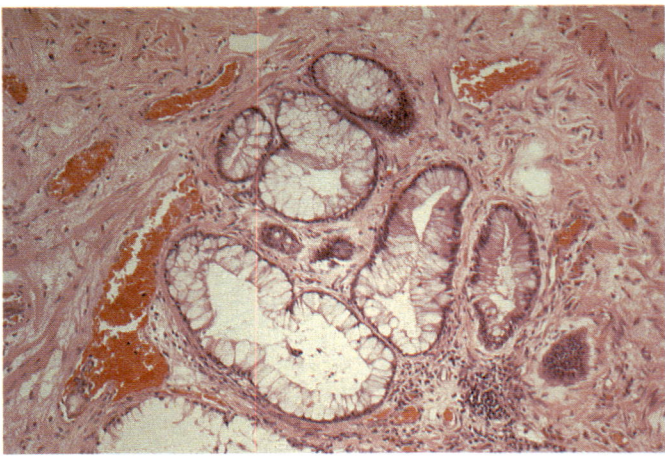

Fig. 19.71 Glandular metaplasia found on the lateral wall of the bladder of a man aged 35 years. The numerous goblet cells give an appearance very much like that of colonic mucosa.

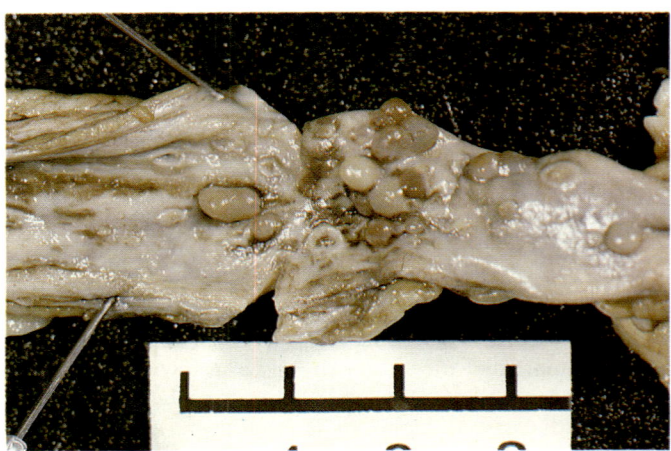

Fig. 19.72 Ureteritis cystica; the cysts project into the lumen (this was an autopsy finding in the ureter and was associated with an ipsilateral hydronephrosis).

Iatrogenic cystitis

Catheter cystitis An indwelling urinary catheter always pro-duces some degree of inflammation of the bladder. Usually this is limited to mild mucosal congestion, but prolonged catheter-ization can lead to *polypoid* or *papillary cystitis*, and the occa-sional allergic reactions to the catheter may be responsible for *eosinophilic cystitis*.

Radiation cystitis. Some degree of radiation cystitis always fol-lows therapeutic radiation for bladder tumours, and also follows radiation to other organs if part of the bladder is included in the field. Radiation injures both the epithelium directly and blood vessels of the bladder wall. In *acute radiation cystitis* there is mucosal ulceration with cytological atypia of the surviving epithelium. Vessels in the lamina propria show endothelial hy-perplasia, fibrinoid necrosis, and focal thrombosis. Bizarre giant cells can usually be seen in the connective tissue (Fig. 19.73). In *a later stage*, larger vessels show gross intimal thickening with loose mucoid connective tissue or fibrosis, leading to luminal occlusion. The associated ulceration, muscle atrophy, and fibrosis is largely due to ischaemia. Radiation also reduces the regenerative potential of the epithelium, leaving it slow to heal and susceptible to infection. A dangerous complication of both early and late radiation cystitis is severe haemorrhage from the ulcerated surface and disordered vasculature.

Drug-induced cystitis *Cyclophosphamide*, an alkylating agent, is associated with a severe cystitis in a proportion of patients treated. The drug and its metabolites are excreted in the urine and have a direct toxic effect on the mucosa. Histologically, there is mucosal oedema and ulceration with haemorrhage into the lamina propria. Additionally, patients with cystitis, and some receiving the drug who do not have cystitis, show cytological atypia of the transitional epithelium that can be confused with carcinoma *in situ*. The cyclophosphamide-induced change usually regresses after treatment is ceased. A late effect of previous cyclophosphamide treatment is the development of transitional cell carcinomas.

Some drugs can rarely be associated with an allergic reaction in the bladder. The pathological features are usually those of eosinophilic cystitis.

Malakoplakia

Malakoplakia is a granulomatous condition of uncertain aetiology that can affect many body tissues but is most commonly found in the urinary tract, and particularly the bladder (Stanton and Maxted 1981; McClure 1983). It occurs at all ages, with a peak incidence of about 50 years of age, and there is, for bladder disease at least, a 4 : 1 female preponderance. The initial clinical features are usually non-specific but usually include a non-specific chronic cystitis. Concurrent chronic infection, malignancy, or a history of immunosuppression is common, and persistent urinary tract infection is almost always found.

Macroscopically, there are soft yellow–brown plaques in the urothelial mucosa, often with central ulceration. With advancing disease these enlarge to become confluent and can spread as tumour-like masses to involve and destroy adjacent tissues. Histologically, the plaques are characterized by sheets of large histiocytic cells with abundant granular cytoplasm (*von Hansemann cells*) associated with numerous intra- and extracellular laminated and calcified spherules measuring 5–10 μm in diameter (*Michaelis–Gutmann bodies*) (Fig. 19.74). The presence of Michaelis–Gutmann bodies is considered pathognomonic of the condition. In prolonged disease there may be fibrosis and healing, leading to scars. Following surgical excision there is a high rate of recurrence; this is a particular problem in the immunosuppressed, and these patients have a high mortality. The precise nature of the condition is unknown. Urinary-tract infection is obviously involved: over 95 per cent of patients have an infection with *E. coli*; there is good evidence that the Michaelis–Gutmann bodies are *mineralized phagolysosomes*, and other phagolysosomes in the von Hansemann cells contain partly degraded bacteria. In addition, the disease progresses if the infection is uncontrolled and may partially regress if the infection is eliminated. However, *E. coli* and other organisms found are common pathogens whereas malakoplakia is a rare condition. Current theories have centred on the host response; one suggestion is that patients with malakoplakia have an acquired defect of macrophage function. This is supported by evidence that macrophages from patients with malakoplakia exhibit normal phagocytosis but a reduced capacity to kill *E. coli*. The cause of the defect is not known.

Amyloidosis

Amyloid involvement of the bladder is rare; it occurs most commonly as an isolated finding, although it has been recorded with systemic amyloid. Typically, patients present with severe haematuria. Macroscopically, nodules are present in the mucosa, these ulcerate and bleed and can be mistaken for

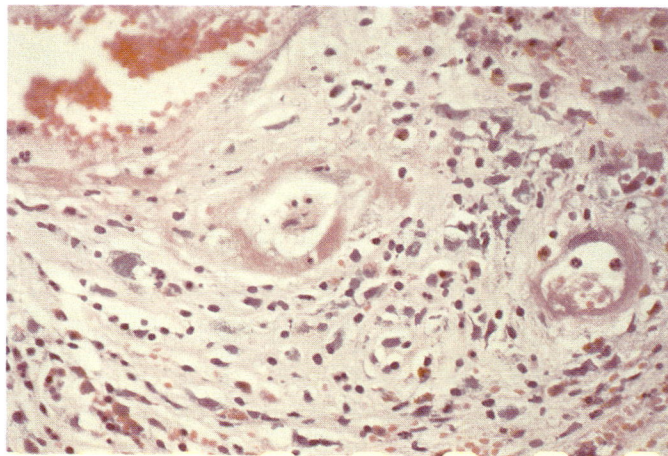

Fig. 19.73 Radiation cystitis; the blood-vessel shows fibrinoid necrosis of its wall, while giant fibroblasts are present in the connective tissue. These changes were associated with severe ulceration.

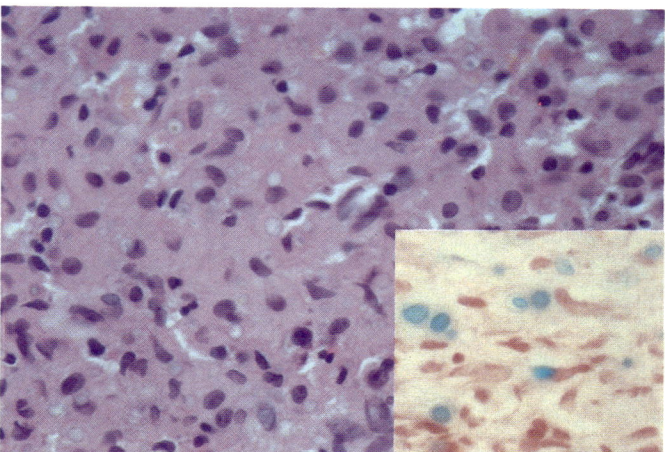

Fig. 19.74 Malakoplakia. The von Hansemann cells have granular eosinophilic cytoplasm. (H & E.) Inset: Michaelis–Gutmann bodies are laminated and contain iron. (Blue-staining with Pearls Prussian blue).

tumours. Microscopically, amyloid is present in the lamina propria, muscularis, and around blood vessels.

Papillary and polypoid cystitis

This form of cystitis is characterized by inflammation, vascular congestion, and oedema of the lamina propria, which throws up the transitional mucosa into papillary, polypoid, or bullous lesions protruding into the bladder lumen. Widespread papillary cystitis is most commonly seen following *prolonged insertion of a urinary catheter*. Similar lesions can also be found after other instrumentation of the urinary tract, particularly *transurethral prostatic resection,* and may rarely be found without previous instrumentation. Catheter-associated disease usually regresses spontaneously following removal of the catheter (Ekeuland *et al.* 1983). The main clinical significance of the lesions is that they can be mistaken for papillary carcinoma, both cystoscopically and histologically. The main distinguishing features are the *abundant inflamed fibrous stroma* in the polyps, the presence *of focal ulceration* and *haemorrhage*, and the *absence of significant epithelial dysplasia* (Fig. 19.75). (Young 1988).

Nephrogenic adenoma

These lesions are found as single or multiple discrete nodules (or more rarely as a diffuse infiltration of the bladder wall). Small lesions may not be uncommon, but lesions more than a few millimetres in diameter are distinctly rare. Histologically, there are *numerous tubular structures* within the lamina propria that are made up of regular flat or cuboidal cells. The overlying surface epithelium usually consists of similar cells, and is often thrown up into papillary fronds. An associated inflammatory infiltrate is common (Fig. 19.76). The histogenesis of the lesion is unknown, but most cases have been described in a background of chronic inflammation so the majority are believed to represent *a reactive metaplasia* rather than a neoplastic process (Gonzalez 1988). The condition can recur but true malignant change has never been reported.

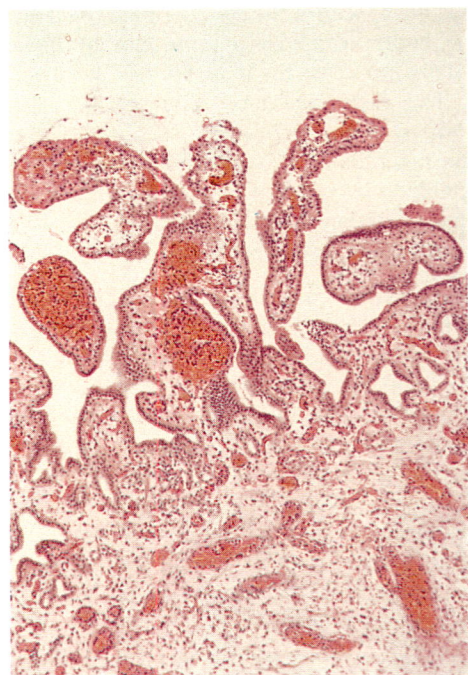

Fig. 19.76 Nephrogenic adenoma. Single-layered tubules in the lamina propria are associated with a papillary surface with flat cuboidal epithelium. Inflammatory cells and dilated blood-vessels are present in the lamina propria.

Others

Fibro-epithelial polyps are polyps of oedematous connective tissue covered with urothelium and are occasionally found in the renal pelvis, ureter, or urethra, where they sometimes cause obstruction. They are most common in the 10–30 year age-group and are thought to be hamartomatous.

Rarely, sarcoma-like *spindle-cell nodules* are found in the urogenital tract following surgery, or occasionally spontaneously. They are thought to be a reactive phenomenon, possibly related to proliferative fasciitis (Nochomovitz and Orestein 1985; Young and Scully 1987).

19.13.4 Urinary-tract obstruction

Causes of urinary-tract obstruction

By far the most common cause of urinary-tract obstruction is enlargement of the prostate in men. Other important causes and the typical sites at which they occur are listed in Table 19.12.

Idiopathic retroperitoneal fibrosis

The syndrome of idiopathic retroperitoneal fibrosis (RPF) consists of progressive fibrosis of the retroperitoneal tissues, involving the ureters and great vessels and causing, initially, back and flank pain and, eventually, bilateral ureteric obstruction. Most cases are idiopathic but *methysergide*—a drug used for

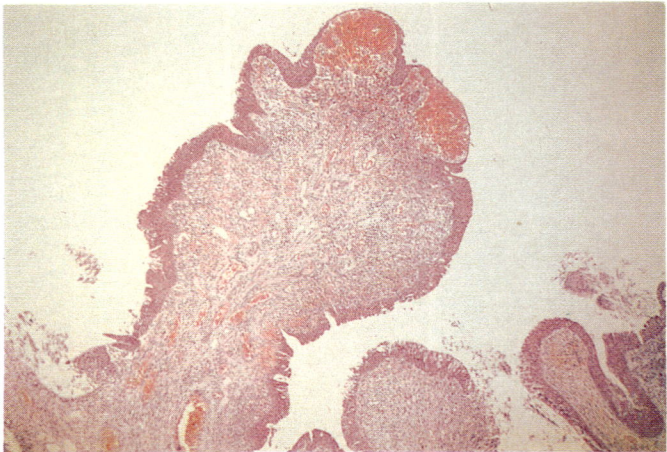

Fig. 19.75 Papillary cystitis; broad-based papilla with an inflamed connective tissue core and dilated blood-vessels (from a patient who had a transurethral resection of the prostate).

Table 19.12 The causes of urinary-tract obstruction

Site	Cause
Pelviureteric junction (PUJ)	Idiopathic PUJ obstruction, calculus, tumour (TCC), TB
Mid-ureter	Calculus, tumour (TCC or secondary), ureteritis cystica, idiopathic retroperitoneal fibrosis
Lower ureter	Calculus, tumour (TCC bladder and SCC of cervix)
Bladder outlet and urethra	Prostate enlargement, stricture, congenital valves, carcinoma, 'functional' obstruction in neurogenic bladder, phimosis

migraine—can cause an apparently identical syndrome. The fibrosis starts around the aorta then spreads laterally to involve the ureters. Histologically, the lesion tends to be zoned: there is an advancing front at the periphery of the lesion, consisting of tissue with a severe chronic inflammatory infiltrate in which lymphocytes predominate; in the central, older, zone mature scar tissue is more prominent. The ureteric obstruction is due to entrapment of the ureters in the fibrotic process; the ureters usually remain patent but peristalsis is inhibited. As the fibrous tissue matures it contracts, drawing the ureters medially.

The aetiology of the condition is not known. In some cases a heavy inflammatory infiltrate is focused on veins, suggesting *a vasculitic process*. Patients with RPF have a higher than expected incidence of the human leucocyte antigen (HLA) B27 and some cases are associated with other idiopathic fibrosing conditions, especially *Reidel's thyroiditis*. The condition is consistently centred on the aorta, which usually shows either *aortitis* or *severe atherosclerosis*, and it is believed that many cases are due to an immune reaction to the extrusion of lipid material, of atheromatous origin, into the aortic intima (Bullock 1988).

Results of urinary-tract obstruction

The results of urinary-tract obstruction are *hydronephrosis*, *hydroureter*, *bladder hypertrophy*, and *diverticula*. The extent and severity of these lesions can largely be predicted from a number of independent factors related to the site and mode of obstruction rather than the specific cause.

Site

Obviously only the parts of the tract proximal to the obstruction show the effects. In unilateral ureteric or PUJ obstruction when the contralateral kidney functions normally, a much more severe hydronephrosis can develop than in bilateral obstruction when declining renal function will usually draw attention to the obstruction.

Rate and severity

In *acute complete obstruction* the renal pelvis distends with urine until the pressure prevents any further net urine production. The kidney may remain morphologically normal for some time despite the complete anuria. In life the distended pelvis can be recognized by ultrasonography. Chronic or intermittent obstruction or unilateral obstruction allows time for hydronephrotic changes to develop in the kidney.

Associated pathology

If obstruction is complicated by urinary-tract infection, this can be particularly severe and can dominate the clinical picture, causing rapid destruction of renal tissue by suppuration to form a *pyonephrosis*. The infection can spread outside the kidney to form a *perinephric abscess*, or may act as a source of *septicaemia*. *Calculi* are also prone to form in partial urinary obstruction; a common combination is chronic upper urinary-tract infection associated with a branching 'staghorn' calculus. This fills the calyces of a hydronephrotic kidney, which will also show the changes of *pyelonephritis* (Fig. 19.77).

Hydronephrosis

The morphological features of hydronephrosis form a continuous spectrum from minor changes of blunting of the renal papillae to severe hydronephrosis where the kidney has been converted into a multiseptate sack with paper-thin walls. In an acutely obstructed kidney there are usually no distinctive macroscopic or microscopic features. As obstruction persists the first morphological changes occur in the tips of the renal papillae, where there is tubular loss and an increase in the amount of interstitial hyaline material. With increasing time the atrophy of the papillae becomes more severe and they become progressively more flattened and fibrosed. This is associated with cortical thinning, due to subcapsular glomerular sclerosis and tubular atrophy, which is probably caused by ischaemia; arteries, even in children with no history of hypertension, show intimal hyperplasia and elastic reduplication. As cortical atrophy progresses, atrophic tubules become filled with proteinaceous casts, giving a striking histological appearance known as *thyroidization*. By this stage there is usually considerable interstitial fibrous tissue and eventually, in end-stage hydronephrosis, the

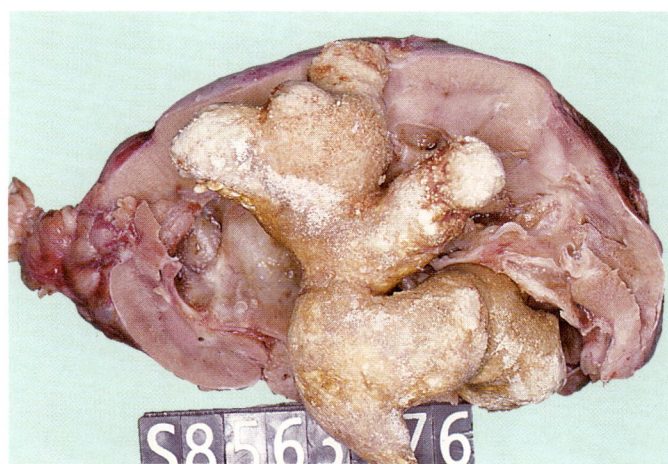

Fig. 19.77 A large staghorn calculus occupying the renal pelvis and calyces; the kidney shows mild hydronephrotic changes.

renal parenchyma becomes a paper-thin rind of fibrous tissue (Fig. 19.78). The renal changes are usually accompanied by expansion of the renal pelvis. Considerable recovery of renal function can occur following the relief of obstruction provided that there is sufficient residual renal parenchyma; unfortunately in many cases, where there is considerable renal loss, function will continue to deteriorate, leading to chronic renal failure. This progressive deterioration is thought to be due to hyperfiltration damaging the surviving glomeruli.

Hydroureter

The ureter usually dilates proximal to an obstruction. In bladder outflow obstruction the ureter and the upper tract is usually partially protected by competence of the valvular mechanism at the ureteric orifices. In severe obstruction this fails, vesico-ureteric reflux develops, and the ureters dilate. The most impressive ureteric dilation occurs in congenital obstruction or reflux, although occasionally such a *megaureter* may be found without evidence of obstruction.

Bladder

Partial bladder outflow obstruction leads initially to an increase in the pressure required for micturition, the bladder compensates for this by hypertrophy of the smooth muscle of the detrusor, leading to a substantial thickening of the bladder wall. In long-standing obstruction there is also an increase in fibrous tissue, both between and within muscle bundles. The broad inner muscular bands of the detrusor are stretched across the inner surface of the bladder, giving it a grossly trabeculated appearance and leaving it susceptible to the formation of diverticula (Fig. 19.79). A chronically obstructed bladder usually fails to expel its full urine volume during micturition. The consequent stasis of the residual volume leads to an increased risk of calculi and infection.

Bladder diverticulum

Acquired bladder diverticula are *pulsion diverticula* due to the

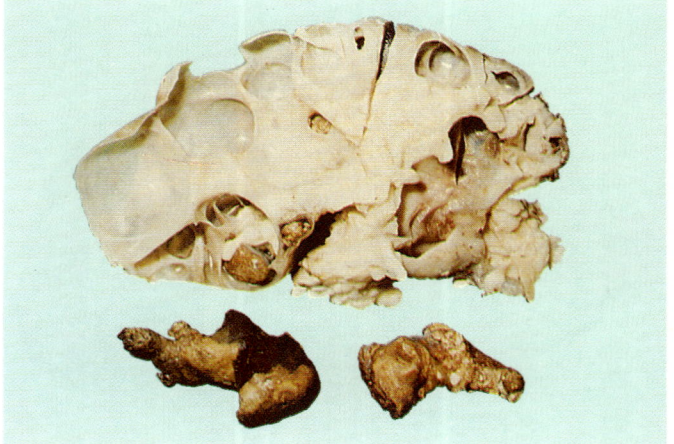

Fig. 19.78 End-stage hydronephrosis; the kidney is reduced to a rind of fibrous tissue; the calculus that obstructed the kidney is present in the pelvis.

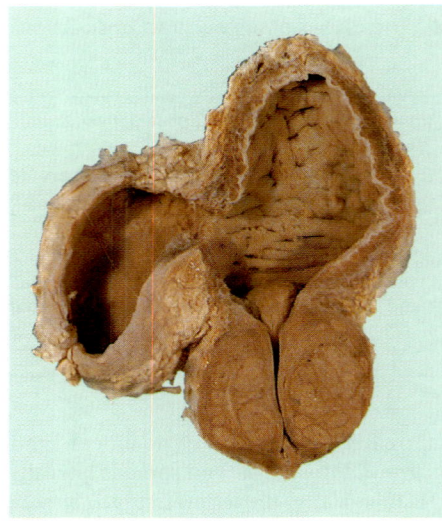

Fig. 19.79 Trabeculated bladder with a thick wall and a diverticulum with a thin wall. Prostatic enlargement is also present.

increased urinary pressure and bladder abnormalities in chronic obstruction. Most arise above and lateral to the ureteric orifices, and originate from an increase in the size of an indentation or sacculation between two adjacent bladder trabeculae. As the indendation enlarges it stretches and displaces more of the deeper layers of the muscularis, reducing further resistance to its formation. Most diverticula are over 5 cm in diameter and have a narrow orifice connecting them to the bladder. As expected, the wall is much thinner than that of the bladder and, while it contains little muscle, there is often a chronic inflammatory infiltrate and fibrosis. Diverticula predispose to calculi and infection but, more seriously, up to 7 per cent may be complicated by epithelial tumours. Most are infiltrative transitional cell carcinomas but squamous carcinomas associated with metaplasia are also common. These tumours will have often spread beyond the thin diverticular wall at diagnosis, so the prognosis is usually poor.

19.13.5   Tumours

The urinary tract can be generally treated as a single entity as far as tumours are concerned. Most tumours are epithelial and originate from neoplastic change in the transitional mucosa. This epithelium has a relatively uniform structure and a similar environment along the urinary tract so the tumours that are found differ little from site to site. Transitional cell carcinoma of the bladder is the most common and important tumour of the urinary tract. It is among the most common cancers in the developed world and provokes interest not only on account of its frequency but also because there is a known relationship with some chemical carcinogens and because even the tumours that do not invade at presentation have a propensity for multiple recurrences. The detection and treatment of these recurrences presents a considerable challenge to the urologist.

Classification

Several different classifications have been offered for bladder cancer (Mostofi *et al.* 1973; Koss 1975; Friedell *et al.* 1980); this probably represents differing interests rather than any fundamental disagreements about the nature of the tumours. The WHO classification is shown in Table 19.13, and this serves most purposes. The main criticism of the WHO system is that it makes little concession to the widely held belief that transitional cell papilloma, transitional cell carcinoma, its variants, and some anaplastic carcinomas make up a continuous spectrum of one type of urothelial neoplasia, nor does it separately define carcinoma *in situ*, which, when it is found without other tumours, presents its own special problem for diagnosis and treatment.

Table 19.13 WHO classification of bladder tumours

I. Epithelial tumours
  A. Transitional cell papilloma
  B. Transitional cell papilloma, inverted type
  C. Squamous papilloma
  D. Transitional cell carcinoma
  E. Transitional cell carcinoma with glandular and/or squamous elements
  F. Squamous cell carcinoma
  G. Adenocarcinoma
  H. Undifferentiated carcinoma
II. Non-epithelial tumours
  A. Benign: leiomyoma, neurofibroma, haemangioma
  B. Malignant: rhabdomyosarcoma, others

Incidence and epidemiology

In England and Wales bladder cancer accounts for about 4 per cent of male and 2 per cent of female cancer deaths. The incidence of the tumour is considerably greater than its mortality. In one registration area (Wales) the age-standardized annual registration rate per 100 000 for males and females was 20 and 7, whereas the equivalent mortality figures were 11 and 4, respectively. This confirms the clinical impression that only about half of those with bladder cancer go on to die of the disease. There are considerable national and regional variations. Some of these variations are due to known aetiological factors. For example, bladder cancer accounts of 11 per cent of cancer in Egypt, where *schistosomiasis* is common, and a high incidence of bladder cancer in Huddersfield, in the UK, was due to a high concentration of dye-manufacturing factories. In other situations the reasons are not clear, e.g. there is a significantly higher incidence in southern Japan than in the north. Like many other epithelial tumours, carcinoma of the bladder is rare below the age of 40 years and increases progressively in incidence after 50 years of age.

Aetiology and pathogenesis

The known aetiological factors related to the development of bladder cancer can be divided into those where chemical carcinogenesis is suspected and those where chronic inflammation and metaplasia are implicated as promoters.

Chemical carcinogenesis

Occupational bladder cancer Bladder cancer was one of the first tumours where a clear link between an exposure to a chemical and the development of a tumour was established (Lower 1982). A dye industry synthesizing dyes from *aromatic amines* started in Germany in the 1860s and was well established by the 1880s. In 1895 a cluster of cases of bladder cancer was reported in a dye factory and by the late 1930s a similar association had been reported in most industrial countries. Bladder cancers had been grown in dogs by feeding them *2-aminonaphthylamine* (β-naphthylamine), thus demonstrating the link between the chemical and the tumour beyond reasonable doubt. This animal model allowed testing of other compounds and also studies to elucidate the mechanism of carcinogenesis. The most potent carcinogens are *benzidine, 2-naphthylamine*, and *4-aminobiphenol*, although other *arylamines*, many of which are, or have been, used in the dye, rubber, or plastics industries, are also active. Exclusion of part of the bladder from the urinary flow by the formation of a pouch protects the epithelium from carcinogenesis, demonstrating that the carcinogens are transported to the bladder epithelium by the urine rather than the bloodstream (McDonald and Lund 1954). The arylamine acts as a *procarcinogen*: liver metabolism converts it to an active carcinogen and then conjugates it with glucuronic acid. The inactive soluble glucuronide is excreted in the urine, where the pH is favourable for glucuronidases to split the conjugate and release the carcinogen, which then acts directly on the epithelium. The major carcinogens are now prohibited or their use is strictly controlled; before control was established heavily exposed individuals had a relative risk of well over one hundred times compared with the unexposed population. With heavy exposure there is a mean latent period of 18 years between first exposure and tumour formation; in industries with lower exposure the latent period increases. The long latent period with low exposure implies that the occupational tumours seen now reflect working practices 30 or more years ago. Current occupational exposure is very much less and large epidemiological surveys are needed to identify groups at risk. Industries where some previous exposure is possible include chemical, rubber, and plastics manufacture and processing, cable manufacture, gas workers, rodent operators, patent fuel manufacture, laboratory work, sewage and water testing, hairdressing, and leather work. The identification of occupationally induced cancers, which depends on an accurate and complete occupational history, remains important, first to locate the source of the exposure to reduce risk to subsequent workers and secondly to ensure that the patient receives any due compensation (Wallace 1988).

Other environmental causes The problem of whether a low level of exposure of populations to carcinogens in the environment, from contamination of plastics, rubber, and dyes is responsible for any tumours, remains to be solved. However, *smoking* is clearly associated with an increased risk of bladder cancer with a relative risk variously estimated as between 1.5 and 4, and it is hence responsible for between 15 per cent and 50 per cent of all bladder cancers. The mechanism is probably similar to that of occupational bladder cancer as cigarette smoke contains 2-naphthylamine.

Cyclophosphamide is an alkylating agent used in the treatment of some malignancies and in severe auto-immune disease. It is excreted in an active form in the urine and may cause a severe acute cystitis. In the longer term, patients who have had high doses are at much increased risk of developing urothelial carcinoma. There is a relatively short latent period of from 5 to 10 years, which is similar to the latent period for exposure to large doses of industrial carcinogens. Even lower doses, used in non-malignant conditions, are now recognized as increasing the risk of urothelial cancer, although the latent period is longer. It has been suggested that these patients should be followed up to detect early bladder tumours.

Analgesics Patients with renal papillary necrosis due to analgesic abuse have a high risk of developing transitional cell carcinoma of the renal pelvis. Phenacetin has usually been implicated: this is an aromatic amide and one proposed mechanism is that it is metabolized into an active carcinogen. However, an increased risk of urothelial carcinoma has also been noted in patients with analgesic nephropathy due to other non-aromatic analgesics, e.g. paracetamol, so some part of the excess risk may be due to the promoting affect of regeneration and hyperplasia of urothelium over the damaged renal medulla as a consequence of the papillary necrosis.

Chronic inflammation

Schistosomiasis There is an increased incidence of bladder cancer in areas where infestation with *schistosoma haematobium* is common. The relative risk of cancer associated with infestation may not be very high, but it is sufficient to make bladder cancer the most common form of death due to malignancy in areas of Egypt where infestation rates are high. The mechanism of carcinogenesis is not known, but over 50 per cent of the tumours are squamous cancers arising in a background of keratinizing squamous metaplasia, and it is widely assumed that regeneration and metaplasia in response to chronic inflammation promotes carcinogenesis. Other factors may also be import-ant: many patients have associated urinary-tract infections and, in some, nitrate-reducing bacteria are responsible for the production of carcinogenic N-nitroso compounds in the urine.

Other aetiological factors

Thorotrast, used in retrograde pyelography, is associated with the development of renal pelvic tumours. Individuals with the *slow acetylator phenotype* have an increased risk of occupational bladder cancer, presumably because of their differing meta-bolism of carcinogens. *Bladder diverticula* also appear at high risk of developing neoplasia. Patients who have *ureterosigmoid-ostomies* are at high risk of tumours at the site of the anasto-mosis: the tumours are adenocarcinomas and it is disputed whether they are colonic or urothelial in origin. Malignant tumours have also been reported in patients with *caecocystoplas-ties*.

Morphological development of urothelial carcinoma

Experimental evidence and clinical observation suggest that invasive bladder cancer can develop through at least two differ-ent morphological pathways (Fig. 19.80). In the first, a *papillary lesion* develops in histologically normal, or hyperplastic, uro-thelium; this papillary tumour can remain non-invasive for a considerable time but eventually epithelial changes occur in some lesions, leading to invasion of the lamina propria. In the alternative pathway, carcinoma *in situ* develops in *flat uro-thelium*; invasion occurs directly from the base of the carcinoma *in situ* without the development of a papillary tumour. In each case, the progression fits well with current theories of the multistep development of cancer; each major morphological change may coincide with the acquisition of a new mutation, taking the neoplastic phenotype further towards that of fully fledged malignant tumour.

Benign epithelial tumours

Transitional cell papilloma

Not all authorities accept the existence of transitional cell papil-lomas, but those that do define them as papillary tumours with fine fibrovascular cores covered with a transitional epithelium of 4–5 nuclei thick and with cells differing little from normal urothelial cells. When these diagnostic criteria are applied strictly, the transitional cell papilloma becomes a very rare

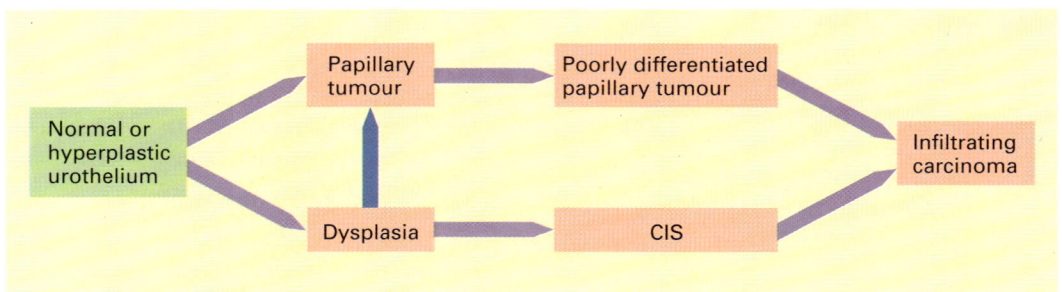

Fig. 19.80 Morphological development of urothelial cancer. CIS, carcinoma *in situ*.

tumour indeed. There is no evidence that these 'papillomas' behave any differently to grade 1 transitional cell carcinomas, and the fact that some are found as small recurrences following resection of a papillary transitional cell carcinoma suggest that they are the well-differentiated end of the spectrum of papillary non-invasive carcinoma.

Transitional cell papilloma, inverted type (inverted papilloma)

Inverted papillomas are rare epithelial tumours which present as smooth-surfaced nodules up to 3 cm in diameter, usually at the bladder neck or trigone, and more rarely elsewhere in the urinary tract. They may be sessile or pedunculated. Histologically, they have a surface of normal urothelium beneath which there are anastomosing cords and columns of regular transitional cells that resemble exaggerated Brunn's nests (Fig. 19.81). These are in continuity with the surface epithelium; foci of squamous metaplasia or of cystic change may be present. The cytology is regular, the lesions are benign, and recurrence is unusual.

Squamous cell papilloma

True squamous cell papillomas of the bladder are very rare. Some probably represent squamous metaplasia in a transitional cell papilloma, while some others may be due to the spread of *condyloma* accuminata from the urethra into the bladder.

Malignant epithelial tumours

Transitional cell carcinoma (TCC)

Staging and grading The macroscopic appearance, microscopic appearance, and the clinical behaviour of individual urothelial tumours are best described with reference to their stage and grade. The *UICC staging system* is widely used and internationally accepted (UICC 1975). This is based on the TNM (tumour, node, metastatis) system and divides the primary tumour into stages (Table 19.14) depending on the nature of the tumour

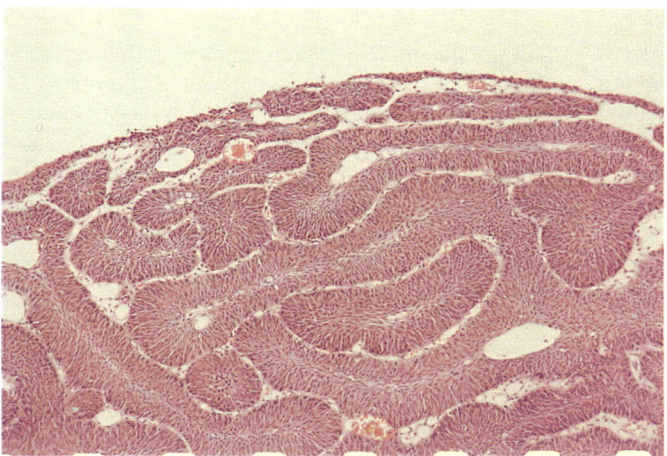

Fig. 19.81 Transitional cell papilloma, inverted type. Thinned surface urothelium covers a tumour of trabeculae and nests of regular transitional cells.

Table 19.14 UICC staging system for bladder cancer—primary tumour (T) stage

Tcis	Carcinoma *in situ*
Ta	Papillary non-invasive carcinoma
T1	Lamina propria invasion only
T2	Invasion of superficial muscle
T3a	Invasion of deep muscle
T3b	Invasion through the bladder wall
T4	Tumour fixed or extending to adjacent structures

and the depth of invasion of the bladder wall. While clinical criteria are given for staging according to the findings at bimanual examination, this has been shown to be inexact, and where possible histological data from resected material should be taken into account when staging is carried out.

While there is wide agreement on the staging of bladder cancer, the same cannot be said for grading. The *WHO grading system* is most widely used and simply divides all transitional carcinomas in three groups, depending on their cellular differentiation: *well-differentiated carcinoma* (G1), *moderately differentiated carcinoma* (G2), and *poorly differentiated or anaplastic carcinoma* (G3); to these three grades a grade for *transitional cell papilloma* (G0) is usually added. Some other grading systems used, e.g. that proposed by Bergkvist (Bergkvist *et al.* 1965), have five stages (G0 to G4). This particular system has the advantage of offering well-defined cytological criteria. Unfortunately, grade is highly dependent on stage and also suffers from considerable inter-observer variation; nevertheless, most studies show that grade correlates well with prognosis. Other measures of cellular differentiation that have also been shown to be good prognostic indicators are cellular DNA content measured by flow cytometry, and reduced expression by tumours of the blood group antigens present on normal urothelial cells (Abel 1988).

Stage is the most reliable prognostic factor (Fig. 19.82) that can be obtained in routine practice, and usually determines the treatment to be given.

Carcinoma in situ (CIS) is often found in flat mucosa adjacent to infiltrating transitional cell carcinomas; less commonly it may be found in the background mucosa of patients with non-invasive papillary carcinoma, when it confers a high risk of subsequent recurrent and invasive disease. Carcinoma *in situ* without evidence of other solid bladder tumours is an uncommon form of bladder cancer that can be found as a cause of asymptomatic microscopic haematuria, or may present with urgency and frequency or macroscopic haematuria. The risk of subsequent invasive disease in these patients has been estimated in follow-up studies to be from 50 per cent to 80 per cent within 5 years. On cystoscopic examination, the bladder mucosa with CIS is often congested and oedematous. Microscopically, the normal urothelium is replaced by cells showing *increased nuclear cytoplasmic ratio, nuclear crowding, hyperchromatism, pleomorphism*, and *frequent mitoses* (Fig. 19.83). The epithelium may vary in thickness and may be thinner than normal epithelium. There is a tendency for the cells to lose their

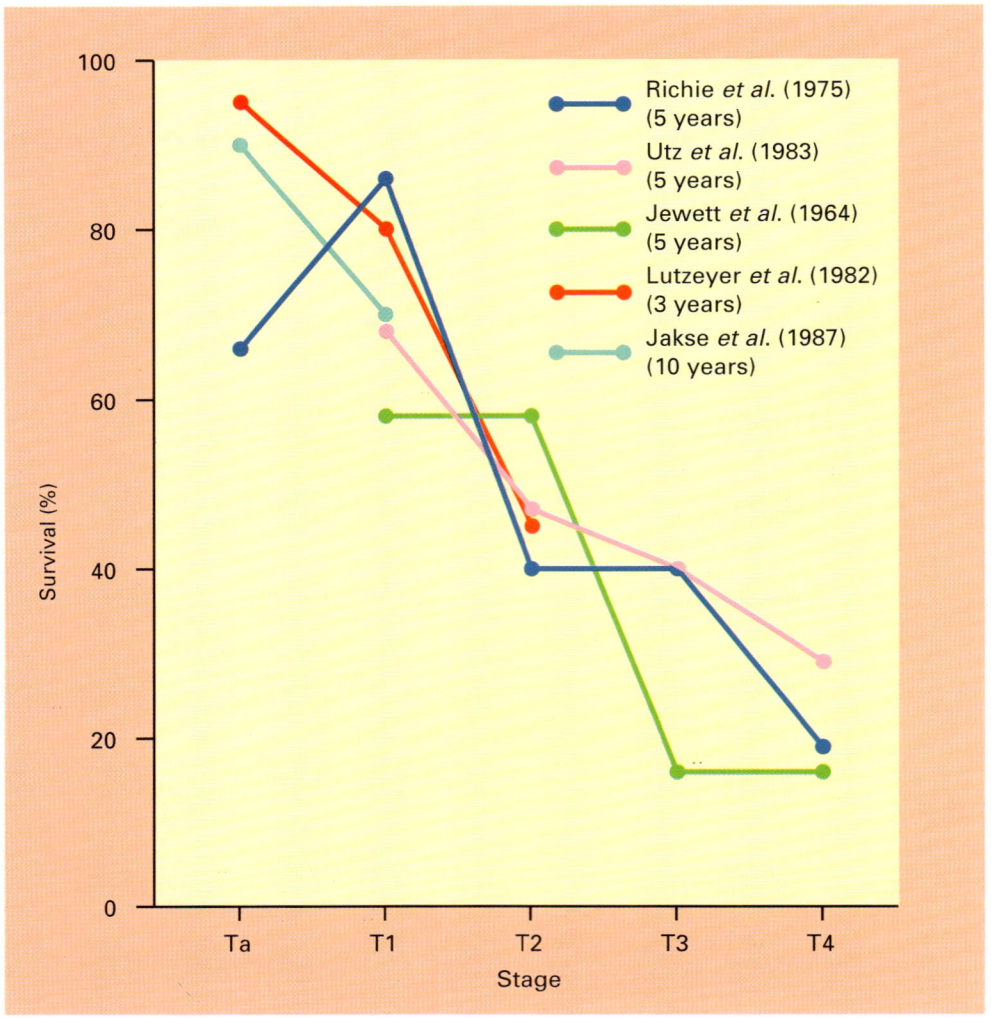

Fig. 19.82 Crude survival rate for bladder cancer related to stage. Five large series: years' survival in parentheses.

cohesion and for the epithelium to become detached from the basement membrane. This can make identification of the disease by biopsy difficult. The cells that have been lost from the epithelium are readily identified by urine cytology, which is a reliable way of confirming the presence of the disease. Carcinoma *in situ* is frequently multifocal, and attempts to eradicate the disease from one site in the urothelium, e.g. by cystectomy or by intravesical chemotherapy, are frequently frustrated by its resurgence in residual urothelium in the ureter or urethra. Spread into the prostatic ducts by carcinoma *in situ*—a common finding in cystoprostatectomy specimens for bladder cancer—may act as a focus for re-establishment of the disease in the bladder following intravesical chemotherapy, and is probably also responsible for the occasional primary invasive TCC in the prostate.

Papillary TCC Most urothelial tumours are discovered after one

or more episodes of haematuria. Macroscopically, the papillary tumours are fronded structures, best appreciated when viewed in fluid (Fig. 19.84), for example at cystoscopy. They can be found anywhere in the urinary tract, but have a predilection for the trigone. Thirty per cent of patients have two or more tumours at presentation and the tumours may be large and 'carpet' large areas of urothelium. The papillary fronds are covered in transitional epithelium. The epithelium may rarely resemble normal urothelium, in which case the grade is G0, or the tumour can be considered a papilloma. More commonly, there is some epithelial hyperplasia with or without nuclear atypia (G1 or G2) (Fig. 19.85), but only rarely is there considerable anaplasia (G3) without evidence of invasion. The tumours often show some variation of their cellular type, and both focal squamous and glandular metaplasia are common findings. About 40 per cent of all bladder tumours are stage Ta at presentation: a quarter of patients with solitary tumours and

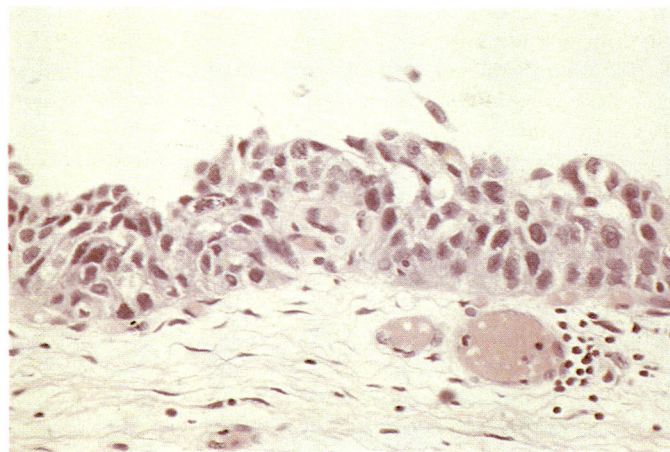

Fig. 19.83 Carcinoma *in situ*. This was found in the background mucosa of a bladder with infiltrating carcinoma.

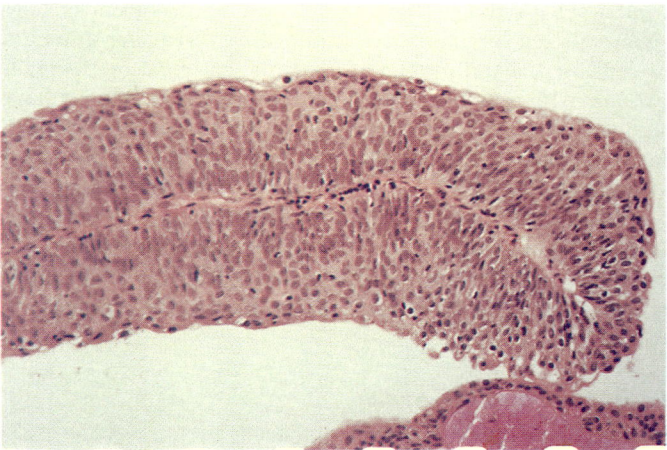

Fig. 19.84 Papillary transitional cell carcinoma. The fronded tumour has spread over a substantial proportion of the bladder. There is no invasion of the bladder wall.

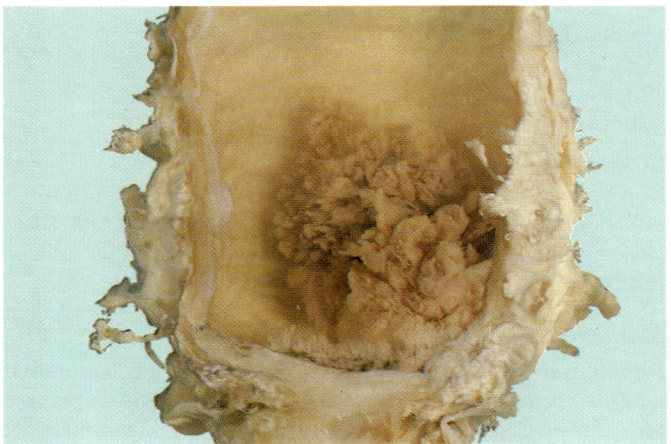

Fig. 19.85 Papillary transitional cell carcinoma. A well-differentiated (G1) tumour showing hyperplastic transitional epithelium covering a papilla that has a fine fibrovascular core.

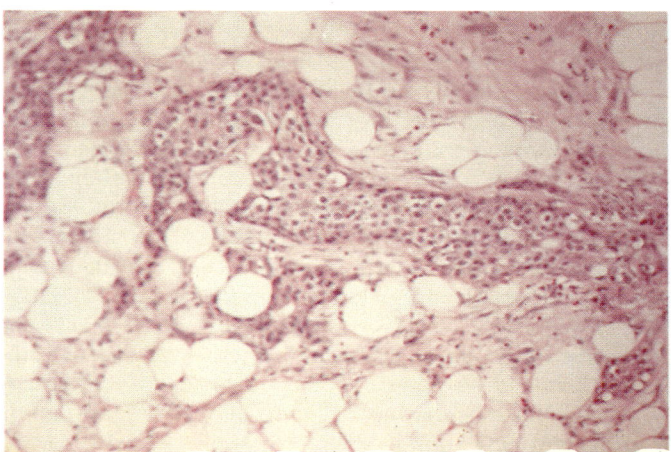

Fig. 19.86 Infiltrating transitional cell carcinoma. An invasive TCC in the extravesical fat.

three-quarters of patients with multiple tumours will have suffered a recurrence within 3 years. After a tumour has recurred once, the risk of further recurrences increases, with some patients suffering multiple recurrences over many years at various sites throughout the urinary tract. The patients who have these multiple recurrences have long been considered to have a diffusely unstable or tumorigenic urothelium. Some have hyperplasia or mild dysplasia of the background epithelium, and, although these are at statistically higher risk of recurrence of their tumours, there are no reliable morphological markers that will allow prediction of recurrence. Recurrences are usually the same stage as the presenting tumour. The risk of recurrences of Ta tumours progressing to muscle invasion is a few per cent only, and subsequent tumour death is a very rare event. If papillary tumours are left untreated, some will invade the bladder wall; most T1 tumours have a surface papillary component, suggesting origin from a pre-existing papillary

tumour. T1 tumours are usually moderately differentiated (G2) but the minority that are poorly differentiated (G3) have a much higher risk of subsequent muscle invasive disease (Birch and Harland 1989). Once a tumour has invaded the lamina propria, its behaviour is similar to that of infiltrating tumours.

Infiltrating TCC The majority of invasive TCCs are invasive from an early stage and are derived from foci of carcinoma *in situ*. Like papillary tumours, they present with haematuria. Macroscopically, they are seen as either an ulcer in the mucosa or as an ulcerating mass protruding into the bladder. The trigone is the most common site and local invasion in this site commonly causes ureteric obstruction, often bilateral.

Microscopically, G2 tumours invade in nests of cells that are readily recognizable as derived from transitional mucosa (Fig. 19.86). G3 tumours are more pleomorphic and cells may invade singularly. *Focal squamous metaplasia* is common and tumours with this feature should not be classified as pure squamous cell carcinomas. Tumours discovered after a solitary episode of haematuria are frequently early stage, whereas patients who present after several months of haematuria have significantly larger tumours of a more advanced stage, suggesting that many infiltrating tumours progress rapidly. Early metastasis from T1 or T2 tumours is uncommon, but tumours that are stage T3 and above regularly metastasize to lymph nodes and via the bloodstream to the liver, the lungs, and bone. Lymphatic or vascular invasion may be identified in histological sections of tumour, in which case the prognosis is significantly worse.

Undifferentiated carcinoma

This group of tumours includes anaplastic tumours of presumed urothelial origin but without any evidence of differentiation, spindle-cell tumours of epithelial origin, and small cell carcinomas. Most present at an advanced stage and have a poor prognosis.

Squamous cell carcinoma

Squamous carcinomas make up about 5 per cent of urothelial malignancy, except where *Schistosoma haematobium* is prevalent, where up to 50 per cent of tumours may be squamous. Occasional tumours may be related to persistent *urinary-tract infections*, *lithiasis*, or *diverticula*. Patients present with haematuria and the tumour is invariably infiltrating and ulcerating. Microscopically, the tumour is identified by the presence of keratin and/or intercellular bridges. It is often associated with *squamous metaplasia* of the adjacent urothelium and this may also show evidence of *dysplasia*. Extravesical spread to adjacent structures, to lymph nodes, and via the bloodstream is common. *Overall, the prognosis is worse than for transitional cell carcinoma*, but much of the difference may be due to the late state of many of the tumours at presentation.

Adenocarcinoma

Most primary adenocarcinomas found in the bladder occur at the dome and are probably of *urachal origin* (see p. 1517); others are of urothelial origin. The urothelial-derived tumours are often related to glandular metaplasia and chronic inflammation, in others the origin is obscure. A variety of histological tumour patterns is seen, including *papillary*, *glandular* (large-bowel-like), *mucinous*, *signet-ring cell type*, and *clear-cell carcinoma*. All are infiltrating at presentation and the prognosis is poor (Gill *et al.* 1989).

Neoplasms at other sites in the urinary tract

Tumours of the renal pelvis and ureter are similar in most respects to bladder tumours, and transitional cell carcinomas at these sites occur concurrently or sequentially with similar bladder tumours in up to 50 per cent of cases. The tumours are graded in a similar manner to bladder tumours, but the staging requires modification because of the differing anatomical relations. In particular, the muscularis propria is thin in these structures and some of the urothelium lies directly on the renal medulla without intervening lamina propria (Eagan 1989). Non-invasive papillary tumours can spread along the urothelium from the renal pelvis into the ureter, causing obstruction and sometimes renal colic. TCCs that invade the renal parenchyma can present with a renal mass in a similar way to renal cell carcinoma. A correct pre- or perioperative diagnosis is important since the appropriate operation for a TCC includes removal of the ureter with a cuff of bladder to avoid ureteric recurrences. Macroscopically, they can be distinguished from renal cell carcinoma by their white or grey colour and by their extensive pelvic involvement. Adenocarcinomas and squamous cell carcinomas in the upper tract are usually associated with chronic inflammation and glandular or squamous metaplasia, due to renal stones or schistosomiasis. In the urethra, TCCs are found in the proximal third, which is lined with transitional mucosa. Tumour-like benign prostatic polyps are sometimes found in the prostatic urethra (Sogbein and Steele 1989). The most common tumour-like lesion found distally is the *condyloma acuminatum*; squamous cancers can also occur and may complicate a *urethral stricture* or a *urethroplasty*.

Other tumours

Benign

Non-epithelial benign tumours are rare; *leiomyomas* are sometimes found in the muscularis and *congenital cavernous haemangiomas* may sometimes be responsible for gross macroscopic haematuria in children.

Malignant

Leiomyosarcoma is the most common bladder sarcoma in adults; it is nevertheless rare, making up less than 0.5 per cent of all bladder tumours. They are usually well-circumscribed tumours that protude into the bladder lumen and have a pale, haemorrhagic or myxoid cut surface. Histologically, they consist of spindle cells in interlacing bundles; survival depends on the degree of differentiation and the extent of spread.

Rhabdomyosarcoma of the bladder or prostate is a rare childhood malignancy, occurring almost exclusively in children under the age of 6 years and most commonly presenting in the first and second years. When they originate in the trigone or prostate they cause urinary-tract obstruction, infection, and haematuria. Macroscopically, they are usually multinodular tumours of glistening gelatinous grape-like structures. Tumours with this typical appearance are called *botryoid-type rhabdomyosarcoma* (from the Greek *botryd*, a bunch of grapes). Histologically, the botryoid tumours are characterized by a zone of undifferentiated cells beneath the epithelium, the *Nicholson cambium layer*; better-differentiated cells, sometimes with rhabdomyoblasts, are found in myxoid tissue in the centre of the nodules. Rhabdomyosarcoma grows rapidly, invading locally and metastasizing to lymph nodes. Recent advances in combination therapy have radically improved the outlook for children with this tumour.

Phaeochromocytoma (paragangliomas) arise from chromaffin cells of the vesical sympathetic plexus. About half are hormonally active, others are small tumours that are sometimes found incidentally. They behave in a similar manner to phaeochromocytomas in the adrenal gland.

Other malignant tumours Tumours in other organs occasionally present as a mass in the bladder. The most common primary sites are the *cervix*, the *prostate*, and the *large bowel*. Metastatic tumours from distant sites are rare, but *lymphomas* can diffusely infiltrate the bladder, either as a manifestation of disseminated disease or, much more rarely, as primary to the bladder.

19.13.6   Bibliography

Abel, P. D. (1988). Prognostic indices in transitional cell carcinoma of the bladder. *British Journal of Urology* **62**, 103–9.

Bergkvist, A., Ljungquist, A., and Moberger, G. (1965). Classification of bladder tumours based on the cellular pattern, preliminary report of a clinical-pathological study of 300 cases with a minimum follow-up of eight years. *Acta Chirurgica Scandinavica* **130**, 371–8.

Birch, B. R. P. and Harland, S. J. (1989). The pT1 G3 bladder tumour. *British Journal of Urology* **64**, 109–16.

Bullock, N. (1988). Idiopathic retroperitoneal fibrosis. *British Medical Journal* **297**, 240–1.

Bullock. P. S., Thoni, D. E., and Murphy, W. M. (1987). The significance of colonic mucosa (intestinal metaplasia) involving the urinary tract. *Cancer* **59**, 2086–90.

Eagan, J. J. (1989). Urothelial neoplasms: renal pelvic and ureter. In *Uropathology*, Vol. 1, (ed. G. S. Hill), pp. 843–72. Churchill Livingstone, New York.

Ekeuland, P., Anderstrom, C., Johansson, S. L., and Larsson, P. (1983). The reversibility of catheter associated polypoid cystitis. *Journal of Urology* **130**, 456–9.

Fall, M., Johansson, S., and Aldenborg, F. (1987). Chronic interstitial cystitis: a heterogeneous syndrome. *Journal of Urology* **137**, 35–8.

Friedell, G., Parija, G., Nagy, G., and Soto, E. (1980). The pathology of human bladder cancer. *Cancer* **45**, 1823–31.

Gill, H. S., Dhillon, H. K., and Woodhouse, C. R. J. (1989). Adenocarcinoma of the urinary bladder. *British Journal of Urology* **64**, 138–42.

Glassberg, K. I., *et al.* (1984). Suggested terminology for duplex systems, ectopic ureters and ureterceles. *Journal of Urology* **132**, 1153–7.

Gonzalez, J. A. (1988). Nephrogenic adenoma of the bladder: report of 10 cases. *Journal of Urology* **139**, 45–7.

Hellstrom, H. R., Davis, B. K., and Shonnard, J. W. (1979). Eosinophilic cystitis. A study of 16 cases. *American Journal of Clinical Pathology* **72**, 777–84.

Hertle, L. and Androulakakis, P. (1982). Keratinizing desquamative squamous metaplasia of the upper urinary tract: leukoplakia-cholesteatoma. *Journal of Urology* **127**, 631–5.

Jakse, G., Loidl, W., Seeber, G., and Hofstadter, F. (1987). Stage T1, grade 3 transitional cell carcinoma of the bladder: an unfavourable tumor. *Journal of Urology* **137**, 39–41.

Jewett, H., King, L., and Shelly, W. (1964). A study of 365 cases of infiltrating bladder cancer: relation of certain pathological characteristics to prognosis after extirpation. *Journal of Urology* **92**, 668–80.

Koss, L. (1975). Tumours of the urinary bladder. In *Atlas of tumour pathology*, fascicle 11, 2nd series. Armed Forces Institute of Pathology, Washington, DC.

Lower G. (1982). Concepts in causality: chemically induced human urinary bladder cancer. *Cancer* **49**, 1056–88.

Lutzeyer, W., Rubben, H., and Dahm, H. (1982). Prognostic parameters in superficial bladder cancer, an analysis of 315 cases. *Journal of Urology* **127**, 250–2.

McClure, J. (1983). Malakoplakia. *Journal of Pathology* **140**, 275–330.

McDonald, D. F. and Lund, R. R. (1954). The role of urine in vesical neoplasm. 1. Experimental confirmation of the urogenous theory of pathogenesis. *Journal of Urology* **71** (5), 560–70.

Mostofi, F., Sobin, L., and Torloni, H. (1973). *International histological classification of tumours. No. 10: Histological typing of urinary bladder tumours.* World Health Organization, Geneva.

Nochomovitz, L. E. and Orestein, J. M. (1985). Inflammatory pseudotumour of the urinary bladder—possible relationship to nodular fasciitis. *American Journal of Surgical Pathology* **9**, 366–73.

Richie, J., Skinner, D., and Kaufman, J. (1975). Radical cystectomy for carcinoma of the bladder. *Journal of Urology* **113**, 186–9.

Ro, J. Y., Ayala, A. G., and El-Naggar, A. (1987). Muscularis mucosa of urinary bladder. Importance for staging and treatment. *American Journal of Surgical Pathology* **11** (9), 668–73.

Sogbein, S. K. and Steele, A. A. (1989). Papillary prostatic epithelial hyperplasia of the urethra: a cause of haematuria in young men. *Journal of Urology* **142**, 1218–20.

Stanton, M. J. and Maxted, W. (1981). Malacoplakia: a study of the literature and current concepts of pathogenesis, diagnosis and treatment. *Journal of Urology* **125**, 139–45.

UICC (1975). *TNM classification of malignant tumours.* International Union Against Cancer, Geneva.

Utz, D., Schmitz, S., and Fugelso, P. (1983). A clinicopathologic evaluation of partial cystectomy for carcinoma of the urinary bladder. *Cancer* **32**, 1075–7.

Wallace, D. M. (1988) Occupational urothelial cancer. *British Journal of Urology* **61**, 175–82.

Weiner, D. P., Koss, L. G., Sablay, B., and Freed, S. Z. (1979) The prevalence and significance of Brunn's nests, cystitis cystica and squamous metaplasia in normal bladders. *Journal of Urology* **122**, 317–21.

Young, R. H. (1988) Papillary and polypoid cystitis. *American Journal of Surgical Pathology* **12**, (7), 542–6.

Young, R. H. and Scully, R. E. (1987). Pseudosarcomatous lesions of the urinary bladder, prostate gland, and urethra. A report of three cases and review of the literature. *Archives of Pathology and Laboratory Medicine* **111**, 354–8.

20

The male generative system

20

The male generative system

20.1 The prostate

I. D. Ansell

20.1.1 Normal structure and function

The prostate gland lies retroperitoneally at the base of the bladder posterior to the symphysis pubis and in close association with the internal and external urethral sphincters. It is traditionally regarded as having the shape of an 'inverted chestnut' and to weigh approximately 20 g. It is composed of a number of tubulo-alveolar glands set in a fibromuscular stroma and is traversed by the prostatic urethra in its more anterior portion. The lumen of this part of the urethra is crescentic in cross-section due to a ridge, the *urethral crest*, on its posterior wall. Towards the superior portion of the urethral crest there is a blind invagination, the *prostatic utricle*; this is the male remnant of the lower fused ends of the Müllerian (paramesonephric) ducts which form the female uterus—hence its alternative name of *uterus masculinus*. The two *ejaculatory ducts* enter the urethra on either side of this structure, which is seen endoscopically as a localized projection, the *verumontanum*. The larger ducts of the anterior, lateral, and posterior parts of the gland drain into the urethra near the urethral crest, whereas the smaller mucosal glands of the upper urethra are arranged around the whole circumference. Like the prostatic utricle, those glands situated superior to it and between the ejaculatory ducts are derived partly from Müllerian tissue and are thus of a different embryological origin than the main glands of the prostate (Fig. 20.1).

The classical description of the lobular architecture of the prostate into anterior, posterior, median, and two lateral lobes has now been abandoned, since these can only be recognized in the embryo. However, one can say that the *median lobe* corresponds to the tissue of Müllerian origin which is situated centrally in the gland, whereas the *anterior, posterior, and lateral lobes* correspond to the true prostate, positioned more peripherally and inferiorly. The different parts of the gland also differ histologically: the acini of the central portion being larger than those of the peripheral. Recognition of these two areas within the prostate is of fundamental importance since the two most common conditions affecting the prostate arise in different areas, *benign nodular hyperplasia* being a condition of the central and superior portions of the gland, whereas *carcinoma* arises in the more peripheral and inferior region. The prostatic acini are lined by a single layer of columnar secretory cells and are often infolded into the lumen to give a pseudopapillary pattern. Surrounding these secretory units is a layer of inconspicuous basal cells (Fig. 20.2); these are *not* myoepithelial cells and are

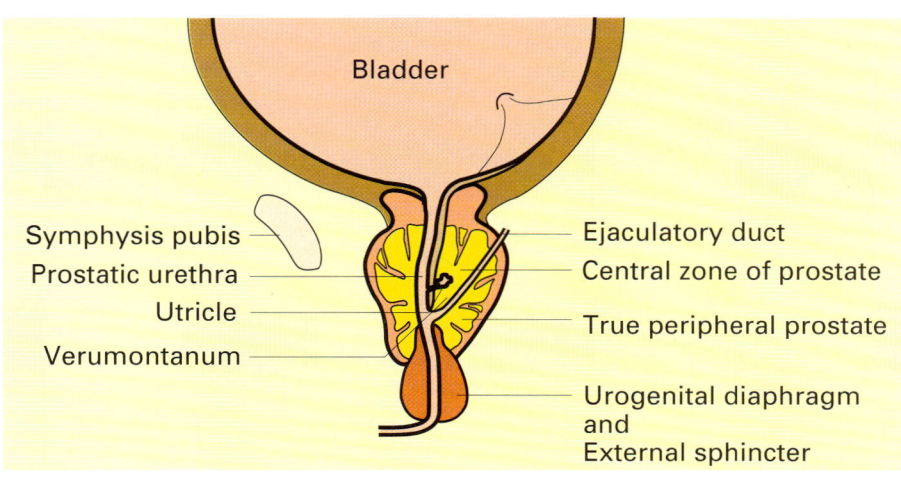

Symphysis pubis
Prostatic urethra
Utricle
Verumontanum

Bladder

Ejaculatory duct
Central zone of prostate

True peripheral prostate

Urogenital diaphragm
and
External sphincter

Fig. 20.1 Sagittal section of the prostate to show the main divisions of the gland.

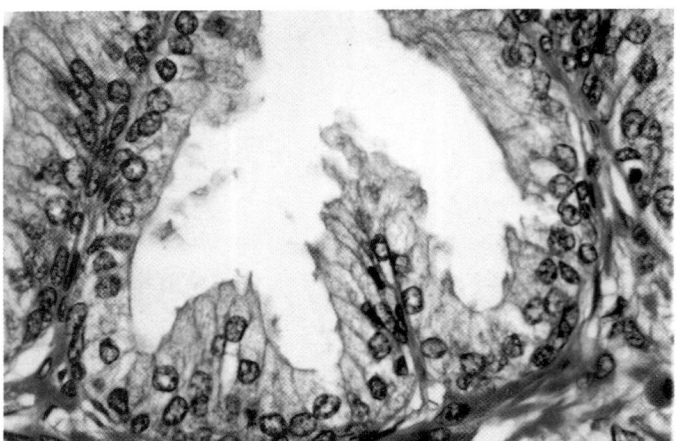

Fig. 20.2 Normal prostatic acinar epithelium with columnar secretory cells and elongate basal cells.

presumed to be the precursors of the secretory cells; they may be demonstrated by the use of specific anti-keratin antibodies and their absence is a helpful feature in the diagnosis of well-differentiated adenocarcinomas. In the older patient many acini contain spherical eosinophilic bodies, *corpora amylaceae*, which are presumed to be composed of inspissated secretion; they are of little pathological significance although, interestingly, they often stain positively for amyloid. The cells lining the prostatic ducts are indistinguishable from acinar cells until the change to the transitional epithelium (or urothelium) which lines the urethra.

Growth and development of the prostate gland are hormone dependent and need the trophic action of both oestrogens and androgens. The gland is immature at birth and only grows to its normal size at puberty when androgen secretion commences. Further growth, atrophy, and neoplasia also appear to be dependent on androgen:oestrogen ratios.

The function of the prostate gland resides in its contribution to seminal fluid at the time of ejaculation. Prostatic secretion contains a number of substances, of which *acid phosphatase* is the best known. This enzyme has been used for many years as a serum marker for disseminated carcinoma of the prostate and, more recently, its demonstration histochemically has proved to be very useful in identifying metastatic deposits as being of prostatic origin. Acid phosphatases are found widely in human tissues and the recent discovery of a protein apparently specific to prostatic cells (*prostate-specific antigen*) has now virtually supplanted prostatic acid phosphatase in clinical usage.

Congenital abnormalities of the prostate are very uncommon, they are rarely of clinical significance and will not be discussed further.

20.1.2   Inflammatory conditions

Prostatitis

Prostatitis is a somewhat confusing entity, for it is not uncommon to see significant numbers of lymphocytes and even neutrophil polymorphs in prostatic tissue removed for benign nodular hyperplasia. Clinical correlation of symptomatic prostatitis to these pathological changes is often non-existent and the presence of small numbers of these cells must be presumed to be associated with the hyperplastic process and not an indication of infection. The term *prostatitis* should thus be restricted to patients with symptoms referrable to the organ. It is conveniently classified into *acute and chronic forms*.

Symptomatic *acute prostatitis* with perineal pain and dysuria is not uncommon in *gonorrhoea* and other venereal conditions in young males; in older men it may complicate urinary tract infections, especially those due to instrumentation. If untreated, acute prostatitis may progress to frank abscess formation—a condition said to be more common in diabetics—or even frank septicaemia.

Chronic prostatitis is a more controversial condition. In some patients it may be a true cause of perineal discomfort and other urinary symptoms. In these patients the diagnosis is made by examining the urine/urethral secretions after digital prostatic massage: if pus is demonstrated then prostatitis is confirmed. It is further subclassified into the *bacterial variety* if coliforms or other bacteria are grown, or abacterial if bacterial cultures are negative—*Chlamydia* are thought to cause a significant number of these infections. However, the role of infective agents in those patients with these symptoms but in whom prostatic secretions are normal is still uncertain as psychosexual abnormalities are common in such individuals, who may be said to have *prostatodynia*.

Granulomatous prostatitis

This term is employed for those prostates in which the degree of interstitial chronic inflammation is sufficient to warrant the term granulomatous. The term granuloma may mean different things to different pathologists but in this context denotes a chronic inflammatory cell infiltrate containing a significant histiocytic and multinuclear giant cell component (Fig. 20.3). The

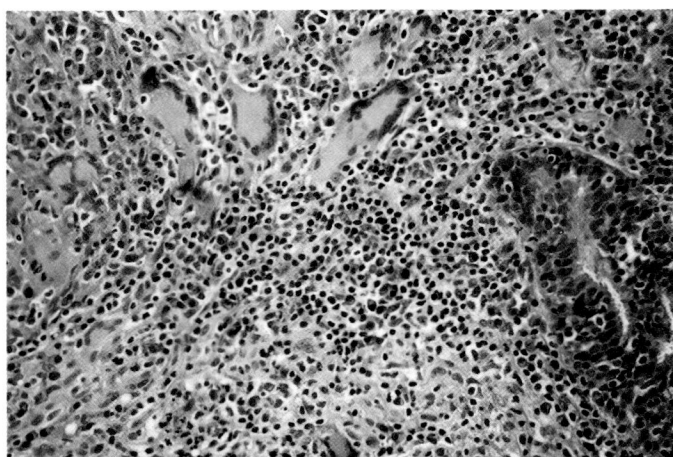

Fig. 20.3 Granulomatous prostatitis: lymphocytes and plasma cells near an inflamed gland with prominent giant cells.

majority of such cases are non-specific; 70 per cent are said to follow a recent urinary tract infection but, in general, the cellular reaction is presumed to be a response to glandular secretions released into the stroma following obstruction to ducts. The associated fibrosis accompanying this inflammation produces a very firm gland which may be mistaken for carcinoma on digital examination and has resulted in unnecessary radical prostatectomies in the past.

An important condition which may give a similar histological picture is *tuberculosis* and this should always be considered and excluded when this picture is present. Typically, tuberculosis will have areas of frank caseous necrosis (Fig. 20.4) and tubercle bacilli will be demonstrable by a Ziehl–Neelsen stain; however, in some there may be little or no caseation, but whenever there is the slightest suspicion of this diagnosis early morning urine should be sent for tubercle culture. Tubercle of the prostate is almost always a complication of urinary tract tuberculosis and the appropriate investigations should be instigated whenever this diagnosis is made (including at the very least an intravenous urogram). Identical granulomas may also be seen in patients receiving *BCG treatment* for flat *in situ* carcinoma of the bladder.

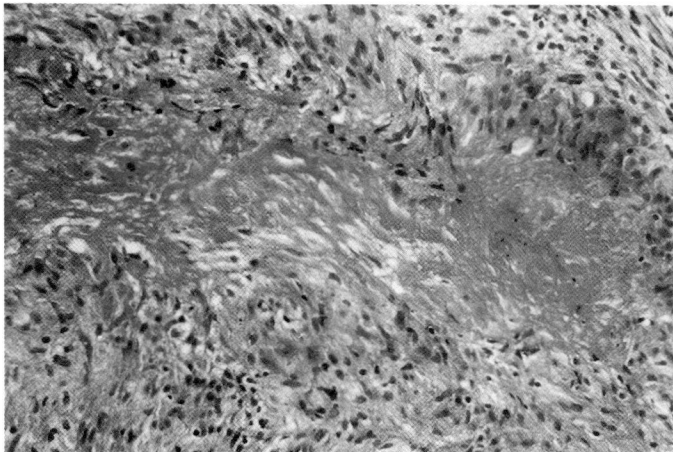

Fig. 20.5 Palisaded granuloma following previous transurethral prostatic resection. Note the resemblance to both tuberculosis and rheumatoid nodule.

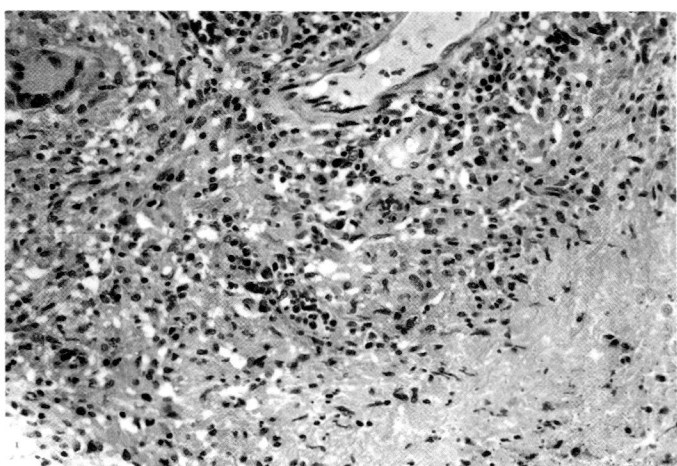

Fig. 20.4 Tuberculous prostatitis: caseation necrosis at bottom right and Langhans giant cell top left.

Post-transurethral resection granuloma

Another more recently recognized entity producing a similar pathological appearance is the *palisaded granuloma* which has a more than passing resemblance to a rheumatoid nodule that is produced by transurethral resection of the prostate; these should produce no diagnostic difficulty if an adequate history of previous surgery is provided (Fig. 20.5). Similar granulomas have been seen in the bladder after transurethral resection and in the cervix after cone biopsy. Previous prostatic transurethral resection may produce a less specific picture of florid inflammatory granulation tissue with numerous eosinophils, although why eosinophils should be so prominent in this situation is

uncertain. It is probable that some of the earlier cases reported as 'eosinophilic prostatitis' were of this origin. Very rarely the histological picture of eosinophilic prostatis is due to exotic parasites, and in a small number of cases is a manifestation of systemic vasculitis or Wegener's granulomatosis.

Malacoplakia

This chronic inflammatory condition is found most commonly in the bladder but is described throughout the urinary tract and indeed, in the gastrointestinal tract and elsewhere. It is characterized histologically by a chronic inflammatory infiltrate containing many plasma cells and large histiocytes with relatively clear cytoplasm. Within the clear cytoplasm of these histiocytes (*von Hansemann cells*) may be seen the pathognomonic targetoid *Michaelis–Gutmann bodies* (Fig. 20.6). These bodies are degenerate calcified lysosomes within which bacteria can be demonstrated ultrastructurally. It is thought that this disease is due to

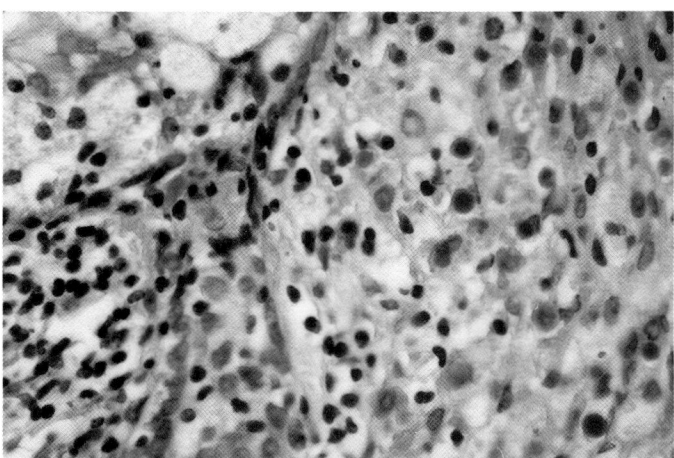

Fig. 20.6 Malacoplakia: pathognomonic target-shaped Michaelis–Gutmann bodies at the centre and on the right.

a defect in lysosomal function in which the normal destruction of engulfed bacteria is defective.

Infarction

Areas of haemorrhagic infarction are not uncommonly seen in prostates resected for benign hyperplasia. They are readily recognized microscopically, even in transurethral resection specimens by the 'ghost-like' acini, focal interstitial haemorrhage, and the not infrequent *squamous metaplasia* of surrounding ductal epithelium (Fig. 20.7). The aetiology of these infarcts is probably multifactorial, with previous *catheterization* and *arteriosclerosis* of the lower aorta and its branches the more important. Their only pathological importance lies in the possibility of the squamous metaplasia being misinterpreted as squamous carcinoma.

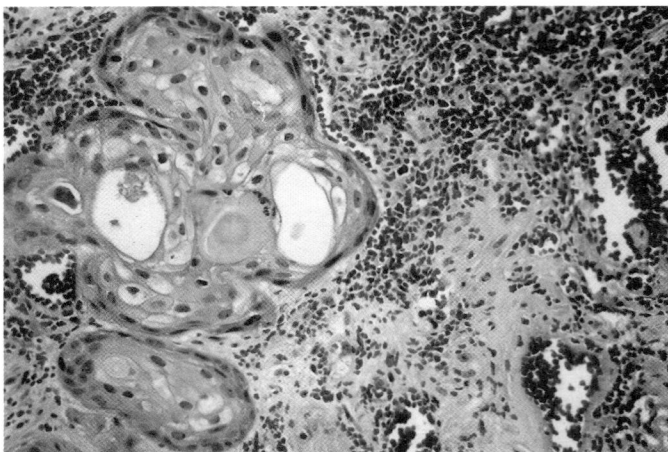

Fig. 20.7 Squamous metaplasia of glandular epithelium at the edge of a haemorrhagic infarct (on the right).

20.1.3   Nodular hyperplasia

Nodular increase in size of the prostate with advancing age may be considered to be a normal occurrence in men; indeed, it is said to reach an incidence of 100 per cent by the tenth decade, although its incidence varies considerably according to the mode of definition. Since a significant proportion of older men in Great Britain now undergo prostatectomy, the condition can certainly be considered to be of considerable significance. The aetiology of this progressive enlargement is unclear. Its absence in men castrated before puberty and its response to anti-androgen therapy indicate an hormonal aetiology, and an increase in dihydrotestosterone has been demonstrated in the stroma of patients with hyperplasia. However, the advent of transurethral resection as an effective and safe treatment of this condition has decreased interest in the use of medical measures. The hyperplasia of the gland is restricted to the central and superior portion between the ejaculatory ducts, which has historically been labelled as the 'median lobe'. Nodular increase in size of the gland distorts and obstructs the prostatic urethra,

compromising normal micturition. The patient's stream thus becomes reduced and difficult to control. Complete emptying of the bladder also becomes difficult, especially if the median lobe reaches proportions sufficient to obstruct the internal urethral meatus at times of detrusor contraction. The rise in pressure required for micturition leads to destrusor hypertrophy and a trabeculated bladder wall (Fig. 20.8) and back pressure up the ureters to the kidneys may lead to obstructive renal failure. Incomplete voiding of urine frequently leads to urinary tract infection with exacerbation of urinary symptoms such as *frequency* and *dysuria*. In the extreme case the patient is unable to void urine at all—acute retention.

The hyperplasia responsible for the increased size of the gland affects all constituent components of the gland—fibrous tissue, smooth muscle, and glands. The hyperplasia is not uniform but gives a distinct nodular appearance on gross inspection (Fig. 20.9). The nodules may consist of smooth muscle and/or fibrous tissue only and these so-called *stromal nodules* are usually situated adjacent to the urethra (Fig. 20.10). Since embryologically it is the stroma that initiates growth and development of the prostatic glandular tissue, these nodules have been considered to be the initial stage in the disease process, their presence stimulating proliferation of adjacent glandular tissue to produce the typical *fibroadenomyomatous nodule*. The acini of these hyperplastic nodules are often dilated such that the cut surface of the gland has a microcystic appearance and may exude prostatic secretions (Fig. 20.11). The hyperplasia

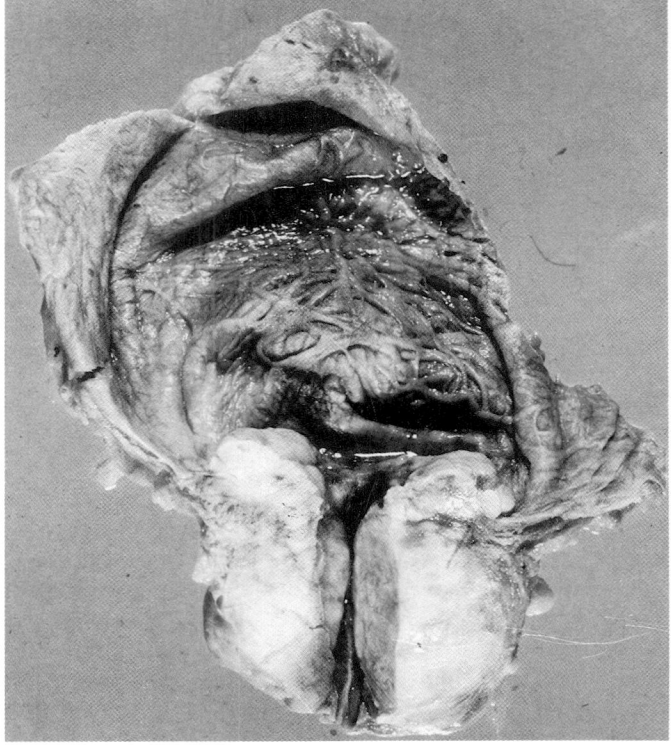

Fig. 20.8 Benign prostatic hypertrophy with massive enlargement of the prostate and trabeculation of the bladder wall.

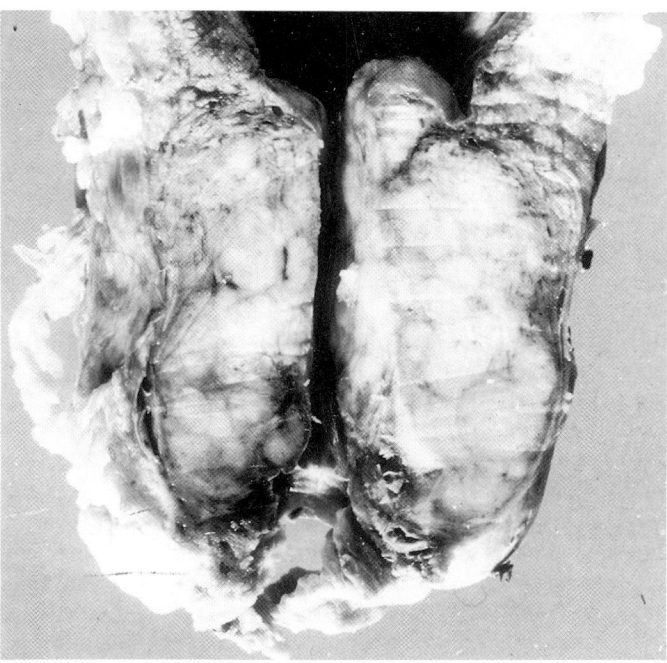

Fig. 20.9 Cut surface of retropubic prostatectomy specimen performed for benign hyperplasia to show marked nodularity.

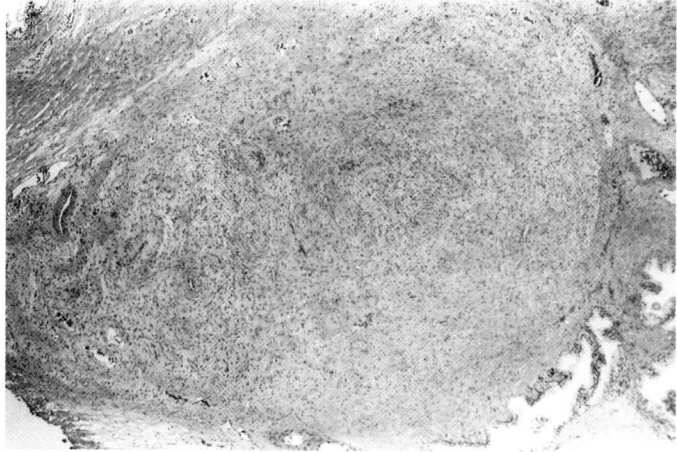

Fig. 20.10 Photomicrograph of a nodule of fibromuscular tissue only in a case of benign prostatic hyperplasia.

may thus be said to produce a spectrum of nodules—*fibromatous, myomatous, fibromyomatous, fibroadenomyomatous*, and occasionally *adenomatous*, although such pathological subclassification has no clinical significance. Although the older literature (and some surgeons) refer to prostatic 'adenomas' current views are that this condition is not neoplastic, and benign tumours such as leiomyomas are considered to be very rare entities to this organ.

There are a number of variants of nodular hyperplasia which have been given a confusing spectrum of names and which, on

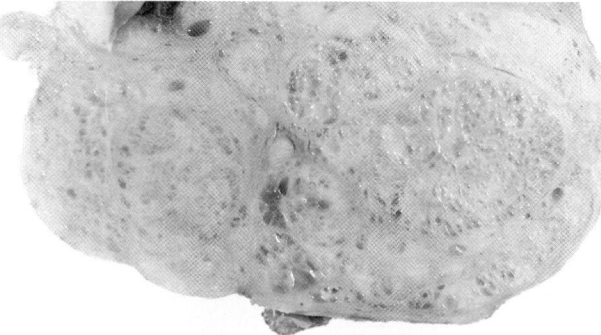

Fig. 20.11 Cut surface of a nodular benign prostatic hyperplasia to show the microcystic appearance.

occasion, may be mistakenly diagnosed as malignant. Hyperplasia affecting predominantly the basal cells produces groups of hyperchromatic cells superficially resembling carcinoma (Fig. 20.12) and proliferation of acinar cells has been termed 'adenosis' or 'atypical hyperplasia'; in some of these the acinar cells have cytological characteristics which could properly be labelled as 'dysplasia' or '*in situ* carcinoma' (Fig. 20.13). However, although dysplasia has been described most commonly in radical prostatectomy specimens removed for carcinoma, convincing evidence that it is truly neoplastic is not available since it is impossible to identify and follow up patients in which these abnormalities are present without removing the lesion under investigation.

20.1.4 Carcinoma

Aetiology and epidemiology

A large majority of prostatic tumours are *adenocarcinomas*, and general discussion on this subject refers to these glandular tumours. Prostatic carcinoma is now the third most important

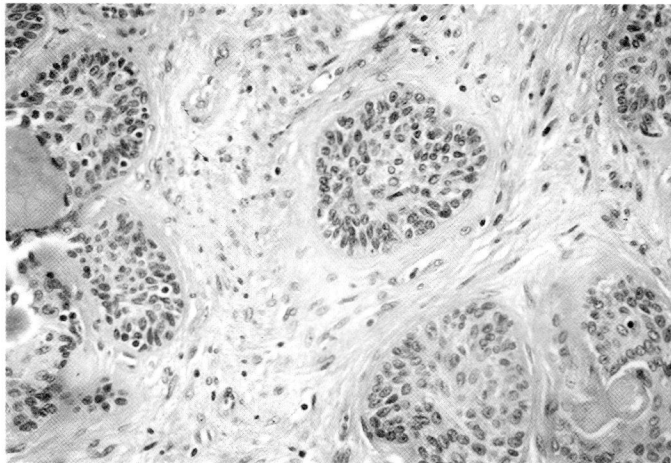

Fig. 20.12 Basal cell hyperplasia of the prostate; this has a passing resemblance to basal cell carcinoma of skin and has been misdiagnosed as carcinoma on occasions.

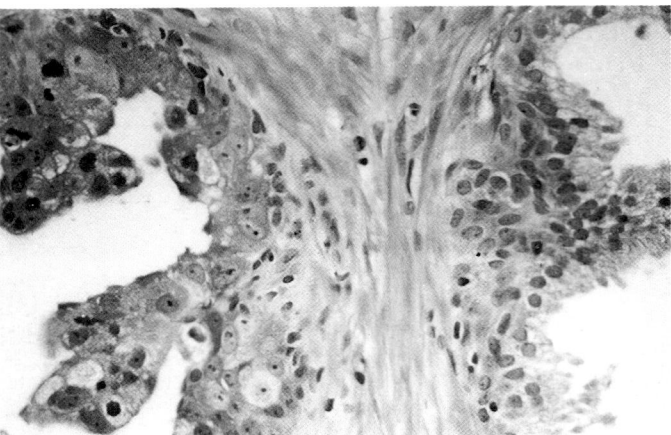

Fig. 20.13 Severe dysplasia of prostatic glandular epithelium. The epithelium on the left shows cytological appearance of *in situ* carcinoma compared to the normal epithelium of the acinus on the right.

malignancy in males in Western communities, with only bronchus and large bowel producing more deaths. Moreover, the incidence of this tumour is much in excess of the death rate for reasons to be explained later.

Post-mortem studies in the 1930s demonstrated a rising incidence of this tumour with age and, of course, the longevity of the Western male continues to increase. It was also recognized at that time that most of these cases of prostatic carcinoma discovered at autopsy were not accompanied by metastatic disease and had produced no clinical symptoms. In a similar way today the increasing frequency of surgery for benign prostatic hyperplasia has resulted in the discovery of histological carcinomas in patients not previously suspected of harbouring a tumour. On further investigation, a proportion of these patients will be found to have evidence of metastatic disease, but in a significant number the tumour appears to be an incidental finding. A clinical classification of the different types of prostatic carcinoma has accordingly evolved. *Clinical* carcinoma denotes those patients with symptoms of both prostatic and metastatic disease, *occult* carcinoma describes those presenting with symptoms of metastatic prostatic cancer but with no symptoms of prostatism, and *latent* carcinoma is the name given to those tumours discovered in tissue removed from patients with symptoms of prostatism only. Today the term *incidental* carcinoma is preferred to *latent*, the latter term being reserved for those non-metastatic tumours discovered at autopsy.

It can be readily understood than any comparison of the incidence of the disease around the world must be extremely careful to compare like with like. Notwithstanding these problems, a high incidence of clinical prostatic cancer has been demonstrated in the USA and Scandinavia, with a low incidence in Japan, Greece, and Mexico. In the USA it has also been shown to be more common in Blacks than in Whites and that Jews are less susceptible to the disease than Protestants. An increased incidence in those Japanese who migrate to the USA suggests an environmental factor, of which diet must be the most likely.

Like benign hyperplasia, prostatic carcinoma is unknown in men castrated before puberty and, since many cases may be controlled by orchidectomy or anti-androgen drugs (such as stilboestrol), the role of androgens in the aetiology of the tumour has been much investigated. However, no convincing conclusions have been produced from these studies, although recent reports of this tumour in men taking anabolic steroids and in butchers (exposed to meat from animals receiving steroid hormones) have awakened interest in this line of investigation.

Histogenesis

Most prostatic carcinomas arise in the peripheral portions of the gland which are not removed by digital retropubic or transvesical prostatectomy. Thus early carcinomas may not be removed by this technique and a previous prostatectomy, either transurethral or by open operation, does not mean that a patient will not develop prostatic cancer. An adequate transurethral resection is much more likely to sample the tumour-bearing area of the gland and most tumours should thus be detected if sufficient tissue is sampled. The actual quantity of resected tissue that should be sampled is contentious, but *five* blocks of tissue have been shown to detect 90 per cent of carcinomas, including all those poorly differentiated tumours with corresponding metastatic potential.

The precursors of prostatic carcinoma are obviously difficult to study in such an inaccessible organ, but nevertheless a number of lesions thought to be precancerous have been described. In the normal course of events the peripheral portions of the gland undergo involution with age, the hyperplastic process that leads to benign nodular hyperplasia occurring in the more central parts of the gland. It is thus a little difficult to explain why these atrophic glands should be the forerunners of malignancy. Early studies described papillary ingrowths into these atrophic glands and suggested that this secondary hyperplasia evolved into carcinoma; later, solid outgrowths of cells were described, infiltrating dense fibrous tissue in this region, a process called *post-sclerotic hyperplasia*. More recently, *dysplasia* or *prostatic intra-epithelial neoplasia* (PIN) has been reported to be present in radical prostatectomy specimens resected for prostatic cancer (see above). As at other sites where the only tissue available for study is that removed at definitive resection of all malignant tissue, definite evidence that such histological entities progress to invasive cancer or that all carcinomas evolve from such abnormalities is difficult, if not impossible to prove. Similarly, the association of carcinoma with benign nodular hyperplasia is controversial and is complicated by problems in the definition of the latter; however, the fact that the two conditions arise from different parts of the gland makes it extremely unlikely that they are in any way related.

Macroscopical appearance and spread

Small carcinomas may be difficult to identify with the naked eye (Fig. 20.14) but larger tumours are recognizable as firm, indistinct white masses obviously infiltrating adjacent tissues, such as bladder base or seminal vesicle (Fig. 20.15), with concomitant blockage of ureters and obstructive renal failure.

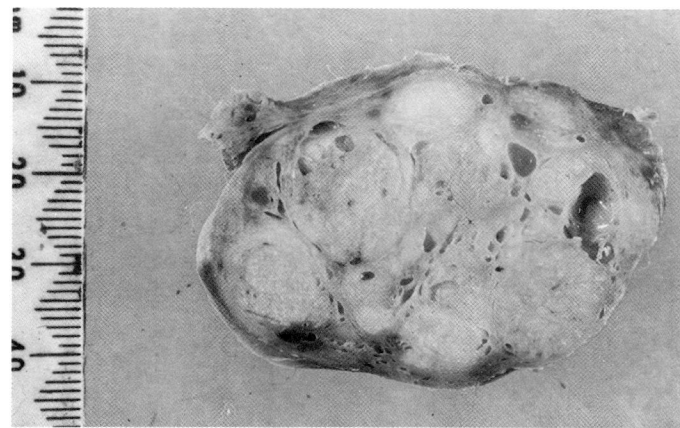

Fig. 20.14 Retropubic prostatectomy specimen. Small focus of indistinct white tissue at top centre proved to be a small carcinoma.

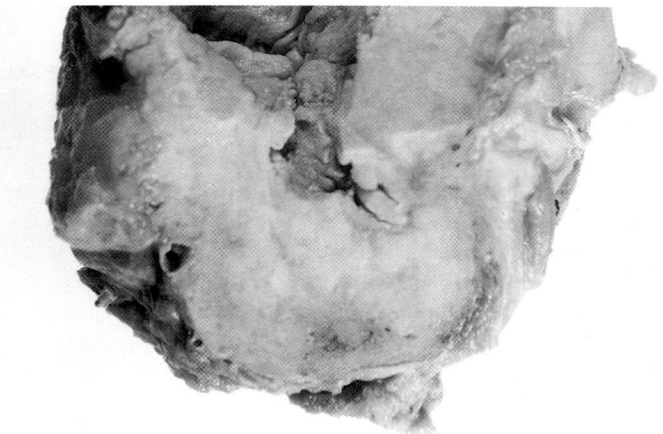

Fig. 20.15 Extensive prostatic carcinoma invading the base of the bladder.

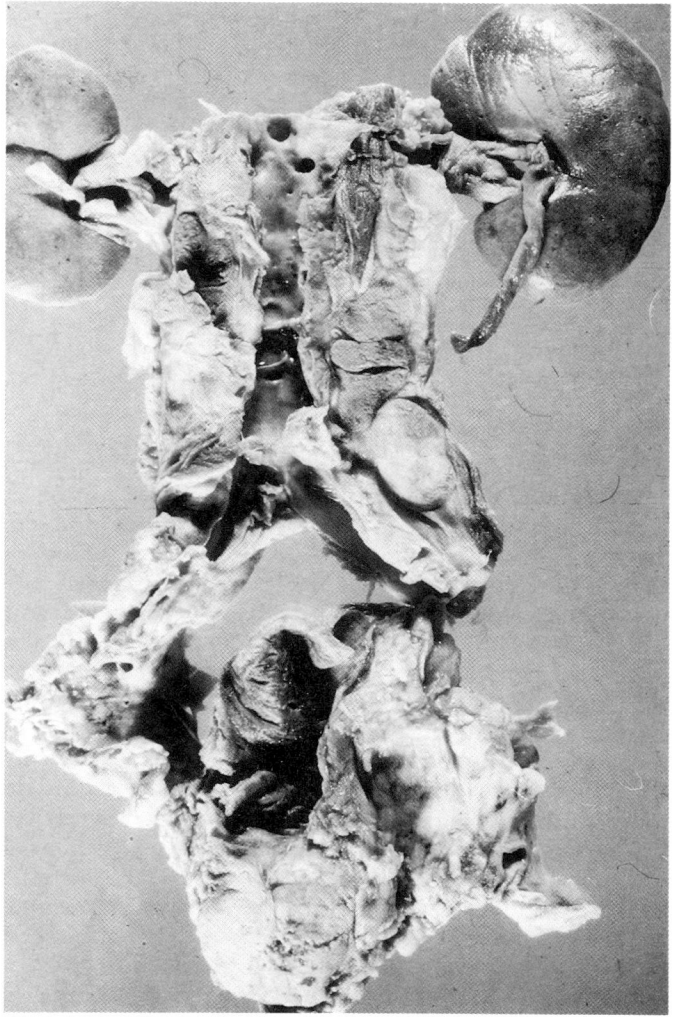

Fig. 20.16 Carcinoma of the prostate with extensive spread to the para-aortic lymph nodes.

Invasion of the rectum is less common as a dense layer of connective tissue, *Dennovillier's fascia*, lies between these two organs. Some tumours contain considerable quantities of lipid and may have a yellowish hue; this characteristic was occasionally used in the past to identify prostatic carcinoma, but is of no real value now except possibly at autopsy.

Prostatic carcinoma spreads principally via the lymphatics, initially to pelvic lymph nodes and thence more widely, such that enlarged para-aortic lymph nodes are commonly found at post-mortem (Fig. 20.16). Haematogenous spread to lungs is also frequently seen at autopsy and bony metastases are also common; very often these osseous secondary deposits are osteoblastic, giving a sclerotic appearance on X-ray (Fig. 20.17). These bony metastases are frequently noted in the lumbar vertebrae in X-rays taken at the time of an intravenous urogram, and for many years it was taught that metastases were of much higher incidence in this region due to retrograde spread along the extensive plexus of venous channels linking

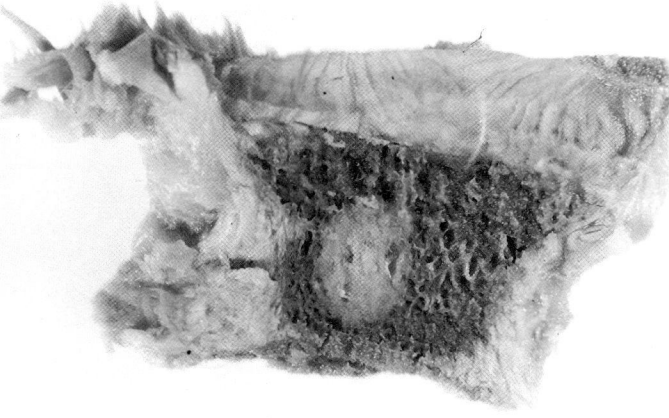

Fig. 20.17 Dense osteosclerostic metastasis of carcinoma of the prostate in a vertebral body.

the pelvis to the lumbar vertebrae (*Batson's plexus*). This concept has now been discredited, the high incidence reported in this region in the past being almost certainly due to this being the area of skeleton most frequently X-rayed in patients with urological disease, and the lumbar vertebrae being the most accessible portions of the skeleton available for examination at routine autopsy. In fact Willis challenged the idea that prostatic secondaries were more common in the pelvic bones many years ago on evidence from his careful extensive autopsies on such cases, where he found no predilection for this site. Recent radiological studies have also failed to demonstrate an excess of metastases in the lumbar vertebrae as compared to the rest of the skeleton.

Microscopical appearances

The majority of carcinomas of the prostate arise from acinar epithelium but they have a wide spectrum of histological appearances due in part to their very varied degree of differentiation. Although a number of defined histological patterns have been described (see below), 90 per cent or more are mere variants of acinar carcinoma and, with the exception of grading (see below), there is no clinicopathological significance in identifying the pattern present. The well-differentiated tumour has a typical acinar configuration (Fig. 20.18), often with an intraglandular papillary structure. Extensive intra-acinar proliferation gives a typical cribriform structure and, if this growth is extensive, central necrosis leads to a comedo-like picture. Less differentiated tumours are not so obviously glandular and have to be distinguished from invasive bladder tumours. Prostatic carcinomas have more prominent nucleoli than transitional cell tumours, although the introduction of immunocytochemistry to demonstrate prostate-specific antigen and prostate-specific acid phosphatase now enables the identification of nearly all poorly differentiated tumours of uncertain origin. Prostatic carcinoma often varies considerably in appearance in different areas (Fig. 20.19) and this has led to some difficulties in the grading of these tumours.

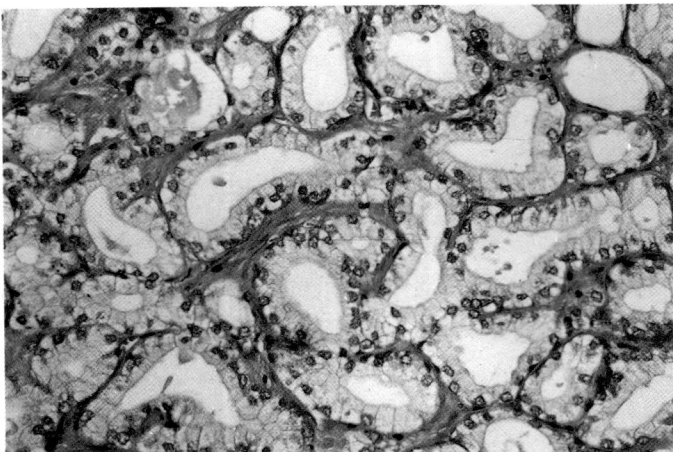

Fig. 20.18 Well-differentiated carcinoma of the prostate composed of closely packed neoplastic glands.

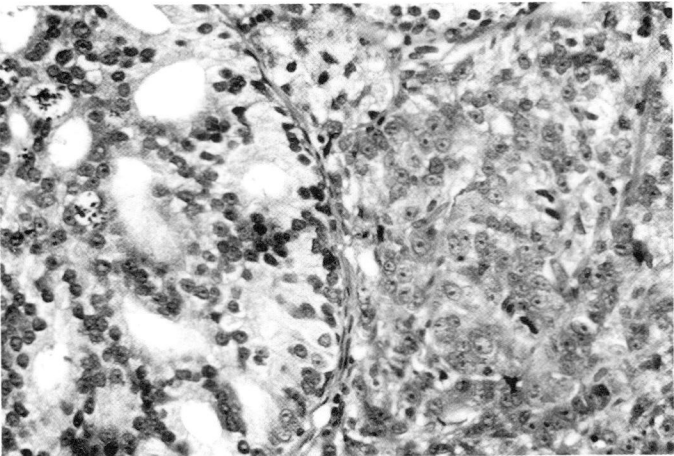

Fig. 20.19 Carcinoma of the prostate with a variable histological pattern. A poorly differentiated tumour can be seen on the right and a cribriform carcinoma on the left.

The prostatic ducts are lined by acinar-like cells until the change to the transitional epithelium of the urothelium. Earlier descriptions of a distinct adenocarcinoma of ductal origin are now largely discredited—these tumours being regarded as mere variants of acinar adenocarcinoma since they have been shown to have identical immunohistochemical features and to behave in a similar manner to typical prostatic carcinoma; this also applies to the so-called *endometrial carcinoma of the verumontanum* which was thought to arise from tissue of a different embryological origin—the uterus masculinus.

Incidental (latent) carcinoma: grading and staging

Earlier, reference was made to the fact that frequently, in both autopsy and surgical practice, prostatic carcinoma is found with no evidence of metastases. Obviously this is of no importance at post-mortem, but what should be done in patients when the tumour is found incidentally after an operation for prostatism? This is of considerable importance since although we know that a good proportion of prostatic cancers respond to hormone manipulation, oestrogen therapy is not without significant risks. A large survey in the USA in the 1960s investigating the effect of oestrogen therapy on prostatic cancer showed convincingly that there was a higher mortality and morbidity in treated patients with small, well-differentiated tumours that had not metastasized, as compared to controls. Subsequent studies reinforced the view that patients with a small, well-differentiated tumour, found incidentally, rarely develop metastatic disease (latent or incidental cancer) and do not require oestrogen therapy with its concomitant risk of atherosclerotic and thromboembolic disease. At the same time, a number of histological grading systems for prostatic cancer have evolved, of which the *Gleason* is the best known. This method attempts to avoid the problem of the well-known variability in degrees of differentiation that may occur in various regions of a single prostatic tumour. Two patterns or degrees of differentiation may be identified and each given a numerical score ranging from 1, the most well differentiated, to 5, the least. In this way scores of between 2 and 10 are obtained (1:1 up to 5:5).

Other studies have found that prostatic cancer may spread to pelvic lymph nodes which are not enlarged on CT scanning. In some specialized centres, particularly in the USA, these lymph nodes are dissected out in order to accurately stage the tumour.

Staging and grading are used predominantly in centres where radical prostatectomy is performed and, as this is rarely done in the UK, such techniques are of limited importance in this country. Thus in clinical practice, in the elderly patient most urologists would not give oestrogen treatment when an incidental carcinoma is found. But for the younger patient the situation is still controversial, since a number of recent long-term follow-up studies in the USA of patients with such tumours has found that some do in fact progress. Since we also know that transurethral resection does not usually remove all the cancer present, the case for radical prostatectomy for this disease in younger men looks quite convincing.

Cytology

For patients with suspected metastatic prostatic cancer, and for those with firm suspicious nodules in the gland but not requiring prostatic resection, the diagnosis of malignancy may be confirmed by two methods. Guided-needle biopsy via the rectum will produce a core of tissue for histological assessment and save the patient the necessity of the anaesthetic required for transurethral resection, as well as being more likely to sample the tumour-bearing area. Alternatively, needle biopsy may be used to produce a sample for cytological assessment; this technique is widely practised on the European continent where it is often combined with flow cytometry.

Rarer tumours

Very rarely, prostatic cancers produce sufficient mucin to warrant the term of *mucoid carcinoma*; more commonly frankly mucin-secreting tumours are likely to be large bowel tumours invading the organ. Similarly, transitional cell carcinoma in the prostate is usually a result of spread from a bladder tumour, although it may occasionally occur as a primary tumour arising from ducts or the prostatic urethra.

Other tumours are distinctly rare; sarcomas occur occasionally, the most common being the *rhabdomyosarcoma* of young men; lymphomas and leukaemias may present with prostatic symptoms or, alternatively, such symptoms develop during the course of the illness.

20.1.5 Further reading

Bostwick, D. G. (1990). *Pathology of the prostate*. Churchill Livingstone, Edinburgh.

Epstein, J. I. (1989). *Prostate biopsy interpretation*. Raven Press, New York.

Murphy, W. M. and Gaeta, J. F. (1989). Diseases of the prostate gland and seminal vesicles. In *Urological pathology* (ed. W. M. Murphy), ch. 3. W. B. Saunders, Philadelphia.

20.2 Seminal vesicles

I. D. Ansell

The seminal vesicles are paired, blind-ending saccular glands which are situated above the prostate and run posteriorly between the bladder and rectum. The *vasa deferentia* pass between them and join with the ducts from the seminal vesicles to form the ejaculatory ducts.

These glands are composed of a single main duct from which arise several subsidiary ducts that terminate in alveoli which are lined by a simple secretory epithelium. The secretory cells contain pigment of lipofuscin type. The glandular tissue is loosely invested by a connective tissue stroma with an outer smooth muscle coat.

The glandular secretion is a mucoid material which is rich in fructose, prostaglandins, and fibrinogen. This secretion is emptied into the ejaculatory duct during ejaculation. It increases the quantity of the ejaculate, the fructose nourishes the spermatozoa on their route to potential fertilization, and the prostaglandins and fibrinogen play a role in enhancing fertilization.

With increasing age a significant number of the lining epithelial cells develop large, hyperchromatic nuclei which have been labelled *monstrous nuclei* (Fig. 20.20). Care should be taken not to confuse these with malignancy, especially in needle biopsies of the prostate.

20.2.1 Developmental abnormalities

Developmental abnormalities of the seminal vesicles are

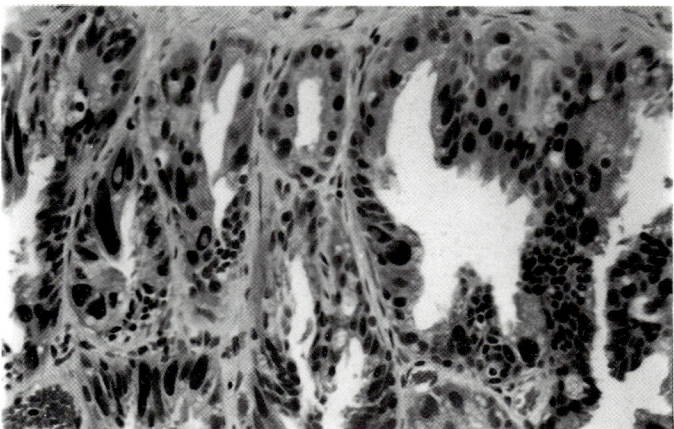

Fig. 20.20 Pleomorphic ('monstrous') nuclei seen in the epithelium of the seminal vesicles.

extremely rare. When they do occur they are usually associated with abnormalities of the ureter and they are cystic in type.

20.2.2   Inflammation

Inflammation of the seminal vesicles is almost invariably associated with inflammation of the prostate. It may be non-specific secondary to instrumentation of the urethra, or it may be secondary to *gonococcal or tuberculous prostatitis*.

20.2.3   Tumours

Tumours of the seminal vesicles are very rare. There are a few reports of cystadenomas. Reported malignant tumours are mainly adenocarcinomas and the bulk of these represent secondary spread from the prostate. To diagnose primary seminal vesicle origin it is necessary to demonstrate an uninvolved prostate gland. Other features in support of primary origin are the presence of lipofuscin pigment within, and the absence of prostatic-specific antigen from the tumour cells. Sarcomas have been reported and a case with both malignant epithelial and stromal elements has been recorded.

20.2.4   Further reading

Guyton, A. C. (1987). *Human physiology and mechanisms of disease* (4th edn), pp. 618–28. W. B. Saunders, Philadelphia.

Mazur, M. T., Myers, J. L., and Maddox, W. A. (1987). Cystic epithelial-stromal tumor of the seminal vesicle. *American Journal of Surgical Pathology* **11**, 210–17.

Warwick, R. and Williams, P. L. (1973). *Gray's anatomy* (35th edn). W. B. Saunders, Philadelphia.

Williamson, R. C. N. (1978). Seminal vesicle tumours. *Journal of the Royal Society of Medicine* **71**, 286–8.

20.3   Testes and appendages

L. Bobrow

20.3.1   Normal structure and function

There is a close relationship between the embryological development of the genital and urinary tracts. The kidneys and the gonads arise from the two urogenital ridges which give origin to the mesonephric and subsequently, in the male, to the genital excretory ducts. At about the third week of embryological development the primitive germ cells migrate from the yolk sac endoderm along the posterior midline of the embryo into the *primitive sex cords*. The primitive sex cords are thought to arise as condensations of mesenchyme with subsequent downgrowths contributed from the overlying coelomic epithelium. The *Sertoli* and *Leydig* cells probably arise from a common precursor cell in the gonadal mesenchyme. *Seminiferous tubules*

develop in the second trimester from the sex cords. The sex cords also give origin to the *tubuli recti*, and *rete testis* which then fuse with the mesonephric tubules. The cephalad mesonephric tubules give rise to the *efferent ductuli* which connect with the *vas deferens*.

The testis normally descends via the inguinal canal to the scrotum sometime during or after the seventh month of fetal development. Testicular descent appears to be closely related to the presence and development of the *gubernaculum* which is a fibrous connection between the epididymis and the scrotum. There is also a muscular component in the gubernaculum which is contributed from the origin of the cremaster around the scrotal ligament.

The testes are not fully developed at birth. They are paired ovoid organs measuring, in the adult approximately $4 \times 3.5 \times 3$ cm each. Each testis is surrounded by a thickened capsule, the *tunica albuginea*, which encloses the coiled seminiferous tubules which are invested by a loose fibrovascular connective tissue containing the interstitial or Leydig cells. The *epididymis* is closely apposed to the posterior and lateral surfaces of the testis. The seminiferous tubules converge and fuse into a group of six or more *ductuli efferentia* which connect with the *caput or head* of the epididymis and then connect via the body to the tail. The epididymi are composed of a loose fibrovascular stroma in which are embedded the epididymal tubules. The epididymis joins the vas deferens almost at the lower pole of the testis. The vas deferens now runs with the nerves and blood vessels of the testis through the inguinal canal as the spermatic cord. Once in the pelvis the vas leaves the spermatic cord and continues to the posterior aspect of the bladder where it is joined by the duct of the seminal vesicle. This fused structure now continues as the ejaculatory duct through the prostate gland to emerge at the verumontanum with the opposite ejaculatory duct into the prostatic urethra.

Normal microanatomy of the testis

Each testis contains approximately 250 lobules which are separated from one another by fibrous septae which take origin from the fibrous capsule surrounding the testis called the tunica albuginea. Each lobule contains 2–4 convoluted seminiferous tubules which run from the capsule inwards to join the tubuli recti. The seminiferous tubules contain the *germinal epithelium* and the *sustentacular or Sertoli cells*. The germinal epithelium is composed of cells in the various stages of spermatogenesis. These are *type A and type B spermatogonia* which, by mitotic division, give rise to *primary spermatocytes*. These in turn, by primary meiotic division, give rise *to secondary spermatocytes* which, following secondary meiotic division, give rise to *spermatids*. The spermatids now undergo a process of maturation, termed *spermiogenesis*, to *spermatozoa*. This orderly development from spermatogonium to spermatozoon is termed the *cycle of the seminiferous epithelium*. Associations of different developmental types represent the stages of the cycle. In man they are less well defined and occupy smaller areas than in laboratory animals, on which much of the published descriptions are based. In man, therefore, sections of testis show tubules in which different associations are seen merging into each other, and occasionally one or more cell type is sparse or lacking (Fig. 20.21).

The Sertoli cells in normal adult seminiferous epithelium lie on the basement membrane of the seminiferous tubule with the nucleus situated close to this structure (Fig. 20.21). The cell extends from the basement membrane to the lumen of the seminiferous tubule and has junctions with adjacent Sertoli cells, thus providing close contact with all elements of the developing germ cells, up to and including the spermatids. The Sertoli cell synthesizes steroids and this function is controlled by *pituitary follicle stimulating hormone* (FSH). They also secrete *FSH-inhibiting factor* and, for a limited period during embryogenesis, a substance called *Müllerian inhibiting substance*. This latter substance causes regression of the Müllerian duct system. The seminiferous tubules are invested by a delicate connective tissue, which contains abundant blood vessels, lymphatics, nerves, reticulin fibres, fibroblasts, and Leydig cells.

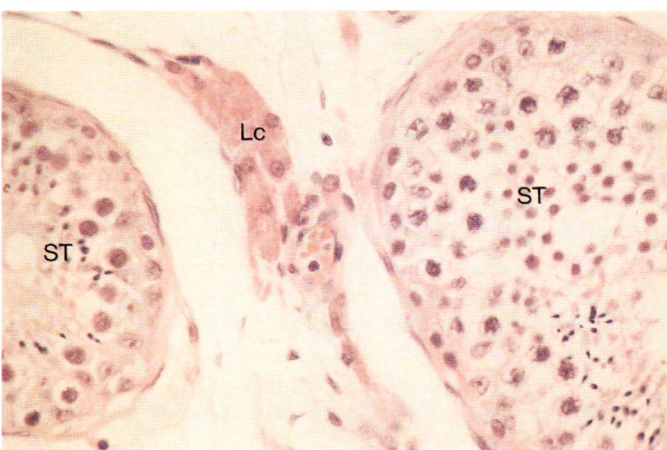

Fig. 20.21 A photomicrograph from a section of normal adult testis showing clumps of Leydig cells (Lc) in close apposition to a capillary lying in the interstices between two seminiferous tubules (ST). The tubules both contain an epithelium showing active spermatogenesis. Some of the different cell associations in spermatogenesis are well illustrated in this section.

The *Leydig or interstitial cells* are scattered singly or in groups usually in close relationship with a capillary (Fig. 20.21) and on section are seen to occupy 3 per cent of the total area. These cells are large and polygonal with eosinophilic cytoplasm and occasionally are seen to contain the characteristic *crystals of Reinke*. Ultrastructurally these cells contain abundant smooth endoplasmic reticulum. They are responsible for the secretion of testosterone under the influence of *pituitary luteinizing hormone* (LH) secretion.

The efferent ducts are lined by an epithelium containing ciliated and non-ciliated cuboidal cells which rest on a basement membrane with an incomplete coat of smooth muscle cells.

The epididymis is composed of a very convoluted tubule which is lined by a columnar epithelium with a microvillous surface. Beneath the basement membrane is a complete circular muscle coat. The vas is also lined by a ciliated columnar epithelium with occasional small, round basal cells. The muscle coat thickens up to three coats around the vas.

The epididymis elaborates a copious secretion which contains hormones, enzymes, and nutrients. Within the epididymis spermatozoa acquire the property of motility. The epididymis also acts as a reservoir for spermatozoa, which can remain here for several months retaining full functional activity.

20.3.2 Developmental anomalies

Persistence of embryonic remnants

Appendix of epididymis

The appendix of the epididymis is a mesonephric remnant which is present in approximately 25 per cent of testes. It is a cystic pedunculated structure which overlies the head of the epididymis. The cyst is lined by a tall columnar epithelium and the surrounding connective tissue coat has an outer covering of mesothelium. The epididymal appendage can undergo torsion.

Appendix of testis (Synonym: hydatid of Morgagni)

The hydatid of Morgagni is a Müllerian remnant which is present in approximately 90 per cent of testes. It is a cystic pedunculated structure which is situated near the antero-superior pole of the testis. The appendix testis can undergo torsion.

Ectopic tissue related to the male gonad

Ectopic adrenal cortex

Ectopic adrenal cortex may be seen anywhere along the course of the spermatic cord or epididymis, or within the substance of the testis or tunica albuginea. Within the testicular parenchyma it must be differentiated from a Leydig cell tumour, which lacks the zoning of cells present in adrenal cortical tissue. The presence of Reinke's crystals within Leydig tumour cells is also a useful parameter in this context.

Ectopic splenic tissue

Ectopic splenic tissue may rarely occur in association with spermatic cord, epididymis, or testis. It is almost invariably left-sided and is frequently associated with other developmental anomalies.

Simple cysts of the testis and the epididymis

See Section 20.3.7.

Atresias of the efferent ducts of the male genital system

Partial or complete atresias of all parts of the efferent ducts in the male genital system have been recorded. Bilateral complete absence of the vasa deferens has been reported in up to 2 per cent of males attending an infertility clinic. More frequently a segmental atresia of this structure is recorded. These segmental atresias are almost always at the epididymal end. Atresias of parts of the excretory duct system are occasionally present in patients with cystic fibrosis. Partial or complete absence of the seminal vesicles and ejaculatory ducts are sometimes seen in association with atresias, particularly those of the vas.

Variation in the number of testes

Absence of both testes (*anorchism*), absence of one testis (*monorchism*), and the presence of more than two testes (*polyorchism*) have all been recorded occasionally. Absence of one or both testes may be associated with absence of the related epididymis, seminal vesicle, or spermatic cord. Three is the largest number of testes recorded in the literature. The extra gonad may be situated anywhere along the normal route of testicular descent. It is usually smaller than a normal testis and, in most instances, has a complete epididymal reduplication associated with it. The supernumerary testis may communicate with the vas of the ipsilateral testis or it may have its own vas. The presence of an undiagnosed extra testis has been reported following the observed persistence of normal sperm counts in a patient following vasectomy. More significant than the above is the possible occurrence of malignancy in an undiagnosed supernumerary testis.

Variations in the position of testes

One or both testes may come to lie at a site not on the normal pathway of testicular descent. These are termed *ectopic testes*.

Ectopic testes

Ectopic testes occur most commonly in the subcutaneous tissues of the perineum and in this site they are particularly liable to injury. Other less common sites of ectopia are the pelvis, overlying the aponeurosis of the anterior abdominal wall, the upper part of the thigh, the root of the penis, and within the contralateral scrotal sac.

Cryptorchidism

Cryptorchidism or true maldescent of the testis is much more common than ectopia. These testes are arrested somewhere along the normal path of testicular descent. The testis normally descends into the scrotum sometime after the sixth month of gestation. In normal full-term deliveries both testes are present in the scrotum at birth in 97 per cent of infants. Descent is delayed in prematurity but by the end of the first year of life the incidence of undescended testes is the same as in the adult. The frequency of undescended testes in adult males is about 0.8 per cent. It is unilateral in most cases but has been reported as bilateral in between 10 and 20 per cent of cases.

Undescended testes are situated most commonly within the inguinal canal. Less commonly they lie more superficially in the inguinal region. A small number are arrested within the abdomen. Failure of testicular descent in a small number of cases is clearly related to pituitary gonadotrophin deficiency. In these cases the maldescent is bilateral and other stigmata of pituitary deficiency are usually apparent. In the vast majority of cases hormonal imbalance or deficiency is not present. Various ana-

tomical abnormalities have been implicated in a proportion of cases. These include absent or abnormal gubernaculum, shortness of the structures in the spermatic cord, incomplete development of the inguinal canal, presence of fibrous bands or adhesions along the route of descent, and complete absence of the external inguinal ring. It has also been suggested that the testis fails to descend normally because it has an underlying primary abnormality. This view is strongly supported by comparative biopsy studies carried out on ectopic and undescended testes at the time of corrective operation. These studies showed that although some of the ectopic testes had evidence of impaired fertility, the undescended testes (as a group) were more frequently abnormal and that these abnormalities always included significant impairment of fertility as judged by the numbers of germ cells per tubule in these biopsies. The opponents of this view argue that the changes observed in these testes are related to the higher temperature these testes are exposed to by virtue of their position; the validity of this argument is supported by the observation that intra-abdominal testes generally show fewer germ cells per tubule than do testes arrested more superficially on their path of descent.

An undescended testis is usually smaller than normal. It is often firmer in consistency due to the laying down of fibrous tissue but the degree of fibrosis will vary depending on the age of the patient. In the pre-pubertal testis the only microscopic abnormality observed is a diminution in the number of germ cells. This change appears to be irreversible. After puberty progressive degenerative changes occur (Fig. 20.22). The diminution in the number of germ cells is reflected in a diminished or absent spermatogenesis. The peritubular basement membrane shows varying degrees of thickening and hyalinization and the tubular diameter becomes decreased. Sertoli cells appear prominent within the tubules because of the diminution or absence of the spermatogenic series. However, eventually they too may disap-

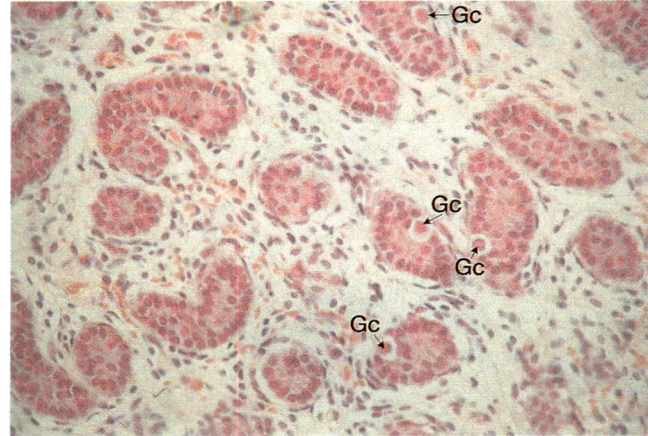

Fig. 20.22 A photomicrograph from a section of an undescended testis removed from an adolescent male. Note the many small seminiferous tubules separated by recently laid-down fibrous tissue. The tubules are largely filled by undifferentiated Sertoli cells. Only four of the 20 tubule cross-sections contain primitive germ cells (Gc). Leydig cells are not identifiable in the interstitium.

pear, leaving a solid hyaline ghost as the only remnant of the testicular tubular structure. The Leydig cells appear morphologically unremarkable but there is an apparent increase in their number because of the shrinkage of the tubular mass. There is frequently a marked increase in interstitial fibrous tissue. The changes described above are commonly associated with infertility, particularly if both testes are affected. Undescended testes are often associated with an inguinal hernia. Patients with undescended testes have a significantly increased chance of developing a germ cell cancer. This risk is not necessarily diminished by surgical placement of the testis in the scrotum, although there is some evidence to suggest that surgical correction of the malposition before 5 years of age may diminish the risk. The contralateral testis is also at increased risk of undergoing malignant change, but the risk is not as great as that in the affected testis. *Seminomas and teratomas* are the types of germ cell neoplasms most commonly encountered in patients with a history of undescended testis. The observation of carcinoma *in situ* in a number of testicular biopsies carried out on males with a history of undescended testis attending an infertility clinic, has been reported. The significance of these observations has been confirmed by several follow-up reports of the development of invasive germ cell malignancies in some of these cases.

20.3.3 Dysgenetic testicular abnormalities

Early in the fifth week of embryonic development, two ridges appear on the posterior coelomic cavity on either side of, and parallel to, the midline. These are the *genital ridges* and they give rise to the definitive gonad. Whether this is a testis or an ovary is determined by the presence or absence of the *testis-determining factor (TDF) gene* which is present on the short arm of the Y-chromosome. TDF exerts its effect on the Sertoli cell and subsequent development of the testicular identity is probably under the control of the Sertoli cell. In the absence of TDF the gonad develops ovarian features.

In the developing testis the medullary portion of the genital ridge proliferates and, with a contribution from the overlying surface epithelium, the primitive sex cords develop. These will ultimately give rise to the seminiferous tubules. The cortical portion of the gonad in the XY fetus involutes at this stage but persists in part in the adult as part of the tunica albuginea.

Hormonal factors play a role in the development of the gonad, as well as being of fundamental importance to the elaboration of the secondary sexual characteristics. Sertoli-cell androgen secretion is important for initiation and maintenance of spermatogenesis in the adult; fetal Sertoli cells secrete Müllerian inhibiting substance which, as its name implies, affects the involution of the Müllerian system. Leydig cell androgen secretion is important in effecting the development of the Wolffian duct system and in initiation and maintenance of the secondary sex characteristics.

Single gene defects

XX male

During meiosis in the male, short regions of the X- and Y-chromosomes pair and exchange material. Occasionally the crossing-over process goes wrong and there is transfer of testis-determining sequences from the Y to the X chromosome. This error gives rise to *XX males*.

These males are generally phenotypically normal although they may have an abnormal hair distribution. Libido may be reduced.

The testicular histology in reported cases shows features of pre-pubertal atrophy.

Testicular feminization

This condition is inherited as an X-linked trait and its incidence is estimated to be 1 per 60 000 males. It arises as a result of a resistance at the cellular level to normal circulating androgens. This aberration is caused by a mutation affecting the *cytosol receptor for androgens*. It is the commonest form of *male pseudohermaphroditism*. In the *complete form* the external genitalia and secondary sex characteristics are female in type. The condition usually presents at puberty with primary amenorrhoea, unless there is a family history. Pubic and axillary hair are scanty, the vagina is short and blind-ending. The uterus, epididymi, vasa deferentia, seminal vesicles, and prostate are absent. The testes are usually intra-abdominal but may be located within the inguinal canal.

The gonads are usually small unless they are involved by tumour. The cut surface is diffuse brownish with one or more small discrete nodules of a lighter yellow-brown colour. A nodular condensation of smooth muscle may be present at one pole of the testis.

Microscopically the diffuse areas are composed of immature solid seminiferous tubules set in a stroma which frequently resembles that of the normal ovary. The tubules may contain spermatogonia but spermatogenesis is not seen. Prominent clumps of Leydig cells are also frequently present. The macroscopic nodules are composed of closely aggregated seminiferous tubules which are lined by very regular immature Sertoli cells and may contain central hyaline material or, on occasion, calcospherites. Clumps of Leydig cells are also sometimes a feature of these nodules. Depending on the different contributions of the above elements, the nodules are termed *hamartomas*, or *Sertoli cell adenomas*. If a pure Leydig cell nodule exceeds 1 cm in diameter the possibility of a Leydig cell tumour should be considered.

Like intra-abdominal testes of other types, these too are at an increased risk of undergoing malignant change. The malignancy is usually a seminoma.

A group of patients with an *incomplete form* of testicular feminization is also recognized. This condition, like the complete form, is also familial and is also transmitted on the X-chromosome.

Chromosomal anomalies

Klinefelter's syndrome

This syndrome, as originally described by Klinefelter and colleagues in 1942, comprised hypogonadism characterized by gynaecomastia, azoospermia, testicular atrophy, and increase in gonadotrophin production. Subsequently it was observed that these cases could be subdivided into *chromatin-positive* and *chromatin-negative* groups. Presently, the designation 'Klinefelter's syndrome' is only used for the chromosome-positive group, i.e. those who have at least one extra X-chromosome. The frequency of the condition thus defined is between 1 per 1000 and 1 per 1400 male live births in the general population. The basic karyotype in these cases is 47XXY but there are cases with more than two X- or one Y-chromosomes and there are also many cases showing mosaicism with at least one cell line containing an extra X-chromosome.

The most consistent clinical features of the syndrome are:

1. *eunuchoidism* of varying degree;
2. *gynaecomastia*, which is present in just over 50 per cent of cases and is usually bilateral;
3. *normal external genitalia* but testes of reduced size;
4. increased excretion of *follicle stimulating hormone* and reduced excretion of *17-ketosteroids*.

A minority of cases show mild mental retardation.

Microscopically the picture seen in these testes is a fairly characteristic one. There is an apparent reduction in the volume of the seminiferous tubules and the majority of those still present are completely hyalinized and usually devoid of elastic fibres. A few small tubules containing immature Sertoli cells only are also frequently seen. The presence of any germ cells, with or without evidence of spermatogenesis, is rare and is believed possibly to indicate the presence of *mosaicism* with a normal 46XY line as part of the mosaic. The Leydig cells are present as large clumps between the shrunken sclerosed tubules and many of them contain an excess of lipofuscin pigment in their cytoplasm. The actual volume of the Leydig cell mass may be decreased, normal, or increased. Where pre-pubertal study of these testes has been possible, the earliest change observed has been a marked deficiency of germ cells.

True hermaphroditism

This is a condition in which ovarian and testicular tissue are present in the same individual. There have been over 300 case reports in the literature of this unusual condition. As defined above, these cases contain both male and female gonadal tissue within them. In approximately a third of the cases the gonads are an ovary plus a contralateral intra-abdominal testis. In about a quarter of the cases the gonads are *bilateral ovotestes*. The remainder comprise ovotestis plus contralateral ovary and testis or bilateral distinct ovary and testis.

Seventy-five per cent of the published cases have a normal karyotype; of these about 80 per cent are female and the remainder are male. The remaining 25 per cent have varying sex-chromosomal mosaicisms.

The external genitalia and secondary sexual characteristics do not necessarily correspond to the chromosomal sex of these cases. Frequently they are ambiguous. The majority present with hypospadias and cryptorchidism. The internal genitalia

have a tendency to differentiate in the same direction as the ipsilateral gonad. Bilateral inguinal herniae are a common complication of this condition.

Microscopically the testicular tissue in these cases has similar features to those seen in abdominally placed testes, except that the recognizable testicular tissue is often very scanty and disorganized by interstitial fibrosis. In very rare cases active spermatogenesis has been observed in some tubules.

XYY syndrome

These patients are phenotypically normal, except that they are, on average, taller than the normal population. The fertility of the group as a whole is slightly diminished so they may first present at an infertility clinic.

The histological appearance can be quite varied, but usually in infertile XYY males there is a tubular abnormality which is either a *spermatogenic arrest* at the primary spermatocyte level or consists of tubules lined by Sertoli cells only.

Duchenne muscular dystrophy

This is an X-linked inherited condition in which there is progressive juvenile muscular dystrophy and, in a proportion of cases, there is a mild associated hypogonadism. The patients rarely reach adulthood so the testicular histology is usually not relevant. The histological changes described are similar to those seen in Klinefelter's syndrome. A post-pubertal type of testicular atrophy is documented in patients with myotonic dystrophy.

20.3.4   Inflammation

Infective

Inflammatory disorders of the testis may be acute or chronic and both forms are frequently associated with epididymitis. The majority are secondary to retrograde spread of urinary tract infections. A small number are due to venous or lymphatic spread of organisms, or as part of septicaemia in the course of acute infection originating elsewhere in the body. The commonest causative agents are Gram-negative organisms but other bacterial species, viruses, fungi, and rickettsiae have all been implicated. Amongst the acute orchitides, those occurring as part of a mumps infection are worthy of separate note.

Mumps orchitis

Mumps is an acute febrile illness of childhood caused by a virus. Usually there is acute swelling and tenderness of the parotid glands. Occasionally other salivary glands, the gonads, or the pancreas are involved. The disease occurs uncommonly in adults, but when it does the incidence of testicular involvement in males is believed to be over 20 per cent. Occasionally it is the only clinical manifestation of the disease. Usually the testicular swelling appears as the salivary gland swelling is subsiding. The swelling is most often one-sided but in about 15 per cent of cases it is bilateral. The testis is extremely tender due to intense oedema involving the whole organ including the tunica vaginalis.

Microscopically there is marked vascular dilation with extravasation of fluid into the tissue compartment. Initially a moderate infiltrate of neutrophils is seen in the interstitium. Later this is replaced by a very dense infiltrate of lymphocytes. Necrosis of the germ cell series is seen. Macrophages and neutrophils are seen within the tubular lumina in relation to the necrosis. Surviving Sertoli cells are also seen intermingled with the inflammatory infiltrate in the seminiferous tubules. With regression of the infection, organization of the exudate occurs and some degree of fibrosis of the interstitium is likely. Regeneration of specialized germ cells occurs only in the tubules where residual viable germ cells still exist. The extent of the fibrosis, atrophy, and germ cell loss is dependent on the severity of the acute phase of the orchitis. All the features of a full-blown post-pubertal atrophy as described in Section 20.3.6 may be present in the late stages of these cases. The persistence of a scattering of interstitial lymphocytes may serve as a clue to the viral aetiology of this atrophy. Significant atrophy following known mumps orchitis is reported in 45 per cent of cases in one series.

Human immunodeficiency virus (HIV) infection

Patients dying from HIV infection almost invariably show pathological changes in their testes. There is diminution in spermatogenesis, usually of a marked degree. Varying degrees of tubular basement thickening and vascular intimal thickening is also seen. Chronic inflammatory cell infiltrates are occasionally present. In a proportion of cases with generalized opportunistic infections direct involvement of the testes also occurs.

There are several forms of chronic orchitis worthy of comment.

Syphilitic orchitis

The testes may be involved in both congenital and acquired syphilis. In both instances the involvement may take the form of diffuse fibrosis with endarteritis obliterans and plasma cell infiltration, or of discrete gummatous lesions. In congenital syphilis the gummatous lesions are unusual and if they do occur they are microscopic in size. In acquired syphilis the testes are involved in the tertiary phase and gummatous lesions are more common than fibrotic lesions. The syphilitic lesion in acquired syphilis may be mistakenly diagnosed as a tumour by the clinician.

The involved testes are painless and may be enlarged or slightly contracted. The cut surface shows areas of firm fibrosis with a single or scattered multiple areas of yellow to grey necrosis, of varying size up to about 3 cm in diameter. The necrosis may extend to the surface and involve the tunica vaginalis. This may be associated with a hydrocoele or with direct extension into the overlying scrotal skin. Microscopically the gummatous areas show necrosis with preservation of the underlying architecture, and the intervening tissue shows the characteristic fibrosis infiltrated by lymphocytes and plasma cells. Occasional multinucleate giant cells may also be present. If the lesion is purely fibrotic, the microscopic picture is as above without the areas of necrosis.

Tuberculous epididymo-orchitis

Tuberculous infection reaches the epididymis by retrograde spread from the urinary tract and is therefore almost invariably associated with tuberculous involvement of the urinary tract, and this is usually secondary to a primary pulmonary focus. Rarely, and usually in advanced disease only, the infection extends into the adjacent testicular tissue. The involved epididymis is usually enlarged, soft and firm, or fluctuant. The ipsilateral cord frequently has palpable bead-like thickenings on it. Caseation may extend outwards to involve the scrotum and thus give rise to sinus formation. Microscopically the lesion shows characteristic caseating granulomata.

Malacoplakia of the testis and epididymis

The term malacoplakia literally means 'soft plaques' and was originally used to refer to lesions with this macroscopic appearance on the bladder mucosa. Microscopically it is a chronic granulomatous lesion which is characterized by the presence within histiocytes of Michaelis–Gutmann bodies. These are concentric, laminated structures which react positively for calcium with the von Kossa technique and also give a positive result in the Perl's reaction for iron.

It is thought to be an unusual response to a Gram-negative bacillary infection. The testis and epididymis are rarely affected by this uncommon condition. When they are, there is almost invariably a concomitant urinary tract infection. The affected testis is slightly enlarged and the cut surface appears either homogeneously yellow or nodular with brown to yellow soft areas interspersed with white firmer fibrous areas. Soft, yellow-brown tissue may extend into the adjacent epididymis and frank abscess formation may also be seen.

Microscopically the lesion is identical to that seen in the bladder.

Non-infective

Idiopathic granulomatous orchitis

This, as the name implies, is an inflammatory condition of unknown aetiology. It is seen in men aged between 30 and 80 years but is most common in the fifth and sixth decades. Preceding trauma to the testis is recorded in a significant number of cases, but whether it is directly causative or whether an already enlarged testis is more prone to injury is not clear. The suggestion that it might have an auto-immune basis is contradicted by the observation that in most instances only one testis is affected. In a proportion of cases, however, the adjacent epididymis contains sperm granulomas. Despite this apparent association, many authors believe these two conditions are unrelated. This view is based on the observation that whereas in the latter condition phagocytosis of spermatozoa is frequently seen, it is never observed in idiopathic granulomatous orchitis.

Macroscopically the testis is enlarged and is covered by a thickened tunica vaginalis. The cut surface shows irregular grey-white indurated areas. Microscopically there are extensive granulomata which appear centred around involved seminiferous tubules. The granulomata are composed of epithelioid cells, with occasional multinucleate giant cells. The involved tubules show early loss of specialized germinal epithelial cells with persistence of Sertoli cells. Eventually the Sertoli cells are also destroyed.

Spermatic granuloma

This lesion is observed in the epididymis and vas deferens and in a significant number of cases is associated with previous vasectomy. Other associations are previous trauma or epididymitis. It has been reported in patients ranging in age from the second to the eighth decade but over 50 per cent occur in men in their twenties. The condition may be asymptomatic or may present with pain and swelling in the affected area.

Macroscopically, nodules of varying size, but usually less than 1 cm in diameter, are seen within the epididymis. The vas deferens may also show nodularity (*vasitis nodosa*). The cut surface of the nodules is soft and creamy white and they are well demarcated from the surrounding healthy tissue.

Microscopically, the features reflect the age of the lesion. In the earliest lesions neutrophils intermingled with extravasated spermatozoa are seen in the subepithelial tissues of the epididymis. As the lesion evolves, granulomata form and histiocytes and lymphocytes replace the neutrophils. Phagocytosis of spermatozoa by histiocytes and occasional multinucleate cells is also seen. In well-established granulomata, sperm may no longer be identifiable but the histiocytes contain abundant ceroid pigment. There is some fibrosis in the surrounding interstitium and the adjacent epithelium shows infiltration with a mixed acute and chronic inflammatory cell infiltrate. Occasionally *squamous metaplasia* of the epithelium is seen in long-standing cases.

Physical agents

Radiation damage

The spermatogenic epithelium is very radiosensitive and is therefore rapidly destroyed following radiation exposure of significant amount. A dose of 300 rad will cause damage to the germinal epithelium of sufficient degree to produce temporary aspermia. The Sertoli and Leydig cells are more radioresistant.

20.3.5   Vascular lesions

Varicocoele

A varicocoele is an abnormally elongated and dilated segment of the *pampiniform plexus*. Its incidence in the general population is reported as varying between 8 and 23 per cent but is somewhat higher amongst patients attending an infertility clinic. It is the most commonly identified cause of male infertility. It is left-sided in over 80 per cent of cases; less frequently it is bilateral, and only rarely do unilateral right-sided cases occur. The vascular anatomy differs on the two sides and this difference is probably responsible for the marked left-sided predisposition, although the precise mechanism has yet to be identified.

The mechanism of the associated infertility in a significant number of cases is poorly understood. Increased scrotal temperature has been put forward as a possible factor. The histological features seen in the testes of these individuals is varied. The most commonly reported abnormalities are partial sloughing of the germinal epithelium, diminished spermatogenesis and peritubular sclerosis, or maturation arrest, with or without associated testicular atrophy of varying degree. Focal small vessel sclerosis is also a commonly observed feature. The abnormalities are usually present bilaterally. The bilaterality of the histological abnormality has been attributed to the possibility of an undiagnosed contralateral varicocoele, or to the existence of anastomatic venous channels between right and left testes.

Testicular infarction

The commonest cause of testicular infarction is torsion of the spermatic cord causing an interruption to the testicular blood flow. This occurs most fequently in the pre-pubertal male but very occasional cases are seen in the neonatal period or in males over the age of 30. The predisposing cause in the vast majority of cases is hypermobility of the testis due to incomplete investment of the testis and epididymis by the tunica vaginalis. This anomaly is developmental and is commonly bilateral.

With complete vascular occlusion the testis appears grossly swollen and haemorrhagic. Microscopically the picture is that of haemorrhagic infarction (Fig. 20.23). The degree of necrosis depends on the duration of the occlusion. If this has been for longer than 10 h, necrosis of the seminiferous epithelium is usually complete and irreversible. With incomplete occlusion, necrosis may be delayed longer and some areas may be spared.

Other rare causes of testicular infarction or haemorrhage include hypercoagulable states, leukaemia, thrombocytopenia, systemic embolization, inferior vena cava thrombosis, and incarcerated inguinal hernia.

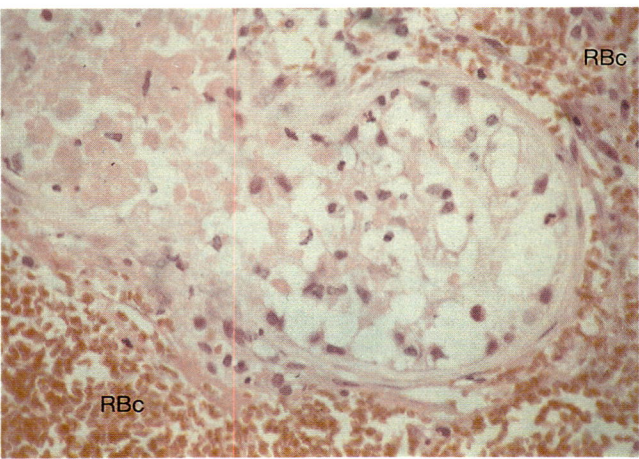

Fig. 20.23 A photomicrograph from a section of a testis which was removed because it had undergone torsion. The interstitium is replaced by red blood cells (RBc). The tubule contains occasional surviving Sertoli cells attached to the basement membrane. All the specialized germ cells have undergone necrosis, as evidenced by the clumped necrotic material within the tubule.

The long-term sequela of infarction without surgical removal of the affected gonad is atrophy of varying degree.

The appendices of either the testis or the epididymis may undergo torsion with or without infarction.

Polyarteritis nodosa

The testes are frequently affected in polyarteritis nodosa. The lesions in the testis are similar to those seen in other organs. The medium-sized arteries show acute vasculitic changes with associated areas of infarction.

20.3.6 Atrophy

Atrophy of the testis may result from many different aetiologies, some of which have already been discussed in the preceding sections on dysgenetic testicular abnormalities, cryptorchidism, inflammation, and vascular abnormalities. Testicular atrophy can occur as a result of hormonal abnormalities resulting from dysfunction of the pituitary, thyroid, or adrenal glands; or from exogenous administration of hormones, e.g. oestrogen treatment of prostatic cancer; an idiopathic group also exists.

The macroscopic appearance of atrophic testis is the same regardless of aetiology. The testes are reduced in volume and of very firm consistency. The cut surface shows loss of the yellow granular consistency, from which it is possible to pluck seminiferous tubules, and replacement by firm, white fibrous tissue. Broadly speaking, atrophy can take two forms. It can be either *pre-pubertal* or *post-pubertal*. In the pre-pubertal type, in the early phases, immature seminiferous tubules may still be identifiable, but in the later phases the changes seen on haematoxylin and eosin sections are indistinguishable from those in the post-pubertal late stage atrophy (Figs 20.24 and 20.25). The tubules are replaced by hyaline ghosts, irregularly disposed in a fibrous stroma. Occasional shrunken tubules with thickened basement membranes and Sertoli cells and occasional degenerate sperma-

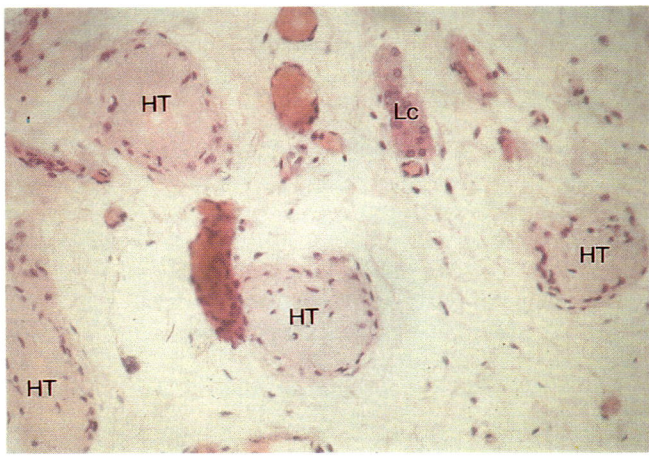

Fig. 20.25 A photomicrograph showing the end stage of testicular atrophy. Scattered hyalinized tubules (HT) separated by fibrous tissue are seen. Occasional dilated blood vessels and scattered collections of Leydig cells (Lc) are contained within the fibrous tissue.

togonia within their lumina may be seen. Clumps of interstitial cells usually persist within the fibrous tissue laid down in the interstitium. They may appear to be increased in volume, but quantitative studies have demonstrated that this is not the case. It is possible to distinguish pre- from post-pubertal atrophy in these late cases by doing an elastic stain. The elastic fibres appear to be laid down in the walls of the seminiferous tubules only when active spermatogenesis occurs. Therefore the absence of elastic fibres from the walls of seminiferous tubules is regarded as a marker of pre-pubertal atrophy.

20.3.7 Cysts and hydrocoele

Two types of cysts are described within the testis. Simple cysts and true epidermoid cysts.

Epidermoid cysts

These occur most commonly and usually affect males between the ages of 20 and 40. They are situated within the testicular parenchyma and contain laminated keratotic debris. The cyst wall is composed of an outer fibrous coat and an inner complete or incomplete lining of keratinizing stratified squamous epithelium. Calcification of parts of the wall is common and ossification is also occasionally present. Absence of dermal adnexal tissue is mandatory for the differentiation of these lesions from teratomatous lesions of the testis.

Simple cyst of the testis

These cysts are extremely rare. They have been reported at all ages. Macroscopically the cyst varies in size from one to several centimetres in diameter and is situated within the testicular parenchyma. The cut surface reveals a unilocular cavity with a smooth inner wall and the fluid contents are clear.

Microscopic examination shows the cyst to be lined by a

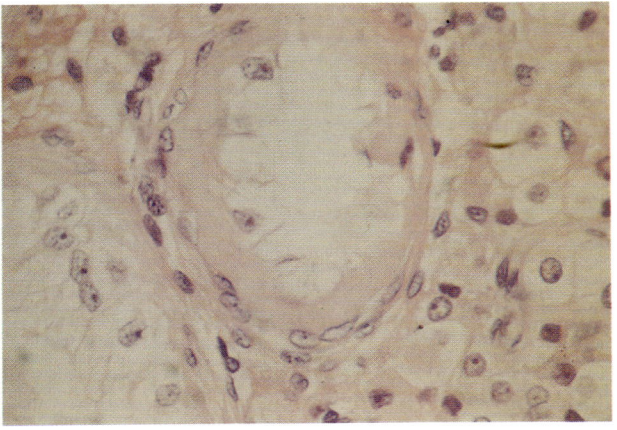

Fig. 20.24 A photomicrograph showing a picture of focal atrophy. The tubule on the left of the picture is lined by Sertoli cells only. The tubule in the centre of the picture shows marked basement thickening and hyalinization. The shrunken lumen contains occasional degenerate Sertoli cells only.

flattened, simple squamous or cuboidal epithelium. The importance of these cysts lies in their distinction from testicular teratoma.

Cysts of the tunica albuginea

These cysts are extremely rare. They have been reported in adult males, particularly in the over-forty age-group. The cysts are situated on the anterolateral surface of the testis. Macroscopically they may be uni- or multilocular and measure up to 4 cm in diameter. They usually have a smooth-walled inner lining and contain clear or bloodstained fluid.

Microscopic examination shows the lining to be composed of a simple squamous or cuboidal epithelium. Mesothelial cell clusters have also been observed within the cyst wall.

Cysts of the epididymis

Cysts of the epididymis are relatively common and are distinguishable from other cysts within this region by the demonstration within them of spermatozoa, hence the other name for epididymal cysts is *spermatocoele*. They arise most commonly from the caput. Macroscopically they may be uni- or multilocular and may measure up to several centimetres in diameter. The cyst wall is usually smooth but occasionally simple papillary projections are seen on the inner surface. The cyst fluid is opalescent.

Microscopically the cysts are lined by a flattened simple epithelium which rests on a fibromuscular stroma. If projections are present they are covered by a single, regular layer of simple cuboidal or columnar epithelium.

The diagnosis is usually made by demonstration of spermatozoa in cystic fluid aspirate.

Hydrocoele

A hydrocoele is an accumulation of serous fluid in the tunica vaginalis. About 6 per cent of neonates have some degree of hydrocoele because of incomplete closure of the *processus vaginalis (congenital hydrocoele)* or because of delayed development of lymphatics in the tunica vaginalis (*infantile hydrocoele*); but most of these have resolved by the end of the first year. The majority of hydrocoeles occur in adults in or after the third decade, and in these acquired cases the aetiology is usually an inflammatory lesion of the testis or, more frequently, the epididymis, within the affected tunica. It may also occur as a complication of varicocoelectomy or, occasionally, be associated with an underlying tumour.

Hydrocoele of the cord is an encysted hydrocoele which results from an enclosed segment of the processus vaginalis remaining patent.

Hydrocoeles may become secondarily infected or haemorrhage may occur into them.

Macroscopically, the sac from an uncomplicated hydrocoele appears smooth and glistening. If complicated by infection or tumour, the sac may be irregularly thickened and dull.

Microscopically, the tissue is fibrous and acellular with or without infiltration by inflammatory or tumour cells. Mesothelial cells may also be seen.

20.3.8   Infertility

In the developed world 10–15 per cent of couples are infertile. Where a cause can be identified, male factors are invoked in approximately half the cases. Testicular biopsy is usually only resorted to after a full clinical investigation, including estimation of plasma hormone levels, has been carried out. Thus many untreatable pretesticular and testicular causes will have been excluded. The group presenting for biopsy are usually therefore azoo- and oligo-spermic males with normal male habitus and normal hormonal status.

Microscopically, the following set of appearances may be encountered in testicular biopsy material:

1. normal histology;
2. decreased spermatogenesis;
3. developmental arrest;
4. sloughing and disorganization of spermatogenic epithelium;
5. maturation arrest;
6. Sertoli cell only pattern;
7. testicular atrophy.

Normal histology is most commonly seen in males with *bilateral obstruction* somewhere along the excretory duct system. The commonest site of obstruction is the distal part of the epididymis and/or the adjacent part of the vas. In the majority of cases the obstruction is post-inflammatory but in some it is congenital or post-traumatic. It occurs in cystic fibrosis due to failure of the normal development of the vas but the testicular histology in these cases is almost invariably abnormal, there being either a maturation arrest or some degree of atrophy. Obstruction occurring at the proximal end of the epididymis, associated with normal testicular histology has been reported in men suffering from Young's syndrome (chronic sinusitis, bronchitis, or bronchiectasis believed to be due to impaired mucociliary clearance), a condition attributed to mercury intoxication (Pink's disease) in infancy.

Infertile males with varicocoeles may occasionally have normal histology.

Decreased spermatogenesis

Decreased spermatogenesis, as the term implies, is a defect limited to the seminiferous epithelium. All the normal spermatogenic elements are present in normal proportions but their absolute number is diminished to a greater or lesser degree. The lesion can be graded according to quantitative criteria described by Johnsen (1970) and then expressed as a *Johnsen count*. In most cases no aetiological agent is apparent, although some patients with varicocoele fall into this category.

Development arrest

In these cases testicular biopsy from an adult male shows the histological features of a pre-pubertal testis. These patients usually have raised plasma androgen levels and a pituitary aetiology should be excluded.

Sloughing and disorganization of the spermatogenic epithelium

This appearance is seen within seminiferous tubules of normal shape and size. The interstitium is usually unremarkable but may occasionally show mild focal fibrosis. Spermatogenesis is seen to be proceeding in all tubules, but there is some distortion in the normal sequence and the lumina are obliterated by sloughed immature cells which may or may not show features of degeneration. The importance of this appearance as a true pathologic entity is disputed by some authors, since these appearances can be produced by poor fixation and crushing of biopsy material.

Maturation arrest

There is an interruption of spermatogenesis at any point in its cycle. Arrest occurs most commonly at the primary spermatocyte phase but it can occur at the secondary spermatocyte or spermatid stage. Arrest is usually complete but occasionally a few cells progress through to full maturation. No other abnormalities are seen in these testes. This pathological picture can be seen in men recovering from fevers or suffering from debilitating diseases. It is also occasionally seen in association with chromosome abnormalities or in patients with cystic fibrosis or a varicocoele. The vast majority of cases, however, have no demonstrable aetiology.

Sertoli cell only syndrome or Del Castillo's syndrome

This is a condition in which there is complete absence of germinal elements but a normal compliment of Sertoli cells within seminiferous tubules of slightly diminished diameter. Occasionally, isolated tubules showing spermatogenesis may be present. This appearance was initially believed to be due to a congenital failure of migration of the primitive germ cells from the yolk sac endoderm to the gonads. Although some cases may be congenital in origin, others appear to be acquired. The above picture in association with genuine Leydig cell hyperplasia and tubular basement membrane thickening is described in cases with 17-ketosteroid dehydrogenase or reductase deficiency.

In testicular atrophy, focal areas showing Sertoli cell only appearance are sometimes seen.

Testicular atrophy either pre- or post-pubertal in type

As described previously (Section 20.3.6), testicular atrophy may be seen in patients with a history of preceding infectious episode, maldescent, varicocoele, with an associated chromosomal abnormality, or in patients with cystic fibrosis or myotonic muscular dystrophy. Most cases, however, are idiopathic.

20.3.9 Further reading

Bartsch, G., Frank, S. T., Marberger, H., and Mikuz, G. (1980). Testicular torsion: late results with special regard to fertility and endocrine function. *Journal of Urology* 124, 375–8.

Brothers, L. R. and Feldtman, W. (1981). Abdominoscrotal hydrocele: youngest case report and review of the literature. *Journal of Urology* 126, 842–7.

Ceccacci, L. and Tosi, S. (1981). Splenic gonadal fusion: case report and review of the literature. *Journal of Urology* 126, 558–9.

Chabon, A. B., Stenger, R. J., and Grabstald, H. (1987). Histopathology of testis in Acquired Immune Deficiency syndrome. *Urology* 29, 658–63.

de la Chappelle, A. (1972). Analytic review: nature and origin of males with XX sex chromosomes. *American Journal of Human Genetics* 24, 71–105.

Clermont, Y. (1963). The cycle of the seminiferous epithelium in man. *American Journal of Anatomy* 112, 35–45.

Cos, L. R. and Cockett, A. T. K. (1982). Genitourinary tuberculosis revisited. *Urology* 20, 111–17.

Del Castillo, E. B., Trabucco, A., and De La Balze, F. A. (1947). Syndrome produced by absence of germinal epithelium without impairment of the Sertoli or Leydig cells. *Journal of Clinical Endocrinology* 7, 493–5.

Denning, C. R., Sommers, S. C., and Quigley, H. J. (1968). Infertility in male patients with cystic fibrosis. *Pediatrics* 41, 7–17.

Drucker, W. D., Blane, W. A., Rowland, L. P., Grumbach, M. M., and Christy, N. P. (1963). The testis in myotonic muscular dystrophy. A clinical and pathological study with a comparison with Klinefelters Syndrome. *Journal of Clinical Endocrinology and Metabolism* 23, 59–75.

Dubin, L. and Hotchkiss, R. S. (1969). Testis biopsy in subfertile men with varicocoele. *Fertility and Sterility* 20, 50–8.

Fawcett, D. W. (1986). *Bloom and Fawcett. A textbook of histology* (11th edn). W. B. Saunders, Philadelphia.

Ferguson Smith, M. A. (1959). The prepubertal testicular lesion in chromatin positive Klinefelter's Syndrome as seen in mentally handicapped children. *Lancet* 1, 219–22.

Ferrie, B. G. and Rundle, J. S. (1983). Tuberculous epididymo orchitis. A review of 20 cases. *British Journal of Urology* 55, 437–9.

Guyton, A. C. (1987). *Human physiology and mechanisms of disease* (4th edn), pp. 618–28. W. G. Saunders, Philadelphia.

Hendry, W. F., Levison, D. A., Parkinson, M. C., Parslow, J. M., and Royle, M. G. (1990). Testicular obstruction; clinicopathologic studies. *Annals of the Royal College of Surgeons of England* 72, 396–407.

Honore, L. H. (1979). Testicular biopsy for infertility: a review of 68 cases with a simplified histologic classification of lesions. *International Journal of Fertility* 24, 49–52.

Johnsen, S. G. (1970). Testicular biopsy score count-A method for registration of spermatogenesis in human testes: normal values and results in 335 hypogonadal males. *Hormones* 1, 2–25.

Kleinman, S. Z., Robinson, D. N. and Simon, S. A. (1983). Malakoplakia of the testis. *Urology* 22, 194–7.

Klinefelter, H. F., Jr, Reifenstein, E. F., Jr, and Albright, F. (1942). Syndrome characterised by gynaecomastia. aspermatogenesis without a-Leydigism, and increased excretion of follicle stimulating hormone. *Journal of Clinical Endocrinology* 2, 615–17.

Leonard, J. M., Paulsen, C. A., and Ospina, L. F. (1979). The classification of Klinefelter's syndrome. In *Genetic mechanisms of sexual development* (ed. H. L. Vallet and I. H. Porter), pp. 407–23. Academic Press, San Diego.

Mack, W. S., Scott, L. S., and Ferguson Smith, M. A. (1961). Ectopic testis and true undescended testis: a histological comparison. *Journal of Pathology* 82, 439–43.

McLeod, J., Hotchkiss, R. S., and Sitterson, B. W. (1964). Recovery of male fertility after sterilisation by nuclear radiation. *Journal of the American Medical Association* **187**, 637–41.

Malek, R. S., Rosen, J. S., and Farrow, G. M. (1986). Epidermoid cysts of testis. *British Journal of Urology* **58**, 55–9.

Manuel, M., Ktayama, K. P., Jones, H. W. Jr (1976). The age of occurrence of gonadal tumours in intersex patients with a Y chromosome. *American Journal of Obstetrics and Gynecology* **124**, 293–300.

Morris, J. M. (1953). The syndrome of testicular feminisation in male pseudohermaphrodites. *American Journal of Obstetrics and Gynecology* **65**, 1192–211.

Mostofi, F. K. and Price, E. G. (1973). Tumours of the male genital system. In *Atlas of tumor pathology*, Fascicle 8, 2nd Series, p. 165. AFIP, Washington, DC.

Mowad, J. J., Baldwin, B. D., and Young, J. (1971). Periarteritis presenting as a mass in the testis. *Journal of Urology* **105**, 109.

Muller, J. (1984). Morphology and histology of gonads from 12 children and adolescents with the androgen insensitivity (testicular feminisation) syndrome. *Journal of Clinical Endocrinology and Metabolism* **59**, 785–9.

Muller, J., Skakkebaek, N., and Nielsen, O. H. (1984). Cryptorchidism and testis cancer: atypical infantile germ cells followed by carcinoma *in situ* and invasive carcinoma in adulthood. *Cancer* **54**, 629–34.

Neville, A. M. and Grigor, K. M. (1975). Structure, function and the development of the human testis. *Pathology of the testis* (ed. R. C. B. Pugh). Blackwell Scientific Publications, Oxford.

van Niekerk, W. A. (1974). *True hermaphroditism. Clinical, morphologic and cytogenetic aspects*. Harper and Row, Hagerstown.

Nistal, M., Paniagua, R., and Diez-Pardo, J. A. (1980). Histological classification of undescended testes. *Human Pathology* **11**, 666–74.

Pelander, W. M., Luna, G., and Lilly, J. R. (1978). Polyorchidism: case report and literature review. *Journal of Urology* **119**, 705–6.

Pesce, C., Reale, A., and Sanguineti, G. (1986). The pathology of testicular atrophy. *Pathological and Immunopathological Research* **5**, 500–11.

Rolnick, D., Kawanoue, S., and Szanto, P. (1968). Anatomical incidence of testicular appendages. *Journal of Urology* **100**, 755.

Rosi, P., Carini, M., Gambacorta, G., Mottola, A., and Selli, C. (1984). Granulomatous orchitis: clinical and pathological aspects. *European Urology* **10**, 130–2.

Rugh, R. (1960). In *Mechanism in radiobiology*, Vol. II (ed. M. Errera and A. Forsberg). Academic Press, New York.

Schmidt, S. S. (1979). Spermatic granuloma: an often painful lesion. *Fertility and Sterility* **31**, 178–81.

Schulze, C., Holstein, A. F., and Schirren, C. (1976). On the morphology of the human Sertoli cells under normal conditions and in patients with impaired fertility. *Andrologia* **8**, 167–78.

Schulze, W. and Rehder, U. (1984). Organisation and morphogenesis of the human seminiferous epithelium. *Cell and Tissue Research* **237**, 395–407.

Scott, L. S. (1960). Mumps and male infertility. *British Journal of Urology* **32**, 183.

Scott, R., Rourke, A., and Yates, B. (1976). The results of 100 small tissue biopsies of testis in male infertile patients. *Postgraduate Medical Journal* **52**, 693–6.

Simpson, E., Chandler, P., Goulmy, E., Disteche, C. M., Ferguson-Smith, M. A., and Page, D. C. (1987). Separation of the genetic loci for the H–Y antigen and for testis determination on the human Y chromosome. *Nature* **326**, 876–8.

Skakkebaek, N. E., Hulten, M., Jacobsen, P., and Mikkelsen, M. (1973). Quantification of human seminiferous epithelium. II. Histological studies in eight 47XYY men. *Journal of Reproduction and Fertility* **32**, 391–401.

Takihara, H., Valao, J. R., and Tokuhara, M. (1982). Intratesticular cysts. *Urology* **20**, 80–2.

Wilson, J. D., Griffin, J. E., Leshin, M., and George, F. W. (1981). Role of gonadal hormones in development of the sexual phenotypes. *Human Genetics* **58**, 78–84.

Warner, K. E., Noyes, D. T., and Ross, J. S. (1984). Cysts of the tunica albuginea testis. A report of three cases with review of the literature. *Journal of Urology* **132**, 131–2.

20.4   Tumours of the testis

L. D. True and J. Rosai

20.4.1   Introduction

Testicular tumours are relatively rare, having an incidence of 1 per 100 000 US males and causing 0.2 per cent of male cancer deaths. In the United States in 1986, 5100 new cases of testicular cancer were predicted. In 1990, 350 died of this tumour in the USA, and an estimated 1 in 250 boys developed this disease.

This chapter will focus on germ cell tumours, which represent over 95 per cent of testicular neoplasms, and which have an importance disproportionately greater than their incidence:

1. They are the most common neoplasm in males 15–35 years of age. As death from disease is rare at these ages, the impact is greater than that of many other neoplasms.

2. Germ cell tumours are one of few tumour types for which modern combination chemotherapy has produced a dramatic improvement in survival.

3. As these tumours manifest an unusually wide range of morphological and functional differentiation, they have served as models for the investigation of various aspects of tumour biology, both in patients and animals, including the association between tumour differentiation and tumour behaviour, and the correlation between serum markers, and tumour histology and extent of spread.

20.4.2   Germ cell tumours

Epidemiology

There is significant geographical heterogeneity in incidence. For example, Whites in North America and Scandinavia have an incidence up to eight times that of native Japanese (Table 20.1). Although high socio-economic status is associated with an increased risk, no other environmental factor of significance has been identified.

The preponderance of cases are sporadic; only rare individuals have a familial history of testicular cancer, and the occurrence in identical twins is quite rare.

Table 20.1 Testicular neoplasia, incidence in selected countres (expressed as cases per 10^5 total population)

Denmark	8
Norway	5
United States	4
Finland	2
India	1
Japan	1

Risk factors

In addition to epidemiological factors, genitourinary abnormalities, particularly cryptorchidism and gonadal dysgenesis, and history of a prior testicular germ cell tumour, increase risk. The risk associated with cryptorchidism reflects less the physical nature of the abnormality than the presence of inherently abnormal tissue. Thus, a normally descended testis contralateral to a cryptorchid testis is at risk for neoplasia, and early re-location of a cryptorchid testis decreases, but does not abolish, the risk of germ cell neoplasia. No other factors, including a history of scrotal trauma or exposure to known carcinogens, have been associated with a significant risk.

Histogenesis

The precursor lesion of germ cell tumours is thought to be an *in situ* proliferative cellular abnormality termed *intratubular germ cell neoplasia* (ITGCN). ITGCN is defined as replacement of the normal cells of seminiferous tubules by a proliferation of atypical cells which morphologically resemble undifferentiated germ cells (Figs 20.26, 20.27). The following observations are evidence that ITGCN is the precursor lesion to invasive germ cell tumours:

1. ITGCN is found, at least focally, adjacent to virtually all germ cell tumours.

2. The presence of ITGCN in a cryptorchid testis and in testicu-

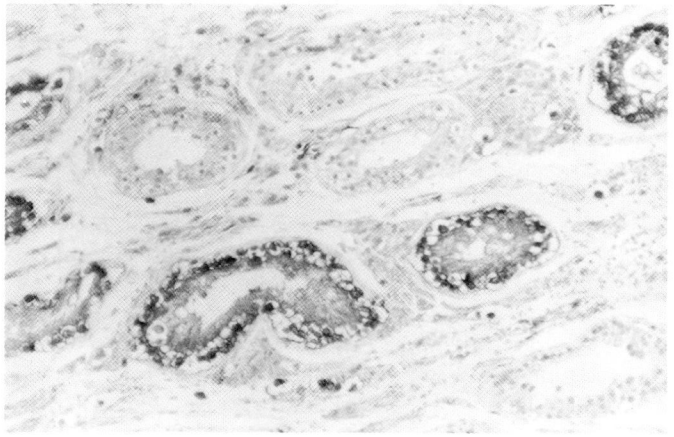

Fig. 20.26 The replacement of germinative elements of seminiferous tubules by large, undifferentiated germ cells is characteristic of ITGCN.

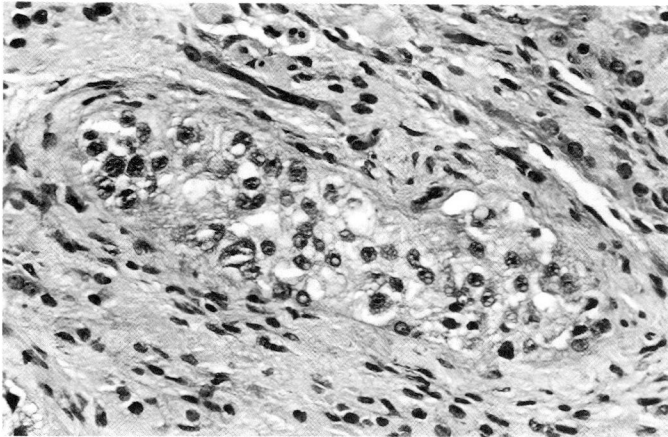

Fig. 20.27 The cells of ITGCN synthesize placental alkaline phosphates, which can be detected by immunohistochemistry.

lar biopsies taken from infertile men is associated with a significantly increased risk of subsequent invasive germ cell tumour.

3. The finding of continuity between ITGCN and some invasive germ cell neoplasm suggests that invasion arose from a precursor state of ITGCN.

Although the cell of origin of testicular tumours has been a subject of prior debate, current evidence favours the concept that these tumours have a common histogenesis from germ cells since:

1. The undifferentiated cells of ITGCN both precede and co-exist with testicular tumours of all histological types.

2. The frequent admixture and combination of all histological types of testicular tumours strongly suggests a common cell of origin. The further observation that both locally recurrent and metastatic neoplasm can have a histology different than that of the primary is further evidence of multipotentiality.

3. That these tumours, as teratomas, can have a histology resembling normal tissues of all three basic cell lines—ectoderm, mesoderm, and endoderm—indicates the presence of *totipotential cells.*

4. Animal experiments further support the totipotential nature of a subpopulation of malignant tumour cells. The implantation of single embryonal carcinoma cells into the subcutaneous tissue of mice produces teratomas.

5. There is direct evidence, in animal models, that germ cells need to be present for the development of a germ cell tumour. Implantation of the genital ridges of fetal mice into adult testes produce teratocarcinomas in 75 per cent of cases. In contrast, only 3 per cent of the implanted genital ridges of a strain of mouse which virtually lacks germ cells results in germ cell tumours.

Types of germ cell tumours

The categorization of germ cell tumours is based upon their

histopathology and structural similarity to non-neoplastic tissues. Further justifications for this nomenclature include the following:

1. the *demographic characteristics* of the tumour types characteristically differ;

2. *tumour function*, particularly the production of such tumour markers as *α-fetoprotein (AFP)* and *chorionic gonadotrophin (HCG)*, is associated with specific cell types;

3. the *behaviour of tumours*, including the likelihood of distant dissemination, the pattern of spread, and the response to different therapies, vary with histological type.

Two classification schemes are current used. The one adopted by the *World Health Organization* (WHO), and the more generally accepted of the two, hypothesizes that all testicular tumours represent various paths of differentiation of malignant germ cells (Fig. 20.28). The scheme adopted by the British Testicular Tumour Panel presumes that the cell of origin of non-seminomatous tumours is a primitive multipotential cell, histogenetically distinct from the seminoma cell. Although these schemes differ in terminology, there is a direct correspondence between tumour types (Table 20.2).

In usage, the WHO classification names the histological components which comprise a tumour. Although two-thirds of tumours contain only one component, the remainder are *mixed*, and are named according to the components present. By convention, tumours consisting of *embryonal carcinoma* and *teratoma* are termed *teratocarcinomas*. For patient management, the most important histological distinction to make is between *seminoma* and *non-seminoma*. The frequencies of histological subtypes of germ cell tumours is similar in different countries (Table 20.3).

Table 20.2 Classifications of germ cell tumours of testis

WHO	British Testicular Tumour Panel
Seminoma typical spermatocytic	Seminoma classical spermatocytic
Embryonal carcinoma	Malignant teratoma, undifferentiated
Embryonal carcinoma with teratoma ('teratocarcinoma')	Malignant teratoma, intermediate
Teratoma, mature	Malignant teratoma, differentiated
Choriocarcinoma	Malignant teratoma, trophoblastic
Yolk sac tumour	Yolk sac tumour

Table 20.3 Incidence of germ cell tumours by histological type (%)

Seminoma classical	52
spermatocytic	1
Pure embryonal carcinoma	10
Pure teratoma	3
Pure choriocarcinoma	0.2
Pure yolk sac tumour	0.3
Mixed non-seminomatous tumour	21
Mixed tumours, with seminoma	13

Seminoma

The usual gross appearance is a well-circumscribed mass of uniform texture and white to tan colour with little haemorrhage or necrosis (Fig. 20.29). Named in 1906 for its resemblance to seminiferous epithelium, seminomas consist of sheets of cells histologically resembling undifferentiated germ cells (Fig. 20.30). The primitive nature of these cells is also true ultrastructurally and functionally; they contain abundant glycogen and exhibit little organellar specialization. Classical seminomas produce neither AFP nor HCG.

The stroma is composed of fibrous bands infiltrated by lymphocytes, predominantly T-cells. In 10 per cent of cases, there are syncytiotrophoblastic-like multinucleated giant cells. These cells are a source of serologically and immunohistochemically detectable HCG (Fig. 20.31). However, the biology of this vari-

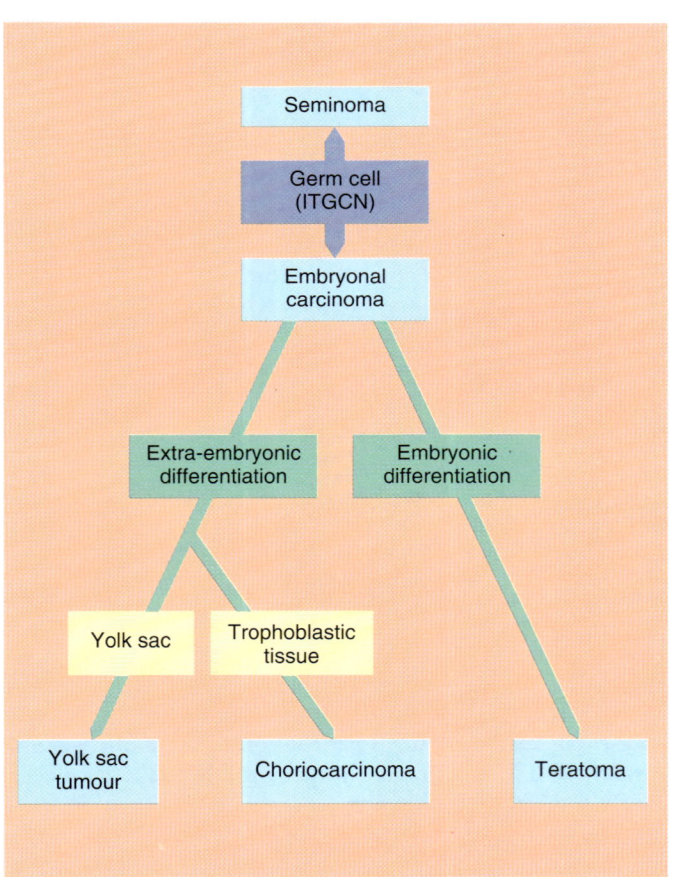

Fig. 20.28 Histogenetic origin of testicular germ cell tumours.

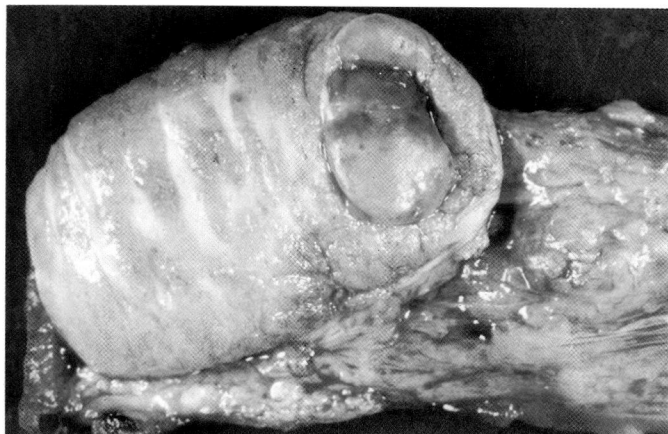

Fig. 20.29 This typical seminoma is a non-encapsulated, tan to white, homogeneous mass, well demarcated from testicular parenchyma, and with no gross haemorrhage or necrosis.

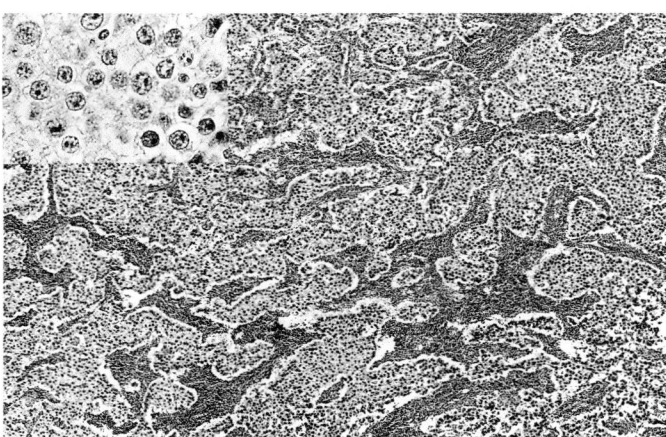

Fig. 20.30 Seminomas are composed of sheets of tumour cells compartmentalized by fibrous trabeculae, which usually contain a mononuclear inflammatory cell infiltrate. Inset: tumour cells have distinct cell borders, which impart a cobblestone appearance, a clear cytoplasm, reflective of their large content of glycogen, and large nuclei with one to two prominent nucleoli.

ant is otherwise identical to that of the typical seminoma. Placental alkaline phosphatase is the only other tumour marker synthesized by seminomas. The finding of excess AFP production is strongly suggestive of a non-seminomatous component.

Seminomas tend to occur in a slightly older age-group than do non-seminomatous germ cell tumours, and are the most common tumours developing in cryptorchid testes. About 10 per cent occur in undescended testes. Pure seminomas represent 40 per cent of all germ cell tumours. The 'anaplastic seminoma' is a histological variant of classical seminoma. However, there is at present a question about whether the behaviour of this variant is distinctive.

Spermatocytic seminoma This is a distinctive variant of eminoma, with a typical clinical setting and biology. The median

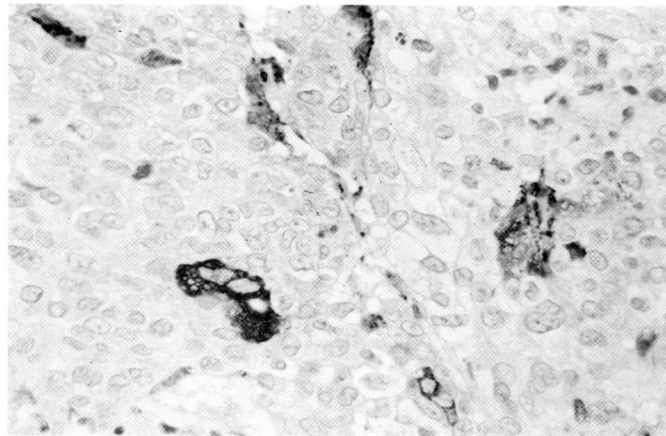

Fig. 20.31 Using an immunoperoxidase stain, antibodies specific to the β-chain of chorionic gonadotrophin are localized to syncytiotrophoblastic cells in this seminoma.

patient age of 55 years is the oldest of patients with germ cell tumours. Grossly, spermatocytic seminomas are irregular masses with a focally soft and spongy texture and a variegated, tan to grey, gelatinous surface. They are composed of sheets of cells which histologically display a spectrum of spermatocytic-like differentiation (Fig. 20.32).

Always occurring as pure tumours, and representing up to 5 per cent of germ cell tumours, spermatocytic seminomas usually have a benign clinical course, only exceptionally upset by the event of sarcomatous transformation.

Embryonal carcinoma

This presents as an irregular mass with, typically, multifocal necrosis and haemorrhage (Fig. 20.33). These tumours are composed of cytologically anaplastic cells which can grow either as sheets of cells or as tubular or reticular structures. Embryonal carcinoma cells are regarded as the progenitor cells

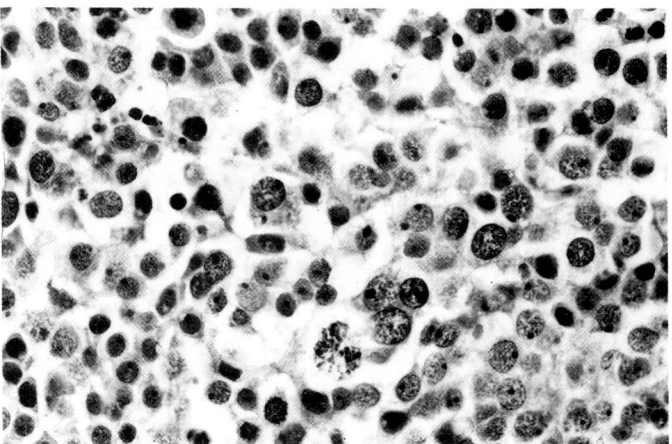

Fig. 20.32 Three cell types comprise spermatocytic seminomas—small, lymphocyte-like cells, intermediate cells, and large cells, which may have a prominent filamentous pattern of chromatin, resembling the 'spireme' arrangement of chromatin in spermatogonia.

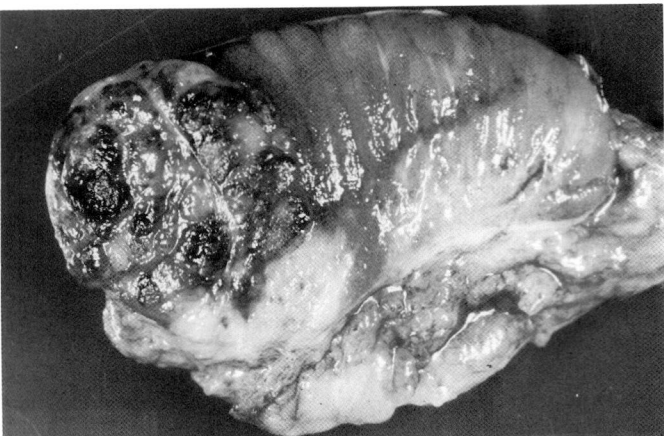

Fig. 20.33 This embryonal carcinoma is an irregular, multifocally haemorrhagic and necrotic mass with a variegated cut surface.

of all non-seminomatous germ cell tumours (Fig. 20.34). AFP and/or HCG can be immunohistochemically localized to some cells in embryonal carcinomas. The presence of these proteins does not change the classification of this tumour.

Teratomas

These are composed of cell types which reflect the three basic germ cell types of the normal, developing mammal—ectoderm, mesoderm, and endoderm. These cells have a benign cytology. Although any histological elements may be present, the most common components are skin, glial tissue, bronchial and gastrointestinal-type mucosa, smooth muscle, cartilage, and fat (Fig. 20.35). The formation of lumina imparts the typical gross appearance of a multicystic mass (Fig. 20.36). The presence of necrosis or haemorrhage raise the possibility of an embryonal cell or choriocarcinoma component.

Teratomas can be sub-classified by degree of differentiation as

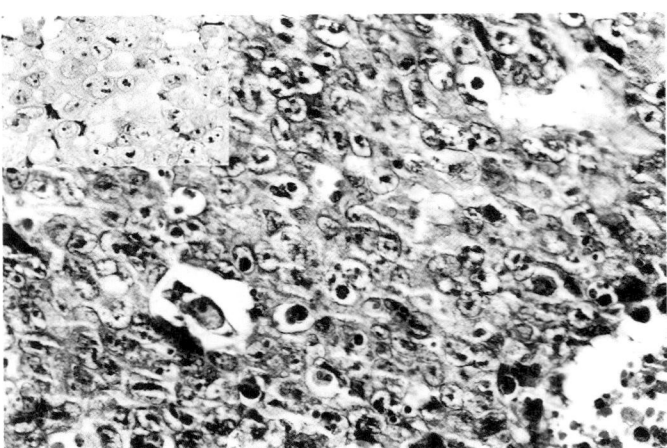

Fig. 20.34 Growing as sheets of cells, this embryonal carcinoma contains a focus of necrosis. Inset. The tumour cells are markedly anaplastic, with multiple, large, and irregular nucleoli in prominent, often overlapping nuclei.

mature or immature. *Monodermal teratomas*, composed of only one cell type, i.e. *carcinoid*, are a third subtype. In about 15 per cent of germ cell tumours, only mature teratoma is found. Although one would expect the behaviour of such histologically bland tumours to be benign, that is not always the case. Only in pre-pubertal patients do mature teratomas apparently lack malignant potential. In adults, teratomas have a malignant potential even when wholly differentiated. This behaviour contrasts with ovarian teratomas, which are usually benign in adults. The difference between ovary and testis in timing of normal germ cell replication provides a possible explanation for this gender-specific difference in malignancy. Assuming that full malignant potential requires homozygosity for a recessive gene, which results from a post-gestational mutation, the germ cells of the ovary, which replicate *in utero*, are far less likely to be homozygous for the putative malignant gene than are male germ cells, which replicate in adolescence.

Yolk sac tumour

Yolk sac tumour, or endodermal sinus tumour, has an architecture considered similar to that of the fetal yolk sac. The most characteristic structures are the *glomeruloid, or Schiller–Duval, bodies* (Fig. 20.37). Analogous to the fetal yolk sac, these cells produce α-fetoprotein, which collects in large, cytoplasmic, eosinophilic globules.

Yolk sac tumour virtually never exists as the sole cell component of germ cell tumours in adults, although it is a component of 45 per cent of adult tumours. In contrast, 40 per cent of childhood testicular tumours are pure yolk sac tumour. In children under 2 years of age, the behaviour of these tumours is markedly more benign than in either older children or adults.

Choriocarcinoma

Histologically and functionally, choriocarcinoma mimics trophoblastic tissue. Both syncytiotrophoblastic and cytotrophoblastic cells are present (Fig. 20.38). The former are the major source of HCG production, which is elevated in the serum of patients with a choriocarcinoma element, and which can be detected by immunohistochemistry. Grossly, areas of choriocarcinoma are always bloody. Pure choriocarcinoma is extremely rare, representing less than 1 per cent of germ cell tumours. More commonly, choriocarcinoma is an element in 2–5 per cent of maligant germ cell tumours.

Clinical features

The majority of tumours present either as scrotal masses, or with localized pain. In only a small minority of patients is there enough endocrine function to be symptomatic, manifesting as gynaecomastia, loss of libido, or infertility. Two-thirds of patients present with tumour localized to the scrotum; in only 15 per cent of patients is identifiable tumour found beyond regional, retroperitoneal lymphatics at presentation (Table 20.4).

Tumour biology

The progression of untreated germ cell tumours follows a

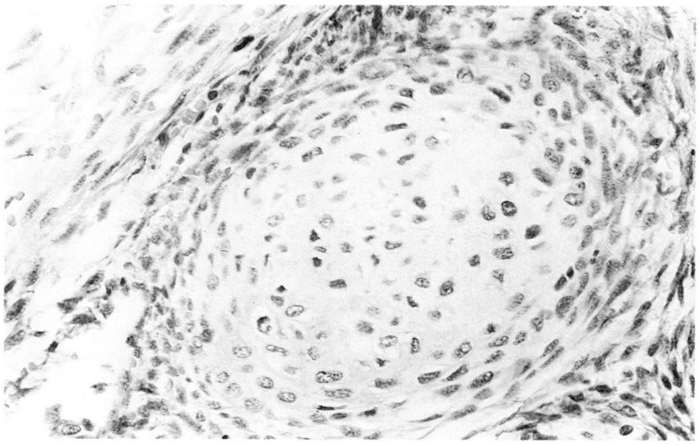

(a)

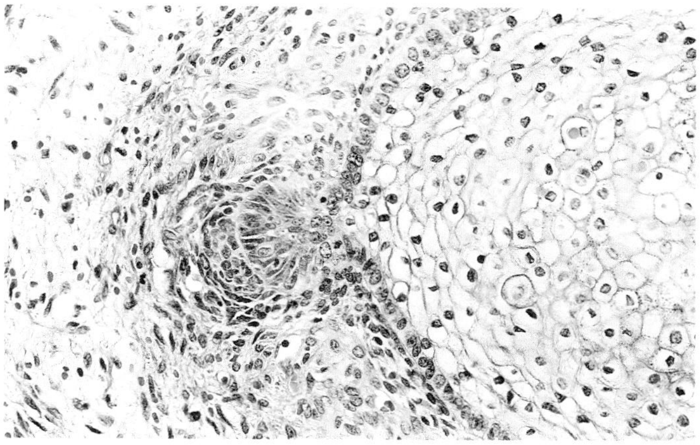

(b)

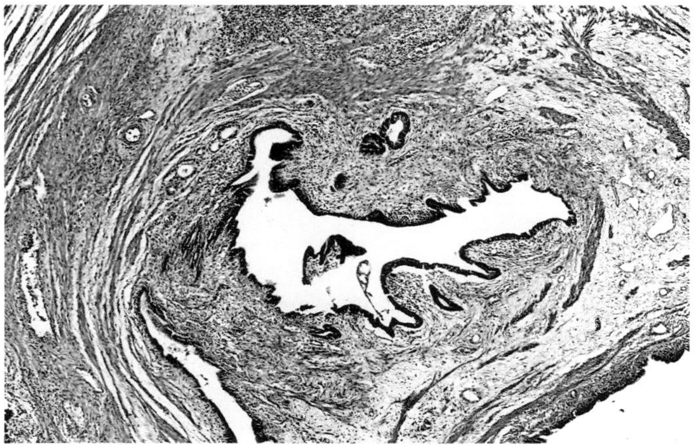

(c)

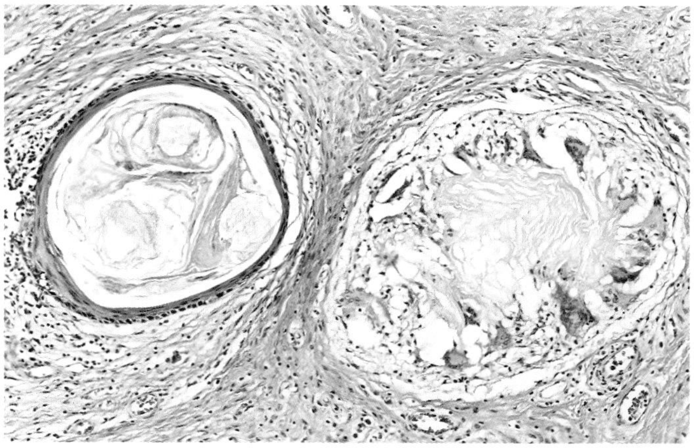

(d)

Fig. 20.35 These elements are commonly present in teratomas. Immature hyaline cartilage contains orderly spaced chondrocytes (a). An immature pilosebaceous unit arises from the basal layer of keratinizing stratified squamous epithelium (b). This cytologically benign cystic structure resembles a hollow viscus. A pseudostratified, columnar epithelium, respiratory in type, lines the tubular structure. Circumferential layers of smooth muscle, characteristic of a bronchus, surround the epithelium (c). One of two adjacent keratinous cysts is infiltrated by inflammatory cells, including foreign-body-type histiocytes (d).

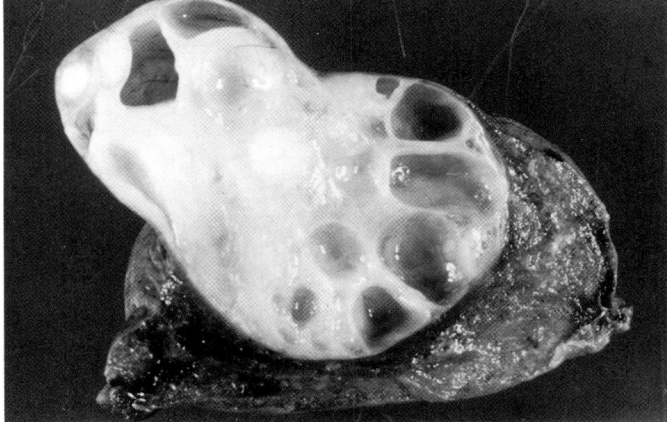

Fig. 20.36 As a lung metastasis, this teratoma is a well-circumscribed, multicystic mass. Islands of cartilage and bone can often be identified grossly.

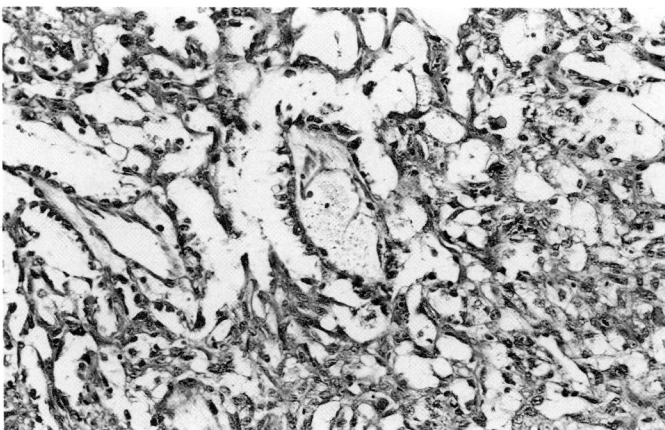

Fig. 20.37 Infantile yolk sac tumours generally contain a uniform population of cytologically malignant tumour cells in a reticular pattern. A Schiller–Duval body is present.

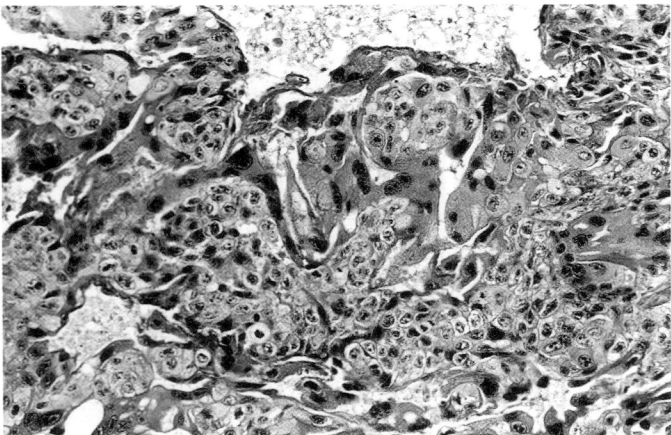

Fig. 20.38 Multinucleated malignant syncytiotrophoblasts partially surround uninuclear malignant cytotrophoblasts. This architecture resembles the trophoblastic tissue of chorionic villi.

Table 20.4　Stage at initial diagnosis as percentage of tumours

Stage	Seminoma	Non-seminoma
I	40	26
II	10	13
III	2	8

relatively predictable pattern. Spread beyond the testicular parenchyma is initially via local lymphatics to retroperitoneal lymph nodes, usually only those which are ipsilateral. There is little lymphatic drainage to inguinal nodes, which are only rarely involved with tumour. And local invasion of the scrotal wall is unusual. From retroperitoneal nodes, the tumour characteristically spreads to supradiaphragmatic nodes—mediastinal and supraclavicular—and to the lungs. Systemic, blood-borne metastatic disease follows in the untreated patient.

Given this somewhat predictable pattern of tumour spread, the likelihood of the patient being cured of tumour can be estimated from tumour stage (Tables 20.5, 20.6). As most patients undergo primary surgical resection of localized (stage I) tumour, the likelihood of recurrence and the behaviour of recurrent tumour can be estimated from tumour features, the most important being whether or not the tumour is a pure seminoma, the presence of embryonal carcinoma and/or vascular invasion, and the status of serum markers AFP and HCG (Table 20.7).

Prior to the 1970s, non-seminomatous germ cell tumours

Table 20.5　Clinical staging of malignant neoplasms of the testis

Stage	Extent of tumour
I	Tumour confined to scrotum
II	Tumour metastatic only to retroperitoneal lymph nodes
III	Tumour has distant metastases

Table 20.6　Classification of testicular neoplasia by TNM system

Primary tumour
　T1　Limited to testicular parenchyma
　T2　Tumour invades through tunica albuginea
　T3　Tumour extends to rete testis or epididymis
　T4　Tumour invades spermatic cord or wall of scrotum

Status of lymph nodes
　N0　Nodes free of tumour
　N1　No more than one regional node involved
　N2　Multiple regional nodes contain tumour
　N3　Nodal involvement produces a palpable mass

Status of distant metastases
　M0　No identifiable distant metastases
　M1　Distant metastases are present

Table 20.7　Tumour markers; percentage predictability for relapse of non-seminomatous tumours (%)

Marker	Sensitivity	Specificity	Positive predictive value
HCG	59	98	87
AFP	36	100	100

This study exemplifies the value of using serum tumour markers to assess recurrence of non-seminomatous germ cell tumours.

were regarded as some of the most malignant tumours affecting men. Patients with tumours which were not resectable by orchiectomy typically died of metastatic tumour within two years of diagnosis. The presence of choriocarcinoma or of yolk sac tumour elements was associated with an especially virulent course of tumour progression. Seminomas were associated with a significantly better prognosis. Even when seminomas spread to regional retroperitoneal lymph nodes, their responsiveness to radiotherapy led to cures. Non-seminomatous tumours are not radiosensitive, nor, in the 1960s, was an effective chemotherapy available.

The introduction of combination chemotherapy, which typically included cisplatin, bleomycin, and vinblastine, produced cures in many patients with disseminated tumours (Table 20.8). Recent substitution of the epipodophyllotoxin *etoposide* for vinblastine has further improved survival of patients with disseminated tumour—both seminomas and non-seminomatous tumours—with fewer side-effects. The prognosis

Table 20.8　Survival; all germ cell tumours (expressed as percentage of patients surviving)

Stage	Time period	5-year	10-year
Localized	1940–1949	65	58
	1970–1979	94	92
Regional	1940–1949	51	51
	1970–1979	77	76
Distant	1940–1949	5	5
	1970–1979	37	36

of disseminated germ cell tumours is little influenced by tumour composition. Even disseminated seminoma is more responsive to the chemotherapy regimen used for non-seminomatous tumours than to radiation therapy.

Current research attempts to cure tumours of all stages by the following approaches:

1. *More aggressive chemotherapy* of bulky metastatic disease, since the extent of tumour is correlated with the probability of cure.

2. *Resection and characterization of metastatases*, when small in number and amenable to surgery. This surgery is justifiable since resection of metastases may be curative, and histological characterization of the resected metastasis from a treated patient may guide further therapy. The risk of recurrent tumour is smaller in those patients whose metastases consist only of necrosis with fibrous tissue, compared with those who have residual tumour. The nature of residual tumour also indicates the biological potential of tumour still in the patient. Metastases consisting only of teratoma behave more benignly than those consisting of embryonal carcinoma.

3. *The development of different types of chemotherapeutic agents.* Agents which might take advantage of the differentiative potential of germ cell tumours by inducing terminal differentiation and, thereby, arrest of growth, is an appealing theoretical approach.

20.4.3   Sex cord-stromal tumours

Constituting about 2 per cent of testicular neoplasms, these tumours are comprised of cells which structurally and functionally resemble *gonadal stromal cells* (Fig. 20.39). Although they typically present as testicular masses, a minority of these tumours synthesize enough hormone to clinically manifest as either precocious masculinization in children, or, more rarely, as feminization. In contrast to germ cell tumours, the majority of these tumours are benign; metastases occur in fewer than 10 per cent of patients. These tumours can be further subclassified by histology into *Leydig cell tumours* and a *non-Leydig cell tumour*

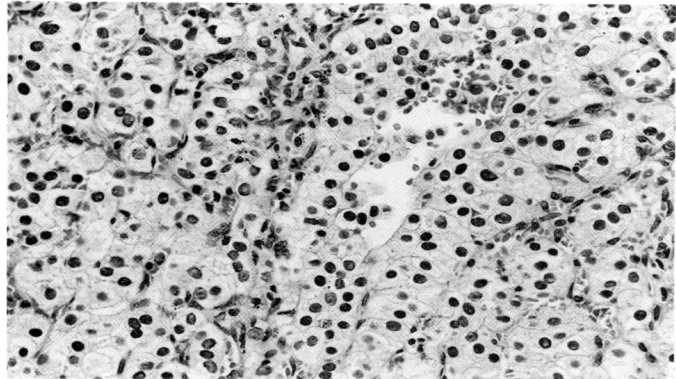

Fig. 20.39   Leydig cell tumours grow as solid sheets of cells having an eosinophilic cytoplasm and round nuclei of generally uniform size.

class, in which the most frequent type is the *Sertoli cell tumour*. In contrast to Leydig cell tumours, Sertoli cell tumours grow as cords, nests and/or tubules of cells.

20.4.4   Haemopoeitic tumours

The most common testicular neoplasm of men older than 55 is *lymphoma*. Virtually all are *non-Hodgkin's lymphomas of B-cell derivation*. In most patients, presentation of a testicular mass is the first sign of a tumour which is already systemic. The gross appearance of lymphoma as a homogeneous mass with a smooth, white to tan surface, resembles seminoma. Microscopically, lymphoma diffusely infiltrates testicular parenchyma (Fig. 20.40). Although clinical staging identifies tumours involving extratesticular tissues in one-half of patients who present with what clinically is thought to be a primary neoplasm of the testis, a higher percentage already have disseminated disease. And up to 40 per cent of individuals have bilateral testicular involvement.

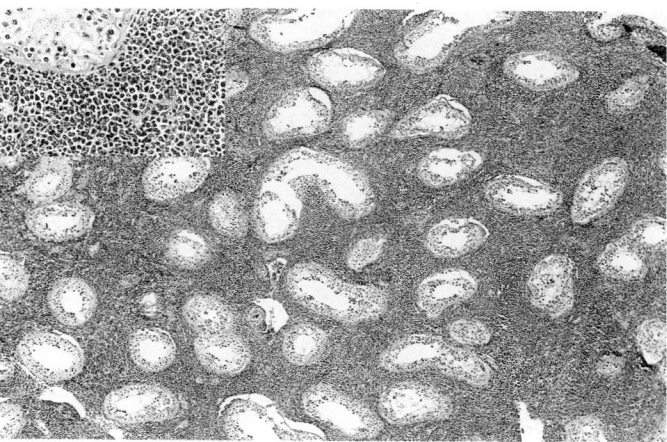

Fig. 20.40   A sheet of lymphoma cells characteristically infiltrates the interstitium between intact seminiferous tubules. Inset: the large, pleomorphic lymphoma cells usually spare tubules.

Despite the success of chemotherapy in producing remissions, with temporary disappearance of the mass, few patients are cured of lymphoma. The five-year survival rate is only 12 per cent. In the few survivors, the tumour was apparently present only in the testis and was thus successfully resected by orchidectomy.

Leukaemia often involves the testis. This can complicate the management of acute leukaemia, particularly of acute lymphoblastic leukaemia, of childhood, where the testis may serve as a reservoir site, harbouring occult malignant cells. For this reason the testis is biopsied, and irradiated if leukaemic cells are found.

20.4.5   Adnexal tumours

The most common adnexal tumour is the *benign adenomatoid*

tumour. Usually located in the epididymis or tunica vaginalis, these are firm, white nodules composed of flattened mesothelial cells, which has been demonstrated, both ultrastructurally and immunohistochemically. Once excised, these neoplasms pose no further clinical problem.

Sarcomas of the testis are virtually non-existent, and those of the adnexae are quite rare. The most common is *rhabdomyosarcoma*, which is most frequent in children. These tumours have a highly malignant potential, requiring aggressive therapy.

The *cystadenoma of the epididymis* is a distinctive benign tumour, readily cured by local excision. It is associated with neoplasms and disease processes of other organs, particularly with haemangiomas in the von Hippel–Lindau syndrome, and with cutaneous and central nervous system abnormalities in tuberous sclerosis.

20.4.6   Secondary tumours

The testis only rarely serves as a clinically significant site of metastatic tumour. Excluding haemopoietic neoplasia, the tumours which most frequently manifest clinically as testicular metastases are *carcinomas of the prostate and lung*.

20.4.7   Further reading

General

Pugh, R. C. B. (ed.) (1976). *Pathology of the testis*. Blackwell, Oxford.

Mostofi, F. K. and Price, E. M. Jr (1973). Tumors of the male genital system, *Atlas of tumor pathology*, 2nd series, Fascicle 8. Armed Forces Institute of Pathology, Washington, DC.

Multi-authored (1987). National Conference of Urologic Cancer—1986. *Cancer (Suppl.)* **60**, 437–718.

Talerman, A. and Roth, L. M. (ed.) (1986). *Pathology of the testis and its adnexa*. Churchill Livingstone, New York.

Specific

Giwercman, A., Brunn, E., Frimodt-Moller, C., and Skakkebaek, N. E. (1989). Prevalence of carcinoma-in-situ and other histopathologic abnormalities in testes of men with a history of cryptorchidism. *Journal of Urology* **142**, 998–1002.

Kleinsmith, L. J. and Pierce, G. B. (1964). Multipotentiality of single embryonal carcinoma cells. *Cancer Research* **24**, 1544–67.

Mintz, B. and Illmensee, K. (1975). Normal genetically mosaic mice produced from malignant teratocarcinoma cells. *Proceedings of the National Academy of Sciences, USA* **72**, 3585–9.

Myers, M. H. and Ries, L. A. G. (1989). Cancer patient survival rates: SEER program results for 10 years of follow-up. *CA* **39**, 21–39.

Riley, P. A. and Sutton, P. M. (1975). Why are ovarian teratomas benign whilst teratomas of the testis are malignant? *Lancet* **1**, 1360–2.

Silverberg, E., Boring, C. C., and Squires, T. S. (1990). Cancer statistics. *CA* **40**, 9–18.

Srigley, J. R., Mackay, B., Toth, P., and Ayala, A. (1988). The ultrastructure and histogenesis of male germ cell neoplasia with emphasis on seminoma with early carcinomatous features. *Ultrastructural Pathology* **12**, 67–86.

von der Maasa, H., Giwercman, A., Mueller, T., and Skakkebaek, N. E. (1989). Management of carcinoma-in-situ of the testes. *International Journal of Andrology* **10**, 209–20.

True, L. D., Otis, C. N., Delprado, W., Scully, R. E., and Rosai, J. (1988). Spermatocytic seminoma of testis with sarcomatous transformation. *American Journal of Surgical Pathology* **12**, 75–82.

Williams, S. D., Birch, R., Einhorn, L. H., Irwin, L., Greco, F. A., and Loehrer, P. J. (1987). Treatment of disseminated germ-cell tumors with cisplatin, bleomycin, and either vinblastine or etoposide. *New England Journal of Medicine* **316**, 1435–40.

Williams, S. D., Loehrer, P. J., Nichols, C. R., Roth, B. J., and Einhorn, L. H. (1989). Disseminated testicular cancer: current chemotherapy strategies. *Seminars in Oncology* (Suppl. 6) **16**, 105–9.

21

The female genital tract and ovaries

H. Fox and C. H. Buckley

21

The female genital tract and ovaries

H. Fox and C. H. Buckley

21.1 Introduction

The female genital tract differs from most other tissues in the body in so far as it does not, throughout life, show a static morphological appearance. The genital tract of a premenarchal girl differs from that of a woman who is in her reproductive years, the appearances in these latter women again changing as they become post-menopausal. Furthermore, during the reproductive era the morphology of the female genital tract is in a repetitive state of flux, the tissues of the tract reflecting faithfully the regular rhythm of ovarian endocrine function. Much of the pathology of the female genital tract is indicative of either an abnormal response to normal ovarian endocrinological stimulation or is a reflection of abnormal ovarian function. Abnormality of ovarian function may be primary or secondary to a fault in the pituitary–hypothalamic axis and it can thus be seen that the female genital tract is at the base of a hierarchical system which runs from the hypothalamus to the anterior pituitary and from there via the ovary to the genital tract. Feedback mechanisms operate, of course, from the ovaries to the hypothalamus but the female genital tract plays a purely passive role in this endocrinological interplay.

The female genital tract is, of course, also subject to all the other pathological processes that can affect more static tissues but is, furthermore, the specific site of sexually transmitted infections, some of which may be of aetiological importance in female genital tract neoplasia.

The ovaries are also unique, for they are the only human organs which cease to function well before the death of the individual. They differ markedly in this respect from their exact male homologue, the testes, and their limited life-span reflects their restricted content of germ cells, total loss of these resulting in cessation of ovarian function.

21.2 Normal development and malformations of the female genital tract

21.2.1 Development of the female genital tract

The primordial gonads appear, at about the fourth week of embryonic life, as a pair of longitudinal gonadal ridges, formed by a proliferation of the coelomic epithelium and a condensation of the underlying mesenchyme, situated just caudal and lateral to the developing mesonephros, the gonadal and mesonephric ridges tending to form a conjoined structure known as the *nephro-genital ridge*. The mesonephroi are connected to the cloaca by the *Wolffian (mesonephric) ducts* and by the sixth week of development the *Müllerian (paramesonephric) ducts* are formed: these latter arise as longitudinal invaginations of the coelomic epithelium on the anterolateral surfaces of the gonadal ridges.

The Müllerian ducts run parallel to the Wolffian ducts for most of their course and the latter appear to act as a scaffolding for the later development of the Müllerian ducts. The cranial parts of the two Müllerian ducts remain separate but caudally they grow medially, the ducts from each side coming into contact in the midline and, after being initially separated by a septum, eventually fusing to form the uterine canal. Further caudal growth of the fused Müllerian ducts brings them into contact with the posterior wall of the urogenital sinus: the two Wolffian ducts remain separate from each other and also open into the urogenital sinus.

The unfused cranial portions of the Müllerian ducts form the Fallopian tubes whereas the caudal fused portions develop into the uterus. In the female embryo the Wolffian ducts play no further role in development, vestiges of these ducts persisting, however, as Gartner's ducts in the broad ligament and in the lateral wall of the uterus.

The vagina is originally a solid cylindrical structure, the *vaginal plate*, which is probably formed as a result of cellular proliferation at the caudal end of the fused Müllerian ducts: this solid structure later becomes cavitated and it is thought that this process of canalization is due to an ingrowth from the urogenital sinus which displaces the Müllerian tissue. Whether the urogenital sinus gives rise only to the mucosa of the vagina or to the entire wall of the organ is still a matter of dispute.

21.2.2 Malformations of the female genital tract

By convention, the term 'malformation', when applied to the female genital tract, refers to anatomical abnormalities of the tract in women who otherwise have no phenotypic, sex chromosomal, gonadal, or endocrinological abnormality.

Classification and types

Female genital tract malformations can be divided, perhaps rather artificially, into four main groups:

1. *aplasias*;
2. *fusion defects*;
3. *failure of septum dissolution*;
4. *failures of canalization*.

Aplasia

Total aplasia of the Müllerian ductal system is extremely rare whilst unilateral aplasia, which results in a hemi-uterus, is very uncommon. The most frequently encountered form of aplasia is that in which there is an aplasia of the vagina together with an absent or rudimentary uterus and either poorly formed or normal Fallopian tubes. This condition, known as the *Rokitansky–Küster–Hauser syndrome*, is due to failure of development of the caudal Müllerian ductal system: there is a high incidence of accompanying abnormalities of the urinary tract and this suggests that the basic defect may be a Wolffian duct abnormality, the absence, or inadequate development, of this structure resulting in the lack of a scaffolding for subsequent Müllerian ductal development.

Fusion defects

Total failure of fusion of the two Müllerian ducts (Fig. 21.1) results in the formation of two uterine bodies, two cervices, and two vaginas (*uterus didelphys*). Progressively lesser degrees of Müllerian ductal fusion failure result in a *uterus bicornis bicollis*, in which there are two uterine bodies and cervices but only one vagina (Fig. 21.2), or a *uterus bicornis unicollis* (bicornuate uterus), characterized by the presence of two uterine bodies (or 'horns') with a single cervix and vagina (Fig. 21.3). The most minor form of fusion defect is the *arcuate uterus* in which the fundus of the uterine body has a midline notch, the uterus hav-

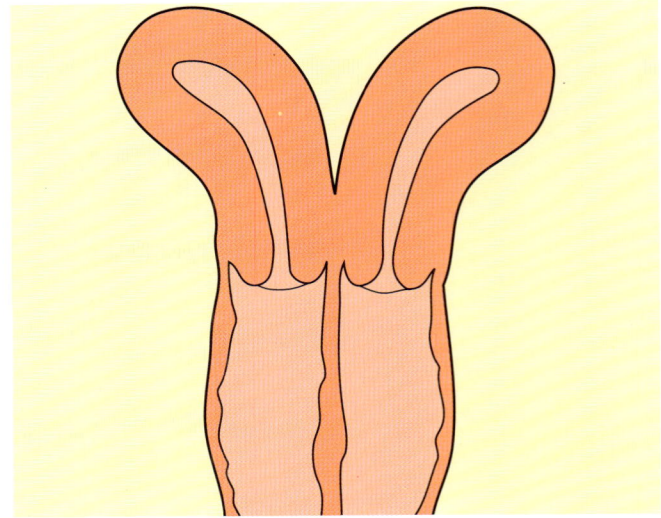

Fig. 21.1 A schematic representation of uterus didelphys with septate vagina. (Drawn after *Pathology for gynaecologists*, 2nd edn., 1991, Fox and Buckley, by kind permission of Edward Arnold.)

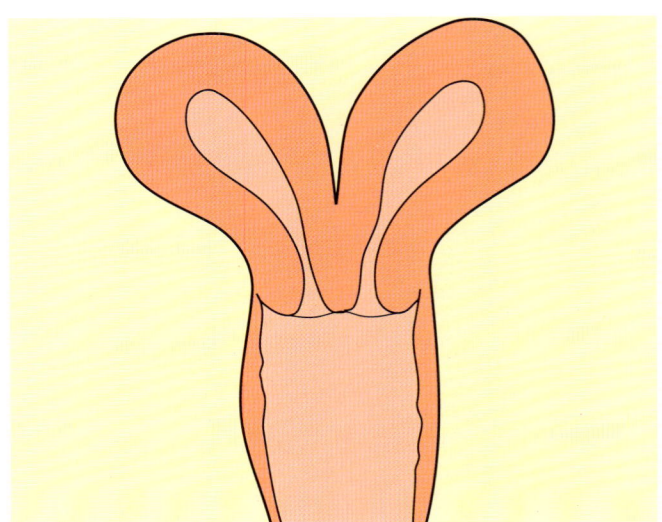

Fig. 21.2 A schematic representation of a uterus bicornis bicollis. (Drawn after *Pathology for gynaecologists*, 2nd edn, 1991, Fox and Buckley, by kind permission of Edward Arnold.)

ing a shape which resembles that of the heart as it is portrayed on a playing card (Fig. 21.4).

Variations of this relatively common theme of Müllerian fusion defects, always most marked cranially, are quite common. Thus in a bicornuate uterus, one horn may be rudimentary, solid, or detached and sometimes does not communicate with the main uterine cavity (Fig. 21.5).

Failures in septum dissolution

These can result in a fully or partially septate uterus (Fig. 21.6), a septate cervix, or a septate vagina. The first two of these anomalies are due to a failure of dissolution of the septum

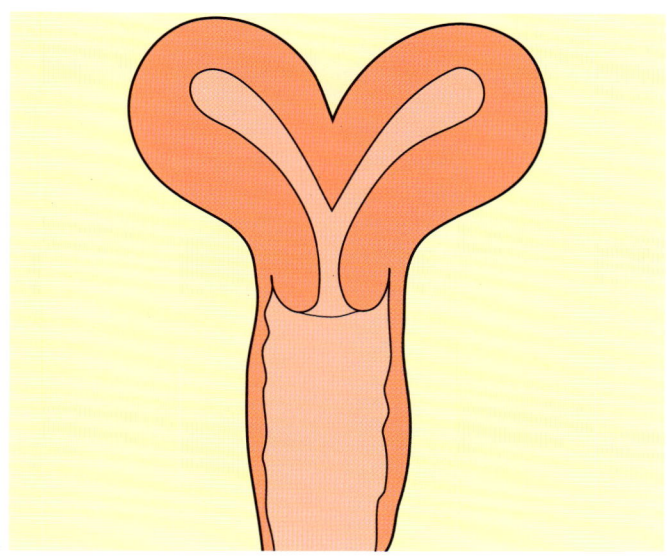

Fig. 21.3 A schematic representation of a uterus bicornis unicollis. (Drawn after *Pathology for gynaecologists*, 2nd edn, 1991, Fox and Buckley, by kind permission of Edward Arnold.)

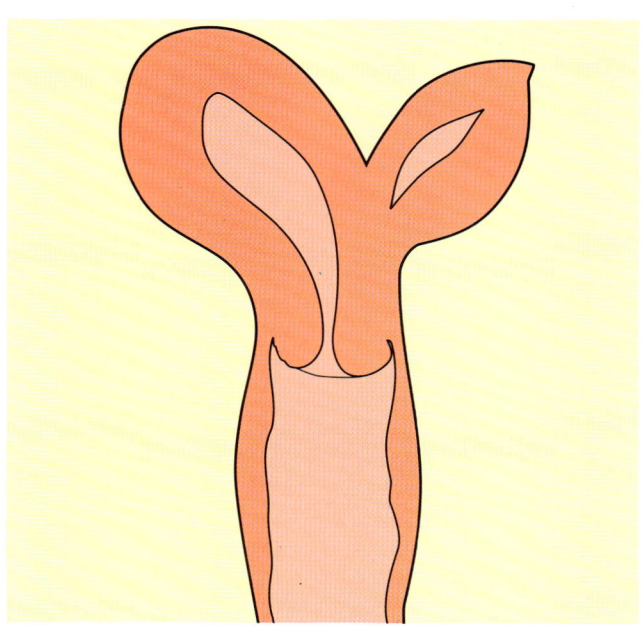

Fig. 21.5 A schematic representation of a bicornuate uterus with a non-communicating rudimentary horn. (Drawn after *Pathology for gynaecologists*, 2nd edn, 1991, Fox and Buckley, by kind permission of Edward Arnold.)

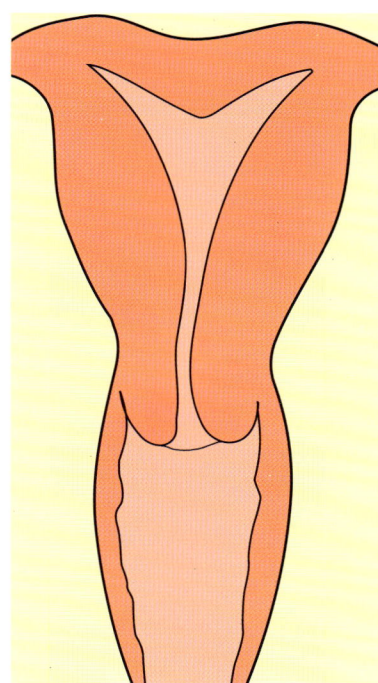

Fig. 21.4 A schematic representation of an arcuate uterus. (Drawn after *Pathology for gynaecologists*, 2nd edn, 1991, Fox and Buckley, by kind permission of Edward Arnold.)

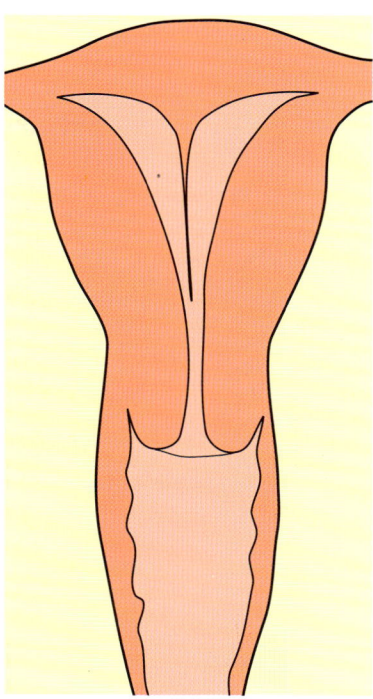

Fig. 21.6 A schematic representation of a septate uterus. (Drawn after *Pathology for gynaecologists*, 2nd edn, 1991, Fox and Buckley, by kind permission of Edward Arnold.)

between the two fused Müllerian ducts, whereas the last is probably due to a similar failure of septum dissolution between the two arms of the early urogenital sinus.

Failures of canalization

Vaginal aplasia, when associated with a normal uterus, is probably due to a failure of canalization of the originally solid vaginal plate because of inadequate ingrowth from the urogenital sinus. This may be because of a failure of fusion of the caudal fused ends of the Müllerian ducts with the urogenital sinus or because of a defect in urogenital sinus formation.

Aetiology and pathogenesis

Genetic factors may play a role in the development of some genital tract anomalies for there are well-documented examples of familial fusion defects and aplasia. Familial persistence of the vaginal plate has been noted in a number of Amish families, while uterine fusion defects are an integral component of the genetically determined *hand–foot–uterus syndrome*.

There is no association between sex chromosomal abnormalities and genital tract malformations, but trisomy 13 is characteristically accompanied by uterine fusion defects, and genital tract malformations have been noted in cases of trisomy 18. Prenatal exposure to thalidomide can cause severe genital tract malformations but the only other teratogen known to produce genital tract abnormalities is diethylstilboestrol (DES), prenatal exposure to this compound resulting in a high incidence of abnormalities, often multiple but usually of a subtle nature.

It has been suggested that many Müllerian duct anomalies are the end result of an interaction between genetic and environmental factors. A plausible suggestion is that a fusion defect results from a slight physical separation of the two Müllerian ducts at a critical stage of development, possibly because of a genetically determined abnormal shape of the embryonic pelvis.

Incidence and clinical features

The exact incidence of genital tract malformation is unknown but a reasonable estimate is that a malformation of greater or lesser degree is found in between 0.25 and 0.5 per cent of women. About one-third of women with a fusion defect have a normal reproductive history but the remainder have an unusually high incidence of abortion, premature labour, abnormal birth presentation, and uterine rupture: fusion defects are also associated with menorrhagia, dysmenorrhoea, and infertility.

21.3 Normal and abnormal sexual development

21.3.1 Normal sexual development

During early embryonic life the gonad is of an indifferent nature

and capable of developing into either a testis or an ovary. Differentiation along one or other of these alternative pathways is determined by the sex chromosomal constitution of the embryo: if the embryo is XY the germ cells migrating to the gonad from the yolk sac will contain the HY antigen which will induce differentiation of the gonad into a testis. If the fetus is XX the gonad will develop into an ovary.

If the gonad develops along a testicular pathway the Sertoli cells secrete a protein, known as *Müllerian inhibiting factor* (MIF), which acts locally to inhibit ipsilateral Müllerian duct development: thus MIF secreted by a left-sided developing testis inhibits Müllerian ductal development on the left side but has no effect on the development of the right-sided duct. MIF is not secreted by a developing ovary and in the absence of this substance there is a passive development of the Müllerian ductal system, no stimulatory factor being required.

The embryonic testis begins to secrete *testosterone* at about the 65th day of life and this hormone acts locally on the ipsilateral Wolffian duct system to induce differentiation into epididymis, vas deferens, and seminal vesicle; in the absence of testosterone, that is, when the gonad is developing into an ovary, the Wolffian duct system will regress and atrophy. Testosterone is also responsible for masculinization of the external genitalia, though for this action to occur the testosterone must first be converted in the target tissue to *dihydrotestosterone* by the enzyme 5-α-reductase. In the absence of dihydrotestosterone the external genitalia will develop along female lines.

Consideration of the control mechanisms of sexual development allow for the defining of two general principles:

1. Control of sexual development is hierarchical, with chromosomal sex determining gonadal sex and gonadal sex determining somatic sex.

2. The ovary does not play any role in normal sexual development and a neuter embryo will always develop along female lines, deviation into a male pattern of somatic development being dependent upon testicular secretion of MIF and testosterone.

21.3.2 Classification of abnormalities of sexual development

Sex can be defined in terms of chromosomal constitution, gonadal structure, phenotypic form, or gender identity; therefore abnormalities of sexual development can be defined and categorized at many different levels. Because, however, the fundamental determinant of sex is the remit of the X and Y chromosomes, it seems logical to regard the chromosomal constitution as a basis for the primary classification of these abnormalities, further subclassification being dependent on the type of gonad present and, to a lesser degree, phenotype.

1. *Disorders associated with normal sex chromosomes*
   (a) With macroscopically normal gonads
       (i) XX chromosomal constitution with bilateral macroscopically normal ovaries;

(ii) XY chromosomal constitution with bilateral macroscopically normal testes.

(b) With macroscopically abnormal gonads
   (i) XX chromosomal constitution with streak gonads;
   (ii) XX chromosomal constitution with ovary and testis;
   (iii) XY chromosomal constitution with streak gonads;
   (iv) XY chromosomal constitution with ovary and testis;

2. *Disorders associated with abnormal sex chromosomes*
  (a) Non-mosaic forms
    (i) XO chromosomal constitution with streak gonads;
    (ii) XXY chromosomal constitution with hypoplastic testes.
  (b) Mosaic forms
    (i) XO/XX chromosomal constitution with streak gonads;
    (ii) XO/XY chromosomal constitution with streak gonad and testis;
    (iii) XO/XY chromosomal constitution with ovary and testis;
    (iv) XX/XY chromosomal constitution with ovary and testis.

It will be realized that this classification simplifies, but not unduly, a very complex subject and does not cover all eventualities: this applies particularly to the chromosomal mosaic abnormalities which are extremely numerous, only the most common being included.

Disorders associated with normal sex chromosomes

With macroscopically normal gonads

XX chromosomal pattern with bilateral macroscopically normal ovaries Individuals with a 46XX chromosomal constitution and normal ovaries who have been exposed to androgen excess during fetal life will show partial masculinization of their external genitalia (Fig. 21.7): the term 'female pseudohermaphroditism' is often applied to this syndrome.

The commonest cause of female pseudohermaphroditism is *congenital adrenal hyperplasia* in which there is a congenital deficiency of one or other of the chain of enzymes necessary for the synthesis of corticosteroids with a consequent accumulation of intermediate androgenic steroids (see Section 26.4).

Administration of androgens or progestagens to the mother of a female infant during pregnancy will also induce masculinization of the external genitalia, though the degree of virilization is usually less profound than that found in congenital adrenal hyperplasia and there is no progression in the degree of genital abnormality after birth.

The presence during pregnancy of a maternal virilizing tumour is a rare cause of female pseudohermaphroditism. Most women with such neoplasms fail to conceive but some have achieved pregnancy and there have been a few reports of rather mild masculinization of the external genitalia of female children resulting from such pregnancies. The least rare virilizing lesion

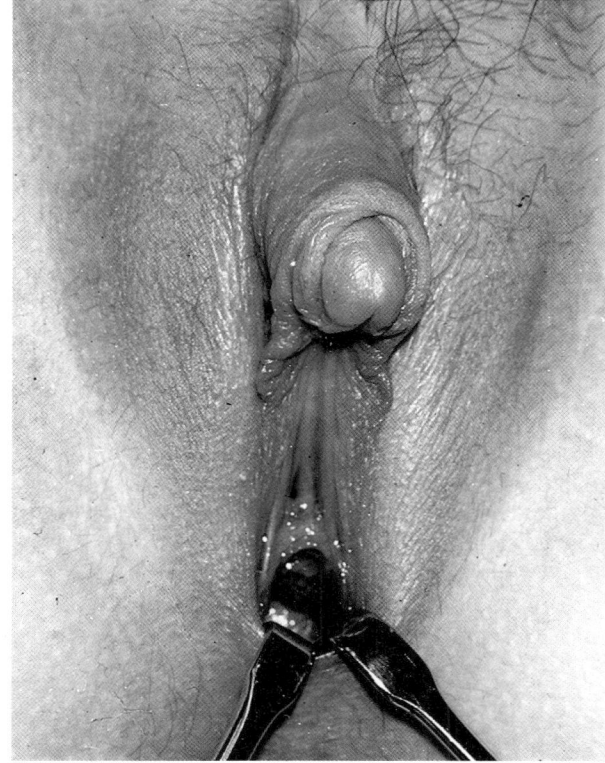

Fig. 21.7 External genital appearances in a partially masculinized 12-year-old girl. (Reproduced by kind permission of Sir John Dewhurst and Churchill Livingstone from *Obstetrical and gynaecological pathology* (ed. H. Fox), Haines and Taylor, 1987.)

occurring during gestation is the luteoma of pregnancy (see p. 1618).

XY chromosomal pattern and bilateral macroscopically normal testes Individuals with a 46XY chromosomal constitution and bilateral macroscopically normal testes who, because of a relative or absolute androgen deficiency during fetal life, have poorly masculinized or female external genitalia are often grouped together as examples of 'male pseudohermaphroditism'.

The *androgen resistance syndrome* is the most important form of this anomaly because it is usually associated with a fully female phenotype and gender identity: nevertheless, most patients with this syndrome not only have a 46XY chromosomal constitution and bilateral testes but also high or normal plasma testosterone levels, and it has become clear that the failure of their external genitalia to masculinize is due to an end-organ insensitivity to the effects of androgens. It will be recalled that testosterone is partially converted peripherally to dihydrotestosterone by the enzyme 5-α-reductase: both hormones bind to the same receptor protein in the target cells and the testosterone–receptor complex is believed to regulate Wolffian duct development, gonadotrophin secretion, and spermatogenesis, whereas the dihydrotestosterone–receptor complex is responsible for external virilization during embryogenesis and for much of the development of secondary sex characteristics at puberty. This system can break down if there is a deficiency of 5-α-reductase, an abnormality of the androgen-receptor protein, or a failure of the cells to respond to the receptor–hormone complex.

An androgen-receptor protein defect is responsible for the clinical syndrome of testicular feminization. Patients with this abnormality have an XY karyotype and female external genitalia. The vagina is short and blind and internal genitalia are absent, apart from bilateral testes which may lie in the abdomen, inguinal canal, or labia majora. At puberty, affected individuals undergo breast development and feminization; their fully female appearance (Fig. 21.8) is combined with a completely female gender identity and patients present either because of primary amenorrhoea or with bilateral inguinal swellings that are often thought to be hernias. These clinical features suggest a complete absence of androgens (but not of MIF), but, nevertheless, plasma levels of both testosterone and dihydrotestosterone are either normal or high; the patients are also completely refractory to exogenous androgens and it is now clear that this syndrome is due to a familial defect or deficiency

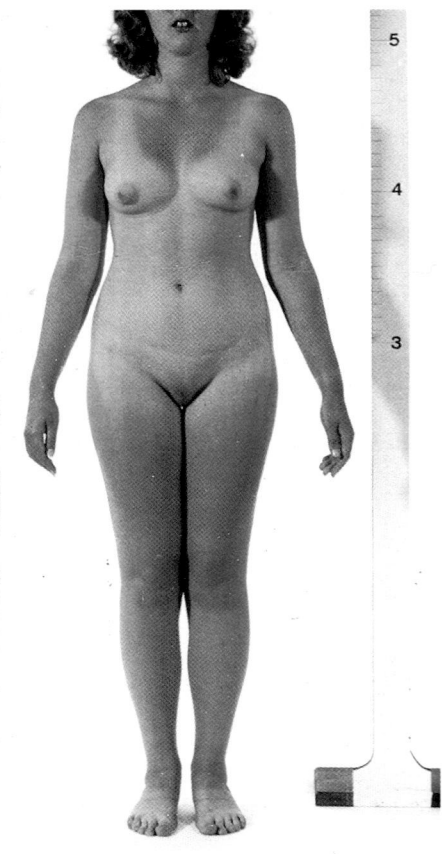

Fig. 21.8 A phenotypic female with a 46XY karyotype and complete androgen resistance syndrome. (Reproduced by kind permission of Sir John Dewhurst and Churchill Livingstone from *Obstetrical and gynaecological pathology* (ed. H. Fox), Haines and Taylor, 1987.)

of androgen-receptor protein. Because the receptor deficiency also involves the hypothalamic centres, the androgen feedback mechanism is inoperative and luteinizing hormone (LH) levels are elevated: synthesis of oestrogens is therefore increased and the high levels of these hormones are responsible for the complete pubertal feminization and for the well-marked breast development. The testes of these patients are particularly prone to develop a germ-cell neoplasm, but there is virtually no risk of this occurring before the age of puberty and it is usual to delay castration until after the patient has undergone pubertal feminization.

A small proportion of patients with an androgen-receptor deficiency have a predominantly male phenotype and present as inadequately virilized males: this condition, known as *Reifenstein syndrome*, appears to be due to a partial deficiency of androgen-receptor protein.

A rare condition is that of *receptor-positive androgen resistance* in which patients with all the clinical features of the complete testicular feminization syndrome are found to have normal amounts of androgen receptor and normal nuclear localization of the receptor–hormone complex: this condition may be due to a nuclear unresponsiveness to the receptor–hormone complex.

The final form of androgen resistance is that due to 5-α-reductase deficiency. This is a rare condition in which XY males with bilateral inguinal or labial testes are of female phenotype at birth but have fully developed Wolffian duct structures (epididymis, vas deferens, seminal vesicles) that terminate in the vagina (Fig. 21.9). At the time of puberty there is a degree of virilization of the external genitalia, some growth of pubic and axillary, but not facial, hair and, occasionally, a switch in gender identity from female to male. These features are those which would be expected if there were a deficiency of dihydrotestosterone, but not of testosterone, during development and, indeed, these individuals have been shown to have high plasma testosterone values and low levels of plasma dihydrotestosterone. These abnormalities reflect the inability of target tissues that are deficient in 5-α-reductase to convert testosterone to dihydrotestosterone, this deficiency being due to the homozygous state of an autosomal recessive gene.

With macroscopically abnormal gonads

Instances are encountered of individuals with normal XX chromosomal patterns but who have either bilateral streak gonads or have both an ovary and a testis. The latter group is one variant of *hermaphrodite* (a condition discussed later) whereas the former are classed as examples of *pure gonadal dysgenesis*. Patients with pure gonadal dysgenesis have normal, but infantile, internal and external genitalia, are of normal stature, and have none of the physical stigmata of Turner's syndrome. These cases are sometimes familial, do not have any predisposition to gonadal neoplasia, and may be due to a specific failure of a hypothetical gonadal 'inductor' substance.

Individuals with 46XY chromosomal constitution may have bilateral streak gonads or even completely absent gonads. Such cases were previously referred to as 'pure XY gonadal dysgenesis', 'anorchia', or 'Swyer's syndrome' but are now

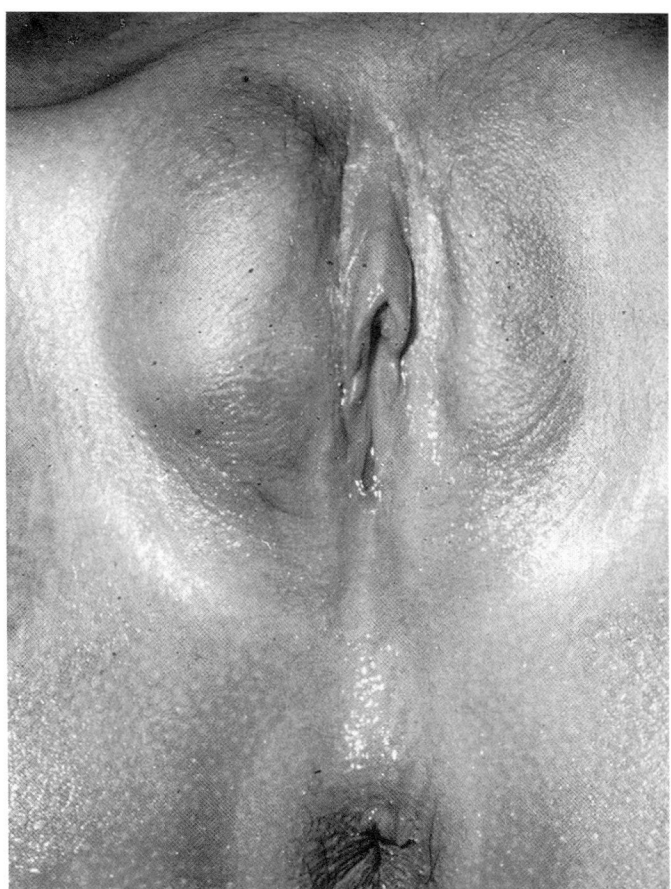

Fig. 21.9 The external genital appearance in a 46XY child aged 9 years and with 5-α-reductase deficiency. Masculinization of the genitalia is minimal, but the child's right testis is readily seen and the left easily brought down from the groin into the labial tissue. Her sister, aged 10, was also affected. (Reproduced by kind permission of Sir John Dewhurst and Churchill Livingstone from *Obstetrical and gynaecological pathology*, Haines and Taylor, 1987.)

thought to represent the *testicular regression syndrome*, in which, for reasons as yet unknown, the testes regress at some stage of fetal life. This results in a very wide spectrum of abnormalities, the nature of which depends upon the timing of gonadal regression relative to the secretion of MIF and testosterone. At one end of this spectrum the external genitalia are female in type, the internal organs are absent, and the gonads are either absent or are streaks, this condition being due to gonadal regression at a very early stage of embryogenesis before differentiation of the Wolffian and Müllerian duct systems. At the other extreme are phenotypic males with normal internal genitalia and infantile or nearly normal external genitalia, such cases being due to testicular regression in late fetal life.

Individuals with 46XY type with both an ovary and a testis represent yet another form of true hermaphroditism (see later).

Disorders associated with abnormal sex chromosomes

Individuals with a sex chromosomal abnormality may have a pure karyotype, e.g. 45XO, or may be chromosomal mosaics, e.g. 45XO/46XX. The possible chromosomal and clinical permutations are many but, in very general terms, most cases of sex chromosomal abnormality fall into one of four clinical groups, namely, *Turner's syndrome, Klinefelter's syndrome, mixed gonadal dysgenesis*, or *true hermaphroditism*.

Turner's syndrome

The vast majority of patients with this syndrome have a 45XO chromosomal constitution, although a small minority are XO mosaics (usually either 45XO/46XX or 45XO/47XXX). In its classical form, the syndrome consists of sexual infantilism and streak gonads (Fig. 21.10) in a phenotypic female of short stature, but a number of other physical abnormalities, collectively known as *Turner's stigmata*, may or may not be present; these include neck webbing, lymphoedema, high palate, shield chest, increased cubital carrying angle, coarctation of the aorta, etc.

The internal genitalia are of normal female form, though infantile, and the gonads are represented by white fibrous streaks, 2–3 cm long and about 0.5 cm in diameter, in the site normally occupied by the ovaries. During embryonic life, the

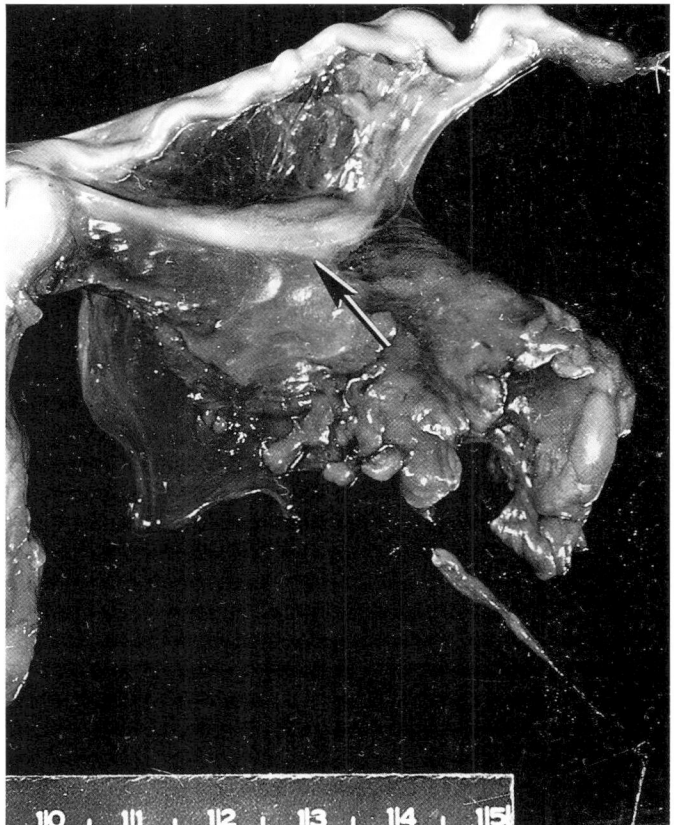

Fig. 21.10 Streak gonad in Turner's syndrome. (Reproduced by kind permission of Dr S. Robboy and Churchill Livingstone from *Obstetrical and gynaecological pathology*, Haines and Taylor, 1987.)

gonad of an XO individual contains a normal complement of germ cells but these rapidly degenerate, are almost all lost by the time of birth and have completely disappeared well before puberty. It has been suggested, therefore, that two X-chromosomes are necessary for the control of granulosa cell development and that in the absence of two such chromosomes the granulosa cells will fail to differentiate, with subsequent degeneration of the germ cells. Patients with an XO mosaicism may retain a few germ cells into adult life and occasionally menstruate, some even becoming pregnant. Patients with Turner's syndrome do not have any tendency to develop gonadal neoplasms.

Klinefelter's syndrome

Patients with this condition are phenotypic males with a 47/XXY chromosomal constitution: exceptionally, there is an XXY mosaicism. The syndrome is characterized by azoospermia, gynaecomastia, and atrophic testes: most patients have sparse body and facial hair, unduly long legs and, often but not invariably, are of rather low intelligence. The testes rarely exceed 2 cm in diameter and show marked hyalinization and degeneration of the seminiferous tubules with an apparent, but not actual, increase in the number of Leydig cells.

Mixed gonadal dysgenesis

Individuals with this abnormality have asymmetrical sexual development, usually having a streak gonad on one side and a testis, albeit one often showing some degree of immaturity and disorganization, on the other side. The chromosomal constitution is variable but is most commonly a 45XO/46XY mosaicism. There is a considerable range of development of internal and external genitalia but most patients present as phenotypic females with partially masculinized external genitalia. Both Müllerian and Wolffian duct structures are commonly present and the gender identity is more often female than male. These patients tend to virilize at puberty and run a high risk of developing germ cell neoplasms of their gonads: hence gonadectomy before the time of puberty is usually advised.

True hermaphroditism

Hermaphrodites have both ovarian and testicular tissue and the term is applied independently of chromosomal constitution. The majority of patients (about 60 per cent) have a 46XX chromosomal constitution but a minority have a 46XY chromosomal pattern or are either 46XX/46XY or 45XO/46XY mosaics: there may be an ovary on one side and a testis on the other or there may be bilateral combined ovotestes. The patients most often present as predominantly phenotypic males with ambiguous external genitalia, though a minority have a predominantly female phenotype. A variety of complex combinations of internal duct development may be encountered but most true hermaphrodites will have a uterus, a minority menstruating and even, on rare occasions, becoming pregnant.

The basic abnormality in most cases of hermaphroditism, particularly those with an XX chromosomal pattern, is unknown but it has been shown that XX hermaphrodites are often HY-antigen positive: indeed, the ovarian tissue may be HY-antigen negative whereas the testicular tissue is HY-antigen positive, this suggesting that there may be a mosaic primordium irrespective of apparent karyotype.

The gonads of a true hermaphrodite have some tendency to develop germ cell neoplasms, though the risk is much lower than in cases of mixed gonadal dysgenesis. Gonadectomy is therefore generally recommended and, in those individuals brought up as females, this operation is performed before puberty so as to prevent pubertal virilization.

21.4   The vulva

The external female genitalia include the mons pubis, labia minora and majora, clitoris, and the vestibule into which open the vagina, urethra, and the ducts of Skene's and Bartholin's glands.

The *mons pubis* is the fatty pad which lies over the pubic symphysis and the muscles of the lower abdominal wall; it is covered by hair-bearing skin.

The *labia majora*, which are the paired soft tissue folds forming the lateral margins of the vulva, are continuous anteriorly with the mons pubis and posteriorly with each other and with the perineum: they enclose the *labia minora* and the *vestibule*. The labia minora, which are also paired, normally lie in close apposition to each other and to the inner surfaces of the labia majora. They unite posteriorly to form the *fourchette*, which is broken during childbirth, and anteriorly divide into lateral parts which unite in the midline to form the *prepuce* of the clitoris and medial parts which form the *frenulum* of the clitoris.

The labia majora are composed of fibro-fatty muscular tissue covered on their outer surfaces by hair-bearing skin in which there are sebaceous glands and both eccrine and apocrine sweat glands: their inner surfaces are smooth and lack hair. The labia minora are devoid of adipose tissue but their connective tissue is particularly rich in elastic fibres and blood vessels: the covering pigmented skin contains sebaceous glands and, immediately adjacent to the clitoris, a small number of mucus-secreting glands.

The squamous epithelium of the vestibule is continuous medially with the transitional epithelium lining the urethra and the glycogenated non-keratinizing squamous epithelium which lines the vagina.

The clitoris lies anteriorly in the midline. It is composed of erectile tissue and covered by a stratified squamous epithelium which is poorly keratinized and lacks sebaceous glands, sweat glands, and hair.

The vulva is supplied by the internal pudendal artery and by the external pudendal branches of the femoral artery; the venous drainage accompanies the arteries. Lymphatic drainage is to the superficial inguinal lymph nodes.

Bartholin's glands are paired, mucus-secreting glands which lie deep in the posterior parts of the labia majora and open into the vestibule. They are composed of lobules of glandular acini, lined by cuboidal epithelium, which drain via ducts lined by a transitional epithelium. The latter not infrequently undergoes metaplasia to a squamous epithelium, particularly if the gland has been infected.

21.4.1 Dermatological disorders

The vulvar skin is part of the body integument and is therefore subject to all the disorders that can affect the skin elsewhere in the body, such as, for example, psoriasis, pemphigus, or lichen planus. Two conditions, lichen simplex and lichen sclerosus et atrophicus, do, however, merit special attention, partly because they occur with some frequency in the skin of the vulva and partly because these two disorders have, until recently, been regarded, rather illogically, as falling into a separate category of 'vulvar dystrophies'.

Lichen simplex (Fig. 21.11), previously classed as 'hyperplastic dystrophy' appears as circumscribed areas of thickened red or white skin, usually on the labia majora. Histologically, the squamous epithelium is thickened, and shows acanthosis, elongation of the rete pegs, parakeratosis, and hyperkeratosis: there is a non-specific chronic inflammatory cell infiltrate of the dermis. In the absence of superimposed intraepithelial neoplasia, lichen simplex is not associated with any increased risk of vulvar carcinoma.

Lichen sclerosus (LS) can occur in any part of the skin but has a particular predilection for the genital area. The skin lesions are papular and occur singly or in confluent patches. Extreme pallor of the tissues, thin fragile epithelium with telangiectasia and gradual loss of the vulval contours may accompany the chronic phase and the tissues become parchment-like (Fig. 21.12). In the early lesions bullae may form due to liquefaction degeneration of the basal layer of the epithelium and dermal

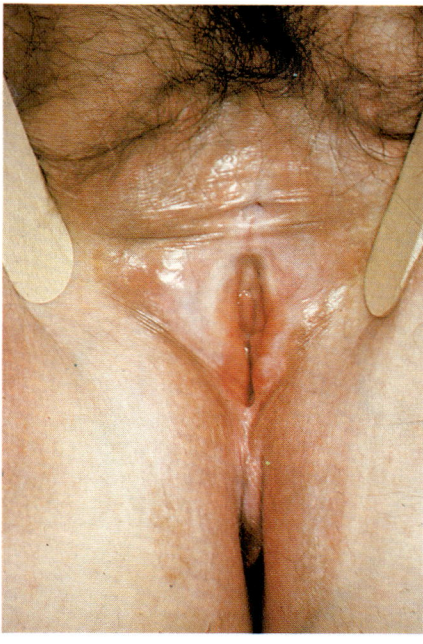

Fig. 21.12 Lichen sclerosus of the vulva: extensive atrophy and loss of substance with erythema and telangiectasia. (Reproduced by courtesy of Dr C. M. Ridley and Churchill Livingstone from *The vulva*, ed. C. M. Ridley, 1988.)

oedema: in childhood, rupture of these bullae may give a false impression of sexual abuse. The lesions of LS are associated with intractable itching and soreness, and pain may accompany the fissuring typical of the chronic phase. Histologically, the epidermis is flat and thin but hyperkeratotic: there is striking hyalinization of the upper dermis and a non-specific chronic inflammatory cell infiltrate of the lower dermis (Fig. 21.13). LS may show *secondary lichenification*, this combination being previously classed as a 'mixed dystrophy'. There has been much

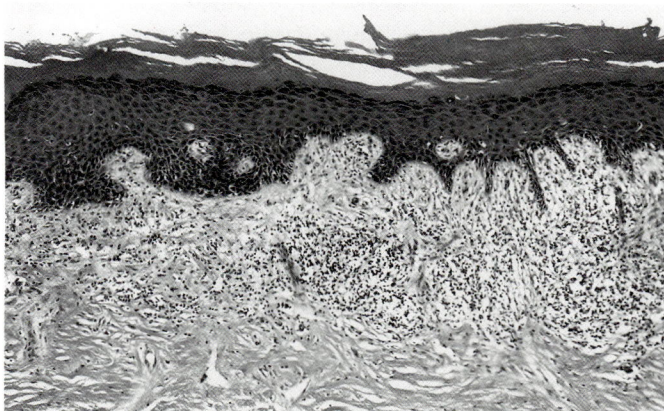

Fig. 21.11 Lichen simplex of the vulva. The epidermis is covered by a thick layer of keratin and the epithelium is mildly thickened (acanthotic). The underlying dermis is infiltrated by chronic inflammatory cells.

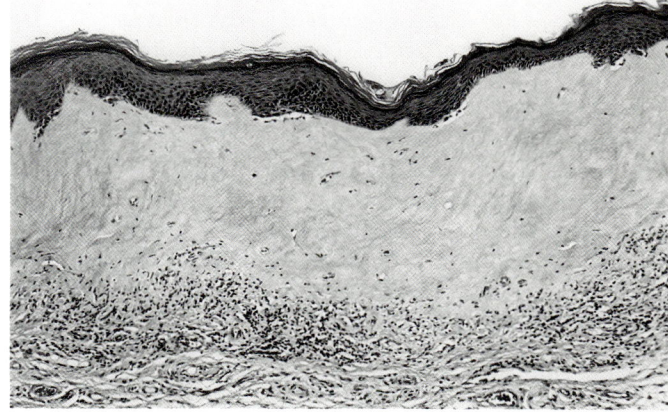

Fig. 21.13 Lichen sclerosus of the vulva. The epidermis is shallow, mildly hyperkeratotic, and there is loss of the rete ridges. The superficial part of the underlying dermis is hyalinized whereas its deeper layers are infiltrated by lymphocytes.

debate as to whether LS, which is essentially an atrophic disorder, is associated with an increased incidence of vulvar carcinoma: the current view is that there probably is a slightly increased risk of squamous cell carcinoma, although the neoplasm does not necessarily develop in that part of the vulva affected by LS.

21.4.2   Inflammation of the vulva

Non-infective vulvitis

Non-infective inflammation of the vulva may be evoked by irritants such as soap, scents, or deodorants, and excessive washing, especially if combined with the liberal use of antiseptics, may aggravate, rather than alleviate, inflammation. Incontinence of urine, a copious vaginal discharge, or excessive sweating can all be irritant to vulvar skin, and a severe vulvitis may follow exposure to radiotherapy.

Infective vulvitis

Herpes virus infection

Herpetic vulvitis is not uncommon, is acquired through sexual contact and occurs particularly in young women. The initial lesions are vesicular and usually painless: later the patient presents with a painful ulcerative vulvitis. The histological features of the infection tend to be rather non-specific and specific diagnosis is dependent upon serological studies or viral culture. Some women infected by the virus develop no signs or symptoms and can transmit the disease in the absence of clinical infection.

Human papilloma virus infection

This results in the development of condylomata and, possibly, vulvar intra-epithelial neoplasis, these subjects being considered later in this section.

Granuloma inguinale

This disease, possibly sexually transmitted, is due to infection with the Gram-negative organism *Calymmatobacterium granulomatis* and is largely encountered in tropical countries. Primary lesions occur on the vulva as painful papules or nodules which break down to form a spreading ulcer with exuberant granulation tissue in its base. Healing of the lesion is by dense fibrosis which leads to extensive scarring: this may cause lymphatic obstruction with resultant brawny vulvar oedema. Histologically there is a luxurious production of non-specific granulation tissue with an infiltrate of plasma cells and histiocytes: the latter contain the rounded or rod-like Donovan bodies which are diagnostic of this disease.

Lymphogranuloma venereum

This is a venereal infection with *Chlamydia trachomatis* and is most prevalent in the tropics and sub-tropics. The primary lesion is a self-healing vulvar papule or shallow ulcer which is later followed by a suppurative inguinal lymphadenitis: the large painful nodes become matted together and liquefy to form

fluctant buboes which drain through the skin via indolent sinuses. In a proportion of cases the primary lesions do not heal and progress to a chronic spreading destructive ulceration which may involve the vulva, vagina, and rectum, leading eventually to vaginal and rectal stenoses. Histologically, characteristic features are present only in the lymph nodes where stellate abscesses are seen.

Syphilis

The vulva is a site of predilection for the primary lesion of syphilis, the chancre appearing as a painless, hard, brownish red nodule with, often, surface erosion: this heals spontaneously after a few weeks. The typical silvery-grey snail-track ulcers of the secondary stage of syphilis can occur on the vulva, whereas elevated moist plaques, known as *condylomata lata*, may involve not only the vulva in secondary syphilis but also the adjacent perineum, peri-anal region, and upper thighs.

Chancroid

This is a sexually transmitted acute infection with *Haemophilus ducrei*. The primary lesions develop on the labia as painful nodules, often multiple, which break down to form small erosions, these tending to coalesce to form large ragged irregular ulcers with an excavated margin. The infection commonly spreads to the inguinal nodes to produce a painful lymphadenitis which may evolve into fluctuant masses that discharge through the skin. The histological appearances are of non-specific granulation tissue.

Condyloma acuminatum

These lesions, also known as venereal or genital warts (Fig. 21.14), occur most commonly in young women and their incidence has been increasing in recent years. The condylomas occur, typically, along the edges of the labia minora, between the labia minora and majora, and around the introitus: they are usually multiple and often confluent. Macroscopically they appear as papillary or verrucous lesions which may be predunculated or sessile. Histologically, complex fibrovascular cores are covered by acanthotic squamous epithelium which shows parakeratosis and, often, hyperkeratosis. Multinucleation, premature individual cell keratinization and koilocytosis are usually present.

Condylomata acuminata are sexually transmitted and are due to infection with *human papilloma virus* (HPV): Southern blot analysis of the viral DNA in these lesions has shown that the warts are usually due to HPV strains 6 or 11. They do not show any tendency to undergo neoplastic change but are, nevertheless, associated with a high incidence of concomitant vulvar and cervical intra-epithelial neoplasia.

Sometimes vulval skin which appears normal to naked eye examination may have histological features similar to those seen in the epithelium covering a condyloma acuminatum. Such lesions are called *flat condylomas*, or subclinical human papilloma virus infection, and have their counterparts on the cervix (see p. 1588). Their significance lies in the fact that they, too, may be associated with vulvar and cervical intra-epithelial

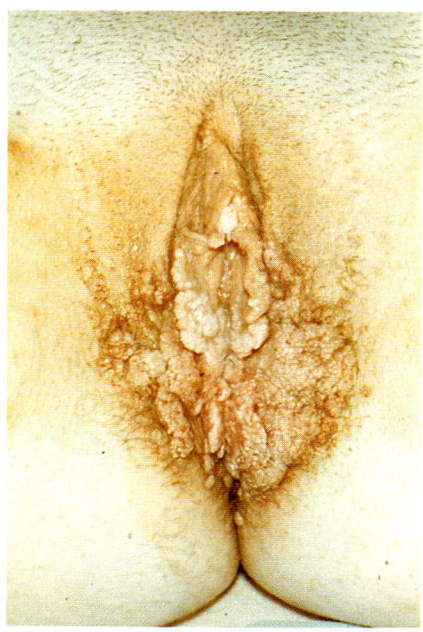

Fig. 21.14 Condylomata acuminata affecting particularly the lower part of the labia minora and the perianal region. (Reproduced by kind permission of Professor V. R. Tindall and Wolfe Medical Publications Ltd.)

neoplasia but may escape detection during ordinary clinical examination. Their diagnosis depends upon an awareness of their occurrence and the undertaking of appropriate cytological studies or histological sampling of the tissue.

21.4.3 Non-invasive, intra-epithelial neoplastic lesions

Vulvar intra-epithelial neoplasia

All cases of intra-epithelial squamous cellular atypia in the vulva are now grouped together into the single category of vulvar intra-epithelial neoplasia (VIN), a term encompassing all lesions previously described as 'vulvar atypia' and 'vulvar carcinoma *in situ*'. This form of nomenclature indicates that VIN is an intra-epithelial squamous neoplasm which may show varying degrees of differentiation, it being now realized that even cases of 'mild atypia' are commonly aneuploid.

VIN is characterized by a disturbance of normal cellular stratification and by abnormalities of cell differentiation. Mitotic figures, often of abnormal form, are found above the basal layers of the epithelium, while nuclear pleomorphism, a high nucleo-cytoplasmic ratio, and irregular clumping of nuclear chromatin are other typical features. VIN is often graded into *well-differentiated* (VIN I), *moderately well-differentiated* (VIN II), and *poorly differentiated grades* (VIN III) in the same way as is cervical intra-epithelial neoplasia (CIN) (see below). In this system, when abnormal, poorly differentiated cells are limited to the lower third of the epithelium, the lesion is classed as VIN I; extension of undifferentiated cells into the middle third of the

epithelium puts the lesion into the category of VIN II; whereas the presence of such cells in the upper third of the epithelium leads to a diagnosis of VIN III, this diagnosis also being applied to those cases in which undifferentiated cells occupy the full thickness of the squamous epithelium (Fig. 21.15). In practice, however, application of this system to vulvar intra-epithelial neoplasia is more difficult than for cervical lesions, as a simple failure of cellular differentiation is not always a prominent feature. Even when nuclear atypia is pronounced, cellular maturation, as judged by cytoplasmic maturation, may seem normal. VIN may be diagnosed, therefore, when there is little or no general failure of cellular differentiation but when cells with abnormal nuclei or containing atypical mitoses are present.

Clinical aspects

The incidence of VIN has increased dramatically in recent years, particularly in young women: patients with VIN have also a high incidence of associated cervical intra-epithelial neoplasia (CIN) and of sexually transmitted diseases. The lesions of VIN may be discrete, though often multifocal, but can involve the entire vulva; they tend to be slightly raised or papular and may be red, white, or brown. Many patients have no symptoms, the condition being detected incidentally during treatment of CIN or a sexually transmitted disease, but a minority of women suffer vulvar pruritis.

Aetiology and natural history

There is strong evidence for an association between HPV infection and VIN, though whether the virus plays a direct aetiological role in the development of the intra-epithelial neoplasm is still a matter for dispute. Southern blot hybridization studies have shown the presence of *HPV strain 16* in the vast majority of cases of VIN.

VIN has many similarities with CIN but, nevertheless, has a quite different natural history. Thus, there is a very low rate of progression of VIN into an invasive squamous cell carcinoma, an invasive neoplasm developing only in, at the most, about 5 per cent of cases and progression tending to occur predominantly in elderly women or in patients who are immunosuppressed. Conversely, about 6 per cent of cases of VIN regress spontaneously. Because of the relatively small risk of development of an invasive carcinoma there is an increasing tendency to treat all cases of VIN by local conservative measures, such as laser therapy.

Paget's disease

Vulvar Paget's disease is rare and occurs most commonly in post-menopausal women in whom it presents as poorly demarcated, often multiple, erythematous areas in any part of the vulvar skin. Histologically (Fig. 21.16), there are large, round or oval cells with pale cytoplasm, lying singly or in nests within the epidermis: glandular differentiation is seen in a few cases. The Paget cells contain mucus and are PAS positive after diastase digestion, characteristics which help to differentiate them from melanocytes.

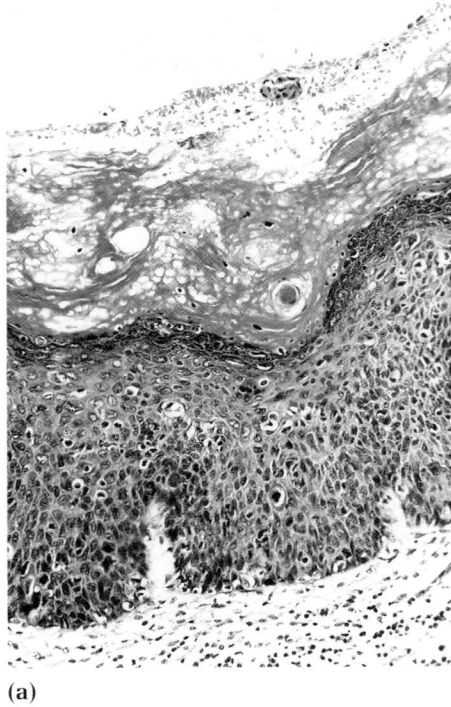

(a)

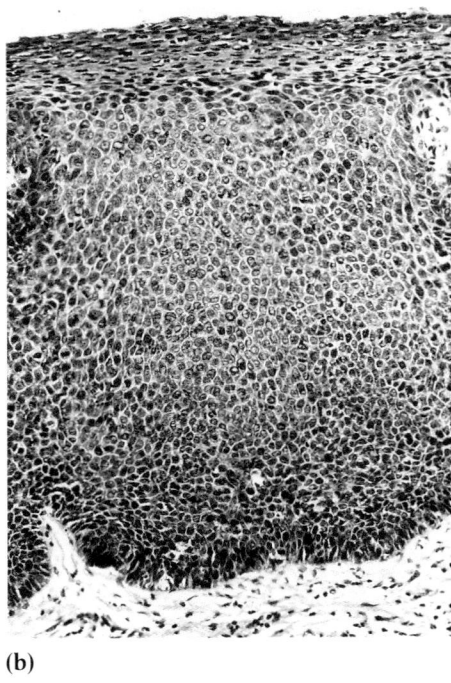

(b)

Fig. 21.15 Vulvar intra-epithelial neoplasia. (a) Bowenoid pattern. The epidermis is hyperkeratotic and there is a gross disturbance of normal stratification. Large numbers of mitoses are seen and individually keratinized cells are present. (b) In contrast to the epithelium shown in (a), the epidermis is parakeratotic and the full thickness is occupied by cells showing little or no differentiation.

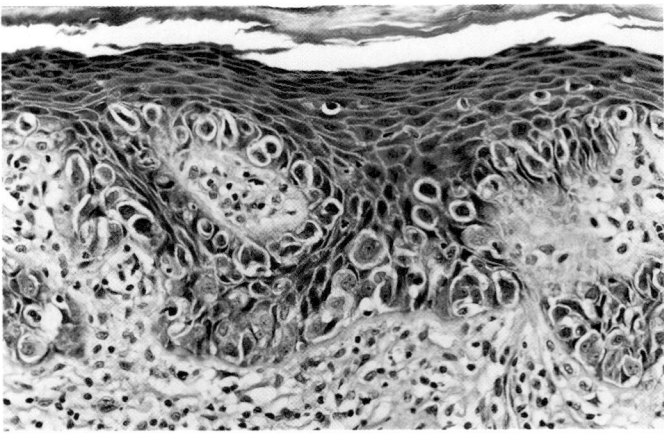

Fig. 21.16 Paget's disease of the vulva. Within the mildly hyperkeratotic epidermis, most markedly in the basal layers, there are groups of large Paget's cells with pale cytoplasm.

Paget's disease of the vulva can arise in two different ways. In some cases, a minority, there is a subjacent adnexal adenocarcinoma, the Paget cells representing an extension, or a metastasis, from this to the epidermis. In most patients, however, there is no associated adenocarcinoma, the Paget cells developing *in situ* from pluripotential undifferentiated cells in the basal layers of the vulvar epithelium; under these circumstances the Paget cells represent an intra-epithelial adenocarcinoma, which can occasionally progress to an invasive lesion.

21.4.4 Non-neoplastic cysts

Several types of non-neoplastic vulval cyst are recognized. They may arise in developmental remnants, may follow the blockage of gland ducts or may be the result of epithelial inclusions; they may also develop in endometriosis.

Cysts typical of those forming in developmental remnants are those of *mesonephric duct* or *peritoneal* origin. The former develop in the lateral part of the labium major and are lined by a cuboidal epithelium; they contain clear serous fluid. Cysts of peritoneal origin develop from the fragment of peritoneum which may accompany the round ligament into the vulva; the resulting cyst is lined by mesothelium, contains clear watery fluid, and lies in the upper part of the labium major.

Epidermoid cysts, which are lined by stratified squamous epithelium and contain laminated keratinous debris, occur most commonly in the labia majora, where they probably develop in the ducts of sebaceous glands, and in the perineal area where they occur in obstetric scars.

Obstruction of one of the minor mucus-secreting glands in the vestibule leads to the formation of a mucous cyst lined by a cubo-columnar, mucin-secreting epithelium. The largest and only individually named gland of this type is Bartholin's gland. Cysts developing in the gland duct (Fig. 21.17) lie in the postero-lateral part of the labium major and most commonly follow obstruction due to post-inflammatory fibrosis or inspissa-

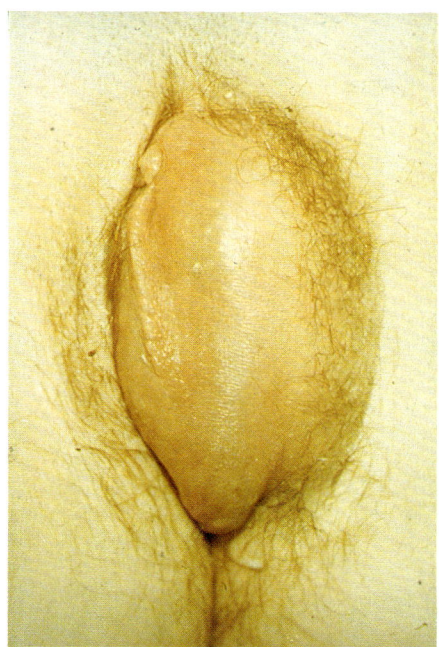

Fig. 21.17 Bartholin's gland abscess. Infection of a left Bartholin's gland cyst has resulted in oedema of the labium minor. (Reproduced by kind permission of Professor V. R. Tindall and Wolfe Medical Publications Ltd.)

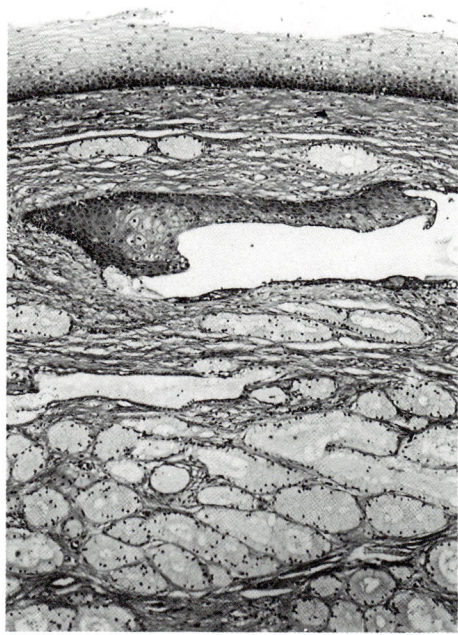

Fig. 21.18 Bartholin's gland cyst. The cyst is lined (above) by a layer of stratified squamous epithelium and, within the wall, there are groups of secretory acini and a further duct lined partly by stratified squamous epithelium.

tion of secretions. The cysts are lined by squamous, transitional, or columnar epithelium (Fig. 21.18) depending upon the level at which the obstruction occurred.

21.4.5 Benign tumours

Benign epithelial tumours of the vulva are more common than benign mesenchymal neoplasms, which are rare.

Epithelial tumours develop from the epidermis and the skin appendages. The most common of the epidermal tumours are the squamous papilloma, the fibro-epitheliomatous polyp, basal cell papilloma, and keratoacanthoma; occasionally intradermal or compound naevi are seen. *Squamous papillomas* and *fibro-epitheliomatous polyps* (skin tags) are of similar appearance and consist of vascular connective tissue covered by mildly acanthotic and hyperkeratotic squamous epithelium; they are most common in the middle aged and elderly.

Basal cell papillomas (seborrhoeic keratoses) are small, exophytic, pigmented lesions which appear to be stuck on the skin. They are composed of sheets of small, regular cells resembling the normal basal cells of the epidermis: in many there are keratin-containing cysts.

Keratoacanthomas are rapidly growing, self-limiting neoplasms which may be of viral origin. They consist of lobules of well-differentiated squamous cell masses arranged around a central keratin-plugged crater.

Tumours may also develop from the sweat glands, one of the commonest of these in the vulva being the *papillary hidraden-*

oma. Hidradenomas are small, painless, subcutaneous swellings, usually on the labia majora, and have a complex tubular, acinar, and papillary histological pattern (Fig. 21.19).

Rarely, adenomas may develop in Bartholin's gland or heterotopic vulvar breast tissue.

Vulval mesenchymal tumours have a tendency to become pedunculated (Fig. 21.20). Fibromas, leiomyomas, lipomas, haemangiomas, neurofibromas, neurilemmomas, and granular cell tumours occur.

21.4.6 Malignant tumours

Squamous cell carcinoma

Tumours of this type account for 90 per cent of all malignant neoplasms of the vulva and for about 5 per cent of female genital tract cancers.

Aetiology and pathogenesis

Some vulvar squamous cell carcinomas develop from pre-existing VIN, but the proportion of invasive neoplasms which arise from such a background is unknown: it is, however, virtually certain that not all squamous cell carcinomas are preceded by a non-invasive neoplasia. Chronic granulomatous diseases of the vulva, such as syphilis, granuloma inguinale, and lymphogranuloma venereum, appear to predispose to vulvar carcinoma, and in countries where such diseases are common, squamous cell carcinoma of the vulva occurs with undue frequency and, often, at an unusually young age. The belief in

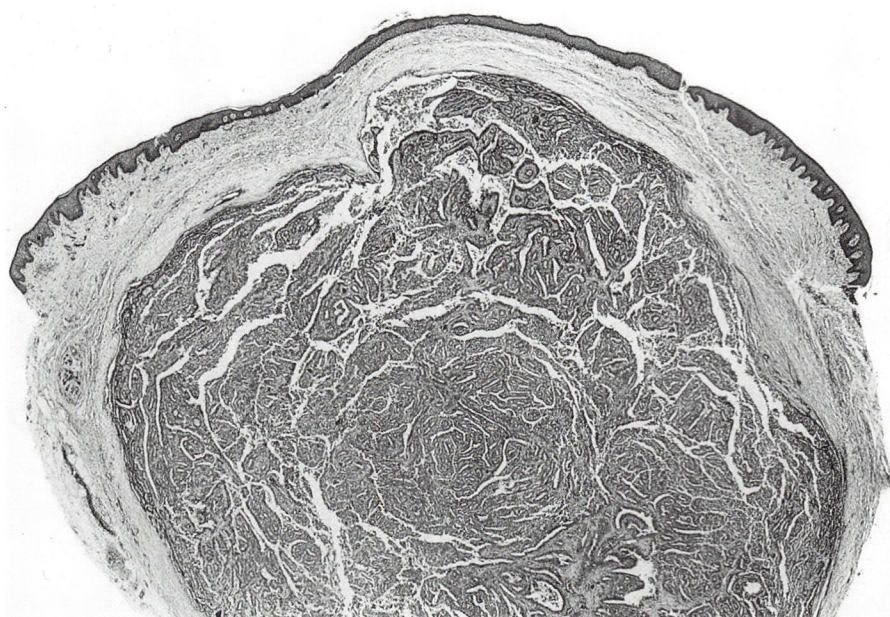

Fig. 21.19 Hidradenoma of the vulva. Within the dermis there is a well-circumscribed nodule composed of closely packed glandular acini. The covering epidermis is intact. (Reproduced by kind permission of Dr C. M. Ridley and Churchill Livingstone from *The vulva*, ed. C. M. Ridley, 1988.)

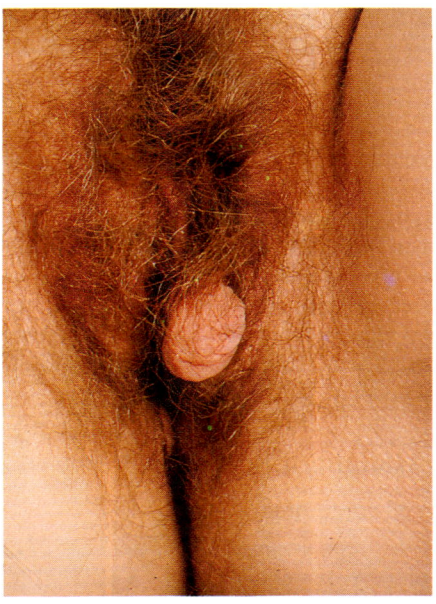

Fig. 21.20 A fibro-epitheliomatous polyp of the vulva. (Reproduced by kind permission of Dr C. M. Ridley and Churchill Livingstone from *The vulva*, ed. C. M. Ridley, 1988.)

an association of vulvar carcinoma with obesity, hypertension, and diabetes mellitus has not been upheld in controlled studies, but a statistical association has been proved between vulvar carcinoma and cigarette smoking, this being attributed to contamination of the vulva by urine containing a carcinogen derived from cigarette smoke. There is a general, though partially anecdotal, belief that women who practice poor vulvar hygiene are particularly prone to develop vulvar carcinoma.

Clinical features

Vulvar squamous cell carcinoma is a disease of relatively elderly women, the peak incidence being between 63 and 65 years and one-third of patients being aged more than 70 years. The usual symptoms are of pruritis, awareness of a vulvar ulcer or nodule, bleeding, or pain: in women with VIN the onset of an overtly malignant tumour may be very insidious.

Pathological features

Most squamous cell carcinomas develop on the labia, the clitoris being the second commonest site. The naked-eye appearances (Fig. 21.21) are usually of an indurated ulcer with raised, rolled edges, but the tumour may take the form of a plaque or a papillary nodule. The neoplasm is usually well differentiated (Fig. 21.22) with tongues and cords of squamous cells which extend down into the dermis and subcutaneous tissue and form well-marked keratinizing epithelial pearls.

Spread and prognosis

The carcinoma may spread directly to involve much of the vulva, and can extend to the perineum and anal margin. Metastasis to lymph nodes is common and often occurs early in the course of the disease. Lymphatic spread is first to the inguinal nodes and thence to the deep pelvic nodes. Blood-borne dissemination occurs late and is principally to the liver, lungs, and bones.

The clinical staging of vulvar carcinoma takes into account both the size of the tumour and the extent of spread:

Stage I   Lesion is less than 2 cm in diameter and no palpable groin nodes.

Stage II   Lesion is greater than 2 cm in diameter and no palpable groin nodes.

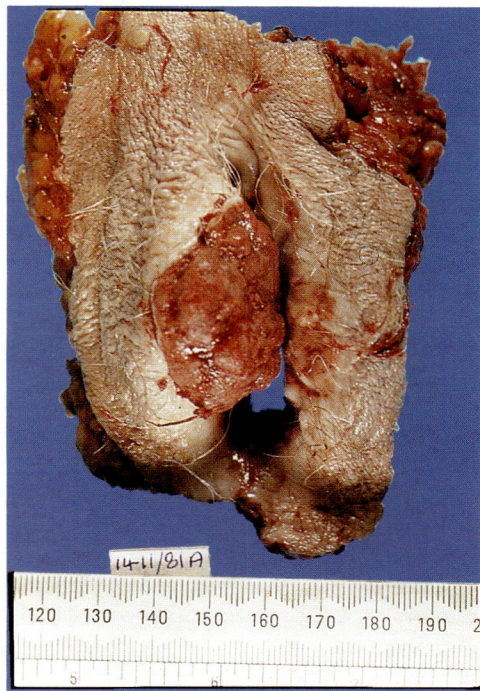

Fig. 21.21 Squamous carcinoma of the vulva. A vulvectomy specimen. An ulcerated carcinoma replaces the right labium minor and part of the right labium major.

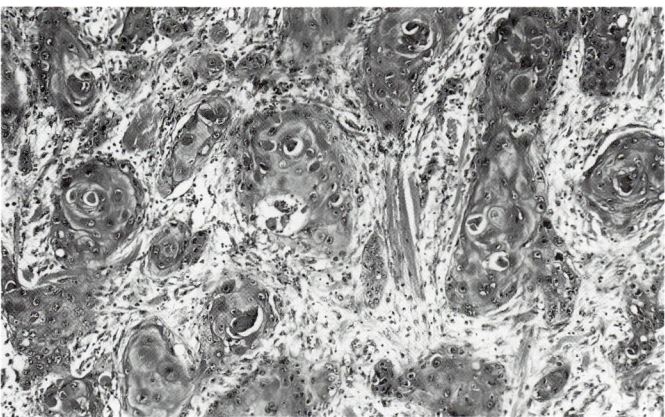

Fig. 21.22 Well-differentiated squamous carcinoma of the vulva. The tumour is composed of infiltrating islands of neoplastic cells forming epithelial pearls.

Stage III   Lesion extends beyond the vulva, with no palpable groin nodes; *or* lesion of any size, with unilateral groin node metastases.

Stage IV   Lesion extends beyond the vulva, with bilateral positive groin nodes; *or* lesion involves mucosa of bladder, rectum, or urethra; *or* all cases with deep pelvic or distant metastases.

Treatment of vulvar squamous cell carcinoma is primarily surgical and the overall five-year survival rate is about 70 per cent. For women with no lymph node involvement this figure is 90 per cent but the survival rate drops to 65 per cent if inguinal node metastases are present and to 25 per cent if there is spread to pelvic nodes.

Verrucous carcinoma

This is a rare but distinctive variant of a squamous cell carcinoma. The tumour presents, usually in the post-menopausal years, as a slowly growing, bulky, fungating, cauliflower-like mass (Fig. 21.23). Histologically these neoplasms have a remarkably bland appearance with little evidence of cellular atypia or mitotic activity. The base of the tumour is well circumscribed with bulbous rete ridges which appear to be compressing, rather than invading, the underlying tissues.

These tumours rarely metastasize to lymph nodes but tend to show a relentless local invasiveness and commonly recur after excision. Treatment is by surgery and they respond to radiotherapy by assuming an even more aggressive stance.

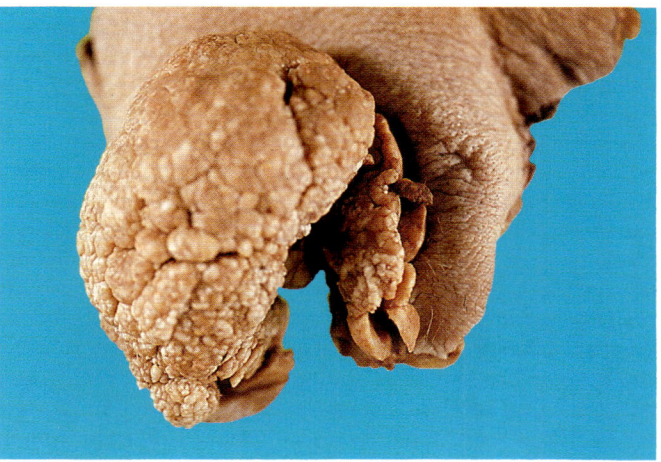

Fig. 21.23 Verrucous carcinoma of the vulva. The right labium major is replaced by an exophytic, cauliflower-like mass which extends on to the left side of the vulva.

Malignant melanoma

Between 3 and 5 per cent of malignant melanomas in women occur in the vulvar skin, a surprisingly high incidence in so far as the vulva accounts for only 1 per cent of the skin surface and is rarely exposed to sunlight. Such neoplasms constitute between 4 and 5 per cent of all malignant vulvar tumours and occur predominantly in the sixth decade of life, about one-third of patients being menopausal. The labia majora, labia minora, and clitoris are involved with about equal frequency, and the melanoma may be of the superficial spreading, nodular, or acral lentiginous type.

The overall five-year survival rate for patients with a malignant melanoma of the vulva is about 30–40 per cent, the tumour tending to spread early to the inguinal nodes and to be widely disseminated via the bloodstream. The prognosis for tumours still localized to the vulva depends upon the thickness of the neoplasm and its depth of invasion: as with malignant melanomas elsewhere in the skin, both Clark's levels and Breslow's thickness measurements are of value in assessing the prognosis.

Basal cell carcinoma

Basal cell carcinomas account for only between 2 and 10 per cent of vulvar neoplasms and tend to develop on the labia majora in the elderly. Their aetiology is uncertain, although 20 per cent of patients have a second malignant neoplasm.

The tumours often present with pruritis, serous or blood-stained discharge, and a polypoidal or plaque-like ulcerated mass may be noted. The vulvar tumours are of a similar histological pattern and clinical behaviour to those encountered elsewhere in the body. About a fifth recur locally after excision but lymph node metastases are exceptional.

Malignant adnexal (skin appendage) neoplasms

Malignant adnexal tumours are rare, those which develop on the vulva being largely confined to the labia majora and interlabial sulcus. In contrast to epithelial tumours they tend to lie entirely within the dermis and form firm, slow growing, non-ulcerated, painless or only mildly tender, nodules. The tumours present a wide variety of histological patterns and they develop from both apocrine and eccrine sweat glands and sebaceous glands. *Adenocarcinomas* of tubular, myxoid, and spindle cell form, *apocrine adenocarcinomas* resembling breast carcinoma, *adenosquamous carcinomas*, *mucoid carcinoma*, and *sebaceous carcinomas* are all recognized. The outcome depends upon the histological differentiation of the neoplasm and the extent to which the tumour has spread at the time of diagnosis. Whilst local recurrence, rather than metastasis, is the pattern of disease elsewhere in the body, and a protracted course is not uncommon, vulvar adnexal carcinomas seem to metastasize unduly frequently although this may be a false impression given by the rarity of their occurrence.

Carcinoma of Bartholin's gland

Carcinomas of Bartholin's gland are rare and tend to occur in a relatively young age-group: the peak age is at about 50 years and a majority of patients are premenopausal. The tumour usually presents as a vulvar nodule or mass which tends eventually to ulcerate through the overlying skin. Most of the neoplasms are either *adenocarcinomas* or *squamous cell carcinomas* (the latter probably arising from foci of metaplastic squamous epithelium within the ducts) but about 15 per cent are *adenoid cystic carcinomas*.

Adenocarcinomas and squamous cell carcinomas tend to avail themselves of the rich lymphatic drainage of Bartholin's gland and metastasize first to the inguinal nodes and then to the deep pelvic nodes, the five-year survival rate for patients with these tumours being only about 30 per cent. Adenoid cystic carcinomas show less tendency to metastasize but are locally highly aggressive, invading extensively and recurring with considerable frequency.

Urethral carcinoma

Urethral carcinoma, although rare, is more common in women than men, affecting particularly old or elderly women. Its incidence is not clearly defined because it is usual to describe as vulval or vaginal any large neoplasm developing at the meatus or involving the introitus.

Tumours of the distal urethra are more common than those in the proximal, or posterior, urethra. A wide variety of symptoms can occur, ranging from haematuria and dysuria to vaginal discharge or urethrovaginal fistula, depending upon the extent of disease at the time of presentation.

In the distal urethra tumours are usually *squamous or transitional*, whereas in the proximal urethra *adenocarcinomas* also occur. Patients in whom disease is limited to the distal urethra have an excellent prognosis but tumours involving the whole urethra or only its proximal portion do particularly badly because in many such cases metastases have already occurred at the time of diagnosis.

Metastatic tumours

The possibility that rare tumours in the vulva, such as adenocarcinomas, might be metastases should always be borne in mind as the vulva is not an uncommon site of metastases from the cervix, endometrium, vagina, ovary, urethra, kidney, breast, rectum, and lung. Their presence is almost invariably associated with a poor prognosis indicating, as they do, disseminated malignancy.

21.5   The vagina

The vagina extends from the vestibule to the uterus, running at an angle of 90 degrees to the uterus and measuring approximately 7 cm along its anterior wall and 9 cm along its posterior wall: it lies posterior to the bladder and anterior to the rectum. The upper part of the vagina surrounds the lower part of the cervix and forms vault-like *vaginal fornices* between its cervical attachment and its lateral wall.

The blood supply of the vagina is largely from branches of the internal iliac artery although it may also receive branches from the uterine and middle rectal arteries: venous drainage is to the internal iliac veins. The lymphatic drainage of the upper three-quarters of the vagina is to the internal and external iliac nodes whereas that of the lower quarter is to the femoral, inguinal, and pelvic nodes.

The vagina is lined by a non-keratinized, glycogenated squamous epithelium, and its wall is formed by smooth muscle and adventitial fibro-elastic tissue. Growth and maturation of the vaginal squamous epithelium is under oestrogenic control and its thickness therefore varies not only at different stages of a woman's life but also throughout the menstrual cycle. Thus the epithelium is thin before the menarche and after the menopause: during the reproductive years the epithelium reaches its maximal thickness just before ovulation, when oestrogen levels are at their highest, whereas squamous maturation and growth are inhibited during the luteal phase by the rising levels of progesterone.

The vagina has an abundant bacterial flora in which there is a very finely balanced microecology. The predominant organism in the normal vagina is the lactic acid-producing bacillus *Lactobacillus acidophilus* which utilizes the glycogen in the vaginal epithelial cells as its substrate. This bacillus tends to inhibit the proliferation of other organisms and its acid-producing capacity is an important factor in maintaining the low pH of the normal vagina.

21.5.1 Vaginal inflammation

Non-infective inflammation

Non-infective vaginal inflammation may complicate trauma, surgery, irradiation, the introduction of foreign bodies, the application of chemical substances, or the wearing of a pessary.

Infective inflammation

Infective vaginitis is common and is characterized clinically by a vaginal discharge which is often malodorous: the discharge is usually irritant to the vulva and many patients complain principally of vulvar itching and discomfort.

Most vaginal infections are sexually transmitted but it is far from certain how the infecting organisms become established in the vagina and overcome the dual threats posed by the normal vaginal flora and the acidity of the vaginal fluids. It is probable that changes in oestrogen or progesterone levels are an important factor in the establishment of an infection in so far as oestrogen deficiency or progesterone excess will result in diminished epithelial growth, a reduction in the supply of glycogen, and restriction of the ability of lactobacilli to flourish, thus allowing invading organisms to gain an ascendancy.

Gardnerella vaginitis

The Gram-negative bacillus, *Gardnerella vaginalis*, either acting singly or in combination with anaerobic organisms, is now recognized to be the cause of the vast majority of cases previously designated as 'non-specific vaginitis': the organism is sexually transmitted. *Gardnerella* vaginitis is associated with a thin, watery, highly malodorous vaginal discharge but the organism is only a surface parasite and does not invade the vaginal tissues or evoke any inflammatory reaction. Because of this lack of an inflammatory response, *Gardnerella* infection is often classed as a 'vaginosis' rather than as a true vaginitis.

Candidiasis

Candida albicans may exist in the vagina without causing any signs or symptoms. The fungal organism can, however, change from a saprophyte to a pathogen if the host is immunosuppressed or if growth of the normal vaginal flora is inhibited by, for example, the use of broad-spectrum antibiotics. Once allowed to proliferate freely, *Candida albicans* penetrates focally into the vaginal epithelium and initiates a vaginitis which is characterized clinically by a vaginal discharge which is highly irritant to the vulva, most patients complaining principally of pruritis vulvae. The vaginal epithelium is congested and whitish plaques may be seen on the vaginal surface; these are easily removed to expose a reddened 'raw' area.

Trichomoniasis

The unicellular protozoal parasite *Trichomonas vaginalis* is one of the commonest causes of a vaginitis; the parasite is usually sexually transmitted but can, on occasion, be transmitted via fomites. The acute stage of the infection is characterized by a frothy vaginal discharge and the vaginal mucosa has a reddish granular appearance (Fig. 21.24). Histologically, congestion, oedema, and a lymphoplasmocytic infiltrate of the subepithelial papillae are characteristic features; the inflammatory infiltrate may extend into the epithelium and form small intra-epithelial abscesses. The infection may progress into a chronic state, although some women become symptomless carriers of the parasite.

Gonorrhoea

The thick squamous epithelium of the adult vagina is resistant to gonococcal infection. In children, however, the thin epithelium is permeable to the organism, which can produce a vaginitis.

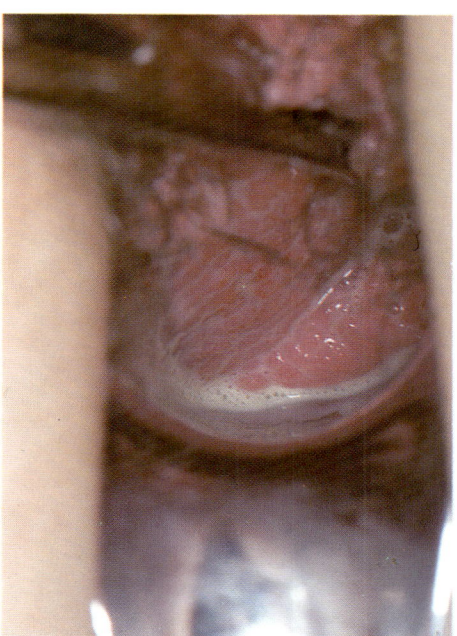

Fig. 21.24 Trichomoniasis of the vagina. The vaginal epithelium is inflamed and there is a copious creamy white frothy discharge. (Reproduced by kind permission of Professor N. A. Bleischer, Melbourne, Australia.)

Syphilis

The vagina is an uncommon site for a chancre but the mucosal 'snail-track' ulcers and condylomata lata of secondary syphilis occur with some frequency in the lower vagina. Tertiary-stage lesions are only rarely encountered in the vagina.

21.5.2 Vaginal adenosis

This condition, which is usually asymptomatic but occasionally associated with a vaginal discharge, is characterized by the presence of glandular structures in the lamina propria of the vagina (Fig. 21.25), some opening on to the vaginal surface. The glands are most commonly lined by a mucinous, endocervical-type epithelium but may have a lining of endometrial or tubal type. The glands have a marked tendency to undergo squamous metaplasia, and eventually, in older women, may be completely replaced by squamous tissue.

Vaginal adenosis is thought to be due to sequestration of Müllerian elements during vaginal embryogenesis and is indicative of a disturbance in the orderly replacement of the lower parts of the Müllerian ducts by the squamous epithelium of the urogenital sinus. The condition may occur spontaneously but is particularly common in girls who have been exposed prenatally to *diethylstilboestrol* (DES). This hormone was administered to many pregnant women in the 1940s and 1950s as a means of preventing spontaneous abortion: the drug proved therapeutically useless in this respect but was transferred across the placenta to the fetus where it apparently modulated the normal interation between Müllerian and urogenital sinus tissues, vaginal adenosis being found in 70 per cent of girls exposed to DES during the first eight weeks of fetal life.

Vaginal adenosis is not, in itself, of any major clinical importance but is of considerable significance as a precursor of the *clear-cell adenocarcinoma of the vagina* (see below).

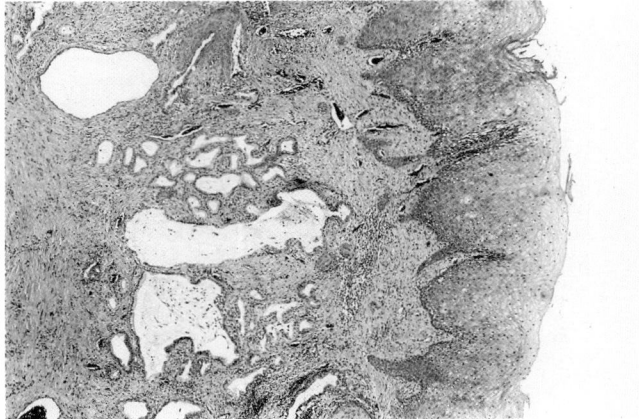

Fig. 21.25 Vaginal adenosis. The vaginal lumen, to the right, is lined by a layer of stratified squamous epithelium. The underlying stroma contains a series of glands, some of which are lined by mucus-secreting epithelium and some of which are lined by endometrial-type epithelium.

21.5.3 Vaginal fistulae

Fistulous communications between the vagina and neighbouring organs, such as the bladder or large bowel, are not uncommon. Vesico-vaginal fistulae are usually due to obstetric trauma, and intestino-vaginal fistulae may complicate diverticular disease of the bowel, Crohn's disease, pelvic surgery, neoplasia, or irradiation.

21.5.4 Vaginal intra-epithelial neoplasia (VAIN)

VAIN has been studied much less intensively than has VIN or CIN and its natural history is poorly understood. The lesion, which is often multifocal, is usually asymptomatic and is discovered only on routine examination, when it is seen either as an area of increased vascularity or as a whitish patch. A very high proportion of women with VAIN have been previously treated for either intra-epithelial or invasive neoplasia of the cervix and it is thought that the aetiological factors for VAIN are similar to those for CIN (see later).

The histological appearances of VAIN are similar to those of both VIN and CIN and include delayed maturation of the squamous cells, disturbances in polarity, an increased nucleocytoplasmic ratio, nuclear pleomorphism, the finding of mitotic figures above the basal layers, and the presence of abnormal mitotic figures. It is usual to grade the lesion into *VAIN 1*, in which undifferentiated cells are confined to the lower third of the epithelium; *VAIN 2*, in which undifferentiated cells extend into the middle third of the epithelium; and *VAIN 3*, in which undifferentiated cells either extend into the upper third of the epithelium or occupy its full thickness.

VAIN is widely regarded as a precursor of an invasive squamous cell carcinoma of the vagina but neither its invasive potential nor its quantitative importance as a precursor of a malignant vaginal neoplasm have been adequately defined.

21.5.5 Vaginal neoplasms

Malignant neoplasms of the vagina are rare, accounting for only about 1 per cent of cancers of the female genital tract. Indeed, a malignant neoplasm in the vagina is more likely to be a metastasis, from sites such as the colon, endometrium, or kidney, than a primary vaginal tumour.

Squamous carcinoma

Neoplasms of this type account for 95 per cent of malignant tumours, and occur predominantly in women in their sixth or seventh decades. Squamous carcinomas develop most commonly in the posterior wall of the upper third of the vagina, usually present as an exophytic fungating mass and are often moderately well differentiated (Fig. 21.26). The tumour invades, at a relatively early stage, adjacent structures such as the cervix, paravaginal tissues, bladder, and rectum. Lymphatic spread from tumours in the upper vagina is to the iliac and

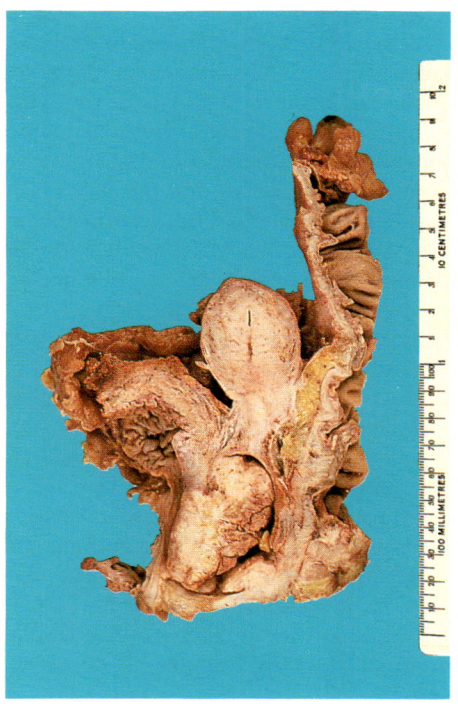

Fig. 21.26 Squamous carcinoma of the vagina. A large infiltrating squamous carcinoma arises in the anterior vaginal wall and protrudes into and distends the vaginal lumen.

obturator nodes whereas that from neoplasms in the lower vagina is to the femoral and inguinal nodes.

The prognosis for women with a squamous cell carcinoma of the vagina depends upon the stage of the disease at the time of initial diagnosis. Staging is as follows:

Stage I   Tumour confined to the vaginal wall.

Stage II Tumour extends into the paravaginal tissues but does not reach the pelvic wall.

Stage III Tumour extends to the pelvic wall.

Stage IV Tumour is invading the bladder or rectum or has extended beyond the pelvis.

The five-year survival rate for women with Stage I disease is approximately 70 per cent but this survival rate falls precipitously to 47, 25, and 8 per cent, respectively, for Stages II, III, and IV disease.

The aetiology of vaginal squamous carcinoma is unknown but it has been suggested that long-standing procidentia or the prolonged wearing of a pessary may be of some aetiological importance: this may well be true but these factors are of little importance in current practice. The role of HPV infection in the aetiology of vaginal carcinoma is currently undetermined.

Clear-cell adenocarcinoma

Neoplasms of this type used to be of extreme rarity. Some years ago it became apparent, however, that there was, in the United States, a significant increase in the incidence of clear-cell adeno-

carcinomas of the vagina, this increase being entirely in young girls who had been exposed prenatally to DES: a similar increase has since been encountered, to a lesser extent, in other parts of the world. Approximately one in 1500 women exposed to DES during the first eighteen weeks of their prenatal life will develop a clear-cell adenocarcinoma, the tumour usually becoming apparent between the ages of 14 and 23 years, most commonly in girls aged 17–19 years. The tumour almost certainly originates in pre-existing vaginal adenosis and is therefore of Müllerian origin.

A clear-cell adenocarcinoma usually develops in the upper third of the vagina and may form a polypoid, nodular, or papillary mass. Histologically (Fig. 21.27) there is a complex mixture of solid, papillary, tubular, and cystic patterns, the solid areas being formed by sheets of cells with clear cytoplasm and the tubules being lined by 'hobnail' cells which have large nuclei that protrude into the tubular lumen.

The tumour spreads by local invasion, the lymphatics, and the bloodstream, and, although the pelvic nodes are commonly the site of metastases, there is a surprisingly high incidence of spread to the supraclavicular nodes: blood-borne dissemination is principally to the lungs. Treatment is by radical surgery and the overall five-year survival rate is 80 per cent. Patients with Stage I disease have a 90 per cent five-year survival rate, this falling to 70, 30, and 20 per cent for those with, respectively, Stage II, III, and IV disease.

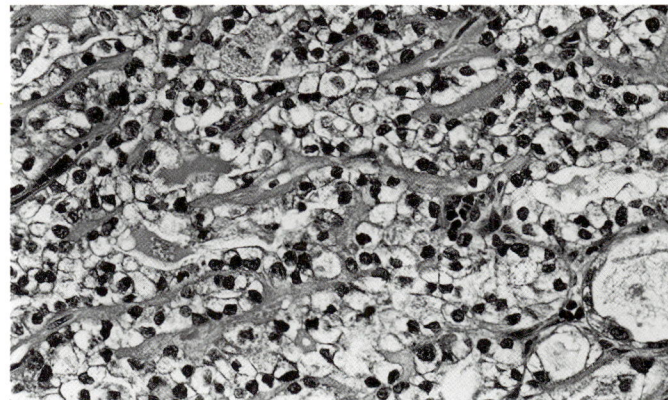

Fig. 21.27 Clear-cell adenocarcinoma of the vagina. The tumour is composed of large cells with well-defined cell margins and clear cytoplasm.

Sarcoma botyroides

This term is applied to the rare *embryonal rhabdomyosarcoma* of the vagina, a tumour which most commonly occurs in the first 5 years of life. The neoplasm arises from the connective tissues of the vaginal wall and tends to form a polypoid mass of greyish-red haemorrhagic tissue which may fill, and protrude from, the vagina. Histologically, there is typically a widely dispersed population of pleomorphic immature mesenchymal cells, rhabdomyoblasts, and striated muscle cells set in an abundant oedematous or myxoid stroma. The epithelium covering the tumour is bland and the neoplastic cells tend to be condensed below this to form a 'cambium' layer.

A vaginal sarcoma botyroides infiltrates locally into the pelvic tissues and has a poor prognosis.

21.6   Uterine cervix

21.6.1   The normal cervix

The cervix, which is basically cylindrical, is that part of the uterus lying below the *isthmus* or *internal os*. It is 2.5–3 cm long in the adult and projects through the upper part of the anterior wall of the vagina. The upper, or supravaginal, part of the cervix lies above the vaginal vault and is surrounded by connective tissue which, anteriorly, separates it from the bladder and laterally extends into the broad ligaments. It is covered posteriorly by the peritoneum of the pouch of Douglas. The lower, or vaginal, part of the cervix is convex, its surface being surmounted by the external os which, in the nulliparous woman, is circular or oval, becoming slit-like and coronal in parous women. The portions of the cervix lying anterior and posterior to the external os are termed the *anterior* and *posterior lips*, respectively. The *endocervical canal* communicates with the vagina, via the external os, below and is continuous above with the uterine cavity.

The blood supply to the cervix is from the descending branches of the uterine arteries which reach the lateral walls of the cervix along the margin of the paracervical ligaments. There is a well-developed capillary network in the cervical stroma, which is particularly prominent immediately below the surface epithelium. The venous drainage parallels the arterial supply and there are communications between the cervical venous plexuses and those at the neck of the bladder.

There are two lymphatic systems, one submucosal and the other deep in the cervical stroma. Both systems collect in two lateral plexuses in the region of the uterine isthmus and give rise to four efferent channels which drain respectively to the external iliac and obturator lymph nodes, the hypogastric and common iliac nodes, the sacral nodes, and the nodes on the posterior wall of the bladder.

The nerve supply of the cervix comes from the pelvic autonomic system via the superior, middle, and inferior hypogastric plexuses and is chiefly limited to the endocervix and the peripheral deep part of the ectocervix. Hence the ectocervix is relatively insensitive to touch and pain.

The cervical stroma is mainly fibrous, containing only a small amount of elastic tissue and smooth muscle, which is chiefly limited to the endocervix. There is virtually no muscle in the vaginal part of the cervix.

The vaginal part of the cervix is covered by a non-keratinizing stratified squamous epithelium which is continuous at the vaginal fornices with the epithelium lining the vagina and at the external os with that lining the endocervical canal. The epithelium is replaced every 4–5 days by a process of surface de-squamation and regrowth from below. Oestrogen promotes maturation of the epithelium and speeds epithelial turnover whereas progesterone inhibits maturation; therefore regular cyclical changes can be detected which mirror ovarian hormonal activity. In the reproductive years glycogen is present in the cytoplasm of the cells in the middle and upper zones of the stratified squamous epithelium, and intracytoplasmic keratin forms in the superficial layers. In the post-menopausal woman the epithelium is shallow, cells mature only to the intermediate or even parabasal state, and there is an absence or paucity of glycogen. This epithelium is fragile, its surface lacks the keratin necessary to form a protective layer, and it is easily traumatized and susceptible to infection.

The endocervix is lined by a tall, mucus-secreting columnar epithelium which is continuous with that lining the endocervical crypts or clefts which extend into the cervical stroma, from the canal, for up to 7 mm. A small number of non-secretory ciliated cells are usually seen but they are inconspicuous.

The transition from squamous to columnar epithelium is usually abrupt and in the majority of cases this transition occurs at the external cervical os. This is not, however, a constant relationship: it varies at different times in life and under different hormonal states (see below).

21.6.2   Cervical mucus

One of the principal functions of the cervix is to secrete mucus. Cervical mucus plays a key role in regulating sperm entry into the uterine cavity, in protecting sperm from the acid environment of the vagina, and in sperm capacitation: furthermore, the mucus forms a barrier which protects the uterus from organisms ascending from the vagina.

Cervical mucus secretion is under both oestrogenic and progestational control and the type of mucus, and its biophysical nature, vary throughout the various phases of the menstrual cycle. The physical characteristics of the mucus are such that sperm ascent occurs most easily in the immediately post-ovulation period of the cycle, movement of sperm through the mucus being much more difficult during the later part of the luteal phase.

Inadequate secretion of mucus by the cervix may be a reflection of inadequate hormonal stimulation, as in oestrogen deficiency states, or may be due to either a congenital or iatrogenic deficiency of mucus-secreting epithelium, as occurs, for instance, in *congenital cervical hypoplasia* or after an overenthusiastic cone biopsy. The chronically inflamed cervix tends to secrete an abnormal mucus, partly because of production of subunits or partial components of normal mucus and partly because of an acquired insensitivity to hormonal control. Insufficient or abnormal mucus secretion by the cervix may hinder sperm movement and can be an important factor in infertility.

21.6.3   Physiological changes in the cervix

Ectopy or ectropion

In the pre-pubertal girl the squamo-columnar junction lies

around the external os or on the ectocervix (Fig. 21.28). At the time of puberty, in pregnancy (particularly the first one), and in many steroid contraceptive users, changes in the hormonal milieu result in an alteration in the shape, and an increase in the bulk, of the cervix, which results in eversion of the endocervical epithelium, the squamo-columnar junction thus being carried passively further out on to the anatomical ectocervix. This rim of endocervical tissue forms an ectopy or ectropion exposed around the external os (Fig. 21.29). The ectopy is red and velvety because the underlying capillary network shows through the thin covering epithelium and the surface is villous: clinically an ectopy is often, but incorrectly, called an 'erosion'.

The exposure of the delicate endocervical epithelium to the acid environment of the vagina leads to squamous metaplasia, the squamous epithelial cells differentiating from pluripotential uncommitted cells. Squamous metaplasia is a protective mechanism in which relatively fragile endocervical columnar epithelium is replaced by a more robust squamous epithelium.

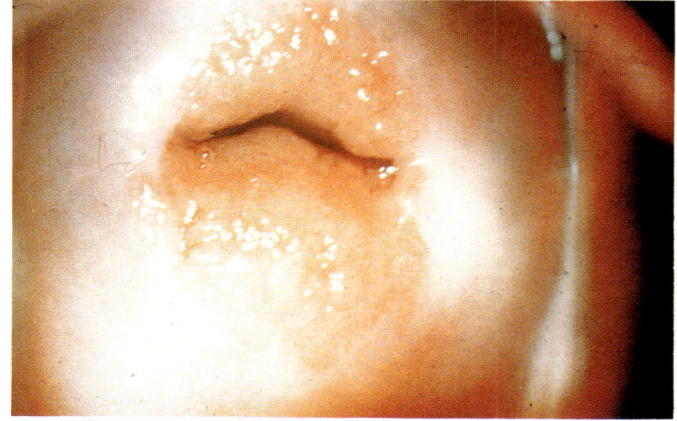

Fig. 21.29 A cervical ectopy. The external os is surrounded by an area of single-layered columnar epithelium through which the underlying capillary vasculature can be seen as a pink area. (Reproduced by kind permission of Professor V. R. Tindall and Wolfe Medical Publications Ltd.)

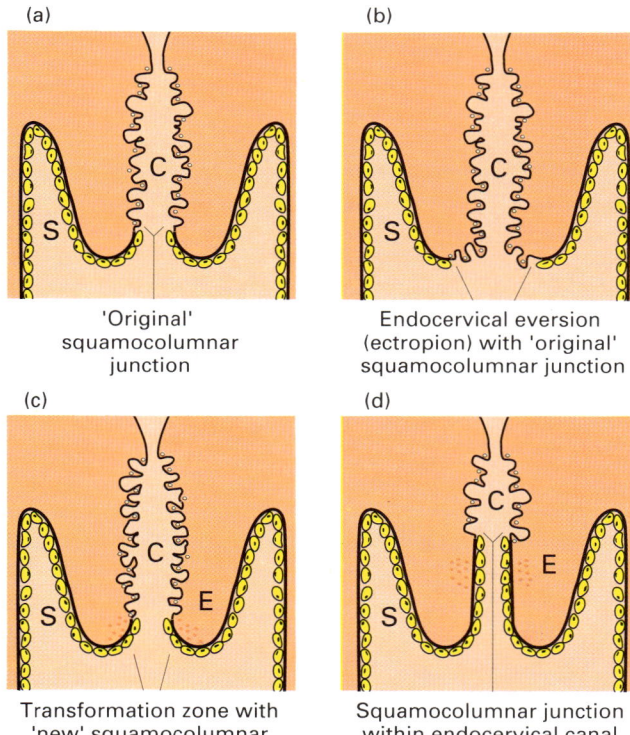

(a) 'Original' squamocolumnar junction

(b) Endocervical eversion (ectropion) with 'original' squamocolumnar junction

(c) Transformation zone with 'new' squamocolumnar junction

(d) Squamocolumnar junction within endocervical canal after menopause

S = Squamous epithelium
C = Columnar epithelium
E = Endocervical glands deep to metaplastic squamous epithelium

Fig. 21.28 Diagram showing the stages in the development of the transformation zone and the changing location of the squamo-columnar junction (a) before puberty, (b) after puberty and pregnancy, (c) during the reproductive life, (d) after the menopause. (Drawn after Coleman and Evans 1988, with permission.)

The metaplastic squamous epithelium occludes the mouths of the endocervical crypts with the resultant formation of *retention cysts* or *Nabothian follicles*. This process also restores the position of the squamo-columnar junction to the external os. The area of squamous metaplasia is termed the *transformation zone* and is the site at which the majority of cervical neoplasms arise. An understanding of its position in the cervix is important to those concerned with the taking of cervical smears and the management of intra-epithelial and invasive neoplasia of the cervix (see below). In the young woman the transformation zone lies where it develops, on the ectocervix, but after the age of 30 years there is an increasing tendency, because of shrinkage of the soft tissue of the cervix, for the squamo-columnar junction to be retracted and come to lie within the endocervical canal; hence, that area of epithelium which formed the transformation zone is also withdrawn to within the canal. An endocervical squamo-columnar junction is a virtually constant finding after the menopause.

Pregnancy

In pregnancy, in addition to the development of an ectopy, there is spongy enlargement of the cervix because of congestion and oedema. Surface maturation of the squamous epithelium is absent because of progesterone predominance of the hormonal milieu and focal decidualization of the stroma is common. The columnar epithelium of the ectopy or endocervical canal often undergoes a form of hyperplasia to form tightly packed glands or tubules lined by flattened or cuboidal cells. This condition of *microglandular hyperplasia* is in most cases only a microscopic change, though it may, on rare occasions, form polypoid nodules which bleed on touch. Postpartum, laceration of the cervix during delivery may radically alter its contours and expose the endocervical tissues.

Genital prolapse

The term prolapse is used to describe the abnormal descent of the vagina and uterus. The prolapse may involve mainly the vaginal walls and, according to the tissues that are affected, it is variously described as a *cystocoele* (upper anterior vaginal wall, involving the bladder), *urethrocoele* (lower anterior vaginal wall, involving the urethra) or *rectocoele* (posterior vaginal wall, involving the large bowel). When the uterus prolapses, the degree of descent is covered by the terms first, second, and third degree. In *first degree prolapse* the uterus remains within the vagina, in second degree prolapse the cervix descends to the level of the introitus, and in *third degree prolapse*, or *procidentia*, the uterus and part or all of the inverted vagina lie outside the vaginal introitus.

Prolapse is associated with urinary incontinence or, if the urethra is angulated, urinary tract infection or difficulty in emptying the bladder; faeces may also be retained in the pouch of bowel within the rectocoele. The cervix is frequently elongated and congested, and there may be keratinization of the vaginal and cervical squamous epithelium with, particularly in procidentia, ulceration of the prolapsed tissues. Although carcinoma of the cervix or vagina is often described as a complication of a prolapse, it is in fact rare.

There is no single cause of prolapse. A congenital weakness of the uterine supports is postulated in those in whom prolapse occurs without apparent cause, and damage to the innervation of the pelvic floor musculature following parturition is believed to play a more important part than simple obstetric trauma. If these predisposing factors are present, increased abdominal pressure, associated with chronic constipation, ascites or cough, or increase in uterine weight, associated with the presence of a uterine tumour, may precipitate a prolapse.

21.6.4　Inflammatory diseases of the cervix

Cervicitis may occur as an isolated lesion or as part of a more widespread inflammatory process in the genital tract: the histological appearances are, however, remarkably stereotyped and often give no clue as to the aetiology (Fig. 21.30).

Inflammation may be acute, active chronic, or chronic; chronic inflammation may be granulomatous or non-granulomatous. There is a normal population of plasma cells and lymphocytes in the stroma adjacent to the external cervical os and these often lead to an unwarranted diagnosis of cervicitis. Hence, the recognition of an inflammatory process depends upon the presence not only of inflammatory cells but also on the finding of associated changes such as a reduction in mucus secretion, infiltration of the epithelium by inflammatory cells, ulceration, the formation of granulation tissue, fibrosis, the development of lymphoid follicles with germinal centres, or granuloma formation.

Acute inflammation is characterized by oedema and congestion, the presence in the stroma and crypts of polymorphonuclear leucocytes and by the outpouring of an acute inflammatory exudate: in severe cases there may be abscess

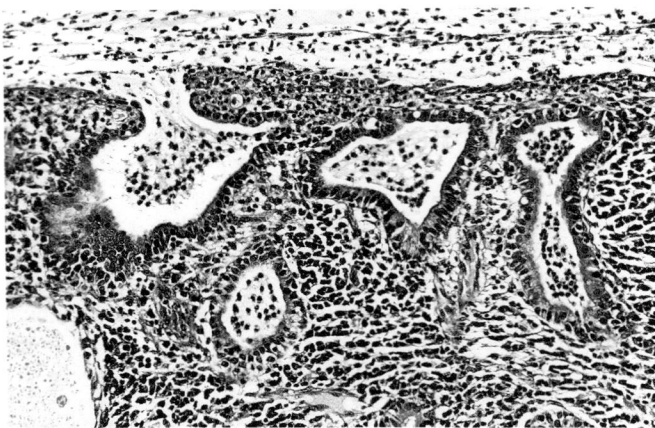

Fig. 21.30 Severe cervicitis. The cervical crypts are distended by an acute inflammatory exudate; there is ulceration of the surface epithelium and the stroma is infiltrated by plasma cells, lymphocytes, and macrophages.

formation and ulceration of the surface epithelium. In persistent or *active chronic inflammation* the infiltrate becomes plasma-lymphocytic and histiocytic with scanty polymorphonuclear leucocytes, whilst in some chronic infections lymphoid follicles or granulomas are a characteristic feature.

Non-infective inflammation

Inflammation occurs following surgery, parturition, cryosurgery, laser therapy, cautery, the use of douches or ointments, and in association with the wearing of an intra-uterine contraceptive device. Bleeding from cervical endometriosis may also elicit a local inflammatory response. The cervix often becomes inflamed if there is a prolapse, and this is particularly marked if ulceration occurs.

Infective inflammation

Many infections of the cervix are of a non-specific polymicrobial nature. Bacterial infections tend particularly to involve the endocervix or an ectopy, partly because the deep crypts afford a safe harbour to the bacteria and other organisms, partly because the columnar epithelium in these sites offers less resistance to infection than does the stratified squamous epithelium of the ectocervix, and partly because organisms sequestrated in the cervical crypts may not be affected by either systemic or local therapeutic agents. Chronic cervical inflammation occurs particularly when there is obstruction to, and stasis of, cervical secretions and is therefore encountered when the vagina is obstructed by a foreign body or tumour or when the endocervical canal is blocked by a neoplasm, polyp, or stricture: the resultant scarring and fibrosis leads to further crypt distortion, thus increasing the obstruction and perpetuating the inflammatory process. The organisms most commonly isolated in such circumstances include coliforms, commensals, *Mycoplasma*, *Gardnerella vaginalis*, and *Chlamydia*, but their role in initiating the inflammation is uncertain.

Infection may also occur following parturition or abortion and may complicate any of the conditions that predispose to non-infective inflammation.

Specific infections

Viral infections

Herpes simplex virus type 2 Herpetic infection of the cervix is most common in teenagers and young adults and is usually associated with infection of the vulva and vagina. Symptoms develop 3–7 days after inoculation and are most severe in primary infections. Although healing is usually rapid and complete, recurrences are frequent and an asymptomatic infected state may develop.

Focal necrosis of the squamous epithelium of the cervix leads to the development of shallow ulcers and, rarely, to the development of a necrotizing cervicitis or a chronic inflammatory mass which may be mistaken for a carcinoma.

Human papilloma virus (HPV) Cervical infection by this sexually transmitted organism is increasingly common. HPV infection can result in condylomata or flat 'warty' lesions and is being increasingly regarded as being of aetiological importance in cervical neoplasia (see sections on condylomata and neoplasia).

Bacterial infection

Neisseria gonorrhoea The squamous epithelium of the ectocervix is relatively resistant to infection by this highly contagious organism. *N. gonorrhoea* can, however, pass through the columnar epithelium of the endocervix to elicit an *acute exudative endocervicitis* characterized by stromal congestion and oedema and a seropurulent exudate: the columnar epithelium becomes focally degenerate and ulcerated.

Infection may clear, become chronic or spread to the endometrium and Fallopian tubes. A proportion of patients become asymptomatic carriers, whilst in others a *chronic gonococcal cervicitis* with pericryptal fibrosis, crypt distortion, and stasis of cervical secretions develops: this tends both to perpetuate the disease and predispose to secondary infection.

Chlamydial infection of the cervix is characterized by the development of a *follicular cervicitis* which can be detected at colposcopy, in a cervical smear, or on histological examination (Fig. 21.31).

The inflammatory infiltrate, which is often very heavy, is composed of plasma cells and lymphocytes which form lymphoid follicles with germinal centres. Intra-epithelial abscesses and ulceration of the overlying epithelium may develop in severe cases. Intracellular organisms are difficult to demonstrate, even with the use of immunohistochemical techniques.

Spirochaetal infection The primary lesion of syphilis occurs in the cervix in up to 40 per cent of cases, where it may be small or form a typical hard, ulcerated chancre; occasionally multiple small ulcers, resembling those seen in herpetic cervicitis, form and, rarely, a fungating mass resembling a neoplasm may de-

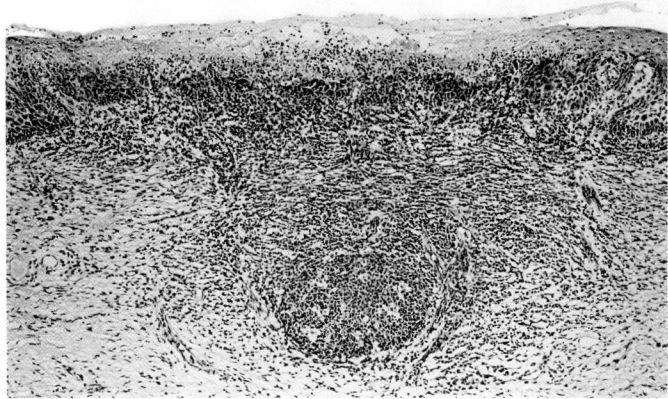

Fig. 21.31 Follicular cervicitis. In addition to the diffuse chronic inflammatory cell infiltrate there is a lymphoid follicle with a germinal centre in the centre of the field. The appearances are suggestive of a chlamydial infection.

velop. When the chancre lies in the endocervix the entire cervix may become indurated and oedematous.

The characteristic histological findings are a dense, subepithelial plasma cell infiltrate, a perivascular infiltrate of lymphocytes with endothelial hyperplasia, and, in long-standing cases, endarteritis.

The mucous patches, but not the condylomata lata, of the secondary stage of syphilis may occur on the cervix but this is an exceptionally rare site for a gumma.

Fungal infections

Candida albicans *Candida* is a commensal in the vagina but in pregnancy, in diabetics, and in patients using steroids or immunosuppressives it may become pathogenic. Characteristically, thick white material adheres to the cervix. The mucosa beneath the patches is reddened and may be ulcerated. Histological examination may reveal fungal hyphae penetrating the epithelium and infiltrating the underlying stroma where there is a polymorphonuclear leucocyte infiltrate.

Protozoal infections

Trichomonas vaginalis Infection of the vagina and cervix by *T. vaginalis* are inseparable. The mucosa of the infected cervix is reddened and the underlying vessels are ectatic, appearing as red spots and leading to the descriptive term, a 'strawberry' cervix. The epithelium is infiltrated by polymorphonuclear leucocytes and is partly desquamated: the underlying stroma contains chronic inflammatory cells.

In many cases the infection resolves following treatment but in others it may become chronic, the endocervical crypts acting as a reservoir of infection.

Schistosomiasis In the United Kingdom schistosomiasis of the cervix is rarely seen but it is a common genital tract pathogen in those areas of the world in which this disease is endemic. Cervical infection leads to the development of a bulky indurated cervix, or a polypoidal mass, and there is a granulomatous response to the ova. Progressive fibrosis may cause gross cervical distortion.

21.6.5   Cervical polyps

These are common and arise, in 95 per cent of cases, from the endocervix. An endocervical polyp represents a focal overgrowth of hyperplastic endocervical epithelium and its underlying stroma: the cause of this overgrowth is unknown.

The polyps form pedunculated, round or ovoid, masses of pinkish tissue which grow into the endocervical canal (Fig. 21.32). Histologically, they have a surface epithelium of columnar endocervical-type epithelium which forms crypt-like infold-

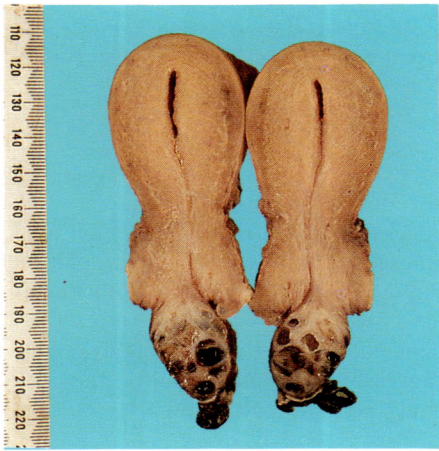

Fig. 21.32   Cervical polyp. A uterus bisected to demonstrate a large, dependent cervical polyp in which there are blood-filled, distended crypts. The patient complained of irregular vaginal bleeding.

ings into the stroma of the polyp (Fig. 21.33). Squamous metaplasia of the surface epithelium is common.

Endocervical polyps occur most frequently in women aged 30–50 years and can present with a vaginal discharge, because of hypersecretion of mucus from the hyperplastic epithelium, or bleeding, due to ulceration of the tip of the polyp. There is no risk of malignant change.

21.6.6   Condylomas of the cervix

Cervical warts, or *condyloma acuminata*, have been long recognized but it is only in recent years that the flat condyloma (also known as 'warty atypia', 'condyloma planum', and 'noncondylomatous cervical wart virus infection') has been identified. Both lesions are due to a sexually transmitted infection with human papilloma virus (HPV) and it is now realized that flat condylomas account for over 90 per cent of HPV infections of the cervix.

Condyloma acuminata are seen as fleshy, pointed papules which are often multiple and sometimes confluent. A flat condyloma is, by contrast, not visible to the naked eye and, although often suggested by an abnormal cervical smear, is detectable only on colposcopy and histology. Histologically, the hallmark of an HPV infection is the presence, within squamous epithelium, of *koilocytes*: these cells have enlarged, irregular, hyperchromatic nuclei with a prominent clear perinuclear space (or 'halo') and margination of the cytoplasm. Multinucleation and premature individual cell keratinization (*dyskeratosis*) are other typical features of HPV infection.

Condylomas occur most commonly in the squamous epithelium of the transformation zone of young women and HPV strains 6, 11, 16, and 18 have been identified, by Southern blot hybridization studies, in a very high proportion of these lesions.

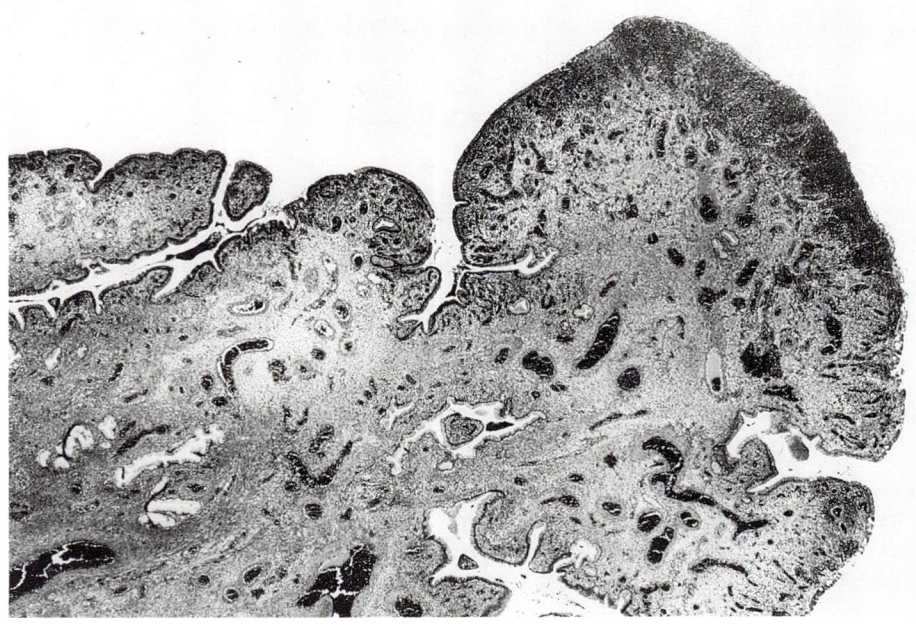

Fig. 21.33   Cervical polyp. The polyp is composed of endocervical tissue containing congested blood vessels and is ulcerated at its tip (to the right).

Condylomas due to infection with HPV-6 or HPV-11 almost invariably pursue a benign course: some regress spontaneously while the remainder may persist, in the absence of treatment, in an unchanged state for many years. Condylomas due to HPV strains 16 and 18 are, however, frequently complicated by a superimposed cervical intra-epithelial neoplasia; it should be noted that condylomas due to these strains of HPV are always of the *flat* variety. The incidence of supervening cervical intra-epithelial neoplasia (CIN) is not known with accuracy for these specific lesions but is believed to be at least 10 per cent.

21.6.7   Cervical neoplasms

Squamous carcinomas, *adenocarcinomas*, and *adenosquamous carcinomas* all occur in the cervix but squamous tumours predominate to the extent that there is a tendency to think of cervical cancer only in terms of squamous carcinoma: this undoubtedly blurs our understanding of the aetiology, pathogenesis, and development of the different tumours.

Squamous neoplasia

Both pre-invasive and invasive squamous neoplasms occur. The condition of cervical intra-epithelial neoplasia (CIN) is thought to represent an intra-epithelial neoplasm and this term is used to encompass those abnormalities previously described as *dysplasia* and *carcinoma in situ*. This lesion occurs, in the vast majority of cases, in that area of metaplastic squamous epithelium which was the transformation zone. CIN may, therefore, develop on the anatomical ectocervix or within the endocervical canal, and is a recognized precursor of invasive squamous carcinoma.

Aetiology

Invasive and intra-epithelial squamous neoplasia of the cervix have, as might be expected, aetiological factors in common and it is convenient, therefore, to discuss the aetiology of both conditions together. Some adenocarcinomas and adenosquamous carcinomas appear to share common aetiological factors with squamous carcinomas but other adenocarcinomas have different aetiological correlates and these are discussed below.

During the process of metaplasia the immature squamous epithelium of the transformation zone appears to be particularly susceptible to oncogenic stimuli, and various factors have been identified which may be of aetiological importance in the development of pre-invasive and invasive neoplasia of the cervix, although final proof of their significance is still lacking. They can be divided into epidemiological factors and causative agents.

It is almost unknown for CIN or invasive squamous carcinoma of the cervix to develop in women who have never had coitus, and there appears to be a direct relationship between coitus and neoplasia of the cervix. The greater the number of partners that the woman, or her consort, has had and the younger her age at first coitus, the greater her risk of developing carcinoma. There is also a direct relationship between carcinoma, early age of first marriage, early age of first pregnancy,

and an unstable marital history. A higher frequency of sexually transmitted disease is reported in women with cervical neoplasia but this may simply be related to the greater number of sexual partners. Patients with invasive carcinoma are more likely to come from the lower than the upper socio-economic groups, though whether this reflects differences in sexual behaviour, age at first intercourse, hygienic measures, or a failure to take advantage of medical advice during the pre-invasive stage of the disease is uncertain: it is interesting to note, however, that CIN is no more common in the lower than in the upper socio-economic groups.

Women who smoke cigarettes are at greater risk of developing both CIN and invasive carcinoma than are those who do not smoke, and when smoking is discontinued the risk falls: it should be noted that smoking is an independent risk factor and is unrelated to other aetiological factors. The effects of smoking may be due to the excretion of chemicals derived from cigarette smoke in the cervical mucus: these are not only capable of exerting a carcinogenic effect but also appear to cause local immunosuppression. Women who use barrier contraceptives are at lower risk of developing cervical neoplasia than those who use non-barrier techniques: this may be because exposure of the cervix to the immunosuppressive effects of seminal plasma promotes the development of carcinoma but could also reflect the fact that barrier contraception prevents the transmission of an aetiological agent. Possibly, women who select barrier techniques form a distinct group with a pattern of sexual behaviour which differs from that of non-barrier contraceptive users.

Evidence that circumcision of the male partner reduces the incidence of cervical carcinoma has not been substantiated, and the lower incidence of cervical squamous carcinoma in women from the orthodox Jewish community probably depends more on ethnic sexual practices than upon circumcision of Jewish men.

All the epidemiological data indicates that a sexually transmitted agent is implicated in the aetiology of cervical carcinoma and that the timing of its transmission may be important. Many suggestions have been made about the nature of this factor or factors. Smegma, spermatozoa, or the protein content of semen have each had their proponents, as has herpes virus simplex type 2. Currently, however, evidence supporting an aetiological role of *human papilloma virus* (HPV) is accumulating, for certain strains of this virus, notably *strains 16 and 18*, have been shown to be present, either in episomal or integrated forms, in many cervical neoplastic lesions, both intra-epithelial and invasive, the viral genome having been detected by both immunocytochemical and *in situ* hybridization techniques. The aetiological role of HPV should not, however, be taken as proven: this virus is present in the histologically normal cervical epithelium of a surprisingly high proportion of women and has been detected in many other epithelia, sometimes in integrated form. It is possible, therefore, that HPV is simply a 'passenger' virus which tends to localize in proliferating epithelia and is more easily integrated into neoplastic than into normal cells. Certainly HPV does not, by itself, *cause* cervical carcinoma, and other factors, such as the carcinogenic effects of cigarette smoking and the local immunosuppression produced by exposure to both metabolites of cigarette smoke and seminal plasma may be of equal, or greater, importance.

Generally speaking, CIN occurs at a younger age than does squamous carcinoma, which has its peak incidence in women over the age of 45 years. In recent years, although the incidence of carcinoma in women between the ages of 35 and 45 has declined, the incidence in women under the age of 35 has increased, and there has been little change in incidence in women over the age of 45 years. There are still approximately 2000 deaths a year from cervical cancer in England and Wales and the incidence of CIN has shown a dramatic increase.

Cervical intra-epithelial neoplasia

Pathological features

CIN is a single disease process: it begins at one end of the spectrum as a *well-differentiated squamous intra-epithelial neoplasm* (CIN 1) and ends with *invasive carcinoma*. There are intermediate grades of *moderately well-differentiated squamous intra-epithelial neoplasia* (CIN 2) and *poorly differentiated intra-epithelial neoplasia* (CIN 3). CIN is recognized histologically by a failure of the normal process of maturation in the squamous epithelium of the transformation zone. CIN 1 (Fig. 21.34) is recognized by an absence of maturation in the lower third of the epithelium, though cytoplasmic maturation occurs in the upper two-thirds of the epithelium. CIN 2 (Fig. 21.35) is characterized by a failure of the cells to mature in the lower one- to two-thirds of the epithelium and CIN 3 (Fig. 21.36) is diagnosed when undifferentiated cells extend into the upper third of the epithelium or occupy its full thickness. The cells that are shed from the surface of this abnormal epithelium closely reflect the abnormality in the underlying epithelium and their examination is the basis of the *cervical smear test*.

Features indicative of HPV infection are present in many cases, these being the presence of kiolocytes, epithelial multinucleation, and individual cell keratinization. These abnormal-

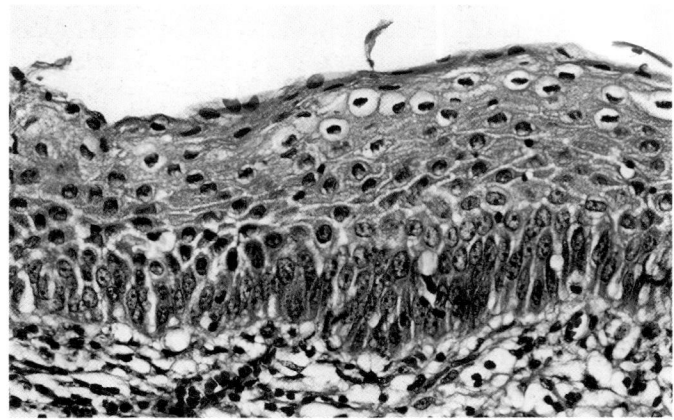

Fig. 21.34 Cervical intra-epithelial neoplasia, CIN 1: the lower third of the epithelium is occupied by cells with large nuclei, high nucleo-cytoplasmic ratios, and lacking differentiation.

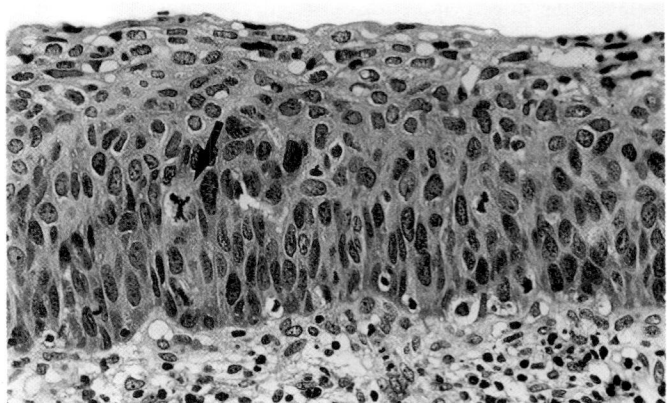

Fig. 21.35 Cervical intra-epithelial neoplasia, CIN 2: the lower half of the epithelium is occupied by cells lacking differentiation. Note the abnormal, tripolar mitosis (arrow).

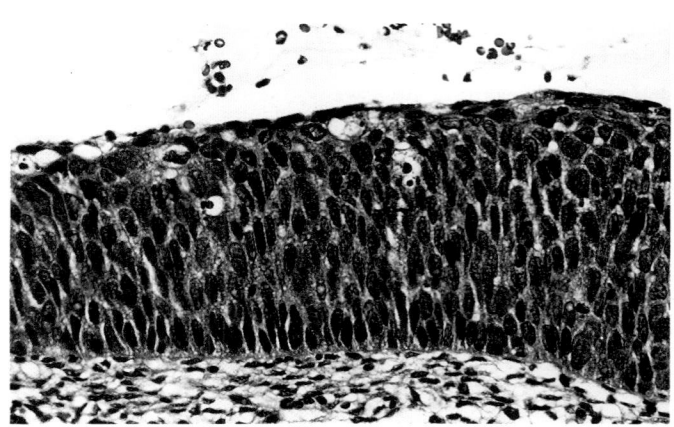

Fig. 21.36 Cervical intra-epithelial neoplasia, CIN 3: the epithelium is occupied by cells which show no evidence of differentiation. The cells have large, hyperchromatic nuclei and high nucleo-cytoplasmic ratios.

ities are most evident in CIN 1 and 2 and are least apparent in CIN 3 in which integration of the viral genome into the DNA of the epithelial cell nucleus has become complete.

CIN 3 is usually assumed to be a *squamous intra-epithelial neoplasm* but can be closely mimicked by a very poorly differentiated *adenocarcinoma in situ*, which can be recognized only by the use of a mucin stain.

The differentiation of the CIN is rarely uniform throughout the affected area of the transformation zone. Generally it is better differentiated at the outer ectocervical margin, adjacent to the ectocervical squamous epithelium, and less well differentiated centrally.

In the transformation zone, metaplasia is not always limited to the surface epithelium and, similarly, CIN may also extend into the underlying endocervical crypts.

When invasion occurs from CIN, it may occur from the surface epithelium or from crypts, and although the epithelium from which invasion has occurred most commonly has the features of CIN 3, invasion may also, less commonly, occur from CIN 1 or 2.

Clinical aspects and prognosis

CIN is asymptomatic and can be detected only by the examination of cervical smears: confirmation of the diagnosis is by colposcopy and biopsy.

CIN is a precursor of invasive squamous cell carcinoma but not all, or even most, cases of CIN will progress to an invasive neoplasm: it is probable that approximately 35–40 per cent of cases of CIN 3 will evolve into an invasive squamous cell carcinoma within 20 years of diagnosis if untreated. The long-term risk of invasive neoplasia in cases of CIN 1 and 2 is less well defined but, in any individual patient, either of these better-differentiated forms of CIN carries the risk of eventual squamous cell carcinoma. Hence, all cases of CIN must, irrespective of grade, be treated in the same manner and it is not the grade of CIN but rather its extent that is of greatest importance for an individual patient. CIN is treated by local ablative techniques, such as laser therapy, cryotherapy, coagulation, or cone biopsy, the latter technique being obligatory if the limits of the abnormal epithelium within the endocervical canal cannot be defined on colposcopy.

Microinvasive carcinoma

Invasion is first recognized by an increase in the amount of cytoplasm and eosinophilia of the cytoplasm in one or more cells in the basal layer of the squamous epithelium covering the surface of the cervix or lining one or more of the crypts. Subsequently the deep margin of the epithelium becomes irregular and jagged as tongues of infiltrating cells penetrate the underlying stroma (Fig. 21.37) where they evoke an inflammatory cell infiltrate and reactive fibrosis.

Microinvasive carcinoma is the term used to describe a degree of invasion which is not associated with any risk of nodal metastasis and is sufficiently small to treat by local or conservative means. It may be multifocal or limited to a single focus. It must be less that 500 mm^3 in volume, must not exceed 1.0 cm in its greatest horizontal axis and must not penetrate the stroma for more than 0.5 cm. With the smallest lesions, those under 200 mm^3, a minor degree of lymphatic permeation in the immediate vicinity of the neoplasm does not exclude the lesion from this category. Earlier descriptions of microinvasive carcinoma in terms only of its depth of penetration are now regarded as having little value and, in some cases, as being misleading and potentially dangerous, there being a clear risk of underestimation of their malignant potential.

Invasive squamous cell carcinoma

Squamous carcinomas constitute about 70 per cent of all malignant cervical noeplasms. They can occur at any age from 17 to 70 years but, although their incidence in young women appears to be increasing, develop most commonly in women in their sixth decade.

Clinical features

Small invasive tumours are usually asymptomatic and identifiable only by a combination of examination of cervical smears, colposcopy, and biopsy. The cardinal symptom of larger lesions is abnormal vaginal bleeding, commonly post-coital, intermenstrual, or post-menopausal: some patients experience a serosanguineous discharge, while pain is a late symptom and indicative of advanced disease. In the late stages of the disease symptoms may be centred around the urinary tract with ureteric obstruction, urinary tract infection, and uraemia. Vesicovaginal or recto-vaginal fistulae may develop.

Pathological features

Squamous carcinoma (Fig. 21.38) may develop either on the ectocervix, where it tends to grow in a predominantly exophytic

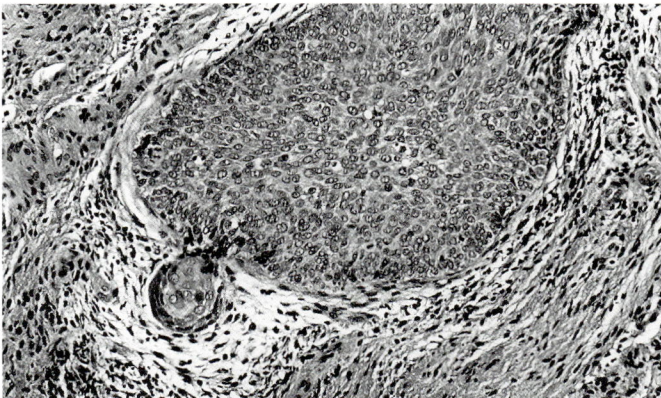

Fig. 21.37 Microinvasive carcinoma of the cervix (early stromal invasion). A crypt, lined by epithelium with the features of CIN 3, lies at the top of the field and from its lower border there arises a bud of superficially invasive squamous carcinoma.

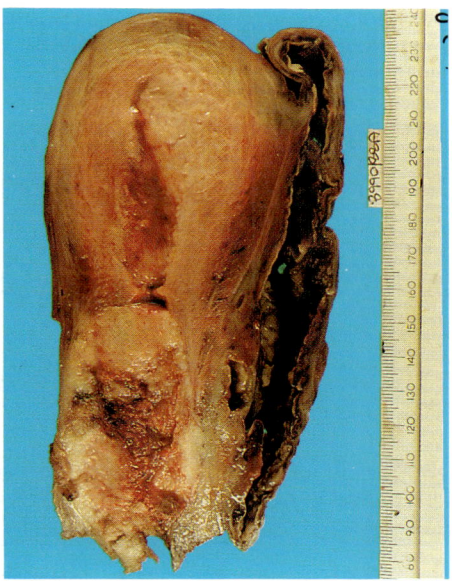

Fig. 21.38 Invasive carcinoma of the cervix. The barrel-shaped cervix, left, is expanded by a centrally necrotic carcinoma.

manner to form a papillary or polypoidal mass, or in the endo-cervical canal, where it commonly expands the cervix to form a hard barrel-shaped mass. Ulceration and necrosis are common features and the tumour often bleeds on touch.

Histologically, squamous cell carcinomas infiltrate the cervical stroma as a network of anastomosing bands which appear on cross-section as irregular islands with spiky or angular margins. The tumours may be well differentiated (the *large-cell keratinizing type*) (Fig. 21.39), moderately differentiated (*large-cell focally keratinizing type*) or poorly differentiated (*large- or small-cell non-kenatinizing types* (Fig. 21.40) but 80 per cent are either moderately or poorly differentiated tumours, well differentiated neoplasms being the exception rather than the rule.

Spread and prognosis

Squamous cell carcinomas spread locally to invade the *uterine body*, *vagina*, *bladder*, and *rectum*: spread occurs along the *paracervical ligaments* to the *lateral side walls of the pelvis*, surround-

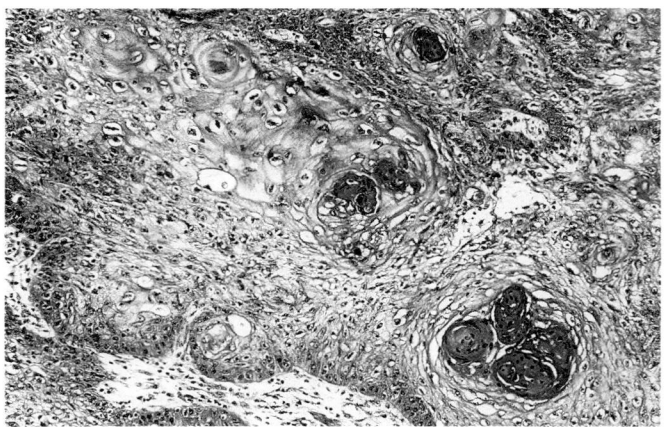

Fig. 21.39 Well-differentiated, keratinizing, squamous carcinoma of the cervix. The tumour is composed of well-differentiated malignant cells which are forming epithelial pearls.

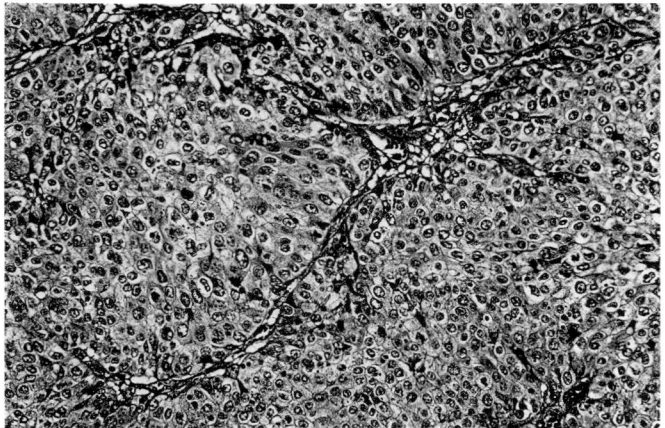

Fig. 21.40 Poorly differentiated, large-cell, non-keratinizing squamous carcinoma of the cervix. The tumour is composed of solid sheets of cells which, in this field, show little or no squamous differentiation.

ing and compressing the *ureters* as they traverse the *paracervical region*. Lymphatic spread is to the *paracervical, iliac, obturator,* and *para-aortic nodes* but dissemination by this route does not occur methodically and an absence of metastases from the iliac nodes is no guarantee that tumour will not be present in para-aortic nodes. Blood-borne spread is a late phenomenon and is principally to the *liver, lungs,* and *skeleton.*

The prognosis for a patient with a cervical squamous cell carcinoma is linked to the stage of the disease at the time of initial diagnosis:

Stage I Invasive carcinoma is confined to the cervix.

Stage II Carcinoma extends outside the cervix but has not reached the pelvic wall: involvement of the vagina is limited to the upper two-thirds.

Stage III Tumour extends to either lateral pelvic wall and/or involves the lower third of the vagina.

Stage IV Tumour is invading the bladder or rectum or extends beyond the true pelvis.

The overall survival rate for women with this neoplasm is only 50 per cent at 5 years, the survival rate ranging from over 90 per cent for patients with Stage I disease to only 10 per cent for those with tumours in Stage IV. Histological grading of the neoplasm bears little relationship to prognosis.

Adenocarcinoma

Both *adenocarcinoma in situ* and *invasive adenocarcinoma* of the cervix are recognized but the relationship between these two conditions is much less clearly defined than is that between CIN and squamous carcinoma of the cervix. Adenocarcinomas currently constitute between 12 and 16 per cent of all cervical neoplasms and this proportion is rising. Whether this reflects a genuine increase in the incidence of these tumours or is due to a reduction in the number of squamous carcinomas is uncertain.

Aetiology

Many adenocarcinomas are found in women with aetiological factors similar to those for squamous carcinoma, and *HPV strains 16 and 18* have been identified in adenocarcinomas. There are, however, two groups of women in whom adenocarcinoma develops and in whom the aetiological factors differ significantly. These are, first, the nulliparous woman or women of low parity who has a history of infertility or dysfunctional hormonal problems and tends, on the whole, to be older than the woman with squamous carcinoma and, secondly and rarely, the girl or young woman who was exposed, *in utero*, to diethylstilboestrol and subsequently, in a small proportion of cases, develops clear-cell carcinoma of the cervix and/or vagina.

Adenocarcinoma in situ

Adenocarcinoma *in situ* occurs in the mucus-secreting columnar epithelium on the surface of a cervical ectopy, within the endocervical canal, or within endocervical crypts. It is recognized histologically by stratification of the epithelial cells, loss of nuclear polarity, loss of mucin-secreting capacity, an increase in nucleo-cytoplasmic ratios, cellular pleomorphism, nuclear hyperchromatism and the presence of numerous, sometimes atypical, mitoses (Fig. 21.41): an increasing complexity of the glandular pattern is often, though not invariably, present. The least well-differentiated forms come to resemble squamous CIN 3. Lesser degrees of epithelial abnormality are recognized, to which the term *cervical glandular intra-epithelial neoplasia (CGIN)* is sometimes applied. This is intended to make the terminology comparable to that of the squamous lesions but it is not yet in common usage.

The relationship between adenocarcinoma *in situ* and invasive adenocarcinoma of the cervix is not established. In certain cases, the origin of an adenocarcinoma from an *in situ* lesion can be traced but an accompanying adenocarcinoma *in situ* is not necessarily identified adjacent to all adenocarcinomas.

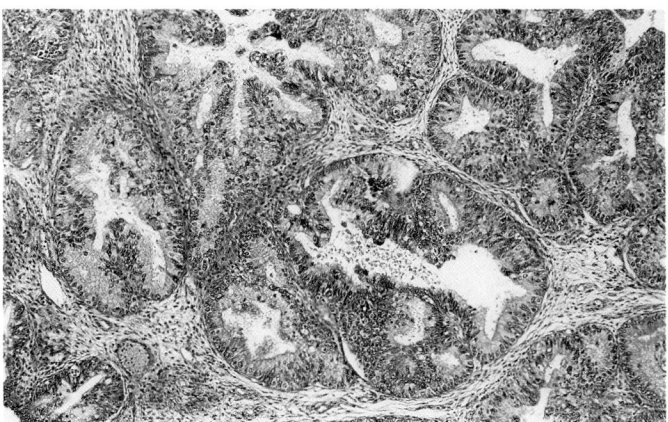

Fig. 21.42 Well-differentiated adenocarcinoma of the cervix. The tumour is composed of well-formed glandular acini lined by tall, mucus-secreting columnar epithelium similar to that which lines the normal endocervix.

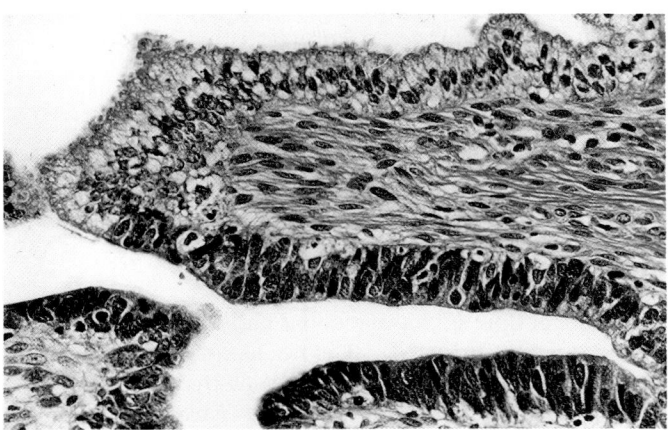

Fig. 21.41 Adenocarcinoma *in situ* of the cervix. The crypt at the top of the field is lined by a single layer of normal mucus-secreting columnar epithelium. In contrast, the lower crypt is lined by a stratified epithelium which is composed of cells with high nucleo-cytoplasmic ratios, large, hyperchromatic nuclei, and diminished mucin secretion.

Adenocarcinoma

There are several histological types of adenocarcinoma, of which the most common is the so-called *endocervical type*: the constituent cells resemble those of the normal endocervix.

The lesion is macroscopically indistinguishable from squamous carcinoma, the diagnosis being made only on histological examination.

Endocervical adenocarcinomas may be well, moderately well, or poorly differentiated. The well-differentiated tumours form glandular acini and branching clefts and crypts and the cells resemble those of the endocervix to a greater or lesser extent (Fig. 21.42). Loss of differentiation is characterized by the loss of the glandular pattern and mucus-secreting capacity. The least well-differentiated forms assume a solid rather than a glandular pattern and thus come, histologically, to resemble a squamous carcinoma with which they may be confused.

Clear-cell carcinoma Cervical neoplasms of this type are iden-

tical to the clear-cell adenocarcinoma of the vagina and although occurring typically in DES-exposed girls, are by no means limited to this group.

Endometrioid adenocarcinoma This term is used to describe carcinomas which are identical histologically with those adenocarcinomas that develop in the endometrium. They are an unusual finding in the cervix.

Prognosis There is a general consensus that adenocarcinomas of the cervix have a poorer prognosis, in general, than do squamous carcinomas.

Carcinoma of mixed pattern

About 8–10 per cent of cervical carcinomas show evidence of differentiation along more than one cell line. Most commonly these are adenosquamous carcinomas (Fig. 21.43) and the diagnosis is made only when histological examination of the tumour is carried out, as they are similar in gross appearance to squamous and adenocarcinomas.

These are aggressive neoplasms with a poor prognosis and a marked tendency to metastasize widely, even when the primary neoplasm is of only small size.

21.6.8   Cervical cytology screening

Cytopathology is the study of disease processes, usually neoplastic conditions, by examination of the individual cells from a lesion. It thus differs from histopathological diagnosis, in which changes in the structure and form of the tissues can be evaluated. The technique is applied in many fields of pathological investigation and diagnosis but is perhaps best known as the basis of the cervical smear test which was introduced to detect the pre-invasive phase of cervical carcinoma, cervical intra-epithelial neoplasia (CIN), thus allowing for removal of the lesion and preventing the development of an invasive carcinoma.

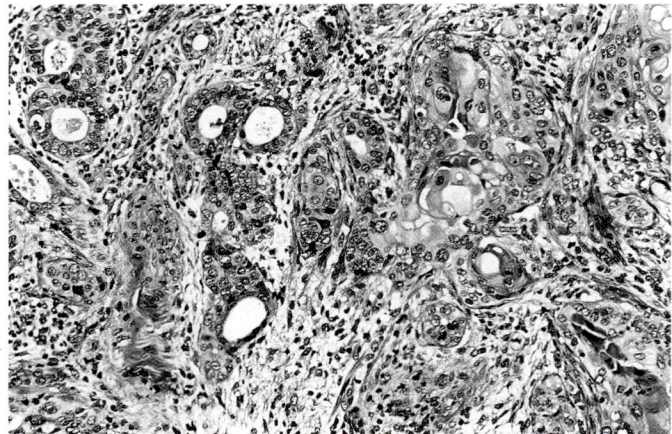

Fig. 21.43 Adenosquamous carcinoma of the cervix. The tumour has two distinct, though intermingled, components. To the left, there are well-formed infiltrating glandular acini and, to the right, focally keratinizing squamous cell carcinoma.

The detection of CIN by the cervical smear technique depends upon the fact that the cells which are desquamated from the surface of a stratified squamous epithelium accurately reflect the abnormalities in the underlying cellular layers: as neoplastic cells show poor cohesion, they are preferentially removed from the surface of the epithelium as a spatulum is scraped over its surface.

It will be recalled that CIN usually develops in that area of the cervix which undergoes metaplasia, the transformation zone, and this is the area from which cells must be taken. To be certain that this area has been adequately sampled the smear should, ideally, also include squamous cells from the ectocervix and columnar cells from the endocervical canal, between which the transformation zone lies. This becomes increasingly difficult as the woman becomes older because the transformation zone is withdrawn to within the endocervical canal and may be out of reach of the operator. This being so, and as the least well-differentiated forms of CIN lie at the endocervical margin of the transformation zone, a cervical smear test may underestimate the degree of abnormality.

The nomenclature which is used for desquamated cells differs from that which is used for the histological lesions, but none the less it is possible, from the character of the cells identified in the smear, to suggest the type of epithelial abnormality which can be anticipated. Cells that have been shed from an epithelium showing CIN have large, somewhat irregular and hyperchromatic nuclei, delayed cytoplasmic maturation, and higher nucleo-cytoplasmic ratios as compared with normal surface cells. They are described as *mild*, *moderately*, or *severely dyskaryotic*, these corresponding respectively to CIN 1, CIN 2, and CIN 3 for invasive carcinoma. In addition, abnormal keratinization, dyskeratosis, may be seen and this suggests the possibility of wart virus infection or carcinoma. Dyskeratosis is also found in a variety of non-neoplastic conditions of which hyperkeratosis is a feature, e.g. prolapse.

The cervical smear test is designed primarily to identify abnormalities of the squamous epithelium of the cervix but the columnar cells of the cervix may also show dyskaryosis and the smear may also, therefore, detect the presence of adenocarcinoma *in situ* or adenocarcinoma of the cervix.

Examination of the smear may, quite incidentally, reveal cervical and vaginal infection by, for example, *Trichomonas vaginalis*, *Candida* or *herpes simplex*. The test is not appropriate for detection of endometrial carcinoma and the finding of cells shed from such lesions should be regarded as fortuitous.

The aim of a cervical cytology screening programme is to reduce the incidence of cervical carcinoma and to decrease the death rate from this form of cancer. Its application, until recently, on an *ad hoc* basis in the United Kingdom has meant that the hoped for reduction in death rate from cervical carcinoma has not occurred. It could be argued, however, that in a period of time when the incidence of CIN has risen sharply it is only the use of the cervical smear test that has prevented a marked increase in deaths from cervical carcinoma.

21.7   Endometrium

21.7.1   The normal endometrium

The endometrium is the functional lining of the body of the uterus. It is continuous above, at the uterine cornua, with the mucosa of the interstitial segments of the Fallopian tubes and below, at the uterine isthmus, with the endocervical epithelium.

The endometrium is composed of simple tubular glands set in a delicate vascular stroma and has two components. There is a basal layer which is shallow, does not respond to hormonal stimulation in the normal cycle and is present throughout life, and a superficial, functional layer which normally develops only during the reproductive years and is exquisitely sensitive to the hormones secreted by the ovary.

Physiological changes

Most tissues in the body have a similar appearance throughout life, but the endometrium of any individual woman varies with her hormonal status. The menstrual cycle represents the recurrent priming of the endometrium in anticipation of conception, and menstruation is the shedding of the functional layer of the endometrium at the end of a cycle in which conception does not occur. The normal cycle lasts for between *21 and 34 days* and, by convention, the first day of menstruation is defined as the first day of the cycle.

Menstruation lasts for approximately 5 days after which, under the influence of oestrogen secreted by the developing ovarian follicle, the endometrium enters a growth phase which lasts for between 4 and 16 days, this being known as the *proliferative or follicular phase*. This endometrial phase corresponds to the development of the ovarian follicle and is characterized by the growth of the endometrial glands and stroma and the induction of progesterone receptors. Shortly after ovulation the endometrium enters the *secretory or luteal phase*. This is characterized, on the one hand, by the cessation of oestrogen-driven endometrial growth and, on the other, by glandular secretion, differentiation of the spiral arteries in preparation for the development of a materno-fetal circulation, and changes in the endometrial stroma known as *decidualization*. These features represent the endometrial response to the progesterone secreted by the corpus luteum and are dependent upon there having been adequate prior oestrogenic stimulation, and hence progesterone receptor induction, in the proliferative phase.

If conception does not occur, the corpus luteum decays, there is a rapid drop in both oestrogen and progesterone levels, and menstruation ensues with necrosis and shedding of most of the functional layer of the endometrium. Regrowth occurs from the residuum of the functional layer and from the basal endometrium. It is worth noting that menstruation is not an essential component of this recurrent cycle, since certain primates have similar cycles but do not menstruate. Necrosis of the endometrium, and hence menstruation, is a consequence of very rapid regression of the endometrium at the end of the cycle, the abruptness of this change being due to a precipitous decline in oestrogen levels as the corpus luteum decays. If oestrogen levels declined more slowly, as is the case in certain species, endometrial regression would be more gradual and necrosis with menstrual loss avoided, but only at the cost of prolonging the cycle. Menstruation is therefore the price that women pay for the shortening of their menstrual cycle which allows for a greater number of possible conceptions during their limited years of fertility.

If conception does occur during a cycle the corpus luteum persists, being sustained by chorionic gonadotrophin secreted by the developing placenta, and menstruation is inhibited; secretory activity continues, spiral artery growth becomes more marked, and decidualization of the stroma is enhanced. A hypersecretory state is normal at this stage and in extreme cases this is known as the *Arias–Stella change*. The finding of this appearance within the endometrium indicates that the patient is pregnant, although the pregnancy may be in the uterine cavity or in an ectopic site (see below).

After the cessation of ovarian activity at the menopause, cyclical changes in the endometrium cease and the uterus becomes lined only by basal endometrium. The tissues retain, however, a capacity to respond to oestrogen stimulation even many years after the menopause and thus may still proliferate if exposed to oestrogens.

Histology of the endometrium

During the menstrual cycle

During the follicular phase of the menstrual cycle (Fig. 21.44) when oestrogen levels are high, the various elements of the functional layer of the endometrium proliferate. The glands are at first straight and narrow but become slightly tortuous during the latter part of this phase, when the rate of glandular growth

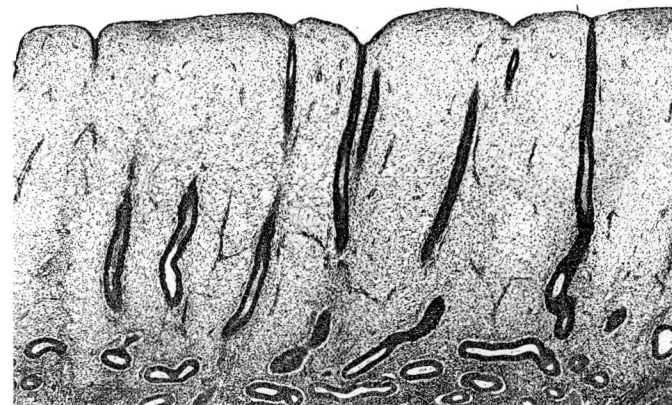

Fig. 21.44 Endometrium in the early proliferative phase. The glands, which are straight and narrow, are set in a delicate cellular stroma. (Reproduced by kind permission of Chapman and Hall from *Biopsy pathology of the endometrium*, Buckley and Fox, 1989.)

outstrips that of the stroma; the glands are lined by columnar cells with basally situated nuclei and there may be a minor degree of multilayering in the late proliferative phase. The stroma is cellular and because the stromal cells have little cytoplasm often presents a 'naked-nuclei' appearance. Mitotic figures are present, in both glands and stroma, throughout the proliferative phase.

In the average cycle, ovulation occurs at about the fourteenth day, the endometrium then entering, under the influence of the rising progesterone levels, the early secretory phase. The morphological changes that characterize the early secretory phase take, however, 24–36 h to develop, although during this period the glands increase slightly in diameter and become somewhat more tortuous: mitotic figures are still present in the glandular epithelium but decrease progressively in number as progesterone exerts its anti-oestrogen effect. The defining feature of the early secretory phase, clearly apparent 48 h after ovulation, is the appearance of *glycogen-containing subnuclear vacuoles* in the glands (Fig. 21.45): these vacuoles,

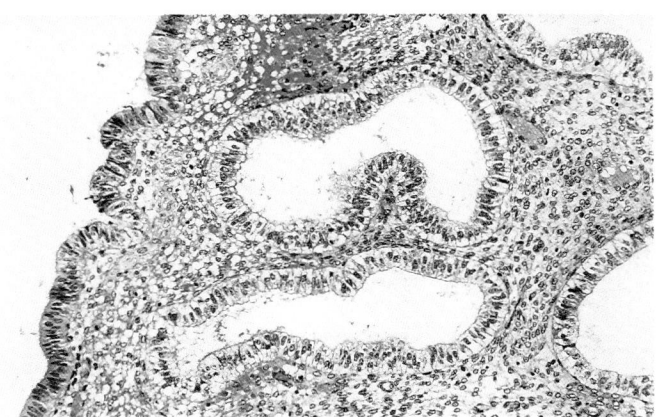

Fig. 21.45 Endometrium in the early secretory phase. There are clear, subnuclear vacuoles in the glandular epithelial cells.

when numerous and prominent, are taken as being definite evidence that ovulation has occurred. The early secretory phase lasts for about 4 days and between the fifth and ninth post-ovulatory days the endometrium is in the mid-secretory phase of the cycle (Fig. 21.46): the subnuclear vacuoles move to a supranuclear position and secrete their contents into the gland lumina, the nuclei of the glands returning to a basal position. Glandular secretion is at a peak during this period and the glands become increasingly dilated and tortuous. During the mid-secretory phase the stroma is markedly oedematous, largely because of the hormonally induced increases in both blood flow through, and hydrostatic pressure in, the endometrial capillary complexes.

At the eleventh post-ovulatory day the endometrium passes into the late secretory phase (Fig. 21.47). Glandular secretion diminishes and the glands tend to collapse and become increasingly tortuous. The stromal oedema regresses and the stromal

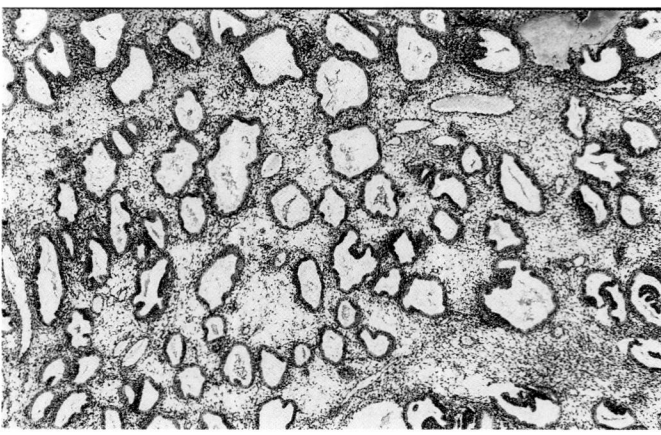

Fig. 21.46 Endometrium in the mid-secretory phase. The glands are distended by secretion and are rather angular: the stroma is oedematous. (Reproduced by kind permission of Chapman and Hall from *Biopsy pathology of the endometrium*, Buckley and Fox, 1989.)

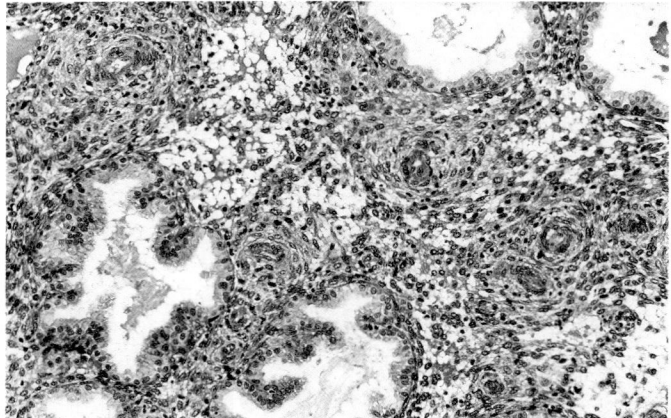

Fig. 21.47 Endometrium in the late secretory phase. The glands are serrated in outline, having collapsed after secreting their contents, and the spiral arteries, which are cuffed by decidualized stromal cells, are well muscularized.

cells take on a pre-decidual appearance, becoming plump with abundant acidophilic cytoplasm and small nuclei. The pre-decidual cells appear first as a mantle around the spiral arteries which, after being previously inconspicuous, are now well developed and prominent. Later, pre-decidual change is seen in the cells surrounding the glands and in those lying directly below the surface epithelium. Towards the end of the late secretory phase the stroma consists largely of sheets of pre-decidual cells which are infiltrated by neutrophil polymorpho-nuclear leucocytes and by *granulated lymphocytes (K-cells)*. The leucocytes increase in number as the endometrium undergoes menstrual changes, characterized by crumbling, necrosis, glandular collapse, and haemorrhage.

It will be appreciated that throughout the proliferative phase of the cycle the endometrium shows a rather consistent pattern and thus an accurate estimation of the day of the menstrual cycle is not possible: after ovulation the endometrium shows an orderly pattern of time-related changes which allow for a relatively precise estimate, to within 24–48 h, of the stage of the cycle.

After the menopause

Oestrogen levels diminish quite abruptly in many women at the time of the menopause and this results in endometrial atrophy, the endometrium becoming shallow, the glands small and inactive and the stroma compact (Fig. 21.48). In some women, however, oestrogen levels show a more gradual decline and there may be a rather irregular pattern of proliferation, with mitotic activity still being discernible for up to two years after cessation of ovulation. Gradually, however, this low-grade stimulation ceases and the presence of mitotic figures in the endometrium more than three years after the menopause is a clear indication of either an abnormal source of endogenous oestrogens or the administration of exogenous oestrogens.

In a high proportion of post-menopausal women the endometrial glands are, either focally or diffusely, cystically dilated (Fig. 21.49), such glands being lined by a single layer of flattened epithelial cells. The incidence of such cystic change in-

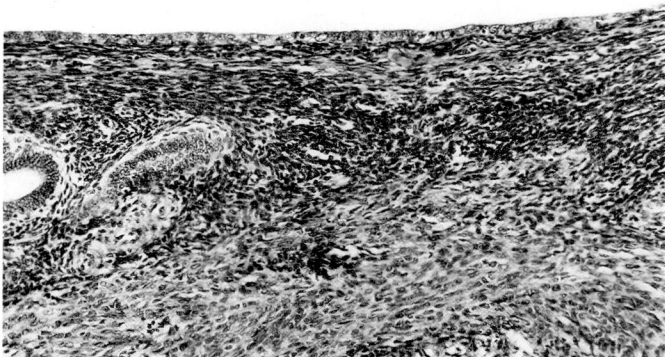

Fig. 21.48 Post-menopausal, atrophic endometrium. There is neither secretory nor proliferative activity. The glands are narrow and the stroma compact and cellular.

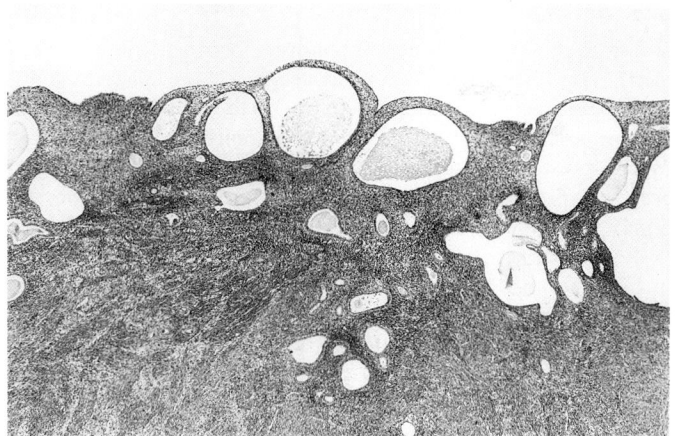

Fig. 21.49 Senile cystic atrophy of the endometrium. Some of the glands are cystically dilated but there is neither proliferative nor secretory activity and the stroma is compact.

creases progressively with advancing age, and it is clear that this is because of blockage of gland ducts during the process of endometrial atrophy and condensation, there being no evidence that this change is indicative of a 'regressed' perimenopausal hyperplasia. The cystically dilated glands may, on occasion, become polypoid.

21.7.2 Functional abnormalities of the endometrium

It is usual to distinguish between those abnormalities of endometrial morphology which are secondary to hormonal disturbances and are sometimes known as functional disorders of the endometrium, although the term has little to commend it, and those in which there is a primary disease process within the endometrium.

Functional abnormalities of the endometrium fall into two main groups, those in which there are inadequacies of hormonal stimulation and those in which such stimulation is excessive.

Low oestrogen states

In the absence of ovarian follicular development there is no oestrogen secretion and hence an absence of endometrial growth and proliferation. In such women, the endometrium is shallow and inactive and the uterus is lined only by endometrium of basal type. This is normal after the menopause but is seen in such pathological processes as *gonadal dysgenesis, premature menopause, 17-hydroxylase deficiency, gonadotrophin-resistant ovary syndrome*, and *hypogonadotrophic hypogonadism*.

High oestrogen states

The secretory phase of the menstrual cycle is remarkably constant at 14 days and most variation in cycle length is due to changes in the length of the proliferative or follicular phase, which is considered to be abnormally long only when it exceeds

21 days. The endometrium in such cycles may be of normal appearance or show nothing more than an increased stratification of the glandular epithelium and a mild increase in the volume of the endometrium; there are no significant consequences of these minor changes. There will, however, be less frequent menstruation than normal and the periods may be irregular. The condition is sometimes associated with subfertility.

In some circumstances ovarian follicular development is not followed by ovulation and, as a consequence of continued oestrogen secretion by the developing follicle or follicles, the endometrium will continue to grow in an uninterrupted fashion and will eventually become hyperplastic. This condition is discussed in more detail below.

Low progesterone states

Low progesterone states are a natural consequence of failure of normal follicular maturation and of ovulation. In some women, however, less profound deficiencies occur; normal ovulation is followed by inadequate development of the corpus luteum with resulting progesterone deficiency. These patients, described as having 'luteal phase insufficiency' or 'inadequate secretory phase', complain of a variety of symptoms, amongst which the most common are premenstrual spotting (the loss of small amounts of blood), prolonged menstruation, and infertility.

Progesterone deficiency may affect the endometrium in several ways. There may be a delay in the development of secretory changes following ovulation, so that the endometrium appears to be less mature than suggested by the date of the woman's cycle; there may be a discrepancy between the maturation of the glands and stroma, with the stroma appearing to be more mature than the glands; or there may be a variable degree of secretory change in different glands in the same tissue, this latter condition being known as 'irregular ripening' (Fig. 21.50).

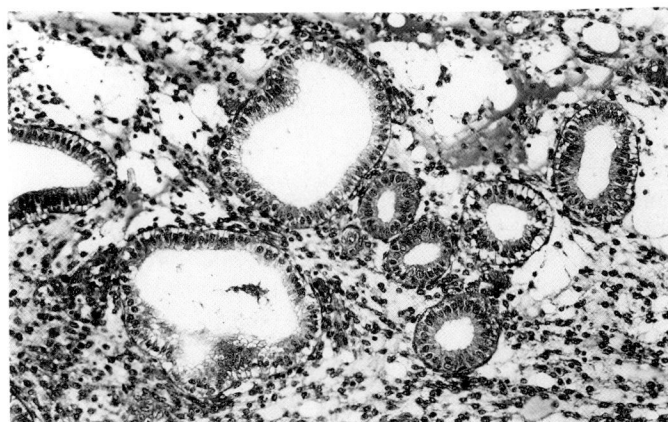

Fig. 21.50 Luteal phase insufficiency: irregular ripening. The glands in this field vary in their degree of maturation. Those to the left are large, and there is subnuclear vacuolation of the glandular epithelium, the appearances are consistent with the fourth to fifth post-ovulatory day. The glands to the right are small, three show no evidence of secretory change and two are small but show early secretory changes.

A low progesterone state can often be diagnosed by examination of the endometrium during the luteal phase, but infertility in women with low progesterone levels is not due only to the endometrial abnormalities but to the effect of the hormone deficiency on the cervical mucus and on Fallopian tube function.

21.7.3 Exogenous hormone effects

Many of the functional abnormalities of the endometrium may be mimicked by exogenous hormones given to a patient for therapeutic or contraceptive purposes. Thus the administration of oestrogens as hormone replacement therapy for the treatment of menopausal symptoms, uninterrupted by progesterone, may result in the development of endometrial hyperplasia of simple, complex, or atypical form, or even of carcinoma.

Progestagens given for the control of symptoms associated with endometriosis or for contraceptive purposes may so inhibit endogenous oestrogenic activity that the endometrium can, after an initial response, become shallow and atrophic.

The changes in the endometrium which accompany the use of a combined steroid contraceptive, the contraceptive 'pill', vary greatly according to the dose of hormone administered, the relative potency of the steroids included in the combination, and their duration of use. The appearances may mimic those of luteal phase insufficiency or resemble those seen after administration of a progestagen.

21.7.4 Inflammation and infection in the endometrium

The endometrium normally contains a population of lymphocytes and, at the time of menstruation, polymorphonuclear leucocytes: the presence of such cells in the endometrium is therefore not indicative of an inflammatory process. *Plasma cells, eosinophils, tissue breakdown associated with a polymorphonuclear leucocyte infiltrate at times other than at menstruation, granulomas, and lymphoid aggregates with germinal centres* are, however, not normally found in the endometrium and are regarded as hallmarks of *inflammation*.

Non-infective inflammation

Inflammation which is not infective in origin may be physiological, such as that which accompanies the remodelling of the decidua in the early stages of pregnancy or follows delivery, or it may be pathological. The latter type occurs when there is abnormal tissue breakdown in the uterine cavity, e.g. when there is torsion of a polyp (see below), in association with an intra-uterine contraceptive device, when there is prolonged and frequent heavy bleeding, or in the presence of neoplasms. These non-infective causes of inflammation are more common than infections in the endometrium. It should be emphasized, however, that infective and non-infective endometritis cannot be regarded as entirely separate entities, for many of the conditions associated with non-infective inflammation of the endometrium also predispose to the development of infection.

Infection of the endometrium

Endometrial infections are uncommon because the establishment of an infective lesion is discouraged by the efficient downwards drainage of the uterine cavity, by the regular shedding of the endometrium which occurs in the reproductive years, and by the presence of an effective cervical mucus barrier which prevents the ascent of most organisms into the uterus from the cervix and vagina.

If, however, these natural protective mechanisms are disturbed, *endometritis* may supervene. Thus, drainage from the uterine cavity may be partly or completely obstructed by polyps, neoplasms or retained products of conception within the uterine cavity, by acute flexion of the uterus, by scarring of the cervix following surgery, obstetric trauma, or radiotherapy, or by a cervical neoplasm. Disruption of the cervical mucus barrier occurs in patients with chronic cervical infection, in whom the mucus may be infected or secretion impaired; in women in whom previous cervical surgery has removed much of the mucus-secreting tissue; and in women who have had operative procedures involving dilatation or biopsy of the cervix. The mucus barrier does not offer complete protection, for certain organisms, of which *N. gonorrhoea* is an example, are capable of penetrating it. Interruption of endometrial shedding, for reasons other than pregnancy, does not, in itself, predispose to infection but permits any infection that may occur to become established.

The uterus has little natural protection against those infections which spread via the bloodstream or descend from the Fallopian tubes.

Pathological features of endometrial inflammation

Inflammation may be *acute, subacute,* or *chronic*: chronic inflammatory lesions may be *granulomatous* or *non-granulomatous*.

Acute endometritis is recognized by the presence, in the endometrium, of polymorphonuclear leucocytes associated with tissue destruction at times other than at menstruation. Acute infections are usually polymicrobial and occur most commonly following abortion: an acute endometritis may, however, be due to gonococcal infection.

In an *active chronic endometrial inflammation* (Fig. 21.51) plasma cells, polymorphonuclear leucocytes, lymphocytes, and histiocytes are found in the stroma and polymorphonuclear leucocytes are present in the glandular lumens. If inflammation is particularly severe, there may be disturbances in the induction of hormone receptors, as a consequence of which the tissues may fail to reflect the normal cyclical hormonal changes.

The incidence of *chronic non-granulomatous endometritis* is difficult to determine and almost certainly underestimated because of the difficulty in distinguishing an abnormal diffuse chronic inflammatory cell infiltrate from the normal lymphocytic population of the endometrium. When the inflammatory infiltrate is predominantly histiocytic the term *histiocytic or xanthomatous endometritis* is sometimes used. The presence of lymphoid follicles with germinal centres is also regarded by most pathologists as indicative of chronic inflammation.

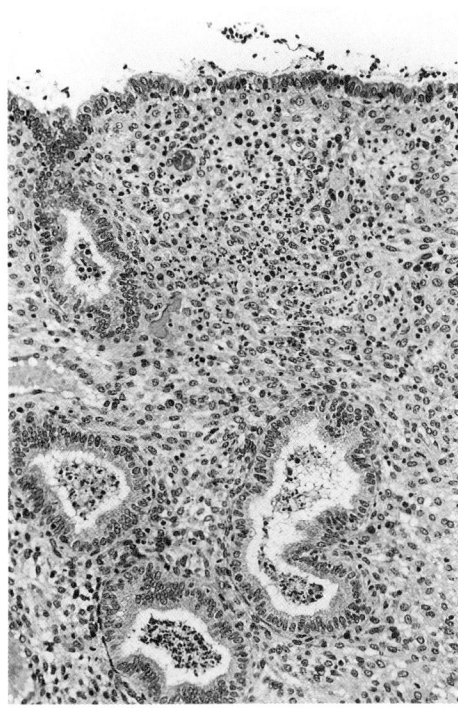

Fig. 21.51 Active chronic inflammation of the endometrium. The endometrial stroma is infiltrated by neutrophil polymorphs, plasma cells, and lymphocytes, and the glands contain an acute inflammatory cell exudate.

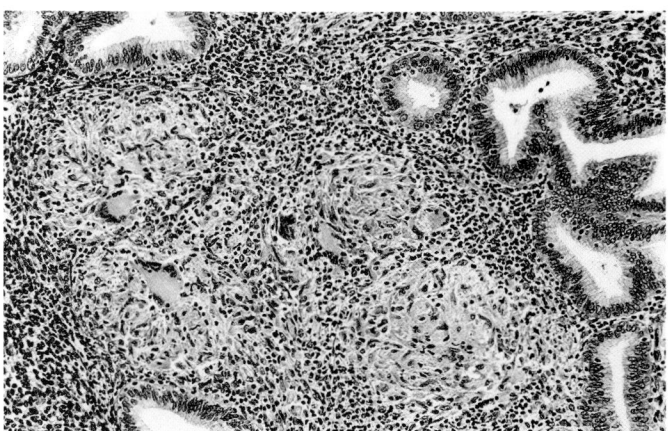

Fig. 21.52 Endometrial tuberculosis. There are non-caseating granulomas with epithelioid macrophages and Langhan's giant cells centrally, with a peripheral cuff of lymphocytes. (Reproduced by kind permission of Chapman and Hall from *Biopsy pathology of the endometrium*, Buckley and Fox, 1989.)

Chronic granulomatous inflammation in the endometrium is regarded as being due to *tuberculosis* until otherwise proven and, indeed, non-tuberculous granulomatous inflammation is extremely uncommon. Endometrial tuberculosis is almost always secondary to infection in the Fallopian tubes, from which site there is repeated inoculation of the endometrial surface. The regular menstrual shedding of the endometrium tends to prevent establishment of infection and, because the shedding of the endometrium occurs at about the same interval as the time taken for a granuloma to be recognizable histologically, granulomas tend to be small and poorly developed (Fig. 21.52): caseation is rarely seen unless endometrial shedding has been incomplete, when caseating granulomas may be seen in the basal endometrium, or after the menopause when extensive, confluent, caseating endometrial tuberculosis may be encountered.

Clinical presentation

Inflammation is present in approximately 4 per cent of the endometria examined routinely. In most cases the diagnosis is made only following histological examination of the tissue and is clinically asymptomatic.

When acute infection occurs, particularly in the postpartum period or following spontaneous abortion, there may be local symptoms of vaginal discharge and uterine tenderness and systemic disturbances such as pyrexia and malaise.

When the endometritis is only one facet of more extensive pelvic infection, the symptoms of endometritis may well be masked by the severity of symptoms localized to the Fallopian tubes or pelvic peritoneum. In less severe infections the presenting complaint may be one of infertility or irregular vaginal bleeding.

Consequences of endometrial inflammation

Acute inflammation has no long-term adverse effects upon the patient's well-being or fertility unless infection persists, there is secondary infection, or infection spreads to the Fallopian tubes. Active early therapy of postpartum and postoperative infections is therefore mandatory. The majority of non-infective inflammatory processes resolve when the initiating cause is treated.

When inflammation is so severe that there is structural damage to the basal layers of the endometrium, tissue regrowth may be hampered. The stroma may be extensively replaced by fibrous tissue, intra-uterine adhesions may be formed, and the glands may be unresponsive to normal hormonal stimulation: this is the condition known as *Asherman's syndrome*. It may play a part in the development of infertility or, should the woman become pregnant, abnormal adherence of the placenta.

21.7.5   Endometrial metaplasia

The tissues of the Müllerian system, that is, the Fallopian tubes, uterus, and endocervix, retain into adulthood a capacity to differentiate into one or more of the tissues to which the paracoelomic epithelium, the embryonic precursor of the Müllerian tract, gives rise during fetal development. This takes the form, in the adult, of epithelial metaplasia which, in the endometrium, is characterized by replacement of the epithelial lining of one or more glands, completely or partly, by a *squamous*, *serous*, or *mucinous epithelium* (Fig. 21.53). This is most common in hyperoestrogenic states and in the elderly, post-menopausal

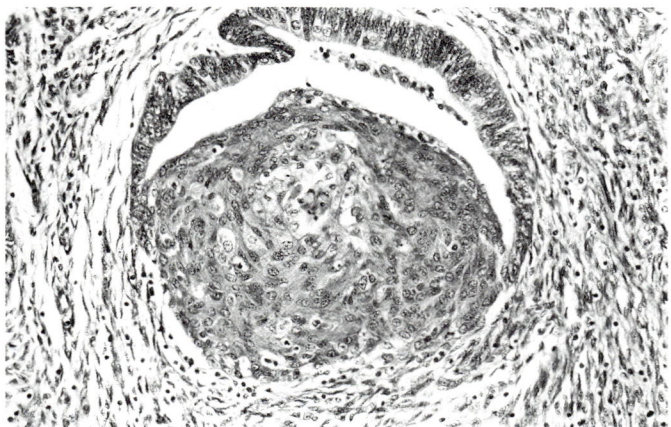

Fig. 21.53 Intraglandular squamous metaplasia of the endometrium. A focus of bland metaplastic squamous epithelium replaces part of the lining of this endometrial gland and protrudes into the lumen.

woman. In older patients with cervical obstruction and intra-uterine infection, the uterus may become lined only by squamous epithelium, a condition known as 'ichthyosis uteri' (Fig. 21.54) and one which may occasionally give rise to a squamous cell carcinoma. *Focal intraglandular squamous metaplasia* also occurs in adenocarcinomas of the endometrium and is discussed below. *Endometrial stromal metaplasia*, with bone, cartilage, or smooth muscle formation, also occurs but is extremely uncommon.

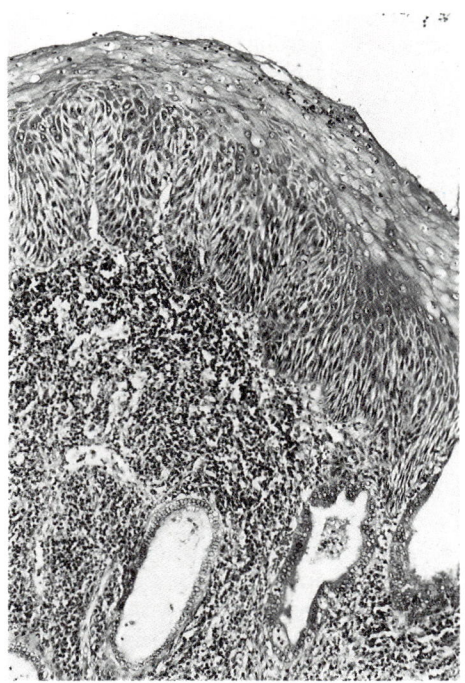

Fig. 21.54 Ichthyosis uteri. The surface epithelium of the endometrium is replaced by stratified squamous epithelium and beneath this inactive, post-menopausal glands, set in a compact chronically inflamed stroma, are visible.

21.7.6   Endometrial polyps

The term 'endometrial polyp' could be used to describe any polypoidal lesion protruding into the uterine cavity. By convention, however, the term is restricted to non-neoplastic pedunculated or sessile nodules composed either of functional or basal endometrium or a combination of the two.

Endometrial polyps develop as a consequence of focal stromal and glandular overgrowth. It is believed that a focal hypersensitivity to oestrogen or lack of sensitivity to progesterone may allow a portion of endometrium to remain unshed at the end of menstruation. This focus continues to grow in each successive cycle until it protrudes into the uterine cavity. Polyps do not occur before the menarche, are most common in the fifth decade, and are sometimes encountered in the post-menopausal woman.

Pathological features

Endometrial polyps vary greatly, ranging from small lesions discovered incidentally during routine biopsy examination of the endometrium, to large masses which protrude from the cervical os: they may be sessile or pedunculated (Fig. 21.55). In the reproductive years they are usually composed either of non-functional basal endometrium, or have a central core of basal-type endometrium, containing thick-walled arteries, covered by a layer of functional endometrium of variable thickness (Fig. 21.56). The latter is frequently out of step with the endometrium elsewhere in the uterine cavity, for example showing only weak proliferative activity during the follicular phase and either lacking secretory features or showing only weak or patchy secretory activity in the luteal phase. The tip of a polyp is often congested, even to the naked eye, and focally inflamed: *ulceration* may occur and the surface epithelium may undergo squamous metaplasia, this being seen particularly in those polyps protruding from the cervical os or developing from the uterine isthmus. On rare occasions predunculated polyps may undergo torsion and infarction.

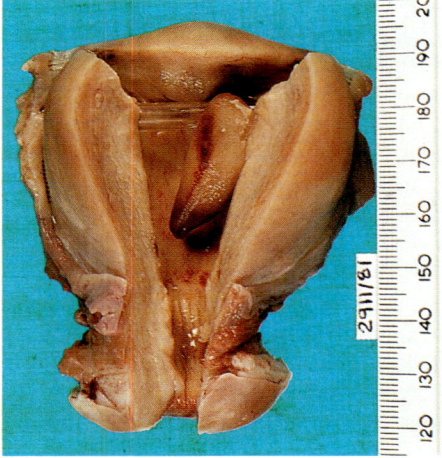

Fig. 21.55 Endometrial polyp. The uterine cavity has been opened to show a polyp, the tip of which is congested, arising from the left cornu.

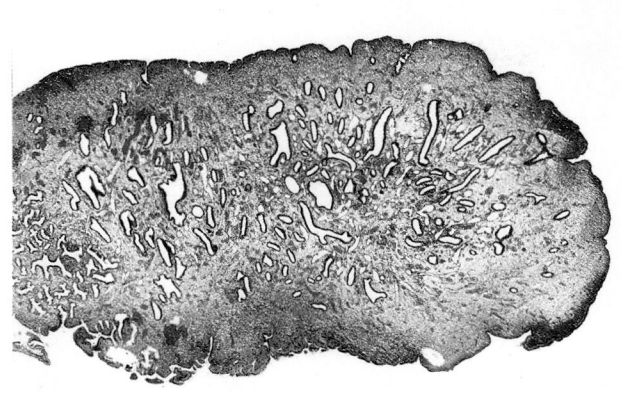

Fig. 21.56 Endometrial polyp. The polyp is composed of endometrial tissue in which the glands are clearly visible. (Reproduced by kind permission of Chapman and Hall from *Biopsy pathology of the endometrium*, Buckley and Fox, 1989.)

Polyps in post-menopausal women may be formed either of inactive basal type endometrium or of senile cystic endometrium with a fibrous stroma.

Clinical features

Many polyps are asymptomatic and discovered only by chance when examining a hysterectomy specimen. Others are associated with irregular or heavy bleeding: they are also a recognized, but uncommon, cause of post-menopausal bleeding. Whether in the latter case the polyp is in fact the direct cause of the bleeding or is simply incidental to bleeding from another cause may be difficult to determine unless there is clear evidence that the polyp is composed of hyperplastic endometrium.

Polyps commonly recur, presumably because they have been incompletely removed or because the underlying defect persists. Polyps do not predispose to the development of a carcinoma: malignant change can, very occasionally, occur in a polyp but most apparent instances of this phenomenon have been, in reality, adenocarcinomas growing in a polypoidal fashion.

21.7.7   Endometrial hyperplasia

Endometrial hyperplasia is widely regarded as a possible precursor of endometrial adenocarcinoma. The term 'endometrial hyperplasia' encompasses, however, several quite different conditions and it is important to distinguish between those types of hyperplasia associated with a significant risk of evolving into an adenocarcinoma and those devoid of any such risk. The defining, and only, feature of an endometrial hyperplasia which is indicative of a propensity for malignant change is *cytological atypia*, and any hyperplastic lesion of the endometrium showing this abnormality is classed as 'atypical hyperplasia of the endometrium'. Hyperplastic conditions that lack cytological atypia are divided into 'simple' and 'complex' forms.

Simple endometrial hyperplasia

Simple hyperplasia (also often, but incorrectly, called cystic glandular hyperplasia) is a relatively common condition and represents the physiological response of the endometrium to prolonged, unopposed oestrogenic stimulation, being in fact only one component of a generalized hyperplasia of all the uterine tissues. The endometrium is thickened and often polypoidal: the entire endometrium is involved and, histologically, there is a loss of the normal distinction between basal and functional zones. The endometrial glands show a proliferative pattern but vary markedly in calibre, some being unusually wide, others of normal calibre, and yet others unduly narrow (Fig. 21.57). The glandular epithelium is formed by plump cuboidal or low columnar cells with basophilic cytoplasm and round, centrally, or basally situated nuclei. The endometrial stroma shares in the hyperplastic process and hence the gland-to-stroma ratio is normal with no glandular crowding. The stroma appears hypercellular whilst mitotic figures, present in both glands and stroma, may be sparse or abundant but are invariably of normal form.

Simple hyperplasia may complicate *exogenous oestrogen therapy*, *oestrogenic ovarian tumours*, or the *polycystic ovary syndrome*: the commonest cause of the condition is, however, a series of *anovulatory cycles* in which oestrogen production by persistent ovarian follicles is not opposed by any luteal secretion of progesterone. Hence this type of hyperplasia occurs most commonly in the perimenarchal and perimenopausal years, when anovulatory cycles are common: patients usually present with irregular, prolonged, or heavy bleeding and it is assumed, perhaps oversimplistically, that these symptoms are due either to intermittent waning of the oestrogen levels or to the endometrium achieving a bulk that exceeds the supportive capacity of the oestrogens. If ovulatory cycles are resumed, or if a progestagen is administered, a simply hyperplasia will regress and the endometrium will return to its normal state.

Simple endometrial hyperplasia is not a precursor of, and

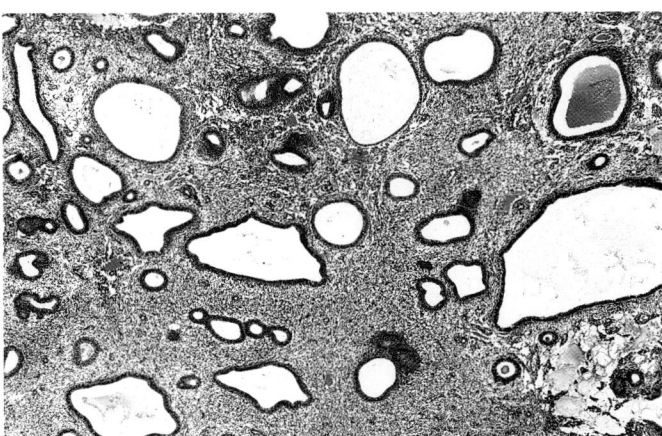

Fig. 21.57 Simple hyperplasia of the endometrium. The endometrium contains glands which are small, and of normal calibre, and others which are cystically dilated. (Reproduced by kind permission of Chapman and Hall from *Biopsy pathology of the endometrium*, Buckley and Fox, 1989.)

does not evolve into, atypical endometrial hyperplasia, and is not associated with any increased risk of developing an adeno-carcinoma.

Complex hyperplasia

This endometrial abnormality may occur under the same circumstances as does simply hyperplasia, i.e. in an endometrium exposed to unopposed oestrogenic stimulation, but can also develop in a normally cycling or atrophic endometrium. A complex hyperplasia is restricted to the glandular component of the endometrium and does not involve the stroma; furthermore it is usually focal or multifocal in nature, involving only a group, or groups, of glands. The hyperplastic glands are variable in size, but often larger than normal, and are crowded together with a reduction in the amount of intervening stroma. The involved glands show an abnormal pattern of growth with outpouchings or buddings of the glandular epithelium into the stroma to give a 'finger-in-glove' pattern (Fig. 21.58): intraluminal epithelial tufting is also common. The glandular epithelium is regular and formed of cuboidal or columnar cells with basal or central nuclei; there is no cytological atypia.

The risk of a complex hyperplasia evolving into an adenocarcinoma has not been fully determined but is almost certainly extremely low.

Atypical hyperplasia

This lesion develops under the same circumstances as does a complex hyperplasia, some cases being 'oestrogen-driven' and others occurring in the absence of undue oestrogenic stimulation of the endometrium. As with a complex hyperplasia, only the glands are hyperplastic and the lesions are either focal or multifocal.

In the hyperplastic areas (Fig. 21.59) there is crowding of the glands with a marked reduction in intervening stroma, and in severe cases the glands show a 'back-to-back' pattern, the stroma between the glands being reduced to a thin wisp or completely obliterated. The glands are usually irregular in shape and are lined by cells showing varying degrees of atypia. In the milder forms of atypical hyperplasia the epithelial nuclei tend to be ovoid with retention of polarity and of a near normal chromatin pattern; the nucleo-cytoplasmic ratio is, however, increased. In more severe cases the nuclei are round and enlarged, nuclear polarity is lost, nucleoli are increased in size, and there is an abnormal chromatin pattern. With progressing severity of atypia there is an increasing degree of *epithelial multilayering* and of *intraluminal tufting*.

An atypical hyperplasia can undoubtedly evolve into an endometrial adenocarcinoma; the exact magnitude of this risk is not adequately defined, but a reasonable estimate would be that approximately 25 per cent of cases of atypical endometrial hyperplasia will eventually give rise to an invasive endometrial adenocarcinoma. When considering this progression from an atypical hyperplasia to an invasive neoplasm it is widely assumed that the controlled proliferation of a hyperplastic process may 'slip over' into the cellular anarchy of neoplasia. It must be doubted, however, if this is a viable concept and there

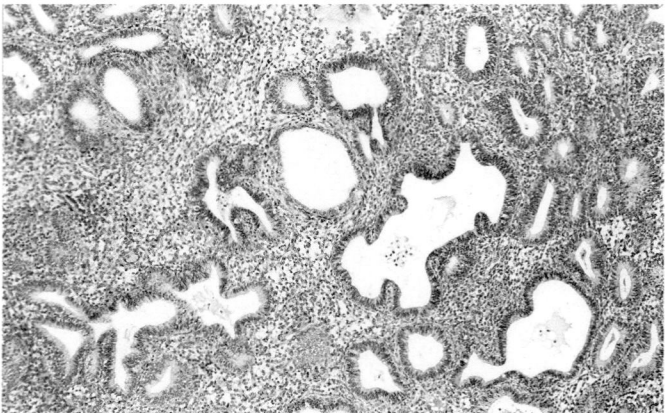

Fig. 21.58 Complex hyperplasia of the endometrium. The endometrial glands are more closely packed than normal and irregular in outline.

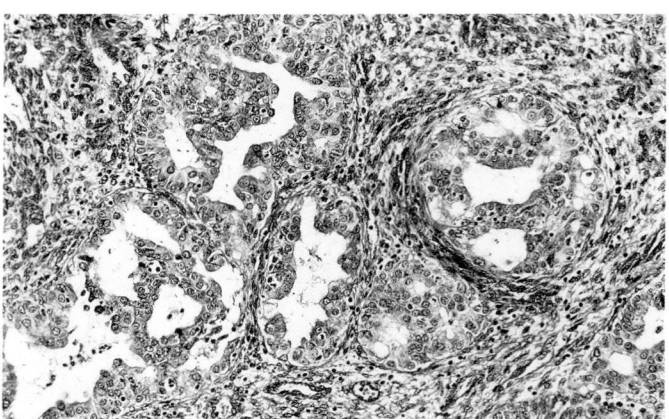

Fig. 21.59 Atypical hyperplasia. The endometrial glands are closely packed, irregular in outline, and lined by cells which are abnormal, that is, their nuclei are enlarged, they have lost their polarity, are stratified, and form bridges across the lumen of the glands. (Reproduced by kind permission of Chapman and Hall from *Biopsy pathology of the endometrium*, Fox and Buckley, 1989.)

are good grounds for believing that the lesion classed as an atypical hyperplasia of the endometrium is, in reality, a form of intra-endometrial neoplasia, comparable in many respects to cervical intra-epithelial neoplasia. The fact that many cases of atypical hyperplasia will regress if treated with a progestagen does not conflict with this hypothesis.

21.7.8   Malignant epithelial tumours of the endometrium

Adenocarcinoma

The vast majority of endometrial neoplasms are adenocarcinomas, which develop most commonly during the sixth decade, many patients being in the early post-menopausal years. Endometrial adenocarcinoma tends to occur unduly frequently in women of high socio-economic status and it is perhaps not surprising that this tumour, relatively common in the Western world, is rare in developing countries. The neoplasm invariably presents with abnormal, usually post-menopausal, vaginal bleeding.

Aetiology and pathogenesis

It is traditionally maintained that women who develop endometrial adenocarcinoma are commonly *nulliparous*, often have an unusually *late menopause*, and have a high incidence of *hypertension*, *diabetes mellitus*, and *obseity*. The association of this neoplasm with nulliparity and a late menopause has withstood the test of case control studies but there is considerable doubt as to whether there is any real link with either hypertension or diabetes: it is certain, however, that obese women have a significantly increased risk of developing an endometrial adenocarcinoma.

The role of oestrogens in the pathogenesis of endometrial adenocarcinoma has been much debated but it is now well established that the administration of *exogenous eostrogens*, either as post-menopausal hormone replacement therapy or as a therapeutic measure for individuals with gonadal dysgenesis, is associated with a greatly increased risk of developing endometrial adenocarcinoma. In the United States, the rise in incidence of the neoplasm which occurred after the introduction of widespread hormonal replacement therapy occurred very rapidly and this suggests that under these circumstances oestrogens were acting as a promoter substance, exposure to a presumed initiator mechanism being therefore very common.

It is thus established that oestrogens can be implicated in the pathogenesis of some endometrial adenocarcinomas: it remains uncertain, however, whether an overproduction of endogenous oestrogen is of aetiological importance in those women, the vast majority, who develop endometrial adenocarcinoma in the absence of exogenous hormones. It is certainly true that patients with *oestrogen-secreting ovarian tumours* have a notably high incidence of associated endometrial adenocarcinoma, but such cases represent only a tiny minority. Many women with endometrial adenocarcinoma have, however, an increased ability to convert *androstenedione*, of adrenal origin, into *oestrone*; this conversion occurs principally in the fat cells of the body and it is probable that this is why obese women, with their excess number of fat cells, are particularly subject to endometrial neoplasia. A similar oestrone excess would, of course, result as a consequence of a primary overproduction of androstenedione and it is therefore of particular note that women with *untreated polycystic ovary syndrome*, in which there is excessive ovarian synthesis of androstenedione, suffer not only a high incidence of adenocarcinoma but tend to develop the neoplasm at an unusually early age.

Simply to look at total oestrogen levels in these patients is, however, far too simplistic an approach for there are many other, largely unexplored, mechanisms by which endometrial cells could be subjected to excessive oestrogenic stimulation: thus the proportion of *free plasma oestrogens*, which are probably the only form of the hormone available for target tissue uptake, may be increased because of a *deficiency of sex-hormone-binding globulin*, the uptake of oestrogens by endometrial cells may be excessive because of increased receptor density, or the enzymatic conversion of oestrogens within the endometrial cells may be abnormal.

Even taking into account the above factors, it is clear that by no means all endometrial adenocarcinomas are oestrogen-related. A significant proportion of these neoplasms arise in an atrophic endometrium and these are probably not oestrogen-driven. The pathogenesis of such tumours is obscure, but it is of note that they often appear to be more aggressive than are those which occur in a setting of hyperoestrogenism.

Pathological features

An endometrial adenocarcinoma may appear as a localized plaque, polyp, or nodule, usually in the upper part of the uterus. More commonly the tumour presents as a diffuse nodular or polypoidal thickening of the uterine lining or as a bulky friable mass (Fig. 21.60) which fills, or even distends, the uterine cavity.

Histologically, most endometrial adenocarcinomas show a greater or lesser degree of endometrial differentiation and are classed as 'endometrioid adenocarcinomas'; many are well differentiated and bear a resemblance, albeit an anarchic one, to normal proliferative endometrium (Fig. 21.61). They are formed of irregular, tightly packed, convoluted glandular acini lined by columnar cells showing a variable degree of pleomorphism, nuclear hyperchromatism, and mitotic activity; irregular multilayering and intraluminal tufting are common. The stroma is scanty and, in many areas, obliterated; foci of necrosis, haemorrhage, and leucocytic infiltration are common, and there may be a noteworthy accumulation of foamy stromal histiocytes.

Less well-differentiated endometrioid adenocarcinomas grow in more solid fashion, and grading of these neoplasms is based

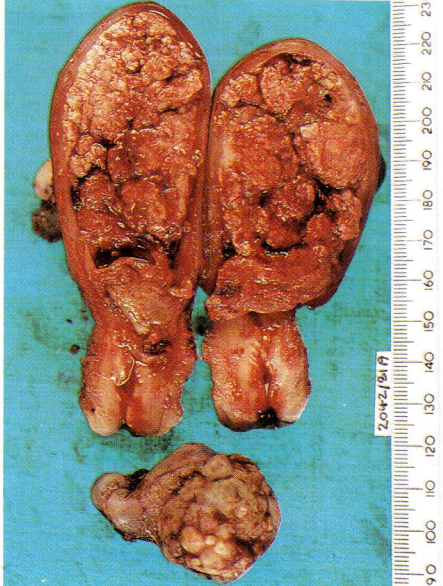

Fig. 21.60 Endometrial carcinoma. The uterine cavity is expanded by a focally necrotic, focally haemorrhagic endometrioid adenocarcinoma.

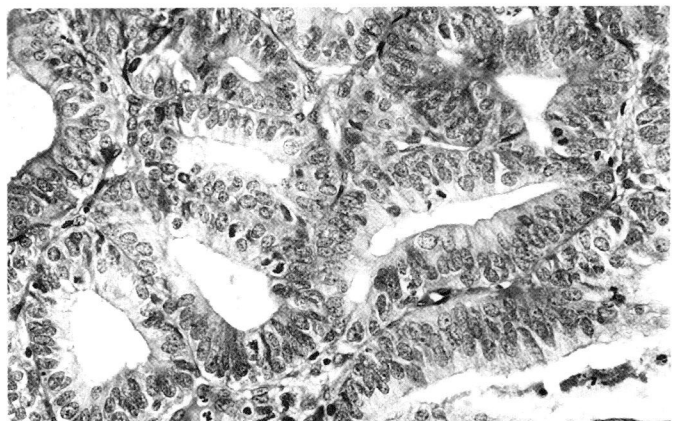

Fig. 21.61 Well-differentiated endometrioid adenocarcinoma of the endometrium. The neoplasm is composed of well-formed, closely packed glandular acini lined by highly abnormal cells in which mitoses are frequent.

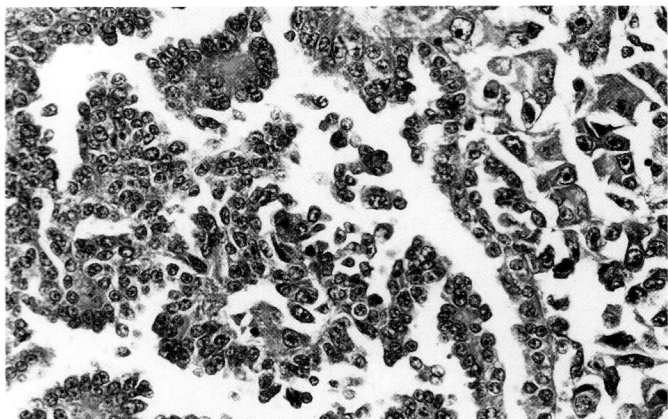

Fig. 21.62 Serous papillary adenocarcinoma of the endometrium. The tumour is composed of papillary, and more solid, areas formed by cells which are poorly differentiated but of tubal type. (Reproduced by kind permission of Chapman and Hall from *Biopsy pathology of the endometrium*, Buckley and Fox, 1989.)

upon a consideration of both the proportion of the tumour showing a solid growth pattern and the degree of cytological atypia.

A number of histological variants of endometrial adenocarcinoma merit attention. Many, indeed most, endometrioid adenocarcinomas contain foci of *bland squamous metaplasia* and it has been suggested that those tumours in which such metaplasia is a prominent feature should be put into a separate category of 'adenoacanthoma'. The frequency with which squamous metaplasia occurs, the subjectivity in deciding what is meant by 'prominent', and the fact that squamous metaplasia, even if widespread, does not alter the prognosis for any given adenocarcinoma, have led to the abandonment of the adenoacanthoma as a diagnostic category.

Some endometrial adenocarcinomas, the *papillary serous carcinomas* (Fig. 21.62), resemble a tubal adenocarcinoma; neoplasms of this type may arise in foci of *endometrial tubal metaplasia* or from uncommitted Müllerian cells which pursue a tubal, rather than an endometrial, pathway of differentiation. These latter cells can also differentiate along endocervical lines and thus give rise to the rare *mucinous adenocarcinomas of the endometrium*.

Clear-cell adenocarcinomas, identical histologically to clear-cell neoplasms of the vagina and ovary (Fig. 21.63), also occur in the endometrium.

Spread and prognosis

Well-differentiated endometrioid adenocarcinomas tend to be slowly growing and often remain within the confines of the uterus for a considerable time, spreading initially by direct invasion of the myometrium and cervix. Later the neoplasm may penetrate the uterine serosa and seed into the *pouch of Douglas* and on to the *pelvic peritoneum*. Cornual carcinomas commonly extend into the Fallopian tubes and tumour cells may pass through the tubal ostia to be deposited on the *ovaries* and *pelvic peritoneum*. Local spread may, of course, also involve the *broad*

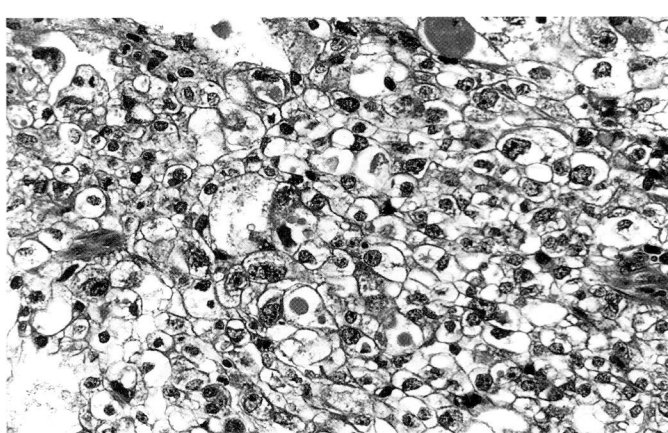

Fig. 21.63 Clear-cell adenocarcinoma of the endometrium. The tumour is composed of sheets of cells with well-demarcated cell margins, large nuclei, and copious clear cytoplasm. (Reproduced by kind permission of Chapman and Hall from *Biopsy pathology of the endometrium*, Buckley and Fox, 1989.)

ligament and the *parametrium*. Lymphatic spread occurs to *pelvic and para-aortic nodes*, whilst haematogenous dissemination to *lungs*, *liver*, *adrenals*, and *bones* occurs late. It should be stressed that this slow pattern of growth is only a feature of the well-differentiated endometrioid adenocarcinomas; poorly differentiated endometrioid tumours, serous papillary adenocarcinomas, and clear-cell carcinomas pursue a much more aggressive course with early deep penetration of the myometrium and spread to *para-aortic nodes*.

The prognosis for patients with an endometrial adenocarcinoma is clearly related to stage, these tumours being staged in the following fashion:

Stage I   The tumour is confined to the uterine body.

Stage II   The tumour has spread to involve the cervix.

Stage III   Carcinomas has extended beyond the uterus but not outside the true pelvis.

Stage VI   The carcinoma has extended beyond the pelvis or is involving the mucosa of the rectum or bladder.

The overall five-year survival for women with endometrial adenocarcinoma is about 65 per cent. For Stage I cases the survival rate is 85 per cent, but this drops to about 50 per cent for women with Stage II tumours and to 35 per cent for Stage III neoplasms, few women with Stage IV tumours surviving 5 years. Stage is thus clearly of prognostic importance but other features related to survival are the *grade of the neoplasm* and the *histological type*, papillary serous tumours and clear-cell adeno-carcinomas having, as already remarked, a poor prognosis. Other prognostic factors to be taken into account are those indicative of a poor outlook, namely, *deep invasion of the myo-metrium*, the presence of *tumour cells in vascular spaces*, a *lack of oestrogen and progesterone receptors*, and an *aneuploid DNA pattern*. A further point of some importance is that tumours arising from a background of atypical hyperplasia have a better prognosis than do those developing in an atrophic endometrium.

Adenosquamous carcinoma

These tumours, which account for about 5 per cent of endometrial neoplasms, contain an admixture of both adenocarcinoma and squamous cell carcinoma (Fig. 21.64). They differ from an adenocarcinoma with squamous metaplasia in so far as the squamous tissue is clearly malignant and invasive. Adenosquamous carcinomas tend to occur at a relatively late age and run an aggressive course, the five-year survival rate being below 40 per cent.

Squamous cell carcinoma

The endometrium is a rare site for this type of neoplasm, which usually develops in elderly women with pyometra and complete squamous metaplasia of the surface epithelium (ichthyosis uteri). In younger patients CIN may spread upwards into the uterine body where it replaces the surface epithelium and can give rise to a squamous cell carcinoma. The prognosis for a squamous cell carcinoma of the endometrium is extremely poor.

21.7.9   Endometrial stromal sarcoma

Sarcomas of the endometrial stroma are rare. Low-grade sarcomas can form localized tumour masses but have a particular tendency to infiltrate extensively the vascular and lymphatic channels of the myometrium; cords of tumour tissue may therefore protrude from the cut surface of the uterus, giving it a 'comedo' or 'rough towel' appearance. Histologically (Fig. 21.65) the neoplasms are formed of sheets of spindle-shaped cells which tend to resemble the endometrial stromal cells of the normal proliferative phase. These neoplasms have *fewer than 10*

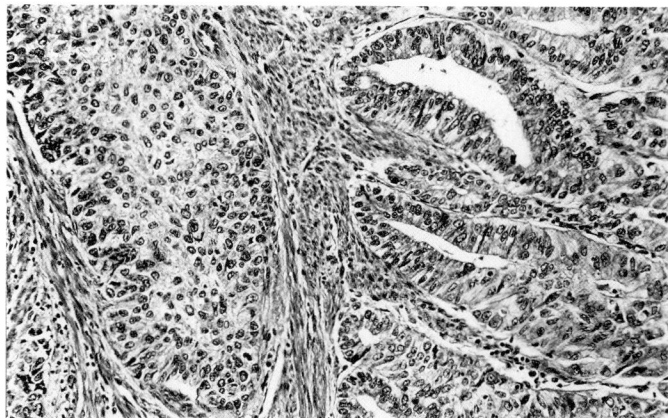

Fig. 21.64 Adenosquamous carcinoma of the endometrium. Two distinct areas of tumour are seen. To the left the neoplasm shows squamous differentiation, whereas to the right there is adenocarcinomatous differentiation. (Reproduced by kind permission of Chapman and Hall from *Biopsy pathology of the endometrium*, Buckley and Fox, 1989.)

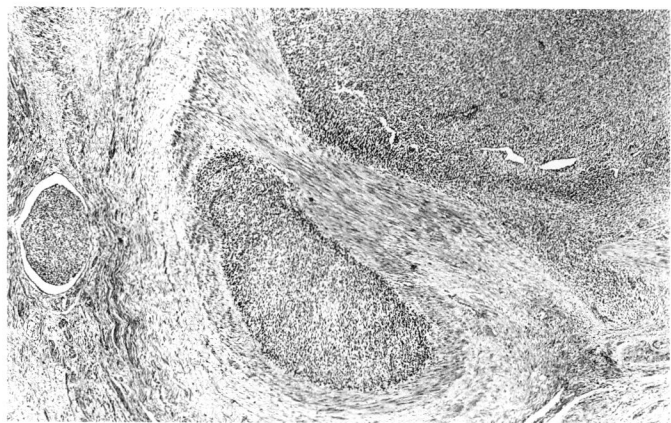

Fig. 21.65 Low-grade endometrial stromal sarcoma of the uterus. The vascular spaces in the myometrium are permeated by a tumour composed of fairly regular, uniform cells resembling those of the normal endometrial stroma. This pattern of infiltration is typical of low-grade stromal sarcoma.

mitotic figures per 10 high-power microscopic fields. Low-grade endometrial stromal sarcomas run an indolently malignant course, tend to spread into the parametrium and often recur locally, sometimes as long as 20 years after removal of the primary tumour. Approximately 20 per cent of patients with these neoplasms will eventually succumb, usually after an extremely protracted course.

High-grade endometrial stromal sarcomas form white, soft, or fleshy masses protruding into the uterine cavity. They are highly cellular, show considerable pleomorphism, have an abundance of mitotic figures, spread rapidly to the parametrium, mesentery, and lungs, and are associated with a very low five-year survival rate.

21.7.10   Mixed tumours

Müllerian cells can differentiate along either epithelial or mesenchymal pathways and although most endometrial neoplasms are either purely epithelial or solely mesenchymal, a few show a dimorphic pattern and contain both epithelial and non-epithelial tissues. Such neoplasms, often classed as 'mixed Müllerian tumours', may be of low-grade malignancy and contain a benign epithelial component and a malignant mesenchymal element (*adenosarcomas*) or can be of high-grade malignancy with both epithelial and mesenchymal elements being malignant (*carcinosarcoma*). The epithelial component of a mixed tumour is usually of a type normally found in the Müllerian system but although the mesenchymal component commonly differentiates into either smooth muscle or endometrial stromal-like cells (i.e. into tissues which are *homologous* for the uterus) it can also differentiate into tissues normally alien to the uterus, the most common of such *heterologous* elements being striated muscle, bone, and cartilage.

Mixed tumours of high-grade malignancy, *carcinosarcomas*, are of unknown aetiology, occur principally in elderly women, and form bulky, fleshy polypoid masses which fill the uterine cavity, sometimes extending into the endocervical canal and occasionally protruding through to the vagina. Histologically they consist of an admixture of carcinomatous and sarcomatous tissues (Fig. 21.66), the adenocarcinomatous element usually resembling an endometrioid adenocarcinoma and the sarcomatous element being either undifferentiated or resembling an endometrial stromal sarcoma; *heterologous tissues* may be present (Fig. 21.67) but they are of no diagnostic or prognostic significance. Endometrial carcinosarcomas are highly aggressive neoplasms which rapidly spread outside the uterus and metastasize by the bloodstream, the prognosis being very poor.

Mixed tumours of low-grade malignancy, *adenosarcomas*, resemble macroscopically the carcinosarcomas but have a

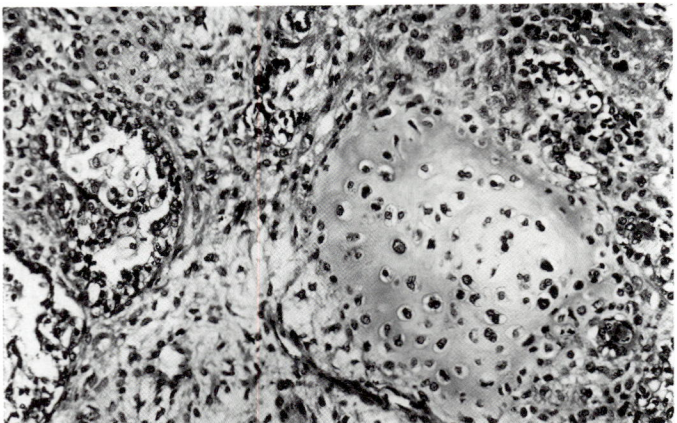

Fig. 21.67 Carcinosarcoma of the endometrium with heterologous elements. An adenocarcinomatous gland is present on the left and the sarcomatous tissue, to the right, contains a focus of chondrosarcoma. (Reproduced by kind permission of Chapman and Hall from *Biopsy pathology of the endometrium*, Buckley and Fox, 1989.)

benign epithelial component, of endometrial, endocervical, or tubal type, set in a stroma resembling an endometrial stromal sarcoma; heterologous elements may be present. These neoplasms spread outside the uterus in only about 50 per cent of cases, and distant metastases are very uncommon: even women with pelvic spread may survive for prolonged periods as this tumour pursues an indolently malignant course.

21.8   Myometrium

The myometrium is the muscular wall of the uterus. Of considerable thickness, it undergoes quite marked atrophy after the menopause. During pregnancy the myometrium undergoes striking alterations in size and contractility.

21.8.1   Adenomyosis

This condition is characterized by the presence of endometrial tissue deep within the myometrium; there is almost invariably an associated hypertrophy of smooth muscle around the ectopic islands of endometrium. The foci of endometrial tissue may be distributed diffusely within the myometrium, in which case the uterus shows a roughly symmetrical enlargement, or can be focal, forming a poorly defined tumour-like, asymmetrical thickening of the myometrium (Fig. 21.68): this localized form is often known as an 'adenomyoma', an unfortunate term because of its misleading connotation of neoplasia. Histologically, foci of adenomyosis consist of both endometrial glands and stroma (Fig. 21.69); the glands are usually of basal type and thus do not show cyclical activity. Less commonly the

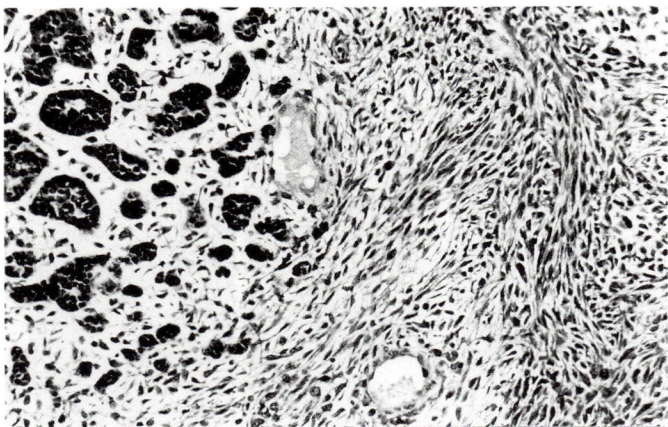

Fig. 21.66 Carcinosarcoma of the endometrium. There is poorly differentiated adenocarcinoma to the left and poorly differentiated sarcoma to the right. (Reproduced by kind permission of Chapman and Hall from *Biopsy pathology of the endometrium*, Buckley and Fox, 1989.)

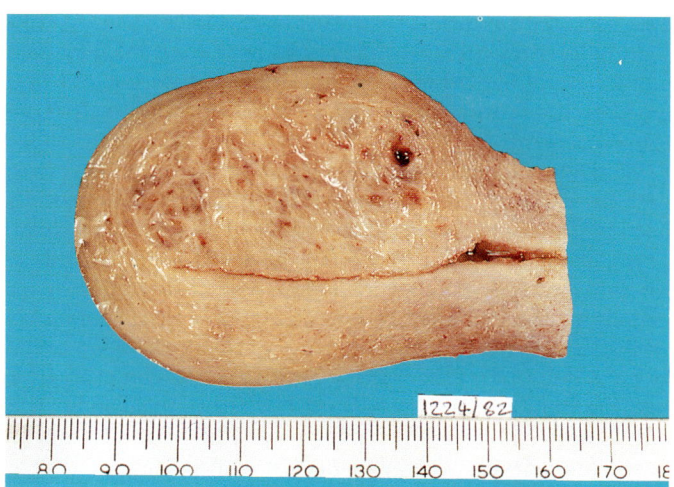

Fig. 21.68 Adenomyosis. The uterine wall is thickened by grey-white whorled tissue in which there are small blood-filled cysts.

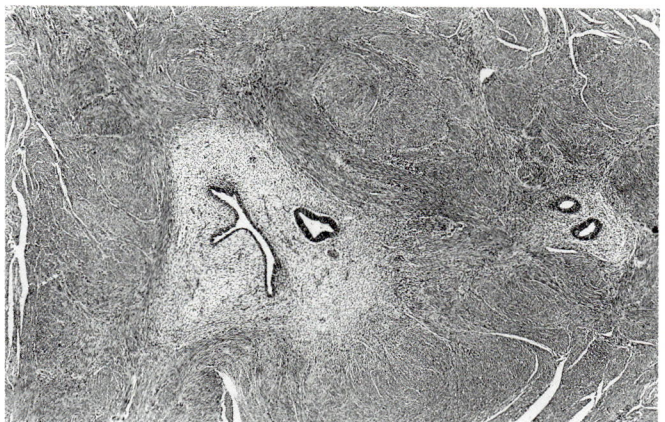

Fig. 21.69 Adenomyosis. Within the myometrium there are two islands of endometrial tissue of basal type, both of which contain glands and stroma.

glands are sensitive to oestrogens but unresponsive to progestagens, thus tending to undergo simple, or occasionally atypical, hyperplasia. True cyclical changes in adenomyotic foci are distinctly uncommon.

Adenomyosis is due to a downgrowth of basal endometrium into the myometrium, and serial sectioning shows a continuity between the basal endometrium and foci of adenomyosis. The aetiology of this *diverticular disease* is, however, obscure, for although both curettage and oestrogenic stimulation have been proposed as aetiological factors, there is no real proof that either is of causal significance.

The clinical importance of adenomyosis is also uncertain; menorrhagia and dysmenorrhoea are often cited as symptoms of this disorder but there is no clear relationship between the presence of adenomyotic foci and symptoms of this nature.

21.8.2 Benign tumours

Leiomyoma

These neoplasms are tumours of the smooth muscle cells of the myometrium. There is commonly an intermingling with fibrous tissue and the tumours are often inaccurately known as 'fibroids'. Myometrial leiomyomas are extremely common, being present in at least 25 per cent of women above the age of 35, and there is considerable circumstantial evidence that *oestrogenic stimulation* plays a role in their pathogenesis; thus, they develop only during the reproductive years, enlarge both during pregnancy and in women using contraceptive steroids, and tend to shrink after the menopause.

The tumours are usually multiple (Fig. 21.70) and vary in size from tiny 'seedlings' to huge masses which fill the abdomen. They may be within the uterine wall, i.e. *intramural*, in a *submucosal* site immediately below the endometrium, or lie just below the peritoneal covering of the uterus in a *subserosal* site. Submucosal leiomyomas tend to bulge into, and distort, the uterine cavity, with thinning of the overlying endometrium. They sometimes become polypoid (Fig. 21.71) to form a mass which cannot only fill the uterine cavity but can also extend through the endocervical canal into the vagina. Subserosal tumours may grow out from the uterine surface and can extend into the broad ligament; they may also become pedunculated, and such a neoplasm may, very rarely, become attached to the omentum or pelvic peritoneum where, after losing its stalk, it derives a new blood supply and flourishes as a *parasitic leiomyoma*.

Uterine leiomyomas have a well-defined regular outline with a surrounding pseudocapsule of compressed muscle fibres; on section they have a firm, bulging, white, whorled or trabeculated appearance. Histologically they consist of smooth muscle fibres arranged in bundles and whorls (Fig. 21.72); the cells are elongated with spindle- or cigar-shaped nuclei. Some tumours, known as *cellular leiomyomas*, contain densely packed cells with elongated nuclei while, rarely, the smooth muscle cells are

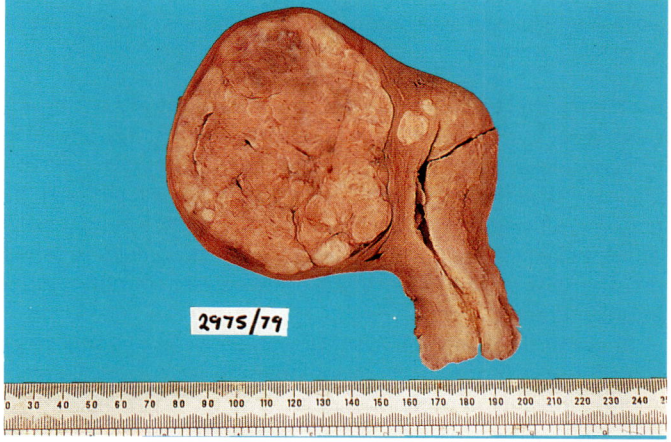

Fig. 21.70 Uterine leiomyomata. The myometrium contains well-demarcated, discrete nodules composed of uniform, rather whorled grey-white tissue.

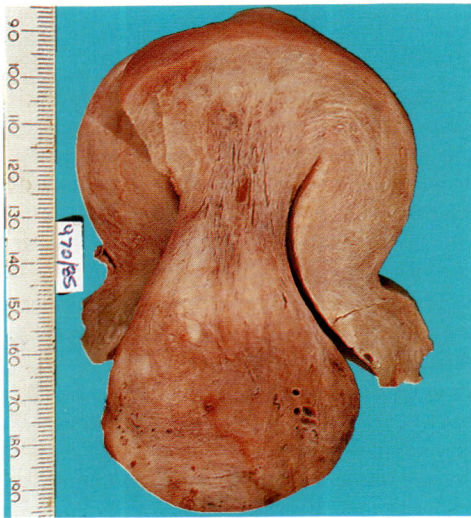

Fig. 21.71 Polypoidal leiomyoma of the uterus. A submucous leiomyoma, which has formed at the uterine fundus, has become so pedunculated that it dilates the uterine cavity and protrudes through the external cervical os.

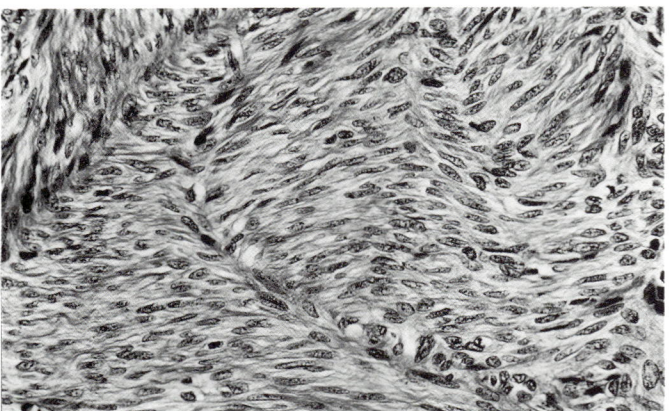

Fig. 21.72 Uterine leiomyoma. The tumour is composed of interweaving bands of elongated smooth muscle cells. There is no mitotic activity or cellular atypia.

rounded with central nuclei and clear cytoplasm; tumours containing such cells being classed as *epithelioid leiomyomas*. Other variants of the usual pattern include the *neurilemmoma-like leiomyoma*, in which the nuclei show a pallisaded pattern; the *bizarre leiomyoma*, characterized by the presence of bizarre multinucleated cells; and the *leiomyoma with tubules* in which an otherwise typical smooth muscle neoplasm contains epithelial-like tubules.

In all but the smallest leiomyomas degenerative changes tend to occur which are due to the neoplasm outgrowing its blood supply; thus, hyaline change, cystic change, myxoid degeneration, patchy necrosis, and calcification are common. A pedunculated submucosal tumour may undergo torsion and infarction, whilst a specific form of necrosis, seen, particularly but not only, in pregnancy, is 'red degeneration', characterized by a dull, beefy red appearance of the tumour which may also have a slightly fishy odour—this change can be accompanied by pain and fever and the presence of thrombosed vessels suggests that it represents haemorrhagic infarction of an extensively hyalinized neoplasm.

Malignant change occurs very rarely in uterine leiomyomas. Certain variants of a leiomyoma, although histologically benign, do, however, appear to behave in an invasive fashion. Thus, in the condition of *intravenous leiomyomatosis* cords of smooth muscle are found in uterine and para-uterine veins, usually in association with more conventional leiomyomas elsewhere in the myometrium: the plugs of tumour cells occasionally extend as far as the inferior vena cava and can even grow into the right atrium. It is not clear whether this condition is due to a special form of leiomyoma which, despite its benign nature, invades veins, or whether the tumours arise from the vein walls. A not dissimilar condition is *benign metastasizing leiomyoma*, in which histologically benign uterine leiomyomas appear to be associated with pulmonary metastases which show no malignant features; such cases probably represent the simultaneous independent development of pulmonary and uterine leiomyomas. In *disseminated peritoneal leiomyomatosis*, small leiomyomatous nodules are found scattered in the peritoneum and omentum in association with uterine leiomyomas: it is thought, however, that these extra-uterine nodules arise *in situ* from the submesothelial mesenchyme of the peritoneum.

Small uterine leiomyomata are asymptomatic but larger neoplasms can cause pelvic discomfort and are often associated with heavy and prolonged menstrual bleeding. Whether the neoplasms are actually responsible for the abnormal bleeding or whether both tumours and symptoms are causally dependent upon a common endocrinological disturbance is a moot point.

Other benign tumours

Fibromas, lipomas, and haemangiomas can all occur in the myometrium but the only other benign myometrial neoplasm which is not of extreme rarity is the *adenomatoid tumour*. Neoplasms of this type are present in 1 per cent of uteri and appear as small, rather poorly delineated, masses in the cornual region, usually in an immediately subserosal site. Histologically (Fig. 21.73), they are formed of complex multiple gland-like spaces which are lined by a flattened or low cuboidal epithelium and are separated from each other by strands of fibromuscular tissue. Adenomatoid tumours are benign, almost invariably asymptomatic and are derived from the serosa, having the ultrastructural, histochemical, and immunocytochemical characteristics of a benign mesothelioma.

21.8.3 Malignant neoplasms

Leiomyosarcoma

These are rare, accounting for only 1 per cent of malignant uterine neoplasms; they occur most commonly in the fifth and sixth decades and the patients present with abnormal vaginal bleeding, pelvic pain, or awareness of a mass. The tumours are

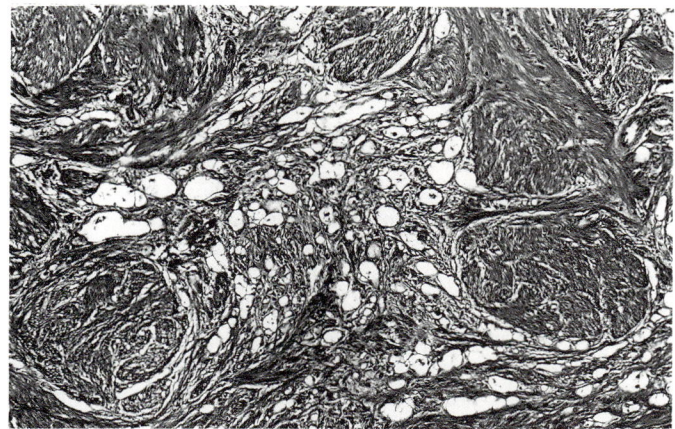

Fig. 21.73 Adenomatoid tumour of the myometrium. The centre of the field is occupied by small gland-like spaces set in a fine fibrous connective tissue stroma: this is an adenomatoid tumour. The surrounding myometrium is normal.

less well demarcated than are leiomyomas, often show areas of haemorrhage or necrosis, and are characterized histologically by their cellularity, pleomorphism, and high mitotic counts (Fig. 21.74). Myometrial leiomyosarcomas spread locally to invade the pelvic organs but it is uncommon for lymph node metastases to occur: blood-borne spread to the lungs, liver, and kidneys is common. The five-year survival rate for women with a neoplasm of this type is only 20–30 per cent.

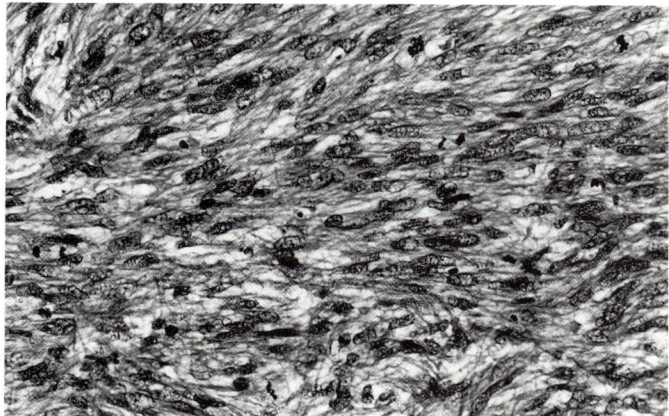

Fig. 21.74 Leiomyosarcoma of the uterus. The neoplasm is composed of closely packed smooth muscle cells with pleomorphic, hyperchromatic nuclei in which there are numerous mitoses.

21.9 The Fallopian tube

The Fallopian tubes are paired, rather convoluted, narrow tubular structures which are 8–10 cm long during the repro-ductive years, and lie in the upper, free border of the broad ligament. They extend from the uterine cornua medially to the ostia laterally where they open into the peritoneal cavity.'

Four anatomical zones are described, the *interstitial segment*, *isthmus*, *ampulla*, and *infundibulum*. The interstitial segment is that part of the tube that traverses the myometrium, lies within the wall of the uterus and leads from the uterine cornu to the uterotubal junction where it is continuous with the isthmus. The isthmus, which is the narrowest part of the tube, is 2–3 cm long, is thick-walled, and leads to the longest segment, the ampulla, which is wider and between 5 and 8 cm long. The most lateral part of the tube is funnel-shaped, approximately 1.0 cm long, and terminates via the fimbriated abdominal ostium.

The tube is lined by a mucosa which is continuous at the uterine cornu with the endometrium and is thrown into a series of longitudinal folds or *plicae* (Fig. 21.75). The plicae are few, short, and simple in the isthmus and interstitial segment of the tube and longer, more numerous, and more complex in the ampulla; the fimbria are covered by mucosa. The junction between the endometrium and tubal mucosa may be gradual or abrupt and does not always correspond precisely with the uterine cornu but may lie in the tube. The mucosal epithelium (Fig. 21.76) contains three types of cell, *secretory cells*, *ciliated cells*, and *intercalary cells*, the latter being exhausted secretory cells. The proportion of each cell type varies in the different parts of the tube, so that ciliated cells are most frequent in the fimbria and in the ampulla and least common in the isthmus and interstitial segments of the tube. The epithelium shows subtle cyclical changes during the reproductive years—increasing in height in the follicular phase, whereas secretory and cilial activity reach a maximum at midcycle, at the time of ovulation, when the cilia beat synchronously in waves towards the uterus. The epithelium is shallow and partly deciliated at the time of menstruation and in pregnancy, and becomes gradually atrophic after the menopause; there are a small number of intra-epithelial lymphocytes. The mucosal lamina propria, which is a delicate vascular connective tissue, contains little collagen in

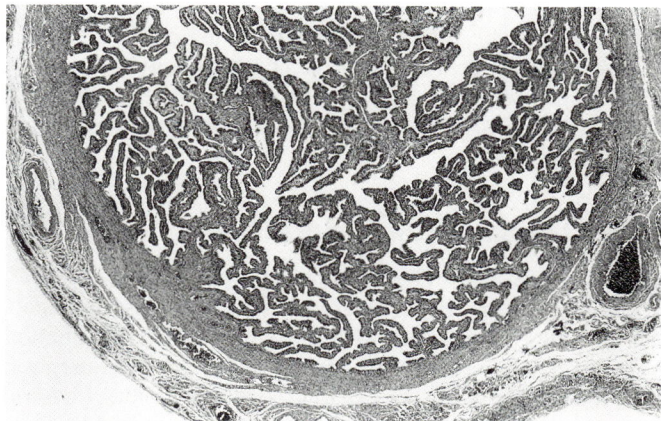

Fig. 21.75 Normal Fallopian tube. The mucosa is thrown into fine, complex folds which fill the lumen of the tube.

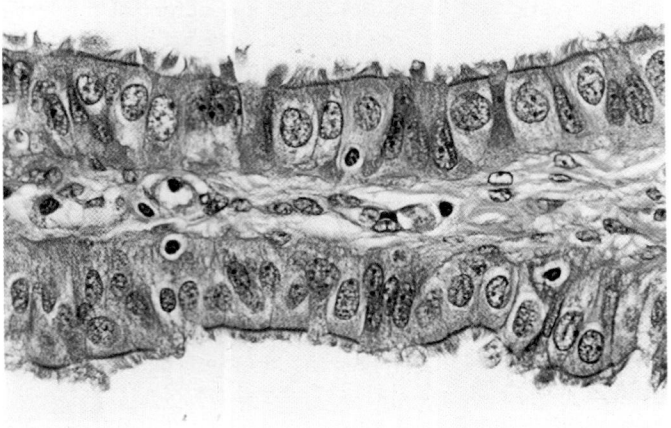

Fig. 21.76 Normal Fallopian tube. The mucosa is composed of cells with large, vesicular nuclei, which bear cilia on their surface, and tall cells with narrow nuclei lying perpendicular to the basement membrane; occasional intra-epithelial lymphocytes are present.

the reproductive years but this increases with age, being most conspicuous after the menopause. It contains a scanty population of histiocytes and mast cells with occasional lymphocytes. There is little stroma in the interstitial and isthmic segments of the tube but it is more abundant in the ampulla and fimbria. In pregnancy the stromal cells may become *decidualized*, the latter change being focal or multifocal and rarely extensive.

The muscular coat of the tube has three layers, an outer longitudinal layer and an intermediate circular layer, which are present throughout the tube, and an inner longitudinal layer which is present only in the isthmic and interstitial segments.

The blood supply to the interstitial segment and the inner two-thirds of the tube is provided by the tubal branch of the uterine artery, which anastamoses with the tubal branches of the ovarian artery which supply the outer part of the tube. The venous drainage of the tube, in general, follows the arteries, from the medial portions of the tubes to the internal iliac veins, and from the lateral parts of the tube to the inferior vena cava on the right and to the renal vein on the left.

The sympathetic innervation of the tube derives from the aortic and pelvic plexuses via fibres which accompany the arteries, and the parasympathetic supply is from vagal fibres in the aortic plexus and from sacral fibres in the pelvic plexus. Their function is uncertain.

21.9.1 Inflammation of the Fallopian tube

Inflammation of the Fallopian tube, or *salpingitis*, is a common, serious disorder of the reproductive years. It is almost invariably infective, although minor degrees of irritative inflammation may occur as a response to the presence of necrotic tissue or blood in the tube due to, for example, menstrual reflux, bleeding from endometriotic foci, or the presence of an ectopic gestation; there may also be a mild inflammatory response to foreign bodies, such as those used in sterilization procedures.

It is difficult to determine accurately the true incidence of infective salpingitis as most cases are not confirmed either histologically or bacteriologically at the time they present, and depend only upon clinical criteria for their diagnosis, particularly in the acute phase.

The term 'pelvic inflammatory disease' (PID) is used by clinicians to encompass signs and symptoms due to inflammation centred on the Fallopian tube, but extending, in many cases, to involve the ovary, mesosalpinx, parametrium, uterine serosa, and uterine ligaments. In the acute phase the clinical features are of an acute febrile illness associated with pelvic pain, vaginal discharge, and tenderness over the Fallopian tube. Chronic or subacute salpingitis may be recognized only when investigations for infertility are undertaken, this being a common complication of the disorder. It should be emphasized that the term PID refers only to a clinical concept and is one that should not be used as a pathological diagnosis, being too imprecise.

Infection reaches the tube by one of three routes, each of which produces a characteristic pattern of inflammation. The inflammation, however, may be so severe that it masks the underlying pattern, or infection may reach the tube by more than one route. The following descriptions represent the typical or stereotyped picture and it should be remembered that, in practice, the findings are not always so clear-cut.

Most commonly, infection ascends from the lower genital tract along the mucosal surface of the tube, causing an *endosalpingitis*. Less commonly, it may spread via the lymphatics to the wall of the tube from the uterus, or other adjacent organs, causing an *interstitial salpingitis*, and least commonly it may be *blood-borne*. The inflammation may be non-granulomatous or granulomatous, the former being very much more common.

Ascending infection

Infection that spreads from the uterine cavity along the mucosal surface of the uterus and Fallopian tube is characteristic of, for example, *N. gonorrhoea*, chlamydial infection, and infection associated with the presence of an intra-uterine contraceptive device (UCD), but most cases are of a non-specific polymicrobial nature. The typical patient is young and sexually active.

In an *acute endosalpingitis*, the tube is tense and swollen, the serosa congested and the subserosal tissues oedematous; in severe infections the serosa may be covered by a fibrinous exudate. The mucosa is oedematous, hyperaemic, and focally haemorrhagic. The lumen contains pus which may leak from the ostium, and the fimbria, as they become inflamed and 'sticky', tend to undergo agglutination and invagination until, finally, the ostium may be occluded. In ascending infections, as might be expected, the mucosa bears the brunt of the damage.

The oedematous tubal plicae are infiltrated by polymorphonuclear leucocytes and the lumen contains an acute inflammatory exudate and tissue debris (Fig. 21.77). In severe infections, there is mucosal ulceration and the inflammatory infiltrate may extend through the wall to the peritoneum causing a *local peritonitis*. In repeated or chronic infections plasma cells, lymphocytes, and histiocytes predominate; the latter may, in very longstanding cases, be the main cell type.

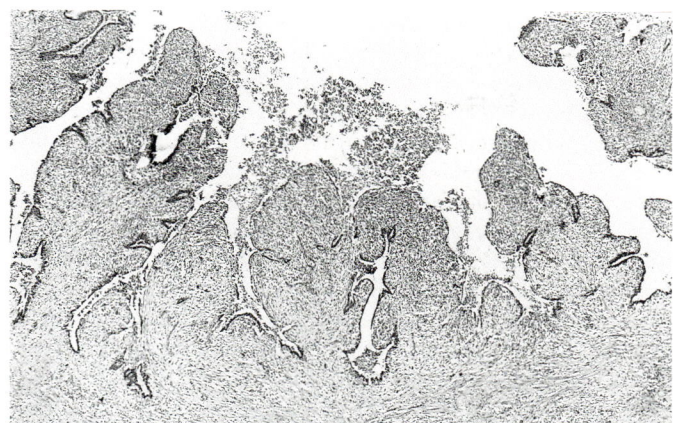

Fig. 21.77 Acute endosalpingitis. The mucosal folds are swollen and oedematous and infiltrated by acute inflammatory cells. The tube lumen contains a trace of purulent exudate.

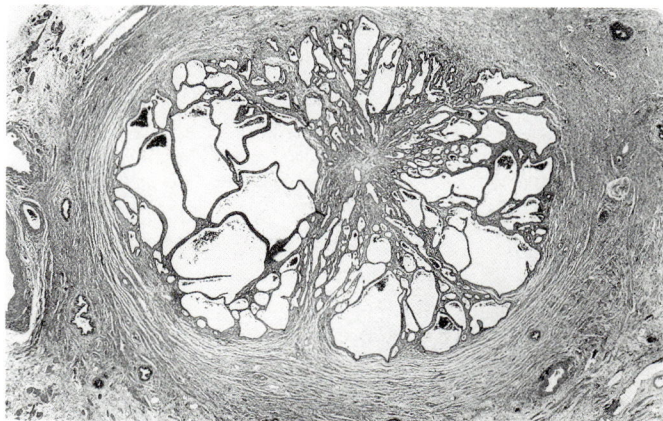

Fig. 21.78 Follicular salpingitis. The mucosal folds are extensively fused forming a mesh across the lumen of the tube. There is very little active inflammation: the appearance is the consequence of a previous endosalpingitis.

If inflammation subsides rapidly or is only mild, there may be little or no residual tubal damage but, unfortunately, an attack of salpingitis predisposes to further attacks, and with each succeeding episode full recovery becomes progressively less likely and the risk of permanent damage, leading to infertility or sterility, more certain. Indeed, tubal damage accounts for between 20 and 30 per cent of cases of infertility.

The sequelae of endosalpingitis may be immediate and complicate the acute inflammatory phase or there may be long-term effects. Their severity depends upon the nature of the infection, its severity, and the response of the host.

Severe inflammation may be complicated by local or generalized peritonitis, extension of infection to the adjacent ovary, the development of a tubo-ovarian abscess, or a pelvic abscess. Systemic dissemination of infection can occur, particularly in gonococcal infections, and may cause an arthritis or endocarditis. During an attack of acute endosalpingitis, the fimbria tend to become agglutinated as pus exudes from the ostium into the abdominal cavity and as a consequence the ostium may be occluded. Subsequent or recrudescent infection may then lead to the development of a *pyosalpinx* (a pus-filled Fallopian tube) in which there is usually extensive ulceration of the mucosa. Such a severe degree of damage is, of course, irrecoverable.

Long-term sequelae of an endosalpingitis may be minimal and limited to minor fibrous scars in the mucosa or the musculature, or they may be major. As the ulcerated mucosa, particularly in the ampulla, heals, there may be fusion of the plical folds across the lumen of the tube to produce a mesh, this being known as *follicular salpingitis* (Fig. 21.78). Plical fusion of this type may also be seen in a tube which is, in addition, distended by clear watery fluid and in which the ostium is occluded: this is the condition known as a *follicular hydrosalpinx*. A hydrosalpinx may also occur in the absence of mucosal fold fusion, and in such cases the tube assumes a retort shape and the wall is thin and translucent (Fig. 21.79); the mucosa is characteristically intact but rather flattened. Conversely, after prolonged or severe tubal inflammation the tube may be thick-walled and

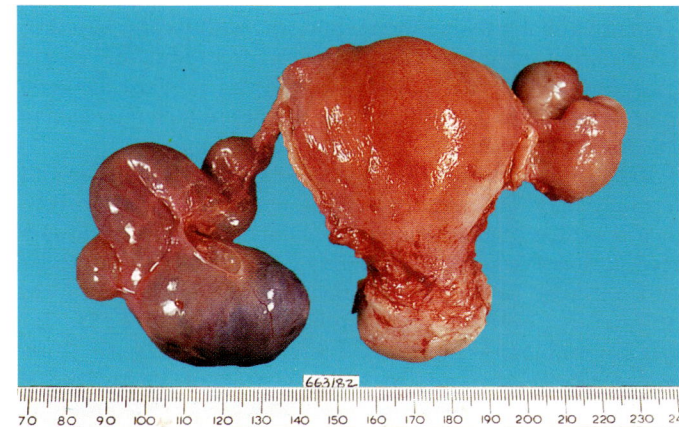

Fig. 21.79 Hydrosalpinx. The Fallopian tube is distended, the distension being maximal in the outer half of the tube, and the wall is thin.

rather rigid as a consequence of intramural and subserosal fibrosis.

Inflammation in the tubal isthmus tends to be more destructive than in the ampulla because the lumen is so narrow. If the mucosa ulcerates, there may, as healing occurs, be total obliteration of the lumen. Changes may also occur in the isthmus as a consequence of damage, usually associated with some degree of obstruction in the outer part of the tube. *Diverticula*, associated with muscular hypertrophy, develop in the isthmus, a condition known as *salpingitis isthmica nodosa* because of the nodules which can be seen or felt in the wall of the isthmus (Fig. 21.80). This condition appears to be secondary to an increase in intraluminal pressure and is, in our experience, not encountered when the remainder of the tube is normal. It is not, as has been previously suggested, a direct, but rather an indirect, effect of inflammation.

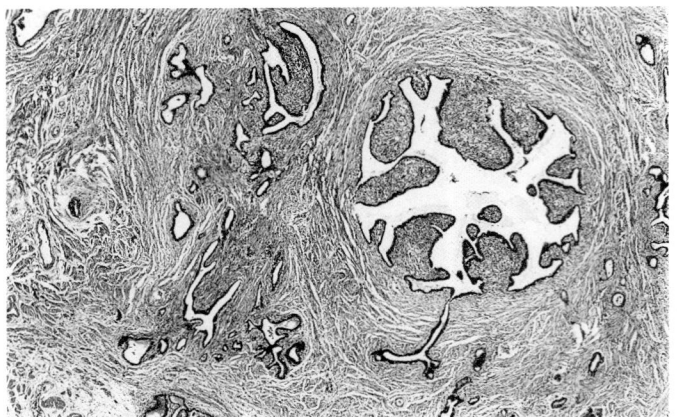

Fig. 21.80 Salpingitis isthmica nodosa, diverticular disease of the Fallopian tube. There are numerous glandular spaces within the muscle layer of the tube wall and, in the lower left, continuity between the lumen of the tube and a diverticulum can be seen clearly. (Reproduced by kind permission of Edward Arnold from *Pathology for gynaecologists*, Fox and Buckley, 2nd edn, 1990.)

Finally, tubal inflammation associated with local peritonitis, either due to salpingitis or pelvic sepsis from another source, e.g. acute appendicitis, may heal leaving fine or dense fibrovascular adhesions around the tube and ovary, which may lead to deformity of the tube.

All these sequelae have an impact on fertility, which depends normally upon a healthy, patent, undeformed Fallopian tube and, as a consequence, women with scarred and distorted tubes have an increased risk of infertility and, particularly in those with follicular salpingitis or salpingitis isthmica nodosa, an increased risk of tubal ectopic pregnancy (see p. 1635). One attack of salpingitis is estimated to cause infertility in 10 per cent of patients, two attacks will render about 25 per cent of women infertile, and three or more attacks will cause infertility in at least 60 per cent of sufferers.

Lymphatic infection

This is the form of infection which classically follows postpartum or postabortive infection and is uncommon nowadays. The interstitial tissues of the tube are the main focus of the inflammatory assault, with relative sparing of the tubal mucosa. As a consequence, the lumen may remain patent and infertility due to mechanical obstruction of the tube is an unlikely outcome. However, inflammation is rarely limited to the tube wall and it is usual to find a co-existing endosalpingitis which may result in any of the problems outlined above.

Blood-borne infection

This is typified by *tuberculosis* which, although it may spread directly to the tube from the peritoneal cavity, urinary tract, or gastrointestinal tract, or via the lymphatics from the intestinal tract, is more likely to arise as a consequence of blood-borne infection from a distant focus.

At the time of diagnosis, the tube has often become converted into a retort-shaped, fibrotic sac which may be focally calcified and contain caseous material. Classically the tubal ostium remains patent and the fimbria relatively normal. Histological examination (Fig. 21.81) shows a *chronic endosalpingitis* with caseating, or non-caseating, intramucosal granulomas, the latter more closely resembling sarcoid-like granulomas than the tuberculous granulomas encountered in tuberculosis elsewhere in the body. In long-standing disease the tube may be lined only by focally calcified fibrous tissue in which it may be difficult to find specific tubercular features. Tuberculosis is an uncommon cause of infertility in the United Kingdom nowadays but, ironically, our improved capacity for treating the disease may limit, but not prevent, tubal damage, thus reducing the risk of permanent sterility but increasing the risk of an ectopic gestation.

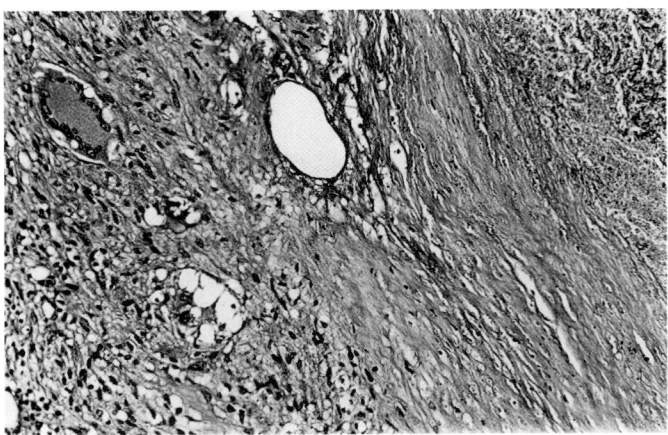

Fig. 21.81 Tuberculosis of the Fallopian tube. In this fibro-caseous tuberculosis, the lumen, to the right, is filled with caseous material and the wall, to the left, is composed of fibrous tissue in which a Langhans cell can be seen.

21.9.2 Cysts

A variety of cysts are commonly found in the tissues surrounding the Fallopian tube. The majority develop in Müllerian duct remnants (*paramesonephric cysts*) or Wolffian duct remnants (*mesonephric cysts*). In the majority of cases they are asymptomatic, small (1–2 cm), and are incidental findings. Only very rarely, for example when they undergo torsion or reach an unusually large size, do they become clinically apparent.

The majority of these cysts are thin-walled, often translucent, and may be pedunculated. Those of Müllerian origin, which include the extremely common *hydatid of Morgagni*, which is pedunculated and attached to the fimbria, are lined by epithelium of tubal type, and those of Wolffian origin are lined by a single layer of cubo-columnar cells. Their walls are fibrous and those of paramesonephric origin tend to contain more muscle than do those of Müllerian origin. On very rare occasions epithelial neoplasms may develop within these cysts.

The tubal serosa commonly exhibits focal transitional, or uro-epithelial, metaplasia, so-called *Walthard's rests* (Fig. 21.82), which may also undergo cystic change. They rarely

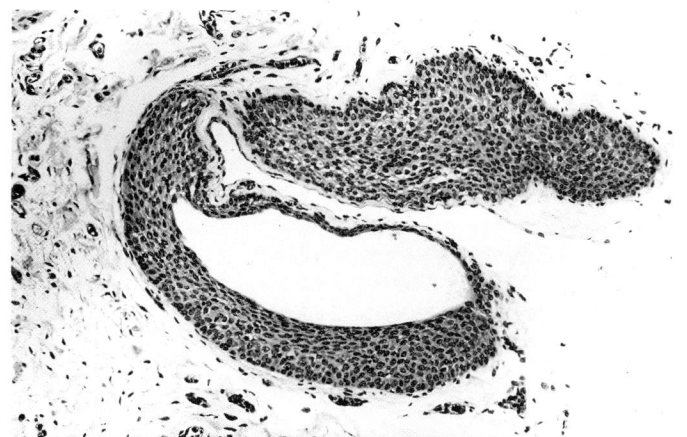

Fig. 21.82 Walthard's rest. The peritoneal surface of the Fallopian tube has undergone metaplasia to uro-epithelium; one of the foci has become cystic.

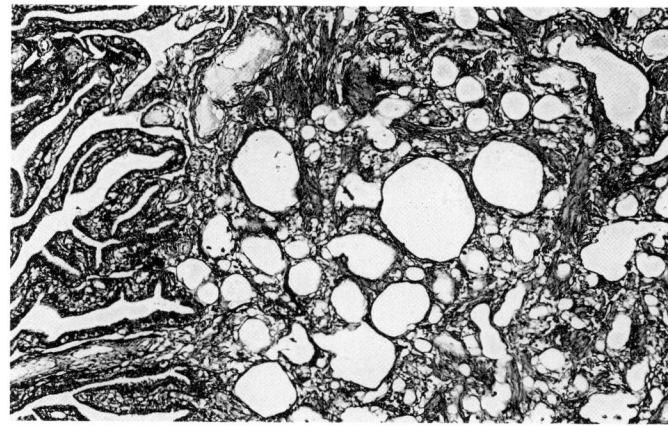

Fig. 21.83 Adenomatoid tumour of the Fallopian tube. Immediately deep to the mucosa of the Fallopian tube, which lies to the left, there is a collection of closely packed, small cystic spaces lying in a fine connective tissue stroma. This is an adenomatoid tumour and the site, within the tube wall, is typical.

become more than a few millimetres in diameter and appear as yellow-grey specks or pinhead-sized granules on the serosal surface of the tube. *Mesothelial inclusion cysts* are also encountered on the surface of the tube. Mesothelial or peritoneal cysts may also form within adhesions around the tube in patients who have had previous peritonitis or surgery.

21.9.3   Tumours of the Fallopian tube

Neoplasms of the Fallopian tube are distinctly uncommon and only very occasionally are they suspected prior to surgery or to examination of a surgical resection specimen. Carcinomas, which are the most common of these rare tumours, constitute only 0.3 per cent of malignant gynaecological tumours.

Benign neoplasms

Benign intraluminal epithelial tumours of the tube may be sessile or polypoidal and typically form small *adenofibromas*. In the interstitial segment of the tube they are usually composed of endometrial tissue, whereas in the remainder of the tube they have a fibrous stroma and the epithelium is of tubal type. It has been suggested that their presence in the narrow areas of the tube, that is, the interstitial and isthmic segments, may be associated with infertility but this is not a universally held belief.

Adenomatoid tumours, which are of mesothelial origin, may develop in the tubal lumen but more commonly grow eccentrically in a subserosal site, locally invaginating the tube wall. They appear as small, usually not exceeding 1–2 cm, round to ovoid, firm, grey to yellow-white, well-circumscribed nodules. Histologically (Fig. 21.83) they are composed of tubules and gland-like spaces lined by a flattened cuboidal epithelium set in a fibrous stroma; they are not encapsulated.

Other very rare benign neoplasms of the Fallopian tube include lipomas, which are generally subserosal, leiomyomas, fibromas, haemangiomas, and neurilemmomas. The majority are asymptomatic but occasionally a leiomyoma may attain a

size sufficient to present as a pelvic mass or cause pain if it undergoes torsion. Mature cystic terotomas have also, exceptionally, been described in the Fallopian tube.

Malignant neoplasms

The commonest primary malignant neoplasms are *adenocarcinomas*. Most cases occur in older women, the average age being in the sixth decade, and more than 50 per cent of patients being post-menopausal. There is often a history of nulliparity, infertility, or 'one-child sterility'. In only very rare instances is the primary site of the neoplasm correctly anticipated clinically, because the presentation is non-specific with abnormal uterine bleeding, an abdominal mass, vaginal discharge, intestinal symptoms, or pelvic discomfort. The classical picture of a serosanguineous, watery or yellow vaginal discharge, pelvic mass, and cramp-like iliac fossa pain occurs in less than 20 per cent of cases. The aetiology is unknown.

The majority of tumours are unilateral, only between 10 and 20 per cent being bilateral. The lesion starts as a small plaque, nodule, or polypoidal lesion within the lumen (Fig. 21.84), most commonly at the junction of the middle and outer thirds of the tube, but usually by the time of diagnosis the tube is distended by tumour. The tube becomes retort-shaped and grossly resembles a hydrosalpinx or pyosalpinx, but unless there has been preceding inflammation it is usual for the fimbria to be normal and the ostium patent. It is unusual for a tumour to have penetrated the wall of the tube.

Most carcinomas are *well-differentiated papillary adenocarcinomas* and closely resemble serous carcinomas of the ovary (Fig. 21.85). Less well-differentiated tumours have a mixed alveolar-papillary pattern and the least well-differentiated neoplasms tend to grow in a solid fashion. Other histological variants are described but they are rare.

The tumour spreads directly via the tubal ostium to the *peritoneum*, via the uterine ostium into the *uterus*, and directly

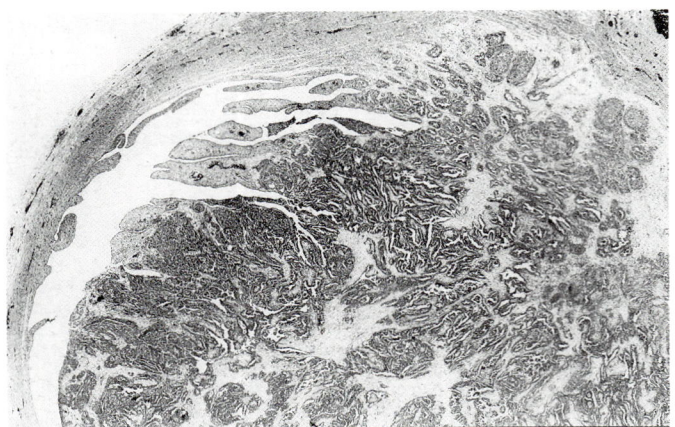

Fig. 21.84 Adenocarcinoma of the Fallopian tube. The tube lumen is distended by a polypoidal adenocarcinoma which arises from the mucosa (at the upper right) and bulges into the lumen.

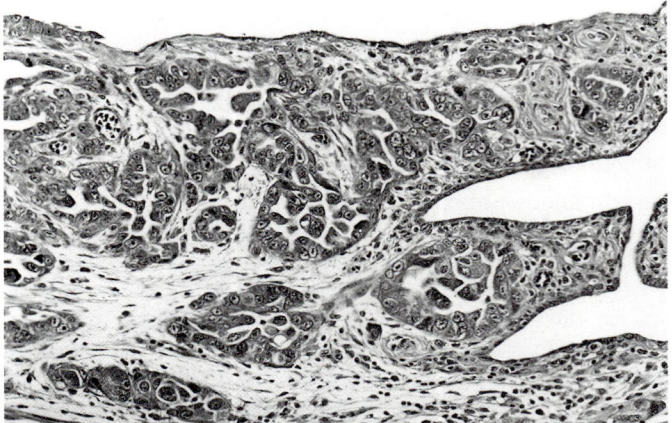

Fig. 21.85 Adenocarcinoma of the Fallopian tube. The mucosa is infiltrated by small neoplastic acini which are lined by rather pleomorphic cells of serous type.

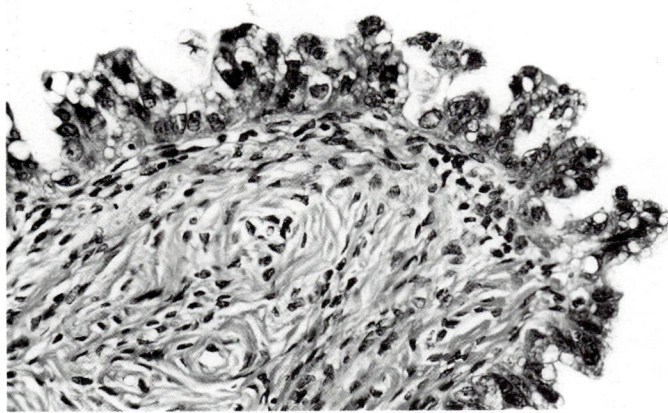

Fig. 21.86 Adenocarcinoma *in situ* of the Fallopian tube. The plica is covered by a stratified epithelium which is composed of cells with large pleomorphic nuclei and which form papillary tufts.

through the tube wall to the *adjacent structures*. Lymphatic spread occurs to the *uterus*, *ovary*, and the *iliac and para-aortic lymph nodes*.

The average survival at 5 years for women with a tubal carcinoma is only about 15 per cent, the majority having remained asymptomatic until late in the course of the disease.

Tubal carcinomas have to be distinguished clinically and histologically from tumours which have metastasized to the tube, for example, from the ovary or uterus. Such a distinction is facilitated by identifying an area of *carcinoma in situ* within the residual tube epithelium (Fig. 21.86) from which the carcinoma can be seen to arise.

21.10   The ovary

The ovaries lie on the posterior surface of the broad ligaments, adjacent to the lateral wall of the pelvis, in the ovarian fossae. Each ovary is attached anteriorly, by a fold of peritoneum (*the mesovarium*), to the broad ligament, medially to the uterine cornu via the *utero-ovarian ligament*, and laterally by the *suspensory ligament* to the Fallopian tube; the posterior border of the ovary lies free.

The ovarian artery arises directly from the aorta, reaches the ovary via the suspensory ligament and enters the ovary at the hilum, along the attachment of the mesovarium, where it divides. In the hilum and medulla, the arterial branches are coiled and hence the ovarian medulla appears highly vascular in tissue sections. The arteries then pass through the medulla to the cortex, giving off arterioles which anastomose freely.

Veins drain from the ovary into a plexus at the hilum, where they unite to form the ovarian vein. The left ovarian vein drains into the left renal vein and the right into the inferior vena cava.

Lymph vessels from the ovary unite with those from the Fallopian tube and uterine fundus to form the *subovarian lymphatic plexus* which lies under the ovarian hilum. Efferent vessels pass to the *upper para-aortic lymph nodes* at the level of the renal arteries.

The histological appearance of the ovary varies throughout life. There is a *cortex* in which, during the reproductive years, are found *ovum-containing follicles* in varying stages of development, a *medulla*, composed mainly of blood and lymphatic vessels but containing a small amount of *ovarian stroma*, and a *hilum*.

In the neonate the ovarian cortex is packed with oocytes and there is relatively little stroma. During the reproductive years the cortex contains follicles in different stages of development, whereas after the menopause follicles are absent and the ovarian cortex becomes narrow, usually measuring no more than 2 mm in depth.

The ovarian surface is covered by an epithelium which is continuous at the mesovarium with the peritoneum: this is a single layer of flattened cuboidal cells. These surface cells have a capacity to undergo 'metaplasia' or differentiation, along any of the epithelial cell lines seen in the genital and urinary tract, and they are the ultimate source of most epithelial neoplasms of the ovary.

In the ovarian hilum, amongst the leash of vessels, are found *hilus cells* and the *rete ovarii*.

The ovarian follicles are described as *primordial*, *primary*, *secondary*, or *tertiary* according to their degree of development. *Primordial follicles* (Fig. 21.87) consist of an oocyte surrounded by a single layer of flattened pregranulosa cells. The development of the *pregranulosa cells* into cuboidal *granulosa cells* marks its transition to a *primary follicle*. Under the influence of *FSH*, the granulosa cells multiply, become layered, and are separated from the ovum by a homogenous eosinophilic band, the *zona pellucida*: this is the *secondary follicle*. In the *tertiary*, or *antral*, *follicle* (Fig. 21.88) a cleft develops in the granulosa cells and the ovum lies at one pole of the follicle within a mound of granulosa cells, the *cumulus ovaricus*. It is from such a tertiary follicle that, under the influence of *LH*, ovulation will occur with subsequent transformation of the follicle into a *corpus luteum*. The corpus luteum is frequently cystic, the size of the cyst depending upon the degree of haemorrhage that occurs at the time of ovulation. In time the corpus luteum is replaced by a fibrous scar, the *corpus albicans*.

Not all follicles develop fully, many being lost at different stages of their development by a process of *atresia*. When this occurs at an early stage of their development the follicle may disappear and leave no histological residue of its existence, but when atresia occurs later small cysts and scar-like *corpora fibrosa*, which are the end result of such atretic follicles, are formed.

In pregnancy, the corpus luteum not only persists for several weeks after conception but develops further to form a conspicuous yellow nodule in the ovary. This corpus luteum of pregnancy can be distinguished from an ordinary corpus luteum not only by its size, which is not a reliable feature, but by the pres-

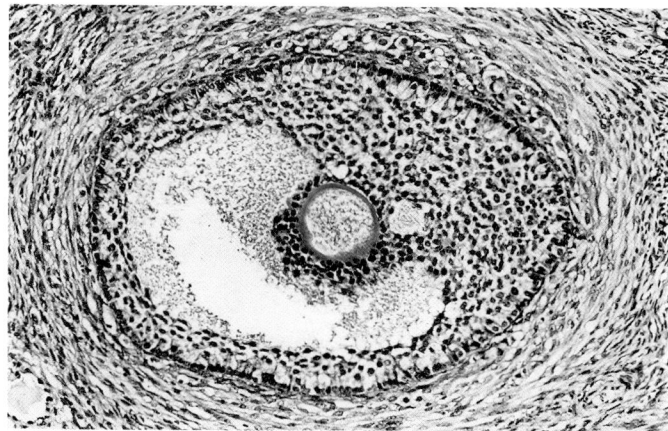

Fig. 21.88 Normal ovary. An antral or tertiary follicle. The ovum, in the centre of the field, has a mantle of small, darkly staining granulosa cells, the cumulus ovaricus. A cleft, the antrum, filled with faintly granular proteinous fluid, lies to the left of the ovum and the entire follicle is surrounded by stromal cells which form a concentric lamina, the theca interna.

ence both within and between *the heavily luteinized granulosa cells* of *eosinophilic hyaline globules* (Fig. 21.89). It is also usual to find luteinization of the ovarian stroma and of follicles which have previously undergone atresia but are still capable of responding to gonadotrophins.

The menopause occurs when the ovarian content of germ cells is totally depleted and hence after the menopause there is an absence of follicles and follicular structures, although corpora fibrosa and corpora albicantia, some occasionally calcified, are still seen. The cortex becomes narrow in most women but in some there is a minor degree of hyperplasia which may be nodular or diffuse.

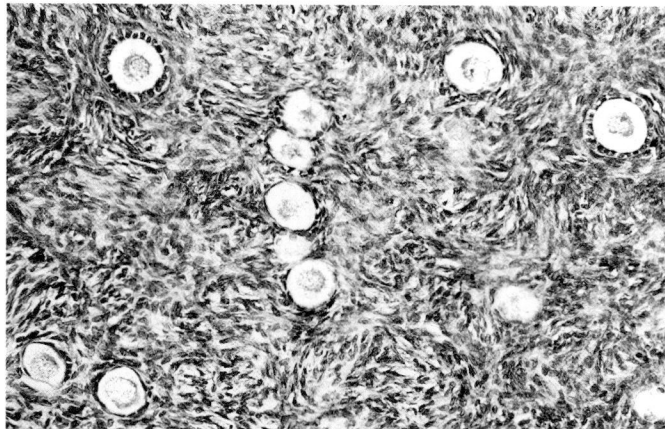

Fig. 21.87 Normal ovary. Primordial and primary follicles are present in the ovarian cortex.

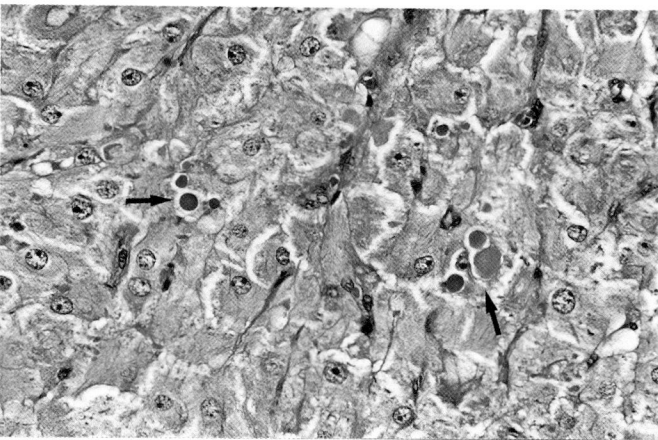

Fig. 21.89 Corpus luteum of pregnancy. The granulosa cells in the corpus have copious eosinophilic cytoplasm, and between the cells are more darkly staining, homogenous globules of proteinous material; the latter are typical of the corpus luteum of pregnancy.

21.10.1 Non-neoplastic diseases of the ovary

Inflammation

Non-infective inflammation

This is not common but may occur as a response to bleeding from *endometriotic foci* and is also seen in ovaries that have undergone torsion. A granulomatous inflammatory response may occur to starch granules from surgical gloves, to keratin derived from ruptured mature cystic teratomas, or to hystero-salpingographic contrast material.

Infective inflammation

Most infections of the ovary are non-specific in nature and poly-microbial in origin. Infection may be secondary to appendicitis, diverticular disease of the colon, or salpingitis, and is rarely due to blood-borne infection from remote foci.

In the acute phase the ovary is reddened and oedematous. A polymorphonuclear infiltrate is present in the superficial cortex and there may be a fibrinous exudate on the ovarian surface. It is rare for infection to extend deeply into the ovary but when it does there may be abscess formation (Fig. 21.90). The chronic phase is characterized by fibrosis of the ovarian surface epithelium and the formation of *peri-ovarian adhesions* (Fig. 21.91).

Non-neoplastic cysts

Non-neoplastic cysts of the ovary may develop from the *surface epithelium*, the *follicles*, *endometriotic foci*, or may, occasionally, be the end result of an *abscess*. Most, whatever their origin, are asymptomatic but some become clinically apparent because of their large size, their undergoing torsion, or their hormonal activity.

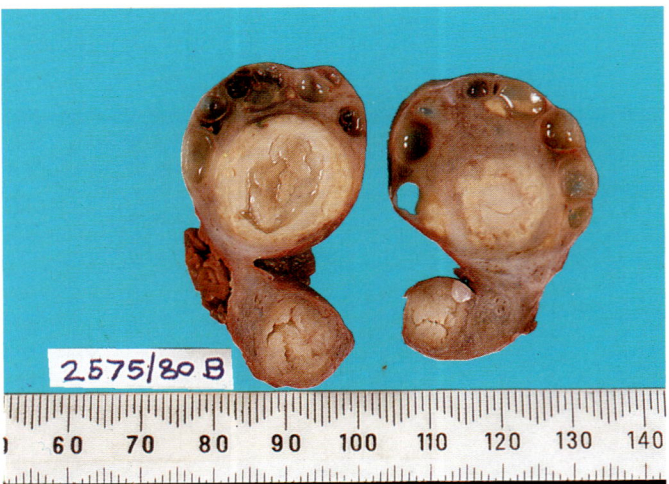

Fig. 21.90 Ovarian abscess. The picture shows the ovary, to the left, and the adjacent Fallopian tube, on the right. In the centre of the ovary there is a cyst, containing yellowish material surrounded by layers of granulation tissue and fibrous tissue. This is an abscess in a woman who had worn an inert intra-uterine contraceptive device for several years. There is also an active endosalpingitis.

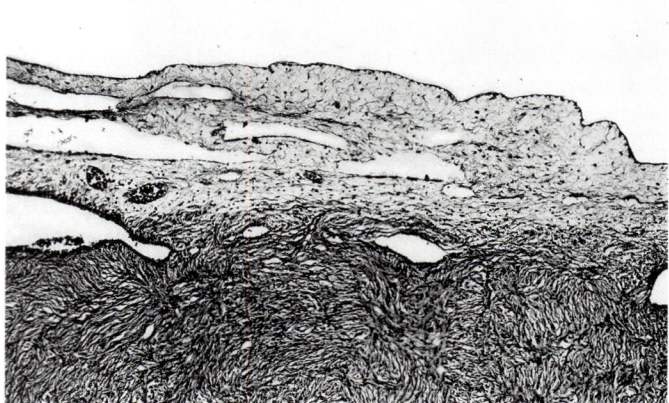

Fig. 21.91 Chronic perioophoritis. The ovarian surface is covered by fine, fibrovascular connective tissue adhesions. These are the consequence of an earlier peritonitis.

Cysts derived from the surface epithelium

The most common of these are the hormonally inactive *epithelial*, or *serous*, *inclusion cysts* which develop as a consequence of invagination of the surface epithelium of the ovary into the stroma, particularly at the site of ovulation. The invaginations lose their connection with the surface epithelium and, because of secretion of fluid, become cystic. These cysts may be single or multiple and can occur at any age. They may lie deep or superficially in the cortex and vary in size from a few millimetres to several centimetres; by convention, although perhaps illogically and incorrectly, cysts measuring more than 3 cm in diameter are classed as *benign cystic neoplasms*. The epithelium lining the cysts is usually *tubal* in nature but may, less commonly, be *endometrioid or endocervical* in type.

Cysts derived from the follicles

Follicular cysts are common but those measuring less than 2.5 cm in diameter are regarded as being physiological and are classed as *cystic follicles* rather than as follicular cysts. Within this definition, follicular cysts are usually single, although multiple cysts of this type are encountered in the *ovarian hyperstimulation* and *polycystic ovary syndromes*.

Solitary follicular cysts can occur at any age and are thin-walled and unilocular. They range in size from 3 to 10 cm (Fig. 21.92) and are lined by an inner layer of granulosa cells and an outer layer of thecal cells. Most follicular cysts are asymptomatic but some appear to be oestrogenic and are associated with symptoms such as precocious puberty or menstrual disturbances, and, occasionally, a follicular cyst may rupture and cause a haemoperitoneum.

Corpus luteum cysts (Fig. 21.93) are again distinguished from cystic corpus luteums by their size. Cysts of this type have a convoluted lining of large luteinized granulosa cells and smaller luteinized thecal cells with an innermost layer of fibrous tissue. Such cysts probably occur when the central cavity of a ruptured

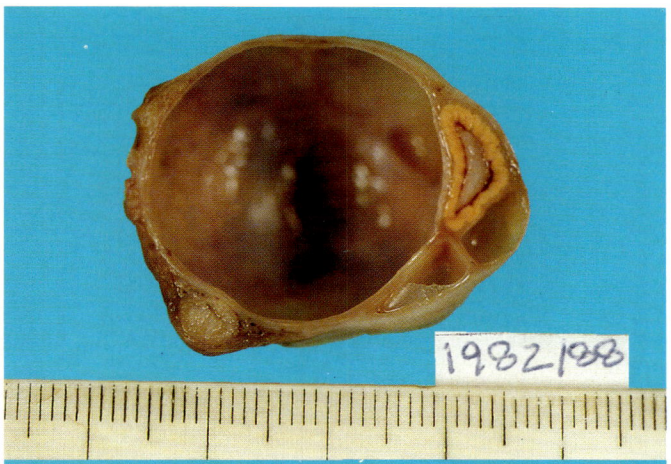

Fig. 21.92 Follicular cyst of the ovary. To the left, the ovary contains a thin-walled, unilocular follicular cyst, and to the right there is a yellow focus which is an old corpus luteum.

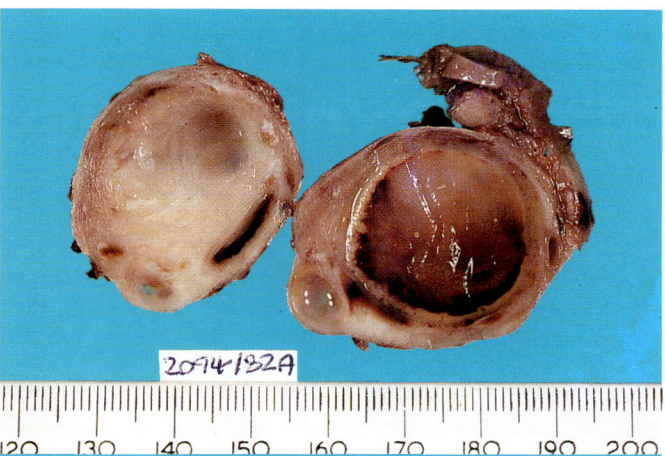

Fig. 21.93 Corpus luteum cyst of the ovary. The ovary has been opened to show the interior of a cystic corpus luteum. The cyst is unilocular and the wall, which is thin, contains a layer of pale yellow tissue.

follicle is unusually large, or when there is excessive intrafollicular haemorrhage at the time of ovulation.

Ovarian hyperstimulation syndrome

This condition is characterized by the presence of *multiple theca-lutein cysts* in the ovaries; these are usually bilateral and may cause considerable ovarian enlargement. The cysts are of follicular origin but have a lining in which the theca interna cells are hyperplastic and heavily luteinized with granulosa cells being either absent or markedly luteinized. Cysts of this type are due to excessive stimulation of the ovary by human chorionic gonadotrophin and may occur in *normal pregnancy*, in *multiple pregnancy*, in patients with a *hydatidiform mole* or a *choriocarcin-*

oma, or in women undergoing *artificial stimulation of the ovary* as part of the treatment of infertility.

There is an increased tendency for ovaries containing multiple theca-lutein cysts to undergo *torsion* (Fig. 21.94) and the patients may present with abdominal pain; some become mildly virilized because of production of androgens by the theca-lutein cysts and ascites is occasionally encountered. The cysts usually regress after removal of their cause.

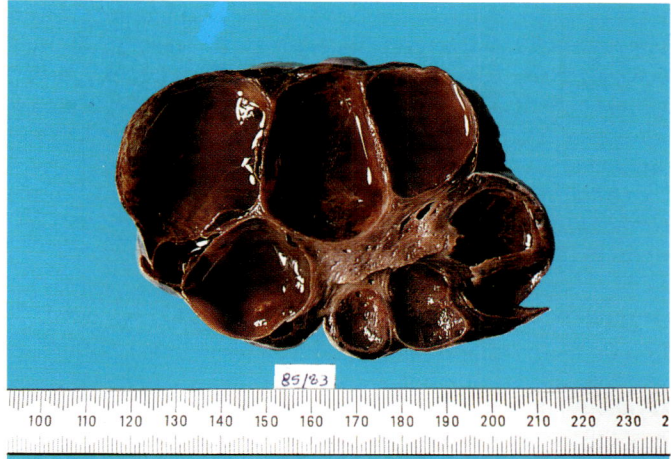

Fig. 21.94 Ovarian hyperstimulation syndrome, infarction. The ovary is expanded by a series of thin-walled, unilocular theca-lutein cysts. It has undergone torsion about its pedicle and, as a consequence, has become infarcted. This explains the intensely haemorrhagic state of the tissue.

Polycystic ovary syndrome (PCO)

The term 'polycystic ovary syndrome' covers an overlapping range of disorders which have in common the presence of *multiple follicular cysts* in the ovaries, *inappropriate gonadotrophin secretion*, *high circulating levels of androgens*, and *increased peripheral conversion of androgens to oestrogens*.

The clinical spectrum associated with PCO is very wide: at one extreme are patients whose sole complaint is of infertility and at the other extreme are women with the features of the *Stein–Leventhal syndrome*, a condition characterized by *oligo- or amenorrhoea*, *anovulation*, *infertility*, *obesity*, and *hirsuties*.

The typical polycystic ovary is enlarged and contains *multiple follicular cysts* which, characteristically, have a prominent outer layer of *luteinized thecal cells*. Other features are more variable, but there is commonly an increased amount of collagen in the superficial layers of the ovarian cortex together with stromal hyperplasia and luteinization. Numerous corpora fibrosa are usually present and corpora lutea are found in 30 per cent of cases.

The pathophysiology of PCO is complex but a constant abnormality is the presence of high, non-cyclic, levels of luteinizing hormone (LH), either because of an increased pituitary sensitivity to luteinizing hormone releasing factor (LHRH) or because of increased secretion of LHRH. The high LH levels stimulate the theca interna cells to produce androstenedione, which is converted in the fat cells of the body into oestrone, the resulting high oestrone levels then inhibiting the release of follicle stimulating hormone (FSH). Because of the low levels of FSH, follicular growth is impaired and the granulosa cells have reduced levels of aromatase and hence a decreased ability to convert androgens to oestrogens. The elevated androgen levels in the ovary are thought to be responsible for the fibrous thickening of the superficial ovarian cortex, while the high circulating levels of the peripherally produced oestrone increase pituitary sensitivity to LHRH and thus perpetuate the cycle. The high oestrone levels are also responsible for the development, in a proportion of these patients, of endometrial hyperplasia of simple, complex, or atypical type, which may progress to an endometrial adenocarcinoma.

Ovarian malfunction is not, however, the only factor in the hormonal disturbance of PCO, for in some patients there is also an excess production of androstenedione by the adrenals.

Stromal hyperplasia and hyperthecosis

Stromal hyperplasia is characterized by varying degrees of non-neoplastic proliferation of ovarian stromal cells. Frequently associated with this is stromal hyperthecosis, in which there is focal luteinization of the stromal cells.

Stromal hyperplasia results in a varying degree of diffuse or nodular ovarian enlargement, occurs most commonly in the immediately post-menopausal years, and is frequently asymptomatic. Some women, particularly those with associated hyperthecosis, show evidence of mild virilization, or, less commonly, there may be hyperoestrogenism because of peripheral conversion of androgens to oestrone.

Massive oedema of the ovary

This term refers to a tumour-like enlargement of one or both ovaries as a result of accumulation of oedema fluid within the ovarian stroma.

Affected ovaries may measure up to 25 cm in diameter and when cut exude watery fluid. Histologically the oedema is diffuse but usually spares the superficial cortex.

Patients with massive oedema of the ovary are usually young and present with abdominal or pelvic pain, menstrual irregularities, or abdominal distension. Some patients are mildly virilized, this being due to the presence of luteinized stromal cells within the oedematous ovary.

Massive oedema of the ovary is thought to result from intermittent torsion of the ovary on its pedicle with partial obstruction of venous and lymphatic drainage. In some cases the torsion appears to be secondary to a *fibromatosis of the ovary*.

Luteoma of pregnancy

Luteomas of pregnancy are non-neoplastic, tumour-like, solid, yellow-brown lesions of the ovary (Fig. 21.95) which develop from either luteinized follicular thecal cells or from luteinized non-follicular stromal cells. The luteomas may be multiple and

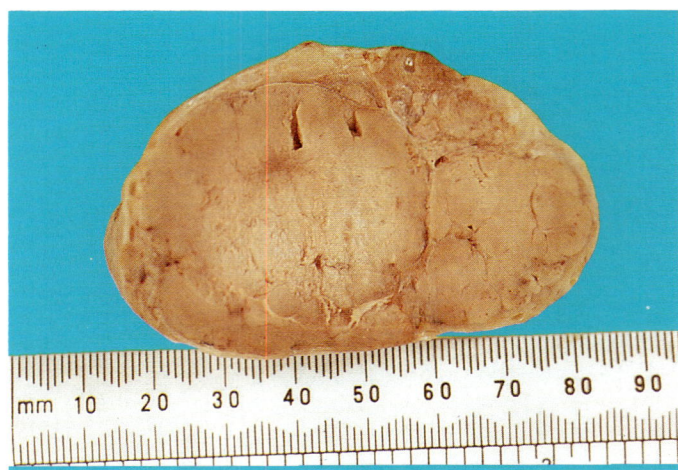

Fig. 21.95 Luteoma of pregnancy. This solid, soft, yellow mass was removed from the ovary of a woman who was noted to have an ovarian mass early in the postpartum period.

bilateral and may be of microscopic size only or reach up to 20 cm in diameter. Most pregnancy luteomas are discovered incidentally at Caesarean section but a few are androgenic and associated with masculinization of a female fetus or virilization of the mother. Luteomas of pregnancy regress spontaneously during the postpartum period.

Premature ovarian failure

This term is applied to those patients in whom there is a cessation of ovarian function before the age of 35–40 years, this occurring despite normal, or elevated, gonadotrophin levels.

True premature menopause

These patients have high gonadotrophin levels and small ovaries in which there is a complete absence of primordial or developing follicles; stigmata of prior ovulation are present.

This condition is thought to be due to a primary paucity of germ cells, possibly because of inadequate migration of germ cells into the developing gonad during embryogenesis. A few cases are secondary to the use of cytotoxic drugs or radiotherapy, both of which can cause destruction of germ cells.

Gonadotrophin-resistant ovary syndrome

This syndrome may be congenital or acquired and is characterized by anovulation, low oestrogen values, and high levels of gonadotrophins. The ovary contains numerous primordial follicles, sometimes showing degenerative changes, but with no evidence of follicular ripening (Fig. 21.96). There is no ovarian response to the administration of exogenous gonadotrophins, even in massive doses.

This syndrome has been variously attributed to a deficiency of ovarian gonadotrophin receptors, to the presence of anti-gonadotrophin receptor antibodies, and to a post-receptor defect.

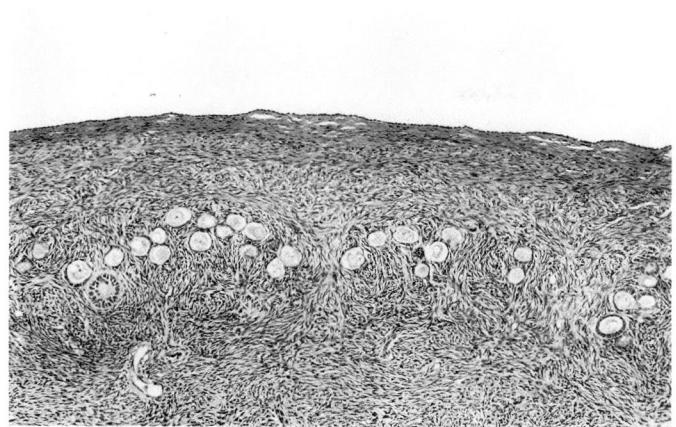

Fig. 21.96 Gonadotrophin-resistant ovary. The ovarian cortex contains large numbers of primordial and primary follicles but there is no evidence of follicular maturation.

Auto-immune oophoritis

Antibodies directed against ovarian steroid-synthesizing cells are found in a proportion of women with auto-immune Addison's disease; these antibodies cross-react with steroid-synthesizing cells in the adrenal glands. Patients with such antibodies present with anovulatory infertility, and histologically there is a lymphocytic infiltrate around secondary or tertiary follicles.

Vascular disorders

Ovarian haemorrhage

Rupture of a *corpus luteum* or a *corpus luteum cyst* may occasionally result in bleeding into the peritoneal cavity, this occurring particularly in women receiving anticoagulant therapy. The clinical picture in these patients resembles that of acute appendicitis.

Ovarian torsion

Torsion of the ovary usually occurs when the gonad is enlarged by the presence of a cyst or tumour, but can also develop when the ovary is normal but the patient has an unusually long mesovarium.

The patients present either with symptoms similar to those of acute appendicitis or with recurrent episodes of abdominal pain and a swollen, haemorrhagic, sometimes infarcted, tubo-ovarian mass is found to be twisted on its pedicle.

Luteinized unruptured follicle syndrome

In this condition the follicle ripens normally but fails to release the ovum; luteinization of the granulosa and theca layers proceeds normally and an ovum-containing corpus luteum is formed. Hormonal activity within the ovary appears to be undisturbed, for secretory changes occur in the endometrium and there thus appears to be a primary defect in the ovum-releasing mechanism. This syndrome can be suspected if normal endometrial cyclical activity is not accompanied by

stigmata of ovulation on laparoscopic examination of the ovarian surface.

21.10.2 Tumours of the ovary

There is a huge range and variety of ovarian tumours. A simplified classification of these neoplasms defines, however, six main groups:

1. *epithelial tumours*;
2. *sex cord stromal tumours*;
3. *germ cell tumours*;
4. *tumours of the non-specialized tissues of the ovary*;
5. *miscellaneous unclassified tumours*;
6. *metastatic tumours*.

Epithelial tumours

These neoplasms constitute 60 per cent of all primary ovarian tumours and 90 per cent of those that are malignant. All are thought to originate from undifferentiated cells in the surface, or serosal, epithelium of the ovary, either arising directly from that epithelium or from epithelial fragments which have become sequestrated into the ovarian cortex to form 'epithelial inclusion cysts'. The ovarian serosa is the direct descendant, and adult equivalent, of the coelomic epithelium which, during embryonic life, overlies the nephrogenital ridge and from which are derived the Müllerian ducts and the structures to which they give rise, namely the endocervical, endometrial, and tubal epithelia. It is believed that undifferentiated cells in the ovarian surface epithelium retain a latent competence to differentiate along the same pathways as do their embryonic predecessors and that a neoplasm derived from these cells can, therefore, differentiate along various Müllerian pathways. Thus those epithelial tumours differentiating along a tubal pathway constitute the *serous group of neoplasms*, those differentiating along endocervical lines form the *mucinous tumours*, and yet others, which pursue an endometrial course, are classed as *endometrioid tumours*. The *Brenner tumour* also usually develops from the ovarian serosa but this type of neoplasm is formed of uro-epithelium, identical in all respects to that found in the urinary tract; tumours of this type are therefore differentiating along Wolffian rather than Müllerian lines, it being not surprising that cells tracing their origin back to the coelomic epithelium of the nephrogenital ridge retain a residual capacity for differentiation along this line. The final member of the group of epithelial ovarian neoplasms is the *clear-cell tumour*. This is identical in appearance to the clear-cell vaginal tumours that occur in DES-exposed girls, and is certainly of a Müllerian nature, although admittedly not bearing a resemblance to any adult tissue of Müllerian origin.

The epithelial tumours of the ovary appear to have in common, therefore, a derivation from the ovarian serosa. This unitary concept is, however, too all-embracing, for a minority of epithelial ovarian neoplasms appear to have a quite different histogenesis. Thus some mucinous tumours are formed, not of endocervical-type epithelium, but of gastrointestinal type epithelium: some such neoplasms may arise from areas of *gastro-intestinal metaplasia* within the ovarian surface epithelium, but some appear to be *monophyletic teratomas*. Further, a proportion of both endometrioid and clear-cell neoplasms originate from pre-existing foci of *ovarian endometriosis*, whilst some Brenner tumours develop in the hilum of the ovary, possibly being derived from structures of Wolffian origin, such as the epoophoron or epigenital tubules.

Despite these exceptions, the vast majority of epithelian neoplasms are derived from the surface epithelium and each type can exist in a benign or malignant form, the various malignant tumours sharing many common characteristics and being considered collectively as 'ovarian adenocarcinomas'. In addition to the benign and malignant types of each neoplasm there exists a third form, namely, tumours of *borderline malignancy* (also known as 'tumours of low malignant potential' and as 'proliferating tumours').

Serous tumours

Most benign serous neoplasms are cystic, taking the form of either a simple or papillary serous cystadenoma. Serous cystadenomas (Fig. 21.97) are thin-walled, usually unilocular, smooth-walled cysts, measuring from 3 to 30 cm in diameter and containing clear, straw-coloured fluid. In the papillary form of this tumour, papillae are present on one or both surfaces of the cyst: these may be few, sessile, and small; or numerous, large, fleshy, and pedunculated. Solid serous tumours are less common and occur either as *surface serous papillomas*, in which finger-like papillae project from the surface of the ovary, or as *serous adenofibromas*, which form hard, knobbly, solid masses. *Serous cystadenomas* are usually lined by a single layer of flattened or cuboidal cells, but in a few instances the tubal nature of the lining epithelium may be more apparent (Fig. 21.98). Certainly, the true nature of the epithelium is usually more overt in

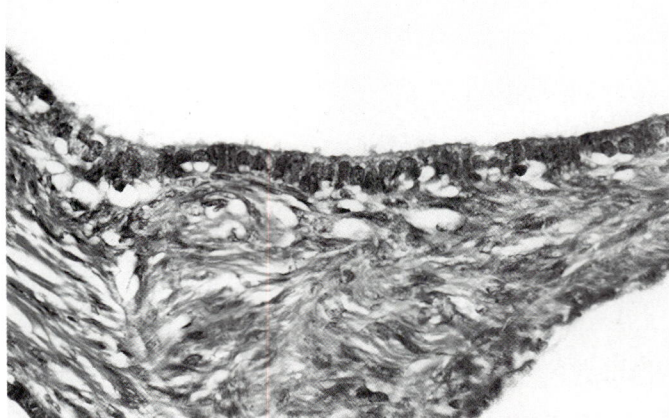

Fig. 21.98 Serous cystadenoma of the ovary. The cyst is lined by a single layer of epithelium similar to that which lines the normal Fallopian tube.

the papillary neoplasms, where the central core of the papillae, formed of loose fibrous tissue, is covered by an epithelium remarkably similar to that of the Fallopian tube, with secretory, ciliated, and peg cells. The serous cystadenoma is a predominantly fibrous tumour containing small cysts, gland-like spaces, or slits lined by tubal-type epithelium.

Serous adenocarcinomas are usually large and are essentially a malignant form of the papillary serous cystadenoma, most being partially cystic and partially solid. The solid areas are formed of closely packed, or merged, papillae, which often penetrate through the outer capsule of the neoplasm (Fig. 21.99). Foci of necrosis or haemorrhage are common and any fluid present in the cystic portion of the tumour is commonly blood-stained. Histologically, well-differentiated serous adenocarcinomas retain a papillary pattern but the epithelium shows multilayering, irregular tufting, nuclear hyperchromatism,

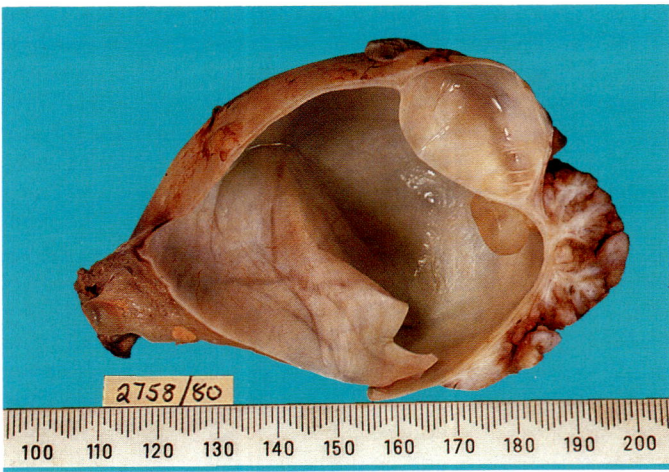

Fig. 21.97 Serous cystadenoma and serous surface papilloma of the ovary. The cyst, to the left, is unilocular and thin-walled; the lining is smooth. To the right, the surface of the ovary bears a shallow, surface papillary neoplasm.

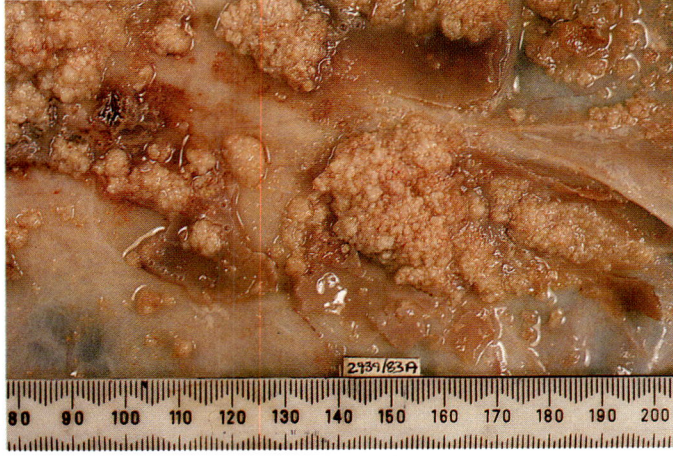

Fig. 21.99 Serous carcinoma of the ovary. This cystic neoplasm has been opened to expose its inner surface. The lining is covered by small papillary excrescences.

pleomorphism, and mitotic activity, whilst stromal invasion is readily apparent (Fig. 21.100). From this clearly papillary form there is a spectrum of differentiation extending through to the diffuse pattern in which the tumour grows in solid sheets of cells.

Mucinous tumours

Benign mucinous tumours are almost invariably cystic, taking the form of a mucinous cystadenoma. These cystic neoplasms commonly measure between 15 and 30 cm in diameter but can attain a huge size and fill the abdominal cavity. The cysts have a thick, parchment-like wall and are usually multilocular, the locules characteristically containing clear, tenacious mucoid material (Fig. 21.101). Histologically, the walls of the locules are formed of fibrous tissue and the cyst is lined by a single layer of tall, mucus-containing cells (Fig. 21.102). In many tumours the epithelium is identical to that of the endocervix, but in a

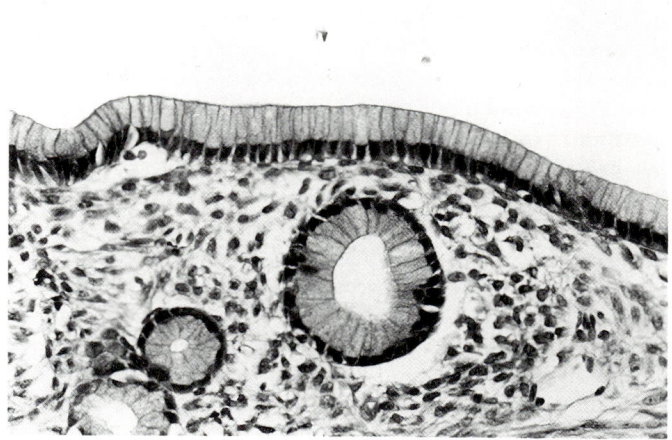

Fig. 21.102 Mucinous cystadenoma of the ovary. The cyst is lined by a single layer of tall, columnar, mucin-secreting epithelium; similar epithelium lines the glands in the cyst wall.

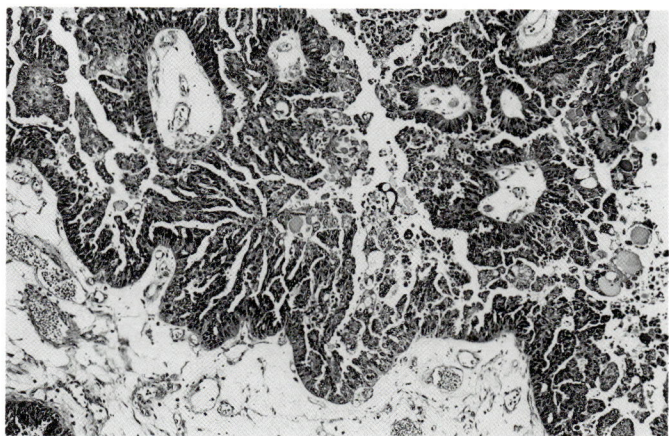

Fig. 21.100 Serous carcinoma of the ovary. The neoplasm is composed of papillary processes covered by an epithelium which shows extensive proliferation and budding.

significant proportion the epithelium is of enteric type, containing goblet cells, argyrophil cells and, occasionally, Paneth cells.

Mucinous adenocarcinomas are usually either partially or wholly solid; areas of necrosis or haemorrhage are common and mucoid material often exudes from their cut surface. These neoplasms show a wide spectrum of differentiation, ranging from a well-marked acinar or glandular pattern (Fig. 21.103) to one in which the tumour is formed largely of solid sheets of cells in which, however, intracellular mucus is usually present.

In any type of mucinous neoplasm there may be seepage out from the tumour of mucus which forms pools in the ovarian stroma, a condition known as *pseudomyxoma ovarii*. There may also be spillage into the abdominal cavity, because of either spontaneous or surgical perforation, to produce a *pseudomyxoma peritoneii*, a condition characterized by accumulation of jelly-like mucoid material in the peritoneal cavity. Whether this

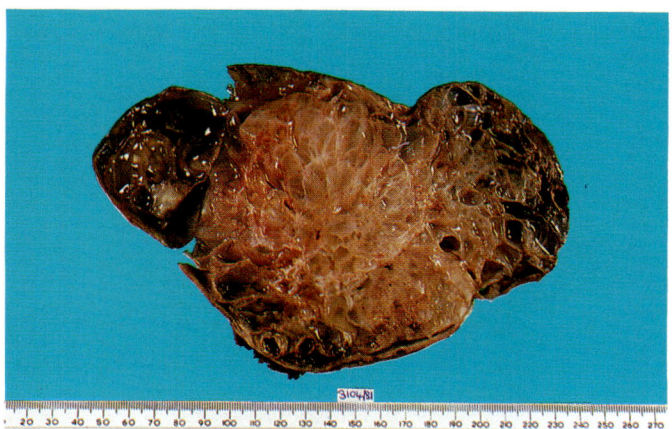

Fig. 21.101 Mucinous cystadenoma of the ovary. The mass is finely multicystic, the locules containing mucus and having smooth linings.

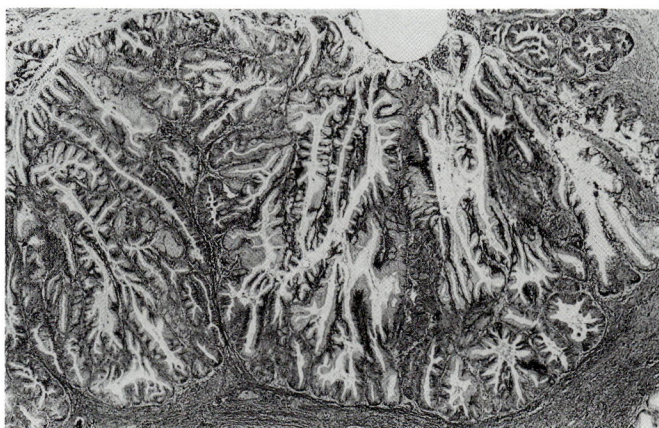

Fig. 21.103 Well-differentiated mucinous adenocarcinoma of the ovary. The neoplasm consists of glandular acini lined by a mucus-secreting columnar epithelium which resembles that seen in the endo-cervix.

is because of implantation and growth of tumour fragments in the peritoneal cavity or because of mucinous metaplasia in the peritoneal serosa is uncertain. Pseudomyxoma peritoneii can also complicate a mucocele of the appendix and some patients with this condition have both an appendicular mucocele and a mucinous ovarian tumour, circumstances in which it is impossible to identify the primary lesion.

Endometrioid tumours

Benign endometrioid tumours appear to be very rare, although occasional examples of an *endometrioid adenoma*, which tends to resemble an endometrial polyp, or of an *endometrioid adenofibroma*, a neoplasm resembling the serous adenofibroma but in which the enclosed glands are lined by an endometrial-type epithelium, are encountered. This apparent paucity of benign endometrioid tumours may, however, be more apparent than real, for it is possible that many of the lesions classed as *endometriotic cysts* of the ovary are, in reality, *benign endometrioid cystadenomas*.

Endometrioid adenocarcinomas may be solid (Fig. 21.104), partially cystic, or wholly cystic, the latter variety usually showing abundant papillary ingrowths. The defining histological feature of an endometrioid adenocarcinoma is that it mimics exactly an endometrial adenocarcinoma (Fig. 21.105); most are well differentiated and have an acinar pattern, but in a minority there is a predominantly sheet-like pattern of growth. Many endometrioid adenocarcinomas contain foci of *squamous metaplasia*, and a clear-cell appearance is sometimes encountered. It is worth noting that any neoplasm that occurs in the endometrium can also arise in the ovary as a variant of an endometrioid adenocarcinoma; thus *carcinosarcomas*, *adenosarcomas*, and *endometrial stromal sarcomas* can all occur in the ovary as forms of endometrioid neoplasia.

Brenner tumours

The majority of Brenner tumours are benign and occur as

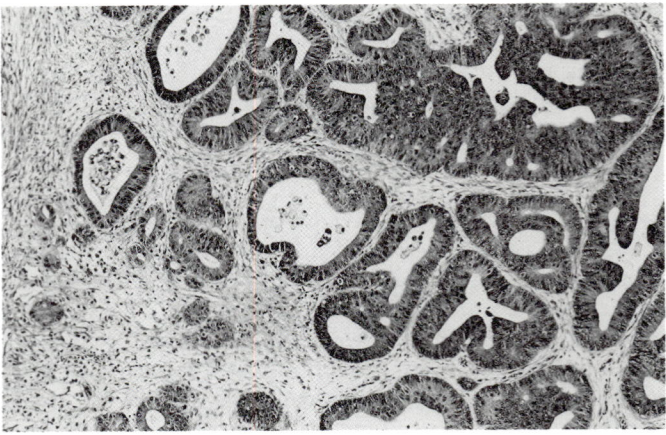

Fig. 21.105 Well-differentiated endometrioid adenocarcinoma of the ovary. The tumour is similar in appearance to the adenocarcinoma arising in the endometrium (Fig. 21.61).

small, solid, well-circumscribed nodules with a smooth or bosselated surface and a hard, whorled, greyish-white, cut surface. Histologically, the Brenner tumour is characterized by well-demarcated nests and branching columns of epithelial cells set in a fibrous stroma (Fig. 21.106). The epithelial nests are formed of round or polygonal cells with distinct limiting membranes, abundant cytoplasm, and ovoid or round nuclei which are often prominently grooved. Cystic change in the centre of the cell nests is common and these cystic spaces may be lined by flattened, cuboidal, or columnar cells.

Malignant Brenner tumours may resemble architecturally a benign Brenner neoplasm but show a marked overgrowth of the epithelial component with nuclear hyperchromatism, cytological atypia, mitotic activity, and stromal invasion. Some malignant Brenner tumours develop, however, as *pure transitional cell carcinomas* (Fig. 21.107), identical in all respects to their counterparts in the urinary tract.

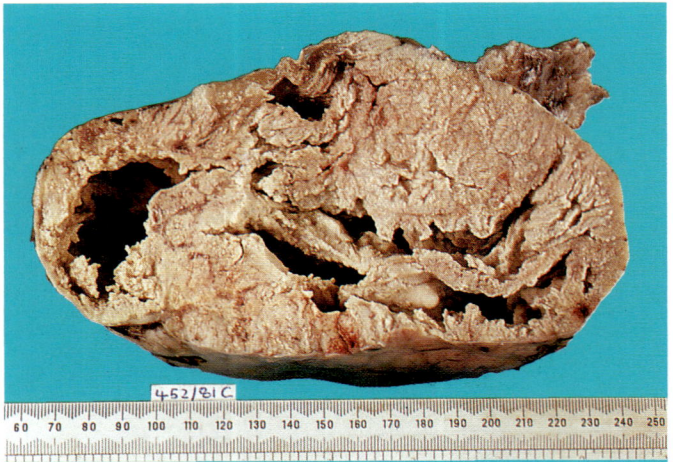

Fig. 21.104 Endometrioid adenocarcinoma of the ovary. The ovary is replaced by a partly solid, partly cystic mass in which there are areas of necrosis.

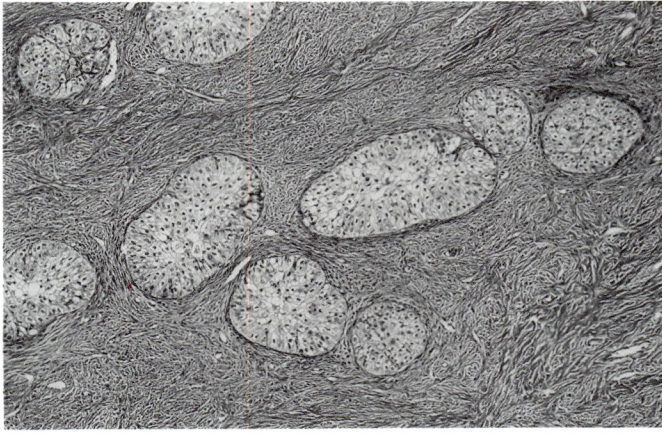

Fig. 21.106 Brenner tumour of the ovary. The neoplasm is composed of dense fibrous tissue in which there are nests of epithelium of transitional type. The nests may become cystic and may then be lined by mucus-secreting epithelium.

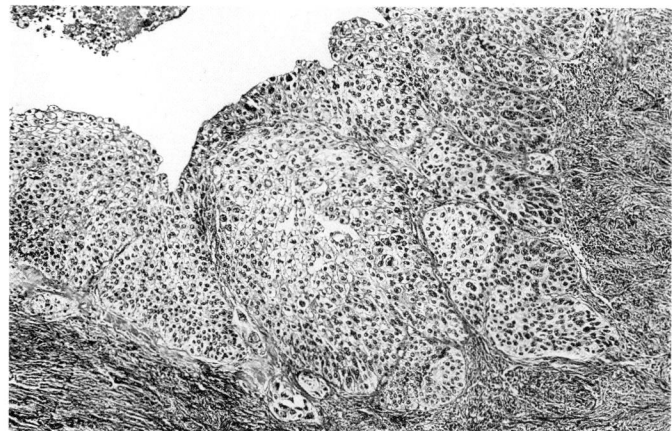

Fig. 21.107 Malignant Brenner tumour of the ovary. The cyst, to the left, is lined by a highly abnormal transitional epithelium which is also infiltrating the cyst wall.

Clear-cell tumours

Benign clear-cell neoplasms are distinctly uncommon and take the form of *clear-cell adenofibromas* in which gland-like spaces set in fibrous tissue are lined by cells with clear cytoplasm and *hobnail nuclei.*

Most clear-cell tumours are adenocarcinomas; these are usually large and only a minority are solid, most being cystic with solid areas. The solid areas tend to be soft and fleshy whereas the cystic portions are commonly multilocular and often contain mucoid material. These neoplasms have a complex histological appearance, showing an admixture of papillary, cystic, glandular, and solid growth forms (Fig. 21.108). The cysts and acini tend to be lined by cells with clear cytoplasm and large, deeply-staining nuclei which protrude into the lumen (hobnail nuclei).

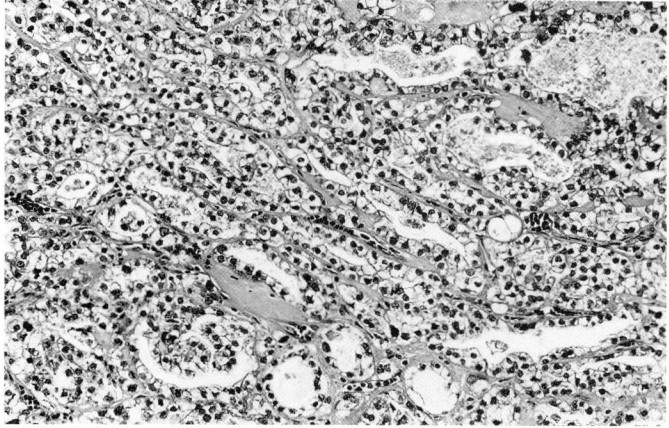

Fig. 21.108 Clear-cell carcinoma of the ovary, consisting of acini and tubules lined by malignant cells with large hyperchromatic nuclei and clear cytoplasm.

Ovarian adenocarcinoma

The malignant forms of the various epithelial tumours of the ovary are, in clinical practice, usually grouped together into the single entity of ovarian adenocarcinoma. These neoplasms tend to occur in women aged 45–60 years and are commonly asymptomatic until they have achieved a considerable bulk, the most common complaints being an increasing abdominal girth, lower abdominal pain or discomfort, and an awareness of a pelvic mass; urinary or bowel symptoms, due to pressure on the bladder or rectum, occur with some frequency.

Serous and endometrioid tumours form the bulk of ovarian adenocarcinoma; mucinous tumours are less common, whereas clear-cell carcinoma and malignant Brenner tumours are relatively rare.

It has been widely believed that tumour type is of some prognostic significance with, for example, serous adenocarcinomas pursuing a more malignant course than do their endometrioid counterparts. Multivariate analysis has, however, shown this not to be true, the only two significant prognostic factors being the clinical stage at the time of diagnosis and the histological grade of the neoplasm.

Staging of ovarian adenocarcinomas is dependent upon a knowledge of their mode of spread. Local spread is by direct seeding on to the *peritoneum* with implantation of secondary deposits in the pouch of Douglas, on the surface of the *uterus*, and in the *omentum*. Malignant cells are also seeded into the small amount of fluid that is normally present in the peritoneal cavity. This fluid tends to circulate upwards along the *paracolic gutters* and, whereas on the left side the circulation of the fluid is dammed by the *phrenico-colic ligament*, there is no such bar on the right side of the abdomen and fluid reaches the under surface of the *right leaf of the diaphragm*. Tumour cells are thus carried into the paracolic gutters and to the right leaf of the diaphragm, these being sites of early metastasis. Lymphatic spread is to the *pelvic nodes* and also occurs, at a relatively early stage in the growth of the tumour, to the *para-aortic nodes*. Blood-borne spread is a late and uncommon event and is usually to the liver and lungs.

The staging system of ovarian carcinomas is rather complex, but for practical purposes can be simplified into:

Stage 1   *Tumour is confined to the ovaries.*

Stage 2   *Tumour is confined to the pelvis.*

Stage 3   *Tumour is confined to the abdominal cavity.*

Stage 4   *Tumour is present outside the abdomen or within the liver.*

Currently, ovarian adenocarcinoma has a gloomy prognosis, the overall five-year survival rate being only in the region of 25 per cent. Unfortunately, little is known of the aetiology of this lethal form of neoplasia. It has been suggested that the ground is prepared for eventual neoplastic change in the surface epithelium by the repetitive minor trauma of ovulation, a view lent credence by the finding that both oral contraception and pregnancy, each associated with inhibition of ovulation, decrease the risk of developing ovarian adenocarcinoma. The protective effect of pregnancy is cumulative but, nevertheless, simple inhibition of ovulation is not the entire explanation for these effects, for one pregnancy offers the same degree of protection as does three years' use of oral contraceptives. Certainly there are grounds for believing that an external carcinogen is also involved in ovarian neoplasia. Particulate matter placed in the lower female genital tract is rapidly transported up into the uterus and through the tubes to reach the surface of the ovaries, and an indication that this route of carcinogenic exposure may be of importance lies in the finding that hysterectomy substantially lessens the risk of ovarian adenocarcinoma. The exogenous carcinogen has not been identified but suspicion has fallen on *talc*. This substance is present in many vaginal toilet preparations, is used to coat barrier contraceptives, and talc crystals have been detected in ovarian carcinomas; further, women using talc-containing perineal dusting powders have an increased risk of developing ovarian carcinoma. Talc has, however, not been shown to be a carcinogen, though it is of note that many commercial talc preparations were, until recently, contaminated by *asbestos*, a potent carcinogen.

Epithelial tumours of borderline malignancy

These neoplasms, also known as 'tumours of low malignant potential' or 'proliferative tumours', lie in the grey area between clearly benign and overtly malignant epithelial ovarian neoplasms. It is largely the serous and mucinous borderline tumours which have been clearly defined, borderline endometrioid, Brenner, and clear-cell neoplasms forming a more controversial group. Borderline mucinous and serous tumours are relatively common and macroscopically resemble closely their fully benign counterparts. Histologically (Figs 21.109, 21.110) the epithelial component of these neoplasms shows some, or indeed all, of the characteristics of malignancy, such as multilayering, irregular budding, cytological atypia, nuclear hyperchromatism and pleomorphism, and mitotic activity; there is, however, no stromal invasion, and this lack of invasiveness is both a defining feature of these neoplasms and an

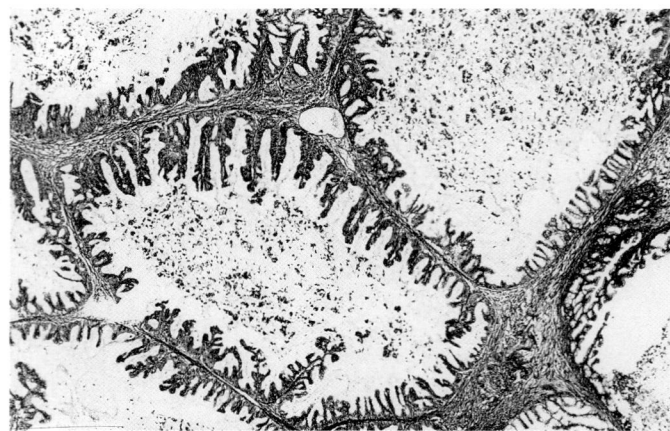

Fig. 21.110 Mucinous tumour of borderline malignancy. The neoplastic locules are lined by a columnar, mucin-secreting epithelium which forms tufts and irregular papillae.

indication of their unique biological status. The tumours, particularly those of serous type, may shown a homogeneously borderline pattern throughout, or there may be an admixture, within a single neoplasm, of clearly benign epithelium and of epithelium showing borderline characteristics. It must be stressed that the diagnosis of a tumour of borderline malignancy is a positive one that is based on the histological findings, and that the use of this term is not indicative of any indecision on the pathologist's part as to whether the tumour is benign or malignant.

In most patients with a tumour of borderline malignancy the neoplasm is confined to the ovary at the time of diagnosis and the majority of patients are cured by an oophorectomy. Unfortunately, a proportion of borderline tumours have spread beyond the ovary at the time of diagnosis to recur after oophorectomy; these neoplasms tend to pursue a leisurely, indolent, but progessive, malignant course and it is currently a matter of concern to identify this subset of tumours with a poor prognosis. It should be noted that apparent extraovarian spread, particularly in the case of serous tumours, is not always due to metastatic spread, for these neoplasms can be associated with concomitant foci of *endosalpingiosis*, a form of benign Müllerian metaplasia, in the subserosal connective tissues of the omentum and pelvic peritoneum.

Sex cord-stromal tumours

These neoplasms contain *granulosa cells*, *Sertoli cells*, *thecal cells*, *Leydig cells*, or *fibroblasts of specialized stromal origin*, or the precursors of these cells, either singly or in any combination. It has been thought that all these cells are ultimately derived from the mesenchyme of the genital ridge, but it is more likely that both granulosa and Sertoli cells differentiate from the sex cords of the developing gonad, cords which probably originate from the coelomic epithelium rather than from mesenchyme. It is believed that sex cord cells can, depending on the nature of the developing gonad, differentiate into either Sertoli or granulosa

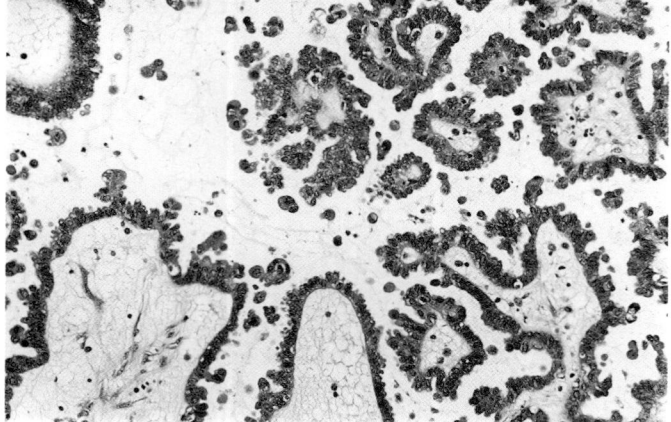

Fig. 21.109 Serous tumour of borderline malignancy. The cyst is lined by cells which are multilayered, rather pleomorphic, and show irregular budding into the cyst lumen.

cells, and that this bisexual potentiality is retained in undifferentiated sex cord cells in the adult gonad, granulosa cell tumours and Sertoli cell neoplasms thus being homologous with each other. Neoplasia of these cells is often accompanied by a reactive stromal proliferation which, in the case of a granulosa cell tumour, often shows thecomatous differentiation and in Sertoli cell neoplasms shows Leydig cell differentiation. Pure stromal neoplasms, thecomas, and Leydig cell tumours can, however, also occur.

There are many experimental techniques for producing sex cord stromal tumours, usually of granulosa cell type. All induce oocyte depletion with consequent granulosa cell degeneration and a subsequent rise in gonadotrophin levels, the latter being considered as the driving force for sex cord-stromal neoplasia. These experimental techniques mimic, therefore, the situation encountered in immediately post-menopausal women, in whom granulosa cell neoplasms predominantly occur. These studies provide no clues, however, to the origin of those granulosa cell neoplasms, a significant proportion, which develop prior to the menopause.

Granulosa cell tumours

These are usually solid neoplasms (Fig. 21.111) which may be hard or rubbery; their cut surface is white, yellow, or grey and their average size is about 12 cm in diameter. A proportion of granulosa cell neoplasms are, however, partially cystic and a few are wholly cystic, resembling a cystadenoma.

Histologically, the cells in a granulosa cell tumour are small, round, or polygonal, having little cytoplasm and indistinct cell boundaries (Fig. 21.112); their large, round or ovoid, pale nuclei characteristically show longitudinal grooving. The cells are arranged in a variety of patterns and, although in any individual neoplasm a particular pattern may predominate, there is usually an admixture of cellular arrangements. In the *insular pattern* the cells are arranged in compact masses or islands whereas in the *trabecular pattern* the cells form anastomosing

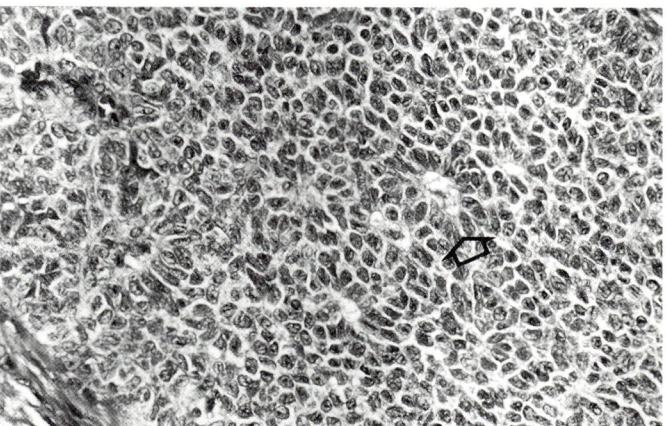

Fig. 21.112 Granulosa cell tumour of the ovary. The solid neoplasm is composed of uniform oval cells with regular darkly staining nuclei which are grooved. In places the cells have a pseudoacinar arrangement, the so-called Call–Exner bodies (arrow).

ribbons or cords (Fig. 21.113). Alternatively, the cells may be arranged in sheets to give a *diffuse pattern*. In the *microfollicular* pattern, granulosa cells are arranged around small spaces containing nuclear fragments, these being the *Call–Exner bodies*, whilst a *macrofollicular pattern* is due to liquefaction within islands of granulosa cells. In *cystic granulosa cell tumours* the cyst lining resembles that of a Graafian follicle but usually contains microfollicles.

A granulosa cell tumour may produce non-specific pelvic tumour symptoms, but about 75 per cent of patients with such neoplasms have symptoms indicative of oestrogen secretion by the neoplasm. Thus, in young girls these tumours commonly result in *isosexual precocious pseudopuberty*, whereas in women of reproductive age complaints of irregular menstruation or menorrhagia are common; in post-menopausal patients granulosa cell tumours cause post-menopausal vaginal bleeding and, sometimes, a resurgence of libido. *Endometrial changes*, such as *simple or atypical hyperplasia*, are commonly found in association

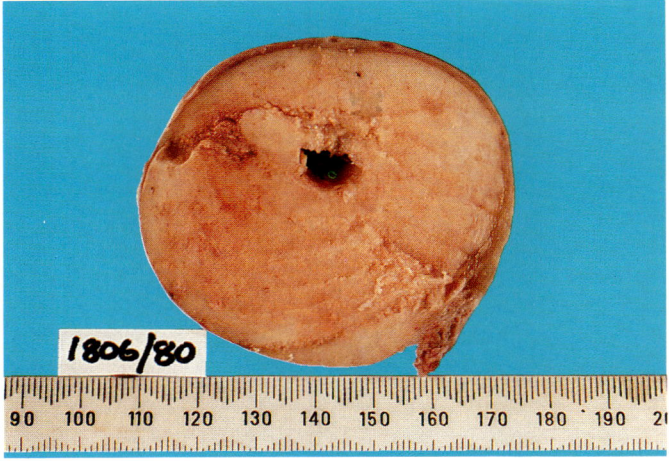

Fig. 21.111 Granulosa cell tumour of the ovary. The tumour is predominantly solid with only small cystic areas. It is uniformly yellow-grey.

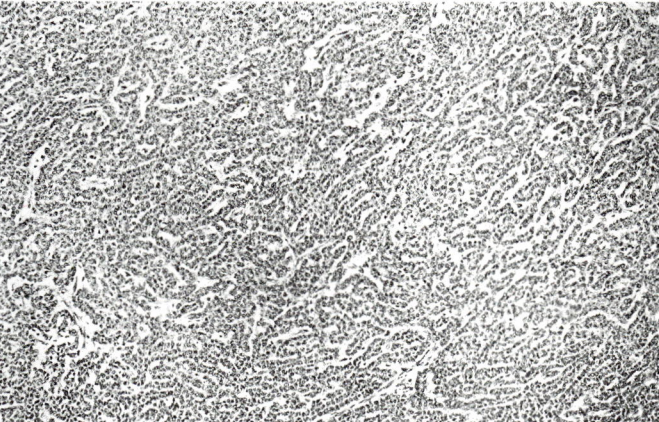

Fig. 21.113 Granulosa cell tumour of the ovary. The cells are arranged in a fine trabecular pattern.

with granulosa cell tumours, whilst an endometrial adenocarcinoma occurs in 6–10 per cent of cases. A few granulosa cell tumours, particularly those which are cystic, appear to be androgenic rather than oestrogenic.

All granulosa cell tumours should be considered as potentially malignant, although the degree of malignancy is often very low and the course pursued by the tumour is frequently very indolent. Recurrences or metastases tend to occur late, commonly after 5 years, not infrequently after 10 years, and sometimes after 20 years. The histological pattern of the tumour is of no prognostic importance; it is indeed doubtful if there are any prognostic indicators apart from extraovarian spread. The long-term survival rate for patients with this neoplasm is between 50 and 60 per cent.

Juvenile granulosa cell tumour

This is a histological variant of a granulosa cell tumour which occurs predominantly in patients aged less than 20 years, although some neoplasms of this type arise in older women. The tumours (Fig. 21.114) contain follicles and cysts lined by granulosa cells, together with solid areas showing a haphazard admixture of granulosa and thecal cells which, not uncommonly, show a striking degree of luteinization. The neoplastic cells lack the nuclear grooving characteristic of an adult-type granulosa cell tumour, and there is often a moderate degree of cytological atypia and mitotic activity.

About 5 per cent of juvenile granulosa cell tumours behave in a malignant fashion, these tending to recur rapidly and disseminate widely throughout the abdominal cavity within 2 years of initial diagnosis, a pattern of malignant behaviour quite unlike that of an adult granulosa cell tumour.

Thecomas (fibrothecoma)

These are solid tumours (Fig. 21.115) which are formed of plump, pale, ovoid, or spindle-shaped cells with indistinct borders which are arranged in interlacing bundles or anastomosing trabeculae (Fig. 21.116). These neoplasms arise from the ovarian mesenchyme and occur most commonly in postmenopausal women; they are oestrogenic and produce symptoms similar to those noted in patients with granulosa cell tumours. Some thecomas show focal luteinization and such neoplasms may be weakly androgenic.

Thecomas are, with rare exceptions, benign; malignant thecomas are not distinguishable from fibrosarcomas.

Fibromas

Neoplasms of this type probably arise from ovarian gonadal stroma rather than from non-specific fibrous tissue within the ovary and therefore merit inclusion within the sex-cord-stromal group of neoplasms. These tumours are similar to fibromas elsewhere in the body, but it is of note that a proportion of ovarian fibromas are, for unknown reasons, accompanied by ascites and a hydrothorax (*Meig's syndrome*). Ovarian fibromas also tend to occur in association with the *basal cell naevus*, or *Gorlin's, syndrome*, under which unusual circumstances the tumours tend to be bilateral, multifocal, and calcified.

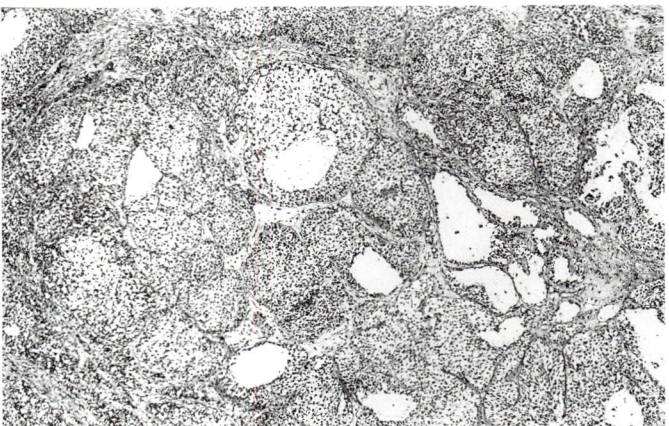

Fig. 21.114 Juvenile granulosa cell tumour of the ovary. The characteristic feature is the numerous gland-like cysts, the macrofollicles.

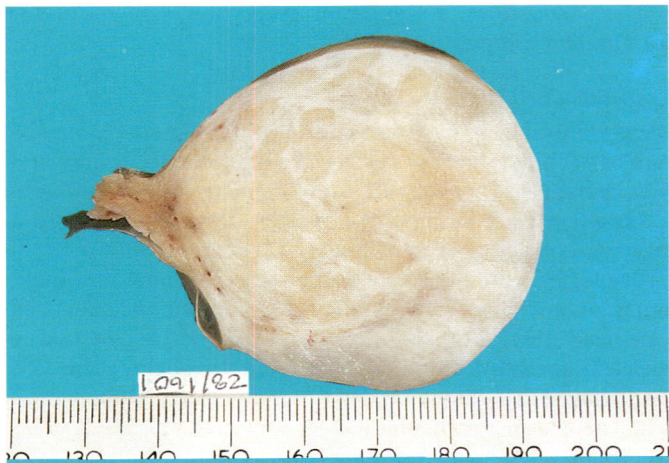

Fig. 21.115 Fibrothecoma of the ovary. The neoplasm is grey-white, solid, and has a whorled appearance. In some areas it has a yellowish appearance, the latter corresponding to areas of luteinization.

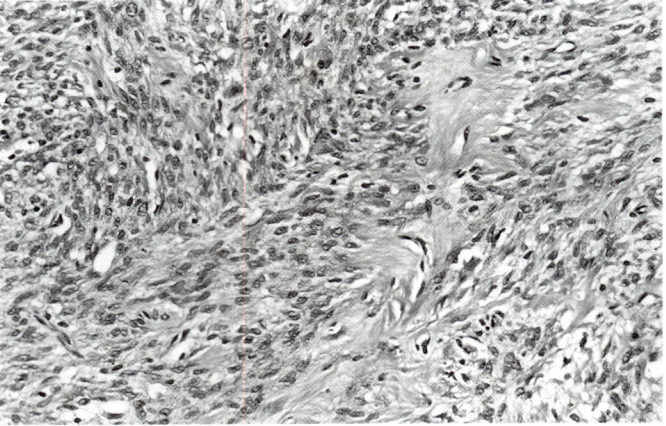

Fig. 21.116 Fibrothecoma of the ovary. The tumour cells are spindle- or oval-shaped and the nuclei pale. There are bands of hyalinized fibrous tissue.

Fibromas are benign but a few show increased cellularity, pleomorphism, and mitotic activity, tumours showing these features to only a mild degree being classed as cellular fibromas, which will recur if incompletely removed, and those with more marked atypia and mitotic activity being classed as fibrosarcomas, highly aggressive neoplasms with a poor prognosis.

Androblastoma

Androblastomas are neoplasms composed of *Sertoli cells*, *Leydig cells*, or a *combination* of the two cell types.

Pure Sertoli cell neoplasms are rare and occur as small, solid, yellowish masses. Histologically (Fig. 21.117) the tumours show highly differentiated tubules lined by a single layer of radially orientated Sertoli cells which commonly contain lipid droplets and are occasionally distended and vacuolated by fat. Sertoli cell neoplasms are, with very rare exceptions, benign, and about 50 per cent appear to be oestrogenic, the remainder lacking any obvious endocrinological activity.

Leydig cell neoplasms may arise either from stromal cells or from pre-existing hilar cells. The tumours are small, yellowish-brown, and consist of Leydig cells arranged in sheets or solid cords (Fig. 21.118). The cytoplasm of the Leydig cells is markedly eosinophilic and their nuclei are large and centrally placed. *Reinke's crystals*, slender rod-shaped bodies with rounded, tapering, or square ends, are present in about 50 per cent of these neoplasms but are irregularly distributed and often difficult to detect.

Leydig cell tumours are nearly always *virilizing*, although occasional oestrogenic or endocrinologically inert examples are encountered; the vast majority (95 per cent) are benign but exceptional tumours of this type give rise to metastases, a possibility not predictable on any histological grounds.

Sertoli–Leydig cell tumours are generally solid neoplasms which show a wide range of histological differentiation. *Well-differentiated neoplasms* are formed of tubules lined by Sertoli cells with variable numbers of Leydig cells between the tubules. In *less well-differentiated tumours* the Sertoli cells are arranged in

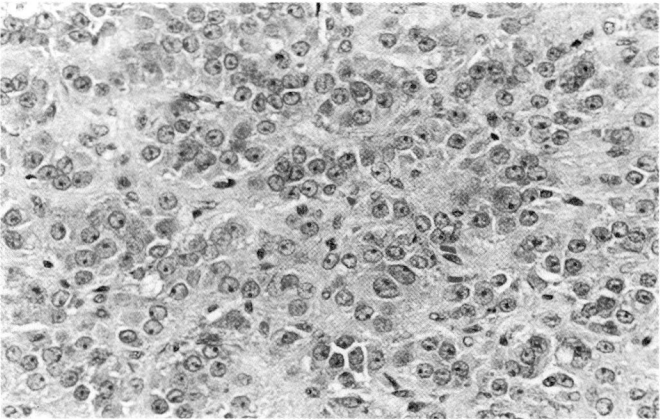

Fig. 21.118 Leydig cell tumour of the ovary. The tumour cells are remarkably uniform in shape and size but notice that the nuclei are grouped and irregularly dispersed.

cords, solid tubules, or trabeculae (Fig. 21.119), these being set in a mesenchymal stroma containing clusters or nodules of Leydig cells. *Poorly differentiated Sertoli–Leydig neoplasms* (Fig. 21.120) consist largely of sheets of spindle-shaped cells in which occasional irregular cord-like structures or imperfectly formed tubules may be recognized, Leydig cells also being present in small clusters.

Sertoli–Leydig cell neoplasms can occur at any age but the majority develop in women aged between 10 and 35 years. These tumours are usually androgenic and produce virilization. The well-differentiated neoplasms always behave in a benign fashion but between 10 and 40 per cent of the less well-differentiated tumours behave in a malignant fashion, this being particularly the case for the poorly differentiated tumours.

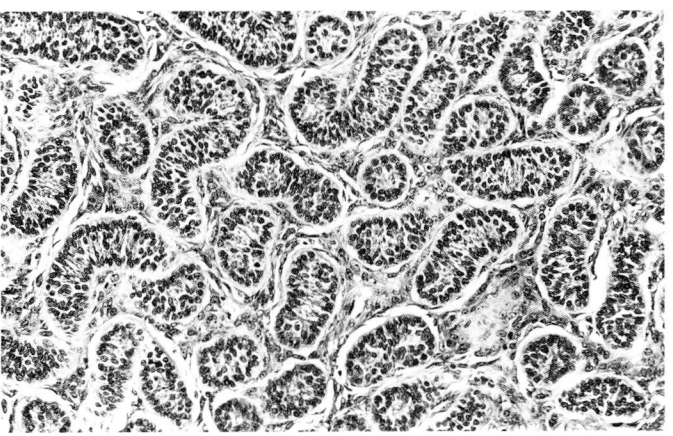

Fig. 21.117 Sertoli cell tumour of the ovary. The neoplasm is composed of narrow tubules lined by cubo-columnar cells set in a fibrous stroma.

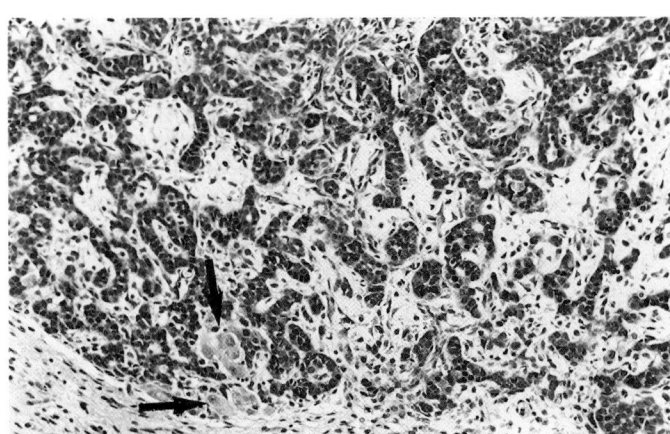

Fig. 21.119 Moderately differentiated Sertoli–Leydig cell tumour of the ovary. The neoplasm is composed of cords of darkly staining cells, resembling sex cords, set in a fibrous stroma in which there are small numbers of large cells with copious pale-staining cytoplasm (arrows), the latter are the Leydig cells. (Reproduced by kind permission of Edward Arnold from *Pathology for gynaecologists*, Fox and Buckley, 2nd edn, 1991.)

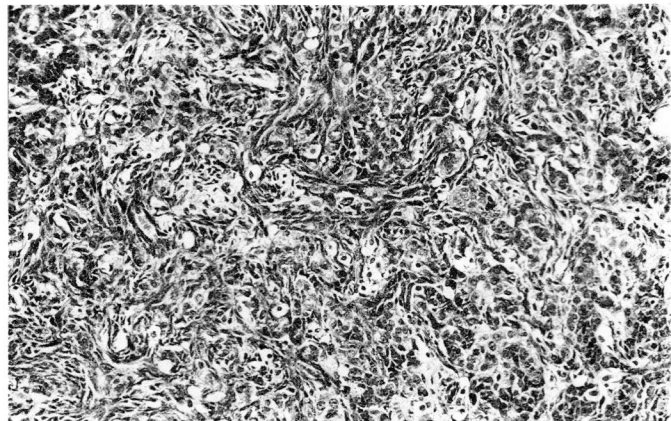

Fig. 21.120 Poorly differentiated Sertoli–Leydig cell tumour. The neoplasm is solid and consists of bundles of spindle cells intermingled with larger, paler cells, the Leydig cells.

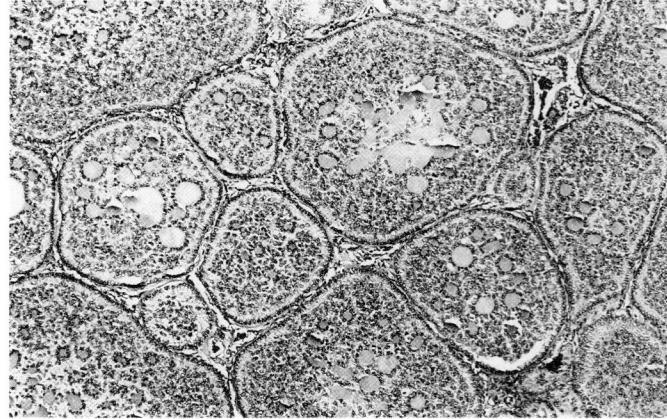

Fig. 21.121 Sex cord tumour with annular tubules. This very striking neoplasm is composed of discrete islands of cells arranged around amorphous, pale-staining material.

Recurrence or metastases, characteristically to the omentum, abdominal lymph nodes, or liver, are usually apparent within one year of initial diagnosis.

Gynandroblastoma

This term has been loosely applied to *virilizing granulosa cell tumours*, to *oestrogenic androblastomas*, and to those *sex cord-stromal neoplasms* which are difficult to classify clearly as either granulosa or Sertoli cell tumours. A true gynandroblastoma must contain an admixture of areas showing unequivocal granulosa cell differentiation and of others in which there is equally incontrovertible Sertoli cell differentiation. Such tumours reflect clearly the ability of undifferentiated sex cord-stromal cells to differentiate into either granulosa or Sertoli cells and are extremely rare, a fact which means that their pattern of behaviour is still largely undetermined.

Sex cord tumour with annular tubules

This uncommon, but histologically distinctive, tumour contains rounded nests in which epithelial-like cells surround hyaline bodies (Fig. 21.121). The epithelial-like cells, which are thought to be immature sex cord cells, are palisaded along the periphery of the cell nests and around the hyaline bodies. About one-third of these tumours are associated with the Peutz–Jeghers syndrome and in such circumstances the lesions are usually bilateral, of microscopic size only, calcified, and benign. The tumours unassociated with the Peutz–Jeghers syndrome are unilateral, large, uncalcified, often show an overgrowth of either granulosa or Sertoli cells, and behave in a malignant fashion in about 20 per cent of cases.

Germ cell tumours

Tumours derived from germ cells may show no evidence of differentiation into either embryonic or extra-embryonic tissues, can differentiate into embryonic tissues, or may differentiate along extra-embryonic pathways into trophoblast or yolk sac structures.

Very little, indeed nothing, is known about the aetiology of germ cell neoplasms. Extensive studies of naturally occurring gonadal teratomas in highly inbred genetic strains of mice and of experimentally induced murine teratomas have, however, indicated that teratomas arise from *parthogenetic pregnancies* (i.e. in which there has been no fertilization of the ovum) which undergo a short period of embryogenesis and then break up to yield a neoplasm. Studies of human ovarian teratomas suggest strongly that these tumours arise in a similar manner.

Dysgerminoma

This neoplasm is formed of cells which closely resemble primordial germ cells, showing no evidence of differentiation into either embryonic or extra-embryonic structures; as such the tumour is identical to the *seminoma of the testis*. Dysgerminomas commonly arise in patients aged between 10 and 30 years, their development usually being announced by non-specific tumour symptoms, although *isosexual precocious pseudopuberty* is sometimes seen in young girls. These neoplasms have a particular tendency to arise in patients with *developmental abnormalities of the gonads*; nevertheless the vast majority of dysgerminomas occur in otherwise fully normal individuals.

The tumours are solid (Fig. 21.122) and usually measure about 12 cm in diameter. Histologically (Fig. 21.123) the neoplastic cells are large, uniform, round, oval, or polyhedral, with well-defined limiting membranes, abundant cytoplasm, and large vesicular nuclei. The cells are commonly arranged in solid nests separated by delicate fibrous septa but may form cords or strands embedded in a fibrous stroma. A lymphocytic infiltration of the stroma, sometimes aggregated into follicles with germinal centres, and small stromal granulomas are characteristic features.

Dysgerminomas are malignant: rupture of their enveloping

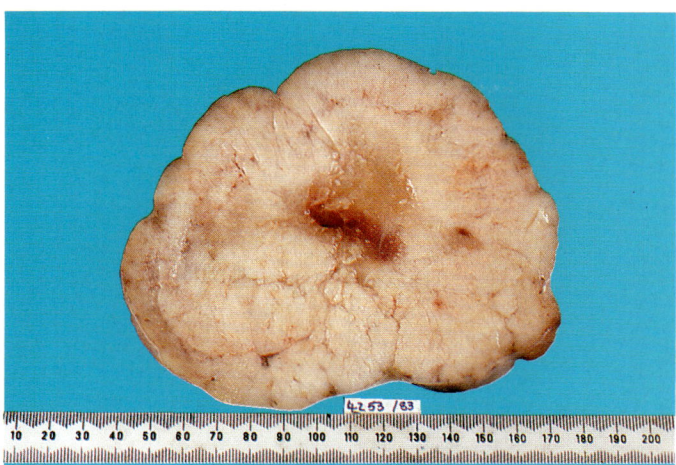

Fig. 21.122 Dysgerminoma of the ovary. The neoplasm is solid with central areas of degeneration and pseudocyst formation. It has a distinctly lobular pattern.

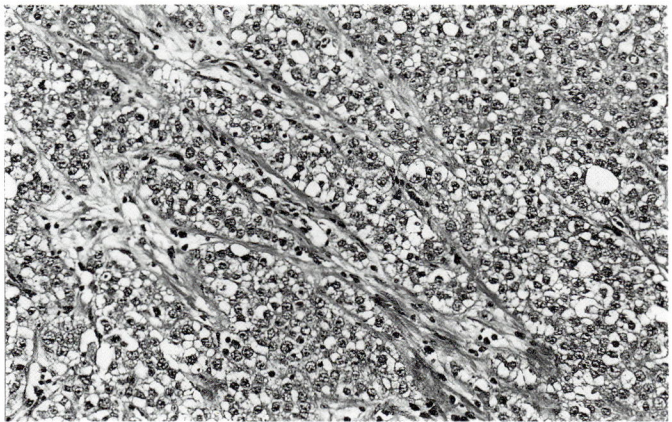

Fig. 21.123 Dysgerminoma of the ovary. The neoplasm is composed of undifferentiated germ cells, which are large cells with vesicular nuclei and clear cytoplasm arranged in cords, trabeculae, and islands. A scattering of lymphocytes lies between the tumour cords.

'capsule' often leads to direct implantation of tumour on to the pelvic peritoneum and omentum, and lymphatic spread occurs relatively early to the *para-aortic*, *retroperitoneal*, *mediastinal*, and *supraclavicular nodes*. *Haematogenous spread*, to *liver*, *lungs*, *kidney*, and *bone*, occurs at a late stage. These tumours are, however, highly radiosensitive and the *five-year survival rate is over 90 per cent*.

Choriocarcinoma

These are germ cell tumours showing *trophoblastic differenti-ation*: they are often combined with other malignant germ cell elements but pure ovarian choriocarcinomas are occasionally encountered. In women of reproductive age it is usually imposs-ible to tell whether such a neoplasm is *a germ cell tumour*, a metastasis from *a uterine choriocarcinoma*, or a tumour arising

from the *placental tissue of an ectopic ovarian pregnancy*. In pre-menarchal and post-menopausal patients this problem does not arise and here an origin from ovarian germ cells can be readily accepted. The histological appearances of such tumours are identical to those of *gestational uterine choriocarcinomas* and both *cytotrophoblast* and *syncytiotrophoblast* are present; these tumours secrete hCG and may therefore induce *precocious isosexual pseudopuberty* in young girls, this hormone also serving as an excellent tumour marker for monitoring response to therapy. Ovarian choriocarcinomas respond poorly to the chemotherapeutic regime which is so successful for uterine gestational choriocarcinomas and they are associated with *a very poor prognosis*.

Yolk sac tumours

These rare neoplasms, also known as *endodermal sinus tumours*, represent neoplastic germ cell differentiation along extra-embryonic lines into *mesoblast* and *yolk sac endoderm*; they share with yolk sac structures the ability to secrete *α-fetoprotein* (AFP).

Yolk sac tumours form large masses showing conspicuous haemorrhage, necrosis, and microcystic change. Their histo-logical appearances are very complex (Fig. 21.124) but there is characteristically a loose, vacuolated labyrinthine network containing microcysts lined by flattened cells together with *Schiller–Duval bodies*, these having a mesenchymal core con-taining a central capillary and an epithelial investment of cu-boidal or columnar cells. A glandular pattern is often seen and there may be *hepatoid* or *endodermal differentiation*. *Eosinophilic hyaline droplets* are present in nearly all yolk sac tumours and these consist predominantly of AFP.

Yolk sac tumours occur predominantly in girls aged between 4 and 20 years, present solely with non-specific tumour symp-toms, and are highly aggressive neoplasms which spread rapidly within the abdomen and to distant sites. Their pre-viously appalling prognosis has been much improved by the

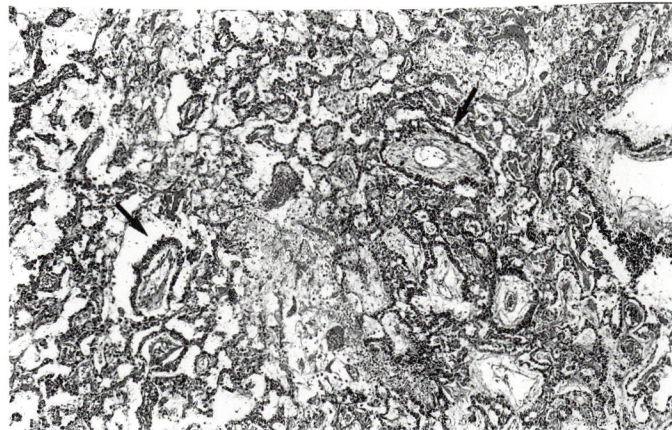

Fig. 21.124 Yolk sac tumour of the ovary. In this area there are several of the typical vascular structures, the Schiller–Duval bodies, which are characteristic of this neoplasm (arrows). Elsewhere the neoplasm forms a delicate mesh and small cystic structures.

introduction of effective chemotherapy and the prognosis is now relatively hopeful in a substantial proportion of cases. The progress of the tumour, its response to chemotherapy, and the development of recurrences can all be monitored by serial estimations of serum AFP levels.

Teratomas

These are germ cell neoplasms showing differentiation along embryonic lines. In most there is a *melange* of tissues but in some, known as *monophyletic teratomas*, there is differentiation along only a single tissue pathway, e.g. solely into thyroid tissue. The terms 'benign' and 'malignant' are not truly applicable to teratomas, for the prognosis of any individual neoplasm is determined not by the usual criteria of malignancy but by the degree of maturity of its constituent tissues, those in which all the components are fully mature behaving in a benign fashion and increasing degrees of tissue immaturity being associated with a progressive tendency towards the neoplasm running a malignant course. Hence teratomas are classed as either 'immature' or 'mature', the term 'malignant' being reserved for those cases in which true malignant change has occurred in a mature teratoma, as, for instance, applies when a squamous cell carcinoma develops in a mature cystic teratoma.

The vast majority of ovarian teratomas are mature and cystic, such neoplasms, often known as 'dermoids', accounting for between 10 and 20 per cent of all ovarian tumours and for 97 per cent of ovarian teratomas, these being usually cystic. Just over 10 per cent of mature cystic teratomas are bilateral, most measure between 5 and 15 cm in diameter and some are pedunculated. They are round or ovoid with a smooth or slightly wrinkled outer surface. On opening, the teratomas are usually unilocular and have a smooth or granular inner surface; there is commonly a focal hillock-like protuberance into the cyst lumen, this being usually known as *Rokitansky's tubercle* or the *mamillary body*. The cysts nearly always contain greasy sebaceous material and hair; *teeth* are present in about a third and may lie loose in the cyst, be embedded in the wall (Fig. 21.125), or can be attached to a rudimentary jaw bone. Histologically, the cyst is almost invariably lined by squamous epithelium and skin appendages are also very common (Fig. 21.126); fat, respiratory-type epithelium, bone, cartilage, neural tissue, gastrointestinal-type epithelium, thyroid, and salivary gland tissue are frequent components. Breast or pituitary tissue is uncommonly encountered and some tissues, such as kidney, pancreas, and spleen, are noticeable for their almost complete absence; there is currently no explanation for this apparent selectivity.

Ninety per cent of mature cystic teratomas are found in women of reproductive age and most are asymptomatic incidental findings. However, some patients suffer complications such as torsion or rupture, both of which present as an acute abdominal emergency. Sometimes a rupture is less acute and slow leakage of cyst contents produces a *chronic chemical peritonitis*. Occasional patients present with a haemolytic anaemia due, it is believed, to the presence of tumour antigens which evoke antibodies that cross-react with erythrocytic antigens.

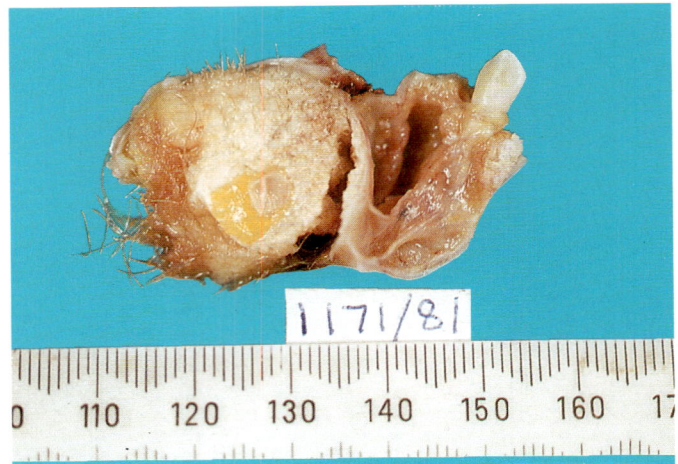

Fig. 21.125 A mature cystic teratoma of the ovary which has been opened to demonstrate a tooth (to the right) and a nodule of yellow adipose tissue covered by hair-bearing skin, to the left.

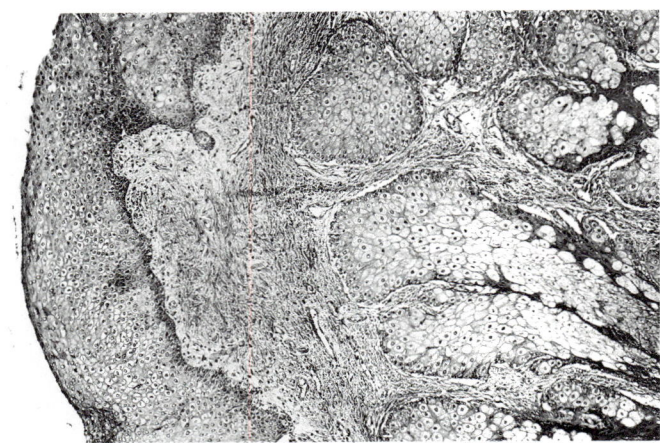

Fig. 21.126 Mature cystic teratoma of the ovary. The cyst is lined by stratified squamous epithelium (to the left) and the wall contains sebaceous glands.

True malignant change occurs in between 1 and 2 per cent of patients with a mature cystic teratoma, this usually taking the form of a squamous cell carcinoma.

A small proportion of mature teratomas are solid rather than cystic but *most solid teratomas are of the immature variety*. These are rare neoplasms which occur principally during the first two decades of life: microscopic examination of such neoplasms reveals an admixture of both mature and immature tissues although immature mesenchyme or neuro-epithelium (Fig. 21.127) tend to be dominant features. Immature teratomas behave in a malignant fashion, implanting on to pelvic peritoneum, metastasizing to retroperitoneal and para-aortic lymph nodes, and being disseminated via the bloodstream to the lungs and liver. The previously extremely poor prognosis of these neoplasms has been transformed by chemotherapy, with approximately 60 per cent of patients now surviving.

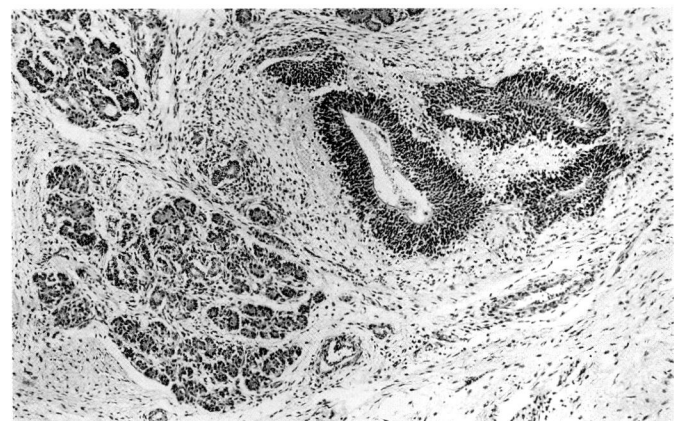

Fig. 21.127 Immature teratoma of the ovary. To the right of the field there are rosette-like structures of immature neuro-epithelial tissue and to the left there are immature glandular structures. The tissues all resemble those that might be seen in the fetus or embryo.

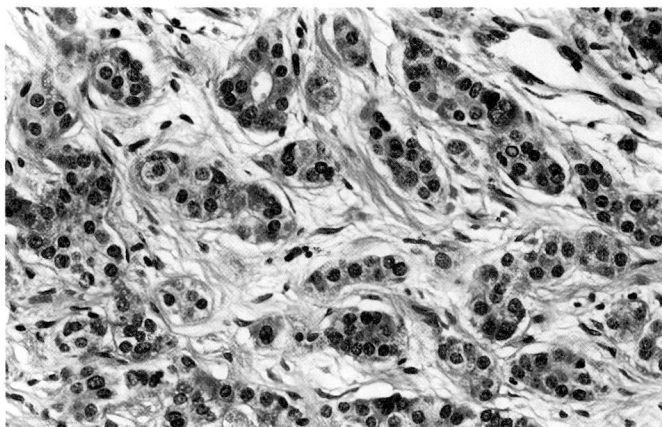

Fig. 21.129 Carcinoid tumour of the ovary. Uniform cells with round nuclei form trabeculae between which there is fibrous tissue.

Monophyletic teratomas, in which differentiation is into only one tissue, are characterized by the *struma ovarii* which consists solely of tissue that is histologically, physiologically, and pharmacologically identical to normal cervical thyroid (Fig. 21.128). This ovarian thyroid tissue may function autonomously to produce a 'pelvic' hyperthyroidism, can show the changes of a lymphocytic thyroiditis, and sometimes undergoes malignant change with a resulting thyroid adenocarcinoma which can metastasize to lymph nodes, liver, and lungs.

Many *carcinoid tumours* of the ovary occur in a mature cystic teratoma, in association with gastrointestinal- or respiratory-type epithelium, but a few are pure and not admixed with any other tissues, these being regarded as *monophyletic teratomas*. Ovarian carcinoid tumours are similar to those that occur in the gastrointestinal tract, usually showing either an insular or a trabecular pattern (Fig. 21.129), but are associated with a high incidence of a typical carcinoid syndrome, this reflecting the ability of these tumours to secrete products directly into the systemic, rather than the portal, circulation.

A *strumal carcinoid* is a rare neoplasm that combines the features of a struma ovarii and a carcinoid tumour. It is thought that the carcinoid component of these neoplasms is derived from the *parafollicular cells* and that it is thus homologous with the *medullary carcinoma of the thyroid gland*.

Tumours of non-specialized ovarian tissue

The only common ovarian tumours of this type are fibromas (already discussed) and leiomyomas.

Steroid cell tumours

These are neoplasms which have an endocrine-type architecture and are formed of cells which resemble *adrenocortical cells*, *Leydig cells*, or *luteinized stromal cells*; all are thought to derive from the ovarian stroma and all may be accompanied by evidence of virilization. Some of the adrenal-like tumours are associated with clinical features suggestive of *Cushing's syndrome* (Fig. 21.130).

Metastatic tumours of the ovary

The ovary is a common site of metastasis, particularly from primary sites in the breast, gastrointestinal tract, and uterus. Thus, ovarian metastases are found in approximately one-third of women dying of malignant disease, and between 10 and 20 per cent of ovarian tumours which appear originally to be primary to that site eventually turn out to be metastatic in nature.

Ovarian metastases are often bilateral, and commonly show extensive areas of haemorrhage and necrosis (Fig. 21.131). Histologically there tends to be a multinodular pattern and the metastases usually reiterate the appearances of the primary tumour.

A particular form of metastatic ovarian neoplasm is the *Krukenberg tumour*. These neoplasms are usually bilateral and solid. The metastatic carcinoma cells occur singly, in clumps or

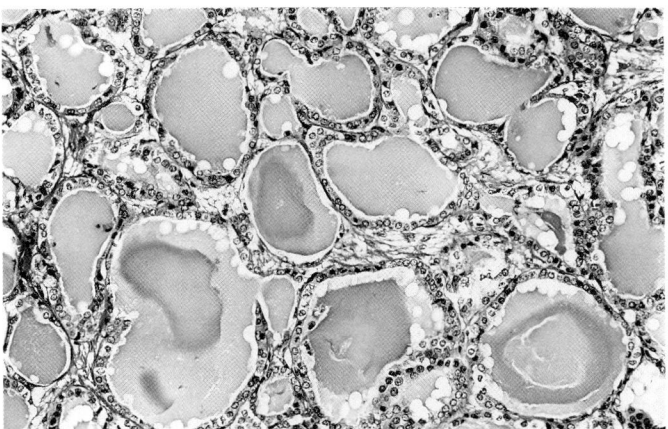

Fig. 21.128 Struma ovarii. The entire mass is composed of mature thyroid tissue.

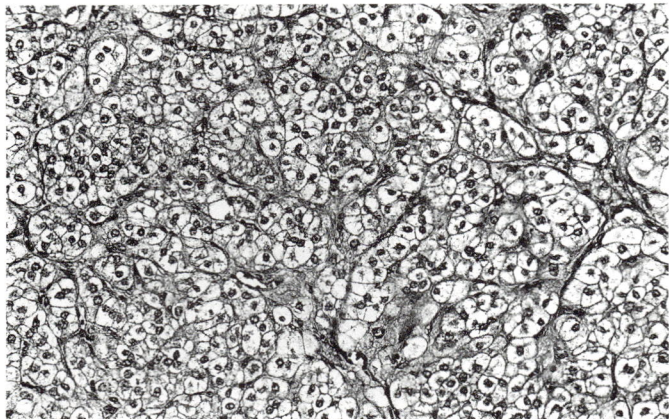

Fig. 21.130 Adrenal-like tumour of the ovary. The entire neoplasm is composed of sheets and islands of cells with round vesicular nuclei and clear, or slightly granular, cytoplasm.

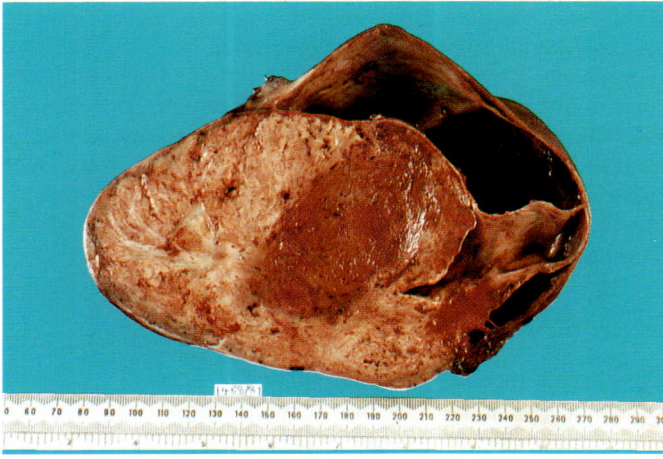

Fig. 21.131 Krukenberg tumour of the ovary. The ovary contains a haemorrhagic, predominantly solid tumour.

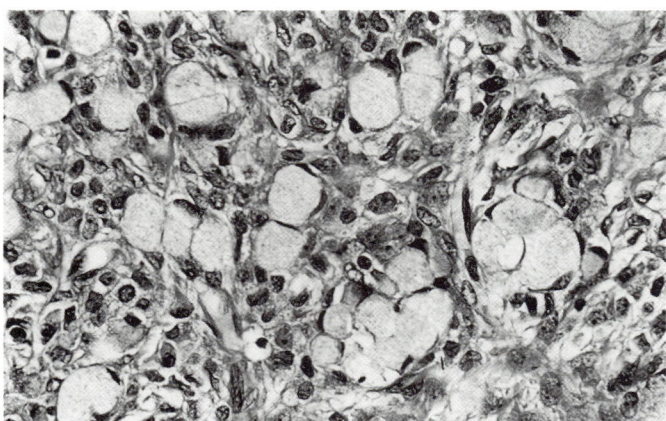

Fig. 21.132 Krukenberg tumour of the ovary. The fibrous ovarian stroma is infiltrated by single cells and cell clusters with eccentric nuclei and vacuolated cytoplasm, so-called signet-ring cells.

sheets, or may form tubules, and a proportion are mucus-containing and have their nuclei displaced laterally to give a 'signet-ring' appearance (Fig. 21.132). The non-neoplastic stromal cells show a degree of pleomorphism and mitotic activity and are often, incorrectly, described as having a pseudo-sarcomatous appearance. Krukenberg tumours are usually metastases from either *gastric or colonic carcinomas*, and the view that gastric carcinomas metastasize to the ovaries by transcoelomic spread is now giving way to the belief that such tumours spread to the ovaries *via the lymphatics*.

21.11 Endometriosis and lesions of the secondary Müllerian system

Tissues normally found in the female genital tract may occur in the peritoneum and subjacent mesenchyme of the pelvis and lower abdomen. The peritoneal mesothelium and the underlying mesenchyme in these areas have the same embryological derivation from coelomic epithelium as does the Müllerian ductal system: hence it is not surprising that these tissues, often called the *secondary Müllerian system*, can differentiate into Müllerian structures.

The most common type of Müllerian tissue found in the pelvic peritoneum is endometrium, but it is by no means certain that endometriotic foci develop *in situ*. Nevertheless the topic of endometriosis will be considered in this section.

21.11.1 Endometriosis

Endometriosis is the presence of ectopic endometrial tissue in an extra-uterine location, and is both common and important. The ectopic tissue occurs most frequently in the ovaries, pouch of Douglas, uterine ligaments, pelvic peritoneum, rectovaginal septum, cervix, appendix, inguinal hernial sacs, and the bowel. Foci of endometriosis are occasionally encountered in surgical scars, in the vulva, at the umbilicus, in the bladder, or in the skin, and exceptional instances of lesions occurring in lymph nodes, kidney, limbs, pleura, and lungs have been recorded.

The pathogenesis of endometriosis is still uncertain but one possible mechanism for its development is the reflux of endometrial tissue through the Fallopian tubes as a result of *retrograde menstruation*, with subsequent implantation on, and growth in, the ovaries, pelvic peritoneum, and uterine ligaments. It has been argued that retrograde menstruation is extremely uncommon and that the shed tissue fragments are dead and thus incapable of further growth; nevertheless, the following facts may be marshalled to support this concept.

1. Retrograde menstruation is, in fact, quite common and is frequently observed at laparoscopy.

2. The distribution of endometriosis in the pelvis is that which would be expected if the endometrial tissue were regurgitated via the tube.

3. Women with congenital obstruction of the lower genital tract tend to have severe endometriosis; in patients with a bifid uterus with drainage from one side only obstructed, endometriosis tends to occur only on that side in which outflow is dammed back.

4. Animal experiments have shown that endometrial tissue shed through an artificially created uteropelvic fistula implants and grows on the pelvic peritoneum.

5. Scar endometriosis following uterine surgery appears to be clearly an implantation phenomenon.

An alternative, but not mutually exclusive, view is that, in the pelvis at least, endometriosis arises as a result of *endometrial metaplasia of the peritoneal serosa*. This is a feasible hypothesis and it may well be that, in fact, such metaplasia is induced by contact with regurgitated fragments of endometrium which, after initiating the metaplastic process, subsequently die and are absorbed. The existence of endometriotic foci in lymph nodes and in distant sites, such as the lung, can clearly not be explained by this mechanism and hence lymphatic or haematogenous dissemination of endometrium must be invoked in such cases. It is, indeed, almost certain that there is no single pathogenetic mechanism that applies to all cases of endometriosis.

If, however, retrograde menstruation occurs in most women, the question arises as to why some women develop implants and others do not. There is increasing, although largely circumstantial, evidence that immunological malfunction may be involved in this selectivity, and there may also be a genetic factor.

The pathology of endometriosis is, in essence, simple, for the only diagnostic criterion is the presence of histologically recognizable endometrial glands and stroma in an ectopic site (Fig. 21.133). Unfortunately, however, the situation is complicated by the tendency towards haemorrhage that is so characteristic a feature of endometriosis. Bleeding into the lesion itself can cause considerable damage and a 'self-destruction' of the endometrial tissue, thus destroying the specific histological findings. Furthermore, haemorrhage into the surrounding tissues releases free iron which is intensely fibrogenic and promotes dense adhesions that tend to obscure the primary lesion.

The early stages of ovarian endometriosis appear to the naked eye as reddish-blue surface implants, which may be raised or dimpled and can measure from 1 to 5 mm across. It is usual for tiny cysts to appear and these progressively enlarge and grow into the ovarian tissue, usually reaching a size of 2–5 cm across but occasionally attaining a diameter of up to 10 cm. The cysts have a smooth or granular lining which is brownish-yellow and their walls, originally thin, become eventually thick and fibrotic: their content of old, semi-fluid or inspissated, blood commonly has a dark brown or black appearance, a feature which has led to the use of the terms 'chocolate' or 'tarry' cyst (Fig. 21.134). There is a marked tendency for blood to leak out from endometriotic cysts and this results in the formation of firm adhesions which bind the enlarged ovary down to the posterior surface of either the broad ligament or the uterus; any attempt at separating the ovary from these structures leads to an escape of brown or black cyst contents. Peritubal adhesions are frequently seen and the tubes may be kinked and distorted; the tubal ostia are, however, usually patent and the tubal lumen is rarely obstructed.

The histological diagnosis of ovarian endometriosis is readily made if endometrial glands and stroma are still present in recognizable form in the lesion. It is, however, by no means unusual for the endometrial lining of the cysts either to be so attenuated as to be unrecognizable as such, or to be largely or completely lost (Fig. 21.135). If the endometrial lining has been totally destroyed, the appearances will be those of a simple haemorrhagic cyst lined by granulation tissue and with a fibrous wall in which aggregates of iron-containing macrophages are usually present. Under these circumstances it is justifiable to conclude that the appearances are 'compatible with a diagnosis of endometriosis' or even to make a diagnosis of 'presumptive endometriosis'. Any endometrial tissue that is present may show the full range of normal cyclical changes but can appear either to be

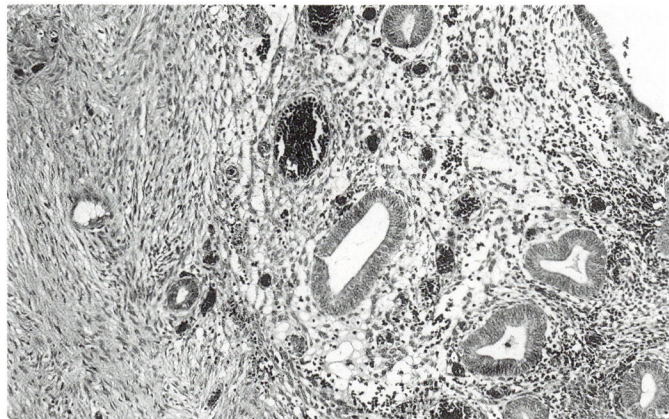

Fig. 21.133 Endometriosis of the ovary. There is a focus of inactive endometrial tissue on the ovarian surface.

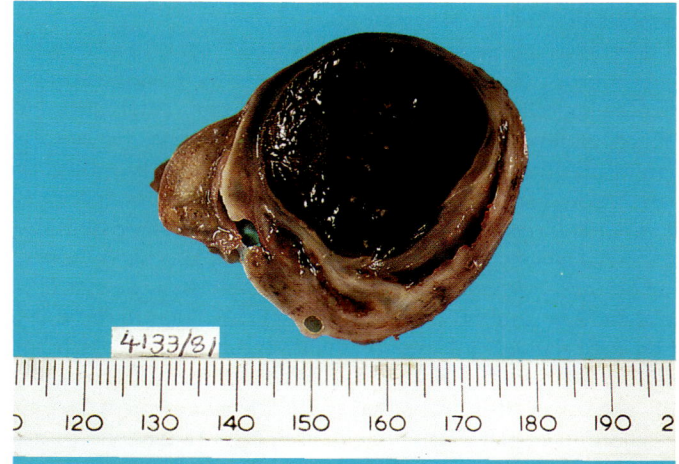

Fig. 21.134 Endometriosis of the ovary. The ovary contains a classical 'chocolate cyst' filled with tarry, altered blood.

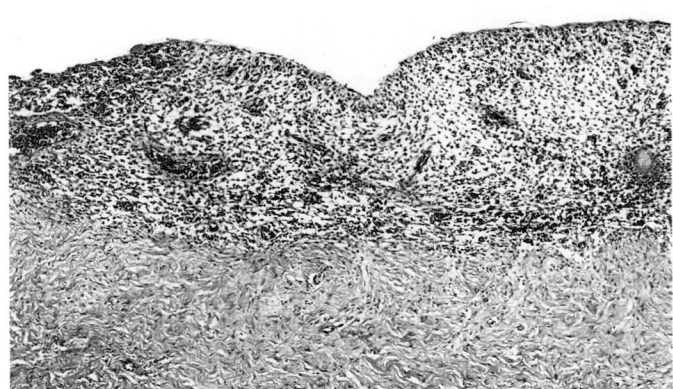

Fig. 21.135 The wall of an endometriotic cyst. The cyst is lined by non-specific granulation tissue and endometrial stroma, and the wall, below, is composed of fibrous tissue.

inactive or to show only proliferative activity; under the latter circumstances there may be a progression to a simple or atypical hyperplasia.

Extraovarian pelvic endometriosis, e.g. in the uterosacral and round ligaments, pouch of Douglas, rectovaginal septum, or on the surface of the uterus, is seen as multiple bluish-red nodules, patches, or cysts, almost invariably with accompanying fibrous adhesions. The lesions are usually small but ligamentous foci may attain a size sufficient to be easily palpable, and endometriotic foci in the rectovaginal septum cannot only lead to fixation of the rectum but can extend into the vaginal vault or the rectum to form small haemorrhagic nodules or polypi.

Women with endometriosis commonly complain of pelvic and back pain just before and during the menstrual period, deep pain on sexual intercourse, and rectal discomfort or bleeding. Recurrent hormonally induced swelling of foci in the uterosacral ligaments is thought to account for the perimenstrual pain, whereas similar swelling and engorgement of lesions in the rectovaginal septum are considered to be responsible for dyspareunia and rectal symptoms.

Infertility is common, occurring in 30–40 per cent of women with the disease. The mechanisms by which endometriosis reduces reproductive capacity are, however, enigmatic, for even a minimal degree of endometriosis is associated with a significant incidence of infertility. Tubal kinking, deformity, or obstruction, because of either *perisalpingeal adhesions* or *fibrosis of intramural endometriotic foci*, is the exception rather than the rule, most women with endometriosis having fully patent tubes. Furthermore, although tubo-ovarian adhesions may cause fimbrial fixation and thus impair access of the ovum to the tube, these are relatively uncommon findings. A disturbance of tubal motility has been invoked as a causal factor in reducing fertility, this being variously attributed to muscle spasm secondary to dyspareunia or pelvic irritation, perisalpingeal adhesions, or the secretion of prostaglandins by ectopic foci of endometrium.

This failure to find an obvious mechanical factor responsible for reducing fertility in women suffering from endometriosis

has, in recent years, directed attention to the possibility of ovarian malfunction. There is little doubt that virtually all women with endometriosis show normal cyclical changes in their endometrium, but it has been suggested that many who are infertile suffer from the 'luteinized unruptured follicle syndrome'. However, others have found this abnormality to occur no more frequently in women with endometriosis than in those not suffering from this disease. Most recently an auto-immune hypothesis has been invoked, it being argued that ectopic foci of endometrium expose the body to tissue antigens which are normally lost during menstruation, with consequent formation of *anti-endometrial antibodies*.

Whether an auto-immune endometritis actually exists in cases of endometriosis, and the possible relationship of such an endometritis to infertility, are questions still being explored. Recently attention has also been paid to the peritoneal macrophages as a cause of infertility in women with endometriosis. In patients with pelvic lesions these macrophages are unduly numerous and have an unusual avidity for ingesting spermatozoa. It has been argued that these cells enter the tubes and engulf the spermatozoa.

Endometriosis can undergo malignant change and in ovarian foci this change is preceded by atypical hyperplasia; very occasionally, an *in-situ adenocarcinoma* is encountered. Overt malignant change gives rise to an *endometrioid adenocarcinoma*, which is usually of the conventional variety, though any of the many morphological variants of this type of neoplasm can also arise in endometriotic foci. Extraovarian endometriosis can also, uncommonly, undergo neoplastic change and give rise to an endometrioid type of adenocarcinoma in such sites as the uterine ligaments, pouch of Douglas, rectovaginal septum, or bladder.

21.11.2   Endosalpingiosis

Small cystic nodules lined by tubal-type epithelium and often containing *psammoma-bodies* may be found scattered on the surface of the uterus, on the pelvic peritoneum, and in the omentum (Fig. 21.136). This condition of endosalpingiosis has been attributed to the displacement of tubal tissue, but it is more probable that it is due to *multifocal tubal metaplasia of the mesothelium*. The principal significance of endosalpingiosis is that the lesions may be misinterpreted as metastases from a serous adenocarcinoma of the ovary, a mistake that can be avoided by noting the benign nature of the epithelium. Proliferative changes can, however, occur in foci of endosalpingiosis and these can progress to a *primary serous adenocarcinoma* in the peritoneum or omentum.

21.11.3   Endocervicosis

Cysts lined by endocervical-type epithelium are occasionally found in the pelvic peritoneum. These can, very rarely, give rise to benign or malignant mucinous neoplasms which are histologically identical to their more common ovarian counterparts.

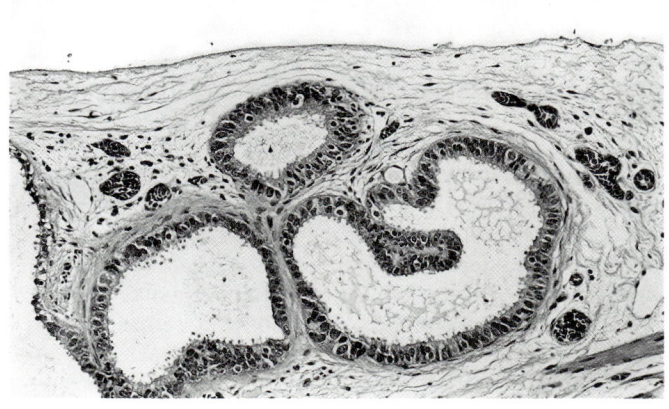

Fig. 21.136 Endosalpingiosis of the peritoneum. A cluster of glands lined by epithelium of tubal type lying within the subserosal connective tissue. Note the absence of stroma which characterizes endometriosis.

21.12 Abnormalities related to pregnancy

21.12.1 Abortion

Any pregnancy which terminates spontaneously during the early months of gestation is considered as an abortion, between 10 and 15 per cent of established conceptuses being spontaneously aborted.

The aetiology of abortion is still poorly understood but factors such as genital tract infection and congenital uterine abnormalities are closely correlated with a high risk of abortion. Psychological stress, submucous leiomyomas, uterine retroversion, occupational exposure to toxins, alcohol ingestion, and endocrine disturbances have all been implicated, with varying degrees of conviction, as causal factors in abortions. In some women who abort repetitively there may be an immunological fault in so far as they appear to be unable to produce blocking antibodies which inhibit the effect of maternal cytotoxic lymphocytes against placental antigens of paternal origin. It has been suggested that this is because of an unusual degree of sharing of HLA antigens between the mother and father, to a degree that the mother fails to recognize the paternal antigens as being alien and does not therefore mount a protective immune response.

It is, however, becoming increasingly clear that in most early abortions the fetus is abnormal. The incidence of obvious fetal malformation is much higher in aborted fetuses than in full-term infants and, indeed, some embryos are so malformed that they appear only as nodules or cylinders. Quite apart from malformations, however, a very high proportion (50–60 per cent) of abortions during the first 8 weeks of pregnancy are of chromosomally abnormal fetuses, the most important chromosomal abnormalities in this respect being XO monosomy, trip-loidy, tetraploidy, and autosomal trisomy. It must be realized, however, that neither a fetal malformation nor a chromosomal abnormality causes an abortion, for it is quite possible for an abnormal fetus with, for example, anencephaly or XO monosomy, to be delivered at term. Fetal abnormalities therefore predispose to, but do not cause, abortion.

21.12.2 Ectopic pregnancy

In approximately 1 per cent of all recognized pregnancies the conceptus implants in a site other than the uterine cavity. The vast majority (95–97 per cent) of such ectopic gestations occur in the Fallopian tube (Fig. 21.137), less common sites being the ovary, cervix, and peritoneal cavity; occasional cases of implantation occur in the vagina, liver, or spleen.

Tubal pregnancies are predisposed to by any factor which impairs the ability of the tube to transport the fertilized ovum. Hence, congenital abnormalities of the tube, failed tubal sterilization, the use of a progesterone-only contraceptive pill, salpingitis isthmica nodosa, reconstructive tubal surgery, and, most importantly, post-inflammatory tubal damage are all associated with an increased incidence of tubal pregnancy. In about 50 per cent of such pregnancies the tube is, however, fully normal. It has been argued that in such cases conception occurred during a cycle in which there was delayed ovulation and a short, inadequate luteal phase: hence, when the fertilized ovum reached the uterine cavity it had not yet developed to a stage when it was secreting enough hCG to prevent decay of the corpus luteum and was, during the subsequent menstrual bleeding, flushed back into the tube by a reflux of menstrual blood. This hypothesis is supported by the fact that tubal gestation occurs only in species which menstruate, and by the not uncommon finding of the corpus luteum of pregnancy on the opposite side to that of a tube containing a pregnancy. This latter phenomenon could, however, also be due to transuterine or transperitoneal migration of the fertilized ovum into the contralateral tube

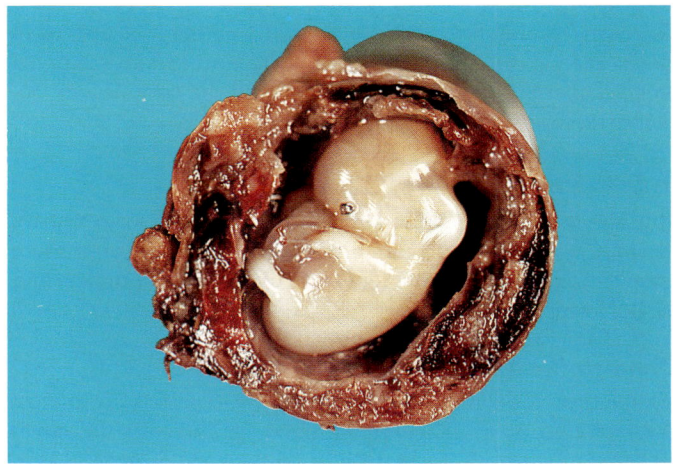

Fig. 21.137 Ectopic gestation. A Fallopian tube which has been opened to show an intraluminal early pregnancy.

where, because of its relatively advanced stage of development, it implants.

If pregnancy occurs in a woman wearing an intra-uterine contraceptive device it will tend to be ectopically situated. This is not because such a device *causes* an ectopic pregnancy: it simply fails to prevent extra-uterine implantation as effectively as it inhibits implantation within the uterus.

Within the tube, the fertilized ovum implants most commonly in the *ampulla*. Implantation occurs in exactly the same manner in the tube as it does in the uterus but, nevertheless, a high proportion of tubal pregnancies abort at an early stage. This may be because the conceptus has implanted on the *plicae*, which offer an inadequate site for placentation, or because trophoblastic invasion of the tubal vessels leads to intramural and intraluminal haemorrhage. Following early abortion the products of conception may be retained in the tube as a form of 'chronic ectopic', be expelled via the uterus, or be gradually absorbed.

Tubal rupture complicates about 50 per cent of tubal pregnancies and appears to be due partly to the limited distensibility of the tube and partly to transmural spread of invading extravillous trophoblast with serosal penetration. Rupture is usually acute and is accompanied by intraperitoneal bleeding and the clinical features of an acute abdomen. Less commonly there is a slow leakage of tubal contents and blood from the tube, which results in a gradually enlarging *peritubal haematoma* and causes dense adhesions between the tube and surrounding structures such as omentum and intestines; occasionally the ureters are obstructed by involvement in this peritubal mass.

Tubal rupture is usually accompanied by fetal death but occasionally the fetus retains sufficient attachment to its blood supply to maintain its viability; the trophoblast grows out through the rupture site and forms a secondary placental site in the abdomen or broad ligament. A secondary abdominal pregnancy of this type may proceed virtually to term.

21.12.3   Trophoblastic disease

The term 'trophoblastic disease' should, in theory, be applied to all disorders of the trophoblast but is, by convention, restricted to *hydatidiform moles*, *choriocarcinoma*, and the *placental site trophoblastic tumour*.

Hydatidiform mole

This aberrant form of pregnancy has been known for centuries but only within recent years has it been recognized that there are two fundamentally different types of mole, the complete and partial forms.

Complete hydatidiform mole

Complete moles complicate about 1 in 1500 gestations in most Western countries but are encountered, for currently unknown reasons, much more frequently in many parts of Africa, Asia, and Latin America. They occur particularly at the two extremes of the reproductive era, in women aged less than 18 or more than 40 years, and usually present either as an abortion or as first trimester vaginal bleeding. Unduly rapid uterine enlargement, excessive morning sickness, and the development, during the first trimester, of a pre-eclampsia-like syndrome are other characteristic features.

A complete hydatidiform mole (Fig. 21.138) forms a bulky mass, sometimes weighing as much as 2000 g, which, when *in situ*, fills and distends the uterine cavity; no fetus is present and no normal placental tissue is seen, all the chorionic villi being swollen and distended to give a 'bunch of grapes' appearance. Histologically (Fig. 21.139), the villi are devoid of fetal vessels and are markedly oedematous, many showing central liquefaction. A constant, indeed defining, feature is atypical hyperplasia of the villous trophoblast; some pleomorphism is often apparent in the proliferating trophoblast but it is the pattern, rather than the degree, of proliferation of trophoblastic cells which is atypical, this being either *circumferential or multifocal* in nature rather than, as in the normal first trimester placenta, polar.

Cytogenetic studies have shown that 85 per cent of complete

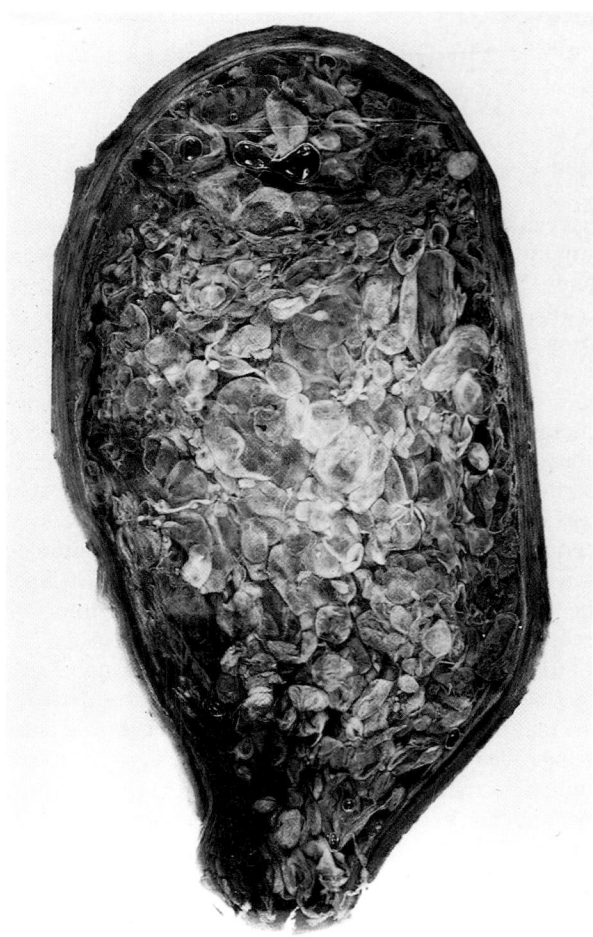

Fig. 21.138 A complete hydatidiform mole. A uterus which has been opened longitudinally to show the 'bunch of grapes-like' structure of a complete hydatidiform mole.

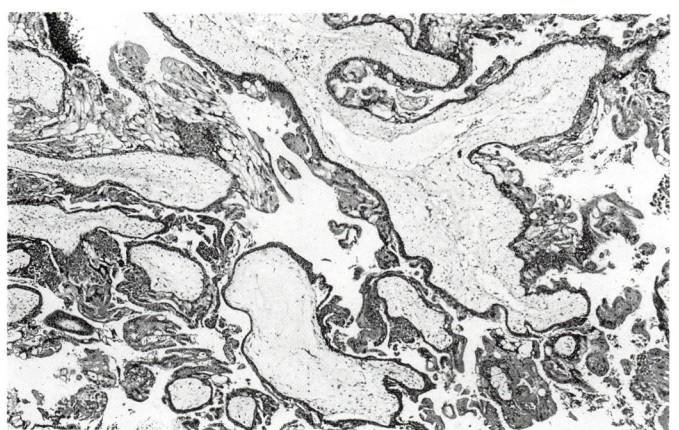

Fig. 21.139 A complete hydatidiform mole. All the villi are abnormal, being surrounded by proliferating trophoblast, and the two largest contain central cisterns, that is, they are vesicular.

hydatidiform moles have a *46XX chromosomal constitution, both X chromosomes being of paternal (androgenetic) origin*: it is thought that this is the result of penetration of a 'dead' ovum, lacking functional maternal DNA, by a single haploid X sperm which then duplicates without cytokinesis. Fifteen per cent of complete moles have, however, a *46XY chromosomal constitution*, both chromosomes again being derived from the father: it is believed that this type of complete mole results from the entry of *two haploid sperms*, one X and the other Y, into an abnormal ovum with subsequent fusion and replication. All XY moles are therefore dispermic (or 'heterologous') and it is now clear that although the vast majority of 46XX moles are *monospermic (homozygous)*, a small proportion resemble the XY moles in being *dispermic*, presumably because of the entry of two, rather than one, haploid X sperms into a defective ovum. This division of complete moles into *heterozygous* and *homozygous forms* is of more than academic interest for it has been shown that the dispermic moles are more likely to be followed by sequelae such as persistent trophoblastic disease (see below) than are their monospermic counterparts.

Hydatidiform moles are a particular form of abortion rather than, as is often implied, a benign neoplasm. Nevertheless, women who have had a complete mole have a much greater risk of subsequently developing a choriocarcinoma (in the region of 2–3 per cent) than do women who have had a normal pregnancy. Attempts have been made to identify those moles most likely to be followed by a choriocarcinoma by grading the degree of trophoblastic hyperplasia, it being maintained that the more marked the degree of trophoblastic proliferation the greater is the risk of eventual choriocarcinoma. Attempts to apply this principle in practice have, however, failed to confirm that the histological features of a complete mole are of any prognostic value and, indeed, reliance upon morphological criteria is potentially dangerous, leading to a false sense of security in some cases and to overtreatment in others. It is now agreed that all women should, after evacuation of a mole be followed up

with serial estimations of human chorionic gonadotrophin (hCG) levels, surveillance being maintained until, and for up to two years after, levels of this placental hormone have returned to normal.

Women in whom hCG values remain elevated, or increase, during follow-up are classed as having 'persistent trophoblastic disease'. This condition may be due to the persistence of residual molar villi, or proliferating trophoblast, the development of an invasive mole (see below), or the development of a choriocarcinoma. In most cases no attempt is made to establish a specific diagnosis and the patients are treated, empirically but successfully, with a short course of chemotherapy.

Partial hydatidiform mole

In a partial mole, vesicular change affects only a proportion of the villous population of a placenta. The macroscopic appearances are therefore those of a largely normal placenta in which, however, a variable number of distended villi are apparent (Fig. 21.140); a gestational sac and a fetus are often, though not invariably, present. Histologically (Fig. 21.141), only a proportion of the villi are distended by oedema fluid, these being intermingled with fully normal villi. The scattered vesicular villi have a markedly irregular outline and show atypical trophoblastic proliferation, usually multifocal in nature and commonly less marked than that seen in a complete mole.

The majority of partial hydatidiform moles are associated with a *fetal triploidy*, a minority having a *tetraploid, trisomic,* or *diploid chromosomal constitution*. Not all triploid conceptions result in moles, and it is now known that if the additional chromosomes are of maternal origin a normal placenta is more likely to result, whereas if the excess chromosomal load is paternally derived a partial mole will probably develop.

The natural history of a partial mole and the magnitude of the risk of subsequent choriocarcinoma have not yet been adequately defined, but it is now clear that a partial mole can be

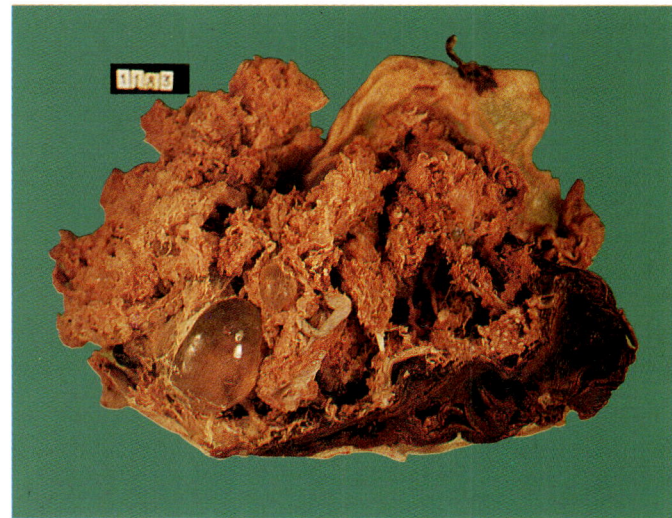

Fig. 21.140 A partial hydatidiform mole. Most of the placental tissue is unremarkable but to the lower left there is a single vesicular villus.

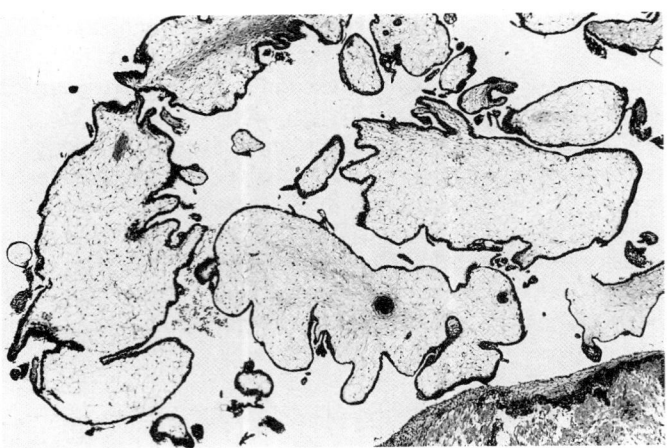

Fig. 21.141 A partial hydatidiform mole. The villi vary in size, some being normal and some large and irregular in outline, the so-called 'Norwegian fjord' appearance.

invasive and that the incidence of persistent trophoblastic disease following evacuation of a partial mole is as high as that after a complete mole. Hence women who have had a partial mole should be followed up in exactly the same way as those with complete moles.

Invasive hydatidiform mole

In 5–10 per cent of moles, either complete or partial, molar villi invade the myometrium, sometimes even penetrating the uterine wall to extend into the broad ligament. Myometrial vessels may also be breached by the invasive villous tissue. A deeply invasive mole usually becomes clinically apparent several weeks after apparently complete evacuation of a mole from the uterus, the patient commonly presenting with haemorrhage. Hysterectomy at this stage will reveal intramyometrial haemorrhagic foci and, on microscopy, vesicular villi are seen in the uterine wall and within myometrial vessels. The villous tissue within the vessels can be transported as emboli to sites such as the lung or vagina where they may continue to grow, pulmonary nodules usually being only apparent radiologically but vaginal lesions presenting as haemorrhagic submucosal nodules. Biopsy of these extra-uterine lesions will show molar villi, a finding which excludes a diagnosis of choriocarcinoma.

An invasive mole is not a maligant lesion. Normal placental villi can penetrate deeply into the myometrium, as in the condition of *placenta increta*, and trophoblastic transportation to extra-uterine sites occurs in every pregnancy. An invasive mole simply represents, therefore, a molar version of placenta increta with associated trophoblastic deportation.

In practice, the diagnosis of an invasive mole is now largely obsolete, for patients with this type of mole are usually diagnosed as having persistent trophoblastic disease, prior to development of symptoms, and are treated by chemotherapy.

Choriocarcinoma

This is a *malignant neoplasm of trophoblast* and has a unique status because, being of fetal origin, it is the only human tumour which is, in effect, an *allograft*. Choriocarcinoma is extremely rare in Western countries, complicating approximately 1 in 45 000 pregnancies, although, as with hydatidiform mole, it is much more common in many parts of Africa, Asia, and South America. Approximately 50 per cent of choriocarcinomas follow a hydatidiform mole, 30 per cent develop after an abortion, and 20 per cent occur after a normal pregnancy. The time-interval between the antecedent pregnancy and the development of a choriocarcinoma is very variable, ranging from a few months to 15 years. Most choriocarcinomas occur, however, in women aged less than 35 years.

A choriocarcinoma forms single or multiple haemorrhagic nodules within the uterus. These are well delineated and consist of a central area of haemorrhagic necrosis and a peripheral rim of viable tumour tissue. The central necrosis is due to the fact that a choriocarcinoma has no intrinsic blood supply, relying for its oxygenation and nutrition on its ability to invade and permeate the maternal vasculature. Histologically (Fig. 21.142) the tumour has a pattern which recapitulates that of the early implanting blastocyst, central cores of *cytotrophoblastic cells* being surrounded by a peripheral rim of *syncytiotrophoblast*. The trophoblastic cells do not differ significantly from those of a normal blastocyst and mitotic activity is rarely excessive. Villi are not present in a choriocarcinoma and, indeed, the presence of villous structures refutes this diagnosis.

A malignant trophoblast's capacity to invade vessels offers an adequate implantation for the *primarily vascular dissemination* of this tumour, spread occurring at an early stage to the *brain*, *lungs*, *liver*, *kidney*, and *gastrointestinal tract*. It is therefore not surprising that choriocarcinoma was, in the past, a highly lethal neoplasm with a mortality little short of 100 per cent and death occurring in months rather than in years. For no other neoplasm, however, has the advent of chemotherapy more radically altered the prognosis, 85 per cent of patients now being permanently cured with cytotoxic drugs.

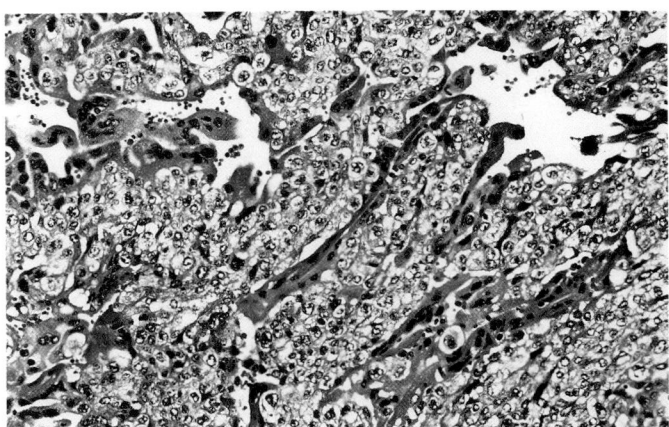

Fig. 21.142 Choriocarcinoma. The neoplasm is composed of two types of cell, the darkly staining syncytiotrophoblast and the cytotrophoblast in which the cytoplasm is pale-staining.

Placental site trophoblastic tumour

This neoplasm originates from the extravillous trophoblastic cells which are normally present in the decidua and myometrium of the placental bed, these forming the *placental site reaction*. A placental site trophoblastic tumour usually occurs after a normal gestation and symptoms such as abnormal bleeding or amenorrhoea become apparent months or years after the pregnancy.

The tumour forms a nodular tan or yellow mass which shows little necrosis or haemorrhage. Histologically (Fig. 21.143), trophoblastic cells, predominantly of the mononuclear cytotrophoblastic type, infiltrate between myometrial fibres in sheets, cords, and islands; some multinucleated cells are usually present but the bilaminar pattern of a choriocarcinoma is not seen. Vascular permeation by tumour cells is seen but the massive intravascular growth typical of a choriocarcinoma is not apparent.

Most of these tumours are cured by simple hysterectomy, but about 10 per cent extend beyond the uterus and behave in a malignant fashion. In general, neoplasms with an abundance of mitotic figures are most likely to pursue a malignant course but there are no histological features that can predict malignant behaviour with certainty. Treatment of malignant cases is currently unsatisfactory, for these neoplasms do not respond well to the therapeutic regime that has met with such success in the treatment of choriocarcinoma.

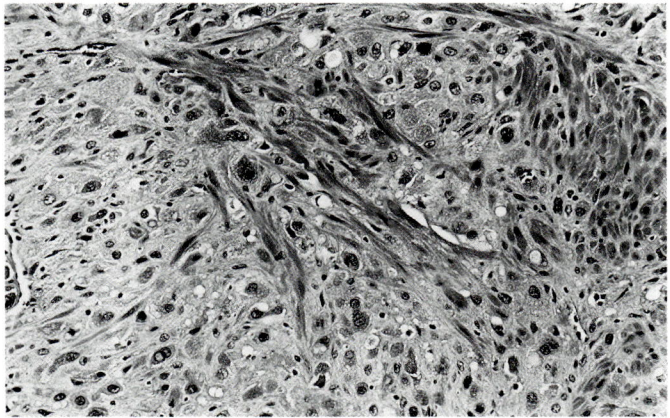

Fig. 21.143 Placental site trophoblastic tumour. The myometrium is infiltrated by cords and sheets of a large extravillous trophoblast. Note the absence of necrosis and haemorrhage.

21.13   Further reading

The literature on this field of pathology is vast and it would be invidious to select individual papers. Those wishing to pursue this subject in greater depth are referred to a number of monographs.

Buckley, C. H. and Fox, H. (1989). *Biopsy pathology of the endometrium.* Chapman and Hall, London.

Coleman, D. V. and Evans, D. M. D. (1988). *Biopsy pathology and cytology of the cervix.* Chapman and Hall, London.

Fox, H. (ed.) (1987). *Haines and Taylor: Obstetrical and gynaecological pathology* (3rd edn). Churchill Livingstone, Edinburgh.

Fu, Y. S. and Reagan, J. W. (1989). *Pathology of the uterine cervix, vagina and vulva.* Saunders, Philadelphia.

Kurman, R. J. (ed.) (1987). *Blaustein's pathology of the female genital tract* (3rd edn). Springer-Verlag, New York.

Ridley, C. M. (ed.) (1988). *The vulva.* Churchill Livingstone, Edinburgh.

Russell, P. and Bannatyne, P. (1989). *Surgical pathology of the ovaries.* Churchill Livingstone, Edinburgh.

Wilkinson, E. J. (ed.) (1987). *Pathology of the vulva and vagina.* Churchill Livingstone, Edinburgh.

22

The breast

22

The breast

22.1 Breast structure, biology, and pathology

Thomas J. Anderson and David L. Page

22.1.1 Introduction

The human breasts are non-functional and physically not prominent in men, while in women they represent motherhood, sexuality, and infant nutrition. These special features heighten the tragedy and challenge of treating breast cancer, a major cause of death for women in their forties in Europe and North America. Although a full range of infectious diseases and unique benign diseases affect the breasts, it is the various aspects of breast cancer and its many mimickers which dominate breast disease. Indeed, most benign breast conditions are of interest because they may mimic cancers, not because of any intrinsic infringement on the quality of life. Other conditions have attracted interest because they are related to an elevated tendency for the development of cancer. Note that emphasis on the dominance of cancer in the concerns of breast disease ignores the huge role of the breast in human infant nutrition. Milk is considered elsewhere: it is important in paediatric nutrition (Chapter 10), and in immunology because the antibodies present in mothers' milk have a role in infant health, most evidently in imparting passive immunity in the neonatal period (see Chapter 4).

Accentuating the psychological impact of both the fear and actuality of breast cancer are a unique combination of features that are central to a woman's confrontation with the threat of that cancer, and the therapeutic decisions which attend the diagnosis. As in few other malignancies, many more women are frightened by the likelihood of having or getting breast cancer than actually contract it. This is largely because breast cancer is relatively common, and because cosmetic concern relevant to the breasts is frequent. Most women know someone who has had breast cancer, so that it is part of the personal experience of most women. With fear of death on one hand, and fear of mutilation with loss of a symbol of feminity on the other, decisions about therapy which involves complete or partial removal of the breasts are both personally threatening and challenging to the decision-making process. Secondly, whereas decision-making in the treatment of breast cancer was oversimplified for many years, there are now many options. For over 70 years, until the 1970s, the only treatment for carcinoma of the breast, thought to be one disease, was mastectomy, with some medical centres adding radiotherapy. Currently various types of partial mastectomy and combinations of radiotherapy and chemotherapy are available, often with no critically demonstrable differences in their survival efficacy.

Of all the major carcinomas affecting women, breast cancers begin to take a toll at an earlier age, are the major cause of death for women at ages 35–54, and kill 30–50 per cent of those so diagnosed (Miller 1987). When controlled for age, breast cancer accounts for about 27 deaths per 100 000 women per year in western Europe and North America (Fig. 22.1). The incidence has been much lower in other parts of the world, but is rising in many countries, such as Japan. With this magnitude of risk of mortality and morbidity, coupled with the concern of deformity and threat to body image, it becomes clear why there is a dominance of concern for cancer, its mimickers, and its correlates in diseases of the breast. Although the specifics will be repeated below, it is appropriate to emphasize here that breast cancer is not a homogeneous disease entity, rather there are many types of breast cancer which differ at the least in

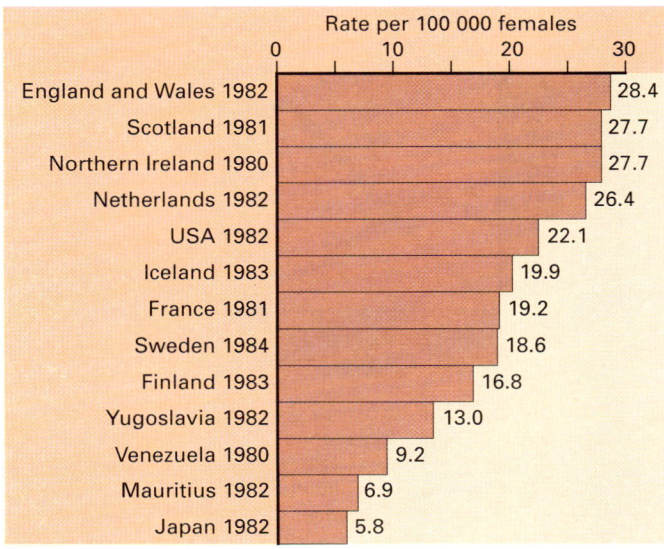

Fig. 22.1 Standardized breast cancer mortality rates for a number of countries. (Source: *Breast cancer screening: Forrest Report* 1986.)

their threat of life. This acknowledges a recurring theme in oncology: it is not enough to characterize a given patient with the basic diagnosis of cancer. Rather, the type, size, extent of spread, etc. are vital to predicting prognosis and affecting therapeutic approaches. Thus, each tale has a beginning and an end, but few are similar one to another.

Clinical presentations of breast diseases are pain, presence of a dominant lump, or abnormal nipple discharge. Diffuse pain, present in both breasts, in a cyclical pattern related to the menses is relatively common. Local pain may be associated with some benign conditions noted below, but has no favoured relation to cancer. However, rarely, pain may be noted as the presenting symptom of a carcinoma. The palpation of a lump in the breast may be related only to the irregularity of placement of elements varying in density within the breast, and the lump may vary with the menstrual cycle. However, any dominant mass in the breast is suspect of being a carcinoma and should be biopsied if it remains unchanged or enlarges over a short period of time. This biopsy may be surgical or by a needle aspiration. Other than female sex, age is a determinant in many mammary conditions. The importance of age for carcinoma is detailed below, but another factor of the interaction of age and breast disease is the likely diagnosis of dominant lumps within the breast. These are most likely fibroadenoma in the third decade, fibrocystic change in the fifth decade, and carcinoma in the seventh decade (Fig. 22.2).

Radiography of the breast (mammography) is not an absolute way of determining the nature of a palpable lump because 10–20 per cent of clinically palpable carcinomas do not appear suspicious for carcinoma by mammography. Mammography is useful in further characterizing most lesions detected by palpation as well as surveying the rest of the breast, but the major role of mammography is the detection of lesions undetectable by other means. Thus it is not seen primarily as a tool of diagnosis, but rather as a means of detecting lesions that are not palpable. This process of finding lesions not detectable by symptoms and

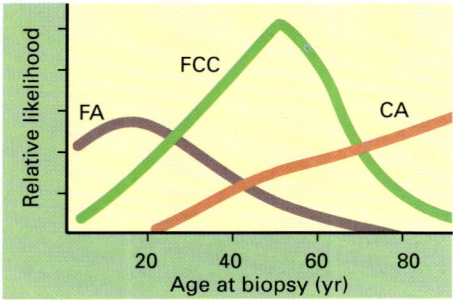

Fig. 22.2 Age incidence of benign and malignant breast disease. Relative incidence of fibrocystic change (FCC), fibroadenoma (FA), and carcinoma (CA) of the breast related to age. Absolute numbers are not given because they depend on the frequency of breast biopsy; the ratio of benign to malignant rises when suspicion of cancer in poorly defined lumps is high and incidence of biopsy is high. The graph is intended to demonstrate the age dependency of these diagnostic possibilities. (Drawn after Page 1987, with permission.)

signs of physical examination is termed 'screening'. The characteristics of carcinomas detected by screening programmes with mammography differ from those found in the usual clinical manner, i.e. by palpation either by patient or physician (see Section 22.2). Many may be called 'occult' because they were not detected by the usual means, but note that *occult* is a relative term, defined by the modalities of detection being discussed. 'Small' and 'early' are also terms of little use because they do not recognize other more useful variables in qualifying carcinomas for prognostic purposes which are discussed below. Thus, the mammographically detected lesions may be smaller than palpable cancers on the average, but their rates of growth, depth within the breast, and relative tendency to metastasize are the major determinants of useful individual characterization.

Another major clinical presentation of breast disease is nipple discharge which is usually benign and most frequently presents as a bilateral condition related to recent pregnancy. When present in middle life, unilateral, and confined to a single ductal opening, nipple discharge when blood-containing is most often associated with ductal papilloma.

22.1.2 Normal breast anatomy, development, and pathophysiology

Anatomy

The breast may be considered at its simplest as a modified sweat gland, but in reality it is an organ of complex arrangement. It is liable to modulation as a result of various physiological stimuli affecting its parenchymal and stromal elements. The basic structure consists of ramifying ducts emanating from the nipple on the skin surface and extending radially outward into a variably contoured fibrous mammary disc enclosed in fat (Fig. 22.3). The ducts have an inner epithelial lining and an outer myoepithelial layer resting on a basement membrane, that is in turn surrounded by fibroblasts, elastin, and collagen. Arising from the ducts are lobules composed of multibranched blind-ending smaller channels enclothed in a loose stroma. These constitute the functioning unit of the breast, the terminal duct lobular unit (TDLU), and usually measure under 1 mm in the mature resting state (Fig. 22.4).

Human beings are unique among mammals in that the organ reaches full resting development of mature lobular components without the stimulus of copulation or pregnancy. These berry-like lobules, numbering many thousands, progress on full differentiation to form the collection of milk-producing acini that empty into the terminal and main branches of the duct system leading to the nipple. The duct system is best considered from its central region at the nipple, where there may be up to 20 or more orifices opening on to the surface. Collected within the core of the nipple, these main ducts descend into more distended collecting sinuses beneath the areola, before continuing more deeply into the breast fat, or more frequently the fibrous tissue element. The mainly dichotomous branching occurs as the ducts extend radially, but the irregularity and overlapping

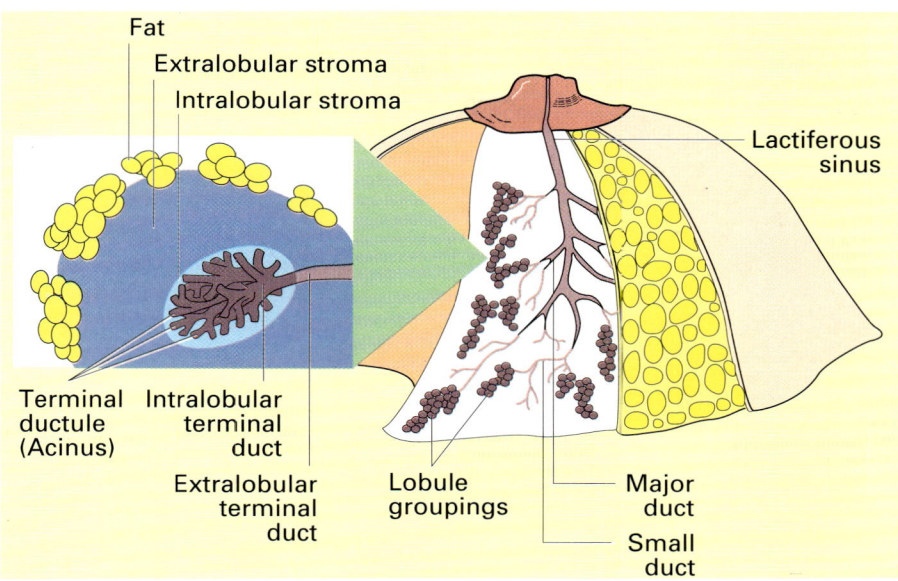

Fig. 22.3 A schematic diagram of the mature breast components, giving a 'window' view of the duct and lobular system connecting with the nipple areolar complex. A blow-up view depicts the resting lobular unit, distinguishing intralobular and extralobular stroma.

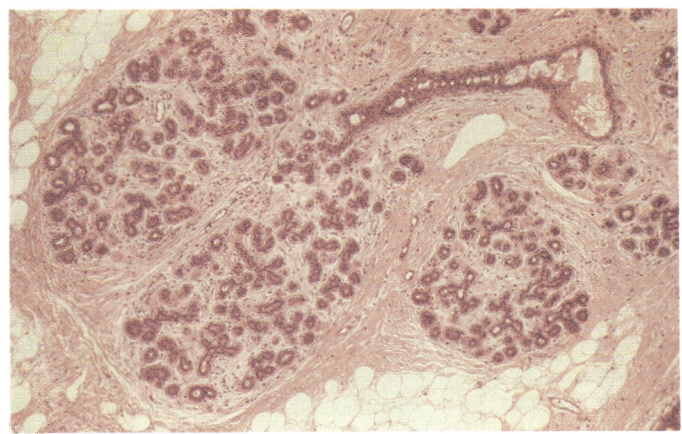

Fig. 22.4 Histological appearance of mature resting breast to illustrate the relationship of terminal duct, lobules, fibrosis, and fat.

nature of this branching process, together with a degree of lobular out-pouching at several levels, results in a highly variable and uneven parenchymal distribution within the mammary disc.

Some consider it convenient to imagine the breast in segments or lobes extending out from the axis of the nipple, but this is only relatively correct, for the duct branchings are frequently overlapping as they swirl and curve in many directions. Perhaps the parenchymal structure is better imagined as an inverted deciduous tree, for in addition to exemplifying the branching complexity, the effect of the seasons can also be likened to the stages of breast alteration through life: development and puberty (spring) maturation, differentiation, and

lactation (summer), involution (autumn), and finally senile atrophy (winter). The complexities of the interrelationship between epithelium and stroma, as well as the precise manner of regulation by hormones and other growth factors is only partially understood (Miller and Anderson 1988). The winter season entails sequential loss of lobular units as the fundamental event in senile involution. The true ducts are relatively spared but even they disappear in the eighth and ninth decades, leaving only fat.

Development

Abnormal development of the breasts, which may produce breasts that are misshapen or of greatly different sizes is unusual. Much more common, but of little concern, is the occasional occurrence of extra-numerary breasts (rare) or nipples (relatively common, and termed 'polythelia'). These extra mammary structures are usually small, having the appearance of small blemishes. They occur in the milk line, from the axilla, along the chest and abdomen, to the upper inguinal area. The milk line is the region where the multiple breasts of other mammals develop.

While recognizing the essential dependence on ovarian function for the development and maturation of the breast, the role of oestrogen and progesterone as the principle regulators is being increasingly questioned in the light of current knowledge. Breast parenchymal structures require a considerably more complex cocktail of stimulants in order to reach and sustain mature development. Menstrual cycles do elicit fluctuating changes in breast epithelial cell appearance and proliferation, but these are distinctly different in character and timing from the endometrial responses to oestrogen and progesterone. Most importantly, mitoses take place in the latter part of the menstrual cycle, long after their disappearance in the endometrium. Also, various steroid hormones affect the breast differently (Anderson *et al.* 1989). However, the variation through the cycle in expression of receptors for these hormones within the epithelial cells confirms their involvement, but suggests a permissive rather than deterministic role. A list of compounds known to influence breast parenchymal development, growth, and differentiation is given in Table 22.1.

Also, modern biological acceptance that autocrine and paracrine mechanisms may be operating leads to awareness that the complete system of control remains to be determined. This realization is particularly relevant when considering the alterations of normal structure that result in disease, the nature of which we are attempting to define and describe. The extent and degree of any alteration is critical to the definition of disease, since the changes exhibit a spectrum that extends from the physiological through to the overtly pathological. Unfortunately, the borders separating them have never been well defined. Nevertheless, elegant studies using subgross stereomicroscopy of chemically cleared breast slices have been instructive (Wellings *et al., 1975*). They have confirmed that most pathological alterations arise from the TDLU and its surroundings, whereas only a few conditions, notably papillomas and duct ectasia, arise solely from the major ducts.

Nomenclature in breast pathophysiology

Discrimination is important between disease and the minor alterations of breast structure that should be considered within the limits of physiological range, either because of minor degree or frequency of occurrence. It is, however, complicated by the varied histopathological nomenclature that has been applied in the past, often regrettably with little discrimination, to the conditions collectively termed 'benign breast disease'. The nomenclature and categorization of breast histopathology terms are therefore appropriate and unavoidable concerns as an introduction to the next section. The variable approaches in current use are either simplistic or elaborate. Although the simplistic approach has the advantage of more rapid assimilation, it has the disadvantage of ignoring the variables that exist to confound such 'artificial' man-made categories, and which may be necessary to facilitate communication between clinicians. It is hoped that a diagrammatic representation of the two approaches might enable a clear appreciation of what consti-

tutes the spectrum of diseases and the overlapping relationships between them as well as with physiological changes. These diagrams depict not just the similar groupings but also provide more detailed identification of various pathological entities, giving some indication of the relationships between them. This latter arrangement offers a broader framework in which the following comments should be considered. Figure 22.5 depicts the first approach and provides the basis for the comments contained in this section. However, the more complex categorization outlined in Fig. 22.6 and glossary will provide a practical perspective of the various patterns and processes found in breast tissue; these constitute the spectrum of separately identifiable conditions from normal, and variants thereof, through benign disorders to the various malignant conditions. It is intended to give an awareness of how they are related or may have affiliations, but must not be regarded as an established 'pedigree' of development or progression. The controversy between 'lumpers' and 'splitters' (simplifiers v. acceptors of the complex) in disease classification (compare Fig. 22.5 with Fig. 22.6) is resolving through awareness of the basic biological processes that result in 'pathological' changes, in contradistinction to mild changes accepted as within normal boundaries (Hughes *et al.* 1989).

22.1.3   Benign conditions

Sclerosing conditions

The lesions described in this section share the feature of excessive activity of the stromal elements, associated in varying degree with increased epithelial cellularity. Consequently, the tissue architecture and consistency are considerably distorted and irregular (mainly on account of the fibrous elements). Such characteristics may lead to suspicion of malignancy, particularly where there is associated calcification on mammography. Naked-eye appearance of surgically removed tissue will depend on the stage of development and the admixture of components, including cystic foci, but is regularly stellate, white and gritty on section. The more creamy-yellow streaks of elastin are characteristic at the centre of radial scars (Fig. 22.7) which are described below.

Sclerosing adenosis

The microscopic appearance of this lesion is perceived at low power as 'lobulocentric', i.e. involving whole lobular units, the extent of the lesion reflecting the number of involved units, with the larger aggregates reaching over 2 cm and giving rise to the term 'adenosis tumour'. Higher-power microscopy reveals the compressed, distorted, and elongated tubules to have the normal two-cell population, at least focally, as well as a distinct basement membrane. Occasionally extension into adjacent perineural spaces will be seen, but is not sinister. Small foci of sclerosing adenosis may be found as an incidental microscopic feature of a biopsy, and are difficult to distinguish from lobules undergoing physiological sclerosis. Discrimination can usually be achieved through assessment of the degree of distortion and

---

Table 22.1   Breast tissue growth factors

General	Specific	Local
Somatomedins	Oestrogen	Prostaglandins
Insulin	Progesterone	EGF
Thyroxine	Androgen	IGF (I and II)
(Parathormone)	Prolactin	TGF (α and β)

EGF, Epidermal growth factor; IGF, insulin-like growth factor; TGF, transforming growth factor.

complexity of the involved units. The mechanism of formation involves an overactivity of fibroblasts and collagen production. Women affected are mostly from the child-bearing and perimenopausal years. Despite the relief that is engendered by the recognition and reporting of this process as the reason for biopsy, there is now accumulating evidence that such cases are associated with a slight (approximately doubled) increased risk of subsequent cancer (Jensen *et al.* 1989).

Radial scars and complex sclerosing lesions (CSL)

These are considered together for they basically have the same components but differ in size (Anderson and Battersby, 1985). Various synonyms have been applied to these tissue processes as they became recognized by pathologists in different countries, namely: sclerosing papillary (or ductal) proliferation, scleroelastic lesion, infiltrating epitheliosis, indurative mastopathy. We prefer radial scar, the original term, for lesions of 10 mm or less, and CSL for the larger varieties. Unlike sclerosing adenosis, there may be cystic and prominently hyperplastic elements, with the centre of the radial structure displaying plentiful elastosis (Fig. 22.8) together with a disordered array of distorted tubules.

Study of the earlier stages discloses inflammation and frequent myofibroblast activity, a feature usual in wound healing, thus accounting for the central contraction and elastin deposition of older lesions. The frequency of subclinical changes and lack of specific associations encourages the view that the process is physiological, yet some still hold that it carries a risk of cancer and may even represent precursor lesions. To some extent this concept arises from close similarities of mammographic, gross, and microscopic appearances with tubular cancers, but conclusive evidence is lacking and judgement is presently reserved. Certainly, the collision and complexity of both parenchymal and stromal elements suggests that the causal mechanisms should incorporate local production of growth factors that stimulate both components. Centred on the smaller ducts and the roots of terminal duct branchings, the process in many situations would be short and self-limiting, but for the larger lesions (CSL) progressive accumulation of adjacent structures seems likely.

Sclerosing papillomatosis

This lesion has many features in common with CSL but usually occurs centrally, affecting larger ducts with a dominant papillary process, frequently causing mammographic densities with calcification. The major importance attached to this and the above group of conditions rests in the discrimination from cancer, which they closely resemble in greater or lesser degree by every clinical diagnostic modality.

Obliterative mastitis

In older postmenopausal women, collagenous overgrowth and obliteration of the lumen of medium-sized ducts may be seen (termed 'obliterative mastitis'). The alteration may extend over some length of the ducts, occurring in regions of the breast where the lobules have atrophied. Associated fibrosis may cause a palpable irregularity and accompanying calcification; both or either prompting biopsy. The lesion represents an end-stage of periductal chronic inflammatory activity.

Hyperplasia

Hyperplasias are recognized as increased numbers of cells above the basement membrane in glandular or ductal spaces. Hyperplasia, not otherwise specified, may be taken to refer to epithelial hyperplasia in the breast. This is because the increases in connective tissue as well as combined increases in connective and epithelial elements are either separately named or are of no known significance.

Mild hyperplasia

The presence of 3–4 cells above the basement membrane (the normal is two) is recognized as mild hyperplasia, and is a relatively common event of no practical significance. The follow-up of women with such changes reveals that they have no increased incidence of carcinoma (Dupont and Page 1985) when compared to women of similar age, followed for equal numbers of years. This is also true of women lacking any hyperplastic changes or other elements of proliferative disease. This large group of women with no increased risk of later breast cancer may be qualified as having no proliferative disease (including those with mild hyperplasia). They may have cysts, fibrosis, or uncomplicated apocrine change and constitute 50–70 per cent of women who undergo biopsy.

Moderate/severe hyperplasia

More developed or quantitatively large examples of hyperplasia are termed moderate, severe, or florid, depending on the degree or extent of involvement by the same cell populations as those noted above. The hyperplastic cells bridge and often fill distended spaces. The usual, or most common pattern of hyperplasia may be termed 'hyperplasia of usual type', and has some specific features. These consist of a mild variation of cytologic pattern with both oval and round nuclei, irregular and frequently slit-like spaces between the cell groups, and a tendency for cells to have subtle intercellular arrangements, giving an appearance of swirling or streaming (Fig. 22.9). Such usual hyperplastic patterns of moderate degree or greater are found in about 20 per cent of breast biopsies. When such women are followed for over a decade after biopsy, they are found to have a slight elevation of breast cancer risk (Dupont and Page 1985). The relative magnitude of this risk is only 1.5–2 times (50 to 100 per cent increase) that of the general population.

Note that this elevation of risk, although slight, may be taken to indicate an abnormality, and thus a disease. Such women may be said to have proliferative disease without atypia. 'Proliferative' indicates histopathology, while 'disease' notes the slight risk of cancer, and 'without atypia' informs that a higher risk indicator is absent. Such lesions have been termed 'papillomatosis' or 'epitheliosis', terms with ambiguous histopathological definition.

Although it is widely thought that some hyperplasias are

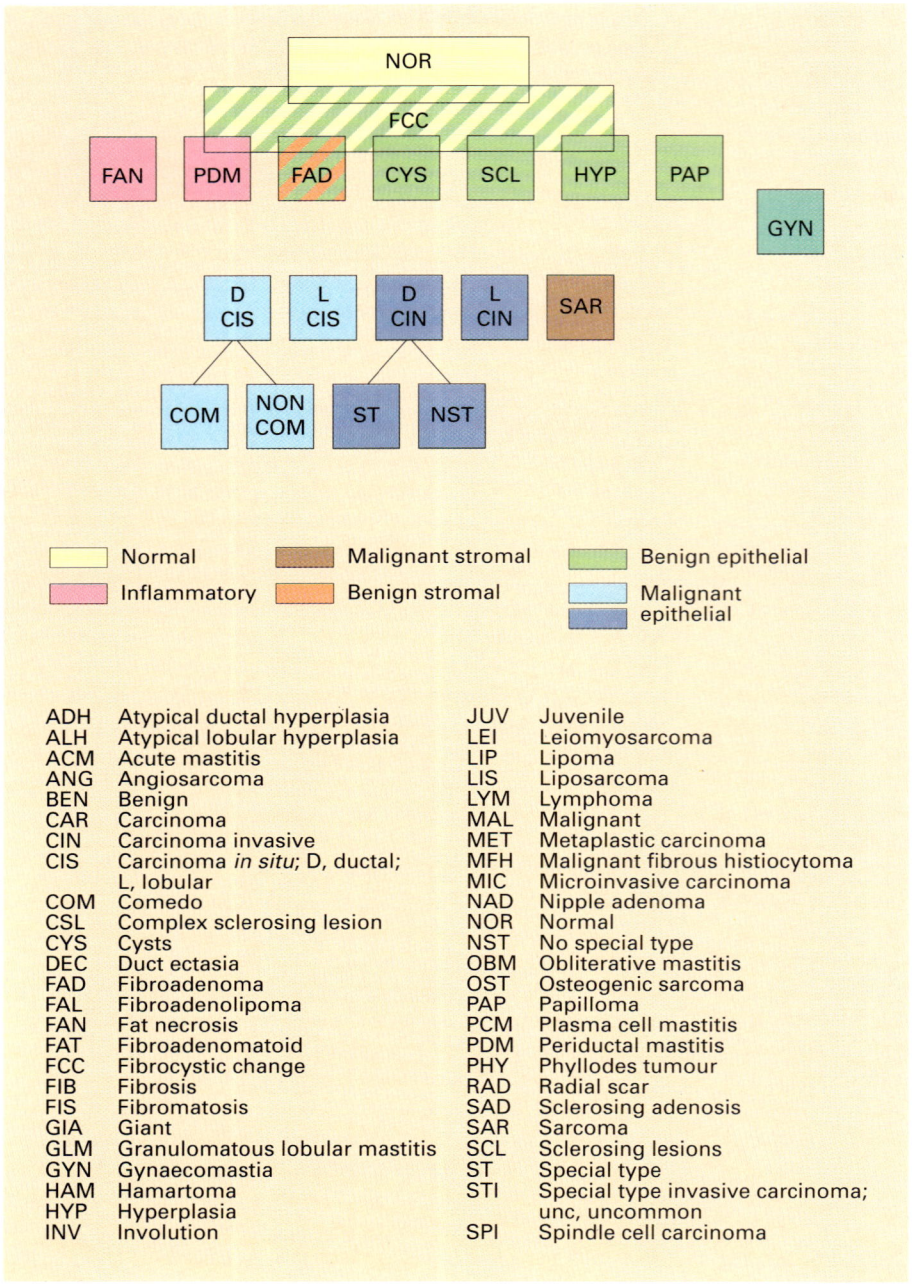

Fig. 22.5 A simplified scheme of breast benign nomenclature.

ADH	Atypical ductal hyperplasia	JUV	Juvenile
ALH	Atypical lobular hyperplasia	LEI	Leiomyosarcoma
ACM	Acute mastitis	LIP	Lipoma
ANG	Angiosarcoma	LIS	Liposarcoma
BEN	Benign	LYM	Lymphoma
CAR	Carcinoma	MAL	Malignant
CIN	Carcinoma invasive	MET	Metaplastic carcinoma
CIS	Carcinoma *in situ*; D, ductal; L, lobular	MFH	Malignant fibrous histiocytoma
		MIC	Microinvasive carcinoma
COM	Comedo	NAD	Nipple adenoma
CSL	Complex sclerosing lesion	NOR	Normal
CYS	Cysts	NST	No special type
DEC	Duct ectasia	OBM	Obliterative mastitis
FAD	Fibroadenoma	OST	Osteogenic sarcoma
FAL	Fibroadenolipoma	PAP	Papilloma
FAN	Fat necrosis	PCM	Plasma cell mastitis
FAT	Fibroadenomatoid	PDM	Periductal mastitis
FCC	Fibrocystic change	PHY	Phyllodes tumour
FIB	Fibrosis	RAD	Radial scar
FIS	Fibromatosis	SAD	Sclerosing adenosis
GIA	Giant	SAR	Sarcoma
GLM	Granulomatous lobular mastitis	SCL	Sclerosing lesions
GYN	Gynaecomastia	ST	Special type
HAM	Hamartoma	STI	Special type invasive carcinoma; unc, uncommon
HYP	Hyperplasia		
INV	Involution	SPI	Spindle cell carcinoma

intermediate stages through which malignant neoplasms arise, in human beings they should be understood as conditions which indicate a raised level of risk for later carcinoma. Thus, they may be merely markers, and not the actual cell populations which eventuate in cancers with metastatic capability. Analogy to experimental rodent systems (Cardiff 1988; Medina 1988) certainly would support the fact that hyperplastic lesions are more easily altered to produce true neoplasms, but not necessarily so. In follow-up or cohort studies of women with various lesions, the status of histopathological lesions as markers has been established, and the relative level of risk has been identified with many lesions. These epidemiological data of women followed after biopsy establish information of potential practical importance. However, the lesions identified are removed by biopsy, which renders our knowledge of the biological behaviour of these putative precursors of cancer quite indirect.

Atypical hyperplasia

The atypical hyperplasias (AH) are recognized by their resemblance to carcinoma *in situ* (CIS), both in histopathological features (see below) and in their risk of invasive carcinoma, which

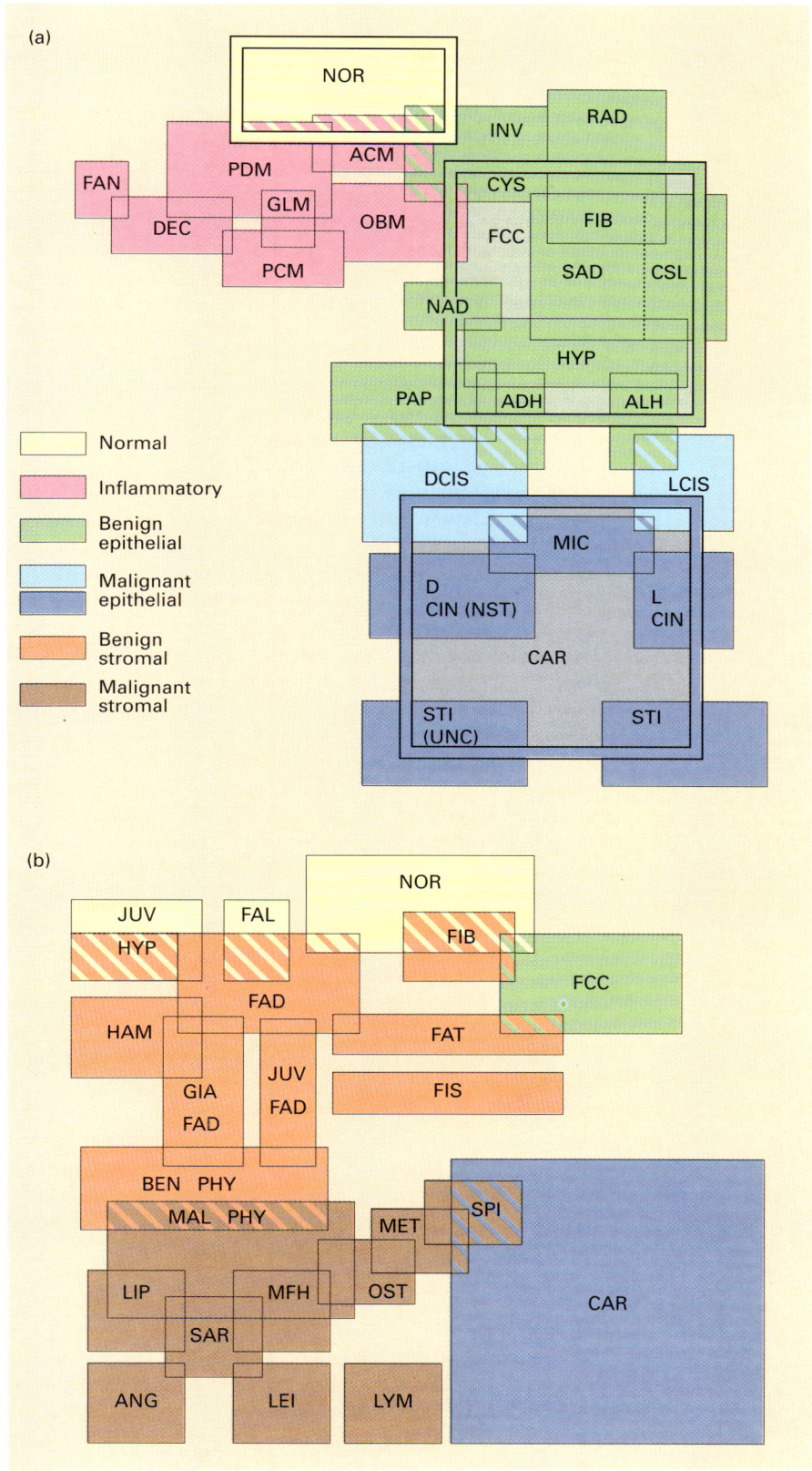

Fig. 22.6 Comprehensive categorization of breast benign and malignant nomenclature. (a) The abnormalities of epithelial derivation; (b) the abnormalities of predominantly stromal derivation.

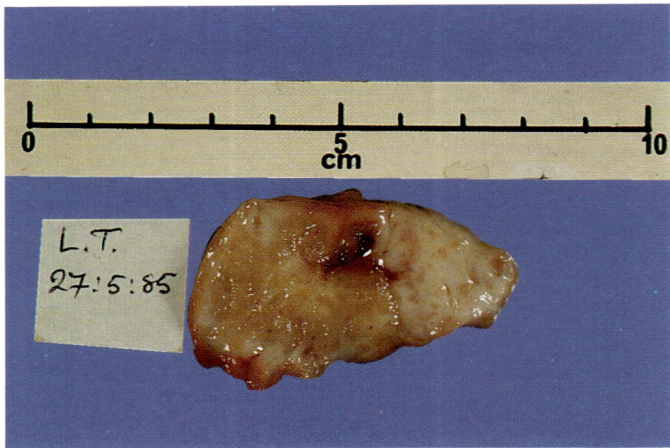

Fig. 22.7 A radial scar/complex sclerosing lesion to show the contrast with adjacent normal breast tissue. The haemorrhage is due to preceding fine-needle aspiration.

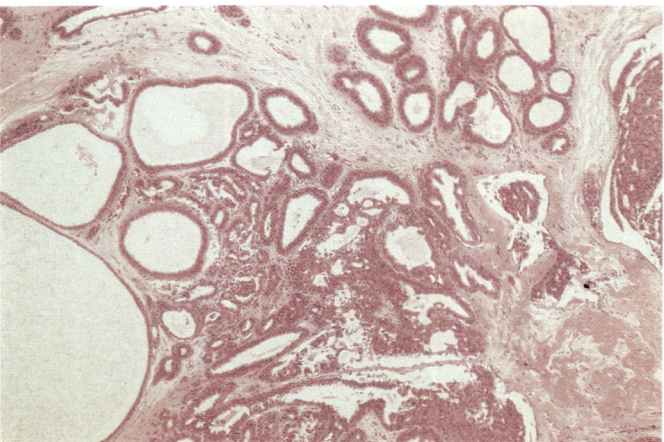

Fig. 22.8 A radial scar to illustrate the association of cystic, hyperplastic, and elastotic areas.

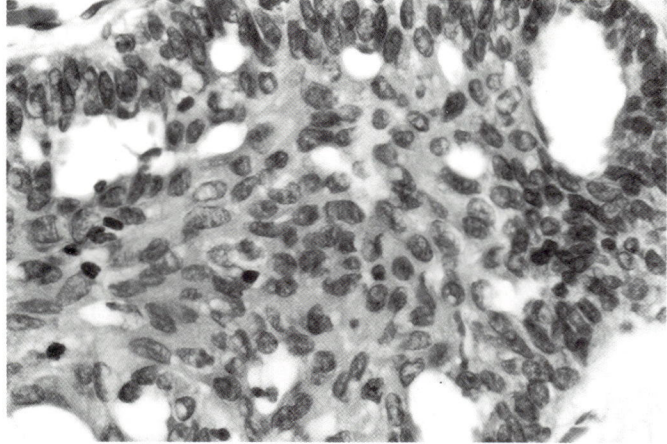

Fig. 22.9 An area of hyperplasia of usual type to show central swirling and peripheral palisading of regular nuclei.

is intermediate between that of the usual hyperplasias and CIS. This level of risk recognized by AH is usually characterized as moderate. Two types of atypical hyperplasia are recognized by analogy to CIS lesions. These lesions, termed atypical ductal hyperplasia (ADH) and atypical lobular hyperplasia (ALH), represent histopathological lesions having some similarity to the analogous CIS lesions without being completely developed (Page *et al*. 1985). In the case of atypical lobular hyperplasia the lobular units are not so completely filled or distended as those seen in lobular carcinoma *in situ,* but the cells constituting the lesions are the same. In ADH, the lesions are usually small in extent and often do not fill an entire basement membrane-bound space with a uniform population of neoplastic-appearing cells. Note that there is not an atypical hyperplasia which is analogous to comedo carcinoma *in situ*: any lesion having such advanced features of nuclear atypicality is considered carcinoma *in situ*. These latter lesions also are regularly aneuploid and have a high growth fraction (Meyer 1986).

The predictability of later invasive carcinoma development after identification of these atypical hyperplasias at surgical biopsy is 4–5 times that of the general population. Although this may appear quite high, it translates in absolute terms to a risk of 10 per cent in 10–15 years for women identified in their late thirties to early fifties. This magnitude of risk is similar to that attributed to the contralateral breast after primary treatment for breast carcinoma in one breast; and, as with that contralateral risk, falls after 10–15 years (Dupont and Page 1989), i.e. the risk is not constant with time. Each breast is at risk after the identification of atypical hyperplasia in either breast. In most aspects, ADH and ALH are similar except that carcinoma develops on average 8 years after ADH and 12 years after ALH are diagnosed at biopsy. Also, ALH is rare in women under the age of 35 and over the age of 55. The combined incidence of the AH lesions is somewhat greater than 5 per cent of benign breast biopsies, and is higher in mammographically indicated biopsies. It is important to emphasize that these atypical hyperplastic lesions are identified in biopsies almost by chance. No known signs or symptoms are present to indicate their presence prior to biopsy. These lesions have been defined by epidemiological studies as a borderline between the ordinary hyperplasias and the carcinomas *in situ* (Dupont and Page 1985; Tavassoli and Norris 1990). There are also some studies that have indicated that tumour-associated antigens, particularly oncogene products and surface glycoprotein tumour-associated antigens, have a favoured association with atypical hyperplasias, again intermediate between those of the hyperplastic lesions and carcinomas (Ohuchi *et al*. 1987).

Fibrocystic change

Predominantly during the early years of middle age, largely the decade prior to the menopause, women often develop an increase in the tendency toward the breast to be palpably lumpy. Occasionally dominant lumps are produced, which most frequently are well-formed and fluid-filled cysts. There is also an associated increase in fibrous tissue with an irregular distribution within the breast. As this is occurring at a time when the firm glandular tissue of the breast is beginning to recede and being replaced by softer fat, it is quite clear how this lumpiness may be produced. Because fat is easily malleable, the remaining fibrous tissue and cysts are usually somewhat firmer than the 'normal' breast tissue. It has long been held that, because of the perimenopausal age at which these occur, they may be related in some way to involution, or the beginnings of that phenomenon. Following the menopause this irregular lumpiness recedes, as do cysts.

The precise mode of formation of cysts is unknown, but it is likely that they occur by the inflation of individual acini and lobular units. Thus as the branching system of acini and terminal ductules inflate, then unfold, fewer and larger spaces are present. Whether larger cysts occur by recruiting adjacent lobular units or through some other mechanism is unknown. Cysts are usually lined by a characteristic epithelium mimicking that found in the apocrine sweat glands. This so-called apocrine change is of unknown clinical significance, although it might indicate a greater likelihood for multiplicity of cysts than indicated by so-called 'simple' cysts which have a flattened or inapparent epithelial lining (Dixon *et al.* 1985). Coloured compounds related to blood pigments or epoxides of various lipids are frequently present within cysts, giving them a bluish or brown colour on direct vision, and regularly a blue colour when viewed intact (blue-domed cysts of Bloodgood).

Cysts are common lesions, particularly in the decade preceding the menopause. Their frequency and greater incidence in geographically defined populations at high risk for carcinoma (Bartow *et al.* 1987) has made cysts of great interest for their possible link with cancer risk. However, cysts are not indicative of cancer risk elevation in prospective studies within populations of geographically determined higher risk, such as North America (Dupont and Page 1985). Cysts remain an important clinical problem because of their presentation as mass lesions, and their varied histopathological and biochemical components merit further study (Bartow *et al.* 1982).

Fibroadenomas and related lesions

Fibroadenomas are smoothly delimited, benign, new growths of fibrous and glandular tissue. They constitute the most common mass lesions of the female breast in the early post-menarchical years, and are most common in women in their twenties. Regularly presenting as a freely movable masses, their benign nature may be confirmed by needle aspiration cytology. Histopathologically, the relationship of the stroma and glandular elements has led to the description of many patterns. For the most part, the association of the two major elements is regular through the lesion, and may seem glandular, or have elongated tubular, or leaf-like arrangements. In any case, the microscopic patterns are benign, although the epithelium may be proliferated in the manner of hyperplasia elsewhere in the breast. The stroma may be quite cellular, hyalinized, or myxoid. Larger and more cellular variants may be termed 'giant'; juvenile or other terms have no certain clinical importance other than to name unusual cli-

nical presentations. Most fibroadenomas develop to a greatest diameter of 1–3 cm and then remain stable in size (Wilkinson *et al.* 1989). It is their detectability within the breast which brings them to clinical attention, particularly when superficial within the breast; they may go undetected for decades when present more deeply within the breast. At least 10 per cent of fibroadenomas are multiple, presenting simultaneously or found subsequent to an initial diagnosis (Fechner 1987). Histological pattern and not size should define the phyllodes tumour, occurring in benign and malignant forms (see below), which is also a tumour of combined stromal and epithelial elements. The closely related benign phyllodes tumour is recognized by a densely cellular stroma with occasional mitoses and deformed epithelial elements presenting in a leaf-like fashion. Malignant transformation in a phyllodes tumour is suggested by: rapid enlargement; invasion of surrounding breast tissue by 'malignant' stroma; increased stroma cellularity; anaplasia of stromal cells; and increased mitotic rate. Even lesions with these features remain localized but can recur after excision. Metastases occur in about 15 per cent of cases. The generic term 'phyllodes tumour' should be used to guard against over-diagnosis and over-treatment, because none of the features given are diagnostic of malignant behaviour.

Papilloma

The mammary papilloma is strictly defined as a lesion of ducts, having a branching fibrovascular supporting structure upon which a benign epithelium resides. These lesions are of clinical note primarily because they usually present with a bloody discharge from a single lactiferous ductal opening in the nipple. The lesion may be inapparent to clinical examination and may even be difficult to find at the time of surgical extirpation. Most papillary tumours are solitary and occur in the large subareolar ducts. The latter lesions may produce irregular and expanding lesions at the nipple surface and are a combination of hyperplasia, sclerosis, and adenosis. These solitary, truly papillary lesions are most common in young middle life, peaking in incidence between fibroadenomas and carcinomas; this is coincident with the age distribution of cysts. The papillomas are frequently complex in anatomy, with areas of sclerosis, epithelial hyperplasia, and organizing regions of infarction; the latter giving rise to the nipple discharge. When large, papillomas may extend along a dilated duct or may produce a rounded palpable mass within an altered duct. In the latter case the lesion may appear to be encysted. Note: the term 'papillomatosis' has been variously used and is intrinsically confusing. Most often 'papillomatosis' has been used to indicate what is here termed the usual pattern of hyperplasia. Peculiar hyperplastic and sclerotic lesions of the nipple collectively termed 'nipple adenoma' or 'subareolar papillomatosis' have mixed microscopic features. A further benign mass lesion is 'ductal adenoma' (Lammie and Millis 1989) with mixed histopathological features.

Papillary or branched patterns of epithelial proliferation are common in the breast, leading to some difficulties in terminology, but there is another condition which is properly termed papilloma, i.e. the peripheral or multiple papilloma. These occur in smaller, more peripheral ducts, tend to be multiple and to recur after local excision. They also are more frequently associated with a florid epithelial proliferation between the stromal fronds of the lesion and in the adjacent lobular units. These epithelial proliferations are frequently atypical or qualify as CIS (Ohuchi *et al.* 1984). Their association with carcinoma both concurrently (Papotti *et al.* 1984) and subsequently (Haagensen 1986) has been documented. This quantitative association is not known precisely, but should occasion treating such complex and extensive truly papillary lesions with care. As they have a tendency to travel along the ducts, their excision should take into account the radial anatomy of the breast ducts.

Miscellaneous benign conditions

Most of the remaining benign breast lesions of clinical importance are of interest because of their mimicry of carcinoma. Some also have an underlying inflammatory nature, the aetiology of which is not understood.

Duct ectasia

This is one of many terms given to a poorly understood condition associated with a segmental involvement of large and intermediate-sized ducts. The involved ducts are characteristically dilated and filled with a grumous material probably representing the shards resulting from years of inflammation and epithelial cell turnover. A dense periductal fibrosis gives rise to palpable masses, and contraction probably also produces the acquired nipple inversion which may attend this disorder. Dystrophic calcification occurring in this fibrous tissue occasionally produces characteristic linear calcifications appreciated by radiography.

Fat necrosis

This may produce large and sclerosing masses which almost perfectly mimic carcinomas in the firmness and irregularity of the affected area. The evolution of this alteration from areas of devitalized fat through inflammation to scarring with 'oil cysts' (free fat surrounded by reacting histiocytes) is similar here to its occurrence elsewhere in the body. In the breast, trauma is probably the major causative factor.

Fibrous mastopathy

Palpable lumps in the breast may be determined histopathologically to consist only of relative increases in more dense fibrous tissue compared to glandular and fatty elements (see Section 22.1.2). This obviously produces a firmer area in the breast and in the absence of aetiologic information is descriptively termed 'fibrous mastopathy' and other related terms.

Granulomatous lesions

Various conditions, e.g. tuberculosis, sarcoidosis, etc., may present within the breast as a granulomatous mastitis. Also, an idiopathic variety may occur, perhaps related to a reaction to secretions or having an autoimmune base.

22.1.4   Non-invasive (*in situ*) carcinoma

The concept of *in situ* carcinoma was first applied formally to the breast in the 1940s. The commonly held belief was that these lesions, which had the appearance of invasive carcinoma but were confined within the spaces where the originating cells were normally present, would lead inevitably to invasive, clinically malignant disease. More recently it has become evident that such lesions may not only progress, but may be static or even capable of regression. Now that the malignant potential of these lesions is not considered a solitary possibility, concepts and therapy have become dynamic, changing, and varied.

Comedo carcinoa in situ is the most familiar of CIS lesions. It is considered a special type of ductal cancer *in situ* (DCIS). Since the end of the nineteenth century these lesions have been accepted as carcinoma and have occasioned the full measure of therapy for carcinoma. They are characterized by an extremely pleomorphic population of cells with nuclei which are large, bizarre, and hyperchromatic (Fig. 22.10). Necrotic foci are characteristic and often calcify, leading to frequent detection by mammography. The extensive use of mammography has greatly raised the incidence of these lesions and resulted in the detection of smaller, non-palpable lesions. Prior to the availability of mammography these lesions regularly became large enough to be palpable and were treated by mastectomy. Of the palpable lesions left untreated, as many as 50 per cent evolve into invasive carcinoma within 3 years. It is frequently difficult to ascertain if there are microscopic foci of invasion in complex and extensive lesions. These most malignant of CIS lesions also have a higher growth rate and frequent overexpression of the *c-erb B2* oncogene (see below) as contrasted with other CIS lesions.

Non-comedo carcinomas in situ of ductal type have long been recognized to occur with the comedo variety, but each frequently occurs in pure form. There is a strong tendency at the

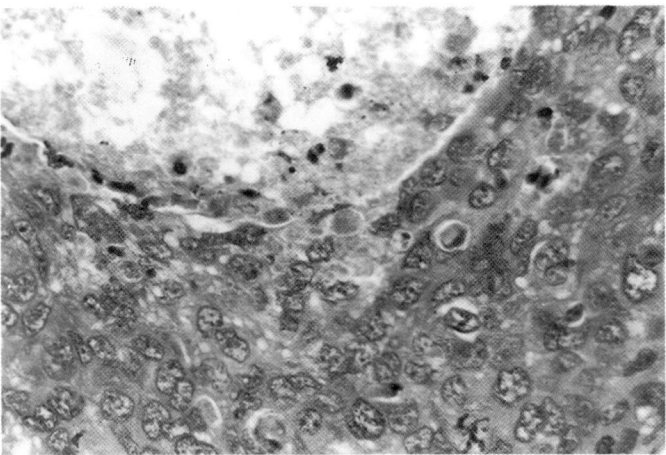

Fig. 22.10 *In situ* carcinoma with comedo necrosis, to illustrate the compact arrangement of pleomorphic cells around the central necrotic comedo.

moment to separate these comedo and non-comedo elements, which were previously grouped under the heading of ductal carcinoma *in situ* (DCIS). This trend recognized that the non-comedo ductal carcinomas *in situ* have greatly increased in frequency with the advent of screening programmes. Both major types of DCIS is some series now make up to 20 per cent of detected carcinomas, with non-comedo cases more frequent. Previously (before the advent of mammography) the incidence of ductal carcinoma *in situ,* with the comedo type predominating, was between 1 and 5 per cent in different series of patients (Connolly *et al.* 1989).

The natural history of these non-comedo lesions of ductal type is best demonstrated by following women who have had these lesions detected at biopsy without having further therapy. This is obviously not an 'untrammelled' natural history, but is of great practical utility because it speaks precisely to the clinical situation in which these lesions are found, i.e. what is the likely clinical outcome if such lesions are left untreated after diagnosis. When 'microscopic' lesions of non-comedo DCIS are found at biopsy and no further therapy is performed, approximately 30 per cent of women will develop invasive carcinoma during the following 10–15 years (Page *et al.* 1982). These lesions will occur in the same area as the previously diagnosed CIS. Also, it seems that very few invasive carcinomas will appear after the ten-year period. Because of this local implication for recurrent and evolving disease, it is becoming more accepted that local therapy with careful attention given to margins may be acceptable therapy for these diseases (Lagios *et al.* 1989). Histopathologically, non-comedo ductal carcinomas *in situ* are characterized by having sculptured and crisply defined formations of evenly placed hyperchromatic cells. These patterns are usually present either as micropapillae of solid cells or as a network of cells separated by sharply defined, circular, secondary spaces. The latter pattern is known as cribriform and the former as micropapillary (Patchefsky *et al.* 1989) and the two patterns often coexist (Fig. 22.11).

Lobular carcinoma in situ (LCIS) was described histopathologically in the 1940s, but not widely accepted until the late 1960s and 1970s (Rosen *et al.* 1978). The reason is that understanding of its natural history was needed before wide acceptance of the lesion could be expected. Histopathologically, each ductule in lobular units is greatly distended and distorted by a uniform population of cells with characteristic cytological features. When this is present in well-developed form, the appearance is inescapable as an example of LCIS (Fig. 22.12). The true incidence of LCIS is unknown because it does not produce detectable signs or symptoms, nor does it produce detectable signs on mammography. As determined by percentage of biopsies performed, LCIS is most frequently found in the perimenopausal age-group, becoming quite uncommon with advancing age. It is therefore widely believed that these lesions are dependent upon the hormonal milieu present during the child-bearing years.

Multifocality is the hallmark of LCIS (Frykberg *et al.* 1987). When it is detected in one breast, the likelihood of finding it in

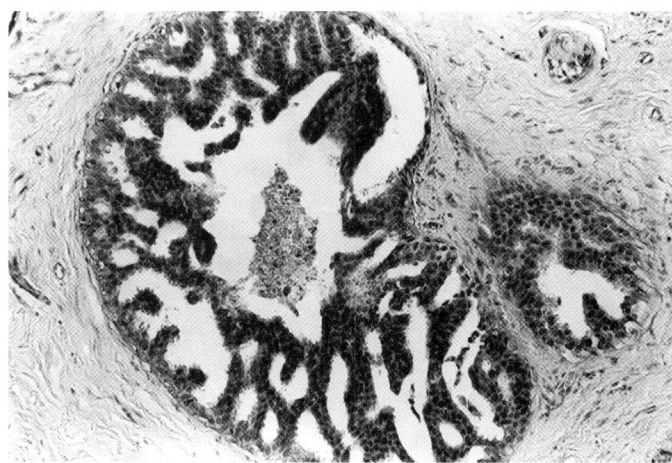

Fig. 22.11 An illustration of the combined cribriform and micropapillary structure that can be found in carcinoma *in situ.* Note the central necrosis.

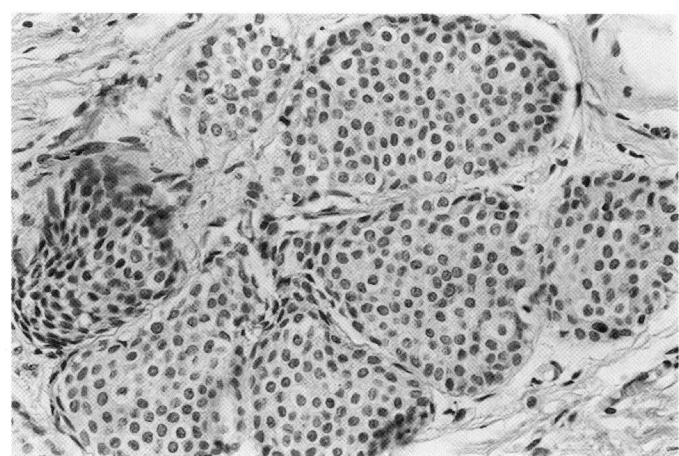

Fig. 22.12 In this example of lobular carcinoma *in situ* the uniform population of cells is seen to completely fill and distend the involved spaces.

the other at biopsy is 25–40 per cent. This is approximately one-half the likelihood of finding the lesion in the remainder of the breast originally biopsied. If women are followed after biopsy alone for LCIS, their likelihood of developing invasive carcinoma is about 10 times greater than that of the general population. The site of later invasive carcinoma development is almost equally divided between either breast, slightly favouring the breast in which LCIS was detected originally. The absolute magnitude of this risk is about 20–25 per cent in 15 years. What might occur beyond that time is not clear, but because of the many competing causes of death operative in advanced ages, it is likely that this risk will fall as a woman approaches the age of 70 and beyond. Treatment options vary from close surveillance to removal of most of the breast tissue and makes the condition frustrating to patients and physicians. It is evident, however, that LCIS is not a cancer in the full or usual definition.

In summary, the mammary carcinomas *in situ* have different natural histories. LCIS is different from DCIS in that subsequently developing invasive carcinomas occur anywhere in either breast, while in DCIS the later carcinomas are regularly in the same area as the initial DCIS. This indicates that DCIS is a more committed precursor-like lesion, and LCIS is more of a marker or indicator of greatly increased likelihood of later carcinoma.

22.1.5   Invasive carcinoma

The dominant characteristic of breast carcinoma is its heterogeneity. The age-adjusted death rate belies breast cancer's exquisite dependence on age. Note that advancing age beyond the menopause is associated with increasing incidence of breast cancer only in high-risk populations; and that with advancing age the likelihood of dying from breast cancer decreases although incidence increases. This is largely because of increasing, competing causes of death from other diseases (Dupont and Page 1989). Apart from these general considerations, the practitioner should focus on characterization of each individual case, because prognostic and therapeutic concerns are varied and should be individualized. Epidemiological concerns are presented below, here we will highlight the varieties of breast cancer and the relationship and characteristics of classification with the prognosis.

In the nineteenth century, women presented with locally advanced disease, i.e. large masses in the breast and relatively frequent local metastases to lymph nodes of the axillae. At the end of that century, *en bloc*, wide excision of the entire breast, and adjacent skin and axilla was introduced as the therapy of choice. The theory of disease behaviour which underpinned this therapeutic approach was that cancer began locally and spread in a direct and centrifugal fashion, largely through local lymphatic channels, to local lymph nodes. Distant spread was held to occur after involvement of the local lymph nodes. Thus, cure could be effected by *en bloc* excision including the local lymph nodes, and was aided by not disturbing the cancer or early elements of local spread. While this theory supported extended operations (which included removal of local lymph nodes of the internal mammary chain under the sternum), others in the field favoured less extensive surgical removal (breast only) with local radiation therapy (McWhirter 1955). The realization in the 1970s that any of these approaches gave similar survivals at 5–10 years after treatment, led to another and diametrically opposed paradigm. This more modern model held that breast cancer was systemically disseminated from its inception. Thus it was the later behaviour of these micrometastases that determined the subsequent morbidity and mortality of patients. The most appropriate, currently accepted paradigm holds that there are at least two kinds of breast cancer: one which remains localized to the breast for prolonged periods of time and rarely spreads, while the other has distant micrometastases at the time of clinical diagnosis (Hellman and

Harris 1987). One cannot understand the theory underlying any therapeutic approach to breast cancer without considering in parallel which of these paradigms provides the theoretical basis of the approach.

Hormonal features

Oestrogen receptor (ER) and progesterone receptor (PR) proteins are indicators of breast cancer prognosis and predictors of response to hormonal manipulation therapy. As with other steroid hormones, oestrogen and progesterone enter the cell and are bound to the binding proteins there, inducing changes in the ER which enhances its ability to induce DNA transcription in the nucleus. The measurement of these proteins may be accomplished by quantitative binding techniques using labelled oestradiol (E_2) and measuring the amount of oestradiol bound per mg of protein in tissue. This produces valuable information with about two-thirds of invasive carcinomas having positive ER. Slightly over 50 per cent of women with ER-positive carcinomas will respond to hormonal therapy, and somewhat less than 10 per cent of women negative for ER determination will respond. This conclusion is largely derived from biochemically determined data. Immunohistochemical determination may also be done, although it gives a qualitative answer. This last approach uses a labelled antibody to the ER and identifies localization of the antibody to the nuclei of the neoplasm. The predictability of response to hormonal manipulation increases directly with quantitative ER values. Thus, breast cancers with very high levels of oestrogen receptor are particularly likely to be responsive to hormonal manipulation.

Metastatic behaviour

Breast cancer kills by spread from the breast, usually by haematogenous routes. As is noted above, this is variably preceded by development of disease in the breast and adjacent lymphatic channels. It is generally held that the presence of regional metastases in the lymph nodes of the axilla indicates the distant metastic potential of an individual breast cancer. This is true in a quantitatively predictive manner, i.e. the more involvement there is in the axillary lymph nodes, the more likely the carcinoma is to be distantly metastatic and lead to the death of the patient. During the course of a complete axillary dissection, 20–30 lymph nodes are removed. The low or proximal lymph nodes are closer to the breast, and more easily removed because of their surgical proximity to the primary tumour. The distant, or high, axillary lymph nodes are found adjacent to the axillary and subclavian veins. In the era before mammography, when breast cancers were generally of much larger size, the twenty-year survival for patients without axillary lymph-node metastases was 65 per cent (Berg and Robbins 1966; Fisher *et al.* 1984). Women who had involvement of the low lymph nodes only had a 38 per cent survival, while those with extensive axillary involvement had only 12 per cent survival. More recently, reported groups of patients have been characterized by the number of lymph nodes involved in the axilla. It is usually the case that when few nodes are involved, they are confined to the low axilla. The ten-year survival for women with 1–3 lymph nodes involved is about 60 per cent, while those with four or more nodes involved have a survival at 10 years of about 20 per cent. Largely because of the demands of protocols used for clinical trials, much of this quantitative information has been simplifed to: lymph-node positivity v. lymph-node negativity. Approximately 25–35 per cent of women with lymph-node involvement will survive 10 years while, conversely, only about 25 per cent of all women without lymph-node involvement will experience distant metastatic disease or die within 10 years of the initial diagnosis.

Distant metastases are most commonly to the lung, bones, and liver. Importantly, one or more of these sites may be dominant, and each will produce quite different morbid events. For example, many women with initial presentation of metastatic disease in the bones may have prolonged clinical courses, often greater than 10 years following the identification of metastases. The extreme variations of disease are also evidenced by the differences between patients with dominant involvement of a single metastatic site such as the lung. While some patients will have few symptoms and small numbers of mass lesions in the lung, which may be endobronchial, others will have diffuse lymphangitic spread in the lungs and severe pulmonary impairment. Brain metastases are quite unusual, with many of the intracranial metastases presenting in the pituitary with the resultant syndrome of inappropriate secretion of antidiuretic hormone (ADH). Characteristic clinical presentation may include meningeal carcinomatosis or the appearance of diffusely infiltrating tumour in the intestinal tract. The latter two presentations are evidently more common with the lobular histopathological pattern of breast cancer. Another frequent pattern of metastasis may be by continuity, following the old paradigm, namely involvement of pleural and pericardial cavities.

Types of invasive carcinoma

Carcinoma not otherwise specified (NOS) is taken to mean invasive carcinoma. Classically, carcinoma of the breast is separated into different histopathological types. The reasons for this are historical and practical: it is how it has been done; and it is useful in predicting clinical behaviour. Other useful, and possibly useful, measures are found in Table 22.2, and are discussed as prognostic measures.

Table 22.2 Measures of prognosis in breast cancer

Size and contour
Histopathology: tumour type and grade
Metastasis: vascular and lymph nodes
DNA quantitation
Growth fraction
Hormone receptors ER,* PR,* others
Oncogenes: amplification and expression
Chromosomal alterations

* ER, oestrogen receptor; PR, progesterone receptor.

Table 22.3 Special types of invasive breast cancer

Major
   Tubular and cribriform
   Medullary
   Lobular
   Mucinous
Minor
   Adenoid cystic, secretory

Mammary cancer, NOS

Specific or special features characterize some breast cancers, while the remainder lack these special features and are termed 'mammary carcinoma, NOS (not otherwise specified)', or no special type (NST) of ductal carcinomas. The latter term is in general usage as a logical counterpart to the so-called lobular type and other special types of carcinoma (Table 22.3).

Carcinoma of NST comprises about 70 per cent of invasive breast cancers, and any general comments about breast cancer NOS should be understood to refer to them. These carcinomas usually occur with well-delimited masses, although the shapes vary from round to spiculated (Fig. 22.13). Most of the spiculated forms have a dense fibrous stroma and have been termed scirrhous, a term which should now be used in a descriptive rather than a defining sense. This hardness produces palpability, which of course varies depending on the firmness of the surrounding breast as well as the depth within the breast of the tumour.

The stroma may contain clumps of elastic-like tissue, which are visible in the gross specimen as chalky dots. Foci of similarly appearing tumour necrosis may also be seen grossly, and may be present within intraductal disease. DCIS often coexists with invasive tumours, and its extensiveness is a determinant of the likelihood of treatment failure after local removal and radiotherapy (Connolly and Schnitt 1988; Holland et al. 1990). The

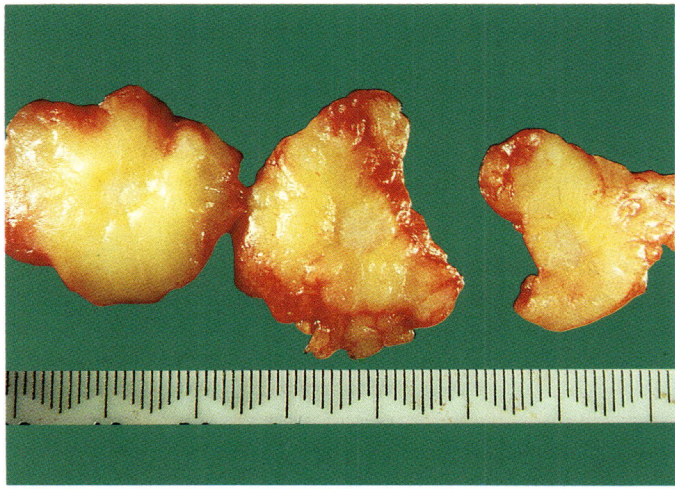

Fig. 22.13 A macroscopic view of a carcinoma. Note the irregular border and the distinct orange-yellow coloration of the fat around the lesion.

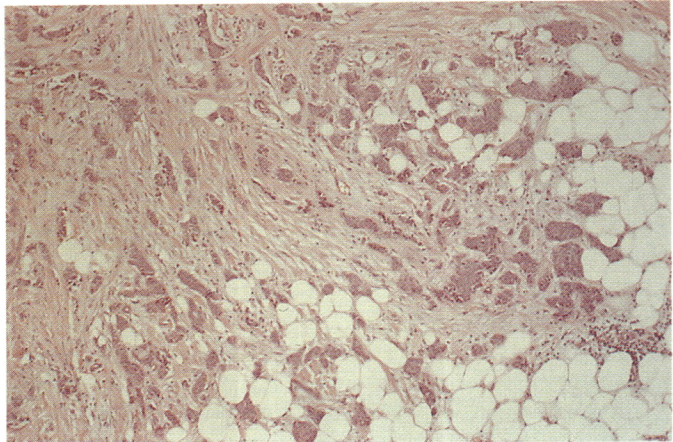

Fig. 22.14 Histological appearance of invasive carcinoma of no special type (NST). The disordered infiltration extends from the fibrous tissue into the fat.

invasive component is as varied as any patterns of adenocarcinoma elsewhere in the body. Gland formation, sheets of cells, reticular formations, and tight clumps or islands of tumour cells (Fig. 22.14) are present in mixed or relatively pure form. Mucin substances and various milk products are found in the cytoplasm. Many mammary carcinomas also have a degree of squamous appearance and/or the appearance of apocrine cytoplasmic differentiation with its large cytoplasmic compartment richly endowed with eosinophilic granules (mitochondria and secretory vacuoles). These, and many other cytoplasmic features such as clear appearance or lipid content, are without known prognostic implication.

The cytological features of many breast carcinomas are remarkably bland, with small, regular nuclei and sparse mitoses. However, other carcinomas of the breast, all of which reside in this largest diagnostic compartment, have frequent mitoses and large, irregular nuclei. These latter features identify breast cancers with a poor prognosis as do other measures discussed below. The extent of gland formation as well as the degree of nuclear atypia and density of mitotic figures have been utilized successfully for prognostication in a system of histopathological grading. Tumours with no gland formation, increased mitosis, and advanced nuclear atypia are termed 'high grade' and have a poor prognosis (Elston 1987).

Tubular carcinoma

This special type of carcinoma rarely kills and should be understood to represent a special subset of low-grade breast carcinomas. They are often small, but probably average about 1 cm in diameter in most series. When histologically pure, not intermixed with other patterns, the prognosis indicates a vanishingly small likelihood of distant metastasis. This is true even in the presence of 1–3 positive lymph nodes which are present in about 10 per cent of tubular carcinomas. If more positive lymph nodes are identified, the primary tumour usually has an intermixed element of higher grade, also not an uncommon event.

The stroma of tubular carcinomas is usually abundant and has well-formed infiltrating glands with a single-cell lining and little cytological atypia.

A variant of invasive tubular carcinoma may be recognized in which the infiltrating epithelium develops complete secondary lumina, resembling cribriform carcinoma *in situ*. Whether this pattern is recognized separately as 'invasive cribriform carcinoma' or as a variant of tubular carcinoma is immaterial. It is important that the excellent prognosis of these lesions, reflecting that of tubular carcinoma, should be recognized.

Medullary carcinoma

When carefully defined, women with medullary carcinoma have an improved 5–10 year prognosis over that of women with the common breast cancer of similar size. These lesions have smooth, rounded contours and may suggest a benign mass on mammogram. Composed of large, bizarre cells with little stroma, these carcinomas are also soft. Characteristically, there is a rich infiltrate of lymphocytes and plasma cells. The major importance of this special type is that it would be categorized as a high-grade lesion by general principles of grading (see above); but this tumour definitely has a better prognosis than the mammary carcinomas (NOS) be they high grade or otherwise.

Carcinomas which are reminiscent of medullary type, but with some aberrant features such as foci of infiltration into adjacent stroma, may be termed atypical medullary carcinomas or medullary variants. The somewhat improved prognosis of the classic type may not be guaranteed in such lesions. Like the classic type, however, these variants are more common in young women.

Lobular carcinomas of invasive type (ILC)

These make up somewhat over 10 per cent of invasive breast cancers and are characterized by several anatomic and prognostic features. Note that this type of carcinoma, as well as the tubular type, is less common in geographical areas of low incidence (Stalsberg *et al.* 1989).

The defining histopathological features are two:

1. cytologic—the cells are relatively small, regular, and not bizarre; and

2. pattern of infiltration—diffuse, widespread, characterized by single-cell infiltration, often in single file, arranged between bundles of collagen (Fig. 22.15).

When both features are present, the pure type of ILC is present; variants are recognized when a more solid or alveolar pattern of cytologically characteristic cells are present. The pure type is associated with an improved prognosis (Dixon *et al.* 1982; Di Costanzo *et al.* 1990).

A unique feature of this cancer type is that the collagen may be increased, in which case a *scirrhous* cancer may be produced with a firm texture to palpation. Otherwise, this diffuse pattern of infiltration may produce little change in the texture of the breast because of its diffuse infiltration. In the latter case, mammography may also be little altered by an extensive carcinoma.

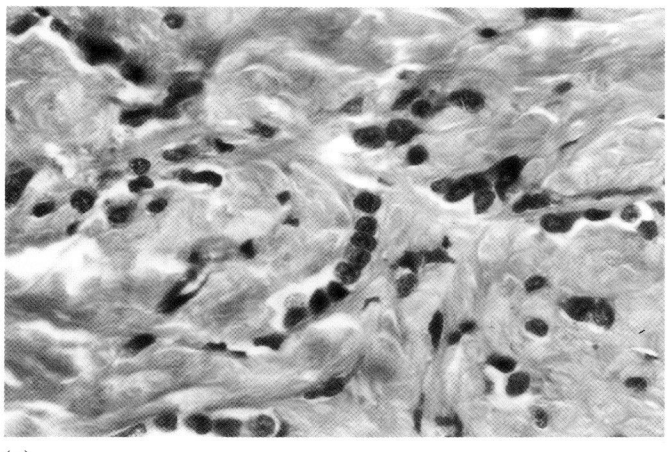

(a)

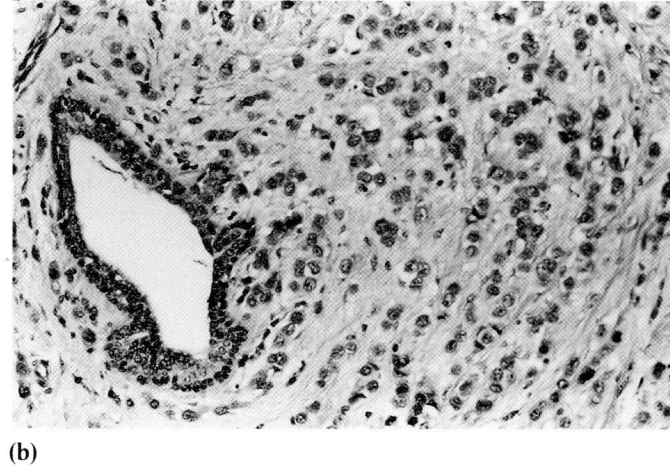

(b)

Fig. 22.15 Characteristic patterns of lobular invasive carcinoma (ILC) are illustrated by these high-power views to illustrate (a) single-file infiltration and (b) diffuse infiltration around a normal parenchymal duct structure.

About 60 per cent of carcinomas with the classic pattern of lobular carcinoma have associated *in situ* carcinoma of the lobular type. This association with LCIS is also present for variants of ILC which have more solid and alveolar patterns. These tumour patterns are associated with increased bilateral occurrence of cancer (Dixon *et al.* 1983).

Mucinous cancer

The synonym 'colloid' also aptly describes this classic special type of breast cancer. It is characterized by the gross presentation of a soft mass made up predominately of mucin in which floats a relatively sparse population of cancer cells, arranged in groups. When present in pure form, i.e. not intermixed with others, this pattern indicates an excellent prognosis. Patients with these lesions tend to be over 60 years old, lack lymph node metastasis, and seldom develop distant metastases. This extracellular production of mucin may be present in only a portion of a carcinoma. In the latter case, excellent prognosis is not assured, and the mixed tumour should be regarded as better categorized by the component with the worse prognosis.

Other rare cancer types

Having an incidence of approximately 1 per 1000 invasive breast cancers, the adenoid cystic and secretory types merit but brief recording. Their special significance is that they rarely, if ever, kill. The adenoid cystic lesion shows resemblance to its namesake having origin in the salivary glands (see Chapter 14). Secretory carcinomas are more frequent in the young, and have been termed 'juvenile'.

Metaplastic carcinomas These comprise less than 1 per cent of malignant neoplasms of the breast, and present largely as sarcomas. Portions of the tumours may be definable as carcinomas, and it is currently assumed by most observers that the mesenchymal or spindle-cells portion is a metaplastic alteration of the carcinoma. These lesions are more common in older women, and may have portions of the tumour differentiating into cartilage or bone. When most of the tumour appears as a sarcoma, the prognosis and behaviour is largely that expected of a similarly appearing pure soft-tissue sarcoma. The implications and attendant observations are that there are few lymph nodal metastases and that distant metastases are frequent.

Other malignant tumours of the breast

Any soft-tissue malignancy may present within the breast. This includes the locally invasive fibromatosis as well as any type of sarcoma occurring elsewhere in soft tissue. These lesions are quite rare within the breast, particularly when the metaplastic sarcomas are recognized as noted above. One specific sarcoma has a special importance for the breast: the angiosarcoma. Although unusual, as in any location, they may be subtle in presentation within the breast and complete removal for histopathological evaluation of vascular tumours within the breast is indicated. This does not mean that benign vascular tumours are not seen in the breast; actually, microscopic perilobular haemangiomas are quite common.

Malignant tumours presenting within the breast may be determined to have metastasized from a primary malignancy at another site. Although this is a clinically rare occurrence, it is of evident importance for the individual patient. Usually the patient is known to have had a previous malignancy. This is the clinical setting for the presentation of most cases within the breast and includes lung carcinomas, melanomas, and ovarian carcinomas, as well as others. Carcinoid tumours and medullary carcinoma of the thyroid may be followed by an apparent primary lesion in the breast, and there are some recorded cases of intestinal carcinoid tumours which first presented clinically as distant metastases within the breast. Special studies are indicated, such as tests for immunolocalization of calcitonin and other markers of specific differentiation. Sarcomas and lymphoid neoplasms may also involve the breast, as may leukaemic infiltrates.

Histopathologically, the secondary tumour masses in the breast may be assumed to closely approximate those of the primary tumour and/or other metastases. Most metastatic tumours are multinodular and seem separate from the breast parenchyma. Special studies are useful in the identification of some of these tumours. In males, particularly useful are the tissue immunochemical markers of prostate-specific antigen and/or prostate-specific acid phosphatase (see Chapter 20) to separate the histopathologically similar breast carcinoma from the probability of a metastasis from the prostate carcinoma.

Unusual presentations of breast carcinoma

Paget disease of the nipple

This condition is not important as a contendable type of breast cancer, but rather because it may be a subtle clinical clue to the presence of underlying breast cancer. Although widely recognized as a separate disease entity, the presence of Paget disease of the nipple actually only indicates that intraductal carcinoma in the ducts beneath the nipple has spread to the nipple surface. The clinical presentation is with a moist, erythematous surface to the nipple, which may spread to the surrounding areola. This clinical resemblance to eczema is produced because the carcinoma cells intermix with and replace the normal squamous cells, producing a nipple surface that is permeable to fluid and easily irritated. The classic histopathological appearance is with large, rounded carcinoma cells interspersed within the stratified keratinocytes. Glandular, cytological, and cell-surface markers are maintained. Complete replacement of the squamous epithelium may also be seen.

The extent of disease in the underlying breast is quite varied. Paget disease may be an indicator of localized, curable disease as well as the first clinical indication of carcinomas of poor prognosis. About 50 per cent of women with breast cancer presenting with an eczematous nipple have palpable masses of invasive carcinoma as well as extensive ductal carcinoma in situ. Only about 10 per cent of women presenting with this diagnostic sign have in situ disease confined to the immediate region of the nipple.

Inflammatory carcinoma

Although frequently cited as a special type of mammary carcinoma, it may be best understood as a special presentation of carcinomas with a poor prognosis. The greatest clinical importance of this uncommon presentation is that it may be mistaken for other, benign conditions which produce a similar clinical appearance of a locally or diffusely swollen, hot, erythematous breast. Fat necrosis, duct ectasia with active inflammation, and especially an abcess may be mimicked clinically.

The clinical features at presentation largely define the inflammatory carcinoma: redness, swelling, and heat are usually extensive. The great majority of these cases will be further identified by the presence of widespread and easily detectable lymphatic metastases. These are usually identified by microscopic examination of the dermal lymphatics in the overlying skin. The histopathological and cytological features of the carcinomas presenting in this fashion are surprisingly diverse, but most are poorly differentiated. Only about 1 per cent of breast cancers have this presentation. The dismal prognosis attending these cancers prior to the advent of currently available therapeutic regimens has been greatly altered by more intensive chemotherapy. Currently, some small series have reported as many as 50 per cent five-year survivors.

22.1.6   Gynaecomastia and male breast cancer

Breast disease only seems to be a condition confined to women because diseases of the breast in men are a minor and unusual consideration. Virtually all of the conditions which occur within the female breast may occur within the male. However, they occur rarely.

The most common disease of the male breast is gynaecomastia, which indicates simply an enlargement of the male breast. This may be unilateral or bilateral and is characterized by an increase in the mass of ducts present in the male breast as well as their ensheathing fibrous tissue. Because the enlargement is a combined change of epithelium and fibrous tissue, the lesion mimics fibroadenoma somewhat (Bland and Page 1991). This mimicry is incomplete however, as the entire tissue of the breast seems to be involved. It more closely resembles the very rare condition in adolescent girls termed 'juvenile hypertrophy'. In both conditions a loose specialized fibrous tissue surrounds small elements which appear to be ducts, without the clustering of glandular elements characteristic of lobules. Also, both conditions have their major occurrence at the time of onset of secondary sexual characteristics. Gynaecomastia is also relatively frequent in men over 70 years of age, presumably because of a relative decrease in androgens as compared to oestrogens and other changes in sex steroid status. Alterations of sex hormones and related substances as occur with many drug regimens may also result in gynaecomastia.

Carcinoma occurs in the male breast with an incidence of one-hundredth that seen in females. This sex ratio of male to female is remarkably constant in both high- and low-incidence populations. The carcinomas occuring in the male are remarkably similar in anatomic patterns and biological behaviour to those seen in the female, although special types are less frequent, particularly the lobular type and its variants. The natural history of breast cancer occurring in males closely resembles that of the disease in women if controlled for stage at presentation (Adami et al. 1989) as well as for sex differences in death from other causes.

22.1.7   Prognostic indicators in breast cancer

The many comments about relative killing capacity, good prognosis, etc. in the preceding sections should be taken as an appropriate comment on the dominance of prognosis as a concern in qualifying breast cancers, individually and in groups. This section highlights this concern arising from the variability of clinical course, and offers comments on the approach to qualifying the individual cancer in the individual patient for reasons of therapeutic decision-making as well as prognosis. Specifically, we hope to identify patients with a poor prognosis who may benefit from chemotherapy which may be toxic.

There are many systems and competing methodologies for the prognostication of breast cancer. The amazing point is that so many indicators have some ability in this regard.

In general terms we recognize all examples of non-invasive carcinoma or carcinoma *in situ* as of no threat to life at the time of their identification.

There is also a group of lesions we call cancer that rarely kill and prognostically are inseparable from the general population controlled for age. These may be recognized as special-type cancers histopathologically as well as by combinations of other measures.

Then there are carcinomas about which our ability to predict is poor, and in general their ability to kill is about that of the average of all breast cancers.

These are followed by a group of breast cancers which are more likely to kill than the rest of the cancers and which may be termed a poor prognosis group.

In general, both size and lymph-node status are the most readily available, reproducible, and useful as prognostic indicators. This information may be combined with other measures as found in Table 22.2 (see above). Studies still in progress are continually analysing prognostic capabilities of these and other variables. The major recent development which has focused attention on this area is the development of varied therapeutic options, particularly local excision plus radiation as an option to total mastectomy, and the acceptance that chemotherapeutic regimens have efficacy. Selection of the appropriate treatment option involves careful characterization of a patient's cancer. For example, extensive ductal carcinoma *in situ* accompanying invasive disease is an indicator of a high likelihood of local treatment failure after radiation of the concerned breast (Holland *et al.* 1990). With so many measures, evaluation of competing strategies by multiple parameter analysis is mandatory.

DNA quantitation is most frequently performed in a flow cytometer which analyses dyes binding to DNA in a quantitative fashion (see Section 30.6). This produces graphic plots identifying the peaks of normal (*2n*) and dividing (*4n*) cells of a diploid population (Fig. 22.16a) in contrast to the abnormal cell population, or 'stem line', with an irregular compliment of DNA, classified as aneuploid (Fig. 22.16b). The aneuploid tumours might arguably be expected to behave aggressively (Clark *et al.* 1989). Whether the prognostic promise that was hoped for from DNA cytometry will be achieved has yet to be revealed with convincing consistency (Koss *et al.* 1989). Two factors that impair its utility are the lack of standardization in techniques or methodology of assessment, and also the meagre understanding of what precisely determines or accounts for the cells with abnormal DNA content that characterizes the aneuploid cell population. The technique has considerable potential to enlarge our understanding of tumour biology but may require some modification of current concepts of its application to

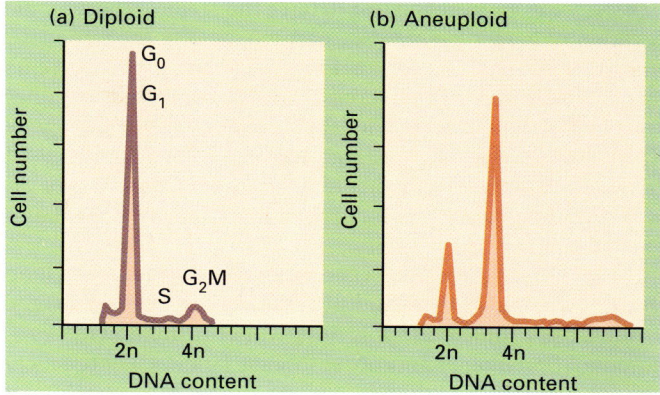

Fig. 22.16 Diagrammatic appearances of flow cytometry of (a) diploid and (b) aneuploid breast tumours. The appropriate phases of the cell growth cycle are shown in relation to the appropriate cell population and its DNA content.

reveal its full potential. It must also be remembered that the prognostic information that these techniques provide can also be obtained more easily by critical evaluation of optimally processed histopathological material, and the value of multiple parameter analysis is emphasized (Uyterlinde *et al.* 1990). See Section 22.1.11 for a fuller description of specific prognostic factors.

22.1.8 Epidemiology

The occurrence of breast carcinoma is strongly related to life events that are unique to females, and are unevenly clustered with regard to geographical and social factors, age and familial associations (Kelsey and Berkowitz 1988). Of these, age, country of residence, family history, and the presence of carcinoma in one breast are the factors that may attain a magnitude of risk greater than four times that of the general population or another reference population. An anatomic factor, determined by histopathological pattern of atypical hyperplasia at biopsy has a similar magnitude of risk elevation, but considering how few women undergo breast biopsy, it is not readily available information.

The epidemiology of breast cancer and other cancers is discussed in Chapter 9 under the general topic of cancer, and provides most of our knowledge as to the settings in which breast carcinoma is more likely to occur and therefore give clues as to the aetiology of the disease. These features are usually related as a relative risk, thus necessitating a reference population. For example, the female sex as compared to the male has a relative risk of 100, or 100 times the rate of breast cancer experienced by males. This specific risk factor, or differential risk between men and women, is remarkably consistent in both high- and low-incidence areas of the world. The descriptive, geographic epidemiology reveals remarkable differences in incidence between various parts of the world (see Fig. 22.1). Breast cancer is the most frequent carcinoma among women in most of Europe, in North America and much of Latin America, and in Australia (Parkin *et al.* 1984).

Of the life events that appear to have the greatest effect on the elevation of breast cancer risk, parity is among the strongest. Women who have children before the age of about 20 years have a decreased risk of breast cancer compared to other women. Those who first complete pregnancies after the age of 30, or who do not have children will experience an increased risk of carcinoma development. Breast feeding may have an additional risk-lowering effect beyond that of parity alone, but it is small.

The familial aggregation of carcinomas of the breast has long been known, and despite intensive research, the precise genetic or other basis underlying this observation is unknown. Chromosome 17 anomalies may occur in some families. For practical purposes, women with histories of carcinoma in close relatives are at an increased risk of developing the disease themselves at a rate about twice that of the general population. This rate increases with the intensity of the history; with the premenopausal occurrence of the cancer in relatives; and with the unusual occurrence of bilateral carcinoma in a relative.

Exposure to ionizing radiation has been shown to increase the risk of subsequent breast carcinoma (Miller 1987). This has been demonstrated in studies of women treated with X-rays for acute postpartum mastitis as well as women exposed to greatly excessive numbers of fluoroscopic examinations, and women exposed to radiation from atomic bomb explosions in Japan. It is evident that this carcinogenic effect of radiation is most evident at young ages, primarily in the second decade, and has little effect when received after age 30.

It must be understood that these risk factors have little effect on clinical management because they rarely indicate prophylactic action due to very high risk. Also, they have never indicated a group of such low risk that they need not be considered for screening or need not have a lump biopsied with the concern that it might be carcinoma. Careful, continuing surveillance by mammography when possible is indicated for most women, particularly those with identifiably increased risk of cancer.

Screening for breast cancer has changed all aspects of clinical practice relative to breast disease (Stewart *et al.* 1991). For practical purposes screening indicates that radiography of the breast (mammography) is performed on women without regard to the presence of some suspicion of carcinoma, including both the sign of a lump as well as the presence of a high-risk indicator such as family history of breast cancer (see Section 22.2).

Age is the most important determinant of breast cancer incidence: 99 per cent of breast carcinomas occur after the age of 30 years; the combined incidence for the decade between the ages of 40 and 50 is approximating 1.5 per cent, i.e. averaging 1.5/1000/yr; and the yearly rate doubles between the ages of 50 and 60. Incidence is also strongly influenced by place of residence: natives of North America and western Europe have the highest breast cancer risk; incidence rates in Asia and parts of South America and Africa are the lowest. The magnitude of these differences are five times or more (Stalsberg *et al.* 1989). However, the effect changes with migration as the risk of breast cancer in second- and third-generation Americans after migrating from Japan begins to approximate that of the native

population. Note also that while the postmenopausal incidence continues to rise in high-risk areas, the incidence plateaus or falls after the menopause in low-incidence regions (Miller 1987). Some of these differences may be accounted for by diet, obesity, and early age at menarche in high-risk areas, but precise reasons are not known. Diet has some effects on risk of breast cancer; high fat, particularly saturated fat, is implicated from animal studies and some epidemiological surveys, but specifics are currently unclear (Willett 1989). Alcohol has been found to be associated with a slight risk elevation in most studies, but related factors are not comprehensively investigated and a biological explanatory rationale is not apparent. Coffee and many other dietary elements have been pursued and found unassociated with cancer risk.

Hormonal theories to explain the aetiology of breast cancer have been frequently espoused, and seldom proved. There is strong support for a hormonal element in causation of this cancer because of such observations as the great lowering of breast cancer risk with ovariectomy in the fourth decade of life. Also, the presence of growth stimulation of many breast cancers by oestrogen supports a role for these hormones in cancer progression. Unfortunately, the specifics of this association are not proven, although endogenous hormone determinations, including those associated with luteal phase dysfunction and androgen production by ovary and adrenal, are under careful scrutiny. Thus the specific hormone(s) and their relative roles are unknown, although constitutionally and reproductively defined risk factors (Pike and Ross, 1984; Henderson *et al.* 1988) remain the main support for an endogenous hormonal hypothesis in mammary carcinogenesis.

22.1.9   Molecular biology of breast cancer

The molecular events that underlie carcinogenesis and the various events that characterize the malignant behaviour of a neoplasm, e.g. cell motility, cell-surface changes, interaction with stroma, growth factors, angiogenesis, etc. have been widely pursued in the 1970s and the 1980s (see Chapter 9.6). Much of this information has been assembled from experimental research models *in vitro* and in animals, yet most awaits demonstration in humans. Most of the methodology developed in these decades has been applied to human tissues. These advances have not yet had a major impact upon the clinical management of breast disease. However, they have elucidated some steps in the aetiology and biological mechanisms of breast cancer and provide promise of diagnostic and therapeutic advances of utility. The most notable advances have been those identifying genetic and molecular changes, considered as either:

1. karyotypic alterations in individual chromosomes;
2. mutations, deletions, or translocations of gene loci; and
3. abnormal expression of proto-oncogene activities.

Genomic alterations in human breast cancers are another area of intensive research. Again, the variability between breast cancers is evident. The conventional metaphase analysis of karyotype has provided little information in breast cancer largely due to the difficulty of growing most breast cancer cells *in vitro* to produce these preparations. Some deletions as well as overrepresentation (amplification) of a portion of chromosomes have been described. Many of these are similar to those seen in other solid tumours and thus may, like some of these other abnormalities, represent epiphenomena associated with the development of growth or other characteristics of malignancy rather than fundamental to its cause. Deletion of genetic material and amplification of genes have also been identified by the application of techniques of molecular biology to specific genes. Besides the additions and subtractions, gene rearrangements, which may disrupt coding sequences, have been described occasionally, as have point mutations. Another interesting finding is the deletion of some alleles, so that while the host may be heterozygous for a specific locus, the neoplasms may be homozygous. The *Rb* gene, first described in retinoblastoma, is an example of such a situation. Homozygous deletions of parts of, or the entire, *Rb* gene, as well as partial gene reduplications, have been described in as many as 27 per cent of primary breast tumours tested. This phenomenon of loss of heterozygosity is diverse and remarkably common. Its role in the causation sequence is unknown. It is quite possible that it will be quantitatively related to measures of tumour burden.

Although several alterations have been recorded, no consistent karyotypic abnormality has been associated with breast cancer (Bodmer 1988). Stimulated by the positive evidence for tumour suppressor genes, supporting Knudson's 'two-hit' hypothesis as the basic mechanism involved in familial and spontaneous forms of retinoblastoma (chromosome 13) and colon cancer (chromosome 5) (reviewed by Spandidos and Anderson 1989), there has been considerable interest in similar deletions in breast cancer. Allelic losses have indeed been consistently identified on chromosomes 11, 13, and 17, yet positive relationships with tumour size suggest that these events may not be related to the initiation and development of cancers. Recent work has focused attention on both the short and long arm of chromosome 17. Loss of heterozygosity for genes on 17p occurs in about 60 per cent of breast cancers. This may or may not be associated with mutations of the p53 gene on 17p (Steele *et al.* 1991).

The activities of the proto-oncogenes (non-mutated oncogenes) belonging to the *ras*, *myc*, and *neu* families have been the major focus of attention in breast cancer. Overactivity of these genes has been documented frequently, not necessarily in mutated form. However, it is the *neu* oncogene, also known as c-*erb* B2 or Her-2neu located on the long arm of chromosome 17, which has received the most recent concentrated attention. This is because of reported capacities for 'single-step' carcinogenesis in transfection studies with rodents (Muller *et al.* 1988), and also because of its prognostic association with established breast cancers (Slamon *et al.* 1989; Wright *et al.* 1989). Overexpression, associated with amplification of gene copy number, is correlated with bad prognosis. So far unexplained is the lack of significance in node-negative cancers and the more frequent overexpression in non-invasive breast cancers. The product of c-*erb* B2 is a presumed growth-factor receptor and over-expression is common also to tumours of brain, ovary, and stomach.

Awareness of other growth factors, especially transforming growth factor α (TGF-α) and β (TGF-β) (see Table 22.1, above), and insulin-like growth factor I (IGF-I) and II, have stimulated interest in autocrine and paracrine mechanisms of modulating growth (Kraus *et al.* 1988, Roberts *et al.* 1988). Although *in vitro* models with breast cell lines are informative, applications to the *in vivo* situation are so far elusive. Epidermal growth factor (EGF) receptor is also important and it is of interest that the inverse relationship with oestrogen receptor, found so consistently for breast cancers and portending a bad prognosis, does not apply in benign breast tissue when both elements can be present together (Barker *et al.* 1989). This is taken to indicate a switch in regulatory mechanisms associated with malignant transformation or clone selection, or both (see Section 22.1.11).

One factor that is believed to give aggressive metastatic advantage to breast cancer cells is (lack of occupancy of) laminin receptor sites on the cancer cell membranes, discouraging adhesion to basal lamina and encouraging motility. Recent work links variation in laminin production with hormone responsiveness to oestrogen and progesterone, thereby providing an explanation for the observed difference in clinical aggression of cancers according to receptor positivity for these hormones. It is, however, no longer acceptable to retain a simplified concept of cancer cell growth modulation by endocrine stimulation, since autocrine and paracrine mechanisms may be more important determinants of clonal selection.

The precise specificity and ease of generation of monoclonal antibodies (MAbs) has changed the speed with which specific tumour-associated antigens may be detected (Thor *et al.* 1986). Several monoclonal antibodies against human mammary carcinomas have been reported. Each one must be characterized, as they differ with regard to binding characteristics and their relative ability to be both sensitive and specific with regard to recognizing malignant cell lines (cells from carcinomas growing *in vitro*) as well as tissue of mammary origin. Many of these surface antigens are related to the milk-fat globule membrane which is found in milk and is a glycoprotein of the mammary epithelial cell surface. Most of these monoclonal antibodies generated by hybridoma technology react with antigens also found on cells from other neoplasms, for instance carcinomas of pancreatic or pulmonary origin. There is a great deal of antigenic heterogeneity in the expression of tumour antigen determinants, both among cells within an individual tumour and between different tumour masses in different patients (McCarty *et al.* 1988). This incredible variability, as well as the fact that cancer cells established in culture often seem to have few determinants in common with 'native' carcinomas, indicate both the promise and difficulties for the diagnostic and therapeutic development of these special tools. The variability means that the uses of MAbs in diagnosis and therapy will demand careful determination of specificity. This applies to serum assays, to targeting of antibodies for their visualization after localization in occult tumour masses, as well as to subcategorization of carcinomas to determine prognostic information. The utilization of these various antibodies in a diagnostic setting involves a certain knowledge of their pitfalls, and relative failures and strengths of sensitivity and specificity. For example, many antibodies are quite specific for epithelial neoplasms and therefore may be used in the differentiation of a lymphoma from a carcinoma. However, if it were not initially certain that the lesion was malignant, the staining for differentiation will not evaluate malignancy. The variety of antigens that may be of utility include: oncogene products (e.g. c-erb-B2), tumour-associated antigens, differentiation antigens (fetal v. adult as well as organ and organ regions), and surface proteins associated with metastatic capability.

Eventually the ability to control critical elements of the molecular events governing breast cancer will allow manipulation and possible control of cancer growth.

22.1.10   Bibliography

Adami, H. O., et al. (1989). The survival pattern in male breast cancer: an analysis of 1429 patients from the Nordic countries. Cancer 64, 1177–82.

Anderson, T. J. and Battersby, S. (1985). Radial scars of benign and malignant breast: comparative features and significance. Journal of Pathology 147, 23–32.

Anderson, T. J., Battersby, S., King, R. J. B., McPherson, K., and Going, J. J. (1989). Oral contraceptive use influences resting breast proliferation. Human Pathology 20, 1139–44.

Barker, S., Panahy, C., Puddefoot, J. R., Goode, A. W., and Vinson, G. P. (1989). Epidermal growth factor receptor and oestrogen receptors in the non-malignant part of the cancerous breast. British Journal of Cancer 60, 673–7.

Bartow, S. A., Black, W. C., Waeckerlin, R. W., and Mettler, F. A. (1982). Fibrocystic disease: A continuing enigma. In Pathology annual, Vol. 17, Part 2 (ed. P. P. Rosen and R. E. Fechner), pp. 93–101. Appleton Lange, Norwalk.

Bartow, S. A., Pathak, D. R., Black, W. C., Key, C. R., and Teaf, S. R. (1987). Prevalence of benign, atypical and malignant breast lesions in populations at different risk for breast cancer. Cancer 60, 2751–60.

Berg, J. W. and Robbins, G. F. (1966). Factors influencing short and long term survival of breast cancer patients. Surgery, Gynecology and Obstetrics 122, 1311–16.

Bodmer, W. (1988). Somatic cell genetics and cancer. Cancer Surveys 7, 239–50.

Bland, K. I. and Page, D. L. (1991). Gynecomastia. In The breast (ed. K. I. Bland and E. M. Copeland), pp. 135–68. W. B. Saunders, Philadelphia.

Breast cancer screening: Forrest report (1986). HMSO Publications, London.

Callahan, R. and Campbell, G. (1989). Mutations in human breast cancer: an overview. Journal of the National Cancer Institute 81, 1780–6.

Cardiff, R. D. (1988). Cellular and molecular aspects of neoplastic progression in the mammary gland. European Journal of Cancer and Clinical Oncology 24, 15–20.

Clark, G. M. and McGuire, W. L. (1989). New biologic prognostic factors in breast cancer. Oncology 3, 49–54.

Clark, G. M., Dressler, L. G., and Owens, M. A. (1989). Prediction of relapse or survival in patients with node-negative breast cancer by DNA flow cytometry. New England Journal of Medicine 320, 627–33.

Connolly, J. L. and Schnitt, S. J. (1988). Evaluation of breast biopsy specimens in patients considered for treatment by conservative surgery and radiation therapy for early breast cancer. In Pathology annual, Vol. 23, Part 1 (ed. P. P. Rosen and R. E. Fechner), pp. 1–23. Appleton Lange, Norwalk.

Connolly, J. L., et al. (1989). In situ carcinoma of the breast. Annual Reviews of Medicine 40, 173–80.

Di Costanzo, D., Rosen, P. P., Gareen, I., Franklin, S., and Lesser, M. (1990). Prognosis in infiltrating lobular carcinoma: an analysis of 'classical' and variant tumours. American Journal of Surgical Pathology 14, 12–23.

Dixon, J. M., Anderson, T. J., Page, D. L., Lee D., and Duffy, S. W. (1982). Infiltrating lobular carcinoma of the breast. Histopathology 6, 149–61.

Dixon, J. M., et al. (1983). Infiltrating lobular carcinoma of the breast: An evaluation of the incidence and consequence of bilateral disease. British Journal of Surgery 70, 573–6.

Dixon, J. M., Scott, W. N., and Miller, W. R. (1985). Natural history of cystic disease: the importance of cyst type. British Journal of Surgery 72, 190–2.

Dongen, J. A. van, et al. (1989). In situ breast cancer: The EORTC consensus meeting. Lancet ii, 25–7.

Dupont, W. D. and Page, D. L. (1985). Risk factors for breast cancer in women with proliferative breast disease. New England Journal of Medicine 312, 146–51.

Dupont, W. D. and Page, D. L. (1989). Relative risk of breast cancer varies with time since diagnosis of atypical hyperplasia. Human Pathology 20, 723–5.

Elston, C. W. (1987). Grading of invasive carcinoma of the breast. In Diagnostic histopathology of the breast (D. L. Page and T. J. A. Anderson), pp. 300–11. Churchill Livingstone, Edinburgh.

Ethier, S. P. and Heppner, G. H. (1987). Biology of breast cancer in vivo and in vitro. In Breast diseases (ed. J. R. Harris, I. C. Henderson, S. Hellman, and D. W. Kinne). Lippincott, Philadelphia.

Fechner, R. E. (1987). Fibroadenoma and related lesions. In Diagnostic histopathology of the breast, (D. L. Page and T. J. Anderson), pp. 72–85. Churchill Livingstone, Edinburgh.

Fisher, E. R., et al. (1984). Pathological findings from the national adjuvant project for breast cancers (Protocol no. 4). X. Discriminants for tenth year treatment failure. Cancer 53, 712–23.

Frykberg, E. R., Santiago, F., Betsill, W. L., and O'Brien, P. H. (1987). Lobular carcinoma in situ of the breast. Surgery, Gynecology and Obstetrics 164, 285–301.

Gompel, C., Faverly, D., and Silverberg, S. G. (1990). The breast. In Principles and practice of surgical pathology (2nd edn) (ed. G. Silverberg). Churchill Livingstone, Edinburgh.

Haagensen, C. D. (1986). Diseases of the breast (3rd edn). Saunders, Philadelphia.

Hellman, S. and Harris, J. R. (1987). The appropriate breast cancer paradigm. Cancer Research 47, 339–42.

Henderson, B. E., Ross, R., and Bernstein, L. (1988). Estrogens as a cause of human cancer: The Richard and Hilda Rosenthal Foundation Lecture. Cancer Research 48, 246–53.

Holland, R., et al. (1990). The presence of an extensive intraductal component (EIC) following a limited excision correlates with prominent residual disease in the remainder of the breast. Journal of Clinical Oncology 8, 113–18.

Hughes, L. E., Mansel, R. E., and Webster, D. J. T. (1989). Benign disorders and diseases of the breast. Baillière Tindall, London.

Jensen, R. A., Page, D. L., Dupont, W. D., and Rogers, L. W. (1989). Invasive breast cancer (IBC) risk in women with sclerosing adenosis. Cancer 64, 1977–83.

Kelsey, J. L. and Berkowitz, G. S. (1988). Breast cancer epidemiology. Cancer Research 48, 5615–23.

Koss, L. G., Czernick, B., Herz, F., and Wersto, R. P. (1989). Flow cytometric measurements of DNA and other cell components in human tumors. *Human Pathology* **20**, 528–48.

Kraus, M. H., *et al.* (1988). Mechanisms by which genes encoding growth factors and growth factor receptors contribute to malignant transformation. *Annals of the New York Academy of Science* **551**, 320–35.

Lagios, M. D., Margolin, F. R., Westdahl, P. R., and Rose, M. R. (1989). Mammographically detected duct carcinoma *in situ*. *Cancer* **63**, 618–24.

Lammie, G. A. and Millis, R. R. (1989). Ductal adenoma of the breast: a review of fifteen cases. *Human Pathology* **20**, 903–8.

McCarty, K. S., Jr, Kinney, R. B., and Bast, R. C., Jr (1988). Epithelial 'Tumor' markers in lesions of the breast. In *Progress in cancer research and therapy* (ed. F. Bresciani, R. J. B. King, M. E. Lippman, and J. P. Raynaud), pp. 282–9. Raven Press, New York.

McWhirter, R. (1955). Simple mastectomy and radiotherapy in the treatment of breast carcinoma. *British Journal of Radiology* **28**, 128–39.

Medina, D. (1988). The preneoplastic state in mouse mammary tumorigenesis. *Carcinogenesis* **9**, 1113–19.

Meyer, J. S. (1986). Cell kinetics of histologic variants of *in situ* breast carcinoma. *Breast Cancer Research and Treatment* **7**, 171–80.

Miller, A. B. (1987). Breast cancer epidemiology, etiology and prevention. In *Breast diseases* (ed. J. R. Harris, I. C. Henderson, S. Hellman, and D. W. Kinne). Lippincott, Philadelphia.

Miller, W. R. and Anderson, T. J. (1988). Oestrogen and progestogins and the breast. In *The menopause* (ed. J. W. W. Studd and M. I. Whitehead), pp. 234–46. Blackwell, London.

Millis, R. R. and Girling, A. C. (1989). The breast. In *Diagnostic surgical pathology* (ed. S. S. Sternberg). Raven Press, New York.

Muller, W. J., Sinn, E., Pattengale, P. K., Wallace, R., and Leder, P. (1988). Single-step induction of mammary adenocarcinoma in transgenic mice bearing the activated c-*neu* oncogene. *Cell* **54**, 105–15.

Ohuchi, N., Rikiya, A., and Kasi, M. (1984). Possible cancerous change of intraductal papillomas of the breast: a 3D reconstruction study of 25 cases. *Cancer* **54**, 605–11.

Ohuchi, N., *et al.* (1987). Expression of tumor-associated antigen (DF3) in atypical hyperplasias and *in situ* carcinomas of the human breast. *Journal of the National Cancer Institute* **79**, 109–17.

Page, D. L. (1987). Benign disorders of the breast. In *Internal medicine* (2nd edn) (ed. J. H. Stein). Little, Brown and Co., Boston.

Page, D. L. and Anderson, T. J. (1987). *Diagnostic histopathology of the breast*. Churchill Livingstone, Edinburgh.

Page, D. L., Dupont, W. D., Rogers, L. W., and Landenberger, M. (1982). Intraductal carcinoma of the breast: follow-up after biopsy only. *Cancer* **49**, 751–8.

Page, D. L., Dupont, W. D., Rogers, L. W., and Rados, M. S. (1985). Atypical hyperplastic lesions of the female breast. *Cancer* **55**, 2698–708.

Papotti, M., Gugliotta, P., Ghiringhello, B., and Bussolati, G. (1984). Association of breast carcinoma and multiple intraductal papillomas: an histological and immunohistochemical investigation. *Histopathology* **8**, 963–75.

Parkin, D. M., Stjernsward, J., and Muir, C. S. (1984). Estimates of the world wide frequency of twelve major cancers. *Bulletin of the World Health Organization* **62**, 163–82.

Patchefsky, A. S. *et al.* (1989). Heterogeneity of intraductal carcinoma of the breast. *Cancer* **63**, 731–41.

Petrakis, N. L., Ernster, V. L., and King, M. C. (1982). Breast. In *Cancer epidemiology and prevention* (1st edn) (ed. D. Schottenfeld and J. F. Fraumeni). W. B. Saunders, Philadelphia.

Pike, M. C. and Ross, R. K. (1984). Breast cancer. *British Medical Bulletin* **40**, 351–4.

Roberts, A. B., Thompson, N. L., Heini, U., Flanders, C., and Sporn, M. B. (1988). Transforming growth factor B: possible role in carcinogenesis. *British Journal of Cancer* **57**, 594–600.

Rosen, P. P., Lieberman, P. H., Braun, D. W., Jr, Kosloff, C., and Adair, F. (1978). Lobular carcinoma *in situ* of the breast: detailed analysis of 99 patients with average follow-up of 24 years. *American Journal of Surgical Pathology* **2**, 225–51.

Slamon, J., *et al.* (1989). Studies of the HER-2/*neu* proto-oncogene in human breast and ovarian cancer. *Science* **244**, 707–12.

Spandidos, D. A. and Anderson, M. L. M. (1989). Oncogenes and oncosuppressor genes; their involvement in cancer. *Journal of Pathology* **157**, 1–10.

Stalsberg, H., Thomas, D. B., and Noonan, E. A. (1989). WHO Collaborative Study of Neoplasia; histological types of breast carcinoma in relation to international variation and breast cancer risk factors. *International Journal of Cancer* **44**, 399–409.

Steel, G. M., Thomson, A. M., and Clayton, J. (1991). Genetic aspects of breast cancer. *British Medical Bulletin* **47**, 504–18.

Stewart, H. J., Anderson, T. J., Forrest, A. P. M. (eds) (1991). Breast disease: new approaches. *British Medical Bulletin* **47** (2).

Tavassoli, F. A. and Norris, H. J. (1990). A comparison of the results of long-term follow-up for atypical intraductal hyperplasia and intraductal hyperplasia of the breast. *Cancer* **65**, 518–29.

Thor, A., Weeks, M. O., and Schlom, J. (1986). Monoclonal antibodies and breast cancer. *Seminars in Oncology* **13**, 393–401.

Uyterlinde, A. M., Baak, J. P. A., Schipper, N. W., Peterse, H., Matze, E., and Meijer, C. J. L. (1990). Further evaluation of the prognostic value of morphometric and flow cytometric parameters in breast cancer patients with long follow-up. *International Journal of Cancer* **45**, 1–7.

Wellings, S. R., Jensen, H. M., and Marcum, R. G. (1975). An atlas of subgross pathology of the human breast with special reference to possible precancerous lesions. *Journal of the National Cancer Institute* **55**, 231–73.

Wilkinson, S., Anderson, T. J., Rifkind, E., Chetty, U., and Forrest, A. P. M. (1989). Fibroadenoma of the breast: A follow-up of conservative management. *British Journal of Surgery* **76**, 390–1.

Willett, W. (1989). The search for the causes of breast and colon cancer. *Nature* **338**, 389–94.

Wright, C., *et al.* (1989). Expression of c-erbB-2 oncoprotein: a prognostic indicator in human breast cancer. *Cancer Research* **49**, 2087–90.

22.1.11 Prognosis and tumour markers

Elizabeth R. Horak and James O'D. McGee

Introduction

General statements about prognosis in breast cancer are made in Section 22.1.7. This section deals more specifically with those parameters which are used in the design of treatment schedules for individual patients. Breast cancer is a heterogeneous set of neoplasms, with diverse clinical course and fatality (Section 22.1.5). The most lethal aspect of malignant tumours is their ability to metastasize. While primary tumours are usually controlled by surgery, it is metastatic disease which leads to the individual's death. The stage of metastasis formation, however, is reached after different periods, and the length of time from the first surgical treatment until the development of metastases ('tumour-free survival') can be used as a clinical measure of the tumour's aggressiveness. Ultimately, the behaviour is characterized by the overall survival of the individual.

Knowledge of the expected behaviour of a malignant tumour is necessary for decision-making concerning optimal treatment of individual tumours. The recent use of restricted surgery (lumpectomy) with local radiation instead of total mastectomy, and especially the wide choice of new chemotherapeutic regimes underlies the need for accurate prognostication. Cytotoxic chemotherapy is a double-edged tool. On the one hand, it can increase life expectancy in advanced malignant disease as an adjunct to other therapy but, on the other hand, it is a hazardous and potentially lethal form of treatment. It is the responsibility of the management team to separate cases which benefit most from this form of therapy from those who will obtain minimal additional life expectancy. No perfect prognostic marker is available, and it is generally agreed that a multifactorial assessment is the best choice at the moment.

Tumour categories with prognostic implications

The empirical approach of histopathologically classifying tumours defines tumour groups with a statistically comparable clinical course. Non-invasive tumours represent a separate category in this classification, in that they have no metastatic capacity, and bear no threat to life if eradicated by complete excision.

Invasive tumours are usually stratified into three, prognostically distinct groups as follow.

1. **Favourable prognosis.** This group includes malignant tumours with a low risk of causing death. Certain histopathological types belong to this group, but some invasive cancers also have a similar clinical course, especially if treated in their early stages. For these tumours, no adjuvant therapy is required.

2. **Intermediate prognosis.** The majority of breast cancers belong to this category. For decisions on adjuvant therapy, further selection criteria are desirable.

3. **Poor prognosis.** Tumours with a highly malignant course, marked by a short disease-free interval and overall survival, form this group. Adjuvant therapy is routinely used in their treatment.

Assigning tumours to the first group according to their clinico-pathological features can be a straightforward task. For example, the long overall survival of tubular carcinomas can be predicted from their histopathological features (Section 22.1.5). For the assessment of tumours in the second and third groups, some indication of the expected behaviour can be derived from the clinico-pathological features. Although these factors are still the most widely used guidelines, it has been realized that their prognostic value is limited and a finer delineation of the expected prognosis is needed.

It is usually the selection of tumours for chemotherapy which needs the most careful consideration. Lymph node negative tumours, are considered to have a good prognosis, yet a proportion of these tumours have a highly malignant course, marked by rapidly developing of metastases. These tumours would probably benefit from early implementation of chemotherapy. Selecting out these latter tumours is the main target of new prognostic markers.

Histopathological parameters of prognostic significance

Tumour type

As has been discussed in Section 22.1.5, there are certain morphological types of breast cancer which have a distinct, favourable clinical course. Tubular or cribrifom carcinomas, even in the presence of lymph node metastases, have an excellent prognosis, with a low risk of mortality. Similarly, the prognosis of medullary and mucinous cancer is favourable.

In situ cancer component The presence of an extensive *in situ* component within an invasive tumour is associated with a higher likelihood of recurrences (Holland *et al.* 1990). The reason for this association is not clear, but possible explanations include the presence of more extensive disease outside of the resected lesion, or increased resistance to radiation among tumours with a large *in situ* component.

Neovascularization In experimental systems, tumour growth beyond a certain size requires angiogenesis, and penetration of vessels is an important step in the process of metastasis formation. It has been shown that the density of newly formed microvessels correlates with the risk of metastasis (Weidner *et al.* 1991). The angiogenic capacity seems to be independent of local invasion, i.e. it is present in some *in situ* tumours. This promises to be a morphological factor of prognostic significance in early tumours, which will be explored in future studies.

Tumour size and lymph node status

Both increased primary tumour diameter and the number of lymph nodes involved have an inverse correlation with survival. Analysis of data from 24 740 breast cancer patients showed that the size of the primary tumour and the lymph node status can be used as independent markers of 5 year prognosis (Fig. 22.17) (Carter *et al.* 1989). There is a linear correlation between the two markers. Whilst only 20 per cent of invasive cancers under 0.5 cm have metastatic tumour in the axillary lymph nodes, the proportion of metastasis increases for larger tumours, reaching 70 per cent in tumours larger than 5 cm (Fig. 22.18). Although tumour size and lymph node status usually go together, the presence or absence of lymph node metastases is paramount. Positive lymph node status reduces the otherwise excellent survival prospects of small (<0.5 cm) tumours to 60 per cent 5-year survival. The number of involved lymph nodes is significant: 5-year survival is significantly better for those patients with three or fewer positive nodes (Fig. 22.19). The decisive role of lymph node metastases has been shown by many clinical trials, and today the lymph node status is accepted as the most significant prognostic factor.

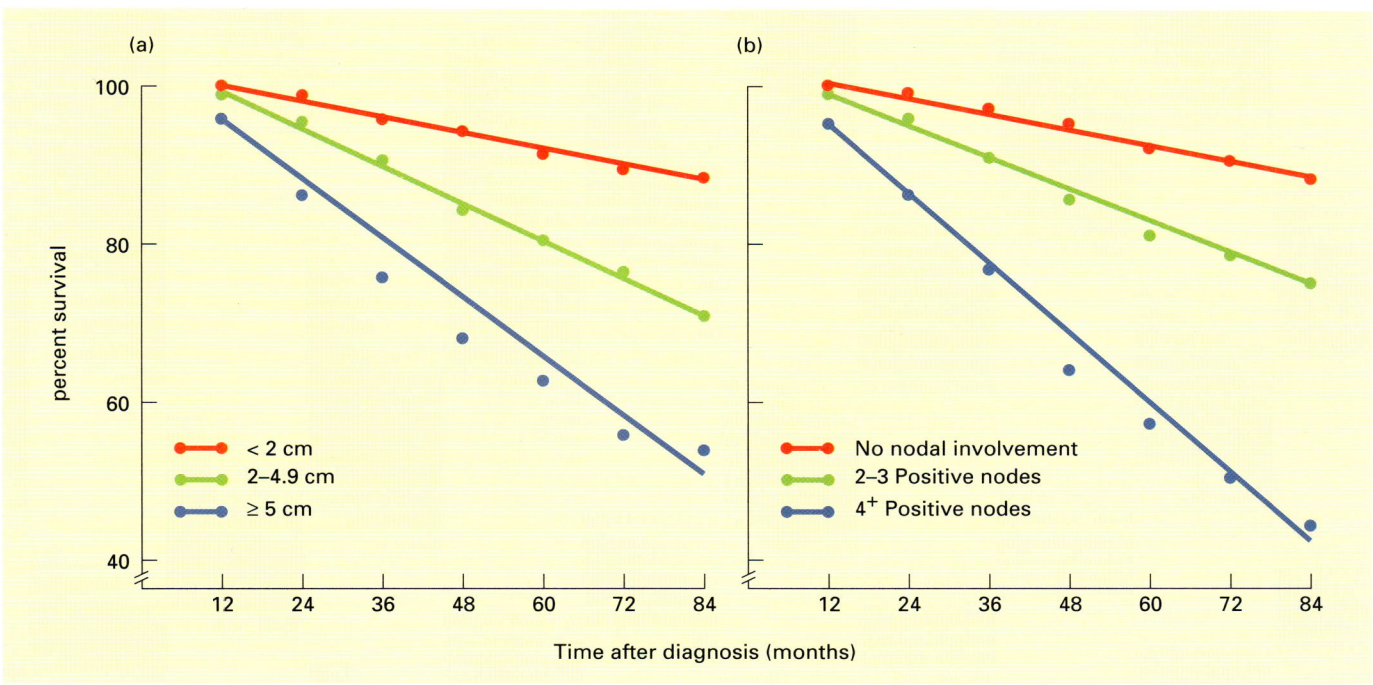

Fig. 22.17 (a) Relative survival of 27 740 breast cancer patients as a function of primary tumour diameter and (b) axillary lymph node status. (Drawn after Carter *et al.* 1989, with permission of the American Cancer Society, Inc., J. B. Lippincott Co.)

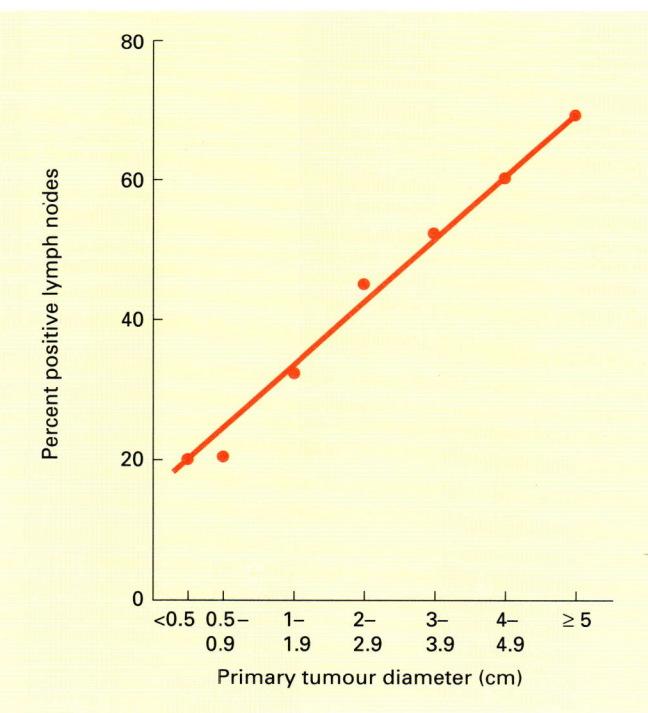

Fig. 22.18 Positive axillary lymph nodes as a function of primary tumour diameter. (Drawn after Carter *et al.* 1989, with permission of the American Cancer Society, Inc., J. B. Lippincott Co.)

The significance of micrometastases in bone marrow Occult tumour cells (single or small islands undetectable by routine microscopy) in the bone marrow can be detected by immuno-histochemistry using monoclonal antibodies against epithelial markers. In 307 women with breast cancer, tumour cells were found in 26 per cent, and these cases were associated with other poor prognostic factors, such as tumour size and lymph node metastasis (Mansi *et al.* 1987). Both relapse-free survival and overall survival were shorter in positive cases, and the presence of occult tumour cells predicted development of skeletal secondaries (but not extra-skeletal metastases). However, the efficiency, benefit, and cost-effectiveness of this method has been widely debated, and some studies do not find its predictive value significant. The latter statement also applies to micrometastases in axillary lymph nodes.

Complex clinico-pathological prognostic assessment

Tumour grade Many morphologic criteria have been used for decades to describe the aggressiveness of breast tumours. Amongst these, the histopathological type of tumour, the degree of nuclear pleomorphism, the presence or absence of an inflammatory response, blood-vessel and/or lymphatic invasion are most frequently used.

For histological grading of breast cancer, the method described originally by Bloom and Richardson in 1957 is widely used. Although the original method has been modified by various authors, the principle is preserved: viz. the mitotic rate,

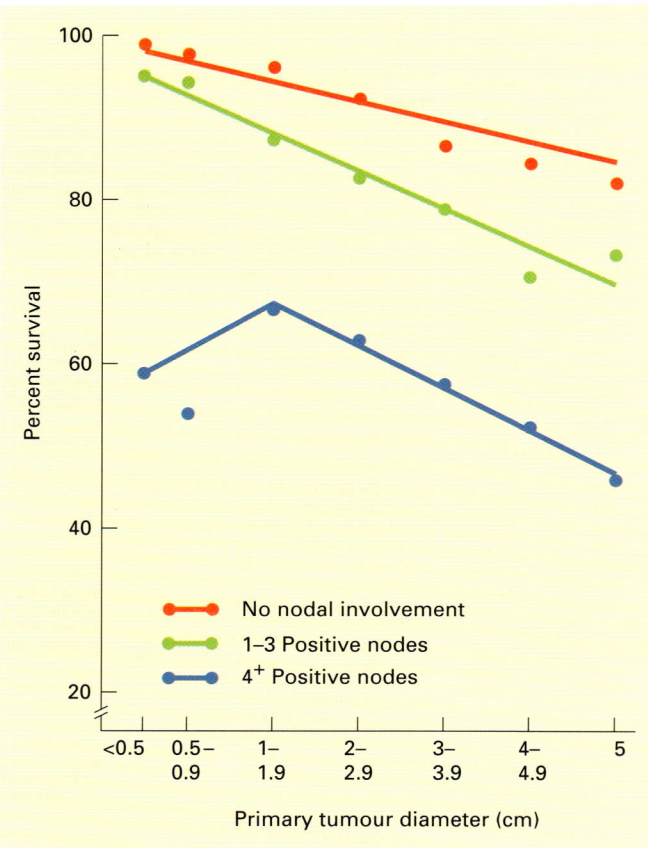

Fig. 22.19 Relation of tumour diameter and lymph node status to 5 year relative survival. (Drawn after Carter *et al.* 1989, with permission of the American Cancer Society, Inc., J. B. Lippincott Co.)

nuclear pleomorphism, and the presence or absence of tubule formation are all individually scored from 1 to 3. The sum of these scores determines the grade of the tumour (see Table 22.4). This method gives reproducible results, and when employed by different investigators, the distribution of grade categories is similar in various cohorts.

Tumour stage In clinical decision-making, the practical approach is to summarize the basic characteristics of a tumour by staging. The *stage* of tumour development, derived from tumour size, lymph *n*ode status and distant *m*etastases (TNM),

together with the morphological *grade*, summarize the basic clinico-pathological aspects of the tumour. This provides a concise and clinically meaningful formula for assessing the tumour's presumed behaviour. However, staging does not make allowance for the different value of each factor in contributing to overall prognosis.

Prognostic index The significance of the clinico-pathological variables is different, and using a multiple regression analysis technique a coefficient can be derived for each factor. This indicates the extent to which they contribute to adverse behaviour, e.g. shorter survival. Employing the respective coefficients to clinico-pathological factors, a prognostic index (PI) has been derived (Haybittle *et al.* 1982), which allows each factor to be considered according to its value.

$$PI = (0.17 \times size) + (0.76 \times lymph\ node\ stage)$$
$$+ (0.82 \times tumour\ grade)$$

Applying this index, a better separation of the best and worst prognostic groups was achieved than with methods using tumour size or lymph node metastases alone. This study confirmed that while lymph node status is the best single prognostic indicator, assessment of multiple factors gives a better indication of poor prognosis.

Practical use of clinico-pathological markers: the shortcomings Tumour size, grade of differentiation, presence or absence of lymph node metastases, and the presence of occult tumour cells or gross metastases are prognostic markers for relatively advanced tumours only. Unfortunately, the use of these factors is still not fully satisfactory for three reasons.

1. Negative lymph node status does not automatically guarantee a favourable outcome: some of these cases will do poorly either with early recurrences or with short survival.

2. Though they are important predictors of survival, the contribution of clinico-pathological markers seems to be restricted to predicting the first 5 years of survival. Studies of cases who survived more than 20 years after the diagnosis of the disease were unable to establish significant clinico-pathological differences between these and those with shorter survival (Fentiman *et al.* 1984). They concluded that lymph node status is a predictor of 5-year survival, rather than of the overall outcome of the disease.

3. Since the introduction of breast screening (see Section 22.2) more tumours are being detected in their earlier stages. The prognostic value of clinico-pathological features in these 'early' tumours is limited.

There is a clear need for markers applicable to 'early' and other tumours, and molecular biology promises some progress. Tumour markers may be generated from an understanding of growth regulation in normal and malignant breast epithelium. Molecular mechanisms involved in growth control may help to identify key steps in the regulatory process and provide insight into the mechanisms involved in progression of a given tumour.

Table 22.4. Grading according to Bloom and Richardson (1957)*

Score	Grade
3, 4, 5	1
6, 7	2
8, 9	3

* See text.

Biological features as prognostic indicators

Cell kinetics and DNA ploidy

Normal cells are fastidious in maintaining their euploid DNA content and standard mitotic rate, characteristic of that tissue. In experimental tumour models, the rate of proliferative activity is a reliable marker of tumour growth, and it can be anticipated that data on cell kinetics and DNA content reflect the growth rate and aggressiveness of malignant tumours.

DNA ploidy is most frequently determined by flow cytometry (see Section 22.1.7). Tumour DNA distribution plots are compared with the 2n and 4n DNA content of normal cells (see Fig. 22.16). According to the DNA distribution, euploid and aneuploid tumours are distinguished. Euploid tumours comprise cell populations with DNA of two- and four-fold diploid values, while the DNA distribution of aneuploid tumours is irregular. DNA ploidy and cell population kinetics are related: euploid tumours have a low S phase compartment, and aneuploid tumours are more likely to have a faster growth, characterized with a higher S phase rate.

DNA distribution plots can be used to derive the proportion of tumour cells in S phase. Other methods of growth fraction assessment are also available. Labelling with ³H-thymidine or with bromodeoxyuridine (BUdR) give a direct indication of the number of cells actively synthetizing DNA. Antibodies (such as Ki67) used against nuclear antigens expressed only in G1, S, G2, and M phases, give comparable results. The immunohistochemical methods are simple and rapid.

Several reports have shown some correlation between DNA ploidy, tumour grade, and oestrogen receptor expression. Aneuploidy and high S phase fraction may be associated with a shorter relapse-free interval and overall survival. However, these findings are not consistent and the results show considerable interlaboratory variability, depending on technical factors and methods of assessment. It is still to be seen whether DNA cytometry, one of the first methods of cell biology offered for prognostication, will fulfil the initial expectations it raised; in the authors' view this is doubtful (Koss *et al.* 1989).

Oestrogen receptor and regulation of tumour growth

Hormone dependence of normal breast development and of breast cancer has been recognized for more than half a century. Some forms of hormonal intervention, such as oophorectomy, adrenalectomy, or steroid hormones, have been used in the treatment of breast tumours for several decades. More recently, oestrogen antagonists have been used for primary treatment of advanced breast cancer, as a single treatment for the elderly, or as an adjuvant to primary surgery.

Regulation of tumour growth by oestrogen hormones Several excellent reviews are available on this subject (Henry *et al.* 1989; Pritchard and Sutherland 1989), therefore only a short summary is given here. Oestrogen stimulation of cells takes place through binding of the hormone to the oestrogen receptor, a 66 kDa nuclear protein. It is followed by coupling the hormone-receptor complex to regulatory DNA regions, which initiate transcription of various genes. The full scale of oestrogen-regulated products is not known, but it includes production of numerous proteins, many of which are involved in the regulation of DNA synthesis and cell growth. Examples of these regulatory proteins are enzymes, such as thymidylate synthetase, thymidine kinase, and DNA polymerases.

Oestrogens may stimulate tumour proliferation via growth factors as 'second messengers'. In some cell lines, the production of TGFα, insulin-like growth factor I (IGF-I), and platelet-derived growth factor (PDGF) are under oetrogen regulation. PDGF is a 'competence' factor, which is necessary to allow cells to enter G1 phase, while IGF-I and TGFα, together with EGF are 'progression' factors, which stimulate transmission from G1 to S phase. In experimental systems, the growth of oestrogen-dependent cell lines can be maintained in the absence of oestradiol, if the cell is supplied by growth factors which are normally induced by oestrogen.

Many more proteins are regulated by oestrogen; these include the precursors of cathepsin B, progesterone receptor, and tissue type plasminogen activator (TPA). Levels of TPA in human breast cancer correlate with oestrogen and progesterone receptor levels, and the expression of this protein has been reported to be associated with a better prognosis.

Antioestrogens The effect of oestrogen antagonists on tumours results in inhibition of the production of autocrine stimulatory factors, thus impeding tumour growth. However, the other function of antioestrogens is equally important; they stimulate the secretion by tumour cells of TGFβ, a potent inhibitor of proliferation of epithelial cells.

In tumours which lose oestrogen dependence, growth factor production and autocrine stimulation become independent of oestrogen, and cannot be controlled by antioestrogen administration. After the loss of oestrogen dependence, continued progression of tumour growth is associated with failure to produce, or respond to growth inhibitory substances. TGFβ, the production of which is stimulated by antioestrogens in oestrogen sensitive tumours, is an example.

Oestrogen receptor and endocrine treatment The proportion of breast tumours which are oestrogen receptor (ER) positive varies between 40 per cent and 80 per cent. The presence of ER indicates that the tumour may be expected to respond to antioestrogen treatment. However, ER expression without functional integrity does not guarantee a good response to endocrine treatment. Indeed, in various studies only 50 per cent of oestrogen receptor positive cases respond to antioestrogen therapy. In ER positive tumours, the expression of progesterone receptor, which is also oestrogen-regulated, gives a better prediction of oestrogen responsiveness.

In experimental tumours, ER positive tumour cells lose their ability to be inhibited by antioestrogens, if they are unable to secrete TGFβ. Although the mechanism has not been demonstrated *in vivo*, this model gives a possible explanation of absent response to antioestrogen treatment in oestrogen-positive tumours.

Paradoxically, 5–10 per cent of the ER negative tumours respond well to endocrine therapy. This phenomenon is not fully explained. It is possible that the existing ER assays are not sensitive enough, or a negative result is the consequence of non-representative sampling in a heterogeneous tumour. It might be possible that the antioestrogen also binds to an unknown site distinct from ER.

Oestrogen receptor and prognosis Most studies agree that expression of ER is a marker of favourable prognosis and patients have an overall survival advantage (Blamey *et al.* 1986; Hawkins *et al.* 1987). This is based on the response of these patients to endocrine therapy, and the association of ER-positive status with other prognostic variables. There is a positive correlation between tumour differentiation, absence of lymph node metastases and positive ER status (Parl *et al.* 1984). Size and type of tumour are also important: smaller tumours and certain histological types, such as lobular carcinoma, are more likely to be receptor positive. ER levels are usually higher and incidences are usually more frequent in postmenopausal patients.

The association between ER expression and disease-free interval is not clear. Some studies report a longer disease-free interval for ER-positive cases; others do not find such an association.

Immunohistochemistry can be used to detect oestrogen receptor expression in breast cancer. Positive tumours show distinct nuclear staining with antibodies against this receptor (Fig. 22.20), and immunohistochemistry shows good correlation with ligand-binding assays.

EGF receptor (EGFr)

Epidermal growth factors (EGF) is one of the polypeptide factors that regulate cell growth. EGF shares 35 per cent amino-acid homology with TGFα, and both factors act as substrate for the same cell-surface receptor, EGFr. EGFr has an external, ligand-binding domain, a transmembrane part, and a cytoplasmic section which is a tyrosine kinase. Ligand binding to the receptor induces an early effect of short-term phosphorylation of tyrosine

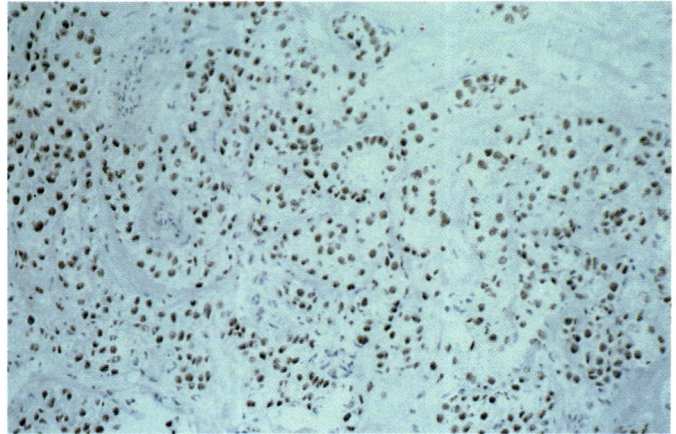

Fig. 22.20 Immunohistochemical detection of ER on a frozen section. This receptor (a nucleoprotein) shows distinct nuclear localization.

residues, and a rapid induction of c-*myc* and c-*fos* expression. A long-term effect is initiated by the internalization of the receptor, which is followed by the induction of DNA synthesis and an increased rate of cell division. Since tyrosine kinase is the only known intrinsic enzyme activity associated with EGFr, it is probable that tyrosine kinase activity is the triggering mechanism for all of these cellular responses. Ligand binding to EGFr may induce activation of the c-erb-B2 coded protein (p185^{neu}), followed by tyrosine phosphorylation through the erb-B2 pathway, thus multiplying the effect of ligand binding.

Activation of EGFr In most squamous tumours, overexpression of EGFr is the consequence of gene amplification, but in breast cancer this is rare. High expression is due to enhanced transcription or translation of the normal gene. EGFr overexpression results in higher binding affinity to EGF, and a higher mitogenic responsiveness to relatively low concentrations of the ligand. EGFr might also be involved in autocrine stimulation of cell proliferation. It has been shown in breast cancer cell lines that tumour cells can release TGFα, which by binding to the receptor on the same cells, stimulates its growth in an autocrine fashion.

Overexpression of EGFr shows an inverse relationship with ER expression (Sainsbury *et al.* 1987), indicating that increased EGFr expression occurs when tumours lose their oestrogen hormone regulation. The overexpression of this receptor is a marker of adverse prognosis (Nicholson *et al.* 1991). Tumours which are positive for EGFr have a shorter tumour-free survival and shorter overall survival (Fig. 22.21).

Antibodies have been raised against various peptide sequences of this receptor. In breast cancer cells, the overexpressed EGF receptor can be detected by immunohistochemistry using these antibodies (Fig. 22.22).

c-erb-B2

Human c-erb-B2 is a cellular gene which codes for a receptor transmembrane glycoprotein of 185 kDa (p185^{neu}), and is a member of the tyrosine kinase family. The protein has close sequence homology with the intracellular domain of EGFr. Despite this close relationship, the two receptors differ in chromosomal localization, in mRNA transcripts, and in molecular weights of their products as shown in Table 22.5. The two receptors have distinct ligands; the substrate for p185^{neu} is now being identified. p185^{neu} oncoprotein and EGFr are expressed independently in malignant tumours.

Tyrosine phosphorylation is an important step in malignant transformation of cells, and takes place through activation of the tyrosine kinase system. Tyrosine kinase activity of the c-erb-B2 protein is regulated by the substrate binding to the extracellular domain of the receptor. However, increased phosphorylation might be stimulated through transregulation of the p185^{neu} receptor by EGF binding to its receptor.

p185^{neu} might also form heterodimers with EGFr, which (similarly to the homodimers of EGF receptor), result in increased affinity and more stable binding to ligands. Heterodimers double the EGF effect: tyrosine kinase activation takes place through both the EGFr and the p185^{neu} pathway. In fact,

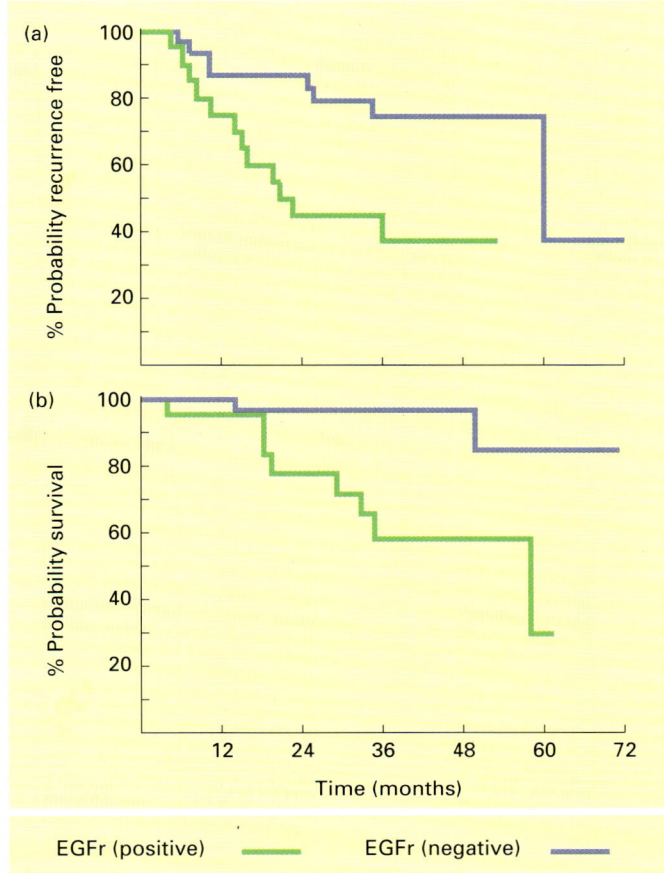

Fig. 22.21 Survival of patients with histopathologically negative axillary nodes stratified by tumour EGF receptor content: (a) relapse-free and (b) overall survival. (Drawn after Nicholson *et al.* 1991, with permission from The Macmillan Press Ltd.)

Table 22.5 Comparison of c-erb-B2 and EGFr

	c-erb-B2	EGFr
Chromosomal localization	17q21	7
mRNA transcript	4.8 kb	5.8/1p kb
Molecular weight of product	185 000	170 000

binding of either EGF or $p185^{neu}$ substrate activates both systems and ensures incresed tyrosine phosphorylation, resulting in markedly increased growth. Heterodimer formation in human breast cancer cell lines results in growth advantages (Goldman *et al.* 1990).

Amplification of the c-erb-B2 oncogene with concomitant overexpression is associated with poor prognosis (Slamon *et al.* 1987). Correlation has also been reported between amplification of the c-erb-B2 gene, positive lymph node status, and tumour differentiation. Studies comparing results obtained by different methods show that although gene amplification results in mRNA and $p185^{neu}$ overexpression, DNA amplification is certainly not the only mechanism by which c-erb-B2 is overexpressed. There are many tumours (10 to 30 per cent) with a single copy of the gene, showing overexpression of mRNA or $p185^{neu}$.

Immunohistochemistry of c-erb-B2 product Antibodies have been raised against various sequences of this oncogene product. Positive immunohistochemistry shows a heterogeneous distribution of membrane staining, on more than 50 per cent of tumour cells (Fig. 22.23). Immunohistochemistry gives higher numbers of positive cases than gene amplification analysis. Comparison of immunohistochemistry with prognosis is controversial. Immunohistochemistry is, however, dependent on many factors, such as varying sensitivity of antibodies raised against different domains of the antigen, different specificity of the antibody, and variations in tissue preservation. Assessment

EGFr (positive) ——— EGFr (negative) ———

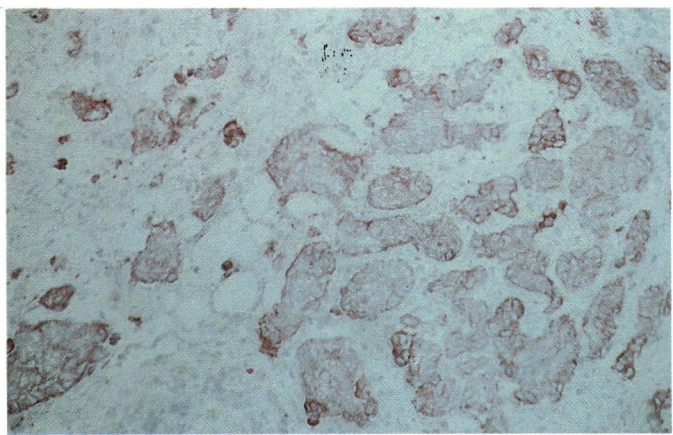

Fig. 22.22 EGFr, detected by EGF-1 monoclonal antibody. This antibody produces membrane staining in the tumour cells, in keeping with the transmembrane localization of this receptor.

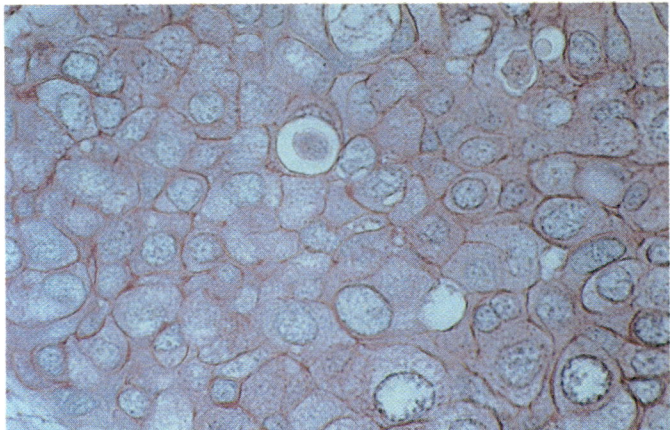

Fig. 22.23 The c-erb-B2 product is localized in the cytoplasmic membrane. The monoclonal antibody NCL CB11 gives clear membrane staining in approximately 20 per cent of tumours when paraffin sections are used.

of immunohistochemistry also involves a subjective component: different investigators might accept various results as positive. Consequently, authors using immunohistochemistry report somewhat different results concerning the association of c-erb-B2 expression to recurrence-free interval and overall survival. Because of this controversy, results of immunohistochemistry are best standardized in relation to gene amplification, at least for now.

Cathepsin D

Enhanced secretion of various forms of cathepsin have been reported in breast cancer. In 1979, a 52 kDa glycoprotein was described, which was secreted by both hormone independent and hormone dependent breast cancer cell lines. In hormone-dependent tumours, its secretion was stimulated by oestrogens and inhibited by antioestrogens. The glycoprotein was identified as the precursor of cathepsin D, a lysosomal acid protease and was named as 52 kDa cathepsin D (CD).

Normal cells secrete only traces of this precursor, which is normally processed by lysosomes to a mature form comprising a 34 and a 14 kDa chain. This double-chain is ubiquitous in lysosomes of normal cells. Cathepsins have acidic proteolytic activity, resulting in degradation of extracellular matrix and basement membranes. CD also has a mitosis-stimulating activity, and can act as an autocrine growth promoter. Both the proteolytic and mitogenic capabilities of this enzyme might influence the outcome of malignant tumours.

The amount of CD detected in breast cancer varies between 10 and 250 pmol/mg cytosol protein. When assessing tumours, most authors use a two-tail system, distinguishing 'high' and 'low' CD content, although in different investigations, the cut-off point varies between 35 and 70 pmol/mg.

No association was found between tumour size, lymph node involvement, histopathological grade, age, or progesterone receptor status, and the level of CD content in primary breast cancer. There was some correlation in premenopausal patients between oetrogen receptor status and CD level of tumours. In other studies, high CD levels were significantly more frequent in tumours with an aneuploid DNA content, and in those with c-*myc* amplification.

Some authors contend that patients with breast tumours containing high CD levels have shorter recurrence-free survival and have a trend towards shorter overall survival (Tandon *et al.* 1990). In multivariate analysis, CD was found to be an independent prognostic factor of approximately the same importance as lymph node status. As this factor is independent of lymph node status, its value may be additional to that of lymph node metastases (Brouillet *et al.* 1990).

Assessment of tumour markers in progression

The process of establishing a marker as prognostically significant includes investigation of the factor on numerous, well documented and followed-up cases, preferably in multiple clinical trials. This process is time consuming and usually there is a lapse between the discovery of a putative marker and recognition of its significance in prognosis. Numerous studies are presently addressing the problem, and the search for new features predicting the outcome of the disease has become one of the most important fields of current breast cancer research.

22.1.12   Bibliography

Blamey, R. W. *et al.* (1980). Relationships between primary breast tumor receptor status and patient survival. *Cancer* **46**, 2765–9.

Bloom, H. J. G. and Richardson, W. W. (1957). Histological grading and prognosis in breast cancer. *British Journal of Cancer* **11**, 359–77.

Brouillet, J.-P. *et al.* (1990). Cathepsin D assay in primary breast cancer and lymph nodes: relationship with c-myc, c-erb-B2 and int-2 oncogene amplification and node invasiveness. *European Journal of Cancer* **26**, 437–41.

Carter, C. L. *et al.* (1989). Relation of tumour size, lymph node status, and survival in 24,740 breast cancer cases. *Cancer* **63**, 181–7.

Fentiman, I. S. *et al.* (1984). Which patients are cured of breast cancer? *British Medical Journal* **289**, 1108–11.

Goldman, R. *et al.* (1990). Heterodimerization of the erbB-1 and erbB-2 receptors in human breast carcinoma cells: a mechanism for receptor transregulation. *Biochemistry* **1990**, 11024–8.

Haybittle, J. L. *et al.* (1982). A prognostic index in primary breast cancer. *British Journal of Cancer* **45**, 361–6.

Hawkins, R. A. *et al.* (1987). Prognostic significance of oestrogen and progestogen receptor activities in breast cancer. *British Journal of Surgery* **74**, 1009–13.

Henry, J. A. *et al.* (1989). Oestrogen receptor and oestrogen regulated proteins in human breast cancer. *Keio Journal of Medicine* **38**, 241–61.

Holland, R. *et al.* (1990). The presence of an extensive intraductal component (EIC) following a limited excision correlates with prominent residual disease in the remainder of the breast. *Journal of Clinical Oncology* **8**, 113–20.

Koss, L. G. *et al.* (1989). Flow cytometric measurements of DNA and other cell components in human tumours. *Human Pathology* **20**, 528–48.

Mansi, J. E. *et al.* (1987). Micrometastases in bone marrow in patients with primary breast cancer: evaluation as an early predictor of bone metastases. *British Medical Journal* **295**, 1093–6.

Nicholson, S. *et al.* (1991). Epidermal growth factor receptor (EGFr); results of a 6-year follow-up study in operable breast cancer with emphasis on the node negative subgroup. *British Journal of Cancer* **63**, 146–50.

Parl, F. F. *et al.* (1984). Prognostic significance of estrogen receptor status in breast cancer in relation to tumor stage, axillary node metastasis, and histopathologic grading. *Cancer* **54**, 2237–42.

Pritchard, K. I. and Sutherland, D. J. A. (1989). The use of endocrine therapy. *Hematology/Oncology Clinics of North America* **3**, 765–805.

Sainsbury, J. R. C. *et al.* (1987). Epidermal-growth-factor receptor status as predictor of early recurrence of and death from breast cancer. *Lancet* **i**, 1398–402.

Slamon, D. J. *et al.* (1987). Human breast cancer: correlation of relapse and survival with amplification of the her-2/neu oncogene. *Science* **235**, 177–82.

Tandon, A. K. *et al.* (1990). Cathepsin D and prognosis in breast cancer. *New England Journal of Medicine* **322**, 297–302.

Weidner, N. *et al.* (1991). Tumour angiogenesis and metastasis—correlation in invasive breast carcinoma. *New England Journal of Medicine* **324**, 1–8.

22.2 Mammography and breast screening

Basil J. Shepstone

22.2.1 Introduction

Lumps in the breast can either be detected clinically or by various diagnostic imaging procedures, the most important of which is X-ray mammography. After localization, such lumps may then be submitted to fine-needle aspiration or open biopsy, or both, to establish their cellular nature by cyto/histopathology. While most lumps are easily identified by any of the modalities used, others remain obscure, with the different methods of approach yielding conflicting answers. A common example of the latter situation is that of the clinically impalpable mass which is visible only on the mammogram and which has to be localized stereotactically before fine-needle aspiration or biopsy can be carried out. The whole thrust of the recent Forrest report (1986) has, in fact, been to detect impalpable cancers by open-access mammography in the 50–64 year age group in a UK National Breast Screening Programme. It should also be remembered that as common and daunting as breast cancer is, most patients presenting with breast lumps have benign disease. It would seem that there are few organs as versatile as the breast in producing an enormous spectrum of both benign and malignant disease.

This section details the mammographic appearances of breast disorders. As breast screening programmes in the West develop, it will be important for pathologists to become expert in mammographic interpretation, so that radiological and biopsy evidence can be evaluated together in arriving at the most accurate diagnosis for individual patients.

22.2.2 Identification of breast lumps

Notwithstanding the finer cytological and histopathological aspects of breast disease discussed in Section 22.1.7, the initial clinical and radiological assessment of breast lumps must consider the entities set out in Table 22.6.

Table 22.6 Potential causes of breast lumps

Benign	Malignant
Fibrous masses	Primary carcinoma
Fibroadenoma	Lymphoma
Cysts	(Phyllodes tumour)
Traumatic fat necrosis	Metastases
Haematoma; abscess; hamartoma	
Phyllodes tumour	
Scar tissue; implant	
Lipoma/fibrolipoma/adenolipoma	
Duct papilloma	
Skin lesions	

22.2.3 Clinical diagnosis of a clinically palpable breast lump

A lump is often found incidentally by the patient herself, her consort, or a medical adviser. With the recent promotion of breast self-examination, more lumps have certainly been detected by patients, but unfortunately without much impact on the detection of carcinoma itself. The history is often helpful in pointing towards implants, haematoma, traumatic fat necrosis, abscess, and papillomata (which often present with nipple discharge or bleeding), but generally there is little to differentiate the benign conditions clinically. Fibroadenoma tends to be rubbery and mobile and are often referred to as 'breast mice'. Large cysts, lipomata, haematomata, and abscesses may be fluctuant. Abscesses are obviously painful, with overlying, reddened skin. Fibrocystic disease often presents with breast pain or tenderness, usually superolaterally and often worse on the left; pain may only occur during certain phases of the menstrual cycle. Malignant lumps are usually hard and can involve the overlying skin (*peau d'orange* and thickening or skin dimpling, often noticed on movement). There may be axillary lymphadenopathy. Lymphoma, besides the associated lymphadenopathy, can present with a diffusely enlarged breast, often also with skin thickening. In the post-menopausal patient, breast pain should always be taken seriously and investigated.

22.2.4 Mammography

The technique of mammography relies on low-kilovoltage radiation directed through the compressed breast in the oblique lateral and craniocaudal directions. Compression is necessary to get better tissue differentiation and to reduce the absorbed radiation dose to the breast. On the whole, mammography in women under 35 years is discouraged because of the inherent risk of radiation. Also, as the common causes of breast lumps in this younger group are fibrocystic disease or fibroadenoma, they should be managed clinically in the first instance. However, it is said that a sharply defined, 1 cm nodular density—which is usually a fibroadenoma—has an approximately 2 per cent chance of being malignant.

Differentiation between benign and malignant

The accepted distinctions between benign and malignant breast opacities on mammography are set out in Table 22.7. However, as in all clinical situations, there are no hard and fast rules and many cancers look benign and vice versa. No one can be absolutely sure, and this is manifested in the sensitivity and specificity of mammography, which are respectively 80–90 per cent and 95 per cent. Another salutary fact worth remembering is that the average breast carcinoma reputedly takes about 10 years to become 1 cm in diameter!

Benign disease of the breast

It should be pointed out that, although these appearances may be well-recognized histopathologically, they cannot of course always be distinguished as such by radiologists, who are

Table 22.7 Distinctions between benign and malignant breast opacities on mammography

Benign	Malignant
Smooth	Irregular
Homogeneous	Heterogeneous
Low density	High density
Relatively coarse or symmetrical calcification; usually smooth and rounded	Microcalcification: usually clustered, angular and irregular, often branching
	Lymphadenopathy
	Skin thickening or tethering
Clinical and mammographic size similar	Clinical size greater than mammographic size

therefore encouraged to use only such terms as 'benign change' or, perhaps, 'benign cystic change' in their reports. This approach is also encouraged by the realization that not all the entities described constitute disease, but are simply variations of normal development and involution. Several authorities have, in fact, encouraged the use of the acronym ANDI to cover 'Aberrations of Normal Development and Involution'.

Normal breast

Normal mammograms are shown in Fig. 22.24. These should be compared with the abnormal mammograms shown on p. 1673 *et seq*.

Fibrocystic change

Individual cysts are round or ovoid opacities with smooth, discrete margins. Sometimes they are slightly irregular or lobulated. A cyst may compress the surrounding fat into a thin

radiolucent halo—the so-called 'halo of safety' (Fig. 22.25a). Multilocular cysts are less frequent. Numerous small cysts with marked epithelio-fibrous proliferation give a generalized nodular pattern (Fig. 22.25b). Calcification of cysts can occur as curvilinear calcification of the walls (Fig. 22.25c). Fibrous tissue proliferation gives the mammogram a diffuse, dense stroma, with or without cysts. Occasionally fibrous-tissue conglomerations may mimic carcinoma (Fig. 22.25d). Terminalduct hyperplasia and adenosis can give a nodular appearance. In the more advanced situations this may be associated with scattered, bilateral fine calcifications and is known as sclerosing adenosis. Ultrasound is very useful in distinguishing cystic from solid lesions.

Fibroadenoma

This (Fig. 22.26a) also has a smooth, well-defined margin and is often indistinguishable from a cyst. The larger ones are more lobulated. In 10–20 per cent of cases they are multiple and they can also calcify. Characteristically, the latter is of the 'pop-corn' variety (Fig. 22.26b).

Juvenile fibroadenoma These (Fig. 22.26c) can grow very large. Mammographically they are identical to fibroadenomata.

Phyllodes tumour Small tumours are indistinguishable from fibroadenomata, but when they become very large this diagnosis and giant fibroadenoma should be considered (Fig. 22.26d). The tumour may recur after excision and the rare malignant varieties may metastasize.

Lipomata

These (Fig. 22.27a) have well-defined, thin, connective-tissue

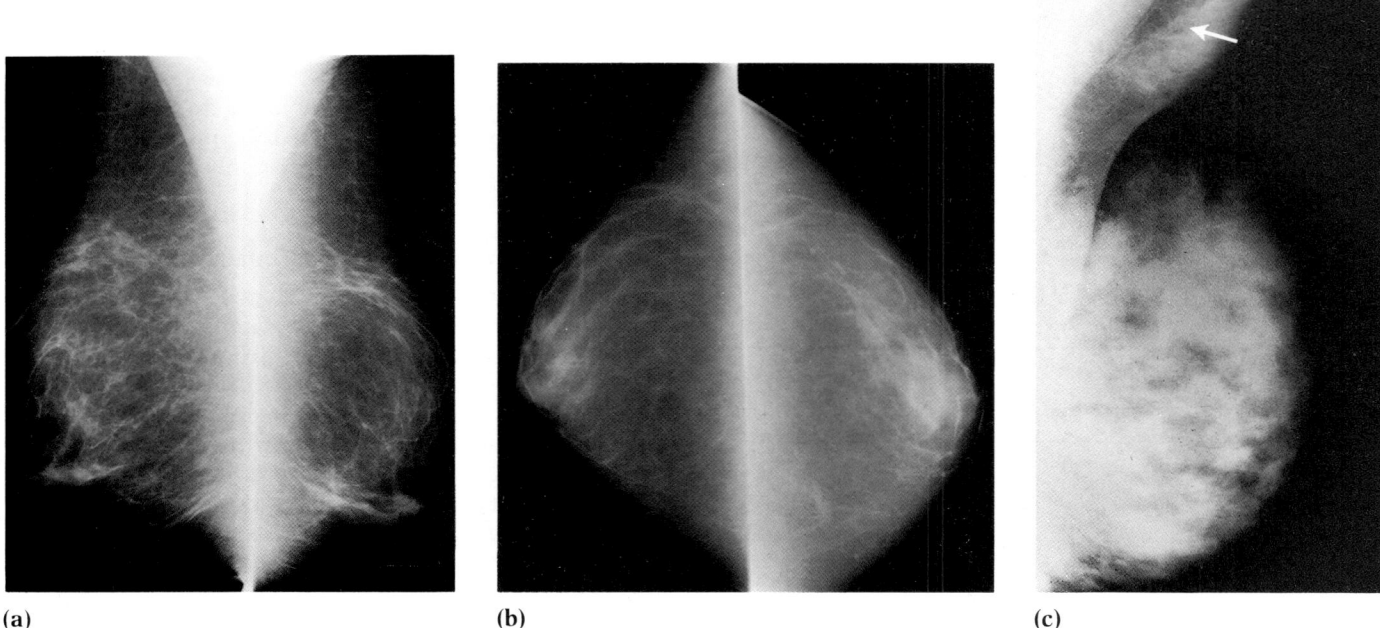

(a)   **(b)**   **(c)**

Fig. 22.24 (a) Normal mammograms, lateral-oblique views. (b) Normal mammograms, craniocaudal views. (c) Normal lactating breast showing coalescing parenchymal densities. Notice that these have extended not only into the left axillary tail but distally into the upper arm (arrow).

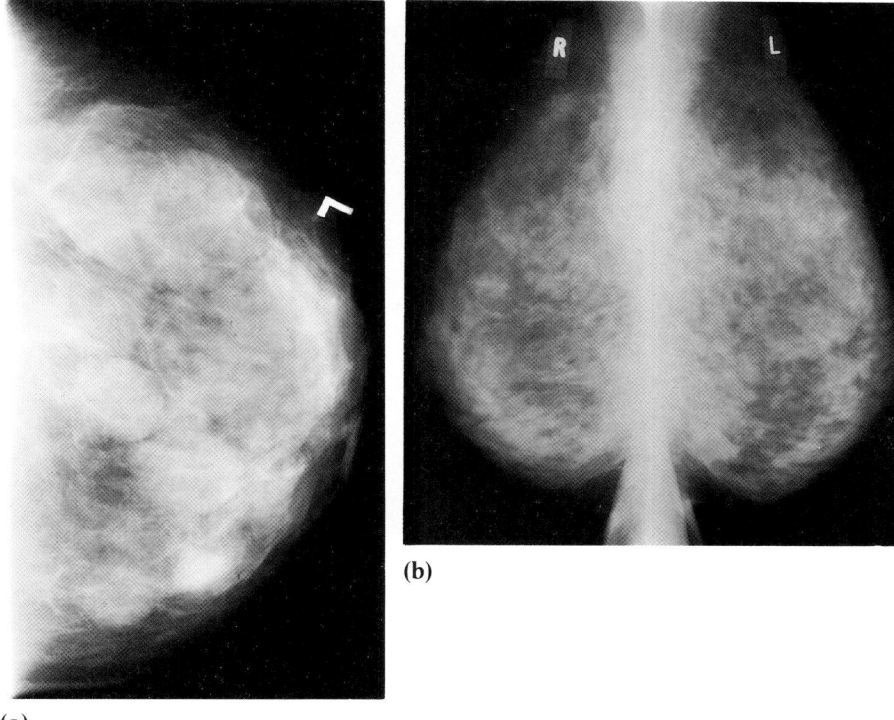

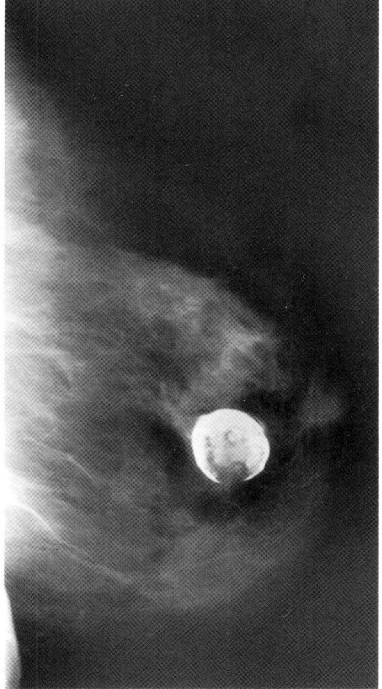

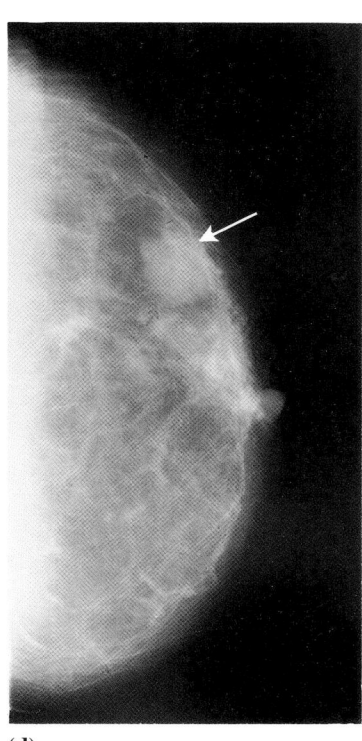

Fig. 22.25 (a) Multiple benign cysts, some showing a surrounding halo of compressed fat. (b) Numerous small cysts with epithelio-fibrous proliferation, giving a generalized nodular pattern; this is a very common appearance and has recently been called 'benign change' and 'benign cystic change'. (c) A calcified cyst; a calcifying fibroma can look very similar to this. (d) A conglomeration of fibrous tissue mimicking a carcinoma (arrow).

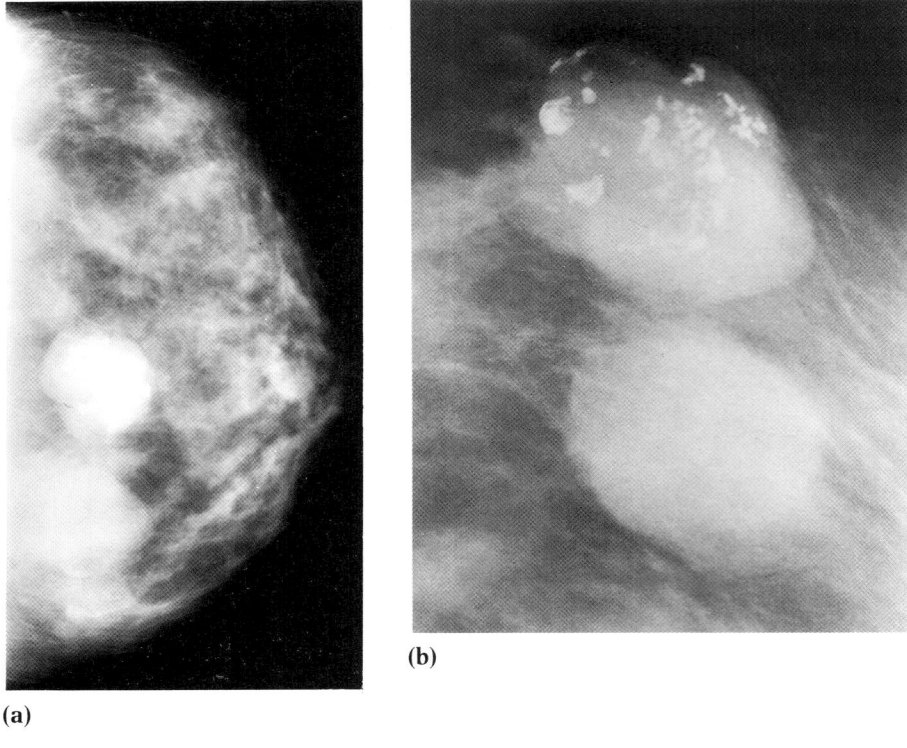

(a)

(b)

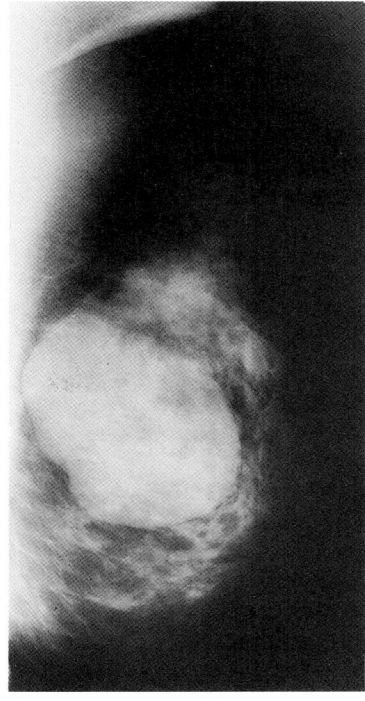

(c)

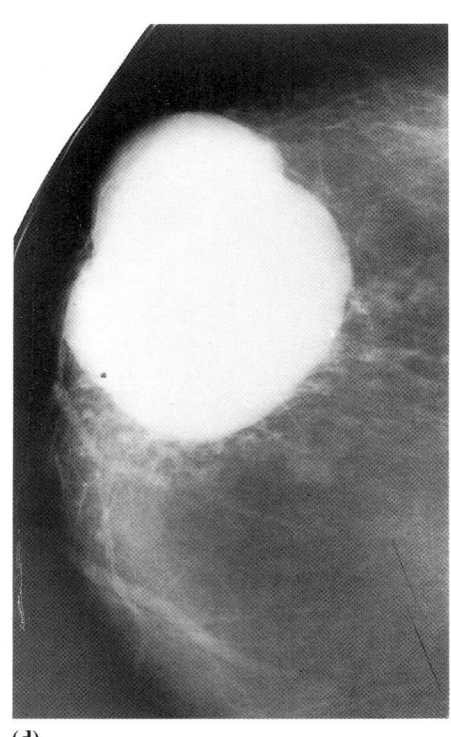

(d)

Fig. 22.26 (a) Two fibroadenomata seen on the craniocaudal view, one of which shows characteristic 'pop-corn' calcification. (b) Detail of the fibroadenomata, but as seen on the lateral oblique view. (c) Juvenile fibroadenoma with well-defined margins and looking very similar to the fibroadenoma in (a), but larger. (d) A phyllodes tumour, the appearances of which are not dissimilar from those of the juvenile fibroadenoma.

capsules surrounding radiolucent fatty tissue and are better seen in glandular breasts than in fatty breasts. Fatty lobules do not have capsules which are as clear along their whole circumference as do lipomata.

Fat necrosis

This is associated with trauma (including biopsy) and may vary in mammographic appearance from a discrete fatty lobule to an irregular mass resembling a carcinoma. It can look very similar to lipomata, but unlike the latter, the walls may calcify. The lobules are often called 'lipoid cysts' (Fig. 22.27b).

Haematoma

These (Fig. 22.27c) produce an ill-defined mass or may just enhance stromal density. On the other hand, a haematoma may be indistinguishable from a cyst.

Abscess

Acute mastitis is limited to the lactational period and usually poses no problem. It should be noted in passing, however, that lactating breast tissue has a formidable appearance on mammography with dense, confluent opacities, often extending to the axilla (see Fig. 22.24c). Chronic abscesses are easily confused with malignant disease as they can be irregular and ill-defined with overlying skin thickening, lymphadenopathy, and nipple retraction. Also, they often do not respond to antibiotics.

'Secretory disease'

This has various appearances. Inspissated secretions may lead to duct dilatation (Fig. 22.28a) and intraductal calcification (Fig. 22.28b; see Section 22.1.3, Duct ectasia). The latter are often tiny and spherical. In the 'plasma-cell mastitis' of older women there may be nipple retraction and skin thickening, besides the mass-like density due to dilated ducts. Galactoceles may appear as small circumscribed radiolucent opacities, similar to fat necrosis.

Gynaecomastia

This is the commonest lesion of the male breast (Fig. 22.29), found in the pubertal and climacteric age-groups and considered by some to be due to disturbance of the androgen/oestrogen ratio. It can also be induced by drugs. Usually the male breast resembles that of a pre-pubertal female, but in gynaecomastia it displays an increased number of ducts with marked intraductal epithelial proliferation and a cellular, vascular, oedematous stroma. The latter may become more fibrous with time. Carcinoma *in situ* does develop in the male breast and then is similar to that described in the female (see below).

Malignant disease of the breast

The mammographic features of breast cancer are given in Table 22.8. Except for radiolucent lipid lesions, it is impossible to state with certainty that any given mammographic opacity is benign.

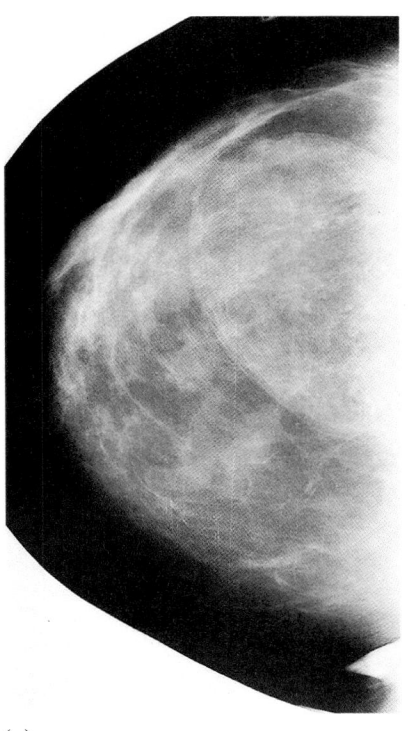 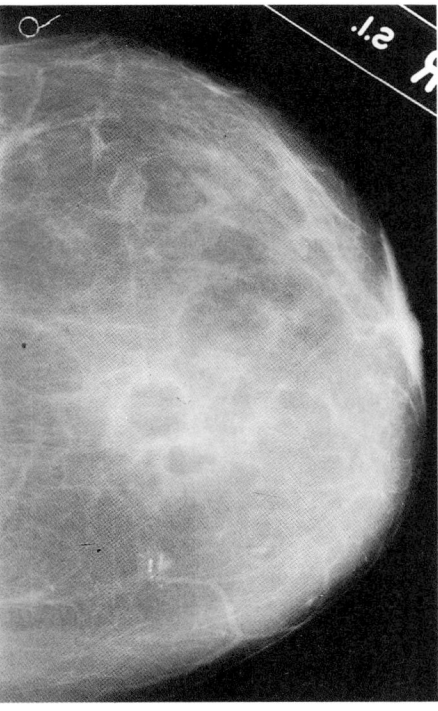 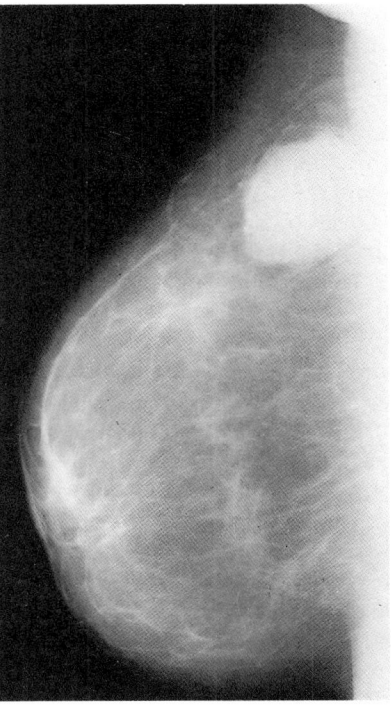

(a)   (b)   (c)

Fig. 22.27 (a) A large, relatively translucent lipoma with a well-defined connective-tissue capsule occupying a large part of the craniocaudal image. (b) A small 'lipoid cyst' consisting of a central translucent area surrounded by a thick rim of connective tissue. (c) A large haematoma resulting from a crush injury to the breast.

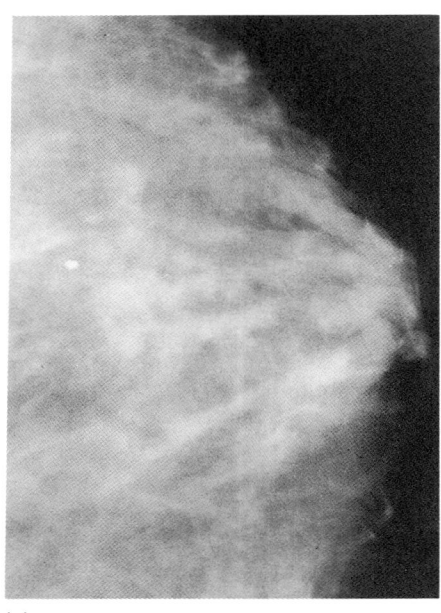

(a)

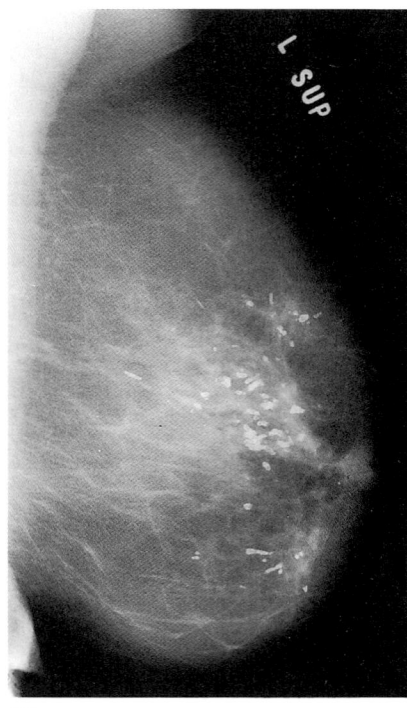

(b)

Fig. 22.28 (a) A close-up of the left retro-areolar cone showing dilated ducts in secretory disease. (b) Calcified inspissated secretions ('secretory granules') in a patient with duct ectasia.

The classic carcinoma is a spiculated density (Fig. 22.30a,b) and the palpable mass usually feels larger than it looks on mammography. However, the border may be ragged or even smooth. Medullary and colloid carcinomata often present as well-demarcated, benign-looking opacities (Fig. 22.30c), but in general mammography cannot distinguish different histopathological types.

Clustered microcalcifications are the single most common sign of early breast cancer and are often the only one (Fig. 22.31). Certainly they occur in benign disease (e.g. fibroadenoma, secretory disease), but they are found in association with 40 per cent of malignant masses and, conversely, 60 per cent of cancers may be found to have calcification. While experts debate the nuances of the appearance of tumour calcification, it is felt on the whole that no discrete microcalcific cluster of any description should be left uninvestigated. On the other hand, calcifications spread symmetrically throughout both breasts are likely to be benign.

Skin changes may include retraction of the skin, nipple, or areola, all of which are visible both clinically and radiologically. Skin thickening, often associated with a diffuse increase in parenchymal densities, is often seen in association with blocked lymph nodes, which may also be visible (Fig. 22.32). However, skin thickening may be seen in inflammatory situations, acromegaly, diffuse fat necrosis, and various skin problems. In Paget disease of the nipple there may be no radiological findings, but occasionally there is thickening of the areolar or nipple skin, or both.

Table 22.8   Mammographic features of breast cancer

Primary signs	Secondary signs
Dominant mass; ragged, spiculated, or smooth contour	Asymmetrical fibroglandular pattern Distortion of architecture, especially 'tenting' due to tissue retraction Microcalcification; usually irregular and angular; often branching Asymmetrical ducts or vessels Lymphadenopathy Skin changes

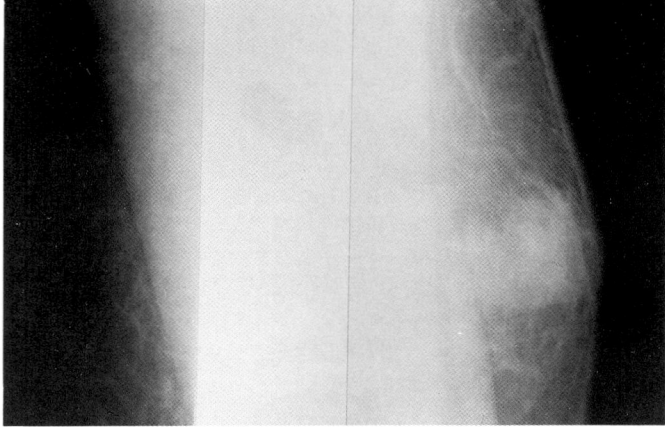

Fig. 22.29 Gynaecomastia of the right breast, compared with a normal male breast on the left.

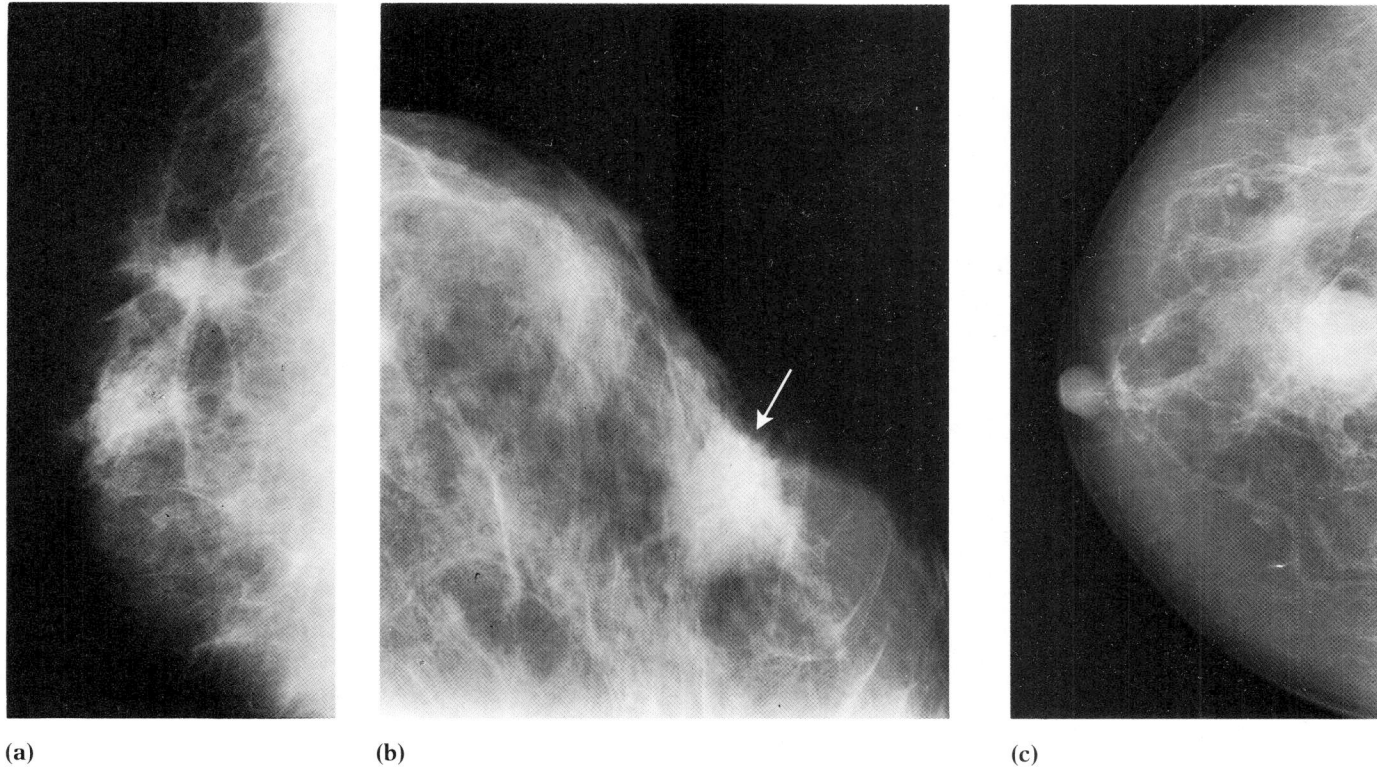

(a)   (b)   (c)

Fig. 22.30 (a) A typical spiculated carcinoma just above the right nipple. (b) Another carcinoma giving rise to local distortion of architecture described as 'tenting' and due to retraction of overlying tissues (arrow). (c) A solitary medullary carcinoma, presenting as a well-defined opacity and not dissimilar from a cyst.

Vascular asymmetry is a very soft sign, but visible axillary nodes may be important. Metastatic nodes are usually dense and large (greater than 1 cm) and sometimes matted together (Fig. 22.33a). One can only be sure that a node is benign is if it has a lucent, fatty centre (Fig. 22.33b).

22.2.5 The Wolfe classification

The mammographic appearance of the connective and epithelial tissues (or their absence) has been suggested by Wolfe as an indicator of the risk of cancer development in the breast. Four categories are described (Fig. 22.34):

N1 Breast composed primarily of fat; often with a trabeculated appearance.

P1 Prominent small-nodular, but linearly arranged duct pattern, corresponding histopathologically to periductal and perilobular fibrosis, covering a quarter or less of the area of the mammogram.

P2 Prominent ducts as described above, occupying more than a quarter of the area of the mammogram.

DY Sheet-like areas of increased density interspersed with collections of fat, but without nodularity or linearity, corresponding to severe mammary 'dysplasia' (fibrous mastopathy).

Women with mammograms falling into the N and P1 categories are reckoned to correlate with a low risk of developing cancers; those having P2 or DY patterns with a high risk. Most articles show these trends to be age-related, being especially applicable to premenopausal women. The scheme has both its adherents and sceptics and more research needs to be done. A common-sense view would seem to be that the denser the parenchyma, the harder it is to recognize small cancers.

22.2.6 Screening

It would seem that the only method at present available for reducing the number of deaths from breast cancer is to detect it mammographically before symptoms arise. The basis for this conclusion is the result of the following studies:

1. The Health Insurance Plan of Greater New York (HIP Study) was a randomized controlled trial over a 20-year period. It showed that breast cancer mortality was reduced by 30 per cent for up to 10 years among women aged 40–64 years at the time of screening. A significant beneficial effect has persisted for 18 years.

2. The Swedish Two-Counties Study, which is also a randomized controlled trial, showed that in the first 7 years breast

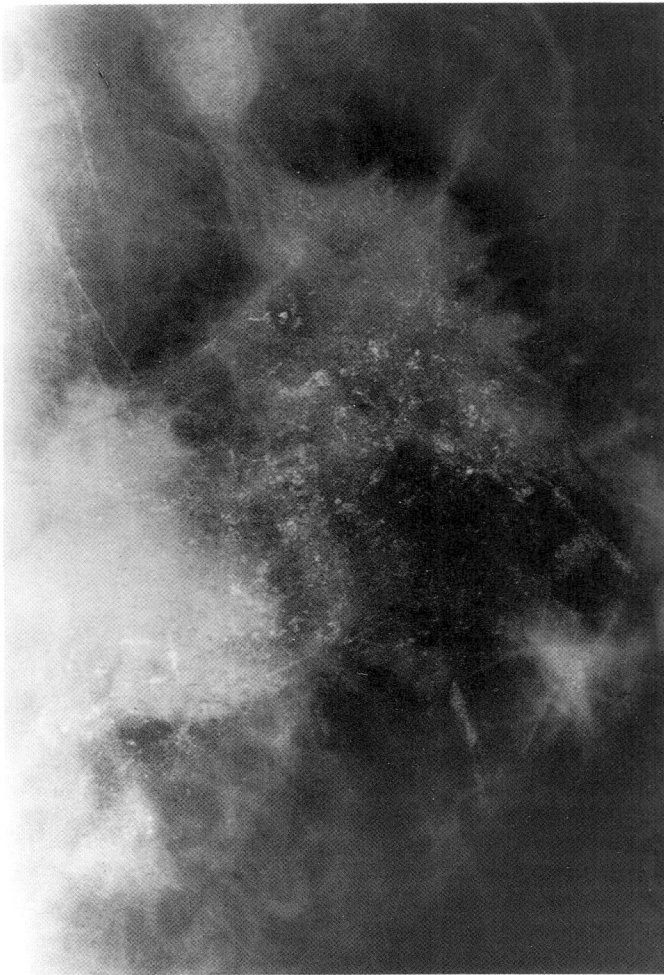

Fig. 22.31 Close-up of a multifocal carcinoma with widespread malignant microcalcification.

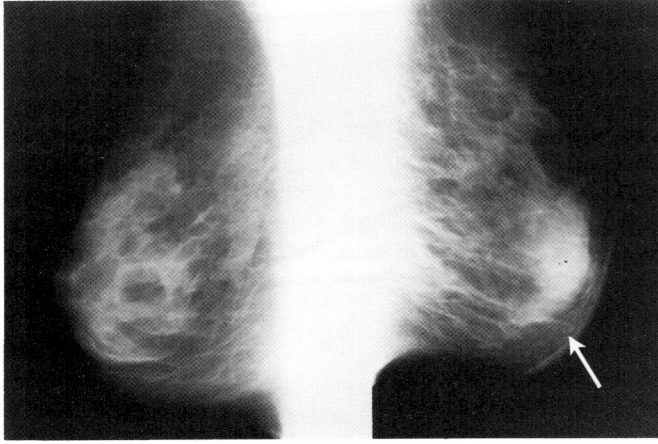

Fig. 22.32 The left breast is diffusely infiltrated and the fibroglandular tissue is denser than on the right. The important sign here is, however, the obvious skin thickening (arrow).

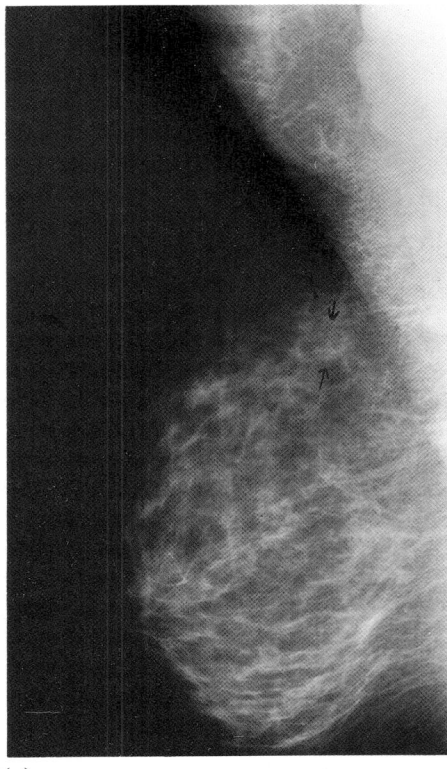

(a)

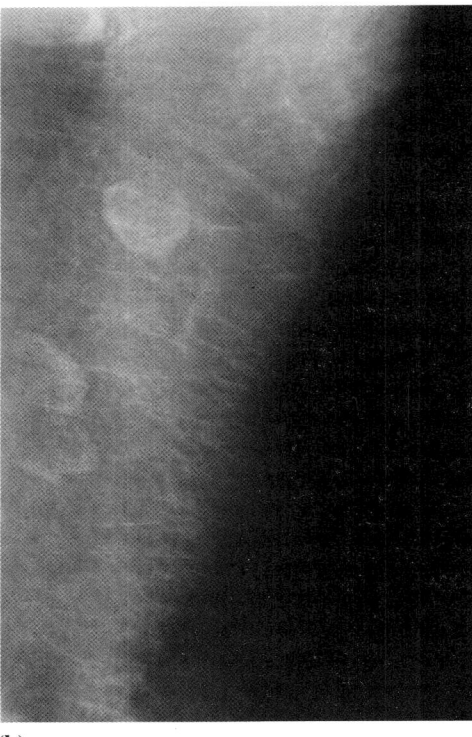

(b)

Fig. 22.33 (a) A large malignant lymph node (or mass of nodes) in the right axilla. (b) Three benign lymph nodes in the right axilla, all showing central replacement by more translucent fat.

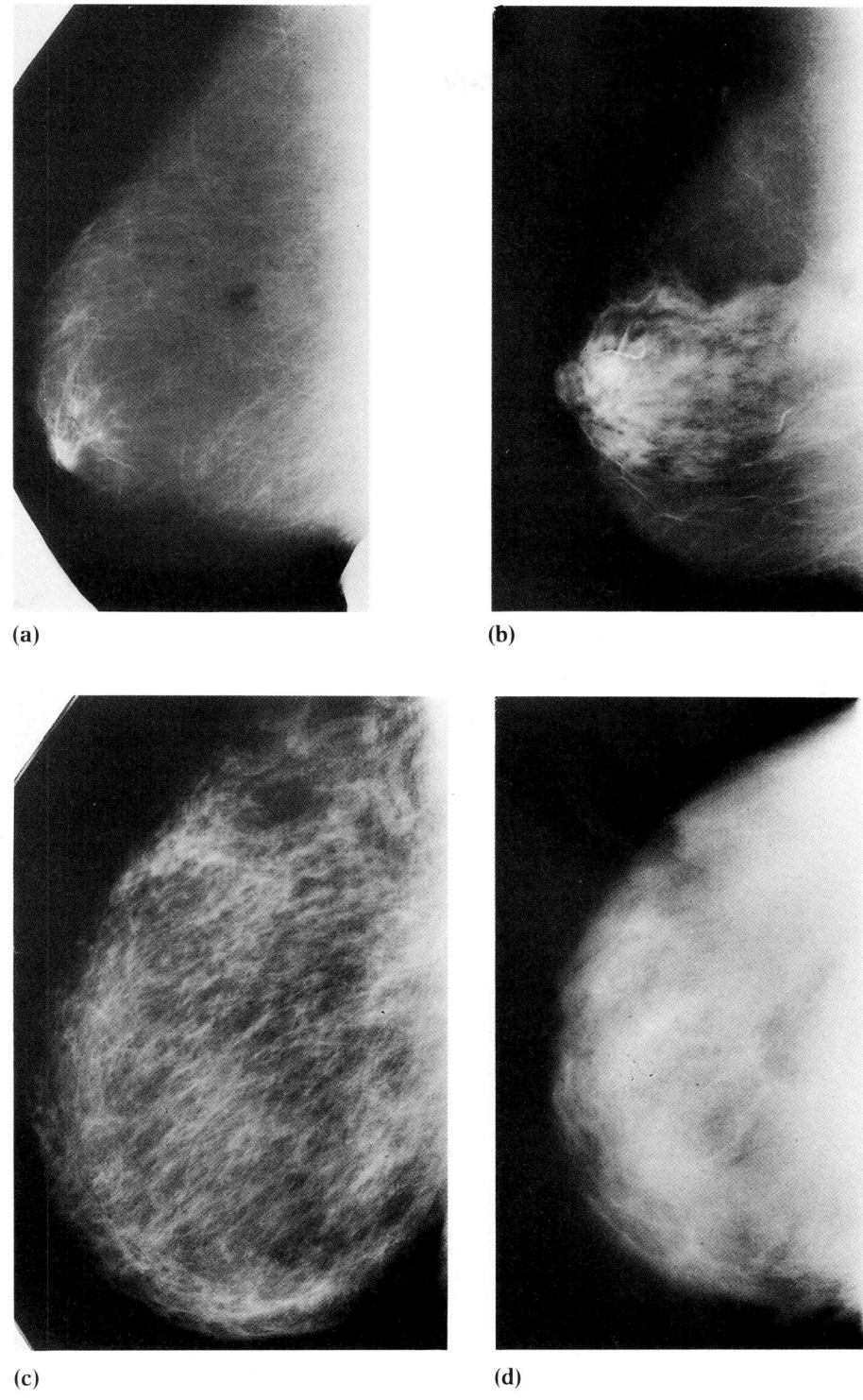

(a)

(b)

(c)

(d)

Fig. 22.34 Wolfe parenchymal patterns. (a) NI pattern: composed primarily of fat. (b) P1 pattern: prominent small-nodular, but linearly arranged duct pattern covering a quarter or less of the mammogram (some vessel calcification is also present). (c) P2 pattern: prominent ducts occupying more than a quarter of the area of the mammogram. (d) DY pattern: sheet-like areas of increased density, interspersed with fat, but without nodularity or linearity.

cancer was reduced by 31 per cent in the study group compared with the control group.

3. The Nijmegen and DOM Projects in The Netherlands are both case-control studies comparing the mortality of screened and unscreened women. The conclusions were that the chances of a screened woman dying were between 0.5 and 0.67 of that of an unscreened woman. A criticism of these studies is that they are biased by the self-selection of screened women with a low risk of dying of the disease into the group.

In 1985 the UK Ministry of Health established a working party under the chairmanship of Professor Sir Patrick Forrest. The two reports of the group published in 1986 state that 'The information that is already available from the principle overseas studies demonstrates that screening by mammography can lead to the prolongation of the lives of women aged 50 years and over with breast cancer. There is a convincing case, on clinical grounds, for a change in UK policy on the provision of mammographic facilities and the screening of symptomless women.'

While the Forrest Reports are consensus documents which have critics as well as proponents, the Secretary of State for Health accepted the reports and announced in February 1987 that the screening by mammography for all women aged 50–64, with recall every 3 years, would be introduced throughout the UK.

The latest reports on the UK Breast Screening Programme estimate that after about 10 years, about 1250 breast cancer deaths are expected to be prevented each year in the United Kingdom and, on average, each of the women in whom death from breast cancer is prevented, will live about 20 years more. Thus by the year 2000, the screening programme is expected to prevent about 25 per cent of the deaths from breast cancer in the population of women *invited* for screening. This translates into about 25 000 extra years of life gained annually in this country. The reduction in mortality in women who *accept the invitation* for screenings could be about 40 per cent!

22.2.7 Techniques other than mammography in breast cancer

These include sonography, thermography, transillumination, magnetic resonance imaging, computed tomography, immunodetection, and digital radiography. The last three methods employ ionizing radiation.

It is a fact of clinical life that lesions that can be easily detected clinically will also be visualized by most, if not all, of the above methods and, of course, by X-ray mammography. However, as implied above, it is the detection of early impalpable lesions that is important and if this can be effected using non-ionizing radiation, so much the better.

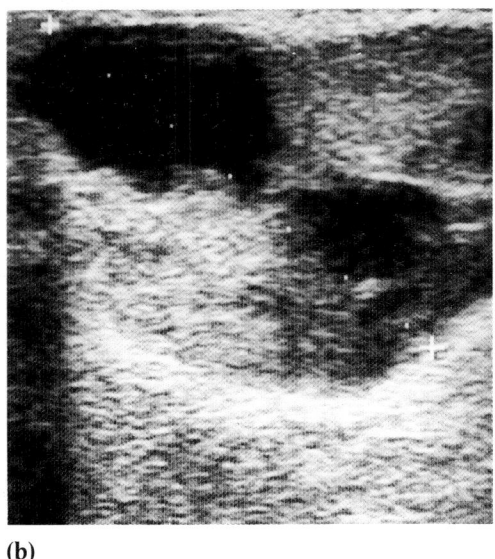

(a) **(b)**

Fig. 22.35 (a) An ultrasonogram showing a round, anechoic area (arrow) due to a cyst. (b) Another ultrasonogram showing detail of a bilocular, necrosing carcinoma with irregular edges and a number of internal echoes.

This being the case, it is really only sonography that has a limited role in the differentiation of cystic from solid masses and as a guide for aspiration and pre-operative localization of selected breast lesions (Fig. 22.35). Of the ionizing methods, computed tomography could be useful in detecting the spatial correlation of lesions. The other methods mentioned are still under assessment.

22.2.8   Further reading

HMSO Publications (1986). *Breast cancer screening: Forrest report.* London.
Wolfe, J. N. (1976). Risk for breast cancer development determined by mammographic parenchymal pattern. *Cancer* **37**, 2486–92.